fourteenth edition

Maxcy-Rosenau-Last

Public Health & Preventive Medicine

fourteenth edition

Maxcy-Rosenau-Last

Public Health & Preventive Medicine

Editor

Robert B. Wallace, MD, MSc

Associate Editor

Bradley N. Doebbeling, MD, MS

Editor Emeritus

John M. Last, MD, DPH

Section Editors

Elizabeth L. Barrett-Connor, MD • Katie Baer, MPH • Jonathan E. Fielding, MD, MPH, MBA
Mark L. Rosenberg, MD, MPH • Arnold J. Schecter, MD, MPH • F. Douglas Scutchfield, MD
Carl W. Tyler, Jr., MD • Richard P. Wenzel, MD, MSc

McGraw-Hill

Medical Publishing Division

New York St. Louis San Francisco Auckland Bogotá Caracas Lisbon London
Madrid Mexico City Milan Montreal New Delhi San Juan
Singapore Sydney Tokyo Toronto

McGraw-Hill

A Division of The ***McGraw-Hill*** *Companies*

Maxcy-Rosenau-Last Public Health & Preventive Medicine, Fourteenth Edition

Chapter 3 was previously published in Last JM. *Public Health and Human Ecology*. 2nd ed. Stamford, CT: Appleton & Lange, 1998.

2 3 4 5 6 7 8 9 0 KGP/KGP 0 9 8 7 6 5 4 3 2 1

ISBN: 0-8385-6185-3 (domestic)

Notice

Medicine is an ever-changing science. As new research and clinical experience broaden our knowledge, changes in treatment and drug therapy are required. The authors and the publisher of this work have checked with sources believed to be reliable in their efforts to provide information that is complete and generally in accord with the standards accepted at the time of publication. However, in view of the possibility of human error or changes in medical sciences, neither the authors nor the publisher nor any other party who has been involved in the preparation or publication of this work warrants that the information contained herein is in every respect accurate or complete, and they disclaim all responsibility for any errors or omissions or for the results obtained from use of the information contained in this work. Readers are encouraged to confirm the information contained herein with other sources. For example and in particular, readers are advised to check the product information sheet included in the package of each drug they plan to administer to be certain that the information contained in this work is accurate and that changes have not been made in the recommended dose or in the contraindications for administration. This recommendation is of particular importance in connection with new or infrequently used drugs.

Library of Congress Cataloging-in-Publication Data

Maxcy-Rosenau-Last public health & preventive medicine / [edited by] Robert B. Wallace. — 14th ed.
p. cm.
Includes bibliographical references and index.
ISBN 0-8385-6185-3 (alk. paper)
1. Public health. 2. Medicine, Preventive. I. Maxcy, Kenneth Fuller, 1889– . II. Rosenau, M. J. (Milton Joseph), 1869–1946. III. Last, John M., 1926– . IV. Wallace, Robert B., 1942– .
[DNLM: 1. Public Health. 2. Preventive Medicine. WA 100 M4635 1998]
RA425.M382 1998
614.4′4—dc21
DNLM/DLC
for Library of Congress 97-53116

Acquisitions Editor: Michael P. Medina
Managing Editor, Development: Kathleen McCullough
Production Service: York Production Services

ISBN: 0-8385-6184-5 (international)

The editors wish to make the following dedications:

Robert B. Wallace: To Maureen

Bradley N. Doebbeling: To Caroline

John M. Last: To Wendy

Elizabeth Barrett-Connor: To James, Jon, Carol, and Steven Connor

Jonathan E. Fielding: To Karin, Andrew, and Preston

Arnold J. Schecter: To Martha-Jean, Ben, Dave, and Anna Beth

F. Douglas Scutchfield: To Phyllis and Alex

Carl W. Tyler, Jr.: To Ginny, Laurie, and Jeff Tyler and Cindy Crenshaw

Richard P. Wenzel: To Jo Gail

In addition, this book is dedicated to all others
who sustained and inspired the contributors.

Preparation of this edition was sponsored by the Association of Teachers of Preventive Medicine (ATPM), Washington, DC. ATPM is the national professional association dedicated to advancing individual and community health promotion and disease prevention in the education of physicians and other health professionals. ATPM individual members are teachers, researchers, practitioners, administrators, residents, and students. ATPM institutional members include preventive medicine and related departments in medical schools, schools, and graduate programs in public health and preventive medicine, other health professions schools, and various health agencies. For more information about ATPM, call 202/463-0550, e-mail *info@atpm.org*, or visit the www homepage of *http://www.atpm.org/atpm.htm*. Members of the ATPM Publications Committee included the following:

David L. Rabin, MD, Chairman
Erica Frank, MD
Kathleen M. Rest, PhD
Carlos Valbona, MD
Kevin Patrick, MD, MS
F. Douglas Scutchfield, MD

Officers of ATPM:
Dorothy S. Lane, MD, MPH
President
Association of Teachers of Preventive Medicine

Barbara J. Calkins, MA
Executive Director
Association of Teachers of Preventive Medicine
Washington, D.C.

Contributors

J. Alberto Abreu
Research Assistant
Department of Psychiatry
University of Iowa College of Medicine
Veterans Administration Center
Iowa City, Iowa

Joseph L. Annest, MD
Director
Office of Statistics and Programming
National Center for Injury Prevention and Control
Centers for Disease Control and Prevention
Atlanta, Georgia

Thomas J. Armstrong, PhD, MPH
Professor
Division of Occupational Health
Department of Environmental and Industrial Health
University of Michigan
Ann Arbor, Michigan

Michael D. Attfield, MD
Division of Respiratory Disease Studies
Epidemiological Investigations Branch
National Institute for Occupational Safety and Health
Morgantown, West Virginia

Katie Baer, MPH
Health Communication Specialist
Division of Violence Prevention
National Center for Injury Prevention and Control
Centers for Disease Control and Prevention
Adjunct Instructor
Rollins School of Public Health of Emory University
Atlanta, Georgia

Patricia A. Baird, MD, CM, FRCP(C), FCCMG
Professor
Department of Medical Genetics
University of British Columbia
Vancouver, British Columbia, Canada

James F. Bale, Jr., MD
Professor
Division of Pediatric Neurology and Infectious Diseases
University of Utah
School of Medicine
Primary Children's Medical Center
Salt Lake City, Utah

Jennifer L. Balfour, PhD (Canad)
Doctoral Candidate
Department of Epidemiology and Public Health Biology
University of California at Berkeley
Berkeley, California

William H. Barker, MD
Associate Professor
Department of Community and Preventive Medicine
University of Rochester Medical Center
Attending Physician
Department of Medicine
Monroe Community Hospital
Rochester, New York

Elizabeth L. Barrett-Connor, MD
Professor and Chief
Department of Family and Preventive Medicine
Division of Epidemiology
University of California at San Diego School of Medicine
La Jolla, California

George Bekesi, MD, PhD
Director of Clinical Immunology
Professor of Medicine
Department of Medicine
Mount Sinai School of Medicine
New York, New York

Renate Belville, MA
Department of Community Health
Mount Sinai School of Medicine
Brooklyn, New York

Stephan A. Billstein, MD, MPH
Attending Dermatologist
Saint Michael's Hospital
Newark, New Jersey
Medical Director

Sandoz Pharmaceuticals
Dermatology/Metabolism
East Hanover, New Jersey

Eula Bingham, PhD
Professor
Department of Environmental Health
University of Cincinnati College of Medicine
Cincinnati, Ohio

Robert E. Black, MD, MPH
Professor and Chair
Department of International Health
Johns Hopkins University School of Hygiene and Public Health
Baltimore, Maryland

Peter B. Bloland, DVM, MPVM
Medical Epidemiologist
Division of Parasitic Diseases
National Center for Infectious Diseases
Centers for Disease Control and Prevention
Atlanta, Georgia

Paul W. Brandt-Rauf, MD, ScD, DrPH
Professor and Director of Occupational and Environmental Health Sciences
Department of Environmental Sciences
New York, New York

Robert F. Breiman, MD
Director
National Vaccine Program Office
Centers for Disease Control and Prevention
Atlanta, Georgia

Evelyn J. Bromet, PhD
Professor
Division of Epidemiology
Department of Psychiatry
State University of New York at Stony Brook
Stony Brook, New York

Claire V. Broome, MD
Deputy Director
Centers for Disease Control and Prevention
Atlanta, Georgia

Fabrizio Bruschi, MD
Associate Professor
Istituto di Patologia
University of Perugia
Perugia, Italy

Joanna Burger, PhD, MSc
Professor of Biology
Division of Environmental and Occupational Sciences
Department of Cell Development and Neurobiology
Rutgers University
Piscataway, New Jersey

Ann W. Burgess, DNsc, CS, FAAN
University of Pennsylvania School of Nursing
Philadelphia, Pennsylvania

Jay C. Butler, MD
Chief
Epidemiology Section
Respiratory Disease Branch
Division of Bacterial and Mycotic Diseases
Centers for Disease Control and Prevention
Clinical Assistant Professor
Department of Medicine
Emory University
Atlanta, Georgia

Willard Cates, Jr., MD, MPH
Senior Vice-President of Biomedical Affairs
Family Health International
Durham, North Carolina

Stephen L. Cochi, MD, MPH
Acting Deputy Director
Polio Eradication Activity
National Immunization Program
Centers for Disease Control and Prevention
Atlanta, Georgia

Denny G. Constantine, DVM, MPH
Former Chief
Southwest Rabies Investigation Station
Centers for Disease Control and Prevention
US Public Health Service
University Park, New Mexico
Retired Public Health Veterinarian
State of California Public Health Services
Berkeley, California

John B. Conway, MPH, PhD
Professor of Environmental Health and Toxicology
Associate Dean and Director of Professional Education Program
New York State University at Albany
Rensselaer, New York

Brian L. Cook, DO
Director
Chemical Dependency Services
University of Iowa Hospitals and Veterans Administration Medical Center

Associate Professor
Department of Psychiatry
University of Iowa College of Medicine
Iowa City, Iowa

David B. Coultas, MD
Professor of Internal Medicine
University of New Mexico School of Medicine
Chief
Division of Epidemiology and Preventive Medicine
University of New Mexico Health Sciences Center
Albuquerque, New Mexico

Robert B. Craven, MD
Chief
Epidemiology and Ecology Section
National Center for Infectious Diseases
Arbovirus Diseases Branch
Division of Vector-Borne Infectious Diseases
Centers for Disease Control and Prevention
Fort Collins, Colorado

Alan W. Cross, MD
Professor
Department of Social Medicine and Pediatrics
University of North Carolina at Chapel Hill School of Medicine
Chapel Hill, North Carolina

John H. Cross, MD
Professor
Division of Tropical Public Health
Department of Preventive Medicine and Biometrics
Uniformed Services University of the Health Sciences
Bethesda, Maryland

Mark R. Cullen, MD
Professor
Departments of Internal Medicine and Epidemiology and Public Health
Yale University School of Medicine
Director
Occupational and Environmental Medicine Program
Yale–New Haven Hospital
New Haven, Connecticut

James W. Curran, MD, MPH
Dean and Professor of Epidemiology
Rollins School of Public Health of Emory University
Atlanta, Georgia

Roy L. DeHart, MD, MPH
Professor and Chairman
Department of Family Medicine and Preventive Medicine
University of Oklahoma College of Medicine
Oklahoma City, Oklahoma

David T. Dennis, MD, PhD
Chief
Bacteriologic Zoonoses Branch
National Center for Infectious Diseases
Division of Vector-Borne Infectious Diseases
Centers for Disease Control and Prevention
Fort Collins, Colorado

James S. Dickson, PhD
Co-Department Executive Officer and Associate Professor
Department of Microbiology, Immunology, and Preventive Medicine
Iowa State University
Ames, Iowa

Bradley N. Doebbeling, MD, MS
Associate Professor
Division of General Internal Medicine
Departments of Internal Medicine and Preventive Medicine and Environmental Health
University of Iowa College of Medicine
Iowa City, Iowa

Janice S. Dorman, PhD
Director
Department of Molecular Epidemiology
University of Pittsburgh
Associate Professor
University of Pittsburgh Graduate School of Public Health
Pittsburgh, Pennsylvania

D. Peter Drotman, MD, MPH
Acting Associate Director for Epidemiologic Science
National Center for Infectious Diseases
Centers for Disease Control and Prevention
Clinical Assistant Professor
Department of Family and Preventive Medicine
Atlanta, Georgia

Maureen S. Durkin, PhD, DrPH
Assistant Professor of Public Health
Division of Epidemiology
School of Public Health
Sergievsky Center
Columbia University
Research Scientist
New York State Psychiatric Institute
New York, New York

Michael P. Eriksen, ScD
Office on Smoking and Health
Centers for Disease Control and Prevention
Atlanta, Georgia

Laverne K. Eveland, PhD
Professor
Division of Biological Sciences

California State University at Long Beach
Long Beach, California

Diana C. Farrow, PhD
Assistant Professor
Department of Epidemiology
University of Washington
Affiliate Investigator
Program in Epidemiology
Fred Hutchinson Cancer Research Center
Seattle, Washington

John E. Ferguson, PhD, MSN
Iowa City, Iowa

Kristi J. Ferguson, PhD
Associate Professor
Department of Preventive Medicine and Environmental Health
University of Iowa
Iowa City, Iowa

Nancy Fiedler, PhD
Associate Professor
Division of Occupational Health
Department of Environmental and Community Health
University of Medicine and Dentistry of New Jersey
Robert Wood Johnson Medical School
Piscataway, New Jersey

Jonathan E. Fielding, MD, MPH, MBA
Professor of Health Services and Pediatrics
University of California at Los Angeles Schools of Public Health and Medicine
Los Angeles, California

Larry J. Fine, MD, DrPH
Director
Division of Surveillance, Hazard Evaluations and Field Studies
National Institute for Occupational Safety and Health
Centers for Disease Control and Prevention
Cincinnati, Ohio

David Finkelhor, PhD
Co-Director
Family Research Laboratory
University of New Hampshire
Durham, New Hampshire

Alf Fischbein, MD
Professor
Division of Environmental and Occupational Health
Department of Life Sciences
Sar Ilan University
Ramat Gan, Israel

Anne H. Flitcraft, MD
Director
Domestic Violence Training Project
New Haven, Connecticut
Associate Professor of Medicine
University of Connecticut Health Center
Farmington, Connecticut

Arthur L. Frank, MD, PhD
Professor
Departments of Occupational and Environmental Medicine
Topperman Professor of Medical Education
University of Texas Health Science Center at Tyler
Tyler, Texas

David W. Fraser, MD
Education Director
International Clinical Epidemiology Network
Philadelphia, Pennsylvania

Jack K. Frenkel, MD
Professor Emeritus
Department of Pathology and Laboratory Medicine
University of Kansas School of Medicine
Kansas City, Kansas
Adjunct Professor
Department of Biology
University of New Mexico
Albuquerque, New Mexico

Andrew Friede, MD, MPH
Physician Executive
Cerner Corporation
Atlanta, Georgia

Cindy R. Friedman, MD
Medical Epidemiologist
Department of Foodborne and Diarrheal Diseases
Division of Bacterial and Mycotic Diseases
National Center for Infectious Diseases
Centers for Disease Control and Prevention
Atlanta, Georgia

Howard Frumkin, MD, DrPH
Associate Professor and Chair
Department of Environmental and Occupational Health
Rollins School of Public Health of Emory University
Atlanta, Georgia

Cedric F. Garland, DrPH
Associate Professor
Department of Family and Preventive Medicine
University of California at San Diego School of Medicine
La Jolla, California

Frank C. Garland, PhD
Department of Family and Preventive Medicine
University of California at San Diego School of Medicine
La Jolla, California

Kristine M. Gebbie, DrPH, RN
Elizabeth Standish Gill Assistant Professor of Nursing
Columbia University School of Nursing
New York, New York

Michael Gochfeld, MD, PhD
Clinical Professor
Division of Occupational Medicine
Department of Environmental and Community Medicine
Environmental and Occupational Health Sciences Institute
University of Medicine and Dentistry of New Jersey
Robert Wood Johnson Medical School
Piscataway, New Jersey

James Godbold, PhD
Pediatric and Adolescent Injury Prevention Program
Kentucky Injury Prevention and Research Center
University of Kentucky
Chandler Medical Center
Lexington, Kentucky

Leon Gordis, MD, DPH
Professor and Chairman
Department of Epidemiology
Johns Hopkins University School of Hygiene and Public Health
Baltimore, Maryland

Edward D. Gorham, MPH
Department of Family and Preventive Medicine
University of California at San Diego School of Medicine
La Jolla, California

Philippe Grandjean, MD, PhD
Professor and Chairman
Institute of Community Health
Department of Environmental Medicine
Odense University
Odense, Denmark

Lawrence W. Green, DrPH
Professor and Head
Department of Health Care and Preventive Medicine
University of British Columbia
Director
Institute of Health Promotion Research
Vancouver, British Columbia, Canada

Dalya Guris, MD
Medical Epidemiologist
Division of Epidemiology and Surveillance
National Immunization Program
Centers for Disease Control and Prevention
Atlanta, Georgia

W. Rodney Hammond, PhD
Director
Division of Violence Prevention
National Center for Injury Prevention and Control
Centers for Disease Control and Prevention
Atlanta, Georgia

Lee H. Harrison, MD
Associate Professor of Epidemiology and Medicine
University of Pittsburgh Graduate School of Public Health and School of Medicine
Pittsburgh, Pennsylvania

Carol B. Hartman, RN, CS, DNSc
Hyde Park, Massachusetts

Rebecca L. Hegeman, BSN, MD
Clinical Assistant Professor
Division of Nephrology
Department of Internal Medicine
University of Iowa Hospital and Clinics
Iowa City, Iowa

Robert F. Herrick, ScD
Department of Environmental Health
Harvard School of Public Health
Boston, Massachusetts

Alan R. Hinman, MD, MPH
Senior Consultant for Public Health Programs
The Task Force for Child Survival and Development
Adjunct Professor of Epidemiology
Rollins School of Public Health of Emory University
Atlanta, Georgia

King K. Holmes, MD, PhD
Director
Center for AIDS and STD
University of Washington
Seattle, Washington

Donald R. Hopkins, MD, MPH
Senior Consultant
The Carter Center
Atlanta, Georgia

Douglas B. Hornick, MD
Associate Professor
Division of Pulmonary, Critical Care and Occupational Medicine
Department of Internal Medicine
University of Iowa College of Medicine
Iowa City, Iowa

James Huff, BS, MS, PhD
Toxicologist/Pharmacologist
Division of Intramural Research

National Institute of Environmental Health Sciences
Research Triangle Park, North Carolina

James M. Hughes, MD
Director
National Center for Infectious Diseases
Centers for Disease Control and Prevention
Atlanta, Georgia

Corinne G. Husten, MD, MPH
Acting Branch Chief
Epidemiology Branch
Office on Smoking and Health
Centers for Disease Control and Prevention
Atlanta, Georgia

S. Patrick Kachur, MD, MPH
Medical Epidemiologist
Malaria Epidemiology Section
Epidemiology Branch
Division of Parasitic Diseases
National Center for Infectious Diseases
Centers for Disease Control and Prevention
Atlanta, Georgia

Arnold F. Kaufmann, DVM, MS
Captain
US Public Service (Retired)
Stone Mountain, Georgia

C. William Keck, MD, MPH
Director
Division of Community Health Sciences
Northeastern Ohio Universities College of Medicine
Rootstown, Ohio

Jennifer L. Kelsey, PhD
Professor
Division of Epidemiology
Department of Health, Research and Policy
Stanford University School of Medicine
Stanford, California

W. Monroe Keyserling, PhD
Professor
Department of Industrial and Operations Engineering
University of Michigan
Ann Arbor, Michigan

Jay S. Keystone, MD, MSc (ctm), FRCPC
Staff Physician
Center for Travel and Tropical Medicine
Division of Infectious Diseases
Department of Medicine
The Toronto Hospital
Professor
Department of Medicine
University of Toronto
Toronto, Ontario, Canada

M. Marlyne Kilbey, PhD
Professor and Chairperson
Department of Psychology
Wayne State University
Detroit, Michigan

Edwin M. Kilbourne, MD
Director
Data Management Division
National Immunization Program
Centers for Disease Control and Prevention
Atlanta, Georgia

Kaye H. Kilburn, MD
Ralph Edgington Professor of Medicine
Division of Pulmonary Medicine
Department of Internal Medicine
University of Southern California School of Medicine
Los Angeles, California

Dean G. Kilpatrick, PhD
Crime Victims Center
Medical University of South Carolina
Charleston, South Carolina

Louis V. Kirchhoff, MD, MPH
Professor
Division of Infectious Diseases
Department of Internal Medicine
University of Iowa
Iowa City, Iowa

Amy Klion, MD
Laboratory of Parasitic Diseases
National Institute of Allergy and Infectious Disease
National Institutes of Health
Bethesda, Maryland

Jess F. Kraus, PhD
Director
Southern California Injury Prevention Center
Professor
Department of Epidemiology
University of California at Los Angeles School of Public Health
Los Angeles, California

Lewis H. Kuller, MD, PhD
Professor and Chair
Department of Epidemiology
University Professor of Public Health
University of Pittsburgh Graduate School of Public Health
Pittsburgh, Pennsylvania

Richard S. Kurz, PhD, MHA
Professor and Dean
School of Public Health
St. Louis University
Saint Louis, Missouri

Darwin R. Labarthe, MD, PhD
James W. Rockwell Professor of Public Health
University of Texas Health Science Center at Houston
Houston, Texas

John C. Lammers, PhD
Associate Professor
Department of Communication
University of California at Santa Barbara
Santa Barbara, California

Philip J. Landrigan, MD, MSc
Ethel H. Wise Professor and Chair
Division of Environmental and Occupational Medicine
Department of Community Medicine
Mount Sinai School of Medicine
New York, New York

Ronald E. LaPorte, PhD
Professor of Epidemiology and Pediatrics
Graduate School of Public Health
University of Pittsburgh
Pittsburgh, Pennsylvania

John M. Last, MD, DPH
Emeritus Professor of Epidemiology
Department of Epidemiology and Pediatrics
University of Ottawa
Ottawa, Ontario, Canada

Carl B. LeBuhn, MD
Staff Physician
Department of Internal Medicine
University of Iowa Hospitals and Clinics
Assistant Professor
University of Iowa College of Medicine
Iowa City, Iowa

James W. LeDuc, PhD
Associate Director for Global Health
National Center for Infectious Diseases
Centers for Disease Control and Prevention
Atlanta, Georgia

Llewellyn J. Legters, MD, MPH
Professor Emeritus
Preventive Medicine and Biometrics
Uniformed Services University of the Health Sciences
Bethesda, Maryland

Stephen M. Levin, MD
Assistant Professor
Division of Environmental and Occupational Medicine
Department of Community Medicine
Mount Sinai School of Medicine
New York, New York

Ruth Lilis, MD
Professor Emeritus
Division of Environmental and Occupational Medicine
Department of Community Medicine
Mount Sinai School of Medicine
Adjunct Attending Physician
Department of Community Medicine
Mount Sinai Medical Center
New York, New York

Scott R. Lillibridge, MD
Associate Director
Emergency, Refugee, and International Health
National Center for Environmental Health
Centers for Disease Control and Prevention
Atlanta, Georgia

Leo X. Liu, MD, DTMH
Assistant Professor of Medicine
Division of Infectious Diseases
Department of Medicine
Harvard Medical School
Attending Physician
Division of Medicine
Beth Israel Hospital
Boston, Massachusetts

Russell V. Luepker, MD, MS
Professor
Division of Epidemiology
University of Minnesota Hospitals and Clinics
Professor and Head
University of Minnesota School of Public Health
Minneapolis, Minnesota

Harold S. Margolis, MD
Chief
Hepatitis Branch
National Center for Infectious Diseases
Centers for Disease Control and Prevention
Atlanta, Georgia

Lauri E. Markowitz, MD
National Immunization Program
Centers for Disease Control and Prevention
Atlanta, Georgia

Douglas L. Marshall, PhD
Associate Professor
Department of Food Science and Technology
Mississippi State University
Mississippi State, Mississippi

Yoshito Masuda, PhD
Professor
Division of Physical Analysis
Department of Pharmacy
Daiichi College of Pharmaceutical Sciences
Fukuoka, Japan

Jeffrey L. Meier, MD
Department of Internal Medicine
University of Iowa
Iowa City, Iowa

James A. Merchant, MD, DrPH
Head
Department of Preventive Medicine and Environmental Health
University of Iowa College of Medicine
Iowa City, Iowa

James A. Mercy, PhD
Associate Director for Science
Division of Violence Prevention
National Center for Injury Prevention and Control
Centers for Disease Control and Prevention
Atlanta, Georgia

Jonathan H. Mermin, MD
Fellow
Epidemic Intelligence Service
Foodborne and Diarrheal Diseases Branch
National Center for Infectious Diseases
Centers for Disease Control and Prevention
Atlanta, Georgia

Karen Messing, PhD
Professor
CINBIOSE
Department of Biological Sciences
University of Quebec at Montreal
Montreal, Quebec, Canada

Eric D. Mintz, MD, MPH
Chief
Diarrheal Diseases and Epidemiology Section
Foodborne and Diarrheal Diseases Branch
Division of Bacterial and Mycotic Diseases
National Center for Infectious Diseases
Centers for Disease Control and Prevention
Atlanta, Georgia

Aage R. Møller, PhD, DMedSci
Professor
Department of Neurological Surgery
University of Pittsburgh School of Medicine
Pittsburgh, Pennsylvania

Arnold S. Monto, MD
Professor
Department of Epidemiology
University of Michigan School of Public Health
Ann Arbor, Michigan

Marion Moses, MD
Pesticide Education Center
San Francisco, California

Nancy R. Mudrick, PhD
Professor
School of Social Work
Syracuse University
Syracuse, New York

K. Darwin Murrell, PhD
Director
Beltsville Agricultural Research Center
United States Department of Agriculture
Beltsville, Maryland

Kenrad E. Nelson, MD
Professor
Division of Infectious Diseases
Department of Epidemiology
Johns Hopkins University
Baltimore, Maryland

Marion Nestle, PhD, MPH
Professor and Chair
Department of Nutrition and Food Studies
New York University
New York, New York

Eli H. Newberger, MD
Assistant Professor
Department of Pediatrics
Harvard Medical School
Director
Family Development Study
Children's Hospital
Boston, Massachusetts

Patrick W. O'Carroll, MD, MPH
Special Assistant to the Director
Public Health Practice Program Office
Centers for Disease Control and Prevention
Atlanta, Georgia
Clinical Associate Professor
Department of Epidemiology and Health Services
University of Washington School of Public Health and Community Medicine
Seattle, Washington

Dawn M. Oh, MS
PhD Candidate and Research Assistant
Division of Epidemiology
Department of Preventive Medicine and Environmental Health
University of Iowa
Iowa City, Iowa

Kean T. Oh, MD
Resident
Department of Ophthalmology
University of Iowa Hospitals and Clinics
Iowa City, Iowa

Trevor J. Orchard, MBBCh, MMedSci
Professor of Epidemiology, Medicine and Pediatrics
Medical Director
Nutrition Lipid Program
Division of Diabetes and Lipid Research
Department of Epidemiology
Rangos Research Center
University of Pittsburgh
Pittsburgh, Pennsylvania

Walter A. Orenstein, MD
Director
National Immunization Program
Centers for Disease Control and Prevention
Atlanta, Georgia

Stephen M. Ostroff, MD
Associate Director for Epidemiologic Sciences
National Center for Infectious Diseases
Centers for Disease Control and Prevention
Atlanta, Georgia

K. Michael Peddecord, DrPH
Professor
Health Services Administration
Graduate School of Public Health
San Diego State University
San Diego, California

Corinne Peek-Asa, PhD
Adjunct Assistant Professor of Epidemiology
Southern California Injury Prevention and Research Center
University of California at Los Angeles School of Public Health
Los Angeles, California

Bradley A. Perkins, MD
Chief
Meningitis and Special Pathogens Branch
National Center for Infectious Diseases
Division of Bacterial and Mycotic Diseases
Centers for Disease Control and Prevention
Atlanta, Georgia

Herbert B. Peterson, MD
Chief
Women's Health and Fertility Branch
Division of Reproductive Health
Center for Chronic Disease Prevention & Health Promotion
Centers for Disease Control and Prevention
Atlanta, Georgia

Michael A. Pfaller, MD
Professor
Division of Medical Microbiology
Department of Pathology
University of Iowa College of Medicine
Iowa City, Iowa

Karl Pillemer, PhD
Associate Professor
Department of Human Development and Family Studies
Cornell University
Ithaca, New York

Susan H. Pollack, MD
Pediatric and Adolescent Injury Prevention Program
Kentucky Injury Prevention and Research Center
University of Kentucky
Chandler Medical Center
Lexington, Kentucky

Lloyd B. Potter, PhD, MPH
Team Leader
Youth Violence Prevention
Division of Violence Prevention
National Center for Injury Prevention and Control
Centers for Disease Control and Prevention
Atlanta, Georgia

D. Rebecca Prevots, PhD, MPH
Epidemiologist
National Immunization Program
Centers for Disease Control and Prevention
Atlanta, Georgia

Shannon D. Putnam, MS
Division of Epidemiology
Department of Preventive Medicine and Environmental Health
University of Iowa College of Medicine
Iowa City, Iowa

M. Patricia Quinlisk, MD, MPS
Medical Director/State Epidemiologist
Iowa Department of Public Health
Adjunct Associate Professor
Department of Preventive and Environmental Health
University of Iowa
Des Moines, Iowa

Katharine C. Rathbun, MD, MPH
Regional Medical Consultant
Social Security Administration
Disability Quality Branch
Kansas City, Missouri

Robert L. Rausch, DVM, PhD
Professor Emeritus
Department of Comparative Medicine/Pathobiology
University of Washington School of Medicine
Seattle, Washington

Jonathan I. Ravdin, MD
Nesbitt Professor and Chair
Department of Internal Medicine
University of Minnesota
Minneapolis, Minnesota

Stephen C. Redd, MD
National Immunization Program
Division of Epidemiology and Surveillance
Centers for Disease Control and Prevention
Atlanta, Georgia

Susan E. Reef, MD
Medical Epidemiologist
National Immunization Program
Division of Epidemiology and Surveillance
Centers for Disease Control and Prevention
Atlanta, Georgia

Arthur L. Reingold, MD
Clinical Professor
Division of Clinical Epidemiology
Department of Medicine
University of California at San Francisco
San Francisco, California
Professor and Head
Division of Public Health Biology and Epidemiology
School of Public Health
University of California at Berkeley
Berkeley, California

Edward P. Richards III, JD, MPH
Professor
University of Missouri at Kansas City School of Law
Kansas City, Missouri

Mark L. Rosenberg, MD, MPH
Director
National Center for Injury Prevention and Control
Centers for Disease Control and Prevention
Visiting Professor
Morehouse and Emory Medical Schools
Harvard and Emory Schools of Public Health
Atlanta, Georgia

R. Gary Rozier, DDS, MPH
Professor
Department of Health Policy and Administration
School of Public Health
University of North Carolina at Chapel Hill
Chapel Hill, North Carolina

Thomas G. Rundall, PhD
Professor of Health Policy and Management
University of California at Berkeley School of Public Health
Berkeley, California

Jonathan M. Samet, MD, MS
Professor and Chairman
Department of Epidemiology
Johns Hopkins University
Baltimore, Maryland

Julius Schachter, PhD
Professor
Chlamydia Research Laboratory
Department of Laboratory Medicine
University of California at San Francisco
San Francisco, California

Peter M. Schantz, VMD, PhD
Epidemiologist
Division of Parasitic Diseases
National Center for Infectious Diseases
Centers for Disease Control and Prevention
Atlanta, Georgia

Helen H. Schauffler, PhD, MSPH
Associate Professor
Division of Health Policy and Administration
School of Public Health
University of California at Berkeley
Berkeley, California

Arnold J. Schecter, MD, MPH
Professor of Preventive Medicine
Clinical Campus at Binghamton
State University of New York Health Science Center–Syracuse
Binghamton, New York
Special Expert
National Institute of Environmental Health Sciences—National Institutes of Health
Research Triangle Park, North Carolina
Adjunct Professor of Epidemiology
School of Public Health
University of North Carolina
Chapel Hill, North Carolina

Nicole Schupf, PhD, DrPH
Research Scientist
Laboratory of Epidemiology

New York State Institute for Basic Research in Developmental Disabilities
Staten Island, New York

C. Roberts Schuster, PhD
Director
Clinical Research Division on Substance Abuse
Professor
Department of Psychiatry
Wayne State University School of Medicine
Detroit, Michigan

Charles R. Scriver, MDCM
Alva Professor of Human Genetics
Biochemical Genetics Department
McGill University
Montreal, Quebec, Canada

F. Douglas Scutchfield, MD
Professor
University of Kentucky
Medical Center
Lexington, Kentucky

Jane F. Seward, MBBS, MPH
Medical Epidemiologist
National Immunization Program
Epidemiology and Surveillance Division
Centers for Disease Control and Prevention
Atlanta, Georgia

Trueman W. Sharp, Commdr USMC, MD, MPH
Officer in Charge
US Naval Medical Research Institute Detachment
Lima, Peru
Adjunct Assistant Professor
Division of Preventive Medicine and Biometrics
Uniformed Services University of the Health Sciences
Bethesda, Maryland

Robert E. Shope, MD
Professor of Pathology
Center for Tropical Diseases
Department of Pathology
University of Texas Medical Branch
Galveston, Texas

Ellen K. Silbergeld, PhD
Professor
Department of Epidemiology and Preventive Medicine
University of Maryland Medical School
Baltimore, Maryland

Louis Slesin, PhD
Editor
Microwave News
New York, New York

Laurence Slutsker, MD
Medical Epidemiologist
Foodborne and Diarrheal Disease Branch
Division of Bacterial and Mycotic Diseases
National Center for Infectious Diseases
Centers for Disease Control and Prevention
Atlanta, Georgia

Jeremy Sobel, MD
Epidemic Intelligence Service
Foodborne and Diarrheal Diseases Branch
National Center for Infectious Diseases
Centers for Disease Control and Prevention
Atlanta, Georgia

Richard A. Spiegel, DVM, MPH
Research Epidemiologist
National Center for Infectious Diseases
Division of Bacterial and Mycotic Diseases
Centers for Disease Control and Prevention
Atlanta, Georgia

Evan Stark, MSW, PhD
Co-Director
Domestic Violence Training Project
New Haven, Connecticut
Associate Professor of Public Administration and Social Work
Rutgers University
Newark, New Jersey

Zena A. Stein, MB, BCh
Professor Emeritus of Public Health and Psychiatry
G.H. Sergievsky Center
Columbia University
Director
Division of Epidemiology of Brain Diseases
New York State Psychiatric Institute
New York, New York

Peter M. Strebel, MBChB, MPH
Chief
Infant Immunization Activity
Epidemiology and Surveillance Division
National Immunization Program
Centers for Disease Control and Prevention
Atlanta, Georgia

Judy A. Streit, MD
Associate in Internal Medicine
University of Iowa College of Medicine
Associate in Internal Medicine
University of Iowa Hospitals and Clinics
Iowa City, Iowa

William A. Suk, PhD, MPH
Director
Office of Program Development
National Institute of Environmental Health Sciences
Research Triangle Park, North Carolina

Mervyn W. Susser, MD
G.H. Sergievsky Professor Emeritus and Special Lecturer
G.H. Sergievsky Center
Columbia University
New York, New York

Roland W. Sutter, MD, MPH&TM
Deputy Chief for Technical Affairs
Polio Eradication Activity
National Immunization Program
Centers for Disease Control and Prevention
Atlanta, Georgia

S. Leonard Syme, PhD
Emeritus Professor of Epidemiology
School of Public Health
University of California at Berkeley
Berkeley, California

David B. Thomas, MD, DrPH
Division of Public Health Sciences
Department of Epidemiology
Fred Hutchinson Cancer Research Center
Seattle, Washington

James C. Torner, PhD
Professor and Director
Division of Epidemiology
Department of Preventive Medicine and Environmental Health
Iowa City, Iowa

Theodore F. Tsai, MD, MPH
Medical Officer
Center for Infectious Diseases
Division of Vector-Borne Infectious Diseases
Fort Collins, Colorado

Margaret A. Turk, MD
Medical Director
Rehabilitation Services
Saint Camillus Health and Rehabilitation, Syracuse
Associate Professor
Department of Physical Medicine and Rehabilitation
State University of New York Health Science Center at Syracuse
Syracuse, New York

Carl W. Tyler, Jr., MD
US Public Health Service (Ret.)
Formerly, Assistant Director for Academic Programs
Public Health Practice Program Office
Centers for Disease Control and Prevention
Atlanta, Georgia

Arthur C. Upton, MD
Clinical Professor
Environmental and Community Medicine
University of Medicine and Dentistry of New Jersey
Robert Wood Johnson Medical School
Piscataway, New Jersey

Dushyanthi Vimalachandra, MPH
Staff Research Associate
Southern California Injury Prevention Research Center
University of California at Los Angeles School of Public Health
Los Angeles, California

Charles R. Vitek, MD
Medical Epidemiologist
Child Vaccine Preventable Diseases Branch
National Immunization Program
Centers for Disease Control and Prevention
Atlanta, Georgia

Judith M. Von, PhD
Licensed Clinical Psychologist
Mount Pleasant, South Carolina

Gregory R. Wagner, MD
Director
Division of Respiratory Disease Studies
National Institute for Occupational Safety and Health
Centers for Disease Control and Prevention
Morgantown, West Virginia

E. Darryl Walker, MD, MPH
Assistant Professor
Department of Community Health and Preventive Medicine
Morehouse School of Medicine
Atlanta, Georgia

Mark R. Wallace, MD
Fellow
Division of Infectious Disease
Naval Medical Center
San Diego, California

Robert B. Wallace, MD, MSc
Professor and Head
Department of Preventive Medicine and Environmental Health
University of Iowa
Iowa City, Iowa

Charles W. Warren, PhD
Research Demographer
National Center for Chronic Disease Prevention and Health Promotion
Centers for Disease Control and Prevention
Atlanta, Georgia

Steven G.F. Wassilak, MD
World Health Organization
Regional Office for Europe
Copenhagen, Denmark

Robert J. Weber, MD
Director
University Hospital at Syracuse
Professor and Chairman
Department of Physical Medicine and Rehabilitation
State University of New York Health Science Center at Syracuse
Syracuse, New York

Jonathan B. Weisbuch, MD, MPH
Maricopa County
Department of Health
Phoenix, Arizona

Jay D. Wenger, MD
Medical Officer
Expanded Programme on Immunization
World Health Organization
Geneva, Switzerland

Richard P. Wenzel, MD, MSc
Professor and Chairman
Department of Internal Medicine
Medical College of Virginia
Virginia Commonwealth University
Richmond, Virginia

S. Benson Werner, MD, MPH
Lecturer
Division of Epidemiology
Department of Biomedical and Environmental Health Sciences
University of California at Berkeley School of Medicine
Chief
Disease Investigations Section
Division of Communicable Disease Control
State of California Department of Health Services
Berkeley, California

Melinda Wharton, MD
National Immunization Program
Division of Epidemiology and Surveillance
Centers for Disease Control and Prevention
Atlanta, Georgia

Richard J. Whitley, MD
Loeb Eminent Scholar in Pediatrics
Professor of Pediatrics, Microbiology, and Medicine
Division of Virology
Department of Pediatrics
University of Alabama at Birmingham
Birmingham, Alabama

Valerie A. Wilk, MS
Health Policy Analyst
Department of Public Policy
American Federation of State, County and Municipal Employees
Washington, DC

Stephen J. Williams, ScD
Professor and Head
Division of Health Services Administration
Graduate School of Public Health
College of Health and Human Services
San Diego State University
San Diego, California

Mary E. Wilson, MD
Associate Professor
Division of Infectious Diseases
Department of Internal Medicine
University of Iowa
Iowa City, Iowa

Rosalie S. Wolf, PhD
Executive Director
Institute on Aging
Memorial Hospital
Assistant Professor
Department of Family and Community Medicine
University of Massachusetts Medical Center
Worcester, Massachusetts

Mary S. Wolff, MD
Division of Environmental Health and Occupational Medicine
Department of Community Medicine
Mount Sinai School of Medicine
New York, New York

Robert G. Yaeger, PhD
Professor of Medicine, Retired
Tulane University School of Medicine
Professor of Tropical Medicine, Retired
Tulane University School of Public Health and Tropical Medicine
New Orleans, Louisiana

Contents

Acknowledgments

Many persons gave generously of their time in the preparation of the fourteenth edition of *Public Health & Preventive Medicine*. The scientific contributors were most responsive to comment and editorial suggestions, and many had colleagues, too numerous to mention, who skillfully gave of their time in facilitating manuscript preparation and in communicating with the section editors and the editorial office. Particular appreciation is noted for LaRae Rudin, who provided high-quality clerical support for assembling the many contributions to this volume. Kathleen McCullough and Michael Medina at Appleton & Lange also gave invaluable support, advice, and assistance in the assembly of this book. Finally, John M. Last has provided unparalleled advice and support for this increasingly complex endeavor.

Preface

Public Health & Preventive Medicine is in its ninth decade of existence having been first published in 1913, and it therefore contains much of the lore of public health and preventive medicine over the twentieth century. With each edition, selecting the appropriate information to include has become increasingly difficult for several reasons. Nearly all the same public health and prevention themes and issues continue to be with us, and new knowledge, research, and practice information for public health and preventive medicine grows at a rapid rate. New diseases are being discovered and our knowledge of existing ones is constantly being refined and expanded. New microorganisms of public health import continue to be discovered. Behavioral science has helped us better understand how to promote healthful, hygienic behaviors. Science and engineering have created occupational and other environmental exposures never before experienced. The increased survivorship of the populations of industrialized nations has heightened the importance of degenerative diseases, complex medical care programs, and the opportunities for prevention of disease. The population growth of our finite and frail planet may be causing present and future public health dilemmas that are yet incompletely understood. There has been increasing attention to the social and "unnatural" causes of human suffering and the recognition of human conflict as a public health problem. The increased convergence of public health practice and the delivery of clinical health services has created and elevated several topics that must be given some prominence.

Every attempt has been made to update the information and acquire new knowledge in this fourteenth edition of *Public Health & Preventive Medicine*. Although several new topics have been introduced in this edition, such as public health information systems, inevitably certain issues could not be fully considered. In particular, to keep this textbook at a reasonable size, there is somewhat less emphasis on the issues of developing countries. Although most of the more than 200 contributors to this textbook are from North America, most of the themes presented here have universal application and the lore comes from scientists and practitioners worldwide.

Robert B. Wallace
Iowa City

Historical Note

Milton J. Rosenau was a Harvard man, as was his principal collaborator, George C. Whipple. His successor, Kenneth Maxcy, moved to Johns Hopkins University. When Maxcy was in turn succeeded as editor by Philip E. Sartwell and the size of the writing team began to grow, the center of gravity of "Maxcy-Rosenau" was decisively located in Baltimore: twenty of the thirty-nine contributors to the tenth edition were on the Johns Hopkins staff, and all but two or three contributors were associated with schools of public health. In 1976, the Publisher invited the Association of Teachers of Preventive Medicine (ATPM) to assume responsibility for the eleventh and subsequent editions. After a search, John M. Last, from the University of Ottawa, was selected as editor. Under his leadership, "Maxcy-Rosenau-Last" evolved in several ways, becoming more comprehensive and international and with an increased number of contributors. Under the auspices of the ATPM, the thirteenth edition was coedited by Last and Robert B. Wallace, from the University of Iowa. The current fourteenth edition has been edited by Wallace with the assistance of Bradley N. Doebbeling, also of the University of Iowa. More than 200 authors from diverse disciplines and geographic situations have contributed to this edition.

I

Public Health Methods

Edited by John M. Last and Carl W. Tyler, Jr.

1

Public Health and Preventive Medicine: Trends and Guideposts

Robert B. Wallace

There have been rapid and important advancements in public health and preventive medicine. Some have come as a result of inexorable achievements in productive science, and others were prodded by special public health emergencies and problems, or organizational changes in the delivery of preventive and curative health services. Many advancements in both practice and knowledge have been evolutionary, but in a few instances there have been fundamental enhancements to our knowledge of the universe and their applications to the public health sciences. While there may be quarrels about what these achievements have been, and indeed some may not yet be fully recognized, the past several years have witnessed several striking and rapidly advancing trends.

Increased incorporation of business and administrative practices into prevention and public health service delivery. While general administrative principles and practices have long been a part of public health education and program delivery, the administrative and business emphasis that has swept through most sectors of Western society has also had a clear impact on public health practice. The further application of "industrial standards" (1), quality improvement techniques, outcome measures, and complex accounting practices have changed the vocabulary and skills requisite for modern public health practice.

Changes in the definition of the group or population, the fundamental unit of public health. In general, "the population" that is both the target of preventive and public health programs and interventions has been historically defined as referring to geographic boundaries, due to the encompassing nature and concordance with governmental jurisdictions. That is, of course, still the case, but there has also been a trend toward increasing delivery of comprehensive clinical services to large groups of individuals defined administratively rather than geographically, often referred to as "managed care." With the health and programmatic information available on these groups and the increasing ability to apply and evaluate public health and preventive services to them, the fundamental public health target group is no longer solely defined in the spatial sense. This has led to the need and opportunity for new partnerships among various private and public health organizations and agencies in order to deliver more effective and efficient public health services (2). In certain respects, this phenomenon has further blurred the boundaries between community-based programs and clinical preventive and curative services. Thus, there is an increasing need to update and redefine the tasks necessary for complete public health and prevention service delivery. However, the emergence of these new groups that are programmatically important and for whom health information is available has probably served to heighten public health program accountability to a higher proportion of the general population than ever before.

Enhanced definition and measurement of health status. This has taken several forms and, while not totally new, has been increasingly incorporated into health status assessment. Perhaps the most important is the increased use of the so-called "quality-of-life" (QOL) measures (3). While the scope and measures of QOL techniques are not consensual, the supplementation of traditional measures of morbidity and mortality with measures and indices of symptoms and syndromes, less well defined clinical conditions and entities, physical function and disability, affective states and the behavioral manifestations of mental diseases, social functions within and outside the family, economic well-being and risk status irrespective of health status have added importantly to the understanding of health and optimization of health status.

In keeping with the theme of enhanced administration in public and preventive services, health status measures for groups and individuals increasingly have become intertwined with the "health" status of preventive and curative programs and service delivery units. That is, the health of members (consumers) of various administered health care units (providers) can be partially assessed or inferred by process measures of the programs themselves, such as rates of vaccine delivery or early disease detection programs.

Increased codification and interpretation of scientific findings relevant to prevention and public health. One of the early important exercises in defining the scientific and evidentiary basis for clinical preventive practices was performed by the Canadian Task Force on the Periodic Health Examination (4) followed by the report of the U.S. Preventive Services Task Force (5) and many others. Making explicit the scientific basis for preventive practices and interventions and using this evidence to structure practice guidelines has had many important effects, including a) placing greater priority on effective interventions, b) educating health practitioners on the strengths and limitations of various interventions, c) providing one basis for program evaluation of these effective interventions and d) identifying the research gaps in these preventive and public health interventions. Parallel tracks of creating guidelines for curative medicine, often called "evidence-based medicine" (6) have made similar and important contributions. More recently, a similar effort has been explored for community-based public health programs (7).

More emphasis on outcome measures. The emphases on both practice guidelines and evidence-based practice has yielded a further orientation toward both traditional and new outcome measures as indicators of community health. More sophisticated measures are in development, and more comprehensive attempts at program performance monitoring are occurring (8). As more sophisticated, detailed and measurable outcomes are developed, this monitoring may not only evaluate specific public health or community programs, but may also work toward assessing the entire public health, health education and clinical service structure within a community.

Establishment of goals for communities to attain improvement in health status. This exercise has been a part of strategic program planning for a long time, but in the past decade has been elevated to explicit goal setting for communities and larger jurisdictions. While national goals for health status improvement (9) may be useful at the local level, most public health officials and community organizations would rather have goal setting performed at the local level. This allows engagement of local professionals and other citizens and takes greater account of local priorities, needs and perceptions of the most compelling health problems to which limited resources should be allocated.

Application of more advanced community health information systems. This takes many forms, but accurate, comprehensive, and timely community health data are an essential requisite of goal-setting and program performance monitoring. Clinical and public health information are both essential and interrelated, raising special issues of ethics and privacy, as well as access. However, the information revolution should allow better program management and assessment, and with appropriate controls should serve the prevention and public health communities in ways not previously possible.

In summary, the current era has been a time of clear change for both preventive medicine and public health. This book attempts to capture and review these changes for the practitioner and student of these strategically important disciplines.

▶ REFERENCES

1. American Public Health Association, Association of Schools of Public Health, Association of State and Territorial Health Officials, National Association of County Health Officials, United States Conference of Local Health Officers, Department of Health and Human Services, Public Health Service, Centers for Disease Control, 1991 *Healthy Communities 2000: Model Standards.* 3rd Edition, Washington, DC, APHA
2. Stoto MA, Abel C, Anne Dievler A, *Eds.* Healthy Communities: New Partnerships for the Future of Public Health. Institute of Medicine, National Academy Press, Washington, DC, 1996
3. Lohr KN, Aaronson NK, Alonso J, Burnam MA, Patrick DL, Perrin EB, Roberts JS: Evaluating quality-of-life and health status instruments: development of scientific review criteria. Clinical Therapeutics 18:979–92, 1996
4. Canadian Task Force on the Periodic Health Examination: Canadian Guide to Clinical Preventive Health Care Ottawa, Canada Communication Group, 1994
5. DHHS: 1996 *Guide to Clinical Preventive Services* (Second Edition): A Report of the US Preventive Services Task Force. Washington, DC: DHHS
6. Maynard A. Evidence-based medicine: an incomplete method for informing treatment choices. Lancet 349:126–128, 1996
7. Council on Linkages Between Academia and Public Health Practice 1995. *Practice Guidelines for Public Health: Assessment of Scientific Evidence, Feasibility and Benefits.* Albany, NY: Public Health Practice Guidelines Development Project, 1995
8. Durch JA, Bailey LA, Stoto MA, *Editors.* Summary. Improving Health in the Community: A Role for Performance Monitoring. Institute of Medicine: National Academy Press, Washington, DC: 1997
9. DHHS 1991 *Healthy People 2000: National Health Promotional and Disease Guidelines.* Washington, DC: DHHS

2

Epidemiology

Carl W. Tyler, Jr. • John M. Last

Epidemiology is the basic science and most fundamental practice of public health and preventive medicine. We can study health and disease by observing their effects on individuals, by laboratory investigation of experimental animals, and by measuring their distribution in the population. Each of these ways of investigating health and disease is used by the epidemiologist. Epidemiology is therefore the scientific foundation for the practice of public health.

The word "epidemiology" comes from epidemic, which translated literally from the Greek means "upon the people." Historically, the earliest concern of the epidemiologist was to investigate, control, and prevent epidemics. This chapter deals with the scientific principles that are the foundation of epidemiology. We then address the sources and characteristics of information used to assess the health of populations. Next we discuss the ways this information can be analyzed. Finally, we show how to use epidemiology in controlling and preventing health problems.

▶ HISTORY

Epidemiology has roots in the Bible and in the writings of Hippocrates, as does much of Western medicine. The Aphorisms of Hippocrates (fourth to fifth century B.C.) contain many generalizations based on prolonged and careful observation of large numbers of cases. The introductory paragraph of "Airs, Waters, Places" offers timeless advice on good environmental epidemiology:

> Whoever would study medicine aright must learn of the following subjects. First he must consider the effect of each season of the year and the differences between them. Secondly he must study the warm and the cold winds, both those that are common to every country and those peculiar to a particular locality. Lastly, the effect of water on the health must not be forgotten. When, therefore, a physician comes to a district previously unknown to him, he should consider both its situation and its aspect to the winds. Similarly, the nature of the water supply must be considered. . . . Then think of the soil, whether it be bare and waterless or thickly covered with vegetation and well-watered, whether in a hollow and stifling, or exposed and cold. Lastly consider the life of the inhabitants themselves, are they heavy drinkers and eaters and consequently unable to stand fatigue or, being fond of work and exercise, eat wisely but drink sparely?[1]

Epidemics of infection seriously concerned physicians in ancient times, although often they could do little more than observe the victims and record mortality. Their limited knowledge rarely permitted effective intervention. Until the Renaissance physicians based their approach more on impressions than real numbers. John Graunt is often regarded as the founder of vital statistics. He first published his numerical methods for examining health problems in *Natural and Political Observations on the Bills of Mortality* in 1662. He was the first to attempt this approach.

Epidemiology was first applied to the control of communicable diseases and public health through quarantine and isolation, even though ideas about disease transmission and microbiology and epidemiology were rudimentary. Johann Peter Frank, a physician who became "director-general of public health" (in modern terminology) to the Hapsburg Empire, systematized and codified many rules for personal and communal behavior in the eighteenth century. His work contributed to public health and is published in *System einer vollstandigen medicinischen Polizey* (1779).

Careful clinical observation, precise counts of well-defined cases, and demonstration of relationships between cases and the populations in which they occur all combine in the method upon which epidemiology depends. This method was first developed in the nineteenth century. Modern epidemiologists hold John Snow[2] in high esteem. He painstakingly collected the facts about sources of drinking water that he related to mortality rates from cholera in London. This proved a classic demonstration of the mode of transmission about 30 years before Koch isolated and identified the cholera *Vibrio*. Snow's great contemporary, William Farr,[3] defined and clarified many basic ideas of vital statistics and epidemiology. Among his most important contributions were the following: *(a)* the scope of epidemiology, *(b)* the concept of person-years, *(c)* the relationship between mortality rate and probability of dying, *(d)* standardized mortality ratios, *(e)* dose-response relationships, *(f)* herd immunity, *(g)* the relationship between incidence and prevalence, and *(h)* the concepts of retrospective and prospective study. He also developed the first effective classification of disease, the direct ancestor of the nosology that we still use today. *Vital Statistics* (1885), an edited volume of excerpts from Farr's annual reports to the registrar-general, is perhaps the best textbook of epidemiology ever written, graced by beautiful writing and well-chosen tables to illustrate the text.

Methods of epidemiological investigation have evolved since the mid-nineteenth century. The case-control study reentered medicine from the social sciences in the third decade of the twentieth century. The cohort study came into use after World War II, as a means of identifying risks associated with heart disease, lung cancer, and other emerging public health problems. Epidemiological "experiments" as now conducted in randomized trials are essentially modern innovations. Statistical methods and the electronic computer add greatly to the power of epidemiological analysis. Present indications suggest expanding potential and an exciting future for epidemiology. Population-based medicine makes community assessment and diagnosis important for determining the need for health services. An increasingly broad interface between clinical medicine and epidemiology is called clinical epidemiology. Molecular epidemiology promises to let epidemiologists link genetic biological markers to health condition, thereby creating new potential approaches to intervention. Case-control studies are adding rapidly to our understanding of cause-effect relationships in many chronic and disabling disorders. Epidemiological methods can also help in evaluating health services.

What does this brief history of epidemiology teach? First, the community and environment influence the health of humans, as do our own inherited characteristics. Second, knowing how a disease is transmitted permits us to control and prevent it, even though we may not know the causal agent. Third, even the simplest information about vital events, illnesses, and populations can detect and analyze epidemiological problems. Finally, epidemiology can help find, investigate, analyze, control, and prevent a wide range of health problems.

► DEFINITION

Epidemiology is both the basic science of public health and its most fundamental practice. Therefore we need to examine both aspects of its meaning.

Science

Epidemiology was originally defined as the scientific study of epidemics. An epidemic is the occurrence in excess of normal of an illness, health event, or health-related behavior that occurs in a specific place or among a group. Reports of cholera by John Snow and childbed fever by Holmes are among the classic examples. In recent years excessive use of tobacco, called by some "the brown plague," and the acquired immunodeficiency syndrome (AIDS) are examples of modern epidemics.

Because the word "epidemic" may lead to chaotic, unreasoned responses to health problems, journalists use the term more often than epidemiologists. Other words, such as outbreak and cluster, are employed by practicing public health professionals to avoid unreasoned public response.

In current use, however, the definition of epidemiology is broader and recognizes the application of this basic science of public health to the control and prevention of health problems. The following definition, recently agreed upon by an international panel, is widely accepted:

> Epidemiology is the study of the distribution and determinants of health-related states and events in specified populations and the application of this study to the control of health problems.[4]

Some terms in this definition require discussion. *Distribution* relates to time, place, and person. The relevant population characteristics include location, age, sex, and race; occupation and other social characteristics; living places; susceptibility; and exposure to specific agents. In addition, the distribution of the exposed cases needs to examine time as a factor. Relationships in time reveal information about trends, cyclic or secular patterns, clusters, and intervals from exposure to inciting factors to the onset of disease.

Determinants include both causes and factors that influence the risk of disease. Many diseases have a single necessary cause. When the agent of disease causes a single, specific condition, as occurs with the tubercle bacillus or the lead in lead-based paint, we know the necessary cause. In addition, there are usually many other determinants. They fall into two broad groups *(a)* host factors that determine the susceptibility of the individual and *(b)* environmental factors that determine the host's exposure to the specific agent. Host factors include age, sex, race, genetic or constitutional makeup, physiologic state, nutritional condition, and previous immunologic experience. Environmental factors include all conditions of living. Among these factors are family size and composition; crowding; hygienic conditions; occupation; and geographic, climatic, and seasonal circumstances. Characteristics of individuals or populations, identified by the term "lifestyle," may include such factors as use of tobacco, alcohol, and automobiles. Past and present environment—including the period of intrauterine life—may influence exposure and susceptibility to disease.

Practice

The practice of a science is best defined by what the scientist does. Langmuir points out that, "the basic operation of the epidemiologist is to count cases and measure the population in which they arise."[5] The practice of epidemiology therefore is the scientific process that detects, investigates, and analyzes health problems, followed by applying this information to the control and prevention of these problems. This practice requires health problems to be the subject of public health surveillance, epidemiological investigation, and analysis. The findings of this analysis linked to health policy can lead to the control and prevention programs intended to resolve the health problem. Evaluation of control and prevention is also the responsibility of the practicing epidemiologist as is the clear and persuasive communication of the scientific findings to the public, policy makers, and program staff.

Uses of Epidemiology

The most important use for epidemiology is to improve our understanding of health and disease—a goal shared by all the disciplines and branches of the biomedical sciences. Morris[6] defined seven uses of epidemiology: historical study, community assessment, working of health services, individual risks and chances, completing the clinical picture, identification of syndromes, and the search for causes (Table 2-1). Each deserves brief comment.

Historical Study

The classic question "Is health improving?" can be answered only by comparing experience (rates) over time; this is one essential routine activity in all health services. Sometimes when the data are closely examined, unexpected trends appear. For example, asthma deaths increased unexpectedly in children and young adults in Britain and other countries in the 1950s and continued to increase into the mid-1960s, before the cause—self-use of isoprenaline nebulizers—was discovered. Removing the offending product from the market halted the unfortunate trend.

Community Assessment

What are the health problems? This question can be answered in many ways. For example, what proportion of school children have become regular cigarette smokers by various stages of their progress through school? Or what proportion of people always or never use seat belts when driving or riding in cars? Answers to such questions have prognostic and also diagnostic value. Community assessment makes it possible to predict the impact of future health problems by known effects of many risk factors.

TABLE 2-1. USES OF EPIDEMIOLOGY

Historical study: Is community health getting better or worse?
Community assessment: What actual and potential health problems are there?
Working of health services
Efficacy
Effectiveness
Efficiency
Individual risk and chances
Actuarial risks
Health hazard appraisal
Completing the clinical picture: Different presentations of a disease
Identification of syndromes: "Lumping and splitting"
Search for causes: Case control and cohort studies
Evaluation of presenting symptoms and signs
Clinical decision analysis

The Search for Causes

This is the most obvious use for epidemiology. Most hypothesis-testing studies (discussed later) have the primary aim of identifying causal factors, or at least of risk factors for disease. This chapter cites many examples of such studies.

Working of Health Services

Are all needed services available, accessible, and used appropriately? Are children receiving necessary immunizations? Can pregnant women begin prenatal care before the end of the first trimester of pregnancy? Do known contacts of persons with sexually transmitted diseases receive follow-up and treatment? Information on these and many other questions is often gathered routinely or by special survey. Health service administrators should not only think always of these simple routine questions, but should be alert to less obvious potential gaps in coverage. For example, the census will state the numbers of elderly persons who live alone. Is all or only a small portion of these known to the public health nurses and others who provide home surveillance and care?

Individual Chances

What is the risk that a person will die before the next birthday? Actuaries who evaluate the risks for persons seeking life insurance have calculated answers based on probabilities derived from experience. This has become a prominent activity of epidemiologists who work on risk assessment and has led to many new insights, for example, about occupational and environmental risks and the hazards associated with immunizations.[7]

Identification of Syndromes

Epidemiologists are called "lumpers and splitters" because epidemiological investigations sometimes make it possible to group together several differing manifestations of a condition or to separate seemingly identical diseases into more than one category. The latter are more common than the former; examples include the differentiation of hepatitis A from hepatitis B and the distinction between several varieties of childhood leukemia. Examples of "lumping" include the identification of many manifestations of tuberculosis. Once each group of symptoms and signs had a different name, such as phthisis, consumption, or pleurisy. Addiction to tobacco is the underlying cause of a variety of outcomes. Among them are respiratory cancers, chronic obstructive pulmonary disease, and a portion of the risk of coronary heart disease. All these conditions could result from "tobaccoism."

Completing the Clinical Picture

One of Morris' original illustrations of this use for epidemiology was the demonstration that myocardial infarction occurs commonly in women as well as in men. An important difference is that this condition occurs in women at older ages and presents more often as "ruptured ventricle"; this causes sudden death. Last used the technique of "completing the clinical picture" to construct a model[8] of what might occur in the average general practice population. In the course of a year, facts known and seen by the physician may be amplified by epidemiological study even though they might be unidentified, undiagnosed, or in a single practitioner's experience and only the submerged part of the iceberg of disease.

Other Uses

Clinical epidemiologists have defined other uses for epidemiology that do not fit any of Morris's original seven uses. One important use is the evaluation of presenting symptoms and signs of disease. Analyzing the data in hospital charts and relating symptoms and complaints to final diagnoses makes it possible for an epidemiologist to produce clinical algorithms. These analyses can show the probability that a particular cluster of presenting symptoms and signs is related to a specific group of underlying disease processes. A related use is clinical decision analysis.[9] This technique is a rigorous quantitative method used to decide the best method of managing patients with particular diseases. This procedure involves the use of decision trees. Decision trees are algorithms in which the probability of an outcome for each different decision is predicted based on clinical experience.

Epidemiological Method

Epidemiologists use a wide range of scientific information, including clinical findings, laboratory data, and field observations. In the end, it is the reasoning of the epidemiologist that ties these facts together. This reasoning is the logic behind disease control and prevention measures.

Epidemiological reasoning is fundamental and straightforward. First, we define events or clinical cases using careful, specific, and objective observations. Next, we count these events or cases and orient them to time, place, and person. Then we determine the population at risk and calculate rates of occurrences for the events or clinical cases. This requires the use of nothing more complicated than long division. We put the events or cases in the numerator according to their relevant characteristics. The next step involves using a denominator of the portion of the population at risk and characterizing this group in the same way as those in the numerator are characterized. At this point we calculate rates of occurrence in the group of cases. These rates are then compared with the rates of occurrence in other population groups. Finally, using this information, we draw inferences about the events that define the health problem and the agent or agents that cause it. These rates also provide information about the host and the environmental factors that influence the risk of occurrence and the transmission of the health problem. Using this information and collaborating with other health professionals, we propose control measures and then continue the observations required to assess the control program.

In identifying a health problem or case, many kinds of clinical examination may be employed. The patient's history may reveal information about exposure to risk, incubation period, susceptibility, occupation, residence, course of disease, or other factors. Physical examination can classify individuals not only about whether they have the condition under study, but as to type, stage, and duration of disease. Laboratory tests are valuable for a similar purpose. In addition, they are essential in revealing clinically inapparent cases, and they often shed light on the pathogenesis of the condition. Field observations are the sine qua non of the epidemiological method.

Viral hepatitis is an example of the ways that clinical, laboratory, and field studies can interlock. Epidemic jaundice, mentioned by Hippocrates, has occurred in wars from ancient times to the present. Medical investigators used needle biopsies, a technique developed in the 1940s, to show generalized parenchymal inflammation accompanied the acute disease. Epidemiological study soon distinguished hepatitis A ("infectious hepatitis") from hepatitis B ("syringe jaundice"). Both were shown to be due to filterable agents, presumably viruses. However, hepatitis A had the epidemiological features of a fecal-oral transmission. Hepatitis B, on the other hand, was clearly blood borne and transmitted by inadequately sterilized hypodermic needles or other medical equipment. No cross-immunity protected people with one form of hepatitis from the other. Subsequent studies showed further differences. Hepatitis A had a shorter incubation period, was more contagious, and had a briefer period of abnormal serum transaminase activity than did hepatitis B.[10] Later epidemiological studies revealed the pattern of sexual transmission of hepatitis B among male homosexuals. In 1965, Blumberg and colleagues found Australia antigen in the serum of patients who had multiple transfusions and, in 1967, this was unequivocally associated with hepatitis B.[11] Subsequently, Blumberg received the Nobel Prize for his work. In 1970, Dane and coworkers[12] identified and described the virus, and in 1971, Almeida and colleagues[13] found that the surface particles, hepatitis B surface antigen (HBsAg), represented Australia antigen. HBsAg was extremely valuable in screening carriers for hepatitis B and in developing a vaccine. Vaccines developed independently in the late 1970s in France and in the United States have been rigorously tested in laboratory and field trials. Both are of proven efficacy and safety in preventing hepatitis B in susceptible individuals. Among their uses are for patients as those in renal dialysis units, infants born to mothers carrying hepatitis B, and male homosexuals. The virus of hepatitis A was identified in 1973 and successfully grown in tissue culture in 1979. This led to preparation of hepatitis A viral antigen, paving the way for serological tests for hepatitis A antibody. Detection of this antibody, found in some 70% of adult urban Americans, suggested a high prevalence of subclinical cases. Vaccine preparation was made possible by such advances. As hygiene and sanitation improve, infants and children are spared. The result is that more serious cases occur among adults in contrast to the previous pattern of subclinical and mild cases among children. Vaccination against the disease is therefore more desirable than ever.

Epidemiological features of hepatitis B among homosexual males have been a useful model to follow in the investigation of AIDS. Both conditions have the same pattern of distribution in this subset of the population. Case-control studies have shown that many persons who contract AIDS, like hepatitis B, are male homosexuals who engage in anal intercourse and have many partners.[14]

The tools employed in this illustration of the epidemiological method are clinical, immunological, microbiological, pathological, demographic, sociological, and statistical. None of these approaches is uniquely epidemiological; it is their employment in particular ways with particular objectives that is the epidemiological method.

In epidemiology, unlike in clinical medicine, the concern is not with individual cases but with all the cases in a defined population. Furthermore, the entire range of manifestations of the condition must be considered in relation to the population from which the cases arise.

Epidemiological Sequence

An orderly sequence characterizes epidemiology: observing, counting cases, relating cases to the population at risk, making comparisons, making scientific inferences, developing the hypothesis, testing the hypothesis, experimenting and intervening, and evaluating. This sequence describes the actions we take whenever a "new" condition occurs. The relationship between cigarette smoking and lung cancer illustrates the stages in this epidemiological sequence.

1. *Observing.* Scientific observations on smoking and cancer appeared in the *Journal of the American Medical Association*[15] in 1920 and in the *New England Journal of Medicine*[16] in 1928. In the following decade, *Science* documented that smokers had a shorter life expectancy than did nonsmokers.[17]
2. *Counting Cases or Events.* Vital statistics trends showed an increase in deaths caused by lung cancer in the United States beginning in the 1930s.
3. *Relating Cases or Events to the Population at Risk.* Increased death rates from lung cancer reported in national vital statistics attracted the attention of health department officials. Registrars of vital statistics in countries where smoking was an established lifestyle characteristic reported a similar trend.
4. *Making Comparisons.* Studies of British physicians reported by Doll and Hill[18] and of contacts of American Cancer Society volunteers reported by Hammond and Horn[19] in the 1950s provided definitive comparisons between smoking and lung cancer. (In addition to identifying this threat to the health of the public, the studies of Doll and Hill established the contemporary criteria for epidemiological associations.[20])
5. *Developing the hypothesis.* Since cigarette smoke contains more than 2,500 chemical components, some of which are carcinogenic in animals,[21] only a small logical step was required to go from inference to hypothesis.
6. *Testing the Hypothesis.* The hypothesis that smoking caused lung cancer lent itself to testing by means of a case control study. A small case control study done in Germany during 1938–1939 was overlooked in the turmoil of World War II. Epidemiological studies designed to test the hypothesis were conducted in postwar Britain by Doll and Hill[18] and in the United States by Hammond and Horn.[19] Both studies showed consistent relationships between the present occurrence of lung cancer and a history of cigarette smoking, with a dose-response relationship. Subsequent case control studies produced similar results. Reports of cohort studies soon followed. Both kinds of investigations confirmed the association and demonstrated other adverse effects.[22]
7. *Making Scientific Inferences.* Several observations led to valid scientific inferences about the association of tobacco smoking and lung cancer. Among them were *(a)* clinical observations, *(b)* national trends in mortality from several countries associated with the increased prevalence of cigarette smoking, *(c)* epidemiological comparisons made in large groups representing different segments of national populations in more than one country, and *(d)* the biological effects of tobacco smoke. All of these observations led to the inference that smoking increased the risk of dying from this disease.
8. *Conducting Experimental Studies.* Laboratory animal studies with beagles show that exposure to tobacco smoke produces the precancerous lesions followed by squamous cell carcinoma in both animals and humans.
9. *Intervening and Evaluating.* Action by public health and voluntary health agencies reduced cigarette smoking rates. A decline in mortality trends in smoking-related causes in the United States and other countries followed this reduction. One of the most important steps in this process was the issuance in 1964 of the Surgeon General's *Report on Smoking and Health*, which commemorated its twenty-fifth issue in 1989.

► FOUNDATIONS OF EPIDEMIOLOGICAL PRACTICE

Putting the epidemiological method into practice requires skill in a unique set of tasks.

Surveillance

Surveillance as an element of epidemiological practice is "the ongoing systematic collection, analysis, and interpretation of health data essential to the planning, implementation, and evaluation of public health practice, closely integrated with the timely dissemination of these data to those who need to know. The final link in the surveillance chain is the application of these data to prevention and control." This definition is part of the plan for the national coordination of disease surveillance of the Centers for Disease Control and Prevention (CDC).[23] It is based in part on the one proposed by Langmuir in 1963.[24]

The surveillance of public health problems is the first important task for the practicing epidemiologist, because it is the means for detecting problems for the life of the surveillance system. Public health surveillance uses established data collection procedures and sets. This approach uses a minimum of data items and is intended to detect changes in the occurrence of health events in time to control and prevent the health problem. Health problems can therefore be detected and confirmed quickly and intervention initiated. Surveillance focuses on descriptive information that is analyzed according to time trends and the rates of occurrence estimated. These findings are fed back to the health personnel who originated the data. Health policymakers who need this information also receive reports of these findings.

Investigation

Surveillance information can trigger epidemiological investigations by public health surveillance reports. Epidemiological investigations can begin because of any of a number of other initiating events, such as news articles, phone calls, or other health departments or colleagues with similar responsibilities.

The investigation of an epidemiological problem, whether it is an epidemic of acute infection or a long-term condition such as cancer, begins with careful observation and a detailed description. The basic steps of an epidemiological investigation are discussed below.

Analysis

The analysis of epidemiological data goes through a series of orderly steps beginning with a careful and detailed description of cases or events. The description ought to include direct observations of persons influenced by the health event. In addition, the environment in which they live and work, the risk factors related to the event, and information about the agents that might have caused the health problem require careful description. The observations need to be quantified. The analysis progresses to comparison groups. The epidemiologist then compares occurrence rates among groups according to specific characteristics of the groups, that is, looking for a dose-response relationship, and may ultimately reach the point of complex and sophisticated quantitative analysis.

Evaluation

Evaluation addresses well-defined problems, such as the effectiveness of a drug or vaccine. It involves the assessment of problem-solving action. Consequently, the first essential step is a detailed description of the problem and the action intended to solve it. Evaluation includes the assessment of the effectiveness of specific agents. In addition, evaluation can assess contraceptive effectiveness, smallpox eradication, or the effectiveness of screening for cervical cancer.

Other Essential Tasks

Communication, management, including team building and human relations, and consultation are essential but not unique to the practice of epidemiology.

Communication

Communicating epidemiological information clearly and persuasively is essential to effective practice. Just as a clinician must persuade a patient to take pills or undergo surgery, an epidemiologist must persuade professional colleagues, public officials, and the public that epidemiological findings warrant action to control and prevent a health problem.

Management and Teamwork

Epidemiologists also need to develop management skills because they rarely work alone. Even in the investigation of a small outbreak, the assistance of a public health nurse may be essential. Subsequent analytic work often requires collaboration with statistical personnel, computer staff, or secretarial professionals. In these circumstances, epidemiologists need to understand the basic concepts of management, beginning with planning and including organizing, team building, directing, and evaluating management.

Human relations are a key part of every management process. Epidemiologists cannot ignore these relationships. Practice and observation are the best ways to learn these skills. Many health professionals deal with human relations in a clinical, patient-to-professional situation. Epidemiological practice requires working in teams, although essential team members may not be professionals. Nonetheless, their skills are indispensable to conducting epidemiological work, and they deserve respect.

Consultation

Consultation with colleagues in epidemiology, other fields of public health, clinical medicine, or public groups is part of the professional practice. Consultation requires a special kind of communication skill; it is difficult to offer scientifically sound advice in a persuasive yet dispassionate manner.

Presentation Skills

The ability to present epidemiological information to professional and public groups is as much a part of epidemiology as doing a case count or computing a relative risk. This skill differs from that of consultation because a presentation is most often a single event in which an epidemiologist discussed the investigation, often presenting complex information orally and visually to a large group. Consultation, on the other hand, is a process that requires information gathering, often involves interviewing, and may conclude with a presentation. Distinguishing between these two is important because of the emphasis of skill in presentation. Without this skill, important epidemiological work may have little health or scientific impact.

Relationship to Other Public Health Professions

The unique discipline of epidemiology interacts with a host of other professions.

Statistics

Statistics is closely allied to epidemiology. Epidemiologists need to know enough statistics to calculate rates and to decide how likely it is that differences in comparison groups could be due to chance. Statisticians support epidemiological studies in many ways, for example, helping determine sample size, choosing samples, ensuring data quality, selecting the correct approach to complex analysis, and interpreting findings.

Laboratory Science

Laboratory science is often the key to correctly identifying a disease agent and an environmental exposure. Microbiologists, immunologists, toxicologists, biochemists, and behavioral and survey research scientists all contribute to epidemiological investigations. Laboratory determinations help characterize host susceptibility and assess carrier and preclinical disease states. Perhaps most important, the laboratory provides the greatest predictive capability possible in arriving at a case definition.

Health Policy

Epidemiologists optimize their contribution to public health when the problems they address influence health policy. Policy decisions often seem remote from the practice of epidemiology because epidemiologists may equate policy with politics. However, epidemiologists influence policy to some degree almost every time they issue a report.

Health Service and Program Management

Epidemiology often provides health service programs and provides the information that sets the standards of care. Epidemiological evaluation of effectiveness may determine the product used in nationwide programs and the schedule for administering preventive agents, such as vaccines, or conducting screening examinations, such as cervical cytology.

▶ SURVEILLANCE

Definition

Because it often marks the beginning of the epidemiological sequence, the definition of surveillance warrants reinforcement. "Surveillance is the ongoing systematic collection, analysis, and interpretation of health data essential to the planning, implementation, and evaluation of public health practice, closely integrated with the timely dissemination of these data to those who need to know."[23] Implicit in this definition is a link between surveillance and prevention and control efforts. This link leads to the formation of a cycle. This cycle brings together the evaluation of prevention and control and the detection of subsequent epidemics through the continued collection, analysis, and interpretation of data into a system of public health surveillance.

While the concept of surveillance in epidemiology goes back centuries—at least to Graunt and Farr—the practice of surveillance continues to evolve. Its most important modern milestone was the clear and precise definition given to this practice by Langmuir in 1963. He stated that surveillance was "the continued watchfulness over the distribution and trends of occurrence through the systematic collection, consolidation, and evaluation of morbidity and mortality reports and other relevant data,"[24] and the reporting of this information to all of those who needed to know, implicitly including health officials, clinical physicians, and the public.

One instance in which surveillance influenced public health and helped control an epidemic is AIDS as it was discovered in Los Angeles County. A more detailed account at the end of this section describes how a health department epidemiologist detected the first cluster of cases reported from that area.

Surveillance is not the same as epidemiological research. The CDC definition explicitly points out the need for timeliness and for dissemination, while it clearly links surveillance to public health action. While surveillance may identify problems in need of research, it is a problem-finding process with an immediate relationship to public health action, rather than a problem-solving process.

Surveillance systems provide information for urgent as well as routine action. In that sense they also differ from health information systems. Health information systems include the registration of births and deaths, the routine abstraction of hospital records, and general health surveys. Most often these systems differ from surveillance systems. Health information systems may report findings episodically, rather than at regular intervals. In addition, reports of this information may describe events not related to specific deadlines, or they may not relate to the prevention or control of a specific health problem. Nonetheless, data from health information systems are important components of the practice of surveillance depending on how the information is used. Birth weight recorded on a birth certificate, for example, is important, because it is essential information in doing surveillance for the birth of premature infants.

Purpose

In the practice of epidemiology and public health, surveillance has the following three generic purposes: *(a)* surveillance may identify public health problems, *(b)* surveillance may stimulate public health intervention, and *(c)* surveillance may suggest hypotheses for epidemiological research. More specifically, surveillance data can serve a host of important public health functions. Among them is the detection of epidemics, including significant individual cases, such as botulism, in which a single event triggers public health action. In addition, surveillance data can pick up changes in long-term trends. The use of laboratory data for surveillance can detect changes in disease agents. Intervention programs often use surveillance data to plan and set program priorities and to evaluate the effects of public health programs. Information from surveillance systems helps to project the occurrence of health problems in the future, as has been reported concerning the HIV/AIDS epidemic.

To ensure that a surveillance system fulfills its purpose, the problem a surveillance system addresses needs a clear definition. Objectives for the system should establish the case (or the event) definition and the times and details for issuing surveillance reports. Because of its role in initiating public health action, Thacker and Berkelman propose that this practice be called "public health surveillance"[25] rather than epidemiological surveillance.

Surveillance Cycle

Public health surveillance embodies a systematic cycle of public health actions. The cycle includes *(a)* collection of pertinent data in a regular, frequent, and timely manner; *(b)* its orderly consolidation, evaluation, and descriptive interpretation; and *(c)* prompt distribution of the findings (Table 2-2). Dissemination must focus on the distribution of information. Two groups must receive these data. Of first importance are those who provided the data. They will need to confirm or correct the data. Next are those who take action on the data. The cycle is ongoing. Updating and correcting the data is essential because new information may require a change in the response of the public health system. Under rare circumstances, surveillance may be ended, as was done when smallpox was eradicated, because the public health problem under surveillance is resolved.

TABLE 2-2. THE SURVEILLANCE CYCLE

- Collection of data
  - Pertinent
  - Standardized
  - Regular
  - Frequent
  - Timely
- Consolidation and interpretation
  - Orderly
  - Descriptive
  - Evaluative
  - Timely
- Dissemination
  - Prompt
  - All who need to know
    - Data providers
    - Action takers
- Action to control and prevent

The surveillance cycle is applicable to a wide range of public health problems, depending on the purpose and objective of the system. Initially, surveillance focused on the detection of epidemics and the characterization of seasonal fluctuations in infections. Now, the surveillance cycle is also used for injury control, a select group of cancers, certain cardiovascular diseases, and high-risk and unintended pregnancies, to cite a few illustrations.

Characteristics of a Surveillance System

An effective system of public health surveillance has seven essential attributes:

1. Simplicity
2. Acceptability
3. Sensitivity
4. Timeliness
5. High predictive value positive
6. Flexibility
7. Representativeness

What do these terms mean when put in the day-to-day practice of epidemiology? *Simplicity* is the characteristic of being clear and easily understood, rather than complex and difficult to understand. Uncomplicated data are easier to maintain, aggregate, interpret, and distribute promptly. *Acceptability* refers to the attribute of being straightforward and free from unintended emotional content. This is a special problem for health problems such as surveillance of abortion or sexually transmitted infections. Acceptability is essential because most public health surveillance systems rely on the cooperation of individuals and organizations to provide objective, unbiased data. *Sensitivity* is a term most often used in connection with screening tests, such as Pap smears. Sensitivity measures the likelihood that a diagnosis of a health problem is correct. This is important in the practice of surveillance because public health surveillance serves as a way to screen for health problems in a community. Just as screening tests must be highly sensitive if they are to detect abnormalities, a public health surveillance system must be highly sensitive. A sensitive system can detect and characterize epidemics, as well as seasonal and long-term trends. A surveillance system must also have a *high predictive value positive*. Predictive value positive (PVP) is another term associated with screening. PVP, when used for a surveillance system, means that those persons reported to have the condition under surveillance have a very high probability of actually having that condition. A system with a low predictive value positive wastes valuable public resources by collecting inadequate data and by requiring unproductive effort on incorrectly identified epidemics. *Timeliness* refers to the fact that data are reported promptly after they are gathered. Surveillance data are important and cannot remain at the point of collection without being sent to the place where data are being edited and analyzed. This is a key characteristic of a surveillance system for two reasons. First, reports based on information obtained need distribution with a very short lag time. Prompt action is necessary to halt additional morbidity or mortality quickly. Second, data collection and processing must be regular and prompt. Punctual editing and revision improve the quality and consistency of the data that are essential to decision-making information. *Flexibility* refers to the need for a surveillance system to be versatile and adaptable. This characteristic is important because such systems are often called upon to adapt to new health problems. For example, when penicillinase-producing *Neisseria gonorrhoeae* infections were first detected and the first clusters of AIDS cases discovered, surveillance documented the spread and transmission of these new epidemics. Finally, surveillance systems must accurately *represent* the health status of the community, that is, the system needs to be *representative*. Data collected by the system need to correctly portray the occurrence of health events over time. They must characterize geographic distribution and characterize the problem in the population.[26]

Data Sources

Vital Statistics

Information about births and deaths, that is, vital events, has been collected, classified, and published at least since the middle of the seventeenth century in several European countries. Now the *International Statistical Classification of Diseases and Related Health Problems*[27] provides the standard nomenclature that categorizes causes of death, disease, and injury.

Mortality. Death is, for the epidemiologist, the least equivocal measure of ill health. A death certificate is a public document of legal, medical, and health importance. It provides information about time, date, and place of death; place of residence; sex, race, birth date, birthplace; marital status and usual occupation; and also cause of death for each individual. It is the basic document for determining the number of deaths, calculating death rates, and estimating the probability of mortality and life expectancy by each variable included on the death certificate.

In developed countries, the occurrence of mortality in a population is almost completely reported, but specific items on the death certificate may not be accurate. Sex and age are recorded with close to 100% accuracy, but race, marital status, and occupation are not. The greatest problems arise in certifying the cause of death. While most people who die of an injury or of cancer have their cause of death correctly certified, persons who die of other causes may not. Cause-of-death certification may change according to current medical interests, perceptions, and philosophies. Moreover, autopsy information received after the death certificate is completed may not appear on the official certificate. The result is that secular and international comparisons are difficult. Some conditions may be difficult to study unless the cause of death is confirmed by interviewing individuals who know the decedent. Other conditions require a review of medical records, or verification of death certificate information through comparison with autopsy reports.

Fertility. Information from birth certificates is increasingly important as epidemiologists turn more to the reproductive health problems. These documents characterize births by sex of the infant, place of residence, place of occurrence, birth date, birth weight, length of gestation, and other characteristics of both parents. Birth data are essential to estimating pregnancy rates and perinatal, neonatal, and infant mortality. They are also often the most appropriate denominators in estimating the occurrence of events, such as rates of birth defects.

Birth registration is more complete than death registration. Nonetheless, some items are not as well reported as others. Information that is not reported fully deserves special care when used for epidemiological study. Among these items are race, ethnicity, marital status, and length of gestation.

Other Certified Events. Marriage and divorce are legally certifiable events that are often related to health. They describe changing characteristics of human populations and human relationships.

Vital Record Linkage. Vital record linkage provides a broad base of information important to the practice of public health. By linking birth and infant or maternal death certificates, for example, describing trends in detail is possible. Record linkage enables trends to be examined over long periods and broad geographic areas.

In the past, health data for individuals in one set could not be related to individuals in a population in another data set. For example, hospital discharge statistics cannot be linked to death certificates. Thus, information for patients receiving a new treatment might be lost unless hospital discharge data were linked to death certificates. In working with birth certificates, relating information in birth certificates to information on infant death certificates is often impossible. This can be true of infants even when birth and death both occur on the same day, let alone when it occurs many months later. A method is needed to assemble and connect, or link, data in different sets. If, for example, data in medical charts were connected with data in birth and death certificates, epidemiological studies of birth factors associated with premature mortality might be possible. This procedure must ensure that the same individual is counted only once. The term *record linkage* describes this method and procedure.[28]

The result is among the most powerful tools available for epidemiological studies. There are three prerequisites. They are: *(a)* the unique identification of individuals even if they change their names, *(b)* a method of abstracting and storing relevant health and vital information, and *(c)* a technique for matching information from different sites and settings over long periods. The final step is output of statistical tables. Record linkage systems with these qualities have been operational for many years in the Oxford region of England, in Scotland, in Sweden, and in Canada.

A record linkage system makes it possible to relate significant health events that are remote from one another in time and place. For example, a patient who received a particular antibiotic drug may be treated elsewhere at some future time for a blood dyscrasia caused by the antibiotic. In a different situation, a worker employed for a short time in the nuclear energy industry may die of cancer. The death may occur many years and several occupations later. As an isolated sequence this would have no significance. However, if appropriate analytic techniques are used to analyze large data files in a comprehensive linked record system, many such sequences can be identified. Record linkage makes it possible to discover significant associations between events and their underlying cause. An important advantage of epidemiological studies that use record linkage is the very large numbers of observations available.

Record linkage studies have successfully identified previously unknown or doubtful occupational cancers,[29] and can assess other occupational risks, for example, exposure to formaldehyde.[30] They have made it possible to calculate the risks associated with exposure to ionizing radiation, both in medical and in occupational settings.[31,32] The epidemiological method is a form of historical cohort study (see below). The investigation usually begins by using personal identifiers to identify those individuals in a population exposed to the risk that is under examination. Past medical records or records from places people have worked can determine the kind and level of exposure. The computer file mortality database is searched to find the causes of death of these individuals whose cause-specific death rates can then be calculated. Computer files for death certificates can verify the identity of individuals in the study. This and certain other aspects of the method require access to personal information that is normally strictly confidential. Access to this information is limited to staff who have signed an oath to preserve the confidentiality of the documents.

In Canada, the national mortality database is the central element in many successful record linkage studies. Details of all deaths in Canada since 1950—personal identifying information and cause of death—have been coded and stored electronically. All the death certificates are preserved.

Canada has made effective use of record linkage, in part, by using simple, standard, readily available documents for the origin of the data. If all items of information are available from two sources, for example, a past medical record or employment history and a death certificate, the two can be matched precisely. This gives an extremely high probability that they relate to the same individual.

Similar procedures to set up a national mortality database began in the United States in 1979. The system in the United States, the National Death Index (NDI), uses magnetic tapes of death records sent to the National Center for Health Statistics by the individual states. These tapes contain standard identifying information. Among the items are the decedent's first and last names and middle initials, father's last name (especially for females), social security number, birth date, sex, state of birth and of residence, marital status, race, and age at death. Names can be matched with other records to be linked with NDI records either by exact spelling or Soundex Code. Soundex is a system based upon phonetic spelling that is effective in other record linkage systems.

Health Reports

Estimates of morbidity, particularly those for infectious disease reporting, are based on a national system of notifiable diseases that has operated in the United States since 1920. Reports from physicians sent through health departments to CDC make up most of the entries in this database, but information provided by hospitals and laboratories is also important. This approach to surveillance has proved effective in characterizing seasonal trends, showing temporal relationships to explain trends, and detecting epidemics although notification of this kind is incomplete. The current program of measles elimination proves this point in its use of surveillance to detect and control outbreaks. Thacker and Berkelman[25] cite a series of national surveillance systems that include some of those mentioned above and also others that are based on information from medical examiners, emergency rooms, and public clinics.

Hospital Records

More than 100 years have passed since Florence Nightingale[33] effectively used hospital statistics to point out the serious problems faced by patients in hospitals. Subsequently, hospital records have proved essential to the acquisition of clinical data, demographic information, sociological data, information about the quality of medical care, economic data, and administrative information such as the site of care and type of service. Few data sources offer such a rich spectrum of information.

Nonetheless, hospital records have unique problems. Items of key importance to studies of past events may not have been collected consistently or at the same level of detail for each subject. Moreover, some information recorded may not be legible. Of greatest seriousness, however, is that in some institutions retrieving the entire record for a given individual may not be possible.

Summary information about hospital discharges can be analyzed from survey data. The National Hospital Discharge Survey (NHDS) has been published in the United States every year since 1965.[34] Nongovernmental organizations are also useful sources of data on hospital discharges. Among the best known are the Commission on Professional and Hospital Activities (CPHA), which is responsible for the Professional Activity Study (PAS),[35] and McAuto, a hospital discharge abstract system operated by the McDonnell-Douglas Corporation. These systems have their own special set of problems, particularly regarding their representation of a definable population. NHDS is based on a stratified probability sample of discharges. Since not all strata are represented in the same way, interpretation of NHDS reports requires a detailed understanding of sampling procedures. Other hospital discharge abstraction systems also exist. Data from programs managed by the Health Care Financing Administration (HCFA) are based on financial information taken from hospital bills. Because each state in the United States has an individual plan for each of these programs, data from HCFA programs must be interpreted based on a detailed understanding of the database.

Registries

There are two kinds of registries: *(a)* population-based and *(b)* disease registries. Population-based registries provide the data most useful for epidemiological purposes. This kind of registry has information about all cases of specific disease in a geographically defined area that relates to a specific population. Data of this kind can be used to calculate rates of occurrence and are also useful for estimating survival rates and rates of disease progression and of mortality from a specific cause. The Surveillance, Epidemiology, and End Results (SEER) centers supported by the National Cancer Institute illustrate this kind of population-based registry for cancer.

Disease-case registries are most often kept at a hospital or treatment facility. They provide detailed documentation of diseases cared for in that facility, but they are not usually population-based for two reasons. First, rarely does a single facility discover all of the cases that occur in a specific area. In addition, a population residing in the catchment area for a health care facility is even more rarely counted or characterized in detail.

Health Surveys

Health surveys provide extremely valuable information. In the United States, CDC's National Center for Health Statistics (NCHS) has conducted nationwide household interview surveys since 1957. These interviews are taken from a probability sample of the civilian population of the United States who are not residing in institutions. They are carried out on a recurring basis and gather a core of information on disability, the characteristics of health problems, and the kinds of care the respondent has undergone. In addition, detailed questions are added to each survey to explore health problems related to a specific system of the body or group of diseases in greater depth.[36]

In 1959 NCHS augmented its household interview surveys by conducting a series of health examination surveys. These surveys involved physical and biological measurements such as height, weight, blood pressure, visual acuity, and hemoglobin. In 1970, a nutrition examination survey was included in the NCHS battery of periodic sample surveys.

Recognizing the importance of information about health care, NCHS now conducts the National Ambulatory Medical Care Survey (NAMCS), the National Hospital Discharge Survey (NHDS), and the National Nursing Home Survey. Information about health care facilities, including family planning clinics, and surveys of the health care workforce are now part of the spectrum of NCHS surveys.[37]

The need for information about risk factors related to chronic diseases led the CDC to initiate the Behavioral Risk Factor Surveillance System (BRFSS).[38] This system uses telephone interviews to collect information about chronic disease risk factors such as obesity, treatment for blood pressure, alcohol use, and exercise. The monthly collection of information about these risk factors permits the characterization of seasonal variations and long-term trends. Perhaps most important, this system gives health professionals and the public current information about these risk factors.

The National Survey of Family Growth (NSFG) conducted by NCHS assesses the use of family-planning services, contraceptive practice, and surgical sterilization.[39] It also gathers information about the determinants of family size and composition. Information from this survey has proved useful in epidemiological studies of human reproduction and the safety of widely used methods of fertility control.

Data Collection

Public health surveillance relies on three approaches to data collection.

1. The first is used in urgent situations, such as an active and ongoing epidemic. Under these circumstances, health agencies initiate surveillance by contacting those data sources most likely to have current information. Called by some "active" surveillance, this approach ensures that reporting will be timely and characterized by simplicity, acceptability, and sensitivity. This approach has the possibility of sacrificing representativeness by weighting responses toward a preselected group of reporting sources. It may also limit the predictive value if reporters need to identify cases before the diagnostic workup is complete, thereby leading to the reporting of cases that do not fulfill the definition.
2. Provider-based data collection is the approach most frequently used by the national notifiable disease surveillance system. Referred to by some as "passive" surveillance, this approach is simple, acceptable, and flexible. It is rarely as sensitive as health agency-based surveillance, and it may not be timely or representative. Nonetheless, its value in describing seasonal and long-range trends and promoting the detection of epidemics has withstood the test of time for public health professionals.
3. Finally, the sentinel approach has its roots in the surveillance of occupational health problems and is now being applied more widely. The use of birds to detect lethal levels of odorless gases, such as carbon monoxide in mines, may have been the earliest form of sentinel surveillance. Concern about epidemic infections has led to the use of sentinel animal flocks to detect arthropod-borne viruses that cause encephalitis and herald the occurrence of epidemics of this infection in humans. Rutstein and his colleagues have proposed that this concept be extended to a broader range of occupational health problems[40] and to the health care system more generally.[41]

Computers and electronic telecommunications permit surveillance information to be transmitted widely, in great detail, and on a timely basis. For decades notifiable disease reporting relied on information reported on postcards. These cards gave the aggregate numbers of cases of infectious diseases. Health departments mailed the cards each week. Computers now permit cases to be characterized individually yet confidentially. Telecommunication ensures that the information is available on a timely basis. Computer networks have the potential of making this information available to a wide range of skilled epidemiological analysts and of eliciting a timely public health response. CDC has developed a software package called Epi Info.[42] This software helps with the collection, recording, and transmission of surveillance information. It is also an important tool for field investigations and epidemiological surveys. A computer telenetwork, the National Electronic Surveillance System (NETSS),[43] now reaches state and many major local health departments, providing electronic surveillance reports. The Information Network for Public Health Officials (INPHO) now permits a wide range of reports, as well as data, to reach health officials to support their policy decisions.

Data Quality

The quality of health data is an increasingly important issue as information plays a more significant role in detecting epidemics, discovering new public health problems, and developing health policy. Just as epidemiologists are concerned about the quality of information they receive from others, they also want to know that the data they collect themselves are of good quality. Four dimensions of data quality are especially important.

1. Data input must be of high quality. In a one-dimensional check of data input, all variables should be within an appropriate range. A surveillance system concerned with childhood lead poisoning, for example, ought not to include a person 50 years old. A two-dimensional check of input would ensure that pairs of variables were reasonable. For example, a surveillance system for the nutritional status of pregnant women should not to include a 17-year-old woman with 10 children. Moreover, data should be logically consistent so that a child with measles reported to have begun on November 1, *1988*, ought not to have had a birth data in *1998*.
2. Management of data records is essential to ensuring data quality. Records will need to be uniquely identified and carefully tracked so that they can be retrieved and verified. The status of record completion will need to be documented, particularly in household and telephone interview surveys. Confidentiality is a point of tension in records management. Striking the balance between ensuring the privacy of an individual and permitting a public agency to meet an urgent public need will always be difficult to resolve. The current AIDS epidemic demonstrated this problem repeatedly. Many conflicts may be resolved by using identification numbers instead of names. However, some events will be rare enough that individuals might be identified simply by knowing the disease they have, their age, sex, and county of residence, especially if the county is not a populous one.
3. Data output must be of excellent quality. One-dimensional, two-dimensional, and logic checks are as important in handling data output as they are in checking data entry. Computer programs that produce the output should create totals for columns and rows added up for each table rather than being brought forward from an earlier computation. Imputation procedures deserve critical examination so that they are relevant to the way the output will be interpreted and used. In short, epidemiologists need to examine every piece of relevant data and to ask "Will this make sense to the people who need this information?"
4. Data archives are the final dimension of data quality. Keeping an archive of public health information requires more than the final output. It also requires enough of the intermediate computations that questions can be answered quickly and intelligently. These inquiries may come from other researchers, the media, or the public. In keeping an archive of epidemiological data, two questions need to be addressed. First, how will the issues of public accountability and individual confidentiality be addressed? Second, if an important question comes up, can the answer be retrieved in 3 seconds? An hour? 2 days? Not at all? Ultimately, data collected by public agencies are in the public domain. Nevertheless, an epidemiologist must consider the measures appropriate for a public agency to use in preserving individual privacy and making data accessible to others. Among those likely to need public data are researchers, journalists, and individual citizens.

Data Reporting

The reporting of public health surveillance data needs to consider four approaches. The first is descriptive. A typical issue of the *Morbidity and Mortality Weekly Report (MMWR)* illustrates this point.[44] The *MMWR* reports case counts of the diseases that are nationally notifiable. Aggregated case reports are entered into tables for each state and a few additional major reporting areas, such as the District of Columbia, each week.

Second, graphs of surveillance data permit a visual analysis. A histogram that shows the distribution of cases of a given disease in a specific area over a stated period is often called an "epidemic curve" (Fig. 2-1). Line graphs that display cases over time help characterize temporal relationships in disease occurrence as shown in Figure 2-2 that displays surveillance data for malaria in the United States. Graphs that display historical data can signal changes in disease trends, as shown in Figure 2-3.

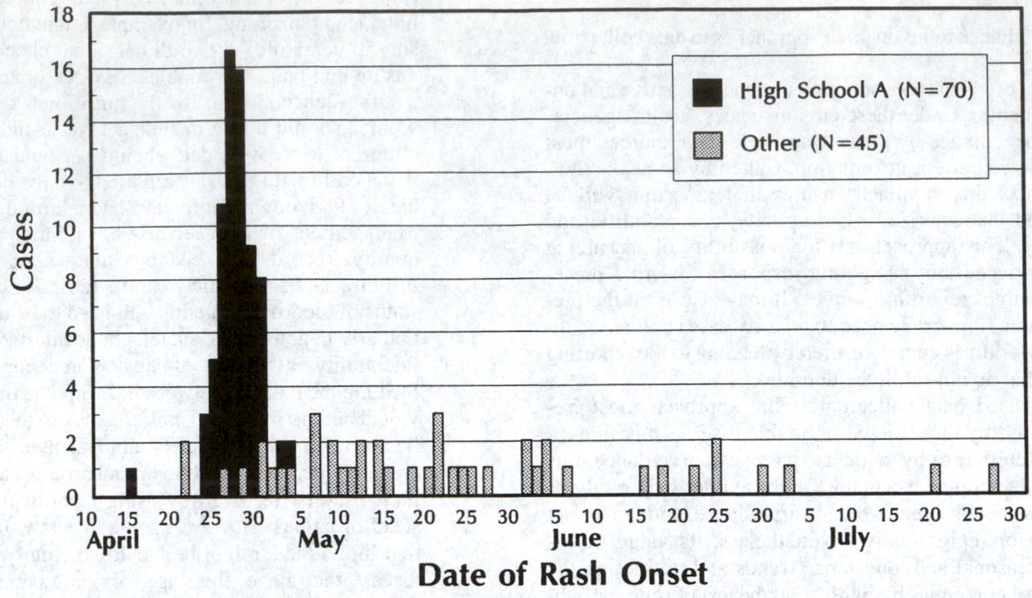

Figure 2-1. Reported measles cases by date of rash onset, Elgin, Illinois, April 15 to July 28, 1985

Third, maps often provide an effective graph of the geographic distribution of a disease (Fig. 2-4). Spot maps illustrate the distribution of individual, or small groups, of cases. The use of shading differentiates the relative intensity with which a disease or other public health problem occurs over a wide area. Sequences of maps illustrate changing disease distributions over time. Three-dimensional maps may also show differing intensities of health problems over an area. Computer mapping using data that describe cases by county of occurrence and residence helps determine whether epidemics are being transmitted across jurisdictional boundaries.

Finally, quantitative analysis of surveillance data may help detect important changes in the trends of health events. Using a moving average in analyzing national trends in fertility is a regular part of the monthly *Vital Statistics Report*[45] published by NCHS. Epidemics can be detected using time series analysis. Analyzing trends in excess mortality graphically using periodic regression or auto-regressive, integrated-moving-averages are time honored ways of identifying influenza epidemics.[46] Excess mortality among the aged during periods of unusual heat waves can also be detected with these methods.[47]

Dissemination

The findings from public health surveillance must be distributed to two groups immediately: *(a)* those who provide data so that it can be verified and *(b)* those responsible for public health actions. When surveillance detects urgent public health problems, such as an epidemic, an immediate telephone response is required. For years, CDC has sent data on notifiable disease surveillance and on epidemic field investigations to state and local health officials before the information is published in the *MMWR*.

Surveillance information is now disseminated in a series of reports based on the *MMWR*. Besides the weekly publication, CDC

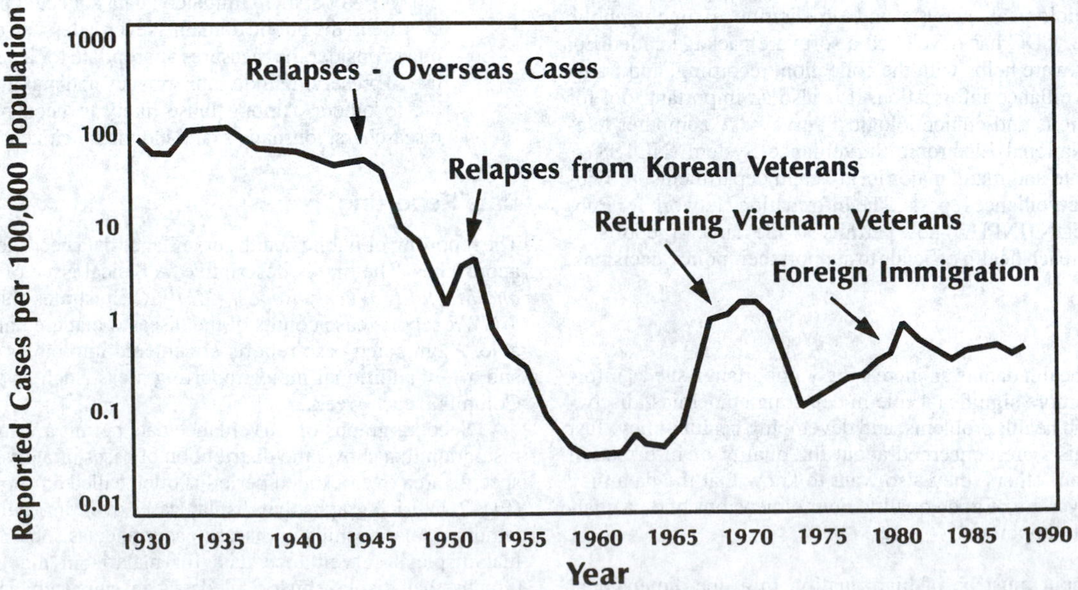

Figure 2-2. Malaria, by year, United States, 1930–1988

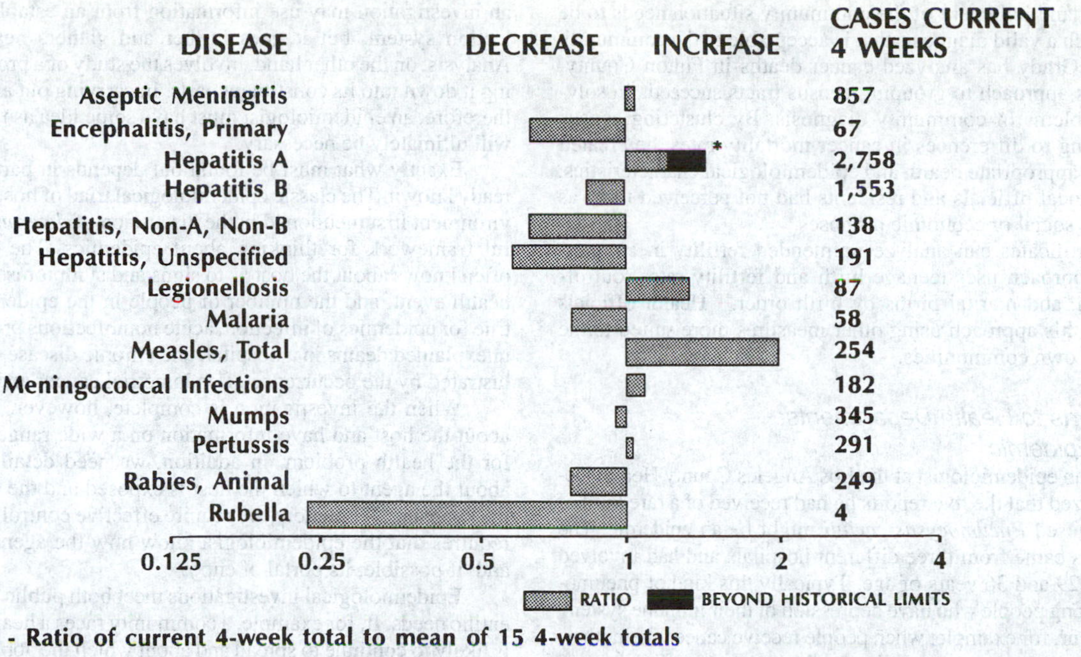

Figure 2-3. Notifiable-disease reports; comparison of 4-week totals, ending 11/25/89, with historical data, United States

issues other special *MMWR* reports and an annual summary of notifiable diseases.[48] CDC also publishes public health and epidemiological findings in many refereed professional journals. Surveillance data characterize historical trends and project those trends into the future. Recently CDC compiled its guidelines for prevention into a single publication that is supplemented with additional details on an electronic compact disc.[49] The World Health Organization (WHO) maintains a worldwide reporting system. The information in this system appear in the *WHO Weekly Epidemiological Record*. These reports are augmented by quarterly, annual, and occasional special supplements.

Applying Public Health Surveillance: Two Case Studies

Using Vital Data: Community Diagnosis Based on Mortality Registration

Community diagnosis assesses health problems of a specific population in a defined geographic area using public health surveillance data. Vital records are often used as the first approach. Holland and colleagues' *European Community Atlas of Avoidable Death* (2nd edition)[50] is an excellent, readily accessible publication that illustrates this use of vital data.

Community diagnosis, carried out in detail and directed at intervening in a health problem, is a stepwise process, as follows:

1. Defining the condition to be diagnosed
2. Estimating the size, characteristics, and occurrence of the condition
3. Refining the diagnosis based on additional data
4. Estimating and characterizing the population in need of service
5. Reevaluating the diagnosis

Vital data can also help diagnose problems for communities smaller than the European community. In addition, community diagnosis for small areas often needs to examine data that cannot be evaluated using statistical testing. In these instances, detailed knowledge

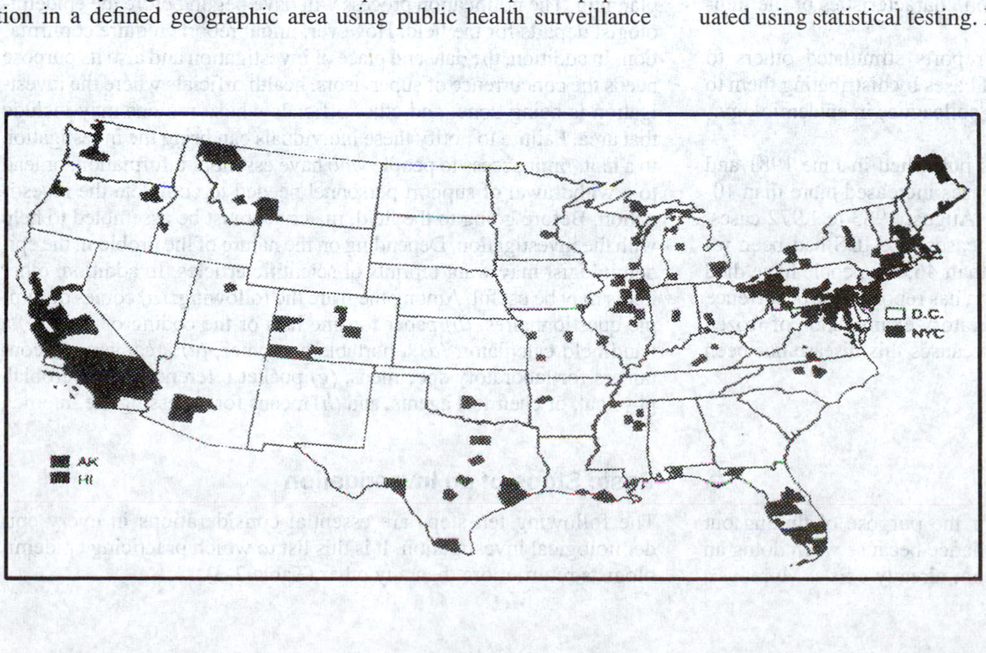

Figure 2-4. Measles (rubeola), counties reporting cases, United States, 1988

of the locality and judgment of the community situation needs to be applied to reach a valid diagnosis that is acceptable to the community members. McGrady has analyzed cancer deaths in Fulton County, Georgia.[51] His approach to grouping census tracts succeeds in solving some problems of community diagnosis. By clustering census tracts according to differences in cancer mortality rates, he created areas that had appropriate health and epidemiological characteristics, even though local officials and residents had not perceived them as such for other social or economic purposes.

Birth certificates can analyze unintended fertility in communities. One approach uses teenage birth and fertility rates, out-of-wedlock birth, and marital births by birth order.[52] Health officials have adapted this approach using other measures more suited to the needs of their own communities.

Using Reports to Health Departments: The AIDS Epidemic

In mid-1981, an epidemiologist at the Los Angeles County Health Department realized that the five reports he had received of a rare kind of pneumonia caused *Pneumocystis carinii* might be an epidemic. The disease reports came from three different hospitals and had involved men between 29 and 36 years of age. Typically this kind of pneumonia occurs among people who have depression of their immune system, which can occur, for example, when people receive cancer chemotherapy. At one hospital, a large university medical center, the clinician caring for these patients had already recognized this unusual occurrence.[53]

A month later, a report from another part of the United States documented the occurrence of this same kind of pneumonia. In addition, some patients had other unusual infections and a rare form of cancer, Kaposi's sarcoma. This group of 26 individuals ranged in age from 26 to 51 years. Twenty of them lived in New York City, six in California; eight had died within 24 months after diagnosis of Kaposi's sarcoma; all were male homosexuals.[54] Within the next year, CDC received 355 additional case reports. Five states—California, Florida, New Jersey, New York, and Texas—accounted for 86% of the reported cases. This was the beginning of the AIDS epidemic.

A cluster of people with an unusual infection that affected previously well individuals was picked up by an astute clinician and an observant epidemiologist. The epidemiologist knew that even five cases of this kind represented an unusual occurrence, perhaps even an epidemic. He took the following four key actions:

1. He confirmed each case.
2. Next, he provided a clear, brief (no more than seven lines of text in the original report) description to a central public agency (CDC, in this instance).
3. Third, he identified the common characteristics of the individuals.
4. Finally, he ensured that the reports stimulated others to search for additional clusters of cases by distributing them to health professionals, including colleagues in epidemiology.

The original group of five reports published in June 1981 and augmented a month later by 26 more cases increased more than 10-fold by June 1982 to 355 cases and by August 1983 to 1,972 cases. As of December 1988, almost 83,000 cases of AIDS had been reported in the United States, and more than 46,000 people have died of AIDS. The World Health Organization has reported the occurrence of AIDS from all over the world. Laboratory examination of frozen human serum shows that the virus that causes this disease has been present in humans at least since 1959.

► INVESTIGATION

An investigation is an examination for the purpose of finding out about something. It differs from surveillance because when doing an investigation one assumes that a problem already exists. Moreover, an investigation may use information from an established data collection system, but it goes farther and gathers new information. Analysis, on the other hand, involves the study of a problem by breaking it down into its constituent parts. In carrying out an investigation, therefore, an epidemiologist must have some idea as to what analysis will ultimately be necessary.

Exactly what must be found out depends in part on what is already known. The classic epidemiological triad of host, agent, and environment first mentioned in the discussion of *determinants*, is a useful framework for thinking about epidemics. The epidemiologist often knows about the host as to signs and symptoms of an illness, or health event, and the number of people in the epidemic. This holds true for epidemics of infection, acute noninfectious problems, such as unexplained deaths in a hospital, and chronic disease problems, as illustrated by the occurrence of endometrial cancer and estrogen use.

When the investigation is complete, however, we must know about the host and have information on a wide range of risk factors for the health problem. In addition, we need detailed information about the agent to which the host is exposed and the environment of the exposure. Ultimately, we require effective control measures. This requires that the epidemiologist know how the agent is transmitted and, if possible, its portal of entry.

Epidemiological investigations meet both public service and scientific needs. If, for example, a community faces a health problem that is likely to continue to spread and about which the approach to control is uncertain, then the epidemiologist has an important role. Epidemics of viral infections that occur in presumably immunized young people, as has been the case of measles epidemics on college campuses, illustrate this problem. Moreover, public concern may also require the epidemiologist to provide assurance that no epidemic exists and none is threatening. Concern about transmission of AIDS by exposure to medical waste in public places is one such example, even though this environmental problem is not a real hazard for transmitting disease.

Scientific need is a second important reason for an epidemiologist to do a detailed field investigation. This kind of investigation recently led to the discovery of Lyme disease and Legionnaire's disease. Field investigation also identified the causal association between vinyl chloride exposure and angiosarcoma of the liver, as it was for oral contraceptive use and hepatocellular adenoma, and a wide range of other health conditions.

Preparing for an Investigation

Preparation for an epidemiological field investigation has three general elements: *(a)* notification of essential people and organizations, *(b)* identification of materials needed for the investigation, and *(c)* travel planning. The notification process will have begun before the epidemiologist departs for the field. However, initial reports require confirmation. In addition, the date and place of investigation and also its purpose needs the concurrence of supervisors, health officials where the investigation is being done, and other officials whose regions may include that area. Failure to notify these individuals can bring the investigation to a halt, limit access to people who have essential information, or lead to a withdrawal of support personnel needed to complete the investigation. Before going to the field, materials must be assembled to help with the investigation. Depending on the nature of the problem, the epidemiologist may want reprints of scientific articles. In addition, other items may be useful. Among them are the following: *(a)* copies of sample questionnaires, *(b)* paper for line lists or the coding of data, *(c)* a hand-held calculator, *(d)* a portable computer, *(e)* a camera, *(f)* containers for laboratory specimens, *(g)* pocket references on microbial, physical, or chemical agents, and *(h)* means for accessing the Internet.

Basic Steps of an Investigation

The following ten steps are essential considerations in every epidemiological investigation. It is this list to which practicing epidemiologists return more than any other (Table 2-3).

TABLE 2-3. STEPS IN AN EPIDEMIOLOGICAL INVESTIGATION

1. Determine the existence of an epidemic
2. Confirm the diagnosis
3. Define and count the cases
4. Orient the data in terms of time, place, and person
5. Determine who is at risk of having the health problem
6. Develop and test an explanatory hypothesis
7. Compare the hypothesis with the proven facts
8. Plan a more systematic study
9. Prepare a written report
10. Propose measures for control and prevention

1. *Ensure the existence of an epidemic.* The first important decision is to decide if an epidemic exists. A preliminary count of people with similar symptoms is often the first criterion for this decision. Laboratory confirmation may be absent. It may even be inappropriate because of the urgent need to begin an investigation.
2. *Confirm the diagnosis.* The epidemiologist needs to know the diagnosis of the health problem being addressed. The number of cases is sometimes too great to do a history and physical examination on every person. Collection of laboratory specimens must then follow quickly, although decisions about epidemic control are often made before laboratory confirmation is available. Using this preliminary information, the epidemiologist must formulate a case definition of the health problem. The symptoms for the case definition are written down, as are the essential physical signs. Measurements of levels of severity of the health problem, or disease, must be determined. Confirming each reported case may not be possible, and laboratory specimens may be obtained on only 15 to 20 percent of the cases. In some large epidemics, a sample of cases gave the essential information about the agent, the host, the method of transmission, the portal of entry, and the environment of the disease. This proved to be the only way to deal with one epidemic in 1985 when *Salmonella* contaminated milk processed in Illinois and involved more than 200,000 individuals.[55] Epidemiologists set up control measures more quickly using this approach than by an exhaustive detection of every ill individual.
3. *Estimate the number of cases.* Case finding often begins with a single report or a small cluster of cases. Initially, the epidemiologist casts a wide net, using a preliminary case definition that is sensitive and excludes as few true cases as possible. After making a preliminary estimate, the epidemiologist must make a key judgment. Should all cases be studied or is the epidemic so large that investigating a sample will lead to a decision more quickly? If only a sample is selected, then only the most severe cases should be studied because they are the ones of most value. Outlying observations deserve special attention because explaining their relationship to the epidemic is often the key to understanding its mode of spread.

   Given a workable definition, the epidemiologist must count the cases and collect data about them. Once the ill persons are identified, the characteristics of the illness from beginning to the present and the demographic characteristics of each individual need to be determined. Next, data on the places where the ill people live, work, and have traveled to, and the possible exposures that might lead to health impairment all must be documented. Among the questions the epidemiologist may want to answer are the following: What signs and symptoms are the most important? Are any of them pathognomonic? What is the laboratory test most likely to confirm the diagnosis? Can both the exposure to the presumed source and the severity of the illness be characterized at different levels? What must be done to identify the people with these problems should long-term follow-up be necessary? Are there any inapparent or subclinical cases? What role do they play in determining the future size of this epidemic or the susceptibility of the people in this community?
4. *Orient the data as to time, place, and person.* Data on each case must include the date of onset of the illness, the place where the person lives and/or became ill, and the characteristics of each individual, including age, sex, and occupation. A simple histogram, often called "the epidemic curve," shows the relationship between the occurrence of cases and their time of onset (Fig. 2-1).[56] The spatial relationships of cases are often shown best on a spot map. Maps, for instance, help show that the cases occurred in proximity to a body of water, a sewage treatment plant, or its outflow. Characterizing individuals by age, sex, and other relevant attributes permits the epidemiologist to estimate rates of occurrence and compare them with other appropriate community groups.
5. *Determine who is at risk of having the health problem.* The epidemiologist will calculate rates at which a health problem, or disease, occurs using the number of the population at risk as the denominator, while the number of those individuals with the problem form the numerator. If the original reports of an illness come from a state surveillance system, then the first estimations of rates may be based on a state's population. If the epidemic occurs only in school-age children from a particular school, however, the population at risk may be only the children who attend that school. Those not ill must be characterized by the same attributes as those who are ill, that is, age, sex, grade in school, or classroom.
6. *Develop an explanatory hypothesis.* During a field investigation comparing the rates of occurrence among those at greatest risk with other groups helps the epidemiologist develop hypotheses to explain the cause and transmission of a health problem. Besides examining rates, other approaches to developing hypotheses of cause include further, more detailed interviews with ill individuals or with local health officials and residents, careful examination of outlying cases, or describing the epidemic in more detail. Depending on the extent of the epidemiologist's field library, reference to current and historical literature can stimulate new hypotheses.
7. *Compare the hypothesis with the established facts.* The hypothesis that explains the epidemic must be consistent with all the facts the epidemiologist knows. If the hypothesis does not do so, then it must be reexamined. It should do more than just strengthen speculation explaining the cases at the peak of the epidemic. The epidemiologist may need to repeat the interview of case subjects, reassess medical records, gather additional laboratory specimens, and repeat calculations.
8. *Plan a more systematic study.* When the initial field investigations and preliminary calculations are complete, the investigator may need to conduct one or more case control studies (see below). The data for such studies may be in hand, but more often additional information will be needed. It may be collected by either interviewing subjects in more detail or surveying the population. Sometimes, a serological survey or extensive sampling of the environment for chemical or biological agents will generate new facts. Sometimes a visual record helps, requiring extensive photography or video taping of a work process. If there is a food-borne infection, a detailed food history is necessary. If a water-borne infection is suspected, a food and liquid intake history stimulates additional causal associations. For example, a water-borne epidemic may be discovered by knowing the number

of glasses of water drunk by each person, thereby permitting the epidemiologist to estimate a dose-response relationship. An occupational illness might be determined by a specific machine that each worker used and the number of hours that each one used it.

9. *Prepare a written report.* Preparing a written document is an essential step in any epidemiological investigation. An epidemic report need not be a publishable paper. However, it should be a benchmark in the conduct of an investigation, just as a hospital discharge summary is for patient care or a thesis is for the advancement of a scholar. The epidemic report is an essential public health document. It may be the basis for action by health officials who may close a restaurant or face a major industry's attorneys in court. For the public, it may provide information for those concerned about the epidemic, its spread, and the likelihood that others will be involved. A report may have scientific epidemiological importance in documenting the discovery of a new agent, a new route of transmission, or a new and imaginative approach to epidemiological investigation. Moreover, many investigative reports are useful in teaching.
10. *Propose measures for control and prevention.* The ultimate purpose of an epidemiological investigation is to control a health problem in a community. The epidemiologist is part of the team that develops the approach to control and prevention.

The establishment of a surveillance system for the population at risk is an important element in ensuring the effectiveness of the control program. This is an essential element of an epidemiologist's responsibility in fulfilling a public need and carrying out a scientific study.

Designing an Investigation

Descriptive Study

Epidemiological investigations often start with case reports, evolve to become a series of cases, and then go on to include ecological studies, cross-sectional studies, or surveys. Working with information from case reports or a series of cases is often the first step in a field or community investigation. For an epidemiologist concerned with the clinical details of an illness, the causal agent, the environmental, and other risk factors, added information will be needed. Demographic, social, and other behavioral characteristics and possible exposures to biological, physical, or chemical agents are also essential.

Ecological Studies

Ecological studies compare the frequency of events that occur in different groups. This type of study compares data and examines correlations useful in generating hypotheses association. The association of increased dietary fat intake and increased occurrence of breast cancer is one important hypothesis generated through an ecological study. Because ecological studies compare groups, rather than individuals, caution is required in drawing conclusions and identifying associations. The hazard found in interpreting studies of this kind is labeled "the ecological fallacy."[57] It is a bias or error in inference that occurs when an association observed between variables on an aggregate level is assumed to exist at an individual level. This fallacy is exemplified in the correlation of membership in the Baptist religion with the occurrence of eclampsia during pregnancy. While this study illustrates this kind of misinterpretation, this kind of fallacy has also been found in studies of the quality of drinking water and mortality from heart disease. This correlation is not a causal association because the criteria for such an association (which are discussed later in the section titled *Analysis*) were not fulfilled. On the other hand, ecological studies are usually quick, easy to do, use existing data, and generate or support new hypotheses.

Cross-Sectional Studies

Cross-sectional studies simultaneously evaluate exposure and outcome in a population. This approach is another important step to developing evidence for a causal association. As an illustration, consider the possibility that a group of women had cervical cytology done during the same examination when a culture for herpes simplex virus was taken. If a statistically significant association existed between premalignant cervical cells and the recovery of herpesvirus from cultures, this finding would be an important step toward a causal association. However, a cross-sectional study would not permit the epidemiologist to decide if the virus was present before the cells became premalignant or if premalignant cells are highly susceptible to viruses. This approach is often useful at the time of an epidemic investigation. It helps to determine the extent of the epidemic in a population and to assess the susceptibility of those in the population at risk. This approach is not an appropriate way to study rare events, events of short duration, or events related to rare exposures. Moreover, cross-sectional studies are not appropriate for assessing the temporal relationship between exposure and health event or outcome.

Analytical Studies

Analytical studies may be observational or experimental. In an observational study, the epidemiologist assigns subjects to case and comparison groups. This assignment may take place after an event has occurred (retrospectively) or before an event has happened (prospectively). The investigation of an epidemic, such as infections following childbirth, or a study based on clinical observation, such as the occurrence of angiosarcoma of the liver in vinyl chloride workers, is typically observational and retrospective. In these instances, the epidemiological study had to be confined to observations about events that had already taken place. Moreover, the epidemiologists used data that had already been collected and assigned people to groups based on the presence of disease or exposure that had already occurred. If cases of postpartum infection had been carefully defined and assigned to case (of postpartum infection) or control (no infection) groups, the study would be observational and prospective.

In an experimental study, on the other hand, subjects are observed under predetermined conditions. Random clinical trials are examples of experimental epidemiology. Both the case definition and the experimental conditions would be carefully defined before the study began. Carefully designed approaches to data and specimen collection and the observations to be made are specified and categorized before the study begins. The individuals being observed in an experimental study may be allocated to different groups on a probabilistic basis.

This section addresses the design of epidemiological studies, only mentioning analytical approaches. The following section, Analysis, deals with analytical issues in more detail and gives examples of ways in which they might be handled.

Observational Studies

Observational studies are categorized as case-control or cohort. In a case-control study, the risk of exposure to a presumed cause by those with a health problem (the case group) is compared with that of those who do not have that problem (the control group). The frequency with which the exposure occurs is compared in the two groups, and the strength of association is measured as an odds ratio. The epidemiologist evaluates the likelihood that such an association could occur because of chance using statistical confidence intervals.

Case-Control Studies

Case-control studies begin with a case group of individuals who have the health problem under investigation. The outcomes typically studied using this design are those that are rare or have a long latent, or incubation, period, such as cancer. Conditions that require detailed records are well suited to study using this design. Among these records are hospital charts, pathology reports and specimens, and laboratory documentation, such as, electrocardiograms, x-rays, or other imaging techniques. For health problems that are rare, or develop over long periods, the case-control design yields findings in a short time and with a minimum resource requirement. One example is the Cancer and Steroid Hormone Study. This collaborative investigation evaluated the association between oral contraceptives and cancer in some key sites of the female reproductive system.[58] This study illustrates the use of the case-control study design in dealing with an important, worldwide public health problem.

Cohort Studies

Cohort studies begin with a case group made up of individuals exposed to the hypothesized cause of a health problem. The comparison group is one that is not so exposed, but has similar demographic, behavioral, and biological characteristics. The groups are compared and characterized using the rates with which the health problem occurs in each group. The strength of association is measured using relative rates; its occurrence due to chance is evaluated statistically by stating the P value, and the precision of the relative risk or odds ratio is shown by the confidence intervals.

Retrospective, or historical, cohort studies may look back in time by reviewing recorded events, or they may require that subjects be observed during the future. Those done by reconstructing records of exposure and health outcomes are called retrospective cohort studies because they look back over time. Those that follow similar groups with different exposures into the future are called prospective cohort studies. The study of American veterans of the Vietnam War who were exposed to Agent Orange is an example of a retrospective cohort study.[59] On the other hand, many reports on cardiovascular disease in Framingham, Massachusetts, illustrate prospective cohort studies.[60] The most difficult problems that cohort studies pose for epidemiologists is, if the study is retrospective, finding records that are comparable for both the exposed and unexposed subjects. If the study is prospective, finding the resources and motivating the staff is usually the greatest challenge. Conducting studies of this kind is difficult because the need for meticulous recording is required for a long time, usually years, and often decades.

The advantages and disadvantages of these two study designs is shown in Table 2-4. Case control studies are advantageous when the epidemiologist is studying a rare condition (for example, a condition that occurs no more often than once in every 100 people in the population under study). In addition, this approach can evaluate an association between disease and exposure relatively quickly. Moreover, it is especially useful if the investigator has limited resources and is dealing with a health problem that has a long latency or incubation period. Of the advantages for cohort studies, on the other hand, three are especially important. The first is that a cohort study provides an opportunity to describe the natural history of a health problem. In addition, the epidemiologist can directly estimate the rate at which the health problem is occurring and take the findings to people who are not epidemiologists.[61]

Bias can distort the findings of any study, whatever its design. Bias is the "deviation of results, or inferences from the truth, or processes leading to such deviation."[4] Bias can occur in any approach to study design. The most generic categories of this kind of deviation are selection bias and information bias. Selection bias occurs when comparison groups differ from each other in some systematic way that influences the outcome or exposure that is being investigated. This form of bias is a more frequent problem in case-control studies, but it can occur in both approaches to study design. A study of oral contraceptive effectiveness in women using two different kinds of pills illustrates this point. Such a study might be biased if the group taking one kind of pill included only women who had given birth (confirming their ability to become pregnant) with another group, none of whom had been pregnant. This selection of subjects leads to a bias that might distort the comparison of effectiveness of the two agents.

The role of information bias is important when an exposure or health outcome is measured systematically in different ways for subjects in the case and control groups. This can be related to the inability to collect comparable information, to systematically different approaches to observing the two groups, or to differences in the quality of the information collected. A comparison of surgical complications in two groups, one of which underwent surgery in a hospital with another that had the operation done in an ambulatory facility, helps illustrate information bias. People in hospitals are often observed hourly overnight and for a day or more thereafter. On the other hand, people undergoing ambulatory surgery are observed only during the first four hours after surgery. In this instance the bias favors the detection of more postoperative complications in the hospitalized subjects than in the others.

Gathering Information

Data gathering is an essential part of "finding out about something." Investigations most often involve interviewing and record review. Anytime an interview is required, a friendly, persuasive introduction should precede questioning. Training of interviewers therefore should include practicing both the introduction and the questions.

The form in which the information is gathered may differ from one investigation to another. In field investigations of epidemics or in surveys, such as childhood immunization surveys, a line listing may suffice. An illustration of this approach is shown in Table 2-5. More complex investigations may need a detailed interview form, sometimes using visual aids for memory, such as pictures of medication packages.

Identifying the respondent, and recording information for follow-up or record retrieval are among the first items gathered. If follow-up or verification of information is needed, then information about family, friends, and neighbors may also be important.

TABLE 2-4. COMPARISON OF ADVANTAGES AND DISADVANTAGES OF CASE-CONTROL AND COHORT STUDIES

	Case Control Studies	*Cohort Studies*
Advantages	Excellent way to study rare *diseases* and diseases with long latency	Better for studying rare *exposures*
	Relatively quick	Provides complete data on cases, stages
	Relatively inexpensive	Allows study of more than one effect of exposure
	Requires relatively few study subjects	Can calculate. Compare rates in exposed, and unexposed
	Can often use existing records	Choice of factors available for study
	Can study many possible causes of a disease	Quality control of data
Disadvantages	Relies on recall or existing records about past exposures	Need to study large numbers
	Difficult or impossible to validate data	May take many years
	Control of extraneous factors incomplete	Circumstances may change during study
	Difficult to select suitable comparison group	Expensive
	Cannot calculate rates	Control of extraneous factors may be incomplete
	Cannot study mechanism of disease	Rarely possible to study mechanism of disease

TABLE 2-5. ILLUSTRATIVE PARTIAL LINE LISTING MEASLES EPIDEMIC IN A HIGH SCHOOL

Case No.	*Identifier*	*Grade*	*Sex*	*Date of Onset*
1	SA041870	09	M	April 24
2	DA101666	12	F	April 22
3	LB020570	09	F	April 25
4	DB061470	09	M	April 27
5	SB040569	10	F	April 22

Responses to questions, both for interview and record abstraction, should be simple and in a form that is easy to code. Initial data collection of items, such as age, should be gathered in terms of individual years; grouping of these items is better done at the time of tabulation and analysis. Avoiding open-ended questions as much as possible reduces the difficulties in tabulating and analyzing the resulting information.

Pretesting the data gathering form or interview is essential. Simulating an interview with a respondent or abstracting a chart that represents a typical case should be followed by simulating some of the unlikely circumstances.

Case finding, that is, searching for and gathering information from subjects for the case and comparison groups, is essential to an investigation. Initially, a study should include a wide range of those at risk of the health problem. Being sure that the entire population at risk is being considered at the beginning of the investigation is generally easier than it is to make a second trip to the community.

If members of the comparison group are matched to specific individuals in the case group, then the forms for both case and comparison individuals must be able to be linked for analysis. Choosing comparison groups is not easy. The epidemiologist must think carefully before selecting the easiest way. If the cases, for example, are all hospitalized, the question of using control subjects from the hospital or from the neighborhoods where the cases normally lived deserves careful study because both groups should come from the environment where exposure occurred.

Case Example: Unexplained Deaths in Hospital[62]

Case Data

Four infants on a pediatric cardiology intensive care service in a 700-bed university-affiliated hospital died unexpectedly. They were found to have unusually high tissue levels of digoxin, a medication used to treat heart failure. This drug had never been prescribed for any of these infants. High tissue levels of digoxin were later found in three additional infants. Hospital authorities sought consultation with several epidemiologists and also specialists from other fields.

Descriptive Epidemiology

Time. The epidemiological investigators determined that for a five-year period before the epidemic there were 49 deaths on the cardiology ward and the death rate had been 11.0 per 10,000 patient days. For the nine months defined as the epidemic period, however, there were 34 such deaths. The resulting rate of 43.1 per 10,000 patient days, gave a relative risk of death equal to 3.9 (the 95 percent confidence intervals ranged from 2.6 to 5.9).

Place. Three months before the epidemic period, the cardiology service had been moved from a single ward to two adjacent wards. Twenty-six of the deaths occurred on one new ward (74.5 per 10,000 patient days). Only eight infant deaths (18.2 per 10,000 patient days) occurred on the other, giving a relative risk of 4.1 with a 95 percent confidence interval ranging from 2.0 to 8.5.

Person. Most (92 percent) of the deaths occurred in children younger than one year of age. Moreover, a large proportion had begun to deteriorate clinically during the midnight to 6:00 A.M. period, and a significant proportion were receiving intravenous fluids during this time. An expert consultant cardiologist judged that a significant number of deaths among 1 year olds cared for on this ward were unexpected. He found these deaths inconsistent with their clinical conditions during the epidemic period as compared with the nonepidemic period. In addition, there was a particularly strong association of clinical digoxin intoxication during the epidemic period. Because these infants were cared for by nursing teams, identifying a specific individual who might be associated with the unexpected deaths during the epidemic period was extremely difficult.

Systematic Study. Nonetheless, by imaginative use of payroll log sheets, duty rosters, call schedules, and also hospital records, the epidemiologists computed relative risks for each member of the nursing team. One nurse in particular was associated with a very high relative risk of death, although another nurse had been the subject of criminal charges.

When this investigation began, the epidemiologists knew of the epidemic, and the cases had clinical diagnoses confirmed by laboratory findings. The investigators could define the epidemic period, calculate mortality rates, and identify the specific hospital ward and age group of patients in which the epidemic had occurred. In this instance, determining the population at risk (patients in the pediatric cardiology wards in a large university-affiliated hospital) was easy. Since criminal charges had already been made, formulating a causal hypothesis had already begun. Comparing this hypothesis with the facts required creativity, good judgment, and courage because the epidemiological and legal evidence led to different conclusions. (One epidemiologist on the team was questioned by more than 20 lawyers.) Using carefully documented data sources (payroll records, duty rosters, and call schedules) was ingenious. Assessment of cardiology ward mortality deaths using relative risks derived from incidence rates showed skill and judgment of a very high level. Nonetheless, the epidemiologists were in a particularly difficult situation because they knew that their findings would be part of legal proceedings.[63] Careful observation and meticulous data collection made an important contribution to this investigation.

Using Judgment in Field Investigations

The judgment of experienced epidemiologists regarding field investigations rests on a series of questions. The first is: When do you do a field investigation? Public need and scientific importance are the most frequent determinants of this answer. A community faced with a health problem of uncertain cause that cannot be controlled or that has created public alarm can be a public health emergency. The community's urgent need may be satisfied only by an immediate, competent epidemiological investigation. Scientific importance, while rarely isolated from public need, is more often determined by the nature of the problem. This was the case in Legionnaire's disease,[64] the initial studies of penicillinase producing *Neisseria gonorrhoeae* infection,[65] and the more recent epidemic of Brazilian purpuric fever. A form of *Haemophilus aegypticus* with a new plasmid type caused this new condition.[66] In each of these instances, the etiologic agent required that an epidemiological investigation be done in the field with intensive and highly technical laboratory support.

Once in the field, when does an epidemiologist ask for help? Since a single health professional rarely carries out an epidemic investigation, key questions must be asked before the field work begins. Among the foremost are: Will there be enough people available to ensure a successful investigation? Will these people have the necessary skills? What are the technical support requirements, in terms of data collection and analysis, specimen gathering, computer science, and laboratory science? Since the answers to these questions will change as the investigation evolves, the epidemiologist must re-examine each of them repeatedly.

How detailed should an investigation be? This question is best answered by considering the reasons for undertaking the investigation.

Responding to public need is the principal determinant. This needs to include recommendations for control measures and addressing public information requirements, even if the epidemiologist is not communicating with the media personally. After fulfilling this obligation, the epidemiologist needs to assess the value of the investigation regarding changes in health policy for a larger population. Finally, the epidemiologist must evaluate the overall scientific importance of the field work.

Before leaving the site of a field investigation, the epidemiologist should have affirmative answers to four questions:

1. Is it possible to do a quantitative analysis of the data?
2. Is the analysis sufficient to permit the epidemiologist to make preliminary recommendations about control measures to the local officials?
3. Is it possible to give local officials a report that would permit them to initiate control measures and provide a credible explanation of the occurrence of the health problem to the public?
4. Will the person responsible for supervising the investigation from its institutional base find the report of the investigation acceptable?

If the epidemiologist cannot answer these questions satisfactorily, the investigation must continue. Epidemiologists who do field investigations should always be prepared to *go back for the facts*, but it is best to get all of the facts in the first place.

Communicating the investigative findings clearly is essential, particularly when the epidemiologist completes the field work. Who needs to know these findings? As a rule, the epidemiologist informs those who reported the first cases in the epidemic first. They are the practitioners who will know if the facts are correct and the public health actions are sensible. If the official and professional personnel responsible for control of the health problem are not part of this group, then they, too, must receive a report. This report describes both the field investigation and the scientific rationale control and prevention. Then those who permitted, enabled, or facilitated the field work should be told of the findings and proposed actions. This group deserves the courtesy of hearing from the investigator, rather than the public media. Finally, the public and the media must be informed. The control and prevention actions are the responsibility of public officials in that community because these measures will occur in their community. Therefore, it is those officials rather than the investigating epidemiologist who should discuss the problem, the investigative findings, and the approach to control and prevention to the community and the media.

▶ ANALYSIS

Epidemiological analysis is the identification and logical separation of the component parts of a health problem, followed by the careful study of each, using statistical analysis and logical inference. Analysis requires correct identification of each component and determining the relationships of these parts. Analysis builds on a foundation of careful *investigation.* However, analysis goes beyond investigation in that analysis focuses on comparisons and relationships while investigation emphasizes careful observation. In some cases, analysis identifies the need to return to vital statistics, or another source of existing health information, or additional field investigation. The process of analysis can be applied to descriptive studies, case-control studies, and cohort studies.

The process of analysis must be orderly. It interacts with the investigation of an epidemiological problem and anticipates the issues that arise during the analytical process of an epidemiological study.

Analysis proceeds from the simple to the complex. Starting with careful description by counting cases, analysis proceeds to percent distributions, risk and rate estimation, and comparison. Only then should an analyst begin to apply more sophisticated, quantitative techniques.

Description

Detailed description is the foundation of epidemiology. Characterizing the individuals who are the cases in an epidemic or who have health problem needs to include the clinical characteristics of the condition and information on time, place, and person. This is important because these cases are essential in calculating rates and risks needed to solve an epidemiological problem. A line listing (Table 2-5) that shows relevant characteristics of the cases also helps determine how to characterize the population at risk. A graphic description of the cases will strengthen the description. One way to do this uses an "epidemic curve" (Fig. 2-1). This graph helps visualize the epidemiological attributes of health problems with a short latent period, or time trends for those with a longer latent period.

The population at risk provides the denominator for calculating rates. Estimating rates is essential to make comparisons between the case groups and other groups. The population at risk will need to be categorized by the same characteristics, using the same intervals as the cases in the numerator of the rate estimates. The first estimate, therefore, usually requires putting the number of cases, or events, that occurred in a given time and in a given population within a geographic area in the numerator. The number of those in the population at risk for the same time and area is the denominator.

The population at risk needs to be determined as precisely as possible. In an epidemic reported from a large area, the initial estimate of the population at risk is likely to include many people who are not really at risk of the reported infection. Subsequent study of the communities in that area is likely to identify one in which almost all who are ill reside. Additional inquiry may show that only the ones who attend a particular school or work in a single factory are really at risk. If, for example, the epidemiologist detects an unusual cancer, then the people with this tumor need characterization. If the only individuals with this unusual cancer do a specific job, such as working with vinyl chloride, then only people who work with that chemical are cases in the epidemiological investigation.

Selection of a comparison group, usually part of the study design and investigative process, warrants review during analysis. An initial study that covers a community may not be sufficiently sensitive, or even appropriate, if those with the health problem under analysis prove to reside in a specific area of the community. For example, if all the ill people live downwind from an industrial effluent, then they decide the area for study. Under such circumstances, omitting data from the analysis may be necessary although it may seem a waste of effort or a risk of losing statistical power.

The two measures most frequently used are cumulative incidence and incidence density. Cumulative incidence, often called the attack rate in an epidemic, is the proportion of a population initially free of a health problem which then develops the health problem. When applied to an epidemic, the cumulative incidence refers to the average population at risk and to a specified period of time, usually that time in which the epidemic occurred. Cumulative incidence is a measure of the probability, or risk, of developing a particular condition during a specified period for the individuals in the population observation.

An explosive epidemic of 70 persons with measles illustrates how to measure cumulative incidence. Figure 2-1 shows how to use a graph of the "epidemic curve." In this outbreak the person who was the index case experienced the onset of rash on April 15. Investigation in the school revealed that 70 students met the case definition (that is, rash, fever, and at least one other symptom). Enrollment data showed that the school had 1,873 students. During the epidemic there was an average of 150 absentees each day, and an average attendance of 1,723. For this epidemic the cumulative incidence was (70/1,723) × 100 = 4.1%.[56]

Incidence density, on the other hand, is a measure that includes *population and time*. Incidence density is a measure of the rate at which those in a population initially free of a health problem develop that particular problem during a given time. The measure most often used is person years. Incidence density is often calculated for annual periods using standard health information. The data used include vital statistics and notifiable disease reports in the numerator, and midyear population for the denominator. Alternatively, estimates of incidence density may be made in a cohort study. In this instance, enrollment in the study to a predetermined point in time, such as the onset of the health problem, defines the time period for the measure.

A particular type of incidence density, the case fatality rate, is estimated, using the number of deaths as the numerator, and the total number of cases in the denominator. During the years 1970–1986, for example, an estimated 790,500 ectopic pregnancies occurred in women who live in the United States; 752 of them died. The case-fatality for ectopic pregnancy during this period is, therefore, 9.5 per 10,000 ectopic pregnancies.[67]

In dealing with the unexplained deaths in a neonatal intensive care unit cited earlier,[62] the epidemiologists used incidence density (that is, deaths per 10,000 patient-days). They reasoned that those at risk of death included newborn infants whose risk of exposure varied. Some infants were born recently, others were discharged after varying lengths of stay in the unit, and still others died. On the other hand, cumulative incidence was the appropriate measure in the measles outbreak in a school. The epidemiologists used this measure because the same group of students was at risk each day during a brief epidemic period.

The unexplained neonatal deaths, moreover, were spread out over a period of nine months. In that period of nine months, or 274 days, an average of 28.8 newborns was in the unit each day, and 34 infants died. The incidence density was therefore, 34/(274 days × 28.8 patients) × 10 = 43.1 per 10,000 patient-days. These epidemiologists compared the risk of death during the epidemic period with the same risk during the preceding five years and six months. They found the incidence density ratio was 3.9, a figure significantly beyond the limits of chance.

Comparison

Calculating and comparing rates is the key to analyzing the cause of a problem and determining the strength of association between a risk factor and health problem. Realizing that rates do not describe the magnitude of a problem is important. Case counts state the size of a health problem. Rates describe the intensity, or severity, and the relative frequency with which events occur. Comparing rates for different geographic areas helps identify the place in which a health problem is most intense. Comparison of age- and sex-specific rates characterizes the age and gender groups at greatest risk of having the disease or health problem in a population.

Quantitative comparisons of rates and risks are easier when using the 2 by 2 tables (Table 2-6). These tables summarize data by distributing it into the four cells. This is done according to the relevant exposure and the health problem or disease. Examining data this way enables the epidemiologist to assess the occurrence of disease in relation to exposure using a number of measures.

Arranging data in a 2 by 2 table (shown in Table 2-6) makes analysis easier by displaying the information needed to calculate incidence rates. These rates compare the risk that an individual will experience the health problem under investigation depending on that person's exposure to the presumed risk factor. Calculating the ratio of the rates in the exposed and unexposed groups gives the relative rate, or relative risk. When the relative rate is equal to 1.0, then there is no evidence of an association between health problem and exposure. However, if it is greater than one, the epidemiologist has evidence that there may be an association between exposure and event. Estimating the confidence intervals surrounding the ratios that do not include one gives added information about the significance and precision of the finding. If, on the other hand, the ratio is significantly less than one, presumably the exposure protects against the occurrence of the health problem.

In the measles epidemic in a school, the index case was a student in the 10th grade as were a total of 474 other students, 21 of whom were ill. The cumulative incidence for measles in the class with the index case is, therefore, 21/474, or 4.4 percent, as shown in Table 2-7. Hypothesizing that students in this class might have greater risk of measles than those in the other classes is reasonable. This latter group includes 49 students with measles and a total of 1,356 in the three other classes. The cumulative incidence in the other classes is 49/1,356, or 3.6 percent. The ratio of the cumulative incidence for these two groups of students is 1.2 (4.4/3.6 = 1.2), a figure that could have occurred because of chance, since the confidence interval (0.7, 2.0) includes 1.0. Being a classmate of the person who is the index case is therefore not a risk factor.

TABLE 2-6. FEATURES OF THE 2 BY 2 TABLE

		Health Event or Disease		
		Present	***Absent***	***Total***
Exposure	*Present*	a	b	a + b
	Absent	c	d	c + d
	Total	a + c	b + d	a + b + c + d

a = Those with both disease and exposure
b = Those exposed who have no disease
c = Those diseased but not exposed
d = Those neither diseased nor exposed
a + c = All those with disease
a + b = All those with exposure
b + d = All those free of disease
c + d = All those without exposure
a + b + c + d = All those at risk

Comparisons in case-control studies use the odds ratio. This measure compares the risk of exposure in a group with a health problem to the risk of the same exposure in a population that does not have the problem. Confidence limits are interpreted for odds ratios as they were for relative rates. Those ratios greater than 1.0 with confidence limits that do not include 1.0 indicate that an association is likely. Those that are significantly less than 1.0 indicate a protective effect.

The use of this measure to show both a causal and a protective effect is illustrated by studies of oral contraceptive (OC) use and tumors in women. A study of OC use in women with benign tumors of the liver by Rooks and her colleagues[68] shows a causal association. Of the 79 women with this rare tumor, 72 had used OCs at some time in their lives. In a group of 220 control subjects, however, 99 had ever taken OCs. These data appear in Table 2-8, panel A. The odds ratio of 12.6 is significantly greater than one, and it has confidence limits that are greater than 1.0.

A study of OC use concerned with ovarian cancer uses the same measure to show a protective effect.[69] Of women with ovarian cancer, 242 had not used OCs for even as long as three months, while 197 had used OCs for more than three months. Of the control subjects, 1,532 had never used OCs, and 2,335 had used them. Table 2-8, panel B, shows that the odds ratio is 0.5, a figure significantly lower than 1.0. This indicates a protective effect by OCs against ovarian cancer.

Comparisons can estimate the potential impact of a health problem. The *risk difference*, also called attributable risk or excess risk, can measure impact as well as the strength of association. The risk difference is the risk in the exposed group minus the risk in the unexposed group. The use of this measure is illustrated in applying it to the lung cancer and smoking data of Doll and Hill[18] (Table 2-9). These data show that lung cancer occurred in three individuals who did not smoke cigarettes. These three people are the numerator for the measure. The study included 42,800 person-years of observation of people who did not smoke tobacco. The lung cancer rate in these subjects is 7 per 100,000 person-years. Among individuals who smoked cigarettes, 133 developed lung cancer in 102,600 person-years, an incidence density of 130 per 100,000 person years. Since the risk dif-

TABLE 2-7. FEATURES OF A COHORT STUDY IN A 2 BY 2 TABLE USING DATA FROM A MEASLES EPIDEMIC IN A SCHOOL

		Disease (Measles)		
		Present	*Absent*	*Total*
Exposure	*Present (10th grade)*	*21 (a)*	*423 (b)*	*474 (a + b)*
	Absent (Not 10th grade)	*49 (c)*	*1,307 (d)*	*1,356 (b + d)*

• ***Cumulative Incidence in the Exposed Group***

$$\frac{a}{a+b} = \frac{21}{21+453} = 0.044 \text{ or } 4.4 \text{ per } 100$$

• ***Cumulative Incidence in the Unexposed Group***

$$\frac{c}{c+d} = \frac{49}{49+1,307} = 0.036 \text{ or } 3.6 \text{ per } 100$$

• ***Relative Risk*** $= \frac{a/(a+b)}{c/(c+d)} = \frac{21/474}{42/1,356} = \frac{0.044}{0.036} = 1.2$

ference is the risk in the exposed (smokers) minus the risk in those not exposed, the attributable risk for smoking and lung cancer in this study is 123 (130 – 7 = 123).

Other measures of potential impact include the attributable risk percent, the population attributable risk, and the population attributable risk percent. The *attributable risk percent* is a measure of the percent of all deaths that can be attributed to the exposure being studied. This measure is also called the etiologic fraction and sometimes the attributable proportion. Using the lung cancer and smoking data of Doll and Hill,[18] the attributable risk divided by the risk in those who smoke (then multiplied by 100) calculate's this measure. The attributable risk percent of smoking for death caused by lung cancer therefore is 95% (123/130) × 100 = 95%. The data from this study means that 95 percent of all deaths due to lung cancer can be attributed to cigarette smoking.

The *population attributable risk* is a measure of the excess disease rate in the total population. It can be estimated by subtracting the incidence density in the population not exposed to a causal risk from the incidence density for the total population. For example, if the risk of death from smoking for lung cancer is 54 per 100,000 population, and the risk of death from lung cancer is 7 per 100, the population attributable risk of death from lung cancer caused by smoking is 47 per 100,000 (54 – 7 = 47). These illustrative data are recent estimates for the United States[70] and estimates reported by Doll and Hill.[18]

The *population attributable risk percent* is the proportion of the rate of a disease that exists in a community, or population, because of a specific exposure. In the case of lung cancer deaths and smoking in the United States, for example, the population attributable risk is estimated to be 47. The death rate caused by lung cancer is 54 per 100,000. Using these data, the population attributable risk percent is 87 percent ((47/54) × 100 = 87). This percent differs from attributable risk percent. The attributable risk percent considers the characteristics of exposure, that is, smoking rates, in the entire population rather than that of a special group of individuals who are the subjects of a study.

TABLE 2-8. FEATURES OF CASE CONTROL STUDIES IN A 2 BY 2 TABLE

• ***A. Causal, or Positive Association***

		Disease (Liver Tumor)	
		Present	**Absent**
Exposure (Oral Contraception)	Present	72 (a)	99 (b)
	Absent	7 (c)	121 (d)

$$\text{Odds ratio} = \frac{a/c}{b/d} = \frac{ad}{bc} = \frac{(72)(121)}{(99)(7)} = 12.6^a$$

• ***B. Protective, or Negative Association***

		Disease (Ovarian Tumor)	
		Present	**Absent**
Exposure (Oral Contraception)	Present	197 (a)	2,335 (b)
	Absent	242 (c)	1,532 (d)

$$\text{Odds ratio} = \frac{(197)(1,532)}{(2,335)(242)} = 0.5^b$$

[a] 95% confidence interval is between 5.5 an 28.6, $P < 0.0001$.
[b] 95% confidence interval is between 0.4 and 0.7, $P < 0.0001$.

TABLE 2-9. MEASURES OF ASSOCIATION AND IMPACT, AN ILLUSTRATION BASED ON SMOKING AND LUNG CANCER

Cigarettes Smoked Daily	*Lung Cancer Cases*	*Person-Years of Risk*	*Incidence Density (per 100,000 person-years)*
None	3	42,800	7
1–14	22	38,600	57
15–24	54	38,900	139
25+	57	25,100	227
All smokers	133	102,600	130
Total	136	145,400	94

These measures, their formulas, and examples are discussed in more detail in textbooks on epidemiology.

Epidemiological analyses measure the strength of the association between exposures and outcomes. These associations are characterized as direct and causal if they are positive, or direct, but protective, if negative. Associations that appear direct, but are the result of the interaction with another variable are indirect; they are often the result of confounding. Associations may also be artifactual. Distinguishing these different forms of association requires knowledge of confounding, effect modification, and chance, and also the other criteria for judging epidemiological associations.

Bias

Some authorities identify many forms of bias;[71] however, most bias falls into two major groups: selection bias or information bias.

Selection Bias

Selection bias may occur when systematic differences exist between those selected for study and those who are excluded. Refusal to participate in a study or respond to a questionnaire may introduce selection bias. This bias occurs when those who refuse or are not able to respond differ in exposure pattern and disease risk from those who do. Selecting case and comparison subjects from hospitalized groups may also introduce bias if, for example, the hospitalized patients used as control subjects do not represent the population from which those with illness have come. In addition, comparing subjects who have died with others who are still living may introduce bias. Selection bias includes, and is sometimes used synonymously with, ascertainment bias, detection bias, sampling bias, or design bias.

Information Bias

Information bias occurs when there are systematic differences in the way data are gathered from controls and cases. For example, if one set of questions is used to evaluate the exposure in the control subjects, and another set is used for the case subjects, the information about the groups may differ systematically. This could easily lead to distorted inferences. If, in a clinical study, one group is observed more frequently than another, the probability of making an observation will be greater in the one observed more frequently. This kind of bias could occur in a study comparing the effectiveness and safety of two approaches to patient care. If one approach was used for subjects seen in an ambulatory clinic while the other required hospitalization, those in the hospital might be seen more frequently than those in the clinic. Information bias may include observer, interviewer, measurement, recall, or reporting bias. Definitions of these terms are discussed in detail in other writings.

Confounding

Comparisons may differ from the truth and therefore be biased when the association between exposure and the health problem varies because a third factor confounds the association. A confounding factor may distort the apparent size of the effect under study. Confounding may occur when a factor that is a determinant of the outcome is unequally distributed among the exposed and unexposed groups being compared. For example, age can confound the findings of a study if the age distribution of two populations differs. Age adjustment, or stratification, evaluates the confounding effect of age differences, as it can for other confounding factors. For example, the effects of occupational exposure upon respiratory disease are often confounded by tobacco smoking.

TABLE 2-10. EVALUATING COMPARISONS BIASED BY CONFOUNDING: AN ILLUSTRATION USING MORTALITY DATA FROM FLORIDA

• ***A. Overall Comparison with Confounding Population***

	Dead	*Alive*	*Total*
Pinellas County	5,726	368,939	374,665
Dade County	8,332	926,725	935,047

Mortality Rate[a]

Pinellas County 15.3

Dade County 8.9

Relative rate = 15.3/8.9 = 1.7

• ***B. Stratified Comparison Adjusted for Confounding***

Age Range: Birth to 54 years

	Dead	*Alive*	*Total*
Pinellas County	737	228,461	229,198
Dade County	2,463	745,572	748,035

Mortality Rate[a]

Pinellas County 3.2

Dade Country 3.3

Relative rate = 3.2/3.3 = 1.0

Age Range: 55 years and older

	Dead	*Alive*	*Total*
Pinellas County	4,989	140,158	145,147
Dade County	5,898	182,087	187,985

Mortality Rate[a]

Pinellas County 34.4

Dade County 31.2

Relative rate = 34.4/31.2 = 1.1

[a] Deaths per 100,00 population.

An example of confounding in mortality rates is shown in death and population data from two counties in Florida (Table 2-10, panel A, Overall Comparison with Confounding Population). The cumulative incidence of mortality is 70 percent greater in Pinellas County than in Dade County, as indicated by the relative risk of 1.7. When the relative risk is adjusted for age, however, it approximates 1.0. This is a better representation of the risk of mortality. This kind of difference occurs because at each age interval these two areas have substantial differences in their age structures.

Stratification of data helps evaluate the effect of a third factor may have on an epidemiological association. In using stratification to assess the effects of confounding, the epidemiologist constructs two or more 2 by 2 tables. One table usually includes subjects and controls who have almost no exposure to the confounding factor. The other 2 by 2 table includes subjects exposed to the confounding factor or having varying levels of exposure to it. Stratification thereby controls the effects of confounding. Using the Florida example and developing separate 2 by 2 tables shows how stratification adjusts for confounding (Table 2-10, panel B, Stratified Comparison Adjusted for Confounding).

Effect Modification

Effect modification is a change in the measure of association between a risk factor and the epidemiological outcome under study by a third variable. The third variable is an effect modifier. An effect modifier provides added information about an association by helping to describe an association in more detail.

Effect modification is illustrated by the association between intentional injury and the sex of the children and adolescents in a study from Massachusetts.[72] The data for individuals younger than 20 years of age in Massachusetts, the incidence density for intentional injury, is half as great for girls as for boys. The top panel of Table 2-11 shows these data. Nonetheless, age modifies this main effect, as shown in the bottom panel of Table 2-11. For children younger than age 5, girls have an incidence density 60% greater than that for boys. In the age interval 5 to 9 years, the rate for girls becomes just one-third of that for boys. The overall association, or main effect, that is, intentional injury associated with male sex, therefore, is not uniform for all age intervals in this study. The effect is modified by age.

Although effect modification and confounding both occur because of the way a third variable influences an epidemiological association, these two concepts are different. While effect modification gives more information about the association, confounding distorts the association. Effect modification is inherent in the nature of the association; confounding is not. A confounding factor is not a consequence of exposure to the risk factor and can occur even in the absence of the risk. A confounding factor exerts its influence by being unevenly distributed between the study groups. It is possible therefore for a variable to be an effect modifier, a confounding factor, both, or neither. Moreover, a single variable may both modify and confound the same main effect in a single study.

TABLE 2-11. EVALUATING COMPARISONS WITH EFFECT MODIFICATION: AN ILLUSTRATION USING INTENTIONAL INJURIES AMONG CHILDREN AND ADOLESCENTS IN MASSACHUSSETS

Effects	*Female*	*Male*	*Relative Risk*
• ***By incidence Density***[a]			
All Ages	53.6	97.9	0.5
• ***By Age (years)***			
0–4	17.0	10.6	1.6
5–9	7.4	21.8	0.3
10–4	40.5	59.7	0.7
15–19	131.0	259.8	0.5

[a] Intentional injuries per 100,000 person-years.

Stratifying an epidemiological analysis by an effect modifier adds knowledge about the association because it describes the effects of such a factor. Statistical testing to determine the probability that the study population contains groups that differ from the total population helps to validate the presence of effect modification. Stratification also adjusts for, or neutralizes, the effects of a confounding factor.

Many analyses require the epidemiologist to stratify for a number of effect modifiers or confounding factors. Analytical complexities of this kind require the use of multivariate analysis. This analytical approach permits the epidemiologist to adjust simultaneously for a number of potential confounding variables. It uses regression analysis that involves multiple factors. Multivariate analysis may assume an additive, straight-line relationship between variables and involve the use of multiple linear regression. Alternatively, the multivariate approach may assume a multiplicative relationship between variables and use multiple logistic regression analysis. Other, more specialized textbooks deal with these analytic approaches in more detail.

Chance

Chance can play two roles in epidemiology. It may account for an apparent association and make it appear real when it is not. (This may be called a type I, or alpha, error.) Alternatively, chance may lead to an association being overlooked, or missed, when it truly exists. (This may be called a type II, or beta, error.) Statistical *significance testing* helps evaluate the role of chance by permitting an epidemiologist to determine the probability that an association actually exists. Assessing *statistical power* helps evaluate the probability that an association would be detected if it were present.

In epidemiology as in other sciences, we must often decide whether a difference between observations is statistically significant. Two questions arise: What does "statistically significant" mean? How can we test for statistical significance? A complete answer to these questions demands a thorough understanding of statistics. Other, more detailed books on statistics cover this subject. The reference list at the end of this chapter gives the titles of some of these textbooks. The following discussion is all that space permits in such a book as this. We assume that the reader is familiar with the terms and concepts of elementary statistics.

When data have a normal or Gaussian distribution, 5 percent of observations lie more than two standard deviations from the mean or central value. Conventional practice, therefore, is that the 5 percent level is a suitable point to set for observed differences that are judged statistically significant. In the conventional notation, the probability of an observation falling in this range is less than 5 percent, or $P < 0.05$. This level of statistical significance is suitable for many purposes in epidemiology. However, we are sometimes justified in insisting upon higher levels, for example, a difference that could occur by chance less often than once in 100 times, that is, $P < 0.01$, or less often than once in 1000, that is, $P < 0.001$. When we set a 5 percent level, that is, $P < 0.05$, one observed difference in 20 can occur just by chance and, therefore, be statistically significant. When many comparisons are being made in sets of data (for example, in multivariate analysis) 1 in 20 of the correlations will, on the average, be statistically significant due to chance alone.

Statistical Testing

The most widely used tests of statistical significance in epidemiology are the χ^2 (chi squared), *t* test, and analysis of variance. A detailed description of ways to perform these tests and their underlying mathematical theory can be found in the reference books listed at the end of this chapter. The following is a brief, and simplified account of the use of statistical testing.

The chi-squared test is used to determine whether two or more series of proportions or frequencies are significantly different from one another or whether a single series of proportions differs from a theoretically expected distribution. There are a number of variations on the chi-squared test. The Mantel-Haenszel test is widely used in epidemiology to test differences in 2 by 2 tables when confounding variables are present.

The *t* test is used to compare the means of two or more populations or groups of data in which the standard deviation is not known. This occurs most often when dealing with small numbers. The *t* test is based on the assumption that the data are normally distributed. In many biomedical data sets, the distribution is skewed rather than normal. However, if the skewness is not extreme, the assumption of normal distribution is considered valid.

The correlation coefficient is used to detect a trend in the relationship of two variables. For example, comparing national per capita consumption of dietary fats and mortality rates from coronary heart disease or cancer of the large bowel has been evaluated using this approach. These relationships are often represented visually as scatter diagrams. These diagrams reveal how two variables are related, although they do not fully describe the nature of the statistical relationship. This information is provided by calculating the correlation coefficient.

If we know the means of two or more distributions, we can use analysis of variance to compare these and detect statistical differences or similarities. When we use analysis of variance, we can search for close similarity or parallelism of trends. In interpreting the results of these tests, one must remember that observed parallelism of trends does not necessarily imply a causal relationship. For example, the death rate from coronary heart disease in the United States rose in the period from the 1940s to the mid-1960s. This increase occurred at about the same rate as the number of licensed automobiles per thousand population. However, this does not mean that automobile use causes coronary heart disease. There are many such "nonsense correlations." Knowledge of the underlying biology and common sense as well as logic must be brought to bear in interpreting data and the results of statistical significance tests.

Confidence Intervals

A confidence interval is the computed interval with a stated probability (usually 95 percent) that the true value of a variable, such as the mean, proportion, or rate, falls within the interval. This measure has two benefits when interpreting data. First, it informs the epidemiologist of the precision of an estimate. The narrower a confidence interval, the more precise the estimate. In addition, the confidence interval tells the epidemiologist about the significance of the estimate. That is, it tells the investigator if the estimate could differ from the expected value because of chance. The work of Doll and Hill[18] on smoking and lung cancer illustrates these points. They observed the distribution of cigarette smoking in the cases and controls shown in Table 2-12 (male patients only). The probability of this distribution occurring by chance, according to Fisher's exact test, was 0.00000064. However, this level of statistical significance means less than the confidence intervals derived from an estimate of relative risk. Using the odds ratio to estimate risk of lung cancer among smokers compared with nonsmokers is 14. Stated another way, smokers had a risk of lung cancer that was 14 times the risk of lung cancer for nonsmokers. The exact confidence intervals are between 3.5 and 122.2. An interval as wide as this must be interpreted with caution. Fortunately, subsequent studies confirmed and verified these findings. The relationship of confidence intervals to sample size, shown Table 2-13, is such that the interval becomes more narrow as the sample size increases, showing that the estimate is more precise.

TABLE 2-12. CASE CONTROL STUDY OF LUNG CANCER AND PAST HISTORY OF SMOKING

History of Smoking	*Cases of Lung Cancer*	*Controls*
Yes	647	622
No	2	27
Total	649	649

Several authorities have argued cogently that scientific papers must show the confidence intervals rather than, or in addition to, the p values derived from statistical significance testing. Methods of calculating confidence intervals vary according to the nature and quality of the data. This is a branch of applied statistics beyond the scope of this book. Details are given in some of the references cited at the end of this chapter. Anyone who has to calculate confidence intervals should be able to use the appropriate statistical methods, and if unable to do so, should consult a statistician.

Statistical Power

It is possible that real difference exists between case and control groups that is not detected by statistical analysis. This is called a type II, or beta, error. Statistical power states the probability that this chance occurrence will be avoided and is expressed as (1-beta), the complement of the type II, or beta, error. Its use is appropriate only when the confidence interval of the measure of association does not include 1.0. Conventional practice is to seek a sample size for the presumed level of risk that will give a type II, or beta, error of 0.10 or 0.20. Conventional practice also includes seeking a sample size that yields a type I, or alpha, error of 0.05, given the hypothesized risk for the exposed group.

Interpretation

Interpreting epidemiological data requires that causal associations between exposure and outcome be correctly identified using specific objective criteria. Although we have focused on the measurement of as-

TABLE 2-13. INFANT MORTALITY RATE: SAMPLE SIZE AND CONFIDENCE INTERVALS

Sample Size: Number of Persons	*Number of Births Observed*	*Number of Infant Deaths Observed*	*Infant Mortality Rate (IMR)*	*95% Confidence Interval for the IMR*
1,000	40	4	100	4–196
5,000	200	20	100	58–142
10,000	400	40	100	70–130
50,000	2,000	200	100	87–113
100,000	4,000	400	100	91–109
250,000	10,000	1,000	100	94–106
500,000	20,000	2,000	100	96–106

Adapted for Development of Indicators for Monitoring Progress Towards Health for All by the Year 2000. Geneva World Health Organization, 1981.

sociation, the identification of bias, and the role of chance up to this point, these criteria include, but go beyond, measurement and chance. The initial criteria used to distinguish causal associations from indirect and artifactual ones were applied to a study of epidemic infections by Koch[73] and can be stated as follows:

1. The causative agent must be recovered from all individuals with the disease,
2. The agent must be recovered from those with the disease and grown in pure culture, and
3. The organism grown in pure culture must replicate the disease when introduced into susceptible animals.

Such rigorous criteria ensure that studies adhering to them are very likely to identify causal associations correctly. Nonetheless, they are restrictive, and, had they been adhered to inflexibly, some important epidemiological associations would not have been found. The association of smoking and lung cancer is one.

In the mid-1960's, criteria more suited to contemporary health problems became the topic of heated scientific debate. Sir Austin Bardford Hill[20] in his first Presidential Address to the section of Occupational Medicine of the Royal Society of Medicine in England proposed a set of criteria more suited to contemporary health problems. Serious objections to the work of Hill and Sir Richard Doll were raised by many respected scientists, including Sir Ronald Fisher. In the United States the Surgeon General of the U.S. Public Health Service convened an Advisory Committee on Smoking and Health. This committee promoted use of criteria similar to those proposed by Hill. These criteria can be summarized as follows:[74]

1. *Chronological relationship:* Exposure to the causative factor must occur before the onset of the disease.
2. *Strength of association:* If all those with a health problem have been exposed to the agent believed to be associated with this problem and only a few in the comparison have been so exposed, the association is a strong one. In quantitative terms, the larger the relative risk, the more likely the association is causal.
3. *Intensity or duration of exposure:* If those with the most intense or longest exposure have the greatest frequency or severity of illness while those with less exposure are not as ill, then the association is likely to be causal. This can be measured by showing a biological gradient or a dose-response relationship.
4. *Specificity of association:* If an agent, or risk factor, can be isolated from others and shown to produce changes in the frequency of occurrence, or severity of the disease, the likelihood of a causal association is increased.
5. *Consistency of findings:* An association is consistent if it is confirmed by different investigators, in different populations, or using different methods of study.
6. *Coherent and plausible findings:* This criterion is met when a plausible relationship between the biological and behavioral factors related to the association support a causal hypothesis. Evidence from experimental animals, analogous effects created by analogous agents, and information from other experimental systems and forms of observation are among the kinds of evidence to be considered.

Interpreting epidemiological data, therefore, requires two major steps. One, the criteria for a causal association must each be carefully evaluated. The second is an equally careful assessment of the association to identify bias and evaluate the role of chance. Undue emphasis may be given to the role of chance. As a result, Sir Austin Bradford Hill in speaking to the Royal Society said of tests of statistical significance "such tests can, and should, remind us of the effects that the play of chance can create, and they will instruct us in the likely magnitude of those effects. Beyond that they contribute nothing to the 'proof' of our hypothesis."[20]

Illustrative Epidemiological Study

Less than a decade after oral contraceptives received FDA approval, a report of seven women with a benign but extremely rare tumor of the liver appeared in the medical literature. Every one of these women used oral contraception. Considering this report, Rooks and her colleagues[68] hypothesized an association between oral contraceptive use and the occurrence of this tumor, hepatocellular adenoma. A review of the literature in 1944 reported only 67 histologically confirmed cases as of that date. However, records at the Armed Forces Institute of Pathology (AFIP) documented 105 such tumors in females during the 20 years following 1957. No similar increase was found for males.

Collaborating with the AFIP, Rooks and coworkers identified 79 women for whom histological confirmation of this tumor was on file. They matched each subject with three women of similar age who lived in the same neighborhood. They were each interviewed about exposures that might influence their risk of liver disease, including liver tumors, and about their obstetric history and contraceptive use. The interview provided a detailed description of both case and control women.

The analysis of this case-control study showed a very strong association between the exposure, oral contraceptive use, and the health problem, hepatocellular adenoma. An overall odds ratio derived from the analysis of a 2 by 2 table was 12.6 (Table 2-8). Separating the level of exposure to oral contraceptive use (measured by months of use) into five levels showed that the odds ratio increased as months of oral contraceptive use increased. The odds ratio estimation retaining the matching of cases with their controls showed an even greater relative risk. This risk was such that, when oral contraceptive use was seven years or longer, the relative risk changed from 49 for the unmatched analysis to more than 500 for the matched analysis (see Table 2-14).

This study meets each criterion for a causal association between oral contraceptive use and the occurrence of hepatocellular adenoma in women. The interviews ensured that oral contraceptive use started before any signs or symptoms of liver disease appeared. The strength of association documented by the odds ratio was so great that statistical testing was hardly necessary. Separating oral contraceptive use into five different levels by duration of use showed that as the degree of exposure increased so did the risk of disease, that is, there was a strong dose-response relationship. Interview information permitted Rooks and her colleagues[68] to identify oral contraception as the specific agent, rather than some other agent used during the same time. Further analysis showed that low-potency oral contraceptive hormones were associated with a lower risk of disease, while high-potency preparations had a higher relative risk, thereby supporting the specificity of this association. This association was consistent with the original case series and with other scientific reports. Moreover, it was coherent and plausible because animal studies also showed that hormones of the kind used in oral contraceptives led to an increased frequency of liver tumors in rats. In addition, two women in the series of Rooks and her colleagues and also nine others reported elsewhere experienced regression of their tumors when they stopped using oral contraception.

TABLE 2-14. ODDS RATIO BY DURATION OF ORAL CONTRACEPTIVE USE ASSOCIATED WITH BENIGN LIVER TUMORS

Duration of Use (Months)	*Cases*	*Controls*	Odds Ratios *Unmatched*	*Matched*
0–12	7	121	(Referrent)	(Referrent)
13–36	11	49	4	9
37–60	20	23	15	116
61–84	21	20	16	129
>84	20	7	49	503
Total	79	220		

Further analysis of potentially confounding variables did not influence risk estimates, and all of these estimates were unlikely to have occurred from chance alone. Moreover, bias was not a likely explanation for these findings because of the use of neighborhood controls, uniform interviewing methods, and a special recall aid, that is, pictures of oral contraceptive packages. The evidence for this association between oral contraceptive use and the occurrence of hepatocellular adenoma in women, is therefore causal and not likely to be due to chance or bias.

Using Judgment in Analysis

The following points are important when applying judgment to epidemiological analysis. They are:

1. Start with data of good quality and know the strength and weakness of the data set in detail.
2. Make careful description the first step.
3. Determine the population at risk as precisely as possible.
4. Selecting the comparison, or control, group is one of the most difficult judgment to make. As a rule, try to choose subjects for comparison who represent the case group and come from the place where the exposure under study is most likely to have occurred.
5. Reduce the data analysis to a 2 by 2 table.
6. The strongest case for an epidemiological association is one that meets all of the causal criteria.
7. Carefully determine the role that bias, including confounding, may have played in distorting an association.
8. In assessing an association, do not rely on tests of statistical significance alone. Remember the words of Sir Austin Bradford Hill. He stated . . . "there are innumerable situations in which they [tests of statistical significance] are totally unnecessary—because the difference is grotesquely obvious, because it is negligible, or because, whether it be formally significant or not, it is too small to be of any practical importance."[20]

▶ EVALUATION

Evaluation for an epidemiologist is the scientific process of determining the effectiveness and safety of a given measure intended to control or prevent a health problem. Evaluation can involve a clinical trial that tests effectiveness of a drug, vaccine, or medical device and the occurrence of adverse side effects. Evaluation also assesses intervention programs in communities, as was done with the fluoridation of water on the prevention of dental caries. Evaluation may also assess the effectiveness of measures to control an epidemic.

Those who work in evaluation make a distinction between the terms effectiveness, efficacy, and efficiency. The effectiveness of a therapeutic or preventive agent or an intervention procedure is determined during its use in a defined population. Efficacy, on the other hand, is evaluated in terms of the benefit that such an agent or procedure produces under the conditions of a carefully controlled trial. Efficiency evaluation assumes that therapeutic or preventive agents and intervention procedures are effective and safe. Efficiency, therefore, concerns the assessment of resources in terms of money, human effort, and time.

Characteristics of Epidemiological Evaluation

The epidemiological evaluation of a health problem has special characteristics. First, the health problem is usually well defined. This means that the epidemiologist does not need to be deeply concerned with questions such as "Is there an epidemic?" Second, because the problem definition is clearer, epidemiological evaluation customarily has specific and explicit objectives that can be quantified. Third, a case definition for the health problem has often been formulated in detail before the epidemiologist begins field work. Finally, careful planning of an evaluation study is often essential, so that a complex set of study design issues need to be carefully addressed.

Epidemiologists evaluate a wide range of issues. An epidemic of an infection, such as measles, may require an evaluation of vaccine effectiveness. An unusual cluster of abnormal cytology reports may suggest either an unusual cluster of cancer cases or a problem with screening procedures for this condition. The epidemiologist may also evaluate therapeutic and preventive measures in carefully designed clinical trials. Such measures may include an assessment of the effectiveness of a surgical procedure such as contraceptive sterilization.[75] In addition, a formal field study of vaccine effectiveness, as was done with polio vaccine,[76] is an epidemiologist's responsibility because immunization is an important official and public health function. More recently, a team of epidemiologists evaluated the effects of low-dose acetyl salicylate on the occurrence of myocardial infarction.[77] Epidemiologists may also evaluate programs intended to improve the health of entire communities, despite the specific method of intervention used, as is done in program evaluation. Worthwhile efforts like this have been made in controlling epidemics of infection and with programs to prevent unplanned pregnancy. In addition, carefully organized community trials have been used to evaluate the prevention of cardiovascular disease, nutritional deficiencies, and dental health problems.

The need for carefully designed clinical and community trials to evaluate prevention programs and agents has led some writers to characterize this as "experimental epidemiology."[78] The scientific desirability of carrying out randomized, blinded, controlled clinical trial of a therapeutic or preventive intervention is undeniable. Nonetheless, epidemiologists may need to evaluate health problems in communities that exist because a presumably effective form of intervention did not adequately prevent or treat a health problem. This topic is discussed in connection with vaccine efficacy during outbreaks when a randomized trial is not feasible either in terms of resources or the urgency of the immediate problem.

Meta-analysis

Meta-analysis is the systematic process of combining the results of different research studies using statistical methods to obtain a numerical estimate of an overall effect. Its primary aim is to enhance the statistical power of research findings when numbers in the available studies are too small. It is more objective and quantitative than a narrative review. In public health and clinical medicine meta-analysis is often applied by pooling results of small randomized controlled trials when no single trial has enough cases to show statistical significance.

The steps in carrying out a meta-analysis begin with an explicit and detailed definition of the problem for which research studies are to be reviewed. Thacker[79] recently reviewed the full sequence of steps given in Table 2-15. Meta-analysis is a term that originated in the field of educational psychology. More recently behavioral and policy scientists have used meta-analysis. It is the topic of several recent books. Applications of this approach have made important contribu-

TABLE 2-15. STEPS IN META-ANALYSIS

1. Define the problem
2. Establish the criteria for including individual studies in the meta-analysis
3. Locate the individual research studies
4. Classify and code each study by characteristics relevant to the meta-analysis
5. Aggregate the results of the individual studies
6. Relate the aggregated results to the characteristics of the meta-analysis
7. Report the results of the meta-analysis

tions to the use of ultrasound[80] and of fetal monitoring in obstetrics,[81] the use of beta blockers[82] in cardiology, and in defining the role of adjuvant therapy for women with breast cancer.[83]

Although meta-analysis is an important new tool for the epidemiologist, it has some pitfalls. First, the problems of bias take on new dimensions. One, called publication bias, results from the tendency of authors and editors to put studies into print that have positive findings in preference to those that show no association. In addition, authors tend to select or emphasize studies that confirm their own viewpoint by applying the criteria for inclusion in a meta-analysis that varies from one study to another, thereby supporting their own beliefs.

Ensuring the meticulous use of the methods and procedures of each meta-analysis is essential, as it is in the individual studies that are the subject of a meta-analysis. If there are uncertainties about comparability of individual studies, the original investigators may be of help in providing more details about research procedures or access to unpublished data. Nonetheless, it may be better to include studies of uncertain methodology in a different category of studies than to group their findings with those for which the methods have been published in detail.

The process of aggregation, or pooling, follows the classification of all the individual studies eligible for inclusion in the meta-analysis. Pooled data are then analyzed by applying appropriate statistical methods to evaluate the association under investigation. As with any epidemiological analysis, it is as important to search for bias and assess the role of chance as it is to evaluate the strength of the association.

Design Issues

Two issues in the design of epidemiological evaluation warrant explicit mention. They are restriction and randomization. Restriction minimizes potential confounding by limiting the study to a group with characteristics for which a confounding variable is either absent or can be clearly identified and measured. In evaluating the effectiveness of a vaccine, for example, those included in the evaluation might be restricted by age. The youngest age at which a child would be included would be that at which children first became eligible for vaccination. The older age limit would be that at which natural immunity was so prevalent that the role of vaccine-induced immunity is negligible. Restriction of this kind reduces confounding by natural immunity. Similarly, a study of the association between the use of hormones and a tumor might restrict admission by age, depending on how the hormone was used. The work of Rooks and her colleagues on oral contraception and liver tumor is a case in point.[68] Restriction has one important limitation. By restricting the population studied, the findings cannot be generalized beyond that population.

Randomization is the probabilistic allocation of eligible participants into study and control groups. It minimizes both selection bias and confounding and ensures the comparability of the two groups being studied. Randomization is a powerful strategy. Its use controls selection bias, but it does not replace the need for blinding observers or using a placebo control group to reduce observation bias.

Analytic Approaches

Measuring the preventive effect of an agent or program can be done by computing the prevented fraction in the exposed group. Comparing the cumulative incidence, or attack rate, of the condition to be prevented in the group receiving the preventive procedure with that for the group which did not permits estimation of the relative risk. Setting the cumulative incidence in the comparison group equal to one and subtracting from it the relative risk of occurrence in the population receiving the intervention gives the prevented fraction. A more detailed and specific discussion of this topic as it applies to vaccine efficacy is given by Orenstein and his colleagues,[84] and by Miettinen.[85]

The uses of modified approaches to the life table are often important for epidemiological evaluation. Studies of contraceptive use and effectiveness focusing on the intrauterine device illustrate this method. It permits estimates to be made of effectiveness and also of specific reasons for discontinuing the use of a device. In addition, the use of ordinal months permits study subjects to be admitted on different dates and to be excluded when lost to follow-up.

Program or Community Evaluation

Program or community intervention evaluation differs from clinical trials in important ways. Community interventions address an intervention approach introduced into a population group, while a clinical trial involves the treatment of individual, usually carefully selected subjects. The evaluation of water fluoridation on dental caries compared the communities of Newburgh (the trial community) and Kingston (the comparison community), New York. This ensured that the public health policy for fluoridation of water to improve dental health had a solid epidemiological basis.[86]

Case Example. Epidemiological evaluation is called for almost any time a new approach to prevention is to have widespread use. The introduction of new plastics and the global concern about uncontrolled fertility led to new developments in intrauterine contraception. While this approach to fertility control was not new, it had never been evaluated for either effectiveness or safety. Under the direction of Christopher Teitze, MD, a network of researchers from around the world began a trial of plastic intrauterine devices (IUDs) to assess their effectiveness, side effects, and continuation of use. A report on nine such devices describes their work.[87] The trial was restricted to women of childbearing age who stated that they were sexually active. Each woman was characterized by age, parity, outcome of last pregnancy, date IUD use began, and clinical center attended. Effectiveness was measured in terms of pregnancies that occurred while an IUD was in place. Side effects were categorized as expulsions, removals, and also pregnancies. The removals were further classified as done for bleeding and/or pain, other medical reasons, planning pregnancy, or other personal choice. The dates on which expulsions and removals occurred and on which pregnancies were diagnosed were recorded. The use of life table techniques permitted the investigators to report the average duration of IUD use and the reason for discontinuing use. (Discontinuing use is analogous to dying, while doing so for a particular reason is analogous to dying from a particular cause, such as heart disease. This is called a multiple decrement life table.) After two years the researchers had accumulated a total of more than 380,000 woman-months of IUD use, ranging from 7,000 to 136,000 for each device. Their results showed that pregnancy rates ranged from 2.2 to 16.1 per 100 woman-months of use depending on the device (Table 2-16). Expulsion rates had a range of 1.8 to 33.4, while removals fell between 11.9 and 20.5. Overall continuation rates did not differ significantly among the devices, and the Lippes loop D was judged to offer the best overall combination of pregnancy prevention and lack of serious side effects. It subsequently became the most widely accepted IUD in the world. More recent trials compared the Lippes loop D and copper-carrying IUD, applying a similar but more refined life table method.

The international evaluation of IUD effectiveness and safety makes important points about using restriction in the design of a study of this kind. It also shows the imaginative use of life table analysis. Restricting study participants to sexually active, reproductive-age women reduces distortion that would result if women not yet able to become pregnant or postmenopausal women were included. Life table analysis enables researchers to use as much of their data as possible and to interpret it precisely and quantitatively. Using ordinal months of study participation and the careful categorization of events are important attributes of this analytic approach. In subsequent reports these workers calculated standard errors for the life table rates.

TABLE 2-16. NET CUMULATIVE RATES OF EVENTS AND CLOSURES PER 100 CASES, BY TYPE OF TERMINATION: ALL DEVICES BY TYPE AND SIZE, TWO YEARS OF USE

	Loops				Spirals		Bows		
Type of Termination	*A*	*B*	*C*	*D*	*Small*	*Large*	*Small*	*Large*	*Steel Ring*
Events									
Pregnancies	9.3	4.8	4.0	4.1	4.5	2.2	16.1	7.1	9.0
Expulsions									
First	22.9	17.7	15.1	11.0	33.4	23.5	4.7	1.8	18.1
Later	4.9	4.4	5.7	4.2	10.0	7.1	1.3	1.1	4.5
Removals									
Bleeding and/or pain	13.0	16.8	15.1	16.5	13.2	20.5	16.5	15.7	11.9
Other medical	6.7	6.3	4.7	5.7	5.5	11.4	4.1	5.6	3.2
Planning pregnancy	4.0	2.2	3.3	2.8	3.4	3.0	4.4	2.6	4.3
Other personal	6.6	2.9	2.4	3.8	12.1	5.8	7.0	3.0	3.3
Closures									
Pregnancies	8.0	4.6	3.7	3.5	3.2	1.7	13.7	6.0	8.2
Expulsions									
First	6.9	4.7	4.1	3.4	9.7	7.6	1.0	0.7	5.3
Later	2.5	2.1	2.1	2.2	3.5	2.1	0.3	0.4	2.2
Removals									
Bleeding and/or pain	8.6	15.3	13.6	14.6	8.8	13.8	9.5	13.3	10.1
Other medical	3.1	4.8	3.6	4.1	3.9	6.3	3.2	4.6	2.9
Planning pregnancy	2.3	2.2	3.0	2.2	1.8	2.6	4.1	2.2	3.4
Other personal	5.1	2.7	2.3	3.4	10.0	4.7	6.2	2.6	3.2
Total Closures	36.5	36.4	32.4	33.4	40.9	38.8	38.0	29.8	35.3
Active at End of 2nd Year	63.5	63.6	67.6	66.6	59.1	61.2	62.0	70.2	64.7
Woman-months of Use	13,428	8,045	43,474	109,946	5,883	28,890	18,987	40,411	25,163

Using Judgment

Standards of Conduct and Doubt

Standards of conduct and scientific doubt are the base from which epidemiological judgment on evaluation must begin. The most fundamental decision is determining the need for an epidemiological evaluation of the kind done for IUD effectiveness, water fluoridation, or polio vaccine use. Nonetheless, the entire body of scientific knowledge needs careful consideration (thus the need for meta-analysis) if this judgment is to be acceptable to scientists and to the public. This contrast is highlighted by the fact that, while these studies were instrumental in setting public health policy, no similar trial of smallpox vaccine effectiveness and safety was ever carried out. Despite this smallpox is still the only disease eradicated using an organized public health program.[88]

Establishing rules for concluding evaluation studies before their scheduled completion also poses ethical problems. If the intervention being evaluated is so effective that the outcome of the trial is obvious before its scheduled completion, what must be done? On the other hand, if the intervention has unexpected problems concerning its safety, how will the decision be made about continuing the trial? More particularly, what should be done if the adverse effects are only mild ones, or if they are extremely rare, but unexpectedly serious? The role of a scientifically competent, publicly acceptable advisory group becomes very important under circumstances of this kind. (See Chapter 3 for further discussion.)

Selection of the Study Population

The selection of subjects for study is critical to both clinical and community trial. The following three factors are among the most important. First, the experimental subjects must be sufficiently representative of the larger population to be influenced by the findings of the trial. Policy change based on epidemiological findings must be scientifically acceptable and credible to the public. Second, the number of subjects estimated to be eligible for and likely to consent to the study must be sufficient that interpretable results will be produced. Finally, the health problem under investigation must occur frequently enough in the subjects being studied that the results will be statistically significant or powerful.

Ascertainment of Outcome

The outcome of concern in an epidemiological evaluation needs to meet clear and explicit criteria. Moreover, it must be as free of observer bias as possible. Mortality is, therefore, a more desirable endpoint for study than morbidity. The availability of the National Death Index in the United States now permits on a regular and complete basis for the nation the identification of persons who die of a specified cause. Morbidity is not similarly indexed, so subjects may be lost to follow-up more often. Moreover, morbidity may recur so that duplication of data entries and analytic problems become more complex.

▶ APPLYING EPIDEMIOLOGY TO PUBLIC HEALTH

Epidemiology, as the scientific basis for the practice of public health, has important applications to resolving high-priority contemporary health problems. This closing section highlights three illustrative case studies on this topic.

Epidemic Control

Epidemiology applied to the control of epidemics is still relevant to contemporary public health practice. While the AIDS pandemic is well recognized, not everyone is aware that epidemics still occur. A recent estimate, for example, indicated that several thousand epidemics occur in the United States each year.

The occurrence of a mumps epidemic in 1986, afflicting 840 persons in one metropolitan area almost 20 years after licensing of the mumps vaccine, illustrates the importance of applying epidemiology to the control of disease outbreaks. In this incident the epidemiologists showed that 332 students from a single public high school acquired mumps at a pep rally held early in the school year. The infection also involved an additional 126 students in middle schools, and 28 elementary school students in feeder schools to that high school. Moreover, 15 private school students had disease that was probably related to living in the same household as a high school student with mumps. Fifty-five high school students required hospital visits and 12 had complications of mumps, such as orchitis, meningitis, or pancreatitis. The administration of vaccine through a high school-based immunization clinic proved effective in bringing the epidemic under control.[89]

Program Operations

Preventive health service programs that affect the health of large population groups and geographic areas are also influenced by the work of epidemiologists. The package inserts for oral contraceptive pills have information for women in their reproductive years that is taken directly from the findings of epidemiological studies. Safeguards against the risks of environmental and occupational exposures, such as those of radon, asbestos, vinyl chloride, and tobacco smoke, are based on epidemiological research. Immunization policy also rests on the scientific work of epidemiologists.

The events that followed the mumps epidemic discussed earlier illustrate how epidemiology may influence the direction of public health programs. Analysis of surveillance data for the entire state for 1986 showed that several other counties spread across the state had high rates of mumps. Moreover, most cases occurred in the group between the ages of 10 and 19 years, rather than in the 5- through 9-year age group, as was the case in most areas. Detailed studies showed that the mumps problem was related, not to vaccine failure, but failure to vaccinate. In addition, nationwide data indicated that mumps epidemics were confined to states, like this one, which did not have laws requiring proof of immunity for school attendance.

In 1987 the total number of mumps cases in the state declined, but epidemics still occurred in specific areas. In one county, for example, more than 10 percent of the population in the 15- to 19-year age group caught mumps. This is a rate almost 100 times greater than that for all state residents in the same age range. This epidemic came under control through immunization with mumps vaccine. Shortly after that, the public media reported more information about the problem and commented on it editorially.[90] Public officials responded effectively, using extraordinary means to add $300,000 to the state immunization program's funds. There are no reports of unexpected recurrences of this disease. What began as a single epidemic investigation at a high school culminated in a statewide change in an important preventive health service program. This solved a problem that kept children from school, parents from work, and caused serious yet preventable complications of a virus infection that might have been avoided.

Policy Development

Epidemiology is essential to the developing of scientifically responsible public health policy. Within the past decade and a half, the countries of North America have analyzed the health problems faced by their citizens and proposed important new approaches to policy development, focusing on nationwide health objectives.[91,92] If these objectives are to be met, professionals throughout public health and preventive medicine will play essential parts. The role of epidemiology and its practicing professionals is, however, not always clearly recognized. Nonetheless, epidemiologists will be involved in carrying out every essential task of the profession. *Surveillance* will be required to provide a baseline description of the epidemiology of each health problem and the ways in which it changes and evolves. *Investigations* will be carried out in communities as unexpected clustering occurs of uncontrolled infections. In addition, emerging new infections, automotive and other vehicular injuries, suicides, homicides, workplace fatalities, disabling exposures to chemical and physical agents, and persisting problems of neoplasia and cardiovascular diseases continue to limit the quality of life. *Analysis* will uncover previously unknown risk factors and ineffective prevention measures. *Evaluation* will lead to the development of new community preventive services and improved clinical treatment. Effective communication will be increasingly important to epidemiology as complicated scientific studies influence the behavior of individuals and the laws and regulations that govern communities.

What evidence is there that epidemiology can have this kind of impact on the health of a population? The eradication of smallpox from our planet is one such bit of evidence. The role of epidemiology in this worldwide effort is now well documented. The development of the Planned Approach to Community Health (the PATCH process)[93] and of APEX/PH[94] has already begun to show how communities can use public health surveillance to define the baseline of the health problems they face. The provision of epidemic and epidemiological assistance by local, state, and national public health agencies illustrates the ways in which investigations influence public health. The elegant analyses of complicated health risks, such as the relationship between ovarian cancer and oral contraceptive use, are likely to influence important groups of people favorably. The epidemiological evaluation of practices, such as low-dose acetyl salicylate administration on myocardial infarction, will lengthen life expectancy. How the sum of all these actions influences health and the quality of living will be determined by the policies, programs, and practices through which they act. Epidemiology plays an important part in developing the scientific base for this kind of societal change. It seems fitting that epidemiologists also play a role in seeing that the outcome of these changes is a desired one.

▶ REFERENCES

1. Lloyd GER (ed): Hippocratic Writings. Harmondsworth, England: Penguin, 1978
2. Snow J: On the Mode of Transmission of Cholera. 2nd ed. London: Churchill, 1855 (reprinted New York: Commonwealth Fund, 1936)
3. Farr W: Vital Statistics. In Humphreys NA (ed): London, The Sanitary Institute, 1885 (reprinted New York: New York Academy of Medicine, 1975)
4. Last JM (ed): A Dictionary of Epidemiology. 3rd ed. New York: Oxford University Press, 1995
5. Langmuir AD: The territory of epidemiology: pentimento. J Infect Dis 155:3, 1987
6. Morris JN: Uses of Epidemiology. 3rd ed. Edinburgh, London: Churchill-Livingstone, 1975
7. Task Force on Health Risk Assessment: Determining Risks to Health: Federal Policy and Practice. Dover, MA: Auburn, 1986
8. Last JM: The iceberg completing the clinical picture in general practice. Lancet 2:28–31, 1963
9. Weiss NS: Clinical Epidemiology: The Study of Illness Outcome. New York: Oxford University Press, 1986
10. Krugman S, Giles JP, Hammon J. Infectious hepatitis: evidence for two distinctive clinical and immunological types of infection. JAMA 200:365–373, 1967
11. Blumberg BS et al: A serum antigen (Australia antigen) in Down's syndrome, leukemia and hepatitis. Ann Intern Med 66:924–931, 1967
12. Dane DS, Cameron CH, Briggs M: Virus-like particles in serum of patients with Australia-antigen-associated hepatitis. Lancet 1:695–698, 1970
13. Almeida JD, Rubenstein D, Stott EJ: New antigen-antibody system in Australia-antigen-positive hepatitis. Lancet 2:1225–1226, 1971
14. Jaffe HW et al: National case-control study of Kaposi's sarcoma and *Pneumocystis carinii* pneumonia in homosexual men. Part I. Epidemiologic results. Ann Intern Med 99:145–151, 1983
15. Broders AC: Squamous-cell epithelioma of the lip: a study of five hundred and thirty-seven cases. JAMA 74:10, 1920

16. Lombard HL, Doering CR: Cancer studies in Massachusetts. 2. Habits, characteristics and environment of individuals with and without cancer. N Engl J Med 198:10, 1928
17. Pearl R: Tobacco smoking and longevity. Science 87:2253, 1938
18. Doll R, Hill AB: The mortality of doctors in relation to their smoking habits: a preliminary report. Br Med J 1:1451–1455, 1954
19. Hammond EC, Horn D: Smoking and death rates: report on forty-four months of follow-up of 187,783 men. II. Death rates by cause. JAMA 166:1159–1172; 1294–1308, 1958
20. Hill AB: The environment and disease: association or causation? Proc R Soc Med 58:295–300, 1965
21. US Department of Health, Education, and Welfare: Smoking and Health: A Report of the Surgeon General. Washington, DC: US Department of Health, Education, and Welfare, Public Health Service, US Government Printing Office, 1979
22. US Department of Health and Human Services: Reducing the Health Consequences of Smoking: 25 Years of Progress: A Report of Surgeon General. DHHS Publication No. (CDC) 89-8411, 1989
23. Centers for Disease Control: Comprehensive Plan for Epidemiologic Surveillance. Atlanta Centers for Disease Control, 1986
24. Langmuir AD: The surveillance of communicable diseases of national importance. N Engl J Med 268:182–192, 1963
25. Thacker SB, Berkelman RL: Public health surveillance in the United States. Epidemiol Rev 10, 1988
26. Centers for Disease Control: Guidelines for evaluating surveillance systems. MMWR 37(Suppl S-5), 1988
27. World Health Organization: International Statistical Classification of Diseases and Related Health Problems (ICD-10). 10th rev. Geneva: World Health Organization, 1992
28. Acheson ED: Medical Record Linkage. London: Oxford University Press, 1967
29. Smith ME, Newcombe HB: Use of the Canadian mortality data base for epidemiological follow-up. Can J Public Health 73:39–46, 1982
30. Acheson ED et al: Formaldehyde in the British chemical industry. Lancet 1:611–616, 1984
31. Epidemiology of radiogenic breast cancer. In Boice JD, Fraumeni JF (eds): Radiation Carcinogenesis: Epidemiology and Biological Significance. New York: Raven Press, 1984, pp 119–130
32. Hewitt D: Radiogenic Lung Cancer in Ontario Uranium Miners, 1955–74. In Ham JR (Commissioner): Report of the Royal Commission on the Health and Safety of Workers in Mines. Toronto: Ministry of the Attorney-General of Ontario, 1976
33. Nightingale F: Notes on Hospitals. London: JW Parker, 1859
34. National Center for Health Statistics. Vital and Health Statistics, Series 1, 13. Washington, DC: US Department of Health, Education and Welfare (published annually)
35. Length of Stay in PAS Hospitals. Ann Arbor, MI: Commission on Professional and Hospital Activities (published annually)
36. National Center for Health Statistics. Vital and Health Statistics, Series 1, 10. Washington, DC: US Department of Health, Education and Welfare (published annually)
37. National Center for Health Statistics. Vital and Health Statistics, Series 1, 11. Washington, DC: US Department of Health, Education and Welfare, 1971
38. Centers for Disease Control: Behavioral risk factor surveillance, 1981–1983. MMWR CDC Surveillance Summaries 33:1SS, 1984
39. National Center for Health Statistics, Series 1, 23. Washington, DC: US Department of Health, Education and Welfare (published annually)
40. Rutstein DD et al: Sentinel health events (occupational): a basis for physicians' recognition. Am J Public Health 75:11, 1985
41. Rutstein DD et al: Measuring the quality of medical care (second revision of tables, May 1980): A clinical method. N Engl J Med 294:582–588, 1976
42. Dean AD, Dean JA, Burton AH, Dicker RC: Epi Info, version 5: a word processing, database, and statistics program for epidemiology on microcomputers. Atlanta: Centers for Disease Control, 1990
43. Graitcer PL, Burton AH: The epidemiologic surveillance project: a computer-based system for disease surveillance. Am J Prev Med 3:123–127, 1987
44. Centers for Disease Control: Table I. MMWR 44(7):738, 1995
45. National Center for Health Statistics Monthly Vital Statistics Report 45(6):1–2, 1996
46. Choi K, Thacker SB: An evaluation of influenza mortality surveillance, 1961–1979. Am J Epidemiol 113:3, 1980
47. Jones TS et al: Morbidity and mortality associated with the July 1980 heat wave in St. Louis and Kansas City, Mo. JAMA 247:24, 1982
48. Centers for Disease Control and Prevention: Summary of notifiable diseases, United States, 1995 MMWR 44(53): 1996
49. Friede A et al: (eds) CDC Prevention Guidelines, a Guide for Action. Baltimore: Williams & Wilkins, 1997
50. Holland WW (ed): European Community Atlas of Avoidable Death. Oxford: Oxford University Press, 1988
51. McGrady G. Community Atlas of Cancer Mortality, Fulton County, Georgia, 1989–1991. Report to the Association of Minority Health Professions' Schools Foundation. Atlanta: Centers for Disease Control and Prevention, 1993
52. Center for Disease Control: Training for Family Planning Program Evaluators: Course Manager's Manual. Atlanta: Center for Disease Control, Public Health Service, US Department of Health, Education, and Welfare, 1980
53. Centers for Disease Control: *Pneumocystis* pneumonia—Los Angeles. MMWR 30:250–252, 1981
54. Centers for Disease Control: Kaposi's sarcoma and *Pneumocystis* pneumonia among homosexual men—New York City and California. MMWR 30:305–308, 1981
55. Ryan CA et al: Massive outbreak of antimicrobial-resistant salmonellosis traced to pasteurized milk. JAMA 258:22, 1987
56. Chen RT et al: An explosive point-source measles outbreak in a highly vaccinated population, modes of transmission and risk factors for disease. Am J Epidemiol 129:1, 1989
57. Morgenstern H: Uses of ecologic analysis in epidemiologic research. Am J Public Health 72:12, 1982
58. Wingo PA et al: The evaluation of the data collection process for a multicenter, population-based, case-control design. Am J Epidemiol 128:1, 1987
59. Centers for Disease Control: Serum 2,3. 7,8-tetrachlorodibenzo-*o*-dioxin levels in US army Vietnam-era veterans. JAMA 260:9, 1988
60. Kennel WB, Wolf PA, Garrison RJ (eds): The Framingham Study: an epidemiologic investigation of cardiovascular disease. Section 35. Washington, DC: National Technical Information Service, 1988. (DHHS Publication No (NIH) 88-2969.)
61. Schlesselman JJ: Case Control Studies New York. Oxford University Press, 1982
62. Buehler JW et al: Unexplained deaths in a children's hospital; an epidemiologic assessment. N Engl J Med 313:4, 1985
63. Grange SGM: Report of the Royal Commission of Inquiry into Certain Deaths at the Hospital for Sick Children and Related Matters. Ontario: Ontario Ministry of the Attorney General, Canada, 1984
64. Fraser DW, McDade JE: Legionellosis. Sci Am 241:4, 1979
65. Centers for Disease Control: Penicillinase-producing *Neisseria gonorrhoeae*—United States, worldwide. MMWR 28:8, 1979
66. Fleming DW, Berkeley SF, Harrison LH, the Brazilian Purpuric Fever Group: Epidemic purpura fulminans associated with antecedent purulent conjunctivitis and *Haemophilus aegypticus* bacteremia in Brazilian purpuric fever. Lancet 2:757–763, Oct. 3, 1987
67. Centers for Disease Control. CDC Surveillance Summaries. MMWR 38(SS-2), 1989
68. Rooks JB et al: Epidemiology of hepatocellular adenoma: the role of oral contraceptive use. JAMA 242:7, 1979
69. Lee NC et al: The reduction in risk of ovarian cancer associated with oral-contraceptive use. N Engl J Med 316:11, 1987

70. National Center for Health Statistics Monthly Vital Statistics Report 39:2, 1990
71. Sackett DL: Bias in analytic research. J Chron Dis 32:51–63, 1979
72. Guyer B et al: Intentional injuries among children and adolescents in Massachusetts. N Engl J Med 321:23, 1989
73. Koch R: Uber bacteriologische Forschung, Verh Ten Internat Med Cong Berlin 1:35, 1891
74. US Department of Health, Education and Welfare: Smoking and Health: A Report of the Surgeon General. Washington, DC: US Government Printing Office, 1964
75. Peterson HB, Grubb GS, DeStefano F: Complications of tubal sterilization. In Siegler AM (ed): The Fallopian Tube: Basic Studies and Clinical Contributions. Cincinnati: Futura Publications, 1986, pp 329–346
76. Francis T et al: Evaluation of the 1954 Field Trial of Poliomyelitis Vaccine. Ann Arbor: University of Michigan Press, 1957
77. Steering Committee of the Physicians' Health Study Research Group: Final report of the aspirin component of the ongoing physicians' health study. N Engl J Med 321:129, 1989
78. Lilienfeld DE, Stolley PD: Foundations of Epidemiology. 3rd ed. New York: Oxford University Press, 1994
79. Thacker SB: Meta-analysis: a quantitative approach to research integration. JAMA 259:11, 1988
80. Thacker SB: Quality of controlled clinical trials: the case of imaging ultrasound in obstetrics: a review. Br J Obstet Gynaecol 92:437–444, 1985
81. Thacker SB: The efficacy of intrapartum electronic fetal monitoring. Am J Obstet Gynecol 156:1, 1987
82. Blackburn BA, Smith H, Chalmers TC: The inadequate evidence for short hospital stay after hernia for varicose vein stripping surgery. Mt Sinai J Med 49:383–390, 1982
83. Himel HN et al: Adjuvant chemotherapy for breast cancer: a pooled estimate based on published randomized control trials. JAMA 256:1148–1159, 1986
84. Orenstein WA, Verner RH, Hinman AR: Assessing vaccine efficacy in the field; further observations. Epidemiol Rev 10:212–241, 1988
85. Miettinen OS: Theoretical Epidemiology: Principles of Occurrence Research in Medicine. New York: John Wiley & Sons, 1985
86. Dunning JM: Principles of Dental Public Health. Chap 16. Cambridge, MA: Harvard University Press, 1986
87. Tietze C, Lewit S: Evaluation of intrauterine devices: ninth progress report of the cooperative statistical program. Stud Fam Plann 55: 1–40, 1970
88. Fenner F et al: Smallpox and Its Eradication. Geneva: World Health Organization, 1988
89. Wharton M et al: A large outbreak of mumps in the postvaccine era. J Infect Dis 158:6, 1988
90. Milner L: Prevention's the cure officials should seek. Sunday Tennessean, Jan. 17, 1988
91. Lalonde M: A New Perspective on the Health of Canadians: A Working Document. Ottawa: Government of Canada, 1974
92. Department of Health and Human Services, Public Health Service: Healthy People 2000: National Health Promotion and Disease Prevention Objectives. DHHS Publication No. (PHS) 91-50212 Washington, DC, US Government Printing Office, 1991
93. Fuchs JA: Planning for community health promotion: a rural example. Health Values 12:6, 1988
94. National Association of County Health Officials, US Conference of Local Health Officers, Association of State and Territorial Health Officials, American Public Health Association, Association of Schools of Public Health, and Centers for Disease Control and Prevention: Assessment Protocol for Excellence in Public Health. Washington, DC. National Association of County Health Officials, 1991

General References

Biostatistics

Colton T: Statistics in Medicine. Boston: Little, Brown, 1984

Fleiss JL: Statistical Methods for Rates and Proportions. 2nd ed. New York: John Wiley & Sons, 1981

Kahn HA, Sempos CT: Statistical Methods in Epidemiology. New York: Oxford University Press, 1989

Epidemiology

Farr W: Vital Statistics: A Memorial Volume of Selections from the Reports and Writings of William Farr, with an Introduction by Mervyn Susser and Abraham Adelstein. Metuchen, NJ: Scarecrow Press, 1975 (published under auspices of New York Academy of Medicine)

Frost WH: Collected Papers. Maxcy KF (ed). New York: The Commonwealth Fund, 1941

Greenwood M: Medical Statistics from Graunt to Farr. Cambridge, England: Cambridge University Press, 1935

Gordis L: Epidemiology. Philadelphia: WB Saunders, 1996

Gregg MB: Field Epidemiology. New York: Oxford University Press, 1996

Hennekens CH, Buring JE, Mayrent SL (eds): Epidemiology in Medicine. Boston: Little, Brown, 1987

Kelsey JL et al: Methods in Observational Epidemiology. 2nd ed. New York: Oxford University Press, 1996

Lilienfeld DE, Stolley PD: Foundations of Epidemiology. 2nd ed. New York: Oxford University Press, 1994

Miettinen OS: Theoretical Epidemiology: Principles of Occurrence Research in Medicine. New York: John Wiley & Sons, 1985

Morris JN: Uses of Epidemiology. 3rd ed. London: Churchill-Livingstone, 1975

Panum PL: Observations Made During the Epidemic of Measles on the Faroe Islands in the Year 1846. Hatcher AS (trans). New York: American Public Health Association, 1940

Schlesselman JJ: Case-Control Studies—Design, Conduct, Analysis. New York: Oxford University Press, 1982

Snow J: The Mode of Communication of Cholera (1855) (reprinted New York: The Commonwealth Fund, 1936)

Terris M: Goldberger on Pellagra. Baton Rouge: Louisiana State University Press, 1964

3

Ethics and Public Health Policy

John M. Last

Ethics is the set of philosophical beliefs and practices concerned with distinctions between right and wrong; with values, human rights, dignity and freedom; with duties to others and to society. We all distinguish between what we regard as acceptable ("right") and unacceptable ("wrong") conduct, although standards and criteria of right and wrong vary greatly. Almost all human cultures observe a taboo against incest. In many other respects, values, ethical norms, behavior, and policies differ widely over time and from one nation or culture to another. In our culture, rules about many aspects of acceptable conduct are derived from ancient roots such as the Ten Commandments, whence evolved laws to protect society from harm caused by violations.

▸ VALUES, ETHICS, MORALITY, AND LAW

Values are what we believe in, what we hold dear, what binds us to others of our kind; values are the foundation of morality. The law, which is based on morality, tells us what we are allowed to do; ethics tells us what we *ought* to do. The distinctions between ethics, morality, and law are based on the intellectual and emotional level at which we accept or abhor behavior: whether we regard conduct as "right" or "wrong" depends upon our ethics. Societal values are the basis for many laws, whether enacted by legislation or based on decisions in a law court.

Community standards are also influenced by social values, which vary over time and among groups in society. An example is changing American values regarding alcohol, which led to the constitutional amendment on prohibition, then to its repeal.

In the past 150 years there have been striking changes in health-related values as a direct result of advances in public health science. In the second half of the 19th century, in a time of improved literacy and plentiful newspapers, the discoveries of epidemiologists and bacteriologists soon became part of general knowledge and popular culture, epitomized in the term "filth diseases" (Milton Rosenau credits Murchison [1858] with the first use of this term.[1]) Values changed, and so did public health policy and law. The results were improved standards of personal hygiene and food handling and sanitary disposal of sewage. Since the 1950s, many epidemiologic studies demonstrating the relationship between tobacco and cancer have transformed other values and behavior. Now smoking is socially unacceptable for most of us and has been legislated or regulated out of existence in elevators, airplanes, cinemas, and many restaurants across America and in other nations. When the mode of transmission of AIDS was worked out, public discussion of sexual practices became socially acceptable. Words like "condom" and "anal intercourse" began to appear in newspapers, and condoms began to be advertised on television and in magazines. The transformation of values and behavior regarding human sexuality since the 1980s has been remarkable and is a triumph of effective health education, spearheaded in the United States by former Surgeon General C. Everett Koop.[2]

Reflecting on these changing values in my lifetime led me to suggest a necessary sequence for the control of any public health problem:[3]

- The awareness that the problem exists
- The understanding of what causes the problem
- The capability to deal with the problem
- A sense of values that the problem matters
- The political will to control the problem

Vickers,[4] discussing the progress of public health, described the final two necessary steps as "redefining the unacceptable."

Laws usually uphold the values of society, but some actions that are legal may be unethical. It is illegal in most jurisdictions for a physician to assist a suicidal act, but it is ethical for a physician to act in a way that avoids needlessly prolonging the distress sometimes associated with the process of dying.

▸ FOUNDATIONS OF BIOMEDICAL ETHICS

Many of our ideas about ethics have descended to us from Aristotle, whose *Ethics*[5] (written in the fourth century B.C.) discussed actions aimed at achieving good or desirable ends. The biblical precepts of the Old Testament and the teachings of Jesus of Nazareth were the source of other fundamental beliefs and values. Hence we sometimes speak of Greco-Judeo-Christian ethics.

▸ ETHICAL THEORY

Much of modern bioethics is founded on four principles enunciated by Beauchamp and Childress:[6] respect for autonomy, non-maleficence, beneficence, and justice.

Respect for autonomy means concern about human dignity and freedom and the rights of individuals to make choices and decisions for themselves, rather than having others decide for them.

Non-maleficence is the principle of not harming, derived from the ancient medical maxim, *primum non nocere* (first do no harm); this may have had greater force in former times when medical care was often hazardous, but it remains relevant today.

Beneficence is the principle of doing good, which members of the professions related to public health believe to be the purpose of our work (a view shared by those in many other callings).

Justice in the ethical sense means social justice or distributive justice—fairness, equity, and impartiality.

Another approach to biomedical ethics is through the **virtues**, many of which were defined by Aristotle. This approach to health care ethics is based mainly on four virtues: prudence, compassion, trustworthiness, and integrity. All obviously should be upheld by public health workers.

We adhere to Beauchamp and Childress's four principles as far as we can in many aspects of health care, but the principles sometimes conflict. For example, we invoke the principles of beneficence and justice in control of communicable diseases, but we must sometimes restrict individual freedom by imposing quarantine on persons who have been in contact with contagious disease. New situations have arisen in modern medical practice. Some are a consequence of advancing medical science and technology, for example the problems presented by organ and tissue transplants, intensive care life support systems, genetic engineering, and new reproductive technologies.

Troubling problems arise from conflicting values. An example with important implications for medical ethics relates to female reproductive behavior and health. Should women have the right to choose whether to become or remain pregnant, or have imposed upon them a view they may not share—that it is sinful to interfere with natural reproductive processes, whether to reduce the risk of pregnancy or to terminate an unwanted pregnancy? There is wide variation in the extent to which individuals and groups regard interference with pregnancy as tolerable, sinful, or criminal; the variation is related to conflict between two values, "right to life" and "freedom of choice." These alternatives seem to be irreconcilable in the United States, where advocates for the two extremes have polarized opinions and the issues have become politicized to a greater extent than in nations where tolerance of the views and behavior of others is more highly valued.

Some ethical problems encountered in public health practice are as difficult to resolve as any encountered in clinical practice. There may be no "right" or "wrong" answer. In the absence of an unequivocal answer, it helps to apply logically the principles of biomedical ethics.

► INDIVIDUAL RIGHTS AND THE NEEDS OF OTHERS: COMMUNICABLE DISEASE CONTROL

The concept of contagion has been recognized for centuries. The usual reaction has been to identify "contagious" persons and sometimes to segregate or isolate them. These customs date from the biblical leper's bell and the medieval lazaretto. In the 14th century, the Venetians added the practice of quarantine; this restricted the freedom of movement of apparently healthy people who had been in contact with persons thought to be suffering from certain infectious diseases.

Identifying persons with communicable diseases means that they are labeled, and this can stigmatize them. Isolation and quarantine restrict freedom. Individuals, families, even entire communities may be identified and stigmatized, isolated, or quarantined—and shunned by their neighbors. During an outbreak of Ebola virus disease in Kikwit, Zaire, in 1995, some of those who had been in contact with infected persons were attacked, even shot at, and denied help by neighbors who feared this deadly infection—a modern echo of the ancient fear of contagion.

Identifying and isolating cases is an accepted feature of communicable disease control, held to be necessary to protect the population. The need to protect society has been recognized as a higher imperative than the rights of an individual patient or contact. When smallpox, cholera, polio, typhoid, diphtheria, and other contagious diseases were prevalent, few people questioned the actions of public health authorities who notified and isolated patients and quarantined contacts, often severely infringing the freedom and dignity of entire families. In polio epidemics in the early 20th century, public health authorities in New York exercised the "police power" of public health to search private homes and detain family members who had been in contact with polio patients.[7] During both world wars, prostitutes and "loose" women suspected of transmitting venereal disease to servicemen were arrested and imprisoned.[8] Some diseases, for example tuberculosis and scabies, have long carried a social stigma because of a supposed connection to drunkenness, lawlessness, dirtiness, or fecklessness.

► ETHICAL RESPONSES TO HIV DISEASE

Reactions to human immunodeficiency virus (HIV) disease have been different. The first wave of the acquired immune deficiency syndrome (AIDS) epidemic in the United States hit an already stigmatized group: male homosexuals who had just begun to overcome age-old prejudice against them. Hostile attitudes to persons with AIDS often were aggravated by homophobia and repugnance for anal intercourse, the main mode of transmission of the virus among gay men. Eloquent and effective advocacy for gay rights, combined with the rising demand for equity and justice for minority groups, heightened awareness of the need to provide health care for all without discrimination. Widely publicized victimization of people with AIDS—gay men hounded out of their jobs, hemophiliac children rejected by schools, even rejected by communities—aroused public opinion in favor of compassionate and humane approaches. A second wave of the HIV epidemic affected intravenous drug abusers, who attracted less sympathy, although their HIV-infected infants have generally been regarded as innocent victims. Even if HIV infection is a consequence of behavior that many public health workers might abhor, we have an ethical duty to apply our professional skills impartially and nonjudgmentally.

Societal reactions to AIDS and HIV infection have provoked much discussion about the ethics of management and control. Informed consent to testing is a sine qua non: both voluntary testing and communicating the results of a positive test must be accompanied by counseling of all persons concerned, and their sexual partners.[9] It is important to protect the privacy of HIV-positive persons and to safeguard the confidentiality of their medical records to minimize the risk of disclosing information that could harm them or members of their families. Health workers have an ethical duty not to discriminate against persons infected with HIV. The duty to care for them is no less than the duty to care for persons with any other communicable diseases. HIV infection is much less contagious than tuberculosis or streptococcal infection, from which in former times many physicians and nurses died after being infected by patients. Health workers who argue for the right to know the HIV status of their patients so they can take precautions should be aware that the risk of occupationally acquired HIV infection is about 1000 times smaller than the risk of hepatitis B or C. As of 1993, fewer than 100 cases of AIDS worldwide out of an estimated 13 to 14 million had been confirmed as occupationally acquired; the risk of infection following episodes of accidental needlestick is about 3 per 1000 episodes.[10] Furthermore, applying the ethical principle of justice, if health workers have the right to know the HIV status of patients or clients, then clients or patients have the right to know the HIV status of health workers.

For epidemiologic surveillance, public health authorities need data on the prevalence of HIV infection. The World Health Organization (WHO) and many national authorities agree that unlinked anonymous HIV testing is the best way to generate prevalence data.[11] The WHO recommendations regarding anonymous unlinked HIV tests for surveillance purposes have been adopted in most nations.

The rules for testing and reporting of HIV infection are a variant on rules and procedures for identifying, notifying, and initiating control measures for other sexually transmitted diseases, or indeed for many other communicable diseases. HIV infection, in contrast to AIDS, is not notifiable in most countries. With the exception of Cuba, where HIV-positive persons have been subject to quarantine (although with weekend leave and marital visiting rights), there have been no serious intrusions on personal liberty. There are, however, other harms: restrictions on medical and life insurance, employment, and freedom to move from one nation to another. Although it makes no epidemiologic sense and violates human rights, most HIV-positive persons are denied entry visas to many countries, including the United States.[12]

► INDIVIDUAL RIGHTS AND COMMUNITY NEEDS: ENVIRONMENTAL HEALTH

Most nations have laws or regulations aimed at protecting people against tainted foodstuffs, unsafe working conditions, and unsatisfactory housing, although the strength of such laws and regulations is variable and enforcement is often lax. Community values and standards have lately shifted toward greater control over environmental hazards to health, reflecting growing concern about our deteriorating environment. In Canada, the Law Reform Commission proposed laws to protect the public from the consequences of "crimes against the environment,"[13] but adherence to environmental ethics would be a better solution for those who pollute the environment harm themselves as well as others; it is in everybody's interest to uphold standards such as those proposed in the European Charter on Environment and Health.[14]

Sometimes health is adversely affected by environmental conditions, but correcting these conditions may have undesirable economic repercussions such as massive unemployment and may be opposed by the people whose health is threatened. Public health officials are then in the situation dramatized by the character Dr. Albert Stockmann in Ibsen's play "An Enemy of the People," reviled for actions aimed at protecting health. Control of the public health hazard ought to have highest priority and is clearly the best course of action in such situations, but if this leads to massive economic loss (in itself harmful to health), the principles of beneficent truth-telling, justice, and nonmaleficence are helpful: what are the full facts about the situation, who will be helped, which of the competing priorities will harm the fewest people?[15]

▸ BENEFITS, COSTS, HARMS, AND RISKS

Faced with an outbreak of smallpox in 1947, the public health authorities of the City of New York vaccinated 5 million people in a period of about 6 weeks. The human costs were 45 known cases of postvaccinial encephalitis and four deaths[16]—an acceptable risk in view of the enormous benefit, the safety of a city of 8 million among whom thousands would have died had the epidemic struck, but a heavy price for the victims of vaccination accidents and their next of kin.

Similar risk-benefit ratios must be calculated for all immunizing agents—indeed, for all forms of health care. Consider measles: there may be a risk, perhaps less than one in 5 million, of subacute sclerosing panencephalitis as an adverse effect of measles vaccination.[17] Measles is close to being eliminated in North America. If we continue to immunize infants against measles after it has been eliminated, there will be occasional harmful consequences, perhaps an episode with fatal cases of septicemia due to a contaminated batch of vaccine. This fact, and the cost of measles vaccination in the face of competing claims for other uses of the same funds, are incentives to stop vaccinating against measles; but the risk of stopping measles vaccination is the return later of epidemic measles, perhaps not until there is a large population of virgin susceptibles. History could repeat itself: mortality rates of over 40 percent occurred when measles was introduced into the Americas by European colonists. High death rates would be unlikely in the era of antibiotics, but the morbidity and complication rates would be troublesome in an unimmunized population.

The risks of adverse reactions to other immunizing agents are greater than the risks of measles vaccine, but the risks of not immunizing are almost always much greater[18] (Table 3-1).

One duty of all who conduct immunization campaigns is to ensure that everybody is aware of the risks as well as having the benefits clearly explained to them; in short, informed consent is essential. This is very important when children are not admitted to school without evidence of immunization; that is, when immunization is mandatory rather than voluntary.

▸ MASS MEDICATION

Risk-benefit calculations are required for all forms of mass medication, not only immunizations. The possibility of adverse effects or idiosyncratic reaction always exists. Opposition to fluoridation of drinking water is based in part on the unfounded fear that fluoride can cause cancer or some other dread disease. Epidemiologic analysis shows no association between fluoridation and cancer.[19] Opposition to fluoridation is more a political than a public health issue, in which the catch-phrase of the antifluoridation movement, "keep the water pure," is difficult to rebut. Another political argument is that fluoridation is a paternalist measure, imposed on the population whether they like it or not. According to the ethical principle of respect for autonomy, individuals in a free society should have the right to choose for themselves whether they want to drink fluoridated water. Responsible adults can choose, but for infants and small children, fluoridated drinking water makes the difference between healthy and carious teeth. Applying the ethical principle of beneficence, public health officials argue that infants and small children should receive fluoride to ensure that their dental enamel can resist cariogenic bacteria.

Some people conscientiously object to mass medication such as fluoridation of drinking water and immunization of their children against communicable diseases. Opting out can be difficult. Opting out of fluoridation means the trouble and expense of using special supplies of bottled water. To opt out of immunization can mean exclusion of one's children from schools that make entry conditional on producing a certificate testifying to successful immunization. The argument for immunization is strengthened by reports of epidemics of paralytic polio among members of religious sects opposed to immunization.[20] Children, it can be argued, should not be exposed to risks because of their parents' beliefs. Often courts have intervened to save the lives of infants and children requiring blood transfusions that their parents object to for religious reasons; but the circumstances are different when immunizations are offered to healthy children to protect them against diseases that are rare anyway. This is a difficult dilemma when the immunizing agent has adverse effects. The principles of beneficence and non-maleficence appear to cancel each other out; there remains another argument based on the principle of justice: all infants deserve the protection of vaccines, even though a few may be harmed by adverse effects.

TABLE 3-1. ESTIMATED RATES OF ADVERSE REACTIONS TO IMMUNIZATIONS

Vaccine	*Reaction*	*Rate per 100,000*
BCG	Disseminated infection	<0.1
	Osteomyelitis	<0.1–30
	Suppurative adenitis	100–4000
DPT	Convulsions	0.3–90
	Encephalitis	0.1–3
	Brain damage	0.2–0.6
	Death	0.2
Measles	Convulsions	30
	Encephalitis	0.0–0.03

Adverse Outcomes of Pertussis and Immunization

Effect (Birth–6 months)	Cases per Million *With Immunization*	*Without*
Hospitalization	1,060	11,098
Death	12.5	130.6
Encephalitis	2.4	25.5
Residual defect	0.8	8.5
(6 months-5 years)		
Cases of pertussis	34,048	356,566
Hospitalizations	6,529	38,787
Deaths	44	457
Encephalitis	162	87
Residual defects	54	29

▶ PRIVACY AND HEALTH STATISTICS

Proponents of computerized medical record storage and retrieval systems assert that computerized records are more secure than paper records; but if unauthorized access does occur, many people's privacy, not just one person's, can be violated. Moreover, computers can "crash," and a whole library of records may be lost or become inaccessible. Other arguments rest on the premise that personal privacy rights can be violated no matter how the records are stored: people have the right to keep to themselves such facts as the nature of their diseases. This argument, and the powerful emotional reaction against invasions of privacy in formerly totalitarian regimes, set public opinion in the European Union (EU) strongly against maintaining or creating national disease registries. Proposed EU directives would have made it illegal to compile or store medical data for longer than the immediate need in treating sick people, and would have prohibited use of medical records for any purpose other than that for which the records were originally collected, without the explicit consent of the persons whose records would be accessed for epidemiologic research, record linkage studies, etc. European societies of epidemiologists and public health specialists successfully argued against this;[21] the 1995 EU Directive[22] supports epidemiologic surveillance and research, whereas earlier versions would have made many forms of it illegal.

Computer storage and retrieval of health-related information greatly enhances the power of analysis to reveal significant associations between exposures and outcomes.[23] Much recently acquired knowledge about many causal relationships has come from routine analyses of health statistics and from epidemiologic studies that have used existing medical records. Examples include the associations between rubella and birth defects, cigarette smoking and cancer, exposure to ionizing radiation and cancer; adverse drug reactions such as the thromboembolic effects of the oral contraceptive pill; excessive child deaths due to use of certain antiasthmatic drugs; and increased risk of hypertension in middle age among low-birthweight and premature infants.[24] Community benefit outweighs any harm attributable to invasion of privacy, especially as the harm is theoretical—confidentiality and personal integrity remain intact. In some nations (for example Sweden, Australia, and Canada), government-appointed guardians of privacy oversee the uses of medical and other records when these are requested for research purposes.

Resistance to use of routinely collected medical records for epidemiologic analysis has come not only from the grassroots and the guardians of privacy, but also from special interest groups who would prefer that inconvenient facts should not be disclosed. Industrial corporations have tried to prevent disclosure of adverse effects of occupational or environmental exposures to toxic substances which it has not been in their interest to have widely known. Even governments that ought to have the public interest as their highest priority have attempted to suppress information derived from analyses of health statistics when it is politically inconvenient for such information to be publicized. Out-of-court settlements of class action suits (for example in tort claims against chemical companies that pollute underground aquifers) have been awarded on condition that the medical records be sealed in perpetuity—a pernicious form of censorship of information that it would be in the public interest to divulge. Public health workers and epidemiologists must be alert to the risk of these forms of censorship and must be prepared to defend access to these sources of health-related information.

Applying the principle of beneficence, it is desirable not only to maintain data files of health-related information, but to expand them: available ideas as well as available information should be used for the common good. Statistical analysis of health-related information has been so convincingly demonstrated to be in the public interest that there is no rational argument against continuing on our present course and further expanding the scope of these activities. This argument applies with particular force to the use of linked medical records, potentially the most powerful method of studying diseases that are rare or have long incubation times, or both.

Health workers have an ethical duty to protect the confidentiality of the records that they use. Irresponsible disclosure of confidential details that can harm individuals is not only unethical but can arouse public opinion against collection and use of such material. Properly used, health statistics and the records from which they are derived do not invade individual privacy.

▶ CONFIDENTIALITY AND THE LAW

Sometimes the law reinforces this ethical position—that the use of health records does not constitute invasion of personal privacy—while respecting autonomy by safeguarding privacy. A U.S. Court of Appeals ruled in favor of preserving the confidentiality of medical records used by the Centers for Disease Control and Prevention in an epidemiologic study of toxic shock syndrome attributed to the use of certain varieties of vaginal tampon. Lawyers for the manufacturer of these tampons had tried to subpoena the records so that they could call the women as witnesses and presumably challenge their testimony. The court ruled that it would not be in the public interest to establish a precedent whereby records of epidemiologic importance could be used in an adversarial situation: this would be a deterrent to future epidemiologic studies and to participants in such studies.[25] However, in 1989 a U.S. Circuit Court granted a tobacco company access to clinical records (albeit stripped of personal identifiers) that had been the basis for another epidemiologic study.[26] In 1996 in a product liability suit against manufacturers of silicon breast implants, plaintiffs were denied access to epidemiologic records from the "Nurses' Health Study" on the grounds that this would jeopardize future cycles of this valuable ongoing study.[27] The variation in rulings is confusing. The issue of confidentiality of medical records, and their subsequent use for epidemiologic analysis, remains open; the threat that courts may allow access by hostile interest groups could be a deterrent to future epidemiologists unless this aspect of law is clarified.

In 1990, the Society for Epidemiologic Research agreed, after much debate, that research data should be shared with outside parties who might wish to reanalyze raw data.[28] Reasons for reanalysis should not influence the right of access.

▶ ETHICAL GUIDELINES FOR EPIDEMIOLOGISTS

These and other problems have preoccupied epidemiologists, who have identified ethical issues and formulated appropriate responses. In addition to the Society for Epidemiologic Research, the Industrial Epidemiology Forum,[29] the Swedish Society of Public Health Research Workers, the International Epidemiological Association,[30] and others have developed guidelines. In 1991, the Council for International Organizations of the Medical Sciences (CIOMS) published *International Guidelines for Ethical Review of Epidemiological Studies*,[31] and in 1992 CIOMS revised its *International Guidelines for Ethical Review of Research Involving Human Subjects*.[32] The 1993 revision of the National Institutes of Health (NIH) *Institutional Review Board Guidebook*[33] has a section on the special circumstances of epidemiologic and public health studies. Research funding agencies in other countries have been concerned about the same issues.

The American College of Epidemiology has had a committee on ethics and standards of practice since 1991; this committee has explored the feasibility of developing a formal code of conduct and has conducted a survey of epidemiologists to determine the nature and frequency of ethical problems that they encounter. Similar initiatives have been taken by the American Public Health Association and other national societies. None so far adequately address the "gray area" between formal (hypothesis-testing) research and routine surveillance. In public health practice and in such settings as cancer registries it can be difficult to say when routine practice ends and research begins.

All epidemiologic studies, whether for surveillance or for research, involve human subjects and must therefore abide by the Helsinki Declaration[34] and its revisions, respecting autonomy and human dignity. Research and surveillance must not harm people,[35] and informed consent is a sine qua non, as important in public health practice as in clinical medicine.

▸ INFORMED CONSENT

The process and procedures for obtaining informed consent[36] should be clearly understood by all health workers. The process consists of transfer of information and understanding of its significance to subjects of medical interventions, followed by explicit consent of the subjects (or responsible proxies) to take part in the intervention. The task of informing should be conducted by somebody senior and responsible, not delegated to a junior nurse or a medical student. Consent is usually active, i.e., agreement to take part; sometimes it is passive, i.e., people are regarded as research subjects unless they explicitly refuse. Consent need not be written. Concepts of autonomy vary: in some cultures, patients regard their personal physician as responsible for all decisions about their health, including participation in research. In other cultures a village headman, tribal elder, or religious leader is considered to have responsibility for the group, in which individuals may not perceive themselves as autonomous. Nevertheless, each individual in such a group should be asked to give consent to whatever procedure is being conducted as part of a public health intervention or epidemiological research project.

▸ VARIATIONS FROM INFORMED CONSENT RULES IN EPIDEMIOLOGIC STUDIES

The 1993 CIOMS Guidelines list ten items of information that must be communicated to and understood by potential research subjects before informed consent is regarded as valid. The latest edition of the NIH Institutional Review Board handbook and the Canadian counterpart of this add another five items (Table 3-2).

Epidemiologists must respect these rules and the Helsinki Declaration, but when studying very large populations it is not feasible to obtain the informed consent of every individual whose records contribute to the statistical analysis.[37] Sometimes the records are those of deceased persons. Epidemiologists then abide by the code of conduct of the International Statistical Institute for official statisticians.[38] This is made formal by requiring those who work with official records to take an oath of secrecy, i.e., never to divulge personal information they see in the course of their work. This protection of privacy extends to communities and groups that would be identifiable in the context of routine reporting: statistical tables are published in a form that precludes identification of small or local jurisdictions.

In the European Union, there has been public and political concern about access to and use of official statistics such as death certificate and hospital discharge data. There have even been proposals to respect the privacy of the dead by withholding from death certificates the cause of death when the cause carries a stigma such as syphilis or AIDS.

Although respect for privacy is important in surveillance and research, sometimes privacy must be invaded, for example when sexual partners must be traced as part of control measures for sexually transmitted diseases. Epidemiologists attempt to obtain informed consent to these invasions of privacy.

▸ IMPARTIALITY AND ADVOCACY

Epidemiology, like all science, is objective, so it ought to be impartial. Can it be "value-neutral"? Epidemiologic findings sometimes reveal dangers to health that require active campaigns aimed at changing the status quo, perhaps in opposition to established custom and social, economic, commercial, industrial, and political interests and institutions. The discovery that smoking causes lung cancer is a good example: public health scientists who identified this massive public health problem sometimes became advocates for better health and opponents of the tobacco industry and of the institutions of society that encouraged the use of tobacco. Advocacy and scientific objectivity are uneasy bedfellows, but most public health research workers believe their duty to protect the public health is a higher imperative than to remain "value-neutral." In many situations since the early days of debate about smoking and lung cancer, epidemiologists have had to wrestle with the problem of reconciling scientific objectivity and impartiality with advocacy of measures to enhance health.

▸ RESEARCH INTEGRITY

Consider the data in Table 3-3. Such distributions could come from a case-control study or a randomized controlled trial. The distributions on the left side of the table do not quite reach a level of statistical significance at the 5 percent level; those on the right side do, just barely. A scientist eager to achieve a "significant" result might yield to the temptation to exclude an observation, perhaps on the grounds that it is an outlier; or find reasons to move an observation from one cell to another in the table. This may seem to be almost a venial sin, but it is not. It is to be hoped that it is rare. It becomes more serious when data are altered after the fact, when some observations in a series are deliberately discarded, and when data are fabricated. Violations of research ethics are coming to light increasingly often; they range from sloppy research design to scientific fraud and misrepresentation. Pressure to get results that will lead to publications required to ensure promotion

TABLE 3-2. INFORMED CONSENT: WHAT MUST BE COMMUNICATED (CIOMS GUIDELINES)

Aims, methods of research
Duration of research
Benefits for subjects and others
Foreseeable risks, harms
Possible advantageous alternatives
Confidentiality details
Extent of responsibility to provide care
Treatment for research-related harm
Compensation for research-related harm
Freedom to refuse or withdraw

Additional NIH Communication Details for Informed Consent

Circumstances allowing investigator to terminate
Possible costs to subject
Consequences of subject's decision to withdraw
Research findings will be communicated to subject
Approximate number of subjects in study

TABLE 3-3. HOW TO ACHIEVE "STATISTICAL SIGNIFICANCE"

	"Not Significant" Differences		***"Significant" Differences***	
	+	−	+	−
+	20	30	20	31
−	30	20	30	19
Total	50	50	50	50
	$P > 0.05$ (= 0.072)		$P < 0.05$ (= 0.045)	
	+	−	+	−
+	6	14	5	14
−	44	36	45	36
Total	50	50	50	50
	$P > 0.05$ (= 0.080)		$P < 0.05$ (= 0.041)	

In each of the above distributions, moving one observation achieves a level of "statistical significance" at the 5 percent level.

or tenure encourage some in academia to depart from impeccable scientific standards. There has been enough concern about serious violations to prompt the Institute of Medicine of the National Academy of Sciences[39] to issue guidelines that include a mandatory requirement to faithfully observe preset protocols, maintain and preserve research logbooks, and adhere to other measures aimed at eliminating unethical and dishonest conduct.

▶ CONFLICTS OF INTEREST, CENSORSHIP AND SECRECY IN PUBLIC HEALTH SCIENCE

Conflicts of interest have worried several professional associations, especially in the United States. Research that had been completed and submitted for publication has been "leaked" to an industrial corporation or pharmaceutical company, which has then hired its own scientists and paid for negative criticism aimed at discrediting the work. Attempts have been made to prevent even casual dissemination (let alone publication) of results that might be damaging to commercial interests. It is impossible to know how often original research results have been suppressed altogether because of intimidation, bribery, or more subtle pressure, because if suppression is completely successful no one outside the immediate circle of those involved will hear about it. This and related problems have preoccupied biomedical science editors.[40] This problem may be more widespread and more serious than crimes like scientific fraud and plagiarism.

▶ HEALTH PROMOTION

Health promotion is the process of enabling people to increase control over and improve their health. Health advocates regard it as a step toward autonomous decision-making for people who were formerly passive recipients of public health measures like purifying drinking water, mass vaccination programs, dietary additives, tuberculin tests, and other routine public health interventions. Health promotion ought to be an entirely beneficent activity; but Abelin[41] has identified some possible untoward consequences. The population may not all share the same values as those who offer health promotion programs and may be made to feel alienated. Prolongation of life as an end in itself ignores the quality of that life. Health promotion may be more effective among educated professionals than uneducated working-class people, so it may widen gaps in health status between socioeconomic groups. Advocates for health promotion programs need to be aware of these and other potential drawbacks.

▶ HEALTH EDUCATION

What could be more beneficent than spreading information about risks to health and actions that can be taken to reduce these risks? Health education encourages all to take greater responsibility for their own health. Often laws or regulations are synergistic with health education about immunizations and admonitions against tobacco addiction. But other issues arise when health educators, with or without the help of laws or regulations, seek to control addiction to tobacco or alcohol use. Some civil libertarians hold that everyone has a right to use alcohol or tobacco. This may be true so long as their use does not harm others, such as the fetus or child of smoking parents or road users who may be killed or maimed by impaired drivers. Economic interests in communities dependent on the alcohol and tobacco industries, it is argued, also must be considered when deciding how to deal with public health problems associated with tobacco and alcohol use and abuse. These are complex economic, political, and ethical questions. No cash crop is as lucrative as tobacco; but in many parts of the developing world as well as in the United States, tobacco has replaced food crops; in Africa, trees are depleted to provide fuel for flue-cured tobacco, contributing to the advance of deserts.[42] These facts, and the worldwide toll of tobacco-related premature deaths, support the argument that the economic well-being of tobacco-producing communities is best ensured by converting to food crops. The ethical principles here are beneficence and justice.

Another concern is that those who fall ill after ignoring health education messages may be blamed for their illnesses or made to feel guilty. It is important for health workers to be nonjudgmental when this possibility exists.

▶ POPULATION POLICIES, FAMILY PLANNING PROGRAMS, AND REPRODUCTIVE FREEDOM

National population policies range from encouragement of couples to have or refrain from having children (often with related laws on access to and use of contraceptives) to vaguely visualized policies implied by the appearance in newspapers and women's magazines of articles on birth control that contain statements about the efficacy of contraceptive methods. Most western nations provide funds from taxation or other revenue for support of family planning clinics that are accessible without charge to low-income women—but not always to sexually active unmarried teenage girls in the United States.

There are many variations in constraints on access to such clinics by girls around the age of puberty who are or may soon become sexually active. There are also great variations in the nature and extent of sex education, especially education about contraception, and in access to effective contraception. These variations are associated with corresponding variations in unwanted teenage pregnancy rates, which are up to ten times higher in the United States than in almost all other nations of the Organization for Economic Cooperation and Development (OECD).[43]

The arguments for early and honest education about sexuality are compelling. Children become sexually mature in their early teens and at the same age begin to question and rebel against parental authority. The tactics of the religious right wing—pious statements ("just say no") and authoritarian orders forbidding sexual activity and denying access to contraception—are a sure way to increase the risks of early teen-age pregnancy and to spread sexually transmitted disease.

Some nations, notably India and China, and one of the most crowded, Singapore, have provided economic incentives or have introduced coercive measures such as enforced sterilization or abortion, aimed at restricting the rate of population growth. Other nations have adopted pro-natalist policies, often because of a perceived threat of being overwhelmed by extraneous population groups.

In nations that have government-supported family planning programs, public health workers are responsible for managing and implementing government policies. Even if population policies are implicit rather than explicit, their general direction is usually clear. In a free society, public health workers have an ethical duty to consider each patient or client as an individual with her own unique life situation, problems, and requests—not as a "case" to whom the official policies necessarily apply. The aspirations of women and couples to have or refrain from having children are powerful and very personal. Staff members of family planning clinics have an ethical duty to offer advice and treatment, and an equally important duty not to enforce their own or official views on individual clients.

Difficult questions arise when we have to balance mothers' rights and those of the fetus. At one extreme are those who would prohibit alcohol and substance use altogether during pregnancy and would indict smoking parents or pregnant women for child or fetal abuse. Law courts have occasionally forced pregnant substance abusers to submit to treatment, which some feminists regard as upholding the view that women exist merely as containers for a fetus. Debates about maternal and fetal rights often reveal irreconcilable differences, and there is no consensus on the "correct" ethical response.

▶ EQUITY AND JUSTICE IN RESOURCE ALLOCATION

Public health is inherently concerned with social justice, with fair and equitable distribution of resources to protect, preserve, and restore health. Public health workers therefore frequently become advocates for health care systems that provide access to needed services without economic or other barriers. Historically, public health workers have often provided the impetus to establish a social security system with unimpeded access to health care for all members of society regardless of income, with access based only on need. In nations that have social security systems, public health workers are prominent among the organizers and administrators. If personal health services are offered to population groups that do not attract fee-for-service practice, these are often run by staff from public health services. When analysis of health statistics reveals regions or districts and population groups that have unmet needs, public health workers often take the initiative to meet these needs.

The principles of equity and justice go further. The allocation of health care budgets is often based on political or emotional grounds and on the ability of eloquent spokespersons for high-technology diagnostic and therapeutic services to promote these interests. Funds sometimes are allocated for expensive equipment and devices, while much-needed public health services such as water purification plants in need of renovation, or logistic support for immunization programs, go without funds. It is an ethical imperative for public health workers to be as aggressive as circumstances require in obtaining an equitable share of resources and funds for public health services.

▸ INTERNATIONAL HEALTH

International health is concerned with the interdependent relationships among all the people and nations on earth. For many years the rich nations have provided support for health care, public health, and medical research in the poorer nations. Until recently, few questioned this; it was regarded as mutually beneficial. There has been concern about the "brain drain"—the hemorrhage of talent from poor nations that send their best and brightest young people abroad for advanced training and lose many of them permanently to the rich nations. This has been regarded as a necessary price for development assistance. Now other difficulties are perceived. Questions have been raised about the appropriateness of technology transfer from rich to poor countries, about "ethical imperialism"[44]—the use by research workers from rich countries of the large populations and the challenging unsolved health problems of the poor countries, with the aim of addressing priorities as perceived in rich countries, but without regard for problems and priorities in the poor nations.

Other problems are associated with the disparity between rich and poor nations. These include the export from rich to poor nations of problems attributable to affluence and industrial development—tobacco addiction, traffic injury, exploitation of workers (often women and children who work for starvation wages), and environmental pollution.

Other problems arise from differing values and behaviors. The status of women may be quite different from that in western industrial nations, and customs such as female genital mutilation, child marriage, and infanticide may exist. Sometimes developing nations are ruled by a repressive military dictatorship without regard for any kind of impartial justice, including equity in health care. International health workers who encounter such phenomena are in a difficult position. To speak out against these customs or against the actions of repressive rulers is unlikely to help the local people and may expose the health worker to the risk of being deported or even arrested, tortured, or imprisoned. Yet it is morally repugnant to remain silent.

International health workers should be able to speak out more forcefully against the export of health-harming practices from industrial to developing nations, such as promotion of infant formula in societies that lack facilities to sterilize infant feeds, dumping of drugs that have not been approved for use in industrial nations, and advertising of tobacco.

▸ PATERNALISM AND PUBLIC HEALTH

Beneficence is the dominant ethical principle of public health. We believe in doing good, and historically we have an impressive record—the sanitary revolution, the control of almost all major communicable diseases, the elimination of many such diseases from large areas they formerly dominated, worldwide eradication of smallpox. The new challenges presented by the "second epidemiological revolution"[45]—coronary heart disease, many cancers, traffic injury, etc., as the main causes of premature death and chronic disability—have led us to respond by aiming to change human behavior. Many of the behaviors we seek to change are pleasurable to those who practice them, and our efforts to initiate change are often resented. If we wish to promote better health, we should be sure that our advice and recommendations are based on solid evidence of efficacy. There is a long tradition of advocacy by public health workers, but in the past this may have been as often associated with preaching as with teaching. The aim of public health services ought to be to enlighten the people about risks to health and to assist people in gaining greater control over environmental, social, and other conditions that influence their own health. We have an ethical duty to work with people, empowering them, doing whatever may be necessary to promote better health—doing things with, not to, people. This is the main thrust of the Ottawa Charter for Health Promotion.[46]

▸ IS THERE A "RIGHT TO HEALTH?"

Social activists proclaim the concept of health as a human right, but there are problems with this view. If there is a right to health, there must be a duty to provide this right; whose duty is it? The answer may be that it is the duty of the individual whose health is the "right" in question—but this encourages victim-blaming when health is impaired. A further difficulty is defining what we mean by "health." There is confusion between health and quality of life. Nobody would describe the theoretical physicist Stephen Hawking as healthy; he has been afflicted with amyotrophic lateral sclerosis for many years, but they have been very productive years, and judging from his own testimony,[47] they have been happy years. There are innumerable examples of severely disabled people whose lives have been happy and productive—and as many "healthy" people who lead miserable lives. Public health workers might be wise to avoid discussing the "right to health." However, it is beneficent for public health workers to strive for economic, environmental, social, and political conditions that will maximize good health, as by implementing the Ottawa Charter for Health Promotion, or the "Targets" document of the European Region of the WHO.[48]

▸ METHODS IN ETHICS

How should we deal with the ethical problems that arise in public health practice and research? Essentially the answer is the same in public health as in clinical practice. Several books provide guidance,[49] although often there is no easy answer. Often we must decide what to do while being aware that some will be unhappy or even harmed by our decision (for instance, when we must trace contacts of sexually transmitted diseases). Decisions can be very difficult. An orderly and systematic approach is therefore essential.

First, we should clearly identify the problem(s). We should identify the available options and decide whose problem(s) we are dealing with—particular persons, communities, health care workers, organizations, institutions, etc. We must gather all the available information and evaluate it carefully, trying as far as possible to set priorities among the options that have to be considered. We must also consider the consequences of the decisions that have to be taken, relating these to prevailing values, beliefs, community standards, etc. Having done all these, we must choose among the options and act. Finally, we must evaluate or review the consequences, often on an ongoing basis—remembering that often there is no "right answer," but a series of alternatives, each of which is in some way both satisfactory and unsatisfactory. One of the most difficult aspects of biomedical ethics is that the more securely we may think we grasp the philosophical principles, the harder it may become to arrive at a satisfactory answer to the problem. Ethical problem-solving often requires high tolerance of ambiguity.

▶ THE PHILOSOPHICAL BASIS FOR PUBLIC HEALTH

All public health workers should ask themselves "Why am I doing this?" The aims of public health are to promote and preserve good health, to restore health, and to relieve suffering and distress. We often judge our success by reduction of infant mortality rates and increased life expectancy, but we seldom try to measure, record, and analyze data on relief of distress (e.g., associated with chronic unemployment or homelessness). Clinicians responsible for intensive care services and for care of the elderly have been obliged to consider the question of quality of life when life-prolonging measures are used. There is growing concern about the quality of death as well as with the quality of life.[50] In public health, a similar reorienting of focus is to use less tangible outcome measures than life expectancy. A set of health expectancy indicators[51] has been suggested as one useful approach. We must also consider the impact of "improved" human reproductive performance on other living creatures with which we share the earth.[52] Human reproductive success is endangering planetary ecology and therefore our own survival as a species: health must be sustainable for other species, not merely for humans.[53]

Spectacular gains in infant mortality have been achieved from the expanded program on immunization, oral rehydration therapy, growth monitoring, etc. Innumerable infants and small children who would have died just a few years ago are living. What will become of them? Will they fall victim to the demographic trap[54]—starve, because there are so many more mouths to feed? Will they get an education? Will they have a lifetime of meaningful work? Will they die eventually, rich in years and experience, surrounded by a loving family? The answers to these questions will depend on our response to challenges more subtle than reduction of infant and child mortality rates.

▶ CONCLUSION

This review hints at the range and complexity of ethical issues in public health practice and research. It does not address the relationship between person-oriented and population-oriented ethics, where there is dissonance in our values and priorities. We spare no effort or expense in striving to prolong the lives of infants with incurable liver disease, by finding donors for liver transplants; we maintain indefinitely on life-support systems some patients who are in a persistent vegetative state from which they cannot recover.[55] Yet we do little to prevent many diseases that commonly take the lives or destroy the joy of life for much larger numbers of people, such as infants who are the victims of fetal alcohol syndrome and young adults who are permanently brain-damaged by serious injuries in traffic crashes. In many states in the United States, the freedom of individuals to ride motorcycles without wearing crash helmets is considered more important than the right of society to protect its resources by reducing the risk that these individuals, mostly young men, will not become a drain on public resources if they sustain head injuries in traffic crashes that leave them permanently brain damaged. We spend large amounts and invest much effort in interventions for advanced coronary heart disease, but devote little intellectual effort or money to measures that might reduce the magnitude of this public health problem.

This raises philosophical questions about the dissonant aims of medicine and public health, questions that go to the heart of the values, beliefs, and meaning of our culture. Similar questions are raised now by critics of environmental development policies that rely on exploitation rather than on learning to live an interdependent existence with other living creatures on our planet.

▶ REFERENCES

1. Rosenau M: Preventive Medicine and Hygiene. New York: Appleton, 1913, p 684
2. Report of the Presidential Commission on the Human Immunodeficiency Virus Epidemic. Washington, DC: June 1988
3. Last JM: The Future of public health. Jpn J Public Health 38:10 (Suppl 1):58–95, 1991
4. Vickers G: What sets the goals of public health? Lancet 1:599–604, 1958
5. Aristotle: Ethics (Translated by JAK Thomson, translation revised by Hugh Tredennick). New York: Viking Penguin, 1976
6. Beauchamp TL, Childress JF: Principles of Biomedical Ethics. 4th ed. New York: Oxford University Press, 1994
7. Paul JR: A History of Poliomyelitis. New Haven, CT: Yale University Press, 1971, pp 148–152
8. Brandt AM: No Magic Bullet; A Social History of the Venereal Diseases in the United States since 1880. New York: Oxford University Press, 1987
9. Ontario Ministry of Health: Testing and Reporting for AIDS and HIV Infection. Toronto: Ontario Ministry of Health, 1989
10. Fitch KM, Alvarez LP, Medine RA, Morrondo RN: Occupational transmission of HIV in health care workers; a review. Eur J Public Health 5:175–186, 1995
11. World Health Organization, Global Programme on AIDS: Guidelines for Monitoring HIV Infection in Populations. Geneva World Health Organization, 1989
12. Duckett M, Orkin AJ: AIDS-related migration and travel policies and restrictions; a global survey. AIDS 3:(Suppl):S231–S252, 1989
13. Law Reform Commission of Canada: Crimes Against the Environment. Working Paper No. 44. Ottawa: Law Reform Commission of Canada, 1985
14. European Charter on Environment and Health. Copenhagen: World Health Organization, Regional Office for Europe, 1989
15. Last JM, Parkinson MD: Health officials and their responsibilities. In Beauchamp D et al (eds): Encyclopedia of Bioethics. 2nd ed. New York: Macmillan, 1995; 2:1113–1116
16. Greenberg M, Appelbaum E: Postvaccinian encephalitis, a report of 45 cases in New York City. Am J Med Sci 216:565–570, 1948
17. WHO Weekly Epidemiological Record 3:13–15, 1984
18. US Department of Health and Human Services Task Force: Pertussis: CPS, a case study. In Determining Risks to Health—Federal Policy and Practice. Dover, MA: Auburn, 1986
19. Kinlen L: Cancer incidence in relation to fluoride level in water supplies. Br Dent J 138:221–224, 1975
20. White FMM, Lacey BA, Constance PDA: An outbreak of poliomyelitis infection in Alberta, 1978. Can J Public Health 72:239–244, 1981
21. Allebech P: New regulations on databases. Epidemiology Monitor, November 1993, vol 3
22. On the Protection of Individuals with Regard to the Processing of Personal Data and on the Free Movement of Such Data. Directive 95/46/EC. Luxembourg: European Parliament and Council, 24 October 1995
23. Newcombe H: Handbook of Record Linkage. New York: Oxford University Press, 1987
24. Barker DJP, Martyn CN, Osmond C, Hales CN, Fall CHD: Growth in utero and serum cholesterol concentrations in adult life. Br Med J 307:1524–1527, 1993
25. Curran WJ: Protecting confidentiality in epidemiologic investigations by the Centers for Disease Control. N Engl J Med 314: 1027–1028, 1986
26. US Court of Appeals, Second Circuit 89-7317: American Tobacco Company, RJ Reynolds Tobacco Company and Philip Morris Inc. versus Mount Sinai School of Medicine and the American Cancer Society
27. US District Court, Northern District of Alabama: CV-92-P-10000-S
28. Epidemiology Monitor 1990, May 11:5:1–2

29. Fayerweather WE, Higginson J, Beauchamp TL (eds): Ethics in Epidemiology. New York: Pergamon Press, 1991 44:(Suppl 1) 1991
30. Last JM: Guidelines on ethics for epidemiologists. Int J Epidemiol 19:226–229, 1990
31. Bankowski Z, Bryant JH, Last JM (eds): Ethics and Epidemiology, International Guidelines. Geneva: Council for International Organizations of the Medical Sciences, 1991
32. International Guidelines for Ethical Review of Biomedical Research Involving Human Subjects. Geneva: Council for International Organizations of the Medical Sciences, 1992
33. National Institutes of Health, Office of Extramural Research, Office for Protection from Research Risks: Protecting Human Research Subjects, Institutional Review Board Guidebook. Washington DC: National Institutes of Health, 1993
34. World Medical Association: Declaration of Helsinki, adopted by the 18th World Medical Assembly, Helsinki, Finland, June 1964, amended by the 29th World Medical Assembly, Tokyo, Japan, October 1975, the 35th World Medical Assembly, Venice, Italy, October 1983 and the 41st World Medical Assembly, Hong Kong, September 1989
35. Last JM: Obligations and responsibilities of epidemiologists to research subjects. J Clin Epidemiol 44(Suppl 1):95S–102S, 1991
36. Faden RR, Beauchamp TL: A history and theory of informed consent. New York: Oxford University Press, 1986
37. Last JM: Epidemiology and ethics. In Bankowski Z, Bryant JH, Last JM (eds): Ethics and Epidemiology; International Guidelines. Geneva: Council for International Organizations of Medical Sciences and the World Health Organization, 1991, pp 14–28
38. International Statistical Institute: Declaration on professional ethics. Int Stat Rev 54:227–242, 1986
39. Institute of Medicine, National Academy of Sciences: Report of a Study on the Responsible Conduct of Research in the Health Sciences (Chairman: A. H. Rubenstein). Washington DC: National Academy of Sciences, Institute of Medicine, 1989
40. Guarding the guardians. Proceedings of the First International Congress on Peer Review in Biomedical Publication. JAMA 263: 1317–1441, 1990
41. Abelin T: Health promotion. In Holland WW, Detels R, Knox G (eds): Oxford Textbook of Public Health. 2nd ed. New York: Oxford University Press, 1991, vol 3, pp 558–589
42. McNamara RS: The challenges for Sub-Saharan Africa. Washington DC: Consultative Group on International Agricultural Research, 1985
43. Jones EF et al: Teenage Pregnancy in Industrialized Countries. New Haven, CT: Yale University Press, 1986
44. Angell M: Ethical imperialism? Ethics in international collaborative research. N Engl J Med 319:1081–1083, 1988
45. Terris M: The complex tasks of the second epidemiologic revolution: the Joseph W. Mountin lecture. J Public Health Policy 4:8–24, 1983
46. World Health Organization: A charter for health promotion (the Ottawa Charter). Can J Public Health 77:425–430, 1986
47. Hawking S: A Brief History of Time. New York: Bantam, 1988
48. Targets for Health for All 2000. Copenhagen: World Health Organization Regional Office for Europe, 1985
49. Gillon R (ed): Principles of Health Care Ethics. New York: John Wiley & Sons, 1995
50. Saunders C: The dying patient. In Gillon R (ed): Principles of Health Care Ethics. New York: John Wiley & Sons, 1995, pp 775–782
51. Robine JM, Mathers CD, Bucquet D: Distinguishing health expectancies and health-adjusted life expectancies. Am J Public Health 83:797–798, 1993
52. Last JM et al: Homo sapiens—a suicidal species? World Health Forum 12:2:129–139, 1991
53. Last JM: Redefining the unacceptable. Lancet 346:1642–1643, 1995
54. King MH: Health is a sustainable state. Lancet 336:664–667, 1990.
55. Annas GJ et al: Bioethicists' statement on the U.S. Supreme Court's Cruzan decision. N Engl J Med 323:686–687, 1990

Additional Readings

Wikler D: Presidential address: bioethics and social responsibility. Bioethics 11(3–4):185–192, 1997

McArthur JH, Moore FD: The two cultures and the health care revolution: commerce and professionalism in medical care. JAMA 277(12): 985–989, 1997

McCormick J: Medical hubris and the public health: the ethical dimension. J Clin Epi 49(6):619–621, 1996

Stone DH, Stewart S: Screening and the new genetics: a public health perspective on the ethical debate. J Pub Health Med 18(1):3–5, 1996

Strader JK: Criminalization as a policy response to a public health crisis. John Marshall Law Review 27(2):435-447, 1994

Konner M: The Trouble with Medicine: Dilemmas of the Medical Revolution. New York: Penguin Books, 1993

Downie RS (ed): Medical Ethics. Dartmouth Publishing Co., Brookfield, VT, 1996

Light DW: The rhetorics and realities of community health care: the limits of countervailing powers to meet health care needs of the twenty-first century. J Health Politics, Policy & Law 22(1):105–145, 1997

Emanuel EJ. Emanuel LL: Preserving community in health care. J Health Politics, Policy & Law 22(1):147–184, 1997

Gaylin W, Jennings B: The Perversion of Autonomy: The Proper Uses of coercion and Constraints in a Liberal Society. Free Press. New York, NY, 1996

Seabright P: John Roemer: distributing health: the allocation of resources by an international agency. Nussbaum Martha C.; Sen, Amartya, eds. The Quality of Life. New York: Oxford University Press, 1996

Daniels N, Light DW, Caplan RL: Benchmarks of Fairness for Health Care Reform. Oxford University Press. New York, 1996.

Grubb A, Mehlman MW, eds. Justice and Health Care: Comparative Perspectives. New York: Wiley. 1995

4

Public Health and Population

Carl W. Tyler, Jr. • Charles W. Warren

Public health focuses on health issues in populations. Carrying out the mission of public health and achieving its goals therefore depend on the factors that change the size and characteristics of the population whose health is at stake.

The relationship between health and population dynamics guides the need for changes in public health practice. Changes in health influence vital events, that is, births and deaths, that lead to population change. Migration, the movement of people from place to place, is a third demographic force that leads to new health issues and problems.

Four such issues illustrate the relationship between public health and population:

1. *Teenage pregnancy:* Teenage pregnancy is a serious public health issue. It creates preventable health problems for both infant and mother. Teenage pregnancies are often unintended. In addition, they may interfere with education, personal development, and socioeconomic advancement for the young mother and father, and therefore the infant. In addition, teenage pregnancies have an important demographic impact on future generations.
2. *Aging:* As the death rate declines in most parts of the world, life expectancy increases, and the number and ages of older people increase. Moreover, when low or declining fertility accompanies the decline in mortality, the proportion of older persons also increases and the median age of the population increases. The result for public health is that the spectrum of health problems and health care needs become drastically different.
3. *Urbanization:* In 1950 fewer than 30 percent of the world's population lived in cities. By the year 2000, more than 40 percent will reside in an urban area.[1] Urbanization creates health problems related to the need for housing and sanitation, improved food supply, better urban transportation, and the redistribution of preventive and other health services.
4. *Refugees and other migrants:* An estimated 15 million refugees are dispersed throughout the world.[2] Refugees and other migrants may bring with them serious public health problems such as severe malnutrition and infections. In addition, their encampments may have unexpected levels of violence.

This chapter should enable a public health practitioner to carry out the following tasks:

1. Identify useful sources of information about *population and vital statistics,*
2. Calculate basic measures of population change,
3. Identify determinants of population change, and
4. Understand four contemporary critical issues related to population change.

▸ POPULATION DATA AND MEASUREMENTS

Data Sources

Population data are essential to defining and measuring public health problems and the groups of people in which they occur. Nonetheless, public health practitioners often find that, while the need for information of this kind is great, their knowledge of existing data sources prevents them from calculating the measurements required to evaluate public health problems. Census, survey, and vital registration statistics are the most fundamental sources of data about populations.

Census

A census is an enumeration of a population that has these essential characteristics:

- Each individual is enumerated separately.
- The characteristics of each individual are recorded separately.
- Those enumerated reside in a precisely defined area.
- Enumeration takes place within a defined and reasonably brief period and in reference to a well-defined time period.
- Enumeration is repeated at regular intervals.[3]

In the United States the census enumerates people first by mail and later by personal interviews of those not responding to mail inquiry. It covers the nation and its territories and makes data public for areas as small as groups of city blocks. (There are certain limits on the information provided in these tabulations because of the need to protect the privacy of individuals.) By law, the census is conducted every 10 years. Because of its importance to political representation, as specified in the Constitution, and because of public concern about use of data by governing bodies, the census in the United States has been a source of controversy. Nonetheless, its importance to the health of the public is undiminished.

Population-Based Surveys

A survey differs from a census in that it is not an enumeration of individuals, and it need not include all members of the population. Nonetheless, most surveys characterize individuals separately rather than in groups, and the sample represents a precisely defined group of people from a specific area. The distinction between a census and a survey is not always sharply delineated. In some instances, a sample of those included in an enumeration must respond to more questions than the total population, and the sample is still considered part of the census. In other cases, data from a national census may be used to establish the sampling frame for surveys at a later time. The topics of these surveys cover such issues as health, fertility, the use of health services, employment, and education.

Current Population Surveys. A series of national population-based surveys, called the Current Population Survey, is conducted each month in the United States. Although this series focuses more on economic than on other issues, its information describes important characteristics of the national population. Among them are such issues as family composition (including births and ages of children), mobility, school enrollment, marital status, living arrangements, work experience, and multiple job holdings.

Health Surveys. In the United States, the National Center for Health Statistics (NCHS) of the Centers for Disease Control and Prevention (CDC) conducts the National Health Care Survey. This survey has four components. The respondents are *(a)* health care providers (see the National Master Facility Inventory), *(b)* hospital and surgical care (see the National Hospital Discharge Survey), *(c)* ambulatory care (see the National Ambulatory Medical Care Survey), and *(d)* long-term care (see the National Nursing Home Survey), and will provide data based on patient follow-up. In addition, NCHS provides data to health officials, their agencies, researchers, and the public through a series of population-based surveys. These include *(a)* the National Health Interview Survey (NHIS; reported annually and based on surveys that began in 1957); *(b)* the National Medical Care Utilization and Expenditure Survey (NMCUES; first conducted in 1980 and 1981); *(c)* the National Health and Nutrition Examination Survey (NHANES; a series of surveys, the first of which was done in 1960–1962); and *(d)* the Hispanic Health and Nutrition Examination Survey (HHANES; conducted since 1984). Each survey measures a different aspect of health in the population of the nation. NHIS gathers information using interview responses. NHANES makes use of physical measurements and laboratory testing, as well as interviews. NHDS reviews hospital records and the accompanying diagnoses and surgical procedures. Plans have been formulated for surveys of follow-up and long-term care on a sample of individual, consenting respondents to these surveys. In addition, the National Survey of Family Growth (NSFG) gathers information on family formation, determinants of infant health, and health practices of women between and during pregnancies. Other surveys, such as the National Maternal and Infant Health Survey, cover samples from the national vital registration system and assess fetal, neonatal, and infant health.[4]

Health behavior is the specific topic of two surveillance systems initiated by the National Center for Chronic Disease Prevention and Health Promotion (NCCDPHP) of CDC. The Behavioral Risk Factor Surveillance System (BRFSS) gathers information about cigarette smoking, seat belt use, cardiovascular risk factors, and alcohol use by people age 18 years and older. The BRFSS began as a one-time survey of 28 states and the District of Columbia in 1981; it was repeated in 1983. Now it is a series of ongoing random digit dialed telephone surveys done in an increasing number of states that began with 15 in 1984 and included 45 states in 1990.[5] The second system monitors health risks in youth and young adults who range in age from 12 to 21 years. Named the Youth Risk Behavior Surveillance System (YRBSS), this system gathers information about six categories of behavior as follows: *(a)* risk factors for injury, both intentional and unintentional; *(b)* tobacco use, including smoking and oral use; *(c)* alcohol and other drug use; *(d)* sexual behavior that is a risk for unintended pregnancy and the transmission of sexually transmitted infection; *(e)* diet; and *(f)* physical activity. This system samples younger Americans in two settings: *(a)* high school students in the 9th through 12th grades and *(b)* people in households who are between 12 and 21 years of age.[6]

Others. Internationally, the World Fertility Survey (WFS), the Demographic and Health Surveys,[7] and the Contraceptive Prevalence Surveys (CPS)[8] have collected data from many (mostly developing) countries around the world. They focus on interview responses form women in their childbearing years and sample the population's reproductive-age women in each country. By 1985 the WFS covered 41 countries in Asia, Africa, the Middle East, and Latin America, gathering information on fertility, family planning, and their determinants. The CPS series included 43 countries, focusing on family planning programs and services. Taken together, these two groups of surveys included more than one-third of the global population, although China and India were not part of either WFS or CPS. Data collection is confined to a few months. A recent survey report for Ghana characterized vital rates, population growth, life expectancy, economic and social status, childbearing desires and accomplishments, and contraceptive use.[7]

Vital Data (Birth, Death, Marriage and Divorce)

The registration of vital events, specifically births and deaths, provides important data for defining public health problems at almost every level of society, including cities, counties, states, nations, and the world. In the United States, vital registries are maintained at the national level by NCHS. At the state level, state health departments and state centers for health statistics perform this function. In some metropolitan areas, vital statistics are gathered and analyzed by the health departments for the immediate jurisdiction, for example, New York City. The registration of other events of health and social importance, specifically marriage and divorce, is also done at the national, state, and local levels.

Other Sources

Migration is an important determinant of population size and distribution. Census information is often available to study internal migration and evaluate its effects. Assessing international migration is, however, more complex. In the United States, annual reports from the Immigration and Naturalization Service provide the official information. For a wider range of countries, special studies by the United Nations and certain issues of the *Demographic Yearbook* give useful data. Unfortunately, the rules for movement across geographic boundaries, especially international borders, make the collection of reliable data much more difficult than that done by census, survey, or vital registration.

Some areas of the world, such as northern and eastern Europe, maintain national population registries based on unique individual identification numbers assigned to each person at birth. This type of registry offers opportunities to study problems that require knowledge of the demographic, social, and economic events experienced by individuals over their lifetimes.

Demographic Measures

The relation between health problems and the populations in which they occur require assessment if they are to be controlled and prevented.

Rates

A rate is a quotient in which time is an essential element and a distinct relationship exists between the numerator and denominator.

Crude Rates. A crude rate is one in which all of the events that occurred in a given time and population are in the numerator. The population of the area at the midpoint of that time period is the denominator. By convention, it also contains a constant multiplier of 1,000. A death rate, for example, might have a numerator of 75 people who died during a given year, and the denominator of the midyear population, 10,000, of the community in which they lived. In this instance the death rate for the community in that year would be 7.5/1,000 population. This rate is the crude death rate (CDR). If the same community had 150 births during the same year, the crude birth rate (CBR) would be 15.0/1,000. The crude rate of natural increase (CRNI) is equal to the CBR minus the CDR; in this illustration the CRNI would be 7.5/1,000, or 0.75 percent.

Standardized Rates. Comparing rates among different populations is often difficult if the demographic characteristics are not known in detail. Following the trend in mortality for the United States over several decades beginning in 1940 illustrates this point (Fig. 4-1).

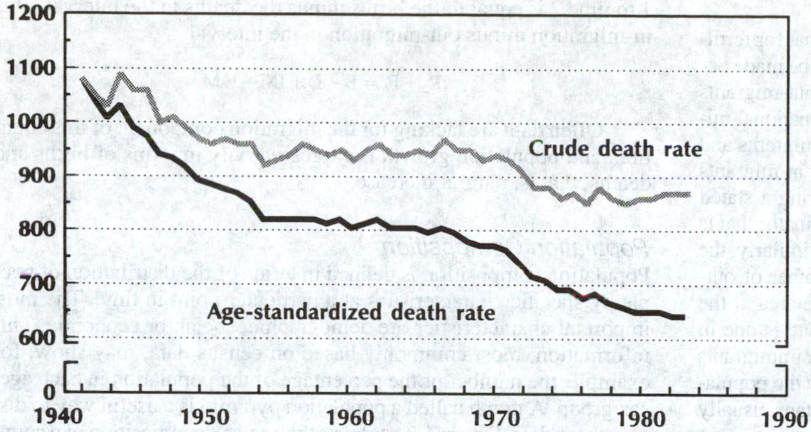

Figure 4-1. Crude and age-standardized death rates, United States, 1940–1987. Rates are for the total population. They have been calculated as deaths per 100,000 population and are standardized on the United States population of 1940. Vertical axis: Rate per 100,000.

The CDR was nearly 10.8/1,000 population at the beginning of that period and decreased to 8.78 by 1980. This comparison, however, masks the real decline in mortality over the 40-year period. Because the U.S. population had an older age composition in 1980, more people were exposed to the high mortality rates of older ages than they were in 1940.

By using a population with the same age composition as that in 1940 as the standard of comparison, the age standardized death rate for the United States in 1980 is 5.85. Comparing standardized rates more accurately reflects the mortality decline in the United States that occurred in all age groups since 1940. However, it is less apparent when looking at the CDR because of the change in age composition, that is, a higher proportion of older people in the more recent years. Other references deal with standardization in more detail.[9]

Period and Cohort Rates. A period rate is one in which the events of concern occur in the population being observed during a specified time interval. The CDR for the United States in the year 1987 of 5.36/1,000 population is an example of a period rate. Most often the period for demographic rates is one year. Figure 4-1 shows the trend of mortality in the United States since 1940 using period rates.

A cohort is a group of people who experience a major event in the same short, clearly defined, time period, usually a year. The most common demographic cohorts are birth cohorts and marriage cohorts. Cohort rates measure events that occur (subsequent to the defining event) to a cohort of people over many periods of time. Population studies are often based on birth cohorts, as was done in the cohort analysis of fertility reported by the National Center for Health Statistics.[10] The analysis of fertility by marriage cohorts helps us to understand changes in fertility or family structure. Epidemiologists use cohort analysis to study groups according to their exposure to a specific agent hypothesized to cause, or prevent, a health problem. If the problem relates to occupational exposure, the cohort may be analyzed by date of employment. Frost's study of mortality caused by tuberculosis is a classic public health report using cohort analysis.[11]

Fertility

The CBR, which uses all births in the numerator and the total population (regardless of gender or age) in the denominator, is the most fundamental fertility measure. The general fertility rate (GFR) also uses all births in the numerator. However, the denominator is women of childbearing age, most often defined as women 15 to 44 years of age. Some authorities prefer to use 49 years as the older age limit. The age-specific fertility rate (ASFR) is calculated using births to women in a specific age interval (usually 5 years, but sometimes single years of age) as the numerator and women in the same age interval in the denominator. Each of these measures is a period rate and is customarily multiplied by a constant of 1,000.

The total fertility rate (TFR) is the sum of all of the age-specific fertility rates by single years of age. This measure characterizes a synthetic cohort of women of reproductive age. By using data for a short period, usually one year, it addresses the question, "If the women in this population continued to have children at the rate they did this year, how many would they have, on average, when they finished bearing their children?" If the sum of age-specific fertility rates totaled 3,000 live births per 1,000 women in a given year, each woman would average 3 children. This assumes that these rates continue unchanged for the remainder of her reproductive years. (The total fertility rate may be expressed per 1,000 women or per 1 woman.) The true cohort rate for fertility is referred to as the completed fertility rate. This measure is customarily based on surveys rather than vital data.

Mortality

The CDR, which uses all deaths in the numerator and the total midyear population in the denominator, is the most fundamental mortality rate. The age-specific death rate (ASDR) is calculated using deaths that occur among those in a specific age interval as the numerator. The population in the same age interval is the denominator. Each of these measures is a period rate and is customarily multiplied by a constant of 1,000. Rates for specific causes of death add an important dimension to mortality analysis. Most often the cause of death is based on vital registration and the International Classification of Diseases (ICD) coding system. Using this coding, deaths are classified by cause and are the numerator of the rate. The population, or an appropriate segment of the population, is the denominator. The rate is usually multiplied by a constant of 100,000.

Some special measures that are not true rates deserve mention. Among them are the infant mortality rate (IMR) and maternal mortality rate (MMR). The IMR is the number of children who die before their first birthday in a year divided by the number of live births in that year. The MMR indicates the risk of death from causes associated with childbirth. Deaths during pregnancy, labor and delivery, or postpartum in a year make up the numerator, and live births in the same year are the denominator. These measurements have been defined succinctly elsewhere.[12]

A life table employs ASDRs converted to probabilities of death for each age interval. Life table data describe the mortality or survival of a person or a group over a lifetime. Life table analysis addresses the question, "What would be the mortality experience and life expectancy of a group of people who had these probabilities of death at each age for the rest of their lives?" Using ASDRs for a specific period (usually 1 year) permits a current, or period, life table to be calculated for a synthetic cohort. Using ASDRs over the lifetime of a group born in the same year, or interval (often 5 years), permits the construction of a real (rather than synthetic) cohort life table. Cohort life tables are more often referred to as generation, or longitudinal, life tables.

Migration

The measurement of migration is conceptually similar to that for fertility and mortality. Defining terms requires that a distinction be made between internal migration (movement by in-migrants and out-migrants across borders that are within a nation's bounds) and international migration (movement across international boundaries by immigrants and emigrants). The crude in-migration rate has the number of in-migrants or immigrants who enter a specified geographic area during a stated time interval in the numerator. This is divided by a denominator that is the population of the area at the midpoint of that interval. Similarly, the crude out-migration rate is the measure in which the number of out-migrants or emigrants is divided by the population of the area at the midpoint of the time interval. The crude net migration rate is one in which the difference between the number of in-migrants or immigrants and out-migrants or emigrants is the numerator divided by the population of the area. All these rates are multiplied by a constant, usually 1,000. Rates constructed using age, gender, and national origin are appropriate for analyzing migration. These rates analyze changes caused by the movement of people in the same way as measures of fertility and mortality analyze changes related to birth and death.

Population Growth

Population growth is a function of births, deaths, and migration. Growth measured by births and deaths alone is referred to as natural increase, it is measured by the CRNI, such that

$$\text{CPNI} = \text{CBR} - \text{CDR}$$

The equation that includes changes in population size resulting from migration, as well as fertility and mortality is called the Demographic Equation. It states that the difference in population from time 1 to time 2 is equal to the births minus the deaths in the interval, plus in-migration minus out-migration in the interval.

$$P_2 - P_1 = B - D + IM - OM$$

Often data are lacking for the migration component of this equation, and population growth is expressed only in terms of births and deaths, that is, natural increase.

Population Composition

Population composition is defined in terms of the distribution of people by specific characteristics at a particular point in time. The most important characteristics are demographic, social, or economic. This information, most commonly based on census data, may show, for example, the number or the percentage of the population in each age-sex group. A graph called a population pyramid is a useful way to display these data. Figure 4-2 contrasts the age-sex composition of a country with low fertility and a long life expectancy (*upper panel, Sweden*) with that of one with high fertility and a shorter life expectancy (*lower panel, Mexico*), showing them as population pyramids.

A brief summary of demographic measures appears in Table 4-1.

► FERTILITY

Fertility is important to public health, population change, and the quality of human life. The role it plays in determining the size, composition, and growth of populations is a powerful factor governing the course of population change. In addition, fertility change influences the health of women, their offspring, their families, and therefore public health practice.

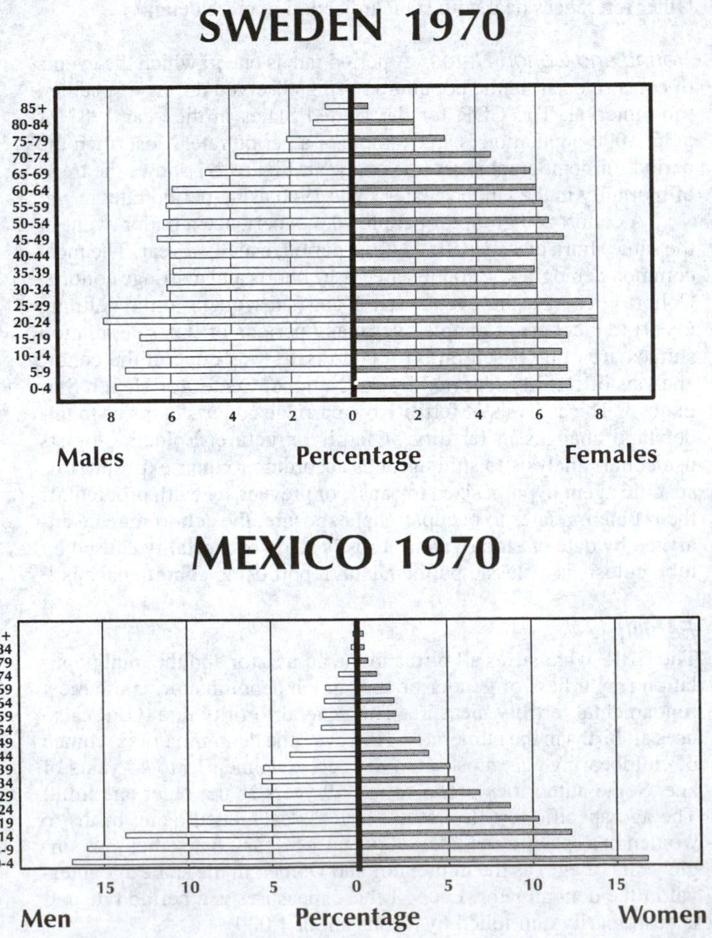

Figure 4-2. Percentage distribution of populations of Sweden (*upper panel*) and Mexico (*lower panel*) by age and sex in 1970. Vertical axis: Age.

TABLE 4-1. BASIC FERTILITY AND MORTALITY MEASURES

Measurement	*Numerator*	*Denominator*	*Constant*[a]
CBR	All births	Total population	1,000
GFR	All births	Women aged 15–44	1,000
ASFR	Birth in age group	Women in age group	1,000
CDR	All deaths	Total population	1,000
ASDR	Death in age group	Population in age group	100,000
IMR	Infant deaths in year	All births in same year	1,000
MMR	Maternal deaths in year	All births in same year	10,000 or 100,000

Abbreviations: CBR, crude birth rate; GFR, general fertility rate; ASFR, age-specific fertility rate; CDR, crude death rate; ASDR, age-specific death rate; MMR, maternal mortality rate.

[a] The constants shown in this column are those used most often. Others may be used in special demographic or public health reports.

Fertility, in its most specific sense, refers to the actual birth of living offspring. Natality is often used synonymously for fertility. Additionally, the capacity to bear children is termed fecundity, and the probability of conceiving in a given month is called fecundability. Natural fertility describes the level of fertility found in populations that use neither contraception (temporary or permanent) nor induced abortion.

The determinants of fertility in a population are both biological and behavioral. They can be aggregated into a structure that permits a quantitative appraisal of the factors influencing fertility change in a population.

Biological Determinants

Menarche and Menopause

Menarche is the beginning of menstruation. It defines the youngest end of the age limit within which women begin to ovulate and are able to conceive. The age of menarche is becoming younger in developed countries. Menopause is the cessation of menstruation. It signals the end of the reproductive years. The age for menopause has increased slightly in recent decades in developed countries. Some societies have experienced a widened span of reproductive years that is caused by a decline in the age at menarche and an increase in the age of menopause. Since these are modernized societies that control fertility with contraception, abortion, and sterilization, changes in the age of menarche or of menopause are not important determinants of present-day fertility.

Ovulation

In demographic terms, ovulation influences fertility most by influencing waiting time until conception, or ovulatory interval. This interval is greatest at the extremes of the reproductive years, either when regular ovulation is not established or when it is waning. While this aspect of ovulation is not a consequential determinant of current fertility levels, the delay in ovulation after childbirth is. The length of postpartum anovulation may vary from 1.5 months to as long as 2 years depending on the frequency and duration of lactation.[13]

Age within Reproductive Span

Once intercourse is an established practice, natural fertility declines with age. Data from several societies with differing fertility levels confirm this observation. Figure 4-3 (*left panel*) illustrates this by showing marital fertility rates by age for two societies with high fertility (Hutterites and Nepal). One society with low fertility (United States) and a standard model population (Coale and Trussel standard schedule) show the same pattern, although the shape of the curves may differ. Figure 4-3 (*right panel*) shows the same data; in this graph, the fertility level for women 20 to 24 years of age is set at an index of 100 for four different populations.[14]

Spontaneous Intrauterine Mortality

The influence on fertility of spontaneous abortions, or miscarriages, and stillbirths is difficult to assess because of the problems in ascertaining these events in a representative population. Nonetheless,

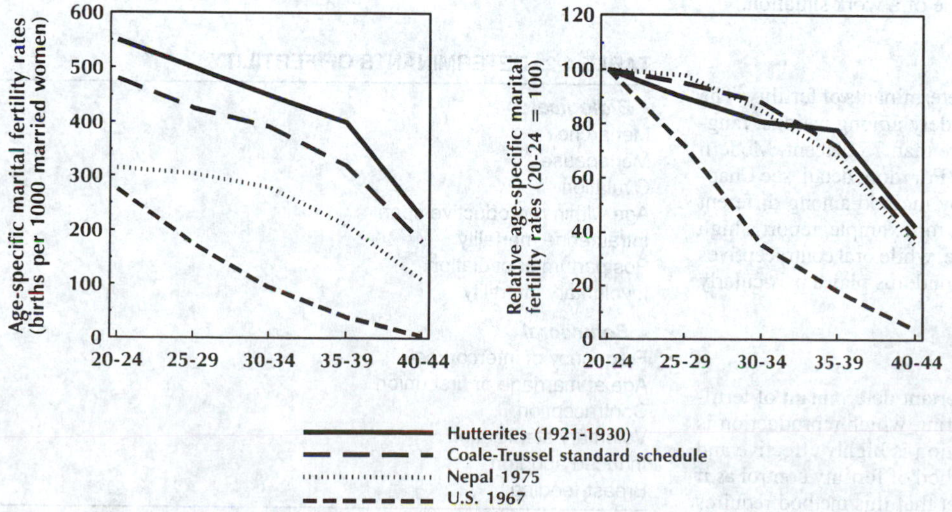

Figure 4-3. Absolute and relative age-specific marital fertility rates of selected populations. Horizontal axis (*both panels*): Age. (From Bongaarts J, Potter RG: Fertility, Biology, and Behavior: An Analysis of the Proximate Determinants. New York: Academic Press, 1983).

current evidence indicates that the risk of spontaneous pregnancy loss is greatest early in pregnancy and declines steadily throughout. It is probably greatest among women in their later childbearing years. Since the evidence suggests little variation from community to community in this biological factor, it is not likely to be a major determinant of differing levels of fertility.

Involuntary Infertility

Involuntary infertility is also called sterility or infecundity. It is measured, in demographic terms, as the inability of a woman to bear a living child during the span of reproductive years. (Although involuntary infertility in males is a serious health concern, it does not influence fertility in a population.) Involuntary infertility in women has several causes. It may result from anatomical abnormalities of the reproductive tract or malfunction of ovulation. When ovaries malfunction, conception does not occur. Recurrent intrauterine loss of pregnancy, or specific diseases associated with infertility, such as gonorrhea and genital tuberculosis, also cause involuntary female infertility.[15] The first three categories are presumed to occur to a similar extent in all populations, although the evidence for this is not entirely satisfactory. The last group, that is, specific diseases such as gonorrhea and tuberculosis, is presumed to account for the occurrence of a high proportion of childlessness. This is especially true among groups in Africa where fertility is otherwise quite high.[16]

Behavioral Determinants[14,17]

Marriage or Sexual Union

Age at first marriage or consensual union is a principal determinant of the number of children a woman will bear. It marks the beginning of socially approved exposure to the probability of conception. The association between increase in the age at marriage and concurrent decline in fertility has been shown in several societies.

Frequency of Intercourse

Frequency of sexual intercourse is directly related to the capacity to bear children, assuming that the menstrual cycle is ovulatory and insemination occurs in mid cycle. Nonetheless, there are very few studies of the frequency of intercourse (not including abstinence) and probability of ovulation in a specific cycle. Therefore, evidence is insufficient to suggest that these factors account for differences in fertility levels from one population to another.

Abstinence, whether voluntary or involuntary, is an important determinant of fertility. In some cultures abstinence is required during lactation. In others, lactation and religious beliefs are related, influencing the role an individual or group plays within a religion. In economic circumstances that require couples to separate because of employment, abstinence may result because of a work situation.

Contraception

Contraceptive use is one of the principal determinants of fertility. The prevalence of contraceptive use varies widely among nations, ranging from approximately 10 percent to more than 75 percent. Modern contraception is highly effective and safe. (For more detail, see Chapter 71.) The variation in patterns of use by method among different countries is substantial. Surveys of China, for example, report a high prevalence of intrauterine device (IUD) use, while oral contraceptives are widely used in the United States and condoms play a particularly important role in Japan.[18]

Voluntary Sterilization

Voluntary surgical sterilization is an important determinant of fertility because it limits the span of years during which reproduction is possible. This approach to fertility regulation is highly effective and safe. Although some studies treat this method of fertility control as if it were a method of contraception, the fact that this method requires surgery makes it more appropriate to identify sterilization separately for health practitioners.

Induced Abortion

Induced abortion is one of the principal determinants of human fertility. In some countries abortion is legally prohibited and the practice of abortion is rarely acknowledged.[19] Elsewhere abortion is permitted virtually on request, and women may experience on average between 2 and 3 during the reproductive years.[20]

Breast-Feeding

Breast-feeding is an important determinant of fertility. Lactation stimulated by a nursing infant influences the duration of anovulation after childbirth. In the United States and other developed countries the practice of breast-feeding has little influence on the level of fertility. However, in less developed areas, groups are found in which infants are breast fed very frequently. Some infants are fed on demand because these nurslings have almost no other source of nutrition. Although the mothers of these babies use no other form of fertility control, they have fertility levels nearly the same as developed countries.

Table 4-2 shows the determinants of fertility.[14]

Status and Trends

United States

Official birth statistics for the twentieth century show that the United States reached an annual peak number of births early in the 1960s of more than 4.25 million. Thereafter, the United States experienced a decline to less than 3.25 million in the early 1970s. The annual number of births increased to 4.16 million in 1990 and then declined during the first 4 years of the decade. The number of births in 1994 was 3.95 million. The CBR was over 30.0 early in this century, but had a peak of 25.0 in 1955, the high point since 1950. The low point, 14.6, for the century was in the 1970s; the CBR reported as 15.2 in 1994 reached its lowest point since 1978.[21]

Estimates of the TFR by scholars indicate that this measure of fertility declined throughout the history of the United States until the 1947–1961 period. These years are referred to as the Baby Boom. Official vital statistics show that the TFR increased from 2.3 in 1940 to 3.7 in 1960. The TFR remained more than 3.0 until 1965, then declined to below 2.0 in 1973, remaining at this level for 15 years. Although the TFR is now above 2.0, it is still low enough that each mother will not replace herself with a daughter. If these fertility levels continue and are accompanied by current trends in migration, growth of the national population will continue. Moreover, this growth will be determined more by migration than by the increase from fertility.

TABLE 4-2. DETERMINANTS OF FERTILITY

• Biological
Menarche
Menopause
Ovulation
Age within reproductive span
Intrauterine mortality
Postpartum anovulation
Involuntary infertility
• Behavioral
Frequency of intercourse
Age at marriage or first union
Contraception
Voluntary sterilization
Induced abortion
Breast-feeding

International
Fertility around the world has undergone striking changes in the last several decades. Because the TFR is standardized for age and the age structure of individual countries differs substantially, the most informative comparisons use the TFR. In the 40 years from 1950 to 1990 the estimated TFR for the world decreased from 5.0 to 3.4, a decline of 32 percent. Despite this, individual regions continue to show fertility that ranges from below replacement (TFR = 1.7 for established market economies) to almost 4 children per woman (TFR = 3.8 for demographically developing nations). Some areas, such as sub-Saharan Africa (TFR = 6.4), continue to have very high fertility. The change in China where the TFR was reduced by half in a peace-time period of 15 years is without historic precedent. On the other hand, many African countries and other major areas, notably Bangladesh, Pakistan, and most Arab countries, experienced a negligible decline in TFR.[22,23] Overall, world fertility remains higher than that of the United States, and the global TFR is estimated to be 3.4 children per 1,000 women aged 15 to 44 years.

▸ MORTALITY

Public health traditionally focuses on preventing death. Measures of mortality describe both the likelihood of dying in any specific time interval and the expectation of survival.

Determinants
The factors that determine differences and changes in the levels of mortality among populations are biological or behavioral.

Age
Age is a principal determinant of mortality. Starting at a high level in infancy, mortality declines precipitously in childhood, remains at a low level through adolescence and early adulthood, and then increases inexorably in adulthood and older ages. This pattern holds true for both males and females in both developed and developing countries and is illustrated by data from the United States in Figure 4-4.

Sex
Throughout life, and perhaps even from conception, males have a higher risk of mortality than females. Figure 4-4 illustrates this point. For this reason, published life tables separate computations for each sex.[24] Exceptions to this point exist under special circumstances, for example, in societies that may value the survival of male offspring over females, and situations of low levels of economic development where childbearing increases the risk of mortality for women of reproductive age. Specific causes of death, as illustrated by breast cancer, may also carry greater risk for women than they do for men. Nonetheless, when all causes of death are considered together, the risk of mortality is less, the likelihood of survival is greater, and life expectancy is longer for females than for males.

Race/Ethnicity
Differences in racial and ethnic characteristics within a population are often associated with differences in mortality. These differences are recognized in population data from major regions of the world including Asia, Africa, and North America and in large part are considered to be the result of social and economic differences between racial or ethnic groups in a population. In the United States differences in the mortality for blacks and whites are sufficiently important that official life tables are published for all causes of death by race, as well as by sex, and official public health policy focuses on approaches to resolve these differences.

Region/Area
Mortality may differ by geographic region both within and across national boundaries. This can be most readily recognized by reviewing United Nations publications, especially the *Demographic Yearbook.* Model life tables constructed to estimate mortality in areas where population data are incomplete reflect this fact by having four sets of models based on regional differences in the risk of death.[25] In North America, data published by region, province, or state show differences in key parameters of mortality such as life expectancy.[21] The reasons for these differences are presumably related to social, economic, and health service factors.

Cause of Death
Although the specific cause of death is important to each individual and often to a specific public health program, population changes are determined by the spectrum of disease causes prevalent in a community and whether the means are available to control such causes. Diarrheal diseases, for example, are an important cause of mortality in developing countries, while cardiovascular disease deaths are more prevalent in modernized nations. One important development is the global occurrence of human immunodeficiency virus (HIV) infections. These viral infections are transmitted by a variety of mechanisms, such as sexual contact, blood products, and needles contaminated with blood from infected individuals. (The current status of this global epidemic is dealt with in detail in a separate chapter.) Patterns of causes of death and their influence on population change is discussed in more detail in the section, Determinants of Population Group: The Epidemiologic Transition.

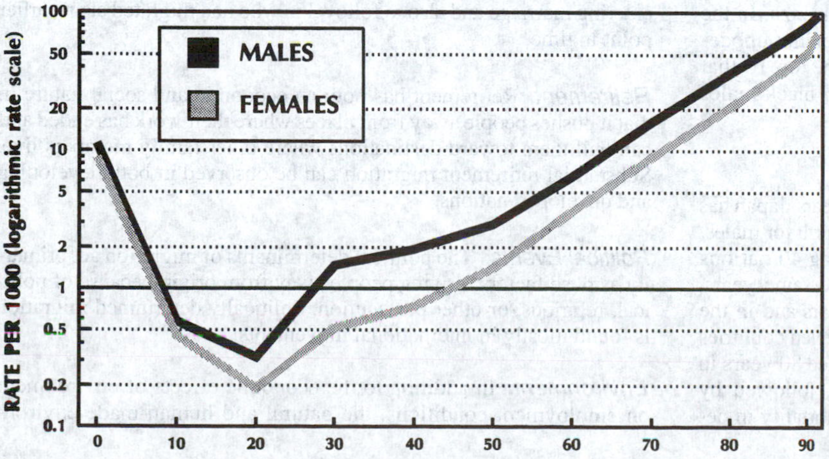

Figure 4-4. Death rates from all causes for females and males, United States, 1976. Rates are deaths per 1,000 population, by age at death, and shown on a logarithmic scale. Horizontal axis: Age.

Social and Economic Conditions

Economic development, measured by per capita national income and other indicators of economic advancement, is related to the increase in life expectancy in most parts of the world; moreover, this one factor accounts for between 10 and 25 percent of the improvement in life expectancy depending on the region and time period over which the change occurred.[26] The mortality decline of the nineteenth century is ascribed to improvements in living standard, diet, sanitation, and improved working conditions.[27]

Public Health

Public health measures have played a leading role in reducing mortality through preventing the transmission of infection. Even before the discovery of specific microorganisms, epidemiologists identified the ways in which diseases, such as childbed fever and cholera, were transmitted and promoted measures for prevention. In recent decades, immunization has led to the worldwide eradication of smallpox[28] and brought about a substantial decline in measles in the United States.[29] Studies of tobacco use and its attendant health problems have led to a reduction in cigarette smoking.[30] Screening for cervical cancer has in all likelihood presumably led to a decline in mortality caused by this condition.[31] More recent improvements in mortality, the likely result of collective individual modifications in lifestyle, such as dietary improvements and exercise, have been aided by public health promotion efforts.

Medicine and Technology

Medical and technological discoveries are important determinants of mortality, although their contribution is reflected in changes during the twentieth century rather than in earlier times. The discovery of insecticides and antibiotics, the introduction of anesthesia, the control of hospital-acquired infection, and the organization of health services are all presumed to have made important contributions to improving mortality.

Status and Trends

United States

Life expectancy at birth has improved substantially over the past century, from 47 years to 76 years. Although life expectancy reached an historic high point (79.8 years in 1992) for white females, this measure for black males crested in 1984 at 65.3 years; provisional data show a life expectancy of 64.9 for this group in 1994. In the past two decades the CDR has declined steadily, and the age-standardized death rate has decreased even more. For the most recent year available (1993) the age-standardized rate is lowest for white females, next lowest for black females, and highest for black males. The ranking of death rates by cause during the mid-1980s consistently shows diseases of the heart to be the leading, albeit a declining, cause of death. It is followed by malignant neoplasms (all organ systems taken together), cerebrovascular diseases, accidents and adverse effects, and pneumonia and influenza. In the national population overall death resulting from human immunodeficiency virus infection is the only cause ranked in the top 10 that has advanced its rank third leading cause of death for black males and the tenth for the nation.[21]

International

Mortality for the world is generally declining. In recent years, Japan has become the country with the highest life expectancy at birth for males, reaching 75.9 years in 1987 and 76.3 by 1992, among 40 nations for which current information is available. (For these same years, male life expectancy in Canada was 73.3 and 74.9 years and in the United States was 71.4 and 72.3 years). For females, eleven countries reported life expectancy at birth that reached or exceeded 80 years in 1992. Of these, Japan was the highest (82.5 years), followed by France (82.3), and Switzerland (81.7).[21] In contrast, mortality in developing countries is at much higher levels. Some of the highest mortality rates are found in Africa. Life expectancy for both sexes combined in 1990, for example, is 43 years in Mozambique, 38 in Sierra Leone and Niger, and 44 in Rwanda and Guinea.[23]

► MIGRATION

Migration is an important component of population change. However, it is often neglected in calculations of population growth because of the difficulty in measuring and collecting accurate migration information. Migration may be defined as movement of people involving a change of residence between two clearly defined geographic units.[32] The definition of residence and the choice of geographic units vary depending on the particular use of the migration data.

The study of migration is divided into two subdisciplines: internal migration and international migration. Internal migration refers to changes of residence within national borders, and the movers are called in-migrants and out-migrants. International migration refers to residence changes across national boundaries, with movers termed immigrants and emigrants.

Determinants

Lee's push-pull Theory[33] theorizes that migration comes about as the result of individuals responding to negative or "push" factors at place of origin and positive or "pull" factors at place of destination. In addition to the positives and negatives at origin and destination, the decision of the potential migrant will also take into account "intervening obstacles," which are factors associated with the migration process itself, such as distance, financial or psychic costs of the move, immigration laws, etc. The determinants of migration can therefore be divided into two groupings: (*a*) characteristics associated with the places of residence and (*b*) characteristics of the migrants themselves.

Characteristics of Places of Origin or Destination

Economic Conditions. Most migration, whether internal or international, occurs in response to economic conditions. Of these, *employment* is the most important factor. In a less developed setting, peasants leave the farm for the city because of poor income, loss of work, or soil depletion. In developed countries, professional workers make inter-urban moves seeking better jobs. *Education* is also considered an factor in that it represents an investment in human capital that will bring later reward in the marketplace. In both less and more developed societies, adolescents and young adults migrate for access to educational institutions.

Family and Kinship. Family and kinship factors are important determinants in less developed countries, but can also be found in developed settings. In many parts of the world people migrate upon entering marriage and also to follow kin who had migrated at an earlier point in time.

Retirement. Retirement has both an economic and social nature in that it pushes people away from places where their work has ended and can pull them toward destinations where other family members live. Substantial retirement migration can be observed in both developing and developed nations.

Political Events. The political determinants of migration act primarily as push factors, driving people away from origin because of political, religious, or other persecution. Politically determined migration is found mostly in international movements.

Environment. In addition to the economic effects of environment on employment conditions, the natural and human-made environments also play an important role as they affect the psychological or physical well-being of people. Migration as a response to purely environmental factors is found primarily in developed societies, where people can afford to make "consumption-oriented" moves.[34]

Characteristics of Migrants

Age. Age is the single characteristic that is found to have a universal association with migration. Throughout the world, peak migration rates are found between the ages of 15 and 29. In less developed countries, the age of men and women at migration clusters around 15 to 24, in more developed countries, the peak age is found between 20 and 29.

Marital Status. In many societies migration is associated with the event of marriage, but this is not consistent across cultures. Migration may be necessary, in certain traditional settings, when marriage occurs between people from different towns or villages. In more modern cultures marriage may precipitate a migration to obtain improved employment or living conditions. In much of the world, however, migration is more frequent among unmarried persons who find it easier to move without the encumbrance of a family.

Socioeconomic Status. The socioeconomic status of migrants varies by level of development of a society. In less developed countries, migrants tend to be among the lower strata of the population, frequently rural peasants moving to urban areas. In more developed countries migrants predominate among the upper educational and occupational groups, where they tend to circulate within the urban sector of society.

Status and Trends

United States

International migration to the United States in the nineteenth and early twentieth centuries has been one of the most significant international movements of population in the history of the world. At the turn of the century, one in ten Americans were born outside of the Untied States. The immigration rate into the Untied States peaked in 1901–1910 at 10.4 per 1,000 population, when 92 percent of the immigrants were from European origins. As a result of restrictive immigration laws, migration into the United States later declined. Today, the legal immigration rate is 2.5 per 1000, with 85 percent arriving from Asian and Latin American countries. In addition, demographic estimates of illegal migration suggest that the United States receives 100,000 to 300,000 "permanent" illegal immigrants annually.[35]

International

In addition to the movement to the United States, nineteenth and twentieth century European migration to South America and Australia was also significant. Other, more recent, major international migrations include the movement of populations between India and Pakistan after the partitioning of the Indian subcontinent, the movement of Chinese into Hong Kong, the migration of Jews and Palestinians into and out of Israel, Southeast Asian refugee movements, and both political and environmental refugees in Africa.[36] As with movements within countries, age, socioeconomic status, and marital status create differences among groups that move from place to place and those that do not. Migration across national borders, however, is influenced disproportionately by armed conflict and political forces.

Internal migration is probably of greatest impact in less developed countries, where the pace of movement into urban areas is often too rapid for the urban infrastructure to absorb the new residents. In developed countries, internal migration is not viewed as a problem because it tends to be more balanced across many urban areas and involves movement of people who have the resources for successful adaptation to the new place of residence.

▶ DETERMINANTS OF POPULATION GROWTH

The determinants of demographic change for the world's population, that is, fertility and mortality, have been the subject of theoretical concepts at least since Malthus published his first *Essay on the Principle of Population As It Affects the Future Improvement of Society* in 1798.[37] Subsequently, careful examination of population data have led to the formulation of other concepts of population change.

Theory of Demographic Transition

The original theory of the demographic transition describes the historical experience of population growth of Western countries that accompanied economic development.[38] The transition can be divided into three stages. During the first stage, birth and death rates both are high but at similar levels so that population growth is minimal. This stage is referred to as the stage of high growth potential because, if mortality were to decline without a concurrent decline in fertility, the size of the population would increase rapidly. The second stage is called the transition stage because it describes the transition from high to low birth and death rates that result from economic development. It is characterized by an initial decline in mortality while fertility remains high, followed by a decline in fertility until both fertility and mortality meet at low levels. During the first part of this stage the high growth potential is realized, while at the latter part of this stage growth has tapered off. The third and final stage of the theory is called incipient decline and describes both birth and death rates at low and relatively stable levels with fertility at times falling below death rates and thus at times producing a decline in population.

Although the classic theory of the demographic transition provides a perspective for interpreting the historical change in Western populations, it does not describe or explain patterns of population change in non-Western societies nor those in developing countries.[39,40] Over the years, the theory has been examined and reexamined in light of new data and knowledge of variation in cultural conditions.[41,42] Today, reformulated versions of the theory that depend more on social structural explanations for changes in birth and death rates are being considered. The basic relationship between mortality decline, fertility decline, and population growth, however, is still used as a framework for comparing population trends.

Epidemiologic Transition

In 1971 the theory of epidemiologic transition was proposed which built upon that of demographic transition. Accepting the assumption that mortality is a fundamental factor in population change, this theory identified three stages through which the causes of mortality evolved: the first was a period of widespread epidemics and famine, the second was a stage of receding epidemics associated with increasing population growth, and the third was a stage of degenerative diseases and those related to individual lifestyle. In terms of fertility, this concept identified a classic, or Western, model in which change is related to social factors, an accelerated model in which change is related to medical factors (including antibiotics, steroids, contraceptive pills, and induced abortion), and a delayed model in which mortality is influenced by the medical factors of the accelerated model, but fertility decline is delayed.[27]

This theory is susceptible to some of the same criticisms as demographic transition theory because both have difficulty adapting to less developed countries and they ignore migration. Moreover, the epidemiologic transition model has not been subject to the detailed scholarly review given the theory of demographic transition. The concept of epidemiologic transition, however, is an important idea that builds appropriately on the theory of demographic transition.

Relative Role of Determinants in the United States

If demographic trends were evaluated for the United States to assess its status in terms of demographic and epidemiologic transitions, it would be in the latest stage of each model. The population of the United States, estimated to be 257.7 million in 1993, grew by nearly

31 million people since the 1980 census. Natural increase accounts for most (74 percent) of this change, and the remaining portion is due to migration. Mortality is caused in greatest part by chronic, degenerative diseases (diseases of the heart, cerebrovascular diseases, and malignant neoplasms). Fertility is maintained at a low level for more than a decade, and in 1993 the TFR was 2.05.[21]

Relative Role of Determinants Internationally

Examining demographic trends for the world in terms of the demographic and epidemiologic transitions is not as easy. Population growth is persistent; the planet's population reached 2.5 billion in 1950, and 5.8 billion in 1996. The rate of increase reached a peak of 2.2 percent between 1965 and 1973 and has declined since; it is estimated to be 1.7 percent between 1980 and 1990. Nonetheless, the downturn has not been sufficiently great to be associated with a decrease in the absolute number of people being added to the world's population. Indeed, the downturn does not reflect a universal decline in growth rates. Most of the decline is a result of low growth and even negative growth in developed countries that have passed through the demographic transition and have been in the final stage for several decades. Applying the demographic transition model to less developed countries would place most of them in the middle stage, where death rates are declining and birth rates are declining less rapidly or not declining at all. Thus, the world growth rate in 1991 of 1.7 percent reflects a growth rate of 0.6 percent for high-income countries and 2.0 percent for middle and low income countries. (The growth rate for the Middle East and North Africa was estimated at 3.2 percent, and for Sub-Saharan Africa, excluding South Africa, it was estimated at 3.1 percent between 1980 and 1990.)[23]

A decline in global mortality is taking place. Between 1950–1955 and 1980–1985 the estimated life expectancy at birth increased worldwide more than 17 years, reaching 65 years of age. Demographically, developing countries increased by 23 years, while established market economy countries increased 11 years to a total of 76 years of life expected at birth.[22,23] Given the success in eradicating smallpox and reducing the burden of other infections, such as malaria, polio, and measles, the transition from mortality resulting from acute infectious diseases to chronic diseases and injuries should continue.

▶ CONSEQUENCES OF POPULATION GROWTH

Projecting Change

Projecting population growth in terms of size and composition is an important starting point in trying to determine the consequences of population change. Using age- and sex-specific probabilities of death, age-specific fertility probabilities and the sex ratio at birth, and reported or assumed migration rates permits demographers to project, but not to forecast, population into the future. The distinction between projecting and forecasting is important because a projection uses an explicit set of assumptions and is intended to be an illustrative calculation based on these assumptions. A forecast, on the other hand, includes an element of subjective judgment to set the levels of mortality, fertility, and migration for specific times in the future. Projections are usually made based on a single set of mortality probabilities. Fertility, on the other hand, because it varies over shorter intervals, is often projected using 3 or 4 different sets of assumed probabilities, thereby generating different projections. Migration is based on current data and estimates; projections of migrants are usually assumed to remain stable unless specific changes in policy or other determinants of population mobility are known.

Projections based on the assumptions judged by the Bureau of the Census to be most likely to hold true in the near future indicate that by the year 2000 the population of the United States will be 267.7 million people, which will increase to 282.1 million by 2010. While the largest proportion of the population will live in the South, the most rapid increase is projected for the West (13.7 percent). Growth in the Northeast (2.4 percent) and Midwest (–0.3 percent) is calculated to be negligible. Most of the increase is expected to be the result of natural increase (72 percent) rather than net migration (28 percent). The median age is projected to increase from 33.0 years in 1990, to 36.5 in 2000, and 39.0 by 2010; the median age in the Northeast is anticipated to exceed 40 years by 2010 for the first time in any major region of the United States.[43]

Population Growth and Economic Change

The role of population growth in relation to economic change is a central global concern, especially of bodies such as the World Bank and the United Nations Fund for Population Activities (UNFPA). The work of Coale and Hoover in 1958 was instrumental in pointing out that "A reduction in fertility would make the process of modernization more rapid and more certain. It would accelerate the growth in income, provide more rapidly the possibility of productive employment, . . . make the attainment of universal education easier—and . . . [provide] women of low-income countries some relief from constant pregnancy, parturition, and infant care."[44] Pursuing a course of lower fertility would, according to these scholars, create this advantageous effect by reducing the number of dependent children, i.e., those age 15 years and younger, with only minor effects on the size of the labor force or its increase until 30 years later.

Reviewing this work 30 years later, Coale emphasized, as he had stated in his earlier writings, that no relationship existed between the rate of growth of the total population and an increase in the rate of per capita income, but current data did show that annual per capita income increased as TFR decreased in developing countries.[45] In addition, he pointed to a positive relationship between the rate of growth in per capita income and increase in life expectancy at birth. Moreover, productive employment is a more realistic prospect in those countries that immediately initiate measures to reduce high rates of fertility. The importance of these observations has not been lost on most world leaders.

Population, the Environment, Resources, and Food

Around the beginning of the 19th century Malthus recorded his views on population growth and its consequences, specifically inadequate food supplies. In more recent years others have emphasized and extended these observations, linking environmental degradation to uncontrolled population growth. Among the most important contributions to this debate was the publication of *The Limits to Growth* in 1972.[46] Supported by an informal group of international professionals who called themselves The Club of Rome, a research team at the Massachusetts Institute of Technology investigated the state of the world in terms of population growth, agricultural productivity, environmental pollution, industrial output, and nonrenewable resources. After determining the status of each factor and the trends of change from 1900 to 1970, they projected the effects of these trends into the future and reached the following conclusions: *(a)* If these trends persist unchanged, the limits to growth on the earth would be reached within the next 100 years; *(b)* the trends could all be altered so that economic and ecological stability might be reached and sustained; and *(c)* the sooner governments and citizens around the world undertake the measures to alter current trends in all five of these areas of social and ecological concern, the greater would be the chances of attaining global equilibrium. A flurry of criticism followed the publication of *The Limits to Growth*. Nonetheless, it heightened the intensity of debate over global issues important to the present and future of human well-being, and many of the issues, including continued population growth, remain important today.

Concern about the environment and its importance to humanity has rekindled awareness of population growth.[1] Ehrlich and colleagues have reemphasized the gravity of environmental degradation as a consequence of population growth. Specifically, they draw attention to the human impact on land use, desertification, deforestation of most tropical areas, and "anthropogenic climate change."[47] In the United States, citizen groups concerned about these issues, such as the National Audubon Society, have also become more active.[48–50]

▶ PUBLIC HEALTH ISSUES

Teenage Fertility

Teenage pregnancies are a profound population issue because children born to young women may lead to unanticipated momentum in population growth by increasing total family size over a lifetime and by shortening the time between generations of future children. Moreover, they are a serious public health problem because teenage pregnancies may be at high risk of preventable infant mortality, and pregnancies in very young women of reproductive age are often not intended. (See Chapter 71).

Demographic Trends and Effects. In the United States the number of births to women 15 to 19 years of age decreased from an estimated 644,700 in 1970 to a low of 461,900 in 1986, and then increased to 521,800 in 1990. By 1994, this age group had 505,500 live births. Moreover, this estimate does not include the legal abortions (232,000 in 1973, 418,000 in 1982, and 256,000 in 1994) that women in this age group underwent.[51,52] However, pregnancy rates for sexually experienced teenage women declined 12 percent between 1980 and 1991, as did the proportion of teenage women reported to have legal abortion.

Birth rates for teenage women in the United States have declined by 26 percent between 1970 and 1986. Subsequently some of that decrease was lost when teenage fertility increased 17 percent between 1986 and 1994 to 58.9 births to women age 15 to 19 years.[53] Compared with other nations for which data on teenage pregnancy are available, the United States rate (95 pregnancies per 1,000 women age 15 to 19) is among the highest. The pregnancy rate for Canada (46) is less than half that for the United States, while the Netherlands has a teenage pregnancy rate of 15, the lowest reported.[18]

These patterns have important demographic implications. Age at first sexual union is a principal determinant of lifetime fertility and family size. Women who begin having children at an early age, therefore, are likely to have larger families, births at shorter intervals, and contribute disproportionately to increasing growth of a community or population than women who begin having children at later ages. In terms of long-term demographic change, couples who have offspring while the mother is still in her teens have a short generation. The result is that the female offspring of these couples are at risk of childbearing in a shorter span of years than are the female children of mothers who defer childbearing until their 20s or 30s.

Health Effects. While the children of teenage mothers are at higher risk of death than are children of women in their 20s, the risk to the health of pregnant women under age 20 is more difficult to assess because first births and births to women in social minorities are thought to carry a higher risk of mortality. Nonetheless, the most recent analysis of maternal mortality by age of mother for the United States did not show any appreciable differences in age-specific mortality ratios.[54] The reasons for the greater risk among minorities are not entirely clear, but they may bear a relationship to marital disruption, access to care, compliance with care standards, or the unintendedness of pregnancies to women in their teen years.

Urbanization

The movement of people to cities (urbanization) is one of the dominant characteristics of population change of the twentieth century. At the beginning of the century, fewer than 1 of every 7 persons in the world lived in a city; as we near the year 2000, more than 40 percent of the world's population is found in an urban area.[1]

The growth of cities is determined by three factors: *(a)* migration; *(b)* natural increase, i.e., the number of births in excess of the number of deaths; and *(c)* the reclassification of areas from rural to urban as they rapidly become more populous. Urban growth at the global level has been 2.5 percent annually in recent years, or about 50 percent greater than that of the total population. Urbanization is most profound in developing countries where the annual urban growth rate is 4.4 percent. As a result, Sao Paulo, Brazil, is projected to have 25.8 million residents, and Mexico City 31.0 million by the year 2000.[55]

The health problems of city life are not so directly caused by urban living as much as they are by the extent to which the infrastructure of society is overwhelmed by the size of the population. Rapid urban growth resulting primarily from rural to urban migration creates health problems related to the need for housing and sanitation, improved food supply, transportation within the city, and the distribution of preventive and curative health services. In many developing countries the vast numbers of people leaving rural areas for urban places reside in the unsanitary conditions of shantytowns or squatter settlements on the fringe of the capital cities, where public health problems are exacerbated.

Refugees and Other Migrants

An estimated 15.2 million refugees are dispersed throughout the world.[2] While most are in Africa (5.2 million) and have come from other countries on that continent, refugees can be found in almost every nation. Although many such people leave their homelands because of civil conflict and other political reasons, others do so for reasons that have led some experts to identify them as "ecological refugees."[36] Jacobson[36] cites food shortages and sharp increases in food prices, generally or for specific staples, as events that trigger ecological refugee movements. In other situations migrants move to find better employment opportunities and an improved quality of life. Nonetheless, even in areas where people from other nations are welcome, or when migration takes place within a single country, the difficulties of geographic displacement may be augmented by occupational displacement, environmental change, social disruption, and economic hardship.

Refugee movements may bring with them serious public health problems such as severe malnutrition as is the case in Africa. In other instances refugees and other migrants may carry infections to areas in which such diseases are under control, or where they have not previously existed, thereby necessitating new or intensified public health screening efforts followed by treatment or other control measures. In some areas violence related to historical ethnic conflicts is a serious problem.

Health problems are also encountered by migrants as a consequence of their move to a new environment. Psychological stress and physical deprivation associated with living in an unfamiliar environment, such as a refugee camp or squatter settlement, can bring about high levels of violence, including suicide, homicide, and rape. Language and other cultural differences between refugees or migrants and their place of destination produce serious barriers to health care information and services at the new location.

Aging

As the death rate declines in most parts of the world, life expectancy increases, and the number and ages of older people increase. This change is more characteristic in developed countries where life expectancy often exceeds 70 years. A shift in the age of a population has important implications for the health problems a society must face and the health services that must be provided.

The United States illustrates how aging has become an important issue and how it is developing momentum for the future. From 1950 to 1980, the world population growth created alarm as it increased at the rate of approximately 2 percent each year, portending a doubling of the global population every 30 years. During this same time the number of people age 65 and older increased 2.3 percent annually; the number of those age 85 years and older increased at a rate of 4.2 percent yearly. By 1992 the number of people in this country age 65 and older increased to 32 million (compared with 3 million in 1900), and those 85 and older numbered 3 million. (In 1900 only 122,000 Americans were in this age group).[21] The combined demographic dynamics of an increase in life expectancy and a decline in fertility has profoundly changed the proportion of the United States population that is age 65 and older. Recent estimates indicate that people who are 65 years and older comprised 13 percent of the national population in 1992; in 1900 they were 4 percent of the nation's people. Current projections show this trend will persist into the next century. Between 1990 and 2010 the number of people 65 and older is likely to increase by at least 7 million, while those between 25 and 44 could decrease by 9 million. By 2030 there is likely to be 59.2 million Americans age 65 and older; 6.3 million of them will be 85 years old and older.[56]

The spectrum of health problems facing the public with an aging population will change profoundly. Heart disease, cancer, and cerebrovascular disease, which account for 60 percent of the deaths in the United States, will continue to be prevalent. Chronic obstructive pulmonary disease is now ranked fourth as a cause of death nationwide and is increasing in older age groups. For the first time Alzheimer's disease is on the list of important causes of mortality. This condition accounted for 16,754 deaths in 1993, two-thirds of which were in women.[57] The need to prevent disability and injury in the aging, intensified needs for long-term care, and other special health services has reached a new level of importance that will persist well into the next century. A survey of people in the United States who were between 55 and 74 years of age showed that more than half (54 percent) had difficulty walking a quarter of a mile; more than three-fifths of them had difficulty lifting 25 pounds (62 percent) or stooping, kneeling, or crouching (65 percent). Moreover, health reasons were given for retirement from the workforce by 1 of every 6 respondents, and the role of health became increasingly important as the age of the respondents increased. Health measures, public policy on retirement, and the desire of the older members of the population to continue working will be important determinants of the quality of living in the future.[58] While research on genetics and diseases, such as diabetes and Alzheimer's disease, hold great promise for the future, their impact is unlikely to be felt on the population of the United States for more than a decade.

▶ REFERENCES

1. World Commission on Environment and Development: Our Common Future. Oxford, England: Oxford University Press, 1987
2. US Committee for Refugees: World Refugees Survey, 1996. Washington, DC: Immigration and Refugees Services of America, 1996
3. United Nations. Principles and recommendations for the 1970 population censuses. Statistical papers, Series M, No. 44, 3–4, 1967
4. Kovar MG: Data systems of the national center for health statistics. Hyattsville, MD: National Center for Health Statistics, March 1989; DHHS Publication No (PHS) 89-1325. (Vital and health statistics; Series 1; No. 23)
5. Remington PL, Smith MY, Williamson DF, Anda RF, Gentry EM, Hogelin GC: Design, Characteristics, and Usefulness of State-based Behavioral Risk Factor Surveillance: 1981–87. Public Health Reports 103:366–375, 1988
6. Kann L, Kolbe LJ, Collins JL, eds: Measuring the Health Behavior of Adolescents: The Youth Risk Behavior Surveillance System. Public Health Reports 106 (suppl) 1993
7. Brown GF, Bongaarts J, Churchill EP, et al (eds): Ghana 1988: Results from the Demographic and Health Survey. Studies in Family Planning. New York: Population Council 21(4):236–240, 1990
8. Population Reports. Fertility and Family Planning Surveys; An Update. The Population Information Program Series M. No. 8, 13(4): M291–293, September–October 1985. Baltimore: Johns Hopkins University, 1985
9. Palmore JA, Gardner RW: Measuring mortality, fertility, and natural increase: a self-teaching guide to elementary measures. Honolulu: East-West Center, 1983
10. Heuser RL: Fertility tables for birth cohorts by color: United States, 1917–73. Rockville, MD: National Center for Health Statistics, 1976; DHEW Publication No. (HRA) 76-1152
11. Frost WH: The age selection of mortality from tuberculosis in successive decades. Am J Hyg 30:90–96, 1939
12. Peavy JV, Dyal WW, Eddins DL: Descriptive statistics rates, ratios, proportions and indices. Atlanta: United States Department of Health and Human Services, Centers for Disease Control, 1989
13. Leridon H: Human fertility: the basic components. Chicago: The University of Chicago Press, 1977
14. Bongaarts J, Potter RG: Natural fertility and its proximate determinants. In: Fertility, biology, and behavior: New York: an analysis of the proximate determinants. Academic Press, 1983
15. Mishell DR: Infertility. In: Droegemueller W, Herbst AL, et al (eds): Comprehensive Gynecology. St. Louis: CV Mosby, 1987
16. Brass W: The demography of French-speaking territories covered by special sample inquiries: Upper Volta, Dahomey, Guinea, North Cameroon, and other areas. In: Brass W, Coale AJ, Demeny P, et al (eds): The Demography of Tropical Africa. Princenton, NJ: Princeton University Press, 1968, pp 342–449
17. Davis K, Blake J: Social structure and fertility: an analytic framework. Econ Dev Cult Change 4:211–235, 1956
18. Hatcher RA, Kowal D, Guest F, et al: Contraceptive technology: international edition. Atlanta: Printed Matter, 1989
19. Jacobson JL: The Global Politics of Abortion: Worldwatch Paper 97. Washington, DC: Worldwatch Institute, 1990
20. Tietze C: Induced abortion: a world review 1981. In: A Population Council Fact Book. New York: The Population Council, 1986
21. National Center for Health Statistics: Health, United States, 1994. Hyattsville, MD: US Public Health Service, 1995
22. Demeny P: The world demographic situation. In Menken J (ed): World Population and U.S. Policy—The Choices Ahead. New York: WW Norton, 1986, pp 27–66
23. The World Bank: World Development Report 1993: Investing in Health. The International Bank for Reconstruction and Development. New York: Oxford University Press, 1993
24. Lancaster HO: Expectations of Life: A Study in the Demography, Statistics, and History of World Mortality. New York: Springer-Verlag, 1990
25. Coale AJ, Demeny P, Vaughan B: Regional model life tables and stable populations. 2nd ed. New York: Academic Press, 1983
26. Preston SH: Mortality patterns in national populations. New York: Academic Press, 1976
27. Omran AR: Epidemiologic transition in the United States—the health factor in population change. Washington, DC: Population Reference Bureau. Popul Bull 32(2): 1980
28. Fenner F, et al: Smallpox and Its Eradication. Geneva: World Health Organization, 1988
29. Centers for Disease Control: Summary of notifiable diseases, United States, 1995. MMWR 44(53): 1996
30. US Department of Health and Human Services: Reducing the Health Consequences of Smoking: 25 Years of Progress. A Report of the Surgeon General. US Department of Health and Human Services, Public Health Service. DHHS Publication No. (CDC) 89-8411, 1989
31. Worth AJ: The Walton report and its subsequent impact on cervical cancer screening programs in Canada. Obstet Gynecol 63: 135–139, 1984
32. Shryock HS, Siegel JS, et al: The Methods and Materials of Demography. Washington, DC: US Bureau of the Census, 1971
33. Lee ES: A theory of migration. Demography 3:47–57, 1966
34. Kuznets SS: Introduction. In Eldridge HT, Thomas DS (eds): Demographic Analyses and Interrelations. Population Redistribution and Economic Growth United States, 1870–1950. Philadelphia: American Philosophical Society, 1964, vol 3
35. Bouvier LF, Gardner RW: Immigration to the US: The Unfinished Story. Washington, DC: Population Reference Bureau, Popul Bull 41(4): 1986
36. Jacobson JL: Abandoning homelands. In Brown LR et al (eds): State of the World, 1989. New York: WW Norton, 1989

37. Malthus TR: On population. Himmelfarb G (ed). New York: Random House, 1960
38. Notestein FW: Population—the long view. In Schultz TW (ed): Food for the World. Chicago: University of Chicago Press, 1945
39. Hauser PM, Duncan OD: Demography as a body of knowledge. In Hauser PM, Duncan OD (eds): The Study of Population: An Inventory and an Appraisal. Chicago: University of Chicago Press, 1959
40. Notestein FW, Kirk D, Segal S: The problem of population control. In Hauser PM (ed): The Population Dilemma. Englewood Cliffs, NJ: Prentice-Hall, 1963
41. Coale A: The Demographic Transition. Proceedings of the International Population Conference, vol I. Liege, Belgium: International Union for the Scientific Study of Population, 1973
42. Caldwell J: Toward a restatement of demographic transition theory. Popul Dev Rev 2(3–4):321–366
43. Wetrogan SI: Projections of the Population of States, by Age, Sex, and Race: 1988 to 2010. Current Population Reports, Series P-25; No. 1017. Washington, DC: US Bureau of the Census, 1988
44. Coale AJ, Hoover E: Population growth and economic development in low-income countries. Princeton, NJ: Princeton University Press, 1958
45. Coale AJ: Population trends and economic development. In Menken J (ed): World Population and U.S. Policy—The Choices Ahead. New York: WW Norton, 1986, 96–104
46. Meadows DH, Meadows DL, Randers J, Behrens WW: The Limits to Growth. New York: Potomac Associates, 1972
47. Ehrlich PR, et al: Global change and carrying capacity implications for life on earth. In DeFries RS, Malone TF (eds): Global Change and Our Common Future. Washington, DC: National Academy Press, 1989
48. Baldi PA, Spivey-Weber F, Snyder K, et al: A Message to Congress on Sustainable Developments in United States Foreign Assistance. Washington, DC: National Audubon Society, 1989
49. Maize KP: Blueprint for the Environment; Advice to the President-Elect from America's Environmental Community. Washington, DC: Blueprint for the Environment, 1988
50. Bender W, Smith M: Population, Food, and Nutrition. Washington, DC: Population Reference Bureau, Popul Bull 51(4):1–48, 1997
51. Henshaw SK, Kenney AM, Somberg D, Van Vort J: Teenage Pregnancy in the United States: The Scope of the Problem and State Responses. New York: The Alan Guttmacher Institute, 1989
52. Centers for Disease Control and Prevention: Abortion surveillance: preliminary data—United States, 1994. MMWR 45(51–52):1123–1127, 1997
53. Ventura SJ et al: Trends in pregnancies and pregnancy rates: estimates for the United States, 1980–1992. Monthly Vital Statistics Report 43(11(S)):1–10, May 25, 1995
54. Centers for Disease Control: Maternal mortality surveillance, United States, 1980–1985. In: CDC Surveillance Summaries. MMWR 37: 19–29, 1988
55. World Bank: World Bank Development Report, 1984. International Bank for Reconstruction and Development. New York: Oxford University Press, 1984
56. Spencer G: Projections of the population of the United States, by age, sex, and race: 1988 to 2080. Current Population Reports, Series P-25, No 1018. Washington, DC: US Bureau of the Census, US Government Printing Office, 1989
57. Gardner P, Hudson BL: Advance Report of Final Mortality Statistics, 1993. Monthly Vital Statistics Report 44(7(S)):1–73, February 29, 1996
58. Kovar MG, LaCroix AZ: Aging in the eighties, ability to perform work-related activities. Data from the supplement on aging to the national health interview survey, United States, 1984. Advance Data from Vital and Health Statistics. No. 136. DHHS Publication No. (PHS) 87-1250. Hyattsville, MD: Public Health Service, 1987

5

Public Health Informatics

Andrew Friede • Patrick W. O'Carroll

Public health informatics (PHI) is the application of information science and technology to public health practice and research.[1] Its practice involves developing computerized information systems that support the mission of disease prevention and health promotion. Practical PHI work, ideally guided by professionals who are trained and experienced in both information technology and public health, involves bringing together specialists in both fields to conceptualize new ways of applying information technology to solve public health problems. The practice of public health informatics goes beyond applying known computer science. Rather, it involves synthesizing knowledge from public health and information science, as well as from many components of business, including business case analysis, project management, marketing, training, and customer relations. If done well, it should lead to new ways of thinking about and practicing public health.

This chapter is not a catalog of PHI systems, as it would be outdated at publication; however, a listing of such CDC systems has been created[2] and there is a relatively recent bibliography for the field.[3] Many systems are described in a review.[1] Rather, we provide an overview of public health informatics and place it in the larger context of medical informatics. We then work through an example of a real public health problem and show how PHI techniques can help. Finally, we discuss some of the practical—and timeless—conundrums involved in buying and building information systems.

▶ WHY PUBLIC HEALTH INFORMATICS?

Until recently, the world of health was often artificially divided into public health (the health of populations, especially poorer ones) and private health (the health of the individual, often called simply "medicine" or "medical care"). University training programs, faculty appointments, and careers followed one track or another, and subspecialties were similarly compartmentalized. This trend was further accentuated when the diseases of poverty (e.g., tuberculosis) became more concentrated in one class. Recent changes in the ecology of disease and organization of health care have prompted a change in this thinking. First, HIV/AIDS forced many to realize that the better-off population would no longer be spared from epidemic infectious diseases. Second, the major controllable causes of morbidity and mortality have come to be understood to be some of the traditional interests of public health, namely, smoking, alcohol and drug abuse, injuries, and a poor diet (including overeating).[4] Finally, the advent of managed care and capitation made payers cognizant of the *populations* they were contracting to protect. The equation of medicine has changed: formerly, medical services providers made more money when their clients were sick and needed services; now they make more money when they are well. Suddenly, prevention is attractive, as it is usually cheaper than treatment, and public health is now in the mainstream of medicine. The combination of the burgeoning interest in the health of populations (created, ironically, by managed care) and the advent of the information age represents an opportunity to bring public health thinking into the daily practice of medicine.

This integration of medicine and public health has multiple implications for the integration of medical informatics and PHI. Medical informatics has traditionally focused on hospital, ambulatory, and home-care clinical records; linkage of laboratory, pharmacy, and radiology data to clinical data; computerized diagnostic and therapeutic systems (including alerts); biomedical engineering; patient and student education; and automation of the medical library.[5] There has usually been a strong focus on accessing data about *individuals* and their treatment.

Public health informatics is focused on systems devoted to data and information that describes *populations* and on dissemination of knowledge to support public health practice. Examples include: surveillance systems and disease registries, which might help a county health officer estimate the number of doses of measles vaccine needed for an outbreak; data integration systems that might facilitate a regional planning commission's efforts to integrate census, surveillance, and hospitalization data to project the occupancy of AIDS hospice beds for a city and prepare related funding requests for the state legislature; program assistance data that an epidemiologist might use to study malnutrition among homeless children and the impact of nutrition programs in different regions; and distance learning programs that train public health staff in infection control or factory inspections.

These are not the kinds of systems that have been hitherto developed by the medical informatics community, although that is already changing, and will change more rapidly, for reasons discussed below. For example, Columbia University and the New York City Department of Health have collaborated on the development of a tuberculosis (TB) registry for northern Manhattan; and Emory University and the Georgia Department of Public Health have built a similar system for TB monitoring and treatment in Atlanta. It is not by chance that these two cities have each developed TB systems; rather, TB is a perfect example of a what was once a "public health" problem (i.e., one that affects the poor and underserved) coming into the mainstream population, as a result of an emerging infectious disease (HIV infection/AIDS), immigration, increased travel, multidrug resistance, and our exploding prison population. Hence, the changing ecology of disease and revolutionary changes in how health care is managed and paid for are combining to cause the line between public health and more traditional "medicine" to be blurred; this will have a parallel effect on the distinction between public health and medical informatics. These fields will come to be more correctly seen to lie along a continuum.

However, it is still true that, because computer systems developed for traditional medical informatics applications or business often lack features required for public health, PHI specialists have often had to develop their systems de novo. For example, standard statistical packages cannot easily be used to perform standardization, fit mathematical models to disease patterns, or calculate sample sizes for case-control studies; commonly available data-entry programs cannot handle the very long or complex questionnaires common in public health; general-purpose graphing programs make bar and pie charts but not histograms or county maps. Epi Info, developed for public health; can carry out most of these functions.[6] There is still no mapping system that contains the boundaries of public health jurisdictions in the United States. (CDC is working on a plan to develop one.)

Furthermore, public health data files often contain many millions of records, and quickly accessing these large files requires special database designs.[7] Finally, there is an increasing need to search the full contents of massive text databases such as publications, reports and recommendations, tables of summary data, information about the Healthy People 2000 Objectives, etc. Typically, these documents do not provide keywords, and their diversity, dynamic nature, and the unavailability of appropriate keywords in the Medical Subject Headings (MeSH) system would preclude doing so. One of the challenges for public health informatics is to develop streamlined ways to access complex textual data.[1]

CDC and other government health agencies increasingly consider information processing and dissemination to be central to their mission. In recognition of this, in 1992 the CDC initiated the Information Network for Public Health Officials (INPHO), which is a 14-state consortium of state-based public health information systems.[8] INPHO started with the building of a statewide information network in Georgia, funded by a $5 million grant from the Woodruff Foundation, which until that time had focused largely on funding "medical" research. The participants in this model public-private partnership included Emory University School of Public Health, the Georgia Center for Advanced Telecommunications Technology, the Georgia Institute of Technology, the Georgia Department of Health, the Medical College of Georgia, and CDC.[9] To date, 12 states have received specific CDC and/or foundation funding for this work, and two others have used other monies.

The principal thrust of INPHO is to help state and local health departments to better perform their public health functions via improved use of modern information technology. Primarily, states have used the monies to improve their fundamental computer infrastructure by integrating existing stand-alone systems, which can be hard or impossible to do with categorical (disease-specific) funding that typically specifies that computer X can be used only for disease Y. Increasingly, state health departments need to spend categorical monies on integrated information systems; these systems frequently serve disease prevention programs that cut across traditional departmental organizational lines. In recognition of this fact, CDC is working with state and local grantees to develop a business-model-based mechanism for states to spend a proportion of those formerly categorical monies on integrated information systems.

Other projects have included building basic infrastructure that supports many health department functions (e.g., a Web site; departmental e-mail); providing Internet access to health departments at all levels; forging closer ties among different departments and agencies within government and among government and private providers (especially for immunization registries); training local health agency staff in information technology; and developing patient information systems for public health clinics. A great deal of day-to-day PHI activities focus on developing these clinical systems, and several states have multimillion dollar, multiyear projects under way. In the era of managed care, when more and more government agencies are moving away from the direct provision of services, we very much question the wisdom of this activity. Even if these systems are needed, the advisability of developing systems in-house is uncertain, because they tend to go beyond the abilities of most agencies, and support issues loom large. A number of these systems have failed. On the other hand, many state and local health departments have elected to purchase commercial systems, again, often at high initial costs. These costs are often later further increased by the inevitable need to integrate them into existing systems or to modify them to fit local needs (see "Buy or Build?" below).

In summary, the proper application of public health informatics will let public health practitioners carry out the study and protection of populations more effectively and efficiently. In particular, it can enhance the investigation of outbreaks; improve the timeliness and efficiency of all data collection and analysis; promote rapid dissemination of new information within the public health community and to the public; and help provide services, such as clinic appointments for childhood immunizations. Moreover, as clinicians incorporate epidemiology and public health principles into clinical medicine and come to see the patient as part of a community, public health informatics will make important contributions to the work of practicing physicians.[10] We will now illustrate some of these principles in practice.

► PUBLIC HEALTH INFORMATICS IN ACTION

As an applied science, public health informatics can be illustrated through a practice-based example. This section illustrates the utility of some of the more important extant public health information systems.

The Case. You are a local health officer in a semirural county, managing a health department staff of 50 people. Being a progressive health officer, you have ensured that personal computers in your health department are connected to each other via a local area network (LAN) and that your LAN is connected to the Internet. You and your staff have been trained in the use of the World Wide Web (WWW) and have accounts providing access to the National Library of Medicine's MEDLINE bibliographic system.

You are notified on a Tuesday morning that an elementary school in your district has more than two dozen children who have been complaining of headaches, upper respiratory symptoms, and nonspecific malaise. No common etiology has been identified by the various physicians who have seen the children, and different children are receiving different kinds of medical treatment. Worried parents have been calling the school principal, who now is requesting that the health department investigate. She has heard of "sick building syndrome" and wonders if that is the problem. The PTA is to meet on Friday and expects the health department to present its findings, or at least its investigative plans, at that time. The principal informs you that some of the parents have demanded that the school be closed until the investigation is completed.

At this early stage of an investigation, the value of modern information systems technology is to update you quickly on the general topic and related issues. For example, a search of MEDLINE for articles related to "sick building syndrome" yields dozens of references, a number of which describe epidemics similar to yours. A search of the World Wide Web (using any of a number of free on-line search tools) will likely yield some usefully summarized information, but some of this will be of questionable authority and not necessarily relevant to the particular issue that you are facing. However, you would find authoritative information on indoor air pollution and sick building syndrome at CDC (www.cdc.gov) and EPA (www.epa.gov). At this early stage, the most important technology tool at your disposal may be e-mail, which you can use to poll your public health colleagues, both locally and at national and international agencies, regarding their experiences with similar challenges.

The Case, continued. Your environmental health scientist does an on-site investigation and determines that all of the classrooms in which children became ill were substantially water-damaged, with a black moldy substance staining the damaged walls. Samples of this mold are sent for testing to the state laboratory. You are notified via e-mail the next afternoon (Wednesday) that the mold has been identified as *Stachybotrys atra*, an organism with which you are not familiar.

The public health laboratory in your state uses the CDC's Public Health Laboratory Information System[11] to help manage data internally and report it to other state agencies (in this case, you) and to CDC. It is based on Epi Info, a database program, which was also developed by the CDC.[6] Most state laboratories now have some kind of computerized information system, which helps promote communications between the laboratories and department of epidemiology.

Unfamiliar with *S. atra*, you turn once again to MEDLINE. This time your search yields more than a dozen articles on *S. atra*, including a few that review the growing evidence that exposure to its spores is associated with pediatric upper respiratory symptoms, nonspecific neuromyalgias, and even hemosiderosis.[12] With the rapid pace of scientific advance, textbooks can no longer meet all the information needs of public health practice. As of early 1997, there is very little information in textbooks about this newly recognized pathogen, and most of the MEDLINE citations are from 1996. You use CDC WONDER on the Internet at http://www.wonder.gov[13] to look up *S. atra* and find on-line the full text of a *Morbidity and Mortality Weekly Report* article from January 1997 that has quite a bit of recent information.[12] You copy the article to your computer and keep it in electronic form for later use (see below).

You are tempted to close the school at this stage, but unsure if the science to date warrants it. To seek expert guidance on this question, you turn once again to e-mail. However, instead of spending hours trying to identify national experts on this pathogen, you send a message to ProMed, an Internet-based, automated mailing list.[14] Subscribers to the mailing list receive all postings by other subscribers through their regular e-mail software. ProMed, internationally used, focuses on, and fosters on-line discussions of, emerging infectious diseases. Through this single e-mail message, you are able to rapidly communicate with thousands of potential "consultants," experts whom you have never met but who have identified themselves as interested in this issue by virtue of subscribing to ProMed. Such instantaneous consultation was impossible prior to the widespread use of e-mail and the international connections among scientists via the Internet.

The Case, continued. Based on consultations with scientists in your state health department, at CDC and EPA, and via ProMed, you determine that it is necessary to close the school until the problem is abated. This causes great consternation, not only to the parents of children in the affected school, but to other parents as well. Your office is inundated with requests for more information.

When faced with the need to distribute rapidly changing information and updates to a broad and undefined audience, traditional methods (e.g., paper publishing, telephone conversations, etc.) are inefficient. The WWW, however, is a powerful tool for such information dissemination. In this case, for example, you could add a new electronic "page" to your health department WWW site entitled, "Latest Information on the Mold Infestation and School Closing." You could add the full electronic text of the *MMWR* article that you saved, which you could use to formulate the background to a press release that you distribute via e-mail to your entire staff for continuing education. You could distribute the on-line address of this page to your local media, parents, and school officials and update it as often as necessary. There would be essentially no marginal cost for such an effort, apart from the time it takes to compose and update the briefing material and the clerical costs of adding it your Web site.

This leads to the question of whether those who need and want this information will have access to the WWW themselves. Many, of course, will not. Nevertheless, representatives of print and broadcast media outlets in your county probably will, and they can distribute the news through traditional channels, being sure of the timeliness of their information, freeing you from interviews, and allowing you to move onto prevention activities, such as disease monitoring.

The Case, conclusion. To assess whether this problem is confined to this one school, you consider setting up a public health surveillance system for *S. atra*.

Surveillance systems need not be electronic to be effective, in fact, one of the most innovative immunization registries in the United States is in Oregon, which uses paper labels and bar codes on postcards to quickly capture and transmit information. Electronic systems usually provide a much faster and usually a much more secure way of exchanging information than does the mail. On the other hand, a crisis is not the best time to set up such a system, although it can be done.[15]

As discussed elsewhere in this textbook, the key to surveillance is to determine the easiest source for acquiring the highest quality information. In our particular case study, as in many real cases, laboratories would seem a likely source for the kind of high quality and reasonably centralized information that will meet your surveillance needs, especially when the laboratories are electronically connected. In our scenario, if we assume that your information dissemination efforts have produced a local public that is sensitized to the health threat posed by this mold and informed about the need to do environmental testing of water-damaged buildings, then daily calls by health department staff to the few state laboratories that might test for *S. atra* would probably be an adequate interim surveillance system.

However, this case study does illustrate the need to establish a better surveillance infrastructure for responding to future outbreaks. For routine work, the CDC does have electronic reporting of about 60 notifiable diseases via its National Electronic Telecommunications System for Surveillance;[16] the French have been doing this for more than 10 years,[17] in part because of the widespread penetration of the Minitel system. As the United States as a whole enters the information age, it will become easier to conduct electronic surveillance from a wide variety of public and private information providers, including private laboratories, hospitals and long-term care facilities, physicians offices, the workplace, schools, and ultimately, the home.

▸ BUYING, DESIGNING, AND BUILDING INFORMATION SYSTEMS

This section provides guidance to the public health professional who is participating in the development of an information system, either as an end-user, a nontechnical analyst, or someone who is charged with procuring a ready-made system, modifying one, or arranging for the design of one from scratch. The most important point to be borne in mind is that the days of the stand-alone public health information system are over. As the lines between medicine and public health blur, and as managed care organizations increasingly offer prevention and treatment services to traditional public health clients, the ability of all these kinds of systems to share information will be the sine qua non of their viability. Whether it is sharing data on clients, transmitting surveillance data, providing recommendations, or tracking outbreaks, public health information systems will be only as valuable as their ability to interact with the myriad providers and agencies who will be moving into and out of the health care arena.

Buy or Build?

Despite all protestations to the contrary, the decision to buy, modify, or build will often be made with little information, as requirements are hard to specify in advance of testing and implementation. Hence, system flexibility must be the cornerstone of any decision. While it might seem obvious to say so, it cannot be too strongly stated that the true features of any system to be acquired or modified must be evaluated firsthand, by both the information technology staff and the public health professional end-users. Repeatedly decisions are made by reading specifications and talking to vendors; there is no substitute for physically trying the system and talking to current clients (outside the hearing of the vendor).

Outside consultants can best be used to help the public health agency be clearer about its own needs and to provide insights into the general reputation and long-term capacities of vendors. Although they are often engaged for what they know, good ones enhance the decision process by facilitating communications about subjects everyone knows about already, but about which everyone is reluctant to speak. Because new information systems often threaten to disrupt current work practices, discussing them may surface long-buried political and personnel issues. Thus, an important part of the consultant's skill set is the ability to enhance communications within your agency and between your agency and potential vendors; hence, it is vital to select someone whom you can trust and with whom you can be very frank. The ideal consultant will be knowledgeable about public health (and preferably how your agency practices public health). Consultants may charge handsomely; again, the best way to select one is to talk with their other clients; good consultants can be well worth it.

There is a strong inclination to buy an existing system and then modify it, in the hope that you can get the best of both worlds. In practice, the opposite is often true: you get the worst of both worlds—the rigidity of a fixed system and all the expense and delays associated with development. We have seen this happen repeatedly. However, the latest systems are designed to be more modifiable than were those from the previous generation, but this must be carefully verified by your own hands-on testing and by confirming the experience of other clients. Systems should never be purchased on a promise of future modifiability or features (unless there is an escape clause in the contract); even the most earnest developers may run into delays caused by factors beyond their control.

There tends to be a strong bias among computer specialists toward developing their own systems. Although one may be tempted to think that this stems from selfish interest, it is often based on their own disappointing experience in buying systems, for themselves or for the agency, that failed to meet expectations. On the other hand, for all but the very smallest projects, development costs and time lines are almost universally underestimated by factors of 3–10. This stems from a variety of factors discussed below; but whatever the causes and remedies, we urge extreme caution in taking on the development of new systems, especially if there is not an expert development group with a strong track record available (directly or on contract).

Developing New Systems

During the past 20 years, there have been numerous studies of the quality and efficiency of the design processes for building information systems, and the results are stunningly disappointing. The majority of major projects are either grossly over budget, years behind schedule, or fail utterly[18, 19]; the bigger the project, the greater likelihood of problems. One often reads of the failures of military systems; as they tend to be huge and so attract attention, but there have been similar fiascoes in business, science, and in medicine. Many a hospital and public health information system has been installed, never to be used. In 1996, the Federal Aeronautics Administration announced its canceling of the revision of the national air traffic control system, which is currently based on computers that use vacuum tubes. The redesign failed completely, and they are starting from scratch: $2 billion in development costs are being written off. Similarly, in 1997 the Internal Revenue Service made an announcement of its plans to revise the IRS's computer system, writing off $4 billion in development costs. Why does this happen, and how can it be prevented? Imagine that you are an architect and contractor, hired to design and build a house. The clients are strangers to you and do not know what their family needs. They are unsure of their budget and are vague with you because this is their first house and they are afraid of overpaying. The couple has two children, but may have more children. The wife is considering asking her aged parents to move in, and the husband may want to work from home so he may want a home office. You are afraid to push them too hard to be more specific because you do not want to risk losing their business. They want the house as soon as possible. Now imagine that this is your first commission.

That is the state of most information systems projects: unclear and evolving requirements (user needs), vague budgets, inexperienced personnel, and unclear deadlines. Moreover, consider that information technology is changing every day. What if new and much better building materials were being introduced half-way through typical housing construction projects, and clients insisted on having them? Or, suppose that you know that, if you don't use the latest materials, your work will look shoddy in 2 years. These are some of the conditions that contribute to the failure of so many computer system designs.

What has been learned about improving this process? There have been a series of schools of thought on this subject. The earliest systems were built with relatively little input from users; they were engineer-driven, and users were expected to adapt or be trained. After many systems were rejected by clients and users, designers began to slowly include users. The earliest attempts to include users involved them somewhat peripherally, passively, and often too late in the process to allow for major design modifications. Users were asked to react to prototypes, and their feedback was usually sought on functional and cosmetic issues rather than on workflow issues. In later evolutions of "involving users in design," users were asked to define their needs, the assumption being that they knew their needs and could express them in ways engineers could understand and translate into systems. Systems developed under this scenario also often failed. Users blamed the engineers. ("That's not what we asked for, you did not listen.") Engineers blamed the users. ("They never know what they want; they can't even describe their jobs.")

The next school of design involved having users and engineers sit together to design projects cooperatively. IBM even trademarked the name Joint Application Design and trained thousands in its techniques. Diligent efforts were made on all sides to really understand the work to be automated and to build practical systems. However, the key underlying assumptions were unchanged: large-scale systems could be successfully designed if the system could be accurately specified in advance. Again, many failures resulted.

What has been going wrong? First, technology is changing faster than anyone can design and deliver large systems. For example, many systems designed in the early 1990s contained built-in communications systems that were not compatible with the Internet; these systems may soon be obsolete. Second, just as in our house example, the users' needs were changing as the computer system was being written, so it was often irrelevant at delivery. This is being driven by the rapidly changing nature of work in America. Computer systems were often being designed for the regimented, hierarchical, predictable workflow of the first assembly plants. But the needs of, for instance, a public health clinic are subject to massive fluxes from external sources: changing patterns of disease caused by newly emerging infectious agents, new environmental toxins, and drug resistance; new populations such as immigrants, the elderly, long-term survivors of chronic diseases; and changes in our social fabric, such as the advent of managed care, capitated Medicaid and Medicare populations, and increasing poverty among our nation's children. Big, rigid information systems are doomed in this environment, no matter how cleverly they are designed, and no matter how completely the requirements were specified *last year*.

What are the characteristics of successfully developed information systems? First, they are flexible with respect to (*a*) data content and data relations and (*b*) underlying technology. Second, they are created by development groups and have specific characteristics.

Flexibility in Data Content and Data Relations

At first, it may seem that all computer systems have built-in flexibility in data content and flow. The content may seem flexible, as most of them have "fill-in-the-blank" fields, so it appears that almost any content is allowed. The relationship between data elements (for instance, the number and sequence of tasks to be performed) seems to be similarly flexible (that is, the tasks can be reordered by the user). In truth, most systems have a huge amount of built-in rigidity, which is often hidden from users and is based on assumptions in the minds of the designers.

A simple example will suffice to illustrate hidden rigidity in content and relations. Imagine designing a surveillance system to measure the long-term effects in children of exposure to *Stachybotrys atra*, as a follow-up to the outbreak described above. You wish to describe the child's family in the database. A traditional place to start would be to specify fields for "Father: First Name," "Father: Last Name," and "Mother: First Name," "Mother: Last Name." What if the biological father dies, the mother remarries, and her new husband adopts the child? Suddenly, you are short four fields (Biological Father: First Name, Last Name and Adoptive Father: First Name, Last Name), and there are two superfluous fields. What if the mother's new husband has chosen not to adopt the child, but they all live together: what do you call him? Perhaps the him is a her, namely, that the mother has taken a female partner. How will your database handle the child who lives in foster care, with grandparents, in an orphanage, or is in a shared custody situation, i.e., some mixture of the above, depending on the day of the week or time of year?

In fact, content and relations, often described as distinct, are not easy to keep in their own boxes, as the above example illustrates. As the content changes, so might the relationship. The other element of design scenarios—namely, processes—are also not so tidily separable, as mutable data content and relations may dictate a different kind of process. To continue our example, if our process is "call home in a month to see if child is still well," but the child lives in several homes or is homeless, the process has certainly been derailed by the data.

How does the sophisticated systems analyst deal with such a complex world? In fact, medical systems tend to be far more complex than many systems that have been traditionally considered to be very complex, such as airline reservations systems, in part because biological and social systems tend to be far more complex than human-made ones. In practice, engineers are often tempted to simplify medical and public health systems as a way of dealing with this kind of messy complexity. For example, one might be tempted to abandon the notion of family in the system, but then valuable information could be lost to someone who is studying, for instance, the problems that a group of related children might have with a common exposure. A better approach would be to design a program called "lives with child X under Y relationship" and execute it every time you look-up X. That way you can enter all the relations you want for child X and have their nature change over time. Hence, you are building a complex *function* that deals with relatively simple data, rather than trying to specify every eventuality into the data. Also, note that over time you can modify this function (for instance, by adding another dimension to it, for example, "for time Z") rather than modifying the entire database.

Another way to deal with complexity is to design and build systems in *small* increments and iteratively: design, build, demonstrate, revise, start the cycle over. There is an almost irresistible temptation to design too much at first, especially because many schools still teach the "systems analysis" approach to information systems design. If you are building a house or a rocket, you may very well want to design the whole thing before you cut a single piece of lumber or titanium—not so in computer systems. There are no material costs in information systems design, so it's easy to throw things away, especially at first; once the first steps are completed, it becomes exponentially harder to make changes; hence, it is critical that the foundation be done correctly. Do not be afraid to start over many times, again, especially at first. If the system is hard to explain to users or extensive training is required, it may very well be at variance with their usual work style, and they are unlikely to adopt it. Getting into the "mental model" of the end-user is the key to successful design.

This principle of flexibility and extensibility also means granting the end-user (or his or her local expert) the right—and responsibility—to make changes to the system. No designer of a medical or public health system, no matter how clever, can be expected to anticipate all conditions, their causes, and all the reports that health practitioners and researchers will need. Again, this is especially important in our era of new exposures and new diseases. For example, if a public health laboratory wishes to report the presence of a new species, it should have the ability to add the name to the system rather than depend on a central office to send new software. Although this may seem to tend toward entropy, the alternative is worse: the new species is reported by telephone (or not at all), and the information is harder to retrieve. The alternative is to allow the local laboratory to add the species, but make clear its provenance ("species S from lab L") and have it officially added to the larger system at a later time.

Importantly, this kind of design is not well-handled with the relatively simple database systems that are designed for tracking inventory, which is the typical example used in many database textbooks, nor can they be managed by short programs; medical and public health systems are notoriously complex. The complexity of computer programs is often described in the number of lines of code they contain. Although this is a crude metric, as the number of lines of code to perform a given function varies greatly from language to language, it serves as a starting point. Systems for small businesses tend to have approximately 10^3 lines of code; systems for larger businesses, 10^4. Complex engineering systems, such as the launch sequence for the space shuttle, may have 10^5 lines; complete medical records systems currently under development have 10^6 lines of code. Anyone charged with developing public health information systems must be educated about this complexity.

Flexibility in Underlying Technology

What kinds of computer technology can be used to foster the kind of flexibility described above? The principles here apply equally well to systems to be bought, modified, or built from scratch. Many vendors of information technology (ranging from development tools to off-the-shelf systems) offer "integrated" solutions, with a tight binding of the database, interface, and communications architecture. While this may be appealing in a stand-alone environment, public health systems rarely operate in isolation; rather, they often need to exchange data with private providers, state laboratories, and state and national surveillance systems. Hence, any integrated solution needs to have entry points ("hooks") to allow data exchange with other systems and the components need to be locally modifiable.

Another reason to be wary of tightly integrated solutions is that one can become the captive of a vendor. For example, you may need to change only one part of the system; the vendor may be able to make the change only if you change the whole system. Finally, tightly integrated solutions are often by their nature relatively difficult to modify. For example, a system that has the communications architecture integrated into the database system may be inaccessible via the Internet, which uses a particular communications protocol (language). A better approach is to have stand-alone modules that communicate with each other in a simple, nonproprietary language.[20] Another advantage of the modular approach is that it may allow you to be more consonant with other standards in your organization. For example, if the design allows you to use database system B as easily as A, and everyone in your agency is also using B, then using B may facilitate acquiring technical support, knowledgeable programmers, and discounted pricing.

On the other hand, hooking together systems from different vendors can also be a nightmare of complexity, especially if the components were not designed to be woven into other systems, but are cleaved from other integrated systems. This is the potential fallacy of the "best of breed" approach, i.e., using, for example, Company A's laboratory system and Company B's patient registration system. Again, there is no substitute for talking to agencies that have tried to use a given system as part of a larger whole. Moreover, even if systems from different firms can be technically integrated, there are important issues of obtaining support from different firms, training on multiple systems, and the inevitable finger-pointing when things go wrong.

Finally, let us add a word about computer languages. There are dozens of languages, many specialized for specific hardware or databases, but we do not discuss their selection here. What is important for the public health professional to understand is that it has been traditionally taught that there is a direct relationship between the difficulty of writing programs in a given language and the flexibility and power and speed of the resultant program. While this relationship is still generally valid, the newest development environments enable programmers to craft excellent and flexible programs with much less effort than is required in the older languages. Many programmers insist on using older languages, as that is what they know. Management must carefully evaluate if an elephant gun is being used to kill a flea.

The Successful Development Group

Although most public health professionals will probably not be charged with developing information systems, it is more than likely that during your career you will participate in designing one, at least as an end-user. This section is designed to acquaint you with some of the characteristics of the successful development group and help you identify roadblocks. It is based on the authors' experiences in developing CDC WONDER[7,13,21] and insights gleaned from the classic text in this field, *The Mythical Man-Month: Essays on Software Engineering*.[18] Although written in 1975, this book is still fresh, insightful, and a pleasure to read as a text on general management.

The most important point to be made about developing information systems is that there must be one person who has a vision of the final product and can articulate that vision. By vision, we mean literally "something that can be seen," not merely a vague set of desires. From this flows the requirement that there be a chief architect, someone who oversees the whole project, because the image of the final result lies clearly in his or her mind. This person need not necessarily be involved in the day-to-day details, rather, the architect should have a bird's-eye view.

The selection of staff is one of the most important decisions the manager will make. As in so many areas of intellectual endeavor, a few gifted individuals make almost all the important contributions. The stereotype of antisocial "nerd" sitting alone in a cubicle is outdated; today, programmer/analysts must be able to communicate smoothly with subject-matter experts and each other and must be open to new ideas and new technologies. We have found that training in computer science per se is not as predictive of performance as native intellectual talents and a mature personality. Brooks[18] notes that the productivity of computer programmers often varies by orders of magnitude, i.e., the best will be 10 or 100 times more productive than their average colleagues; and we have found this to be absolutely true. Often that productivity comes not from the most clever program, but from making the most intelligent use of productivity-enhancing tools (including reusing existing code) and from understanding the mental model of users. Hence, the trick is to identify a few good people, not a multitude.

Developing information systems is mentally demanding, as many factors must be kept in mind at once. Hence, it is best done by smart people who are working in a quiet, supportive atmosphere, free from distractions (especially unnecessary meetings), supplied with the best workstations you can possibly afford. This is in marked contrast to the environment that is frequently found: noisy cubicles, frequent unscheduled meetings, and the "boss" having the latest equipment, which is used for word processing, if at all.

Another reason to keep the development group small is to facilitate intragroup communications. The title of *The Mythical Man-Month* stems from that author's experience of having production *slowed* by adding new programmers ("man-months"), and conversely, having it speeded up by shrinking the staff. Convincing management to pay a few people more is an ongoing challenge, especially in the public sector.

The leadership (and ideally the staff, too) of a development group should contain both information technology professionals and subject-matter experts. Involving users peripherally is the usual poor substitute; having a user centrally involved changes the whole nature of the process. Three of CDC's largest computer systems, namely, Epi Info,[6] CDC WONDER,[13] and the AIDS Reporting System were led by a medical epidemiologist or health statistician, with excellent results. In fact, both NIH's and CDC's information technology offices have been successfully led by physicians with a thoroughgoing understanding of their agencies' missions, and increasingly, the chief information officers of health care agencies are health professionals. Public health agency information technology offices are more frequently employing public health professionals in key management positions. The Kansas Health Foundation and the Foundation for the Centers for Disease Control and Prevention have developed a fellowship in public health informatics designed to train future leaders in this field; similar programs are sorely needed to help fill the shortage of public health professionals trained in informatics.

The actual management should be entrusted to whomever is most adept, but, at the risk of stereotyping, the best information technology professionals are rarely good managers, as they tend to be more cerebral than practical. More importantly, they ought to be left alone to do their work. Many development groups are dominated by former programmers who have risen through the ranks and are often untrained for, and have little interest in, strategic planning, business decisions, personnel issues, corporate politics, etc. The frequent turnover of staff, so rampant in development groups, and which contributes greatly to lost productivity, is often attributable to poor management.

Finally, it may be appropriate to conclude with a word about why it is so hard to bring projects to closure. First, a system can always be enhanced, but "creeping embellishments" must be put off until the next version. Second, no project will be using the latest technology at completion, as it was—by definition—unavailable when the work began. This must be accepted by users, management, and staff. Finally, computer programmers may love their work so much and be so deeply invested in their projects that they simply do not want them to end. Management must often step in and bring things to completion.

▶ REFERENCES

1. Friede A, McDonald MC, Blum H: Public health informatics: how information-age technology can strengthen public health. Annu Rev Public Health 16:239–252, 1995
2. Friede A, O'Carroll PW: CDC/ATSDR information resources for public health officials. J Public Health Manage Pract 2:10–24, 1996
3. Selden C, Humphreys B, Friede A, Geisslerova Z: Public Health Informatics, January 1980 through December 1995: 471 selected citations. Bethesda, MD: National Institutes of Health, National Library of Medicine, 1–21, 1996
4. McGinnis JM, Foege WH: Actual causes of death in the United States. JAMA 270(18):2207–2212, 1993
5. Greenes RA, Shortliffe EH: Medical informatics, an emerging academic discipline and institutional priority. JAMA 263:1114–1120, 1990
6. Dean AG, Dean JA, Burton AH, Dicker RC: Epi Info: a general purpose microcomputer program for public health information systems. Am J Prev Med 7:178–182, 1991
7. Friede A, Reid JA, Ory HW: CDC WONDER: a comprehensive online public health information system of the Centers for Disease Control and Prevention. Am J Public Health 83:1289–1294, 1993
8. Baker EL, Friede A, Moulton AD, Ross DA: CDC's Information Network for Public Health Officials (INPHO): A framework for integrated public health information and practice. J Public Health Manage Pract 1:43–47, 1995
9. Chapman KA, Moulton AD: The Georgia Information Network for Public Health Officials (INPHO): a demonstration of a CDC INPHO concept. J Public Health Manage Pract 1:39–43, 1995
10. Greenlick MR: Educating physicians for population-based clinical practice. JAMA 267:1645–1648, 1992
11. Bean NH, Martin SM, Bradford H: PHLIS: an electronic system for reporting public health data from remote sites. Am J Public Health 82:1273–1276, 1992
12. CDC: Update: pulmonary hemorrhage/hemosiderosis among infants—Cleveland, Ohio, 1993–1996. MMWR 46:33–35, 1997
13. Friede A, O'Carroll PW, Thralls RB, Reid JA: CDC WONDER on the Web. Proceedings of the 1996 AMIA Annual Fall Symposium (formerly SCAMC) 408–412, 1996

14. Woodall J: Stalking the next epidemic: ProMED tracks emerging diseases. Public Health Rep 112:78–82, 1997
15. O'Carroll PW, Friede A, Noji EJ, Lillebridge SR, Atchison CG, Fries D: The rapid implementation of a statewide emergency health information system during the 1993 Iowa flood. Am J Public Health 85:564–567, 1995
16. CDC: National Electronic Telecommunications System for Surveillance—United States, 1990–1991. MMWR 40:502, 1991
17. Valleron A-J, Bouvet E, Garnerin P, et al: A computer network for the surveillance of communicable diseases: the French experiment. Am J Public Health 76:1289–1292, 1986
18. Brooks FP: The Mythical Man-Month: Essays on Software Engineering. Reading, MA: Addison-Wesley, 1975; reprinted with corrections, 1982
19. Gibbs WW: Software's chronic crisis. Sci Am 86–95, 1994
20. Friede A, O'Carroll PW, Nicola RM, Oberle MW, Teutch SM: The CDC Prevention Guidelines. Baltimore: Williams & Wilkins, 1997
21. Friede A, Rosen DR, Reid JA: CDC WONDER/PC: cooperative processing for public health informatics. J Am Med Informatics Assoc 1:303–312, 1994

II

Communicable Diseases

Edited by Richard P. Wenzel

6

Control of Communicable Diseases

Overview

Richard P. Wenzel

The most important function of public health in its broadest sense is to seek an optimal harmony between groups of people in society and their environment. This goal can be approached in three ways *(a)* by methods to improve host resistance of populations to environmental hazards; *(b)* by effective plans to improve the safety of the environment; and *(c)* by improving health care systems designed to increase the likelihood, efficiency, and effectiveness of the first two goals. With respect to infectious diseases there are special elements within each of the three categories (Table 6-1). One might then view communicable diseases as an imbalance in the relationship of people and their environment which favors microbial dominance in populations.

It is often argued that improved host resistance is the purview of clinical medicine and that both environmental safety and public health systems are public health efforts. However, improved resistance in populations cannot be divorced from necessary educational and effective health delivery systems. For that reason it may be considered an essential component of public health. In this schema of public health, the infectious agent is considered not as a separate focus but as one important component of the environment. This organization is designed to integrate the schema with a concept of health, and of public health in particular. The implication is that the organism is a necessary but not sufficient cause of ill health; it is only one of many risk factors. Moreover, humans constantly encounter myriads of potential microbial pathogens, and removing all such organisms is untenable. It seems more fruitful to develop effective barriers between humans and problematic environmental microbes or at the very least to create pathways for peaceful coexistence. In addition, to many authors it has seemed that public health has focused excessively on environmental controls and too little on the health care system. Yet all of these categories are interrelated; a change in any aspect of the three areas perturbs the entire system and has a direct effect on public health.

With respect to improved host resistance, McKeown[1] has argued that improved nutrition, personal hygiene, and public sanitation have more to do with the control of infectious diseases than vaccines and health care. There is no question, however, that vaccines and new antibiotics have greatly reduced morbidity and mortality from infectious diseases.[2] For example, with respect to smallpox, the vaccine—in concert with a public health system for identifying and isolating cases and contacts—was essential for its eradication.[3]

Recently it has been proposed that exercise may improve both mental and physical health[4,5] and that there may be important interactions between psychological factors and immunity.[6] Lastly, with the explosion of activities in the field of molecular biology and the prospect of cloning the human genome,[7] it is not far-fetched to think that, within a decade, genetic alteration of cells will enable us to enhance host resistance to adverse environmental challenges.[8]

The environment has long been a primary focus of public health, with efforts to improve the cleanliness of food and water, upgrade public sanitation, and clean the air of toxic pollutants. Efforts to remove infectious agents by reducing animal reservoirs and vectors or efforts to reduce their numbers have been another focus for public health in general and in veterinary medicine in particular. Recently many have postulated that adequate personal space is important for prevention of many urban problems. It has long been recognized that control of streptococcal infections in the military could be minimized by increasing space between the bunks of recruits and that crowding is a major risk factor.[9] In addition, since large droplets are known to be important for many viral respiratory agents,[10] it is generally accepted that spatial considerations are important for the prevention and control of communicable diseases.

A third method for public health control of infectious diseases involves the systems approach or management aspects. The social, economic, legal, and administrative forces important for health must operate in the interest of the public. Progress toward such goals must begin with access not only to health care but also to preventive health services and to health education. To do that, resources must be made available and important public health problems given sufficient priority—usually a political process—to demand necessary resources. Proper management at federal, state, and local levels needs to be operative for efficiency, effectiveness, and cost-effective delivery of care and education. Moreover, surveillance needs to be developed and maintained to detect new problems, new epidemics, and the efficacy of control measures.[11]

▸ MAJOR PROBLEMS

There is always risk in attempting to prioritize the most important infectious agents, and readers may construct a different list from that of the author (Table 6-2). Nevertheless, the agents listed are important and serve as a focus for discussion of public health issues. An example of how one might apply the proposed schema to a communicable disease is discussed below with the example of acquired immunodeficiency syndrome (AIDS).

There is no question that AIDS—caused by the human immunodeficiency viruses 1 and 2 (HIV-1 and HIV-2)—is the principal viral problem today. It is a global epidemic that affects the young in our society. Therapy is in its infancy, there is no cure in sight, and it involves the strongest of human emotions. Few drugs are available to assist in its control, and only one was known to prolong life;[12] the efficacy of educational programs, until recently, has not been proven, and many problems have been related to health care delivery. With respect to improving host resistance, prophylactic aerosolized pentamidine or oral trimethoprin-sulfametnoxazole have been shown to reduce the incidence of *Pneumocystis* infections, but no effective drugs directly affecting the immune system are available. Most patients attempt to maintain a high level of nutrition and personal hygiene, and some engage in exercise, support groups, and reading, which appear to provide a positive psychological outlook. New hope has emerged with the

TABLE 6-1. METHODS OF IMPROVED PUBLIC HEALTH CONTROL OF COMMUNICABLE DISEASES

- ***Improved Resistance to Environmental Hazards***

Hygiene
Nutrition
Immunity
Antibiotics
Psychological factors
Exercise
Genetic alteration

- ***Improved Environmental Safety***

Sanitation
Air
Water
Food
Infectious agents
Vectors
Animal reservoirs

- ***Public Health Systems***

Access
Efficiency
Resources
Priorities
Containment
Contact tracing for prophylaxis and therapy
Education
Social forces
Laws
Measurement of problems and of the efficiency and effectiveness of control

availability of treatment with protease inhibitors. In terms of availability, however, the White House backed away from a plan for Medicaid to cover the cost of AIDS drugs. (*NY Times*, December 6, 1997, PA 14)

With respect to improved environmental safety, the office of the surgeon general of the United States has recommended barrier protection, that is, safer sexual practices, and the Centers for Disease Control has recommended universal precautions for health care workers to minimize transmission in hospitals and clinics.[13] Since patients with HIV infection are at high risk for infections of all kinds, especially intracellular parasites, obviously it is prudent for them to avoid environments with high risk (e.g., exposure to tuberculosis, *Legionella*, or obviously infected people and animals). Nevertheless, specific guidelines are not yet available.

From a public health systems point of view, a great deal of discussion has occurred regarding access to medical care for AIDS victims and efficient testing of new drugs, and there has been unprecedented political pressure by activists for continued priority and use of national resources to prevent and control this infection. Similar pressures have been applied to create equitable and compassionate laws

TABLE 6-2. CHIEF INFECTIOUS DISEASES IN THE LATE 1990s

Infectious Disease Class	*Major Problem*	*Other Major Problems*
Virus	AIDS	Measles Hepatitis
Bacterium	Staphylococci	Streptococci Nosocomial infections Pathogens
Spirochete	Lyme disease	Syphilis
Parasite	Malaria	Onchocerciasis Leishmania

to protect the interests of high-risk groups and infected patients. One can apply the proposed paradigm to HIV infection (Table 6-1) and understand not only the illness but also the disease in populations as a function of the three components of public health control.

Other illnesses needing special attention in the next decade (Table 6-2) are discussed elsewhere in this text. One could easily expand the list and include other classes of agents such as fungi (which include *Pneumocystis*). Little work has been done internationally on the rickettsial infections despite continuing problems with several species, and much remains to be learned about Q fever, the newly recognized problem with *Ehrlichia* species,[14] and the pathogenesis of the so-called spongiform encephalopathies.[15] Within each infectious disease class one might easily include other agents that have recently caused public health problems.

▶ A NEW ROLE FOR PUBLIC HEALTH

With the spiraling costs of medical care and the corresponding interest in cost containment and accountability,[16] it is reasonable to avoid duplications. We need a closer link of clinical and public health disciplines and activities. In medical schools it is propitious for these disciplines to develop curricula and research projects collaboratively.

In the health service arena, closer ties between clinicians and public health officials will be efficient and effective for the good of the population. A special role for public health officials could be to "translate" important epidemiological data for clinicians giving primary care. This could be particularly important and useful in enhancing prevention. Examples of useful data would be the risk ratios for becoming an alcohol abuser for persons with and without a family history of abuse; cigarette smoking for the smoker, those nearby, and the unborn fetus; and for fatal versus nonfatal injury in persons driving with and without a seat belt. In the field of communicable diseases it is useful to know the risk of AIDS in those practicing intravenous drug abuse or unprotected sexual activities, the relative risk of Lyme disease in those using effective insect repellents versus those not using such agents, and the relative risk of hepatitis B in health care workers who have received the vaccine and those who have not. An epidemiological approach to communitywide education about local health risks, perhaps with a well-designed periodical, would further link the clinician and public health official. The Centers for Disease Control (CDC) has done this successfully with *Morbidity and Mortality Weekly Report*. A communitywide modification for consumption by local practitioners would be helpful. Such networking is feasible and desirable.

Networking with schools, businesses, health clubs, and senior citizen groups might increase compliance with behavior designed to enhance resistance to environmental hazards. Fundamentals of general and dental hygiene, nutrition, exercise, and stress control would be essential components. It would be reasonable to reinforce such basic principles as maintaining immunizations and proper use of antibiotics. In summary, we need a proactive and integrative role in education, one that involves networking with clinicians and the public directly.

Improving environmental safety has been the focus and strength of public health. Essentially, the goal has been to reduce the microbial hazards to humans. For the most part, this is carried out by systematic measurement or a series of inspections of the environment. Good general sanitation and safe air, water, and food are hallmarks of public health. Environmental activist groups have heightened interest in environmental safety. This is an opportune time to build a coalition between informed public health officials and interested and energetic activists genuinely concerned with improving the environment.

From an infectious diseases point of view, an important goal would be to reduce the degree of exposure while preserving the vitality of the ecosystem. The government of Brazil was reported to have instituted a $200 million program to control malaria in the Amazon region by spraying dichlorodiphenyltrichloroethane (DDT) in thousands of rain forest huts. As McCoy[17] pointed out, however, the chemical has been banned in over 40 countries because of its lethal effect on birds and fish. Moreover, in India, although it had a remarkable short-term effect initially (75 million annual cases of malaria reduced in the 1950s to 50,000), the number of cases rose to 65 million by 1976, the result of resistance in mosquito vectors. Moreover, bottled milk sampled in India in April 1990 had 10 times the permissible limit of DDT. DDT is fat soluble and has been carried in food chains to countries all over the world.[17] The lesson we have learned from the Russian nuclear accident at Chernobyl, the AIDS epidemic, and the DDT experience is that radiation, viruses, and pollutants respect no national borders.

The response to such lessons needs to be an enhanced commitment by individuals, communities, and nations to solve the problems of others and to view the world as a global village. Limiting the survival of important infection agents, their animal reservoirs, or hosts requires careful examination of the implications of such approaches in collaboration with veterinarians, entomologists, and toxicologists.

► PUBLIC HEALTH SYSTEMS

Of the 10 proposed public health systems important for control of communicable disease (Table 6-1), containment, contact tracing for prophylaxis and therapy, education, and measurement (surveillance) have been the mainstay of public health. Public health should become more involved with the rest as well.

The Centers for Disease Control and Prevention (CDC) has taken the lead by suggesting an epidemiological approach to priorities, listing adjusted mortality rates for various conditions and years of productive life lost (YPLL) for leading causes of death.[18,19] Ideally there would also be separate measures of morbidity and economic burdens so that, in a country with limited resources, leaders of the public health system could make more informed decisions and have the general community "buy into" their decisions.

It would seem prudent and desirable to have public health become more visible in terms of medical care access and efficiency of care. Great optimism can be appreciated, however, by the effort of the CDC to show the real risk of AIDS and the low (but not zero) probability of incurring an infection while taking care of an AIDS patient. Surely this contributes to the access of AIDS victims to the health care system.

With respect to efficiency of care, it has primarily been a function of the individual physician and more recently of hospitals interested in cost containment. Such activities are often subsumed under the umbrella term "quality assurance."[20] Accrediting agencies in the United States such as the Joint Commission for Accreditation of Healthcare Organizations (JCAHO) also are interested in the efficiency of health care services. It is not unreasonable to expect that public health officials, working with hospital epidemiologists and staff of "managed care" systems, would lend their expertise to this aspect of quality care of populations.

The legal process is paying attention to epidemiological data. Public health workers may need to "translate" public health findings that may have an impact on the legal system in a beneficial way for the population. Finally, social forces are often more effective than education alone in beneficially modifying health-related behavior. The facts on the hazards of smoking have been available for decades, but only in the last 15 years have substantial numbers of the population in the United States avoided smoking. It has become socially unacceptable in many situations to smoke; applause is often heard when the pilot of a commercial airline announces a smoke-free flight. In addition, lucrative business enterprises have made healthy behavior and exercise fashionable. These social forces need to be exploited and tested for use in control of infectious diseases. Patients in hospitals could be advised to request that all their health care providers wash their hands before touching them. This would reduce nosocomial infection rates, especially those due to staphylococci. It is not far-fetched to imagine safer sex as a result of social pressure to ask a partner to use barrier protection. Similar social pressures are operating when both passengers and drivers use their seat belts or when friends drive an intoxicated friend home after a party. Such social forces are powerful.

A corollary would be a suggestion for marketing good public health. An effective marketing campaign was carried out by former Surgeon General of the United States C. Everett Koop. He was perceived as caring, knowledgeable, and honest. An expanded approach to increasing the acceptance of vaccines, avoiding unsafe travel, and avoiding unsafe sex could be promoted just as consumer products are promoted—by use of effective peer groups and role models. This is a testable hypothesis for the 1990s.

In summary, a unified approach to public health is suggested involving clinicians, public health officials, and interested members and groups in the community. Networking, clarity in the presentation of epidemiologically important data, and a sense of the global community at risk with its environment are important. A sensitivity for the side effects of public health measures is essential and the use of effective education, social forces, and marketing practices may be the new tools of public health.

Emerging Infectious Diseases

Stephen M. Ostroff • James H. Hughes

> One can think of the middle of the twentieth century as the end of one of the most important social revolutions in history, the virtual elimination of the infectious disease as a significant factor in social life. . . .
>
> —Sir McFarland Burnet, 1962

> Emerging infectious diseases present one of the most significant health and security challenges facing the global community. . . . We are committed to ensuring that American citizens have the best protection possible from emerging infectious diseases, and that means a coordinated, comprehensive approach at both the national and international levels.
>
> —Vice President Albert Gore, 1996

These two quotes serve to illustrate the conundrum of emerging infectious diseases in the last half of the twentieth century. During the period of the 1950s through the 1970s, there was a widespread belief that infectious diseases were largely vanquished. The optimistic scenario conveyed by Nobel Laureate Sir McFarland Burnet was echoed by others. This conviction arose from experiences with recently developed antimicrobial agents such as penicillin and streptomycin coupled with successes from use of effective vaccines for childhood diseases such as polio and measles. In the United States, substantial declines in the incidence of infectious conditions as diverse as tuberculosis, polio, diphtheria, and typhoid fever (to name but a few)[1] fueled a perspective that all of the major issues regarding the control and prevention of infectious diseases had been identified and solved.

However, these predictions proved to be remarkably shortsighted. Today infectious diseases remain the leading cause of death

TABLE 6-3. LEADING INFECTIOUS CAUSES OF DEATH WORLDWIDE, 1995

Disease Category	*Number of Deaths*
Acute respiratory infections	4.4 million
Diarrheal disease	3.1 million
Tuberculosis	3.1 million
Malaria	2.1 million
Measles	1.1 million

Source: World Health Organization: World Health Report, 1996. Geneva: World Health Organization, 1996.

throughout the world (Table 6–3).[2] The leading global causes of infectious disease mortality include acute respiratory infections, diarrheal diseases, tuberculosis, and malaria. These diseases have a disproportionate impact on the developing nations of the world. Infectious diseases are also an important cause of mortality in developed countries such as the United States, where studies have demonstrated that overall deaths from infectious etiologies increased by 58 percent between 1979 and 1992.[3] As an example, mortality from acquired immunodeficiency syndrome (AIDS), a disease not recognized until 1981 in Los Angeles and New York City,[4] escalated rapidly throughout the 1980s and by 1994 became the leading cause of death among persons 25 to 44 years of age in the United States.[5] The rapid global emergence of AIDS demonstrates the extreme volatility of infectious diseases and the need to maintain an appropriate infrastructure for their identification, investigation, control, and prevention.

In 1992, a committee established by the Institute of Medicine of the National Academy of Science examined issues related to emerging infectious diseases. The committee, which was co-chaired by Drs. Joshua Lederberg and Robert Shope, produced a report entitled *Emerging Infections: Microbial Threats to Health in the United States*.[6] The authors of this report defined an emerging infection as one that has increased in incidence in the past two decades or that threatens to increase in the near future. This definition, or some variation on this definition, has been widely adopted by scholars and public health authorities working in the field of infectious diseases. The report documents the complacency that had developed concerning infectious diseases, describes the threats posed by microbial agents, identifies major factors that contribute to disease emergence and reemergence, and stresses the need for heightened domestic and global awareness and vigilance for timely recognition of, and response to, new threats.

The Institute of Medicine report highlights important examples of emerging infections, including the global emergence of AIDS in the early 1980s. More recent examples cited by the committee include the resurgence of measles in the United States in 1989–1991,[7] the reemergence of tuberculosis beginning in the mid-1980s,[8] and the detection of multidrug-resistant forms of tuberculosis in the early 1990s linked to outbreaks in institutional settings.[9]

▸ FACTORS CONTRIBUTING TO DISEASE EMERGENCE

Six major factors are thought to contribute to the emergence of infectious agents, according to the Institute of Medicine committee. They include changes in human demographics and behavior, industrial and technologic development, economic development and changes in the patterns of land use, expanding international commerce and travel, microbial adaptability, and failure to implement public health measures tied to a general deterioration in the public health infrastructure.[6] The deteriorating public health infrastructure can be tied to financial and human resource constraints; these constraints have been well documented at the state level.[10] It is often difficult to single out any one of these six factors with the emergence or reemergence of an infectious disease. Instead, it is the complex interplay among the various factors that leads to disease emergence. This interplay can be seen in a number of examples of diseases currently posing challenges to clinicians, microbiologists, and public health officials in the United States and abroad.

▸ EXAMPLES OF EMERGING INFECTIONS IN THE UNITED STATES

Within a few months of publication of the Institute of Medicine report in late 1992, a series of emerging infectious disease challenges occurred in the United States. The first was an interstate food-borne outbreak of hemorrhagic colitis and hemolytic uremic syndrome in several western states. This outbreak was due to *Escherichia coli* O157:H7, a food-borne bacterium that was first recognized as a human pathogen during simultaneous outbreaks of hemorrhagic colitis in Oregon and Michigan in 1982.[11] As was the case with the initial outbreaks, the 1993 multistate outbreak was linked to undercooked hamburgers served at outlets of a fast-food restaurant chain.[12] At least 700 persons became ill, with four fatalities. This outbreak highlights our increasing vulnerability to widespread food-borne disease outbreaks resulting from technologic changes that permit large-scale food production and distribution and from behavioral changes favoring foods prepared out of the home.

A few months after the *Escherichia coli* O157:H7 outbreak, the largest water-borne disease outbreak in United States history occurred in Milwaukee, Wisconsin. It has been estimated that over 400,000 persons became ill with diarrhea caused by the parasitic agent, *Cryptosporidium parvum*.[13] *C. parvum* was first recognized as a human pathogen in 1976 and has emerged not only as an important cause of water-borne disease outbreaks but as a major opportunistic pathogen of HIV-infected persons.[14] It has an animal reservoir, particularly cattle, and can be frequently isolated from water sources. The Milwaukee outbreak resulted from lapses in the function of the municipal water system. The emergence of cryptosporidiosis is in part related to factors that include changing farming patterns and practices, human demographic changes with expanding populations of immunocompromised hosts, and breakdown of public health measures for the supply of safe drinking water.

In May 1993, an outbreak of adult respiratory distress syndrome was recognized in the Four Corners area of the southwestern United States.[15] The disease mainly affected previously healthy young adults and was associated with high fatality rates. Initial symptoms included a flulike illness followed by abrupt onset interstitial pulmonary edema, hypoxia, and cardiac and respiratory failure.[16] Initially suspected diagnoses could not be confirmed in the laboratory. In early June, serologic assays provided the first clue to the etiology, which was a previously unrecognized member of the hantavirus family. Primers were then designed to amplify hantavirus-specific RNA from tissues and potential animal reservoirs. Extensive investigations in the affected area implicated the deer mouse *(Peromyscus maniculatus)* as the principal reservoir for the newly recognized pathogen, which is now referred to as Sin Nombre virus.[17] Identification of hantaviral antigens in capillary endothelium of the lung using immunohistochemical techniques provided an important pathogenic link to the pulmonary edema observed in persons with the disease.[18] Prevention strategies were developed and implemented even before the virus was finally isolated in cell culture months later.[19] Retrospective studies of stored autopsy materials and rodent tissues demonstrated that the virus has been present in the western United States for decades, if not for centuries.[20] Surveillance for human disease and surveys of rodents indicate that Sin Nombre virus is widespread in North America, and additional pathogenic hantaviruses in other rodent vectors have been found.[21] Local environmental and climatologic factors are thought to play an important role in the distribution and timing of hantavirus infection.

▶ EMERGING FOOD-BORNE DISEASES

In addition to *Escherichia coli* O157:H7, other food-borne pathogens are also emerging in the United States. In 1994, the Minnesota Department of Health identified an outbreak caused by *Salmonella* serotype Enteritidis when the state public health laboratory noticed an increase over the expected number of isolates of this serotype. Prompt epidemiologic investigations identified the vehicle as contaminated ice cream produced in Minnesota by one company and distributed in 48 states. The product was immediately removed from distribution. Surveillance identified culture-confirmed cases in 41 states with an estimate of 250,000 cases having occurred nationwide.[22]

Cases of food-borne illness associated with two contaminated, widely distributed products were detected in 1995 by the Public Health Laboratory Information System used for the reporting and analysis of data from state public health laboratories to the Centers for Disease Control and Prevention.[23] The first outbreak involved cases of *Salmonella* serotype Agona infection associated with a contaminated snack food imported from Israel. The cases were detected in the United States following the identification of the outbreak in England through investigations conducted by the Communicable Disease Surveillance Center.[24] The second outbreak involved cases of *Salmonella* serotype Stanley infection in several different states. Epidemiologic investigations implicated contaminated alfalfa sprouts from a single United States distributor as the source. The seeds were imported from Europe, where similar outbreaks also occurred.[25]

In 1996, a large outbreak of diarrhea due to the parasitic agent *Cyclospora cayatenensis* occurred in 18 eastern states and Canada.[26] *Cyclospora* was first recognized as a human pathogen in the late 1970s, and previously only local outbreaks had been observed. Investigations of case clusters and sporadic illnesses occurring during the spring outbreak period implicated raspberries imported from Guatemala as the likely source. Later in 1996, another multistate outbreak of *E. coli* O157:H7 occurred. This outbreak was linked to widely distributed unpasteurized apple juice.[27] Previous outbreaks of this infection linked to apple cider, and outbreaks during 1996 associated with lettuce mixes, suggest that food vehicles other than ground beef are becoming an important source for this pathogen.

Recent experiences with food-borne disease outbreaks demonstrate two themes. First, large-scale food production and distribution technology can result in large, multistate (and multinational) disease outbreaks if problems occur. Second, increasing global commerce, particularly in raw fruits and vegetables, from locations with varying levels of hygiene and sanitation can enhance the potential for outbreaks due to known pathogens as well as those not commonly associated with food-borne disease in this country. New strategies to address the evolving nature of food-borne disease and food-borne pathogens are required.[28]

▶ EMERGING VECTOR-BORNE DISEASES

Lyme disease was first recognized as a distinct entity in 1976 during the investigation of a cluster of suspected juvenile arthritis in Connecticut.[29] Since then, the disease has been reported with increasing frequency in the western, north-central, and eastern United States and elsewhere in the world.[30] It is now recognized as the most common tick-borne infection in this country. The recognition of Lyme disease fueled renewed interest in the study of tick-borne diseases.

In the mid-1980s, human monocytic ehrlichiosis was first reported in the United States.[31] This disease, which results in a nonspecific febrile illness similar to Rocky Mountain spotted fever, is produced by the rickettsial agent *Ehrlichia chaffeensis*. More recently a second variant of ehrlichiosis (human granulocytic ehrlichiosis) was identified in the upper midwest.[32] Both forms of the disease are increasingly recognized over a widening geographic area.[33] The principal tick vector for human monocytic ehrlichiosis is the deer tick *(Ixodes scapularis)* which is also the major vector for Lyme disease and also for babesiosis. Simultaneous infections with these agents have been reported.[34]

Tropical vector-borne diseases have been identified in the United States in the last several years. Dengue fever cases were recognized in south Texas in 1995 in association with a large outbreak in adjacent areas of Mexico.[35] Since 1993, small numbers of cases of locally acquired malaria have occurred in New York City, Houston, Michigan, south Florida, and Georgia.[36–39] In 1996, the first case of imported yellow fever since 1924 was identified in a Tennessee resident who had visited the Amazon basin.[39a]

Factors associated with emerging vector-borne diseases include human behaviors (such as increased outdoor activities), changing land use patterns (an important factor in Lyme disease, particularly the spread of suburban locales), international travel (imported vector-borne agents), and failure to implement public health prevention measures (for example, mosquito control and use of personal protective measures).

▶ EMERGING ZOONOTIC DISEASES

Recognition of hantavirus pulmonary syndrome has led to a reawakened interest in zoonotic disease threats. During the 1990s, wildlife rabies has reached historically high levels in the United States.[40] Much of this increase is attributable to the continued northward spread of a raccoon rabies epizootic in the northeastern states which began in the late 1970s. Coyote rabies in south Texas also poses an increasing threat among domestic animal populations and humans.[41] During the 1990s there has also been an increase in human rabies cases in the United States when compared to the previous two decades.[42] Subtyping of strains from these human cases show most are of bat origin. Since a history of bat bite has been largely absent from these human cases, the bat exposure is cryptogenic. This has led to the liberalization of criteria for rabies prophylaxis after bat contact.[42]

▶ EMERGING DRUG-RESISTANT INFECTIONS

Drug-resistant infections represent a major challenge to the public health, clinical, and research communities in the United States and other countries.[43] Drug resistance has the potential to profoundly impact morbidity and mortality from infectious diseases and to escalate health care costs due to inadequately treated infections and their complications and the need to use more expensive therapeutic alternatives.[44] Drug resistance is now a serious problem among nosocomial and community-acquired infections.[45]

An example of a rapidly emerging nosocomial drug-resistant infection is caused by the vancomycin-resistant enterococcus (VRE). First detected in the late 1980s in the United States, data from the National Nosocomial Infections Surveillance System show that the incidence of VRE in hospitalized patients has risen dramatically and has become geographically dispersed.[46] VRE are often resistant to all of the available antimicrobial agents, rendering infections with these strains essentially untreatable. Concerns have also been raised that the genes mediating vancomycin resistance could be transferred to *Staphylococcus aureus*, the most common nosocomial pathogen.[47] For methicillin-resistant *S. aureus*, vancomycin is currently the only therapeutic option. In 1997, strains of *S. aureus* with reduced susceptibility to vancomycin (known as vancomycin-intermediate *S. aureus*, or VISA) were identified in Japan and the United States.[47a]

Surveillance for drug-resistant community-acquired infections in the United States has been limited to sentinel systems and periodic surveys for selected pathogens such as *Shigella* and *Salmonella* species. Recent experiences with multidrug-resistant tuberculosis (MDRTB)[9] and the emergence of drug-resistant *Streptococcus pneumoniae* (DRSP)[48] demonstrates the need for more comprehensive systems to monitor drug resistance. Increasing levels of DRSP are of concern since *S. pneumoniae* is a leading cause of pneumonia, bacteremia, bacterial meningitis, and otitis media in the United States. The frequency of high-level penicillin resistance in sterile site isolates of *S. pneumoniae* from patients in 13 hospitals increased more than 60-fold from 0.02 percent in 1987 to 1.3 percent in 1991 to 3.2 percent in 1993–1994.[48–50] In 1994, active population-based surveillance for sterile-site DRSP isolates in the Atlanta metropolitan area showed even higher rates (7.1 percent) of high-level penicillin resistance.[51]

Several of the major factors associated with disease emergence apply to the problem of drug resistance. Human behavioral factors include patient expectations for, and abuse of, antimicrobial agents, and inappropriate prescribing practices by clinicians. Industrial uses of antibiotics, particularly as growth promoters in animal husbandry, also contribute. International travel promotes the spread of drug-resistant strains. Acquisition of drug resistance is among the most obvious examples of microbial adaptation. Failure to apply public health measures such as infection control contribute to nosocomial drug resistance, and breakdown of tuberculosis control programs resulting in failure to assure therapeutic compliance was a major factor in the development of drug-resistant tuberculosis. As the problem of drug resistance is multifactorial, solutions will require a coordinated effort on the part of clinicians, microbiologists, researchers, and public health personnel. Programs to improve antimicrobial use must be implemented to help preserve the effectiveness of these valuable drugs since few new antimicrobial agents are being introduced.

▶ EMERGING INFECTIONS OUTSIDE THE UNITED STATES

Other parts of the world have also been affected by emerging infectious diseases. In 1991, cholera reappeared in South America for the first time in the twentieth century and rapidly spread throughout all of Latin America.[52] The following year, a new epidemic strain of *Vibrio cholerae* (serotype O139) was detected in India and Bangladesh.[53] This represents the first non-O1 *Vibrio cholerae* capable of producing epidemic disease. In 1994, pneumonic plague occurred in India and, although the apparent number of cases was small, the episode had worldwide ramifications and resulted in substantial losses to the Indian economy.[54] In 1995, Ebola hemorrhagic fever struck the city of Kikwit, Zaire, resulting in 317 cases with a 77 percent mortality rate.[55] This was the first outbreak of Ebola hemorrhagic fever in 16 years and heralded additional outbreaks in nearby Gabon the following year.[56] The natural reservoir for Ebola virus is unknown. In the Western hemisphere in 1995, epidemic Venezuelan equine encephalitis reappeared in Venezuela and Colombia for the first time in almost two decades,[57] and in Nicaragua an epidemic of febrile illness and pulmonary hemorrhage was eventually diagnosed as leptospirosis.[57]

During 1996, a tentative link between bovine spongiform encephalopathy (BSE) and a variant form of Creutzfeldt-Jakob disease (v-CJD) was established in Great Britain.[58] BSE was first recognized in British cattle in 1986 but rapidly increased in frequency by the end of the decade. The announcement of the tentative link between BSE and v-CJD produced widespread bans on export of British beef.

Also in 1996, an outbreak of hantavirus pulmonary syndrome (HPS) was reported in Argentina, following an outbreak 1 year earlier in Paraguay.[59] Cases of HPS have also been recognized in Canada. The largest outbreak of *Escherichia coli* O157:H7 infection was reported in Japan, affecting almost 10,000 persons, principally school children.[60] Significant *E. coli* O157:H7 outbreaks were also reported in Germany and Scotland, demonstrating the increasing global spread of this pathogen. A new rabieslike *Lyssavirus* was recognized in fruit bats in Australia, and the first fatal human case was detected in that country late in 1996.[61] Finally, epidemic o'nyong-nyong fever, an arboviral infection, was identified in southwestern Uganda for the first time in over three decades.[62]

These examples demonstrate that emerging infectious diseases are recognized in both developing and developed countries. They can significantly impact morbidity and mortality, have the potential to divert scarce public health resources, and can rapidly spread to other countries. They can also have considerable political and economic ramifications. These factors make it imperative for a coordinated international response to address the emerging infectious disease threat.

▶ STRATEGIES FOR ADDRESSING EMERGING INFECTIOUS DISEASES

In 1994, the CDC, in consultation with outside experts in clinical infectious diseases, microbiology, and public health, developed a strategic plan to address emerging infectious diseases.[63] The strategy contains four major goals, including strengthening surveillance and response capacity, enhancing applied research in priority areas, developing and implementing control and prevention strategies, and improving the local, state, and federal public health infrastructure.

Effective implementation of the CDC plan requires partnerships with other federal, state, and local agencies, clinicians, microbiologists, academic institutions, industry, professional societies, and global partners such as the World Health Organization and its regional affiliates.[64] CDC has begun graded implementation of the emerging infections plan, including development of active population-based surveillance for high priority diseases and pathogens through state-based Emerging Infections Programs (EIPs). These programs represent an example of effective partnerships between federal and state health departments and academic institutions. Each site performs a core set of disease monitoring activities, and each performs site-specific surveillance and investigation projects of high priority to their area (an example is investigations of coccidioidomycosis in the California EIP). The EIPs monitor both known pathogens and unknown ones through intensive investigations of unexplained deaths that are potentially of an infectious etiology.[65]

CDC has also initiated national sentinel provider networks that include infectious disease specialists through the Infectious Disease Society of America, a consortium of emergency departments and travel health specialists. An Emerging Infectious Disease Laboratory Fellowship Program has been developed in collaboration with the Association of State and Territorial Laboratory Directors, and a peer reviewed journal, *Emerging Infectious Diseases*, has been created. The journal is also posted on the Internet (http://www.cdc.gov) for more rapid information dissemination.

▶ ADDRESSING EMERGING INFECTIOUS DISEASES AROUND THE WORLD

Recent outbreaks, such as the plague episode in India, Ebola hemorrhagic fever in Zaire, and leptospirosis in Nicaragua, highlight the limited global capacity to rapidly diagnose and respond to emerging disease threats. In 1995, there were only six operational maximum containment laboratories in the world capable of handling agents like Ebola hemorrhagic virus; personnel from three of these six laboratories participated in the Zaire investigation. For many other emerging agents, limited global diagnostic capability is also an issue.

Responding to the global threat of emerging diseases requires a coordinated global response with development of expertise in epidemiology, laboratory science, behavioral science, and disease control. To address this issue, in 1995 a working group on Emerging and Re-Emerging Infectious Diseases was established by the National Science and Technology Council's Committee on International Science, Engineering, and Technology (CISET). The working group included participants from 17 United States government agencies and organizations. The group considered ways for the various agencies to collaborate and coordinate their domestic and international efforts and how best to support WHO's programs to combat infectious diseases. The working group published their recommendations in September 1995.[66] The recommendations focus on the need for a global infectious disease surveillance and response system, enhanced domestic infectious disease surveillance, improved response capacity through collaboration with the private sector, assistance to other countries to strengthen their national surveillance systems, and enhanced authority of United States agencies to make the most effective use of their expertise to address emerging infectious disease threats.

In 1995, the World Health Assembly passed a resolution expressing concern about the emerging infectious disease threat and urging member states to make surveillance and control a priority consideration.[67] The resolution encouraged national active surveillance programs, improved routine diagnostic capacity, improved communications and reporting, routine antimicrobial susceptibility testing and rational antibiotic use, increased epidemiologic and laboratory investigative personnel, and fostering of applied research in diagnostics, standards, and prevention strategies. In response, WHO developed plans to enhance their ability to support national efforts to combat emerging diseases and created an organizational unit to coordinate this effort called Emerging and other Communicable Diseases Surveillance and Control.[68] In addition to improving WHO outbreak response capacity, assessing and expanding the WHO Collaborating Center network, and providing rapid communication of suspected and confirmed disease outbreaks, the unit has been involved in updating the International Health Regulations governing communicable disease control.[69]

TABLE 6-4. EXAMPLES OF EMERGING INFECTIONS DURING 1996

• ***United States***	
Ebola Reston subtype in nonhuman primates	Texas
Raccoon rabies	Ohio
Cyclospora gastroenteritis	Multiple states
Indigenous malaria	Georgia and Florida
Intrinsic contamination of albumin	Multiple states
Yellow fever (imported)	Tennessee
E. coli O157:H7 in apple juice	Multiple states
• ***Other Countries***	
Meningococcal meningitis	Africa
Ebola hemorrhagic fever	Gabon
Lassa fever	Sierra Leone
Streptococcus iniae infection	Canada
Variant Creutzfeldt-Jakob syndrome	Great Britain
E. coli O157:H7 infections	Japan, Germany, and Scotland
Dengue hemorrhagic fever	India
West Nile fever	Romania
O'nyong-nyong fever	Uganda

▶ CONCLUSIONS

Infectious diseases are important, evolving, complex public health problems. Their prevention and control requires the application of sophisticated epidemiologic, biologic, statistical, and behavioral approaches and technologies and the integration of epidemiologic and laboratory science. Ensuring information exchange and technology transfer is critical if future infectious disease threats are to be promptly recognized so that cost-effective control and prevention measures can be implemented. As noted in the Institute of Medicine report, "Pathogenic microbes can be resistant, dangerous foes. Although it is impossible to predict their individual emergence in time and place, we can be confident that new microbial diseases will emerge."

While it is difficult to predict future challenges posed by infectious agents, the experience in the United States and elsewhere (Table 6-4) indicates that we will continue to be confronted by national and international outbreaks, new syndromes caused by recognized microbial agents, and increasing problems of drug resistance. The challenge is to implement effective programs to minimize the impact and associated costs, morbidity, and mortality associated with these threats.

Health Advice for International Travel

Jay S. Keystone

It is estimated that each year more than 40 million Americans work and travel internationally in search of exotic vacation destinations or to conduct business, government, or missionary activities in remote areas of the world. Studies show that between 50 and 75 percent of short-term travelers to the tropics or subtropics report some health impairment, usually caused by an infectious agent.[1,2] Although infectious diseases are the major causes of morbidity associated with travel, they account for only 1 to 4 percent of deaths among travelers.[3] Cardiovascular disease and injuries are the most frequent causes of death, accounting for approximately 50 and 22 percent of deaths, respectively. Although mortality due to cardiovascular disease is similar to that of nontravelers, injury deaths, mostly from motor vehicle accidents, drowning, and aircraft accidents, are several times higher among travelers.[4]

By and large, travel-related illnesses are preventable by immunizations, prophylactic medications, and appropriate pretravel health education. Health recommendations for international travel are based primarily on individual risk assessment and any requirements mandated by public health authorities of the countries that the traveler plans to visit.[5] The risk of acquiring illness depends on the area of the world visited, the length of stay, activities and location of travel within these areas, and the underlying health of the traveler. It is essential for the health advisor to know the travel itinerary and the sequence in which countries will be visited and transited, the length of stay in each country, whether travel will be rural or urban, the style of travel (first class hotels versus local homes), the reason for travel, whether the traveler has any underlying health problems, allergies, or previous immunizations, and in the case of a female traveler, whether or not she is planning pregnancy or is pregnant.

▶ IMMUNIZATIONS

Immunizations for international travel can be categorized as *(a)* routine, childhood and adult immunizations (e.g., diphtheria/tetanus, polio/measles/mumps/rubella (MMR)); *(b)* required, those needed to cross international borders as required by international health regulations (e.g., yellow fever and meningococcus); and *(c)* recommended, according to risk of illness (e.g., typhoid, hepatitis A, rabies).

Routine Immunizations

Travel is an excellent opportunity for the practitioner to update an individual's "childhood" or adult immunizations such as diphtheria/tetanus, measles, mumps, polio, rubella, *Haemophilus influenzae*, and influenza. These immunizations are discussed in the guide for adult immunization[6] and the recommendations of the immunization practices advisory committee.[7]

Required Immunizations

Each year the World Health Organization (WHO) updates a list of required immunizations by country, which is subsequently included in "Health Information for International Travel," published annually by the Centers for Disease Control (CDC).[8] Required vaccinations must be recorded in the document "International Certificate of Vaccination" in accordance with international health regulations and validated by a stamp issued by state health departments. Yellow fever vaccine, and under specific circumstances, meningococcal vaccine, are the only two immunizations that WHO designates as vaccinations required for entry into specific countries. Although the World Health Organization eliminated the requirement for cholera vaccine for travelers in 1988, some unscrupulous health officials at international borders may still seek evidence of immunization. Countries requiring immunization against any of the above infections could refuse the right of entry to travelers who do not have a recorded valid immunization or (in some cases) a written statement by a physician indicating why immunization was not given. No vaccinations are required for U.S. residents to re-enter the United States.

Yellow Fever

Yellow fever, limited to tropical Africa and Central and South America, can be prevented by a single subcutaneous injection of a live attenuated virus vaccine. A certificate of yellow fever vaccination is valid for 10 years after a 10-day waiting period, although protection probably lasts for life. The vaccine is not recommended for infants less than 9 months of age. Like all other live virus vaccines, it should be avoided during pregnancy and in immunocompromised patients. However, pregnant women and HIV-positive individuals with CD4 counts greater than 200 should be immunized if they are at high risk of infection. Because the vaccine is grown in chick embryos, it should not be given to persons hypersensitive to eggs. If patients cannot be immunized safely, they should receive a physician's letter stating that the immunization is contraindicated.

Cholera

Cholera remains an important cause of severe diarrheal disease globally, especially with its recent spread into Central and South America. However, cholera among travelers is extremely rare (1:500,000 travelers).[9] There is some recent anecdotal evidence that in Latin America cholera may be playing a greater role in travelers' diarrhea. The standard phenol-killed whole cell cholera vaccine requires two injections for a maximum protection of only 50 percent for 3 to 6 months. New oral vaccines, not yet available in the United States, provide 80 percent protection for about 6 months to 1 year, but are not effective against the new sero type 0139, which is spreading rapidly through Asia.[10] For those countries that still require proof of cholera vaccination for entry, one dose, preferably 0.2 mL intradermally, will meet international requirements. The intradermal route causes fewer reactions than the subcutaneous route. After a 6-day waiting period, the cholera vaccination certificate is valid for 6 months. The vaccine is recommended only for health care workers and other volunteers working in high endemic areas (e.g., refugee camps) who are likely to be exposed to infection. The vaccine is not recommended or required for infants less than 6 months of age.

Meningococcal Meningitis

Vaccination against meningococcal meningitis is required for entry to Saudi Arabia for those attending the annual hajj (see recommended immunizations).

Recommended Immunizations

Tetanus

Serosurveys in the United States indicate that at least 50 percent of adults over the age of 60 lack protective levels of tetanus antitoxin and are therefore not adequately protected against tetanus. These same studies show that 40 to 80 percent of adults over 60 may be susceptible to diphtheria.[11] Tetanus immunization must be kept up-to-date; it is protective for at least 10 years. Because diphtheria is endemic in many countries, and is currently showing a resurgence in Eastern Europe, tetanus immunization should be given in combination with diphtheria vaccine, either as tetanus and diphtheria (DdT) for adults or diphtheria-pertussis-tetanus (DPT) vaccine for children less than 6 years of age. Some physicians vaccinate adult travelers at 5- to 10-year intervals so as to avoid the need for a booster or tetanus immune globulin if a person has a tetanus-prone wound within 5 years. This approach reduces the traveler's likelihood of receiving an injection in a developing country where the sterility of needles may be in question.

Poliomyelitis

Although poliomyelitis has recently been eradicated from the western hemisphere, it remains endemic in many other parts of the world. All travelers to developing countries should be immunized adequately. Individuals who have completed the primary series of three doses require only one lifetime booster dose of enhanced potency inactivated polio vaccine or the oral live attenuated vaccine. Since oral poliomyelitis vaccine recipients have a small (1:11,000,000 doses) risk of vaccine-induced paralysis, adults with an uncertain history of immunization and immunocompromised patients and their families should receive the parenteral vaccine.

Measles

In recent years measles has seen a resurgence in the United States and remains a major problem overseas where travelers could be exposed. More than ¼ of United States cases have been imported or epidemiologically linked to international travel; half were in returning residents and the other half in foreign visitors. Therefore, measles vaccine is recommended for all persons traveling abroad including those who are infected with HIV or who have AIDS. Children may be immunized as early as 6 months of age with the monovalent measles vaccine. In such cases, they should receive measles-mumps-rubella vaccine at 15 months and again when they reach school age. In adults, no immunity from natural infection is likely in those born after 1956, nor is acquired immunity common in those vaccinated before 1980 or those who have received live vaccine before 15 months of age. These individuals should also be immunized. Pregnant women and other immunocompromised patients (with the exception of HIV-infected individuals) should not be given the measles vaccine.

Hepatitis A

Hepatitis A is the most frequent vaccine-preventable infection of travelers. The incidence of symptomatic infections during a 1-month stay in a developing country ranges from 3 to 6 cases per 1,000 in resort areas to 20 per 1,000 for those who stray from the usual tourist routes.[12] Mortality from hepatitis A increases with age and reaches 2.1 percent of those over the age of 40.[13] Although most infants and young children are asymptomatic when infected, they do pose a health risk to others due to the ease of fecal-oral spread of this virus. Hepatitis A vaccination is recommended for all long-stay travelers to the developing world, those straying from the usual tourist routes, and repeated short-stay travel to areas of the world where food and water purity cannot be guaranteed. Two new, well-tolerated parenteral hepatitis A vaccines are highly efficacious, with seroconversion rates of almost 100 percent by the second dose.[14,15] Within 2 weeks of the first dose, between 70 and 85 percent of vaccinees will have protective antibodies. Although the CDC recommends simultaneous administration of immunoglobulin when travel is imminent, peak antibody levels may be lowered, potentially interfering with long-term protection. In view of the rapidity of vaccine-induced seroconversion and the long incubation period for hepatitis A, travel advisors in many countries, including Canada, do not recommended simultaneous administration of immune serum globulin even for travel that is imminent. Both inactivated hepatitis A vaccines require two doses 6 to 12 months apart. Studies of antibody decline suggest that these vaccines will provide at least 10 years and perhaps 20 or 30 years of protection.

Hepatitis B

The monthly incidence of hepatitis B infection, both symptomatic and asymptomatic, is 80 to 240 cases per 100,000 for long-stay overseas workers who are at considerable risk for hepatitis B, in part because of unprotected sexual contact with high-risk partners.[16] Currently available recombinant vaccines are highly effective and may provide lifetime protection. Hepatitis B immunization is recommended for health care or laboratory workers, long-stay travelers (more than 3 months) in countries with a high prevalence of hepatitis B surface antigenemia, and for those whose activities or health might place them at risk (e.g., those engaged in casual sex, dangerous sports, or those whose underlying health might put them at risk of receiving injections or intravenous medications). High-risk areas for hepatitis B include parts of southeast Asia, sub-Saharan Africa, and the Amazon basin of South America. Many now feel that hepatitis B vaccine should be recommended universally, regardless of travel, independent of an individual's risk of infection. The two recombinant hepatitis B surface antigen vaccines are given in two doses, 1 month apart, with a third dose 5 months after the second; some protection is probably afforded by fewer doses if time constraints are present. At present, no booster dose is recommended after the primary series.

Typhoid Fever

More than half of the approximately 500 cases of typhoid fever reported each year in the United States are acquired during foreign travel. The risk of typhoid fever has been estimated to be one case per 30,000 per month of stay in the developing world; however, attack rates have been documented to be 10-fold higher in India, Senegal, and North Africa.[17] Typhoid vaccination is highly recommended for those traveling off usual tourist routes, those returning to their homeland to visit and stay with relatives and friends, and those who plan to stay abroad for prolonged periods (more than 3 months), even in highly developed urban centers. The most frequently recommended typhoid vaccines are the live, attenuated multidose oral vaccine developed from the Ty21a strain of *Salmonella typhi* and the Vi capsular polysaccharide vaccine (ViCPS) administered intramuscularly in a single dose. A third, parenteral, heat-phenol–inactivated vaccine has been widely available for years but has significantly greater adverse reactions. All three vaccines have been shown to protect 50 to 80 percent of recipients, depending in part on the degree of exposure to the organism. The oral vaccine is administered as one capsule on alternate days for four doses with a booster required after 5 to 7 years. The oral vaccine should not be given concurrently with chloroquine or mefloquine. Because vaccine administration is undertaken by the recipient, there may be associated compliance problems. The parenteral, polysaccharide vaccine is administered in a single dose with a booster required at 3 years. For the older, less well-tolerated parenteral vaccine, two doses 4 weeks apart are recommended. When not contraindicated, either the oral Ty21a or parenteral ViCPS vaccine is preferable.

Meningococcal Disease

Meningococcal meningitis poses a sporadic or epidemic risk—most notably to trekkers in Nepal, travelers to Saudi Arabia during the hajj, and travelers to sub-Saharan Africa, Kenya, Tanzania, Burundi, and Mongolia. Although the risk of meningococcal disease has not been quantified, it appears to be greatest among travelers who live with indigenous populations in overcrowded conditions in high-risk areas. A single dose of quadrivalent A/C/Y/W-135 vaccine appears to be protective for about 3 years in adults and older children. Meningococcal vaccine is not effective in children less than 2 to 3 years of age.

Rabies

A few cases of rabies have been reported in travelers, but there are no data on the risk of infection. Preexposure rabies vaccine is appropriate for adults and children planning extended stays in much of the developing world and for persons who might be at occupational risk of exposure (veterinarians, spelunkers, etc.) in areas where rabies is a significant threat. Children may be at particular risk of rabies because of their usual cavalier attitude toward petting stray animals. The human diploid cell culture vaccine, a killed vaccine that is more immunogenic and less reactogenic than earlier rabies vaccines, is given on days 1, 7, and 28. Since the three-dose series almost always yields a satisfactory antibody level, routine measurement of titers is no longer recommended after the third vaccine dose. Travelers should be advised that pre-exposure vaccine eliminates the need for rabies immune globulin after rabies exposure, but does not eliminate the need for additional postexposure rabies vaccinations. In addition, travelers should be counseled on the avoidance of animals, particularly dogs, and prompt and thorough cleansing of animal bite wounds. The intradermal route should be completed more than 30 days before travel and should not be used when chloroquine or mefloquine are being taken concurrently.

Japanese Encephalitis

Japanese B encephalitis is a mosquito-borne, viral encephalitis found throughout much of the rural Indian subcontinent and southeast Asia. The risk of Japanese encephalitis is 1:5,000 per month of stay in an endemic area. The infection has been reported in 24 travelers over the 15-year period from 1978 through 1992.[18] Although most infections are asymptomatic, among those who develop clinical disease the case fatality rate may be as high as 30 percent, with severe neurological sequelae occurring in half of survivors. The vaccine should be reserved for those traveling in endemic areas for more than 3 weeks, especially when there is rural exposure in areas of rice and pig farming during summer months. The primary series consists of three injections 1 week apart with a booster dose at 12 to 18 months, and then every 4 years if risk continues.

Plague

Immunization against plague is recommended rarely except in rural southeast Asia and parts of South America for those whose occupation puts them at particular risk (e.g., exposure to rodents). Three injections of the formaldehyde-inactivated vaccine are given at 4-week intervals, with boosters every 6 to 12 months. Plague vaccine should not be given to infants less than 12 months of age. The vaccine is not readily available in North America.

Typhus

Since typhus is rarely seen in travelers, routine immunization is not recommended. Typhus vaccine is not available in the United States.

Tuberculosis

Tuberculosis has now become the number one infectious disease killer globally with estimates of 3 million new cases per year for the next 10 years. Persons who will live for prolonged periods in developing countries and those who will have close contact with locals are at increased risk of exposure. The efficacy of the Bacille Calmette-Guérin (BCG), a live vaccine derived from a strain of *Mycobacterium bovis*, is still debated in the United States. In developing countries, the vaccine appears to be most effective in preventing severe complications of tuberculosis in children. Most European countries recommend BCG vaccine for persons with a negative tuberculin skin test who are planning an extensive stay in a developing country. Side effects, ranging from draining abscesses at the site of immunization (common) to disseminated infection (rare), must be weighed against the risk of exposure to active tuberculosis for the traveler—a risk that varies directly with the intimacy and duration of contact with the indigenous population. If BCG vaccine is not administered, long-stay travelers (more than 6 months) should have a baseline tuberculin skin test placed before travel and repeated at 1- to 2-year intervals if risk continues.

Many travelers come to the physician only a short time before their anticipated date of departure. When necessary, inactivated vaccines can be administered simultaneously at separate sites using separate syringes. Theoretically, live vaccines should be administered 30 days apart because of possible impairment of the immune response. However, this does not apply to oral polio vaccine (OPV) and MMR, which may be given together. Ideally, immunoglobulin administration should be delayed until after the administration of certain live attenuated vaccines because of the possible reduction in antibody response. This caveat does not apply to OPV or yellow fever vaccines but does apply especially to MMR and its component vaccines. It should be remembered that killed or inactivated vaccines usually pose no danger to the immunocompromised host, although the immune response to these vaccines may be suboptimal; also, they are not usually a contraindication during pregnancy. Regardless of the duration of an interruption of a vaccination schedule, there is no need to restart a primary series of immunizations. It is sufficient to continue where the series was interrupted. Finally, all immunizations should be recorded in the international certificate of vaccination booklet and carried with the passport.

▶ MALARIA PROTECTION

More than 30,000 North American and European travelers develop malaria each year.[19] The risk of malaria is highest in sub-Saharan Africa and Oceania (1:50 to 1:1000), intermediate (1:1000 to 1:12,000) for travelers to Haiti and the Indian subcontinent, and low (less than 1:50,000) for travelers to southeast Asia and to Central and South America.[20] With the worldwide increase in chloroquine and multidrug-resistant falciparum malaria, decisions about chemoprophylaxis have become more difficult. In addition, the spread of primaquine- and chloroquine-resistant *Plasmodium vivax* has added further complexity to the issue of malaria prevention and treatment. Compliance with antimalarial chemoprophylaxis regimens and use of personal protection measures to prevent mosquito bites are keys to the prevention of malaria. Travelers must be educated about the risk of malaria, personal protection measures against mosquito bites, appropriate chemoprophylaxis, symptoms of the disease, and measures to be taken in case of suspected malaria during travel. In order to make the above determinations, travel medicine advisors must conduct a careful review of the itinerary, whether urban and/or rural areas will be visited, the length of stay, style of travel, and medical history including allergies and the likelihood of pregnancy. Current information on malaria transmission by country is provided by the World Health Organization and by the Centers for Disease Control in the United States through a fax and telephone system:

WHO Fax: 41-22 791 07 46; Tel: 011-41-22-791-4510

CDC Fax: 404-488-4427; Tel: 404-639-3311.

Personal Protection Measures

Anopheles mosquitoes, the vectors of malaria, are exclusively nocturnal in their feeding habits; protection from mosquito bites from dusk to dawn is highly effective in reducing infection. Travelers should wear protective clothing such as long-sleeved shirts and long pants when outside during evening hours. The most effective method to prevent mosquito bites is to combine a pesticide such as permethrin on clothing with an insect repellent containing DEET (NN-diethylmethyltoluamide) to exposed skin.[21] Where possible, travelers should use a bed net impregnated with permethrin, which has an efficacy of up to 80 percent in the prevention of malaria.[22] A pyrethroid-based flying insect spray should be used to clear the bed net and room of mosquitoes. Where bed nets are not available, mosquito coils and other preparations of vaporized pyrethrum have been shown to reduce mosquito bites.

Chemoprophylaxis

Personal protection measures greatly reduce but do not eliminate risk of malaria. Most antimalarials are only suppressives, acting on the erythrocytic stage of the parasite beyond the liver phase, thereby preventing the clinical symptoms of disease but not infection. No drug guarantees protection against malaria. For this reason, travelers must be informed that any febrile illness that occurs during or soon after travel to a malaria-endemic area should be evaluated immediately by a health care professional. Since in only one-third of patients in the United States who died from malaria was the diagnosis considered before death, it is incumbent upon febrile returned travelers to inform their health care provider of the risk of malaria and the need to have it ruled out regardless of the malaria prophylactic used.

Most antimalarials should be started 1 to 2 weeks prior to entry into a malarious area, during exposure, and for 4 weeks after departure. Beginning antimalarials early assures an adequate blood concentration of the drug and enables travelers to switch to alternative drugs should adverse effects occur. The postexposure period of prophylaxis is particularly important to enable the antimalarial to eradicate any organisms that have been released from the liver into the bloodstream after departure from a malarious area.

Chloroquine is still recommended for travelers to Central America, Haiti, and parts of the Middle East. However, the global spread of chloroquine-resistant falciparum malaria has necessitated the use of alternative regimens for most areas of the world. Chloroquine should be taken with meals to reduce gastrointestinal side effects. Chloroquine can be given safely to children and pregnant women. However, since the difference between a prophylactic dose and a potentially fatal toxic dose is relatively small, the tablets and pediatric elixir should be kept in closed, childproof containers. Nonallergic, intense pruritus is well documented, almost exclusively in black Africans. Chloroquine is administered to adults weekly as two 250-mg tablets.

Mefloquine is the drug of choice for travelers to Africa, South America, Asia, and southeast Asia (with the exception of Thailand). As a result of reports of severe neuropsychiatric reactions and the media response, mefloquine has acquired a bad reputation. Mefloquine nevertheless remains the drug of choice for the above-mentioned areas. Prospective and retrospective studies suggest that the risk of severe neuropsychiatric reactions (seizures and psychosis) is 1:13,000, whereas milder but disabling adverse events (anxiety, irritability, depression, nightmares, and insomnia) appear to occur in approximately 1:200 users.[23,24] Gastrointestinal side effects can be reduced by taking the drug with food. Mefloquine is administered to adults as a 250-mg tablet weekly. It is contraindicated for those with a history of seizures, psychosis, or cardiac conduction defects. It is no longer contraindicated in pregnancy, for those whose occupation requires fine coordination (such as airline pilots), or for newborn infants.

Fansidar, a fixed combination of pyrimethamine and sulfadoxine, is no longer recommended except as self-treatment, because of severe adverse cutaneous reactions.[25] Fansidar resistance is widespread; therefore, as a self-treatment regimen (3 tablets taken at once for a febrile illness that occurs in an area where medical attention is not available), it should be restricted to those areas of the world where the malaria parasite is still sensitive.

Doxycycline is the drug of choice for malaria chemoprophylaxis along the Thai-Cambodian and Burmese (Myanmar) borders, where *P. falciparum* malaria is resistant to both chloroquine and mefloquine. Doxycycline is administered 1 to 2 days prior to travel, daily (100 mg in adults) during exposure, and for 4 weeks after departure from the malarious area. The side effects of doxycycline, gastrointestinal upset, exaggerated sunburn, and vaginal candidiasis, can be reduced or managed by taking the drug with food, using a sunscreen containing a UVA blocker, and carrying a topical antifungal cream for self-treatment, respectively. The drug is contraindicated during pregnancy and in children under 8 years of age.

Primaquine, which has in the past been used to prevent relapses of *P. vivax* malaria, has recently been shown to be a very effective antimalarial when taken daily.[26,27]

Regardless of the chemoprophylactic regimen recommended, it is important for travel health advisors to inform travelers that *(a)* globally there is no uniformity concerning malaria chemoprophylaxis recommendations and *(b)* they are likely to meet fellow travelers and health care providers overseas who give conflicting advice as to the optimal regimen for malaria chemoprophylaxis. Individuals who are unable to tolerate effective antimalarials, who are in an area where drug resistance is frequent, and who are unable to obtain medical care in less than 48 hours may consider carrying a self-treatment regimen. Unfortunately, those who carry self-treatment regimens often use them inappropriately. The drugs used for self-treatment are the same agents used for malaria treatment (quinine plus doxycycline, mefloquine, halofantrine, atovaquone plus proguanil and fansidar). The global spread of drug-resistant malaria has stimulated the search for new approaches to prevention and treatment of malaria. Azithromycin, atovaquone/proguanil, pyronaridine, WR238, 605, and primaquine are in the clinical trial stage as promising alternatives to our present armamentarium.

▶ TRAVELERS' DIARRHEA

Diarrhea is the most frequent health problem among visitors to developing countries, affecting one-third to one-half of all travelers.[28,29] Although travelers' diarrhea is a self-limited illness, usually caused by enterotoxigenic *E. coli* (ETEC), among those who become ill, 30 percent will remain in bed and another 40 percent will have to curtail their activities.[30] When counseling travelers about diarrhea, several issues must be considered: food and water precautions, chemoprophylaxis, self-treatment of illness, and immunization.

Food and Water Precautions

Unpeeled fruits, uncooked vegetables, food that has been cooked or stored at insufficient temperatures, unpurified water and ice cubes made from it are believed to be the main sources of enteric pathogens for the traveler. Tap water, ice cubes, and unpasteurized milk and milk products should be avoided, tea or coffee is safe when consumed hot, and commercially bottled, carbonated beverages are highly recommended. If safe beverages are not available, travelers may need to disinfect water by bringing it to a boil or by using commercial iodine or chlorine tablets for chemical disinfection or using purification devices. Raw foods are best avoided. Vegetables and fruits should be eaten only if they can be peeled by the traveler.

Chemoprophylaxis/Self-Treatment

If one considers the standard food and water precautions outlined above, it is clear that flawless observance may be virtually impossible, particularly among vacationers, who, wanting to relax and indulge in local cuisine, are likely to be noncompliant with food precautions.[31] For this reason, the concepts of chemoprophylaxis and self-treatment have gained popularity in recent years. Since bacterial pathogens account for the majority of episodes of travelers' diarrhea, antibiotics and bismuth subsalicylate have been the focus of testing for both treatment and prevention. The overriding principle in the management of travelers' diarrhea is the maintenance of adequate fluid and electrolyte balance. Fluids can be replenished with bottled soft drinks, juices, or electrolyte-containing oral rehydration solutions. Because of damage to the intestinal lactase-producing cells by enteric pathogens, dairy products should be avoided during illness.

Most travel advisors recommend that travelers should carry an antimotility agent (such as imodium or lomotil) and an antibiotic for self-treatment of diarrhea that occurs during travel.[32] Many studies have shown that antimicrobial therapy leads to symptomatic improvement and reduction in the duration of illness, particularly among those infected with ETEC and *Shigella*. Widespread resistance of enteric pathogens to trimethoprim-sulfamethoxazole, ampicillin, and doxycycline have, for the most part, rendered these drugs ineffective. The drugs of choice for treatment of travelers' diarrhea are the quinolone antibiotics. Standard therapy with ciprofloxacin (500 mg), norfloxacin (400 mg), and ofloxacin (300 mg) consists of one dose twice daily for 3 days.[33] Recent data have shown that single-dose therapy with ciprofloxacin (500 mg to 1 g), and norfloxacin (800 mg), with or without an antimotility agent, can be as effective as the standard 3-day course of treatment.[34,35] Travelers should be cautioned that antibiotic resistance is on the rise globally. In Thailand, for example, *Campylobacter* isolates from U.S. troops with diarrhea showed 70 and 30 percent resistance to ciprofloxacin and azithromycin, respectively.[36]

Prophylactic antimicrobials are not generally recommended because of the potential for increasing antibiotic resistance and the risk of untoward drug reactions or superinfection with more pathogenic microorganisms. Bismuth subsalicylate (Pepto-Bismol), two tablets four times daily, has shown a protective effect of up to 65 percent. Antibiotic agents, on the other hand, have shown up to 90 percent efficacy in protecting against travelers' diarrhea, particularly a single daily dose of ciprofloxacin (500 mg), norfloxacin (400 mg), or ofloxacin (300 mg).[37,38] Some authors recommend prophylactic therapy with bismuth subsalicylate or a quinolone antibiotic for travel less than 3 weeks for those who repeatedly develop diarrhea during travel, those with diminished protective gastric acidity, those who cannot afford incapacity for even 1 day (e.g., athletes, military personnel) and those with an underlying medical disorder for whom travelers' diarrhea might be poorly tolerated, e.g., those suffering from inflammatory bowel disease, insulin-dependent diabetes mellitus, chronic renal failure, or AIDS.

Recent studies have shown that the oral cholera B subunit whole cell vaccine provides short-lived protective efficacy against ETEC bacteria responsible for travelers' diarrhea. On the horizon are new antibacterial vaccines against ETEC, *Salmonella*, and *Shigella* species.

▶ VECTOR-BORNE DISEASES

Although malaria is the most important vector-borne infection in travelers, there are others that require attention. Of these, dengue fever is an increasing problem as noted by a dramatic rise in the infection globally, particularly in the Caribbean, Central and South America, and southeast Asia. Dengue fever is transmitted by the *Aedes* mosquito which prefers an urban and often indoor habitat. This mosquito bites during the day, particularly in the hours of the early morning and late afternoon. Therefore, it is important to take insect precautions during the day to prevent dengue as well as between dusk and dawn to prevent malaria. In addition to insect precautions, some vector-borne diseases can be prevented by prophylactic medication. For example, loiasis can be prevented by taking 300 mg (adult dose) of diethylcarbamazine once each week while in a very heavily infested area such as Central or West Africa. Tick- and mite-borne typhus, relapsing fever, bartonellosis, and plague can be prevented by using doxycycline prophylaxis, 100 mg daily, during exposure. For the most part, prophylaxis of these latter infections is not recommended except for a very select group of individuals at high risk for infection.

▶ SEXUALLY TRANSMITTED DISEASE

During international travel, individuals often feel the sense of anonymity, may be less sexually inhibited, and may therefore put themselves at greater risk for the acquisition of sexually transmitted disease. The risk is increased by exposure to multiple or professional partners. Safer sexual practices, including the use of condoms throughout intimacy, are particularly important in the era of AIDS. Immunization against hepatitis B is a must for those who intend to engage in casual sex while abroad.

▸ SOIL- AND WATER-BORNE DISEASES

Schistosomiasis, a helminthic disease that infects over 200 million people worldwide in parts of South America, the Caribbean, Africa, the Middle East, and southeast Asia can be avoided by advising travelers to stay out of slow moving, fresh water in these areas of the world. Swimming in the ocean or fresh water pools without snails is safe. Barefoot walking exposes the traveler to a variety of hazards including tungiasis (sand flea), snake bites, cutaneous larva migrans from dog and cat hookworms, human hookworm infection, and strongyloidiasis. Sandals provide only partial protection, whereas closed footwear should be fully protective.

▸ ADAPTATION TO THE ENVIRONMENT

Excessive sun exposure can cause erythema and sunburn, chemical hypersensitivity, eye damage, bleaching of the skin, and predisposition toward skin cancers including malignant melanoma. Sunscreens with an SPF factor of 15, offer 93 percent protection. Adaptation to a hot climate can take from one to several weeks depending on the ambient temperatures and humidity. Clothing should be made of natural fibers such as cotton and linen to allow air to circulate. Light colors reflect light and are preferable to dark fabrics. Since sweat contains both water and salt, it is important to replace salt by eating salty foods or adding extra salt to food. In hot weather and in the absence of strenuous exercise, the average person must replace at least 1½ liters of fluid per day.

▸ SPECIAL RISK TRAVELERS

It is beyond the scope of this review to cover health issues related to pregnant and infant travelers, the chronically ill, or HIV-infected individuals. Excellent recent reviews are available on these subjects.[39–42]

▸ ILLNESS AFTER RETURN

It is more the exception than the rule that physicians ask "where have you been?" of travelers who become ill after their return. Therefore, before departure travelers should be warned that, if they become ill on return, regardless of how carefully they have followed recommended precautions, they should immediately inform their physician that they have traveled recently. This is particularly important for febrile travelers since no antimalarial drug guarantees protection against malaria.

Infectious and Chronic Diseases Epidemiology: The Distinction Wanes

Lewis H. Kuller • Lee H. Harrison

Epidemiologists often describe their work as either chronic or infectious disease epidemiology. The fundamental differences between the study of infectious and so-called chronic diseases relate mainly to the incubation periods of the disease.[1] In the past, most infectious diseases had a short incubation period, and chronic disease had a longer one. A second difference between many infectious and chronic diseases relates to the mode of transmission. Although there are important examples of common-source infectious diseases,[2] many infectious diseases are transmitted person-to-person. Major chronic diseases, on the other hand, are often consistent with a common source, such as diet or environmental pollutants, or have an unknown mode of transmission.

Infectious disease epidemiology has focused more on traditional concepts of host, agent, and environment. The shorter defined incubation period and, often, a better definition of disease has resulted in a greater emphasis on measures of traditional epidemics, including time, place, and person. Chronic disease epidemiologists have had to face the problems of poor definition of an onset of disease and the time point of initial exposure to an agent (i.e., the interrelationship between diet and the percentage of calories from specific saturated fat and risk of coronary heart disease).

A major difference between the study of infectious and chronic diseases has been the notion that the etiologies of these two groups of diseases were mutually exclusive. However, medical discoveries in the past decade or so have taught us that this is clearly untrue. There are now numerous examples of chronic diseases that have infectious etiologies and the list is likely to grow.

The Koch-Henle postulates were put forth to determine when infectious agents caused a specific disease process:[3]

1. The parasite occurs in every case of the disease in question and under circumstances that can account for the pathological changes and clinical course of the disease.
2. It occurs in no other diseases as a fortuitous and nonpathogenic parasite.
3. After being fully isolated from the body and repeatedly grown in pure culture, it can produce the disease anew.

Recent advances have forced a rethinking of these postulates because they are no longer consistent with our understanding of both the infectious and noninfectious etiologies of most diseases. Evans, in his book on the *Causation of Disease: A Chronological Journey*,[3] described the changes in the guidelines for establishing causation in an infectious disease epidemic:

1. The agent should be isolated from the majority of cases involved in the epidemic.
2. The agent should be isolated more commonly in sick than in well persons (but a high incidence of subclinical infectious may obscure this difference).
3. The incubation period of the agent isolated should correspond to that of the disease.
4. Antibody to the agent should appear during illness, or a 4-fold or greater rise in titer should occur, or an agent-specific IgM antibody should be demonstrated.
5. Intervention measures that abolish the source of exposure to the agent, or interrupt its means of transmission, or which protect the host by agent-specific active or passive immunization should control the epidemic. Treatment or prophyl-

axis with an antibiotic or antiviral agent to which the organism is sensitive that halts epidemic spread is indirect evidence of a causal association but is usually not agent-specific.

6. The disease can be reproduced in susceptible experimental animals with evidence of spread by a similar route of transmission.
7. No other agent should show the same causal associations, unless it is the rare instance in which two infectious agents are needed to produce the clinical picture. (HIV and the opportunistic infections of AIDS is an example.)

Chronic disease epidemiology initially evolved from studies of infectious diseases that had relatively long natural history such as tuberculosis and syphilis. In the classic Muskegee County Study, Comstock used similar techniques for estimating the prevalence of tuberculosis infection and the prevalence of hypertension in a defined population and the association with selected risk factors.[4] Blood pressure levels and definition of hypertension were equated with prevalence of positivity of a tuberculin skin test or the presence of clinical tuberculosis based on a chest radiograph.

The modern generation (probably from the 1970s on) of chronic diseases epidemiology became strongly linked with biostatistical methodology and the social/behavioral sciences. The concepts of causality of chronic diseases were rooted in statistical associations such as the consistency, strengths, and specificity of associations, the temporal relationships, and the coherence of the association as enunciated in the 1964 Surgeon General's report.[5] Interest in the possible infectious etiology of important chronic diseases such as cancer also lost favor as investigators were unsuccessful in identifying specific infectious agents as causes of cancer in humans, such as carcinoma of the breast, leukemia, and lymphoma.

Epidemiologists studying chronic diseases soon recognized that, except in unusual circumstances, the etiology of the disease could be quantified at different levels—from social/behavioral attributes (i.e., social class, education) to environmental factors or broadly defined agents and, in few circumstances, to the specific agent and mode of transmission.

Four recent events have dramatically changed the interrelationship between infectious and chronic disease epidemiology. The first was the development of new microbiologic techniques to identify etiologic infectious agents of disease, including those that could not be isolated in culture, and to identify infectious agents as causes of specific diseases. For example, hepatitis B and C viruses were found to be etiologic agents of liver cancer.[6] Similarly, improved microbiological laboratory methods led to the probable association of Epstein-Barr (EB) virus and Hodgkin's disease[7] using seroepidemiologic methodology in nested case-control studies. In addition, human T-lymphotropic virus type I (HTLV-I) was shown to cause adult T-cell leukemia/lymphoma and HTLV-I associated myelopathy.[8,9]

Second, the epidemic of HIV and AIDS resulted in a great expansion of research in immunology and virology, a marked improvement in laboratory methods of identifying the specific organisms and, most important, the recognition of the interrelationship between infectious diseases, immunology, and the development of chronic diseases, such as the high rates of Kaposi's sarcoma and non-Hodgkin's lymphoma among patients with AIDS.

Third, the observation that an infectious agent could be causally related to a chronic disease received a very high boost with the observation that *Helicobacter pylori* infection of the gastrointestinal tract was probably the primary cause of peptic ulcer and gastric cancer and that antibiotic therapy is part of the treatment of peptic ulcer.[10,11]

The fourth and most recent major change has been the recognition of the possible epidemic of Creutzfeldt-Jakob disease associated with, perhaps, a prion agent that is transmitted from cattle, i.e., bovine spongiform encephalopathy (BSE) to humans. This and other recent observations suggest that other infectious agents may cross species barriers and cause human disease.[12,13]

The identification of infectious etiologies of chronic diseases is a field that is exploding.[14] This is due, in part, to the utilization of new molecular biologic approaches that allow organisms to be identified that have not been isolated in culture.[15] For example, Relman et al. discovered one of the agents of bacillary angiomatosis, a vascular proliferative process associated with human immunodeficiency virus (HIV) infection, by amplifying highly conserved and other ribosomal RNA sequences from diseased tissue using polymerase chain reaction.[16] The agent, a bacterium now known as *Bartonella henslae*, has also been shown to be the cause of cat-scratch disease.[17] In addition, Choo et al. used an interesting approach to discover the hepatitis C virus, previously a major cause of posttransfusion hepatitis.[18] The investigators constructed gene products of complementary DNA from RNA taken from an infected chimpanzee's blood, then used serum from a patient with hepatitis of unknown etiology to screen the products and identify the virus.

The potential to identify a specific infective agent in the etiological pathology of a chronic disease could result in reduction of incidence of disease by modifying the transmission chain of infection, specific drug therapy against the agent, or modification of the host immune response. There are several mechanisms by which an infectious agent can be linked to a chronic disease:

1. An infectious agent may be the direct cause of a chronic disease. For example, hepatitis B is likely an etiologic agent of hepatocellular carcinoma.
2. An infectious agent may be part of the causal pathway of the chronic disease if it causes immunosuppression. For example, patients with HIV-induced immunodeficiency have an increased incidence of non-Hodgkin's lymphoma. In addition, there are examples of chronic diseases in which mechanisms 1 and 2 both play a role. For example, Kaposi's sarcoma requires HIV-induced immunosuppression for expression in most patients and appears to have a viral etiology (see below). Similarly, group B streptococcal bacteremia is more common among individuals who have diabetes mellitus or other chronic diseases associated with alterations in immune function.[19]
3. An infectious agent can be an important precipitant of chronic disease or substantially affect the natural history of the chronic disease. Pneumonia, due to a variety of organisms, is probably an important risk factor for acute exacerbations of congestive heart failure among individuals with cardiac dysfunction. Acute infectious diseases may possibly precipitate myocardial infarction.
4. An infectious disease could result in a nonspecific inflammatory response. Activation of various cytokines and acute phase proteins can upregulate the risk of thrombosis. The higher risk of thrombosis could then be associated with arterial or venous thrombosis and chronic disease.

How have infectious agents been linked to long-incubation-period chronic diseases? First, traditional epidemiology methods may link higher incidence of a specific infectious disease (i.e., hepatitis B and C) and incidence of chronic disease (i.e., liver cancer) among populations. Second, a model of the disease, either in humans or animals, may be consistent with similar diseases of unknown etiology in humans, such as the transmissible spongiform encephalopathies. Third, the potential etiological agent may be identified with specific pathology, such as human papilloma virus type 16 with cervical cancer and *H. pylori* with gastric and duodenal ulcer. Fourth, seroepidemiological studies demonstrate an association of an infectious agent, such as higher titers to EB virus and lymphoma, and disease and mode of transmission, and epidemiology consistent with a causal association. Fifth, the development of a specific chronic disease may be linked with a prior infection among higher risk individuals, viral infection, superantigens, specific genetic susceptibility, and development of insulin-dependent diabetes mellitus (IDDM).

▶ EXAMPLES OF POSSIBLE ETIOLOGIC ASSOCIATIONS BETWEEN INFECTIOUS AND CHRONIC DISEASES

Coronary Heart Disease

Do infectious agents play an important role in the etiology or in the natural history of coronary heart disease or stroke?[20,21] The epidemiological evidence to support an association between infectious disease and risk of coronary heart disease begins with the higher mortality of coronary heart disease and stroke in the winter. Temperature changes, as well as higher risk of infectious diseases in the winter, have long been suggested as probable determinants of the seasonality. Epidemiological studies have reported a higher prevalence of respiratory infection prior to the onset of a myocardial infarction.[22]

There may be a biological basis for the association of infectious agents and coronary artery disease. Macrophages, derived from blood monocytes, play a very important role in the development of the atherosclerotic plaque. Inflammation within an atherosclerotic plaque may be important in the pathogenesis leading to ruptured plaque, thrombosis, occlusion of the blood vessel, myocardial infarction, and sudden death.

Libby and coworkers[23] have noted that monocytes bond to leukocyte adhesion receptors on the endothelial surface. The monocytes accumulate lipids and are transferred to macrophage-foam cells. The macrophages can produce pro-coagulants, such as tissue factor, as well as cytokines. Fatty streaks develop into complex atherosclerotic plaques that contain smooth muscle cells, extracellular matrix, and extracellular lipid core. The collagen breakdown of the fibrous atherosclerotic plaque is primarily affected by macrophage-degrading enzymes.

In prospective studies, higher white blood cell count is a risk factor for heart attack.[24] Decreased pulmonary function, possibly due (in part) to increased respiratory infections such as chlamydia and pneumoniae (TWAR), has been linked to an increased risk of coronary heart disease.

Infectious diseases are associated with an increase in acute phase proteins such as fibrinogen and c-reactive protein and, possibly, with an increased risk of thrombosis. Higher levels of acute-phase protein have been linked to risk of coronary heart disease in both case-control and longitudinal studies.[25–28]

It is possible that inflammation, secondary to infection, within an atherosclerotic plaque or infection at other sites, may result in elevated acute-phase proteins and increased risks of cardiovascular disease.[25]

Some studies have suggested an association between periodontal disease and severity and risk of both coronary disease and stroke.[29] Periodontal diseases are Gram-negative infections and may be an unrecognized risk factor for atherosclerosis and thromboembolic events. An underlying inflammatory response secondary to periodontal disease stimulates inflammatory cytokines and endotoxins, which may exacerbate atherosclerosis and thrombotic events. In the Normative Aging and the Dental Longitudinal studies, mean bone loss scores and, worse, probing pocket depth scores per tooth, were associated with about a 2-fold increased risk of coronary heart disease and stroke.[29]

Brunner and colleagues have shown higher fibrinogen levels (an acute-phase protein), possibly a secondary response to infection, among lower socioeconomic class as compared with upper socioeconomic class children and hypothesized that the socioeconomic gradient in coronary heart disease could be, in part, related to elevated fibrinogen and other acute-phase proteins among lower socioeconomic children.[30] Many infections have much higher prevalence in lower socioeconomic class and contribute to the higher risks of coronary heart disease.

At least four infectious agents have been linked to the risk of coronary heart disease: cytomegalovirus (CMV), herpes simplex, *Chlamydia pneumoniae* and *Helicobacter pylori*. Although a causal role has not been proved for any of these organisms, intriguing data suggest that they may play a role in coronary heart disease.

Recent studies have noted a possible important role of CMV and restenosis following coronary atherectomy and angioplasty and also in graft atherosclerosis following heart transplantation.[31–34] Prior infection with CMV is a strong independent risk factor for restenosis after coronary atherectomy. Studies have linked specific CMV protein and high amounts of P-53. CMV protein binds to P-53 and may abolish its ability to transcriptionally activate a reporter gene. CMV and its related proteins may inhibit P-53 function and contribute to the development of restenosis.[33]

The causes of restenosis are excessive accumulation of smooth muscle cells and vascular remodeling. CMV is present in vascular smooth muscle cells and interacts with smooth muscle cell P-53 to interfere with its suppressive functions. The angioplasty or atherectomy results in injury to the vessel wall and reactivation of latent CMV. Monocytes may be the source of the latent CMV. These monocytes are recruited to the site of the injury, at which time the CMV can be activated, leading to CMV-mediated neointimal proliferation.[33] Whether this model of CMV and restenosis is related to the development of atherosclerosis and thrombosis in the general population is unknown. Other prospective studies have shown higher titers of CMV among individuals who have more atherosclerosis in the carotid arteries[35,36] based on ultrasound examination. Epidemiological studies have also shown that antibodies against CMV have been elevated significantly in patients with angiographically defined coronary heart disease compared with controls.[37]

Chlamydia pneumoniae has also been associated with potential risk of coronary heart disease. *Chlamydia pneumoniae* is an important cause of pneumonia, bronchitis, sinusitis, and other acute respiratory infections.[38] It is transmitted by the respiratory route and can be treated with antibiotic therapy. Pathologic studies have identified *Chlamydia pneumoniae* organisms in atherosclerotic lesions in the carotid and coronary arteries.[39,40] Higher titers were associated with angiographically demonstrated coronary artery disease.[41] In prospective nested case-control studies, higher *Chlamydia pneumoniae* titers are a risk factor for coronary heart disease.[42]

Coronary heart disease subjects are also more likely to be *H. pylori* seropositive than are control subjects.[43] Seropositive patients for *H. pylori* have been reported to have higher fibrinogen levels and lower high density lipoprotein cholesterol (HDLc) and higher blood pressure.[44,45]

All of these infectious agents, possibly associated with coronary artery disease, are very prevalent in the population. As with antibodies to many infectious agents, seropositivity increases with age and, in older age groups, approaches 50 to 80 percent of the population. There is no evidence that the geographic variation of the prevalence of infection is related to the known substantial geographic variations in coronary heart disease. It is unlikely that these infectious agents alone are the primary cause of coronary artery disease. However, in combination with other cardiovascular risk factors, the infectious agents may play an important role in both the early development of the atherosclerotic lesions and, most likely, in the progression of atherosclerosis to clinical disease such as myocardial infarction, unstable angina pectoris, sudden death, and possibly the incidence of stroke.

Kaposi's Sarcoma

Among the best recent examples of new methods to identify an infectious cause of a chronic disease is the identification of the likely infectious etiology of Kaposi's sarcoma (KS), a neoplasm commonly associated with HIV infection, renal transplantation, and certain ethnic populations.[46,47] The epidemiology of KS had long led investigators to conclude that this entity was due to an infectious etiology.[48] Several years ago, Chang and coworkers identified the DNA of a herpes virus in tissue from patients with KS by using a method called representational difference analysis (RDA).[49] This method is polymerase chain reaction–based and relies on identifying DNA in diseased tissue that is not present in healthy tissue from the same individual. Subsequently, the virus has been isolated and characterized as a herpes virus, commonly referred to as KS-associated herpesvirus (KSHV).[50]

As outlined above, the finding of an infectious agent in diseased tissue does not prove that it has a causative role in the disease. For example, based on extensive epidemiologic evidence, *Herpes simplex* virus type 2 was long thought to cause cervical carcinoma.[51] However, it is now clear that this virus is an innocent bystander and that human papilloma virus is the true etiologic agent.[52]

Substantial effort has gone into determining whether KSHV has a casual role in KS. Initial studies investigated the presence of KSHV in appropriate case and control tissues. These studies demonstrated that KSHV sequences were present in over 90 percent of KS tissues from AIDS patients, 15 percent of samples of non-KS tissue from AIDS patients, and none in tissue samples from patients without AIDS or KS.[49] In addition, KSHV has been found in all forms of non-AIDS–associated KS, indicating that this agent is not simply an opportunistic infection in HIV infection.[53,54]

Serologic studies have also helped clarify the role of KSHV in KS. For example, 80 percent of AIDS-associated KS patients were found to be positive for antibodies against KSHV antigens versus only 18 percent of homosexual men without KS.[55] In addition, no seropositives were found among a sample of blood donors and hemophilia-associated HIV-infected men without KS. Most importantly, seroconversion to KSHV was shown to predate the onset of KS lesions in over half of AIDS-associated KS patients.

More recent studies have focused on the biologic plausibility of KSHV having an etiologic role in KS. KSHV encodes multiple known oncoproteins and cytokines that play important roles in preventing apoptosis and promoting cell proliferation that may be involved in KS pathogenesis and related neoplastic disorders. However, a great deal of additional study is needed to carefully define the role, if any, of these proteins in the pathogenesis of KS (PS Moore, personal communication).[56–59]

The importance of infectious etiologies of chronic disease is now firmly established. It is likely, at least in the United States and other developed countries, that the contributions of infections to the etiology of so-called chronic diseases may have a greater impact on morbidity and mortality than classic infectious diseases. The infectious agents are not the only cause of the "chronic" disease. The interaction of the agent, infectious organism, host, genetic susceptibility, environment, diet, environmental chemicals, and psychosocial factors probably determine the incidence and natural history of specific diseases.

▸ REFERENCES

Overview

1. McKeown T: The Role of Medicine: Dream, Mirage, or Nemesis? Oxford: Basil Blackwell, 1979
2. Plotkin SA (ed): Vaccines. Philadelphia: WB Saunders, 1994
3. Imperato PJ: Smallpox and measles in Mali: contrasting control strategies and outcomes. Caduceus 12(1):61–72, 1996
4. Ransford HE, Palisi BJ: Aerobic exercise, subjective health and psychological well-being within age and gender subgroups. Soc Sci Med 42(11):1555–1559, 1996
5. Blair SN, Horton E, Leon AS et al: Physical activity, nutrition, and chronic disease. Med Sci Sports Exerc 28(3):335–349, 1996
6. Locke S: Mind and Immunity. New York: Praeger: Institute for the Advancement of Health, 1985
7. Watson JD: The human genome project: past, present and future. Science 248:44–48, 1990
8. Friedmann T: Human gene therapy—an immature genie, but certainly out of the bottle. Nat Med 2(2):144–147, 1996
9. Quinn RW: Streptococcal infections. In Evans AS, Feldman HA (eds). Bacterial Infections of Humans, Epidemiology and Control. New York: Plenum, 1982, pp 538–539
10. Knight V: Airborne transmission and pulmonary deposition of respiratory viruses. In Viral and Mycoplasma Infections of the Respiratory Tract. Philadelphia: Lea & Febiger, 1973, pp 1–9
11. Murphy FA: Problems in the surveillance and control of viral diseases with special reference to the developing world. Infect Agents Dis 4(4):171–177, 1995
12. Brouwers P, Hendricks M, Lietzau JA, et al: Effect of combination therapy with zidovudine and didanosine on neuropsychological functioning in patients with symptomatic HIV disease—a comparison of simultaneous and alternating regimens. AIDS 11(1):59–66, 1997
13. Centers for Disease Control: Update: universal precautions for prevention of transmission of human immunodeficiency virus, hepatitis B virus, and other bloodborne pathogens in health-care settings. MMWR 37(24):377–387, 1988
14. Dumler JS, Bakken JS: Human granulocytic ehrlichiosis in Wisconsin and Minnesota—a frequent infection with the potential for persistence. J Infect Dis 173(4):1027–1030, 1996
15. Collee JG, Bradley R: BSE—a decade on Part 2. Lancet 349(9053): 715–721, 1997
16. Relman AS: Assessment and accountability: the third revolution in medical care. N Engl J Med 319:1220–1222, 1988
17. McCoy TM: Brazil enlists DDT against malaria outbreak. World Watch 3:9–10, 1990
18. Anonymous: Cigarette smoking-attributable mortality and years of potential life lost—United States, 1990. MMWR 42(33):645–649, 1993
19. Anonymous: Years of potential life lost before age 65—United States, 1990 and 1991. MMWR 42(13):251–253, 1993
20. McGowan JE Jr: Success, failures and costs of implementing standards in the USA—lessons for infection control. J Hosp Infect 30:76–87, 1995

Emerging Infectious Diseases

1. Centers for Disease Control and Prevention: Summary of Notifiable Diseases, United States, 1995. MMWR 44(53):1–87, 1995
2. World Health Organization: World Health Report, 1995 Geneva: World Health Organization, 1996.
3. Pinner RW, Teutsch SM, Simonsen L, et al: Trends in infectious disease mortality in the United States. JAMA 275:189–193, 1996
4. Centers for Disease Control: Kaposi's Sarcoma and *Pneumocystis* pneumonia among homosexual men—New York City and California. MMWR 30:305–308, 1981
5. Centers for Disease Control and Prevention: HIV/AIDS surveillance report. Atlanta: US Department of Health and Human Services, Public Health Service 3–4, 30–33 (vol 8, No. 1), 1996
6. Institute of Medicine: Emerging infections: microbial threats to health in the United States. Washington, DC: National Academy Press, 1992
7. Centers for Disease Control: Measles outbreak—New York City, 1990–1991. MMWR 40:305–306, 1991
8. Snider DE, Roper WL: The new tuberculosis. N Engl J Med 326:703–705, 1992
9. Edlin BR, Tokars JI, Grieco MH, et al: An outbreak of multidrug-resistant tuberculosis among hospitalized patients with the acquired immunodeficiency syndrome. N Engl J Med 326:1514–1521, 1992
10. Osterholm MT, Birkhead GS, Meriwether RA: Impediments to public health surveillance in the 1990s: the lack of resources and the need for priorities. J Public Health Manag Pract 2:11–15, 1996
11. Griffin PM, Tauxe RV: The epidemiology of infections caused by *Escherichia coli* O157:H7, other enterohemorrhagic *E. coli*, and the associated hemolytic uremic syndrome. Epidemiol Rev 13:60–98, 1991
12. Bell BP, Goldoft M, Griffin PM, et al: A multistate outbreak of *Escherichia coli* O157: H7-associated bloody diarrhea and hemolytic uremic syndrome from hamburgers: the Washington experience. JAMA 272:1349–1353, 1994
13. MacKenzie WR, Hoxie NJ, Proctor ME, et al: A massive outbreak in Milwaukee of *Cryptosporidium* infection transmitted through the public water supply. N Engl J Med 331:161–167, 1994

14. Juranek DD: Cryptosporidiosis: sources of infection and guidelines for prevention. Clin Infect Dis 21(Suppl 1):S57–61, 1995
15. Centers for Disease Control and Prevention: Outbreak of acute illness—southwestern United States, 1993. MMWR 42:421–424, 1993
16. Duchin JS, Koster F, Peters CJ, et al: Hantavirus pulmonary syndrome: a clinical description of 17 patients with a newly recognized disease. N Engl J Med 330:949–955, 1994
17. Nichol ST, Spiropoulou CF, Morzunov S, et al: Genetic identification of a Hantavirus associated with an outbreak of acute respiratory disease. Science 262:914–917, 1993
18. Zaki SR, Greer PW, Coffield LM, et al: Hantavirus pulmonary syndrome: pathogenesis of an emerging infectious disease. Am J Pathol 146:552–579, 1995
19. Centers for Disease Control and Prevention: Hantavirus infection—southwestern United States. Interim recommendations for risk reduction. MMWR 42(RR-11):1–13, 1993
20. Zaki SR, Khan AS, Goodman RA, et al: Retrospective diagnosis of hantavirus pulmonary syndrome, 1978–1993: implications for emerging infectious diseases. Arch Pathol Lab Med 120:134–139, 1996
21. Khan AS, Khabbaz RF, Armstrong LR, et al: Hantavirus pulmonary syndrome: the first 100 U.S. cases. J Infect Dis 173:1297–1303, 1996
22. Hennessy TW, Hedberg CW, Slutsker L, et al: A national outbreak of *Salmonella enteritidis* infections from ice cream. N Engl J Med 334:1281–1286, 1996
23. Bean NH, Martin SM, Bradford H: PHLIS: an electronic system for reporting public health data from remote sites. Am J Public Health 82:1273–1276, 1992
24. Killalea D, Ward LR, Roberts D, et al: International epidemiologic and microbiologic study of outbreak of *Salmonella agona* from a ready to eat savoury snack—I: England and Wales and the United States. Br Med J 313:1105–1107, 1996
25. Mahon BE, Pönkä A, Hall WN, et al: An international outbreak of *Salmonella* infections caused by alfalfa sprouts grown from contaminated seeds. J Infect Dis 175:876–882, 1997
26. Herwaldt BL, Ackers ML, Cyclospora Working Group: An outbreak in 1996 of cyclosporiasis associated with imported raspberries. N Engl J Med 336:1548–1556, 1997
27. Centers for Disease Control and Prevention: Outbreak of *Escherichia coli* O157:H7 infections associated with drinking unpasteurized commercial apple juice—British Columbia, California, Colorado, and Washington, October 1996. MMWR 45:975, 1996
28. Department of Agriculture, Department of Health and Human Services, Environmental Protection Agency: Food safety from farm to table: a National Food-Safety initiative. Washington, DC, 1997
29. Steere AC, Malawista SE, Snydman DR, et al: Lyme arthritis: an epidemic of oligoarticular arthritis in children and adults in three Connecticut communities. Arthritis Rheum 20:7–17, 1977
30. Steer AC: Lyme disease. N Engl J Med 321:586–596, 1989
31. Maeda K, Markowitz N, Hawley RC, Ristic M, Cox D, McDade JE: Human infection with *Ehrlichia canis*, a leukocytic *Rickettsia*. N Engl J Med 316:853–856, 1987
32. Bakken JS, Dumler JS, Chen SM, Eckman MR, Van Etta LL, Walker DH: Human granulocytic ehrlichiosis in the upper Midwest United States: a new species emerging? JAMA 272:212–218, 1994
33. Dumler JS, Bakken JS: Ehrlichial diseases of humans: emerging tick-borne infections. Clin Infect Dis 20:1102–1110, 1995
34. Centers for Disease Control and Prevention: Human granulocytic ehrlichiosis—New York, 1995. MMWR 44:593–595, 1995
35. Centers for Disease Control and Prevention: Dengue fever at the U.S.—Mexico border, 1995–1996. MMWR 45:841–844, 1996
36. Layton M, Parise ME, Campbell CC, et al: Mosquito-transmitted malaria in New York City, 1993. Lancet 346:729–731, 1995
37. Centers for Disease Control and Prevention: Local transmission of *Plasmodium vivax* malaria—Houston, Texas, 1994. MMWR 44: 295–303, 1995
38. Centers for Disease Control and Prevention: Mosquito-transmitted malaria—Michigan, 1995. MMWR 45:398–400, 1996
39. Centers for Disease Control and Prevention: Probable locally acquired mosquito-transmitted *Plasmodium vivax* infection—Georgia, 1996. MMWR 46:264–267, 1996
39a. McFarland JM, Baddour LM, Nelson JE, et al: Imported yellow fever in a United States citizen. Clin Infect Dis 25:1143–1147, 1997
40. Krebs JW, Strine TW, Smith JS, Noah DL, Rupprecht CE, Childs JE: Rabies surveillance in the United States during 1995. J Am Vet Med Assoc 208:2031–2044, 1996
41. Centers for Disease Control and Prevention: Human rabies—Alabama, Tennessee, and Texas, 1994. MMWR 44:269–272, 1995
42. Centers for Disease Control and Prevention: Human rabies—Kentucky and Montana, 1996. MMWR 46:397–400, 1997
43. Tenover FC, Hughes JM: The challenges of emerging infectious diseases; development and spread of multiply-resistant bacterial pathogens. JAMA 275:300–304, 1996
44. Holmberg SD, Solomon SL, Blake PA: Health and economic impacts of antimicrobial resistance. Rev Infect Dis 9:1065–1078, 1987
45. Cohen ML: Epidemiology of drug resistance: implications for a post-antimicrobial era. Science 257:1050–1055, 1992
46. Frieden TR, Munsiff SS, Low DE: Emergence of vancomycin-resistant enterococci in New York City. Lancet 342:76–79, 1993
47. Centers for Disease Control and Prevention: Nosocomial enterococci resistant to vancomycin, United States, 1989–1993. MMWR 42: 597–599, 1993
47a. Centers for Disease Control and Prevention. Update: *Staphylococcus aureus* with reduced susceptibility to vancomycin-United States, 1997. MMWR 46:813–815, 1997
48. Breiman RF, Butler JC, Tenover FC, Elliott JA, Facklam RR: Emergence of drug-resistant pneumococcal infections in the United States. JAMA 271:1831–1835, 1994
49. Spika JS, Facklam RR, Plikaytis BD, Oxtoby MJ: Antimicrobial resistance of *Streptococcus pneumoniae* in the United States, 1979–1987. J Infect Dis 163:1273–1278, 1991
50. Butler JC, Hofmann J, Cetron MS, et al: The continued emergence of drug-resistant *Streptococcus pneumoniae* in the United States: an update from the Centers for Disease Control and Prevention's Pneumococcal Sentinel Surveillance System. J Infect Dis 174:986–993, 1996
51. Hofmann J, Cetron MS, Farley MM, et al: The prevalence of drug-resistant *Streptococcus pneumoniae* in Atlanta. N Engl J Med 333: 481–486, 1995
52. Tauxe RV, Mintz ED, Quick RE: Epidemic cholera in the New World: translating epidemiology into new prevention strategies. Emerg Infect Dis 1:141–146, 1995
53. Cholera Working Group: Large epidemic of cholera-like disease in Bangladesh caused by *Vibrio cholerae* O139 synonym Bengal. Lancet 342:387–390, 1993
54. Campbell GL, Hughes JM: Plague in India: a new warning from an old nemesis. Ann Intern Med 122:151–153, 1995
55. Butler JC, Kilmarx PH, Jernigan DB, Ostroff SM: Perspectives in fatal epidemics. Infect Dis Clin North Am 10:917–937, 1996
56. Georges-Courbot MC, Sanchez A, Lu CY, et al: Isolation and phylogenetic characterization of Ebola viruses causing different outbreaks in Gabon. Emerg Infect Dis 3:59–62, 1997
57. Brandling-Bennett AD, Pinheiro F: Infectious diseases in Latin America and the Caribbean: are they really emerging and increasing? Emerg Infect Dis 2:59–61, 1996
58. Will RG, Ironside JW, Zeidler M, et al: A new variant of Creutzfeldt-Jacob disease in the United Kingdom. Lancet 347:921–925, 1996
59. Wells RM, Estani SS, Yadon ZE, et al: An unusual hantavirus outbreak in southern Argentina; person-to-person transmission? Emerg Infect Dis 3:171–174, 1997
60. World Health Organization: Food safety, enterohaemorrhagic *Escherichia coli* infection. Wkly Epidemiol Rec 30:229–230, 1996
61. Fraser GC, Hooper PT, Lunt RA, et al: Encephalitis caused by a lyssavirus in fruit bats in Australia. Emerg Infect Dis 2:327–331, 1996

62. Rwaguma EB, Lutwama JJ, Sempala SDK, et al: Emergence of epidemic o'nyong-nyong fever in southerwestern Uganda, after an absence of 35 years. Emerg Infect Dis 3:77, 1997
63. Centers for Disease Control and Prevention: Addressing emerging infectious disease threats: a prevention strategy for the United States. Atlanta: Centers for Disease Control and Prevention, Public Health Service, US Department of Health and Human Services, 1994
64. Satcher D: Emerging infections: getting ahead of the curve. Emerg Infect Dis 1:1–6, 1995
65. Perkins BA, Flood JM, Danila R, et al: Unexplained deaths due to possibly infectious causes in the United States: defining the problem and the design of surveillance and laboratory approaches. Emerg Infect Dis 2:47–52, 1996
66. Committee on International Science, Engineering, and Technology (CISET): Report of the NTSC CISET Working Group on emerging and reemerging infectious diseases. Washington, DC: National Science and Technology Council, 1995
67. World Health Assembly: Communicable diseases prevention and control: new, emerging, and re-emerging infectious diseases. WHO Doc WHA 48.13, May 12, 1995
68. LeDuc JW: World Health Organization strategy for emerging infectious diseases. JAMA 275:3318–3320, 1996
69. World Health Assembly: Revision and updating of the International Health Regulations WHO Doc WHA 48.7, May 12, 1995

Health Advice for International Travel

1. Steffen R, Rickenbach M, Wilhelm U, et al: Health problems after travel to developing countries. J Infect Dis 156:84–91, 1987
2. Cossar JH, Reid D, Fallon RJ, et al: A cumulative review of studies on travellers, their experience of illness and the implications of these findings. J Infect 21:27–42, 1990
3. Hargarten SW, Baker TD, Guptill K: Overseas fatalities of United States citizen travellers: an analysis of deaths related to international travellers. Ann Emerg Med 20:622–626, 1991
4. Prociv P: Deaths of Australian travellers overseas. Med J Aust 163:27–30, 1995
5. Hill D: Immunizations. Infect Dis Clin North Am 6:291–312, 1992
6. ACP Task Force on Adult Immunization and Infectious Diseases Society of America: Guide for Adult Immunization. 2nd ed. Philadelphia: American College of Physicians, 1990
7. Advisory Committee on Immunization Practices (ACIP), Centers for Disease Control. *General recommendations on immunization.* MMWR 43(Suppl):1–86, 1994
8. Centers for Disease Control: Health Information for International Travel. Atlanta: U.S. Dept. of Health and Human Services, Public Health Service, 1995. HHS Publication No. (CDC) 95-8280
9. Snyder JD, Blake PA: Is cholera a problem for U.S. travelers? JAMA 247:2268–2269, 1982
10. Arya SC: Cholera and typhoid vaccines: a review of current status. Clin Immunother 6:28–38, 1996
11. Karzon DT, Edwards KM: Diphtheria outbreaks in immunized populations. N Eng J Med 318:41–43, 1988
12. Steffen R, Kane MA, Shapiro CN, et al: Epidemiology and prevention of hepatitis A in travelers. JAMA 272:885–889, 1994
13. Centers for Disease Control: Hepatitis surveillance. MMWR 51(suppl):1–26, 1987
14. Clemens R, Safary A, Hepburn A, et al: Clinical experience with an inactivated hepatitis A vaccine. J Infect Dis 171(suppl 1):S44–49, 1995
15. Nalin DR: VAQTA, Hepatitis A vaccine, purified, inactivated. Drugs Future 20:24–29, 1995
16. Steffen R: Risk of hepatitis B for travellers vaccine. 8:31–32, 1990
17. Steffen R, Lobel HO: Epidemiologic basis for the practice of travel medicine. J Wilderness Med 5:56–66, 1994
18. Centers for Disease Control: Inactivated Japanese Encephalitis Virus Vaccine. Recommendations of the Advisory Committee on Immunization Practices (ACIP). MMWR 42:(RR-1)1–15, 1993
19. Hoffman SL: Diagnosis, treatment and prevention of malaria. Med Clin North Am 76:1327–1355, 1992
20. Lobel HO: Malaria and the use of prevention measures among United States travelers. In Steffen R, Lobel HO, Haworth J, Bradley OJ (eds): Travel Medicine. Berlin: Springer-Verlag, 1989 pp 81–89
21. Gupta RK, Rutledge LC: Role of repellents in vector control and disease prevention. Am J Trop Med Hyg 50(suppl)82–86, 1994
22. Choi HW, Breman JG, Teutsch SM: The effectiveness of insecticide-impregnated bed nets in reducing malaria infection: a meta-analysis of published results. Am J Trop Med Hyg 52:337–382, 1995
23. Steffen R, Heusser R, Mächler R: Malaria chemoprophylaxis among European tourists in tropical Africa: use, adverse effects and efficacy. Bull World Health Organ 68:313–322, 1990
24. Phillips-Howard PA, terKuile F: CNS adverse events associated with antimalarial drugs. Drug Safety 12:370–383, 1995
25. Phillips-Howard PA, West LJ: Severe adverse drug reactions to pyrimethamine-sulphadoxine, pyrimethamine-dapsone and to amodiaquine in Britain. J R Soc Med 83:82–85, 1990
26. Baird JK, Fryauff DJ, Basri H, et al: Primaquine for prophylaxis against malaria among non-immune transmigrants in Irian Jaya, Indonesia. Am J Trop Med Hyg 52:479–484, 1995
27. Fryauff DJ, Baird JK, Basri H, et al: Randomised placebo-controlled trial of primaquine for prophylaxis of falciparum and vivax malaria. Lancet 346:1190–1193, 1995
28. Steffen R: Epidemiologic studies of travelers' diarrhea, severe gastrointestinal infections and cholera. Rev Infect Dis 8(suppl 1): S122–S130, 1986
29. Steffen R, Boppart I: Travellers' diarrhea. Baillieres Clin Gastroenterol 1:361–376, 1987
30. Gorbach SL: Travelers' diarrhea. N Engl J Med 307:881–883, 1982
31. Kozicki M, Steffen R, Schär M: "Boil it, Peel it, Cook it or Forget it." Does this rule prevent travelers' diarrhea? Int J Epidemiol 14: 169–172, 1985
32. Gorbach SL, Carpetier CC, Graysion R, et al: Consensus Development Conference Statement. Rev Infect Dis 8(suppl 2):S227–S233, 1986
33. DuPont H, Khan FM: Travelers' diarrhea: epidemiology, microbiology, prevention and therapy. J Trav Med 1:84–93, 1994
34. Petrucelli BP, Murphy GS, Sanchez JL, et al: Treatment of travelers' diarrhea with ciprofloxacin and loperamide. J Infect Dis 165: 558–560, 1992
35. Salam I, Katelaris P, Leigh-Smith S, et al: Randomized trial of single dose ciprofloxacin for travellers' diarrhoea. Lancet 334: 1537–1539, 1994
36. Kuschner RA, Trofa AF, Thomas RJ, et al: Use of azithromycin for the treatment of *Campylobacter* enteritis in travelers to Thailand, an area where ciprofloxacin resistance is prevalent. Clin Infect Dis 21:536–541, 1995
37. Taylor DN: Quinolones as chemoprophylactic agents for travelers' diarrhea. J Trav Med 1:119–121, 1994
38. DuPont HL: Travelers' diarrhea: which antimicrobial? Drugs 6: 910–917, 1993
39. Wilson ME, von Reyn CF, Fineberg HV: Infections in HIV-infected travelers: risks and prevention. Ann Intern Med 114:582–592, 1991
40. Bia FJ: Medical considerations for the pregnant traveler. Infect Dis Clin North Am 6:371–388, 1992
41. Barry M: Medical considerations for international travel with infants and older children. Infect Dis Clin North Am 6:389–404, 1992
42. Bia FJ, Barry M: Special health considerations for travelers. Med Clin North Am 76:1295–1312, 1992

Infectious and Chronic Disease Epidemiology: The Distinction Wanes

1. Norden CW, Kuller LH: Identifying infectious etiologies of chronic disease. Rev Infect Dis 6:200–213, 1984
2. Stolley PD, Lasky T: Investigating Disease Patterns. The Science of Epidemiology. New York: Scientific American Library, 1995

3. Evans AS: Causation and Disease: A Chronological Journey. New York: Plenum, 1993
4. Comstock GW: An epidemiologic study of blood pressure levels in a biracial community in the southern United States. Am J Epidemiol 141:584–628, 1995
5. The Surgeon General's Advisory Committee on Smoking and Health: Smoking and Health. Report of the Advisory Committee to the Surgeon General of the Public Health Service. US Department of Health, Education and Welfare. 1964. Public Health Service Publication No. 1103
6. Tsukuma H, Hiyama T, Tanaka S, Nakao M, Yabuuchi T, Kitamura T, Nakanishi K, Fujimoto I, Inoue A, Yamazaki H, Kawashima T. Risk factors for hepatocellular carcinoma among patients with chronic liver disease. N Engl J Med 328:1797–1801, 1993
7. Evans AS, Mueller NE: Viruses and cancer. Causal associations. Ann Epidemiol 1:71–92, 1990
8. Yoshida M, Miyoshi I, Hinuma Y: Isolation and characterization of retrovirus from cell lines of human adult T-cell leukemia and its implication in the disease. Proc Natl Acad Sci USA 79:2031–2035, 1982
9. Poiesz BJ, Ruscetti FW, Gazdar AF, Bunn PA, Minna JD, Gallo RC: Detection and isolation of type-C retrovirus particles from fresh and cultured lymphocytes of patients with cutaneous T-cell lymphoma. Proc Natl Acad Sci USA 77:7415–7419, 1980
10. Mobley HLT: Defining *Helicobacter pylori* as a pathogen: strain heterogeneity and virulence. Am J Med 100:2S–11S, 1996
11. NIH Consensus Development Panel on *Helicobacter pylori* in Peptic Ulcer Disease: *Helicobacter pylori* in peptic ulcer disease. JAMA 272:65–69, 1994
12. Will RG, Ironside JW, Zeidler M, et al: A new variant of Creutzfeldt-Jacob disease in the U.K. Lancet 347:921–925, 1996
13. Hsich G, Kenney K, Gibbs CJ Jr, Lee KH, Harrington MG: The 14-3-3 brain protein in cerebrospinal fluid as a marker for transmissible spongiform encephalopathies. N Engl J Med 335:924–930, 1996
14. Lorber B: Are all diseases infectious? Ann Intern Med 125:844–851, 1996
15. Gao SJ, Moore PS: Molecular approaches to the identification of unculturable infectious agents. Emerg Infect Dis 2:159–167, 1996
16. Relman DA, Loutit JS, Schmidt TM, Falkow S, Tompkins LS: The agent of bacillary angiomatosis. An approach to the identification of uncultured pathogens. N Engl J Med 323:1573–1580, 1990
17. Regnery RL, Tappero J: Unravelling the mysteries associated with cat-scratch disease, bacillary angiomatosis, and related syndromes. Emerging Infectious Diseases 1:16–21, 1995
18. Choo QL, Kuo G, Weiner AJ, Overby LR, Bradley DW, Houghton M: Isolation of a cDNA clone derived from a blood-borne non-A, non-B viral hepatitis genome. Science 244:359–362, 1989
19. Jackson, LA, Hildson R, Farley MM, Harrison LH, Reingold AL, Plikaytis BD, Wenger JD, Schuchat A: Risk factors for B streptococcal disease in adults. Ann Intern Med 123:415–420, 1995
20. Lopes-Virella MF, Virella G: Immunological and microbiological factors in the pathogenesis of atherosclerosis. Clin Immunol Immunopathol 37:377–386, 1985
21. Buja LM: Does atherosclerosis have an infectious etiology? Circulation 94:872–873, 1996
22. Penttinen J, Valonen P: The risk of myocardial infarction among Finnish farmers seeking medical care for an infection. Am J Public Health 86:1440–1442, 1996
23. Libby P, Geng YJ, Aikawa M, Schoenbeck U, Mach F, Clinton SK, Sukhova GK, Lee RT: Macrophages and atherosclerotic plaque stability. Curr Opin Lipidol 7:330–335, 1996
24. Belch JJF: The relationship between white blood cells and arterial disease. Curr Opin Lipidol 5:440–446, 1994
25. Kuller LH, Tracy RP, Shaten J, Meilahn EN for the MRFIT Research Group: Relation of c-reactive protein and coronary heart disease in the MRFIT nested case-control study. Am J Epidemiol 144:537–547, 1996
26. Liuzzo G, Biasucci LM, Gallimore JR, et al: The prognostic value of c-reactive protein and serum amyloid A protein in severe unstable angina. N Engl J Med 331:417–424, 1994
27. Ernst E: Fibrinogen as a cardiovascular risk factor—interrelationship with infections and inflammation. Eur Heart J 14:82–87, 1993
28. Biasucci LM, Vitelli A, Liuzzo G, Altamura S, Caligiuri G, Monaco C, Rebuzzi AG, Ciliberto G, Maseri A: Elevated levels of interleukin-6 in unstable angina. Circulation 94:874–877, 1996
29. Beck J, Garcia R, Heiss G, Vokonas PS, Offenbacher S: Periodontal disease and cardiovascular disease. J Periodontol 67:1123–1137, 1996
30. Brunner E, Smith GD, Marmot M, Canner R, Beksinska M, O'Brien J: Childhood social circumstances and psychosocial and behavioural factors as determinants of plasma fibrinogen. Lancet 347:1008–1013, 1996
31. Zhou YF, Leon MB, Waclawiw MA, Popma J, Yu ZX, Finkel T, Epstein SE: Association between prior cytomegalovirus infection and the risk of restenosis after coronary atherectomy. N Engl J Med 335:624–630, 1996
32. Speir E, Modali R, Huang E-S, Leon MB, Shawl F, Finkel T, Epstein SE: Potential role of human cytomegalovirus and p53 interaction in coronary restenosis. Science 265:391–393, 1994
33. Epstein SE, Zhou YF, Guetta E, Leon M, Finkel T: The role of infection in restenosis and atherosclerosis: focus on cytomegalovirus. Lancet 348:s13–17, 1996
34. Grattan MT, Moreno-Cabral CE, Starnes VA, Oyer PE, Stinson EB, Shumway NE: Cytomegalovirus infection is associated with cardiac allograft rejection and atherosclerosis. JAMA 261:3561–3566, 1989
35. Nieto FJ, Adam E, Sorlie P, Farzadegan H, Melnick JL, Comstock GW, Szklo M: Cohort study of cytomegalovirus infection as a risk factor for carotid intimal-medial thickening, a measure of subclinical atherosclerosis. Circulation 94:922–927, 1996
36. Sorlie PD, Adams E, Melnick SL, Folsom A, Skelton T, Chambless LE, Barnes R, Melnick JL: Cytomegalovirus/herpesvirus and carotid atherosclerosis: the ARIC Study. J Med Virol 42:33–37, 1994
37. Adam E, Melnick JL, Probtsfeld JL, Petrie BL, Burek J, Bailey KR, McCollum CH, DeBakey ME: High level of cytomegalovirus antibody in patients requiring vascular surgery for atherosclerosis. Lancet 2:291–293, 1987
38. Grayston JT: *Chlamydia pneumonia*, strain TWAR pneumonia. Annu Rev Med 43:317–323, 1992
39. Grayston JT, Kuo C-C, Coulson AS, Campbell LA, Lawrence RD, Lee MJ, Strandness ED, Wang S-P: *Chlamydia pneumonia* (TWAR) in atherosclerosis of the carotid artery. Circulation 92:3397–3400, 1995
40. Muhlestein JB, Hammond EH, Carlquist JF, Radicke E, Thomson MJ, Karagounis LA, Woods ML, Anderson JL: Increased incidence of *Chlamydia* species within the coronary arteries of patients with symptomatic atherosclerotic versus other forms of cardiovascular disease. J Am Coll Cardiol 27:1555–1561, 1996
41. Thorn DH, Grayston JT, Siscovick DS, Wang S-P, Weiss NS, Daling JR: Association of prior infection with *Chlamydia pneumoniae* and angiographically demonstrated coronary artery disease. JAMA 268:68–72, 1992
42. Saikku P, Leinonen M, Tenkanen L, Linnanmäki E, Ekman M-R, Manninen V, Mänttäri M, Frick MH, Huttunen JK: Chronic *Chlamydia pneumoniae* infection as a risk factor for coronary heart disease in the Helsinki Heart Study. Ann Intern Med 116:273–278, 1992
43. Scragg RKR, Fraser A, Metcalf PA: *Helicobacter pylori* seropositivity and cardiovascular risk factors in a multicultural workforce. J Epidemiol Commun Health 50:578–579, 1996
44. Patel P, Mendall MA, Carrington D, Strachan DP, Leatham E, Molineaux N, Levy J, Blakeston C, Seymour CA, Camm AJ, Northfield TC: Association of *Helicobacter pylori* and *Chlamydia pneumoniae* infections with coronary heart disease and cardiovascular risk factors. Br Med J 311:711–714, 1995

45. Lip GYH, Wise R, Beevers G: Association of *Helicobacter pylori* infection with coronary heart disease. Study shows association between *H. pylori* infection and hypertension [Letter]. Br Med J 312:250–251, 1996
46. DiGiovanna JJ, Safai B: Kaposi's sarcoma. Retrospective study of 90 cases with particular emphasis on the familial occurrence, ethnic background and prevalence of other diseases. Am J Med 71: 779–783, 1981
47. Safai B, Johnson KG, Myskowski PL, Koziner B, Yang SY, Cunningham-Rundles S, Godbold JH, Dupont B: The natural history of Kaposi's sarcoma in the acquired immunodeficiency syndrome. Ann Intern Med 103:744–750, 1985
48. Beral V, Peterman TA, Berkelman RL, Jaffe HW: Kaposi's sarcoma among persons with AIDS: a sexually transmitted infection? Lancet 335:123–128, 1990
49. Chang Y, Cesarman E, Pessin MS, Lee F, Culpepper J, Knowles DM, Moore PS: Identification of herpesvirus-like DNA sequences in AIDS-associated Kaposi's sarcoma. Science 265:1865–1869, 1994
50. Moore PS, Gao S-J, Dominguez G, Cesarman E, Lungu O, Knowles DM, Garber R, Pellett PE, McGeoch DJ, Chang Y: Primary characterization of a herpesvirus-like agent associated with Kaposi's sarcoma. J Virol 70:549–558, 1996
51. Pacsa AS, Kummerländer L, Pejtsik B, Pall K: Herpesvirus antibodies and antigens in patients with cervical anaplasia and in controls. J Natl Cancer Inst 55:775–781, 1975
52. Lungu O, Sun XW, Felix J, Richart RM, Silverstein S, Wright TC Jr: Relationship of human papillomavirus type to grade of cervical intraepithelial neoplasia. JAMA 267:2493–2496, 1992
53. Moore PS, Chang Y: Detection of herpesvirus-like DNA sequences in Kaposi's sarcoma in patients with and without HIV infection. N Engl J Med 332:1181–1185, 1995
54. Dupin N, Grandadam M, Calvez V, Gorin I, Aubin JT, Havard S, Lamy F, Leibowitch M, Huraux JM, Escande JP: Herpesvirus-like DNA sequences in patients with Mediterranean Kaposi's sarcoma. Lancet 345:761–762, 1995
55. Gao SJ, Kingsley L, Hoover DR, Spira TJ, Rinaldo CR, Saah A, Phair J, Detels R, Parry P, Chang Y, Moore PS: Seroconversion to antibodies against Kaposi's sarcoma-associated herpesvirus-related latent nuclear antigens before the development of Kaposi's sarcoma. N Engl J Med 335:233–241, 1996
56. Chang Y, Moore PS, Talbot SJ, Boshoff CH, Zarkowska T, Goddenkent D, Paterson H, Weiss RA, Mittnacht S: Cyclin encoded by KS herpesvirus. Nature 382:410, 1996
57. Cesarman E, Nador RG, Bai F, Bohenzky RA, Russo JJ, Moore PS, Chang Y, Knowles DM: Kaposi's sarcoma-associated herpesvirus contains G protein-coupled receptor and cyclin D homologs which are expressed in Kaposi's sarcoma and malignant lymphoma. J Virol 70:8218–8223, 1996
58. Russo JJ, Bohenzky RA, Chien M-C, Chen J, Yan M, Maddalena D, Parry JP, Peruzzi D, Edelman IS, Chang Y, Moore PS: Nucleotide sequence of the Kaposi sarcoma-associated herpesvirus (HHV8). Proc Natl Acad Sci USA 93:14862–14867, 1996
59. Moore PS, Boshoff C, Weiss RA, Chang Y: Molecular mimicry of human cytokine and cytokine response pathway genes by KSHV. Science, 274:1739–1744, 1996

7

Diseases Controlled Primarily by Vaccination

Measles

Walter A. Orenstein • Stephen C. Redd • Lauri E. Markowitz • Alan R. Hinman

Measles has been recognized as a distinct clinical disease for more than 10 centuries and in the developing world is associated with high mortality rates in early childhood. The epidemiology of measles is markedly affected by population size, density, movement, and social behavior. In the absence of vaccination, the disease infects essentially everyone at some time during life except in isolated populations. Beginning in 1963 the availability and increasing use of live attenuated measles vaccines have made prevention possible. Countries in the Americas and Europe have undertaken the elimination of measles.[1,2]

Measles is one of the most contagious of infectious diseases. Mathematical models suggest that in a totally susceptible population the average case of measles may result in transmission of measles to 12 to 18 persons.[3] Thus it is estimated that the immunity level needed to interrupt transmission is on the order of 94 percent or higher. Contact rates vary substantially by age group and affect the age-specific level of immunity needed to prevent transmission. Although a vaccination coverage rate of 80 percent has been found adequate to prevent transmission in some preschool-aged populations, sustained transmission has been documented in school-age populations with 96 percent immunity levels, documented by serology.[4,5] Although high levels of immunity substantially reduce the likelihood that susceptible persons within a population will be exposed to disease, there is no level of immunity short of 100 percent that will absolutely guarantee absence of transmission.

Clinical Characteristics

Following an incubation period averaging 10 to 12 days (range, 8 to 16 days) the patient typically has fever and malaise, followed shortly thereafter by cough, coryza, and conjunctivitis.[6] An enanthem, characterized by small bluish-white spots on a red background (Koplik's spots), may be seen on the buccal mucosa within the 2 days before and after the onset of rash. The characteristic maculopapular rash of measles usually appears an average of 14 days after infection begins and typically 2 to 4 days after the onset of the prodromal symptoms. The exanthem classically starts on the face and hairline and then spreads to the trunk and extremities. The patient's temperature usually peaks 1 to 3 days following the onset of rash. The rash, areas of which fade in order of appearance, typically lasts 5 to 7 days, and the illness is entirely gone by 10 to 14 days after the onset of symptoms. Clinically apparent primary infections are the rule.

The patient is infectious during the prodromal period and for the first few days of rash. The infectious period is usually considered to stretch from 4 days before to 4 days after the onset of rash. Measles is usually transmitted in large respiratory droplets, requiring close contact between patients and susceptible persons. However, measles virus can survive for at least 2 hours in fine droplets, and airborne spread has been documented.[7,8] Neither a long-term infectious carrier state nor an animal reservoir is known.

Complications

The risk of complications and death is highest in young children and adults. The most common complications of measles are otitis media and pneumonia, which occur in 5 to 9 percent and in 1 to 6 percent of cases, respectively. Pneumonia, the most common cause of death, may be caused by the measles virus itself or by secondary bacterial infection.[9] These complications frequently require specific antibiotic therapy. Secondary viral infections may play a prominent role in measles pneumonia-related deaths in the developing world.[10] Severe diarrhea and malnutrition may result from measles infection, particularly in the developing world.[11] A substantial proportion of patients in less developed countries who survive during the first month after measles succumb during the ensuing year.[12]

Measles encephalitis, which occurs typically 4 to 7 days after the onset of rash (range, generally 1 to 15 days), is reported approximately once in every 1,000 cases of measles, but since cases tend to be more underreported than the deaths, the true death to case ratio is probably lower.[13] Approximately 15 percent of patients with measles encephalitis die, and another 25 to 35 percent have permanent neurologic residua. Less common complications include bronchiolitis, sinusitis, mastoiditis, myocarditis, keratoconjunctivitis, mesenteric adenitis, hepatitis, and thrombocytopenic purpura. In the United States, the reported death-to-case ratio has been 1 to 3 deaths per 1000 cases. In contrast, the death-to-case ratio in the developing world, particularly where malnutrition and crowding are common, frequently ranges from 5 to 10 percent or higher.[14]

Atypical measles syndrome, characterized by high fever, pneumonia, pleural effusions, edema of the hands and feet, hepatic abnormalities, and an unusual rash, is a rare manifestation of measles infection sometimes seen in persons who received killed measles vaccine in the past and who were subsequently exposed to measles virus. An estimated 600,000 to 900,000 persons in the United States received the killed vaccine between 1963 and 1967.

Measles infection during pregnancy is associated with spontaneous abortion and with delivery of low-birth weight infants.[15] Although there have been rare reports of congenital malformations associated with measles infection during the first trimester, there is no good evidence for the existence of a congenital measles syndrome.

In addition to the acute complications noted above, approximately once in every 100,000 cases, measles virus can cause a degenerative disorder of the central nervous system known as subacute sclerosing panencephalitis (SSPE).[16] This illness begins insidiously an average of 7 years following the initial infection and is characterized by progressively severe personality changes, myoclonic seizures, motor impairment, coma, and death over the course of several months to years. There is no convincing evidence of a causal association between measles and multiple sclerosis.

Occurrence

Prevaccine Period. Before the introduction and widespread use of measles vaccine, measles infection was essentially universal in the United States. Approximately 95 percent of persons living in urban areas were infected by age 15 years.[17] The disease typically appeared in cycles, with major peaks every 2 to 3 years. A marked seasonal pattern was apparent, with peaks during the late spring months. The highest reported age-specific incidence rates were in children 5 to 9 years old. In the decade from 1950 to 1959, an annual average of more than 500,000 cases was reported. The true number of infections was estimated to be nearly 10 times as high. During the same period, nearly 500 measles deaths were recorded each year.

Postvaccine Period. The licensure and widespread use of live virus vaccine, beginning in 1963, have brought about both a dramatic reduction in the reported occurrence of measles and a substantial alteration in its epidemiologic characteristics. By 1968 the reported level dropped by 95 percent, reaching a low of 22,231 cases (Fig. 7-1). Between 1968 and 1978 the reported occurrences varied from a low of 22,094 cases to a high of 75,290 cases. In 1978 an effort began to eliminate indigenous measles in the United States. Between 1981 and 1988, reported measles incidence averaged about 3,100 cases annually, ranging from a low of 1,497 cases in 1983 to a high of 6,282 in 1986.[18] Between 1989 and 1991, the United States experienced a resurgence of measles, peaking in 1990 with 27,786 cases and 64 deaths. During the 3-year period 55,622 cases, 11,252 hospitalizations, and 123 deaths were reported. The epidemic disproportionately affected members of racial and ethnic minority groups and children living in inner cities.[19] The major cause was failure to achieve high levels of immunization coverage during the second year of life, with measles coverage in 2-year-old children in some cities as low as 52 percent.[19,20]

Since the mid-1980s in the United States, three major patterns of measles transmission have been identified: preschool, school, and college.[21] The preschool pattern consists of high proportions of cases in unvaccinated preschoolers (primarily in the inner cities), many of whom are younger than the routine age for measles vaccination. In the school-age pattern, the majority of patients generally have histories of receipt of at least one dose of measles vaccine. In the larger outbreaks among school-age children, up to 90 percent of patients have histories of vaccination on or after the first birthday. Most of these vaccine failures are thought to result from an initial seroconversion failure (primary vaccine failure), although in some cases seroconversion may have occurred but immunity was lost later (secondary vaccine failure).[22] Characteristics of college outbreaks are similar to school-age outbreaks.

After 1991, reported measles incidence declined dramatically, with fewer than 1,000 cases annually since 1993. A record low of 309 cases was set in 1995. Indigenous measles transmission appears to have been interrupted in 1993. No indigenous cases were reported for 6 consecutive weeks. Further, analysis of the gene sequences of the hemagglutinin (H) and nucleoprotein (N) genes of measles viruses isolated in the United States since 1993 documented that they are significantly different from strains circulating between 1989 and 1992 and that they are related to strains isolated elsewhere in the world.[23] All measles in the United States today is believed to be due to recent international importations.

Recent outbreaks have also been reported among religious groups opposed to vaccination and in noninstitutionalized community settings involving multiple age groups, especially young adults. The latter outbreaks tend to be small.

Etiologic Agent, Immunology, and Diagnosis

Measles is caused by a single-stranded RNA virus of the paramyxovirus group. It is very sensitive to acid conditions, drying, and light, but can survive well in aerosolized droplets. Three membrane proteins appear to play critical roles in the pathogenesis. The hemagglutinin protein (H), which projects from the virion, attaches to cell surfaces. The fusion (F) protein allows cell-to-cell spread. Finally, the matrix (M) protein, associated with the inner surface of the viral envelope, appears to be important for successful generation of intact viral particles. Abnormalities in the synthesis of these proteins have been postulated to play an important role in the pathogenesis of SSPE.[24]

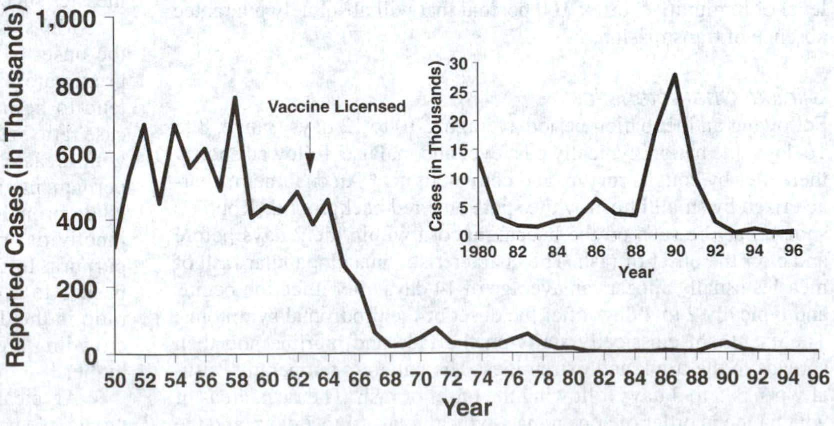

Figure 7-1. Reported measles cases, United States, 1950–1989 (1989 provisional data).

Measles virus infection induces the production of a variety of antibodies. The most frequently used assays to detect measles antibodies include enzyme immunoassay (EIA), neutralization (Nt), hemagglutination inhibition (HI), and immunofluorescence (IF). Antibodies identified with Nt and HI tests tend to appear with rash onset and peak 2 to 4 weeks later.[25] In the absence of re-exposure with subclinical reinfection and titer boosts, HI antibodies, measured by standard assays (screening dilution 1:8 to 1:10) persist in approximately 85 percent of patients for at least 16 years.[26] Nt testing is laborious and generally confined to research settings. HI testing requires a supply of monkey erythrocytes. Because of the widespread availability and ease of use, EIA tests are increasingly being used to detect measles antibodies. EIA tests have been developed to measure IgM and IgG. Persons who have lost detectable antibody by EIA or HI usually have measurable antibody detectable by more sensitive Nt tests. IgM antibodies are detectable in approximately 80 percent of cases within the first 72 hours after rash onset and in nearly 100 percent of cases thereafter.[27] IgM antibodies peak between 7 and 14 days after rash onset and decline to undetectable levels approximately 1 to 2 months later. Immunity following measles disease appears to be lifelong.

Measles virus can be cultured from respiratory secretions or urine, but the clinical diagnosis is more easily confirmed by documenting IgM antibodies in a single serum specimen or a significant rise in antibody in paired serum specimens. A radioimmunoassay to detect IgM in saliva has been developed in the United Kingdom and is routinely used to confirm measles there. Sensitivity is 92 percent and specificity is 98 percent for the saliva assay compared with serologic testing as the "gold standard."[28] Recent developments in isolating measles virus, using the marmoset lymphocyte B95a cell line, and in automated processes to determine the genetic sequence of the measles virus proteins have brought the tools of molecular epidemiology to measles control efforts.[23] Using these techniques, different lineages of measles virus have been identified, allowing the source of outbreaks often to be determined. Obtaining viral isolates from each chain of transmission and each isolated measles case is recommended.

Immunization

Passive Immunity. Passive immunity against measles disease can be induced by the administration of commercially prepared immune globulin (IG) (formerly called immune serum globulin [ISG]), which typically has a high measles antibody titer. Administration of 0.25 mL of IG per kilogram (maximum dose, 15 mL) can modify or prevent the development of measles in the exposed person.[29] The IG preparation is most effective if administered within 6 days of exposure, preferably as soon after the exposure as possible. IG is particularly indicated for susceptible household contacts, especially those who are immunocompromised. Persons in the latter groups are at greatest risk of complications from measles.

Almost all infants acquire passive immunity against measles from the transfer of maternal antibodies across the placenta. Such infants are usually immune to measles for at least the first 6 months of life. Immunity gradually wanes thereafter, and by 12 to 15 months essentially 100 percent of infants are susceptible. Children born to younger mothers who presumably have vaccine-induced antibodies tend to become seronegative earlier than infants born to older mothers who have had natural infection.[30] Natural infection induces higher levels of antibodies than measles vaccines.

"Modified" measles is a mild form of illness occasionally seen in persons with passively acquired antibody. The incubation period may be prolonged up to 20 days. Immunity after modified measles is believed to be permanent.

Active Immunity. In 1963, two types of measles vaccine were licensed in the United States. One was a vaccine prepared from live attenuated virus grown in chick embryo tissue culture (Edmonston B strain). Because there was a high rate of reactions to this vaccine, including fever, rash, and catarrhal symptoms, the concomitant administration of IG was recommended.[29]

A second vaccine used the same virus, but the virus had been inactivated (killed) by formaldehyde. Immunity to the killed measles virus vaccine (KMV), or to KMV followed by live measles vaccine within 3 months, was short lived and induced hypersensitivity to measles virus in some persons, resulting in atypical measles syndrome (see above).

Beginning in 1965, vaccines prepared from further attenuated strains of measles virus and not requiring the concomitant administration of IG became available and quickly became the most common vaccines in use in the United States (Schwarz strain, licensed in 1965, and Moraten strain, licensed in 1968). From 1963 through 1996 more than 294 million doses of live measles vaccines have been distributed in the United States.

The age at which measles vaccine is administered represents a balance between the ability of the vaccinee to respond to vaccination and the risk of measles. The proportion of vaccine recipients who developed antibodies to measles virus is inversely related to the age at administration up to 15 months of age, presumably because of the persistence of passively acquired maternal antibodies in the infant and young child.[31] Infants born to mothers whose immunity is secondary to vaccination have lower antibody levels at birth and become seronegative at an earlier age than infants born to mothers with natural infection.[30] When measles vaccine was first introduced, it was administered at 9 months of age because of the high risk of measles, even though seroconversion rates were not optimal. As the risk of measles declined, the age at administration was raised to 12 months (1965) and 15 months (1976) to ensure maximal seroconversion rates. Recent studies, performed when an increasing proportion of infants are born to mothers with vaccine-induced immunity, indicate seroconversion rates at 12 months are comparable to rates at 15 months.[32] Thus, in 1994 the Advisory Committee on Immunization Practices (ACIP) recommended that the first dose of measles vaccine as part of measles, mumps, rubella (MMR) could be administered any time between 12 and 15 months of age.[33] Earlier administration is particularly important in inner cities where children might be exposed at earlier ages than in other settings. Administration of further attenuated live measles vaccine to children at 12 to 15 months of age or older can be expected to produce measurable circulating antibodies in 95 percent or more of recipients.[26] During measles outbreaks, vaccine can be given to children as young as 6 months of age with subsequent revaccination. The vast majority of persons with seroconversion have long-term, probably lifelong, immunity, although waning immunity may occur in a small percentage.[22]

Measles vaccine is indicated for all persons without contraindications who are at least 12 months of age, who were born after 1956, and who lack documented proof of the receipt of live measles vaccine on or after the first birthday, proof of physician-diagnosed measles, or laboratory evidence of immunity.[29] Whenever such proof is lacking, persons should be vaccinated. Vaccination causes no harm if the person is already immune to measles.

Because measles transmission had been documented among the 2 to 5 percent of persons who did not respond to a first dose of measles vaccine, in 1989 both the Committee on Infectious Diseases of the American Academy of Pediatrics (AAP) and the ACIP recommended a change from a one-dose schedule to a routine two-dose schedule for measles vaccination.[29,34] The two-dose schedule was generally implemented in one age group at a time, although some localities elected to revaccinate multiple age groups to achieve more rapidly the goal of vaccinating all school children with two doses. The ACIP has established a goal of ensuring that all children from kindergarten through 12th grade receive a second dose of measles-containing vaccine by 2001.[35] In addition to routine revaccination at entry to kindergarten or first grade, all children should be checked at the adolescent visit at 11 to 12 years of age to ensure they have received a second dose. Both recommended doses should be combined measles-mumps-rubella vaccine (MMR). The primary purpose of the second dose is to induce immunity in persons who failed to mount an adequate immune response to the first dose. Waning of vaccine-induced immunity, while documented, appears to play only a limited role in sustaining measles transmission among vaccine failures.[22] Approximately 95 percent of persons who failed to respond to the first dose make a primary immune response, characterized by IgM antibody, following a second dose.[36]

Both the AAP and the ACIP recommend that college entrants document having received two doses of measles vaccine or provide other evidence of measles immunity (i.e., documented prior physician-diagnosed measles or laboratory evidence of immunity). In addition, in controlling school-based outbreaks, both groups recommend that school-age persons and school staff at risk be revaccinated if they have not previously received two doses of live vaccine on or after the first birthday or do not have other evidence of measles immunity.

Fever of 103°F (39.4°C) or higher and fleeting rash are reported in 5 to 15 percent of recipients of measles vaccine.[29] Encephalitis has been reported after the use of measles vaccine. Comparing the number of cases reported to have occurred within the 30 days after immunization to the number of doses distributed in the United States yields an estimate of approximately one case of encephalitis per million doses of vaccine distributed.[16] This rate is similar to that of reported encephalitis of unknown cause seen in a comparable period in the general population in the same age group. Recently, the Institute of Medicine has concluded that available evidence is not sufficient to prove that vaccination causes encephalopathy or encephalitis.[37] SSPE has been reported in recipients of measles vaccine, but the incidence rate is approximately 5 percent of that following natural illness. Case-control and cohort studies have not suggested any relationship between measles vaccine and SSPE.[16]

It had been recommended that measles vaccine should not be given to persons with anaphylactic hypersensitivity to eggs (hives, swelling of the mouth and throat, difficulty breathing, hypotension, or shock). However, a recent study and review of the available information suggested that children with such histories had little risk of anaphylaxis following vaccination and that skin tests were not useful in distinguishing those who would develop anaphylaxis from those who would not.[38] Thus, children with anaphylactic reactions to egg ingestion may be vaccinated without prior skin testing. They should be observed for 30 minutes before releasing to ensure they do not develop severe allergic reactions. Children with allergies to eggs that are not anaphylactic may be vaccinated without problems. Persons with a history of anaphylactic hypersensitivity to neomycin or gelatin should not be vaccinated, because measles vaccine contains neomycin and gelatin. On theoretical grounds, vaccine should not be administered to a woman known to be pregnant.

Measles vaccine is contraindicated in persons with immunodeficiency or immunosuppression. However, it should be administered to persons with asymptomatic human immunodeficiency virus (HIV) infection, since measles disease may be severe or fatal in such persons. Recently, a 20-year-old man with hemophilia and HIV infection was reported to have been hospitalized with giant cell pneumonia, determined to be caused by the vaccine strain of measles virus. He had been vaccinated 11 months before this episode of pneumonia and had a CD4 T lymphocyte cell count of "too few to enumerate." These data suggest that severely immunocompromised persons with HIV infection should not be vaccinated.[35,39] Severe immunosuppression is defined as (*a*) $CD4^+$ T lymphocyte counts less than 750 for children younger than 12 months, less than 500 for children 1 to 5 years, or less than 200 for persons 6 years old or older; or (*b*) $CD4^+$ T lymphocytes less than 15 percent of total lymphocytes for children younger than 13 years.

Measles vaccination causes clinically evident thrombocytopenia in 1 : 30,000 to 1 : 40,000 vaccinations. Because persons with a history of idiopathic thrombocytopenic purpura (ITP) may be at increased risk for thrombocytopenia following measles vaccination, a history of ITP is a contraindication to measles vaccination.[40]

Vaccination of persons who received IG, whole blood, or other antibody-containing blood products should be postponed for 3 to 7 months or longer, depending on the product and dose received, to avoid potential interference with seroconversion.[33] Vaccination should be postponed in persons with severe febrile illnesses. Persons with mild illnesses such as upper respiratory tract infections may be vaccinated.[41]

Measles Elimination in the United States

The United States has made three attempts to eliminate indigenous measles transmission beginning in 1966. The current elimination strategy has four components: (*a*) achieving and maintaining high immunization levels, (*b*) careful surveillance, (*c*) aggressive outbreak control, and (*d*) working to improve the global control of measles. The most important component is high immunization levels. The enactment and enforcement of comprehensive school immunization laws covering all students, from kindergarten through high school, have been instrumental in achieving high levels. States with strict enforcement policies had significantly lower incidence rates than states without such policies.[42] Careful surveillance includes establishing active surveillance systems in which persons likely to see persons with measles are queried periodically, particularly in inner-city hospitals. A national case definition has been instituted. A probable case of measles is defined as an illness with (*a*) fever (101°F [38.3°C] or above, if measured), (*b*) generalized rash of 3 or more days' duration, and (*c*) either cough, coryza, or conjunctivitis. A confirmed case is any case with laboratory confirmation, or one that meets the clinical definition given above and that is epidemiologically linked to a laboratory-confirmed case. Aggressive outbreak control consists of defining zones of risk for transmission, establishing a target population, and vaccinating that population. In school-based outbreaks, exclusion of students lacking proof of immunity has played a key role in terminating transmission.[16] All students should have evidence of receipt of two doses of measles-containing vaccine on or after the first birthday, at least 1 month apart, a history of physician-diagnosed measles disease, or laboratory evidence of measles immunity.

Measles elimination has proved to be more difficult than initially anticipated. However, surveillance and molecular epidemiologic information indicate that indigenous measles transmission was probably interrupted in late 1993 and subsequently in 1995 and 1996.[43,44] Sustained elimination will require implementation of the full strategy, including high coverage with the first dose in preschool populations, a second dose for all school-age children, improved surveillance with greater laboratory confirmation of suspected cases, and aggressive response to cases. The fourth component of the strategy—to improve the global control of measles—is needed, because all measles today in the United States is believed to be due to recent importations. Efforts to improve measles control in other countries are necessary to sustain elimination in the United States.

Worldwide Control and Elimination

Measles poses a substantial health problem in both the developing and the developed world. Factors predisposing infected persons to complications and death are young age, crowding, malnutrition, and coincident respiratory or gastrointestinal illness. Before immunization, almost 2.5 million children died from measles or measles-related complications annually.[45] About 1 million deaths still occur each year. In the developed world, measles vaccine is usually recommended during the second year of life, typically at 12, 15, or 18 months of age, depending on the country. In contrast, in the developing world, measles vaccine is generally administered in a single dose at 9 months of age. This younger age was chosen for two reasons. First, measles attack and complication rates are often high during the first year of life in the developing world. Waiting until the second year would result in substantial morbidity and mortality. Second, seroconversion rates after measles vaccination at 9 months of age are higher in developing countries than in developed countries.

In developing countries it is particularly important to vaccinate sick children. Often, they are at greatest risk of measles complications, and nosocomial spread of disease is common.

A major problem with measles in the developing world is its occurrence in infancy, when standard Schwarz and Moraten vaccines are not maximally effective because of interference by maternal antibody. While preliminary data showed that high-titer measles vaccines (titers 10- to 100-fold greater than standard doses) could overcome maternal antibody inhibition, subsequent follow-up in several studies revealed higher mortality than expected, primarily in females who received the high-titer vaccines.[46] Use of these vaccines is no longer recommended.

In 1994, the 24th Pan American Sanitary Conference established a goal of eliminating measles from the Western Hemisphere by the year 2000.[1] The strategy for Latin America and the English-speaking Caribbean consists of mass vaccination of children 9 months to 14 years of age regardless of prior vaccination status, high routine immunization coverage, and careful surveillance. In addition, to sustain elimination, periodic mass vaccination campaigns are undertaken to prevent the accumulation of susceptible persons. These latter campaigns seek to immunize children born subsequent to the initial campaign, regardless of prior vaccination status, and take place once the number of susceptible children exceeds the number of children born in a single year. The number of susceptible children is determined from the proportion of children not vaccinated routinely each year and the proportion of those vaccinated annually who will not be protected (i.e., the vaccine failure rate). This accumulation generally takes 3 to 5 years. The strategy has led to the virtual elimination of measles in many countries in Latin America.

A recent expert group concluded that (*a*) worldwide measles eradication was feasible, (*b*) a single-dose strategy was inadequate and that mass campaigns like those used in Latin America and the United Kingdom (or two-dose strategies with targeting of high-risk populations) were necessary, and (*c*) a goal should be set in the next few years for global measles eradication between 2005 and 2010.[47]

Mumps

Melinda Wharton

Hippocrates described mumps (epidemic parotitis) as a distinct clinical entity in the fifth century B.C. Knowledge of the clinical illness has improved over the past two centuries with the awareness that orchitis and meningoencephalitis are relatively common complications. Isolation of the virus and development of a safe, effective vaccine have led to a dramatic decline in mumps-associated morbidity and mortality rates in the United States. When given in combination with measles and rubella vaccines, mumps vaccine reduces the costs associated with mumps by more than 86 percent.[1]

Etiologic Agent, Immunology, and Diagnosis

Mumps is caused by an RNA virus of the paramyxovirus group. Humans are the only known reservoir. Transmission occurs after direct contact with, or droplet spread from, an infected person. The incubation period ranges from 14 to 21 days, with an average of 18 days. Virus may be excreted from 7 days before to 9 days after the clinical onset of disease. Less than half of mumps infections result in parotitis; in other cases, infection is asymptomatic or results in mild respiratory illness.[2] Immunity is long lasting; reports of second attacks have lacked epidemiologic, virologic, or serologic confirmation.

Although diagnosis has frequently been made on clinical grounds, recent experience in the United States suggests that laboratory confirmation should be obtained in sporadic cases of parotitis, as these are now unlikely to be due to mumps.[3] The enzyme-linked immunosorbent assay (EIA) is widely available commercially and is more sensitive than the complement fixation, hemagglutination inhibition, or radial hemolysis assay. IgM antibodies are detectable within the first few days of illness, reach a maximum level about a week after the onset of symptoms, and remain elevated for several weeks or months. False-positive IgM results by immunofluorescent antibody (IFA) assays have been reported.[4] Recently, techniques have been developed to distinguish vaccine from wild mumps viruses.[5,6]

Clinical Characteristics

Mumps is a generalized viral infection. The most common clinical manifestations are mild to moderate fever and painful unilateral or bilateral parotic gland swelling.[7] Prodromal symptoms—including anorexia, headache, vomiting, and myalgia lasting for 12 to 48 hours—are present in some cases. Inflammation of other salivary glands may occur alone or in combination with the parotitis. The usual uncomplicated illness resolves completely in approximately 10 days. Other viruses (such as parainfluenza and coxsackievirus) and bacteria may cause parotitis, but these occur sporadically; other infectious agents are not known to cause epidemic parotitis.

Complications

Among the reported mumps-associated complications, strong epidemiologic and laboratory evidence for an association with meningoencephalitis, deafness, and orchitis has been reported.[8] Aseptic meningitis occurs in up to 4 to 6 percent of clinical cases and typically is mild.[2,9,10] Reported rates of mumps encephalitis range as high as 5 cases per 1,000 reported mumps cases, and adults are at higher risk than children. Permanent sequelae are rare, but the reported encephalitis death-to-case ratio has averaged 1.4 percent. Although the overall mortality is low, death caused by mumps infection is more likely to occur in adults; about half of mumps-associated deaths have been in persons 20 years of age or older.[8] Sensorineural deafness associated with mumps infection may be bilateral, sudden in onset, and permanent. Orchitis (usually unilateral) has been reported as a complication in up to 38 percent of clinical mumps cases in postpubertal males.[7,10] Some testicular atrophy may occur following mumps orchitis, but sterility rarely occurs. Symptomatic involvement of other organs has been observed less frequently. There are limited experimental, clinical, and epidemiologic data suggesting that mumps infection may rarely result in permanent pancreatic damage.[11] Further research is indicated to determine whether mumps infection contributes to the pathogenesis of diabetes mellitus. Mumps infection during the first trimester of pregnancy may increase the rate of spontaneous abortion (reported to be as high as 27 percent).[12] There is no evidence that mumps during pregnancy causes congenital malformations, although mumps virus has been shown to cross the placenta and infect the fetus.

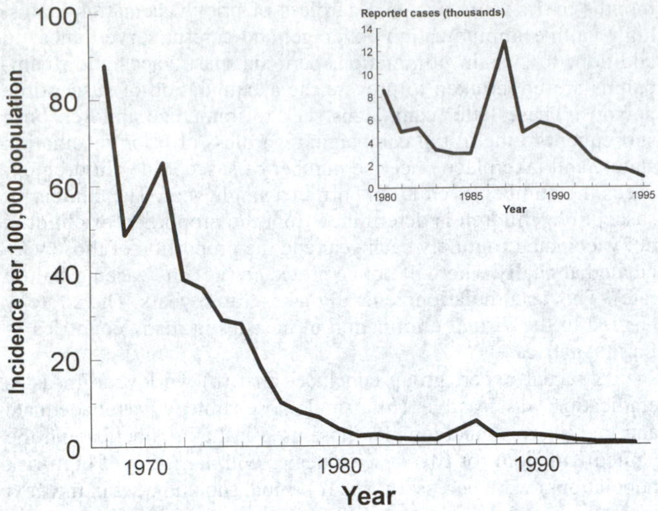

Figure 7-2. Reported mumps incidence per 100,000 population, United States, 1968–1995, and reported cases of mumps (in thousands of cases), United States, 1980–1995.

Occurrence

There appear to be no geographical differences in the clinical presentation or epidemiology of mumps infection. Cases follow a seasonal pattern, with peak occurrences in winter and spring. After the introduction of the live mumps virus vaccine in 1967 and recommendation of its routine use in 1977, there was a steady decrease in the incidence rate of reported mumps cases in the United States until 1986–1987, when a relative resurgence of mumps occurred. In the late 1980s, mumps incidence again began to decrease in the United States, and in 1995 a record low of 906 cases were reported, representing more than a 99 percent decline from the 185,691 cases reported in 1967 (Fig. 7-2).

In the prevaccine era, the majority of reported mumps cases occurred among school-aged children (5 to 14 years of age).[13] Although reported cases of mumps decreased dramatically following the introduction of the live attenuated mumps vaccine in 1967, mumps remained a disease with highest incidence among children 5 to 9 years of age until 1986. During the period 1986 to 1991, the peak incidence rate shifted from 5- to 9-year-old children to 10- to 14-year-old children.[14,15] During this period the increased occurrence of mumps in susceptible adolescents and young adults was demonstrated in outbreaks in high schools,[16–19] on college campuses,[20] and in occupational settings.[21] Both the shift in risk to older persons and the relative resurgence of reported mumps activity noted during the period 1985 to 1987 are attributable primarily to the relatively underimmunized cohort of children born between 1967 and 1977.[22] However, outbreaks were reported among well-immunized populations, suggesting an additional contribution of primary vaccine failure. Because mumps vaccine is less than 100 percent effective (estimates of vaccine effectiveness have ranged from 75 to 91 percent),[16–18,22–24] the occurrence of disease in vaccinated persons is anticipated. Although recent vaccination has been found to be more protective than earlier vaccination in some studies, mumps infection following the waning of vaccine-induced immunity has not been demonstrated to be of epidemiologic importance.[17,19] The large decrease in mumps incidence in the 1990s is likely due to the change in the recommendation for use of measles-mumps-rubella vaccine (MMR) in 1989. The implementation of the two-dose MMR vaccination schedule, with the second dose given at 4 to 6 years or at 11 to 12 years, likely decreased mumps incidence further by immunizing children who failed to respond to the first dose of mumps vaccine.

Lower incidence rates have been demonstrated in states with laws requiring mumps immunization for school attendance. In 1987 the lowest incidence rates (1.1 cases per 100,000 population) were reported from the District of Columbia and from the 14 states with comprehensive laws requiring proof of immunity to mumps for school attendance from kindergarten through grade 12, and the highest rates (11.5 cases per 100,000 population) were in the 14 states that had no requirements for mumps vaccination.[12] These trends persisted but were much less dramatic as disease incidence decreased in the United States during the period 1988 to 1993.[15]

Strategy for Prevention

Based on the epidemiology of mumps infection and the biological properties of the mumps virus, mumps virus is considered potentially eradicable. Nonetheless, there is no worldwide agreement regarding the necessity of preventing mumps infection, and there are insufficient data on the health impact of mumps in developing countries to establish mumps elimination as a priority globally.[25] The principal strategy employed in the United States to remove the burden of mumps illness is through achieving and maintaining high immunization levels with MMR, routinely administered in a two-dose schedule.

A killed-virus vaccine was developed in 1948 but did not provide lasting protection. In 1967 the Jeryl Lynn strain of live attenuated vaccine was licensed in the United States.[26] It induced seroconversion in more than 95 percent of recipients in clinical trials and was found to be noncommunicable and safe. Minimal side effects were reported during large-scale field trials. In clinical trials, vaccine efficacy was 95 percent.[26] In field studies of vaccine effectiveness performed after licensure, vaccine effectiveness has been somewhat lower, ranging from 75 to 91 percent.[16–18,22–24] Vaccine-induced immunity is expected to be lifelong.[27,28] Although the Jeryl Lynn strain is the only mumps vaccine now licensed in the United States, other live attenuated mumps vaccines are in use in other countries.

In the United States, mumps vaccine is usually administered in combination with measles and rubella vaccines as MMR. The first dose of MMR vaccine is recommended for routine administration at 12 to 15 months of age, and the second dose at 4 to 6 years, before a child enters kindergarten or first grade. The preadolescent health visit at age 11 to 12 years can serve as a catch-up opportunity to verify vaccination status and administer MMR vaccine to children who have not yet received two doses of MMR. Adults born in 1957 or later who do not have a medical contraindication should receive at least one dose of MMR vaccine unless they have documentation of vaccination with at lest one dose of measles-, rubella-, and mumps-containing vaccine or other acceptable evidence of immunity to these diseases. Persons can be considered immune to mumps if they (*a*) have documentation of vaccination with live mumps virus vaccine on or after their first birthday, (*b*) have laboratory evidence of mumps immunity, (*c*) were born before 1957, or (*d*) have documentation of physician-diagnosed mumps.

There is no evidence that vaccination with mumps vaccine given after exposure provides protection in persons already infected, nor is there any contraindication to the vaccine's use. However, persons who were exposed but not infected may be protected. The vaccine has not been observed to increase the severity of disease, and if the exposure did not result in infection, it should induce protection against subsequent infection. IG given after exposure to mumps will not reliably prevent infection or viremia and is not recommended. Mumps IG is not available or licensed for use in the United States.

Contraindications to vaccination include pregnancy, recent administration of IG, altered immunity, severe febrile illnesses, and anaphylactic allergy to components of the vaccine (including gelatin and neomycin). Persons with a history of anaphylactic reactions following egg ingestion were previously considered to be at increased risk of serious reactions after receipt of measles or mumps vaccine, which are produced in chick embryo fibroblasts. However, recent studies suggest that most anaphylactic reactions to measles and mumps vaccines are not associated with hypersensitivity to egg antigens but to other components of the vaccines.[29,30]

Although the mumps vaccine is well tolerated, adverse events including parotitis following mumps vaccination have been reported. Aseptic meningitis has rarely been reported following receipt of the

Jeryl Lynn strain of mumps vaccine. In contrast, in several countries where the Urabe strain has been used for mumps vaccination, aseptic meningitis following vaccination has been well documented.[31]

In Finland, high coverage with two doses of MMR has resulted in virtual elimination of mumps.[32] In the United States, a goal of 500 or fewer cases of mumps has been established for the year 2000.[33] In 1995, 906 cases were reported in the United States. Further decline in mumps incidence can be achieved by maintaining high immunization levels in infants and young children and by vaccination of all school children with two doses of MMR. Increased use of laboratory confirmation of suspected mumps cases is likely to result in further reductions in reported cases of mumps in the United States.

Rubella

Susan E. Reef

In 1941 an epidemic of congenital cataracts in Australia was observed in the wake of a large outbreak of rubella.[1] A usually mild and self-limited illness assumed new importance because of its ability to induce congenital defects in infants of women who acquire rubella during pregnancy. Subsequent success in developing and making available an effective vaccine to prevent rubella has been a major public health achievement. Because vaccine has not been administered to all susceptible persons (including persons born in countries that do not have a routine rubella vaccination program), a low level of congenital rubella infection, with its full array of long-term sequelae, persists in the United States. Elimination of indigenous transmission of rubella and congenital rubella syndrome (CRS) in the United States will require collaboration with other countries to develop and implement national rubella vaccination policies.

Etiologic Agent, Immunology, and Diagnosis

Rubella (German or 3-day measles) is caused by an RNA virus of the togavirus group. Other agents in this group include eastern and western equine encephalomyelitis viruses, yellow fever virus, and dengue virus. Humans are the only known reservoir. Rubella is highly communicable but less so than measles or varicella. Virus is transmitted by the respiratory route, and infection usually occurs as a result of contact with nasopharyngeal secretions of infected persons by droplet spread.

Primary rubella infection induces lifelong immunity. Viremia and infection of nasopharyngeal tissues with limited viral shedding has rarely been detected after reinfections with rubella virus in persons with either natural or vaccine-induced immunity.[2] However, there is no demonstrable risk of communicability, and such reinfection in a pregnant woman apparently poses minimal risk to the unborn fetus.[3]

Clinical diagnosis is often unreliable, because symptoms (including rash) are absent in up to one-half of persons infected with rubella. A history of exposure to rubella may be helpful in the absence of the full complement of clinical signs and symptoms. Culture of virus is difficult and not widely available. Serologic confirmation remains the definitive means of diagnosing rubella. Antibodies to the virus (initially, both IgM and IgG) appear after the onset of illness. IgM antibodies generally do not persist more than 4 to 5 weeks after the onset of illness, whereas IgG antibodies usually persist for the lifetime of the patient. Many rubella antibody assay methods are available, such as enzyme-linked immunosorbent assay (EIA), latex agglutination (LA), and fluorescent immunoassay (FIA).

Approximately 90 percent of all neonates with congenital rubella infection have virus in most of their accessible extravascular fluids (e.g., cerebrospinal fluid, tears, urine) and in the posterior portion of the oropharynx.[4,5]

Because IgM antibody normally does not cross the placenta, the presence of rubella-specific IgM antibody in cord blood is evidence of congenital infection. The presence and persistence of rubella-specific IgG postpartum at higher levels than expected (the half-life of maternal antibodies is 1 month) are also suggestive of intrauterine infection.

Clinical Characteristics

Postnatal Infection. Rubella is an acute, mild disease in children and young adults. The first symptoms occur after an incubation period ranging from 14 to 21 days. Communicability begins about 7 days before the onset of rash and persists at least 4 days after rash onset. The cardinal manifestations of the disease are a nonspecific maculopapular rash lasting 3 days or less (hence the term "3-day measles") and generalized lymphadenopathy, particularly of the postauricular, suboccipital, and posterior cervical lymph nodes. However, asymptomatic infections are common: up to 50 percent of infections occur without rash. The rash, which is often the first sign of illness, appears first on the face and then spreads downward rapidly to the neck, arms, trunk, and extremities; pruritus is not unusual. In adolescents or adults, the rash may be preceded by a 1- to 5-day prodrome of low-grade fever, headache, malaise, anorexia, mild conjunctivitis, coryza, sore throat, and lymphadenopathy. The manifestations rapidly subside after the first day of the rash. Exanthems comparable to that observed with rubella infection have been described in infections with echovirus and coxackievirus, fifth disease (parvovirus), other enteroviral infections, and mild measles; these infections, however, are not commonly associated with postauricular or suboccipital adenopathy.

Prenatal Infection. The major disease burden of rubella virus is congenital infection. Primary rubella infection during pregnancy, whether clinical or subclinical, carries a significant risk of fetal infection. Congenital rubella is often associated with a disseminated and chronic infection that may persist throughout fetal life and for many months after birth. Spontaneous abortion, stillbirth, or CRS can result from chronic infection and inhibition of cell multiplication in the developing fetus. Delayed and deranged organogenesis and hypoplastic organ development lead to the characteristic structural defects; Table 7-1 lists manifestations associated with congenital rubella infection. Transplacental infection is not always reflected by immediately apparent disease; up to 50 to 70 percent of infants with congenital rubella infection may appear normal at birth. Deafness is commonly diagnosed later when it is the sole manifestation. Other, relatively less frequent effects, including delayed developmental milestones to learning and speech, behavioral, and psychiatric disorders, have been described.[6] Endocrinopathies such as thyroiditis with hypothyroidism or hyperthyroidism, diabetes mellitus, and Addison's disease have also been occasionally reported to be late sequelae.

Congenital infection is not inevitable, however, and the fetal response to infection is not uniform; the gestational age of the concep-

TABLE 7-1. MANIFESTATIONS OF CONGENITAL RUBELLA INFECTION

Spontaneous abortions
Stillbirths
Bone lesions
Cardiac defects
Patent ductus arteriosus
Pulmonary stenosis and coarctation
Myocardial necrosis
CNS defects
Encephalitis
Mental retardation
Microcephaly
Progressive panencephalitis
Psychomotor retardation
Spastic quadriparesis
Hearing impairment (deafness)
Endocrinopathies
Adrenal disorders
Diabetes mellitus
Precocious puberty
Growth retardation
Growth hormone deficiency
Eye defects
Cataracts
Glaucoma
Microphthalmos
Retinopathy
Genitourinary defects
Hematologic disorders
Anemia
Thrombocytopenia
Immunodeficiencies
Hepatitis
Interstitial pneumonitis
Psychiatric disorders

tus at the time of primary maternal infection is the principal factor influencing the outcome of pregnancy. The risk of CRS as a consequence of maternal infection in the first trimester may be as high as 85 percent,[7] but the risk decreases sharply after the eighth week and is absent after the twentieth week of gestation.

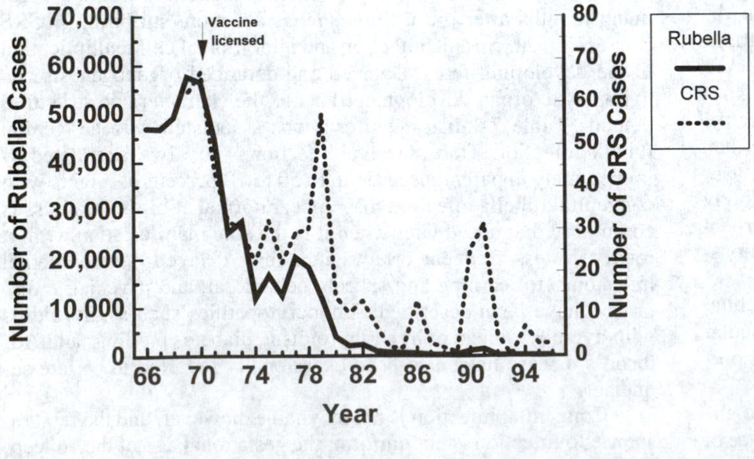

Figure 7-3. Incidence rates of reported rubella and congenital rubella syndrome (CRS) cases, United States, 1966–1996.

Complications

Although rubella is a mild disease in children, it may be more significant with complications in adults.[8] Arthralgia and arthritis may occur in adults, particularly women, at a reported rate as high as 70 percent. Joint involvement usually occurs after the rash fades and typically lasts 5 to 10 days. Rare complications include optic neuritis, thrombocytopenic purpura, and myocarditis. Postinfectious encephalitis of short duration may occur 1 to 6 days after the appearance of rash; its incidence rate is estimated at 1 in 5,000 to 16,000 cases.

Occurrence

In temperate climates, rubella is endemic year-round, with a regular seasonal peak during springtime. In tropical areas, rubella is widespread. Before the advent of rubella vaccination, major epidemics of rubella tended to occur at 6- to 9-year intervals. The last major epidemic of rubella in the United States occurred in 1964 and 1965 (Fig. 7-3) and resulted in an estimated 12,500,000 cases of rubella and an estimated 31,000 cases of congenital rubella syndrome; of these CRS cases, 11,000 resulted in fetal death or therapeutic abortion and 20,000 infants were born with CRS. However, the incidence of rubella has declined by more than 99 percent since 1969, the year that rubella vaccine was licensed. Long-term trends of rubella incidence indicate that rates have declined by 95 percent or more for all age groups, with the greatest decreases occurring among persons less than 15 years of age. Since 1994, three-fourths of reported rubella cases occurred among persons aged 15 to 44 years, a substantial increase from the years 1966 to 1968, when only 23 percent of reported rubella infections occurred among persons aged 15 years or older. In 1996 a total of only 238 cases of rubella were reported.[9] As of May 1, 1997, only three cases of CRS in children born in 1996 were reported, although the actual number of undiagnosed or unreported CRS cases may be as much as 10-fold higher.[10] Despite the marked drop in incidence, it is estimated that up to 15 percent of adolescents and young adults remain susceptible.[11–13] Transmission of rubella has continued to occur in the postpubertal population, with more than half of all cases occurring among persons 20 years of age or older in recent years.[9]

Strategy for Prevention

Since licensure of live attenuated rubella virus vaccines in 1969, efforts to control rubella in the United States have been directed primarily at preschool and elementary school children of both sexes. It was reasoned that, in addition to protection of children, circulation of the virus would be greatly reduced or interrupted, and susceptible pregnant women would be protected indirectly by virtually eliminating the risk of exposure. As noted above, this strategy has substantially reduced the incidence of rubella and congenital rubella infection in the United States; however, this program did not reduce susceptibility among persons more than 15 years old. In 1977 the Advisory Committee on Immunization Practices (ACIP) recommendations were modified to include the vaccination of susceptible postpubertal females. With combined routine childhood and vaccination of women of childbearing age, cases of rubella and CRS are at a record low in the United States. Another approach initially implemented elsewhere (e.g., in the United Kingdom) prescribed immunization of young adolescent girls at approximately 11 to 14 years of age, accompanied by vaccination of all susceptible adult women of childbearing age. It was anticipated that this approach would not reduce the total number of cases of rubella but would have a direct protective effect as these girls entered their childbearing years. Indeed, there was little change in the reported occurrence of rubella and CRS in the United Kingdom through the mid-1980s, and major epidemics occurred in 1978, 1979, 1982, and 1983; nonetheless, serologic evidence indicates that the proportion of young adult women who are susceptible has declined in recent years. However, because the vaccine is less than 100 percent efficacious and immunization coverage is less than 100 percent in girls, cases of rubella in women of childbearing age do occur.[14] In the United Kingdom, MMR vaccine was introduced in 1988 as part of the routine childhood immunization schedule, resulting in dramatic decreases in the incidence of rubella.[15]

In 1969, three rubella vaccines were licensed for use in the United States: the HPV-77 strain, prepared in duck embryo cell culture; the HPV-77, prepared in dog kidney cell culture; and the Cendehill strain, prepared in rabbit kidney cell culture. In 1979 the RA 27/3 strain, which is prepared in human diploid cells, was introduced and has since been the only rubella vaccine that is distributed in the United States. In at least 95 percent of vaccinees, all these vaccines induce antibodies that have been shown to persist for more than 16 years,[16] indicating that immunity is durable and probably lifelong. However, two studies have documented that there may be waning of rubella antibodies in adolescents who were vaccinated with rubella vaccine 9 to 14 years earlier.[17,18] In recent years, outbreaks of rubella have occurred in young adults, with few cases occurring among persons with documented previous vaccination. This suggests that waning of antibody levels is not associated with loss of protection. Most of the persons who lack detectable antibody by standard tests have been shown to have antibody by more sensitive tests. When exposed to either natural disease or revaccination, such persons typically do not develop an IgM response and do not have detectable viremia.

In the United States, rubella vaccine is recommended for all susceptible persons 12 months of age and older, unless vaccination is contraindicated.[19] Rubella vaccination is most cost-effective when offered as MMR vaccine. Persons should be considered susceptible to rubella unless they have documentation of (*a*) adequate immunization with rubella virus vaccine on or after their first birthday or (*b*) laboratory evidence of immunity. Persons who are unsure of their rubella disease or vaccination history or both should be vaccinated. *With the exception of women who might become pregnant*, birth before 1957 generally can be considered acceptable evidence of immunity. Adults born before 1957 may receive MMR vaccine unless it is otherwise contraindicated.

Rubella vaccine given after exposure may not provide protection, but there is no contraindication to its use. The vaccine has not been observed to increase the severity of disease, and if the exposure did not result in infection, it should induce protection against subsequent infection. Immune globulin (IG) given after exposure to rubella will not reliably prevent infection or viremia but may only modify or suppress symptoms. Infants with congenital rubella have been born to women given IG shortly after exposure. The routine use of IG for postexposure prophylaxis of rubella in early pregnancy is not recommended unless termination would not be considered under any circumstances.

Adverse events following vaccination include low-grade fever, rash, and lymphadenopathy. As many as 40 percent of vaccinees in large-scale field trials had joint pain, usually of the small peripheral joints, but frank arthritis has generally been reported in fewer than 2 percent of subjects. As with natural disease, vaccine-associated arthralgia and transient arthritis occur more frequently and tend to be more severe in women than in men or children. As many as 3 percent of susceptible children have been reported to have arthralgia, and arthritis has been reported only rarely in these vaccinees; in contrast, 10 to 15 percent of susceptible female vaccinees have been reported to have arthritis-like symptoms. With both natural and vaccine-associated disease, these symptoms usually have not caused disruption of activities and most often have not persisted. However, rubella infection in adults is associated with a higher incidence, greater severity, and more prolonged duration of joint manifestations than are seen after rubella immunization. During the mid-1980s, investigators from one institution reported persistent or chronic arthropathy in 5 to 11 percent of adult females following rubella vaccination.[20] In 1991, Institute of Medicine concluded that, "Evidence is consistent with a causal relation between the currently used rubella vaccine strain (RA27/3) and chronic arthritis in adult women, although the evidence is limited in scope and confined to reports from one institution."[21] However, data from studies in the United States and experience from other countries using the RA 27/3 strain rubella vaccine have not supported this finding, suggesting that such occurrences are rare and may not be causally related to administration of rubella-containing vaccines.[22,23] Transient peripheral neuritic complaints, such as paresthesias and pain in the arms and legs, have also very rarely occurred. Reactions such as these usually occur only in susceptible vaccinees; persons who are already immune to rubella, due to either previous rubella vaccination or natural infection, are not at increased risk of local or systemic reactions following the receipt of rubella vaccine.[22,23,24]

Although use of rubella vaccine is contraindicated in pregnant women or women planning pregnancy within 3 months, inadvertent administration of the vaccine to pregnant women does occur. To evaluate the risk to the fetus of exposure to attenuated rubella vaccine virus, outcomes of pregnancy in 1,238 women who inadvertently received rubella vaccine within 3 months before or 3 months after their presumed date of conception were determined between 1971 and 1989. All 290 infants born to 538 women vaccinated during pregnancy with either Cendehill or HPV-77 rubella vaccine through April 1979 were free of defects compatible with CRS, although eight infants had serologic evidence of intrauterine infection. By April 1989 when the registry was discontinued, the vaccination of 700 women with the RA 27/3 rubella vaccine within 3 months of conception was also reported. Among the 289 women who were known to be susceptible at the time of vaccination, outcomes of pregnancy are known for 275 (94 percent); 83 percent delivered living infants, all 229 of whom were free of defects associated with CRS. Rubella-specific IgM was detected in three infants, but all three were normal on physical examination. These data are consistent with results reported from other countries, suggesting that if live attenuated rubella vaccine causes defects associated with CRS, it does so at a very low rate (less than 1.6 percent).

In view of the importance of protecting women of childbearing age from rubella, reasonable practices for avoiding vaccination of pregnant women in a rubella immunization program should include (*a*) asking women if they are pregnant, (*b*) excluding from the program those who say they are, and (*c*) explaining the theoretical risks to the others before vaccinating. The vaccine should also not be given to those with immunodeficiency diseases or compromised immune systems as a result of disease or treatment because of the theoretical possibility that replication of the vaccine virus can be potentiated. Other contraindications to vaccination are recent administration of IG, and severe febrile illness.

The goal of elimination of indigenous rubella and congenital rubella syndrome in the United States has been established for the year 2000. The effectiveness of rubella prevention efforts in the United States is reflected by the dramatic decline in reported cases compared with the prevaccine era, and the low annual average number of cases since 1991. All 50 states have enacted laws requiring rubella vaccination at school entry, and in 41 states and the District of Columbia the students at all grade levels are included. With the increasing proportion of cases among persons 15 years of age and older, vaccination activities should include adolescents and young adults. Vaccination of women not known to be pregnant and without a history of vaccination is justifiable without serologic testing, particularly when the costs of testing are high and follow-up of identified susceptible women for vaccination is not ensured. Programs to identify and vaccinate high-risk groups include premarital screening and vaccination of susceptible women, prenatal screening followed by postpartum vaccination of susceptible women, establishment of requirements for proof of rubella immunity for college entry, and routine vaccination of all hospital employees, volunteers, trainees, and physicians, both male and female.

Rubella remains uncontrolled in much of the developed as well as the developing world.[24] Combinations of strategies have been undertaken in some countries, with vaccination of all children at age 1 year, combined with vaccination of adolescent girls to reduce rubella transmission and to provide future protection of those about to enter the childbearing period. Other countries have combined vaccination of children of both sexes at age 1 year and at ages 6 to 12 years to shorten the period necessary to achieve high immunity among children and to interrupt transmission.

Over the last few years, cases of rubella and CRS reported in the United States have been epidemiologically linked to areas in Mexico, Asia, Europe, and Central and South America. In 1996, approximately 40 percent of the reported rubella cases were associated with importation of the rubella virus into the United States. A molecular technique to characterize rubella isolates has recently been developed, and geographic strain variation has been documented.[25] This technique is now being used to define which strains—if any—are circulating in the United States and to identify the likely origin of imported strains. This is important (*a*) to confirm the interruption of indigenous strains and (*b*) to identify the countries of origin in order to establish additional priorities for rubella control. Elimination of indigenous rubella in the United States will require collaboration with other countries to develop and implement national rubella vaccination policies.

Pertussis

Peter M. Strebel • Dalya Guris • Steven G.F. Wassilak

Pertussis is a highly communicable, vaccine-preventable disease that lasts for many weeks and is typically manifested in children with spasms of severe coughing, whooping, and posttussive vomiting. It is caused by infection with *Bordetella pertussis*, a bacillus first isolated in 1906 by Bordet and Gengou. Because other etiologic agents may also cause the symptom complex suggestive of pertussis and because clinical pertussis is frequently not confirmed by laboratory testing, the constellation of symptoms is often referred to as the "whooping cough syndrome." Whooping cough also may be caused infrequently by *Bordetella parapertussis* and by the animal pathogen *Bordetella bronchiseptica*. Adenoviruses, *Mycoplasma pneumoniae*, and *Chlamydia pneumoniae* should be included in the differential diagnosis.

Clinical Characteristics

The main clinical feature of classic pertussis is episodic and paroxysmal coughing (i.e., the sudden onset of repeated violent coughs without intervening respirations). The onset of illness is insidious. During the first 1 or 2 weeks of illness, coryza is accompanied by shallow, irritating, nonproductive coughing, which gradually changes into episodes of paroxysmal coughing. The patient generally remains well and free from cough between episodes. As the coughing attacks become more severe, they are commonly followed by inspiratory whooping or vomiting. After a week or so of paroxy-smal coughing, the disease peaks in severity and begins to subside, although convalescence is protracted, lasting for up to 3 months in some cases. In young unvaccinated children, leukocytosis and lymphocytosis are generally present during the early paroxysmal stage of the disease.

Adults, partially immunized persons, and infants younger than 6 months of age do not commonly have the repeated typical paroxysms or experience whooping, but a clinical diagnosis may be suggested by a history of a persistent cough before or after exposure to a known case. Although boosting of pertussis antibodies occurs in a majority of household contacts of a patient, asymptomatic infection, demonstrated by bacterial culture, occurs only in a small minority of household contacts. Long-term carriage is thought not to occur.

Complications

The major complications, including hypoxia, pneumonia, malnutrition, seizures, and encephalopathy, are most common in younger patients. The following rates of complications were estimated from a large population-based study in the United Kingdom.[1] Fifteen percent of children younger than 5 years of age with pertussis are hospitalized (60 percent of those younger than 6 months). Pneumonia (primary or secondary) complicates the course of at least 2 percent of patients; seizures, possibly caused by hypoxia or toxin-mediated events or both, occur in 0.4 percent. Encephalopathy occurs in 2 to 6 per 10,000 patients. Patients who die of encephalopathy generally had evidence of hypoxic damage or hemorrhage without inflammation. Death occurs in 0.17 percent of patients (0.7 percent of patients younger than 1 year of age). In an active surveillance project conducted in Kenya in the mid-1970s, 4 percent of pertussis patients developed pneumonia and 1.2 percent died; the case-to-fatality rate among infants was 3.2 percent.[2]

Long-term complications include residual neurologic deficits and, both in the preantibiotic era and currently in the developing world, substantial permanent lung damage.

Bacteriology and Pathogenesis

B. pertussis is a small, fastidious, Gram-negative coccobacillus. Isolation requires a complex medium that contains blood or charcoal or both, on which it appears as a small, pearly colony. The presence of agglutinogens permits serotyping of *B. pertussis* strains. The possible role of agglutinogens as virulence factors and in the acquisition of immunity against pertussis is controversial. Fimbriae possessing the agglutinogen are apparently responsible for the specific attachment of *B. pertussis* organisms to the site of infection.

Pathologically, pertussis is a superficial respiratory infection, primarily of the subglottic respiratory tract. The organism is found attached to mucosal cells and inside alveolar macrophages. Systemic invasion does not occur. Pathologic specimens from patients demonstrate local bronchial epithelial necrosis and inflammation. Pertussis appears to be a toxin-mediated disease resulting from local infection.[3] The products or antigens of *B. pertussis* that may be responsible for the local or systemic pathophysiological events, or both, include pertussis toxin (PT), endotoxin, dermatonecrotic toxin, tracheal cytotoxin, extracytoplasmic adenylate cyclase, filamentous hemagglutinin (FHA), and pertactin (a 69-kilodalton outer-membrane protein). PT is an inhibitor of cellular adenylate cyclase and is considered responsible for the lymphocytosis and hypoglycemia that may be seen in whooping cough. PT and adenylate cyclase are considered important mediators of altered immunologic and phagocytic function. FHA and pertactin may mediate its attachment to respiratory epithelial cells.

Characterization of different strains of *B. pertussis* using molecular methods (e.g., pulsed-field gel electrophoresis) may be a useful tool for identifying chains of infection in epidemiologic investigations and in the study of the bacterial genome itself.

Diagnosis

Laboratory confirmation of the clinical diagnosis can be difficult. Culture specimens are obtained either by a nasopharyngeal aspirate or by passing a fine wire tipped with Dacron or calcium alginate through the patient's nose to the posterior portion of the nasopharynx. Swabs are streaked on Bordet-Gengou, Regan-Lowe, or other appropriate agar medium. A selective antimicrobial agent such as cephalexin greatly enhances recognition of pertussis colonies by suppressing the overgrowth of normal flora. The plates must be incubated for at least 3 to 5 days.

Recovery of *B. pertussis* from patients is affected by prior vaccination or antimicrobial therapy and by the stage of illness.[4] If nasopharyngeal specimens are collected from children during the early stages of the disease and cultured on proper media, an experienced laboratory technician can isolate *B. pertussis* from up to 80 percent of patients with clinical disease who have had no prior vaccination or antimicrobial therapy. The frequency of positive cultures diminishes rapidly after the onset of paroxysmal cough. Cultures obtained 21 or more days after cough onset are usually negative.

During acute infection, increases in antibody titer of agglutinins (antibodies to the specific surface agglutinogens of *B. pertussis*) or of class-specific antibodies (as measured by EIA) to several cellular components—including PT, FHA, and pertactin—can be useful in diagnosis. However, the first of paired serum specimens must be collected soon after cough onset for these tests to exhibit a significant antibody increase.[5] Diagnosis of pertussis on the basis of a single high antibody level is being increasingly used but requires information from a healthy, age-matched control population.[6]

Polymerase chain reaction (PCR) methods have been developed for *B. pertussis* and are being increasingly used in research and for routine diagnosis. Compared with culture, PCR testing is more rapid and more sensitive. However, laboratory contamination may cause false-positive test results, and PCR does not provide a bacterial isolate, which may be needed for antimicrobial sensitivity testing or molecular characterization.

Direct fluorescence antibody (DFA) staining of mucus smears from nasopharyngeal swabbing is also used for laboratory diagnosis. Specific adsorbed antisera, the inclusion of positive and negative controls, and experienced personnel are needed to maximize the reliability of this method. However, rates of false positivity and false negativity can be high; for this reason DFA should be considered a screening, rather than confirmatory, diagnostic test.

Immunity

The mechanism of immunity in pertussis is not well understood. After natural infection, a rise in serum antibody level in most patients can be observed by agglutination testing or EIA measurement of class-specific antibodies to PT, FHA, or pertactin. The timing of the appearance of humoral antibody and local IgA corresponds roughly to the disappearance of culturable organisms from the nasopharynx. Studies in mice support a role for cell-mediated immunity in protection against pertussis. Immunity against clinical whooping cough induced by natural infection is believed to be long lasting; however, frequent exposures to the organism ("street car boosting") during an individual's lifetime may be required to maintain protection. Neonates are apparently generally susceptible to pertussis, suggesting either low levels of maternal antibody or ineffective protection from immunoglobulins that cross the placenta.

The components of *B. pertussis* that induce protective antibody in humans have not been precisely identified. The protective effect of whole-cell pertussis vaccine in humans, as measured by its effect on the secondary attack rate in household contacts, correlates moderately well with its potency in protecting mice against intracerebral challenge with the organism. In the mouse potency test, mice are inoculated intraperitoneally with dilutions of the vaccine being tested or with the U.S. standard pertussis vaccine. Fourteen days later the mice are challenged intracerebrally with live pertussis bacteria and then observed for 14 days. Protection is determined by comparing the survival rate among recipients of the test vaccine with that among recipients of the standard vaccine.

Persons with titers of circulating agglutinins of 1:320 or higher are usually protected against pertussis. However, persons with lower or undetectable titers may also be protected, suggesting that other humoral and cell-mediated mechanisms may be important. One theory about immunity is that protective antibody may either prevent attachment of *B. pertussis* to ciliated epithelial cells by combining with surface components such as FHA, or may neutralize circulating PT or other toxin(s) produced by virulent organisms.

Experience gained in recent field trials of different acellular pertussis vaccines has provided new information regarding immunity to pertussis.[7–10] Inactivated pertussis toxin is an essential component of all acellular pertussis vaccines tested and may account for most of their efficacy. The addition of FHA, pertactin, or agglutinogens (fimbriae) may increase efficacy by 10 to 15 percent. Vaccines containing attachment factors may have the added benefit of inhibiting colonization and thereby potentially enhancing herd immunity.

Transmission

Pertussis is spread from person to person by respiratory droplets or by direct contact with secretions from the respiratory tract. It is highly contagious, with secondary attack rates in unimmunized susceptible household contacts as high as 90 percent. The incubation period is usually 7 to 10 days (range, 4 to 21 days). The period of communicability begins approximately 1 week after effective exposure. A person is considered most infectious during the early stages of the disease. By 3 weeks after the onset of coughing, culture positivity rapidly declines.

Occurrence

Pertussis occurs worldwide. With immunization coverage of 80 percent, the Expanded Program on Immunization of the World Health Organization (WHO) estimates a global total of 39 million cases of pertussis per year, with approximately 350,000 deaths. In countries without an immunization program, the WHO estimates that 80 percent of surviving newborn infants acquire pertussis in the first 5 years of life. In communities with high vaccination levels, the reported numbers of cases of severe disease and deaths attributable to pertussis are substantially reduced, usually by more than 95 percent compared with the prevaccine era.

Before the introduction of pertussis vaccines in the late 1940s in the United States, morbidity and mortality rates for pertussis had already begun to decline, indicating that other factors (e.g., household crowding) may affect the occurrence of pertussis (Fig. 7-4). Despite the achievement of high preschool (more than 90 percent) and school-entry (more than 95 percent) immunization levels in the United States, transmission of *B. pertussis* appears to continue uninterruptedly, as evidenced by the persistence of an interepidemic interval of 3 to 5 years and isolation of the organism in almost all states every year. Pertussis is widely underrecognized and underreported in the United States.[11] During the period from 1992 to 1995, an average of 5,000 cases were reported annually, of which approximately one-third were confirmed by culture. An investigation of pertussis deaths reported in the United States during 1992 and 1993 found that, of 23 patients who died, 70 percent were less than 3 months of age, 78 percent had received no doses of pertussis vaccine, and all but one had pneumonia as a complication.[12] Among pertussis cases reported in the United States during 1992 to 1995, the case-to-fatality ratio was 0.2 percent overall; for infants younger than 6 months of age, the ratio was 0.6 percent. Of patients whose age was known, 40 percent were less than 1 year of age and 20 percent were 1 to 4 years of age. The proportion of pertussis patients aged 10 years old and older has increased from 19 percent between 1980 and 1989 to

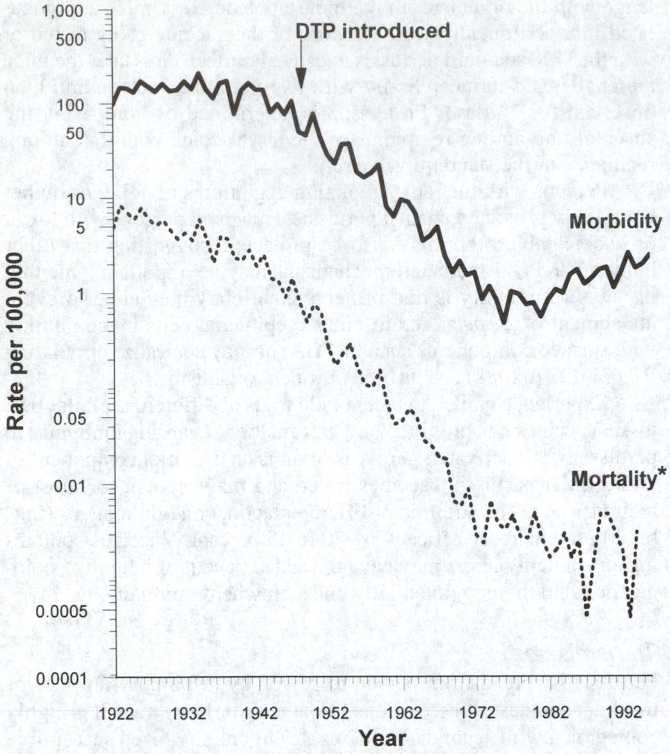

*Mortality data not available for 1995 and 1996
DTP = Combined diphtheria and tetanus toxoids and whole-cell pertussis vaccine

Figure 7-4. Reported morbidity and mortality rates for pertussis per 100,000 population, United States, 1922–1996.

30 percent between 1992 and 1995. This increase has been most marked in states such as Massachusetts where awareness and laboratory testing for pertussis in adolescents and adults has become widespread.[13]

With the introduction and widespread use of vaccine, the age-specific incidence and clinical manifestations of reported pertussis have changed; the incidence of disease is now highest in infants too young to receive adequate immunization (i.e., at least three doses) or in adolescents whose immunity from childhood vaccination has waned. Studies of selected populations suggest that pertussis is an important cause of acute cough illness of more than 7 days' duration in adolescents and adults, with 12 to 26 percent of such patients having serologic evidence of recent infection with *B. pertussis*.[14,15] In addition, recent outbreaks in institutions such as schools and hospitals have highlighted the important role that older children and adults play in transmitting the agent. In communities with high childhood vaccination coverage, adolescents and adults are often the primary case in the household, whereas in settings with low vaccination levels young children are most frequently the primary case.[16]

Strategy for Prevention and Control

Active Immunization. Active immunization is the most effective method for the prevention of pertussis. The first generation of pertussis vaccines were developed and tested in the 1940s and consist of formaldehyde-treated whole-cell preparations of *B. pertussis* combined with diphtheria and tetanus toxoids (DTP). These vaccines have been used worldwide since the 1950s and have substantially reduced pertussis morbidity and mortality. Concerns about the safety of whole-cell pertussis vaccines led to the development of acellular vaccines that contain purified antigenic components of *B. pertussis* combined with diphtheria and tetanus toxoids (DTaP) and are much less likely to provoke common adverse events. Acellular pertussis vaccines have been in use in Japan since the early 1980s and were initially administered to children 2 years of age and older. In 1991, acellular pertussis vaccines were licensed in the United States for use as the fourth and fifth doses of the pertussis vaccination series but were not licensed for use in infants because of the absence of data on efficacy in this age group.

Eight different acellular pertussis vaccines and four whole-cell vaccines were recently evaluated in large field studies for safety and efficacy when administered to infants (Table 7-2).[7–10,17–19] Because of differences in study design, clinical case definition, and laboratory method used to confirm the diagnosis, comparison of efficacy estimates from these studies should be made with caution. All the acellular vaccines evaluated were associated with fewer local (pain, redness, and swelling at the site of injection) and systemic (fever and fussiness) adverse reactions than whole-cell vaccines. The protective efficacy of the acellular vaccines against moderately severe pertussis disease ranged from 59 to 85 percent. Vaccine efficacy for the four whole-cell vaccines ranged from 36 to 98 percent. One whole-cell vaccine, manufactured and distributed in the United States, had unexpectedly low vaccine efficacy when used as a three-dose series in studies conducted in Sweden and Italy.

The efficacy of immunization with whole-cell pertussis vaccines for preventing disease is good initially (70 to 90 percent)[20] but apparently begins to wane over several years. One study showed efficacy to be 79 percent in the first 3 years, 53 percent after 4 to 7 years, 35 percent after 8 to 11 years, and essentially nil 12 years after immunization.[21] Preliminary data indicate that protection by acellular pertussis vaccines lasts at least several years; long-term efficacy is not yet defined. When pertussis does occur in immunized persons, it tends to be milder, with coughing of shorter duration than in the unimmunized.[22]

In a randomized double-blinded study ($n = 2,200$ infants) of the adverse reactions following administration of 13 different acellular pertussis vaccines and one whole-cell vaccine at 2, 4, and 6 months of age, all the acellular vaccines were associated with substantially fewer local and systemic reactions than the whole-cell vaccine.[23] Pain at the site of injection occurred in 10 percent of DTaP recipients compared with 40 percent of DTP recipients; swelling occurred in 61 percent and 20 percent, and fever (temperature 38°C or above) in 5 percent and 16 percent of DTaP and DTP recipients, respectively. More severe adverse reactions following primary vaccination also appear to be less frequent following administration of acellular compared with whole-cell vaccines. In the Italian efficacy study ($n = 15,601$ infants), hypotonic hyporesponsive episodes within 2 days of vaccination occurred at a rate (per 10,000 doses of vaccine administered) of 6.7 and 0.7, and seizures at a rate of 2.2 and 0.7 for whole-cell and acellular vaccine recipients, respectively.[8] It is currently unknown whether DTaP vaccines may cause the most severe and very rare adverse event (i.e., encephalopathy) associated with whole-cell pertussis vaccines.

Although pertussis vaccines are less immunogenic in younger infants than in older infants, it is recommended that immunization begin at 6 to 8 weeks of age because the disease is most often life-threatening in young infants. The WHO recommends three doses of diphtheria and tetanus toxoids combined with whole-cell pertussis vaccine (DTP) at 6, 10, and 14 weeks of age. Booster doses in the second year of life or at school entry are optional and depend on the epidemiology of diphtheria, tetanus, and pertussis in the country as well as the coverage achieved with the first three recommended doses. In the United States, five doses of diphtheria, tetanus, and pertussis vaccine are recommended, three primary doses at 2, 4, and 6 months of age, a booster dose in the second year of life (15 to 18 months), and a second booster dose at school entry (4 to 6 years).[24] Because acellular pertussis vaccines are effective when administered to infants and are associated with fewer local and systemic reactions that may follow administration of DTP, acellular pertussis vaccines are recommended for all doses in the schedule in the United States. As the transition from DTP to DTaP for routine vaccination of infants is being made, whole-cell pertussis vaccines remain an acceptable alternative for pertussis vaccination in the United States. Because of high inci-

TABLE 7-2. ABSOLUTE EFFICACY OF DTaP AND WHOLE-CELL DTP VACCINES WHEN ADMINISTERED AS A THREE-DOSE PRIMARY SERIES TO INFANTS ACCORDING TO STUDY SITE, VACCINE COMPOSITION, VACCINATION SCHEDULE, AND CASE DEFINITION USED IN THE STUDIES

Site of Study	*Vaccine Composition*				*Age at Vaccination (months)*	*Case Definition*	*Vaccine Efficacy, % (95% CI)*	
	PT	*FHA*	*Pn*	*Fim*			*DTaP*	*DTP*
Randomized controlled studies:								
Stockholm, Sweden[7]	+	+	+	+	2, 4, 6	≥21 days of paroxysmal cough[a]	85 (81-89)	48 (37-58)[b]
	+	+			2, 4, 6	≥21 days of paroxysmal cough[a]	59 (51-66)	48 (37-58)[b]
Italy[8]	+	+	+		2, 4, 6	≥21 days of paroxysmal cough[a]	84 (76-90)	36 (14-52)[b]
	+	+	+		2, 4, 6	≥21 days of paroxysmal cough[a]	84 (76-89)	36 (14-52)[b]
Göteborg, Sweden[9]	+				3, 5, 12	≥21 days of paroxysmal cough[a]	71 (63-78)	Not studied
Observational studies[c]:								
Erlangen, Germany[17d]	+	+	+	+	3, 5, 7, 17	≥21 days of cough and paroxysms or whoop or vomiting and confirmation by culture or serology or link to culture-positive household contact	73 (51-86)[e] 85 (76-90)[f]	83 (65-92)[e] 94 (89-97)[f]
Mainz, Germany[10]	+	+	+		3, 4, 5	≥21 days of paroxysmal cough[a]	89 (77-95)	98 (83-100)[g]
Senegal[18d]	+	+			2, 4, 6	≥21 days of paroxysmal cough[a]	85 (66-93)	96 (87-99)[g]
Munich, Germany[19]	+	+			3, 5, 7	≥21 days any cough and confirmation by culture or link to culture-positive household contact	80 (59-90)	95 (81-99)[g, h]

Abbreviations: PT, pertussis toxin; FHA, filamentous hemagglutinin; Pn, pertactin; Fim, fimbriae.
[a]With culture or serologic confirmation. In Stockholm, Göteborg, and Senegal, patients with link to a culture-confirmed household contact were also considered confirmed; in Senegal, polymerase chain reaction (PCR) was also used for confirmation of the cases.
[b]Distributed by Connaught Laboratories, Inc., and licensed for use in the United States.
[c]Wyeth-Lederle DTaP was tested in a prospective cohort study; SmithKline Beecham DTaP and Pasteur Mérieux DTaP, in household contact studies; and Connaught-Biken DTaP, in a case-control study.
[d]In Erlangen and Senegal, children were randomly given DTaP or DTP; however, recruitment of DT recipients was not randomized.
[e]Efficacy after three doses; whole-cell DTP distributed by Wyeth-Lederle Vaccines and Pediatrics, and licensed for use in the United States.
[f]Efficacy after four doses; whole-cell DTP distributed by Wyeth-Lederle Vaccines and Pediatrics, and licensed for use in the United States.
[g]Whole-cell DTP used in Mainz and Munich, Germany, was manufactured by Behringwerke; whole-cell DTP used in Senegal was manufactured by Pasteur Mérieux.
[h]DTaP and whole-cell DTP vaccine efficacy estimates are not directly comparable due to differences in recruitment of children in the study.

dence of local reactions, whole-cell vaccines are not recommended for use in persons 7 years of age or older in the United States.

Limitations of both whole-cell and acellular pertussis vaccines restrict their usefulness in controlling outbreaks among unvaccinated children. A single dose of DTP or DTaP vaccine does not confer protection, but rather three or more doses are believed necessary to reliably confer protection. In the United States, during pertussis outbreaks, the first three doses may be given at 6, 10, and 14 weeks of age to provide protection as early as possible.

Passive Immunization. Controlled studies have shown that human pertussis IG given for postexposure prophylaxis does not alter the incidence or severity of illness.

Treatment and Chemoprophylaxis. Erythromycin is the drug of choice for treatment of pertussis (children: 40 to 50 mg/kg per day in four divided doses; adults: 1 to 2 g/day). The recommended duration of therapy is 14 days. Among the three oral erythromycin formulations (estolate, ethylsuccinate, and stearate), erythromycin estolate achieves the highest concentrations in serum and respiratory secretions and is preferred by some experts.[25] Trimethoprim-sulfamethoxazole (children: trimethoprim 8 mg/kg per day, sulfamethoxazole 40 mg/kg per day in two divided doses; adults: trimethoprim 320 mg per day, sulfamethoxazole 1,600 mg per day) is an alternative for patients who do not tolerate erythromycin. Pertussis symptoms may be ameliorated when effective antimicrobial therapy is started during the catarrhal stage or within 2 weeks of cough onset. However, once the paroxysmal stage has begun, antimicrobial therapy has no clear effect on the course of illness. One study found that high-dose specific pertussis IG administered to young children with whooping cough early in the course of their disease reduced the severity of disease.[26]

The major role for antimicrobial agents is to decrease communicability and thereby shorten the period of isolation. In general, untreated children may return to school 21 or more days after cough onset; children treated with effective antimicrobial agents become noninfectious after 5 days of therapy. Health care workers symptomatic with pertussis should be excluded from patient contact for 7 days while on effective antimicrobial treatment.[27]

Household studies and a recent clinical trial suggest that erythromycin and trimethoprim-sulfamethoxazole may be effective for chemoprophylaxis of susceptible persons exposed to pertussis. Generally, chemoprophylaxis is recommended for all close contacts of a pertussis patient, especially if the contact is an unvaccinated child or is known to have contact with infants.

Antimicrobial Resistance. The first and only known case of pertussis caused by a strain of *B. pertussis* resistant to high concentrations of erythromycin was reported from Arizona in June 1994.[28] The case occurred in a 2-month-old infant who failed to respond to sequential oral and intravenous erythromycin therapy. After initiation of therapy with trimethoprim-sulfamethoxazole, the infant's condition improved rapidly and the strain was subsequently shown to be fully sensitive to trimethoprim-sulfamethoxazole. Although antimicrobial resistance does not appear to be an impediment to pertussis treatment and control at this time, surveillance for resistant organisms is needed.

Future Perspectives

Acellular pertussis vaccines are currently under evaluation for use in adolescents and adults as booster doses. A recent study found that an acellular pertussis vaccine combined with adult-formulation tetanus and diphtheria toxoids was well tolerated and resulted in good antibody responses.[29] This suggests that adults who receive a booster dose of acellular pertussis vaccine may be protected for a period of time; however, the impact this would have on preventing transmission to young unvaccinated infants is unknown. Further evaluation of the health impact of pertussis in adults and the effectiveness and cost-effectiveness of adult vaccination will be required before a recommendation for routine use of acellular pertussis vaccine for adolescent or adult booster vaccination can be made. In the future, if acellular pertussis vaccines are licensed for use among persons 7 years of age or older in the United States, they will likely be recommended initially for health care workers and for outbreak control in institutions (e.g., schools).

New antimicrobial agents (e.g., azithromycin and clarithromycin) are being increasingly used for treatment of pertussis because of reduced gastrointestinal side effects and simpler dosage regimens.[30] However, additional data from clinical studies may be required before these agents can be recommended for routine treatment or chemoprophylaxis.

In developing countries, routine infant immunization with whole-cell pertussis vaccine and early diagnosis and treatment of severe clinical cases with erythromycin will likely remain the primary tools for pertussis control into the twenty-first century.

Tetanus

D. Rebecca Prevots • Roland W. Sutter

Although tetanus is not transmissible from one person to another, its prevention has high public health priority throughout the world because the causative agent is ubiquitous, the disease has a high case-to-fatality ratio, and because, with the wide availability of an effective safe toxoid, it is almost completely preventable. Following the introduction and widespread use of tetanus toxoid, tetanus has become an uncommon disease in developed countries but is still common in developing countries, particularly among neonates.[1,2]

Etiologic Agent, Pathogenesis, and Diagnosis

Clostridium tetani, an anaerobic, Gram-positive rod that exists in both vegetative and sporulated forms, is the causative organism of tetanus. The spores are highly resistant to heat and chemical agents but can be destroyed by sterilization procedures.

Tetanus spores can survive for years if not exposed to deleterious influences. As a result, spores are ubiquitous in nature and are found in soil, dust, animal feces (and, less commonly, human feces), and on human skin. Germination and multiplication of tetanus bacilli are favored by the presence of necrotic tissue and the lack of oxygen at the site of inoculation.

The *C. tetani* bacillus produces an exotoxin, tetanospasmin, a potent selective neurotoxin responsible for clinical tetanus. Tetanospasmin travels along motor nerves generally after being disseminated through the bloodstream. It fixes to gangliosides in skeletal muscle, the spinal cord, the brain, and the autonomic nervous system. The quantity of toxin that causes disease may not be sufficient to induce an immune response. Consequently, tetanus infection may not confer immunity.

The diagnosis of tetanus depends on clinical signs and symptoms and not on bacteriologic confirmation. Isolation of *C. tetani* is neither sensitive nor specific: it is infrequently recovered from the contaminated wound or may be isolated from patients who do not have tetanus. The following case definition has been recommended by the Council for State and Territorial Epidemiologists (CSTE) since 1990: "Acute onset of hypertonia and/or painful muscular contractions (usually of the muscles of the jaw and neck) and generalized muscle spasms without other apparent medical cause (as reported by a health professional)."[3] Sera collected before tetanus immune globulin (TIG) is administered can demonstrate susceptibility of a patient to the disease.

Clinical Characteristics

The interval from trauma to the onset of clinical manifestations is variable, ranging from 2 days to 3 weeks or longer, but generally from 6 to 8 days. Clinical disease is a result of the effect of the neurotoxin on various receptors. Generalized tetanus is the most common form. Early signs and symptoms include stiffness or cramps in muscles around a wound, deep tendon hyperreflexia (particularly in the wounded extremity), stiffness of the neck and jaw, facial pain, and a change of facial expression (risus sardonicus). These may progress to include sudden contractions of muscle groups, causing opisthotonos. Spasms of laryngeal, diaphragmatic, and intercostal muscles may produce acute respiratory failure. Instability of the autonomic nervous system is a relatively common complication. Recovery from the acute episode of tetanus may require several weeks and is often complicated by pneumonia and difficulty in maintaining adequate nutrition. In general, the risk of death is related not only to the quality of supportive care provided but also to the patient's age and immunization status. Localized tetanus is occasionally seen; it is characterized by stiffness and rigidity around the site of injury. Localized tetanus may resolve without sequelae or may progress to generalized tetanus. Cephalic tetanus is a rare manifestation of the disease that is generally associated with lesions of the head or face, especially in the distribution of the facial nerves and orbits. In contrast to the other forms of tetanus, which are characterized by generalized spasms, cephalic tetanus is associated with atonic nerve palsies.

Neonatal tetanus results from *C. tetani* infection of the umbilical stump, at or following delivery, of a child born to a mother who did not possess sufficient circulating antitoxin to protect the infant passively by transplacental transfer.[4] Contamination of the umbilical stump usually occurs in the circumstance of an unattended delivery or one attended by an untrained midwife. In some areas of the world, the cord is cut with an unclean object or the umbilical stump is traditionally covered with contaminated materials.

Occurrence

Tetanus can occur as a complication of puncture wounds, compound fractures, abrasions, burns, injections, surgery, animal bites or scratches, gastrointestinal infections, abortions, childbirth, and infections of the umbilical stump. Puncture and deep wounds, especially those associated with necrotized tissue, are more hazardous than superficial abrasions. Abscesses and chronic skin ulceration may permit infection and lead to tetanus. Illicit injection drug use carries a risk of this disease. Tetanus has occurred after innocent-appearing wounds and in instances where no wound could be recalled.

The incidence rate of tetanus in the United States declined substantially from 1947 through the early 1970s.[5] Since then, the incidence has leveled off. The incidence rate of 0.02 cases per 100,000 population during the period from 1991 to 1994 remained unchanged from the incidence of 0.02 per 100,000 population between 1987 and 1990.[5-7] Tetanus remains a severe disease of older adults who are unvaccinated or inadequately vaccinated. A total of 201 cases were reported with onset between 1991 and 1994, for an average of 50 cases per year; 54 percent of cases occurred in persons 60 years of age or older, and 5 percent in persons less than 20 years of age. Overall, only 12 percent of cases had a history of three or more doses of tetanus toxoid, and 57 percent of these received their last booster dose more than 10 years prior to the onset of illness. The case-to-fatality ratio has declined in the last decade but remains 25 percent in reported cases, with a poorer prognosis for tetanus in elderly patients, particularly those with underlying medical conditions, and in neonates.[7]

Data obtained from a national population-based serosurvey conducted in the United States between 1988 and 1991 indicate that the prevalence of immunity to tetanus declines with increasing age from more than 80 percent among persons ages 6 to 39 years to 28 percent among persons 70 years of age or older. The lower prevalence in older age groups likely reflects a combination of a lower likelihood of having completed a primary series of tetanus vaccination (in part due to birth after initiation of routine childhood immunization with tetanus toxoid) as well as to waning immunity with time since the last dose. Seroprevalence was lower among the lower socioeconomic group and among persons born outside of the United States.[8]

Neonatal tetanus (NT) is a leading cause of death in many parts of the world and is second only to measles among the vaccine-preventable diseases as a cause of childhood mortality. In 1994, an estimated 490,000 neonatal deaths were attributed to NT, with an estimated global mortality rate from NT of 6.5 per 1,000 live births.[1] In the United States, NT is virtually eliminated. The last case of neonatal tetanus occurred in 1995, in an infant delivered in a hospital using standard aseptic practices, to a mother who had immigrated from Mexico 8 years previously. She had a history of receipt of one dose of tetanus toxoid at age 12 and had received prenatal care for this pregnancy (Centers for Disease Control and Prevention, unpublished data). The last prior case of neonatal tetanus in the United States occurred in 1989 in an infant born at home to an unvaccinated mother[6] who was born outside of the United States.

Prevention

Preexposure Vaccination. Preexposure active immunization with tetanus toxoid offers the best and most efficient method of preventing tetanus. Tetanus toxoid is one of the most effective of the immunobiologic agents and has been used on an increasing scale since the mid-1930s. The results of active immunization of U.S. Army personnel during World War II demonstrated the effectiveness of the toxoid. Only 12 cases occurred among 2.73 million wounded or injured personnel (0.44/100,000), compared with 70 cases among 0.52 million wounded or injured during World War I (13.4/100,000).[9]

Both aluminum phosphate adsorbed and fluid single-antigen tetanus toxoid (TT) preparations are available. The adsorbed preparations are more immunogenic. Tetanus toxoid, adsorbed, is available combined with diphtheria toxoid and acellular pertussis vaccine (DTaP), or with diphtheria toxoid and whole-cell pertussis vaccines (DTP). Adsorbed preparations without pertussis antigens are available as DT, for use in children less than 7 years of age, or with less than 2 Lf of diphtheria toxoid as Td for use in adults. The adsorbed toxoid preparations are currently recommended for primary immunization and booster doses. In general, tetanus toxoid should be given as DTaP, DTP, DT, or Td to provide concurrent protection against diphtheria with or without protection against pertussis.

In the United States, five doses of DTaP are recommended for routine childhood immunization, with three primary doses at 2, 4, and 6 months of age, a booster dose in the second year of life (15 to 18 months), and a second booster dose at school entry (4 to 6 years). DTaP is preferred for all doses of the pertussis vaccination series, but whole-cell pertussis vaccines remain acceptable alternatives.[10] The World Health Organization (WHO) recommends three doses of diphtheria and tetanus toxoids combined with whole-cell pertussis (DTP) at 6, 10, and 14 weeks of age. Booster doses in the second year of life are optional but recommended in many developing countries.

DTaP, DTP, or DT are not routinely recommended for persons 7 years of age or older because of the declining risk of serious cases of pertussis and the increasing frequency and severity of reactions to diphtheria toxoid with increasing age. Unimmunized individuals 7 years of age or older should receive a primary series with Td; for such persons a primary series consists of three doses, the first two given at an interval of 4 to 8 weeks and the third 6 to 12 months later. Booster doses are recommended at 10-year intervals. There is no need to restart a primary series regardless of the time elapsed between doses.

Available evidence indicates that a complete primary series with a tetanus toxoid–containing preparation provides long-lasting protective levels of circulating antitoxin—10 years or more—in most recipients. Rarely has a case of tetanus been reported in a person with a documented primary series of toxoid injections. Consequently, after complete primary tetanus immunization, booster doses of tetanus need be given only once every 10 years.[11] Although alternative booster schedules have been proposed,[12–14] the 10-year booster remains the recommended public health strategy for tetanus prevention in the United States. Recently, the Advisory Committee on Immunization Practices has lowered the age for the first Td booster dose to ages 11 to 13 years (e.g., adolescent immunization visit) and recommended an adult immunization visit at age 50 years to review past vaccination histories and to assess the need for and administer any other recommended vaccine.

Although severe systemic reactions to tetanus toxoid occur infrequently, if an anaphylactic reaction to a previous dose is suspected, a history of such a reaction should be confirmed by skin testing with appropriately diluted toxoid before a decision is made to discontinue further tetanus toxoid immunization.[15] Major local reactions have been reported, particularly in adults who have received doses more frequently than is generally recommended.[16]

Wound Management. The management of wounds includes adequate wound cleaning and débridement, evaluation of the wound, and evaluation of immunization status.[17,18] The need for tetanus toxoid (active immunization) with or without TIG (passive immunization) depends on both the condition of the wound and the patient's vaccination history. A careful attempt should be made to determine how many doses of toxoid a person has received previously. The major obstacle to appropriate prophylaxis in wound management is the difficulty of obtaining an accurate immunization history. Patients with unknown or uncertain previous immunization histories should be considered to have received no previous tetanus toxoid. Patients who have not completed a primary series require tetanus toxoid at the time of wound cleaning and débridement and may require passive immunization (depending on the type of wound and whether it appears contaminated), preferably with human tetanus immune globulin (TIG) (Table 7-3).[17]

If the patient has completed a primary series or received a booster dose within the preceding 10 years, and if the wound is judged to be clean and minor, no further toxoid is necessary. A small proportion of vaccines do not maintain a protective level of antitoxin for 10 years. If a patient sustains a wound that is judged to be other than clean and minor, and if the tetanus toxoid primary series was completed or a booster dose was received more than 5 years before, a booster dose is required. Persons with a clean, minor wound and fewer than three known previous doses of toxoid need only a dose of toxoid at the time of initial treatment. For patients with wounds with an increased risk of tetanus and fewer than three known previous doses of toxoid, appropriate passive immunization is indicated at the time of wound treatment in addition to a dose of toxoid. Subsequently, all inadequately immunized patients should receive complete primary immunization.[17]

When passive protection is indicated, 250 to 500 units of TIG given intramuscularly and concurrently with tetanus toxoid is an appropriate regimen for protection against tetanus.[19] Tetanus toxoid and TIG should be given at separate sites. Protection from TIG can be expected to last about 3 weeks. The use of equine antitoxin has serious disadvantages compared with the use of the human product, including short-lived protection, serum sickness, and occasionally anaphylaxis. Since the TIG of human origin has become widely available, there is little justification for the use of equine antitoxin for postexposure prophylaxis and treatment.

The treatment of tetanus includes administration of TIG in dosages of 3,000 to 6,000 units intramuscularly to neutralize circulating tetanus toxin, administration of antibiotics, and débridement to help eliminate the organism and thereby prevent further toxin production. In addition, intensive primary medical and supportive care is critical. Because tetanus disease may not induce immunity to tetanus, all persons with tetanus should start or complete a primary immunization series.

Neonatal Tetanus Prevention

The goal of global elimination of tetanus was adopted by the World Health Assembly in 1989.[20] The key strategies are (*a*) achievement and maintenance of high vaccination coverage levels for at least two doses of tetanus toxoid among women of childbearing age in high-risk areas, and (*b*) promotion of clean delivery and cord care practices.[1,2,21] Active immunization of unimmunized pregnant women with two doses of appropriately timed toxoid prevents tetanus neonatorum. Additional doses can be given with each pregnancy. Five adult doses are likely to provide lifelong protection against neonatal tetanus, and is currently the schedule recommended by the WHO for neonatal tetanus prevention.[22] A recent review of TT production in

TABLE 7-3. SUMMARY GUIDE TO TETANUS PROPHYLAXIS IN ROUTINE WOUND MANAGEMENT, 1991

History of Adsorbed Tetanus Toxoid (doses)	Clean Minor Wounds		All Other Wounds[a]	
	Td[b]	*TIG*	*Td*[b]	*TIG*
Unknown or fewer than three	Yes	No	Yes	Yes
Three or more[c]	No[d]	No	No[e]	No

[a]Such as, but not limited to, wounds contaminated with dirt, feces, soil, and saliva; puncture wounds; avulsions; and wounds resulting from missiles, crushing, burns, and frostbite.
[b]For children less than 7 years old DTaP or DTP (DT, if pertussis vaccine is contraindicated) is preferred to tetanus toxoid alone. For persons 7 years of age and above, Td is preferred to tetanus toxoid alone.
[c]If only three doses of fluid toxoid have been received, then a fourth dose of toxoid, preferably an adsorbed toxoid, should be given.
[d]Yes, if more than 10 years since the last dose.
[e]Yes, if more than 5 years since the last dose. (More frequent boosters are not needed and can accentuate side effects).

developing countries has identified the need for monitoring of local TT production and field effectiveness in these countries to ensure compliance with WHO standards.[2] Neonatal tetanus is currently rare in the United States because the vast majority of deliveries are appropriately attended and because routine immunization in childhood for several decades has resulted in a high percentage of immunized women of childbearing age.[21]

Summary

All persons should receive active primary tetanus immunization, preferably combined with diphtheria toxoid (and, if appropriate for age, pertussis vaccine), and booster doses once every 10 years. Health care providers should use every encounter a person has with a health service to evaluate immunization status and administer needed immunizations.

Diphtheria

Charles Vitek

In the course of the twentieth century, diphtheria has evolved from being a major childhood killer to a clinical curiosity in developed countries because of the development and wide use of an effective and safe toxoid vaccine. However, a massive diphtheria epidemic in the countries of the former Soviet Union since 1990 following decades of good control has illustrated the potential for this vaccine-preventable disease to reemerge. Diphtheria also continues to be an important cause of disease and death in developing countries.

Etiologic Agent, Pathogenesis, and Diagnosis

Corynebacterium diphtheriae is a Gram-positive, nonmotile bacillus and an obligate parasite of humans that was first described as the etiologic agent of diphtheria by Loeffler in 1884. The organism is killed if held at 60°C for 20 minutes but survives freezing and desiccation for months when enclosed in proteinaceous materials. Some strains of *C. diphtheriae* contain a bacteriophage coding for the production of a polypeptide exotoxin; non-toxin-producing strains can be converted to toxin production if infected by the bacteriophage. Although there are three biotypes of *C. diphtheriae* (gravis, mitis, and intermedius), toxin-producing strains of all three biotypes produce an identical exotoxin, and no consistent difference in pathogenicity has been demonstrated between the three biotypes.

Diphtheria is a distinct clinical syndrome caused by the phage-induced toxin; infections with non-toxin-producing strains of *C. diphtheriae* are not associated with diphtheria but can cause localized inflammation and, rarely, other syndromes.[1] The syndrome is initiated by a superficial infection and toxin production by *C. diphtheriae* usually on pharyngeal mucosa or other respiratory mucosa. The toxin binds to a wide range of mammalian cells, including epithelial, nerve, and muscle cells, interfering enzymatically with protein synthesis, and leading to cell damage and death. Local effects include severe tissue inflammation and the formation of a pseudomembrane composed of necrotic debris, exudate, and bacteria. Progressively greater systemic absorption of the toxin occurs as the pseudomembrane enlarges and local inflammation increases.

Diphtheria transmission is generally by droplet spread from either active cases or carriers. Untreated, a patient generally remains infectious for 2 weeks or less. Chronic carriage may occasionally occur, rarely even after antimicrobial therapy. Transmission from cutaneous cases can be a result of environmental contamination or of direct skin contact.

Clinical diagnosis is usually based on the presence of diphtheritic pseudomembrane in a patient with a febrile pharyngitis. Specific diagnosis depends on the recovery of the organism and confirmation of toxigenicity and is possible in the majority of cases if specimens are taken before administration of antibiotics. If clinical specimens cannot be immediately transported to the laboratory, they should be sent in a transport medium or, if a long delay is anticipated, in silica gel. Culture requires the use of selective media, with a tellurite-containing medium being best for primary isolation. Toxigenicity of the diphtheria organism can be determined by in vivo (guinea pig) or in vitro (Elek) tests of isolates. Testing of clinical specimens with a recently developed polymerase chain reaction for the gene coding for toxin has been shown to be useful for laboratory confirmation in isolated situations where the organism is difficult to recover, but this is currently available only at certain reference laboratories.[2] Molecular analysis of *C. diphtheriae* strains shows considerable promise in aiding epidemiologic investigations and is available at some reference laboratories.[3,4]

Clinical Characteristics

The clinical syndrome known as diphtheria usually develops insidiously over 1 to 2 days after an incubation period of 1 to 5 days following infection with *C. diphtheriae* in the respiratory tract, or, rarely, of the skin or other sites (such as the eye, ear, or genitalia). The syndrome usually presents as a febrile, membranous pharyngitis, associated with signs of systemic toxicity such as weakness, tachycardia, and agitation disproportionate to the degree of fever, which is usually mild throughout the illness. In severe cases, especially with delays in obtaining medical care, neck edema, airway obstruction, myocarditis, or polyneuritis may be present at presentation.

Respiratory forms of diphtheria include pharyngotonsillar, laryngotracheal, or nasal forms, either singly or in combination. Patients with pharyngotonsillar diphtheria usually have a sore throat, difficulty in swallowing, and low-grade fever at presentation. Examination of the throat may show only mild erythema, localized exudate, or a pseudomembrane. The membrane may be localized to a patch of the posterior pharynx or tonsil, may cover the entire tonsil, or, less frequently, may spread to cover the soft and hard palates and the posterior portion of the pharynx. In the early stage or in patients who have been partially or fully immunized, a membrane may be whitish and may wipe off easily. However, in inadequately immunized patients, the membrane may extend and become thick, blue-white to gray-black, and adherent. Attempts to remove the membrane result in bleeding. Marked mucosal erythema surrounds and underlies the membrane. Patients with severe disease may have marked edema of the submandibular areas and the anterior portion of the neck, which, along with lymphadenopathy, gives a characteristic "bull-neck" appearance. Pharyngitis with a pseudomembrane may also occur in infectious mononucleosis, viral pharyngitis (rarely), and streptococcal or monilial pharyngitis.

Laryngotracheal diphtheria is most often preceded by pharyngotonsillar disease, is usually associated with hoarseness and a croupy cough at presentation, and, if the infection extends into the bronchial tree, is the most severe form of disease. Initially it may be clinically indistinguishable from viral croup or epiglottitis. Nasal diphtheria, the mildest form of respiratory diphtheria, is usually localized to the septum or turbinates of one side of the nose. Occasionally a membrane may extend into the pharynx.

Nonrespiratory mucosal surfaces (i.e., the conjunctivae and genitals) may also be sites of infection. Severe diphtheria can occasionally result.

Cutaneous infection with toxigenic *C. diphtheriae* is common in tropical areas; in temperate zones, cutaneous diphtherial infections are frequently associated with poor hygiene and low socioeconomic status. The clinical syndrome of diphtheria rarely results from isolated cutaneous diphtherial infections, even in inadequately immunized individuals. Cutaneous infections often result from a secondary infection of a previous skin abrasion or infection. The presenting lesion, often an ulcer, may be surrounded by erythema and covered with a membrane.

Complications

With the exception of airway obstruction, the serious complications result from the systemic effects of toxin absorption and include myocarditis, polyneuritis and, rarely, renal failure, thrombocytopenia, or shock with disseminated intravascular coagulation. Airway obstruction can result from extension or sudden displacement of the membrane into the larynx or the bronchial tree. Myocarditis and polyneuritis caused by the toxin are the most common serious complications; myocarditis and mechanical airway obstruction are the major causes of death. Antitoxin therapy has significantly reduced the rates of complications and death, which are directly related to the delay before antitoxin treatment and the extent of the local lesion (although even mild illness can occasionally produce complications), and inversely related to the adequacy of previous vaccination.

Myocarditis may begin in the first through the sixth week of clinical illness. Electrocardiographic changes are present in as many as one-fourth of the patients; clinically evident cardiac impairment or congestive heart failure is present in a smaller proportion. Recovery usually is complete, but persistent cardiac abnormalities may result.

Cranial or peripheral neuritis, primarily involving motor loss, usually develops 1 to 8 weeks or longer after the onset of disease, although isolated paralysis of the soft palate may be present at disease onset. Loss of visual accommodation, diplopia, nasal-sounding voice, and difficulty in swallowing are the most frequent manifestations of cranial nerve involvement. Complete recovery of neurologic impairment is the rule.

Treatment

The administration of serum containing high titers of antibody against diphtheria antitoxin dramatically lowers the death rate from diphtheria, as was first reported in 1893 by von Behring. Treatment should not be delayed for bacteriologic confirmation of the diagnosis, as increasing intervals between onset and treatment are correlated with higher rates of complications and death.[5] The dosage of antitoxin depends on this interval and the severity of disease and ranges between 20,000 and 100,000 units. Currently, no U.S. licensed diphtheria antitoxin product is available. A diphtheria antitoxin licensed in Europe (Pasteur Mérieux, Lyon, France) is available on a case-by-case basis through the Centers for Disease Control and Prevention (CDC) under an Investigational New Drug Protocol with the FDA to treat suspected diphtheria cases.

All commercially available diphtheria antitoxin products are produced from serum obtained from hyperimmunized horses and can produce severe or fatal anaphylaxis in sensitized individuals. The treatment of a patient with suspected diphtheria requires treatment with diphtheria antitoxin as soon as possible after testing for hypersensitivity to horse serum; desensitization should be performed if necessary.

In addition to anaphylaxis, adverse effects of antitoxin treatment include febrile reactions occurring shortly after administration and serum sickness, which occurs in approximately 5 percent of patients receiving antitoxin, usually 7 to 14 days after treatment. The risk of febrile reactions and serum sickness is not predicted by hypersensitivity testing.

In addition to antitoxin treatment, antibiotic treatment with penicillin or erythromycin is also needed to eliminate the organism, stopping toxin production and limiting transmissibility. In addition, patients should receive any doses of diphtheria toxoid needed to complete a primary series or bring booster doses up to date.

Occurrence

Developed Countries. The occurrence of diphtheria in the United States has fallen dramatically from more than 147,000 cases and 13,000 deaths in 1920 to an annual average of three reported cases of respiratory diphtheria from 1980 through 1995. Thirty of the 43 cases reported in the United States during 1980 through 1995 affected persons 20 years of age or older, most of whom lacked a history of up-to-date vaccination. Limited serosurveys in the 1970s and 1980s in the United States indicated that 40 percent or more of adults lacked protective levels of circulating antibodies against diphtheria. A similar pattern has been seen in many other developed countries, where vaccination programs have greatly reduced the circulation of toxigenic *C. diphtheriae* and adults do not receive routine booster immunizations.[6]

Diphtheria Resurgence in the Newly Independent States of the Former Soviet Union (NIS). A gap in adult immunity has been a major factor in the diphtheria epidemic in the NIS, where diphtheria had been reduced to very low levels since the early 1960s due to highly successful childhood immunization programs but where more than 125,000 cases and 4,000 deaths, primarily among adults, have been reported between 1990 through 1995.[7]

Additional factors that may have contributed to the resurgence include lowered childhood immunization due to misperceptions among the population and physicians of the relative risks and benefits of vaccination, increased population movement due to the breakup of the Soviet Union, and socioeconomic hardship.[8] A change in the *C. diphtheriae* organism as represented by the appearance of an epidemic clone of gravis strains in Russia may also have contributed to the epidemic;[4] however, large outbreaks with mitis strains have also occurred during this epidemic, supporting a major role for the human population factors.

Effective control of the epidemic has required raising childhood vaccination levels and achieving unprecedentedly high adult vaccination coverage.[9] Control strategies have included concerted efforts to decrease the resistance to vaccination among physicians and the population and organizing mass vaccination campaigns for adults and children in all of the NIS. In a very successful response to a perceived international public health emergency, an international coalition of public health donors, led by the World Health Organization (WHO), mobilized the large amounts of vaccine and other supplies needed by all of the NIS except Russia, which remains self-sufficient for vaccines. Very few imported cases and no secondary outbreaks have been reported from neighboring European countries.

Developing Countries. In developing countries, a steady decrease in diphtheria incidence has occurred since the introduction of diphtheria toxoid into the WHO Expanded Programme on Immunization in most of these countries in the late 1970s. In 1974, developing countries contributed 97 percent of the more than 70,000 cases reported to the WHO, while in 1992 they contributed 79 percent of the 20,444 cases reported.

Even prior to the introduction of immunization programs, developing countries rarely experienced large outbreaks of diphtheria, although reporting many cases of diphtheria among very young children. The lack of outbreaks is thought to result from widespread natural immunity from high rates of skin infections with *C. diphtheriae* in early childhood. Recently, outbreaks of diphtheria have occurred in many developing countries that have had effective childhood immunization programs for 5 to 10 years, with a shift in the affected age groups to older children and young adults. The introduction of additional routine booster doses into immunization programs may be needed to prevent outbreaks in these age groups.[6]

Prevention and Control

In 1918, New York City initiated an immunization program for children using a mixture of antitoxin and toxin; the results provided the first large-scale demonstration that such a program could decrease diphtheria incidence and mortality. The subsequent improvements in efficacy and safety of immunization from the introduction of toxoid (formalin-treated toxin) by Ramon in 1923, and then alum-precipitated toxoid in 1931, led to the establishment of programs for childhood vaccination against diphtheria in the United States and many other developed countries in the 1930s and 1940s.[10]

Active Immunization. Active immunization provides individual protection by inducing and maintaining adequate levels of circulating antitoxin. These levels will limit the extent of local invasion of the organism and neutralize unbound absorbed toxin, thus preventing life-threatening systemic complications. A three-dose series of diphtheria toxoid is highly immunogenic in all age groups and significantly reduces both the risk of diphtheria and the severity of clinical illness. In addition to individual protection, high levels of population vaccination appear to have decreased diphtheria transmission in the United States and other developed countries, even though toxoid is not thought to prevent carriage of the organ-ism in the pharynx or on the skin. Booster doses of diphtheria toxoid are required to maintain immunity in the absence of "natural" boosting from circulating diphtheria as vaccine-induced antibody levels wane over time; the duration of immunity depends on multiple factors, including the timing and antigenic content of the primary series.[6]

The global WHO recommendations for diphtheria immunization are for delivery of a primary series (three doses of a high-antigenic content preparation) in infancy and maintenance of immunity throughout life. Strategies to achieve this will vary by country depending on the capacity of immunization services and epidemiologic pattern of diphtheria.[11] Currently few developing countries provide routine booster doses to older children or adults. Global coverage for children with a primary series of three doses of diphtheria toxoid has exceeded 80 percent since 1990; coverage rates are high in most of the developing countries outside of Africa.

In recent years, the number of doses of diphtheria toxoid-containing vaccine in the recommended vaccine schedule in the United States has remained constant, although the licensure of new combination vaccines has created a greater choice of preparations, and further licensure of new combination vaccines is expected. Diphtheria toxoid is available in combination with pertussis vaccine (whole cell or acellular) or tetanus toxoid or both as DTP, DTaP, and DT for use in children less than 7 years of age; the antigenic content of these preparations ranges from 6.7 to 15 Lf. Another preparation, Td, containing less than 2 Lf of diphtheria toxoid, is intended for use in older children and adults.

The current schedule in the United States recommends three doses of diphtheria toxoid-containing vaccine (DTaP, DTP, or DT) at 4- to 8-week intervals beginning, when possible, at 2 months of age. A fourth dose is recommended approximately 6 to 12 months after the third dose, and a fifth dose at 4 to 6 years of age.[12,13] Because with increasing age the frequency and severity of local reactions increase, unimmunized individuals 7 years of age or older should receive a primary series with Td; for such persons a primary series consists of three doses, the first two given at an interval of 4 to 8 weeks and the third 6 to 12 months later. Booster doses are recommended at 10-year intervals. There is no need to restart a primary series regardless of the time elapsed between doses.

Management of Contacts of Patients with Suspected Disease. All household contacts and other close contacts should be cultured and receive prophylactic antibiotics and any needed vaccination.[14] Vaccination with a dose of an age-appropriate diphtheria toxoid-containing vaccine should be done unless less than 5 years has elapsed since completion of a primary series or the last booster dose. After cultures are taken, antibiotic treatment with a single dose of intramuscular penicillin (600,000 units for persons less than 6 years old and 1.2 million units for those 6 years old and older) or a 7- to 10-day course of oral erythromycin (30 to 50 mg/kg; maximum, 2 g/day) is recommended for all persons exposed to diphtheria, regardless of vaccination status. Persons found to be carriers of *C. diphtheriae* should have cultures repeated a minimum of 2 weeks after completion of antibiotics; persistent carriers should receive an additional 7- to 10-day oral course of erythromycin.

Conclusion

Routine diphtheria vaccination has been highly successful in greatly reducing the once devastating burden of this disease. However, the recent diphtheria epidemic in the former Soviet Union underlines the need to maintain high levels of immunization in both children and adults in the United States and other countries to provide both individual protection and high population immunity. Health care providers should use every patient encounter to review and recommend any needed vaccination.

Influenza

Bradley N. Doebbeling

Influenza is an acute febrile respiratory illness caused by influenza virus A, B, or C. Although typically a mild or asymptomatic disease, influenza can be severe and even fatal. Influenza A or B usually occurs in outbreaks most winters. Worldwide outbreaks, which occur less frequently, are termed pandemics. Type C influenza is uncommon and has not been associated with epidemics. Unlike several other classic viral diseases which have been eradicated or greatly controlled, influenza remains uncontrolled. Importantly, vaccination decreases the attack rate and severity of disease. However, since the virus regularly alters its two major surface proteins, elimination of the disease through vaccination directed at these antigens is at present unachievable.

History

Recurrent epidemics of influenza occur on average once every 1 to 3 years and can be traced back hundreds of years. As early as the twelfth century, widespread outbreaks of rapidly spreading febrile respiratory diseases with a high attack rate and frequent cough were likely influenza outbreaks. The term "influenza" resulted from an epidemic in 1357, which Buonissequi referred to as the "grande influenza."[1] The Italian word for "influence" was used as a collective term for various causes of widespread epidemics. Among them, cold weather, "influenza di freddo," was regarded as a causal factor for many years. Although conjecture on origin was lively when influenza was prevalent, interest waned between the major epidemics.

The first clearly described pandemic occurred in 1580; 31 have been subsequently described. The pandemic of 1918–1919 demonstrated the potential devastation of influenza. Worldwide, an estimated 500 million persons were infected and 21 million persons died, including 549,000 in the United States. In the era of AIDS, it is easily forgotten that influenza caused the most deadly epidemic of disease in recorded history. Although this pandemic is the foremost example, many other epidemics show the severe impact of influenza on public health and economics.

The rapidity of the spread of influenza was probably best documented in the epidemic of 1957. A distinctive strain of influenza A was recovered in Hong Kong and Singapore in early April. The virus spread rapidly through the South Pacific, Southeast Asia, and the Middle East by June, and into Europe and North America by midsummer. By the end of 1957 the "Asian" strain of the virus had spread worldwide. In the United States, primary and secondary waves of cases resulted in nearly 70,000 deaths.

In contrast to earlier epidemics, the epidemic of the "Russian" strain of influenza A in 1977–1978 was remarkable in that the illness was largely confined to persons born after about 1955. Most adults in 1977 appeared to have possessed immunity as a result of infection with similar strains that had been present beginning in the late 1940s. Even so, major outbreaks occurred in children and young adults in the rest of the world during the next few months, and the rate of spread was parallel to that of earlier pandemic viruses.

A series of important discoveries led to the modern understanding of the virus and its epidemiology. The first influenza virus isolated was a type A virus from ferrets in 1933 by Smith et al.[2] Influenza B was first isolated in 1939 by Francis,[3] and influenza C in 1950 by Taylor.[4] Burnet's discovery in 1936 that the virus could be grown in embryonated chickens' eggs facilitated the study of viral characteristics and the development of inactivated vaccines.[5] Hirst's discovery of hemagglutination in 1941 led to improved measures of the virus and specific antibody.[6] Public health control measures such as widespread use of inactivated vaccines began in the 1950s. Since then, vaccines have been directed at selected segments of the population considered to be at risk. Chemotherapy and prophylaxis with amantadine began in the United States in 1966.

The difficulties of epidemiologic forecasts and the complexities of developing a national influenza-prevention strategy were demonstrated in 1976 when a focal outbreak of "swine" influenza A occurred in a New Jersey military camp. Since this strain resembled the one thought to have caused the great epidemic of 1918 and 1919, scientists promptly agreed on the need for a national vaccination program using a swine influenza-specific vaccine. Congress voted funds for vaccine production and program development and eventually insured manufacturers against vaccine-associated risks so that the program could be implemented. The vaccination program for swine influenza begun in December 1976 was a major undertaking, distributing 85.4 million doses of vaccine. In that program, 38 percent and 32 percent of elderly and young high-risk patients, respectively, were vaccinated.

Although expected to become widespread, the swine influenza outbreak did not reach epidemic proportions. Furthermore, the vaccination program had to be abandoned after 3 months when there appeared to be an excessive number of cases of Guillain-Barré syndrome after vaccination. The remarkable achievement of implementing a coordinated national influenza immunization program (conducted at the state and local health department level) was overshadowed by challenges to the soundness of scientific judgment and public health policy in responding to the prospects of epidemic influenza.

Etiologic Agent

Influenza virus is a medium-sized virus (80 to 120 nm) and is a member of the family *Orthomyxoviridae*. Usually spherical, the virus consists of single-stranded ribonucleic acid (RNA) enclosed in a helical protein shell, or nucleocapsid. The virus is covered by a lipid envelope with surface projections or spikes. Influenza viruses can be divided into three distinct types—A, B, and C—on the basis of their ribonucleoprotein (RNP), or soluble protein. Influenza A viruses have been isolated from humans, horses, swine, and avian species. Types B and C are almost exclusively recovered from humans, although type C influenza has now been isolated from pigs in China. Influenza C virus, which almost always causes an upper respiratory (common cold-like) illness, differs biochemically from types A and B and may eventually be assigned to another genus.

Projecting from the surface of the envelope are two distinct types of polypeptide spikes, 8 to 14 nm long, both of which are highly antigenic. The more common of the spikes, the hemagglutinin (HA), is named for its ability to cause agglutination of erythrocytes (hemagglutination). HA serves as the attachment site of the virus to host cells before phagocytosis, and specific antibody to it prevents the initiation of infection. Neuraminidase (NA), the second type of spike, occurs less frequently on the viral surface than HA and is an enzyme that splits neuraminic acid from mucoproteins. Neuraminidase is involved in releasing newly formed viruses from the host cell surface, although whether it provides other functions for the virus is less clear. Both HA and NA can be subdivided into distinct subtypes.

Immunity

Antibodies to surface antigens of the influenza viruses are important in preventing infection. Most patients convalescing from influenza develop specific antibodies in 2 to 4 weeks. Whereas adults have a high degree of resistance to reinfection with the same virus strain or its subsequent variants for many years, children can be reinfected frequently. Immunity to influenza is a complex function of antibody, host resistance, and changes in the biological and antigenic characteristics of prevalent viruses.

Antibody against the hemagglutinin is the primary mechanism for virus neutralization, and its relative abundance provides the best index of protection. Nonetheless, antibody against neuraminidase also plays a role in ameliorating disease and decreasing virus transmission. The roles of secretory antibody in local immunity and of cytotoxic T cells in cell-mediated immunity are not yet fully understood.

Clinical Characteristics

Influenza usually occurs as an abrupt respiratory illness with fever, chills, fatigue, headache, myalgias, malaise, anorexia, and nonproductive cough. Fever is the most characteristic finding, appearing early (within 12 to 24 hours) and possibly reaching 40°C (104°F) or higher. Headache and myalgias are often the most distressing symptoms and are related to the degree of fever elevation. Early laboratory studies reveal a normal leukocyte count with a relative lymphopenia (low lymphocyte count in relation to the total white blood cell count). The chest x-ray film usually shows only enlarged hilar shadows. Typically, fever lasts 3 days, occasionally as long as 8 days, after which systemic symptoms begin to resolve and respiratory symptoms (cough, nasal obstruction, discharge) become more prominent. Recovery is usually rapid, although cough sometimes persists for weeks.

Complications

Complications of influenza, although relatively uncommon, are usually pulmonary in nature. Either primary influenza virus pneumonia or a complicating (secondary) bacterial pneumonia can occur, both of which can be severe, with a high mortality rate. Risk factors for primary influenza viral pneumonia include cardiac disease, especially rheumatic heart disease, other chronic disorders, and pregnancy.[7] Complicating bacterial pneumonias are reported in fewer than 1 percent of all patients with influenza. Risk factors for them include advanced age and chronic pulmonary, cardiac, metabolic, or other disease. Pneumococci, *Staphylococcus aureus*, and *Haemophilus influenzae* are the most common causes of secondary bacterial pneumonias. Other milder pulmonic syndromes may occur, including acute tracheobronchitis, localized viral pneumonia, mixed viral and bacterial bronchopneumonia, croup, or exacerbations of chronic pulmonary disease.[7]

Nonpulmonary complications are less common. Cardiac complications, including pericarditis and myocarditis, although unusual, occur primarily in patients with pneumonia. Neurologic syndromes such as encephalitis, transverse myelitis, and Guillain-Barré syndrome have followed influenza; however, no definitive causal relationship has been established. Children will occasionally acquire myositis after influenza. Reye's syndrome has been associated with influenza B more commonly than with influenza A.[8] The effects of influenza infection on the fetus are controversial. Information regarding congenital defects and spontaneous abortion suggests that the fetus may be at increased risk, although the exact risk is unknown. The case-to-fatality ratio during pregnancy has been reported to be increased.

Influenza Virus Surveillance

Because of frequent changes in the surface antigens of the influenza virus and the resultant epidemics, the WHO established an international network in 1947 to collect and disseminate laboratory and epidemiologic data on the virus. The laboratory surveillance effort is aimed primarily at (*a*) monitoring influenza infection in humans and animals, (*b*) characterizing antigenic changes in prevalent viruses to trace their evolution, and (*c*) detecting antigenic changes that may signal the need for an updated formulation of influenza vaccines. Current approaches to surveillance include a system of collaborating laboratories that report influenza isolation, a network of sentinel physicians, monitoring of the proportion of hospital pneumonia and influenza discharges, and monitoring rates of school and work absenteeism. Recent data demonstrate that school-based surveillance is an acceptable, simple, timely, and sensitive system for detecting influenza outbreaks by monitoring absenteeism rates.[9]

Virus can be isolated from throat swabs, nasal swabs, nasal washes, and sputum. Cultures can be grown in primary monkey kidney cell culture and in certain continuous cell lines. Successful virus recovery is dependent on early collection of specimens (within 72 hours of the onset of illness), proper transport to the laboratory, and correct culture techniques. The isolation can be confirmed with hemadsorption inhibition, hemagglutination inhibition, or serum neutralization. Direct or indirect fluorescent antibody staining of nasal mucosal cells aspirated from patients have also been used for rapid diagnosis. Serologic tests are available and consist of type-specific complement fixation tests using ribonucleoprotein antigen, and strain-specific hemagglutination inhibition tests employing selected viral antigens. Positive serologic test results require a 4-fold risebetween paired acute and convalescent serum drawn 2 to 3 weeks apart. Since such tests require a delay in processing, serologic findings are not helpful in making an early diagnosis. Thus, influenza is usually a clinical diagnosis based on history, physical examination, season, and presence of documented influenza in the community.

Epidemiology

General Characteristics. Influenza occurs worldwide. In the tropics, influenza occurs year round in an endemic pattern; nevertheless, epidemics can also occur in any season. In temperate climates, cases usually occur in an epidemic pattern in winter and early spring. Physical conditions such as ambient temperature, low humidity, relative intactness of mucous membranes, and closeness of personal contact are believed to contribute to the seasonality of influenza. Pandemics can occur at any time following a major antigenic shift.

Influenza A epidemics are more common than influenza B epidemics, due to the slower rate of antigenic variation of type B strains. The virus is transmitted by respiratory secretions via an airborne route. The incubation period is short, just 1 to 2 days. Viral shedding usually begins 1 to 2 days before onset of symptoms and generally lasts about 1 week.

Attack rates during outbreaks may be as high as 10 to 40 percent. Although attack rates are higher among children than adults, the frequency of complications is lower. Even though most often a self-limited disease, influenza can cause death. It has a low case-to-fatality ratio, about 1 or 2 deaths per 2,000 cases; however, in selected groups such as the chronically ill and elderly, the case-to-fatality ratio can be as high as 30 percent.

Influenza infects susceptible persons, primarily children and young adults, who in turn spread the infection to adults in their homes and in the community. Transmission between adults occurs but is less important than spread from younger to older persons, except possibly when distinctly new strains appear.

The first evidence of influenza in a community is often an explosive outbreak in a school or nursing home. The outbreak is often preceded by sporadic cases or clusters of cases either overlooked or unrecognized. Often a dramatic increase in the number and geographic extent of reported outbreaks and visits to physicians or hospital emergency clinics for medical care confirms the spread of the disease. In circumscribed geographic areas, epidemics reach peak levels within 2 to 3 weeks and resolve over the next month.

Attack rates range from 10 to 25 percent of those in a community during mild to moderately brisk epidemics. Some population subgroups have markedly differing experiences, however, because of enhanced susceptibility or increased chances of exposure. Children play an important role in the acquisition and spread of influenza. For example, while 40 to 60 percent or more of children who ride crowded school buses may develop influenza, suburban adults without children can appear to be completely uninvolved in the same outbreak. There is evidence for the importance of herd immunity in nursing homes, since outbreaks occur more often in larger homes and in those with lower rates of vaccine acceptance.[10]

In the Northern Hemisphere, the "influenza season" usually lasts 3 to 4 months, typically beginning in mid-November. Sporadic cases of influenza occur throughout the summer. However, occasionally outbreaks of influenza A may occur and should be considered in outbreaks of acute, febrile respiratory illness.[11] At times the season is prolonged or shortened depending on the causative viruses or cocirculation of both A and B strains.

Antigenic Variation

The ability of the influenza virus to frequently change its surface antigens is unrivaled; this capability is referred to as antigenic variation. Antigenic variation occurs approximately yearly in influenza A and is responsible for the nearly annual epidemics. Although antigenic variation occurs in type B influenza, it happens less frequently. Antigenic variation has not been identified in influenza C. Alteration of the antigen structure leads to exposure to viral strains to which the population may have little or no immunity, resulting in an epidemic.

Antigenic Drift

Minor changes in either the HA or NA antigen within an influenza subtype is termed antigenic drift. Each subtype is referred to by its HA and NA. There have been three hemagglutinins (H1, H2, and H3) and two neuraminidases (N1 and N2) recognized in humans. Strains within the subtype are identified by the site and year of viral isolation. The nomenclature classification system for influenza virus in general use was developed by the World Health Organization (WHO). It includes, in order, the virus type, geographic origin, laboratory reference number, and year of isolation. For example, the first type B strain isolated in Oregon in 1965 would be designated B/Oregon/1/65. Among influenza A viruses, a parenthesized description of the HA and NA antigens follows the strain designation: A/Mississippi/1/85/H3N2. The WHO system is periodically revised as necessary to accommodate new information.[12] Antigenic drift is attributed to a mutation or mutations affecting the RNA segment coding for either the HA or NA.

Antigenic Shift

Major antigenic changes of type A strains are termed antigenic shift and occur prior to worldwide pandemics. Importantly, these viruses appear to be unique strains to which the population has little or no immunity. Because there is typically little or no serologic relatedness between these two strains, each receives a different HA and NA classification. For example, the 1957 pandemic occurred when type A "Asian" (H2N2) replaced type A (H1N1) influenza. Three new hemagglutinins and two new neuraminidases have emerged in the last century. The mechanism of antigenic shift has been attributed to genetic reassortment of RNA, resulting in a new surface glycoprotein.

After the emergence of a new HA or NA subtype, antigenic drift occurs infrequently. New variants appear more and more frequently until the next major change or antigenic shift occurs. Antigenic drift has been attributed to selection of preexisting mutants because of pressure from increasing immunity in the population to circulating strains. When there is sufficient immunity in the population as a result of minor viral changes (antigenic drift) to allow the virus to escape the immunity, then major antigenic changes (antigenic shift) occur with a resultant pandemic. The most popular explanation of antigenic shift is a genetic recombination of human and animal strains.

Migrating waterfowl and shorebirds throughout the world are two partly overlapping reservoirs of influenza A.[13] These species contain influenza viruses of all known hemagglutinin and neuraminidase subtypes, although avian virus genes show far less variation than mammalian virus gene lineages. Periodic exchanges of influenza virus genes or whole viruses occur, giving rise to pandemics of disease among humans, animals, and birds. It has been suggested that pigs serve as a site for reassortment between influenza viruses from mammalian and avian hosts.

Newer strains may "replace" older strains in a continual, linear fashion. For example, H1N1 strains were commonly isolated until 1957, when H2N2 strains appeared. The H2N2 strains were the predominant strains isolated until they were replaced in 1968 by H3N2 strains. Recently, however, several strains have coexisted at the same time, and mixed infections have occurred, albeit infrequently. The virus may also "recycle" its surface antigen by having a previously predominant strain that has disappeared return as the prevalent isolate.[14] However, there is no evidence that recycling is predictable.

Epidemic-Pandemic Potential

Influenza occurs in epidemics and pandemics because of the high mutability of the surface antigens of the virus and the prevalence of susceptible persons in the population. Thus, the ability of any new variant strain to cause infection depends on the novelty of the strain with respect to the immunologic experience of the exposed groups.

Public Health Implications

Estimates of the morbidity and mortality directly attributable to influenza have been problematic, due to the difficulty in separating out the effects of different respiratory pathogens circulating in the population at the same time. There are relatively few data on the average cost of a case of influenza. Estimates of total U.S. expenditures on influenza range from $1 billion to $3 billion per year.[15] Industrial absenteeism generally increases by less than 1 to 2 percent during the average epidemic; however, it can be extremely disruptive at times. Of particular concern are cases of influenza in nursing homes, where attack rates up to 80 percent and case-to-fatality rates of 30 percent have been reported.

In the United States, an excess 13.8 to 16.0 million respiratory illnesses occur each year among those under 20 years of age, whereas the older population experience 4.1 to 4.4 million excess illnesses each year.[16] Similarly, it has been estimated that among those under 20, there are 152.0 to 176.4 million excess respiratory ill days; among those 20 years old or older, there are 65.7 to 70.6 million excess respiratory ill days. These illnesses are not inconsequential, with the population under age 20 experiencing 47.1 to 54.7 million excess bed and restricted-activity days, versus 16.6 to 17.6 million for the older population.

In the United States each year an excess 10,000 to 20,000 deaths are attributed to influenza, primarily in elderly persons. Deaths caused by pneumonia and influenza average about 5 to 6 percent of the total U.S. deaths and peak in the winter.[17] When deaths from pneumonia and influenza exceed the threshold for epidemics, influenza is almost always the cause (Fig. 7-5). Estimates of excess mortality due to influenza are currently based on time-series analysis of mortality data from the National Center for Health Statistics.[18] When influenza and pneumonia deaths exceed the epidemic threshold, excess mortality is almost always due to influenza A, or occasionally to influenza B. Deaths occur both in pandemic and interpandemic periods, with mortality of the interpandemic periods exceeding that of the pandemic years.[18]

Control

Traditional efforts to control epidemics on a global or community scale, such as quarantine, isolation, or travel restrictions, are generally impractical and not worthwhile due to the rapid spread, short incubation period, and shedding of virus with subclinical disease. Environmental approaches such as ultraviolet irradiation and air-purifying or sterilizing techniques have either not been tested or are too inefficient to be put into practical use. Efforts to control influenza have been successful in two areas: (*a*) vaccination and (*b*) chemotherapy or chemoprophylaxis with amantadine or rimantadine.

Influenza Vaccines

Commercially available vaccines are prepared from allantoic fluids of infected embryonated hens' eggs. Viruses are formalin inactivated and purified by a variety of means. Vaccines may contain whole virions, "split" virus products, or purified surface antigens created by disrupting the viruses with detergents or lipid solvents. Live attenuated vaccines are in use in several countries but remain experimental in the United States. Vaccines work by inducing production of serum antibodies against the H and N antigens.

Recent experience with live attenuated, cold-adapted influenza A vaccines indicates that when given intranasally to infants the vaccines appear to be safe and immunogenic and offer some protection.[19] Data from infants under 6 months of age suggest that two doses may be needed to achieve protection.[20]

The WHO makes recommendations yearly to the Centers for Disease Control and Prevention and the vaccine manufacturers on the formulation of the vaccine.[21] The purpose of this effort is to ensure that the proposed vaccine contains antigens similar to those of strains already in circulation elsewhere. Thus the formulations are necessarily changed frequently. Data such as the recent and expected strains in the community, antigenicity of strains, and in vitro strain similarities are used to determine which viral strains to include in the vaccine. Recently, antigenically similar strains with good growth characteristics have been substituted for strains with poor growth to ensure adequate production of strains for manufacture of the vaccine. The most common recent vaccines are trivalent and have contained two A strain viruses and one B strain virus. Data suggest that current inactivated vaccines provide protection against even antigenically drifted influenza A strains.[22]

Vaccination is protective against both disease and death in a wide range of hosts. Influenza vaccination protects even healthy, working adults; recipients had 25 percent fewer episodes of upper respiratory illness, 43 percent fewer days of sick leave due to upper respiratory illness, and 44 percent fewer visits to physicians' offices for upper respiratory illness.[23] A meta-analysis of studies in the elderly demonstrates that the influenza vaccine has an efficacy (1-odds ratio) of approximately 56 percent in preventing respiratory illness, 53 percent in preventing pneumonia, and 50 percent in preventing hospitalization.[24]

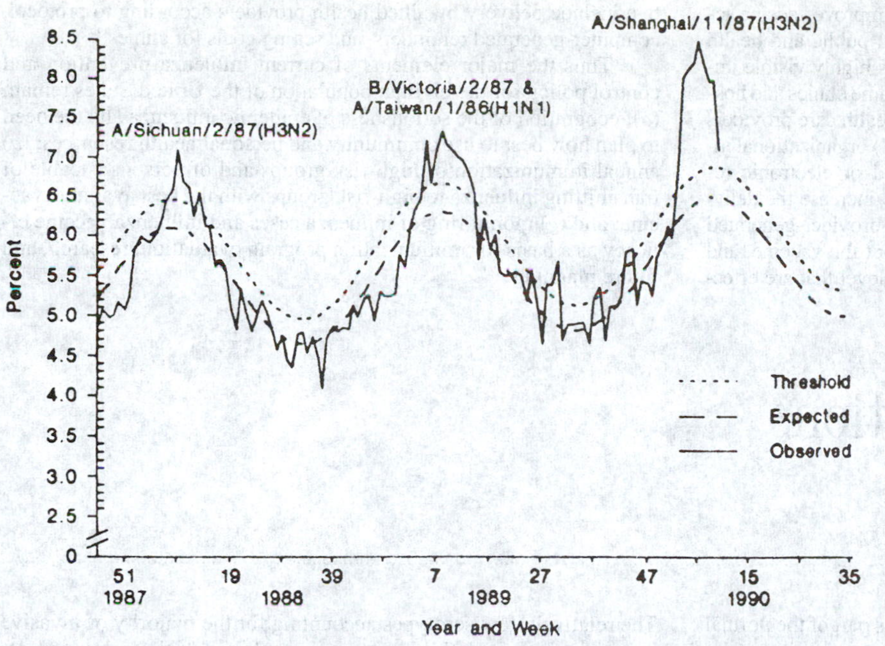

Figure 7-5. Pneumonia and influenza deaths as a percentage of total deaths in the United States, from October 1988 to March 3, 1990. Data were reported to the Centers for Disease Control from 121 U.S. cities. Pneumonia and influenza deaths include all deaths for which pneumonia is listed on the death certificate as a primary or underlying cause or for which influenza is listed on the death certificate. The predominant strains are shown above the peak mortality rate for each season. The epidemic guideline (threshold) for each season is 1.645 standard deviations above the expected baseline, estimated by using a periodic regression model applied to observed percentages since 1983. This baseline was estimated by using a robust regression procedure.

Influenza vaccine is also effective in reducing mortality from influenza, with even greater efficacy after repeated annual vaccination.[25] Among the elderly, vaccination reduces mortality by approximately two-thirds (68 percent).[24] Annual influenza vaccination provides important cost savings per year for each vaccinated person.[23,24,26]

The side effects of inactivated vaccines are almost always minor and are typically local, rather than systemic.[27] Side effects are most common in persons younger than 20 years and in those given whole-virus vaccines. During general use of a "swine" influenza virus vaccine in 1976 in the United States, the Guillain-Barré syndrome (GBS) was reported to affect one in 120,000 vaccinees. Recomputation of attributable risk data suggests that there was in fact a lesser degree of association (4.0 to 5.9 cases per million vaccinees).[28] An increased incidence of GBS has not been observed with influenza vaccines administered since 1976.

Antiviral Drugs

Amantadine hydrochloride and its analog rimantadine hydrochloride are available in the United States for treatment or prophylaxis of influenza A.[29] Neither is effective against influenza B. They are most effective when given before exposure and reduce both the frequency of infection (attack rate) and the severity of illness. When used prophylactically, from 70 to 90 percent of cases can be prevented. For therapy of a new infection, symptoms such as fever are reduced by approximately 50 percent if administration begins within 48 hours of the onset. Studies continue to accumulate showing the efficacy of amantadine and rimantadine in specialized situations, including protection of high-risk patients in acute care hospitals and long-term care facilities.[29,30] Current recommendations call for administration of one of these agents to all nursing home residents without specific contraindications at the beginning of an apparent outbreak to control disease.[29,31] Prophylaxis may also be useful in the event of a major immunologic change in the circulating virus from the strains covered by the current vaccine.

Amantadine has a higher frequency of neurologic side effects than rimantadine and should be used cautiously in persons with renal failure or pre-existing neurologic or neuropsychiatric disorders. Rimantadine is favored in most instances because of its lower incidence of side effects; however, it should be used cautiously in patients with severe hepatic dysfunction or renal failure. Use of an antiviral agent may lead to drug resistance and prolonged excretion of resistant organisms from immunodeficient hosts.[10]

Current Recommendations

The Advisory Committee on Immunization Practices of the Centers for Disease Control and Prevention makes recommendations for the use of influenza vaccine in the United States.[32] Generally, the goals of vaccine use are to reduce influenza-associated mortality rates. Traditionally this program has recommended that the vaccine be given annually to persons at greatest risk of death: persons of all ages with chronic cardiovascular, bronchopulmonary, renal, or metabolic diseases; residents of nursing homes; persons older than 65 years of age; immunosuppressed persons, including those with HIV infection, and persons who are receiving long-term aspirin therapy and are therefore at risk of Reye's syndrome. The recommendations were expanded in 1984 to include the immunization of persons capable of transmitting influenza to those high-risk patients: all health care workers of acute and long-term care facilities, members of high-risk patients' households, and providers of home care to high-risk persons.

Influenza immunization practices vary in different countries. In the United States, inactivated vaccines are generally recommended only for those at greatest risk of severe and fatal consequences of disease; in Japan, inactivated vaccines are widely used for schoolchildren in an attempt to reduce transmission of the virus.

Currently it is thought that immunizing the entire U.S. population is neither feasible nor desirable for technical and logistical reasons and because of costs. Despite evidence showing the vaccines' efficacy in reducing morbidity and mortality rates in certain populations, such data do not support their use in the general population.

Despite the existence of an effective, safe, and reasonably inexpensive vaccine, many populations of persons for whom the vaccine was recommended are not adequately immunized.[25,33] Influenza vaccination programs within health maintenance organizations, for example, have been effective in immunizing up to 85 percent of chronically ill elders.[34] In Canada, 45 percent of the elderly are routinely immunized.[35] One of the most important factors in influencing patients to receive the vaccine is the recommendation of a physician or other health care provider.[35] Reasons for not receiving the vaccine include perceptions that the individual is not at risk or fear of side effects.

Studies have generally suggested four ways to improve vaccine acceptance: (*a*) educational programs for the general public and health care providers, (*b*) administrative direction, such as highly visible immunization programs or mandated vaccination for some clinics and hospitals, (*c*) financial incentives or disincentives for health care providers by institutions and reimbursement providers, and (*d*) organizational interventions to provide vaccine through automated or electronic reminders. Some of the most effective approaches to increase the delivery of influenza vaccine to patients have included provider-generated recruitment letters, availability of information about the vaccine, and open vaccine clinics. Interventions at the provider level that are effective include delivery by allied health providers according to protocol, computer-generated reminders, and setting goals for clinics.[34,36]

Thus the major elements of current influenza prevention and control policy for the civilian population of the United States remain (*a*) recognition of the seriousness of epidemic influenza and the need to plan how best to use community and personal health resources; (*b*) annual immunization of high-risk groups and of persons capable of transmitting influenza to high-risk groups with the best available vaccine; and (*c*) monitoring of influenza cases and influenza vaccine efficacy as a basis for immunization program evaluation, research, and future planning.

Pneumococcal Infections

Carl B. LeBuhn • Bradley N. Doebbeling

The pneumococcus (*Streptococcus pneumoniae*) is part of the normal bacterial flora of the human nasopharynx and often exists in a commensal relationship with its host. Injury to any region of the respiratory epithelium may disturb this equilibrium, leading to tissue penetration, organism replication, immune system activation, and the development of clinical illness. The pneumococcus was first identified in France and was found in the United States in 1881.[1,2] Subsequently, data on its recovery from all five continents were reported in 1939, indicating a wide geographic distribution.[3] Despite intensive research, widespread antibiotic use, and vaccination, the morbidity and mortality of pneumococcal infections remain significant. *S. pneumoniae* remains the most common cause of bacterial pnemonia[4,5] and otitis media[6] worldwide and is a major cause of bacterial meningitis. Each year, in the United States alone, there are approximately 3,000 cases of meningitis, 50,000 bacteremias, 500,000 cases of pneumonia, and 7 million cases of otitis media caused by the pneumococcus.[7] Pneumococcal infections result in an estimated 40,000 deaths[8] and the expenditure of over $4 billion annually in the United States.[9] The public health impact of infections due to this pathogen is only likely to increase with the spread of penicillin-resistant and multidrug-resistant strains.

Pneumococcal Types

Currently 90 different pneumococcal capsular types have been identified.[10] The composition and quantity of the capsular polysaccharide has an impact on virulence,[11] and as a result, not all serotypes are equally invasive and the majority of infections are due to a relatively small number of serotypes. Approximately one-half of invasive infections are caused by six types, an additional one-fourth by six additional types, and an additional one-eighth by six other types. The distribution of pneumococcal types causing infection has remained fairly stable but does tend to vary somewhat by age, geographic areas, and time.

The distribution of pneumococcal serotypes that cause invasive disease in children is more limited than in adults. As part of ongoing national surveillance, the Centers for Disease Control and Prevention (CDC) recently evaluated 3,570 pneumococcal isolates collected between 1978 and 1994 from blood or cerebrospinal fluid (CSF) of children less than 6 years of age.[12] Seven serotypes accounted for 80 percent of invasive pneumococcal infections. Listed in descending order of frequency of occurrence, the serotypes are 14, 6B, 19F, 18C, 23F, 4, and 9V. The development of immunologic responsiveness to capsular antigens of many of these types later in life than the immune response to other capsular antigens may explain this distribution. In children older than 2 years of age, the serotypes causing invasive disease are more similar to the strains causing disease in adults.[13] The relatively few serotypes accounting for the majority of invasive infections in young children may be exploited in the continued development of protein-conjugated pneumococcal vaccines. Although conjugated vaccines may contain antigens for only a limited number of serotypes, unlike the polysaccharide vaccine, they are immunogenic in persons less than 2 years old. A protein-conjugated vaccine containing the seven serotypes listed above could potentially prevent as many as 86 percent of pneumococcal bacteremias, 83 percent of pneumococcal meningitis cases, and 65 percent of pneumococcal otitis media cases.[12]

Compared to infants and young children, a slightly wider range of serotypes account for the majority of invasive pneumococcal infections in the adult population. Blood and CSF isolates collected by the World Health Organization (WHO) from persons more than 14 years of age between 1982 and 1987 revealed that 12 serotypes accounted for approximately 65 percent of invasive infections (listed in descending order: 3, 1, 14, 7F, 4, 8, 23F, 9V, 19F, 6B, 12F, and 19A).[14] In the United States, serotyping of blood and CSF isolates collected between 1978 and 1992 from 2,322 unvaccinated persons more than 6 years of age as part of the CDC's national surveillance program revealed that 65 percent of invasive infections were caused by 10 different serotypes (listed in descending order: 4, 14, 23F, 9V, 12F, 6B, 3, 8, 1, and 9N).[15] When compared with younger children and with patients from other parts of the world, a slightly different distribution in rank order and capsular types can be appreciated. In North America infections with type 1 pneumococci occur less frequently than in other parts of the world. Infections with type 2 and 5 pneumococci, which are relatively common in South America, Africa, and Asia, occur only rarely in the United States.[11] Twenty-five years ago, organisms of capsular types 1, 3, 4, 7, 8, and 12 caused the majority of invasive disease. Continued close monitoring of the serotypes responsible for invasive infections in both children and adults will remain important in the formulation and distribution of newer conjugate vaccines.[12]

Epidemiologic data suggest that genetic constitution may influence susceptibility to infection with certain pneumococcal types. Infections with capsular types 45 and 46 have been frequent among black gold miners in South Africa, whereas they have been isolated only rarely from white persons in the same region.

Penicillin resistance was first identified in a type 1 pneumococcus through in vitro experiments performed by Eriksen in 1945.[16] In 1967, a penicillin-resistant type 23 pneumococcus was isolated from the sputum of a patient with hypogammaglobulinemia and bronchiectasis who had received multiple prior courses of antibiotics.[17] In 1971, type 4 resistant isolates were recovered from multiple patients in New Guinea who were participating in a trial of prophylactic penicillin use.[18] Further data from Australia and New Guinea published in 1974 identified penicillin resistance in 10 different serotypes.[19] Although antibiotic resistance is independent of capsular type, it tends to be found most often in strains that most frequently cause infection in children (6B, 9V, 14, 19A, 19F, and 23F).[20]

Pneumococcal Colonization

S. pneumoniae can be found in the nasopharynx in 5 to 10 percent of adults and 20 to 40 percent of children without signs or symptoms of clinical disease. Although organisms can be recovered from the nasopharynx of healthy children and adults throughout the year, colonization is seasonal, with an increase in the midwinter period.[21] Infants tend to acquire their first pneumococcal type at a mean age of 6 months, but colonization may begin as early as the day of birth. In this setting the type acquired is usually the type carried by the mother.[13,22] The majority of children will have carried at least one type of pneumococcus by the age of 2 years.[13] In the first years of life, rates of pneumococcal carriage are high, and children have been found to be colonized sequentially with as many as 12 distinct serotypes.[23] Carefully executed studies have shown approximately half of all children carry two pneumococcal types simultaneously, and simultaneous carriage of as many as four serotypes has been demonstrated.[24] The mean duration of carriage in children seems to range between 2.7 and 4.2 months, but carriage of a single serotype for more than 1 year has been demonstrated.[13] Duration of carriage varies somewhat both by serotype and by age. The younger the infant at the time of acquisition, the longer the strain is likely to be carried.[13] In adults, carriage of a single serotype usually lasts for 1 to 2 months, but carriage of a single type for longer than 3 years has been demonstrated.[25] Few data are available concerning the acquisition of new types by adults with the passage of time, but limited findings suggest the number to be one or two per year.[26] Rates of pneumococcal carriage tend to decline with age.

Colonization with a given pneumococcal type may be followed by the development of type-specific anticapsular antibody in the absence of overt signs of clinical illness.[27] The presence of circulating anticapsular antibody will not eliminate an established carrier state, but it will reduce the likelihood of being colonized with the same strain by approximately one-half.[28] The ability of antimicrobial drugs to eliminate the pneumococcal carrier state seems limited.[29] Neither penicillin, sulfonamides, nor a variety of other antimicrobial agents have been successful in ridding the nasopharynx of pneumococci from all carriers. In fact, the use of prophylactic antibiotics and frequent antibiotic use has been linked to colonization and infection with penicillin/multidrug-resistant strains.[20,30] In one study, rifampin was used in an outbreak setting in a Houston day care center. Although nasal carriage of a multiply resistant strain was reduced by 70 percent, rifampin treatment did not prevent new acquisition of the organism by three children and one family member.[31] Attempts to eradicate carriage with topical antibiotics, such as mupirocin, have also failed.[32]

Organisms are spread from person to person in settings that promote close personal contact over prolonged periods. Day care centers have become a well-recognized area of both increased rates of pneumococcal colonization and infection.[31] The high carriage rates of pneumococci in children, the selective pressure of antibiotics prescribed for the treatment of otitis media, and crowded conditions make day care centers an optimum environment for the development and spread of penicillin/multidrug-resistant pneumococci.[33] Increased rates of colonization and infection have also been demonstrated in certain work environments. Outbreaks have been described among adults living in crowded conditions such as military camps, prisons, and homeless shelters.[34] Nosocomial outbreaks have been reported as well.[35,36]

Risk Factors for Invasive Disease

Invasive pneumococcal disease develops when the normal balance between organism colonization and host defense is tipped in favor of disease. Risk factors for invasive pneumococcal disease can be divided into three main categories: (*a*) factors increasing or altering the normal carrier state, (*b*) diseases that alter antibody formation or phagocytosis, and (*c*) multifactorial causes that result in either decreased antibody formation or increased overall susceptibility to infection.

Injury to the epithelial lining of the respiratory tract can disrupt the normal commensal relationship between the organism and the host, causing the development of symptomatic disease. The predisposing injury is usually viral in etiology due to either influenza or another upper respiratory tract pathogen.[21] Studies in experimental animals have shown both the normal lung and the normal middle ear to be resistant to pneumococcal infection, but both areas are vulnerable to bacterial multiplication when viral injury has antedated exposure to the bacterium.[37] Current and prior tobacco use also increases the risk of invasive pneumococcal disease, presumably from injury to the respiratory lining or impaired mucociliary clearance of organisms.[38] Inflammatory conditions of the airways such as asthma and COPD are also risk factors for pneumococcal disease. As mentioned previously, crowded living conditions can also increase the risk of colonization and thus lead to increased rates of disease when the appropriate conditions or host factors are present.

Diseases such as agammaglobulinemia, IgG subclass deficiency, multiple myeloma, chronic lymphocytic leukemia, lymphoma, and defective complement increase the risk of developing pneumococcal disease, primarily through impaired antibody production. These reduce available opsonizing antibody and diminish the effectiveness of phagocytosis. Neutropenia, either primary or drug-induced, also limits the effectiveness of phagocytosis. A history of splenectomy or autosplenectomy from sickle cell disease increases the risk of pneumococcal infection through impaired clearance of pneumococcal bacteremia. Other conditions that predispose to pneumococcal disease include hospitalization, malnutrition, cirrhosis, alcoholism, renal insufficiency, and glucocorticoids. Individuals at extremes of age (infants and elderly) are also at increased risk of pneumococcal infection. Infection with the human immunodeficiency virus (HIV) has become a major risk factor for pneumococcal infection. Pneumococcal pneumonia is 10 times and bacteremia 100 times more frequent in patients with HIV infection than in an age-matched population.[39] *S. pneumoniae* is also the leading cause of invasive bacterial respiratory disease in adults infected with HIV.[40]

Risk factors for colonization and/or infection are similar for penicillin-resistant and multidrug-resistant strains. Risk factors include extremes of age (less than 2 years old or 70 years old and older), previous β-lactam antibiotic treatment, and children and staff in day care centers.[41] Other studies have identified as risk factors frequent antibiotic use, use of prophylactic antibiotics for prevention of otitis media, and recent hospitalization in institutions where resistant strains have been introduced.[20]

Pneumococcal Infections

The pneumococcus remains the most common cause of community-acquired bacterial pneumonia worldwide.[4] The clinical features of the disease have been described in detail by Heffron[3] and have also been recently reviewed.[38] Because of the difficulty in establishing the cause of bacterial pneumonia in the absence of bacteremia, the exact incidence of pneumococcal pneumonia is unknown.[42] Most cases of pneumococcal bacteremia in adults are due to pneumonia, and there are an estimated three to four cases of nonbacteremic pneumococcal pneumonia for every bacteremic case. On the basis of available evidence, the incidence of pneumococcal pneumonia in developed countries is estimated to be between 1 and 5 per 1,000 persons per year. Retrospective assessment of pneumococcal bacteremia in the United States has yielded rates of approximately 10 per 100,000 persons per year,[43] but passive prospective surveillance suggests an overall minimum rate of 25 to 30 per 100,000 persons per year.[42] Certain populations have a higher rate of infection. In Alaska, a bacteremia rate of 105 per 100,000 persons per year has been reported in persons of all ages in the native population.[44] A study performed in South Carolina demonstrated that there is a marked difference in bacteremia rates with respect to age; 160 per 100,000 infants and children, 5 per 100,000 young adults, and 70 per 100,000 elderly (age greater than 70 years).[45] Pneumococcal bacteremia rates of 940 per

100,000 persons per year have been reported in patients infected with HIV.[46] Case-to-fatality rates of bacteremic pneumococcal pneumonia remain approximately 20 percent, even with optimal antibiotic therapy.[47] Mortality rates as high as 60 percent have been reported in the elderly.[8]

S. pneumoniae, Neisseria meningitidis, and *Haemophilus influenzae* type b appear to be capable of invading the epithelium of the nasopharynx and spreading to the regional lymph nodes, where, if unchecked, they can reach the systemic circulation and lead to bacteremia. Pneumococcal bacteremia, in the absence of an identifiable focus of infection, is now a well-recognized syndrome in infants, and, more recently, has been identified in adults.[48]

The pneumococcus is a common cause of acute sinusitis and is the most common cause of otitis media, a disorder that afflicts three-fourths of American children at least once in their first 6 years of life. Although rarely followed by serious or lethal sequelae, pneumococcal otitis media is the cause of considerable morbidity and expenditures for medical services. Recurring attacks caused by a succession of pneumococcal types are not infrequent.[6] Otitis media that is not responsive to antimicrobial therapy is becoming more frequent with the increased prevalence of antibiotic-resistant pneumococci in the day care environment.[33]

Pneumococcal meningitis can arise from bacteremia, from contiguous spread of infection involving the paranasal sinuses, or as a local complication of mastoiditis. It remains one of the three most common causes of bacterial meningitis in both infants and adults. The case-to-fatality rate is high, exceeding 40 percent in persons over 40 years of age.

Pneumococcal Resistance to Antimicrobial Drugs

The first drug-resistant pneumococcus recovered from a human was isolated from a patient being treated with Optochin in 1916.[49] Penicillin resistance was first noted in vitro and in vivo as early as 1943, approximately 15 years after it was first discovered; however, clinical resistance to penicillin was not reported again until 1965.[50] In the late 1960s and early 1970s an increasing number of resistant strains were identified in New Guinea, Australia, and South Africa. Penicillin interacts with penicillin-binding proteins located in the bacterial cell wall. This interaction impairs the normal synthesis of the cell wall and eventually causes cell death. Resistance to penicillin and cephalosporins develops when genes that encode for penicillin-binding proteins are remodeled with DNA from resistant strains or with DNA from other organisms. This process alters the structure of penicillin-binding proteins, decreasing their affinity for penicillin. Successive mutations are required in the development of penicillin resistance, which may be one reason why, at least initially, penicillin resistance was somewhat slow to develop in the clinical arena.[51] According to the National Committee for Clinical Laboratory Standards (NCCLS), penicillin susceptibility and resistance is currently defined in the following way: isolates with a minimum inhibitory concentration (MIC) of 0.06 μg/mL or less are considered fully susceptible; isolates with an MIC between 0.12 and 1 μg/mL are considered intermediate; and isolates with an MIC of 2 μg/mL or above are considered highly resistant. Isolates that show high-level resistance to penicillin often manifest resistance to other classes of antibiotics as well. Similarly to penicillin, resistance to sulfonamide drugs was recognized within a few years of the advent of sulfapyridine. Since the late 1970s, multiply resistant strains of pneumococci (defined as resistance to at least three antibiotics) have emerged and spread across a wide geographic area.[52,53]

The first infection in the United States due to a penicillin-resistant pneumococcus was reported in 1974. During the 1980s, reports of drug-resistant pneumococci appeared from a wide geographic area, suggesting the rapid spread of resistance. Over the past decade, there has been a steady increase in the prevalence of penicillin-resistant strains. In Spain, the prevalence of penicillin resistance increased from 8.8 percent between 1979 and 1981 to 44 percent in 1989.[53] In England and Wales, the prevalence of intermediate or full resistance to penicillin increased from 1.5 percent in 1990 to 3.9 percent in 1995.[54] Susceptibility testing performed on 5,459 isolates from the United States collected between 1979 and 1987 revealed only one (less than 0.02 percent) with high-level penicillin resistance. In 1991–1992, seven of 567 isolates (1.3 percent) collected by the CDC showed high-level resistance.[20] In Dallas, the prevalence has increased from 8 percent between 1981 and 1983 to 19 percent in 1993.[55] A 1994–1995 surveillance study involving 1,527 clinically significant isolates from 30 U.S. centers found an overall prevalence of penicillin resistance (intermediate and high level) of 23.6 percent,[56] although significant variability in prevalence continues to exist between different communities.[57] The overall prevalence of penicillin-resistant strains may reach 40 to 50 percent by the year 2000.[56]

Multidrug-resistant pneumococci were first isolated in South Africa in 1977. Subsequently, a high prevalence of multidrug-resistant pneumococci was identified in Spain. In 1991, Munoz et al examined several isolates (serotype 23F) from Spain and Ohio using multilocus enzyme electrophoresis and gene-restriction endonuclease profiles.[58] They were able to demonstrate the apparent intercontinental spread of this resistant clone. Using similar techniques, McDougal et al were able to show that this same clone had been disseminated across a wide area of the United States.[59] Evidence also exists for the intercontinental spread of a multidrug-resistant serotype 6B between Spain and Iceland in 1989.[60] The areas of highest prevalence continue to be South Africa and Spain, although over the past 15 years pneumococci manifesting the multidrug-resistant phenotype have been identified from numerous different places. The prevalence of multidrug-resistant strains has shown a steady increase. In one recent study of invasive pneumococcal disease in the Atlanta area, 11 percent of isolates demonstrated resistance to three or more antimicrobial drugs or drug classes.[9] Currently, multiple antibiotic resistance occurs primarily in four serotypes (6B, 14, 19, and 23F),[30] although one study demonstrated evidence that in vivo capsular transformation may be a potential mechanism by which the multidrug-resistant phenotype could extend to new serotypes.[61]

The drug-resistant *Streptococcus pneumoniae* (DRSP) Working Group has recently published a strategy to help minimize the impact of the increasing problem with resistance.[7] They recommend focusing on four different areas: (*a*) development and implementation of an electronic laboratory-based surveillance system to aid in reporting and providing feedback to clinicians, (*b*) continuing studies to identify risk factors and assess outcomes of DRSP infections, (*c*) increasing the use of the 23-valent pneumococcal vaccine, and (*d*) continued promotion of more judicious antimicrobial drug use.

Treatment of Pneumococcal Infections

The treatment of pneumococcal infections has been recently reviewed.[30,62] Treatment decisions should be based primarily on the site of infection, the prevalence of resistant strains in the community or facility, and the actual antibiotic susceptibility pattern of the organism as soon as it is available. In patients without a history of hypersensitivity to β-lactam antibiotics, penicillin remains the treatment of choice for invasive pneumococcal disease caused by a fully susceptible organism (MIC less than 0.1 μg/mL). A recent review evaluated the clinical outcomes of patients with pneumococcal pneumonia due to resistant strains. The authors of this study concluded that high-dose penicillin may be adequate in the treatment of pneumococcal pneumonia due to strains with intermediate resistance.[63] Cefotaxime, ceftriaxone, vancomycin, and imipenem-cilastin are treatment alternatives for pneumococcal pneumonia due to strains with intermediate or high-level penicillin resistance, provided that susceptibility testing shows appropriate MICs to these antibiotics. No pneumococci that manifest resistance to vancomycin have been isolated to date. Meningitis remains the most difficult pneumococcal infection to treat in the setting of resistance because of the poor penetration of many antibiotics into the cerebrospinal fluid. Cefotaxime or ceftriaxone should be used as the initial empiric therapy for suspected pneumococcal meningitis, but vancomycin should be added when high-level penicillin or cephalosporin resistance is suspected. Some authors recommend including vancomycin in all initial regimens for the treatment of pneumococcal meningitis, since local prevalence data are often unavailable and patients may have recently traveled to other areas with a higher prevalence of resistant strains.[30] In the treatment of pneumococcal meningitis, the combination of cefotaxime or ceftriaxone and vancomycin may be more effective than either drug alone.[64] Other treatment options for pneumococcal meningitis include vancomycin plus rifampin or imipenem-cilastin. Treatment failures have been reported with all of these regimens. Thus it is important to obtain rapid and accurate susceptibility data, follow patients very closely clinically, and consider early reevaluation of cerebrospinal fluid in patients with meningitis.[62]

Immunoprophylaxis of Pneumococcal Infections

The high prevalence of pneumococcal infections in all populations, the high mortality unlikely to be further reduced by antimicrobial agents, the high cost of treating pneumococcal infections, and the dissemination of resistant strains provide the basis for immunoprophylactic measures to prevent pneumococcal infections.

The human infant is immunologically immature at birth and demonstrates only a transient IgM response to purified polysaccharide antigens. However, a successful conjugate vaccine for *Haemophilus influenzae* type b has been developed that, when administered to infants, has markedly decreased the incidence of invasive *Haemophilus* infections. Conjugate pneumococcal vaccines incorporating capsular types responsible for the majority of invasive disease in children have also been under development.[65] When administered to infants and toddlers, these newer vaccines appear to elicit a good antibody response (IgM and IgG) and show evidence of boosting on repeated vaccination.[66] Conjugate pneumococcal vaccines also show promise in certain higher-risk populations.[67]

Probably because of exposure and colonization with the more common pneumococcal types during childhood, adults respond to many purified pneumococcal polysaccharide antigens with the formation of IgM and IgG antibodies. Initially a 14-valent pneumococcal vaccine was developed, but this was replaced by a 23-valent vaccine in 1983. The 23-valent vaccine remains in use today and contains 25 μg of each of the following capsular types: 1, 2, 3, 4, 5, 6B, 7F, 8, 9N, 9V, 10A, 11A, 12F, 14, 15B, 17F, 18F, 19F, 19A, 20, 22F, 23F, and 33F. These 23 serotypes cause 88 percent of invasive pneumococcal infections in both children and adults in the United States.[68] Importantly, 95 percent of infections due to multidrug-resistant strains are by serotypes included in the current vaccine. In assessing the efficacy of a vaccine of this complexity, it is important to recognize that the vaccine is designed to prevent 23 immunologically distinct infections, thus its aggregate efficacy can never equal that of a monovalent vaccine.

Several methods have been used to assess the aggregate efficacy of polyvalent pneumococcal polysaccharide vaccines, including randomized, double-blind, controlled trials, quasi-cohort studies, and case-control studies.[15,69–73] Trials of all three designs have found the aggregate efficacy of polyvalent pneumococcal vaccines to be between 60 and 80 percent. Efficacy is variable, depending on the patient population evaluated. Some authors have questioned whether the vaccine should be strongly encouraged in groups in which efficacy has been less clearly demonstrated. Pneumococcal vaccine is rarely accompanied by untoward reactions, and no permanent injuries or deaths have resulted from its administration. Limited studies in older children and in adults of all ages so far have found no age-related differences in the vaccine's aggregate efficacy. Limited data have also not revealed a decline in protection by the vaccine in the 6 years following immunization.[15]

The 23-valent pneumococcal polysaccharide vaccine remains an underutilized preventive health measure, despite good evidence for vaccine efficacy, particularly in the prevention of pneumococcal bacteremia. Data from the 1993 National Health Interview Survey reported vaccination rates of 25 to 30 percent for persons 65 years of age or older.[74] Although this is an improvement from the 10.7 percent rate in 1985, it remains far below the National Health Objective of a 60 percent vaccination rate of at-risk patients by the year 2000.[75] Missed opportunities to vaccinate patients during contacts with the health care system, lack of vaccine delivery systems in different settings, patient and provider concerns of vaccine side effects, provider questions concerning vaccine efficacy, and lack of awareness among both patients and providers of the importance of vaccine-preventable diseases have all been suggested as reasons for the relatively low vaccination rate.[76,77] There is a strong rationale for developing hospital-based delivery systems, since two-thirds of people admitted with pneumococcal bacteremia have had a previous admission within the past 4 years.[78] Successful hospital-based strategies (both inpatient and outpatient) using physician reminders, prevention teams, and educational campaigns have been reported.[79,80]

The pneumococcal vaccine appears to be cost effective, relative to other preventive health services, and may in fact be cost saving. In the management of pneumococcal pneumonia, the Office of Technology Assessment study determined that pneumococcal vaccination would cost $3,795 (in 1992 dollars) to achieve 1 quality-adjusted life-year (QALY), assuming a duration of vaccine efficacy of 3 years.[81] If the actual duration of protection is 8 years, then pneumococcal vaccination is a cost-saving measure. In the prevention of invasive pneumococcal disease for which vaccine efficacy data is strongest, the cost-effectiveness estimates are between $5,000 and 10,000 per QALY.[81] This compares very favorably with other preventive services. In examining hospitalized patients with pneumonia, Fedson et al. estimated that vaccinating 100 people age 65 or greater at the time of discharge would prevent one readmission for pneumonia over the next 5 years.[78] This study estimated that the benefit-cost ratio of vaccination would exceed 3:1 (i.e., the cost of vaccination would be one-third the costs of hospital care for patients eventually readmitted with pneumonia). The vaccine also appears to be cost-effective in HIV-infected individuals, especially if administered when the CD4 count is greater than 200.[82]

Recommendations for the administration of pneumococcal vaccine have been published by the Advisory Committee on Immunization Practices of the CDC and by the American College of Physicians in its *Guide for Adult Immunization*.[47] The vaccine should be administered to all persons 65 years of age and older and to those over 10 to 15 years of age with any of a variety of chronic systemic illnesses associated with increased risk of a fatal outcome from bacteremic pneumococcal infection. Although the vaccine may be given to immunocompromised persons at increased risk of pneumococcal infection, it must be administered with the understanding that its efficacy will be limited in those whose antibody responses are impaired. All persons with anatomic or functional asplenia, including recipients of 14-valent pneumococcal vaccine, should be given the 23-valent pneumococcal vaccine because of their high risk of death if infected with any pneumococcal type. Repeated vaccination after 6 years is now recommended in some high-risk groups.[47]

Haemophilus influenzae Infections

Jay D. Wenger • David W. Fraser • Claire V. Broome

Haemophilus influenzae was advanced by Pfeiffer in 1892 as the etiologic agent of influenza because of its recovery from the respiratory tract of many persons with that disease. Although later shown not to cause influenza, it was identified as a major cause of invasive bacterial disease in children and of significant morbidity in adults with chronic respiratory disease. The most virulent strain of this organism—*Haemophilus influenzae* type b (Hib)—was the most common cause of bacterial meningitis and invasive bacterial disease in children in the United States, but, in a major public health triumph, infection with this strain has been practically eliminated in many countries through routine infant immunization with a new type of vaccine.

Bacteriology

H. influenzae usually appears as a small, pleomorphic, Gram-negative coccobacillus on Gram-stained clinical specimens. However, it can be difficult to stain and may occasionally appear as Gram-positive diplococci in the spinal fluid.

H. influenzae strains may be either encapsulated or nonencapsulated. Among the encapsulated strains there are six distinct capsular types, designated a, b, c, d, e, and f. Most invasive *H. influenzae* disease—defined as disease in which the bacteria was cultured from the blood, cerebrospinal fluid, or other body fluid in which bacteria are not usually found—is caused by type b encapsulated strains.

Until recently, *H. influenzae* consistently demonstrated in vitro susceptibility to ampicillin and chloramphenicol. Since plasmid-mediated ampicillin resistance associated with β-lactamase activity was first reported in 1974, resistance among *H. influenzae* organisms has become widespread. In 1986, 33 percent of *H. influenzae* strains isolated from persons with invasive disease were resistant to ampicillin.[1] Resistance to chloramphenicol is much rarer but has been observed in type b and nonencapsulated strains.

Clinical Characteristics and Pathophysiology

Meningitis is the most common life-threatening illness caused by *H. influenzae* and is caused almost exclusively by encapsulated type b strains. Bacteremia has been documented in about 70 percent of meningitis cases but probably occurs in all as a necessary step as the bacteria pass from the nasopharynx to seed the meninges.[2] The case-to-fatality rate averages 3 to 6 percent; 20 to 30 percent of survivors may have significant residual neurologic deficits, including blindness, severe retardation, hydrocephalus, seizures, or hearing loss.

Acute epiglottitis—with cellulitis and edema of the epiglottis, aryepiglottic folds, and surrounding soft tissue—is most commonly caused by Hib. Because of respiratory obstruction, it can be rapidly fatal.

H. influenzae and the pneumococcus are the major causes of severe acute respiratory infection (ARI) in the developing world. ARI is the single largest cause of death in children less than 5 years of age in these areas; a recent study suggests that up to 20 percent of all hospitalized cases of chest radiograph-documented pneumonia in children less than 5 years of age in the Gambia may be caused by Hib.[3] Nontypeable *H. influenzae* strains are a common cause of pneumonia or exacerbations of chronic bronchitis in adults with chronic lung disease; bacteremia is uncommon in such cases.

H. influenzae and the pneumococcus are the two most common causes of acute otitis media. Ninety-five percent of *H. influenzae* strains causing otitis media are nonencapsulated. *H. influenzae* may cause facial or orbital cellulitis, septic arthritis, or bacteremia without a detectable focus.

Diagnosis of *Haemophilus* infection is by culture of the organism from normally sterile body fluids or by demonstration of capsular antigens in those fluids by counterimmunoelectrophoresis, latex particle agglutination, or staphylococcal coagglutination. Nasopharyngeal cultures are of limited assistance in making a specific diagnosis, because this organism can frequently be found in the absence of disease.

Initial therapy for life-threatening *H. influenzae* infections may include both ampicillin and chloramphenicol or a third-generation cephalosporin; antibiotic therapy can be simplified when it is shown that the infecting strain does not produce β-lactamase. Otitis media is best treated with ampicillin unless it is refractory; trimethoprim-sulfamethoxazole is a useful alternative.

Immunity

In 1933 Fothergill and Wright described an inverse relationship between serum bactericidal activity against Hib and the incidence of *H. influenzae* meningitis at various ages. A nadir in bactericidal activity from age 3 months to 2 years corresponded to the age of peak incidence of *H. influenzae* meningitis. The prevalence of antibody to polyribosylribitol phosphate (PRP), the type b capsular material, correlates inversely with age-specific incidence. Experimental studies have shown that anti-PRP antibodies are protective against *H. influenzae* type b infection in animal models and in humans.

Protective antibodies can be induced by exposure of older children and adults to the organism through nasopharyngeal carriage or systemic disease, or by parenteral administration of PRP. However, in children less than 2 years of age, those at highest risk of disease, none of these exposures reliably induces an immune response. The polysaccharide antigen does not elicit a response from the immature immune system of infants and young children and does not, in contrast to protein antigens used in children of the same age, induce T-cell activity. Researchers subsequently employed a novel technology to chemically conjugate immunogenic protein antigens (such as the diphtheria or tetanus toxoids) to PRP to create a new generation of effective vaccines that stimulate anti-PRP antibody production in these children.[4]

Transmission

H. influenzae is carried primarily in the nasopharynx. *H. influenzae* strains can be isolated frequently from children (often from 50 percent or more of children less than 6 years of age). However, Hib carriage is less common and was identified in 2 to 6 percent of children in most studies before the introduction of conjugate vaccines.[5] Hib carriage was most prevalent in 3- and 4-year-olds.

Little is known about the dynamics of the spread of *H. influenzae* from one person to another, although it probably occurs via contact with respiratory secretions or respiratory droplets. Culture surveys of family or day care center contacts of children with Hib disease have generally shown high rates of carriage of the organism. Whether the index case is usually the cause or the victim of active transmission has not been defined.

Occurrence

Before widespread use of Hib conjugate vaccines, invasive *H. influenzae* disease occurred most commonly in children. Ninety-five percent of *H. influenzae* meningitis cases occurred in children less than 5 years of age, and nearly all of these cases were caused by Hib. That age group had an average incidence of meningitis of about 40 per 100,000 per year in the U.S. The peak incidence (150/100,000 per year) was in children 6 to 7 months old. Epiglottitis is distinctive among illnesses caused by encapsulated strains in that most cases occur in children 2 to 5 years of age. Pneumonia caused by nonencapsulated strains is probably most common in older adults. Incidence was as much as 3 times higher in blacks, but subsequent studies suggested most of the increased risk was associated with risk factors such as crowding and day care attendance rather than genetic factors.[6] Similarly, rates 10 times the U.S. average were identified in native Alaskan and aboriginal Australian populations, which may, at least in part, also be due to socioeconomic or behavioral factors. The incidence of *H. influenzae* infection is lowest in the summer, with peak incidence from October to December and a second peak in March and April.[7]

Children with disorders of immunoglobulin synthesis are at increased risk of *H. influenzae* disease, as apparently are those with sickle cell disease. Chronic lung disease has been mentioned as predisposing patients to pneumonia caused by nonencapsulated strains.

Large epidemics of *H. influenzae* disease have not been observed, although clusters of cases are seen in households, day care centers, and facilities for the care of chronically ill children. The risk of systemic *H. influenzae* disease in household contacts during the month after the onset of *H. influenzae* meningitis in an index case has been estimated as 0.3 percent overall, and 2 percent in contacts younger than 4 years of age. Other studies have suggested that the risk of disease in day care classroom contacts younger than 2 years of age may be as high as 1 percent.

Prevention

Initial efforts to develop a vaccine for prevention of *H. influenzae* disease focused on evaluation of a purified PRP antigen. A randomized double-blind field trial in Finland showed 90 percent efficacy of a PRP vaccine in children 2 years of age and older, and, consistent with immunogenicity data, no efficacy in younger children.[8] The vaccine was licensed for use in U.S. children at 18 to 24 months of age, but most postmarketing studies showed only moderate efficacy in this country.[9]

In the meantime, efforts continued to develop vaccines that would be more immunogenic, especially in younger children. The most promising candidate vaccines were prepared by covalently binding PRP with a protein carrier. Immunogenicity studies of several of these conjugate vaccines showed marked increases in anti-PRP antibody in children immunized at 18 months of age, and in 1988, three conjugate vaccines were licensed for use in 18-month-olds. In 1990, trials of two of these conjugate vaccines given to infants in the United States at the same time as DTP were completed and both showed efficacy against invasive disease.[10,11] Both vaccines were licensed and recommended for routine infant immunization in late 1990. Figure 7-6 shows the impact of Hib vaccines on *H. influenzae* meningitis in the United States.[12] Although the PRP vaccine had little effect on meningitis rates, soon after introduction of the first Hib conjugate vaccines in 18-month-olds, disease rates began to fall, and by 1995, after introduction of infant immunization,[13] rates of *H. influenzae* meningitis had dropped by more than 95 percent.[14] The dramatic reduction in disease was due in part to the effect of the vaccine in reducing carriage of the organism.[15] In several populations in which the vaccine was widely given, asymptomatic carriage of the organism was practically eliminated, reducing exposure of the general population to the pathogen and thus "protecting" even the unimmunized. This "herd immunity" effect caused declines in disease in excess of vaccine coverage and is likely to play a major role in the remarkable success of these vaccines.

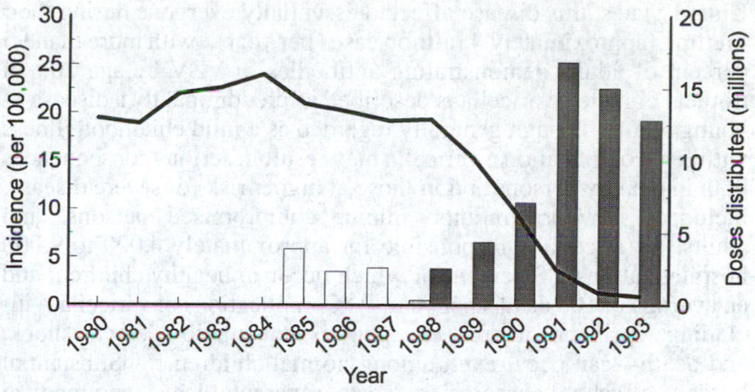

Figure 7-6. Incidence of *H. influenzae* meningitis reported to the National Bacterial Meningitis and Bacteremia Reporting System, and the number of doses of Hib polysaccharide vaccine (*clear bars*) and Hib conjugate vaccine (*shaded bars*) distributed.

Although secondary cases (those occurring in persons with close contact with an initial case of disease, such as day care classmates or siblings) represent only 1 to 3 percent of *H. influenzae* disease, the elevated rate in such contacts indicates the need for effective prophylaxis. Several studies during the prevaccine era support the effectiveness of chemoprophylaxis for household and day care contacts. Therefore, chemoprophylaxis with rifampin is recommended for all household contacts if there are any children less than 4 years old in the household who are not fully vaccinated, and for all day care classmates and teachers if there are any children less than 2 years of age who are not fully vaccinated in the classroom.

The Hib conjugate vaccines have demonstrated their effectiveness for prevention of invasive Hib disease in every industrialized country in which they have been used and in several developing nations. A recent study in the Gambia showed they can also prevent severe pneumonia caused by Hib in developing areas.[3] Although developing countries have a vastly greater burden of disease, due largely to pneumonia, wider use of the Hib conjugate vaccines in these areas is limited by price. Nevertheless, the new Hib conjugate vaccines represent a modern public health triumph, and hold forth promise of virtual elimination of Hib disease worldwide.

Varicella and Herpes Zoster

Jane F. Seward • Melinda Wharton

Varicella

Public Health Significance

Varicella (chickenpox) and herpes zoster (shingles) are two distinct disease entities caused by the varicella zoster virus (VZV). Varicella is the clinical manifestation of the primary infection caused by VZV, which, like other herpes viruses, is capable of maintaining latency in the human body and reactivating to result in the secondary or reactivated form of disease known as herpes zoster or shingles. In temperate climates, varicella is a common, highly communicable childhood illness characterized by fever and a generalized pruritic exanthem. Prior to the availability of a vaccine for prevention of varicella in the

United States, this disease affected essentially everyone during their lifetime (approximately 4 million cases per year),[1] with more than 95 percent of adults demonstrating antibodies to VZV by age 20.[2] In tropical climates, varicella is described as predominantly a disease of young adults. Though generally regarded as a mild childhood illness with few complications, varicella may result in serious consequences both in healthy persons and in those at higher risk for severe disease, including newborn infants, immunocompromised persons, and adults.[3,4] Varicella is responsible for approximately 4,000 to 9,000 hospitalizations, 80 percent of which occur in healthy children, and an average of 100 deaths per year.[1,5,6] Complications of varicella—including sepsis, pneumonia, encephalitis, coagulation defects, shock, and death—can occur even among normal children.[3–5,7] Substantial burdens of school absenteeism, costs of parental leave, and medical costs are associated with childhood chickenpox, with net cost-benefit estimates for a routine childhood vaccination program calculated as $5.40[8] and $66.47.[9] A varicella vaccine was licensed for use in the United States in 1995, making prevention of this disease possible.

Etiology

The varicella-zoster virus is a DNA virus of the herpes family. Humans are the only source of infection for this highly contagious virus. Although the etiologic agent responsible for varicella and zoster was not identified and named until the 1950s, herpes zoster was described in the very early medical literature. Varicella, however, was frequently confused with another "pox" illness, smallpox (variola), until the end of the nineteenth century. It was not until the early 1900s that the association between varicella and zoster was suggested when von Bokay reported on the occurrence of varicella following cases of zoster in two families. The association was confirmed experimentally by demonstration that inoculation of vesicular fluid from persons with herpes zoster produced varicella in susceptible volunteers in 1925. It was not until 1943 that it was first suggested that zoster was due to a reactivation of a latent agent that had been originally acquired during varicella. Weller, in 1953, confirmed that varicella and herpes zoster have a common etiology by isolating and propagating the etiologic agent from both diseases in vitro. He and colleagues then demonstrated that the viruses were morphologically and serologically identical and the agent was named varicella-zoster virus in 1958.[10]

Immunology

The VZV induces both humoral and cell-mediated immune responses. Cell-mediated immunity to VZV is believed to be particularly important in preventing recurrences of varicella after reexposure, in maintaining the latent state of the virus in dorsal root ganglia, and in preventing the occurrence of herpes zoster. Infection usually produces a typical clinical illness; clinically inapparent or asymptomatic primary infection is estimated to occur in no more than 5 percent of susceptible children.[11] Lifelong protective immunity usually occurs following one attack of varicella. However, rarely, recurrence or reinfection of chickenpox has been reported in immunocompetent individuals with documented VZV immunity.[12,13] Reexposure to wild-type varicella frequently results in reinfection that boosts immunity without causing clinical illness or detectable viremia.

Laboratory Tests

Laboratory tests are available to confirm varicella in atypical disease presentations, to type varicella strains, and to assess immune status. Because varicella is an easily identified distinct clinical entity, laboratory confirmation is not indicated in mild and uncomplicated cases. However, in severe cases of suspected varicella or herpes zoster, especially when presentation is disseminated or atypical, rapid laboratory confirmation using sensitive and specific viral identification techniques is essential in order to initiate appropriate antiviral therapy. Such therapy provides the maximum benefit when instituted as soon as possible after disease onset. Serologic tests, which may take several days or weeks (for paired samples of acute and convalescent sera) for test results are appropriate for the diagnosis of disease in mild, atypical cases in which confirmation is necessary and for identifying the immune status of individuals whose history of varicella is negative or uncertain and who may be candidates for varicella-zoster immune globulin (VZIG) or vaccination. Viral typing or strain identification is used to distinguish wild varicella-zoster virus from the vaccine strain in the United States. These tests are discussed in the following sections.

Serology. Serologic tests are available for IgG and IgM antibodies to VZV. Testing for IgM antibody is not useful clinically, since available methods lack sensitivity and specificity. False-positive results are common in the presence of high IgG levels.[14] Many tests have been used to detect IgG antibody to VZV.[15] Rising IgG antibody levels from paired acute and convalescent sera taken 2 to 3 weeks apart is evidence of infection with VZV. Single IgG assays are used to screen or verify an individual's immune status. Prior to the availability of varicella vaccine, the fluorescent antibody to membrane antigen (FAMA) test was considered the "gold standard" test, although it was not widely available. With automation of testing equipment and high-volume testing in the laboratory setting, the enzyme-linked immunosorbent assay (ELISA) test using total VZV antigen has replaced both latex agglutination (LA) and FAMA as the most common serologic test available. In immunologically competent persons, the presence of antibody detectable by one of these assays may be considered evidence of past infection with VZV and hence evidence of immunity. Commercial ELISAs are highly specific but less sensitive than FAMA; 10 to 15 percent individuals who are immune may be identified as susceptible.[14] Because history of disease is highly predictive of serologic immunity, a reliable history of varicella is accepted as evidence of immunity. In adults in the United States, 97 to 99 percent of those with a positive history are seropositive. The majority of adults with a negative or uncertain history are also seropositive (71 to 97 percent).[16–18]

Levels of antibody following vaccination may be lower than those following natural varicella infection and may not be detected by commercially available tests. A highly sensitive gpELISA test, using purified viral glycoproteins as antigen, was developed for testing of immunogenicity in vaccine clinical trials but is not commercially available at the present time.[19] The interpretation of test results in vaccinees should take into account the fact that low levels of antibody may not be detected using currently commercially available ELISA tests.[15]

Virologic Laboratory Tests. Methods for diagnosis of VZV infections detect infectious virus, viral antigen, or viral protein in clinical specimens. In cases of severe disease or an atypical clinical presentation, diagnosis must be confirmed as rapidly as possible. In these instances, rapid antigen detection tests are the preferred method. The most commonly available and widely used test is the direct fluorescence antibody (DFA) test, which is rapid (results are available in several hours), sensitive, and highly specific. The DFA test uses immunofluorescence procedures to label polyclonal or monoclonal antibodies that bind to VZV antigens to allow the rapid identification of VZV proteins in cells from the base of skin lesions. Polymerase chain reaction (PCR) and enzyme immunoassay (EIA) methods can also be used to detect VZV proteins in swab specimens from skin lesions and other clinical specimens. Direct and indirect immunofluorescence methods may detect VZV-infected cells in tissue sections of lung, liver, brain, and other organs in patients with disseminated primary or recurrent VZV infection.

Cultures for VZV, though confirming unequivocally the diagnosis of VZV infection, require a minimum of 2 days, more frequently 7 days or longer, to detect infectious virus in cell culture. More rapid culture techniques using Shell vials and special procedures may yield results within 2 or 3 days. VZV can be cultured from many clinical specimens, including fluid from vesicles, urine, nasal secretions, blood, throat swabs, urine, cerebrospinal fluid (CSF), bronchial washings, and joint fluid, and at autopsy from lungs, heart, liver, pancreas, gastrointestinal tract, and eyes.

PCR and restriction fragment length polymorphism (RFLP) techniques are used to distinguish wild VZV from the vaccine (Oka/Merck) strain in the United States.[20] Viral typing or strain identification is labor intensive, costly, and time consuming and is usually undertaken only in clinical circumstances with severe or unusual disease occurrence after vaccination to distinguish the wild virus from the vaccine virus. Such situations include a severe rash, suspected secondary transmission of the vaccine virus and herpes zoster, or any serious adverse event after vaccination.

Clinical Characteristics

Varicella is highly contagious, with secondary infection rates in susceptible household contacts approaching 90 percent.[21,22] Transmission occurs from person to person by direct contact from patients with either varicella or zoster lesions or by airborne spread from respiratory secretions. Indirect exposure may occur through contact with articles soiled by discharges from an infected person. In hospitals, airborne transmission has been documented in the absence of direct contact between the index case and the susceptible patients who contracted varicella.[23] The path of entry of the virus is assumed to be the upper respiratory tract. The incubation period for varicella ranges from 10 to 21 days, most commonly 14 to 16 days. This period may be shorter in immunocompromised patients and prolonged (for up to 28 days) in recipients of VZIG.[18,24,25] A low-level primary viremia occurs 4 to 6 days after infection, which enables the virus to infect and replicate in the liver, spleen, and possibly other organs. This is followed by a secondary viremia 10 to 20 days after infection, which results in a prodrome of fever and constitutional symptoms that may precede the rash by 1 to 3 days. The prodrome in children is milder than in adults. Fever (approximately 38° to 39°C [100° to 102°F]) is present during the peak of rash evolution and disappears by the time all the vesicles have either dried or crusted over.

The characteristic rash is pruritic, appears in successive crops, and quickly evolves from macules to papules to clear, fluid-filled vesicles approximately 2 to 4 mm in diameter. Early in the illness all stages of the rash can coexist. The vesicles are initially surrounded by an erythematous base, which fades during the process of crusting. The vesicles sequentially become purulent and dry and crust over. Drying starts at the center of the lesion, giving it an umbilicated appearance. The crust, which is not infectious, may remain for 1 to 3 weeks. The rash is distributed centrally, with more lesions occurring on the face, scalp, and trunk than on the extremities. Lesions are not confined to the skin and can develop on any mucosal surface, including inside the mouth and vagina. They can also develop on the cornea[26] and tympanic membranes. A person with varicella is contagious from 1 to 2 days before the rash appears until all of the vesicles have crusted, usually 5 to 6 days after the onset of rash. Patients with altered immunity may have a prolonged period of infectivity because new lesions may develop for an extended period.

Complications

Though generally a benign disease in childhood, varicella may be followed by complications, which are most likely to occur among immunocompromised persons, neonates, and adults.[4,5,27] Serious complications include secondary bacterial infections, pneumonia, postinfectious encephalitis, cerebellar ataxia, Reye's syndrome, and death.[4,28,29,30] Rarer complications include nephritis, arthritis, Guillain-Barré syndrome, thrombocytopenia, and clinical hepatitis. Though clinical hepatitis occurs rarely, evidence of subclinical hepatitis is frequent.[14]

Complications from varicella vary by age. In healthy children with varicella, secondary bacterial infections are the most common complications requiring hospitalization, followed by encephalitis and pneumonia.[30] There is concern that serious complications caused by invasive group A β-hemolytic streptococcus (GABHS) organisms have increased over the last decade.[28,31–34] This is consistent with reported changes in the epidemiology of GABHS infections, with more frequent isolation of more invasive and lethal strains (M-types 1, 3, and 18) in recent years.[35] Reports of life-threatening or lethal GABHS infections include cellulitis, necrotizing fascutis, septic arthritis, osteomyelitis, septicemia, and toxic shock syndrome.

Neurologic complications are the second most common indication for hospitalization for healthy children with varicella. Central nervous system (CNS) complications—meningoencephalitis and cerebellar ataxia—are more frequent in children younger than 5 years and in adults 20 years of age and older.[36] Varicella-associated encephalitis, a postinfectious condition similar to that seen after measles, is estimated to occur in one to four per 10,000 reported chickenpox cases, with a case-to-fatality ratio similar to that of post-measles encephalitis.[36] Symptoms generally begin 2 to 6 days after the appearance of the rash, although cases of encephalitis and ataxia have been reported preceding the rash.[37] Varicella encephalitis is usually transient, resolving within 24 to 72 hours.[14] Cerebellar ataxia occurs in approximately 35 percent of encephalitis cases and may persist for longer, but usually resolves completely. The risk of fatal CNS complications is difficult to determine, with estimates ranging from 5 to 18 percent.[14] VZV was the cause of encephalitis in 13 percent of cases with known etiology in cases reported by the CDC during the period from 1972 to 1977.[3,36] Reye's syndrome has become a rare complication following the marked decline in the use of salicylates among children with varicella.[38]

A higher rate of complications occurs in adults. Systemic involvement is more prominent, with primary varicella pneumonia the most common life-threatening complication.[30] Pneumonia most frequently occurs 1 to 6 days after the onset of rash, with presentation of cough and shortness of breath. Estimates of the frequency of pneumonia complicating varicella in healthy adults have varied widely from 0.3 to 50 percent, with wide ranges also in fatality from pneumonia of 9 to 50 percent.[39–41] The increased morbidity and mortality associated with varicella in adults is primarily due to the higher risk of varicella pneumonia in these patients.[39,42] In Stockholm in the 1980s, pneumonia was the most common complication (12 percent) requiring hospitalization in healthy adults with varicella, but only four of 36 patients required intensive care and there were no deaths.[41] Hemorrhagic complications occur more commonly in adults than in healthy children. These may include thrombocytopenia associated with bleeding into skin lesions, petechiae, purpura, hematuria, and gastrointestinal hemorrhage, which may proceed to disseminated intravascular coagulopathy, shock, and death. Some studies have indicated that pregnant women have a higher risk of complications than do nonpregnant adults of childbearing age. In a reported series of 118 cases of varicella in pregnant women in the United States, 24 of them developed pneumonia and 11 died.[43]

Deaths. Both varicella and herpes zoster are listed as underlying causes of death every year in the United States. The mortality attributed to varicella averaged 100 deaths per year in the 1970s; the rate decreased to a level of 47 deaths in 1986 and has increased to an average of 104 deaths per year from 1990 to 1994[3] (CDC, unpublished data). Septic complications, pneumonia, and encephalitis are the usual causes of death in children, whereas pneumonia is most often the cause of death in adults.[3,42] Encephalitis deaths accounted for approximately 10 percent of all deaths due to varicella between 1972 and 1978. The more severe course of varicella infection in normal adults is reflected in a higher case-to-fatality ratio in adults than in children.[3] The estimated death-to-case ratio in previously healthy patients (without cancer or other underlying cause of immune system dysfunction) is approximately 20 to 40 times higher in adults than in children[6] (CDC, unpublished data). Case-to-fatality rates of 7 to 14 percent have been reported for immunocompromised children, but the case-to-fatality rate has decreased with the use of antiviral agents to treat chickenpox in this group and the availability of a vaccine for children with leukemia.[44]

Immunocompromised Patients. In immunocompromised patients, all expressions of the infection may be markedly enhanced.[14,24,25] In such patients, atypical presentations of varicella may be difficult to distinguish from disseminated herpes zoster. Severe disseminated varicella or zoster and serious complications have been described in many situations associated with an immunocompromised state, including leukemia and other cancers, HIV/AIDS, disorders of the immune system, and immunosuppression secondary to the use of steroids or cancer chemotherapeutic drugs.[45,46] Numerous studies suggest that an impaired cellular immune state is the major contributing factor.[47] Feldman has reported several studies of varicella in children with cancer. Of 77 cancer patients with varicella, 32 percent of the children who were receiving cancer chemotherapy when they developed varicella had visceral dissemination and 7 percent died.[48] At St. Judes Children's Research Hospital during the period from 1962 to 1985, 5 percent of patients had one or more episodes of varicella. Mortality was 7 percent among 127 untreated patients before the advent of effective antiviral therapy.[49] VZV pneumonitis developed in 28 percent of untreated patients and was associated with a 25 percent mortality. Use of antiviral therapy and passive immunization for children with cancer and vaccination for children with leukemia has significantly decreased morbidity and mortality from this disease in children with malignancies.[49,50]

Among persons with human immunodeficiency virus (HIV) infections, varicella may be severe with serious complications, disseminated, and may result in death.[51–53] In a large series of 391 HIV-infected children in Romania, over a 15-month period in 1991–1992, 10 percent of the children had varicella and 2 percent had herpes zoster. The duration of varicella was prolonged (mean duration, 13.5 days) in more than 50 percent of the children and the rate of complications (40 percent) was higher than that reported in healthy children hospitalized with varicella. The most common complications were skin infections (26 percent) and pneumonia (24 percent). Two children (5 percent) died of pneumonia. Acyclovir was not available for treatment in Romania at that time.[54]

Neonatal Varicella. Prior to the advent of antiviral therapy, as many as 30 percent of infected infants whose mothers had a chickenpox rash within 5 days before delivery died of the disease. The risk of serious illness is highest when maternal onset of varicella is from 5 days before delivery to 2 days afterward, because the baby does not acquire passive immunity transplacentally. Disease earlier in pregnancy is associated with the passage of protective maternal antibody to the fetus.[55]

Congenital Varicella Syndrome. Maternal infection within the first 20 weeks of gestation can lead to congenital varicella syndrome, a recognized constellation of congenital defects including hypoplasia of an extremity, cicatricial skin scarring, localized muscular atrophy, encephalitis, microcephaly, cortical atrophy, ocular abnormalities, mental retardation, and low birth weight. This syndrome has been estimated to occur in about 0.4 percent of infections that occur from weeks 0 to 12 and 2.0 percent of infections that occur from weeks 13 to 20.[56] Other researchers have suggested that milder atypical cases may also occur that may be more difficult to diagnose. Gestational varicella is associated with an increased risk of zoster occurring at an early age.[55]

Epidemiology

In temperate climates, varicella is a disease of childhood, with 80 to 90 percent of cases occurring before 10 years of age.[1,22,26,57] Chickenpox is endemic in the United States and has a striking seasonal distribution with peak incidence in the winter and spring. Nationally reported cases to the CDC represent only an estimated 4 to 6 percent of the actual number of cases that occur. Assuming that virtually all persons are infected by adulthood, the equivalent of a birth cohort (approximately 4 million) of persons is infected annually. The highest reported annual incidence rate has typically been described in 5- to 9-year-old children, followed by the 1 to 4 year age group.[1,3,11] However, recent studies reporting the highest incidence among 1- to 4-year-old children indicate that the disease may be shifting to younger children, perhaps because of the earlier and more frequent attendance at preschools and child care centers.[57,58] By adulthood, 95 percent of the U.S. population are immune to varicella. Among 20- to 29-year-olds, the prevalence of antibody is 96 percent, increasing to 99 percent among 30- to 39-year-olds (CDC, unpublished data). Among U.S. Navy and Marine Corps recruits, higher varicella susceptibility (13.6 percent) has been reported in male African Americans than in whites (6.5 percent).[59] Among U.S. Army recruits, 14.2 percent of African Americans and 6.0 percent of whites were found to be seronegative.[60] This suggests differences in exposure during early childhood. However, the fact that this pattern of disease is also seen in Singapore argues in favor of climate being the major factor affecting transmission.

In tropical regions, varicella is less common among children, with more frequent and serious disease occurring among adults. In a serosurvey in St. Lucia, West Indies, very few children less than 10 years old were seropositive; 10 percent had infections before the age of 15 years; and 50 percent of the population were seropositive by age 35. The reasons for this difference in the age-specific incidence of varicella in tropical than in temperate climates are unclear but may include higher ambient temperatures and differences in population size, population density, and crowding, resulting in decreased transmission in the tropics.[61] In the USA, outbreaks of varicella among Army recruits from Puerto Rico have highlighted the increased susceptibility of this adult population. Forty-two percent of 810 recruits from Puerto Rico tested were seronegative, a much higher percentage than that described in U.S.-born recruits.[62]

Changes in the epidemiology of varicella in the United States are expected to occur following implementation of a national program for universal vaccination of all infants.[1,63] Although disease incidence will decline overall, the age distribution of the remaining cases of varicella will shift to older age groups, among whom the disease is more severe. However, based on a mathematical model, a net decrease in hospitalizations is expected because of the decrease in cases among children.[8,64] If susceptible adolescents and adults are also vaccinated, as recommended, the pool of individuals subject to severe disease should diminish markedly.[63] In England and Wales, where vaccine for healthy persons is not yet available, there has been an upward shift in the age distribution of varicella cases over the last 20 years, with an increase in proportion of cases in the 15- to 44-year-old age group.[65] This change has not been documented in the United States with serial analysis of population base data. Age-specific incidence from National Health Interview Survey data in the United States for the periods 1972 to 1978 and 1980 to 1990 were remarkably constant (CDC, unpublished data).

Strategies for Control and Prevention

Active Immunization: Varicella Vaccine. With licensure of the varicella vaccine in 1995, varicella became a vaccine-preventable disease in the United States. The virus was originally isolated from a healthy child with varicella in Japan. A live attenuated viral vaccine (Oka/Biken) has been available in Japan and Korea since the 1980s for use in healthy and immunocompromised persons (although it is not recommended for routine infant vaccination), and another vaccine (Oka/SB Bio) is licensed for use among immunocompromised children in nine countries in Europe.[44] The Oka/SB Bio vaccine has been reformulated to facilitate its use for general vaccination in healthy children, and efficacy studies in the United States are currently being conducted.[66]

The live attenuated varicella vaccine (Oka/Merck strain) was licensed for use in the United States in March 1995, with recommendations for its use published by the Advisory Committee on Immunization Practices (ACIP),[18] the American Academy of Pediatrics (AAP),[66] the American Academy of Family Physicians (AAFP),[67] and the American College of Physicians (ACP)[68] in 1995 and 1996. Clinical trials to test the safety, immunogenicity, and efficacy of this vaccine in the United States began as early as the 1970s among immunocompromised children with leukemia in remission. Phased trials testing different formulations of the vaccine strain were conducted among healthy children and adults between 1982 and 1991. The formulation licensed for use in the United States contains a minimum of 1,700 plaque-forming units (PFU). The clinical trials varied greatly in the amounts of live virus given, the numbers of doses, the proportions of live to killed virus, and the ages of vaccinees, which led to noncomparability of immunogenicity, safety, and efficacy estimates between trials.[44]

Varicella vaccine is approved for use in healthy susceptible children aged 12 months or more and in susceptible adolescents and adults. The ACIP and the AAP recommend that all children be routinely vaccinated between 12 and 18 months of age, and that all susceptible children ages 19 months to 13 years be vaccinated by their 13th birthday. The vaccine may be administered at any time during childhood but should be given at the 11- to 12-year-old adolescent visit if the child is still susceptible at that time. Children 13 years old and younger receive one 0.5-mL dose, administered subcutaneously. For persons 13 years old and above, priority groups for vaccination include susceptible persons who have close contact with persons at high risk for serious complications (e.g., health care workers and family contacts of immunocompromised persons); vaccination should be considered for susceptible persons who are at high risk of exposure (e.g., teachers of young children, college students, military personnel) nonpregnant women of childbearing age and international travelers. Vaccination is desirable for other susceptible adolescents and adults. Two doses of vaccine administered 4-8 weeks apart are required for persons of age 13 years and above. The AAFP and the ACP recommend vaccination of all susceptible adults, with priority groups established by the ACP for those at highest risk of disease or exposure. Vaccination is recommended for all susceptible health care workers.[18,69]

Immunogenicity and Duration of Immunity. The vaccine produces both humoral and cell-mediated immune responses detected 6 to 8 weeks after vaccination. The antibody response is dependent on the age at vaccination, the dose of virus and the number of doses of vaccine administered, the length of follow-up, and the cutoff point for seroconversion. With a cutoff point of 0.3 units or greater (by gpELISA titer) and a dose of 950 PFU or greater, the vaccine produces an antibody response in 95 to 99 percent of healthy children after one dose[70–72] and in 94 to 99 percent of healthy adults after two doses.[73–75] The vaccine is also well tolerated and highly immunogenic when administered as a two-dose series in immunocompromised children with leukemia. Although the vaccine is not licensed for use in this population, it may be used as an investigational agent.[18] Humoral immunity has been shown to persist for more than 20 years in Japan and for up to 6 to 10 years in the United States among 95 to 100 percent of adult and 93 to 100 percent of child and adolescent vaccinees in the presence of wild virus circulating in the community.[76,77] Persistence of immunity in the absence of exposure to the wild virus and natural boosting of immunity is unknown. Ongoing studies and surveillance will determine the need for a second dose in the future. Cell-mediated immunity is also induced and shows strong persistence in 94 percent of vaccinated children for the 6 years of follow-up that have been completed.[76]

Trials were also conducted in children and adults with a negative history of varicella but who demonstrated antibody to VZV. Among the children immunized, the vaccine led to more than a 4-fold boost in humoral immunity in more than 95 percent of children, which was maintained for 9 to 12 months. A boost in cellular immune response was also noted among all children tested. Among adults, one dose of vaccine boosted either humoral and/or cellular immunity in 66 percent of persons.[74] These findings have led to larger-scale evaluation of the use of this vaccine in immune elderly persons and its potential for boosting immunity for the prevention of herpes zoster.

Efficacy. The varicella vaccine is highly effective in preventing varicella. Clinical trials prior to licensure demonstrated vaccine efficacies ranging from 70 to 100 percent depending on the age at vaccination, dosage, number of doses given, type of exposure (household or community), length of follow-up, and outcome of disease studied (i.e., severity of disease). Adults have a lower degree of protection than children.[73] With 5 to 10 years of follow-up of vaccinated children and adolescents, reported vaccine efficacies have ranged from 83 to 95 percent.[70,71,78] The vaccine is more than 95 percent effective in preventing severe disease after household exposure in both children and adults. Breakthrough disease (varicella due to wild-type virus in a vaccinated person) is usually mild with shorter duration of disease, absence of fever, and fewer than 50 skin lesions. The incidence of breakthrough infections is approximately 2 to 3 percent of vaccinees per year and does not appear to increase with time since vaccination.[71,78]

Postexposure efficacy studies indicate that varicella vaccine given within 3 days of exposure is more than 90 percent effective in preventing secondary cases of varicella among susceptible contacts in the household setting.[74,79] Although the efficacy of postexposure vaccination in controlling outbreaks in larger closed settings such as child care centers and schools has not been established, vaccination in these settings might protect those recently infected as well as confer immunity in susceptible persons not yet infected.

Safety. The vaccine is well tolerated in healthy individuals. Local pain and/or redness at the injection site, fever, and generalized varicella-like rash may occur. From prelicensure clinical trials, the reported incidence of rash at the injection site after vaccination was approximately 3 to 4 percent among children, adolescents, and adults following the first dose. For generalized rash these rates are 4 percent for children and 6 percent for adolescents and adults, respectively. The median number of lesions was low: two at the injection site and five for generalized rash. Vaccine-related rashes are more common (up to 50 percent) after vaccination of immunocompromised persons.[50] Secondary transmission of the vaccine virus was documented in clinical trials from immunocompromised to healthy siblings. Post-marketing surveillance has documented a case of secondary transmission from a healthy vaccinee to a healthy susceptible contact. [79a] Transmission has not been confirmed in the absence of a rash after vaccination. The vaccine virus is capable of reactivating to cause herpes zoster in an immunocompromised host,[44] and since licensure of the vaccine, this has also been documented rarely in healthy children (Merck & Co., Inc., unpublished data). Data from clinical trials among immunocompromised children demonstrate that zoster incidence is lower in vaccinees than in children who had natural varicella.[80] Post-marketing surveillance data in healthy children are supportive of these findings.

Severe adverse reactions are very rare after vaccination, but encephalitis, ataxia, Bell's palsy, anaphylaxis, erythema multiforme, thrombocytopenia, meningitis, purpura, paresthesia, and Stevens-Johnson syndrome have been reported as temporally related to use of this vaccine. There is no evidence of a causal association. Pneumonia due to the vaccine virus in a child with undiagnosed HIV/AIDS and other cases of pneumonitis following vaccination have been reported (Merck & Co., Inc., unpublished data).

Contraindications and Precautions. Contraindications and precautions to vaccination include pregnancy (women should avoid becoming pregnant for 1 month after receiving a dose of varicella vaccine); allergy to vaccine components (vaccine contains neomycin but does not contain egg protein or preservatives); recent administration of blood, plasma, or immune globulin, altered immunity, including malignant conditions; primary or acquired immunodeficiency, including HIV/AIDS; and conditions that require steroid therapy (more than 2 mg/kg/day or a total of 20 mg/day of prednisone or its equivalent). The vaccine manufacturer, in collaboration with the CDC, has established the VARIVAX Pregnancy Register[81] to monitor the outcomes of pregnant women who are inadvertently vaccinated 3 months before or at any time during pregnancy [telephone, 800-969-8999]. No adverse events associated with the use of salicylates after varicella vaccination have been reported. However, the vaccine manufacturer recommends that vaccine recipients avoid using salicylates for 6 weeks after receiving varicella virus vaccine because of the association between aspirin use and Reye's syndrome following varicella. The vaccine is available for use, through a research protocol, in children with acute lymphoblastic leukemia in remission. The safety and immunogenicity of varicella vaccine virus in HIV-infected children is currently being studied.

Passive Immunization. Varicella-zoster immune globulin (VZIG) is available for postexposure prophylaxis in susceptible persons at high risk for developing severe disease who have been exposed to either varicella or zoster. VZIG has been shown to be effective in reducing the severity of varicella when given up to 96 hours after exposure. It should, however, be given as soon as possible after exposure. The decision to administer VZIG to a person exposed to varicella should be based on (*a*) whether the person is susceptible, (*b*) whether the exposure is likely to result in infection, and (*c*) whether the patient is at greater risk for complications than the general population. Identified high-risk groups include newborn infants whose mothers developed varicella around the time of delivery (less than 5 days before to 2 days after delivery), immunocompromised persons including those on immunosuppressive medications and steroids, susceptible pregnant women, hospitalized premature infants of 28 weeks or longer gestation or more than 1000 g whose mother has no history of varicella and/or antibodies to VZV, and premature infants of less than 28 weeks gestation or less than 1000 g regardless of the mother's history of varicella. The recommended dose is one vial (125 U) per 10 kg body weight given by intramuscular injection.[18,82]

Isolation Guidelines. Isolation of individuals with varicella until all lesions have crusted is a routine outbreak control measure. Isolation is also recommended for exposed susceptible individuals who may be in contact with persons at high risk of serious complications (e.g., health care workers and families of immunocompromised persons). Such isolation is required for the duration of the period of communicability; that is, from the 10th until the 21st day after exposure or until the 28th day if the exposed individual receives VZIG.[25]

Therapy. A variety of antiviral drugs are now available for treatment of varicella and herpes zoster. Antiviral therapy has dramatically changed the prognosis for VZV infections in immunocompromised persons. Acyclovir is a synthetic nucleoside analog that inhibits replication of human herpes viruses, including the varicella-zoster virus; it is available in both oral and intravenous forms and is most effective when administered *within 24 hours of rash onset.*[18,82,83] Oral acyclovir is not recommended *routinely* for the treatment of uncomplicated varicella in healthy children but is recommended for treatment of primary varicella among certain groups at increased risk of severe disease or its complications. This includes healthy adolescents and adults, children older than 12 months with a chronic cutaneous or pulmonary disorder, those receiving long-term salicylate therapy, and those receiving long-term, short, intermittent, or aerosolized courses of corticosteroids.[18,82] Since oral acyclovir is poorly absorbed, IV acyclovir is recommended for the treatment of severe primary varicella and/or serious complications of varicella in healthy or immunocompromised individuals and for recurrent zoster in immunocompromised persons. The newer generation of acyclovir analogs licensed for treatment of herpes zoster—famciclovir and valacyclovir—have improved bioavailability and may offer improved treatment of severe primary varicella in the future. Another nucleoside analog, sorivudine, was recently assessed in a placebo-controlled trial for the treatment of varicella in healthy adults. The drug significantly shortened the clinical course of adult varicella in a dose-dependent fashion and, in contrast to acyclovir, was effective in patients who presented more than 24 hours after rash onset.[84] VZV resistance to acyclovir has not proved to be a problem in immunocompetent hosts. In immunocompromised hosts, acyclovir-resistant VZV infections have been reported and may become an increasing problem with the use of prolonged acyclovir therapy for patients with chronic or recurrent herpes zoster infections. For such patients, the best alternative therapy is foscarnet. Interferon is now rarely used for VZV therapy.[83,85]

Herpes Zoster

Clinical Characteristics and Complications

Herpes zoster, or shingles, is a localized disease with a painful vesicular rash that results from reactivation of VZV after latency within sensory ganglia following an earlier attack of varicella.[24,47,86,87] The rash is characterized by a unilateral dermatomal distribution in 1 to 3 sensory dermatomes. Herpes zoster may present as a disseminated, generalized rash in immunocompromised patients. The varicella-zoster virus may be transmitted from patients with herpes zoster to susceptible individuals, resulting in varicella. The latent virus is more likely to become reactivated under certain conditions, most notably advancing age, following varicella acquired in utero or during the first year of life, malignancy, and immunosuppression.[24,47,86,87] Because this reactivation can occur in the presence of circulating antibodies against the varicella-zoster virus, and the majority of predisposing conditions are associated with declining or relatively absent cell-mediated immunity, cell-mediated immunity is considered to play an important role in this process. The incidence and severity of zoster, as well as the incidence and severity of complications, increase markedly with age, and decreased cell-mediated immunity to VZV has been demonstrated in the elderly. Complications from herpes zoster occur in almost 50 percent of elderly individuals (more than 65 years of age). The most frequent complication in this age group is post-herpetic neuralgia (PHN), a syndrome of pain, allodynia, dysesthesia, and hyperesthesia that persists or develops after the dermatomal rash has healed.[87] PHN may be prolonged and disabling. Other complications include cranial or peripheral nerve palsies, sensory loss, deafness, ocular complications, transverse myelitis, and disseminated infection with pneumonitis, hepatitis, pericarditis, or arthritis.[24]

In immunocompromised hosts, herpes zoster results in more severe disease, which can be disseminated and life-threatening. Individuals who suffer from lymphoproliferative malignancies or require bone marrow transplantation are at unusually high risk for disseminated herpes zoster with visceral complications, particularly pneumonia.[88]

Epidemiology

In the United States, herpes zoster is a significant cause of hospitalization and morbidity among elderly adults[87] and was listed as the underlying cause for an average of 145 deaths annually between 1968 and 1994 (CDC, unpublished data). Studies in the United Kingdom have described an overall incidence of 3.4 cases per 1,000 person-years, with incidence of 6.8 per 1,000 person-years in persons 60 to 69 years of age and 11.0 per 1,000 person-years for persons 80 years of age or older.[86] The strong association with age has been noted in all studies. Data from the United States in the 1970s showed an annual incidence rate of 1.3 per 1,000 person-years in a population in Minnesota, with the highest rates reported for older adults (more than 4 per 1,000 person-years for persons older than 75 years).[89] A population-based study in children and adolescents showed that the incidence increased with age from 20 cases per 100,000 person-years in children less than 5 years to 63 cases per 100,000 person-years in those aged 15 to 19 years.[90] A study of incident and recurrent zoster in an HMO population in Massachusetts between 1990 and 1992 reported a 2-fold increase in the age-adjusted incidence compared with data from 30 years ago.[91] This increase was not due to an increase in persons with immunosuppressive conditions, although recurrences of zoster were associated with such conditions. Data from a longitudinal study in an elderly population (more than 64 years) in North Carolina has demonstrated an annual incidence rate of 7.1 per 1,000 person-years, with striking increases with age and significant differences in the occurrence of herpes zoster by race. African Americans were one-fourth as likely (adjusted OR = 0.25, 95% CI, 0.18–0.35) to have experienced herpes zoster after controlling for age, cancer history, female gender, education, and urban residence.[92]

Treatment

Early and vigorous treatment with antiviral agents has been demonstrated to shorten time to healing of skin lesions and may shorten the duration of postherpetic neuralgia.[84,93] Acyclovir, famciclovir, and valacyclovir have been approved for treating herpes zoster in immunocompetent persons and are most effective in reducing the duration of rash and the incidence and duration of postherpetic neuralgia if given within 48 to 72 hours of the onset of rash.[14,84,93] The newer-generation drugs, famciclovir and valacyclovir, are more bioavailable when administered orally than acyclovir and require less frequent administration.[94] It is anticipated that they will be effective for treatment of immunocompromised patients on the basis of experience in immunocompetent patients. Foscarnet and interferon (IFN-α), both antiviral drugs licensed for the treatment of herpes zoster, may be useful for acyclovir-resistant strains.

Future Research Directions

Studies of the effectiveness of the varicella vaccine in boosting humoral and cellular immunity have been conducted among children and young and elderly adults.[74,95] It has been demonstrated that waning VZV-specific cell-mediated immunity in elderly persons can be stimulated by varicella vaccine to levels typical of those observed in younger persons, among whom herpes zoster is less common and less severe.[95] A large placebo-controlled clinical trial is planned to test the hypothesis that restoration of waning cell-mediated immunity to VZV will reduce the incidence and severity of herpes zoster and its complications in the elderly.

Poliomyelitis

Roland W. Sutter • Stephen L. Cochi

Poliomyelitis, or infantile paralysis, is an acute infectious disease characterized by fever, flaccid paralysis, and muscle atrophy as a result of the destruction of motor neurons in the spinal cord and brainstem; three different serotypes of poliovirus can cause an infection that ranges in severity from inapparent illness to flaccid paralysis and death. Flaccid paralysis may resolve or lead to permanent disability and deformity. Decades after the acute episode, new paralysis or weakness may appear. This clinical entity is referred to as post-polio syndrome.[1] Poliomyelitis probably has afflicted mankind for thousands of years; however, only in 1789 was the disease first described in the medical literature. Epidemic poliomyelitis became an emerging public health problem in the United States and Northern Europe in the late nineteenth and early twentieth centuries, with tens of thousands of cases reported annually.

Etiology

In 1908, Landsteiner and Popper experimentally induced paralytic disease in monkeys by intraperitoneal inoculation of spinal cord material from a patient with fatal poliomyelitis. However, it was not shown until the early 1940s in other experiments that the infectious agent was usually present in stools of the patients with symptomatic disease and their symptom-free contacts.

In 1931, Burnet and Macnamara established that more than one virus strain can cause poliomyelitis. A major typing effort headed in 1951 by the Committee on Typing of the National Infantile Paralysis Society determined that there were only a total of three serotypes of polioviruses, designated as poliovirus types 1, 2, and 3.[2] These closely related but antigenically distinct viruses are classified as picornaviruses belonging to the enterovirus group.[3] A major laboratory breakthrough occurred in 1949 when Enders, Weller, and Robbins successfully propagated poliovirus for the first time in human embryonic nonnervous tissue; at the same time, these investigators documented viral growth directly in cell cultures (i.e., "cytopathogenic effect") and thus eliminated the need for in vivo methods (e.g., monkeys) to confirm viral replication.[4] These accomplishments were essential to pave the way for efficient growth of virus for the ultimate production of vaccines.

Pathogenesis

After ingestion into the oral cavity, polioviruses replicate initially in the oropharyngeal mucosa and the Peyer's patches in the ileum after gaining access into cells at specific receptor sites.[5] Viremia may ensue and central nervous system (CNS) infection may follow; in the latter instance, the virus specifically targets the motor neuron of the spinal cord and occasionally also the brainstem. Viral replication in the motor neurons results in cell destruction and flaccid paralysis of the muscles they innervate. Death is usually a result of bulbar involvement with respiratory paralysis.

Infections with only limited involvement of the CNS may not produce the characteristic flaccid paralysis of poliomyelitis. Rather, they may cause illness with fever and evidence of meningeal irritation—stiff neck and back and elevated protein and leukocyte levels in the spinal fluid—followed by complete recovery. This syndrome is clinically identical to aseptic meningitis caused by other viral agents such as mumps virus, echovirus, and coxsackie viruses. The vast majority of infected persons, however, have no infection of the CNS and are symptom free or have nonspecific, mild illness consisting of any combination of fever, malaise, headache with nausea, vomiting, constipation, diarrhea, and sore throat. The ratio of asymptomatic infection to paralytic disease in most studies has varied between 100:1 to 1,000:1, presumably because of differences in neurovirulence among serotypes, with type 1 being the most neurovirulent virus.

Epidemiology

Following the development and widespread use of effective poliovirus vaccines in the United States and other industrialized countries, paralytic poliomyelitis has largely been eliminated as a public health concern.[6] The same success has yet to be achieved in much of the developing world, however, where an estimated 70,000 cases occurred in 1995.[7] Most of these cases are reported from tropical and subtropical regions, where crowding, poor sanitation, inadequate hygiene, and other factors are believed to facilitate transmission of wild polioviruses and other enteric pathogens.

Humans are the only known reservoir of poliovirus infection and excrete the agent in pharyngeal secretions and feces. The incubation period is most commonly 7 to 24 days, with a range of 3 to 36 days. Patients can be infectious before symptoms develop; virus is subsequently excreted in pharyngeal secretions for a few days and in the stool for several weeks. Transmission occurs via the fecal-oral route, particularly in settings where sanitation and personal hygiene are poor, and via the oral-oral route in settings with good hygiene. Boys are affected more often than girls. In developing countries, poliomyelitis primarily afflicts infants less than 2 years of age, while in industrialized countries members of groups objecting to vaccination are now at highest risk for poliomyelitis.

During the past several years, considerable information has been obtained on the epidemiologic features of poliovirus transmission using molecular techniques.[8] In contrast to influenza viruses, which tend to spread globally on an annual basis, most polioviruses appear to circulate within relatively limited geographic areas, with occasional instances of spread to adjacent countries and infrequently across continents. The more widespread use of genomic sequencing in recent years has provided an effective tool to monitor the circulation of poliovirus genotypes, to document the spread of poliovirus from endemic areas to nonendemic areas, and to substantiate the gradual elimination of different lineages of poliovirus genotypes in polioendemic areas. Recombinant mouse cell lines cloned with the human poliovirus receptor gene will facilitate the isolation of poliovirus because these cell lines are relatively resistant to supporting other enterovirus growth. The use of these cell lines and/or application of polymerase chain reaction (PCR) will allow for enhanced detection of wild virus in sewage, water, and other environmental samples as an additional means of surveillance at the national, regional, and global levels as global eradication of poliomyelitis approaches.

After an interval of 30 to 40 years, many persons (25 to 40 percent) who contracted paralytic poliomyelitis in their childhood may experience muscle pain and exacerbation of existing weakness or may develop new weakness or paralysis. This disease entity is referred to as post-polio syndrome. To date, this syndrome has been described only in persons infected during the era of wild poliovirus circulation. Factors that enhance the risk of post-polio syndrome include (*a*) increasing length of time since acute poliovirus infection; (*b*) presence of permanent residual impairment after recovery from the acute illness; and (*c*) female gender. The pathogenesis of post-polio syndrome is thought to involve late attrition of oversized motor units that developed during the recovery process of paralytic poliomyelitis.[1]

Prevention and Control

Vaccine Development and Use. After Enders' successful propagation of poliovirus in human nonembryonic nonnervous tissue culture, Salk used this method to prepare an inactivated poliovirus vaccine (IPV), which, after major field trials in 1954, was shown to be highly effective in preventing paralytic disease.[9] Sabin and others soon developed live, attenuated strains of the three poliovirus types, which were ultimately incorporated into an orally administered, trivalent vaccine (OPV). Because of the ease of administration of OPV and improved effectiveness in preventing gut infection with wild polioviruses, Sabin's vaccine largely supplanted IPV for use in the United States beginning in the early 1960s.

The apparent elimination of the indigenous spread of wild-poliovirus infections in the United States during the past 18 years can be attributed to the high degree of effectiveness of widespread immunization with poliovirus vaccines. After licensure of IPV in 1955, more than 450 million doses were administered to children and adults during the next 5 years. During this period the incidence of poliomyelitis declined precipitously from 18 cases per 100,000 total population to fewer than two cases per 100,000. After licensure of OPV in 1961, the incidence of poliomyelitis declined rapidly in the United States and most other industrialized nations, as well as in a number of developing countries that have achieved high levels of coverage with three or more doses of OPV.[10]

Reliance on OPV probably achieved elimination of indigenous wild poliovirus genotypes in the United States in the 1960s. Subsequently, only three outbreaks of poliomyelitis occurred in the 1970s; all of these outbreaks presumably were due to imported virus. Thus, the only forms of poliomyelitis reported in the United States since 1979 are the 8 to 10 cases annually of vaccine-associated paralytic poliomyelitis (VAPP), in addition to approximately one poliomyelitis case classified as imported each year.

Vaccine-Associated Paralytic Poliomyelitis. In spite of the apparent elimination of naturally occurring poliovirus infection in the United States and other industrialized nations, an epidemiologically distinct but rare clinical occurrence of vaccine-associated poliomyelitis has been observed since the introduction of OPV. Although the absolute number of vaccine-recipient or contact-associated cases has remained small—no more than 14 per year, with an average of approximately 8 to 10 cases per year since 1980—such cases now account for the vast majority of all reported cases of poliomyelitis in the United States.[6] Moreover, it is probable that some additional unreported cases of VAPP occur.[11] Although the exact risk of contracting vaccine-associated poliomyelitis is not known, it has been estimated that one case of vaccine-associated disease occurs for every 2.4 million doses of OPV distributed.[12] However, the relative frequency of paralysis associated with the first dose in the OPV series appears to be higher (one case per 750,000 doses) than for subsequent doses (one case per 5.1 million doses distributed). The type 3 strain causes paralysis most frequently, followed by type 2 and, more rarely, type 1.

Current U.S. Polio Vaccination Policy. Reevaluation of the national poliomyelitis vaccination policy in the United States was prompted by the continued occurrence of VAPP cases, as well as the progress of the polio eradication initiative in the Americas, where the last cases were reported in 1991; the entire hemisphere was certified as free of indigenous wild poliovirus by an international commission in 1994. After an extensive process that considered all aspects related to a change in vaccination policy in the United States, the Advisory Committee on Immunization Practices of the Centers for Disease Control and Prevention adopted the use of a sequential schedule of two doses of IPV administered at ages 2 and 4 months, followed by two doses of OPV at 12 to 18 months and 4 to 6 years of age, for implementation beginning in 1997.[13] This change capitalizes on the strength of IPV (inducing humoral immunity without the risk of VAPP) while maintaining the proven benefits of OPV in inducing mucosal immunity and spread of vaccine-virus to unvaccinated contacts of vaccinees. The sequential schedule is expected to prevent at least half of the VAPP cases occurring each year. In addition, the new schedule should maintain high levels of population immunity to polioviruses to prevent poliomyelitis outbreaks should wild poliovirus be reintroduced. Nonetheless, a sequential schedule must be considered an interim recommendation (3 to 5 years) until worldwide global eradication is achieved. At that time, or when combination vaccines that reduce the need for multiple simultaneous vaccine injections are available, an IPV-only schedule will likely be recommended.

A schedule relying exclusively on IPV is recommended primarily for persons with congenital or acquired immunodeficiency disorders.[13] A primary series of IPV consists of three doses, which are usually administered according to the same schedule as the OPV schedule. A supplemental dose of IPV should be given at school entry, unless the third dose of IPV was administered on or after the fourth birthday. The need for routine administration of additional doses of OPV or IPV has not been established, but immunity after a complete series of OPV is believed to be lifelong. However, one dose of either vaccine should be given to previously immunized adults who may be at increased risk of exposure to wild poliovirus.

Global Poliomyelitis Eradication Initiative. In 1988 the World Health Assembly adopted the goal of global polio eradication by the year 2000.[14] The initiative relies exclusively on the use of OPV and promotes the following strategies to accomplish the eradication target: (*a*) achievement and maintenance of high routine vaccination coverage levels among children with at least three doses of OPV, (*b*) development of sensitive systems of epidemiologic and laboratory surveillance, including the use of standard case definitions; (*c*) administration of supplementary doses of OPV to preschool-aged children (generally age less than 5 years) during National Im-

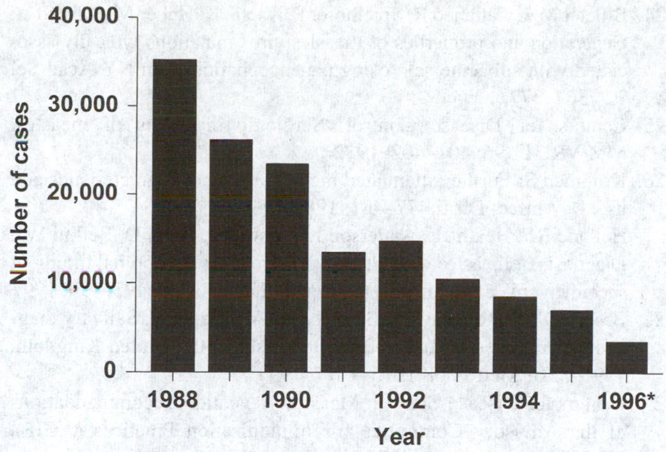

Figure 7-7. Number of reported poliomyelitis cases, globally, 1988–1996 (*1996 data preliminary).

munization Days (NIDs) to rapidly interrupt poliovirus transmission; and (*d*) "mopping-up" vaccination campaigns—localized campaigns targeted at high-risk areas where poliovirus is most likely to persist at low levels. To date, extraordinary progress has been achieved toward polio eradication. The incidence of reported poliomyelitis cases has declined by 90 percent (from 35,251 in 1988 to a provisional total of 3,996 in 1996) (Fig. 7-7). In 1991, the last case of poliomyelitis associated with wild poliovirus in the Western Hemisphere was detected in Peru, and in 1994 an international commission certified the hemisphere free of indigenous wild poliovirus. In the vast population of China indigenous wild poliovirus has not been isolated in more than 2 years despite substantial improvements in surveillance. The entire Western Pacific Region of the World Health Organization—a region populated by 1.6 billion people—appears to be on the brink of achieving polio eradication.[7] Progress has also been reported from many other parts of the world. Countries in the Americas and in Europe, Central Asia, the Middle East, and South Asia pioneered collaboration in conducting synchronized National Immunization Days. Bangladesh, Bhutan, India, Myanmar, Nepal, Pakistan, and Thailand followed their example in December 1996 and January 1997. By the end of 1996, all polio-endemic countries of Europe and Asia had conducted National Immunization Days, as well as 28 countries in Sub-Saharan Africa[15] (Fig. 7-8). Globally, nearly three-quarters of the world's children less than 5 years of age received supplemental doses of OPV through National Immunization Days in 1996. National Immunization Days have been the occasion for the largest single public health events in recorded history. In India, 119 million children were vaccinated in one day. Concurrently, surveillance systems have been strengthened in virtually all of these countries, and a global laboratory network has been established to provide virologic support for the initiative in all regions. In the vast majority of the participating countries, these achievements were associated with improvements in routine coverage with OPV and other vaccines. Although the goal is an ambitious one, the global poliomyelitis eradication initiative remains on target for complete eradication of naturally occurring poliovirus infection by the year 2000.

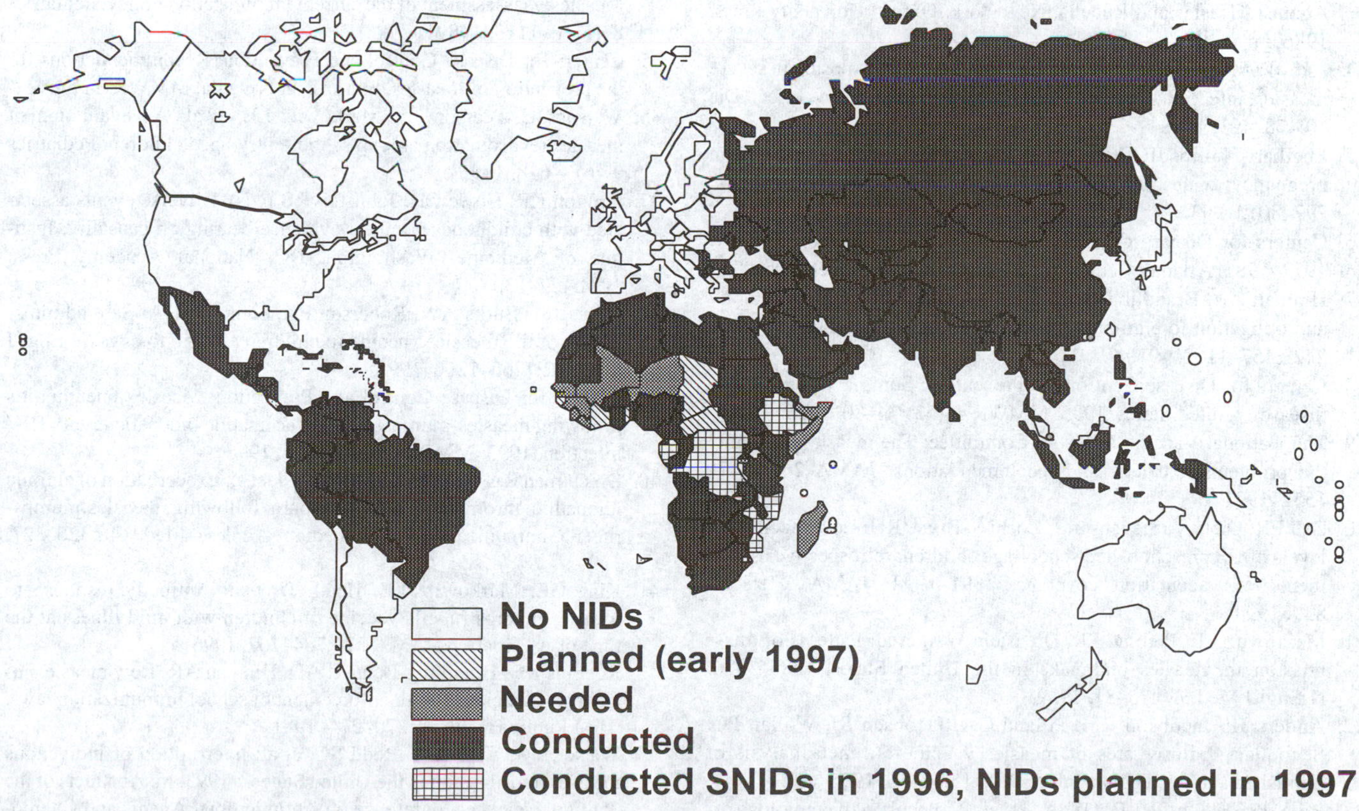

Figure 7-8. National Immunization Days, by country, 1996. NIDs, National Immunization Days; SNIDs, Sub-National Immunization Days.

► REFERENCES

Measles

1. de Quadros CA, Olivé JM, Hersh BS, et al: Measles elimination in the Americas. JAMA 275:224–229, 1996
2. Centers for Disease Control: The feasibility of measles elimination in Europe. MMWR 32:523–524, 530, 1983
3. Anderson RM, May RM: Directly transmitted infectious diseases: control by vaccination. Science 215:1053–1060, 1982
4. Schlenker TL, Bain C, Baughman AL, Hadler SC: Measles herd immunity. JAMA 267:823–826, 1992
5. Gustafson TL, Lievens AW, Brunell PA, et al: Measles outbreak in a fully immunized secondary school population. N Engl J Med 316: 771–774, 1987
6. Robbins FC: Measles: clinical features. Am J Dis Child 101: 266–272, 1962
7. DeJong JG, Winkler KC: Survival of measles virus in air. Nature 201:1054–1055, 1964
8. Bloch AB, Orenstein WA, Ewing WM, et al: Measles outbreak in a pediatric practice: airborne transmission in an office setting. Pediatrics 75:676–683, 1985
9. Barkin RM: Measles mortality: analysis of the primary cause of death. Am J Dis Child 129:307–309, 1975
10. Kaschula ROC, Druker J, Kipps A: Late morphologic consequences of measles: a lethal and debilitating lung disease among the poor. Rev Infect Dis 5:395–404, 1983
11. Morley D: Severe measles: some unanswered questions. Rev Infect Dis 5:460–462, 1983
12. Hull HF, William PJ, Oldfield F: Measles mortality and vaccine efficacy in rural West Africa. Lancet 1:972–975, 1983
13. Bloch AB, Orenstein WA, Wassilak SG, et al: Epidemiology of measles and its complications. In Gruenberg E, Lewis C, Goldston SE (eds). Vaccinating Against Brain Syndromes: The Campaign Against Measles and Rubella. New York: Oxford University Press, 1986, pp 5–20
14. Aaby P: Malnutrition and overcrowding/intensive exposure in severe measles infection: review of community studies. Rev Infect Dis 10:478–491, 1988
15. Eberhart-Phillips JE, Fredrick PD, Baron RC, Mascola L: Measles in pregnancy: a descriptive study of 58 cases. Obstet Gynecol 82: 797–801, 1993
16. Centers for Disease Control: Measles surveillance report. No. 11, 1977–1981. Atlanta: Centers for Disease Control, September 1982
17. Hinman AR, Brandling-Bennett AD, Nieburg PI: The opportunity and obligation to eliminate measles from the United States. JAMA 242:1157–1162, 1979
18. Centers for Disease Control and Prevention: Summary of notifiable diseases, United States, 1995. MMWR 44(53):74–80, 1996
19. The National Vaccine Advisory Committee: The measles epidemic: the problems, barriers, and recommendations. JAMA 266:1547–1552, 1991
20. Zell ER, Dietz V, Stevenson J, Cochi S, Bruce RH: Low vaccination levels of US preschool and school-age children: retrospective assessments of vaccination coverage, 1991–1992. JAMA 271:833–839, 1994
21. Markowitz LE, Preblud SR, Orenstein WA, et al: Patterns of transmission in measles outbreaks in the United States, 1985–1986. N Engl J Med 320:75–81, 1989
22. Anders JF, Jacobson RM, Poland GA, Jacobsen SJ, Wollan PC: Secondary failure rates of measles vaccines: a metaanalysis of published studies. Pediatr Infect Dis J 15:62–66, 1996
23. Rota JS, Heath JL, Rota PA, et al: Molecular epidemiology of measles virus: identification of pathways of transmission and implications for measles elimination. J Infect Dis 173:32–37, 1996
24. Billeter MA, Cattaneo R, Spielhofer P, Kaelin K, Huber M, Schmid A: Generation and properties of measles virus mutations typically associated with subacute sclerosing panencephalitis. Ann NY Acad Sci 724:367–377, 1994
25. Centers for Disease Control: Serologic diagnosis of measles. MMWR 31:396, 401–402, 1982
26. Krugman S: Further attenuated measles vaccine: characteristics and use. Rev Infect Dis 5:477–481, 1983
27. Helfand RF, Heath JL, Anderson LJ, Maes EF, Guris D, Bellini WJ: Diagnosis of measles with an IgM capture EIA: the optimal timing of specimen collection after rash onset. J Infect Dis 175:195–199, 1997
28. Brown DWG, Ramsay MEB, Richards AF, Miller E: Salivary diagnosis of measles: a study of notified cases in the United Kingdom, 1991–3. Br Med J 308:1015–1017, 1994
29. Centers for Disease Control: Measles prevention: recommendations of the Advisory Committee for Immunization Practices (ACIP). MMWR 38(S-9):1–18, 1989
30. Markowitz LE, Albrecht P, Rhodes P, et al: Changing levels of measles antibody titers in women and children in the United States: impact on response to vaccination. Pediatrics 97:53–58, 1996
31. Orenstein WA, Markowitz LE, Preblud SR, Hinman AR, Tomasi A, Bart KJ: Appropriate age for measles vaccination in the United States. Dev Biol Stand 65:13–23, 1986
32. King G, Markowitz L, Burns S, Heath J, Nordin J, Bellini W: A comparison of seroconversion rates to measles vaccine of children vaccinated at 9, 12, or 15 months of age. In: Abstracts of the 34th Interscience Conference on Antimicrobial Agents and Chemotherapy. Washington, DC: American Society for Microbiology, 1993, Abstract no. H108
33. Centers for Disease Control and Prevention: General Recommendations on immunization: recommendations of the Advisory Committee on Immunization Practices (ACIP). MMWR 43(RR-1):1–48, 1994
34. American Academy of Pediatrics Committee on Infectious Diseases: Measles: reassessment of the current immunization policy. Pediatrics 84:1110–1113, 1989
35. Centers for Disease Control and Prevention: Recommendations for the prevention of measles, mumps, and rubella. MMWR, in press
36. Watson JC, Pearson JA, Markowitz LE, et al: An evaluation of measles revaccination among school-entry-aged children. Pediatrics 97:613–618, 1996
37. Stratton KR, Howe CH, Johnston RB (eds): Adverse events associated with childhood vaccines: evidence bearing on causality. Institute of Medicine. Washington, DC: National Academy Press: 1994:122–130
38. James JM, Burks AW, Roberson PK, Sampson HA: Safe administration of the measles vaccine to children allergic to eggs. N Engl J Med 332:1262–1266, 1995
39. Centers for Disease Control and Prevention: Measles pneumonitis following measles-mumps-rubella vaccination of a patient with HIV infection, 1993. MMWR 45:603–606, 1996
40. Drachtman RA, Murphy S, Ettinger LJ, et al. Exacerbation of chronic idiopathic thrombocytopenic purpura following measles-mumps-rubella immunization. Arch Pediatr Adolesc Med 148:326–327, 1994
41. King GE, Markowitz LE, Heath J, et al: Antibody response to measles-mumps-rubella vaccine of children with mild illness at the time of vaccination. JAMA 275:704–707, 1996
42. Robbins KB, Brandling-Bennett AD, Hinman AR: Low measles incidence: association with enforcement of school immunization laws. Am J Public Health 71:270–274, 1981
43. Watson, JC, Vitek CR, Redd SC, et al: Interruption of indigenous measles transmission in the United States—1993. In: Abstracts of the 35th Interscience Conference on Antimicrobial Agents and Chemotherapy. Washington, DC: American Society for Microbiology, 1995, Abstract No. K11

44. Centers for Disease Control and Prevention: Measels eradication: recommendations from a meeting cosponsored by the World Health Organization, Pan American Health Organization and CDC. MMWR 1997; 46: (No. RR-11)[1-22]
45. Henderson RH, Keja K, Hayden G, et al: Immunizing the children of the world: progress and prospects. Bull World Health Organ 66:535–543, 1988
46. Halsey NA: Increased mortality after high titer measles vaccines: too much of a good thing. Pediatr Infect Dis J 12:462–465, 1993
47. World Health Organization: Feasibility of measles eradication. Wkly Epidemiol Rec 41:305–309, 1996

Mumps

1. Koplan JP, Preblud SR: A benefit-cost analysis of mumps vaccine. Am J Dis Child 136:362–364, 1982
2. Falk WA, Buchan K, Dow M, Garson JZ, Hill E, Nosal M, Tarrant M, Westbury RC, White FMM: The epidemiology of mumps in southern Alberta, 1980–1982. Am J Epidemiol 130:736–749, 1989
3. Pelosi JW, Besselink LC: Reducing mumps morbidity in Texas. Abstracts of the 30th Immunization Conference, Washington, DC, April 9–12, 1996, Abstract No. 213
4. Schluter WW, Reef SE, Dykewicz CA, Jennings CE: Pseudo-outbreak of mumps—Illinois, 1995. Abstracts of the 30th Immunization Conference, Washington, DC, April 9–12, 1996, Abstract No. 338
5. Forsey T, Mawn JA, Yates PJ, Bentley ML, Minor RD: Differentiation of vaccine and wild mumps viruses using the polymerase chain reaction and dideoxynucleotide sequencing. J Gen Virol 71:987–990, 1990
6. Cusi MG, Bianchi S, Valassina M, Santini L, Arnetoli M, Valensin PE: Rapid detection and typing of circulating mumps virus by reverse transcription/polymerase chain reaction. Res Virol 147:227–232, 1996
7. Philip RN, Reinhard KR, Lackman DB. Observations on the mumps epidemic in a "virgin" population. Am J Hyg 69:91–111, 1959
8. Centers for Disease Control: Mumps surveillance, January 1977–December 1982. Atlanta: Centers for Disease Control, September 1984
9. Reed D, Brown B, Merrick R, Sever J, Feltz E: A mumps epidemic on St. George Island, Alaska. JAMA 199:113–117, 1967
10. McGuinness AC, Gall EA: Mumps at Army camps in 1943. War Med 1944;5:95–104
11. Hyöty H, Hiltunen M, Reunanen A, Leinikki P, Vesikari T, Lounamaa R, Tuomilehto J, Akerblom HK, the Childhood Diabetes in Finland Study Group: Decline of mumps antibodies in Type 1 (insulin-dependent) diabetic children and a plateau in the rising incidence of Type 1 diabetes after introduction of the mumps-measles-rubella vaccine in Finland. Diabetologia 36:1303–1308, 1993
12. Siegel M, Fuerst HT, Peress NS: Comparative fetal mortality in maternal virus diseases: a prospective study on rubella, measles, mumps, chickenpox, and hepatitis. N Engl J Med 274:768–771, 1966
13. Collins SD: Age incidence of the common communicable diseases of children. Public Health Rep 44:763–826, 1929
14. Centers for Disease Control: Mumps in the United States—1985–1988. MMWR 38:101–105, 1989
15. Centers for Disease Control and Prevention: Mumps surveillance—United States, 1988–1993. MMWR 44(SS-3):1–14, 1995
16. Wharton M, Cochi SL, Hutcheson RH, Bistowish JM, Schaffner WA: A large outbreak of mumps in the post-vaccine era. J Infect Dis 158:1253–1260, 1988
17. Hersh BS, Fine PEM, Kent WK, Cochi SL, Kahn LH, Zell ER, Hays PL, Wood CL: Mumps outbreak in a highly vaccinated population. J Pediatr 119:187–193, 1991
18. Cheek JE, Baron R, Atlas H, Wilson DL, Crider RD: Mumps outbreak in a highly vaccinated school outbreak: evidence for large-scale vaccination failure. Arch Pediatr Adolesc Med 149:774–778, 1995
19. Briss PA, Fehrs LJ, Parker RA, Wright PF, Sannella ED, Hutcheson RH, Schaffner W: Sustained transmission of mumps in a highly vaccinated population: assessment of primary vaccine failure and waning vaccine-induced immunity. J Infect Dis 169:77–82, 1994
20. Sosin DM, Cochi SL, Gunn RA, Jennings DE, Preblud SR: The changing epidemiology of mumps and its impact on university campuses. Pediatrics 84:779–784, 1989
21. Kaplan KM, Marder DC, Cochi SL, Preblud SR: Mumps in the workplace. JAMA 260:1434–1438, 1988
22. Cochi SL, Preblud SR, Orenstein WA: Perspectives on the relative resurgence of mumps in the United States. Am J Dis Child 142: 499–507, 1988
23. Chaiken BP, Williams NM, Preblud SR, Parkin W, Altman R: The effect of a school entry law on mumps activity in a school district. JAMA 257:2455–2458, 1987
24. Kim-Farley R, Bart S, Stetler H, Orenstein W, Bart K, Sullivan K, Halpin T, Sirotkin B: Clinical mumps vaccine efficacy. Am J Epidemiol 121:593–597, 1985
25. Centers for Disease Control: Recommendations of the International Task Force for Disease Eradication. MMWR 42(RR-16):1–27, 1993
26. Hilleman MR, Buynak EB, Wiebel RE, Stokes J Jr: Live, attenuated mumps-virus vaccine. N Engl J Med 278:227–232, 1968
27. Weibel RE, Buynak EB, McLean AA, Hilleman MR: Follow-up surveillance of antibody in human subjects following live attenuated measles, mumps, and rubella virus vaccines. Proc Soc Exp Biol Med 162:328–332, 1979
28. Weibel RE, Buynak EB, McLean AA, Roehm RR, Hilleman MR: Persistence of antibody in human subjects for 7 to 10 years following administration of combined live attenuated measles, mumps, and rubella virus vaccines. Proc Soc Exp Biol Med 165:260–263, 1980
29. Kelso JM, Jones RT, Yunginger JW: Anaphylaxis to measles, mumps, and rubella vaccine mediated by IgE to gelatin. J Allergy Clin Immunol 91:867–872, 1993
30. James JM, Burks AW, Roberson PK, Sampson HA: Safe administration of the measles vaccine to children allergic to eggs. N Engl J Med 332:1262–1266, 1995
31. Miller E, Goldacre M, Pugh S, Colville A, Farrington P, Flower A, Nash J, MacFarlane L, Tettmar R: Risk of aseptic meningitis after measles, mumps, and rubella vaccine in UK children. Lancet 341:979–982, 1993
32. Peltola H, Heinonen OP, Valle M, Paunio M, Virtanen M, Karanko V, Cantell K: The elimination of indigenous measles, mumps, and rubella from Finland by a 12-year, two-dose vaccination program. N Engl J Med 331:1397–1402, 1994
33. Healthy People 2000: National Health Promotion and Disease Prevention Objectives. Washington, DC: US Department of Health and Human Services, 1991

Rubella

1. Gregg NM: Congenital cataract following German measles in the mother. Trans Ophthalmol Soc Austr 3:35, 1941
2. Balfour HH Jr, Groth KE, Edelman CK, et al: Rubella viremia and antibody responses after rubella vaccination and reimmunization. Lancet 1:1078–1080, 1981
3. Robinson J, Lemay M, Vaudry WL: Congenital rubella after anticipated maternal immunity: two cases and a review of the literature. Pediatr Infect Dis J 13:812–815, 1994
4. Preblud SR, Serdula MK, Frank JA Jr, et al: Rubella vaccination in the United States: a ten-year review. Epidemiol Rev 2:171–194, 1980
5. Cooper LZ, Krugman S: Clinical manifestations of postnatal and congenital rubella. Arch Ophthalmol 77:434–439, 1967
6. Ziring PR: Congenital rubella: the teenage years. Pediatr Ann 6:762–70, 1977
7. Miller E, Cradock-Watson JE, Pollock T: Consequences of confirmed maternal rubella at successive stages of pregnancy. Lancet 320:781–785, 1982

8. Preblud SR, Alford CA: Rubella. In Remington JS, Klwin JO (eds): Infectious Diseases of the Fetus and Newborn Infant. 3rd ed. Philadelphia: WB Saunders, 1991
9. Centers for Disease Control and Prevention: Summary of Notifiable Diseases, United States: 1996. MMWR 45:8, 1997
10. Cochi SL, Edmonds LE, Dyer K, et al: Congenital rubella syndrome in the United States, 1970–1985: on the verge of elimination. Am J Epidemiol 129:349–361, 1989
11. Crowder M, Higgins HL, Frost JJ: Rubella susceptibility in young women of rural East Texas: 1980 and 1985. Texas Med 83:43–47, 1987
12. Bart KJ, Orenstein WA, Preblud SR, Hinman AR: Universal immunization to interrupt rubella. Rev Infect Dis 7(Suppl 1):S177–S184, 1985
13. Centers for Disease Control and Prevention: Unpublished data
14. Best JM, Welch JM, Baker DA, Banatvala JE: Maternal rubella at St Thomas' Hospital in 1978 and 1986: support for augmenting the rubella vaccination programme. Lancet 2:88–90, 1987
15. Miller E, Tookey P, Morgan-Capner P, Hesketh L, Brown D, Waight P, Vurdien J, Jones G, Peckham C: Rubella surveillance to June 1994: third joint report from the PHLS and the National Congenital Rubella Surveillance Programme. Commun Dis Rep CDR Rev 4:R146–R152, 1994
16. Chu SY, Bernier RH, Stewart JA, et al: Rubella antibody persistence after immunization: sixteen-year follow-up in the Hawaiian Islands. JAMA 259:3133–3136, 1988
17. Orenstein WA, Herrman KL, Holmgreen P, Bernier R, Bart KJ, Eddins DL, Fiumara NJ: Prevalence of rubella antibodies in Massachusetts school children. Am J Epidemiol 124:290–298, 1986
18. Johnson CE, Kumar ML, Whitwell J, Staehle BO, Rome LP, Dinakar C, Hurni W, Nalin DR: Antibody persistence after primary measles-mumps-rubella vaccine and response to second dose given at four to six vs eleven to thirteen years. Pediatr Infect Dis J 15:687–692, 1996
19. Centers for Disease Control: Rubella prevention: recommendation of the Immunization Practices Advisory Committee (ACIP) MMWR 39(RR-15), 1990
20. Mitchell LA, Tingle AJ, Shukin R, Sangeorzan JA, McCune J, Braun DK: Chronic rubella vaccine-associated arthropathy. Arch Intern Med 153:2268–2274, 1993
21. Evidence concerning rubella vaccines and arthritis, radiculoneuritis, and thrombocytopenic purpura. In Howson CP, Howe CJ, Fineberg HV (eds): Adverse Effects of Pertussis and Rubella Vaccines: A Report of the Committee to Review the Adverse Consequences of Pertussis and Rubella Vaccines. Institute of Medicine. Washington DC: National Academy Press, 1991
22. Slater PE, Ben-Zvi T, Fogel A, Ehrenfeld M, Ever-Hadani S: Absence of an association between rubella vaccination and arthritis in underimmune postpartum women. Vaccine 13:1529–1532, 1995
23. Frenkel LM, Nielsen K, Garakian A, Jin R, Wolinsky JS, Cherry JD: A search for persistent rubella virus infection in persons with chronic symptoms after rubella and rubella immunization and in patients with juvenile rheumatoid arthritis. Clin Infect Dis 22: 287–294, 1996
24. Ray P, Black S, Shinefield H, Dillon A, Schwalbe J, Holmes S, Hadler S, Chen R, Cochi S, Wassilak S. Risk of chronic arthropathy among women after rubella vaccination. JAMA 278(7):551–556, 1997
25. Frey TK, Abernathy ES: Identification of strain-specific nucleotide sequences in the RA 27/3 rubella virus vaccine. J Infect Dis 168: 854–864, 1993

Pertussis

1. Miller CL, Flectcher WB: Severity of notified whooping cough. Br Med J 1:117–119, 1976
2. Voorhoeve AM, Muller AS, Schulpen TWJ, 'tMannetje W, Van Rens M: Machakos Project Studies: agents affecting the health of mother and child in a rural area of Kenya. VI: The epidemiology of pertussis. Trop Geogr Med 30:125–139, 1978
3. Pittman M: Pertussis toxin: the cause of the harmful effects and prolonged immunity of whooping cough—a hypothesis. Rev Infect Dis 1:401–412, 1979
4. Strebel PM, Cochi SL, Farizo KM, Payne BJ, Hanauer SD, Baughman AL: Pertussis in Missouri: evaluation of nasopharyngeal culture, direct fluorescent antibody testing, and clinical case definitions in the diagnosis of pertussis. Clin Infect Dis 16:276–285, 1993
5. Onorato IM, Wassilak SGF: Laboratory diagnosis of pertussis: the state of the art. Pediatr Infect Dis J 6:145–151, 1987
6. Van der Zee A, Agterberg C, Peeters M, Mooi F, Schellekens J: A clinical validation of *Bordetella pertussis* and *Bordetella parapertussis* polymerase chain reaction: comparison with culture and serology using samples from patients with suspected whooping cough from a highly immunized population. J Infect Dis 174:89–96, 1996
7. Gustafsson L, Hallander HO, Olin P, Reizenstein E, Storsaeter J: A controlled trial of a two-component acellular, a five-component acellular, and a whole-cell pertussis vaccine. N Engl J Med 334(6): 349–355, 1996
8. Greco D, Salmaso S, Mastrantonio P, Giuliano M, Tozzi AE, Anemona A, Ciofi Degli Atti ML, Giammanco A, Panei P, Blackwelder WC, Klein DL, Wassilak SGF, Progetto Pertosse Working Group: A controlled trial of two acellular vaccines and one whole-cell vaccine against pertussis. N Engl J Med 33:341–348, 1996
9. Trollfors B, Taranger J, Lagergard T, Lind L, Sundh V, Zackrisson G, Lowe CU, Blackwelder W, Robbins JB: A placebo-controlled trial of a pertussis-toxoid vaccine. N Engl J Med 333:1045–1050, 1995
10. Schmitt HJ, Wirsing von Konig CH, Neiss A, Bogaerts H, Bock HL, Schulte-Wisserman H, Gahr M, Schult R, Folkens JU, Rauh W, Clemens R: Efficacy of acellular pertussis vaccine in early childhood after household exposure. JAMA 275:37–41, 1996
11. Sutter RW, Cochi SL: Pertussis hospitalizations and mortality in the United States, 1985–1988: evaluation of the completion of national reporting. JAMA 267:386–391, 1992
12. Wortis N, Strebel PM, Wharton M, Bardenheieir B, Hardy IRB: Pertussis deaths: report of 23 cases in the United States, 1992 and 1993. Pediatrics 97:607–612, 1996
13. Marchant CD, Loughlin AM, Lett SM, Todd CW, Wetterlow LH, Bicchieri R, Higham S, Etkind P, Silva El, Siber GR: Pertussis in Massachusetts, 1981–1991: incidence, serologic diagnosis, and vaccine effectiveness. J Infect Dis 169:1297–1305, 1994
14. Mink CM, Cherry JD, Christenson P, et al: A search for *Bordetella pertussis* infection in university students. Clin Infect Dis 14: 464–471, 1992
15. Nennig ME, Shinefield H, Edwards KM, Black SB, Fireman BH: Prevalence and incidence of adult pertussis in an urban population. JAMA 275:1672–1674, 1996
16. Wirsing von Konig, CH, Postels-Multani S, Bock HL, Schmitt HJ: Pertussis in adults; frequency of transmission after household exposure. Lancet 346:1326–1329, 1995
17. Lederle Laboratories: ACEL-IMUNE package label
18. Simondon F, Preziosi M, Yam A, Kane C, Chabirand L, Iteman I, Sanden G, Mboup S, Hoffenbach Knudsen K, Guiso N, Wassilak S, Cadoz M. A randomized double-blind trial comparing a two-component acellular to a whole-cell pertussis vaccine in Senegal. Vaccine 1997; 15:1606–1612
19. Connaught Laboratories Inc. Tripedia package label
20. Fine PE, Clarkson JA: Reflections on the efficacy of pertussis vaccines. Rev Infect Dis 9:866–883, 1987
21. Lambert HJ: Epidemiology of a small pertussis outbreak in Kent County, Michigan. Public Health Rep 80:365–369, 1965
22. Farizo KM, Cochi SL, Zell ER, et al: Epidemiological features of pertussis in the United States, 1980–1989. Clin Infect Dis 14: 708–719, 1991

23. Decker MD, Edwards KM, Steinhoff MC, Rennels MB, Pichichero ME, Englund JA, Anderson EL, Deloria MA, Reed GF: Comparison of 13 acellular pertussis vaccines: adverse reactions. Pediatrics 96(Suppl):557–566, 1995
24. Centers for Disease Control and Prevention: Pertussis vaccination: use of acellular pertussis vaccines among infants and young children. Recommendations of the Immunization Practices Advisory Committee (ACIP). MMWR 1997, in press
25. Pertussis. In Peter G (ed): 1994 Red Book: Report of the Committee on Infectious Diseases. 23rd ed. Elk Grove Village, IL: American Academy of Pediatrics, 1994, p 356
26. Granstrom M, Olinder-Nielsen AM, Holmblad P, Mark A, Hanngren K: Specific immunoglobulin for treatment of whooping cough. Lancet 338:1230–1233, 1991
27. Garner JS, Simmons BP, Williams WW: CDC guideline for isolation precautions in hospitals and CDC guideline for infection control in hospital personnel. Infect Control 4(Suppl):245–325, 1983
28. Lewis K, Saubolle MA, Tenover FC, Rudinsky MF, Barbour SD, Cherry JD: Pertussis caused by an erythromycin-resistant strain of *Bordetella pertussis*. Pediatr Infect Dis J 14:388–391, 1995
29. Edwards KM, Decker MD, Barney S, et al: Adult immunization with acellular pertussis vaccine. JAMA 269:53–56, 1993
30. Aoyama T, Sunakawa K, Iwata S, Takeuchi Y, Fujii R: Efficacy of short-term treatment of pertussis with clarithromycin and azithromycin. J Pediatr 129:761–764, 1996

Tetanus

1. World Health Organization: The "high-risk" approach: the WHO-recommended strategy to accelerate elimination of neonatal tetanus. Wkly Epidemiol Rec 71:33–36, 1996
2. Dietz V, Milstien JB, van Loon F, Cochi S, Bennett J: Performance and potency of tetanus toxoid: implications for eliminating neonatal tetanus. Bull World Health Organ 74:619–628, 1996
3. Centers for Disease Control: Case definitions for public health surveillance. MMWR 39(RR-13):1–43, 1990
4. Wassilak SGF, Orenstein WA, Sutter RW: Tetanus toxoid. In Plotkin SA, Mortimer EA (eds): Vaccines. Philadelphia: WB Saunders, 1994, pp 57–90
5. Centers for Disease Control: Summary of notifiable diseases, United States, 1987. MMWR 36(54):41, 1988
6. Prevots R, Sutter R, Strebel PM, Cochi S, Hadler S: Tetanus surveillance—United States, 1989–1990. MMWR 41(SS-8):1–9, 1992
7. Izurieta HS, Sutter RW, Strebel PM, Bardenheier, Prevots DR, Wharton M, Hadler SC: Tetanus surveillance—United States 1991–1994. MMWR 46(SS-2):15–25, 1997
8. Gergen PJ, McQuillan GM, Kiely M, Ezzati-Rice TM, Sutter RW, Virella G: A population-based serologic survey of immunity to tetanus in the United States. N Engl J Med 332:761–766, 1995
9. Long AP, Sartwell PE: Tetanus in the U.S. Army in World War II. Bull US Army Med Dept 7:371–85, 1947
10. Centers for Disease Control and Prevention: Recommended childhood immunization schedule—United States, 1997. MMWR 46:35–40, 1997
11. Peebles TC, Levine L, Eldred MC, Edsall G: Tetanus toxoid emergency boosters: a reappraisal. N Engl J Med 280:575–581, 1969
12. Simonsen O, Badsberg JH, Kjeldsen K, Moller-Madsen B, Heron I: The fall-off in serum concentration of tetanus antitoxin after primary and booster vaccination. Acta Pathol Microbiol Immunol Scand 94:77–82, 1986
13. Balestra DJ, Littenberg B: Should adult tetanus immunization be given as a single vaccination at age 65? A cost-effectiveness analysis. J Gen Intern Med 8:405–412, 1993
14. Bowie C: Tetanus toxoid for adults—too much of a good thing [Letter]. Lancet 348:1185–1186, 1996
15. Jacobs RL, Lowe RS, Lanier BQ: Adverse reactions to tetanus toxoid. JAMA 247:40–42, 1982
16. Edsall G, Elliot MW, Peebles TC, Levine L, Eldred MC: Excessive us of tetanus toxoid boosters. JAMA 202:111–113, 1967
17. Centers for Disease Control: Diphtheria, tetanus, and pertussis: recommendations for vaccine use and other preventive measures. MMWR 40(RR-10):1–28, 1991
18. Brand DA, Acampora D, Gottlieb LD, Glancy KE, Frazier WH: Adequacy of antitetanus prophylaxis in six hospital emergency rooms. N Engl J Med 309:636–640, 1983
19. McComb JA: The prophylactic dose of homologous tetanus antitoxin. N Engl J Med 270:175–178, 1964
20. Resolution 42.32. Handbook of Resolutions and Decisions of the World Health Assembly and the Executive Board. 3rd ed. (1985–92). Geneva: World Health Organization, 1993, vol 3
21. Hinman AR, Foster SO, Wassilak SGF: Neonatal tetanus: potential for elimination in the USA and the world. Pediatr Infect Dis J 6:813–816, 1987
22. Expanded Program on Immunization: A vision for the world: global elimination of neonatal tetanus by the year 1995—plan of action. WHO document EPI/GAG/89/WP.9. Geneva: World Health Organization, 1989

Diphtheria

1. Tiley SM, Kociuba KR, Heron LG, Munro R: Infective endocarditis due to nontoxigenic *Corynebacterium diphtheriae*: report of seven cases and review. Clin Infect Dis 16:271–275, 1993
2. Mikhailovich VM, Melnikov VG, Mazurova IK, Wachsmuth IK, Wenger, JD, Wharton M, Nakao H, Popovic T: Application of PCR for detection of toxigenic *Corynebacterium diphtheriae* strains isolated during the Russian diphtheria epidemic, 1990 through 1994. J Clin Microbiol 33:3061–3063, 1995
3. Zoysa A, Efstratiou A, George R, et al: Molecular epidemiology of *Corynebacterium diphtheriae* from northwestern Russia and surrounding countries studied by using ribotyping and pulsed-field gel electrophoresis. J Clin Microbiol 33:1080–1083, 1995
4. Popovic T, Kombarova SY, Reeves MW, et al: Molecular epidemiology of diphtheria in Russia, 1985–1994. J Infect Dis 174:1064–1072, 1996
5. Naiditch MJ, Bower AG: Diphtheria: a study of 1,433 cases observed during a 10-year period at Los Angeles County Hospital. Am J Med 17:229–245, 1945
6. Galazka AM, Robertson SE: Diphtheria: changing patterns in the developing world and the industrialized world. Eur J Epidemiol 11: 107–117, 1995
7. Hardy IR, Dittmann S, Sutter RW: Current situation and control strategies for resurgence of diphtheria in Newly Independent States of the former Soviet Union. Lancet 347:1739–1744, 1996
8. Galazka A, Robertson S, Oblapenko G: Resurgence of diphtheria. Eur J Epidemiol 11:95–105, 1995
9. Centers for Disease Control and Prevention: Update: diphtheria epidemic—New Independent States of the former Soviet Union, January 1995–March 1996. MMWR 45:693–697, 1996
10. Dolman C: Landmarks and pioneers in the control of diphtheria. Can J Public Health 64:317–336, 1973
11. Galazka A: Diphtheria: The Immunological Basis for Immunization. WHO document WHO/EPI/GEN/93.12. Geneva: World Health Organization, 1993
12. Centers for Disease Control and Prevention: Pertussis vaccination: use of an acellular pertussis vaccine among infants: recommendations of the Advisory Committee on Immunization Practices (ACIP). MMWR 1997, in press
13. Centers for Disease Control: Diphtheria, tetanus, and pertussis: recommendations for vaccine use and other preventive measures: recommendations of the Immunization Practices Advisory Committee (ACIP). MMWR 40(RR-10):1–28, 1991

14. Farizo KM, Strebel PM, Chen RT, et al: Fatal respiratory disease due to *Corynebacterium diphtheriae*: case report and review of guidelines for management, investigation, and control. Clin Infect Dis 16:59–68, 1993

Influenza

1. Skinner HA: The Origin of Medical Terms. Baltimore: Williams & Wilkins, 1949, pp 191–192
2. Smith W, Andrews CH, Laidlaw PP: A virus obtained from influenza patients. Lancet 2:66, 1933
3. Francis TJ: A new type of virus from epidemic influenza. Science 92:405, 1940
4. Taylor RM: A further note on 1233 ("influenza C") virus. Arch Gesamte Virusforsch 4:485, 1951
5. Burnet FM: Influenza virus on the developing egg: I. Changes associated with the development of an egg-passage strain of virus. Br J Exp Pathol 17:282, 1936
6. Hirst GK: The agglutination of red cells by allantoic fluid of chick embryos infected with influenza virus. Science 94:22, 1941
7. Betts RF: Influenza virus. In Mandell GL, Bennett JE, Dolan R (eds): Principles and Practice of Infectious Diseases. 4th ed. New York: Churchill Livingstone, 1996, pp 1546–1567
8. Varma RR, Riedel DR, Komorouski RA, et al: Reye's syndrome in non-pediatric age groups. JAMA 242:1373, 1979
9. Lenaway DD, Ambler A: Evaluation of a school-based influenza surveillance system. Public Health Rep 110:333–337, 1995
10. Arden N, Monto AS, Ohmit SE: Vaccine use and the risk of outbreaks in a sample of nursing homes during an influenza epidemic. Am J Public Health 85:399–401, 1995
11. Kohn MA, Farley TA, Sundin D, Tapia R, McFarland LM, Arden NH: Three summertime outbreaks of influenza type A. J Infect Dis 172:246–249, 1995
12. World Health Organization: A revision of the system of nomenclature for the influenza viruses: A WHO memorandum. Bull World Health Organ 58:585–591, 1980
13. Webster RG, Sharp GB, Claas EC: Interspecies transmission of influenza viruses. Am J Respir Crit Care Med 152:S25–S30, 1995
14. Masurel N, Marine WM: Recycling of Asian and Hong Kong influenza A virus hemagglutinin in man. Am J Epidemiol 97:44–49, 1973
15. Schoenbaum SC: Economic impact of influenza: the individual's perspective. Am J Med 82:26–30, 1987
16. Sullivan KM, Monto AS, Longini IM, Longini IM Jr: Estimates of the U.S. health impact of influenza. Am J Public Health 83: 1712–1716, 1993
17. Centers for Disease Control and Prevention: Influenza—United States, 1989–90. MMWR 39:157–159, 1990
18. Centers for Disease Control: Influenza—Respiratory Disease Surveillance Report. Atlanta: Centers for Disease Control, 1973, p 88
19. Gruber WC, Belshe RB, King JC, et al: Evaluation of live attenuated influenza vaccines in children 6–18 months of age: safety, immunogenicity, and efficacy. J Infect Dis 173:1313–1319, 1996
20. Clements ML, Makhene MK, Karron RA, et al: Effective immunization with live attenuated influenza A virus can be achieved in early infancy. J Infect Dis 173:44–51, 1996
21. Centers for Disease Control: Recommendations of the Immunization Practices Advisory Committee (ACIP): prevention and control of influenza. 1. Vaccines. MMWR 38:297–311, 1989
22. Sugaya N, Nerome K, Ishida M, Matsumoto M, Mitamura K, Nirasawa M: Efficacy of inactivated vaccine in preventing antigenically drifted influenza type A and well-matched type B. JAMA 272: 1122–1126, 1994
23. Nichol KL, Lind A, Margolis KL, et al: The effectiveness of vaccination against influenza in healthy, working adults. N Engl J Med 333:889–893, 1995
24. Gross PA, Hermogenes AW, Sacks HS, Lau J, Levandowski RA: The efficacy of influenza vaccine in elderly persons. A meta-analysis and review of the literature. Ann Intern Med 123:518–527, 1995
25. Ahmed AE, Nicholson KG, Nguyen-Van-Tam JS: Reduction in mortality associated with influenza vaccine during 1989–90 epidemic. Lancet 346:591–595, 1995
26. Nichol KL, Margolis KL, Wuorenma J, Von Sternberg T: The efficacy and cost effectiveness of vaccination against influenza among elderly persons living in the community. N Engl J Med 331:778–784, 1994
27. Govaert TM, Dinant GJ, Aretz K, Masurel N, Sprenger MJ, Knottnerus JA: Adverse reactions to influenza vaccine in elderly people: randomised double blind placebo controlled trial. Br Med J 307:988–990, 1993
28. Langmuir AD, Bregman DJ, Kurland LT, Nathanson N, Victor M: An epidemiologic and clinical evaluation of Guillain-Barré syndrome reported in association with the administration of swine influenza vaccines. Am J Epidemiol 119:841–879, 1984
29. Monto AS: Using antiviral agents to control outbreaks of influenza A infection. Geriatrics 49:30–34, 1994
30. Couch RB, Kasel JA, Glezen WP: Influenza: its control in persons and populations. J Infect Dis 153:431–440, 1986
31. Centers for Disease Control and Prevention: Prevention and control of influenza: recommendations of the Advisory Committee on Immunization Practices (ACIP). MMWR 44:1–22, 1995
32. Centers for Disease Control: Prevention and control of influenza: recommendations of the Immunization Practices Advisory Committee. Ann Intern Med 107:521–525, 1987
33. Doebbeling BN, Edmond MB, Davis CS, Woodin JR, Zeitler RR: Influenza vaccination of health care workers: evaluation of factors that are important in acceptance. Prev Med 1997, in press
34. Pearson DC, Thompson RS: Evaluation of Group Health Cooperative of Puget Sound's senior influenza immunization program. Public Health Rep 109:571–578, 1994
35. Duclos P, Hatcher J: Epidemiology of influenza vaccination in Canada. Can J Public Health 84:311–315, 1993
36. Nichol KL, Korn JE, Margolis KL, Poland GA, Petzel RA, Lofgren RP: Achieving the national health objective for influenza immunization: success of an institution-wide vaccination program. Am J Med 89:156–160, 1990

Pneumococcal Infections

1. Pasteur L: Note sur la maladie nouvelle provoquee par la salive d' un enfant mort de la rage. Bull Acad Natl Med (Paris) 10:94, 1881
2. Sternberg GM: A fatal form of septicaemia in the rabbit produced by subcutaneous injection of human saliva: an experimental research. Natl Bd of Health Bull 2:781, 1881
3. Heffron R: Pneumonia, with Special Reference to Pneumococcus Lobar Pneumonia. New York: Commonwealth Fund, 1939. [Reprinted, Cambridge, MA.: Harvard University Press, 1979]
4. Macfarlane J: Community-acquired pneumonia. Br J Dis Chest 81:116–27, 1987
5. Anonymous: Community-acquired pneumonia in adults in British hospitals in 1982–1983: a survey of aetiology, mortality, prognostic factors and outcome. The British Thoracic Society and the Public Health Laboratory Service. Q J Med 62:195–220, 1987
6. Austrian R, Howie VM, Ploussard JH: The bacteriology of pneumococcal otitis media. Johns Hopkins Med J 141:104–11, 1977
7. Jernigan DB, Cetron MS, Breiman RF: Minimizing the impact of drug-resistant *Streptococcus pneumoniae* (DRSP). A strategy from the DRSP Working Group. JAMA 275:206–209, 1996
8. Haglund LA, Istre GR, Pickett DA, Welch DF, Fine DP: Invasive pneumococcal disease in central Oklahoma: emergence of high-level penicillin resistance and multiple antibiotic resistance. Pneumococcus Study Group. J Infect Dis 168:1532–1536, 1993

9. Hofmann J, Cetron MS, Farley MM, et al: The prevalence of drug-resistant *Streptococcus pneumoniae* in Atlanta. N Engl J Med 333: 481–486, 1995
10. Henrichsen J: Six newly recognized types of *Streptococcus pneumoniae*. J Clin Microbiol 33:2759–2762, 1995
11. Austrian R: Some observations on the pneumococcus and on the current status of pneumococcal disease and its prevention. Rev Infect Dis 3(Suppl):S1–S17, 1981
12. Butler JC, Breiman RF, Lipman HB, Hofmann J, Facklam RR: Serotype distribution of *Streptococcus pneumoniae* infections among preschool children in the United States, 1978–1994: implications for development of a conjugate vaccine. J Infect Dis 171:885–889, 1995
13. Gray BM, Converse GM, 3d, Dillon HC Jr: Epidemiologic studies of *Streptococcus pneumoniae* in infants: acquisition, carriage, and infection during the first 24 months of life. J Infect Dis 142:923–933, 1980
14. Nielsen SV, Henrichsen J: Capsular types of *Streptococcus pneumoniae* isolated from blood and CSF during 1982–1987. Clin Infect Dis 15:794–798, 1992
15. Butler JC, Breiman RF, Campbell JF, Lipman HB, Broome CV, Facklam RR: Pneumococcal polysaccharide vaccine efficacy. An evaluation of current recommendations. JAMA 270:1826–1831, 1993
16. Eriksen KR: Studies on induced resistance to penicillin in a pneumococcus Type I. Acta Pathol 22:398–405, 1945
17. Hansman D, Bullen MM: A resistant pneumococcus (Letter). Lancet 264–265, 1967
18. Hansman D, Glasgow H, Sturt J, Devitt L, Douglas R: Increased resistance to penicillin of pneumococci isolated from man. N Engl J Med 284:175–177, 1971
19. Hansman D, Devitt L, Miles H, Riley I: Pneumococci relatively insensitive to penicillin in Australia and New Guinea. Med J Aust 2:353–356, 1974
20. Breiman RF, Butler JC, Tenover FC, Elliott JA, Facklam RR: Emergence of drug-resistant pneumococcal infections in the United States. JAMA 271:1831–1835, 1994
21. Hodges RG, MacLeod CM, Bernhard WG: Epidemic pneumococcal pneumonia. III. Carrier studies. Am J Hyg 44:207–243, 1946
22. Gundel M, Schwarz FKT. Studien über die Bakterienflora der oberen Atmungswege Neugeborener (im Vergleich mit der Mundhöhlenflora der Mutter und de Pflegepersonals) unter besonderer Berucksichtigung ihrer Bedeutung für das Pneumonie-problem. Z Hyg Infectionskir 113:411, 1932
23. Loda FA, Collier AM, Glezen WP, Strangert K, Clyde WA Jr, Denny FW: Occurrence of *Diplococcus pneumoniae* in the upper respiratory tract of children. J Pediatr 87:1087–1093, 1975
24. Gundel M, Okura G: Untersuchungen über das gleichzeitige Vorkommen mehrer Pneumokokkentypen bei Gesunden und ihre Bedeutung fur die Epidemiologie. Z Hyg Infektionskr 114:678, 1933
25. Webster LT, Hughes TP: The epidemiology of pneumococcus infection: the incidence and spread of pneumococci in the nasal passages and throats of healthy persons. J Exp Med 53:535, 1931
26. Bliss EA, McClaskey WD, Long PH: A study of pneumococcus carriers. J Immunol 27:95, 1934
27. Gwaltney JM Jr, Sande MA, Austrian R, Hendley JO: Spread of *Streptococcus pneumoniae* in families. II. Relation of transfer of *S. pneumoniae* to incidence of colds and serum antibody. J Infect Dis 132:62–68, 1975
28. MacLeod CM, Hodges RG, Heidelberger M: Prevention of pneumococcal pneumonia by immunization with specific capsular polysaccharides. J Exp Med 82:445, 1945
29. Austrian R: Some aspects of the pneumococcal carrier state. J Antimicrobial Chemother 18(Suppl A):35–45, 1986
30. Lonks JR, Medeiros AA: The growing threat of antibiotic-resistant *Streptococcus pneumoniae*. Med Clin North Am 79:523–535, 1995
31. Rauch AM, O'Ryan M, Van R, Pickering LK: Invasive disease due to multiply resistant *Streptococcus pneumoniae* in a Houston, Tex, day-care center. Am J Dis Child 144:923–927, 1990
32. Klugman KP, Coffey TJ, Smith A, Wasas A, Meyers M, Spratt BG: Cluster of an erythromycin-resistant variant of the Spanish multiply resistant 23F clone of *Streptococcus pneumoniae* in South Africa. Eur J Clin Microbiol Infect Dis 13:171–174, 1994
33. Reichler MR, Allphin AA, Breiman RF, et al: The spread of multiply resistant *Streptococcus pneumoniae* at a day care center in Ohio. J Infect Dis 166:1346–1353, 1992
34. Mercat A, Nguyen J, Dautzenberg B: An outbreak of pneumococcal pneumonia in two men's shelters. Chest 99:147–151, 1991
35. Berk SL, Gage KA, Holtsclaw-Berk SA, Smith JK: Type 8 pneumococcal pneumonia: an outbreak on an oncology ward. South Med J 78:159–161, 1985
36. Gould FK, Magee JG, Ingham HR: A hospital outbreak of antibiotic-resistant *Streptococcus pneumoniae*. J Infect 15:77–79, 1987
37. Doyle MG, Morrow AL, Van R, Pickering LK: Intermediate resistance of *Streptococcus pneumoniae* to penicillin in children in day-care centers. Pediatr Infect Dis J 11:831–835, 1992 [published erratum appears in Pediatr Infect Dis J 12:32, 1993]
38. Musher DM: Infections caused by *Streptococcus pneumoniae* clinical spectrum, pathogenesis, immunity, and treatment. Clin Infect Dis 14:801–807, 1992
39. Janoff EN, Breiman RF, Daley CL, Hopewell PC: Pneumococcal disease during HIV infection. Epidemiologic, clinical, and immunologic perspectives. Ann Intern Med 117:314–324, 1992
40. Burack JH, Hahn JA, Saint-Maurice D, Jacobson MA: Microbiology of community-acquired bacterial pneumonia in persons with and at risk for human immunodeficiency virus type 1 infection. Implications for rational empiric antibiotic therapy. Arch Intern Med 154:2589–2596, 1994
41. Caputo GM, Appelbaum PC, Liu HH: Infections due to penicillin-resistant pneumococci. Clinical, epidemiologic, and microbiologic features. Arch Intern Med 153:1301–1310, 1993
42. Austrian R: Pneumococcal pneumonia. Diagnostic, epidemiologic, therapeutic and prophylactic considerations. Chest 90:738–743, 1986
43. Broome CV, Facklam RR, Allen JR, Fraser DW, Austrian R: Epidemiology of pneumococcal serotypes in the United States, 1978–1979. J Infect Dis 141:119–123, 1980
44. Davidson M, Schraer CD, Parkinson AJ, et al: Invasive pneumococcal disease in an Alaska native population, 1980 through 1986. JAMA 261:715–718, 1989
45. Filice GA, Darby CP, Fraser DW: Pneumococcal bacteremia in Charleston County, South Carolina. Am J Epidemiol 112:828–835, 1980
46. Redd SC, Rutherford GW 3d, Sande MA, et al: The role of human immunodeficiency virus infection in pneumococcal bacteremia in San Francisco residents. J Infect Dis 162:1012–1017, 1990
47. Pneumococcal infections. In ACP Task Force on Adult Immunization and Infectious Diseases Society of America: Guide for Adult Immunization. 3rd ed. Philadelphia: American College of Physicians, 1994, pp 107–114
48. Austrian R: Untreated pneumococcal bacteraemia of cryptic origin in the human adult with spontaneous recovery. S Afr Med J October 11(Suppl):46–49, 1986
49. Moore HF, Chesney AM: A study of ethylhydrocuprein (Optochin) in the treatment of acute lobar pneumonia. Arch Intern Med 19:611, 1917
50. Kislak JW, Razavi LMB, Daly AK, Finland M: Susceptibility of pneumococci to nine antibiotics. Am J Med Sci 54:261–268, 1965
51. Jabes D, Nachman S, Tomasz A: Penicillin-binding protein families: evidence for the clonal nature of penicillin resistance in clinical isolates of pneumococci. J Infect Dis 159:16–25, 1989
52. Appelbaum PC: World-wide development of antibiotic resistance in pneumococci. Eur J Clin Microbiol 6:367–377, 1987
53. Appelbaum PC: Antimicrobial resistance in *Streptococcus pneumoniae:* an overview. Clin Infect Dis 15:77–83, 1992
54. Johnson AP, Speller DC, George RC, et al: Prevalence of antibiotic resistance and serotypes in pneumococci in England and Wales:

results of observational surveys in 1990 and 1995. Br Med J 312: 1454–1456, 1996
55. Friedland IR, Klugman KP: Antibiotic-resistant pneumococcal disease in South African children. Am J Dis Child 146:920–923, 1992
56. Doern GV: Trends in antimicrobial susceptibility of bacterial pathogens of the respiratory tract. Am J Med 99:3S–7S, 1995
57. Spika JS, Facklam RR, Plikaytis BD, Oxtoby MJ: Antimicrobial resistance of *Streptococcus pneumoniae* in the United States, 1979–1987. The Pneumococcal Surveillance Working Group. J Infect Dis 163:1273–1278, 1991
58. Munoz R, Coffey TJ, Daniels M, et al: Intercontinental spread of a multiresistant clone of serotype 23F *Streptococcus pneumoniae*. J Infect Dis 164:302–306, 1991
59. McDougal LK, Facklam R, Reeves M, et al: Analysis of multiply antimicrobial-resistant isolates of *Streptococcus pneumoniae* from the United States. Antimicrob Agents Chemother 36:2176–2184, 1992
60. Soares S, Kristinsson KG, Musser JM, Tomasz A: Evidence for the introduction of a multiresistant clone of serotype 6B *Streptococcus pneumoniae* from Spain to Iceland in the late 1980s. J Infect Dis 168:158–163, 1993
61. Barnes DM, Whittier S, Gilligan PH, Soares S, Tomasz A, Henderson FW: Transmission of multidrug-resistant serotype 23F *Streptococcus pneumoniae* in group day care: evidence suggesting capsular transformation of the resistant strain in vivo. J Infect Dis 171: 890–896, 1995
62. Friedland IR, McCracken GH Jr: Management of infections caused by antibiotic-resistant *Streptococcus pneumoniae*. N Engl J Med 331:377–382, 1994
63. Pallares R, Gudiol F, Linares J, et al: Risk factors and response to antibiotic therapy in adults with bacteremic pneumonia caused by penicillin-resistant pneumococci. N Engl J Med 317:18–22, 1987
64. Friedland IR, Paris M, Ehrett S, Hickey S, Olsen K, McCracken GH Jr: Evaluation of antimicrobial regimens for treatment of experimental penicillin- and cephalosporin-resistant pneumococcal meningitis. Antimicrob Agents Chemother 37:1630–1636, 1993
65. Siber GR: Pneumococcal disease: prospects for a new generation of vaccines. Science 265:1385–1387, 1994
66. Kayhty H, Ahman H, Ronnberg PR, Tillikainen R, Eskola J: Pneumococcal polysaccharide-meningococcal outer membrane protein complex conjugate vaccine is immunogenic in infants and children. J Infect Dis 172:1273–1278, 1995
67. Chan CY, Molrine DC, George S, et al: Pneumococcal conjugate vaccine primes for antibody responses to polysaccharide pneumococcal vaccine after treatment of Hodgkin's disease. J Infect Dis 173:256–258, 1996
68. Gardner P, Schaffner W: Immunization of adults. N Engl J Med 328:1252–1258, 1993
69. Austrian R, Douglas RM, Schiffman G, et al: Prevention of pneumococcal pneumonia by vaccination. Trans Assoc Am Physicians 89:184–194, 1976
70. Broome CV, Facklam RR, Fraser DW: Pneumococcal disease after pneumococcal vaccination: an alternative method to estimate the efficacy of pneumococcal vaccine. N Engl J Med 303:549–552, 1980
71. Shapiro ED, Clemens JD: A controlled evaluation of the protective efficacy of pneumococcal vaccine for patients at high risk of serious pneumococcal infections. Ann Intern Med 101:325–330, 1984
72. Shapiro ED, Berg AT, Austrian R, et al: The protective efficacy of polyvalent pneumococcal polysaccharide vaccine [see comments]. N Engl J Med 325:1453–1460, 1991
73. Bolan G, Broome CV, Facklam RR, et al: Pneumococcal vaccine efficacy in selected populations in the United States. Ann Intern Med 104:1–6, 1986
74. Centers for Disease Control and Prevention: Increasing pneumococcal vaccination rates among patients of a national health-care alliance—United States, 1993. MMWR 44:741–744, 1995
75. Centers for Disease Control and Prevention: Influenza and pneumococcal vaccination coverage levels among persons aged ≥65 years—United States, 1973–1993. MMWR 44:506–515, 1995
76. Fedson DS: Clinical practice and public policy for influenza and pneumococcal vaccination of the elderly. Clin Geriatr Med 8: 183–199, 1992
77. Williams WW, Hickson MA, Kane MA, Kendal AP, Spika JS, Hinman AR: Immunization policies and vaccine coverage among adults. The risk for missed opportunities. Ann Intern Med 108:616–625, 1988 [published erratum appears in Ann Intern Med 109:348, 1988]
78. Fedson DS, Harward MP, Reid RA, Kaiser DL: Hospital-based pneumococcal immunization. Epidemiologic rationale from the Shenandoah study. JAMA 264:1117–1122, 1990
79. Herman CJ, Speroff T, Cebul RD: Improving compliance with immunization in the older adult: results of a randomized cohort study. J Am Geriatr Soc 42:1154–1159, 1994
80. Clancy CM, Gelfman D, Poses RM: A strategy to improve the utilization of pneumococcal vaccine. J Gen Intern Med 7:14–18, 1992
81. Fedson DS, Shapiro ED, LaForce FM, et al: Pneumococcal vaccine after 15 years of use. Another view. Arch Intern Med 154: 2531–2535, 1994
82. Rose DN, Schechter CB, Sacks HS: Influenza and pneumococcal vaccination of HIV-infected patients: a policy analysis. Am J Med 94:160–168, 1993

Haemophilus influenzae Infections

1. Wenger JD, Hightower AW, Facklam RR, Gaventa S, Broome CV, the Bacterial Meningitis Study Group: Bacterial meningitis in the U.S., 1986: report of a multistate surveillance project. J Infect Dis 162:1316–1323, 1990
2. Moxon ER, Glode MP, Sutton A, Robbins JB: The infant rat as a model of bacterial meningitis. J Infect Dis 136(Suppl):S186–S190, 1977
3. Mulholland EK, Hilton S, Adegbola R, et al: *Haemophilus influenzae* type b tetanus protein conjugate vaccine prevents pneumonia and meningitis due to *Haemophilus influenzae* type b in Gambian infants. Lancet 1997, in press
4. Schneerson R, Barrera O, Sutton A, Robbins JB. Preparation, characterization, and immunogenicity of *H influenzae* type b polysaccharide-protein conjugates. J Exp Med 152:361–376, 1980
5. Mohle-Boetani JC, Ajello G, Breneman E, et al: Carriage of *Haemophilus influenzae* type b in children after widespread vaccination with *Haemophilus influenzae* type b vaccines. Pediatr Infect Dis J 12:589–593, 1993
6. Cochi SL, Fleming DW, Hightower AW, et al: Primary invasive *Haemophilus influenzae* type b disease: a population-based assessment of risk factors. J Pediatr 108:887–896, 1986
7. Schlech WF, Ward JI, Band JD, Hightower AW, Fraser DW, Broome CV: Bacterial meningitis in the United States, 1978 through 1981: the National Bacterial Meningitis Surveillance Study. JAMA 253:1749–1754, 1985
8. Peltola H, Kayhty H, Virtanen M, Makela PH: Prevention of *Haemophilus influenzae* bacteremia infections with the capsular polysaccharide vaccine. N Engl J Med 310:1561–1566, 1984
9. Ward JI, Broome CV, Harrison LH, Shinefeld H, Black SB: *Haemophilus influenzae* type b vaccine: lessons for the future. Pediatrics 81:886–893, 1988
10. Black SB, Shinefeld HR, Fireman B. et al: Efficacy in infancy of oligosaccharide conjugate *Haemophilus influenzae* type b (HbOC) vaccine in a United States population of 61,080 children. Pediatr Infect Dis J 10:97–104, 1991
11. Santosham M, Wolff M, Reid R, et al: The efficacy in Navajo infants of a conjugate vaccine consisting of *Haemophilus influenzae* type b polysaccharide and *Neisseria meningitidis* outer membrane protein complex. N Engl J Med 324:1767–1772, 1991

12. Adams WG, Deaver KA, Cochi SL, et al: Decline of childhood *Haemophilus influenzae* type b (Hib) disease in the Hib vaccine era. JAMA 269:221–226, 1993
13. Centers for Disease Control and Prevention: Recommendations for use of *Haemophilus* b conjugate vaccines and a combined diphtheria, tetanus, pertussis *Haemophilus* b vaccine. MMWR 42(RR13): 1–15, 1993
14. Centers for Disease Control and Prevention: Progress toward elimination of *Haemophilus influenzae* type b disease among infants and children—United States, 1987–1995. MMWR 45:901–906, 1996
15. Takala AK, Eskola J, Leinonen M, et al: Reduction of oropharyngeal carriage of *Haemophilus influenzae* type b (Hib) in children immunized with Hib conjugate vaccine. J Infect Dis 164:982–986, 1991

Varicella and Herpes Zoster

1. Wharton M: The epidemiology of varicella-zoster virus infections. Infect Dis Clin North Am 10 (3):571–581, 1996
2. Van Loon F, Markowitz L, McQuillan G, et al: Varicella seroprevalence in US population. In: 33rd Interscience Conference on Antimicrobial Agents and Chemotherapy. Washington, DC: American Society for Microbiology, 1993, p 359
3. Preblud SR, Orenstein WA, Bart JJ: Varicella: clinical manifestations, epidemiology, and health impact. Pediatr Infect Dis 3:505–509, 1984
4. Preblud SR: Varicella: Complications and costs. Pediatrics 78: S728–S735, 1986
5. Guess HA, Broughton DD, Melon LJ, et al: Population-based studies of varicella complications. Pediatrics 78:S723–S727, 1986
6. Wharton M, Fehrs L, Cochi SL, et al: Health impact of varicella in the 1980s. In: Abstracts of the 30th Interscience Conference on Antimicrobial Agents and Chemotherapy. Washington, DC: American Society for Microbiology, 1990
7. Weller TH. Varicella: historical perspective and clinical overview. J Infect Dis 174(Suppl 3):S306–S309, 1996
8. Lieu TA, Cochi SL, Black SB, et al: Cost-effectiveness of a routine varicella vaccination program for US children. JAMA. 271:375–381, 1994
9. Huse DM, Meissner C, Lacey MJ, Oster G: Childhood vaccination against chickenpox: an analysis of benefits and costs. J Pediatr 124:869–874, 1994
10. Weller TH, Witton HM, Bell EJ: The etiological agents of varicella and herpes zoster. Isolation, propagation and cultural characteristics in vitro. J Exp Med 108:843–868, 1958
11. Gordon JE: Chickenpox: an epidemiologic review. Am J Med Sci 224:362–389, 1962
12. Gershon A, Steinberg SP, Gelb L: Clinical reinfection with varicella-zoster virus. J Infect Dis 149:137–142, 1984
13. Junker AK, Angus E, Thomas EE: Recurrent varicella-zoster virus infections in apparently immunocompetent children. Pediatr Infect Dis J 10(8):569–575, 1991
14. Arvin AA: Varicella-zoster virus. Clin Microbiol Rev 9(3):361–381, 1996
15. Krah D: Assays for antibodies to varicella-zoster virus. Infect Dis Clin North Am 10(3):507–527, 1996
16. McKinney WP, Horowitz MM, Battiola RJ: Susceptibility of hospital-based health care personnel to varicella-zoster virus infections. Am J Infect Control 17:26–30, 1989
17. Alter SJ, Hammond JA, McVey CJ, Myers MG: Susceptibility to varicella-zoster virus among adults at high risk for exposure. Infect Control 7(9):448–451, 1986
18. Centers for Disease Control and Prevention: Prevention of varicella: recommendations of the Advisory Committee on Immunization Practices (ACIP). MMWR 45(RR-11):1–36, 1996
19. Wasmuth EH, Miller WJ: Sensitive enzyme-linked immunosorbent assay for antibody to varicella zoster using purified VZV glycoprotein antigen. J Med Virol 32:189–193, 1990
20. LaRussa P, Lungu O, Hardy I, et al: Restriction fragment length polymorphism of polymerase chain reaction products from vaccine and wild-type varicella-zoster virus isolates. J Virol 66:1016–1020, 1992
21. Ross AH: Modification of chickenpox in family contacts by administration of gamma globulin. N Engl J Med 267:369–376, 1962
22. Hope-Simpson RE: Infectiousness of communicable diseases in the household (measles, chickenpox and mumps). Lancet 2:549–554, 1952
23. Leclair JM, Zaia JA, Levine MJ, et al: Airborne transmission of chickenpox in a hospital. N Engl J Med 302:450–453, 1980
24. Rockley PF, Tyring SK: Pathophysiology and clinical manifestations of varicella zoster viral infections: a review. Int J Dermatol 33(4): 227–232, 1994
25. Varicella-zoster infections. In: 1994 Red Book: Report of the Committee on Infectious Diseases. 23rd ed. Elk Grove Village, IL: American Academy of Pediatrics, 1994, pp 510–517
26. Jordan DR, Noel L-P, Clarke WN: Ocular involvement in varicella. Clin Pediatr 23:434, 1984
27. Fleisher G, Henry W, Sorley M, et al: Life-threatening complications of varicella. Am J Dis Child 135:896–899, 1981
28. Aebi C, Ahmed A, Ramilo O: Bacterial complications of primary varicella in children. Clin Infect Dis 23:698–705, 1996
29. Jackson MA, Burry VF, Olson LC: Complications of varicella requiring hospitalization in previously healthy children. Pediatr Infect Dis J 11:441–445, 1992
30. Choo PW, Donahue JG, Manson JE, Platt R: The epidemiology of varicella and its complications. J Infect Dis 172:706–712, 1995
31. Doctor A, Harper MB, Fleisher GR: Group A beta-hemolytic streptococcal bacteremia historical overview, changing incidence, and recent association with varicella. Pediatrics 96(3):428–433, 1995
32. Vugia DJ, Peterson CL, Meyers HB, et al: Invasive group A streptococcal infections in children with varicella in Southern California. Pediatr Infect Dis J 15:146–150, 1996
33. Cowan MR, Primm PA, Scott SM, et al: Serious Group A betahemolytic streptococcal infections complicating varicella. Ann Emerg Med 23:818–822, 1994
34. Brogan TV, Nizet V, Waldhausen JHT, et al: Group A streptococci; necrotizing fasciitis complicating primary varicella: a series of fourteen patients. Pediatr Infect Dis J 14:588–594, 1995
35. Schwartz B, Facklam RR, Breiman RF: Changing epidemiology of group A streptococcal infection in the USA. Lancet 336:1167–1171, 1990
36. Preblud SR: Age-specific risks of varicella complications. Pediatrics 68:14–17, 1981
37. Liu TA, Finker LJ, Sorel ME, Black SB, Shinefield HR: Pre-eruptive varicella encephalitis and cerebellar ataxia. Pediatr Neurol 8:69–70, 1992
38. Remington RL, Rowley D, McGee H, et al: Decreasing trends in Reye's syndrome and aspirin use in Michigan. Pediatrics 77:93–98, 1986
39. Krugman S, Goodrich CH, Ward R: Primary varicella pneumonia. N Engl J Med 257:843–848, 1957
40. Feldman S: Varicella-zoster virus pneumonitis. Chest 106(Suppl 1): 22S–27S, 1994
41. Nilsson A, Örtqvist Å: Severe varicella pneumonia in adults in Stockholm County 1980–1989. Scand J Infect Dis 28:121–123, 1996
42. Gogos, CA, Bassaris HP, Vagenakis AG: Varicella pneumonia in adults. A review of pulmonary manifestations, risk factors and treatment. Respiration 59:339–343, 1992
43. Gershon AA: In Remington JS, Klein JO (eds): Infectious Diseases of the Fetus and Newborn Infant. 3rd ed. Philadelphia: WB Saunders, 1990, pp 395–445
44. Krause PR, Klinman DM: Efficacy, immunogenicity, safety, and use of live attenuated chickenpox vaccine. J Pediatr 127:518–525, 1995
45. Dowell SF, Bresee JS: Severe varicella associated with steroid use. Pediatrics 92(2):223–228, 1993
46. Reiches NA, Jones JF: Commentary: steroids and varicella. Pediatrics 92(2):288–289, 1993

47. Weller TH: Varicella and herpes zoster: changing concepts of the natural history, control, and importance of a not-so-benign virus (second of two parts). N Engl J Med 309(23):1434–1440, 1983
48. Feldman S, Hughes WT, Daniel CB: Varicella in children with cancer: seventy-seven cases. Pediatrics 56:388–397, 1975
49. Feldman S, Hughes WT, Daniel CB: Varicella in children with cancer: impact of antiviral therapy and prophylaxis. Pediatrics 80: 5472–5474, 1987
50. LaRussa P, Steinberg S, Gershon AA: Varicella vaccine for immunocompromised children: results of collaborative studies in the United States and Canada. J Infect Dis 174(Suppl 3):S320–S323, 1996
51. Wallace MR, Hooper DG, Pyne KM, et al: Varicella immunity and clinical disease in HIV-infected adults. South Med J 87:74–76, 1994
52. Cohen PR, Grossman ME: Clinical features of human immunodeficiency virus-associated disseminated herpes zoster virus infection: a review of the literature. Clin Dermatol 14:273–276, 1989
53. Perronne C, Lazanas M, Leport C, et al: Varicella in patients infected with human immunodeficiency virus. Arch Dermatol 126:1033–1036, 1990
54. Leibovitz E, Cooper D, Giurgiutiu D, at el: Varicella-zoster virus infection in Romanian children infected with the human immunodeficiency virus. Pediatrics 92(6):838–842, 1993
55. Brunell PA: Fetal and neonatal varicella zoster infections. Semin Perinatol 7:47–56, 1983
56. Enders G, Miller E, Cradock-Watson J, Bolley I, Ridehalgh M: Consequences of varicella and herpes zoster in pregnancy: prospective study of 1739 cases. Lancet 343:1548–1551, 1994
57. Finger R, Hughes JP, Meade BJ, et al: Age-specific incidence of chickenpox. Public Health Rep 109(6):750–755, 1994
58. Yawn BP, Yawn RA, Lydick EJ: The community impact of childhood varicella infections. J Pediatr 1997, in press
59. Struewing JP, Hyams KC, Tueller JE, Gray GC: The risks of measles, mumps and varicella among young adults: a serosurvey of US Navy and Marine Corps recruits. Am J Public Health 83: 1717–1720, 1993
60. Kelley PW, Petruccelli BP, Stehr-Green P, et al: The susceptibility of young adult Americans to vaccine-preventable infections. A national serosurvey of US Army recruits. JAMA 266(19):2724–2728, 1991
61. Garnett GP, Cox MJ, Bundy DAP, Didier JM, St. Catherine J: The age of infection with varicella-zoster virus in St, Lucia, West Indies. Epidemiol Infect 110:361–372, 1993
62. Longfield JN, Winn RE, Gibson RL, et al: Varicella outbreaks in Army recruits from Puerto Rico. Arch Intern Med 150:970–974, 1990
63. Plotkin SA: Varicella vaccine [Commentary]. Pediatrics 97(2): 251–253, 1996
64. Halloran ME, Cochi SL, Lieu TA, Wharton M, Fehrs L: Theoretical epidemiologic and morbidity effects of routine varicella immunization of preschool children in the United States. Am J Epidemiol 140:81–104, 1994
65. Fairley CK, Miller E: Varicella-zoster virus epidemiology—a changing scene? J Infect Dis 174(Suppl 3):S314–S319, 1996
66. Meurice F, De Bouver JL, Vandevoorde D, et al: Immunogenicity and safety of a live attenuated varicella vaccine (Oka/SB Bio) in healthy children. J Infect Dis 174(Suppl 3):S324–S329, 1996
67. Committee of Infectious Diseases, American Academy of Pediatrics: Recommendations for the use of live attenuated varicella vaccine. Pediatrics 95(5):791–796, 1995
68. American Academy of Family Physicians: Summary of Policy Recommendations for Periodic Health Examination. Kansas City, MO: American Academy of Family Physicians, November 1996
69. Gardner PG, Eickhoff T, Poland GA, et al: Adult immunizations. Ann Intern Med 124(1):35–40, 1996
70. Kuter BJ, Weibel RE, Guess HA, et al: Oka/Merck varicella vaccine in healthy children: final report of a 2-year efficacy study and 7-year follow-up studies. Vaccine 9:643–647, 1991
71. Clements DA, Armstrong CB, Ursano AM, et al: Over five-year follow-up of Oka/Merck varicella vaccine recipients in 465 infants and adolescents. Pediatr Infect Dis J 14:874–879, 1995
72. White C, Kute B, Isganitis K, et al: Varicella vaccine in healthy children and adolescents: results from clinical trials, 1987–1989. Pediatrics 97(5):604–610, 1991
73. Gershon AA, Steinberg SP, LaRussa P, et al: Immunization of healthy adults with live attenuated varicella vaccine. J Infect Dis 158 (1):132–137, 1988
74. Arbeter AA, Starr SE, Plotkin SA. Varicella vaccine studies in healthy children and adults. Pediatrics 78(Suppl):748–756, 1986
75. Weibel RE, Neff BJ, Kuter BJ, et al: Live attenuated varicella virus vaccine: efficacy trial in healthy children. N Engl J Med 310: 1409–1415, 1985
76. Watson B, Gupta R, Randall T, et al: Persistence of cell-mediated and humoral immune responses in healthy children immunized with live attenuated varicella vaccine. J Infect Dis 169:197–199, 1994
77. Asano Y, Suga S, Yoshikawa T, et al.: Experience and reason: twenty-year follow-up of protective immunity of the Oka strain live varicella vaccine. Pediatrics 94(4 Pt 1):524–526, 1994
78. Watson B, Piercy S, Plotkin S, et al: Modified chickenpox in children immunized with the OKA/Merck varicella vaccine. Pediatrics 81:17–22, 1993
79. Asano Y, Hirose S, Iwayama S et al: Protective effect of immediate inoculation of a live varicella vaccine in household contacts in relation to the viral dose and interval between exposure and vaccination. Biken J 25:43–45, 1982
79a. Salzman, MB, Sharrar RG, Steinberg S, LaRussa P: Transmission of varicella-vaccine virus from a healthy 12-month-old to his pregnant mother. J Pediatrics 131: 151–154, 1997
80. Hardy I, Gershon AA, Steinberg SP et al: The incidence of zoster after immunization with live attenuated varicella vaccine. N Engl J Med 325:1545–1550, 1991
81. Centers for Disease Control and Prevention: Establishment of VARIVAX® Pregnancy Registry. MMWR 45:239, 1996
82. Centers for Disease Control: Varicella zoster immune globulin for the prevention of chickenpox. MMWR 33:84–90, 95–100, 1984
83. Committee on Infectious Diseases, AAP. The use of oral acyclovir in otherwise healthy children with varicella. Pediatrics 91:674–676, 1993
84. Balfour HH: Current management of varicella zoster virus infections. J Med Virol 1:74–81, 1993
85. Wallace MR, Chamberlin CJ, Sawyer M, et al: Treatment of adult varicella with Sorivudine: a randomized, placebo-controlled trial. J Infect Dis 174:249–255, 1996
86. Hope-Simpson RE: The nature of herpes zoster: a long term study and a new hypothesis. Proc R Soc Lond 58:9–20, 1965
87. Oxman MN: Immunization to reduce the frequency and severity of herpes zoster and its complications. Neurology 45(Suppl 8): S41–S46, 1995
88. Whitley RJ: Therapeutic approaches to varicella-zoster infections. J Infect Dis 166(Suppl 1):S51–S57, 1992
89. Donahue JG, Choo PW, Manson JE, Platt R: The incidence of herpes zoster. Arch Intern Med 155:1605–1609, 1995
90. Ragozzino MW, Melon L., Kurland LT, et al: Population-based study of herpes zoster and its sequelae. Medicine 61:310–316, 1982
91. Guess HA, Broughton DD, Melton LJ, Kurkland LT: Epidemiology of herpes zoster in children and adolescents: a population-based study. Pediatrics 76(4):512–517, 1985
92. Schmader K, George LK, Burchett BM, et al: Racial differences in the occurrence of herpes zoster. J Infect Dis 171:701–704, 1995
93. Wood MJ, Kay R, Dworkin RH et al: Oral acyclovir therapy accelerates pain resolution in patients with herpes zoster: a meta-analysis of placebo-controlled trials—a review. Clin Infect Dis 22:341–347, 1996
94. Famciclovir for herpes zoster. Med Lett Drugs Ther 36:97–98, 1994
95. Gershon A and Silverstein S: Live attenuated varicell vaccine for prevention of Herpes Zoster. Biologicals 25:227–230, 1997

96. Levin MJ, Murray M, Rotbart HA, et al: Immune response of elderly individuals to a live attenuated varicella vaccine. J Infect Dis 166: 253–259, 1992

Poliomyelitis

1. Ramlow J, Alexander M, LaPorte R, Kaufman C, Kuller L: Epidemiology of post-polio syndrome. Am J Epidemiol 136:769–786, 1992
2. Paul JR: A History of Poliomyelitis. New Haven, CT: Yale University Press, 1971
3. Evans AS (ed): Viral Infections of Humans: Epidemiology and Control. 3rd ed. New York: Plenum Medical Book Company, 1991
4. Enders JF, Weller TH, Robbins FC: Cultivation of the Lansing strains of poliomyelitis virus in cultures of various human embryonic tissue. Science 109:85–87, 1949
5. Mendelsohn CL, Wimmer E, Racaniello VR: Cellular receptor for poliovirus: molecular cloning, nucleotide sequence, and expression of a new member of the immunoglobulin superfamily. Cell 56: 855–865, 1989
6. Strebel PM, Sutter RW, Cochi SL, et al: Epidemiology of poliomyelitis in the United States one decade after the last reported case of indigenous wild virus-associated disease. Clin Infect Dis 14: 568–579, 1992
7. Centers for Disease Control and Prevention: Progress toward global eradication of poliomyelitis, 1995. MMWR 45:565–568, 1996
8. Rico-Hesse R, Pallansch MA, Nottay BK, Kew OM: Geographic distribution of wild poliovirus type 1 genotypes. Virology 160:311–322, 1987
9. Francis T, Napier JA, Voight RB, et al: Evaluation of the 1954 Field Trial of Poliomyelitis Vaccine. Ann Arbor, MI: Edward Brothers, Inc., 1957
10. Cochi SL, Hull H, Sutter RW, Wilfert C, Katz S (eds): Status report on the global poliomyelitis eradication initiative. J Infect Dis 175: S1–S292, 1997
11. Prevots DR, Sutter RW, Strebel PM, Weibel RE, Cochi SL: Completeness of reporting for paralytic poliomyelitis, United States, 1980 through 1991: implications for estimating the risk of vaccine-associated disease. Arch Pediatr Adolesc Med 148:479–485, 1994
12. Centers for Disease Control and Prevention: Paralytic poliomyelitis—United States, 1980–1994. MMWR 46:79–83, 1997
13. Centers for Disease Control and Prevention: Poliomyelitis prevention in the United States: introduction of a sequential vaccination schedule of inactivated poliovirus vaccine followed by oral poliovirus vaccine. Recommendations of the Advisory Committee on Immunization Practices (ACIP). MMWR 46(RR-3):1–25, 1997
14. World Health Assembly: Global eradication of poliomyelitis by the year 2000 (Resolution WHA 41.28). In: Resolutions of the 41st World Health Assembly. Geneva: World Health Organization, 1988
15. Okwo-Bele JM, Lobanov A, Biellik R, et al: Overview of poliomyelitis in African region and current regional plan of action. J Infect Dis 175:S10–S15, 1997.

8

Sexually Transmitted Diseases

Willard Cates, Jr. • King K. Holmes

The field of sexually transmitted diseases (STDs) has been a truly dynamic area of public health. During the past two decades, this discipline has evolved from one emphasizing the traditional venereal diseases of gonorrhea and syphilis, to one concerned with the bacterial and viral syndromes associated with *Chlamydia trachomatis*, herpes simplex virus (HSV), and human papilloma virus (HPV), to one dominated by the fatal systemic infection caused by human immunodeficiency virus (HIV).[1,2] In addition, since 1980, eight sexually transmitted pathogens were either newly identified or newly recognized to be sexually transmitted.[2] Over 20 organisms (Table 8-1) and countless syndromes (Table 8-2) are now recognized as being sexually transmitted. All these STDs are historically, biologically, behaviorally, economically, and programmatically interrelated.[3]

Four key long-term health consequences make controlling these infections a crucial public health priority: *(a)* STD-related neoplasia, *(b)* reproductive health problems, *(c)* adverse outcomes of pregnancy for both women and infants, and *(d)* increased risk of HIV transmission. Regarding cancer, several key subtypes of sexually acquired HPV cause nearly all cancers of the cervix, vagina, vulva, anus, and penis. Moreover, hepatitis B virus causes hepatocellular carcinoma, and human herpes virus type 8 probably causes Kaposi's sarcoma. Regarding reproductive consequences, upper genital tract infections related to chlamydia, gonorrhea, and anaerobic bacteria lead to tubal infertility and/or ectopic pregnancy. Regarding adverse outcomes of pregnancy, both bacterial vaginosis and trichomoniasis are the most important infectious causes of preterm delivery and low–birth weight infants. Moreover, pregnant women with STDs may transmit the infection to their fetus or newborn child. Such infections as congenital syphilis, neonatal herpes, HBV, and HIV account for a large percentage of perinatal infection worldwide. Finally, the role of both ulcerative and nonulcerative STDs in facilitating the HIV epidemic has been confirmed through both epidemiologic studies and intervention trials. Thus, controlling STDs becomes one of the nation's highest priorities as cost-effective investment in preventing many long-term health consequences.

▶ HISTORY OF STDs AND PUBLIC HEALTH

Social Attitudes

Throughout history, STDs have caused society to wrestle with its moral feelings about this public health problem. In recent years, the human tragedies suffered by the persons with STD have led to more effective social and political responses designed to interrupt transmission and reduce complications, rather than to stigmatize those with disease.

Before 1900, physicians were known to withhold treatment for STD, fatalistically regarding infection as evidence of (and even punishment for) "promiscuous" behavior.[14] Prior to World War I, the increasing professionalization of medicine coincided with the rise of venereology as an established specialty. Syphilis became the disease upon which the skills of twentieth-century physicians were judged. Knowledge in this field rapidly progressed from acceptance of the germ theory, to fascination with serologic tests, to use of toxic cures. The foundations were laid for a medical, rather than a moralistic, approach to STD control.

In the New Deal era, Surgeon General Thomas Parran seized an opportunity to dramatize the plight of those with STD. With the availability of penicillin and the higher national imperative of winning a war, the image of STD shed a portion of its stigmatic cloak during the 1940s. The diagnosis and treatment of sexually transmitted infections could be performed on an outpatient basis, thus allowing a more positive attitude toward finding and treating both patients and partners alike.

Finally, during the most recent decades, the changing social role of women and minorities and the greater acceptance of homosexuality have been accompanied by a slow shift in the nation's attitude toward human sexuality. The population at risk of STD increased, creating a growing constituency that demanded personal and public health solutions. Feminists, realizing that women and children bear the brunt of the sexually related complications, played an increasingly active role in politics. At Cairo in 1994, STD became an integral part of the global reproductive health agenda. Homosexual organizations, spurred by the availability of a hepatitis B vaccine and the tragedy of HIV and acquired immunodeficiency syndrome (AIDS), lobbied for a greater share of political resources being directed to their health concerns. In addition, groups interested in minority health and international health have increasingly acknowledged STD and HIV as priorities for their constituency. Thus, society has become more concerned about STD as the scope of the problem increased and public health interventions have become more available.

Control Programs

Our current public health approaches to STD and HIV greatly resemble those we used for syphilis in the preantibiotic era. National programs to control STD were established in the United States during the early days of World War I.[4] For the next half century, the focus was almost exclusively on the control of syphilis and its complications. Diagnosis was complex, and treatments were dangerous. This stimulated the continued development of the specialty of venereology. Federal grants to support venereal disease control initiatives were begun in 1939. Rapid treatment centers for syphilis and gonorrhea were established during World War II.

After World War II, the widespread availability of penicillin led to a dismantling of the rapid treatment centers and a decline of the clinical specialty of venereology. However, particularly during the 1960s, federal assistance continued to support sex partner tracing, serologic testing for syphilis, and health education of patients. The

TABLE 8-1. SEXUALLY TRANSMITTED PATHOGENS AND THE DISEASES THEY CAUSE

Agent	*Associated Disease or Syndrome*
• ***Bacteria***	
Neisseria gonorrhoeae	Urethritis, epididymitis, proctitis, cervicitis, endometritis, salpingitis, perihepatitis, bartholinitis, pharyngitis, conjunctivitis, prepubertal vaginitis, ?prostatitis, accessory gland infection, disseminated gonococcal infection (DGI), chorioamnionitis, premature rupture of membranes, premature delivery, amniotic infection syndrome
Chlamydia trachomatis	All of above except DGI. Also, otitis media, rhinitis, and pneumonia in infants; and Reiter's syndrome
Mycoplasma hominis	Postpartum fever, ?salpingitis
Ureaplasma urealyticum	Nongonococcal urethritis, ?chorioamnionitis, ?premature delivery
Treponema pallidum	Syphilis
Gardnerella vaginalis	Bacterial ("nonspecific") vaginosis (in conjunction with *Mycoplasma hominis* and vaginal anaerobes, such as *Mobiluncus* spp)
Haemophilus ducreyi	Chancroid
Calymmatobacterium granulomatis	Donovanosis (granuloma inguinale)
Shigella spp	Shigellosis in homosexual men
Campylobacter spp	Enteritis, proctocolitis
Group B streptococcus	Neonatal sepsis, neonatal meningitis
• ***Viruses***	
Human immunodeficiency virus, types 1 and 2	AIDS
Herpes simplex virus	Initial and recurrent genital herpes, aseptic meningitis, neonatal herpes
Human papilloma virus (more than 70 separate types identified)	Condyloma acuminata, laryngeal papilloma, cervical intraepithelial neoplasia and carcinoma, vaginal carcinoma, anal carcinoma, vulvar carcinoma, penile carcinoma
Hepatitis B virus	Acute hepatitis B, chronic active hepatitis, persistent (unresolved) hepatitis, polyarteritis nodosa, chronic membranous glomerulonephritis, ?mixed cryoglobulinemia, ?polymyalgia rheumatica, hepatocellular carcinoma
Hepatitis A virus	Acute hepatitis A
Hepatitis C virus	Acute hepatitis C
Cytomegalovirus	Heterophil-negative infectious mononucleosis; congenital CMV infection with gross birth defects and infant mortality, cognitive impairment (e.g., mental retardation, sensorineural deafness); protean manifestations in the immunosuppressed host
Molluscum contagiosum virus	Genital molluscum contagiosum
Human T-lymphotrophic retrovirus, type 1	Human T-cell leukemia or lymphoma
Human herpes virus type 8	Kaposi's sarcoma, lymphoma
• ***Protozoa***	
Trichomonas vaginalis	Trichomonal vaginitis
Entamoeba histolytica	Amebiasis in men who have sex with men
Giardia lamblia	Giardiasis in men who have sex with men
• ***Fungi***	
Candida albicans	Vulvovaginitis, balanitis
• ***Ectoparasites***	
Phthirus pubis	Pubic lice infestation
Sarcoptes scabiei	Lice
	Scabies

STD "epidemiologist" emerged as a central figure in syphilis control efforts, focusing on locating and treating individuals exposed to syphilis.

By the late 1960s, officials became concerned with the rapidly escalating number of gonorrhea cases. The gonorrhea epidemic, together with the development of selective culture media for isolating the gonococcus, stimulated the implementation of a national gonorrhea control strategy.[5] Beginning in 1968, pilot projects had been initiated to evaluate case-finding of infected women both by using culture diagnosis and also by identifying sex partners of infected men. During the remainder of the 1970s gonorrhea control gradually received a larger portion of the STD federal dollar, at the expense of syphilis control. By 1980, expenditures for gonorrhea control accounted for almost three-quarters of federal STD grant dollars.

Simultaneously, the growing variety and recognition of other syndromes causing patients to seek STD care produced a need for major improvements in clinical skills, clinic services, and physical facilities. This upgrading was necessary both to encourage infected individuals to obtain treatment and to provide additional capability to diagnose the broad array of STDs. Once again, technological change required hard choices. In the 1980s, increased availability of laboratory diagnostic testing for chlamydial infection created opportunities for chlamydia control, requiring further tradeoffs among resources primarily directed to gonorrhea and syphilis control. By the late 1980s, the provision of counseling and testing for HIV infection in STD clinics placed additional demands on STD personnel and facilities, which contributed to a delay in implementing chlamydia control programs.

TABLE 8-2. SELECTED SYNDROMES AND COMPLICATIONS WITH ASSOCIATED SEXUALLY TRANSMITTED AGENTS[a]

Agent	Associated Sexually Transmitted Agents
• Men	
AIDS	Human immunodeficiency virus, types 1 and 2
Urethritis	*Neisseria gonorrhoeae, Chlamydia trachomatis*, herpes simplex virus, *Ureaplasma urealyticum*
Epididymitis	*C. trachomatis, N. gonorrhoeae*
Intestinal infections	
Proctitis	*N gonorrhoeae*, herpes simplex virus, *C. trachomatis*
Proctocolitis or enterocolitis	*Campylobacter* spp, *Shigella* spp, *Entamoeba histolytica*
Enteritis	*Giardia lamblia*
Hepatitis	Hepatitis A, B, and C viruses, cytomegalovirus, *Treponema pallidum*
• Women	
AIDS	Human immunodeficiency virus, types 1 and 2
Lower genitourinary tract infection	
Vulvitis	*Candida albicans*, herpes simplex virus
Vaginitis	*Trichomonas vaginalis, C. albicans*
Vaginosis	*Gardnerella vaginalis, Mobiluncus* spp, other anaerobes, *Mycoplasma hominis*
Cervicitis	*N gonorrhoeae, C. trachomatis*, herpes simplex virus
Urethritis	*N gonorrhoeae, C. trachomatis*, herpes simplex virus
Pelvic inflammatory disease	*N. gonorrhoeae, C. trachomatis, M. hominis*, anaerobes, Group B streptocococcus
Infertility	*N. gonorrhoeae, C. trachomatis, ? M. hominis*
Postsalpingitis, postobstetrical, postabortion	
Pregnancy morbidity	Several STDs have been implicated in one or more of these conditions
Chorioamnionitis, amniotic fluid infection, prematurity, premature rupture of membranes, preterm delivery, postpartum endometritis, ectopic pregnancy	
• Men and Women	
Neoplasia	
Cervical, vulvar, vaginal, anal, and penile intraepithelial neoplasia, carcinoma	Human papilloma virus
Hepatocellular carcinoma	Hepatitis B virus
Kaposi's sarcoma, non-Hodgkin's lymphoma	Human immunodeficiency virus, types 1 and 2
Genital ulceration	Herpes simplex virus, *T. pallidum, Haemophilus ducreyi, Calymmatobacterium granulomatis, C. trachomatis* (LGV strains)
Acute arthritis with urogenital or intestinal infection	*N. gonorrhoeae, C. trachomatis, Shigella* spp, *Campylobacter* spp
Genital warts	Human papilloma virus
Molluscum contagiosum	Molluscum contagiosum virus
Ectoparasite infestations	*Sarcoptes scabiei, Pthirus pubis*
Heterophil-negative mononucleosis	Cytomegalovirus, Epstein-Barr virus (some evidence for sexual transmission)
• Neonates and Infants	
TORCHES syndromes[b]	Cytomegalovirus, herpes simplex virus, *T. pallidum*
Conjunctivitis	*C. trachomatis, N. gonorrhoeae*
Pneumonia	*C. trachomatis, ?U. urealyticum*
Otitis media	*C. trachomatis*
Sepsis, meningitis	Group B streptococcus
Cognitive impairment, deafness	Cytomegalovirus, herpes simplex virus, *T. pallidum*

[a] For each of the syndromes, some cases cannot yet be ascribed to any cause and must currently be considered idiopathic.
[b] TORCHES is an acronym for toxoplasmosis, rubella, cytomegalovirus, herpes, and syphilis. The syndrome consists of various combinations of encephalitis, hepatitis, dermatitis, and disseminated intravascular coagulation (DIC).

In the 1990s, STD control strategies matured to their present form.[5] Spurred on by the need for HIV prevention, community-based planning became woven into state and local STD prevention activities. Embraced by women's advocacy groups, and supported by empiric evidence of the pilot program in the Pacific Northwest, chlamydia control efforts received an increasing share of STD control resources under the banner of "infertility prevention." Regional programs emulating those on the West Coast spread eastward. Moreover, based in part on inferences drawn from models of STD transmission dynamics, a greater appreciation emerged of the inextricable links between both biomedical and behavioral interventions to achieve effective STD control.[6] Together with a realization of the value of both population-level and individual-level STD control strategies, health advocates began taking a more sophisticated look at the variety of synergistic STD prevention and control activities. Finally, a landmark report by the Institutes of Medicine has provided a blueprint for addressing the "hidden epidemic" of STD in the United States.[3] Key strategies laid out by this document will form the foundation for national STD control policies into the twenty-first century.

▶ INFRASTRUCTURE FOR CONTROLLING STD/HIV

Governmental Responsibilities for STD Control and HIV Prevention

National, regional, and local tiers of government have different responsibilities for STD control and HIV prevention.[1] At the federal level, in the United States, the Centers for Disease Control and Prevention (CDC) coordinates STD (including HIV) control strategies, provides surveillance for STD/HIV/AIDS, and undertakes epidemiologic and laboratory research.[7] The National Institutes of Health (NIH) supports both basic science and applied clinical investigations.

State and local health departments have the statutory responsibility for control of many communicable diseases, including STDs. States (and the largest metropolitan areas) receive federal project grants (numbering 63 in 1996) from CDC for STD control activities, including disease reporting, health promotion, training, and program evaluation. They also receive support through federal cooperative agreements for HIV surveillance and prevention. Local health departments are charged with providing direct clinical services, which include diagnosis, treatment, patient counseling, and sex partner notification activities.

These different responsibilities require federal, state, and local health officials to cooperate closely to help ensure an integrated STD/HIV prevention program. Crucial factors include *(a)* identification of local priorities based on well-defined epidemiologic indicators, and *(b)* application of prevention and control strategies with the greatest potential for preventing disease. Unfortunately, well-designed studies to evaluate standard STD interventions are lacking. Moreover, each of the three governmental tiers has increasingly had to create a matrix of activities both within and outside the traditional health sphere to gain further leverage on preventing STD/HIV. For example, STD control programs require close integration with programs for family planning, maternal and child health, and adolescent health; and school health and education programs have required collaboration with education officials, substance abuse programs with law endorsement officials, and so on.

Resources for STD Control and HIV Prevention

National budgets allocated to preventing STD other than HIV have not kept pace with the worsening problem in most countries. For example, in the United States, after adjusting for effects of inflation, the peak year for funding STD control programs was 1947. In that year, over $130 million (in 1996 dollars) were focused on the control of a single STD, syphilis. By 1973, even with the boost of a national gonorrhea control program, *total* federal grant resources for these two diseases was $64 million. By 1996, this aggregate amount had risen to $105 million, although it was spread across the full spectrum of STDs described earlier.[7]

The level of funding from state and local governments for STD-related programs is unknown. Moreover, based on selected surveys, wide variation exists in the capacities of state and local health departments to underwrite STD-control programs. Some regions spend more than double the amount they receive from CDC, whereas others provide little supplementation to the federal resources. In 1994, an informal CDC survey of state and local health departments found the aggregate contribution was approximately $125 million; this is approximately 25 percent more than the federal investments for non-HIV STD prevention.[2]

Resources for HIV prevention have grown rapidly throughout the world, especially after the HIV antibody test was developed. Prior to 1985, the U.S. government had invested less than $50 million in AIDS research and prevention. However, since mid-1985, federal spending for HIV/AIDS prevention and research has risen every year, to more than $1 billion in 1996; approximately 30 percent of this is allocated for HIV surveillance and prevention activities coordinated by CDC. State and local health departments are also increasing their resources for HIV prevention; in 1994, an estimated $525 million was available from state and local legislatures for a variety of programs, including surveillance, prevention, research, and patient care.[2]

STD Clinical Preventive Services

The phrase usually goes "an ounce of prevention is worth a pound of cure"—for a 1:16 ratio. However, in the STD arena, cure is part of prevention. Proper treatment of persons infected with curable STD serves several preventive functions.[8] First, reservoirs for sexual transmission are eliminated; this represents primary prevention. Second, the more severe complications are prevented; this represents secondary prevention. Third, patients can be counseled to reduce high-risk sexual behavior and to refer sex partners for treatment (primary and secondary prevention). Fourth, treatment of curable STDs (e.g., syphilis and chancroid) may reduce concurrent transmission of certain incurable STD, such as HIV infection.

For these reasons, STD prevention strategies employ approaches—such as diagnosis and treatment—that have typically been considered in the realm of the clinician rather than that of the public health practitioner. Simplified diagnosis of persons with symptoms ensures rapid treatment; the Gram stain for gonorrhea is an example. Single-dose therapy reduces problems with compliance; ceftriaxone for gonorrhea and metronidazole for *Trichomonas* infection are examples. Attractive clinical settings allow those with stigmatizing conditions to obtain dignified health care. Thus, curative and preventive medicine are complementary in STD control.

Public STD services vary in both focus and quality. In 1995, a stratified, random sample of 800 local health departments were surveyed to ascertain their STD-related clinical services.[9] Approximately half of the nearly 3,000 local health department clinics provided treatment for STDs. Three-quarters integrated their STD-related services with those for HIV. Nineteen of 20 local health departments provided HIV counseling or testing as part of STD-related clinical services. Over one-third of local health departments (predominantly those in small, rural counties without an extensive STD problem) integrate their STD-related clinical services with other categorical programs such as family planning or maternal and child health.

The largest STD clinics, representing a small minority of facilities, serve the majority of public STD clients and offer a limited array of public health services. Fourteen percent provide only STD services in dedicated sessions; these represent predominantly metropolitan areas with the largest number of reported STDs. As expected, the clinics offering dedicated versus integrated STD-related services differ when it comes to providing for holistic client needs: those in large metropolitan areas were less likely to offer a spectrum of other preventive services including contraceptive counseling, cervical cancer screening, or advice on immunization practices.

To assist clinicians in deciding which STD services might be most useful for their patients, the U.S. Preventive Services Task Force[10] has provided recommendations for preventing STD (Table 8-3). Screening cultures and serologic tests are primarily recommended only for those patients practicing high-risk behaviors. Prophylactic treatment for a sex partner of someone known to be infected has a strong scientific basis for efficacy and should be integral to clinical practice. While the evidence supporting other STD interventions is less conclusive, those providing clinical preventive services should be aware of the role of such strategies as STD reporting, partner notification, and patient education.

Public Interest in STD

Because the public's perception of the STD problem influences both policymakers and program planners, it has a strong impact on the resources available for STD control. However, the public's interest in STD has varied. The press has ignored (or denied) the importance of these infections in some years and then has overreacted

TABLE 8-3. RECOMMENDATIONS FOR PREVENTION OF SEXUALLY TRANSMITTED DISEASES

Diseases	*Intervention*	*Grade of Evidence*[a]	*Recommendations*[b]
General recommendations	Epidemiological treatment	I	A
	Contact tracing	II-2	B
	Disease reporting	III	B
	Barrier methods	II-3	B
	Patient education	III	C
Gonorrhea			
Gonococcal ophthalmia neonatorum	Erythromycin	I	A
	Ophthalmic ointment		
	Postpartum		
	Culture of pregnant women	III	C
Gonorrhea	Culture of high-risk group members	II-1	A
Syphilis			
Syphilis	Epidemiological treatment of sexual contacts of established infection	I	A
	VDRL testing of high-risk group members	III	B
Congenital syphilis	VDRL testing of pregnant women	II-3	Risk group B No risk group C
HIV infection	HIV antibody testing	III	Risk group B No risk group C Pregnant women B
	Use of heat-treated blood products	II	A
	Blood and needle precautions for persons exposed to infected secretions	II	A
Hepatitis A	Immune serum globulin	I	A
Genital warts	Physical examination of risk group members	III	C
Neonatal herpes	Cesarean section in women with active genital herpes during labor	III	B
Chlamydia trachomatis			
Ophthalmia neonatorum	Erythromycin eye ointment	I	A
Neonatal chlamydial infection	Culture screening of pregnant women	III	Risk group B

[a] Effectiveness of interventions:
I: Evidence obtained from at least one properly randomized controlled trial.
II-1: Evidence obtained from well-designed controlled trials without randomization.
II-2: Evidence obtained from well-designed cohort or case-control analytic studies, preferably from more than one center or research group.
II-3: Evidence obtained from multiple time series studies with or without the intervention. Dramatic results in uncontrolled experiments could also be regarded as this type of evidence.
III: Opinions of respected authorities, based on clinical experience, descriptive studies, or reports of expert committees.
[b] Classification of recommendations:
A: There is good evidence to support the recommendation that the condition be specifically considered in a periodic health examination.
B: There is fair evidence to support the recommendation that the condition be specifically considered in a periodic health examination.
C: There is poor evidence regarding the inclusion of the condition in a periodic health examination, but recommendations may be made on other grounds.

in others. In part because of these media vicissitudes, knowledge and awareness of STDs among Americans is low.[2] Almost two-thirds of women 18 to 60 years of age surveyed in 1995 knew nothing or little about STDs other than HIV. One-third could not even name any other STD. In addition, respondents seriously underestimate their risk of acquiring an STD: among those with self-admitted behaviors that placed them at high risk for STDs, about three-quarters of women and men were not concerned about becoming infected. Without any widespread perception of susceptibility to sexually acquired infections, the public cannot be mobilized to advocate for resources and/or programs to help prevent these infections and their consequences.

Different interest groups also affect public policy. Only one national nonprofit organization, the American Social Health Association, has as its sole mission advocacy to prevent STD. Other public health organizations are now recognizing the necessity of controlling STD at both the national level and in their own communities and have been organized by the American Social Health Association into the coalition to fight STD. Increased networking among private health-interest organizations, AIDS-service groups and other community-based organizations serving minorities, and the federal/state/local government will help generate an increasing public interest in STD.

▶ TRENDS IN SEXUALLY TRANSMITTED INFECTIONS

Measures of STDs

Estimates of the incidence and prevalence of STDs in developed countries vary according to the source of data and the methods used to detect infections.[11] Sources generally include *(a)* reportable infections (e.g., gonorrhea and syphilis), *(b)* visits to office-based practices, *(c)* national surveys of representative populations, and *(d)* data on patients attending specialized health facilities (e.g., STD clinics, family planning clinics, etc.).

STD surveillance data for the United States are collected by the Centers for Disease Control and Prevention through formal surveillance systems based in the states.[12] Data may vary in accuracy, depending upon the priorities of STD control programs. These morbidity data tend to be more accurate in states that have laws that require reporting of positive STD tests. Data on infections in the private sector can be derived from three key sources: *(a)* the Hospital Discharge Survey of the National Center for Health Statistics (NCHS), which includes 7,500 randomly selected hospitals from throughout the United States; *(b)* the National Ambulatory Medical Care Survey of NCHS, which is a probability sampling of the diagnoses of 1,900 physicians; and *(c)* the National Disease and Therapeutic Index (NDTI), which is a private survey of a random sample of office visits to U.S. physicians in office-based practices.

Unfortunately, each of these sources has limitations. Data on reported infections are affected by differences in the completeness of reporting between public and private health care sources. Because infections diagnosed in public facilities are reported more frequently, these data are susceptible to biases related to the characteristics of individuals who tend to use public clinics. Likewise, data from private clinicians' practices are often affected by the absence of diagnostic validation. National surveys are limited by their sporadicity and the superficial nature of the analytic variables. Moreover, the private sector databases include relatively small numbers of STDs in the samples, which leads to wide confidence intervals in subpopulations. Finally, data from specific health facilities suffers from the problem of patient selection bias, as well as from geographic variation.

A cascading set of circumstances must occur for STDs to be measured accurately by public health authorities. For symptomatic infections, the symptoms must be initially perceived as abnormal by the individual and must be severe enough to cause the person to seek health care. The STD must then be diagnosed and reported to appropriate health authorities by clinicians. For asymptomatic infections, screening programs must be available at health services routinely used by infected persons.

Data on specific STDs also varies by the type of infection,[12] depending on whether current or cumulative infection is being measured. Symptomatic viral infections (measured by physician visits) occur less frequently than serologic or cytologic indicators of the cumulative number of infected persons. Thus, care must be used in making comparisons among the different estimates of STDs, and differences between incident and prevalent infections should be kept in mind.

► BACTERIAL AND PROTOZOAL INFECTIONS

Syphilis

Syphilis remains an important sexually transmitted organism because of *(a)* its public health heritage; *(b)* its effect on perinatal morbidity and mortality; *(c)* its association with HIV transmission; *(d)* its concentration among underserved populations, minority heterosexuals; and *(e)* its capacity for prevention. After the introduction of penicillin in the late 1940s, the number of cases of primary and secondary syphilis in the United States declined by 99 percent.[5] However, in recent years, infectious syphilis trends have followed specific patterns (Fig. 8-1). During the second half of the 1980s, infectious syphilis increased dramatically to its highest level in 40 years.[12] This increase largely occurred in low-income, minority heterosexual populations (Fig. 8-1). An important contributor to this rise was the exchange of sexual services for drugs, especially crack cocaine.

In the 1990s, with increasing efforts redirected to syphilis control, infection rates and numbers declined again. Syphilis rates decreased in 1995 to its lowest level in many years. However, it remains an important problem in certain geographical areas and among subpopulations, particularly in the South and among African Americans.[12] For example, while primary and secondary syphilis declined in all regions of the United States in 1995, the rate of 12.1 cases per 100,000 population in the South was more than twice as high as the nearest other region, the Midwest. Moreover, in 1995, the rate among African Americans of 46.2 cases per 100,000 population was nearly 60 times greater than the rate for non-Hispanic whites. These dramatically higher rates of syphilis among underserved populations remain a challenge for current STD control efforts.

Trends in congenital syphilis (CS) reflect both recent heterosexual syphilis rates and also varying definitions of the condition. While steady declines in incidence of CS occurred in the 1950s and 1960s, substantial increases have been reported in recent years.[12] Part of the rise observed since 1984 may be attributed to changing surveillance definitions—particularly for stillbirths. In addition, increased vertical transmission may also be related to underutilization and inadequacy of prenatal care. With high rates of female syphilis occurring in selected areas of the United States, early prenatal care and serologic testing in both the first and third trimester must be encouraged.

Gonorrhea

Recent gonorrhea trends reveal two major themes: *(a)* a sustained decrease in cases caused by penicillin-sensitive organisms; and *(b)* the continued increase in the number and variety of antibiotic-resistant

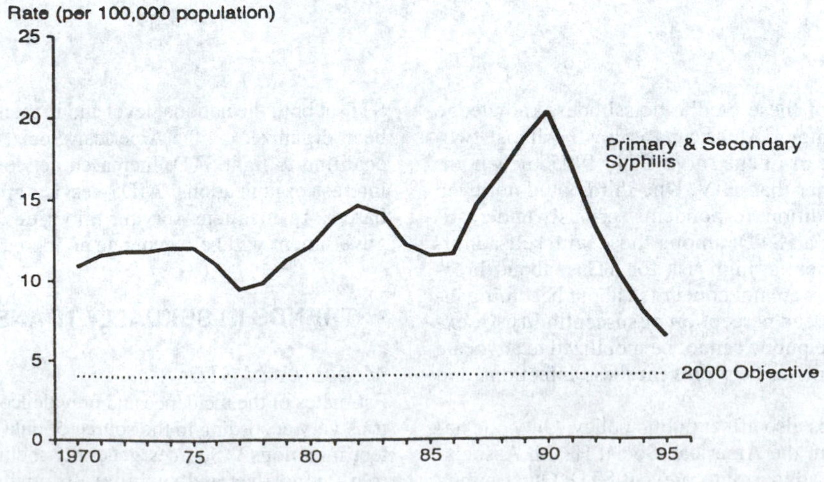

Figure 8-1. Primary and secondary syphilis—Reported rates: United States, 1970 to 1995, and the Healthy People Year 2000 Objective.

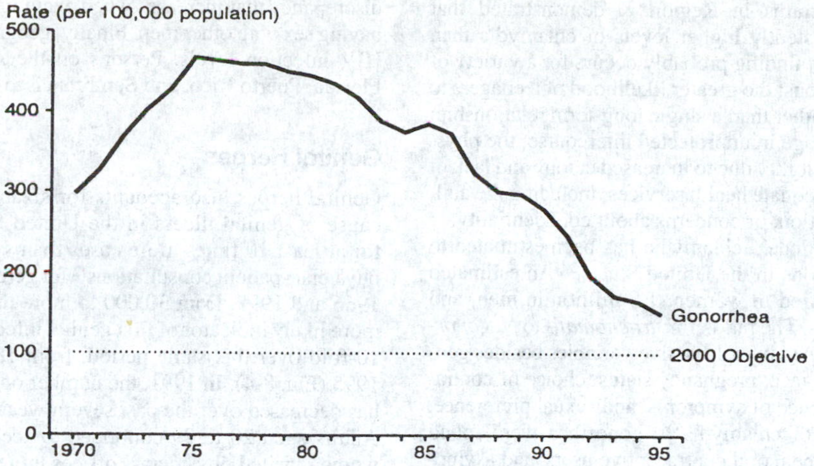

Figure 8-2. Gonorrhea—Reported rates: United States, 1970 to 1995, and the Healthy People Year 2000 Objective. Note: Georgia was excluded in 1994.

strains. From 1975 to 1995, reported gonorrhea in the United States has declined to less than half its former level, with nearly all the decrease occurring since 1981 (Fig. 8-2). In 1995, fewer than 400,000 cases of gonorrhea were reported.[12] Like syphilis, gonorrhea rates decreased in all regions of the United States, with the South continuing to have a higher rate than other regions. Rates in all racial groups also declined, but rates among African Americans remain almost 40 times greater than the rates for non-Hispanic whites. Gonorrhea among young adults remains a concern. Overall, the 15- to 19-year-old age group had higher rates than any other. In addition, awareness of antimicrobial resistance patterns remains crucial to treating gonorrhea. In 1995, nearly one-third of isolates collected by CDC were resistant to penicillin, tetracycline, or both.

Part of the decrease in gonorrhea may be an artifact of evolving tradeoffs in our gonorrhea control strategy. First, in the interests of cost-effectiveness, we have focused gonorrhea screening on the populations that have yielded the highest percentage of positive cultures. This focusing of effort has decreased the overall number of asymptomatic persons tested, and thus reduced the total number of infected persons identified. Second, as a cost-saving measure, a number of public STD clinics have either shut down satellite facilities and/or shortened the hours of their central clinics. Finally, because the amount of clinical care required for a typical STD patient in 1997 is greater than it was a decade earlier (e.g., HIV counseling, pelvic examinations, Pap smears, therapy for genital warts), fewer symptomatic persons can be evaluated in the same interval of time. As a result, fewer of those with gonorrhea are being diagnosed, further contributing to an artifactual decline.

In the face of the generally declining rates—whether real or artifactual—gonorrhea trends in teenagers and racial minorities are disturbing.[12] Adolescents have not shared proportionately in the two decades-long gonorrhea decrease. The disturbing disease rates among the teenage population may mean that gonorrhea control programs are having difficulty reaching this key risk group.

Gonococcal antibiotic resistance further clouds the gonorrhea scene. The discovery of β-lactamase-producing *Neisseria gonorrhoeae* in 1976 marked the beginning of an accelerated trend toward greater antibiotic resistance. Since the emergence of this strain, clinically significant resistance has been described for most of the widely used classes of drugs—including the penicillins, tetracyclines, aminoglycosides, and cephalosporins. Furthermore, the variety of mechanisms involved is cause for increasing concern.

Chlamydia

Genital infections caused by *Chlamydia trachomatis* are the most commonly reported sexually transmitted syndromes in the United States today.[12] Despite this dubious distinction, surveillance for chlamydial infections remains incomplete in many areas of the country. A variety of factors hinders adequate documentation of the incidence and prevalence of genital chlamydial infection: the large reservoir of asymptomatic persons who can be detected only through screening programs; the limited (though increasing) resources to support widespread chlamydial screening activities; and incomplete information systems for surveillance of new chlamydia cases. Thus, although high, the number of reported chlamydia cases reflects more the degree of local interest in chlamydia as a public health problem rather than the true chlamydial disease trend.

Nonetheless, from 1984 to 1995, reported rates of chlamydia increased dramatically from 3.2 to 182.2 cases per 100,000 population (Fig. 8-3). These trends continue to reflect the increased screening of asymptomatic infection mainly in women. In 1995, rates of chlamydia were highest in the West and Midwest, where sizable resources had been committed for organized screening programs in family planning clinics. In those regions where effective screening programs have been in place for several years, the chlamydia rates far exceed the gonorrhea rates. For similar reasons, reported rates of chlamydia in women are much higher than those in men, in 1995 nearly 6-fold higher. The low rates in men suggests that many of the sex partners of women with chlamydia are not being diagnosed and/or reported.

The level of chlamydial infections in adolescents and young adults is particularly of concern. Numerous investigations of chlamydial prevalence in a variety of clinic populations have shown that sexually active adolescents have high rates of chlamydial infection.[13]

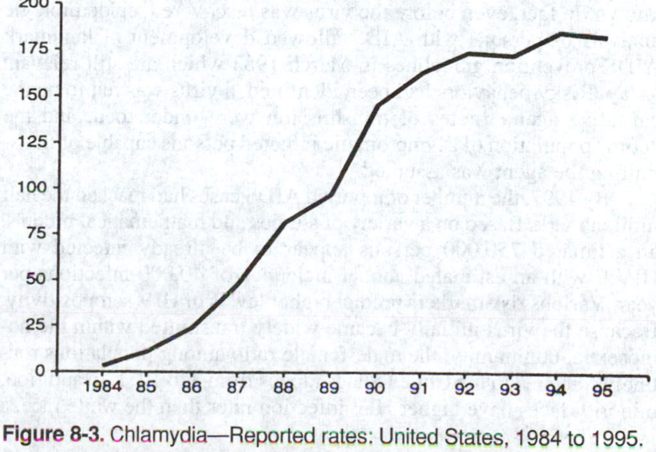

Figure 8-3. Chlamydia—Reported rates: United States, 1984 to 1995.

Large-scale screening programs in Region X demonstrated that younger women have consistently higher levels of chlamydia than older women. This persistent finding probably occurs for a variety of behavioral and biologic reasons: the greater likelihood of teenagers to have multiple sex partners rather than a single long-term relationship; the greater likelihood to engage in unprotected intercourse; the physiologically increased susceptibility due to increased ectopy and lack of immunity; and the lack of adequate health services, including the ability to pay, lack of transportation, or concerns about confidentiality.

Using gonorrhea as an index, chlamydia has been estimated to cause over 4 million infections in the United States.[14] An estimated 2.6 million infections occurred in women, 1.8 million in men, and one-quarter million in infants. The ratio of *C. trachomatis* to *N. gonorrhoeae* infection was influenced by at least five variables besides gender and age. These included race, pregnancy status, choice of contraception, the presence or absence of symptoms, and sexual preference. Considerably higher ratios of chlamydia to gonorrhea were found among whites, pregnant women, oral contraceptive users, and asymptomatic individuals; lower ratios were found among homosexual men.

Efforts to control chlamydia using strategies similar to those for gonorrhea have been successful. National chlamydia control guidelines were developed by CDC in 1985.[5] To make maximum use of then limited STD funds, recommendations for chlamydia control were primarily based on treating syndromes rather than specific infections. As chlamydia screening became more widespread, decreasing prevalence occurred among those receiving care at these facilities. In areas with the capacity to provide a full range of chlamydia clinical services such as diagnosis, screening, and partner notification, measurable declines in sexually transmitted chlamydial infections have occurred.[12] Moreover, screening programs to detect cervical chlamydia have produced lower levels of pelvic inflammatory disease (PID) in women effectively treated.[15]

Trichomoniasis

Trichomonal infections are the most common curable STD in the world, and probably also in the United States.[16] Based on estimates made from studies of the prevalence of *Trichomonas vaginalis* in selected populations, these vaginal and urethral organisms may cause upwards to 3 million infections annually in the United States. However, comprehensive surveillance data are not available. Ongoing trend information can be gleaned from estimates of visits to physicians' office practices provided by the National Disease and Therapeutic Index.[12] Based on this measure, the trend in diagnosed trichomonal infections has been declining over the last several decades, especially compared to the diagnosis of other vaginal infections.

▶ PERSISTENT VIRAL INFECTIONS

Human Immunodeficiency Virus

The epidemiology of HIV—and its fatal sequela AIDS—is well known. In fact, even before the virus was discovered, epidemiologic analysis of persons with AIDS allowed development of landmark AIDS prevention guidelines in March 1983 which are still relevant today. Risky behaviors had been identified, a virus was felt to be the causative agent, routes of transmission were understood, and the "core" population of asymptomatic infected persons capable of transmitting the agent was assumed.

By 1997, the number of reported AIDS cases had reached the half million mark. Based on a variety of studies and mathematical models, an estimated 750,000 persons appear to be already infected with HIV,[17] with an estimated annual incidence of 40,000 infections per year. Various risk markers predict higher levels of HIV seropositivity. Because the virus initially became widely transmitted within the homosexual community, the male-female ratio among populations routinely screened in the United States ranges from 3 to 10 : 1. In addition, minority races have higher HIV infection rates than the white race, a discrepancy that increases when excluding men who acquired HIV by having sex with other men. Finally, geography also strongly influences HIV infection levels. Persons on the Atlantic Coast and in South Florida, Puerto Rico, and San Francisco have higher rates.

Genital Herpes

Genital herpes also accounts for sizable morbidity. It is the main cause of genital ulcers in the United States, probably accounting for at least 10 times more cases than syphilis. The total number of physician-patient consultations[12] for genital herpes increased between 1966 and 1995, from 30,000 to more than 400,000. Initial visits—a more likely indicator of first genital infections—also increased nearly 10-fold over this same period, from 18,000 in 1966 to 175,000 in 1995 (Fig. 8-4). In 1991, the number of initial infections peaked, but has decreased over the past several years to levels seen in the 1980s. Adults aged 20 to 29 continued to account for most consultations; women visited physicians' offices more frequently than did men for genital herpes.

Symptomatic genital herpes infections are merely a tip of the iceberg. Only one-fourth of those with antibodies to HSV-2 give histories compatible with genital herpes infection.[18] Based on data from a national sample in 1990, over 40 million Americans are probably infected with HSV-2 today. African Americans are more likely to have HSV-2 antibodies than are whites. HSV-2 antibody prevalence was higher in women than in men.

Asymptomatic individuals are primarily responsible for sexual transmission of HSV. Three-fourths of those who had been the sources of infection for patients with documented primary HSV-2 infections gave no histories of genital lesions at the time of contact. Although all source contacts had HSV antibodies indicative of prior infection, only one-third had ever noticed any symptoms compatible with genital herpes.

Infection with HSV-2, as with syphilis, has been linked to higher risks of acquiring HIV infection. Presumably this is due to either genital or anorectal herpetic lesions (both recognized and unrecognized), which act as the portal of entry (or egress) for HIV.

Genital Human Papilloma Virus Infections

The frequency of consultations for symptomatic genital warts is more frequent than that for genital herpes,[19] and the key consequence associated with this infection, cervical neoplasia, more severe. In the United States, the number of physician-patient consultations for genital warts increased between 1966 and 1995, from 179,000 to about 1 million. Initial visits also increased[12] over the same period from 54,000 in 1966 to 250,000 in 1995 (Fig. 8-5). Persons from 20 to

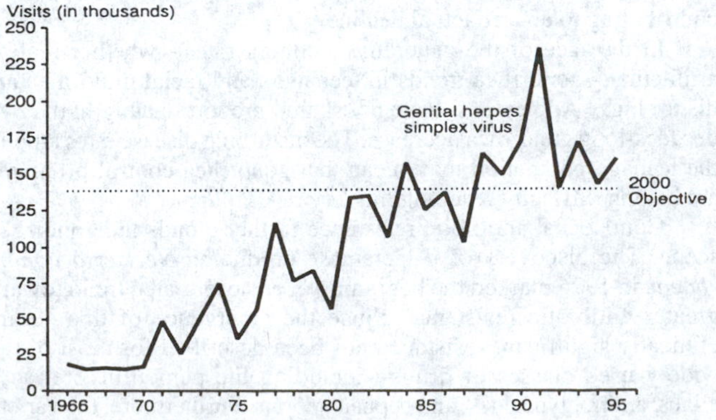

Figure 8-4. Genital herpes simplex virus infections—Initial visits to physicians' offices: United States, 1966 to 1995, and the Healthy People Year 2000 Objective. *(Source: National Disease and Therapeutic Index, IMS America, Ltd.)*

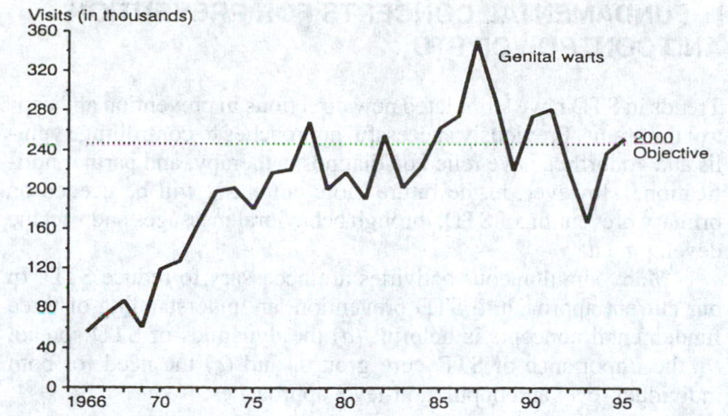

Figure 8-5. Human papilloma virus (genital warts)—Initial visits to physicians' offices: United States, 1966 to 1995, and the Healthy People Year 2000 Objective. *(Source: National Disease Therapeutic Index, IMS America, Ltd.)*

24 years of age had more frequent consultations for genital warts than did patients in other age groups; visits for women outnumbered those for men.

Even more than for genital herpes, genital warts represent only the symptomatic tip of the iceberg of HPV infections. As physician awareness and availability of diagnostic methods increase, subclinical papilloma virus infections of the male and female genital tract are becoming commonly recognized.[19] At present, serologic tests are still under development, and the virus cannot be grown in cell culture. HPV is now being detected by the polymerase chain reaction (PCR) in the cervix of a much higher percentage of sexually active women, many of whom have had normal cervical cytologic smears.

By 1995, more than 70 types of HPV had been described, each type differing on DNA homology by more than 50 percent determined by hybridization. At least 10 HPV types are associated with genital infection, of which types 16 and 18 are most closely associated with cervical cancer. Even these so-called high-risk types seem to be highly prevalent. For example, HPV type 16 has been detected by PCR in cervical specimens from over 10 percent of college students and over 20 percent of STD clinic patients in Seattle. The prevalence of HPV infection in men has been less well studied, but subclinical penile infection is thought to be common. Subclinical penile HPV infection has been detected by non-PCR DNA hybridization methods in nearly 10 percent of young healthy men.

Hepatitis B Virus Infections

Nationwide, the incidence of hepatitis B virus (HBV) has not declined appreciably in spite of both effective blood screening programs and the availability of a vaccine. Approximately 100,000 new HBV infections are caused by sexual transmission each year.[20] Nearly half of those infected suffer symptomatic acute hepatitis. However, the more serious concerns involve the effects of chronic HBV infection. Between 6 and 10 percent of those infected with HBV become chronic carriers. Chronic active hepatitis develops in more than 25 percent of carriers, and studies in Taiwan of persons infected at birth have shown a high risk of progression to cirrhosis and hepatocellular carcinoma. The natural history of HBV infection acquired sexually by adults has not yet been well studied.

Most HBV infections in the United States with known routes of transmission result from sexual exposure. Unfortunately, our vaccination programs have not successfully reached the populations that account for most HBV cases[20]—intravenous drug users, persons acquiring the disease through heterosexual exposure, and homosexual men. These groups have also been responsible for spreading the most HBV infection. Therefore, vaccination of seronegative members of these risk groups would be the most efficient method of interrupting transmission.

▸ TRENDS IN SYNDROMES CAUSED BY STD

Pelvic Inflammatory Disease

Pelvic inflammatory disease is one of the most severe complications of lower genital tract infections in women and has major public health consequences. Trends in PID have been similar to trends in gonorrhea in women.[12] Results of two national databases generated from physician office visits have demonstrated a consistent slow falloff from the peak number of PID cases in the mid-1970s. Unlike as in gonorrhea, the decline was greater among women of black and other races than among white women. The pace of decline of outpatient PID has picked up in the last several years. Initial visits for PID to physicians' offices declined from 1993 to 1995 (Fig. 8-6). In 1993, an estimated 313,000 women age 15 to 44 years were diagnosed with PID in emergency departments.

Hospitalized PID has followed a different course. Overall, rates increased slightly during the decades of the 1970s, with nearly all the increase occurring in young white women. However, beginning in the 1980s, hospitalized PID rates have fallen in all age and racial categories. This is consistent with trends in hospitalization for all causes during the same interval. One hypothesis for these trends is that the changing spectrum of sexually transmitted organisms (i.e., a decline in the incidence of gonorrhea relative to the incidence of chlamydial infection) has led to a greater proportion of subclinical PID. While chlamydial PID is less clinically severe, it smolders to produce subsequent tubal damage and reproductive sequelae.

The cumulative impact of PID affects a substantial portion of the female population. One in seven American women of reproductive age reported having had PID. The syndrome was reported twice as frequently among blacks as among whites; one in four black women and one in eight white women reported having received treatment for PID. As expected, the condition increased with age up to 35, and then plateaued.

Infertility

Involuntarily infertility, as well as requests for infertility services, also increased during the 1970s, but stabilized thereafter. The exact proportion of those infertile couples whose status is secondary to the consequences of STD is unknown; estimates have ranged from 15 to 30 percent, depending upon the populations involved and the types of infertility attributed to STD. Extrapolating from the number of PID cases, and assuming a 15 percent risk of infertility due to tubal occlusion after PID, between 100,000 and 150,000 women would be rendered involuntarily infertile each year because of pelvic infection

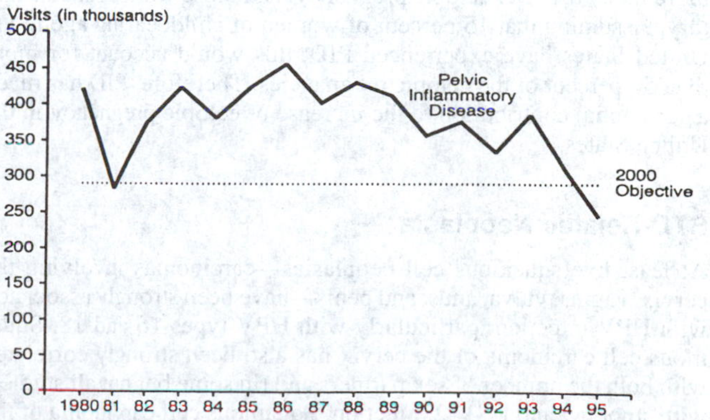

Figure 8-6. Pelvic inflammatory disease—Initial visits to physicians' offices by women 15 to 44 years of age: United States, 1980 to 1995, and the Healthy People Year 2000 Objective. *(Source: National Disease Therapeutic Index, IMS America, Ltd.)*

after STD. This estimate does not include causes of infertility that might also be related to STD (e.g., cervical factor infertility, chronic endometritis, epididymal occlusion).

Reproductive Outcomes

Prenatal STD also produce adverse effects on both pregnancy outcome and maternal infant health. The obstetrical consequences of syphilis are well known. Nearly 40 percent of pregnant women with recently acquired but untreated syphilis suffer a spontaneous abortion, a stillbirth, or a perinatal death. About half the infants who survive will be infected with *Treponema pallidum* and develop congenital syphilis. Gonococcal infection during pregnancy has been associated with an increased risk of chorioamnionitis, premature rupture of membranes, and prematurity in several retrospective studies.

The effects of other bacterial and protozoal STDs on pregnancy outcome are becoming clearer. For example, both bacterial vaginosis (BV) and trichomoniasis in pregnant women are associated with premature delivery of a low–birth weight infant. Women with BV were 40 percent more likely to deliver a premature infant compared with women without this condition;[21] women with trichomoniasis were slightly less likely, but still significantly greater than uninfected pregnant women.[22] Because these conditions are so common, their attributable risk for producing complications of pregnancy is higher than their other bacterial STD counterparts.

Finally, genital HSV and systemic HIV infection influence both pregnancy management and outcome. The risk of neonatal herpes is greatest when the mother experiences an initial attack of genital herpes at the time of delivery. In women with visible ulcers at the time of labor, cesarean deliveries have been recommended to reduce the risk of neonatal herpes. Although a large proportion of neonatal herpes cases occur without any history of genital lesions in the mother, screening prior to delivery for genital HSV shedding by the mother is not a cost-effective way to prevent neonatal herpes. Moreover, cesarean delivery solely for the purpose of preventing neonatal herpes is not indicated for asymptomatic women with only a history of genital herpes. Primary HSV infection during pregnancy has also been associated with spontaneous abortion.

Ectopic Pregnancy

Ectopic pregnancy increased dramatically during the 1970s and 1980s. Since 1965, the number of ectopic pregnancies quadrupled in the United States. Although some of this alarming rise may be attributable to improved detection of subclinical ectopic pregnancies, the data are consistent with a cumulative effect of PID causing tubal scarring, which eventually leads to an ectopic implantation should conception occur. Women with a history of PID are over eight times more likely to suffer ectopic pregnancy than those without such a history. Assuming that 15 percent of women of childbearing age in the United States have experienced PID, this would account for more than 50 percent of the ectopic pregnancies. Therefore, PID has made a substantial contribution to the increase of ectopic pregnancy in the United States.

STD-Related Neoplasia

At least five squamous cell neoplasias—carcinomas involving the cervix, vagina, vulva, anus, and penis—have been strongly associated with HPV infection, particularly with HPV types 16 and 18. Squamous cell carcinoma of the cervix has also been strongly correlated with both the number of sex partners and (in some but not all studies) with smoking and HSV-2 infection. Squamous cell carcinoma of the anus is greatly increased among homosexual men. Hepatocellular carcinoma is usually caused by hepatitis B virus, another sexually transmitted virus. Finally, Kaposi's sarcoma and non-Hidgkin's lymphomas themselves have a viral etiology and their clinical course may be accelerated by HIV immunosuppression.

► FUNDAMENTAL CONCEPTS FOR PREVENTION AND CONTROL OF STD

Trends in STD have stimulated new directions in prevention and control programs. Previously successful approaches to controlling syphilis and gonorrhea have relied on diagnosis, therapy, and partner notification.[5] However, in the future more emphasis will be needed on primary prevention of STD, through behavioral messages and vaccine development.

Many simultaneous activities are necessary to reduce STD. In our current approach to STD prevention, an understanding of three fundamental concepts is helpful: *(a)* the dynamics of STD spread, *(b)* the importance of STD core groups; and *(c)* the need for both individual-level and population-level approaches.

STD Transmission Dynamics

The forces responsible for sustaining transmission of any sexually transmitted infection can be represented in a simple equation, $R_0 = \beta \times C \times D$.[23] R_0 represents the reproductive rate of an infection, i.e., the number of new infections produced by an infected individual. β is the average probability that an infected individual will infect a susceptible partner given exposure. C is the average number of new partners acquired by an infected individual per unit of time. D is the average duration of infectiousness of the specific infection. Public health interventions to prevent STD are targeted at reducing the magnitude of β, C, or D by *(a)* reducing the probability of infecting a susceptible partner; *(b)* limiting the number of partners who have sex with infected persons; and *(c)* reducing the duration of infectiousness.

The probability of infecting a susceptible partner can be reduced by promoting condom use and safe sex practices (e.g., masturbation is the most safe and receptive anal intercourse is the most unsafe with respect to acquiring HIV or hepatitis B). The efficiency of transmitting HIV can also be reduced by controlling ulcerative and nonulcerative STDs. Promoting circumcision might reduce the acquisition of chancroid in countries where chancroid is now endemic. Prophylactic antibiotics can protect susceptible partners, and vaccination can lower the susceptibility of the available partner pool.

The average number of new partners acquired by an infected individual can be lowered if everyone in the population chose to have fewer sexual partners. Alternatively, reducing exposures by those with high-risk behaviors who are likely to be infected would more specifically target this behavioral approach. In the case of chronic, incurable viral STD, identifying those who are infected and encouraging them to have fewer partners, as well as to employ measures to reduce the efficiency of STD transmission, is essential.

The duration of infectiousness, for the curable STD, can be reduced by early diagnosis and curative treatment. This in turn can be improved by screening for asymptomatic infections; by improving recognition of STD symptoms; by motivating early health care seeking; by increasing access to good health care; and by notifying and treating sex partners.

STD "Core Groups"

The role of "core groups" (involving "high-frequency transmitters") in sustaining the spread of STD within a community is crucial.[24] In terms of the above equation, such subgroups of individuals may be less effective users of condoms, may have larger numbers of sex partners, and may have longer duration of infection (because of inadequate health care). Clearly, preventing a case of STD in a high-frequency transmitter[6] will have a greater impact on reducing subsequent transmission of STD in communities than preventing a case in individuals who are not high-frequency transmitters. Thus, public health interventions should include efforts to identify and reach members of STD core groups.

The concept of core groups extends beyond simply an aggregation of individuals to involve the complex dynamics of sexual networks.[25] In fact, definitions of "core groups" vary considerably depending upon whether the perspective is clinical-epidemiologic, mathematical, or sociocultural.[24] For example, the traditional STD clinical-epidemiologic core group perspective is drawn predominantly on individuals coming to an STD clinic and is prevention based on clinical STD management; those with repeat infections are seen as the "empiric core." From a mathematical perspective, however, core populations are defined as those infectious subgroups who transmit STDs to susceptible populations. Though useful for forecasting the potential effect of STD interventions, this mathematical view of core groups is less practical for identifying populations for targeted interventions. From the sociocultural perspective, core groups are defined through high levels of risky behaviors that increase the rate of STD transmission in a community. Such occupations as sex workers, truck drivers, migrant workers, or military personnel connote situations with high risks of STD transmission. These groups can be best accessed for preventive interventions outside of STD clinics. Moreover, specific interventions can be targeted to either reduce risky behaviors and/or reduce high prevalence of infections.

Finally, our approach to core populations has involved an increased understanding of the structure of sexual networks.[25] The increased rates of sexual interaction among people with a high prevalence of infection leads to extensive dissemination of STD within the population, rather than its being confined to specific subgroups.[5] So-called "spread networks" occur in groups marked by *(a)* higher rates of concurrent sexual relationships *(b)* many sexual exposures within that same subpopulation, and *(c)* moderate sexual "bridging" to other populations. Therefore, what has traditionally been referred to as separate core groups are in reality a variety of diverse sexual and social networks that contribute to STD epidemics through a complex set of sexual and health care behaviors. In this light, core populations are quite dynamic, representing a constantly changing ecology that demands different and creative interventions.

Individual-Level Versus Population-Level Approaches

As our understanding of the factors involved in both transmitting infections between individuals and their spread within populations has become more sophisticated, the realization of the differences in distinguishing between individual-level and population-level interventions has become integral to STD prevention strategies.[6] Both the individual- and the population-levels can be considered both as determinants of spread and as targets of prevention strategies. Thus, they provide approaches to intervention, as well as levels for measuring the impact of that intervention.

Depending upon whether STD prevention strategies are viewed from the individual or population perspective, a different emphasis emerges (Fig. 8-7). The objective of prevention from an individual perspective is to prevent acquisition of infection, to relieve symptoms, and to prevent further disease progression to more severe complications. However, from a population perspective, the object is to prevent transmission of infection and to intervene with those who are most likely to spread infection within a community. Therefore, the individual-level intervention would emphasize treating the exposed partner, but the population perspective would treat the "source partner" to reduce further transmission. Likewise, from an individual perspective, screening programs would be directed to individuals, and treatment would be provided for those found to be infected. From a population perspective, the prevalence of STD in specific groups would be determined, and mass treatment could be offered depending on the prevalence threshold.

Using syphilis as the ultimate STD paradigm, an individual-level approach would be to either detect and treat late syphilis or screen pregnant women to avoid congenital infection.[6] From a population perspective, detecting and treating early syphilis in its infectious stage eliminates the risk of community transmission, while screening female sex workers for syphilis focuses interventions on source populations capable of infecting many. Finally, from an individual perspective, promoting use of condoms with a primary partner reduces the risk of STD within this dyad; from a population viewpoint, promoting the use of condoms with nonprimary partners emphasizes reducing spread more widely within the population.

The importance of considering STD prevention from both an individual- and a population-level perspective allows policymakers to design reinforcing strategies for reducing *both* the transmission and the sequelae of STD. Individual-level activities are usually conducted in clinical settings where clients at increased risk might be found: STD clinics, family planning clinics, drug treatment centers, and other primary care facilities. Population-level interventions are delivered more broadly, using media communications to affect social norms. The sexual behaviors in the community at large are the target. These population-level "structural interventions," also called "en-

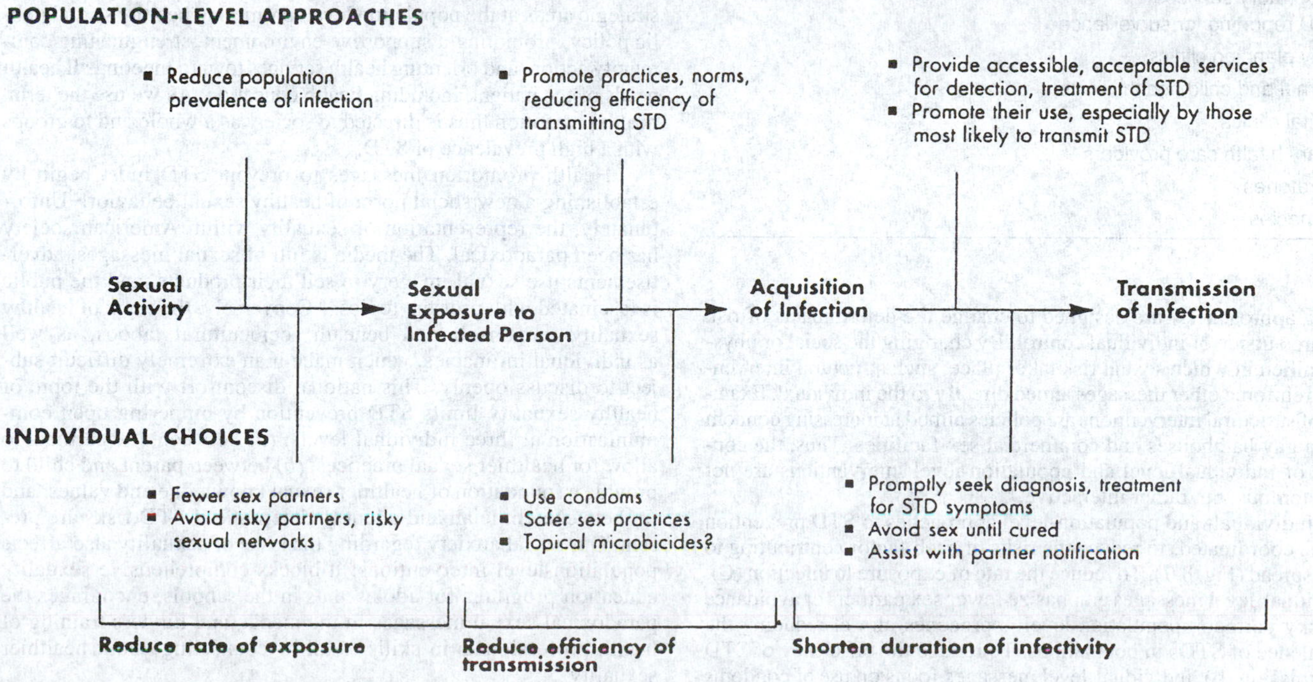

Figure 8-7. Individual-level and population-level approaches to STD prevention.

TABLE 8-4. ORGANIZATION AND LEVEL OF FUNCTIONAL RESPONSIBILITIES OF AN STD CONTROL PROGRAM

- ***SINGLE ADMINISTRATIVE DIRECTOR FOR STD/HIV***
- ***STD/HIV Program Management and Planning***

Set quantifiable objectives and plan for STD/HIV program (e.g., 3–5 years)
Coordinate planning with managers of related programs
Develop STD program guidelines for:
- Health promotion/behavioral intervention
- Laboratory services
- Patient management
- Counseling, testing, partner notification
- STD surveillance
- Surveillance of risk behaviors
- Evaluation, replanning of STD program, including all components of the program (e.g., health services)

Coordinate community involvement, coordinate training program
Resource-development and financial management, public relations

- ***Model STD/HIV Centers***

Implementation and feedback reporting to management
Health promotion
Clinical services (diagnosis and treatment), consultations
Laboratory services
Training (clinicians, technicians, counselors, managers)
Surveillance
Operational research
- Monitor treatment outcome
- Monitor antimicrobial resistance
- Evaluate new diagnostic tests
- Evaluate new treatments
- Evaluate health promotion

- ***Other STD/HIV Services***

STD clinics
- Health promotion
- STD diagnosis and treatment
- Counseling and partner notification
- Contraceptive counseling and services
- Laboratory services
- STD reporting for surveillance

Family planning clinics
Maternal and child health clinics
Hospital clinics
Primary health care providers
Laboratories
Pharmacies

abling approaches," are designed to change the determinants of risk that are outside of individual control. By changing the social or physical milieu in which sexual risk takes place, such structural interventions reinforce other messages aimed directly to the individual. Examples of structural interventions are policies aimed at increasing condom use in gay bathhouses and commercial sex facilities. Thus, the concepts of individual-level and population-level interventions are not dichotomous, but rather interactive.

Individual- and population-level approaches to STD prevention can be coordinated[8] to reduce the risks of each factor contributing to STD spread (Fig. 8-7). To reduce the rate of exposure to infection (C), individual-level messages emphasize fewer sex partners or avoidance of risky partners; population-level approaches aim at reducing the prevalence of STDs in populations. To reduce the efficiency of STD transmission (β), individual-level messages focus on use of condoms and safer sex practices; population-level approaches try to change social norms so that condom use becomes acceptable within different peer groups. Finally, to shorten the duration of infection (D), individual approaches emphasize prompt diagnosis and treatment if persons are symptomatic; population-level approaches make clinical services more accessible in communities and promote their use among high-prevalence sexual networks.

All the public health interventions we discuss should be designed and delivered differently, according to target groups. Health promotion and behavioral intervention messages can move from generalities to greater specificity as one approaches the target groups at highest risk.

▶ PREVENTION AND CONTROL STRATEGIES FOR STD

We will group the available strategies for STD prevention into eight somewhat overlapping categories: organization of STD control, health promotion, clinical skills, STD detection, STD treatment, patient counseling, partner notification, and use of vaccines.

Organization, Implementation, and Evaluation of an STD Control Program

At all levels of government where STD control programs are part of the health bureaucracy, the overall organization of the program, and the levels of specific functional responsibilities, must be clearly defined. A model program would include a program manager, one or more special STD centers, and a health care infrastructure that must provide STD program interventions (Table 8-4). The program manager is responsible for setting quantifiable objectives for the program, developing an overall strategy for STD control, and for participating in the evaluation of the program at regular intervals. This involves setting both process indicators (e.g., are services being provided at the level indicated?) and outcome indicators (e.g., is the incidence of STD falling?).

Health Promotion

Health promotion is an integral part of STD intervention activities. This concept is based on three principles: advocacy, enabling, and mediating. Broadly defined, health promotion encompasses four strategic areas at the population level: promoting healthy sexual public policy, promoting a supportive environment, strengthening community action, and orienting health services toward meeting all health needs of the patient, including health education. As we use the term, health promotion thus is directed to society as a whole and to groups with a high prevalence of STD.

Health promotion messages to prevent STD must begin by establishing a new social norm of healthy sexual behavior.[2] Unfortunately, the representation of sexuality within American society has been paradoxical. The media is full of sexual messages, advertisements use sexual imagery to sell their products, and the public is fascinated with prurient topics.[26] Conversely, the topic of healthy sexuality remains buried beneath sociocultural taboos, as well as individual intimacies, which make it an extremely difficult subject to discuss openly. This national discomfort with the topic of healthy sexuality limits STD prevention by hindering open communication at three individual levels: *(a)* between sex partners to allow for healthier sexual practices; *(b)* between parent and child to provide a foundation of healthier sexual knowledge and values; and *(c)* between clinician and client to determine if STD risks are present. Our social anxiety regarding the issue of sexuality also affects population-level interventions: it blocks comprehensive sexuality education programs for adolescents in the schools, encourages the paradoxical sexual messages in the media, and hinders training of health professionals in skills to allow counseling about healthier sexuality.

Traditional STD community health education efforts have usually encouraged primary prevention (preventing acquisition of an STD) in persons at risk. Through experience, we have found judgmental messages are not an effective method of changing behavior. In fact, stigmatizing infected individuals by widespread social disapproval may even hinder STD control through delaying care or increasing denial of high risk behaviors. Given concerns about HIV, public health officials are continually trying to balance their messages between creating excessive fear or excessive reassurance.[2] While fear can provide necessary stimulation for preventive actions, it can also lead to less rational responses, which undermine constructive programs.

School education strategies to increase the students' knowledge of the full spectrum of STD (including HIV) have gained momentum. Unfortunately, our past heritage of teaching about "VD" in high schools has generally consisted of didactic biomedical lectures concentrating only on syphilis and gonorrhea. To correct this situation, prototype school AIDS and STD curriculum materials for both teachers and students in grades 6 through 12 have been widely circulated. These curricula use a self-instructional format and emphasize behavioral skill building. Well-designed evaluations are under way to assess their impact on knowledge, behaviors, and STD/HIV outcomes.

National hotlines in the United States for both STD and AIDS provide general information and specific answers to questions of all callers. These hotlines are funded by the Centers for Disease Control and Prevention and operated by the American Social Health Association. In 1996, more than 1.5 million calls were answered on both the STD hotline and the AIDS hotline. A large proportion of callers are referred to confidential medical services in either the public or private sector. Many state and local hotlines for AIDS and STD are also operated throughout the United States and AIDS hotlines are being used in other countries.

In the future, we need to make better use of the mass media for promoting healthy sexuality as a national objective. Awareness of AIDS is widespread largely because of the attention given these conditions by the media. Teenagers are a special audience for the broadcast media; they spend an average of 23 hours a week listening to radio or watching television.[26] Public service announcements are increasingly being aired to encourage condom use in high-risk settings and to publicize hotline numbers for further questions.

STD Clinical Training

Medical schools in the United States have responded slowly to the increasing magnitude of the STD/HIV problem. A survey conducted in 1991 showed more than three-quarters of American medical schools had increased the amount of STD clinical training for their students.[17] This occurred just when American physicians need STD training the most; the majority enter specialties requiring knowledge of STD diagnosis and treatment. In 1996, nearly two-thirds of first-year residents chose internal medicine, pediatrics, obstetrics and gynecology, family practice, emergency medicine, and dermatology. Without training in STD problems, the medical community cannot be effectively mobilized to support control programs.

While an increasing percentage of American medical students appear to be receiving some training in STD clinical care, the quality of this training remains a problem. For example, the 1991 survey showed that links to a dedicated STD clinic existed in less than half of medical schools providing training, and only one-third offered students a full clinical elective in STD/HIV. Because typical primary care ambulatory settings allow only infrequent encounters with STD clients, adequate clinical skills in diagnosis and treatment may be limited. Moreover, even though the American Medical Association has developed guidelines for improving clinical communication skills in assessing STD risks, relatively few schools have included such sensitive sexual history-taking techniques into their typical primary care training. Therefore, the current system for clinical training of health care professionals is less than ideal for producing primary care providers effective in managing STD.

Most clinicians are incapable of taking an adequate sexual history; inquiring about the intimate details of their patient's sexual practices and partners does not come naturally. These skills must be taught. Clinicians could include a brief sexual history while patients are being asked about such behaviors as smoking, alcohol and other drugs, exercise, sleep patterns, etc. Eliciting a history of prior STD is important as an index of sexual risk-taking behavior. The need for reinforcing safer sexual messages to help prevent the curable bacterial STD to incurable viral STD makes it particularly important that clinicians shift their emphasis toward helping clients to adopt a healthy sexual lifestyle.

Recent STD training initiatives have taken three approaches. First, to respond to immediate needs, clinical practice guidelines have been developed by CDC and the World Health Organization (WHO) to assist active STD services in improving patient management. For STD clinicians, national STD treatment recommendations are regularly reviewed to reflect changing diagnostic capabilities, antibiotic susceptibilities, and pharmaceutical innovations.[28] In addition, a variety of useful clinical publications have been produced aimed at primary care physicians to allow a syndromic approach to STD patient management.[28a]

Second, federally funded regional STD prevention and training centers integrate a university medical school with a model public STD clinic for purposes of providing training for midcareer clinicians, as well as for medical, nursing, and paramedical students. Training curricula are updated annually and include management of the HIV-infected patient. By 1996, nine such multidisciplinary centers were in operation; over 15,000 clinicians have been trained in these facilities since 1979.[7]

Third, clinical and research training support has been provided directly by CDC, NIH, and the American Social Health Association to medical schools. These funds help train a cadre of medically qualified clinicians and researchers who have a career commitment to the STD discipline. Faculty role models and challenging clinical clerkships are the most important influences on students' choice of their specialty. Once interested in STD, these individuals are able to establish their own STD academic programs, thus multiplying the effect of the training efforts. However, despite these efforts, as of 1995, STD research and/or STD clinical training centers existed in less than 10 percent of American medical schools.

STD Detection

Early detection of infection is crucial to STD intervention strategies. Early detection affects primary prevention (by decreasing the duration of infectiousness) and secondary prevention (by leading to treatment before complications). Case-finding methods include presumptive clinical diagnosis based on symptoms and signs, confirmatory laboratory testing in patients with suggestive symptoms or signs, targeted laboratory diagnostic testing in individuals at high risk, broader screening without regard to likelihood of STD (e.g., premarital testing, testing of blood donor), and locating sex partners of persons with STD.

Whether for making specific diagnoses in those with symptoms or for screening persons without symptoms, tests for STD should ideally be inexpensive, rapid, simple, and accurate. Our current methods for diagnosing the common STD incorporate these principles (Table 8-5). However, for many less-developed countries, constraints on expense and simplicity are so great that few of these tests can be used, except in specialized central laboratories. Therefore, use of STD risk assessment and syndrome management has been encouraged. Even in more developed countries, constraints on expense have delayed introduction of some diagnostic tests—for example, *C. trachomatis*—despite situations where such tests are cost-effective.

The usual parameters for assessing diagnostic techniques—sensitivity, specificity, and predictive value—have certain unique implications for STD control. STD treatment is generally shorter

TABLE 8-5. CURRENT METHODS FOR DIAGNOSING COMMON SEXUALLY TRANSMITTED DISEASES

Presumptive Diagnosis	*Definitive Diagnosis*
• ***Neisseria gonorrhoeae***	
Microscopic identification of typical Gram-negative intracellular diplococci on smear of urethral exudate (men) or endocervical material (women) or Growth on selective medium demonstrating typical colonial morphology, positive oxidase reaction, and typical Gram-stain morphology.	Growth on selective medium demonstrating typical colonial morphology, positive oxidase reaction, and typical gram-stain morphology; confirmed by sugar utilization, coagglutination, or antigonococcal fluorescent antibody (FA) testing. A definitive diagnosis is required if specimen is (*a*) extragenital, (*b*) from a child, or (*c*) medicolegally significant.
• ***Chlamydia trachomatis***	
Mucopurulent cervicitis The presence of yellow mucopurulent endocervical exudate or the finding of this exudate on a white cotton-tipped swab of endocervical secretions. In women without visible mucopus, the presence of >10 polymorphonuclear leukocytes per ×1000 field on a Gram-stained specimen of endocervical mucus (without contamination by vaginal cells) also allows a presumptive diagnosis.	Definitive diagnosis is made by growth on cycloheximide-treated McCoy cells. Fluorescent monoclonal antibody stains or enzyme-linked immunoassay (ELISA) tests are also widely available. If confirmatory tests are not available, empirical therapy can be given on clinical grounds
Nongonococcal urethritis (NGU) Symptomatic men are presumed to have NGU when their gonorrhea tests are negative and they have either white blood cells on Gram's stain of urethral discharge or sexual exposure to an agent known to cause NGU. Asymptomatic men with negative gonorrhea tests are also presumed to have NGU if they have >4 polymorphonuclear leukocytes per ×1000 field on an intraurethral smear.	Same as above.
• ***Treponema pallidum***	
Primary: Patients have typical lesion(s) and newly positive serological test for syphilis (STS), or their present STS titer is at least 4-fold greater than the last, or there has been syphilis exposure within 90 days of lesion onset. *Secondary:* Patients have the typical clinical presentation and a strongly reactive STS. *Latent:* Patients have serological evidence of untreated syphilis without clinical signs.	Primary and secondary syphilis are definitively diagnosed by demonstrating *T. pallidum* with darkfield microscopy or FA techniques in material from a chancre, regional lymph node, or other lesion. A definitive diagnosis of latent syphilis cannot be made under usual circumstances.
• ***Herpes Simplex Virus***	
When typical genital lesions are present or a pattern of recurrence has developed, herpes infection is likely. A presumptive diagnosis is further supported by direct identification of multinucleated giant cells with intranuclear inclusions in a clinical specimen prepared by Pap or other histochemical stain, by typical HSV morphology by electron microscopy, or by detection of HSV antigens by monoclonal or polyclonal antibody detection systems.	An HSV virus tissue culture demonstrates the characteristic cytopathogenic effect (CEP) following inoculation of a specimen from the cervix, the urethra, or the base of a genital lesion. The isolates can be identified as type 1 or type 2 by FA, neutralization, or other serological techniques.
• ***Human Papilloma Virus***	
A diagnosis may be made on the basis of the typical clinical presentation. Colposcopy may also aid in the diagnosis of certain cervical lesions. Exclude the possibility of condylomata lata by obtaining a darkfield or serological test for syphilis.	A biopsy, although usually unnecessary, is required to make a definitive diagnosis. Very atypical lesions, where neoplasia is a consideration, should be biopsied before initiating therapy. A Pap smear of cervical lesions shows typical cytological changes.
• ***Human Immunodeficiency Virus***	
A presumptive diagnosis of HIV infection usually is based on clinical evidence.	A diagnosis of asymptomatic HIV infection usually is made on the basis of a repeatedly reactive ELISA test followed by a reactive supplemental test (e.g., Western blot or immunofluorescent assay or indirect FA) Polymerase chain reaction (PCR) is a gene amplification technique that has been used as a research tool to detect infection before detectable levels of antibody are found by ELISA or Western blot techniques. Although isolation of the virus from body fluids is the most highly specific means to make a definitive diagnosis of HIV infection, such testing is not widely available.

and safer than therapy for many chronic conditions. Moreover, as discussed earlier, curing STD in one individual frequently prevents infection in others. Consequently, achieving high sensitivity by reducing false negatives becomes a priority. Achieving high specificity by reducing false positives is less important from the public health perspective when treatment is safe, simple, and inexpensive. However, if false-positive tests trigger provider-based partner notification, additional expenses must be considered. Furthermore, from the individual's perspective, the emotional costs of erroneously stigmatizing someone as having an STD means specificity cannot be ignored.

Deficiencies in *sensitivity* of STD tests cause particular problems in populations with a high prevalence of a curable infection with serious morbidity. For example, a new test for chlamydia with a sensitivity of 80 percent in women would fail to identify 20 percent of infected women. If the prevalence of chlamydia in women at an STD clinic is 30 percent, then 6 women of 100 tested would not be identified, and would be at risk for both developing salpingitis and spreading the infection.

Deficiencies in *specificity* of STD tests can also cause difficulties, especially in low-prevalence populations. For example, a new test for *C. trachomatis* with a specificity of 90 percent and sensitivity of 100 percent, when used in a low-prevalence population (1 percent), would produce almost 10 times as many false-positive tests as true-positive tests. Referring and evaluating 11 individuals and their sex partners to identify just a single infected person and that person's exposed partner(s) would tax clinical personnel and cause unnecessary anxiety. In public health terms, testing 20,000,000 women using the new test would increase the follow-up burden from approximately 200,000 with culture diagnoses to 2,200,000 individuals from the new test. Such an increase could overwhelm clinical resources.

Even with highly specific tests (specificity ≥99 percent), screening for STD of very low prevalence (<0.1 percent) creates many false positives. Thus, tests such as the fluorescent treponemal antibody-absorption (FTA-ABS) or *Treponema pallidum* hemagglutination (TPHA) test for syphilis, although highly specific and having high positive predictive value in patients with positive reagin tests for syphilis, are not recommended for screening the general population for syphilis. In the United States, the prevalence of syphilis has become so low in many areas that the cost-effectiveness of serologic screening and case-finding with the less expensive and less specific reagin tests (e.g., in premarital examinations, blood banking services, and new admissions to hospitals) is being abandoned. Because yield and cost considerations are particularly important to screening activities, selection of the target population directly influences these factors.

To make most effective use of resources, targeted case-finding and screening has been recommended *(a)* in high prevalence groups such as commercial sex workers, homosexual men, and illicit drug users; *(b)* in facilities (jails, emergency rooms) where high levels of STD might be expected; and *(c)* in pregnant women in whom STD could cause adverse pregnancy outcomes. In the United States, testing sex workers for syphilis, chancroid, and resistant gonorrhea has proved particularly useful for stemming specific outbreaks in Los Angeles and New York City. Experience using mobile vans to provide STD screening to those visiting crack houses in Philadelphia has also been encouraging.

STD Treatment

Treatment based on presumptive diagnosis should be inexpensive, simple, safe, and effective. Early and adequate treatment of patients and their sexual partners is an effective means of preventing the community spread of STD. National treatment recommendations are an essential part of STD control strategies worldwide.[28] Initially, in the United States these recommendations covered syphilis and gonorrhea, but have been expanded in the 1980s and 1990s to include more than 20 other sexually transmitted organisms and syndromes. Current regimens for treating common STDs have been derived from clinical consensus among a group of experts (Table 8-6).

Selective prophylactic (preventive or "epidemiological") treatment of individuals also has a major role in STD control strategies. In certain clinical instances, as with many other infectious diseases, it is preferable to offer treatment to clients on the basis of presumptive diagnosis or sexual exposure, before the specific diagnosis is

TABLE 8-6. CURRENT REGIMENS FOR TREATING COMMON SEXUALLY TRANSMITTED DISEASES

Recommended Treatment
• ***Neisseria gonorrhoeae***
Cefixime, 400 mg, orally in a single dose or 725 mg IM once, *plus* doxycycline, 100 mg orally 2 times a day for 7 days or azithromycin, 1 gm orally in a single dose.
• ***Chlamydia trachomatis***
Doxycycline, 100 mg orally 2 times a day for 7 days, azithromycin, 1 gm orally in a single dose.
• ***Traponema pallidum***
Primary, secondary, or early syphilis of less than 1 year's duration: Benzathine penicillin G, 2 4 million units IM. Syphilis of indeterminate length or of more than 1 year's duration. Benzathine penicillin G, 7.2 million units total, administered as 2.4 million units IM given 1 week apart for 3 consecutive weeks. Neurosyphilis [inpatient therapy recommended; see STD Treatment Guidelines for outpatient regimen]. Aqueous crystalline penicillin G, 12–24 million units total, administered as 2–4 million units q4h IV, for 10–14 days.
• ***Herpes Simplex Virus***
No known cure. Systemic acyclovir treatment may reduce symptoms and signs of herpes episodes and may accelerate healing but does not eradicate the infection or effect subsequent recurrence.
First Clinical Episode of Genital Herpes
Acyclovir, 200 mg orally 5 times daily for 7 to 10 days or until clinical resolution occurs.
Recurrent Episodes
Acyclovir, 200 mg orally 5 times daily for 5 days initiated within 2 days of onset, *or* acyclovir, 800 mg orally 2 times a day for 5 days.
Suppression of Recurrent Genital Herpes Infection
Continuous treatment reduces the frequency of active disease by at least 75% among patients with frequent [at least 6/y] recurrences. Dosage must be individualized for each patient. Acyclovir 200 mg orally 2 to 5 times daily, *or* acyclovir, 400 mg orally 2 times daily.
• ***Human Papilloma Virus***
Cryotherapy with liquid nitrogen [or cryoprobe for external genital/perianal warts].
Alternative Treatments for External Genital/Perianal/Vaginal Warts
Podophyllin, 10%–25% in compound tincture of benzoin, trichloroacetic acid, 80%–90%. Note: For women with cervical warts, dysplasia must be excluded before treatment is begun. Management should therefore be carried out in consultation with an expert.
• ***Human Immunodeficiency Virus***
For persons with HIV infection, combination antiviral therapy including zidovudine (ZDV, formerly called AZT), other nucleoside reverse transcriptase and protease inhibitors have been shown to be effective in reducing viral load and preventing the clinical conditions associated with AIDS. In persons with AIDS, it has been shown to prolong life. Aerosolized pentamidine has been shown to be effective in preventing *Pneumocystis carinii* pneumonia. Both of these drugs have serious side effects and require careful monitoring by knowledgeable clinicians. For persons in whom AIDS has been diagnosed, standard therapy consists of treating opportunistic diseases aggressively as they occur. See JAMA 276: 146-154, 1996

confirmed. In addition, based on epidemiological indications, antibiotics can be administered to high-risk individuals when infection is considered likely, in the interest of public health gains. This philosophy underlies the CDC recommendation for giving azithromycin concurrently with penicillin to patients with confirmed gonococcal infections, since a relatively high proportion are likely to be harboring coexistent *C. trachomatis*. This presumptive treatment approach offers three main advantages: *(a)* it interrupts the chain of transmission and prevents complications that might occur between the time of testing and treatment; *(b)* it ensures treatment for infected individuals with false-negative laboratory tests; and *(c)* it guarantees treatment for those who might not return when notified of positive tests.

At the population level, an analogous strategy of selective preventive treatment has helped to limit outbreaks of syphilis, resistant gonorrhea, and chancroid in metropolitan areas of the United States. Within certain communities with high prevalence of infection, mass antibiotic treatment has been useful. In Rakai, Uganda, a community-based randomized controlled trial of biannual mass prophylaxis has produced encouraging results. Single-dose treatments with azithromycin, ciprofloxacin, and metronidazole were provided to the intervention communities, whereas the comparison communities received mass antihelminth treatment, iron/folate, and referral for STD treatment. Preliminary data revealed that community-based mass STD treatment is feasible and that significant reductions in genital ulcer disease, syphilis, and trichomoniasis occurred in the intervention communities.[29]

Counseling of Patients

Because of HIV and other incurable viral STDs, individual counseling (e.g., educating) of patients to facilitate changes in their behavior has taken on a new importance. Clients with an STD in any clinical setting are a crucial target group. Because of their own or their partner's behavior, they need both treatment and preventive counseling. The key behaviors to emphasize to those already infected include: *(a)* responding to disease suspicion by promptly seeking appropriate medical evaluation, *(b)* taking oral medications as directed, *(c)* returning for follow-up tests when applicable, *(d)* promoting concern for sex partners and assuring examination and treatment of partners when indicated, *(e)* avoiding future sexual exposure while infectious, and *(f)* preventing exposure by using condoms in high-risk settings.

Risk-reduction counseling to prevent acquisition or transmission of STD has become ingrained as a standard part of STD clinical care, whether provided in public STD clinics, other public health facilities, or private physician offices. In those areas of the world where health care is provided by nurses, pharmacists, and traditional practitioners (e.g., traditional birth attendants, who attend the majority of deliveries in rural areas in developing countries), these individuals also should be trained to provide such counseling. The emergence of persistent viral infections has lessened the role of curative treatment and simultaneously raised the need for risk reduction counseling (primary prevention). The need for "safer sex" has captured worldwide attention because of HIV infection.

Risk-reduction counseling is much more than emphasizing condom use. If they are to reduce their risks, patients need to understand the importance of inquiring about the risk behaviors of their partners. They need to know which sexual practices reduce the potential risk of infection and which practices carry highest risk. They should be introduced to the social skills essential to negotiating safer behaviors with their partners. Counselors need to maintain nonjudgmental attitudes in discussing potential lifestyle changes. Unrealistic recommendations will either be ignored or will lead to only short-term changes. Patients must find the counseling messages comprehensible, acceptable, and attainable.

Partner Notification

Traditionally, STD control programs in the more developed countries have emphasized active intervention by the health providers to interview the client, to identify the sex partners, and to assure that these exposed individuals are evaluated and treated. The privacy of original index patients and their partners is rigorously protected. During the 1970s in the United States, due to the expanded spectrum of infections, a process of active notification was modified in many settings to encourage the client to assume responsibility for locating and referring his or her sex partners.

This client referral method actively involves them in the disease control effort, is relatively inexpensive, is acceptable to many patients, and reserves scarce staff time for targeted provider referral. Potential shortcomings of client referral methods, however, include *(a)* limited effectiveness with noncompliant clients, and *(b)* difficulty in evaluating its outcomes.

Active provider referral (i.e., partner notification by the public health staff) is more labor-intensive, time-consuming, and expensive; therefore, active provider referral frequently concentrates on high-yield cases or on high-risk "core" environments. Despite the initial costs, provider referral can be cost-beneficial because of its greater yield of infected persons and because most of these sex partners are high-frequency transmitters of STD. Special situations where this strategy has been useful include: *(a)* partners of persons infected with HIV who might not otherwise realize that they have been exposed to infection; *(b)* introduction of a serious disease (e.g., syphilis or resistant gonorrhea infection) into a community previously unaffected; *(c)* men and women with repeated STD infections; and *(d)* STD infections in children.

Clinicians providing clinical preventive services may find it especially difficult to notify the sex partner(s) of their long-standing clients. Not only do such issues as infidelity, homosexuality, and/or child abuse generate human anxieties, but also the potential need for marital counseling may require skills and time that the clinician does not have. More training in this delicate area is necessary to provide private clinicians with skills and justification for partner notification.

Vaccines

Hepatitis B virus vaccine has been available for a decade and a half, but has not yet been efficiently deployed to prevent sexual transmission of HBV.[20] Since sexual transmission has been implicated as the principal route of transmission of the virus in the more developed countries, vaccination strategies for preventing sexual transmission have been developed.

During the 1980s, hepatitis B vaccine had been initially recommended for persons at high risk of acquiring HBV infection, including men who have sex with men and those attending STD clinics. However, in the early 1990s, public health officials realized that this strategy was having little effect on the overall incidence of hepatitis B in the United States. Awareness of the difficulties in identifying and immunizing high-risk persons focused on the problems of initial acceptance of the vaccine, as well as compliance with the full three-dose schedule. This recognition led to a change to a longer-term 3-fold strategy to reduce HBV infection: *(a)* prevention of perinatal transmission; *(b)* routine immunization of infants, and *(c)* "catch-up" vaccination of children, adolescents, and high-risk adults not previously immunized.

Vaccines against other STDs have been disappointing. Apart from hepatitis B, trials of immunizing agents against both bacterial and viral STDs have shown at best only short-term elevations in correlates of immunity. Little individual or communitywide immunity was found in the larger trials of gonorrhea or HSV vaccines. Moreover, hopes for an HPV vaccine have gone unrealized. Finally, despite the heightened attention for an HIV vaccine, only phase I and phase II clinical trials are currently under way. No realistic expectations for a new STD vaccine should be entertained until the twenty-first century.

► STD IN DEVELOPING COUNTRIES

Magnitude of the Problem

While population-based information on STD is generally lacking, sexually transmitted infections are common problems in nearly all developing countries.[30] Health care visits for lower genital tract complaints are extremely numerous, adding more stress to the already overburdened health care services of resource-poor nations. As in the United States, HIV commands center stage as the "international STD." Trichomoniasis, chlamydia, gonorrhea, syphilis, and chancroid are also of great concern because they are curable conditions and because they contribute to HIV spread.[16]

In developing countries, few nations have rudimentary surveillance systems; therefore, STD incidence is usually derived from attendance at health care facilities. STD prevalence is typically extrapolated from studies performed on selected high-risk populations. While these data provide useful estimates, they must be viewed with even more caution than reports from the developed world.

WHO has used a simple prevalence model to estimate the magnitude of curable STD worldwide.[16] Using the available information on STD prevalence from developing countries, including Africa, Asia, Latin America, and the Caribbean, prevalence rates of gonorrhea, chlamydial infection, syphilis, and trichomoniasis were estimated by gender and by United Nation region. The 1995 regional "denominator" was calculated using midyear population estimates of adults 15 to 49 years of age. Next, the duration of each curable infection was estimated by gender and by region. These duration estimates were based on the probability that a symptomatic or asymptomatic person received treatment of her or his STD. Regional STD incidence in adults was then calculated by dividing the estimated prevalence by the estimated duration of each disease. Although based on broad assumptions, this WHO approach provides a standardized mechanism to make global estimates for public health purposes.

The epidemiology of STDs in developing countries differs greatly from the situation in industrialized nations.[31] Overall, STDs are a more frequent health problem in developing countries. WHO estimates that at least 333 million new cases of curable STD will occur globally in 1995.[16] The bulk of these will be in developing countries. STDs are among the top five causes of consultation at health services in Cameroon, representative of many African countries; and among adults, STD is the leading diagnosis. In Zimbabwe, up to 10 percent of the population had a documentable STD. Intensive studies of women in India, Bangladesh, Uganda, and Egypt have found STD rates ranging from 52 to 92 percent, less than half of which were recognized by the women as abnormal.[32,33] Further, among STD syndromes, the etiology of genital ulcer infection apparently differs from that in the developed world. Syphilis and chancroid are the major causes of genital ulcers in tropical countries, with genital herpes accounting for a smaller proportion of the asymptomatic conditions.

Syphilis in developing countries remains at levels seen half a century ago in industrialized nations. The interpretation of serological tests for syphilis is difficult since seropositivity could be due to sexually transmitted infection or to previous infection with nonvenereal treponematosis. Realizing these limitations, past syphilis infections among prenatal populations in the developing countries have ranged from 1 percent in Saudi Arabia to 33 percent in Swaziland. In one population of rural Somalia, nearly one-quarter of men and women in the general population had past evidence of syphilis. WHO estimates that in 1995 approximately 12 million new cases of adult syphilis will occur worldwide, with the greatest number in South Asia and sub-Saharan Africa.[16] Thus, syphilis is highly prevalent in developing countries, and considerable risk for congenital syphilis exists in many areas.

In the developing world, gonorrhea, like syphilis, is more prevalent than in industrialized countries. Estimates for large cities in Africa suggest an annual gonorrhea rate of between 3,000 and 10,000 cases per 100,000 inhabitants.[31] These frequencies have been extrapolated mainly from attendance at general health care centers or from special surveys of prevalence in population groups that may not be representative. Surveys of gonorrhea in pregnant women have ranged from less than 1 percent in Malaysia to 40 percent in Uganda. Among women attending family planning clinics, rates have ranged from 2 percent in Swaziland to 17 percent in Kenya. In 1995, WHO estimates that approximately 62 million new cases of gonorrhea will have occurred among adults worldwide; as with syphilis, the greatest number will be transmitted in South Asia and sub-Saharan Africa.[16]

Genital chlamydial infections in the developing world have a similar prevalence to those in the developed world, both occurring at high levels. Among pregnant women, chlamydial infections are more frequent than are gonococcal infections, with rates ranging from 6 percent in Nigeria to 29 percent in Kenya. Among men with symptoms of urethritis, rates of chlamydial infection (as measured by nongonococcal urethritis) appear to be lower than in the developed world. However, because chlamydia causes less symptomatic infections, patients may not be motivated to seek treatment in resource-poor areas where health care is difficult to obtain. In 1995, WHO estimates that approximately 89 million new cases of chlamydia will occur among adults worldwide; and again, as with syphilis and gonorrhea, the greatest number will be transmitted in South Asia and sub-Saharan Africa.[16]

Chancroid is highly endemic in many tropical countries, particularly in Southeast Asia and Eastern and Southern Africa.[30] The global incidence of chancroid is probably equivalent to that of syphilis, with a resurgence of interest occurring due to the availability of new methods for detecting the causative organism, *Haemophilus ducreyi*. As in the developed world, commercial sex workers and their clients play a crucial role in the spread of chancroid within developing nations.

Based on extrapolations from selected local studies, WHO estimates that trichomoniasis is the most common curable STD.[16] Prevalence rates among women attending antenatal clinics range from 12 percent in Kenya to 47 percent in Botswana. Though trichomonal infection is frequently asymptomatic in men, cross-sectional screening has found this infection in nearly one-quarter of Nigerian male and female adolescents. In 1995, WHO estimates 170 million new cases of trichomoniasis will occur among adults worldwide, especially in developing countries.[16]

Though even fewer data are available on sexually transmitted *viral* infections in the developing nations, their levels are quite high. Serologic studies have found that asymptomatic herpes simplex type 2 infections are frequently more common than evidence of past syphilis. Likewise, HPV has been the most prevalent STD found in selected studies, even when compared to vaginal bacterial infections. Finally, in Asia and elsewhere, hepatitis B virus (HBV) is widespread; this virus is transmitted not only among sexual partners, but also from mothers to their newborns.

HIV infection in the developing world has been predominantly transmitted through heterosexual behaviors.[8] As of 1996, an estimated 32 million persons were infected worldwide, of whom 14 million were in sub-Saharan Africa.[34] The HIV epidemic emerged later in Asia; however, rapid increases have occurred in both South and Southeast Asia. A striking increase in the percentage of HIV-infected commercial sex workers in Thailand and India, for example, provides a harbinger of future levels of HIV infection among the general population in these countries. It is hoped that the encouraging recent trends in Thailand of both STD and HIV declining, attributed to the success of the country's 100 percent condom policy, will be the model for other countries to follow.[34–36]

The level of so-called endogenous STD among women in developing countries is typically even higher than the traditional STDs. In rural India, upon careful physical examination and laboratory investigation, 92 percent of women were found to have genital infections.[24] Less than half of these women had reported any STD symptoms when interviewed prior to being examined. Similar situations were found both in Egypt, in another region in India, and in Uganda. The type of dominant endogenous infection varied among the populations, although bacterial vaginosis and candidiasis were both common.

Determinants of Global STD

Into the twenty-first century continued demographic and behavioral factors will further influence STD in developing countries. The number of young people—the group at highest risk for STD—and their proportion in the population will increase because of the existing high fertility levels. In developing countries, approximately half the population is under the age of 15. Thus, this population is entering the age when they are beginning sexual activity and the age group with the highest STD prevalence. This will drive the number of STD cases even higher in developing countries, further exacerbating their STD problems.

Other determinants of global STD epidemiology are important to developing countries. For example, decreases in infant and childhood mortality rates from successful immunization and diarrhea control programs will reinforce the population growth trend. Population shifts from rural to urban areas, where STD rates are higher, have proceeded rapidly in most of the developing world. The growing use of contraceptives that do not protect against STD may further alter patterns of sexual behavior, particularly among women. In addition, increasing educational opportunities for women in some developing countries may delay marriage, also increasing STD risks.

Worldwide communication and transportation patterns affect STD. The rapid social transition in developing countries has produced corresponding changes in values between generations. Diffusion of cultural values from developed countries to developing countries introduces new social concepts. Migration, particularly temporary labor migration, expanded mass communications, and educational exchanges are substantial and further broaden the generation gap since youth are more receptive to riskier sexual values.

STD Clinical Management

In developing countries, comprehensive case management of STDs, the cornerstone of STD control, is limited by the available technologies and resources. Specific constraints include: *(a)* lack of access to the laboratory methods necessary for making specific etiologic diagnoses of STDs; *(b)* shortages of well-trained staff; and *(c)* high work loads with limited staff time available for each client.

In these resource-poor settings, appropriate diagnostic tools should be modified to enable health care workers to maximize their chances of making the correct diagnosis in most cases. Since 1990, a syndromic approach to STD case management has allowed health care workers to make diagnoses without sophisticated laboratory tests.[37] This approach is based on defining a group of recognizable symptoms and convenient signs (e.g., a syndrome) associated with a number of clearly identified STD organisms. Once this syndrome has been detected, treatment can be provided for the majority of organisms responsible for that syndrome.

Clinical flowcharts have been established for several STD syndromes, allowing them to be managed easily and rapidly. These clinical algorithms (also called decision trees) portray pathways of clinical diagnostic reasoning. Standardized medical decision-making has many advantages: *(a)* it simplifies STD data collection and analysis, which in turn helps in planning for drugs and supplies; *(b)* it assists in STD surveillance, making reports from different health facilities comparable; *(c)* it facilitates training and supervision of health care workers because a similar approach to STD management is used in each case; and *(d)* it ensures that STD clients receive the same treatment for each group of symptoms/signs.

Extensive experience to date with syndromic management has produced mixed reviews.[8] In general, those flowcharts addressing genital ulcers or male urethral discharge appear to have adequate clinical predictability. However, those for vaginal discharge and female upper genital tract infection have been less sensitive and specific. Therefore, recommendations have been made to adjust each of these syndromic management algorithms to the particular etiologic agent most prevalent in the local community. Moreover, using standard STD risk assessment tools determine the prognostic value of risk markers has been useful in some settings (e.g., for gonococcal and chlamydial cervicitis), but less so for others (e.g., organisms causing vaginitis). Ongoing validation and acceptability studies will further demonstrate the advantages of adding STD risk assessment scores compared to using the traditional clinical approach.

Even with syndromic diagnosis, effective treatment remains a problem. Unfortunately most effective antimicrobial agents (e.g., spectinomycin, newer cephalosporins) are either prohibitively expensive or not available in developing countries. This is especially true at the primary health care level. The majority of women seen for symptoms of gonorrhea or chlamydial infection in Africa probably do not receive effective treatment for either of these infections. Even if such economic and administrative barriers could be overcome with altered national or international pharmaceutical policies, practical issues of how to distribute the new drugs and how to ensure that they are used effectively must be solved.

STD Control in Developing Countries

Because of the documented relation between STD and transmission of HIV,[38] increased attention is being given to establishing effective STD control programs in developing countries. Thus, the time is ripe for creative strategies.[8] The goals of STD control in resource-poor settings should be oriented toward *(a)* eliminating the principal reservoirs of bacterial STD infection, so costly to the countries themselves and so important to the spread of HIV; and *(b)* decreasing maternal and perinatal infection to create an atmosphere where fecundability and life expectancy are sufficiently great that voluntary family planning will be acceptable.

Not all of the STD control strategies currently used in the developed countries are appropriate for the developing world. Limited resources and rudimentary health facilities do not allow the type of intensive intervention efforts through categorical STD programs that can be applied in developed countries. Simplified STD services must be provided at the primary health care level and other sources of health care (e.g., family planning clinics, pharmacies) to ensure that effective management of the greatest number of cases is achieved. Such management limits further disease transmission and reduces STD complications. These providers can also perform important preventive services by encouraging treatment of steady sex partners and informing communities about the health effects of, and ways to avoid, STD, including HIV infection.

The highest priority for prevention of serious consequences of STD in developing countries should be given to those programs that are least expensive and most effective. For example, clinicians concerned with maternal and child health in developing countries should be providing effective ocular prophylaxis against gonorrhea in all neonates and serologic testing for syphilis in all pregnant women.

A number of new antimicrobial agents broadens the options for treatment of resistant gonococcal and chancroid infections. For example, safe, effective, and affordable alternatives to the penicillins for treatment of gonorrhea are being used in Africa and Asia. Hepatitis B vaccines are effective and safe and are increasingly available in the developing world economies.

Finally, STD control activities provide an opportunity for enhancing other, high-priority health programs. For example, HIV prevention strategies are partly based on controlling other STDs.[38] In addition, provision of optimal diagnosis and treatment for gonorrhea and chlamydia in family planning clinics will prevent infertility. Conversely, interaction with the young adult population who have STD can be used to promote acceptance of immunization and diarrhea treatment programs for children and contraceptive programs for young adults.

▶ FUTURE DIRECTIONS

First, reducing the transmission of HIV through effective STD control programs will become even more integral to global public health and preventive medicine. STD/HIV public health activities will evolve over time from emphasis on public and professional education to actual disease intervention through person-to-person HIV counseling/testing and confidential partner notification. Physician skills will increasingly involve supportive counseling to assist those dealing with consequences of persistent and potentially lethal infections and the need for maintaining safer sexual behaviors.

Second, through the pervasiveness of managed care organizations, the private medical sphere will increasingly underwrite the costs and delivery of modern STD diagnostic and therapeutic methods for private patients.[2] STD care will be paid for by private insurance and understood by patients and providers alike to be cost-effective. As emphasized earlier, with STD, curative medicine equals preventive medicine.

Third, clinicians practicing in other facilities beyond STD clinics will increasingly provide STD services to the high-risk populations, e.g., drug treatment centers, adolescent health, maternal and child health, and family planning clinics. Diagnosis and treatment of STD in these settings will be funded by public and private resources and will be justified as part of essential medical services provided to these population groups.

Fourth, through community planning efforts, the public will increasingly understand the pervasive medical problems of STD. This will generate improvement in compliance with therapeutic recommendations and the responsibility toward informing sex partners of infected patients.

Fifth, clinicians must improve their ability to take and provide an accurate sexual history. STD/HIV management will become part of routine medical examinations. Medical school and postgraduate education programs will increasingly involve developing skills in client counseling and community appreciation.

▶ CONCLUSION

In the United States today, over 12 million new cases of STD occur in our young adult population each year. Globally, the number exceeds 330 million per year (Fig. 8-8). Up to 40 million persons in the United States are currently infected with HSV, so the cumulative prevalence of all STD is much higher. Estimates of the total cost of STD to the United States approach $10 billion annually. Internally, the human and financial costs are exponentially higher. Moreover, the magnitude of the STD problem appears to be expanding. We have an urgent need for both the public and private medical sectors to recognize the implications of the STD problems confronting us in the late 1990s. The growing complexity and incidence of viral STD requires all those providing clinical care to employ the most current diagnostic and treatment methods. The entrenchment of STD in inner city "core" populations, already succumbing to urban decay and illicit drugs, makes client involvement a herculean task. Moreover, rates of traditional STD remain elevated in rural, southern areas of the United States. Without stronger international support and simultaneous involvement of the public and private health care sectors, the incidence of STD will continue to increase. The Institute of Medicine has called for a revamped national system to prevent STD in the United States. The opportunity for promoting health, preventing human suffering, and reducing societal costs is great.

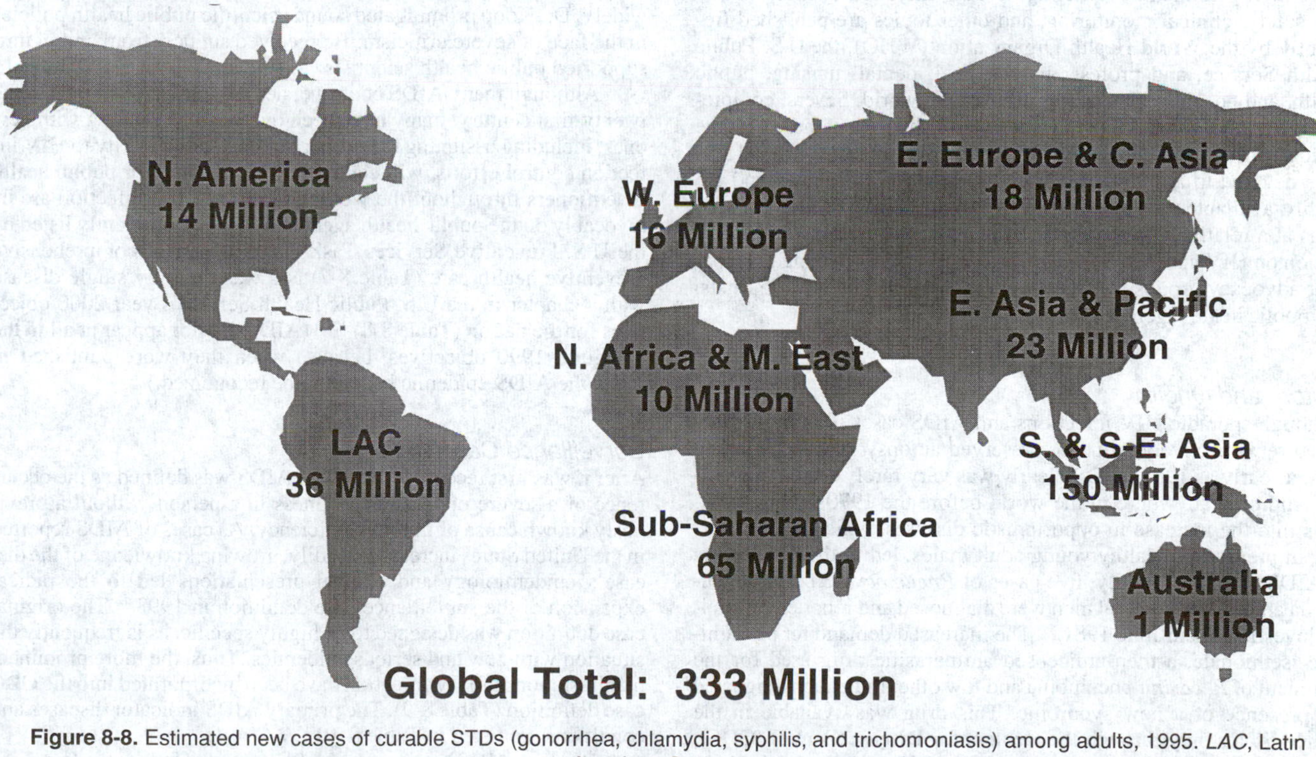
N. America
14 Million
W. Europe
16 Million
E. Europe & C. Asia
18 Million
E. Asia & Pacific
23 Million
N. Africa & M. East
10 Million
LAC
36 Million
S. & S-E. Asia
150 Million
Sub-Saharan Africa
65 Million
Australia
1 Million
Global Total: 333 Million

Figure 8-8. Estimated new cases of curable STDs (gonorrhea, chlamydia, syphilis, and trichomoniasis) among adults, 1995. *LAC*, Latin American Countries.

Epidemiology and Prevention of Human Immunodeficiency Virus Infection and Acquired Immunodeficiency Syndrome

D. Peter Drotman • James W. Curran

Acquired immunodeficiency syndrome (AIDS) emerged as the chief public health issue of the late twentieth century, not only because it became a leading cause of morbidity and mortality throughout the world, but also because it involved topics that captured the public's attention and imagination such as fear of contagion, sex, premature death, and intimate personal relationships. The AIDS epidemic has prompted changes in public health departments, private clinical practice, and research and has had an impact on the financing of medical care and social services. No textbook chapter can adequately address all the biomedical, social, economic, political, legal, and other issues that AIDS encompasses, especially since they change so rapidly in response to new data, research findings, and public attitudes. Therefore, knowing sources of information that are both reliable and current is as important as knowing the basic principles of human immunodeficiency virus (HIV)/AIDS virology and epidemiology. This raises yet another topic that the AIDS epidemic has seriously affected: health communications.

HIV infection and AIDS are among the most heavily researched topics of our time, with hundreds of scientific reports being published monthly in biomedical and other professional or academic journals, including several devoted entirely to AIDS. Recommendations for prevention, treatment, counseling, testing, infection control, laboratory safety, clinical monitoring, and other topics are published frequently by the World Health Organization (WHO), the U.S. Public Health Service, and professional medical, dental, nursing, public health, and hospital associations all over the world. Several comprehensive textbooks on AIDS have been published,[1,2] but these become dated rapidly. Computer-based information storage and retrieval systems devoted to AIDS and HIV citations have proliferated and are readily available to users with appropriate hardware and minimal skills at a relatively low cost. The Internet is a rich source of information on HIV and AIDS from a variety of sources ranging from patient advocacy groups to educational institutions, medical journals, and public health agencies.

History and Origin

Although sporadic HIV infections and AIDS cases have been diagnosed retrospectively by using preserved autopsy specimens dating from as early as 1968, AIDS clearly was very rarely seen as a medical syndrome anywhere in the world before the 1970s.[3,4] Investigations into the increase in opportunistic diseases, which were occurring in previously healthy young adult males, led to the first reports of AIDS in 1981. Initially, five cases of *Pneumocystis carinii* pneumonia among homosexual men were diagnosed and reported by clinical investigators in June 1981.[5,6] The increased demand for pentamidine isethionate, a then-unlicensed antiparasitic drug used for the treatment of *P. carinii* pneumonia and few other indications, signaled the presence of a new syndrome. This drug was available in the United States only through the Centers for Disease Control (CDC). Reviews of requests for pentamidine from 1965 to 1980 revealed only one request for the drug to treat an adult without an underlying immune disorder.[7] Shortly afterward, cases of Kaposi's sarcoma, a neoplasm that previously had been reported in the United States only rarely, were reported in young homosexual men.[8,9] Extensive surveillance for fatal opportunistic infections and Kaposi's sarcoma in the United States revealed relatively few cases prior to 1981, and those were in New York and San Francisco.[7]

By 1985, a basic understanding of the etiology, immunopathogenesis, and epidemiology of HIV infection and AIDS had been developed as the result of immense research efforts directed to this syndrome.[10] The origin of HIV remains undocumented, but it likely can be traced to African nonhuman primates. How and when an "ancestor" simian immunodeficiency virus (SIV) "jumped species" are unknown.

Both social and biological factors explain why AIDS became a worldwide epidemic during the 1980s. Among these were changes in sexual behavior, particularly increases in numbers of sexual partners and sexually transmitted diseases among substantial numbers of gay men, high rates of injection drug use (both opiates and cocaine), and the development of technology to use large plasma pools with thousands of donors for the manufacture of clotting factor concentrates. These factors represented amplification systems that, in combination with the long incubation period for AIDS, allowed extensive transmission of HIV to occur even before the first cases were discovered.

Former Surgeon General of the U.S. Public Health Service, C. Everett Koop, MD, deserves considerable credit for promoting understanding of both the disease and persons afflicted with HIV infection and AIDS. By preparing his 1986 *Surgeon General's Report on AIDS* to be readable by the lay public and then distributing it widely, Dr. Koop promulgated sound scientific public health policies in the face of severe criticism. He received support from and in turn supported public health scientists.

Although many AIDS controversies are likely to persist into the twenty-first century, many have been overcome.[11] Dealing with new ones, including assigning the proper public health priority to HIV infection control efforts, will continue to be an issue for public health practitioners throughout the world. AIDS and HIV infection are irrevocably on the public health agenda. AIDS is prominently listed by the U.S. Preventive Services Task Force as part of comprehensive preventive health care (Table 8-7) and was the only single disease with a chapter in the U.S. Public Health Service's year 2000 objectives for the nation (Table 8-8).[12,13] (AIDS did not appear at all in the inaugural 1990 objectives, because when they were published in 1980, the AIDS epidemic had yet to be recognized.)

Surveillance Case Definition

After it was first recognized in 1981, AIDS was defined as the occurrence of a severe opportunistic illness in a person without a previously known cause of immunodeficiency. As cases of AIDS reported in the United States increased steadily, growing knowledge of the disease's epidemiology and clinical presentations led to the radical expansion of the surveillance case definition in 1993.[14] The original case definition was designed to be highly specific, as is frequently the situation with new and serious epidemics. Thus, the more prominent manifestations of HIV infection have been incorporated into the CDC case definition (Table 8-9). The primary AIDS indicator diseases and conditions are listed in Table 8-10.[15]

Because AIDS cases are now often reported before the first diagnosis of an opportunistic disease, the most important indicator condition on the list is severe immunodeficiency as measured by enumerations of CD4 cells (T helper lymphocytes). Despite its being largely preventable by prophylaxis, *P. carinii* pneumonia remains the most frequently reported severe opportunistic disease, due to failure to diagnose HIV infection, failure to receive prophylaxis, as well as failure of prophylaxis.[16] AIDS cases are only the tip of an iceberg repre-

TABLE 8-7. CLINICAL INTERVENTIONS FOR HIV RECOMMENDED BY THE U.S. PREVENTIVE SERVICES TASK FORCE

- ***Counseling and testing for HIV should be offered to:***

Persons seeking treatment for sexually transmitted diseases

Homosexual and bisexual men

Past or present injecting drug users

Persons with a history of prostitution or multiple sexual partners

Women and men whose past or present sexual partners were HIV-infected, bisexual, or injecting drug users

Persons with a history of transfusion between 1978 and 1985 in the U.S.

Women who are pregnant or contemplating pregnancy

- ***Routine screening for HIV is reasonable for:***

Infants born to high-risk mothers

Prisoners

Runaway youths

Homeless persons

Persons with long-term residence or birth in an area with high prevalence of HIV infection

Testing should not be performed in the absence of informed consent and pretest counseling, which should include the purpose of the test, the meaning of reactive and nonreactive results, measures to protect confidentiality, and the need to notify persons at risk.

A positive test requires at least two reactive enzyme-linked immunosorbent assay tests and a follow-up Western blot test. Clinicians should have these tests performed only at qualified laboratories that perform frequent test runs, use appropriate controls, and receive regular external proficiency testing.

Persons found to be seropositive for the first time should have a second specimen tested.

HIV-infected patients should receive information regarding the meaning of the results, the distinctions between casual nonsexual contact and proven modes of HIV transmission, measures to reduce risk to themselves and others, symptoms requiring medical attention, and the availability of medical treatment—including experimental therapies—and community resources to provide psychological counseling, support groups, and other forms of assistance.

Seropositive persons should be evaluated for severity of immune dysfunction and screened for other infectious diseases, particularly tuberculosis. The latest U.S. Public Health Service guidelines for HIV treatment should be consulted. Arrangements for follow-up medical care are especially important for injecting drug abusers, who may require assistance in achieving entrance to a drug-treatment program.

All seropositive individuals should be encouraged to notify sexual partners, persons with whom injecting drug needles have been shared, and others at risk of exposure. Seropositive cases should be reported confidentially or anonymously to public health officials.

Persons with nonreactive test results should be informed that the risk of acquiring subsequent HIV infection can be prevented by maintaining monogamous sexual relationships with uninfected partners. Other measures to reduce the risk of infection, such as using condoms, and not using unsterilized needles and syringes, should be specifically mentioned. Drug-using patients should be informed of available resources for sterile injection equipment, including needle/syringe exchange programs. The frequency of repeat testing of seronegative individuals is a matter of clinical discretion. In persons with recent (less than 3 months) high-risk exposure, repeat testing is warranted to rule out an initial false-negative result from low antibody titers.

Adapted from U.S. Preventive Services Task Force. Guide to Clinical Preventive Services. 2nd ed. Alexandria, VA: International Medical Publishing, 1996

senting the full clinical spectrum of infection with HIV. This spectrum includes asymptomatic HIV infection; mild illness with such nonspecific symptoms as fever, fatigue, loss of appetite and weight, diarrhea, and lymphadenopathy; and other conditions not always associated with AIDS, such as idiopathic thrombocytopenic purpura.

The case definition has proved very useful in public health surveillance in the United States and other industrialized countries. The consistent use of a specific case definition resulted in accurate trend monitoring from 1981 until 1993, when the definition was expanded to reflect current clinical practice and to encourage early HIV diagnosis and treatment. Since 1993, several statistical adjustments for reporting delay and clinical status have been necessary to visualize trends clearly and consistently (Figs. 8-9 and 8-10). AIDS has always represented the most severe end of a very wide clinical spectrum, but the restrictive (highly specific) case definition caused the magnitude of this HIV disease epidemic to be underestimated. To address this issue, the CDC has expanded surveillance approaches beyond AIDS and has revised the AIDS case definition several times to reflect more accurately the range of severe morbidity due to HIV infection and to maintain consistency with contemporary diagnostic practice. These changes have increased both the sensitivity of the case definition (by including such conditions as HIV encephalopathy and wasting syndrome in 1987 and tuberculosis, recurrent pneumonia, invasive cervical cancer, and severe immunodeficiency in 1993) and its specificity (by encouraging laboratory diagnosis of HIV infection).[14,17–20]

Etiologic Agent and Natural History

By discerning that the main modes of transmission of the causative agent of AIDS in adults were sexual contact, sharing contaminated needles, and receipt of blood or certain blood products, epidemiologists provided direction for laboratory investigators seeking the etiology of the disease. In 1983 and 1984, researchers at the Institut Pasteur (Paris) and the National Cancer Institute isolated HIV, a retrovirus, and demonstrated it to be the cause of AIDS.[21–25] In 1985, a genetic variant of the AIDS virus was isolated, which has been named HIV-2.[26,27] Serologic tests to detect antibody to HIV were developed rapidly. HIV-1 has been subtyped by using genetic markers into subtypes, at this writing designated A through I (with others likely to be identified), as well as a group of "outliers" designated as group O.[28] This information is important in ensuring that diagnostic and screening tests are sensitive for all strains of HIV-1 as well as in molecular epidemiologic studies.

HIV preferentially infects CD4 lymphocytes because a glycoprotein (gp) of the viral envelope (termed gp120 because of its molecular weight of about 120 kilodaltons) strongly binds to the CD4 molecule, a marker found on the surface of CD4 lymphocytes and a few other cell types. HIV is an RNA virus, which replicates by a process known as reverse transcription. Viral genetic material is incorporated into the host cell's DNA, and the cell then becomes a "factory" for viral particles, thus completing HIV's life cycle and eventually destroying the host cell. This destruction results in the characteristic decrease in CD4 cell and total lymphocyte counts and the immunodeficiency that characterize AIDS.[29] Although the immune system is extraordinarily resilient and regenerative, HIV reproduces at a rate of 10 billion new virions per day in an infected person.[30]

Potential manifestations occupy a wide clinical spectrum, ranging from life-threatening opportunistic illnesses to asymptomatic HIV carriers. Classification systems have been proposed to assist in clinical management, prognosis, and epidemiologic study of the natural history of HIV infection. Because clinical decisions regarding the use of antiviral drugs and chemoprophylaxis for opportunistic infections correlate best with estimates of the number of HIV virions present in the patient's blood as well as declining absolute CD4 lymphocyte counts, clinically useful systems are heavily dependent on laboratory measures of immune status and viral replication.[31,32] These classification systems are often impractical for use in surveillance or

TABLE 8-8. NATIONAL HEALTH PROMOTION AND DISEASE PREVENTION OBJECTIVES FOR THE YEAR 2000 FOR SPECIAL POPULATION TARGETS

• ***Health Status Objectives***

1. *Confine annual incidence of diagnosed AIDS cases to no more than 98,000 cases. [Baseline: An estimated 44,000 to 50,000 diagnosed cases in 1989.]*

Diagnosed AIDS Cases	1989 Baseline	2000 Target
Homosexual and bisexual men	26,000–28,000	48,000
Blacks	14,000–15,000	37,000
Hispanics	7,000–8,000	18,000

NOTE: Targets for this objective are equal to upper bound estimates of the incidence of diagnosed AIDS cases projected for 1993.

2. *Confine the prevalence of HIV infection to no more than 800/100,000. [Baseline: An estimated 400/100,000 in 1989.]*

Estimated Prevalence of HIV Infection [per 100,000]	1989 Baseline[a]	2000 Target
Homosexual men	2,000–42,000[b]	20,000
Intravenous drug abusers	30,000–40,000[c]	40,000
Women giving birth to live-born infants	150	100

• ***Risk Reduction Objectives***

3. *Reduce the proportion of adolescents who have engaged in sexual intercourse to no more than 15% by age 15 and no more than 40% by age 17. [Baseline: 27% of girls and 33% of boys by age 15 and 50% of girls and 66% of boys by age 17 were reported in 1988.] Baseline data sources: National Survey of Family Growth; National Survey of Adolescent Males.*

4. *Increase to at least 50% the proportion of sexually active, unmarried people who used a condom at last sexual intercourse. [Baseline: 19% of sexually active, unmarried women aged 15 through 44 reported that their partners used a condom at last sexual intercourse in 1988.]*

Use of Condoms	1988 Baseline[d]	2000 Target
Sexually active young women [by their partners] aged 15–19	26%	60%
Sexually active young men aged 15–19	57%	75%
IV drug abusers	—	60%

Baseline data sources: National Survey of Family Growth; National Survey of Adolescent Males.

NOTE: Strategies to achieve this objective must be undertaken sensitively to avoid indirectly encouraging or condoning sexual activity among teens who are not yet sexually active.

5. *Increase to at least 50% the estimated proportion of all IV drug abusers who are in drug abuse treatment programs. [Baseline: An estimated 11% of opiate abusers were in treatment in 1989.] Baseline data source: National Institute on Drug Abuse.*

6. *Increase to at least 50% the estimated proportion of IV drug abusers not in treatment who use only uncontaminated drug paraphernalia ["works"]. [Baseline: 25% to 35% of opiate abusers in 1989.] Baseline data source: National Institute on Drug Abuse.*

7. *Reduce the risk of transfusion-transmitted HIV infection to no more than 1/250,000 units of blood and blood components. [Baseline: 1/40,000 to 150,000 units in 1989.]*

• ***Service and Protection Objectives***

8. *Increase to at least 80% the proportion of HIV-infected people who have been tested for HIV infection. [Baseline: An estimated 15% of approximately 1 million HIV-infected people had been tested at publicly funded clinics in 1989.] Baseline data source: Center for Prevention Services.*

9. *Increase to at least 75% the proportion of primary and mental health care providers who provide age-appropriate counseling on the prevention of HIV and other STDs. [Baseline: 10% of physicians reported that they regularly assessed the sexual behaviors of their patients in 1987.]*

HIV Counseling by	1987 Baseline	2000 Target
Primary care and mental health care providers who practice in areas of high AIDS and STD incidence	—	90%

NOTE: Primary care providers include physicians, nurses, nurse practitioners, and physician assistants. Areas of high AIDS and STD incidence are cities and states with incidence rates of AIDS cases, HIV seroprevalence, gonorrhea, or syphilis that are at least 25% above the national average.

10. *Increase to at least 95% the proportion of schools that have age-appropriate HIV education curricula for students in grades 4 through 12, preferably as part of quality school health education. [Baseline: 66% of school districts required HIV education, and 5% of school districts required HIV education in each year for grades 7 through 12 in 1989. Data source: General Accounting Office.]*

NOTE: Strategies to achieve this objective must be undertaken sensitively to avoid indirectly encouraging or condoning sexual activity among teens who are not yet sexually active.

11. *Provide HIV education for students and staff in at least 90% of colleges and universities. [Baseline data available in 1995.]*

12. *Increase to at least 90% the proportion of cities with populations over 100,000 that have outreach programs to contact drug abusers [particularly IV drug abusers] to deliver HIV risk reduction messages. [Baseline data available in 1995.]*

NOTE: HIV risk reduction messages include messages about reducing or eliminating drug use, entering drug treatment, disinfection of injection equipment if still injecting drugs, and safer sex practices.

13. *Increase to at least 50% the proportion of family planning clinics, maternal and child health clinics, STD clinics, tuberculosis clinics, drug treatment centers, and primary care clinics that screen, diagnose, treat, counsel, and provide [or refer for] partner notification services for HIV infection and bacterial STDs [gonorrhea, syphilis, and Chlamydia] [Baseline: 40% of family planning clinics for bacterial STDs in 1989. Data source: State Family Planning Directors.]*

14. *Extend to all facilities where workers are at risk for occupational transmission of HIV regulations to protect workers from exposure to blood-borne infections, including HIV infection. [Baseline data to be available in 1992.]*

NOTE The Occupational Safety and Health Administration [OSHA] is expected to issue regulations requiring worker protection from exposure to blood-borne infections, including HIV, during 1990. Implementation of the OSHA regulations would satisfy this objective.

[a] Data from Centers for Disease Control and Prevention [CDC].
[b] Per 100,000 homosexual men aged 15 through 24 based on men tested in selected STD clinics in unlinked surveys; most studies find HIV prevalence of between 2,000 and 21,000/100,000.
[c] Per 100,000 IV drug abusers aged 15 to 24 in the New York City vicinity; in areas other than major metropolitan centers, infection rates in people entering selected drug treatment programs tested in unlinked surveys are often under 500/100,000.
[d] Data from Center for Biologic Evaluation and Research, U.S. Food and Drug Administration.

TABLE 8-9. AIDS CASES BY AGE GROUP, EXPOSURE CATEGORY, AND SEX, REPORTED JULY 1995 THROUGH JUNE 1996, JULY 1996 THROUGH JUNE 1997; AND CUMULATIVE TOTALS, BY AGE GROUP AND EXPOSURE CATEGORY, THROUGH JUNE 1997, UNITED STATES

Adult/Adolescent Exposure Category	Males				Females				Totals					
	July 1995–June 1996		*July 1996–June 1997*		*July 1995–June 1996*		*July 1996–June 1997*		*July 1995–June 1996*		*July 1996–June 1997*		*Cumulative Total*[1]	
	No.	*(%)*	*No.*	*(%)*	*No.*	*(%)*	*No.*	*(%)*	*No.*	*(%)*	*No.*	*(%)*	*No.*	*(%)*
Men who have sex with men	29,773	(52)	24,146	(48)	—	—	—	—	29,773	(42)	24,146	(38)	298,699	(49)
Injecting drug use	13,701	(24)	11,576	(23)	5,219	(37)	4,574	(33)	18,920	(27)	16,150	(25)	154,664	(26)
Men who have sex with men and inject drugs	3,528	(6)	2,684	(5)	—	—	—	—	3,528	(5)	2,684	(4)	38,923	(6)
Hemophilia/coagulation disorder	366	(1)	250	(0)	27	(0)	15	(0)	393	(1)	265	(0)	4,567	(1)
Heterosexual contact:	3,249	(6)	3,357	(7)	5,940	(43)	5,459	(40)	9,189	(13)	8,816	(14)	54,571	(9)
Sex with injecting drug user	*969*		*794*		*2,078*		*1,666*		*3,047*		*2,460*		*22,890*	
Sex with bisexual male	—		—		*400*		*298*		*400*		*298*		*2,768*	
Sex with person with hemophilia	*11*		*5*		*37*		*36*		*48*		*41*		*390*	
Sex with transfusion recipient with HIV infection	*37*		*33*		*69*		*40*		*106*		*73*		*867*	
Sex with HIV-infected person, risk not specified	*2,232*		*2,525*		*3,356*		*3,419*		*5,588*		*5,944*		*27,656*	
Receipt of blood transfusion, blood components, or tissue[2]	323	(1)	245	(0)	274	(2)	244	(2)	597	(1)	489	(1)	8,075	(1)
Other/risk not reported or identified[3]	6,497	(11)	8,385	(17)	2,479	(18)	3,422	(25)	8,976	(13)	11,807	(18)	44,677	(7)
Adult/adolescent subtotal	57,437	(100)	50,643	(100)	13,939	(100)	13,714	(100)	71,376	(100)	64,357	(100)	604,176	(100)

(continued)

TABLE 8-9. AIDS CASES BY AGE GROUP, EXPOSURE CATEGORY, AND SEX, REPORTED JULY 1995 THROUGH JUNE 1996, JULY 1996 THROUGH JUNE 1997; AND CUMULATIVE TOTALS, BY AGE GROUP AND EXPOSURE CATEGORY, THROUGH JUNE 1997, UNITED STATES (Continued)

	Males		Females		Totals		
Pediatric (<13 Years Old)	*July 1995–June 1996*	*July 1996–June 1997*	*July 1995–June 1996*	*July 1996–June 1997*	*July 1995–June 1996*	*July 1996–June 1997*	*Cumulative Total*[1]
Exposure Category	***No. (%)***	***No. (%)***	***No. (%)***	***No. (%)***	***No. (%)***	***No. (%)***	***No. (%)***
Hemophilia/coagulation disorder	2 (1)	3 (1)	— —	1 (0)	2 (0)	4 (1)	232 (3)
Mother with/at risk for HIV infection[3]	331 (93)	291 (91)	335 (95)	261 (90)	666 (94)	552 (91)	7,157 (91)
Injecting drug use	*96*	*79*	*92*	*61*	*188*	*140*	*2,878*
Sex with an injecting drug user	*55*	*36*	*44*	*36*	*99*	*72*	*1,304*
Sex with a bisexual male	*4*	*7*	*7*	*4*	*11*	*11*	*161*
Sex with person with hemophilia	—	2	*1*	—	*1*	*2*	*27*
Sex with transfusion recipient with HIV infection	—	—	—	—	—	—	*26*
Sex with HIV-infected person, risk not specified	60	*59*	*62*	*58*	*122*	*117*	*982*
Receipt of blood transfusion, blood components, or tissue	*2*	*5*	*1*	*5*	*3*	*10*	*150*
Has HIV infection, risk not specified	*114*	*103*	*128*	*97*	*242*	*200*	*1,629*
Receipt of blood transfusion, blood components, or tissue[2]	10 (3)	2 (1)	2 (1)	3 (1)	12 (2)	5 (1)	375 (5)
Risk not reported or identified[3]	13 (4)	24 (8)	16 (5)	24 (8)	29 (4)	48 (8)	138 (2)
Pediatric subtotal	356 (100)	320 (100)	353 (100)	289 (100)	709 (100)	609 (100)	7,902 (100)
Total	**57,793**	**50,963**	**14,292**	**14,003**	**72,085**	**64,966**	**612,078**

From Centers for Disease Control and Prevention: HIV/AIDS Surveillance Report 9(1):8, 1997.

[1] Includes 11 persons known to be infected with human immunodeficiency virus type 2 (HIV-2). See *MMWR* 1995;44:603-06

[2] Thirty-seven adults/adolescents and 3 children developed AIDS after receiving blood screened negative for HIV antibody. Twelve additional adults developed AIDS after receiving tissue, organs, or artificial insemination from HIV-infected donors. Four of the 12 received tissue, organs, or artificial insemination from a donor who was negative for HIV antibody at the time of donation. See *N Engl J Med* 1992;326: 726–32.

[3] "Other" also includes 63 persons who acquired HIV infection perinatally but were diagnosed with AIDS after age 13. These 63 persons are tabulated under the adult/adolescent, not pediatric, exposure category.

TABLE 8-10. AIDS-INDICATOR CONDITIONS REPORTED IN 1996, BY AGE GROUP, UNITED STATES

	Adults/Adolescents		***Children <13 Years Old***	
AIDS-Indicator Conditions	***No.***	***(%)***	***No.***	***(%)***
AIDS-defining opportunistic illness[1]	29,227	(43)	678	(100)
Bacterial infections, multiple or recurrent	*NA*[2]		*138*	*(20)*
Candidiasis of bronchi, trachea, or lungs	*654*	*(2)*	*20*	*(3)*
Candidiasis of esophagus				
Definitive diagnosis	*2,708*	*(9)*	*42*	*(6)*
Presumptive diagnosis	*1,621*	*(6)*	*45*	*(7)*
Carcinoma, invasive cervical	*120*	*(0)*	*NA*[3]	
Coccidioidomycosis, disseminated or extrapulmonary	*122*	*(0)*	*1*	*(0)*
Cryptococcosis, extrapulmonary	*1,455*	*(5)*	*1*	*(0)*
Cryptosporidiosis, chronic intestinal	*555*	*(2)*	*20*	*(3)*
Cytomegalovirus disease other than retinitis	*1,363*	*(5)*	*37*	*(5)*
Cytomegalovirus retinitis				
Definitive diagnosis	*801*	*(3)*	*7*	*(1)*
Presumptive diagnosis	*428*	*(1)*	*3*	*(0)*
Herpes simplex, with esophagitis, pneumonitis, or chronic mucocutaneous ulcers	*1,676*	*(6)*	*31*	*(5)*
Histoplasmosis, disseminated or extrapulmonary	*247*	*(1)*	—	—
HIV encephalopathy (dementia)	*1,680*	*(6)*	*114*	*(17)*
HIV wasting syndrome	*5,592*	*(19)*	*100*	*(15)*
Isosporiasis, chronic intestinal	*29*	*(0)*	—	—
Kaposi's sarcoma				
Definitive diagnosis	*1,789*	*(6)*	—	—
Presumptive diagnosis	*630*	*(2)*	—	—
Lymphoid interstitial pneumonia and/or pulmonary lymphoid hyperplasia				
Definitive diagnosis	*NA*[2]		*71*	*(10)*
Presumptive diagnosis	*NA*[2]		*70*	*(10)*
Lymphoma, Burkitt's (or equivalent term)	*176*	*(1)*	*3*	*(0)*
Lymphoma, immunoblastic (or equivalent term)	*624*	*(2)*	*6*	*(1)*
Lymphoma, primary in brain	*230*	*(1)*	*1*	*(0)*
Mycobacterium avium *or* M. kansasii, *disseminated or extrapulmonary*				
Definitive diagnosis	*1,485*	*(5)*	*34*	*(5)*
Presumptive diagnosis	*257*	*(1)*	*7*	*(1)*
M. tuberculosis, *disseminated or extrapulmonary*				
Definitive diagnosis	*460*	*(2)*	*1*	*(0)*
Presumptive diagnosis	*80*	*(0)*	—	—
M. tuberculosis, *pulmonary*				
Definitive diagnosis	*1,310*	*(4)*	*NA*[3]	
Presumptive diagnosis	*227*	*(1)*	*NA*[3]	
Mycobacterial disease, other, disseminated or extrapulmonary				
Definitive diagnosis	*324*	*(1)*	*4*	*(1)*
Presumptive diagnosis	*74*	*(0)*	*3*	*(0)*
Pneumocystis carinii *pneumonia*				
Definitive diagnosis	*7,473*	*(26)*	*119*	*(18)*
Presumptive diagnosis	*3,888*	*(13)*	*43*	*(6)*
Pneumonia, recurrent				
Definitive diagnosis	*1,267*	*(4)*	*NA*[3]	
Presumptive diagnosis	*374*	*(1)*	*NA*[3]	
Progressive multifocal leukoencephalopathy	*286*	*(1)*	*1*	*(0)*
Salmonella septicemia, recurrent	*87*	*(0)*	*NA*[4]	
Toxoplasmosis of brain				
Definitive diagnosis	*695*	*(2)*	*1*	*(0)*
Presumptive diagnosis	*673*	*(2)*	*1*	*(0)*
Immunosuppression, severe HIV related[5]	39,246	(57)	NA[3]	
Total	**68,473**	**(100)**	**678**	**(100)**

From Centers for Disease Control and Prevention: HIV/AIDS Surveillance Report 9(1):18, 1997.

[1] Percentages for individual AIDS-defining opportunistic illnesses are based upon 29,227 adults/adolescents and 678 children reported to CDC in 1996, with at least one of the illnesses listed above. The sum of percentages is greater than 100 because some patients are reported with more than one illness. Of persons reported with AIDS-defining opportunistic illnesses, 69 percent also were reported with severe HIV-related immunosuppression.

[2] Not applicable as indicator of AIDS in adults/adolescents.

[3] Not applicable as indicator of AIDS in children.

[4] Tabulated above in "bacterial infections, multiple or recurrent."

[5] Defined as CD4+ T-lymphocyte count of less than 200 cells/μL or a CD4+ percentage less than 14 in adults/adolescents who meet the AIDS surveillance case definition. In 1996, 59,284 adults/adolescents were reported with severe HIV-related immunosuppression. The 39,246 adults/adolescents presented on this table are those persons reported with immunosuppression as their only AIDS-indicator conditiion. These persons may also have other AIDS-indicator conditions that are unreported.

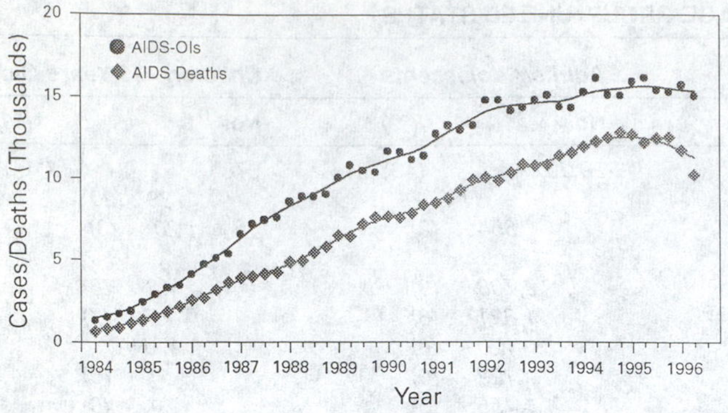

Figure 8-9. Estimated incidence of AIDS-opportunistic illnesses (AIDS-OIs) and estimated deaths among persons with AIDS (AIDS deaths), adjusted for delays in reporting, by quarter year of diagnosis/death, United States, 1984–June 1996. Estimates of AIDS deaths include persons aged less than 13 years. Points represent quarterly incidence; lines represent "smoothed" incidence. Estimates are not adjusted for incomplete reporting of diagnosed AIDS cases. *(From Centers for Disease Control and Prevention: Trends in AIDS incidence, death, and prevalence—United States, 1996. MMWR 46:165–173, 1997.)*

HIV reporting, especially in developing countries or in other areas where access to health care or laboratory services is lacking.

In the United States, all persons with HIV should be considered for treatment with a combination of antiretroviral agents.[33] Observations before the era of combination antiretroviral therapy suggested that at least 50 to 70 percent of HIV-seropositive homosexual men developed AIDS within 10 years of HIV infection. Current therapies and prophylaxis against opportunistic infections have improved this outlook by several years in many persons.[16,33,34] Because early treatment of HIV-infected persons seems to present the greatest promise for a good prognosis, early diagnosis of HIV infection and access to medical care (particularly to drugs and laboratory tests that are sophisticated and expensive) will remain key issues for the foreseeable future.

Infection with HIV, as with all retroviruses, is presumed to be lifelong. Rare reports of persons (mainly young children) having a loss of HIV infection[35] have yet to be corroborated. The virus titer and potential infectiousness of HIV in a given individual may vary according to many factors, including the infected person's clinical and treatment status, duration of HIV infection, the CD4 lymphocyte count, and possibly the strain of the infecting virus.

Relatively little is known about what determines rates and risks of severe clinical outcomes of HIV infection. Factors that may contribute to variations in the development of clinically severe manifestations of HIV infection include increasing age of the patient, basic health and nutritional status of the host, route of exposure to the virus, and exposure to possible environmental or infectious cofactors.[36] For instance, Kaposi's sarcoma, an opportunistic tumor that is far more common among homosexual male AIDS patients than others with AIDS, is strongly associated with a human herpesvirus known as Kaposi's sarcoma–associated herpesvirus or human herpesvirus 8 (HHV-8).[37]

Modes of Transmission and Distribution of Infection

HIV has been recovered from peripheral blood, semen, vaginal secretions, and numerous other body fluids and anatomical sites.[38,39] It is transmitted sexually or through injection or transfusion of infected blood or its components or untreated concentrates of clotting factors VIII and IX. Epidemiologic observations and controlled studies have confirmed these routes of transmission in homosexual and bisexual men,[40] heterosexual men and women,[41] and injecting drug users.[42] The previously documented risks to persons with hemophilia[43–45] and transfusion recipients[46] have been remarkably well controlled by educating donors, by testing all donations of blood and plasma for HIV-1 and HIV-2 antibody and HIV-1 antigen, and by developing safe clotting factor concentrates.[47,48]

AIDS has been recognized in infants as a result of transmission of HIV from infected mothers before, at, or shortly after birth.[49] The rate of transmission of HIV infection to such infants has been about 25 percent in the United States, but this route of transmission is reduced to less than 10 percent when antiviral drugs are given to HIV-infected pregnant women and their newborns and when infected women avoid breast feeding.[50] All pregnant women should be offered HIV testing, and past experience has shown that nearly all accept the offer as a routine part of prenatal care.[51] The implementation of these recommendations represents a breakthrough in prevention and has resulted in more than a 40 percent decline in HIV transmission to newborns in the United States.[52] However, simpler and less expensive regimens are needed to prevent perinatal HIV transmission in developing countries.[53]

Health care and laboratory workers have been infected through occupational exposure to blood or specimens from HIV-infected patients. Risk of infection following parenteral exposures was about 0.3 percent in several long-term prospective studies.[54,55] Well-documented reports of seroconversion and HIV infection following skin or mucous membrane exposure to HIV-infected blood indicate that these can occur, but the risk is much lower than that following parenteral exposures. Because of this risk and the uncertainty and ineffectiveness of trying to identify every infected patient, health care workers should always follow standard precautions (previously referred to as "universal precautions") to minimize exposures to HIV, hepatitis B and C viruses, and other blood-borne pathogens. Standard precautions entail the use of appropriate barrier protection (such as gloves, masks, gowns, or goggles) whenever contact with blood or nonintact tissue seems likely.[56] Postexposure prophylaxis with a course of antiretroviral agents is recommended for workers who sustain percutaneous or mucous membrane exposure to HIV-infected materials.[57,57a] Reviews of recommended precautions and guidelines for hospital settings are available from the National Institute for Occupational Safety and Health or from the Occupational Safety and Health Administration, U.S. Department of Labor, which regulates health care workplaces regarding exposure to HIV and other blood-borne pathogens. In 1990, transmission of HIV to patients from an infected dentist was documented, and transmission from a surgeon to a patient was reported in 1997.[58,59] The possibility that HIV can be transmitted from infected dentists or surgeons to their patients has prompted further revisions in guidelines for infection control during invasive procedures.

A series of retrospective seroprevalence surveys using frozen serum samples from a high-risk cohort of homosexual men in San Francisco documented a rapid increase in seroprevalence rates from 0.3 percent in 1978 to 28 percent in 1981 before plateauing at about 50 percent by 1983.[60] In New York City, 57 percent of IV drug users had antibody detected by 1987.[61] Of 860 hemophilia A patients tested in California, 62 percent were infected with HIV.[62] Seroprevalence rates in childbearing women ranged from 0.02 percent in New Mexico to 1.40 percent in New York City in blinded surveys.[61]

There is no evidence that HIV is spread by air, water, food, or casual contact. If such modes of transmission did exist, the epidemiology of HIV and AIDS would be much different, with clusters occurring in schools, nursing homes, and households. Only a small fraction of the reported cases do not fall readily into a characteristic patient group. This fraction includes patients from whom information was not available because of severe illness, rapid death, or refusal to cooperate and patients for whom further investigation is incomplete.[63] Extensive follow-up of household contacts of both adults and children with AIDS has failed to demonstrate evidence of HIV transmission via shared living space, kitchens, or bathrooms or through casual contact.[64] However, rare instances of HIV transmission in households where direct care of AIDS patients was the risk factor indicate that

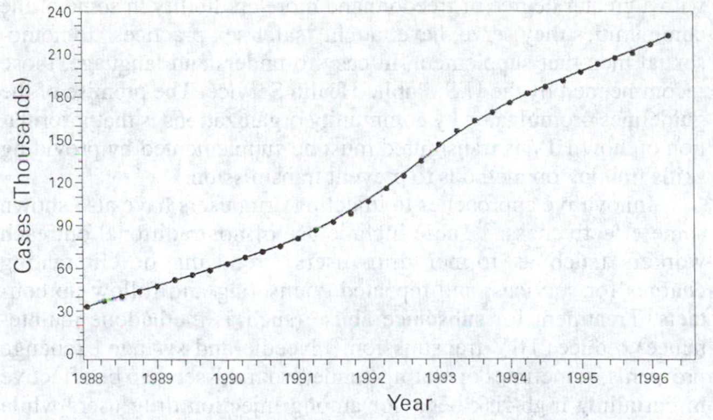

Figure 8-10. Number of prevalent AIDS cases among persons aged more than 13 years, adjusted for delays in reporting, by quarter year, United States, 1988–June 1996. Points represent quarterly prevalence; the line represents "smoothed" prevalence. Estimates are not adjusted for incomplete reporting of diagnosed AIDS cases or AIDS deaths. *(From Centers for Disease Control and Prevention: Trends in AIDS incidence, death, and prevalence—United States, 1996. MMWR 46:165–173, 1997.)*

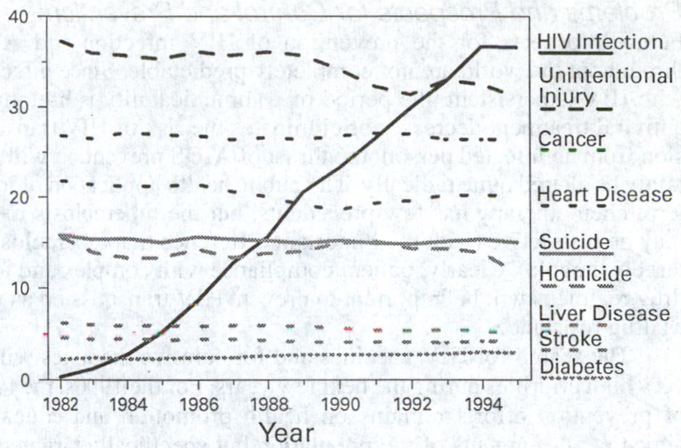

Figure 8-11. Death rates (per 100,000 population) for leading causes of death among persons aged 25 to 44 years, by year, United States, 1982–1995. Based on underlying cause of death reported on death certificates, using final data for 1982–1994 and preliminary data for 1995. *(From Centers for Disease Control and Prevention: Trends in AIDS incidence, death, and prevalence—United States, 1996. MMWR 46:165–173, 1997.)*

the standard precautions originally developed for use in hospitals should apply to home health care as well.[65]

Although the number of patients with AIDS has increased markedly and steadily in the United States since the first cases were reported in 1981 through 1996 (Fig. 8-9), the epidemiologic pattern has evolved somewhat gradually. AIDS has become a major public health issue in minority communities. In 1995, the incidence rates of AIDS (with opportunistic illness) were about 7-fold greater in the African American community and 3-fold greater in Hispanic populations than among whites.[66] The CDC estimated the number of persons living with AIDS in the United States to be 223,000 in 1996 (Fig. 8-10). This represented a sharp increase over previous years. The explanation for this increase was not that incidence increased (it had stabilized at about 60,000 cases per year), but that the death rate declined from about 50,000 per year to less than 45,000 per year (Fig. 8-9).[66] Even so, AIDS remained the leading cause of death among persons aged 25 to 44 years through 1995 (Fig. 8-11).[66] The decline in AIDS mortality accelerated in 1996 and was attributed to the effect of newer antiretroviral therapies.[66a]

International Patterns

The geographic origin of HIV is not proven, but sub-Saharan Africa seems to fit most observations.[67] When AIDS first occurred has not been established, but from the limited data available, it has been hypothesized that HIV may have evolved no more recently than the 1940s.[68] Large numbers of AIDS cases and HIV infections are now being diagnosed in many countries around the world. In Africa, Latin America, and most of Asia, the male-to-female ratio of patients is about equal, in contrast to the male preponderance seen in industrialized countries. While homosexual transmission and injecting drug use are significant factors for the spread of HIV in the latter countries, heterosexual transmission accounts for the vast majority of HIV infections in the developing world. An epidemic in intravenous drug use and prostitution in Southeast Asia and India has allowed HIV to gain a foothold on that populous part of the world, and millions of new infections have already occurred.[69]

At the end of 1997, the Joint United Nations Programme on HIV/AIDS (UNAIDS) estimated aver 30 million persons had been infected with HIV throughout the world. In the industrialized nations of Western Europe, clinical and epidemiologic patterns are similar to those seen in the United States. Since the opening of Eastern Europe, HIV has been noted as a public health problem there, where it is most often transmitted through sexual contact and injecting drug use and in health settings where transfusions are not screened and injection equipment is reused. Most notable was the major epidemic of HIV and AIDS among children in Romania reported in 1989. Over 1,000 children and infants apparently acquired HIV while living in overcrowded orphanages and other health facilities, probably largely through receipt of unscreened blood transfusions and the reuse of injection equipment.[70]

Therapy

Prospects for effective treatment for patients with AIDS or HIV infection are steadily improving. Zidovudine (ZDV) (formerly known as azidothymidine, or AZT) was licensed in the United States and other countries in 1987. ZDV, which inhibits reverse transcriptase, an enzyme key to HIV replication, became the first mainstay of antiviral therapy. By 1997, well over a dozen antiretroviral agents were available or in clinical trials.[33,71] Clinical trials showed that patients taking combinations of two reverse-transcriptase inhibitors and one protease inhibitor have fewer opportunistic illnesses and survive longer, with evidence of remarkable viral suppression. Although the long-term impact of current combination therapies is unknown, further progress in therapy may be expected from trials using different dosage schedules and various combinations of antiretroviral agents and immune modulators, such as cytokines and interferons, in patients with different stages of infection.

Monitoring asymptomatic HIV-infected patients with serial CD4 lymphocyte counts and other clinical and laboratory markers has been the standard of care in developed nations. In 1996, quantitating viral concentration in plasma became possible by using several different assays.[31,32] Use of prophylactic antibiotics (trimethoprim-sulfamethoxazole orally) to prevent *P. carinii* pneumonia, as well as central nervous system toxoplasmosis and bacterial pneumonia, and prevention of active tuberculosis are recommended for persons with depressed immune function.[16]

As more HIV-infected persons perceive the specific medical benefits of early HIV diagnosis, the medical care system may be faced with the costs and challenges of caring for over half a million infected persons in the United States alone. This has become a serious issue for health care services and those who allocate economic resources in many cities where HIV and AIDS are highly prevalent.

As yet, there are no documented "cures," and HIV infection must be considered to be an ultimately fatal infection. Although survival is likely to lengthen as more and better treatments are developed, the severe clinical course of AIDS, the uncertain outcome of treatment, and the costs and toxicity of available treatments will remain major concerns.

Problems and Prospects for Control and Prevention

Future prospects for the prevention of HIV infection and AIDS throughout the world are not completely predictable. Since infection with HIV is persistent, the period of communicability is lifelong. If antiviral treatment decreases or eliminates the risk of HIV transmission from an infected person, the thrust of AIDS prevention will certainly be altered quite radically. The public health application of long-term chemotherapy has few precedents, but the tuberculosis model may be instructive (with the important difference that tuberculosis is largely curable). Clearly, patient compliance with complex and toxic drug regimens will be important to prevent HIV transmission as well as drug resistance.

The search for HIV vaccines and for curative therapies will be very high priorities during the next few years. For the 1990s, the focus of prevention efforts remains on health promotion and education aimed at all segments of the population but specifically targeted toward infected individuals and youth at increased risk. Evidence that many homosexual men changed their sexual practices in the early 1980s to avoid infection with HIV was indicated by a decline in the incidence of sexually transmitted diseases (STDs) with short incubation periods, such as syphilis and rectal gonorrhea.[72] This eventually led to a decline in AIDS among gay men in the mid-1980s despite the very high prevalence of HIV and continued high risk of infection. This behavior change may not be uniform, since HIV transmission rates remain unacceptably high among gay youths.[73] Well-planned community-level interventions can favorably influence persons at risk for HIV infection to change their sexual and needle-using behavior and thus reduce their risk.[74]

Serologic tests to screen donated blood and to aid in the diagnosis of patients were licensed for use in the United States in March 1985. Sensitive and specific antibody tests on both serum and oral fluid specimens are now standardized and part of clinical prevention-oriented practices and public health services throughout the United States. In 1996, home collection kits were licensed, with anonymous results reported by telephone by trained counselors. Additional tests, perhaps including tests for viral antigens or nucleic acid sequences, may become more widely available, but acceptance may vary widely by population.[75]

Many concerns about misuses of HIV test results remain. Will seropositive individuals be unjustly excluded from employment or housing? How well can the confidentiality of test results be ensured? What are the benefits versus costs of requiring reporting of serologic test results by name to health departments? The availability of improved therapies and the need to counsel infected persons regarding transmission to others will be weighed against individual privacy and discrimination concerns.

AIDS differs from other public health problems in the degree of public concern it has generated over a prolonged period. This concern has resulted in public support for research, public information programs, and school health education. Some concern, however, has been misplaced, resulting in fear, panic. prejudice, and discrimination. Public health personnel have expended considerable effort to sidetrack nonproductive approaches and allay inappropriate concerns. Increased testing for HIV antibodies may raise issues of discrimination anew, especially in communities with few reported AIDS cases.

On first consideration, the recommendations for preventing HIV infection are deceptively easy: avoid sex with others known or thought to be infected, stop using injecting drugs or avoid sharing drug administration equipment, and eliminate infectious blood from use in transfusions or blood products. Changing sexual behavior can be extraordinarily difficult, however, and changing sexual practices or giving up drugs are often beyond an individual's control without strong social support systems. Not surprisingly, the greatest progress has occurred in influencing changes in sexual practices among homosexual men in cities where AIDS was first recognized, such as New York and San Francisco, with a corresponding leveling off of new AIDS cases among gay men years later.[76] Independent community-based organizations, often working with official health agencies, but with a greater degree of freedom and more credibility in some of the communities they serve, have taught "safer sex practices" to homosexual men that supplement, in easy-to-understand language, those recommended by the U.S. Public Health Service. The premise of the guidelines promulgated by community organizations is that information on how HIV is transmitted must be supplemented by providing skills training on methods to prevent transmission.

Innovative approaches to injecting drug users have also shown some effectiveness.[77] These include use of nontraditional outreach workers (such as former drug users), reducing or eliminating charges for services, and repeated counseling and follow-up contacts. Treatment for substance abuse (such as methadone maintenance) reduces HIV transmission.[78] Needle and syringe exchange programs, sometimes operating "underground," seem to be effective in curtailing high-risk behavior among injection drug users while not increasing drug abuse.[79] Because these and other prevention approaches are controversial, current and proposed health promotion activities must be assessed and their ability to prevent HIV infection evaluated carefully before they are widely adopted. In addition, resources for prevention efforts that focus on sexual transmission or injecting drug use are scarce, often resulting in competition with other public health programs.

Internationally, preventing HIV and AIDS is an enormous challenge because the problem is increasing rapidly, while the resources to address it are not. A landmark study in rural Mwanzaa, Tanzania, showed that treating "traditional" STDs was useful in preventing HIV transmission.[80] Most notably, massive efforts in Thailand (including a campaign for 100 percent condom use in brothels and other strategies) have been effective in slowing the spread of HIV in that country.[81,82]

In the nearly two decades since its discovery, AIDS has generated extraordinary interest and sustained publicity, often characterized by fear and hysteria. There are many reasons for this reaction, including the public's fear and prejudice toward the groups comprising nearly all of the first AIDS patients and the misperception that AIDS was highly contagious. Fear also resulted from the belief that little was known about the disease, although AIDS was characterized clinically, epidemiologically, immunologically, etiologically, and serologically within 3 years of its discovery. More and better health communication strategies and products are needed. School health education guidelines have been promulgated.[83] Their application holds the best hope for the future of HIV prevention. Future progress in treatment and prevention can be anticipated. Now and in the future, public health officials at all levels will continue to be called on for leadership and direction in attempts to control HIV infection and AIDS. There remains much for all of us to do.[84]

▶ REFERENCES

1. Holmes KK, Sparling PF, Mardh P-A, et al (eds): Sexually Transmitted Diseases. 3rd ed. New York: McGraw-Hill, 1997
2. Eng TR, Butler WT (eds): The Hidden Epidemic: Confronting Sexually Transmitted Diseases. Washington, DC: National Academy Press, 1997
3. Cates W Jr: The "other STDs"—do they really matter? JAMA 259:3606–3608, 1988
4. Brandt AM: No Magic Bullet: A Social History of Venereal Disease in the United States since 1880. New York: Oxford University Press, 1985
5. Wasserheit JN, Aral SO: The dynamic topology of sexually transmitted disease epidemics: implications for prevention strategies. J Infect Dis 174(Suppl 2):S201–213, 1996
6. Aral SO, Holmes KK, Padian NS, Cates W Jr: Overview: individual and population approaches to the epidemiology and prevention of sexually transmitted diseases and human immunodeficiency virus infection. J Infect Dis 174(Suppl 2):S127–133, 1996

7. Centers for Disease Control and Prevention, Division of Sexually Transmitted Diseases: Annual Report, 1996. Atlanta: Centers for Disease Control and Prevention, 1997
8. Dallabetta G, Laga M, Lamptey PR (eds): Control of sexually transmitted diseases: a handbook for the design and management of programs. Arlington, VA: AIDSCAP/Family Health International, 1996
9. Landry DJ, Forrest JD: Public health departments providing sexually transmitted disease services. Fam Plann Perspect 28:261–268, 1996
10. US Preventive Service Task Force: Guide to Clinical Preventive Services. 2nd ed. Baltimore: Williams & Wilkins, 1996
11. Rothenberg RB: Analytic approaches to the epidemiology of sexually transmitted diseases. In Holmes KK, Mårdh P-A, Sparling PF, Wiesner PJ, Cates W Jr, Lemon SM, Stamm WE (eds): Sexually Transmitted Diseases. 2nd ed. New York: McGraw-Hill, 1990, pp 37–42
12. Centers for Disease Control and Prevention, Division of Sexually Transmitted Diseases: Sexually Transmitted Diseases Surveillance, 1995. Atlanta: Centers for Disease Control and Prevention, 1996
13. Centers for Disease Control and Prevention: Recommendations for the prevention and management of *Chlamydia trachomatis* infections. MMWR 42(RR-12):1–39, 1993
14. Washington AE, Johnson RE, Sanders LL, et al: Incidence of *Chlamydia trachomatis* infections in the United States: Using reported *Neisseria gonorrhoeae* as a surrogate. In Oriel D, Ridgway G, Schachter J, et al (ed.): Chlamydial Infections. Cambridge, England: Cambridge University Press, 1986, p 487
15. Scholes D, Stergachis A, Heidrich FE, Andrilla H, Holmes KK, Stamm WE: Prevention of pelvic inflammatory disease by screening for cervical chlamydial infection. N Engl J Med 334:1362–1366, 1996
16. World Health Organization: Global Programme on AIDS: An Overview of Selected Curable Sexually Transmitted Diseases. Geneva: WHO/GPA, August 1995
17. Rosenberg PS: Scope of the AIDS epidemic in the United States. Science 270:1372–1375, 1995
18. Johnson RE, Lee F, Hadgu A, McQuillan G, Aral SO, Keesling S, Nahmias A: U.S. genital herpes trends during first decade of AIDS: prevalences increased in young whites and elevated in blacks. Sex Transm Dis 21:S109, 1994
19. Koutsky LA, Galloway DA, Holmes KK: Epidemiology of genital human papillomavirus infection. Epidemiol Rev 10:122–163, 1988
20. Lemon SM, Thomas DL: Vaccines to prevent viral hepatitis. N Engl J Med 336:196–204, 1997
21. Hillier SL, Nugent RP, Eschenbach DA, et al: Association between bacterial vaginosis and preterm delivery of a low-birth-weight infant. N Engl J Med 333:1737–1742, 1995
22. Cotch MF, Pastorek JG II, Nugent RP, et al: *Trichomonas vaginalis* associated with low birth weight and preterm delivery. Sex Transm Dis 1997, 24:353–360, 1997
23. May R, Anderson R: Transmission dynamics of HIV infection. Nature 326:137–142, 1987
24. Thomas JC, Tucker MJ: The development and use of the concept of a sexually transmitted disease core. J Infect Dis 174(Suppl 2): S134–143, 1996
25. Rothenberg RB, Potterat JJ, Woodhouse DE: Personal risk taking and the spread of disease: beyond core groups. J Infect Dis 174(Suppl 2):S144–149, 1996
26. Brown JD, Childers KW, Waszak CS: Television and adolescent sexuality. J Adolesc Health Care 11:62–70, 1990
27. McKay HT, Toomey KE, Schmid GP: Survey of clinical training and STD and HIV/AIDS in the United States [Abstract 281]. Proceedings of the IDSA Annual Meeting, September 6–18, 1995, San Francisco
28. Centers for Disease Control and Prevention: 1997 Sexually transmitted diseases treatment guidelines. MMWR 1997, in press
29. Wawer MJ, Sewankambo NK, Gray RH, et al: Community-based trial of mass STD treatment for HIV control, Rakai, Uganda: preliminary data on STD declines [Abstract Mo.C.443]. Program and Abstracts of the XI International Conference on AIDS, July 7–12, 1996, p. 39 Vancouver, Canada
30. Adler M: Sexually transmitted disease control in developing countries. Genitourin Med 72:83–88, 1996
31. Over M, Piot P: Human immunodeficiency virus infection and other sexually transmitted diseases in developing countries: public health importance and priorities for resource allocation. J Infect Dis 174(Suppl 2):S162–175, 1996
32. Bang RA, Bang AT, Baitule M, Chaudhury Y, Sarmukaddam S, Tale O: High prevalence of gynaecological diseases in rural Indian women. Lancet 1:85–87, 1989
33. Zurayk H, Khattab H, Younis N, Kamal O, El-Helw M: Comparing women's reports with medical diagnoses of reproductive morbidity conditions in rural Egypt. Stud Fam Plann 26:14–21, 1995
34. World Health Organization: HIV/AIDS: the global epidemic—December 1996. Wkly Epidemiol Rec 72:17–21, 1997
35. Hanenberg RS, Rojanapithayakorn W, Kunasol P, Sokal DC: Impact of Thailand's HIV-control Programme as indicated by the decline of sexually transmitted diseases. Lancet 344:243–245, 1994
36. Nelson KE, Celentano DD, Eiumtrakol S, et al: Changes in sexual behavior and a decline in HIV infection among young men in Thailand. N Engl J Med 335:297–303, 1996
37. Vuylsteke B, Meheus A: STD syndrome management. In Dallabetta GA, Laga M, Lamptey PR. (eds): Control of sexually transmitted diseases. A handbook for the design and management of programs. Arlington, VA: AIDSCAP/Family Health International, 1996, pp. 149–168
38. Grosskurth H, Mosha F, Todd J, Mwijarubi E, Klokke A, Senkoro K, et al: Impact of improved treatment of sexually transmitted diseases in HIV infection in rural Tanzania: randomized controlled trial [see comments]. Lancet 346:530–536, 1995b

Epidemiology and Prevention of HIV Infection and AIDS

1. Wormser GP, ed: AIDS and Other Manifestations of HIV Infection. 3rd ed. New York: Raven Press, in press
2. Mandel GL, Mildvan D (eds): Atlas of Infectious Diseases. 2nd ed. Philadelphia: Churchill Livingstone, 1997, vol 1, AIDS
3. Huminer D, Rosenfeld JB, Pitlik SD: AIDS in the pre-AIDS era. Rev Infect Dis 9:1102–1108, 1987
4. Garry RF, Witte MH, Gottlieb AA, et al: Documentation of an AIDS virus infection in the United States in 1968. JAMA 260:2085–2087, 1988
5. Centers for Disease Control: *Pneumocystis* pneumonia—Los Angeles. MMWR 30:250–252, 1981
6. Gottlieb MS, Schroff R, Schanker HM, et al: *Pneumocystis carinii* pneumonia and healthy homosexual men. N Engl J Med 305: 1425–1431, 1981
7. CDC Task Force on Kaposi's Sarcoma and Opportunistic Infections: Epidemiologic aspects of the current outbreak of Kaposi's sarcoma and opportunistic infections. N Engl J Med 306:248–252, 1982
8. Centers for Disease Control: Kaposi's sarcoma and *Pneumocystis* pneumonia among homosexual men—New York City and California. MMWR 30:305–308, 1981
9. Hymes K, Cheung T, Greene JB, et al: Kaposi's sarcoma in homosexual men. Lancet 2:598–600, 1981
10. Scientific American: The Science of AIDS. New York: W.H. Freeman, 1989
11. Fauci AS: AIDS in 1996: much accomplished, much to do. JAMA 276:155–156, 1996
12. U.S. Preventive Services Task Force. Guide to Clinical Preventive Services. 2nd ed. Alexandria, VA: International Medical Publishing, 1996
13. U.S. Public Health Service: Healthy People 2000: National Health Promotion and Disease Prevention Objectives. Washington, DC: U.S. Public Health Service, 1990, pp 476–491

14. Centers for Disease Control and Prevention: 1993 revised classification system for HIV infection and expanded surveillance case definition for AIDS among adolescents and adults. MMWR 41(RR-17): 1–19, 1992
15. Centers for Disease Control and Prevention: HIV/AIDS Surveillance Report 8(2):1–39, 1996
16. Centers for Disease Control and Prevention: U.S. Public Health Service/IDSA guidelines for the prevention of opportunistic infections in persons infected with human immunodeficiency virus: a summary. MMWR 44(RR-8):1–34, 1995
17. Centers for Disease Control: Revision of the CDC surveillance case definition for acquired immunodeficiency syndrome. MMWR 36:1–15S, 1987
18. Selik RM, Buehler JW, Karon JM. Chamberland ME, Berkelman RL: Impact of the 1987 revision of the case definition of acquired immunodeficiency syndrome in the United States. J Acquir Immune Defic Syndr 3:73–82, 1990
19. Centers for Disease Control and Prevention: Update: impact of the expanded AIDS surveillance case definition for adolescents and adults on case reporting. MMWR 43:160–161, 167–170, 1994
20. Centers for Disease Control and Prevention: Update: trends in AIDS diagnosis and reporting under the expanded AIDS surveillance case definition for adolescents and adults—United States, 1993. MMWR 43:826–831, 1994
21. Barre-Sinoussi F, Chermann JC, Rey F, et al: Isolation of a T-lymphotropic retrovirus from a patient at risk for acquired immunodeficiency syndrome (AIDS). Science 220:868–871, 1983
22. Popovic M, Sarngadharan MG, Read E, et al: Detection, isolation, and continuous production of cytopathic retroviruses (HTLV-III) from patients with AIDS and pre-AIDS. Science 224:497–500, 1984
23. Gallo RC, Salahuddin SZ, Popovic M, et al: Frequent detection and isolation of cytopathic retroviruses (HTLV-III) from patients with AIDS and at risk for AIDS. Science 224:500–503, 1984
24. Schupbach J, Popovic M, Gilden RW, et al: Serological analysis of a subgroup of human T-lymphotropic retroviruses (HTLV-III) associated with AIDS. Science 224:503–505, 1984
25. Sarngadharan MG, Popovic M, Bruch L, et al: Antibodies reactive with human T-lymphotropic retroviruses (HTLV-III) in the serum of patients with AIDS. Science 224:506–508, 1984
26. Barin F, M'Boup S, Denis F, et al: Serological evidence for virus related to simian T-lymphotropic retrovirus III in residents of West Africa. Lancet 2:1387–1389, 1985
27. Clavel F, Guetard D, Brun-Vezinet F, et al: Isolation of a new human retrovirus from West African patients with AIDS. Science 233:343–346, 1986
28. Hu DJ, Dondero TJ, Rayfield MA, et al: The emerging genetic diversity of HIV: the importance of global surveillance for diagnostics, research, and prevention. JAMA 275:210–216, 1996
29. Fauci AS: The human immunodeficiency virus: infectivity and mechanisms of pathogenesis. Science 239:617–622, 1988
30. Ho DD, Neumann AU, Perelson AS, Chen W, Leonard JM, Markowitz M: Rapid turnover of plasma virions and CD4 lymphocytes in HIV-1 infection. Nature 373:123–126, 1995
31. Mellors JW, Rinaldo CR Jr, Gupta P, White RM, Todd JA, Kingsley LA: Prognosis in HIV-1 infection predicted by the quantity of virus in plasma. Science 272:1167–170, 1996
32. Saag MS, Holodniy M, Kuritzkes DR, et al: HIV viral load markers in clinical practice. Nat Med 2:625–629, 1996
33. Carpenter CJC, Fischl MA, Hammer SM, et al: Antiretroviral therapy for HIV infection in 1996: recommendations of an international panel. JAMA 276:146–154, 1996
34. Ward JW, Bush TJ, Perkins HA, et al: The natural history of transfusion-associated infection with human immunodeficiency virus: factors influencing the rate of progression to disease. N Engl J Med 321:947–952, 1989
35. Bryson YJ, Pang S, Wei LS, et al: Clearance of HIV infection in a perinatally infected infant. N Engl J Med 332:833–838, 1995
36. Buchbinder SB, Katz MH, Hessol NA, O'Malley PM, Holmberg SD: Long-term HIV-1 infection without immunologic progression. AIDS 8:1123–1128, 1994
37. Moore P, Chang Y: Detection of herpesvirus-like DNA sequences in Kaposi's sarcoma lesions from persons with and without HIV infection. N Engl J Med 332:1181–1185, 1995
38. Ho DD, Schooley RT, Rota TR, et al: HTLV-III in the semen and blood of a healthy homosexual man. Science 226:451–453, 1984
39. Bernard DZJ, Leibowitch J, Safai B. et al: HTLV-III in cells cultured from semen of two patients with AIDS. Science 226:449–451, 1984
40. Auerbach DM, Darrow WW, Jaffe HW, et al: Cluster of cases of acquired immunodeficiency syndrome: patients linked by sexual contact. Am J Med 76:487–492, 1984
41. Peterman TA, Stoneburner RL, Allen JR, et al: Risk of human immunodeficiency virus transmission from heterosexual adults with transfusion-associated infections. JAMA 259:55–58, 1988
42. Guinan ME, Thomas PA, Pinsky PF, et al: Heterosexual and homosexual cases of acquired immunodeficiency syndrome: a comparison of surveillance, interview, and laboratory data. Ann Intern Med 100:213–218, 1984
43. Centers for Disease Control: *Pneumocystis carinii* pneumonia among persons with hemophilia A. MMWR 31:365–367, 1982
44. Stehr-Green JS, Holman RC, Jason JM, Evatt BL: Hemophilia-associated AIDS in the United States, 1981 to September 1987. Am J Public Health 78:439–442, 1988
45. Goedert JJ, Kessler CM, Aledort LM, et al: A prospective study of human immunodeficiency virus type I infection and the development of AIDS in subjects with hemophilia. N Engl J Med 321:1141–1148, 1989
46. Curran JW, Lawrence DL, Jaffe HW, et al: Acquired immunodeficiency syndrome (AIDS) associated with transfusions. N Engl J Med 310:69–75, 1984
47. Ward JW, Holmberg SD, Allen JR: Transmission of human immunodeficiency virus (HIV) by blood transfusions screened as negative for HIV antibody. N Engl J Med 318:473–477, 1989
48. Centers for Disease Control and Prevention: U.S. Public Health Service guidelines for testing and counseling blood and plasma donors for human immunodeficiency virus type 1 antigen. MMWR 45(RR-2):1–9, 1996
49. Rogers MF, Ou C-Y, Rayfield M, et al: Use of the polymerase chain reaction for early detection of the proviral sequences of human immunodeficiency virus in infants born to seropositive mothers. N Engl J Med 320:1649–1654, 1989
50. Connor EM, Sperling RS, Gelber R, et al, for the Pediatric AIDS Clinical Trials Group Protocol 076 Study Group: Reduction of maternal-infant transmission of human immunodeficiency virus type 1 with zidovudine treatment. N Engl J Med 331:1173–1180, 1994
51. Centers for Disease Control and Prevention: Recommendations of the U.S. Public Health Service Task Force on the use of zidovudine to reduce perinatal transmission of human immunodeficiency virus. MMWR 43(RR-11):1–20, 1994
52. Centers for Disease Control and Prevention: U.S. Public Health Service recommendations for human immunodeficiency virus counseling and voluntary testing for pregnant women. MMWR 44(RR-7): 1–15, 1995
53. Mansergh G, Haddix AC, Steketee RW, et al: Cost-effectiveness of short-course zidovudine to prevent perinatal HIV type 1 infection in a sub-Saharan African developing country setting. JAMA 276: 139–145, 1996
54. Tokars JI, Marcus R, Culver DH, et al: Surveillance of HIV infection and zidovudine use among health care workers after occupational exposure to HIV-infected blood. Ann Intern Med 118: 913–919, 1993
55. Henderson DK: HIV-1 in the health care setting. In Mandel GL, Bennett JE, Dolan R (eds): Principles and Practice of Infectious Diseases. 4th ed. New York: Churchill Livingstone, 1995, pp 2632–2656

56. Centers for Disease Control: Update: universal precautions for prevention of transmission of human immunodeficiency virus, hepatitis B virus, and other bloodborne pathogens in healthcare settings. MMWR 37:377–388, 1988
57. Centers for Disease Control and Prevention: Update: provisional recommendations for chemoprophylaxis after occupational exposure to human immunodeficiency virus. MMWR 45:468–472, 1996
57a. Cardo DM, Culver DH, Ciesielski CA, et al: A case-control study of HIV seroconversion in health care workers after precutaneous exposure. N Engl J Med 337:1485–1490, 1997.
58. Centers for Disease Control: Possible transmission of human immunodeficiency virus to a patient during an invasive dental procedure. MMWR 39:489–493, 1990
59. Dorozynski A: French patient contracts AIDS from surgeon. Br Med J 314:250, 1997
60. Hessol NA, Lifson AR, O'Malley PM, Doll LS, Jaffe HW, Rutherford GW: Prevalence, incidence, and progression of human immunodeficiency virus infection in homosexual and bisexual men in hepatitis B vaccine trials, 1978–88. Am J Epidemiol 130:1167–1175, 1989
61. Centers for Disease Control: AIDS and human immunodeficiency virus infection in the United States: 1988 update. MMWR 38(S-4): 1–38, 1989
62. Holman RC, Gomperts ED, Jason JM, Abildgaard CF, Zelasky MT, Evatt BL: Age and human immunodeficiency virus infection in persons with hemophilia in California. Am J Public Health 80:967–969, 1990
63. Centers for Disease Control and Prevention: HIV/AIDS Surveillance Report, 8(1):1–33, 1996
64. Friedland G, Kahl P, Saltzman B, et al: Additional evidence for lack of transmission of HIV infection by close interpersonal (casual) contact. AIDS 4:639–644, 1990
65. Human immunodeficiency virus transmission in household settings—United States. MMWR 43:347, 353–6, 1994
66. Centers for Disease Control and Prevention: Update: trends in AIDS incidence, deaths, and prevalence—United States, 1996. MMWR 46:165–173, 1997
66a. Centers for Disease Control and Prevention: Update: Trends in AIDS incidence–United States, 1996. MMWR 46:861–867, 1997
67. Osmond D: AIDS in Africa. In Cohen PT, Sande MA, Volberding PA (eds): The AIDS Knowledge Base: A Textbook on HIV Disease from the University of California, San Francisco, and the San Francisco General Hospital, Waltham. MA: The Medical Publishing Group, 1990, pp 1.1.4:1–10
68. Smith TF, Srinivasan A, Schochetman G, Marcus M, Myers G: The phylogenetic history of immunodeficiency viruses. Nature 333: 573–575, 1988
69. Mann, JM, Tarantola D (eds): AIDS in the World. Oxford, England: Oxford University Press, 1996, vol 2
70. World Health Organization: Acquired immunodeficiency syndrome (AIDS): surveillance update to 31 March 1990 in the WHO European Region and analysis of transfusion-associated cases to 31 December 1989. Wkly Epidemiol Rec 65:239–243, 1990
71. Deeks SG, Smith M, Holodniy M, Kahn JO: HIV-1 protease inhibitors: a review for clinicians. JAMA 277:145–153, 1997
72. Centers for Disease Control: Declining rates of rectal and pharyngeal gonorrhea among males—New York City. MMWR 33:295–297, 1984
73. Lemp GF, Hirozawa AM, Givertz D, et al: Seroprevalence of HIV and risk behaviors among young homosexual and bisexual men: The San Francisco/Berkeley Young Men's Survey. JAMA 272:449–454, 1994
74. Centers for Disease Control and Prevention: Community-level prevention of human immunodeficiency virus infection among high-risk populations: The AIDS community demonstration projects. MMWR 45(RR-6):1–24, 1996
75. Irwin KL, Valdiserri RO, Holmberg SD: The acceptability of voluntary HIV antibody testing in the United States: a decade of lessons learned. AIDS 10:1707–1717, 1996
76. Centers for Disease Control: Update: acquired immunodeficiency syndrome—United States, 1989. MMWR 39:81–86, 1990
77. Centers for Disease Control: Update: reducing HIV transmission in intravenous-drug users not in drug treatment—United States. MMWR 39:529, 535–538, 1990
78. National Institutes of Health: National Institutes of Health consensus development conference statement: interventions to prevent HIV risk behaviors. Bethesda, MD: National Institutes of Health, February 1997
79. Lurie P, Reingold AL, Bowser B, et al: The public health impact of needle exchange programs in the United States and abroad. San Francisco: University of California, 1993, vol 1
80. Grosskurth H, Mosha F, Todd J, et al: Impact of improved treatment of sexually transmitted diseases on HIV infection in rural Tanzania: a randomized controlled trial. Lancet 346:530–536, 1995
81. Ungphakorn J, Sittitrai W: The Thai response to the HIV/AIDS epidemic. AIDS 8(Suppl 2):S133–S163, 1994
82. Moodie R, Aboagye-Kwarteng T: Confronting the HIV epidemic in Asia and the Pacific: developing successful strategies to minimize the spread of HIV infection. AIDS 7:1543–1551, 1993
83. Centers for Disease Control: Guidelines for effective school health education to prevent the spread of AIDS. MMWR 37(S-2):1–14, 1988
84. Valdiserri RO: Preventing AIDS: The Design of Effective Programs. New Brunswick, NJ: Rutgers University Press, 1989

9

Diseases Spread by Close Personal Contact

Acute Respiratory Infections

Arnold S. Monto

Acute respiratory diseases are the most common illnesses suffered by humans. In the developing world, acute respiratory infections are principal causes of death in young children, but in industrialized countries illness alone is the usual consequence of infection. The Health Interview Survey has estimated that more than 122 million respiratory episodes that involve restricted activity or medical consultation occur annually in the United States. The pathogens involved are multiple, and reinfection with the same agent is common. In this chapter, the situation in developed countries and the principal pathogens involved there are discussed. Infection with influenza virus is discussed on pages 107 to 112. Agents reviewed in detail are parainfluenzaviruses, respiratory syncytial virus (RSV), the rhinoviruses, coronaviruses, adenoviruses, *Mycoplasma pneumoniae*, and *Chlamydia pneumoniae*. Additional agents, such as *Coxiella burnetti*, the cause of Q fever, and a number of other viruses, such as coxsackie and echoviruses, are less frequent or limited causes of acute illness. These pathogens and other agents, such as the measles virus, which produce respiratory manifestations as one component of a more generalized disease, are considered elsewhere.

Although there are certain well-defined clinical syndromes associated with specific agents, such as croup or bronchiolitis, it is not possible on the basis of clinical characteristics of most illnesses to classify them etiologically in the absence of laboratory tests. An illustration of the situation is seen in Figure 9-1. In each portion of Figure 9-1 is shown the frequency with which individuals, infected with a particular agent, exhibit a specific respiratory symptom or restriction of daily activity. The agents are those most frequently encountered in a normal population. No clearly distinguishing characteristics are present. In spite of the overlap, however, certain differences are apparent. With the exception of coryza, symptoms are less abundant with the rhinoviruses. RS virus and parainfluenza-associated illnesses are similar in characteristics, although cough is more common with the parainfluenzaviruses, and activity restriction is more common with RS virus. Hemolytic streptococcal illness is included for completeness, and as expected, sore throat is its most prominent symptom. Influenza produces the most severe illnesses, with a greater frequency of symptoms and activity restriction for type A than for type B.

Because of the inability to determine etiology on clinical grounds, it is usual for illnesses to be enumerated simply as common or undifferentiated respiratory disease. The distribution of these illnesses has been defined in a number of different populations, and determinants of their frequency have been identified. Illness rates are highest in youngest children and decrease with increasing age, except in the third decade of life when young adults are exposed to infection by their own young children. The actual number of illnesses reported per year has varied not only with age but also with the population studied and the methods used to ascertain their occurrence. In the Cleveland family study,[1] which was carried out in a group of upper middle class households, infants had more than four such annual episodes. In the Tecumseh study,[2] in which a larger number of households of all social groups were followed, this number was 6.1. In young adults age 20 to 24 years, it was 2.8. The difference is related not only to social group, since better educated people are known to perceive more illness as occurring than less well educated individuals, but also to the method of ascertainment. In Cleveland, illness was recorded by medical personnel who visited the household, but in Tecumseh, frequency and characteristics of acute episodes were determined by a weekly telephone call.

Illness frequency is affected by sex as well as by age and social group: adult women experience more illness than men. This observation has been confirmed by laboratory investigations documenting that infections are more common in women. The greater exposure of women to small children may be responsible for this. Although there has been disagreement about the small sex difference in frequency of illness and infection in older children, there is agreement that in young children, especially under age 3 years, boys are affected more often and more severely.

Familial factors also influence the frequency of respiratory illnesses. Schoolchildren, including preschoolchildren, most often introduce infection into the family, fathers least often. The position of children in the family also determines their frequency of infection. Youngest children suffer more frequent illness earlier in life than their siblings did, mainly because of exposure to and introduction of infection by their older siblings.

The discussion of the principal agents involved focuses on their microbiology, the pathogenesis and spectrum of diseases they cause, the potential severity and frequency of these diseases, and the possibility of prevention and control. The order selected for consideration is not based simply on the relative importance of an agent but rather on a combination of factors, including potential severity and prospects for prevention.

▶ RESPIRATORY SYNCYTIAL VIRUS

Characteristics, Pathogenesis, and Distribution

This virus was isolated originally from chimpanzees and was termed the "chimpanzee coryza agent." When it was associated with disease

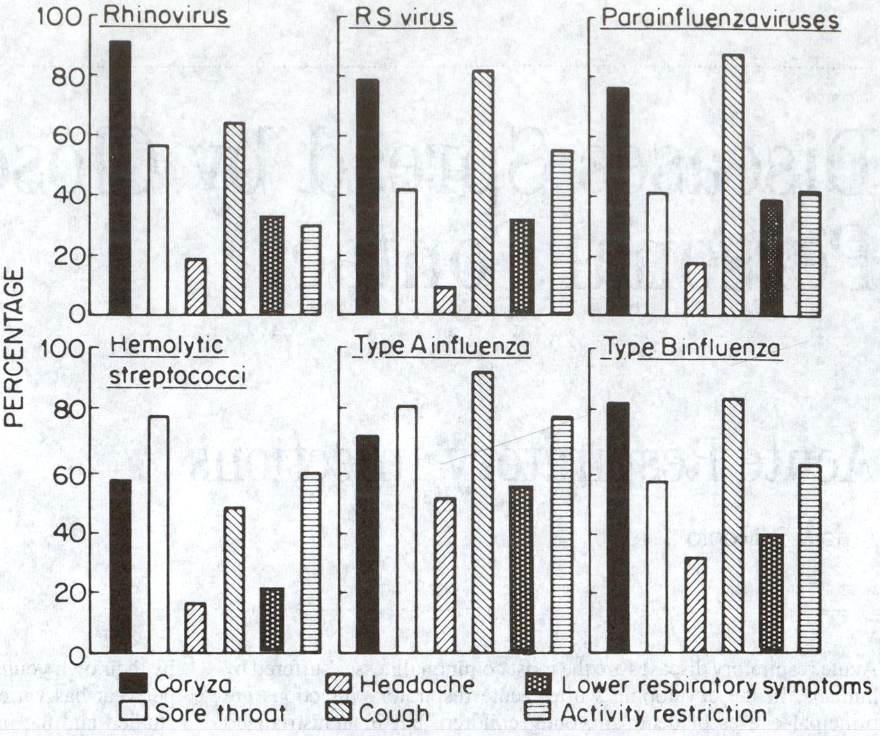

Figure 9-1. Characteristics of illnesses associated with isolation of viruses and hemolytic streptococci; percentage of those infected experiencing five symptoms and activity restriction.

in humans, it was renamed respiratory syncytial virus (RSV) on the basis of the appearance of its cytopathic effect in cell culture. It is a medium-sized (120 to 200 nm), lipid-containing pleomorphic RNA virus and has been classified as a member of the pneumovirus group. The virion possesses spikelike projections, which in similar viruses would be associated with a hemagglutinin. However, RSV virus never has been found to hemagglutinate, and identification of the virus and antibody against it must rely on different methods, such as complement fixation, neutralization, and enzyme-linked immunosorbent assay (ELISA). The virus can be identified directly by the last technique and by fluorescent antibody methods. Minor antigenic variation among RSV isolates has been recognized for many years.[3] Monoclonal antibody has permitted separation into two groups, generally termed A and B. The significance of this diversity in terms of cross-protection is unclear.[4] Other techniques such as the polymerase chain reaction have also been used to group isolates and to identify further antigenic diversity.[5]

RSV is considered the most important agent of respiratory infection among infants and young children because of its capacity to cause life-threatening bronchiolitis and pneumonia. In a number of large cities in different parts of the world, it is possible to determine when RSV transmission is occurring simply by observing the sharp increase in pediatric admissions for lower respiratory disease.[6] A number of theories have been offered to explain the pathogenesis of the disease. Since all except young children have been infected many times in life by RSV, mothers always pass RSV antibodies transplacentally to their children. RSV-associated bronchiolitis and pneumonia are more severe when they occur in the first 6 months of life, when infants usually still have detectable circulating IgG antibodies against RSV. Thus, it was postulated that these antibodies, through antigen-antibody complex formation, are involved, at least in part, in the pathogenesis of the disease. The theory was difficult to prove epidemiologically, and it has now been discounted, since maternally derived antibody actually is protective when present at sufficient titer.[7,8] The evidence is so strong that immunization of mothers is a suggested approach to prevention of disease in young children.

Certain facts about RSV illnesses are well documented. The virus is transmitted mainly during the winter and spring, and the duration of this transmission period is longer in large cities than in small communities.[9] Major outbreaks occur in the winter of alternate years. Then, in the next year, a smaller outbreak takes place in the spring.[3,6] Although a small proportion of young children when initially infected become ill enough to be hospitalized or seek medical attention, by age 4 or 5 years, all have antibodies against RSV, indicating that infection with the agent has occurred. Severe manifestations of the initial infection are more common among residents of densely populated urban areas, probably as a result of crowding and greater likelihood of infection early in life.[10] Severe illnesses are more common in small boys than in girls. Protection is relative, and reinfection with the virus throughout life is common, occurring at least every 5 years in childhood and less frequently thereafter. When reinfection occurs in partially immune adults or older children, it may result in asymptomatic infection that can be detected only serologically or mild illness that does not resemble the severe disease in infants. However, it is these individuals who frequently are responsible for transmitting severe infection to young children in a family group or introducing infection in newborn nurseries.

Prevention and Control

RSV was given high priority for attempts at prevention by immunization after recognition of its association with severe lower respiratory illness in infants. It was decided first to use a formalinized concentrated cell culture preparation because of the known protective value of inactivated influenza vaccine. Not only did this vaccine not prevent infection when infants and children subsequently were naturally exposed to wild virus, but the disease they experienced was more severe than otherwise would have been expected.[11] The vaccine had stimulated production of high levels of circulating IgG antibodies. A number of theories have been developed to explain this phenomenon, including an antibody response not balanced between the F and G glycoprotein antigens of the virus.

As a result of this experience, efforts at development turned toward a live attenuated vaccine, usually for intranasal inoculation. A live vaccine would be more similar to natural infection, without the danger of inducing a paradoxical antibody response. The intent would be to modify, not necessarily to prevent, the first infection in life so that it would resemble in severity that seen on reinfection. More recently, recombinant technology has been employed to produce preparations containing F and G glycoproteins, those antigens thought to be associated with protection. Work has proceeded with caution, based in part on past adverse experience with inactivated vaccines. Another problem with any kind of vaccine is that the target age group, young infants, may have difficulty in mounting a good antibody response. In view of the importance of RSV in potentially lethal disease of infants, further evaluation of candidate vaccines is of great importance.

It has been found that ribavirin may modify the severity of RSV disease when administered by aerosol. The effect appeared most marked in children with preexisting illnesses or disabilities.[12] However, the value of the drug is now in question, especially following several observational studies.[13] Also in early use are approaches involving prophylaxis with immune globulin.[13]

▸ PARAINFLUENZA VIRUSES

Characteristics and Pathogenesis

These viruses are members of the paramyxovirus group. The virions contain RNA, and essential lipids are relatively large and pleomorphic, with spikelike projections. Each spike incorporates both the hemagglutinin and neuraminidase enzyme of the virus. There are four different types of parainfluenzaviruses. Their presence in cell culture usually is detected through the hemadsorption technique, the result of viral budding from the cell surface. Type 1 and type 3 viruses originally were detected by hemadsorption, the latter originally called HA (hemadsorption agent) 1 and the former HA 2.[15] Type 2 parainfluenzavirus was first detected by virtue of its cytopathic effect, and it previously was called the croup-associated, or CA, virus. Type 4 viruses were described somewhat later and have been divided into two subtypes, type 4A, originally called M25, and type 4B, originally called 19503. Although it is relatively easy to separate isolates of the parainfluenzaviruses into types, it is difficult to determine serologically the specific virus involved in an illness, other than very early in life during primary infection.

As with RSV, initial infections with parainfluenzavirus are more likely to produce severe disease than are subsequent reinfections in later years. However, in these initial infections, the different parainfluenzavirus types produce quite distinct syndromes. Both types 1 and 2 are responsible for a large proportion of croup (laryngotracheobronchitis) in the first years of life, type 1 more frequently than type 2. In contrast, type 3 is more likely to produce bronchiolitis and pneumonia in infants.[16] Type 4 viruses normally do not produce severe disease at all and have been associated mainly with mild upper respiratory infection. Recent reports suggest that severe illness can occassionally result, similar in characteristics to that seen with types 1, 2, and 3.[17] The pathogenesis of the severe infections with types 1 and 2 and that with type 3 appear to differ. As with RSV, bronchiolitis seen with type 3 parainfluenzavirus occurs in the first 6 months of life. In contrast, initial infection with types 1 and 2 usually is delayed until at least past the first 4 months of life.

Occurrence of Infection

The seasonality of the different parainfluenzavirus types is not uniform. Type 3 virus is transmitted year around, usually with a late autumn and sometimes a spring peak. Type 2 is transmitted for a limited period in the late autumn into the winter. Parainfluenza type 1 participates with type 3 in the autumn peak of infection. However, two patterns of occurrence of this virus have been observed. In the early 1960s, parainfluenza 1 virus was isolated year around, resembling parainfluenza type 3. In the late 1960s into the 1970s, type 1 virus began to exhibit a different prevalence and, like type 2, was isolated only during a period each year. In fact, for a period, type 1 virus was being seen every other year, and in the alternate years, type 2 virus was being transmitted. It is not clear why the change in viral prevalence occurred, but it has been repeated in recent years.[10,18,19]

Reinfection of older children and adults with the parainfluenzaviruses is at least as common as with RSV. When infections were evaluated serologically, it was found that each year 28.6 percent of individuals were reinfected with one or more of the parainfluenzaviruses. This rate varied from 42.9 percent in children 5 to 9 years of age to 16.1 percent in adults. A most important feature of these reinfections is that they serve as a means to introduce the infection into a family group, so that mild or asymptomatic infection in an adult may have as its consequence severe croup or pneumonia in an infant.[18]

Prevention and Control

Vaccines for parainfluenza types 1, 2, and 3 are currently under development. Type 4 has not been included because it is involved only with mild sporadic disease. As with RSV, the aim of vaccine prophylaxis would be to make an initial infection in an infant or small child more like a reinfection. Thus, the intent is not to prevent the infection but rather to modify it. Inactivated vaccines, similar to those produced against influenza, were studied initially. They induced high levels of antibody but neither protected against infection nor made the subsequent disease more severe.[12] There appears to be an essential difference between parainfluenza types 1 and 2 and parainfluenza type 3 in time of occurrence. With the former agents, initial infection is not frequent until after the first 4 to 6 months of life. This observation means that immunization against types 1 and 2 can be delayed, but immunization for type 3, like that for RSV, would have to be given to an infant shortly after birth. A variety of methods, including live attenuated and recombinant antigens, are being tested.[20] The development of immunoprophylaxis is encouraged by evidence that vaccine against the bovine parainfluenza virus, related to type 3 virus, is associated with protection in calves.

▸ RHINOVIRUSES

The Agent and Its Pathogenesis

Although similar to the previously described agents in possessing RNA, the rhinoviruses are different in being small, capsomeric viruses without essential lipid. They are members, along with the enteroviruses, of the picornavirus family. The rhinovirus genus is made up of a very large number of serotypes. The total number of types is unknown but is in excess of 110. However, an isolate can be identified as a rhinovirus by its growth characteristics in cell culture and its acid and ether lability without the necessity of actually typing it. This is of some importance, since sera to most types are not readily available. There is some evidence of cross-reactions among certain types,[21] but protection appears mainly to be type specific, and, thus, sequential infection with different rhinoviruses occurs throughout life. As with most respiratory viruses, antibody is only partially protective against reinfection. The higher the titer of antibody, the greater the likelihood of protection.[22]

Rhinoviruses are the principal etiological agent of common colds in all age groups. There is no evidence that disease caused by initial infection in small children is more severe than that observed later in life. Minor alterations in lung function values can be seen in healthy individuals, but only in persons with altered host defenses, such as those with chronic bronchitis or asthma, is rhinoviral infection associated with symptomatic disease of the lower respiratory tract.[23] The major site of viral replication appears to be in the nasal mucosa, where extrusion of ciliated epithelial cells is observed. The resulting symptoms of sneezing and nasal obstruction are well-known characteristics of the common cold. Secretory IgA antibody, if present in sufficient titer in nasal secretion, protects against infection. In the absence of antibody, a very small dose of infectious virus, about the lowest amount that can be detected by the most sensitive cell culture system, is sufficient to initiate infection. When infection does occur, it is accompanied by disease in approximately 70 percent of cases.

Distribution of Infection

Rhinoviruses are the most commonly involved viruses in respiratory infections. This relationship holds not only in adults, where other agents such as the parainfluenzaviruses are not frequently isolated, but also in young children, who actually have the highest rhinoviral isolation rates. For this reason, many of the observations made on total respiratory illnesses not of specified etiology apply directly to the rhinoviruses. Infection rates are highest in the younger age groups and fall with increasing age. School and home are important sites for transmission of rhinoviral infection. Rhinoviruses can be isolated year round but peak in frequency in the autumn. After the opening of school, there is typically a sharp increase in respiratory illness in general, which is accompanied by a parallel increase in rhinoviral isolations. This increase is not restricted to one type of rhinovirus, but instead up to 20 different types can be recovered during this period.[24] Transmission in the school clearly is responsible for the mixing of the different types and their subsequent introduction into the home, where secondary cases then occur. Secondary cases are more frequent in more crowded surroundings, and mothers experience more infections than fathers, presumably because of closer contact with their infected children. The mechanisms that have been suggested for rhinoviral transmission are large droplet and indirect contact via autoinoculation. The relative importance of these two mechanisms has been a matter of debate.[25]

The existence of multiple serotypes is a major problem both in describing the epidemiology of the rhinoviruses and in developing strategies for control. Sera must be prepared for each type in order to identify and track occurrence of a strain. Thus only a limited number of investigations have been carried out on the relative importance of each type. It appears that some may cause more infections than others. There also have been suggestions that new rhinoviral types may be evolving or that old strains never before identified are recycling, but more recent evidence suggests that this may not be the case.[26]

Protection and Control

An important portion of common colds is rhinoviral in origin, and it is useful to consider prevention of rhinoviral infection as prevention of the common cold. The technology is available for production of vaccines against a single rhinoviral type, and such a vaccine would be protective. However, the multiplicity of different rhinoviral types makes the feasibility of immunoprophylaxis questionable. Certain rhinoviruses are encountered more commonly than others, and there may be more sharing of antigens than previously realized. Both of these factors might make the development of vaccines more attractive.

Rhinoviruses are sensitive to interferon, and it has been shown experimentally that intranasal interferon at relatively low doses can prevent rhinoviral infection. However, this approach has been limited by the occurrence of side effects as have more recent efforts with certain antiviral agents.[27] Chemoprophylaxis of rhinoviral infections also has been studied, and, although there have been some encouraging results with certain compounds, large-scale trials have not yet demonstrated efficacy and safety. The attractiveness of chemoprophylaxis is that a suitable compound ideally would be effective against many or all rhinoviral types.

Vitamin C has been used for common cold prophylaxis, and, as noted above, most common colds are rhinoviral in origin. The data from controlled trials to date have not been conclusive, especially in those involving viral isolation.[28] There remains the possibility of environmental control. When schoolchildren have a cold, it is common sense to keep them at home, but whether doing so limits the transmission to other children is debatable. It is also common sense for adults to absent themselves from work when they have a cold. Again, the value of thus limiting contact in controlling the spread of infection is uncertain.

► CORONAVIRUSES

The Virus and Occurrence of Disease

The coronaviruses are another group of RNA-containing agents heavily involved in the etiology of respiratory infections. The name of the group was adopted to describe the typical fringelike projection seen on electron microscopy. This appearance clearly distinguishes them from the paramyxoviruses with which they were initially confused because both are approximately of the same size and possess essential lipid. Coronaviruses infect a number of domestic animals, and the entire group originally was designated the infectious bronchitis-like viruses, named after the prototype coronavirus of chicken.

The greatest problem with the human viruses is that, aside from one strain, 229E, they cannot be isolated in cell culture. One additional strain, OC43, although originally isolated in organ culture, has been adapted to growth in a number of cell systems.[29,30] The majority of the human strains can be isolated and propagated in human embryonic tracheal organ culture, with subsequent visualization of the virus on electron microscopy. This fact has hampered the determination of the number of types of coronaviruses, their behavior, and relative importance in human infections. Much of the work on epidemiology of the agents has been carried out by serological studies using 229E and OC43 as antigens. Molecular studies of the viruses themselves generally have used the animal agents.

The animal coronaviruses are similar to the human strains from a virological standpoint and cause a variety of disease syndromes, including hepatitis, gastroenteritis, and encephalitis. In contrast, the human agents have as yet not been associated convincingly with any illnesses except those involving the respiratory tract. The disease is generally similar to that produced by the rhinoviruses, with more profuse nasal discharge and somewhat less frequent sore throat. The mean duration of coronaviral colds is shorter, 6½ days, than that seen with rhinoviruses, 9½ days. There is no clear evidence that coronaviruses are involved in lower respiratory tract infection in infants and young children. There have been reports of identification of the virus in association with a few instances of lower respiratory diseases in both hospitalized children and military recruits, but these associations should be viewed as tentative. Infection is associated with production of clinical disease in approximately 50 percent of cases.

All information on the behavior of coronaviruses in human populations is based on serological studies using two strains, OC43 and 229E. Occurrence of infection by age is similar to that seen with the other respiratory agents, with the highest rates of infection in children, decreasing in frequency with increasing age. Reinfection in the face of preexisting antibody has been demonstrated. In contrast to the rhinoviruses, a single coronavirus type is capable of producing outbreaks of infection in a community over a limited period of time, which suggests that coronaviruses may be transmitted by the small droplet or airborne route. The principal season of such transmission is late winter and early spring, at the time when rhinoviral isolation rates decrease but respiratory illnesses in general still are occurring at relatively high frequency. A particular coronaviral type exhibits a cyclical pattern of occurrence. The 229E-virus reappears every 2 to 3 years, but with OC43, although cycling does occur, its periodicity is difficult to define. This problem is related to the existence of other, as yet not properly studied, coronaviruses that are serologically related to OC43. Such viruses have been identified in investigations using organ culture.[31] The cycling phenomenon and the involvement of coronaviruses in outbreaks have led to the conclusion that, as compared to the rhinoviruses, there are a relatively limited number of coronaviral serotypes.

Prevention and Control

It is premature to think in terms of prevention or control of coronaviral infections. The initial need is not control but rather the development of techniques for isolation and cultivation of the coronaviruses so that more can be determined on the epidemiological behavior. Data now suggest that ELISA techniques might be used for recognition of these noncultivable viruses.[32,33] Until this is accomplished, it is impossible to plan for vaccine or chemoprophylaxis. From animal data, it appears that vaccine can be protective.

▸ ADENOVIRUSES

Characteristics and Resultant Diseases

Unlike all previously described viruses, the adenoviruses contain DNA, which is double stranded. The size of the virion is 60 to 90 nm, and it is capsomeric in structure. Adenoviruses are much more stable to acid pH and adverse environmental conditions, a fact that has important implications for transmission patterns. They can be isolated easily in a number of cell systems, and infection can be identified serologically using a common antigen that all share. The adenoviruses are divided into more than 40 types, which can be grouped together by virtue of the species of red cells that they hemagglutinate and nucleic acid homology. Adenoviruses of different types behave epidemiologically in very different fashions, so that such identification is of great importance, especially when outbreaks are being investigated. Certain adenoviral types cause enteric, not respiratory, disease and are described below.

The clinical types of respiratory illness produced by adenoviruses are summarized in Table 9-1. Several of the lower numbered types produce common respiratory disease in family settings. It has been estimated that about 5 percent of all respiratory disease occurring under age 5 can be attributed to adenoviruses. No clear syndromes, such as croup or bronchiolitis, are associated in this situation with adenoviruses, but a portion of these infections do involve the lower respiratory tract, with infrequent production of pneumonia.[34] All adenoviruses can infect the intestinal as well as the respiratory tract and may be shed in the stool for prolonged periods. Fecal-oral transmission often is of considerable importance in acquisition of infection by young children. Secondary spread in this situation can take longer than would be expected if only respiratory transmission were involved.[35] Few infections can be documented during the first 6 months of life, indicating that passively acquired maternal antibody exerts a protective effect. Initial infection is acquired during the first years of life, especially in crowded situations and in East Asia, and is associated half of the time with symptomatic disease.

Acute respiratory disease (ARD) is an entity confined to military recruits in many nations of the world. In North American forces, it has been an important cause of morbidity, second only to influenza. Clinical characteristics include fever, sore throat, cough, headache, and chest pain. Pulmonary infiltrates in chest x-ray have been found in approximately 10 percent of those with typical illness. Deaths from the syndrome have been rare, but they do occur.[36] Transmission is by the respiratory route. Of great concern to the military is the high attack rate over a short period of time and the incapacity that results.

TABLE 9-1. CHARACTERISTICS OF ADENOVIRUS-ASSOCIATED DISEASE

Disease	*Principal Types Involved*	*Characteristics*
Common respiratory disease	1, 2, 5, 3, 6	Endemic infections of childhood
Acute respiratory disease	4, 7, 21, 14, 3	Febrile disease of military recruits
Epidemic kerato-conjunctivitis	8	"Shipyard eye," iatrogenic spread
Pharyngoconjunctival fever	3, 7	Epidemic spread; may involve water
Pneumonia	7, 12	Unusual

Epidemic keratoconjunctivitis (EKC) was described during World War II in Hawaii and on both coasts of the U.S. mainland.[37] Outbreaks have since been observed in families, especially in East Asia and in crowded settings. In the United States, iatrogenic spread also has occurred, usually involving improperly sterilized tonometers in ophthalmologists' offices. This suggests that direct inoculation of the agent into the eye is the important route of transmission. Typically, clinical keratitis is produced, and the conjunctivitis may be follicular.

The clinical features of pharyngoconjunctival fever are incorporated into the name of the syndrome. It was initially described in 1955 in association with adenovirus type 3.[38] It may occur in sporadic or in epidemic form in children and their families. However, it is most dramatically associated with common source outbreaks involving swimming pools and small lakes. Children directly exposed to the water usually exhibit the most severe disease. Secondary spread to contacts does occur, generally resulting in milder illness. The fact that common source outbreaks are possible with the adenoviruses is a good indication of their relative stability.

Prevention and Control

Unlike the previously described viruses, there is clear evidence that vaccines can protect against adenoviral infection. However, vaccine development and use have been limited to situations in which the illness produced is viewed as being of particular importance. Military recruits are an identifiable population at high risk of ARD, a disease of high morbidity. Thus, it was decided early to be worthy of prevention. Initial inactivated vaccines against types 4 and 7 were used extensively and were protective. However, for reasons not related to efficacy, their use was discontinued, and ARD returned to recruit camps. Subsequently, live preparations of types 4 and 7 have been administered orally in enteric-coated capsules. The route of inoculation is possible in view of the ability of adenovirus to multiply in the intestinal tract.[39] This unusual approach has again been successful in prevention of ARD.

A number of candidate vaccines have been developed against the adenoviral types involved in common respiratory disease of children, but there is some question as to the need for these preparations because of the low frequency of illness of significant severity. Prevention of EKC in ophthalmologists' offices can be accomplished easily by proper sterilization of equipment. Pharyngoconjunctival fever can be prevented by proper chlorination of pools and monitoring of other places used for swimming. Bacteriological testing can be used as an indirect indication of the safety of water.

▸ MYCOPLASMA-PNEUMONIAE

This agent and *Chlamydia pneumoniae*, although not viruses, are included in a discussion of acute respiratory disease because both can produce an undifferentiated upper respiratory tract illness and lower respiratory illness previously called "viral pneumonia." As a mycoplasma, *M. pneumoniae* can be grown in artificial media, but for efficient isolation, there are rather rigid cultural requirements. In addition, *M. pneumoniae* is susceptible to a number of antibiotics that sometimes are incorporated into media used for collecting specimens for viral isolation. Needless to say, these must be omitted.[40]

Mycoplasma pneumoniae is the agent principally responsible for primary atypical pneumonia (PAP). The responsible pathogen formerly was called Eaton agent and was thought to be a virus.[41] The clinical description of the pneumonic disease has remained unchanged. Typically, there is abrupt onset and a protracted course. Symptoms of fever, cough, headache, chills, and malaise may be present for 5 days before x-ray evidence of pneumonitis develops. The nonspecific cold agglutinin test, when positive in a person with pneumonic disease, correlates well with laboratory confirmation of true *M. pneumoniae* infection. However, in only half of cases of PAP documented to be of mycoplasmal etiology is the cold agglutinin test positive. As the laboratory tests for identification of the agent became available, it was quickly realized that, as with other respiratory pathogens, there was a wide spectrum of clinical manifestations associated with *M.-pneumoniae* infection. This varies from asymptomatic infection through a common coldlike syndrome to lower respiratory illness. Reinfection with the agent also was identified, and the question of the role of antibody in the pathogenesis of the condition was investigated.

The distinct patterns of behavior of *M. pneumoniae* can be identified, that observed in families and the community and that seen in the military and in closed populations. Infections move slowly through families because, unlike the situation with most other respiratory pathogens, the incubation period of *M. pneumoniae* infection is relatively long, from 14 to 21 days. By seroepidemiology, the age groups most frequently involved are children and adolescents, indicating again the importance of school-age children in introducing infections to the family. Most of the infections seen in the family are mild, but it has been estimated that pneumonitis of some degree occurs in approximately 10 percent of infections. *M. pneumoniae* does not exhibit any clear seasonality, but there is, at least in certain geographic areas of the United States, cyclical waxing and warning of prevalence. In the eastern and central portions of the country, periods of near absence of the agent have been observed, but in the Seattle area, such a pattern has not been seen.[42]

In the military, *M. pneumoniae* has been involved in periodic outbreaks of illness with a relatively high attack rate. Such outbreaks were carefully documented at Camp Lejeune, North Carolina, in the 1960s. Often, they occurred at the same time as outbreaks of ARD caused by adenoviruses, and it was difficult to differentiate between them clinically. Outbreaks have been documented in other military situations and in civilian institutions.[43] The hypothesis has been advanced that crowding is responsible for the different frequency of transmission from that seen in families.

Prevention and Control

An inactivated vaccine was developed against *M. pneumoniae* primarily for use in the military, where the agent may be a serious problem. It was shown to protect, but the protective efficacy was approximately 50 percent, which limited its practical usefulness.[44] Because of the nature of disease in the civilian population, no serious efforts at prevention have been attempted. As a bacterium, *M. pneumoniae* is susceptible to certain broad-spectrum antibiotics. The drugs in use such as erythromycin and tetracycline, are effective in speeding recovery from this usually protracted illness. Once the drug is stopped, however, it is common for the agent to return and persist in the now asymptomatic individual. Thus, drug therapy has only limited usefulness in control of further transmission.[45]

▶ CHLAMYDIA PNEUMONIAE

Chlamydia pneumoniae strain TWAR can now be considered an important cause of infections similar in general characteristics to those produced by *Mycoplasma pneumoniae*. The species designation is new, and the strain designation comes from the combined laboratory identification numbers of two original isolates, one of which was recovered in Taiwan in 1965.[46] The exact nature of the organism and its relation to disease remained in question for so long because of the problem of cross-reaction with other chlamydia, resolved only with the availability of monoclonal antibodies. It can be grown in cell culture. The most satisfactory line has been found to be HL cells, by chance also used to identify RSV. The organisms are identified by the fluorescent antibody technique. Most epidemiological studies have relied on serological tests, and for this purpose, the microimmunofluorescent method is most sensitive and specific. This technique allows recognition of two kinds of antibody response, one associated with primary infection and the second with reinfection.

Knowledge of the behavior of *C. pneumoniae* strain TWAR in populations is not as complete as with other agents because of its relatively recent characterization. It clearly is an important cause of pneumonia, accounting for 6 to 10 percent of those hospitalized with the diagnosis. The characteristics of these illnesses do not allow recognition of the etiological agent on clinical grounds, since so much overlap in symptoms exists. There are insufficient data to determine the organism's importance in milder illness in the community, although it appears to be involved in producing bronchitis and pharyngitis. Asymptomatic or nonpneumonic infection must be common, since by age 20, half of the population can be shown to have acquired antibodies.[47]

The transmission is clearly person to person, not involving birds (as with *Chlamydia psittaci*, a much less common cause of pneumonia) or other animal reservoirs. No seasonality has been demonstrated, but there may be cycling over a period of years. Outbreaks among military recruits have been documented in Finland, lasting over periods of months.[48]

Prevention and Control

No vaccines are available for this agent, nor are any likely to be developed in the near future. Work on prevention of diseases caused by other chlamydia, however, ultimately may have implications for *C. pneumoniae*. No controlled trials of treatment have been carried out, but as with other chlamydia infections, antibiotics are useful in therapy. Tetracycline and erythromycin are the drugs of choice, and therapy must be at high dosage and maintained for up to 2 weeks.

Development of new techniques for detection of the agent itself, such as PCR, will help in moving understanding of its behavior forward.[49]

Viral Hepatitis

Harold S. Margolis

Certain forms of jaundice or hepatitis have been recognized as infectious entities for many centuries. Five viruses have been characterized, each belonging to a different taxonomic family, whose common characteristic is primary replication in the liver. Those hepatitis viruses transmitted by the fecal-oral route (hepatitis A virus (HAV), hepatitis E virus (HEV)) produce acute, self-limited infections, while those hepatitis viruses transmitted by blood and body fluids (hepatitis B virus (HBV), hepatitis C virus (HCV), hepatitis D virus (HDV)) have the ability to produce a persistent infection and chronic liver disease. In addition, there remain cases of hepatitis whose epidemiologic characteristics suggest an infectious etiology.

Historically, two major forms of hepatitis were described based on their means of transmission. "Infectious hepatitis" produced large epidemics in various settings and was transmitted by the fecal-oral route through food, water, and person-to-person contact. It appears that this disease entity was primarily caused by HAV infection, but may have also included epidemics caused by HEV. The injection of medicinal products produced from human lymph or serum resulted in outbreaks of "serum hepatitis" that were primarily due to HBV infection but probably also included HCV.

Human volunteer studies conducted in the mid-1940s and early-1950s firmly established the viral etiology, clinical picture, and routes of transmission of the two major type of hepatitis and determined the mutually exclusive specificity of the immunity produced by each type of infection. Studies conducted by Krugman and colleagues[1] showed that short incubation period (31 to 38 days) hepatitis could be transmitted either orally or parenterally using a serum pool (MS-1) collected from a patient prior to the onset of illness. A second serum pool (MS-2) obtained from the same patient following a second episode of hepatitis was shown to transmit disease only when inoculated parenterally, and this disease had a longer incubation period (41 to 83 days). Subsequently, MS-1 hepatitis was shown to be caused by HAV; and MS-2 hepatitis, by HBV.

In 1965, Blumberg and coworkers studying the production of isoantibodies in Australian aborigines, identified an antigen that they called "Australian antigen," which was subsequently found to be the hepatitis B surface antigen (HB_sAg).[2,3] Characterization of the antigens and antibodies produced during HBV infection led to the development of diagnostic tests, the routine screening of blood for HB_sAg to prevent HBV-related posttransfusion hepatitis, and the development and licensure of hepatitis B vaccines.

In 1973, HAV was identified in the stools of persons involved in a food-borne outbreak of hepatitis and in the stools of the volunteers inoculated with MS-1.[4,5] These findings led to the development of diagnostic tests that could differentiate acute from past infection, the propagation of HAV in cell culture, and the development and licensure of hepatitis A vaccines.

In 1977, Rizzetto and colleagues described second episodes of hepatitis in patients chronically infected with HBV and characterized a new antigen in the liver of these patients.[6] Subsequent studies showed that this form of hepatitis was transmitted only in the presence of acute or chronic HBV infection and that HDV was a defective virus that required HB_sAg to produce infection.[7]

By the mid-1970s, another type of blood-borne hepatitis was characterized because of the availability of serologic tests to identify HAV and HBV infection and the occurrence of posttransfusion hepatitis in spite of donor testing for HB_sAg.[8] Population-based surveillance studies showed that most parenterally transmitted non-A, non-B (PT-NANB) hepatitis occurred outside of the transfusion setting,[9] and in 1989, HCV was characterized by molecular cloning and found to be the primary cause of PT-NANB hepatitis.[10]

The ability to make the serologic diagnosis of acute HAV infection led to the identification of enterically transmitted NANB (ET-NANB) hepatitis, a disease that produced large epidemics and was transmitted by the fecal-oral route.[11] Although the virus associated with ET-NANAB hepatitis was identified in 1983, HEV was not characterized until 1989,[12] with the subsequent development of diagnostic tests and prototype vaccines.

Worldwide, there continues to be considerable morbidity and mortality attributable to the acute and chronic sequelae of viral hepatitis. However, at a time when control, prevention, or elimination of most forms of viral hepatitis are attainable, the recent interest in emerging infectious diseases has the potential to direct attention away from these major public health problems. In fact, each etiologic form of viral hepatitis meets the Institute of Medicine's definition of an emerging infectious disease.[13] In the United States alone, over 12,000 persons die annually of viral hepatitis-related acute or chronic liver disease (Table 9-2), and except for hepatitis E, each of these diseases has emerged or reemerged in the United States over the past two decades. We have adequate knowledge to prevent or control most types of viral hepatitis. The challenge is to turn this knowledge into effective prevention programs.

▸ HEPATITIS A

Etiologic Agent

HAV is a 27-nm, nonenveloped single-stranded, positive-sense RNA virus whose genomic organization and replication scheme are similar to that of polio virus and other members of the family Picornaviridae. HAV has an icosohedral capsid configuration, with each structural unit comprised of three polypeptides. However, when compared to other picornaviruses, HAV is more resistant to inactivation by heating, to $pH < 3$, to drying at ambient temperature, and to low concentrations of free chlorine or hypochlorite.[14,15] HAV remains infectious in feces or on environmental surfaces for several weeks, is only partially inactivated by pasteurization (60°C for 1 hour), but is completely inactivated by formalin or heating at 100°C for 5 minutes.[14,15] HAV grows poorly in cell culture, where it requires a long adaptation period (up to 1 month), rarely produces a cytopathic effect, and rapidly becomes attenuated.[14,15] Although previously classified in the genus *Enterovirus*, HAV has been placed in a new genus (*Heparnavirus*) because of the large number of characteristics that distinguish it from other enteroviruses.[14]

Humans appear to be the only natural host of HAV; however, a number of nonhuman primates (chimpanzees, tamarins, macaques) are susceptible to experimental infection. In addition, several genetically distinct strains of HAV have been identified in Old World monkeys, but these viruses have not been identified in humans and they produce only an attenuated infection in the chimpanzee model of human HAV infection.[16–18] Antibody binding studies indicate that there is only a single HAV serotype. HAV isolates from diverse geographic areas are recognized by polyclonal antibody generated against capsid proteins (anti-HAV), and by neutralizing monoclonal antibodies to human HAV. Old World monkey HAV is recognized by polyclonal human anti-HAV but not by neutralizing monoclonal antibodies to human HAV, suggesting phenotypic differences in these viruses. Although HAV has little phenotypic diversity, enough genetic diversity exists in the capsid region to define several genotypes and allows for studies of molecular relatedness.[17]

Clinical Illness, Pathogenesis, and Immune Response

Manifestations of HAV infection include fecal shedding of virus, viremia, age-dependent expression of clinical illness (i.e., jaundice), the occasional occurrence of fulminant liver failure, and absence of

TABLE 9-2. EPIDEMIOLOGIC FEATURES OF VIRAL HEPATITIS AS AN EMERGING INFECTIOUS DISEASE IN THE UNITED STATES

Agent	*Change in Incidence (years)*	*Acute Cases/ Year*	*Chronic Infections (total)*	*Deaths/Year*
Hepatitis A virus	Increase 1988–1991	150,000	None	100–150
Hepatitis B virus	Increase 1979–1985	260,000	1–1.25 million	5,000
Hepatitis C virus	Increase 1987–1989	120,000	3.9 million	8,000–10,000
Hepatitis D virus	Unknown	10,000	70,000	1,000
Hepatitis E virus	Unknown	Unknown	None	Unknown

chronic liver disease. Children under 6 years of age generally have mild, nonspecific symptoms that include malaise, nausea, vomiting, diarrhea, fever, and dark urine. Jaundice is uncommon in this age group, being present in less than 5 percent of children under age 3 and in 10 percent of children age 4 to 6 years.[19] Among adolescents and adults infected with HAV, the majority have classic signs or symptoms, including jaundice, fever, malaise, nausea, vomiting, loss of appetite, and dark urine.[20]

Clinical symptoms due to hepatitis A are indistinguishable from those due to other types of viral hepatitis and should not be used to establish an etiologic diagnosis. The risk of fulminant hepatitis is 0.1 to 0.5 percent; the highest case fatality rate is among persons over age 40 years (1.3 to 2.2 percent) and is often associated with underlying chronic liver disease.[21,22] HAV infection or hepatitis A does not cause chronic liver disease or persistent infection, although 15 to 20 percent of patients may have a relapse of clinical illness.[23]

The pathogenetic events that occur during the course of infection have been determined from experimental infections in chimpanzees and naturally acquired infections in humans (Fig. 9-2). The incubation period for HAV infection has ranged from 14 to 45 days, with a median of 28 days.[14,15] Virus is found in hepatocytes throughout the course of infection and is excreted in the bile and feces in high concentrations 7 to 10 days prior to the onset of clinical illness. Virus excretion begins to decline at the onset of symptoms, and most adult patients (66 percent) have no detectable virus 1 week following the onset of clinical illness.[24,25] However, children may excrete virus for longer periods than do adults.[25,26] Viremia occurs for 10 to 15 days, beginning in the incubation period and continuing into the early part of the clinical illness (Fig. 9-2). Available data suggest that the pathogenesis of liver injury is immune mediated rather than due to direct cytotoxicity and probably involves cell-mediated immune responses. A specific IgM antibody response to HAV capsid proteins (IgM anti-HAV) develops prior to the onset of clinical illness, and neutralizing IgG antibodies are usually detectable at or before the onset of clinical illness. The IgM anti-HAV response is also accompanied by a nonspecific rise in the concentration of serum IgM.[14,15]

Diagnosis

Acute HAV infection is diagnosed by the detection of IgM anti-HAV using commercially available immunoassays. This antibody response is usually detectable 1 week prior to the onset of symptoms and remains detectable for 3 to 6 months after infection (Fig. 9-2). Previous HAV infection is diagnosed by the detection of IgG anti-HAV, which persists for life. Commercially available immunoassays detect only total anti-HAV (IgG and IgM). In a well person, a positive test for total anti-HAV indicates a previous infection. However, if the person is suspected of having an asymptomatic, acute infection, he or she should also be tested for IgM anti-HAV.

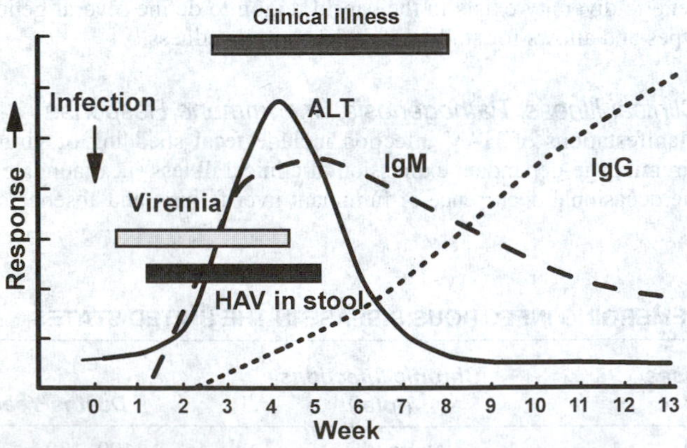

Figure 9-2. Clinical pattern and immunologic and virologic events during hepatitis A virus infection. (Adapted from Cromeans T, Nainan OV, Fields HA, Favorov MO, Margolis HS: Hepatitis A and E viruses. In Hui YH, Gorham JR, Mucell KD, Cliver DO (eds): Foodborne Disease Handbook. New York: Marcel Dekker, 1994.)

IgG anti-HAV is produced following an acute infection and following immunization with hepatitis A vaccine. Serologic testing following hepatitis A vaccination is not recommended and most commercially available tests, unless modified, cannot detect the lower range of vaccine-induced antibody.[27] However, anyone found to be anti-HAV positive with currently available tests should be considered to have protective levels of antibody (i.e., >20 mIU/mL).[27] IgM anti-HAV is detected only rarely during the month following hepatitis A vaccination, and presence of this antibody should be considered evidence of an acute infection.[27] Detection of antibodies to the nonstructural proteins of HAV have the potential to differentiate immunized persons from persons with HAV infection. However, attempts to develop assays with an adequate level of sensitivity have not been successful.

Methods to detect HAV are generally limited to research laboratories. HAV antigen can often be detected in feces, cell culture, and some environmental specimens by enzyme immunoassay.[14] Growth in cell culture requires a long period of adaptation and changes the genetic makeup of the virus.[14] Amplification of HAV RNA by the polymerase chain reaction (PCR) is the most sensitive means to detect HAV in feces, blood, cell culture, or environmental samples.[14] However, unless PCR is performed by initially capturing the virus particle with anti-HAV, the detection of HAV RNA may not be equated with infectivity.

Epidemiology

Hepatitis A is an important cause of illness throughout the world and there exist several patterns of infection endemicity (Fig. 9-3). Endemicity of infection is directly related to hygienic standards and inversely related to socioeconomic conditions. In areas with a high endemicity of HAV infection, almost all adults have been infected, usually as children before 10 years of age.[28] In countries that have had significant changes in socioeconomic levels over the past several decades (i.e., Greece, Taiwan, Italy, parts of China), improved sanitation and living standards have significantly reduced the endemic rate of HAV infection. In such countries or regions, a significant decrease in the prevalence of HAV infection has occurred among young children. However, HAV infection continues to occur among older children and young adults, and a paradoxical increase in the incidence of hepatitis A may occur because of the greater likelihood of symptomatic infection. In addition, the potential remains for epidemics to occur as long as HAV is present in the population or the environment, including food sources. Shifts in infection patterns were recently observed in Shanghai, China, when over 300,000 young adults became ill when shellfish contaminated with HAV were sold in the marketplace and subsequently prepared in a traditional manner at temperatures that did not kill the virus.[29]

Low endemic rates of HAV infection are found in the United States, western Europe, and Australia where the prevalence of past infection varies from 30 to 70 percent in adults and is less than 10 percent in young children (Fig. 9-3). In the United States, disease incidence varies among racial/ethnic groups, with the highest rates in American Indians/Alaskan Natives and Hispanics; these high rates of infection are most likely related to low socioeconomic level.[27] About 60 percent of cases occur in persons age 15 to 39 years and 25 percent occur in children under 15 years of age.[21]

In both low and high endemic populations, HAV infection behaves like most other acute infectious diseases, producing periodic epidemics as the pool of susceptible individuals increases. Most disease in the United States occurs within the context of community wide epidemics that primarily affect young persons of low socioeconomic status.[27,30] Communities can be generally classified into those with high, intermediate, or low rates of disease.[27] High rates of disease generally occur in small communities on Indian reservations, in Alaskan Native villages, around the United States-Mexican border,

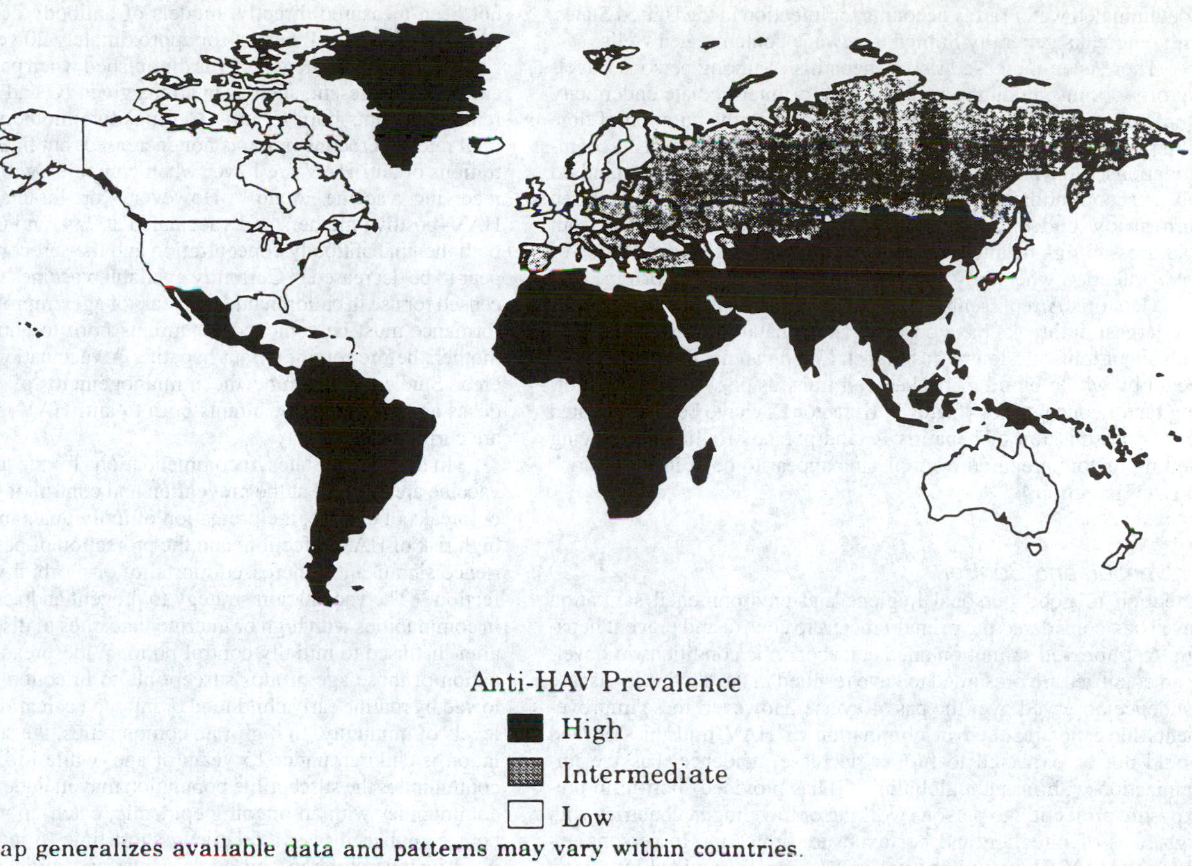

Figure 9-3. Patterns of hepatitis A virus infection (endemicity) worldwide. (From Centers for Disease Control and Prevention: Prevention of hepatitis A through active or passive immunization. Recommendations of the Advisory Committee on Immunization Practices. MMWR 45 (RR-15):1, 1996.)

or in religious communities. A high prevalence of infection is present throughout the community, most infections occur among children under 10 years of age, and epidemics occur with regular periodicity.[31–33] Intermediate rates of disease generally occur in larger cities, and the pattern of infection is more variable throughout the community. Highest rates of infection are often found among children identified by race/ethnicity or socioeconomic level living in certain neighborhoods or census tracts. In addition, high rates of disease may occur in young adults who are often drug users or in their contacts.

In some communities, the sources of HAV infection may change between epidemic and nonepidemic periods, with certain risk groups (i.e., drug users, homosexual men) contributing to the increased number of cases. However, in all settings, contact with an infected person is the most important source of new infections. Contact with a person known to have hepatitis A in the household setting is the source of infection for 12 to 25 percent of cases in the United States.[21] Contact with children in a day care center is reported for an additional 11 to 16 percent of cases. However, this source of infection may be overestimated since serologic testing was not required to identify HAV infection in the day care center.[21] Other sources of infection include travel to a country with a high or intermediate endemicity of infection (5 to 7 percent), injection or noninjection drug use (2 to 16 percent), homosexual activity (7 percent), or an outbreak attributable to contaminated food or water (2 to 5 percent). The source of infection cannot be identified in approximately 40 percent of cases.[21]

Hepatitis A outbreaks in child care centers involve transmission not only among children, but to adult contacts who often compose 70 to 80 percent of the recognized cases.[34] However, day care attendance per se does not place a child at increased risk of infection. The age-specific prevalence of HAV infection among children having attended day care is the same as among children who were not enrolled in day care.[27] Generally, an increased risk of infection occurs only when HAV is introduced into a day care center, and day care centers are infrequently the source of epidemics in communities. In general, day care providers are not at increased risk of infection.[35]

Susceptible household contacts have a 10 to 50 percent risk of acquiring disease from a family member with acute illness. During communitywide epidemics of hepatitis A, contact with children under 6 years of age appears to be a risk factor for infection. Among adults with no known source of infection, approximately 40 percent of children under 6 years of age living in their households have been found to have serologic evidence of asymptomatic infection, suggesting that they were the source of the infection in the adult.

HAV is also transmitted through sexual contact, especially among men who have sex with men.[27,36] HAV infection is common among injection and noninjection drug users and the mode of transmission probably includes both parenteral and person-to-person exposures.[27]

Common source outbreaks due to contaminated food or water continue to occur, but appear to account for a small proportion (2 to 5 percent) of cases in the United States, although it is not known to what extent these sources account for sporadic cases. Implicated foods are generally eaten raw and have been contaminated during growing, harvest, final processing, or preparation.[14] Foods contaminated during preparation have included salads, sandwiches, and glazed or iced pastries. Shellfish associated outbreaks have been due to eating raw or partially cooked oysters, clams, or mussels harvested from contaminated waters.[14,37] Fruits or vegetables contaminated during harvest or packing and eaten raw (i.e., lettuce, strawberries, raspberries) have accounted for some outbreaks.[14,38,39]

Contaminated water rarely accounts for infection in the United States, with outbreaks generally limited to sewage contaminated wells.[14]

There is an increased risk of hepatitis A among persons traveling or working in countries with a high or intermediate endemicity of infection, and risk of infection increases with the duration of time in the country.[40] Persons traveling outside of general tourist accommodations (i.e., hikers, campers) and persons staying in standard tourist accommodations are at increased risk of infection. Children born in low endemic areas whose parents have immigrated from countries of high or intermediate endemicity are at increased risk of HAV infection when they visit their parent's country of origin.

Hepatitis A represents a rare cause of posttransfusion hepatitis. The largest outbreaks have occurred in neonatal intensive care units with silent transmission to hospital staff and parents from infants infected by whole blood or packed cell transfusions.[26] Recently, clotting factor concentrates (factor VIII, factor IX) have been implicated in the transmission of hepatitis A, and persons routinely receiving clotting factors prepared from plasma appear to be at increased risk of HAV infection.[41,42]

Prevention and Control

Attention to good personal hygiene and environmental sanitation have been considered the primary means to control and prevent hepatitis A. Improved sanitation and socioeconomic conditions in developed countries are presumed to have resulted in the decline in disease incidence observed over the past 40 years. However, these improvements have not resulted in elimination of HAV transmission and would not be expected to further decrease incidence. Passive immunization with immunoglobulin (IG) has provided short-term preexposure protection to persons working or traveling in countries with high rates of infection and postexposure protection to persons exposed to HAV. However, the use of IG has not provided long-term protection from HAV infection and has rarely interrupted ongoing communitywide epidemics. The recently licensed inactivated hepatitis A vaccines are highly immunogenic and produce long-term immunity that makes the control, prevention, or elimination of HAV transmission an achievable goal.

Numerous studies have confirmed that preparations of human immunoglobulin that contain anti-HAV are 75 to 85 percent effective in preventing symptomatic HAV infection if given before or within 2 weeks of exposure.[27,43] When given prior to exposure, IG appears to prevent infection. When given following exposure, passive-active immunization often occurs from an infection that produces little or no symptoms and limited virus shedding.[43] With the availability of hepatitis A vaccines, IG is primarily recommended for preexposure immunization of children under 2 years of age traveling to countries with a high or intermediate endemicity of HAV infection (Fig. 9-3).[27] However, IG remains the mainstay of postexposure prophylaxis and should be given to household and sexual contacts of persons with hepatitis A within 2 weeks of exposure and to children and staff exposed in day care or certain other institutional settings.[27] In the chimpanzee model of HAV infection, hepatitis A immunization appears to provide limited protection and to reduce virus shedding when given soon after exposure.[44] However, the efficacy of active postexposure immunization has not been evaluated in clinical trials.

The currently licensed hepatitis A vaccines are produced from cell culture adapted virus that is formalin inactivated and adsorbed on an alum adjuvant.[45] These vaccines have been shown to be highly immunogenic in children, adolescents, and adults using a two-dose vaccination schedule.[27] While other prototype vaccines have been developed and evaluated (i.e., live attenuated vaccines), it is not clear whether they will offer distinct advantages over the current licensed vaccines.[45]

In controlled clinical trials, preexposure vaccination with inactivated hepatitis A vaccine has been shown to be more than 95 percent effective in preventing hepatitis A and HAV infection.[46,47] Although the duration of immunity provided by hepatitis A immunization has not been measured directly, models of antibody decay predict that protective levels will persist for approximately 20 years.[27]

Vaccine immunogenicity is diminished when passively acquired anti-HAV is present, such as in adults given IG and vaccine concurrently or infants born to anti-HAV positive mothers.[27] In adults the final rate of seroconversion is not decreased, but final serum concentrations of anti-HAV are lower when compared with that in persons receiving vaccine alone.[27] However, for infants born to anti-HAV–positive mothers and vaccinated at 2, 4, and 6 months of age, both the final antibody concentration and the seroconversion rate appear to be decreased.[27] Currently available vaccines have not been licensed for use in children under 2 years of age. Improved vaccine performance must be achieved for infants born to anti-HAV–positive mothers before routine infant hepatitis A vaccination can be considered. Studies to examine the immunogenicity of various vaccine doses and schedules for infants born to anti-HAV–positive mothers are currently under way.

In the United States, recommendations for the use of hepatitis A vaccine are directed at the prevention and control of communitywide outbreaks of disease, the protection of individuals in those groups at high risk of HAV infection, and the protection of persons who experience significantly increased mortality or morbidity from HAV infection.[27] The vaccination strategy to prevent and control hepatitis A in communities with high or intermediate rates of disease is patterned after that used to initially control polio. Widespread catch-up vaccination of those age groups susceptible to infection is required, followed by routine early childhood or infant vaccination to sustain high levels of immunity. In high-rate communities, the susceptible population is children under 15 years of age, while in intermediate rate communities the susceptible population may include young adults. In communities with an ongoing epidemic, catch-up vaccination must be accomplished over a relatively short time (6 months to 1 year), must include children and adolescents, and might have to include older age groups. Maintenance of active disease surveillance and analysis of surveillance data with respect to demographic characteristics and risk factors for infection is essential to tailor hepatitis A vaccination programs and evaluate their effectiveness.

Epidemics in a number of smaller (high-rate) communities have been interrupted using this recommended approach.[48] However, in larger (intermediate rate) communities, experience is limited due to the logistical considerations of rapidly vaccinating large numbers of children outside of routine health care encounters. As was the case for polio, integration of hepatitis A vaccine into the routine infant vaccination schedule will be required to effectively maintain a reduction in disease incidence.

Persons (adults and children) traveling or working in countries with a high or intermediate endemicity of HAV infection (Fig. 9-3) should be vaccinated prior to departure.[27] If the child traveler is under 2 years of age, IG should be used for preexposure immunization since the currently available vaccines are not licensed for use in this age group.[27] Although immunogenicity studies show a high rate of seroconversion 2 weeks following receipt of the first vaccine dose, vaccination should be completed 1 month prior to travel to ensure adequate protection.[27] Vaccination is recommended for persons in other groups at high risk of infection, including drug users (injection and non injection), men who have sex with men, and hemophiliacs.[27] In addition, vaccination is recommended for persons with chronic liver disease because of their increased risk of mortality and morbidity from hepatitis A.[27]

When vaccinating adults or persons in groups at high risk of HAV infection, consider that many will already have been infected with HAV. Because of the relatively high vaccine cost, prevaccination testing might be considered if the cost of the vaccine is greater than the cost of testing and the follow-up visits.[27] Based on the prevalence of HAV infection, prevaccination testing could be considered in persons over 40 years of age, persons of any age who were born in a country of high or intermediate endemicity of infection, drug users, and men who have sex with men. Postvaccination testing is not warranted.

▸ HEPATITIS B

Etiologic Agent

Hepatitis B virus (HBV) is a member of the family Hepadnaviridae, which includes viruses that infect woodchucks, ducks, ground squirrels, and herons. HBV has a small (3.2-kilobase) genome with a circular DNA that is partly single stranded and a retroviral replication strategy with an RNA intermediate. The genome codes for a surface glycoprotein, nucleocapsid protein, DNA polymerase, and the "x" protein which may be involved with transformation.[49] The liver is the primary site of replication of the Hepadnaviridae. All cause persistent infection and have the potential for integration into host cells where they are oncogenic. The complete HBV virion (Dane particle) is 42 nm in diameter and composed of the outer hepatitis B surface antigen (HB_sAg) glycoprotein and the inner nucleoprotein or hepatitis B core antigen (HB_cAg). Besides being associated with the whole virion, HB_sAg exists independently and circulates as 22-nm spheres and tubules. HBV has been shown to retain infectivity for at least 1 month when stored at either room temperature or frozen. Infectivity is destroyed at 90°C after 1 hour.[50] The only natural host of HBV appears to be humans. Propagation in cell culture has generally been unsuccessful; however, HBV is easily purified from the plasma of infected hosts and a number of antigen and antibody systems have been characterized that identify the various stages of infection (Table 9-3). HB_sAg is the most useful marker of viral presence, and subtypes of HB_sAg have been used in epidemiologic studies to identify patterns of disease transmission.[51]

Although HBV cannot be consistently propagated in cell culture, its molecular biology has been extensively characterized. This has resulted in the production of antigens for vaccines and immunodiagnostic tests, the development of infectious clones, and the development of transgenic mouse models of persistent infection. The retroviral-like (RNA) intermediate that is produced during HBV replication produces a relatively high mutation rate for this DNA virus. Identified mutations include those in the region of HB_sAg that binds neutralizing antibody (the *a* determinant), and those in the nucleocapsid that result in the lack of production of hepatitis B e antigen (HB_eAg).[52] These mutations may exist as either the dominant virus population or as subpopulations in persons with chronic HBV infection. While there has been speculation that these variants influence the clinical outcome of infection or produce a loss of vaccine efficacy, no epidemiologic studies confirm this speculation.

TABLE 9-3. HEPATITIS B VIRUS TERMINOLOGY

HBV	Hepatitis B virus: a 42-nm DNA virus, originally known as the Dane particle
HB_sAg	Hepatitis B surface antigen: the surface glycoprotein coat of HBV; also exists free of virus as 22-nm, spherical and tubular particles; the antigen in hepatitis B vaccine; positive serologic test for HB_sAg indicates HBV infection
HB_cAg	Hepatitis B core antigen: the nucleocapsid antigen of HBV
HB_eAg	Hepatitis B e antigen: soluble antigen that indicates level of infectivity; associated with high levels of HBV DNA
anti-HBs	Antibody to hepatitis B surface antigen: present after resolved infection or hepatitis B immunization; positive serological test usually indicative of protection against infection
anti-HBc	Antibody to hepatitis B core antigen: present after resolved infection or during chronic infection; IgM anti-HBc indicates acute HBV infection
anti-HBe	Antibody to hepatitis B e antigen: present after resolved infection and in persons with chronic infection but of low infectivity

Clinical Illness, Pathogenesis, and Immune Response

Acute HBV infection can be asymptomatic, cause clinically evident hepatitis, or result in fulminant hepatitis and death. Acute hepatitis B cannot be differentiated from other types of viral hepatitis on the basis of signs or symptoms, the correct diagnosis being made only by serologic testing. The clinical onset of hepatitis B is usually insidious, with malaise, weakness, and anorexia being the most common findings. Myalgia and arthralgia without other clinical signs have been described in 10 to 30 percent of patients, and in one-third an urticarial or maculopapular rash appears, often along with joint symptoms. Jaundice develops in 20 to 30 percent of infected adults and may persist for several weeks. Liver enzyme elevations usually occur prior to the onset of jaundice. Acute HBV infection is rarely symptomatic (1 to 10 percent) in infants and young children.[53]

During acute infection, HB_sAg may become detectable 1 to 2 months prior to the onset of clinical symptoms and is soon followed by the appearance of IgM anti-HBc. In late convalescence, there is a transition period ("window phase") when the concentration of HB_sAg declines and the concentration of antibody to HB_sAg (anti-HBs) increases. As these markers reach equivalency, neither may be detectable because they form immune complexes; however, both IgG anti-HB_c and IgM anti-HB_c remain detectable. For infections that resolve, HB_sAg disappears from circulation and anti-HBs becomes detectable along with anti-HBc.

Among individuals in whom HBV infection persists, both HB_sAg and anti-HBc remain detectable, usually indefinitely. During the early part of chronic HBV infection, HB_eAg is present and indicates a high level of viral replication and infectivity. Each year approximately 10 percent of persons with chronic HBV infection will lose HB_eAg, a modest proportion will lose HBV DNA, and up to 1 to 2 percent per year may naturally lose HB_sAg.[54] Persons with chronic HBV infection are at risk of chronic liver disease (i.e., chronic active hepatitis, cirrhosis, liver failure) and primary hepatocellular carcinoma (PHC). The majority of HBV-infected persons remain well and will not die from HBV-related diseases. However, prospective studies have shown that 25 percent of persons who acquired chronic HBV infection as infants or young children will die as adults (average age 45 years) from HBV-related PHC or chronic liver disease.[55,56] Among persons who acquire chronic HBV infection as adults, it is estimated that 15 percent will die from HBV-related chronic liver disease at an average age of 55 years.[57] In addition, HBV infection is associated with extrahepatic disease such as vasculitis and membranoproliferative glomerulonephritis.[58]

HBV must gain access to the circulation and arrive in the liver for primary replication in hepatocytes. Access occurs through direct percutaneous inoculation, breaks in the skin that allow inapparent inoculation, or passage through mucous membranes. Although HB_sAg has been detected in tissues other than the liver, there is little evidence to suggest sustained replication at these sites. The number of hepatocytes affected during the acute phase of replication is variable and can reach almost 100 percent. During persistent infection, approximately 10 percent of hepatocytes remain infected.

There is strong evidence that the hepatocellular injury that occurs during HBV infection is immune mediated. Cell-mediated injury is targeted at hepatocytes through a combination of human leukocyte antigen (HLA) molecules and HBV antigens.[59] The precise mechanism(s) that lead to viral persistence are unknown, but may include the induction of immune tolerance by HB_eAg.

Diagnosis

Solid-phase immunoassays are commercially available for the detection of HB_sAg and have a high degree of sensitivity and specificity when used according to the manufacturer's directions. When used for screening in low prevalence populations (i.e., routine testing of blood donors or pregnant women), test manufacturers recommend confirmation of initially positive results by repeat testing and neutralization of the repeatedly positive specimen. A serum sample positive for HB_sAg indicates the presence of HBV infection, but does not fully determine the stage of the disease. An individual is classified as having a chronic infection if HB_sAg remains detectable for more than 6 months or if he or she is HB_sAg positive and IgM anti-HBc negative. All HB_sAg-positive persons should be considered infectious. However, a higher degree of infectivity is ascribed to persons who are positive for HB_eAg or HBV DNA.

Detection of anti-HBs is not routinely performed during diagnostic testing but may be used in certain instances to determine a person's immune status following vaccination. Postvaccination testing is recommended for persons in a number of categories, including:[60] (*a*) health care workers at continued risk of needlestick or other percutaneous exposures, (*b*) immunocompromised persons at continued risk of HBV exposure, (*c*) the sexual partner of a chronically infected person, and (*d*) infants who have received postexposure prophylaxis because they were born to an HB_sAg-positive mother. Anti-HBs concentrations in serum are expressed as milli-international units/mL based on a World Health Organization standard.[61] Concentrations of anti-HB_s greater than 9.9 mIU/mL have been shown to protect against chronic HBV infection.[60]

The diagnosis of acute HBV infection is best made by the detection of HB_sAg and IgM anti-HBc. During acute infection, IgM anti-HBc becomes detectable almost coincident with the appearance of HB_sAg, persists for 2 to 6 months, and is present during the "window phase" of convalescence. While IgM anti-HBc can be detected in low levels among persons with chronic HBV infection, commercially available tests are configured in such a manner as to minimize the likelihood of a positive result in this situation.[62]

Epidemiology

The endemicity of HBV infection varies greatly throughout the world (Fig. 9-4).[63] Endemicity is considered high in those areas where the prevalence of chronic infection is 8 percent or more and where 60 to 90 percent of the population has serologic evidence of previous infection. In these areas, infection during the perinatal period and early childhood account for high rates of chronic infection and its sequelae. In most developed countries, the prevalence of HBV infection is low, with rates of HB_sAg positivity being less than 1 percent. In these areas, most infections occur among adults and certain high-risk populations that include injection drug users, persons with multiple homosexual or heterosexual partners, household or sexual contacts of persons with chronic HBV infection, patients on hemodialysis, persons with occupational exposure to blood or body fluids, residents of institutions for the developmentally disabled, and persons receiving clotting factor concentrates or frequent blood transfusions.[60] However, within areas of low endemicity the prevalence of infection can vary widely. For example, within North America there reside Eskimo populations with a high endemicity of HBV infection and first-generation immigrant populations from high endemic areas (e.g., Asia, Africa, Middle East, former Soviet Union) that continue to have high rates of HBV transmission.[64,65] In those parts of the world with an intermediate endemicity of HBV infection, transmission in infancy, early childhood, and adulthood maintains the level of chronic infection.

The principle modes of HBV transmission are shown in Table 9-4. Direct transmission via blood or blood products has been eliminated in those countries that routinely screen donors for HB_sAg and require viral inactivation of clotting factor concentrates. In developed countries, nosocomial transmission of HBV from inadequately sterilized medical instruments or reuse of injection equipment has not been a significant problem. However, occasional outbreaks continue to occur from the contamination of multiple dose vials, fingerstick, and other medical devices.[66] Sharing needles and other injection equipment among drug users accounts for a large proportion of cases in the United States (Fig. 9-5).[67] In developing countries, nosocomial

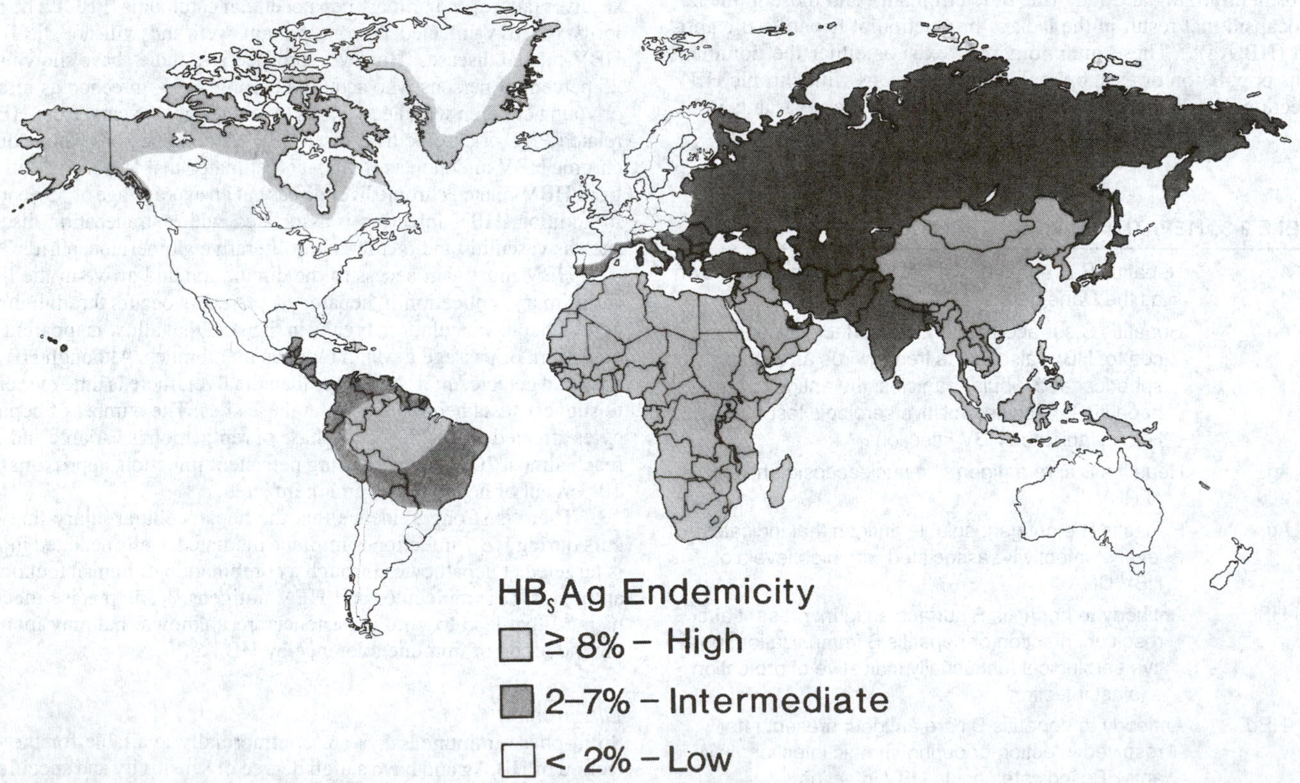

Figure 9-4. Patterns of chronic hepatitis B virus infection (endemicity) worldwide. (Adpated from Maynard JE, Kane MA, Hadler SC: Global control of hepatitis B through vaccination: role of hepatitis B vaccine in the Expanded Programme on Immunization. Rev Infect Dis 11:s574, 1989.)

TABLE 9-4. MECHANISMS OF HEPATITIS B VIRUS TRANSMISSION

Mode	*Examples*
Direct percutaneous	Blood transfusion, infusion of blood products, use of contaminated needles or medical instruments, human bites (saliva)
Inapparent percutaneous	Contamination of cuts, scratches, sores, dermatitis, pyoderma, insect bites with blood or serous fluid; shared razors; shared washcloths; contamination of open sores from contaminated surfaces
Permucosal	Conjunctiva contaminated by blood or body fluid; shared toothbrushes; premastication of food; sexual contact

transmission of HBV from transfusion of unscreened blood, inadequate sterilization of medical and dental instruments, and unsafe injection practices continues to be a problem and may account for a majority of infections among older children and adults.

Perinatal HBV transmission is one of the most efficient modes of infection. Women with an active HBV infection (acute or chronic) can transmit infection to their newborn either in utero (rare) or after delivery from mucous membrane exposure to blood (common). The primary determinant of infection is a high concentration of maternal HBV DNA, as indicated by the presence of HB$_e$Ag.[68–70] However, up to 20 percent of HB$_e$Ag-negative mothers have moderately high levels of HBV DNA and may infect their newborns during the perinatal period.[70] Infants born to HB$_s$Ag-positive mothers and not infected at birth remain at high risk of infection during the first 5 years of life.[71]

HBV in semen and vaginal secretions provides the means for transmission through homosexual and heterosexual activity. Since the late 1980s, sexual transmission has been the most frequently identified source of HBV infection in the United States, accounting for approximately 50 percent of cases of hepatitis B (Fig. 9-5).[67] Having more than one partner in a 6-month period or having a sexually transmitted disease is associated with an increased risk of HBV infection, and risk increases significantly with increasing number of partners.[67]

Person-to-person transmission can occur in settings where nonsexual interpersonal contact occurs over a long period of time, such as from mother to infant, between siblings, and between adults. Approximately 30 percent of children living in a household with an HB$_s$Ag-positive person become infected, and in areas of high HBV endemicity it is estimated that 50 percent of infections in young children are acquired from contact with HB$_s$Ag-positive persons living outside of the child's household.[60,65] While the precise mechanisms of transmission are unknown, transmission is presumed to occur when secretions such as blood or saliva contaminate nonintact skin or repeatedly contact mucous membranes. Sharing personal articles such as razors, washcloths, and toothbrushes is associated with HBV infection. In addition, widespread HB$_s$Ag contamination of surfaces has been demonstrated in homes of persons with chronic infection.[72]

Frequent contact with blood in the occupational setting poses a risk for HBV infection. Prior to the routine use of barrier precautions and hepatitis B vaccination, health care workers were at significantly increased risk of infection.[73,74] While an increased frequency of exposure to blood or body fluids occurs in a number of other occupations (e.g., police, firefighters, correctional officers), increased rates of HBV infection have not been found.[75]

Epidemics of hepatitis B are unusual and usually signal transmission through direct parenteral exposure. Outbreaks have been reported among injection drug users, occasionally in association with HDV infection.[76] Outbreaks of nosocomial hepatitis B continue to occur and usually represent lapses in infection control practices or the failure to vaccinate groups at high risk of infection, such as hemodialysis patients.[77] Chronically infected health care workers performing invasive procedures may on rare occasions transmit infection. Risk factors associated with these infections have been high levels of HBV DNA in the health care worker and the blind palpation of suture needles.[78,79]

Control and Prevention

Elimination of HBV transmission, chronic HBV infection, and HBV-related chronic liver disease is the primary objective of any prevention and control program. Hepatitis B vaccination is the most effective means to prevent HBV infection, and elimination of HBV transmission through widespread vaccination is an attainable goal.[80] The finding that HB$_s$Ag could serve as an immunogen and that anti-HBs protected against infection led to the development of vaccines using HB$_s$Ag purified from the plasma of chronically infected individuals. These plasma-derived vaccines have been produced in a number of countries, including the United States, France, Japan, China, and Korea and continue to be widely used today.[81] However, it was soon shown that HB$_s$Ag could be expressed using recombinant DNA technology and that vaccines produced with recombinant expressed antigen were immunogenic and conferred protection at a rate comparable to that achieved with the plasma-derived vaccines.[82]

Initially, strategies for the use of hepatitis B vaccine were based solely on the endemicity of HBV infection within a given country or region. For areas with a high or intermediate endemicity of infection, routine infant vaccination was recommended to interrupt perinatal or early childhood transmission that produced high rates of chronic infection.[63,83] In areas of low endemicity of infection, selective vaccination was recommended because the majority of infections occurred among adolescents and adults in various risk groups.[83] However, a decade after the development of these recommendations it was evident that, while routine vaccination of infants was feasible, selective vaccination of adults had met with little success. In 1992, the World Health Assembly recommended that all countries routinely vaccinate infants against hepatitis B to prevent perinatal, infant, early childhood, and eventually adolescent and adult transmission of HBV.[84]

For populations with a high or intermediate endemicity of HBV infection, prevention of perinatal and early childhood infection can be achieved by initiating vaccination within 24 hours of birth and integrating the remainder of the vaccine series into the routine childhood vaccination schedule. Such a schedule provides effective active postexposure prophylaxis for infants born to HB$_s$Ag-positive mothers, including infants born to HB$_e$Ag-positive mothers,[69,85] and preexposure immunization for all other infants. However, in some

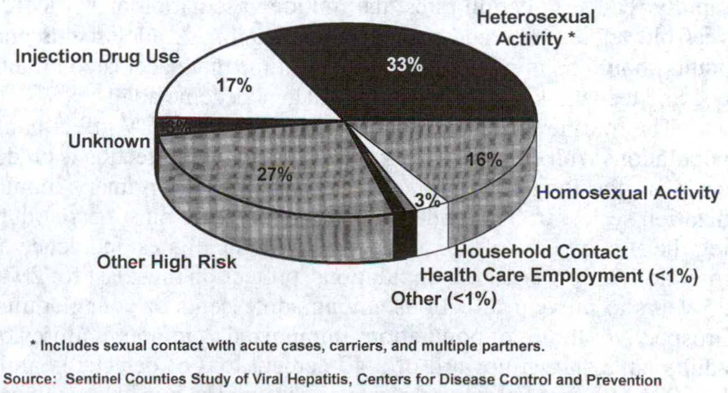

Figure 9-5. Risk factors for acute hepatitis B in the United States, 1995. Persons with "other high risk behaviors" include a history of previous injection drug use, incarceration, homosexual activity that occurred outside of the incubation period for HBV infection. (Adapted from Alter MJ, Hadler SC, Margolis HS, et al: The changing epidemiology of hepatitis B in the United States; need for alternative vaccination strategies. JAMA 263:1218, 1990 and Centers for Disease Control and Prevention, unpublished data.)

countries it is not feasible to deliver hepatitis B vaccine soon after birth because most births do not occur in the hospital. In some instances, birth attendants have been trained to carry hepatitis B vaccine and vaccinate soon after birth, which is possible because hepatitis B vaccine remains immunogenic when stored at 37°C. Otherwise, the first dose of hepatitis B vaccine should be given at the first medical or immunization encounter, which usually occurs at 4 to 6 weeks of age. While late vaccination will not prevent perinatal HBV transmission, it can prevent 80 to 90 percent of infections, since in most of these areas there is a low prevalence (less than 20 percent) of HB_eAg among pregnant women (i.e., in Africa).[86]

The effectiveness of routine infant vaccination in eliminating HBV transmission has been demonstrated in population-based studies worldwide. Dramatic reductions (80 to 90 percent) in chronic HBV infection have occurred in populations where immunization is begun soon after birth[87–89] or at 1 to 2 months of age.[90] In addition, recent data from Taiwan indicate a significant reduction in the incidence of PHC in young children within 15 years of the introduction of routine infant immunization.[91]

In areas of low endemicity of HBV infection, selective vaccination of adults and children at high risk of infection has not been implemented for a number of reasons.[60] In countries such as the United States, it became evident that there existed large populations with high rates of childhood infection who were not being immunized.[65,92] By the late 1980s, hepatitis B vaccination of children as part of the routine childhood immunization schedule was suggested as the most effective approach to eliminate transmission of HBV. In 1991, the United States developed a strategy to eliminate HBV transmission[60] that included (*a*) routine screening of pregnant women for HB_sAg to identify infants who required postexposure prophylaxis to prevent perinatal HBV infection; (*b*) routine vaccination of infants to produce cohorts of adolescents and adults immune to HBV infection; (*c*) catch-up vaccination of children at high risk of HBV infection (i.e., Alaskan Natives, Pacific Islanders, children whose parents immigrated from areas of high or intermediate endemicity of infection); (*d*) catch-up vaccination of adolescents through routine vaccination at 11 to 12 years of age or vaccination of older adolescents in high risk groups; and (*e*) vaccination of at-risk adults.

In the United States, routine vaccination of infants is cost-effective, and because of the large number of young children who acquire chronic HBV infection, this strategy is preferable over a strategy of routine vaccination beginning in adolescence.[57,60] Routine infant vaccination has been well accepted, with a high level of three-dose completion achieved within 3 years after the introduction of the program.[93] However, it will take many decades for routine infant vaccination to lower the incidence of HBV infection, since the majority of infections continue to occur among young adults. To more rapidly reduce infection rates, the routine vaccination of 11- to 12-year-old adolescents and vaccination of high-risk adolescents and adults should be implemented until such time that vaccinated infants become teenagers and vaccinated teenagers become adults.[60,94]

The routine vaccination of infants to prevent HBV infection in populations with either a high or low endemicity of infection is predicated on the long-term protection afforded by the primary immunization series. In high endemic areas, protection must persist during the first 5 years of life, the period with the highest incidence of infection. In low endemic populations, protection must last for 20 to 25 years to prevent infections among adolescents or young adults. Prospective studies of populations immunized as infants, children or adults have shown upward of a 40 percent loss of detectable anti-HB_s 7 to 10 years later, but the rate of chronic HBV is low to nonexistent. However, a low (less than 1 percent/year) rate of asymptomatic infection occurs as defined by anti-HBc seroconversion.[60] In addition, among immunized persons who have lost antibody, revaccination produces a rapid return of detectable anti-HBs, indicating the presence of intact immune memory.[60]

Two decades of experience have shown that hepatitis B vaccination is a safe and cost-effective means to prevent HBV infection and its acute and chronic consequences. Large-scale, population-based infant immunization projects have shown that transmission of HBV infection can be effectively eliminated in areas of high endemicity of infection. However, only 50 percent of the nations of the world have implemented this immunization strategy and there are 1 million deaths annually from HBV-related chronic liver disease and PHC. The current challenge is to mobilize the resources required to effectively provide routine hepatitis B vaccination and eliminate this major public health problem.

In spite of the implementation of effective hepatitis B vaccination programs, there remain a large number of persons with chronic HBV infection. Antiviral therapy with alpha-interferon has been shown to have sustained effect in eliminating HBV replication in 25 to 40 percent of patients.[95] In addition a number of other antiviral agents have shown promise in the treatment of chronic HBV infection and are currently under evaluation. In the United States and many other developed countries, a large number of persons with chronic HBV infection are identified through screening of pregnant women and blood donors and during diagnostic testing. Vaccination of all household members and sexual contacts of these persons is indicated to prevent further HBV transmission.[60] In addition, persons with chronic HBV infection should be evaluated as potential candidates for antiviral therapy to minimize the impact of chronic liver disease and to reduce the reservoir of persons with chronic HBV infection.[96]

▶ HEPATITIS C

Etiologic Agent

Hepatitis C virus has been shown to be the primary etiologic agent of parenterally transmitted non-A, non-B (PT-NANB) hepatitis worldwide.[10] HCV has a single-stranded, positive-sense RNA genome with an organization and replication strategy similar to that found in the family Flaviviridae, which includes yellow fever virus, St. Louis encephalitis virus, and West Nile virus. However, HCV has been classified in its own genus, hepacivirus, because of similarities to both flavivirus and pestivirus genomic organization. The 5′ end of the genome contains an untranslated region that is highly conserved across geographically and epidemiologically distinct isolates.[97,98] The single translated polyprotein contains putative structural proteins (envelope (E1, E2), and nucleocapsid (core)) at the 5′ end and continues with nonstructural proteins (protease (NS3), helicase (NS3), polymerase (NS5), and unknown functions (NS2, NS4)).[97,99]

Portions of the HCV genome display a high degree of variability as a result of mutations that occur during viral replication.[97] Comparative sequence analysis of a large number of HCV isolates suggests the existence of at least six distinct genotypes and a large number of subgroups. In addition, within a single infected individual there usually exists a population of viruses produced over time (quasispecies) that are heterogeneous but closely related. It is postulated that the rapid evolution of genetic variation within an individual represents an immune escape mechanism that facilitates viral persistence.[97,98]

During the course of active HCV infection, antibodies are produced to most viral proteins. However, antibody to no single antigen is associated with resolution of HCV infection. Antibodies to nonstructural and core proteins are used for diagnostic immunoassays and cannot differentiate an active from a resolved infection. While HCV-Ag has been detected in the liver of infected persons,[100] circulating virus-associated antigens have not been detected during the course of infection. This has limited the detection of active HCV infection to the identification of HCV RNA by nucleic acid amplification methods such as the PCR.

HCV has not been propagated in cell culture except for what appear to be abortive replication cycles and it has not been ascribed a physical structure because it has not been visualized by electron microscopy. Native proteins have not been purified from any sources; however, infectious clones of HCV have been recently reported and should provide the best means to further characterize this important viral infection.

Clinical Illness, Pathogenesis, and Immune Response

The spectrum of illness ranges from an asymptomatic infection (most common) to acute fulminant hepatitis (very rare). The incubation period for acute, symptomatic HCV infection (hepatitis C) following a known exposure (i.e., transfusion, needlestick) averages 6 to 7 weeks, with a range of 2 to 26 weeks.[101,102] Most persons with acute HCV infection are asymptomatic (60 to 80 percent) and only 15 to 30 percent become jaundiced.[103] The clinical illness in persons with acute hepatitis C is similar to that observed in hepatitis of other viral etiologies, and the diagnosis of hepatitis C can be made only with appropriate serologic testing.

In the experimentally infected chimpanzee, HCV is detectable in liver and serum within 72 hours of inoculation, and in human recipients of infectious blood transfusions, HCV RNA is detectable 1 to 2 weeks after exposure.[100,104] Anti-HCV is detectable in approximately 40 percent of infected persons 10 weeks after exposure, in 80 percent at 15 weeks, and in virtually all infected persons by 6 months following exposure.[105]

The striking feature of acute HCV infection is that a persistent infection develops in more than 85 percent of adults and children and may occur with or without evidence of chronic hepatitis. Of persons with chronic HCV infection, an average of 67 percent (range 58 to 81 percent) develop chronic hepatitis with elevated liver enzymes (alanine aminotransferase (ALT)) within 6 months after the onset of their acute infection, and no clinical or epidemiologic features of patients appear to be predictive of the progression to chronic infection or hepatitis.[105–107] Among patients with biopsy-proven HCV-related chronic hepatitis there are a wide spectrum of ALT patterns, ranging from persistent elevations to prolonged periods (12 months) of normal activity. This variable pattern of disease activity requires that patients with acute HCV infection receive long-term follow-up to ascertain the extent of their disease.

The progression or course of chronic liver disease associated with chronic HCV infection is not completely known, having been inferred from short-term prospective studies of patients beginning with their acute infection and retrospective cross-sectional studies of persons with chronic HCV infection. In addition, studies that examine only disease outcome may underestimate the severity or progression of HCV infection since persons with biopsy-proven liver disease that is relatively severe (i.e., cirrhosis, chronic active hepatitis) may be totally asymptomatic for many years, except for fatigue. Long-term studies (16 to 23 years) of cohorts of patients with transfusion-acquired HCV infection have shown that 3 to 5 percent died of HCV-related chronic liver disease and up to 33 percent had evidence of cirrhosis.[106,108,109] Among patients followed prospectively from the onset of acute hepatitis C acquired from a variety of sources, 26 to 50 percent had chronic active hepatitis and 3 to 26 percent had cirrhosis on liver biopsy within 5 years of the acute infection.[105,110] On the other hand, among a cohort of women who became infected from HCV-contaminated Rh_o immune globulin, approximately 33 percent had biochemical evidence of chronic hepatitis, 2 percent had histologic evidence of cirrhosis, and none had died after 17 years of follow-up.[111] Thus, it is clear that a large proportion of HCV-infected persons are at risk of some form of chronic liver disease, but precise estimates of the long-term mortality and morbidity associated with this infection must await the outcome of ongoing studies.

A variety of factors may be associated with the outcome or progression of HCV-related chronic liver disease and include genotype, alcohol use, older age at infection, male gender, acquisition of infection by blood transfusion, and immunodeficiency. However, most of these factors have been identified in studies that suffer from a lack of adequate control groups or selection bias and it remains to be seen if they remain as independent predictors of disease outcome.

Case-control studies have shown a 5- to 50-fold increased risk of PHC among anti-HCV–positive persons, compared with that among anti-HCV–negative persons.[112] However, in areas of high HBV endemicity, chronic HBV infection remains the primary risk factor for PHC.[113]

HCV infection is also associated with extrahepatic diseases, including essential mixed (type II) cryoglobulinemia,[114] membranoproliferative glomerulonephritis,[115] and sporadic porphyria cutanea tarda.[116] A number of other nonhepatic diseases have been attributed to HCV infection (e.g., autoimmune thyroiditis, lichen planus, idiopathic pulmonary fibrosis), but definitive associations have not been established.

The immunologic factors associated with the pathogenesis of persistent HCV infection and HCV-related chronic liver disease are not known because of the lack of experimental systems such as cell culture, small-animal models, and well-characterized transgenic mouse models of infection. What is known comes from the chimpanzee model of infection and studies in humans. The high rate of persistent infection in the face of antibodies produced to various viral epitopes suggests that these are not neutralizing antibodies. Experiments in chimpanzees have shown that rechallenge with the same or different strains of HCV resulted in the reappearance of viremia, and early postexposure administration of HCV immune globulin did not prevent infection.[117–119] In the chimpanzee model, high titer antibodies to recombinant capsid proteins (E2) appear to provide short-term protection against chronic infection with the homologous virus, but do not appear to provide long-term protection upon rechallenge.[120] The role of cell-mediated immunity in virus clearance and liver injury has not been defined at this time.

Diagnosis

The current enzyme immunoassay (EIA-2) for anti-HCV is comprised of recombinant proteins from the core and nonstructural regions (NS3, NS4). The EIA-2 is highly sensitive and identifies 90 to 95 percent of HCV-infected persons.[121,122] However, as with all immunoassays used for diagnostic or screening purposes, the predictive value of a positive test depends on the prevalence of the condition in the population being tested. Although a true confirmatory test is not available for EIA-2 since native HCV proteins have not been identified, a supplemental assay (Recombinant Immunoblot Assay, RIBA™, Ortho Diagnostic Systems) has been produced from synthetic HCV proteins. Where the prevalence of HCV infection is low (e.g., blood donor screening), repeatedly reactive anti-HCV–positive specimens should be confirmed by supplemental testing. However, among persons with liver disease, a repeatedly reactive anti-HCV–positive specimen probably does not require supplemental test confirmation.[122]

The diagnosis of acute HCV infection is limited by the lack of a sensitive and specific immunoassay, such as IgM anti-HCV. The diagnosis of acute infection can be made in rare instances where the patient has a documented anti-HCV seroconversion, with or without signs or symptoms of disease. Among patients with signs or symptoms of acute viral hepatitis, serologic tests must be obtained to rule out acute HAV (IgM anti-HAV) and acute HBV (IgM anti-HBc and HB_sAg) infection along with a test for anti-HCV. In addition, if the initial anti-HCV result is negative, it should be repeated since upward of 20 percent of persons with acute hepatitis C are anti-HCV negative at the time of initial presentation.[105,121]

A positive test for anti-HCV is indicative of HCV infection among persons with symptomatic chronic liver disease. For these patients, further diagnostic evaluations should include liver function testing to determine the degree of impairment and might include testing to determine the presence of viremia (i.e., HCV RNA). Persons with no symptoms who are found anti-HCV positive through blood donor screening or testing because of a history of risk factors for HCV infection are most likely to have a false-positive result. If their test result is repeatedly reactive, it should be confirmed by supplementary testing.

A number of tests have been developed that amplify nucleic acid to detect HCV RNA, with some being more sensitive than others.[123] Nucleic acid amplification by PCR is very sensitive but suffers from high cost and lack of standardization; a recent worldwide study to asses reliability among laboratories showed that only 16 percent obtained faultless results.[124] Practitioners considering the use of nucleic acid amplification to detect HCV RNA should know their laboratory, its methods, and the best means to collect specimens to avoid contamination.

Epidemiology

It is apparent that HCV has a worldwide distribution, that in some countries or populations within a country the rates of infection are higher than the general population, and that HCV infection is a major cause of chronic liver disease. In the United States, hepatitis C has accounted for an average of 15 percent of cases of acute viral hepatitis over the past 15 years.[107,121,125] Although early studies focused on transfusion of blood and clotting factors as the primary source of PT-NANB hepatitis, population-based surveillance studies demonstrated that most infections were not transfusion associated (Fig. 9-6).[105] Risk factors for acute hepatitis C are primarily related to direct parenteral exposures to blood and have included injection drug use (30 to 50 percent of cases), occupational exposure (1 to 2 percent), blood transfusion or receipt of clotting factor concentrates (1 to 15 percent), hemodialysis (1 to 2 percent) and multiple heterosexual partners (3 to 9 percent).[105] During the 1980s, the overall incidence of acute hepatitis C remained constant, but has declined by more than 80 percent since 1989, apparently due to changes in disease transmission patterns.[121]

The risk of transfusion associated HCV infection has declined from an estimated 5 percent per transfused unit prior to 1970 to 0.01 to 0.001 percent per unit in 1992. This change has occurred in a stepwise fashion beginning with the elimination of paid blood donors in the early 1970s, donor screening for human immunodeficiency virus (HIV) infection beginning in 1985, and anti-HCV testing of donors that was begun in 1990.[121] Prior to 1987 when heat-inactivated clotting factor concentrates were widely introduced, most hemophiliacs became infected with HCV and most older patients suffered from chronic liver disease. However, since the introduction of viral inactivation methods, the incidence of HCV infection has dropped dramatically in persons who require clotting factor infusions, and anti-HCV screening of donors has diminished the risk of infection among persons who receive multiple blood transfusions. Immunoglobulin preparations, either for intramuscular injection or intravenous infusion, have not been associated with infection, until a recent outbreak of HCV infection among recipients of intravenous immunoglobulin emphasized the need for viral inactivation of these products.[126]

In the United States, most of the recent decline in disease incidence appears to be associated with a decline in cases associated with drug use. The highest prevalence of infection is found among injection drug users (60 to 90 percent), although intranasal cocaine use has been associated with HCV infection. Even persons with a history of "recreational drug use" or "one-time injection" should be considered at high risk of infection, since HCV infection is acquired more rapidly among injection drug users than either HBV or HIV infection.[127] However, the reason for the recent decline in disease incidence is not known, but may represent saturation of the susceptible population with HCV infection and/or a decrease in new injection drug users.

Parenteral drug abuse	30–50%
Occupational exposure	1–2%
Hemodialysis	1–2%
Multiple heterosexual partners	3–9%
Other/unknown exposures	40–60%

Figure 9-6. Risk factors for acute hepatitis C in the United States, by mutually exclusive groups, 1995. (Adapted from Alter MJ, Hadler SC, Judson FN, et al: Risk factors for acute non-A, non-B hepatitis in the United States and association with hepatitis C virus infection. JAMA 264:2231, 1990 and Centers for Disease Control and Prevention, unpublished data.)

Persons with occupational exposure to blood are not at increased risk of HCV infection when compared with the general population, in contrast to the risk of HBV infection. However, persons with direct percutaneous (e.g., needlestick) exposures from HCV-infected persons are at risk of infection.[74,121,128] Nosocomial transmission of infection appears to be infrequent in the United States, except in the hemodialysis setting where there continues to be a low rate of infection, along with occasional outbreaks. However, in countries without routine blood donor screening or with poor infection control or injection practices, there appears to be a high rate of nosocomial HCV transmission that accounts for high rates of infection in the general population.

Heterosexual transmission of HCV infection occurs at a frequency that is lower than that observed for HBV and HIV infection.[105,121] While transmission appears to be low in most studies of monogamous partners and among nondrug-using men who have sex with men, persons with multiple sexual partners and persons seen in sexually transmitted disease (STD) clinics continue to have a somewhat increased risk of infection.[107,121]

In the United States, the prevalence of HCV infection as measured by anti-HCV positivity in the general civilian population is 1.8 percent, or an estimated 3.9 million persons. The highest prevalence of infection occurs in the 30- to 45-year-old age group.[107] In addition, several population-based studies have shown that 40 to 60 percent of persons with symptomatic chronic liver disease are infected with HCV, that 9 to 12 percent have chronic HBV infection, that 15 to 25 percent have excessive alcohol use, and that 10 to 15 percent have no attributable etiology for their disease. HCV-related chronic liver disease is responsible for an estimated 8,000 to 12,000 deaths each year and medical and work loss costs of $680 million.

Control and Prevention

Currently, there is little evidence that a vaccine to prevent acute or chronic HCV infection will be available in the foreseeable future. A high degree of genetic diversity, a high mutation rate, and little evidence for the existence of a durable neutralizing antibody suggest that the development of effective pre-exposure or postexposure prophylaxis may require innovative approaches. While high-titer antibodies to recombinant envelope proteins have been shown to afford short-term protection to a homologous virus challenge in the chimpanzee model, there does not appear to be long-term protection.[120] In addition, postexposure prophylaxis with specially prepared hepatitis C immune globulin has not been shown to protect against infection in the chimpanzee model of infection.[119] However, until such time as an effective immunoprophylactic measure becomes available, prevention of HCV infection must rely on (*a*) elimination of risk behaviors that facilitate transmission; (*b*) screening of blood, solid organ, and tissue donors; (*c*) the use of standard and universal precautions to prevent occupational and nosocomial transmission; and (*d*) identification of infected persons for counseling and possible treatment.

Until recently, little attention has been directed at the prevention of new HCV infections other than screening of blood, organ, or tissue donors. The presumption is that efforts directed at the prevention of injection drug use to prevent HIV infection would prevent HCV infection. Because HCV infection is rapidly acquired after sharing needles or injection "works," it is important to include this information in prevention and education messages for the public and health care providers. In addition, needle exchange programs have been shown to reduce significantly the risk of HCV infection among participating drug users.[129] While the primary goal is to prevent injection drug use, a secondary goal is to prevent chronic HCV infection and chronic liver disease among those who might experiment with or regularly inject drugs. Injection drug use currently accounts for the largest proportion of new cases of HCV infection (Fig. 9-6). Prevention of viral hepatitis (HCV and HBV) must be added to the disease prevention aspects of the drug prevention message.

The screening of donors for anti-HCV with EIA-2 has significantly reduced the risk of infection from blood transfusion and organ transplantation. In addition, the addition of viral inactivation steps to the production of certain blood products has significantly reduced the risk of transmission among persons with certain medical conditions. The current estimated risk of HCV infection from a whole blood transfusion is 0.01 to 0.001 percent per unit.

All persons with HCV infection should be considered infectious and should be counseled concerning available measures to prevent transmission of HCV infection to others.[96] They should not donate blood, semen, body organs, or other tissues. Cuts or skin lesions should be kept covered and personal articles such as toothbrushes, razors, or other items that could be contaminated with blood should not be shared. Although there are no recommendations for changes in sexual practices for persons with a steady sex partner, infected persons should be informed of the potential risk of sexual transmission so they can decide if they should take precautions. Persons with multiple sex partners should follow safe sex practices and use barriers to prevent contact with body fluids.[96]

Alpha-interferon is licensed for the treatment of chronic hepatitis C, and treatment is generally recommended for anti-HCV–positive persons with abnormal liver enzymes and compensated chronic hepatitis on liver biopsy.[130] Approximately 50 percent of treated patients have a complete response at the end of treatment, with normalization of liver enzymes and a loss or decrease in HCV RNA, and 25 percent have a sustained response one or more years after therapy.[130] While treatment is not considered a primary means of prevention of HCV transmission, a sustained treatment response probably has some secondary benefit by reducing the reservoir of HCV-infected individuals.

▶ DELTA HEPATITIS

Etiologic Agent

The hepatitis delta virus (HDV) is a 35- to 38-nm enveloped particle containing a small, circular, single-stranded RNA, the delta antigen, and an outer coat of HB_sAg.[131,132] HDV appears most closely related to the satellite viruses of plants (viriods) and requires HB_sAg as a surface protein to replicate.[132,133]

Clinical Illness, Pathogenesis, and Immune Response

There are three forms of HDV infection: (*a*) an acute coinfection that occurs with HBV, (*b*) superinfection of a person with chronic HBV infection, and (*c*) latent infection in persons who receive a liver transplant for HBV-HDV liver disease and in whom HDV infection occurs without evidence of HBV infection.[7,132] Coinfection follows exposure to an inoculum containing both HBV and HDV, has an incubation period similar to HBV infection and produces a biphasic illness in 15 to 20 percent of cases—something not observed in most other forms of viral hepatitis. HDV replication is limited by the resolution of HBV infection, with chronic HDV infection occurring only when the patient acquires a chronic HBV infection. HDV superinfection may appear within 2 to 6 weeks after exposure of a person with chronic HBV infection to an HDV inoculum.[7,132] Acute HDV infection may partially suppress HBV replication and occasionally allows a patient to eliminate a chronic HBV infection. However, the majority of persons with chronic HBV-HDV superinfection have chronic hepatitis and persistent infection with both viruses.[132] Latent HDV infection does not cause liver disease unless HBV infection recurs, in which case acute and chronic hepatitis may occur.

The spectrum of clinical disease in acute HDV coinfection or superinfection varies from no illness to fulminant hepatitis. In general, HDV infection augments the severity of both acute and chronic HBV infection, with 50 to 70 percent of acute infections (coinfection or superinfection) resulting in an episode of clinical hepatitis with jaundice, compared with 30 percent of HBV infections. The risk of fulminant hepatitis may reach 10 percent for clinically apparent HBV-HDV coinfections and 20 percent in HDV superinfections.[76,132] HDV infection has been found in 30 to 50 percent of cases of HBsAg-positive fulminant hepatitis.[134] During coinfection, serologic markers of acute HBV infection are accompanied by detectable HDV antigen (HDV-Ag) and antibodies to HDV (IgG or IgM anti-HDV). HDV-Ag is usually present during the early part of the acute illness, while IgM anti-HDV appears within days to weeks after onset of symptoms.[132] The antibody response to HDV is not strong, and accurate diagnosis is best accomplished during the acute illness or early convalescence. In acute superinfection, serologic markers of chronic HBV infection are present, HDV-Ag may be present early in the illness, and IgG and IgM anti-HDV appear rapidly. In fulminant hepatitis, serum markers of HDV infection may be negative in spite of detectable HDV-Ag in the liver.[132] In chronic HDV hepatitis, HB_sAg is present along with IgM anti-HDV and HDV-Ag in the liver.

Chronic HDV infection can be asymptomatic, manifest as chronic active hepatitis, or progress rapidly to cirrhosis and death due to liver failure.[135] HDV superinfection markedly increases the risk of chronic liver disease, and it is estimated that 50 to 90 percent of these patients develop chronic hepatitis. There is conflicting evidence concerning HDV infection and the risk of PHC, with some studies finding an increased rate of cancer among younger HDV-infected persons and others failing to find HDV infection among HB_sAg-positive cases of PHC.

Diagnosis

Both IgM and IgG antibodies develop during the course of HDV infection; however, the only serologic tests commercially available in the United States detect total antibody (IgG and IgM) to HDV and may result in underdiagnosis of HDV infection. Tests for HDV-Ag in serum are also available, are only positive during the acute phase of the illness, and have modest sensitivity because they require the detergent treatment of the specimen to disrupt the HB_sAg coat of the virus particle. Immunoperoxidase and immunofluorescence assays for HDV-Ag in liver are more sensitive and can be used to verify infection in liver biopsies from cases of chronic hepatitis. Hybridization assays for HDV-RNA in serum have proven more sensitive than assays for HDV-Ag and appear useful in determining the potential infectivity of persons with chronic HDV infection.[132]

The diagnosis of acute HBV-HDV coinfection is made by the presence of serologic markers of acute HBV infection (IgM anti- HBc and HB_sAg) and either serum HDV-Ag or total and/or IgM anti-HDV. Acute HDV superinfection is diagnosed by the presence of either HDV-Ag or total and/or IgM anti-HDV in a patient with acute hepatitis and serologic evidence of chronic HBV infection (HB_sAg positive and IgM anti-HBc negative). However, in cases of fulminant HDV hepatitis, serologic markers of HDV infection may be negative, but HDV-Ag should be present in liver tissue.

Patients with chronic HDV infection have serologic evidence of chronic HBV infection (HB_sAg positive and IgM anti-HBc negative) and HDV infection (total anti-HDV positive or HDV-RNA positive). Often IgM anti-HDV is present and HDV-Ag is present in the liver.

Epidemiology

The epidemiology of HDV infection parallels that of HBV infection. The highest concentrations of HDV are found in the blood of persons with acute or chronic infection, and HDV is presumed to be present in serum-derived body fluids such as wound exudates. However, its presence in other body fluids has not been confirmed. Transmission of HDV, like HBV, occurs by percutaneous or mucous membrane exposure to blood or body fluids either directly, indirectly, or by sexual contact. Perinatal transmission from mother to infant can occur, but is of minimal importance as a means of disease transmission. Like HBV, casual contact does not result in virus transmission, but HB_sAg-positive nonsexual household contacts of persons with chronic HDV infection are at significant risk of superinfection over long periods of time.

The age-specific risk of HDV infection closely parallels that of HBV infection, with several notable exceptions. In areas with a low endemicity of HBV infection such as the United States or western

Europe, the prevalence of HDV infection among persons with chronic HBV infection is low (0 to 5 percent), but reaches 10 to 25 percent among persons with HBV-related chronic liver disease. Among persons with chronic HBV infection in certain risk groups (e.g., injection drug users, hemophiliacs), there is a high prevalence (30 to 50 percent) of HDV infection. However, the prevalence of HDV infection is much lower among homosexual men (5 percent), persons with multiple heterosexual partners, and household contacts of persons with chronic HBV infection.[132] These data suggest that HDV is transmitted less efficiently by sexual contact than by blood exposure. In the United States, HDV infection is found in about 5 percent of cases of acute hepatitis B and in up to 25 percent of cases of fulminant hepatitis.[132]

The highest prevalences of HDV infection are found in the Amazon basin, parts of Africa, and Romania, where 20 percent of persons with chronic HBV infection and up to 90 percent of patients with HBV-related chronic liver disease have HDV infection. In other areas of intermediate and high HBV endemicity (i.e., southern Italy, parts of Eastern Europe, the Middle East, Africa, some Pacific Island group, the Central Asian Republics of the former Soviet Union), HDV prevalence tends to be higher, infecting 15 percent of persons with chronic HBV infection and 30 to 50 percent of patients with HBV-related chronic liver disease. HDV has been identified as the cause of an endemic form of fulminant hepatitis in northern Colombia that has been recognized since the 1930s and is the cause of Labrea hepatitis, which is endemic in the Amazon basin.[136] Curiously, the prevalence of HDV infection is low in eastern and southeastern Asia despite the high endemicity of chronic HBV infection in this region.[137]

Outbreaks of HDV infection have been recognized among drug abusers and in certain populations with a high endemicity of HBV infection. Outbreaks among drug abusers usually involve coinfection with HBV and HDV, may cause high mortality due to fulminant hepatitis, and result in secondary transmission to sexual contacts.[76] Outbreaks of HDV superinfection in populations with a high endemicity of chronic HBV infection have been recognized in Brazil, Venezuela, Colombia, and the Central African Republic.[138] These epidemics characteristically affect children and young adults, cause high mortality among persons with acute disease, and produce high rates of chronic liver disease. Transmission occurs primarily via open skin wounds and sores and through sexual contact. Risk is highest for those persons with chronic HBV infection who live with an index case and accounts for familial clustering of cases of fulminant hepatitis observed in these regions.[138]

Control and Prevention

Prevention of HDV infection is dependent on the prevention of HBV infection. Vaccination to prevent acute and chronic HBV infection is the best protective measure against HDV coinfection. Routine vaccination of infants and catch-up vaccination of older children in areas with previous outbreaks of delta hepatitis have eliminated the transmission of both HBV and HDV infection. However, persons with chronic HBV infection continue to remain at risk of HDV superinfection. General measures that include attention to sterilization and safe injection practices to prevent nosocomial transmission and screening of blood and blood products for HB_sAg are effective in preventing both HBV and HDV infection. Otherwise no specific prevention measures can be offered for persons at risk of superinfection other than counseling to avoid contaminated needles and occupational or sexual exposure to HBV-HDV–infected persons.

Antiviral treatment with alpha-interferon of persons with chronic HBV infection is moderately effective (40 percent) in eliminating the chronic infection and the HB_sAg carrier state.[139] Treatment of HDV-infected persons with high doses of alpha-interferon may produce a 25 to 70 percent remission of chronic liver disease, but many persons relapse when treatment is discontinued. However, following discontinuation of antiviral therapy, up to 33 percent of patients become HDV RNA and HB_sAg negative with cessation of chronic liver disease.[139,140]

▶ HEPATITIS E

Etiologic Agent

The development of specific serologic tests for acute HAV infection resulted in the retrospective determination that large outbreaks of hepatitis in developing countries and with a fecal-oral mode of transmission were not hepatitis A.[141] This new form of non-A, non-B hepatitis was initially called epidemic NANB hepatitis, then enterically transmitted (ET) NANB hepatitis, and then hepatitis E. Laboratory investigations identified HEV in the feces of cases or experimentally infected cynomolgus macaques.[142] HEV is a 32- to 34-nm icosohedral, nonenveloped RNA virus that has been cloned and fully sequenced.[12,142,143] The genome has approximately 7.5 kilobases with three open reading frames.[143] There is a modest degree of genetic variability between isolates from various geographic regions, but there appears to be serologic cross-reactivity among isolates. Although the physical structure of HEV resembles that of caliciviruses, the genomic organization is similar to that of rubella virus, and HEV has not been specifically classified.

Clinical Illness, Pathogenesis, and Immune Response

The incubation period of hepatitis E is longer than that of hepatitis A with a range of 22 to 60 days and mode of 40 days. A prodromal phase lasting 1 to 10 days has been described, followed by nausea (40 to 85 percent), dark urine (92 to 100 percent), abdominal pain (41 to 87 percent), vomiting (50 percent), pruritus (13 to 55 percent), joint pain (28 to 81 percent), rash (3 percent), and diarrhea (3 percent). Fever and hepatomegaly have been present in over 50 percent of patients.[142]

Clinical signs and symptoms or serum chemistries cannot differentiate hepatitis E from hepatitis A. A human volunteer study showed that transmission of HEV could occur via the enteral route in a person immune to HAV infection.[144] In the human volunteer study and the nonhuman primate model of infection, the relationship of virus excretion in feces to liver enzyme elevations was similar to that observed in hepatitis A; the peak of shedding occurred prior to the onset of illness.[144,145] Histopathologic examination of liver biopsies from nonfulminant cases of hepatitis E have shown a cholestatic form of hepatitis with glandlike transformation and a preserved lobular structure. Liver cell necrosis has varied from single cell degeneration to bridging necrosis.[146]

The ratio of clinical to subclinical infection has not been determined, but it appears that children may have a lower rate of symptomatic infection.[142] A high case-fatality rate among pregnant women has been a consistent feature of hepatitis E and has ranged from 5 to 25 percent.[14,142] A high perinatal death rate among infants of mothers with fulminant hepatitis has been observed, but termination of pregnancy does not improve the clinical status of the mother. Most persons with hepatitis E have a self-limited disease, and follow-up studies of persons with hepatitis E indicate that chronic liver disease is not an outcome.

Diagnosis

The key to diagnosis is an increased awareness that the disease may exist in particular regions of the world (Fig. 9-7) and the serologic work-up of all cases of hepatitis. Immunoassays to detect antibody to HEV (anti-HEV) are available worldwide, but commercially produced assays are available to only a limited degree in the United States.[14] All assays are constructed from synthetic HEV antigens derived from ORF 2 epitopes, and some include ORF 3 epitopes. In general, all assays identify persons with acute hepatitis E with a high level of sensitivity and specificity. In the United States, the very low rate of HEV infection does not warrant HEV serologic testing of every person with acute hepatitis. However, those patients remaining after exclusion of acute hepatitis A, hepatitis B, and hepatitis C should be tested for hepatitis E.

Immunoassays to detect HEV in stool specimens are not available. However, HEV-RNA can be detected in feces or serum after nucleic acid amplification by PCR.[14] HEV antigen can be visualized in liver biopsies.[147]

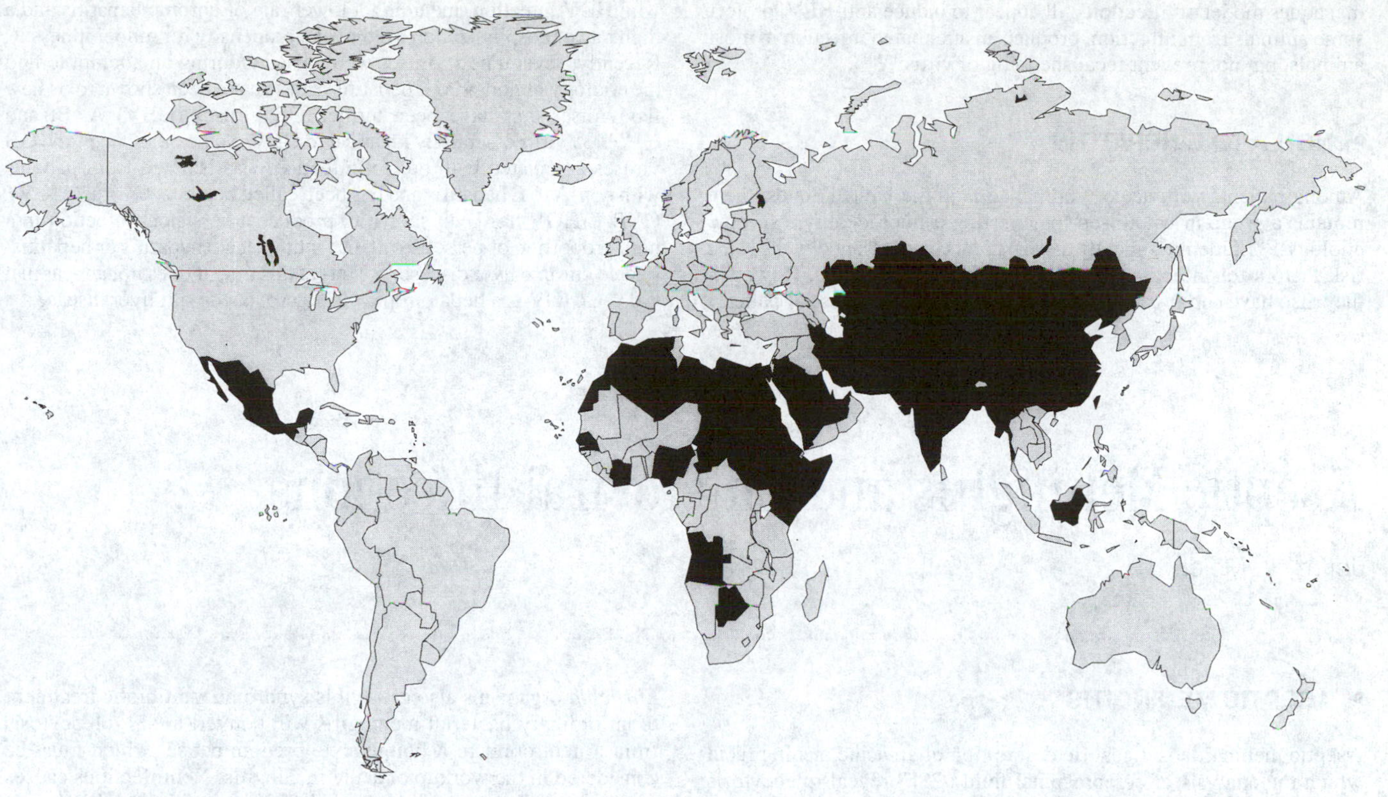

Figure 9-7. Areas with high endemic rates of hepatitis E as defined by the occurrence of an epidemic or more than 25 percent of sporadic cases of non-A-C hepatitis being serologically positive for acute HEV infection. (From Centers for Disease Control and Prevention, unpublished data.)

Epidemiology

Worldwide, the identification of numerous outbreaks of hepatitis E and of high rates of sporadic cases in some regions of the world (Fig. 9-7) has been the result of more widespread IgM anti-HAV testing of cases of acute hepatitis and an increased awareness of this disease. Epidemics of hepatitis E have been reported worldwide, and hepatitis E is endemic in many parts of the world (Fig. 9-7), almost always where HAV infection is also highly endemic. Disease identification requires a high index of suspicion, but several epidemiologic features distinguish hepatitis E from hepatitis A, and include a high attack rate among adults and an unusually high case-fatality rate among pregnant women.[14,142] The mean age of infection is 29 years and the highest prevalence of infection is observed in persons 20 to 30 years of age.[14,142] Although asymptomatic infections occur among children, seroprevalence studies in high endemic areas have not identified high rates of infection in this age group, which is in contrast to HAV infection, in which approximately 90 percent of children under 15 years of age have been infected.

HEV is primarily transmitted by the fecal-oral route. In endemic areas, the primary source of infection is fecally contaminated drinking water, although food-borne transmission has been suggested but not proven.[142,148,149] Person-to-person transmission is rare and secondary attack rates in households are low, ranging from 0.7 to 2.2 percent, which is in contrast to the approximately 30 percent household secondary attack rate observed for hepatitis A. Person-to-person nosocomial transmission has been reported in endemic areas, but bloodborne transmission from the viremic stage of infection has not been documented. In nonendemic areas, travel to endemic areas is the primary source of acute cases of hepatitis E. The source of asymptomatic infections has not been determined, but secondary household transmission from known acute cases has not been reported.

The reservoir for HEV is unknown. While fecally contaminated water is the source of most infections, the source of the HEV contamination is not known. The stability of HEV is not known, but it is unlikely that persistence in the environment is the major reservoir of infection, especially since epidemics occur following intervals of little or no disease activity. While serial transmission among susceptible individuals could sustain HEV in a population and result in periodic outbreaks, the low rate of infection among children tends not to support this model for persistence. Another possibility is that HEV infection is primarily zoonotic, with humans being an end or inadvertent target. Experimental infection has been reported in pigs and sheep, and a high prevalence of anti-HEV has been deteced among domestic animals (i.e., pigs, cattle, sheep) from endemic areas, compared with low rates found in age-matched animals from nonendemic areas. Recently, HEV was isolated from domestic pigs in the United States and HEV RNA has been identified in pigs in an endemic area.

Control and Prevention

The most important means to prevent hepatitis E is protection of water systems from contamination with fecal material. Epidemiologic evidence indicates that boiling water will interrupt HEV transmission. Data concerning chlorination of water are not available, although chlorination of water should be attempted in epidemic situations. Because of the significant adverse consequences of HEV infection in pregnant women, they should be advised to pay particular attention to water sanitation. Travelers to areas endemic for HEV infection should be particularly cautious concerning their drinking water.

Prevention of hepatitis E by immunization may be possible. Studies of postexposure immunization using immunoglobulin prepared from plasma collected in endemic areas has generally not had a protective effect.[150,151] However, cynomolgus macaques given preexposure immunization with immunoglobulin prepared from previously infected animals were protected from symptomatic infection.[152] Several prototype vaccines have been evaluated in the cynomolgus macaques model of infection. All appear to induce anti-HEV, protect some animals from infection, produce an attenuated infection in most animals, but not prevent fecal shedding of virus.[152,153]

▶ NON-A TO E HEPATITIS

Among patients with acute viral hepatitis in the United States, there remains a group in whom serologic testing cannot identify a specific etiology.[125] Epidemiologically these patients have essentially the same risk factors for infection as persons with HCV infection. However, they also have certain characteristics that differ from those of patients with HCV infection, including a lower rate of chronic hepatitis and a high rate of hospitalization in spite of a propensity for milder illness.[125] Recently, several new viruses were isolated during an attempt to find the etiology of non-A to E hepatitis. These have been shown to be new flaviviruses that have been termed GB viruses (GBV) A, B, and C.[154,155] A virus essentially identical to GBV-C, the only one of the GB viruses associated with human infection, was isolated from patients with non-A to E hepatitis and has been called hepatitis G virus (HGV). GVB-C/HGV has been shown to produce a persistent infection in a high proportion of persons with or without acute hepatitis or hepatitis-related chronic liver disease.[125] Thus at this time it does not appear that GBV-C/HGV is a hepatotropic virus associated with liver disease.

Aseptic Meningitis and Enteroviral Infections

Jeffrey L. Meier

▶ ASEPTIC MENINGITIS

Aseptic meningitis is a generic description of an acute meningitis in which the analysis of cerebrospinal fluid (CSF) reveals pleocytosis but no bacteria or fungi on standard microbiologic stains and cultures.[1,2] This syndrome often clinically manifests as fever, headache, photophobia, and stiff neck. There are both infectious and noninfectious causes of aseptic meningitis, although the latter category is infrequent. The incidence rate of aseptic meningitis is about 11 per 100,000 person-years, based on a large retrospective study of cases in Olmstead County, Minnesota, from 1950 to 1981.[3]

Viruses cause most cases of aseptic meningitis. Nonpolio enteroviruses are responsible for at least 80 to 90 percent of the cases of aseptic meningitis in which an etiologic agent is identified.[2,4,5] Among the many members of this viral group that may provoke aseptic meningitis are several types of the ECHO viruses and Coxsackieviruses, as well as enterovirus type 71.[4–7] Of the Coxsackieviruses, the B group viruses are most often culpable. Aseptic meningitis may also result from infection with the mumps virus, lymphocytic choriomeningitis (LCM) virus, herpes simplex virus (HSV), poliovirus, or certain arboviruses (e.g., St. Louis encephalitis and California encephalitis group viruses).[1] Aseptic meningitis may also be part of the acute retroviral syndrome caused by human immunodeficiency virus (HIV). Attention to accompanying clinical and epidemiologic features of the aseptic meningitis episode helps in distinguishing between the viral etiologies. However, these viruses do not appreciably differ in their abilities to produce a lymphocytic pleocytosis in the CSF, although neutrophils may predominate within the first 48 hours of some viral infections. CSF protein amount is usually mildly-to-moderately elevated. CSF glucose is often normal, but may be low in episodes involving the mumps virus, LCM virus, HSV, or poliovirus. Standard viral culture methods may detect HSV, mumps virus, poliovirus, and some nonpolio enteroviruses. Serological studies are useful to evaluate infections with LCM virus, mumps virus, arboviruses, poliovirus, and HIV, but may require a comparison of acute and convalescent results so that the etiologic agent is identified only in retrospect. Polymerase chain reaction (PCR)-based methods will likely assume a greater role in the rapid diagnosis of viral etiologies in the future. The investigational use of this methodology has detected nonpolio enteroviruses in the CSF of nearly two-thirds of persons who have aseptic meningitis but negative viral cultures.[4]

Aseptic meningitis may also be produced by spirochetes that cause Lyme disease, syphilis, and leptospirosis.[1] *Rickettsia* and *Ehrlichia* organisms also cause this syndrome. Antibiotic treatment of an ordinary bacterial meningitis will convert a CSF pleocytosis from a neutrophil to a lymphocyte predominance, which must be considered in the workup of acute meningitis. Noninfectious causes of aseptic meningitis include systemic lupus erythematosus, Behçet's syndrome, sarcoidosis, and meningeal carcinomatosis. Drugs are infrequent causes of aseptic meningitis. Nonsteroidal antiinflammatory agents, orthoclone (OKT3), and trimethroprim-sulfamethoxazole are examples of drugs that may produce such episodes.

▶ ENTEROVIRUSES

Humans are the only natural host for the human enteroviruses. The *Enterovirus* genus includes the polioviruses (3 types), groups A (23 types) and B (6 types) coxsackieviruses, ECHO viruses (31 types), and enterovirus types 68–71.[7] These nonenveloped RNA viruses are resistant to stomach acid and to several kinds of disinfectants such as 5 percent Lysol, 70 percent alcohol, and 1 percent quaternary ammonium compounds, and various detergents. They are variably inactivated by 0.3 percent formaldehyde, chlorine, and drying. Enteroviruses are thermolabile and are destroyed by autoclaving. Despite their relative resiliency, the enteroviruses are believed to be spread primarily by person-to-person contact. Nonetheless, some types of enteroviruses can be cultured from sewage and fomites, potentially providing additional modes of transmission. Enterovirus 70, the cause of epidemic hemorrhagic conjunctivitis, is readily transmitted by fomites, including contaminated ophthalmologic instruments.[8]

This chapter discusses the nonpolio enteroviruses because the polioviruses are addressed in Chapter 7. The nonpolio enteroviruses are distributed worldwide and the specific virus types that predominate vary with geographic region and time.[6,7,9] Regional outbreaks of infection with these viruses occur frequently, while large epidemics or pandemics happen infrequently. Infection rates depend on season and geographic location, as well as the socioeconomic status and age of the population. Infection is more common in summer and autumn months in temperate climates, whereas this seasonal periodicity in infection rate is not observed in tropical climates. The majority of nonpolio enteroviral infections occur in children, with infants under 1 year of age having the highest infection rates. Only about 16 to 20 percent of infections in the United States involve persons over 20 years of age.[10] Living in a low socioeconomic setting correlates with an increased prevalence and early acquisition of enteroviral infections.

Nonpolio enteroviral infections are usually self-limited. However, they may persist in persons with dysfunctional or deficient B lymphocytes, which are essential for viral clearance and immunity. Immunity to enteroviruses is type-specific and appears to be lifelong. Acute infection generally results in viral shedding from the upper respiratory and gastrointestinal tracts. Of these two anatomic sites, virus is shed from the gastrointestinal tract for substantially longer periods that may last many days to several weeks, depending on virus type and host factors. This finding likely accounts for the predominant fecal-oral route of enteroviral transmission, although some respiratory-oral spread may also be involved. Some exceptions to this generality include coxsackievirus A21, which is spread primarily by respiratory secretions, and enterovirus 70, which is transmitted by fingers and fomites. Secondary attack rates in susceptible family members are about 75 percent for Coxsackieviruses and less than 50 percent for echoviruses.[11] The period of maximum viral shedding into feces corresponds to the period of maximum contagiousness.

The incubation period for enteroviral illness is usually 3 to 5 days, but ranges from 2 days to 2 weeks.[6,7] At least 50 to 80 percent of nonpolio enteroviral infections are asymptomatic. Most symptomatic episodes present as a nonspecific febrile illness, which may be accompanied by upper respiratory symptoms. These episodes last a few days. However, some nonpolio enteroviral infections may result in distinct clinical syndromes.[6,7] The likelihood of developing a particular clinical syndrome depends on virus type and host factors, such as age and gender. The clinical syndromes are categorized as acute aseptic meningitis, encephalitis, paralysis, exanthems (e.g., rubelliform, roseoliform, herpetiform, or petechial rashes), hand-foot-and-mouth disease, herpangina, pleurodynia, epidemic hemorrhagic conjunctivitis, and myopericarditis. The latter three syndromes occur frequently but not exclusively in adolescents and young adults, whereas the other clinical syndromes often affect children. Neonates are susceptible to overwhelming infection, which may involve life-threatening myocarditis, encephalitis, and hepatitis. Most neonatal infections result from vertical transmission during the perinatal period. Infected mothers and health care workers have been sources of outbreaks of enteroviral infections in neonatal nurseries, which likely result from spread by the hands of personnel in direct contact with an infected neonate.[6]

The definitive diagnosis of nonpolio enteroviral infection generally requires the detection of the virus in CSF, throat washings, or feces.[6,7] Virus can be recovered by standard cell culture methods in about two-thirds of cases of nonpolio enteroviral aseptic meningitis.[4,6] In most of these cases, virus is cultured from CSF; in the remainder of cases, it is recovered only in throat washings or feces. Some members of the group A coxsackieviruses do not grow in cell culture, but are infrequent causes of aseptic meningitis.[4,5] PCR-based methods that enable the detection of nucleic acids of nearly all of the nonpolio enteroviruses are under evaluation to rapidly diagnose enteroviral infection; the sensitivity and specificity of this approach is expected to be excellent.[4] In general, serological evaluation of nonpolio enteroviral infection is not feasible, given the multiplicity of serotypes.

The management of nonpolio enteroviral infections is primarily supportive.[4,6] Neither antiviral drugs nor vaccines are currently available. Passive immunization is considered in selected circumstances, such as in a virulent nursery outbreak or in susceptible persons with profound humoral immunodeficiency. Large doses of immunoglobulin may be beneficial in the treatment of neonatal enteroviral disease and of persistent enteroviral infections in persons with deficient humoral immunity. The combined practice of universal (standard) precautions, handwashing, and appropriate disposal of infected secretions and feces is usually sufficient to prevent transmission of nonpolio enteroviruses in the hospital setting. More rigorous precautions are applied to infants and young children who are in diapers or incontinent.[12] These infected individuals should be isolated in a private room or together, and persons in direct contact with them should wear gloves and gowns.

Epstein-Barr Virus and Infectious Mononucleosis

Jeffrey L. Meier

Epstein-Barr virus (EBV) is a member of the *Herpesviridae* family. Humans are its only natural host. EBV infection is lifelong and most often inconsequential. Infectious mononucleosis is the most common illness caused by EBV in developed countries. The virus is also associated with a variety of other illnesses. For instance, EBV is the cause of oral hairy leukoplakia in persons with human immunodeficiency virus (HIV) infection. EBV sometimes produces a life-threatening lymphoproliferative disorder in persons with acquired or congenital cellular immunodeficiency. A strong epidemologic association exists between EBV infection and nonkeratinizing nasopharyngeal carcinoma and the African form of Burkitt's lymphoma.

Pathogenesis

EBV is an enveloped virus that contains linear DNA.[1–3] The receptor for EBV is also that for the C3d component of complement and is borne primarily by B lymphocytes (B cells) and oropharyngeal epithelial cells. Oropharyngeal epithelial cells permit the production of infectious viral progeny. Replication and packaging of the linear viral genome requires the sequential expression of viral early and late genes. The viral early and late gene product groups compose the early antigen (EA) and viral capsid antigen (VCA), respectively, which are used in serological testing of EBV infection. The viral thymidine kinase is an early gene product that renders a productive EBV infection susceptible to inhibition by acyclovir.

Most B cells support a latent EBV infection, in which the viral genome persists as circular extrachromosomal DNA (episome).[1–3] EBV uses one of three programs of latent gene expression, and each differs from that used in productive infection. Two of these programs restrict viral gene expression to help the virus elude cellular immune surveillance. The unrestricted program activates and transforms the infected B cell, but risks susceptibility to cellular immune defenses. As these EBV-immortalized B cells proliferate, the viral episome replicates and partitions with daughter B cells using mechanisms that are unaffected by acyclovir. The Epstein-Barr nuclear antigens (EBNA) that are employed in serological testing are examples of viral latency gene products. Stimulation of the latently infected B cell can trigger EBV reactivation to yield infectious virus.

EBV is shed intermittently from oropharyngeal and salivary duct epithelium into saliva.[1–3] Close oral contact with infectious saliva can transmit EBV to oropharyngeal epithelium of susceptible individuals. This acquisition yields a primary infection that extends to the B cells. Infection is largely curtailed by the host cellular immune system, although neutralizing antibodies may limit the spread of cell-free virus. Cytotoxic $CD8^+$ T cells control the proliferation of

EBV-immortalized B cells, but virus persists in a small population (1 in 10^5 to 10^6) of circulating B cells. As EBV reactivates from these cells, it may reinfect oropharyngeal epithelial cells to temporarily reinstate viral shedding.

Infectious mononucleosis reflects an exuberant immune response to a primary EBV infection.[2,3] Expansion of the activated T-cell population results in the atypical lymphocytosis in peripheral blood and the hypertrophy of lymphoid tissues that are hallmarks of the illness. The cytokines produced from this immune activation may contribute to clinical manifestations. Only about 0.1 to 1 percent of circulating B cells contain EBV. These infected cells generate polyclonal antibodies, which include the heterophile antibodies and sometimes autoantibodies. Heterophile antibodies agglutinate sheep and horse red blood cells, lyse beef red blood cells, and fail to bind to guinea pig kidney cells. They do not bind to EBV-specific antigens and their amounts do not correlate with severity of illness. The EBV-immortalized B cell population can proliferate excessively and even evolve into frank malignancy in persons who have a major deficiency in cytotoxic T-cell function.

Nonkeratinizing nasopharyngeal carcinomas and African Burkitt's lymphomas usually contain clonal copies of the latent EBV episome displaying restricted gene expression.[2,3] The malignant potential of these cells is mostly conferred by host cell chromosomal abnormalities. In Burkitt's lymphoma, for example, there is chromosomal translocation leading to dysregulation of the cellular oncogene c-*myc*. EBV's role in promoting these kinds of malignancies is unclear.

Epidemiology

Serological surveys conducted virtually worldwide have shown that EBV is ubiquitous and that almost 95 percent of all persons, regardless of gender, acquire EBV infection by the end of their third decade of life.[3,4] Persons living in developing countries or in areas of low socioeconomic standing where poor personal hygiene is pervasive usually acquire EBV in childhood. For instance, EBV seroprevalance among children 5 years or younger exceeds 95 percent in Africa and China, 80 percent in the Amazon Basin, and 90 percent on the Aleutian Islands.[4] Acquisition of EBV is more likely to be delayed until adolescence or early adulthood in persons living in developed countries or among an affluent population, where sexual intimacy becomes a factor in EBV transmission. This delay is exemplified in a prospective serologic study of college freshmen at Yale University that found antibodies to EBV in only half of the students at the time of enrollment, but 13 percent of susceptible students acquired infection within 9 months.[5] In another study of cadets entering a United States Military Academy, 63.5 percent of individuals were EBV seropositive.[6] The annual seroconversion rates among susceptible cadets during the ensuing 4 years were 12.4, 24.4, 15.1, and 30.8 percent. Many of these newly acquired infections were subclinical.

Infectious mononucleosis results from a primary EBV infection, following a 30- to 50-day incubation period. It occurs most often in adolescents and young adults with ages ranging from 15 to 25 years.[4,7,8] This is because infants and children usually do not display manifestations of infectious mononucleosis when acutely infected and most older adults are no longer susceptible to EBV, although they retain the ability to develop the illness. Accordingly, the incidence of infectious mononucleosis largely depends on the number of EBV-seronegative adolescents and young adults in a given population. The incidence of infectious mononucleosis in the United States is 45 to 100 cases per 100,000 persons.[7,8]

EBV is spread by close oral contact with infectious saliva.[3,4,9] Blood products or donor tissues containing latent EBV can occasionally be the source of transmission. Persons with infectious mononucleosis may shed EBV into saliva for many months; 55 percent of such persons shed virus for 6 months after the onset of illness. However, secondary spread of EBV among susceptible household contacts is infrequent. Susceptible roommates of college students with infectious mononucleosis acquire EBV no more frequently than other students. Most seropositive healthy persons intermittently shed EBV in their saliva. EBV can be cultured from the saliva of about 15 to 20 percent of randomly selected healthy seropositive persons. In one study of hospital patients and staff, 17 percent of staff members were found to shed EBV.[10] The rate of viral shedding increases in groups of persons with concomitant malignancy or cellular immune deficiency. EBV has not been cultured from fomites, reflecting its liability in the ambient environment.

Clinical Presentation

The diagnosis of infectious mononucleosis is made when the characteristic findings of fever, pharyngitis, and cervical lymphadenopathy; absolute peripheral lymphocytosis; atypical lymphocytosis greater than 10 percent of the differential; and heterophile antibodies are present.[3,9,11] The probability of EBV as the cause of a mononucleosis-like illness decreases as these criteria are relaxed. Atypical episodes are more likely to occur in infants, young children, the elderly, and immunosuppressed persons. In these cases, the diagnosis of acute EBV infection can be established with EBV-specific serological testing.

Infectious mononucleosis commonly produces symptoms of sore throat, mild headache, sweats, fatigue, and malaise. Most of these symptoms subside within 1 to 2 weeks, although fatigue and malaise may resolve gradually over a longer period. Common signs of infectious mononucleosis include exudative tonsillopharyngitis, anterior and posterior cervical lymphadenopathy, splenomegaly, and fever less than 40°C. Rash is infrequent unless evoked by ampicillin or amoxicillin. Laboratory studies often reveal mild hepatitis and thrombocytopenia. Most cases of infectious mononucleosis are uneventful, but a wide range of complications can occur. For instance, extreme lymphoid hyperplasia in tonsillar tissue may result in airway obstruction, and the enlarged spleen is susceptible to traumatic rupture. Autoantibodies can form to produce severe hemolytic anemia, neutropenia, or thrombocytopenia. Fatalities caused by complications of infectious mononucleosis are rare and largely the result of encephalitis, hepatic failure, myocarditis, splenic rupture, or bacterial infection associated with neutropenia.[3,9,11]

Infectious mononucleosis may evolve into a life-threatening lymphoproliferative disorder in persons with profound acquired or congenital cellular immunodeficiency. Fulminant infectious mononucleosis occurs as a rare hereditary disorder of young males, termed the X-linked lymphoproliferative disorder. Survivors of the acute illness develop aplastic anemia, dysgammaglobulinemia, and lymphoma. EBV rarely causes chronic infectious mononucleosis, which manifests as interstitial pneumonitis, marrow failure, dysgammaglobulinemia, Guillain-Barré syndrome, uveitis, and massive lymphadenopathy and hepatosplenomegaly. In contrast, the chronic fatigue syndrome is not caused by ongoing EBV activity, although the misinterpretation of EBV-specific serological tests to suggest such an association remains a problem.

Heterophile antibodies develop in 90 to 95 percent of typical episodes of infectious mononucleosis and are only seldom seen in viral hepatitis, primary HIV infection, and lymphoma. They resolve in 3 to 6 months following the onset of infectious mononucleosis and do not reappear. The appearance of EBV-specific anti-VCA immunoglobulin (Ig)M substantiates the diagnosis of primary EBV infection. These antibodies are usually detectable when patients present with infectious mononucleosis, but vanish in weeks to months and do not reappear. Anti-VCA IgG titers are usually near their peak when patients present with infectious mononucleosis. Thus a comparison of paired acute and convalescent anti-VCA IgG titers is generally unhelpful in diagnosing infectious mononucleosis. These antibodies persist for life and are useful for determining past EBV infection. Anti-EA antibodies are often induced in infectious mononucleosis and their amounts wane over time. The persistence of these antibodies at low titers has no clinical significance. Anti-EBNA antibodies are not detected by the immunofluorescence assay during acute infectious mononucleosis, but appear in convalescence and persist. Caution should be used when comparing EBV-specific antibody titers, since results generated at different times, in different places, or with different assays may be misleading.[3,9,11]

The differential diagnosis of a mononucleosis-like syndrome also includes primary infections with cytomegalovirus, toxoplasma, HIV, rubella, viral hepatitis (e.g., hepatitis A and B viruses), as well as streptococcal pharyngitis. While each of these other causes may have distinguishing clinical features, their definitive diagnosis usually rests on the results of specific laboratory tests. EBV ought not be forgotten as a potential cause of heterophile-negative mononucleosis.[9,12]

EBV infection is associated with a variety of other disorders.[3,9] EBV causes oral hairy leukoplakia in HIV-infected persons. This disorder is characterized by an exophytic growth of epithelial cells of the tongue and buccal mucosa that accompanies productive EBV replication and resolves with acyclovir treatment. Unbridled EBV-driven expansion of B cells is believed to be the cause of most post-transplant lymphoproliferative disorders. EBV is also associated with some B-cell lymphomas and rare T-cell lymphomas. In persons with acquired immunodeficiency syndrome (AIDS), about one-third of all B-cell lymphomas contain the EBV genome, while this frequency approaches 100 percent for such tumors originating in the brain. The EBV genome is present in more than 90 percent of Burkitt's lymphomas in persons from Africa, but is found in only 20 percent of these lymphomas occurring in persons from the United States. Virtually all nonkeratinizing nasopharyngeal carcinomas, which are prevalent in persons from southern China and certain Native Americans, contain the EBV genome. The viral genome is also found in smooth-muscle tumors of children who have AIDS or received organ transplantation. The association of EBV with Hodgkin's disease is less clear.

Treatment

Infectious mononucleosis is managed with general supportive care, such as rest, hydration, antipyretics, and analgesics. Activity is restricted in proportion to degree of symptoms. Contact sports are suspended for 1 month or until absence of splenomegaly is verified. Treatment of uncomplicated infectious mononucleosis with empiric antibiotics or glucocorticoids is inadvisable. More than 85 percent of persons with infectious mononucleosis who are treated with ampicillin or amoxicillin will develop rash. Therefore, these antibiotics should not be used for treatment of a concurrent bacterial infection. Throat cultures containing *S. pyogenes* should be treated with 10 days of penicillin or erythromycin, since as many as 30 percent of such cases later exhibit serologic evidence of streptococcal infection. While acyclovir can effectively suppress viral shedding, no appreciable clinical benefit is conferred. Additional treatment measures may be required for the complications of infectious mononucleosis. For instance, airway obstruction necessitates intubation or tracheostomy, and critical anemia or thrombocytopenia requires transfusions. Glucocorticoid therapy is useful in protracted severe illness, autoimmune hemolytic anemia and thrombocytopenia, and impending airway obstruction from tonsillar enlargement. This therapy is also considered in EBV-related aplastic anemia, encephalitis, myocarditis, and pericarditis. There is no compelling evidence that antiviral agents, such as acyclovir, provide clinical improvement in complications of infectious mononucleosis.[3,9,12] Treatment of the other EBV-related disorders is beyond the scope of this text.

Prevention

There is currently no vaccine to prevent EBV infection and its disorders, although candidate vaccines are undergoing development.[3] Transmission of EBV can be reduced by restricting intimate contact, but this is usually impractical and may delay virus acquisition to an age when symptoms are more likely. Nonetheless, this restriction is reasonable when the consequences of infection would be devastating. Such persons who require blood products or tissue allografts would ideally benefit from receipt of irradiated blood products or EBV-negative tissues to obviate risk of EBV transmission. The practice of standard (universal) precautions and handwashing is sufficient to prevent nosocomial transmission of EBV. Therefore, persons with infectious mononucleosis generally need not be placed in isolation.[13]

Herpes Simplex Virus

Richard J. Whitley[a]

Herpes simplex virus (HSV) is one of the most common infections encountered by humans worldwide. As a member of the herpesvirus family, it shares the unique biologic characteristic of being able to exist in a latent state and recur periodically, if not chronically, serving as a reservoir for transmission from one person to another. Herpes simplex virus exists as two distinct antigenic types, HSV-1 and HSV-2. HSV-1 is usually associated with infections above the belt, namely involving the oropharynx and lips; however, increasing numbers of genital infections attributed to this virus have been recognized. HSV-2 infections more commonly cause infection below the belt, involving the genitalia, buttocks, and infrequently the lower extremities. In addition, HSV-2 is a cause of infection of the newborn. The spectrum of disease caused by HSV ranges from benign and nuisance infections to those that can be life threatening.[1]

▸ EPIDEMIOLOGY

Herpes simplex virus infection is transmitted by direct contact. The epidemiology of infection can best be defined according to seroprevalence of HSV-1 and HSV-2. By adulthood, the majority of adults have experienced HSV-1 infections (70 to 90 percent).[2] Primary HSV-1 infections usually occur in the young child, under 5 years of age, and are most often asymptomatic. The prevalence of HSV-1 infection increases to a peak in the seventh decade of life, affecting approximately 80 percent in the United States. Geographic location, socioeconomic status, and age influence the occurrence of HSV infection, regardless of the mode of assessment. In developing countries and in lower socioeconomic communities, primary infection occurs early in life. In some areas of the world, the seroprevalence to HSV-1 is in excess of 95 percent, as is the case in Spain, Italy, Rwanda, Zaire, Senegal, China, Taiwan, Haiti, Jamaica, and Costa Rica. Most of these infections are asymptomatic.

[a]*Studies performed by the author were initiated and supported under Contract NO1-AI-65306 from the Antiviral Research Branch of the National Institute of Allergy and Infectious Diseases, Program Project Grant PO1 AI 24009, an unrestricted grant in infectious diseases from Bristol-Myers Squibb, and by grants from the General Clinical Research Center Program (RR-032), and the State of Alabama.*

Acquisition of HSV-2 usually occurs in association with onset of sexual activity. Acquisition of HSV-2 is a function of the number of lifetime sexual partners. Overall, seroprevalence to HSV-2 in the United States is approximately 35 percent in the mid-1990s, reflecting a 30 percent increase since the early 1980s. Among heterosexual men, the seroprevalence approaches 80 percent for individuals with more than 50 lifetime sexual partners.[2] In contrast, for women with a similar number of sexual partners, the prevalence of HSV-2 exceeds 90 percent. In general, women acquire HSV-2 infection more frequently than do men, irrespective of the number of partners. For pregnant women, approximately 1 percent will excrete virus at the time of delivery. Nevertheless, the incidence of neonatal HSV infection is only approximately 1 in 2,500 to 1 in 5,000 liveborn infants in the United States, implying a relative degree of protection of the newborn.

Nosocomial HSV infection has been documented both in newborn nurseries as well as in intensive care units.[1] In addition, the occurrence of herpetic Whitlow, as a consequence of exposure has been documented.[1]

Pathogenesis

The pathogenesis of HSV infections is dependent upon the requirement for intimate contact between a person who is shedding virus and a susceptible host. After inoculation of HSV onto the skin or mucous membrane, an incubation period of 4 to 6 days is required before there is evidence of clinical disease. Herpes simplex virus replicates in epithelial cells. As replication continues, cell lysis and local inflammation ensue, resulting in characteristic vesicles on an erythematous base. Regional lymphatics and lymph nodes become involved; viremia and visceral dissemination may develop, depending upon the immunologic competence of the host. In all hosts, the virus generally ascends peripheral sensory nerves and reaches the dorsal root ganglia. Replication of HSV within neural tissue is followed by retrograde axonal spread of the virus back to other mucosal and skin surfaces via the peripheral sensory nerves. Virus replicates further in the epithelial cells, reproducing the lesions of the initial infection, until infection is contained through both systemic and mucosal immune responses.

Latency is established when HSV reaches the dorsal root ganglia after anterograde transmission via sensory nerve pathways. In its latent form, intracellular HSV DNA cannot be detected routinely unless specific molecular probes are used.

Rarely HSV can infect the central nervous system and cause encephalitis.[3] The focality and temporal lobe affinity suggest direct extension of virus along neural tracts. Encephalitis caused by HSV is characterized by necrosis of the inferior medial portion of the temporal lobe, initially unilaterally and then contralaterally. This necrotic process accounts for the high morbidity and mortality of infection. Infection of the neonate is usually the consequence of direct contact with infected maternal genital secretions, accounting for approximately 85 percent cases of neonatal herpes. The remaining 15 percent are caused by in utero infection, secondary to viremia, or postnatal acquisition whereby the baby comes in contact with infectious virus in the environment.

▸ CLINICAL MANIFESTATIONS

Mucocutaneous Infections

Gingivostomatitis

Mucocutaneous infections are the most common clinical manifestations of HSV-1 and HSV-2. Gingivostomatitis is usually caused by HSV-1 and occurs most frequently in children under 5 years of age. It is characterized by fever, sore throat, pharyngeal edema and erythema, followed by the development of vesicular or ulcerative lesions of the oral or pharyngeal mucosa. Recurrent HSV-1 infections of the oropharynx frequently manifest as herpes simplex labialis (cold sores), and appear on the vermilion border of the lip. Intraoral lesions as a manifestation of recurrent disease are uncommon in the normal host but do occur frequently in the immunocompromised host.

Genital Herpes

Genital herpes is most frequently caused by HSV-2 but an ever increasing number of cases are attributed to HSV-1.[4] Primary infection in women usually involves the vulva, vagina, and cervix. In men, initial infection is most often associated with lesions on the glans penis, prepuce, or penile shaft. In individuals of either sex, primary disease is associated with fever, malaise, anorexia, and bilateral inguinal adenopathy. Women frequently have dysuria and urinary retention due to urethral involvement. As many as 10 percent of individuals will develop an aseptic meningitis with primary infection. Sacral radiculomyelitis may occur in both men and women, resulting in neuralgias, urinary retention, or obstipation. The complete healing of primary infection may take several weeks. The first episode of genital infection is less severe in individuals who have had previous HSV infections at other sites, such as herpes simplex labialis.

Recurrent genital infections in either men or women can be particularly distressing. The frequency of recurrence varies significantly from one individual to another. It has been estimated that one-third of individuals with genital herpes have virtually no recurrences, one-third have approximately three recurrences per year, and another third have more than three per year. By applying polymerase chain reaction to genital swabs from women with a history of recurrent genital herpes, virus DNA can be detected in the absence of culture proof of infection.[5] This finding suggests the chronicity of genital herpes as opposed to a recurrent infection.

Herpetic Keratitis

Herpes simplex keratitis is usually caused by HSV-1 and is accompanied by conjunctivitis in many cases.[4] It is considered among the most common infectious causes of blindness in the United States. The characteristic lesions of herpes simplex keratoconjunctivitis are dendritic ulcers best detected by fluorescein staining. Deep stromal involvement has also been reported and may result in visual impairment.

Other Skin Manifestations

Herpes simplex virus infections can manifest at any skin site. Common among health care workers are lesions on abraded skin of the fingers, known as herpetic whitlows. Similarly, because of physical contact, wrestlers may develop disseminated cutaneous lesions known as herpes gladiatorum.

Neonatal Herpes Simplex Virus Infection

Neonatal HSV infection is estimated to occur in approximately 1 in 2,500 to 1 in 5,000 deliveries in the United States annually.[6] Approximately 70 percent of cases are caused by HSV-2 and usually result from contact of the fetus with infected maternal genital secretions at the time of delivery. Manifestations of neonatal HSV infection can be divided into three categories: (*a*) skin, eye and mouth disease; (*b*) encephalitis; and (*c*) disseminated infection. As the name implies, skin, eye, and mouth disease consists of cutaneous lesions and does not involve other organ systems. Involvement of the central nervous system may occur with encephalitis or disseminated infection and generally results in a diffuse encephalitis. The cerebrospinal fluid formula characteristically reveals an elevated protein and a mononuclear pleocytosis. Disseminated infection involves multiple organ systems and can produce disseminated intravascular coagulation, hemorrhagic pneumonitis, encephalitis, and cutaneous lesions. Diagnosis can be particularly difficult in the absence of skin lesions. The mortality rate for each disease classification varies from zero for skin, eye, and mouth disease to 15 percent for encephalitis and 60 percent for neonates with disseminated infection. In addition to the high mortality associated with these infections, morbidity is significant in that children with encephalitis or disseminated disease develop normally in only approximately 40 percent of cases, even with the administration of appropriate antiviral therapy.

Herpes Simplex Encephalitis

Herpes simplex encephalitis is characterized by hemorrhagic necrosis of the inferomedial portion of the temporal lobe. Disease begins unilaterally, then spreads to the contralateral temporal lobe. It is the most common cause of focal, sporadic encephalitis in the United States today and occurs in approximately 1 in 150,000 individuals. Most cases are caused by HSV-1. The actual pathogenesis of herpes simplex encephalitis is unknown, although it has been speculated that primary or recurrent virus can reach the temporal lobe by ascending neural pathways, such as the trigeminal tracts or the olfactory nerves.

Clinical manifestations of herpes simplex encephalitis include headache, fever, altered consciousness, and abnormalities of speech and behavior. Focal seizures may also occur. The cerebrospinal fluid formulae for these patients is variable, but usually consists of a pleocytosis of monocytes. The protein concentration is characteristically elevated and glucose is usually normal. Historically, a definitive diagnosis could be achieved only by brain biopsy, since other pathogens may produce a clinically similar illness. However, the application of polymerase chain reaction (PCR) for detection of virus DNA has replaced brain biopsy as the standard for diagnosis.[7] The mortality and morbidity are high, even when appropriate antiviral therapy is administered. At present, the mortality rate is approximately 30 percent 1 year after treatment. In addition, approximately 70 percent of survivors will have significant neurologic sequelae.

Herpes Simplex Virus Infections in the Immunocompromised Host

Herpes simplex virus infections in the immunocompromised host are clinically more severe, may be progressive, and require more time for healing. Manifestations of HSV infections in this patient population include pneumonitis, esophagitis, hepatitis, colitis, and disseminated cutaneous disease. Individuals suffering from human immunodeficiency virus infection may have extensive perineal or orofacial ulcerations. Herpes simplex virus infections are also noted to be of increased severity in individuals who are burned.

▶ DIAGNOSIS

The diagnosis of HSV infections is usually predicated on clinical evaluation of mucocutaneous manifestations. However, confirmation of the diagnosis requires isolation of HSV in appropriate cell culture systems or the detection of viral gene products or, alternatively, the detection of viral DNA by PCR. Herpes simplex virus grows readily in tissue culture, producing cytopathic effects within a few days in a wide variety of mammalian cell lines. The routine typing, namely distinguishing HSV-1 from HSV-2, of the isolate is not usually required unless epidemiologic studies are being performed.

Polymerase chain reaction has become a useful method for diagnosing HSV infections, particularly those involving the central nervous system, specifically neonatal HSV infection and herpes simplex encephalitis. The detection of HSV DNA by PCR in the CSF has replaced brain biopsy as a method of diagnosis of central nervous system infections.

Type-specific serologic assays are not commercially available. The utilization of immunoblot detection of specific glycoproteins that distinguish HSV-1 from HSV-2, namely, glycoprotein (g) G-1 and gG-2, are available in research laboratories for determining prior exposure to HSV-1 and HSV-2 infections. Likely, in the near future, a commercially available assay that distinguishes HSV-1 from HSV-2 will become available.

Historically, Tzanck smears have been used to diagnose HSV infections. Tzanck smears are not sensitive enough for routine diagnostic purposes. However, immunofluorescent staining of cell trap preparations from lesions is both sensitive and specific for the diagnosis for HSV infections.

▶ TREATMENT

Infections due to HSV are the most amenable to therapy with antiviral drugs. Acyclovir has proved useful for the management of specific infections caused by HSV. At present, acyclovir is the treatment of choice for mucocutaneous HSV infections in the immunocompromised host and for herpes simplex encephalitis, neonatal HSV infections, and HSV infections caused by HSV-2 involving the genital tract. Intravenous administration is the preferred therapy for individuals with life-threatening disease. Immunocompromised individuals with mucocutaneous HSV infections that are not life threatening can be given oral acyclovir. Caution must be exercised when acyclovir is used intravenously, because it may crystallize in renal tubules when administered too rapidly or to dehydrated patients. Recently, both valacyclovir and famciclovir have been licensed for the treatment of genital herpes. The advantages of these medications over acyclovir is unclear.

Topical therapy with one of several antiviral ophthalmic preparations is appropriate for HSV keratoconjunctivitis. However, the treatment of choice is viroptic or trifluorothymidine. Secondary choices include vidarabine ophthalmic or topical idoxuridine.

▶ PREVENTION AND CONTROL

At the present, there is no licensed vaccine for the prevention for HSV infections. Indeed, one glycoprotein vaccine under development has been abandoned for the lack of efficacy. This vaccine included glycoproteins to the two major immunodominant glycoproteins of HSV, namely, gB and gD. In the absence of efficacy, even to the slightest extent, with this experimental vaccine, efforts for further vaccine development will proceed slowly. If any vaccine will be successful, it will likely be one that is attenuated and genetically engineered. As a consequence, the prevention of HSV infections resides in the most part on knowledge of the mechanisms of transmission, both person to person as well as in the hospital environment. Individuals with known recurrent HSV infections should be counseled on the possibility of transmission of infection while lesions are present. The use of condoms for individuals with recurrent genital herpes is encouraged in that detection of HSV DNA by PCR can occur even in the absence of lesions. Similarly, for individuals who have recurrent herpes labialis, kissing should be discouraged.

There is a risk of nosocomial transmission of HSV within the hospital environment. Since many individuals excrete HSV in the absence of clinical symptoms, it is impossible to exclude all workers from the hospital environment who could transmit infection. Thus, many authorities simply recommend strict handwashing and covering of lesions, should they exist.

Finally, no data exist on the prevention of neonatal HSV infection. The anticipatory administration of acyclovir to babies delivered through an infected birth canal may prove of value, particularly for women who have first episode genital herpetic infection. However, no data exist to substantiate this hypotheses. Since over 1 percent of all women at delivery excrete HSV and the rate of neonatal HSV infection is only 1 in 2,500 to 1 in 5,000 liveborn infants as noted earlier, the routine administration of acyclovir to all children born to HSV-positive women is not reasonable. Alternative approaches, namely administration of acyclovir to known HSV-2–infected women is under investigation.[8] This latter study, at least, will consider the consequences of acyclovir administration on cesarean section and its complications.

Cytomegalovirus Infections

James F. Bale, Jr

Human cytomegalovirus (CMV), a member of the herpesvirus family, can produce life- or sight-threatening infections when the virus infects the developing fetus or persons who are receiving immunosuppressive therapy or have immunocompromising medical conditions, such as the acquired immunodeficiency syndrome (AIDS).[1–5] Studies worldwide indicate that 0.5 to 2.5 percent of infants excrete CMV at birth, and most adults over 40 years of age have serologic evidence of prior CMV infection. Fortunately, the majority of infected persons do not experience serious complications of CMV infection.

Approximately 30 to 40 percent of the pregnant women who undergo primary CMV infection transmit the virus to their fetuses.[6] Of the infected newborns, 5 to 10 percent have a multisystemic disorder characterized clinically by petechial rash, jaundice, hepatosplenomegaly, microcephaly, or chorioretinitis. Surviving infants have a 90 percent risk of sequelae consisting of sensorineural hearing loss, visual loss, seizures, or developmental and intellectual delays.[7] Silently infected infants have a 10 to 15 percent risk of sensorineural hearing loss, but have very low rates of other neurologic or ophthalmologic complications.

Acquired CMV infection can cause a heterophil-negative infectious mononucleosis syndrome that resembles disease to the Epstein-Barr virus.[4] Infected persons have malaise, low-grade fever, lymphadenopathy, pharyngitis, hepatitis, or occasionally, pneumonitis. Although the course of CMV-induced mononucleosis can be protracted, immunocompetent persons typically recover without sequelae.

By contrast, CMV can be an especially virulent pathogen in immunocompromised hosts, causing fatal pneumonitis, severe gastroenteritis, necrotizing retinitis, polyradiculopathy, or disseminated encephalitis.[2,3] Conditions associated with severe CMV infections include congenital immunodeficiency syndromes, immunosuppression for solid organ or bone marrow transplantation, chemotherapy for malignancy or connective tissue disorders, and AIDS.[3] CMV infections develop in 30 to 60 percent or more of bone marrow or solid organ transplant recipients as a result of primary infection, reactivated latent infection, or reinfection.[2] CMV affects 40 percent or more of persons with AIDS, making CMV one of the most frequently recognized opportunistic infections in such patients.[3]

In infected persons CMV can be detected in urine, saliva, circulating leukocytes, breast milk, semen, or cervical secretions.[2,5] Ingestion of CMV-infected breast milk or contact with the saliva or urine of infected playmates or family members accounts for most acquired infections in infants and young children.[5] After puberty, sexual contact with CMV-infected persons contributes to transmission.[8] Infected persons excrete CMV in saliva or urine for extended periods, several years after congenital infection and as long as 1 year after acquired infections. Reinfection with new CMV strains also occurs.[9,10]

CMV can be acquired via transfusion of blood products or transplantation of organs or tissues from CMV-seropositive blood or organ donors. The risk of infection after transfusion, greatest when patients receive blood from multiple donors, ranges from 0.14 to 2.7 percent per unit transfused.[11] Solid organs, bone marrow, or skin from seropositive donors can transmit CMV, with seronegative recipients being at greatest risk of CMV infection and invasive disease.[2,12]

Culturing the urine or other body fluids using the shell vial assay remains the most widely used and specific means to confirm CMV infection.[4] CMV infection can also be established by identifying antigenemia, a relatively rapid diagnostic method that detects CMV pp65 antigens in leukocytes,[13] or by identifying CMV nucleic acids in body fluids or tissues using the polymerase chain reaction (PCR) or nucleic acid hybridization methods.[14] CMV isolates can be studied using PCR and other molecular techniques to compare CMV strains[10,15] or to detect DNA mutations that confer resistance to ganciclovir or foscarnet.[14] Seroconversion or detection of CMV-specific IgM supports recent infection, although serologic methods generally have reduced sensitivity when compared with culture, antigenemia assay, or DNA detection.[4]

Prevention and Therapy

Congenital or acquired CMV infections cannot currently be prevented by immunization. Several candidate vaccines have been studied during the past two decades, and although some appear to induce cellular, humoral, or neutralizing immune responses against CMV,[4,16] none have, as yet, proceeded beyond clinical trials. Studies using subunit vaccines prepared from immunodominant CMV proteins, such as glycoprotein B, are ongoing.

The factors that contribute to CMV transmission, such as size of the virus inoculum or the duration of contact, have not been determined precisely.[2] Thus, measures that uniformly interrupt natural routes of CMV transmission have not been established. When compared with other viral pathogens, however, CMV is not highly contagious. Because infection appears to require contact with fresh, CMV-infected fluids, attention to hygienic principles, such as handwashing or avoiding oral contact, and adoption of standard precautions diminish the risk of CMV transmission. Condoms reduce the risk of sexual transmission.

Fomites may contribute to CMV transmission in child care centers or nursery environments,[17] and the potential for CMV transmission can be reduced by prompt disposal of soiled diapers or decontamination of environmental surfaces. In child care environments, mouthing toys can be disinfected by immersion in a bleach and water solution, prepared fresh daily by adding ¼ cup of household bleach to 1 gallon of water.[18] Items that cannot be immersed should be air-dried thoroughly.

Young, toddler-age children who attend child day care centers have high rates of CMV infection and frequently transmit CMV to their playmates, parents, or other adult care providers.[19–21] Although child-to-child transmission of CMV poses little or no risk to young children, CMV transmission to a nonimmune pregnant woman can have serious consequences for the developing fetus. Thus, women who have contact with young children and intend to become pregnant should assess their CMV serologic status prior to pregnancy. Seronegative pregnant women should attempt to reduce their risk of CMV infection by washing their hands after contact with diapers or body fluids, avoiding oral contact with young children, and refraining from sharing food or eating utensils with young children, including their own. The virus poses little or no risk to healthy women who are CMV-seropositive.

In seronegative bone marrow or solid organ transplant recipients, the risk of primary CMV infection, the most serious form of infection, can be reduced by transfusing CMV seronegative or leukocyte-depleted blood products.[22,23] CMV seronegative blood products should be administered also to premature infants or infants undergoing large volume exchange transfusions. Matching of seronegative recipients with organs from seronegative donors, although an effective means to prevent primary CMV infection, cannot be accomplished easily because of the limited availability of CMV seronegative organ donors.[23]

Several strategies, including passive immunotherapy and antiviral chemotherapy, alone or in combination, may prevent CMV infection or reduce the severity of CMV disease in high-risk patients, such as transplant recipients who are CMV seronegative and receive tissues from CMV-seropositive donors.[22,23] Because preventive or therapeutic approaches to invasive CMV infections continue to evolve, however, we caution that infectious disease or transplant experts should be consulted to obtain updated information regarding CMV prophylaxis or treatment in immunocompromised patients.

Potential prophylactic immunologic strategies include the expansion of CMV-specific cytotoxic T-lymphocyte populations or the administration of CMV hyperimmune globulin. The former approach remains experimental, whereas the latter strategy has become an important component of protocols designed to reduce the potential for CMV infection and to treat certain diseases in high-risk transplant patients.[22,23]

Meta-analysis of several published studies suggests that immunoglobulin enriched for CMV-IgG antibodies diminishes the rates of infection or death among CMV seronegative bone marrow or solid organ transplant recipients.[24] Common to the regimens is an attempt to provide CMV immunoglobulin during the high-risk period for CMV infection, typically the first 3 to 4 months after transplantation.[24,25] CMV immunoglobulin is initiated 4 to 10 days before marrow transplantation or within 72 hours of solid organ transplantation and is continued at intervals for 2 to 4 months posttransplantation. Side effects of immunoglobulin therapy consist of headache, fever, flushing, nausea, vomiting, or allergic reactions.

Acyclovir, ganciclovir (9-((1,3-dihydroxy-2-propoxy)methyl) guanine (DHPG)), and foscarnet (trisodium phosphonoformate) have been used to prevent or treat invasive CMV infections.[26,27] In some studies of bone marrow or renal transplant recipients, acyclovir begun orally or intravenously before transplantation and continued orally for several weeks after transplantation has reduced the incidence of CMV infection or severity of CMV disease.[28] Acyclovir has been ineffective, however, when used to treat active CMV disease. Ganciclovir, the first effective antiviral agent for invasive CMV infections,[26] given intravenously prior to and after solid organ or bone marrow transplantation, also reduces the incidence and severity of CMV disease.[23]

Ganciclovir, a 2′-deoxyguanosine analog that inhibits CMV DNA synthesis, has efficacy when used to treat CMV pneumonitis, retinitis, gastroenteritis, or neurologic complications in a wide range of immunocompromised patients.[26,29,30] In persons with AIDS and CMV retinitis, a sight-threatening disorder, ganciclovir halts disease when given at a dose of 5 mg/kg intravenously twice daily for 14 to 21 days. To prevent relapses, however, the drug must be continued indefinitely thereafter using intravenous (5 mg/kg once daily) or oral routes.[26,31] Potential adverse effects include neutropenia (the most common toxic manifestation), anemia, azoospermia, thrombocytopenia, nausea, or vomiting. Patients with CMV retinitis require frequent ophthalmologic monitoring.

Successful therapy of CMV disease in bone marrow and solid organ transplant recipients remains a distinct clinical challenge.[2,22,23] Current management includes pre-emptive therapy, a strategy by which antiviral agents, such as ganciclovir and CMV immunoglobulin, are initiated in high-risk transplant patients, e.g., CMV-seropositive donor and CMV-seronegative recipient, as soon as CMV is detected at any site by culture, antigenemia assay, or PCR.[23] Invasive disease in solid organ transplant recipients may respond favorably to ganciclovir 5 mg/kg twice daily for 14 days or longer, but the drug alone has generally been ineffective for CMV pneumonitis in lung or bone marrow transplant recipients.[2] Several studies indicate, however, that combined therapy with ganciclovir and CMV immunoglobulin improves survival in patients with CMV pneumonitis.[32,33]

Ganciclovir has also been used to treat serious CMV infections of congenitally infected newborns and other immunocompetent patients. Uncontrolled case studies suggest that congenitally infected infants may benefit from postnatal ganciclovir therapy,[34] but widespread application of this therapeutic strategy awaits the results of placebo-controlled trials. Considerations of ganciclovir use in immunocompetent hosts must balance the severity of the clinical syndrome and the toxicities of the drug. The drug must be used cautiously in patients receiving other myelosuppressive agents.

Foscarnet, generally reserved for CMV infections that fail to respond to ganciclovir, inhibits CMV replication by binding with the viral DNA polymerase.[27] CMV-infected bone marrow or solid organ transplant recipients, treated with foscarnet in doses ranging from 60 to 300 mg/kg/d intravenously for 1 to 4 or more weeks, have shown favorable clinical responses.[27] Foscarnet has therapeutic efficacy comparable to that of ganciclovir for AIDS-associated CMV retinitis and can be used in combination with ganciclovir to treat serious CMV disease in person with AIDS.[35] The major side effects associated with foscarnet therapy include nephrotoxicity, anemia, seizures, and alterations in calcium homeostasis.[27] Foscarnet must be used cautiously in patients receiving other potentially nephrotoxic drugs.[27]

Acute Gastrointestinal Infections

Arnold S. Monto

Enteric illnesses are second only to respiratory illnesses in causing acute disease in the U.S. population. Based on the Household Interview Survey, it has been estimated that 21 million episodes involving restricted activity or medical attention occur annually. Enteric disease is of even greater consequence in the developing countries. There, in an interplay with malnutrition and acute respiratory infection, it was responsible for a major portion of infant mortality, but has responded dramatically to use of oral rehydration therapy. In developed country populations the common enteric illnesses are self-limited diseases with symptoms of vomiting, diarrhea, and abdominal pain, alone or in combinations. Studies of frequency and patterns of occurrence were delayed because of the lack of knowledge of the principal etiological agents involved. Now, an increasing number of viral and bacterial pathogens have been identified as etiological agents, and greater attention is being paid to the problem.

As with respiratory disease, enteric illnesses are most common in young children, and incidence falls with increasing age. The actual annual number of episodes experienced has varied from study to study, depending on population evaluated and methods used to ascertain occurrence. In the Cleveland Family Study, it was found that children under the age of 10 years experienced approximately two episodes a year, whereas young adults had somewhat more than one such acute attack each year. School attendance was associated with an increase in illness frequency, as was increasing family size.[1] In the Tecumseh Study, with different methods of ascertaining occurrence of illness and a broader population group, illness frequency again varied with age. Mean annual incidence was 1.9 in the under 5 year olds, 1.2 in the 5- to 19-year age group, and 1.0 in adults.[2] The episodes occurred mainly in the colder months of the year, with 28.3 percent occurring in autumn, 36.7 percent in winter, 18.3 percent in spring, and 16.7 percent in summer.

In Tecumseh, as in Cleveland, a problem in interpretation arose from the overlap of respiratory and gastrointestinal symptoms in the same illness. Approximately 25 percent of people with gastrointestinal illness observed during 6 years of study in Tecumseh also had respiratory symptoms, with the highest overlap in children under 5 years of age. In the Cleveland Study, the combined respiratory-gastrointestinal syndrome made up 20 percent of all cases of gastrointestinal illness, and the frequency of association of the two types of symptoms in the same illness was much higher than would be expected by chance alone. Thus, it appears that certain specific agents may be responsible for this combined illness.

Studies of the common enteric illnesses have determined if specific agents can be associated with particular syndromes or certain seasons of the year. It is now known that at least three groups of viruses, the rotaviruses, the Norwalk-like agents, now recognized to be calicivirus and certain adenoviruses, are significantly involved in such illnesses. The adenoviruses are discussed elsewhere as etiological agents of respiratory disease. The ones involved in gastrointestinal disease were identified by electron microscopy more often from hospitalized children with enteric illness than from control subjects. These viruses could not be grown in standard cell culture.[3] Other studies confirmed the etiological role of these agents, which have been identified also in a number of outbreaks, especially among infants. These particular adenoviruses belong to a limited number of serotypes, share nucleic acid characteristics in common (subgroup F), and have been grown in a special cell culture.[4]

Other viruses, including astroviruses, reoviruses, and coronaviruses, have been reported in some enteric illnesses and outbreaks. In most cases, they have been identified by electron microscopy from cases of illness. It is not yet clear if any or all of them are truly etiologically associated with disease, since the necessary controlled or experimental investigations have yet to be performed. However, association with disease has been most convincingly demonstrated with the astroviruses and caliciviruses. Certain bacteria, other than the salmonella and shigella, are known to be involved in enteric illnesses. These are toxigenic, invasive, and enteropathogenic strains of *Escherichia coli*. They are described in Chapter 10.

▶ ROTAVIRUSES

The rotaviruses are double-stranded RNA-containing viruses belonging to the family *Reoviridae*. The name "rotavirus" was suggested for the group on the basis of the wheel-like appearance of complete virions on electron microscopy. They can be distinguished on the basis of morphology and other characteristics from true reoviruses and orbiviruses and have been variously termed in earlier descriptions human reovirus-like agents and duoviruses. The rotaviruses cause diarrhea in humans and in several species of domestic animals.[5,6] The animal agents can be grown readily in a number of generally available cell systems. However, this is not true of the human rotaviruses, which are difficult to grow in cell culture except under special circumstances, such as pretreatment of specimens with trypsin. Other methods must, therefore, be employed in most laboratories to detect the human agents. Initially, all studies used electron microscopy to identify the virus. It is now known that this was possible because it is so abundant in stool, with a titer of 10^8 or 10^9 particles per gram. A number of alternate techniques have been developed for detection of virus. The enzyme-linked immunosorbent assay (ELISA) has the greatest use, since it is sensitive and can be done without special equipment.[7] It is also useful, with modification, for detection of antibody.

Much of the information on the pathogenesis of the disease comes from work with animal agents because of the ability to collect appropriate specimens.[8] Microscopically, the sides and tips of the villi are most affected, especially in the lower part of the small intestine. In severe cases, there is almost complete destruction of the villi. Damage to the brush-bordered epithelium produces a local decrease in disaccharidases, which results in accumulation of lactose and other disaccharides in the bowel. Fluids accumulate in the lumen osmotically, resulting in diarrhea and a degree of malabsorption. Immunity to rotaviruses is acquired at an early age and is transmitted transplacentally. Infants in newborn nurseries are infected frequently but usually do not experience disease, even if not breast fed, which suggests that circulating IgG antibody may protect.[9]

The rotavirus genome contains 11 segments. The genes coding for the various antigens of biological importance have been identified, and the complex antigenic structure of the virus has been clarified. This structure is of importance in view of work in vaccine development. There is a group antigen, as well as subgroup and serotype antigens. Most rotaviruses of humans are in group A. Four serotypes, determined by the glycoprotein of the virus, are of importance in human disease.[10] Non–group A viruses have been isolated in China from outbreaks of unusual characteristics.[11]

Distribution of Disease

Aside from the outbreaks described above, rotavirus diarrhea is mainly a disease of infants and small children. Characteristically, the children ill enough to be hospitalized are febrile, and half have vomiting in addition to diarrhea. Dehydration is a typical feature of these illnesses. The incidence of diarrheal disease associated with rotaviruses resulting in a visit to a physician can be estimated to be 15/100 children under the age of 1 year.[12] It is also known that in developed countries close to 50 percent of children age 1 to 3 years, hospitalized for severe diarrhea, are infected with rotaviruses.[13] A similar frequency of rotaviruses in severe dehydrating diarrhea has been found in several developing countries. Since the total incidence of such illnesses is higher there than in developed countries and the events are associated with mortality and malnutrition, it is apparent that rotaviruses are of critical importance in the third world.[14]

In the temperate zone, rotaviruses exhibit a distinct seasonal pattern, with infections most common in the colder months of the year. During peak months, more than 75 percent of children hospitalized with diarrhea are infected with the agent.[15] Studies in families have not been carried out extensively, but it is already clear that transmission does occur, with reinfection of older children and adults.[16]

Prevention and Control

Rotaviruses are stable agents, relatively resistant to adverse environmental conditions. They are not inactivated by lipid solvents, are acid stable, and can remain on surfaces and in water for prolonged periods. Since fecal-oral transmission is the likely method of acquisition, interruption of this mechanism by appropriate interventions is a possible means of prophylaxis, recognizing the possible persistence of the agent. Since rotaviruses possess a segmented genome, it should be possible through reassortment recombination to create an attenuated variant for vaccine purposes. Vaccines prepared by this method and those using viruses of animal origin are currently being licensed. These studies, although generally encouraging, occasionally have produced conflicting results, in part reflecting prior antibody status of diverse populations. Most recently, clear evidence of efficacy of a quadravalent vaccine was demonstrated when severe, rather than total, diarrheal disease was used as the preventive endpoint.[17] Such a vaccine could be especially useful in the developing countries where, interacting with malnutrition, the virus is responsible for considerable childhood mortality.

Norwalk-like Agents

Characteristics, Pathogenesis, and Distribution

This distinct group of agents is responsible for outbreaks of enteric disease with diarrhea, vomiting, and systemic symptoms. Disease has occurred among residents of institutions and individuals of all ages living in families. The etiological agents have never been grown in cell culture but have been visualized on electron microscopy. On the basis of appearance and size, they were termed the 27-nm, or Norwalk, agent, the latter name referring to an outbreak from which the most thoroughly studied strain was isolated.[18] Most recently the viruses have been cloned and are clearly of the *Caliciviridae* family, although they lack classic appearance under electron microscope.[19] The viruses are acid and ether stable and relatively resistant to heat.[20] Thus it is not surprising that they have been involved in waterborne outbreaks.

There are at least four serotypes of the agent[21] that are quite distinct antigenically from the others[22] plus others that might be related. No animal strains with shared antigens have been identified. These facts have presented great difficulties in the study of the behavior of the agents in population groups. In addition, the virus is present in relatively small quantities in the stool. Thus it may not be visualized easily without the use of immune serum for clumping of the virus (immune electron microscopy).[23] It also means that stool is not as rich a source of virus for use as a reagent in seroepidemiology; this problem has recently been overcome by cloning of the virus.[23]

In spite of the problems posed by these observations, valuable information has been gathered on the Norwalk-like agents. Antibody is not acquired very early in life, as is the situation with the rotaviruses. Its later acquisition indicates that widespread exposure to these viruses is somewhat delayed. In keeping with this finding, when adults are challenged experimentally, disease often results. Typically, illness consists of combinations of diarrhea, vomiting, low-grade fever, abdominal cramps, and malaise. Upper gastrointestinal symptoms usually predominate, and the illness has a relatively short duration. Microscopically, in the proximal intestine, there is mucosal inflammation, villous shortening, crypt hypertrophy, and absorptive cell abnormalities.[24] When a group of volunteers was challenged with this virus, half experienced self-limited illness with characteristic vomiting or diarrhea or both after an incubation period of approximately 1 to 2 days. On rechallenge of the same volunteers 2 or more years later, the same individuals who had initially experienced illness again were sick. On further rechallenge 4 to 8 weeks thereafter, most of those who previously had developed illness were protected.[25] Thus, immunity to the Norwalk-like agents is complicated, and the reagents now available following cloning of the virus will help in explaining the observations.

Prevention and Control

Work with these viruses has been hampered by technical difficulties, and any conclusions on control must be regarded as tentative. The principles of environmental control discussed for the rotaviruses probably apply to the Norwalk-like agents. These viruses do affect adults and are stable, and they have occurred in familial and institutional-propagated outbreaks. They also have been associated with waterborne outbreaks in which large numbers of cases have occurred. In the former situation, prevention of the opportunity for fecal-oral transmission will be useful. In the latter, proper handling of sources of water has been associated with cessation of outbreaks. Coliform counts can be useful as an indication of the effectiveness of treatment of the water. Until more is known of the precise nature of the virus and until it can be cultivated in some way, vaccine development will be impossible.

Trachoma and Inclusion Conjunctivitis

Julius Schachter

Trachoma, a chronic inflammation of the mucous membranes lining the eyelid and eyeball, is the leading cause of preventable blindness in the world. Inclusion conjunctivitis is an acute infection of newborns and sexually active adults that usually heals spontaneously without sequelae even if not treated. Trachoma and inclusion conjunctivitis may, in fact, be two forms of eye diseases caused by the same organism or may be different aspects of the same clinical spectrum. These two diseases, however, have different epidemiological patterns and present very real differences in terms of relevance to public health and control measures.

Etiology

The etiological agents of trachoma and inclusion conjunctivitis, formerly referred to as the "TRIC" agents and originally believed to be viruses, now are classified as chlamydiae. Some human chlamydial diseases, such as trachoma, have been known since antiquity, but the recognized clinical spectrum still is expanding. The current human diseases attributed to chlamydiae are summarized in Table 9-5.

Trachoma and inclusion conjunctivitis are caused by *Chlamydia trachomatis*. This species also includes the causative agent of lymphogranuloma venereum (LGV). These organisms are obligatory intracellular bacteria that are placed in an order (Chlamydiales) separated from other microorganisms because of a unique developmental cycle. The other organisms in the same genus are *Chlamydia psittaci*, the causative agent of psittacosis and a variety of mammalian and avian infections; *Chlamydia pneumoniae*, a human respiratory pathogen; and *Chlamydia pecorum*, a pathogen of sheep and cattle.

Chlamydia trachomatis may be separated into 18 related serovars. Three (designated L1, L2, and L3) compose the LGV strains, which may be differentiated from the others by biological properties. Trachoma in the endemic and blinding form has been associated with types A, Ba, B, and C, whereas types D, E, F, G, H, I, J, and K have been associated with inclusion conjunctivitis and genital tract disease. It is not known whether these differentiations represent sampling limitations or geographical distribution or reflect biological properties of the organism. The trachoma-associated serotypes are rarely, and in some cases have never been, recovered from genital tract infections. The genital strains have been associated with eye disease (inclusion conjunctivitis) and, in some instances, with a disease clinically indistinguishable from trachoma.

Extraocular infections with trachoma organisms do occur, and many children in endemic trachoma areas have infections of the upper pulmonary or gastrointestinal tracts. Relevance of this observation to pathogenesis of trachoma or to *C. trachomatis*–induced extraocular disease is not clear. Persistence of extraocular infection may well have implications for the efficacy of topical chemotherapy.

▸ TRACHOMA

Distribution and Public Health Significance

Trachoma is usually more severe in poorer populations. With increased economic development, it becomes milder and may disappear in time. Blinding trachoma is a major public health problem in

TABLE 9-5. HUMAN DISEASES CAUSED BY *CHLAMYDIA*

Species	Serovar[a]	Disease
Chlamydia psittaci	Many unidentified serovars	Psittacosis
Chlamydia trachomatis	L1, L2, L3	Lymphogranuloma venereum
	A, B, Ba, C	Hyperendemic blinding trachoma
	D, E, F, G, H, I, J, K	Inclusion conjunctivitis (adult and newborn), otitis, nongonococcal urethritis, cervicitis, salpingitis, proctitis, epididymitis, and pneumonia of newborns
Chlamydia pneumoniae	One	Pneumonia, other respiratory disease

[a] Predominant but not exclusive association of serotype with disease.

developing countries in North Africa, sub-Saharan Africa, the Middle East, and the drier regions of the Indian subcontinent and Southeast Asia. Small areas with blinding trachoma are recognized in Australia, the Pacific Islands, and Latin America.

Trachoma was once a major problem in the United States. The last pockets of blinding trachoma were found on the American Indian reservations. Control programs and improved environmental conditions have reduced the consequences, but mild trachoma can still persist. Active trachoma cases may be imported from endemic areas, and although they should be treated, they are not a major public health problem because hygienic conditions in the United States are not conducive to spread.

Clinical Description

In areas where blinding trachoma is endemic, the onset of the disease is usually in young children. Trachoma is a chronic follicular conjunctivitis with varying degrees of papillary hypertrophy and inflammatory infiltration of the conjunctiva and corneal pannus. Bacterial superinfection contributes significantly to the pathogenesis of the disease. As trachoma progresses, scarring of the conjunctiva may develop, with progression from fine linear scars to broader confluent scars. As a result of scarring, the major potentially blinding sequelae slowly develop. These lesions, called trichiasis and entropion (distortion of the lids in the inward direction so that the eyelashes abrade the cornea), cause the corneal damage that ultimately results in visual loss. The end result of blindness usually develops many years after active inflammatory disease has waned. Active disease peaks in the early childhood years, whereas the blinding lesions resulting from contraction of scars and tear deficiencies may occur 25 or more years later.

Classification

Trachoma cases usually are classified in stages according to the McCallan classification, which scores conjunctival findings of follicles and scars. This classification has not been useful in evaluating the impact of trachoma on a community, since it does not identify the potentially disabling lesions. A modification that classifies intensity of active inflammatory diseases and potentially disabling, irreversible lesions recently has come into use.

Transmission

Trachoma usually is transmitted from child to child and occurs in families. Concomitant bacterial infections increase the severity of the disease and the quantity of ocular discharges. These discharges are spread by contact and also by moisture-seeking flies, which act as mechanical vectors of chlamydiae in traveling from eye to eye.

Treatment and Control

Trachoma responds more to improved hygiene, sanitary conditions, and economic development than to specific measures. In hyperendemic areas, virtually all children are infected in the first months of life, and active disease progresses for several years. It is almost impossible to institute mass systemic treatment with any antichlamydial drug under such conditions. Thus, the thrust of trachoma control has been not to eradicate the disease but to prevent blinding complications. Periodic intermittent topical treatment with tetracyclines has been recommended by the World Health Organization (WHO) as the method of choice. This probably works in reducing the load of *Chlamydia* as well as minimizing the secondary bacterial infections, thus decreasing the severity of the disease and minimizing the development of blinding sequelae.

The topical treatment regimen will undoubtedly be replaced by oral administration of azithromycin. A single oral dose of this drug has been shown to be at least as effective as the long-term courses of topical antibiotics.

▶ INCLUSION CONJUNCTIVITIS

Distribution and Public Health Significance

Inclusion conjunctivitis occurs in two distinct age groups and generally is considered to be a sporadic disease occurring in industrialized societies. The disease, which is not considered a cause of blindness, affects neonates and sexually active adults. The incidence of inclusion conjunctivitis is a reflection of the larger genital tract reservoir of the agent. Incidence of the adult form is not known, but it is considered one of the most common forms of follicular conjunctivitis. Cohort studies indicate that 30 to 50 percent of infants exposed to the organism during the birth process will develop chlamydial conjunctivitis. Prevalence rates in maternal cervix cover a wide range, with rates from 2 to 30 percent being reported.

Clinical Description

The adult form (AIC) is an acute follicular conjunctivitis that is usually self-limited. Keratitis is common, and occasionally the disease is chronic. In infants, inclusion conjunctivitis of the newborn (ICN) is usually a mucopurulent conjunctivitis that occurs 1 to 2 weeks after birth. The disease generally is considered to be self-limiting, although conjunctival scarring may develop, and chronic forms, with visual debility resulting later in life, have been identified.

Transmission

AIC results from inoculation of the conjunctiva with infective genital tract discharges. Before the introduction of chlorination this was one of the forms of swimming pool conjunctivitis. ICN results from infection of the neonate during passage through an infected birth canal. The chlamydiae are spread through the population by sexual activity. Genital tract infections are very common, eye disease is relatively uncommon, and eye-to-eye transmission is rare.

Treatment and Control

Inclusion conjunctivitis in the infant is not prevented by Crede prophylaxis (silver nitrate drops), used for the prevention of gonococcal ophthalmia neonatorum. Programs involving screening of pregnant women and treatment of those infected have been shown to prevent transmission of chlamydia to the infant.

Inclusion conjunctivitis in adults always calls for systemic treatment because the individuals almost always have genital tract infection. Three-week courses with tetracycline, erythromycin, or sulfonamides at full doses are recommended. Neonatal inclusion conjunctivitis may be treated topically, although high failure rates are observed. It is not known whether this failure is due to inadequate administration of the drug or reflects inadequate treatment. With the recent recognition that *C. trachomatis* is a cause of pneumonia in infants, it seems prudent to recommend systemic treatment with erythromycin (50 mg/kg in divided doses given four times daily for 2 weeks).

Chlamydial Pneumonia

Julius Schachter

Chlamydia trachomatis is a common sexually transmitted pathogen. It is the major identifiable cause of nongonococcal urethritis in men and is commonly found in the cervices of sexually active women. The infant born through an infected birth canal is at risk of acquiring the infection. A neonatal conjunctivitis (inclusion conjunctivitis of the newborn) has been recognized since early in this century. Only since 1975 has it been known that the same agent is capable of producing systemic disease in such exposed infants.

A characteristic pneumonia syndrome in infants has been shown to be caused by these organisms. The disease is characterized by a chronic afebrile course, a staccato cough (without the inspiratory whoop of pertussis) and tachypnea, marked elevation of immunoglobulins, and a relative eosinophilia. Chlamydial pneumonia is found often in infants infected with other potential pulmonary tract pathogens.

History or presence of inclusion conjunctivitis of the newborn (ICN) is common. Minor upper respiratory signs often precede the development of pneumonia. Some of the children have otitis. These infants do not appear to be severely ill, although x-rays may show the appearance of extensive interstitial pneumonia. Biopsies have demonstrated both interstitial pneumonitis and a rather severe necrotizing bronchiolitis. The disease usually develops in the second month of life, although incubation periods ranging from 3 weeks to 4 months have been observed. In the absence of treatment, the course tends to be prolonged, but ultimately the infants recover. Systemic treatment with sulfonamides or erythromycin does not provide dramatic response but does result in more rapid recovery. Most infected infants have decreased respiratory function and many become asthmatic.

This disease appears to be relatively common. Preliminary surveys indicate it may represent 30 to 50 percent of pneumonias seen in infants less than 6 months of age.

Approximately 10 to 20 percent of the exposed infants do develop pneumonia. Chlamydial pneumonia can be prevented by treatment of the infected pregnant woman. Screening programs, which involved testing women for cervical infection and treating those found to be infected, have been shown to prevent perinatal infection.

Streptococcal Disease

Leon Gordis

Streptococcal infections are among the most frequent bacterial infections in human populations. Their importance lies in both the immediate morbidity associated with these infections and in the nonsuppurative sequelae they produce—acute rheumatic fever and glomerulonephritis. Over the past decades, as both morbidity from streptococcal infections and incidence of rheumatic fever diminished, streptococcal infections were increasingly considered a problem of the past in developed countries. However, in recent years, this complacency has been shattered in the United States by the re-emergence of severe and occasionally fatal streptococcal infections and the occurrence of outbreaks of rheumatic fever.[1]

▸ BIOLOGY OF THE STREPTOCOCCUS

A basic understanding of the biology of the streptococcus is essential for understanding the epidemiology of these infections and of their nonsuppurative sequelae and for developing a rational program of treatment and prevention. Streptococci are classified as hemolytic or nonhemolytic. When grown on blood agar plates, β-hemolytic strains are surrounded by a clear zone of hemolysis, whereas α-hemolytic strains are surrounded by green zones of hemolysis. The β-hemolytic strains can be subdivided into groups designated A, B, C, and so on, on the basis of serologically specific carbohydrates in their cell wall. Over 90 percent of human streptococcal infections are caused by group A strains. Current evidence indicates that rheumatic fever can follow only group A streptococcal infections.

As seen in Figure 9-8,[2] the cell wall of the streptococcus is a three-layered structure: the outer layer contains the protein antigens; the middle layer, the group-specific carbohydrates; and the inner layer, the peptidoglycan (mucopeptide). The cell wall encloses a central core of cytoplasm surrounded by a distinct cytoplasmic membrane.

The protein layer of the cell wall contains M, T, and R proteins. The M protein is most important for several reasons. It is antigenic and immunologically distinct and stimulates production of type-specific antibodies in the infected person. The M protein appears to be localized in hairlike fimbriae that may facilitate the adherence of

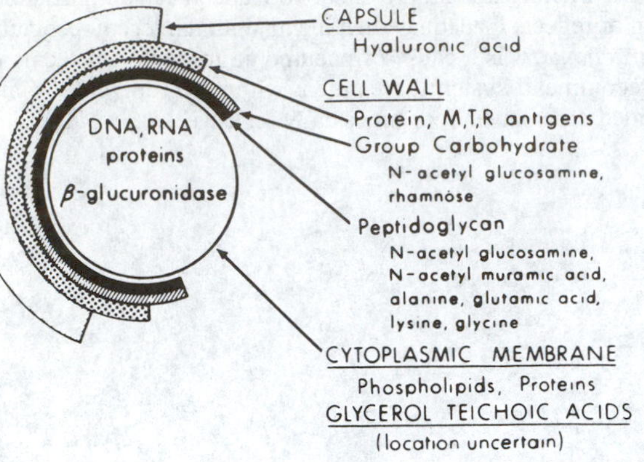

Figure 9-8. Schematic representation of cellular components of β-hemolytic streptococci. (From Krause RM: Symposium on relationship of structure of microorganisms to their immunologic properties. IV. Antigenic and biochemical composition of hemolytic streptococcal cell wall. Bacteriol Rev 27:369, 1963.)

the streptococcus to epithelial linings. On the basis of their M proteins, the group A strains can be subdivided into serologic types, and these types are designated types 1, 2, 3, and so on. Well over 80 types have now been identified. The antibodies produced in response to the M antigen of each type are type-specific bactericidal antibodies that confer long-lasting immunity, possibly for life, to the particular serologic type causing the infection. Since the antibodies are type-specific, they do not protect against infection with other types. Consequently, successive streptococcal infections in the same person are usually caused by different serologic types, although under certain circumstances, there may be cross-protection. Finally, certain M types of streptococcus have been found to be associated with rheumatic fever or nephritis. However, recent studies indicate that virulence may be more associated with certain strains than with serologic types and advances in molecular biology permit the genetic characterization of such strains.[3]

The group A streptococci secrete a number of important extracellular products, including streptolysin O, streptolysin S, erythrogenic toxin, NADase, several DNAses, hyaluronidase, streptokinase, and proteinase. Several of these are antigenic and can, therefore, be used in antibody tests for streptococcal infections. For example, streptolysin O is the basis for the anti-streptolysin O (ASO) test, which is the best standardized antibody test for streptococcal infections thus far available. The anti-DNAse B test is another useful serologic test for detecting streptococcal infections. Erythrogenic toxin is the cause of the rash of scarlet fever and stimulates a specific antitoxin. There is no evidence to suggest that any of the specific extracellular products produced by the streptococcus is the etiologic factor in rheumatic fever. However, new importance has been attached to streptococcal toxins, which are involved in the invasive streptococcal infections seen increasingly in recent years.

The human oropharynx appears to be the main natural reservoir for hemolytic streptococci. Streptococci have also been transmitted from nasal, anal, and vaginal streptococcal carriers. The incubation period is approximately 24 to 48 hours. After infection, antibodies to the antigenic extracellular products of the streptococcus develop relatively rapidly and reach a maximum level at about 3 to 4 weeks, following which they gradually decline. The type-specific antibodies to M proteins take longer to rise and persist for protracted periods of time.

In many of the early reports of streptococcal transmission through food outbreaks, milk and milk products were responsible. Foods contaminated during preparation, such as egg salad, also have been implicated. Droplet transmission does not appear to play a major role in person-to-person transmission. Infection is caused primarily by intimate or direct contact.

▶ STREPTOCOCCAL PHARYNGITIS

Streptococcal pharyngitis has been called "an occupational disease of schoolchildren." In addition, as the number of day care centers has increased in recent years, the group A streptococcus has been shown to be an important pathogen in this setting as well.[4]

The sudden onset of fever, pain, swelling, or beefy redness of the pharynx, with exudate and tender cervical nodes, represents a characteristic syndrome of the streptococcal sore throat. A scarlatinal rash is diagnostic when it occurs, but it is much less frequent today than it was in the past. The classic findings of streptococcal disease are more likely to be present during epidemics, and the diagnosis of streptococcal pharyngitis during endemic periods is extremely difficult on a clinical basis. The diagnosis is even more difficult when tonsils are absent and when the patient is seen only once during the course of the illness. Several studies have shown that physicians can correctly diagnose streptococcal infections clinically in 55 to 75 percent of cases.

A major problem is in distinguishing mild streptococcal illnesses from viral infections of the upper respiratory tract. Conjunctivitis, coryza, hoarseness, and tracheitis are more likely to be caused by viral infections. Pharyngeal redness alone is not enough to distinguish a streptococcal infection. Even an exudate may not be a sufficiently reliable sign, since exudative pharyngitis also has been described in adenoviral and Coxsackie viral infections. Appropriate laboratory tests must, therefore, be carried out for diagnosing streptococcal infections.

Throat cultures are an important technique for diagnosing streptococcal infection. Although such cultures are often available in public health laboratories, they can be readily done also in the physician's office using inexpensive prepared media and a low cost incubator. Sheep blood agar is superior for recognizing β-hemolytic streptococci and is available in disposable plastic plates from many commercial laboratories. When necessary, swabs well moistened with pharyngeal secretions may be kept for several hours at room temperature before inoculation. The plates can be read after overnight incubation at 37°C. β-Hemolytic streptococci hemolyze the blood cells in the medium completely and are, therefore, completely surrounded by a clear halo in contrast to the greenish area visible around α-streptococci.

Grouping is generally not necessary, since most streptococcal infections are caused by group A organisms, but when grouping is indicated, several approaches are possible. Antisera are available commercially for grouping streptococci by the Lancefield precipitin method. Fluorescent antibody techniques also are available. A simple practical method for identifying group A involves applying a 0.02-unit bacitracin disk to a culture of streptococci growing on blood agar. The bacitracin will inhibit group A but not nongroup A strains. The fluorescent antibody technique and the bacitracin disk method are 90 percent accurate when compared with the Lancefield method.

In recent years several rapid group A streptococcal antigen detection tests have become commercially available. Such tests are generally highly specific but have limited sensitivity, especially when the amount of streptococcal antigen present is small.[5] Consequently, a common approach is to accept a positive result of such a test as evidence of group A streptococcal infection, but to follow a negative antigen detection test with a throat culture for group A streptococci. Technology in this area is progressing rapidly, so that these tests may be of considerable value in the diagnosis and prevention of streptococcal infections and their sequelae. Physicians should be encouraged to take and read the throat cultures of their own patient. Not only is this approach economical, but a number of studies have shown that physicians can read such cultures with considerable accuracy after minimal training. This approach also eliminates the delay inherent in sending cultures to a laboratory and waiting for the report. When this is not feasible, however, state and other laboratories should be used appropriately.

In recent years, as the nonsuppurative sequelae of group A streptococcal infections have generally declined, the value of throat cultures has been called into question. However, a negative throat culture has a high negative predictive value and thus can contribute to avoiding needless use of antibiotic treatment in children with acute pharyngitis. Furthermore, in view of the reported outbreaks of rheumatic fever in several U.S. cities in recent years, as well as the high risk in many developing countries, throat cultures remain important for the prompt diagnosis of streptococcal infection and the prevention of rheumatic fever.

In addition to attempting to isolate streptococci from throat cultures of individuals suspected of having had streptococcal infections, it is possible to obtain serological confirmation of streptococcal infections even when the organism can no longer be isolated from the throat or the skin. The most frequently employed antibody test is the ASO test, which has been well standardized. The antigen, streptolysin O, is readily available commercially, and the procedure can be performed by most laboratories with reliable results. The highest dilution of the patient's serum that inhibits lysis of red blood cells by 1 unit of streptolysin O is the endpoint. The ASO titer is expressed in units as the reciprocal of the endpoint dilution. The series of dilutions most commonly used results in the following progression of titers: 12, 50, 100, 125, 166, 250, 333, 500, 625, 833, 1250, and 2500.

The ASO titer increases from infancy, and highest levels are found in school-age children. Titers as high as 250 units are common in well children ages 6 to 14 years in the north temperate part of the United States. In this age group, a single titer of 333 units is considered borderline, and a titer of 500 units is considered indicative of a recent streptococcal infection. A single low or borderline titer does not exclude a streptococcal infection. Regardless of the initial level, a rise or fall in titer of two or more increments (tube dilutions) in serial specimens is considered significant. It is best to perform the test on serial specimens simultaneously. In cases where the ASO is negative, additional antistreptococcal antibody determinations may be useful. These include the anti-DNAse B and the antihyaluronidase tests.

▸ STREPTOCOCCAL PYODERMA

Although pharyngitis is one of the most common manifestations of streptococcal infection, streptococcal pyoderma and, specifically, impetigo skin infections have been shown to precede the development of glomerulonephritis. Impetigo is primarily a disease of the summer, a time when respiratory infections are infrequent. It often will follow some type of skin trauma. Streptococci can be transferred to the skin from the respiratory tract but rarely in the reverse direction. Different serologic types can coexist in the skin lesions and in the throat. Streptococcal infections of the skin differ in a number of ways from streptococcal pharyngitis, as shown in Table 9-6.

Since it appears that treatment of pyoderma, even when effective, may not prevent subsequent glomerulonephritis, attempts have been made at prophylaxis of skin infections. However, such attempts have produced only temporary control of streptococcal infections at best, so that mass prophylaxis does not appear feasible.

TABLE 9-6. GENERAL FEATURES OF STREPTOCOCCAL INFECTIONS AT DIFFERENT SITES

Feature	*Streptococcal Pharyngitis and Tonsillitis*	*Streptococcal Impetigo and Pyoderma*
■ ***Clinical***		
Erythema	Usually present and generalized	Often minimal and localized to immediate area around lesion
Vesicular stage	Absent	Type of early lesion but transient
Pustular stage	Patchy exudate—sometimes confluent	Usually discrete, flora often mixed
Crusted stage	Absent	Frequent and characteristic
Local pain	Common—may be intense	Usually absent
Systemic reaction	Fever, headache, and malaise occur commonly	Unusual
Regional adenitis	Common	Less common, but adenopathy frequently seen
Course	Typically acute, except in infants	Often chronic
■ ***Laboratory***		
Leukocytosis	Usually present	Often absent
Bacteriological species	Group A streptococci usually predominate	Often also contain large numbers of staphylococci
Serological types of group A streptococci	Many different types	Few types predominate
Antistreptolysin O response	Common	Uncommon
■ ***Epidemiology***		
Seasonal occurrence	Winter and spring	Late summer and early fall
Common source epidemics	May occur	Not described
Geographical distribution	More common in temperate or cold climates	Common in hot or tropical climates
Age	Young school-age children	Children of preschool age
Sex	Equal	Equal
Transmission	Direct spread from human reservoirs, particularly nasal carriers	Unknown; insects may be mechanical vectors
Carrier state	Common in pharynx of many populations	Unusual in skin, except in certain situations
Preceding trauma	Not present	May predispose to natural or experimental infection
■ ***Complications***		
Acute nephritis	Occurs; preventability unknown	Occurs; preventability unknown
Acute rheumatic fever	Occurs; preventable	Does not occur
■ ***Treatment***		
Local	Not important	Removal of crusts and scrubbing with hexachlorophene soap
Systemic	Single injection of intramuscular benzathine penicillin or oral penicillin for 10 days	May not be necessary; extensive lesions may require intramuscular benzathine penicillin

Adapted from Wannamaker LW: N Engl J Med 282:23–31, 78–85, 1970.

▶ SCARLET FEVER

Scarlet fever results from infection with strains of β-hemolytic streptococci that produce erythrogenic toxin. The illness occurs primarily in children between the ages of 2 and 8 years. It is most frequent during the winter and spring months. The clinical findings generally include those symptoms seen in streptococcal sore throat plus a classic skin rash. The rash usually is erythematous and punctate and blanches on pressure. The rash is often most visible on the neck, chest, and skin folds and does not involve the face. Desquamation of the skin, particularly the tips of the fingers and the toes, is characteristic during convalescence. In the United States, the incidence of scarlet fever seems to have declined in recent years, and in particular the severity of the disease has decreased. As with other forms of streptococcal infection, nonsuppurative sequelae may follow this condition.

▶ INVASIVE STREPTOCOCCAL INFECTIONS

For many years, streptococci generally have not caused very serious infections in developed countries, but in the past decade severe invasive streptococcal infections have been observed in the form of streptococcal septicemia, streptococcal fasciitis, and streptococcal toxic shock–like syndrome. The elderly and those with chronic medical conditions are at greatest risk, and transmission within households and health care institutions is frequent.[6] The increased prevalence of distinctly mucoid strains often considered to be characteristic of virulent infections suggest that specific group A strains rather than M serotypes may be responsible for the increase in severe group A streptococcal infections.[7] The factors that account for the emergence of these virulent infections in recent years are not known.

Necrotizing Fasciitis

Necrotizing fasciitis is a deep infection of the subcutaneous tissue in which both fascia and fat are destroyed. The clinical picture was described as early as 1924 and called "acute hemolytic streptococcal gangrene," but in recent years both the incidence and reporting of this condition have dramatically increased. Necrotizing fasciitis is characterized by rapidly spreading inflammation and tissue necrosis and is associated with case-fatality rates approaching 50 percent. Shock and organ failure are common, and many patients present with the toxic shock–like syndrome described below.[8] The frequent rapid progression of this disease has led to tremendous public concern, which has been reflected in the use by the media of the term "flesh-eating bacteria." Mucoid streptococcal strains are frequently isolated from the patients. Early diagnosis of the condition is essential, and treatment often requires aggressive surgical treatment including débridement or at times amputation, together with antistreptococcal therapy. In early stages, penicillin may be adequate, but when the invasive infection has become established, addition of an agent such as clindamycin, which will prevent further toxin production, may be indicated.

Streptococcal Toxic Shock–like Syndrome

In the late 1980s, severe streptococcal infections producing a toxic shock–like syndrome were reported, characterized by shock and organ failure. About half the patients manifest necrotizing fasciitis. Cone and associates[9] reported two patients with such a syndrome in California, and Stevens and colleagues[10] reported 20 cases of streptococcal infection in the Rocky Mountain region that were characterized by considerable tissue destruction and systemic disease, including renal impairment and a respiratory distress syndrome with a high case fatality rate. The disease seems to be linked to a streptococcal pyrogenic exotoxin and has again focused attention on the extracellular toxic products of the streptococcus that for many years attracted relatively little interest. The appearance of this condition over a relatively short period of time suggests that there has been an increase in the virulence of the streptococcal strains prevalent in many communities. Schwartz et al reported that, from 1972 to 1988, the proportions of M-types 1, 3, and 18 increased significantly.[11] These types were more likely to be invasive, to cause fatal infections, and to occur in clusters of infections than were other serologic types.

▶ TREATMENT

The principal aim of treating streptococcal infections is to eliminate the organism from the nasopharynx. Clinical recovery alone is not sufficient and may occur even when the organism persists in the nasopharynx. The basic principles of antistreptococcal therapy are (*a*) selecting an appropriate antimicrobial agent, (*b*) administering it in sufficient dosage, and (*c*) maintaining therapeutic blood levels for 10 days. Penicillin is the drug of choice, and erythromycin is a satisfactory substitute when penicillin sensitivity precludes its use. Although sulfonamides have been shown to be effective in preventing streptococcal infection, they are not effective in treating streptococcal infection and should not be used for this purpose.

The most effective treatment procedure is a single intramuscular injection of benzathine penicillin, 600,000 to 900,000 units in children and 1.2 million units in adolescents and adults.[12] Such treatment will eliminate the streptococci in 95 percent of patients. Since benzathine penicillin may cause painful local reactions, it is useful to combine it with procaine penicillin. When this is done, it is essential that the total dose the patient receives contain the full recommended amount of benzathine penicillin G.

Oral penicillin, 200,000 to 250,000 units four times daily, also may be used, or twice-daily doses of 400,000 units for a full 10 days. Although the oral preparations of different penicillins appear to be equally effective when given in proper dosages, it is generally recommended that oral penicillin G be taken only under fasting conditions. When patients are allergic to penicillin, erythromycin in a dose of 125 to 250 mg four times daily for 10 days is effective. Tetracyclines should probably be avoided because of reports of increasing numbers of tetracycline-resistant strains of group A streptococci.

Although oral medication has a number of advantages—it can be stopped if the culture is negative or if there is an allergic reaction, it is less likely to produce an allergy, and it is preferred by many patients over an injection—it has a major disadvantage, and that is the potential problem of patient noncompliance. A number of studies have shown that many children prescribed 10 days of penicillin failed to complete the course of therapy. It is, therefore, essential that each patient and family be individually assessed regarding the likelihood that the patient will comply for a full 10 days. If the patient seems unlikely to comply, the intramuscular route should probably be selected.

Streptococcal Carriers

In certain patients, streptococci may persist in the nasopharynx for a long period after an untreated infection and occasionally even after several courses of antibiotics. Such carriers are usually only lightly colonized and not dangerous to others and also are unlikely to develop complications themselves. Such carriers, however, have posed therapeutic dilemmas in view of the failure of different antibiotic regimens to eradicate the organism. Because of the generally declining risk of nonsuppurative sequelae of streptococcal infections in developed countries, it would appear wise not to pursue the treatment of streptococcal carriers vigorously unless they are members of a family with a prior history of rheumatic fever.

Treatment of Family Contacts. A number of studies have shown that there is a relatively high rate of spread of streptococci when there is an active infection in a household. Although some physicians prescribe prophylactic doses of penicillin for several days for children and adults who have been in contact with the infected individual, some of these family contacts often already have positive cultures at the time the diagnosis is made in the index case. Consequently, prophylactic doses of penicillin in such individuals would be potentially dangerous, since they might suppress an overt infection but not eradicate the organism.

Although it might be desirable ideally to culture all members of the family, this often is not possible, particularly when patients lack a continuous relationship with a physician. Antibiotic therapy should be considered for asymptomatic siblings in low-income families since the risk of secondary cases has been shown to be higher in such families.

► OBTAINING MASS THROAT CULTURES FROM SCHOOLCHILDREN

A number of projects have been undertaken in various cities in the United States to obtain cultures of the throats of schoolchildren, identify infected individuals, and exclude them from school until a negative culture is obtained.[13] Although there is some appeal to the idea of identifying such children in school populations and thereby preventing transmission to other children in order to prevent rheumatic fever and nephritis as well as the morbidity associated with streptococcal infections themselves, there does not appear to be sufficient justification for communitywide programs for obtaining throat cultures from schoolchildren in most areas of the United States today. A case might be made, however, for conducting such programs on a limited basis in certain high-risk populations, such as inner-city schools, if they are shown to have had high streptococcal infection rates during the preceding years. In any such program, it is essential that obtaining the cultures go hand in hand with the provision of follow-up services and that an ongoing evaluation of the effectiveness of such a program be an integral component.

► INFECTIONS WITH NONGROUP A ORGANISMS

Although the group A streptococci are by far the most important from the standpoint of human infections, particularly the subsequent development of rheumatic fever and nephritis, in recent years infections with streptococci of other serologic groups have gained increasing prominence. Group B streptococci have been recognized to be important human pathogens.[14] Group B infections in early infancy are particularly serious. Neonatal meningitis as a result of group B infection is a major concern. Neonatal sepsis is another complication of group B infection. Aggressive antibiotic treatment is essential, and intravenous γ-globulin may be a useful adjunct.

Infection in early infancy seems to be associated with maternal colonization, prematurity, low–birth weight, and prolonged rupture of the membranes. In one study, 19 percent of nonpregnant women were found to be vaginal carriers of group B organisms, and the carrier rate in pregnancy in another study was 28 percent. Group B streptococci have been isolated also from the throat, perianal skin, and urethra of the mothers. There is evidence that neonatal group B infections can be prevented in infants receiving an intramuscular injection of 50,000 units of aqueous penicillin immdiately upon delivery.[15] Although it is potentially possible to develop a polyvalent vaccine, this does not appear to be a practical solution in the immediate future. Group C streptococci also have been found to colonize newborns and to produce neonatal meningitis. Glomerulonephritis has been reported following group C streptococcal infection.

► NONSUPPURATIVE SEQUELAE OF GROUP A STREPTOCOCCAL INFECTIONS

Rheumatic Fever

A major sequel of group A streptococcal infections is rheumatic fever. In the past, the attack rate of rheumatic fever following streptococcal infections was about 3 percent in military populations and 0.3 percent in populations of schoolchildren. In the United States today, the attack rate may be much lower, but valid data are not available.

The diagnosis of rheumatic fever is made using the modified Jones criteria, which were first proposed by Dr. T. Duckett Jones in 1941. Although today the criteria play a major role in the clinical diagnosis of rheumatic fever, it is interesting that Jones originally proposed them for three purposes: (*a*) to provide a uniform diagnostic reference for prevention and treatment studies; (*b*) to educate the medical and lay communities about the diagnosis of rheumatic fever; and (*c*) to collect more accurate data on the incidence of rheumatic fever. The criteria were revised in 1992 and for the first time are now specifically designed for use only in the diagnosis of initial attacks[16] (Table 9-7). It is important to emphasize that the diagnosis is suspect in the absence of evidence of a preceding streptococcal infection. The lack of serologic response to streptococcal antigens, combined with the lack of microbiologic evidence of pharyngeal group A streptococci, makes the diagnosis of acute rheumatic fever extremely unlikely. Most cases of rheumatic fever in the United States today are manifested by arthritis. Since carditis is the only manifestation that can lead to permanent sequelae, interest in prevention of rheumatic fever largely focuses on this manifestation. The arthritis seen in rheumatic fever invariably clears without any permanent damage. The carditis, on the other hand, may often lead to the development of rheumatic heart disease, particularly of the mitral valve.

There is no satisfactory animal model for rheumatic fever, and usually the streptococcus can no longer be isolated from the patient by the time acute rheumatic fever develops, since there is a latent period of several weeks between the streptococcal infection and the development of rheumatic fever. The evidence linking the streptococcus to rheumatic fever is of three general types.[17] First, epidemiological data suggest that outbreaks of streptococcal infection often are followed by outbreaks of rheumatic fever. Second, if the sera of children with acute rheumatic fever are examined for at least three streptococcal antibodies, evidence of a recent streptococcal infection can be obtained in 95 percent. Third, chemotherapeutic agents that prevent β-hemolytic streptococcal infections have been observed also to reduce the attack rate of acute rheumatic fever.

The epidemiology of rheumatic fever results from an interaction of the agent, the group A streptococcus, a susceptible host, and the environment. Available data suggest that the environment operates primarily by facilitating transmission of the streptococcus from one person to another primarily through crowding.[18] No genetic characteristics have been consistently found in children who develop rheumatic fever. A familial pattern is observed in rheumatic fever, but

TABLE 9-7. GUIDELINES FOR THE DIAGNOSIS OF INITIAL ATTACK OF RHEUMATIC FEVER (JONES CRITERIA, 1992 UPDATE)[a]

■ ***Major Manifestations***
Carditis
Polyarthritis
Chorea
Erythema marginatum
Subcutaneous nodules

■ ***Minor Manifestations***
Clinical findings
  Arthralgia
  Fever
Laboratory findings
  Elevated acute phase reactants
    Erythrocyte sedimentation rate
    C-reactive protein
  Prolonged PR interval

Supporting Evidence of Antecedent Group A Streptococcal Infection
Positive throat culture or rapid streptococcal antigen test
Elevated or rising streptococcal antibody titer

[a] If supported by evidence of preceding group A streptococcal infection, the presence of two major manifestations or of one major and two minor manifestations indicates a high probability of acute rheumatic fever.

in contrast to glomerulonephritis, multiple cases in the same family are rarely seen simultaneously. Both the familial pattern and the high rates seen in childhood could be due either to increased exposure to streptococcal infections or to an increased susceptibility to their rheumatogenic potential once they have occurred.

It is difficult to obtain reliable data regarding temporal changes that have taken place in the incidence of rheumatic fever. In developed countries, morbidity rates are far more important than mortality rates as indices of rheumatic fever. Because of a variety of problems, including incomplete ascertainment of cases, inclusion of diseases other than rheumatic fever, and the highly selected populations that often are studied, valid incidence rates are difficult to generate. However, a study of rheumatic fever in Nashville, Tennessee, from 1963 to 1965, using intensive case finding yielded an estimated incidence of 12.6 per 100,000 population of all ages. Rates among blacks were almost twice as high as rates among whites. A study in Baltimore from 1960 to 1964 yielded annual attack rates of 13.3 per 100,000 for initial attacks, 2.3 for recurrences, and 15.6 for all attacks for the age group 5 through 19. Rheumatic fever rates were two and one-half times as high in blacks as in whites and appeared highest in low-income areas. These observations appeared to be due primarily to increased crowding in these groups.

Despite all the methodological difficulties, it seems quite clear that both the incidence and the severity of rheumatic fever have significantly declined in the United States. A comparison of data from the National Health Survey from 1935–1936 and the data from Baltimore in 1960–1964 shows a decline in the incidence of both first and recurrent attacks of rheumatic fever, with the greatest drop being seen in recurrent attacks. This may be attributable to a change in the disease itself over time, or more likely to the effectiveness of secondary prevention programs.

Studies of the changing incidence rates of rheumatic fever in Baltimore from 1960–1964 to 1968–1970, showed a dramatic decline in incidence in black children in Baltimore, but during this time the rates in white children remained relatively unchanged. Analysis of these comparative data indicated that the declining incidence in Baltimore resulted entirely from a reduction in preventable cases that were preceded by clinically overt pharyngitis. The findings suggested that comprehensive care programs were the critical factor in reducing the incidence of rheumatic fever in the inner city during this period.[19] From 1968–1970 to 1977–1981, incidence rates in Baltimore declined dramatically in both blacks and whites to a rate of only 0.5 per 100,000 in both races.[20] (Figs. 9-9 and 9-10). These findings appear comparable to the experience in most areas of the United States.

The clinical spectrum of the disease also has changed, so that chorea, for example, is a highly unusual clinical finding today. In addition, the disease appears to be generally milder in the United States. Studies of the prevalence of rheumatic heart disease in schoolchildren have shown significant declines over time. Whereas prevalence rates varied from 4.3 to 5.0 per 1,000 in New York, Boston, and Philadelphia in the 1920s and 1930s, later studies in Chicago, Michigan City, and Los Angeles reported prevalence rates of 0.7 and 0.5 per 1,000.

In the mid-1980s, however, rheumatic fever outbreaks unexpectedly were reported from communities in many parts of the United States, including Utah, Ohio, and Pennsylvania, and from several military installations.[21] The Centers for Disease Control and Prevention reported a doubling of incidence rates in 6 of 24 states with passive surveillance for rheumatic fever. The epidemiological characteristics of these new outbreaks are of particular interest, since the disease was found to occur not in impoverished urban minority populations as in the past but rather in white, middle-class children, with access to medical care. Although the explanation for these outbreaks is not completely clear, a mucoid type 18 streptococcus has been implicated. In any case, the most reasonable explanation is that the observed outbreaks are the result of some biological change in the organism that led to the emergence of rheumatogenic strains of streptococci in these populations. The incidence of rheumatic fever in the intermountain area of the United States has been declining from the peak reached in 1985, but continues at rates comparable to those of the 1960s.[22] It is not clear at this time whether these outbreaks portend a general resurgence of rheumatic fever in the United States or whether these outbreaks are only relatively isolated phenomena in the face of a continuing general decline in rheumatic fever incidence.

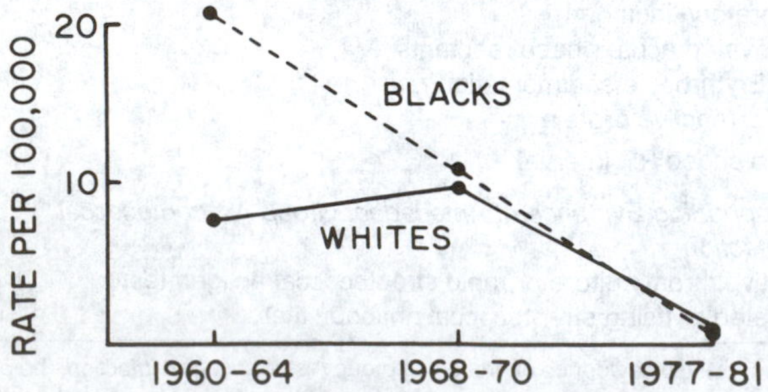

Figure 9-9. Average annual incidence of first attacks of rheumatic fever for ages 5 to 19, by race, in Baltimore from 1960 to 1981.

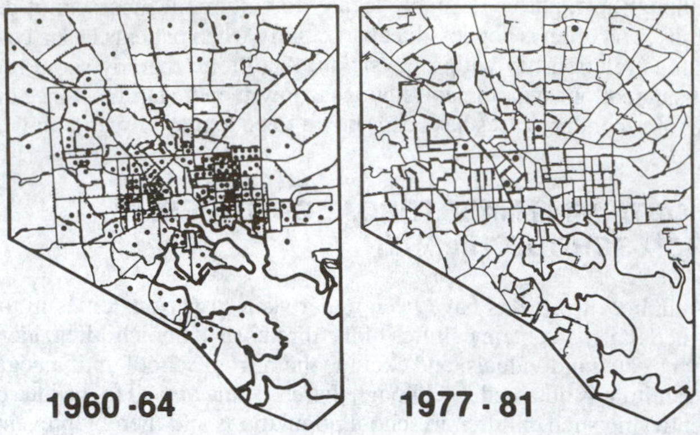

Figure 9-10. Spot maps showing distributions of residence of hospitalized cases of rheumatic fever in Baltimore in 1960 to 1964 and 1977 to 1981.

Mortality rates from rheumatic fever have also declined. Although mortality rates from rheumatic heart disease have not shown as sharp a drop, any decline in these rates resulting from improved treatment of streptococcal infections would be expected to follow the decline in rheumatic fever death rates by several decades, since in the past, most mortality from acute rheumatic fever has occurred in childhood and that from rheumatic heart disease has occurred in adult life. Thus, if the members of a given birth cohort benefit from antistreptococcal treatment, reduction of mortality from rheumatic fever would occur when they are children and from rheumatic heart disease when they reach adult life.

Rheumatic fever is a worldwide disease, which, although more prevalent in temperate climates, is also found in tropical areas. Thus countries with warm climates, such as Egypt and India, have relatively high incidence rates of rheumatic fever, and this fact may well reflect inadequate living conditions of much of the population in developing countries.

The incidence of rheumatic fever is highest in children. There is a seasonal pattern to rheumatic fever occurrence. The peak in the eastern United States is in March and April, and on the west coast of the United States, the peak appears to be in January and February. The seasonal pattern appears to parallel the seasonal pattern of streptococcal pharyngitis and differs from that of poststreptococcal glomerulonephritis (Fig. 9-11).

A latent period occurs between the acute pharyngitis and the clinical appearance of acute rheumatic fever or glomerulonephritis. The latent period for nephritis is shorter than that for rheumatic fever, and although the difference in length of latent period probably is related to the pathogenetic mechanisms involved, the nature of such mechanisms is not yet understood (Fig. 9-12). It is important to em-

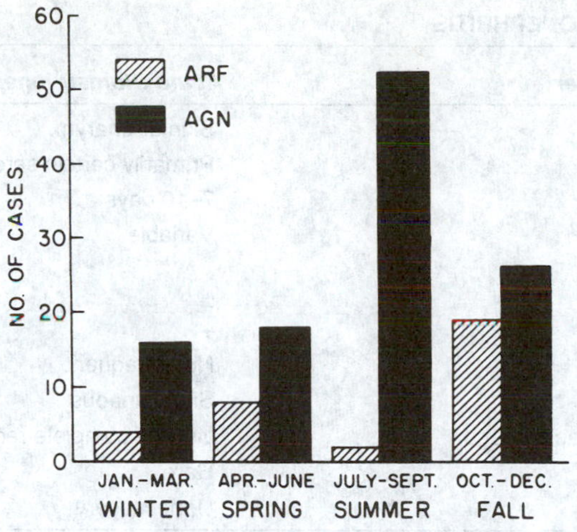

Figure 9-11. Seasonal distribution of acute rheumatic fever (*ARF*) and acute glomerulonephritis (*AGN*) admission at the City of Memphis Hospital from September 1965 to August 1968. (From Bisno AL et al: N Engl J Med 2B3:561–565, 1970.)

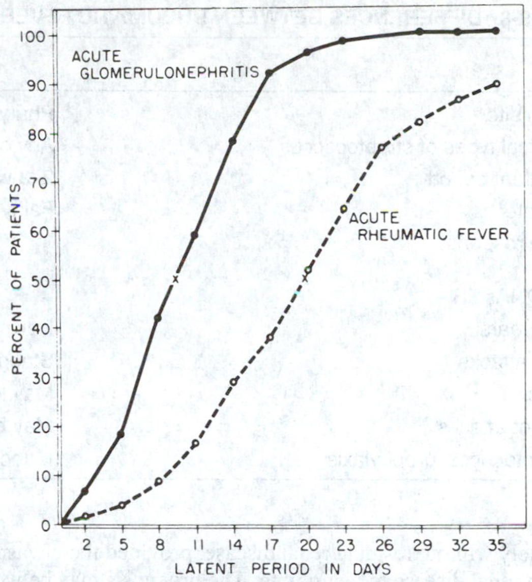

Figure 9-12. Latent period between onset of acute pharyngitis and clinical appearance of acute glomerulonephritis and acute rheumatic fever.

phasize, however, that while streptococcal infections are contagious, there is no communicability of rheumatic fever or nephritis.

Rheumatic Fever Recurrences

One of the most striking characteristics of rheumatic fever is its tendency to recur. Before the introduction of preventive measures, 60 to 75 percent of patients with an initial attack of rheumatic fever had one or more recurrences. In recent years, the recurcence rate appears to have dropped significantly. Virtually every recurrence of rheumatic fever appears to be associated with a preceding streptococcal infection. The risk of a recurrence after streptococcal infection appears related to the magnitude of the immune response. Recurrences are more common when the initial attack occurs early in life, when this attack includes carditis, and when the interval since the last attack is short. Recurrences are more frequent in childhood than in adult life, and the risk of recurrences rises in proportion to the number of previous recurrences and the severity of heart disease.

Because of the concern over recurrent attacks of rheumatic fever and particularly because of the likelihood of a recurrence aggravating the cardiac damage from preceding attacks, continuous antistreptococcal prophylaxis is essential. This can be accomplished by using oral penicillin, the recommended prophylactic dose being 200,000 units (125 mg) twice daily. If oral penicillin G is used, it should be given before meals. Sulfadiazine may be used in doses of 0.5 g daily for patients weighing 27 kg (60 lb) or less and 1.0 g daily for patients weighing over 27 kg. An alternate route is to use a single monthly intramuscular injection of 1.2 million units of benzathine penicillin G. Hypersensitivity reactions to benzathine penicillin G occur at a rate of less than 1 percent in adults and even lower in children.

All children and adolescents who have had a documented attack of rheumatic fever or chorea or who have rheumatic heart disease should be started on prophylactic treatment as soon as the diagnosis is made. Most investigators believe that every rheumatic individual should be started on prophylaxis whether or not carditis is demonstrated. The American Heart Association has suggested that the safest general procedure is to continue prophylaxis indefinitely, particularly if rheumatic heart disease is present. At a very minimum, prophylaxis should be maintained for 5 years after the most recent attack, and individuals with a high risk of exposure to streptococcal infection, such as young men in military service, mothers of young children, school teachers, physicians, nurses, and allied medical personnel, should be protected. In addition, individuals with high recurrence rates of streptococcal infection, including those with rheumatic heart disease, those with a recent previous attack of rheumatic fever, or those with multiple attacks, also should receive prophylaxis. Low socioeconomic groups are at high risk, and special efforts should be made to ensure that regular prophylaxis is maintained in all these groups.

Adolescents are particularly likely to be delinquent in their prophylaxis, so that careful follow-up of compliance is essential in this age group, and intramuscular prophylaxis should be strongly considered. The reader should consult the excellent statements issued by the American Heart Association regarding prevention of rheumatic fever and methods for culturing β-hemolytic streptococci from the throat.

Historically, registries of patients who have had rheumatic fever or currently have rheumatic heart disease and require continuous antistreptococcal prophylaxis were established in many communities in the United States. The main purpose of such registries was to facilitate follow-up of rheumatic fever patients so that regular prophylaxis could be maintained. All too often, however, registries remained lists of names without any follow-up program. Reporting was often inadequate, and invalid cases were often reported. Thus, overascertainment and underascertainment of cases occurred simultaneously. These problems, together with the marked decline in the incidence of rheumatic fever and in the prevalence of rheumatic heart disease in the United States, have led to the discontinuation of many community registries, although the concept of registries may still be of value in developing countries where rheumatic fever remains a major problem.

▸ ACUTE GLOMERULONEPHRITIS

Acute glomerulonephritis may follow a group A β-hemolytic streptococcal infection but may also be associated with bacterial endocarditis, pneumococcal lobar pneumonia, staphylococcal infections, viral infections, systemic diseases, and drug exposures. The poststreptococcal form of the disease follows the infection after a latent period that is shorter than that of rheumatic fever (Fig. 9-12). Nephritis is characterized by hematuria, proteinuria, and red blood cell casts. Edema and hypertension are frequent. Acute heart failure, hypertensive encephalopathy, and convulsions may occur. The disease is of sudden onset, and serological evidence of a recent streptococcal infection can generally be obtained. Although the ASO response is generally weak, responses to DNAse B often can be demonstrated.

Although the data are equivocal, available evidence suggests that the vast majority of patients with acute glomerulonephritis recover

TABLE 9-8. DIFFERENCES BETWEEN RHEUMATIC FEVER AND GLOMERULONEPHRITIS

	Rheumatic Fever	*Acute Glomerulonephritis*
Infection site	Pharynx	Skin or pharynx
Serological types of streptococcus	Any of over 60	Primarily certain serotypes
Usual latent period	2–3 wk	7–10 days
Attack rate	Fairly constant	Variable
Immune response		
ASO	+	±
Anti-DNAse B	+	+
Age <3 years	Rare	Not infrequent
Familial attacks	Staggered	Simultaneous
Prognosis	May leave residual cardiac damage	Usually complete recovery
Recurrent attacks	May be frequent	Rare
Antistreptococcal prophylaxis	Mandatory	Unnecessary

completely without residual renal disease, provided there was no underlying renal disease to begin with. The prognosis may be worse in adults who contract nephritis than in children.

In contrast to rheumatic fever, acute poststreptococcal glomerulonephritis is seen in epidemic form. Large epidemics have been seen in hot areas, such as Israel, Trinidad, and the southern United States, generally following skin infections rather than pharyngitis or tonsilitis. Heat, humidity, arthropod bites, and crowded living conditions are all important risk factors. Streptococcal pyoderma is often seen in low-income families with many children. There appears to be a male preponderance over age 6, and this may be a result of increased trauma to the skin.

In many areas today, most cases of poststreptococcal glomerulonephritis occur after skin infections rather than throat infections. This accounts for the observation that the anti-DNAse B response is present whereas the ASO response is weak. Nephritis follows infections with specific serologic types of streptococci. It is seen after respiratory infections with types 1, 4, 12, 49, and possibly other types. Skin infections with types 2, 49, 52, 55, 57, 59, 60, and 61 are also followed by nephritis. Since there are specific nephritogenic strains, epidemics of nephritis associated with outbreaks of streptococcal infections due to specific strains are observed.

It has been shown that *prophylaxis* of streptococcal infections can prevent acute glomerulonephritis. When military recruits were routinely administered 1.2 million units of benzathine penicillin upon arrival at a naval base, nephritis was virtually eliminated. However, there is insufficient evidence to suggest that prompt *treatment* of streptococcal infections will also prevent nephritis. Further studies are needed to document such a possible effect.

Persons who have had glomerulonephritis do not require continuous antistreptococcal prophylaxis because nephritis is caused by relatively few serologic types. Patients who have been infected by another nephritogenic strain and have developed type-specific immunity are unlikely to be infected by another nephritogenic strain to which they are susceptible and, therefore, are at low risk of developing a second attack of glomerulonephritis. This is in contrast to the situation in rheumatic fever, where there is no clear-cut evidence to indicate that only a few types of streptococci are rheumatogenic. Consequently, any serological type of streptococcus may cause rheumatic fever, and a patient who has had an acute attack of rheumatic fever may be at high risk for a recurrent attack on infection with another strain of streptococcus of any type. Some of the major contrasts between rheumatic fever and glomerulonephritis are seen in Table 9-8.

► DISEASE REPORTING

For many years, there was a policy of requiring reporting of streptococcal infections and of rheumatic fever in many communities in the United States. With the decline in rheumatic fever incidence and that of other serious complications of streptococcal infections, there generally has been a relaxation of reporting policy. It would be difficult to justify routine reporting of streptococcal infections and rheumatic fever today in the United States. In a recent 5-year period in Baltimore, for example, only five new hospitalized cases of rheumatic fever could be documented. Although this probably represents an underestimate of the true number of cases of rheumatic fever, the small number reported and the lack of any concerted program of action in response to reporting would raise serious questions about the justification for such a continued requirement. On the other hand, a stronger case probably can be made for reporting glomerulonephritis. Since much of the glomerulonephritis seen in the United States is associated with the nephritogenic strains of streptococci, a sudden increase in reported cases of glomerulonephritis could alert health departments to outbreaks of nephritogenic streptococcal infection. If such outbreaks were ascertained, vigorous prophylactic and therapeutic measures could be undertaken to prevent glomerulonephritis.

Meningococcal Disease

Bradley A. Perkins • Jay D. Wenger

Vieusseux provided the first definite description of epidemic cerebrospinal meningitis as it occurred in Geneva, Switzerland, in 1805. In 1887, Weichselbaum demonstrated that *Neisseria meningitidis* was the cause of this disease. The high mortality and epidemic potential of meningococcal disease has led to intensive study of means for its control and prevention since the early part of this century.

Bacteriology

Neisseria meningitidis is a nonmotile, nonspore-forming Gram-negative coccus. The organisms usually are arrayed in pairs that are flattened along the axis joining them. Isolation of meningococci from the nasopharynx in Mueller-Hinton agar is facilitated by addition of vancomycin, colistin, and nystatin, to which they are resistant. Addition of blood or other detoxicants in agar also facilitates growth, as does incubation in 5 percent of 10 percent CO_2. All *Neisseria* species are oxidase positive. The meningococcus can be differentiated from other *Neisseria* by its fermentation of glucose and maltose but not of sucrose or lactose, by its lack of pigmentation, and by its failure to grow at room temperature.

Strains of *N. meningitidis* are serologically classified based on immunologic reactivity of their capsular polysaccharides (serogroup), class 2 or 3 outer membrane proteins (serotype), class 1 outer membrane protein (serosubtype), and lipopolysaccharides (immunotype). The standard nomenclature listed serogroup, serotype, serosubtype, and immunotype, each separated by a colon (e.g., B:4:P1.15:L3, 7,9).[1] Serogrouping of strains is accomplished easily by agglutination with specific antisera. Other strains lack capsular polysaccharide and cannot be serogrouped. The vast majority of cases of invasive meningococcal disease are caused by groupable strains, with serogroups A, B, C, Y, and W-135 accounting for almost all invasive disease. Application of multilocus enzyme electrophoresis typing has allowed estimates of genetic relatedness between strains of meningococci. Studies using this method have demonstrated that highly related, or clonal, groups of meningococci are responsible for epidemic meningococcal disease.[2]

Clinical Characteristics

The most common infection caused by *N. meningitidis* is of the oropharynx or nasopharynx and is primarily asymptomatic. Specific immunity may be induced, but carriage is not eradicated by the serologic response.

In an occasional person, meningococci penetrate respiratory epithelium and cause bacteremia. Clinical manifestations then vary according to the intensity of bacteremia, the organs seeded from the blood, and perhaps the strain involved. Overwhelming septicemia can cause death within 2 to 8 hours of the first symptoms and can be associated with vasculitis; irregular petechial, purpuric, or maculopapular skin eruption; cutaneous infarction; and bilateral adrenal hemorrhage (Waterhouse-Friderichsen syndrome).

Although arthritis, pericarditis, and pneumonia occur, meningitis is the most common systemic manifestation of meningococcal disease. The incubation period is often difficult to assess but apparently ranges from 2 to 10 days. Symptoms of meningitis include sudden onset of malaise, followed rapidly by fever, headache, nausea, vomiting, and stiff neck.

The diagnosis of acute fulminant meningococcemia often can be made clinically, although bloodstream infection with other bacteria or rickettsiae can be close mimics. Specific diagnosis can be made by recovery of meningococci from blood, spinal fluid, or other normally sterile sites or by detection of capsular polysaccharide in those sites by latex agglutination. A presumptive diagnosis may be made by demonstration of Gram-negative diplococci in Gram-strained smears of blood buffy coat or normally sterile body fluids. However, these observations do not exclude the role of *Neisseria gonorrhoeae* or other organisms of similar appearance.

Currently, penicillin is the drug of choice for meningococcal disease except for persons who are allergic to it. Up to 20 million units per day (300,000 U/kg/d for children) may be given intravenously in divided doses. Clinical isolates with intermediate resistance to penicillin (minimal inhibitory concentration (MIC), 0.1 to 1.0 μg/mL) have been isolated in Europe, South Africa, and the United States.[3,4] For patients who have inadequate clinical response to penicillin therapy, strains should be tested for susceptibility to penicillin, and therapy should be changed to ceftriaxone (or cefotaxime).

Carriers

Pharyngeal carriage of meningococci is common. The proportion of carriers may vary from 5 to 80 percent, depending on the population, season, age, and living conditions.[5] Carriage tends to be greatest in the winter and spring and under crowded conditions, such as among military recruits.

In many populations, carriage of nongroupable strains is more common than that of groupable strains. Carriage tends to persist for a long time. In one study, the average was 10 months. The carriage rate in a population is of little value in predicting whether an outbreak will occur, probably because of the great variation in virulence of strains, susceptibility of the population, and the difficulty in assessing incidence of infection from a prevalence measurement, such as the carriage rate.

Immunity

Immunity to the meningococcus is mediated primarily by bactericidal antibodies directed against capsular or noncapsular antigens. Goldschneider and colleagues showed that bactericidal antibody probably resulted most commonly from asymptomatic meningococcal infection in the nasopharynx.[6] The presence of serum bactericidal antibodies is common in neonates, reflecting transplacental transfer of maternal antibodies, and decreases rapidly in the first 3 months of life, increasing again toward the end of the first year. The prevalence of bactericidal antibodies thus mirrors the incidence of meningococcal disease, which peaks at 6 to 7 months of age for endemic disease. Following asymptomatic infection or disease, antibodies commonly develop to capsular polysaccharide—although less strikingly to group B than to other serogroup antigens—and to outer membrane protein antigens. The presence of complement is necessary for the full protection of bactericidal antibody.

A number of bacteria share antigens with various strains of meningococci and may be important inducers of protective antibody. Serogroup A meningococcal polysaccharide cross-reacts with certain strains of *Bacillus pumilis* and enterococcus, group B polysaccharide with *Escherichia coli* K1, and group C polysaccharide with other *E. coli* strains. Meningococci can cleave secretory IgA, but whether this function assists pathogenesis is unknown.

Transmission

Meningococci are found only in humans. They are spread from the nasopharynx of one person to that of another, probably by respiratory droplets, although airborne spread may play a role under certain conditions.[7] Transmission is most intense in closed, crowded conditions—in the home, barracks, or jail.[8] In sub-Saharan Africa, where seasonal epidemics are typical, disease occurs primarily in the dry season and decreases abruptly with the first rains.[9] However, transmission of carriage occurs during both the dry and rainy seasons. A study of a Nigerian village has shown high rates of seroconversion to serogroup A during an epidemic period, even among people without clinical disease.[10]

Studies of meningococcal carriage in case contacts have shown that persons who sleep overnight in the house of a person with meningococcal disease are more likely to be colonized than those who visit only during the day or are neighbors.[11] Roommates are no more likely than other family contacts to carry the organism. Typically, the meningococcus is introduced into the household by an adult and spreads first to older children and then to infants.[12] Hospital contacts are colonized infrequently.

Occurrence

Meningococcal disease occurs endemically at a rate of 1 to 3 cases per 100,000 population per year, with a peak in late winter and early spring.[13] Serogroups B and C have been responsible for most endemic disease, although variations in the proportion of disease due to each serogroup are observed. The peak incidence is at 6 to 7 months of age. Group B is relatively more common in cases in young infants. Race and economic level do not appear to be major risk factors for endemic disease. The risk of meningococcal disease is increased 1,000-fold among household contacts of a person with meningococcal disease. In endemic periods, 0.4 percent of such contacts, if not given chemoprophylaxis, develop meningococcal disease in the month after the index case.[14]

Most large epidemics of meningococcal disease are caused by serogroup A, although epidemics of group B or C have been observed in recent years.[9] Epidemics may be communitywide or confined to only parts of the population. In the latter situation, crowded or impoverished groups seem particularly susceptible, for example, military recruits, prisoners, and skid row residents. Until 1945, major meningococcal epidemics occurred about every 10 years in the United States. For unknown reasons, these major epidemics stopped but clusters of serogroup C meningococcal disease have been occurring more frequently in the United States since 1991, and a serogroup B epidemic was recognized in Oregon in 1994.[15–17] Periodic large epidemics continue to occur in sub-Saharan Africa, where incidence rates may increase to more that 1,200 cases per 100,000 population per year. Although introduction of new strains, concurrent viral infections, socioeconomic status, and other factors may be important in epidemic disease, additional study is needed to define the relative importance of these factors.[18–20]

Prevention

Antimicrobial chemoprophylaxis of close contacts of sporadic cases of meningococcal disease is the primary means for prevention of meningococcal disease in the United States.[21] Close contacts include household members, day care center contacts, and anyone directly exposed to the patient's oral secretions (e.g., through kissing, mouth-to-mouth resuscitation, endotracheal intubation, or endotracheal tube management). Rifampin is administered twice daily for 2 days (600 mg bid for adults, 10 mg/kg bid for 2 days for children over 1 month of age, and 5 mg/kg bid for 2 days for neonates). In addition to rifampin, other antimicrobial agents are effective in reducing nasopharyngeal carriage of *N. meningitidis*. Single doses of ciprofloxacin (500 mg orally) or ceftriaxone (an intramuscular dose of 250 mg for adults and 125 mg for children) are reasonable alternatives to the multidose rifampin regimen. Respiratory isolation of patients with meningococcal disease is widely practiced but is of unproven value, and secondary cases in hospital contacts are rare.

Serogroup C vaccine was first tested in military recruits, for whom it was 90 percent effective in preventing disease.[22] A subsequent study in Brazil has showed it to be effective in children as young as 2 years of age. Serogroup A vaccine was first shown to be effective in Egyptian schoolchildren.[23] In widespread immunization of the Brazilian population to control an outbreak, the vaccine appeared to be effective in children as young as 1 year of age. A trial of group A meningococcal vaccine in children 3 months to 5 years of age in Finland also showed efficacy, but the numbers of cases observed were too few to permit a judgment as to whether the vaccine was effective for children less than 1 year of age to whom a booster had been given to improve immunogenicity.[24] A subsequent study in Burkina Faso demonstrated substantial protective efficacy for as long as 3 years after a single dose of group A meningococcal vaccine given to persons older than 4 years. However, protective efficacy declined rapidly in children vaccinated at less than 4 years of age. Efficacy in this group was estimated to be 8 percent 3 years after vaccination.[25]

In the United States, a licensed vaccine for groups A, C, Y, and W-135 is available. Use is recommended for control of localized outbreaks known to be due to serogroups included in the vaccine. Specific recommendation has recently been made for evaluation and management for suspected serogroup C meningococcal outbreaks in the United States.[26] These recommendations suggest that when three or more confirmed cases of serogroup C meningococcal disease occur in a defined community or organization over 3 months or less and result in an attack rate of greater than 10 cases per 100,000 population (about 20 times greater than the endemic rate of serogroup C disease in the United States), mass vaccination of the affected population should be considered. Group A vaccine is used for control of epidemic meningococcal meningitis in sub-Saharan Africa. Vaccine also has been used with some success in protecting household contacts of group A meningococcal cases in the 5 weeks after onset of the index case.[27]

Since immunogenicity of groups A and C vaccines in very young children is poor and, in children less than 4, of short duration, researchers are attempting to develop new meningococcal vaccines. To enhance the immunogenicity and protective efficacy of A and C polysaccharides in infants and young children, methods similar to those used for *Haemophilus influenzae* type b conjugate vaccines have been applied to produce conjugate A and C meningococcal vaccines.[28–30] Although these vaccines appear promising, efficacy has not been demonstrated in humans.

Because the serogroup B capsular polysaccharide is poorly immunogenic in humans, vaccine development for serogroup B meningococci has focused on use of the outer membrane proteins of specific epidemic strains as potential immunogens. The immunogenicity and protective efficacy of several outer membrane protein vaccines have been evaluated recently. These evaluations have revealed estimated efficacies ranging from 57 to 83 percent in older children and adults.[31–33] However, a subsequent study on one of these vaccines did not document efficacy in children under 4 years of age, the group often at highest risk for disease.[34] None of the currently available serogroup B meningococcal vaccines are licensed for use in the United States.

Tuberculosis

Douglas B. Hornick

Tuberculosis (TB) has been an affliction of humankind since before recorded history. TB inspired writers such as John Bunyan to aptly describe this deadly and mysterious disease in 1660 as "the captain of all these men of death that came against him to take him away, was the consumption for it was that brought him down to the grave."[1] As with the classic works of literature, tuberculosis endures. In spite of the much heralded medicinal cures developed in the 1940s and 1950s, which proved very successful through the mid-1980s, tuberculosis has come surging back from what appeared to some as ripe for final elimination from Western populations. Aspects of the pathogenesis of this disease still remain shrouded with mystery. *Mycobacterium tuberculosis*, the agent of tuberculosis, has become increasingly more resistant to first-line antimycobacterial medications and has been especially virulent among those suffering from acquired immunodeficiency syndrome (AIDS). These are disturbing trends as tuberculosis returns to the forefront among the deadly infections of humankind.

The Microbiology of M. tuberculosis

M. tuberculosis is classified within the *M. tuberculosis* complex: Closely related members of the *M. tuberculosis* complex are *Mycobacterium bovis*, and two very uncommon species *Mycobacterium microti* and *Mycobacterium africanum*.[2] *M. tuberculosis* and *M. bovis* along with *Mycobacterium leprae* cause communicable disease, which sets these species apart from the multiple other species of *Mycobacteria*, which are referred to as nontuberculous mycobacteria (NTM).

M. tuberculosis organisms exhibit a bacillary morphology and produce an impervious waxy cell wall. The cell wall excludes most antimicrobial agents and is resistant to alkali and acid. The latter property is taken advantage of by the acid-fast stains (e.g., Ziehl-Neelsen, Kinyoun, fluorochrome). *M. tuberculosis* organisms can be killed relatively easily by ultraviolet (UV) light at 254-nm wavelength, sunlight, heat, and specific disinfectants such as tricresol and phenol.

Mycobacteria divide every 18 to 24 hours compared to every 2 to 3 hours for most other bacterial pathogens. Mycobacteria have traditionally been cultured on egg-potato–based solid media, Lowenstein-Jensen (L-J) slants, or Middlebrook 7H10 or 7H11 agar-based solid media. Following a 3- to 4-week incubation, an array of biochemical tests and additional growth on artificial media have been necessary traditionally to distinguish *M. tuberculosis* from the other multiple species of mycobacteria.[2] Final identification by these methods can take 6 to 8 weeks.

Antimycobacterial Resistance. Resistant mutations occur spontaneously to the first-line medications such as isoniazid (INH) and rifampin. Genetic data have shown that deletion of the gene encoding for catalase and peroxidase results in INH resistance.[3] Mutations within the region encoding β subunit of RNA polymerase cause rifampin resistance.[4] The probability of spontaneous resistance is estimated at 10^{-6} for isoniazid and 10^{-8} for rifampin, and the probabilities for resistance to the other first-line medications fall within the same range.[5] The occurrence of these mutations is an unlinked phenomenon, so the probability that a single organism will be resistant to both INH and rifampin is the product of the probability of each mutation or 10^{-14}. The estimated burden of organisms in a patient varies as follows: 10^3 bacteria for a latent infection, 10^4 to 10^5 bacteria per gram of tissue for noncavitary pulmonary disease, and 10^9 to 10^{11} organisms per gram of tissue for cavitary pulmonary disease. The use of INH alone in a patient with latent TB infection is not believed to risk selection of resistant strains. The use of INH alone in a patient with cavitary pulmonary disease, however, allows spontaneously resistant strains to grow selectively. Resistance to multiple medications can develop with time if other antimycobacterial medications are added sequentially. Resistance that develops in this fashion is defined as *acquired* (or *secondary*) *drug resistance*.

Drug resistance that is discovered in an isolate from a patient who has not previously received antituberculous medications is called *primary drug resistance*. Primary resistance is usually found in patients who have been infected by transmission from another individual with drug-resistant TB. *M. tuberculosis* isolates that exhibit simultaneous resistance to at least INH and rifampin are referred to as *multidrug-resistant tuberculosis* (MDRTB).[6,7] The rationale for specific definition of this term is that treatment is dramatically compromised when the two most potent first-line medications, INH and rifampin, are ineffective.

Pathogenesis and Transmission of M. tuberculosis

M. tuberculosis infects the human host following inhalation of small infectious particles called *droplet nuclei*.[8,9] Infectious droplet nuclei measure approximately 1 to 5 μm in diameter, deposit in the terminal bronchioles and alveoli of the host, and theoretically may contain as few as one viable organism. The bacteria may multiply briefly at the site of deposition but eventually are ingested by pulmonary macrophages. *M. tuberculosis* interact with macrophages mainly via complement receptors, but with mannose receptors as well in a cooperative manner. Following phagocytosis, *M. tuberculosis* inhibit phagolysosomal fusion, allowing the organism to survive and multiply intracellularly within lysosomes.[10]

The infected macrophages then initiate the cellular immune response that in most individuals eventually contains the infection. During this initial phase of infection and multiplication, the inflammatory response can be of sufficient intensity to cause a localized pneumonitis. In general the host is asymptomatic or minimally symptomatic. This form of the disease is called *primary tuberculosis*. During this phase, also, the organisms are carried into the regional lymphatics, then into the hilar and mediastinal lymph nodes.[11] Lymphohematogenous dissemination occurs with deposition of the bacteria at multiple extrapulmonary sites, where further multiplication may continue. After the primary infection and during dissemination, cellular immunity then matures and further multiplication and dissemination of the organism is halted in the majority of healthy individuals.[12] Thus, the infection remains subclinical.

The cellular immune response takes approximately 4 to 8 weeks to mature in the naive host, and it is manifested in the human host by the Mantoux skin test response. The response results from an intradermal injection of *tuberculin* or purified protein derivative (PPD) of *M. tuberculosis* culture extract. Also, the cellular immune response to *M. tuberculosis* produces the caseous necrosis and granulomatous inflammation that one sees under the microscope when examining tissues that have been infected.

The specific attenuation of the cellular immune response, which allows continuous intracellular survival of the organism, is still not well understood.[12] The *M. tuberculosis* organisms can remain latent within the reticuloendothelial system both within pulmonary and extrapulmonary sites. Approximately 10 percent of individuals with a latent infection later progress to active disease. About half of this group do so in the first 2 years after the initial infection and the remaining half develop active disease at less predictable times during the remaining years of life.

Factors listed in Table 9-9 affect the cellular immune response or reflect an increased burden of latent infection, resulting in more risk for progressing to active disease.[13] The rate of progression among human immunodeficiency virus (HIV) patients is 8 to 10 percent annually, much higher compared with all others hosts.[14,15] HIV coinfection increases the risk of progression by greater than 100-fold.[16] The other factors listed increase risk for progression to active disease between 3- and 7-fold.[17,18]

Transmission of Tuberculosis. Transmission of tuberculosis to other human hosts is strictly via droplet nuclei. *M. tuberculosis* within secretions or droplet nuclei that have deposited on a surface lose the potential for infection. Patients with pulmonary or laryngeal TB

TABLE 9-9. RISK FACTORS FOR DEVELOPING ACTIVE TB SUBSEQUENT TO INFECTION

HIV or AIDS

One or more of the following medical conditions:

- Intravenous drug users that are HIV negative
- Diabetes mellitus
- Silicosis
- Renal failure
- Immunosuppressive therapy (e.g., steroids, chemotherapy)
- Hematologic malignancy (e.g., leukemia, Hodgkin's disease)
- Head and neck malignancy
- Chronic malabsorption syndrome or body weight 10% below ideal
- Intestinal bypass or gastrectomy

TB infection documented in the previous 2 years

History of active TB in the past, but treatment incomplete or inadequate produce infectious droplet nuclei.[19,20] Those with extrapulmonary tuberculosis do not, unless the site of TB infection is manipulated in such a way that an aerosol is generated. Transmission of infection to another human host is generally a function of the concentration of infectious droplet nuclei, duration of contact with the infectious case, and the susceptibility of the host exposed. The data from the Centers for Disease Control and Prevention (CDC) show that approximately 21 to 23 percent of individuals in close contact to patients with infectious tuberculosis become infected.

Classic experiments examining droplet nuclei concentration and infection were done in the late 1950s and early 1960s by Riley and investigators in the Baltimore City veterans hospital.[9] In theses studies, air from a room containing patients with active pulmonary tuberculosis was diverted to either a UV light chamber then a control group of guinea pigs, or directly past a test group of guinea pigs. By monitoring the rate of guinea pig infections and the volume of air circulated over the study period, the average concentration of infectious units was calculated at approximately 1 per 15,000 to 20,000 cubic feet of air. If an adult person ventilates approximately 18 cubic feet of air per hour, the probability of infection for an hour of exposure would be approximately 1 in 800 to 1,000, which is comparable to risk data from other studies examining nosocomial tuberculosis transmission.

The guinea pig investigations also demonstrated significant variation in the concentration of infectious units or droplet nuclei.[21] The variation depended upon clinical characteristics of TB in the source patient and whether or not the patient was on antituberculosis therapy. Transmission dropped rapidly after the source patient was started on antimycobacterial treatment.

Most patients with active pulmonary disease produce droplet nuclei by coughing, sneezing, or speaking. In two modern studies, one from New York City and the other from San Francisco, the investigators showed that approximately 1 patient in 10 was responsible for transmitting tuberculosis to others.[22,23] Both studies used restriction fragment length polymorphism (RFLP) methodology or DNA fingerprinting to precisely track the *M. tuberculosis* isolates from active cases. While consistent in demonstrating that few active cases are effective at transmitting disease, the factors that made that subgroup more likely to transmit infection were not identified.

Specific characteristics can predict when a patient with TB will be more likely to transmit the disease to others, although the science is not exact. Cavitary disease increases the probability of infection among contacts because of the large number of organisms in the sputum from these patients. A study from Finland even suggested that the probability of active tuberculosis was also higher among contacts of patients who produced sputum smears that contained a high number of organisms.[24] At the other end of the spectrum, patients who produce a low concentration of organisms in sputum, those who are smear-negative, but culture-positive, are the least likely to transmit infection, yet transmission does occur at low levels.[25]

The behavior of the infectious patient also affects the concentration of droplet nuclei released. When a patient with active pulmonary disease cooperates in covering their nose and mouth when coughing or sneezing, or in wearing an ordinary surgical mask, the large droplets with the potential to form infectious droplet nuclei are captured and inactivated.[19] The effect as a physical barrier rather than the filtration properties are what is important with such techniques.

Environmental factors also affect the concentration of droplet nuclei in the air.[19] The volume of air common to the source and the contact is one such factor. The smaller the room, the more concentrated the droplet nuclei. The amount of outside air ventilated into a room is another factor, since fresh air will dilute the number of droplet nuclei. Modern buildings are engineered for air recirculation. The closed heating and air conditioning systems increase the concentration of droplet nuclei since not much outside air is introduced into such a system. Engineering controls that reduce contamination include passage of recirculated air across a UV light source or across high-efficiency particulate air (HEPA) filters.

Duration of exposure and immune status of the close contact of an infectious case also affect the probability of transmission. The longer the duration of exposure, the greater the probability of inhaling a critical number of droplet nuclei and exceeding the threshold for infection. Naive hosts who are immunosuppressed or at the extremes of age (under 5 or over 65) are more likely to become infected when they are in close contact with a patient with a positive sputum smear. In contrast, close contacts who have been infected previously, demonstrable by a positive PPD skin test, are very unlikely to be reinfected as long the immune and health status is intact.[26]

Clinical Aspects of Tuberculosis

Active TB is suspected in specific clinical settings. The confirmation of active TB still relies on the time-consuming process of culture of sputum or infected tissue followed by identification of the organism. The promise of new and faster diagnostic tests, however, is more genuine now than in years past. The additional standard tests such as the sputum smear, the PPD skin test, and chest x-ray, also help identify those patients with active disease.

Characteristics of Patients with Tuberculosis. Primary TB precedes all infections and usually is asymptomatic or is a minimally symptomatic bronchopneumonia. The majority of primary infections (approximately 90 percent) result in healing and granuloma formation. The organism then becomes dormant and the infection remains latent. Individuals with latent infection are completely asymptomatic and are detected only by a positive PPD skin test reaction. These individuals cannot transmit tuberculosis to others and represent the most prevalent form of tuberculosis.

Active tuberculosis in the nonimmunocompromised host is generally infectious because it presents as a pulmonary infection in 85 percent of the cases. Symptoms are insidious in onset and develop over several weeks or months. The typical pulmonary symptoms are a productive cough of small or scant amounts of a nonpurulent sputum, hemoptysis, and vague chest pain. Patients also have systemic symptoms such as chills, night sweats, fever, easy fatigue, loss of appetite, and/or weight loss. A physical examination of patients with active pulmonary tuberculosis usually contributes little to the diagnosis of tuberculosis.

Patients with active tuberculosis and HIV or AIDS co-infection, present differently than the nonimmunosuppressed patient. Atypical chest findings or extrapulmonary disease is far more common in HIV hosts. Extrapulmonary disease can occur in up to 70 percent of patients.[27] The probability of an atypical presentation increases as the CD4+ T-cell count falls. Sputum samples and PPD tests also are less reliable adjuncts to diagnosis. The reaction to the PPD skin test is often blunted and as many as 40 percent of HIV patients with active TB will not react to the PPD.[28] A recent study showed that 100 percent of AIDS patients with CD4+ T-cell counts below 100 and active TB had a negative PPD.[29] Furthermore, histologic samples from patients infected with TB may not demonstrate a mature granuloma. In general, specific diagnosis of tuberculosis in patients with AIDS often requires a high index of suspicion, a comprehensive search for site of infection, and biopsy to demonstrate and identify the organisms in the tissue site.

Culture of Clinical Specimens. Recent developments in culture techniques and DNA technology have cut the time for culture and identification from up to 8 weeks to approximately 3 weeks. For example the BACTEC radiometric culture system uses a selective liquid media, Middlebrook 7H12 containing ^{14}C-labeled palmitic acid and an automated detector system for $^{14}CO_2$, a by-product of growth. After 14 to 20 days, a sufficient growth index is achieved and enough DNA can be harvested from the organisms for hybridization with DNA probes for *M. tuberculosis* complex. Antibiotic susceptibilities for the first-line medications have been adapted to this rapid culture process so that notification of resistant isolates can be available in as little as an additional 5 days.

Sputum Examination. The standard sputum acid-fast smear is less sensitive and not specific compared to culture for detecting *M. tuberculosis*. To detect organisms in a sputum smear, the concentration needs to exceed approximately 10,000 organisms/mL.[30,31] Only 50 to 80 percent of patients with active pulmonary TB will have a positive acid-fast smear. Acid-fast smears also cannot distinguish *M. tuberculosis* from acid-fast staining NTM.

The latest technology for interpreting sputum smears uses nucleic acid amplification techniques based upon polymerase chain reaction (PCR). PCR techniques improve the specificity of the sputum smear and in the future promise to improve the sensitivity as well. Recently, commercial PCR kits have been approved by the Food and Drug Administration (FDA), but with the caution that these kits may not reliably identify *M. tuberculosis* when acid-fast bacilli are not detectable by microscopic examination. The real advantage of these kits lies in the immediate confirmation that the acid-fast organisms seen on smear are *M. tuberculosis*.[32]

Chest Radiography. The chest x-ray in active pulmonary tuberculosis typically demonstrates infiltrates within the apical and/or posterior segments, and often the infiltrates contain variably sized cavities. In immunocompromised and particularly HIV patients, the chest x-ray may be normal or exhibit only hilar or mediastinal adenopathy or infiltrates in any lung zone. Also, cavities within infiltrates are uncommon.

The Mantoux Skin Test. The standard Mantoux skin test is 5 tuberculin units (TU) of PPD injected intradermally. The test identifies persons who have been previously infected with *M. tuberculosis* and have developed the specific cellular immune response. Infected individuals will develop induration at the site of injection at 48 to 72 hours. The diameter of induration is measured to determine whether the test is positive or negative. The modern classification of a positive Mantoux tuberculin skin test depends upon the pretest probability that the person was infected with *M. tuberculosis*.[13,33]

False-positive reactions rarely arise from subclinical infection by other similar organisms such as NTM, which express antigens that cross-react with *M. tuberculosis*. False-positive results have the greatest impact in populations with a low incidence of tuberculosis. For persons living in regions of low tuberculosis incidence, such as those in rural parts of the United States, a higher cut point set at 15 mm of induration minimizes the possibility of a false-positive test misidentifying someone as having tuberculosis.

The cut point is established at 5 mm of induration for those persons with a high probability of being infected and who may exhibit an attenuated cellular immune response. HIV-infected persons, close contacts of an active case of tuberculosis, and individuals with a chest x-ray compatible with old or healed tuberculosis lesions are those in which the smaller reaction is still considered positive.

The standard cut point of 10 mm of induration effectively identifies all other patient populations where the incidence of TB is significant. These groups include foreign-born persons (Africa, southeast Asia, Pacific Islands, and Central and South America), medically underserved and low-income populations, intravenous drug abusers, residents of long-term care facilities, and individuals with medical conditions (other than HIV) known to increase the risk of TB (Table 9-9).

Pitfalls in PPD Skin Test Interpretation. The *booster phenomenon* should be taken into consideration when screening congregate populations, particularly those containing a significant proportion of elderly people. An insignificant skin test reaction may be exhibited by a person who was infected in the distant past, because the cellular immune response to *M. tuberculosis* wanes with time. Within a week, however, a boosted reaction can be seen upon placing a second PPD. The first PPD induces a recall of the immune response so that the second test should be classified as a true-positive result. The boosted response can last up to a year, so that it potentially can be confused with a PPD conversion. Therefore two tests separated by 1 to 2 weeks, or *two-step* testing, is recommended for screening populations that contain a significant number of persons infected in the distant past (e.g., at a long-term care facility).[19]

TB vaccination (bacillus Calmette-Guérin (BCG)) is used in many parts of the world and may confound the interpretation of the PPD skin test reaction when screening foreign-born populations for tuberculosis infections. Prior BCG vaccination can induce a PPD skin test reaction ranging from 0 to 19 mm of induration. A larger reaction cannot be used reliably to differentiate those also infected with *M. tuberculosis*.[34] Recent data indicate that a positive PPD remains the best tool for finding those infected by *M. tuberculosis* among individuals who were previously vaccinated and have immigrated from parts of the world where TB is prevalent. Thus, the CDC recommends that a significant skin test reaction be considered indicative of *M. tuberculosis* infection in an individual from a high TB prevalence area regardless of whether they were previously vaccinated with BCG.[13,35]

Reporting a Verified Case of Tuberculosis. Active tuberculosis cases must be reported to the CDC as part of ongoing public health surveillance. Specific criteria have been established to generate a valid report of a verified case of tuberculosis (RVCT).[36] Case definition for an RVCT relies on laboratory and clinical criteria. The laboratory criteria require identification of *M. tuberculosis* from a clinical specimen or demonstration of acid-fast bacilli on smear when a culture has not or cannot be obtained. In the absence of laboratory data, a valid case must meet the following clinical criteria: (*a*) a positive PPD skin test, (*b*) signs and symptoms compatible with active TB (e.g., clinical evidence of active disease, changing chest x-ray), (*c*) treatment with two or more antituberculous medications, and (*d*) completed diagnostic evaluation.

Treatment of Tuberculosis

Treatment of tuberculosis requires identifying patients with active disease from those with a latent infection. The current approach to treatment of active TB in particular, reflects the evolving epidemiology of tuberculosis. More emphasis is placed on ensuring adherence to treatment to head off the development of secondary resistance. Also, the recommendations for using INH to prevent a latent infection from progressing to active disease, and for using BCG vaccination as primary prevention, have both been updated in the last decade.

Treatment of Active Tuberculosis. The basic principles of therapy are to provide a safe, cost-effective medication regimen in the shortest period of time. Multiple drugs are used in the initiation phase of treatment to rapidly reduce the number of viable organisms. Also, steps are taken to ensure adherence to treatment.

To treat pulmonary and most forms of extrapulmonary tuberculosis in nonimmunosuppressed patients as well as those co-infected with HIV, four of the following five first-line medications are used during the first 2 months: isoniazid, rifampin, pyrazinamide, ethambutol, or streptomycin.[13] Ethambutol or streptomycin need not be given if the probability of resistance is extremely low (less than 4 percent in the regional population) or susceptibility data indicates that the organism is susceptible to all first-line medications. Following the multidrug induction phase, INH and rifampin are given for an additional 4 months. This four-medication regimen has been shown to be highly effective. CDC data for the United States indicate that 95 percent of patients treated by this regimen will receive at least two drugs to which the infecting organism is susceptible. Also, patients who default before completing this regimen are more likely to be cured than those receiving fewer medications at the onset.

The duration of respiratory isolation for a patient who has started on treatment remains a contentious issue. It is known from the guinea pig studies cited earlier that, once treatment is started, the risk of transmission of infection rapidly diminishes, and by approximately 2 weeks of effective treatment, the risk approaches zero.[21] The sputum smear and culture from patients on therapy, however, may remain positive well beyond 2 weeks. For example, in the study by

Cohn et al,[37] which achieved a 98.4 percent cure rate, the median time to culture negativity was 4.6 weeks, and 25 percent of the patients had sputum samples still culture positive at 8 weeks. The persistently positive sputum often raises concern for continued contagion. Conservative recommendations come from the CDC, which state that a patient should remain in respiratory isolation until three successive sputum samples are smear-negative.[13,19]

Most patients with active tuberculosis are not severely ill, and treatment can be initiated safely in the outpatient setting. Temporary hospitalization for isolation of an active pulmonary case may be necessary while treatment is initiated, if household members include highly susceptible contacts such as HIV-positive individuals or children under 5 years of age. Miliary tuberculosis or tuberculous meningitis are examples of serious extrapulmonary TB that require inpatient management. Enforcement of compliance for a patient who has been repeatedly noncompliant with treatment as an outpatient is another reason to use the inpatient setting for treatment.

INH-resistant bacteria can be treated successfully with the four-medication regimen noted above.[37,38] MDRTB strains, however, pose a more complicated treatment problem. The treatment is generally extended much longer than 6 months. At least three medications to which the organism is susceptible need to be provided. Often second-line medications are required, which are less effective generally and carry a higher side effect and intolerance profile.

Compliance Issues for Treating Patients with Active TB. Adherence to therapy is essential for successful outcome and to prevent the development of resistance. Nonadherence to tuberculosis therapy is common with standard self-administered regimens. Approximately 25 percent of patients with active tuberculosis fail to complete the 6-month standard regimen by 12 months. In homeless and substance-abusing patients, the number approaches 90 percent.[39] In addition, the ability of physicians to predict nonadherence is generally poor.[40] A study in a tuberculosis clinic showed that only 68 percent of patients nonadherent to therapy were identified as such.

Physicians can improve upon their ability to anticipate nonadherence through continuing education that teaches them the most reliable predictors. A history of poor adherence to therapy, for example, has been shown to be among the best predictors. Other predictive factors include homelessness, substance abuse, emotional disturbance, and lack of family and social support.[41] Cultural factors also influence adherence to tuberculosis therapy. For example, Hispanic patients with active TB risk rejection by their family.

The modern approach to tuberculosis treatment incorporates interventions aimed at minimizing some of these problems so that patient adherence to therapy is improved. Supervised or directly observed therapy (DOT) is at the core of most of the more successful approaches. The advantages of DOT have been proven in several studies. A prospective study in Tarrant County, Texas, demonstrated that DOT, compared to standard self-administered therapy, decreased relapse rates and decreased incidence of drug-resistant strains of *M. tuberculosis*.[42] In New York City, prior to introducing a DOT program, a dismal 35 percent of the patients returned for follow-up appointments, with an overall 11 percent adherence to therapy. After a DOT program was introduced, 88 percent of patients were adherent to treatment and all sterilized their sputum. Relapses became rare and only in those with primary drug resistance.[43] Data such as these have led the Advisory Council for Elimination of Tuberculosis (ACET) to strongly recommend widespread or universal use of DOT for all patients with active pulmonary tuberculosis.[33]

Treatment of Latent Tuberculosis. The indications for treatment of latent tuberculosis are based on the relative risk for progression to active disease balanced against the risk of INH hepatotoxicity, which increases with patient age, pre-existing liver disease, or the concurrent ingestion of certain medications and/or alcohol.[13] INH daily for 6 to 9 months is 65 to 80 percent effective in preventing a nonimmunosuppressed individual from developing active tuberculosis.[13,44] Preventive INH treatment in an HIV patient with a latent infection also reduces the risk of developing active TB from 4.7 cases per 100 patient-years to 1.6 cases per 100 patient-years.[45]

HIV patients, patients whose HIV status is unknown but suspected, close contacts of a newly diagnosed person with tuberculosis, persons exhibiting recent tuberculosis skin test conversion from negative to positive (less than 2 years), and persons with certain non-HIV medical conditions that are known to increase the risk of active tuberculosis (Table 9-9) are all groups of patients in whom the risk for developing active tuberculosis clearly outweighs the risk of developing hepatitis from INH.

Epidemiologic data also has identified individuals in whom the incidence of tuberculosis infection is relatively high. These persons, however, do not exhibit a significant increased risk for developing active disease from a latent infection. Therefore, the risk of INH hepatitis becomes a consideration. Immigrants to the United States from high TB prevalence countries, medically underserved individuals, residents of long-term care facilities, and staff of schools, correctional, health, and child care facilities are population groups that have a relatively high prevalence of TB infection, but the risk of progression to active disease is low. The risk of hepatitis from INH treatment, although very low, exceeds the benefit of treatment for those in this group who are older than 35 years of age.

Efficacy of the BCG vaccine. An *M. bovis* strain was continuously subcultured by Calmette and Guerin from 1908 to 1922 to produce the live attenuated strain named for them, bacillus Calmette-Guérin (BCG). BCG has been used as the basis for the live attenuated vaccine against tuberculosis since 1922. BCG is still the best available TB vaccine today and is used in many parts of the world.

Assessment of efficacy of the BCG vaccine has been clouded by multiple variables, which include the variability of BCG strains from which vaccines have been prepared, method and route of administration, characteristics of populations studied, and endpoints selected. Two recent meta-analyses of best studies dating back to 1950 indicate that the vaccine's efficacy is more than 80 percent in preventing TB meningitis and miliary TB in children.[46,47] These meta-analyses were unable to unravel the disparate data regarding prevention of pulmonary TB in adults. It is likely that the BCG vaccine does not prevent infection in adults, but possibly decreases the probability of progression to active TB.

The CDC has recommended that BCG be used rarely because of the questions surrounding its efficacy and the issues relative to PPD skin test interpretation and because the overall risk for TB exposure in the United States is low compared with elsewhere in the world. Infants and young children at high risk of repeated TB exposure are the main indication for BCG use in the United States.[35]

Epidemiology of Tuberculosis

Crowded conditions, poverty, and host susceptibility facilitate the spread of this disease within populations. These situations have evolved over the past millennium and over the past decade effecting the trends in TB incidence in the United States, the rest of the world, and specific subpopulations.

Tuberculosis Trends through History. Anthropological data suggest that *M. bovis* may have caused ancient forms of tuberculosis. *M. bovis* was endemic to animals before humans evolved, and probably was transmitted from prey to predator. After humans evolved, *M. bovis* may have been transmitted in an analogous way, from animals killed for food.[48] Active infections, which would be similar to tuberculosis as it is known today, probably remained sporadic and uncommon because *M. bovis* is poorly adapted to transmission between humans. Evidence for tuberculosis in ancient civilizations has come from the remains of ancient Egyptians, early Hindu writings referring to a disease called consumption, and ancient Greek medical literature referring to tuberculosis as phthisis.

More compelling documentation comes from granulomata in a 1,000-year-old pre-Columbian Peruvian mummy. The granulomata contain DNA compatible with *M. tuberculosis* by amplification studies, although the authors could not exclude *M. bovis*.[49] Also, spinal and psoas abscesses, along with a lung granuloma containing acid-fast staining bacilli were found in another Peruvian mummy dated to 700 A.D.[50] *M. bovis* human infections perhaps became more prevalent in Europe and the Middle East as humans began to domesticate animals and drink animal milk. At that point, mutation to the closely related and more human-adapted pathogen, *M. tuberculosis*, may have occurred.[48]

Tuberculosis became widespread after 1600 A.D. with the onset of the Industrial Revolution in Europe.[48,51] Crowded conditions, poor sanitation, and poor nutrition were all features of rapidly expanding cities. Conditions were ideal for transmission of tuberculosis and it became epidemic. At its peak, 100 percent of western European urban dwellers may have been infected and the mortality rate was extremely high.[48] Tuberculosis struck predominantly the young people. Those that survived to reproductive age are believed to have had a selective advantage. After several generations, a degree of natural immunity and a greater prevalence of chronic infection developed. The higher prevalence of chronic infection, however, facilitated transmission of infection. TB naturally followed the Europeans to the Americas, where the immunologically naive Native Americans were extremely susceptible to tuberculosis upon first exposure. The same can be said for the peoples in the interior of Africa, where the disease arrived with western culture around 1910. Similar transmission to naive populations occurred in New Guinea in 1950 and in the deep Amazon region of South America in the 1970s.[52]

During the twentieth century before the development of effective antituberculosis treatment in 1945, TB mortality in the United States and Europe continuously declined, probably in part because of the continued development of natural immunity. In the United States from 1900 to 1945, the number of new cases dropped from 194 to 40 per 100,000.[53] Improved socioeconomic conditions and public health interventions are other factors that likely contributed to the decline in incidence.[51] The public health interventions for finding active cases included the widespread use of fluorography, skin testing, and chest x-ray for patients with a positive PPD. The patients with active disease were removed from society and placed into sanitaria, which helped break the transmission cycle. Sanitaria-focused care was the state-of-the-art for tuberculosis management prior to the development of effective antimycobacterial medications. In the sanitaria, patients received rest and fresh air therapy supplemented by surgical lung collapse and resection. Mortality remained as high as 50 percent.

Widespread use of effective drug treatment finally reduced TB mortality to nearly zero in the United States during the 1950s through the early 1980s. The decline in incidence of TB disease continued over the same period, but the rate of decline did not change or accelerate. The most plausible explanation is that socioeconomic conditions and public health measures have had the predominant effect on TB incidence, while treatment improvements have affected mortality rates. It is disconcerting to realize that in the United States and the rest of the world over the last decade, the incidence of tuberculosis has risen and antituberculosis drugs are becoming less effective.

Modern Tuberculosis Trends within the United States. In 1984, the incidence of new cases of tuberculosis had declined to 9.4 per 100,000 and mortality was low at 0.7 per 100,000. Federal funding for TB control was also declining rapidly, and different public health needs had moved to the forefront, diverting money away from TB programs. City and state governments downgraded their TB control and treatment supervision programs. With this decline in attention, there was a unanticipated upswing in TB incidence from 1985 to 1992. Incidence peaked at 10.5 cases per 100,000 population and there were 51,700 excess new cases of tuberculosis.[28,54] Other factors contributing to the resurgence in tuberculosis, besides the failure of public health surveillance, included the exponential growth in the AIDS epidemic, the development of drug-resistant strains of tuberculosis, the influx of immigrants from countries with high TB prevalence, the increase in homelessness in urban centers, and the increase in substance and drug abuse.

The combination of AIDS and drug-resistant TB made treatment and control of infections more difficult and allowed for more prolonged transmission of infection. The greatest upswing in cases were in geographically restricted, congested urban centers such as New York City, Miami, and San Francisco, where AIDS and drug-resistant tuberculosis were most prevalent.[55] The drug resistance problem in particular was a by-product of the failing public health system (e.g., poor case management, poor patient compliance with treatment) and the importation of drug-resistant *M. tuberculosis* with immigrants.

By 1993, the infusion of money from the U.S. government for TB control programs had increased substantially and was targeted to the urban centers where the most significant outbreaks were occurring. The trend in the incidence of new cases since has been downward. In 1995, the incidence of new cases was down to 8.7 per 100,000.[56] The success of these increased financial resources has been due to improving containment of active cases and improving compliance with prescribed treatment (e.g., widespread DOT), which resulted in interrupting TB transmission.

HIV and Tuberculosis. HIV impairs cell-mediated immunity and the host's ability to resist tuberculous infection. The resurgence of TB in the United States has been closely interwoven with the HIV epidemic.[57,58] Approximately 57 percent of the excess cases of tuberculosis from 1986 through 1991 have been attributable to HIV co-infection.[59] Several other facts provide further evidence for the close link between HIV and tuberculosis. The AIDS epidemic and the resurgence of TB have followed similar time courses. Persons in the 25 to 44 age group have exhibited the highest increase in TB and included the majority of AIDS cases.[60,61] The geographic distribution of the two epidemics has correlated closely.[60] AIDS and tuberculosis cases have clustered in a few urban areas such as New York City, Newark, and Miami. These urban TB clinics have found a high prevalence of HIV among the TB cases, approximately 30 percent, and up to 58 percent. On a state-by-state analysis as well, the percentage increases in tuberculosis cases have correlated closely with increases in AIDS cases.

Many persons within populations with a high incidence of HIV are independently at high risk for exposure to tuberculosis.[16,58] For example, many HIV-positive individuals living in urban areas in the Eastern United States are more likely to be exposed to others with active TB. TB infection among HIV-positive individuals is 50 to 200 times the rate of that seen in the general U.S. population. A positive PPD in these areas is more likely to represent recent infection.[45] The frequency of primary disease among new cases of active tuberculosis is approximately 60 percent in New York City.[22]

AIDS patients with active tuberculosis will acquire a new infection exogenously, which is extremely uncommon in the nonimmunocompromised host. Investigators monitored the RFLP patterns of *M. tuberculosis* isolates from patients with AIDS and active tuberculosis who were responding poorly to antituberculosis treatment.[62] The data indicated that relapses on therapy or after successful completion of therapy in a significant proportion of the group was caused by infection with a new *M. tuberculosis* strain, identifiable by the distinct RFLP pattern. Thus infectious TB patients who also have AIDS not only require isolation for public health reasons, but also to be protected from others with active TB.

Beyond the United States, increasing HIV and TB co-infection is a troublesome trend in developing countries of the world (see Global Tuberculosis below).

Drug-Resistant Tuberculosis—U.S. Data. The number of drug-resistant cases of tuberculosis increased dramatically during the last decade. The theoretical explanations for how drug resistance develops (see earlier text) have been borne out in epidemiologic data. Patients with cavitary pulmonary TB were 4-fold more likely to exhibit resistant isolates compared with those with noncavitary disease. Also, among *M. tuberculosis* isolates from patients who relapsed after previous treatment, resistance was demonstrated 4.7 times more frequently compared with those with no history of prior treatment. The combination of cavitary disease and prior treatment produced a risk of resistance that was additive.[63]

Errors in prescribing treatment are a too frequent reason for development of drug resistance.[64] Inappropriate use of monotherapy for active TB, failure to provide an adequate medication regimen at time of TB diagnosis, failure to ensure adherence to treatment, and failure to recognize and treat medication failure are the typical prescribing errors. Patient errors are also a significant factor and follow a similar theme.[65] Without supervision or sufficient education, patients may take partial doses or only some of the drugs prescribed. Malabsorption of some of the drugs is an issue that is of theoretical concern in HIV patients and could predispose these individuals to a greater risk for acquired resistance.[66]

The greatest concentrations of drug-resistant cases were found in urban populations, particularly New York City. In 1982 the CDC national survey revealed that single drug resistance was at 6.9 percent and two or more drug resistance was at 2.3 percent.[67] By 1991 these numbers had risen to 14.2 percent and 6 percent, respectively. Rifampin resistance appeared at a significant rate for the first time in the 1991 data. More disturbing was the rapidly emergent trend for MDRTB, with resistance to both INH and rifampin present in 3.5 percent of all cases surveyed.[68] The New York City region accounted for 63 percent of these MDRTB cases, while only 1 percent of the other counties surveyed reported MDRTB. The New York City TB Control Bureau reported in 1991 that 26 percent of *M. tuberculosis* isolates exhibited resistance to INH and 19 percent exhibited multidrug resistance.[69] The results of subsequent aggressive efforts to ensure appropriate treatment, compliance, and effective isolation of infectious TB cases, particularly in New York City, indicate that the trend of rising numbers and spread of resistant *M. tuberculosis* strains has moderated.[70]

The dramatic impact of several MDRTB outbreaks that displayed overlapping chains of transmission within eight hospitals and one prison in the upstate New York region during the early 1990s has been chronicled in several CDC publications.[6,7,14,15,71] Approximately 300 individuals, including 17 health care workers developed active MDRTB and most were co-infected by HIV. A high attack rate, short incubation time, and rapid progression to active disease and death were among the most striking characteristics and were a function of the high prevalence of patients with AIDS and tuberculosis. The mortality rate in most of the hospitals approached 100 percent, with a median time from diagnosis to death of 4 weeks.

The upstate New York MDRTB outbreaks also demonstrated clear evidence for nosocomial transmission between patients, prisoners, and health care workers (HCWs) and provided the impetus behind government efforts to tighten isolation procedures for health care facilities (discussed below under Guidelines for Protection of Health Care Workers).

Global Tuberculosis. The figures for tuberculosis incidence and mortality among third world countries are reaching staggering proportions. Approximately one-third of the world's population is infected with tuberculosis and two-thirds of the populations of developing countries are infected with tuberculosis.[72] There will be 90 million new cases of tuberculosis worldwide in the decade that ends with the millennium.[73] The numbers of new cases annually are predicted to continue to increase from 7.5 million in 1990 to 12 million new cases in the year 2005.[74] Ninety-five percent of the cases of tuberculosis occur in developing countries and 80 percent are in African nations. The highest rates of tuberculosis in the world occur in the sub-Sahara region of Africa at about 225 cases per 100,000 population. It is estimated that 75 to 85 percent of sub-Saharan Africans are infected with tuberculosis. Analogous to western Europe during the Industrial Revolution, the youthful population has been hit hardest. Approximately 75 percent of those infected with tuberculosis are under the age of 50.[75] Approximately one-third of those infected worldwide during this decade will die if the rate of treatment success remains at the level seen in 1990. Almost 98 percent of the deaths from tuberculosis occur in developing countries and account for 25 percent of avoidable adult deaths in these countries.[76]

The pandemic of HIV infection and the development of drug-resistant tuberculosis are the two major factors contributing to the increases in tuberculosis in the developing countries of the world.[77] In 1994 the estimated worldwide prevalence of HIV was 13 to 14 million individuals. Ninety percent of the world's AIDS cases occur in developing countries and mostly affect young adults and children. The impact of AIDS and HIV, therefore, is greatest on the same population in whom tuberculosis prevalence is the greatest. The rate of progression to active disease from a latent infection in persons co-infected with HIV worldwide is similar to the rate in the United States, about 8 to 10 percent annually. There were 5.6 million cases of TB/HIV co-infection in 1994. The majority, 3.8 million, were in sub-Saharan Africa, which represented 20 to 40 percent of the TB cases in that region. Southeast Asia contributed the next largest number of TB and HIV co-infections at 1.15 million, of which 9 to 26 percent of the TB cases were co-infected. Brazil, Mexico, and Haiti combined contributed a smaller proportion, 0.45 million cases of TB and HIV co-infection.

A significant prevalence of drug-resistant tuberculosis is the other major factor contributing to the increase in TB worldwide. The extent of the prevalence cannot be accurately assessed because few countries keep track of these data reliably. Southeast Asia is one of the areas where both acquired and primary drug resistance are very high due to failure of the national TB program to achieve high compliance and cure rates.[78] In other parts of the world, drug resistance has resulted from the misguided policy of including isoniazid in over-the-counter cough syrups.

Tuberculosis rates will probably continue to grow rapidly worldwide. HIV is anticipated to play an even larger role in the tuberculosis epidemic.[73] By the year 2000 the proportion of tuberculosis associated with HIV is anticipated to rise to 13.8 percent, up from 4.2 percent in 1990. Likewise, the proportion of tuberculosis deaths attributable to HIV co-infection will rise to 14 percent in the year 2000, up from 4.6 percent in 1990. As the HIV problem expands, drug resistance is likely to continue to be an increasing problem as well. Other factors such as famine, war, and natural disasters will also contribute to the spread of tuberculosis because of the impact of crowding large populations of displaced, malnourished individuals.

The World Health Organization in 1993 declared that tuberculosis was a global health emergency. Strategies for control were developed and were published in 1994.[79] This document established the following targets for tuberculosis control: first, to cure 85 percent of newly detected smear-positive tuberculosis cases, and second, to find at least 70 percent of existing cases by the year 2000. The key elements in this control program emphasized the administration of the standard short-course therapy with a very strong effort toward supervised treatment, adequate drug supplies, and effective program management and evaluation. Despite these well-intentioned targets, the World Health Organization is still strapped by financial constraints that remain a major obstacle to completely instituting this plan.

Tuberculosis in Foreign-Born Immigrants to the United States. Foreign-born immigrants are having an increasing impact on the new cases of tuberculosis in the United States. According to the 1990 census data, the foreign-born population in the United States increased by more than 40 percent during the preceding decade.[80] Also, the proportion of United States TB cases that is comprised of the foreign-born population increased from 22 to 36 percent over the period of 1986 to 1995.[56,80] Mexico, the Philippines, Vietnam, China, and Korea are the top five countries of origin for new immigrants. Tuberculosis rates for these countries average above 125 per 100,000 per year, approximately 10 to 30 times greater than the U.S. rate. Also, conversion from latent to active disease among these immigrants is as high as 100 to 200 times the U.S. rate.[81] Another potential contributor to the tuberculosis rate, which is difficult to measure, are the 15 million nonimmigrant, foreign arrivals per year that are in the United States as tourists, business visitors, and students.[72] These people do not receive any sort of screening for tuberculosis before they arrive.

Most cases of tuberculosis in the foreign-born population have occurred in Latin American (44 percent) and Southeast Asian (35 percent) immigrants. Approximately 35 to 53 percent of these individuals are PPD-positive upon arrival in this country.[82,83] The case rate for active tuberculosis among these persons after they arrive in the United States is about 30.6 per 100,000 or almost four times the U.S. rate. Most of the cases of active tuberculosis (55 percent) are diagnosed during the first 5 years in the United States.[80]

Although direct data on HIV rates are lacking, HIV co-infection does not appear to be contributing to the high rate of tuberculosis in the immigrant population.[84] The two main reasons are that HIV infection rates in the country of origin are lower compared with that of the population in the cites where the immigrants settle, and the U.S. laws bar immigration to anyone who has HIV. Transmission of tuberculosis among the foreign-born population also seems to be lower compared with that of nonimmigrant populations, which contain a larger proportion of HIV co-infection.[23] Active tuberculosis in the foreign-born population most often arises from activation of a prior infection.

Tuberculosis in Correctional Institutions. More people are in jail, and recidivism occurs at a greater rate, than ever before.[85] The number of people incarcerated increased from 1 of every 453 people in 1980 to 1 of 189 in 1994. The rate of recidivism in 1994 was 61 percent. A correctional institution is a congregate setting that is ideal for transmission of tuberculosis between inmates and/or the correctional workers. Also, evidence indicates that prisoners released into the communities extend transmission, particularly to children in the home.[85,86]

Tuberculosis is more prevalent in prison populations compared with its prevalence in the general population. Fourteen to 25 percent of inmates have a positive PPD skin test.[87,88] The probability of tuberculosis infection increases directly with the length of incarceration, which indicates that transmission of tuberculosis must occur in prisons.[86,89] The rate of tuberculosis in prisoners compared with that in the general population varies depending on the prison location. For example, in New York State, the rate of TB in the prisons is 6.3 times the rate for that state's general population, whereas in New Jersey and California the values are even higher at 11- and 10-fold, respectively.[85,90]

Multiple factors contribute to the high rates of tuberculosis in correctional institutions.[85] Many state and federal facilities operate up to 25 percent above design capacity. Overcrowding, coupled with typically poor ventilation in the prison environment, facilitates aerosol transmission of tuberculosis. The high rate of HIV infection is another factor, which is highlighted by a recent study showing that the HIV-seropositive rate in the prison population was approximately 50 times greater than that in a matched population of military recruits.[54] In the absence of HIV infection, history of intravenous drug abuse is associated with a higher risk of tuberculosis. In a survey of 20,000 state and federal prisoners from 45 states, 25 percent of the inmates had a history of IV drug abuse. Also, the prison population represents a lower socioeconomic group, a segment of the population that is more commonly infected with tuberculosis. All of these factors taken together help explain the higher rates of tuberculosis among individuals housed in correctional institutions.

Nosocomial Transmission of Tuberculosis. The major causes of tuberculosis transmission within hospitals are from those cases where it is not suspected, the diagnosis is delayed, or the respiratory isolation procedure breaks down.[91,92]

The following unusual example of extrapulmonary tuberculosis aptly illustrates these aspects of nosocomial transmission.[93] A deep thigh abscess, not suspected to be tuberculous, was surgically débrided in an Arkansas hospital, then irrigated daily for approximately 2 weeks using a Water Pik–type device. Eventually, of the 70 HCWs either directly exposed to or working on the same hallway as this patient 63 percent became infected and 14 percent developed active tuberculosis between 9 to 12 weeks after the exposure. The high rate of transmission resulted from the combined effect of the following factors: (*a*) unsuspected, high concentration of *M. tuberculosis* in the abscess tissues; (*b*) unrecognized generation of aerosol densely contaminated with *M. tuberculosis* because of wound irrigation (perhaps further facilitated by the high intensity of the water stream produced by the irrigating device); and (*c*) unanticipated positive air pressure in the patient's room so that the contaminated air circulated outside the room and up and down the hallways.

Medical students, pathologists, and assistants working in an autopsy room exhibit a higher risk for tuberculosis infection and active disease.[94,95] The autopsy suite stands out as one of the hospital sites where the heaviest exposure to tuberculosis may occur for several reasons. When cutting infected lung or bone with a knife or oscillating saw, an aerosol with a high density of bacteria is likely to be generated. Recent data show that the concentration can be as high as 1 infectious unit per 3.5 cubic feet of air,[96] a far more dense concentration when one considers that on a tuberculosis ward the concentration measures approximately 1 infectious unit per 24,000 cubic feet of air.[9] Also, autopsy workers are more frequently exposed to patients unsuspected of having tuberculosis antemortem, so adequate respiratory protection may not be in place.

The extensive MDRTB outbreaks that occurred in eight hospitals and a New York state prison illustrated several common characteristics of nosocomial transmission.[6,7,14,15,71] Delayed diagnosis, delay in effective treatment, lack of effective isolation procedures, and a high proportion of patients with severe AIDS (CD4+ lymphocytes less than 100/mL) were all common features. Severe AIDS altered the clinical picture of active TB and contributed significantly to the delayed diagnosis. The laboratory confirmation of *M. tuberculosis* was also delayed for several of the following reasons: TB went unsuspected, so confirmation tests were not done; acid-fast bacilli (AFB) present on smears of clinical specimens were assumed to be *M. avium* complex instead of *M. tuberculosis*; and the mean time between specimen collection and identification of *M. tuberculosis* was 6 weeks. The realization that the *M. tuberculosis* strain isolated was resistant was further delayed because the task of susceptibility testing required at least an additional 6 weeks. All of these factors together resulted in extended opportunities for transmission of MDRTB in the hospitals, outpatient clinics, and among the prisoners. Over 150 HCWs were directly exposed and 27 percent became infected. Seventeen of these developed active MDRTB, eight were co-infected with HIV, and four of those persons died from MDRTB. Three others died, one of whom may also have been immunosuppressed as a result of a malignancy.

Guidelines for Protection of Health Care Workers. The resurgence of tuberculosis, and in particular the lessons learned from the MDRTB outbreaks reviewed above, drove the process for reevaluating the 1990 CDC guidelines for tuberculosis containment in the hospital environment.[97,98] These efforts culminated in detailed, broad guidelines published by the CDC and the National Institute for Occupational Safety and Health (NIOSH) at the end of 1994.[99] The guidelines encompass three specific areas: administrative controls, environmental controls, and respiratory protection. The recommendations also recognize the geographic variation in TB prevalence and that the majority of hospitals in the United States are not faced with an overwhelming number of new cases. Therefore, a risk assessment for tuberculosis transmission is recommended for each institution. The level of risk classifications are associated with a hierarchy of recommendations for control steps.

The administrative and environmental controls portion of the guidelines recognize the value of applying the traditional tuberculosis infection control practices. The development of a written tuberculosis control policy that includes specific plans for early identification, treatment, and isolation of patients with infectious tuberculosis are examples of issues addressed under the administrative controls portion of the guidelines. The engineering control recommendations are aimed at reducing the concentration of droplet nuclei within the patient's room. They focus primarily on mechanisms for negative-pressure ventilation in hospital rooms.

A contentious issue was determining appropriate respiratory protection.[98] In 1992, NIOSH took the stance that the risk to HCWs had to be completely eliminated and therefore all who were at risk for exposure to TB patients should wear HEPA-filtered, powered, personal respirators and participate in a mandatory respirator fit-testing program. These recommendations were put forward even though there was no specific data to support the necessity of such a drastic upgrade from the standard surgical masks. Subsequent revision of the guidelines released a year later in the *Federal Register* by both the CDC and NIOSH recommended HEPA-filtered disposable particulate respiratory protection and fit-testing, yet adequate data to support this recommendation was still not available. After reviewing the extensive public criticism (2,700 responses) to those revised guidelines, the CDC and NIOSH agreed to accept the use of disposable personal particulate respirators that met the less stringent specifications of 95 percent efficiency at filtering 1-μm particles (N95 classification). Fit-testing was still required to ensure that the appropriate-size mask works properly in at least 90 percent of individuals at risk for exposure. This final revision of the guidelines attempted to merge scientific and theoretical data, yet recognized that additional research was necessary to determine what is adequate respiratory protection.[99]

Several recent studies have demonstrated that various infection control plans successfully arrest nosocomial transmission. For example, a study by Wenger et al[100] demonstrated that even strict implementation of the 1990 CDC tuberculosis control guidelines substantially reduced transmission of MDRTB to HCWs and among HIV-positive inpatients. Characteristic of studies such as this is that multiple factors were tested simultaneously, making it difficult to determine which component of the infection control practices is most essential. Blumberg et al[101] evaluated a broad upgrade of administrative controls, engineering controls, and respiratory protection. The administrative controls specifically were an expanded isolation policy mandating discharge from isolation only after three sputums were AFB smear negative, an expanded infection control department, increased HCW education, and more frequent PPD screening of workers at risk for TB exposure. The engineering controls included simply introducing negative-pressure ventilation via a window fan installation in isolation rooms so that air was vented directly to the outdoors. And for respiratory protection, the hospital switched to a disposable personal particulate respirator from the standard surgical mask. The result of these changes was a significant reduction in nosocomial transmission. Maloney et al[97] demonstrated that the combination of early isolation and treatment of patients with tuberculosis, the use of techniques more rapid for identifying *M. tuberculosis* in specimens, configuration of isolation rooms with negative-pressure ventilation, and molded surgical masks for HCWs greatly reduced transmission within the hospital studied. Taken together these studies confirm that stricter adherence to standard infection control measures greatly reduce nosocomial transmission of tuberculosis, but do not provide data to evaluate the impact of individual control measures.

Tuberculosis in IV Drug Abusers. The IV drug abuse population has a higher incidence of tuberculosis than does the general population in areas of the United States where tuberculosis is prevalent.[102] Higher rates of HIV co-infection within the IV drug abuse population increases the risk of a tuberculosis infection and the development of active disease in this population. The data is somewhat conflicting regarding whether drug abuse in absence of co-infection with HIV is an independent risk factor for tuberculosis.[103,104] Recent data suggest that non-HIV–infected drug abusers may exhibit lower levels of cellular immunity, and PPD testing is less reliable in this population.[105]

Other risk factors for tuberculosis are prevalent among populations of drug abusers. Drug abusers as well as alcohol abusers have a poor record of compliance with tuberculosis therapy.[106] They frequent similar spots, so they are more likely to transmit to others within the cohort. They are a mobile population that is difficult to hold onto in tuberculosis treatment programs. Thus they are also at higher risk for acquired drug resistance because they often do not complete therapy or take therapy on an irregular basis.

Tuberculosis in the Elderly. Analogous to that in the foreign-born population, the majority of tuberculosis cases in the elderly population are a result of activation of a prior infection, and only approximately 10 to 20 percent of active cases are due to primary infection.[107,108] Into the 1930s, approximately 80 percent of the U.S. population was infected by tuberculosis once they reached the age of 30. About 20 to 25 percent of this cohort is still alive today. In a study of 43,000 nursing home residents from Arkansas, it was found that the rate of positive PPD was 13.2 percent.[109]

Pulmonary infection occurs in 75 percent of active cases in the elderly in contrast to 85 percent of a younger cohort.[107] A higher proportion of elderly patients present with disseminated tuberculosis, tuberculous meningitis, and skeletal tuberculosis. Signs can be nonspecific and the PPD skin test may be nonreactive.[110] Consequently, active tuberculosis in the elderly has a greater probability of going undiagnosed for an extended period of time with the increased risk of transmission to other individuals.

Transmission of Tuberculosis during Airline Flights. The risk of *M. tuberculosis* transmission to other passengers during airline flight is not greater than in any other confined spaces. Several studies have even shown that passengers with documented cavitary pulmonary disease did not infect other passengers.[111,112] These data may have been confounded by the fact that the investigations were initiated many weeks to months following the flight, which limited contact finding and the effectiveness of the tuberculosis skin test to detect conversions.

Airplane ambient air is relatively sterile.[113,114] The fresh air is compressed and passed through the jet engines, where it is heated to 250°C and then cooled at high pressures (450 pounds per square inch). Since the 1980s, however, airplanes have not used 100 percent fresh air circulation. About 50 percent of the air is recirculated. The air is introduced as vertical laminar sheets from the top of the cabin to the floor and is recirculated every 3 to 4 minutes. This is more frequent than the standard of 5 to 12 minutes that is seen in offices and homes. In newer airplanes, the recirculated air passes across a HEPA filtration unit. Investigators have shown that the usual bacteria contamination of airplane air is less than 100 colony-forming units (CFUs) per 160 L, which is significantly less than the approximately 1000 CFUs per 160 L found in city buses, shopping malls, or even airline terminals. These data suggest that transmission risk may be lower within airplanes.

A recent CDC report identifies three critical factors necessary to increase the probability that others may be infected during flight.[111,115] Clear-cut evidence of infectiousness at the time of the flight (e.g., cavitary disease, laryngeal TB, evidence of household transmission prior to flight), prolonged flight time (probably exceeding 8 hours), and proximity to the active case (risk is measurable within 15 rows of the active case).

Bovine Tuberculosis

M. bovis most commonly causes extrapulmonary disease such as lymphadenitis, genitourinary tract infections, or bone and joint infections, but it may also cause pulmonary infection.[116] *M. bovis* is closely related to *M. tuberculosis*. DNA from *M. bovis* is almost 100 percent homologous to DNA from *M. tuberculosis*. Clinical laboratories using standard nucleic acid probes cannot distinguish *M. tuberculosis* from *M. bovis*. Distinguishing one from the other has clinical relevance because *M. bovis* is normally resistant to pyrazinamide, one of the first-line medications for tuberculosis.

Pulmonary infection due to *M. bovis* is clinically indistinguishable from pulmonary tuberculosis. Up to 3 percent of the mycobacteria respiratory isolates in San Diego are *M. bovis*, and most are from

Hispanic adult immigrants to the United States.[116] This form of bovine tuberculosis probably results from livestock (usually a cow)-to-human and human-to-human aerosol transmission and indicates that bovine tuberculosis has not been effectively eliminated from domestic cattle herds. In fact, *M. bovis* remains endemic in beef and dairy cattle herds in many regions of Mexico and Central America.

The cervical lymphadenitis form of *M. bovis* is also clinically indistinguishable from *M. tuberculosis*.[117] Cervical adenitis due to *M. bovis* occurs more often in children and usually results from the ingestion of unpasteurized milk from contaminated cows.

In general, the problem of bovine tuberculosis can be solved by removing the infected cows from the herd and pasteurizing the milk.

Leprosy

Kenrad E. Nelson

Leprosy (also called Hansen's disease) is a chronic infectious disease involving primarily the peripheral nervous system, skin, eyes, and mucous membranes. It is endemic in many countries in Asia, Africa, the Pacific Islands, Latin America, southern Europe, and the Middle East. There are endemic areas of infection in the United States as well, particularly in Louisiana, Texas, and California. The major sequelae of leprosy are physical deformities involving the extremities, face, and eyes due primarily to damage to the sensory nerves from *Mycobacterium leprae* infection and the immune reaction to the organism. The resultant deformities often lead to stigmatization that continues after the infection becomes inactive and the patient is noninfectious.

Since several effective antileprosy drugs are now available, new cases of leprosy can be treated effectively and rendered noninfectious. Leprosy should not pose a significant public health problem once treatment is instituted. In fact, despite the recognized importation of over 100 cases annually in the United States for the last few decades, indigenous secondary transmission from these imported cases to their contacts after immigration to this country has not been documented.

Etiologic Agent

Leprosy is caused by *M. leprae*, a weakly acid-fast organism. The organism can be found in tissues using a modified acid-fast stain, the Fite-Faraco stain. The bacterium was originally identified in 1873 by Gerhard Henrik Armauer Hansen but it has not yet been successfully cultivated in vitro. *M. leprae* has one of the slowest replication cycles of any known bacteria. It divides only every 10 to 12 days during the log phase of growth. The organism replicates in mouse footpads,[1] in thymectomized mice or rats, nude mice, severe combined immunodeficient mice (SCID) mice, the nine-banded armadillo, and in several nonhuman primate species.[2] Naturally occurring leprosy infections have been documented in nine-banded armadillos,[3] chimpanzees, and sooty mangabeys.[4] Currently a collaborative scientific effort is under way to completely sequence and characterize the entire genome of *M. leprae*. These genetic data on the causative organism could yield a more thorough understanding of important issues in the pathogenesis of leprosy, such as the very slow replication of the organism, its preferential growth in cooler areas of the body, its neurotropism, and the nature of the immune response in humans and experimental animals.[5]

Clinical Manifestations

The clinical manifestations of leprosy are variable. The clinical presentation and course of the disease depend on the interactions between the *M. leprae* bacterial load and the host immune system, especially the cellular immune system. The most widely used system for clinical-immunologic classification of leprosy is that developed by Ridley and Jopling,[6] which subdivides leprosy into five general classes: polar lepromatous leprosy (LL), borderline lepromatous (BL) leprosy, midborderline (BB) leprosy, borderline tuberculoid (BT) leprosy, and polar tuberculoid (TT) leprosy. In addition, a very early form of leprosy, which is not readily classified into any of the above groups, is called indeterminate (I) leprosy. Indeterminate leprosy is the earliest clinical evidence of infection and often resolves spontaneously without specific therapy. However, it may progress to one of the five classes. Leprosy is often divided into only two groups: multibacillary leprosy (MB), consisting of LL, BL, and BB leprosy, and paucibacillary leprosy (PB) consisting of BT and TT leprosy. These broader groupings are useful for therapeutic decisions.

There is a good correlation between the clinical appearance, the number of organisms and distribution and type of skin lesions, and the patient's classification according to the Ridley-Jopling criteria. Patients with paucibacillary leprosy have well-defined macular skin lesions with distinct borders that are few in number and distributed asymmetrically. The lesions increase in number and become more diffuse and smaller as the disease moves toward the lepromatous end of the spectrum. Patients with BL or LL leprosy have ill-defined, sometimes nodular, skin lesions without clear borders. Loss of eyebrows or hair and deformities of the pinna of the ear are common in patients with lepromatous disease. Another characteristic of leprosy is anesthesia of the skin lesions. The skin lesions of leprosy generally spare the warmer intertriginous areas of the body. Enlargement and nodularity of the peripheral nerves, especially the ulnar, posterior tibial, and great auricular nerves, are characteristic. Patients may have corneal anesthesia and keratitis or lagophthalmos due to involvement of the facial nerve. Damage to the hands, feet, and eyes is characteristic of lepromatous disease. Trophic ulcers and resorption of digits may result from the sensory nerve damage and repeated trauma that these patients undergo. Early involvement of large sensory nerves is characteristic of tuberculoid leprosy.

An important clinical feature of leprosy is leprosy reactions, which are of two types: type 1, which are reversal (or downgrading) reactions that represent an increase (or decrease in the case of downgrading reactions) in cell-mediated immune responses to the organisms; and type 2, erythema nodosum leprosum (ENL) reactions, which are believed to be mediated largely by humoral immune responses to *M. leprae* leading to immune complexes. Nearly half of all leprosy patients experience a reaction during the first few years after their diagnosis.[7] Type 1 (reversal) reactions can occur in any patient with borderline (BL, BB or BT) leprosy; they are not seen in patients with polar lepromatous or tuberculoid leprosy. Type 2 (ENL) reactions are characteristic of and limited to patients with multibacillary leprosy. Clinically type 1 reactions consist of acute inflammation of pre-existing leprosy lesions, including superficial nerves, with fever and systemic symptoms that begin gradually and have a natural course of several weeks or months. Early recognition and aggressive therapy of type 1 reactions is especially important to prevent irreversible deformity from nerve damage. Type 2 reactions consist of the sudden appearance of crops of tender, erythematous nodules in areas of the skin that had not had leprosy lesions previously, along with fever, malaise, and sometimes acute neuritis, arthritis, orchitis, iritis, glomerulonephritis, myalgia, and peripheral edema. Type 2 reactions typically have a sudden onset and may subside in several days to a few weeks, though they may result in severe nerve damage in that time. Type 2 reactions may recur over the course of a year or more, especially in patients treated with anti-inflammatory agents, when these drugs are withdrawn or tapered.

Diagnosis

The diagnosis of leprosy is usually made clinically. Skin lesions that are anesthetic to light touch, enlarged nerves to palpation, lagophthalmos, and distal stocking-glove anesthesia are characteristic of leprosy. The diagnosis should be confirmed by skin biopsy and slit-skin smears whenever possible. When taking a punch biopsy, it is important to include specimens of the entire dermis at the active border of a lesion, because the organisms are often deeply located in the skin. They often are not seen in the epidermis and there may be a "clear zone" at the dermal-epidermal junction in multibacillary disease. The histopathologic features of leprosy correlate well with the clinical presentation of the disease. Patients with lepromatous disease have many organisms in their lesions and lack a well-developed granulomatous response due to their ineffective cellular immunity to the organism. In contrast, tuberculoid patients have few (or no detectable) organisms with a well-organized granulomatous infiltrate. Consultation for the interpretation and classification of skin biopsies or for therapeutic decisions can be obtained from the National Hansen's Disease Center at Baton Rouge, Louisiana (Phone: 504-642-4740), or the Armed Forces Institute of Pathology, Washington, D.C.

The Mitsuda lepromin skin test is not useful in making a diagnosis of *M. leprae*. The main use of the lepromin test is in classifying patients once the diagnosis has been made. Patients with polar lepromatous leprosy will have no induration at 3 to 4 weeks after the intradermal injection of Mitsuda lepromin. Patients with tuberculoid leprosy, and many with no history of clinical leprosy or exposure to leprosy, will have a positive Mitsuda skin test.[8] The Mitsuda skin test measures the ability to respond to *M. leprae* antigens, hence its usefulness in classifying patients with leprosy.

A phenolic glycolipid has been isolated from the cell wall of *M. leprae* that is antigenic and specific.[9] However, serodiagnosis is insufficiently sensitive to be useful as a routine diagnostic adjunct, since not all untreated multibacillary patients and only 20 to 30 percent of paucibacillary patients are antibody positive.[10]

Distribution

Leprosy has existed in eastern Mediterranean and Asian populations since ancient times. During the Middle Ages, leprosy became widespread in Europe. It declined in most of Europe after the sixteenth century but peaked in Norway during the nineteenth century, followed by a rapid decline during the late nineteenth and early twentieth centuries. The last known endemic case in Norway had onset about 1950.[11] The disease was introduced into the northern United States and Canada by European settlers from Norway, France, and Germany. It persisted in several clearly defined foci and within certain family groups for several decades and then disappeared.[12]

Currently the disease is primarily epidemic in certain tropical countries in Africa, Southeast Asia, India, some Pacific Islands, and Latin America. The disease remains a significant endemic problem in 84 countries worldwide. However, five countries, namely, India, Brazil, Nigeria, China, and Sudan, accounted for nearly 80 percent of the cases registered with the World Health Organization (WHO) in 1993.[13] The prevalence rates have declined substantially in the last 15 years, since the WHO recommended in 1982 that the disease be treated with a course of multiple drugs.[14] The WHO recommended the routine treatment of all active cases with multidrug therapy (MDT) containing dapsone, rifampin, and clofazimine for a fixed time period, rather than indefinite treatment with dapsone alone, as was common practice until then.

While 12 million leprosy cases were estimated to be present worldwide in 1982, estimates in 1992 are between 3.1 and 5.0 million cases.[15] The substantial decline in the global numbers of leprosy cases probably is related in part to the widespread use of supervised MDT in accordance with WHO recommendations for active cases in most countries where the disease is epidemic. Multidrug therapy may have rendered most leprosy cases noninfectious sooner after the start of therapy in comparison to the previous experience of monotherapy with dapsone, a bacteriostatic drug to which some organisms are resistant. It is believed by some experts that better compliance with shorter drug regimens may have decreased the rates of relapse, as well as interrupted the transmission cycle.[16] However, another factor that clearly has affected the estimated current prevalence of leprosy is the acceptance of a defined course of therapy for patients on MDT and the release of patients from the registry of active cases after this therapy has been completed. Previously, dapsone monotherapy had been recommended for life for multibacillary cases, and patients were never dropped from the registry even after they became inactive, or "cured." So, the decreased leprosy prevalence rates are due in part to a change in the definition of what constitutes an "active case."[17]

Leprosy apparently was introduced into the Americas through African and European immigration. Leprosy was reported in French Polynesia as the eighteenth century ended. Trade links among these islands, Easter Island, and Hawaii probably helped spread the disease.[18] North American endemic foci are now limited to Louisiana, Texas, and California. New cases in North America now occur primarily among immigrants, which occur 5 to 10 times more commonly than infections acquired among U.S. residents. Many cases in the United States come from Southeast Asia, and some come from Mexico and other countries in Latin America or Africa where leprosy is endemic.

One of the most impressive epidemics of leprosy was reported from the island of Nauru, in the South Pacific.[19] A single case of leprosy was introduced into a population of approximately 1,200 persons in 1912 and this led to an epidemic that eventually affected 30 percent of the population over the next 30 years. It is of interest that nearly all of the leprosy cases on Nauru were of the tuberculoid type, and only about 1 percent were multibacillary. The marked predominance of tuberculoid leprosy in hyperendemic populations led Newell to suggest that lepromatous leprosy occurs only in persons with specific genetic immunological deficits to the organism, a view subsequently supported by several genetic studies.[20]

Epidemiology

Transmission

Mycobacterium leprae is believed to be transmitted from person to person by close contact. However, some debate continues about the exact means of transmission. Only about 30 to 40 percent of patients with clinical leprosy who live in endemic areas have a history of close personal or household contact with a known leprosy case.[21] However, the indolent nature and the long incubation period of the disease could have led to failure to recognize or recall this exposure in many cases.

In contrast with tuberculosis, a primary site of infection in the respiratory tract has not been documented. Nevertheless, many experts believe that the infection is most often transmitted from contact with the nasal secretions of an infectious case. Studies of the nasal discharge of multibacillary cases have estimated that 10^7 bacilli per day may be contained in these secretions.[22] Recently investigators have used the polymerase chain reaction to amplify *M. leprae* DNA to confirm the presence of the organism in the nasal secretions of leprosy cases and their household contacts.[23,24]

In contrast with these findings, the organism is not found in the epidermis of the intact skin, although it may be present in ulcerated lesions, usually in much lower numbers than found in nasal secretions. The organism has also been found in high concentration in the blood of lepromatous cases[25] and in the breast milk of patients with active disease.[26] Some investigators speculate that *M. leprae* may be infectious by direct skin contact. The more common occurrence of the initial leprosy lesions on exposed areas of skin is sometimes cited as evidence for this site of entry of the organisms.[27] However, since the organisms is known to grow better in cooler, exposed areas of the skin, this could influence the distribution of lesions. There are reports of inoculation of *M. leprae* by tattooing or bacillus Calmette-Guérin (BCG) injection, leading to clinical leprosy at the site of inoculation, but many years later.[21] Some special exposures in some populations (e.g., Micronesia) in which leprosy is epidemic, such as sharing of bamboo sleeping mats with an active case, could result in the transmission of *M. leprae* by direct inoculation of organisms from an infectious case into the skin (J. Douglas, personal communication).

Reservoir

Viable *M. leprae* have been recovered from arthropods including mosquitoes and bed bugs who have fed on lepromatous patients.[28] Cochrane noted that, even when malaria prevalence was equal in adjacent villages in India, leprosy prevalence differed significantly, suggesting that, at least anopheline transmission of *M. leprae* was not important.[29] It is also possible that organisms could enter humans through the gastrointestinal tract, as does *Mycobacterium avium* complex organisms, but no evidence for this route of entry has been published. Some investigators have suggested that the site of the original entry of *M. leprae* could condition the host immune response to the organism; skin or upper respiratory penetration could more readily provoke a TH-1–type lymphocyte response, whereas the lower respiratory or oral route could lead to a TH-2–type lymphocyte response and progression of infection to lepromatous disease.[30]

Infectious human cases almost certainly are the only important reservoir of *M. leprae* for human infections. Nevertheless, there are reports of isolation of noncultivatable mycobacteria resembling *M. leprae* from several environmental sites, including soil, sphagnum moss, and thorns;[31] also, leprosy infections are endemic in feral armadillos.[32]

Prevalence and Incidence

The prevalence of leprosy varies widely in different populations but generally involves 0.01 to 2.0 percent of the population in areas where the disease is endemic. Although leprosy may occur in infants and young children, the disease is rare in children under 7 years of age. This is likely due to the long incubation period between exposure and the onset of clinical symptoms. The length of the incubation period has been estimated among military personnel and missionaries who have returned to the United States or Europe from endemic areas. These data indicate that the incubation period is longer for lepromatous (median of 8 to 12 years) than it is for tuberculoid disease (median of 2 to 5 years).[33] These studies are also the basis for the estimate that only approximate 5 percent of the adult population may be susceptible.

The incidence of leprosy peaks between the ages of 10 and 29 years.[21,34,35] The rates of new cases are at least 5- to 10-fold higher in persons with a close contact in the household.[21,34,35] Leprosy incidence rates rarely exceed 2 per 1,000 persons per year, except in persons with a household contact with an active case. A recent prospective study in Malawi found the incidence to be 1.2 per 1,000 persons per year and the rates were significantly higher (65 percent) in persons who had not had BCG vaccination.[36]

Household crowding and low socioeconomic status of a population are important factors promoting the transmission of *M. leprae* and the development of clinical leprosy. A recent prospective study in Malawi found a lower incidence of leprosy in persons with less household crowding and higher levels of education.[37] Improvement in the standards of living may have been critical in the spontaneous disappearance of leprosy from several countries, such as Norway, where the disease had been endemic in the nineteenth and early twentieth centuries.[38]

It is likely that genetic susceptibility may be one of the important factors contributing to the risk of leprosy and in the type of leprosy that develops after exposure. A twin study found higher concordance rates for leprosy among 62 monozygotic twin pairs (60 percent) than among 40 dizygotic twin pairs (20 percent).[39] However, this important study may have been affected by recruitment bias, since more monozygotic than dizygotic twins were studied. Several studies of human lymphocyte antigen (HLA) distributions of leprosy patients have found significant associations with certain HLA haplotypes.[40–43] A segregation analysis of leprosy in families with multiple cases has suggested that the genetic susceptibility may differ between tuberculoid and lepromatous disease.[44]

The proportion of leprosy cases that are multibacillary and paucibacillary in different populations has been observed to differ considerably geographically. A much higher proportion of lepromatous cases has been observed in southeast Asia than in Africa, where most cases are tuberculoid.[45] Whether these differences are due to host differences (such as genetic or nutritional factors), epidemiological factors influencing the route or age at the time of exposure, the size of the inoculum, or to differences in the strains of *M. leprae* in different areas of the world is not known. The inability to culture the organism and the lack of a good animal model that develops a disease similar to that seen in humans has hindered investigations of these important scientific questions.

Interaction of HIV and Leprosy

The pandemic of human immunodeficiency virus (HIV) infection and acquired immunodeficiency syndrome (AIDS) has resulted in a markedly increased incidence of several mycobacterial infections, particularity *Mycobacterium tuberculosis* and *Mycobacterium avium-intracellulare*. This has led to concerns that HIV infection might also increase the rates of leprosy in areas of the world where both HIV and *M. leprae* are epidemic. Immunosuppression from HIV could affect the transmission of *M. leprae* by increasing the prevalence of multibacillary forms of leprosy, which could be more readily transmitted. Theoretically, the interaction between HIV infection and leprosy could produce a higher proportion of multibacillary cases, a greater incidence, and more frequent relapses after a course of therapy.[46]

Several studies of the interaction between HIV and *M. leprae* have been reported recently from areas of the world where both leprosy and HIV infections are common. Most of these studies have not found HIV infections to have a significant impact on leprosy. Case-control studies in Malawi,[47] Uganda,[48] and Yemen[49] have failed to show a significantly higher HIV antibody prevalence among leprosy patients than in control subjects. Also, these studies did not find a higher proportion of multibacillary leprosy cases among patients infected with HIV than in those who were HIV uninfected. However, a small hospital-based study in Zambia found a higher HIV prevalence rate in leprosy patients than control subjects.[50] A larger community-based case-control study in Tanzania, in which leprosy cases and control subjects were matched by their geographic areas of residence, found an association between HIV infection and leprosy in those from rural areas and in those with multibacillary leprosy.[51]

The different findings in these studies could be explained by several factors. The HIV epidemic in different countries varies in duration and severity. It is possible that the effect of HIV immunosuppression on leprosy might be manifest at more severe levels of immunosuppression than for tuberculosis. Also, the rates of leprosy are higher in rural populations, whereas HIV infections often are concentrated among urban populations. Therefore, overlap between the epidemics of leprosy and HIV/AIDS may not have occurred yet in some countries where both diseases are epidemic. While the effects of HIV infection certainly are not as evident for leprosy as they have been for tuberculosis, further evaluation of this interaction is warranted before definite conclusions are drawn.

No data have been published on whether active leprosy accelerates the progression of HIV infection. However, there are data that suggest that patients with HIV infection who develop active tuberculosis have more rapid progression of their HIV-related immunosuppression than do tuberculosis uninfected patients.[52] One intriguing study[53] in rhesus monkeys who were inoculated with *M. leprae* suggested that those monkeys who were co-infected with Simian Immunodeficiency Virus (SIV) were more likely to progress to lepromatous leprosy.

Treatment and Rehabilitation

Antileprosy Drugs

At present three drugs are commonly used for the treatment of leprosy: dapsone, rifampin (Rifadin), and clofazimine (Lamprene). The use of ethionamide-prothionamide (Trecator) has been abandoned due to its hepatotoxicity and the availability of better alternative drugs. Dapsone and clofazimine have weak bactericidal activity against *M. leprae*, and rifampin has potent bactericidal activity against nearly all strains of the organism. However, a few strains of *M. leprae* that are resistant to rifampin have been reported. Other drugs have recently been shown to have good antibacterial activity against *M. leprae*. Included are ofloxacin (Floxin), sparfloxacin, minocyline (Minocin), and clarithromycin (Biaxin). Isoniazid (INH), which is an important first-line drug for the treatment of tuberculosis, is ineffective for treating leprosy.

Dapsone. The usual dose is 100 mg daily for adults and 1.0 mg per kg per day for children. It is a safe, cheap, and effective drug for treating all types of leprosy. Strains of *M. leprae* that are fully sensitive to dapsone have a minimal inhibitory concentration (MIC) of about 0.003 mg per mL, as determined in the mouse footpad assay. Although doses of 100 mg per day of dapsone exceed the MIC by a factor of nearly 500-fold, the increasing prevalence of mild, moderate, or complete resistance to dapsone among *M. leprae* organisms, either in untreated leprosy (primary resistance) or emergence of resistance during treatment (secondary resistance), and the relatively weak bactericidal action of the drug have dictated the current recommendation for treatment at the 100 mg daily dosage. Because of the problem of dapsone resistance, the drug should always be used in combination with rifampin and/or clofazimine for the treatment of active leprosy[14] (Table 9-10).

The most common side effect of dapsone therapy is anemia. However, this is usually very mild and well tolerated, unless the patient has a complete glucose-6-phosphate dehydrogenase (G6PD) deficiency, in which case the anemia may be more severe. Therefore, it is useful to screen patients to detect complete (G6PD) deficiency prior to instituting therapy with dapsone. More serious but, fortunately, very rare side effects of dapsone include agranulocytosis, exfoliative dermatitis, hepatitis, and a syndrome termed the "dapsone syndrome," which includes hepatitis and a generalized rash and can progress to exfoliation. Since these more serious toxic effects generally occur soon after initiation of therapy, patients should be seen periodically, and complete blood counts and liver enzymes should be measured after therapy is begun.

Rifampin. Because of its excellent bactericidal activity against *M. leprae*, rifampin is included in the therapy of leprosy patients. Patients with lepromatous leprosy who are treated with a drug regimen that includes rifampin will become noncontagious after only 2 to 3 weeks, or less, of treatment. The usual adult dose is 600 mg daily; children should be treated with 10 to 20 mg per kg, not to exceed 600 mg per day. The cost of daily administration of rifampin is prohibitive for leprosy control programs in the developing world. However, the very slow replication of *M. leprae* permit administration of the drug once monthly. The alternative regimen recommended by WHO for leprosy control programs in developing countries includes administration of 600 mg of rifampin at monthly intervals as directly observed therapy. This regimen of once monthly administration of rifampin has been shown to be equivalent to daily doses of the drug. The major toxic side effect of rifampin is hepatotoxicity. Generally, rifampin should be discontinued if the alanine transaminase (ALT) (SGPT) or aspartate transaminase (AST) (SGOT) levels increase to more than 2.5 to 5.0 times the upper limit of normal. Rifabutin, a drug licensed for therapy of *M. avium* complex infections, also has bactericidal activity against *M. leprae*.

Clofazimine. Clofazimine is an iminophenazine dye with antimycobacterial activity roughly equivalent to that of dapsone. It is a useful drug for the treatment of leprosy, since it also has some anti-inflammatory activity, which is useful for the control of leprosy reactions. The usual adult dose is 50 to 100 mg daily. Higher doses of 200 to 300 mg daily have more pronounced anti-inflammatory activity but are more likely to lead to gastrointestinal toxicity with chronic use. Also, clofazimine has been used in doses of 100 mg three times weekly for the chronic treatment of leprosy. The drug is deposited in the skin and slowly released, thus providing a repository effect in chronic therapy.

The most frequent side effect of therapy with clofazimine is reddish-black pigmentation of the skin. The degree of pigmentation is dose related. However, the pigmentation tends not to be uniform in many patients but is concentrated in the areas of the lesions, producing a blotchy pigmentation that many patients consider to be unsightly. Since virtually all fair-skinned patients will have some pigmentation with clofazimine therapy, it also serves as a useful marker of drug compliance. The pigmentation is slowly cleared 6 to 12 months or more after therapy is discontinued.

Aside from pigmentation, the major side effects of clofazimine therapy involve the gastrointestinal tract. Patients may develop abdominal cramps, sometimes associated with nausea, vomiting, and diarrhea. On high doses of clofazimine (over 100 mg daily), these symptoms are common after more than 3 to 6 months of therapy. Radiographic studies of the small bowel may show a pattern compatible with malabsorption. Fortunately, these symptoms usually are reversible upon discontinuation of the drug.

Other side effects include anticholinergic activity, which may result in diminished sweating and tearing. Since patients with lepromatous leprosy may have autonomic nerve involvement from their disease, they commonly have ichthyosis from their decreased sweating, and this problem may be intensified by clofazimine.

Ofloxacin. A number of fluoroquinolones have been developed; many of these drugs, such as ciprofloxacin, are not active against *M. leprae*. Among those that are active against *M. leprae* are ofloxacin[54,55] and sparfloxacin.[56] These drugs interfere with bacterial DNA replication by inhibiting the enzyme DNA gyrase. They have been shown in animal and short-term human experiments to have good bactericidal activity against *M. leprae*. Ofloxacin is well absorbed orally and is generally given in a dose of 400 mg once daily. A trial is currently under way to determine whether a combi-

TABLE 9-10. WORLD HEALTH ORGANIZATION RECOMMENDATIONS FOR MULTIDRUG THERAPY FOR LEPROSY

Drug	Dose
■ ***Multibacillary Leprosy***[a]	
Rifampin	600 mg once a month, supervised
Dapsone	100 mg/day, self-administered
Clofazimine	300 mg once a month, supervised
Clofazimine	50 mg/day, self-administered
Therapy should be continued for 2 years or until leprosy is inactive.	
■ ***Paucibacillary Leprosy***	
Rifampin	600 mg once a month, supervised
Dapsone	100 mg/day, self-administered

[a] Any of the following three drugs can be substituted for one of the above drugs in cases of drug intolerance: Ofloxacin 400 mg/day, minocyline 100 mg/day, or clarithromycin 500 mg/day.

nation of rifampin and ofloxacin, with or without minocyline, can reduce the treatment period of multibacillary leprosy significantly, i.e., to 1 to 3 months.[57,58]

Minocyline. Minocyline is the only member of the tetracycline group of antibiotics that has significant bactericidal activity against *M. leprae*.[59] The standard dose is 100 mg daily, which gives a peak serum level that exceeds that MIC of minocyline against *M. leprae* by a factor of 10 to 20. Clinical trials are under way to determine optimal usage of the drug. The drug is relatively well tolerated, although vestibular toxicity has been reported in some patients.

Clarithromycin. Among the macrolide antibiotics, clarithromycin (Biaxin) is the only drug shown to have significant bactericidal activity against *M. leprae*. When given in a dose of 500 mg once daily to patients with lepromatous leprosy, 99 percent of bacilli were killed within 28 days and 99.9 percent were killed by 56 days.[60] The drug is relatively nontoxic, however gastrointestinal irritation, nausea, vomiting, and diarrhea are the most common side effects.

Treatment Regimens

The standard therapy for leprosy should include MDT for all forms of the disease.[14] Prior to the early 1980s patients were often treated with dapsone alone. This led to the emergence of dapsone resistance and rendered further dapsone therapy ineffective in many areas. In 1981 a WHO study group met to recommend new treatment regimens for leprosy control programs. The WHO study group reviewed the data on the resistance of *M. leprae* organisms to dapsone and their sensitivity to rifampin and clofazimine and recommended that multidrug therapy be used to treat all active cases of leprosy (Table 9-10). The WHO recommended the treatment of patients with paucibacillary disease with 100 mg (1 to 2 mg per kg) of dapsone daily, unsupervised, and 600 mg of rifampin once a month as directly observed therapy for 6 months. Patients with multibacillary leprosy are to be treated with dapsone 100 mg daily, clofazimine 50 mg daily, both self-administered, and rifampin 600 mg once monthly and clofazimine 300 mg once monthly, both supervised for at least 2 years or until the disease becomes inactive. Patients in whom acid-fast organisms were identified on their slit-skin smears or skin biopsies prior to treatment should be treated with the regimen for multibacillary disease. Also, patients with currently "inactive" leprosy who have had only monotherapy with dapsone should be given MDT to prevent relapse. Relapse rates of 1.0 percent or less have occurred in the 5 to 9 years after completion of these regimens in patients who were successfully treated. Patients should be followed at frequent intervals after treatment is started. Follow-up should include examination for new skin lesions, new areas of anesthesia, new motor deficits, enlargement or tenderness of nerves, and clinical evidence of reactions. In addition, annual skin biopsies are useful in documenting changes in disease status. Slit-skin smears are helpful in estimating the bacillary load of acid-fast organisms remaining in the skin. These smears are done by pinching the skin to reduce bleeding, cleaning with alcohol, and making a superficial skin slit through the epidermis with a scalpel blade and transferring the subepidermal fluid to a circular area 5 to 6 mm in diameter on a clean glass slide. Slit-skin smears are taken from six or more sites (e.g., earlobe, eyebrow, trunk, elbow, thigh, and knee) at 6- to 12-month intervals and stained using the Fite-Faraco acid-fast stain. The bacteriologic index (BI) is a semiquantitative logarithmic estimate of the number of organisms in the skin (Table 9-11). With effective therapy of lepromatous patients, the average BI should decrease at a rate of about 1/2 to 1 log each year. Failure of the BI to fall suggests poor compliance with therapy or infection with drug-resistant organisms. The National Hansen's Disease Center at Carville, Louisiana, will stain and examine slides prepared by the slit-skin smear technique. Inactivity of leprosy is defined as a BI of zero on slit-skin smear, no active lesions on skin biopsy, and no clinical evidence of disease activity for at least 1 year. In cases of intolerance to one of the primary drugs (i.e., dapsone, clofazimine, or rifampin) or drug-resistant organisms one of the other antileprosy drugs can be substituted (i.e., ofloxacin, minocycline, or clarithromycin).

Treatment of Reactions

Reactions are common during leprosy treatment and complicate the outcome of therapy. Educating patients to recognize and seek prompt treatment for reactions is essential for a successful therapeutic outcome. Such reactions, especially those involving major nerves or the eyes, can cause permanent incapacitation if they are not promptly recognized and properly treated.

Type 1 Reactions. The most important goals in the treatment of type 1 reactions (reversal reactions) are to prevent nerve damage and to control severe inflammation and prevent necrosis of skin lesions. Antileprosy chemotherapy should not be interrupted during the reaction. In mild reactions, especially those without neuritis or facial lesions, treatment with analgesics and close observation may suffice. However, any reaction where there is evidence of acute neuritis with pain, tenderness, or loss of nerve function should be treated with steroids, starting with prednisone in doses of 40 to 60 mg per day. It should be noted that the metabolism of prednisone is accelerated in patients who are also receiving rifampin. The patient may need hospitalization and should be closely observed with frequent voluntary muscle tests (VMTs) to evaluate nerve weakness. The dose of prednisone may be reduced by 5 to 10 mg every 1 to 2 weeks until a maintenance dose of 20 to 25 mg is reached. It can then be reduced slowly over the course of 6 months or more while repeating VMT and observing for recurrence of the reaction. Careful management of type 1 reactions is essential to prevent long-term sequelae.

Type 2 Reactions. Although type II (ENL) reactions are important because of their frequency and the potential for organ damage, mild ENL reactions sometimes can be managed with anti-inflammatory agents, such as salicylates or nonsteroidal anti-inflammatory agents. However, severe or persistent ENL often requires therapy with corticosteroids, thalidomide, or clofazimine singly or in combination. Commonly, prednisone in doses of 40 to 60 mg are given and the patient is started on 400 mg per day of thalidomide. Steroids can be reduced or withdrawn, and the ENL can be controlled in some cases with thalidomide alone. Although thalidomide often is effective in controlling ENL reactions, it cannot be given to women of child-bearing age, unless they are following a fool-proof method of contraception, since the drug is highly teratogenic. Clofazimine in doses of 100 to 300 mg per day has anti-inflammatory effects, but gastrointestinal toxicity is common when the drug is continued at this dose for more than 2 to 3 months. Some patients will require chronic steroid therapy to suppress their ENL reaction, which can persist for several months.

Iridocyclitis. Iridocyclitis commonly accompanies type II reactions and may cause blindness in leprosy; another cause of visual damage in leprosy is keratitis secondary to facial nerve damage causing lagophthalmos. Acute iridocyclitis should be treated with mydriatics, such as 1 percent atropine or 0.25 percent scopolamine, and anti-inflammatory drugs, such as 1 percent hydrocortisone.

TABLE 9-11. THE BACTERIAL INDEX

BI	*Number of Organisms*
0	No bacilli in 100 OIF[a]
1+	1–10 bacilli per 100 OIF
2+	1–10 bacilli per 10 OIF
3+	1–10 bacilli per OIF
4+	10–100 bacilli per OIF
5+	100–1,000 bacilli per OIF
6+	Over 1,000 bacilli per OIF

[a] OIF, oil immersion fields.

Other Complications

Important complications of leprosy, such as neuritis, iridocyclitis, orchitis, and glomerulonephritis, may occur during reactions. Therefore it is important that leprosy patients be carefully monitored at frequent intervals, especially while the disease is active. Baseline slit lamp examination of the eyes is wise, if available.

Patients should be trained to avoid injuries to anesthetic areas and to report injuries promptly, even in the absence of pain. Sensory loss (to the point of compromise of protective sensation) is often more severe than is generally appreciated.[61] Frequent inspection of the feet and hands and construction of special footwear to prevent permanent damage to deformed and anesthetic feet are important aspects of the care of leprosy patients. Reconstructive surgery, such as tibialis posterior muscle transfer to correct footdrop, and temporalis muscle transplant to correct lagophthalmos, may be important in treating some patients. Patients who have ocular problems should be seen by an ophthalmologist.

Control and Prevention

Three basic approaches have been used to control and prevent leprosy, namely:

1. Early detection and supervised chemotherapy of active cases, as described above;
2. Preventive treatment of household contacts, especially children, of infectious cases;
3. Immunization with BCG.

Active case finding is an important activity for leprosy control in areas where the disease is endemic. Especially important is periodic screening and follow-up of household contacts of newly diagnosed cases. Training of health care professionals in leprosy endemic areas in the recognition and treatment of leprosy is important. Health care facilities, such as general or skin disease clinics, can provide screening and appropriate leprosy therapy in an atmosphere that is not stigmatizing. Screening of special populations, such as schoolchildren, laborers, or military populations can be useful in detecting early leprosy in some highly endemic populations.

Prophylaxis with dapsone, 50 mg daily for 3 years, has been recommended for persons under the age of 25 who have a household contact with a patient with active multibacillary leprosy.[62] Children with close contact with someone with paucibacillary (tuberculoid) leprosy are also at some increased risk; however, their risk is less, so they should be examined every 6 to 12 months for several years after this exposure, and biopsies should be obtained of any suspicious lesions in order to detect and institute treatment soon after clinical disease appears. The rate of leprosy in household members in the 10 years after close household contacts with someone with untreated lepromatous leprosy was reported to be about 11 percent after 10 years follow-up in careful studies by Worth and Hirschy in Hawaii[63] and Hong Kong.[64] When the index case had tuberculoid leprosy, the incidence in household contacts was reported to be 0.5 percent. A randomized controlled study of dapsone prophylaxis using a 50 mg daily dose for 3 years in household contacts found a 52.5 percent reduction in leprosy in the 12 years after exposure in those who received dapsone.[65]

The initial experimental evidence for the possible preventive efficacy of BCG was reported by Shepard in 1966.[66] He found that vaccination of mice with BCG prevented experimental infection from footpad inoculation with viable *M. leprae*. Subsequently, several randomized trials of BCG in human populations were done. A trial in Uganda, where most leprosy is tuberculoid, showed an 80 percent protective efficacy of BCG.[67] Another trial in Karimui, New Guinea, found an efficacy of 48 percent.[68] A third trial in Burma found an efficacy of 20 percent; however, the efficacy was 38 percent in children from 0 to 4 years of age and when a second more immunogenic lot of freeze-dried BCG was used.[69] A more recent trial of BCG in Malawi found a 50 percent reduction in the incidence of leprosy associated with a second inoculation of BCG, but no additional efficacy was associated with the inclusion of heat-killed *M. leprae* with BCG.[70] In summary, these controlled studies of BCG, together with several case-control studies,[71,72] suggest that BCG affords significant protection against leprosy in most populations.

The widespread use of effective multidrug therapy for leprosy under direct supervision, the earlier diagnosis of leprosy, the reduction of the stigma previously associated with this disease in many societies, and the routine use of BCG in many leprosy endemic countries have led to a decline in new cases of leprosy in recent years.[13,73] Many experts are cautiously optimistic that this trend will continue in the future and that the public health importance of leprosy will continue to decline,[13,74,75] as long as the effort to control this important disease persists. The long-term outlook for the control of leprosy as a public health problem is good, as long as the effective prevention efforts are not abandoned prematurely.

▶ REFERENCES

Acute Respiratory Infections

1. Dingle JH, Badger GF, Jordan WS Jr: Illness in the Home: a Study of 25,000 Illnesses in a Group of Cleveland Families. Cleveland: The Press of Western Reserve University, 1964
2. Monto AS, Ullman BM: The Tecumseh study. Acute respiratory illness in an American community. JAMA 227:164–169, 1974
3. Monto AS, Bryan ER, Rhodes LM: The Tecumseh study of respiratory illness. VII. Further observations on the occurrence of respiratory syncytial virus and *Mycoplasma pneumoniae* infections. Am J Epidemiol 100:458, 1975
4. Mufson MA, Belshe RB, Orvell C, Norrby E: Respiratory syncytial virus epidemics: variable dominance of subgroups A and B strains among children, 1981–1986. J Infect Dis 157:143–148, 1988
5. Van Milaan AJ, Sprenger MJ, Rothbarth PH, Brandenburg AH, Masurel N, Class EC: Detection of respiratory syncytial virus by RNA-polymerase chain reaction and differentiation of subgroups with oligonucleotide probes. J Med Virol 44:80–87, 1994
6. Mufson MA, Levine HD, Wasil RE, et al: Epidemiology of respiratory syncytial virus infection among infants and children in Chicago. Am J Epidemiol 98:88, 1973
7. Glezen WP, Paredes A, Allison JE, et al: Risk of respiratory syncytial virus infection for infants from low-income families in relationship to age, sex, ethnic group, and maternal antibody level. J Pediatr 98:708, 1981
8. Chanock RM, Kapikian AZ, Mills J, et al: Influence of immunological factors in respiratory syncytial virus disease. Arch Environ Health 21:347, 1970
9. Kim HW, Arrobio JO, Brandt CD, et al: Epidemiology of respiratory syncytial virus infection in Washington, DC. I. Importance of the virus in different respiratory tract disease syndromes and temporal distribution of infection. Am J Epidemiol 98:216, 1973
10. Glezen WP, Denny FW: Epidemiology of acute lower respiratory disease in children. N Engl J Med 288:498, 1973
11. Chin J, Magoffin RL, Shearer LA, et al: Field evaluation of a respiratory syncytial virus vaccine and a trivalent parainfluenza virus vaccine in a pediatric population. Am J Epidemiol 89:449, 1969
12. Hall CB, McBride JT, Walsh EE, et al: Aerosolized ribavirin treatment of infants with respiratory syncytial viral infection. A randomized double-blind study. N Engl J Med 308:1443, 1983
13. Ohmit SE, Moler FW, Monto AS, Khan AS: Ribavirin utilization and clinical effectiveness in children hospitalized with respiratory syncytial virus infection. J Clin Epidemiol 49:963–967, 1996
14. Groothusis JR, Simoes EA, Hemming VG: Respiratory syncytial virus (RSV) infection in preterm infants and the protective effects of RSV immune globulin (RSVIG). Respiratory syncytial virus immune globulin study group. Pediatrics 95:463–467, 1995

15. Chanock RM, Parrott RH, Cook K, et al: Newly recognized myxoviruses from children with respiratory disease. N Engl J Med 258: 207, 1958
16. Chanock RM, Parrott RH, Johnson KM, et al: Myxoviruses: Parainfluenza. Am Rev Respir Dis 88:152, 1963
17. Rubin EE, Quennec P, McDonald JC: Infections due to parainfluenza virus type 4 in children. Clin Infect Dis 17:998–1002, 1993
18. Monto AS: The Tecumseh study of respiratory illness. V. Patterns of infection with the parainfluenza viruses. Am J Epidemiol 97:338, 1973
19. Knott AM, Long CE, Hall CB: Parainfluenza viral infections in pediatric outpatients: seasonal patterns and clinical characteristics. Pediatrics Infect Dis J 13:269–273, 1994
20. Karron RA, Wright PF, Hall SL, et al: A live attenuated bovine parainfluenza virus type 3 vaccine is safe, infectious, immunogenic, and phenotypically stable in infants and children. J Infect Dis 171:1107–1114, 1995
21. Cooney MK, Kenny GE, Tam R, Fox JP: Cross relationships among 37 rhinoviruses demonstrated by virus neutralization with potent monotypic rabbit antisera. Infect Immun 7:335, 1973
22. Hendley JO, Edmondson WP Jr, Gwaltney JM Jr: Relationship between naturally acquired immunity and infectivity of two rhinoviruses in volunteers. J Infect Dis 125:243, 1972
23. Minor TE, Dick EC, De Meo AN, et al: Viruses as precipitants of asthmatic attacks in children. JAMA 227:292, 1974
24. Monto AS, Cavallaro JJ: The Tecumseh study of respiratory illness. IV. Prevalence of rhinovirus serotypes, 1966–1969. Am J Epidemiol 96:352, 1972
25. Hendley JO, Wenzel RP, Gwaltney JM Jr: Transmission of rhinovirus colds by self-inoculation. N Engl J Med 288:1361, 1973
26. Monto AS, Bryan ER, Ohmit S: Rhinovirus infections in Tecumseh, Michigan: Frequency of illness and number of serotypes. J Infect Dis 156:43–49, 1987
27. Hayden FG, Hipskind GJ, Woerner DH, et al: Intranasal pirodavir (R77,975) treatment of rhinovirus colds. Antimicrob Agents Chemother 39:290–294, 1995
28. Coulehan JL, Eberhard S, Kapner L, et al: Vitamin C and acute illness in Navajo schoolchildren. N Engl J Med 295:973, 1976
29. Hamre D, Beem M: Virologic studies of acute respiratory disease in young adults. V. Coronavirus 229E infections during six years of surveillance. Am J Epidemiol 96:94, 1972
30. McIntosh K, Becker WB, Chanock RM: Growth in suckling-mouse brain of "IBV-like" viruses from patients with upper respiratory tract disease. Proc Natl Acad Sci U S A 58:2268, 1967
31. Monto AS, Lim SK: The Tecumseh study of respiratory illness. VI. Frequency of and relationship between outbreaks of coronavirus infection. J Infect Dis 129:271, 1974
32. McNaughton MR: Occurrence and frequency of coronavirus infections in humans as determined by enzyme-linked immunosorbent assay. Infect Immun 38:419, 1982
33. Gill EP, Dominguez EA, Greenberg SB, et al: Development and application of an enzyme immunoassay for coronavirus OC43 antibody in acute respiratory illness. J Clin Microbiol 32:2372–2376, 1994
34. Benyesh-Melnick M, Rosenberg HS: The isolation of adenovirus type 7 from a fatal case of pneumonia and disseminated disease. J Pediatr 64:83, 1964
35. Fox JP, Brandt CD, Wassermann FE, et al: The virus watch program: A continuing surveillance of viral infections in metropolitan New York families. VI. Observations of adenovirus infections: Virus excretion patterns, antibody response, efficacy of surveillance, patterns of infection, and relation to illness. Am J Epidemiol 89:25, 1969
36. Dudding BA, Wagner SC, Zeller JA, et al: Fatal pneumonia associated with adenovirus type 7 in military trainees. N Engl J Med 286:1289, 1972
37. Jawetz E: The story of shipyard eye. Br Med J 1:873, 1959
38. Bell JA, Rowe WP, Engler JI, et al: Pharyngoconjunctival fever: epidemiological studies of a recently recognized disease entity. JAMA 175:1083, 1955
39. Top FH Jr, Grossman RA, Bartelloni PJ, et al: Immunization with live types 7 and 4 adenovirus vaccines. I. Safety, infectivity, and potency of adenovirus type 7 vaccines in humans. J Infect Dis 124:148, 1971
40. Slotkin RI, Clyde WA Jr, Denny FW: The effect of antibiotics on *Mycoplasma pneumoniae* in vitro and in vivo. Am J Epidemiol 86: 225, 1967
41. Eaton MD, Meiklejohn G, Van Herick W: Studies on etiology of primary atypical pneumonia. I. Filterable agent transmissible to cotton rats, hamsters and chick embryos. J Exp Med 79:649, 1944
42. Foy HM, Kenny GE, McMahan R, et al: *Mycoplasma pneumoniae* pneumonia in an urban area. Five years of surveillance. JAMA 214: 1666, 1970
43. Sawyer R, Sommerville RG: An outbreak of *Mycoplasma pneumoniae* infection in a nuclear submarine. JAMA 195:958, 1966
44. Wenzel RP, Craven RB, Davies JA, et al: Field trial of an inactivated *Mycoplasma pneumoniae* vaccine. I. Vaccine efficacy. J Infect Dis 134:571, 1976
45. Smith CB, Friedewald WT, Chanock RM: Shedding of *Mycoplasma pneumoniae* after tetracycline and erythromycin therapy. N Engl J Med 276:1172, 1967
46. Grayston JT, Kuo CC, Campbell LA, Wang SP: *Chlamydia pneumoniae* sp. nov. for *Chlamydia* sp. strain TWAR. Int J Syst Bacteriol 39:88–90, 1989
47. Grayston JT, Campbell LA, Kuo C-C, et al: A new respiratory tract pathogen: *Chlamydia pneumoniae* strain TWAR. J Infect Dis 161: 618, 1990
48. Kleemola M, Saikku P, Visakorpi R, et al: Epidemics of pneumonia caused by TWAR, a new *Chlamydia* organism, in military trainees in Finland. J Infect Dis 157:230–236, 1988
49. Gaydos CA, Roblin PM, Hammerschlag MR, et al: Diagnostic utility of PCR-enzyme immunoassay, culture, and serology for detection of *Chlamydia pneumoniae* in symptomatic and asymptomatic patients. J Clin Microbiol 32:903–905, 1994

Viral Hepatitis

1. Krugman S, Giles JP, Hammond J: Infectious hepatitis: Evidence for two distinctive clinical, epidemiological and immunological types of infection. JAMA 200:365, 1967
2. Blumberg BS, Alter HJ, Visnich S: A "new" antigen in leukemia sera. JAMA 191:541, 1965
3. Prince AM: An antigen detected in the blood during the incubation period of serum hepatitis. Proc Natl Acad Sci U S A 60:814, 1968
4. Feinstone SM, Kapikian AZ, Purcell RH: Hepatitis A: detection by immune electron microscopy of a virus-like antigen association with acute illness. Science 182:1026, 1973
5. Gravelle CR, Hornbeck CL, Maynard JE, Schable CA, Cook EH, Bradley DW: Hepatitis A: report of a common-source outbreak with recovery of a possible etiologic agent. II. Laboratory studies. J Infect Dis 131:167, 1975
6. Rizzetto M, Canese MC, Arico S, et al: Immunofluorescence detection of a new antigen-antibody system (delta/anti-delta) associated to the hepatitis B virus in the liver and in the serum of HBsAg carriers. Gut 18:997, 1977
7. Rizzetto M, Canese MC, Gerin JL, London WT, Sly ID, Purcell RH: Transmission of the hepatitis B virus associated delta antigen to chimpanzees. J Infect Dis 141:590, 1980
8. Purcell RH, Walsh JH, Holland PV, et al: Seroepidemiological studies of transfusion-associated hepatitis. J Infect Dis 123:406, 1971
9. Alter MJ, Gerety RJ, Smallwood L, et al: Sporadic non-A, non-B hepatitis: frequency and epidemiology in an urban United States population. J Infect Dis 145:886, 1982

10. Choo QL, Kuo G, Weiner AJ, Overby LR, Bradley DW, Houghton M: Isolation of a cDNA clone derived from a bloodborne non-A, non-B viral hepatitis genome. Science 244:359, 1989
11. Melnick JL: A water-borne urban epidemic of hepatitis. In Hartman FW, LoGrippo GA, Matffer JG, Barron J (eds): Hepatitis Frontiers. Boston: Little, Brown, 1957
12. Reyes GR, Purdy MA, Kim JP, et al: Isolation of a cDNA from the virus responsible for enterically transmitted non-A, non-B hepatitis. Science 247:1335, 1990
13. Committee on Emerging Microbial Threats to Health: Factors in emergence. In Lederberg J, Shope RE, Oaks SCJ (eds): Emerging Infections: Microbial Threats to Health in the United States. Washington, DC: National Academy Press, 1992
14. Cromeans T, Nainan OV, Fields HA, Favorov MO, Margolis HS: Hepatitis A and E viruses. In Hui YH, Gorham JR, Mucell KD, Cliver DO (eds): Foodborne Disease Handbook. New York: Marcel Dekker, 1994
15. Lemon SM: Type A viral hepatitis: new developments in an old disease. N Engl J Med 313:1059, 1985
16. Nainan OV, Margolis HS, Robertson BH, Balayan M, Brinton MA: Sequence analysis of a new hepatitis A virus naturally infecting cynomolgus macaques (*Macaca fascicularis*). J Gen Virol 72:1685, 1991
17. Robertson BH, Jansen RW, Khanna B, et al: Genetic relatedness of hepatitis A virus strains recovered from different geographical regions. J Gen Virol 73:1365, 1992
18. Emerson SU, Tsarev SA, Govindarajan S, Shapiro M, Purcell RH: A simian strain of hepatitis A virus, AGM-27, functions as an attenuated vaccine for chimpanzees. J Infect Dis 173:592, 1996
19. Hadler SC, McFarland L: Hepatitis in day care centers: epidemiology and prevention. Rev Infect Dis 8:548, 1986
20. Benenson MW, Takafuji ET, Bancroft WH, Lemon SM, Callahan MO, Leach DA: A military community outbreak of hepatitis type A related to transmission in a child care facility. Am J Epidemiol 112:471, 1980
21. Centers for Disease Control and Prevention: Hepatitis Surveillance Report No. 56. Atlanta: Centers for Disease Control and Prevention, 1996
22. Akriviadis EA, Redeker AG: Fulminant hepatitis A in intravenous drug users with chronic liver disease. Ann Intern Med 110:838, 1989
23. Sjogren MH, Tanno H, Fay O, et al: Hepatitis A virus in stool during clinical relapse. Ann Intern Med 106:221, 1987
24. Carl M, Kantor PJ, Webster HM, Fields HA, Maynard JE: Excretion of hepatitis A virus in the stools of hospital patients. J Med Virol 9:125, 1982
25. Tassopoulos NC, Papaevangelou GJ, Ticehurst JR, Purcell RH: Fecal excretion of Greek strains of hepatitis A virus in patients with hepatitis A and in experimentally infected chimpanzees. J Infect Dis 154:231, 1986
26. Rosenblum LS, Villarino ME, Nainan OV, et al: Hepatitis A outbreak in a neonatal intensive care unit: risk factors for transmission and evidence of prolonged viral excretion among preterm infants. J Infect Dis 164:476, 1991
27. Centers for Disease Control and Prevention: Prevention of hepatitis A through active or passive immunization. Recommendations of the Advisory Committee on Immunization Practices. MMWR 45(RR-15):1, 1996
28. Hadler SC: Global impact of hepatitis A virus infection changing patterns. In Hollinger FB, Lemon SM, Margolis HS (eds): Viral Hepatitis and Liver Disease. Baltimore: Williams & Wilkins, 1991
29. Halliday ML, Kang Lai-Y, Zhou T, et al: An epidemic of hepatitis A attributable to the ingestion of raw clams in Shanghai, China. J Infect Dis 164:852, 1991
30. Shaw FE Jr, Sudman JH, Smith SM, et al: A community-wide epidemic of hepatitis A in Ohio. Am J Epidemiol 123:1057, 1986
31. Shaw FEJ, Shapiro CN, Welty TK, Dill W, Reddington J, Hadler SC: Hepatitis transmission among the Sioux Indians of South Dakota. Am J Public Health 80:1091, 1990
32. Williams R: Prevalence of hepatitis A virus antibody among Navajo school children. Am J Public Health 76:282, 1986
33. Bulkow LR, Wainwright RB, McMahon BJ, Middaugh JP, Jenkerson SA, Margolis HS: Secular trends in hepatitis A virus infection among Alaska Natives. J Infect Dis 168:1017, 1993
34. Shapiro C, Hadler S: Significance of hepatitis in children in day care. Semin Pediatr Infect Dis 1:270, 1990
35. Jackson LA, Stewart LK, Solomon S, et al: Risk of infection with hepatitis A, B, C, cytomegalovirus, varicella or measles among child care providers. Pediatr Infect Dis J 15:584, 1995
36. Corey L, Holmes KK: Sexual transmission of hepatitis A in homosexual men. N Engl J Med 302:435, 1980
37. Desenclos JA, Klontz KC, Wilder MH, Nainan OV, Margolis HS, Gunn RA: A multistate outbreak of hepatitis A caused by the consumption of raw oysters. Am J Public Health 81:1268, 1991
38. Rosenblum LS, Mirkin IR, Allen DT, Safford S, Hadler SC: A multifocal outbreak of hepatitis A traced to commercially distributed lettuce. Am J Public Health 80:1075, 1990
39. Niu MT, Polish LB, Robertson BH, et al: A multistate outbreak of hepatitis A associated with frozen strawberries. J Infect Dis 166:518, 1992
40. Steffen R, Kane MA, Shapiro CN, Billo N, Schoellhorn KJ, van Damme P: Epidemiology and prevention of hepatitis A in travelers. JAMA 272:885, 1994
41. Centers for Disease Control and Prevention: Hepatitis A among persons with hemophilia who received clotting factor concentrate—United States, September–December 1995. MMWR 45:29, 1996
42. Mah MW, Royce RA, Rathouz PJ, et al: Prevalence of hepatitis A antibodies in hemophiliacs: preliminary results from the Southeastern Delta Hepatitis Study. Vox Sang 67(Suppl 1):21, 1994
43. Winokur PL, Stapleton JT: Immunoglobulin prophylaxis for hepatitis A. Clin Infect Dis 14:580, 1992
44. Robertson BH, D'Hondt EH, Spelbring J, Tian HW, Krawczynski KZ, Margolis HS: Effect of postexposure vaccination in a chimpanzee model of hepatitis A virus infection. J Med Virol 43:249, 1994
45. Siegl G, Lemon SM: Recent advances in hepatitis A vaccine development. Virus Res 17:75, 1990
46. Innis BL, Snitbhan R, Kunasol P, et al: Protection against hepatitis A by an inactivated vaccine. JAMA 271:1328, 1994
47. Werzberger A, Mensch B, Kuter B, et al: A controlled trial of formalin-inactivated hepatitis A vaccine in healthy children. N Engl J Med 327:453, 1992
48. Centers for Disease Control and Prevention: Hepatitis A vaccination programs in communities with high rates of hepatitis A. MMWR 46:600, 1997
49. Tiollais P, Charnay P, Vyas GN: Biology of hepatitis B virus. Science 213:406, 1981
50. Kobayashi H, Tsuzuki M, Koshimuzu K, et al: Susceptibility of hepatitis B virus to disinfection or heat. J Clin Microbiol 20:214, 1984
51. Bancroft WH, Holland PH, Mazzur S, Courouce AM, Madalinski K: The geographical distribution of HBsAg subtypes. Bibl Haematol Basel 42:42, 1976
52. Brown JL, Carman WF, Thomas HC: The clinical significance of molecular variation within the hepatitis B virus genome. Hepatology 15:144, 1992
53. McMahon BJ, Alward WLM, Hall DB, et al: Acute hepatitis B virus infection: relation of age to the clinical expression of disease and subsequent development of the carrier state. J Infect Dis 151:599, 1985
54. Alward WLM, McMahon BJ, Hall DB, Heyward WL, Francis DP, Bender TR: The long-term serological course of asymptomatic hepatitis B virus carriers and the development of primary hepatocellular carcinoma. J Infect Dis 151:604, 1985

55. Beasley RP, Hwang L-Y: Overview on the epidemiology of hepatocellular carcinoma. In Hollinger FB, Lemon SM, Margolis HS (eds): Viral Hepatitis and Liver Disease. Baltimore: Williams & Wilkins, 1991, pp 532–535
56. Beasley RP: Hepatitis B virus. The major etiology of hepatocellular carcinoma. Cancer 61:1942, 1988
57. Margolis HS, Coleman PJ, Brown RE, Shiengold SH, Mast EE, Arevalo JA: Control of hepatitis B virus infection in the United States by routine infant vaccination: an economic analysis. JAMA 274:1201, 1995
58. McMahon BJ, Bender TR, Templin DW, et al: Vasculitis in Eskimos living in an area hyperendemic for hepatitis B. JAMA 244: 2180, 1980
59. Penna A, Chisari FV, Bertoletti A, et al: Cytotoxic T lymphocytes recognize an HLA-A2-restricted epitope within the hepatitis B virus nucleocapsid antigen. J Exp Med 174:1565, 1991
60. Centers for Disease Control: Hepatitis B virus: a comprehensive strategy for eliminating transmission in the United States through universal childhood vaccination. Recommendations of the Immunization Practices Advisory Committee (ACIP). MMWR 40:(RR), RR 13, 1–25, 1991
61. Hollinger FB, Dienstag JL: Hepatitis viruses. In Lannete EH, Balows A, Hausler WH Jr, Shadomy HJ (eds): Manual of Clinical Microbiology. 4th ed. Washington, DC: American Society for Microbiology, 1985
62. Chau KH, Hargie MP, Decker RH, Mushahwar IK, Overby LR: Serodiagnosis of recent hepatitis B virus infection by IgM class anti-HBc. Hepatology 3:142, 1983
63. Maynard JE, Kane MA, Hadler SC: Global control of hepatitis B through vaccination: role of hepatitis B vaccine in the Expanded Programme on Immunization. Rev Infect Dis 11:s574, 1989
64. Schreeder MT, Bender TR, McMahon BJ, et al: Prevalence of hepatitis B in selected Alaskan Eskimo villages. Am J Epidemiol 118:543, 1983
65. Franks AL, Berg CJ, Kane MA, et al: Hepatitis B infection among children born in the United States to southeast Asian refugees. N Engl J Med 321:1301, 1989
66. Polish LB, Shapiro CN, Bauer F, et al: Nosocomial transmission of hepatitis B virus associated with a spring-loaded fingerstick device. N Eng J Med 326:721, 1992
67. Alter MJ, Hadler SC, Margolis HS, et al: The changing epidemiology of hepatitis B in the United States; need for alternative vaccination strategies. JAMA 263:1218, 1990
68. Stevens CE, Neurath RA, Beasley RP, Szmuness W: HBeAg and anti-HBe detection by radioimmunoassay: correlation of verticle transmission of hepatitis B virus in Taiwan. J Med Virol 3:237, 1979
69. Xu ZY, Liu CB, Francis DP, et al: Prevention of perinatal acquisition of hepatitis B virus carriage using vaccine: preliminary report of a randomized double-blind placebo-controlled and comparative trial. Pediatrics 76:713, 1985
70. Lee S-D, Lo K-J, Wu J-C, et al: Prevention of maternal-infant hepatitis B transmission by immunization: The role of serum hepatitis B virus DNA. Hepatology 6:369, 1986
71. Beasley RP, Hwang L-Y: Postnatal infectivity of hepatitis B surface antigen-carrier mothers. J Infect Dis 147:185, 1983
72. Petersen NJ, Barrett DH, Bond WH, et al: Hepatitis B surface antigen in saliva, impetiginous lesions, and the environment in two remote Alaskan villages. Appl Environ Microbiol 32:572, 1976
73. Hadler SC, Doto IL, Maynard JE, et al: Occupational risk of hepatitis B infection in hospital workers. Infect Control 6:24, 1985
74. Shapiro CN: Occupational risk of infection with hepatitis B and hepatitis C viruses. Surg Clin North Am 75:1047, 1995
75. Woodruff BA, Moyer LA, O'Rourke KM, Margolis HS: Blood exposure and risk of hepatitis B virus infection in firefighters. J Occup Med 35:1048, 1993
76. Lettau L, McCarthy JG, Smith MH, et al: An outbreak of severe hepatitis due to delta and hepatitis B viruses in parenteral drug abusers and their contacts. N Engl J Med 317:1256, 1987
77. Centers for Disease Control and Prevention: Outbreaks of hepatitis B virus infection among hemodialysis patients—California, Nebraska, and Texas, 1994. MMWR 45:285, 1996
78. Harpaz R, Von Seidlein L, Averhoff FM, et al: Transmission of hepatitis B virus to multiple patients from a surgeon without evidence of inadequate infection control. N Engl J Med 334:549, 1996
79. Tassopoulos NC, Papaevangelou GJ, Sjogren MH, Roumeliotou-Karayannis A, Gerin JL, Purcell RH: Natural history of acute hepatitis B surface antigen-positive hepatitis in Greek adults. Gastroenterology 92:1844, 1987
80. Centers for Disease Control and Prevention: Recommendations of the International Task Force for Disease Eradication. MMWR 42(No. RR-16):12, 1993
81. Sitrin RD, Wampler DE, Ellis RW: Survey of licensed hepatitis B vaccines and their production processes. In Ellis RW (ed): Hepatitis B Vaccines in Clinical Practice. New York: Marcel Dekker, 1993
82. Hadler SC, Margolis HS: Hepatitis B immunization: vaccine types, efficacy, and indications for immunization. In Remington JS, Swartz MN (eds): Current Clinical Topics in Infectious Diseases. Boston: Blackwell Scientific Publications, 1990, vol 12
83. World Health Organization: Progress in the control of viral hepatitis: memorandum from a WHO meeting. Bull WHO 66:443, 1988
84. World Health Assembly: Immunization and Vaccine Quality. Agenda Item 18 Document WHA 45.17. Forty-fifth World Health Assembly, Geneva
85. Andre FE, Zuckerman AJ: Review: protective efficacy of hepatitis B vaccines in neonates. J Med Virol 44:144, 1994
86. Hadler SC, Margolis HS: Epidemiology of hepatitis B virus infection. In Ellis RW (ed): Hepatitis B Vaccines in Clinical Practice. New York: Marcel Dekker, 1993
87. Xu ZY, Margolis HS: Determinants of hepatitis B vaccine efficacy and implications for vaccination strategies. In Wen YM, Xu ZY, Melnick JL (eds): Viral Hepatitis in China: Problems and Control Strategies. Monographs in Virology. Basel: Karger, 1992, vol 19
88. Chen D-S: Control of hepatitis B in Asia: mass immunization program in Taiwan. In Hollinger FB, Lemon SM, Margolis HS (eds): Viral Hepatitis and Liver Disease. Baltimore: Williams & Wilkins, 1991
89. Mahoney FJ, Woodruff BA, Erben JJ, et al: Effect of hepatitis B vaccination program on the prevalence of hepatitis B virus infection. J Infect Dis 167:203, 1993
90. Chotard J, Inskip HM, Hall AJ, et al: The Gambia hepatitis intervention study: follow-up of a cohort of children vaccinated against hepatitis B. J Infect Dis 166:764, 1992
91. Chang MH, Chen CJ, Lai MS, et al: Universal hepatitis B vaccination in Taiwan and the incidence of hepatocellular carcinoma in children. N Engl J Med 336:1855, 1997
92. Mahoney FJ, Lawrence M, Scott C, Le Q, Lambert S, Farley TA: Continuing risk of hepatitis B virus transmission among Southeast Asian infants in Louisiana. Pediatr 96:1113, 1995
93. Centers for Disease Control and Prevention: Status report on the Childhood Immunization Initiative: national, state, and urban area vaccination coverage levels among children aged 19–35 months—United States, 1996. MMWR 46:657, 1997
94. Centers for Disease Control and Prevention: Update: Recommendations to prevent hepatitis B virsus transmission—United States. MMWR 44:574, 1995
95. Perrillo RP, Schiff ER, Davis GL: A randomized controlled trial of interferon alfa-2b alone and after prednisone withdrawal for the treatment of chronic hepatitis B. N Engl J Med 323:295, 1990
96. Centers for Disease Control: Public Health Service interagency guidelines for screening donors of blood, plasma, organs, tissues

and semen for evidence of hepatitis B and hepatitis C. MMWR 40 (RR-4):1, 1991
97. Bukh J, Miller RH, Purcell RH: Genetic heterogeneity of hepatitis C virus: quasispecies and genotypes. Semin Liver Dis 15:41, 1995
98. Purcell RH: Hepatitis C virus: historical perspective and current concepts. FEMS Microbiol Rev 14:181, 1994
99. Bradley DW, Beach MJ, Purdy MA: Recent developments in the molecular cloning and characterization of hepatitis C and E viruses. Microb Pathog 12:391, 1992
100. Krawczynski K, Beach MJ, Bradley DW, et al: Hepatitis C virus antigen in hepatocytes: immunomorphologic detection and identification. Gastroenterology 103:622, 1992
101. Koretz RL, Brezina M, Polito AJ, et al: Non-A, non-B posttransfusion hepatitis: comparing C and non-C hepatitis. Hepatology 17:361, 1993
102. Marranconi F, Mecenero V, Pellizzer GP, et al: HCV infection after accidental needlestick injury in health-care workers. Infection 20: 111, 1992
103. Aach RD, Stevens CE, Hollinger FB, et al: Hepatitis C virus infection in post-transfusion hepatitis. An analysis with first- and second-generation assays. N Engl J Med 325:1325, 1991
104. Negro F, Pacchioni D, Shimizu Y, et al: Detection of intrahepatic replication of hepatitis C virus RNA by in situ hybridization and comparison with histopathology. Proc Natl Acad Sci U S A 89:2247, 1992
105. Alter MJ, Margolis HS, Krawczynski K, et al: The natural history of community-acquired hepatitis C in the United States. N Engl J Med 327:1899, 1992
106. Seef LB, Buskell-Bales Z, Wright EC, et al: Long-term mortality after tranfusion associated non-A, non-B hepatitis. N Engl J Med 327:1992, 1992
107. Alter MJ: Epidemiology of hepatitis C in the West. Semin Liver Dis 15:5, 1995
108. Koretz RL, Abbey H, Coleman E, et al: Non-A, non-B post-transfusion hepatitis: looking back in the second decade. Ann Intern Med 119:110, 1993
109. Di Bisceglie AM, Goodman ZD, Ishak KG, et al: Long-term clinical and histopathological follow-up of chronic posttransfusion hepatitis. Hepatology 14:969, 1991
110. Conry-Cantilena C, VanRaden M, Gibble J, et al: Routes of infection, viremia, and liver disease in blood donors found to have hepatitis C virus infection. N Engl J Med 334:1691, 1996
111. Crowe J, Doyle C, Feilding JF, et al: Presentation of hepatitis C in a unique uniform cohort 17 years from inoculation. Gastroenterology 108:A1054, 1995
112. Yu MC, Tong MJ, Coursaget P, Ross RK, Govindarajan S, Henderson BE: Prevalence of hepatitis B and C viral markers in black and white patients with hepatocellular carcinoma in the United States. J Natl Cancer Inst 82:1038, 1990
113. Kaklamani E, Trichopoulos D, Tzonou A, et al: Hepatitis B and C viruses and their interaction in the origin of hepatocellular carcinoma. JAMA 265:1974, 1991
114. Agnello V, Chung RT, Kaplan LM: A role for hepatitis C virus infection in type II cryoglobulinemia. N Engl J Med 327:1490, 1992
115. Johnson RJ, Gretch DR, Yamabe H, et al: Membranoproliferative glomerulonephritis associated with hepatitis C virus infection. N Engl J Med 328:465, 1993
116. Fargion S, Piperno A, Cappellini MD, et al: Hepatitis C virus and porphyria cutanea tarda: evidence of a strong association. Hepatology 16:1322, 1992
117. Farci P, Alter HJ, Govindarajan S, et al: Lack of protective immunity against reinfection with hepatitis C virus. Science 258:135, 1992
118. Farci P, Alter HJ, Wong DC, et al: Prevention of hepatitis C virus infection in chimpanzees after antibody-mediated in vitro neutralization. Proc Natl Acad Sci U S A 91:7792, 1994
119. Krawczynski K, Alter MJ, Tankersley DL, et al: Effect of immune globulin on the prevention of experimental hepatitis C virus infection. J Infect Dis 173:822, 1996
120. Farci P, Orgiana G, Purcell RH: Immunity elicited by hepatitis C virus. Clin Exp Rheumatol 13 (Suppl 13):S9, 1995
121. Alter MJ: The detection, transmission, and outcome of hepatitis C virus infection. Infect Agents Dis 2:155, 1993
122. Alter MJ: Review of serologic testing for hepatitis C virus infection and risk of posttransfusion hepatitis C. Arch Pathol Lab Med 118: 342, 1994
123. Gretch DR, delaRosa C, Carithers RL Jr, Willson RA, Williams B, Corey L: Assessment of hepatitis C viremia using molecular amplification technologies: correlations and clinical implications. Ann Intern Med 123:321, 1995
124. Damen M, Cuypers HT, Zaaijer HL, et al: International collaborative study on the second EUROHEP HCV-RNA reference panel. J Med Virol 58:175, 1996
125. Alter MJ, Gallagher M, Morris TT, et al: Acute non-A-E hepatitis in the United States and the role of hepatitis G virus infection. N Engl J Med 336:741, 1997
126. Bresee JS, Mast EE, Coleman PJ, et al: Hepatitis C virus infection associated with administration of intravenous immune globulin. JAMA 276:1563, 1996
127. Garfein RS, Vlahov D, Galai N, Doherty MC, Nelson KE: Viral infections in short-term injection drug users: the prevalence of hepatitis C, hepatitis B, human immunodeficiency and human T-lymphotropic viruses. Am J Public Health 86:655, 1996
128. Shapiro CN, Tokars JI, Chamberland ME, American Academy of Orthopedic Surgeons Serosurvey Study Committee: Use of hepatitis-B vaccine and infection with hepatitis B and C among orthopaedic surgeons. J Bone Joint Surg 78-A:1791, 1996
129. Hagan H, Jarlais DC, Friedman SR, Purchase D, Alter MJ: Reduced risk of hepatitis B and hepatitis C among injection drug users in the Tacoma syringe exchange program. Am J Public Health 85:1531, 1995
130. National Institutes of Health: National Institutes of Health Consensus Development Conference Statement on Management of Hepatitis C, March 24–27, 1997. Bethesda, MD: National Institutes of Health, 1997
131. Bonino F, Hoyer BH, Shih JW, Rizzetto M, Purcell RH, Gerin JL: Delta hepatitis agent: structural and antigenic properties of the delta associated particle. Infect Immun 43:1000, 1984
132. Polish LB, Gallagher M, Fields HA, Hadler SC: Delta hepatitis. Molecular biology and clinical and epidemiological features. Clin Microbiol Rev 6:211, 1993
133. Wang K-S: Structure, sequence and expression of the hepatitis delta viral genome. Nature 323:508, 1986
134. Smedile A, Farci P, Verme G, et al: Influence of delta infection on the severity of hepatitis B. Lancet 2:9, 1982
135. Rizzetto M, Verme G, Recchia S, et al: Chronic hepatitis in carriers of hepatitis B surface antigen with intrahepatic expression of the delta antigen. An active and progressive disease unresponsive to immunosuppressive treatment. Ann Intern Med 8:437, 1981
136. Maynard JE, Hadler SC, Fields HA: Delta hepatitis in the Americas: an overview. Prog Clin Biol Res 234:493, 1986
137. Ponzetto A, Forzani B, Parravicini PP, Hele C, Zanetti A, Rizzetto M: Epidemiology of delta virus infection. Eur J Epidemiol 1:257, 1986
138. Hadler SC, De Monson M, Ponzetto A, et al: Delta virus infection and severe hepatitis. An epidemic in the Yucpa Indians of Venezuela. Ann Intern Med 100:339, 1984
139. Hoofnagle JH, Di Bisceglie AM: Therapy of chronic delta hepatitis: overview. In Hadziyannis SJ, Taylor JM, Bonino F (eds): Hepatitis Delta Virus. Molecular Biology, Pathogenesis, and Clinical Aspects. New York: Wiley-Liss, 1993
140. Van Thiel DH, Faginoli S, Wright HI: Liver transplantation and viral hepatitis: the current situation. In Hadziyannis SJ, Taylor JM,

Bonino F (eds): Hepatitis Delta Virus. Molecular Biology, Pathogenesis and Clinical Aspects. New York: Wiley-Liss, 1993
141. Wong DC, Purcell RH, Sreenivasan MA, Prasad SR, Pavri KM: Epidemic and endemic hepatitis in India: evidence for non-A/non-B hepatitis virus etiology. Lancet 2:876, 1980
142. Mast EE, Purdy MA, Krawczynski K: Hepatitis E. Baillieres Clin Gastroenterol 10:227, 1996
143. Bradley DW, Krawczynski K, Beach MJ, Purdy MA: Non-A, non-B hepatitis: toward the discovery of hepatitis C and E viruses. Semin Liver Dis 11:128, 1991
144. Balayan MS, Andjaparidze AG, Savinskaya SS, et al: Evidence for a virus in non-A, non-B hepatitis transmitted via the fecal-oral route. Intervirology 20:23, 1983
145. Bradley DW, Krawczynski K, Cook EH Jr, et al: Enterically transmitted non-A, non-B hepatitis: serial passage of disease in cynomolgus macaques and tamarins, and recovery of disease-associated 27 to 34 nm viruslike particles. Proc Natl Acad Sci U S A 84:6277, 1987
146. De Cock KM, Bradley DW, Sandford NL, Govindarajan S, Maynard JE, Redeker AG: Epidemic non-A, non-B hepatitis in patients from Pakistan. Ann Intern Med 106:227, 1987
147. Krawczynski K, Bradley DW: Enterically transmitted non-A, non-B hepatitis: identification of virus-associated antigen in experimentally infected cynomolgus macaques. J Infect Dis 159:1042, 1989
148. Centers for Disease Control: Enterically transmitted non-A, non-B hepatitis—East Africa. MMWR 36:241, 1987
149. Kane MA, Bradley DW, Shrestha SM, et al: Epidemic non-A, non-B hepatitis in Nepal: recovery of a possible etiologic agent and transmission studies to marmosets. JAMA 252:3140, 1984
150. Centers for Disease Control: Enterically transmitted non-A, non-B hepatitis—Mexico. MMWR 36:597, 1987
151. Joshi YK, Baku S, Sarin S, Tandon BN, Gandhi BM, Chaturvedi VC: Immunoprophylaxis of epidemic non-A, non-B hepatitis. Indian J Med Res 81:18, 1985
152. Tsarev SA, Tsareva TS, Emerson SU, et al: Successful passive and active immunization of cynomolgus monkeys against hepatitis E. Proc Natl Acad Sci U S A 91:10198, 1994
153. Purdy M, McCaustland K, Krawczynski K, et al: An expressed recombinant HEV protein that protects cynomologus macaques against challenge with wild-type hepatitis E virus. In: Immunobiology and Pathogenesis of Persistent Virus Infections. Amsterdam: Elsevier Science Publishers, 1992
154. Simons JN, Leary TP, Dawson GJ, et al: Isolation of novel virus-like sequences associated with human hepatitis. Nat Med 1:564, 1995
155. Linnen J, Wages J Jr, Zhang-Keck Z-Y, et al: Molecular cloning and disease association of hepatitis G virus: a transfusion-transmissible agent. Science 271:505, 1996
156. Alter MJ, Hadler SC, Judson FN, et al: Risk factors for acute non-A, non-B hepatitis in the United States and association with hepatitis C virus infection. JAMA 264:2231, 1990

Aseptic Meningitis

1. Tunkel AR, Scheld MW: Acute meningitis. In Mandell GL, Bennett JE, Dolin R (eds): Mandell, Douglas, and Bennett's Principles and Practices of Infectious Diseases. New York: Churchill Livingstone, 1995, pp 831–865
2. Rotbart HA: Viral meningitis and the aseptic meningitis syndrome. In Scheld WM, Whitley RJ, Durack DT (eds): Infections of the Central Nervous System. New York: Raven Press, 1991, pp 19–40
3. Nicolosi A, Hauser WA, Beghi E, Kurland LT: Epidemiology of central nervous system infections in Olmstead County, Minnesota, 1950–1981. J Infect Dis 154:399–408, 1986
4. Rotbart HA: Enteroviral infections of the central nervous system. Clin Infect Dis 20:971–981, 1995
5. Berlin LE, Rorabaug ML, Heldrich F, Roberts K, Doran T, Modlin JF: Aseptic meningitis in infants <2 years of age: diagnosis and etiology. J Infect Dis 168:888–892, 1993
6. Modlin JF: Coxsackieviruses, echoviruses, and newer enteroviruses. In Mandell GL, Bennett JE, Dolin R (eds): Mandell, Douglas, and Bennett's Principles and Practices of Infectious Diseases. New York: Churchill Livingstone, 1995, pp 1620–1636
7. Melnick JL: Enteroviruses: polioviruses, coxsackieviruses, echoviruses, and newer enteroviruses. In Fields BN, Knipe DM, Howley PM (eds): Fields Virology. Philadelphia: Lippincott-Raven, 1996, pp 655–712
8. Yin-Murphy M: Acute hemorrhagic conjunctivitis. Prog Med Virol 29:23–44, 1984
9. Modlin JF: Picornaviridae. Introduction. In Mandell GL, Bennett JE, Dolin R (eds): Mandell, Douglas, and Bennett's Principles and Practices of Infectious Diseases. New York: Churchill Livingstone, 1995, pp 1606–1614
10. Strikas RA, Anderson LJ, Parker RA: Temporal and geographic patterns of isolates of nonpolio enteroviruses in the United States, 1970–1986. J Infect Dis 153:346–351, 1986
11. Kogan A, Spigland I, Frothingham TE, Elveback L, Williams C, Hall CE, Fox JP: The virus watch program. A continuing surveillance of viral infections in metropolitan New York families. Am J Epidemiol 89:51–61, 1969
12. Garner J, Hospital Infection Control Practices Advisory Committee: Guideline for isolation precautions in hospitals. Infect Control Hosp Epidemiol 17:53–80, 1996

Epstein-Barr Virus and Infectious Mononucleosis

1. Kieff E: Epstein-Barr virus and its replication. In Fields BN, Knipe DM, Howley PM (eds): Fields Virology. Philadelphia: Lippincott-Raven, 1996, pp 2343–2396
2. Rickinson AB, Kieff E: Epstein-Barr virus. In Fields BN, Knipe DM, Howley PM (eds): Fields Virology. Philadelphia: Lippincott-Raven, 1996, pp 2397–2446
3. Straus SE, Cohen JI, Tosato G, Meier JL: Epstein-Barr virus infections: biology, pathogenesis, and management. Ann Intern Med 188:45–58, 1993
4. Straus SE, Fleisher GR: Infectious mononucleosis epidemiology and pathogenesis. In Schlossberg D (ed): Infectious Mononucleosis. New York: Springer-Verlag, 1989, pp 2–28
5. Sawyer RN, Evans AS, Niederman JC, et al: Prospective studies of a group of Yale University freshmen. I. Occurrence of infectious mononucleosis. J Infect Dis 123:263–270, 1971
6. Hallee TJ, Evans AS, Niederman JC, et al: Infectious mononucleosis at the United States Military Academy. Yale J Biol Med 47: 182–195, 1974
7. Henke GE, Kurland LT, Elveback LR: Infectious mononucleosis in Rochester Minn., 1950–1969. Am J Epidemiol 98:483, 1973
8. Heath CW, Brodsky AL, Potolsky AI: Infectious mononucleosis in a general population. Am J Epidemiol 95:46–52, 1972
9. Schooley RT: Epstein-Barr virus (infectious mononucleosis). In Mandell GL, Bennett JE, Dolin R (eds): Mandell, Douglas, and Bennett's Principles and Practices of Infectious Diseases. New York: Churchill Livingstone, 1995, pp 1364–1377
10. Strauch B, Siega N, Andrews LL, et al: Oropharyngeal excretion of Epstein-Barr virus by renal transplant recipients and other patients treated with immunosuppressive drugs. Lancet 1:234–237, 1974
11. Chervenick PA: Infectious mononucleosis: the classical clinical syndrome. In Schlossberg D (ed): Infectious Mononucleosis. New York: Springer-Verlag, 1989, pp 29–34
12. Meier JL: Epstein-Barr virus and other causes of the infectious mononucleosis syndrome. In Schlossberg D (ed): Current Therapy of Infectious Disease. St. Louis: Mosby-Year Book, 1996, pp 488–494

13. Garner J, Hospital Infection Control Practices Advisory Committee: Guideline for isolation precautions in hospitals. Infect Control Hosp Epidemiol 17:53–80, 1996

Herpes Simplex Virus

1. Whitley RJ: Herpes simplex virus. In Fields BN, Knipe DM, Howley PM, et al (eds): Fields Virology. Philadelphia: Lippincott-Raven, 1996, p 2297
2. Nahmias AJ, Lee FK, Bechman-Nahmias S: Sero-epidemiological and sociological patterns of herpes simplex virus infection in the world. Scand J Infect Dis 69:19, 1990
3. Whitley RJ: Herpes simplex virus. In Scheld WM, Whitley RJ, Durack DT (eds): Infections of the Central Nervous System. Philadelphia: Lippincott-Raven, 1996, p 73
4. Corey L, Spear P: Infections with herpes simplex virus. N Engl J Med 314:749, 1986
5. Wald A, Zeh J, Barnum G, et al: Suppression of subclinical shedding of herpes simplex virus type 2 with acyclovir. Ann Intern Med 124:8, 1996
6. Whitley RJ, Schlitt M: Encephalitis caused by herpesviruses, including B virus. In Scheld WM, Whitley RJ, Durack DT (eds): Infections of the Central Nervous System. New York: Raven Press, 1991, p 41
7. Lakeman FD, Whitley RJ, National Institute of Allergy and Infectious Disease CASG: Diagnosis of herpes simplex encephalitis: application of polymerase chain reaction to cerebrospinal fluid from brain biopsied patients and correlation with disease. J Infect Dis 171:857, 1995
8. Scott LL, Sanchez PJ, Jackson GL, et al: Acyclovir suppression to prevent cesarean delivery after first-episode genital herpes. Obstet Gynecol 87:69, 1996

Cytomegalovirus Infections

1. Weller TH: The cytomegaloviruses: ubiquitous agents with protean clinical maninfestations. N Engl J Med 285:203–214, 267–274, 1971
2. Ho M: Cytomegalovirus: Biology and Infection. New York: Plenum, 1982
3. Drew WL: Cytomegalovirus infection in patients with AIDS. J Infect Dis 158:449–456, 1988
4. Alford CA, Britt WJ: Cytomegalovirus. In Fields BN, Knipe DM, et al (eds): Virology. 2nd ed. New York: Raven Press, 1990
5. Demmler G: Summary of a workshop on surveillance for congenital cytomegalovirus disease. Rev Infect Dis 13:315–329, 1991
6. Stagno S, Pass RF, Cloud GA, et al: Primary cytomegalovirus infection in pregnancy. Incidence, transmission to fetus, and clinical outcome. JAMA 256:1904–1908, 1986
7. Pass RF, Stagno S, Myers GT, et al: Outcome of symptomatic congenital cytomegalovirus infection: results of long-term longitudinal follow-up. Pediatrics 66:758–762, 1980
8. Sohn YM, Oh MK, Balcarek KB, et al: Cytomegalovirus infection in sexually active adolescents. J Infect Dis 163:460–463, 1991
9. Chou S: Acquisition of donor strains of cytomegalovirus by renal transplant recipients. N Engl J Med 314:1418–1423, 1986
10. Bale JF Jr, Petheram SJ, Souza IE, Murph JR: Cytomegalovirus reinfection in young children. J Pediatr 128:347–352, 1996
11. Tegtmeirer GE: Transfusion-transmitted cytomegalovirus infections: significance and control. Vox Sang 51 (Suppl 1):22–30, 1986
12. Kealey GP, Rosenquist MD, Lewis RW, Strauss R, Bale JF Jr: Skin allograft transmission of cytomegalovirus to burn patients. J Am Coll Surg 182:201–205, 1996
13. The TH, van der Bij W, van der Berg AP, van der Giessen M, Weits J, et al: Cytomegalovirus antigenemia. Rev Infect Dis 12:S737–S744, 1990
14. Spector SA, Hsia K, Wolf D, Shinkai M, Smith I: Molecular detection of human cytomegalovirus and determination of genotypic ganciclovir resistance in clinical specimens. Clin Infect Dis 21 (Suppl 2): S170–S173, 1995
15. Chou S: Differentiation of cytomegalovirus strains by restriction analysis of DNA sequences amplified from clinical specimens. J Infect Dis 162:738–742, 1990
16. Plotkin SA, Friedman HM, Fleisher GR, et al: Towne-vaccine induced prevention of cytomegalovirus disease after renal transplantation. Lancet 1:528–530, 1984
17. Hutto C, Little EA, Ricks R, et al: Isolation of cytomegalovirus from toys and hands in a day care center. J Infect Dis 154:527–530, 1986
18. Andersen RD, Bale JF Jr, Blackman JA, Murph JR: Infections in Children. 2nd ed. Rockville, MD: Aspen, 1994
19. Pass RF, August AN, Dworsky M, Reynolds DW: Cytomegalovirus infection in a day care center. N Engl J Med 307:477–479, 1982
20. Adler SP: Cytomegalovirus and child day care: evidence for an increased infection rate among day care workers. N Engl J Med 321: 1290–1296, 1989
21. Murph JR, Baron JC, Brown KC, Ebelhack CL, Bale JF Jr: The occupational risk of cytomegalovirus infection among day care providers. JAMA 265:602–608, 1991
22. Goodrich JM, Boeckh M, Bowden R: Strategies for the prevention of cytomegalovirus disease after marrow transplantation. Clin Infect Dis 19:287–298, 1994
23. Patel R, Snydman DR, Rubin RH, Ho M, Prescovitz M, Martin M, Paya CV: Cytomegalovirus prophylaxis in solid organ transplant recipients. Transplantation 61:1279–1289, 1996
24. Wittes JT, Kelly A, Plante KM: Meta-analysis of CMV-Ig studies for the prevention and treatment of CMV infection in transplant patients. Transplant Proc 28:1–8, 1996
25. Snydman DR, Werner GB, Heinze-Lacey B, et al: Use of cytomegalovirus immune globulin to prevent cytomegalovirus disease in renal transplant recipients. N Engl J Med 317:1049–1054, 1987
26. Crumpacker CS: Ganciclovir. N Engl J Med 335:721–729, 1996
27. Wagstaff AJ, Bryson HM: Foscarnet. Drugs 48:199–226, 1994
28. Balfour HH Jr, Chace BA, Stapleton JT, et al: A randomized, placebo controlled trial of oral acyclovir for the prevention of cytomegalovirus disease in recipients of renal allografts. N Engl J Med 320: 1381–1387, 1989
29. Verheyden JPH: Evolution of therapy for cytomegalovirus infection. Rev Infect Dis 10 (Suppl 3):S477–S489, 1988
30. Buhles WC, Mastre BJ, Tinker AJ, et al: Ganciclovir treatment of life or sight threatening cytomegalovirus infection: experience with 314 immunocompromised patients. Rev Infect Dis 10 (Suppl 3):S495–S506, 1988
31. Drew WL, Ives D, Lalezari JP, Crumpacker C, et al: Oral ganciclovir as maintenance treatment for cytomegalovirus retinitis in patients with AIDS. N Engl J Med 333:615–620, 1995
32. Emanuel D, Cunningham I, Jules-Elysee K, et al: Cytomegalovirus pneumonia after bone marrow transplantation successfully treated with the combination of ganciclovir and high dose immune globulin. Ann Intern Med 109:777–782, 1988
33. Reed EC, Bowden RA, Dandliker PS, et al: Treatment of cytomegalovirus pneumonia with ganciclovir and intravenous cytomegalovirus immunoglobulin in patients with bone marrow transplants. Ann Intern Med 109:783–788, 1988
34. Nigro G, Scholz H, Bartmann U: Ganciclovir therapy for symptomatic congenital cytomegalovirus infection in infants: a two-regimen experience. J Pediatr 124:318–322, 1994
35. Jacobsen MA: Current management of cytomegalovirus disease in AIDS. AIDS Res Hum Retroviruses 10:917–923, 1994

Acute Gastrointestinal Infections

1. Dingle JH, Badger GF, Jordan WS Jr: Illness in the Home: a study of 25,000 Illnesses in a Group of Cleveland Families. Cleveland: The Press of Western Reserve University, 1964
2. Monto AS, Bryan ER, Rhodes LM: The Tecumseh study of respiratory illness. VII. Further observations on the occurrence of respiratory

syncytial virus and *Mycoplasma pneumonaie* infections. Am J Epidemiol 100:458, 1975
3. Brandt CK, Hyun WK, Rodriguez WJ, et al: Pediatric viral gastroenteritis during eight years of study. J Clin Microbiol 18:71, 1983
4. Takiff HE, Straus SE, Garon CF: Propagation and in vitro studies of previously noncultivable enteral adenoviruses in 293 cells. Lancet 2:832, 1981
5. Bishop RF, Davidson GP, Holmes IH, Ruck BJ: Virus particles in epithelial cells of duodenal mucosa from children with acute nonbacterial gastroenteritis. Lancet 2:1281, 1973
6. Flewett TH, Woode GN: The rotaviruses: brief review. Arch Virol 57:1, 1978
7. Yolken RH, Kim HW, Clem T, et al: Enzyme-linked immunosorbent assay (ELISA) for detection of human reovirus-like agent of infantile gastroenteritis. Lancet 1:263, 1977
8. Hall GH, Gridger JC, Chandler RL, Woode GN: Gnotobiotic piglets experimentally inoculated with neonatal calf diarrhea reovirus-like agent (rotavirus). Vet Pathol 13:197, 1976
9. Murphy AM, Albrey MB, Crewe EB: Rotavirus infections of neonates. Lancet 2:1149, 1977
10. Mattion NM, Cohen J, Estes MK: The rotavirus proteins. In: Kapikian AZ (ed): Viral infections of the gastrointestinal tract. New York: Marcel Dekker, 1994, pp 169–249
11. Wang S, Cai R, Chen J, et al: Etiologic studies of the 1983 and 1984 outbreaks of epidemic diarrhea in Guangxi. Intervirology 24:140, 1985
12. Koopman JS, Turkish VJ, Monto AS, et al: Patterns and etiology of diarrhea in three clinical settings. Am J Epidemiol 119:114, 1984
13. Birch CJ, Lewis FA, Kennett ML, et al: A study of the prevalence of rotavirus infection in children with gastroenteritis admitted to an infectious diseases hospital. J Med Virol 1:69, 1977
14. Paniker CKJ, Mathew S, Dharmarajan R, et al: Epidemic gastroenteritis in children associated with rotavirus infection. Indian J Med Res 66:525, 1977
15. Kapikian AZ, Kim HW, Wyatt RG, et al: Human reovirus-like agent as the major pathogen associated with "winter" gastroenteritis in hospitalized infants and young children. N Engl J Med 294:965, 1976
16. Monto AS, Koopman JS, Longini IM, Isaacson RE: The Tecumseh study. XII. Enteric agents in the community. J Infect Dis 148:284, 1983
17. Kapikian AZ, Hoshino Y, Chanock RM, Perez-Schael I: Efficacy of a quadrivalent rhesus rotavirus-based human rotavirus vaccine aimed at preventing severe rotavirus diarrhea in infants and young children. J Infect Dis 174:S65–S72, 1996
18. Thornhill TS, Kalica AR, Wyatt RG, et al: Pattern of shedding of the Norwalk particle in stools during experimentally induced gastroenteritis in volunteers as determined by immune electron microscopy. J Infect Dis 132:28, 1975
19. Jiang X, Graham DY, Wang K, Estes MK: Norwalk virus genome cloning and characterization. Science 250:1580–1583, 1990
20. Dolin R, Blacklow NR, DuPont H, et al: Biological properties of Norwalk agent of acute infectious nonbacterial gastroenteritis. Proc Soc Exp Biol Med 140:578, 1972
21. Parker SP, Cubitt WD, Jiang X, Estes MK: Efficacy of a recombinant Norwalk virus protein enzyme immunoassay for the diagnosis of infection with Norwalk virus and other "candidate" caliciviruses. J Med Virol 41:108–118, 1993
22. Wyatt RG, Dolin R, Blacklow NR, et al: Comparison of three agents of acute infectious non-bacterial gastroenteritis by cross-challenge in volunteers. J Infect Dis 129:709, 1974
23. Thornhill TS, Wyatt RG, Kalica AR, et al: Detection by immune electron microscopy of 26- to 27-nm viruslike particles associated with two family outbreaks of gastroenteritis. J Infect Dis 135:20, 1977
24. Schreiber DS, Blacklow NR, Trier JS: The mucosal lesion of the proximal small intestine in acute infectious nonbacterial gastroenteritis. N Engl J Med 288:1318, 1973
25. Parrino TA, Schreiber KDS, Trier JS, et al: Clinical immunity in acute gastroenteritis caused by Norwalk agent. N Engl J Med 297:86, 1977

Trachoma and Inclusion Conjunctivitis

General References

Dawson CR, Jones BR, Darougar S: Blinding and non-blinding trachoma: assessment of intensity of upper tarsal inflammatory disease and disabling lesions. Bull World Health Organ 52:279–282, 1975

Jones BR: The prevention of blindness from trachoma. Trans Ophthalmol Soc UK 95:16–33, 1975

Schachter J: Chlamydial infections. N Engl J Med 298:428–435, 490–495, 540–549, 1978

Schachter J, Dawson CR: Human Chlamydial Infections. Littleton, MA: Publishing Sciences Group, 1978

Chlamydial Pneumonia

General References

Schachter J, Lum L, Gooding CA, Ostler B: Pneumonitis following inclusion blennorrhea. J Pediatr 87:779–780, 1975

Beem MO, Saxon EM: Respiratory-tract colonization and a distinctive pneumonia syndrome in infants infected with *Chlamydia trachomatis*. N Engl J Med 296:306–310, 1977

Harrison HR, English G, Lee K, Alexander R: *Chlamydia trachomatis* infant pneumonitis (comparison with matched controls and other infant pneumonitis). N Engl J Med 298(13):702–708, 1978

Schachter J: Chlamydial infections. N Engl J Med 298:428–435, 490–495, 540–549, 1978

Streptococcal Disease

1. Bronze MS, Dale JB: The reemergence of serious group A streptococcal infections and acute rheumatic fever. Am J Med Sci 311: 41–54, 1996
2. Krause RM: Symposium on relationship of structure of microorganisms to their immunologic properties. IV. Antigenic and biochemical composition of hemolytic streptococcal cell wall. Bacteriol Rev 27:369, 1963
3. Bessen DE, Sptor CM, Readdy TL, et al: Genetic correlates of throat and skin isolates of group A streptococci. J Infect Dis 173:896–900, 1996
4. Smith TD, Wilkinson V, Kaplan EL: Group A *Streptococcus*-associated upper respiratory tract infections in a day-care center. Pediatrics 83:380–384, 1989
5. Kaplan EL: The rapid identification of group A beta-hemolytic streptococci in the upper respiratory tract—current status. Pediatr Clin North Am 35:535–542, 1988
6. Davies HD, McGeer A, Schwartz B, et al: Invasive Group A streptococcal infections in Ontario, Canada. N Engl J Med 335:547–554, 1996
7. Kaplan EL, Johnson DR, Rehder CD: Recent changes in group A streptococcal serotypes from uncomplicated pharyngitis: a reflection of the changing of epidemiology of severe group A infections? J Infect Dis 170:1346–1347, 1994
8. Bisno AL, Stevens DL: Streptococcal infections of skin and soft tissue. N Engl J Med 334:240–245, 1996
9. Cone LA, Woodard DR, Schlievert PM, Tomory GS: Clinical and bacteriologic observations of a toxic shock-like syndrome due to *Streptococcus pyogenes*. N Engl J Med 317:146–149, 1987
10. Stevens DL, Tanner MH, Winship J, et al: Severe group A streptococcal infections associated with a toxic shock-like syndrome and scarlet fever A. Infectious Disease Service, Veterans Administration Medical Center, Boise, Idaho. N Engl J Med 321:1–7, 1989

11. Schwartz B, Facklam RR, Breiman RF: Changing epidemiology of group A streptococcal infection in the USA. Lancet 336:1167–1171, 1990
12. Taranta A, Markowitz M: Rheumatic Fever. 2nd ed. Boston: Kluwer Academic Publishers, 1989, p 87
13. Jackson H: Streptococcal control in grade schools. Am J Dis Child 130:273–279, 1976
14. Wilkinson HW: Group B streptococcal infection in humans. Annu Rev Microbiol 32:41–57, 1978
15. Baker CJ: Group B streptococcal infection in neonates: is prevention possible? South Med J 69:1527, 1976
16. Special Writing Group of the Committee on Rheumatic Fever, Endocarditis and Kawasaki Disease of the Council on Cardiovascular Disease in the Young of the American Heart Association: Guidelines for the diagnosis of rheumatic fever, Jones Criteria, 1992 update. JAMA 268:2069–2073, 1992
17. Markowitz M, Gordis L: Rheumatic Fever. 2nd ed. Philadelphia: WB Saunders, 1972, p 222
18. Gordis L, Lilienfeld A, Rodriguez R: Studies in the epidemiology and preventability of rheumatic fever. II. Socioeconomic factors in the incidence of acute attack. J Chronic Dis 21:655, 1969
19. Gordis L: Effectiveness of comprehensive-care programs in preventing fever. N Engl J Med 289:331–335, 1973
20. Gordis L: The virtual disappearance of rheumatic fever in the United States: lessons in the rise and fall of disease. T. Duckett Jones Memorial Lecture. Circulation 72:1155–1162, 1985
21. Bisno AL: The resurgence of rheumatic fever in the United States. Annu Rev Med 41:319–329, 1990
22. Veasy LG, Tani LY, Hill HR: Persistence of acute rheumatic fever in the intermountain area of the United States. J Pediatr 124:9–16, 1994

Meningococcal Disease

1. Frasch CE, Zollinger WD, Poolman JT: Proposed schema for identification of serotypes of Neisseria meningitidis. In Schoolnik GK (ed): The Pathogenic Neisseria. Washington DC: American Society for Microbiology, 1985, pp 519–524
2. Olyhoek T, Crowe BA, Achtman M: Clonal population structure of *Neisseria meningitidis* serogroup A isolated from epidemics and pandemics between 1915 and 1983. Rev Infect Dis 9:665–692, 1987
3. Jackson LA, Tenover FC, Baker C, et al: Prevalence of *Neisseria meningitidis* relatively resistant to penicillin in the United States, 1991. J Infect Dis 169:438–441, 1994
4. Quagliarello VJ, Scheld WM: Treatment of bacterial meningitis. N Engl J Med 336:708–716, 1997
5. Broome CV: The carrier state: *Neisseria meningitidis*. J Antimicrob Chemother 18 (Suppl A):25–34, 1986
6. Goldschneider I, Gotschlich EC, Artenstein MS: Human immunity to the meningococcus. I. The role of humoral antibodies. J Exp Med 129:1307–1326, 1969
7. Ghipponi P, Darrigol J, Skalova R, Cvjetanovic B: Study of bacterial air pollution in an arid region of Africa affected by cerebrospinal meningitis. Bull World Health Organ 45:95–101, 1971
8. Tappero JW, Reporter R, Wenger JD, et al: Meningococcal disease in Los Angeles County, California, and among men in the county jails. N Engl J Med 335:833–840, 1996
9. Riedo FX, Plikaytis BD, Broome CV: Epidemiology and prevention of meningococcal disease. Pediatr Infect Dis J 14:643–657, 1995
10. Blakebrough IS, Greenwood BM, Whittle HC: The epidemiology of infections due to *Neisseria meningitidis* and *Neisseria lactamica* in a Northern Nigerian community. J Infect Dis 146:626–637, 1982
11. Munford RS, Taunay ADE, Morais JS: Spread of meningococcal infection within households. Lancet 1:1275–1278, 1974
12. Greenfield S, Sheehe PR, Feldman HA: Meningococcal carriage in a population of "normal" families. J Infect Dis 123:67–73, 1971
13. Jackson LA, Wenger JD: Laboratory-based surveillance for meningococcal disease in selected areas, United States, 1989–1991. MMWR 42(SS-2):21–30, 1993
14. The Meningococcal Disease Surveillance Group: Analysis of endemic meigococcal disease by serogroup and evaluation of chemoprophylaxis. J Infect Dis 134:201–204, 1976
15. Jackson LA, Schuchat A, Reeves MW, Wenger JD: Serogroup C meningococcal outbreaks in the United States. An emerging threat. JAMA 273:383–389, 1995
16. Centers for Disease Control and Prevention: Serogroup B meningococcal disease—Oregon, 1994. MMWR 44:121–124, 1995
17. Fischer M, Perkins BA: *Neisseria meningitidis* serogroup B: emergence of the ET-5 complex. Seminars in Pediatric Infectious Diseases 8:50–56, 1997
18. Moore PS, Hierholzer J, DeWitt W, et al: Respiratory viruses and mycoplasma as cofactors for epidemic group A meningococcal meningitis. JAMA 264:1271–1275, 1990
19. Moore PS, Reeves MW, Schwartz B, Gellin BG, Broome CV: Intercontinental spread of an epidemic group A *Neisseria meningitidis* strain. Lancet 2:260–263, 1989
20. Pinner RW, Onyango F, Perkins BA, et al: Epidemic meningococcal disease in Nairobi, Kenya—1989. J Infect Dis 166:359–364, 1992
21. Centers for Disease Control and Prevention: Control and prevention of meningococcal disease: recommendations of the Advisory Committee on Immunization Practices (ACIP). MMWR 46:1–10, 1997
22. Artenstein MS, Gold R, Zimmerly JG, Wyle FA, Schneider H, Harkins C: Prevention of meningococcal disease by group C polysaccharide vaccine. N Engl J Med 282:417–420, 1970
23. Wahdan MH, Rizk R, El-Akkad AM: A controlled field trial of a serogroup A meningococcal polysaccharide vaccine. Bull World Health Organ 48:667–673, 1973
24. Peltola H, Makela PH, Kayhty H, et al: Clinical efficacy of meningococcus group A capsular polysaccharide vaccine in children three months to five years of age. N Engl J Med 297:686–691, 1977
25. Reingold AL, Broome CV, Hightower AW, et al: Age-specific differences in duration of clinical protection after vaccination with meningococcal polysaccharide A vaccine. Lancet 2:114–118, 1985
26. Centers for Disease Control and Prevention: Control and prevention of serogroup C meningococcal disease: evaluation and management of suspected outbreaks. MMWR 46:13–21, 1997
27. Greenwood BM, Hassan-King M, Whittle HC: Prevention of secondary cases of meningococcal disease in household contacts by vaccination. Br Med J 1:1317–1319, 1978
28. Lieberman JM, Chiu SS, Wong VK, et al: Safety and immunogenicity of a serogroups A/C *Neisseria meningitidis* oligosaccharide-protein conjugate vaccine in young children. JAMA 275:1499–1503, 1996
29. Twumasi PAJ, Kumah S, Leach A, et al: A trial of a group A plus group C meningococcal polysaccharide-protein conjugate vaccine in African infants. J Infect Dis 171:632–638, 1995
30. Leach A, Twumasi PA, Kumah S, et al: Induction of immunologic memory in Gambian children by vaccination in infancy with a Group A plus Group C meningococcal polysaccharide-protein conjugate vaccine. J Infect Dis 175:200–204, 1997
31. Sierra GVG, Campa HC, Varcacel NM, et al: Vaccine against group B *Neisseria meningitidis:* protection trial and mass vaccination results in Cuba. NIPH Annu 14:195–207, 1991
32. Bjune G, Hoiby EA, Gronnesby JK, et al: Effect of an outer membrane vesicle vaccine against group B meningococcal disease in Norway. Lancet 338:1093–1096, 1991
33. Boslego J, Garcia J, Cruz C, et al: Efficacy, safety, and immunogenicity of a meningococcal vaccine group B (15:P1.3) outer membrane protein vaccine in Iquique, Chile. Chilean National Committee for Meningococcal Disease. Vaccine 13:821–829, 1995

34. Moraes JC, Perkins BA, Camargo MCC, et al: Protective efficacy of a serogroup B meningococcal vaccine in Sao Paulo, Brazil. Lancet 340:1074–1078, 1992

Tuberculosis

1. Dubos R, Dubos J: The White Plague: Tuberculosis, Man, and Society. New Brunswick, NJ: Rutgers University Press, 1952
2. Wayne LG, Kubica L: Genus *Mycobacterium*. In Sneath (ed): Bergey's Manual of Systematic Bacteriology. vol 2. Baltimore: Williams & Wilkins, 1986
3. Zhang Y, Heym B, Allen B, Young D, Cole S: The catalase-proxidase gene and isoniazid resistance of *Mycobacterium tuberculosis*. Nature 358:591–593, 1992
4. Telenti A, Imboden P, Marchesi F, Lowrie D, Cole S, Colston MJ, et al: Detection of rifampicin-resistant mutations in *Mycobacterium tuberculosis*. Lancet 341:647–650, 1993
5. Iseman M, Madsen LA: Drug-resistant tuberculosis. Clin Chest Med 10:341–349, 1989
6. Pearson ML, Jereb JA, Frieden TR, Crawford JT, Davis BJ, Dooley SW, Jarvis WR: Nosocomial transmission of MDRTB: a risk to patients and health care workers. Ann Intern Med 117:191–196, 1992
7. Beck-Sague C, Dooley SW, Hutton MD, Otten J, Breeden A, Crawford JT, Pitchenik AE, Wookley C, Cauthen G, Jarvis WR: Hospital outbreak of multidrug resistant tuberculosis infections: factors in transmission to staff HIV related patients. JAMA 268:1280–1286, 1992
8. Wells WF, Ratcliffe HC, Crumb C: On the mechanics of droplet nucleii infection. Am J Hyg 47:11–28, 1948
9. Riley RL, Mills CC, Nyka W, Weinstock N, Storey PB, Sultan LU, Riley MC, Wells WF: Aerial dissemination of pulmonary tuberculosis. A two year study of contagion in a tuberculosis ward. Am J Hyg 70:185–196, 1959
10. Schlesinger LS: The role of mononuclear phagocytes in tuberculosis. In Lipscomb MF, Russell SW (eds): Lung Macrophages and Dendritic Cells in Health and Disease. New York: Marcel Dekker, 1997
11. Harmsen AG, Muggenburg BA, Snipes MB, Rice DE: The role of macrophages in particle translocation from the lungs to the lymph nodes. Science 230:1277–1280, 1985
12. Cooper AM, Flynn JL: The protective immune response in *Mycobacterium tuberculosis*. Curr Opin Immunol 7:512–516, 1995
13. American Thoracic Society, Centers for Disease Control and Prevention: Treatment of tuberculosis and tuberculosis infection in adults and children. Am J Respir Crit Care Med 149:1349–1374, 1994
14. Centers for Disease Control and Prevention: Nosocomial transmission of multidrug resistant tuberculosis among HIV-infected persons—Florida and New York, 1988–1991. MMWR 40:585–591, 1991
15. Edlin BR, Tokars JI, Grieco MH, Crawford JY, Williams J, Sordillo EM, Ong KR, Kilburn JO, Dooley SW, Castro KG, Jarvis WR, Holmberg SD: An outbreak of multidrug resistant tuberculosis among hospitalized patients with acquired immunodeficiency syndrome. N Engl J Med 326:1514–1521, 1992
16. Markowitz N, Hansen NI, Wilcosky TC, Hopewell PC, Glassroth J, Kvale PA, et al: Tuberculin and anergy testing in HIV-seropositive and -seronegative persons: Ann Intern Med 119:185–193, 1993
17. Comstock GW: Epidemiology of tuberculosis. Am Rev Respir Dis 125:8–15, 1982
18. Reider HL, Cauthen GM, Comstock GW, Snider DE: Epidemiology of tuberculosis in the United States. Epidemiol Rev 11:79–98, 1989
19. American Thoracic Society, Centers for Disease Control and Prevention: Control of tuberculosis in the United States. Am Rev Respir Dis 146:1623–1633, 1992
20. Braden CR: Infectiousness of a university student with laryngeal and cavitary tuberculosis. Clin Infect Dis 21:565–570, 1995
21. Riley RL, Mills CC, O'Grady F, Sultan LU, Wittstadt F, Shivpuri DN: Infectiousness of air from a tuberculosis ward. Ultraviolet irradiation of infected air: comparative infectiousness of different patients. Am Rev Respir Dis 85:511–525, 1962
22. Alland D, Kalkut BE, Moss AR, McAdam RA, Hahn JA, Bosworth W, Drucker E, Bloom BR: Transmission of tuberculosis in New York City. An analysis of DNA fingerprinting and conventional epidemiologic methods. N Engl J Med 330:1710–1716, 1994
23. Small PM, Hopewell PC, Singh SP, Paz A, Parsonnet J, Ruston DC, Schecter GV, Daley CL, Schoolnik GK: The epidemiology of tuberculosis in San Francisco. A population based study using conventional and molecular methods. N Engl J Med 330:1703–1709, 1994
24. Lippop KK, Kulmala K, Tal EOJ: Focusing on tuberculosis contact tracing by smear grading of index cases. Am Rev Respir Dis 148: 235–236, 1993
25. Grzybowski S, Barnett GD, Sylblo K: Contacts of cases of active pulmonary tuberculosis. Bull Int Union of Tuberculosis 50:92–106, 1975
26. Stead WW: Management of health care workers after inadvertent exposure to tuberculosis: a guide for the use of preventive therapy. Ann Intern Med 122:906–912, 1995
27. Chaisson RE, Slutkin G: Tuberculosis and human immunodeficiency virus. J Infect Dis 159:96–100, 1989
28. Centers for Disease Control and Prevention: Tuberculosis morbidity: United States, 1992. MMWR 42:696–704, 1993
29. Jones BE, Young SMM, Antoniskis D, Davidson PT, Kramer F, Barnes PF: Relationship of the manifestations of tuberculosis to CD4 cell counts in patients with human immunodeficiency virus infection. Am Rev Respir Dis 148:1292–1297, 1993
30. Yeager H, Racey J, Smith LR, Lemaistre CA: Quantitative studies of mycobacterial populations in sputum and saliva. Am Rev Respir Dis 95:998–1002, 1967
31. Hoppy GL, Holman AP, Iseman MD, Jones JM: Enumeration of tubercle bacilli in sputum of patients with pulmonary tuberculosis. Antimicrob Agents Chemother 4:94–99, 1973
32. Centers for Disease Control and Prevention: Nucleic acid amplification tests for tuberculosis. MMWR 45:950–952, 1996
33. Centers for Disease Control and Prevention: Screening for tuberculosis and tuberculosis infection in high risk populations. Recommendations of the advisory council for the elimination of tuberculosis (ACET). MMWR 44:19–34, 1995
34. American Thoracic Society, Centers for Disease Control: The tuberculin skin test. Am Rev Respir Dis 124:356–363, 1981
35. Centers for Disease Control and Prevention: The role of BCG vaccine in the prevention and control of tuberculosis in the United States. MMWR RR-45:1–18, 1996
36. Centers for Disease Control: Case definitions for public health surveillance. MMWR RR-39:39–40, 1990
37. Cohn DL, Catlin BJ, Peterson KL, Judson FN, Sbarbaro JA: A 62-dose, 6-month therapy for pulmonary and extra-pulmonary tuberculosis. Ann Intern Med 112:407–415, 1990
38. Combs DL, O'Brien RJ, Ctiter LJ: USPHS TB short-course chemotherapy trial 21: effectiveness, toxicity, and acceptability. The report of final results. Ann Intern Med 112:397–406, 1990
39. Brudney K, Dobkin J: Resurgent tuberculosis in New York City. Am Rev Respir Dis 144:745–749, 1991
40. Sbarbaro JA: Tuberculosis in the 1990s. Epidemiology and Therapeutic Challenge. Chest 108:58S–62S, 1995
41. Sumartojo E: When tuberculosis treatment fails. A social account of patient adherence. Am Rev Respir Dis 147:1311–1320, 1993
42. Weis SE, Slocum PC, Blais FX, King B, Nunn M, Matney GB, Gomez E, Foresman BH: The effect of directly observed therapy on

the rates of drug resistance and relapse in tuberculosis. N Engl J Med 330:1179–1184, 1994
43. Schleuger N, Cotoli C, Cohen D, Johnson J, Rom WN: Comprehensive tuberculosis control for patients at high risk for noncompliance. Am J Respir Crit Care Med 151:1486–1490, 1995
44. Ferebee SH, Mount FW: Tuberculosis morbidity in a controlled trial of the prophylactic use of isoniazid among household contacts. Am Rev Respir Dis 85:490–510, 1962
45. Markowitz N, Hansen NI, Hopewell PC, Glassroth J, Kvale PA, Mangura BY, Wilcosky TC, Wallace JM, Rosen MJ, Reichman LB: The pulmonary complications of HIV infection study group. Incidence of tuberculosis in the U.S. among HIV-infected persons. Ann Intern Med 126:123–132, 1997
46. Colditz GA, Brewer TF, Berkey CS, Wilson ME, Burdick E, Fineberg HV, Mosteller F: Efficacy of BCG vaccine in the prevention of tuberculosis. Meta-analysis of the published literature. JAMA 271:698–702, 1994
47. Rodriques LC, Diwan VK, Wheeler JG: Protective effect of BCG against tuberculosis meningitis and miliary tuberculosis. Int J Epidemiol 22:1154–1158, 1993
48. Bates JH, Stead WW: The history of tuberculosis as a global epidemic. Med Clin North Am 77:1205–1217, 1993
49. Salo WL, Aufderheide AC, Buikstra J, Holcomb TA: Identification of *Mycobacterium tuberculosis* DNA in pre-Columbian Peruvian mummy. Proc Natl Acad Sci 91:2091–2094, 1994
50. Allison MR, Medoza O, Pezziea A: Documentation of a case of tuberculosis in pre-Columbian Peruvian America. Am Rev Respir Dis 107:985–991, 1972
51. Blower SM, McLean AR, Porco TC, Small PM, Hopewell PC, Sanchez MA, et al: The intrinsic transmission dynamics of tuberculosis epidemics. Nature Med 1:815–821, 1995
52. Black FL: Infectious disease in primitive societies. Science 187: 515–518, 1975
53. Pinner M: Pulmonary Tuberculosis in the Adult: Its Fundamental Aspects. Springfield, IL: Charles C Thomas, 1945
54. Centers for Disease Control and Prevention: Expanded tuberculosis surveillance in tuberculosis morbidity—U.S., 1993. MMWR 43: 361–366, 1994
55. Centers for Disease Control: Tuberculosis morbidity: United States, 1990. MMWR 40:23–70, 1991
56. Centers for Disease Control and Prevention: Tuberculosis morbidity: United States, 1995. MMWR 45:365–369, 1996
57. Daley CS, Small PM, Schecter GF, Schoolnik GK, McAdam RA, Jacobs WR, Hopewell PC: An outbreak of tuberculosis with accelerated progression among persons infected with the human immunodeficiency virus: An analysis using restriction-fragment-linked polymorphisms. N Engl J Med 326:231–235, 1992
58. Selwyn PA, Hartekl D, Lewis VA, et al: A prospective study of the risk of tuberculosis among intravenous drug users with HIV infection. N Engl J Med 320:545–550, 1989
59. Bloom BR, Murray CJL: Tuberculosis: commentary on a reemergent killer. Science 257:1055–1064, 1992
60. HIV/AIDS Surveillance Report 1992. Atlanta: Centers for Disease Control, 1993
61. Cantwell MF, Snider DE, Cauthen GM, Onorato IM: Epidemiology of tuberculosis in the United States, 1985–1992. JAMA 272:535–539, 1994
62. Small PM, Shafer RW, Hopewell PC, Singh SP, Murphy MJ, Desmond E, Sierra MF, Schoolnik GK: Exogenous reinfection with multidrug resistant tuberculosis in patients with advanced HIV infection. N Engl J Med 328:1137–1144, 1993
63. Ben-Dov I, Mason GR: Drug-resistant tuberculosis in a Southern California hospital: trends from 1969 to 1984. Am Rev Respir Dis 135:1307–1310, 1987
64. Mahmoudi A, Iseman M: Pitfalls in the care of patients with tuberculosis. JAMA 270:265–268, 1993
65. Kopanoff DE, Snider DE, Johnson M: Recurrent tuberculosis: why do patients develop disease again? Am J Public Health 78:30–33, 1988
66. Peloquin CA, MacPhee AA, Berning SE: Malabsorption of antimycobacterial medications. N Engl J Med 329:1122–1123, 1993
67. Centers for Disease Control: Primary resistance to anti-tuberculosis drugs—United States. MMWR 32:521–522, 1983
68. Bloch AR, Cauthen GM, Onorato IM, Dansbury KG, Kelly GD, Driver CR, Snider DE: Nationwide survey of drug-resistant tuberculosis in the United States. JAMA 271:665–671, 1994
69. Frieden TR, Sterling T, Pablos-Mendez A, Kilburn JO, Cauthen GM, Dooley SW: The emergence of drug-resistant tuberculosis in NYC. N Engl J Med 328:521–526, 1993
70. Frieden TR, Fujiwara PI, Washko RM, Hamburg MA: Tuberculosis in New York City—turning the tide. N Engl J Med 333:229–233, 1995
71. Valway SE, Richard SB, Kovacovich J, et al: Outbreak of MDRTB in a New York State prison. Am J Epidemiol 140:113–122, 1994
72. Raviglione MC, Snider DE, Kochi A: Global epidemiology of tuberculosis: morbidity and mortality of a worldwide epidemic. JAMA 273:220–226, 1995
73. Dolin PJ, Raviglione MC, Kochi A: Global tuberculosis incidence and mortality during 1990–2000. Bull World Health Organ 72: 213–220, 1994
74. Centers for Disease Control and Prevention: Estimates for future global tuberculosis morbidity and mortality. MMWR 42:961–964, 1993
75. Sudre P, Ten Dan G, Kochi A: Tuberculosis: a global overview of the situation today. Bull World Health Organ 70:149–159, 1992
76. Murray CJL, Styblo K, Rouillon A: Tuberculosis in developing countries: burden, intervention, and cost. Bull Int Union Tuberculosis and Lung Disease 65:6–24, 1990
77. World Health Organization Global Program on Aids: The current global situation of the HIV/AIDS pandemic. Wkly Epidemiol Rec 69:189–196, 1994
78. Kochi A, Vareldzis B, Styblo K: Multidrug resistant tuberculosis and its control. Res Microbiol 144:104–110, 1993
79. World Health Organization: WHO Tuberculosis Programme: Framework for Effective Tuberculosis Control. (Publication WHO/TB/94.179) Geneva: World Health Organization, 1994
80. McKenna MT, McGray E, Onorato I: Epidemiology of tuberculosis from foreign-born persons in the United States, 1986–1993. N Engl J Med 332:1071–1076, 1995
81. Syblo K: Overview in epidemiologic assessment of the current global tuberculosis situation with an emphasis on control in developing countries. Rev Infect Dis 11:S339–S346, 1989
82. Nolan CM, Elarth AM: Tuberculosis in a cohort of Southeast Asian refugees: five year surveillance study. Am Rev Respir Dis 137: 805–809, 1988
83. Blum RN, Polish LD, Tapy JM, Catlan BJ, Cohn DL: Results of screening for tuberculosis in foreign born persons applying for adjustment of immigration status. Chest 103:1670–1674, 1993
84. Onorato I, McCray E: Prevalence of HIV infection among patients attending tuberculosis clinics in the United States. J Infect Dis 165: 87–92, 1992
85. Centers for Disease Control and Prevention: Prevention and controlled tuberculosis in correctional facilities. MMWR RR-45:1–27, 1996
86. Stead WW: Undetected tuberculosis in prison (source of infection for the community at large). JAMA 240:2544–2547, 1978
87. Spencer SS, Morton AR: Tuberculosis surveillance in a state prison system. Am J Public Health 79:507–509, 1989
88. Centers for Disease Control and Prevention: Tuberculosis prevention in drug-treatment centers and correctional facilities—selected U.S. sites, 1990–1991. MMWR 42:210–213, 1993

89. Bellin EY, Fletcher DD, Safyer SM: Association of tuberculosis infection with increased time in or admission to the New York City jail system. JAMA 2228–2231, 1993
90. Centers for Disease Control and Prevention: Probable transmission of multidrug resistant tuberculosis in a correctional facility—California. MMWR 42:48–51, 1993
91. Kantor HS, Poblete R, Pusateri SL: Nosocomial transmission of tuberculosis from unsuspected disease. Am J Med 84:833–839, 1988
92. Schwartzman K, Loo V, Pasztor J, Menzies D: Tuberculosis infection among health care workers in Montreal. Am J Respir Crit Care Med 154:1006–1012, 1996
93. Hutton MD, Stead WW, Cauthen GM, Bloch AB, Ewing WM: Nosocomial transmission of tuberculosis associated with a draining abscess. J Infect Dis 161:286–295, 1990
94. Morris LI: Tuberculosis as an occupational hazard during medical training. Am Rev Tuberculosis 54:140–157, 1946
95. Reid DD: Incidence of tuberculosis among workers in medical laboratories. Br Med J 2:10–14, 1957
96. Templeton GL, Illing LA, Young L, Cave D, Stead WW, Bates JH: The risk for transmission of *Mycobacterium tuberculosis* at the bedside during autopsy. Ann Intern Med 122:922–925, 1995
97. Maloney SA, Pearson ML, Gordon NT, Del Castillo R, Boyle JF, Jarvis WR: Efficacy of control measures in preventing nosocomial transmission of multidrug resistant tuberculosis to patients and health care workers. Ann Intern Med 122:90–95, 1995
98. Jarvis WR, Bolyard EA, Bozzi CJ, Burwen DR, Dooley SW, Martin LS, Mullan RJ, Simone PM: Respirators, recommendations, and regulations: the controversy surrounding protection of health care workers from tuberculosis. Ann Intern Med 122:142–146, 1995
99. Centers for Disease Control and Prevention: Guidelines for preventing the transmission of tuberculosis in health-care facilities. MMWR RR-43:1–132, 1994
100. Wenger PN, Otten J, Breeden A, Orfas D, Beck-Sague CM, Jarvis W: Control of nosocomial transmission of MDRTB among health-care workers and HIV-infected patients. Lancet 345:235–240, 1995
101. Blumberg HM, Watkins DL, Berschling JD, Antle A, Moore P, White M, Hunter N, Green B, Ray SM, McGowan JE: Preventing the nosocomial transmission of tuberculosis. Ann Intern Med 122:658–663, 1995
102. Pearlman DC, Salomon N, Perkins MP, Yancovitz S, Paone D, Des Jarlais DC: Tuberculosis in drug users. Clin Infect Dis 21:1253–1264, 1995
103. Reichman LD, Felton CP, Edaall JR: Drug dependence, a possible new risk factor for tuberculosis disease. Arch Intern Med 139: 337–339, 1979
104. Friedman LN, Sullivan GM, Bevilaqua RP, Loscos R: Tuberculosis screening in alcoholics and drug addicts. Am Rev Respir Dis 136:1182–1192, 1987
105. Graham NMH, Nelson KE, Solomon L, Bonds M, Rizzo RT, Scavoto J, Asteborski J, Vlahov D: Prevalence of tuberculin positivity and skin test anergy in HIV-seropositive and -seronegative intravenous drug users. JAMA 267:369–373, 1992
106. Nazar-Stewart V, Nolan CM: Results of a directly observed intermittent isoniazid preventive therapy program in a shelter for homeless men. Am Rev Respir Dis 146:57–60, 1992
107. Stead WW, Dutt AK: Tuberculosis in elderly persons. Annu Rev Med 42:267–276, 1991
108. Stead WW, Lofgren JP, Warren E, Thomas C: Tuberculosis as an epidemic nosocomial infection among the elderly in nursing homes. N Engl J Med 312:1483–1487, 1985
109. Stead WW, To T: The significance of tuberculin skin test in elderly persons. Ann Intern Med 107:837–842, 1987
110. Battershill JH: Cutaneous testing in the elderly patient with tuberculosis. Chest 77:188–189, 1980
111. Centers for Disease Control and Prevention: Exposure of passengers and flight crew to *Mycobacterium tuberculosis* on commercial aircraft, 1992–1995. MMWR 44:137–140, 1995
112. McFarland JW, Hickman C, Osterholm MT, MacDonald KL: Exposure to *Mycobacterium tuberculosis* during air travel. Lancet 342:112–113, 1993
113. Wick RL, Irvine LE: The microbiological composition of airline or cabin air. Aviat Space Environ Med 66:220–224, 1995
114. Wenzel RP: Air travel and infection. N Engl J Med 334:981–982, 1996
115. Kenyon TA, Valway SE, Ihle WW, Onorato IM, Castro KG: Transmission of multidrug resistant *Mycobacterium tuberculosis* during a long airplane flight. N Engl J Med 334:933–938, 1996
116. Dankner WM, Waecker JN, Essey MA, Moser K, Tompson N, Daves CE: *Mycobacterium bovis* infections in San Diego: a clinical epidemiologic study of 73 patients and a historical review of a forgotten pathogen. Medicine 72:11–37, 1993
117. Colville A: Retrospective review of culture positive mycobacterial lymphadenitis cases in children in Nottingham, 1979–1990. Eur J Clin Microbiol Infect Dis 12:192–195, 1993

Leprosy

1. Shepard CC: The experimental disease that follows the injection of human leprosy bacilli into foot-pads of mice. J Exp Med 112:445–454, 1960
2. Walsh GP, et al: Experimental leprosy, workshop 5. Int J Lepr 61, 4(Suppl):733–736, 1993
3. Kirchheimer WF, Storrs CC: Attempts to establish the armadillo (*Dasypus novemcinctus*) as a model for the study of leprosy. Int J Lepr 39:693–702, 1971
4. Gormus BJ, Wolf RH, Baskin GB, et al: A second sooty mangabey monkey with naturally acquired leprosy. Int J Lepr 56:61–65, 1988
5. Cole ST: The genome of *Mycobacterium leprae*. Int J Lepr 62:122–125, 1994
6. Ridley DS, Jopling WH: Classification of leprosy according to immunity; a five-group system. Int J Lepr 34:255–273, 1966
7. Scollard DM, Smith T, Bhoopat L, Theetranont C, Rangdaeng S, Morens DM: Epidemiologic characteristics of leprosy reactions. Int J Lepr 62:559–567, 1994
8. Shepard CC, Saitz CW: Lepromin and tuberculin reactivity in adults not exposed to leprosy. J Immunol 99:637–642, 1967
9. Hunter SW, Brennan PJ: A novel glycolipid from *Mycobacterium leprae* possibly involved in immunogenicity and pathogenicity. J Bacteriol 147:725–735, 1981
10. Chanteau S, Glaziou P, Plichert C, Luquiaud P, Plichart R, Faucher JF, Cartel JL: Low predictive value of PGL-1 serology for the early diagnosis of leprosy in family contacts: results of a 10-year prospective field study in French Polynesia. Int J Lepr 61:533–541, 1993
11. Irgens LM: Leprosy in Norway—an epidemiological study based on a national patient registry. Lepr Rev 51 (Suppl):1–130, 1980
12. Feldman RA, Sturdivant M: Leprosy in the United States 1950–1969: an epidemiologic review. South Med J 69:920–929, 1976
13. Jesudasan K, et al: Workshop 8: approaches to epidemiology, prevention and control. Int J Lepr 61, 4(Suppl):742–743, 1993
14. WHO Study Group: Chemotherapy of leprosy for control programs. (Tech Rep Ser 675). Geneva: World Health Organization, 1982.
15. Nordeen SK: Elimination of leprosy as a public health problem. Int J Lepr 62:278–283, 1994
16. Jesudasan K, Vijayakumaran P, Pannikarvk, Christian M: Impact of MDT on leprosy as measured by selective indicators. Lepr Rev 59:215–233, 1988
17. Bechelli LM: Prospects of global elimination of leprosy as a public health problem by the year 2000. Int J Lepr 62:284–292, 1994
18. Vigneron E: The epidemiological transition in an overseas territory: disease mapping in French Polynesia. Soc Sci Med 28:913–922, 1989

19. Wade HW, Ledowski V: The leprosy epidemic at Naura: a review with data on the status since 1937. Int J Lepr 20:1–29, 1952
20. Newell KW: An epidemiologists' view of leprosy. Bull World Health Organ 34:827–857, 1966
21. Fine PM: Leprosy: the epidemiology of a slow bacterium. Epidemiol Rev 4:161–188, 1982
22. Davey TF, Rees RJW: The nasal discharge in leprosy: clinical and bacteriological aspects. Lepr Rev 45:121–134, 1974
23. Pattyn SR, Ursi D, Ieven M, Grillone S, Raes V: Detection of *Mycobacterium leprae* by the polymerase chain reaction in nasal swabs of leprosy patients and their contacts. Int J Lepr 61:389–393, 1993
24. Gillis TT, Williams DL: Polymerase chain reaction and leprosy. J Lepr 59:311–316, 1991
25. Drutz DJ, Chen TSN, Lu WH: The continuous bacteremia of lepromatous leprosy. N Engl J Med 287:159–164, 1972
26. Pedley JC: The presence of *M. leprae* in human milk. Lepr Rev 38:239–242, 1967
27. Leiker DL: On the mode of transmission of mycobacterium leprae. Lepr Rev 48:9–16, 1977
28. Kirchheimer WF: The role of arthropods in the transmission of leprosy. Int J Lepr 44:104–107, 1976
29. Cochrane RA: Epidemiology. In: A Practical Textbook of Leprosy. London: Oxford University Press, 1947, pp 10–22
30. Challacombe SJ, Tomasi TB: Systemic tolerance and secretory immunity after oral immunization. J Exp Med 152:1459–1472, 1980
31. Blake LA, West BC, Cary CH, Todd JR: Environmental non-human sources of leprosy. Rev Infect Dis 9:562–577, 1987
32. Walsh GP, Storrs LE, Burchfield HP, Cottrell EH, Vidrine MF, Binford CH: Leprosy-like disease occurring naturally in armadillos. J Reticuloendothelial Soc 18:347–351, 1975
33. Brubaker MC, Binford CH, Trautman JR: Occurrence of leprosy in US veterans after service in endemic areas aboard. Public Health Rep 84:1051–1058, 1969
34. Doull JA, Guinto RS, Rodriquez JN, et al: The incidence of leprosy in Cordova and Talisey, Philippines. Int J Lepr 10:107–131, 1942
35. Doull JA, Guinto RS, Rodriquez JN, Bancroft H: Risk of attack on leprosy in relation to age at exposure. Int J Lepr 13:435–439, 1945
36. Ponnighaus JM, Fine PEM, Sterne JAC, Bliss L, Wilson RJ, Malema SS: Incidence rates of leprosy in Karonga district, Northern Malawi: patterns by age, sex, BCG status and classification. Int J Lepr 62:10–22, 1994
37. Ponnighaus JM, Fine PEM, Sterne JAC, Malema SS, Bliss L, Wilson RJ: Extended schooling and good housing conditions are associated with reduced risk of leprosy in rural Malawi. Int J Lepr 62: 345–352, 1994
38. Irgens LM, Skjerven R: Secular trends in age at onset, sex ratio, and type of index in leprosy observed during declining incidence rates. Am J Epidemiol 122:695–705, 1985
39. Chakravarti MR, Vogel F: A twin study on leprosy. Top Hum Genet 1:1–123, 1973
40. DeVries RRF, Fat RFMI, Nijenhnis LE, et al: HLA-linked genetic control of host response to mycobacterium lerpae. Lancet 2:1328–1330, 1976
41. Fine PEM, Wolf E, Pritchard J, et al: HLA-linked genes and leprosy: a family study in a south Indian population. J Infect Dis 140:152–161, 1979
42. DeVries RRP, Van Eden W, Van Rood JJ: HLA-linked control of the course of *M. leprae* infections. Lepr Rev 52(Suppl):109–119, 1981
43. Schauf V, Ryan S, Scollard DM, Vithayasai V, Nelson KE: Leprosy is associated with HLA-DR2 and DQW1 in the population of northern Thailand. Tissue Antigens 26:243–247, 1985
44. Wagener DK, Schauf V, Nelson KE, Scollard D, Brown A, Smith T: Segregation analysis of leprosy in northern Thailand. Genet Epidemiol 5:95–105, 1988
45. Bryceson A, Pfaltzgraff RE: In: Leprosy. 2nd ed. New York: Churchill Livingstone, 1979, Chapter 3, Symptoms and Signs
46. Turk JL, Rees RJW: AIDS and leprosy. Lepr Rev 59:193–194, 1988
47. Ponninghaus JM, Mwanjasi LJ, Fine PEM, Shaw MA, Turner AC, Oxborrow S, et al: Is HIV infection a risk factor for leprosy? Int J Lepr 59:221–228, 1991
48. Kuwama HJS, Bwire R, Adatu-Engwau F: Leprosy and infection with the human immunodeficiency virus in Uganda: a case-control study. Int J Lepr 62:521–526, 1994
49. Leonard G, Sangare A, Verdier M, et al: Prevalence of HIV infection among patients with leprosy in African countries and Yemen. J Acquir Immune Defic Syndr 3:1109–1113, 1990
50. Meeran K: Prevalence of HIV infection among patients with leprosy and tuberculosis in rural Zambia. Br Med J 298:364–365, 1989
51. Borgdorff MW, VandenBroek J, Chum HJ, Klokke AH, Graf P, Barougo LR, et al: HIV-1 infection as a risk factor for leprosy: a case-control study in Tanzania. Int J Lepr 61:556–562, 1993
52. Whalen C, Horsburgh CR, Hom D, Lahart C, Simberkoff M, Ellner J: Accelerated course of human immunodeficiency virus infection after tuberculosis. Am J Respir Crit Care Med 151:129–135, 1995
53. Gormus BJ, Murphey-Corb M, Martin LN, et al: Interactions between simian immunodeficiency virus and *Mycobacterium leprae* in experimentally inoculated rhesus monkeys. J Infect Dis 160:405–413, 1989
54. Grosset JH, Guelpa-Laorus C, Peraai EG, N'Dell L: Clinical trials of pefloxacin and ofloxacin in the treatment of lepromatous leprosy. Int J Lepr 58:281–286, 1990
55. Ji B, Perani EG, Petinom C, N'Dell L, Grosset JH: Clinical trials of ofloxacin alone and in combination with dapsone plus clofazimine for treatment of lepromatous leprosy. Antimicrob Agents Chemother 38:662–667, 1994
56. Chan GP, Garcia-Ignacio BY, Chavez VE, Livelo JB, Jimenez CL, Parrilla MR, Franzblau SG: Clinical trial of sparfloxacin for lepromatous leprosy. Antimicrob Agents Chemother 38:61–65, 1994
57. Grosset JH: Progress in the chemotherapy of leprosy. Int J Lepr 62:268–277, 1994
58. Pattyn SR: Search for effective short-course regimens for the treatment of leprosy. Int J Lepr 61:76–81, 1993
59. Gelber RH, Murray CP, Siu P, Tsaang M, Rea TH: Efficacy of minocycline in single dose and at 100 mg twice daily for lepromatous leprosy. Int J Lepr 64:568–573, 1994
60. Franzblau SG, Hastings RC: In vitro and in vivo activities of macrolides against *Mycobacterium leprae*. Antimicrob Agents Chemother 34:229–231, 1990
61. Bell-Krotoski J: A study of periperal nerve involvement underlying physical disability of the hand in Hansen's disease. J Hand Ther 5:1–10, 1992
62. Filice GA, Fraser DW: Management of household contacts of leprosy patients. Ann Intern Med 88:538, 1978
63. Worth RM, Hirschy ID: A test of the infectivity of tuberculoid leprosy patients. Hawaii Med J 24:116–119, 1964
64. Worth RM: Is it safe to treat the lepromatous patient at home? Int J Lepr 36:296–302, 1968
65. Nordeen SK: Chemoprophylaxis in leprosy. Lepr India 41:247–254, 1969
66. Shepard CC: Vaccination against human leprosy bacillus infections of mice: protection by BCG given during the incubation period. J Immunol 96:279–283, 1966
67. Stanley SJ, Howland C, Stone MM, Sutherland I: BCG vaccination of children against leprosy in Uganda: final results. J Hyg 87: 233–248, 1981
68. Bagshawe A, Scott GC, Russell DA, Wigley SC, Merianos A, Berry G: BCG vaccination in leprosy: final results of the trial in Karimui, Pagon New Guinea, 1963–79. Bull World Health Organ 67:389–399, 1989
69. Lwin K, Sundaresan T, Gyi MM, Bechelli LM, Tamondong C, Garbajosa PG, Sansarricq H, Nordeen SK: BCG vaccination of children

against leprosy: fourteen year findings of the trial in Burma. Bull World Health Organ 63:1069–1078, 1985

70. Karonga Prevention Trial Group: Randomized controlled trial of single BCG, repeated BCG, or combined BCG and mycobacterium leprae vaccine for prevention of leprosy and tuberculosis in Malawi. Lancet 348:17–24, 1996
71. Convit JC, Smith PG, Zuniga M, Simpson C, Ulrich M, Plata JA, et al: BCG vaccination protects against leprosy in Venezuela: a case-control study. Int J Lepr 61:185–191, 1993
72. Muliyil JP, Nelson KE, Diamond EL: Effect of BCG on the risk of leprosy in an endemic area: a case-control study. Int J Lepr 59:229–236, 1991
73. Smith TC, Richardus JH: Leprosy trends in northern Thailand: 1951–1990. Southeast Asian J Trop Med Public Health 24:3–10, 1993
74. Bechelli LM: Prospects of global elimination of leprosy as a public health problem by the year 2000. Int J Lepr 62:284–292, 1994
75. Fine PEM: Reflections on the elimination of leprosy. Int J Lepr 60:71–80, 1992

10

Diseases Spread by Food and Water

Typhoid Fever

Jonathan H. Mermin • Eric D. Mintz

Typhoid fever is an acute, life-threatening, febrile illness caused by the bacterium *Salmonella*, serotype Typhi. Because humans are the only known natural host for *S.* typhi, fecal-oral transmission through contaminated food and water is the most common mode of infection. In the United States about 400 cases are reported each year, and the majority of these are acquired while traveling internationally.[1,2]

Bacteriology

S. Typhi, like other *Salmonella* species, is a Gram-negative, flagellated, non–lactose-fermenting bacillus. It is identified by its biochemical properties and somatic (O) and flagellar (H) antigens. Most freshly isolated strains have a capsular (Vi) antigen. In the Kauffman-White schema, *S.* typhi is a member of *Salmonella* group D, characterized by O antigens 1, 9, and 12. The organism survives well in water and sewage but is readily killed by pasteurization.[3]

S. Typhi is most frequently isolated from blood during the first week of illness, but it can also be present during the second and third weeks of illness, during the first week of antimicrobial therapy, and during clinical relapse. Fecal cultures are positive in approximately half the cases during the first week of fever, but the largest number of positive cultures occurs during the second and third weeks of disease. Bone marrow cultures are frequently positive (90 percent of cases) and are more likely to yield *S.* Typhi than are cultures from any other site, especially when the patient has already received antimicrobial therapy.[4] Organisms can also be isolated from duodenal aspirates, from rose spots (see below), and infrequently from urine cultures.[4,5]

Clinical Characteristics

Typhoid fever has an insidious onset characterized by fever, headache, constipation, malaise, chills, and myalgia.[3] Many patients cough for the first few days of illness, and some report sore throat or joint pain. Splenomegaly, leukopenia, and abdominal distention and tenderness are generally present. Early in the illness, small, discrete, rose-colored spots caused by bacterial emboli in the skin capillaries may appear on the trunk. Confusion, delirium, intestinal perforation, and death may occur in severe cases. Diarrhea is uncommon, and vomiting is not usually severe. In children, the disease presentation is often atypical, and respiratory symptoms and diarrhea are often present.[6]

In studies of volunteers, as few as 10^5 bacteria have caused clinical illness, with ingestion of 10^7 organisms resulting in 50 percent of subjects becoming ill.[7] Incubation periods have been as short as 3 days and as long as 56 days; a higher inoculum is associated with shorter incubation periods. The median incubation period for a dose of 10^5 organisms was 9 days; for 10^7 organisms, 7 days; and for 10^9 organisms, 5 days.[7] Partial immunity follows clinical illness, but reinfection and illness can occur after a large oral dose. Antibody titers are not correlated with resistance to reinfection or occurrence of relapse.

Treatment

Effective antimicrobial therapy reduces morbidity and mortality from typhoid fever. Without therapy, the illness may last for 3 to 4 weeks, and death rates range between 12 and 30 percent.[3,5] With appropriate treatment, clinical symptoms subside within 2 days, fever recedes within 5 days, and in the United States mortality is approximately 1 percent.[2] Relapses, characterized by a less severe but otherwise typical illness, occur in 10 to 20 percent of patients with typhoid fever, usually after an afebrile period of 1 to 2 weeks. Relapses may still occur despite antimicrobial therapy.[3]

Intestinal hemorrhage, perforation, and other complications of typhoid fever are less likely if effective antimicrobial therapy is begun early. Organisms resistant to antimicrobial agents (including amoxicillin, trimethoprim-sulfamethoxazole, and chloramphenicol) have increasingly been reported from foreign countries and from within the United States.[2,8] Determining antimicrobial resistance patterns is essential in recommending treatment. Quinolones and third-generation cephalosporins are probably the best choice for empiric treatment of typhoid fever, although rare quinolone resistance has been reported in isolates from the Indian subcontinent.[9–11]

Serologic Diagnosis

In typhoid fever, serologic responses to O, H, and Vi antigens usually occur by the end of the first week of illness. The Widal test, which measures antibody responses to H and O antigens, can suggest the diagnosis, but the results are not definitive and must be interpreted with care because titers may be elevated in a number of other infections. Single high-titer serum specimens from adults in areas of endemic disease have little diagnostic value. Even when paired sera are used, the results must be interpreted in light of the patient's history of typhoid immunization and previous illness, the stage of the illness when the first serum specimen was obtained, the use of early antimicrobial therapy, and the reagents used.[12]

Carriers

Following treated or untreated infection, carriage of *S.* Typhi in the stool often persists for 1 to 2 months. The likelihood of a chronic carrier state—excretion of the organism for more than 1 year—is related to age at the onset of disease and sex of the patient. Women are three times more likely than men to become chronic carriers. For both men and women whose illness begins when they are under 20 years of age, chronic enteric carriage is infrequent (0.3 percent), whereas for women with disease onset over 40 years of age, chronic enteric carriage is more common (13.3 percent).[13] Antimicrobial treatment of typhoid fever may not significantly decrease the occurrence of chronic fecal carriage. Urinary excretion is common in the first months after illness, but chronic urinary carriage is usually associated with preexisting pathologic changes in the kidneys or bladder, such as occur in patients with schistosomiasis and in the elderly. Elimination of a chronic carrier state requires prolonged use of antimicrobial agents in high doses.[5] Orally administered quinolones have had reported cure rates of approximately 80 percent.[14] In patients with chronic gallbladder or urinary tract disease, antimicrobial agents alone may be ineffective, and surgery may be necessary.

Antibody to the Vi antigen is often present in high titers in serum samples from persons who are chronic carriers and can be used as a screening test for identification of chronic carriers in certain high-risk groups and during investigation of sporadic cases and outbreaks.[15–17]

Transmission

Since *S.* Typhi has no known animal reservoir other than humans, isolated cases and outbreaks must originate from a human infection. Most typhoid outbreaks are traced to ingestion of food or water contaminated with human waste; however, the sources of the majority of sporadic cases acquired in the United States are unexplained.[1] Working in a microbiology laboratory has been associated with increased risk of acquiring infection, but working in a sewage collection or treatment plant has not been associated with increased risk.[18] Studies of common-source outbreaks have rarely revealed secondary spread in families.

Historically, health departments have developed routine methods of monitoring known chronic typhoid carriers. These persons are asked to supply periodic stool specimens for culture, are instructed concerning personal hygiene, and are prohibited from preparing food for anyone except family members. However, termination of the carrier state through antimicrobial therapy or surgery may be a more practical strategy.

Occurrence

Typhoid fever has worldwide distribution but varies widely in incidence, seasonality, and vehicles of infection. An estimated 16 million cases of typhoid fever and 600,000 deaths occur worldwide.[19] The steady decrease in incidence of the disease in western Europe and the United States in the first half of the twentieth century was associated with the development of protected water supplies, pasteurization of milk, and improved sewage systems. In the United States, approximately 400 clinical cases are reported each year, of which 72 percent are associated with foreign travel, especially travel to the Indian subcontinent, Southeast Asia, Africa, and Latin America.[2] Occasionally, large food-borne outbreaks do occur in the United States, frequently due to contamination by asymptomatic food handlers.[20]

Prevention

Travel-associated typhoid fever is largely preventable. Travelers to less industrialized countries should be encouraged to take routine precautions in selecting and preparing foods and beverages: cooked foods should be eaten hot, raw fruits and vegetables should be peeled by the traveler, and only low-risk beverages should be consumed, such as hot drinks, carbonated beverages without ice, and water that has been boiled or chemically disinfected. In addition, vaccination against typhoid fever is recommended for travelers visiting countries with endemic disease.[21] Vaccines against typhoid fever have been available for more than 80 years.[22] Studies of volunteers have shown that vaccine-induced immunity is protective (65 to 70 percent effective) against low to moderate infecting doses, but, like natural immunity, it provides little protection against very large challenge doses.[7] Three vaccines are licensed for use in the United States: the parenteral killed bacterial vaccine, the live oral vaccine, and an improved parenteral vaccine licensed in 1995 (Table 10-1). The oral vaccine—a live, attenuated *S.* Typhi strain (Ty2la) that lacks the enzyme UDP-galactose-4-epimerase[23]—and the new single-dose parenteral vaccine (ViCPS)—a polysaccharide formula based on purified Vi antigen—are equally effective and rarely cause adverse reactions.[21] Microbiology laboratory workers are at risk for typhoid fever and should be vaccinated if they anticipate having contact with specimens from patients with typhoid fever or with isolates of *S.* Typhi.

The incidence of typhoid fever in the United States depends closely on its incidence in other countries. Travelers can lower their risk of typhoid fever by carefully selecting foods and beverages and by vaccination. However, the elimination of typhoid fever in the United States will ultimately depend on improving health and sanitation throughout the world.

TABLE 10-1. TYPHOID FEVER VACCINATION

Vaccine Name	How Given	Number of Doses Necessary	Time Between Doses	Total Time Needed to Set Aside for Vaccination	Minimum Age for Vaccination	Booster Needed Every
Ty21a (Vivotif Berna, Swiss Serum and Vaccine Institute)	1 capsule by mouth	4	48 hours	2 weeks	6 years	5 years
ViCPS (Typhim Vi, Pasteur Mérieux)	Injection	1	—	1 week	2 years	2 years
Inactivated Typhoid Vaccine (Wyeth-Ayerst)	Injection	2 (1 if booster)	4 weeks	5 weeks	6 months	3 years

Shigellosis

Jeremy Sobel • Eric D. Mintz

Lack of safe piped water and sewage disposal, absence of personal hygiene, and crowding underlie epidemics of dysentery caused by *Shigella* species. These epidemics have occurred primarily among the military, displaced persons, and crowded urban and rural poor populations experiencing these conditions.[1] The term "bacillary dysentery," used to describe a diarrheal illness with fever, abdominal pain, and blood and pus (leukocytes) in the stool, is often used as a synonym for diarrhea caused by *Shigella*. Since the "sanitary revolution" of the late nineteenth century, shigellae no longer cause epidemic dysentery in the United States, but they do commonly cause outbreaks and sporadic cases of diarrhea.

Bacteriology

At the end of the nineteenth century, bacillary dysentery was clearly distinguished from dysentery caused by amoebae. At that time the bacillary illness was found to be caused by a fairly homogeneous group of aerobic, nonmotile, non–lactose-fermenting, Gram-negative bacilli, divided serologically and biochemically into four species. These species are named and given an alphabetical serologic designation. *Shigella dysenteriae* (group A) has 13 serotypes; type 1 (the Shiga bacillus) remains a cause of epidemic severe dysentery in the developing world. *Shigella flexneri* (group B) has six serotypes, some of which are subdivided. *Shigella boydii* (group C) is divided into 18 serotypes. *Shigella sonnei* (group D) has only one serotype. Determinations of serotypes and subtyping by means of antibiotic resistance profiles, phage types, plasmid profiles, colicin types, and pulsed-field gel electrophoresis patterns have been useful in epidemiologic studies.

Many *Shigella* organisms are present in the intestinal mucus or feces early in the illness. When feces are alkaline, the bacilli may survive for days, whereas in acidic stools they remain viable for only a few hours. Therefore, if direct inoculation of culture media is not possible, placing fecal material or rectal swabs in Cary-Blair transport medium is suggested. Isolation of *Shigella* organisms from the blood is rare.

Antimicrobial resistance has increased markedly in recent years. Strains of *S. dysenteriae* type 1 resistant to ampicillin, chloramphenicol, nalidixic acid, streptomycin, sulfonamides, tetracycline, and trimethoprim-sulfamethoxazole are increasingly common in Africa.[2,3] Resistance of *Shigella* to ampicillin and trimethoprim-sulfamethoxazole has been reported worldwide, and ciprofloxacin resistance has recently emerged in the Indian subcontinent.[4] Multiple drug resistance is increasingly common in the United States as well.[5,6]

Clinical Characteristics

Shigellosis often begins with fever, abdominal pain, and watery diarrhea without blood. At this stage the diarrhea is difficult to distinguish from that caused by other agents. With invasion of the colonic mucosa, stools often become bloody, mucoid, and of low volume. The usual incubation period is about 48 hours but ranges from less than 12 hours to 6 days. The clinical illness associated with *S. dysenteriae* type 1 (Shiga bacillus) is often severe. In a major outbreak in Central America in the late 1960s, case-to-fatality ratios were 8 to 15 percent among untreated persons.[7] The death rate was highest among children up to 4 years of age.

Extraintestinal infections are rare, but the disease has some important noninfectious extraintestinal manifestations. Convulsions may occur in children, but the mechanism has not been established.[8] Reiter's syndrome is a late complication of *S. flexneri* infection, especially in persons with the genetic marker HLA-B27. Hemolytic-uremic syndrome can occur after *S. dysenteriae* type 1 infection.[9]

Asymptomatic infections occur, but an asymptomatic excreter is less likely than a clinically ill person to transmit infection.[10] Prolonged carriage is uncommon in healthy people, but carriage for more than 1 year has been reported.[11] With repeated infections by the same serotype, clinical illness becomes milder or absent. In volunteers, prior infection has resulted in reduced proliferation of virulent organisms, apparently because of local gut immunity.

Treatment and Diagnosis

Treatment with appropriate antimicrobial agents reduces the duration of symptoms and the excretion of shigellae;[12–14] however, *Shigella* organisms are often resistant to first-line antimicrobial agents. Resistance to ampicillin or trimethoprim-sulfamethoxazole is increasing in the United States, and strains acquired outside the United States are significantly more resistant. Monitoring local antimicrobial resistance patterns in a community with endemic disease can help guide selection of effective agents with which to begin therapy. Since the illness is often mild and self-limited, in areas with endemic shigellosis a policy of reserving antimicrobial treatment for very ill and high-risk persons may delay the emergence of resistant strains. Without a positive culture, diagnosis is often difficult. In a study of Bolivian children, crying during defecation, temperature above 38.4°C, five or more stools per 24 hours, and more than 50 leukocytes per high-power field on microscopic fecal examination were associated with *Shigella* infection.[15]

Transmission

The primary reservoir for *Shigella* organisms is humans, although shigellae occasionally infect other primates. A small inoculum (10 to 200 organisms) is sufficient to cause infection. As a result, person-to-person spread can easily occur by the fecal-oral route and occurs more frequently than transmission by food and water. In the United States, groups with an increased risk of shigellosis include children in day care centers[16] and persons in custodial institutions, where personal hygiene is difficult to maintain;[14,17] Native Americans;[5] orthodox Jews;[18] travelers;[19] homosexual men;[20] and those in homes with inadequate water for handwashing. Secondary attack rates are high in homes of preschool children with clinical shigellosis.

Outbreaks are infrequently caused by contaminated food.[21,22] The most common vehicle in food-borne *Shigella* outbreaks in the United States is salad; its contamination is usually attributed to poor hygiene practices of the food handler.[23] Drinking or swimming in contaminated water has also led to outbreaks.[24,25]

Occurrence

Shigella infections are most common in preschool children, reflecting their lack of hygiene, but may occur at any age. In the United States the highest attack rates are among children 1 to 4 years of age, with the peak rate in 2-year-olds. Raw numbers of isolates show a female predominance in the age groups 10 to 29 and 60 to 79 years.[26] The seasonality of infections varies from country to country; in the United States, *S. sonnei* infections are common in the late summer. The serotype pattern of *Shigella* isolates changes as a region develops, with *S. dysenteriae* being replaced by *S. flexneri* and in turn by *S. sonnei*. In recent years in the United States, *S. sonnei* has been isolated more than four times as frequently as *S. flexneri*.[26] Isolation of *S. dysenteriae* and *S. boydii* is infrequent in the United States; these species are common in developing countries. Epidemics of multiply resistant *S. dysenteriae* type 1 infections with considerable mortality occur in developing areas, most notably in recent years in Africa.[2,3,27,28] In the United states, modes of transmission of the various *Shigella* serotypes are reflected in the mean age of patients. The mean age of patients with *S. sonnei* infections is 7 years, reflecting the predominance of day care transmission. The mean age of patients with *S. flexneri* infections is 17 years, probably reflecting in part anal-oral transmission among adult male homosexuals.[20] The mean age of patients with *S. dysenteriae* infections is 29 years, reflecting importation of this infection by adults returning from overseas travel.[19]

Prevention and Control

Outbreaks of shigellosis are difficult to control.[18,29] Interrupting the fecal-oral transmission cycle is the key objective, and handwashing with soap and running water is the most effective intervention. Additionally, efforts have included isolation of patients, improved sanitation, antimicrobial treatment of ill persons and occasionally those with asymptomatic infection, and, rarely, prophylactic treatment of all members of a household or closed institution. Shigellosis outbreaks in day care centers, the most common setting in the United States, are associated with preparation of food by workers who also changed diapers, provision of group transportation to young children, and high child-to-toilet ratios.[16] Cohorting is a key element in controlling day care outbreaks. Recovering children who no longer have diarrhea may return to day care but are kept in a separate room with a separate toilet and cared for by dedicated staff until they have a negative stool culture. This practice is preferable to barring clinically recovered but still infectious children from the day care center, because it does not encourage parents to send their children to other facilities without reporting the antecedent infection.[29] Attempts to control outbreaks with antimicrobial agents may be compromised by the development of antimicrobial-resistant strains. Control of outbreaks requires unflagging insistence on handwashing, with supervision, if required; prevention rests on inculcating individuals with a consciousness of hygiene and sanitation. Efforts have been directed to the development of *Shigella* vaccines, but an effective commercially available vaccine is still years in the future.[30,31]

Shigella infections are least common in communities and institutions where treated water is readily available and used frequently for handwashing and where an adequate system exists for disposal of human wastes. Handwashing is an effective control measure even in areas with poor sanitation.[32] Protected food supplies and adequate refrigeration are important in reducing the possibility of common-source infection.

Cholera

Robert E. Black

Cholera, an acute infection of the small intestine by *Vibrio cholerae*, is manifested as watery diarrhea. It has been known and feared for centuries because of its propensity to occur in epidemics, resulting in high mortality and social disruption.

History

Cholera has probably afflicted humankind since prehistoric times but was not clearly distinguished from other diarrheal illness in ancient medical writings. As a result, the ancestral home of the cholera vibrio is unclear, although Portuguese explorers' descriptions of diarrhea epidemics in India from the late fifteenth century suggest that the Bengal region of India and Bangladesh has been a continuous endemic region for cholera.[1]

The worldwide spread of cholera began in 1817, and by 1823 the first pandemic of cholera had spread from the Ganges River delta to much of Asia and Africa. During the nineteenth century, cholera repeatedly spread along routes of trade and travel from India to Europe, Africa, and North America. Five periods of pandemic spread occurred before 1900: from 1817 to 1823; from 1826 to 1837; from 1846 to 1862; from 1864 to 1875; and from 1887 to 1896. In each country involved, thousands were affected, with case-to-fatality rates often approaching 50 percent. The fear of this disease can be appreciated from a description written in 1831:

> [Its victims] were in a manner stricken down at once, and exhibited more the appearances of a corpse than a living being; with the eyes sunk in the sockets, the skin dark as if from nitrate of silver, the toes and fingers shriveled, and the tendons standing out like rigid cords along the limbs; while the very breath was cold, and the pulse scarcely to be felt.[2]

The sixth pandemic (1902 to 1923) also involved severe epidemics, especially in Asia, but outbreaks in Africa and Europe were more limited than in previous pandemics, and the Western Hemisphere was not involved. The sixth pandemic and presumably the previous pandemics were due to the classic biotype of *V. cholerae*. This biotype decreased in frequency of isolation in the 1960s and has largely disappeared except in Bangladesh, where it reemerged in epidemic form in 1982.[3]

The seventh pandemic, which still continues, is generally considered to have started in 1961. The causative agent of this pandemic was first isolated in 1905 by Gotschlick from pilgrims returning from Mecca at the El Tor quarantine camp in Egypt. Although this organism was initially considered nonpathogenic, outbreaks of severe disease between 1937 and 1958 confirmed its ability to cause epidemics.[4] An outbreak caused by *V. cholerae* biotype El Tor in Sulawesi in 1961 was the beginning of the seventh pandemic. From there it quickly spread to Java, Sarawak, Borneo, the Philippines, and most of Southeast Asia. Between 1963 and 1969 this organism continued its spread across the Asian mainland. The El Tor biotype eventually replaced classic *V. cholerae* in Asia. In 1970 the pandemic continued its westward progression and involved the Middle East and the Soviet Union, and resulted in serious outbreaks in Spain, Portugal, and Italy. From 1970 to the present nearly all countries in Africa have been involved with cholera outbreaks, and there was a recrudescence in 1991 when 20 countries were affected.

North America had no indigenous cases of cholera in this century until a single case was detected in Texas in 1973. In August 1978 a case in Louisiana led to an investigation that ultimately detected infection in 11 persons.[5] In this outbreak *V. cholerae* El Tor serotype Inaba was recovered from sewage and canal water and from crabs, which were implicated as the vehicle of infection. In 1981 cholera was found in two residents of the Gulf Coast of Texas and another 16 persons on an oil rig in the gulf near Texas. Investigations of these outbreaks determined that they were due to a unique strain of *V. cholerae* that apparently persisted in the environment. This observation and other evidence has led to the conclusion that cholera is indigenous to the Gulf Coast area of the United States, where the organism has a persistent environmental reservoir. Other than in the United States, no recent cases of cholera were recognized in any country of North, Central, or South America until 1983 when a U.S. tourist apparently became infected with *V. cholerae* while visiting the Caribbean coast of Mexico and developed cholera after returning home. The strain causing this infection was the same as the U.S. Gulf Coast strains, suggesting that the environmental reservoir may also run south around the Gulf of Mexico. It appears that Australia also has a similar environmental reservoir, in this case freshwater rivers instead of brackish water of the Gulf estuaries, resulting in a small number of cases or small outbreaks.

Latin America was spared from cholera epidemics since the end of the last century until early 1991 when cholera appeared in Peru.[6] The outbreak, which began in a number of cities along a 900-km coastal area, subsequently spread throughout Peru, with more than a half million cases reported in 1991–1992. The source of the initial contamination is unknown, but subsequent transmission was shown to be related to both water and foods.[6,7] Cholera spread rapidly throughout Latin America, with Bolivia, Brazil, Colombia, Ecuador, El Salvador, Guatemala, and Mexico each reporting more than 10,000 cases between 1991 and 1993.[8] In countries other than Peru, where cities were the major focus of the epidemic, rural areas were more affected than urban areas; native cultures appear to have been at especially high risk. Although about 7,000 deaths were reported due to cholera between 1991 and 1993, the case-to-fatality rate was less than 1 percent, probably reflecting the effectiveness of rehydration therapy widely available in Latin America.

All epidemic cholera in previous pandemics had been due to *V. cholerae* serotype O1, although other strains appear to have caused sporadic cases. In October 1992 cases of cholera associated with a *V. cholerae* strain that did not agglutinate with O1 antisera were reported from Madras, India, and subsequently other cities in southern and eastern India and Bangladesh.[9] This strain, ultimately designated serotype O139, caused epidemic disease throughout Bangladesh, and cases occurred in Malaysia, Nepal, Pakistan, and Thailand. After the initial outbreaks the rates of disease have decreased in Bangladesh, but the strain persists along with *V. cholerae* O1. These outbreaks clearly demonstrate the potential for strains other than serotype O1 to cause epidemic cholera and appear to represent the beginning of a new pandemic of cholera.

Agent and Pathogenesis

In 1883 Koch first isolated *V. cholerae* from the stools of patients with cholera. It is a small, curved, motile aerobic Gram-negative organism best identified by inoculating stool into taurocholate-tellurite-gelatin agar (TTGA) or thiosulfate-citrate-bile salts-sucrose (TCBS) agar. *V. cholerae* colonies are relatively small on TTGA after 24 hours and are translucent with a dark center and a cloudy zone surrounding the colonies. On TCBS agar *V. cholerae* are easily recognized as large yellow colonies on a blue-green medium. The species is identified on the basis of cultural and biochemical tests; the O group determination requires agglutination with type-specific antisera.[10] A variant colonial morphology termed "rugose" has been described for *V. cholerae*. These organisms remain virulent and are more resistant to killing by chlorine than the usual smooth *V. cholerae*.[11]

Cholera vibrios, which have been associated with pandemic disease, are assigned to O serogroups 1 and 139. They are further separated into three serotypes—Ogawa, Inaba, and Hikojima—based on three somatic, or O antigens. Closely related vibrios that do not agglutinate in cholera antiserum are assigned to other O groups. They may be isolated from persons with sporadic and even epidemic diarrhea but have not occurred in pandemics as have *V. cholerae* O groups 1 and 139. *V. cholerae* O1 El Tor is differentiated from classic *V. cholerae* by its ability to agglutinate chick cells and by its resistance to phage IV and to polymyxin.[12]

V. cholerae produces a protein enterotoxin that increases the activity of adenylate cyclase in the intestinal mucosa, resulting in increased levels of cyclic 3′,5′ adenosine monophosphate (cAMP). This in turn leads to inhibition of sodium chloride absorption by villus cells and secretion of chloride and bicarbonate by secretory cells in the crypts of Lieberkuhn. The bacteria do not invade or structurally damage the intestinal mucosa.

Clinical Characteristics

The clinical spectrum of cholera is broad, ranging from inapparent infection to cholera gravis, which may be fatal in a few hours. The incubation period of 24 to 48 hours is followed by an abrupt onset of watery, generally painless diarrhea. Vomiting often follows the diarrhea in the early stages of illness.

In severe cases the loss of diarrheal stool can be extreme. The appearance of the stool as a nonoffensive, sometimes fishy-smelling, clear fluid with flakes of mucus has resulted in the descriptive term "rice water stool."

The symptoms and signs of cholera are entirely due to the loss of large volumes of isotonic fluid and resultant depletion of intravascular and extracellular fluid, metabolic acidosis, and hypokalemia. In addition to the diarrhea and vomiting, symptoms include lightheadedness, anxiety, thirst, and muscle cramps. Signs include cyanosis, tachycardia, hypotension, tachypnea, and loss of skin turgor. In those who survive, the disease subsides spontaneously in 2 to 7 days. Excretion of the organism may continue for days and occasionally weeks after recovery from the illness; a chronic gallbladder carrier state is rare. Both the duration of diarrhea and the persistence of the organism can be reduced by tetracycline therapy.[13] However, the emergence of *V. cholerae* strains resistant to multiple antibiotics, including tetracycline, in East Africa and Asia complicates antimicrobial therapy.

The severity of illness caused by classic and El Tor *V. cholerae* differs greatly. In classic cholera about 60 percent of infections are inapparent but 20 percent of infected persons have severe cholera requiring hospitalization. In El Tor cholera 80 percent of infections are inapparent and fewer than 3 percent are severe. This milder disease has important public health implications, because for each severe case many more undetected infections are present in the community.

Therapy has improved dramatically during the last 20 years, so that with prompt treatment few persons die of cholera, regardless of severity. Therapy is based simply on the prompt and complete replacement of water and electrolytes. This can be done intravenously or more simply by the oral route in those not vomiting.[14] Intravenous therapy is necessary for patients in shock and for those with an exceptionally high rate of stool output. In these settings, the rapid administration of a large volume of fluid may be lifesaving. Since glucose-facilitated sodium absorption is not disturbed in cholera, all but the most severe disease can be treated with oral administration of glucose (or even sucrose) electrolyte solution. The oral solution currently recommended by the World Health Organization (WHO) contains (in milliequivalents or millimoles per liter) sodium 90, potassium 20, chloride 80, citrate 30, and glucose 111. This oral therapy has great importance, because in many areas where cholera occurs, a sufficient supply of intravenous fluid is too expensive or too difficult to obtain. The ingredients for oral rehydration can be readily packaged, transported, and reconstituted on site. In the absence of any immediately available method of prevention in many areas of the world that are infected with cholera, this simplified treatment is critically important.

Susceptibility and Immunity

Lower socioeconomic groups have a higher incidence of cholera for a variety of reasons: (*a*) occupational exposures (e.g., boatmen in several areas have a high incidence of cholera, probably because they often drink raw river water or eat seafood); (*b*) unsanitary conditions in low-income housing areas, primarily reflected in inadequate sewage disposal and contaminated water sources; and (*c*) high population density in low-income areas, increasing the risk of introduction of *V. cholerae* and possibly enhancing transmission of the organism after it has been introduced. Malnutrition among low-income people may aggravate the risk of infection. Although some studies suggest that poor nutrition increases the duration of diarrhea from *V. cholerae*, there is no convincing evidence of an increased incidence of disease.[15]

Many studies have demonstrated an increased rate of infection among the household contacts of persons with cholera.[16] Although the techniques varied in sensitivity, these studies reveal that 6 to 27 percent of family contacts are also infected with *V. cholerae* within 10 to 14 days after the person whose disease was initially recognized. The onset of disease at almost the same time in the initial patient and household contacts suggests that the family contacts have "co-primary" cases; that is they are infected from the same common source rather than by "secondary" infection from the first patient.

Studies in India, Italy, Israel, and Bangladesh, as well as volunteer challenge studies, have shown that diminished gastric acid increases the risk of infection and of more severe illness.[17] The protection afforded by gastric acid is probably due to the sensitivity of *V. cholerae* to the low pH. In addition, for unknown reasons severe disease is more common in persons with blood group O. The relationship between age and cholera has been extensively studied. In newly infected areas, cholera characteristically affects more adults than children. The earliest cases often occur in men, who may have more frequent exposure because of their greater mobility. In endemic areas such as Bangladesh, cholera has a higher attack rate in children than in adults, with a peak incidence in the 2- to 9-year-old group.[18]

One possible explanation for the difference in age distribution of cholera between newly infected and endemic areas is acquired immunity. Studies in Bangladesh demonstrated that, with increasing age and a fall in cholera incidence, the serum vibriocidal titer rises. Serum vibriocidal antibody is thought to reflect the immune state but does not itself provide protection. Animal experiments and volunteer challenge studies suggest that immunity to *V. cholerae* is long lasting and is mediated by the local intestinal immune system.[19] The way in which these defenses operate is not yet clearly understood, but intensive work is being aimed at exploiting these mechanisms for the development of a more protective cholera vaccine.

Breast feeding protects infants against cholera in areas of both endemic and epidemic disease.[18] Breast feeding, especially exclusively, reduces exposure to *V. cholerae* in food or water. In addition, IgA antibodies in breast milk protect children from diarrhea, although not from infection.

Seasonality

Cholera occurs in a seasonal pattern; however, the season differs among countries and even among regions of the same country. Moreover, the season may change with time in the same area. Thus, the waning of an epidemic may be a natural occurrence and not the result of control measures.

Pattern of Spread

The spread of cholera during the seventh pandemic has been facilitated by modern transportation. Now, as observed in 1931, "It travels as man travels, stops where he stops, and proceeds again at the time, and in the direction, in which he resumes his journey."[1]

Humans are the usual reservoir of *V. cholerae*. These organisms reach the environment through the stool of infected persons, but *V. cholerae* poorly tolerates exposures such as drying and sunlight. On moist, fecally contaminated clothing *V. cholerae* El Tor survives 1 to 3 days, but on dry surfaces it dies quickly; thus, fomites are not a dangerous vehicle of cholera. Cholera vibrios may remain viable for up to 7 days on the surface of fruits, vegetables, and meat under favorable conditions, and for up to 3 weeks in nonacidic fish and shellfish.[20]

In water the survival time is enhanced by a temperature of 18° to 23°C (60° to 70°F), pH between 6 and 9, and sodium chloride content between 1 and 4 percent. Many other factors, such as the presence of nutrients and the deposition of a large number of organisms, may favor survival. In contrast, competitive organisms, sunlight, chemicals such as chlorine and iodine, and rapidly flowing water shorten survival. *V. cholerae* El Tor probably does not survive for more than 4 weeks when deposited in water and usually survives for less than 1 week. On the other hand, *V. cholerae* can be an autochthonous resident of brackish or even fresh water, apparently in a viable but nonculturable state. These dormant organisms are capable of transforming into a culturable and presumably fully virulent state if environmental conditions are favorable. *V. cholerae* in a nonculturable state may associate with phytoplankton or zooplankton or with blue-green algae, and "blooms" of these organisms may lead to reemergence of *V. cholerae* and its transmission to humans.[21]

Since the investigations of John Snow (see Chapter 2) and the water-borne epidemic in Hamburg in 1892, water has been considered an important vehicle in the transmission of cholera. Water is probably the primary vehicle of infection in endemic areas such as Bangladesh.[22] Even in this setting, however, the exposures are varied and complex. Epidemiologic studies in rural Bangladesh have failed to demonstrate lower cholera infection rates in persons taking drinking water from bacteriologically safe tube wells than in persons drinking contaminated surface water. This unexpected finding has led to the speculation, supported by several studies, that the protection afforded by drinking better-quality water may be overwhelmed by frequent exposure to polluted surface water through bathing, food preparation, and utensil washing.[23] Avoidance of tube well water by children, who have a high incidence of cholera, may also contribute to the apparent lack of protection noted in these areas when such safe drinking water was provided.

In endemic areas, outbreaks can sometimes be related to a common food source. In addition, contaminated foods have been the source of explosive outbreaks in newly infected areas. During the seventh pandemic, careful epidemiologic investigation of outbreaks has frequently led to the identification of a responsible food item. These have included mussels in Italy (1973), salted fish in Guam (1974), raw cockles and commercially bottled water in Portugal (1974), raw shellfish in the Gilbert Islands (1977), and inadequately steamed crabs in Louisiana (1978). Non-seafood items that have been implicated include millet gruel in Mali (1984), leftover cooked rice in Guinea (1986), raw pork in Thailand (1987), and frozen coconut milk in Maryland (1991). In Latin America seafood, cooked rice, raw vegetables and fruit, and street vendor food were implicated in transmission (1991). The commonly implicated shellfish either come from polluted water or are "freshened" with contaminated water before being sold. In arid inland areas of Africa that should be hostile to marine vibrios the organism seems to survive better than predicted. Person-to-person transmission can occur under special circumstances. For example, transmission during burial ceremonies has been reported, particularly in Africa. In these settings transmission may be from person to person, although it could also be via food or drinks served at the time of the burial. Hospitals are another setting in which person-to-person spread has been reported. Although flies may transport a small number of vibrios from excreta to food, the lack of multiplication of vibrios in such contaminated food and the necessary high infectious dose makes it unlikely that flies play an important role in transmission. Fomites probably play only a limited role in transmission, although fecally contaminated bed linen or clothing may pose a risk if measures to avoid further contaminating the environment are not taken during laundering.

Prevention

The provision of safe water and adequate disposal of excreta would reduce the high rate of cholera and other diarrheal diseases in many developing countries. Certainly in an epidemic, steps should be taken to ensure uncontaminated or treated water and proper disposal of feces.

Surveillance, including systematic identification, investigation, and reporting of cases, is a vital aspect of any cholera control program. Appropriate use of laboratory diagnostic tests facilitates identification of cases. A rectal swab or stool sample should be obtained from persons with suspected cholera to confirm the presence of *V. cholerae*. Communities threatened by cholera can easily institute bacteriologic surveillance for the introduction of *V. cholerae* by culturing feces from the community sewage system. Complete reporting of cases and suspected cases to appropriate public health authorities is important. Repressive control measures such as quarantine should be avoided, since they serve little purpose and may inhibit reporting of cases. Epidemiologic investigation of cases and analysis of information are critical for the formulation of specific control measures.

Surveillance also suggests where to establish treatment facilities in an affected area. With proper warning and preparation, supplies can be ordered and staff trained or shifted to the area. This must remain the first priority of a control effort, because adequate treatment can prevent deaths from cholera.

Antibiotic prophylaxis of household contacts of persons with cholera decreases the risk of disease. However, such an approach has little application for the community at large, where individual risk of infection is much lower, is harder to define, and is spread over a longer period. Treating hundreds of persons would be necessary to prevent a single case.

Mass immunization with parenteral cholera vaccine, although frequently done, offers little in a cholera control program. The current vaccine does not prevent transmission of the organism, and the 50 to 60 percent protection, lasting for less than 5 months, that is conferred is not enough to justify the cost and difficulty of its delivery. Thus an immunization program may create a false sense of security among both recipients and health administrators and should not supplant more effective control measures. The WHO no longer recommends cholera vaccine as a requirement for travel from country to country in any part of the world. New killed or live *V. cholerae* vaccines may offer greater efficacy and/or duration of protection. An oral vaccine consisting of killed vibrios resulted in 52 percent efficacy for preventing cholera cases over a 3-year period in Bangladesh; addition of the B subunit of cholera toxin to the vaccine, with the intention of stimulating antitoxic immunity, did not enhance protection.[24] A live attenuated strain of *V. cholerae* that has shown high-level efficacy in volunteer studies is being evaluated in a large field trial in Indonesia.[25] Further consideration of the cost-effectiveness of using such vaccines for cholera control is warranted.

Escherichia coli Diarrhea

Robert E. Black

Escherichia coli is a Gram-negative bacillus that can be found in the normal intestinal flora of humans and animals but is also an important cause of enteric illness.[1] *E. coli* can be typed biochemically and serologically. The serotypes are described by letter and number on the basis of three antigenic groups, O, K, and H (e.g., *E. coli* O111, K58, and H12).

E. coli organisms are important causes of diarrhea in residents and visitors in developing countries, but *E. coli*–associated diarrhea is relatively uncommon in the United States and northern Europe. *E. coli* can cause diarrhea by a wide variety of pathogenic mechanisms, including the production of toxins (enterotoxigenic), invasion of gut mucosa (enteroinvasive), cytotoxin-induced tissue damage (enterohemorrhagic) or adherence to the membrane of the enterocyte, resulting in destruction of the microvilli (enteroadherent).

Enteropathogenic Escherichia coli

Nursery epidemics of watery diarrhea associated with *E. coli* were first reported in the 1940s. The *E. coli* identified in these outbreaks commonly belonged to specific serotypes that subsequently became known as "enteropathogenic" serotypes.[2] Nursery epidemics associated with enteropathogenic serotypes have decreased in the United States in recent years but continue to be reported in other countries, such as the United Kingdom.

Enteropathogenic serotypes of *E. coli* rarely produce the enterotoxins associated with enterotoxigenic *E. coli*. The ability of some enteropathogenic *E. coli* isolated during an outbreak to cause diarrhea when given to volunteers suggested that other mechanisms of action existed. In fact, with the recent discovery that many of the *E. coli* belonging to the so-called enteropathogenic serotypes adhere in a seemingly pathognomonic way to the intestinal epithelium (see the discussion of enteroadherent *E. coli*) or have other mechanisms of action, this category of enteropathogenic *E. coli* based on serotype should no longer be used.

Enterotoxigenic Escherichia coli

In the late 1960s it was first recognized that some *E. coli* strains produced enterotoxins that caused diarrhea in many animals and in humans. Research in the following decade led to the recognition that these organisms are a major cause of diarrhea in developing countries. The illness caused by enterotoxigenic *E. coli* ranges from mild diarrhea to a dehydrating cholera-like illness but is usually characterized by watery, nonbloody diarrhea lasting from 1 to 7 days and little or no dehydration. Replacement of water and electrolytes by either the oral or the parenteral route is the only treatment usually required.

Enterotoxigenic *E. coli* organisms are now known to produce two plasmid-mediated enterotoxins: one heat labile and the other heat stable. The heat-labile toxin is structurally similar to cholera toxin and causes loss of fluid and electrolytes in the intestine as a result of adenylate cyclase stimulation. The heat-stable toxin acts in a similar way through stimulation of guanylate cyclase.[3] The relative frequency with which *E. coli* produces the heat-labile toxin, the heat-stable toxin, or both varies in different regions of the world. Analysis of *E. coli* from various areas suggests that strains producing both toxins are largely restricted to a small number of serotypes that are different from the so-called enteropathogenic serotypes. The ability to produce only heat-stable toxin or only heat-labile toxin seems to occur in a broader range of serotypes. Colonization factors, also plasmid mediated, appear to be essential for the *E. coli* to establish itself in the small intestine.

Enterotoxigenic *E. coli* have been shown to cause diarrhea worldwide but are more common in developing countries. In 17 community-based studies in children in developing countries, a median of 14 percent of diarrheal episodes were associated with enterotoxigenic *E. coli*.[4] The incidence of diarrhea is highest during the first 2 years of life. Although enterotoxigenic *E. coli* diarrhea also occurs in adults, partial immunity does appear to develop after early childhood in endemic areas, and the incidence declines after the first 2 years of life.[5]

Transmission of enterotoxigenic *E. coli* is thought to be primarily through water and food. Water was the vehicle for an outbreak in a national park in the United States.[6] Food-borne outbreaks have also been reported in a hospital nursery and on a cruise ship, and enterotoxigenic organisms have been isolated from foods in Bangladesh and the United States. Rarely, person-to-person transmission occurs, particularly in hospital nurseries.

Because of the association of contaminated water and food with occurrence of this disease, avoidance of fecally contaminated water and attention to hygienic food handling help prevent illness. More specific prevention measures, including immunizations, may be possible after further epidemiologic and laboratory studies.

Travelers' Diarrhea

Travelers' diarrhea, or "turista," commonly affects travelers within 1 to 2 weeks after they arrive in a foreign country, particularly a developing country. The illness usually consists of watery diarrhea with abdominal cramps; vomiting and high fever are unusual. The diarrhea lasts from 1 to 7 days and is self-limited in most cases.

Diarrhea in travelers may be caused by a variety of bacteria (such as shigellae, salmonellae, and vibrios), viruses (such as calicivirus and rotavirus), and parasites (such as *Giardia lamblia* and *Entamoeba histolytica*). Enterotoxigenic *E. coli* strains appear to cause most cases, however.[7] Travelers apparently acquire the *E. coli* from fecally contaminated water or food, such as salads containing raw vegetables.

Travelers should be advised to avoid water and ice of dubious safety, uncooked foods, and partially cooked shellfish and meats. Perishable or cooked foods that have been left at room temperature should also be avoided. Raw fruits the traveler peels are generally safe, but raw leafy vegetables (if consumed at all) should be disinfected in chlorine solution. Drinking water may be purified by boiling or by adding 2 to 4 drops of 5 percent chlorine bleach or 5 to 10 drops of 2 percent tincture of iodine per quart of water 30 minutes before drinking. Carbonated drinks may be considered safe, but noncarbonated drinks should be avoided.

Daily prophylaxis with doxycycline or trimethoprim-sulfamethoxazole prevents most travelers' diarrhea, primarily by preventing infection with enterotoxigenic *E. coli*. Norfloxacin is also effective in preventing travelers' diarrhea. The antibiotics, however, may have side effects and may promote the emergence of bacteria with multiple drug resistance. Prophylactic use of antibiotics is not generally recommended, but might be considered if disruption of travel plans would cause severe problems.

Iodochlorhydroxyquin (Entero-Vioform) should not be used in therapy for diarrhea; it is of dubious value and is dangerous (associated with subacute myelooptic neuropathy). Limited studies have shown little or no value in using most antidiarrheal agents, such as kaolin-pectin or diphenoxylate-atropine, to treat diarrheal illness. Preparations containing bismuth subsalicylate (e.g., Pepto-Bismol), however, may reduce gastrointestinal fluid loss. Furthermore, several studies with trimethoprim-sulfamethoxazole or other drugs indicate that antibiotic treatment of diarrhea caused by enterotoxigenic *E. coli* decreases the duration of illness and reduces the total volume of diarrheal fluid lost. Although replacement of stool fluid and electrolyte losses during enterotoxigenic *E. coli* diarrhea is usually sufficient, as in cholera, antibiotic therapy may be indicated for persons with particularly severe diarrhea or those with cardiac, renal, or other diseases, in whom management of fluid and electrolyte imbalance is difficult.[8] Some other types of diarrhea occurring in travelers, such as shigellosis, giardiasis, and amebiasis, may require more specific antimicrobial treatment.

Enteroinvasive Escherichia coli

In 1971 an outbreak of disease caused by enteroinvasive *E. coli* involved almost 400 persons in the United States. This outbreak was caused by imported French cheese contaminated with *E. coli* O124:B17.[9] These *E. coli* organisms, similar to *Shigella* species, cause a dysenteric diarrheal illness with tenesmus, fever, abdominal cramps, and sometimes bloody stools. The *E. coli* strains associated with this illness produce keratoconjunctivitis in guinea pigs, which serves as a marker for the capability of these organisms to invade the intestinal mucosa.

The global importance of enteroinvasive *E. coli* organisms as a cause of disease is unknown, but they have not been common in several studies in the United States, Bangladesh, and other areas of the world. Because of limited knowledge about the transmission, specific preventive measures are unknown.

Enterohemorrhagic Escherichia coli

In 1982 two outbreaks of illness characterized by severe abdominal cramps, grossly bloody diarrhea, and little or no fever occurred.[10] The outbreaks were due to *E. coli* of a rare serotype (O157:H7), which was acquired from inadequately cooked, contaminated ground beef eaten at a fast food restaurant. The *E. coli* strains were not invasive or toxigenic by standard tests but produced a cytotoxin similar to Shiga toxin of *Shigella dysenteriae* type 1 that is involved in the pathogenesis of the bloody diarrhea. Since these outbreaks, sporadic cases and other outbreaks of hemorrhagic colitis associated with O157:H7 *E. coli* have been reported in many areas of the world.[11] These infections have also been associated with hemolytic-uremic syndrome and thrombotic thrombocytopenic purpura.

In the United States most outbreaks have been caused by foods of bovine origin, especially ground beef; however, outbreaks have also been related to unchlorinated water, unpasteurized apple juice contaminated with bovine feces, and raw vegetables, among other vehicles. Person-to-person transmission has been the mode in a number of outbreaks among children in day care centers, elderly adults in nursing homes, and in institutions for the mentally retarded. While this organism is not part of the normal bowel flora, asymptomatic infections can occur and contribute to spread. An animal reservoir in cattle is also important in its epidemiology.

There is no proven specific therapy for disease due to enterohemorrhagic *E. coli*; the results of trials of antibiotic therapy have been inconclusive. Prevention is a challenge and must encompass control measures in farming, cattle raising, and animal slaughtering and processing as well as thorough cooking or pasteurization of beef, milk, apple juice and vegetables, chlorination of water, and hygienic practices to reduce person-to-person spread.[12] Surveillance for this organism and prompt epidemiologic investigation can also help to limit the scope of outbreaks.

Enteroadherent Escherichia coli

This group of pathogens can be recognized by their ability to adhere in one of three characteristic patterns to cells in tissue culture. They include the "locally adherent" *E. coli* that encompass many of the previously designated enteropathogenic *E. coli*, and these strains are clearly associated with diarrhea. These strains cause a characteristic lesion in the intestine with close adherence to the enterocyte membrane with cupping around the organisms and destruction of the microvilli.[13] Another type, the enteroaggregative *E. coli*, have a "stacked brick" pattern of adherence to tissue culture cells and glass slides.[14] These organisms have been associated with acute and persistent diarrhea in children of developing countries and in travelers and have generally caused diarrhea in healthy U.S. adult volunteers.[15–17] A number of possible mechanisms of action have been postulated. Strains of *E. coli* manifesting a diffuse pattern of adherence to tissue culture cells have been described. Their association with diarrhea has been variable and their mechanism of pathogenicity unclear.[15–17]

Illness associated with these organisms is characterized by fever and malaise, and by vomiting and diarrhea with fecal mucus but not gross blood. Control measures, as for other forms of *E. coli*–associated diarrhea, consist of limiting fecal-oral transmission.

Yersiniosis

M. Patricia Quinlisk

Although they were first described in 1934, it is over the past 30 years that *Yersinia enterocolitica* and *Yersinia pseudotuberculosis* have been increasingly recognized as significant pathogens.

Clinical Characteristics

Two-thirds of acute *Yersinia* infections present as enterocolitis and are characterized by a febrile diarrhea with abdominal pain lasting more than a week. The diarrhea can be bloody, especially in children less than 5 years old. In older children and adolescents, acute infection more often presents as an acute mesenteric lymphadenitis with leukocytosis, which can be clinically indistinguishable from acute appendicitis and may result in unnecessary laparotomies. In Scandinavia, between 10 and 30 percent of adults with *Y. enterocolitica* infection develop a reactive polyarthritis, which begins a few days to a month after the onset of diarrhea. Most of these patients have the HLA-B27 gene type and are asymptomatic by 12 months after onset.

Erythema nodosum occurs in up to 30 percent of Scandinavian cases, with women outnumbering men two to one. Symptoms occur 2 to 20 days after the onset of fever and abdominal pain and usually resolves within 1 month. Both of these manifestations have also been reported following *Y. pseudotuberculosis* infection, but mesenteric adenitis is the most common presentation. Less frequently reported manifestations are exudative pharyngitis, septicemia, and abscesses. *Yersinia enterocolitica* sepsis has been reported after blood transfusion from asymptomatic and mildly symptomatic donors.[1] Convalescent carriage of *Yersinia* is common and can be prolonged, but secondary spread is rare. There is increasing evidence that chronic complaints may not be uncommon following *Yersinia* infection.[2,3]

Bacteriology

Yersinia enterocolitica can be isolated using routine techniques for stool cultures; however, the colonies are small after 24 hours and can be easily overgrown. Most laboratories in the United States culture specifically for *Y. enterocolitica* only on request because it is not cost-effective to routinely include selective media for this low-prevalence organism and since the majority of clinically significant infections can by identified without it. The use of selective media like cefsulodin irgasan novobiocin (CIN) with incubation at lower than usual temperatures increases the probability of isolating of *Yersinia* species (including nonpathogenic strains) and may be of particular use in persons with low numbers of organisms in their stool, such as convalescent patients. *Yersinia* spp. can be isolated from blood using standard blood culture media. Serologic tests (agglutination tests or enzyme-linked immunosorbent assays) can be useful for diagnosis, particularly in culture-negative cases, but availability is limited.

More than 50 serotypes of *Y. enterocolitica* have been described; serotypes O3, O8, O9, and O5,27 are most frequently associated with human illness. Although type O8 has been associated with most of the U.S. outbreaks in the past, O3 became more common in the 1990s.[4] Isolates in Europe are usually types O3 or O9. Approximately 80 percent of *Y. pseudotuberculosis* infections are caused by O-group I strains.

In these *Yersinia* species a 70-kb plasmid encodes several virulence factors, including a secreted protein kinase. Some isolates of *Y. enterocolitica* produce a heat-stable enterotoxin, similar to that produced by *E. coli*, at 25°C but not at 37°C, and therefore is probably not of clinical significance.

Epidemiology

Yersinia enterocolitica has been only infrequently isolated as a cause of gastroenteritis in the United States, Africa, Asia, and South America. However, in parts of Northern Europe, Japan, and Canada it may be as common as or more common than other enteric pathogens, such as *Shigella* or *Salmonella*. Most cases occur in the cold months, and although susceptibility is general, children are more likely to be infected.

A wide variety of animals have been found to be asymptomatically infected with *Y. enterocolitica*, including domestic dogs, cats, sheep, cattle, and pigs. Although this bacterium has been isolated from a variety of foods, most of these isolates are nonpathogenic. In Northern Europe this bacterium is frequently found in the pharynx of pigs, with many of the strains isolated from raw pork and pork products being pathogenic. These foods have often been implicated as a source of human disease.[5] Since this organism grows at 4°C, raw or partly cooked refrigerated meats may play a major role in sporadic cases as well as in outbreaks.[6] Recently in the United States, illness in black infants has been associated with pork chitterlings (intestines) being prepared in the infant's home.[7] Outbreaks have also been associated with ingestion of milk, contaminated tofu, and bean sprouts prepared in unchlorinated well water. Few cases have been associated with water even though this organism has been found in rivers, lakes, and drinking water. Secondary cases are rare, but nosocomial and intrafamilial transmission have been reported. The incubation period is generally 4 to 7 days, and it is estimated that the dose needed for infection may be as high as 10^9.

Infection caused by *Y. pseudotuberculosis* is rare in humans but can be found in wild and domesticated birds and mammals. Most human infections occur in young males.

Prevention

At the present time in the United States, these organisms do not appear to play a major role in food-borne illness; however, their incidence and prevalence are probably underestimated. Several suggestions have been made to prevent and control these infections: (*a*) during the butchering of pigs, steps should be taken to prevent contamination of the pork with the bacteria in the pharynx (irradiation would also reduce the number of bacteria), (*b*) pork should be used promptly to minimize the time kept at refrigerator temperatures, (*c*) all meat should be properly cooked prior to consumption, (*d*) steps should be taken to minimize the possibility of milk being contaminated after pasteurization, and (*e*) prospective blood donors with recent history of gastroenteritis should be deferred and/or blood handling practices should be modified.[8]

Legionellosis

Robert F. Breiman • Jay C. Butler

Legionellosis occurs most often as either of two clinically and epidemiologically distinct syndromes: Legionnaires' disease, a serious, potentially fatal disease that often includes pneumonia, and Pontiac fever, a self-limited, influenza-like disease without pneumonia.[1] Legionellosis was first recognized during an epidemic of pneumonia that largely affected persons attending an American Legion convention in Pennsylvania in 1976.[2] Five months after the outbreak, McDade identified the etiologic agent, *Legionella pneumophila*, a bacterium that had not been recognized as a cause of human disease.[3] Testing of stored specimens associated with earlier investigations demonstrated that sporadic cases and epidemics of pneumonia occurring as early as 1947 were caused by species in the genus *Legionella*. Since the initial description of legionellosis, considerable knowledge has been gained about the causal bacteria and the epidemiology, treatment, and prevention of the disease.

Bacteriology

Since the recognition of the first species of *Legionella* in 1977, at least 39 species and 61 serogroups have been identified from clinical and environmental specimens.[4] Members of the genus have common characteristics, including failure to grow on blood agar and a nutritional requirement for L-cysteine. *L. pneumophila* accounts for more than 75 percent of reported cases of documented legionellosis. Although 15 serogroups of *L. pneumophila* have been described, serogroup 1 causes the greatest number of clinical infections, followed by serogroups 4 and 6. Other legionellae associated most frequently with clinical infections include *Legionella micdadei, Legionella dumoffii, Legionella bozemanii, Legionella feeleii*, and *Legionella longbeachae*.[5]

Legionella species are widely distributed in water, both in natural sites such as lakes and ponds and in human-made sources such as cooling towers and plumbing systems. The bacteria do not survive desiccation, and while they have been isolated from certain potting soils,[6,7] they have never been isolated from dry soil.

Legionella grows slowly on agar media supplemented with ferric salts and L-cysteine but not at all on most other bacteriologic media. Buffered charcoal yeast extract agar supports growth particularly well. The ideal temperature range for growth of *Legionella* is 25° to 42°C. *L. pneumophila* is a facultative intracellular bacterium because it multiplies avidly inside certain human cells, including monocytes and alveolar macrophages,[8,9] as well as within ciliated protozoa and amoebae, and it does not multiply if supporting cells are removed from tissue culture medium.[10] Amoebae, also ubiquitous in water supplies, appear to support *Legionella* multiplication in aquatic environments where the bacteria's strict nutritional requirements cannot otherwise be met.

Clinical Characteristics

Legionnaires' disease begins with headache, myalgia, and fever. The disease often progresses rapidly (over 1 to 3 days) with chills (often rigors), cough, and pleuritic chest pain, which may be accompanied by diarrhea or obtundation. The physical examination typically shows few abnormalities except pulmonary rales and sometimes confusion. The white blood cell count is mildly elevated but there may be a preponderance of immature polymorphonuclear cells suggestive of a pyogenic bacterial (e.g., pneumococcal) infection. Proteinuria and microscopic hematuria are common. Chest roentgenograms taken early in the course of the disease show patchy alveolar infiltrates that may progress to nodular or diffuse consolidation. While pleural effusions are common, they are usually not clinically significant. Lung abscess with cavitation occasionally develops, particularly in immunocompromised persons. Renal failure with or without antecedent shock occurs in some cases; temporary dialysis has been necessary for about 3 percent of patients.

Since the clinical presentation of Legionnaires' disease is not distinct from that of pneumonia caused by other bacterial pathogens, the diagnosis must be confirmed by laboratory evidence of infection. Laboratory tests for *Legionella* infection include (*a*) recovery of *Legionella* spp. from lung tissue or respiratory secretions, or use of a direct fluorescent antibody (DFA) test to demonstrate reacting bacteria, (*b*) detection of *L. pneumophila* serogroup 1 antigens in urine by means of a radioimmunoassay or enzyme immunoassay, or (*c*) a 4-fold rise in paired acute- and convalescent-phase serum antibody reciprocal titer to 128 or greater by use of an indirect immunofluorescent antibody (IFA) assay. Although culture is the "gold standard" and appears to be 100 percent specific, sensitivity depends greatly on the quality, handling, and processing of the specimen. The DFA test generally is not sensitive (25 percent), and specificity depends on the level of experience of personnel performing the test and on the reagents used.[11] Urinary antigen assays are highly specific (greater than 99 percent) and are 50 to 60 percent sensitive for *L. pneumophila* serogroup 1 infections.[11–13] For infection caused by *L. pneumophila* serogroup 1, the sensitivity of the IFA assay is 75 percent and the specificity is 99 percent if *L. pneumophila* serogroup 1 is the only antigen used but is lower if additional antigens are used.[13] While serology is useful for epidemiologic purposes, its clinical utility is limited because in most patients it takes 3 to 6 weeks to mount at least a 4-fold rise in antibody titer, and single acute-phase serologic titers have low predictive value.[12] The sensitivity and specificity of diagnostic tests for legionellae other than *L. pneumophila* serogroup 1 are not well defined.

Macrolides (erythromycin, azithromycin, or clarithromycin) with or without rifampin are generally effective therapy. Quinolone agents (including ofloxacin, ciprofloxacin, and levofloxacin) also appear effective, but they have been evaluated in only a small number of patients with Legionnaires' disease.[13] Other antibiotics with activity against *Legionella* include doxycycline and trimethoprim-sulfamethoxazole. However, azithromycin, dipithromycin, leuofloxacin, and trovofloxain currently have an indication by the U.S. Food and Drug Administration for treatment of Legionnaires' disease.

Death from progressive pneumonia or shock occurs in 10 to 15 percent of patients.[5] Extreme fatigue and chronic respiratory symptoms may persist for several months after recovery from acute infection. Exposure to *L. pneumophila* has been shown to provide protective immunity against a subsequent lethal dose of the bacteria in an animal model.[14] However, subsequent episodes of legionellosis have been reported for severely immunocompromised patients.[15]

Pontiac fever is a self-limited illness in which fever, headache, and myalgia are prominent symptoms; pleuritis has been observed, but not pneumonia.[1] Illness generally resolves within 5 days without antibiotic therapy.

Legionella infections that do not fit the clinical syndromes of Legionnaires' disease or Pontiac fever have also been reported and include endocarditis, peritonitis, and skin and soft tissue infections.[13] Extrapulmonary disease generally occurs in immunosuppressed patients.

Transmission

Legionellosis is transmitted to persons who inhale *Legionella* organisms in respirable droplets of water from aerosol-producing devices. Cooling towers and evaporative condensers, heat-rejection devices that produce sizable volumes of aerosol, have been sources of several outbreaks.[16–18] Ducts and vents of air-conditioning systems can be conduits for the passage of aerosol containing *Legionella* organisms from nearby contaminated cooling towers. Most studies have indicated that aerosol from contaminated cooling towers can transmit disease within a limited range (less than 200 m); however, in certain circumstances, cooling towers may transmit *Legionella* to persons several miles away.[19] Air-conditioning systems based on direct exchange of heat from refrigerant to air, without use of water evaporation (such as window and most other home air-conditioning units and automobile air-conditioners) are not intrinsically capable of transmitting disease.

Use of showers that produce droplets of respirable size containing *L. pneumophila* serogroup 1 was epidemiologically linked to Legionnaires' disease in one outbreak[20] and has probably played a role in others.[21,22] Whirlpool spas can transmit disease to persons who are exposed to their contaminated aerosols (including persons who are nearby but do not enter the spas).[23,24] An ultrasonic humidifier, contaminated with *L. pneumophila* serogroup 1 and used as a misting machine for produce in a grocery store, was implicated in a large community-wide outbreak.[25] The role of home humidifiers in sporadic cases of Legionnaires' disease is unknown. Respiratory therapy equipment containing contaminated tap water has been shown to transmit disease.[26] A large outbreak of Pontiac fever at an automobile engine assembly plant resulted from aerosolization of an industrial grinding fluid containing *L. feeleii*.[27] The infectious dose for *L. pneumophila* is unknown, but data from an outbreak investigation suggest that disease can be transmitted to susceptible persons exposed to one colony-forming unit of bacteria per 50 L of air.[17]

Legionellosis resulting from aspiration of upper respiratory secretions or gastric contents may occur among certain hospitalized patients.[28] Transmission of extrapulmonary *L. dumoffii* infection by direct inoculation of surgical wounds with colonized tap water during bathing or dressing changes has been reported.[29] No evidence has shown person-to-person transmission or persistent colonization of humans with the bacteria. Although early epidemiologic studies suggested an association between Legionnaires' disease and exposure to construction sites, transmission has not been demonstrated to occur via inhalation of dust.

Occurrence

Between 600 and 1,500 cases of Legionnaires' disease are reported annually in the United States. However, the actual incidence is probably much higher, because fewer than 10 percent of cases are detected and reported.[5] In one population-based study, the incidence of legionellosis was 6.0/100,000 adults per year.[30] Though the incidence rates are likely variable, Legionnaires' disease has been shown to occur worldwide, in areas where diagnostic tests are available. *Legionella* species are the etiologic agents in 1 to 5 percent of community-acquired pneumonias in adults.[30–33]

Legionnaires' disease occurs predominantly in middle-aged and elderly adults, cigarette smokers, and persons who have underlying medical conditions, including chronic renal failure, organ transplantation, use of immunosuppressive agents (e.g., corticosteroids), malignancy, HIV infection, chronic pulmonary disease, diabetes mellitus, and alcohol addiction. The incubation period is generally 2 to 10 days. In outbreaks of disease the attack rate is often 1 to 5 percent, reflecting the importance of host susceptibility to developing disease. In contrast, Pontiac fever often occurs in young, healthy people, has a brief (12 to 48 hours) incubation period, and has a very high (up to 100 percent) attack rate. The basis for the divergence of the two syndromes is not established; however, one possibility is that Pontiac fever represents a toxic or inflammatory response to nonviable *Legionella* antigens or other antigens (e.g., amoebae) that may be inhaled along with *Legionella*. This theory is based on the observation that Pontiac fever does not progress to systemic *Legionella* infection but consistently has a self-limited course. Legionnaires' disease occurs in both epidemic and sporadic form. Most cases are sporadic and are not linked to recognized epidemics. Some epidemics have been brief and explosive, whereas others have smoldered for several years. Explosive outbreaks occur most commonly in summer months and are often associated with point sources, such as cooling towers or evaporative condensers. Prolonged outbreaks have often been documented in institutional settings, such as hospitals and hotels, and have frequently been attributed to contaminated potable water. While the sources of infection for sporadic cases are generally unknown, it is likely that the modes of transmission for these cases are similar to those that occur in epidemic settings. Pontiac fever is recognized only in epidemic form, sporadically occurring disease would probably be misclassified as influenza or other viral syndrome.

Prevention and Control

An intensive epidemiologic investigation is frequently necessary to identify the source of a legionellosis outbreak. Interviews with patients can help generate hypotheses about possible exposure risks, and case-control or cross-sectional studies are necessary to evaluate the hypotheses. Since the bacteria are often found in aquatic environments, identification of *Legionella* species in the water in an aerosol-producing device alone does not implicate that device as the source of disease. Particle-sizing microbial air samplers can help to demonstrate that a device suspected of transmitting *Legionella* is capable of generating an aerosol containing viable bacteria within droplets of respirable size (1 to 5 μm in diameter).[17,20] Comparing isolates from patients and from aerosol-producing devices by molecular subtyping techniques, including monoclonal antibody subtyping, pulsed-field gel electrophoresis, and arbitrarily primed polymerase chain reaction, can support epidemiologic findings by demonstrating that isolates from patients are similar to isolates from suspected sources of transmission.[34–36] However, these tests alone cannot reliably implicate a source without epidemiologic data, because the distribution of isolates of various subtypes in the environment is unknown.

Once a source of bacteria-laden aerosol is identified, intervention by decontamination procedures depends on the type of source and the institution in which it is located. For a potable water source (e.g., tap water, showers, or hot water heaters), flushing the entire system with superheated (above 60°C) or hyperchlorinated (more than 10 mg free residual chlorine per liter) water may reduce the concentration of *Legionella* spp. to undetectable levels and prevent transmission.[37,38] In addition, contaminated water heaters require drainage and mechanical cleaning, particularly if they contain sediment. These procedures must be followed by a regular maintenance program to decrease the likelihood that *Legionella* will recolonize the system. Possible strategies include continuous infusion of chlorine (generally 1 to 2 mg free residual chlorine per liter), maintenance temperatures above 50°C, or intermittent superheating or hyperchlorination. Drawbacks to these approaches include expensive damage to plumbing fixtures as a result of persistent exposure to chlorine[39] and the risk of scalding, particularly among elderly persons and young children. Although they are still being evaluated, commercially available maintenance systems that rely on the bactericidal activity of silver and copper ions appear promising.

Cooling towers and evaporative condensers that are sources of legionellosis should be drained, mechanically cleaned with a dispersant (such as automatic dishwasher detergent), and hyperchlorinated.[40] Maintenance strategies include regular cleaning and infusion of chlorine or other biocides that inhibit *Legionella* growth.

After decontamination procedures, monitoring the source of transmission for the presence of the bacteria and surveillance for new cases of legionellosis are necessary for at least 6 to 12 months to evaluate the effectiveness of the intervention and make changes in the maintenance strategy.

The value of routine bacterial monitoring and maintenance of natural and human-made water systems in preventing epidemics of legionellosis has not been shown, in part because legionellae are so widespread and frequently do not cause disease. The bacteria have been found in water of aerosol-producing devices without being associated with known cases of disease, even in hospital settings where susceptible persons are potentially exposed. Use of biocides in conjunction with periodic drainage and cleaning recommended for efficient operation of cooling towers and evaporative condensers may prevent proliferation of legionellae to high concentrations in those devices. Some institutions maintain hot water temperatures above 50°C. Silver-copper ionization, ultraviolet light, and ozone in potable water systems are promising approaches that require further study to evaluate their effectiveness. Whirlpool spas and humidifiers should be drained and cleaned regularly, although their role in sporadic and epidemic legionellosis is not fully defined. Whirlpool spa filters should be inspected and cleaned or changed regularly. Several studies have demonstrated that tap water should not be used in the operation, rinsing, or cleaning of respiratory care equipment.[26,41]

The Hospital Infection Control Practices Advisory Committee (HICPAC) has made recommendations for the control of legionellosis in hospital settings.[42] The American Society of Heating, Refrigerating, and Air-Conditioning Engineers (ASHRAE) is in the process of developing guidelines for minimizing the risk of legionellosis in public places. Regulations with this objective are in force in several other countries, including the United Kingdom, Australia, and Japan.

Better understanding of the relationship between *Legionella* and amoebae may lead to exciting new approaches in prevention and control. Sampling water from aerosol-producing devices for the presence of both *L. pneumophila* and certain species of amoebae may detect sites likely to support *Legionella* multiplication to high concentrations. Based on available information, interventions should focus on eliminating both amoebae and *Legionella* from the outbreak source and on altering environmental factors that promote their interaction.

Erythromycin chemoprophylaxis of immunosuppressed patients at a hospital with a high incidence of nosocomial Legionnaires' disease due to colonization of the hot water distribution system resulted in protection against Legionnaires' disease.[43] However, in view of the generally low attack rate during outbreaks and the potential of eliminating the source of the organism, chemoprophylaxis is seldom indicated. Vaccination of susceptible persons represents an entirely different approach for prevention of Legionnaires' disease. Two vaccine preparations provide protective immunity in animals but have not yet been tested in humans.[44,45] However, their development will require a substantial change in the way immunizations are viewed and used for prevention of infectious disease in adults.

Amebiasis and Amebic Meningoencephalitis

Jonathan I. Ravdin

▸ AMEBIASIS

Amebiasis refers to human infection by the enteric protozoan *Entamoeba histolytica*. *E. histolytica* and nonpathogenic *Entamoeba dispar* infect 10 percent of the earth's population, with the percentage higher in poor developing areas. *E. histolytica* is estimated to be the third leading parasitic cause of death worldwide.[1] Infection with *E. histolytica* or *E. dispar* readily follows ingestion of the cyst form; however, only approximately 10 percent of those infected with *E. histolytica* manifest the symptoms of invasive amebiasis, colitis, and liver abscess. *E. dispar* infections are always asymptomatic. Recognition of amebic infection requires knowledge of the epidemiology of the parasite, the varied clinical presentations, and the available diagnostic methods. Therapy for amebiasis requires use of multiple antiparasitic drugs that act against amebae in the bowel lumen or invading host tissues. Prevention of amebic infection depends on adequate sanitation with availability of safe water supplies and avoidance of direct fecal-oral contamination among family members or sexual partners.

Life Cycle and Epidemiology

Infection is contracted by ingestion of the cyst form, which by virtue of its chitinous cell wall resists desiccation in the environment and destruction by stomach acid. Cysts contain one to four nuclei; excystation occurs in the small bowel, and the trophozoite form proceeds downstream to colonize the colon. Encystment of trophozoites followed by fecal excretion of cysts completes the life cycle; trophozoites rapidly disintegrate in the environment and if immediately ingested would most likely be killed by the acid pH of the stomach.

Risk factors for acquisition of *E. histolytica* infection and increased susceptibility to aggressive invasive amebiasis are summarized in Table 10-2. Infection is most prevalent in developing areas of the world such as Mexico, Africa, India, and South America. In developed countries, amebic infection and disease are concentrated in high-risk groups, such as those with prior exposure to an endemic environment or more likely to have direct fecal-oral contamination because of unhygienic living conditions or sexual practices. Although *E. histolytica* is one of the treatable causes of diarrhea in patients with the acquired immunodeficiency syndrome (AIDS),[2] aggressive fulminant amebiasis has not been reported in this group, despite their profound defects in host immunity. Severe invasive amebiasis with increased mortality has been reported in the very young, during pregnancy, in association with corticosteroid administration, and in malnourished individuals. A careful epidemiological history is essential for recognition of amebic disease.

Pathogenesis and Host Immune Response

The low frequency of invasive clinical disease complicating widespread *E. histolytica* infection appears to be due to the existence of distinct pathogenic and nonpathogenic species (*histolytica* and *dispar*, respectively)[3,4] and a complex interplay between parasite and host factors that regulate expression of invasive pathogenic activities. Isoenzyme

TABLE 10-2. EPIDEMIOLOGIC RISK FACTORS THAT APPARENTLY PREDISPOSE TO *ENTAMOEBA HISTOLYTICA* INFECTION AND INCREASED SEVERITY OF DISEASE

■ ***Increased Prevalence***
Lower socioeconomic status in endemic area, including crowding and lack of indoor plumbing
Immigrants from endemic area
Institutionalized population, especially mentally retarded
Communal living
Promiscuous homosexual men

■ ***Increased Severity***
Children, especially neonates
Pregnancy and postpartum states
Corticosteroid use
Malignancy
Malnutrition

Reproduced with permission from Ravdin JI [ed]: Amebiasis Human Infection by *Entamoeba histolytica*. New York: Churchill Livingstone, 1988, p 496.

analysis of *E. histolytica* isolates was first used to demonstrate electrophoretic patterns uniquely associated with invasive amebiasis or asymptomatic noninvasive infection.[5] Asymptomatic intestinal infection with *E. histolytica* does occur and is distinguished from *E. dispar* infection by the presence of serum antiamebic antibodies during pathogenic infection.[6] In addition, serum antigenemia occurs during *E. histolytica* and not *E. dispar* infection.[7] Mucosal antiamebic IgA responses are more prominent in infection with *E. histolytica* than with *E. dispar*.[8]

Pathogenesis of invasive amebiasis requires adherence of amebae to the colonic mucus blanket, disruption of the colonic epithelial barrier, parasite attachment to and lysis of host epithelial and acute inflammatory cells, and resistance of trophozoites to host humoral and cell-mediated immune defense mechanisms present in tissues.[9] Amebic adherence to colonic mucins is mediated by a surface lectin inhibitable by galactose or *N*-acetyl-D-galactosamine (Gal/GalNAc); binding of this Gal/GalNAc-inhibitable adherence lectin to cell surface carbohydrates is required for *E. histolytica* cytolytic activity. Amebic proteinases can degrade epithelial basement membranes and cell-anchoring proteins, disrupting epithelial cell layers. Amebae lyse responding host neutrophils, resulting in release of neutrophil nonoxidant constituents that are toxic to host tissues. *E. histolytica* cytolytic activity is apparently regulated by a parasitic protein kinase C enzyme, involves amebic phospholipase A enzyme and acid pH vesicles, and results from an irreversible toxic increase in target cell free intracellular calcium ion concentration, possibly mediated by an amebic pore-forming protein.[10] The amebic pore-forming protein has been well-defined; bearing genetic hemology to bee venom proteins such as melliten, it apparently mediates the parasite's host defense against ingested bacteria.[11] Purified pore-forming protein can lyse nucleated cells in vitro, but may not be directly involved in amebic cytolysis of human cells. Invasive *E. histolytica* trophozoites are resistant to the lytic effects of complement, despite their activation of both alternative and classic pathways. This is apparently due to an inhibitory binding effect of the lectin-heavy subunits, preventing formation of lytic complement complexes.[12] In a nonimmune host, *E. histolytica* trophozoites are capable of killing host lymphocytes and macrophages.

In humans, asymptomatic *E. histolytica* infection usually ends within 8 to 12 months; whether this results from a specific host mucosal immune response or is associated with even brief immunity to subsequent intestinal infection is unknown. In contrast, cure of invasive amebiasis in humans or experimental animals is followed by resistance to a recurrence of invasive amebic disease. This is apparently due to development of an amebicidal cell-mediated immune response, although antibodies that block the amebic adherence lectin are also present in the serum and mucosal secretions of immune individuals.[10] Immunization of experimental animals with total amebic protein, purified Gal/GalNAc-inhibitable adherence lectin, and a 52-kDa recombinant lecith subunit provides effective immunity against liver abscess through amebicidal cell-mediated mechanisms.

Clinical Characteristics

The clinical syndromes associated with *E. histolytica* infection are listed in Table 10-3. As discussed, up to 90 percent of individuals infected with *E. histolytica* are asymptomatic and without evidence of ill health related to the parasite. Many infected persons have nonspecific gastrointestinal symptoms, such as abdominal pain, bloating, or watery diarrhea, but are without evidence of invasive disease. Although the reason for their complaints may not be clear or detectable, their amebic infection should be eradicated. Amebic dysentery has a subacute onset over days to weeks and is manifest as abdominal pain and bloody diarrhea; only a minority of patients are febrile.[13] Stool almost always contains occult blood; despite the inflammatory nature of the lesion, fecal leukocytes may not be present because the trophozoites can lyse neutrophils. The differential diagnosis includes invasive bacterial causes of colitis such as *Campylobacter, Shigella*, and *Salmonella* infection or toxin-mediated *Clostridium difficile* colitis.

Amebic colitis may be fulminant, especially in the high-risk groups summarized in Table 10-2, with high fever, peritonitis, and colonic perforation resulting in a high mortality. Conversion of amebic dysentery to toxic megacolon is clearly associated with corticosteroid administration, often resulting from the misdiagnosis of amebic colitis as idiopathic inflammatory bowel disease. A chronic nondysenteric syndrome is characterized by intermittent bouts of inflammatory diarrhea over a period of years. These patients have invasive amebic colitis that can be diagnosed by biopsy and the presence of serum antiamebic antibodies, yet their disease is frequently mistaken for idiopathic ulcerative colitis.[14] Ameboma is a chronic segmental lesion, usually in the cecum or ascending colon, that is characterized by abdominal pain and mass and is often confused with colonic carcinoma. Perianal ulcerative amebic lesions may develop

TABLE 10-3. CLINICAL SYNDROMES ASSOCIATED WITH *ENTAMOEBA HISTOLYTICA* INFECTION

■ ***Intestinal Disease***
Asymptomatic infection
Symptomatic noninvasive infection
Acute rectocolitis (dysentery)
Fulminant colitis with perforation
Toxic megacolon
Chronic nondysenteric colitis
Ameboma
Perianal ulceration

■ ***Extraintestinal Disease***
Liver abscess
Liver abscess complicated by
  Peritonitis
  Empyema
  Pericarditis
Lung abscess
Brain abscess
Genitourinary disease

Reproduced with permission from Mandell GL, Douglas RG Jr, Bennett JE [eds]: Principles and Practice of Infectious Diseases, 3rd ed. New York: Churchill Livingstone, 1989.

in patients with skin maceration caused by diarrhea; squamous epithelium is usually resistant to amebic invasion.

Extraintestinal disease is overwhelmingly due to liver abscess and its spread to contiguous body spaces. Common symptoms of amebic liver abscess are acute right upper quadrant pain and fever, necessitating differentiation from biliary tract disease. Alternatively, liver abscess may become manifest over a period of weeks with pain and weight loss but without fever, a presentation more suggestive of abdominal malignancy.[15] Knowledge of epidemiological risk factors and early use of hepatic imaging are essential for diagnosis. The risk of amebic liver abscess manifesting in patients returning from an endemic area is greatest in the first 3 months and rarely, if ever, is observed after 6 months unless infection is acquired locally. Occasionally an amebic liver abscess, especially an abscess of the left lobe, which may be less symptomatic, ruptures into the peritoneum. The liver abscess can also penetrate through the diaphragm into the pleural space, resulting in an empyema. Extension of a left lobe abscess into the pericardium is a rare but often fatal complication that usually occurs because the clinical presentation is fulminant and confusing. Lung and brain abscesses are rare examples of hematogenous dissemination; amebiasis of the penis and of the uterine cervix has been reported.

Diagnosis

Diagnosis of intestinal amebiasis usually rests on microscopic findings of *E. histolytica* in the stool. The occurrence of invasive colitis is indicated by the finding of trophozoites (often containing ingested erythrocytes) in stool, a positive serological test for antiamebic antibodies, and the presence of ulcerative mucosal lesions observed by lower gastrointestinal endoscopy.[16] For reliable exclusion of amebic disease from the diagnosis, at least three separate stool samples should be examined using permanently stained slides; alternatively, total colonoscopy with biopsy is highly sensitive and definitive. At minimum, serological tests for *E. histolytica* should be performed before a diagnosis of idiopathic inflammatory bowel disease leads to use of corticosteroids. New diagnostic methods include detection of amebic lectin antigen in feces and serum. Use of epitope-specific monoclonal antibodies to the 170-kDa lectin subunit in enzyme-linked immunosorbent assay (ELISA) is an effective research tool to detect and differentiate *E. histolytica* and *E. dispar* intestinal infection. Antigen-detection ELISA methodology is commercially available for clinical application. Gastrointestinal barium roentgenograms are useless and make parasitological examinations of the stool unreliable for weeks.

Patients with a clinical syndrome and epidemiological risk factors consistent with amebic liver abscess should immediately undergo ultrasonography to look for a nonhomogeneous defect in the liver or evidence of biliary tract disease. Ultrasonography is highly sensitive, nontoxic, and relatively inexpensive; computed tomography (CT) and magnetic resonance imaging are not more specific and are only slightly more sensitive.[17] Amebic liver abscess is difficult to distinguish from bacterial liver abscess or hepatoma by imaging but usually a correct clinical diagnosis is possible. Amebic liver abscess may occur at any age in persons who do not have the risk factors commonly associated with pyogenic abscess or hepatoma; however, if amebic serological testing is unavailable, ultrasonography or CT-guided fine-needle aspiration can be helpful. Gram's stain and culture for bacteria establish the diagnosis; in amebic abscesses a yellow proteinous debris without white blood cells is found. Trophozoites are not usually seen in the abscess aspirate, since they commonly reside in tissue only at the lesion's periphery. Virtually all persons with amebic liver abscess develop serum antiamebic antibodies but often not until the seventh day of symptoms.[15] Thus an initial negative serological test for *E. histolytica* can be misleading early in the course of the abscess. *E. histolytica* trophozoites or cysts can be found in the stool of only a small number of patients with amebic liver abscess.

Treatment

Therapy for *E. histolytica* infection is complicated by the necessity for different agents to treat intraluminal and tissue infestation. Tables 10-4 and 10-5 summarize the drugs in use, their respective sites of activity, and recommendations for drug dosage and duration of therapy. In a nonendemic area, most experts would treat asymptomatic cyst passers, especially given the difficulty differentiating *E. histolytica* from *E. dispar* isolates. I recommend that, in a highly endemic area, asymptomatic infection be treated only if serum antiamebic antibodies are present or fecal antigen test is positive for *E. histolytica*. Diloxanide furoate is highly efficacious and relatively nontoxic; unfortunately, in the United States this drug is available only from the Centers for Disease Control Drug Service in Atlanta.[18] Paromomycin is a nonabsorbable aminoglycoside that is efficacious and often better tolerated than the combination of tetracycline and diiodohydroxyquin.[19]

The nitroimidazoles are the drugs of choice for treatment of invasive amebiasis; metronidazole is the only one available in the

TABLE 10-4. ANTIMICROBIAL AGENTS FOR USE IN TREATING AMEBIASIS

■ ***Luminal Agents***
Diloxanide furoate
Paromomycin
Diiodohydroxyquin

■ ***Tissue Agents***
Bowel wall only
  Tetracycline
  Erythromycin
Liver only: chloroquine

■ ***Agents Active in All Tissues***
Metronidazole
Tinidazole
Emetine hydrochloride
2-Dehydroemetine

Reproduced with permission from Mandell GL, Douglas RG Jr, Bennett JE [eds]: Principles and Practice of Infectious Diseases, 3rd ed. New York: Churchill Livingstone, 1989.

TABLE 10-5. THERAPEUTIC REGIMENS FOR TREATMENT OF AMEBIASIS[a]

■ ***Cyst Passers***
Diloxanide furoate 500 mg tid × 10 d
Paromomycin 30 mg/kg/d in 3 divided doses × 5–10 d
Tetracycline 250 mg qid × 10 d then diiodohydroxyquin 650 mg tid × 20 d
Metronidazole 750 mg tid × 10 d

■ ***Invasive Rectocolitis***
Metronidazole 750 mg tid × 5–10 d or 2.4 gr qd × 2–3 d or 50 mg/kg × 1 dose plus diloxanide furoate or paromomycin
Tetracycline 250 mg qid × 15 d plus chloroquine [base] 600 mg, 300 mg, then 150 mg tid × 14 d
Dehydroemetine 1–1.5 mg/kg/d × 5 d plus diloxanide furoate or paromomycin

■ ***Liver Abscess***
Metronidazole 750 mg tid × 5–10 d or 2.4 mg qd × 1–2 d plus diloxanide furoate or paromomycin
Dehydroemetine 1–1.5 mg/kg/d × 5 d plus diloxanide furoate or paromomycin
Chloroquine [base] 600 mg qd × 2 d, 300 mg base qd × 2–3 w [can be added to other regimens]

[a] All dosages are for oral administration except that of dehydroemetine, which is given intramuscularly; metronidazole can be given intravenously. Reproduced with permission from Mandell GL, Douglas RG Jr, Bennett JF [eds]: Principles and Practice of Infectious Diseases, 3rd ed. New York: Churchill Livingstone, 1989.

United States. In the regimens outlined in Table 10-5, metronidazole is highly effective in treating amebic colitis or liver abscess; however, treatment with an intraluminal agent should follow to ensure that intestinal infection is eradicated. Use of metronidazole may be limited by side effects such as nausea and vomiting and by concerns regarding carcinogenesis and teratogenesis. Long-term clinical follow-up has not indicated a carcinogenic effect of metronidazole, but if possible the drug should be avoided during pregnancy. The emetines are second-line agents rarely used in the United States. Adding these cardiotoxic agents to metronidazole has not been found to enhance clinical outcome. Patients with amebic liver abscess respond to metronidazole with gradual defervescence and decreased symptoms over a 3- to 5-day period. Progression of symptoms during therapy or failure of metronidazole treatment is an indication for drainage of the liver abscess by needle aspiration and continued treatment with metronidazole.[20] Open surgical drainage or addition of emetine therapy usually is not indicated but may be considered. Some authorities routinely add chloroquine to metronidazole in treatment of liver abscess, but I know of no studies that support this practice.

Prevention

Prevention of *E. histolytica* infection rests on availability of safe water supplies, adequate disposal of fecal material, and avoidance of practices that promote direct fecal-oral contamination. Boiling of water is the only certain means of killing *E. histolytica* cysts; use of halide tablets is generally inadequate. No vaccine or reasonable form of chemoprophylaxis is available; however, recent research on pathogenesis and host immunity has suggested that numerous amebic proteins are viable candidates for vaccine development.

▶ AMEBIC MENINGOENCEPHALITIS

Amebic meningoencephalitis is a rare clinical syndrome caused by acquisition of free-living amebae from the environment. *Naegleria fowleri* causes a primary amebic meningoencephalitis (PAM) in otherwise healthy individuals; infection with *Acanthamoeba* spp. is manifest as a subacute granulomatous amebic encephalitis (GAE) in patients already having serious underlying diseases. The diagnostician must be familiar with the epidemiology and clinical manifestations of amebic meningoencephalitis to avoid overlooking this infection in the differential diagnosis of patients at risk, despite the low frequency of occurrence. Diagnosis ultimately rests on finding the amebae in cerebrospinal fluid or brain tissue. Unfortunately, treatment is usually ineffective for either syndrome if it is diagnosed, or the diagnosis is not made until postmortem examination.

Life Cycle and Epidemiology

N. fowleri can exist in a trophozoite or a flagellate form; cell division is restricted to trophozoites. The organism grows best at higher temperatures (46°C) and is acquired from fresh water.[21] Encystment does occur and allows prolonged survival of the parasite at low temperatures. PAM is a rare disease despite the frequent occurrence of warm fresh water exposure during swimming, diving, or boating. The disease occurs in all areas of the world, especially in tropical regions.

Acanthamoebae exist in only the trophozoite and cyst forms, grow best at normal ambient temperatures (25 to 35°C), and may be transmitted by an airborne or a droplet route.[22] As with *Naegleria*, despite broad exposure to the *Acanthamoeba* species, *A. culbertsoni*, *A. polyphaga*, and *A. rhysodes*, GAE is found mainly in individuals with serious underlying conditions such as diabetes mellitus, AIDS, or recent organ transplantation.

Pathogenesis and Host Immune Response

N. fowleri apparently enters the central nervous system by penetrating the nasal mucosa and cribriform plate. Trophozoites can be found in nerves and perivascular spaces.[22] Amebic cell lytic activity has been demonstrated in vitro. Invasion of gray matter results in purulent meningitis. Trophozoites are susceptible to complement-mediated lysis, which is potentiated by agglutinating antibody to *N. fowleri*. Humoral and cell-mediated mechanisms limit the occurrence of PAM despite the ubiquitous exposure to this parasite.

In GAE, granulomatous lesions can occur throughout the central nervous system, suggesting a hematogenous route of dissemination. Further evidence for this route of spread is the frequent occurrence of skin lesions before spread to the nervous system and other organ systems. *Acanthamoeba* can be differentiated from *Naegleria* by the presence of cysts in tissue. The opportunistic nature of *Acanthamoeba* infection suggests that cell-mediated mechanisms are important in resistance to disease; however, GAE in immunologically competent hosts has been reported.

Clinical Characteristics

PAM is often first manifest as alterations in taste or smell, followed by abrupt onset of headache, fever, and meningismus.[21,22] A fulminant illness ensues with depressed mental status and focal neurologic signs ending in death within 1 week. Other than the olfactory involvement in PAM, the disease is difficult to distinguish from community-acquired bacterial meningitis.

GAE is a subacute disease that becomes manifest over a period of weeks with focal neurologic signs, mental status changes, seizures, headache, and fever.[23] The occurrence of nodular or ulcerative skin lesions containing *Acanthamoeba* can be helpful in establishing the diagnosis. Most patients do not have meningismus, and the disease must be differentiated from brain abscess or other opportunistic infection such as toxoplasmosis.

Diagnosis

PAM is characterized by a neutrophilic cerebrospinal fluid (CSF) pleocytosis; elevated protein levels in the CSF and hypoglycorrhachia are not uncommon. A Gram stain of CSF negative for bacteria and an India ink test negative for cryptococcal disease in a young healthy person should suggest the need to examine the CSF for motile *N. fowleri* trophozoites, which are 10 to 30 μm in diameter. In contrast, in GAE, amebae are not found in the CSF, and brain biopsy is necessary for diagnosis. CT scans of the brain reveal nonspecific findings in PAM but may show focal lucencies in GAE.[24] In GAE the CSF undergoes nonspecific changes such as lymphocytic pleocytosis and alterations in protein and glucose levels. A biopsy specimen should be obtained from any suspect skin lesion and examined for *Acanthamoeba*.

Treatment

No effective treatment for amebic meningoencephalitis has been established. Known survivors of PAM were treated with systemic and intrathecal amphotericin B.[17] One patient also received systemic rifampin, sulfisoxazole, and miconazole by the intravenous and intrathecal routes. Successful therapy for GAE also is undetermined; *Acanthamoeba* is generally susceptible in vitro to ketoconazole, miconazole, 5-flucytosine, and pentamidine, although isolates vary substantially,[25] systemic and intrathecal miconazole, and rifampin and sulfisoxazole. If GAE is diagnosed, in vitro susceptibility should be studied, and therapy with the above agents and amphotericin B considered.

Prevention

PAM and GAE are such rare infections that, in general, preventive measures are unnecessary. A small risk of PAM may be associated with repeated episodes of having water forced into the nose under pressure, as in diving or waterskiing in warm freshwater lakes. However, the level of risk is impossible to define. Opportunistic infections other than GAE are more common and of paramount importance in immunocompromised individuals.

Giardiasis

Mary E. Wilson

Giardia lamblia is a flagellated protozoan that causes subacute or chronic diarrheal disease in humans. Giardiasis occurs worldwide, particularly where people do not adhere strictly to good hygienic standards. In the United States giardiasis has been documented as a cause of waterborne outbreaks, epidemics in day care centers, and sporadic disease of overseas travelers, family members, and campers or hikers who ingest untreated surface water. The disease can be associated with acute or chronic malabsorption and may be a cause of failure to thrive in children.

Life Cycle

The life cycle of *G. lamblia* includes two stages: the cyst and the trophozoite. Giardiasis is acquired by ingestion of the dormant cyst from contaminated environmental sources. The parasite excysts while passing through the acidic stomach environment, and out of each cyst emerge two trophozoites that colonize the proximal portion of the small intestine. As the parasite passes through to the proximal colon, it once again encysts and undergoes one cell division before it is passed in the stool. Trophozoites are fragile motile forms with four pairs of flagellae, a ventral surface disc involved in attachment to intestinal mucosa, central axonemeas, and two nuclei, which give the parasite a facelike appearance. Cysts are oval and thin walled with four nuclei. During severe bouts of diarrhea both stages of the parasite can be seen in fresh stool specimens because of rapid transit of bowel contents. Often, however, only cysts are detected in stool samples.

Several aspects of the parasite's life cycle are important determinants in the epidemiology of the disease. First, *G. lamblia* cysts are immediately infectious for humans when passed in the stool, allowing person-to-person transmission of infection in settings of frequent interpersonal contact. This accounts for epidemic outbreaks in day care centers and institutions and for transfer of infection between family members. Second, *Giardia* cysts can survive for long periods in the environment, up to 16 days at 8°C, so that waterborne spread of infection or spread by fomites is possible. Third, most infected patients are asymptomatic carriers, providing a large reservoir of infection in some populations. In combination these factors produce efficient fecal-oral spread of the organism, particularly where hygienic practices are poor.

Pathogenesis and Clinical Characteristics

The spectrum of giardial infection includes asymptomatic cyst passage; subacute, noninflammatory, usually self-limited diarrhea; and a chronic diarrheal syndrome with malabsorption and weight loss. The incubation period is 1 to 2 weeks, after which typical symptoms of abdominal bloating, flatulence, eructation, crampy abdominal pain, malaise, and greasy foul-smelling diarrhea may develop. Tenesmus, vomiting, and fever are less common, and leukocytes are generally absent from the stool. The symptoms are often present for a prolonged period, averaging 17 days in one study, and approximately half of patients have a significant weight loss of approximately 10 lbs. Laboratory examinations may reveal increased fecal fat content, as well as impaired absorption of D-xylose, lactose, and vitamin B_{12}. Protein-losing enteropathy and vitamin A deficiency have also been documented.[1]

Histological studies often show flattening of intestinal villi and varying degrees of cellular infiltration. According to one study these changes relate to symptoms and are reversible with eradication of the organism. Assays of brush-border disaccharidases show deficient levels in patients with giardiasis, leading to theories that enzymatic deficiencies, abnormal lipolysis, and other factors may contribute to the pathogenesis of disease.[1] Host immune responses seem to provide partial protection against giardiasis. This has been established in animal models, but appears relevant during human disease since many adults residing in endemic regions appear less susceptible to symptomatic disease than do children or visitors. Individuals with common variable immunodeficiency and children with X-linked agammaglobulinemia are more susceptible than healthy individuals to giardiasis, indicating the importance of humoral responses in clearance of infection. Serum IgM and IgG antibodies to *G. lamblia* antigens develop during giardiasis, but the most important isotype appears to be IgA secreted locally in the gut. IgA is not in itself cytotoxic for the parasite, and IgA-mediated protection likely occurs by preventing trophozoite adherence to gut endothelium. Cellular elements are also important in clearing *G. lamblia* from infected mice. These include $CD4^+$ T lymphocytes that may provide help for IgA production, and macrophages that ingest and present *G. lamblia* antigens to T cells.[2]

Several factors in human breast milk provide partial protection against giardiasis in children. The level of secretory IgA in breast milk correlates with protection of African children against infection,[3] and of Mexican children against symptomatic disease.[4] Additionally fatty acids[2] and peptides derived from lactoferrin[5] are cytocidal for the organisms.

A major target antigen for the humoral immune response belongs to a heterogeneous set of variant-specific surface proteins (called VSPs) on the surface of *G. lamblia* trophozoites.[6] These molecules range from 30 to 200 kDa in size, but they share a conserved cysteine-rich motif and a 34–amino acid homologous peptide at their C-termini. Host antibody responses are generated to variable and semi conserved portions of the VSP proteins, but not to the 34–amino acid conserved C-terminal peptide. There is evidence for switching between VSP types in individual *G. lamblia* isolates, raising the possibility that humoral responses to one VSP induces expression of a distinct VSP.[7] Other targets of humoral immunity are heat shock proteins and other structural proteins.[2]

Diagnosis

Three methods are available for diagnosis of giardiasis: microscopic examination of stool samples for ova and parasites, microscopic examination after staining with fluorescent antibodies to *G. lamblia* and *Cryptosporidium*, and enzyme-linked immunosorbent assay (ELISA) examination of the stool for a 65-kDa *G. lamblia* antigen. When technician time for the former two assays is considered, all are comparable in cost. The sensitivity of microscopic examination increases from 50 to 70 percent on one stool sample to >90 percent after three examinations and offers the advantage that other pathogens can also be detected. When *G. lamblia* is the primary diagnostic consideration, however, such as in individuals who obtained their exposure through day care centers or by hiking in endemic regions of the United States, specific examination for *G. lamblia* may be in order. In such a setting, the immunofluorescence assay (Merifluor DFA, Meridian Diagnostics, Inc., Cincinnati, OH) has been reported with 55 to 100 percent sensitivity and 99.8 to 100 percent specificity and has the advantage that another cause of chronic diarrhea, *Cryptosporidium*, can also be detected. The ELISA (ProSpecT Giardia EZ Microplate Assay, Alexon, Inc., Sunnyvale, CA) is 91 to 97 percent sensitive and has 98 to 99.8 percent sensitivity and is quicker to perform. Several other companies offer alternate ELISA and indirect fluorescent antibody (IFA) detection kits. The sensitivity of any of the above tests increases with repeated examinations.[2,8,9]

Although stool examinations are almost always adequate for diagnosis of symptomatic giardiasis, other methods allow examination of duodenal contents for the organism. The least invasive is the Enterotest (HDC Corp., San Jose, CA) comprised of a capsule containing a weighted string that extends into the duodenum when swallowed. After recovering the string, mucus from the duodenum is examined microscopically for trophozoites. Upper endoscopy with aspiration of duodenal contents and/or small bowel biopsy can also be used to detect *G. lamblia* and simultaneously examine for other causes of chronic malabsorption (e.g., bacterial overgrowth, sprue). Giardiasis does cause a systemic antibody response, but since IgG remains for a long period after infection, this is not as useful for diagnosis as for epidemiologic surveys. Other tools that are currently of use for epidemiologic or research purposes include DNA fingerprinting of individual *G. lamblia* isolates and polymerase chain reaction (PCR) diagnosis of infection.

Treatment

Treatment of giardiasis has changed now that quinacrine, a previously used agent, is no longer manufactured in the United States. Because of familiarity and the fact that it is well tolerated, most physicians choose to treat with metronidazole 250 mg tid for 5 to 7 days. This meets with 80 to 95 percent success rates. Tinidazole, a nitroimidazole that is not marketed in the United States, is as effective as metronidazole (90 percent) in a single dose of 2 gr orally. Alternates include furazolidone 100 mg qid for 7 to 10 days (80 percent efficacy), a medication favored for use in children because it is available in suspension form. There is not a recommended means of treating pregnant women due to theoretic adverse effects of the above agents. An option is to delay treatment until after delivery. Paromomycin, a nonabsorbed aminoglycoside with about 60 to 70 percent efficacy against giardiasis, may have a therapeutic role if this is not possible.[1,10]

Other medications that are effective against *G. lamblia* in vitro include Albendazole, mebendazole, thiabendazole, and azithromycin. Albendazole at a dose of 400 mg tid for 5 days was comparable in efficacy to metronidazole in one study of infected children in Bangladesh. There is limited or no experience in use of these four agents for treating human infection.

Epidemiology

Transmission of giardiasis occurs by the fecal-oral route, either through direct contact with an infected individual or by ingestion of contaminated water or (less often) food. Giardia infection is more common in young children, probably both because of their poorer hygienic practices and in highly endemic situations due to the development of partial immunity. Prevalence rates for the organism vary widely depending on location. In the United States 3.9 percent of stool specimens submitted for examination have contained the organism, and prevalence among 1- to 3-year-olds in Washington State was 7.1 percent. The prevalence of cyst carriage in day care centers ranges from 0 to 50 percent at different centers, with many children remaining asymptomatic.[11] Children in Queensland, Australia, were found to harbor the organism in 5.7 and 2.1 percent of random stool samples from households serviced by septic tanks or city sewage lines, respectively.[12] In South Australia 2.1 percent of 100 adults undergoing upper endoscopy and 9 percent of 200 adults in Pakistan were positive for *G. lamblia*.[13,14] The annual incidence of symptomatic disease has been 9.8, 11.6, and 45.7 per 100,000 population in Minnesota, Colorado, and Vermont, respectively.[15] Prevalence rates were higher in developing countries, estimated at 19.4 percent in Zimbabwe and 42 percent in rural Egypt.[16] Surveillance of travelers to the Soviet Union revealed that 22.8 percent of 1419 tourists were ill with giardiasis and that infection was strongly associated with consumption of tap water in Leningrad.[17]

Cases of giardiasis can be divided into those occurring sporadically in high-risk individuals and those associated with outbreaks. The former group includes travelers to countries where the organism is endemic and hikers or campers who ingest untreated surface water in areas where the streams and lakes are contaminated, such as Minnesota or Colorado. Up to 20 percent of homosexual men harbored the organism in surveys of stool examinations, presumably because of habits that facilitate fecal-oral transmission. The presence of the organism in this population, however, does not correlate well with symptomatic disease and there does not seem to be an increase in symptomatic giardiasis in the AIDS population.[2] In addition up to 50 percent of children who attend day care centers pass giardial cysts, and rates of giardiasis among household contacts of infected children range from 12 to 27 percent.

Several large outbreaks of giardiasis have resulted from contamination of municipal water supplies with human waste. One such outbreak, affecting 11.3 percent of 1094 skiers, occurred in an Aspen ski resort during the 1965–1966 season when well water was contaminated with leaking sewage.[18] A large outbreak in Rome, New York, affected 10.6 percent of the population (5300 persons). This outbreak was possibly due to contamination of the water supply with human waste from settlements in the watershed area. Investigators discovered a *G. lamblia* cyst in a water sediment sample from a city water inlet.[19] In addition, in several waterborne outbreaks human waste was not thought to be the source of contamination. Notably, a Camas, Washington outbreak was traced to the city water supply, and cysts were found in three beavers in the watershed area for the water system, implying that they might constitute a reservoir for the parasite.[20] During another outbreak in Pittsfield, Massachusetts, *Giardia* cysts were found in one of three city reservoirs, and again the surrounding area contained *Giardia*-positive animals that may have been the source.[21] Although chlorine may be sufficient to kill *Giardia* cysts in the laboratory, other factors such as temperature, pH, and contact time with chlorine may result in less than optimal killing of cysts in water treatment systems that use chlorination alone. Thus, of 21,990 cases of waterborne giardiasis caused by contaminated surface water sources in the United States between 1965 and 1984, 10.1 percent were due to cross-contamination of water supplies with sewage lines and 54.6 percent of cases (56 percent of outbreaks) occurred in water sources treated with chlorination alone. In contrast, only 33.8 percent of cases (21 percent of outbreaks) were associated with water supplies that had also undergone filtration. Thus systems that include a filtration step as well as chlorination seem to be most effective in eliminating the organism.[18]

Outbreaks of symptomatic giardiasis in day care centers have affected between 17 and 47 percent of the children attending. In general, ambulatory diapered children harbor the organism most frequently.[22] Several recurrent outbreaks have been documented, sometimes despite extensive efforts to improve personal and environmental hygiene among children and staff.[23] One study documented that 16 percent of asymptomatic children harbored *G. lamblia* cysts, although no caregivers were infected other than those whose children were also infected. Thus fastidious hygiene can prevent infection of workers, but children and family members are still at risk. In the same study, *G. lamblia* cysts were recovered from chairs and tables in day care centers, indicating a possible route of transfer of cysts between the children.[11] Other situations that have facilitated outbreaks of giardiasis include a contaminated cistern providing water to several families and a swimming pool contaminated by feces of a mentally retarded child. Finally, several food-borne outbreaks have been documented, usually traced to a dish consumed by the majority of affected individuals. These usually have occurred when food was mixed by the bare hands of an individual carrying *G. lamblia* cysts.[24]

Humans are the main reservoir of *G. lamblia*; thus giardiasis is often a cosmopolitan disease. However, several animal hosts also harbor the organism and may constitute a reservoir for human outbreaks. These include most notably beavers, but *G. lamblia* cysts have also been found in muskrats, cows, goats, and sheep. Gerbils, dogs, and cats can be experimentally infected. Whether any or all of these hosts serve as a reservoir in nature, and whether strains found in these animals are pathogenic for humans, is not clear.[2]

Control measures for giardiasis include identification and treatment of colonized or infected individuals and screening of their household members for cyst passage. Treatment of water supplies by both chlorination and filtration is most effective for clearing the organism. In addition, water supplies should be routinely screened for coliform bacteria and turbidity to monitor for contamination with sewage or other sources. Treatment of asymptomatic cyst passers is desirable due to the possibility that they will develop symptoms or that they will pass the infection to family members. However, in situations where the infection is highly endemic, such as in most developing countries and in some day care centers, this may not be practical. In these situations the question of treatment must be individualized.

Dracunculiasis

Donald R. Hopkins

Dracunculiasis (Guinea worm disease), caused by infection with the parasite *Dracunculus, medinensis*, has affected humans for centuries. Definitive evidence of the disease has been found in the 3,000-year-old mummy of an Egyptian girl. The ancient practice of "treating" the infection by slowly wrapping the emerging adult worm around a stick or twig is thought by some medical historians to have been the inspiration for the caduceus and the Staff of Aesculapius—symbols of the healing arts. Although dracunculiasis is not usually fatal, it causes enormous socioeconomic damage in affected rural populations, which is the main reason why this disease is now being eradicated.

The Parasite and Its Life Cycle

People are infected with *D. medinensis* when they drink water from contaminated ponds or step wells in which larvae of the parasite are found in tiny water fleas (copepods). When gastric juices kill the copepods, the larvae escape to migrate through the wall of the stomach into the abdominal cavity. Three or four months later, the parasites mate, after which the male worm dies, and the female worms continue to grow. Approximately 1 year after the infection began, adult female worms measuring about 1 meter long migrate toward the skin, often on a lower limb, and produce a painful blister. When the blister ruptures, usually upon immersion of the affected limb in water, the gravid female worm, which resembles an ivory-colored strand of spaghetti, spews hundreds of thousands of larvae into the water. Diminishing numbers of larvae are spilled into the water by the same worm over the next several days as the wound is reimmersed in water.

Only immature larvae that are eaten by a receptive species of copepod within a few days of being released into the water survive. In the copepod, they undergo two molts within about 2 weeks, after which they are infective to humans who drink water containing the infected copepod. The larvae themselves are too small to be seen by the naked eye, but copepods are barely visible as moving specks if such water is held up to the light in a glass or jar. There is no known animal reservoir of *D. medinensis*.

Clinical Disease, Diagnosis, and Treatment

Infections are asymptomatic during most of the year-long incubation period. Shortly before a worm emerges, patients may experience nonspecific fever, nausea, or aching, but often the first sign of infection is a painful blister or appearance of the worm under the skin. No inflammatory reaction to the worm is apparent before the blister appears, but thereafter white blood cells surround the body of the emerging worm and create resistance to its removal. Although most victims suffer only one worm that usually emerges through the skin on the lower leg, ankle, or foot, this parasite may emerge from any part of the body, and some especially unfortunate persons have had more than a dozen worms emerge at the same time. Diagnosis is facilitated by the striking appearance of such a worm emerging through the skin, since no other infection of humans is manifested in that way. Often the ulcer surrounding an emerging worm becomes secondarily infected with various bacteria, which sometimes results in fatal complications of tetanus. Most commonly, the painful infection incapacitates a person for periods averaging 2 months. An estimated 0.5 percent of victims are permanently crippled each year as a result of infections or secondary complications that involve a major joint. People do not become immune to reinfection.

At best, modern medicine can offer infected persons only relief from pain and secondary infections by providing analgesics and antibiotics when indicated, cleaning wounds, and applying topical antiseptics. Providing or updating tetanus immunization is also advisable. Some anthelmintics such as niridazole, thiabendazole, and metronidazole may facilitate removal of the worm by reducing associated inflammation. Physical removal of the worm by slowly wrapping it around a stick over several days or weeks, or surgical removal of an accessible worm, can shorten the duration of suffering. Great care must be taken, however, to avoid breaking the worm, since withdrawal of a broken worm into the body spills larvae in the tissues and causes a severe inflammatory reaction. Dead worms may be absorbed by the body or they may calcify, producing unusual patterns on x-ray.

Epidemiology and Prevention

Because they drink larger amounts of water, working-age adults, especially farmers, are most affected by dracunculiasis. Many children are unable to attend school at certain times of the year in endemic areas because they cannot walk due to dracunculiasis. In some communities, more than half of the village's population may be affected at the same time. Depending on the local ecology, the peak transmission season, which is when the disease is most prevalent, often coincides with the planting or harvest season. Because of the association with contaminated surface sources of drinking water, most affected areas consist of remote rural villages with poor inhabitants, but distribution of the disease in a given country is usually sporadic. In recent years the infection has occurred in India, Pakistan, Yemen, and 16 countries in sub-Saharan Africa. It is estimated that about 3.3 million persons were infected in 1986.

Incapacitation of farmers, mothers, and schoolchildren in large numbers year after year for periods averaging about 8 weeks during the harvest or planting season is devastating in affected communities. As a result, dracunculiasis has significant adverse effects on agricultural production, school attendance, and the care and nutrition of uninfected infants, in addition to its direct effects on the health of those who are infected. Thus the combined socioeconomic impact of dracunculiasis greatly exceeds what one might otherwise expect of a disease that is not usually fatal.

While there is no curative treatment for dracunculiasis, there are several ways to prevent the disease. Providing a safe source of drinking water such as from a borehole well that is not subject to contamination by persons with emerging Guinea worms is the preferred preventive measure, since it also helps prevent other water-borne diseases and may reduce the time and energy required to collect water for household use. But providing borehole wells is relatively expensive and slow.

Educating persons at risk to understand that the infection comes from their drinking water is another intervention. Demonstrating copepods swimming in their drinking water is particularly effective in conveying that insight to villagers. Corollary teaching of villagers not to enter sources of drinking water when a worm is emerging from their body helps reduce contamination of the water. Although boiling of the water kills copepods and Guinea worm larvae as well as other undesirable pathogens, most villagers at risk of dracunculiasis are too poor to afford enough fuel to boil their drinking water regularly. The intervention used most commonly in recent years has been to teach villagers to filter their drinking water through a finely woven cloth to remove the copepods.

Applying temephos (Abate) to ponds at 4-week intervals during the transmission season is an effective means of vector control that may also be used in some circumstances to kill the copepods. At the recommended concentration of one part per million, Abate is tasteless, colorless, and odorless, does not harm fish or plant life, and has a wide margin of safety for humans.

The Eradication Campaign

The international campaign to eradicate dracunculiasis got under way in 1980, just before the beginning of the International Drinking Water Supply and Sanitation Decade (1981–1990). One of the goals of that Decade, which was sponsored by United Nations agencies and other development organizations, was to provide safe drinking water to all unserved populations. Although that overall goal was not achieved, the backers of the Decade had accepted eradication of dracunculiasis as one of the Decade's sub-goals, and by the end of the "Water Decade," half of the known infected countries (only Yemen was discovered to have current cases in 1994) had established national Guinea Worm Eradication Programs.

In 1988, African ministers of health resolved to eradicate dracunculiasis by the end of 1995. The same goal was endorsed by the World Health Assembly in 1989 and 1991, making dracunculiasis the next disease after smallpox to be officially targeted by the World Health Organization (WHO) for eradication globally. Although the strategy for eradication of dracunculiasis was at first based mainly on providing safe drinking water to affected populations, because of the slow pace and expense of that approach, primary emphasis later shifted to health education and use of cloth filters, with vector control by means of Abate employed in certain appropriate areas. After programs reduced the prevalence of dracunculiasis by over 80 percent using those village-based interventions, the eradication effort recently began stressing an even more intensive "case containment" strategy, which focuses on preventing transmission from each infected person.

Only about 150,000 cases of dracunculiasis were reported globally in 1996, in about 10,000 endemic villages (more than 23,000 villages were known to be endemic in 1993). More than three-fourths of the cases in 1996 were in Sudan, where a 13-year-old civil war has hampered implementation of control measures. This is a reduction of over 95 percent in the incidence of dracunculiasis from the estimated total of 3.3 million cases in 1986. Approximately 25 percent of the remaining cases outside of Sudan in 1996 were in Nigeria, formerly the most highly endemic country, which reduced its cases from over 653,000 reported in 1989 to about 12,000 cases reported in 1996. Outside of Sudan, the numbers of reported cases are being reduced by more than 50 percent per year, and nearly two-thirds of the cases reported in 1996 are believed to have been fully contained.

Thus dracunculiasis was not eradicated by the end of 1995 as targeted, but it is well on the way to becoming extinct. By the end of 1996, Pakistan had reported no cases of dracunculiasis for more than 3 years, Kenya had reported no indigenous cases for over 2 years, and five other endemic countries (Cameroon, Chad, India, Senegal, and Yemen) had reported 100 cases or fewer during the entire year. The WHO's International Commission for the Certification of Dracunculiasis Eradication began reviewing the status of formerly endemic countries in 1997, and certified Pakistan as drancunculiasis-free.

Human Enteric Coccidial Infections

Judy A. Streit

Enteric protozoa of the phylum Apicomplexa, subclass Coccidiasina, are recognized as important agents of diarrhea in both immunocompetent and immunocompromised persons. Appreciation of the pathogenicity of the agents *Cryptosporidium parvum, Isospora belli*, and *Cyclospora cayetanensis* for humans has been enhanced or newly established over the past 2 decades.[1–4] The organisms may be common pathogens worldwide. Generally a higher incidence of infection is found in developing countries and is likely affected by the adequacy of sanitation. Distinguishing characteristics of the epidemiology of disease are discussed below under the appropriate headings.

These three coccidia share several important biological, clinical, and epidemiologic features.[5] All are spore-forming agents and cause intracellular infections. Transmission occurs after ingestion of infectious oocysts (also known as spores), and only small numbers of organisms are necessary for the production of disease. The ingested oocysts release sporozoites, which invade enterocytes, primarily in the small bowel. Asexual and sexual stages of multiplication and development occur in the epithelial cells, and as the infected host cells die, cysts are shed.[6] Infection is associated with intestinal inflammation, villous blunting, and malabsorption. The secretory nature of the diarrhea that occurs suggests that a toxin is involved, though this has not been established.

The clinical spectrum of disease varies from asymptomatic infection to life-threatening diarrhea. The most prominent symptom encountered in immunocompetent persons is acute, watery diarrhea that is prolonged (longer than 2 weeks) in a significant percentage of cases and can be recurrent.[7,8] Nausea, occasional vomiting, abdominal pain, fever, and malaise are accompanying symptoms. In contrast to diarrhea caused by enteroinvasive bacteria and protozoa such as *Entamoeba*, erythrocytes and leukocytes are not found in the stool.

Immunodeficient patients experience either transient or chronic infection. A small number of asymptomatic infections are reported, but patients usually suffer more severe and prolonged disease than their immunocompetent counterparts.[9–12] Large-volume diarrhea and significant weight loss are more frequent with profound immune deficiencies. The acquired immunodeficiency syndrome (AIDS) is an important risk factor worldwide for disease caused by these coccidians, but other alterations in immune function such as IgA deficiency, receipt of chemotherapy for malignancy, and malnutrition are associated with clinical infection as well.[13,14] In addition to intestinal infection, biliary infection by *Cryptosporidium* and *Isospora* can lead to obstruction and dilatation of intrahepatic and extrahepatic bile ducts or acalculous cholecystitis.[15–17] Cryptosporidium has been isolated from respiratory secretions in AIDS patients with pulmonary symptoms as an isolated organism or together with typical lung pathogens.[18]

Cryptosporidia

Of the coccidial species under discussion, *C. parvum* is the only agent that infects both humans and other mammals. Transmission occurs by ingestion of oocysts excreted in the feces of infected humans and animals. A distinguishing feature of this organism is that the newly excreted oocysts are infectious and can remain so for months in a cool, moist environment. Direct sources of infection can be surface waters or food con-taminated by excrement, contact with domestic animals that have high levels of oocyst excretion such as young calves and lambs, or person-to-person transmission. Newborn puppies and kittens have been shown to excrete the organism, but documented transmission from these pets to humans is limited. Ready transmission of the organism has been shown by outbreaks that occurred in day care centers, hospitals, and households.[19]

Several large outbreaks of disease due to *C. parvum* have been attributed to municipal waters in the United States that were treated by usual methods of disinfection and filtration.[20] This demonstrates that oocysts can withstand usual levels of chlorine in treated water and are not completely removed by filtration systems used in developed areas. There is evidence that low-level transmission of *C. parvum* from drinking water occurs in the United States and other developed nations, though the health risk is unclear.

The frequency of occurrence of *C. parvum* in the stools of symptomatic patients varies with geographic region and immunologic status of the patients evaluated. Prevalence rates from surveys in Europe and North America of patients with diarrhea have been from 0.6 to 4.3 percent. Rates from Asia, Africa, and Central and South America have been from 3 to 20 percent.[6] Some studies report that the organism was the most common parasite found or the most significant of all detected enteropathogens among patients with diarrhea.[21] A higher prevalence of infection is usually reported for children than adults, especially in youngsters less than 2 years of age. Infections are more common in warm, wet months. Other risk factors include crowded housing conditions and large numbers of domestic animals capable of transmitting the infection near the home. Seroprevalence data in Europe and North America typically demonstrate prior infection in 25 to 35 percent of people evaluated, though levels of 58 percent have been reported for U.S. adolescents.[22,23] Populations of children or children and adults in South America have seroprevalence rates near 65 percent.[24]

The prevalence of *C. parvum* infection in AIDS patients has varied with the reporting institution, but it has ranged from 2 to 15 percent in the United States and was reported as 21.2 percent in France.[25–27] Among Haitian AIDS patients with chronic diarrhea, 30 percent had stools that contained *C. parvum*.[28]

Recommendations for prevention of *C. parvum* infection depend on the principal means of transmission for a given group of people. This is especially important for those at particular risk of severe and chronic disease, such as patients with AIDS. However, data are not available to ascribe relative risks to the known modes of transmission in immunocompromised patients. Such people are advised to avoid ingestion of water from lakes, rivers, or recreational sites (e.g., swimming pools), as oocysts are not killed by the usual levels of chlorination. The risk of infection imparted by consumption of municipal tap water varies with conditions such as whether a filtration system is used, the season, and presence of local animal reservoirs. The oocysts can be killed by boiling water for 1 minute. Filters that are effective in removing oocysts are those labeled as "absolute" 1-micron filters and those that meet National Sanitation Foundation Standard No. 53 for "cyst removal."[19] Careful use of these filters according to the manufacturer's instructions is needed. Cooking and freezing also kill oocysts. In the hospital, risk of person-to-person spread warrants the use of standard precautions (handwashing and wearing gloves and gowns) by staff when caring for affected patients, and private rooms if diarrhea is severe. Immunodeficient people should minimize exposure to newborn animals with diarrhea, especially calves and lambs, but also puppies and kittens.

Cyclospora

Cyclospora cayetanensis has not yet definitively been shown to have an animal reservoir. In contrast to *Cryptosporidium*, freshly excreted oocysts have not yet sporulated and are not infectious. Thus, person-to-person transmission is not an important means of acquisition. Instead, contaminated food and water are the likely sources for spread of disease. These organisms have been detected worldwide in the feces of immunocompetent and immunocompromised patients with diarrhea. Many of those affected are residents of developing nations or are travelers who have visited these areas. Reports from travelers to Nepal revealed that 11 percent of those with diarrhea had *Cyclospora* in their stools.[29] Peruvian children who submitted stools every week for 18 to 24 months had a 6 to 8 percent rate of passage of oocysts during this time, although a minority were symptomatic.[30] Additionally, studies in Peru show that both *Cyclospora* and *Cryptosporidium* tend to infect children aged 1 to 2 years, primarily in the summer months. This suggests a common mode of spread for the two organisms.

Urban outbreaks have occurred in association with a contaminated water supply or are likely caused by ingestion of contaminated imported food. An endemic prevalence rate for *Cyclospora* in immunocompetent patients with diarrhea in developed countries has been reported as 0.2 percent.[31]

Prevalence data from immunocompromised patients show higher rates for those who live in developing nations than for people in developed areas. This is demonstrated by an 11 percent detection rate for *Cyclospora* in Haitian AIDS patients with chronic or intermittent diarrhea, but infrequent reports of detection in U.S. AIDS patients with diarrhea.[28]

Preventive measures are limited to obvious recommendations of avoiding food or water that is possibly contaminated by human excrement. The risk of contamination is higher for those living in areas with poor sanitation or for those who consume fresh food imported from such areas.

Isospora

Isospora belli infection follows the consumption of food or water contaminated with human excrement. This species of *Isospora* has only been demonstrated to infect humans; animal reservoirs are not known to exist. Oocysts have not yet sporulated when passed in human feces, so person-to-person transmission is unlikely. Infection is endemic in broad regions of South America, Asia, and Africa, although exact prevalence rates are not known.[32] This endemicity is attributed to poor sanitary conditions. Sporadic outbreaks among immunocompetent patients have occurred in day care centers and among the institutionalized in the United States.[33,34] Among AIDS patients in developing nations of Africa, South America, and the Caribbean, rates of *Isospora* isolation from diarrheal stools has varied from 10 to 16 percent.[30,35,36] This compares to a frequency of 0.2 percent among AIDS patients in the United States.[10] Prevention of *Isospora* infection is similar to that stated for *Cyclospora*.

▶ REFERENCES

Typhoid Fever

1. Ryan CA, Hargrett-Bean NT, Blake PA: *Salmonella typhi* infections in the United States, 1975–1984: increasing role of foreign travel. Rev Infect Dis 2:1–8, 1988
2. Mermin JH, Townes JM, Gerber M, Dolan N, Mintz ED, Tauxe RV. Typhoid fever in the United States, 1985–1994: changing risks of international travel and increasing antimicrobial resistance. Archives of Internal Medicine 1998, in press.
3. Christie AB: Infectious Diseases: Epidemiology and Clinical Practice. 4th ed. New York: Churchill Livingstone, 1987
4. Gilman RH, Terminel M, Levine MM, et al: Relative efficacy of blood, urine, rectal swab, bone-marrow, and rose-spot cultures for recovery of *Salmonella typhi* in typhoid fever. Lancet 1:1211–1213, 1975

5. Edelman R, Levine MM: Summary of an international workshop on typhoid fever. Rev Infect Dis 8:329–349, 1986
6. Mahle WT, Levine MM: *Salmonella typhi* infection in children younger than five years of age. Pediatr Infect Dis J 12:627–631, 1993
7. Hornick RB, Greisman SE, Woodward TE, et al: Typhoid fever: pathogenesis and immunologic control. N Engl J Med 283:686–691, 739–746, 1970
8. Gupta A: Multidrug-resistant typhoid fever in children: epidemiology and therapeutic approach. Pediatr Infect Dis J 13:134–140, 1994
9. Alam MN, Haq SA, Das KK, et al: Efficacy of ciprofloxacin in enteric fever: comparison of treatment duration in sensitive and multidrug-resistant *Salmonella*. Am J Trop Med Hyg 53:306–311, 1995
10. Smith MD, Duong NM, Hoa NT, et al: Comparison of ofloxacin and ceftriaxone for short-course treatment of enteric fever. Antimicrob Agents Chemother 38:1716–1720, 1994
11. Rowe B, Ward LR, Threlfall EJ: Ciprofloxacin-resistant *Salmonella typhi* in the UK. Lancet 346:1302, 1995
12. Levine MM, Grados O, Gilman RH, et al: Diagnostic value of the Widal test in areas endemic for typhoid fever. Am J Trop Med Hyg 27:795–800, 1978
13. Ames WR, Robbins M: Age and sex as factors in the development of the typhoid carrier state, and a method for estimating carrier prevalence. Am J Public Health 33:221–230, 1943
14. Rodriguez-Noriega E, Andrade-Villanueva J, Amaya-Tapia G: Quinolones in the treatment of *Salmonella* carriers. Rev Infect Dis 11:S1179–S1187, 1989
15. Nolan CM, White PCJ, Feeley JC, et al: Vi serology in the detection of typhoid carriers. Lancet 1:583–585, 1981
16. Engleberg NC, Barrett TJ, Fisher H, et al: Identification of a carrier by using Vi enzyme-linked immunosorbent assay serology in an outbreak of typhoid fever on an Indian reservation. J Clin Microbiol 18:1320–1322, 1983
17. Lanata CF, Ristori C, Jimenez L: Vi serology in detection of chronic *Salmonella typhi* carriers in an endemic area. Lancet 2:441–443, 1983
18. Blaser MJ, Hickman FW, Farmer JJ, et al: *Salmonella typhi*: the laboratory as a reservoir of infection. J Infect Dis 142:934–938, 1980
19. Ivanoff B, Levine MM, Lambert PH: Vaccination against typhoid fever: present status. Bull World Health Organ 72:957–971, 1994
20. Birkhead GS, Morse DL, Levine WC, et al: Typhoid fever at a resort hotel in New York: a large outbreak with an unusual vehicle. J Infect Dis 167:1228–1232, 1993
21. Centers for Disease Control and Prevention: Typhoid immunization: recommendations of the Advisory Committee on Immunization Practices. MMWR 43:1–7, 1994
22. Levine MM, Taylor DN, Ferreccio C: Typhoid vaccines come of age. Pediatr Infect Dis J 8:374–381, 1989
23. Levine MM, Ferreccio C, Black RE, et al: Progress in vaccines against typhoid fever. Rev Infect Dis 11:S552–S567, 1989

Shigellosis

1. Felsen J: Bacillary Dysentery Colitis and Enteritis. Philadelphia: WB Saunders, 1945
2. Ries AA, Wells JG, Olivola D, et al: Epidemic *Shigella dysenteriae* type 1 in Burundi: panresistance and implications for prevention. J Infect Dis 169:1035–1041, 1994
3. Aragon M, Barreto A, Chambule J, Noya A, Tallarico M: Shigellosis in Mozambique: the 1993 outbreak rehabilitation—a follow-up study. Trop Doct 25:159–162, 1995
4. Thirunarayanan MA, Jesudason MV, Jacob JT: Resistance of *Shigella* to nalidixic acid & fluorinated quinolones. Indian J Med Res [A]97:239–241, 1993
5. Griffin PM, Tauxe RV, Redd SC, Puhr ND, Hargrett-Bean N, Blake PA: Emergence of highly trimethoprim-sulfamethoxazole-resistant *Shigella sonnei* in a Native American population: an epidemiologic study. Am J Epidemiol 129:1042–1051, 1989
6. Cook K, Boyce T, Puhr N, Tauxe R, Mintz E: Increasing antimicrobial-resistant *Shigella* infections in the United States [Abstract E-20]. In: Abstracts of the 36th Interscience Conference on Antimicrobial Agents and Chemotherapy (New Orleans). Washington, DC: American Society for Microbiology, 1996, p 84
7. Mendizabal-Morris CA, Mata LJ, Gangarosa EJ, Guzman G: Epidemic Shiga-bacillus dysentery in Central America: derivation of the epidemic and its progression in Guatemala, 1968–1969. Am J Trop Med Hyg 20:927–933, 1971
8. Barrett-Connor E, Connor JD: Extraintestinal manifestations of shigellosis. Am J Gastroenterol 53:234–245, 1970
9. Butler T, Islam MR, Azad MAK, Jones PK: Risk factors for development of hemolytic uremic syndrome during shigellosis. J Pediatr 110:894–897, 1987
10. Ross AI: The role of the symptomless excreter in the spread of Sonnei dysentery. Monthly Bulletin of the Ministry of Health 16:174–179, 1957
11. Levine MM, DuPont HL, Khodabandelou M, Hornick RB: Long-term *Shigella* carrier state. N Engl J Med 288:1169–1171, 1973
12. Nelson JD, Kusmiesz H, Shelton S: Oral or intravenous trimethoprim-sulfamethoxazole therapy for shigellosis. Rev Infect Dis 4:546–550, 1982
13. Gotuzzo E, Oberhelman RA, Maguina C, et al: Comparison of single-dose treatment with norfloxacin and standard 5-day treatment with trimethoprim-sulfamethoxazole for acute shigellosis in adults. Antimicrob Agents Chemother 33:1101–1104, 1989
14. Mahoney FJ, Farley TA, Burbank DF, Leslie NH, McFarland LM: Evaluation of an intervention program for the control of an outbreak of shigellosis among institutionalized persons. J Infect Dis 168:1177–1180, 1993
15. Townes JM, Quick R, Gonzales O, et al: Etiology of bloody diarrhea in Bolivian children: implications for empiric therapy. J Infect Dis, 1997;175:1527–30.
16. Mohle-Boetani JC, Stapleton M, Finger R, et al: Communitywide shigellosis: control of an outbreak and risk factors in child day-care centers. Am J Public Health 85:763–764, 1995
17. DuPont HL, Gangarosa EJ, Reller LB, et al: Shigellosis in custodial institutions. Am J Epidemiol 92:172–179, 1970
18. Sobel J, Cameron D, Ismail J, et al. A prolonged outbreak of Shigella sonnei infections in traditionally observant Jewish communities in North America caused by a molecularly distinct bacterial subtype. J Infect Dis 1998, in press.
19. Parsonnet J, Greene KD, Gerber AR, Tauxe RV, Aguilar OJV, Blake PA: *Shigella dysenteriae* type 1 infections in US travelers to Mexico, 1988. Lancet 2:543–545, 1989
20. Tauxe RV, McDonald RC, Hargrett-Bean N, Blake PA: The persistence of *Shigella flexneri* in the United States: increasing role of adult males. Am J Public Health 78:1432–1435, 1988
21. Cook K, Boyce T, Langkop C, et al: A multistate outbreak of *Shigella flexneri* 6 traced to imported green onions [Abstract K72]. In: Abstracts of the 35th Interscience Conference on Antimicrobial Agents and Chemotherapy (San Francisco, CA). Washington, DC: American Society for Microbiology, 1995
22. Kapperud G, Rorvik LM, Hasseltvedt V, et al: Outbreak of *Shigella sonnei* infection traced to imported iceberg lettuce. J Clin Microbiol 33:609–614, 1995
23. Black RE, Craun GF, Blake PA: Epidemiology of common-source outbreaks of shigellosis in the United States, 1961–1975. Am J Epidemiol 108:47–52, 1978
24. Keene WE, McAnulty JM, Hoesly FC, Williams LP, et al: A swimming-associated outbreak of hemorrhagic colitis caused by *Escherichia coli* 0157:H7 and *Shigella sonnei*. N Engl J Med 331:579–584, 1994
25. Centers for Disease Control and Prevention: *Shigella sonnei* outbreak associated with contaminated drinking water—Island Park, Idaho, August 1995. MMWR 45:229–231, 1996

26. Centers for Disease Control and Prevention: *Shigella* Surveillance, Annual Tabulation Summary, 1993–1995. Atlanta: Centers for Disease Control and Prevention, 1996
27. Ebright JR, Moore EC, Sanborn WR, Schaberg D, Kyle J, Ishida K: Epidemic Shiga bacillus dysentery in Central Africa. Am J Trop Med Hyg 33:1192–1197, 1984
28. Tuttle J, Ries AA, Chimba RM, Perera CU, Bean NH, Griffin PM: Antimicrobial-resistant epidemic *Shigella dysenteriae* type 1 in Zambia: modes of transmission. J Infect Dis 171:371–375, 1995
29. Tauxe RV, Johnson KE, Boase JC, Helgerson SD, Blake PA: Control of day care shigellosis: a trial of convalescent day care in isolation. Am J Public Health 76:627–630, 1986
30. Formal SB, Hale TL, Kapfer C: *Shigella* vaccines. Rev Infect Dis 11:S547–S551, 1989
31. Ashkenazi S, Cohen D: An update on *Shigella* vaccines. Isr J Med Sci 30:495–497, 1994
32. Khan MU: Interruption of shigellosis by hand washing. Trans R Soc Trop Med Hyg 76:164–168, 1982

Cholera

1. Pollitzer R: Cholera Monograph No. 43. Geneva: World Health Organization, 1959
2. Schoenberg BS, Mann RJ, Kurland LT: Snow on the water of London. Mayo Clin Proc 49:680–684, 1974
3. Samadi AR, Huq MI, Shahid N, et al: Classical *Vibrio cholerae* biotype displaces El Tor in Bangladesh. Lancet 1:805–807, 1983
4. Glass R, Black RE: Epidemiology of cholera. In Barna D, Greenough WB III (eds): Cholera. New York: Plenum Medical Book Co., 1992, pp, 129–154
5. Blake PA, Allegra DT, Snyder JD, et al: Cholera—a possible endemic focus in the United States. N Engl J Med 302:305–309, 1980
6. Swerdlow DL, Mintz ED, Rodriguez M, et al: Waterborne transmission of epidemic cholera in Trujillo, Peru: lessons for a continent at risk. Lancet 340:28–32, 1992
7. Ries AA, Vugia DJ, Beingolea L, et al: Cholera in Piura, Peru: a modern urban epidemic. J Infect Dis 166:1429–1433, 1992
8. Tauxe R, Seminario L, Tapia R, Libel M: The Latin American epidemic. In Wachsmuth IK, Blak PA, Olsvik O (eds): *Vibrio cholerae* and Cholera. Molecular to Global Perspectives. Washington, DC: American Society for Microbiology, 1994
9. Cholera Working Group: Large epidemic of cholera-like disease in Bangladesh caused by *Vibrio cholerae* O139 synonym Bengal. Lancet 342:387–390, 1993
10. Wachsmuth IK, Morris GK, Feeley JC: *Vibrio*. In Lennette EH, Balows A, Hausler WJ, Truant JP (eds): Manual of Clinical Microbiology. 3rd ed. Washington, DC: American Society for Microbiology, 1980
11. Morris JG, Sztein MB, Rice EW, et al: *Vibrio cholerae* O1 can assume a chlorine-resistant rugose survival form that is virulent for humans. J Infect Dis 174:1364–1368, 1996
12. Bart KJ, Huq Z, Khan M, Mosley WH: Seroepidemiologic studies during a simultaneous epidemic of infection with El Tor Ogawa and classical Inaba *Vibrio cholerae*. J Infect Dis 121:S17–S24, 1970
13. Greenough WB, Gordon RS, Rosenberg IS, et al: Tetracycline in the treatment of cholera. Lancet 1:355–357, 1964
14. Black RE: The prophylaxis and therapy of secretory diarrhea. Med Clin North Am 66:611–621, 1982
15. Palmer DL, Koster FT, Alam AKMJ, Islam MR: Nutritional status: a determinant of severity of diarrhea in patients with cholera. J Infect Dis 134:8–14, 1976
16. Oseasohn R, Ahmen S, Islan MA, Rahman ASMM: Clinical and bacteriologic findings among families of cholera patients. Lancet 1:340–341, 1966
17. Nalin DR, Levine RJ, Levine MM, et al: Cholera, nonvibrio cholera, and stomach acid. Lancet 2:856–859, 1978
18. Glass RI, Srennerholm A-M, Stoll BJ, et al: Protection against cholera in breast-fed children by antibodies in breast milk. N Engl J Med 308:1389–1392, 1983
19. Levine MM, Black RE, Clements ML, et al: Duration of infection-derived immunity to cholera. J Infect Dis 143:818–820, 1981
20. Colwell RR, Brayton PR, Grimes DJ, et al: Viable, but non-culturable *Vibrio* cholerae and related pathogens in the environment: implications for release of genetically engineered microorganisms. Biol Technology 3:817–820, 1985
21. Islam MS, Draser BS, Sack RB: The aquatic environment as a reservoir of *Vibrio cholerae*: a review. J Diarrhoeal Dis Res 1194: 197–206, 1993
22. Spira WM, Khan MU, Saeed A, Sattar MA: Microbiological surveillance of intra-neighbourhood El Tor transmission in rural Bangladesh. Bull WHO 58:731–740, 1980
23. Hughes JM, Boyce JM, Levine RJ, et al: Epidemiology of El Tor cholera in rural Bangladesh: importance of surface water in transmission. Bull World Health Organ 60:395–404, 1982
24. Clemens JD, Sack DA, Harris JR, et al: Field trial of oral cholera vaccines in Bangladesh: results from three-year follow-up. Lancet 1:270–273, 1990
25. Levine MM, Herington D, Losonsky G, et al: Safety, immunogenicity, and efficacy of recombinant live oral cholera vaccines, CVD 103 and CVD 103-HgR. Lancet 2:467–468, 1988

Escherichia coli Diarrhea

1. Gorbach SL: Intestinal microflora. Gastroenterology 60:1110–1129, 1971
2. Robins-Browne RM: Traditional enteropathogenic *Escherichia coli* of infantile diarrhea. Rev Infect Dis 9:28–53, 1987
3. Richards KL, Douglas SD: Pathophysiological effects of *Vibrio cholerae* and enterotoxigenic *Escherichia coli* and their exotoxins in eucaryotic cells. Microbiol Rev 42:592–613, 1978
4. Black RE, Lanata CF: Epidemiology of diarrheal diseases in developing countries. In Blaser MJ, Smith PD, Ravdin JI, Greenberg HB, Guerrant RL (eds): Infections of the Gastrointestinal Tract. New York: Raven Press, 1995, pp 13–36
5. Black RE, Brown KH, Becker S, et al: Longitudinal studies of infectious diseases and physical growth of children in rural Bangladesh. II. Incidence of diarrhea and association with known pathogens. Am J Epidemiol 115:315–324, 1982
6. Rosenberg ML, Kaplan JP, Wachsmuth IK, et al: Epidemic diarrhea at Crater Lake from enterotoxigenic *E. coli*: a large waterborne outbreak. Ann Intern Med 86:714–718, 1977
7. Black RE: Epidemiology of travelers diarrhea and relative importance of various pathogens. Rev Infect Dis 12:S73–S79, 1990
8. Black RE: The prophylaxis and therapy of secretory diarrhea. Med Clin North Am 66:611–621, 1982
9. Marier R, Wells JG, Swanson RC, et al: An outbreak of enteropathogenic *Escherichia coli*: foodborne disease traced to imported French cheese. Lancet 2:1376–1378, 1973
10. Riley LW, Remis RS, Helgerson SD, et al: Hemorrhagic colitis associated with a rare *Escherichia coli* serotype. N Engl J Med 308:681–685, 1983
11. Griffin PM, Tauxe RV: The epidemiology of infections caused by *Escherichia coli* O157:H7, other enterohemorrhagic *E. coli*, and the associated hemolytic uremic syndrome. Epidemiol Rev 13:60–98, 1991
12. American Gastroenterological Association: Consensus conference statement: *Escherichia coli* O157:H7 infections—an emerging national health crisis, July 11–13, 1994. Gastroenterology 108: 1923–1934, 1995
13. Ulshen MH, Rollo JL: Pathogenesis of *Escherichia coli* gastroenteritis in man—another mechanism. N Engl J Med 302:99–101, 1980
14. Vial PA, Robins-Brown R, Lior H, et al: Characterization of enteroadherent-aggregative *Escherichia coli*, a putative agent of diarrheal disease. J Infect Dis 158:70–79, 1988
15. Baqui AH, Sack RD, Black RE, et al: Enteropathogens associated with acute and persistent diarrhea in Bangladeshi children <5 years of age. J Infect Dis 166:792–796, 1992

16. Cravioto A, Tello A, Navarro A, et al: Association of *Escherichia coli* Hep-2 adherence patterns with type and duration of diarrhoea. Lancet 1:337:262–264, 1991
17. Levine MM, Ferreccio C, Prado V, et al: Epidemiologic studies of *Escherichia coli* diarrheal infections in a low socioeconomic level peri-urban community in Santiago, Chile. Am J Epidemiol 138: 849–869, 1993

Yersiniosis

1. Centers for Disease Control: Update: *Yersinia enterocolitica* bacteremia and endotoxin shock associated with red blood cell transfusions—United States, 1991. MMWR 40:176–178, 1991
2. Saebo A, Lassen J: Acute and chronic gastrointestinal manifestations associated with *Yersinia enterocolitica* infection. Ann Surg 215: 250–255, 1992
3. Yli-Kerttula T, Tertti R, Toivanen A: Ten-year follow up study of patients from a *Yersinia pseudotuberculosis* III outbreak. Clin Exp Rheumatol 13:333–337, 1995
4. Lee LA, Taylor J, Carter GP, et al: *Yersinia enterocolitica* O:3: an emerging cause of pediatric gastroenteritis in the United States. J Infect Dis 163:660–663, 1991
5. Tauxe RV, Vandepitte J, Wauters G, et al: *Yersinia enterocolitica* infections and pork: the missing link. Lancet 1:1129–1132, 1987
6. Ostroff SM, Kapperud G, Hutwagner LC, et al: Sources of sporadic *Yersinia enterocolitica* infections in Norway: a prospective case-control study. Epidemiol Infect 112:133–141, 1994
7. Lee LA, Gerber AR, Lonsway DR, et al: *Yersinia enterocolitica* O:3 infections in infants and children, associated with the household preparation of chitterlings. N Engl J Med 322:984–987, 1990
8. Butler T: *Yersinia* infections: centennial of the discovery of the plague bacillus. Clin Infect Dis 19:655–663, 1994

Legionellosis

1. Glick RH, Gregg MB, Berman B, et al: Pontiac fever—epidemic of unknown etiology in a health department: clinical and epidemiologic findings. Am J Epidemiol 107:149–160, 1978
2. Fraser DW, Tsai TF, Orenstein W, et al: Legionnaires' disease: description of an epidemic of pneumonia. N Engl J Med 297: 1189–1197, 1977
3. McDade JE, Shepard CC, Fraser DW, et al: Legionnaires' disease: isolation of a bacterium and demonstration of its role in other respiratory disease. N Engl J Med 297:1197–1203, 1977
4. Dennis PJ, Brenner DJ, Thacker WL, et al: Five new *Legionella* species isolated from water. Int J Syst Bacteriol 43:329–337, 1993
5. Marston BJ, Lipman HB, Breiman RF: Surveillance for Legionnaires' disease: risk factors for morbidity and mortality. Arch Intern Med 154:2417–2422, 1994
6. Steele TW, Langser J, Sangster N: Isolation of *Legionella longbeachae* serogroup 1 from potting mixes. Appl Environ Microbiol 56:49–53, 1990
7. Hughes MS, Steele TW: Occurrence and distribution of *Legionella* species in composted plant material. Appl Environ Microbiol 60:2003–2005, 1994
8. Horwitz MA, Silverstein SC: Legionnaires' disease bacterium (*Legionella pneumophila*) multiplies intracellularly in human monocytes. J Clin Invest 66:441–450, 1980
9. Nash TW, Libby DM, Horwitz MA: Interaction between the Legionnaires' disease bacterium (*Legionella pneumophila*) and human alveolar macrophages. J Clin Invest 74:771–782, 1984
10. Fields BS, Sanden GN, Barbaree JM, et al: Intracellular multiplication of *Legionella pneumophila* in amoebae isolated from hospital hot water tanks. Curr Microbiol 13:131–137, 1989
11. Edelstein PH: Laboratory diagnosis of infections caused by legionellae. Eur J Clin Microbiol 6:4–10, 1987
12. Plouffe JF, File TM, Breiman RF, et al: Reevaluation of the definition of Legionnaires' disease: use of the urinary antigen assay. Clin Infect Dis 20:1286–1291, 1995
13. Edelstein PH: Legionnaires' disease. Clin Infect Dis 16:741–749, 1993
14. Breiman RF, Horwitz MA: Guinea pigs sublethally infected with aerosolized *Legionella pneumophila* develop humoral and cell-mediated immune responses and are protected against lethal aerosol challenge. J Exp Med 164:799–811, 1987
15. Leverstein-van Hall MA, Verbon A, Huisman MV, Kuijper EJ, Dankert J: Reinfection with *Legionella pneumophila* documented by pulsed-field gel electrophoresis. Clin Infect Dis 19:1147–1149, 1994
16. Dondero TJ, Rentdorff RC, Mallison GF, et al: An outbreak of Legionnaires' disease associated with a contaminated air-conditioning cooling tower. N Engl J Med 302:365–370, 1980
17. Breiman RF, Cozen W, Fields BS, et al: Role of air-sampling in an investigation of an outbreak of Legionnaires' disease associated with exposure to aerosols from an evaporative condenser. J Infect Dis 161:1257–1261, 1990
18. Keller DW, Hajjeh R, DeMaria A, et al: Community outbreak of Legionnaires' disease: an investigation confirming the potential for cooling towers to transmit *Legionella* species. Clin Infect Dis 22: 257–261, 1996
19. Addiss DG, Davis JP, LaVentura M, et al: Community-acquired Legionnaires' disease associated with a cooling tower: evidence for longer-distance transport of *Legionella pneumophila*. Am J Epidemiol 130:557–568, 1989
20. Breiman RF, Fields BS, Sanden G, Volmer L, Meier A, Spika J: An outbreak of Legionnaires' disease associated with shower use: possible role of amoebae. JAMA 263:2924–2926, 1990
21. Hanrahan JP, Morse DL, Scharf VB, et al: A community hospital outbreak of legionellosis; transmission by potable hot water. Am J Epidemiol 125:639–649, 1987
22. Tobin JO, Dunnill MS, French M, et al: Legionnaires, disease in a transplant unit: isolation of the causative agent from shower baths. Lancet 2:118–121, 1980
23. Jernigan DB, Hofmann J, Cetron MS, et al: Outbreak of Legionnaires' disease among cruise ship passengers exposed to a contaminated whirlpool spa. Lancet 347:494–499, 1996
24. Centers for Disease Control and Prevention: Legionnaires' disease associated with a whirlpool spa display—Virginia, September–October, 1996. MMWR 46:83–86, 1997
25. Mahoney FJ, Hoge CW, Farley TA, et al: Communitywide outbreak of Legionnaires' disease associated with a grocery store mist machine. J Infect Dis 165:736–739, 1992
26. Mastro TD, Fields BS, Breiman RF, Campbell J, Spika JS: Nosocomial Legionnaires' disease and use of medication nebulizers. J Infect Dis 163:667–671, 1991
27. Herwaldt LA, Gorman GW, McGrath T, et al: A new *Legionella* species, *Legionella feeleii* species nova, causes Pontiac fever in an automobile plant. Ann Intern Med 100:333–338, 1984
28. Johnson JT, Yu VL, Best MG, et al: Nosocomial legionellosis in surgical patients with head and neck cancer: implications for epidemiological reservoir and mode of transmission. Lancet 2:298–300, 1985
29. Lowry PW, Blankenship RJ, Gridley W, Nancy RN, Troup NJ, Tompkins LS: A cluster of *Legionella* sternal wound infections due to postoperative topical exposure to contaminated tap water. N Engl J Med 324:109–113, 1991
30. Marston BJ, Plouffe JF, File TM, Hackman B, Salstrom SJ, Lipman HB, Breiman RF: Incidence of community-acquired pneumonia requiring hospitalization: results of a population-based active surveillance study in Ohio. Arch Intern Med, 157:1709–1718, 1997
31. Fang G-D, Fine M, Orloff J, et al: New and emerging etiologies for community-acquired pneumonia with implications for therapy: a prospective multicenter study of 359 cases. Medicine 69: 307–316, 1990

32. Ruf B, Schürmann D, Horbach I, Fehrenbach FJ, Pohle HD: Prevalence and diagnosis of *Legionella* pneumonia: a 3-year prospective study with emphasis on application of urinary antigen detection. J Infect Dis 162:1341–1348, 1990
33. Marrie TJ, Durant H, Yates L: Community-acquired pneumonia requiring hospitalization: 5-year prospective study. Rev Infect Dis 11:586–599, 1989
34. Barbaree JM: Selecting a subtyping technique for use in investigations of legionellosis epidemics. In Barbaree JM, Breiman RF, DuFour AP (eds): *Legionella*: Current Status and Emerging Perspectives. Washington, DC: American Society for Microbiology; 1993, pp 169–172
35. Gomez-Luz P, Fields BS, Benson RF, Martin WT, O'Connor SP, Black CM: Comparison of arbitrarily primed polymerase chain reaction, ribotyping, and monoclonal antibody analysis for subtyping *Legionella pneumophila* serogroup 1. J Clin Microbiol 31:1940–1942, 1993
36. Pruckler JM, Mermel LA, Benson RF, et al: Comparison of *Legionella pneumophila* serogroup 1 isolates by arbitrarily primed PCR and pulsed-field gel electrophoresis: analysis from seven epidemic investigations. J Clin Microbiol 33:2872–2875, 1995
37. Bartlett CLR, Macrae AD, MacFarlane JT: Surveillance, control, and prevention. In: *Legionella* Infections. London: Edward Arnold, 1986, pp 134–138
38. Sanden GN, Fields BS, Barbaree JM, Feeley JC: Viability of *Legionella pneumophila* in chlorine-free water at elevated temperatures. Curr Microbiol 18:61–65, 1989
39. Helms CM, Massanari RM, Wenzel RP, et al: Legionnaires' disease associated with a hospital water system: a five-year progress report on continuous hyperchlorination. JAMA 259:2423–2427, 1988
40. Control of *Legionella* in cooling towers—summary guidelines. Madison: Wisconsin Department of Health and Human Services, 1987
41. Arnow PM, Chou T, Weil D, Shapiro EN, Kretzschmar C: Nosocomial Legionnaires' disease caused by aerosolized tap water from respiratory devices. J Infect Dis 146:460–467, 1982
42. Centers for Disease Control and Prevention: Guidelines for prevention of nosocomial pneumonia. MMWR 46(RR-1):1–79, 1997
43. Vereerstraeten P, Stolear JC, Schoutens-Serruys E, et al: Erythromycin prophylaxis for Legionnaires' disease in immunosuppressed patients in a contaminated hospital environment. Transplantation 41:52–54, 1986
44. Blander SJ, Horwitz MA: Vaccination with the major secretory protein of *Legionella pneumophila* induces cell-mediated and protective immunity in a guinea pig model of Legionnaires' disease. J Exp Med 169:691–705, 1989
45. Blander SJ, Breiman RF, Horwitz MA: A live avirulent mutant *Legionella pneumophila* vaccine induces protective immunity against lethal aerosol challenge. J Clin Invest 83:810–815, 1989

Amebiasis and Amebic Meningoencephalitis

1. Walsh JA: Prevalance of *Entamoeba histolytica* infections. In Ravdin JI (ed): Amebiasis: Human Infection by *Entamoeba histolytica*. New York: Churchill Livingston, 1988, pp 93–105
2. Smith PD, Lane HC, Gill VJ, et al: Intestinal infections in patients with the acquired immunodeficiency syndrome (AIDS): etiology and response to therapy. Ann Intern Med 108:328–333, 1988
3. Tannich E, Horstmann RD, Knobloch J, Arnold HH: Genomic differences between pathogenic and nonpathogenic *Entamoeba histolytica*. Proc Natl Acad Sci USA 86:5118, 1989
4. Diamond LS, Clark CG: A redescription of *Entamoeba histolytica* Shaudinn 1903 (amended Walker 1911) separating it from *Entamoeba dispar* (Brumpt 1925). J Eukaryot Microbiol 40:340, 1993
5. Sargeaunt PG: The reliability of *Entamoeba histolytica* zymodemes in clinical diagnosis. Parasitol Today 3:40–43, 1987
6. Ravdin JI, Jackson TFHG, Petri WA, Murphy CFM, Unger BLP, Gathiram V, Skilogiannis J, Simjee AE: Association of serum anti-adherence lectin antibodies with invasive amebiasis and asymptomatic pathogenic *Entamoeba histolytica* infection. J Infect Dis 162: 768–772, 1990
7. Abd-Alla M, Jackson TFHG, Gathirim V, El-Hawey AM, Ravdin JI: Differentiation of pathogenic from nonpathogenic *Entamoeba histolytica* infection by detection of galactose-inhibitable adherence protein antigen in sera and feces. J Clin Microbiol 31: 2845–2850, 1993
8. Abou-El-Magd I, Soong CG, El-Hawey AM, Ravdin JI: Humoral and Mucosal IgA antibody response to a recombinant 52-kDa cysteine-rich portion of the *Entamoeba histolytica* galactose-inhibitable lectin correlates with detection of native 170-kDa lectin antigen in serum of patients with amebic colitis. J Infect Dis 174:157–162, 1996
9. Ravdin JI: Amebiasis, "state of the art." Clin Infect Dis 20:1453–1466, 1995
10. Ravdin JI: *Entamoeba histolytica*: pathogenic mechanisms, human immune response, and vaccine development. Clin Res 38:215–225, 1990
11. Leippe M, Andra J, Muller Eberhard HJ: Cytolytic and antibacterial activity of synthetic peptides derived from amoebapore, the pore-forming peptide of *Entamoeba histolytica*. Proc Natl Acad Sci USA 91:2602, 1994
12. Braga LL, Ninomiya H, McCoy JJ, et al: Inhibition of the complement membrane attack complex by the galactose-specific adhesin of *Entamoeba histolytica*. J Clin Invest 90:1131, 1992
13. Adams EB, MacLeod IN: Invasive amebiasis I. Amebic dysentery and its complications. Medicine (Baltimore) 56:315–323, 1977
14. Schleupner CJ, Barritt AS III: Differentiation and occurrence of amebiasis in inflammatory bowel disease. In Ravdin JI (ed): Amebiasis: Human Infection by *Entamoeba histolytica*. New York: Churchill Livingstone, 1988, pp 582–593
15. Katzenstein D, Rickerson V, Braude A: New concepts of amebic liver abscess derived from hepatic imaging, serodiagnosis, and hepatic enzymes in 67 consecutive cases in San Diego. Medicine (Baltimore) 61:237–246, 1982
16. Ravdin JI: Intestinal disease caused by *Entameoba histolytica*. In Ravdin JI (ed): Amebiasis: Human Infection by *Entamoeba histolytica*. New York: Churchill Livingstone, 1988, pp 495–509
17. Ralls PW, Henley DS, Colletti PM, et al: Amebic liver abscess: MR imaging. Radiology 165:801–804, 1987
18. Drugs for parasitic infections. Med Lett 30:15–24, 1988
19. Sullam PM, Slutkin G, Gottlieb AB, et al: Paromomycin therapy of endemic amebiasis in homosexual men. Sex Transm Dis 13:151–155, 1986
20. Thompson JE Jr, Forlenza S, Verma R: Amebic liver abscess: a therapeutic approach. Rev Infect Dis 7:171–179, 1985
21. Sotelo-Avila C: *Naegleria* and *Acanthamoeba:* Free-living amebas pathogenic for man. Perspect Pediatr Pathol 10:51–85, 1987
22. Martinez AJ: Free-Living Amebas: Natural History, Prevention, Diagnosis, Pathology and Treatment of Disease. Boca Raton, FL: CRC Press, 1985
23. Martinez AJ: Is *Acanthamoeba* encephalitis an opportunistic infection? Neurology 30:567–574, 1980
24. Wiley CA, Safin RE, Davis CE, et al: *Acanthamoeba* meningoencephalitis in a patient with AIDS. J Infect Dis 155:130–133, 1987
25. Duma RJ, Finley R: In vitro susceptibility of pathogenic *Naegleria* and *Acanthamoeba* species to a variety of therapeutic agents. Antimicrob Agents Chemother 10:370–376, 1976
26. Seidel JS, Harmatz P, Visvesvara GS, et al: Successful treatment of primary amebic meningoencephalitis. N Engl J Med Vol 36 Issue #6, 346–348, 1982
27. Brown RL: Successful treatment of primary amebic meningoencephalitis. Arch Intern Med 151:1201–1202, 1991
28. Anderson K, Jamieson A: Primary amoebic meningoencephalitis. Lancet I:902–903, 1972

Giardiasis

1. Hartong WA, Gourley WK, Arvanitakis C: Giardiasis: clinical spectrum and functional-structural abnormalities of the small intestinal mucosa. Gastroenterology 77:61–69, 1979
2. Hill DR: *Giardia lamblia*. In: Mandell GL, Douglas RG, Bennett JE (eds): *Principles and Practice of Infectious Diseases*. 4th ed. New York: Churchill Livingstone, 1995, pp 2487–2493
3. Gendrel D, Lenoble DR, Kombila M, Gendrel C, Baziomo JM Giardiasis and breast-feeding in urban Africa. Pediatr Infect Dis J 8: 58–59, 1989
4. Walterspiel JN, Morrow AL, Guerrero ML, Rjiz-Palacios GM, Pickering LK: Secretory anti-*Giardia lamblia* antibodies in human milk: protective effect against diarrhea. Pediatrics 93:28–31, 1994
5. Turchany JM, Aley SB, Gillin FD: Giardicidal activity of lactoferrin and N-terminal peptides. Infect Immun 63:4550–4552, 1995
6. Nash TE, Mowatt MR: Variant-specific surface proteins of *Giardia lamblia* are zinc-binding proteins. Proc Natl Acad Sci USA 90: 5489–5493, 1993
7. Müller N, Stäger S, Gottstein B: Serological analysis of antigenic heterogeneity of *Giardia lamblia* variant surface proteins. Infect Immun 64:1385–1390, 1996
8. Aldeen WE, Hale D, Robison AJ, Carroll K: Evaluation of a commercially available ELISA assay for detection of *Giardia lamblia* in fecal specimens. Diagn Microbiol Infect Dis 21:77–79, 1995
9. Zimmerman SK, Needham CA: Comparison of conventional stool concentration and preserved-smear methods with Merifluor *Cryptosporidium/Giardia* direct immunofluorescence assay and ProSpecT Giardia EZ microplate assay for detection of *Giardia lamblia*. J Clin Microbiol 33:1942–1943, 1995
10. Drugs for parasitic infections. Med Lett 37:99–108, 1995
11. Cody MM, Sottnek HM, O'Leary VS: Recovery of *Giardia lamblia* cysts from chairs and tables in child day-care centers. Pediatrics 94: 1006–1007, 1994
12. Boreham PFL, Dondey J, Walker R: Giardiasis among children in the city of Logan, South East Queensland. Aust Pediatr J 17:209–212, 1981
13. Kerlin P, Ratnaike RN, Butler R, Gehling N, Grant AK: Prevalence of giardiasis: a study at upper-gastrointestinal endoscopy. Dig Dis 23: 940–942, 1978
14. Qureshi H, Zuberi SJ, Baqai R: *Giardia lamblia* in patients undergoing upper GI endoscopy. Am J Gastroenterol 89:459–460, 1994
15. Birkhead G, Vogt RL: Epidemiologic surveillance for endemic *Giardia lamblia* infection in Vermont. Am J Epidemiol 129:762–768, 1989
16. Sullivan PS, DuPont HL, Arafat RR, Thornton SA, Selwyn BJ, El-Alamy MA, Zaki AM: Illness and reservoirs associated with *Giardia lamblia* in Egypt: the case against treatment in developing world environments of high endemicity. Am J Epidemiol 127:1272–1281, 1988
17. Brodsky RE, Spencer AC, Schultz MG Giardiasis in American travelers to the Soviet Union. J Infect Dis 130:319–323, 1974
18. Fishel S, Webster J, Jackson P, Faratian B: Waterborne giardiasis in the United States 1965–84. Lancet 2:513–514, 1986
19. Shaw PK, Brodsky RE, Lyman DD, Wood BT, Hibler CP, Healy GR, MacLeod KIE, Stahl W, Schultz MG: A community-wide outbreak of giardiasis with evidence of transmission by a municipal water supply. Ann Intern Med 87:426–432, 1977
20. Dykes AC, Juranek DD, Lorenz RA, Sinclair S, Jakubowski W, Davies R: Municipal waterborne giardiasis: an epidemiologic investigation. Ann. Intern Med 92:165–170, 1980
21. Kent GP, Greenspan JR, Herndon JL, Mofenson LM, Harris JS, Eng TR, Waskin HA: Epidemic giardiasis caused by a contaminated public water supply. Am J Public Health 78:139–143, 1988
22. Pickering LK, Woodward WE: Diarrhea in day care centers. Pediatr Infect Dis 1:47–52, 1982
23. Steketee RW, Reid S, Cheng T, Stoebig JS, Harrington RG, Davis JP: Recurrent outbreaks of giardiasis in a child day care center, Wisconsin. Am J Public Health 79:485–490, 1989
24. Common-source outbreak of giardiasis—New Mexico. MMWR 38: 405–407, 1989

Dracunculiasis

General References

Hopkins DR: Dracunculiasis: an eradicable scourge. Epidemiol Rev 5:208–219, 1983

Hopkins DR, Ruiz-Tiben E: Strategies for dracunculiasis eradication. Bull World Health Org 69:533–540, 1991

Watts SJ: Dracunculiasis in Africa in 1986: its geographic extent, incidence, and at risk population. Am J Trop Med Hyg 37:119–125, 1987

World Health Organization: Dracunculiasis: global surveillance summary, 1996. Wkly Epidemiol Rec 72:133–139, 1997.

Human Enteric Coccidial Infections

1. Soave R, Dubey JP, Ramos LJ, Tummings M: A new intestinal pathogen? Clin Res 34:533A, 1986
2. Soave R, Armstrong D: *Cryptosporidium* and cryptosporidiosis. Rev Infect Dis 8:1012–1023, 1986
3. Nime FA, Burek JD, Page DL, Holscher MA, Yardley JH: Acute enterocolitis in a human being infected with the protozoan *Cryptosporidium*. Gastroenterology 70:592–598, 1976
4. Whiteside ME, Barkin JS, May RG, Weiss SD, Fischl MA, MacLeod CL: Enteric coccidiosis among patients with the acquired immune deficiency syndrome. Am J Trop Med Hyg 33:1065–1072, 1984
5. Goodgame RW: Understanding intestinal spore-forming protozoa: cryptosporidia, microsporidia, isospora, cyclospora. Ann Intern Med 124:429–441, 1996
6. Current WL, Garcia LS: Cryptosporidiosis. Clin Microbiol Rev 4:325–358, 1991
7. Berlin OGW, Novak SM, Porschen RK, Long EG, Stelma GN, Schaeffer FW III: Recovery of *Cyclospora organisms* from patients with prolonged diarrhea. Clin Infect Dis 18:606–609, 1994
8. Soave R, Johnson WD Jr: *Cryptosporidium* and *Isospora belli* infections. J Infect Dis 157:225–229, 1988
9. Centers for Disease Control: Cryptosporidiosis: assessment of chemotherapy of males with acquired immune deficiency syndrome (AIDS). MMWR 31:589–592, 1982
10. DeHovitz JA, Pape JW, Boncy M, Johnson WD Jr: Clinical manifestations and therapy of *Isospora belli* infection in patients with the acquired immunodeficiency syndrome. N Engl J Med 315: 87–90, 1986
11. Wurtz R: Cyclospora: a newly identified intestinal pathogen of humans. Clin Infect Dis 18:620–623, 1994
12. Wittner MW, Tanowitz HB, Weiss LM: Parasitic infections in AIDS patients: cryptosporidiosis, isosporiasis, microsporidiosis, cyclosporiasis. Infect Dis Clin North Am 7:569–586, 1993
13. Jacyna MR, Parkin J, Goldin R, Baron JH: Protracted enteric cryptosporidial infection in selective immunoglobulin A and *Saccharomyces opsonin* deficiencies. Gut 31:714–716, 1990
14. Sallon S, Deckelbaum RJ, Schmid II, Harlap S, Baras M, Spira DT: Cryptosporidium, malnutrition, and chronic diarrhea in children. Am J Dis Child 142:312–315, 1988
15. Schneiderman DJ, Cello JP, Laing FC: Papillary stenosis and sclerosing cholangitis in the acquired immunodeficiency syndrome. Ann Intern Med 106:546–549, 1987

16. Hinnant K, Schwartz A, Rotterdam H, Rudski C: Cytomegaloviral and cryptosporidial cholecystitis in two patients with AIDS. Am J Surg Pathol 13:57–60, 1989
17. Benator DA, French AL, Beaudet LM, Levy CS, Orenstein JM: *Isospora belli* infection associated with acalculous cholecystitis in a patient with AIDS. Ann Intern Med 121:663–664, 1994
18. Hojlyng N, Jensen BN: Respiratory cryptosporidiosis in HIV-positive patients [Letter]. Lancet 1:590–591, 1988
19. Juranek DD: Cyryptosporidiosis: sources of infection and guidelines for prevention. Clin Infect Dis 21(Suppl 1):S57–S61, 1995
20. Hayes EB, Matte TD, O'Brien TR, et al: Large community outbreak of cryptosporidiosis due to contamination of a filtered public water supply. N Engl J Med 320:1372–1376, 1989
21. Fayer RL, Ungar BLP: *Cryptosporidium* spp. and cryptosporidiosis. Microbiol Rev 50:458–483, 1986
22. Casemore DP: The antibody response to *Cryptosporidium* development of a serological test and its use in a study of immunologically normal persons. J Infect 14:125–134, 1987
23. Kuhls TL, Mosier DA, Crawford DL, Griffis J: Seroprevalence of cryptosporidial antibodies during infancy, childhood, and adolescence. Clin Infect Dis 18:731–735, 1994
24. Ungar BLP, Gilman RH, Lanata CF, Perez-Schael I: Seroepidemiology of *Cryptosporidium* infection in two Latin American populations. J Infect Dis 157:551–556, 1988
25. Navin TR, Hardy AM: Cryptosporidiosis in patients with AIDS. J Infect Dis 155:150, 1987
26. Laughon BE, Druckman DA, Vernon A, et al: Prevalence of enteric pathogens in homosexual men with and without acquired immunodeficiency syndrome. Gastroenterology 94:984–993, 1988
27. Rene E, Marche C, Regnier B, et al: Intestinal infections in patients with acquired immunodeficiency syndrome. A prospective study in 132 patients. Dig Dis Sci 34:773–780, 1989
28. Pape JW, Verdier R, Boncy M, Boncy J, Johnson WD Jr: *Cyclospora* infection in adults infected with HIV: clinical manifestations, treatment, and prophylaxis. Ann Intern Med 121:654–657, 1994
29. Ortega YR, Sterling CR, Gilman RH, Cama VA, Diaz F: *Cyclospora* species—a new protozoan pathogen of humans. N Engl J Med 328: 1308–1312, 1993
30. Hoge CW, Shlim DR, Rajah R, et al: Epidemiology of diarrhoeal illness associated with coccidian-like organism among travellers and foreign residents in Nepal. Lancet 341:1175–1179, 1993
31. Wurtz RM, Kocka FE, Peters CS, Weldon-Linne CM, Kuritza A, Yungbluth P: Clinical characteristics of seven cases of diarrhea associated with a novel acid-fast organism in the stool. Clin Infect Dis 16:136–138, 1993
32. Faust E, Giraldo L, Caciedo G, Bonfante R: Human isosporiasis in the Western hemisphere. Am J Trop Med Hyg 10:343–350, 1961
33. Pape JW, Johnson WD Jr: *Isospora belli* infection. Prog Clin Parasitol 2:119–127, 1991
34. Jeffrey G: Epidemiologic considerations of isosporiasis in a school for mental defectives. The American Journal of Hygiene 67: 251–255, 1958
35. Sauda FC, Zamarioli LA, Ebner Filho W, Mello L de B: Prevalence of *Cryptosporidium* sp. and *Isospora belli* among AIDS patients attending Santos Reference Center for AIDS, Sao Paulo, Brazil. J Parasitol 79:454–456, 1993
36. Conlon CP, Pinching AJ, Perera CU, Moody A, Luo NP, Lucas SB: HIV-related enteropathy in Zambia: a clinical, microbiologic, and histological study. Am J Trop Med Hyg 42:83–88, 1990

11

Food Poisoning

S. Benson Werner

Although the expression "food poisoning" is generally applied to any disease caused by food, a more appropriate rubric is "foodborne disease." This designation includes not only true "poisonings," such as from the metabolic products (toxins) produced by certain microorganisms while they multiply in food (e.g., *Staphylococcus aureus*), but also foodborne "infections" such as salmonellosis.

The potential for large-scale foodborne outbreaks has never been greater. A major reason is our increasing reliance on massive, centralized food production and processing, combined with extensive distribution. Any contamination in that chain, even low-level or infrequent contamination, could result in the exposure of thousands, whereas contamination of foods processed in the home, where foods were primarily processed generations ago, exposed relatively few individuals. The technological advances in industry that freed homemakers from food production and processing have not always been coupled with advances that assured food safety.

In addition, the epidemiology of foodborne diseases has changed in recent years: there is (*a*) increasing globalization of our food supplies, (*b*) increasing consumption of raw or minimally processed foods, particularly of fruits, vegetables, and grains (and less consumption of meat and other high fat foods), and (*c*) increasing consumption of food outside the home, in fast-food and other restaurants.[1] As the production/processing/distribution/preparation of foods has grown in complexity, so too have the opportunities for contamination. When contamination occurs today, sporadic illnesses tend to be widely dispersed, whereas the proverbial church supper outbreak of the past (but still occurring today, of course) caused high attack rates in localized settings.

The consuming public has also changed: (*a*) the population of elderly persons has increased markedly in absolute numbers (and in older age there is decreased resistance to infection through waning immunity and less stomach acid) and (*b*) there is an ever-expanding population of other individuals who are immunocompromised (by AIDS, cancer, chemotherapy for a number of conditions, diabetes mellitus, and others). Such individuals are susceptible to a greater range of microorganisms and become ill with smaller doses. It is for these reasons that humans have become the "ultimate bioassay" for low-level contamination of pathogens in our food supply.

▸ CLASSIFICATION OF FOODBORNE DISEASES

The extensive variety of foodborne diseases can be classified into several major categories based on the type of agent that causes illness. These are outlined below:

1. *Infection, bacterial:* Salmonellosis is an example. As with other infections, and in contrast to poisons, fever is common.
2. *Poisons, bacterial:* Staphylococcal or botulinal toxin poisoning. As with other poisons, these produce no fever.
3. *Infection, viral:* Hepatitis A and Norwalk viruses are examples.
4. *Infection, parasitic:* Trichinosis, taeniasis, and anisakiasis.
5. *Poisons, chemical:* Salts and oxides of such chemicals as arsenic, antimony, copper, and lead. Gastrointestinal symptoms generally begin just minutes after ingestion.
6. *Poisons, plant and fungal origin:* Mushroom poisoning, ergot alkaloids, hemlock poisoning, jimsonweed.
7. *Poisons, animal (including marine) origin:* Ciguatera (ichthyosarcotoxism), scombroid, and paralytic shellfish poisoning.
8. *Radionuclides:* Strontium-90 from nuclear weapon testing.

Bryan's monograph[2] reviews the many etiological agents; their nature, sources, and important reservoirs; epidemiology; foods frequently involved; specimens to study; and control measures.

▸ SURVEILLANCE AND INVESTIGATION OF FOODBORNE DISEASES

The surveillance of foodborne diseases has traditionally aimed at disease control through (*a*) identification and removal of contaminated products from the commercial market, (*b*) identification and correction of improper food handling practices both in commercial establishments and in the home, (*c*) the identification and treatment of cases and carriers of foodborne disease, and (*d*) knowledge of disease causation, trends, new etiologic agents, and their food vehicles.

In the data published by the Centers for Disease Control and Prevention (CDC) summarizing foodborne diseases in the United States in recent years, about 500 outbreaks have been reported annually. In only about 40 percent of these was a cause identified; of these, it has been bacterial about 75 percent of the time, chemical 20 percent, parasitic 3 percent, and viral 2 percent of the time. Most outbreaks of unknown etiology have had incubation periods of more than 15 hours and many had secondary cases, suggesting an infectious cause; many of these were probably viral but laboratory capability to diagnose Norwalk-like agents is still not widely available. Most cases of bacterial origin involve *Salmonella, Staphylococcus*, and *Clostridium perfringens*. Accordingly, an appreciation of the different clinical features and incubation periods of these three diseases (Table 11–1) is important in the investigation of foodborne outbreaks. If a judgment as to probable cause can be made early in an epidemic investigation, then one can better decide on the most appropriate specimens and methods to select for study, and how far back in time to inquire about food exposures.

Procedures for the investigation of foodborne disease outbreaks are detailed in a monograph published by the International Association of Milk, Food, and Environmental Sanitarians, Inc.[3] Some

TABLE 11-1. DISTINCTIVE FEATURES OF THREE COMMON CAUSES OF FOODBORNE ILLNESS[a]

Entity	*Incubation Period (hrs.)*	*Fever*	*Vomiting*	*Diarrhea*
Staphylococcal poisoning	3	−	+	±
Clostridium perfringens poisoning	12	−	−	+
Salmonella infection	24	+	±	+

[a]Applicable as a group phenomenon; no great reliance as to probable etiology should be placed on a single case of illness.

Note: These features offer practical guidelines for provisional identification of the etiology in foodborne disease outbreaks; they help to decide the most appropriate specimens for study, whether they should be studied aerobically or anaerobically, and how far back to inquire about food exposure. Laboratory confirmation is necessary for definitive diagnosis.

general points merit emphasis. Interviews with food handlers, patients, and control subjects should be conducted as soon as possible: memories fade, people scatter, and the suspect foods may be discarded and unavailable for study or, worse, consumed by others. The investigator should appreciate the urgent necessity to collect the facts and materials that may not be practical or sometimes even possible to obtain at a later time.

In a relatively small outbreak, an effort should be made to question all who were exposed, whether ill or not, for symptoms and food consumption history. To identify the responsible food(s), a retrospective cohort study design is commonly used (see Chapter 2). Rates of illness in those who ate specific food items (the "attribute" or "characteristic") are calculated and compared with the rates of illness in those who did not eat those items (Table 11–2). The implicated foods generally have the highest attack rates. More important, however, is that when rates for eaters and noneaters are compared, the implicated foods show the greatest differences in attack rates. The difference is called the "attributable risk," or the rate of disease that can be attributed to the food under consideration. Alternatively, "relative risks" may be calculated (see Chapter 2) by comparing, as a ratio, the rate of illness in those exposed to specific foods to the rate of illness in those not exposed. If the relative risk is significantly greater than 1.0, there may be an association between food exposure and illness. CDC has developed a popular software program called Epi Info for analyzing data collected in foodborne and other outbreak investigations.[4] In Table 11–2, barbecued chicken appears to be implicated (see last column), while those eating fried chicken might appear to have been spared from illness (probably by choosing that item instead of barbecued chicken). The necessity of interviewing well people in order to incriminate a particular food is illustrated by the item root beer, which might have been suspected as the cause of the outbreak. More ill people had root beer than any other item; in fact, all ill people had drunk some. However, it is evident that root beer was also consumed by nearly all those who remained well. The reason it was so popular is that it was the only drink available.

One might think that the association of illness with a particular implicated food should be "perfect" (i.e., all those who ate it must have become sick, and all those who got sick must have eaten it), but there are several reasons why this is rarely so:

1. The implicated food may not be contaminated throughout.
2. Host susceptibility varies.
3. Dosage (the quantity consumed) varies.
4. Food histories may contain reporting errors through faulty recall, uncertainty, or lying; there may also be errors in recording.
5. Those who report illness but no exposure to the incriminated food may have coincidental, unrelated illness or secondary infection when the outbreak is due to infection (e.g., *Salmonella*); alternatively, illness may be due to trace contamination of other foods or utensils by the implicated food.

If an outbreak is large and it is not possible to interview all participants, a random sample should be selected and questioned for symptoms and food exposure history. The data can be arranged in prospective fashion, as in Table 11–2, and similarly analyzed.

On the other hand, outbreaks can also be studied in a case-control fashion; and, in fact, there may be no alternative to case-control studies when the overall attack rate is low. In such situations

TABLE 11-2. DIFFERENCES IN FOOD-SPECIFIC ATTACK RATES IN AN OUTBREAK OF FOODBORNE ILLNESS

	Persons Who Ate Specified Food				Persons Who Did Not Eat Specified Food				
	(a)[a] Ill	*(b)[a] Well*	*Total*	*Attack Rate (%)*	*(c)[a] Ill*	*(d)[a] Well*	*Total*	*Attack Rate (%)*	*Difference in Attack Rates*
Shrimp salad	8	4	12	67	15	21	36	42	+25
Olives	19	13	32	59	5	13	18	28	+31
Fried chicken	10	33	43	23	4	2	6	67	−44
Barbecued chicken	17	1	18	94	3	27	30	10	+84
Baked beans	12	13	25	48	12	10	22	55	−7
Potato salad	17	20	37	46	8	6	14	57	−11
Macaroni salad	9	15	24	38	15	10	25	60	−22
Root beer	23	23	46	50	0	2	2	0	+50
Bread	8	9	17	47	18	13	31	58	−11
Neapolitan cream pie	1	2	3	33	21	21	42	50	−17

[a]To see how this table relates to the classic 2 by 2 table, refer to Table 2–6.

the frequencies with which specific food items were selected by patients are compared with the frequencies in controls; that is, the so-called "food preference" rates are compared and odds ratios calculated (see Chapter 2). Food preference rates can also be effectively used when recall for specific food items is compromised, as can occur in patients ill with diseases that have especially long incubation periods, such as hepatitis A.[5]

The remainder of this chapter describes the most frequently encountered foodborne diseases and comments briefly on newly identified ones.

▶ STAPHYLOCOCCAL FOOD POISONING

History

The work of Dack et al.[6] in 1930 established staphylococci as a cause of food poisoning. They isolated *Staphylococcus aureus* in pure culture from a cake implicated in an outbreak; when cell-free filtrates prepared from broth cultures of the isolate were fed to volunteers, symptoms like those in the outbreak resulted. Eight enterotoxins have been identified, and a ninth may exist. These toxins easily resist boiling for 30 minutes or more. It is the heat-stable, preformed toxin, not *S. aureus* organisms per se, that causes staphylococcal food poisoning. The target organ is the gut.

Symptoms

Symptoms usually appear 2 to 4 hours after ingestion; the range is 1 to 6 hours. Onset is generally abrupt and may be violent. Salivation, nausea, vomiting, abdominal cramps, prostration, diarrhea (diarrhea less often than vomiting), and occasionally hypertension occur. There is generally no fever or chills, but patients may experience a subjective feeling of fever from the flushing and perspiration that accompany vomiting, and a subsequent chilly sensation as perspiration evaporates. Acute gastrointestinal symptoms commonly last several hours but generally less than a day; weakness may persist for another 1 or 2 days. Death in otherwise healthy individuals is rare. The intensity of symptoms has prompted surgical exploration (for suspected appendicitis) in sporadic, severe cases.

Diagnosis

Staphylococcal food poisoning is generally suspected when a number of people develop acute, predominantly upper gastrointestinal tract symptoms a few hours after eating some food item in common. Isolation of coagulase-producing staphylococci from epidemiologically implicated food, vomitus, or stool specimens confirms the diagnosis. Rarely, coagulase-negative *S. aureus* and other staphylococcal species (e.g., *S. intermedius*) have been implicated. The implicated food generally contains at least 10^6 *S. aureus* organisms per gram to produce sufficient enterotoxin to cause human disease. A small amount of *S. aureus* in food is not unusual, and so it is incumbent on the investigator to refrigerate food specimens promptly and maintain refrigeration until testing can be done, so that any *S. aureus* present will not multiply to levels that did not exist when the food was obtained. On the other hand, if staphylococci are not recovered from the epidemiologically implicated food, the food may have been heated by someone apprised of an imminent visit by local public health authorities and aware that heating can destroy bacteria. In this case a Gram stain may be useful in demonstrating sheets of Gram-positive cocci, and an assay is available at special laboratories to identify the presence of heat-resistant enterotoxin. Isolates of *S. aureus* from patients and from foods can be compared to those recovered from food handlers, either by antibiogram typing or by phage typing, to complete the epidemiological connection.

Sources of Contamination

Staphylococci are widely distributed in nature, and humans are a natural reservoir. *S. aureus* can colonize normal, healthy skin as well as the normal oronasopharynx, but the organism can be especially abundant in purulent discharges of an infected finger, hangnail, cut, burn, eye, or chronic infections of the nasal sinuses. Individuals with acne, boils, carbuncles, and common colds may be heavy shedders as well. Cows with infected udders also pose a health hazard if their milk is not promptly refrigerated. Foods implicated in staphylococcal food poisoning generally require much handling and are characteristically rich in protein (e.g., custards and cream fillings, sliced and chopped meats). Occasionally, surprising foods are implicated such as the extensive, widespread 1989 outbreak due to canned mushrooms imported from the People's Republic of China.

Prevention

The three principal requirements for the production of sufficient enterotoxin to cause disease are: (*a*) the food must be contaminated with enterotoxin-producing staphylococci; (*b*) the food must be a good growth medium, and (*c*) the food must be held at an improper temperature (such as ambient room) for several hours. Prevention depends on eliminating sources of contamination and practicing safe food handling: workers with purulent discharges, common colds, etc., should be excluded from food preparation. The actual food handling time should be reduced to an absolute minimum. Foods should be at room temperature no longer than necessary, preferably under 1 hour, and then should be kept hot (≥140°F, 60°C) or cold (≤40°F, 4°C), and covered to exclude dust.

▶ *SALMONELLA* INFECTION

The epidemiology of salmonellosis is discussed in Chapter 14; this discussion will focus on aspects of salmonellae as a cause of food-borne disease. Salmonellae are among the most prevalent of zoonotic infectious agents. Raw meat and raw meat products frequently harbor salmonellae (poultry more commonly than pork; pork more commonly than beef). Food-borne *Salmonella* infection, however, can be prevented by adequate heating to destroy these pathogens and avoidance of cross-contamination after heating. On the other hand, raw produce such as sprouts have caused *Salmonella* outbreaks; and, sprouts are not commonly washed in homes or restaurants. The ultimate sources of such contaminations have not been identified but may relate to contact of sprout seeds or plants with animals or their wastes. Occasionally, infected food handlers are implicated in outbreaks as sources of contamination, but more often they represent additional cases, having eaten the same foods as their customers. Any "responsibility," however, lies in their not having eradicated (through proper heating, etc.) the salmonellae introduced into their establishments in the raw meat and meat products that were implicated.

While low-level contamination of foods with *S. aureus* is unavoidable and, in itself, poses no threat, there can be no tolerance of any level of *Salmonella* contamination in foods ready for serving.

The infective dose for *Salmonella* infection is most commonly given as 10^5 organisms but can be as high as 10^9 or 10^{10}, depending on the serotype and the host. However, past volunteer studies to determine the infectious dose were limited by several factors: they were often done on healthy young males with laboratory strains that could have lost their virulence; they failed to assess minimal infective doses; and they used few volunteers at the lower dose levels. Much lower infective doses, of $\leq 10^3$ total organisms ingested, have been estimated from observations in the "more natural" setting of recent food-borne outbreaks. Specifically, 60 to 2300 organisms per 100 g of food were estimated in raw hamburger that caused *S. newport* infection,[7] less than 100 organisms per 100 g of chocolate candy that caused *S. eastbourne* infection,[8] less than 10 organisms per 100 g in Schwan's ice cream in the 1994 *S. enteritidis* outbreak estimated to have affected more than 200,000 persons nationwide,[9] and less than 1 organism per 100 g of cheddar cheese that caused *S. heidelberg* infection.[10] A comprehensive review of the infective dose of *Salmonella* in both volunteers and outbreak settings has been published.[11]

It is recognized that gastric acid protects against ingested enteric pathogens such as salmonellae. This can explain why infants (and the aged) can be infected by relatively low doses: they may normally lack stomach acid. The reason why the foods listed above may have caused disease in presumably healthy, young adults despite low-level *Salmonella* contamination probably relates to their high fat content, which protects the salmonellae from gastric acid and allows salmonellae to reach the less hostile, alkaline duodenum. Milk (and ice cream) have high fat content and, if contaminated, pose an additional risk. Since these are fluids, they quickly pass into the duodenum (unless consumed with solid food) and escape acid contact. The large Riverside, California, waterborne outbreak of 1965[12] was due to low-level contamination (MPN of 17 salmonellae per liter) of water which, as a fluid, could similarly reach the duodenum after short gastric contact time.

▸ *CLOSTRIDIUM PERFRINGENS* FOOD POISONING

History

While it was suggested earlier in this century that *C. perfringens* (*C. welchii*) caused food-borne disease, it was not until the classic paper by Hobbs et al. in 1953[13] that *C. perfringens* received attention. Since then it has become recognized as one of the most common foodborne diseases in developed countries.

The organism is a common, anaerobic, spore-forming rod that exists widely in nature and can frequently be recovered from raw meats and meat products. Five toxicological types (A to E) are recognized; types A and C cause human gastroenteritis. Type A also causes gas gangrene, and type C, necrotic enteritis ("pigbel"). Of the several toxins and enzymes produced by *C. perfringens* type A, the important one appears to be alpha toxin, which includes the enzyme lecithinase. *C. perfringens* produces both heat-resistant spores and heat-sensitive spores; the latter predominate in nature, but it is the heat-resistant strains that are most often associated with outbreaks of food-borne poisonings.

Typical Setting of C. Perfringens Poisoning

With rare exceptions the implicated food is a meat dish prepared in advance, and in bulk, for a large group such as a banquet or institutional population, in such a way that anaerobic and thermal conditions existed to permit germination of spores that survived initial cooking. These spores are heat shocked (activated) to germinate as soon as the cooling mass reaches a suitable temperature. Young vegetative cells continue to multiply, depending on temperature, storage time, and the nature of the food (liquid masses of meat such as stews can provide especially good anaerobic conditions). With generation times as short as 9 minutes under optimal conditions, a critical dose of disease-producing *C. perfringens* (several million organisms or a concentration of organisms $\geq 10^5$/g of food) can readily result. If the mass is too large to cool quickly during subsequent refrigeration, multiplication can continue in the refrigerator and can also resume on subsequent rewarming if not carried out at temperatures inhibitory to growth (≥140°F, 60°C). In summary, the cooking of meats and poultry in huge quantities, prolonged storage at room temperature, slow cooling, and insufficient reheating are typical features in *C. perfringens* outbreaks.

The Disease

After an incubation period of approximately 12 hours (range: 6 to 24), abdominal cramps and diarrhea develop. Occasionally, nausea is reported, but vomiting and fever are typically absent. The disease is so mild that medical consultation is rarely sought; for most, the illness lasts only a day or less. In elderly debilitated patients, however, the disease can be severe, and deaths have been reported.

Diagnosis

As in any foodborne outbreak, laboratory study of the epidemiologically implicated food is most important; for *C. perfringens*, the organism concentration criterion is $\geq 10^5$/g. A direct smear of the implicated food typically shows square-ended, Gram-positive bacilli almost exclusively. Stool cultures could be obtained from patients and control subjects for quantitative determination of *C. perfringens*. Although healthy adults may harbor *C. perfringens* in their intestinal tracts, many different serotypes are represented and the concentration of *C. perfringens* is much less than in those who are ill. *C. perfringens* enterotoxin can also be detected in the feces of patients but not in the feces of control subjects. Environmental cultures from the kitchen and fecal cultures from food handlers are not encouraged. Since *C. perfringens* is so commonly found in raw meat and poultry, the human carrier or unsanitized kitchen equipment and working surfaces represent relatively unimportant sources of contamination.

Prevention

Outbreaks of *C. perfringens* foodborne disease would not occur if cooked foods were eaten after initial cooking, while still hot. If it is absolutely necessary to prepare large amounts of food several hours or days before its intended use, the cooked food should not be held at room temperature to cool. Instead, it should be chilled rapidly to a temperature of 40°F (4°C), preferably in a walk-in refrigerator with forced air circulation. To speed the cooling process, the meat, gravy, or stew should be placed in a freezer compartment or divided into shallow containers to induce more rapid heat transfer in the refrigerator. The meat may be served cold, but if it is to be served hot, it should be rewarmed to 165°F (74°C) as quickly as possible. Cold meat slices may be covered with boiling-hot gravy immediately before serving, but the habit of pouring warm gravy on sliced meat and putting both in a warming oven with temperature below 140°F (60°C) is to be condemned. The expression "Keep hot foods hot and cold foods cold" is worth emphasizing for *C. perfringens*, as well as for other organisms responsible for foodborne diseases.

▸ BOTULISM

History

Botulism was first recognized as a disease entity early in the nineteenth century and was named for sausage (from the Latin *botulus*), which was often implicated in the earliest outbreaks. Since then a host of other improperly preserved foods (fish, vegetables, fruit) have caused disease, but the name has been retained. Van Ermengem first identified the causative organism in 1895. Its neurotoxins (simple proteins) are among the most deadly of all known poisons.

Three forms of botulism are now recognized according to the site of toxin production by *Clostridium botulinum* (although a fourth category, "undetermined," exists for those cases not easily categorized):

1. Classic foodborne botulism, the form with which most health workers are familiar, results from the ingestion of preformed botulinal toxin in improperly preserved food. Interest in foodborne botulism far exceeds its importance as a cause of extensive illness (less than 2000 cases reported in the United States since 1900 and only about 10 cases per year in recent decades).
2. Wound botulism results from local tissue infection and in situ toxin production by *C. botulinum*; it was first reported in 1951. This form of botulism is rarely documented; approximately 100 cases have been reported worldwide through 1995. California, alone, has reported 80 of those cases, and most of those related to injecting drug use (particularly of Mexican "black tar" heroin) in the 1990s.
3. Infant botulism results from colonization of the gut lumen by *C. botulinum* with subsequent in vivo production of toxin. This third form of botulism was first recognized in 1976 and, by 1995, more than 1400 cases had been identified world-

wide. Some "undetermined" cases of botulism in adults have been considered adult forms of infant botulism, occurring particularly in those who have had altered intestinal anatomy and physiology.[14]

Clostridium botulinum is a Gram-positive, strictly anaerobic, spore-forming bacillus whose natural habitat is the soil. Eight toxigenic types have been identified but, in humans, the disease is almost always caused by A, B, or E toxins and rarely by F or G. These toxins prevent the release of acetylcholine at cholinergic synapses. The most notable effect is flaccid paralysis because of the interruption of nerve impulses at the myoneural junction. The spores of *C. botulinum* are ubiquitous, and except for those infants who develop infant botulism for reasons still unknown, the spores are not otherwise dangerous when ingested. Indeed, since spores are so widely distributed in soil and dust, they could be ingested every time fresh produce is eaten. Toxin is elaborated, however, when spores that survive improper food preservation germinate in anaerobic conditions. Botulinal toxin, once formed, is readily destroyed by boiling, but most botulinum spores are not promptly destroyed by boiling; they require temperatures of 240°F (116°C) for destruction.

The Disease

In foodborne botulism, signs and symptoms of intoxication appear 6 hours to 8 days (most typically 12 to 48 hours) after ingestion of contaminated food. Those with the shortest interval to onset (less than 24 hours) generally are most severely affected. The initial symptoms are frequently ptosis, blurred or double vision, and dry, sore throat. Progressive descending paralysis, usually but not always symmetrical, may then develop. After impairment of cranial nerve function (which causes diplopia and poor accommodation, dysphagia, dysphonia, and inability of neck muscles to support the head), paralysis of the respiratory muscles and of the extremities may ensue. Conspicuously absent are objective sensory abnormalities, altered mental status, and fever. Gastrointestinal symptoms are frequently but not necessarily present and may precede or accompany neurological symptoms; constipation is common after paralysis develops. The case fatality ratio for classic foodborne botulism was formerly about 60 percent, but in recent years it has been less than 30 percent. Respiratory paralysis is generally the immediate cause of death. If vital functions can be maintained, full neurological recovery can be expected, although convalescence may be slow and weakness may last for months.

The clinical picture in *wound* botulism is like that in foodborne botulism, but there is more likely to be fever (secondary to wound infection) and less likely to be early gastrointestinal complaints. With some exceptions, cases to date have primarily involved wounds of an extremity, and the median interval between injury and symptoms of botulism has been 6 days. An increasing proportion of recent cases has been reported in injecting drug users, particularly by "skin popping" or by intramuscular injections. The resulting abscess formation and associated devitalized/scar tissue provide a favorable milieu for the establishment and multiplication of injected anaerobes such as *C. botulinum*.

In the typical case of *infant* botulism requiring hospitalization, the child is 3 months old, and the first symptom is usually constipation, followed by lethargy, poor sucking and swallowing, and then generalized weakness and hypotonia. The infant appears "floppy." The case fatality rate in children hospitalized for infant botulism in the United States is less than 3 percent; however, it has been shown that some cases of sudden infant death syndrome (SIDS) can be attributed to infant botulism.

Foods Involved

Most cases of foodborne botulism are caused by home-preserved foods that received some preliminary heat treatment as by canning or smoking. More recently, however, major restaurant-associated outbreaks have involved foods that were not preserved in the usual sense, for example, previously baked potatoes used for potato salad, chopped garlic in oil, and sauteed fresh onions. Store-bought refrigerated foods that were not kept refrigerated after purchase have also caused botulism outbreaks. Inadequately rewarmed foods have also been implicated, such as commercial potpies and home-prepared meat loaf that were kept in gas ovens, with only the pilot light on, for many hours after initial cooking. Despite the publicity given to commercial foods, about 90 percent of all outbreaks in recent years have been due to improper home canning rather than commercial canning. Home canning at temperatures insufficient to destroy spores is the usual problem. For vegetables, a pressure cooker that can reach temperatures of 240°F (116°C) is necessary. Resistance of spores to heat sterilization is reduced at a low pH, and this is why highly acid fruits are rarely implicated in outbreaks and why acidification of home-canned vegetables (with vinegar or lemon juice) is recommended before pressure cooking as an extra measure of protection.

In the United States, most botulinal poisonings are due to home-canned vegetables or fruits, rarely meats; but in Europe, most cases are due to sausages, smoked or preserved meats, and fish. Foods spoiled by some types of *C. botulinum* are frequently foul smelling and vile tasting, especially when proteolytic strains of the organism are involved. Jar lids or can tops may be swollen from gas produced by *C. botulinum*, but this is not invariably the case.

For those infants who develop botulism, it is likely that there are multiple sources of gastrointestinal colonization since botulinal spores are ubiquitous in the environment. To date, toxin has not been found in any food fed to infants with botulism. *C. botulinum* spores, however, have been found in up to 10 percent of honey samples surveyed and in honey that had been fed to patients.

Distribution

Spores of *C. botulinum* exist in soil throughout the world. In nations where home canning is discouraged (e.g., England) or where fresh fruits and vegetables are available year round and there is little home canning (as in tropical Third World countries), botulism outbreaks are rare. Additionally, some cases may go undiagnosed in some developed and in most developing countries because laboratory tests to diagnose the disease are not generally available.

In the United States, more than 50 percent of outbreaks have been reported from five western states. California alone has reported 33 percent of the national total. There is a distinct geographical distribution of botulinal toxin types: type A outbreaks predominate west of the Mississippi River, type B occurs primarily in eastern states, and type E is reported primarily from Alaska and the Great Lakes area. This correlates with the types of spores found in these respective regions. Most outbreaks in Europe are due to type B, and in Japan most are due to type E.

Wound botulism has been reported primarily from the United States which has reported more than 90 percent of the world's cases. The diagnosis should be considered when characteristic features of botulism develop in a person with a wound, particularly of an extremity (not necessarily suppurative), where food cannot be incriminated.

Infant botulism, as of December 1996, has been recognized on all inhabited continents except Africa. More than 1300 of the world's 1400+ laboratory-confirmed cases have been identified in the United States, where it was first recognized. As medical awareness of this disease entity increases throughout the world, the incidence and importance of infant botulism worldwide will probably exceed that of classic foodborne botulism, as it has in the United States.

Diagnosis

Botulism is confirmed by demonstrating that the patient's serum, gastric aspirate, stool, or wound material contains a heat-labile substance toxic for mice that is specifically neutralized by botulinal antitoxin. Parallel studies should be performed on leftover, suspect food or, if none is available, on food from the same lot or batch. Stool cultures for *C. botulinum* should also be obtained. Despite the routine ingestion of *C. botulinum* spores on fresh fruits and vegetables, neither *C. botulinum* organisms nor its toxins are normally found in feces. For this reason the presence of *C. botulinum* toxin or organisms in the stools of patients with suspected foodborne botulism can be considered diagnostic. In wound botulism an effort should be made to study the wound for evidence of *C. botulinum* organisms and toxin. In recent years, the California Department of Health Services demonstrated, for the first time, that free toxin could be demonstrated in wedge resections of abscessed tissue from wound botulism cases (J McGee, unpublished data).

Electromyography is a useful diagnostic tool. In botulism the muscle action potential is diminished after a single nerve stimulus, but repetitive stimulation at rates of 20 to 50 per second can result in facilitation (augmentation) of the action potential. This may not be present early, however, and it is not pathognomonic. In infant botulism a characteristic electromyographic pattern termed "brief, small, abundant, motor unit action potentials" (BSAPs) can be observed and has been seen to persist for as long as clinical evidence of blocked neuromuscular transmission is present.[15]

Treatment

Most important in all forms of botulism is high-quality supportive care with immediate access to an intensive care unit, so that respiratory failure—the usual cause of death—can be anticipated and promptly treated. Polyvalent antitoxins of equine origin are available that neutralize circulating toxin but not the toxin already fixed to nerve tissue. If treatment is clinically indicated, antitoxin should be administered without delay and without waiting for results of mouse bioassay (which are usually not available for at least 24 hours). The role of antitoxin in infant botulism, however, is not clear: circulating toxin has been demonstrated only rarely, and virtually all hospitalized patients have recovered completely without antitoxin treatment. A study to evaluate the efficacy of botulism immune globulin (of human origin) in infants is nearing completion in California. Antibiotics have not been of value in either foodborne or infant botulism. Antibiotics certainly have not prevented continued excretion of *C. botulinum* toxin and organisms. In foodborne botulism the gastrointestinal tract should be emptied of still unabsorbed toxin by emesis or gastric lavage with activated charcoal (if foods were eaten recently) and by cathartics and high enema (if ileus is absent). In those who are suspected of having ingested contaminated food but are not symptomatic, evacuation of gastrointestinal contents as described is also indicated. In wound botulism, thorough débridement, wound irrigation, and antibiotic therapy are indicated along with administration of antitoxin which should, ideally, be administered before the wound is disturbed. Trivalent botulinal antitoxin is available around-the-clock from the Centers for Disease Control and Prevention, Atlanta, Georgia at (404)639-2888.

Prevention

For foods canned at home, attention must be given to the necessary time, pressure, and temperature to ensure destruction of *C. botulinum* spores. Vegetables should generally be acidified before they are pressure cooked and should be reboiled for at least 3 minutes, with stirring, before serving. Although the toxin is readily destroyed by boiling, foods with off-odors should not be consumed or "taste tested," and cans or bottles with bulging lids, whether home canned or commercial, should not be opened. Foodborne botulism is a public health emergency; local public health authorities should be notified immediately of any presumed case so that efforts can be initiated to confirm the diagnosis, locate other cases and impending cases, determine the food source, and confiscate all existing food containers. Notification of even suspected cases is a legal requirement in most states. Until the epidemiology of infant botulism is better delineated, no recommendations can be given except that honey should not be fed to infants, especially since this is not an essential food. The only practical way to prevent wound botulism from the injection of illicit drugs is to stop such injections.

▶ MISCELLANEOUS

Other important foodborne diseases deserve comment. *Vibrio parahaemolyticus* is one of the leading causes of foodborne disease in Japan, but it was not identified in the United States until 1969. Most outbreaks have been traced to crustaceans taken from warm coastal marine waters that were either inadequately cooked or subsequently recontaminated by raw shellfish or surfaces and implements that had contact with raw fish or shellfish. The incubation period is about 12 hours; onset is generally acute; and symptoms resemble those of salmonellosis. Recovery is usually complete in 2 to 5 days. Special media (thiosulfate citrate bile salts sucrose agar (TCBS)) should be used when this disease is suspected. Other *Vibrio* species (which contaminate 5 to 10 percent of shellfish in the U.S. market) cause disease too. The most virulent is *V. vulnificus*, which is fatal in more than 50 percent of those who develop bacteremia. At greatest risk of serious *V. vulnificus* infection are those with liver disease (such as from alcoholism), reduced stomach acid (naturally occurring or therapeutically induced), acquired immunodeficiency syndrome (AIDS), and other conditions with compromised immunity. These individuals, especially, should avoid eating raw or undercooked shellfish. Cholera, due to *V. cholerae* serogroup 1, has occurred in the United States from a variety of imported foods that were transported by international travelers; but cases have also been traced to Gulf Coast shellfish.

Scombroid fish poisoning results from the ingestion of spoiled fish, primarily of the suborder *Scombroidei* (e.g., tuna, mackerel). Inadequate or delayed refrigeration at sea of fish taken from temperate and tropical waters results in overgrowth of bacteria (*Proteus morganii,* among others) that normally comprise the microflora of fish. These bacteria metabolize histidine and degrade the protein of fish flesh to produce scombrotoxin, which consists of histamine and other amines. Since orally administered histamine has no effect in humans, perhaps co-contaminants like cadaverine, putrescine, and other products of fish decomposition enhance the toxic action of histamine by inhibiting histaminases in the human intestine.[16] (Similarly, drugs such as isoniazid, which inhibit histamine-detoxifying enzymes, have evoked reactions to low levels of histamine normally found in such foods as cheese). Scombroid fish poisoning is sometimes misdiagnosed as "fish allergy." Symptoms develop about 30 minutes after eating and include a peppery sensation of the tongue, rash, flushing (sometimes urticaria), pruritus, headaches, dizziness, periorbital edema, thirst, nausea, vomiting, diarrhea, and abdominal cramps. Some of these symptoms resemble histamine reaction and respond to antihistamine therapy. Laboratory studies of implicated fish frequently show "honey-combing" (a sign of decomposition), bad odor, and histamine levels ≥50 mg/100 g. Scombrotoxin is heat stable and can withstand the temperatures used in canning; commercially canned fish has been implicated in several international outbreaks.

Ciguatera poisoning can be caused by more than 400 species of fish that are primarily bottom-dwelling shore fish caught near reefs between 35°N and 35°S latitude. In the United States, 90 percent of outbreaks are reported from Hawaii and Florida and are due mostly to grouper, red snapper, and barracuda. Ciguatoxin is actually produced by certain dinoflagellates attached to algae on coral reefs. Small fish feed on the algae and are, in turn, eaten by larger bottom-dwelling shore fish and so on up the food chain. The larger fish are more toxic than smaller ones; organs such as liver, intestines, and gonads are the most toxic parts. The median latency period is 5 hours, and the median duration of symptoms is 8 days. Besides gastrointestinal symptoms of abdominal cramps, nausea, vomiting, and diarrhea, there may be numbness and paresthesia of lips and tongue, paresthesias of the extremities, metallic taste, arthralgia, myalgia, blurred vision, temporary blindness, and paradoxical temperature sensation. In those with life-threatening disease there may be hypotension, bradycardia, cranial nerve palsies, and respiratory paralysis. Therapy is primarily supportive, although intravenous mannitol has been reported to produce dramatic improvement.[17] Tocainide, an orally effective lidocaine analog, has also been reported of value (presumably by blocking the toxic effect of ciguatoxin).[18] Prevention is difficult; ciguatoxic fish do not appear or taste spoiled, and ordinary cooking does not destroy the heat-stable toxin. Unusually large reef fish should be avoided, especially their liver and roe.

Paralytic shellfish poisoning is caused by the ingestion of filter-feeding bivalve mollusks (e.g., mussels and clams) that had previously ingested (without adverse effect) toxic dinoflagellates of *Alexandrium* sp. (formerly *Gonyaulax* sp.) and concentrated the neurotoxin saxitoxin in their tissues. Symptoms in humans usually begin about 30 minutes after eating, with paresthesias of the mouth, lips, face, and fingertips; then, in more severe cases, dysphagia, dysphonia, ataxia, weakness, paralysis, and occasionally respiratory arrest occur. Treatment is supportive and should include efforts to remove unabsorbed toxin from the gut. Fortunately, even in severe cases, symptoms disappear completely in 1 to 2 days. A standardized mouse bioassay is used for demonstrating and quantifying toxin in shellfish. Toxic dinoflagellates bloom in waters above 30°N and below 30°S latitude and sometimes impart a reddish color to the water—the so-called red tide. Regulatory agencies monitor shellfish and impose quarantines on harvesting them, when deemed necessary to protect the public health.

Cyclospora cayetanensis (previously known as blue-green algae, cyanobacteria, and "big *Cryptosporidium*") is a recently characterized coccidian parasite. Before 1996, only three outbreaks (all in the 1990s) had been reported in the United States. In the spring of 1996, however, a great number of outbreaks involving more than 1000 laboratory-confirmed cases occurred in states east of the Rocky Mountains. Investigations implicated fresh raspberries probably imported from Guatemala, but it was not possible to trace back to the farm(s) of origin or identify the mechanism(s) of contamination. Whether animals can serve as sources of infection is also unknown. The usual incubation period is about 1 week and the symptoms and protracted course are reminiscent of giardiasis. Diagnosis is by demonstration of *Cyclospora* oocysts in stool by modified acid-fast stain (the cysts are twice the size of *Cryptosporidia*). Treatment is possible with trimethoprim-sulfamethoxazole. Produce eaten raw should be thoroughly washed but this may not entirely eliminate risk, and some fruits, such as raspberries, don't tolerate washing without becoming macerated.

Bacilius cereus poisoning has been recognized for decades in Europe, but the first fully documented episode in the United States occurred in 1969. At least two clinical syndromes exist. The first is like staphylococcal food poisoning in that it has a median latency period of only 2 hours and produces primarily upper gastrointestinal symptoms. The vehicle for this form has most commonly been fried rice served in Chinese restaurants, where the rice had previously been steamed or boiled and then left unrefrigerated for hours or days before it was mixed with egg or pork and quickly stir-fried before serving. The second syndrome resembles *C. perfringens* poisoning in that it has a median latency period of 10 hours and produces primarily lower gastrointestinal symptoms. A variety of foods has been implicated in this type of illness. In both syndromes, disease is generally mild and lasts only a few hours. Diagnosis can be confirmed by the isolation of $\geq 10^5$ *B. cereus* organisms per gram of food from epidemiologically implicated food and also by fecal culture. The prevalence of *B. cereus* in control subjects will be much less than in patients. The organism produces at least two enterotoxins—one is heat stable and causes vomiting, and the other is heat labile and causes diarrhea. *B. cereus* is widely distributed in soil and in raw, dried, and processed foods. In one survey, 52 percent of 1500 food ingredients were positive for *B. cereus*.[19] Foods with low colony counts (e.g., $\leq 10^3$/g) probably pose no problem if they are handled properly and refrigerated promptly after cooking.

Listeria monocytogenes is commonly found in the environment and in raw food. Studies in the United States and Europe have shown it to be present in 15 to 20 percent of ground beef, in 15 to 80 percent of poultry, and in a small percentage of ready-to-eat processed foods including such dairy products as soft cheeses. Moreover, unlike other foodborne pathogens, this organism continues to grow at refrigerated temperatures (4°C, 39°F), and so the degree of contamination increases with storage. The infectious dose is unknown, but it is presumably less for immunosuppressed persons, pregnant women, and the elderly. Although most cases are sporadic (1 to 10 per million people per year), common-source outbreaks have occurred and have implicated several commercial foods: cole slaw, pasteurized milk, and soft cheeses. Case-control studies have implicated uncooked hot dogs and undercooked chicken. A World Health Organization (WHO) informal working group on food-borne listeriosis has concluded that total elimination of *Listeria* from all food is impractical, if not impossible, but that control procedures should be carried out at all possible points during processing. The group recommended withdrawal of foods from market in two situations: (*a*) when the contents of sealed packages are contaminated despite treatment to eliminate *Listeria* and (*b*) when foods have been implicated in human cases of listeriosis.

Escherichia coli can be grouped into five categories by differences in virulence properties, epidemiology, and clinical syndromes. These are enteropathogenic *E. coli* (EPEC), enteroinvasive *E. coli* (EIEC), enterotoxigenic *E. coli* (ETEC), enteroadherent *E. coli* (EAEC), and enterohemorrhagic *E. coli* (EHEC). The latter is most commonly represented by *E. coli* O157:H7. Symptomatic and asymptomatic human carriers are believed to be a principal reservoir and source of EPEC, EIEC, ETEC, and EAEC strains involved in human illness, whereas the primary reservoir for *E. coli* O157:H7 appears to be dairy cattle. Ground beef (hamburger) and, less commonly rare roast beef, and raw cow's milk, and, recently, even raw apple juice have been implicated in outbreaks due to *E. coli* O157:H7. *E. coli* O157:H7 cannot be identified by routine stool cultures but requires plating on sorbitol-MacConkey agar (SMAC) where this strain cannot ferment sorbitol within 24 hours as most *E. coli* can. Infection with *E. coli* O157:H7 is followed by hemolytic uremic syndrome (HUS) 5 to 10 percent of the time, particularly in children with bloody diarrhea. On the other hand, about 90 percent of cases of HUS probably result from *E. coli* O157:H7 infection. Antibiotic treatment of that infection may be a predisposing factor for developing HUS.[20] Studies of retail meat and poultry in the United States and Canada have revealed *E. coli* O157:H7 in 4 to 30 percent of ground beef and in about 2 percent of pork, poultry, and lamb samples. Accordingly, concern about *E. coli* O157:H7 disease should provide one additional reason to avoid consumption of raw milk and undercooked meats, especially hamburgers. Recent outbreaks from raw, unpasteurized apple juice and from dry, fermented salami indicate the unusual tolerance of *E. coli* O157:H7 to acidic pH values ≤4.6. A huge outbreak in widespread areas of Japan in 1996 that involved more than 10,000, particularly schoolchildren, defied efforts to identify a cause although one or more items in school lunches were suspected and probably responsible. The interstate outbreak from salami in 1994 indicated the infectious dose of *E. coli* O157:H7 can be less than 50 organisms. At such low doses, secondary person-to-person transmission can easily occur, as they have in day care centers and custodial institutions.

Yersinia enterocolitica infection has been recognized for years in other areas of the world, especially Scandinavia and Japan. While outbreaks have suggested the possibility of foodborne transmission, specific food items have not been incriminated until recently. These include not only unprocessed "natural" products such as tofu, raw milk, and raw pork but also pasteurized milk and pasteurized products probably contaminated by the addition of ingredients after pasteurization (chocolate milk). Generally, *Y. enterocolitica* is destroyed by standard pasteurization; but, if it is present in great numbers, some *Yersinia* may survive pasteurization and multiply during refrigeration.[21] In one large multistate outbreak due to pasteurized milk, symptoms in children included abdominal pain (suggestive of acute appendicitis, which prompted appendectomies), fever, and diarrhea; many adults, however, presented with pharyngitis and had throat cultures positive for *Y. enterocolitica*.[22] Since this pathogen grows best at 75 to 77°F (24 to 25°C), it may be missed when stools, foods, and pharyngeal swabs are cultured at the usual 99°F (37°C).

Campylobacter jejuni, formerly known to veterinarians as *Vibrio fetus*, has become recognized as an important cause of enteritis in humans and also of Guillain-Barré syndrome. In developed countries it has been isolated from the stools of 3 to 14 percent of patients evaluated for diarrhea, but it is rarely isolated from healthy individuals.[23] Transmission occurs through contaminated food and water, as well as from person to person. The apparent incubation period is 2 to 10 days. The organism has been found in pets, domestic livestock, and fowl (live and dressed). Investigations in the United States have implicated raw milk, raw clams, raw hamburger, raw and undercooked chicken, untreated water, and even municipal water supplies. The epidemiology of this pathogen is similar to that of *Salmonella* (for which chicken is also a common vehicle), and where reporting is compulsory, the incidence of *C. jejuni* infection commonly surpasses that of salmonellosis. Selective media, vacuum jar, and an incubator set at 109°F (43°C) have made this zoonotic infection an important addition to the growing list of enteric pathogens.

Mushroom poisoning can be produced by 50 species among the 2000 that are known. Even trained mycologists confuse toxic varieties with edible ones because of the extensive variations and intergradations between species; contrary to popular belief, there are no simple field tests to aid in differentiation. Mushroom poisons are conveniently divided into two categories based on their latency period: the delayed onset group and the rapid onset group. The most deadly types tend to have delayed onsets of at least 6 hours. These include *Amanita phalloides*, *Amanita verna*, and certain *Galerina* species, which cause 90 percent of all deaths from mushrooms and produce heat-stable cyclic polypeptides toxic to kidneys and liver. Typically a biphasic illness is seen. There may be sudden onset of severe nausea, vomiting, bloody diarrhea, abdominal pain, and cardiovascular collapse 6 to 20 hours after ingestion. After a short phase of improvement, painful, tender hepatomegaly with jaundice and oliguria may develop. Confusion, coma, and convulsions are common. Death ensues in 30 to 50 percent of cases. There is no specific antidote for *Amanita* intoxication; treatment is mostly supportive but should include purgation and high enemas to remove unabsorbed toxin. Experimental or invasive treatment including hemodialysis or hemoperfusion, repeated doses of activated charcoal given orally, cytochrome *c*, penicillin, corticosteroids, or thioctic acid (which is available from the FDA) have not been subjected to controlled studies to confirm effectiveness.[24] An algorithm for treating mushroom poisoning has been proposed.[25]

The rapid onset group (2 hours or less) includes mushrooms that contain hallucinogens that produce psychotropic, LSD-like effects that begin minutes after eating as well as mushrooms with muscarinic effects of salivation, perspiration, lacrimation, increased bronchial secretions, abdominal pain, miosis, nausea, vomiting, diarrhea, and bradycardia beginning about 1 hour after ingestion. Atropine is a specific antidote for this intoxication. Other mushroom poisons primarily cause gastric irritation, produce disulfiram-like effects, or produce states resembling alcoholic intoxication.

Chemical food poisoning may result from eating foods that have been contaminated accidentally or deliberately with toxic chemicals. The contaminant may be inorganic or organic, naturally occurring or human made. The soluble salts or oxides of such heavy metals as antimony, cadmium, copper, tin, and zinc can cause abrupt and severe gastrointestinal symptoms, typically in a setting where foods or beverages of high acid content have reacted chemically with the metal containers in which they were prepared or stored. The latency period is characteristically short (about 15 minutes). The explosive vomiting that occurs generally eliminates enough of the chemical from the gastrointestinal tract so that systemic toxicity is rarely a problem. Treatment is symptomatic and supportive, antiemetics should be avoided to prevent gastrointestinal retention of toxic ions and potential systemic absorption. A greater threat to life is posed by foods poisoned with *insecticides* and *rodenticides*. These chemicals are all too often kept in kitchens where they are mistaken for flour, salt, sugar, baking powder, and other food ingredients. Such chemicals include arsenic, barium carbonate, sodium fluoride, and silver polishes containing cyanide and mercury. Preventive measures are obvious; such chemicals should be labeled poisonous and kept out of food handling areas and away from children.

Contamination with heavy metal salts occurs occasionally in commercial food items with catastrophic consequences. In 1955 more than 12,000 Japanese children were poisoned by arsenic-tainted Morinaga dry milk, and more than 130 died. A study of survivors 15 years later showed them to be shorter and to have lower IQs, more central nervous system disorders (epilepsy, brain damage, reduced hearing), and other mental and physical defects than control subjects had. Another catastrophic incident due to a commercial product occurred in Morocco in 1960 when 10,000 people became ill (6000 suffered paralysis) after they had consumed cooking oil adulterated with turbo-jet lubricating oil containing 3 percent triorthocresyl phosphate.

Chinese Restaurant Syndrome sometimes follows ingestion by those susceptible to monosodium glutamate (MSG), a flavor enhancer especially popular in Chinese restaurants. Illness typically begins 20 to 30 minutes after exposure and can include a flushed or burning sensation of the neck and face, perspiration, a heavy feeling in the precordial area, palpitations, headache, and lacrimation. Since absorption of MSG is rapid when the stomach is empty, the first course of a meal—typically soup—is a common vehicle. Susceptible individuals, who can be sensitive to just 2 g of MSG, should avoid eating foods containing MSG, especially on an empty stomach.

In 1981 an epidemic of a new illness tentatively designated "toxic oil syndrome" (TOS) occurred in Spain and resulted in 20,000 cases and 300 deaths. It was traced to the ingestion of unlabeled, illegally marketed rapeseed oil that had been denatured with aniline and further treated to remove the aniline before it was fraudulently sold to the public as pure olive oil. As yet unidentified toxic agents were probably produced during the illegal refining process but the resulting disease, which affected multiple organ systems in progression, suggested either a continued body burden of toxin(s) or, more probably, the triggering of a chronic autoimmune process. Unique was the common progression of disease through an initial phase of febrile pneumonia-like symptoms sometimes with rash, followed late in the first month by gastrointestinal problems and striking eosinophilia, and about 100 days after onset in severely affected cases by profound neuromuscular manifestations (myalgia, atrophy of major muscle groups, and contractures). In late 1989 a new disease, designated *eosinophilia-myalgia syndrome* (EMS), was identified. It shares many clinical features of the intermediate and chronic phases of TOS. In EMS a striking association has been found with oral preparations of L-tryptophan-containing products.

The hazard of *methylmercury poisoning* was dramatized in Japan. Those who consumed fish taken from Minamata Bay, which had received direct factory discharges of methylmercury, subsequently developed Minamata disease which was frequently fatal. Methylmercury poisoning may take weeks, months, and possibly even years before symptoms are manifest, and unlike poisoning from inorganic mercury, it primarily affects the central nervous system, especially the cerebellum and cerebrum, where damage is usually irreversible. Symptoms can include paresthesia, ataxia, emotional lability, blindness, deafness, and in those most severely affected, stupor, coma, and death. It is not generally appreciated that discharges of even relatively inoffensive metallic mercury can be converted via biological methylation to methylmercury by bottom-dwelling bacteria. These bacteria are then consumed by plankton, which are consumed by small fish, and these by larger fish, and so on up the food chain until humans fall victim. Human exposure can sometimes be more direct. Alkyl mercury compounds have been used for years as a fungicidal seed dressing. Although such seeds are meant for planting purposes only, they have occasionally been consumed by people who were unaware of the danger or were driven by starvation. In 1971, 80,000 tons of methylmercury-treated wheat and barley were imported by Iraq for planting. Some of the grain was used, however, in the preparation of homemade bread and resulted in 6000 hospital admissions and 400 deaths. Similar outbreaks were reported from Pakistan and Guatemala.

Food-borne viral infections are uncommonly reported. Poliomyelitis appears to have been the first human viral disease for which a food vehicle was reported (in 1914, in association with raw milk), but there have been no polio foodborne outbreaks reported since 1949.[26] Though hepatitis A is an uncommon cause of foodborne disease, a 1988 outbreak associated with raw shellfish from the Shanghai area of China that affected nearly 300,000 gives hepatitis A the distinction of causing the "largest" foodborne outbreak recorded.[27] Other foodborne illnesses of proven viral etiology include tickborne encephalitis virus, ECHO 4, and, most importantly of late, Norwalk agent and other small round structured viruses (SRSVs) in the calicivirus family.[26] The Norwalk group probably caused many past outbreaks previously designated as "gastroenteritis of undetermined etiology" or "acute infectious nonbacterial gastroenteritis (AING)" but was not identified until modern diagnostic methods, particularly immune electron microscopy, became available. But inasmuch as the necessary viral diagnostic capability to detect SRSVs exists at only a few centers and since stools collected only during the first 2 days of illness contain a sufficient number of viral particles to be detected, these important causes of foodborne outbreaks will continue to escape detection, and cases will continue to be passed off as "stomach flu" or "intestinal flu." The incubation period for Norwalk-like viruses is 24 to 48 hours; onset is abrupt; symptoms can include nausea, vomiting, abdominal cramps, diarrhea, headache, and sometimes low-grade fever; the duration is generally 1 to 2 days. The secondary attack rate among contacts of cases is notably higher than in other foodborne infections. While viruses belonging to about seven groups (rotaviruses, parvoviruses, adenoviruses, caliciviruses, enteroviruses, astroviruses, and coronaviruses) commonly cause human gastroenteritis, are shed in stools, and have the potential to contaminate food, it has primarily been the SRSVs of the calicivirus group that have been repeatedly identified in common-source outbreaks of gastroenteritis.[26]

The two basic mechanisms for the contamination of food by viruses that infect the intestinal tract are (*a*) "indirect" contamination by growing of filter-feeding shellfish in fecally contaminated waters or by irrigating or washing produce by polluted water and (*b*) "direct" contamination of food, primarily by feces but sometimes by vomitus, by a food handler with poor personal hygiene. Once contamination has occurred, the question is whether the virus will retain infectivity. Unlike bacterial pathogens, viruses do not multiply (or produce toxins) in food.

▸ REFERENCES

1. Hedberg CW, MacDonald KL, Osterholm MT: Changing epidemiology of food-borne disease: a Minnesota perspective. Clin Infect Dis 18:671–680, 1994
2. Bryan FL: Diseases Transmitted by Foods (A Classification and Summary). 2nd ed. HHS Publication No. (CDC) 83-8237. Atlanta: US Public Health Service, Centers for Disease Control, 1982
3. Committee on Communicable Diseases Affecting Man, Food Subcommittee: Procedures to Investigate Foodborne Illness, 4th ed. Ames, IA: International Association of Milk, Food, and Environmental Sanitarians Inc, 1987
4. Dean AG, Dean JA, Coulombier, et al: Epi Info, Version 6: A Word Processing, Database, and Statistics Program for Epidemiology on Microcomputers. Georgia: Centers for Disease Control and Prevention, 1994
5. Joseph PR, Millar JD, Henderson DA: An outbreak of hepatitis traced to food contamination. N Engl J Med 273:188–194, 1965
6. Dack GM, Cary WE, Woolpert O, Wiggers HJ: An outbreak of food poisoning proved to be due to a yellow hemolytic staphylococcus. J Prevent Med 4:167–175, 1930
7. Fontaine RE, Arnon S, Martin WT, et al: Raw hamburger: an interstate common source of human salmonellosis. Am J Epidemiol 107:36–45, 1978
8. D'Aoust JY, Aris BJ, Thisdele P, et al: *Salmonella eastbourne* outbreak associated with chocolate. J Inst Can Sci Technol Aliment 8:181–184, 1975
9. Hennessy TW, Hedberg CW, Slutsker L, et al: A national outbreak of *Salmonella enteritidis* infections from ice cream. N Engl J Med 334:1281–1286, 1996
10. Fontaine RE, Cohen ML, Martin WT, Vernon TM: Epidemic salmonellosis from cheddar cheese: surveillance and prevention. Am J Epidemiol 111:247–253, 1980
11. Blaser MJ, Newman LS: A review of salmonellosis: I. Infective dose. Rev Infect Dis 4:1096–1106, November–December 1982
12. Collaborative Report: A waterborne epidemic of salmonellosis in Riverside, California, 1965—epidemiologic aspects. Am J Epidemiol 93:33–48, 1971
13. Hobbs BC, Smith ME, Oakley CL, et al: *Clostridium welchii* food poisoning. J Hyg 51:75–101, 1953
14. Bartlett JC: Infant botulism in adults. N Engl J Med 315:254–255, 1986
15. Arnon SS, Midura TF, Clay SA, et al: Infant botulism—epidemiological, clinical, and laboratory aspects. JAMA 237:1946–1951, 1977
16. Taylor SL: Histamine food poisoning: toxicology and clinical aspects. CRC Crit Rev Toxicol 17:91–128, 1986
17. Palafox NA, Jain LG, Pinano AZ, Gulick TM, Williams RK, Schatz IJ: Successful treatment of ciguatera poisoning with intravenous mannitol. JAMA 259:2740–2742, 1988
18. Lange WR, Kreider SD, Hattwick M, Hobbs J: Potential benefit of tocainide in the treatment of ciguatera: Report of three cases. Am J Med 84:1087–1088, 1988
19. Nygren B. Phospholipase C-producing bacteria and food poisoning. Acta Pathol Microbiol Scand 160(Suppl):1–89, 1962
20. Griffin PM, Tauxe RV: The epidemiology of infections caused by *Escherichia coli* O157:H7, other hemorrhagic *E. coli*, and the associated hemolytic uremic syndrome. Epidemiol Rev 13:60–98, 1991
21. Francis DW, Spaulding PL, Lovett J: Enterotoxin production and thermal resistance of *Yersinia enterocolitica* in milk. Appl Environ Microbiol 40:174–176, 1980
22. Tacket CO, Davis BR, Carter GP, et al: *Yersinia enterocolitica* pharyngitis. Ann Intern Med 99:40–42, 1983
23. Blaser MJ, Reller LB. *Campylobacter* enteritis. N Engl J Med 305:1444–1452, 1981
24. Olson KR, Pond SM, Seward J, et al: *Amanita phalloides*-type mushroom poisoning. West J Med 137:282–289, 1982
25. Hanrahan JP, Gordon MA: Mushroom poisoning—case reports and a review of therapy. JAMA 251:1057–1061, 1984
26. Cliver DO: Manual of Food Virology. Geneva: World Health Organization, 1983
27. World Health Organization: Wkly Epidemiol Rec 38:290–291, Sept 22, 1989

12

Control of Infections in Institutions

Nosocomial Infections

Bradley N. Doebbeling

Nosocomial, or hospital-acquired, infections occur at a rate of approximately 5 to 10 per 100 admissions in U.S. hospitals.[1] While precise national mortality data are unavailable, an estimated 30,000 patients die each year as a direct result of nosocomial bloodstream infection.[2] Furthermore, many nosocomial infections are associated with an extended length of stay, substantial morbidity, and prolonged therapy.[2,3] Because of these factors, it was estimated that nosocomial infections had a direct cost of up to $10 billion annually in the United States in 1985.[4] Nosocomial infections also occur in other institutions such as chronic care facilities and prisons, although relatively little is known regarding their epidemiology.

In the era of managed care, hospitals typically receive no additional reimbursement to care for patients with nosocomial infections. Data from the Study on the Efficacy of Nosocomial Infection Control (SENIC) suggested that up to one-third of nosocomial infections could have been prevented in the mid-1970s if effective infection control programs had been in place.[1] Thus there are strong financial incentives and benefits for hospitals to implement and maintain an effective infection control program. Although little data exist on the frequency of nosocomial infections in developing countries, rates may be as high as 65 percent on certain services, with nosocomial diarrhea particularly prevalent.[5] Outbreaks of disease may occur relatively easily in developing countries, particularly those related to parenteral injections and surgery if medical staff are not adequately trained and guidelines developed and monitored.[6] In Third World countries with markedly limited economic resources, the importance of preventing nosocomial infections is even more apparent.

▸ DESCRIPTIVE EPIDEMIOLOGY

An individual's risk of nosocomial infection is determined by the same three factors responsible for other types of infection: the host, the agent, and the environment. First, intrinsic host susceptibility to infection is clearly important and is influenced by characteristics such as age, nutritional status, comorbidities, and severity of underlying disease. Second, a variety of organisms are important nosocomial pathogens by virtue of characteristics such as the ability to colonize and survive within institutional and human reservoirs, as well as their intrinsic virulence. Finally, location within the hospital environment involves a variety of risks. Diagnostic procedures, various medical devices, and medical or surgical therapy may breach the normal host defenses and predispose patients to infections. Potent immunosuppressives, chemotherapeutic agents, and antibiotics may affect the host's normal colonizing flora, cause skin and mucosal membrane breakdown, and impair the function of the immune system. Exposure to infected or colonized patients, asymptomatic colonized or infected health care workers, and other reservoirs of organisms may transmit infecting microorganisms as well.

Currently, relatively little can be done to decrease individual patients' intrinsic susceptibility to infection. Prospective hospital surveillance may identify clusters of a particular type of infection or a specific infectious agent at an early stage. Importantly, investigation of the reservoirs of organisms and modes of transmission may allow effective interventions to be planned and implemented.[7] Appropriate use of diagnostic procedures, invasive devices, and medical therapy, particularly antibiotics, may also decrease the likelihood of nosocomial infection. Similarly, the hospital environment may be modified to prevent nosocomial infections. Strategies to increase proper use of isolation materials, handwashing, and other effective approaches to prevent transmission may be particularly beneficial.

Infection rates differ considerably among hospitals. Referral hospitals generally have higher rates than community hospitals, a difference that has primarily been attributed to the more complex patient mix and more aggressive modes of therapy used at referral centers.[1] Infection rates also differ among hospitals of the same type, however; these differences are probably influenced by a variety of factors, including local work practices as well as the effectiveness of the hospital infection control program.[8] Within an institution, rates also vary by the area of the hospital and the service caring for patients.

Infection Categories

Virtually any infection that occurs in the community may be acquired within the hospital. Certain sites of infection, however, are particularly common because of the unique susceptibility and exposure of the hospitalized patient (Fig. 12-1).

Within the intensive care unit, a high-risk area for nosocomial infections, the most common infections are pneumonia (47 percent), lower respiratory tract infection (18 percent), urinary tract infection (18 percent), and bloodstream infection (12 percent).[9] General risk factors for nosocomial infection within the ICU include prolonged ICU stay (more than 48 hours), mechanical ventilation, diagnosis of trauma, presence of a central vascular (central venous or pulmonary artery) or urinary catheter, and stress ulcer prophylaxis.[9]

Urinary Tract Infections

Urinary tract infections (UTIs) are the most common infections acquired in the hospital and nursing home and constitute one-third of nosocomial infections.[8,10] Most (80 percent) nosocomial UTIs are related to the use of urinary catheters, with another 5 to 10 percent due to urinary tract manipulation.[10,11] The typical UTI prolongs hospital stay by an average of 1.2 days.[12] The daily incidence of bacteriuria in the presence of a catheter ranges from 3 to 10 percent.[13,14] The vast majority of catheterized patients will be bacteriuric at the end of 30 days, the typical cutoff point between short-term and long-term

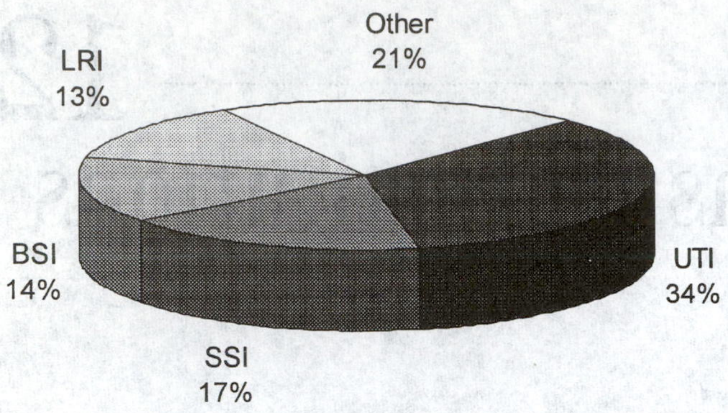

Figure 12-1. Frequency distribution of nosocomial infections at each of the major sites, 1990–1996. These proportions represent percentage distribution of nosocomial pathogens recovered by infection site, Hospital Wide Component. *UTI,* urinary tract infection; *LRI,* lower respiratory tract infection; *SSI,* surgical sites infection; *BSI,* bloodstream infection. (Adapted from Centers for Disease Control and Prevention: National Nosocomial Infections Surveillance [NNIS] system report. Am J Infect Control 24:380–388, 1996.)

catheter use.[10] The indications for short-term catheterization include measurement of urinary output, surgery, urinary retention or obstruction, and incontinence. The major indication for long-term use is urinary retention. The prevalence of bacteriuria during short-term use of a urinary catheter is approximately 15 percent, compared with a prevalence of 90 percent in long-term use.

Risk factors for bacteriuria include duration of catheterization, microbial colonization of the drainage bag, no antibiotic use, female gender, diabetes mellitus, abnormal serum creatinine, errors in catheter care, failure to use a urinometer (drip chamber), and indications other than drainage during surgery or measurement of output.[15,16] Patients catheterized late in their hospitalization have an even higher rate of bacteriuria.[16] Periurethral colonization with a potential uropathogen also increases the risk of bacteriuria more than 3-fold.[17] Duration of catheterization is the most important risk factor for the development of catheter-associated bacteriuria.[14,15] More than 70 percent of catheter-associated bacteriuria cases appear to be due to movement of bacteria up the urethra on the external catheter surface.[14]

The major complications of short-term catheterization are fevers, symptomatic UTI, and bacteremia, although acute pyelonephritis and death may occur. The complications of long-term catheterization include these, as well as catheter obstruction, urinary stones, periurinary infections, renal failure, and bladder cancer.[10] Most episodes of short-term catheter-associated bacteriuria are asymptomatic. Catheter-associated bacteriuria predisposes to surgical wound and intravascular catheter infections due to the same organism.[10,18] Fewer than 5 percent of catheter-associated bacteriuria episodes will be identified as causing bacteremia.[11,13,19] Men appear to be at increased risk for bacteremia secondary to UTI. Certain organisms, such as *Serratia marcescens,* appear to cause bacteremia more frequently than others. Nosocomial UTIs are responsible for up to 15 percent of nosocomial bloodstream infections, making them the single most important source.[11,13,19] The mortality directly attributable to bacteremia from nosocomial bacteriuria is 15 percent or less.[19]

Prevention of UTI can be viewed in three ways: prevention of catheterization, prevention of bacteriuria once catheterized, and prevention of bacteremia once bacteriuric. Avoidance of catheterization, if possible given other constraints to treat the patient optimally, is simple and extremely effective. Consideration of the risks and benefits of catheterization has led to the development of more limited indications for its use.[20] Alternative approaches to catheterization have included patient training and biofeedback, medications, surgery, and the use of special clothes and pads. Specific approaches include intermittent catheterization, use of external collection devices (condom catheters), suprapubic catheterization, and urinary diversions. The relative merits and disadvantages of each approach should be defined in controlled studies. If a urinary catheter must be used, minimizing the duration of catheterization and maintaining the closed drainage system are recommended as measures to prevent bacteriuria. There is no apparent benefit to treating the episodes of asymptomatic bacteriuria of long-term catheterized patients. After bacteriuria develops, there is limited ability to prevent its complications. The single measure most likely to prevent cross-transmission of urinary pathogens is good handwashing after caring for each patient.[21,22]

Surgical Wound Infections

Surgical wound infections (SWIs) or surgical site infections are now the second most common hospital-acquired infections, accounting for at least 17 percent of nosocomial infection.[8] Infection rates vary with the level of contamination of the operative site and disease comorbidity. Operative wounds have traditionally been classified as clean, clean-contaminated, and contaminated based on the degree of bacterial contamination expected during a particular procedure. In the era of routine preoperative administration of antibiotics, infection rates have been 0.8, 1.3, and 10.2 per hundred, respectively, for each of the classes of procedures (listed above) in one large series.[23] More recently, a risk algorithm has been advocated to predict risk more accurately based on consideration of the type of procedure and patient-related factors.

SWIs contribute substantially to patient morbidity, prolonged hospital stay, and increased direct costs.[24] A variety of host factors have been shown to predispose to surgical wound infection: age, obesity, current infection at another site, and prolonged preoperative hospitalization. Although a variety of sources of microbial contamination of the surgical wound have occasionally been implicated, important sources include direct inoculation from the patient's residual flora, contaminated host tissues, and surgical team members' hands at the time of surgery; airborne contamination at the time of surgery; and postoperative drains or catheters.

Effective preoperative measures in preventing wound infection include not shaving the operative site with a razor, disinfection of the skin at the incision site, and appropriate use of preoperative antibiotics when indicated. Perioperative antibiotics started immediately before surgery and continued for up to 24 hours are effective in clean-contaminated and contaminated surgery. Perioperative antibiotics may also be beneficial in certain clean procedures when the occurrence of a postoperative wound infection would be potentially catastrophic (for example, implantation of prosthetic devices and open heart surgery) or when it is consistently shown to be beneficial in prospective trials.[25] Important intraoperative measures include good surgical technique, minimizing the duration of surgery, and, possibly, the appropriate use of surgical drains. Aseptic technique in changing dressings on a postoperative wound left open is also important. Feedback of surgeon-specific infection rates for clean procedures to each member of the surgical staff has been shown to reduce the rates of SWIs, presumably through more meticulous attention to surgical technique.[26]

Lower Respiratory Infections

As a group, lower respiratory infections (LRIs) or pneumonias are responsible for 13 percent or more of nosocomial infections.[8,27] The incidence of nosocomial LRI is estimated to be approximately 6 per 1,000 discharges in acute care hospitals. Nosocomial LRIs are the most common fatal nosocomial infection, with a case-to-fatality rate of 30 percent,[28] ranging from 20 to 50 percent in different series.[27] It has been estimated that nosocomial LRIs are responsible for approximately 15 percent of all hospital-associated deaths.[29]

A matched cohort study of nosocomial pneumonia demonstrated that the pneumonia itself accounts for one-third of the crude mortality observed and is associated with an excess length of stay of 1 week.[28]

Stepwise logistic regression demonstrated that age, time from admission to pneumonia, prior use of mechanical ventilation, and neoplastic disease were significant risk factors for mortality.[28] Similarly, prior mechanical ventilation, posttracheotomy status, nasogastric intubation, immunosuppression or leukopenia, and prior bacteremia were significantly associated with prolonged hospital stay. In another similar recent study of pneumonias in ventilated patients, the attributable mortality was 27 percent and risk of death 2.0, with an attributable length of stay of 13 days.[30] For pneumonias due to either *Pseudomonas* or *Acinetobacter*, the attributable mortality was 43 percent and the risk of death 2.5.

Most nosocomial LRIs occur in intensive care units or postsurgical recovery units. Endotracheal intubation has consistently been shown to predispose to nosocomial pneumonia. Both tracheostomy and endotracheal intubation bypass the normal upper respiratory tract defense mechanisms, lead to drying of the lower respiratory mucosa, and provide a direct portal for the introduction of exogenous microorganisms. Ventilator and other respiratory equipment may also transmit infection. Contaminated aerosols from fluid nebulizers, as well as inadequately cleaned equipment, have been shown to cause nosocomial LRIs.[31] The condensate in disposable ventilator tubing may also become contaminated with bacteria and predispose to LRI. Other risk factors include prior administration of antibiotics, surgery, chronic lung disease, advanced age, and immunosuppression.[29]

Prevention of nosocomial LRI has been approached in several different ways. General hygienic measures encouraging handwashing, the use of barrier isolation materials when appropriate, and routine decontamination of respiratory equipment have been widely used. The normal gastric acidity is an important natural barrier that kills bacteria that otherwise would colonize the upper gastrointestinal tract. Maintenance of the stomach's acidity through avoidance of histamine type 2 blockers and antacids in intubated patients may also be protective.[32] Compliance with glove and gown isolation precautions has been shown to decrease the nosocomial spread of respiratory syncytial virus.[33] Routine changing of ventilator tubing at specific intervals is an example of a measure that was assumed to be protective but has not been shown to be beneficial on careful evaluation.[34] Topical broad-spectrum antibiotics or selective decontamination of the gastrointestinal tract has been used in several European centers and occasionally in the United States in an attempt to prevent nosocomial pneumonia. Although nosocomial pneumonia rates were decreased in several series,[35] results from meta-analyses and concern about the emergence of resistant bacteria has limited the approach in this country.[36] Immune system modulation is the final area of potential intervention. The immunocompromised host is at risk for a broad range of respiratory infections; a large number of preventive measures have been evaluated.[37] The single immunologic measure most likely to decrease nosocomial respiratory infections is annual influenza immunization of patients and hospital staff members.

Diarrhea

Nosocomial diarrhea is a common problem, although relatively little is known of its epidemiology. *Clostridium difficile* is considered the most common pathogen among adults.[38] The organism is found in 10 to 12 percent of hospitalized patients with diarrhea. Risk factors include older age, severe underlying disease, hospitalization of more than 1 week, long stay in intensive care units, and prior antibiotic treatment.

Bloodstream Infections

Perhaps the most important hospital-acquired infections are bloodstream infections (BSIs), which are responsible for up to 14 percent of nosocomial infections.[8] Rates of nosocomial bacteremia have ranged from 1.5 to 4 per 1,000 admissions in most series, although higher rates have occasionally been reported.[2] At least 120,000 episodes of nosocomial bacteremia occur annually in the United States.[39] Data on secular trends of bloodstream infection suggest that they are increasing in frequency, primarily because of increases in infections with Gram-positive bacteria and fungi.[40] The etiologic fraction, or the proportion of deaths in patients with BSI to all deaths, increased from 11 percent in 1981 to 20 percent in 1992.[40] Among neonates in high-risk nurseries, the bloodstream is the most common site of nosocomial infection.[41]

A primary bacteremia is defined as the isolation of a bacterial bloodstream pathogen in the absence of an infection at another site. Secondary bacteremia occurs when bacteria are isolated from the blood during an infection with the same organism at another site; that is, a UTI, SWI, or LRI. Independent predictors of true bacteremia from a prospective cohort of hospitalized patients include temperature of 38.3°C or higher, presence of a rapidly or ultimately fatal disease, shaking chills, intravenous drug abuse, acute abdomen, and major comorbidity.[42] The mortality rate for nosocomial bacteremia is higher than for community-acquired bacteremia and increases with the isolation of more than one organism (polymicrobial) in some series. A controlled study of nosocomial BSI demonstrated that independent predictors of death (excluding parameters of septic shock) included increased age, severity of underlying disease, and infection with either *Pseudomonas aeruginosa* or *Candida* species.[43] The attributable mortality (the crude mortality of infected individuals minus that in carefully matched controls) for nosocomial BSI has ranged from 21 to 31 percent in several studies.[2] The attributable mortality for nosocomial BSI in surgical intensive care unit (ICU) patients was 35 percent; the excess length of stay in the hospital was 24 days; the excess length of stay in the ICU was 8 days; and the excess costs attributable to the infection were $40,000 per survivor.[44]

The chief sources of primary bacteremia or fungemia include IV catheters, intrinsic IV fluid contamination, and multidose parenteral (IV) medication vials. A number of outbreaks of pseudobacteremia have been reported, related either to contamination of the blood culture medium or skin at the bedside or to contamination at different points in the microbiology laboratory. Vascular catheter-related infection appears to be the most important source of BSI and may be due to contaminated antiseptics used to disinfect the skin, contamination from the hands of health care workers, autoinfection following hematogenous seeding, or most importantly due to external colonization of the intravascular catheter. Risk factors for peripheral catheter infection include duration longer than 72 hours, cutdown placement (rather than percutaneous), lower-extremity site, emergent placement, and poor handwashing.

Effective preventive measures have not been well studied. Minimizing the duration of intravascular catheterization appears to be important. The peripheral catheter should be routinely changed to a new site every 72 hours if possible. Vascular catheters should not be routinely changed over a wire, particularly if there is any concern about the possibility of infection. Careful handwashing prior to catheter placement or manipulation, minimizing entry into the system, and careful observation for the development of any signs or symptoms of infection should be performed.

Major Pathogens

The spectrum of microbial organisms causing nosocomial infections continues to evolve. Gram-positive organisms now represent the top three nosocomial bloodstream pathogens: the coagulase-negative staphylococci, *Staphylococcus aureus*, and the enterococci together now account for approximately one-half of nosocomial BSIs (Fig. 12-2). A variety of Gram-negative bacteria remain important causes of nosocomial BSI, UTI, LRI, and SWI. The most common urinary tract pathogen is *Escherichia coli*, although other frequent pathogens include *Pseudomonas aeruginosa, Klebsiella* spp., *Proteus mirabilis, Staphylococcus epidermidis*, enterococci, and *Candida* spp. Other bacteria have been recognized as important causes of nosocomial infection as our ability to isolate organisms improves. For example, *Legionella pneumophila*, the agent of Legionnaire's disease, causes sporadic and occasionally epidemic LRIs in certain hospitals with reservoirs of the organism in the potable water system. The most frequent pathogens in European

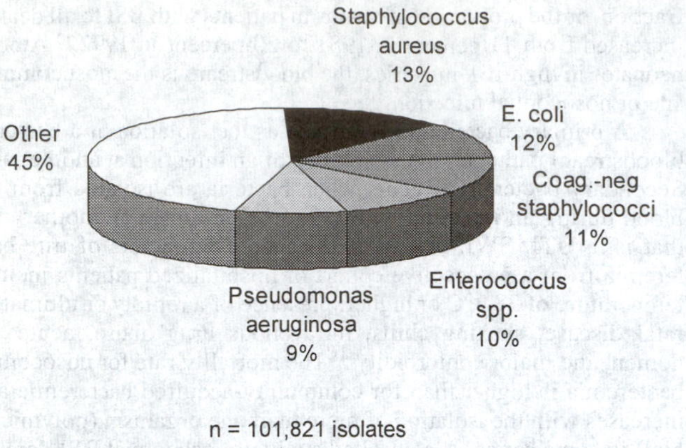

Figure 12-2. Frequency distribution of major nosocomial pathogens causing infections at each of the major sites, 1990–1996. These proportions represent percentage distribution of specific nosocomial pathogens recovered at any infection site, Hospital Wide Component. *Coag.-negative staphylococci,* coagulase-negative staphylococci. (Adapted from Centers for Disease Control and Prevention: National Nosocomial Infections Surveillance [NNIS] system report. Am J Infect Control 24:380–388, 1996.)

ICUs include Enterobacteriaceae (34 percent), *Staphylococcus aureus* (30 percent), *Pseudomonas aeruginosa* (29 percent), coagulase-negative staphylococci (19 percent), and fungi (17 percent).[9] The most common pathogens among neonates in high-risk nurseries include coagulase-negative staphylococci, *Staphylococcus aureus*, enterococci, *Enterobacter* spp., and *Escherichia coli*.[41]

The fungi have emerged as major nosocomial pathogens, primarily as a result of increasing host susceptibility and therapeutic practices in recent years. Chemotherapy and immunosuppression predispose to infections due to a variety of microorganisms. In addition, widespread antibiotic use appears to reduce the host's indigenous flora and predispose to colonization and infection. The *Candida* species as a group have shown the most rapid growth and are now among the most common causes of bloodstream infection.[45] The *Candida* species are responsible for an increasingly large proportion of nosocomial BSIs and have an attributable mortality of approximately 38 percent.

The changing bacterial and fungal spectrum in hospitals presumably reflects increased antibiotic use, particularly of the newer broad-spectrum antimicrobial agents. In addition, the development of antibiotic resistance by certain bacteria, increased use of invasive devices, and profound immunosuppressive agents used have likely also affected the secular trends of microorganisms in hospitals. Multidrug-resistant bacteria and mycobacteria of particular concern within the hospital or long-term care facility include vancomycin-resistant enterococci,[46,47] methicillin-resistant *Staphylococcus aureus* (MRSA),[48] penicillin-resistant pneumococci,[49,50] and multidrug-resistant (MDR) tuberculosis. Vancomycin-resistant enterococci (VRE) are of particular concern because the organism is often resistant to the only other antibiotics that have been shown to be effective in killing it.

Overcrowding and understaffing of particular nursing units have been associated with increased rates of MRSA colonization and infection.[48] Risk factors for BSI with vancomycin-resistant enterococci include severity of illness, underlying disease, particularly hematologic malignancy, neutropenia or AIDS, prolonged hospitalization, and receipt of vancomycin.[47,51] The efficacy of some recommended measures to prevent transmission of these organisms within institutions have recently been evaluated.[36,46,48,52] Perhaps the most common risk factor for development of infection due to a multidrug-resistant bacterium is prior use of broad-spectrum antibiotics; this fact emphasizes the importance of controlling the utilization of antibiotics.

Nosocomial outbreaks of tuberculosis, particularly MDR-TB, have occurred in a number of hospitals and occasionally in prisons. In one outbreak, up to 48 percent of health care workers at a county hospital developed tuberculin skin test conversions, and eight developed active disease.[53] Underlying conditions and performing charting in the nurses' work room were associated with progression to active disease among those infected. Delays of 2.5 months or more in treatment of workers with symptoms or prophylaxis of skin test conversions were also associated with progression. Control measures—including prompt isolation and treatment of patients with tuberculosis and the use of rapid diagnostic techniques for processing specimens, negative-pressure isolation rooms, and molded surgical masks for health care workers—appear to be effective in reducing nosocomial transmission of MDR strains to patients and health care workers.[54–56] Updated guidelines for preventing the transmission of tuberculosis within institutions have recently been published.[57]

Certain viruses—particularly cytomegalovirus, varicella-zoster virus, and herpes simplex viruses—are common causes of infection in immunocompromised hosts. Viral upper respiratory infections have been shown to increase airborne dispersal of MRSA from a colonized worker, which in turn can transmit the organism to patients.[58] The hepatitis viruses—particularly A, B, and C—may be transmitted in the hospital between patients and occasionally to and from health care workers.[59–63] Preventive measures to protect against viral hepatitis, including the use of hepatitis B vaccine, have recently been reviewed.[59]

The acquired immunodeficiency syndrome (AIDS) virus is increasingly prevalent among hospitalized patients, and occasional transmission has occurred. The routine use of standard precautions has been recommended to attempt to decrease the likelihood of exposure to potentially infectious blood and body fluids. Measures designed to decrease the likelihood of exposure from contaminated sharp objects, particularly the routine use of rubber gloves during invasive procedures and avoidance of recapping, should be equally important in the prevention of transmission.

Infection Control

During the late 1960s the need for a more vigorous approach to the prevention and control of nosocomial infections became apparent. A model infection control program, widely publicized by the Centers for Disease Control (CDC), the American Hospital Association, and the Joint Commission on the Accreditation of Healthcare Organizations, was adopted in principle by many U.S. hospitals by the mid-1970s.[64] The CDC conducted the SENIC in the late 1970s to evaluate the effectiveness of hospital infection control programs.[1] The SENIC project evaluated a random sample of 338 hospitals, stratified by size, medical school affiliation, and type of infection control program, and assessed the effect of infection control programs on rates of UTI, LRI, SWI, and BSI in adult patients. The study demonstrated that hospitals with active surveillance and control programs had significantly fewer infections than did hospitals without such programs.[1] The SENIC study also found that four elements were associated with effective programs: (*a*) an active infection surveillance system with reporting of results to staff members, (*b*) the presence of vigorous control measures designed to eliminate recognized hazards, (*c*) at least one full-time infection control practitioner for every 250 beds, and (*d*) a physician on the staff knowledgeable about nosocomial infections who took an active part in the infection control program.

Components of Effective Programs

Surveillance

An infection control program may include surveillance of patient infections, patient care practices, and microbial contamination of the environment. Evaluation of patient disease is the most important activity, because the incidence of nosocomial infection is the ultimate measure of program effectiveness.

Surveillance of patient illness should be conducted prospectively, before patients are discharged. Typical surveillance is conducted by an infection control practitioner who actively seeks nosocomial infections by making regular, frequent visits to patient care areas. The practitioner may review patient care plans, microbiology laboratory results, medical charts, radiographic reports, and lists of patients receiving antibiotics or on isolation precautions.[65] Once an infection is identified, the practitioner uses standard criteria to determine whether it is nosocomial. Other techniques such as questionnaires or surveys may be useful in the evaluation of specific problems or clusters of cases. Retrospective case finding is difficult to perform effectively and does not provide current information upon which to base decisions about intervention. Although some hospitals require that nosocomial infections be listed as discharge diagnoses, surveillance based on these diagnoses is ineffective because of underreporting and failure to use standard criteria for diagnosis.

Infection rates by site, pathogen, specialty service, and patient care area should be calculated at regular intervals, at least monthly. Other analyses, such as surgeon-specific wound infection rates and procedure-specific rates, may be useful. Surveillance data should be analyzed carefully and the resulting analyses reported to members of the hospital staff.[1] Infection rates that lie beyond the 95 percent confidence limits of the baseline rates may identify an outbreak and should be investigated.[7]

Surveillance of patient care practices may also be useful. The hospital, through its infection control committee, is responsible for developing policies and procedures. The infection control practitioner, through frequent visits to patient care areas to review patient care practices, can do much to ensure their implementation.

Microbiological surveillance of the inanimate hospital environment may also be elected. Except for monitoring the effectiveness of sterilization and disinfection procedures or investigating a specific problem, routine microbiological surveillance of the environment adds little to the infection control program and is not recommended.

Control Measures

Most preventable nosocomial infections are related to specific patient care practices. A substantial proportion of urinary tract, respiratory, and bloodstream infections are related to instrumentation, and guidelines are available to minimize their risks.[66] In addition, the hospital should develop and implement policies for isolation of patients with potentially communicable diseases, use of antimicrobial agents, and control of the hospital environment.

Infection Control Practitioner

Hospitals have traditionally employed infection control practitioners to provide day-to-day coordination of surveillance and control programs. Practitioners have occasionally been laboratory technicians, nonphysician epidemiologists, or sanitarians, although over 90 percent of U.S. hospitals have employed nurses to function as infection control practitioners.[1] Their duties have included collecting and analyzing surveillance data, assisting in the development of infection control policies and procedures, and providing education and consultation to other hospital personnel.

The SENIC project demonstrated that the presence of at least one full-time infection control nurse (ICN) for every 250 hospital beds significantly improved the effectiveness of infection control programs.[1] The effectiveness of these programs decreased as the ratio of beds to ICNs increased, suggesting that a single ICN is not sufficient in large hospitals.

Hospital Epidemiologist

A physician who takes responsibility for the infection control program also appears to be integral to the program's success.[1] This physician usually serves as the hospital epidemiologist, although nonphysician epidemiologists have occasionally filled this role. The physician supervises the infection control nurses and practitioners, provides liaison with other members of the medical staff, and provides advice about surveillance methods, analysis of surveillance data, methods of conducting epidemiologic studies, and development of control measures. The physician plays a critical role in advising the hospital's medical staff and administration about the clinical implications of patient care practices, infection problems, and prevention and control measures.

Investigation of Problems

Even in hospitals with exemplary infection control programs, epidemic and endemic infections continue to occur. The infection control committee is responsible for ensuring that problems are investigated effectively. Usually these investigations are conducted by the hospital's infection control team, the infection control practitioner(s), and the hospital epidemiologist. Occasionally, however, outside assistance is required from local or state health departments or the CDC. Most epidemiologic investigations are case-control studies, although other study designs, such as retrospective cohort or cross-sectional studies, are occasionally needed.

▶ RESOURCES FOR NOSOCOMIAL INFECTION CONTROL

The Joint Commission on Accreditation of Healthcare Organizations (JCAHO) requires that accredited hospitals have an active infection control program, an infection control committee, and specific written infection control policies and procedures for each of the hospital's departments. The JCAHO also requires written definitions of nosocomial infections, a system for reporting of infections, laboratory support for infection control, an active employee health program, and review of antibiotic use. The American Hospital Association (AMA) Committee on Infections within Hospitals has published guidelines for establishing infection control programs. The Association of Practitioners in Infection Control and the Society for Healthcare Epidemiology in America (the professional organizations for persons working in infection control) have developed training courses in infection control. Additionally, several state health departments, universities, and the CDC also provide training courses and advice or assistance in conducting epidemiologic investigations. Guidelines on preventing transmission of nosocomial infection to patients and workers have recently been published.[67,68,69]

▶ REFERENCES

1. Haley RW, Culver DH, White J, et al: The efficacy of infection surveillance and control programs in preventing nosocomial infections in U.S. hospitals. Am J Epidemiol 121:182–205, 1985
2. Wenzel RP: The mortality of hospital-acquired bloodstream infections. Int J Epidemiol 17:225–227, 1988
3. Townsend TR, Wenzel RP: Nosocomial bloodstream infections in a newborn intensive care unit: a case-controlled matched study of morbidity, mortality, and risk. Am J Epidemiol 114:73–80, 1981
4. Wenzel RP: Nosocomial infections, diagnosis-related groups, and survey on the efficacy of nosocomial infection control: economic implications for hospitals under the prospective payment system. Am J Med 78(Suppl 6B):3–7, 1985
5. Ponce de Leon S: Nosocomial infection control in Latin America: we have to start now. Infect Control 5:511–512, 1984
6. Fisher-Hoch SP, Tomori O, Nasidi A, et al: Review of cases of nosocomial Lassa fever in Nigeria: the high price of poor medical practice. Br Med J 311:857–859, 1995
7. Doebbeling BN: Epidemics: identification and management. In Wenzel RP (ed): Prevention and Control of Nosocomial Infections. 2nd ed. Baltimore: Williams & Wilkins; 1993, pp 177–205
8. National Nosocomial Infections Surveillance System. National Nosocomial Infections Surveillance (NNIS) report, data summary from October 1986–April 1996, issued May 1996. Am J Infect Control 24:380–388, 1996

9. Vincent JL, Bihari DJ, Suter PM, et al: The prevalence of nosocomial infection in intensive care units in Europe. Results of the European Prevalence of Infection in Intensive Care (EPIC) study. EPIC International Advisory Committee. JAMA 274:639–644, 1995
10. Warren JW: Nosocomial urinary tract infections. In Mandell GL, Bennett JE, Dolin R (eds): Principles and Practice of Infectious Diseases. 4th ed. New York: Churchill Livingstone, 1995, pp 2607–2616
11. Krieger JN, Kaiser DL, Wenzel RP: Urinary tract etiology of blood stream infections in hospitalized patients. J Infect Dis 148:57–62, 1983
12. Dixon RE: Effect of infections on hospital care. Ann Intern Med 89(2):749–753, 1978
13. Garibaldi RA, Mooney BR, Epstein BJ, et al: An evaluation of daily bacteriologic monitoring to identify preventable episodes of catheter-associated urinary tract infection. Infect Control 3:466–470, 1982
14. Garibaldi RA, Burke JP, Dickman ML, Smith CB: Factors predisposing to bacteriuria during indwelling urethral catheterization. N Engl J Med 291:215–219, 1974
15. Platt R, Polk BF, Murdock B, et al: Risk factors for nosocomial urinary tract infection. Am J Epidemiol 124:977–985, 1986
16. Shapiro M, Simchen E, Izraeli S, et al: A multivariate analysis of risk factors for acquiring bacteriuria in patients with indwelling urinary catheters for longer than 24 hours. Infect Control 5:525–532, 1984
17. Garibaldi RA, Burke JP, Britt MR, et al: Meatal colonization and catheter-associated bacteriuria. N Engl J Med 303:316–318, 1980
18. Krieger JN, Kaiser DL, Wenzel RP: Nosocomial urinary tract infections cause wound infections postoperatively in surgical patients. Surg Gynecol Obstet 156:313–318, 1983
19. Bryan C, Reynolds K: Hospital-acquired bacteremic urinary tract infection: epidemiology and outcome. J Urol 132:494–498, 1984
20. Stamm WE: Catheter-associated urinary tract infections: epidemiology, pathogenesis and prevention. Am J Med 91:65S–71S, 1991
21. Doebbeling BN, Stanley GL, Sheetz CT, et al: Comparative efficacy of alternative hand-washing agents in reducing nosocomial infections in intensive care units. N Engl J Med 327:88–93, 1992
22. Casewell M, Phillips I: Hands as route of transmission for *Klebsiella* species. Br Med J 2:1315–1317, 1977
23. Olson M, O'Connor M, Schwartz ML: Surgical wound infections: a five-year prospective study of 20,193 wounds at the Minneapolis VA Medical Center. Ann Surg 199:253–259, 1984
24. Green JW, Wenzel RP: Postoperative wound infection: a controlled study of the increased duration of hospital stay and direct cost of hospitalization. Ann Surg 185:264–268, 1977
25. Platt R, Zaleznik DF, Hopkins CC, et al: Perioperative antibiotic prophylaxis for herniorrhaphy and breast surgery. N Engl J Med 322:153–160, 1990
26. Cruse PJE, Foord R: A five-year prospective study of 23,649 surgical wounds. Arch Surg 107:206–210, 1973
27. Pennington JE: Nosocomial respiratory infections. In Mandell GL, Bennett JE, Dolin R (eds): Principles and Practice of Infectious Diseases. 4th ed. New York: Churchill Livingstone, 1995, pp 2599–2607
28. Leu HS, Kaiser DL, Mori M, Woolson RF, Wenzel RP: Hospital-acquired pneumonia: Attributable mortality and morbidity. Am J Epidemiol 129:1258–1267, 1989
29. Gross PA, Neu HC, Aswapokee P, et al: Deaths from nosocomial infections: experience in a university hospital and community hospital. Am J Med 68:219–223, 1980
30. Fagon JY, Chastre J, Hance AJ, Montravers P, Novara A, Gibert C: Nosocomial pneumonia in ventilated patients: a cohort study evaluating attributable mortality and hospital stay. Am J Med 94:281–288, 1993
31. Pierce AK, Sanford JP, Thomas GP, et al: Long-term evaluation of decontamination of inhalation-therapy equipment and the occurrence of necrotizing pneumonia. N Engl J Med 282:528–531, 1970
32. Driks MR, Craven DE, Celli BR, et al: Nosocomial pneumonia in intubated patients given sucralfate as compared with antacids or histamine type 2 blockers. N Engl J Med 317:1376–1382, 1987
33. Leclair JM, Freeman J, Sullivan BF, et al: Prevention of nosocomial respiratory syncytial virus infections through compliance with glove and gown isolation precautions. N Engl J Med 317:329–333, 1987
34. Kollef MH, Shapiro SD, Fraser VJ, et al: Mechanical ventilation with or without 7-day circuit changes. A randomized controlled trial. Ann Intern Med 123:168–174, 1995
35. Ledingham IM, Alcock SR, Eastaway AT, McDonald JC, McKay IC, Ramsay G: Triple regimen of selective decontamination of the digestive tract, systemic cefotaxime, and microbial surveillance for prevention of acquired infection in intensive care. Lancet 1:785–790, 1988
36. Kollef MH: The role of selective digestive tract decontamination on mortality and respiratory tract infections. A meta-analysis. Chest 105:1101–1108, 1994
37. Doebbeling BN, Wenzel RP: Prevention of respiratory disease in immunosuppressed patients. In Shelhamer J, Pizzo PA, Patillo JE, Masur H (eds): Respiratory Disease in the Immunosuppressed Host. Philadelphia: J.B. Lippincott, 1990
38. Barbut F, Corthier G, Charpak Y, et al: Prevalence and pathogenicity of *Clostridium difficile* in hospitalized patients. A French multicenter study. Arch Intern Med 156:1449–1454, 1996
39. Haley RW, Culver DH, White JW, et al: The nationwide nosocomial infection rate: a new need for vital statistics. Am J Epidemiol 121:159–167, 1985
40. Pittet D, Wenzel RP: Nosocomial bloodstream infections. Secular trends in rates, mortality, and contribution to total hospital deaths. Arch Intern Med 155:1177–1184, 1995
41. Gaynes RP, Edwards JR, Jarvis WR, Culver DH, Tolson JS, Martone WJ: Nosocomial infections among neonates in high-risk nurseries in the United States. National Nosocomial Infections Surveillance System. Pediatrics 98:357–361, 1996
42. Bates DW, Cook F, Goldman L, Lee TH: Predicting bacteremia in hospitalized patients: a prospectively validated model. Ann Intern Med 113:495–500, 1990
43. Miller PJ, Wenzel RP: Etiological organisms as independent predictors of death and morbidity associated with bloodstream infection. J Infect Dis 156:471–477, 1987
44. Pittet D, Tarara D, Wenzel RP: Nosocomial bloodstream infection in critically ill patients. Excess length of stay, extra costs, and attributable mortality. JAMA 271:1598–1601, 1994
45. Beck-Sague C, Jarvis WR: Secular trends in the epidemiology of nosocomial fungal infections in the United States, 1980–1990. National Nosocomial Infections Surveillance System. J Infect Dis 167:1247–1251, 1993
46. Morris JG Jr, Shay DK, Hebden JN, et al: Enterococci resistant to multiple antimicrobial agents, including vancomycin. Establishment of endemicity in a university medical center. Ann Intern Med 123:250–259, 1995
47. Shay DK, Maloney SA, Montecalvo M, et al: Epidemiology and mortality risk of vancomycin-resistant enterococcal bloodstream infections. J Infect Dis 172:993–1000, 1995
48. Haley RW, Cushion NB, Tenover FC, et al: Eradication of endemic methicillin-resistant *Staphylococcus aureus* infections from a neonatal intensive care unit. J Infect Dis 171:614–624, 1995
49. Orenstein JB: Invasive pneumococcal infection in a community hospital, 1993 to 1995. Characteristics of resistant strains. Arch Pediatr Adolesc Med 150:809–814, 1996
50. Reichler MR, Rakovsky J, Slacikova M, et al: Spread of multidrug-resistant *Streptococcus pneumoniae* among hospitalized children in Slovakia. J Infect Dis 173:374–379, 1996
51. Montecalvo MA, Shay DK, Patel P, et al: Bloodstream infections with vancomycin-resistant enterococci. Arch Intern Med 156: 1458–1462, 1996
52. Slaughter S, Hayden MK, Nathan C, et al: A comparison of the effect of universal use of gloves and gowns with that of glove use alone on acquisition of vancomycin-resistant enterococci in a medical intensive care unit. Ann Intern Med 125:448–456, 1996

53. Zaza S, Blumberg HM, Beck-Sague C, et al: Nosocomial transmission of *Mycobacterium tuberculosis*: role of health care workers in outbreak propagation. J Infect Dis 172:1542–1549, 1995
54. Maloney SA, Pearson ML, Gordon MT, et al: Efficacy of control measures in preventing nosocomial transmission of multidrug-resistant tuberculosis to patients and health care workers. Ann Intern Med 122:90–95, 1995
55. Wenger PN, Otten J, Breeden A, Orfas D, Beck-Sague CM, Jarvis WR: Control of nosocomial transmission of multidrug-resistant *Mycobacterium tuberculosis* among healthcare workers and HIV-infected patients. Lancet 345:235–240, 1995
56. Blumberg HM, Watkins DL, Berschling JD, et al: Preventing the nosocomial transmission of tuberculosis. Ann Intern Med 122:658–663, 1995
57. Jarvis WR, Bolyard EA, Bozzi CJ, et al: Respirators, recommendations, and regulations: the controversy surrounding protection of health care workers from tuberculosis. Ann Intern Med 122:142–146, 1995
58. Sheretz RJ, Reagan DR, Hampton KD, et al: A cloud adult: the *Staphylococcus aureus*-virus interaction revisited. Ann Intern Med 124:539–547, 1996
59. Doebbeling BN, Wenzel RP: Nosocomial viral hepatitis and infections transmitted by blood and blood products. In Mandell GL, Bennett JE, Dolin R (eds): Principles and Practice of Infectious Diseases. 4th ed. New York: Churchill Livingstone, 1995, pp 2616–2632
60. Doebbeling BN, Li N, Wenzel RP: An outbreak of hepatitis A among health care workers: risk factors for transmission. Am J Public Health 83:1679–1684, 1993
61. Allander T, Gruber A, Naghavi M, et al: Frequent patient-to-patient transmission of hepatitis C virus in a haematology ward. Lancet 345:603–607, 1995
62. Esteban JI, Gomez J, Martell M, et al: Transmission of hepatitis C virus by a cardiac surgeon. N Engl J Med 334:555–560, 1996
63. Harpaz R, Von Seidlein L, Averhoff FM, et al: Transmission of hepatitis B virus to multiple patients from a surgeon without evidence of inadequate infection control. N Engl J Med 334:549–554, 1996
64. Haley RW, Schachtman RH: The emergence of infection surveillance and control programs in US hospitals: an assessment, 1976. Am J Epidemiol 111:574–591, 1980
65. Mullan, RJ, Baker, EL, Bell, DM, et al: Guidelines for prevention of transmission of the human immunodeficiency virus and hepatitis B virus to health-care and public-safety workers. MMWR 38(S-6): 1–37, 1989
66. Wenzel RP, Osterman CA, Hunting KJ, Gwaltney JM: Hospital acquired infections: 1. Surveillance in a university hospital. Am J Epidemiol 103:251–260, 1976
67. Anonymous. OSHA enforcement policy and procedures for occupational exposure to tuberculosis. Infect Control Hosp Epidemiol 14:694–699, 1993
68. Goldmann DA, Weinstein RA, Wenzel RP, et al: Strategies to prevent and control the emergence and spread of antimicrobial-resistant microorganisms in hospitals. A challenge to hospital leadership. JAMA 275:234–240, 1996
69. Doebbeling BN. Protecting the healthcare worker from infection and injury. In: RP Wenzel (Ed): *Prevention and Control of Nosocomial Infections*. Baltimore, Maryland: Williams & Wilkins, 3rd Edition: 397–435, 1997

13

Diseases Transmitted Primarily by Arthropod Vectors

Viral Infections

Robert E. Shope • Theodore F. Tsai

The term *arbovirus* (a contraction of *arthropod-borne virus*) refers to a group of taxonomically diverse animal viruses that are unified by an epidemiological concept, that of transmission between vertebrate host organisms by the agency of blood-feeding (hematophagous) arthropod vectors, such as mosquitoes, ticks, sandflies, and midges. True arboviruses have the capacity to multiply in arthropod tissues, including the salivary glands; this provides a mechanism for transmission of the virus to susceptible hosts by bite and distinguishes *biological* and *mechanical* transmission, in which virus is simply transported between hosts by insects with externally contaminated mouth parts. A significant delay is required between ingestion of an infectious blood meal and sufficient viral replication in salivary tissues of the vector for transmission to occur; this interval is referred to as the *extrinsic incubation period*. Arboviruses are distinguished from viruses of insects and many viruses of plants, which also replicate in and are transmitted by arthropods, in their capacity to infect vertebrate animal hosts. After infection, vertebrate host species, which are essential to maintenance of the arboviral transmission cycle, circulate virus in their blood at levels (titers) sufficiently high to infect arthropod vectors. The arboviral transmission cycle is determined by important quantitative variables, which include (*a*) the susceptibility of individual vector species or populations to infection and (*b*) the susceptibility of individual vertebrate species to mount an infection-effective viremia. Variables that affect the extent to which arboviruses are amplified in vector-host cycles in natural communities are discussed further below.

Certain vertebrates respond to infection without developing overt signs of illness. If such *inapparent infections* are accompanied by an effective viremia in a high proportion of infected individuals, the species is well suited as an epidemiologically important host in the transmission cycle. In general, the primary hosts for arboviruses have silent infections, representing an evolved and balanced host-parasite relationship. This is not invariably the case, since for some infections (e.g., yellow fever and dengue fever in humans, Venezuelan equine encephalitis in equines) the primary viremic hosts are also clinically involved. Since arthropod vectors rarely confine their blood feeding to single vertebrate species, hosts other than those involved in transmission occasionally become exposed to arboviruses. In this instance, infection may be abortive, resulting in no illness or viremia but often leaving a detectable record in the form of serum antibodies. On the other hand, infection may produce clinically apparent disease, such as encephalitis or febrile illness. Because of the individual variability within host species, severe or medically recognizable disease generally occurs in only a small fraction of the total number infected. The ratio of clinically inapparent or mild to apparent or severe infections is a distinctive and measurable quality of a given arboviral infection and often may be dependent on age.

The disease patterns produced by arboviruses are fairly simple and provide a basis for a classification that is most useful to the epidemiologist. Arboviruses produce infections in clinically susceptible hosts that are characterized predominantly or in their classic form by:

1. *Acute central nervous system disease* (aseptic meningitis, encephalitis, encephalomyelitis).
2. *Undifferentiated febrile illness* with or without rash.
3. *Fever and arthritis* with or without rash.
4. *Hemorrhagic fever* (febrile systemic illness with hemorrhagic manifestations, cardiovascular instability, and varying degrees of hepatic and renal insufficiency).

Specific infections manifested by these syndromes may be transmitted to mosquitoes, ticks, or other arthropod vectors. Arthropod-borne hemorrhagic fevers will be described in another chapter that includes certain nonarthropod-borne (often rodent-associated) zoonotic diseases, most of which produce the hemorrhagic fever syndrome.

▸ ETIOLOGICAL AGENTS

At present more than 520 viruses are registered in the *International Catalogue of Arboviruses*.[1] Of these, only approximately 100 viruses are known to produce disease in humans and only about 25 are known or suspected to cause illness in domestic livestock. Those viruses that are of true medical importance, because the disease produced is either unusually severe or of high incidence, are much fewer in number. It is on these epidemiologically important diseases that we focus in this section; the reader is referred to more exhaustive reviews[2,3] for information about the full spectrum of arboviral infections.

The arboviruses and hemorrhagic fever viruses are divided into families on the basis of morphological and physiochemical properties. Within each family further groupings are made on the basis of shared serological and, in some instances, morphological characteristics. Some ungrouped viruses and serologically related groups of viruses remain taxonomically unclassified. Most medically important viruses are included in seven families of RNA viruses, the *Togaviridae, Flaviviridae, Bunyaviridae, Reoviridae, Arenaviridae, Filoviridae*, and *Rhabdoviridae* (Table 13-1). The virological properties that distinguish these families are reviewed elsewhere.[4–7] Within the

TABLE 13-1. SELECTED ARBOVIRAL INFECTIONS OF EPIDEMIOLOGICAL IMPORTANCE

Predominant Syndrome	Transmission	Etiology: Virus	Etiology: Family (Genus)	Pattern or Frequency of Recognized Human Disease	Associated Animal Disease	Known Geographical Distribution of Virus
Central nervous system infection	Mosquito-borne	Eastern equine encephalitis	*Togaviridae* (alphavirus)	Endemic-epidemic	Equids, penned exotic birds	United States, Canada, Caribbean, South America
		Western equine encephalitis	*Togaviridae* (alphavirus)	Endemic-epidemic	Equids	United States, Canada, Mexico, Guyana, Argentina, Brazil, Uruguay
		St. Louis encephalitis	*Flaviviridae* (flavivirus)	Endemic-epidemic	—	United States, Canada, Mexico, Caribbean, Guatemala, South America
		Japanese encephalitis	*Flaviviridae* (flavivirus)	Endemic-epidemic	Swine, equids	East and Southeast Asia [see text]
		Murray Valley encephalitis	*Flaviviridae* (flavivirus)	Endemic-epidemic	—	Australia
		Rocio encephalitis	*Flaviviridae* (flavivirus)	Epidemic	—	Brazil
		California serogroup viruses (e.g., La Crosse and Jamestown Canyon)	*Bunyaviridae* (bunyavirus)	Endemic	—	United States, Canada
	Tick-borne	Tick-borne encephalitis	*Flaviviridae* (flavivirus)	Endemic	—	Eastern Europe, former Soviet Union, Scandinavia
		Powassan	*Flaviviridae* (flavivirus)	Rare, sporadic	—	United States, Canada, former Soviet Union
		Louping ill	*Flaviviridae* (flavivirus)	Rare, sporadic	Sheep	British Isles
Undifferentiated febrile illness (with or without rash)	Mosquito-borne	Bwamba	*Bunyaviridae* (bunyavirus)	Endemic-epidemic	—	West, East Africa
		Carapuru, Marituba, Oriboca, and five other related viruses	*Bunyaviridae* (group C bunyavirus)	Rare, sporadic	—	Central and South America
		Dengue	*Flaviviridae* (flavivirus)	Endemic-epidemic	—	Worldwide (see text)
		Guama, Catu	*Bunyaviridae* (Guama group bunyavirus)	Rare, sporadic	—	South America
		Orungo	*Reoviridae* (orbivirus)	Endemic-epidemic	—	West, East Africa

		Rift Valley fever	*Bunyaviridae* (phlebovirus)	Epidemic	Sheep, cattle	South Africa, East Africa, Nigeria, Mauritania, Madagascar, Egypt
		Semliki forest	*Togaviridae* (alphavirus)	Epidemic	Equids	Sub-Saharan Africa
		Spondweni	*Flaviviridae* (flavivirus)	Rare, sporadic	—	Africa
		Tataguine	*Bunyaviridae*	Endemic	—	West Africa
		Usutu	*Flaviviridae* (flavivirus)	Rare, sporadic	—	Africa
		Venezuelan equine encephalitis	*Togaviridae* (alphavirus)	Endemic-epidemic	Equids	Venezuela, Colombia, Ecuador, Trinidad, Peru, Central America, Mexico, United States
		Wesselsbron	*Flaviviridae* (flavivirus)	Rare, sporadic	Sheep	South and West Africa, Asia
		West Nile	*Flaviviridae* (flavivirus)	Endemic-epidemic	Equids (rare)	Africa, Asia, Europe
		Zika	*Flaviviridae* (flavivirus)	Rare, sporadic	—	Africa, Asia
	Culicoides-borne	Oropouche	*Bunyaviridae* (bunyavirus)	Endemic-epidemic	—	Brazil, Panama, Guianas, Trinidad, Peru
	Phlebotormine-borne	Phlebotomus fever, Sicilian and Naples	*Bunyaviridae* (phlebovirus)	Endemic-epidemic	—	Mediterranean, Syria, Iran, Pakistan, India, Afghanistan,Sudan, former Soviet Union
		Toscana	*Bunyaviridae* (phlebovirus)	Endemic-epidemic	—	Italy
		Alenquer	*Bunyaviridae* (phlebovirus)	Endemic-epidemic	—	Brazil
		Punta Toro, Chagres, Candiru	*Bunyaviridae* (phlebovirus)	Endemic-epidemic	—	Central America
	Tick-borne	Colorado tick fever	*Reoviridae* (coltivirus)	Endemic	—	United States
	Vector unknown	Vesicular stomatitis	*Rhabdoviridae* (vesiculovirus)	Rare, sporadic	Cattle	North Central and South America
Fever and arthritis	Mosquito-borne	Barmah Forest	*Togaviridae* (alphavirus)	Endemic	—	Australia
		Chikungunya	*Togaviridae* (alphavirus)	Endemic-epidemic	—	Sub-Saharan Africa, Asia
		Mayaro	*Togaviridae* (alphavirus)	Endemic-epidemic	—	South America
		O'nyong-nyong	*Togaviridae* (alphavirus)	Epidemic	—	Sub-Saharan Africa

(continued)

TABLE 13-1. SELECTED ARBOVIRAL INFECTIONS OF EPIDEMIOLOGICAL IMPORTANCE (Continued)

Predominant Syndrome	*Transmission*	Etiology		*Pattern or Frequency of Recognized Human Disease*	*Associated Animal Disease*	*Known Geographical Distribution of Virus*
		Virus	*Family (Genus)*			
		Ross River	*Togaviridae* (alphavirus)	Endemic-epidemic	—	Australia, Oceania
		Sindbis	*Togaviridae* (alphavirus)	Endemic-epidemic	—	Africa, Asia, Europe
Hemorrhagic fever (HF)	Mosquito-borne	Yellow fever	*Flaviviridae* (flavivirus)	Endemic-epidemic	Certain monkey species	Tropical America, Africa
		Dengue HF	*Flaviviridae* (flavivirus)	Endemic-epidemic	—	Southeast Asia, Caribbean
	Tick-borne	Kyasanur Forest disease	*Flaviviridae* (flavivirus)	Endemic-epidemic	Monkeys	India
		Omsk HF	*Flaviviridae* (flavivirus)	Endemic-epidemic	Muskrats	Former Soviet Union
		Crimean-Congo HF	*Bunyaviridae* (nairovirus)	Endemic-epidemic	—	Former Soviet Union, Pakistan, Africa, Iraq, Saudi Arabia, Dubai

Togaviridae the genus *Alphavirus* contains agents among which are the important mosquito-borne encephalitis viruses that cause eastern, western, and Venezuelan equine encephalitides, and the arthritis viruses that cause chikungunya, o'nyong-nyong, Mayaro, and Ross River diseases. The Flaviviridae comprise registered virus infections, including mosquito-borne encephalitides (e.g., St. Louis encephalitis and Japanese encephalitis), undifferentiated febrile illnesses (e.g., dengue fever), and hemorrhagic fevers (e.g., yellow fever), as well as tick-borne diseases characterized by these syndromes. Each of the other major families of arboviruses is similarly represented by medically important viruses within the classification by disease category and arthropod vector (Table 13-1).

▸ EPIDEMIOLOGICAL PATTERNS

Arboviral epidemiological patterns may be simple, as exemplified by dengue and urban yellow fever, which are transmitted in a human-*Aedes aegypti*-human cycle (Fig. 13-1), or more complex, with enzootic cycles involving one or more vector species and wild animal hosts (Fig. 13-2). Many epidemiological, ecological, and biological factors play a role in determining the distribution and incidence of infections.

Geographical Distribution

The distribution of an arbovirus is determined by the presence of competent arthropod vectors, susceptible vertebrate hosts, efficient means of virus survival through periods (winter or dry season) adverse to continued transmission, and other more poorly understood factors. Barriers to spread of a virus may be geophysical (e.g., a water mass or a mountain range) or biological. A possible example of the latter is the absence of yellow fever in Asia despite presence of established vector species (*A. aegypti*), susceptible hosts, and ample opportunities for introduction; possible explanations include cross-protection of the human population by immunity to heterologous flaviviruses, such as dengue fever, or relative insusceptibility of Asian *A. aegypti* to yellow fever viral infection. The distribution of a virus may also be much wider than that of the associated disease. For example, St. Louis encephalitis (SLE) virus is distributed throughout the western hemisphere but causes epidemics only in North America. In this and other examples, one or more explanations may apply: among them (*a*) the vector(s) in the silent, enzootic part of the virus's distribution may be only weakly attracted to clinically apparent hosts (humans); (*b*) the virus may circulate only in remote, inaccessible areas rarely visited by humans or under minimal medical surveillance; or (*c*) viral strains in the epidemiologically silent area have reduced virulence for humans. In general, viruses that have birds as hosts are more evenly distributed than agents with such hosts as small terrestrial mammals that are restricted in their movements and migrations.

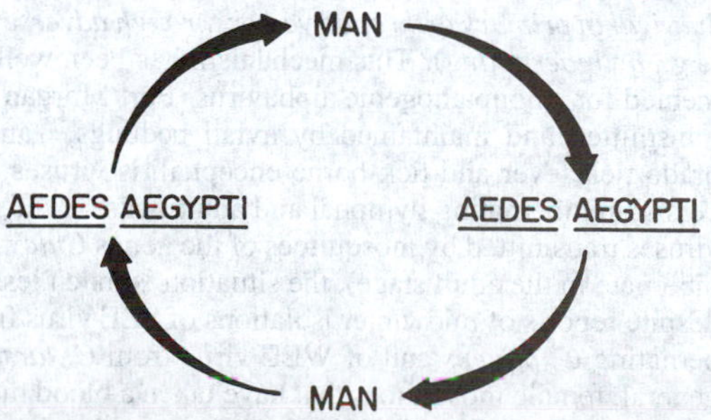

Figure 13-1. Schematic transmission cycle of urban yellow fever and dengue. Humans serve as source of virus for *Aedes aegypti* mosquito vectors.

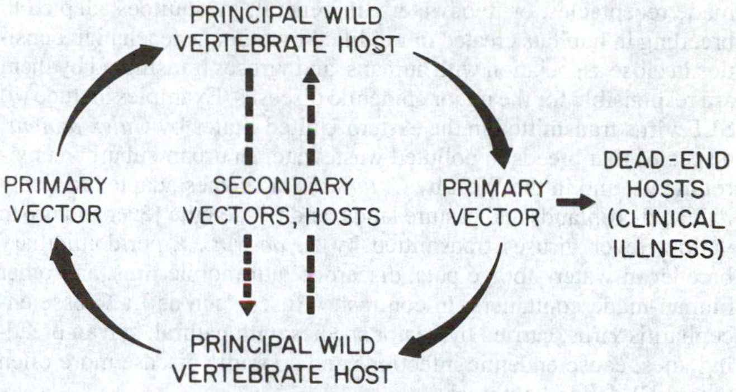

Figure 13-2. Schematic transmission cycle of arboviruses with complex natural histories involving wild vertebrate hosts (birds, rodents, etc.) and hematophagous arthropod vectors. Enzootic transmission occurs during the spring and summer in the silent cycle and may spill over tangentially to (dead-end) hosts (such as humans or horses), which are clinically susceptible but do not serve as a source of infection for vectors.

Seasonal Distribution and Chronology of Epidemics

In the temperate zone, viral transmission is limited to seasons of the year, principally late spring through early fall, when arthropod vectors are active. This period of activity often corresponds to the breeding period and peak population density of immunologically susceptible wild vertebrate hosts, thereby assuring amplification of virus in the natural cycle. In tropical regions, dry seasons with low vector density correspond to wintertime periods in the temperate zone: the transmission cycle is retarded or interrupted, risk of infection of clinically apparent hosts is reduced, and virus survival is challenged. The known and speculative mechanisms for viral recrudescence after adverse seasonal periods are discussed briefly later.

The seasonal distributions of individual arboviral diseases vary. For example, in the western United States, western equine encephalitis (WEE) and SLE viruses share the same mosquito vector (*Culex tarsalis*) and the same wild bird hosts; however, human and equine WEE infections occur in early summer, whereas human SLE cases occur in late summer and fall. The greater temperature dependence of SLE virus for replication and the longer extrinsic incubation period in the vector, plus the lower, briefer, and relatively delayed viremia in avian hosts retard amplification of the virus. In addition, exposure of *C. tarsalis* larvae to high temperatures appears to reduce their ability to transmit WEE but not SLE virus.

In general, since arboviruses with complex transmission cycles (Fig. 13-2) must amplify by progressive and cumulative infection of wild vertebrates and vectors before the virus can spill over to humans or domestic livestock, the appearance of an outbreak reflects intense viral transmission weeks or more earlier. This forms the basis for surveillance of viral activity in the natural cycle.

Viruses transmitted by arthropods often cause sharply defined outbreaks with a rapid accumulation of cases, a relatively sharp peak, and a rapid decline, as conditions unfavorable to vector breeding, host seeking, or survival develop or as susceptible hosts are depleted.

▸ VECTORS AND VERTEBRATE HOSTS: VARIABLES AFFECTING VIRAL TRANSMISSION

The principal vectors and hosts for medically important arboviruses and the reservoir hosts of rodent-borne zoonoses are listed in Table 13-1. General concepts regarding their biology and interactions are presented here, and special references are given in the sections on individual diseases. Mosquitoes require aquatic habitats for oviposition and larval development; the exact requirements vary from species to species and include such diverse conditions as tree holes, human-made receptacles, or floodwaters. In general, mosquitoes adapted to breeding in habitats created or modified by humans reach high densities in close association with humans, and viruses transmitted by them are responsible for the major epidemic diseases. Examples include (*a*) SLE virus transmitted in the eastern United States by *Culex pipiens*, a species that breeds in polluted wastewater in urban-suburban environments, and in the West by *C. tarsalis*, a species adapted to richly irrigated croplands and pasture lands; and (*b*) dengue fever and urban yellow fever viruses transmitted by *A. aegypti*, a peridomiciliary breeder in water-storage pots, discarded automobile tires, and other human-made containers. In contrast, viruses such as La Crosse encephalitis virus, carried by vector species with natural, sylvan breeding sites, cause endemic infections and sporadic disease more often than well-defined outbreaks.

Most mosquito-borne arboviruses are transmitted by one primary vector species or, at most, one primary and several secondary species. This phenomenon probably reflects constraints of evolved and specialized relationships among virus, vector, and reservoir host. However, there are a few examples of viruses that are transmitted by a wide array of taxonomically and ecologically different vectors. These viruses, such as those that cause Venezuelan equine encephalitis and Rift Valley fever, have the common feature of producing exceedingly high viremias in vertebrate hosts, surpassing the threshold for infection of many and diverse arthropod species.

Ticks have terrestrial immature stages that, like the adult, feed on blood; in some species, such as *Dermacentor andersoni*, the vector of Colorado tick fever, the larval, nymphal, and adult stages seek different hosts, adding complexity to the transmission cycle. In general, because of lower vector densities, specialized or focal ecological requirements, and other factors, tick-borne infections are more often endemic than epidemic; certain infections, notably Kyasanur Forest disease and tick-borne encephalitis, nevertheless, reach high incidence in regions conducive to intense viral transmission.

Some tick-borne infections may be amplified by a curious phenomenon that bypasses the need for virus replication in the vertebrate host. Attached, infected ticks may transfer virus (e.g., certain tick-borne orthomyxoviruses, flaviviruses, and nairoviruses) directly to cofeeding uninfected ticks via the host's tissues (lymphatics or macrophages) without the need for viremia or viral replication in vertebrate host tissues.

Several factors related specifically to the vector determine the rate of viral transmission and the risk of epidemics. One of these, *vector abundance*, is also an important variable, in turn dependent on favorable climatic and environmental conditions for breeding and survival. In the western United States, for example, Reeves[8] has shown that human and equine cases of WEE appear only when the density of *C. tarsalis* vectors reaches 10 adult females per light trap night. Yet extremely high vector densities may actually inhibit viral transmission, since host-avoidance behavior is increased or host-selection patterns are altered. *Longevity* of the vector is also a critical factor, since even a brief prolongation may increase the proportion of the vector population capable of transmitting virus and able to take a second blood meal. The *host preference* of vector species is also epidemiologically important; vectors that are strongly attracted to virus reservoir hosts but are also highly anthropophilic are ideal vectors. Host preference may change during the viral transmission season. The vectors of WEE and SLE viruses shift from predominant avian feeding in early summer to mammals (including humans) in late summer, a situation that is obviously ideally suited to amplification and spillover to humans.

Wild birds are important vertebrate hosts in transmission cycles of most of the mosquito-borne encephalitides and several mosquito-borne undifferentiated febrile diseases; some ground-dwelling kinds may also play a role in tick-borne infections. Birds are abundant, often present in large numbers in close association with humans and livestock. Moreover, because they readily move and migrate, they may transport, disseminate, and reintroduce viruses over considerable distances. Nestling birds, present in large numbers during spring and summer, are relatively defenseless against mosquito bites and often support higher viremic infections than do adults; they are considered important hosts for some viruses. In general, birds develop viremia within 18 to 48 hours after being bitten by an infected arthropod; viremia lasts 2 to 5 days and is followed by the appearance of specific antibodies. Antibodies to certain viruses (e.g. SLE) are passed transovarially to hatchlings but wane rapidly. Most avian species show no outward signs of infection. However, in the case of eastern equine encephalitis in exotic penned birds (chukar partridges, pheasants), severe outbreaks sustained by direct bird-to-bird viral transmission through pecking may provide an indication of viral activity in advance of human or equine cases. Clinical disease caused by the eastern equine encephalitis virus in the whooping crane (an endangered species) has caused concern.

Rodents are the principal hosts for (*a*) a number of viruses transmitted by ticks, including tick-borne encephalitis, Colorado tick fever, Powassan encephalitis, Crimean-Congo hemorrhagic fever, and Kyasanur Forest disease viruses; (*b*) viruses that cause some important mosquito-borne infections such as La Crosse encephalitis; and (*c*) viruses responsible for certain zoonotic hemorrhagic fevers. General characteristics of rodent hosts that affect viral transmission rates include high reproductive capacity and population turnover, limited movements and dispersal, and, often, specific requirements for habitat. These factors favor restricted or focal viral transmission, which, however, can be quite intense. In general, rodents are hosts for the larval and nymphal stages of tick vectors, whereas the adult forms generally feed on large animals, including humans.

Domestic animals are effective viremic hosts for a limited number of arboviruses. Those viruses of epidemiological importance (and their amplifying hosts) include those that cause Venezuelan equine encephalomyelitis (*Equidae*), Rift Valley fever (sheep, cattle), and Japanese encephalitis (swine). In each case the hosts show signs of illness in addition to serving as sources of infection for arthropod vectors that may transmit the virus to humans. Since viral amplification in livestock necessarily precedes spillover to humans, occurrence of an epizootic often provides warning of an impending epidemic. Unlike agents with rodent or avian hosts that have high reproductive potential, epizootics caused by these viruses often deplete the population of immunologically susceptible large animal hosts; several more years may be required to attain susceptible host population densities allowing a high rate of viral transmission.

Overwintering is an important concept in the epidemiology of vector-borne diseases, since the annual recrudescence of viral activity after periods (winter, dry season) adverse to continual transmission depends on a mechanism for local survival of virus or its reintroduction from outside the endemic area. To some extent, the risk of a summertime epidemic may be determined by the relative success of virus survival in the local winter reservoir. Since overwinter survival may, in turn, depend on the level of viral activity during the preceding summer and fall, arboviral outbreaks sometimes occur for 2 or more successive years.

For a comprehensive review of the many possible explanations of overwintering, see Reeves.[9] Briefly, the mechanisms for survival of virus may be summarized as follows:

1. *Survival in primary arthropod vector through adverse period (e.g., by hibernating):* This mechanism has been well documented for a nonpathogenic alphavirus (Fort Morgan virus), transmitted and maintained by avian bedbugs,[10] and Colorado tick fever and tick-borne encephalitis viruses, which persist in hibernating nymphal and adult ticks. In the case of viruses transmitted by mosquitoes of the genus *Culex* (which hibernate in the adult stage), the situation is much less clear, despite reports of midwinter isolations of SLE virus from hibernating *C. pipiens* and of WEE virus from *C. tarsalis*. In general, female mosquitoes that have taken a blood meal (required for acquisition of the infection) appear to be physiologically poorly prepared for hibernation and rarely survive the winter. Other observations[11] suggest that this may not always be the case.

2. *Survival in persistently infected vertebrate reservoirs:* Chronic arboviral infections, sometimes spanning periods of hibernation, have been experimentally demonstrated in a variety of vertebrates, including bats (SLE and Japanese encephalitis virus) and small mammals (tick-borne encephalitis and Tahyna virus, a member of the California encephalitis group). Long-term virus persistence and congenital infections have been demonstrated in laboratory models (mice, monkeys) of several flaviviruses. In general, evidence that chronically infected, intermittently viremic animals maintain arbovirus *in nature* is lacking. A possible exception requiring confirmation may be blue tongue, an important pathogen of sheep and cattle, in which congenitally acquired, immunotolerant latent infection may occur. In this instance, viremic relapses may be stimulated nonspecifically by bites of uninfected *Culicoides* gnats. Persistent viral carriage assures the maintenance of some zoonotic infections of rodents in nature. Lymphocytic choriomeningitis virus in *Mus musculus*, Machupo virus in *Calomys callosus*, Lassa fever virus in *Mastomys natalensis*, and several hantaviruses in their rodent hosts are principal examples; moreover, chronic shedding of large amounts of virus in the urine by specific rodents harboring these and related agents is the most important element in transmission of disease to humans (see the following).
3. *Inherited infection in the arthropod vector:* Transovarial infection, first demonstrated for a human pathogen and a dipteran insect vector in the case of vesicular stomatitis virus, has been shown to account for local survival of California encephalitis group viruses in their *Aedes* mosquito vectors. The vector-host relationships of these viruses explain the evolution of this mechanism. The vertebrate hosts for these viruses are small forest rodents unsuited for dispersal or reintroduction of virus from afar, and the vector *Aedes* overwinters only in the egg stage. Transovarial transmission is biologically efficient: a high proportion (70 to 90 percent) of progeny from infected female *Aedes* mosquitoes acquires the virus, and as many as 1 percent of mosquitoes reared from overwintering ova collected in nature have been found infected.[12] Evidence has now been obtained to show that a number of flaviviruses, notably those that cause SLE, Japanese encephalitis (JE), and dengue and yellow fevers, may also be vertically transmitted by *Aedes*. Unlike the California encephalitis group of bunyaviruses, rates of inherited infection are often lower (1:100 or less). Obviously, high rates of summertime amplification are required for the virus to successfully survive the winter as a low-incidence infection of mosquito ova. Certain tick-borne infections (e.g., tick-borne encephalitis and Crimean-Congo hemorrhagic fever) are also transovarially transmitted in their tick vectors.
4. *Reintroduction of virus by migratory vertebrates:* Transport of viruses over long distances by migratory birds has occasionally been documented, but it is generally not considered to be an important mechanism for the annual recrudescence of viral activity.

▶ SURVEILLANCE AND DIAGNOSIS OF VECTOR-BORNE VIRAL DISEASES

Recognition of disease in the community and definition of the incidence, geographical extent, and chronology are essential if control measures are to be applied and their effectiveness assessed. In the case of dengue fever, surveillance of human cases is the only applicable method, but viral infections involving wild vertebrate hosts lend themselves to other approaches. A classic example is jungle yellow fever, which may be monitored in neotropical forests by observing wild monkey populations or sentinel monkeys for deaths or antibody conversions. Similarly, epizootics of encephalitis in equids or epornitics in penned exotic birds may provide warning of human outbreaks of certain equine encephalitides.

Viruses with clinically silent enzootic transmission cycles, such as the SLE virus, require sophisticated studies to determine the level of viral activity in nature. Serologic surveillance of wild bird populations, periodic antibody tests on individually marked, sentinel chickens, determination of vector population density and age structure, and viral assays of vector mosquitoes have all been used to detect viral activity. Experience over the years has allowed quantitative estimates of the risk of an impending human outbreak. For example, cases of human western equine encephalitis in California appear only when adult female *C. tarsalis* mosquitoes are present at densities reflected by 10 captures per light trap night and when minimum infection rates in *C. tarsalis* exceed 3/1000. SLE outbreaks in the eastern United States seem to occur only when the prevalence of antibodies in wild bird populations exceeds about 3 percent.[13]

Surveillance of human or equine cases or of wild hosts and vectors requires the availability of a competent virus laboratory. In the case of human surveillance, the need for laboratory diagnosis is underscored by the nonspecific nature of the clinical illness caused by most arboviruses. Dengue fever may be confused with influenza or rubella; yellow fever, with hepatitis, malaria, leptospirosis, or the other viral hemorrhagic fevers; and acute arboviral infections of the central nervous system, with those caused by enteroviruses or childhood infections.

Diagnosis of arboviral infection (in humans or lower vertebrates) is achieved either directly by viral isolation or antigen detection or indirectly by demonstration of specific serum antibodies. Certain viruses, such as dengue, yellow fever, West Nile, group C bunyaviruses, Rift Valley fever, Lassa, Marburg, Ebola, Crimean-Congo hemorrhagic fever, Argentine hemorrhagic fever, and Venezuelan equine encephalitis (VEE) viruses, may be isolated from serum during the first few days of illness; certain other viruses are not readily recovered, probably because viremia is of low magnitude and occurs only during the incubation period. Similarly, in many of the encephalitides, infectious virus is no longer present in detectable form in brain tissue at autopsy. Viral isolation techniques vary from laboratory to laboratory. Intracerebral inoculation of infant mice has long been a standard method, but cell cultures have come into increased use. Certain viruses are difficult to isolate (because of insensitivity of the usual assay systems), notably dengue virus, the phlebotomus fever viruses, and o'nyong-nyong virus. The advantage of inoculation of live mosquitoes or mosquito cell cultures for isolation of dengue virus from human serum has been recognized.[14] The presence of virus in the assay systems mentioned is detected by the appearance of illness (mice), cytopathic effect or plaques (cell cultures), or specific immunofluorescence (cell cultures or mosquitoes). Viral isolates are further identified and characterized by physicochemical and serologic techniques. Use of specific monoclonal antibody reagents has facilitated this task. Advances in antigen detection in serum by enzyme-linked immunosorbent assay (ELISA) have allowed rapid diagnosis of yellow fever, dengue fever, Crimean-Congo hemorrhagic fever, Ebola, and other virus infections without the need for viral isolation. Recent development of the polymerase chain reaction (PCR) for detecting viral genome in clinical samples provides extremely sensitive and specific diagnostic approaches; application has been reported for detection of dengue, Ebola, VEE, and Dugbe viruses (a nairovirus).

Serological diagnosis is achieved by use of one or more tests, including hemagglutination inhibition (HI), complement fixation (CF), neutralization (N), fluorescent antibody (FA), ELISA, or radioimmunoassay (RIA). The bases for these techniques and their relative sensitivity and specificity are reviewed elsewhere.[15] Generally accepted criteria for the serological diagnosis of a case are as follows:

- *Confirmed case:* A 4-fold or greater rise or fall in antibody titer in appropriately timed paired sera or demonstration of virus-specific IgM antibodies in a single serum.
- *Presumptive cases:* (*a*) High antibody titers in a single convalescent serum, (*b*) stable high serum titers in paired sera

obtained during convalescence, or (*c*) a case that is fatal 5 days or more after onset, with presence of detectable antibody in serum and postmortem findings consistent with the presumed infection.

- *Inconclusive case:* Antibody present but at titers that do not satisfy above criteria.
- *Negative case:* No antibodies, or stable minimally detectable titers in appropriately timed paired sera.

▶ PREVENTION AND CONTROL

Effective vaccines have been produced for a number of arbovirus infections, including yellow fever, tick-borne encephalitis, Japanese encephalitis, Rift Valley fever, Crimean-Congo hemorrhagic fever, Hantaan, dengue, VEE, and western and eastern equine encephalitis, but only two (yellow fever and Japanese encephalitis vaccines) are licensed for human use in the United States. Immunization of equids with VEE, WEE, and eastern equine encephalitis (EEE) vaccines is widely practiced. Both live attenuated and inactivated VEE vaccines are available, and their use is especially relevant, since nonimmune equids are the principal source of VEE virus for arthropod vectors in epizootics or epidemics. Tick-borne encephalitis, Japanese encephalitis, and yellow fever vaccines have been responsible for reduced morbidity in regions where these vaccines have been effectively employed. Since most arboviruses and hemorrhagic fever viruses have transmission cycles involving wild animals, vaccination of clinical hosts must as a rule be continued indefinitely. Immunization of wildlife may, however, be a practical approach in the future.

Prophylaxis of disease in persons accidentally exposed in the laboratory to the viruses included in this section represents a minor, if important, public health problem. Transfusion of plasma or globulin containing specific neutralizing antibodies may successfully abort infection in such cases, especially if given early (within 24 hours) after exposure. Immune globulin is also used for postexposure (tick bite) prophylaxis of tick-borne encephalitis and for treatment of Crimean-Congo hemorrhagic fever.

Prevention of epidemics may be achieved by reduction of arthropod vector populations. In the case of mosquito-borne infections, this is most efficiently done by reducing the sources of vector breeding and by killing the larvae. In the event of an impending outbreak (viral activity at a high level detected in nature) or an established outbreak, measures must be taken to eliminate the adult female mosquitoes themselves, since source reduction and killing of larvae will not rapidly reduce the infected, transmitting segment of the vector population. The use of insecticide space sprays, applied by ground or aerial equipment by the ultralow-volume (ULV) technique, may be effective. It is essential that the effectiveness of such vector control efforts be monitored. Factors to be measured include (*a*) susceptibility of the target vector population to the insecticide used; (*b*) reduction in target vector populations, and (*c*) effects on the viral transmission cycle (vector infection rates, sentinel flock seroconversions, incidence of human disease, etc.).

▶ VIRUSES CAUSING ACUTE CENTRAL NERVOUS SYSTEM INFECTIONS

Mosquito-Borne Viral Infections

The Equine Encephalitides

Viruses causing outbreaks of encephalitis in equids and humans are most important in the Western Hemisphere.

Eastern equine encephalitis occurs in South Dakota, states east of the Mississippi River, in the Caribbean, and throughout much of South America. Epizootics or epidemics have been reported from Massachusetts (1938, 1956, 1973, 1983), Louisiana (1947), Maryland (1968), New Jersey (1959), Michigan (1982), Georgia (1982), Gulf and Atlantic states (1989), the Dominican Republic (1949, 1978), Jamaica (1962), Panama (1969), Venezuela (1977), Mexico (1996), and Argentina (1981). Epornitics in penned exotic birds are a feature of the disease in the United States. Outbreaks in the United States occur in the late summer and early fall. Sporadic equine and human EEE cases occur annually in enzootic areas of the eastern United States (Fig. 13-3). Between 1955 and 1996, 225 human cases have been reported, with fewer than 10 cases in most years (Table 13-2). The clinical disease is severe, with case-fatality rates in humans approaching 50 percent. Young children and elderly persons are primarily affected. The inapparent-apparent infection ratio in these age groups is estimated at 1:10 and 1:20, respectively, but is about 1:50 in young adults. Illness is characterized by fever, signs of severe neurological dysfunction, high cell counts in cerebrospinal fluid with early granulocytic predominance, and a high incidence of residual neurological damage. In the United States the virus is sustained in freshwater swamps in a cycle involving wild birds and *Culiseta melanura* mosquito vectors. This species only rarely bites horses and humans, and the epidemic vectors vary from place to place; *Aedes sollicitans* and *Coquillettidia perturbans* have been implicated in the spread of EEE virus to clinical hosts. Horses apparently contribute to the cycle only rarely as viremic hosts, although this point deserves further study.

The epidemiology in tropical areas is less well known; *C. taeniopus* and wild birds constitute the enzootic cycle in Trinidad, Brazil, and Panama. Two serotypes of the virus are distinguishable, designated North American and South American subtypes. The North American subtype, present in the United States, is also responsible for outbreaks in the Greater Antilles. It is unknown whether this virus is enzootic in these islands or is periodically introduced by southward-migrating birds. A rough coincidence has been noted between outbreaks in the Caribbean and in the Atlantic seaboard states. The overwintering mechanism of EEE virus in the United States is unknown; midwinter isolations of the virus have been made from *C. melanura* larvae and small rodents, but the significance of these observations is disputed. Surveillance techniques applied to detect early EEE viral activity include the use of sentinel fowl, virologic testing of mosquitoes, and indices of vector populations. In coastal New Jersey, the vector potential of *A. sollicitans* is routinely measured by the number of parous mosquitoes landing on human bait in 1 minute.

In pheasants and other penned birds and in equids the disease is controlled with the use of a formalin-inactivated vaccine, usually in the form of a bivalent (EEE/WEE) or trivalent (EEE/WEE/VEE) vaccine. Vector control affords the only available means of controlling established epidemics.

Western equine encephalitis virus is distributed throughout western North America (Fig. 13-4), and the virus has been isolated in Brazil, Argentina, and Guyana. Outbreaks have occurred in the western United States, Canada, Uruguay, and Argentina. Large epizootics/epidemics occurred in the United States in 1941, with more than 3,000 human cases in the north central region and neighboring Canadian provinces, and in 1952 in the Central Valley of California (375 cases). Between 1955 and 1996, 1,034 human cases were officially reported to the Centers for Disease Control in Fort Collins, Colorado (Table 13-2). During this interval, small outbreaks, involving 25 to 68 human cases, occurred in Kansas, Utah, and California (in 1958), western Texas (1963–1964), Colorado (1965 and 1987), and the Red River basin of Minnesota and North Dakota (1975). On a statewide basis, the attack rates in these outbreaks were in the range of 4 to 6 per 100,000 population; however, rates in severely affected counties (such as Kern County, California, in 1952 or Hale County, Texas, in 1963–1964) have been higher, 50 to 125 per 100,000. The disease occurs in midsummer, and the appearance of equine outbreaks often precedes the occurrence of human cases by several weeks. Human factors, including the practice of watching television indoors and the use of screens and air conditioners, have been partly responsible for a declining incidence of infection in the United States.

The virus causes clinical encephalitis in equids and in humans; it is an especially severe infection in infants, producing neurological sequelae. The case-fatality rate approximates 3 percent. Infection most

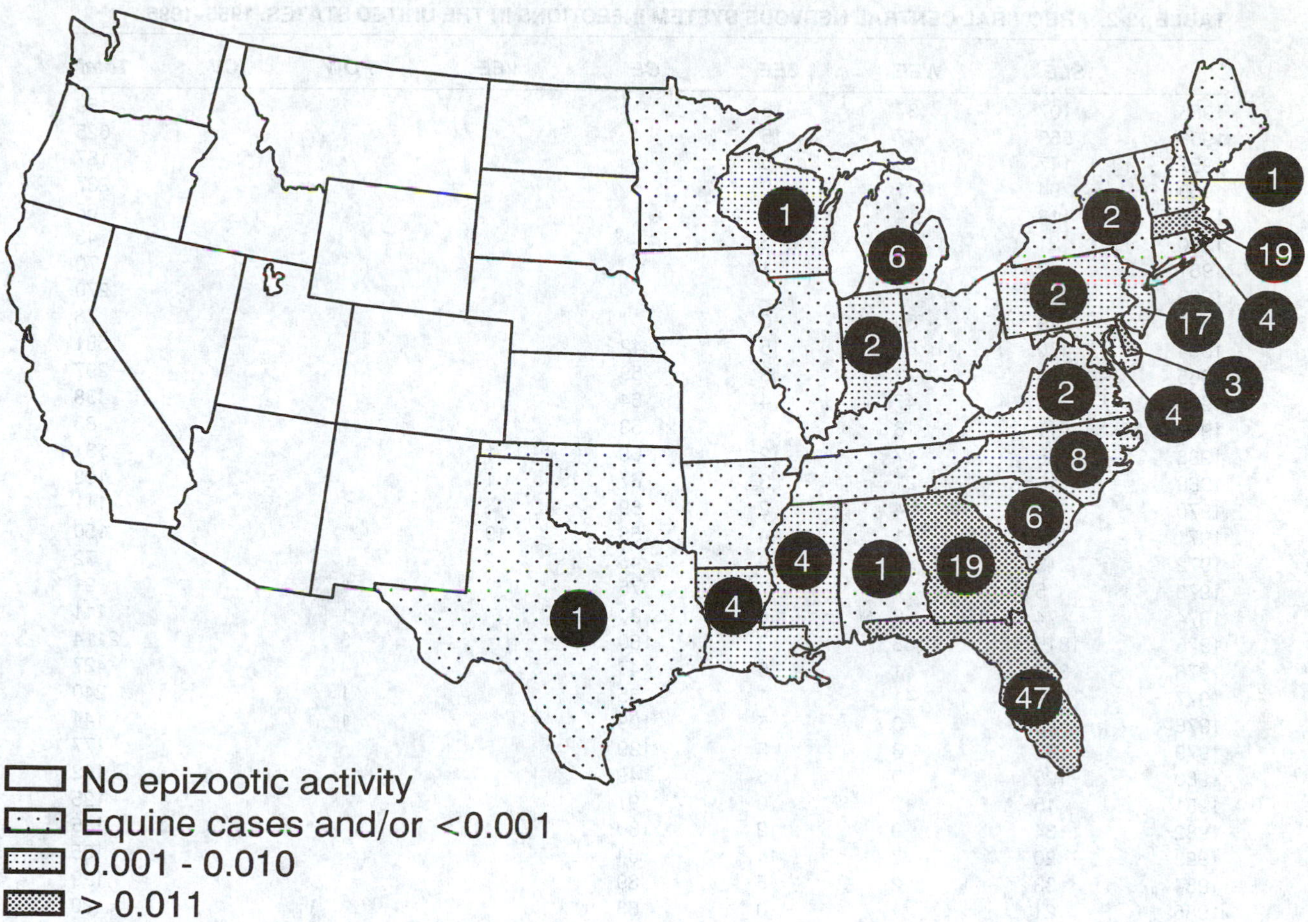

Figure 13-3. Distribution of human cases of eastern equine encephalitis, United States, 1964–1996. Some states report animal cases only, as indicated in legend.

often is abortive or mild and undifferentiated; the ratio of inapparent infection to overt central nervous system infection is approximately 50:1 in children under the age of 5 years and more than 1000:1 in adults. Surveys in endemic areas have demonstrated an antibody prevalence of about 5 percent in young children, rising to 20 percent in adults.

In the western United States, the virus circulates between wild birds (especially house finches and house sparrows) and *C. tarsalis* mosquitoes. Since the primary enzootic vector also bites horses and humans, it is responsible for disease transmission. *Cx. tarsalis* may feed exclusively on birds in the spring and then shift to mammalian hosts in midsummer, coinciding with the appearance of equine and human infections. Horses and humans do not have viremias sufficient to infect mosquito vectors. *C. tarsalis* breeds predominantly in irrigated pastureland, and the incidence of human infections is correlated with rural residence and agricultural pursuits. Flooding of riverine basins, heavy snow melt, and river flows yield high vector populations and may accelerate rates of viral transmission. The WEE viral transmission cycle is shared with that of SLE virus in the western United States; mixed WEE-SLE outbreaks have occurred, although in general one of the two viruses predominates in a given year. In the eastern United States, a virus (Highlands J) closely related to WEE virus is enzootically maintained in freshwater swamps in a cycle identical to that of EEE. Only rare equine and human cases have been reported, and the viral strains in this region may have reduced virulence characteristics.

Various means of surveillance of WEE viral activity have been applied. As previously noted, measurements of adult female *C. tarsalis* populations provide an index of risk, but more direct information on rates of viral transmission may be obtained by use of sentinel fowl or determination of viremia rates in wild nestling house sparrows. The latter indices appear to correlate well with risk of human disease[16] and appear to have predictive value.

Mosquito control provides the only available means of reducing human infections. Survey data on mosquito-breeding sites are used to direct efforts in source-reduction campaigns and the use of biological and chemical agents to eliminate larvae. Aerial ULV applications of chemical adulticides may be used to control outbreaks. An effective formalinized vaccine is licensed for equine use.

Venezuelan equine encephalitis occurs in the form of focal or extensive epizootics and epidemics in northern South America, from Venezuela south to Peru. In 1969 the disease appeared on the Pacific coast of Guatemala, whence it spread southward to Costa Rica in 1970 and northward through Mexico, reaching Texas in 1971. The equine morbidity associated with VEE outbreaks has been high. For example, the 1967 epizootic in Colombia is estimated to have killed more than 100,000 horses and burros; that in 1969 in Ecuador, approximately 30,000; and that in Central America and Mexico between 1969 and 1971, more than 20,000. A total of 1426 horses died in Texas in 1971. The disease in humans is usually mild and grippe-like, characterized by sudden onset, fever, chills, headache, myalgia, and gastrointestinal disturbances; pharyngitis is a feature of the infection in about 25 percent of the cases. The illness lasts 4 to 6 days, but a small proportion of cases have a biphasic illness pattern, with return of signs and symptoms several days to a week after initial onset. Overt signs of encephalitis occur in only about 4 percent of the cases; the incidence of encephalitis is highest in children under 15 years of age. The overall case-fatality rate is under 1 percent, but it is higher (15 percent) among patients with encephalitis. Subclinical

TABLE 13-2. ARBOVIRAL CENTRAL NERVOUS SYSTEM INFECTIONS IN THE UNITED STATES, 1955–1996

	SLE	WEE	EEE	CE	VEE	POW	CV	Total
1955	107	37	15					159
1956	563	47	15					625
1957	147	35	5					187
1958	94	141	2					237
1959	118	14	36					168
1960	21	21	3					45
1961	42	27	1					70
1962	253	17	0					270
1963	19	56	0	1				76
1964	470	64	5	42				581
1965	58	172	8	59				297
1966	323	47	4	64				438
1967	11	18	1	53				83
1968	35	17	12	66	1			131
1969	16	21	3	67	1			108
1970	15	4	2	89		1		111
1971	57	11	4	58	19			150
1972	13	8	0	46	2			72
1973	5	4	7	75				91
1974	74	2	4	30		1		111
1975	1815	133	3	160		3		2114
1976	379	1	0	47				427
1977	132	41	1	65		1		240
1978	26	3	5	109		1		144
1979	32	3	3	139				177
1980	125	0	8	49				182
1981	15	19	0	91				125
1982	34	9	12	130				185
1983	20	7	14	64				105
1984	33	2	5	89				129
1985	21	1	0	68				90
1986	43	7	1	64				115
1987	17	41	3	87				148
1988	4	1	3	41				49
1989	34	0	9	65				108
1990	247	0	6	61				314
1991	78	1	11	41				131
1992	14	0	2	29				45
1993	18	0	5	55				78
1994	20	2	1	76				99
1995	26	0	4	71			1	102
1996	1	0	2	42				45
Total	5575	1034	225	2293	23	7	1	9162

Abbreviations: SLE, St. Louis encephalitis; WEE, Western equine encephalitis; EEE, eastern equine encephalitis; CE, California (La Crosse) encephalitis; VEE, Venezuelan equine encephalitis; POW, Powassan encephalitis; CV, Cache Valley encephalitis.

infections are rare. More than 20,000 human cases have been associated with individual major equine epizootics in South America. The disease appears during the rainy season; equine outbreaks precede epidemics by several weeks or longer.

The epidemiology of VEE is complicated by the existence of multiple antigenic subtypes and varieties, only two of which (designated IAB and IC) have been associated with epizootics.[17] Other, enzootic subtypes are widespread in tropical regions of the hemisphere (including Florida), where they produce a high prevalence of infection but only sporadic disease. The epizootic subtypes (IAB, IC) differ not only in their virulence but also in their vector-host relationships. Equidae are the principal viremic hosts in the cycle, and transmission is effected by a wide variety of mosquito vectors, including species of the genera *Aedes, Psorophora,* and *Mansonia*.[18] In contrast the enzootic subtypes are transmitted in a silent cycle involving primarily small rodents and *Culex (Melanoconion)* mosquitoes. Several enzootic subtypes and varieties (ID, IE, IF, II, III) cause sporadic disease in humans but not in Equidae.

In tropical America, outbreaks occurred at intervals of approximately 10 years, generally in dry tropical forests and coastal plains. The periodicity of outbreaks was in part due to the high infection rates and consequent exhaustion of immunologically susceptible equines. The epizootic IC virus was thought to have disappeared after 1973, but it suddenly reappeared in 1995 in Colombia and Venezuela, affecting an estimated 100,000 people.[19] The maintenance cycle of VEE virus in Colombia and Venezuela during interepizootic periods is believed to involve natural selection of virulent mutants of enzootic ID serotype. IC epizootic virus is phylogenetically very close to ID enzootic virus and is thought to arise (evolve) as a mutant population of the ID variety.[20]

Surveillance techniques are rudimentary in much of tropical America, and specific laboratory diagnosis of equine and human central nervous system infections is rarely achieved. Potentially useful techniques for surveillance of the infection include use of sentinel equines or sentinel laboratory rodents, such as hamsters or guinea pigs.

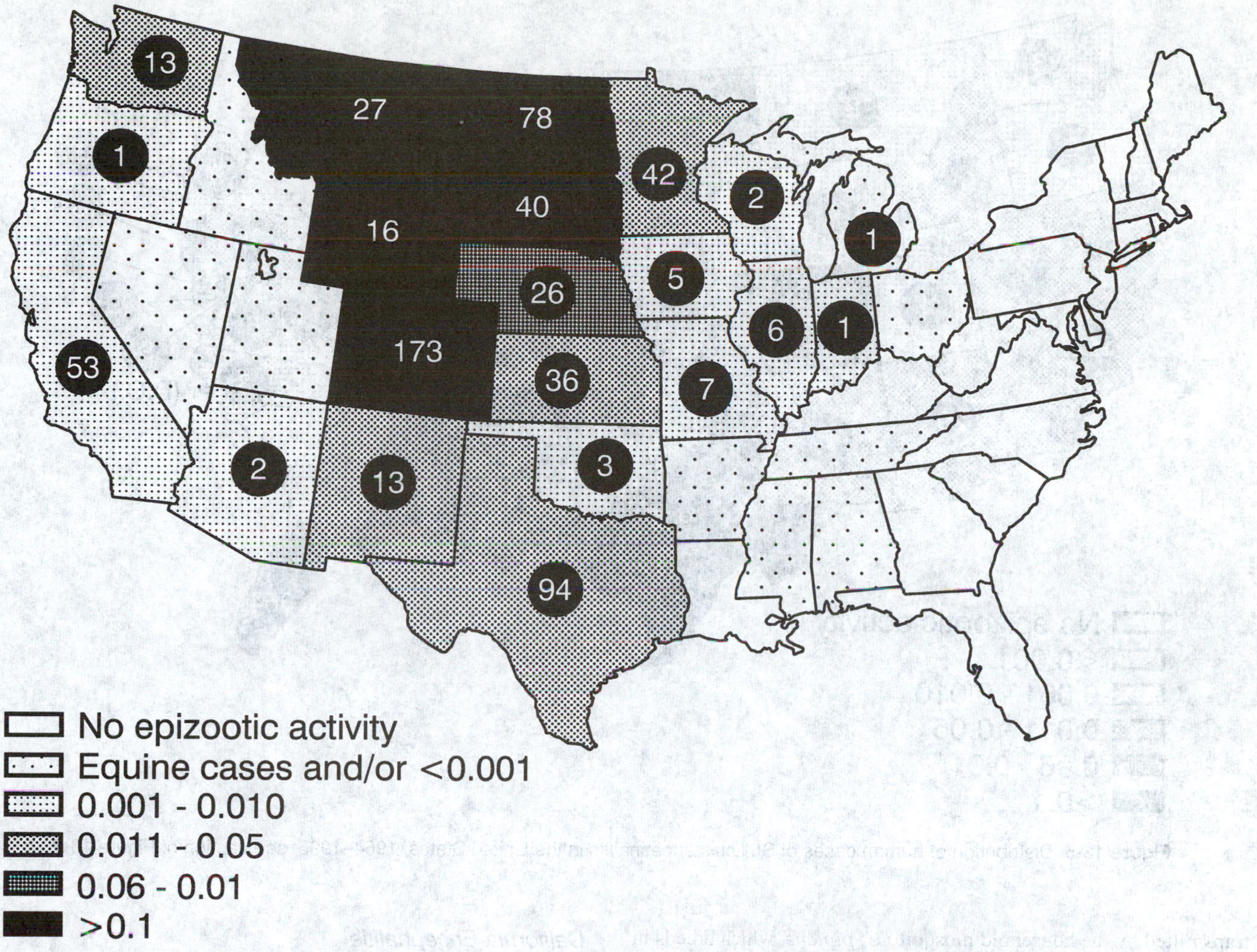

Figure 13-4. Distribution of human cases of western equine encephalitis in the United States, 1964–1996; see caption of Figure 13-3.

Prevention of epizootics and epidemics may be achieved by use of VEE vaccine in Equidae. Both an effective live attenuated vaccine (TC-83) and killed vaccines prepared from TC-83 are available. Development of immunity is rapid following use of the live vaccine, and it therefore has a role in limiting the spread of an ongoing epizootic. Aerial ULV applications of organophosphate insecticide have been used in several outbreaks.

St. Louis Encephalitis

St. Louis encephalitis (SLE) is the most important epidemic arboviral disease in the United States, and it is widely distributed (Fig. 13-5).[21] In certain epidemic years the incidence of SLE exceeds that of all other viral encephalitides of known etiology combined (Table 13-2). Between 1955 and 1996, 5,575 cases of SLE were reported to the Centers for Disease Control, representing 61 percent of the total cases of arboviral encephalitis in the United States. The virus also is widespread in tropical America, but only rare, sporadic clinical infections are recognized.

Two epidemiological patterns of SLE are evident in the United States. In the West, SLE is an endemic infection, generally of low incidence; small epidemics of fewer than 100 cases occur periodically, usually associated with outbreaks of WEE. In 1989 the largest outbreak in California in 30 years struck the Central Valley. Morbidity is generally higher in rural or suburban populations living in irrigated farmland districts than it is in urban populations. Most cases occur in children because older age groups have acquired high levels of immunity. The disease appears to be less severe than in the eastern United States; the case-fatality rate in persons over 60 years of age is about 9 percent, compared to 20 percent in age-matched patients in the East, suggesting a difference between geographic virus strains in human virulence. The virus circulates in a bird-*C. tarsalis*-bird cycle. Human infections occur in late summer. *C. tarsalis* (and possibly *C. pipiens*) are responsible for virus transmission to humans. Horses develop antibodies but not overt signs of illness.

In the eastern United States, the disease occurs in epidemic form at approximately 10- to 20-year intervals. Outbreaks have varied in size from a few clustered cases to more than 2,000 cases in a multifocal pattern throughout the Ohio-Mississippi basin and eastern Texas. Attack rates in individual outbreaks have been as high as 800/100,000. The economic cost of these epidemics has been high; the 1966 Dallas, Texas, outbreak was estimated to have resulted in direct costs (resulting from hospital charges, investigation, and vector control) and indirect costs (loss of work output) of $10 million (1990 dollars). The disease strikes urban-suburban areas and affects primarily older persons. Antibody surveys conducted after outbreaks have shown that this age distribution is due to an increased susceptibility of the elderly to overt encephalitis, rather than to an increased rate of exposure to the virus. The inapparent-apparent infection rate is approximately 800:1 in children under 10 years, 400:1 in young adults, and 80:1 in persons over 60 years. In some large urban outbreaks, attack rates have been highest in predominantly black, low socioeconomic areas of the city. This and other epidemiological features of the disease are based on the virus-vector relationships. SLE in the eastern United States (except Florida) is

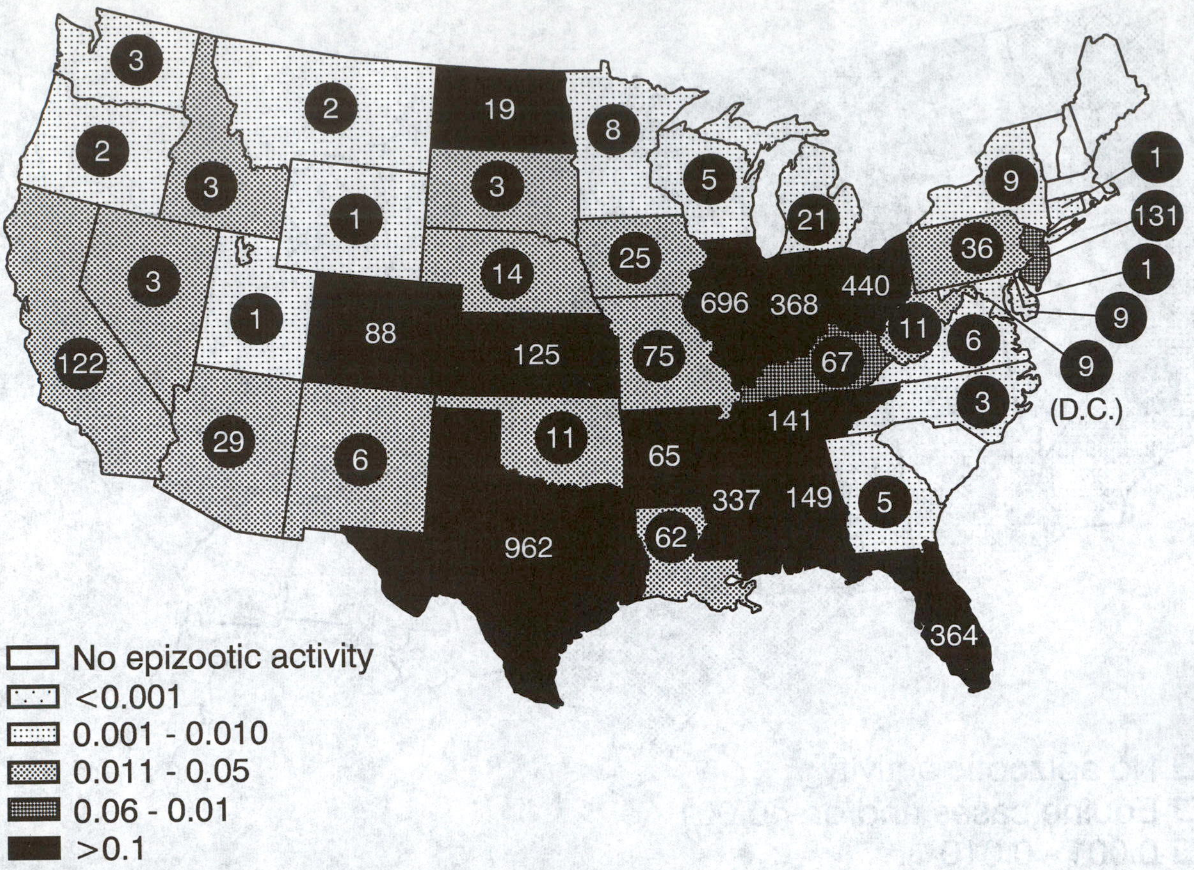

Figure 13-5. Distribution of human cases of St. Louis encephalitis in the United States, 1964–1996; see caption of Figure 13-3.

transmitted by the household mosquito *C. pipiens*, which breeds in polluted wastewater. High vector populations are associated with poor sanitary conditions and weather patterns (low rainfall, high temperatures) that favor pooling and stagnation of water. Wild birds, especially species abundant in the urban-suburban environment (house sparrows, pigeons, blue jays, robins) constitute the principal reservoirs. In Florida the tropical mosquito *Culex nigripalpus* is the vector.

Although many epidemics have been limited to a single year, reappearance of outbreaks in successive years has been a feature of SLE in some localities. The overwintering mechanism of the virus has not been elucidated, but it is likely that these successive occurrences may be caused by "priming" dependent on a high rate of local maintenance of SLE virus during the intervening winter season. SLE virus may be carried through the winter by infected hibernating adult *C. pipiens*.[11] Vertical transmission of virus from infected female *Culex* mosquitoes to their progeny promotes this phenomenon, since mosquitoes may not feed on blood before hibernation.

The interval between the date of onset of the first human case and the recognition of an epidemic has been between 2 and 8 weeks. Much attention has been paid in recent years to development of systems for early detection of SLE viral activity in nature. Monitoring antibody prevalence in juvenile wild birds and serological conversion rates in sentinel fowl have provided reasonably accurate predictions.[13]

No vaccine is available for human use. The principles of prevention and control by reduction of vector populations have been discussed above. Reduction of *C. pipiens* breeding is extremely difficult, and the growth of cities with attendant problems of human-made mosquito breeding sites has increased the potential for outbreaks of this disease in the United States.

California Encephalitis

A group of 11 antigenically distinct but related viruses constitutes the California virus group, of which three (La Crosse, Jamestown Canyon, and California encephalitis viruses) are established human pathogens in the United States. A subtype of La Crosse virus designated snowshoe hare virus is also associated with human disease in North America. La Crosse virus is responsible for nearly all recognized infections. It is an important cause of endemic disease of children under the age of 15 years in the north central states, primarily Ohio, Minnesota, Wisconsin, eastern Iowa, Illinois, and upstate New York. The disease is also reported from the southern and southeastern states and California (Fig. 13-6). From 50 to 75 cases are reported to the Centers for Disease Control in years of average viral activity, and they occur in July, August, and early September. Between 1963 and 1996, 2,293 cases have been reported (Table 13-2). The pattern is one of scattered clinical infections; viral activity tends to be quite focal, associated with residence in small valleys with deciduous hardwood forests. The true clinical disease spectrum is poorly understood, but mild, undifferentiated febrile illness, perhaps with respiratory symptoms, occurs in addition to full-blown encephalitis. Encephalitis may be clinically severe during the acute phase, but full recovery is the rule, and the occurrence of neuropsychiatric sequelae has not been well established, although seizure disorders seem linked to the disease. The case-fatality rate is less than 1 percent. La Crosse virus has been isolated from brain tissue in three fatal cases.

Antibody surveys have shown increasing rates of immunity with age, from 5 percent in children under 5 years to more than 30 percent in adults over 40 years of age. Serosurveys are complicated by the presence of other California group viruses in La Crosse endemic areas, which cause cross-reacting antibody responses. La Crosse virus is transmitted by woodland *Aedes* mosquitoes, primarily *A. triseriatus* and *A. canadensis*. The vectors breed in tree holes and ar-

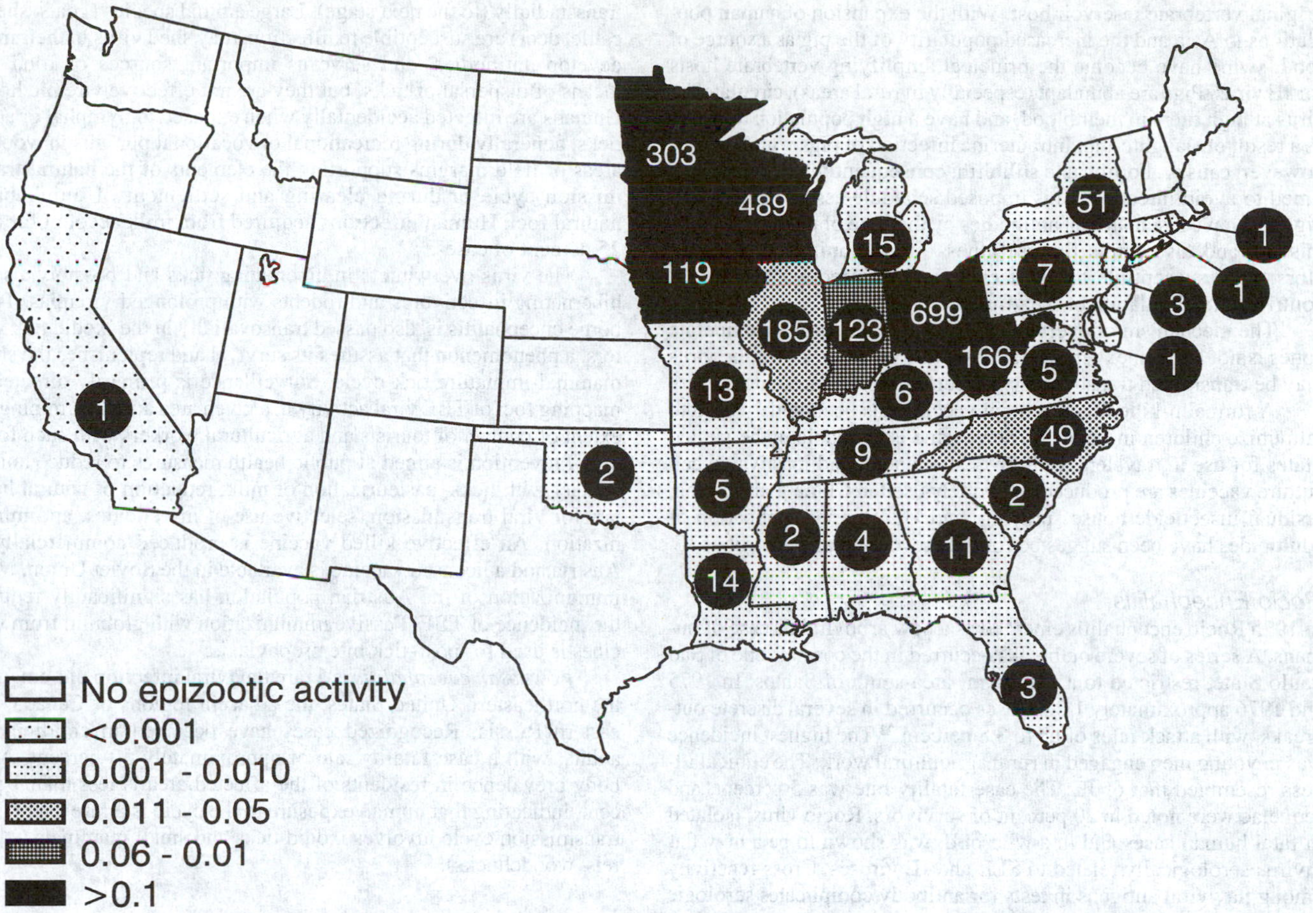

Figure 13-6. Distribution of California encephalitis in the United States, 1964–1996. Most cases are caused by the La Crosse serotype, but others also contribute to human morbidity; see caption of Figure 13-3.

tificial containers (e.g., tires) and transmit the virus to small rodents, such as chipmunks and tree squirrels. La Crosse virus is transovarially transmitted in *A. triseriatus*, and the virus can apparently survive in an area for up to 4 years without amplification by horizontal spread in vertebrate hosts.[12] The phenomenon of vertical transmission through many generations of the mosquito vector assures its survival and undoubtedly contributes to the focality of the human disease.

Surveillance has consisted mainly of human case finding, but detection of the virus with the use of sentinel rabbits is feasible. Control measures are not well established. Elimination of tree holes (by filling with cement) and other sites of vector mosquito breeding (artificial containers) may be locally effective. Because of the sporadic pattern of cases and the vertical transmission of the virus, spraying to reduce adult vector populations would be expected to have limited and transient usefulness.

The Jamestown Canyon serotype has been mainly associated with disease (febrile illness, aseptic meningitis, encephalitis) in adults in the north central United States and Ontario.

California-group viruses have a wide distribution. Snowshoe hare virus has been implicated in human disease in China and Russia, and Tahyna virus with febrile and neurological syndromes in Europe and the former Soviet Union states.

Japanese Encephalitis

Japanese encephalitis (JE) virus, a close relative of SLE virus, causes endemic/epidemic disease in parts of Asia, including Japan, Korea, Taiwan, Okinawa, Guam, China, Vietnam, the Philippines, Malaysia, Thailand, northern Australia, Nepal, and eastern India. Morbidity in some outbreaks has been high, with thousands of cases; case-fatality rates of 50 percent or more have been reported but reflect poor recognition of nonfatal cases. Children and older persons are at higher risk of clinical infections that are young adults; in endemic areas, however, where immunity prevalence increases with age, the disease occurs primarily in preschool children. Since 1960 the disease has declined as a problem in Japan (as a result of immunization and changing agricultural practices that have limited vector breeding), but elsewhere (China, northern Thailand, and India) recurrent outbreaks account for more than 50,000 cases annually. In tropical parts of Asia (e.g., southern Thailand, Indonesia), human infections are prevalent, but only sporadic disease occurs. RNA sequence data indicate that these tropical strains differ genetically, and it is likely that their human virulence may be less than that of epidemic virus strains.

JE is generally a more severe disease than SLE. Neurological sequelae have been noted in as many as 75 percent of survivors and are more severe in affected children under 10 years of age; sequelae include motor disturbances, parkinsonism, and psychiatric abnormalities.

The disease has a summer-fall distribution in temperate areas, but in tropical areas no clear seasonal pattern is evident. The principal epidemic vector differs by geographical region, but overall *Culex tritaeniorhynchus*, a rice paddy breeder, is the most important. This species principally bites large animals but also feeds on birds. Other *Culex* species implicated include *C. pseudovishnui* (in India), *C. gelidus* (Malaysia, Thailand), *C. annulus* (Guam, Taiwan), and *C. fuscocephalus* (Taiwan, Thailand). The virus has also been isolated from certain *Aedes* species, which may play a role in enzootic viral transmission and overwintering. Wild birds, especially black-crowned night herons, are effective viremic hosts in the cycle, may be important in dispersal of the virus, and probably represent its original vertebrate reservoir host. With the expansion of human populations in Asia and the increased popularity of the pig as a source of food, swine have become the principal amplifying vertebrate hosts for JE virus. Pigs are abundant (especially in rural areas), circulate the virus at high titers in their blood, and have a high population turnover as a result of slaughtering. Intrauterine infection of pigs with JE virus, however, causes abortion and stillbirth; consequently, pig breeding is timed to avoid infection. This imposed schedule assures that young pigs will have lost maternal antibodies by the time of peak viral transmission and also limits the usefulness of immunization of sows. Horses are susceptible to overt encephalitic infection but do not contribute to circulation of the virus.

The mechanism of overwinter survival of JE virus in temperate zones is not known; experimental observations suggest that the virus may be transmitted transovarially by certain *Aedes* mosquitoes.

A formalin-killed mouse brain vaccine has been widely used to immunize children in Japan.[22] The vaccine is available in the United States for use in travelers. Both live, attenuated, and inactivated cell culture vaccines are produced and widely used in China. Larviciding, residual insecticide house spraying, and ULV aerial application of adulticides have been suggested for the prevention and control of JE.

Rocio Encephalitis

In 1975 Rocio encephalitis emerged as a new arboviral disease of humans. A series of severe outbreaks occurred in the coastal zone of Sao Paulo State, restricted to a 1,000-km^2 area south of Santos. In 1975 and 1976 approximately 1,000 cases occurred in several discrete outbreaks, with attack rates of up to 3.8 percent.[23] The highest incidence was in young men engaged in rural agricultural work. The clinical illness resembled that of JE. The case-fatality rate was 5 percent, and sequelae were noted in 20 percent of survivors. Rocio virus, isolated in fatal human cases and in a wild bird, was shown to be a new flavivirus serologically related to SLE and JE viruses. Cross-reactivity among flaviviral antigens in tests for antibody complicates serologic diagnosis, since human infections with other viruses (SLE and Ilheus) related to Rocio virus are prevalent in Brazil. Since the distribution of the virus may not be limited to southern Brazil, the diagnosis of Rocio viral infection should be considered in all cases of central nervous system infection from tropical America. The transmission cycle is not known, but birds are believed to be the principal hosts; and *A. scapularis* mosquitoes, the vector.

No vaccine is available. Since the virus-vector relationships are not understood, specific preventive and control measures cannot be formulated accurately, but emergency spraying to reduce mosquito populations would seem warranted in the event of future epidemics.

Tick-borne Viral Infections

Tick-borne encephalitis (TBE), also known as Russian spring-summer encephalitis, central European encephalitis, and diphasic meningoencephalitis, is an important endemoepidemic disease in eastern Europe and Russia; imported infections have been rarely documented in the United States. Between 500 and 1,000 cases are reported annually in Europe, with peak incidence during June and July. Infection is acquired both by tick bite and by ingestion of unpasteurized milk from infected goats or sheep.

The ecology and clinical features of the disease in Europe and far eastern Russia differ. In Europe the typical case has a biphasic course with an early, viremic influenza-like stage, followed in 7 to 8 days by the appearance of signs of meningoencephalitis. The central nervous system disease is generally mild, but occasional severe motor dysfunction and permanent disability are described. The case-fatality rate is 0 to 2 percent. In the far eastern form, severe encephalomyelitis and residual damage are much more frequent and the case-fatality rate is high (20 to 30 percent).

Ixodes ricinus in Europe and *Ixodes persulcatus* in far eastern Russia are the principal vectors. Small mammals, especially rodents and insectivores, and larval and nymphal ticks constitute the basic viral transmission cycle. As infected ticks molt, the virus is passed transstadially (to the next stage). Large animal species (goats, sheep, cattle, deer) are susceptible to infection, may shed virus in their milk, develop antibodies, and serve as important sources of food and means of dispersal of ticks, but they are not effective viremic hosts. Humans are infected accidentally when exposed to nymphal or adult ticks, generally during recreational or vocational pursuits in wooded areas or field margins supporting the elements of the natural transmission cycle or during clearing and settlement of uninhabited natural foci. Human infections acquired from milk account for 8 to 25 percent of cases.

The virus overwinters in hibernating ticks and possibly also in hibernating insectivores and rodents with prolonged viremias. Tick-borne encephalitis is also passed transovarially in the ixodid tick vectors, a phenomenon that assures its survival and replenishes the small mammal-immature tick cycle. Surveillance is primarily directed at mapping foci of TBE viral activity in a given area and determining the extent of contact of tourists and agricultural workers with such foci.

Prevention is aimed at public health measures to reduce human contact with ticks, pasteurization of milk, reduction of natural habitats for viral transmission, selective use of insecticides, and immunization. An effective killed vaccine is produced commercially in Austria and a licensed vaccine is available in the Soviet Union. Mass immunization of the Austrian population has significantly reduced the incidence of TBE. Passive immunization with globulin from vaccines is used for post–tick bite prophylaxis.

Powassan encephalitis is a rare flaviviral infection of humans in the northeastern United States, the adjacent regions of Canada, and eastern Russia. Recognized cases have occurred in children and adults, with a case-fatality rate of approximately 50 percent. Antibody prevalence in residents of the affected area is less than 1 percent, indicating that human exposure to the cycle is a rare event. The transmission cycle involves ixodid ticks and small mammals (squirrels, woodchucks).

▶ VIRUSES CAUSING UNDIFFERENTIATED FEBRILE ILLNESS

Mosquito-Borne Infections

Dengue fever (breakbone fever) outbreaks have occurred on every continent between 30 and 40° north and south of the equator, coinciding with the range of the principal vector mosquito, *A. aegypti*. The disease was a major affliction of troops in the Pacific theater of World War II. In the last two decades pandemics involving millions of cases have occurred in the Caribbean, eastern Africa, southern Asia, and the Pacific Islands. Dengue is not a single virus but, rather, consists of four distinct serotypes (dengue type 1, type 2, etc.) within the *Flavivirus* genus of the Flaviviridae. Infection with one serotype confers long-lasting specific immunity but only incomplete and short-lived cross-protection to infection with heterologous serotypes. Consequently, recurrent outbreaks may occur in a geographical region on introduction of a new serotype.

Classic dengue fever is an acute, self-limited disease characterized by abrupt onset, a biphasic febrile course, anorexia, weakness, prostration, arthralgia, rash, leukopenia, lymphadenopathy, and, in a small proportion of cases, minor hemorrhagic manifestations (petechiae, epistaxis). A prolonged convalescence with asthenia and depression is not uncommon. No fatalities have been recorded. This syndrome is in marked contrast to that of dengue hemorrhagic fever, described in the next part of this chapter.

The public health significance of dengue fever may be appreciated by a brief review of events in the Americas since 1977. Before this time, outbreaks of dengue types 2 and 3 infection had occurred repeatedly in Caribbean islands and major epidemics of type 2 infection had swept the Atlantic coast of Colombia. In March 1977 a dengue type 1 outbreak occurred in Jamaica, the agent possibly being introduced from western Africa or southeast Asia. This virus was spread to other islands by infected humans, reaching Barbados and

Trinidad by late 1977 and coastal Central America by 1978. In the fall of 1980 it arrived in the continental United States at Brownsville, Texas, but failed to cause a major epidemic there or to spread to neighboring cities.[24] A rather similar geographical movement of dengue type 4 virus, which had never been isolated in the region, subsequently occurred. Millions of cases were reported, and attack rates of 500 to 5,000 per 100,000 population were registered. The costs were very high in terms of investigative and vector-control efforts and losses of work and tourist revenues. In Cuba in 1981, dengue hemorrhagic fever occurred in epidemic form for the first time in the Americas, with 116,143 hospitalized cases and 158 deaths. The epidemic followed the introduction of dengue 2 virus 4 years after a major outbreak of dengue 1; the severe form of the disease occurred in persons sustaining sequential infections (see Dengue Hemorrhagic Fever (DHF) in next part of this chapter). Between 1982 and 1985, 25,000 to 68,000 cases of dengue fever were reported in the Americas annually. In 1986 the city of Rio de Janeiro and other areas of coastal Brazil were struck by epidemic dengue 1, with at least 300,000 cases (and perhaps as many as 1 million). Over the next several years, large outbreaks of dengue appeared in Paraguay, Bolivia, Ecuador, and Peru, signaling the recrudescence of *A. aegypti*-borne disease in areas of the Americas from which the vector had long been eradicated. Venezuela experienced an epidemic of DHF in 1989, with 3,108 cases of severe disease and 73 deaths; once again the offending serotype was dengue 2. At present, all four serotypes of dengue (types 1, 2, 3, and 4) are circulating in the Americas, with the near certainty of further outbreaks of DHF.

The virus is transmitted from person to person, principally by *A. aegypti* mosquitoes. Infected humans circulate the virus in their blood for several days. *A. aegypti* is a daytime-biting, peridomiciliary mosquito, which breeds in any container holding fresh water. It is also the urban vector of yellow fever virus, and occurrence of dengue fever outbreaks in the Caribbean and northern South America is prima facie evidence of the receptivity of these areas to introduction and spread of yellow fever from the jungle cycle.

Prevention depends on avoiding mosquito bite (use of screening, repellents, protective clothing) and reduction of *A. aegypti* by elimination of breeding sites and use of larvicides. Eradication of *A. aegypti* has been a goal of member states of the Pan American Health Organization since 1947 and was successful in a few areas, notably Brazil, Argentina, Chile, Paraguay, Uruguay, Peru, and Ecuador. By the 1980s, however, nearly all countries that had succeeded in eradication had become reinfested, with resulting introduction and spread of dengue fever. Areas of the southern United States have high *A. aegypti* populations, but, despite imported cases of dengue fever from the tropics, only limited secondary transmission has occurred. Prophylaxis by immunization is feasible, and experimental live attenuated vaccines are under study. Epidemic measures are based on use of space insecticides applied by the ULV technique.

Colorado Tick Fever

Colorado tick fever (CTF) occurs in mountainous areas of the United States within the distributional range of the vector, *Dermacentor andersoni* (Colorado, Wyoming, Idaho, Montana, Utah, and parts of South Dakota, New Mexico, California, Oregon, Washington, Alberta, and British Columbia). Several hundred human cases are recorded annually, but the actual incidence of the disease is probably 10-fold higher. Infections are acquired during recreational and occupational pursuits that bring humans into contact with infected ticks; campers, foresters, telephone line workers, and the like are thus affected. Infections occur from early spring to October, but the highest incidence is in May and June, representing the seasonal peak of adult tick vector feeding activity. In focal areas of high viral activity, such as some campsites within the Rocky Mountain Park (Colorado), as many as 20 percent of adult tick vectors are found to be infected; the risk of acquiring the disease is approximately one case per 400 camper days.

The clinical illness is characterized by an incubation period of 3 to 6 days, abrupt onset of biphasic febrile course, chills, weakness, prostration, headache, myalgia, photophobia, gastrointestinal complaints, leukopenia, and thrombocytopenia. Rash is uncommon (5 to 10 percent of cases) but may lead to confusion with Rocky Mountain spotted fever. Meningoencephalitis, pericarditis, orchitis, and pleuritis are rare manifestations. Hemorrhagic phenomena have been described in the two reported fatal cases, both involving children.

The virus is amplified in a cycle involving immature *D. andersoni* ticks and small rodents, especially ground squirrels and chipmunks. These species develop prolonged viremias. The virus survives the winter in infected hibernating nymphal and adult ticks, which reinitiate the cycle in the spring. Adult ticks feed on large mammals, including humans, but humans are dead-end hosts and do not serve as a source of tick infection. Infected persons have prolonged viremias, however, and antibodies appear late. Consequently, the possibility of transfusion-induced CTF is recognized.

Viruses Transmitted by Phlebotomine Flies

Phlebotomus (sandfly) fever is caused by at least six serologically distinct viruses (designated Sicilian and Naples phlebotomous fever, Alenquer, Candiru, Chagres, Punta Toro, and Toscana viruses), which belong to a group of 38 related viruses comprising the genus *Phlebovirus*, family *Bunyaviridae* (Table 13-1). Naples and Sicilian viruses cause disease in the Mediterranean region, the Middle East, Iran, India, Pakistan, southern former Soviet Union states, and the Sudan. Immunity rates are generally high, and infection is usually acquired early in life, when disease is mild or escapes notice. Explosive outbreaks with high attack rates have nonetheless occurred, involving as many as 1 million persons. The epidemic disease has occurred with wartime disturbances, displacement of populations, and movements of nonimmune armies. The clinical infection is characterized by a dengue fever–like syndrome but without rash. Toscana virus has been associated with febrile disease and aseptic meningitis in Italy.

Phlebotomus papatasii is the vector. This terrestrial breeding species is mainly nocturnal, is found in close association with humans, and has a very limited flight range. The phlebotomus fever viruses are transmitted transovarially by the vector, and this apparently represents their main means of survival, since adult sandflies do not overwinter. Humans probably contribute little to the transmission cycle (because of low and brief viremias); no other vertebrate reservoir has been unequivocally demonstrated, although serologic evidence suggests that certain rodents (gerbils) may be involved.

Several phleboviruses in tropical America (Alenquer, Candiru, Chagres, Punta Toro viruses) cause sporadic undifferentiated febrile illness in humans but are not of public health consequence. Control is by reduction of vector populations through use of insecticides.

Culicoides-borne Infections

Oropouche fever (febre du Mojui), caused by a bunyavirus of the Simbu group, is responsible for at least 15 major epidemics in cities and towns of the Amazon region of Brazil and Peru, and Panama. As many as 102,000 persons were infected in individual outbreaks, at rates as high as 30 percent. The disease is self-limited, characterized by sudden onset, high fever, severe headache, myalgia, gastrointestinal symptoms, leukopenia, and prostration, sometimes requiring hospitalization. Aseptic meningitis is an uncommon complication. The virus has been isolated from *Culicoides paraensis* gnats (suspected to be the epidemic vector) and from mosquitoes. Experimental studies show conclusively that *Culicoides paraensis* is a biologically competent vector of Oropouche virus.[25] Wild birds, monkeys, or sloths may play a role in the forest transmission cycle. Although the ecological relationships are not completely understood, reduction of *Culicoides* populations appears to be a justifiable approach in future outbreaks.

▶ VIRUSES CAUSING FEVER AND ARTHRITIS

Chikungunya virus (an alphavirus) is a generally benign disease that clinically resembles classic dengue fever. The Swahili name means "that which bends up," referring to the severe arthralgia that accompanies the illness. Deaths and hemorrhagic phenomena are extremely rare and poorly documented features of the disease. The virus is endemic in sub-Saharan Africa and the Asian tropics. Major outbreaks have occurred in Africa and Asia, with high attack rates. The infection is now hyperendemic in areas of Africa and Asia infested with *A. aegypti*, the principal viral vector to humans. An enzootic, sylvan transmission cycle in Africa, however, involves subhuman primates and forest mosquitoes, including *A. furcifer*, and is analogous to that of jungle yellow fever.

Various experimental chikungunya viral vaccines have been investigated, but none are commercially available. Control measures applicable to the epidemic disease are similar to those described for dengue fever.

Viral Hemorrhagic Fevers

James W. LeDuc

Hemorrhagic fevers caused by viruses are generally rare diseases, but as witnessed recently, some, like Ebola, have attracted sufficient attention of press and lay public that they have become part of our normal vocabulary. The clinical condition known as hemorrhagic fever is in fact quite variable and may result from infection with several different viruses or bacteria. In general, they present as a febrile disease that progresses to manifest some degree of hemorrhage, often in the form of increased capillary permeability, which may lead to death in a significant proportion of those clinically ill. The number of distinct viruses able to cause hemorrhagic fevers continues to grow as we recognize new viruses, such as those associated with hantavirus pulmonary syndrome and the arenaviruses of South America (Table 13-3). All hemorrhagic fever viruses, with the possible exception of dengue viruses, are zoonotic agents that exist in nature in a silent cycle that involves nonhuman vertebrate hosts and often arthropod vectors. Transmission to humans is by the bite of an infectious arthropod vector, by small-particle aerosol from infectious urine or feces of infectious rodent host (or occasionally by bite from these hosts), or through nosocomial transmission, often under conditions where routine safe hospital practices are not being followed. Person-to-person transmission may occur, but is usually not the dominant mode of transmission. Hemorrhagic fever viruses do not share a common taxonomic origin; they are found among four different virus families: *Bunyaviridae, Flaviviridae, Arenaviridae,* and *Filoviridae.*

Arenaviruses

Until recently, only three arenaviruses were associated with hemorrhagic fever: Lassa fever caused by Lassa virus of West Africa; Argentine hemorrhagic fever, caused by Junin virus of Argentina; and Bolivian hemorrhagic fever caused by Machupo virus of Bolivia. In the past decade, however, two new pathogenic arenaviruses have been discovered, and it is likely that others will be recognized as humans continue to occupy previously sparsely populated regions of the world (Table 13-4).

TABLE 13-3. VIRAL HEMORRHAGIC FEVERS

Family Virus of Transmission	*Disease*	*Distribution*	*Means*
Arenaviridae			
Lassa	Lassa fever	West Africa	Rodent
Junin	Argentine HF	Argentina	Rodent
Machupo	Bolivian HF	Bolivia	Rodent
Guanarito	Venezuelan HF	Venezuela	Rodent
Sabia	Brazilian HF(?)	Brazil	Unknown
Bunyaviridae			
Rift Valley fever virus	Rift Valley fever	Sub-Saharan Africa	Mosquito
Crimean-Congo HF	Crimean-Congo HF	Africa, Asia, Southern Russia, NIS	Tick
Hantaan and related viruses	HF with renal syndrome	Asia, Balkans, Russia, Europe	Rodent
	Hantavirus pulmonary syndrome	Americas	Rodent
Filoviridae			
Marburg	Marburg HF	Sub-Saharan Africa	Unknown
Ebola	Ebola HF	Sub-Saharan Africa	Unknown
Flaviviridae			
Yellow Fever	Yellow fever	Tropical Americas, Sub-Saharan Africa	Mosquito
Dengue	Dengue fever, dengue HF, shock syndrome	Asia, Africa, Pacific, Americas	Mosquito
Kyasanur Forest disease	Kyasanur Forest disease	India	Tick
Omsk	Omsk HF	Russia	Tick

Abbreviation: NIS, newly independent states.

TABLE 13-4. ARENAVIRUSES KNOWN TO CAUSE HUMAN DISEASE

Virus	*Abbreviation*	*Host*	*Original Isolation*	*Disease*
Lymphocytic choriomeningitis	LCM	*Mus musculus*	United States	Lymphocytic choriomeningitis
Lassa fever	LAS	*Mastomys* sp.	Nigeria	Lassa
Junin	JUN	*Calomys musculinus*	Argentina	Argentine hemorrhagic fever
Machupo	MAC	*Calomys callosus*	Bolivia	Bolivian hemorrhagic fever
Guanarito	GUA	*Zygodontomys brevicauda*	Venezuela	Venezuelan hemorrhagic fever
Sabia	SAB	Unknown	Brazil	Not named

Lassa Fever

First recognized during 1969 in Nigeria, Lassa fever has focused worldwide attention on problems related to the management and control of highly hazardous viruses. This was the result of several West African nosocomial outbreaks in rural hospitals in Nigeria, Liberia, and Sierra Leone, where direct secondary transmission with high mortality occurred. These outbreaks have often devastated rural hospital staffs, claiming physicians and nurses as well as the index patient's families and friends. Moreover, Lassa fever is the most common dangerous viral disease of international travelers, with imported cases reported from England, Japan, the Netherlands, Israel, and the United States.

The disease appears to be restricted to West Africa, occurring principally in savannah landscapes or tropical areas severely modified by human agricultural activity, with the majority of cases seen in Liberia, Sierra Leone, Guinea, and Nigeria, and accounting for 10 percent or more of admissions to some hospitals. In its severe form, Lassa fever is a protean febrile disease attacking many vital organs including heart, lungs, liver, pancreas and kidneys. Jaundice is unusual but pulmonary and peritoneal effusions are commonly observed. A fulminating hemorrhagic picture with shock occurs in only about 20 percent of hospitalized cases. Virus is present in blood and effusions for many days and has been recovered from throat washing and urine. The virus also attacks the human fetus, and abortion with increased mortality is a common feature of infection among pregnant women, with up to 25 percent of maternal deaths due to Lassa in some hospitals. Lassa virus has also been isolated from milk, suggesting that there is a clear risk to nursing infants. Deafness is an important sequela of Lassa fever, with studies in Sierra Leone indicating that approximately one-quarter of prospectively studied Lassa patients developed hearing loss. Antibodies to Lassa virus are also more common in deaf residents of endemic areas. While no specific vaccine is available for Lassa fever, the disease does appear to respond well to treatment with the antiviral drug, ribavirin. Unfortunately, access to this drug is significantly hampered due to lack of availability, cost, and licensure issues.

Lassa virus is maintained by peridomestic rodents of the genus *Mastomys*. Original studies indicated that *Mastomys natalensis* was the principal reservoir host, but this actually represents a complex of sibling species difficult to differentiate by physical characteristics alone. It is now thought that the species most likely to harbor Lassa virus are *Mastomys erythroleucus* and *Mastomys hildebrandtii*, which are distinct from *M. natalensis*. These large mice, which resemble juvenile house rats (*Rattus rattus*), live in close proximity to humans and readily enter households. Indeed, many villages in eastern Sierra Leone may average 1 to 4 *Mastomys* in each house, with as many as 20 percent infected with Lassa virus. Mice are chronically infected and shed virus in their urine for many weeks, leading to infectious aerosol, which may contaminate the environment and foodstuffs or directly lead to infection by inhalation or contact on cuts or mucous membranes. In addition, in some areas these mice are consumed by villagers for food, leading to greater risk of Lassa infection.

Prospective, laboratory-based studies of Lassa fever in eastern Sierra Leone have demonstrated that transmission is endemic, with peak activity in the dry season months of January through May. Attack rates range up to 5 per 1,000 per year, with a case-fatality rate of 18 percent, much lower than reported during earlier outbreaks. Epidemiological investigations conducted in villages, however, showed that up to half the population had been infected with the virus and annual infection rates as high as 8 percent have been documented, giving an infection-case ratio of approximately 16:1. Persons of all ages and both sexes are infected and may suffer severe clinical illness; why only certain individuals become very sick is still not known.

Surveillance for Lassa fever presents a difficult challenge. Geographical surveys in West Africa have disclosed significant foci of infection in areas where the disease has never been clinically detected. Because the clinical spectrum observed in laboratory-documented infection is so wide, it is now clear that only the most severe cases could be clinically suspected, and probably then only if a cluster of such cases occurred with transmission to hospital staff. Thus, specific diagnosis is essential and best done by measurement of virus-specific IgM antibodies, which appear in all patients within 7 to 10 days after onset of symptoms, or by direct measurement of viral antigen or nucleic acids earlier in the course of illness. Mortality in Lassa fever is directly related to virus concentration in blood; consequently, the potential hazards associated with such laboratory work and the paucity of virological laboratories in West Africa have limited the application of these technologies.

Because persons coming from *rural* West Africa may introduce Lassa virus into other countries at any time, it is important that facilities and plans for their isolation and care as well as surveillance of known direct contacts be organized in any nation that has significant commerce with Africa. Clinical and laboratory isolation facilities of a high order are indicated, and these should be designated to provide protection to the medical care team as well as to the general community. Fever surveillance, but not quarantine, for 3 weeks is indicated for all persons in direct face-to-face contact with Lassa patients prior to their effective isolation.

Control of Lassa fever represents a major biological challenge. Vaccine development is hampered by technical problems and the absence of an economically sustainable market. Rodent control is effective in reducing virus transmission to humans, but is likewise difficult to apply or sustain over the broad distribution of *Mastomys*.

Argentine Hemorrhagic Fever

Like Lassa fever, Argentine hemorrhagic fever (AHF) is maintained by a rodent and is transmitted to humans by infectious urine. The disease is caused by Junin virus, first discovered in the 1950s in the rich agricultural pampas of Buenos Aires, Cordoba, and Santa Fe Provinces of Argentina. Until recently, the annual incidence of AHF ranged from 50 to more than 2,000 cases annually during the autumn months of February through July. Adult males compose the great majority of cases, due to their occupational exposure through farming and related agrarian activities. Onset of symptoms is usually gradual with fever and malaise progressing to myalgia, headache, and dizziness and followed by signs of central nervous system (CNS) involvement such as tremor of the limbs and tongue, gastrointestinal symptoms including nausea and vomiting, and indications of vascular instability that may progress to shock. Severely ill patients may bleed from the gums, gastrointestinal tract, or mucosal surfaces, and severe neurological symptoms include coma and convulsions. Case fatality rate is from 5 to 15 percent, and inapparent infections rarely occur. Viremia is sporadic or of low titer and nosocomial infections, although reported, are very unusual. Attack rates may be quite high in circumscribed, small communities, as for example in O'Higgins, Argentina, in 1953 when they reached 10/100.

Chronic viremic and viruric infection of rodents has been shown to be the principal means of virus maintenance and, by strong inference, of transmission to humans. The main host of AHF is the field mouse, *Calomys musculinus*. Similar in size to house mice (*Mus musculus*), this indigenous rodent invades crops during the fall from permanent harborage along roadsides, railways, and other linear habitats. Population densities are highest in fields of maize. Migratory workers harvesting maize by hand were the principal victims during the 1950s and early 1960s, although now combine and truck operators have attack rates estimated as 20 to 50 times those of the earlier migrant laborers. Aerosols as well as blood and fluids from mice crushed in the combines are now thought to be the primary source of infection. Prospective study of *C. musculinus* suggest that most infected animals acquire the virus horizontally after weanling, although vertical transmission clearly occurs.

A live, attenuated vaccine, Candid 1, developed jointly by the Government of Argentina, the Pan American Health Organization, the United Nations Development Programme, and the United States Army Medical Research and Development Command, has recently been evaluated for both safety and efficacy in preventing AHF. Many at risk individuals in the endemic region of Argentina have now received the vaccine, leading to a dramatic drop in AHF incidence.

Bolivian Hemorrhagic Fever

Similar in both the clinical disease produced and the way it is maintained in nature, Bolivian hemorrhagic fever (BHF) is caused by Machupo virus. The disease was first recognized in 1959, and by the early 1960s nearly 500 cases had been recorded, with a case fatality rate of approximately 30 percent. In 1963–1964 a large outbreak occurred in San Joaquin after a population explosion of the primary rodent host, *Calomys callosus* led to hundreds of mice invading the town, resulting in a BHF attack rate among residents of 20/100 per year.

The ecology of BHF is different from that of AHF in several ways. The reservoir host is *C. callosus*, a larger rodent that is naturally found at the edge of riverine forest-savannah formations. When humans cut the forest to plant gardens, *C. callosus* invades these plots and the houses of humans as well. Thus, disease transmission by the continual excretion of virus in the urine of this species occurs in and near homes, resulting in disease among all members of the population. To exemplify this point, in July of 1994 a cluster of BHF cases was identified among a family residing in Magdalena, a small town of about 5,000 inhabitants in the north-central district of Beni near the border with Brazil. Eight of nine family members were infected, and seven, aged 10 months to 50 years, died. In general, BHF is limited to the sparsely populated subtropical savannah of Beni province, where cases occur in adults and children. There is no sex difference in the attack rate, and peak incidence is usually during the late rainy season and early dry season months of February to July. Outbreaks of BHF have been controlled and prevented by vigorous rodent control programs in affected towns and ranches. The live, attenuated Junin vaccine cross-protects against BHF in monkey models and may offer an alternative to rodent control among rural populations at high risk of BHF.

Venezuelan Hemorrhagic Fever

This newly recognized disease was discovered when a cluster of hemorrhagic fever cases was seen in the city of Guanarito in the central Venezuelan state of Portuguesa in 1989. A total of 104 presumptive cases with 26 deaths was recorded, and the causative agent, named Guanarito virus for the city from which it came, was isolated. Clinical disease is similar to that documented for AHF and BHF, although pharyngitis appears to be more common. Both sexes are affected almost equally, but to date the majority of cases have been in persons over the age of 16 years. Most cases have occurred during the dry season of December to March in Portuguesa state, and like AHF and BHF cases, those infected are usually rural residents involved in agricultural activities. The cane mouse, *Zygodontomys brevicauda* appears to be the primary reservoir host, and laboratory studies have demonstrated that this rodent may sustain long-term viremia and viruria.

Sabia Virus

Only three cases of Sabia virus have been recognized, the original fatal infection of a young woman hospitalized in Sao Paulo, Brazil, in 1990 and two subsequent laboratory infections acquired, first in Belem, Brazil, and later in New Haven, Connecticut, by scientists attempting to characterize this new virus. Both survived, with the later cases apparently responding well to treatment with ribavirin administered soon after the diagnosis was suspected. Attempts to identify a rodent host of Sabia virus have to date been unsuccessful, and there is little known about the natural history of the virus, although it is clear from the laboratory infections that it is easily transmitted by aerosol.

Lymphocytic Choriomeningitis

Lymphocytic choriomeningitis (LCM) virus is the prototype member of the family *Arenaviridae*. It is maintained in nature through chronic infections of the peridomestic mouse, *Mus musculus*, and both the virus and vector have been recognized virtually worldwide.

Unlike other arenaviruses discussed above, human disease due to LCM virus is almost never fatal or hemorrhagic. Clinical syndromes range from an acute undifferentiated febrile illness to forms characterized by aseptic meningitis and mild encephalitis, the neurological symptoms and signs usually appearing during a second febrile period that begins 1 to 5 days after termination of an initial febrile episode of 3 to 7 days' duration. Clinical diagnoses of 150 patients, proved to have LCM virus infection during hamster-associated outbreaks, indicated that about half had "flu-like" symptoms; 22 percent were diagnosed as aseptic meningitis; 5 percent, as encephalitis, 1 percent, as myelitis, and 23 percent, as "healthy." LCM virus may also cause abortion in pregnant women or lead to hydrocephalus, chorioretinitis, or mental retardation in the newborn child.

The virus is maintained in nature by chronic infection of feral *Mus* mice, and infection is acquired both vertically from infected parent to progeny and horizontally through contact among individuals of this species. Mice infected in utero or from maternal milk secrete significant quantities of virus in the urine for weeks, months, or throughout their entire lives. Transmission to humans occurs on exposure to infectious rodent urine, most commonly in the form of aerosols associated with nests. An alternate host of significance in recent years in both Europe and the United States is the Syrian hamster. Outbreaks have occurred among personnel in medical research institutions where hamsters were housed, as well as among persons keeping hamsters as pets. These animals are also chronically infected with continuous viruria.

Because of this very specific transmission pattern, attack rates in human populations are almost impossible to determine. Infection is probably more common than is realized, since specific viral techniques are needed to make the diagnosis. Over 30 years ago about 10 percent of aseptic meningitis and encephalitis cases studied in one U.S. center over a period of several years were caused by LCM virus. The accumulated literature suggested that adults are infected more often than children are and that most *Mus*-related infections occur in fall and winter. Between 1965 and 1975, hamster-related outbreaks of 7, 48, and 181 proven cases occurred in New York, California, and 10 other states.

There is no specific treatment and no vaccine is available for LCM infection. Good standards of environmental sanitation and testing of hamster colonies for endemic LCM virus infection represent available methods for avoiding human contact with this agent.

Filoviruses

Among the most severe and mysterious viral pathogens to emerge in this century, Marburg and Ebola viruses have burst on an unprepared world only since 1967. Knowledge of these agents is largely restricted to a few distinct human outbreaks, although recent intense investigations triggered by the Ebola outbreak of Kikwit, Zaire, in 1995 are starting to provide better definition to the problem. Filoviruses are morphologically similar but immunologically distinct. They are long, pleomorphic rods reminiscent of but distinguishable from rhabdoviruses, such as rabies, and are now placed in a new family, the *Filoviridae*. Clinical disease seen during each of the individual cases or outbreaks affecting a total of nearly 1,100 persons by early 1997 was almost always very severe and similar in all instances. The incubation period averaged about 1 week, but on occasion was longer, and fatal infections were uniformly marked by the advent of a hemorrhagic diathesis after 4 to 7 days of generalized symptoms. Disseminated intravascular coagulation was documented in most such cases where it was sought. A maculopapular rash, necrotizing nonicteric hepatitis, and chemical pancreatitis were common findings. Case-fatality rates ranged from 25 to 88 percent, and person-to-person transmission, largely nosocomial, occurred in each major epidemic. Little is known about the ecology of the filoviruses. There is no vaccine for either Ebola or Marburg virus, and no known antiviral drug. Immune horse serum has been produced for Ebola, but its efficacy in treatment or prevention of disease is unknown.

Marburg Virus

Marburg virus was first discovered following the importation of African green monkeys, *Cercopithecus aethiops*, into Germany and Yugoslavia from Uganda. These monkeys were used for production of kidney cells for use in preparation of poliovirus vaccine; the monkeys served as the source of Marburg virus infection for laboratory workers initially, with secondary spread to both medical staff and family members. A total of 31 cases and 7 deaths occurred in Marburg, Germany, and another two in Belgrade, Yugoslavia, both of whom survived. Subsequent investigations failed to disclose any evidence of natural infection in this or other monkey species in the region of their capture in Uganda. Subsequent isolated cases of Marburg infection have sporadically appeared in Zimbabwe and Kenya, and a total of 36 known cases and 10 deaths have now been documented. The ecology of Marburg virus remains virtually unknown.

Ebola Virus

An outbreak involving 318 cases and 280 deaths occurring in Yambuku, Zaire, in 1976 led to the discovery of Ebola virus. Investigations suggested that reuse of contaminated needles served to amplify the outbreak with devastating effects; all those infected by needle died. At nearly the same time, a second outbreak was in progress in Maridi, Sudan, that involved 284 cases and left 151 dead. Surprisingly, when virus isolates from these two outbreaks were compared, they proved *not* to be the same virus. While morphologically similar, they are antigenically and genetically distinct and clearly represented two separate events. These viruses are now referred to as Ebola-Zaire and Ebola-Sudan and both have been associated with subsequent outbreaks: Ebola-Zaire with a fatal case in Tandala, Zaire, in 1977–1978; Nzoia, Kenya, in 1980; Kikwit, Zaire, in 1995; and various locations in Gabon in 1994 and 1996–1997. Ebola-Sudan has reappeared only once, in 1979 in Nzara, Sudan.

In 1990 another Ebola virus was discovered and, like Marburg virus, it was associated with the importation of nonhuman primates for medical research. But rather than originating in Africa, these animals had been imported from the Philippines. Infected monkeys suffered a severe, often fatal hemorrhagic disease, but although there is serological evidence of at least 16 human infections, none were symptomatic. This strain has been named Ebola-Reston for the Virginia city where the first epizootic was discovered.

Ebola-Côte d'Ivoire is the most recently recognized strain and originated from a single human infection acquired when a primatologist studying free-living chimpanzees in the Tai Forest of western Côte d'Ivoire was infected while taking clinical specimens from a chimpanzee that had recently died of a hemorrhagic illness. This animal was one of several that had succumbed during a series of epizootics that had devastated the troop over the course of a few years. The patient suffered a febrile illness with rash, but fully recovered, and it was learned that her infection was due to a new strain of Ebola only after she had been discharged from the hospital. There was no indication of spread to the medical staff.

The major outbreaks of Ebola virus have all been associated with hospitals or clinics where nosocomial transmission was associated with reuse of needles or other unhygienic practices, from intimate contact between patients and caregivers at home, or from burial rituals that facilitated transmission. Recent outbreaks in Gabon appear to have originated following human contact with chimpanzees either killed or found dead and prepared as food. In the Kikwit outbreak, transmission was halted when patients were isolated, strict barrier nursing procedures implemented, and burial rituals controlled. Isolated cases seen in modern, well-equipped medical facilities have not experienced sustained nosocomial transmission; however, a recent importation of an Ebola case from Gabon to South Africa resulted in the fatal infection of a South African nurse and serves as warning that with modern air travel even an outbreak in a remote area represents a risk to all countries. Although the blood of patients contains large amounts of virus, there is little to suggest that infectious aerosols played a major role in these epidemics.

The ecology of Ebola viruses is unknown, although it is clear from observations in Côte d'Ivoire, Gabon, and the Philippines that nonhuman primates encounter the virus in nature. It appears that monkeys and apes suffer a severe disease similar to that seen in humans, and as such are unlikely to be major reservoirs of the virus. Recent experimental infections of various species of plants and animals naturally occurring in areas where Ebola outbreaks have occurred found that fruit and insectivorous bats supported Ebola virus replication and circulation of high titers of virus without becoming ill. It remains to be determined if such infections actually occur in nature and are epidemiologically relevant.

Flaviviruses

Viruses of the family *Flaviviridae* compose some of the most important hemorrhagic fevers known. They include viruses transmitted primarily by mosquitoes, others by ticks, and are found in both the tropics and temperate zones. Dengue hemorrhagic fever is one of the true emerging diseases of the twentieth century, with increases in incidence both in Asia, where it has been endemic since the 1950s, as well as in the American tropics, where the past decade has witnessed massive outbreaks in Venezuela, Brazil, and other countries. Yellow fever is the prototype member of the family.

Dengue Hemorrhagic Fever

In addition to the classic syndrome of breakbone fever, all four dengue virus serotypes are capable of producing a more severe, sometimes fatal syndrome variously called dengue hemorrhagic fever (DHF) or dengue shock syndrome. Although there is historical evidence that this disease occurred during major dengue outbreaks in Greece and Australia more than 70 years ago, it has been recognized since 1948 only in certain areas of Southeast Asia, some islands of the western Pacific Ocean, the Middle East, and with the reinfestation of many parts of the Americas with the principal mosquito vector, *Aedes aegypti*, more frequently in Latin America. This geographical distribution is still far smaller than that of dengue virus infection, but is growing as multiple serotypes of dengue become established.

A fundamental problem is clinical definition of DHF. Persons with dengue virus infections who have a positive tourniquet test reaction have been included in this taxon by some authors. Many patients with otherwise self-limited illnesses may have scattered petechiae in the skin, and these phenomena are frequently recorded during dengue outbreaks in parts of the world where the more serious form of the disease is rare or absent. The fully developed DHF clinical picture consists typically of the abrupt onset, after a 2- to 7-day incubation period, of fever and myalgia, significant thrombocytopenia, hepatomegaly, and various bleeding manifestations, including hemorrhagic petechiae, epistaxis, and gastrointestinal bleeding, There is loss of intravascular protein with attendant hemoconcentration, metabolic acidosis, and in 10 to 40 percent of cases there is both objective and clinical evidence of shock. The mortality rate during the shock crisis ranges from 1 to 20 percent depending on the vigor and efficacy of supportive therapy.

The basic virus cycle, the seasonal pattern of occurrence, and the arthropod vectors of DHF do not differ from those of classic dengue infection; hemorrhagic fever is seen either in annual rainy season outbreaks in large metropolitan areas in Southeast Asia where all dengue serotypes are endemic or during epidemics on islands where a given serotype is introduced after a variable period of absence.

Extensive work on this problem has been done in Bangkok, Thailand, where the primary vector is *A. aegypti*. There the majority of hemorrhagic fever patients are children under 10 years of age. Annual hospitalization rates on an age-specific basis may reach 5 to 8 per 1,000, or about 1 case per 60 to 100 serologically estimated dengue virus infections in this age group. Females are affected more often than males, 1.2:1 to 1.4:1, despite that dengue virus infection rates in this population do not differ by sex. There are no differences in attack rates between the major ethnic groups: Thai and Chinese.

Hemorrhagic fever occurred significantly more often in children with immunological evidence of secondary dengue virus infection than in those who had a primary response. From this observation it has been postulated that DHF is an immunopathological process selectively occurring among persons experiencing a second dengue infection in a rather short interval. Recent work appears to both strengthen and modify this hypothesis. In vitro and in vivo experimental studies demonstrated that dengue virus replication in mononuclear phagocytic cells, the apparent primary target cells for infection, was enhanced in the presence of small amounts of heterologous dengue antibody. Such antibodies have been found in cord blood of infants born in virus-endemic areas of Southeast Asia. In addition, the first recorded epidemic of DHF in the Americas occurred in Cuba in 1981. This outbreak was caused by dengue 2 virus just 4 years after a major epidemic of type 1 infection that was the first dengue experience on that island in more than 30 years. Similar observations have been made in Brazil, Venezuela, Mexico, and other Central, South American, and Caribbean countries in recent years as multiple dengue serotypes were introduced and residents exposed to second dengue infections. It has also been shown that primary dengue infection can cause DHF; however, the risk of DHF following primary infection is 0.25 percent compared with 3.1 percent after secondary infection. Complex variables, including virus strain differences and host genetic factors, remain to be elucidated before a clear understanding of the relative risk factors influencing DHF emerges. In Cuba the risk of contracting DHF was greater in whites than in blacks, despite similar rates of secondary infection with dengue 2 virus.

Methods for surveillance and control of DHF are the same as those described earlier for classic dengue fever. At present there is no vaccine for dengue; however, phase 1 clinical trials are in progress for a live, attenuated tetravalent dengue vaccine. Should this vaccine proved to be safe and efficacious, it will certainly play a significant role in determining how future dengue and DHF epidemics are controlled.

Yellow Fever

Yellow fever is the prototypical viral hemorrhagic fever. It now occurs only in tropical and subtropical regions of Africa and the Americas, but historically it was an important passenger during the burgeoning European colonial period of the eighteenth and nineteenth centuries, causing urban epidemics in major seaport cities of the United States, the United Kingdom, and Europe. Indeed, the roots of our current system of quarantine, infectious disease control, and a now defunct chain of national marine hospitals can be traced to attempts to understand and control yellow fever in the past century. Yellow fever is caused by a flavivirus closely related to the dengue virus and several other arthropod-transmitted agents of the *Flavivirus* genus. A single infection confers lifelong immunity; thus the modern pattern of disease occurrence consists of recurrent outbreaks with intervals of several years in areas where an extra human virus cycle is maintained.

Clinical response to infection with yellow fever virus ranges from mild, undifferentiated fever to severe illness in which hemorrhagic, hepatic, and renal manifestations predominate. In patients who survive or do not manifest an early fulminating hemorrhagic syndrome, jaundice typically develops after 4 to 6 days of illness, when viremia wanes and humoral antibodies appear. Renal tubular necrosis may occur during the second week of illness and, before the advent of peritoneal or hemodialysis, it accounted for nearly one-third of fatalities. Notwithstanding these various clinical forms of disease, it is the clustering of jaundice cases with fatality rates of 10 to 50 percent that usually brings yellow fever outbreaks to public health attention, a feature of fundamental value in differential diagnosis between this disease and most other viral hemorrhagic fevers.

Attack rates during urban epidemics of yellow fever in the eighteenth and nineteenth centuries were often staggering, ranging to 20 cases per 100 persons, with up to a 5 percent mortality rate. In the past 30 years one of the largest epidemics on record was in southwestern Ethiopia, where an estimated 100,000 cases occurred in a population of 2 million, with 30,000 deaths. More recently, an epidemic in Gambia caused 2.5 severe illnesses per 100 inhabitants of nine villages with a case-fatality rate of 19 percent. Serological studies carried out before an emergency immunization campaign revealed that about 12 persons had been infected for each severe clinical case; this ratio was 8:1 where yellow fever infection was the first apparent exposure to a flavivirus, but 45:1 where the infection was secondary to a previous experience with a yellow fever-related virus. Between 1987 and the early 1990s, Nigeria sustained a series of sylvatic and urban outbreaks, with several thousand officially notified cases and a case-fatality rate exceeding 50 percent. A total of 18,735 cases and 4,522 deaths were reported to the World Health Organization from 1987 to 1991, mostly from Africa, and represents the greatest amount of yellow fever activity for any 5-year period since 1948. These figures represent but a fraction of the real burden of yellow fever.

Humans of all ages and both sexes are equally susceptible to yellow fever virus infection. Although frequently suggested, there is no scientific evidence that blacks are more resistant clinically to this virus than members of other races.

Observed patterns of human yellow fever are based on enzootic cycles of virus maintenance; despite decades of investigation, several major ecological mysteries persist. Classic urban yellow fever is transmitted in a human-mosquito cycle by the mosquito, *A. aegypti*, the same vector as for dengue viruses. African in origin, this species has been disseminated throughout the tropics and subtropics of the entire world. Yet yellow fever has never occurred in India or in the densely populated countries of southeast Asia. Control of this mosquito and of urban yellow fever during the 1920s in the Americas led to the recognition of a forest cycle causing "jungle" yellow fever. Each year tens to several hundred cases are reported from the countries composing the Amazon, Orinoco, and Magdalena River systems of South America, and the virus makes additional periodic incursions into Panama, the island of Trinidad, or Bolivia. Mosquito vectors are arboreal, diurnally active species of the genera *Haemagogous* and *Sabethes*, which oviposit in tree holes. Monkeys are the only proven nonhuman vertebrate hosts in this cycle, and certain species incur high mortality, which is frequently an early warning of pending human outbreaks. Although attack rates in humans are usually low, disease is concentrated in adult males involved in road building, lumbering, or agriculture where destruction of forest is in progress. The virus appears to wander about the vast tropical rain forest, returning to cause human disease at intervals of 5 to 10 years.

Yellow fever ecology in Africa is more complex. Monkeys and arboreal *Aedes* species, such as *A. africanus*, appear to maintain enzootic cycles with only scattered cases of human disease in the rain forests of central and eastern Africa. Larger outbreaks in rural and semiurban settings take place in the savannah and savannah-transition belts around the forests with extensions into western Africa. Here human-mosquito cycles are important and vectors include *A. luteocephalus*, *A. simpsoni*, and *A. furcifer*, which breed in tree holes. Recent experimental documentation of transovarial mosquito transmission of virus indicates that many questions concerning yellow fever ecology require reexamination. African monkeys are generally not susceptible to fatal yellow fever virus infection and thus do not provide an early signal of human outbreaks.

There is no specific treatment for human yellow fever, but prevention and control of epidemics can be achieved by use of one of the most successful live attenuated vaccines known to science. The 17D vaccine is highly immunogenic and has a very low incidence of clinical reaction. Rates for serious side effects are so low as not to have been accurately calculated. The vaccine confers long-lasting (perhaps lifetime) immunity, although international requirements for persons traveling to endemic or epidemic areas call for reimmunization every 10 years. No untoward effects on the human fetus have been reported, but in the absence of definitive data, prudence requires due exercise of judgment regarding degree of potential exposure before immunization of pregnant women. In spite of the availability of an excellent vaccine, travelers continue to visit at risk areas without the benefit of vaccination, all too often with devastating results. In 1996, two travelers to the Amazon Basin of Brazil died of yellow fever on return to their homes in Switzerland and the United States. As "ecotourism" and the ease of international travel in general continues to grow, both individual travelers and their health care providers need to remain cognizant of the risk of yellow fever and ensure that proper vaccination is received prior to travel.

Adjuncts to mass vaccine programs during urban epidemics of yellow fever include destruction of *A. aegypti* breeding sites (sanitary engineering and cleanup efforts) and the use of insecticides to reduce both adult and larval mosquito populations. These measure are futile where virus transmission is of the "jungle" type.

Kyasanur Forest Disease

Kyasanur forest disease (KFD) was first recognized in 1957 in a forest area of the state of Mysore in southwestern India. Attention of health authorities was drawn to a dramatic epizootic among monkeys in this forest, and it was feared that yellow fever had at last arrived in India. The causative agent was, indeed, shown to be a flavivirus, but it proved to be immunologically related to tick-borne flaviviruses causing encephalitis and Omsk hemorrhagic fever in the Soviet Union.

The incubation period of human disease is 5 to 8 days. Clinical forms, characterized by gastrointestinal hemorrhage, mild encephalitis, or both are commonly observed. Case-fatality rates vary between 3 and 10 percent and the apparent-inapparent infection rate has been estimated at about 1:1. Within the slowly expanding endemic region in the state of Karnataka, the disease occurs in a strongly focal pattern, and the number of cases recorded annually ranges from 50 to more than 1,000. Attack rates in given villages may reach 5/100 in a given year, but it is clear that variables related to the natural virus cycle, rather than immunity in human populations, are responsible for the large swings in disease occurrence.

KFD is strongly seasonal, most cases being recorded during the intermonsoon drier spring months from February through June. Adults are attacked more commonly than children, males slightly more often than females. This pattern reflects the seasonal activity of both the forest-dwelling tick vectors and humans. Larval and nymphal stages of *Haemaphysalis spinigera* and *Haemaphysali turturis* are most active at this time, and people enter the forest to gather wood and wild plants for food during this annual pause in their agricultural year. Domestic livestock serve as an important source of blood of adult *Haemaphysalis* ticks but do not take part in the virus transmission cycle.

Human infection is most commonly acquired after the bite of tick nymphs. Although there is no evidence of transovarial tick transmission of KFD virus, the agent has been recovered frequently from forest monkeys, rodents, and squirrels. Birds are infected by KFD virus, although there is no conclusive proof that they serve as a source of tick infection. Thus the mechanism of overwintering for this virus has not been elucidated.

Hospital-based surveillance of acute febrile disease with hemorrhagic or neurological manifestations is maintained in the endemic area. Diagnoses are made principally by serologic procedures. An inactivated vaccine was tested in the affected region about 30 years ago. Although the vaccine was not highly immunogenic, a trial in villagers in the state of Karnataka showed efficacy. Research on improved vaccine is required.

Recently a new virus related to KFD and tick-borne encephalitis viruses was recovered from persons working in Saudi Arabia. Two fatal infections were documented in individuals suffering from a hemorrhagic illness; signs and symptoms included fever, hemorrhagic phenomena including epistaxis, ecchymosis at needle puncture sites, extensive subcutaneous bleeding, bloody diarrhea or rectal bleeding, and hematemesis. A total of 9 cases were confirmed serologically or by virus isolation; 3 had rash, and 2 had encephalitis manifested by convulsions, semicoma, and coma. Six others had either unusual irritability or drowsiness. Virus was recovered from specimens taken during the course of the illnesses, and preliminary characterization suggests that virus may represent a new flavivirus; however, additional studies are needed to fully characterize the agent. Epidemiological investigations indicated that all 9 patients were adults, 8 were male, and 6 worked as butchers and 1 was a zoo worker routinely exposed to raw meat. The butchers routinely slaughtered and handled meat of sheep most frequently, but also processed beef and camels. A confirmed route of transmission has not been determined, but several patients had cut their hands during the course of their work. Tick bites were also a possible source of infection. To date, all recognized cases have occurred during the spring or fall of 1994 or 1995. This apparently new flavivirus has yet to be formally named.

Omsk Hemorrhagic Fever

Omsk hemorrhagic fever (OHF) is restricted to the mixed forest-steppe region of western Siberia. First recognized during World War II, clinical cases reported per year ranged from the teens to a few hundred during the next 2 decades but have apparently decreased dramatically in recent years, with only sporadic cases in muskrat trappers and their families. OHF is caused by a virus closely related to that of Russian spring-summer encephalitis, and the geographical areas of occurrence of these agents overlap, rendering many epidemiological aspects of OHF rather imprecise in the absence of a laboratory method for clear differentiation of these infections.

The disease resembles KFD. The incubation period of OHF in humans ranges from 3 to 7 days. Fever is typically present in two distinct waves. During the first interval of 5 to 12 days there are signs of bronchopneumonia and hemorrhagic manifestations, while mild neurological signs appear during the second febrile period of 2 to 7 days. Case-fatality rates are less than 5 percent. No data are available regarding human attack rates or inapparent/apparent infection ratios. Transmission of infection to humans occurs either by tick bite, the principal vector being the adult form of *Dermacentor pictus*, or by direct contact with infected muskrats, *Ondatra*, introduced into this region from Canada about 1929 to generate a fur industry. A variety of small mammals and tick species of the genus *Ixodes* have been blamed by Soviet workers to explain the evidently complex natural virus cycle.

Although there is no doubt that muskrats experience serious disease with high viremia when infected by OHF virus, it is not clear how they acquire the infection. Experimental studies show that this mammal is readily infected orally and that the OHF virus is naturally present in water frequented by muskrats and other rodents. Persons trapping and skinning these animals formerly accounted for many cases during the winter and early spring months, and the possibility of aerosol transmission exists, since several laboratory infections have been recorded from such exposure. Muskrat populations have declined dramatically for unknown reasons in recent years, so that today the few cases reported occur mainly in May, June, and August, are all secondary to tick bite, and affect principally young women who work on farms.

Cross-protection against OHF may be afforded by tick-borne encephalitis vaccines. However, given the low incidence of infection, vaccination is not a practical measure except for laboratory workers and, perhaps, muskrat hunters.

Viruses of the Family *Bunyaviridae*

Viruses of this family are widely distributed, and infection of humans may range from asymptomatic seroconversion to fulminant hemorrhagic disease and death. Many viruses of this family have not yet been associated with human disease. Four major genera include human pathogens; *Bunyavirus, Phlebovirus, Nairovirus,* and *Hantavirus*. Viruses of the genus *Bunyavirus* are most often transmitted by mosquitoes and are not known to cause hemorrhagic disease. Phleboviruses take their name from sandflies (genus *Phlebotomus*) which often serve as vectors; however Rift Valley fever virus, the only phlebovirus to cause hemorrhagic disease in humans, is thought to be transmitted primarily by mosquitoes. Ticks serve as the principal vector for nairoviruses, and the hantaviruses are maintained in nature by chronically infected rodent hosts, similar to the arenaviruses.

Rift Valley Fever

Until 1977, outbreaks of Rift Valley fever (RVF) were limited to small numbers of cases observed in eastern and southern Africa in association with major epizootics among large wild and domestic animals. In that year, however, portions of the lower Nile River delta in Egypt were struck by an explosive epidemic-enzootic in which an estimated 200,000 cases with at least 598 deaths were recorded.

RVF virus is a member of the genus *Phlebovirus*, family *Bunyaviridae*. Clinical illness in humans as observed in eastern and southern Africa is usually an undifferentiated acute febrile illness marked by high but brief fever and no sequelae. Serious complications of clinical ocular serous retinopathy with central scotomata are seen in about 1 percent of cases, and in another 1 percent fulminant acute, usually nonicteric, hepatitis and hemorrhage with death develop. Nothing resembling the Egyptian epidemic had ever occurred before, however. In this outbreak patients with seemingly typical self-limited illnesses suddenly had hemorrhagic manifestations (gastrointestinal and other mucous membrane bleeding and skin petechiae) and died within 1 to 3 days. Infection-morbidity rates were not accurately determined, but it is estimated that up to 20 percent of persons of all ages and both sexes were infected in the Ismailia district. A similar outbreak occurred in 1993, although not as severe as that of 1977–1978, but nonetheless leading to as many as 6,000 human infections in Aswan Governorate and ultimately spreading to Sharkiya and Giza Governorates in the Nile River Delta. A unique characteristic of this outbreak was the preponderance of ocular disease, an infrequent and late manifestation seen during the earlier Egyptian outbreak.

Although the ecology of RVF virus in Africa is still not clear, there is evidence suggesting that biological transmission of the agent may be principally attributed to mosquitoes of the genus *Aedes*. In eastern and southern Africa, the association of RVF maintenance cycles with specific breeding habitats of *A. mcintoshi* (shallow depressions called "dambos") has been elucidated in Kenya. During periods of high rainfall, flooding of dambos results in an abundance of *Aedes* and recrudescence of virus in transovarially infected mosquitoes. The latter initiate infection in domestic livestock, with secondary cycles of virus transmission being affected by *Anopheles, Culex*, and *Erethmapodites* vectors. Mechanical transmission by biting arthropods seems likely in addition because of the very high viremia levels (10^6 to 10^9 infectious units) reached in many domestic animals, and direct transmission to humans handling infected large animals or their carcasses is a recurrent phenomenon. Both contact with infectious blood and infectious aerosols are suspected as mechanisms.

The vectors involved in the Egyptian epidemic-epizootics have not been conclusively elucidated; the principal candidate for the 1977–1978 outbreak is the mosquito *Culex pipiens quinquefasciatus*, which was present in large numbers in houses and environs during the months of October and November, when most cases occurred. This species was likewise abundant in collections made during the 1993 outbreak, but definitive demonstration that this is the principal epidemic vector remains elusive.

Retrospective evidence now suggests that the virus may have reached Egypt from the Sudan, where animal epizootics were documented during the 5-year period before 1977. Subsequent outbreaks involving animals and humans have been reported in Mauritania (1987) and Madagascar (1990), in addition to the recurrence in Egypt in 1993. National and international concern over this emergent disease is not limited to public health workers. RVF virus causes a serious pantropic infection in domestic animals with significant mortality and high rates of abortion. Since it occurs naturally only in Africa, other nations are vitally interested in preventing its introduction into their animal industries. Thus work with this virus in the United States and many other countries is either totally proscribed or limited to facilities with a maximum containment configuration.

To date there is no treatment for the human disease, although the antiviral drug ribavirin, as well as interferon and interferon inducers, shows promise in preclinical studies. Inactivated vaccines provide immunity for 2 years after two or three doses and have been used to immunize livestock. Such products, however, are of little use should an outbreak occur in a previously uninfected country. The dynamics of virus transmission revealed in Egypt are so strikingly similar to those of VEE virus in the Americas that a live vaccine for animals that will confer rapid protection and curtail arthropod virus transmission is urgently needed. A live vaccine developed in South Africa is produced, but has been associated with abortion in sheep. More recently, a live vaccine (MP-12) developed in the United States appears safe and highly effective but requires field testing. Such a vaccine, together with emergency mosquito-control measures, forms a rational armamentarium against a major tragedy, which could strike inside or away from Africa. Killed vaccines for human use have been used to protect laboratory workers and military populations.

Crimean-Congo Hemorrhagic Fever

Although compatible clinical accounts of Crimean-Congo hemorrhagic fever (CCHF) in central Asia date to the thirteenth century, epidemics occurring during World War II in the Crimea provided the first modern recognition and the name of this clinically serious syndrome. The causative agent of the disease was finally isolated in newborn mice in 1968. It was found to be a member of the large *Bunyaviridae* family, genus *Nairovirus*, and, surprisingly, was antigenically indistinguishable from a virus of African origin, Congo virus, originally discovered in 1956. This virus was subsequently proved to be responsible for previously independent nosologic hemorrhagic entities termed Bulgarian and central Asia hemorrhagic fever and has been designated as Crimean-Congo hemorrhagic fever virus.

The clinical disease caused by CCHF outside Africa is one of the most virulent viral hemorrhagic fevers. The incubation period is brief (2 to 9 days), and the onset of fever and nonspecific symptoms is sudden. Hemorrhagic manifestations, often with severe blood loss, appear after 3 to 7 days of illness. There are various mild neurological manifestations as well, and surviving patients occasionally suffer peripheral neuritis, emotional disturbances, or both for months or even years. The disease is acquired by exposure to infected ticks or by close contact with persons who have the disease. Case-fatality rates average 13 to 25 percent for tick-transmitted disease, but nearly 40 percent for contact infection, which is frequently nosocomial where strict isolation of patients and use of protective clothing are not practiced. Attack rates in certain areas of the former Soviet Union have reached 14/1,000 in "epidemic" years. The infection morbidity ratio in the Astrakhan and Rostov regions has been estimated at about 6:1.

Depending on the geographical area, a large variety of tick species has been implicated in the natural cycle and transmission to humans of CCHF virus. In Bulgaria and the valleys of the lower Don and Volga Rivers of the Soviet Union, *Hyalomma marginatum*, a two-host species, is the principal vector. Immature stages parasitize hares, small rodents, and ground-feeding birds, while adults favor large domestic animals, such as cattle and sheep, and also attack humans. Persons engaged in pastoral and agricultural activities are most often attacked, and most cases occur during April to July, the period of peak activity of the adult ticks. Outbreaks of disease in central Asia are less strongly seasonal but tend to occur most often during summer months and are thought to be transmitted by ticks of the genera *Hyalomma*, *Rhipicephalus*, and *Boophilus*, which have life cycles ranging from single to as many as three hosts, most of which are large domestic animals. This epidemiological pattern extends from Dubai, Iraq, and Iran as far east as Pakistan.

To date approximately 70 human cases have been recognized in Africa, including temperate South Africa and tropical areas of eastern, western, and central Africa. The virus has been recovered on numerous occasions from ticks, cattle, and hedgehogs in these areas. The case-fatality rate (30 percent in South Africa) is similar to that in eastern Europe and the Soviet Union, and there is no evidence of a difference in virulence between virus strains.

The dynamics of virus maintenance in nature are not clear. CCHF in the Soviet Union has decreased significantly since 1970, but the biological correlates of this phenomenon were not elucidated. There is good evidence that CCHF virus is maintained serially in *H. marginatum* ticks by overwintering in infected nymphs and by both transstadial and transovarial passage. Hares experience viremia and can, therefore, infect larval and nymphal ticks, but birds apparently serve only as hosts for tick reproduction. Viral biology in ticks and vertebrate hosts in Asia and Africa is even less well known.

Soviet workers state that virus-specific passive antibodies are of value in therapy of CCHF if given during the initial 3 days of illness. An immunoglobulin formulation for intravenous administration is used in Bulgaria, with good results reported. A formalinized mouse brain vaccine has been produced and tested in more than 150,000 persons in Bulgaria, but no definitive conclusions as to efficacy have been reported. Prevention of disease is stressed in the Soviet Union through use of personal measures, such as special clothing, tick repellents, and the systematic dipping of livestock to control adult stages of tick vectors. Whether these measures or natural forces are responsible for the observed decline in disease in the Volga and Don River basins during this decade is not known.

The lack of an animal model of CCHF disease is an obstacle to development of a vaccine and an antiviral drug. Ribavirin may be an effective therapeutic agent. In uncontrolled trials in South Africa, early initiation of intravenous therapy is said to be lifesaving. Given orally, the drug may also be useful for postexposure prophylaxis of case contacts. Future work on this disease is dependent on construction of more maximum containment laboratories since CCHF virus is a class IV pathogen, and it is important to remember that CCHF is the hemorrhagic fever most likely to be confused with a noninfectious cause of acute gastrointestinal hemorrhage, with potentially devastating consequences to patient and medical staff alike.

Hemorrhagic Fever with Renal Syndrome

Hemorrhagic fever with renal syndrome (HFRS) is a general term used to denote a constellation of similar clinical diseases caused by related viruses of the genus *Hantavirus*, family *Bunyaviridae*. Many synonyms exist for this disease, including epidemic hemorrhagic fever, Korean hemorrhagic fever, hemorrhagic nephrosonephritis, nephropathia epidemica, and others. Like arenaviruses, the hantaviruses are maintained in nature by chronic infection of rodent hosts, with humans becoming infected following aerosol exposure to infectious excreta or occasionally by bite. Unlike arenaviruses, nosocomial outbreaks or person-to-person transmission have not been recorded for viruses that cause HFRS (but see hantavirus pulmonary syndrome below). Many different hantaviruses have now been recognized, and each appears to be associated with a specific rodent host (Table 13-5). Consequently, the distribution of individual hantaviruses is dependent upon the distribution of its rodent host, and risks of human infection are directly related to the amount of potential contact existing between these rodents and humans. The prototype hantavirus is Hantaan virus, cause of epidemic hemorrhagic fever in China and Korean hemorrhagic fever in Korea, which occurs in a wide belt across Eurasia from Japan and Korea to the Ural mountains of Russia and including much of China. Hantaan virus is maintained by the striped field mouse, *Apodemus agrarius*, and humans are most frequently infected in the fall and early winter months, when adults in rural areas are exposed as part of harvest activities. Also commonly infected are military populations while on field maneuvers, shepherds, woodcutters, campers, and others involved in outdoor activities. Other hantaviruses causing HFRS include Seoul virus, associated with domestic rats (*Rattus rattus, Rattus norvegicus*) and found virtually worldwide, wherever rats are abundant; Puumala virus, maintained by the bank vole, *Clethrionomys glareolus*, and abundant in western Europe, especially in western Russia and Scandinavia, and Dobrava/Belgrade virus, now known only in the Balkans region of Europe and thought to be hosted by *Apodemus flavicollis*.

Incidence rates of HFRS vary by country, the virus present, and the natural variation in abundance of their principal rodent hosts. In China, approximately 100,000 cases occur annually or about 0.1 per 1,000 population, and rates of about 0.2 to 0.5 per 1,000 have been recorded among the Korean military. The incidence rate of nephropathia epidemica due to Puumala virus is about 0.01 to greater than 0.2 per 1,000, depending upon the abundance of its rodent host. The incidence rates of Seoul and Dobrava/Belgrade viruses are unknown, but likely to be less than those for Hantaan and Puumala.

Classic HFRS has a variable but potentially long incubation period up to 4 weeks. The disease is characterized by five phases: a *febrile phase* of 3 to 7 days' duration with fever, malaise, headache, abdominal

TABLE 13-5. HANTAVIRUSES KNOWN TO CAUSE HUMAN DISEASE

Virus	Virus Abbreviation	Host	Original Isolation	Disease
Hantaan	HTN	*Apodemus agrarius*	Korea	HFRS
Seoul	SEO	*Rattus norvegicus, Rattus rattus*	Korea	HFRS
Dobrava/Belgrade	DOB	*Apodemus flavicollis*	Slovenia	HFRS
Puumala	PUU	*Clethrionomys glareolus*	Finland	HFRS/NE
Sin Nombre	SN	*Peromyscus maniculatus*	New Mexico	HPS
Black Creek Canal	BCC	*Sigmodon hispidus*	Florida	HPS
New York	NY	*Peromyscus leucopus*	Long Island, New York	HPS
Bayou	BAY	*Oryzomys palustris*	Louisiana	HPS
Andes		Unknown (human derived)	Patagonia, Argentina (sequence only)	HPS

Abbreviations: HFRS, hemorrhagic fever with renal syndrome; NE, nephropathia epidemica; HPS, hantavirus pulmonary syndrome.

pain, nausea, vomiting, facial flushing, petechiae, and conjunctival hemorrhage, a *hypotensive phase* of a few hours to 3 days' duration, when hypotension, shock, visual blurring, hemorrhagic signs, and a drop in blood pressure occur, an *oliguric phase* of 3 to 7 days' duration during which oliguria or anuria predominates and hemorrhagic manifestations may worsen, a *diuretic phase* of days' to weeks' duration when polyuria predominates, and a prolonged *convalescence phase* of weeks to months. Mortality rates for classic HFRS due to Hantaan virus range from 1 to 10 percent, varying greatly depending upon the quality of care available. Seoul virus causes a similar but generally milder disease with mortality rates less than 1 percent, as does Puumala virus. Dobrava/Belgrade virus appears to have a mortality rate at least equal to classic Hantaan, although relatively few patients have been documented. Seoul virus has also been associated with outbreaks of HFRS traced to infected laboratory rat colonies. Seoul virus is known to be abundant in urban rats in many large cities, including in the United States, and recent studies among Baltimore residents suggest that past infection with Seoul virus may be associated with subsequent development of hypertensive renal disease.

Diagnosis of HFRS is hampered by the lack of readily available diagnostic tests and that it is not often considered in the differential diagnosis of physicians in nonendemic countries. A placebo-controlled trial of intravenous ribavirin conducted in 1986–1987 in China showed that initiation of treatment early in the course of the disease reduced mortality and the incidence of renal failure and hemorrhage.

Control of HFRS relies primarily on reduction of potential human-rodent contact through good sanitation and waste management, rodent control, and rodent-proofing buildings. It is difficult to reduce exposure to rodents for rural populations, especially for those individuals staying in temporary campsites, but careful management of foods and waste may reduce the number of rodents attracted. A commercially available inactivated vaccine has been marketed in Korea, although its efficacy has yet to be demonstrated. Inactivated vaccines for Hantaan virus are also under field tests in China, and efforts are under way to develop molecularly based vaccines for both Hantaan and Puumala viruses.

Hantavirus Pulmonary Syndrome (HPS)

In 1993 hantavirus pulmonary syndrome (HPS) was first recognized when a cluster of fatal unexplained adult respiratory distress syndrome cases occurred among otherwise healthy young adults in the southwestern United States. The disease is a severe, systemic illness characterized by fever, myalgia, cough, headache, and gastrointestinal symptoms, followed by abrupt onset of noncardiogenic pulmonary edema and shock, often leading to death. Initial investigations determined that the disease was caused by a new hantavirus, subsequently named Sin Nombre virus, and found to be maintained in nature by the deer mouse, *Peromyscus maniculatus*. Approximately 150 cases of HPS have now been documented in the United States, with a mortality rate of about 50 percent. Recently cases of HPS have been seen in individuals residing in areas outside the natural range of *P. maniculatus*, and it is now clear that several other genetically and antigenically related viruses are capable of causing HPS (Table 13-5), including newly recognized hantaviruses found in South America and maintained by field rodents there. A disturbing finding yet to be confirmed is the apparent person-to-person transmission of HPS among individuals infected in Argentina.

Rickettsial Infections

Bradley N. Doebbeling

There are at least 14 major rickettsial diseases of humans, which are caused by six antigenically related groups of organisms (Table 13-6). Most of the rickettsioses are characterized by the syndrome of severe headache, fever, myalgias, and a quite variable rash. There is no rash with Q fever. The epidemiological and public health aspects of rickettsial diseases are emphasized in this account. More comprehensive reviews of the historical, clinical, microbiological, and diagnostic aspects of the rickettsial infections are available elsewhere.[1–6]

The Rickettsiaceae that are pathogenic for humans are classified into five genera: *Rickettsia* (including typhus and spotted fever groups), *Orientia* (scrub typhus), *Rochalimaea, Coxiella*, and *Ehrlichia*. The latter organisms have only recently been shown to be important causes of human disease. Numerous other rickettsiae occur as parasites of vertebrates and arthropods. Although a few of these may be of minor importance as human pathogens, they are not considered here.

Considerable progress has been made in the past decade in clarifying the taxonomy, biochemistry, genetics, and morphology of the Rickettsiaceae. The rickettsiae are obligately intracellular parasites that can propagate only in living cells. They are small coccoid to rod-shaped bacteria, usually 0.3 to 0.5 μm in diameter and up to 2.0 μm in length. The rickettsiae have typical bacterial cell walls and cytoplasmic membranes, contain both DNA and RNA, and divide by binary fission. They may be cultured and isolated in several laboratory animal species, arthropod vectors, embryonated eggs, and some cell cultures; however, this is a time-consuming, expensive, and occasionally dangerous process.

Serology is the mainstay of laboratory diagnosis, although diagnostic titers are not achieved until the second week of illness or later. Indirect fluorescent antibody (IFA) tests are the most widely accepted serological diagnostic techniques; they are now available for all the human rickettsioses. The complement-fixation (CF) test using acute- and convalescent-phase sera and the nonspecific Weil-Felix (WF) reaction for agglutinating antibodies against certain *Proteus* strains are still widely used, although both tests lack sensitivity.[1] A 4-fold rise in titer by any technique other than the WF reaction is considered diagnostic. Immunohistology, if available, may demonstrate *Rickettsia rickettsii* in the skin lesions of Rocky Mountain spotted fever or *Rickettsia conorii* in the lesions of Mediterranean spotted fever. For most rickettsial infections, however, therapy must be initiated on the basis of clinical presentation and epidemiological setting.

The natural life cycles of rickettsiae involve arthropod vectors (lice, fleas, mites, or ticks) and to a lesser extent various vertebrate hosts. In ticks and mites, transovarial transmission of the agent to the offspring frequently occurs. The vector transmits the rickettsiae to animals or humans by direct bite inoculation, fecal contamination of the bite wound, or scratches or other skin breaks; occasionally inhalation of aerosols may occur. Humans are incidental hosts and not important in the life cycle of the rickettsial organism, with the exception of louse-borne typhus. In the latter disease, humans are the major reservoirs.

Rickettsial infections cause a generalized capillary and small-vessel vasculitis, with consequent damage in the host's skin, brain, lungs, and other organs. Chronic infection or late relapse (especially

TABLE 13-6. RICKETTSIAL DISEASES OF HUMANS

Disease	Etiological Agent	Geographical Distribution	Vector(s)	Natural Hosts
■ Typhus Group				
Epidemic typhus	*Rickettsia prowazekii*	Africa, Central and South America, Asia, potentially worldwide	Human body louse [*Pediculus humanus corporis*]	Humans; flying squirrel, others[?]
Brill-Zinsser disease	*Rickettsia prowazekii*	Worldwide	None	Humans[recurrent attacks]
Murine typhus	*Rickettsia typhi* [formerly *L. mooseri*]	Temperate zones, worldwide	Oriental rat flea [*Xenopsylla cheopis*], others[?]	Rats [*Rattus rattus, Rattus norvegicus*], cats, opossums, other peridomestic mammals[?]
■ Scrub Typhus Group				
Scrub typhus	*Orientia tsutsugamushi* (formerly *Rickettsia tsutsugamushi*)	Asia, Australia, Pacific Islands	Larval trombiculid mites [*Leptotrombidium* species]	Small wild rodents, birds
■ Spotted Fever Group				
Rocky Mountain spotted fever (and related spotted fevers)	*Rickettsia rickettsii*	Western hemisphere	Numerous tick species [*Dermacentor, Amblyomma, Rhipicephalus, Haemaphysalis*]	Numerous small mammals [rodents, rabbits, hares and dogs]
Mediterranean spotted fever	*Rickettsia conorii*	Mediterranean region, Black Sea region, Middle East, Africa, India	Numerous tick species [*Rhipicephalus, Hyalomma, Amblyomma, Dermacentor*[?], *Ixodes*[?]]	Small mammals [rodents, dogs], birds[?]
North Asian tick typhus	*Rickettsia sibirica*	Siberia, central Asia, China, Mongolia, Pakistan [?]eastern Europe	Various tick species [*Dermacentor, Haemaphysalis, Rhipicephalus*]	Small mammals [rodents]; domestic animals[?]
Queensland tick typhus	*Rickettsia australis*	Australia	Ticks [*Ixodes holocyclus, Ixodes tasmani*]	Small marsupials, rodents
Rickettsialpox	*Rickettsia akari*	North America, former Soviet Union, Korea, South Africa	Gamasid mite [*Liponyssoides* [= *Allodermanyssus*] *sanguineus*]	House mouse [*Mus musculus*], other rodents[?]
■ Miscellaneous				
Ehrlichiosis	*Ehrlichia canis*	United States, unknown	*Rhipicephalus sanguineus*[?]	Canids
Sennetsu fever	*Ehrlichia sennetsu*	Japan	Unknown	Humans[?]
Q fever	*Coxiella burnetii*	Worldwide	Inhalation, ingestion[?], numerous ixodid and argasid tick species	Cattle, sheep, goats, other domestic animals; numerous wild mammals; birds[?]
Trench fever	*Rochalimaea quintana*	Potentially worldwide	Human body louse [*Pediculus humanus corporis*]	Humans

in epidemic typhus) and long-term persistence of rickettsiae in lymph nodes or other tissues has been documented. Antibiotic treatment with tetracyclines or chloramphenicol is usually effective if started early. The drugs inhibit the organisms' growth rather than kill them; general supportive measures and the host's immune response are important factors in recovery. Prevention and control of rickettsial diseases depend on avoidance of vector-infested sites, vector and vertebrate host control by habitat modification, or use of appropriate pesticides.

▶ TYPHUS GROUP

Epidemic Typhus

Rickettsia prowazekii has been responsible for millions of cases of epidemic or louse-borne typhus (typhus exanthematicus, classic typhus fever) and uncounted deaths throughout history. This disease has disappeared from much of the world except remote areas of Africa, Asia, Central, and South America. It may, however, recur under conditions of famine, war, or other disasters.

Gerhard distinguished the disease from typhoid fever clinically in 1836, and Brill described a milder (recrudescent) form unassociated with body lice in 1910. After an incubation period of 1 to 2 weeks, there is an abrupt onset of fever, chills, malaise, muscle ache, and severe headache. Approximately 5 days later a faint pink macular rash usually develops over the upper trunk. The rash may become darker, maculopapular, and confluent, covering the entire body but usually sparing the face, palms, and soles, or it may gradually fade away. High fever becomes constant early, typically lasting up to 2 weeks, terminating by lysis. Changes in mental status occur frequently, occasionally with delirium or coma. Mortality ranges from 5 to 40 percent if the disease is untreated, increasing with age. Tetracycline or chloramphenicol is usually curative if given early. Recovery is complete, with immunity to reinfection. Epidemic typhus may recur decades later, however, as Brill-Zinsser (BZ) disease, which is usually milder with little or no rash.

Humans are the hosts and long-term reservoirs. The body louse, *Pediculus humanus corporis*, is infected by a blood meal from a rickettsemic patient. *R. prowazekii* replicates in the louse's intestinal tract and then is excreted in its feces within 1 week. After a blood meal, the louse defecates, contaminating the broken skin of the host. Other potential mechanisms of infection include either mucosal contact or inhalation of dried louse feces. The louse dies of its rickettsial infection within a few weeks. *R. prowazekii*, however, may remain viable for months to years in the dried state. Lice can be infected by feeding on persons with BZ disease as well as on those with acute typhus, thus ensuring the perpetuation of *R. prowazekii*. Head lice, crab lice, and some fleas may be experimentally infected, although their role as natural vectors is uncertain. Transmission between humans usually requires close personal contact or exposure to contaminated clothing or bedding. Rickettsiae are not present in human secretions, so there is no direct person-to-person spread.

Extrahuman reservoirs have been suspected in ticks and certain animal species; yet most of the evidence is tenuous. The southern flying squirrel, *Glaucomys volans*, found in the eastern United States, has recently been implicated as an animal reservoir for *R. prowazekii*. Human infections have been linked to the flying squirrel, although the mode of transmission has yet to be demonstrated.[4] This flying squirrel–associated typhus agent may have a lower virulence than the louse-borne variant, although better health and nutritional status, living conditions, and antirickettsial treatment might explain the absence of reported fatalities. While human body lice may be experimentally infected with *R. prowazekii* from flying squirrels, the general scarcity of body lice in the United States may explain the lack of outbreaks in this country.[1]

Certain social factors that predispose to epidemic typhus, including overcrowding, poverty, and infrequent bathing or changing of clothes, are especially common during cold weather or periods of war. Most cases occur in the winter or spring. Epidemic typhus nearly disappeared from Europe, where it was once common, coincident with improved sanitation, delousing measures, antibiotics, and better medical care after World War II. Under international sanitary regulations, louse-borne typhus ceased to be a quarantinable disease in 1971, although the World Health Organization (WHO) continues to monitor the disease because of its epidemic potential. Endemic foci still produce thousands of cases annually in highland areas of central Africa (particularly Rwanda, Burundi, and Ethiopia) and southern Africa, the Himalayas and Asian highlands, Mexico, and Central and South America. Case reporting is incomplete because of inadequate surveillance and often undocumented by specific laboratory tests, particularly in the areas of highest endemicity. The presence of the vector, as determined by social, cultural, and climatic conditions, affects the geographic distribution of cases. No epidemics have occurred in the United States since 1893, and the last recorded small outbreak occurred in 1921. Brill-Zinsser disease is reported sporadically from many countries, particularly in southeastern Europe.

Prevention of epidemic typhus is accomplished primarily by application of residual insecticide powder to the individual, the clothing, and the bedding on which the eggs are laid and lice reside. Several applications may be required periodically, since the eggs are resistant to most insecticides and continue to hatch. A pediculicide, such as DDT or lindane, that is effective on the local body louse population should be used. Alternatively, malathion or carbaryl may be effective in resistant settings. Washing clothes in hot water kills lice and eggs. Head lice and pubic lice should also be eradicated with effective chemical agents. Similar treatment of family or other close contacts is advisable. Once deloused, the patient need not be quarantined, but others who have been exposed should remain under surveillance for the disease for 2 weeks. In epidemics, treatment of the entire community with insecticide is often the most practical and effective approach.

As a secondary measure, immunization of all susceptible persons during an outbreak may also be useful. Although no vaccine is currently available commercially, under epidemic conditions, the live attenuated strain would be acceptable in many situations even though mild typhus occurs in a small portion of vaccine recipients and reversion to virulence has been described.

Murine Typhus

In 1926 Maxcy differentiated murine or endemic typhus (flea-borne typhus, shop typhus, urban typhus) from epidemic typhus in the eastern United States on clinical and epidemiological grounds. The rodent reservoir and flea vector of the agent, *Rickettsia typhi* (formerly *Rickettsia mooseri*), were demonstrated in the early 1930s.

Murine typhus is usually milder than epidemic typhus, with an incubation period of 1 to 2 weeks. Fever lasts 1 to 2 weeks, often accompanied by persistent headache, myalgia, nausea and vomiting, abdominal pains, conjunctivitis, splenomegaly, and pneumonitis; delirium, stupor, or coma occurs rarely. On the fourth day a macular rash usually appears (in 20 to 80 percent of the patients, depending on the darkness of the skin pigmentation) on the chest and abdomen, becoming maculopapular and persisting 4 to 8 days without significant limb involvement. Permanent sequelae are rare, and no BZ-like phenomenon has been observed. Death occurs in approximately 1 percent of cases, and a single attack confers immunity.

Murine typhus occurs in tropical, subtropical, and temperate zones throughout the world, principally in coastal regions of Malaysia, southeast Asia, Africa, Central America, and the Mediterranean region. In the United States, it is most prevalent in Texas and Southern California. During the 15-year period prior to 1946 approximately 42,000 cases occurred. Subsequently, a sharp decrease occurred; this was attributed primarily to reductions in the populations of the Oriental rat flea, *Xenopus cheopis*, by use of DDT, and improved rat control. Fewer than 80 cases are now recorded annually in the United States, although the disease is probably greatly underreported. Murine typhus occurs primarily in seaports, urban areas, and certain rural settings infested by wild rats (e.g., grain-storage facilities). A seasonal incidence peak occurs in late summer and fall, although the disease peaks in late spring and early summer along the Gulf Coast. Cases tend to be sporadic or to occur in clusters or small outbreaks related to common exposure to rat-flea focus. The infection is relatively frequent in southern Texas, particularly among older adults and Hispanics,[7] in a cycle involving cat fleas and opossums, which also maintain a similar pathogenic typhus group organism, *Rickettsia filis*. There is no documented person-to-person spread.

The main life cycle involves a reservoir of rats (*Rattus rattus* and *Rattus norvegicus*) and other rodents and the vector the flea *cheopis*. The rat flea is infected by the blood of a rickettsemic host, remains infected for life, and readily infects other rats and humans. *R. typhi* infects the intestinal tract and feces of the flea, and transovarial transmission may occur. Flea feces or crushed fleas apparently contaminate skin breaks or the mucous membranes; direct flea bites or inhalation of aerosols may also cause infection. The human flea, *Pulex irritans*, and the human body louse may play a role in transmission. Numerous wild vertebrates are natural hosts and may bring infected fleas into close proximity. Dog and cat fleas have been suspected as occasional vectors for humans.

Prevention requires ongoing control of the natural host and vector: rodent-control measures and use of organophosphate or carbamate insecticides. Local public health authorities should be consulted for advice on approved residual-action insecticides to apply to rat habitats. Flea control should be achieved initially, followed by rat poisoning and trapping, rodent-proofing of buildings, and elimination of rodent shelter and food attractants. Failure to control the flea population initially may lead to human outbreaks as the infected fleas move from dying rats to humans. There is no specific vaccine.

Scrub Typhus

Although scrub typhus (tsutsugamushi disease, mite-borne typhus, Japanese river fever, tropical typhus, rural typhus) was described by Li Shi-Zhen in sixteenth-century China, definitive studies were first reported by Japanese workers in the late nineteenth century. The ancient name for scrub typhus in China was *sha shi du*, meaning chigger fever.[8] The disease is known in Japan as tsutsugamushi disease, which, roughly translated, means "noxious mite."[9] Fletcher first differentiated murine typhus and scrub typhus in 1926. A rickettsial agent (*Orientia orientalis*) was described in 1930, and the current name (*Orientia tsutsugamushi*) was assigned in 1931. There is genetic, antigenic, and pathogenic diversity of the agent, with numerous serotypes recognized.

The clinical spectrum of scrub typhus is broad, with most infections of mild to moderate severity. Significant morbidity occurs regularly, however, and mortality rates range from 0 to 30 percent if the disease is untreated. The first sign of disease after an incubation period of 6 to 21 days is a vesicular lesion at the site of mite feeding, which later becomes an eschar or ulcer, with tender lymphadenopathy common. Although an eschar develops in 85 to 90 percent of patients,[9] in its absence the disease may be misdiagnosed as fever of unknown origin.[10] Fever lasts up to 2 weeks, accompanied by headache, myalgia, and occasionally conjunctivitis or cough. In one-third of the patients a central macular rash may appear on the trunk and in the axillary folds around the fifth day, spreading to involve the proximal arms and legs. The rash usually becomes maculopapular, lasting only a few days. Pneumonitis and encephalitis may occur.

Infection with one strain provides only short-term immunity against subsequent infection by others, and immunity even to homologous strains lasts for only 1 to 3 years. Nevertheless, second and even third attacks may be milder or atypical. No person-to-person transmission has been documented. Tetracyclines and chloramphenicol are relatively effective, but relapses are common, after short courses of therapy, often requiring another course of treatment. Doxycycline appears to be particularly reliable, and relapses are rare following its use for a full course.[8]

O. tsutsugamushi strains are widespread throughout much of the Far East and the western Pacific, including southeastern Asia, India, Pakistan, Indonesia, southern China, eastern Russia, Korea, Japan, the Philippines and the South Pacific islands, and northern Australia. It remains a leading cause of illness in indigenous populations throughout endemic areas. World War II brought the disease to the attention of the Western world; 18,000 cases occurred in U.S. troops, with up to a 35 percent mortality rate in some situations. Similarly, scrub typhus was a frequent source of illness in U.S. troops during the Vietnam conflict. Scrub typhus is seen in North America primarily among returning travelers. A well-defined seasonal occurrence that peaks during the hot, wet months occurs in many areas, although the disease may peak in the winter or occur year-round in other regions. Seasonal incidence varies by region but is related to the presence of the larval mite. The incidence of scrub typhus in Japan has markedly increased since 1975, predominantly during the winter.[9]

Larval mites ("chiggers") of the family Trombiculidae, subgenus *Leptotrombidium*, are the vectors and reservoirs. Although approximately 150 species have been described, only a few are known to be important vectors for humans (e.g., *L. deliensis, L. akamushi, L. fletcheri, L. arenicola, L. scutellare, L. pallidum,* and *L. pavlovksyi*). The larval mite feeds just once on the lymph and tissue juice of a mammalian host and transmits the agent by fecal contamination. Other life stages of the mite are free living only; transovarial or vertical transmission occurs regularly, with nearly all offspring affected.[9]

The ecological niches of *R. tsutsugamushi* are highly variable, being especially common in wet tropical and subtropical areas, including equatorial rain forests, along riverbanks and seashores, and occasionally in semideserts, Himalayan alpine meadows, and areas with harsh, cold winters.[8] The agent may persist in hyperendemic foci of vector mites as small as a few square feet.[9] The limited mobility of unfed larvae, the clustering of broods of larvae within a localized area, and the clustering of hundreds of larvae at a few sites on an individual animal, where they may be brushed off at one time, favor the focal distribution of larvae on the ground.[9] Endemic foci usually occur where secondary or transitional vegetation (e.g., abandoned farmland or human-made forest clearings) has created a habitat attractive to the natural hosts of the vector mites, particularly *Rattus* species. The chiggers or mites are not host-specific and will attack any animal, including humans, that invades their limited territory.

Focal areas known to be endemic should be avoided. Alternatively, vertebrate hosts and protective vegetation can be eliminated and the area can be treated with chlorinated hydrocarbons (e.g., lindane, dieldrin, or chlordane). Personal prophylaxis with protective clothing, treatment of clothing with insecticides such as benzyl benzoate, and application of mite repellents (diethyltoluamide) to the skin is useful. Prophylactic antibiotic use for short-term exposures has been shown to be effective. There is no commercial vaccine.

▶ SPOTTED FEVER GROUP

Rocky Mountain Spotted Fever

Rocky Mountain spotted fever (RMSF) is the best-known and most severe of the tick-borne rickettsioses. Although various names are used (São Paulo typhus, fiebre manchada), there is basically a single clinical entity and a single agent, *R. rickettsii*. Closely related species and diseases occur in Europe, Africa, Asia, and Australia (see below). RMSF has been recognized as a distinct entity in the United States since the late 1800s; various workers, most notably Ricketts in Montana (1906), defined the disease and described the natural cycle of the agent.

Illness usually begins abruptly 2 to 12 days after tick exposure. A high, persistent fever of 2 to 3 weeks' duration, severe headache, and myalgias are characteristic, while nausea, vomiting, abdominal pain, and conjunctivitis occur frequently. The maculopapular rash, present in about 90 percent of the cases, usually does not appear until the third day or later. The rash begins on the ankles or wrists and spreads rapidly to the rest of the body; later it becomes petechial in 50 percent of cases, and often is accompanied by edema. Involvement of the palm and soles is quite characteristic but occurs, only half of cases, used as a relatively late event. Headache is typically severe; meningismus or focal neurologic deficits may result, occasionally with permanent neurological sequelae. Necrosis of the skin lesions or gangrene of extremities occurs in only 4 percent of cases. Thrombocytopenia, anemia, coagulopathy, renal failure, pulmonary edema, and involvement of all organ systems may be seen. The overall fatality rate is about 20 percent untreated, higher in adults over 30, in males, in glucose-6-phosphate dehydrogenase–deficient persons, and in persons who are inadequately treated. Treatment should be initiated promptly on the basis of epidemiological setting and clinical suspicion. Immunohistologic examination of skin lesions for rickettsiae, if available, may provide immediate confirmation; however, most laboratory diagnoses are made retrospectively by means of serological studies. Supportive care is important in the management of the complications of RMSF. The disease is not contagious except by direct inoculation of contaminated blood.

Cases have been reported from across the country, with the highest prevalence in the south Atlantic and west-south-central states. Cases also occur in western Canada, from British Columbia to Saskatchewan. *R. rickettsii* produce a very similar disease in Mexico and Central and South America. The incidence of RMSF peaks during late spring and summer, although the disease occurs in temperate climates through the winter at a low incidence. Disease is most common among people exposed occupationally or recreationally to tick-infested areas. However, RMSF has been demonstrated in areas seemingly as unlikely as a public park in New York City.[10]

The vectors and major reservoir of *R. rickettsii* include various ixodid ticks, particularly the dog tick, *Dermacentor variabilis* in the East, and the wood tick, *Dermacentor andersoni* in the West. *Amblyoma cajennense* and *Rhipicephalus sanguineus* have been implicated in Mexico and Central and South America. Ticks on occasion may acquire the agent from a rickettsemic vertebrate hosts (e.g., cotton rat) during feeding. Dogs are also infected, sometimes developing clinical disease, and can readily transport ticks to the close proximity of humans.[11] The tick salivary glands, gut, and tissues become heavily infected with rickettsiae, which are maintained through transstadial (larva, nymph, adult) and transovarial transmission through repeated generations. During attachment and blood feeding, the tick inoculates rickettsiae in tick saliva into the skin. Even contact with crushed ticks may be hazardous since the salivary glands, tissues, and coxal fluid may contain organisms.

No commercial RMSF vaccine is available.

Other Spotted Fever Rickettsioses

The etiological agents and clinical manifestations of spotted fevers in the Eastern Hemisphere are sufficiently different to separate them from RMSF of the Western Hemisphere. Boutonneuse fever, Mediterranean spotted fever (Kenya tick typhus, South African tick-bite fever, Indian tick typhus, Marseilles fever) caused by *Rickettsia conorii*, occurs in the countries of southern Europe (Portugal, Spain, Italy, France), Asia, the Middle East, India, and eastern, northern, and southern Africa. Boutonneuse fever is the most ubiquitous of the spotted fever group of diseases and the most commonly seen rickettsial disease among travelers returning to North America.[12] The disease is transmitted by tick bite. Important vectors include ticks of the genera *Rhipicephalus, Amblyomma*, and *Haemaphysalis*. In the Mediterranean countries, where the disease has seen a recent resurgence, the common dog tick, *Rhipicephalus sanguineus*, is particularly important as both vector and transovarially maintained reservoir.[13,14] Returning travelers usually give a history of exposure to an endemic area with high grass or bush, although the bite of immature tick stages is usually not noticed.[12]

A mild to moderately severe illness, with high fever lasting a few days to 2 weeks, is typical. The name *boutonneuse fever* is derived from the buttonlike maculopapular rash, which is similar in timing and distribution to RMSF. The rash appears on about the third day and is usually generalized. Three fourths of patients develop a characteristic eschar ("tache noir") at the site of tick attachment.[14] Abrupt onset of headache, arthralgia, and myalgia is common. The rash persists 6 to 7 days and is less frequently associated with the progressive, hemorrhagic tendency of RMSF. Antibiotic therapy shortens the course of the illness. Although the disease is usually self-limited, fatal and very severe cases are not uncommon.

North Asian tick typhus (Siberian tick typhus, North Asian tick-borne rickettsiosis) is clinically similar to boutonneuse fever but is caused by a separate species, *Rickettsia sibirica*. It occurs in Siberia, other parts of Asiatic Russia, Mongolia, and China. The vectors include ticks of the genera *Dermacentor*, and *Haemaphysalis*. Various rodents and other wild mammals may play a role in the maintenance of these mainly transovarially passaged rickettsiae in nature. Another rickettsiosis of the spotted fever group caused by a novel rickettsia, *Rickettsia japonica*, has been described in Japan.[15]

North Queensland tick typhus is clinically similar, although the etiologic agent is the distinctive organism *Rickettsia australis*, which has been recognized only in eastern Australia. The natural history involves *Ixodes holocyclus* ticks. Another rickettsiosis caused by *Rickettsia honei* has been identified so far on Flinders Island in the Bass Straits between the continent and Tasmania. Spotted fever rickettsioses of undetermined etiology have been discovered in Thailand, Hong Kong, and Yucatan.

Avoidance of tick bite is the only reliable method for prevention of the tick-borne rickettsioses. Obviously, eradication of the vectors, the natural hosts, or the rickettsiae from their well-established niches in nature is not feasible. Protective clothing, tick repellents on skin or clothing, regular searching of the body for ticks and removal of them with tweezers, and chemically impregnated collars or shampoos for domestic pets are often useful.

Rickettsialpox

Rickettsialpox (vesicular rickettsiosis) was first recognized as a distinct clinical entity in apartment dwellers in New York City in 1946. *Rickettsia akari*, the causative agent, is related to a member of the spotted fever group.

The disease is relatively mild. Early in the incubation period of 7 to 21 days, a firm, red 1- to 3-cm papular lesion with surrounding erythema develops at the site of mite feeding, accompanied by regional lymphadenopathy. The papule ulcerates centrally, forming an eschar and a permanent scar. Systemic symptoms, including fever, chills, sweats, headache, myalgias, and occasionally photophobia, last approximately 1 week. A generalized maculopapular rash develops within a few days of the onset of symptoms on the face, trunk, and extremities. The rash becomes vesicular, eventually healing without scarring. Recovery is complete, and death has not been documented to occur.

Cases were subsequently also detected in Boston, West Hartford, Philadelphia, Cleveland, Pittsburgh, and Utah, with an annual incidence of nearly 200 cases. Recently only a few cases have been confirmed in the United States; the disease may be misdiagnosed as chickenpox or other rash diseases, or it may have actually decreased in frequency. Rickettsialpox has also been recognized in the Ukraine and in Croatia.

The vector in the United States is the mouse mite, *Lipomyssoides sanguineus*, a small colorless parasite of the house mouse, *Mus musculus*. All stages of the mite except the larvae ingest blood through a painless bite. Transstadial and transovarial transmission occur.[16] Residual insecticides and rodent-control measures may limit or eliminate the vector and thus rickettsial transmission to humans.

► TRENCH FEVER

Epidemics of trench fever (Wolhynian fever, 5-day fever, quintana fever) during World Wars I and II in troops living under crowded, unhygienic conditions brought this disease to prominence. Subsequently it has nearly disappeared, although it has been reported in Mexico. The etiological agent is *Rochalimaea* (formerly *Rickettsia*) *quintana*, which is genetically related to the typhus-group agents. *R. quintana* is an unusual species with the ability to grow on blood agar at 37°C (98°F) under 5 percent carbon dioxide. In addition, it can be isolated from feeding lice on the patient (xenodiagnosis).

The incubation period ranges from 9 to 17 days. Trench fever is self-limited, but patients may be severely ill for 6 to 8 weeks. Headache, malaise, myalgias, and single or multiple episodes of fever occur, and splenomegaly is common. A transient, macular rash may develop on the trunk and recur. Trench fever has a striking tendency to relapse, similar to Brill-Zinsser disease, and recurrences 20 to 30 years after primary infection have been documented. Rickettsemia may persist for many months, even when the patient is entirely free of symptoms.

The natural cycle had been thought to involve only humans and the human body louse, *Pediculus humanus corporis*. However, an agent (*Rochalimaea vinsonii*), which is similar or identical to *R. quintana* from a vole in Canada, suggests the possibility of a wildlife cycle. Lice remain infectious for life and appear unharmed by infection. Infected louse feces contaminate breaks in the skin, transmitting infection to humans. Transovarial transmission of *R. quintana* does not occur. Preventive measures include improvement in hygiene and living conditions and delousing if cases occur, as described for epidemic typhus.

► Q FEVER (QUERY FEVER)

In the 1930s, Derrick studied cases of "abattoir fever" in Brisbane, Australia, describing the agent, *Rickettsia burnetii*, now renamed *Coxiella burnetii*. In 1935, an agent isolated from *Dermacentor andersoni* ticks in Montana was found to be identical. *C burnetii* is a pleomorphic organism that differs from the *Rickettsia* species in its ability to grow in host cell acid phagolysosomes rather than in the cytoplasm or nucleus. The unusual resistance of *C. burnetii* to ultraviolet light, drying, heat, and chemical agents and its ability to persist in the environment may be due to its endospore-like differentiation.

Many infections are asymptomatic or mild, self-limited, febrile illnesses. After an incubation period of 2 to 4 weeks, Q fever often manifests as fever, malaise, myalgias, headache, weakness, anorexia, and weight loss, lasting a few days to several weeks or longer. Adult Q fever is a systemic disease frequently accompanied by pneumonitis and hepatic involvement. Convalescence is slow, although mortality is rare. In patients with chronic Q fever, endocarditis is the most frequent form and is often fatal. Tetracyclines and fluoroquinolones are useful but less efficacious in chronic Q fever, in which relapses may occur, requiring repeated treatment. *C. burnetii* may remain latent for years.

The diagnosis of Q fever is usually confirmed serologically. A 4-fold rise in the convalescent titers or a single IFA titer of 256 or greater is usually considered diagnostic. *C. burnetii* can be isolated from blood, sputum, urine, or spinal fluid, but this is rarely practical because of the biohazard posed by this highly infectious agent.

Q fever is essentially worldwide in distribution. *C. burnetii* is the most frequent and important cause of rickettsiosis in many areas, although it is seldom diagnosed in the United States. Q fever caused major epidemics during World War II ("Balkan grippe") in southern and eastern Europe. Sporadic or focal outbreaks occur wherever contact with domestic animals (predominantly cattle, sheep, and goats) occurs, particularly on farms, dairies, and abattoirs.

Many animals and various birds are natural hosts for the agent. Ticks develop a generalized, massive infection and appear to be important vectors. More than 40 species of naturally infected ixodid and argasis ticks are known, particularly of the genera *Amblyomma, Dermacentor, Haemaphysalis*, and *Ixodes*. Domestic animals, including cattle, sheep, and goats, are the main source of human illness. The agent persists in the environment for months or years, particularly in wool, hides, feces, dried placental detritus, dried tick feces, and soil. Inhalation is the usual route of infection for humans. Airborne transmission over long distances or from animal products transported from endemic sites may account for epidemiologically puzzling cases. Raw milk from infected cattle and goats contains *C. burnetii* and may transmit infection. Sheep used in medical research facilities have caused outbreaks, and special control measures have been advised.[17]

Control of the natural life cycles of *C. burnetii* in ticks and wild animals is clearly impossible. However, the main sources of human infection can be partially controlled by aerosol reduction and disinfection and appropriate disposal of infected animal tissues. Milk pasteurization should eliminate that mode of transmission. Vaccines for occupationally exposed workers have been demonstrated to be effective.

▶ EHRLICHIOSIS

There are two *Ehrlichia* species that cause human infections in the United States, *Ehrlichia chaffeensis* and an organism that is very closely related to *Ehrlichia phagocytophila* and *Ehrlichia equi*. The only member of the genus *Ehrlichia* previously known to cause disease in humans was *Ehrlichia sennetsu*, which caused a mononucleosis-like syndrome called Sennetsu fever, described in Japan in 1954. *Ehrlichia canis* was eventually shown to cause a puzzling syndrome of tropical canine pancytopenia in military working dogs in Vietnam, which was often fatal.[18] Other species of *Ehrlichia*, particularly *Ehrlichia risticii* (potomac horse fever), *E. equi* (equine granulocytic ehrlichiosis), and *E. phagocytophilia* (tick-borne fever) have been shown to be animal pathogens. In 1986 an acute febrile syndrome similar to RMSF was first recognized in humans.[18] The ehrlichiae differ from the *Rickettsia* species because they replicate within the host cell phagosome and are tropic for white blood cells.

The human monocytotropic ehrlichioses caused by *E. chaffeensis* usually begins with tick attachment, followed by a mean incubation period of 9 days. Acute onset of fever, malaise, myalgia, fatigue, and headache develops, occasionally with vomiting, cough, or dyspnea. Encephalopathy, coagulopathy, and azotemia occur in severe cases. The clinical presentation is remarkably similar to that of RMSF; however, a macular (nonpetechial) rash is present in less than one-half of the patients and leukopenia is common.[18–20] Diagnosis is based on clinical and epidemiological risk factors. IFA serologic study is usually confirmatory.

Human monocytic ehrlichiosis has been recognized primarily in the south central and southeastern United States, although it has occurred sporadically elsewhere. The disease is tick-borne with a peak incidence in May through July.[19,20] Most patients (75 percent) are male and are exposed occupationally or recreationally to ticks. Human monocytic ehrlichiosis is transmitted by *Amblyomma americanum* and possibly *Dermacentor variabilis* ticks from infected deer to humans.

Preventive measures include avoidance of exposure to ticks, as well as prompt removal of ticks when found.

Plague

Robert B. Craven • David T. Dennis

Human plague, historically known as "the plague" or "the Black Death," continues, in some instances, to produce panic and irrational responses even though the disease is curable and its spread is preventable. The association between rodent deaths, fleas, and human plague was not appreciated until late in the nineteenth century; since then, however, ecological factors have been recognized as crucial in understanding the epidemiology and control of this disease.

History

Three plague pandemics have been recorded in history.[1,2] The first pandemic severely affected the Roman Empire in the sixth and seventh centuries A.D. The second pandemic began in central Asia and spread to Europe in the fourteenth century. It is estimated that one-fourth of the affected populations perished in its early course. In England, as many as half of the total population died. Public health quarantine measures date from this time. The second pandemic waned over several centuries, and plague eventually disappeared from Europe. The third (modern) pandemic era began in China in the late nineteenth century when, in 1894, plague struck Hong Kong and then spread by rat-infested steamships to all inhabited continents. Within a few years of its initial spread, millions of persons had died of plague in India, and outbreaks had occurred in many countries of the world, including the United States.

During the modern pandemic, plague became established in rodent populations in widely scattered foci around the world.[1,3,4] It persisted in some areas for a few years (gulf coastal areas of the United States, Australia), or a few decades (Hawaii and the Philippine Islands), but in many areas it became entrenched. Plague foci are currently found throughout most of the world (Fig. 13-7). Some wild rodent plague foci have apparently receded; others have continued to spread, as has occurred in the western United States. These scattered residual plague foci are not amenable to elimination, and it

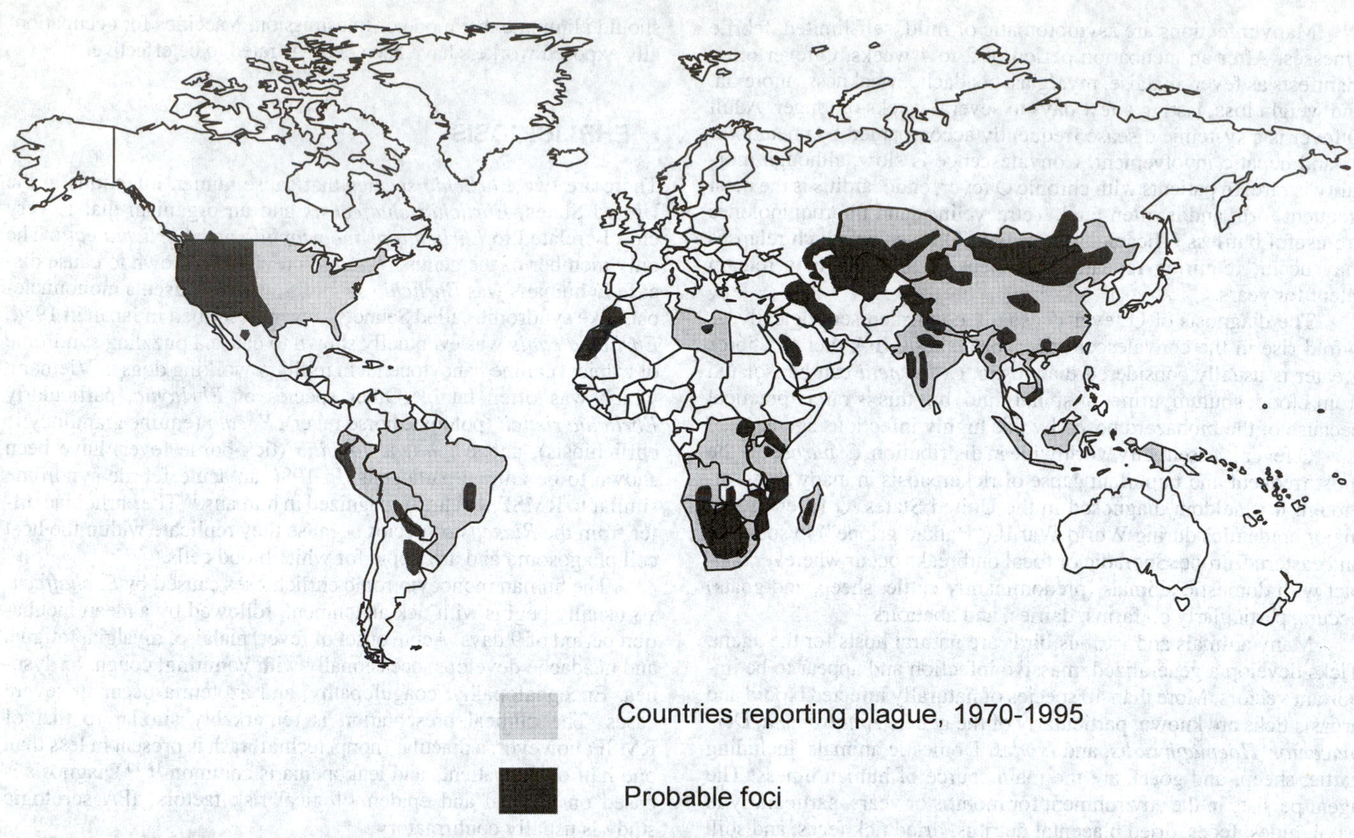

Figure 13-7. Distribution of natural foci of plague. (Compiled from the World Health Organization, the Centers for Disease Control and Prevention, and other sources.)

is unknown whether they will be stable, spontaneously die out, or expand.

Plague in Nature

The causative agent of plague, *Yersinia pestis*, is maintained in a natural reservoir of infected rodents and their fleas.[1,3,5,6] Naturally occurring plague is either enzootic or epizootic. In enzootic plague, *Y. pestis* is maintained in relatively disease-resistant rodent populations and the disease is stable, has a low mortality, and is not readily noticed (silent, quiescent). Enzootic plague is typically associated with a low human risk. In epizootic plague, *Y. pestis* infection is amplified in susceptible rodents and their fleas. The resultant rodent die-off promotes rapid and dangerous spread of plague, since infected fleas leave dead hosts to seek other blood sources, including humans. Rodent die-offs from epizootic plague are likely to be noticed, especially when diurnal rodents, such as prairie dogs, are affected.[3,6]

The Plague Organism

Y. pestis is a Gram-negative, bipolar staining, nonsporulating, nonmotile coccobacillus. It grows slowly in most nutrient bacteriologic media even at the optimum temperature of 28°C (82°F). On agar plates incubated at 37°C (98.6°F), colonies are barely discernible at 24 hours and are small (1 to 3 mm in diameter) at 48 hours. Stained smears of *Y. pestis* grown in a liquid medium may reveal pleomorphic cells occurring singly, in pairs, or in chains. Since other Gram-negative bacilli may appear to be bipolar, identification of *Y. pestis* by staining characteristics alone is unreliable. A positive fluorescent antibody (FA) test to detect the highly specific *Y. pestis* fraction 1 (F1) antigen provides a presumptive identification only, since interpretation of fluorescence is subjective and sometimes inconclusive. Isolation of *Y. pestis* in microbiological media and its lysis by a specific bacteriophage provide definitive (confirmatory) identification of *Y. pestis*.[2,7]

Flea Vectors

Fleas are the only arthropods known to transmit *Y. pestis* in nature.[4,8] The vector efficiency of fleas varies by species and by environmental conditions such as temperature and humidity.[9,10] High vector flea densities (flea indices) on rodent hosts are associated with increased likelihood of spread. Although fleas vary in their propensity to bite humans, any flea species should be considered a potential plague vector. When some highly efficient vectors, such as the oriental rat flea (*Xenopsylla cheopis*) ingest an infected blood meal, plague bacilli multiply to enormous numbers and block the flea's foregut (proventriculus). Starved blocked fleas avidly seek new hosts; attempts to feed result in regurgitation of *Y. pestis* organisms into the bite wound, thus enhancing the probability of transmission. The vector efficiency of the oriental rat flea is markedly decreased at temperatures of 28°C and above, since at these higher temperatures blockages undergo enzymatic lysis.[10,11]

Vertebrate Hosts

Rodents serve as the primary hosts for both enzootic (maintenance) and epizootic (amplification) plague, and their fleas are the primary source of spread. Other naturally involved mammals—such as lagomorphs (rabbits, hares), carnivores (canids, felids, mustellids), and humans—are incidental hosts that only occasionally serve as direct (not flea-mediated) sources of infection to other animals or humans.

Epidemic plague is historically associated with domestic rats (the black or roof rat, *Rattus rattus*, and the brown or Norway rat, *Rattus norvegicus*) and their fleas.[2,3] Epizootics involving these commensal rodents constitute the most serious hazard to humans. Epizootic plague among wild rodents may produce sporadic human infections, but an epizootic among commensal rats is likely to produce multiple human cases, especially since infective exposures occur in persons' living environments, often in circumstances of crowding, and because the oriental rat flea is a highly efficient vector that readily feeds on humans.

Enzootic and epizootic wild rodent plague cycles vary greatly in the rodent and flea species involved and in the environmental characteristics of different foci of infection.[1,3,5,6] The complex interplay between contiguous or overlapping cycles is poorly defined in most areas of the world. In the United States, enzootic plague is thought to occur in a variety of small burrowing rodents, such as voles and deer mice, whereas epizootic plague occurs conspicuously among prairie dogs, various ground squirrels, and chipmunks.[3–6] The most frequent sources of human plague in the United States are thought to be cycles of *Y. pestis* involving the rock squirrel, *Spermophilus variegatus*, and the California ground squirrel, *Spermophilus beecheyi*, and their fleas (especially *Oropsylla montana*).[6] Even when other rodents or domestic pets, such as cats or dogs, are implicated as the source of fleas infecting humans, the ultimate source of the infected fleas often has been these ground squirrels or related species. Wild carnivores or predatory birds may transport infected rodent fleas to susceptible rodent populations, and rodent fleas may be transported to humans by dogs, cats, or other mammals. Humans may also be bitten by infected fleas in the vicinity of abandoned burrows and through contact with infested rodent nest materials.

Humans have become infected by dissecting infected mammals, including lagomorphs, rodents, and carnivores, when the organism apparently gains entry through breaks in the skin.[12,13] Most carnivores, although readily infected by eating infected prey, rarely develop a bacteremia and seldom, if ever, serve as a source of *Y. pestis* to their fleas. Wild and domestic cats, however, may develop severe and fatal plague.[14,15] Cats with oropharyngeal and pneumonic plague can infect humans who come into direct contact with their infective exudates and secretions, and a small but increasing number of fatal primary pneumonic plague cases have resulted from such exposures.[16–19]

Current World Distribution

Plague persists as a public health problem in many areas of the world because of continued human contact with infected rodents and their fleas. In the 15-year period from 1980 to 1994, the World Health Organization (WHO) reported a total of 18,739 cases of plague with 1,852 plague deaths from 20 countries (Table 13-7).[20] The mean annual number of reported cases for the period was 1,249 per year, with relatively minor annual fluctuations in the totals. More than half (10,155) of the total number of cases were reported by countries in eastern and southern Africa, approximately one-third (5,661) by Asia, and the remainder (2,923) by the Americas. Recently, significant plague outbreaks have been reported from India, Madagascar, Mozambique, Myanmar (Burma), Peru, Tanzania, and Vietnam. In 1994, the government of India reported 876 cases of plague and 54 deaths arising from outbreaks of bubonic plague in Maharashtra State in west-central India and an explosive outbreak of apparent pneumonic plague in the city of Surat in neighboring Gujarat State.[20–22] These were the first reports of plague from India in almost 30 years, and they caused international alarm and great cost to India due to disruptions in travel and trade.[23] In formulating a response to a reported large outbreak of plague in another country, officials should consider that (*a*) plague infections respond rapidly to commonly available antibiotics; (*b*) surveillance of international arrivals from an epidemic area should readily detect persons acutely ill with pneumonic plague (the only contagious form of concern) because of its typically severe and fulminant character; (*c*) transmission of pneumonic plague requires close, direct contact with the ill person; and (*d*) interdiction of travel and trade, if warranted at all, should be specific to the actual plague focus and not applied country-wide. Unjustified, punitive responses are likely to inhibit plague reporting. A coordinated national surveillance for pneumonic plague was rapidly implemented in the United States during the recent perceived emergency arising from reports of plague outbreaks in India.[24] Limited outbreaks of urban plague have recently been reported also from Madagascar, Myanmar, and Vietnam without causing alarm and exaggerated responses.[20]

Between 1980 and 1994, the United States reported 229 plague cases (mean of 15 cases per year) and 33 (14 percent) deaths. A high of 40 cases and 6 deaths was reported in 1983. Although wild rodent plague occurs in the 17 contiguous western states that have territory west of the 100th meridian, more than 80 percent of human plague cases arise in the southwestern states of New Mexico, Arizona, and Colorado, and about 10 percent in California. Human plague in the United States is typically sporadic, with only single cases or small common-source clusters in an area, almost always following exposure to fleas of wild rodents. The United States reports all presumptive and confirmed cases of human plague, and its reporting is thought to be complete. In some areas of the world, reported cases may reflect only a part of the total; on the other hand, during plague outbreaks some countries include suspected cases as well as confirmed cases in their reports to the World Health Organization (WHO).

TABLE 13-7. REPORTED CASES OF PLAGUE IN HUMANS, BY COUNTRY, 1980–1994

Continent	*Country*	*No. of Cases*	*No. of Deaths*
Africa	Angola	27	4
	Botswana	173	12
	Kenya	49	10
	Libya	8	0
	Madagascar	1,390	302
	Malawi	9	0
	Mozambique	216	3
	South Africa	19	1
	Tanzania	4,964	419
	Uganda	660	48
	Zaire	2,242	513
	Zambia	1	1
	Zimbabwe	397	31
Total		10,155	1,344
America	Bolivia	189	27
	Brazil	700	9
	Ecuador	83	3
	Peru	1,722	112
	United States	229	33
Total		2,923	184
Asia	China	252	76
	India	876	54
	Kazakhstan	10	4
	Mongolia	59	19
	Myanmar	1,160	14
	Vietnam	3,304	158
Total		5,661	325
World Total		18,739	1,853

From World Health Organization: Human plague in 1994. Wkly Epidemiol Rec 22:165–172, 1996.

Changes in the ecology and epidemiology of plague are to be expected where relatively stable ecological features are disrupted by major industrial and agricultural development. For example, intensive irrigation of deserts for agricultural purposes, particularly for grain production, may produce burgeoning rodent populations close to human habitation, work, or recreational sites. In such settings, exposure of humans may result from the amplification of existing known or even unrecognized wild rodent plague foci, by spread from wild rodent populations to commensal species, or by noncontiguous (per saltum) spread of plague-infected rodents or their fleas in shipments of agricultural products.[1]

Surveillance

According to the *International Health Regulations*, each state's health authorities shall report to the WHO all human plague cases, the presence of the plague bacillus in any part of a country's territory, and a description of the epidemiologic circumstances and of the precautions taken to prevent its spread to other territories.[25] In the United States, it is mandatory to report all suspected human plague cases to local, state, and federal authorities (Centers for Disease Control and Prevention (CDC), Fort Collins, CO).

Each human plague case should, if possible, be epidemiologically investigated. Surveillance of animal plague activity should be carried out in areas where plague has occurred in recent decades. Direct surveillance is accomplished by bacteriological testing of rodents found dead from natural causes. A sensitive indication of epizootic rodent plague may be obtained by surveying carnivores for seropositivity to *Y. pestis*. Further, field reconnaissance may be undertaken to detect rodent die-offs, and rodents and fleas may be collected and processed for evidence of plague infection. The data should then be evaluated to determine the potential risk to humans and whether control measures are needed.[6]

▶ HUMAN PLAGUE

Human plague occurs in primary and secondary forms. The classic primary form of *Y. pestis* infection in humans, bubonic plague, occurs in about 90 percent of cases. Other clinical forms (e.g., septicemic, pneumonic, meningeal) usually occur as complications of bubonic plague. Bubonic plague almost always occurs as the result of a bite by an infected flea, and a small local papule or vesicle is sometimes present at the bite site. Rarely, local ulceration, similar to lesions seen with tularemia (eschar), occurs at the site of entry of *Y. pestis*. In addition to flea bites, entry sites can include mucous membranes of the eye and oropharynx as well as broken skin. The usual incubation period is 2 to 6 days, but it may be longer. Illness is manifested by fever, chills, headache, myalgia and arthralgia, development of pain and tenderness in affected lymph nodes draining the site of inoculation, and eventually lymph node enlargement (the bubo). In untreated, progressive disease, plague septicemia develops. Septicemia in the absence of lymph node involvement is referred to as primary septicemic plague. Plague septicemia, if untreated, generally results in septic shock and rapid death. Blood-borne dissemination to other organs may lead to plague pneumonia, meningitis, multiple lymphadenopathy, endophthalmitis, arthritis, or focal abscesses. In the absence of a bubo as a hallmark, illness in primary septicemic plague may be compounded by delayed diagnosis and by circumvention of the defenses of reactive regional lymph nodes.

Secondary pneumonic plague results from hematogenous spread from bubonic or septicemic plague. In contrast, primary pneumonic plague results from close (within 2 m) contact with a person or animal expelling fine droplets of *Y. pestis* organisms by vigorous coughing. *Y. pestis* does not survive as a saprophyte, and true aerosol or droplet nuclei transmission has not been recognized.

Before antibiotic therapy was available, approximately 5 percent of patients during plague outbreaks were diagnosed as pneumonic plague. In the United States in the early part of the twentieth century, sporadic cases of primary pneumonic plague occurred during bubonic plague outbreaks, and two small pneumonic plague outbreaks occurred in 1919 (Oakland, CA) and 1924 (Los Angeles, CA). From 1925 through 1996, 42 of 400 patients (10.5 percent) developed secondary plague pneumonia, and seven patients had primary pneumonic plague five resulting from domestic cat exposures (CDC, unpublished data). Over 2,000 known or possible contacts of these patients with respiratory plague were given chemoprophylaxis, and no spread to contacts was recognized. A recent increase in the United States of both secondary and primary (cat-related) pneumonic plague cases raises a concern about the possible spread of pneumonic plague to household contacts or medical personnel.[26]

Pharyngeal or tonsillar plague has occasionally been associated with exposure to infected respiratory particles from pneumonic patients or animals and with ingestion of infected animal tissues.[27,28]

Diagnosis and Treatment

A careful epidemiologic history is essential in considering a diagnosis of plague. When plague is suspected, it is imperative to obtain diagnostic specimens promptly and, if the clinical and epidemiologic evidence is sufficiently strong, to initiate specific therapy without awaiting laboratory results. Bubonic plague is best diagnosed by culture of material aspirated from a bubo; if the aspiration is "dry," sterile saline should be injected into the node and then aspirated. Multiple blood cultures and, if indicated, throat and sputum cultures should also be obtained. Materials for culture should be taken before specific antibiotics are given. Paired serum samples obtained at least 3 weeks apart should be tested for antibody to *Y. pestis*. Smears of bubo aspirates, exudates, respiratory secretions, and suspect organisms isolated in bacteriologic media should be stained by a polychromatic stain, such as Wayson's or Giemsa, to demonstrate the characteristic bipolar staining of *Y. pestis*, and by fluorescence antibody directed against the F1 antigen of *Y. pestis*.[2,7] Suspect clinical materials and cultures should be forwarded to reference diagnostic laboratories for confirmatory identification.

The antibiotic of choice for treating *Y. pestis* infection is streptomycin.[29] Gentamicin is an acceptable alternative and is more widely available. Other highly effective drugs include tetracycline and chloramphenicol. The penicillins, cephalosporins, and macrolides, are not suitably effective against *Y. pestis* and should not be used for treating plague. Chloramphenicol, a highly effective drug for *Y. pestis*, is the agent of choice for plague meningitis, pleuritis, or endophthalmitis because of its high tissue permeability. Cotrimoxazole (a combination of trimethoprim and sulfamethoxazole) has been reported to be effective in treating bubonic plague, but the few reports of its efficacy involve a small number of patients, almost all of them adults.[30,31]

Hospital Procedures and Care of Contacts

Because patients with bubonic or septicemic plague may develop secondary plague pneumonia, all patients with suspected plague should be placed in respiratory isolation for at least 48 hours after beginning specific antibiotic therapy. Isolation beyond this is not necessary unless the patient has pulmonary infection or draining exudates. Personnel caring for patients with pneumonic plague must observe strict respiratory droplet precautions, including the use of eye protection. All patients should have an initial pulmonary radiograph to rule out pneumonia.

Household members and others sharing the same environmental circumstances should be placed under surveillance because of the possibility of exposures to the same zootic source as the index case; antibiotic prophylaxis may be indicated when there is a concern about exposure to infected fleas but is not indicated as a routine practice. All persons who have had close contact with a pneumonic plague patient in a previous 6-day period should be given postexposure prophylaxis for 7 days. Tetracycline, doxycycline, or chloramphenicol are acceptable prophylactic agents. Exposed persons should also be kept under close observation, including measurement of body temperature at least twice daily. Should fever develop, the person should be immediately hospitalized in isolation for diagnostic evaluation, and streptomycin should be given if indicated.

Prevention and Control

Surveillance, education, and environmental management are the cornerstones of plague prevention. Public health authorities should identify and monitor active plague foci and maintain a system for rapid identification and evaluation of any suspected human cases or plague epizootics. Persons in known plague foci should protect themselves and their domestic pets from fleas and should maintain a living and working environment free of rodents. Environmental sanitation should include rodent proofing of buildings, removal of other harborage such as wood piles, brush and junk heaps, and removal of any rodent food sources, such as garbage or animal feed. Persons should be instructed to avoid sick or dead animals and to use gloves when handling animals killed by hunting or trapping.

Immunization with the formalin-inactivated plague vaccine USP is thought to provide at least partial protection against bubonic plague. Other than for military personnel, the vaccine is recommended only for persons at high risk of exposure such as laboratory personnel who routinely work with *Y. pestis* and persons whose work brings them into regular contact with potentially infected wild rodents and their fleas.[32] Short-term antibiotic prophylaxis with a tetracycline, chloramphenicol, or trimethoprim-sulfamethoxazole may occasionally be recommended for persons who are unable to avoid an area where a plague outbreak is in progress or who are caring for plague patients.[29,32]

Killing fleas with insecticides is the principal control measure in situations where epizootic plague places persons at risk of exposure. Rodent burrows, rodent runs, and other places where rodents and their fleas may be found should be sprayed or dusted with appropriate insecticides by trained persons. The decision to control plague by killing rodents should be left to health authorities and should be done only when adequate flea control measures are in place. Control of rodents without environmental sanitation may worsen the situation, since the void may be quickly filled by a more susceptible, immature population of rodents.

Malaria

S. Patrick Kachur • Peter B. Bloland

Malaria remains one of the most widespread potentially fatal infectious diseases. It is an important public health concern both in countries where transmission occurs regularly and in areas where transmission has been largely eliminated. Malaria is an extremely complex condition that is manifested differently in different parts of the world depending on a range of variables that include the infecting parasite species and its susceptibility to antimalarial drugs; the distribution and efficiency of insect vectors; climatic and environmental conditions; and the genetic composition, acquired immunity, and behavior of human populations. Children, pregnant women, and nonimmune visitors to malarious areas are at greatest risk of severe or fatal infections. Multiple strategies exist to combat malaria, but none of them are both appropriate and affordable in all malaria-endemic areas. Public health efforts to prevent or control malaria must be carefully tailored to the intensity of local transmission and local conditions of the parasite, vector, environment, and human population as well as the level of resources available. Although the global malaria eradication campaign of the 1950s and 1960s was unsuccessful in many countries, the intense international effort did yield lasting improvements in some areas and provided valuable experience for the integrated malaria control programs recommended today.

Malaria occurs in over 90 countries worldwide. Thirty-six percent of the global population lives in areas where there is risk of malaria transmission. Seven percent of the world's people reside in areas where malaria has never been under meaningful control, but another 29 percent live in areas where malaria was once transmitted at low levels or not at all, but where significant transmission has been reestablished.[1] The development and spread of drug-resistant strains of malaria parasites and insecticide-tolerant strains of the mosquito vector have been identified as key factors in this resurgence. Other important considerations are the shifting patterns of support for malaria-related research and control activities in endemic countries and among international donors, which left many endemic countries without resources or technical capacity for malaria control activities once international support for the eradication campaign disappeared. The World Health Organization (WHO) also lists environmental disruption for agricultural or economic reasons, sociopolitical unrest, and population migration among the probable precipitating causes of the most serious malaria problems.

Each year an estimated 300 to 500 million clinical cases of malaria occur, making it one of the most prevalent infectious diseases. Malaria can be, in certain epidemiologic circumstances, a devastating disease with high morbidity and mortality, demanding a rapid and comprehensive response. In other settings, it can be a more pernicious public health threat. In many malarious areas of the world, especially sub-Saharan Africa, malaria is ranked among the most frequent causes of morbidity and mortality among children and is often the leading identifiable cause. The WHO estimates that more than 90 percent of the 1.5 to 2.0 million deaths attributed to malaria each year occur in African children.[1] In addition to its morbidity and mortality burden, the economic effects of malaria infection can be tremendous. These include direct costs for treatment and prevention, as well as indirect costs such as lost productivity from morbidity and mortality, time spent seeking treatment, and diversion of household resources. The annual economic burden of malaria infection in 1995 was estimated at $US 1.7 billion for Africa alone.[2] This heavy toll can hinder economic and community development activities throughout the region.

Malaria transmission occurs primarily in tropical and subtropical regions in sub-Saharan Africa, Central and South America, the Caribbean island of Hispaniola, the Middle East, the Indian subcontinent, Southeast Asia, and Oceania (Fig. 13-8). In areas where malaria occurs, however, there is considerable variation in the intensity of transmission and risk of malaria infection. Highland regions (those above 1,500 m) and arid areas (those receiving less than 1,000 mm of rainfall per year) typically have less malaria, although they are also prone to epidemic malaria when parasitemic individuals provide a source of infection and climate conditions are favorable to mosquito development.[1] Although urban areas have typically been at lower risk, explosive, unplanned population growth has contributed to the growing problem of urban malaria transmission.[3]

Although sustained malaria transmission in the United States was eliminated in the 1950s, more than 1,000 cases of malaria are reported in the United States each year.[4] In recent years, nearly all of the malaria cases reported in the United States have occurred among immigrants, refugees, and travelers from parts of the world where ongoing transmission persists. A small number of malaria cases are acquired within the United States and its territories. Some of these cases are congenitally acquired, some are unintentionally induced by blood transfusion or organ donation, and a small number of cases appear to be transmitted by local anopheline mosquitoes.[5] These rare instances of mosquito-borne malaria in the United States are of concern because they demonstrate the potential for reintroduction of transmission, even in temperate climates where malaria has been eradicated.

Agent and Life Cycle

In humans, malaria infection is caused by one or more of four species of intracellular protozoan parasite. *Plasmodium falciparum, Plasmodium vivax, Plasmodium ovale*, and *Plasmodium malariae* differ in geographic distribution, microscopic appearance, clinical features (periodicity of infection, potential for severe or complicated disease, and tendency for clinical relapses or recrudescences), and immunogenic potential (Table 13-8). Although *P. vivax* infections are more common,

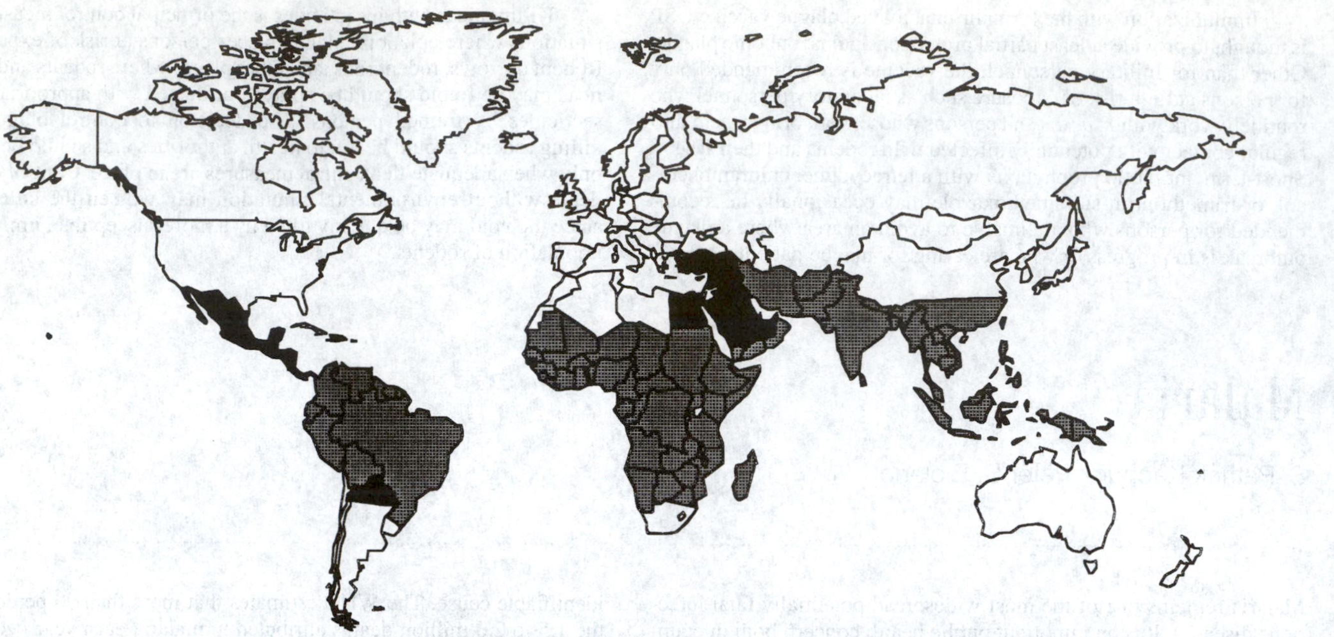

Figure 13-8. Malaria-endemic areas of the world. (Adapted from World Health Organization: World malaria situation in 1993, part I. Wkly Epidemiol Rec 71[1]:17–22, 1996.)

worldwide, *P. falciparum* malaria represents the most serious public health problem because of its tendency toward severe or fatal infections.

Routes of Transmission

Malaria is typically transmitted by the bite of an infective female *Anopheles* sp. mosquito. Mosquito-borne cases are referred to as **autochthonous malaria** to distinguish them from cases transmitted in other ways. **Congenital malaria** refers to infection passed from mother to infant in utero. **Induced malaria** refers to infection that is passed directly from one individual to another through contaminated blood or blood products, injection equipment, or organ transplant. Until the 1950s, induced malaria infection was widely practiced as a treatment for late neurosyphilis.[6] While this treatment has been replaced by effective antibiotics, the practice of malariotherapy has reemerged several times in recent decades, primarily as an alternative medicine practice in economically developed countries.[7] Finally, when a route of transmission cannot be established, even after careful investigation, a case may be classified as **cryptic malaria**.[8]

TABLE 13-8. CHARACTERISTICS OF THE FOUR SPECIES OF HUMAN MALARIA

	Plasmodium falciparum	*Plasmodium vivax*	*Plasmodium ovale*	*Plasmodium malariae*
Exoerythrocytic cycle	6–7 days	6–8 days	9 days	14–16 days
Prepatent period	9–10 days	11–13 days	10–14 days	15–16 days
Incubation period {mean}	9–14 {12} days	12–17 {15} days to 6–12 months	16–18 {17} days or longer	18–40 {28} days or longer
Severity of primary attack	Severe	Mild to severe	Severe	Severe
Duration of primary attack[a]	16–36 hours or longer	8–12 hours	8–12 hours	8–10 hours
Duration of untreated infection[a]	1–2 years	1.5–5 years	1.5–5 years	3–50 years
Relapse	No	Yes	Yes	No
CNS complications[a]	Frequent	Infrequent	Infrequent	Infrequent
Anemia[a]	Frequent	Common	Infrequent	Infrequent
Renal insufficiency[a]	Common	Infrequent	Infrequent	Infrequent
Effects on pregnancy[a]	Frequent	Infrequent	Unknown	Unknown
Hypoglycemia	Frequent	Unknown	Unknown	Unknown

Adapted from Bruce-Chwatt LJ: Essential Malariology. 2nd ed. New York. John Wiley and Sons, 1985.
[a]Influenced by immunity. Documentation of complications for species other than *P. falciparum* is limited.

Life Cycle

Although there are important differences between them, the four human malarias share a common life cycle. Malaria infection begins when an infective female mosquito injects *Plasmodium* sp. sporozoites into the bloodstream while feeding (Fig. 13-9). The sporozoites circulate only momentarily; those that survive host immune defenses infect cells of the liver parenchyma. There they undergo asexual reproduction (exo-erythrocytic schizogony), producing hepatic schizonts. In 6 to 14 days, these schizonts mature and rupture, releasing merozoites into the bloodstream. Merozoites then invade red blood cells, where they undergo a second phase of asexual reproduction (erythrocytic schizogony), developing into rings, trophozoites, and finally erythrocytic schizonts. Once mature, the infected red blood cells rupture, releasing still more merozoites into the bloodstream and starting another cycle of asexual development and multiplication. Clinical symptoms are associated with the rupture of erythrocytic schizonts and usually develop after several cycles of erythrocytic schizogony. The classic clinical presentation of periodic fever occurs when the cycles of erythrocytic schizogony are synchronized. Malaria parasites continue to proliferate until (*a*) immune responses eliminate the infection, (*b*) effective antimalarial drugs kill all the erythrocytic parasites, or (*c*) the host dies from the infection.

Eventually, some merozoites develop into sexual forms called gametocytes. Both male and female gametocytes circulate without causing symptoms and can be ingested by a mosquito during a subsequent blood meal. Sexual reproduction occurs within the mosquito midgut. The fertilized zygote quickly transforms into an amoeboid ookinete, which penetrates the midgut wall and forms an oocyst. After several days to weeks, the oocyst ruptures, releasing sporozoites, which migrate through the celomic cavity to the salivary glands. The life cycle starts again when the infective mosquito bites another human. The mosquito is essential to the development of the malaria parasite as well as its transmission. The sporogonic cycle—the period of time between ingestion of gametocytes and becoming infective to humans—varies among the different species of parasite and anopheline vectors and can be affected by environmental conditions as well.

The timing of events in the life cycle of malaria parasites and the number of merozoites produced from each schizont differ among the four *Plasmodium* species that infect humans. In addition, *P. vivax* and *P. ovale* can produce a dormant form (hypnozoites) that can persist in the liver for months to years, causing periodic relapses of parasitemia and illness (Table 13-8). Hypnozoites result only from primary sporozoite inoculation in mosquito-borne infections and are not present after cases of induced or congenital malaria. While *P. falciparum* and *P. malariae* do not form hypnozoites, infection with these parasites can persist in the blood at subpatent or undetectable levels following resolution of symptoms. This very low-level parasitemia can result in recrudescence of clinical disease. Except in partially immune persons, *P. falciparum* rarely recrudesces more than several months after initial infection. However, recrudescent *P. malariae* infections can occur 40 years or longer after infection.

Clinical Features and Diagnosis

Patients with malaria can present with a wide variety of symptoms and a broad spectrum of severity depending on such factors as the infecting species and the level of acquired immunity in the host. In general, partial immunity to malaria is acquired only after repeated exposure. Individuals who survive repeated malaria infections can tolerate the presence of malaria parasites in their blood with a minimum of symptoms. In areas where malaria transmission is intense, the first exposure to malaria occurs very early in childhood. After many subsequent infections, the likelihood of severe illness or death lessens.

Clinical Presentation

Typical symptoms among nonimmune individuals with malaria include fever, chills, myalgias and arthralgias, headache, diarrhea,

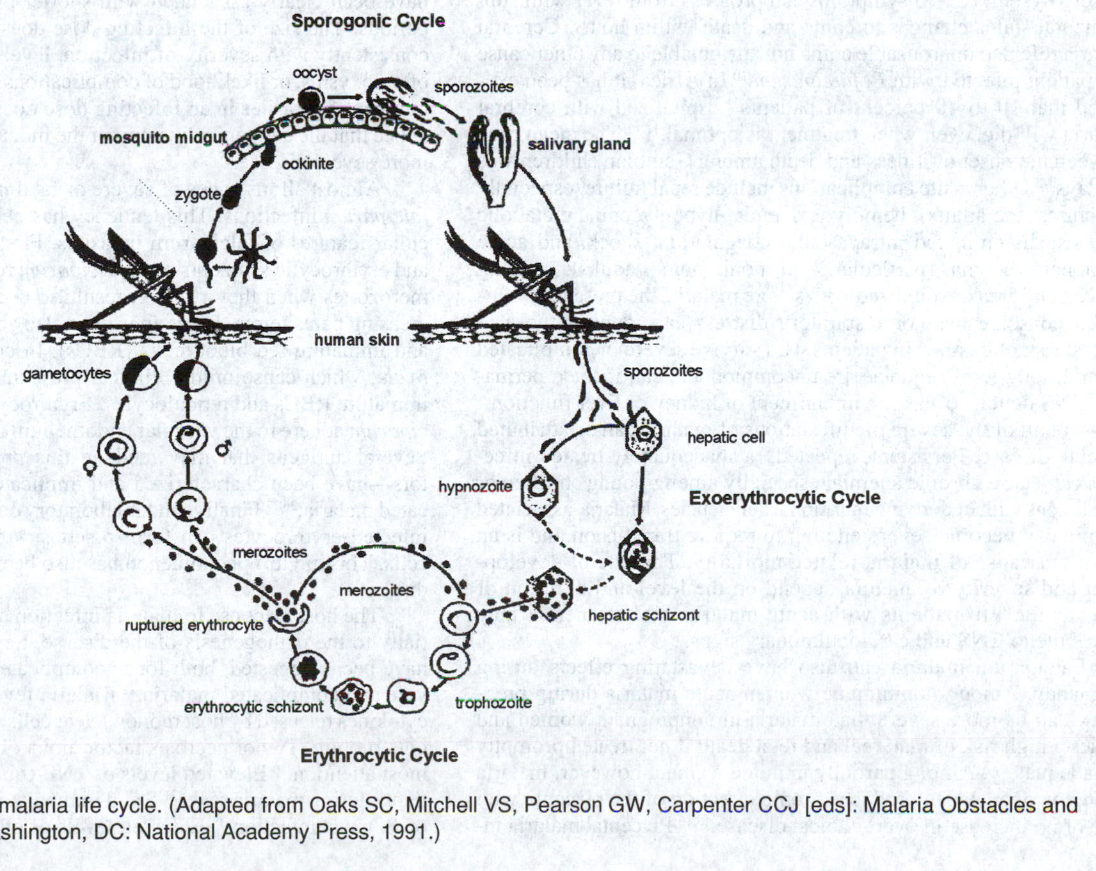

Figure 13-9. The malaria life cycle. (Adapted from Oaks SC, Mitchell VS, Pearson GW, Carpenter CCJ [eds]: Malaria Obstacles and Opportunities. Washington, DC: National Academy Press, 1991.)

vomiting, and other nonspecific signs. Splenomegaly, anemia, thrombocytopenia, pulmonary or renal dysfunction, and neurologic findings may also be present. When synchronous infections (occurring when a majority of schizonts rupture at the same time) develop, each species of *Plasmodium* causes a characteristic pattern of periodic fever. The paroxysms of *P. vivax* and *P. ovale* malaria classically occur every 48 hours, while those of *P. malariae* occur every 72 hours. *P. falciparum* infections often feature a daily or irregular pattern of symptoms. However, this classic presentation with predictably recurring fever and chills is highly variable and may not be present at all, particularly in *P. falciparum* infections, early in the course of an illness, when the patient is taking medications that have antipyretic or antimalarial activity, or when partial immunity exists.

Signs and symptoms of malaria can be greatly modified by the patient's immune status; malaria infections among partially immune individuals range from asymptomatic to severe. The presenting signs and symptoms may be atypical or subtle, especially among infants and young children. The classic presentation of periodic fever sometimes seen in nonimmune individuals with synchronous infections is frequently absent among partially immune individuals. Because the manifestations of malaria illness can be so nonspecific, it is a common practice in malaria-endemic areas to treat all febrile illnesses as malaria, especially in children and pregnant women, who are at greatest risk for severe or fatal disease.

Severe or Complicated Infections

Uncomplicated malaria infection can progress to severe disease or death within hours. The potential for severe and complicated illness is particularly ominous in patients with high levels of parasitemia and without partial immunity from prior exposure to malaria infection. *P. falciparum* is the major cause of severe disease and death; severe or fatal malaria rarely results from infections with *P. vivax*, *P. ovale*, and *P. malariae* unless there is another contributing cause of death or coinfection with *P. falciparum*. An extremely rare exception is splenic rupture, which can occur with acute nonfalciparum malaria.[9]

Neurologic manifestations are the best known potentially fatal complication in nonimmune adults and children. Malaria with central nervous system (CNS) symptoms can progress from fever with subtle mental status changes to coma and death within hours. Cerebral malaria refers to unarousable coma not attributable to any other cause in a patient infected with *P. falciparum*.[10] In Africa, it has been estimated that 10 to 40 percent of patients hospitalized with cerebral malaria will die, even when treatment is optimal.[11,12] The mean time between the onset of illness and death among Gambian children was 2.8 days.[13] Other acute complications include renal failure (especially in nonimmune adults), hemolytic anemia, hypoglycemia, metabolic acidosis, disseminated intravascular coagulation, shock, and acute pulmonary edema (particularly in nonimmune adults). Among African children hospitalized with severe malaria, the presence of impaired consciousness or respiratory distress can identify those at highest risk of death.[14] In patients who survive severe or complicated malaria, long-term sequelae are uncommon and can include permanent CNS deficits or lasting impairment of kidney or liver function.

Not all of the severe manifestations of malaria can be attributed to acute disease. Persistent, repeated, or inadequately treated infections can cause chronic anemia, especially among young children or populations with underlying nutritional deficiencies. Malaria-associated anemia can become severe enough to require transfusion and is an important cause of malaria-related mortality. The rate of development and severity of anemia depend on the level and duration of parasitemia.[10] In patients with acute malaria, severe anemia may contribute to CNS and cardiopulmonary signs.

Falciparum malaria can also have devastating effects during pregnancy. Among nonimmune women acute malaria during pregnancy can be more severe than malaria in nonpregnant women and carries a high risk of maternal and fetal death if not treated promptly and adequately. Among partially immune women, however, malaria during pregnancy can produce chronic infection of the placenta with little or no increase in overt clinical disease.[15,16] Placental malaria infection, in turn, is a cause of low birth weight, the greatest single risk factor for infant mortality.[17,18] In most populations, malaria is most significant during a woman's first and second pregnancies, although in populations with a high prevalence of HIV infection, placental malaria infection can occur in all pregnancies.[19]

Whereas rates of severe disease and mortality among nonimmune populations are typically not age related, there is a disproportionate level of mortality among children in partially immune populations.[20] In Africa, where the majority of malaria-associated deaths occur, the highest mortality affects children less than 5 years of age. In the Gambia, it has been estimated that malaria accounted for 25 percent of all deaths among children less than 5 years of age.[13]

Recent comparisons between malarious areas suggest that disease manifestations, age profile, and severity of illness vary widely with the intensity of malaria transmission.[21,22] The overall or community level of immunity to malaria is highest in areas where malaria transmission is the most intense. In such communities, the burden of malarial illness and death is shifted to the youngest age groups. Additionally, severe malaria tends to manifest itself more frequently as anemia than as cerebral disease in the setting of intense transmission. As transmission intensity decreases, community-level immunity is lessened, illness is seen more frequently in all age groups, and the incidence of cerebral disease increases relative to anemia.

Pathophysiology

The usual incubation period from infective mosquito bite to onset of symptoms ranges from 9 to 30 days or longer, depending on the species of parasite (Table 13-8), host immune status, infecting dose, and use of antimalarial drugs. The clinical symptoms associated with malaria infection are caused by a complex interplay between the parasite and the host immune response. Symptoms are associated with the asexual erythrocytic stage parasites. Exoerythrocytic forms (sporozoites, exoerythrocytic schizonts, and hypnozoites) and gametocytes do not cause clinical symptoms.

In general, higher levels of parasitemia are associated with clinical symptoms in partially immune populations and with severe or complicated disease in nonimmune persons. Larger infecting doses have been clearly associated with shorter prepatent and incubation periods. The size of the infecting dose does not appear to correlate consistently with severity of infection, level of parasitemia, number of paroxysms, or likelihood of complications.[23,24] Even if the absolute number of parasites in an infecting dose does not, there is some evidence that the antigenic diversity of the inoculum does correlate with more severe disease.[25]

Almost all instances of severe or fatal malaria are caused by *P. falciparum* infections. This tendency has been linked to several peculiar features of falciparum parasites. First of all, exoerythrocytic and erythrocytic schizonts of *P. falciparum* release larger numbers of merozoites when they rupture, resulting in a more rapid rate of increasing parasitemia. *P. falciparum* is also able to infect both mature and immature red blood cells (RBCs). In contrast, *P. vivax* and *P. ovale*, which cause milder clinical presentations, selectively infect immature RBCs and reticulocytes. Erythrocytes infected with *P. falciparum* adhere to the vascular endothelium of postcapillary venules. Several antigens that may mediate this property—adherence factors—have been characterized and implicated in severe or complicated malaria.[26,27] Finally, under laboratory conditions, *P. falciparum*-infected erythrocytes can form rosettes with uninfected red blood cells. This in vitro phenomenon has also been correlated with severe disease.[28]

The host response to malaria infection also contributes substantially to the pathogenesis of the disease. Several specific mediators have been suggested, both for uncomplicated infections and for severe and complicated malaria.[29] Malaria fever appears to arise from cytokines released by host mononuclear cells when erythrocytic schizonts rupture. Tumor necrosis factor alpha (TNF-α) has received the most attention.[30] Elevated levels of TNF-α have been detected in patients during malaria fever[31,32] and immediately preceding paroxysms of *P. vivax* infection.[33] Elevated levels of other cytokines, including interferon gamma and interleukins 1 and 6 have also been described and may contribute to fever in malaria infection.[32,34]

While the occurrence of severe and complicated malaria remains unpredictable and incompletely understood,[23] it appears that both direct and immunologic effects play important roles in each of the major complications. Cerebral malaria appears to be caused partly by direct processes—such as the tendency for parasitized erythrocytes to sludge in capillaries and venules of the CNS, reduced deformability of infected RBCs, or adherence of infected cells to vascular endothelium and noninfected erythrocytes—and partly by immunological responses—such as complement activation, immune complex–mediated vasculitis, cytokine release, and nitric oxide. Likewise, malaria-related anemia may evolve from direct effects—such as lysing of infected cells or their removal by the spleen—as well as immunologic effects—including inhibition of erythropoiesis, immune-mediated removal of noninfected RBCs, and autoantibodies to RBC antigens.[35]

Diagnostic Tests

The diagnosis of malaria must be considered in all febrile patients who have traveled to or lived in malaria-endemic areas or who have received blood products, tissues, or organs from persons who have been to such areas. Direct microscopic examination of intracellular parasites on stained blood films is the current standard for definitive diagnosis in nearly all settings. However, several other approaches exist, or are in development, that may be appropriate under special conditions.

Although reliable diagnosis cannot be made on the basis of signs and symptoms alone because of the nonspecific nature of clinical malaria, clinical diagnosis of malaria is common in many malarious areas. In much of the malaria-endemic world, resources and trained health personnel are so scarce that presumptive clinical diagnosis is the only realistic option. Clinical diagnosis offers the advantages of ease, speed, and low cost. In areas where malaria is prevalent, clinical diagnosis usually results in all patients with fever and no apparent other cause being treated for malaria. This approach can identify most patients who truly need antimalarial treatment, but it is also likely to misclassify many who do not.[36] Overdiagnosis contributes to misuse of antimalarial drugs. Clinical diagnosis of malaria can lead health workers to overlook other obvious and treatable causes of fever in a febrile patient.[37] Considerable overlap exists between malaria and other diseases, especially acute lower respiratory tract infection (ALRI) and bacteremia.[38] Attempts to improve the specificity of clinical diagnosis for malaria by including signs and symptoms other than fever or history of fever have met with only minimal success.[39]

A definitive diagnosis of malaria can be made by several approaches, including light microscopy, special staining, rapid antigen detection, and detection of parasite nucleic acid sequences. Definitive diagnosis can decrease the use of antimalarial drugs by patients not needing malaria therapy, improve the ability to identify patients in need of treatment for nonmalarial illnesses, direct antimalarial therapy to specific species of malaria, and monitor the impact of malaria infection and treatment over time. General disadvantages of definitive diagnosis include the cost of equipment and supplies, the time expended training and supervising personnel and conducting the test, and the need for handling blood.

Simple light microscopic examination of stained blood films is the most widely practiced and useful method for definitive malaria diagnosis. With a minimum of equipment and recurring expense, fast and reliable diagnosis of malaria can be obtained even under the most difficult conditions. In areas where *P. falciparum* causes only a portion of malaria infections, microscopic diagnosis allows differentiation between species, a capability not possible at present with some of the newer technologies. Another advantage of this approach is that an experienced microscopist can also quantify the level of infection and distinguish clinically important asexual parasite stages (rings, trophozoites, and schizonts) from the sexual forms (gametocytes), which may persist without causing symptoms. This can be critical for determining whether a given treatment has been effective. While several different stains can be used, Giemsa gives the best results. Specific disadvantages are that slide collection, staining, and reading can be time consuming and microscopists need to be trained and supervised to ensure consistent reliability. Although electricity is not needed as long as there is sunlight, the availability of electricity improves reliability and extends the hours during which diagnosis can be made available. Even when performed correctly, simple microscopic diagnosis does have some important limitations. In partially immune persons, asymptomatic parasitemia may be detected, which can be of limited clinical significance and may cause the clinician to overlook another cause of illness. Conversely, in nonimmune persons, symptoms may develop before there are detectable levels of parasitemia. For this reason, several blood smear examinations are needed to positively rule out a diagnosis of malaria in a symptomatic patient.

A modification of light microscopy, the quantitative buffy coat method (QBC™, Becton Dickinson) was originally developed to screen large numbers of specimens for complete blood cell counts.[40] Adapted for malaria diagnosis, the technique involves the use of a special fluorescent stain to highlight malaria parasites and centrifugation to concentrate parasites at a predictable location on a specially prepared capillary tube.[41] Advantages to QBC are that less training is required to operate the system and the test is typically quicker to perform. Field trials have shown that QBC may be marginally more sensitive than conventional microscopy under ideal conditions.[41–43] Disadvantages are that electricity is always required, special equipment and supplies are needed, the per-test cost is higher than simple light microscopy, and species-specific diagnosis is not reliable. These disadvantages and the limited resources available for diagnosis generally prohibit the widespread use of QBC in many malaria-endemic countries.

A third diagnostic approach involves the rapid detection of parasite antigens, usually through enzyme-linked immunosorbent assay (ELISA) and radioimmunoassay (RIA) techniques. Multiple experimental tests have been developed targeting a variety of parasite antigens.[44–46] One commercially available kit (ParaSight™-F, Becton-Dickinson) detects the histidine-rich protein (HRP-II) of *P. falciparum*. Compared with light microscopy and QBC, this test yielded rapid and highly sensitive diagnosis of *P. falciparum* infection.[47,48] Advantages to this technology are that no special equipment is required, the test and reagents are stable at ambient temperatures, and no electricity is needed. The principal disadvantage is a high per-test cost. The test is specific for falciparum malaria and is nonquantitative. Furthermore, detectable antigen can persist for 10 to 14 days after adequate treatment and cure, and the test cannot adequately distinguish a resolving infection from treatment failure due to antimalarial drug–resistant parasites. Although promising, this particular test cannot replace light microscopy, particularly in settings where infections with non-falciparum species and asymptomatic parasitemias are prevalent.

Detection of parasite genetic material through polymerase chain reaction (PCR) techniques has gained prominence as a research tool. It will almost certainly have a growing role in the diagnosis of malaria. Specific primers have been developed for each of the four species of human malaria. One important use of this new technology is in detecting mixed infections or differentiating between infecting species when microscopic examination is inconclusive.[49] In addition, improved PCR techniques could prove useful for tracing molecular epidemiology in investigations of malaria clusters or epidemics.[50]

Techniques also exist for detecting antimalaria antibodies in serum specimens. Specific serologic markers have been identified for each of the four species of human malaria. Positive studies generally indicate past infection. Serology is not useful for diagnosing acute infections, because detectable levels of antimalaria antibodies do not appear until weeks into infection and persist long after parasitemia has resolved. Moreover, the test is relatively expensive and is not widely available. However, in particular settings, such as screening large numbers of blood donors in the epidemiologic investigation of a transfusion-induced case of malaria, serologic studies can be an appropriate and valuable tool.

Treatment

Antimalarial Drugs

There are only a limited number of drugs that can be used to treat or prevent malaria. Because of rapidly developing and spreading resistance to antimalarials and the relatively slow process of developing new antimalarials, the number of useful drugs is dwindling. All currently available antimalarial drugs are discussed here even though not all are practical or appropriate to use in any given situation.

Quinine. Quinine was first isolated from cinchona bark in 1820 and has since been the fundamental chemotherapeutic agent for the treatment of malaria, especially severe disease. Quinine and its dextroisomer, quinidine, are rapidly acting drugs that target the erythrocytic asexual stages of all malaria parasites. It is available in both oral and parenteral preparations and can be used in infants and pregnant women. Side effects include nausea, dysphoria, blurred vision, and tinnitus and typically resolve after treatment has ended. *P. falciparum* from most areas of the world responds well to quinine; because of this, shortened courses of quinine can be used in conjunction with a second drug to reduce the likelihood of quinine-associated side effects. *P. falciparum* from many areas of Southeast Asia require full-course quinine treatment in conjunction with a second drug (Table 13-9).

Chloroquine. Chloroquine is a 4-aminoquinoline derivative of quinine first synthesized in 1934. Historically, chloroquine has been used as the drug of choice for the treatment of nonsevere or uncomplicated malaria and for chemoprophylaxis. Chloroquine acts primarily against erythrocytic asexual stages, although it has gametocytocidal properties. Because of widespread resistance to this drug, its usefulness is increasingly limited. Where chloroquine retains efficacy, it can be safely used for treatment or prophylaxis of infants and pregnant women. Side effects are uncommon and not generally serious. They include nausea, headaches, gastrointestinal disturbance, and blurred vision. Some patients, especially if dark-skinned, can experience pruritus.

Amodiaquine. Amodiaquine is closely related to chloroquine but has fallen out of favor because of a high incidence of adverse reactions (including agranulocytosis and hepatitis), primarily when used for prophylaxis, and resistance patterns similar to those of chloroquine. Recent reports have suggested that amodiaquine may be useful in limited settings of very low-level chloroquine resistance.[51]

Antifol Combination Drugs. These drugs are various combinations of dihydrofolate reductase inhibitors (proguanil, chlorproguanil, pyrimethamine, and trimethoprim) and sulfa drugs (dapsone, sulfalene, sulfamethoxazole, sulfadoxine, and others). Although these drugs have antimalarial activity when used alone, parasitologic resistance can develop rapidly. When used in combination, they produce a synergistic effect on the parasite and can be effective even in the presence of resistance to the individual components. Typical combinations include sulfadoxine/pyrimethamine (Fansidar), sulfalene-pyrimethamine (metakelfin), and sulfamethoxazole-trimethoprim (cotrimoxazole). Proguanil is often used in combination with chloroquine for prophylaxis in areas of moderate chloroquine resistance, although studies suggest that minimal additional benefit is derived.[52] Side effects are uncommon; however severe allergic reactions can occur. When used prophylactically among American travelers, sulfadoxine-pyrimethamine has been associated with a high incidence of severe cutaneous reactions (1 per 5,000 to 8,000 users) and mortality (1 per 11,000 to 25,000 users).[53] These side effects do not appear to occur as frequently when the drug is used for treatment. Concerns about sulfa drug use during pregnancy are outweighed by the known risks to mother and fetus associated with untreated malaria. The use of folate supplementation may increase the frequency of treatment failure with antifol combination drugs.[54]

Tetracyclines. Tetracycline and derivatives such as doxycycline are very potent antimalarials and are used for both treatment and prophylaxis. In areas where response to quinine has deteriorated, tetracyclines are often used in combination with quinine to improve cure rates. Tetracyclines are also used in conjunction with shortened courses of quinine to decrease the likelihood of quinine-associated side effects. Tetracyclines should not be used during pregnancy or breast feeding, or in children less than 8 years of age, because they can disrupt the development of teeth and bones. Common side effects include nausea, vomiting, diarrhea, *Candida* superinfections, and photosensitivity.

Primaquine. Primaquine, an 8-aminoquinoline, is primarily used as a tissue schizonticide for the purpose of reducing the likelihood of relapse due to hypnozoites of *P. vivax* and *P. ovale*. Recent studies have shown that primaquine has reasonably good efficacy (74 percent against *P. falciparum* and 90 percent against *P. vivax*) when used for prophylaxis.[55] Although it has activity against blood-stage asexual parasites, the concentrations required to achieve blood schizonticidal action are toxic; primaquine is also a potent gametocytocidal drug and has been used in community-based control programs to reduce the prevalence of gametocyte-carrying individuals in the population. People with glucose-6-phosphate dehydrogenase (G6PD) deficiencies can experience severe and potentially fatal hemolytic anemia if treated with primaquine. Individuals with mild to moderate G6PD deficiency (A variant) can tolerate a weekly dosing regimen, but primaquine should be avoided entirely in persons who demonstrate severe deficiency with less than 10 percent residual enzyme activity. The most severe Mediterranean B variant and related Asian variants of G6PD deficiency can occur at high rates among some groups or in certain regions (among Kurdish Jews, 62 percent; in Saudi Arabia, 13 percent; in Myanmar, 20 percent; and in southern China, 6 percent). Migration, mutation, and intermarriage has spread these variants throughout the world. Primaquine should not be used in pregnancy because the drug may cross the placenta and cause hemolytic anemia in a G6PD-deficient fetus.

Mefloquine. Mefloquine is a quinoline-methanol derivative of quinine. It can be used either therapeutically or prophylactically in most areas with chloroquine-resistant malaria. Resistance to mefloquine, however, occurs frequently in western Cambodia and along the Thai-Cambodian and Thai-Burmese borders; in vitro resistance has been reported to occur in areas of Africa and South America.[56] Mefloquine has been associated with a relatively high incidence of neuropsychiatric side effects when used at treatment doses but is otherwise well tolerated. Neuropsychiatric side effects are rare (1 in 10,000 to 1 in 15,000) in persons taking prophylactic doses. Although not licensed for use during pregnancy or in very young infants, mefloquine appears to be both safe and effective in those groups. Mefloquine can be difficult to use in small children because it frequently causes vomiting and because no pediatric formulation is available.

Halofantrine. Halofantrine is a phenanthrene-methanol compound with activity against the erythrocytic stages of the malaria parasite. Its use has been especially recommended in areas with chloroquine-resistant falciparum. Recent studies have indicated, however, that the drug can produce cardiac conduction abnormalities (specifically, prolongation of the PR and QT intervals), which limits its usefulness.[57] A subsequent study suggests that cardiac abnormalities are dose dependent and can be severe in patients with preexisting cardiopathy; the authors suggest electrocardiography be conducted on all patients prior to treatment with halofantrine.[58] A micronized formulation has improved halofantrine's poor oral

TABLE 13-9. DRUGS USED TO TREAT MALARIA

Drug	Adult Dosage	Pediatric Dosage
Uncomplicated *Plasmodium falciparum* in areas **WITHOUT** chloroquine resistance and *Plasmodium malariae*		
(i) Chloroquine phosphate	600 mg (base) immediately, followed by 300 mg (base) in 6–8 hr, then 300 mg (base) daily for 2 days (total of 1500 mg base)[a]	10 mg/kg (base) immediately, followed by 5 mg/kg (base) in 6–8 hr, then 5 mg/kg (base) daily for 2 days (total of 25 mg/kg base)[a]
Plasmodium vivax[b] or *Plasmodium ovale*		
(i) Chloroquine phosphate	As above	As above
AND		
Primaquine phosphate[c,d,e]	15 mg (base) daily for 14 days	0.3 mg/kg (base) daily for 14 days
Uncomplicated *P. falciparum* acquired in areas **WITH** chloroquine resistance		
(i) Quinine sulfate	650 mg (salt) three times daily for 3 to 7 days[g]	
AND		
Tetracycline[f]	250 mg qid orally for 7 days	5 mg/kg qid for 7 days[h]
(ii) Pyrimethamine/sulfadoxine	3 tablets, single dose	<1 yr: ¼ tablet, single dose 1–3 yr: ½ tablet 4–8 yr: 1 tablet 9–14 yr: 2 tablets >14 yr: 3 tablets
(iii) Mefloquine[j]	15 mg/kg, single dose[i]	Same
(iv) Artesunate[k,l]	4 mg/kg stat, followed by 2 mg/kg once daily for 3 days (total of 10 mg/kg over 3 days)	Same
AND		
Mefloquine	15 mg/kg, single dose	Same
Severe *P. falciparum* malaria		
(i) Quinidine gluconate[m]	10 mg/kg (salt) loading dose IV over 1–2 hr, then 0.02 mg/kg/min continuous infusion until p.o. therapy can be started	Same
AND		
Tetracycline[f]	As above	As above[h]

Adapted from Bloland PB, Campbell CC: Malaria. In Rakel RE (ed): Conn's Current Therapy, 1992. Philadelphia: WB Saunders, 1992, pp 82–88.

[a] A standard dosing option: *Adults:* 600 mg (base) once daily for 2 days, followed by 300 mg (base) once on the third day; *Children:* 10 mg/kg (base) once daily for 2 days, followed by 5 mg/kg once on the third day.

[b] Some *P. vivax* parasites from Southeast Asia (Burma, Thailand, Indonesia), India, and South America (Guyana) have been shown to be resistant to chloroquine.

[c] Primaquine is used to eradicate hypnozoites from the liver of infected individuals. Because of the probability of reinfection, routine use of primaquine in endemic areas is generally not recommended. Primaquine is also gametocytocidal; for this reason, some malaria control programs use primaquine therapy to help decrease transmission. The overall efficacy of this practice in most areas is questionable.

[d] Some experts recommend primaquine used at 30 mg/kg daily for 14 days, especially for *P. vivax* infections acquired in Southeast Asia and Oceania.

[e] Patients who require primaquine should be screened for G6PD deficiency prior to therapy. Patients with mild G6PD deficiency (A variant with 10 to 60 percent residual enzyme activity) can be treated with 45 mg (adult dose) once per week for 8 weeks. Severely deficient patients (B variant with less than 10 percent residual enzyme activity) should not be treated with primaquine because of risk of severe and potentially fatal hemolysis. Primaquine should not be used during pregnancy.

[f] Preferred regimen for nonimmune patients. Possible alternatives for very young children or pregnant women include sulfadoxine/pyrimethamine (dose as described above), trimethoprim/sulfamethoxazole, or clindamycin. SP or trimethoprim/sulfamethoxazole regimens may fail in infections from areas with SP resistance. Clindamycin use in nonimmune patients has been associated with high rates of recrudescence.

[g] Quinine sulfate given for 3 days should be used in conjunction with a second drug such as tetracycline for 7 days, or pyrimethamine/sulfadoxine. *P. falciparum* infections from some areas of Southeast Asia, most notably Thailand, should be treated with 7 days of quinine sulfate and 7 days of tetracycline.

[h] The benefits of using tetracycline must be weighed against the known risks of adverse effects in children less than 9 years of age. Alternatives include pyrimethamine/sulfadoxine, trimethoprim/sulfamethoxazole, mefloquine, or clindamycin.

[i] Mefloquine at treatment doses has been associated with a high incidence of serious neuropsychiatric side effects (1/2000 to 1/1200). Incidence was higher among patients treated with 25 mg/kg and much higher (1/173) among patients receiving 25 mg/kg after failing 15 mg/kg. Splitting the dose (15 mg/kg on the first day followed by 10 mg/kg 24 hr later) may reduce side effects of high-dose mefloquine.

[j] In Thailand, response to treatment with 15 mg/kg mefloquine is poor, and even treatment with 25 mg/kg results in low-grade resistance in about 50 percent of cases and high-grade resistance in about 15 percent.

[k] Artesunate and related compounds should not be used except as an adjunct therapy in the treatment of cerebral malaria and treatment of multidrug-resistant *P. falciparum* (such as occurs in Thailand).

[l] Artesunate given for 5 to 7 days appears to be an effective treatment of multidrug-resistant *P. falciparum* malaria. Courses shorter than 5 to 7 days have a high rate of recrudescence and should be used only in conjunction with a second drug (mefloquine). Single-day therapy of 10 mg/kg artesunate and 15 mg/kg mefloquine has recently been shown to be highly effective, although less so than the 3-day regimen given, and improves compliance and reduces risk of adverse reactions associated with high-dose mefloquine therapy.

[m] Quinine dihydrochloride can also be used, if available (it is not available in the U.S.) *Adults:* 600 mg diluted in 300–500 mL normal saline, infused over 1–2 hr. Dose repeated every 8 hr until patient is able to take oral quinine sulfate (as described for p.o. quinine sulfate); *Children:* 25 mg/kg divided into 3 doses per day, infused over 1–2 hr until patient is able to take oral quinine sulfate (as described for p.o. quinine sulfate).

bioavailability; however, it should be given on an empty stomach. Fatty foods dramatically increase absorption, improving the drug's antiparasitic activity but increasing the risk of cardiac complications. Recrudescences can occur with one round of treatment, and (especially when treating nonimmune individuals) a second course should be given 7 days after the first. Retreatment of patients who had failed mefloquine therapy with halofantrine was less successful than primary treatment with halofantrine, suggesting the possibility of clinical cross-resistance between the two drugs.[59,60] Halofantrine therapy after mefloquine or quinine therapy also increases the risk of cardiac problems.

Clindamycin. Clindamycin has only limited antimalarial activity when compared to other available antimalarial drugs. Recrudescence rates are high following treatment with clindamycin alone. Combined with other drugs, such as quinine, clindamycin may be somewhat useful for treatment of pregnant women or very young children; however, more effective drugs are available that can be used in these groups (such as trimethoprim-sulfamethoxazole or mefloquine).

Artemisinin Compounds. A number of sesquiterpine lactone compounds have been synthesized from the plant *Artemisia annua* (artesunate, artemether, artether). These compounds are used for treatment of severe malaria and have shown very rapid parasite clearance times and faster fever resolution than occurs with quinine. Preliminary results of studies to determine if this faster action produces improved survival suggest that there is a quicker improvement of coma following treatment with artemisinins.[61,62] When used alone, especially for durations of 5 days or less, recrudescence rates are high. Artemisinins are most frequently used in combination with mefloquine.[63]

Atovaquone. Atovaquone is a hydroxynaphthoquinone that is currently being used most widely for the treatment of opportunistic infections in immunosuppressed patients. It is effective against chloroquine-resistant *P falciparum*, but because of a high incidence of recrudescence, atovaquone is usually given in combination with proguanil.[64, 65] A new fixed-dose antimalarial combination of 250 mg atovaquone and 100 mg proguanil will be marketed as Malarone™. Treatment is usually with 1,000 mg atovaquone and 400 mg proguanil daily for 3 days. Malarone™ is reportedly effective against erythrocytic forms of all four species of human malaria.[64-66]

Pyronaridine. Pyronaridine is a drug that has been synthesized and used in China for over 20 years. While the drug was reportedly 100 percent effective in one trial in Cameroon,[67] it was only between 63 and 88 percent effective in Thailand.[68] Further testing is required before pyronaridine can be recommended for use.

Treatment of Malaria

The diagnosis of malaria should be considered in any person who has fever and has been in a malarious area within the past 6 months. In addition, reports of induced and reintroduced transmission in the United States should alert clinicians that malaria can cause illness even in patients who have not visited malarious areas.[5] *P. falciparum* infection in a nonimmune person can rapidly develop into severe, complicated or fatal malaria. Therefore, a high index of suspicion and a rapid, accurate diagnosis are critical. The choice of appropriate therapy will depend on the infecting species, the density of infection, the presence or absence of complications, the possibility of drug resistance, and the drugs that are available for treatment. Assistance with diagnosis and treatment recommendations is available in the United States from the Centers for Disease Control and Prevention Malaria Hotline (telephone 770-488-7788). A list of recommended treatment drugs is included in Table 13-9.

Patients infected with *P. vivax*, *P. ovale*, or *P. malariae* and patients with uncomplicated *P. falciparum* infections acquired in areas where drug resistance has not been documented should be treated with a 3-day course of oral chloroquine. A 14-day course of primaquine should also be given to patients infected with *P. vivax* or *P. ovale* to eradicate dormant liver-stage parasites (hypnozoites). This combination of chloroquine and primaquine will prevent relapse in a majority of cases, but some strains of *P. vivax* from Southeast Asia and Oceania appear less susceptible to primaquine and may require larger doses or a longer duration of therapy.[69]

The choice of treatment for uncomplicated *P. falciparum* infections acquired in areas where drug resistance has been documented is more difficult. Recommended regimens include quinine combined with tetracycline or sulfadoxine-pyrimethamine, mefloquine alone, or halofantrine alone. The derivatives of artemisinin and atovaquone-proguanil combination drugs appear to be effective as well, but are not widely available.

Parenteral therapy is recommended for falciparum malaria when CNS or renal complications are present or when there is a high-density infection (more than 5 percent of the RBCs are infected). Infections acquired in areas without chloroquine-resistant *P. falciparum* (CRPF) may be treated with intravenous chloroquine. However, if the infection has been acquired in areas endemic for CRPF, intravenous quinine or quinidine is necessary. In addition to parenteral therapy, exchange transfusion is recommended when cerebral malaria, renal failure, or very high-density (more than 10 percent of RBCs infected) infection is present.[70]

Treatment options are more limited for children and pregnant women.[51] Tetracyclines cannot be used in pregnancy or in children less than 8 years old. Primaquine is contraindicated for pregnant women because of the risk of hemolysis in the fetus. While most of the other antimalarial drugs are well tolerated in children, many are difficult to use because they are not available in pediatric formulations. Experience is limited, but evidence suggests that mefloquine can be used in children who weigh less than 15 kg, although infants may be more likely to vomit following treatment doses.[71] Treatment doses of chloroquine, sulfadoxine-pyrimethamine (SP), quinine, and quinidine are considered safe during pregnancy, but there is a theoretical risk of kernicterus when SP is given in the third trimester. For chloroquine-resistant infections in pregnant women, quinine is preferred, especially in the first trimester. Some experience suggests that mefloquine and artemisinin derivatives may be useful in the second and third trimesters.[72]

Geographic Distribution

Figure 13-8 shows the areas of the world where malaria transmission occurs. The numbers of cases of malaria reported to the World Health Organization by region (for the 10-year period 1984 to 1993) are presented in Table 13-10. These figures reflect considerable underreporting, particularly from African countries, where many cases of malaria go undiagnosed and health information systems are incomplete. It is estimated that more than 90 percent of malaria cases and deaths occur in sub-Saharan Africa. The figures reported to the WHO reflect only a small fraction of the 300 to 500 million cases that occur annually.[1]

Some indication of the geographic distribution of malaria can be gleaned from the numbers of malaria cases imported into the United States, but these figures are also shaped by changing patterns of international travel. Figure 13-10 shows the number of malaria cases reported in the United States by year. The overwhelming majority of these infections are imported and occur in U.S. residents who have traveled to or immigrated from malaria-endemic countries. Small numbers of cases (fewer than 10 per year) are acquired within the United States and its territories. While comparatively few persons travel between the United States and Africa, a disproportionate number of the U.S. cases are acquired on that continent. Surveillance data suggest that a growing proportion of malaria cases imported into the United States occur among immigrants and naturalized citizens who return to their countries of origin to visit friends and relatives.[4]

TABLE 13-10. MALARIA CASES REPORTED BY WHO REGION, 1984–1993[a]

WHO region	*1984*	*1985*	*1986*	*1987*	*1988*	*1989*	*1990*	*1991*	*1992*	*1993*
Africa[b]	4,422	13,207	17,927	20,588	24,712	29,381	12,302	8,994	8,384	2,590
Americas	932	911	951	1,018	1,120	1,114	1,058	1,231	1,188	984
Southeast Asia	3,005	2,502	2,685	2,834	2,791	2,942	2,970	3,087	3,078	3,077
Europe	64	57	47	28	25	21	14	16	22	50
Eastern Mediterranean	335	391	613	608	434	528	586	541	309	292
Western Pacific	1,410	1,177	1,307	1,145	1,002	1,071	1,032	968	733	674
Total, excluding Africa[c]	5,746	5,038	5,603	5,633	5,372	5,676	5,661	5,843	5,329	5,077

Adapted from World Health Organization: World malaria situation in 1993, part I. Wkly Epidemiol Rec 71(1):17–22, 1996.
[a]The information provided does not always cover the entire population at risk.
[b]Mainly clinically diagnosed cases; incomplete figures.
[c]Sums may not equal because of rounding.

Distribution of Four Plasmodium *Species*

Not all species of malaria are transmitted in all malarious areas. While *P. falciparum* is transmitted in nearly all areas where malaria occurs, it accounts for over 90 percent of all malaria infections in sub-Saharan Africa and nearly 100 percent of infections in Haiti. *P. falciparum* causes two-thirds or more of malaria cases in Southeast Asia. *P. vivax* is only rarely transmitted in sub-Saharan Africa because most ethnic groups lack the RBC marker required for invasion by this parasite,[73] but it predominates in Central America, most of malarious South America, and the Indian subcontinent. Recent reports have documented the resurgence of vivax malaria in the Central Asian republics of the former Soviet Union. *P. malariae* has a patchy distribution but may be transmitted in most of the malarious world. In contrast, *P. ovale* transmission is limited to tropical Africa and Papua New Guinea.

Distribution of Drug-Resistant Strains

Chloroquine-resistant *P. falciparum* (CRPF) was first recognized almost simultaneously in Thailand and South America in the late 1950s. CRPF was documented on the east coast of Africa in 1978. In the past 20 to 25 years, CRPF has spread and intensified to the point that only central America northwest of the Panama Canal, the island of Hispaniola (Haiti and the Dominican Republic), and limited regions of the Middle East remain free of chloroquine resistance. In all other endemic areas malaria is, to varying extent, resistant to chloroquine. In some regions, chloroquine resistance has intensified to the point where chloroquine no longer has a significant effect on *P. falciparum* parasites and can no longer be relied on to provide effective treatment or prophylaxis. Finally, there is recent evidence that chloroquine-resistant *P. vivax* has emerged in South America, Southeast Asia, and the Indian subcontinent.[74,75]

Drug resistance is not an all-or-nothing phenomenon. In any given area, a wide range of parasitologic responses can be found, from complete sensitivity to complete resistance. In parts of East Africa, resistance has intensified to the point where 80 to 90 percent of *P. falciparum* infections are moderately to highly resistant.[76] In response to these high rates of resistance, Malawi switched from chloroquine to sulfadoxine-pyrimethamine for first-line therapy for *P. falciparum* in 1993. South Africa, Kenya, and Botswana have adopted similar changes in treatment policy for select districts where resistance is intense. Other nations in eastern and central Africa are currently reevaluating chloroquine efficacy and considering the need for similar changes.

The problem of drug resistance is not limited to chloroquine. In Southeast Asia, falciparum malaria has rapidly developed resistance to one compound after another. After chloroquine was abandoned as

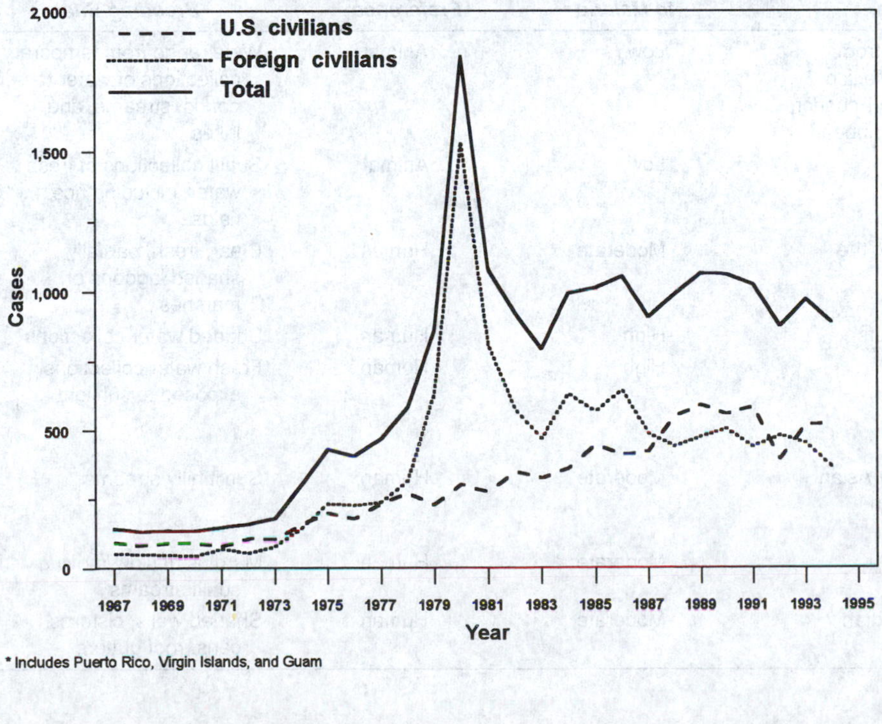

Figure 13-10. Malaria cases reported among civilians, United States, 1967–1994. (Adapted from Kachur SP, Reller ME, Barber A, et al: Malaria surveillance—United States, 1994. MMWR Surveillance Summaries, 1997, in press.)

first-line therapy for malaria in Thailand in 1972 in preference to sulfadoxine-pyrimethamine (SP), resistance to that drug developed and intensified. In 1985, SP was briefly replaced by a combination of SP and mefloquine (Fansimef™).[77] Currently, more than 50 percent of *P. falciparum* infections show resistance to mefloquine (15 mg/kg) in some areas of Thailand.[56] Cure rates were improved to between 70 and 80 percent by increasing the dose of mefloquine to 25 mg/kg, but the incidence of side effects also increased. Increasing the dose of halofantrine from 24 mg/kg to 72 mg/kg over 72 hr improved cure rates from 65 to 99 percent but also increased the toxicity. Currently, multidrug-resistant malaria is being treated with a combination of mefloquine and artemisinin derivatives.

Drug resistance develops rapidly to dihydrofolate reductase inhibitors (such as pyrimethamine and proguanil) when used alone.[78] In Southeast Asia and South America, parasitologic response to quinine has been deteriorating.[79] Resistance to newer antimalarials such as halofantrine has been reported, especially in areas with established mefloquine resistance.[59,60]

Transmission

Human malaria is transmitted by the bite of female mosquitoes belonging to the genus *Anopheles*. Of the 400 or so species of *Anopheles* in the world, approximately 60 are important vectors of malaria. However, a particular species of *Anopheles* may be an important vector in one area of the world and of little or no consequence in another. Table 13-11 lists several of the anophelines that have been incriminated as principal malaria vectors, their geographic distribution, and information on their susceptibility to malaria, preferred hosts, and breeding sites.

There are four stages in the mosquito life cycle: egg, larva, pupa, and adult. Eggs are deposited singly on water in suitable breeding sites where the developing embryo hatches as a larva after 2 or more days. At this stage the mosquito undergoes a complete metamorphosis, emerging as an adult. The length of each developmental stage is temperature dependent. Generation times in the tropics can be as brief as 5 days. The life span of adults under natural conditions is difficult to determine, but in the case of malaria vectors it is clearly longer than the time required to become infective—probably 3 to 4 weeks.

Levels of Transmission and Endemicity

Malariologists have devised a number of systems for characterizing malaria transmission. The stability of transmission has important implications for the clinical features of malarial illness, the degree of population immunity, and the optimal mix of preventive approaches that is relevant in a given area. **Stable** malaria transmission is intense, varies little from season to season, and can be difficult to interrupt. Populations living in areas with stable transmission generally acquire partial immunity; consequently, severe and fatal illness tends to occur only in young children or pregnant women. **Unstable** malaria transmission is intermittent and highly variable. Populations in areas of unstable transmission rarely develop sufficient immunity for protection; as a result, severe and fatal disease can occur in persons of all ages, and there is a high risk for epidemic malaria.[80] In Africa, stability of transmission is also associated with the predominant vector species; the highly efficient vector *Anopheles gambiae* tends to predominate in areas of stable transmission, while *Anopheles arabiensis* is more prevalent in unstable, epidemic-prone areas.

Malaria transmission can also be characterized by its intensity. In **holoendemic** regions there is intense malaria transmission year round and population immunity is high, particularly among adults. While older children and adults may become infected and develop clinical disease in these settings, severe or fatal malaria occur almost exclusively in children between the ages of 1 and 4 years old. In **hyperendemic** areas, malaria transmission is seasonal and the population's level of immunity does not confer adequate protection from disease for all age groups. As a result, severe and fatal malaria infections occur in children and adults. In **mesoendemic** areas there is some malaria transmission and population immunity is low. Finally, in **hypoendemic** areas there is very little transmission and little or no immunity to the parasite. While malaria may constitute a minor public health burden in mesoendemic and hypoendemic communities, the low levels of population immunity leave these areas prone to devastating malaria epidemics.[80] The level of endemicity in a region can be quantified by determining the percentage of chil-

TABLE 13-11. FEATURES OF COMMON MALARIA VECTORS

Species	*Distribution*	*Susceptibility to Malaria*	*Host Preference*	*Typical Breeding Sites*
Anopheles albimanus	Western hemisphere from southeast Texas, Mexico, Central America, to Ecuador, Venezuela, and Caribbean	Low	Animal	Wide range from temporary collections of water to ponds, streams, and lakes
Anopheles culicifacies	Indian subcontinent	Low	Animal	Sunlit collections of fresh water, including rice fields
Anopheles darlingi	South America east of the Andes	Moderate	Human	Clear, fresh, partially shaded lagoons or marshes
Anopheles dirus	Southeast Asian forests	High	Human	Shaded water collections
Anopheles gambiae, Anopheles funestus	Tropical Africa	High	Human	Fresh water collections exposed to sunlight
Anopheles maculatus	Foothills of Southeast Asian countries and Indian subcontinent	Moderate	Human	Sunlit hilly streams
Anopheles minimus	Southeast Asian hills	Moderate	Human	Margins of slow-moving sunlit streams
Anopheles stephensi	Urban areas of the Indian subcontinent	Moderate	Human	Shaded wells, cisterns, cans, roof gutters

TABLE 13-12. LEVELS OF ENDEMICITY BY RATES OF SPLEEN ENLARGEMENT AND PARASITE PRESENCE IN CHILDREN 2–9 YEARS OF AGE

Endemicity	*Spleen Enlarged (%)*	*Parasite Present (%)*
Hypoendemic	0–10	0–10
Mesoendemic	11–50	11–50
Hyperendemic	>50 (>25 in adults)	51–75
Holoendemic	>75 (low in adults)	>75

Adapted from Molineaux L: The epidemiology of human malaria as an explanation of its distribution, including some implications for its control. In Wernsdorfer WH, McGregor I (eds): Malaria: Principles and Practice of Malariology. Edinburgh: Churchill Livingstone, 1988, pp 913–998.

dren (2 to 9 years old) with enlarged spleens and malaria parasites in their blood (Table 13-12).[81] In general, as the level of endemicity decreases, the stability of transmission also declines and the risk of epidemic malaria increases.

Host Factors Affecting Distribution

Several heritable characteristics of human hosts also affect the distribution of the human malarias. Similarly, endemic malaria has influenced the rates of genetic polymorphisms and genetic diseases in many human populations. Genetic factors can influence the hosts' susceptibility to malaria infections and their likelihood of developing severe or complicated malaria.[82] For example, *Plasmodium vivax* invades red blood cells by recognizing the Duffy antigen on their surface. Persons who are genetically Duffy-negative, therefore, will be unable to sustain vivax infections. For this reason, *P. vivax* does not occur among West African populations, who lack this blood group marker.

Perhaps the most well-recognized group of host genetic factors associated with malaria are the hemoglobinopathies. Hemoglobin S in its homozygous state causes sickle cell disease. Although persons with sickle cell disease or its heterozygous carrier state can develop malaria infections, heterozygous individuals are afforded 80 to 95 percent protection from severe or complicated *P. falciparum* infections.[83] Other hemoglobinopathies, including hemoglobins C and E, the α and β thalassemias, and persistence of fetal hemoglobin have also been associated with protection from severe or complicated malaria illness.[84] It appears that falciparum parasites are not able to metabolize these variant hemoglobin molecules. In addition to the hemoglobinopathies, other alterations in RBC structure or function can affect host susceptibility to malaria. Recent studies have demonstrated some protective effect for persons who carry the genes for hereditary ovalocytosis[85] and G6PD deficiency.[86] Studies have also associated resistance to malaria and its severe manifestations with the highly variable human leukocyte antigens (HLA) of the major histocompatibility complex (MHC).[87] In a large case-control study in the Gambia, children with severe malaria were less likely to have the class I antigen HLA B53 or one form of the class II antigen HLA DR13.[83] The association was stronger for severe malaria than for mild infections. Polymorphisms in the gene that codes for tumor necrosis factor α have also been shown to alter the risk of severe malaria.[88,89]

Nutrition

The interaction between undernutrition and malnutrition and malaria is complex and incompletely understood. Some nutritional deficiencies apparently protect against malaria, and others exacerbate malaria infection. Although cerebral malaria was found more commonly among well-nourished children in Nigeria than children with clinical marasmus or kwashiorkor,[90] children in the Gambia had no difference in risk of cerebral malaria[13] or risk of nonsevere malaria infection[91] based on weight-for-age. Iron deficiency in children may protect against malaria infection, and oral or parenteral iron supplementation has been shown in some studies[92–94] to increase malaria prevalence or incidence. Other studies, however, show that hematologic recovery is maximized with a combination of iron supplementation and effective malaria therapy.[54] Parenteral iron supplementation during pregnancy has been shown to increase the risk of malaria infection among primigravid women[95] but not among multigravid women.[96] Zinc and vitamin A deficiency may increase the frequency and severity of malaria in children.[97–100] Concomitant administration of folate or iron with antifol antimalarials (i.e. sulfadoxine-pyrimethamine) has been shown to increase the risk of treatment failure.[54,101]

Malnutrition can also be worsened because of malaria. Malaria causes increased destruction and decreased production of RBCs,[13] exacerbating existing nutritional anemias. In addition, the anorexia and vomiting frequently associated with malaria infection can further limit food intake and contribute to further nutritional deficiency.[102] The effects of malnutrition on immunologic responses to malaria are unclear. The prevalence and degree of parasitologic resistance to both chloroquine and SP was worse among malnourished Rwandan refugees,[103] possibly because of impaired immune function. Malaria can have immunosuppressive effects and can increase the risk of infection with other pathogens, including *Salmonella*.[104]

Social and Behavioral Factors

The relationships between malaria transmission and human behavior are multiple and complex. Many of the human behaviors that favor malaria transmission stem from broad social, cultural, and economic forces. Such factors include poverty, agricultural and industrial development, population mobility, and urbanization.[80] In addition to these broad social forces, malaria transmission and control are invariably affected by local beliefs, attitudes, and practices.

In most malaria-endemic areas, poverty is also deeply entrenched and can influence the distribution of malaria as well as other health conditions. As described above, the undernutrition associated with poverty contributes to malaria mortality, especially in children. Impoverished families often reside in substandard housing that affords little protection from anopheline mosquitoes. In poor communities, inadequate sanitation and drainage control can create ideal breeding sites for some malaria vectors. In addition, the lack of economic resources, at both the national and household levels, leaves residents of highly malarious areas with few options for malaria prevention and control, and limited access to appropriate health care services.[105] Poverty-related medical practices such as misuse and underdosing of antimalarial medications play an important role in the development and spread of drug-resistant malaria.[106]

Agricultural development can contribute to malaria transmission in a number of important ways. Clearing forests for crop production can create ideal breeding sites for anopheline vectors.[107,108] In addition to deforestation, the changes in water use and altered populations of wild and domesticated animals that typically accompany agricultural development can also affect the likelihood of human-mosquito contact and malaria transmission.[109] Finally, it has been suggested that the agricultural use of pesticides may contribute to mosquito resistance to DDT and other insecticides.[110]

Human mobility has had a tremendous effect on the global malaria situation as well. Among 20 countries with high risk of malaria transmission in the Americas, 16 identified human mobility as a major cause of persistence of transmission.[111] Migration has been associated with the spread of drug-resistant malaria in Africa and Southeast Asia.[112,113] Migrant farm workers have been linked to outbreaks of autochthonous transmission of malaria in the United States, raising the concern of the possibility of reestablishment.[5] These outbreaks provide evidence that movements of individuals or small numbers of people can have an effect on malaria. Movements of large populations either into or out of malaria endemic areas, however, carry a much higher risk of disastrous consequences.

In the process of urbanization, construction for new settlements often creates additional anopheline breeding sites.[114] When populations first settle new towns they often choose to locate near water supplies and in recently disrupted local environments. While rural areas are generally considered at greatest risk for malaria, anopheline vectors have become well adapted to conditions in many cities.[115] Moreover, the rapid rates of urbanization in many malarious areas easily outpace the expansion of health and environmental services. As a result, many new urban residents are forced into marginal areas, slums, and squatter settlements where malaria transmission may readily occur.[116] Furthermore, these peripheral peri-urban areas often include populations who migrate between larger settlements and rural areas for employment and might easily introduce malaria. The increasing proportion of residents of malarious countries who live in urban and peri-urban settings demands that additional attention be given to understanding and controlling malaria in these settings.

In addition to these globally determined processes, local social, cultural, and behavioral patterns can influence the transmission of malaria as well as a community's acceptance of and compliance with malaria control activities. Culturally defined patterns of housing and sleeping behavior can reduce or favor malaria transmission and will affect the appropriateness and acceptability of most vector-control strategies.[117,118] Local perceptions of fever, complicated malaria, and their causes[119,120] can influence local acceptance of malaria control activities. Likewise, local attitudes toward antimalarial drugs can affect compliance with treatment and prophylaxis programs.[121,122] Careful involvement of community members can overcome some of these potential problems.[123]

Malaria Control

Historical Perspective

In 1955, the eighth World Health Assembly launched a program to eradicate malaria worldwide.[124] The eradication effort produced dramatic results, especially in temperate climates and island nations. However, throughout the 1950s and 1960s, malaria persisted as a serious health threat in most continental tropical countries.[125] Indeed, sub-Saharan Africa was excluded from the eradication effort altogether.[126] The global program relied heavily on a strategy of focused domestic application of DDT. Since it was anticipated that insecticide resistance would develop, eradication was considered a time-limited activity. From the start, the program placed little emphasis on research, attitudes of local populations, or regional differences in vector behavior.[80]

By 1969, a revised global malaria strategy had evolved. The new approach emphasized malaria control by integrating multiple prevention measures tailored to local conditions. Global funding for malaria declined. By the late 1970s, countries were encouraged to integrate malaria control activities into their basic health service programs, as international health policy shifted, favoring decentralized, horizontal approaches like primary health care and child survival over highly centralized vertical programs like malaria eradication. Ultimately, these changes in international priorities and support, combined with the emergence of drug-resistant parasites and insecticide-resistant vectors, contributed to the resurgence of malaria worldwide.[117,127]

Some early malaria control projects combined two or more preventive strategies, such as residual spraying with mass distribution of drugs,[128] to produce a greater public health impact. Contemporary malaria control efforts aim to reduce malaria-related morbidity and mortality through a combination of multiple interventions that disrupt the parasite-vector-human cycle at several points. This stratified approach is based on the observation that the effectiveness of different malaria control options can depend heavily on local conditions.[129] Some understanding of these conditions is therefore needed in order to develop a malaria control project. First of all, basic malaria surveillance data are necessary to determine the level of endemicity, assess the seasonality of transmission, and identify the level of risk in different population groups. It can be more efficient to target some interventions to population groups at most risk for severe consequences of malaria infection, such as children, pregnant women, and nonimmune visitors to endemic areas. In some areas, drug efficacy testing will be needed to understand the relative prevalence of antimalarial drug-resistant parasites and to develop effective treatment and chemoprophylaxis policies. An understanding of local attitudes and beliefs is also important, since these can affect the acceptability of some interventions, particularly those that depend on changing human behavior. Finally, entomologic studies to identify the principal vectors are necessary for selecting appropriate vector control options. These scientific inputs should be used to devise an integrated malaria control program that will be well suited to local conditions of malaria epidemiology, the vector, climate, geography, and human populations. The array of possible combinations is vast but includes four general types of intervention methods: case management, chemoprophylaxis, personal protection, and vector control measures.

Case Management

Whereas vector control through residual spraying was the principal feature of malaria eradication, case management is the cornerstone of integrated malaria control activities in most endemic areas.[129] Prompt diagnosis and treatment of patients with uncomplicated malaria can prevent severe and complicated illnesses and avert deaths. It can also be a useful tool for controlling transmission. Diagnosis and treatment options vary widely from one endemic area to another depending on the level of transmission, the availability and cost of different antimalarial drugs, local patterns of antimalarial resistance, and the resources available for diagnosis and treatment. In areas of intense sustained transmission, particularly in sub-Saharan Africa, it is commonly recommended that all children with fever receive treatment for malaria. This approach has been adopted in many countries and has been incorporated into the WHO/UNICEF initiative for the integrated management of childhood illness (IMCI).[130] The ideal approach to diagnosis and management of febrile illness is less clear in areas of low malaria endemicity. Furthermore, because of the relative lack of health personnel and resources in many highly endemic areas, even this simple approach to case management is often difficult to implement and sustain.

Unfortunately, the spread of antimalarial drug resistance in recent years has further complicated case management efforts. The presence of multiple drug-resistant malaria in Southeast Asia has necessitated several rapid changes in recommended therapies. However, antimalarial treatment options in many nations still favor chloroquine as the first-line drug, even where it is ineffective in more than half of *P. falciparum* infections. In 1993, Malawi became the first African nation to switch from chloroquine to sulfadoxine-pyrimethamine for first-line therapy of uncomplicated malaria. Similar policy changes have been made for certain districts in South Africa, Kenya, and Botswana and seem imminent in other countries on the continent.

In addition to treating acute infections, some case management strategies in low-transmission or epidemic-prone areas include follow-up treatment with primaquine. This strategy is generally recommended either to reduce the risk of relapse in *P. vivax* or *P. ovale* infections or to eliminate circulating gametocytes in treated patients. Eradicating gametocytes following treatment can be a useful method for blocking further transmission. Primaquine is rarely recommended in settings of intense transmission where reinfection is likely to occur before relapse.

Chemoprophylaxis

Antimalarial drugs are always recommended for prophylaxis of nonimmune travelers visiting malaria-endemic areas. In some instances, chemoprophylaxis can also be an important component of malaria control activities in endemic areas, especially for groups at high risk of severe consequences from malaria, such as pregnant women, young children, and nonimmune migrant populations. Large-scale chemoprophylaxis is generally not practical for whole populations residing long term in endemic areas, and it may favor the development and spread of drug-resistant parasites.

In nonimmune travelers, the choice of drugs for prophylaxis must be made on an individual basis. Providers should consider the traveler's destination, the presence of antimalarial-resistant strains, the type of exposure and accommodations, the timing and duration of travel, and the traveler's age, drug allergies, other medications, and medical history. Recommendations may also differ depending on the source of the advice and the range of antimalarial preparations available in the traveler's home country or destination. The recommendations of the Centers for Disease Control and Prevention (CDC) appear in Table 13-13. For places where chloroquine-resistant malaria has not been documented, weekly chloroquine is the drug of choice. For destinations where chloroquine-resistant *P. falciparum* is transmitted, weekly mefloquine is recommended for prophylaxis. Travelers who cannot take mefloquine should take daily doxycycline. If a traveler to an area endemic for CRPF is unable to take either mefloquine or doxycycline, the only remaining alternative is weekly chloroquine with or without daily proguanil. Because the chloroquine-proguanil regimen is considerably less effective, travelers who rely on it should seek microscopic diagnosis and medical care at the first sign of fever and may be advised to carry a treatment dose of sulfadoxine-pyrimethamine if adequate facilities for diagnosis and treatment are more than 24 hours away. Chemoprophylaxis should be started 1 week before arriving in a malaria-endemic destination (1 or 2 days is sufficient for doxycycline) and should be continued during travel and for 4 weeks after leaving the malarious area.[131,132]

Most of the antimalarial drugs commonly used for chemoprophylaxis act only on intraerythrocytic stages of the parasite. Even when they are effective and used appropriately, these medications do not prevent primary infection, exoerythrocytic schizogony, or the establishment of hypnozoites in the liver. An individual infected with *P. vivax* or *P. ovale* will only rarely develop clinical symptoms of the primary infection while taking effective antimalarial chemoprophylaxis but may become acutely ill weeks or months later when the infection relapses from the dormant liver stage. A 14-day course of primaquine can eliminate hypnozoites in travelers exposed to intense or prolonged *P. vivax* or *P. ovale* transmission even if they have no symptoms. Postexposure prophylaxis with primaquine should not be given to most short-term travelers; it should be reserved for those with long-term rural exposures (such as returned missionaries or Peace Corps volunteers) or travelers returning from areas of intense *P. vivax* transmission (such as Papua New Guinea).[132]

Malaria infection during pregnancy can pose a significant risk to both mother and child. Even partially immune women appear to be more susceptible to malaria when pregnant, especially in their first and second pregnancies. Malaria in pregnancy can cause low birth weight, preterm labor, and intrauterine growth retardation. Preventing these adverse pregnancy outcomes is an important element of many malaria control programs. In endemic areas, chemoprophylaxis during pregnancy is generally recommended. Voluntary compliance with weekly chloroquine prophylaxis programs is often quite poor.[133] In areas with CRPF, intermittent treatment with two or more doses of sulfadoxine-pyrimethamine during the second and third trimesters has been shown to reduce placental malaria infections and reduce the risk associated with malaria in pregnancy.[134]

Personal Protection

There are numerous personal protective measures individuals can use to reduce their own and their household's risk of malaria infection by preventing contact with mosquitoes. Since no antimalarial drug is 100 percent effective for chemoprophylaxis, nonimmune travelers should also be advised to follow personal protective measures that reduce contact with infective mosquitoes. These include wearing protective clothing, using insect repellents, screening windows and doors, and

TABLE 13-13. DRUGS USED FOR CHEMOPROPHYLAXIS OF MALARIA[a]

Drug	*Adult Dosage*	*Pediatric Dosage*
Travel in areas with chloroquine-sensitive *Plasmodium falciparum*		
(i) Chloroquine phosphate	300 mg base (500 mg salt) orally, once a week	5 mg/kg base (8.3 mg/kg salt) orally, once a week; up to maximum adult dose of 300 mg base/week
(ii) Hydroxychloroquine sulfate	310 mg base (400 mg salt) orally, once a week	5 mg/kg base (6.5 mg/kg salt) orally, once a week; up to maximum adult dose of 310 mg base/week
Travel in areas with chloroquine-resistant *Plasmodium falciparum*		
(i) Mefloquine[b]	228 mg base (250 mg salt) orally, once a week	15–19 kg: ¼ tablet weekly 20–30 kg: ½ tablet weekly 31–45 kg: ¾ tablet weekly >45 kg: 1 tablet weekly
(ii) Doxycycline	100 mg orally, once a day	>8 years of age: 2 mg/kg orally, once a day, up to maximum adult dose of 100 mg/day
(iii) Chloroquine phosphate **AND**	300 mg base (500 mg salt) orally, once a week	5 mg/kg base (8.3 mg/kg salt) orally, once a week, up to maximum adult dose of 300 mg base/week
Proguanil[c]	200 mg orally, once a day	<2 years: 50 mg daily 2–6 years: 100 mg daily 7–10 years: 150 mg daily >10 years: 200 mg daily
Prevention of relapses		
Primaquine[d]	15 mg base (26.3 mg salt) orally, once a day for 14 days	0.3 mg/kg base (0.5 mg/kg salt) orally, once a day for 14 days

Adapted from Bloland PB, Campbell CC: Malaria. In Rakel RE (ed): Conn's Current Therapy, 1992. Philadelphia: WB Saunders, 1992, pp 82–88.

[a]Chemoprophylaxis should begin 1 week prior to travel (1–2 days for doxycycline) and should be continued while in the malarious area and for 4 weeks after leaving the malarious area.

[b]Mefloquine is contraindicated for persons with known hypersensitivity to the drug and is not recommended for persons with a history of serious psychiatric or seizure disorder. Small children who are given mefloquine for prophylaxis should receive a weekly dose of 5 mg/kg.

[c]Proguanil is not available in the United States.

[d]Primaquine can cause hemolytic anemia in patients with glucose-6-phosphate dehydrogenase deficiency. Primaquine should not be given during pregnancy.

using insecticide-treated curtains and bed nets. While personal protection measures can be effective at the individual level, their role in population-based control strategies is less clear.

In recent years, however, studies have demonstrated that community-wide distribution of insecticide-treated mosquito nets and curtains can reduce transmission and decrease malaria illness in a wide range of settings.[135] The strategy is best applied in settings where the primary vector bites primarily at night and indoors. In a controlled trial in the Gambia, insecticide-treated bed nets reduced all-cause mortality for children 1 to 4 years old by 63 percent.[136] Later, a nationwide program showed a 25 percent reduction in childhood mortality.[137] These results are encouraging, but it does appear that the intervention may be less effective in areas of more intense transmission.[138,139] While some efficacy questions remain, the greater challenge will be translating these findings into effective, sustainable projects that can be integrated into broader malaria control programs.

Vector Control

Vector control strategies were key elements in the malaria eradication effort and remain an important and valuable component of malaria control activities today. Among the vector control options available are insecticide spraying to kill adult mosquitoes and the use of pesticides and environmental measures to reduce mosquito larvae. In addition, a number of innovative vector control strategies are promising. The aim of vector control is to reduce human-mosquito contact, thereby reducing malaria transmission.

Differences in the behavior patterns of adult mosquitoes have a marked effect on their capacity to transmit malaria as well as on the choice of control methods used. Preferred time of biting, for example, can vary from daytime to late evening. The efficacy of many control measures varies depending on the mosquito activity cycle. For example, mosquito nets, an effective barrier to human-mosquito contact at night, probably have little effect on malaria transmission by daytime biters. Similarly, control measures that are used indoors, such as residual spraying with insecticides, may have little effect on mosquitoes that bite outdoors. Preferred resting sites (after a blood meal, the female "rests" while oogenesis proceeds) may be indoors, where they can be targeted by house spraying, or outdoors, where spraying is not effective. Mosquitoes also exhibit biting preferences that affect their capacity to transmit malaria. Some prefer humans (anthropophilic), while others select animals (zoophilic). Most, however, are opportunists and will bite humans if given a chance. Choosing when and where to implement a given vector control strategy, therefore, requires a thorough understanding of the taxonomy and biology of local vector species.

Wide-scale spraying to kill adult mosquitoes was a prominent component of malaria eradication programs in many parts of the world. Insecticides with residual action lasting up to 6 months, sprayed on the inside walls of houses, are most effective when most human-anopheline contact occurs indoors. In many settings of high transmission, residual spraying is not a realistic option and would be largely ineffective even if high rates of coverage could be achieved and sustained.[140] However, residual spraying can be very valuable in other circumstances, such as in refugee settlements and agricultural and industrial development projects, where large numbers of nonimmune persons are introduced into endemic areas. Residual spraying would also be useful in areas threatened by malaria epidemics.

Chemical application at breeding sites can kill mosquito larvae and, theoretically, reduce malaria transmission. Larger-scale water management projects can also reduce mosquitoes and are credited with eradicating malaria from much of the southern United States. However, in many endemic areas, breeding habitats are too numerous and inaccessible to be treated or eliminated entirely through these approaches. However, the use of larvicides is warranted in some settings, especially in urban areas, where malaria transmission can frequently be linked to a discrete number of accessible breeding sites.

Future Vector Control Options

Although not yet fully operational, a number of innovative strategies for vector control appear promising. Biological control agents and naturally occurring predators can be introduced to reduce the numbers of immature and adult-stage mosquitoes. Aquatic plants and larvivorous fishes can reduce larvae in breeding sites.[141] Alterations of the vector genome may ultimately allow populations of malaria-transmitting mosquitoes to be replaced with genetically transformed mosquitoes that cannot sustain transmission.[142] Finally, vaccines that induce hosts to produce anti-vector antibodies may ultimately be able to alter parasite development and/or reduce the survival of mosquito vectors.[143]

Vaccine Development and Testing

Development of malaria vaccines has proceeded along three lines. Sporozoite vaccines are directed against the stage of the malaria parasite that is injected into the human host when a mosquito takes its blood meal. An effective sporozoite vaccine would protect the recipient from infection and thus from all symptoms of a malarial illness. Merozoite or blood-stage vaccines are directed against the asexual blood stages of the parasite, which are responsible for malaria symptoms. It is likely that such vaccines would mimic naturally acquired immunity to malaria; recipients might continue to have occasional malarial illnesses, but the severity and duration of symptoms would be reduced and malaria-related mortality would be prevented. Transmission-blocking vaccines prevent development of the sexual stages of the malaria parasite in the human host or mosquito vector. Such vaccines would have no impact at all on an individual patient's symptoms but would reduce the level of transmission within the community by rendering mosquitoes noninfective.

Numerous candidate vaccines have been developed, but no clearly effective vaccine has yet been identified. The first field trials of the asexual blood-stage candidate vaccine, SPf 66, showed that it did not afford significant protection from *P. falciparum* malaria,[144,145] despite earlier encouraging results from experimental trials.[146] A recent report demonstrated promising results for a sporozoite vaccine under experimental conditions,[147] but field trials have yet to be conducted.

Conclusion

Between the history of an unsuccessful eradication program and the future promise of an effective vaccine and improved options for treatment and prevention, malaria remains a major public health concern worldwide. A growing number of strategies are currently available for malaria control, but none is universally effective or appropriate. Research is needed to develop additional options as well as to describe the best approaches to implementing existing strategies. At present, the best hope for malaria control in endemic areas is an integrated approach that combines multiple strategies and that is carefully matched to local conditions of the parasite, vector, and human populations.

Lyme Disease

David T. Dennis

Lyme disease is a tick-borne zoonosis caused by infection with the spirochete *Borrelia burgdorferi*. Infection in humans results in a multisystem, multistage inflammatory disease principally affecting the skin, joints, nervous system and heart. Several syndromes constituting Lyme disease (Lyme borreliosis) were recognized in Europe beginning in the late nineteenth century; however, the disease was first comprehensively described in Connecticut in 1977.[1] Rodents and ticks are the principal reservoirs and amplifying hosts of *B. burgdorferi* infection; deer are the usual maintenance hosts for vector ticks; and humans are incidentally infected when they intrude into the natural zootic cycle. The disease occurs throughout the temperate Northern Hemisphere. In the United States, Lyme disease now accounts for more than 95 percent of all reported cases of vector-borne disease, and it is an emerging infection of considerable public health importance. Between 1982 and 1996, the annual reported incidence in the United States increased approximately 30-fold to more than 15,000 cases a year. Although comparable statistical data are not available for Eurasian countries, the annual number of cases there is thought to be several times that of the United States. The ecology and epidemiology of Lyme disease are complex, and practical methods for control at the community level have not yet been found. The disease is slowly expanding its geographic range, and the incidence of human cases continues to increase in both new and established foci of infection.

Agent

After a considerable search for an infectious cause of Lyme disease, novel spirochetes were identified in the midgut of the adult blacklegged tick, *Ixodes scapularis* (*I. dommini*, the deer tick).[2] The spirochete was cultured from ticks in a modified Kelly's medium (BSK), and shortly thereafter cultured from blood, skin, and cerebrospinal fluid of patients with early Lyme disease. The spirochete was described as *Borrelia burgdorferi* in 1984.[3]

Borreliae are flexible helical cells composed of a protoplasmic cylinder surrounded by a cell membrane, seven to 11 periplasmic flagella, and an outer membrane that is loosely associated with the underlying structures. The outer membrane of *B. burgdorferi* and other borreliae is unique in that genes encoding its proteins are located on linear plasmids; these extrachromosomal genes determine the molecular identity of the various strains and genospecies and are responsible for adaptive antigenic variability. *B. burgdorferi* is composed of at least 30 different immunogenic proteins, including three major outer-surface proteins, Osp-A (30 kDa), Osp-B (34 kDa), and Osp-C (23 kDa).[4] A prominent 41-kDa antigen is located on the flagellum. A number of genetic differences have been described within and between *B. burgdorferi* genospecies from Europe and the United States. The strain infecting humans in the United States is designated *B. burgdorferi* sensu stricto, of which strain B31 is the prototype; the two dominant *B. burgdorferi* genospecies in Europe and Asia are *Borrelia garinii* and *Borrelia afzellii* (Group V5461).[5] These genospecies have been found to be associated with somewhat different disease expressions: arthritis appears to occur more frequently following infection with *B. burgdorferi*, neurologic manifestations are more common in infections with *B. garinii*, and cutaneous manifestations occur more frequently in association with *B. afzellii* infection.

Life Cycle

The basic elements in the life cycle of *B. burgdorferi* in North America are as follows: (*a*) small rodents, especially the white-footed mouse and the chipmunk in the northeastern and north-central regions, and the dusky wood rat (pack rat) in the Pacific coastal region, serve as the principal reservoirs of *B. burgdorferi* infection for vector ticks; (*b*) three stages of tick (larva, nymph, adult) are involved in a 2-year life cycle, and each stage normally takes a single blood meal; (*c*) transstadial transmission of *B. burgdorferi* from larva to nymph helps maintain the infective cycle, while transmission from an infected adult female to her eggs rarely occurs; (*d*) the efficiency of the cycle is enhanced in eastern regions of the United States by sequential feeding patterns in which nymphs, feeding in the spring, infect rodents that later in the year serve as sources of infection for larvae, which feed in the summer months; (*e*) deer, especially the white-tailed deer, and other large and medium-sized animals, serve as a mating ground for adult ticks and provide adult female ticks the blood meal required for egg production.[6,7] In Eurasia, the cycle is quite similar, although meadow voles and woodland mice serve as the principal rodent reservoirs of infection, and the roe deer and other cervids typically serve as maintenace hosts for vector ticks.

Humans are incidental hosts of *B. burgdorferi*. In the eastern United States, persons are most often infected by the bite of nymphal-stage ticks, usually in the late spring and early summer, and much less frequently by adult female ticks, which feed mostly in the late fall and winter but also in the early spring. Figure 13-11 is a schematic diagram of the transmission cycle.

The Disease

Lyme disease is an inflammatory process that can be generally categorized into early localized, early disseminated, and late disseminated stages of infection and disease.[8] The portal of entry of *B. burgdorferi* is the dermis, at the site of attachment of the infective tick. Following inoculation, infection spreads by cutaneous, lymphatic, and hematogenous routes. An incubation period of 3 to 30 days (typically 7 to 14 days) occurs between the time of infection and the onset of the characteristic erythema migrans (EM) rash that is the hallmark of early localized infection. This expanding, annular, erythematous rash, which is observed in 70 percent or more of cases, is usually accompanied by mild constitutional symptoms of fever, headache, myalgia, and arthralgia and occasionally by regional lymphadenitis. Not all patients remember a rash or other early manifestations; if untreated, weeks or months may elapse before signs and symptoms of disseminated infection are recognized.

Early disseminated infection usually occurs days to weeks after the onset of localized infection. The skin, nervous system, musculoskeletal system, and heart may be affected. Multiple secondary erythema migrans lesions occur fairly frequently. Some patients manifest neurologic signs and symptoms, most commonly aseptic (lymphocytic) meningitis, cranial neuropathy (especially nerve VII palsy), or radiculoneuritis. Many patients complain in the early disseminated stage of infection of migratory musculoskeletal pains without objective signs, although episodes of swelling and tenderness of one or a few joints may uncommonly occur in this early stage. Rarely, persons with early Lyme disease develop cardiac conduction abnormalities—most often mild, transient atrioventricular block.

Manifestations of late disseminated infection occur weeks to months after infection in untreated patients. The most common late-stage manifestion is intermittent oligarticular arthritis in one or a few joints—usually large, weight-bearing joints such as the knee. Less frequently, persons with late disseminated infection develop a chronic encephalomyelitis with subtle memory deficits or may develop a chronic axonal polyneuropathy.

Untreated and inadequately treated infection may result in microbial persistence, and *B. burgdorferi* has been isolated from skin lesions, myocardium, synovial fluid, and cerebrospinal fluid (CSF) months and

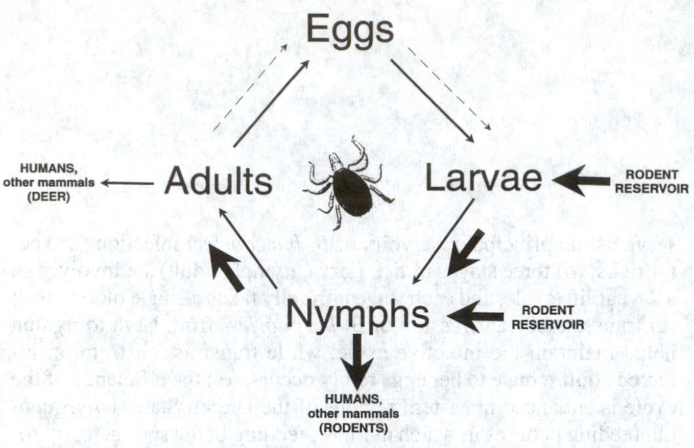

Figure 13-11. Schematic diagram of the zootic cycle of *Borrelia burgdorferi*, showing the force of infection (*heavy arrows*) as ticks advance from one stage to another (*thin arrows*). Infection moves from the rodent reservoir to larval and nymphal stages and transstadially from larva to nymph to adult tick. Transstadial transmission is important, while transovarial transmission is minimal and inconsequential (*dashed arrows*).

years after the onset of symptoms. Asymptomatic and subclinical infection is probably common. Genetic differences in susceptibility to infection have not been described, but chronic, refractory Lyme arthritis is associated with the major histocompatibility antigen HLA-DR4.[9]

Morbidity can infrequently be severe, chronic, and disabling, especially if the disease is not treated in its early stages, but Lyme disease is rarely, if ever, a principal cause of death. There have been no reports of deaths due to Lyme disease that have been confirmed by cultural isolation of *B. burgdorferi* from infected tissues. Similarly, maternal Lyme disease is not a proven cause of intrauterine death or congenital malformations, although this association has been suggested. Epidemiologic studies do not show a correlation between Lyme disease endemicity and rates of adverse events of pregnancy.[10] Concurrent infection with *B. burgdorferi* and *Babesia microti* (the agent of babesiosis) has been associated with a severity and duration of illness greater than expected for either infection alone. A case of fatal Lyme disease pancarditis, in which spirochetes were seen in the myocardium, was reported in a patient who had concurrent babesiosis.[11] The importance of differentiating between illness caused by *Borrelia*, *Babesia*, and *Ehrlichia* species and by other (as-yet unidentified) agents transmitted by the same tick vectors has recently been highlighted.[12,13]

Diagnosis

The diagnosis of Lyme disease is relatively easily made in persons presenting with characteristic manifestations in an endemic area. History of recent tick exposure significantly increases the pretest probability of a true diagnosis of Lyme disease, and laboratory testing is generally unnecessary in persons with typical clinical presentations of early disease and with known endemic exposures. Serodiagnostic testing may be indicated when a presentation is atypical or a history of exposure is not clear. The recommended test approach utilizes a sensitive first test, either enzyme-linked immunosorbent assay (EIA) or indirect fluorescent antibody (IFA) testing, followed by Western blot (WB) of serum specimens found to be equivocal or positive in the first test.[14] Specific WB banding criteria have been recommended for both IgM and IgG antibodies. IgM antibodies to *B burgdorferi* can be detected within 2 weeks after the onset of EM in 40 percent or more of patients and usually peak between the third and sixth weeks of illness; IgG responses may arise early or be delayed for weeks, and occur in about 65 percent of persons with early, localized Lyme disease.[15,16] *B. burgdorferi* can be cultured from 80 percent or more of biopsy specimens taken from early EM lesions, but culture is not a routine procedure. Patients with early disseminated disease, such as cranial neuritis or multiple EM, and with active later-stage disease, such as arthritis, radiculoneuritis, meningoencephalitis, and acrodermatitis chronicum atrophicans, almost always have strong seroreactivity to *B. burgdorferi* antigens. Antibiotic treatment in early localized disease may blunt or abrogate the immune response. Seronegative late-stage Lyme disease rarely occurs. Infection does not confer lasting protective immunity, and more than one occurrence of primary EM is not uncommon among persons at high environmental risk.

▶ ECOLOGY

Arthropod Vectors of B. burgdorferi

Cycles of *B. burgdorferi* are found in the range of *Ixodes ricinus* complex ticks throughout temperate North American and Eurasian regions (Fig. 13-12).[6,7] *I. scapularis* is the principal vector in the eastern United States; *Ixodes pacificus*, the western black-legged tick, transmits *B. burgdorferi* in the western United States; *I. ricinus* is the principal vector in western and central Europe; and *Ixodes persulcatus* is the main vector in central and eastern Russia, China, and Japan. *I. ricinus* and *I. persulcatus* coexist in some areas of eastern Europe, and both tick species also transmit the tick-borne encephalitis (TBE) virus to humans.

In the United States, spirochete rates in nymphal and adult ticks are often 25 to 50 percent in highly endemic areas of the northeastern and mid-Atlantic regions. Spirochete rates are generally 10 to 20 percent in the north-central region, 1 to 2 percent in the Pacific coastal region, and only 0 to 3 percent in the southeastern and south-central areas of the United States. Nymphal ticks are responsible for most Lyme disease in humans. Peak nymphal activity between May and August strongly coincides with the peak incidence of disease onset in humans.

The lone star tick, *Amblyomma americanum*, has been suggested as a potential vector of the Lyme disease spirochete. However, it is an incompetent experimental vector of *B. burgdorferi* and has never been found to maintain a cycle of the spirochete in nature. Although spirochetes thought to be *B. burgdorferi* have been identified in blood-sucking insects such as fleas, mosquitoes, and horseflies, there is no indication that the organism is adapted for survival in these insects or that mechanical transmission has any epidemiologic importance.

Environmental Factors

The ticks that transmit Lyme disease require shade, high humidity in their microenvironment, and ready access to preferred vertebrate hosts. In the United States, *I. scapularis* is most often found in moist coastal or riverine areas. The northeastern coastal and island habitat is characterized by dense brush dominated by scrub oak, pine, and bayberry bush, and the inland northeastern and north-central habitat by mixed deciduous succession forests with sapling understory. A study of tick distribution on large suburban residential properties in Westchester County, New York, found infective black-legged (deer) ticks on 60 percent of properties, with the greatest tick densities occurring in wooded areas, followed by fringe habitat, and much lesser densities among ornamental shrubbery and on lawns.[17] Leaf litter and humus provide a particularly favorable microenvironment for ixodid ticks. The habitat in southern Atlantic coastal and island areas is complex mixed deciduous-conifer woodlands. *I. pacificus* in northern California is typically found in grassy, oak woodland sites. Geographic information services (GIS) data are being used to better define the various ecological parameters associated with enzooticity and geographic spread.[18]

Vertebrate Hosts

In the coastal northeastern United States, the white-footed mouse is the most competent vertebrate reservoir of *B. burgdorferi*. It typically has infection rates of 80 percent or greater in highly endemic foci, maintains infection without apparent ill effects, and serves as the preferred vertebrate host for the immature stages of the tick vector. The chipmunk is also a competent reservoir host in the eastern United States and may be more important than the white-footed mouse in maintaining cycles of infection in the north-central region. Deer appear to be a prerequisite for the establishment of black-legged (deer) tick populations, and the explosive repopulation by white-tailed deer of the eastern United States in recent decades preceded the emergence of *I. scapularis* ticks and Lyme disease in this region. Wherever

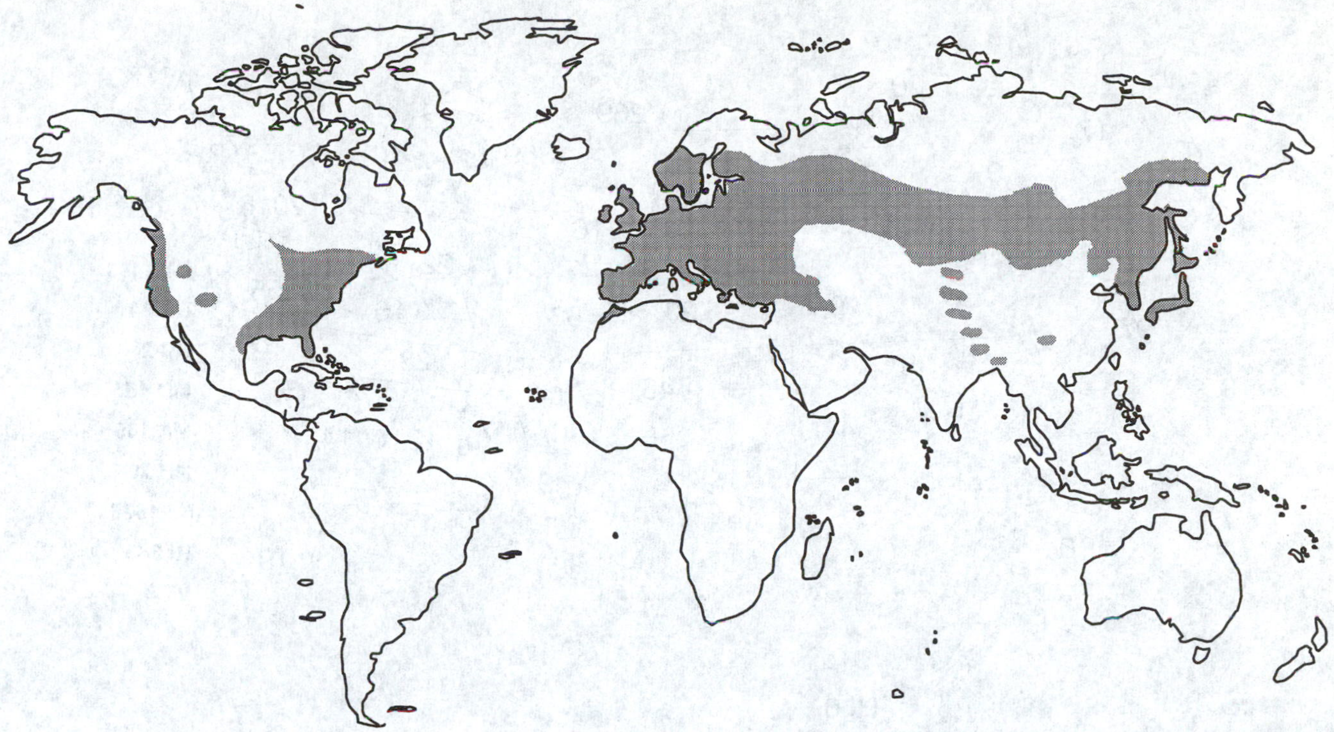

Figure 13-12. The global distribution of *Ixodes* spp. ticks able to transmit the agent of Lyme disease, *Borrelia burgdorferi*. (Modified from Filipova NA [ed]: Taiga tick, *Ixodes persulcatus* [Schulze] [Acarina, Ixodidae]. Leningrad: Nauka Publishers, 1985.)

I. scapularis is found in large numbers, deer are numerous as well. However, *I. scapularis* is found on at least 33 species of mammals and 49 species of birds, and the experimental removal of deer from selected areas results in an important reduction but not elimination of this tick in these areas. Alternate but less favorable tick maintenance hosts include raccoons, skunks, canids, and other medium-sized and large mammals. The low infection rates of *Ixodes* vectors in the southern and western regions of the United States may be partly explained by the preferential feeding of immature stages of the tick there on lizards. Lizards are incompetent reservoirs of *B. burgdorferi* and thus act as zooprophylactic hosts.[6,19]

Several bird species serve as maintenance hosts for vector ticks, and some, such as robins, may serve as lesser reservoir hosts of *B. burgdorferi*. It is probable that migrating birds have been responsible for establishing some new enzootic foci; however, contiguous spread arising from movement of deer and carnivores is the principal factor in geographic spread. Studies mapping the distribution of ticks, reservoir rodent hosts, seropositivity of dogs and deer, and the incidence of human cases over time provide valuable information on the spread of Lyme disease in the United States. Seropositivity of dogs appears to be a sensitive and reliable epidemiologic marker of the geographic distribution of *B. burgdorferi*, and dogs have recently been described as possible reservoirs of *B. burgdorferi* in the peri-residential environment.

▸ EPIDEMIOLOGY

Transmission of Infection to Humans

Lyme disease is transmitted in the saliva of feeding ticks, and possibly by regurgitation into the bite site of tick midgut contents. There is no evidence that *B. burgdorferi* is passed directly from one person to another. Infection is not known to be transmitted by sexual contact or through breast milk. Transplacental infection of the fetus has been suggested by the finding of rare silver-stained spirochetal structures in fetal tissues; however, this has not been confirmed by cultural isolation and bacterial characterization. Although *B. burgdorferi* can be cultured from the blood in a small percentage of patients with early acute infection and is able to survive in stored blood for prolonged periods, transfusion-acquired infection has not been documented.

Global Distribution

Endemic Lyme disease occurs in portions of the United States and Canada; the British Isles; Scandinavia; western and central Europe; the Balkan states; states of the former Union of Soviet Socialist Republics from the Baltics east through northern forested areas of Russia to the Pacific Coast; northern China; Korea, and Japan.[20] The disease is endemic in China in forested northeastern regions and is found in lesser frequency in widely scattered foci elsewhere in China. Sporadic human cases occur in central Japan. In the highly endemic areas of North America and Eurasia, the incidence and epidemiologic patterns of Lyme disease are similar.[21] Suspected cases of Lyme disease have been reported from sub-Saharan Africa, South America, and Australia, but no transmission cycles of *B. burgdorferi* have been identified at these sites and no isolations of the Lyme disease spirochete have been made from suspected cases. In Canada, Lyme disease is thought to be endemic only in southeastern Ontario, although *I. scapularis* is found in limited foci elsewhere in eastern Canada, and *I. pacificus* infected with *B. burgdorferi* have been found in British Columbia.

Surveillance Statistics for the United States

Lyme disease was made a nationally notifiable disease in 1990, a uniform national case definition was adopted for surveillance purposes in 1991,[20] and reporting is now mandatory in all 50 states. Lyme disease accounts for more than 95 percent of all reports of vector-borne infectious disease in the United States. A total of 11,700 cases of Lyme disease were reported by 43 states in 1995, compared with 497 cases by 11 states in 1982 (Fig. 13-13).[22] The national incidence of reported cases was 4.4 per 100,000 population in 1995, ranging from zero in several western states and in Hawaii to 45.6 per 100,000 in Connecticut. The map of the distribution of cases by state clearly shows geographic concentrations in the northeastern region, in the north-central region (Fig. 13-14), and in northern California. Incidences of greater than 4.4 per 100,000 population were reported by only eight states—

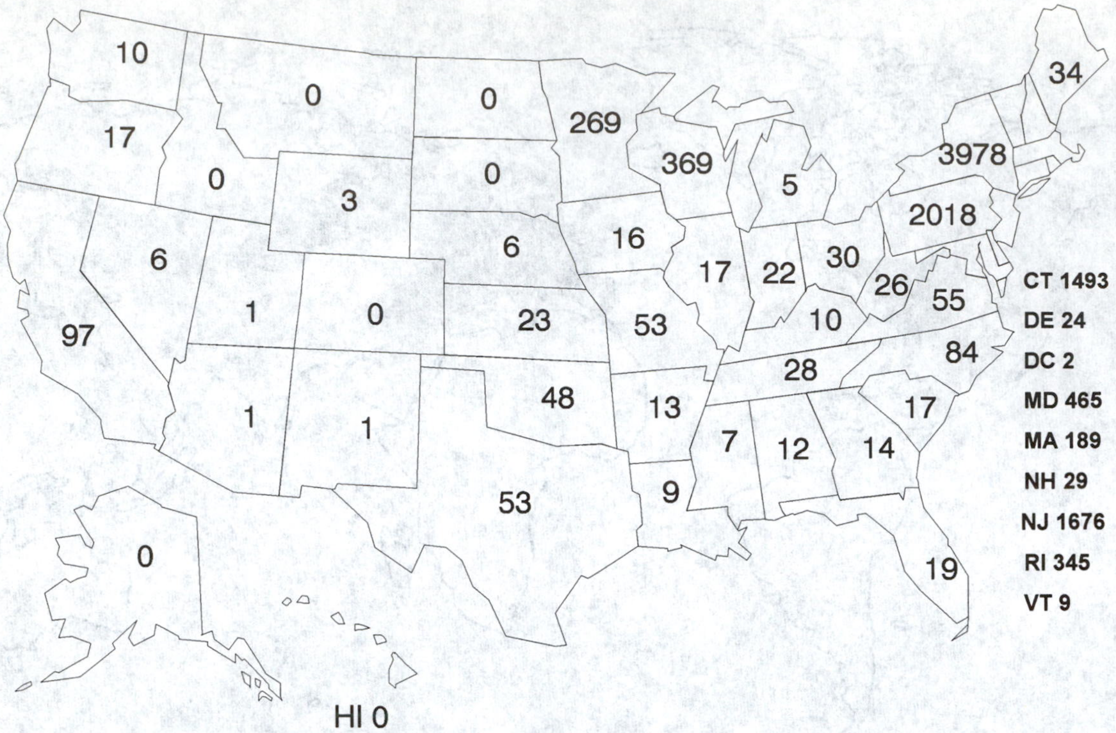

Figure 13-13. Number of reported Lyme disease cases, by state—United States, 1995.

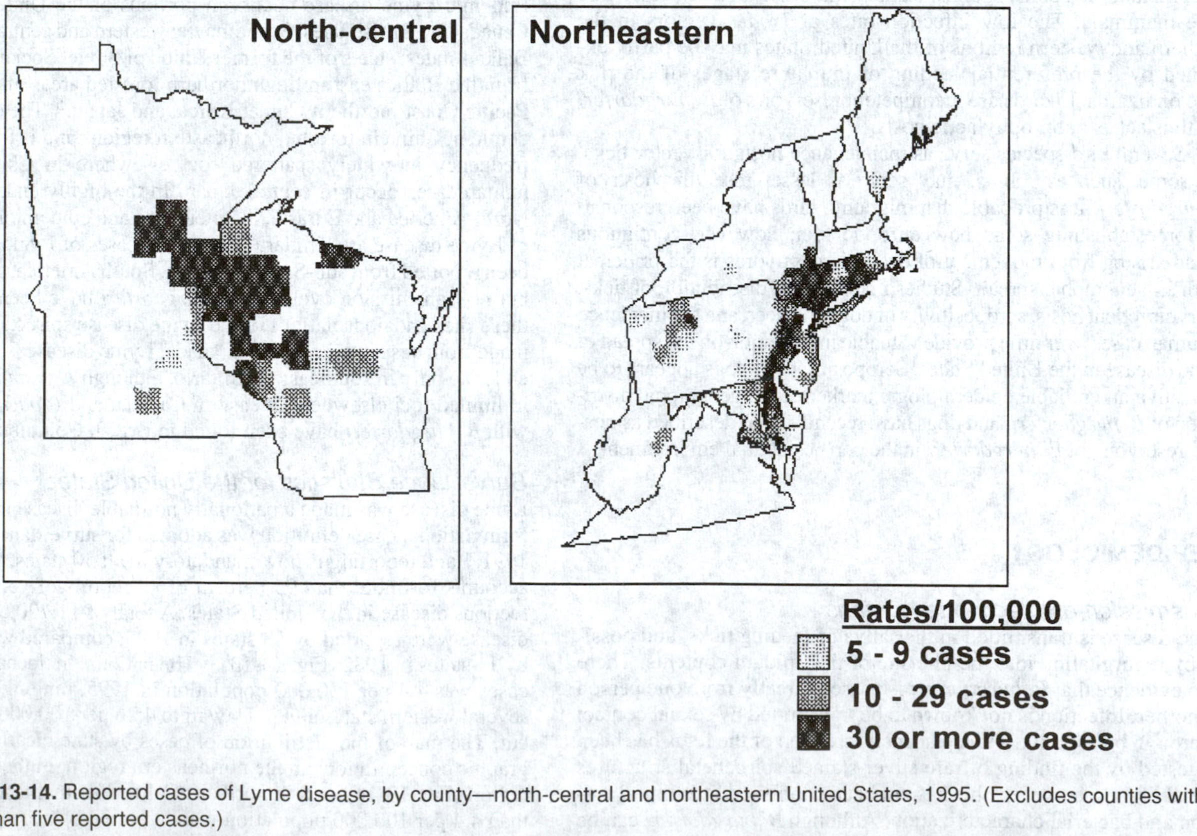

Figure 13-14. Reported cases of Lyme disease, by county—north-central and northeastern United States, 1995. (Excludes counties with fewer than five reported cases.)

Connecticut (45.6), Rhode Island (34.9), New York (21.9), New Jersey (21.1), Pennsylvania (16.7), Maryland (9.2), Wisconsin (7.2), and Minnesota (5.8)—and these states account for more than 90 percent of the total number of reported cases. New York State alone accounted for more than 35 percent of nationally reported cases, mostly from Suffolk and Westchester counties. Clustering of cases by county, by township, and even by neighborhood is highly correlated with the abundance of vector ticks in the environment. Persons at greatest risk are residents of rural or suburban properties that are wooded or are contiguous with wooded tracts inhabited by deer; others at relatively high risk include persons who live or vacation in northeastern coastal areas and in north-central woodlands. Recent findings of *I. scapularis* in deer-inhabited parks in Baltimore, New York City, and greater Philadelphia suggest the potential for a small but emerging urban risk.

Lyme disease affects persons in all age-groups, but the highest rates are found in children less than 15 years of age and in adults 30 years of age and older (Fig. 13-15). Males and females are nearly equally affected. National surveillance data for 1995 provide the following demographic breakdown: males, 51 percent; 0 to 14 years, 24 percent; 35 to 49 years, 24 percent, white, 95.8 percent; black, 2.4 percent; other race, 1.8 percent.[21]

Lyme disease case reporting is fraught with problems of misclassification, misdiagnosis, and underreporting. In 1991–1992 in Connecticut, more than 80 percent of all cases of Lyme disease in the state registry were reported by physicians from four primary care specialties, even though only 7 percent of physicians in these specialties had reported cases. Follow-up interviews with a sample of physicians in the four specialty areas suggested that fewer than 20 percent of all cases diagnosed and treated as incident cases of Lyme disease had been reported.[23] A recent study in Maryland suggested that Lyme disease is underreported by 10- to 12-fold in that state and that many more patients are seen and treated for presumptive Lyme disease and for tick bite alone than patients meeting the case criteria for reporting.[24]

Lyme Disease Emergence

Lyme disease is one of a number of emerging tick-borne diseases in the United States. Several outbreaks of Lyme disease have been described in the eastern United States since 1980.[20] A study on Fire Island, a barrier island off the south coast of Long Island, New York, described a cumulative prevalence of 7.5 percent and a seasonal incidence of 1 to 3 percent among residents of this summer vacation site. A longitudinal study of a community of about 160 persons on Great Island, Massachusetts, found a slow buildup of incidence to a peak of 3 percent per year and a total cumulative prevalence of 16 percent over a 20-year period. A similar restricted population in the northern coastal area of Ipswich, Massachusetts, experienced an outbreak of Lyme disease in the 1980s. The attack rate from 1980 through 1987 was 35 percent among 190 residents living within 5 km of a nature preserve heavily infested with *B. burgdorferi*-infected ticks; the annual incidence reached a peak of 10 percent, and a number of residents became reinfected one or more times. Population-based studies in highly endemic suburban communities in northern Westchester County, New York, described a seasonal attack rate of 2.6 percent and a prevalence of 8.8 percent.

The introduction and buildup of Lyme disease to highly endemic levels within some states and regions over the past two decades is a considerable public health concern, especially since there is no practical strategy to prevent expansion of the zootic cycle. The buildup has been most pronounced in suburban and rural residential areas in northeastern states. A review of surveillance data in Connecticut for the period 1977 to 1985 suggested a 3-fold to 8-fold increase in incidence in the communities where Lyme disease was first described and an extension of disease from one county to all counties within the state. Rapid emergence has also been well documented in New York State.[25] Prior to 1979, vector ticks were known only from eastern Long Island. By 1989, they were recognized in 22 New York counties, and enzootic cycles of *B. burgdorferi* were described in eight adjacent counties in southern New York. The Hudson River Valley appears to be a natural avenue of spread, and the latest count identifies 34 New York counties where *I. scapularis* has been found, including counties bordering on Canada. Endemic Lyme disease extends from southern Maine to Maryland, while enzootic cycles of undetermined public health importance extend farther along the southern Atlantic Coast to northern Florida, with greatest enzootic intensity occurring there on barrier islands. Patterns of disease emergence similar to those in New York have been noted in Pennsylvania, New Jersey, Maryland, and Wisconsin. Enzootic *B. burgdorferi* is found in areas of Minnesota, Illinois, and northern Michigan that are contiguous with known foci in Wisconsin. Lyme disease appears to be more stable in the Pacific coastal region, where the majority of reported human cases occur in a few counties in northern California.

Areas with Unconfirmed Endemicity

The reporting of cases from areas where ticks are not known to transmit *B. burgdorferi* to humans, such as throughout many southern, midwestern, and mountain states, remains enigmatic. In the southern United States, *I. scapularis* has a low *B. burgdorferi* infection rate and rarely feeds on humans. Epidemiologic studies in Missouri of persons with EM-like lesions and of area-matched controls provide evidence that the disease there is associated with the bites of ticks but is not caused by *B. burgdorferi* or other known tick-borne infection.[26] EM-like lesions were noted in this study and by others to occur following bites by the Lone Star tick, *A. americanum*. The Lone Star tick is widely distributed throughout the southern and mid-Atlantic regions, and it is the most common human-biting tick in the South. Spirochetal structures have regularly been seen by dark-field microscopy in the midguts of 5 percent or fewer of adult, questing *A. americanum* ticks. However, *B. burgdorferi* sensu stricto has not been cultivated from *A. americanum* ticks or from biopsies of EM-like lesions of patients in the south-central or southeastern United States. Recent studies using polymerase chain reaction techniques did identify a new, uncultivatable spirochete, *Borrelia lonestari*, sp. nov., in dark field–positive *A. americanum*,[27] but a link of this organism to infection and disease in humans and animals has not been made. Cryptic cycles of *B. burgdorferi* involving *Ixodes dentatus* ticks and rabbits in the eastern and southern United States and *Ixodes spinipalpis* ticks and woodrats in the Rocky Mountain foothills of eastern Colorado are not believed to pose a public health risk, since these ticks rarely feed on humans.

Risk Factors for Infection with the Lyme Disease Spirochete

Lyme disease is a disease of place. The principal risk factor for Lyme disease in the United States is permanent or seasonal residence in an area with high infestation with infected ticks, such as is found in some coastal fringe and island areas of New England, selected wooded residential communities and natural areas of northeastern states, mainly from Massachusetts to Maryland, rural wooded areas of Wisconsin, northern Michigan, and eastern Minnesota, and certain counties of northwestern California. Exposures to infected ticks are most likely in the parts of residential properties and surroundings that are relatively undisturbed, i.e., tall grass, brushy scrub, and wooded tracts. Recreational activities in natural areas, such as hiking, camping, fishing, and hunting, also expose persons to infective tick bites, especially during the late spring and summer months. Outdoor occupations, such as landscaping, brush clearing, forestry, and wildlife and parks management, may place persons at high risk in some areas.

As previously reviewed,[20] a study of employees in New Jersey showed that outdoor workers were more than four times as likely to have had Lyme disease as indoor workers. A comprehensive study of workers in Lyme disease endemic counties of downstate New York showed that persons with a history of outdoor employment were twice as likely to be seropositive as those without such a history. Although this difference was not statistically significant, the seroprevalence rate of outdoor employees was 5.9 times higher than a comparison group of anonymous blood donors from the same region of New York. However, the most important risk factor for Lyme disease in New York workers was a history of spending 30 or more hours of leisure time a week outdoors. Studies in Europe have shown occupational risks associated with forestry occupations, and serologic evidence of high *B. burgdorferi* exposure in forest workers was positively associated with worker's age, history of tick bite, and history of EM.

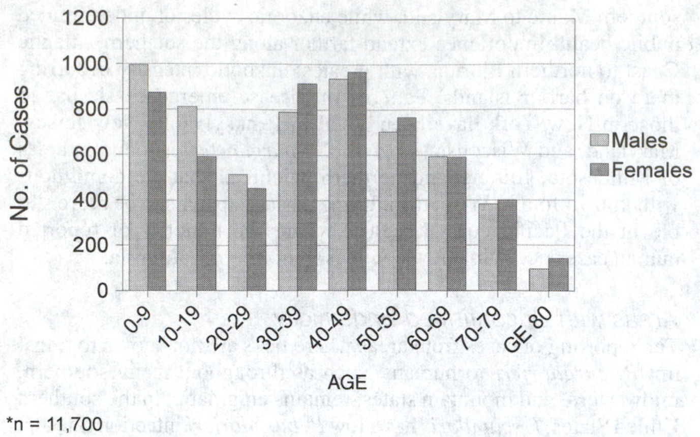

Figure 13-15. Rates per 100,000 population of reported Lyme disease cases by age group and gender, United States, 1995.

Ownership of cats has been found to be associated with an increased risk of acquiring Lyme disease in several small studies, and domestic cats have been observed to bring unattached nymphal ticks into homes. A study of dogs and persons living in the same households in two highly endemic areas in Massachusetts showed that dogs were more likely to have serologic evidence of *B. burgdorferi* infection than their human co-residents and that dog ownership was not associated with an increased risk for their owners.[28]

▶ PREVENTION

Avoidance and Personal Protection

Prevention of Lyme disease is based on avoidance of tick-infested areas, personal protection, environmental management, and early detection and treatment of disease manifestations. The public should be informed of tick-infested areas and avoid risky exposures, especially in spring and summer. Information on the distribution of ticks in an area can usually be obtained from health departments, park personnel, and agricultural extension services.

When in tick-infested areas, persons should wear light-colored clothing so that ticks can be spotted more easily and removed, and they should wear long-sleeved shirts and tuck pants into socks or boot tops to prevent ready access of ticks to skin. Ticks, especially nymphs and larvae, quest close to the ground, and entomologists who work in tick-infested areas find that wearing high rubber boots prevents tick attachment—a simple protection for persons clearing leaf litter and underbrush from their wooded properties. Insect repellents containing deet can be applied to clothes and to exposed skin other than the face, and permethrin compounds (which kill ticks on contact) can be sprayed on clothing.

One of the most important preventive measures is the early detection and proper removal of attached ticks. Tweezers should be used to grasp the tick mouthparts and the tick should be removed by steady, gentle traction. Studies have shown that transmission of *B. burgdorferi* from an infected tick is unlikely to occur before 36 hours of attachment;[29] when in tick-infested areas, a daily check for ticks and their proper removal are an important measures to prevent infection. Antibiotic treatment to prevent Lyme disease after a known tick bite is not routinely warranted; the risk of asymptomatic infection or disease in untreated persons has been found to be less than 3 percent, even when bitten by known vector species in highly endemic areas, and this risk of exposure is, in most circumstances, below the cost-benefit threshold of treatment.[29]

Landscape Management and Tick Control

In endemic residential areas of the northeastern United States, wood lots, stone fences, and unkempt edges of yards pose a significantly greater risk than lawns and ornamental shrubby areas. Removing leaf litter and woodpiles and clearing trees and brush around houses and at the edges of yards to admit more sunlight and remove habitat suitable for deer, ticks, and rodent reservoirs of infection may reduce the numbers of ticks that transmit Lyme disease in the ensuing transmission seasons. Area application of acaricides to residential properties has been found to be highly effective in suppressing vector ticks but raises environmental concerns; the distribution in yards of acaricide-impregnated cotton balls that mice then use for nest building has produced variable results. Excluding deer from properties and maintaining tick-free pets may reduce tick numbers in the immediate peri-residential environment.

There are no known practical measures for controlling tick vectors or rodent reservoirs of infection over large areas. Management of deer populations and control of ticks on deer would seem to be a logical strategy for reducing the intensity of enzootic transmission in already established foci of infection and for limiting spread to new areas. The control of ticks on deer using self-dosing systems for applying topical and systemic acaricides is being evaluated in pilot trials.

Vaccination

Vaccines against infection with *B. burgdorferi* have been developed for both dogs and humans. One commercial canine vaccine contains inactivated *B. burgdorferi*, which in laboratory experiments protects against challenge by inoculated live organisms as well as infected ticks. The vaccines under evaluation for human use, and a recently marketed canine vaccine, use a *B. burgdorferi* recombinant outer surface protein A (Osp-A) as immunogen. This recombinant Osp-A vaccine has been shown in phase 1 and phase 2 human trials to be safe and immunogenic;[30] phase 3 trials of the Osp-A vaccines in humans, involving approximately 20,000 participants and vaccines by two manufacturers, have recently been completed in endemic areas of the north-central and northeastern United States. A unique aspect of the Osp-A vaccine is the killing of *B. burgdorferi* within the midgut of ticks feeding on immunized experimental animal hosts. If the vaccines are found to be safe and efficacious, it is expected that there will be a considerable consumer-driven market for them; care providers and public health practitioners will need to know how to weigh risks of infection, potential benefits, and costs in determining their rational use.

Trypanosomiasis

Louis V. Kirchhoff

▶ AMERICAN TRYPANOSOMIASIS (CHAGAS' DISEASE)

American trypanosomiasis, or Chagas' disease, is caused by the protozoan hemoflagellate *Trypanosoma cruzi*.[1] This parasite is enzootic and endemic in Latin America and the southern and southwestern United States. Only a handful of cases of vector-borne transmission of *T. cruzi* to humans in the United States have been reported. The number of *T. cruzi*-infected persons living here, however, has increased markedly in recent decades as several million Latin Americans have emigrated to the United States. Many thousands of these immigrants are infected with *T. cruzi* and they present diagnostic and therapeutic challenges to the physicians who provide their medical care. Moreover, since most of these infected persons harbor the parasite asymptomatically, they pose a risk of transmission of the parasite in hospitals by blood transfusion, and several such cases have already been described.

Biology and Transmission

Transmission of *T. cruzi* to its mammalian hosts occurs when feces of a blood-sucking insect vector containing infective organisms contaminate mucosal surfaces, the conjunctivas, abrasions, or the bite wound. The parasites penetrate local cells and after multiplying intracellularly are released as the host cells die to invade adjacent cells and the bloodstream. In this manner a cycle is established in the mammalian hosts of *T. cruzi* that alternates asynchronously between nondividing infective forms that circulate in the bloodstream and intracellular multiplying forms. The cycle is completed when an insect vector ingests blood containing the circulating infective forms. Not surprisingly, transfusion of blood from donors who harbor *T. cruzi* frequently results in new infections.[2] In addition, *T. cruzi* can be passed from mother to fetus, causing spontaneous abortion or congenital Chagas' disease,[3] and laboratory accidents resulting in transmission of the parasite occur with disquieting frequency.[4]

Pathology and Clinical Features

Acute Chagas' disease is usually a mild illness with a death rate of less than 5 percent. As parasites spread hematogenously from the site of initial entry and multiplication, they can cause malaise, fever, edema of the face and lower extremities, hepatosplenomegaly, and generalized lymphadenopathy. Muscles are often parasitized, and severe myocarditis develops in a small number of patients with acute infections.[5] The organisms can also invade the central nervous system, and meningoencephalitis is a rare complication.[6] Acute Chagas' disease resolves spontaneously over 4 to 8 weeks, and patients then enter the indeterminate phase of *T. cruzi* infection. This asymptomatic phase is characterized by subpatent parasitemias and easily detectable antibodies to a variety of *T. cruzi* antigens. Most infected persons remain in the indeterminate phase for life, and this sets the stage for transmission of the organism by transfusion.

Years or decades after the resolution of acute *T. cruzi* infection, symptomatic chronic Chagas' disease develops in approximately 10 to 30 percent of infected persons. The heart is most commonly affected, and pathologic changes can include thinning of ventricular walls, biventricular enlargement, mural thrombi, and apical aneurysms. Lymphocytic infiltration, diffuse interstitial fibrosis, and atrophy of myocardial cells are often seen in stained specimens. The conduction system is often affected, typically causing right bundle branch block, left anterior fascicular block, and third-degree atrioventricular block. Associated symptoms reflect the cardiomyopathy, rhythm disturbances, and thromboembolism that gradually develop, and death usually results from heart block or congestive heart failure.[7,8] In some patients megaesophagus and/or megacolon (megadisease) develop and cause regurgitation, dysphagia, repeated aspiration, and constipation.[9] The pathogenesis of the lesions associated with chronic *T. cruzi* infection is not well understood, but it is clear that denervation in affected organs plays an important role. The role of autoimmunity is an issue of considerable debate.[10]

Immunosuppression of patients who harbor *T. cruzi* chronically can cause a recrudescence of the infection, often with features that are atypical of acute Chagas' disease in immunocompetent persons. This is particularly true in Chagas' disease patients who undergo cardiac transplantation,[1] as well as in persons co-infected with *T. cruzi* and the human immunodeficiency virus.[11]

Epidemiology

T. cruzi is found only in the Americas, where it is distributed unevenly from the southern United States to Chile and Argentina in triatomine insect vectors (kissing bugs) and many species of wild and domestic mammals. Humans become part of the cycle of transmission when infected insects take up residence in the primitive adobe, wood, and stone houses that are common in many parts of Latin America. Most new *T. cruzi* infections occur among poor children in rural areas and result from contact with infected vectors, but tens of thousands of people become infected each year in urban areas by transfusion of contaminated blood. The incidence of acute Chagas' disease is unknown because most cases go undiagnosed. An estimated 16 to 18 million persons are chronically infected with the parasite, the majority of whom live in Brazil, Bolivia, Argentina, and Chile. Roughly 50,000 deaths due to chronic Chagas' disease are thought to occur each year.

Acute Chagas' disease is uncommon in the United States. Only four cases of autochthonous transmission have been reported,[5] and three instances of transmission by blood transfusion have been described.[12] In addition, in the past 26 years, 9 imported cases of acute Chagas' disease and seven laboratory-acquired infections have been reported to the Centers for Disease Control and Prevention (CDC). No acute infections among United States tourists returning from endemic areas have been reported. In contrast, the numbers of persons with chronic *T. cruzi* infections in the United States has grown enormously as immigration from Latin America has burgeoned, especially from Central America, where prevalence rates of *T. cruzi* infection are high. In a study conducted in Washington, DC, 5 percent of Nicaraguan and Salvadoran immigrants were found to be chronically infected with *T. cruzi*.[13] Estimates based on this latter finding and on several prevalence studies of blood donors suggest that at least 50,000 *T. cruzi*–infected immigrants now live in the United States.[14]

Diagnosis

Acute Chagas' Disease. The first consideration in diagnosing acute Chagas' disease is establishing that possible exposure to *T. cruzi* has occurred. Exposure can result from residence in an area in which vector-borne transmission of the parasite occurs, a recent blood transfusion in an endemic area, being born to a mother who is at risk of harboring *T. cruzi*, or a laboratory accident involving the parasite.

The diagnosis of acute Chagas' disease is made by detecting parasites, and serological tests are not useful. In immunocompetent patients, examination of blood is the cornerstone of detecting *T. cruzi*. Circulating parasites are highly motile and frequently can be seen in wet preparations of buffy coat or anticoagulated blood. The organisms may also be seen in Giemsa-stained blood smears. In immunocompromised patients suspected of having acute Chagas' disease, other specimens such as bone marrow aspirates, cerebrospinal fluid, pericardial fluid, and lymph nodes should be examined microscopically. If these approaches fail to detect *T. cruzi* in a patient whose epidemiologic and clinical histories suggest that the parasite is present, growing the organism may be attempted. This can be done by xenodiagnosis, a method that involves feeding a patient's blood to laboratory-reared insect vectors, or by culturing blood or other specimens in liquid medium.[15] These two methods take at least a month to complete, however, and this is far beyond the time at which a decision about drug treatment needs to be made. Polymerase chain reaction–based assays have shown promise for diagnosing both acute and chronic *T. cruzi* infections under research laboratory conditions,[16] but the assays are not available commercially.

Chronic Chagas' Disease. Chronic Chagas' disease is usually diagnosed by detection of IgG that binds to specific *T. cruzi* antigens, and parasitologic studies are unnecessary. Several highly specific serologic tests are used widely in Latin America, such as indirect immunofluorescence (IIF), complement fixation (CF), and enzyme-linked immunosorbent assay (ELISA). A persistent problem with these assays, however, is the occurrence of false-positive results, which typically occur with sera from persons having leishmaniasis, malaria, syphilis, collagen vascular diseases, and other parasitic and nonparasitic illnesses. Because of this lack of specificity, most authorities recommend that blood specimens be tested in two or three assays before being accepted as positive.

In the United States, specimens can be sent to the CDC for testing by CF and IIF (770-488-4474). In addition, ELISA-based tests, manufactured by Abbott Laboratories (Abbott Park, IL),[17] Gull Laboratories (Salt Lake City, UT), and Hemagen Diagnostics (Waltham, MA) have been cleared by the Food and Drug Administration for clinical use. Finally, in the author's laboratory (319-335-6786), a radioimmune precipitation test is available. This test was shown to be highly sensitive and specific when used to test a geographically diverse group of sera from patients with Chagas' disease and control subjects.[18]

Treatment

Nifurtimox (Lampit, Bayer 2502) and benznidazole (Radimil, Roche 7-1051) are the only drugs currently recommended for treating patients with Chagas' disease. Nifurtimox can be obtained from the CDC (770-639-3670 (weekdays); 770-639-2888 (off-hours)). Benznidazole is not available in the United States, although it is the drug of choice in endemic countries. Both of these agents reduce the severity and duration of acute Chagas' disease, but they achieve parasitologic cures only in about 50 percent of treated patients. Moreover, they must be taken for extended periods and often cause severe side effects.[19] The parasitologic cure rates of the two drugs are similar in chronically infected patients, but because there is little evidence that they alter the course of chronic Chagas' disease, their use beyond the acute phase of *T. cruzi* infection is controversial. Allopurinol has no place in the treatment of *T. cruzi* infections.

Control

Since drug treatment is problematic and vaccines are not available, reducing *T. cruzi* transmission in Latin America must depend on serologic identification of infected donors in blood banks and on reducing contact with insect vectors through housing improvement and spraying of insecticides. Major successes with these approaches have been achieved in several endemic countries, including Argentina, Brazil, Uruguay, Chile, and Venezuela. United States tourists traveling in areas where *T. cruzi* transmission occurs should avoid sleeping in dilapidated houses in rural areas and should use mosquito nets and insect repellent to reduce exposure to vectors.

In the United States prospective blood donors from endemic countries should be screened serologically for *T. cruzi* infection. Moreover, all immigrants from regions in which Chagas' disease is endemic should be tested, as identification of infected persons should prompt physicians who care for them to perform appropriate diagnostic monitoring and supportive therapy when indicated. Persons who work with *T. cruzi* and infected vectors in the laboratory should wear gloves and eye protection. Cardiac transplantation in patients with end-stage chagasic cardiomyopathy should be approached with caution because the immunosuppression required postoperatively often results in reactivation of *T. cruzi* infection, leading to serious consequences and even death.[1]

▶ AFRICAN TRYPANOSOMIASIS (SLEEPING SICKNESS)

African trypanosomiasis, or sleeping sickness, is caused by two subspecies of trypanosomes, *Trypanosoma brucei gambiense* and *Trypanosoma brucei rhodesiense*, which are found in West and Central Africa and in East Africa, respectively. These flagellated protozoan parasites are transmitted by blood-sucking tsetse flies. The major biological difference between *T. cruzi* and African trypanosomes is that the latter multiply in the bloodstream and perivascular tissues of their mammalian hosts and do not have an intracellular form. In untreated patients these organisms first cause a febrile illness that months or years later is followed by progressive neurologic impairment and death. *T.b. gambiense* and *T.b. rhodesiense* trypanosomiases differ primarily in that the latter follows a much more aggressive course.

Tens of thousands of new cases occur each year in a broad belt across Central and West Africa. In the United States imported cases appear about once every 2 years, usually in tourists who have visited East African game parks. In both acute and chronic African trypanosomiasis the diagnosis is made by detecting parasites, either in blood, in aspirates of lymph nodes or the trypanosomal chancre that can appear at the site of entry, or in cerebrospinal fluid. Treatment is complicated but usually effective and varies from one patient to another depending on the infecting subspecies and on whether or not there is central nervous system involvement.[20]

Control of African trypanosomiasis is based on reducing tsetse populations and drug treatment of infected persons. Major progress in reducing transmission has been made in many areas, but widespread foci of intense transmission still remain. Persons traveling to endemic countries can reduce their risk of acquiring sleeping sickness by avoiding areas known to harbor infected insects, by using insect repellent, and by wearing protective clothing.

Leishmaniasis

Mary E. Wilson

Leishmaniasis refers to a constellation of diseases caused by protozoa belonging to the genus *Leishmania*. The clinical forms of leishmaniasis comprise a wide spectrum, and new entities are being recognized as travel and political conflict bring people from Western countries into endemic regions. Although varied in their clinical manifestations, the different *Leishmania* species share a common life cycle and transmission characteristics. All forms of leishmaniasis are initiated by the bite of a sandfly vector, which deposits the infectious promastigote form of the parasite into the skin of a susceptible mammal. The extracellular flagellated promastigote then attaches to a mononuclear phagocyte, triggering phagocytosis through one or more macrophage receptor molecules. Once intracellular, the parasite retracts its flagellum and transforms to the obligate intracellular amastigote. Thereafter the amastigote survives in the mammalian host as an obligate intracellular parasite of macrophages.

The three major forms of leishmaniasis are cutaneous, visceral, and mucosal (or mucocutaneous) disease. More minor presentations are discussed below. Infections due to each of the *Leishmania* species lead to a characteristic clinical disease syndrome, although case reports are making it clear that there is considerable variability in clinical presentation. The most common form is cutaneous leishmaniasis. Old World cutaneous leishmaniasis occurs in tropical and subtropical Asia, China, India, Africa, and the Middle East, whereas New World cutaneous leishmaniasis is found throughout South and Central America and extends north into southern Texas. Visceral leishmaniasis also occurs widely and affects people in Latin America, Africa, India, Bangladesh, and China, as well as in countries surrounding the Mediterranean Sea, including France, Italy, and Spain. Severe mucosal disease due to *Leishmania braziliensis* occurs in Latin America, although mucosal involvement has been reported with a number of other *Leishmania* species throughout endemic regions. The biochemical differences between parasite species responsible for different clinical manifestations are not entirely clear.[1]

As with any infectious disease, clinical manifestations are determined not only by biological characteristics of the parasite species or strain, but also by differences in the susceptibility of individual hosts. It has been clearly established that there is genetic susceptibility to *Leishmania* infections in experimental mice. Murine susceptibility to *Leishmania donovani* infection maps to a single gene that has been cloned and named *Nramp*, the same gene that governs susceptibility to mycobacterial and *Salmonella* infections.[2] In contrast, murine susceptibility to infection with *Leishmania major* maps to a different locus. Whether there is similar genetic susceptibility to leishmaniasis in humans is not proven, although racial differences in the development of mucosal disease and the finding of familial clustering of visceral leishmaniasis cases suggest that genetic factors may influence severe human disease manifestations.[3,4] Nutritional factors are also critical, demonstrated by the fact that malnutrition predisposes to the development of visceral leishmaniasis in Brazilian children.[5] Thus, the clinical manifestations of disease are determined not only by the species of *Leishmania* that predominate in a region but also by a number of host factors, some of which are not fully defined.

Clinical Disease Syndromes

The *Leishmania* species are divided into the subgenera *Leishmania* (*L.*) and *Viannia* (*V.*). These will be identified the first time each species is mentioned below.

Cutaneous Leishmaniasis. Classic cutaneous leishmaniasis is typically caused by *L (L.) major*, *Leishmania (L.) tropica*, or *Leishmania (L.) aethiopica* in the Old World or by *Leishmania (L.) mexicana*, *Leishmania (V.) panamensis*, *Leishmania (L.) amazonensis*, or *Leishmania (V.) braziliensis* in the New World. The disease onset occurs between 2 weeks and several months after the sandfly bite. Cutaneous lesions begin as papules that gradually increase in size and eventually ulcerate. They often appear as chronic ulcers with raised erythematous borders and a granulomatous base. Metastatic lesions in nearby skin are common, and regional adenopathy can occur particularly with *L. braziliensis* disease. Lesions may last for months to more than a year. New World cutaneous leishmaniasis, particularly that caused by *L. braziliensis*, can take on more severe forms in which ulcers are deep and mutilating, and there is massive lymphadenopathy or chains of enlarged lymph nodes resembling sporotrichosis. Eventually most lesions heal spontaneously, leaving a flat atrophic scar. Although spontaneous healing is common, treatment can speed or ensure recovery. Both during and after recovery from disease, patients usually exhibit strong delayed-type hypersensitivity (DTH) responses to *Leishmania* antigen, found clinically by intradermal administration of a promastigote lysate commonly called the Montenegro or leishmanin test.

Rare chronic forms of cutaneous leishmaniasis include diffuse cutaneous leishmaniasis (DCL) in which there are many localized papules that do not ulcerate. Satellite lesions and metastatic skin lesions arise, usually on the face and extremities. DCL is an anergic form of leishmaniasis, with a negative Montenegro response occurring primarily in South America. In contrast, leishmaniasis recidivans is a relapsing tuberculoid form of cutaneous leishmaniasis, usually caused by *L. tropica* in the Old World, in which lesions on the extremities or face slowly spread outward while healing in the center. This is associated with strong DTH reactivity. Both of these unusual forms of cutaneous leishmaniasis can lead to chronic disease lasting 20 years or more.

Mucosal Leishmaniasis. After cutaneous infections with *L. braziliensis* or occasionally other *Leishmania* species, 2 to 3 percent of individuals can develop recurrent disease at a mucosal site distant from the original cutaneous lesion. This occurs between 1 month and more than 20 years after the original cutaneous ulcer. The disease begins with edema and erythema of mucosal sites in the nose or oropharynx. Progressive granulomatous inflammation can lead to destruction of the nose with perforation of the nasal septum, as well as to lesions involving the lips, tongue or the buccal, pharyngeal, or laryngeal mucosa. Death is rare but occurs due to involvement of the trachea or larynx and subsequent complications such as aspiration. Mucosal leishmaniasis is associated with strong cellular immune responses manifested as positive DTH reactivity and peripheral lymphocyte reactivity. The disease process is likely exacerbated by a hyperergic response to the parasite.

Visceral Leishmaniasis. Visceral disease is generally caused by parasites related to *L. donovani*, including *L (L.) donovani* and *Leishmania (L.) infantum* in the Old World and *Leishmania (L.) chagasi* in the New World. Cases of visceral leishmaniasis due to other species (*L. amazonensis*, *L. tropica*) have been reported. This severe form of leishmaniasis usually begins between 3 and 8 months after the bite of an infected sandfly. Most patients develop the insidious onset of fevers, malaise, and weight loss associated with splenomegaly, hepatomegaly, anemia, leukopenia, thrombocytopenia, and hypergammaglobulinemia. Lymphadenopathy occurs in the Sudan but is not as common in other regions. The disease can lead to progressive suppression of specific and nonspecific cell-mediated responses with absent Montenegro reactivity, and associated bacterial infections causing pneumonia, diarrhea, or tuberculosis are common. These secondary infections contribute to the high mortality seen in untreated symptomatic disease. The spectrum of visceral leishmaniasis ranges from asymptomatic infection, occurring in 86 to 95 percent of infected Brazilians, to fulminant disease that may be fatal. Indeed, most fatalities due to leishmaniasis are due to the visceral form of disease.

Visceral leishmaniasis due to *L. infantum* has been reported in AIDS patients in Spain, France, and Italy as their presenting manifestation of HIV disease. Although most of these patients present with typical disease symptoms, unusual presentations have been documented. In addition, a previously unrecognized form of visceral infection, termed "viscerotropic leishmaniasis," was reported in U.S. troops returning from the Persian Gulf conflict. These individuals had varied symptoms and findings, including fever, chills, malaise, generalized lymphadenopathy, diarrhea, nausea, abdominal pain, and weight loss, although one individual had no symptoms at all. Biopsy and culture of the bone marrow revealed *L. tropica*, a species previously thought only to cause cutaneous disease.[6]

Visceral leishmaniasis can be followed by a syndrome termed post-kala azar dermal leishmaniasis (PKDL). This manifests with generalized skin lesions ranging from hyperpigmented macules to nodules containing numerous organisms. This entity is particularly common in East Africans who do not complete a course of therapy, and in the Indian subcontinent. Since PKDL allows parasites to survive in a cutaneous location, it may be important in allowing humans to serve as a reservoir of visceral disease.[7]

Diagnosis

The diagnosis of either cutaneous or visceral leishmaniasis should be considered in patients from endemic areas who present with typical findings of chronic cutaneous ulcer or fever with hepatosplenomegaly, respectively. Unfortunately, leishmaniasis is often not considered in immigrants or travelers seen by practitioners in countries where these diseases are uncommon. A diagnosis can be established by demonstration of the parasite in infected tissues (parasitologic diagnosis). Cutaneous ulcers can be biopsied at lesion margins, and the parasite found either by histologic examination of sections stained with hematoxylin and eosin or Giemsa or by culture of the parasite in specific media obtained from the Centers for Disease Control and Prevention (CDC). Visceral leishmaniasis is demonstrated by the finding of *Leishmania* in bone marrow biopsy or aspirate, or occasionally in the peripheral blood of patients with concurrent AIDS and visceral leishmaniasis.[8] Practitioners in some endemic countries will demonstrate parasites causing visceral leishmaniasis by fine-needle aspiration of the spleen, although the potential for hemorrhage makes this a less desirable test than a sternal marrow aspirate.

Anti-leishmanial antibodies are frequently elevated in immunocompetent individuals with visceral leishmaniasis, although such tests are unreliable in immunocompromised states such as HIV infection. Antibody tests include indirect fluorescent antibody (IFA) (used by the CDC), enzyme-linked immunosorbent assay (ELISA), and a direct agglutination test (DAT) optimized for use in developing countries. The recent finding that many patients with active visceral leishmaniasis have antibodies to the recombinant antigen k39 may result in the widespread use of an ELISA to this antigen in the future.[9,10] Unfortunately, patients with cutaneous leishmaniasis do not reliably develop antibody responses, so serology is often not helpful in evaluating cutaneous ulcers. In addition, troops with "viscerotropic" leishmaniasis had negative or low antibody titers, making this an unreliable test for this form of visceral disease. Cross-reactive antibodies may occur in patients with Chagas' disease or leprosy, so a positive antibody titer is a sensitive but not specific test for typical visceral disease in areas where these diseases are prevalent.

Delayed-type hypersensitivity responses to intradermally administered *Leishmania* antigen (the Montenegro or leishmanin test) usually develop during uncomplicated cutaneous and mucosal leishmaniasis. The Montenegro test is usually positive in leishmaniasis recidivans and PKDL but negative during diffuse cutaneous leishmaniasis. It is negative during acute visceral leishmaniasis, making the test useful only for epidemiologic purposes. Thus skin testing must also serve as an adjunct to clinical and parasitologic diagnosis. A number of laboratories have reported diagnosis of infection with the different *Leishmania* species by PCR, but these tests are not standardized and therefore cannot be offered other than in a research setting.

Treatment

Although small, inconspicuous cutaneous lesions can resolve without therapy, symptomatic visceral leishmaniasis is potentially fatal and requires treatment. Treatment is also recommended for lesions due to *L. braziliensis* because of their potential to develop into mucosal disease, and for large or cosmetically problematic cutaneous lesions. The mainstays of therapy for visceral leishmaniasis are the pentavalent antimony (Sb^V) compounds sodium stibogluconate and meglumine antimoniate, available through the CDC. These must be administered either intravenously or intramuscularly and are associated with considerable gastrointestinal, liver, pancreatic, and cardiac toxicity, sometimes requiring cessation of therapy. Increasing reports of relapse or treatment failure may reflect drug-resistant parasite isolates. Alternative treatments include amphotericin B or pentamidine. Liposomal amphotericin B has been successful in treating visceral leishmaniasis in recent reports and provides a less toxic alternative.[11] Recombinant interferon gamma has been used successfully as an adjunct to antimony therapy in cases of treatment failure, but this is not available other than for experimental purposes. Unfortunately, all the treatments mentioned above require repeated doses of parenteral therapy and are not optimal for use in many endemic or epidemic situations. Although there are case reports of treatment with ketoconazole or itraconazole, these drugs are not well studied and are not to be relied on for treatment of severe disease.

Cutaneous leishmaniasis can also be treated with antimony compounds, and these are recommended for *L. braziliensis* disease. Again, amphotericin B and pentamidine can be used as alternate drug choices. Other modes of treatment have been used for non-*L. braziliensis* cutaneous disease with varying success. These include local heat therapy, topical antimony, ketoconazole, itraconazole, allopurinol, and immunotherapy with BCG plus leishmania lysate. In adopting these alternate modes one must be careful to use therapy that has been reported helpful for the particular *Leishmania* species in question and to avoid unconventional therapy if *L. braziliensis* may be the causative organism.

Mucosal leishmaniasis also needs to be treated, and antimony compounds are the recommended antibiotic choice. This disease, diffuse cutaneous leishmaniasis, and leishmaniasis recidivans are often difficult to treat, requiring repeated courses of the same or alternate therapies. Antimony, amphotericin B, and pentamidine have all been used in these situations.

Transmission and Epidemiology

The World Health Organization has estimated that 350 million people are at risk for leishmaniasis. The annual incidence of cutaneous leishmaniasis is estimated at 1 to 1.5 million cases, and the incidence of visceral leishmaniasis is estimated to be 500,000 cases per year.[12] Major ongoing epidemics have been found in southern Sudan, eastern India, and urban centers in northeast Brazil. Furthermore, the incidence of HIV and *Leishmania* coinfection in Spain and France is increasingly recognized.[8]

Leishmania are transmitted by phlebotomine sandflies belonging to the genus *Phlebotomus* in the Old World and the genus *Lutzomyia* in the Americas. Female sandflies ingest macrophages containing amastigotes, which transform into infectious promastigotes in the sandfly gut.[13] After 7 to 9 days of development, infectious metacyclic promastigotes in the sandfly proboscis are ready for inoculation into a new host.[14] The different sandfly species are often either susceptible or resistant to infection with particular *Leishmania* species. For example, *Lutzomyia longipalpis* is the natural host for *L. chagasi* but not *L. major*.[15] Sandflies remain within close proximity of their habitat, and mammalian disease occurs when humans or a susceptible reservoir hosts venture into these environments. Depending on whether the particular sandfly species resides in an arid or semi-arid, a sylvatic, or a peridomestic habitat, it feeds on mammals such as desert sand rats, anteaters, opossums, wild rodents, or humans. When cycles are maintained in semi-arid conditions such as in the Middle East, sandflies often inhabit rodent burrows, and the reservoirs of disease are small desert rodents. Thus, Old World cutaneous leishmaniasis is acquired when humans venture near uninhabited areas or villages near the desert where these rodents survive. American cutaneous leishmaniasis is also a zoonosis, maintained in a sylvatic cycle between small forest rodent reservoirs and *Lutzomyia* sp. sandflies.[16] Most human infection occurs in the context of agricultural, settlement, forestry, or military activities. Major deforestation efforts in the tropical forests of South America have led to increases in cutaneous leishmaniasis in many regions.[17]

Visceral leishmaniasis occurs worldwide with a variety of reservoir hosts. The disease is endemic in many regions of Africa, Southern Europe, India, China, and Latin America. There are epidemics occurring in India, the Sudan, and urban areas of northeast Brazil.[7] Endemic disease in East Africa and countries surrounding the Mediterranean Sea is maintained in wild rodent reservoirs. Human infection occurs sporadically in these regions. Canine leishmaniasis is additionally a problem in Spain and France, providing a reservoir close to human habitat. The recent increase in HIV infection has led to a high incidence of visceral leishmaniasis in Spanish and French patients, sometimes caused by parasite zymodemes that rarely cause symptomatic infection in healthy hosts.[18] A high incidence of PKDL in the Sudan makes it possible that humans contribute as reservoir hosts to the ongoing epidemic in the southern part of that country. Also contributing to the epidemic is the fact that the long-standing civil war has led to migration of a large population of nonimmune hosts into endemic regions. No animal reservoir has been identified for visceral leishmaniasis in India, and again the high frequency of PKDL may contribute to the ability of humans to serve as a reservoir. Finally, in Latin America *L. chagasi* infection is sporadic in many rural regions. There are large outbreaks in several urban areas of northeastern Brazil, which reflect adaptation of the sandfly to a peridomestic life cycle. The insects survive in garbage heaps, crevices, and sometimes in the walls of houses. South American visceral leishmaniasis is most common in children, and their adult relatives often exhibit skin test positivity reflecting prior exposure and immunity against infection. Domestic dogs serve as major reservoirs of peridomestic infection in South America,[16] leading the Brazilian government to actively survey for and treat canine leishmaniasis.

Prevention and Control

Difficulties in gaining control over the different forms of leishmaniasis can be thought of in terms of the diseases that are transmitted via anthroponotic versus zoonotic versus peridomestic cycles. All face the fact that many affected persons reside in regions where access to medical care is limited. This is compounded by the fact that the most efficacious drugs require lengthy parenteral administration and cause considerable toxicity, making therapy difficult to administer and monitor. In the case of anthroponotic disease such as that occurring in India and possibly the Sudan, the presence of PKDL allows the disease to be maintained that much longer in the environment. Improved human disease detection and treatment would help diminish the disease. The wild rodent or canid reservoirs of zoonotic leishmaniasis are difficult or impossible to eradicate. Attempts to poison rodents in their burrows are obviously effective only in very limited regions.[19] Peridomestic disease, such as occurs during transmission of South American visceral leishmaniasis, is simpler to tackle in that a major reservoir of disease is the domestic dog, which is available for surveillance and treatment. However, even in the case of *L. chagasi* this is probably not the only disease reservoir. Until living conditions can be improved to remove human habitat from sandfly breeding grounds and to make treatment and early disease recognition more available, the cycle is likely to be maintained. Vector control in the form of insect repellents containing deet and the use of fine mesh netting during sleep is recommended for individual travelers to endemic regions. Attempts at vector eradication to control disease in endemic countries, however, have proved to be impractical. As an illustration, the incidence of leishmaniasis decreased after World War II when there was widespread use of DDT to prevent malaria. However, after the discontinuation of DDT leishmaniasis resurged, indicating the insecticide provided only a temporary measure. Insecticides are expensive, they are environmentally unfriendly, and they select for drug-resistant insects. Thus, they are unlikely to provide a long-term solution to control of these diseases.

Due to the difficulties mentioned above in interrupting the life cycle of *Leishmania* either by vector control or by reservoir eradication or cure, a protective vaccine would be an ideal means of controlling the disease in endemic countries. In theory it should be possible to develop a vaccine, since cure of human leishmaniasis results in long-term immunity against reinfection with the same organism. As proof of this contention, a solution to the high incidence of cutaneous leishmaniasis in the Middle East has been to expose a cosmetically acceptable area of the body to sandflies or live *L. major* promastigotes. Resolution of this purposefully induced disease results in protection against more disfiguring cutaneous leishmaniasis in the future. Despite this naturally occurring protective immunity, however, there is not yet an established protective vaccine. The World Health Organization is orchestrating several trials of killed promastigote vaccines with or without BCG as adjuvant, and prior trials have met with different degrees of success. However, these potential vaccines are still in their early stages of development, and if effective they will at the very least require refinement. Thus, several topics of current interest to the scientific community and the World Health Organization, including the development of a protective vaccine and the search for less toxic and more efficacious treatment modalities, could greatly improve our ability to control these problematic and common infections.

Lymphatic Filariasis

Amy D. Klion

Lymphatic filariasis is a chronic, often debilitating, infection caused by the filarial parasites *Wuchereria bancrofti*, *Brugia malayi*, and *Brugia timori*. More than 120 million people in 73 endemic countries of the tropics and subtropics are afflicted and as many as 900 million residents of endemic areas are at risk for infection.[1] Although the prevalence of lymphatic filariasis is increasing worldwide, mostly as a result of unplanned urbanization, recent advances in filarial diagnosis and treatment are likely to increase the success of ongoing control programs. Consequently, lymphatic filariasis has been targeted by the International Task Force for Disease Eradication as one of six "eradicable" or "potentially eradicable" infectious diseases.[2]

Biology and Life Cycles

Human infection occurs when infective larvae penetrate the skin during the bite of a mosquito vector and migrate to the nearest lymphatic vessel. Over the course of several months, they develop into thread-like adult worms (the males are approximately 40 by 0.1 mm and the females 100 by 0.25 mm in size). The average life span of the adult worms has been estimated at 5 years.[3] Fertilized female worms produce sheathed microfilariae, which are released into the bloodstream. In most areas of the world, these microfilariae are detectable in the peripheral blood only at night (nocturnal periodicity); however, a subperiodic form, in which microfilarial counts are maximal during the day, is found in some regions of the Pacific islands, eastern Malaysia, and Vietnam. Circulating microfilariae, ingested by the appropriate mosquito vector during a blood meal, develop over the course of several weeks into infective larvae, completing the parasite life cycle.

Distribution

The geographic distribution of lymphatic filariasis is determined primarily by the ability of the parasite to adapt to different mosquito vectors. Consequently, *W. bancrofti*, which can be transmitted by a large number of *Anopheles, Culex,* and *Aedes* species, is the most widespread of the agents of lymphatic filariasis, occurring in parts of Africa, Asia, South and Central America, the Caribbean, and the Pacific. Transmitted predominantly by *Mansonia* species, *B. malayi* infection is restricted to areas of south and east Asia. *B. timori* infection has been reported from only two islands in Indonesia (Timor and Flores), where it is transmitted by *Anopheles barbirostris*.

Although experimental infection of nonhuman primates is possible, animals other than humans do not appear to be natural reservoirs of *W. bancrofti* or *B. timori*.[4] In contrast, *B. malayi* is a zoonosis in some parts of Malaysia, where leaf-eating monkeys, wild cats, civets, and pangolins are reservoirs of infection.[4]

Lymphatic filariasis is found predominantly in urban settings, where mosquitoes breed in unsanitary water sources such as abandoned wells and septic tanks, pit latrines, and water storage tanks.[5] In rural foci of infection, swamps and rice paddies provide a suitable environment for mosquito larvae.[6]

Pathologic and Clinical Manifestations

The spectrum of clinical manifestations of lymphatic filariasis is broad and includes asymptomatic microfilaremia, recurrent episodes of acute adenolymphangitis (ADL), chronic lymphedema/elephantiasis, and tropical pulmonary eosinophilia. Whereas differences in the immune response to filarial infection are clearly involved in determining the early clinical response to infection, recent studies have implicated recurrent bacterial infections as an important factor in recurrent episodes of ADL and progression toward chronic lymphedema and elephantiasis.[1,7]

Numerous large population studies have shown that most natives of endemic areas who acquire lymphatic filariasis are asymptomatic with circulating microfilaria detectable in the peripheral blood (microfilaremia).[5,8] However, despite the lack of obvious clinical signs or symptoms, pathologic changes—including alterations in lymphatic flow, as detected by lymphoscintigraphy,[9] and renal abnormalities (hematuria and proteinuria)[10]—have been demonstrated in these individuals.

In contrast to the above-described asymptomatic microfilaremic patients, the majority of visitors to endemic areas who become infected present with signs and symptoms of acute infection.[11] These include recurrent episodes of fever, lymphadenitis, and/or retrograde lymphangitis, sometimes referred to as "filarial fevers." The lower extremities are affected more frequently than the upper extremities and breast, and in *W. bancrofti* infection, the scrotum or female external genitalia may also be involved. Episodes generally last from 3 to 7 days unless they are complicated by abscess formation along the affected lymphatic, in which case healing may take several months. Additional early manifestations of *W. bancrofti* infection include orchitis and inflammation of the spermatic cord, which can lead to permanent thickening of the spermatic cord and/or hydrocele. Genital manifestations are rare in brugian filariasis.[12]

After years of infection, chronic lymphatic obstruction develops in some patients. Recurrent episodes of inflammation and infection lead to irreversible enlargement of the affected area with a thickened, warty appearance of the overlying skin (elephantiasis). In contrast to *W. bancrofti* infection, in which the entire limb is generally involved, the chronic lymphedema of brugian filariasis is characteristically limited to the distal portion of the involved extremity.[12] Although elephantiasis itself is generally painless and well tolerated, ulceration and secondary infection are common and contribute greatly to the morbidity and mortality of lymphatic filarial infection. In the genital region, lymphatic obstruction may lead to rupture of the dilated lymph vessels into the urinary tract and intermittent chyluria.

A minority of patients with lymphatic filariasis present with the hyperresponsive syndrome of tropical pulmonary eosinophilia (TPE).[13] The clinical manifestations of TPE are predominantly pulmonary, consisting of nocturnal wheezing, cough, and dyspnea, although constitutional symptoms may be present. Laboratory studies are notable for marked eosinophilia (both in the peripheral blood and the lower respiratory tract) and elevated serum IgE and antifilarial antibody levels. Chest radiographs typically show diffuse reticulonodular infiltrates, and pulmonary function tests are consistent with a predominantly restrictive pattern. Although most patients with TPE respond rapidly to a 3-week course of diethylcarbamazine (DEC), chronic respiratory tract inflammation and mild interstitial lung disease are not uncommon.[14] Untreated, TPE may progress to irreversible interstitial fibrosis.

Diagnosis

Until recently, definitive parasitologic diagnosis could only be made by demonstration of the characteristic sheathed microfilariae in a Giemsa-stained specimen of peripheral blood or, rarely, by excision of an adult worm. Because the microfilariae in lymphatic filariasis exhibit periodicity in many areas of the world, the timing of blood samples for parasite detection is critical and often inconvenient. Consequently, circulating filaria antigen assays for *W. bancrofti*, which are as sensitive and specific as detection of microfilariae and are unaffected by periodicity, are replacing the more conventional parasitologic methods.[15,16] Unfortunately, comparable assays do not exist for *B. malayi* or *B. timori* infection. Preliminary studies suggest that recently developed DNA-based polymerase chain reaction (PCR) assays for *W. bancrofti* and *B. malayi* are comparable in sensitivity and specificity to the circulating antigen assay for detection of microfilaremia and offer the advantage of tissue diagnosis from biopsy specimens.[17,18] Widespread use of such assays has not been implemented to date, however.

Antifilarial antibody measurement is useful in documenting infection in patients with TPE and in visitors to endemic areas who have symptoms consistent with infection but no detectable microfilariae. However, such assays do not distinguish between the various filarial infections of humans, several of which have overlapping geographic distributions.[19,20] Furthermore, they are often positive in uninfected residents of endemic areas, precluding their widespread use in this population.

Other diagnostic aids include ultrasonography, which has been used to document living adult worms in the lymphatics of patients with hydrocele and their response to therapy,[21] and lymphoscintigraphy.[9]

Treatment

The two drugs available for the treatment of lymphatic filariasis are diethylcarbamazine (DEC) and ivermectin.[22] DEC is a piperazine derivative with excellent microfilaricidal activity at low doses. The mechanism of action of DEC is unknown but appears to depend on the host immune response. Although adult worms are affected by prolonged, high-dose DEC,[21] killing is inefficient and cure is uncommon. Furthermore, the incidence of side effects (nausea, vomiting, anorexia, headache, malaise, arthralgias, and localized swellings along the lymphatics) are dose related. Side effects of low-dose therapy for lymphatic filariasis are generally mild; however, severe reactions may occur in patients with concomitant loiasis or onchocerciasis.[23,24] Consequently, individuals from areas where these infections are co-endemic with lymphatic filariasis should be screened before treatment with DEC. Although there is no direct evidence for the development of drug resistance in lymphatic filariasis, diminished efficacy of DEC treatment in some patients with circulating microfilariae despite adequate drug levels suggests that resistance may occur in some situations.[25]

Ivermectin shows similar activity to DEC against microfilariae of lymphatic-dwelling filariae but has no effect on adult worms.[21] It acts by blocking the neurotransmitter γ-aminobutyric acid (GABA). Ivermectin is usually well tolerated and has a similar side effect profile to low-dose DEC. Since severe reactions have been reported in patients with high levels of circulating *Loa loa* microfilariae,[26] ivermectin should be used cautiously in areas endemic for loiasis.

In view of the recent data demonstrating pathologic changes even in asymptomatic patients, all infected individuals should be treated with the goal of preventing morbidity and decreasing disease transmission. The current recommended therapy for lymphatic filariasis is high-dose treatment with DEC (6 mg/kg/day for 12 days [*W. bancrofti*] or 6 days [*Brugia*]).[22] Potential alternative regimens for asymptomatic microfilarial carriers include intermittent DEC (6 mg/kg)[27] or yearly ivermectin (400 μg/kg),[28] although large comparative studies are lacking. For symptomatic patients, intensive local hygiene and prompt treatment of bacterial or fungal superinfection should be instituted as well.

Once elephantiasis is present, treatment modalities are few. Surgical bypass of affected lymphatic vessels has been performed in some patients, but the technical difficulty and high cost of this procedure has limited its usefulness.[29] Daily administration of coumarin (5,6-benzo-alpha-pyrone) for 1 year has been shown to decrease lymphedema and the incidence of inflammatory episodes in patients with lymphatic filariasis for up to 1 year after the treatment was discontinued;[30] however, the long-term effects of this therapy have not been assessed.

Control and Prevention

A primary goal of current filariasis control programs is the interruption of transmission of infection (infection control). Since vector control measures alone have been generally unsuccessful in decreasing the prevalence of infection, an integrated approach of (*a*) microfilaremia reduction through chemotherapy, (*b*) vector control, and (*c*) reduction of host-vector contact has been advocated. The optimal control strategies for a given endemic area will depend on the particular parasite and vector species involved as well as on the ecological, cultural, and political factors specific to the region.

Although there is no curative chemotherapy for lymphatic filariasis, both DEC and ivermectin have been demonstrated to suppress microfilaremia in infected patients for up to 1 year after therapy is stopped. Several regimens appear to have similar efficacy (90 to 95 percent reduction in microfilaremia for more than 1 year): (*a*) the use of DEC-fortified salt (0.2 to 0.4 percent w/w), (*b*) single annual or semiannual administration of DEC (6 mg/kg body weight), and (*c*) once-yearly administration of ivermectin (400 μg/kg).[31,32] Combination therapy with ivermectin and DEC is slightly more effective (99 percent reduction),[32] but it cannot be used in areas where onchocerciasis or loiasis are endemic. Preliminary data from ongoing studies of combination therapy with albendazole and ivermectin suggest that this combination is safe and at least as effective as DEC and ivermectin, although conclusive evidence is unavailable at this time. Thus, the choice of an optimal regimen depends on the co-endemicity of other filarial parasites, drug availability, cost, and community acceptance.

In general, mass distribution programs are preferred over selective treatment of infected individuals for several reasons, including the cost of screening and the inability of current diagnostic methods to reliably identify prepatent infection (i.e., early infection prior to the release of microfilariae). The length of time that control strategies need to be continued to completely eradicate lymphatic filariasis from an endemic area is unknown, but 5 to 10 years has been suggested for yearly dose regimens and 9 to 12 months for DEC-salt.[1]

Vector control in lymphatic filariasis (as in malaria) has been problematic, primarily because of the widespread distribution of potential mosquito vectors and their ability to adapt to varied ecological conditions.[33] Nevertheless, reduction of vector density could accelerate the interruption of filarial transmission in regions with ongoing chemotherapy-based control programs and contribute to the long-term maintenance of control. Multiple strategies have been employed with varying success. Toxin-producing bacteria such as *Bacillus sphaericus* and *Bacillus thuringiensis*,[34] larvivorous fish,[35] and polystyrene beads (which expand to cover the surface of breeding areas in closed water systems and suffocate developing larvae)[36] have been used to control larvae of *Culex* and *Mansonia* species. The elimination of breeding sites through the construction of improved water and sanitary facilities would be more desirable but is economically unfeasible in most endemic regions. Reduction of host-vector contact can be achieved with the use of insect repellents and protective clothing or, in areas where vector feeding is predominantly indoors, with indoor spraying with pyrethroids and other household measures (including screens, bed nets, and mosquito coils). In most instances, a combination of measures has been most effective.[34,37]

The ability to prevent lymphatic filariasis through immunization would greatly enhance current control strategies by limiting the population at risk for infection. Although the presence of small numbers of long-term residents of filaria-endemic regions who have neither clinical nor laboratory evidence of infection suggests that protective immunity to filariasis may occur naturally, vaccine development has been hampered by the complexity of the human immune response to filarial infection and the lack of clinically relevant nonprimate models of infection. Consequently, a safe and effective vaccine is unlikely to be available in the near future.

An essential part of any successful control program is community participation. For this to occur, there must be a basic understanding of the methods of transmission, prevention, and control of infection. Several studies have demonstrated, however, that the majority of the people living in highly endemic areas are lacking in this basic knowledge.[38,39] That an understanding of the mechanism of disease transmission is associated with a decreased risk of infection is suggested by the finding that 20 percent of the uninfected residents of an endemic area in India, but only 9 percent of infected residents, were aware that mosquitoes transmit filarial infection.[38] Although this association has not been formally proven by prospective longitudinal studies, community-wide education programs targeted at filariasis prevention and control are likely to include information of broad general health benefit (i.e., mosquito prevention and personal hygiene measures) and should be included in all integrated filariasis control programs.

Using combined chemotherapy and vector control programs, lymphatic filariasis has been eliminated from Japan, Taiwan, South Korea, and the Solomon Islands and is approaching eradication in China.[1] However, relaxation of control programs has led to the resurgence of the disease in other regions, including the Nile Delta and French Polynesia.[40] Furthermore, new areas of endemicity will likely continue to arise as global warming, urbanization, and other natural and human-made environmental changes create vector habitats in previously unsuitable locations. Consequently, long-term surveillance must be an integral part of filariasis control. The recent development of sensitive and specific assays that are suitable for large-scale epidemiologic studies of endemic populations and detection of infected vectors (i.e., circulating antigen and DNA-based PCR assays) should facilitate such monitoring, both in areas of ongoing control and in areas at risk of becoming endemic for lymphatic filariasis.

Even if control measures are successful in eliminating transmission of lymphatic filariasis, the prevention of infection-related morbidity will remain a problem in the foreseeable future. Clearly, every effort should be made to promote local hygiene and early treatment of cellulitis in symptomatic patients, since these have been associated with a decrease in the number of episodes of adenolymphangitis. The approach to asymptomatic infected individuals is less straightforward, in view of the lack of long-term studies comparing disease progression in treated and untreated patients with microfilaremia. However, the resolution of hematuria and proteinuria in response to antifilarial chemotherapy has been demonstrated, suggesting that some of the early pathology seen in asymptomatic patients with lymphatic filariasis may be reversible. Since the potential benefits of therapy (i.e., prevention of elephantiasis) are substantial and the risks minimal, it seems prudent to treat all individuals with documented filarial infection regardless of symptoms.

▶ REFERENCES

Viral Infections

1. Karabatos N (ed): International Catalogue of Arboviruses, Including Certain Other Viruses of Vertebrates. 3rd ed. San Antonio: American Society of Tropical Medicine and Hygiene, 1985
2. Monath TB (ed): The Arboviruses: Ecology and Epidemiology, Boca Raton, FL: CRC Press, 1988, vol. I–V
3. Field RN, Knipe DM (eds): Virology. 3rd ed. New York: Raven Press, 1995, vol I–II
4. Elliott RM: Molecular biology of the *Bunyaviridae*. J Gen Virol 71:501–522, 1990
5. Strauss JH, Strauss EG (eds): The *Togavirdae* and *Flaviviridae*. New York: Plenum Press, 1986
6. Elliott RM (ed.): The Bunyaviridae, New York: Plenum Press, 1996.
7. Bishop DHL: The Rhabdoviruses. West Palm Beach, FL: CRC Press, 1979
8. Reeves WC: Factors that influence the probability of epidemics of western equine, St. Louis, and California encephalitis in California. Calif Vector Views 14:13–18, 1967
9. Reeves WC: Overwintering of arboviruses. Prog Med Virol 17:193–220, 1974
10. Hayes RO, Francy DB, Lazuick JS, Smith GC, Gibbs EPJ: Role of the cliff swallow bug (*Oeciacus vicarius*) in the natural cycle of a western equine encephalitis-related alphavirus. J Med Entomol 14:257–262, 1977
11. Bailey CL, Eldridge BF, Hayes DE, et al: Isolation of St. Louis encephalitis virus from overwintering *Culex pipiens* mosquitoes. Science 199:1346–1349, 1978
12. Miller BR, DeFoliart FR, Yuill TM: Vertical transmission of La Crosse Virus (California encephalitis group): transovarial and filial infection rates in *Aedes triseriatus* (*Diptera: Culicidae*). J Med Entomol 14:437–440, 1977
13. Bowen GS, Francy DB: Surveillance. In Monath TP (ed). St. Louis Encephalitis. Washington, DC: American Public Health Association, 1979
14. Rosen L, Gubler D: The use of mosquitoes to detect and propagate dengue viruses. Am J Trop Med 23:1153–1160, 1974
15. Beaty BJ, Calisher CH, Shope RE: Arboviruses. In: Lennette EH, Lennette DA, Lennette ET (eds): Diagnostic Procedures for Viral, Rickettsial, and Chlamydial Infections. 7th ed. Washington, DC: American Public Health Association, 1995, pp 189–212
16. Holden P, Hayes RO, Mitchell CJ, et al: House sparrows, *Passer domesticus* (L.), as hosts of arboviruses in Hale County, Texas. I. Field studies, 1965–1969. Am J Trop Med Hyg 22:244–253, 1971
17. Young NA, Johnson KM: Antigenic variants of Venezuelan equine encephalitis virus their geographic distribution and epidemiologic significance. Am J Epidemiol 89:286–307, 1969
18. Sudia WD, Newhouse VF: Venezuelan equine encephalitis in North America: a summary of virus-vector-host relationship. Am J Epidemiol 101:1–13, 1975
19. Weaver SC, Salas R, Rico-Hesse R, et al: Re-emergence of epidemic Venezuelan equine encephalomyelitis in South America. Lancet 348:436–440, 1996
20. Weaver SC, Bellew LA, Rico-Hesse R: Phylogenetic analysis of alphaviruses in the Venezuelan equine encephalitis complex and identification of the source of epizootic viruses. Virology 191:282–290, 1992
21. Monath TP, Tsai TF: St. Louis encephalitis: lessons from the last decade. Am J Trop Med Hyg 37:40S–59S, 1987
22. Tsai TF, Yu YX. In Plotkin SA, Mortimer EA (eds.): Vaccines, 3rd Ed. Philadelphia, WB Saunders, 1994, pp. 671–714
23. Lopes OS, Sachetta L de A, Coimbra TLM, Pinto GH, Glasser CM: Emergence of a new arbovirus disease in Brazil. II: Epidemiologic studies on 1975 epidemic. Am J Epidemiol 108:394–401, 1978
24. Hafkin B, Kaplan JE, Reed C, et al: Reintroduction of dengue fever into the continental United States. I. Dengue surveillance in Texas, 1980. Am J Trop Med Hyg 31:1222–1228, 1982
25. Pinheiro FP, Travassos da Rosa AP, Gomes ML, LeDuc JW, Hoch AL: Transmission of Oropouche virus from man to hamster by the midge *Culicoides paraensis*. Science 215:1251–1253, 1982

Viral Hemorrhagic Fevers

General References

Anonymous: Ebola haemorrhagic fever, a summary of the outbreak in Gabon. Wkly Epidemiol Rec 72:7–8, 1997

Anonymous: Ebola haemorrhagic fever, Gabon. Wkly Epidemiol Rec 72:71, 1997

Anonymous: Ebola haemorrhagic fever in Zaire, 1976: report of an international commission. Bull World Health Organ 56:271–293, 1978

Anonymous: Ebola haemorrhagic fever, Zaire. Wkly Epidemiol Rec 70:241–241, 1995

Anonymous: Haemorrhagic fever with renal syndrome, Russian Federation. Wkly Epidemiol Rec 68:189–191, 1993

Anonymous: Outbreak of Ebola haemorrhagic fever in Gabon officially declared over. Wkly Epidemiol Rec 71:125–126, 1996

Anonymous: Rift Valley fever, Egypt. Wkly Epidemiol Rec 68:300–301, 1993

Anonymous: Vaccination against Argentine haemorrhagic fever. Wkly Epidemiol Rec 68:233–234, 1993

Duchin JS, Koster FT, Peters CJ, et al: Hantavirus pulmonary syndrome: a clinical description of 17 patients with newly recognized disease. N Engl J Med 330:949–955, 1994

Halstead SB: Observations related to pathogenesis of dengue hemorrhagic fever: hypotheses and discussion. Yale J Biol Med 42:350–362, 1970

Hoogstraal H: The epidemiology of tick-borne Crimean-Congo hemorrhagic fever in Asia, Europe and Africa. J Med Entomol 15:307–417, 1979

Jahrling PB, Geisbert TW, Dalgard DW, et al: Preliminary report: isolation of Ebola virus from monkeys imported to USA. Lancet 335: 502–505, 1990

Kharitonova NN, Leonov YA: Omsk hemorrhagic fever, ecology of the agent and epizootiology. New Delhi: Published for the National Library of Medicine by Amerind Publishing, 1985

LeDuc JW: *Hantavirus* infections. In Porterfield JS (ed): Kass Handbook of Infectious Diseases, Exotic Viral Infections. London: Chapman and Hall, 1995, pp 261–284

LeDuc JW, Childs JE, Glass GE: The hantaviruses, etiological agents of hemorrhagic fever with renal syndrome: a possible cause of hypertension and chronic renal disease in the United States. Annu Rev Public Health 13:79–98, 1992

McCormick JB, Fisher-Hock SP: *Filovirus* infections. In Porterfield JS (ed): Kass Handbook of Infectious Diseases, Exotic Viral Infections. London: Chapman and Hall, 1995, pp 319–328

McCormick JB, Webb PA, Krebs JW, et al: A prospective study of the epidemiology and ecology of Lassa fever. J Infect Dis 155:445–455, 1987

Meegan JM: The Rift Valley fever epizootic in Egypt 1977–1978. I. Description of the epizootic and virological studies. Trans R Soc Trop Med Hyg 73:618–623, 1979

Mills JN, Ellis BA, Childs JE, et al: Prevalence of infection with Junin virus in rodent populations in the epidemic area of Argentine hemorrhagic fever. Am J Trop Med Hyg 51:554–562, 1994

Nasidi A, Monath TP, Vandenberg J, et al: Yellow fever vaccination and pregnancy: a four-year prospective study. Trans R Soc Trop Med Hyg 87:337–339, 1993

Pattyn SR (ed): Ebola Virus Haemorrhagic Fever. Amsterdam: Elsevier/North-Holland, 1978
Peters CJ: Arenaviruses. In Belshi R (ed): Textbook of Human Virology. 2nd ed. St. Louis: Mosby–Year Book 1991, pp 541–570
Peters CJ, LeDuc JW: *Bunyaviridae* bunyaviruses, phleboviruses, and related viruses. In Belshi R (ed). Textbook of Human Virology. 2nd ed. St. Louis: Mosby–Year Book, 1991, pp 571–614
Qattan I, Akbar N, Afif H, et al: A novel flavivirus: Makkah Region 1994–1996. Saudi Epidemiol Bull 3:2–4, 1996
Robertson SE, Hull BP, Tomori O, et al: Yellow fever, a decade of reemergence. JAMA 276:1157–1162
Strode GK (ed): Yellow fever. New York: McGraw-Hill, 1951
Swanepoel R: *Nairovirus* infections. In Porterfield JS (ed): Kass Handbook of Infectious Diseases, Exotic Viral Infections. London: Chapman and Hall, 1995, pp 285–294
Swanepoel R, Leman PA, Burt NA, et al: Experimental inoculation of plants and animals with Ebola virus. Emerging Infect Dis 2:321–325, 1996
Ter Meulen J, Lukashevich I, Sidibe K, et al: Hunting of peridomestic rodents and consumption of their meat as possible risk factors for rodent-to-human transmission of Lassa virus in the Republic of Guinea. Am J Trop Med Hyg 55:661–666, 1996

Rickettsial Infections

1. McDade JE, Fishbein DB. Rickettsiaceae. The Rickettsiae. In Balows A, Hausler WJ Jr, Lennette EH (eds): The Laboratory Diagnosis of Infectious Diseases: Principles and Practice. New York: Springer-Verlag, 1988, vol 2, pp 864–890
2. Krieg NR (ed): Bergey's Manual of Systematic Bacteriology. Baltimore: Williams & Wilkins, 1984, vol 1, pp 687–704
3. Raoult D, Walker DH: *Rickettsia rickettsii* and other spotted fever group Rickettsiae (Rocky Mountain spotted fever and other spotted fevers). In Mandell GL, Douglas RG Jr, Bennett JE (eds): Principles and Practice of Infectious Diseases. 3rd ed. New York: Churchill Livingstone, 1989, pp 1465–1471
4. Saah AJ: *Rickettsia prowazekii* (Epidemic or louse-borne typhus). In Mandell GL, Douglas RG Jr, Bennett JE (eds): Principles and Practice of Infectious Diseases. 3rd ed. New York: Churchill Livingstone 1989, pp 1476–1478
5. Saah AJ: *Rickettsia tsutsugamushi* (Scrub Typhus). In Mandell GL, Douglas RG Jr, Bennett JE (eds):. Principles and Practice of Infectious Diseases. 3rd ed. New York: Churchill Livingstone, 1989, pp 1480–1482
6. Marrie TJ: *Coxiella burnetii* (Q fever). In Mandell GL, Douglas RG Jr, Bennett JE (eds): Principles and Practice of Infectious Diseases. 3rd ed. New York: Churchill Livingstone, 1989, pp 1472–1476
7. Taylor JP, Betz TG, Rawlings JA: Epidemiology of murine typhus in Texas, 1980 through 1984. JAMA 255:2173–2176, 1986
8. Ming-yuan F, Walker DH, Shu-rong Y, Qing-huai L. Epidemiology and ecology of rickettsial diseases in the People's Republic of China. Rev Infect Dis 98:823–840, 1987
9. Rapmund G: Rickettsial diseases of the Far East: new perspectives. J Infect Dis 149:330–338, 1984
10. Salgo MP, Telzak EE, Currie B, et al. A focus of Rocky Mountain spotted fever within New York City: N Eng J Med 318:1345–1348, 1988
11. Gordon JC, Gordon SW, Peterson E, Philip RN. Rocky Mountain spotted fever in dogs associated with human patients in Ohio. J Infect Dis 148:1123, 1983
12. McDonald JC, MacLean JD, McDade JE: Imported rickettsial disease: clinical and epidemiologic features. Am J Med 85:799–805, 1988
13. Mansueto S, Tringali G, Walker DH: Widespread simultaneous increase in the incidence of spotted fever group rickettsiosis. J Infect Dis 154:538–540, 1986
14. Font-Creus B, Bella-Cueto F, Espejo-Arenas E, et al: Mediterranean spotted fever: a cooperative study of 227 cases. Rev Infect Dis 7: 635–642, 1985
15. Uchida T, Tashiro F, Funato T, et al: Isolation of a spotted fever group rickettsia from a patient with febrile exanthematous illness in Shikoku, Japan. Microbiol Immunol 30:1323–1326, 1986
16. Brettman LR, Lewin S, Holzman RS, et al: Rickettsialpox: report of an outbreak and a contemporary review. Medicine 60:363–372, 1981
17. Bernard KW, Parham GL, Winkler WG, Helmick CG: Q fever control measures: recommendations for facilities using sheep. Infect Control 3:461–465, 1982
18. Maeda K, Markowitz N, Hawley RC, Ristic M, Cox D, McDade JE: Human Infection with *Ehrlichia canis*, a leukocytic Rickettsia. N Engl J Med 316:853–856, 1987
19. McDade JE: Ehrlichiosis—a disease of animals and humans. J Infect Dis 161: 609–617, 1990
20. Rohrbach BW, Harkess JR, Ewing SA, Kudlac J, McKee GL, Istre GR: Epidemiologic and clinical characteristics of persons with serologic evidence of *E. canis* infection. Am J Public Health 80: 442–445, 1990

Plague

1. Pollitzer R: Plague. WHO Monograph Series 22:1. Geneva: World Health Organization, 1954
2. Perry RD, Fetherston JD: *Yersinia pestis*—etiologic agent of plague. Clin Microbiol Rev 10:35–66, 1977
3. Poland JD, Barnes AM: Plague. In Steele J (ed): Handbook of Zoonoses. Boca Raton, FL: CRC Press, 1979, pp 515–559
4. Gage KL: Plague. In Collier L, Balows A, Sussman M, Hausler WJ (eds): Topley and Wilson's Microbiology and Microbiological Infections. Vol 3, Bacterial Infections. London: Edward Arnold; 885–903, 1997
5. Pollitzer R, Meyer KF: The ecology of plague. In May JH (ed): Studies in Disease Ecology. New York: Hefner, 1961:433–501
6. Barnes AM: Surveillance and control of bubonic plague in the United States. Symp Zool Soc Lond 50:237–270, 1982
7. Quan TJ: Plague. In Wentworth BB (ed): Diagnostic Procedures for Bacterial Infections. 7th ed. Washington, DC: American Public Health Association, 445–453, 1987
8. Hoogstraal H: The roles of fleas and ticks in the epidemiology of human diseases. In Traub R, Starcke H (eds): Fleas. Rotterdam: A.A. Balkema, 1980, pp 241–244
9. Cavanaugh DC, Marshall JD Jr: The influence of climate on the seasonal prevalence of plague in the Republic of Vietnam. J Wildl Dis 8:85–94, 1972
10. Cavanaugh DC: The specific effect of temperature upon the transmission of the plague bacillus by the oriental rat flea (*Xenopsylla cheopis*). Am J Trop Med Hyg 20:264–272, 1979
11. Hinnebusch BJ, Perry RD, Schwann TG: Role of the *Yersinia pestis* hemin storage (*hms*) locus in the transmission of plague in fleas. Science 273:367–370, 1996
12. von Reyn CF, Barnes AM, Weber NS, Hodgrin UG: Bubonic plague from exposure to a rabbit: a documented case and a review of rabbit-associated plague cases in the United States. Am J Epidemiol 104:81–87, 1976
13. Centers for Disease Control and Prevention: Winter plague—Colorado, Washington, Texas, 1983–1984. MMWR 33:145–148, 1984
14. Eidson M, Thilsted JP, Rollag OJ: Clinical, clinicopathologic, and pathologic features of plague in cats: 119 cases (1977–1988). JAMA 199:1191–1197, 1991
15. Gasper PW, Barnes AM, Quan TJ, et al: Plague (*Yersinia pestis*) in cats: description of experimentally induced disease. J Med Entomol 30:20–26, 1993

16. Kaufman AF, Mann JM, Gardiner TM, et al: Public health implications of plague in domestic cats. J Am Vet Med Assoc 179:875–878, 1981
17. Eidson M, Tierney LA, Rollag AJ, et al: Feline plague in New Mexico: risk factors and transmission to humans. Am J Public Health 78:1333–1335, 1988
18. Doll JM, Zeitz PS, Ettestad P, et al: Cat-transmitted fatal pneumonic plague in a person who traveled from Colorado to Arizona. Am J Trop Med Hyg 51:109–114, 1994
19. Centers for Disease Control and Prevention: Human plague—United States, 1993–1994. MMWR 43:242–246, 1994
20. World Health Organization: Human plague in 1994. Wkly Epidemiol Rec 22:165–172, 1996
21. Anonymous: Plague in India. World Health Organization International Plague Investigative Team Report, December 9, 1994. Geneva: World Health Organization, 1994
22. Ramalingaswami V: An overview of the work carried out by the Technical Advisory Committee on Plague. Curr Sci 71:783–786, 1996
23. Campbell GL, Hughes JM: Plague in India: a new warning from an old nemesis. Ann Intern Med 122:151–153, 1995
24. Fritz CL, Dennis DT, Tipple MA, et al: Surveillance for pneumonic plague in the United States during an international emergency: a model for control of imported emerging diseases. Emerging Infectious Diseases 2:30–36, 1996
25. World Health Organization: International Health Regulations (1969). Geneva: World Health Organization, 1983, pp 10–15
26. Craven RB, Maupin GO, Beard ML, et al: Reported cases of human plague infections in the United States, 1979–1991. J Med Entomol 30:758–761, 1993
27. Marshall JD, Quy DV, Gibson FL: Asymptomatic pharyngeal plague infection in Vietnam. Am J Trop Med Hyg 16:175, 1967
28. Christie AB, Chen TH, Elberg SS: Plague in camels and goats: their role in human epidemics. J Infect Dis 141:724–726, 1980
29. Campbell GL, Dennis DT: Plague and other *Yersinia* infections. In Isselbacher KJ, Braunwald E, Wilson JD, et al (eds): Harrison's Principles of Internal Medicine. New York: McGraw Hill, 975–980, 1997
30. Nguyen VI, Nguyen DH, Pham VD, et al: Co-trimoxazole in bubonic plague. Br Med J 108–109, 1973
31. Butler T, Levin J, Nguyen NL, et al: *Yersinia pestis* infection in Vietnam. II. Quantitative blood cultures and detection of endotoxin in the cerebrospinal fluid of patients with meningitis. J Infect Dis 133: 493–499, 1976
32. Centers for Disease Control and Prevention: Prevention of plague. Recommendations of the Advisory Committee on Immunization Practices (ACIP). MMWR 45(RR-14):1–15, 1996

Malaria

1. World Health Organization: World malaria situation in 1993, part I. Wkly Epidemiol Rec 71(1):17–22, 1996
2. Shepard DS, Ettling MB, Brinkmann U, Sauerborn R: The economic cost of malaria in Africa. Trop Med Parasitol 42(3):199–203, 1991
3. Knudsen AB, Slooff R: Vector-borne disease problems in rapid urbanization: new approaches to vector control. Bull World Health Organ 70(1):1–6, 1992
4. Kachur SP, Reller ME, Barber A, et al: Malaria surveillance—United States, 1994. MMWR Surveillance Summaries, 1997, in press
5. Zucker JR: Changing patterns of autochthonous malaria transmission in the United States. Emerging Infectious Diseases 2(1):37–43, 1996
6. Austin SC, Stolley PD, Lasky T: The history of malariotherapy for neurosyphilis. Modern parallels. JAMA 268(4):516–519, 1992
7. Centers for Disease Control and Prevention: Imported malaria associated with malariotherapy for Lyme disease—New Jersey. MMWR 39(48):667–668, 1990
8. World Health Organization: Terminology of malaria and of malaria eradication. Geneva: World Health Organization, 1963, p 32
9. Zingman BS, Viner BL: Splenic complications in malaria: case report and review. Clin Infect Dis 16(2):223–232, 1993
10. World Health Organization: Severe and complicated malaria. Trans R Soc Trop Med Hyg 84(Suppl 2):1–65, 1990
11. Greenberg AE, Ntumbanzondo M, Ntula N, et al: Hospital-based surveillance of malaria-related paediatric morbidity and mortality in Kinshasa, Zaire. Bull World Health Organ 67(2):189–196, 1989
12. Molyneux ME, Taylor TE, Wirima JJ, Borgstein J: Clinical features and prognostic indicators in paediatric cerebral malaria: a study of 131 comatose Malawian children. Q J Med 71(265):441–459, 1989
13. Greenwood BM, Bradley AK, Greenwood AM, et al: Mortality and morbidity from malaria among children in a rural area of the Gambia, West Africa. Trans R Soc Trop Med Hyg 81(3):478–486, 1987
14. Marsh K, Forster D, Waruiru C, et al: Indicators of life-threatening malaria in African children. N Engl J Med 332(21):1399–1441, 1995
15. Bray RS, Anderson MJ: Falciparum malaria and pregnancy. Trans R Soc Trop Med Hyg 73(4):427–431, 1979
16. Galbraith RM, Faulk MP, Galbraith GMP, et al: The human maternal-foetal relationship in malaria: 1. Identification of pigment and parasites in the placenta. Trans R Soc Trop Med Hyg 74(1):52–72, 1980
17. McCormick MC. Contribution of low birth weight to infant mortality and childhood mortality. N Engl J Med 312(2):82–90, 1985
18. McDermott JM, Wirima JJ, Steketee RW, et al: The effect of placental malaria on perinatal mortality in rural Malawi. Am J Trop Med Hyg 55(1):61–65, 1996
19. Steketee R, Wirima JJ, Bloland PB, et al: Impairment of a pregnant woman's ability to limit *Plasmodium falciparum* by infection with human immunodeficiency virus type 1. Am J Trop Med Hyg 55(1)42–49, 1996
20. Campbell CC: Challenges facing antimalarial therapy in Africa. J Infect Dis 163(6):1207–1211, 1991
21. Snow RW, Bastos de Azevedo I, Lowe BS, et al: Severe childhood malaria in two areas of markedly different *P. falciparum* transmission in East Africa. Acta Trop 57(4):289–300, 1994
22. Slutsker L, Taylor TE, Wirima JJ, Steketee RW: In-hospital morbidity and mortality due to malaria-associated severe anaemia in two areas of Malawi with different patterns of malaria infection. Trans R Soc Trop Med Hyg 88(5):548–551, 1994
23. Greenwood B, Marsh K, Snow R: Why do some African children develop severe malaria? Parasitology Today 7(10):277–281, 1991
24. Glynn JR, Bradley DJ: Inoculum size, incubation period and severity of malaria. Analysis of data from malaria therapy records. Parasitology 110(Pt 1):7–19, 1995
25. Robert F, Ntoumi F, Angel G, et al: Extensive genetic diversity of *Plasmodium falciparum* isolates collected from patients with severe malaria in Dakar, Senegal. Trans R Soc Trop Med Hyg 90:704–711, 1996
26. Staunton DE, Ockenhouse CF, Springer TA: Soluble intercellular adhesion molecule 1-immunoglobulin G1 immunoadhesin mediates phagocytosis of malaria-infected erythrocytes. J Exp Med 176:1183, 1992
27. Aikawa M, Iseki M, Barnwell JW, et al: The pathology of human cerebral malaria. Am J Trop Med Hyg 43(2 Pt 2):30–37, 1990
28. Carlson J, Helmby H, Hill AV, et al: Human cerebral malaria: association with erythrocyte rosetting and lack of anti-rosetting antibodies. Lancet 336(8729):1457–1460, 1990
29. Miller LH, Good MF, Milon G: Malaria pathogenesis. Science 264(5167):1878–1883, 1994
30. Kwiatkowski D: Tumour necrosis factor, fever, and fatality in falciparum malaria. Immunol Lett 25(1–3):213–216, 1990
31. Grau GE, Taylor TE, Molyneux ME, et al: Tumor necrosis factor and disease severity in children with falciparum malaria. N Engl J Med 320(24):1586–1591, 1989
32. Kern P, Hemmer CJ, Van Damme J, et al: Elevated tumor necrosis factor alpha and interleukin-6 serum levels as markers for compli-

cated *Plasmodium falciparum* malaria. Am J Med 87(2):139–143, 1989

33. Karunaweera ND, Grau GE, Gamage P, et al: Dynamics of fever and serum levels of tumour necrosis factor are closely associated during clinical paroxysms in *Plasmodium vivax* malaria. Proc Natl Acad Sci USA 89(8):3200–3203, 1992
34. Kwiatkowski D, Hill AVS, Sambou I, et al: TNF concentration in fatal cerebral, non-fatal cerebral, and uncomplicated *Plasmodium falciparum* malaria. Lancet 336(8725):1201–1204, 1990
35. Playfair JHL: The pathology of malaria: a possible target for immunisation? Immunol Lett 43(1–2):83–86, 1994
36. Olivar M, Develoux M, Abari AC, Loutan L. Presumptive diagnosis of malaria results in a significant risk of mis-treatment of children in urban Sahel. Trans R Soc Trop Med Hyg 85(6):729–730, 1991
37. English M, Punt J, Mwangi I, et al: Clinical overlap between malaria and severe pneumonia in African children in hospital. Trans R Soc Trop Med Hyg 90:658–662, 1996
38. Redd SC, Bloland PB, Kazembe PN, et al: Usefulness of clinical case-definitions in guiding therapy for African children with malaria or pneumonia. Lancet 340(8828):1140–1143, 1992
39. Smith T, Armstrong Schellenberg JRM, Hayes RJ: Attributable fraction estimates and case definitions for malaria in endemic areas. Stat Med 13:2345–2358, 1994
40. Wardlaw SC, Levine RA: Quantitative buffy coat analysis. A new laboratory tool functioning as a screening complete blood cell count. JAMA 249(5):617–620, 1983
41. Spielman A, Perrone JB, Teklehaimanot A, et al: Malaria diagnosis by direct observation of centrifuged samples of blood. Am J Trop Med Hyg 39(4):337–342, 1988
42. Tharavanij S: New developments in malaria diagnostic techniques. Southeast Asian J Trop Med Public Health 21(1):3–16, 1990
43. Rickman LS, Long GW, Oberst R, et al: Rapid diagnosis of malaria by acridine orange staining of centrifuged parasites. Lancet 1(8629):68–71, 1989
44. Mackey LJ, McGregor IA, Paounova N, Lambert PH: Diagnosis of *Plasmodium falciparum* infection in man: detection of parasite antigens by ELISA. Bull World Health Organ 60(1):69–75, 1982
45. Fortier B, Delplace J, Dubremetz F, et al: Enzyme immunoassay for detection of antigen in acute *Plasmodium falciparum* malaria. Eur J Clin Microbiol 6(5):596–598, 1987
46. Khusmith S, Tharavanij S, Kasemsuth R, et al: Two-site immunoradiometric assay for detection of *Plasmodium falciparum* antigen in blood using monoclonal and polyclonal antibodies. J Clin Microbiol 25(8):1467–1471, 1987
47. Shiff CJ et al: The rapid manual ParaSight™-F. A new diagnostic tool for *Plasmodium falciparum* infection. Trans R Soc Trop Med Hyg 87(6):646–648, 1993
48. Uguen C, Rabodonirina M, De Pina JJ, et al: ParaSight™-F rapid manual diagnostic test of *Plasmodium falciparum* infection. Bull World Health Organ 73(5):643–649, 1995
49. Snounou G, Pinheiro L, Goncalves A, et al: The importance of sensitive detection of malaria parasites in the human and insect hosts in epidemiological studies, as shown by the analysis of field samples from Guinea Bissau. Trans R Soc Trop Med Hyg 87(6):649–53, 1993
50. Viriyakosol S, Siripoon N, Petcharapirat C, et al: Genotyping of *Plasmodium falciparum* isolates by polymerase chain reaction and potential uses in epidemiological studies. Bull World Health Organ 73(1):85–95, 1995
51. White NJ: The treatment of malaria. N Engl J Med 335(11): 800–806, 1996
52. Lobel HO, Miani M, Eng T, et al: Long-term malaria prophylaxis with weekly mefloquine. Lancet 341(8849):848–851, 1993
53. Miller KD, Lobel HO, Satriale RF, et al: Severe cutaneous reactions among American travelers using pyrimethamine-sulfadoxine (Fansidar) for malaria prophylaxis. Am J Trop Med Hyg 35(3):451–458, 1986
54. van Hensbroek MB, Morris-Jones S, Meisner S, et al: Iron, but not folic acid, combined with effective antimalarial therapy promotes haematological recovery in African children after acute falciparum malaria. Trans R Soc Trop Med Hyg 89(6):672–676, 1995
55. Baird JK, Fryauff DJ, Basri H, et al: Primaquine for prophylaxis against malaria among nonimmune transmigrants in Irian Jaya, Indonesia. Am J Trop Med Hyg 52(6):479–484, 1995
56. Mockenhaupt FP: Mefloquine resistance in *Plasmodium falciparum*. Parasitology Today 11(7):248–253, 1995
57. Nosten F, ter Kuile FO, Luxemburger C, et al: Cardiac effects of antimalarial treatment with halofantrine. Lancet 341(8852):1054–1056, 1993
58. Monlun E, Le Metayer P, Szwandt S, et al: Cardiac complications of halofantrine: a prospective study of 20 patients. Trans R Soc Trop Med Hyg 89(4):430–433, 1995
59. ter Kuile FO, Dolan G, Nosten F, et al: Halofantrine versus mefloquine in treatment of multidrug-resistant falciparum malaria. Lancet 341(8860):1044–1049, 1993
60. Wongsrichanalai C, Webster HK, Wimonwattrawatee T, et al: Emergence of multidrug-resistant *Plasmodium falciparum* in Thailand: in vitro tracking. Am J Trop Med Hyg 47(1):112–116, 1992
61. Taylor TE, Wills BA, Kazembe P, et al: Rapid coma resolution with artemether in Malawian children with cerebral malaria. Lancet 341(8846):661–662, 1993
62. Salako LA, Walker O, Sowunmi A, et al: Artemether in moderately severe and cerebral malaria in Nigerian children. Trans R Soc Trop Med Hyg 88(Suppl 1):S13–S15, 1994
63. Nosten F, Luxemburger C, ter Kuile FO, et al: Treatment of multidrug-resistant *Plasmodium falciparum* malaria with 3-day artesunate-mefloquine combination. J Infect Dis 170(4):971–977, 1994
64. Looareesuwan S, Viravan C, Webster HK, et al: Clinical studies of atovaquone, alone or in combination with other antimalarial drugs for the treatment of acute uncomplicated malaria in Thailand. Am J Trop Med Hyg 54(1):62–66, 1996
65. Radloff PD, Phillips J, Nkeyi M, et al: Atovaquone and proguanil for *Plasmodium falciparum* malaria. Lancet 347(9014):1511–1513, 1996
66. Radloff PD, Phillips J, Hutchinson D, Kremsner PG: Atovaquone plus proguanil is an effective treatment for *Plasmodium ovale*, and *P. malariae* malaria. Trans R Soc Trop Med Hyg 90:682, 1996
67. Ringwald P, Bickii J, Basco L: Randomised trial of pyronaride versus chloroquine for acute uncomplicated falciparum malaria in Africa. Lancet 347(8993):24–27, 1996
68. Looareesuwan S, Olliaro P, Kyle D, Wernsdorfer W: Pyronaridine [Letter]. Lancet 347(9009):1189–1190, 1996
69. Bunnag D, Karbwang J, Thanavibul A, et al: High dose of primaquine in primaquine resistant vivax malaria. Trans R Soc Trop Med Hyg 88(2):218–219, 1994
70. Miller KD, Greenberg AE, Campbell CC: Treatment of severe malaria in the United States with a continuous infusion of quinidine gluconate and exchange transfusion. N Engl J Med 321(2):65–70, 1989
71. ter Kuile FO, Luxemberger C, Nosten F, et al: Mefloquine treatment of acute falcipaum malaria: a prospective study of nonserious adverse effects in 3,673 patients. Trans R Soc Trop Med Hyg 73:631–642, 1996
72. World Health Organization: The role of artemisinin and its derivatives in the current treatment of malaria: report of an informal consultation convened by WHO in Geneva, 27–29 September 1993 (WHO/MAL/94.1067). Geneva: World Health Organization, 1994
73. Miller LH, McAuliffe FM, Mason SJ: Erythrocyte receptors for malaria merozoites. Am J Trop Med Hyg 26(6 pt 2):204–208, 1977
74. Canessa A, Mazzarello G, Cruciani M, Bassetti D: Chloroquine-resistant *Plasmodium vivax* in Brazil. Trans R Soc Trop Medi Hyg 86(5):570–571, 1992
75. Garg M, Gopinathan N, Bodhe P, Kshirsagar NA: Vivax malaria resistant to chloroquine: case reports from Bombay. Trans R Soc Trop Med Hyg 89(6):656–657, 1995

76. Bloland PB, Lacritz EM, Kazembe PN, et al: Beyond chloroquine: implications of drug resistance for evaluating malaria therapy efficacy and treatment policy in Africa. J Infect Dis 167(4):932–937, 1993
77. Thaithong S, Suebsaeng L, Rooney W, Beale GH: Evidence of increased chloroquine sensitivity in Thai isolates of *Plasmodium falciparum*. Trans R Soc Trop Med Hyg 82(1):37–38, 1988
78. Bjorkman A, Phillips-Howard PA: The epidemiology of drug-resistant malaria. Trans R Soc Trop Med Hyg 84(3):177–180, 1990
79. Bunnag D, Harinasuta T: Quinine and quinidine in malaria in Thailand. Acta Leidensia 55:163–166, 1987
80. Oaks SC, Mitchell VS, Pearson GW, Carpenter CCJ (eds): Malaria Obstacles and Opportunities. Washington, DC: National Academy Press, 1991
81. Molineaux L: The epidemiology of human malaria as an explanation of its distribution, including some implications for its control. In Wernsdorfer WH, McGregor I (eds): Malaria: Principles and Practice of Malariology. Edinburgh: Churchill Livingstone, 1988, pp 913–998
82. Weatherall DJ: Host genetics and infectious disease. Parasitology 112(Suppl):S23–S29, 1996
83. Hill AVS, Allsopp CEM, Kwiatkowski D, et al: Common west African HLA-antigens are associated with protection from severe malaria. Nature 352(6336):595–600, 1991
84. Flint J, Harding RM, Boyce AJ, Clegg JB: The population genetics of the haemoglobinopathies. Clinics in Haematology 6(1):215–262, 1993
85. Jarolim P, Palek J, Amato D, et al: Deletion in erythrocyte band 3 gene in malaria-resistant Southeast Asian ovalocytosis. Proc Natl Acad Sci USA 88(24):11022–11026, 1991
86. Ruwende C, Khoo SC, Snow RW, et al: Natural selection of hemi- and heterozygotes for G6PD deficiency in Africa by resistance to severe malaria. Nature 376(6537):246–249, 1995
87. Hill AVS: Genetic susceptibility to malaria and other infectious diseases: from the MHC to the whole genome. Parasitology 112 (Suppl):S75–S84, 1996
88. McGuire W, Hill AV, Allsopp CE, et al: Variation in the TNF-alpha promoter region associated with susceptibility to cerebral malaria. Nature 371(6497):508–510, 1994
89. D'Alfonso S, Richiardi PM: A polymorphic variation in a putative regulation box of the TNFA promoter region. Immunogenetics 39(2):150–154, 1994
90. Hendrikse RG, Hasan AH, Olumide LO, Akinkunmi A: Malaria in early childhood. An investigation of five hundred seriously ill children in whom a "clinical" diagnosis of malaria was made on admission to the children's emergency room at University College Hospital, Ibadan. Ann Trop Med Parasitol 65(1):1–20, 1971
91. Snow RW, Byass P, Shenton FC, Greenwood BM: The relationship between anthropometric measurements and measurements of iron status and susceptibility to malaria in Gambian children. Trans R Soc Trop Med Hyg 85(5):584–589, 1991
92. Smith AW, Hendrickse RG, Harrison C, et al: The effects of malaria on treatment of iron-deficiency anaemia with oral iron in Gambian children. Ann Trop Paediatr 9(1):17–23, 1989
93. Murray MJ, Murray AB, Murray MB, Murray CJ: The adverse effect of iron repletion on the course of certain infections. Br Med J 2(6145):1113–1115, 1978
94. Oppenheimer SJ, Gibson FD, Macfarlane SB, et al: Iron supplementation increases prevalence and effects of malaria: report on clinical studies in Papua New Guinea. Trans R Soc Trop Med Hyg 80(4):603–612, 1986
95. Oppenheimer SJ, Macfarlane SB, Moody JB, Harrison C: Total dose iron infusion, malaria and pregnancy in Papua New Guinea. Trans R Soc Trop Med Hyg 80(4):818–822, 1986
96. Menendez C, Todd J, Alonso PL, et al: The effects of iron supplementation during pregnancy, given by traditional birth attendants, on the prevalence of anaemia and malaria. Trans R Soc Trop Med Hyg 88(5):590–593, 1994
97. Gibson RS, Heywood A, Yaman C, et al: Growth in children from the Wosera subdistrict, Papua New Guinea, in relation to energy and protein intakes and zinc status. Am J Clin Nutr 53(3):782–789, 1991
98. Bates CJ, Evans PH, Dardenne M, et al: A trial of zinc supplementation in young rural Gambian children. Br J Nutr 69(1): 243–255, 1993
99. Galan P, Samba C, Luzeau R, Amedee-Manesme O: Vitamin A deficiency in pre-school age Congolese children during malarial attacks. Part 2: impact of parasitic disease on vitamin A status. Int J Vitam Nutr Res 60(3):224–228, 1990
100. Sturchler D, Tanner M, Hanck A, et al: A longitudinal study on relations of retinol with parasitic infections and the immune response in children of Kikwawila village, Tanzania. Acta Trop 44(2): 213–227, 1987
101. Nwanyanwu O, Ziba C, Kazembe P, et al: The effect of oral iron therapy during treatment for Plasmodium falciparum malaria with sulphadoxine-pyrimethamine on Malawian children under 5 years of age. Ann Trop Med Parasitol 90(6):589–595, 1996
102. McGregor IA: Malaria: nutritional implications. Rev Infect Dis 4(4):798–804, 1982
103. Wolday D, Kibreab T, Bukenya D, Hodes R: Sensitivity of *Plasmodium falciparum in vivo* to chloroquine and pyrimethamine-sulfadoxine in Rwandan patients in a refugee camp in Zaire. Trans R Soc Trop Med Hyg 89(6):654–656, 1995
104. Mabey DC, Brown A, Greenwood BM: *Plasmodium falciparum* malaria and *Salmonella* infections in Gambian children. J Infect Dis 155:1319–1321, 1987
105. Brown PJ: Culture and the global resurgence of malaria. In Inhorn MC, Brown PJ (eds): The Anthropology of Infectious Disease. New York: Gordon and Breach, 1997
106. Foster SF: The distribution and use of antimalarial drugs: not a pretty picture. In Targett GAT (ed): Malaria: Waiting for the Vaccine. New York: John Wiley and Sons, 1991
107. Coluzzi M, Petrarca V, Di Deco MA: Chromosomal inversion intergradation and incipient speciation in *Anopheles gambiae*. Bolletino di Zoologia 52:45–63, 1985
108. Laderman C: Malaria and progress: some historical and ecological considerations. Soc Sci Med 9(11–12):587–594, 1975
109. Hyma B, Ramesh A, Chakrapani KP: Urban malaria control situation and environmental issues. Ecology of Disease 2(4)321–335, 1983
110. Chapin G, Wasserstrom R: Pesticide use and malaria resurgence in Central America and India. Soc Sci Med 17(5):273–290, 1983
111. Pan American Health Organization: Regional status of malaria in the Americas, 1994. Epidemiol Bull 16(3):10–14, 1995
112. Verdrager J: Epidemiology of the emergence and spread of drug-resistant falciparum malaria in South-East Asia and Australia. J Trop Med Hyg 89(6):277–289, 1986
113. Thimasarn K, Sirichaisinthop J, Vijaykadga S, et al: In vivo study of *Plasmodium falciparum* to standard mefloquine/sulfadoxine/pyrimethamine (MSP) treatment among gem miners returning from Cambodia. Southeast Asian J Trop Med Public Health 26(2): 204–212, 1995
114. Bruce-Chwatt LJ, de Zulueta J: The Rise and Fall of Malaria in Europe. London: Oxford University Press, 1980
115. Bang YH, Shah NK: Human ecology related to urban mosquito-borne disease in countries of South East Asia region. J Commun Dis 20(1):1–17, 1988
116. World Health Organization. Urban vector and pest control. Eleventh report of the WHO Expert Committee on Vector Biology and Control. WHO Technical Report Series No. 767. Geneva: World Health Organization, 1988
117. Brown PJ: Cultural adaptations to endemic malaria in Sardinia. Med Anthropol 5:313–339, 1981
118. Aikins MK, Pickering H, Greenwood BM: Attitudes to malaria, traditional practices and bednets (mosquito nets) as vector control

measures: a comparative study in five West African countries. J Trop Med Hyg 97(2):81–86, 1994
119. Ramakrishna J, Brieger WR: The value of qualitative research: health education in Nigeria. Health Policy and Planning 2:171–175, 1987
120. Jackson LC: Malaria in Liberian children and mothers: biocultural perceptions of illness vs. clinical evidence of disease. Soc Sci Med 20(12):1281–1287, 1985
121. Kaseje DCO, Sempebwa EKN, Spencer HC: Malaria chemoprophylaxis to pregnant women provided by community health workers in Saradidi, Kenya. I. Reasons for non-acceptance. Ann Trop Med Parasitol 81(Suppl 1):77–82, 1987
122. Helitzer-Allen D: Examination of the Factors Influencing the Utilization of the Antenatal Malaria Chemoprophylaxis Program, Malawi, Central Africa. Doctoral dissertation. Johns Hopkins University School of Hygiene and Public Health, Baltimore, Maryland, 1989
123. Krogstad DJ, Ruebush TK: Community participation in the control of tropical diseases. Acta Trop 61(2):77–78, 1996
124. World Health Organization: WHA8.30 Malaria Eradication, from the Ninth Plenary Meeting, May 26, 1995. WHO Official Records No. 63. Geneva: World Health Organization, 1955, pp. 31–32
125. Brown AWA, Haworth J, Zahar AR: Malaria eradication and control from a global standpoint. J Med Entomol 13(1):1–25, 1976
126. Lepes T: Present status of the Global Malaria Eradication Programme and prospects for the future. J Trop Med Hyg 77(4s):47–53, 1974
127. Farid MA: The Malaria Programme—from euphoria to anarchy. World Health Forum 1:8–33, 1980
128. Molineaux L, Gramicca G: The Garki Project, Research on the Epidemiology and Control of Malaria in the Sudan Savannah of West Africa. Geneva: World Health Organization, 1980
129. World Health Organization Study Group on the Implementation of the Global Plan of Action for Malaria Control: Implementation of the Global Malaria Control Strategy. WHO Technical Report Series no. 839. Geneva: World Health Organization, 1993
130. World Health Organization, Division of Diarrhoeal and Acute Respiratory Disease Control: Integrated management of the sick child. Bull World Health Organ 73(6):735–740, 1995
131. Centers for Disease Control and Prevention: Health Information for International Travel, 1995. HHS Publication No. (CDC) 95-8280. Washington, DC: U.S. Government Printing Office, 1995
132. Zucker JR, Campbell CC: Malaria: principles of prevention and treatment. Infect Dis Clin North Am 7(3):547–567, 1993
133. Steketee RW, Wirima JJ, Slutsker L, et al: The problem of malaria and malaria control in pregnancy in sub-Saharan Africa. Am J Trop Med Hyg 55(1):2–7, 1996
134. Schultz LJ, Steketee RW, Macheso A, et al: The efficacy of antimalarial regimens containing sulfadoxine-pyrimethamine and/or chloroquine in preventing peripheral and placental *Plasmodium falciparum* infection during pregnancy. Am J Trop Med Hyg 51(5):515–522, 1994
135. Choi, HW, Breman JG, Teutsch SM, et al: The effectiveness of insecticide-impregnated bed nets in reducing cases of malaria infection: a meta-analysis of published results. Am J Trop Med Hyg 52(5):377–382, 1995
136. Alonso PL, Lindsay SW, Armstrong Schellenberg JRM, et al: The effect of insecticide-treated bed nets on mortality of Gambian children. Lancet 337(8756):1499–1502, 1991
137. D'Alessandro U, Olaleye BO, McGuire W, et al: Mortality and morbidity from malaria in Gambian children after introduction of an impregnated bednet programme. Lancet 345(8948):479–483, 1995
138. Nevill CG, Some ES, Mung'ala VO, et al: Insecticide-treated bednets reduce mortality and severe morbidity from malaria among children on the Kenyan coast. Trop Med Int Health 1(2):139–146, 1996
139. Binka FN, Kubaje A, Adjuik M, et al: Impact of permethrin impregnated bednets on child mortality in Kassena-Nankana district, Ghana: a randomized controlled trial. Trop Med Int Health 1(2):147–154, 1996
140. Trape JF, Rogier C: Combating malaria morbidity and mortality by reducing transmission. Parasitology Today 12(6):236–240, 1996
141. Service MW: Biological control of mosquitoes—has it a future? Mosquito News 43:113–120, 1983
142. Miller LH, Sakai RK, Roumans P, et al: Stable integration and expression of a bacterial gene in the mosquito *Anopheles gambiae*. Science 237(4816):779–781, 1987
143. Ramasamy MS, Ramasamy R: Effect of host anti-mosquito antibodies on mosquito physiology and mosquito-pathogen interactions. In Borovsky D, Spielman A (eds): Host-Regulated Developmental Mechanisms in Vector Arthropods. Vero Beach: University of Florida, 1989, pp. 142–148
144. Nosten F, Luxemburger C, Kyle DE, et al: Randomised double-blind placebo-controlled trial of SPf66 malaria vaccine in children in northwestern Thailand. Lancet 348(9029):701–707, 1996
145. D'Alessandro U, Leach A, Drakeley CJ, et al: Efficacy trial of malaria vaccine SPf66 in Gambian infants. Lancet 346(8973): 462–467, 1995
146. Tanner M, Lengeler C, Lorenz N: Case studies from the biomedical and health systems research activities of the Swiss Tropical Institute in Africa. Trans R Soc Trop Med Hyg 87(5):518–523, 1993
147. Stoute JA, Slaoui M, Heppner G, et al: A preliminary evaluation of a recombinant circumsporozoite protein vaccine against *Plasmodium falciparum* malaria. N Engl J Med 336:86–91, 1997

Lyme Disease

1. Steere AC, Malawista SE, Hardin JA, et al: Erythema chronicum migrans and Lyme arthritis: the enlarging clinical spectrum. Ann Intern Med 86:685–698, 1977
2. Burgdorfer WA, Barbour AG, Hayes SF, et al: Lyme disease—a tick-borne spirochetosis? Science 216:1317–1319, 1982
3. Johnson RC, Schmid GP, Hyde FW, et al: *Borrelia burgdorferi* sp. nov.: etiologic agent of Lyme disease. Int J Syst Bacteriol 34: 496–497, 1984
4. Rosa PA, Schwan TG: Molecular biology of *Borrelia burgdorferi*. In Coyle PK (ed): Lyme Disease. Chicago: Mosby-Year Book, 1993, pp 8–17
5. Baranton G, Postic D, Saint-Girons I, et al: Delineation of *Borrelia burgdorferi* sensu stricto, *Borrelia garinii* sp. nov., and Group V5461 associated with Lyme borreliosis. Int J Syst Bacteriol 42:378–383, 1991
6. Spielman A, Wilson ML, Levine JF, Piesman J: Ecology of *Ixodes dammini*-borne human babesiosis and Lyme disease. Annu Rev Entomol 30:439–460, 1985
7. Lane RS, Piesman J, Burgdorfer W: Lyme borreliosis: relation of its causative agent to its vectors and hosts in North America and Europe. Annu Rev Entomol 36:587–609, 1991
8. Steere AC: Lyme disease. N Engl J Med 321:586–596, 1989
9. Steere AC, Dwyer E, Winchester R: Association of chronic Lyme arthritis with HLA-DR4 and HLA-DR2 alleles. N Engl J Med 323:219–223, 1990
10. Williams CL, Strobino B, Weinstein A, et al: Maternal Lyme disease and congenital malformations: a cord blood serosurvey in endemic and control areas. Paediatr Perinatal Epidemiol 9:320–330, 1995
11. Krause PJ, Telford SR, Spielman A, et al: Concurrent Lyme disease and babesiosis: evidence for increased severity and duration of illness. JAMA 275:1657–1660, 1996
12. Fishbein DB, Dennis, DT: Tick-borne diseases—a growing risk. N Engl J Med 333:452–453, 1995
13. Walker DH, Barbour AG, Oliver JH, et al: Emerging bacterial zoonotic and vector-borne diseases: ecological and epidemiologic factors. JAMA 275:463–469, 1996

14. Centers for Disease Control and Prevention: Recommendations for test performance and interpretation from the Second National Conference on Serologic Diagnosis of Lyme Disease. MMWR 44: 590–591, 1995
15. Dressler F, Whalen JA, Reinhardt BN, et al: Western immunoblotting in the serodiagnosis of Lyme disease. J Infect Dis 167:392–400, 1993
16. Johnson BJB, Robbins KE, Bailey RE, et al: Serodiagnosis of Lyme disease: accuracy of a two-step approach using a flagella-based ELISA and immunoblotting. J Infect Dis 174:346–353, 1996
17. Maupin GO, Fish D, Zultowsky J, et al: Landscape ecology of Lyme disease in a residential area of Westchester County, New York. Am J Epidemiol 133:1105–1113, 1991
18. Glass GE, Amerisinghe FP, Morgan JM, et al: Predicting *Ixodes scapularis* abundance on white-tailed deer using geographic information systems. Am J Trop Med Hyg 51:538–544, 1994
19. Spielman A: Prospects for suppressing transmission of Lyme disease. Ann NY Acad Sci 539:212–220, 1988
20. Dennis DT: Epidemiology. In Coyle PK (ed): Lyme Disease. Chicago: Mosby-Year Book, 1993, pp 27–37
21. Berglund J, Eitrem R, Ornstein K, Lindberg A, et al: An epidemiologic study of Lyme disease in southern Sweden. N Engl J Med 333:1319–1324, 1995
22. Centers for Disease Control and Prevention: Lyme disease—United States, 1995. MMWR 45:481–484, 1996
23. Meek JI, Roberts CL, Smith EV, Cartter ML: Underreporting of Lyme disease by Connecticut physicians, 1992. J Public Health Manage Pract 2:61–65, 1996
24. Coyle BS, Strickland GT, Liang YY, et al: The public health impact of Lyme disease in Maryland. J Infect Dis 173:1260–1262, 1996
25. White DJ, Chang H-G, Benach JL, et al: The geographic spread and temporal increase of the Lyme disease epidemic. JAMA 266: 1230–1236, 1991
26. Campbell GL, Paul WS, Schriefer ME, et al: Epidemiologic and diagnostic studies of patients with suspected early Lyme disease, Missouri. J Infect Dis 172:470–480, 1995
27. Barbour AG, Maupin GO, Teltow GJ, Carter CJ, Piesman J: An uncultivable *Borrelia* sp in the hard tick, *Amblyomma americanum*: a possible agent of a Lyme disease-like disease. J infect Dis 173: 403–409, 1996
28. Eng TR, Wilson MI, Spielman A, et al: Greater risk of *Borrelia burgdorferi* infection in dogs than people. J Infect Dis 158: 1410–1411, 1988
29. Piesman J, Maupin GO, Campos EG, et al: Duration of adult female *Ixodes dammini* attachment and transmission of *Borrelia burgdorferi*, with description of a needle aspiration isolation method. J Infect Dis 163:895–897, 1991
30. Wormser GP: Prospects for a vaccine to prevent Lyme disease in humans. Clin Infect Dis 21:1267–1274, 1995

Trypanosomiasis

1. Kirchhoff LV: American trypanosomiasis (Chagas' disease)—a tropical disease now in the United States. N Engl J Med 329:639–644, 1993
2. Schmunis GA: *Trypanosoma cruzi*, the etiologic agent of Chagas' disease: status in the blood supply in endemic and nonendemic countries. Transfusion 31:547–557, 1991
3. Freilij H, Altcheh J: Congenital Chagas' disease: diagnostic and clinical aspects. Clin Infect Dis 21:551–555, 1995
4. Herwaldt BL, Juranek DD: Laboratory-acquired malaria, leishmaniasis, trypanosomiasis, and toxoplasmosis. Am J Trop Med Hyg 48:313–323, 1993
5. Ochs DE, Hnilica V, Moser DR, Smith JH, Kirchhoff LV: Postmortem diagnosis of autochthonous acute chagasic myocarditis by polymerase chain reaction amplification of a species-specific DNA sequence of *Trypanosoma cruzi*. Am J Trop Med Hyg 34:526–529, 1996
6. Villanueva MS: Trypanosomiasis of the central nervous system. Semin Neurol 13:209–218, 1993
7. Kirchhoff LV, Neva FA: Chagas' disease in Latin American immigrants. JAMA 254:3058–3060, 1985
8. Hagar JM, Rahimtoola SH: Chagas' heart disease in the United States. N Engl J Med 325:763–768, 1991
9. Kirchhoff LV: American trypanosomiasis (Chagas' disease). Gastroenterol Clin North Am 25:517–533, 1996
10. Cunha-Neto E, Duranti M, Gruber A, et al: Autoimmunity in Chagas disease cardiopathy: biological relevance of a cardiac myosin-specific epitope crossreactive to an immunodominant *Trypanosoma cruzi* antigen. Proc Natl Acad Sci U S A 92:3541–3545, 1995
11. Rocha A, Oliveira de Meneses AC, da Silva AM, et al: Pathology of patients with Chagas' disease and acquired immunodeficiency syndrome. Am J Trop Med Hyg 50:261–268, 1994
12. Kirchhoff LV: Is *Trypanosoma cruzi* a new threat to our blood supply? Ann Intern Med 111:773–775, 1989
13. Kirchhoff LV, Gam AA, Gilliam FC: American trypanosomiasis (Chagas' disease) in Central American immigrants. Am J Med 82:915–920, 1987
14. Leiby DA, Read EJ, Lenes BA, et al: Seroepidemiology of *Trypanosoma cruzi*, etiologic agent of Chagas' disease, in U.S. blood donors. J Infect Dis 176:1047–1052, 1997
15. Chiari E, Dias JCP, Lana M, Chiari CA: Hemocultures for the parasitological diagnosis of human chronic Chagas disease. Rev Soc Bras Med Trop 22:19–23, 1989
16. Kirchhoff LV, Votava JR, Ochs DE, Moser DR: Comparison of PCR and microscopic methods for detecting *Trypanosoma cruzi*. J Clin Microbiol 34:1171–1175, 1996
17. Pan AA, Rosenberg GB, Hurley MK, Schock GJ, Chu VP, Aiyappa A: Clinical evaluation of an EIA for the sensitive and specific detection of serum antibody to *Trypanosoma cruzi* (Chagas' disease). J Infect Dis 165:585–588, 1992
18. Kirchhoff LV, Gam AA, Gusmao RD, Goldsmith RS, Rezende JM, Rassi A: Increased specificity of serodiagnosis of Chagas' disease by detection of antibody to the 72- and 90-kilodalton glycoproteins of *Trypanosoma cruzi*. J Infect Dis 155:561–564, 1987
19. Marr JJ, Docampo R: Chemotherapy for Chagas' disease: a perspective on current therapy and considerations for future research. Rev Infect Dis 8:884–903, 1986
20. Pepin J, Milord F. The treatment of human African-trypanosomiasis. Adv Parasite 33:1–47, 1995

Leishmaniasis

1. Herwaldt BL, Arana BA, Navin TR: The natural history of cutaneous leishmaniasis in Guatemala. J Infect Dis 165:518–527, 1992
2. Vidal SM, Malo D, Vogan K, Skamene E, Gros P: Natural resistance to infection with intracellular parasites: isolation of a candidate for *Bcg*. Cell 73:469–485, 1993
3. Cabello PH, Lima AMVMD, Azevedo ES, Krieger H: Familial aggregation of *Leishmania chagasi* infection in northeastern Brazil. Am J Trop Med Hyg 52:364–365, 1995
4. Pearson RD, Wilson ME: Host defenses against prototypical intracellular protozoans, the *Leishmania*. In Walzer PD, Genta RM (eds): Parasitic Infections in the Compromised Host. New York: Marcel Dekker, 31–81, 1989
5. Pearson RD, Cox G, Jeronimo SMB, Castracane J, Drew JS, Evans T, de Alencar JE: Visceral leishmaniasis: a model for infection-induced cachexia. Am J Trop Med Hyg 47(Suppl):8–15, 1992
6. Magill AJ, Gasser RA, Oster CN, Grogl M: Viscerotropic leishmaniasis in persons returning from Operation Desert Storm—1990–1991. MMWR 41:131–134, 1992
7. Pearson RD, Sousa AD: Clinical spectrum of leishmaniasis. Clin Infect Dis 22:1–13, 1996

8. Alvar J: Leishmaniasis and the AIDS co-infection: the Spanish example. Parasitol Today 10:160–163, 1994
9. Burns JM Jr, Shreffler WG, Benson DR, Ghalib HW, Badaro R, Reed SG: Molecular characterization of a kinesin-related antigen of *Leishmania chagasi* that detects specific antibody in African and American visceral leishmaniasis. Proc Natl Acad Sci USA 90:775–779, 1993
10. Singh S, Gliman-Sachs A, Chang K-P, Reed SG: Diagnostic and prognostic value of k39 recombinant antigen in Indian leishmaniasis. J Parasitol 8:1000–1003, 1995
11. Torre-Cisneros J, Villaneuva JL, Kindelan JM, Jurado R, Sanchez-Guijo P: Successful treatment of antimony-resistant visceral leishmaniasis with liposomal amphotericin B in patients infected with human immunodeficiency virus. Clin Infect Dis 17:625–627, 1993
12. Division of Communicable Disease Prevention and Control, Communicable Disease Program, HPC/HCT, and PAHO: Leishmaniasis in the Americas. Epidemiol Bull 15:8–11, 1994
13. Killick-Kendrick R, Wallbanks KR, Molyneux DH, Lavin DR: The ultrastructure of *Leishmania major* in the foregut and proboscis of *Phlebotomus papatasi*. Parasitol Res 74:586–590, 1988
14. Sacks DL, Perkins PV: Development of infective stage *Leishmania* promastigotes within phlebotomine sand flies. Am J Trop Med Hyg 34:456–459, 1985
15. Walters LL: *Leishmania* differentiation in natural and unnatural sand fly hosts. J Protozool 40:196–206, 1993
16. Ward RD: Vector biology and control. In Chang K-P, Bray RS (eds): Leishmaniasis. New York: Elsevier Science Publishers, 199–212, 1985
17. Walsh JF, Molyneux DH, Birley MH: Deforestation: effects on vector-borne disease. Parasitology 106(Suppl):S55–S75, 1993
18. Pratlong F, Dedet JP, Marty P, Portus M, Deniau M, Dereure J, Abranches P, Reynes J, Martini A, Lefebvre M, Rious JA: *Leishmania*—human immunodeficiency virus coinfection in the Mediterranean basin: isoenzymatic characterization of 100 isolates of the *Leishmania infantum* complex. J Infect Dis 172:323–326, 1995
19. Chang K-P, Bray RS: Leishmaniasis. New York: Elsevier, 1985

Lymphatic Filariasis

1. World Health Organization: Lymphatic filariasis infection and disease: control strategies. Report of a consultative meeting held at Universiti Sains Malaysia, Penang, Malaysia, August 1994
2. Centers for Disease Control: Recommendations of the International Task Force for Disease Eradication. MMWR 42:1–38, 1993
3. Vanamail P, Ramaiah KD, Pani SP, et al: Estimation of the fecund life span of *Wuchereria bancrofti* in an endemic area. Trans R Soc Trop Med Hyg 90:119–121, 1996
4. Laing ABG, Edeson JFB, Wharton RH: Studies on filariasis in Malaya: the vertebrate hosts of *Brugia malayi* and *Brugia pahangi*. Ann Trop Med Parasitol 54:92–99, 1960
5. Raccurt CP, Lowrie RC Jr, Katz SP, et al: Epidemiology of *Wuchereria bancrofti* in Leogane, Haiti. Trans R Soc Trop Med Hyg 82:721–725, 1988
6. Sasa, M.: Human Filariasis. Baltimore: University Park Press, 1–819, 1976
7. Pani SP, Yuvaraj J, Vanamail P, et al: Episodic adenolymphangitis and lymphoedema in patients with bancroftian filariasis. Trans R Soc Trop Med Hyg 89:72–74, 1995
8. Weller PF, Ottesen EA, Heck L, et al: Endemic filariasis on a Pacific island. I. Clinical, epidemiologic, and parasitologic aspects. Am J Trop Med Hyg 31:942–952, 1982
9. Freedman DO, Filho PH, Besh S, et al: Abnormal lymphatic function in presymptomatic bancroftian filariasis. J Infect Dis 171:997–1001, 1995
10. Dreyer G, Ottesen EA, Galdino E, et al: Renal abnormalities in microfilaremic patients with bancroftian filariasis. Am J Trop Med Hyg 46:745–751, 1992
11. Wartman WB: Filariasis in American armed forces in World War II. Medicine 26:333–394, 1947
12. Turner LH: Studies on filariasis in Malaya: the clinical features of filariasis due to *Wuchereria malayi*. Trans R Soc Trop Med Hyg 53:154–169, 1959
13. Neva FA, Ottesen EA: Tropical (filarial) eosinophilia. N Engl J Med 298:1129–1131, 1978
14. Rom WN, Vijayan VK, Cornelius MJ, et al: Persistent lower respiratory tract inflammation associated with interstitial lung disease in patients with tropical pulmonary eosinophilia following conventional treatment with diethylcarbamazine. Am Rev Respir Dis 142:1088–1092, 1990
15. Weil GJ, Jain DC, Santhanam S, et al: A monoclonal antibody-based enzyme immunoassay for detecting parasite antigenemia in bancroftian filariasis. J Infect Dis 156:350–355, 1987
16. Chanteau S, Moulia-Pelat JP, Glaziou P, et al: Og4C3 circulating antigen: a marker of infection and adult worm burden in *Wuchereria bancrofti* filariasis. J Infect Dis 170:247–250, 1994
17. McCarthy JS, Zhong M, Gopinath R, et al: Evaluation of a polymerase chain reaction-based assay for diagnosis of *Wuchereria bancrofti* infection. J Infect Dis 173:1510–1514, 1996
18. Lizotte MR, Supali T, Partono F, et al: A polymerase chain reaction assay for the detection of *Brugia malayi* in blood. Am J Trop Med Hyg 51:314–321, 1994
19. Ambroise-Thomas P: Immunological diagnosis of human filariases: present possibilities, difficulties and limitations. Acta Trop 31:108–128, 1974
20. Ottesen EA, Weller PF, Lunde MN, et al: Endemic filariasis on a Pacific island. II. Immunologic aspects: immunoglobulin, complement, and specific antifilarial IgG, IgM and IgE antibodies. Am J Trop Med Hyg 31:953–961, 1983
21. Dreyer G, Addiss D, Noroes J, et al: Ultrasonographic assessment of the adulticidal efficacy of repeat high-dose ivermectin in bancroftian filariasis. Trop Med Int Health 1:427–432, 1996
22. Drugs for parasitic infections. Med Lett Drugs Ther 37:99–108, 1995
23. Carme B, Boulesteix J, Boutes H, et al: Five cases of encephalitis during treatment of loiasis with diethylcarbamazine. Am J Trop Med Hyg 44:684–690, 1991
24. Ottesen EA: Description, mechanisms and control of reactions to treatment in the human filariases. Ciba Found Symp 127:265–283, 1987
25. Eberhard ML, Lammie PJ, Dickinson CM, et al: Evidence of nonsusceptibility to diethylcarbamazine in *Wuchereria bancrofti*. J Infect Dis 163:1157–1160, 1991
26. Ducorps M, Gardon Wendel N, Ranque S, et al: [Secondary effects of the treatment of hypermicrofilaremic loiasis using ivermectin]. Bull Soc Pathol Exot 88:105–112, 1995
27. Ottesen EA: Efficacy of diethylcarbamazine in eradicating infection with lymphatic-dwelling filariae in humans. Rev Infect Dis 7:341–356, 1985
28. Moulia-Pelat Y, Glaziou P, Nguyen LN, et al: Ivermectin 400 mg/kg: long-term suppression of microfilariae in bancroftian filariasis. Trans R Soc Trop Med Hyg 88:107–109, 1994
29. Jamal S: Lymphovenous anastomosis in filarial lymphedema. Lymphology 14:64–68, 1981
30. Casley-Smith JR, Wang CT, Casley-Smith JR, et al: Treatment of filarial lymphoedema and elephantiasis with 5,6-benzo-a-pyrone (coumarin). Br Med J 307:1037–1041, 1993
31. Reddy GS, Venkateswaralu N: Mass administration of DEC-medicated salt for filariasis control in the endemic population of Karaikal, south India: implementation and impact assessment. Bull World Health Organ 74:85–90, 1996
32. Moulia-Pelat JP, Glaziou P, Weil GJ, et al: Combination ivermectin plus diethylcarbamazine, a new effective tool for control of lymphatic filariasis. Trop Med Parasitol 46:9–12, 1995
33. Arata AA: Difficulties facing vector control in the 1990s. Am J Trop Med Hyg 50 (Suppl 6):6–10, 1994
34. Regis L, Silva-Filha MH, de Oliveira CM, et al: Integrated control measures against *Culex quinquefasciatus*, the vector of filariasis in Recife. Mem Inst Oswaldo Cruz 90:115–119, 1995

35. Panicker KN, Jayasree M, Krishnamoorthy KA: A cost benefit analysis of fish culture strategy towards the control of Mansonioides in Shertallai, Kerala state. Indian J Med Res 95:157–160, 1992
36. Maxwell CA, Curtis CF, Haji H, et al: Control of bancroftian filariasis by integrating therapy with vector control using polystyrene beads in wet pit latrines. Trans R Soc Trop Med Hyg 84:709–714, 1990
37. Ault SK: Environmental management: a re-emerging vector control strategy. Am J Trop Med Hyg 50(Suppl 6):35–49, 1994
38. Ramaiah KD, Kumar KN, Ramu K: Knowledge and beliefs about transmission, prevention and control of lymphatic filariasis in rural areas of south India. Trop Med Int Health 1:433–438, 1996
39. Eberhard ML, Walker EM, Addiss DG, et al: A survey of knowledge attitudes and perceptions (KAPs) of lymphatic filariasis, elephantiasis and hydrocele among residents in an endemic area in Haiti. Am J Trop Med Hyg 54:299–303, 1996
40. Harb M, Faris R, Gad AM, et al: The resurgence of lymphatic filariasis in the Nile Delta. Bull World Health Organ 71:49–54, 1993

14

Diseases Transmitted Primarily from Animals to Humans (Zoonoses)

Viruses

Rabies

Denny G. Constantine

Rabies, an acute viral infection of the central nervous system, is known to have occurred in animals and humans since ancient times. The major reservoir of rabies is wildlife, but in much of the world it is a public health hazard because of its endemicity in dogs. Humans are only incidental hosts. The etiologic agent is a bullet-shaped virus that belongs to the Rhabdoviridae, a family that includes over 100 viruses of vertebrates, invertebrates, and plants. Rabies has a worldwide distribution and exists enzootically on every continent except Australia. Many islands or peninsular countries, such as Hawaii, New Zealand, and Cyprus, have never experienced rabies or they have eliminated the infection and remain free of it through the application of rigid control and quarantine measures, as in Japan, Norway, Sweden, the United Kingdom, and Iceland.

Occurrence

The incidence of human rabies in the countries of western Europe, Canada, and the United States has been reduced to none to several cases per year but is much higher in other parts of the world. Each year, about 50,000 persons and millions of animals are said to die of rabies worldwide, and some 3.7 million people take rabies prophylaxis.[1] The diagnosis and reporting of human and animal rabies in developing countries of Asia, Africa, and South America is grossly deficient, and information on the incidence of the disease in these areas is not reliable. Other diseases may cause greater mortality or morbidity, but the impact of rabies remains very significant in most parts of the world, causing great discomfort, sometimes serious side effects, and incalculable anxiety in the individuals and families concerned. The number of persons treated for potential rabies exposure each year in the United States is probably much higher than the 20,000 persons estimated, because this estimation is based on a study of treatment in 21 states, where strict consultation likely reduced the numbers of persons treated to one-fifth (or fewer) of the numbers treated in other states.[2]

Epidemiologic Patterns and Distribution

Rabies in nature exists in two epidemiologic forms: (*a*) the urban type in dogs, and (*b*) wildlife rabies, principally in wild Canidae (jackals, wolves, coyotes, foxes), Viverridae (mongoose, civet cat, meerkat), Mustelidae (weasel, polecat, skunk), Procyonidae (raccoon), and Chiroptera (bats). Urban (canine) rabies is the more noticeable epidemiologic pattern in most parts of the world and usually constitutes the main source of human infections. The true character or extent of the wildlife reservoir in many counties remains unexamined, however.

Fox rabies is a serious problem in North America and has resulted in widespread and current epizootics in Europe since at least 1803. In Africa and Asia, the jackal is a prominent source of virus for other species, and in western Asia, the wolf has long been known as a dangerous source of the virus. The mongoose is an important transmitter of rabies in certain Caribbean islands, India, and South Africa. In Central and South America, the vampire bat is a principal vector of rabies for both humans and domesticated animals and is estimated to cause losses in cattle exceeding $40 million annually. In Canada, where canine rabies was the primary problem from 1920 to 1950, a shift to wildlife rabies, primarily in skunks and foxes, was reported following widespread disease in foxes in Arctic areas.

In the United States, there is a complex epidemiologic pattern of disease, with widespread terrestrial animal rabies (skunk, fox, raccoon) overlaid by the disease in insectivorous bats. A shift in the distribution of rabies cases, by species, has been reported in the United States dur-

TABLE 14-1. REPORTED RABIES CASES IN THE UNITED STATES (1946–1994)

Year	Dogs	Cats	Farm Animals	Foxes	Skunks	Bats	Raccoons	Other Animals	Humans	Total
1946	8,384	455	1,055	—	—	—	—	956	33	10,883
1954	4,083	462	1,032	1,028	547	4	—	118	8	7,282
1962	565	232	614	594	1,449	157	62	52	2	3,727
1970	185	135	399	771	1,235	296	181	71	3[a]	3,276
1978	119	96	254	148	1,657	567	404	49	4	3,298
1986	95	166	255	207	2,379	788	1,576	85	0	3,551
1994	153	267	170	535	1,450	631	4,780	238	6	8,230

[a] One patient recovered.

ing the last 50 years (Table 14-1), but the early lack of surveillance in certain animals, such as bats, may have distorted this recorded pattern. In recent years, skunk rabies constituted over half of all wildlife rabies reports. However, there has been a marked increase in raccoon rabies cases in the eastern portion of the United States since 1982. The decrease in dog and cat cases is a true diminution of the disease in these species and is related to widespread canine immunization and the application of rabies control measures. Cat cases are generally sporadic and peripheral to cycles in dogs and wild carnivores. Although the actual number of reports of rabies-positive bats has increased markedly since the disease was first described in this species in 1953, the proportion of those found to have the disease in comparison to the total number of submitted specimens apparently has not changed. Thus, no real increase in bat disease has occurred. On rare occasions, a rodent has been found infected with rabies virus, but no rodent species has been implicated as a source of the virus for other mammals.

Associated with the decrease of rabies seen in the dog and cat are a marked decrease of the disease in humans and a shift in the species responsible for causing human disease. There were 41 cases of human rabies in the United States between 1976 and 1995. Fourteen, evidently all of dog origin, were imported. Of the remaining 27 indigenous cases, 22 were associated with bats (nine by histories and 13, including a corneal transplant and its donor, by viral strain characterization), three with dogs, one with a skunk, and one (nonfatal but resulting in severe sequelae) with an experimental vaccine being prepared in baits for distribution in nature for immunization of wildlife. Animal rabies in the United States and its territories in 1994 was widespread except in Hawaii, Guam, and the Virgin Islands. The relative importance of different animal species (i.e., fox, skunk, raccoon, and bat) varies according to area, but since 1976, close to 92 percent of all reported animal rabies in the United States has been in wildlife species.[3]

Transmission

Typical rabies virus may be present in saliva 7 days before the onset of symptoms in dogs and for longer intervals in wildlife. Skunks may secrete virus 8 days and bats 12 days before the development of symptoms. The bite route is the main rabies transmission mechanism among animals and from animals to humans, but nonbite routes have been documented. Respiratory transmission of rabies virus was implicated in the deaths of two men who had been working in a bat cave that contained millions of bats.[4] Two laboratory workers contracted rabies, apparently as a consequence of accidentally inhaling aerosolized virus during experimental procedures. Both oral and respiratory transmission routes have been demonstrated experimentally in animals. Whether such nonbite routes play an important role in maintaining the virus in nature is speculative.[5]

The Disease in Animals

Rabies has a prolonged and highly variable incubation period and is remarkable in the variety of symptoms it may evoke in any species of animal. A dog bitten by a rabid animal may develop rabies within 9 days, or it may show no symptoms for 8½ months or longer. The incubation period usually ranges from 20 to 60 days.

The dog manifests symptoms in either or both of two forms: (*a*) furious rabies and (*b*) dumb or paralytic rabies. The form the disease assumes may depend on the dose of the virus, the strain of virus, the resistance of the animal, and the sequence of nerve cells involved as the virus invades the brain and central nervous system. Furious rabies is frequent and is more likely to lead to infection of other animals or humans. During the early stages, the dog may appear more affectionate than usual but is easily irritated and, if picked up, may bite. It exhibits restlessness and a tendency to snap at anything that comes its way.

In dumb rabies, the animal is not observed to be irritable and usually hides and becomes somnolent. Paralysis of the jaw is followed rapidly by general paralysis, and death occurs 1 to 3 days after onset. Dogs with this form of disease present much less of a hazard, but exposure may result from attempting to look in the animal's throat or to administer medication.

Rabid cats may hide and may viciously attack anyone who comes near. The cat's voice becomes hoarse and is soon lost as paralysis sets in. Prostration and death follow in a few days. Most other animals show similar syndromes, with the furious and aggressive behavior slowly giving way to gradually developing incoordination and paralysis.

The disease in bats, including vampire bats, is nearly always paralytic. In the United States, colonial bats, such as the free-tailed bat, show the paralytic form, whereas some noncolonial bat species rarely show furious signs before becoming paralytic. Most human bites result from handling sick or paralyzed bats.

The signs of rabies may resemble those of other infectious diseases or toxic syndromes that affect the central nervous system, and clinical diagnosis is uncertain. Laboratory tests must be performed to be certain of the diagnosis. There is increasing evidence that rabies in animals may not necessarily have a fatal outcome. Live skunks, foxes, and raccoons have been found with serologic evidence of past infection, and clinical rabies has been described in the vampire bat, followed by recovery.[5] Serologic studies in the gregarious free-tailed bats have shown that 15 to 80 percent have evidence of serum antibody but are free of the virus. Abortive clinical rabies has been demonstrated in laboratory animals and has been followed by recovery.[6]

The Disease in Humans

The virus, after inoculation into a wound, travels along the nerves from the peripheral site of inoculation to the central nervous system. The incubation period in humans is highly variable and is determined in part by the location of the bite and the distance the virus must travel to the brain. The incubation period is usually rather short after facial bites and longer after bites on the extremities. The typical incubation period is about 6 weeks, but extremes of 10 days to 15 months and longer have been recorded. In animals and presumably in humans, the incubation period is also influenced by the viral strain, the dose, and the type of tissue exposed.[7]

The disease in humans usually runs its course within 1 week. The term "hydrophobia" derives from the fact that swallowing is difficult and produces painful contraction of the muscles of deglutition, leading to a reflex contraction at the sight of liquids and an aversion to them. There are alternate periods of excitability (sometimes reaching the point of mania) and quiet. Paralytic manifestations are usually late and may not appear. Prolonged survival of up to 133 days has been reported after the use of intensive respiratory care to prevent hypoxia.[8] Four cases are on record of recovery from probable clinical rabies, but only two patients recovered completely.

Diagnosis

The diagnosis of rabies is based on the consideration of as many factors as are available, including the history of exposure, clinical symptoms, and course. If a seemingly healthy dog or cat has bitten someone, it should be held under veterinary supervision for at least 10 days unless clinical symptoms of rabies develop, at which time it may be killed and its brain examined. Ordinarily, symptomatic rabid dogs or cats succumb within 7 days. However, wild rabid animals may live for 18 days or longer after the appearance of disease signs, so wild animals that have bitten humans should be destroyed immediately and tested as quickly as possible.

There should be no delay in submitting the head for diagnosis. Following decapitation, the head should be placed in a water-tight container for shipping. Alternatively, the brain may be removed with aseptic precautions and either quick-frozen in dry ice or preserved in 50 percent glycerol saline. The laboratory diagnosis of rabies may consist of one or more of several types of examinations.

The fluorescent rabies antibody (FRA) test is the test of choice in the United States and many other countries. The test is highly specific and requires only a few hours to perform. It is based on the identification of rabies antigen in a slide of brain or salivary gland tissue by direct staining so as to visualize the antigen-antibody reaction. The FRA test on a corneal smear taken from a living patient is sometimes positive and thus may be useful to confirm a diagnosis of rabies. The demonstration of Negri bodies in brain neurons is a method decreasingly used throughout the world, because the inclusions are not always present or may be atypical or confused with other inclusions.

The mouse inoculation test can take 7 to 14 days or more before results are apparent. The virus can be identified by a positive FRA test or a positive serum virus neutralization test. In comparative trials, the mouse inoculation test and the FRA test proved equally sensitive as diagnostic procedures. Antibody level in blood serum can be determined by serum virus neutralization tests performed either by a mouse inoculation technique or by the rapid fluorescent focus inhibition test (RFFIT), which can measure antibody levels in 24 hours. Because it can be done quickly, the latter is the test of choice for antibody, but its performance requires a well-equipped laboratory and well-trained technicians. A greater than 4-fold rise in titer in the serum neutralization (RFFIT), complement fixation (CF), or indirect FRA tests in patients who have not received rabies vaccine is considered diagnostic of rabies.

Rabies viral strains have been considered similar antigenically, with only minor differences being demonstrable. Recently, certain rabies-related viruses, discovered in African shrews and bats and in bats of mainland Europe, England, and Australia, have been observed to produce rabies-like diseases in humans, dogs, and cats. These viruses may be mistaken for rabies or missed altogether in FRA tests. Rabies vaccines and globulins provide little, if any, protection, and no specific biological agents are available for immunization against these rabies-like viruses.[9]

Postexposure Treatment

Postexposure and preexposure recommendations are derived primarily from the 1991 rabies prevention report of the Advisory Committee on Immunization Practices (ACIP) of the U.S. Department of Health and Human Services,[10] which should be consulted for further details. Prompt and adequate treatment of all skin wounds possibly contaminated with rabies virus is of paramount importance. Local treatment of animal bites and scratches should include thorough cleansing with a 20 percent soap solution or a detergent and flushing of the wound. Although cauterization with nitric acid in puncture wounds has its advocates, there is no available evidence that this procedure is more effective than soap solutions. The wound should not be sutured immediately if this can be avoided. Use of antibiotics and tetanus prophylaxis may be indicated.

Prophylactic Immunization

Pasteur developed a method of postexposure rabies prophylaxis using desiccated nerve tissue in 1883. Agents such as phenol (the basis of Semple vaccine), formalin, and ultraviolet light have been reported to inactivate the virus in brain or spinal cord tissue while allowing it to retain its antigenicity.

Allergic reactions may occur after the administration of vaccine made from such nerve tissue. Much more serious are the occasional neurologic complications—encephalitis, peripheral neuritis, and various paralytic phenomena—that have been attributed to sensitization to brain tissue. These occur more often in persons who have previously received rabies vaccine. The frequency of paralysis during and after administration of a course of Semple vaccine containing nervous tissue has varied considerably in different countries. Some estimates of incidence have ranged between 1:600 and 1:6,000 individuals immunized. Despite these reactions, the Semple vaccine continues to be widely used in many countries. A suckling mouse brain vaccine is used widely in South America. In the United States, a duck embryo vaccine (DEV) was in routine use from 1957 until about 1980–1981. This vaccine was used in a manner similar to the Semple vaccine (14 to 21 doses at daily intervals).

A human diploid cell rabies vaccine (HDCV) became available in the late 1970s; another vaccine, rabies vaccine absorbed (RVA), grown on rhesus diploid cells, became available in 1988. Either vaccine produces a more rapid, high and greater conversion rate of antibody titer than previous vaccines. Moreover, reactions to vaccination are less common and less serious. HDCV has been studied extensively, because it has been available longer and has seen widespread use. Local reactions to HDCV such as pain, erythema, and swelling or itching at the injection site are reported in 30 to 74 percent of recipients. Systemic reactions such as headache, nausea, abdominal pain, muscle aches, and dizziness are reported in 5 to 40 percent of recipients. Three cases of Guillain-Barré syndrome that resolved without sequelae in 12 weeks were reported. A few other subacute central and peripheral nervous system disorders were temporarily associated with HDCV, but no causal relationship was established. Hypersensitivity reactions characterized by general urticaria and sometimes arthralgia, arthritis, angioedema, nausea, vomiting, fever, and malaise were seen in 6 of 98 patients from minutes to 21 days following a booster, but hospitalization was not indicated. The implicated antigen was a β-propiolactone-human serum albumin complex formed during preparation of the vaccine.[11] No reaction has been regarded as life threatening.

The recommended postexposure regimen for either HDCV or RVA is five 1-mL doses, the first dose given as soon as possible and each succeeding dose on days 3, 7, 14, and 28. Each dose is to be given intramuscularly in the deltoid region (or on the anterolateral upper thigh in infants). The gluteal area should never be used.

Use of Rabies Immune Globulin

Rabies immune globulin (RIG) of human origin should be given to all persons bitten by animals in whom rabies cannot be excluded and for nonbite exposures to animals suspected or proved to be rabid. The only exceptions to this recommendation are those persons who have received preexposure rabies immunization. RIG should be given as soon as possible after exposure and should be used regardless of the interval between exposure and the onset of treatment. If RIG was not given when rabies vaccine was started, however, these globulins can be given up to the eighth day after the first vaccine dose was given. Up to half the dose may be given intramuscularly and the rest thoroughly infiltrated around the wound. The first dose of vaccine should be given at the same time at a separate site.

TABLE 14-2. RABIES POSTEXPOSURE PROPHYLAXIS GUIDE, UNITED STATES

Animal Type	*Evaluation and Disposition of Animal*	*Postexposure Prophylaxis Recommendations*
Dogs and cats	Healthy and available for 10 days' observation	Should not begin prophylaxis unless animal develops symptoms of rabies[a]
	Rabid or suspected rabid	Immediate vaccination
	Unknown (escaped)	Consult public health officials
Skunks, raccoons, bats, foxes, and most other carnivores; woodchucks	Regarded as rabid unless geographic area is known to be free of rabies or until animal proven negative by laboratory tests[b]	
Livestock, rodents, and lagomorphs (rabbits and hares)	Consider individually	Consult public health officials. Bites of squirrels, hamsters, guinea pigs, gerbils, chipmunks, rats, mice, other rodents, rabbits, and hares almost never require antirabies treatment

From Centers for Disease Control: Rabies prevention—United States, 1991: recommendations of the Immunization Practices Advisory Committee (ACIP). MMWR (RR-3), 1991.

[a] During the 10-day holding period, begin treatment with RIG and HDCV or RVA at first sign of rabies in a dog or cat that has bitten someone. The symptomatic animal should be killed immediately and tested.

[b] The animal should be killed and tested as soon as possible. Holding for observation is not recommended. Discontinue vaccine if immunofluorescence test results of the animal are negative.

Note: The recommendations in this table are only a guide. They should be applied in conjunction with knowledge of the animal species involved, circumstances of the bite or other exposure, immunization status of the animal, and presence of rabies in the region. Local or state public health officials should be consulted if questions arise about the need for rabies prophylaxis.

General Guide to Postexposure Treatment

The ACIP has published a guide[10] for specific postexposure treatment (Table 14-2). These recommendations are subject to modification depending on the circumstances of the bite, the species of animal involved, the type of exposure, and the prevalence of rabies in the biting species. Knowledge of the last condition requires adequate surveillance.

Preexposure Immunization

For persons with special risks of exposure to rabies, such as veterinarians, laboratory staff working with rabies virus, dog handlers, field naturalists, or those living or working in parts of the world where rabies is a constant threat, it is desirable to provide active immunization in advance of possible exposure. For this purpose, three doses of either HDCV or RVA are recommended on days 0, 7, and 21 or 28. Because the antibody response following the recommended preexposure regimen has been so satisfactory, routine postimmunization serologic study is not generally recommended unless the person is continuously exposed or immunosuppressed (e.g., due to illness or administration of corticosteroids). It needs to be pointed out that preexposure immunization does not eliminate the need for postexposure prophylaxis after an exposure; it only reduces the postexposure regimen. Periodic (every 6 months to 2 years, depending on the degree of risk) antibody testing should be scheduled for those who remain at continued risk of exposure to rabies. A booster dose of vaccine is recommended if the titer falls below 1:5.

Because HDCV is a very expensive vaccine, the intradermal deltoid area route of administration using 0.1 mL per dose of HDCV has been explored and approved for preexposure immunization. Results generally have been good, but the mean antibody response is somewhat lower and may be of shorter duration than with the 1.0-mL dose given intramuscularly. Poor antibody titers resulted when the technique was used on subjects during antimalarial chemoprophylaxis with chloroquine and similar drugs.[11,12] RVA should not be given by the intradermal dose/route.

Animal Vaccines

Vaccines for dogs and cats contain either inactivated virus or modified live virus. Some of these vaccines must be administered annually, whereas the other vaccines, which produce an immunity lasting at least 3 years, are generally vaccines of choice.

A compendium for animal rabies vaccines and recommendations for immunization procedures has been developed and is available through the National Association of State Public Health Veterinarians. This compendium reviews all the licensed animal rabies vaccines and provides information on dosage, species, age at immunization, and reimmunization schedules. For many species, specific contraindications concerning particular vaccines exist, so caution should be used in selecting vaccines for animal use. Although it is uncommon, certain live-virus rabies vaccines have been known to cause rabies in some species, especially wildlife species; these vaccines are no longer available in the United States.

Control

It has been demonstrated in many parts of the world that rabies can be controlled, even eradicated, in limited geographic areas by quarantine measures applied to the dog population, provided wild animals are not involved in the propagation of the disease. Where rabies has become established in wildlife, control depends basically on measures that are directly or indirectly effective in reducing stray dogs below the critical number required to maintain continuous propagation of the virus by serial biting. By the enforcement of ordinances designed to accomplish this reduction, rabies frequently has been temporarily eliminated from urban and suburban communities in the United States.

The prophylactic immunization of dogs is one of the most important methods for rabies control. Where the disease is enzootic in wildlife, routine immunization of both dogs and cats should be practiced. Although it is effective where it is used, such immunization does not reach stray dogs or feral cats, however. Therefore, it is essential to maintain other measures of dog control, designed to "prevent any dog from biting another for a period of the longest latency of the disease."[7] Licensure of dogs and collection of all stray, ownerless, or unwanted dogs should be carried out routinely. Where there is any threat of canine rabies, all dogs in urban areas should be restrained on a leash or kept on the owner's premises. Restraint of cats is indicated as well. Cats bring home the majority of bats that bite or are handled by people. Animal bites should be reported to an official agency, and if rabies is present in a community, any dog or cat biting a person must be confined and observed for signs of rabies. Biting wildlife should be killed and tested without delay.

A permanent solution to the enzootic rabies problem in humans and animals would require the control and eventual elimination of the disease in wildlife. Rabies control in wildlife is exceedingly difficult or impossible, however, depending on the host species. The only proved if temporary method for carnivores is population reduction. This is highly controversial, meeting great resistance from ecologists and conservationists.

Except for vampires, bats should not be killed or molested, since this will likely increase exposures as people and animals handle the fallen animals. House bat colonies do not experience rabies outbreaks. Generally only 0.1 percent are infected, and the infected bat does not bite unless handled. Unwanted colonies should be excluded from buildings after summer, when young bats can fly, by permitting them to leave through check-valve systems, which prevent reentry, followed by sealing the opening.[13] Massive reduction of carnivores (skunks, foxes, coyotes, bobcats) in North America and vampire bats in Latin America has effectively reduced the immediate threat to the local animal or human population. The programs are expensive, however, and unless they are intensively carried out to the extent of at least 80 percent reduction of the target species over a wide area, the effects are short-lived.

For maximum effectiveness, reduction programs should be undertaken only by professional predator-control specialists. The choice of techniques depends on local conditions and may include poisoning or gassing or the more expensive methods of trapping and shooting. In areas where human or domestic animal populations are heavily concentrated, poisoning must be used with great care. Other methods under study include interrupting the reproductive cycles of wild carnivores and the immunization of wildlife populations. The former has been unsuccessful to date, and the latter is undeveloped or controversial. Compared to the cost of trapping and killing predators, immunizing the trapped animals with an inactivated vaccine and releasing them would be more productive in rabies control. The procedure requires a yet-undevised trap, however, that will capture the more wary carnivores without injury. Immunization of foxes (but not other species) by feeding them baits that contain large doses of live attenuated rabies vaccine virus has been used as one method of rabies control in Europe, where foxes constitute the predominant wildlife species. Subsequent declines in cases usually credited to immunization are not readily differentiated from declines in cases that occur due to the population-decimating effect of rabies-outbreak mortality. Native rodents and some nontarget carnivores can develop the infection after consuming these vaccine strains, and they can spread at least one of the strains among themselves. A cat was similarly infected during a field trial. Recombinant oral vaccines show promise of effectiveness in skunks and raccoons, but vaccine efficacy trials in target and nontarget species and extremely extensive safety testing, including the potentially dangerous effects of vaccine virus crossing with other agents, should precede field use.

Until these problems can be resolved, the control of wildlife rabies will continue to be an immense problem and challenge in most areas, and the occasional human case of rabies from this vast reservoir will also continue to occur.

Bacteria

Psittacosis

Julius Schachter

Psittacosis is a zoonosis first described approximately 100 years ago. The causative agent is an obligatory intracellular bacterium, *Chlamydia psittaci*. Virtually all avian species may be naturally infected with *C. psittaci*. When these agents infect humans or psittacine species, the resulting diseases are called psittacosis. Similar infections in other birds are called ornithosis. In infected birds, the infection is mainly in the gastrointestinal tract, with a secondary respiratory involvement. The agent is shed in feces or respiratory secretions and ususally is transmitted to humans in an aerosolized form.

Clinical Description

Human psittacosis usually is described as a severe febrile pneumonitis. It is commonly associated with severe headache, and there often is a pulse rate much lower than would be predicted in patients with high fever. The x-rays show extensive pneumonic involvement even in the absence of severe respiratory symptoms. Although a cough is common, its is dry, hacking, and nonproductive. In addition to the respiratory syndrome, a form of psittacosis without marked respiratory involvement is recognized, in which patients are febrile and appear toxic, often having a severe headache. Hepatosplenomegaly may occur in either form of the disease. Complications, such as hepatitis, myocarditis, endocarditis, and meningitis, are known. Milder flulike disease and asymptomatic infections also occur.

Human psittacosis may be diagnosed by demonstrating rising titers of complement-fixing or fluorescent antibodies to chlamydial antigens in paired acute convalescent sera. Isolation of chlamydiae is feasible, but it is best left to specialized laboratories because of the danger of laboratory infection. Chlamydial infection in birds may be demonstrated by finding characteristic intracytoplasmic inclusions in smears from involved organs.

Public Health Significance

Human psittacosis is relatively uncommon. In recent years, less than 100 cases have been reported in the United States. Because correct diagnosis requires a high index of suspicion by the physician and specialized laboratory tests, it is likely that the true incidence is considerably higher.

Psittacosis is a common occupational hazard to workers in the pet bird industry and in turkey-processing plants. The major threat for mass outbreaks is an industrial one. Sporadic cases commonly are associated with ownership of pet birds. Often, smuggled birds are implicated. Psittacosis occurs worldwide, but reliable data on distribution are not available.

Control and Treatment

As a public health measure, all imported psittacine species are required to undergo a quarantine period, during which they receive a chemoprophylactic regimen of chlortetracycline in their feed for 30 days. Since the efficacy of this program is not monitored, it has been found that infected birds often escape adequate treatment and are released into commerce. Specific methods of treating birds according to the feeding habits of different species have been developed and have been shown to be efficacious both in artificially infected birds and in treatment centers where adequate intake of the chlortetracycline has been documented.

Mass treatment of infected turkey flocks by incorporation of tetracyclines in their feed has been shown to suppress the infection.

For treatment of human psittacosis, tetracycline is considered the drug of choice, and the recommended regimen is 250 mg four times daily for 21 days. Short-term treatment is not indicated and may result in relapse. Response to treatment often is not dramatic, and there may be a prolonged convalescent period. The infection does not confer immunity.

Tularemia

David T. Dennis

Tularemia is an uncommon but potentially severe and fatal bacterial zoonosis caused by the Gram-negative coccobacillus *Francisella tularensis*. The natural cycle of the organism involves amplification in mammalian and tick reservoir hosts. Transmission occurs by several modes, including bites by infective arthropods, direct mucocutaneous contact with or ingestion of contaminated materials, and inhalation of aerosols. The disease is widely distributed in temperate and subarctic regions of North America and Eurasia. Infection in humans results in various clinical presentations depending on the route of inoculation and the virulence of the infecting strain. Most commonly, the disease in humans presents as an indolent ulcer at the site of cutaneous inoculation accompanied by regional lymphadenitis (ulceroglandular form). Other forms include glandular, oculoglandular, oropharyngeal, gastrointestinal, septic, and pneumonic forms. In the United States, fewer than 200 cases annually have been reported in recent years, continuing a steady decline in incidence that has occurred in the 50 years since 1948, when a peak of 1,400 cases was reported (Fig. 14-1).[1]

Agent

F. tularensis (formerly *Pasteurella tularensis*) is a small (0.2 × 0.2 to 0.2 × 0.7 μm), nonmotile, nonsporulating, pleomorphic, Gram-negative coccobacillus. It is a strict aerobe that is fastidious, requiring cysteine, cystine, or other sulfhydryl source for growth. *F. tularensis* grows (slowly) on glucose cysteine blood agar, thioglycollate broth, and buffered charcoal-yeast agar.[2] Inoculated plates should be incubated at 37°C and held for up to 14 days. Colonies are pinpoint after 24 hours of incubation, and may be only 3 mm in diameter at 96 hours. Because of its slow growth, *F. tularensis* may be obscured in culture by more rapidly growing organisms. In specialized laboratories, isolation of pure *F. tularensis* may be obtained from contaminated materials by passage through laboratory mice. The organism has a lipidated capsule and is a hardy saprophyte that survives well in water, moist soil, and decaying animal carcasses. Various strains cannot be distinguished using standard serologic testing methods, but *F. tularensis* may be divided into two main groups by virulence testing, biochemical reactions, and epidemiologic features. Strains of the more virulent form, termed Jellison type A (*F. tularensis* biovar *tularensis*) have an LD_{50} in rabbits of fewer than 10 organisms. They are found only in North America. Jellison type B strains (*F. tularensis* biovar *palaearctica*) have an LD_{50} of more than 10^7 organisms in rabbits. Type B strains occur in North America as well as in Eurasia. Multiple distinct antigens have been described by immunoblotting, including several outer-surface membrane proteins and a lipopolysaccharide endotoxin.[3]

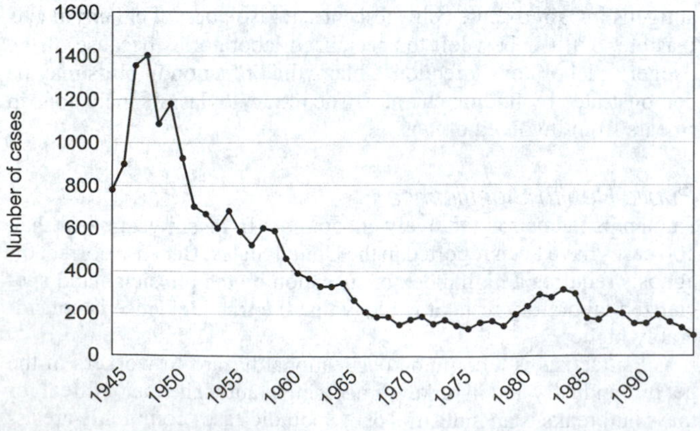

Figure 14-1. Numbers of reported cases of tularemia, United States, 1945–1994.

Life Cycle of F. tularensis

The principal reservoirs of *F. tularensis* are numerous small and medium-sized mammals, especially lagomorphs (rabbits and hares), aquatic rodents (beaver, muskrats, and water voles), and field voles, as well as various hard ticks. In its endemic range, the organism is widespread in nature and has been found in more than 100 species of wild mammals, at least nine species of domestic animals (including cattle, dogs, and cats), 25 species of birds, some amphibians and fish, and more than 50 species of arthropods. However, only mammals and biting arthropods are epidemiologically important.[4] *F. tularensis* is readily isolated from contaminated water and soil. Humans become infected when they intrude into the arthropod-borne cycle and are bitten by infected ticks, biting flies, or mosquitoes; through direct contact with infectious animal tissues, secretions, or exudates; by mucocutaneous contact with or ingestion of contaminated water or soil; or by inhalation of infective aerosols. Person-to-person transmission has not been documented.

Epidemiology

Geographic Distribution

Tularemia is endemic throughout much of the neoarctic and palearctic regions between latitudes 30°N and 71°N. This includes all of North America from the arctic circle to Mexico, and much of Eurasia, including continental Europe, states of the Russian Federation, China, and Japan.[4] In North America, the highest rates of incidence occur in the south-central, Great Plains, and Rocky Mountain regions of the United States;[1] in Eurasia, high incidences occur in Scandinavian countries and Russia.

Populations Affected

Tularemia is a rural disease. It affects persons of all ages and both sexes. It principally affects hunters, trappers, wildlife specialists, and others who handle potentially infected animals; persons in contact with water and soils contaminated by wild animals, especially aquatic mammals; and persons exposed to bites of certain hard ticks and some species of biting flies.[4–6] In the United States, in the early part of the century, the disease was known as "rabbit fever" because of its frequent occurrence in rabbit hunters; similarly, in Japan, the disease was labeled "wild hare disease."

In the United States, 1,409 cases and 20 deaths were reported in the period between 1985 and 1992, for a mean of 171 cases per year and a case-to-fatality rate of 1.4 percent.[1] Of 1,298 cases for which information was available (Centers for Disease Control and Prevention, unpublished data), 942 (72.6 percent) occurred in males, and the excess in males was seen in all age groups. Of 950 evaluatable patients, 88.3 percent were Caucasian, 7.2 percent were Native American, 5.4 percent were black, and 2.3 percent were of other racial or ethnic origins. Tularemia occurred among all age groups, with bimodal peaks in children 0 to 9 years of age and in adults 50 years of age and older. The highest rates occurred in older males. Cases have been reported from all states other than Hawaii; however, the states of Arkansas, Missouri, and Oklahoma regularly report more than half of all cases in the United States. The numbers of cases reported by state for the 10-year period 1985 to 1994 are shown in Figure 14-2.[1,7,8]

Sources of Infection

The principal sources of infection of humans in the United States are bites by ticks or deer flies and contact with infected animals or their carcasses, especially the cottontail rabbit.[5,6] Mosquitoes are important in transmitting the disease to humans in forested Scandinavian and Baltic regions, and mosquito-borne outbreaks have been reported from Sweden and Finland. Hares, aquatic mammals, and contaminated water and soil are the principal sources of infection in humans in most of Eurasia. In Sweden, a large outbreak of pneumonic tularemia occurred among farm workers exposed to hay contaminated by field voles. In Japan, the disease has been historically associated with the hunting and eating of wild rabbits. The seasonal distribution of tularemia cases is related to human and arthropod vector activities in natural areas where the disease is endemic. In the United States, a seasonal peak in the spring and summer months is associated mostly with bites by infected ticks and blood-feeding flies, and the peak in the late fall and winter is associated with direct exposures to infected animals, especially among hunters and trappers of rabbits.[9] Mosquito-borne tularemia in Scandinavia and states of the Russian federation occurs in summer months.

In the United States, several tick species are vectors of tularemia, principally the American dog tick (*Dermacentor variabilis*), the Lone Star tick (*Amblyomma americanum*), and the Rocky Mountain wood tick (*Dermacentor andersoni*).[4,5] Outbreaks of glandular tularemia due to bites by American dog ticks have repeatedly occurred in late spring and early summer among Native Americans in Great Plains states of the United States.[10] Lone Star tick bites are thought to account for most cases in south-central states. The wood tick accounts for scattered human cases across the western United States. Sporadic

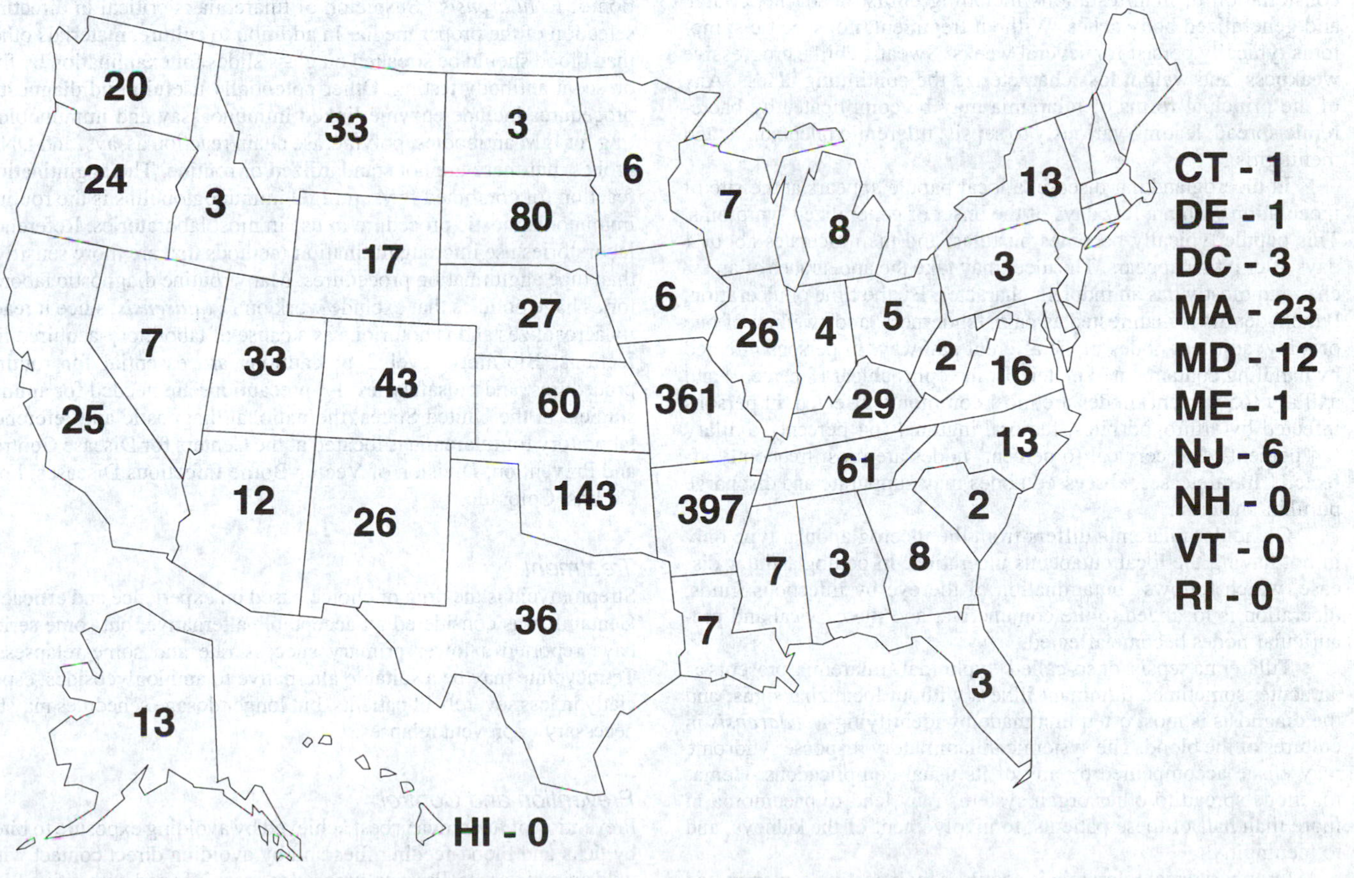

Figure 14-2. Reported cases of tularemia, by state, United States, 1985–1994.

cases and clusters of cases associated with biting flies have been reported from some western states, especially semiarid areas of Utah, Nevada, and California.[11] Direct contact with rabbits still accounts for most cases in the southeastern United States. A number of outbreaks associated with exposure to muskrats, beaver, and contaminated water have been reported, including a large outbreak among trappers in Vermont.[12] Aerosolization of *F. tularensis* occurs and may result in primary pneumonic tularemia; this has been especially problematic among laboratory workers but has also been described following exposures to contaminated stored and freshly mown hay and among factory workers exposed to contaminated water sprays. In the United States, an increasing number of tularemia cases have resulted from bites or scratches by infected cats.[13]

The epidemiology of tularemia in the United States has changed significantly since the 1930s, when the disease had a much higher incidence and when most cases were linked to the hunting and eating wild rabbits and hares rather than to tick bites.[9] In many states, regulations were imposed to restrict rabbit hunting to winter months to reduce the risk of human exposure to infection; further, the harvesting of wild rabbits for food is less common now than it once was.

The Disease

Clinical Manifestations[5,6,14,15]

Tularemia is a plague-like disease. The major clinical forms of tularemia include the following: ulceroglandular (45 to 85 percent of cases); glandular (10 to 25 percent); oculoglandular (fewer than 5 percent); septic (fewer than 5 percent); oropharyngeal (fewer than 5 percent); and, pneumonic (fewer than 5 percent). All forms have similar onset and nonspecific constitutional manifestations. The incubation period is usually 3 to 5 days (range, 1 to 21 days). Onset is sudden. Typically, the patient has fever of 38°C to 40°C and a constellation of manifestations including chills, headache, cough, and generalized body aches. Without treatment, nonspecific symptoms typically persist for several weeks. Sweats, chills, progressive weakness, and weight loss characterize the continuing illness. Any of the principal forms of tularemia may be complicated by bacteremic spread, leading variously to sepsis, tularemic pneumonia, and meningitis.

In ulceroglandular disease, a local papule appears at the site of inoculation within a few days of the onset of generalized symptoms. This papule typically becomes pustular, and then ulcerates about 4 days after it first appears. The ulcer may take the appearance of an eschar and mostly has an indolent character. By the time of ulceration, lymphadenitis is manifested as pain, tenderness, and swelling of one or a few adjacent nodes in the afferent pathway. In persons infected by handling contaminated materials, the epitrochlear (8 percent) and axillary (65 percent) nodes are most commonly affected. In persons infected by arthropod bites, femoral/inguinal (64 percent), axillary (24 percent), and cervical (6 percent) nodes are most frequently affected.[6] In rare cases, abscessed nodes may suppurate and discharge purulent material.

Glandular tularemia differs from the ulceroglandular type only in not having the local cutaneous ulceration. In oculoglandular disease, which follows contamination of the eye by infectious fluids, ulceration is localized to the conjunctiva, and the cervical and preauricular nodes become affected.

Tularemia sepsis, or so-called "typhoidal" tularemia, presents as an acute, sometimes fulminant illness without localizing signs, and the diagnosis is most often first made by identifying *F. tularensis* in cultures of the blood. The systemic inflammatory response syndrome may ensue accompanied by any of its usual complications. Hematogenous spread to other organ systems may lead to pneumonia in more than half of these patients, to involvement of the kidneys, and to meningitis.

Oropharyngeal tularemia is acquired by ingesting contaminated food (almost always inadequately cooked meat) or water. Typically the patient develops exudative pharyngitis or tonsillitis, sometimes with ulceration, and cervical lymphadenopathy. Stomatitis occasionally occurs. Infrequently, the upper gastrointestinal tract may become involved, leading to persistent diarrhea.

Pneumonic plague is a common secondary complication of other forms of tularemia. Infrequently, primary pneumonia arises from exposure to an infective aerosol. Pneumonic infiltrates of varying character may be seen in one or more lobes and are often accompanied by pleural effusion and by hilar lymphadenopathy. Lung abscesses are sometimes seen. Pulmonic manifestations include cough (usually with minimal sputum production), sometimes pleuritic pain, and, rarely, dyspnea.

Prior to the use of antibiotics, the overall mortality from infections with the more severe, Jellison Type A (biovar *tularensis*) strains was in the range of 5 to 10 percent, but with a fatality of 40 to 60 percent for septicemic and pneumonic forms of disease. Infection with biovar *paleoarctic a* strains was associated with a fatality of only 1 to 3 percent. In the United States, the overall fatality rate in recent years has been less than 2 percent.[1]

Diagnosis

The presumptive diagnosis of tularemia is made by clinical findings combined with information on potentially infective exposures. Differential diagnostic possibilities are many: in persons with glandular disease they include plague, sporotrichosis, lymphogranuloma venereum, chancre, and chancroid; in persons with oropharyngeal tularemia, other bacterial and viral causes of stomatitis, pharyngitis, and cervical adenitis must be considered; in persons with pneumonia, the possibilities include Legionnaires' disease, histoplasmosis, and tuberculosis; and in persons with tularemia sepsis, possibilities are typhoid fever and other causes of systemic inflammatory response syndrome. The diagnosis of tularemia is confirmed by isolation of *F. tularensis*.[2] Suspicion of tularemia is critical in directing selection of the proper media. In addition to culture, materials other than blood should be streaked on glass slides for examination by fluorescent antibody testing. Other potentially useful rapid diagnostic procedures include enzyme-linked immunoassay and immunoblotting for IgM antibodies, polymerase chain reaction assays, and DNA probes, but these are not standardized or routine. The agglutination reaction for combined IgM and IgG immunoglobulins is the routine immunodiagnostic procedure in use in most laboratories. Reference laboratories use microagglutination methods that are more sensitive than tube agglutination procedures. Many routine diagnostic laboratories have policies that exclude work on *F. tularensis*, since it readily aerosolizes and is notorious as a cause of laboratory-acquired infections. Biosafety level 2 precautions are essential for routine procedures, and biosafety level 3 precautions are needed for animal studies. In the United States, the national diagnostic and reference laboratory for tularemia is located at the Centers for Disease Control and Prevention, Division of Vector-Borne Infectious Diseases, Fort Collins, Colorado.

Treatment

Streptomycin is the drug of choice based on experience and efficacy. Gentamicin is considered an acceptable alternative, but some series have reported a lower primary success rate and some relapses.[16] Tetracycline may be a suitable alternative to aminoglycosides, especially in less severely ill patients, but longer dosage schedules may be necessary to prevent relapses.

Prevention and Control

Prevention of tularemia is best achieved by avoiding exposure to bites by ticks and blood-feeding flies and by avoiding direct contact with wild animal tissues. Persons exposed to areas infested with biting flies and ticks should when feasible wear protective clothing, tuck pants legs into socks, and apply insect repellents containing deet to skin and clothing as directed by the manufacturer. Permethrin-based acaricides can be applied to clothing to kill ticks on contact. Clothing and skin should be frequently examined for ticks, and attached ticks should be promptly removed. Persons should avoid contact with sick or dead animals, and hunters and trappers should always handle animal carcasses with impervious gloves. To reduce tick infestations in residential areas, pet dogs and cats should be restrained and kept tick-free using appropriate acaricides. A live attenuated vaccine is available for laboratory personnel who routinely work with *F. tularensis* in specialized facilities. Antibiotic prophylaxis is not routinely recommended for persons having exposure to patients with pneumonic tularemia, since person-to-person respiratory spread has not been documented.

Anthrax

Richard A. Spiegel • Arnold F. Kaufmann

Anthrax has been recognized as an infectious disease of humans and animals for many centuries. The term "anthrax" is derived from the Greek word *anthrakos*, which means coal; this refers to the coloration of the eschar associated with cutaneous anthrax.[1] Anthrax has been thought to have been identified as many as 12,000 years ago, around the earliest periods of the domestication of livestock, and has been described in other periods as well, including approximately 6,000 years ago in Mesopotamia and Egypt.[2] A major outbreak of anthrax in Europe in 1613 is reported to have killed 60,000 people and, at that time was referred to as the "black bain." In his description of a disease outbreak, Virgil observed that eating meat or wearing clothes made from wool or hides of infected animals resulted in human anthrax. Unfortunately, Virgil's admonition that the contagion be controlled by burial of carcasses was not widely practiced.

In nineteenth-century Europe, anthrax occurred in epidemic proportions, with the magnitude of the losses of livestock to anthrax creating widespread concern for the future of animal agriculture in Europe. In France, at least 20 to 30 percent of the sheep and cattle died of anthrax each year. The need to control the disease stimulated the work of Davaine and others during the mid-1800s.These researchers demonstrated "bodies" in the blood of ill animals; they also demonstrated that anthrax could be transmitted from one animal to another by inoculating the blood of anthrax-affected sick or dead animals into previously healthy animals and transmitting the disease. The famous Koch's postulates were actually first demonstrated by Robert Koch using the anthrax bacillus. Anthrax also was the first disease conclusively proved to be caused by a microorganism, as well as the first bacterial disease for which an effective vaccine was developed.

The Agent

Bacillus anthracis, the etiologic agent of anthrax, is a large, Gram-positive, nonmotile, spore-forming bacterial rod. The bacillus grows well on a variety of bacterial culture media at 35°C to 37°C. On blood agar plates, the bacillus forms large, nonhemolytic colonies resembling ground glass. The tenacious (sticky) character of these colonies can be demonstrated by lifting a colony with an inoculating loop, and the colonies have been described as standing up like whipped egg white. *B. anthracis* has three primary virulence factors, which are all plasmid mediated: The edema toxin, lethal toxin, and a poly-D-glutamic acid capsule.[3] The edema and lethal toxin share a common binding moiety, which is referred to as protective antigen. The combination of edema factor and protective antigen has been demonstrated to reduce polymorphonuclear neutrophil function, and this may be responsible for increasing host susceptibility to infection with *B. anthracis*. DNA probes for detection of the plasmids can be used for rapid, specific identification of the bacillus.

Diagnosis of anthrax may be made by culture of clinical or autopsy specimens, by visualization of *B. anthracis* on direct Gram-stained smears, or by serologic evaluation. One serologic method is a Western blotting technique referred to as the electrophoretic immunotransblot, which detects antibody to *B. anthracis* toxins.[4] In addition, fluorescent antibody examination of tissues to detect the organism cell wall or its capsule can also be useful. Newer diagnostic tests include a chromatographic assay to detect toxin in clinical specimens as well as PCR to detect the presence of viable or not viable anthrax bacilli. A number of molecular methods exist for identification and characterization of *B. anthracis*, but these are currently limited to research settings.[5]

Human Anthrax

Human anthrax has three major clinical forms: cutaneous, inhalation, and gastrointestinal.[6] Cutaneous anthrax is the result of introduction of the spore through the skin; inhalational anthrax, via the respiratory tract; and gastrointestinal anthrax, through ingestion via the gastrointestinal tract. Cutaneous anthrax is by far the most common manifestation of infection with *B. anthracis*.

Cutaneous anthrax is associated with a characteristic skin lesion developing 2 to 7 days after infection (range: 1 to 12 days). The lesion develops at the site where the anthrax bacillus is introduced beneath the skin; (e.g., by rubbing or through a cut). Most cutaneous anthrax lesions occur on exposed areas of the body. The lesion is usually first noted as a red-brown papule resembling a pimple or insect bite. Blistering or vesiculation of the papule occurs within 3 days, and the vesicle ruptures shortly after its formation, revealing an underlying ulcer. A scab or eschar then develops over the surface of the ulcer. The lesion is usually surrounded by edematous swelling disproportionate to the magnitude of the central lesion. Although death occurs in 5 to 20 percent of untreated patients, treatment with penicillin or other appropriate antibiotics virtually eliminates fatalities associated with the cutaneous form of anthrax. Meningitis can be a complication of cutaneous anthrax.

Inhalational (pulmonary) anthrax usually occurs in persons exposed to certain industries (e.g. processing of goat hair).[7] In 1979, an outbreak of inhalational anthrax reported by Meselson, et al, involving 77 patients and 66 deaths in the community of Sverdlovsk in the former Soviet Union; the outbreak was concluded to be related to an aerosol release of anthrax at a military facility.[8] Inhalational anthrax usually results from inhaling aerosols of anthrax spores generated during certain manufacturing processes. After an incubation period of 1 to 6 days, the initial illness is characterized by low-grade fever; malaise; fatigue; myalgia; nonproductive cough; and occasionally a sensation of precordial oppression. Following the onset of symptoms in the first 3 days, the second stage of acute toxicity begins with sudden onset of dyspnea, cyanosis, and profuse sweating. On x-ray, widening of the mediastinum with pleural effusions caused by swollen lymph nodes and surrounding edema is often apparent. The diagnos of inhalational anthrax is is rarely made before death, unless the history clearly suggests associated risk factors.

Gastrointestinal anthrax is very rare in most areas of the world, although it may occur in explosive outbreaks associated with ingestion of meat from an animal that has become ill or died as a result of anthrax. Gastrointestinal anthrax develops 2 to 5 days after eating meat from infected animals. The clinical course varies. Many patients have fever and cervical and submental swelling, apparently caused by profound cervical lymphadenopathy or subcutaneous edema. Other patients have a gradual onset of nausea, vomiting, anorexia, and fever. This mild prodromal illness is followed by abdominal pain, intensification of vomiting with the vomitus changing to red or black, increasing temperature, and diarrhea that may be blood tinged. In less severe cases, only mild diarrhea and abdominal pain may be noted. The entire clinical course persists 1 to 5 days, and mortality ranges from 25% to 75%. Mortality often results from septicemia and the toxic factors associated with anthrax.

Animal Anthrax

Although anthrax in animals has been reported in all continents, the incidence varies greatly by geographic area. Anthrax frequently occurs in tropical and subtropical areas that experience periods of heavy rainfall. Anthrax has been described as a naturally occurring disease and experimental disease in numerous animal species, but it primarily occurs in cattle, sheep, goats, horses, and pigs.[9] Compared to these animals birds are more resistant to anthrax, except ducks and ostrichs. Anthrax in animals resembles the gastrointestinal form of the disease in humans. The inhalational and cutaneous forms of human anthrax do not occur naturally in animals.

In domestic livestock, the incubation period is typically 3 to 7 days but may range from 1 to>14 days. The clinical course ranges from acute to chronic. Sudden death is common in animals that appeared normal a few hours earlier. In cattle, sheep, and goats, the acute illness is characterized by abrupt onset of fever, variably followed by anorexia, ruminal stasis, signs of abdominal pain, hematuria, and blood-tinged diarrhea. Pregnant animals may abort, and milk production in lactating animals often abruptly decreases, with the milk being abnormal or blood tinged. Subcutaneous edematous swelling may occur, particularly on the ventral side of the neck. Death usually occurs 1 to 3 days after onset. Occasionally animals survive infection without treatment, but this is uncommon. Chronic infection, characterized by localized edematous subcutaneous swelling, rarely occurs in cattle. In swine, the disease is similar to that in ruminants, except that both acute and chronic infections more commonly localize in the tonsils and cervical lymph nodes.

Mode of Transmission

The natural reservoir of *B. anthracis* is soil.[10] The organism is a part of the normal flora of numerous soil types having a pH >6. Spores can remain viable in soil for many decades. Although naturally contaminated soil is the usual reservoir of infection, animal anthrax outbreaks have been traced to a variety of sources, such as animal-origin feed and fertilizer, river water contaminated by wastes from animal product processing, and crops raised on contaminated soil. Anthrax is not communicable directly between animals, although infection can be acquired by scavengers feeding on infected carcasses.

In the United States, animal anthrax is distributed widely but is seen most commonly in the lower Mississippi River valley. Sporadic outbreaks have been reported from many other states, and disease can occur virtually anywhere. Anthrax occurs annually in some areas (usually during periods of high humidity and high temperature), and in other regions intervals of many years between outbreaks are typical.[11] Outbreaks among grazing animals occur primarily when the minimum daily temperature is >16°C (61°F), but documented cases have occurred even during midwinter in cold climates. Epizootics frequently occur after periods of marked climatic or ecological change, such as heavy rainfall, flooding, or drought.

Human anthrax is considered to be secondary to animal anthrax. Infection may occur as an occupational risk of veterinarians and farmers through direct contact with animal tissues at necropsy or during attempts to salvage parts of the carcass (which is particularly problematic in developing countries). The risk for acquiring anthrax occurs when hides, hair, and wool are removed from the carcass and sold for processing, a practice that has made anthrax an occupational disease in the tanning, gelatin, and animal hair and wool-processing industries. Occasional human cases have resulted from contaminated animal-origin products sold at the retail level, such as shaving brushes, yarn, and goatskin-topped drums. Recovery from anthrax will usually result in protective immunity.

Occurrence

Anthrax occurs worldwide but is, more common in widespread areas of Asia and Africa. Fewer than 10 cases have occurred in the United States during the past decade. In some countries, such as Haiti, however, several hundred cases still occur each year, and in Zimbabwe an epidemic of almost 10,000 human cases occurred in the period from 1978 to 1980, when political instability disrupted animal anthrax control activities. Cases associated with industrial processing of animal products may occur at any season. Agriculture-related cases, however, occur in a seasonal pattern parallel to that of animal anthrax in the area. Animal anthrax has a worldwide distribution. In the United States, multiple small outbreaks of animal anthrax occur each year, but epizootics are uncommon.

Prevention and Control

Prevention of human anthrax associated with agriculture is dependent on the control of animal anthrax. Annual vaccinization of livestock in areas of endemic anthrax is recommended. The animal anthrax vaccine that is most commonly used is a live spore suspension of the avirulent Sterne strain.[12] Livestock should be vaccinated 2 to 4 weeks before the season when outbreaks may be expected. Because immunity to the vaccine is short-lived, annual revaccination of livestock is recommended.

Reporting of animal anthrax outbreaks to agriculture and public health officials should be mandatory. Affected premises or areas should be quarantined to prevent infected animals from being marketed, and all susceptible livestock on affected and surrounding premises should be vaccinated. Investigation of sources of infection other than contaminated pastures should be initiated and, if identified, should be eliminated. Carcasses of animals that die from anthrax should be either buried deeply or burned completely. Bedding and other contaminated material should also be burned or buried.

In an outbreak area, dairy herds should be placed under surveillance if the herd has not been vaccinated previously.[13] The rectal temperature of each animal should be determined immediately before milking; a febrile animal should be isolated immediately and its milk discarded. All afebrile animals should be vaccinated when surveillance is initiated. Surveillance can be terminated 10 days after vaccination.

A human anthrax vaccine is available in the United States to protect persons with ongoing risk for infection.[14] The vaccine is recommended for employees of high-risk industries, such as those processing imported animal hides, hair, and wool as well as for laboratory personnel working with *B. anthracis* cultures.

Disinfection of materials and surfaces contaminated with *B. anthracis* is complicated by the resistance of the spore; however, a variety of procedures are effective. These include dry heat, steam under pressure, formaldehyde soaking or vapor exposure, ethylene oxide gas exposure, hypochlorite solution soaking, and gamma irradiation. The potential risks of the disinfection method (use of formaldehyde or ethylene oxide) needs to be weighed against the risk for anthrax infection in considering the decontamination method of choice. Regardless of the procedure used, the effectiveness of disinfection should be verified by appropriate cultures and quality control procedures.

Brucellosis

Richard A. Spiegel • Arnold F. Kaufmann

Brucellosis is an important zoonotic disease with a worldwide distribution.[1] Brucellosis was first recognized as a vague febrile illness occurring in Mediterranean countries. Mediterranean fever, as it was then known, was a major cause of illness in the British soldiers garrisoned on Malta. In 1887, the cause of the illness was first reported to be *Brucella melitensis* by Sir David Bruce, a British army surgeon. Nearly 20 years elapsed before the role of the goat and its milk in the epidemiology of brucellosis was uncovered by Sir Themistokles Zammit, a Maltese physician.

B. abortus and *B. suis* were first isolated from cattle and swine, respectively. In contrast to *B. melitensis*, the ability of *B. abortus* and *B. suis* to cause human disease was seriously questioned until the mid-1920s. Alice Evans, a U.S. Public Health Service bacteriologist, deserves much of the credit for gaining acceptance of the pathogenesis of *B. abortus* and *B. suis* by the medical community. Evans acquired brucellosis during the course of her pioneering work and suffered relapsing illness for approximately 20 years, once being hospitalized for 14 months.

The Agent

Brucella organisms are small, nonmotile, Gram-negative bacilli. The various *Brucella* species are slow-growing, fastidious organisms that vary in their nutrient requirements.[2] All *Brucella* species and biotypes appear to be partially host adapted. The species having known human health significance and their usual reservoir hosts are *B. abortus* (cattle), *B canis* (dogs), *B. melitensis* (goats and sheep), and *B. suis* (swine). *B. melitensis* infection acquired through exposure to sheep and goats is the most important form of brucellosis affecting humans worldwide.

Definitive diagnosis of brucellosis can be made only by culture, and blood cultures are most useful, especially during the acute phase of the disease. Cultures of bone marrow or other infected tissues may be valuable, especially for patients with chronic disease. Automated incubation methods are useful for the growth of *Brucella* sp, but allowance must be made for the slow growth of the organism.[3] Molecular methods using polymerase chain reaction (PCR) appear promising, but need further evaluation.

A variety of serologic tests for brucellosis are available.[2,4] The standard tube agglutination test, which uses a *B. abortus* antigen, is used most commonly in the United States and can detect infections caused by *B. abortus*, *B. melitensis*, and *B. suis*. Detection of *B. canis* antibody requires use of a *B. canis*–specific antigen. Enzyme-linked immunosorbent assay (ELISA) tests for *Brucella* antibody are now available and appear to be more useful than the tube agglutination test in areas of high endemnicity. In the U.S., for example, false positives would vastly outnumber true positives.

The Disease

Human illnesses caused by the various *Brucella* species are similar, however *B. melitensis* and certain *B. suis* biotypes tend to produce more severe disease. The incubation period is highly variable and difficult to determine outside common source outbreaks. A range of 5-60 days will be observed in most cases. The onset of illness often is insidious but can be abrupt.

Brucellosis is most consistently characterized by fever (constant or intermittent), chills, sweats, malaise, weakness, headache, muscle aches, loss of appetite, and loss of weight.[5,6] Pregnant women may abort spontaneously. Less common findings include aching joints, pneumonia, meningitis, epistaxis, and enlarged lymph nodes, spleen, and liver.

The course of illness is variable, ranging from a few days to years in duration. If untreated, the illness often lasts months. Even with treatment, a patient often is ill for a month or more. Relapsing illness is common. Five percent of the patients receiving appropriate therapy have one or more relapses within 3 years of initial onset, and the relapse rate is higher in the absence of appropriate therapy. Death from brucellosis is rare but is more common with *B. melitensis* infections. Chronic brucellosis is rare in appropriately treated patients. Chronic manifestations include spondylitis, osteomyelitis, and granulomas in a variety of sites, such as the liver, spleen, kidney, heart, and abdominal aorta. Prolonged mental depression is an infrequent sequel of brucellosis.

The drugs of choice for treating brucellosis are currently under discussion. The World Health Organization (WHO) recommended treatment for acute brucellosis is 600 to 900 mg of rifampicin and 200 mg of doxycycline daily for at least 6 weeks, however treatment failures have been documented. Others claim that fewer relapses will occur with an aminoglycoside (gentamicin or streptomycin) combined with doxycycline.[7] It should be noted that, although streptomycin is recommended in the literature for treating brucellosis, its availability is much more limited than gentamycin. In many countries, a combination of doxycycline and rifampin has been adopted as the standard therapy.

Brucellosis in animals causes infertility and abortion.[6] When brucellosis is first introduced into a group, an abortion epizootic often ensues. Endemic disease is less dramatic, because abortion occurs primarily in animals experiencing their first pregnancies. The birth of weak offspring, retained placentas, and diminished milk production also may occur. In males, chronic inflammation of the testicle and epididymis may result in infertility. Infection of the bones and joints may occur and may result in chronic lameness and, on occasion, posterior paralysis.

Mode of Transmission

In the animal reservoir hosts, brucellosis is transmitted by several mechanisms. Venereal transmission can occur as the result of infected semen. This is thought to be of minor importance except with artificial insemination, when it could be significant. The most important mechanism of transmission is the shedding of *Brucella* organisms in the uterine discharges after abortion or, on occasion, normal parturition in infected animals. Other animals in the herd become infected by ingesting *Brucella* organisms from the contaminated environment or directly from the infected animal's genitals. Fetal membranes and aborted fetuses may serve as sources of infection. *Brucella* organisms are capable of surviving for months in moist environments and manure.

Brucella organisms also may be shed in milk. This shedding may occur for several months, during multiple successive lactation periods in otherwise apparently healthy dairy cows. The period of shedding is shorter for goats but still lasts for weeks and may recur during the next lactation period.

Human infections result primarily from exposure to *Brucella* organisms by one of three routes: ingestion, direct contact, or inhalation.[8,9] *Brucella* species also vary in their virulence for humans. For example, *B. melitensis* can produce disease with fewer organisms than can *B. abortus* when ingested in dairy products. A study in California determined that 78.7% of cases of brucellosis between the years 1973 and 1992 were due to *B. melitensis*; over 80 percent of these cases occurred in Hispanics who had consumed milk and cheese from Mexico.[10] Worldwide, ingestion of unpasteurized dairy products is the primary source of human brucellosis. Cheese made from raw goat's milk is particularly hazardous.

Contact with infectious materials, such as uterine discharges or blood, is an important source of infection for livestock raisers, veterinarians, and abattoir workers. Intact skin is an effective barrier against invasion by *Brucella* organisms under experimental conditions; however, the persons at primary risk of acquiring infection, frequently have skin abrasions and cuts as a result of their occupation. *Brucella* organisms can readily invade the body through the conjunctiva if infectious material is rubbed or sprayed into the eyes.

Infection via inhalation also occurs under certain circumstances. This route of infection is only slightly less effective than parenteral challenge for inducing brucellosis in laboratory animals. Occupational groups at risk for infection via inhalation include laboratory and abattoir workers. Reports of person-to-person transmission of brucellosis are rare. Transmission via whole blood transfusions has been reported but is very rare.

Occurrence

Brucellosis occurs worldwide. The reporting of cases is far from complete. Nonetheless, appoximately 20,000 cases are reported each year. Brucellosis is considered an important public health problem in Western and Central Asia, the Mediterranean region of Europe and Africa, and a number of countries in Central and South America.

In the United States, the reported incidence of brucellosis increased rapidly from slightly more than 100 cases in 1927 to a peak of appoximately 6,300 cases in 1947. Subsequently, the virtually universal requirement for dairy product pasteurization and efforts to eradicate the disease from livestock have resulted subsequently in a progressive reduction in incidence. Less than 100 cases are now reported annually.

The relative importance of the various reservoir hosts and their associated *Brucella* species differs from region to region. *B. melitensis* infections associated with ingestion of unpasteurized goat cheese and milk remain a serious public health problem in most hyperendemic countries. *B.suis* biotype 4 infections are associated predominantly with ingestion of raw bone marrow and other tissues from caribou in Arctic regions.

In the United States, *B. abortus* infections associated with consumption of raw dairy products or contact with infected cattle constituted the majority of cases until the late 1950s. Subsequently, brucellosis has been primarily an occupational disease of abattoir workers, livestock producers, veterinarians, and laboratory workers. The primary source of infection has changed to swine, and *B. suis* is now the predominant infecting species.[11] Cases associated with ingestion of unpasteurized dairy products continue to be reported, but these are now mostly *B. melitensis* infections associated with eating dairy products while traveling in Mediterranean countries and Mexico.[10]

Brucellosis occurs throughout the year. Seasonal variations in incidence do occur, but the reasons for seasonality are not always clear. In regions where *B. melitensis* infections predominate, peak seasonal incidence coincides with the months when goats give birth. Cases in the United States occur more frequently in April, May, and June and least frequently in November and December.

In the United States, brucellosis usually is a disease of adult males, reflecting their occupational exposure except situations involving foodborne transmission would be expected to have an equal M:F ratio. Adult male predominance, although less marked, also occurs in other countries, reflecting increased risk associated with occupational exposure of livestock raisers.

First reported as a cause of reproductive disease in dogs, *B. canis* now is known to cause human disease. Infections caused by this organism are widespread in the dog and, possibly, the cat populations of many countries. In contrast, only a small number of human infections have been reported. Less than 40 human infections have been reported in the United States through 1989.

Prevention and Control

The ideal method of preventing brucellosis is to eradicate the disease from domestic livestock. Bovine brucellosis reportedly has been eradicated from the British Channel Islands, Norway, Sweden, Finland, Denmark, Czechoslovakia, the Netherlands, Belize, and the Isle of Man. Other countries, including the United States and England, have made substantial progress toward eradicating bovine brucellosis, but the disease persists in swine and other domestic species.

Eradication programs are cost-beneficial to a country's economy in the long term because of increased livestock productivity. However, the short-term capital expenditure and disruption of agricultural routines have reduced enthusiasm for carrying out eradication programs. When eradication is not feasible, control and reduction of incidence in livestock can be achieved with vaccination.

A safe, effective vaccine is not available for use in humans. Persons who have fully recovered from an initial infection are resistant to reinfection. The protection afforded by a prior infection appears to be in the range of 90 percent.[12]

Pasteurization of milk and dairy products is an effective control measure. Pasteurization will simultaneously control other milk-borne diseases, such as salmonellosis and tuberculosis. For persons with occupational exposure, some efforts can be made to reduce risk of infection and ameliorate the impact of the disease. An educational program should inform these persons about the disease, its symptoms, how it is acquired, and the need for early diagnosis and treatment. The use of appropriate protective equipment should be encouraged. For example, shoulder length rubber gloves should be worn during obstetrical procedures on livestock.

Although there is no United States licensed *Brucella* vaccine for use in humans, strain 19 *B. abortus* vaccine and strain RB51 *B. abortus* vaccines are in widespread use in the United States for use in the control of brucellosis in U.S. cattle. Because it is a live vaccine, there is potential for inadvertent inoculation of the veterinarian administering the vaccine to the cattle. Current recommendations for strain 19 exposures are to place the person on 3 weeks' prophylaxis with doxycycline and rifampin if initiated promptly after the inadvertant innoculation. It is not presently clear what the appropriate postexposure prophylaxis should be for strain RB51, because it is considered to be of lower pathogenicity than strain 19 has the characteristic of being rifampin resistant in vitro.[13] In the case of a possible human infection with strain RB51, serologic diagnosis will prove difficult, because infection with this organism cannot be detected using the currently available serologic test for detection of *B. abortus*.[13]

Brucellosis should be considered routinely in the differential diagnosis of febrile illnesses in persons having occupational exposure to the disease. All such persons with fever of unknown origin lasting more than 3 days should be evaluated appropriately to avoid undue delay in diagnosis. As a group, brucellosis patients for whom therapy is initiated within 30 days of onset have a shorter course of illness and fewer complications.

Leptospirosis

Arnold F. Kaufmann • Bradley A. Perkins

Leptospirosis was first recognized in 1883 as an occupational disease of sewer workers, an association that is still true.[1] Soon thereafter, the disease was reported in widely separated geographic areas. Whether leptospirosis was a variant of viral hepatitis or a truly distinct disease soon became a controversial topic. The issue was resolved when the infecting leptospires were isolated in Japan about 1914 and shortly thereafter in Germany.

The initial confusion as to whether leptospirosis and viral hepatitis were distinct diseases was later repeated with yellow fever. The isolation of leptospires from jaundiced patients in areas endemic for yellow fever led to this controversy, which continued until the viral etiology of yellow fever was established in 1928.

The Agent

The genus *Leptospira* comprises pathogenic and saprophytic strains. Although now subdivided into at least 12 species on the basis of DNA relatedness,[2] the older taxonomic system based on the serologic relatedness of strains continues to be used. More that 250 pathogenic serovars are currently recognized. A leptospiral serogroup is a collective term for antigenically related serovars, but members of a serogroup may belong to multiple species as defined by DNA relatedness.

The parasitic leptospires are fastidious, slow-growing spirochetes.[3] They are small, thin, threadlike organisms tightly coiled about their long axis. Actively motile, leptospires rotate on their long axis, often with a whip-like motion.

Most leptospiral serovars have their primary reservoir in wild mammals, although some appear to be adapted to certain domestic and peridomestic animals. For example, *canicola* is associated with dogs; *pomona*, with cattle and swine; and *ballum* and *icterohaemorrhagiae*, with rats and mice.

Leptospirosis is definitively diagnosed by culture of the organism from clinical or autopsy specimens using a semisolid medium. Culture of leptospires from environmental specimens such as water is best done by inoculation of laboratory animals.

In practice, serologic tests, such as the microscopic agglutination procedure, are used more frequently than cultures for diagnostic purposes.[4] A variety of new serologic tests, including a dipstick for use in the field and in developing countries, are being tested.[5,6] A number of PCR-based tests are being developed for the detection of leptospires in clinical specimens.[7–9] Leptospires may also be identified using immunohistochemical regents for examination of affected tissues (e.g., lung).[10] Direct microscopic examination of patient specimens with dark field and fluorescent-antibody techniques is also used but is considered unreliable.

The Disease

Leptospirosis was originally described as a severe disease characterized by fever, jaundice, hemorrhage, and liver and renal failure. Subsequently, leptospirosis was recognized to occur much more frequently in a variety of often mild clinical forms. The protean manifestations of leptospirosis frequently result in its being misdiagnosed. Some common symptoms of the disease include influenza-like illness, fever of unknown origin, generalized enlargement of lymphoid glands resembling infectious mononucleosis, a macular to maculopapular rash, particularly with a pretibial distribution, abdominal pain, and aseptic meningitis and encephalitis.[11]

To some extent, specific clinical syndromes more commonly occur after infection with certain leptospiral serovars. The severe icteric form is associated with *icterohaemorrhagiae* infections, a prominence of gastrointestinal complaints with *grippotyphosa* infections, and aseptic meningitis with *pomona* and *canicola* infection. These associations are generalizations at best, and any leptospiral serovar can cause the various signs and symptoms associated with leptospirosis.

The incubation period is 4 to 19 days, usually 10 days. The illness is often biphasic, with an initial febrile (septicemic) stage lasting 3 to 7 days followed by a second (immune) stage lasting from 0 to 30 days or more.[12] Disease referable to specific organs—such as the kidneys, liver, eye, and meninges—becomes apparent in the immune stage. Mortality is generally low but is higher for older persons and those with jaundice.

Penicillin G (1.5 million units every 6 hours intravenously) or ampicillin (500 to 1000 mg every 6 hours intravenously) are appropriate therapies for severe leptospirosis. In milder cases, when patients can tolerate oral therapy, doxycycline (100 mg twice per day), ampicillin (500 to 750 mg four times per day), or amoxicillin (500 mg four times per day) can be used. Although there are limited data on the effectiveness of antimicrobial therapy for leptospirosis, a recent controlled trail demonstrated benefit among patients with severe or moderately severe leptospirosis.[13]

Animal leptospirosis, as in the human disease, is often subclinical. Leptospirosis in dogs is characterized by febrile jaundice with liver and renal failure or by renal infection alone. In cattle and sheep, hemolytic anemia, hemoglobinuria, abortion, atypical mastitis, and production of thick, yellow, blood-tinged milk are common manifestations. Leptospirosis in swine is a nonspecific illness, with abortions late in pregnancy being the most important single sign.

Leptospiruria, the shedding of leptospires in urine, is a common and epidemiologically important aspect of the disease. Leptospiruria frequently continues for months after initial infection, particularly in animals. Leptospiruria is more transient in humans and seldom lasts more than 60 days.

Mode of Transmission

Human leptospirosis is contracted almost exclusively from direct or indirect exposure to urine of leptospiruric animals. Direct exposure appears to be a mode of transmission for pet owners and certain occupational groups, such as farm workers and veterinarians. Indirect exposure, through such vehicles as contaminated water and soil, is more common, however. Humans are a dead-end host for practical purposes, and person-to-person transmission is rare.

Leptospires can gain entry into the body through breaks in the skin as well as via mucous membranes. Most common-source outbreaks in the United States have been associated with swimming in contaminated water. Persons in occupations that involve exposure to water and mud, such as sewer workers and rice field workers, have a high risk for leptospiral infections. Partial or total immersion in water or mud seems to play a role in facilitating infection.

Milkers are another high-risk group. In herringbone milking parlors, persons milking cows are frequently spattered in the face with urine, with resultant infection via the conjunctiva.

Infections following animal bites are reported occasionally. Most of these cases involve rodent bites. Infection following consumption of contaminated food and water has been reported, and because leptospires cannot survive in the acid gastric environment, the route of infection in these cases presumably is the mucous membranes of the mouth and esophagus.

Occurrence

Leptospirosis occurs worldwide. Epidemic disease may occur in association with flooding.[10] Although it is considered more common in tropical countries, the majority of cases are reported from countries with temperate climates. The geographic distribution of reported cases reflects the availability of diagnostic facilities and the interests of individual investigators.

Of the 1,500 to 2,000 cases reported annually worldwide, about 100 are from the United States. In contrast to many infectious diseases, leptospirosis has been reported with increasing frequency over the past five decades in the United States. Sixteen cases were reported in the period from 1925 to 1934; 230 between 1935 and 1944; 267 between 1945 and 1954; 705 between 1955 and 1964; 791 between 1965 and 1974; and more than 800 between 1975 and 1984.

The incidence of leptospirosis varies by season, with most cases occurring in the late summer and early fall. In the United States, more than 50 percent of cases occur in the months July through October.

In most countries, leptospirosis is predominantly a disease of adult males, reflecting the importance of occupational exposure. In the United States, a trend toward more cases in females and at younger ages has developed. This reflects changing social roles and the increasing importance of exposure during leisure activities. Almost half of the cases in the period from 1978 to 1987 were associated with recreational exposures.

A shift has occurred in the predominant infecting serogroup in the United States. Before 1948, only infections by *icterohaemorrhagiae* (90 percent) and *canicola* (10 percent) were recognized. In the period from 1949 to 1961, infections by members of the *pomona, grippotyphosa, autumnalis, hebdomidis, bataviae, ballum*, and *pyrogenes* serogroups were recognized, and fewer than 40 percent of the cases were ascribed to *icterohaemorrhagiae* infections. In the period from 1978 to 1987, infections by members of all the foregoing serogroups plus *tarassovi, javanica, cynopteri, andamana, australis,* and *shermani* were detected, and only 32 percent of the cases were ascribed to *icterohaemorrhagiae* infections.

Prevention and Control

All leptospirosis cases should be investigated to detect potential common-source outbreaks and to implement appropriate control measures to prevent occurrence of further cases. Control, unfortunately, is not a simple matter.

Human leptospirosis vaccines have been used in countries other than the United States for selected high-risk populations, such as rice field workers in Italy. These vaccines are serovar specific.

A recent field study demonstrated that 200 mg of doxycycline administered once weekly was effective in the prevention of leptospirosis.[14] Chemoprophylaxis is recommended when the exposure period is short term and the expected attack rate is greater than 1 percent.

Animal vaccines are available that protect against illness but not against infection and leptospiruria. Human infections have been acquired from asymptomatic dogs that were immunized but nonetheless shed leptospires in their urine.

Treatment with antibiotics, such as streptomycin and tetracycline, has been recommended as a method of eliminating renal shedding in swine, cattle, and dogs. The effectiveness of this approach is equivocal. In cattle, concurrent administration of streptomycin and vaccine has been recommended to control acute outbreaks.

Use of protective equipment is of value in certain circumstances. The wearing of rubber boots is recommended for sewer workers and agricultural workers who frequently wade in water contaminated with rodent urine. Environmental hygiene measures, such as rodent control and work surface decontamination, may also be of benefit. Swimming should not be permitted in streams where risk of infection is high.

Salmonellosis

Cindy R. Friedman • Laurence Slutsker

The *Salmonella* genus of bacteria was identified in 1885 by Salmon and Smith. There are now over 2,000 specific antigenic types of *Salmonella*, and new ones are still being identified. Salmonellosis is a convenient etiological term to describe a variety of conditions that affect humans and many animal species. The clinical manifestations of *Salmonella* infection in humans range from symptomless carriage to septicemia, with infection often the result of ingestion of contaminated foods. In contrast to *Salmonella* Typhi, infection and illness with the nontyphoid *Salmonella* are increasing in areas with adequate sanitation and are now an important cause of morbidity and expense in many developed and developing countries (Fig. 14-3).

Characteristics of the Bacteria

Bacteria of the genus *Salmonella* are Gram-negative bacilli that have many cultural properties and antigens in common with other members of the family Enterobacteriaceae. Individual serotypes are characterized by their somatic (O) and flagellar (H) antigens. Salmonellae are grouped and subgrouped (A, B, C_1, C_2, C_3, D, E_1, E_2, E_3, E_4, and so on) by O antigens. Within each group, individual serotypes are distinguished by their H antigens. Although over 2,000 serotypes are known, 10 serotypes accounted for approximately 70 percent of the total human isolates reported to the Centers for Disease Control and Prevention in 1995 (Table 14-3).[1]

Temperatures used in routine pasteurization of milk destroy salmonellae. However, salmonellae within meat or other products may survive if cooking temperatures and time of cooking are adequate to cook only the surface of the food. Refrigeration does not destroy this bacterium and growth has been recorded at 10°C (50°F). Once in the environment, salmonellae survive for long periods in water and soil and on or within foods. Phage typing of many individual serotypes is possible and has been used in epidemiological studies.[2] More recently, pulsed-field gel electrophoresis (PFGE) has been used for molecular fingerprinting of certain *Salmonella* serotypes.[3] Use of antimicrobials in animal feeds has led to antimicrobial-resistant salmonellae, often with transferable drug-resistant plasmids, and antimicrobial-resistant salmonellae from animal sources have caused outbreaks in humans.[4] Transfer of antimicrobial resistance from *Salmonella* to other bacteria has been documented.[5] A multidrug-resistant strain of *Salmonella* Typhimurium called definitive type 104 (DT104) has recently emerged as an increasingly important cause of *Salmonella* infections in the United Kingdom and the United States.[6]

Clinical Characteristics

The most frequent symptoms of salmonellosis—diarrhea, abdominal cramps, pain, fever, headache, nausea, and vomiting—do not easily distinguish salmonellosis from many other causes of gastroenteritis. The illness results from bacterial invasion, predominantly of the ileum, which explains the frequent occurrence of fever and generalized symptoms. In addition to gastroenteritis, *Salmonella* infections may occasionally result in a septicemic illness resembling typhoid and described as enteric fever. Persons with human immunodeficiency virus (HIV) infections and other immunocompromising conditions are particularly prone to develop bloodstream infections, which may recur after apparently adequate therapy. Occasionally, localization of the salmonellae may lead to an abscess, meningitis, osteomyelitis, and other inflammatory conditions. Many infections are not associated with clinical illness. Following gastrointestinal infection, the median duration of enteric carriage is approximately 5 weeks.[7] Children, especially infants, have longer periods of carriage than other age groups. Antimicrobials are indicated in the treatment of systemic illness; however, antimicrobial agents are not indicated for uncomplicated gastroenteritis because they do not shorten the illness and actually prolong bacterial shedding.[8] For severe salmonellosis, the most effective antibiotic is a fluoroquinolone, such as ciprofloxacin. In the United States a fluoroquinolone antibiotic has re-

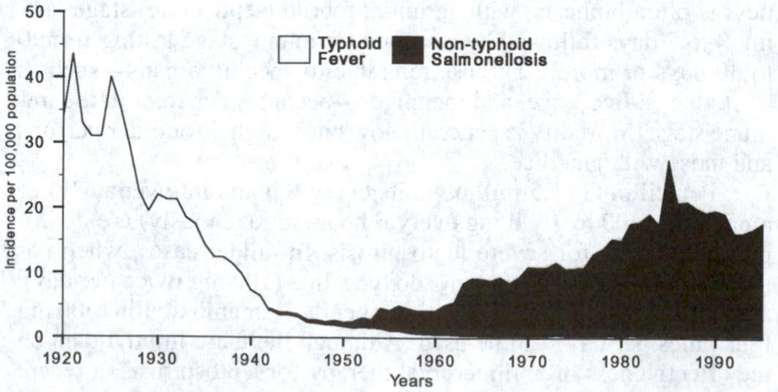

Figure 14-3. Reported combined incidence of typhoid fever and non-typhoid salmonellosis in the United States from 1920 to 1995.

TABLE 14-3. THE 10 MOST COMMON SEROTYPES IDENTIFIED AMONG HUMAN *SALMONELLA* INFECTIONS IN 1980 AND 1995

1980			1995		
Serotype	*No. of Isolates*	*Percentage*	*Serotype*	*No. of Isolates*	*Percentage*
Typhimurium	10,443	34.8	Enteritidis	10,201	24.7
Heidelberg	1,075	6.6	Typhimurium	9,702	23.5
Enteritidis	1,904	6.4	Newport	2,566	6.2
Newport	1,651	5.5	Heidelberg	2,095	5.1
Infantis	1,428	4.8	Hadar	812	2.0
Agona	1,402	4.7	Javiana	758	1.8
Saint Paul	757	2.5	Muenchen	754	1.8
Montevideo	665	2.2	Montevideo	685	1.7
Typhi	605	2.0	Agona	683	1.7
Oranienberg	503	1.7	Thompson	625	1.5
Other	8,671	28.9	Other	12,341	29.9
Total	30,004		Total	41,222	

cently been approved for use in animals; this may lead to the development of fluoroquinolone-resistant *Salmonella* in humans.

Case fatality rates are usually low, but infants, the aged, and the immunosuppressed often become seriously ill. The incubation period is most often between 6 and 48 hours, although long incubation periods (over 10 days) have been documented.

Diagnosis

The laboratory diagnosis is made by culture of feces on one of the standard selective media, followed by determination of biochemical reactions and by specific agglutination with polyvalent and monovalent typing sera by the simplified method described by Edwards and Ewing.[9] In the septicemic, typhoidal, and other extraintestinal forms, the organism may be recovered from the blood or from a site of focal infection. Although serological response may occur to the O and H antigens of the infecting *Salmonella*, they are not useful routinely in diagnosis because of nonspecific cross-reaction with other infectious agents.

Transmission

Infections in humans are often related directly or indirectly to infection in animals. Before its distribution was banned in 1975, the small pet turtle was the single most commonly identified source of salmonellosis in the United States.[10] In recent years, rare serotypes of *Salmonella* have caused illness in young children exposed to pet iguanas, snakes, and other reptiles. In most instances direct contact with these reptiles was not necessary for transmission.[11] Infections in animals may be initiated when animal feed or feed supplements are contaminated with salmonellae. Infections in animals are often restricted to the intestinal tract, but occasionally involve systemic lymph nodes. Contamination of meat before or during slaughter can lead to human infection if meat is cooked only superficially. Infections may be amplified when herds are stressed during moving or holding before slaughter and, subsequently, within the slaughterhouses themselves.[12] Salmonellae infect cattle, pigs, fowl, and other vertebrates and enter the human food chain on raw meat brought into the kitchen. Cross-contamination by uncooked food or inadequate cooking of food may then lead to human infection. Salmonellae often are found in unpasteurized milk.[13] Although eggs, meat, and poultry have traditionally been the most common vehicles, fruits and vegetables have been implicated as the vehicles in several recent salmonellosis outbreaks.[14–16] *Salmonella* serotype Enteritidis has become the most common serotype in the United States; between 1976 and 1994, the proportion of reported *Salmonella* isolates that were this serotype increased from 5 to 26 percent.[17] Consumption of raw and undercooked shell eggs is the dominant source of sporadic and outbreak-associated cases of *Salmonella* Enteritidis infections.[18–20] This serotype can cause a chronic ovarian infection in hens and can invade the egg contents before the shell is formed. A particular subtype of *Salmonella* Enteritidis, phage type 4, has become the endemic strain in Western Europe.[21] It has been suggested that this phage type may be more infectious to chickens, and once introduced into a flock it may replace all other *Salmonella* Enteritidis phage types.[22] In 1993, *Salmonella* Enteritidis, phage type 4 caused two human disease outbreaks in Texas.[23] By 1994, phage type 4 emerged in commercial layer flocks in California and has caused human disease outbreaks in California and Utah.[24–26]

In outbreaks, in which only a small proportion of exposed persons may be infected, the estimated oral dose of *Salmonella* necessary to initiate a human infection has been low ($<10^3$ organisms).[27] However, volunteer studies have suggested that a large dose ($>10^6$ organisms) of *Salmonella* is generally necessary to initiate infection in most persons. This high dose may explain the low frequency of secondary illnesses in households where a primary case is identified. The virulence of the organism, the nature of the vehicle, and host factors, such as underlying disease and reduced gastric acidity in infants and the elderly may increase the risk of infection, even with a low infectious dose. Use of antibiotics for other reasons shortly before or during exposure increases the susceptibility of the host to infection with resistant strains by reducing competitive flora and lowering the infectious dose.[4]

A mean of 110 food-borne outbreaks of salmonellosis was reported to the Centers for Disease Control and Prevention each year during the period 1988 to 1992; 38 percent occurred in restaurants or cafeterias. Eggs, poultry, meat, and dairy products were the most commonly reported food vehicles. These outbreaks typically resulted from mishandled foods of animal origin. Inadequate cooking, cross-contamination, and prolonged holding at inappropriate temperatures were the usual contributing food handling errors.

Although food handlers often are found to be infected in the course of an investigation, this is generally because they ate the contaminated foods; they are more likely to be victims than sources of the contamination.[28]

Nosocomial Salmonellosis

Outbreaks of salmonellosis in hospitals and nursing homes are associated with especially high mortality.[29–31] Such outbreaks appear to have become less common in recent years and, when they occur, are often the result of food-borne transmission. Good routine infection control and handwashing procedures can reduce transmission from caregivers to patients, and thus make person-to-person transmission less likely. Because of the extreme susceptibility of newborns, intensive care patients, and those with immunosuppressive conditions, special precautions are warranted to prevent transmission to these patients.

Salmonellae can spread among patients in a ward, either by person-to-person contact or occasionally by fomites. Fomites have included dust, delivery room resuscitators, bedside tables and cribs, thermometers, waterbaths, suction tubing, and endoscopes. The common vehicles identified in institutional outbreaks are most often foods but occasionally have included medicinal and pharmaceutical products of animal origin, such as carmine dye, pancreatin, pepsin, bile salts, gelatin, vitamins, extracts of various tissues, and transfused platelets. Outbreaks in nurseries often are preceded by an episode of diarrhea in the mother of the index case infant.[32]

Occurrence

Approximately 40,000 *Salmonella* isolations are reported annually in the United States.[1] The highest reported infection rates occur in children 1 to 4 years of age.[1] Approximations of the number of cases actually occurring in the United States, extrapolated from data developed during studies of outbreaks, suggest that there are 30 to 100 persons clinically ill for every *Salmonella* isolate reported.[33] Thus it is probable that 1 to 4 million cases of salmonellosis actually occur annually in the United States.

Regular seasonal changes in the incidence of salmonellosis generally have been observed in all countries studied, but the pattern varies with the serotype, vehicle, mode of spread, and local circumstances.[34] The reasons for seasonality are poorly understood but may include increased transmission among food animals, heavier contamination at slaughter plants, and greater opportunity for rapid bacterial growth should refrigeration be inadequate in the warmer months. The age-specific incidence varies considerably by serotype, probably because different serotypes contaminate different food vehicles.[34] The annual frequency of individual serotypes is not stable, since single serotypes can rapidly gain importance after introduction into the food chain. For example, *Salmonella* serotype Agona emerged as a dominant serotype worldwide after it was introduced into poultry feed on contaminated fishmeal in the early 1970s.[35] *Salmonella* Enteritidis currently is increasing rapidly on four continents as a result of widespread infection of poultry flocks.[36]

Some *Salmonella* serotypes are highly host specific (*Salmonella* Dublin in cattle, *Salmonella* Choleraesuis in pigs, *Salmonella* Pullorum in poultry, and *Salmonella* Typhi in humans), whereas others have very broad host ranges. Some salmonellae are restricted to certain geographical areas, whereas others are global. Some serotypes are frequent in a particular region or state in the United States (e.g., *Salmonella* Weltevreden in Hawaii).

Prevention

Since the majority of human infections occur directly or indirectly through food, control measures are most effective when applied somewhere along the food chain or in preventing *Salmonella* from entering the kitchen.

Salmonellae are frequent contaminants of animal feeds, and efforts have been made to prevent *Salmonella* from infecting food animals. The high cost of such efforts has limited their use in the past except in a few Scandinavian countries, but the steady increase in salmonellosis in many countries has led to increased interest in these methods.[32] Prohibiting the sale of *Salmonella*-contaminated pet turtles in the United States led to reduction in disease associated with this vehicle.[10] However, beyond the pasteurization of milk and the regulation of precooked beef, the control of *Salmonella* contamination in foods has not yet been generally effective in the United States. Attempts to reduce the frequency of antimicrobial-resistant *Salmonella* have been initiated in many countries in Europe by restricting the use of antimicrobials in animal feed.

Inspecting food service areas to ensure that food-handling procedures are well understood, refrigeration is adequate, storage facilities are appropriate, and handwashing is frequent is a critical part of preventing salmonellosis outbreaks. Control of *Salmonella* in food handlers is difficult to achieve because excretion of *Salmonella* may be prolonged, and no treatment regimen has been shown to reduce carriage. Although many health departments recommend special prevention measures, control of salmonellosis by procedures directed at food handlers is probably most effectively addressed by educating them in good personal hygiene and proper food-handling practices. For infected persons working in hospitals, restriction of their contact with patients is prudent, although transmission from hospital personnel to patients is rarely documented. Patients excreting *Salmonella* should be managed with routine enteric precautions.

It is unlikely that the incidence of salmonellosis in humans can be reduced significantly with the control measures currently used. A better understanding of the ecology of *Salmonella* in animals is needed to improve current prevention strategies for human salmonellosis. Studies to determine risk factors for *Salmonella* infection in farm animals and to characterize farms where infected herds are found would be helpful in formulating effective prevention measures. Irradiation of foods of animal origin has also been suggested by the World Health Organization and the U.S. Public Health Service as a future general control measure.[37,38]

Protozoa

Toxoplasmosis

Robert G. Yaeger • Jack K. Frenkel

The etiologic agent of toxoplasmosis is *Toxoplasma gondii*, one of the most common protozoan parasites of humans. Although the organism was described and named early in this century, human infection was not recognized until three decades later. Before 1969, numerous surveys demonstrated that this parasite was found worldwide and in a wide range of warm-blooded hosts. Furthermore, it was shown that infection in humans was highly prevalent in many areas. Yet it was not until 1970 that the taxonomic position and the life cycle of *T. gondii* were elucidated.[1]

Life Cycle and Modes of Transmission

The three forms of the protozoan—the tachyzoite, the bradyzoite, and the sporozoite—are similar in appearance, being crescent shaped and 4 to 8 μm long. The tachyzoites (Fig. 14-4) are the rapidly proliferating intracellular forms seen in many tissues and organs during the acute phase of infection. Bradyzoites occur in cysts (Fig. 14-5) and are formed primarily in brain, eye, heart muscle, and skeletal muscle. Bradyzoites multiply slowly and persist in tissues for many years, possibly for the life of the host. The sporozoite occurs in the mature

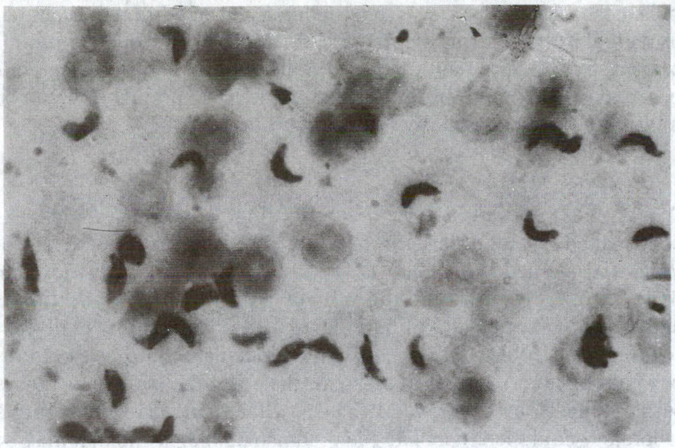

Figure 14-4. Tachyzoites of *Toxoplasma gondii* in smear of mouse peritoneal fluid. (Giemsa stain, ×1200)

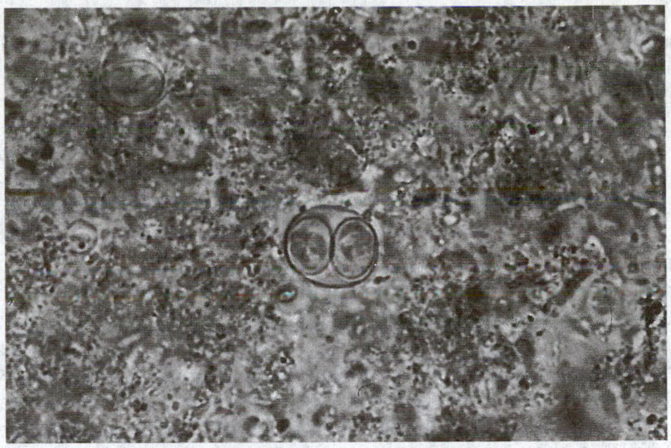

Figure 14-6. Sporulated oocyst of *Toxoplasma gondii* containing two sporocysts, each with four sporozoites. (×1,200)

oocyst (Fig. 14-6). It is the stage resulting from the sexual reproduction phase, which takes place in the small intestine of cats. Tachyzoites and bradyzoites occur in all hosts susceptible to this infection, but oocysts occur only in felines, where they develop during the sexual phase of the enteroepithelial cycle.

Cats usually acquire infection by ingesting bradyzoites in fresh tissues and rarely from tachyzoites or sporulated oocysts. Kittens are more susceptible than older cats. The prepatent period of infection—that is, the time between ingestion of infective stages and the passage of oocysts in the feces—may be as short as 3 to 10 days when bradyzoites are ingested or between 21 and 40 days if either tachyzoites or mature oocysts are eaten. Cats that have recovered from toxoplasmosis may become reinfected if exposed, but their immunity generally arrests the infection before oocyst formation.

Hosts other than cats usually become infected in the same manner—by ingestion of infective stages. However, there is no enteroepithelial cycle leading to the production of oocysts in nonfelines.

After initial infection of the intestinal wall, the parasites spread to extraintestinal sites, where intracellular multiplication of tachyzoites takes place. Rupture of infected cells releases tachyzoites, which infect nearby cells or are carried to other sites by body fluids to repeat the cycle. Hosts whose immune system has not been compromised usually survive the acute phase without specific therapy, whereupon tachyzoites disappear and bradyzoite-containing cysts form in the tissues, mainly the brain and muscle. This chronic or latent infection may persist for the life of the host.

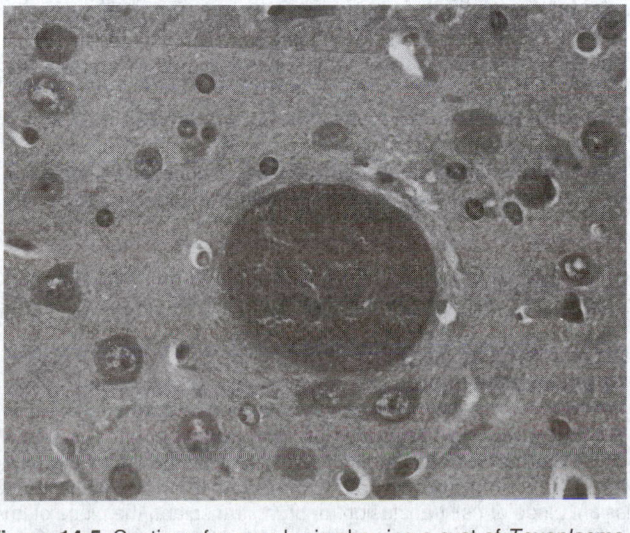

Figure 14-5. Section of mouse brain showing a cyst of *Toxoplasma gondii* containing hundreds of bradyzoites. (Hematoxylin and eosin stain, ×480)

Although ingestion of infective material is the principal mode of transmission for *Toxoplasma* in humans, others are known. In fact, the disease was first recognized in transplacentally infected babies, where it may have serious consequences. Parasitemia occurs primarily during the acute stage of toxoplasmosis, and although transmission via blood transfusion can be considered possible, the risk from normal donors is apparently slight.[1] Acquisition of *T. gondii* infection from donor organs has been reported in transplant recipients and probably resulted from persistent tissue cysts.[2]

Clinical Characteristics

Postnatally acquired toxoplasmosis is usually asymptomatic or has such mild transient manifestations that it goes unrecognized. This is substantiated by the high prevalence of seropositive individuals with no history of a diagnosed infection with this protozoon. The most common feature in the immunocompetent host is local or generalized lymphadenopathy, which must be differentiated from lymphomas such as Hodgkin's disease.[3] Tender cervical nodes are often accompanied by fever, sore throat, myalgia, a maculopapular rash sparing the palms and soles, abdominal pain from enlarged retroperitoneal nodes, hepatosplenomegaly, and atypical lymphocytosis suggestive of infectious mononucleosis. With rare exceptions, symptoms resolve over a period of several weeks without chemotherapy, although lymphadenopathy may persist for many months. Studies in laboratory animals have demonstrated the persistence of cysts in brain and skeletal muscle for long periods after the initial mild acute stage, but data on the proportion of recovered human cases with persistent cysts are not available. In a few instances the acute infection was accompanied by pneumonitis, myocarditis, pericarditis, hepatitis, polymyositis, encephalitis, meningoencephalitis, and ocular manifestations of acute retinochoroiditis. Whether these patients with illness were immunocompetent was not reported in most of these cases. It has been estimated that only 10 to 20 percent of immunocompetent individuals are symptomatic during mild acute infections. In adolescents and adults, retinochoroiditis may be the only manifestation of toxoplasmosis, and most of these infections are believed to have been congenitally acquired. The lesions, which may be unilateral or bilateral, occur as recurrent active infection consisting of an active lesion without a scar, as old scars with active satellite lesions, or as inactive scars.

Congenital toxoplasmosis may occur when a woman acquires her initial infection during pregnancy. Although the infection is usually inapparent in the woman, the lesions in the fetus show a wide degree of severity, depending on the gestational age at which transplacental transmission occurred. Results can be (*a*) a spontaneous abortion of a severely damaged fetus, (*b*) a fully developed stillborn infant with evidence of severe lesions, (*c*) a live infant with classic signs, such as hydrocephalus or microcephalus, cerebral calcifications, and retinochoroiditis, or (*d*) a seemingly normal infant who fails to thrive and in whom retinochoroiditis or other symptoms of central nervous system involvement may develop later.[4] Evidence suggests that if a woman becomes infected a few weeks before conception, it is unlikely that the infant will be born infected. Since physical examinations and antibody titers of infants born to women who acquired *Toxoplasma* infection during pregnancy may be inconclusive, these infants should be observed over a period of up to 10 years for the development of antibody, or for the development of lesions such as retinochoroiditis, or for cerebral calcifications. If a child is found to be infected, prompt therapy should be given to prevent more serious injury to the brain and retina.[5,6]

The persistence of *T. gondii* in the tissues of individuals who have recovered from a primary infection, together with the high percentage of such individuals in many populations, has become another problem for AIDS patients. The development of immunodeficiency in these individuals may result in a recrudescence, and the latent or chronic infection reverts to the acute stage. It has been estimated that toxoplasmic encephalitis will develop in about 30 percent of AIDS patients in the United States who are seropositive for the organism.[7] Furthermore, individuals who acquire HIV infection and who have not been infected previously with *Toxoplasma* are more likely to develop a severe primary infection with this organism. Toxoplasmic encephalitis is a life-threatening complication that has been seen more frequently in AIDS patients in recent years.[7] In some instances the CNS symptoms occurred before a diagnosis of HIV infection was made. Ocular lesions are less common than encephalitis but can lead to blindness. The prognosis is poor if the patient is in a coma when first seen. Involvement of other organs has also been described occasionally.

Epidemiology

Most *Toxoplasma* infections are acquired by the ingestion of infective stages; that is, tissue forms in undercooked meat or oocysts passed into the environment by felines from 4 to 15 days after infection. Cats usually cover their feces, thus protecting the oocysts, which measure 10 by 13 μm and may remain viable for up to a year. An area where cats abound may be continually contaminated with infective oocysts as generations of cats inhabit the area. Although cats can become reinfected, evidence suggests that in subsequent infections oocysts are not passed, or only a few are passed, if a previous infection resulted in oocyst production. Thus cats that had been infected previously have some degree of immunity.

Parasitemia is transient during acute toxoplasmosis. Hence, infection via transfusion of whole blood or cells occurs rarely, if ever. Patients who receive organ transplants may acquire *T. gondii* infection from the donor organ, or they may suffer from recrudescence of their latent infection as a result of antirejection immunosuppressive therapy.[8]

Serologic surveys have shown that up to 95 percent of various populations have been infected with *Toxoplasma*. Such studies have shown that the percentage of seropositive individuals increases with age, indicating continued exposure throughout life. The presence of cats has also been associated with a higher percentage of seropositive individuals. The prevalence of infection is highest in hot, humid climates and lowest in dry or cold climates, as well as at high altitudes. A 10-year study in Panama showed that antibody prevalence rose from 25 percent at 5 years of age to 50 percent at 10 years and increased gradually, reaching 90 percent by 60 years of age.[9] In a collaborative project involving 12 university medical centers located throughout the United States, an analysis of antibody titers to *Toxoplasma* for 22,845 pregnant women was conducted in relation to clinical and laboratory findings in the mothers and children through 7 years of age.[10] Based on more than 900 observations considered for each mother and child, the major findings were in children and included a doubling in predicted frequency of deafness and a 60 percent increase in microcephaly among children born to women with antibody to *Toxoplasma*. A high antibody titer (1:256 to 512) in the mothers was associated with a 30 percent increase in low IQ (below 70).

Toxoplasma is one of the most common protozoan parasites of humans. Survival as a species is ensured because (*a*) it does not usually kill its host; (*b*) it infects a wide range of hosts; (*c*) it can persist in its host for many years so that predators can acquire infection; (*d*) its natural hosts, various members of the cat family, produce millions of oocysts, which remain infective in the environment for long periods; and (*e*) (although of lesser epidemiologic importance) it can be transmitted transplacentally in certain hosts (Fig.14-7).

Diagnosis

A diagnosis can be made by demonstrating the characteristic crescent-shaped zoites in tissue imprints or CSF made from patient material and stained with Giemsa. Biopsies of bone marrow, lymph nodes, brain, placenta, and other involved tissues can be sectioned and stained with hematoxylin to identify the spherical nuclei of *Toxoplasma*. Material from patients can be inoculated into cell cultures or weanling mice in an effort to isolate the protozoa. In most instances serologic tests are employed because of the difficulty of locating a laboratory equipped to isolate the organism and the time that may be required to accomplish this task. The dye test (DT), the conventional indirect fluorescent antibody test (IFAT), and the direct agglutination test (DAT) detect IgG antibody. Titers rise soon and reach higher levels (greater than 1:1,000). Usually, peak titers are reached within 3 months, begin to fall within a year, and reach a stable, low level in 2 or 3 years. Patients from highly endemic areas, such as the low-lying areas of Latin America, maintain higher titers (greater than 1,000) probably because of more frequent reinfections, which in the United States may be misdiagnosed as indicating active infection.

In all suspected cases of acute toxoplasmosis a test for IgM *Toxoplasma* antibody should be performed.[11] If the test is positive and rising, if it is confirmed by an IgG test for *Toxoplasma* antibody, and if the clinical course is compatible with toxoplasmosis, further tests are probably unnecessary. The indirect fluorescent antibody test for IgM (IgM-IFAT) can give false-positive and false-negative results.

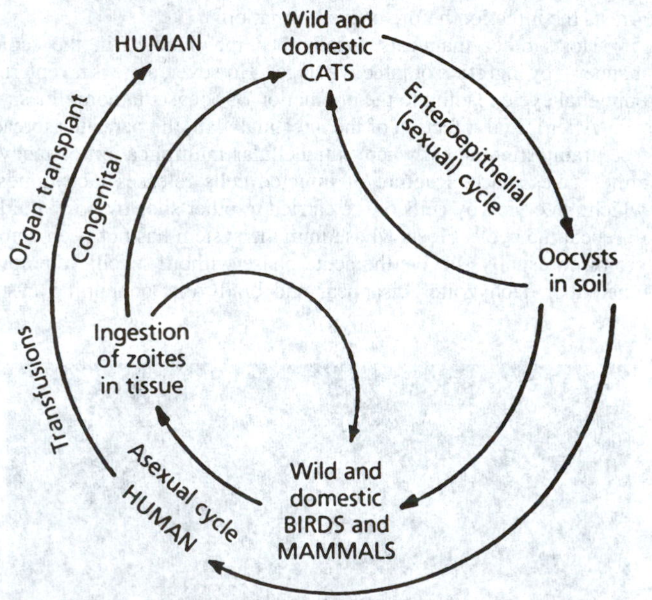

Figure 14-7. Transmission of *Toxoplasma* in nature involves two main cycles: (*a*) from cats to intermediate hosts and back to cats and to humans through fecal contamination of the environment with oocysts that are generated during the enteroepithelial cycle in the cat, mature in the outside environment, and are taken up in contaminated foods or water, and (*b*) from intermediate hosts to cats and to intermediate hosts (and humans) when zoites (tachyzoites and bradyzoites, generally the latter) that are generated in extraintestinal tissues by asexual reproduction (endodyogeny) are ingested. Except for congenital transmission, blood or cell transfusion, or organ transplant, the place of humans in either of these two cycles is that of a dead-end intermediate host. Predation and cannibalism among intermediate hosts, though not essential to enzooticity, are factors of great significance.

An antibody capture test circumvents this problem. The double-sandwich IgM enzyme-linked immunosorbent assay (DS IgM-ELISA) has been recommended for acquired and congenital toxoplasmosis. A modification of the test, claimed to be more sensitive and specific than the immunofluorescence assay, requires only 2 hours to complete.[12] False-negative results may be obtained when rheumatoid factor or antinuclear antibody is present. If the serologic test results are equivocal, the test should be repeated after 2 weeks or more. A serial two-tube or greater rise in titer with any serologic test usually establishes a diagnosis of acute infection. In some instances it may be advisable to submit a serum sample to a reference laboratory.

Serologic tests are unreliable in immunosuppressed patients, and diagnostic tests for Toxoplasma DNA are most useful in such patients. Several *Toxoplasma* primers are available and are quite effective in using the polymerase chain reaction (PCR) technique to detect *Toxoplasma* DNA in involved tissues and fluids.[13,14] However, both positive PCR and serologic results need to be linked to the presence of active infection, because of the persistence of *Toxoplasma* cysts and antibody in asymptomatic chronic latent infections. Histologic study of a tissue biopsy can often help to distinguish active from latent toxoplasmosis.

Treatment

Most immunologically competent individuals recover from the acute phase of toxoplasmosis without chemotherapy. In the presence of illness, combinations of pyrimethamine with either sulfadiazine or trisulfapyrimidines have been shown to be effective. Where these are unavailable, the fixed combination of trimethoprim with sulfamethoxazole has been used. Specific inhibition of the parasite's folate-metabolizing enzymes is the mode of action of these combinations. Frequent differential blood and platelet counts are required to check for bone marrow toxicity. Folinic acid (not folic acid), given in dosages of 5 to 15 mg/d or higher if necessary, has been employed to counteract toxicity without impairing the chemotherapeutic effect.[7] If the patient has a hypersensitivity reaction to the pyrimethamine-sulfonamide combination, most often it is to the sulfonamide component, and pyrimethamine plus clindamycin can be substituted.[15] Treatment during pregnancy and of the newborn and infant have been successfully carried out in immunocompetent individuals, although this treatment does not eliminate the parasite completely.[4,16–18]

In a patient with AIDS, recrudescence or a newly acquired toxoplasmic infection generally requires chemotherapy until significant clinical improvement has been achieved. Thereafter, maintenance therapy in lower doses is necessary for the life of an AIDS patient, or as long as he or she remains immunosuppressed. Reactivation and progression of ocular or cerebral toxoplasmic lesions in AIDS patients after the discontinuation of therapy has been reported.[6] Empirical treatment of suspected *Toxoplasma* encephalitis based on radiographic findings has been satisfactory, thereby avoiding a brain biopsy.[15]

Preventive Measures

Even though clinical toxoplasmosis is likely to be more severe (and therefore prevention more important) in the immunosuppressed patient, the preventive measures are identical for both immunocompetent and immunosuppressed individuals. Although hard freezing of meat kills most *Toxoplasma* stages, there is no assurance that an occasional organism will not survive. Meat can be safe only if it has been thoroughly heated during cooking, until the color changes and the juices are clear. It is essential that meat be completely thawed and that the thicker cuts be sufficiently heated. Women who are seronegative to *Toxoplasma* should take precautions to avoid infection. Pregnant women in particular should not eat raw meat in the belief that it is advantageous to the developing infant. Pregnant women should be admonished to *wash their hands* after contact with meat, soil, and outdoor cats and their litter boxes, and before eating. Because some dogs have the habit of eating or rolling in cat feces, hand washing after contact with dogs should also be recommended.[18] Contact with soil should be avoided by wearing gloves when working in the garden, and thoroughly scrubbing the hands, including under the nails, is advisable.

Cats do not recognize property lines, and a neighbor's cats may use the yard of another, especially if the soil is well cultivated for flowers or vegetables. Children's sandboxes should be covered when not in use. Ideally, cat box litter should be bagged daily for disposal. Only cooked meat, dried food, or canned food should be fed to cats. Stray cats should be controlled. If possible, house cats should wear bells to diminish their chances of catching rodents and birds, becoming infected, and leaving millions of infectious oocysts in yards, flower beds, or children's sandboxes.

Transmission through blood transfusion or organ transplantation should be of concern if the recipient is immunocompromised; donor's and recipient's blood should be serologically tested.

Two types of vaccines have been developed: one to immunize humans (such as seronegative transplant recipients) and meat animals, and another to vaccinate cats against oocyst shedding.[20,21] Both vaccines are live and need to be kept frozen until used. In New Zealand and England a vaccine similar to the first one is used to immunize sheep against abortion from toxoplasmosis. Efforts are under way to develop stable recombinant vaccines.

Helminths

Trichinellosis

K. Darwin Murrell • Fabrizio Bruschi

Trichinellosis is caused by the larval stage of nematodes of the genus *Trichinella*, of which until recently only a single species, *Trichinella spiralis*, was known. Over the past two decades, new knowledge of this disease's epidemiology has been obtained, revealing a transmission pattern that can involve domestic swine, horses, and wild animals. New genetic data have also resulted in the creation of a new taxonomy for *Trichinella*, one that includes five species rather than one (Table 14-4).[1] This revised taxonomy, based on genetic and ecological differences, has helped to increase the understanding of clinical differences in the disease caused by different *Trichinella* species. Although *T. spiralis* remains the most important pork-borne species, a significant proportion of all human cases are derived from wild game and horses; *Trichinella nativa* and *Trichinella britovi* are important species in this epidemiology.[2]

Life Cycle

All stages in the life cycle of *Trichinella* occur in individual mammalian hosts. When skeletal muscle containing the infective larvae is ingested by another mammal, the larvae are released by the action of gastric fluids and pass into the small intestine. There, the parasites molt four times before becoming sexually mature. After copulation, the females begin to expel newborn larvae (NBL) about 6 or 7 days after infection. This process continues for the life of the female. Although it is generally believed that the adult worms may persist in the intestine for only several weeks, there is evidence that they may survive for much longer periods, especially if the host's immune system is compromised.[3] Most of the NBL penetrate into the submucosa and are carried in the circulatory system to various organs, including the myocardium, brain, lungs, retina, lymph nodes, pancreas, and cerebrospinal fluid. However, only the larvae that invade the skeletal muscle survive. They gradually encyst and develop into the infective stage about 21 to 30 days after infection. Larval infectivity can be retained for many years, depending on the species of mammalian host. The larvae appear to be nonpathogenic for the natural hosts (excluding humans) unless very large numbers are involved.

Epidemiology

Trichinosis is a cosmopolitan disease with over 100 different animal species capable of being infected. There are two transmission patterns. Sylvatic trichinellosis is a state in which the parasite cycles among wild carnivores. Domestic trichinellosis cycles among humans, rats, and pigs. The most important source of infection for humans is the flesh of swine, game, and horse meat. Pigs and rats can become infected by feeding on infected pork waste in garbage or by consuming infected animal carcasses (including pigs). The importance of wild animal reservoirs is often underappreciated. In the United States, one-third to one-half of human cases are caused by consumption of infected game; in Europe, nearly all cases are due to wild game. In Asia, human infection may follow the same pattern. For example, in Thailand, infected pork has been the cause of most infections (*T. spiralis*) but in an outbreak in Thailand 59 people were infected with *Trichinella pseudospiralis* after consumption of raw meat from a feral pig. Surprisingly, over the past 20 years, Europe has experienced six large outbreaks due to infected horsemeat, a heretofore unrecognized source of infection.[4] Three outbreaks occurred in France in 1976 (125 patients) and two in 1985 (400 and 980 patients), and one in 1993 (200 patients). Three outbreaks occurred in Italy, one in 1976 (96 patients), one in 1984 (13 patients), and another in 1986 (300 patients).[2] Four of the outbreaks were shown to be due to *T. britovi*, one to *T. nativa*, and one to *T. spiralis*. In the Arctic, *T. nativa* is a common parasite of terrestrial carnivores and, less frequently, of marine mammals (Pinnipedia). As indicated in Table 14-4, this species has the unusual ability to retain its infectivity after long exposure to freezing temperatures. Bear meat is a very common source of infection for humans, and single-source outbreaks due to sharing of large animals are not uncommon.[4,5]

The worldwide incidence of human trichinellosis has declined substantially over the past few decades, but outbreaks are still frequent, especially in developing regions (Table 14-5).[2] In developed countries, the epidemiology of human trichinellosis is typified by urban common-source outbreaks. In the United States, the largest human outbreaks have occurred among ethnic groups with preferences for raw or only partially cooked pork. Infected meat is typically purchased from local supermarkets, butcher shops, or other commercial outlets.

Foreign travelers also account for some cases of human trichinellosis. Twenty-six cases occurred from 1975 to 1989 in the United States, most of them after travel to Mexico or Asia. Globally, the prevalence of *T. spiralis* in domestic swine ranges from less than 0.001 percent (United States) to 25 percent or more (e.g., some regions of China). The global rise in consumer demand for greater quality assurance in food is also normally found in domestic pigs.

The Disease

The severity of the clinical course depends on parasitic factors such as the species involved and the number of larvae ingested and host factors such as sex, age, and ethnic group.[2] Immune status also plays an important role. Prolonged diarrhea in the absence of myalgia, as reported in elderly Inuit people, may be due to an acquired immunity against the parenteral stages of the parasite, and weak intestinal immunity.[6] The disease incubation period ranges from 7 to 30 days, again depending on the severity of infection. When severe, the incubation period may be briefer. The clinical course of the acute period of infection is characterized by two phases, an *enteral phase* in which the parasite alters intestinal function and a *parenteral phase*, which is associated with an inflammatory and allergic response to muscle invasion by the larval parasites.[7]

Gastrointestinal signs appear first, a result of mucosal invasion by the first-generation (ingested) larvae. These signs typically last 2 to 7 days but may persist for weeks. Subsequently, fever, myalgia, periorbital edema, and eosinophilia—which constitute the so-called

TABLE 14-4. BIOLOGICAL AND ZOOGEOGRAPHICAL CHARACTERISTICS OF THE SPECIES OF *TRICHINELLA*

	Trichinella spiralis	*Trichinella nativa*	*Trichinella nelsoni*	*Trichinella britovi*	*Trichinella pseudospiralis*
Infectivity for:					
Humans	High	High	High	Moderate	Moderate(?)
Swine	High	Low	Low	Low	Low
Rats	High	Low	Low	Low	Moderate
Mice	High	Low	Low	Low	Moderate
Chickens	No	No	No	No	Yes
Pathogenicity for humans	High	High	Low	Moderate	Low-Moderate
Resistance to freezing	Low	High	Low	Low	Low
Nurse cell development (in days)	16–37	20–30	34–60	24–42	Absent (no capsule forms around L_1)
Distribution	Cosmopolitan	Arctic	Equatorial Africa	Temperate	Cosmopolitan
Major host reservoirs	Suidae *Rattus*	Ursidae Canidae	Hyaenidae Felidae	Suidae Canidae	Mammals Birds
Availability of diagnostic DNA probes	Yes	Yes	Yes	Yes	Yes
Unique alloenzyme markers	6	2	4	1	12

See Pozio et al[1]

TABLE 14-5. EXAMPLES OF RECENT OUTBREAKS OF HUMAN TRICHINELLOSIS

Country	*Date*	*No. of Cases*	*Source*
USA	1970–90	1820	Pork, game
Canada	1970–85	924	Polar bear, walrus
Argentina	1992	151	Pork
Lebanon	1981–82	1100	Pork
Egypt	1975	51	Pork
Ethiopia	1990	20	Wild boar
China			
Yunnan Pr.	1983	5558	Pork, bear, other?
Henan Pr.	1992	167	Pork
Heilongjiang	1981	147	Mutton?
Thailand	1982–88	3052	Pork
France	1993	200	Horse meat
	1985	1073	Horse meat
Italy	1984–86	582	Wild boar, horse meat
Lithuania	1992	819	Pork, wild boar
Slovakia	1980	77	Wild boar
Poland	1982–86	1427	Pork, wild boar
Yugoslavia (former)	1983–85	1734	Pork

trichinellotic syndrome or general trichinellosis syndrome—begin. However, the acute phase, lasting 1 to 8 weeks, is commonly asymptomatic, especially when the number of larvae ingested is low. The clinical course of infection may be abortive (symptomatology not complete), mild (complete even if mild symptomatology), moderate, or severe (frequently associated with complications). Malaise, anorexia, nausea, vomiting, abdominal pain, fever, diarrhea, or constipation may occur. Diarrhea is more persistent than vomiting and may last up to 3 months and, when excessive, causes dehydration; this and enteritis are occasional causes of death. Muscles are mainly affected during the parenteral phase, but other organs such as the myocardium, central nervous system, lungs, kidney, skin, etc., may also be involved.[2] The trichinellotic or general trichinellosis syndrome is characterized by facial edema, muscle pain and swelling, weakness, and frequently fever; occurring less frequently are anorexia, headache, conjunctivitis, and urticaria. Fever, usually remittent, generally begins at 2 weeks and peaks after 4 weeks, with temperatures up to 40° to 41°C in severe cases. Despite fever, patients may appear in good condition. Ocular signs at this time may help in diagnosis, particularly edema of the eyelids, chemosis, conjunctivitis, conjunctival hemorrhages, disturbed vision, and ocular pain. Periorbital edema is peculiar to trichinellosis, with an occurrence ranging from 17 to 100 percent. The entire face may also be involved, giving the patients a characteristic aspect, often rendering them unrecognizable. At this time the muscles of the rest of the body usually become painful. Extraocular muscles, masseters, tongue and larynx muscles, diaphragm, neck muscles, and intercostal muscles are most frequently infected. The pain may be so severe as to limit the functionality of the arms and legs, inhibiting walking, speaking, moving the tongue, breathing, and swallowing. Weakness is also a consequence of the muscle involvement. The muscles become stiff and hard and present edema. Gastrointestinal symptoms may also extend into this phase.[8]

Neurologic manifestations, more common in severe infections when a great number of living larvae are ingested, occur in 10 to 24 percent of cases. Headache is very common in trichinellosis and is exacerbated by movements of the head. Myocarditis is the most frequent cardiovascular complication, leading sometimes to heart failure or bronchopneumonia; in some cases death occurs between the fourth and the eighth week of infection, although sudden death may occur even earlier. Electrocardiographic alterations are present from the second week and may persist up to the third or fourth week. Blood pressure is usually low during the early phase of infection and may also remain low during convalescence.

After the acute period, convalescence follows (lasting from months to years), usually with complete recovery. Over the succeeding few years, muscle larvae are slowly but completely destroyed, followed by calcification.

Because of improved therapy, death is now rare in trichinellosis. However, it may result from congestive heart failure due to myocarditis, encephalitis, pneumonitis, hypokalemia, adrenal gland insufficiency, and obstruction of blood vessel circulation.[8] In the United States, during the period from 1982 to 1986, of 57 annually reported trichinellosis cases, only three resulted in fatalities.[5]

Diagnosis

Diagnosis is difficult in low-level, sporadic infections because the resulting clinical manifestations are common to many other diseases, including chronic fatigue syndrome.[2,7] Differential diagnosis must be carried out in cases of food poisoning, sinusitis, typhoid fever, influenza, intolerance to pork meat, muscle rheumatism, cerebrospinal meningitis, dermatomyositis, periarteritis nodosa, eosinophilic leukemia, acute alcoholism, etc.[8] Trichinellosis should be considered in the differential diagnosis of myositis in patients with HIV infection. When the infection occurs in epizootic or outbreak form, its diagnosis is easier. Special care must be taken when developing clinical histories; particular attention should be paid to eating habits during the weeks before the onset of symptoms. Exposure to infected meat (raw or incompletely cooked), the presence of gastroenteritis, myalgia, facial edema, hemorrhages, etc., and an increase in blood eosinophils should suggest trichinellosis. Electromyography (EMG) may help in the diagnosis of moderate and severe infections during the acute period, even if the muscle changes are not pathognomonic. With clinical improvement, EMG changes generally disappear within 2 to 3 months, although these alterations may persist for 1 to 8 years.

A definitive diagnosis may be made when larvae are found in a muscle biopsy, generally performed in the deltoid muscle; although in humans other muscles are more infected, the deltoid is preferred because it is more accessible.[2] Muscle biopsy is recommended only in rare and difficult cases, particularly when serology is not clear. A negative result, however, does not exclude the presence of low-level infections. Artificial digestion (1 percent pepsin) of a muscle sample is more sensitive than direct microscopic observation of the tissue specimen, but, importantly, larvae cannot be isolated from muscle before 17 to 21 days of infection, because of their lack of resistance to digestion.

The diagnosis of trichinellosis is difficult in sporadic cases, but it is even more difficult when CNS involvement is present. Neurotrichinosis is sometimes accompanied by multifocal CNS lesions, nodular or ring-like, with diameter of 3 to 8 mm, and, in most of the cases, showing contrast enhancement.[9]

Eosinophilia, leukocytosis, serum muscle enzyme level increases, and an increase in immunoglobulin levels, especially total IgE, are the most characteristic laboratory findings of this disease. Eosinophil levels especially increase dramatically during trichinellosis (up to 8.700 per cubic millimeter).[7] The eosinophilia (based on the absolute number rather than the percentage) occurs in all cases of trichinellosis, even the subclinical; exceptions might be very severe infection with eosinopenia, a prediction of a fatal course of the disease. Eosinophilia may also be absent when bacterial infections complicate the disease.[8] After steroid therapy, eosinophil levels also decrease.[8] Leukocytosis, up to 24,000 cells per cubic millimeter, occurs in very severe infections, usually early in the infection.

Increased creatine phosphokinase (CPK), lactate dehydrogenase (LDH), aldolase, and aminotransferase levels reflect skeletal muscle damage, helping in diagnosis.[4] Serum CPK levels can increase up to more than 17,000 U/L.

Changes in immunoglobulin level may also occur, the most characteristic being increase in total IgE. However, an increase in total IgE level is not a consistent phenomenon, and it is not possible to exclude trichinellosis by its absence.

Many serologic tests are available for diagnosis.[2] Seroconversion usually occurs between the third and the fifth week of infection, and sera may remain positive up to 1 year or more after the cessation of the clinical symptomatology. Antibodies have been detected, however, up to 19 years after the end of the acute phase of infection.[6,9] Antibody levels do not correlate with the severity of the clinical course nor with a particular clinical course.

Indirect hemagglutination, bentonite flocculation, indirect immunofluorescence, latex agglutination, and enzyme-linked immunosorbent assay (ELISA) are the more commonly used tests, the last being the most sensitive.[4] The indirect immunofluorescence test is performed with whole L1 larvae killed in formalin, or with unfixed frozen sections of infected muscles. With this test all specific immunoglobulins can be evaluated. The ELISA method, using excretory/secretory antigens, is preferable to crude extracts of *T. spiralis* muscle larvae for soluble antigen because it is more specific. This is particularly important in tropical regions where cross-reactions with other helminth parasites can give false-positive results.[2]

When a diagnosis must be confirmed, methods such as ELISA-IgG, bentonite flocculation, or indirect immunofluorescence should be used. ELISA-IgG or IgM are also useful for epidemiologic studies.[2]

Treatment and Prognosis

It is difficult to differentiate the efficacy of drug therapy from natural recovery of infection in mild to moderate cases. Factors such as the species of *Trichinella* involved, host response, and the intensity and length of infection can aid in deciding the course of treatment.[8] Symptomatic treatment includes analgesic and antipyretic drugs, bed rest, and administration of corticosteroids (prednisolone at 50 mg per day), especially in severe infections, to prevent shock-like symptoms. Specific treatment with mebendazole (200 to 300 mg three times per day for 5 to 10 days) or albendazole (400 mg/day for 3 days, even followed by 800 mg/day for 15 days), or thiabendazole (50 mg/kg for 5 days) is recommended for intestinal and muscle stages, but light infections do not require treatment. The treatment goal for the very early infection phase is to limit muscle invasion by larvae; when this has already occurred the goal is to reduce muscle damage, responsible for the major clinical manifestations. Therapeutic plasma levels of the drug should be maintained for an extended period, rather than high levels for short periods. The success of treatment is evident from clinical improvement of the patient's symptoms.

Prevention and Control

Control of swine trichinellosis and prevention of human infection has both direct and indirect aspects. Mandatory inspection of pork at slaughter, while common among developed countries, especially Europe, is not required in the United States. In developing countries, testing for trichinellosis as part of routine inspection is rare. Instead, emphasis is placed on educating the consumer on safe handling and cooking of pork and wild game. The U.S. Department of Agriculture (USDA) has established recommended procedures for devitalizing any muscle larvae present in these meats by cooking or freezing. For example, the consumer should cook pork until all pink color has disappeared, which normally occurs at about 137°F; to allow for a margin of error, however, it is recommended that the internal temperature of meat should uniformly reach 160°F throughout.

Fresh pork less than 6 inches thick can be rendered safe if frozen to 5°F (–17°C) for 20 days, –10°F (–23°C) for 10 days, or –20°F (–29°C) for 6 days. Because of the freeze resistance shown by *T. nativa*, freezing of meat from game is not completely reliable.[1] Infection from wild animal meat accounts for an important proportion of human trichinellosis; therefore, the inspection of wild game muscle is to be recommended and is mandatory in some European countries. Consumers should also be warned of the danger and be advised on proper meat handling and preparation procedures.

The control of trichinellosis in swine relies on good general management practices.[10] For example, pork producers are encouraged to observe federal garbage feeding regulations in states where this practice is allowed, to practice stringent rodent control, to avoid exposing pigs to dead animal carcasses of any kind, to ensure that hog carcasses are properly disposed, and to try to establish effective barriers between domestic swine and wild and domestic animals.

Larva Migrans Syndromes

Leo X. Liu

A number of nematode infections in humans are caused by infective larvae of species that are normally parasitic for other carnivorous mammals. Due to the restricted host specificity of parasitic nematodes, under such circumstances these developmentally arrested larvae do not mature to adult worms within the human body, but rather migrate through different tissues or organs, causing local and occasionally severe inflammation. These zoonotic infections include visceral larva migrans due to *Toxocara* roundworms, cutaneous larva migrans due to animal hookworms, and anisakiasis due to marine nematodes.

▸ VISCERAL LARVA MIGRANS

Visceral larva migrans (VLM) is most frequently caused by infective larvae of the canine ascarid nematode *Toxocara canis*, a ubiquitous parasite of dogs in temperate and warm climates. VLM is uncommonly caused by the cat roundworm *Toxocara cati* and has not been associated with a second canine ascarid, *Toxascaris leonina*. When the infective eggs of *T. canis* are ingested by a dog, the larvae hatch and penetrate the intestinal wall, then are carried by the circulation to the liver, lungs, and subsequently other tissues. In most dogs these infective larvae remain developmentally arrested within the tissues. In pregnant female dogs, *T. canis* larvae resume development by migrating across the placenta and infecting all of the fetal pups. After birth, the infective larvae emigrate from the lungs via the trachea and pass through the upper gastrointestinal tract before maturing in the small intestine. Thus, full maturation to gravid adult female *T. canis* worms occurs mainly in unweaned young puppies less than 3 months old and their lactating mothers. Large numbers of eggs that are shed in the dog feces embryonate over weeks in the soil and are quite resistant to environmental stresses.

Humans acquire VLM by accidentally ingesting infective *T. canis* eggs that contaminate sandboxes, playground dirt, or other areas frequented by infected dogs. Thus, VLM is usually a disease of toddlers and young children. The infective *T. canis* larvae are released in the small intestine, after which they migrate extensively through visceral organs. The majority of developmentally arrested larvae localize in the liver, but the lungs, central nervous system, eyes, and other sites may also be invaded. Like other tissue helminths, the larvae provoke a local eosinophilic granulomatous host response. The clinical manifestations of *T. canis* infection depend on the number of infective eggs ingested, site of localization, duration of infection, and other poorly understood factors. Most cases of human toxocariasis are probably relatively mild or asymptomatic, as evidenced by seroprevalence rates that range from 2 percent in an unselected American population to greater than 20 percent among kindergarten children in the United States and England. In full-blown VLM, clinical findings of hepatic or pulmonary involvement include hepatomegaly, bronchopneumonia, febrile episodes, transient anorexia and other gastrointestinal disorders, and other nonspecific constitutional symptoms. Invasion of the central nervous system is a rare but serious complication and may cause muscular weakness, sensory abnormalities, convulsions, and coma. The rarely reported infection by the neurotropic raccoon ascarid *Baylisascaris procyonis* causes a syndrome that is analogous and clinically similar to VLM. Ocular involvement with *T. canis* larvae causes a distinct syndrome referred to as ocular larva migrans (OLM). Curiously, patients with OLM tend to be older children without evidence of other visceral involvement, suggesting an alternate pathogenesis perhaps involving only a few larvae. Granulomatous inflammation of the retina in OLM mimics the appearance of retinoblastoma, which has occasionally resulted in unnecessary enucleation.

Clinical and laboratory findings are important in the diagnosis of all larva migrans syndromes, but as with all uncommon or zoonotic infections the critical first step is to consider the possibility of this diagnosis in the first place. A history of geophagia or pica in a young child, or a close association with young puppies, is helpful in conjunction with clinical findings. Significant and occasionally extremely high peripheral eosinophilia is generally found in VLM but not mild toxocariasis. Enzyme-linked immunosorbent assay (ELISA) of specific antibodies to *T. canis* larval antigens is the most sensitive and specific test to establish the diagnosis of toxocariasis and VLM due to *T. canis*.

There is no specific treatment for VLM, as available anthelminthic agents are largely ineffective against the *T. canis* larval stage. Thiabendazole has been recommended in severe cases of VLM, but its efficacy has not been firmly established and the drug is associated with considerable side effects. Corticosteroids may be beneficial in severe cases to ameliorate local symptoms, which are largely due to host inflammatory responses. Ingestion of *T. canis* eggs can be prevented by high sanitary standards, including measures to minimize dog fecal contamination of public playgrounds and sandboxes. Although canine toxocariasis is common (particularly among stray dogs) in some parts of the United States, in many areas the prevalence of canine roundworm infection has declined due to animal control measures and the widespread veterinary use of broad-spectrum anthelmintics effective against the adult worms, such as the combination of ivermectin and pyrantel.

▶ CUTANEOUS LARVA MIGRANS

Cutaneous larva migrans, or creeping eruption, is a serpiginous skin eruption caused by infective-stage larvae of animal hookworms, usually the dog and cat hookworms *Ancylostoma caninum* and *Ancyclostome braziliense*. First-stage larvae hatch from embryonated eggs passed in animal feces and mature to the third-stage infective larvae in the soil. These larvae invade the skin directly when humans are barefoot or in other direct skin contact with contaminated soil in areas frequented by infected domestic animals. Cutaneous larva migrans is more prevalent among children and in warm, humid climates. After percutaneous invasion, the larvae migrate along the upper dermis, causing inflammatory erythematous lesions to form along their tortuous tracks, which can advance several centimeters in a day. These intensely pruritic lesions are usually confined to the foot and lower extremity but may occur anywhere on the body. Previously sensitized individuals can develop a more severe allergic response, with subsequent vesicle and bulla formation. Animal hookworm larvae do not mature in humans, and left untreated will die out after several weeks with resolution of the skin lesions. The clinical diagnosis is readily made based on the typical skin lesions; a skin biopsy is of little specific diagnostic value. Symptoms can be ameliorated by oral albendazole with high efficacy and few side effects, as well as by oral or topical thiabendazole. An analogous eruption is caused by infective (filariform) larvae of *Strongyloides stercoralis*, which cause an even more rapidly migrating serpiginous eruption called larva currens. However, this phenomenon occurs in chronic autoinfection with *S. stercoralis*, a serious human parasite that always merits anthelminthic treatment in view of its propensity to cause hyperinfection in immunocompromised individuals.

▶ ANISAKIASIS

Anisakiasis is an acute and often severe gastrointestinal disease caused by infective larvae of *Anisakis simplex* and *Terranova* species infesting uncooked saltwater fish. The adult worms of these marine ascarid nematodes parasitize large sea mammals and produce offspring larvae that develop first in minute crustaceans and then in many kinds of fish, where the larvae migrate to the fish musculature. When humans consume raw infected fish, a liberated *Anisakis* larva may immediately penetrate the stomach mucosa, causing violent gastric pain sometimes accompanied by nausea and vomiting. Presenting often as an acute abdomen, the diagnosis can be made by direct visual inspection on upper endoscopy, which can be curative if promptly followed by endoscopic extraction of the offending larva. More distal penetration of the intestine causes the formation over 1 or 2 weeks of focal eosinophilic granulomas, producing a syndrome of intermittent abdominal pain, diarrhea, nausea, or fever that resembles Crohn's disease. Here the diagnosis is usually made only after surgical resection reveals a nematode larva embedded within a granuloma, although the diagnosis can be suggested by focal constriction on barium contrast studies. Like the other zoonotic infections due to nematode larvae of species that are normally parasitic for other mammals, *Anisakis* larvae do not mature in humans, and therefore parasite eggs will not be found on stool examination. Also known as herring worm disease, anisakiasis has most often been reported from Japan but occurs in the Netherlands, Chile, the United States, and anywhere that sushi and other raw fish dishes are consumed. Cooking or freezing of infected marine fish will effectively kill *Anisakis* larvae.

Liver, Lung, and Intestinal Trematodes

Fascioliasis and Paragonimiasis[a]

John H. Cross

▶ FASCIOLIASIS

Liver fluke disease (liver rot) is caused by *Fasciola hepatica*, a cosmopolitan and enzootic parasite of sheep, cattle, goats, and hogs. Human fascioliasis is not infrequent in sheep-raising and cattle-raising areas, where the infection is caused by consumption of raw watercress to which the infective cysts of the fluke, the metacercariae, are attached. In addition to the many reports in the medical literature of sporadic cases, there have been small epidemics of fascioliasis. Major endemic countries are Peru, Egypt, Iran, France, Portugal, Puerto Rico, and Bolivia.[1]

Life Cycle

The relatively large, operculated eggs of *F. hepatica* are excreted in the feces of infected mammals, especially sheep and cattle. When they reach fresh water, the eggs mature within 9 to 15 days. Within 24 hours, the larva, or miracidia, must find snails of the genus *Lymnaea*, especially *Lymnaea truncatula*, and other species of the family Lymnaeidae. Within the snail host, the miracidia multiplies and develops into many mature cercariae, which, after leaving the snail, encyst as metacercariae on aquatic vegetation. A moist environment is favorable for their survival, and even short periods of drying can kill the metacercariae. Ingestion of viable cysts attached to grass and water plants, predominantly free watercress (*Nasturtium officinale*), leads to infection. Humans are accidental hosts. The young fluke migrates through the peritoneal cavity, entering the liver from its surface. It reaches the bile ducts after about 6 to 8 weeks and begins to produce eggs approximately 3 months after the infective cysts were ingested.

Pathology and Symptoms

During the period of invasion the fluke can cause traumatic damage and toxic necrosis along its pathway through the liver. Large amounts of proline produced by adult worms may be related to the fibrotic changes in the bile duct.[2] This may be accompanied by fever and eosinophilia. After reaching the bile ducts, *F. hepatica* causes chronic inflammation leading to symptoms similar to those described for clonorchiasis. In addition, fascioliasis hepatica can cause constitutional and systemic symptoms, including fever, malaise, anemia, and urticaria. There may be night sweats, weight loss, and pain under the right costal margin. Occasionally, severe and persistent coughing may occur. From time to time, the immature as well as mature fluke is recovered from atypical locations such as the lungs, abdominal wall, pleural cavity, orbit, brain, epididymis, and subcutaneous tissues.[3]

Diagnosis

The diagnosis is based on the recovery of the typical eggs in stool specimens. Their similarity to those of *Fasciolopsis buski*, the giant intestinal fluke, and echinostomes can cause difficulties in differential diagnosis. Duodenal intubation and recovery of eggs of *Fasciola hepatica* from bile can help to establish a firm diagnosis. False fascioliasis occurs in individuals who, following the ingestion of livers of sheep, goats, and cattle infected with the trematode, excrete eggs of the fluke in their stools. Serological tests, such as enzyme-linked immunosorbent assay (ELISA) and skin tests with purified antigens from *F. hepatica*, are helpful diagnostic tools. There is eosinophilia and increased erythrocyte sedimentation rate. Even after an outbreak there can be difficulties in reaching a firm diagnosis. In the early stages of an epidemic, many other conditions may be considered in the differential diagnosis, such as diaphragmatic pleurisy, cholecystitis, ambebiasis, and peptic ulcer. The mimicry of fascioliasis ranging from symptom-free cases to severe illness is remarkable.

Community Patterns of Infection

Most infections result from the ingestion of the encysted metacercariae attached to watercress. Because humans are only occasional hosts of this infection, most cases are sporadic. However, epidemics of human fascioliasis have been reported from many countries in the world where the dietary habits of the population favor consumption of raw watercress. The infections occur equally frequently in males and females and involve persons of all ages. Although consumption of watercress as salad greens is the most common means of acquiring the infection, occasionally apples and pears dropped from the trees into ponds and pools and subsequently contaminated with metacercariae can serve as vehicles of infection.

Treatment

Drug treatment of fascioliasis has been unsatisfactory. Bithionol was the drug of choice but is no longer produced and praziquantel has not always been effective. Triclabendazole, a benzimidazole anthelmintic, is active against *F. hepatica* when given in one or two single daily doses of 10 mg/kg. The drug is effective against adult as well as larval flukes.[4]

Prevention and Control

Even where eggs of *Fasciola* are found, one has to make sure that these are not spurious infections of eggs in transit following the ingestion of infected liver of cattle or sheep.

At the present time, radical and fundamental control of fascioliasis, including natural infections in herbivorous animals, is not possible. Triclabendazole in dosages of 10 to 12 mg/kg will kill adult and larval worms in domestic animals. Prevention of human disease can be achieved by omitting watercress and other freshwater plants from the diet, particularly in areas where sheep and cattle are raised and where liver fluke infection is known to occur. Cooking will destroy metacercariae on aquatic vegetation.

[a] *This is a modified version of the sections, authored by Alfred A. Buck, that appeared in this chapter in the previous edition.*

▸ PARAGONIMIASIS

Paragonimiasis (lung fluke disease, endemic hemoptysis, pulmonary distomiasis) is caused by various species of the trematode genus *Paragonimus*. Humans and a great variety of crab-eating and crayfish-eating mammals are definitive hosts and act as reservoirs. Until about 1950, human paragonimiasis was thought to be endemic only in the Far East and in Southeast Asia. Since then, there has been clear evidence of its endemicity in other parts of the world, notably West and Central Africa, South America, and New Guinea. About 22 million people worldwide may have paragonimiasis.[1] Other species of *Paragonimus* infecting humans are *Paragonimus miyazaki*, *Paragonimus heterotremous*, *Paragonimus kellicotti*, *Paragonimus africanus*, *Paragonimus uterobilateralis*, *Paragonimus mexicanus*, and *Paragonimus (Pagumogonimus) skrjabini*.

Life Cycle

All species of *Paragonimus* that infect humans have similar life cycles, which require two intermediate hosts, a snail and a freshwater crab or crayfish. There are now at least eight different species of lung fluke diseases in humans, of which *Paragonimus westermani* is the most widespread in the endemic areas of the Orient.

Infection with the human lung fluke is acquired by ingestion of raw or partially cooked freshwater crabs and crayfish that contain the encysted stages of the parasite, the metacercariae. After ingestion of the viable cysts by the definitive host, excystation occurs in the duodenum. The young worm migrates through the peritoneal cavity, remains in the cavity or enters the abdominal wall for a period of time, and then re-enters the body cavity. The young worms will penetrate the diaphragm, enter the lung, and finally settle down near a bronchiole. The large number of eggs and the metabolites produced by the fluke cause injury to the surrounding lung tissue and walls of the bronchioli. The circuitous migration from the intestinal tract to the lungs provides abundant opportunity for the worms to become sidetracked or to wander into organs and tissues far removed from the typical intrapulmonary residence of the adult worm.

Eggs are excreted either by expectoration or, if swallowed, with the stools. When they reach fresh and clear water, they embryonate and usually hatch within 16 to 20 days. The free-swimming larva, or miracidium, then must enter a suitable snail host of several species of *Semisulcospira*, *Tarebia*, *Thiara*, and *Brotia*, where development to the cercarial stage takes place in approximately 3 months of maturation. The cercariae emerge from the snail and penetrate into the second intermediate host, one of various species of freshwater crabs or crayfish of the genera *Potamon*, *Eriocheir*, *Cambaroides*, *Macrobrachium*, or *Sunddathelphusa*. In the flesh of these crustaceans, they encyst and form metacercariae.

In addition to humans, the other mammalian hosts that serve as reservoirs for human paragonimiasis are cats, dogs, pigs, tigers, leopards, wolves, wildcats, opossums, mongoose, and bandicoots.

Geographic Distribution

Areas of relatively high endemicity of paragonimiasis usually are confined to foci near streams, especially mountain streams, and rivers, where the intermediate hosts are abundant. Endemic areas with a high prevalence of lung fluke disease are in the Far East in Korea, Taiwan, China, and Japan; in Southeast Asia in the Philippines, Indonesia, Thailand, Vietnam, Laos, India, and New Guinea; in Africa in Cameroon, Congo, Chad, Gabon, Guinea, Liberia, Zaire, Nigeria, Senegal, and Gambia; and in South America in Peru, Ecuador, Venezuela, and Colombia. Sporadic cases are reported from Bokina Faso, Ivory Coast, and Solomon Islands. Prevalence rates are decreasing in China, Taiwan, Japan, and Korea due to the implementation of control and educational programs.[2]

Clinical Illness

The clinical picture of paragonimiasis depends on the organs involved and on the extent to which the tissue is parasitized. Paragonimiasis occurs primarily as a chronic lung disease characterized by chronic cough and hemoptysis. Its onset usually is insidious. Later, chest pain, dyspnea, and constitutional symptoms may be present. Pleurisy with effusion, empyema, and pleural adhesions are common complications. Extrapulmonary paragonimiasis occurs more often than is usually thought. Most important are cerebral lesions. Other sites include the liver, mesenteric lymph nodes, genitourinary system, the eye, and the subcutaneous tissue.

Diagnosis and Screening

Recognition is the first step toward prevention. A specific diagnosis can be made readily by the recovery of *Paragonimus* eggs from patients having the typical rusty, blood-tinged sputum. Nevertheless, a correct diagnosis of pulmonary paragonimiasis is often missed, owing to the similarity of the symptoms to those of pulmonary tuberculosis and an inability to find the eggs in the sputum. In extrapulmonary paragonimiasis, surgical means may be the only way to recover the eggs from the tissue lesions. Sputum examination for the presence of acid-fast bacilli by appropriate staining methods can deform and even destroy *Paragonimus* eggs beyond recognition. Therefore, unstained sputum specimens should be examined wherever paragonimiasis is suspected. Recovery of eggs can be improved by including a routine stool examination. *Paragonimus* eggs are large (18–120 by 40–60 μm) and yellow-brown with a thick shell with a visible operculum. Transbronchial brushing and bronchial lavage will often reveal eggs of the parasite.

Chest x-rays may be helpful in making a tentative diagnosis. The use of intradermal and serological tests with purified antigens of *P. westermani* can be regarded as a valuable aid both for the differential diagnosis against tuberculosis and for epidemiological surveys. A highly purified antigen has been produced that does not cross-react with other parasites commonly found in areas where paragonimiasis exists. An ELISA-inhibition test using monoclonal antibodies has been developed.[3]

Community Patterns of Infection

In endemic areas, the prevalence of the disease and the infection continues to rise with age up to about 40 years, when the prevalence levels off. In some areas, as in Korea, there is a significant sex difference, with male preponderance. This is related to the habit of eating raw, marinated, or pickled crabs and crayfish while consuming alcoholic beverages in public bars. The common practice of pickling crabs in wine, vinegar, or brine does not always kill the infective metacercariae of the parasite. By contrast, in some African foci, women are more frequently affected than men because the eating of raw crayfish and crabs is thought to enhance fertility.

In time of famine, the incidence of paragonimiasis often rises significantly because many new infections occur in persons who eat raw freshwater crabs and crayfish when other food is unavailable.

Small, single-source epidemics of paragonimiasis have occurred after the consumption of crab and crayfish meat heavily infected with the metacercariae of *P. westermani*.

The reported frequency of cerebral paragonimiasis appears to be much higher in the Far East than in any of the other endemic foci.

Control and Prevention

There are two effective drugs for treatment of paragonimiasis. They are praziquantel (2-cyclohexylcarbonyl 1,2,3,6,7,11b-hexahydro-pyrazino(2,1-a) isoquinolin-4-a), and menichlopholan (Niclofolan) (2,2′-dihydroxy-3,3′-dinitro-5,5-dichlordiphenyl).[2] Praziquantel is the drug of choice, with close to 95 percent cure rates when given orally in three doses of 25 mg/kg over 3 days.

Temporary control of snails by molluscicides as well as destruction of crabs is feasible but requires careful consideration of the effects of the chemicals on local nontarget fauna. Significant results of controlling paragonimiasis by sanitary disposal of sputum and feces can be expected only if the maintenance of the life cycle of *Paragonimus* does not depend on other mammalian reservoir hosts. Education of people in endemic areas concerning the life cycle of the parasite is one of the most important methods for preventing paragonimiasis. The present method of preparing uncooked crabs and crayfish by keeping them in brine for several days is not sufficient to kill the infective metacercariae, especially when the time of aging in these salt solutions is short. Cooking the crabs and crayfish is a safe way to prevent infection. It requires continued and intensive efforts to convince the people that a change in their food habits is the best safeguard against new infections with the lung fluke.

In Korea, mass treatment of paragonimiasis using a single dose of menichlopholan (Niclofolan) has been effective, with few side effects.[2]

The fertility of the adult trematodes may be as long as 20 years or more, during which eggs may be discharged by the human host. Even after destruction of the mollusks and crustaceans involved in the life cycle of the lung fluke, therefore, transmission may begin again as soon as the intermediary hosts repopulate the rivers and streams in the area.

Clonorchiasis and Opisthorchiasis

Kenrad E. Nelson

Three parasitic trematodes of the family Opisthorchiidae—*Clonorchis sinensis, Opisthorchis viverrini,* and *Opisthorchis felineus*—are responsible for the production of chronic disease of the liver and bile ducts in humans. Infections with these similar trematodes are widely distributed in countries in the Far East and Southeast Asia and countries of the former Soviet Union. They present serious public health problems in certain localized areas of China, Korea, Thailand, Laos, Cambodia, Vietnam, and several countries of the former Soviet Union. The World Health Organization has estimated recently that at least 7 million persons are infected with *C. sinensis* in China and Korea, 2 million persons are infected with *O. felineus* in Russia, and 6 million persons are infected with *O. viverrini* in Southeast Asia.[1] With increased travel and migration of populations at risk and importation of indigenous uncooked foods contaminated with these parasites, infections have also occurred on occasion in nonendemic areas.[2]

Life Cycle

The parasites *C. sinensis, O. viverrini,* and *O. felineus* require two intermediate hosts and a definitive host for the completion of their life cycle. In addition to humans, dogs, cats, rats, and other fish-eating mammals can serve as reservoir hosts. When the eggs are passed with the stools of humans or infected carnivores, they are fully embryonated. However, they do not hatch spontaneously when they reach fresh water. The miracidium is set free only after the eggs are ingested by an operculate snail, the first intermediate host. Species of these snails that can serve as intermediate hosts are from the genera *Parafossarulus, Bulinus, Semisulcospina, Alocinma,* and *Thiara*. In these intermediate hosts, further development from the stage of miracidium to cercariae takes place. The cercariae emerge into water, and on contact with a suitable fresh-water fish of the minnow and carp family (Cyprinidae), they penetrate the skin of the fish, discard their tails, and encyst in the flesh as metacercariae. When infected raw fresh-water fish containing the encysted stages of the parasite are eaten, the larvae are set free in the duodenum of the final host and enter the bile ducts within a few hours after being ingested. In about 4 weeks, the flukes reach maturity and begin to shed eggs into the bile ducts. When the embryonated eggs are passed in the stool and reach fresh water the life cycle of the parasite is completed. The complete life cycle, from one infected person to another, requires at least 3 months.

Geographic Distribution

The geographic distribution of endemic clonorchiasis or opisthorchiasis is determined by three factors: (*a*) the presence of suitable intermediate hosts, (*b*) the preference of the people in these areas to eat raw fish, and (*c*) exposure of these aquatic environments to sewage containing parasite eggs. Infections with *C. sinensis* are common in populations in Korea, China, parts of Japan and Taiwan, the Red River Valley in Indochina, and among refugees from Vietnam and Cambodia. Infections with *O. viverreni* are endemic in Thailand, Laos, Cambodia, and the Philippines; *O. felineus* infections occur among populations in Siberia and other areas of Central Russia and the Ukraine. Clonorchiasis or opisthorchiasis in humans can be long-lived (up to 25 years) if it is not treated. The infection has involved Asians living in all parts of the world. Nevertheless, no new endemic foci are known to have been introduced into this new environment by these migrants, due largely to the absence of suitable intermediate hosts.

Clinical Illness

The flukes cause injury to the bile ducts and produce chronic cholangitis characterized by marked hyperplasia of the cylindrical epithelium, frequently associated with numerous mitoses. Eventually, the nonspecific changes due to chronic inflammation and subsequent reinfections lead to a progressive fibrous thickening of the walls, causing partial or complete obstruction of terminal bile ducts, pressure necrosis of the surrounding parenchyma, and, in severe cases, biliary cirrhosis. Development of cholangitic cirrhosis is enhanced by intermittent acute episodes of complicating bacterial cholangitis, especially from *Escherichia coli* and other gut flora, which produces abscesses that lead to chronic cholecystitis. A causal relationship between chronic clonorchiasis or opisthorchiasis and biliary tract carcinoma (cholangiocarcinoma) has been established.[2–5] Approximately two-thirds of patients from northeastern Thailand having obstructive jaundice secondary to malignant disease have cholangiocarcinoma related to liver flukes.[1] In contrast, carcinoma of the head of the pancreas is by far the most frequent cause of obstructive jaundice secondary to malignant disease in persons living in Western nations.

The signs and symptoms of clonorchiasis and opisthorchiasis are nonspecific. Most infected persons are asymptomatic. Only about one-third of chronic infections are symptomatic. In patients who do have symptoms, gradual onset of discomfort in the upper abdomen, anorexia, indigestion, and abdominal pain or distention can occur. In the late stages obstructive jaundice, portal hypertension, ascites, and gastrointernal bleeding can occur. Recurrent pyogenic cholangitis is the most frequent serious acute complication of clonorchiasis. These episodes can be followed by the formation of biliary stones in the gallbladder and bile ducts.[1]

Diagnosis

Diagnosis is based on recovery of the typical eggs from stool specimens. Field surveys for the eggs in the stool can be made using standard fecal examination techniques, such as the sedimentation or the modified cellophane fecal thick-smear technique (Kato-Katz technique); these are simple and reproducible methods for the detection of trematode eggs. The Kato technique also permits storage of slides for later reexamination for quality control. Sometimes, eggs may be found only in the bile or duodenal contents after intubation and aspiration. The eggs of *C. sinensis* are among the smallest produced by trematodes that are pathogenic for humans and measure only 27 by 16 μm. They are yellow-brown and have a characteristic operculum fitting into the rim of the shell like a lid on a sugar bowl and a small knoblike protuberance located at the opposite pole.

Intradermal and complement-fixation tests with purified antigens prepared from *C. sinensis* or *O. viverreni* are helpful in establishing the diagnosis. Among the modern immunodiagnostic tests, an enzyme-linked immunosorbent assay (ELISA) gives highly predictive results. The test combines a high degree of sensitivity with specificity and is a good tool for epidemiologic investigations.[6,7]

Community Patterns of Infection and Disease

In hyperendemic areas, there is a rapid increase in the prevalence of infection from the age of 1 to about 20 years. Thereafter, the prevalence stabilizes and may fall among persons over 40 years of age. In rural areas of the Republic of Korea, along the Naktong River, it is not unusual to find as many as 80 percent of the villagers infected with *C. sinensis*. Although raw fish is eaten by both sexes, males are more often infected. This sex difference is probably related to local customs of serving raw fish with alcoholic beverages at the many social gatherings, which are attended exclusively by males.

Community studies in rural areas of China, Korea, and Indochina may yield age-specific prevalence rates close to 100 percent. In rural areas of northeastern Thailand and Laos the prevalence of *O. viverrni* infection can be over 80 percent in some populations. The disease has a pronounced focal distribution, depending on the availability and the habit of eating uncooked fish containing the metacercariae of the fluke. Spread of infection has been related to the use of aquaculture to develop sources of fish protein for consumption in areas where sanitary disposal of human waste is not available and consumption of uncooked fish is common.

Liver cancer is one of the most common malignancies in Southeast Asia. In many areas hepatocellular liver cancer, associated with chronic hepatitis B virus infection, are most common. However, in some areas the types and causes of liver cancer differ. Khon Kaen, in northeastern Thailand, has one of the world's highest incidence rates of liver cancer.[1] The high incidence of cholangiocarcinoma, which in many other populations accounts for only a minority of liver cancer cases, is particularly striking. In 1988 in Khon Kaen, 89 percent of liver cancers were cholangiocarcinomas. The age-standardized incidence rates for 1988 were 89.2 per 100,000 males and 35.5 per 100,000 females. In contrast, a cancer registry established in the province of Chiang Mai in northern Thailand, where the prevalence of *O. viverrini* infection is much lower, reported rates of cholangiocarcinoma of 5 per 100,000 males and 3 per 100,000 females. A retrospective study of hospital records in Khon Kaen yielded estimated annual age-standardized incidences of cholangiocarcinoma of 135.4 per 100,000 males and 43.0 per 100,000 females. Nearly all patients with diagnosed cholangiocarcinoma had heavy egg burdens of *O. viverrini* in their stools.

In the central part of the Tyumen region in Russia, where the prevalence of *O. felineus* infection was 45 percent, the rate of cholangiocarcinoma was 49.8 per 100,000 population.[1] In contrast, in the southern part of the Tyumen region only 0.5 percent of the population were infected with *O. felineus*, and the average prevalence of cholangiocarcinoma was reported to be 4.4 per 100,000.[1]

The full public health importance of *C. sinensis* infection in relation to the prevalence and intensity of infection, the frequency of reinfections, and the risks of developing chronic liver disease or cancer of the bile ducts has not been adequately evaluated. Although *C. sinensis* infections and cholangiocarcinoma have been associated, fewer studies of the public health importance of *C. sinensis* infection have been reported.

Treatment and Control

Praziquantel—2-(cyclohexylcarbonyl)-1,2,3,6,7,11b-hexahydro-4*H*-pyrazino[2,1-*a*] isoquinolin-4-one—is the most effective drug for the treatment of human chlonorchiasis or opisthorchiasis. The recommended doses are 25 mg/kg body weight of praziquantel three times daily, ie, 75 mg/kg given in three doses on a single day.[8] Mass treatment with a single dose of 40 mg/kg has been used in public health campaigns in northern Thailand.[1] Cure rates as high as 90 percent have been reported in mass treatment campaigns. Of course, reinfection with the organism can occur readily unless public health practices are instituted that change the preparation and consumption of fish and/or the disposal of contaminated fecal material in endemic areas.

Poverty, pollution, and population growth are the triad of underlying determinants that directly influence the incidence of food-borne trematode infections. Although thorough cooking of all fish in endemic areas is an effective safeguard against infection, shortage of fuel in some poor homes may mandate the consumption of uncooked fish products. Traditional dishes in Southeast Asia that contain fermented freshwater fish may promote the transmission of food-borne trematodes.

Sanitary disposal of contaminated feces using latrines is another important method of public health control of the infection. In areas where night soil is used as a fertilizer in fish ponds, treatment of the feces with a 0.7 percent solution of ammonium sulfate can be used to kill the miracidia in the eggs and interrupt the chain of infection.

In Thailand public health efforts, which involve annual mass treatment of populations with praziquantel and distribution of cooking pots, have been successful in dramatically reducing the prevalence of infection in some populations with high prevalence of infection.[1]

Shipments of dried or pickled fish from endemic areas may be sources of infection in nonendemic areas. Therefore, more effective control of these imported food products is needed.

Cestode Infections

Taeniasis and Cysticercosis

Kenrad E. Nelson

Taeniasis refers to an intestinal infection with the adult stage of the beef tapeworm (*Taenia saginata*) or the pork tapeworm (*Taenia solium*). Cysticercosis is the somatic infection with the larval stage of the pork tapeworm. Both beef and pork tapeworms have been known as parasites of humans since ancient times, but infection of humans by the larval stage of the pork tapeworm was not recognized until the sixteenth century.[1]

Life Cycle

Cestodes of the family Taeniidae complete their cycle in two mammalian hosts, typically a carnivore and an herbivore between which a well-defined predator-prey relationship exits.[1] Humans are the definitive hosts for two species of *Taenia*, *Taenia saginata* and *Taenia solium*. The larval stages of the species occur in cattle (*T. saginata*) and in swine (*T. solium*). The larvae of *T. solium* can develop in dogs and humans also. Humans contract taeniasis through the ingestion of infective cysticerci in raw or undercooked beef, pork, or dog meat. In the small intestine, the cysticercus invests its scolex to attach to the mucosa and develops into the adult worm. Adult *T. saginata* can measure 4 to 12 m in length and can survive up to 30 years in the human intestine. Release of segments containing eggs infective for the intermediate host begins in the human intestine after 8 to 10 weeks for *T. saginata* and 9 to 13 weeks for *T. solium*. A tapeworm carrier releases between 6 and 9 proglottids daily, each containing about 50,000 fertile eggs. Humans acquire cysticercosis by ingestion of *T. solium* eggs, either from exogenous surroundings or from their own stool. Internal autoinfection, in which the eggs of *T. solium* are swept back into the stomach by reverse peristalsis, is also possible.

Distribution

According to recent estimates, about 45 million people worldwide are infected by *T. saginata* and about 3.5 million by *T. solium*. *Taenia saginata* is common in some regions of the former Soviet Union, Southeast Asia, Africa, and some South American countries. The highest rates of human infection have been reported in Africa among nomadic cattle herders.[2] *T. saginata* is uncommon in North America north of Mexico, but its prevalence seems to have increased locally in the southwestern United States. In that region, workers harboring the adult worms may contaminate sewage used in irrigation, which are the sources of infection for cattle.[3,4] *T. solium* is uncommon in most developed countries, but it is relatively common in some regions of Africa, southern Asia, Mexico, and Central and South America.

Clinical Picture

The presence of these cestodes in the human intestine is often asymptomatic. The symptoms, when present, are vague and include abdominal pain, nausea, flatulence, diarrhea, and weight loss. Patients, especially those infected with *T. saginata*, may sense the active migration of proglottids through the anus. *T. solium* proglottids do not migrate spontaneously.

The larval stage of *T. solium* is the cause of cysticercosis in humans. This cestode is unique in the family Taeniidae in that both stages of its cycle are capable of development in a single mammalian host. Larvae in skeletal muscle do not usually develop into mature cysts and generally are not symptomatic unless present in large numbers. However, significant functional disturbances may result when cysticerci localize in tissues of the central nervous system. Neurocysticercosis can be associated with a variety of clinical symptoms. Seizures are by far the most common clinical manifestation and occur in about 80 to 90 percent of cases. Less commonly, patients can present with headache, symptoms of elevated intracranial pressure, depressed mental status (including coma), stiff neck, or focal neurologic findings. The clinical presentation depends on the location, number, and viability of the cysts as well as the host response to their presence.[5,6]

Diagnosis

The diagnosis of taeniasis is made on the basis of the characteristic eggs or proglottids found in the stool. The eggs of *T. solium* and *T. saginata* are indistinguishable, but the species can be differentiated by examination of the gravid proglottids. The number of main uterine branches of *T. saginata* is 15 to 20, and that of *T. solium* is 7 to 13.

The diagnosis of cysticercosis involving the central nervous system is sometimes difficult. Cysticercosis should be considered in the differential diagnosis of epilepsy, basilar meningitis, obstructive hydrocephalus, and other neurologic disorders in patients with a history of residence or travel in regions where *T. solium* is endemic. The cysts are sometimes seen radiologically in skull films after the death and calcification of the larvae. Imaging techniques such as computed tomographic (CT) scanning and nuclear magnetic resonance imaging (MRI) are the main diagnostic tools in neurocysticercosis.[5–9] CT is the best method for detecting calcification associated with a previous infection. Most parenchymal cysts will appear as low-density cysts, with enhancement of the cyst wall or surrounding tissues, usually accompanied by surrounding edema. MRI is more sensitive than CT for revealing cysts in the brain parenchyma or extraparenchymal sites and in basilar cisterns. Cysticerci localized in subcutaneous tissues or skin, where they form palpable nodules, are readily identified by biopsy. Immunodiagnostic tests for cysticercosis are available. Both antibody and antigen have been detected in serum or cerebrospinal fluid by enzyme-linked immunosorbent assay (ELISA) or a combination of other immunochemical techniques based on ELISA.[10–12] Highly purified specific antigens are required for reliable results. The enzyme-linked immunoelectrotransfer blot (EITB) method, using lentil-lectin affinity-purified glycoprotein antigens for immunodiagnosing human cysticercosis, has been reported to be nearly 100 percent sensitive and specific.[13,14] The test is more sensitive with serum than CSF samples.[14] However, the sensitivity is lower in patients with only calcified lesions.[14] Cysticercosis appears to have increased in frequency recently. However, some of this increase in prevalence may be related to more sensitive methods of diagnosis, using ELISA or EITB, coupled with neuroradiologic techniques such as CT scanning and MRI. Also, increased travel from areas of the world where *T. solium* is endemic may have increased the frequency of the disease in the United States and Europe.[6]

Treatment

In the treatment of taeniasis, good results have been obtained with niclosamide and dichlorophen, both of which cause some disintegration of the strobilae. Praziquantel is 100 percent effective against *T. saginata* and other cestodes when administered in a single dose of 10 mg/kg. Transient side effects occur in only a small proportion of patients and are considered to be of negligible importance.

Treatment of parenchymal neurologic cysticercosis has relied on the use of anticonvulsive drugs to control epileptiform attacks. Treatment has been advocated with praziquantel in doses of 50 to 60 mg/kg per day in three daily doses for 15 days or albendazole in doses of 15 mg/kg per day for 8 to 30 days. Some investigators recommend that corticosteroids be used routinely as an adjuvant to the antiparasitic therapy.[15] Others use steroids only in patients who develop symptoms.[16] Controlled trials have suggested that treatment with these antiparasitic drugs is associated with only modest improvement in the rate of resolution of cysts.[17,18] Disorders attributable to interference with the flow of cerebrospinal fluid due to extraparenchymal racemose cysticerci can sometimes be alleviated surgically by removing the cysts or by performing shunting procedures.

Prevention and Control

Requisite conditions for the infection of humans by *T. saginata* and *T. solium* are poor sanitation and consumption of beef and pork insufficiently cooked to kill the cysticerci. The use of raw sewage containing human feces to fertilize crops completes the life cycle of these organisms. The best preventive measures include strict attention to personal hygiene, environmental sanitation, and protection of cattle and hogs from contact with human excretions. Individual infection is prevented by thorough cooking of beef and pork at 55°C or freezing at –17°C for 5 days. In endemic regions, educational programs are needed to alert the public to the risks of eating inadequately cooked beef and pork. In the United States, federal meat inspection includes direct examination for the presence of cysticerci (i.e., looking for "measly" meat). However, interruption of the cycle of infection in animals by good sanitation is a preferable public health approach to prevention.

Other Cestodiases and Diphyllobothriases

Robert L. Rausch • John H. Cross • Alan W. Cross

▶ OTHER CESTODIASES

Hymenolepis nana is a common parasite of humans, estimated to infect about 50 million people worldwide.[1] It differs from almost all other tapeworms in being able to complete its entire life cycle in a single host. *H. nana* is a small, filamentous tapeworm ranging up to about 100 mm in length. When ingested by humans or rodents, eggs disseminated in the feces of the final host hatch in the small intestine. The released embryos penetrate into the villi, where development to the infective larval stage (cysticercoid) takes place within a few days. The cysticercoids then reenter the lumen and attach to the mucosa of the ileum, where the worms develop. Eggs appear in the feces about 30 days after exposure. The cycle may involve an intermediate host if eggs are ingested by grain beetles or larvae of fleas. The embryo penetrates to the hemocoelom of the insect, where the cysticercoid develops. Infection of the final host follows ingestion of insects containing cysticercoids.

Children are infected more commonly by *H. nana* than are adults. The cestodes have little apparent effect when present in small numbers, but infections involving hundreds to thousands of tapeworms are typically symptomatic. Symptoms in patients infected by *H. nana* are reported to include restlessness, diarrhea, abdominal pain, irritability, and anal and nasal pruritus. Eosinophilia exceeded 5 percent in a third of the patients. More severe disorders commonly attributed to infection by *H. nana* include enteritis, epileptiform convulsions, laryngeal spasm, and strabismus.

Infection by *H. nana* is diagnosed by finding the eggs in the feces. Recent trials indicate that a single oral dose of 25 mg/kg of praziquantel is highly efficacious against *H. nana*.

H. nana is a common parasite of humans in warmer regions, wherever poor sanitation, inadequate storage of grain, and an abundance of rats and mice provide the requisite conditions for completion of its life cycle. It is the most common tapeworm infection in North America. It would appear that eggs disseminated on grain products and other foods by murine rodents provide the most important source of infection for humans. The ingestion of small grain beetles, such as *Tribolium*, could result in massive infections because of the lack of immunity conferred by the cysticercoids. Implementation of large-scale measures to control *H. nana* does not now seem practicable in most regions where this cestode is a prevalent parasite of humans.

Cestodes that occasionally or rarely infect humans include *Hymenolepis diminuta*, *Dipylidium caninum*, and species of such diverse genera as *Bertiella*, *Raillietina*, *Inermicapsifer*, and *Mesocestoides*. Infections are usually asymptomatic, and diagnosis depends on identification of the characteristic eggs or gravid segments in the feces. Treatment is as for other cestodes.

▶ INTESTINAL TREMATODES

The most important trematodes that occur in the human intestine are *Fasciolopsis buski*, *Heterophyes heterophyes*, *Metagonimus yokogawai*, *Gastrodiscoides hominis*, and *Echinostoma* species. The eggs of these trematodes are expelled in the feces of the final host, after which the motile miracidium hatches in water. After penetration of the tissues of a snail by the miracidium, a complex process of asexual reproduction leads to the development of cercariae. The cercariae escape from the snail and encyst in a second intermediate host or on vegetation, where the infective metacercariae develop. Use of human excreta to fertilize aquatic vegetation or discharge of sewage into water ensures completion of the cycles of these trematodes.[2]

Fasciolopsis buski is a parasite of humans and pigs in Asia, including China, Thailand, and India. Its occurrence in humans is restricted by the distribution of certain aquatic plants, particularly water caltrop, *Trapa* species, on which the metacercariae encyst. The cultivation of such plants usually involves fertilization with feces of humans or pigs. Humans usually become infected by ingesting metacercarial cysts attached to the seedpods of water caltrop, which are peeled with the aid of the teeth, or to the bulbs or roots of other edible plants. The ingested metacercariae excyst in the intestine and attach to the mucosa of the duodenum and jejunum, where they attain full development in about 3 months. The trematodes may cause ulceration and an inflammatory response at the site of attachment and may produce diarrhea and abdominal pain. When large numbers are present, absorption of metabolic products may cause severe toxic or allergic reactions, manifested by facial or generalized edema, ascites, and other disorders. Diagnosis usually is based on clinical findings and identification of the eggs in the feces. The prognosis is good in light infections, which often are asymptomatic, or when early diagnosis is made. Massive infections may be fatal. The trematodes can be expelled by treatment with praziquantel 75 mg/kg/day in 3 doses.[3]

Heterophyes heterophyes is a very small trematode that may occur in large numbers in the intestine of humans and other fish-eating mammals in southern Asia, Egypt, Turkey, and perhaps in southern Europe. The metacercariae encyst beneath the scales or in the superficial musculature of fishes of various species. Following ingestion by the final host, the metacercariae excyst and attach to the intestinal mucosa, where they attain full development in about a week. Light infections are typically asymptomatic, but large numbers of trematodes may cause mucous diarrhea and abdominal discomfort. The trematodes sometimes penetrate the intestinal wall to the extent that eggs find their way into the systemic circulation. Such eggs may localize in tissues, such as the myocardium or brain, where they seem to act as minute emboli. They evoke little inflammatory response, but focal fibrosis may be observed. Diagnosis of heterophyiasis is best made after treatment, since the eggs in the feces of the host closely resemble those of other trematodes. The trematodes are expelled by treatment with praziquantel 75 mg/kg/day in 3 doses.

Metagonimus yokogawai is another small trematode that occurs in humans as well as in other fish-eating mammals and certain birds in Asia and in the Balkan region. The metacercariae localize in the gills, in the musculature, and on the scales of fishes that serve as second intermediate host. In humans, this trematode typically localizes in the jejunum, where its effects are similar to those of *H. heterophyes*. Diagnosis is best made after treatment, for which praziquantel is suitable.

Gastrodiscoides hominis is a relatively large, thick-bodied trematode that inhabits the caecum and ascending colon of humans. It also occurs in pigs. The cercaria is believed to encyst on vegetation, but the cycle has not been fully elucidated. The trematodes attach firmly by drawing a small mass of mucosa into the ventral sucker, around which a superficial, craterlike lesion is formed. Infections are usually asymptomatic, but large numbers of trematodes may cause a mucoid diarrhea. Diagnosis is made from eggs expelled in the feces. Tetrachloroethylene is recommended for treatment, but praziquantel should also be effective.

Trematodes of the genus *Echinostoma*, including *Echinostoma ilocanum*, *Echinostoma malayanum*, and others, occur in the small intestine of humans in southern Asia and less commonly in other regions, such as southern Europe and the former Soviet Union. Infections are acquired through consumption of mollusk containing the metacercariae. Large numbers of trematodes may cause diarrhea and abdominal pain, but most infections are asymptomatic. Diagnosis depends on identification of eggs in the feces. Treatment is usually with tetrachloroethylene, praziquantel, mebendazole, and albendazole.

Trematodes of several other species occur occasionally of rarely in the human intestine. Most have been recorded from populations among which traditional dietary habits favor exposure to infection by trematodes that occur typically in other animals. Most are of minor medical importance.

▶ DIPHYLLOBOTHRIASIS

Among the members of the cestode genus *Diphyllobothrium*, the most common species occurring in humans are *Diphyllobothrium latum, Diphyllobothrium pacificum, Diphyllobothrium nikonkaiense*, and *Diphyllobothrium dendriticum*.

Life Cycle

The life cycle of these cestodes requires three hosts for completion, but additional paratenic hosts may be involved. After hatching of the egg in water, the motile embryo (coracidium) is ingested by a minute crustacean (copepod), in which the first-stage larva (procercoid) develops. When the copepod containing the procercoid is ingested by the second intermediate host, a fish, further development leads to the plerocercoid, infective for the final host. The site of localization of the plerocercoid in the second intermediate host differs with species of *Diphyllobothrium* and, to some extent, species of fish.

After the final host ingests the plerocercoid, the adult worm develops comparatively rapidly. Depending on species, the adult worm ranges from less than 1 m long to 12 m or more. The largest have thousands of segments, each of which produces large numbers of eggs. Eggs may be present in great numbers in the feces of the final host, but detached spent segments are not often observed. Host specificity is little developed in these cestodes.

Epidemiology

D. latum occurs in most parts of the world but is most prevalent in subarctic and temperate regions of the northern hemisphere, including Scandinavia, Northern Italy, Switzerland, Hungary, parts of Germany, Finland, North America, and the western former Soviet Union. It is found also in the Middle East, Chile, Argentina, Peru, and Japan. In North America, several foci have been known, particularly western Alaska, the lake regions of northern Minnesota, southeastern Manitoba, and the Lake Nippigon district of Ontario, but some of these areas may no longer be endemic.[4] *Diphyllobothrium pacificum* is reported from Chile and Peru, *Diphyllobothrium nikonkaiense* from Japan and *Diphyllobothrium dendriticum* from subartic regions.[4] Plerocercoids are found commonly in a variety of fresh water fish, such as pike, salmon, trout, sugar, ruff, and whitefish. Up to 70 percent of walleye pike found in some small lakes in the northern United States and Canada are infected. Although a number of fish-eating mammals—dogs, bear, cats, martins—may act as reservoir hosts, humans are the primary definitive host and are mainly responsible for establishing and maintaining endemicity in human populations through contamination of water with feces.

Clinical Picture

In a high proportion of human cases, infections are asymptomatic and remain undetected. Conditions, such as weakness, diarrhea, and abdominal discomfort, frequently are attributed to these cestodes. In a small proportion of persons infected by *D. latum* (1 to 2 percent), depletion of vitamin B_{12} produces a macrocytic anemia resembling pernicious anemia. The cestode apparently interferes with absorption of vitamin B_{12} by the host and at the same time takes up a large quantity of the vitamin. Factors contributing to development of the deficiency include inadequate supply of vitamin B_{12} in the diet, deficiency of intrinsic factor attributable to endogenous or exogenous damage to the gastric mucosa, location of the cestodes proximally in the small intestine or the presence of a large mass of worm tissue, and an increased requirement for the vitamin.[5] Other species of *Diphyllobothrium* are not known to be associated with macrocytic anemia. Toxic substances excreted by the worms may affect the central nervous system causing peripheral and spinal nerve degeneration.

Diagnosis

Diagnosis of infection by *D. latum* and other diphyllobothriid cestodes usually depends on finding the eggs in the feces of the host. Clinically, vitamin B_{12} deficiency caused by *D. latum* is diagnosed from the combination of macrocytic anemia with leukopenia, thrombocytopenia, increased hemolysis, signs of neurological disorders, and reduced serum levels of vitamin B_{12}.

Treatment

Of the various anthelmintics used to expel diphyllobothriid cestodes from the human host, a single dose of 2 g of niclosamide or a single oral dose of 25 mg of praziquantel are effective.[6] After expulsion of the cestodes by anthelmintic treatment, therapeutic use of vitamin B_{12} may be indicated.

Prevention and Control

The infection of humans by *Diphyllobothrium* species depends on the consumption of fish containing plerocercoids. Thorough cooking or freezing at –18°C for 24 to 48 hours will make fish safe for consumption. Drying or brine curing also will render the plerocercoid in fish noninfective. Fish from endemic areas should be frozen for at least 24 hours before being shipped. Dumping of human excreta into local ponds and streams and the pumping of raw sewage by ships sailing the waters and hotels along lakes should be prohibited. Proper treatment of sewage can have a major impact on preventing infection. Programs conducted in various countries have been reviewed by von Bonsdorff.[5] It is not practicable to attempt control of diphyllobothrids, for which fish-eating birds and mammals also serve as final hosts.

Hydatid Disease (Echinococcosis)

Peter M. Schantz • Robert L. Rausch

Hydatid disease (echinococcosis) is the infection of humans by the larval stages of taeniid cestodes of the genus *Echinococcus*. Four species of *Echinococcus* are currently recognized, of which three cause distinctive forms of disease: *Echinococcus granulosus* (cystic hydatid disease), *Echinococcus multilocularis* (alveolar hydatid disease), and *Echinococcus vogeli* (polycystic hydatid disease). The fourth species, *Echinococcus oligarthrus*, has only rarely (in fewer than five cases) been identified as a cause of human disease. Diverse subpopulations of *E. granulosus*, distinguished by morphologic and biological characteristics, have long been recognized; the taxonomic significance of these differences remain unresolved and controversial. However, recent demonstrations of consistent genetic differences has prompted calls for splitting this species.[1] As a cause of morbidity in humans, *Echinococcus* species rank high among the helminths.

Life Cycle

The life cycles of *Echinococcus* species involve carnivores as final hosts and herbivores or omnivores as intermediate hosts. In their adult stage, these cestodes are small, ranging from about 2 to 12 mm in length, with three to six segments. They typically localize in the lower duodenum and jejunum of the final host. Embryophores containing infective embryos are expelled in large numbers in the feces of the final carnivorous host. After ingestion by the intermediate host, the embryo is released into the small intestine, which it penetrates, and soon enters the portal circulation. The site of localization and development of the embryo to the larval or hydatid stage differs with species of *Echinococcus* and may be influenced as well by species of the intermediate host. Humans are an incidental intermediate host, since further development of these cestodes depends on ingestion of their larvae (hydatids) by a carnivore.

Distribution and Transmission Patterns

Cystic hydatid disease is caused by the larval stage of *E. granulosus*, of which at least two biologically distinct forms are recognized. The northern form is indigenous to the Holarctic zones of tundra and boreal forest. It is propagated via a sylvatic cycle, which involves the wolf and deer (mainly reindeer and moose) as final and intermediate hosts, respectively. In some regions of North America where the wolf has been extirpated, the cycle is completed in coyotes and deer. Attempts to infect domestic ungulates with cestodes of this form have not been successful. Wild ungulates are an important source of infection for dogs when viscera of animals killed by hunters are fed directly or are discarded in accessible places. This has been an important pattern of transmission to dogs in northern North America, where subsistence hunting is widely practiced. Nonindigenous populations may be at risk in rural areas, as in south-central Alaska.

The other form, or forms, of *E. granulosus* have a nearly cosmopolitan distribution and are propagated via pastoral cycles, which involve almost exclusively synanthropic animals (dogs and domestic ungulates). Subpopulations adapted to sheep, equines, cattle, and swine appear to be genetically distinct, suggesting that the taxon *E. granulosus* is paraphyletic and may require taxonomic revision.[2,3] The cestode is prevalent in broad regions of Eurasia, in several South American countries, and in Africa. *E. granulosus* in sheep-dog cycles is endemic in apparently disjunct regions of the western United States. Populations at risk include Basque Americans in California, Mormons in central Utah, and Navajo and Zuni Indians in New Mexico.[4] Humans become infected through association with dogs that have been fed viscera from slaughtered animals or have had access to carcasses or discarded offal of domestic ungulates in which the larvae are present.

Alveolar hydatid disease is caused by *E. multilocularis*, which has an extensive geographic range in the northern hemisphere. The natural cycle involves foxes and small rodents as final and intermediate hosts, respectively. This cestode appears to have a continuous distribution in the zone of tundra, from the White Sea in the west to Hudson Bay in the east. Alveolar hydatid disease is most prevalent in indigenous populations in the arctic and sub-arctic, with the highest known rates reported in northeastern Siberia. An endemic region exists in central Europe, where the larval stage was first identified in the human liver in 1854. *E. multilocularis* occurs widely at low latitudes in the former Soviet Union and in central and western China; reports of alveolar hydatid disease in India and Tunisia suggest that its occurrence is more extensive than had been realized.[5] This cestode has become established in northern Japan (Hokkaido) and in central North America. Since its recognition in North Dakota in 1964, the cestode has been recorded in twelve of the surrounding states and in the three adjacent provinces of Canada. The first autochthonous case of alveolar hydatid disease in the United States outside Alaska was diagnosed in Minnesota in 1977.[6]

The infection of humans by the larval *E. multilocularis* is often the result of association with dogs and perhaps cats that have eaten infected rodents. Villages within the zone of tundra may constitute hyperendemic foci because of the interaction between dogs and wild rodents that live as commensals in and around dwellings. In central Europe, rodents inhabiting cultivated fields and gardens become infected by ingesting embryophores expelled by foxes and, in turn, may be a source of infection for dogs and cats. In rural regions of central North America, the cycle involves foxes and rodents of the genera *Peromyscus* and *Microtus*. Keeping uncontrolled dogs and cats in these regions may be hazardous.

Polycystic hydatid disease, caused by *E. vogeli*, has been reported infrequently from Central and South America. The natural hosts of this cestode are the bush dog, *Speothos venaticus*, and the paca, *Cuniculus paca*.[1] The larval stage occurs occasionally in rodents of other species. Little is known of the epidemiology of polycystic hydatid disease. The natural final host of *E. vogeli*, the bush dog, is a wary and rarely seen animal that is an unlikely source of infection for humans. The intermediate host, the paca, is widely hunted for food in northern South America, and local hunters routinely feed the viscera of pacas to their dogs; thus, infected dogs may be the primary source of infection for humans.[7]

Clinical Picture

Cystic Hydatid Disease. In humans, hydatid cysts of *E. granulosus* are slowly enlarging masses comparable to benign neoplasms; the clinical manifestations are variable and are determined by the site, size, and condition of the cysts.[8] The larval stages of the two best-defined biological forms, the northern form and the "European" form, exhibit well-defined differences in the human host.[9] That of the northern form occurs almost exclusively in the lungs and liver and, in clinical cases, with a ratio of frequency in the two organs of about 6:4. In the lungs, cysts of this form are relatively small, with an average diameter of about 40 mm. Spontaneous rupture of pulmonary cysts, with evacuation of larval membranes and fluid, occurs rather frequently. Secondary spread after spontaneous rupture or rupture at surgery is unknown, nor have anaphylaxis or other serious complications been observed. The disease in humans is benign and usually asymptomatic and has a low mortality. The larval stage of the European form is more pathogenic. The localization of cysts in clinical cases is different, with a ratio in lungs and liver of about 3:5.5. Cysts in the lungs are larger than with the northern form. In about 15 percent of cases, the cysts occur in organs other than the lungs and liver. In addition to the severe effects produced by larvae in such loci as the cranium, orbit, or myocardium, conditions such as anaphylaxis, secondary spread following rupture, pathologic fracture of bones, infected cysts with empyema, formation of hepatopulmonary fistulae, and other complications are frequent.[9]

Alveolar Hydatid Disease. The embryo of *E. multilocularis* seems to localize invariably in the liver of the intermediate host. Development of the larval *E. multilocularis* is inhibited in humans, so it persists indefinitely in the proliferative phase. As a result, the hepatic parenchyma is gradually invaded and replaced by fibrous tissue in which great numbers of vesicles, many microscopic, are embedded. Proliferation continues peripherally, with the result that an entire hepatic lobe may be replaced over a period of years. As the lesion enlarges, it usually undergoes degenerative changes that lead to central necrosis, often with liquefaction, and abscesses with a volume of several liters may be produced. Uneven calcification of necrotic tissues is typical in lesions of long standing. Hepatomegaly is characteristic and may be extreme. The disease takes a chronic course, with deterioration of health often occurring around middle age. Patients eventually succumb to hepatic failure, invasion of contiguous structures, or, less frequently, metastases to the brain.[10] However, instances of spontaneous death of the cyst during its early stage of development have been reported in people with asymptomatic infection.[11]

Polycystic Hydatid Disease. In human cases, hepatomegaly or tumor-like masses in the liver have been typical findings. Proliferation of vesicles may lead to destruction of much of the liver, and involvement of adjacent structures by extension does not appear to be unusual. The prognosis in polycystic hydatid disease is poor. The known cases have been described by D'Alessandro and associates.[7]

Diagnosis

The presence of a cyst-like mass in liver or lungs of a person with a history of exposure to sheep dogs in areas in which *E. granulosus* is endemic supports the diagnosis of cystic hydatid disease.[8] However, echinococcal cysts must be differentiated from benign cysts, cavitary tuberculosis, mycoses, abscesses, and benign or malignant neoplasms. A noninvasive confirmation of the diagnosis can usually be accomplished with the combined use of radiologic imaging and immunodiagnostic techniques. Roentgenography permits the detection of echinococcal cysts in the lungs; this is the most common means of diagnosis of the northern form, which most commonly localizes in the lungs. In other sites, calcification is necessary for roentgenographic visualization by x-ray. Computerized axial tomography (CT), magnetic resonance, and ultrasound imaging are useful for diagnosing deep-seated lesions in the liver and other organs and are further useful for defining the extent and condition of avascular fluid-filled cysts. The CT image of *E. granulosus* echinococcal cysts typically shows sharply contoured cysts (sometimes with internal daughter cysts) and marginal calcifications.[12]

Serologic tests are useful to confirm presumptive radiologic diagnoses, although some patients with cystic hydatid disease do not develop a detectable immune response.[8] Hepatic cysts are more likely to elicit an immune response than pulmonary cysts; however, it appears that, regardless of location, the sensitivity of serologic tests is inversely related to the degree of sequestration of the echinococcal antigens inside cysts. Enzyme-linked immunosorbent assay (ELISA) or the indirect hemagglutination test are highly sensitive procedures for the initial screening of sera; specific confirmation of reactivity can be obtained by demonstrating echinococcal antigens by immunodiffusion (arc 5) procedures or immunoblot assays (8/12 kD band).[13] Eosinophilia is present in fewer than 25 percent of infected persons.

In seronegative patients, a presumptive diagnosis may be confirmed by demonstrating protoscoleces or hydatid membranes in the liquid obtained by percutaneous aspiration of the cyst. Although previously considered taboo because of the potential for anaphylaxis or dissemination of protoscoleces, with certain precautions percutaneous aspiration for purposes of diagnosis or treatment is now standard procedure. Ultrasound guidance of the puncture, anthelmintic coverage, and anticipation of the possible need to treat an allergic reaction now minimize risks.[14] Protoscoleces can sometimes be demonstrated in sputum or bronchial washings; identification of hooklets is facilitated by acid-fast stains.

Diagnosis of alveolar echinococcosis may be difficult, particularly in regions where its possible occurrence is not known to clinicians and pathologists, as in central North America; the disease is typically seen in persons of advanced age, in whom it closely mimics hepatic carcinoma or cirrhosis. Plain roentgenography shows hepatomegaly and characteristic scattered areas of radiolucency outlined by calcific rings 2 to 4 mm in diameter. The usual CT image of *E. multilocularis* infection is that of indistinct solid tumors with central necrotic areas and perinecrotic plaque-like calcifications.[15] Serologic tests are usually positive at high titers; purified *E. multilocularis* antigens are highly specific, and comparing a patient's titers to both purified-specific and shared antigens permits serologic discrimination between patients infected with *E. multilocularis* and those infected with *E. granulosus*.[16,17] Needle biopsy of the liver may confirm the diagnosis if larval elements are demonstrated. Exploratory laparotomy is often done for diagnosis and delineation of the size and extent of the invasion.

Polycystic echinococcosis has characteristics intermediate between those of the cystic and alveolar forms.[7,18] The relatively large cysts are filled with liquid and contain brood capsules with numerous protoscoleces. The primary localization is the liver, but cysts may spread to contiguous sites or occur in other primary locations. Immunodiagnostic and other techniques useful for diagnosing cystic or alveolar hydatid disease are also of value in diagnosing polycystic hydatid disease. The hydatid cysts of *E. vogeli* can be differentiated from those of other species based on differences in the dimensions of the hooks of the protoscoleces.[7]

Treatment

Until recently, surgery was the only option for treatment of hydatid cysts; however, in the past 15 years chemotherapy has been introduced and evaluated; more recently, combinations of cyst puncture, aspiration, and drainage, with or without injection of chemicals—called percutaneous aspiration, injection, reaspiration (PAIR)—have been evaluated and, increasingly, are seen to supplement or even replace surgery as the preferred treatment.[19] Surgery remains the preferred treatment when cysts are large (more than 10 cm in diameter), secondarily infected, or located in certain organs, i.e., the brain or heart. The aim of surgery is total removal of the cyst while avoiding the adverse consequences of spilling its contents. Pericystectomy is the usual procedure, but simple drainage, capitonnage, marsupialization, and resection of the involved organ may be used, depending on the location and condition of the cyst(s). At times, surgery may be impossible because of the patient's general condition and the extent and location of the cysts. Under such conditions, treatment with benzimidazole drugs may be tried; approximately one-third of patients treated with benzimidazole drugs have been cured of their disease (e.g., complete and permanent disappearance of cysts), and an even higher proportion have responded with significant regression of cyst size and alleviation of symptoms.[20,21] Both albendazole (10 mg per kilogram body weight per day) and mebendazole (40 to 50 mg/kg) have demonstrated efficacy; however, albendazole (because of its superior pharmacokinetic profile, which favors intestinal absorption and penetration into the cysts) is slightly more efficacious. Similar adverse reactions (neutropenia, liver toxicity, alopecia, and others), reversible upon cessation of treatment, have been noted in most patients treated with both drugs. The minimum duration of treatment is 3 months. The long-term prognosis in individual patients is difficult to predict; therefore, prolonged follow-up with ultrasound or other imaging procedures is needed to determine the eventual outcome. A third option for the treatment of echinococcosis cysts in the liver, first used in Italy, is percutaneous puncture under sonographic guidance, aspiration of the liquid contents, and instillation of a protoscolicidal agent (e.g., 95 percent ethanol or cetrimide), followed by reaspiration.[22] To avoid sclerosing cholangitis, this procedure must not be performed in patients whose cysts have biliary communication; the presence of the latter can be determined by testing the cyst fluid for presence of bilirubin or by intraoperative cholangiography. The possibility of secondary echinococcosis resulting from accidental spillage during this procedure can be minimized by concurrent treatment with albendazole; in fact, a recent report suggests that combining PAIR with anthelmintic therapy may improve the results of treatment in comparison with either chemotherapy or PAIR alone.[23] A policy of conservative management has been adopted generally in the treatment of infections by the relatively benign northern form of *E. granulosus*, and surgical intervention is considered only in cases of uncertain diagnosis (i.e., possible neoplasms) or in rare cases of symptomatic disease.

Until recently, surgery has offered the only possibility for treatment of alveolar echinococcosis. The usual procedure has involved removal of the lesion with part or all of the affected hepatic lobe. Cases of advanced disease and those involving multiple lesions are often inoperable. With or without surgery, alveolar hydatid disease has a very high mortality rate. With metastases to the brain, death occurs within a few months after the onset of neurologic disorders. Long-term treatment with mebendazole (50 mg/kg per day) or albendazole (10 mg/kg) inhibits growth of larval *E. multilocularis*, reduces metastasis, and enhances both the quality and length of survival; prolonged therapy may eventually be larvicidal in some patients.[19] Liver transplantation has been employed successfully in otherwise terminal cases.[24]

Experience in the treatment of polycystic echinococcosis is limited.[7,18] Because the lesions are so extensive, surgical resection may be difficult and usually incomplete. A combination of surgery with albendazole is most likely to be successful.

Prevention and Control

Infection of humans by larval cestodes of the genus *Echinococcus* is contingent on ingestion of eggs distributed in the feces of dogs and perhaps other carnivores that harbor the adult worms. Control of hydatid disease in humans depends on the means to prevent or to eliminate infection of dogs. These objectives, so simple in concept, have generally been unattainable and will probably remain so in many regions because of human attitudes and other factors that defy change.

Little effort has been made to control the northern form of *E. granulosus*, in part because of the benign nature of the infection and perhaps also because the disease affects mainly scattered indigenous peoples. The significant decrease in incidence observed in recent years in Alaskan Eskimos and Indians has been attributable mainly to the replacement of dogs by mechanized vehicles for winter travel. Some advantage, however, is being lost with the growing tendency of these people to adopt the European practice of keeping dogs as pets.

Few countries have shown significant accomplishment in attempts to control *E. granulosus* in life cycles involving synanthropic animal hosts. In most regions where hydatid disease is a serious medical and economic problem, the combination of uncontrolled slaughter, indiscriminate disposal of carcasses and offal, and an abundance of free-ranging dogs provides nearly optimal conditions for the completion of the life cycle of this cestode. Large-scale programs of control have had noteworthy success only in Iceland, New Zealand, Australia, Tasmania, and Cyprus, which have in common the features of insularity, literate populations, satisfactory economies, and effective political organizations.[5] In these countries, the programs have been based on public education combined with strict regulations directed particularly toward control of dogs. Nearly complete control of *E. granulosus* in the Greek-controlled area of Cyprus was accomplished during the period between 1971 and 1975 through elimination of excess dogs, destruction of all dogs found to be infected, and regulation of slaughter. Development of the effective echinococcicidal drug praziquantel permitted the effective use of an anthelmintic in conjunction with other measures for the control of hydatid disease. The mass treatment of dogs and strict control of slaughter is effective under some conditions but of little value where early reinfection is probable.

Control of *E. multilocularis* presents a difficult problem of potentially increasing importance. Measures for control of the cestode have involved anthelmintic treatment of dogs and destruction of stray animals. In Alaska, the general reduction of numbers of dogs and improvements in housing have probably had some effect on the prevalence of *E. multilocularis*. The implications of the spread of *E. multilocularis* in central North America are currently not predictable. Since the control of this cestode in its natural hosts does not appear to be possible, preventive measures must be directed toward domestic carnivores. In endemic areas, strict controls on the movement of pet dogs and cats is necessary to prevent ingestion of infected rodents. Regular anthelmintic treatment of such animals might be practicable under some conditions.[25]

▸ REFERENCES

Rabies

1. Kuwert E, Merieux C, Koprowski H, Boegl K (eds): Rabies in the Tropics. Berlin: Springer-Verlag, 1985
2. Helmick GG: The epidemiology of human rabies postexposure prophylaxis, 1980–1981. JAMA 250:1990–1996, 1983
3. Krebs JW, Smith JS, Rupprecht CE, et al: Rabies surveillance in the United States during 1996. J Am Vet Med Assoc 211:1525–1539, 1997
4. Constantine DG: Rabies Transmission by Air in Bat Caves. Public Health Service Publication No. 1617. Washington, DC: U.S. Government Printing Office, 1967
5. Baer GM (ed): The Natural History of Rabies. Boca Raton, FL: CRC Press, 1991
6. Bell JF: Abortive rabies infection. J Infect Dis 114:249–257, 1964
7. Johnson HN: Rabies. In Horsfall FL, Tamm L (eds): Viral and Rickettsial Infections of Man. Philadelphia. JB Lippincott, 1967
8. Emmons RW, Leonard LL, De Gennaro F Jr, et al: A case of human rabies with prolonged survival. Intervirology 1:60–72, 1973
9. WHO Expert Committee on Rabies: Eighth Report. World Health Organ Tech Rep Ser 824, 1992
10. Centers for Disease Control: Rabies prevention—United States, 1991: recommendations of the Immunization Practices Advisory Committee (ACIP). MMWR (RR-3), 1991
11. Fishbein DB, Yenne KM, Dreesen DW, et al: Risk factors for systemic hypersensitivity reactions after booster vaccinations with human diploid cell rabies vaccine: a nationwide prospective study. Vaccine 11:1390–1394, 1993
12. Pappaioanou M, Fishbein DB, Dreesen DW, et al: Antibody response to preexposure human diploid-cell rabies vaccine given concurrently with chloroquine. N Engl J Med 314:280–284, 1986
13. Constantine DB: Batproofing of buildings by installation of valvelike devices in entryways. J Wildl Manage 46:507–513, 1982

Psittacosis

General References

Meyer KF: Ornithosis. In Biester HE, Schwarte LH (eds): Diseases of Poultry. 5th ed. Ames, IA: Iowa State University Press, 1965, pp 675–770

Page LA: Chlamydiosis (ornithosis). In Hofstad MS (ed): Diseases of Poultry. 6th ed. Ames, IA: Iowa State University Press, 1972, pp 414–447

Schachter J, Dawson CR: Human Chlamydial Infections. Littleton, MA: Publishing Sciences Group, 1978

Schachter J, Sugg N, Sung M: Psittacosis: the reservoir persists. J Infect Dis 137: 44–49, 1978

Tularemia

1. Centers for Disease Control and Prevention: Summary of notifiable diseases, United States, 1992. MMWR 41:67–73, 1993
2. Stewart SJ: Francisella. In Murray PR, et al (eds): Manual of Clinical Microbiology. Washington, DC: ASM Press, 1995, pp 545–548
3. Bevanger L, Maeland JA, Naess AI: Agglutinins and antibodies to *Francisella tularensis* outer membrane antigens in the early diagnosis of disease during an outbreak of tularemia. J Clin Micro 26: 433–437, 1988.
4. Hopla CE: The ecology of tularemia. Adv Vet Sci Comp Med 18:25–53, 1974
5. Francis E: Tularemia. JAMA 84:1243–1250, 1925
6. Penn RL: *Francisella tularensis* (tularemia). In Isselbacher KJ, et al (eds): Harrison's Principles of Internal Medicine. New York: McGraw-Hill, 1994, pp 2060–2067
7. Centers for Disease Control and Prevention: Summary of notifiable diseases, United States, 1993. MMWR 42:67–73, 1994
8. Centers for Disease Control and Prevention: Summary of notifiable diseases, United States, 1994. MMWR 43:69–77, 1995
9. Boyce JM: Recent trends in the epidemiology of tularemia in the United States. J Infect Dis 131:197–199, 1975
10. Markowitz LE, Hynes NA, de la Cruz P, et al: Tick-borne tularemia: an outbreak of lymphadenopathy in children. JAMA 254:2922–2925, 1985
11. Klock LE, Olsen PF, Fukushima T: Tularemia epidemic associated with the deerfly. JAMA 226:149–152, 1973
12. Young LS, Bicknell DS, Archer BG, et al: Tularemia epidemic: Vermont, 1968. N Engl J Med 280:1253–1260, 1969

13. Capellan J, Fong IW: Tularemia from a cat bite: case report and review of feline-associated tularemia. Clin Infect Dis 16:472–475, 1993
14. Dienst FT: Tularemia: a perusal of three hundred thirty-nine cases. J La State Med Soc 115:114–127, 1963
15. Evans ME, Gregory DW, Schaffner W, McGee ZA: Tularemia: a 30-year experience with 88 cases. Medicine 64:251–269, 1985
16. Enderlin G, Morales L, Jacobs RF, Cross JT: Streptomycin and alternative agents for the treatment of tularemia: review of the literature. Clin Infect Dis 19:42–47, 1994

Anthrax

1. Whitford HW, Hugh-Jones ME: Anthrax. In Beran GW (ed): Handbook of Zoonoses. Boca Raton, Florida: CRC Press; 1994, pp 61–82
2. Klemm DM, Klemm WR: A history of anthrax. J Am Vet Med Assoc 135:458–462, 1959
3. Turnbull PC: Proceedings of the International Workshop on Anthrax. Salisbury Medical Journal 68:1–105, 1990
4. Sirisanthana T, Nelson KE, Ezzell JW, Abshire TG: Serological studies of patients with cutaneous and oral-oropharyngeal anthrax from northern Thailand. Am J Trop Med Hyg 39:575–581, 1988
5. Carl M, Hawkins R, Coulson N, et al: Detection of spores of *Bacillus anthracis* using the polymerase chain reaction. J Infect Dis 165:1145–1148, 1992
6. Dutz W, Kohout E: Anthrax. [Review]. Pathol Annual 6:209–248, 1971
7. LaForce FM: Woolsorters' disease in England. Bull N Y Acad Med 54:956–963, 1978
8. Meselson M, Guillemin J, Hugh-Jones M, et al: The Sverdlovsk anthrax outbreak of 1979. Science 266:1202–1208, 1994
9. Lincoln RE, Walker JS, Klein F, Haines BW: Anthrax. Adv Vet Sci 9:327–368, 1964
10. Van Ness GL: Ecology of anthrax. Science 172:1303–1307, 1964
11. Fox MD, Kaufmann AF, Zendel SA, et al: Anthrax in Louisiana, 1971: epizootiologic study. J Am Vet Med Assoc 163:446–451, 1973
12. Kaufmann AF, Fox MD, Kolb RC: Anthrax in Louisiana, 1971: an evaluation of the Sterne strain anthrax vaccine. J Am Vet Med Assoc 163:442–445, 1973
13. Tanner WB, Potter ME, Teclaw RF: Public health aspects of anthrax vaccination of dairy cattle. J Am Vet Med Assoc 173:1465–1466, 1978
14. Brachman PS, Gold H, Plotkin SA et al: Field evaluation of a human anthrax vaccine. Am J Public Health 52:632–645, 1997

Brucellosis

1. Corbel MJ: Brucellosis: an overview. Emerg Infect Dis 3:213–221, 1997
2. Joint FAO/WHO Expert Committee on Brucellosis: Sixth Report. Technical Report Series No. 740. Geneva: World Health Organization, 1986
3. Solomon HM, Jackson D: Rapid diagnosis of *Brucella melitensis* in blood: some operational characteristics of the BACT/ALERT. J Clin Microbiol 30:222–224, 1992
4. Araj GF, Kaufmann AF: Determination by enzyme-linked immunosorbent assay of immunoglobulin G (IgG), IgM, and IgA to *Brucella melitensis* major outer membrane proteins and whole-cell heat-killed antigens in sera of patients with brucellosis. J Clin Microbiol 27:1909–1912, 1989
5. Young EJ, Corbel MJ: Brucellosis: clinical and laboratory aspects. Boca Raton, Florida: CRC Press, 1989
6. Spink WW: The Nature of Brucellosis. Minneapolis, Minnesota, University of Minnesota Press, 1956
7. Ariza J, Gudiol F, Pallares R, Rufi G, Fernandez-Viladrich P: Comparative trial of rifampin-doxycycline versus tetracycline-streptomycin in the therapy of human brucellosis. Antimicrob Agents Chemother 28:548–551, 1985
8. Kaufmann AF, Fox MD, Boyce JM, et al: Airborne spread of brucellosis. Ann NY Acad Sci 353:105–114, 1980
9. Anonymous: Brucellosis outbreak at a pork processing plant—North Carolina, 1992. MMWR 43:113–116, 1994
10. Chomel BB, DeBess EE, Mangiamele DM, et al: Changing trends in the epidemiology of human brucellosis in California from 1973 to 1992: a shift toward foodborne transmission. J Infect Dis 170:1216–1223, 1994
11. Fox MD, Kaufmann AF: Brucellosis in the United States, 1965–1974. J Infect Dis 136:312–316, 1977
12. Buchanan TM, Hendricks SL, Patton CM, Feldman RA: Brucellosis in the United States, 1960–1972, an abattoir-associated disease. Part III. Epidemiology and evidence for acquired immunity. Medicine (Baltimore) 53:427–439, 1974
13. Schurig GG, Roop RM II, Bagchi T, Boyle S, Buhrman D, Sriranganathan N: Biological properties of RB51; a stable rough strain of *Brucella abortus*. Vet Microbiol 28:171–188, 1991

Leptospirosis

1. Alston JM, Broom JC: Leptospirosis in man and animals. Edinburgh: Livingstone, 1958
2. Yasuda PH, Steigerwalt AG, Sulzer KR: Deoxyribonucleic acid relatedness between serogroups and serovars in the family Leptospiraceae with proposals for seven new *Leptospira* species. Int J Syst Bacteriol 37:407–415, 1987
3. Turner LH: Leptospirosis. III. Maintenance, isolation and demonstration of leptospires. Trans R Soc Trop Med Hyg 62:623–646, 1970
4. Faine S: Guidelines for the control of leptospirosis, Offset Publication No. 67, World Health Organization Geneva, Switzerland, 1982
5. Pappas MG, Ballou WR, Gray MR, Takafuji ET, Miller RN, Hockmeyer WT: Rapid serodiagnosis of leptospirosis using the IgM-specific dot-ELISA: comparison with microscopic agglutination test. Am J Trop Med Hyg 34:346–354, 1985
6. Gussenhoven GC, van der Hoon MAWG, Goris MGA, et al: LEPTO dipstick: a dipstick assay for the detection of Leptospira-specific immunoglobulin M antibodies in human sera. J Clin Microbiol 35:92–97, 1997
7. Bal AE, Gravekamp C, Hartskeerl RA, Meza-Brewster J, Korver H, Terpstra WJ: Detection of leptospires in urine by PCR for early diagnosis of leptospirosis. J Clin Microbiol 32:1894–1898, 1994
8. Brown PD, Gravekamp C, Carrington DG, et al: Evaluation of the polymerase chain reaction for early diagnosis of leptospirosis. J Med Microbiol 43:110–114, 1995
9. Merien F, Baranton G, Perolat P: Comparison of polymerase chain reaction with microagglutination test and culture for diagnosis of leptospirosis. J Infect Dis 172:281–285, 1995
10. Zaki SR, Shieh WJ, Epidemic Working Group: Leptospirosis associated with outbreak of acute febrile illness and pulmonary haemorrhage, Nicaragua, 1995. Lancet 347:535–536, 1996
11. Feigin RD, Anderson DC: Human leptospirosis. Crit Rev Clin Lab Sci 5:413–467, 1975
12. Turner LH: Leptospirosis I. Trans R Soc Trop Med Hyg 61:842–855, 1967
13. Watt G, Tuazon ML, Santiago E: Placebo-controlled trial of intravenous penicillin for severe and late leptospirosis. Lancet 1:433–435, 1988
14. Takafuji ET, Kirkpatrick JW, Miller RN: An efficacy trial of doxycycline chemoprophylaxis against leptospirosis. N Engl J Med 310:497, 1984

Salmonellosis

1. Centers for Disease Control and Prevention: *Salmonella* Surveillance Annual Tabulation Summary, 1993–1995. Atlanta: Centers for Disease Control and Prevention, 1996
2. Holmberg SD, Wachsmuth IK, Hickman-Brenner FW, Cohen ML: Comparison of plasmid profile analysis, phage typing, and anti-

microbial susceptibility testing in characterizing *Salmonella typhimurium* isolates from outbreaks. J Clin Microbiol 19:100–104, 1984
3. Threlfall EJ, Hampton MD, Ward LR, Rowe B: Application of pulsed-field gel electrophoresis to an international outbreak of *Salmonella agona*. Emerg Infect Dis 2:130–132, 1996
4. Cohen ML, Tauxe RV: Drug-resistant *Salmonella* in the United States: an epidemiologic perspective. Science 234:964–969, 1986
5. Tauxe RV, Holmberg SD, Cohen ML: The epidemiology of gene transfer in the environment. In Levy SB, Miller RV (eds): Gene Transfer in the Environment. New York: McGraw-Hill, 1989, pp 377–403
6. Centers for Disease Control and Prevention: Multidrug-resistant *Salmonella* serotype *typhimurium*—United States, 1996. MMWR 46: 308–310, 1997
7. Buchwald DS, Blaser MJ: A review of human salmonellosis. II: Duration of excretion following infection with nontyphi *Salmonella*. Rev Infect Dis 6:345–356, 1984
8. Asserkoff B, Bennett JV: Effect of antibiotic therapy in acute salmonellosis on the fecal excretion of salmonellae. N Engl J Med 281:636–640, 1969
9. Ewing WH: Edwards and Ewing's identification of Enterobacteriaceae. In: 4th ed. New York, Elsevier Science, Inc, 1986
10. Cohen ML, Potter M, Pollard R, Feldman RA: Turtle-associated salmonellosis in the United States. Effect of public health action, 1970–1976. JAMA 243:1247–1249, 1980
11. Centers for Disease Control and Prevention: Reptile-associated salmonellosis—selected states, 1994–1995. MMWR 44:347–350, 1995
12. Schwabe CW: Veterinary Medicine and Human Health. 3rd ed. Baltimore: Williams & Wilkins, 1984
13. Marth EH: *Salmonellae* and salmonellosis associated with milk and milk products: a review. J Dairy Sci 52:283–312, 1969
14. Mahon BE, Ponka A, Hall WN, Komatsu K, Dietrich SE, Siitonen A, et al: An international outbreak of Salmonella infections caused by alfalfa sprouts grown from contaminated seeds. J Infect Dis 175:876–882, 1997
15. Hedberg CW, MacDonald KL, Osterholm MT: Changing epidemiology of food-borne disease: a Minnesota perspective. Clin Infect Dis 18:671–682, 1994
16. Centers for Disease Control and Prevention: Multistate outbreak of *Salmonella poona* infections—United States and Canada, 1991. MMWR 40:549–552, 1991
17. Centers for Disease Control and Prevention: Outbreaks of *Salmonella* serotype *enteritidis* infection associated with consumption of raw shell eggs—United States, 1994–1995. MMWR 45:737–742, 1996
18. St. Louis ME, Morse DL, Potter M, et al: The emergence of grade A eggs as a major source of *Salmonella enteritidis* infections: new implications for the control of salmonellosis. JAMA 259:2103–2107, 1988
19. Mishu B, Koehler J, Lee LA, Rodrigue D, Hickman-Brenner F, Blake P, et al: Outbreaks of *Salmonella enteritidis* infections in the United States, 1985–1991. J Infect Dis 169:547–552, 1994
20. Hedberg CW, David MJ, White KE, MacDonald KL, Osterholm MT: Role of egg consumption in sporadic *Salmonella enteritidis* and *Salmonella typhimurium* infections in Minnesota. J Infect Dis 167:107–111, 1993
21. Rampling A: *Salmonella enteritidis* five years on. Lancet 342: 317–318, 1993
22. Poppe C, Demczuk W, Mcfadden K, Johnson RP: Virulence of *Salmonella enteritidis* phage types 4, 8 and 13 and other *Salmonella* spp for day-old chicks, hens and mice. Can J Vet Res 57:281–287, 1993
23. Boyce TG, Koo D, Swerdlow DL, Gomez TM, Serrano B, Nickey LN, et al: Recurrent outbreaks of *Salmonella enteritidis* infections in a Texas restaurant: phage type 4 arrives in the United States. Epidemiol Infect 117:29–34, 1996
24. Kinde H, Read DH, Chin P, Bickford AA, Walker L, Ardans A, et al: *Salmonella enteritidis*, phage type 4 infection in a commercial layer flock in Southern California: bacteriologic and epidemiologic findings. Avian Dis 40:665–671, 1996
25. Pissaro DJ, Reporter R, Mascola L, Kilman L, Malcolm GB, Rolka H, et al: Epidemic *Salmonella enteritidis* infection in Los Angeles County, California. The predominance of phage type 4. West J Med 165:126–130, 1996
26. Sobel J, Hirshfeld A, Mctigue K, Nichols C, Burnette C, Mottice S, et al: *Salmonella enteritidis* phage type 4 pandemic reaches Utah. 36th Interscience Conference on Antimicrobial Agents and Chemotherapy 1996, LB27 12 Abstract Washington, DC: American Society for Microbiology
27. Blaser MJ, Newman LS: A review of human salmonellosis. I. Infective dose. Rev Infect Dis 128:1096–1106, 1982
28. Cruickshank JG, Humphrey TJ: The carrier foodhandler and non-typhoid salmonellosis. Epidemiol Infect 98:223–230, 1987
29. Baine WB, Gangarosa EJ, Bennett JV, Barker WH: Institutional salmonellosis. J Infect Dis 128:357–360, 1973
30. Levine WC, Smart JF, Archer DL, Bean NH, Tauxe RV: Foodborne disease outbreaks in nursing homes, 1975 through 1987. JAMA 266:2105–2109, 1991
31. Telzak EE, Budnick LD, Zweig Greenberg MS, Blum S, Shayegani M, Benson CE, et al: A nosocomial outbreak of *Salmonella enteritidis* infection due to the consumption of raw eggs. N Engl J Med 323:394–397, 1997
32. Weikel CS, Guerrant RL: Nosocomial salmonellosis [Editorial]. Infect Control 6:218–220, 1985
33. Chalker RB, Blaser MJ: A review of human salmonellosis III. Magnitude of *Salmonella* infection in the United States. Rev Infect Dis 10:111–124, 1988
34. Martin SM, Hargrett-Bean N, Tauxe RV: An Atlas of *Salmonella* in the United States: Serotype Specific Surveillance, 1968–1986. Stock No. PB89-213441-AS, National Technical Information Service. Atlanta: Centers for Disease Control, 1989
35. Clark GM, Kaufmann AF, Gangarosa EJ: Epidemiology of an international outbreak of *Salmonella agona*. Lancet 2:490–493, 1973
36. Rodrigue DC, Tauxe RV, Blake PA, Rowe B: International increase in *Salmonella enteritidis:* a new pandemic? Epidemiol Infect 105:21–27, 1990
37. World Health Organization Wholesomeness of irradiated foods: Technical Report Series 659, Geneva: World Health Organization, 1981
38. Lee PR: From the Assistant Secretary for Health, US Public Health Service: irradiation to prevent foodborne illness. JAMA 272:261, 1994

Toxoplasmosis

1. Frenkel JK: Toxoplasmosis. Parasite life cycle, pathology, and immunology. In Hammond DM, Long PL (eds): The Coccidia. Baltimore: University Park Press, 1973, pp 343–410
2. Wreghitt TG, Hakim M, Gray JJ, et al: Toxoplasmosis in heart and lung transplant recipients. J Clin Pathol 42:194–199, 1989
3. McCabe RE, Brooks RG, Dorfman RF, Remington JS: Clinical spectrum in 107 cases of toxoplasmic lymphadenopathy. Rev Infect Dis 9:754–774, 1987
4. Desmonts G, Couvreur J: Congenital toxoplasmosis. A prospective study of 378 pregnancies. N Engl J Med 290:1110–1116, 1974
5. Mcauley J, Boyer KM, Patel D, et al: Early and longitudinal evaluations of treated infants and children and untreated historical patients with congenital toxoplasmosis—the Chicago collaborative treatment trial. Clin Infect Dis 18:38–72, 1994
6. Mets MB, Holfels E, Boyer KM, et al: Eye manifestations of congenital toxoplasmosis. Am J Ophthalmol 122:309–324, 1996
7. Dannemann BR, Remington JS: Toxoplasmic encephalitis in AIDS. Hosp Pract 139–154, March 15, 1989

8. Luft BJ, Naot Y, Araujo FG, et al: Primary and reactivated *Toxoplasma* infection in patients with cardiac transplants. Clinical spectrum and problems in diagnosis in a defined population. Ann Intern Med 99:27–31, 1983
9. Sousa OK, Saenz RE, Frenkel JK: Toxoplasmosis in Panama: a 10-year study. Am J Trop Med Hyg 38:315–322, 1988
10. Sever JL, Ellenberg JH, Ley AC, et al: Toxoplasmosis: maternal and pediatric findings in 23,000 pregnancies. Pediatrics 82:181–192, 1988
11. Brooks RG, McCabe RE, Remington JS: Role of serology in the diagnosis of toxoplasmic lymphadenopathy. Rev Infect Dis 9:775–782, 1987
12. Tomasi JP Schlit AF, Stadtsbaeder S: Rapid double-sandwich enzyme-linked immunosorbent assay for detection of human immunoglobulin M anti-*Toxoplasma gondii* antibodies. J Clin Microbiol 24:849–850, 1986
13. Ostergaard L, Nielsen AK, Black FT: DNA amplification on cerebrospinal-fluid for diagnosis of cerebral toxoplasmosis among HIV-positive patients with signs or symptoms of neurological disease. Scand J Infect Dis 25(2):227–237, 1993
14. Filice GA, Hitt JA, Mitchell CD, Blackstad M, Sorensen SW: Diagnosis of *Toxoplasma parasitemia* in patients with AIDS by gene detection after amplification with polymerase chain-reaction. J Clin Microbiol 31(9):2327–2331, 1993
15. Cohn JA, MeMeeking A, Cohen W, et al: Evaluation of the policy of empiric treatment of suspected *Toxoplasma* encephalitis in patients with the acquired immunodeficiency syndrome. Am J Med 86:521–527, 1989
16. Guerina NG, Hsu HW, Meissner HC, et al: Neonatal serologic screening and early treatment for congenital *Toxoplasma gondii* infection. N Engl J Med 330:1858–1863, 1994
17. Roizen N, Swisher CN, Stein MA, et al: Neurologic and developmental outcome in treated congenital toxoplasmosis. Pediatrics 95: 11–20, 1995
18. Frenkel JK, Hassanein KM, Hassanein RS, Brown E, Thulliez P, Quintero-Nuñez R: Transmission of *Toxoplasma gondii* in Panama City: a five-year prospective cohort study of children, cats, rodents, birds, and soil. Am J Trop Med Hyg 53:458–468, 1995
19. Holland GN, Engstrom RE, Glasgow BJ, et al: Ocular toxoplasmosis in patients with the acquired immunodeficiency syndrome. Am J Ophthalmol 106:653–667, 1988
20. Waldeland H, Frenkel JK: Live and killed vaccines against toxoplasmosis in mice. J Parasitol 69:60–65, 1983
21. Frenkel JK, Pfefferkorn ER, Smith DD, Fishback JL: A *Toxoplasma* vaccine for cats using a new mutant. Am J Vet Res 52:759–763, 1991

Trichinellosis

1. Pozio E, LaRosa E, Murrell KD, Lichtenfels R: Taxonomic revision of the genus *Trichinella*. J Parasitol 78:654–659, 1992
2. Murrell KD, Bruschi F: Clinical trichinellosis. In: Sun T (ed): Progress in Clinical Parasitology. 4th ed. Boca Raton, FL: CRC Press, 1994, pp 117–150
3. Jacobson EE, Jacobson HG: Trichinosis in an immunosuppressed human host. Am J Clin Pathol 68:791–794, 1977
4. Dupouy-Camet J, Soule CI, Ancelle T: Recent news on trichinellosis: another outbreak due to horse meat consumption in France in 1993. Parasite 1:99, 1994
5. Bailey TM, Schantz PM: Trends in incidence and transmission patterns of trichinosis in humans in the United States: comparisons of the periods 1975–1981 and 1982–1986. Rev Infect Dis 12:5–11, 1990
6. MacLean JP, Viallet J, Law C, Stuart M: Trichinosis in the Canada Arctic: report of five outbreaks and a new clinical syndrome. J Infect Dis 160:513–520, 1989
7. Capo V, Despommier DD: Clinical aspects of infection with *Trichinella* spp. Clin Microbiol Rev 9:47–53, 1996
8. Gould SE: Clinical manifestations, a symptomatology. In: Trichinosis in Man and Animals. Springfield, IL: Charles C Thomas, 1970, pp 269–306
9. Manhorter SD, Kazura JW: Trichinosis of the central nervous system. Semin Neurol 13:148–161, 1993
10. Murrell KD: Foodborne parasites. Int J Environ Health Res 5:63–85, 1995

Larva Migrans Syndromes

General References

Chaudry A, Longworth D: Cutaneous manifestations of intestinal helminth infections. Dermatol Clin 7:275–290, 1989

Glickman LT, Magnaval JF: Zoonotic roundworm infections. Infect Dis Clin North Am 7:717–732, 1993

Matsui T, Iida M, Murakami M, et al.: Intestinal anisakiasis: clinical and radiologic features. Radiology 157:299–302, 1985

Orihuela A, Torres J: Single dose of albendazole in the treatment of cutaneous larva migrans. Arch Dermatol 126:398–399, 1990

Sugimachi K, Inokuchi K, Ooiwa T, Fujino T, Ishii Y: Acute gastric anisakiasis: analysis of 178 cases. JAMA 253:1012–1013, 1985

Taylor MR, Keane CT, O'Connor P, Mulvihill E, Holland C: The expanded spectrum of toxocaral disease. Lancet 1:692–694, 1988

Fascioliasis and Paragonimiasis

Fascioliasis

1. Chen MG, Mott KE: Progress in assessment of morbity due to *Fasciola hepatica* infection: a review of recent literature. Trop Dis Bull 7:R1–R38, 1990
2. World Health Organization: Control of Foodborne Trematode Infections. Report of a WHO Study Group. WHO Technical Report Series No. 849, Geneva: World Health Organization, 1995
3. Arjona R, Riancho JA, Aguado JM et al: Fascioliasis in developed countries: a review of classic and aberrant forms of the disease. Medicine 74:13–23, 1995
4. Apt W, Aguilera X, Vega F, et al: Treatment of human chronic fascioliasis with triclabendazole: drug efficacy and serologic response. Am J Trop Med Hyg 52:532–535, 1995

Paragonimiasis

1. Toscano C, Yu SH, Nunn P, Mott KE: Paragonimiasis and tuberculosis, diagnostic confusion: a review of the literature. Trop Dis Bull 92:R1–27, 1995
2. World Health Organization: Control of Foodborne Trematode Infections. Report of a WHO Study Group. WHO Technical Report Series No. 849. Geneva: World Health Organization, 1995
3. Yong TS, Seo JH, Yeo IS: Serodiagnosis of human paragonimiasis by ELISA-inhibition test using monoclonal antibodies. Korean J Parasitol 31:141–147, 1993

Clonorchiasis and Opisthorchiasis

1. WHO Study Group: Control of Foodborne Trematode Infections. WHO Technical Report Series No. 849. Geneva: World Health Organization, 1995, pp 1–157
2. Chou ST, Chan CW: Mucin-producing cholangiocarcinoma: an autopsy study in Hong Kong. Pathology 8:321–328, 1976
3. Purtilo DT: Clonorchiasis and hepatic neoplasms. Trop Geogr Med 28:21–27, 1976

4. Shin HR, Lee CH, Park HJ, et al: Hepatitis B and C virus, *Clonorchis sinensis* for the risk of liver cancer: a case-control study in Pusan, Korea. Int J Epidemiol 25:933–940, 1996
5. Anonymous: Infection with liver flukes, *Opisthorchis viverrini*, *Opisthorchis felineus* and *Clonorchis sinensis*, a review: IARC Monographs on the Evaluation of Carcinogenic Risks to Humans 61: 121–175, 1994
6. Fang YY: Epidemiologic characteristics of *Clonorchis sinensis* in Guan Dong Province, China. Southeast Asian J Trop Med Public Health 25:291–295, 1994
7. Lin YL, Chen ER, Yen CM: Antibodies in the serum of patients with clonorchiasis before and after treatment. Southeast Asian J Trop Med Public Health 26:114–119, 1995
8. Loscher T et al: Praziquantel in clonorchiasis and opisthorchiasis. Trop Med Parasitol 32:234–236, 1981

Taeniasis and Cysticercosis

1. Rausch RL: On the ecology and distribution of *Echinococcus* spp (Cestoda: Taeniidae), and characteristics of their development in the intermediate host. Ann Parasitol 42:19–63, 1967
2. Van As AD, Joubert J: Neurocysticercosis in 578 black epileptic patients. S Afr Med J 80:327–328, 1991
3. Slonka GF, Matulich W, Morphet E, et al: An outbreak of bovine cysticercosis in California. Am J Trop Med Hyg 27:101–105, 1978
4. Pawlowski Z, Schultz MG: Taeniasis and cysticercosis (*Taenia saginata*). Adv Parasitol 10:269–343, 1972
5. Cuetler AC, Garcia-Bobadilla JG, Guerra CG, Martinez FM, Kaim B: Neurocysticercosis: focus on intraventricular disease. Clin Infect Dis 24:157–164, 1997
6. White AC Jr: Neurocysticercosis: a major cause of neurological disease worldwide. Clin Infect Dis 24:101–115, 1997
7. Rodriguez-Carbajal J, Boleaga-Duran B, Dorfsman J: The role of computed tomography (CT) in the diagnosis of neurocysticercosis. Childs Nerv Syst 3(4):199–202, 1987
8. Pau A, Turtas S, Brambilla M, et al: Computed tomography and magnetic resonance imagining of cerebral cysticercosis. Surg Neurol 27:548–552, 1987
9. Lotz J, Hewlett R, Albeit B, et al: Neurocysticercosis: correlative pathomorphology and MR imaging. Neuroradiology 30:35–41, 1988
10. Plancarte A, Espinoza B, Flisser A: Immunodiagnosis of human neurocysticercosis by enzyme-linked immunosorbent assay. Childs Nerv Syst 3(4):203–205, 1987
11. Nunez R, Munoz A, Nunez C, Gomerz B: A micro ELISA for the diagnosis of cerebral cysticercosis. J Immunoassay 10(2–3):169–176, 1989
12. Estrada JJ, Estrada JA, Kuhn RE: Identification of *Taenia solium* antigens from patients with neurocysticercosis. Am J Trop Med Hyg 41(1):50–55, 1989
13. Tsang VC, Brand JA, Boyer AE: An enzyme-linked immunoelectrotransfer blot assay and glycoprotein antigens. J Infect Dis 159:50–59, 1989
14. Wilson M, Bryan RT, Fried JA, et al: Clinical evaluation of the cysticercosis enzyme-linked immunoelectrotransfer blot in patients with neurocysticercosis. J Infect Dis 164:1007–1009, 1991
15. DeGhetalidi LD, Norman RM, Louville AW: Cerebral cysticercosis treated biphasically with dexamethasone and praziquantel. Ann Intern Med 99:179–181, 1983
16. Del Brotto OH, Sotelo J, Roman GC: Therapy for neurocysticercosis: a reappraisal. Clin Infect Dis 17:730–735, 1993
17. Sotelo J, Escobedo F, Penagos P: Albendazole versus praziquantel for therapy for neurocysticercosis: a controlled trial. Arch Neurol 45:532–534, 1988
18. Carpio A, Santillon F, Leon P, Flores C, Hauser WA: Is the course of neurocysticercosis modified by treatment with antihelminthic agents? Arch Intern Med 155:1982–1988, 1995

Other Cestodeases and Diphyllobothriasis

1. Pawlowski Z: Cestodiasis; taeniasis, cysticercosis, diphyllobothriasis, hymenolepiasis and others. In Warren K, Mahmoud AF (eds): Tropical and Geographic Medicine. 2nd ed. New York: McGraw-Hill, 1990, pp 490–504
2. World Health Organization: Control of Foodborne Trematode Infections. Report of a Study Group. WHO Technical Report Series No. 849. Geneva: World Health Organization, 1995
3. Drugs for Parasitic Infections. Med Lett 37:99–108, 1995
4. Rausch RL, Scott EM, Rausch VR: Helminths in Eskimos in western Alaska, with particular reference to *Diphyllobothrium* infection and anemia. Trans R Soc Trop Med Hyg 61:351–357, 1967
5. von Bonsdorff B: Diphyllobothriasis in Man. New York: Academic Press, 1997
6. Cross JH: Fish and invertebrate-borne helminths. In Hui YH, Gorham JR, Murrell KD, Cliver DO (eds): Foodborne Disease Handbook: Diseases Caused by Viruses, Parasites and Fungi. New York: Marcel Dekker, 1994, pp 279–329.

Hydatid Disease (Echinococcosis)

1. Rausch RL: Life-cycle patterns and geographic distribution of *Echinococcus* species. In Thompson RCA, Lymbery AJ (eds): *Echinococcus* and Hydatid Disease. Wallingford, United Kingdom: CAB International, 1995, pp 89–134
2. Lymbery AJ, Thompson RCA: Species of *Echinococcus*: pattern and process. Parasitol Today 12:486–491, 1996
3. Thompson RCA, Lymbery AJ, Constantine CC: Variation in *Echinococcus*: towards a taxonomic revision of the genus. Adv Parasitol 35:146–176, 1995
4. Pappaioanou M, Schwabe CW, Sard DM: An evolving pattern of human hydatid disease transmission in the United States. Am J Trop Med Hyg 26:732–742, 1977
5. Schantz PM, Chai J, Craig PS, et al: Epidemiology and control. In Thompson RCA, Lymbery AJ (eds): *Echinococcus* and Hydatid Disease. Wallingford, United Kingdom: CAB International, 1995, pp 233–331
6. Gamble WB, Segal M, Schantz PM, Rausch RL: Alveolar hydatid disease in Minnesota: first human case acquired in the contiguous United States. JAMA 241:904–907, 1979
7. D'Alessandro A, Rausch RL, Cuello C, Aristizabal N: First observation of *Echinococcus vogeli* in man, with a review of human cases of polycystic hydatid disease in Colombia and neighboring countries. Am J Trop Med Hyg 28:303–317, 1979
8. Kammerer WS, Schantz PM: Echinococcal disease. Infect Dis Clin North Am 7:605–618, 1993
9. Wilson JF, Diddams AC, Rausch RL: Cystic hydatid disease in Alaska. A review of 101 autochthonous cases of *Echinococcus granulosus* infection. Am Rev Respir Dis 98:1–15, 1968
10. Wilson JF, Rausch RL: Alveolar hydatid disease: a review of clinical features of 33 indigenous cases of *Echinococcus multilocularis* infection in Alaskan eskimos. Am J Trop Med Hyg 29:340–349, 1980
11. Rausch RL, Wilson JF, Schantz PM, et al: Spontaneous death of *Echinococcus multilocularis* cases diagnosed serologically (by EM2 ELISA) and clinical significance. Am J Trop Med Hyg 36:576–585, 1987
12. Morris DL, Richards KS: Hydatid Disease: Current Medical and Surgical Management. Oxford: Butterworth-Heineman, 1992

13. Maddison SE, Slemenda SB, Schantz PM, et al: A specific diagnostic antigen of *Echinococcus granulosus* with an apparent molecular weight of 8 kDA. Am J Trop Med Hyg 40:337–383, 1989
14. Hira PR et al: Diagnosis of cystic hydatid disease: role of aspiration cytology. Lancet 2:655–658, 1988
15. Didier D, Weiler S, Rohmer P, et al: Hepatic alveolar echinococcosis: correlative US and CT study. Radiology 154:179–186, 1985
16. Gottstein G, Eckert J, Fey H: Serological differentiation between *Echinococcus granulosus* and *E. multilocularis* infections in man. Zeitschrift fur Parasitenkunde 69:347–356, 1983
17. Gottstein B, Jacquier P, Bresson-Hadni S, Eckert J: Improved primary immunodiagnosis of alveolar echinococcosis in humans by an enzyme-linked immunosorbent assay using the Em 2 plus antigen. J Clin Microbiol 31:373–377, 1993
18. Meneghelli UG, Martinelli ALC, Llorach Velludo MAS, et al: Polycystic hydatid disease (*Echinococcus vogeli*). Clinical, laboratory and morphologic findings in nine Brazilian patients. J Hepatol 14:203–210, 1992
19. Anonymous: Guidelines for treatment of cystic and alveolar echinococcosis in humans. Bull World Health Organ 74:231–243, 1996
20. Davis A, Pawlowski ZS, Dixon H: Multicentre clinical trials of benzimidazole carbamates in human echinococcosis. Bull World Health Organ 64:383–387, 1986
21. Davis A, Dixon H, Pawlowski Z: Multicentre clinical trials of benzimidazole carbamates in human cystic echinococcosis (phase 2). Bull World Health Organ 67:503–508, 1989
22. Filice C, Pirola F, Brunetti E, et al: A new therapeutic approach for hydatid liver cysts. Aspiration and alcohol injection under sonographic guidance. Gastroenterology 98:1366–1368, 1990
23. Khuroo MS, Dar MY, Yattoo GN, et al: Percutaneous drainage versus albendazole therapy in hepatic hydatidosis: a perspective, randomized study. Gastroenterology 104:1452–1459, 1993
24. Bresson-Hadni S, Miguet JP, Mantion G, et al: Orthotopic liver transplantation for incurable alveolar echinococcosis of the liver; report of 17 cases. Hepatology 13:1061–1070, 1991
25. Rausch RL, Wilson JF, Schantz PM: A programme to reduce the risk of infection by *Echinococcus multilocularis*: the use of praziquantel to control the cestode in a village in the hyperendemic region of Alaska. Ann Trop Med Parasitol 84:239–250, 1991

15

Opportunistic Fungal Infections

Michael A. Pfaller

Fungal infections, or mycoses, may be broken into two broad categories: (*a*) endemic and (*b*) chiefly opportunistic. The endemic mycoses are those in which susceptibility to the infection is acquired by living in a geographic area constituting the natural habitat of the particular fungus. The most commonly encountered endemic mycoses in North America are due to *Histoplasma capsulatum, Coccidioides immitis, Blastomyces dermatitidis*, and *Sporothrix schenckii*. Infection due to these agents is usually acquired by inhalation of conidia from an environmental source. Although infections with these fungal pathogens are clearly important, a more pressing problem now is that of the opportunistic mycoses, which carry a particularly high mortality and appear to be increasing significantly.

The opportunistic mycoses occur primarily in immunocompromised patients, particularly those with malignancies and acquired immune deficiency syndrome (AIDS) and after major surgery, severe burn injury, and bone marrow and solid organ transplantation. Contributing factors include exposure to broad-spectrum antibacterial agents, adrenal corticosteroids, and cytotoxic chemotherapeutic agents and prolonged use of indwelling catheters. The most important agents of the opportunistic mycoses are *Candida* spp., *Cryptococcus neoformans, Aspergillus* spp., and the Zygomycetes.

The prevention, diagnosis, and therapy of opportunistic mycoses remain extremely difficult. Increased recognition of the importance of these infections has spurred efforts to develop new diagnostic and therapeutic approaches as well as to expand our knowledge of the epidemiology and pathogenesis of the mycoses.

▸ CANDIDIASIS

Clinical and Epidemiologic Features

Candida species are commonly found as part of the endogenous microbial flora of the oropharynx, gastrointestinal tract, and vagina of a variable proportion of normal persons. Although *C. albicans* remains the most common cause of local and disseminated infection, there has been an increase in infections caused by *Candida tropicalis, Candida parapsilosis, Candida krusei, Candida glabrata*, and *Candida lusitaniae*.[1,2]

The clinical manifestations of candidiasis include local mucocutaneous infection and hematogenously disseminated candidiasis. Local mucocutaneous candidiasis is most commonly caused by *Candida albicans* and may involve the oropharynx (thrush) and the entire gastrointestinal tract, including the esophagus, stomach, and large and small bowel. Genitourinary tract involvement includes cystitis and vulvovaginal candidiasis. Superficial infections of the skin are less common but may involve the axillae, groins, inframammary folds, perianal region, and other warm moist areas, particularly following antimicrobial therapy. Although vulvovaginitis commonly occurs in otherwise normal, healthy women, mucocutaneous candidiasis most commonly occurs in immunocompromised patients: neonates, the elderly, patients with AIDS, and patients hospitalized with various malignancies and following organ transplantation and major surgery. Prolonged exposure to multiple broad-spectrum antibiotics may promote mucosal overgrowth of *Candida* spp. and thus predispose these patients to superficial candidiasis.[3,4]

Chronic mucocutaneous candidiasis is a rare syndrome associated with defects in T cell-mediated immunity. These patients have persistent superficial *Candida* infection of skin, scalp, nails, and mucous membranes.[4] Disease onset may begin at any age and may be associated with various endocrinopathies (diabetes mellitus, hypoparathyroidism, hypothyroidism, or hypoadrenalism), and the clinical manifestations may be limited or quite extensive.

Hematogenously disseminated candidiasis is a serious infection of hospitalized and immunocompromised patients that appears to be increasing markedly over the past 10 to 15 years.[1–4] Candidemia and disseminated candidiasis occur most commonly in hospitalized patients with neutropenia, malignancies, and severe burn injuries, and following major surgical procedures.[1–4] Disseminated candidiasis is also a frequent, serious problem in infants hospitalized in neonatal intensive care units. Hematogenously disseminated candidiasis is generally thought to originate from an endogenous, usually gastrointestinal, source and is most commonly caused by *C. albicans* followed by *C. glabrata, C. tropicalis, C. parapsilosis*, and *C. krusei.* Infection of peripheral and central venous catheters may result from endogenous or exogenous contamination of the catheter surface. The infected catheter may serve as a nidus for subsequent hematogenous dissemination. The clinical manifestations of hematogenously disseminated candidiasis are nonspecific, and infection may present with candidemia or focal involvement of specific "target organs" such as skin, liver, lung, bone, eye, or central nervous system.

Crude mortality rates reported for patients with candidemia and disseminated candidiasis have been as high as 90 percent; however, because these infections occur in patients with serious underlying disease, the actual contribution of the infection to the death of the patients has been difficult to estimate. One study has estimated the mortality directly attributable to nosocomial candidemia to be approximately 38 percent.[5] This estimate of attributable mortality is comparable to data reported for primary aerobic Gram-negative bacteremia and is considerably higher than the 13.6 percent reported for nosocomial bloodstream infections due to another opportunistic pathogen, *Staphylococcus epidermidis*.

The identification of risk factors for disseminated candidiasis has been difficult because of the complex nature of the patients at risk for these infections. Significant independent risk factors for disseminated candidiasis identified by multivariate analysis include prior colonization by *Candida* spp., central catheterization (including Hickman catheters), neutropenia, hemodialysis, and chemotherapy for hematologic malignancies.[3,6] These factors may be important in the development of serious candidal infection independent of the underlying disease state or other confounding factors and should serve as the focus for future studies concerning methods of prevention, diagnosis, and therapy.

Microbiology

Candida organisms are small (4 to 6 μm), oval, thin-walled cells that reproduce by budding and may also form pseudohyphae and hyphae in tissue. Although over 80 species of *Candida* have been identified, only a few have been isolated from humans, including *C. albicans, C. tropicalis, C. glabrata, C. parapsilosis, C. krusei, Candida guilliermondii, Candida kefyr*, and *C. lusitaniae*. *Candida* species grow well on most laboratory media and appear as white, creamy colonies and may be smooth, wrinkled, or fuzzy in appearance. Blastospores (yeasts), hyphae, or pseudohyphae may be seen directly in Gram-stained (Gram positive) or potassium hydroxide (KOH)-treated preparations of clinical material. Special stains, such as the Gomori methenamine silver stain, may be used to visualize the organisms in tissue sections. Identification of *Candida* isolates to species level is accomplished by employing a series of biochemical and physiological tests. A number of prepackaged identification kits are commercially available that allow species identification within 48 to 72 hours. The germ tube test is a simple and rapid means of presumptively identifying isolates of *C. albicans*. This test takes advantage of the fact that most *C. albicans*, but not other species of *Candida*, will form germ tubes (hyphal evaginations) within 2 hours in the presence of serum.

Diagnosis

One of the major problems in the prevention and therapy of candidiasis in hospitalized patients is the difficulty in diagnosing infection versus colonization in these frequently complex patients.[1–4] The clinical signs and symptoms associated with both local and disseminated candidiasis are nonspecific and are generally not helpful in distinguishing bacterial from candidal infection. The most common clinical presentation of superficial candidiasis is that of white or gray pseudomembranous plaques overlying the mucosal surface. Removal of the plaques reveals a red, painful base with ulcerations and necrosis. Oropharyngeal and esophageal involvement may be quite painful with considerable dysphagia and pain on swallowing. Vaginal and cutaneous involvement may be both painful and pruritic. Two major clues to diagnosis of hematogenously disseminated candidiasis are the presence of endophthalmitis and macronodular skin lesions. *Candida* endophthalmitis is marked by single or multiple raised, white fluffy chorioretinal lesions, with or without an overlying vitreous haze. The lesions are usually in the macular area and are easily detected by ophthalmoscopic examination. Unfortunately they are rarely observed in neutropenic patients. In addition to endophthalmitis and macronodular skin lesions, several additional clinical presentations of disseminated candidiasis have been described in recent years, including suppurative thrombophlebitis, hepatitis, purpura fulminans and bullous dermatitis, epiglottitis, and osteomyelitis.[1–4]

The laboratory diagnosis of candidiasis has been limited because available methods are insensitive and nonspecific. Superficial infection may be diagnosed by direct microscopic examination of 10 percent KOH-treated or Gram-stained material obtained from infected lesions. The most reliable means of documenting disseminated candidiasis is by histopathologic demonstration of tissue invasion on biopsy or recovery of *Candida* spp. from normally sterile body fluids such as pleural fluid, peritoneal fluid, or cerebrospinal fluid. Isolation of *Candida* spp. from urine or sputum may be helpful but frequently only represents colonization or contamination of the specimen. Isolation of *Candida* spp. from blood is also helpful; however, fungemia may occasionally be transient and is not indicative of widespread dissemination, particularly when associated with a removable intravascular focus such as an infected catheter. Conventional broth blood cultures are positive for *Candida* spp. in fewer than 50 percent of patients with documented disseminated candidiasis and frequently are positive only immediately preceding or after death. Therefore, they are not always helpful in making diagnostic and therapeutic decisions. The usefulness of blood cultures in diagnosing disseminated candidiasis is significantly improved when biphasic media or lysis-centrifugation methods are employed to optimize the detection of candidemia.[7] Serologic methods have also been disappointing.[7] Measurement of antibody titers has been unsuccessful in delineating colonization and local infection from disseminated candidiasis. Likewise, detection of circulating fungal antigens, with few exceptions, has not been successful in providing an accurate, early diagnosis of disseminated infection.

Therapy

Deeply invasive infection such as severe esophagitis and disseminated candidiasis requires systemic therapy with amphotericin B. Prompt removal of potentially contaminated devices such as intravenous catheters is important. The addition of 5-fluorocytosine may provide synergistic candidicidal activity; however, improved clinical efficacy has not been proved in properly designed clinical trials. Although newer antifungal compounds—including a wide array of azole antifungal agents—have been developed, their usefulness in the treatment of disseminated candidiasis remains to be established. Amphotericin B remains the drug of choice. Fluconazole may be a useful alternative for the treatment of candidemia in nonneutropenic patients.[8] Topical antifungal agents such as nystatin, clotrimazole, or miconazole may be useful in the treatment of superficial mucocutaneous infections. Oral therapy with fluconazole has proved extremely useful in the treatment of oral candidiasis in AIDS patients. Attempts at prophylaxis with oral or systemic administration of antifungal agents have met with limited success in preventing invasive disease despite a reduction in the extent of local colonization.

▶ CRYPTOCOCCOSIS

Clinical and Epidemiologic Features

Cryptococcosis is a mycosis caused by the encapsulated yeast *Cryptococcus neoformans* that may present as a localized acute or chronic pulmonary infection or, more importantly, with hematogenous dissemination and meningitis. Although the incidence and prevalence of cryptococcosis is unknown, the disease occurs worldwide.[1–4] Pulmonary infection is most common; however, symptoms may be mild and self-limited and thus less likely to be reported than cryptococcal meningitis. There are four capsular serotypes of *C. neoformans* (A through D), with serotype A being responsible for most disease worldwide.[1] Serotype D is common only in Europe, whereas serotypes B and C are found predominantly in the tropics and subtropics, including a focus in southern California.

C. neoformans serotypes A and D are commonly recovered in large numbers from environmental sources contaminated with the droppings of pigeons and other birds. The only known environmental source of serotypes B and C is *Eucalyptus camaldulensis* (red gum tree). Despite the strong association of *C. neoformans* with pigeon droppings, most patients infected with *C. neoformans* do not give a history of contact with pigeons or other birds. Thus, infection most likely results from inhalation of aerosolized organisms. Infection due to direct implantation has been reported but is extremely rare.

Cryptococcosis, particularly meningitis, commonly occurs in patients with underlying immunodeficiency; however, both local and disseminated infections are observed in patients with no known immunologic defect. Immunosuppressed patients at particular risk for cryptococcal infection include those with lymphoreticular malignancies or sarcoid and those receiving corticosteroid therapy, organ transplants, or immunosuppressive therapy. The most common immunologic defect in patients with cryptococcal infection is a defect in cell-mediated immunity. The importance of cell-mediated immunity as a host defense mechanism is underscored by the fact that cryptococcosis is the fourth most common infection complicating AIDS.[4] It is estimated that 7 to 10 percent of patients with AIDS are infected with

C. neoformans. Because of persistent immunologic defect in patients with AIDS, cryptococcal infection is extremely difficult to manage and generally requires life-long suppressive therapy.

Primary cryptococcal disease is generally considered to occur in the lungs. The presentation of pulmonary cryptococcal infection is variable, ranging from asymptomatic airway colonization without parenchymal invasion to an acute pneumonic process with lobar infiltrates, cough, and fever. Chronic pulmonary infection may occur with progressive involvement over several years. Although only about 10 percent of all patients with pulmonary cryptococcosis have evidence of immunologic deficiency, this group of patients is at high risk for dissemination and development of cryptococcal meningitis.

Central nervous system lesions are the most common and important clinical manifestation of extrapulmonary cryptococcosis. It is estimated that approximately 300 cases of cryptococcal meningitis occur in the United States each year; however, this number is likely to increase dramatically with the increasing number of immunocompromised patients and the emergence of *C. neoformans* as a major pathogen complicating AIDS.[1–4] Central nervous system infection may present as either a focal or a diffuse process, and chronic meningitis with disease presenting over weeks to months has been observed. Although meningitis is the most common manifestation of systemic cryptococcosis, disseminated infection may present with cryptococcemia and involvement of skin and mucous membranes, bone, liver, lung, kidneys, prostate, adrenals, spleen, lymph nodes, or testes with or without clinically apparent central nervous system involvement.

Microbiology

C. neoformans is a ubiquitous encapsulated soil yeast that reproduces asexually by budding. The perfect or sexual stage of *C. neoformans* can be produced by mating the fungus in vitro; however, the role of this stage in infectivity and pathogenesis is unknown. The yeast cell may vary from 4 to 20 μm in diameter and is surrounded by a polysaccharide capsule ranging from 1 to 30 μm. The narrow-based buds are usually single. The capsule may be visualized indirectly by the India ink or nigrosin technique and more specifically in clinical material with mucicarmine, which stains capsular mucopolysaccharide. In tissue, cryptococci stain poorly with hematoxylin and eosin but well with methenamine silver and periodic acid-Schiff.

C. neoformans grows well on most bacterial and fungal media used in the routine clinical microbiology laboratory. A rapid presumptive identification of an encapsulated yeast as *C. neoformans* may be accomplished by demonstration of urease and phenoloxidase enzyme activity.[1,3] *C. neoformans* is strongly urease positive and possesses a membrane-bound phenoloxidase enzyme that converts phenolic compounds to melanin. Phenoloxidase activity is readily demonstrated on media such as birdseed agar or caffeic acid agar, which contains 3,4-dihydroxycinnamic acid. Oxidation of the *O*-diphenol in medium produces dark colonies suggestive of *C. neoformans*. Confirmatory identification is accomplished by employing standard biochemical and physiological tests.

Diagnosis

The clinical presentation of pulmonary cryptococcosis may mimic a number of acute and chronic infectious processes as well as malignancies. Signs and symptoms include fever, malaise, pleuritic pain, cough, scanty sputum, and hemoptysis. Chest roentgenograms may reveal lobar infiltrates, single or multiple nodules, or tumor-like masses. Sputum cultures are positive in only 20 percent of cases, and the diagnosis is frequently made at thoracotomy for suspected malignancy. Patients with pulmonary cryptococcosis should be thoroughly evaluated for systemic infection, with cultures of blood, urine, and cerebrospinal fluid (CSF).

Central nervous system cryptococcosis may present as either meningitis (most common), encephalitis, or a more focal process suggestive of malignancy. Signs and symptoms in patients without AIDS include fever, headache, mental status changes, ocular symptoms, meningismus, nausea, vomiting, cranial nerve palsies, and seizures. Aside from fever and headache these signs and symptoms may be significantly less common in patients with AIDS. The chest roentgenogram may or may not be abnormal in patients with central nervous system or systemic cryptococcosis. Extraneural dissemination may present as cryptococcemia or focal involvement of one of several target organs.

The laboratory diagnosis of cryptococcosis requires the isolation of cryptococci from normally sterile body fluids, histopathology showing encapsulated organisms, or detection of cryptococcal antigen in serum or CSF. A rapid diagnosis of extraneural infection may be facilitated by biopsy and staining with methenamine silver and mucicarmine. Examination of the CSF in patients with meningitis usually suggests a chronic lymphocytic meningitis with a low-grade (less than 500/mm^3) lymphocytic pleocytosis, elevated protein, and low glucose. Microscopic examination of CSF mixed with India ink or nigrosin may reveal encapsulated organisms in approximately 50 percent of cases. Cultures of CSF and other clinical material are usually positive. Occasionally repeated lumbar punctures, cisternal taps, or sampling of large volumes (up to 10 mL) of CSF may be necessary to establish the diagnosis. In patients with AIDS, cryptococci are present in large numbers, but the CSF shows fewer abnormalities.

Detection of cryptococcal antigen in serum and CSF is extremely valuable in the diagnosis of cryptococcal infection. Antigen titers are particularly high in patients with AIDS. Several latex agglutination assays are commercially available and are rapid, sensitive, and specific.[1–3] Antigen is detected in the serum in approximately 50 percent and in CSF in more than 90 percent of patients with cryptococcal meningitis. High titers of cryptococcal antigen in CSF or serum are associated with a poor prognosis. False-positive results are rare but may be due to rheumatoid factor or cross-reactivity in patients infected with *Trichosporon beigelii*.[5]

Therapy

Pulmonary cryptococcosis may not require therapy as long as the process appears to be resolving and the patient is intact immunologically. Long-term follow-up is necessary in patients whose infection is diagnosed at thoracotomy, because there is a 3 to 10 percent risk of meningitis for up to 3 years after surgery. Patients with progressive pulmonary infection, particularly those who are immunocompromised, and all patients with extrapulmonary infection require systemic antifungal therapy. At present such therapy consists of intravenous amphotericin B. The efficacy of fluconazole or other azoles in the treatment of pulmonary cryptococcosis remains to be documented in appropriate clinical trials.

Cryptococcal meningitis and extrapulmonary cryptococcosis always require systemic antifungal therapy. Cryptococcal meningitis is almost universally fatal without therapy, but approximately 80 to 90 percent of patients (non-AIDS) can be cured with current therapeutic regimens. Current therapeutic recommendations are restricted to amphotericin B alone or in combination with 5-fluorocytosine.[1–3] The combination of amphotericin B and 5-fluorocytosine provides synergistic fungicidal activity and is favored by many clinicians; however, the added toxicity of 5-fluorocytosine (bone marrow suppression and gastrointestinal and liver toxicity) may limit its application, particularly in AIDS patients.

Treatment of cryptococcal meningitis in patients with AIDS has been difficult. Initial response to both combination and single-drug therapy has been poor, and relapses are common. Current recommendations include the use of amphotericin B with or without 5-fluorocytosine for acute therapy. Fluconazole is used for acute therapy in only very mild cases or in patients with severe intolerance to amphotericin B.[6] In general, patients with AIDS cannot be cured of their cryptococcal infection and require chronic maintenance therapy with either weekly amphotericin B or fluconazole. Fluconazole is more effective than amphotericin B and is usually preferred for maintenance therapy.[6]

▶ ASPERGILLOSIS

Clinical and Epidemiologic Features

The term *aspergillosis* refers to any one of a number of disease states caused by members of the genus *Aspergillus*. *Aspergillus* species are ubiquitous fungi that may be isolated from a variety of environmental sources, including insulation and fireproofing materials, soil, grain, leaves, grass, and air.[1] The aerosolized conidia are present in large numbers and are constantly being inhaled. Although several hundred species of *Aspergillus* have been described, relatively few are known to cause disease in humans. *Aspergillus fumigatus* remains the most common cause of aspergillosis, followed by *Aspergillus flavus, Aspergillus terreus, Aspergillus niger, Aspergillus glaucus*, and *Aspergillus nidulans*.[1–3]

Aspergillus infections occur worldwide and appear to be increasing in prevalence, particularly among patients with chronic pulmonary disease and among the immunocompromised populations.[2–6] *Aspergillus* species are particularly important causes of nosocomial infections in patients who are immunocompromised secondary to burn injury, malignancy, leukemia, and bone marrow and other organ transplantation. Several major outbreaks of invasive nosocomial aspergillosis have been described in association with exposure to *Aspergillus* conidia aerosolized by hospital construction, contaminated air handling systems, and insulation or fireproofing materials within walls or ceilings of hospital bed units.[6] The crude mortality associated with these infections is high, approximately 90 percent in most series.[2,7]

The clinical manifestations of aspergillosis include pulmonary colonization with bronchitis and aspergilloma formation, allergic syndromes such as allergic bronchopulmonary aspergillosis (ABPA), and invasive aspergillosis.[1–3] Intoxication or neoplasm secondary to ingestion of aflatoxin or other toxins produced by *Aspergillus* spp. contaminating grain and other foods is also a serious problem worldwide.

Pulmonary colonization by *Aspergillus* spp. may involve the bronchial mucosa or may become localized in a preexisting cavity, resulting in the formation of an aspergilloma. Superficial colonization of the tracheobronchial mucosa produces little inflammation and is not associated with tissue invasion. The expectoration of bronchial casts containing mucus and hyphal elements may be observed. Patients in whom mucosal colonization is observed are those with preexisting pulmonary disease, including cystic fibrosis, chronic obstructive pulmonary disease, and chronic asthma requiring administration of corticosteroids.

Aspergillomas are masses of mycelia and amorphous debris localized in preexisting pulmonary cavities, usually in the upper lobes. The cavities are usually lined with modified bronchial epithelium and have been formed secondary to other disease processes such as tuberculosis, infarcts, or neoplasms. There is little surrounding inflammation, and invasion of the pulmonary parenchyma by *Aspergillus* spp. is rare. Aspergillomas may be clinically silent; however, hemoptysis secondary to ulceration of the epithelial lining of the cavity is observed in 50 to 80 percent of cases.[2] The lesions may be stable, grow, or shrink with the surrounding cavity. Spontaneous lysis occurs in approximately 10 percent of cases within 3 years.

The allergic manifestations of aspergillosis are the result of tissue hypersensitivity to conidia or other antigens of *Aspergillus* spp. (almost always *A. fumigatus*).[3] The clinical picture may vary from mild asthma to fibrosis and bronchiectasis secondary to allergic bronchopulmonary aspergillosis. Exposure to aerosolized *Aspergillus* conidia may produce bronchospasm in individuals with atopic asthma. Repeated and heavy inhalation of *Aspergillus* conidia and other antigens may result in extrinsic allergic alveolitis in nonatopic patients. Prolonged exposure may lead to micronodular changes and fibrosis. ABPA is the result of type I (IgE-mediated), type III (immune complex-mediated), and possibly type IV (cell-mediated) hypersensitivity reactions to *Aspergillus* antigens. This condition occurs in up to 20 percent of individuals with asthma and is associated with colonization of the bronchial mucosa by *Aspergillus* spp. These patients experience recurrent bouts of severe asthma, wheezing, fever, weight loss, chest pain, and cough productive of blood-tinged sputum. Eventually the disease becomes chronic, with the development of fibrosis, bronchiectasis, and mucus plugging with subsequent atelectasis or cavitation. This condition may be associated with nasal polyps and chronic sinusitis.

Invasive aspergillosis occurs most commonly in patients who are severely immunocompromised secondary to hematologic and lymphoreticular malignancies. Major risk factors include neutropenia, broad-spectrum antibacterial therapy, and administration of corticosteroids.[1–4] Patients undergoing bone marrow transplantation are at particularly high risk. Although invasive aspergillosis may be acquired either in the community or in the hospital, most cases are nosocomial in origin. The disease process is most commonly localized to the lungs, followed by the paranasal tissues. The infectious process is typified by mucosal ulceration and direct extension of hyphae into surrounding tissues. Vascular invasion results in thrombosis, embolization, and infarction. Hematogenous dissemination occurs in 35 to 40 percent of cases of invasive pulmonary aspergillosis and may involve brain, liver, kidneys, gastrointestinal tract, thyroid, heart, skin, and other sites.[1–5] Extension of paranasal infection into the orbit and brain may mimic rhinocerebral zygomycosis. Although the pulmonary process may occasionally be inapparent, it most commonly presents as a necrotizing, patchy bronchopneumonia with or without hemorrhagic infarction. In all infected foci the infection is characterized by vascular invasion, tissue infarction, and necrosis. Massive hemoptysis, gastrointestinal bleeding, and cerebral infarcts and abscesses may occur.

Chronic necrotizing aspergillosis, a more indolent pulmonary infectious process, occurs predominantly in middle-aged patients with mildly compromised host defenses or preexisting pulmonary lung damage.[8] The locally invasive infection is slowly progressive and results in cavitation and aspergilloma formation. The infectious process is usually confined to the upper lobes but occasionally may involve an entire lung.

Microbiology

Aspergillus species are molds that reproduce by means of spores or conidia. The conidia germinate to form hyphae, which are the forms most commonly found in infected tissue. *Aspergillus* species grow well on most media and are identified to species level based on the microscopic identification of specific morphologic features. Over 600 different species of *Aspergillus* have been described; however, most clinical infections are due to *A. fumigatus* and *A. flavus*.[1] *A. niger* is the most common cause of otomycosis. At present there are no commercially available kits to aid in the identification of *Aspergillus* spp. In tissue, *Aspergillus* hyphae stain well with Gomori methenamine silver stain and are uniform, 2 to 7 μm in diameter, septate, and dichotomously branched with angles of approximately 45°. These features are not diagnostic and are shared by several other opportunistic fungal pathogens.

Diagnosis

The clinical signs and symptoms of pulmonary aspergillosis are nonspecific and range from mild asthma to severe hemoptysis, acute bronchopneumonia, and pulmonary infarction. Extrapulmonary involvement may present as cellulitis, hemorrhage, or infarction depending on the specific site of infection. Chest radiographs may be useful in the diagnosis of aspergilloma with the appearance of a freely movable intracavitary mass surrounded by a crescent of air (Monod's sign). The radiographic appearance of allergic bronchopulmonary aspergillosis varies with the stage and chronicity of the disease but may appear as bronchiectasis with bronchial thickening or dilation, consolidation, and atelectasis. The most common radiographic picture of invasive pulmonary aspergillosis is that of a patchy density or well-defined nodule, which may be single or multifocal with progression to diffuse consolidation or cavitation.

The laboratory diagnosis of aspergillosis is generally unsatisfactory. Definitive diagnosis of invasive aspergillosis usually requires biopsy of the involved tissue. Unfortunately the severe underlying diseases and associated bleeding diatheses commonly seen in these patients often preclude such an invasive approach. Sputum cultures are nondiagnostic and may be positive in patients with simple colonization and negative in patients with the invasive disease.[1–4] The usefulness of surveillance cultures in high-risk patients remains to be confirmed.[6] Blood, urine, and CSF cultures are rarely positive in patients with invasive disease. Detection of *Aspergillus* antigen in blood, urine, and lung washings is a promising noninvasive means of diagnosing invasive aspergillosis but is restricted to the research laboratory at present.[9] Skin tests and demonstration of serum precipitins have been useful in diagnosing ABPA; however, they are of no use in diagnosing invasive infection. Additional laboratory features of ABPA include elevated serum IgE and peripheral blood eosinophilia.

Therapy

Treatment of aspergillosis is difficult and is probably not indicated for aspergilloma unless life-threatening hemoptysis occurs, in which case segmental resection or lobectomy is indicated. Systemic antifungal therapy has been of no value. Likewise, neither systemic nor aerosolized antifungal therapy has been effective in treatment of the allergic syndromes such as ABPA. Corticosteroids are considered the treatment of choice.

Given the high mortality associated with invasive aspergillosis, an aggressive approach to diagnosis and treatment is required. In addition, return of bone marrow function or reversal of neutropenia is essential for survival. Amphotericin B is the only antifungal agent with established activity in this infection. Concomitant reduction or elimination of immunosuppressive therapy may also be necessary. The efficacy of granulocyte transfusions, 5-fluorocytosine, or rifampin in combination with amphotericin B is unproven. The activity of itraconazole against *Aspergillus* species represents a clinically important extension of the antifungal spectrum of the azoles. Itraconazole has been found useful in the treatment of acute and chronic aspergillosis in several small studies and has produced remission in patients who were neutropenic or receiving immunosuppressive therapy.[5]

Prophylaxis of invasive aspergillosis is most important in immunocompromised patients. Laminar airflow facilities provide the only means of preventing this infectious complication. Prophylactic antifungal drugs lack proven efficacy. Intranasal instillation of amphotericin B has been used with promising results; however, more studies will be necessary.

▶ ZYGOMYCOSIS

Clinical and Epidemiologic Features

Zygomycosis is a general term that includes infections caused by fungi in the order Mucorales and order Entomophthorales (class Zygomycetes). The Zygomycetes are ubiquitous worldwide in soil and decaying vegetation. Zygomycosis is not communicable and is acquired by inhalation, ingestion, or contamination of wounds with conidia from the environment. Although *Rhizopus arrhizus* is the most common agent of human zygomycosis, additional species of *Rhizopus, Mucor, Absidia, Mortierella, Cunninghamella*, and *Saksenaea* have been causing infection with increasing frequency.[1–3]

Clinically zygomycosis is a fulminant infectious process that produces rhinocerebral disease in patients with diabetic ketoacidosis; rhinocerebral, pulmonary, or disseminated disease in immunocompromised patients; local or disseminated disease in patients with burns or open wounds; and gastrointestinal disease in patients with malnutrition or preexisting gastrointestinal disorders. In each case, the progression of disease may be rapid, with invasion and destruction of key anatomic structures in a matter of days. This is particularly true with rhinocerebral infection, wherein death may occur within 3 to 10 days in untreated patients.[1–3] Although classically the major risk factor for zygomycosis is diabetic acidosis, it is now clear that neutropenia, hematologic malignancy, and cytotoxic or immunosuppressive therapy place patients at risk for these infections.[1–3]

The hallmark of zygomycosis is vascular invasion with thrombosis, hemorrhage, infarction, and tissue necrosis. The disease usually extends locally across tissue planes; however, hematogenous dissemination may also occur. Mortality is directly related to rapidity of diagnosis (extent of disease), aggressiveness of therapy, and underlying disease state. Estimates of crude mortality in patients with rhinocerebral zygomycosis are 40 percent in patients with diabetes and 80 percent in patients with other underlying diseases (malignancy, organ transplantation, neutropenia). The prognosis is poor in cases of pulmonary zygomycosis: only about 15 patients have been reported to have survived the infectious process.[2,3]

Focal outbreaks of zygomycosis have been related to the use of certain adhesive bandages or tape on open wounds. The resulting cutaneous infections were due to *Rhizopus* species, which were also isolated from the bandage material.[4,5]

Microbiology

The agents of zygomycosis are molds that reproduce by means of spores or conidia. All of the Zygomycetes appear identical in tissue and are seen microscopically following staining with hematoxylin and eosin or Gomori methenamine silver as broad (6 to 50 μm), irregular, branching, usually aseptate hyphae. Definitive identification requires isolation on agar medium and subsequent microscopic examination. Following primary isolation the Zygomycetes grow well on most media; however, primary isolation from clinical material is frequently difficult. Isolates are identified to genus and species level based on the microscopic identification of specific morphologic features.

Diagnosis

The clinical signs and symptoms of zygomycosis are dependent on the site of infection. Rhinocerebral disease may present with nasal stuffiness, blood-tinged nasal discharge, facial swelling, and facial or orbital pain. Major diagnostic clues are the presence of a black eschar on the nasal or palatine mucosa and drainage of "black pus" from the eye.[1–3,5] Radiographic examination of the sinuses may reveal clouding, thickening of the mucous membranes, and bone destruction. Progression of disease is manifested by orbital cellulitis, proptosis, and cranial nerve defects. Cerebral infarction caused by vascular compromise is common. Examination of the CSF may reveal elevated protein, normal glucose, and a modest pleocytosis. Culture and microscopic examination of CSF is uniformly negative. Pulmonary zygomycosis may resemble invasive pulmonary aspergillosis presenting as an acute bronchopneumonia or pulmonary infarction. Radiographic findings are nonspecific and include a patchy, nonhomogeneous infiltrate progressing to consolidation and cavitation. Life-threatening hemoptysis may occur. Gastrointestinal infection may present with abdominal pain, diarrhea, and bleeding. Vascular invasion results in infarction and perforation of the bowel with subsequent hemorrhage and peritonitis. Cutaneous infection may present as chronic ulceration, papules, or black, necrotic areas of infarction.

The fulminant and life-threatening nature of these infections precludes the use of culture in the diagnosis of zygomycosis.[1,3] Cultures are positive in only 20 percent of cases and are rarely positive antemortem. Serologic tests are not reliable, and microscopic examination of sputum or wound drainage is rarely positive for fungal elements. The key to diagnosis is the demonstration of the characteristic hyphae in tissue obtained on biopsy.[3] A negative histopathologic examination does not rule out infection, and additional material should be obtained if clinically indicated.

Therapy

Successful therapy of zygomycosis requires early diagnosis, systemic antifungal therapy with amphotericin B, aggressive surgical débridement of the involved area, and control of the underlying disorder. Local instillation of amphotericin B into infected paranasal sinuses may be useful. There is no proven role for additional antifungal agents such as 5-fluorocytosine or the azoles.

Prevention of zygomycosis involves control of underlying disease and conservative use of immunosuppressive agents. As seen with invasive aspergillosis, the use of laminar airflow facilities may be necessary to protect severely immunocompromised patients from infections with the Zygomycetes.

▸ REFERENCES

Candidiasis

1. Pfaller MA: Epidemiology of candidiasis. J Hosp Infect 30(Suppl): 329, 1995
2. Pfaller MA: Nosocomial candidiasis: emerging species, reservoirs, and modes of transmission. Clin Infect Dis 22(Suppl 2):S89, 1996
3. Fridkin SK, Jarvis WR: Epidemiology of nosocomial fungal infections. Clin Microbiol Rev 9:499, 1996
4. Odds FC (ed): Candida and Candidiasis. 2nd ed. London: Bailliere Tindall, 1988
5. Wey SB, Mori M, Pfaller MA, Woolson RF, Wenzel RP: Hospital-acquired candidemia: the attributable mortality and excess length of stay. Arch Intern Med 148:2642, 1988
6. Wey SB, Mori M, Pfaller MA, Woolson RF, Wenzel RP: Risk factors for hospital-acquired candidemia: a matched case-control study. Arch Intern Med 148:2642, 1989
7. Pfaller MA: Laboratory aids in the diagnosis of invasive candidiasis. Mycopathologia 120:65, 1992
8. Rex JH, Bennett JE, Sugar AM, Pappos PG, Van der Horst CM, Edwards JE, Washburn RG, Scheld WM, Karchmer AW, Dine AP, Levenstein MJ, Webb CD, the Candidemia Study Group, the NIAID Mycoses Study Group: A randomized trial comparing fluconazole with amphotericin B for the treatment of candidemia in patients without neutropenia. N Engl J Med 331:1325, 1994

Cryptococcosis

1. Kwon-Chung KJ, Bennett JE (eds): Medical Mycology. Philadelphia: Lea & Febiger, 1992
2. Patterson TF, Andriole VT: Current concepts in cryptococcosis. Eur J Clin Microbiol Infect Dis 8:457, 1989
3. Perfect JR: Cryptococcosis. Infect Dis Clin North Am 3:77, 1989
4. Powderly WG: Cryptococcal meningitis and AIDS. Clin Infect Dis 17:837, 1993
5. McManus EJ, Jones MJ: Detection of a *Trichosporon beigelii* antigen cross-reactive with *Cryptococcus neoformans* capsular polysaccharide in serum from a patient with disseminated *Trichosporon* infection. J Clin Microbiol 21:681, 1985
6. Powderly WG: Recent advances in the management of cryptococcal meningitis in patients with AIDS. Clin Infect Dis 22(Suppl 2): S119, 1996

Aspergillosis

1. Rinaldi MG: Invasive aspergillosis. Rev Infect Dis 5:1061, 1983
2. Bodey GP, Vartivarian S: Aspergillosis. Eur J Clin Microbiol Infect Dis 8:413, 1989
3. Levitz SM: Aspergillosis. Infect Dis Clin North Am 3:1, 1989
4. Khoo SH, Denning DW: Invasive aspergillosis in patients with AIDS. Clin Infect Dis 19(Suppl 1):S41, 1994
5. Denning DW: Therapeutic outcome in invasive aspergillosis. Clin Infect Dis 23:608, 1996
6. Fridkin SK, Jarvis WR: Epidemiology of nosocomial fungal infections. Clin Microbiol Rev 9:499, 1996
7. Pannuti CS, Gingrich RD, Pfaller MA, Wenzel RP: Nosocomial pneumonia in adult patients undergoing bone marrow transplantation: a 9-year study. J Clin Oncol 9:77, 1991
8. Binder RE, Faling LJ, Pugatch RD, Mahasaen C, Snider GL: Chronic necrotizing pulmonary aspergillosis: a discrete clinical entity. Medicine 61:109, 1982
9. deRepentigny L: Serodiagnosis of candidiasis, aspergillosis, and cryptococcosis. Clin Infect Dis 14(Suppl 1):S11, 1992

Zygomycosis

1. Rinaldi MG: Zygomycosis. Infect Dis Clin North Am 3:19, 1989
2. Parfrey NA: Improved diagnosis and prognosis of mucormycosis: a clinicopathologic study of 33 cases. Medicine 65:113, 1986
3. Sugar AM: Mucormycosis. Clin Infect Dis 14(Suppl 1):S126, 1992
4. Fridkin SK, Jarvis WR: Epidemiology of nosocomial fungal infections. Clin Microbiol Rev 9:499, 1996
5. Mead JH, Lupton GP, Dillavou CL, Odem RB: Cutaneous *Rhizopus* infections: occurrence as a postoperative complication associated with an elasticized adhesive dressing. JAMA 242:272, 1979

16

Other Infection-Related Diseases of Public Health Import

Dermatophytoses

Stephan A. Billstein

Dermatophytosis, commonly known as ringworm, is a general term used to describe superficial mycotic infections of the dead, cornified layers of the skin and its appendages (hair and nails). These infections are not severe ordinarily and rarely become systemic. Because of high prevalence, however, they are of public significance throughout the world, especially in areas with a warm, moist environment and where personal hygiene is poor. These infections will also increase in prevalence in high-density populations and at time of war.

Three genera and a multitude of species of fungi, known collectively as the dermatophytes, are the etiological agents of ringworm. Most human infections are caused by the following species: *Microsporum canis, Microsporum audouinii, Trichophyton rubrum, Trichophyton mentagrophytes, Trichophyton tonsurans, Trichophyton schoenleinii*, and *Epidermophyton floccosum*. A single dermatophyte species can cause a variety of clinical manifestations in different parts of the body, and the same clinical picture may be due to dermatophytes of different species and different genera.

Epidemiology

The incidence of dermatophytosis is a dynamic situation. The patterns of geographic distribution and prevalence are not fixed. They will change continually due to influences of climate, human social and antisocial activities, cultural habits, migration, and developments in diagnosis and therapy.[1,5,6,8]

The endemic or most prevalent species of dermatophyte can differ strikingly from one locality to another. Most often the reasons are not known. Some species are widely distributed, and others have a limited geographic range. The true incidence in a population is also not known as dermatophytosis is not a required reportable disease. The reported incidence in the literature, therefore, reflects the interest of the investigator and the incapacity of the patient.

The incidence and distribution of dermatophyte infections by area, season, age, sex, and race have not been well delineated because extensive epidemiological surveys of these infections have not been carried out. As dermatophytoses are not reportable diseases, most of the available data has been obtained from patients who seek medical care. From these data it has been estimated for developed countries that 5 percent of patients with dermatological conditions have ringworm, and more than 90 percent of the male populations have had at least a transient ringworm infection by the age of 40. Onychomycosis, a ringworm infection of the nails, has been reported to occur at a rate of 5 to 15 percent in a population.[1,8,10] A recent ongoing total population epidemiologic survey of Iceland reveals that at least 10 percent or more of that population have onychomycosis (B. Sigurgeirsson, personal communication.)

Reported epidemics of tinea capitis or corporis occur in school children predominantly. In the United States the dominant causative dermatophyte in these outbreaks is currently *Trichophyton tonsurans* (greater than 90 percent of isolates) for tinea capitis and *Microsporum canis* for tinea corporis. In Europe, both *Trichophyton tonsurans* and *Microsporum canis* are isolated about 50 percent of the time in tinea capitis. In the case of toenail onychomycosis, *Trichophyton rubrum* is the dominant organism in both the United States and in Europe, usually accounting for greater than 90 percent of the isolates.[3,13] The military is another population group in which ringworm epidemics have been prominent. Soldiers especially are prone to acquisition of these infections in hot, humid climates, where hygiene is poor and clothing is inappropriate to climatic conditions.[12] Outbreaks in the military have most often been caused by *Trichophyton mentagrophytes* or *Tricophyton rubrum*.

Clinical Presentation and Pathogenesis

Clinically, ringworm is classified according to the body area involved. The Latin word *tinea*, meaning gnawing worm, is used with the designated site of dermatophyte infection to describe ringworm of the scalp (tinea capitis), body (tinea corporis), feet (tinea pedis), groin (tinea cruris), nails (tinea unguium), and so on. It has been postulated that some ringworm strains are more virulent than others. These may occur naturally or may develop selectively whenever better nutrition is afforded by opportunity for invasion deep into the skin or hair follicles. Dermatophytes seek the areas of newly forming keratin deep in the skin, hair follicles, or nails for maximum development.

Infection with dermatophytes most often appears on the skin as red, scaly patches. These patches become progressively larger if untreated, the border extends while the center area clears, and this process gives rise to a ringlike, wormy-appearing lesion. Although the fungi invade only the dead, keratinized layers of the skin, hair, and nails, the resulting signs and symptoms—which may include erythema, scaling, and vesiculation—are more than would be expected from such a superficial infection. Much of the disease is a result of the host's reaction to the fungus.

Tinea capitis (ringworm of the scalp) is seen in elementary school epidemics. The usual clinical presentation is hair loss, erythema, and scaling. Pruritus is rare.

Tinea corporis (ringworm of the body) presents with erythematous, scaling, round patches on any part of the body. The annular lesions have a central scaly area and an advancing active periphery, which is usually studded with crusting vesicles and pustules. Most lesions are relatively asymptomatic, although some of them cause itching.

Tinea pedis (athlete's foot) most often presents as scaling or cracking between the toes and vesicular lesions on the soles of the feet. The dorsal areas of the feet are rarely involved at the onset. Poor hygiene, hyperhidrosis, inadequate drying of the feet, and immunodeficiency are factors that contribute to disease. Once infection has been acquired, it may remain throughout life and exhibit periods of exacerbation and remission.

Tinea cruris (ringworm of the groin or apposed areas) has a similar pathogenesis to that of tinea pedis. In the apposed areas such as the groin, under the breasts, and in the axillae, the disease will present as scaling or cracking. Poor hygiene, hyperhidrosis, tight-fitting clothing, clothing that does not breathe, and immunoincompetence are factors that will contribute to the onset of this condition. If these conditions are not corrected along with proper treatment, then tinea cruris will exhibit periods of exacerbation and remission throughout one's lifetime.

Tinea unguium or onychomycosis (ringworm of the nails) is characterized by symptoms of pain, pigmentation, thickening, onycholysis, accumulation of subungal debris and brittleness of the nails. The four common types of this disease are distal or lateral subungal, white superficial, proximal white subungal, and that caused by *Candida* species. Distal or lateral subungal onychomycosis is the most common type and will start as an infection in the nail bed underneath the nail plate at the distal end of the toe and progress proximally. The white superficial type pathology begins on top of the nail plate and rarely penetrates to the nail bed. Proximal white subungal onychomycosis will start under the nail plate in the nail bed usually in the area of the nail matrix. It will progress distally under the nail plate. Both the white superficial and proximal white subungal types may be a herald that alerts the clinician that the patient has an immunodeficiency as part of their clinical makeup. Proximal white subungal onychomycosis is often a presenting sign of acquired immunodeficiency syndrome (AIDS). *Candida*-caused onychomycosis often accompanies either disseminated mucocutaneous candidiasis or a disease causing the patient to be immunodeficient such as diabetes mellitus. It is most prevalent in the fingernails. Dermatophytes are the most common etiology of onychomycosis. However, yeasts such as *Candida* and nondermatophytic molds often play a role in a small percentage of cases. Most literature sources support dermatophytes as causing greater than 90 percent of onychomycosis infections.[3,13] Nondermatophytic molds have been cited as possible pathogens in approximately 4 to 10 percent of cases when isolated as sole organisms. *Candida* species of yeasts have played a smaller role, usually associated with 1 percent or less of these onychomycosis infections. On occasion, both yeasts and nondermatophytic molds are present as co-organisms with a dermatophyte isolate. One should be aware that in a culture taken to determine the etiology of onychomycosis, nondermatophytic molds are rapid growers and may overwhelm the dermatophyte growth obscuring it. If this occurs, the true etiology may not be established when one isolates only an organism that is not a true dermatophyte. Hence, it is prudent to repeat the culture that produces organisms other than a dermatophyte to accurately determine the true infecting or causative agent.

Diagnosis

The existence of these fungal infections is often suspected by the morphology of the individual lesions and their anatomical distribution. A presumptive diagnosis can be made by treating scrapings from skin lesions or from the nail bed underneath the nail plate with a 10 percent potassium hydroxide solution and examining this preparation under a microscope for the presence of arthrospores and/or segmented, branched filaments. Confirmation of the diagnosis is made by culture on Sabouraud's agar medium, a procedure requiring 2 to 6 weeks for growth and isolation. The potassium hydroxide preparation cannot differentiate between living and dead organisms. Therefore, it is not a method that can confirm mycologic cure after treatment is completed. The culture must be used.

It has been shown that the technique[11] of rubbing a sterile, moist cotton swab or toothbrush over the surface of a suspected ringworm lesion and then onto the culture medium will produce a similar positive yield of cultures as the scalpel scraping technique. This method will probably not replace the scalpel method for potassium hydroxide examinations, as the scales would have to be removed from the fibers of the cotton swab, a difficult procedure. The cotton swab has the following advantages over the scalpel technique: (*a*) easy availability, (*b*) easy adaptability to lesions of the eyelids, ears, nose, and areas between the toes, (*c*) less frightening to children and adults than the blade, making for a more easily obtainable specimen, and (*d*) less costly.[1]

Examination of the scalp hairs under ultraviolet light (wood's filter) for yellow-green fluorescence is helpful in diagnosing tinea capitis caused by *Microsporum canis* or *Microsporum audouinii*. Ringworm of the scalp caused by *Trichophyton* species will not show fluorescence. It is also important to alert the patient not to shampoo or wash the scalp hair for least 24 hours before presenting to the office for this examination.

Tinea pedis, tinea corporis, and tinea unguium are common in patients with human immunodeficiency virus (HIV) disease. Despite being immunocompromised, an inflammatory response to the fungus is often quite pronounced. Therefore, in patients who present with marked inflammatory lesions that are diagnosed as being dermatophyte infections, it is prudent to evaluate for an underlying disease such as AIDS or diabetes mellitus. As stated previously, an individual who presents with proximal white subungal onychomycosis, would also be someone to evaluate for AIDS.

Source of Infection

The source of human infections can be infected persons (anthrophilic fungi), infected animals (zoophilic fungi), or soil (geophilic fungi). It is speculated that the dermatophytes arose in two or three related genera among the ascomycetes, which grew as saprophytes in the soil. The initial saprophytic species probably used shed hair and dander as preferential nutritional substrates. From these, other species evolved, which acquired progressively greater pathogenicity and dependence on the living skin of animal hosts until, as in the case of *Microsporum audouinii* and *Tricophyton tonsurans*, a high degree of host specificity and an apparently intimate biochemical relationship developed between the parasite and the host.

A multiplicity of sources of dermatophyte infections exists. Fomites such as combs, towels, blankets, and barber shears can disseminate the fungus from the primary source to contacts. Tina capitis, when caused by *M. canis* or *M. audouinii*, usually has as its source a human or an animal host, especially a dog or kitten. The source of tinea corporis due to *M. canis* is frequently a dog or kitten, but this fungus can also be spread from human to human. In addition, various *Trichophyton* species can cause tinea corporis, and these may be animal or human in origin. Tinea pedis is most often caused by *T. rubrum* or *T. mentagrophytes* in the United States, the source of these fungi can be anthropophilic or geophilic. Onychomycosis is associated at least 50 percent of the time with the long-standing presence of a tinea pedis infection.

Prevention and Control

Public health departments usually are not involved in the routine control of dermatophytosis but frequently are called upon when an outbreak is suspected. It is difficult to define an outbreak precisely, because the baseline or endemic level of these infections varies greatly by area and population involved.

Outbreaks of tinea pedis (athlete's foot) are rarely related to a common source. Usually, a noticeable increase in cases results from poor hygiene, coupled with hot, humid climatic conditions. Outbreaks most often occur among persons who participate in vigorous sports and among military personnel who have been on training exercises or in combat conditions where personal hygiene and climate control are poor. Efforts to control tinea pedis are primarily directed toward education of the infected population about the need to maintain strict personal hygiene. Careful drying of the toes after bathing and an application of dusting powder containing an effective fungicide will prevent most infections.

In contrast to the treatment of athlete's foot, topical medications for managing tinea capitis or tinea corporis are usually not effective. These medications often miss incubating lesions, which are not easily visible yet are still contagious. Therefore, griseofulvin has been the treatment of choice for these infections together with a topical agent.[2] Griseofulvin given orally will reach the basal layer of the epidermal skin by dermal-epidermal diffusion within 24 to 48 hours and will grow out with the epidermis and eventually contain the ringworm infection within a period of 2 to 6 weeks. The use of topical peeling agents, dyes, imidazole derivatives, and/or allylamines applied to the overt lesions will help prevent spread from the treated lesions as the systemic therapy takes hold to eradicate them.

Ketoconazole and itraconazole, orally administered imidazoles, have also been used systemically to treat difficult ringworm infections. They have mostly been used when griseofulvin treatment has failed or the patient is unable to take griseofulvin. They differ from griseofulvin in that they both reach peak concentration in the epidermis by both dermal-epidermal diffusion into the basal layer of the epidermis as well as excretion directly into the stratum corneum via the sweat glands. Terbinafine, an orally administered allylamine, has also been used systemically to treat recalcitrant ringworm infections. It reaches peak concentrations in the epidermis by both dermal-epidermal diffusion into the basal layer and direct excretion into the stratum corneum via the sebaceous glands.[4,7] It is important to note that, when one chooses to use one of the newer systemic therapies or even an older one, corrective measures as to controlling or stopping the inciting events such as poor hygiene and improperly fitting clothing is also necessary to not only gain a cure but to prevent recurrence.

Outbreaks of tinea capitis or corporis require the identification and treatment of all infections.[9] In responding to these outbreaks, it is important to inspect all contacts of cases diagnosed initially, that includes family and intimate contacts, as well as their environment, in order to identify and eliminate all possible sources of infection. Identification of the causal dermatophyte species may be useful in directing the search for environmental and animal sources of infection. Some animals, especially kittens, may be inapparent carriers. The public, especially parents, needs to be educated as to the danger of acquiring infection from infected children as well as from dogs, kittens, and other animals. They also need to be instructed as to appropriate hygiene to help effect the cure when the proper medication is prescribed.

Immunization against dermatophytoses has been explored with whole mycelium or crude extracts. It is unlikely, however, that effective vaccines for dermatophytoses will be developed for general use.

Hookworm Disease: Ancylostomiasis, Necatoriasis, Uncinariasis

Laverne K. Eveland

Hookworms cause one of the most important diseases of humans in tropical and subtropical climates throughout the world, infecting nearly one-quarter of humanity, with prevalence estimates between 700,000 and 900,000 per year and deaths between 50,000 and 60,000 annually.[1] This is particularly significant because in endemic areas 60 percent of the hookworms are harbored by less than 10 percent of the people, which theoretically should facilitate control.[2] The disease results in enormous human misery and economic loss, especially in areas where poverty and unsanitary living conditions prevail. Disease prevalence has decreased in areas such as the United States and Puerto Rico, where improvements in socioeconomic conditions have elevated living standards. Although an analysis of 216,000 stool specimens examined in 1987 identified hookworms (1.5 percent), *Trichuris trichiura* (1.2 percent), and *Ascaris lumbricoides* (0.8 percent) as the leading causes of helminth infections in the United States, the highest rates of hookworm infection were in states lacking indigenous transmission.[3]

Infection leads to an iron-deficiency anemia that further hinders nutrition, thus retarding growth and impairing learning and cognitive development.[4] Disease manifestations are insidious and have historically been confused with innate shiftlessness. Although frank disease is usually not apparent in well-nourished persons, disease occurs as protein absorption is impaired,[5] and a significant amount of protein is also lost into the intestinal tract in the form of plasma or tissue protein.[2]

The Parasites

Necator americanus and *Ancylostoma duodenale* are small nematodes, approximately 9 to 13 mm long, with specialized mouthparts resembling teeth or cutting plates for "biting" into the intestinal mucosa. They, along with *A. ceylanicum* in Asia and the Pacific, are the only species that cause hookworm disease in humans, although larvae of zoonotic hookworms, which cannot develop to maturity in humans, cause dermatitis when they migrate through human skin. In northeastern Australia the canine hookworm *A. caninum* is implicated as the cause of enteritis and acute abdominal pain with peripheral blood eosinophilia in humans.[6–9] *N. americanus* and *A. duodenale* differ in their morphology, life cycles, and biology, which has important implications for how they infect and survive in their mammalian hosts and for their control. *A. duodenale* is apparently not as well adapted to its host as *N. americanus*. It is relatively short lived but more pathogenic, as measured by the severity of gastrointestinal symptoms,[10] blood loss, anemia,[11] and its heightened protease profiles.[12] *A. duodenale* increases the probability of contacting its host by producing a greater number of eggs, synchronizing maximal egg output with the season most favorable for free-living development, and having robust larvae capable of infecting orally or percutaneously.[13]

Where the two species are found together, their relative abundance varies geographically with host age, sex, and other factors. *N. americanus* coexists with *A. duodenale* in southern India, Myanmar, Malaysia, the Philippines, Indonesia, Micronesia, Polynesia, and Myanmar Angola, although it is the predominant species in these areas. In coastal Peru and Chile *A. duodenale* predominates.

A. duodenale is also found in southern Europe, northern coastal Africa, northern India, north China, and Japan. It has been described in native Paraguayan Indians, in the hill tribes of Fukien, China, and in the aborigines of western Australia.[14]

The life cycles of the two species are similar but differ in several important ways that influence their epidemiology, pathogenesis, diagnosis, treatment, and control. The eggs, approximately 60 by 40 μm, are usually at the four- to eight-cell stage of development when they are passed in human feces. If they are deposited in suitable moist, shady, sandy soil, they develop and hatch in 1 or 2 days into first-stage rhabditiform larvae (0.25 to 0.30 mm long by 17 μm wide), which have characteristics that distinguish them from *Strongyloides stercoralis* larvae and free-living larvae such as those of *Rhabditis* species. The rhabditi-form larvae grow for 2 or 3 days, feeding on bacteria and organic debris. They then molt into second stage rhabditoid larvae (0.5 to 0.6 mm long), which continue to feed for several days, and then into third stage filariform larvae. The filariform larvae, which infect humans by penetrating the skin, may remain viable in the soil for several weeks under favorable conditions. Both hookworm species are carried to and through the right heart to the lungs, then up the respiratory tree and down the digestive tract into the small intestine where after a final molt they attach to the mucosa of the jejunum and upper levels of the ileum and develop into sexually differentiated adults. The lung migration is essential for the development of *N. americanus* but not for *A. duodenale*. After the worms reach the intestine, eggs of *N. americanus* usually appear in the feces within 40 to 60 days. *A. duodenale* has a much more variable prepatent period, ranging from 43 to 105 days.[15]

A. duodenale larvae can infect by the oral route and develop into adults without lung passage[16] and probably can also infect by the transplacental route.[4] In a study in China many children showed clinical manifestations and eggs in their feces on days 1 to 26 after birth, suggesting transplacental transmission.[17] Although the evidence is indirect, the facts that *A. duodenale* infects nursing infants with no apparent exposure to other routes of infection and that in a number of endemic areas there is a predominance of *A. duodenale* in infants strongly argue for transmammary transmission.[2]

The prepatent period for *A. duodenale* is long because arrested larvae may persist for extended periods in deep tissues. Human patients dewormed as long as 200 days following their initial infection have been reported positive for fourth and fifth stage *A. duodenale* larvae.[18] *A. duodenale* larvae sequester in the muscles of experimental animals,[19] and at least 28-day-old muscle larvae of *A. caninum* develop to adulthood when fed to dogs.[2] These observations indicate that meat-borne *A. duodenale* infection of humans is possible through the ingestion of larvae in paratenic hosts, although no work has been done to explore the actual epidemiological significance of this means of transmission.[2] The duration of infections is highly variable; many worms are eliminated within a year, but records of longevity range from 4 to 20 years for *N. americanus* and 5 to 7 years for *A. duodenale*.[14]

Infection and Disease

The pathogenesis of hookworm disease usually begins when the larvae enter any portion of the skin with which they make contact, producing a stinging sensation of minor or moderate intensity, depending upon the number of larvae penetrating and the sensitivity of the host. Skin reactions vary from erythematous papules lasting 7 to 10 days to vesiculation and edema.[2] Secondary bacterial infections may also occur, especially if the itching lesions are abraded by scratching. This so-called "ground itch" or "dew itch" must be distinguished from the characteristic "cutaneous larva migrans (CLM)" caused by the zoonotic *Ancylostoma braziliense* and other nematodes of the family Ancylostomidae. CLM is characterized by tortuous inflammatory areas in the dermis associated with swelling, erythema, papular dermatitis, and pruritus. *N. americanus* sometimes migrates in the skin and produces a mild CLM, which is of shorter duration than that caused by *A. braziliense*.[14]

Although migrating hookworm larvae do not usually produce pulmonary symptoms, they do produce minute focal hemorrhages when they break out of pulmonary capillaries and may produce clinical pneumonitis in massive infections. Wakana disease, which has been described in Japan, sometimes results following the ingestion of *A. duodenale* larvae, penetration of the larvae into mucous membranes of the mouth and pharynx, and their migration to the lungs. The initial symptoms that occur shortly after the larvae are ingested are pharyngeal itching, hoarseness, salivation, nausea, and vomiting, followed by an illness of several days duration that includes coughing, dyspnea, wheezing, urticaria, nausea, and vomiting.[2] Infiltrations may be visible on chest x-ray films.[14] Because the disease can be produced by heat-killed organisms, it is presumed to be caused by an allergic reaction to the larvae.[20]

Although light infections are usually asymptomatic, acute, heavy hookworm infections can produce gastrointestinal symptoms similar to those of acute peptic ulcer, which include fatigue, nausea, vomiting, and burning and cramping abdominal pain. Blood eosinophilia occurs, and Charcot-Leyden crystals may be present in the feces. The acute disease occurs more frequently with *A. duodenale* than with *N. americanus*.

As the infection progresses, anemia resulting from chronic blood loss may be accompanied by a loss of appetite and congestive heart failure. Geophagia and pica may develop, with constipation resulting from the dietary change. The worms suck blood, but they actually utilize only 40 percent of the ingested erythrocytes that pass through their bodies.[21] However, they also spill a significant amount of blood by lacerating the mucosa during feeding.[21,22] Blood loss from mucosal damage increases disproportionately in heavy infections because the worms attach and reattach more frequently because of mating competition, especially early in the infection.[14] Adult worms also produce anticoagulants, which may enhance blood loss,[23,24] and a neutrophil adhesion inhibitor that is probably used by the hookworm to evade the host's inflammatory response.[25,26]

Classic hookworm disease is an iron-deficiency, microcytic, hypochromic anemia resulting directly from blood loss. Intestinal injury and changes in motility might contribute to disordered absorption of nutrients for the host, but hookworm patients usually are no more malnourished than uninfected subjects.[2,27] In general, good nutrition consisting of iron, other minerals, and animal protein mitigates the disease associated with light to moderate hookworm infections, even though it does not affect the existing hookworm population or protect an individual from infection. In extremely heavy infections, disease cannot be ameliorated by diet alone. Although the disease is usually associated with heavy infections, it has long been a mystery why it occurs in some persons with only light infections while other persons with extremely heavy infections have no signs or symptoms. The answer appears to lie in the availability of dietary iron stores rather than diet per se,[4,21] because in hookworm endemic areas dietary intake of iron appears to be generally adequate.[2] It is likely that those more susceptible to disease cannot absorb sufficient iron for reasons unrelated to their hookworm infection, such as concurrent intestinal diseases.[28]

Remote organs may also be indirectly affected by hookworm infection.[29,30] Thus, chronic anemia of hookworm disease may also be accompanied by increased pulmonary vital capacity, increased tolerance of tissue cells to anoxia, and lowered systolic pressure and peripheral blood flow. The heart may dilate and show increased collateral circulation of coronary arteries with an accompanying decreased risk of myocardial infarction.[14] Changes may occur in bone marrow because of blood loss; retroperitoneal lymph nodes can become enlarged secondary to antigenic stimulation; and the anemia and anoxia of hookworm disease are sometimes associated with fatty deterioration of the heart, liver, and kidneys.[2]

Infections that produce more than 5,000 eggs per (EPG) of feces are considered heavy; 2,000 to 5,000 EPG, moderately heavy; 500 to 2,000 EPG, moderately light; and less than 500 EPG, light. Light infections are usually not of clinical grade, but medium and heavy infections are often associated with significant anemia. Diagnosis is complicated in early infections because hookworm anemia may actually begin before eggs are detectable, when larval and immature hookworms first reach the mucosa and begin to cause blood loss.[4] Hookworm disease should be suspected in a person with a subnormal hemoglobin level, Charcot-Leyden crystals in the feces, and a history of exposure. Specific immunoglobulin E has been reported to be highly specific (96 percent) and sensitive (100 percent) in the serodiagnosis of hookworm infections.[31] Although heavy infections may be detected by direct fecal smears, in light infections (<500 EPG of feces), concentration techniques are usually needed to demonstrate the eggs. Several excellent concentration methods are available, including zinc flotation and several modifications of formalin-ether and formalin-ethyl acetate techniques. Unless anemia is present or the intake of dietary iron is inadequate, light infections are usually not treated. Hookworm eggs may develop and hatch in fecal specimens stored for more than 24 hours at room temperature or above. It is then necessary to distinguish the rhabditiform larvae from those of free-living nematodes and *S. stercoralis*.

Epidemiology

The most favorable conditions for the development of hookworm larvae and completion of the life cycle include loose, moist, shady, sandy humus, promiscuous defecation or the use of improperly treated human feces (night soil) as fertilizer, and the opportunity for humans to come into contact with the soil. An important epidemiological factor appears to be the presence of dung beetles that thrive in such soil and bury human feces efficiently.[14] Rainfall is required to provide adequate moisture for the larvae to migrate, aggregate, and reach human skin on grass or other moist surfaces. Temperature is an important factor in determining which species of hookworm is found, because *A. duodenale* withstands colder temperatures than *N. americanus*, which conversely can tolerate much higher temperatures than *A. duodenale*. The infective larvae may remain viable in the soil for months during periods of drought or low temperatures. Eggs and third-stage hookworm larvae have also been found on the external body and in the gut of certain flies.[32,33]

White males are much more susceptible to infection than females or nonwhites, and evidence suggests that heavily infected persons are genetically predisposed to such levels of infection.[13,34,35] For epidemiological purposes, the amount of hookworm disease in a community depends on both the prevalence and intensity of infection, as measured by egg output.[2] However, people who contribute large numbers of eggs to the environment are not necessarily those who are the greatest source of infection for others, because infective larvae show a high degree of aggregation in the soil.[36]

Prevention and Control

Theoretically, hookworm disease could be reduced by the sanitary disposal of human feces, wearing shoes and protective clothing, the use of ovicides or larvicides, vaccines, and adequate chemotherapy for mass therapy or individual use. However, the mere availability of properly constructed sanitary latrines does not ensure their use, as local habits, customs, or beliefs regarding hygiene may be major obstacles.[3] It has been demonstrated that children, and to a lesser extent adults, fail to use sanitary facilities when they are present, but prefer the convenience of defecating among bushes in backyards or nearby fields.[37] Shoes and protective clothing are not a reasonable expectation because they are expensive, difficult to clean, and can be extremely uncomfortable in hot weather. Health education should encourage people to defecate where free-living stages cannot develop or survive, such as on saline soils, open dry, fallow land, or in flooded fields.[2]

At present no effective vaccines are available. There is little direct evidence that protective immunity to hookworm develops in humans. Based upon epidemiological evidence suggesting immunity, a cDNA clone encoding a specific antigenic protease has been proposed as a candidate immunogen in human beings.[2] However, a study in Papua New Guinea following chemotherapy showed that infection with *N. americanus* returned to pretreatment levels after 2 years and that the predisposition to reinfection did not vary significantly between age or sex classes.[38]

In general, only persons at highest risk for disease as determined by egg output and iron-deficiency anemia should be treated. Little benefit is gained from treating individuals with light infections in endemic areas, as reinfection commonly occurs in such foci. Persons who return from endemic areas to good sanitary conditions and adequate nutrition may not require treatment.[2]

Thiabendazole is larvicidal, and mebendazole is ovicidal and larvicidal. Albendazole kills both preintestinal and intestinal worms, but it is not known whether it affects arrested larvae of *A. duodenale*.[2] Bephenium hydroxynaphthoate is effective against *A. duodenale*, and also against *N. americanus* when combined with tetrachloroethylene, although the latter is difficult to obtain for human use in the United States. Tetrachloroethylene is effective when used alone in higher doses but should not be used if *Ascaris* worms are present. Pyrantel pamoate is useful against both species and is useful for combined infections with *Ascaris*.

The objective of control actions should be to lower the intensity of the infection, which will reduce morbidity and gradually disrupt transmission. To achieve this objective, further research is needed in (*a*) development of species- and stage-specific diagnostic tests, (*b*) investigation of the consequences of arrested development of hookworms, (*c*) study of hookworm transmission in various regions in the context of varied cultural factors, (*d*) quantification of the effects of morbidity on individuals and communities, (*e*) investigation of the relationships between hookworm disease and human nutrition, (*f*) elucidation of the human host response to infection, and (*g*) the search for potential vaccines.

Other Intestinal Nematodes

Mark R. Wallace • Shannon D. Putnam

Intestinal nematodes are the most common parasites in humans, infecting up to one-fourth of the world's population. Most infestations occur in the developing world where warm, moist climates, poverty, and poor sanitation favor transmission. Since most helminths do not multiply in the human host (*Strongyloides stercoralis* and *Capillaria philippinensis* being notable exceptions), the overall worm burden is usually light and symptoms minimal. Heavy worm burdens occur in a sizable minority of infected persons (often children) and may cause severe illness, impaired school or work performance, stunted growth, and a variety of unusual manifestations. Through autoinfection, *S. stercoralis* and *C. philippinensis* have the potential to cause life-threatening hyperinfections.

The intestinal nematodes vary greatly in size, life cycle, and disease manifestations. In this chapter we review the most common intestinal nematodes excluding the hookworms, which are discussed elsewhere. With the exception of *C. philippinensis*, all the intestinal nematodes discussed are primarily pathogens of humans.

Strongyloides stercoralis

Though strongyloidiasis is less prevalent than the other common intestinal nematodes and is often only minimally symptomatic, its potential for autoinfection allows for unusually chronic and/or severe infections.

The Parasite

The life cycle for *S. stercoralis* is similar to that of the hookworms (Fig. 16–1). The adult worm, a parthenogenetic female, lives within the mucosal epithelium of the human small intestine and deposits eggs (usually less than 50 per day) in the mucosa. There they hatch

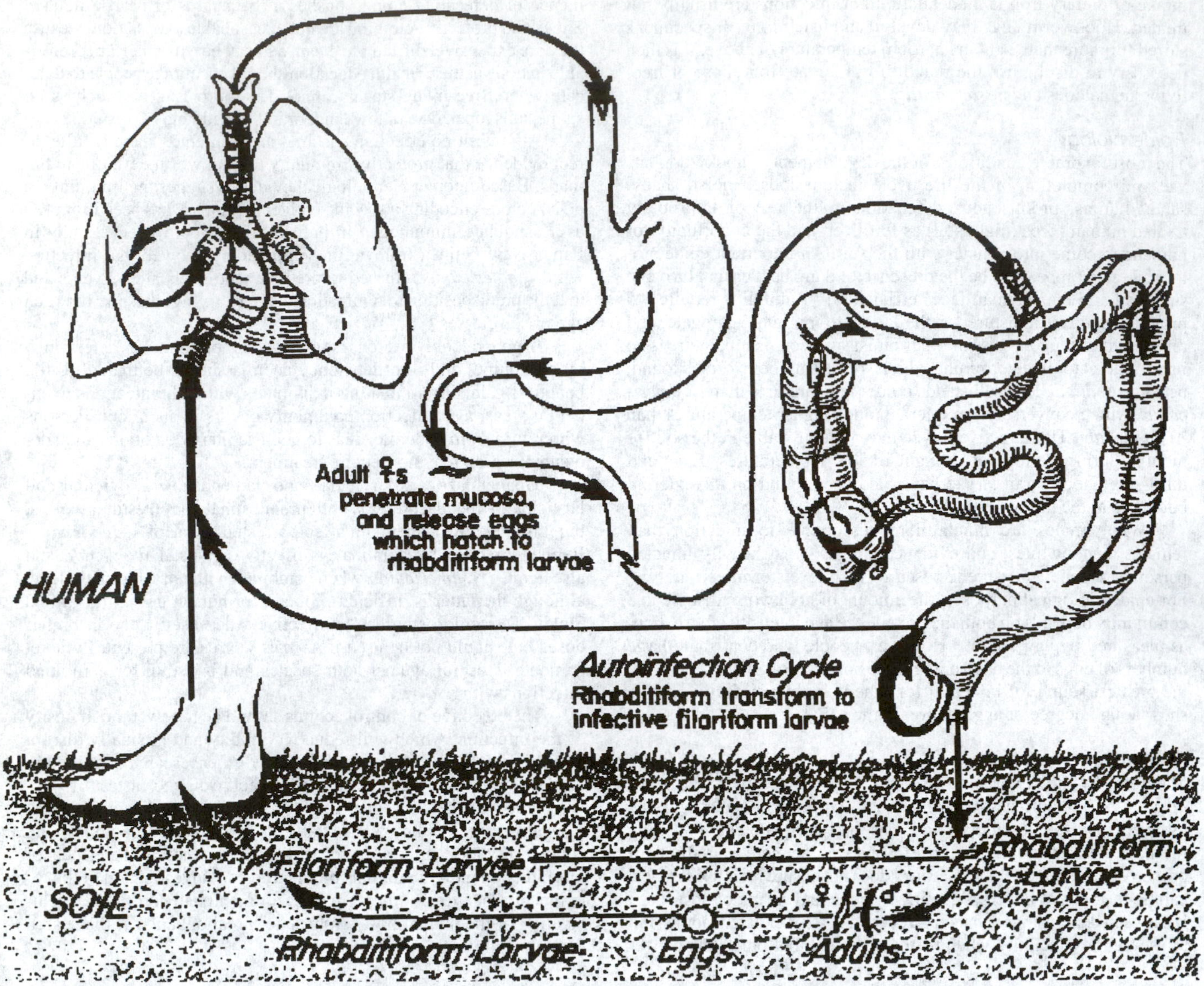

Figure 16-1. Life cycle of *Strongyloides stercoralis.* (Redrawn from Longworth DL, Weller P: Hyperinfection syndrome. In Remington JS, Swartz S, eds; Current Clinical Topics in Infectious Disease. New York, McGraw-Hill, 1986, vol 7.)

into noninfective rhabditiform larvae, migrate into the small intestinal lumen, and are discharged with human feces into the soil. The larvae then develop into either the infective filariform larvae (direct cycle) or adult worms capable of producing additional generations of rhabditiform larvae, which subsequently moult into infective filariform larvae (indirect cycle). Human infection is acquired through skin penetration or (less commonly) ingestion of filariform larvae, which then traverse the venous circulation to the lungs. Once in the lungs, the larvae penetrate capillary walls, enter the alveoli, ascend the trachea to the epiglottis, are swallowed, and eventually reach the upper part of the small intestine where they develop into adult worms.

In the autoinfection cycle, the rhabditiform larvae mature to infective filariform larvae within the human gut and reinvade through the intestinal mucosa or perianal skin. This allows the infection to continue and the parasites to multiply without any additional exposure to soil-borne filariform larvae. Autoinfection accounts for the extremely long-lived infections (sometimes over 50 years) and the possible development of hyperinfection and disseminated strongyloidiasis in immunocompromised hosts.

Epidemiology

Strongyloidiasis is an infection of worldwide importance. It is endemic in the developing world, much of Europe, and the Appalachian region of the United States. The prevalence rates vary greatly between surveys with estimates of up to 100 million cases worldwide. Immigrants, travelers, and military personnel can acquire *S. stercoralis* in endemic areas and then harbor the parasite with few (if any) symptoms for decades through autoinfection. Residents of mental institutions are also at particularly high risk for strongyloidiasis due to fecal-oral transmission and geophagia.

Infection and Disease

The initial entry of the filariform larvae through the skin may produce a transient pruritus similar to that of the hookworms. Cough and wheezing, indistinguishable from that seen in hookworm or *Ascaris* infection, may occur as the larval forms migrate through the respiratory tree. The pulmonary symptoms are usually mild and short-lived, but may be severe in hyperinfection.

Established infection in the immunocompetent host may be asymptomatic or manifested by intermittent vague abdominal pain, indigestion, nausea, anorexia, or diarrhea. The autoinfection cycle may perpetuate strongyloidiasis infection for decades. Patients with ongoing autoinfection may develop larva currens, an urticarial, serpiginous rash. This rapidly moving eruption (up to 5 to 10 cm/hour) is due to autoinfecting filariform larva migrating under the skin after penetrating the perianal surface. Larva currens may last days and recur over months or years; it is said to be pathognomonic of strongyloidiasis. Children may have malabsorption and growth retardation with heavy worm burdens. Severe strongyloidiasis may resemble inflammatory bowel disease and lead to the (disastrous) initiation of immunosuppressive therapy and subsequent hyperinfection.

Hyperinfection and disseminated strongyloidiasis occur when autoinfection is amplified by the presence of immunosuppression or chronic illness. Common predisposing factors include corticosteroid therapy, immunosuppressive chemotherapy, renal failure, malignancy, chronic pulmonary disease, alcoholism, tuberculosis, or malnutrition. Hyperinfection strongyloidiasis may present with severe pulmonary or gastrointestinal symptoms due to the massive parasite load and may also involve other organs as *S. stercoralis* larvae aberrantly migrate to the central nervous system, liver, heart, or other distant sites. Bacteremias may occur as the larvae penetrate the gastrointestinal mucosa and carry gastrointestinal flora into the bloodstream. Hyperinfection should always be considered in immunosuppressed patients with unexplained gastrointestinal or pulmonary processes or recurrent Gram-negative bacteremias. Eosinophilia, prominent in uncomplicated strongyloidiasis, is often absent in these seriously ill patients. Overall mortality of the hyperinfection syndrome is high even with appropriate therapy.

Diagnosis

The diagnosis of *S. stercoralis* infection rests on identifying the larval forms; eggs hatch before exiting and are usually not seen in the stool. Because of the low rate of egg production, examination of a single stool detects only about 30 percent of infections; three or more fresh stools should be examined for the presence of rhabditiform larvae. Various stool concentration methods may improve the yield, and *Strongyloides* stool cultures are available in a few laboratories. Duodenal aspirates or sampling by the "string test" are positive in over 90 percent of infections. When pulmonary symptoms are present, a sputum examination for filariform larvae is indicated. In some cases where strongyloidiasis is suspected but no larval forms can be demonstrated, an enzyme-linked immunosorbent assay (ELISA) serology may be helpful; this is both sensitive and specific. Serologic testing may be used to screen patients from endemic areas prior to the initiation of immunosuppressive therapies.

Therapy

Eradication is the goal of strongyloidiasis therapy. A simple reduction of worm burden is inadequate as it leaves the patient exposed to the risk of subsequent hyperinfection. Thiabendazole has been the traditional therapy of choice for strongyloidiasis and is given for 3 days in uncomplicated cases and 7 (or more) days in hyperinfection syndromes. Cure rates of 90 percent are expected in uncomplicated cases, but are lower in hyperinfected patients. Virtually all patients treated with thiabendazole will develop some toxicity; disorientation, fatigue, and gastrointestinal complaints are the primary side effects. Single-dose ivermectin may be emerging as the drug of choice. In comparison to thiabendazole, it has been found to have similar efficacy with a much improved side effect profile. Cure rates of 80 percent and minimal side effects have been also reported with albendazole.

Prevention and Control

The sanitary disposal of human feces is essential for the control of strongyloidiasis in endemic areas. The wearing of appropriate footwear is a valuable adjunct to prevention, but may be impractical in warmer climates. Hyperinfection syndromes are prevented by the identification and eradication of strongyloidiasis infections.

Ascaris lumbricoides

Ascaris lumbricoides is the largest and most common of all the intestinal geohelminths infecting humans. Though usually asymptomatic, severe clinical manifestations occur in a significant minority of patients. The fecundity of the female ascarid and the prolonged egg survival in the soil guarantee that ascariasis will continue to be among humankind's most prevalent infections for the foreseeable future.

The Parasite

The adult worms are 120 to 400 mm in length and live in the small intestine for 1 to 2 years. The mature female produces approximately 200,000 unembryonated eggs daily. The eggs have a rough, mammillated coat and are discharged into the intestinal lumen and passed with the feces. Once deposited in soil, the eggs embryonate and become infectious, remaining viable for years despite extremes of temperature and moisture. After ingestion via contaminated soil or foods, the eggs hatch into rhabditiform larvae in the small intestine. The larvae penetrate the intestinal mucosa, invade the portal veins, pass through the liver, and continue to the lungs. Once in the lung, they penetrate into the alveoli, are coughed up, swallowed, and return to the small intestine where they develop into the adult worms.

Epidemiology

It is estimated that over 1 billion humans are infected with *Ascaris*. Ascariasis is most common in warmer climates with inadequate human waste facilities, but cases can occur in temperate climates with good sanitation; there are an estimated 4 million cases per year in the United States. Although the usual mode of transmission is usually fecal-soil-oral, egg-contaminated food or inhalation of airborne eggs may also produce infection.

Infection and Disease

Most infections with *A. lumbricoides* are asymptomatic. Clinical disease is most likely in heavily infected individuals, especially children. During the larval migration through the lungs in primary infection, a transient pneumonitis with eosinophilia may be seen, which is indistinguishable from the pulmonary phase of *Strongyloides* and hookworms. Gastrointestinal symptoms of ascariasis are often mild and vague, but wandering ascarids occasionally cause severe pancreatic or hepatobiliary disease. Children with heavy infections may develop bowel obstruction. The role of sustained heavy *Ascaris* burdens in childhood malnutrition and developmental delays is difficult to firmly establish but probably is a contributing factor.

Diagnosis

The diagnosis of ascariasis is easily made by the identification of a large number of eggs in a single stool specimen. Pulmonary ascariasis is occasionally diagnosed by the identification of the larvae in sputum. Adult worms may be found in the stools or emerging from the mouth or nose.

Treatment

Multiple excellent choices are available for the therapy of ascariasis, including mebendazole, albendazole, pyrantel pamoate, and piperazine. Piperazine should be used if intestinal obstruction or "wayward worms" are suspected, as it will cause paralysis of the worms and reduce the risks of additional visceral injury. Mebendazole and albendazole are contraindicated in pregnancy.

Prevention and Control

Proper human waste disposal is essential to the control of ascariasis. Targeted mass treatment aimed at groups at risk for heavy helminthic infections (usually children) are often conducted as a part of preventative medicine programs and may reduce overall morbidity and mortality.

Trichuris trichiura

Trichuriasis is an extremely common infection, with approximately 800 million persons infected worldwide. Many are co-infected with *Ascaris* or hookworm, which share a similar geographic and socioeconomic distribution. Like *Ascaris*, most infections are asymptomatic, but severe disease can occur with massive worm burdens.

The Parasite

Adult *T. trichiura* are approximately 30 to 50 mm long and live for years in the cecal and colonic mucosa. The posterior section of the adult worm appears thick and tapers to a long threadlike anterior structure, resembling a bull whip (hence the name whipworm). The adult male worm's tail is coiled while the female worm's tail is straight. The females are oviparous, producing 2,000 to 10,000 eggs each day, which pass into the environment with the fecal stream. Once in the soil, the eggs mature over the next 2 to 4 weeks developing into infective first-stage larvae. Upon ingestion of fecally contaminated material, the first-stage larvae hatch in the small intestine and migrate to the colon where they develop into mature worms. There is no tissue phase in the whipworm life cycle.

Epidemiology

Trichuris has a cosmopolitan geographic distribution with a preference for warm, moist regions where sanitation facilities are lacking. The use of human waste for fertilizer ("night soil") facilitates *T. trichiura* transmission. Though more common in the developing world, trichuriasis is also found in the southeastern United States and Puerto Rico.

Infection and Disease

Most *T. trichiura* infections are asymptomatic, but abdominal pain, anorexia, and diarrhea can be seen. Heavy infections can produce the *Trichuris* dysentery syndrome with whipworm infiltration of the bowel from the cecum to the rectum. The dysentery syndrome may be so severe as to resemble inflammatory bowel disease and may result in anemia or rectal prolapse. As with other geohelminths, children are most often heavily infected with *Trichuris* and may suffer delayed development. *Trichuris* is usually not associated with eosinophilia.

Diagnosis

Diagnosis is made by the identification of the eggs in the feces. The eggs have a thick, clear shell with distinctive bipolar plugs. More than 10,000 eggs per g. of stool indicates heavy infection. The diagnosis is occasionally made endoscopically through direct visualization of adult worms in the colon.

Treatment

A 3-day course of mebendazole is the optimal therapy for the individual patient, but single doses of either mebendazole or albendazole are often used in the targeted treatment of children in heavily endemic areas. Single-dose therapy results in a 60 to 75 percent cure rate.

Prevention and Control

As with most intestinal nematodes, the primary mode of prevention is to provide for the proper disposal of human feces and to avoid ingestion of soil-contaminated material through careful hand washing and food preparation.

Capillaria philippinensis

Unlike the more common intestinal nematodes infecting humans, capillariasis is not primarily a human disease and almost always results in severe infection.

The Parasite

Capillaria philippinensis is believed to exist primarily in a fish-bird life cycle. Birds, the proposed reservoir host, harbor the adult worms and in turn defecate eggs, which are fed upon by freshwater fish. Larval forms of *C. philippinensis* develop within the fish, which are then consumed by birds to complete the cycle. Humans inadvertently become infected by ingesting raw fish or crustaceans infected with the larval forms; the eggs are not infectious to humans. Following raw fish ingestion, the adult worms develop and reside in the proximal small bowel. Like strongyloidiasis, eggs can hatch into infective larvae within the human gut and produce autoinfection with extremely high parasite burdens and serious illness.

Epidemiology

Since first discovered in the 1960s, most cases of *C. philippinensis* infections have been reported from the Philippines and Thailand. More recently, cases have been reported from Japan, Iran, Taiwan, Egypt, Indonesia, Korea, and India.

Infection and Disease

Infection with *C. philippinensis* usually (if not always) leads to a serious illness characterized by abdominal pain, nausea, vomiting, borborygmi, and voluminous diarrhea. Severe chronic infection can cause malabsorption, electrolyte abnormalities, wasting, and eventual death. The untreated mortality has been estimated at 10 to 30 percent.

Diagnosis

Diagnosis is based on the identification of thick-shelled, striated, bipolar eggs in the feces. The eggs (35 to 45 μm long by 20 μm wide) somewhat resemble those of the closely related *Trichuris*. In chronic cases, larvae and adult worms may also be seen in stool specimens. Examination of small bowel aspirates or biopsies may occasionally be helpful in making the diagnosis when stool examinations are negative.

Treatment

A 10-day course of albendazole is the preferred treatment, as it kills all forms of the parasite. A 20-day mebendazole regimen is the best alternative. The previously used 30-day course of thiabendazole is too toxic for routine therapy. Shorter courses of treatment lead to an unacceptably high relapse rate and should be avoided.

Prevention and Control

Human capillariasis may be entirely prevented by avoiding the consumption of raw fish. When cases occur, prompt treatment is essential to prevent mortality and to limit possible contamination of local waters with feces, which could create local outbreaks. As with all other intestinal nematodes, proper disposal of human waste is essential to disease prevention.

Enterobius vermicularis

Enterobius (human pinworm) is one of the most common parasitic intestinal infections, occurring in both temperate and tropical climates. The worldwide prevalence is difficult to estimate, as the infection is often asymptomatic, but some authorities have speculated that over a billion people are infected. Pinworm infection rarely results in serious illness, but frequently produces considerable morbidity and anxiety among school-age children and their parents.

The Parasite

Adult pinworms are small (females, 8 to 13 mm long with a long pointed tail; males, 2 to 3 mm in length with a blunt tail) and live in the ileum, cecum, colon, and appendix for 1 to 3 months. The typical infection involves a few to several hundred adult worms. The gravid adult female migrates out of the anus at night to lay thousands of eggs in the perianal region. The eggs are elongated, flattened on one side, with a thick clear shell. They are partially embryonated when laid and become infective within 4 to 6 hours at body temperature. Infection occurs when the eggs are ingested, hatch in the small intestine to produce larvae, and pass into the colon where they moult twice as they mature into adult worms.

Epidemiology
Enterobiasis occurs worldwide, affecting all socioeconomic classes. It is the most common nematode infection in the United States, usually involving school-aged children. The condition may spread rapidly within families, day care facilities, institutions, or other crowded situations. Ingestion of infective eggs via contaminated fingers, fomites, or direct oral-anal sexual contact leads to infection.

Infection and Disease
Most infections are asymptomatic. Pruritus or dysesthesia of the perianal and perineal areas are the primary symptoms of infection. Vulvovaginitis and urinary tract infection due to migration of adult worms are sometimes reported in prepubescent girls. Rarely, adult worms may traverse the fallopian tubes or move across breaks in the gut mucosa to gain access to the peritoneum and form granulomas. The pinworm larval forms have been implicated in case reports as a rare cause of eosinophilic colitis resembling the trichuriasis dysentery syndrome. Pinworm infection does not cause eosinophilia or anemia.

Diagnosis
Enterobiasis diagnosis is best made by applying adhesive tape to the perianal region and microscopically examining the tape for *E. vermicularis* eggs or adults. For the highest diagnostic sensitivity, material should be collected in the early morning prior to bathing or defecation. Examination may need to be repeated six times before infection can be conclusively excluded, but three specimens are adequate in most cases. Standard "ova and parasite" stool examination is positive in only 5 to 15 percent of confirmed cases.

Treatment
Single doses of albendazole, mebendazole, or pyrantel pamoate are all highly effective and widely used; a second dose 1 to 2 weeks after initial therapy is often given. Reinfection, whether through self infection or infection from close contacts, is a major problem in *E. vermicularis* therapy. Attention to washing hands after defecation, keeping fingernails cut short and avoiding perianal scratching are the keys to avoiding reinfection. All family members may need to be simultaneously treated to avoid a circle of infection.

Prevention and Control
Enterobiasis infection can be prevented through proper personal hygiene practices including washing hands after defecation and before eating or preparing foods, discouraging bare perianal scratching, changing undergarments and bedding regularly, and providing sanitary human waste disposal.

Schistosomiasis

Amy D. Klion

Schistosomiasis, or bilharziasis, is a chronic debilitating disease with significant morbidity and mortality. It affects more than 200 million people in the endemic area worldwide and is second only to malaria in socioeconomic and public health importance in tropical and subtropical areas.[1] Human disease is caused by five species of blood flukes of the genus *Schistosoma: Schistosoma mansoni, Schistosoma haematobium, Schistosoma japonicum, Schistosoma mekongi*, and *Schistosoma intercalatum.*

Biology and Life Cycles
The schistosome requires an intermediate and a definitive host to complete its life cycle. Asexual reproduction takes place in the molluscan intermediate host and sexual reproduction in the definitive vertebrate host. Free-swimming miracidia hatch from eggs deposited in freshwater during defecation or urination by an infected definitive host. These miracidia penetrate the appropriate snail host and develop into primary sporocysts, each of which produces multiple secondary sporocysts. Each of the secondary sporocysts produces a great number of cercariae, resulting in the production of hundreds to thousands of cercariae from an individual miracidium. The fork-tailed cercariae migrate out of the snail and propel themselves toward the surface of the water. Of note, both miracidia and cercariae have a limited life in the absence of an appropriate host span (6 to 24 hours under experimental conditions).[2] Sporocysts, on the other hand, remain dormant during adverse conditions and are able to resume cercarial production with the return of a favorable environment.

When humans contact schistosome-infested water, cercariae penetrate the skin, lose their tails, and are transformed into schistosomula. After several days, the schistosomula enter a venule or lymphatic vessel and migrate to the right side of the heart, then to the lungs, and finally to the liver sinusoids, where they begin to mature. On reaching maturity, adult male and female worms pair and migrate to their final habitats. There, eggs are deposited in the venules of the intestine or urinary bladder, break through the submucosa and mucosa into the lumen, and are evacuated through the feces or urine, completing the life cycle.

The mature female schistosome measures from 7.2 to 26 mm in length and 0.25 to 0.5 mm in width, whereas the mature male measures from 6.5 to 20 mm in length and 0.5 to 1 mm in width. They remain in copula for their entire lifespan, an average of 5 to 8 years, but sometimes for as long as 30 years.[3] The preferred location of adult worms in the host is different among the schistosome species. *S. japonicum* and *S. mekongi* adult parasites are generally found in the superior mesenteric vein; *S. mansoni* and *S. intercalatum*, in the inferior mesenteric vein; and *S. haematobium*, in the vesicular and pelvic venous plexuses. Daily egg production also varies with the species: from approximately 1,500 to 3,000 eggs/day/worm pair in *S. japonicum* infection to 250 eggs/day in *S. mansoni* and *S. intercalatum* infection and 50 to 100 eggs/day in *S. haematobium* infection. These biological differences between schistosome species are important in determining both the clinical manifestations and transmission rates of infection.

Distribution
Schistosomiasis is endemic in many tropical and subtropical countries.[1] The distribution is dependent on the existence of the appropriate snail host and necessary environmental conditions.[3] *S. mansoni* (intermediate host: *Biomphalaria* spp.) has the most widespread distribution, ranging from the Arabian peninsula to South America and the Caribbean. *S. japonicum* (intermediate host: *Oncomelania* spp.) is confined to the Far East, distributed in parts of China, Indonesia (*S. japonicum*-like), the Philippines, and until recently, Japan. A related species, *S. mekongi* (intermediate host: *Neotricula* spp.), is found in Laos, Cambodia, and Thailand. *S. haematobium* (intermediate host: *Bulinus* spp.) is endemic in the Middle East, Africa, Turkey, and India. Transmitted by the same intermediate host as *S. haematobium, S. intercalatum* is found only in regions of Central and West Africa. Important reservoir hosts for *S. japonicum* include mice, dogs, goats, rabbits, cattle, sheep, rats, pigs, horses, and buffalo.[4] Although natural

infection of nonhuman primates with *S. mansoni* and *S. haematobium* has been described, animals other than humans do not appear to be major reservoirs of infection with these species.[5]

Pathological and Clinical Manifestations

Most of the pathological changes and clinical manifestations of schistosomiasis result from the host's immunological response to the eggs. The severity of the disease depends on the species, strain, location of parasites, intensity and duration of infection, frequency of reinfection, and the host's reactivity. Mild infections without symptoms often occur. The course of infection may be divided into four progressive stages: invasion, maturation, established infection, and chronic infection with its attendant complications.

In the invasion stage, exposure of the sensitized host to cercarial or schistosomular antigens may lead to transient allergic manifestations. Although most infected individuals have no symptoms during cercarial penetration, a localized papular dermatitis ("swimmer's itch") may occur with repeated exposures. A similar, but more intense, reaction is provoked when schistosome species that normally do not infect humans penetrate the skin and die in the dermis, releasing large quantities of parasite antigen.[6] Petechial hemorrhages, foci of eosinophilia, and leukocytic infiltration may be produced in the lung or in the liver when schistosomula migrate through the lungs and reach the liver. During this period, transitional symptoms of fever, malaise, cough, and a generalized allergic reaction may appear. When present, symptoms generally resolve in 5 to 15 days without treatment.

Active schistosomiasis starts with worm maturation and the beginning of egg production. Severe cases of acute schistosomiasis, or Katayama fever, are not uncommon and occur 35 to 40 days after *S. japonicum* or heavy *S. mansoni* infection, coincident with the first 2 weeks of egg production. The clinical manifestations are characterized by a serum sicknesslike syndrome of fever, chills, cough, arthralgias and myalgias, diarrhea, eosinophilia, hepatosplenomegaly, and generalized lymphadenopathy. Recovery usually occurs within several weeks, but fatalities do occur. The syndrome most likely reflects the strong host immune response to egg antigens and the formation and deposition of circulating immune complexes.

In the established stage, intense egg deposition and excretion take place. The intestinal schistosomes (*S. japonicum, S. mekongi, S. mansoni*, and *S. intercalatum*) release eggs into the mesenteric veins. Some of these become lodged in the intestinal submucosa, where they secrete proteolytic enzymes that erode the tissue and break through the intestinal wall. In heavy infection, this may cause diarrhea and blood in the stool. Other eggs may be trapped at the original site or swept back into the portal blood flow and distributed to the liver, spleen, or other ectopic foci, where they provoke an inflammatory tissue response and granuloma formation. This may cause thrombosis of vessels, formation of polyps in the intestinal wall, or hepatosplenic schistosomiasis (see below). In *S. mansoni* infection, the rectum and colon are affected more frequently than other parts of the gastrointestinal tract. The severity of early disease is closely correlated with the number of eggs and their anatomic location. Consequently, *S. japonicum*, which has the highest capacity for egg production and the widest egg distribution, is a more common cause of severe, disseminated disease.

Adult *S. haematobium* in the veins surrounding the urinary bladder deposit eggs into the vesicular plexus. These commonly break through the bladder wall and cause dysuria, urinary frequency, and hematuria. Inflammatory polypoid masses in the bladder or ureteral walls are common early in infection and are a significant cause of obstructive uropathy. Eggs may also be carried by the venous system to the genital organs, gastrointestinal tract, lungs, and liver.

The chronic stage with its attendant complications is generally observed only in heavy infection. The acute symptoms (if present) resolve, and the level of egg secretion becomes stable. Although most individuals with chronic infection are asymptomatic, egg-induced granuloma formation, fibrous proliferation, and vascular obliteration lead to chronic pathology in others (see below). Once initiated, schistosome-induced fibrosis may progress despite resolution of the initial infection.[7]

Chronic intestinal schistosomiasis is characterized by fibrous patches, inflammatory polyps, thickening of the intestinal wall, and adhesions of the thickened mesentery and omentum to the intestine. Complications include secondary bacterial infection and intestinal obstruction. Recurrent *Salmonella* bacteremia is particularly common.[8] In hepatosplenic schistosomiasis, granulomas develop around eggs in the portal venules. Hepatosplenomegaly may be pronounced. Over time, the liver gradually shrinks in size as a result of increasing fibrosis in a periportal distribution, called Symmers' pipestem fibrosis. This may result in blockage of presinusoidal blood flow, leading to portal hypertension, ascites, and esophageal varices. An association between hepatosplenic schistosomiasis and nephrotic syndrome secondary to immune complex glomerulonephritis has been well documented.[9]

Pulmonary schistosomiasis has been reported in all five species of schistosome infection. Eggs may be carried to the lungs by venous shunting through systemic collateral vessels formed as a result of portal hypertension or because of aberrant migration of worms into the vena caval or vertebrate venous systems. The resultant granulomatous arteritis of the pulmonary capillary bed may lead to obliterative arteriolitis, dilation of the pulmonary arteries, and pulmonary hypertension. Rarely, this leads to cor pulmonale with right-sided heart failure.

Fibrosis and calcification of the eggs in the urinary bladder may impair bladder function. Fibrosis of the neck of the bladder and opening of the ureter result in obstruction of urine flow and may lead to the development of hydroureter, hydronephrosis, renal stones, and rarely, renal failure. Chronic ulceration and irritation of the bladder epithelium may in time lead to malignant transformation and the development of squamous cell carcinoma of the bladder.

In cerebrospinal schistosomiasis, ectopic eggs may cause granuloma formation in the central nervous system, resulting in focal damage.[10] Brain involvement is most common in *S. japonicum* infection and may present acutely as meningoencephalitis.[10] In chronic infection, seizures are the predominant manifestations. *S. mansoni* and *S. haematobium* more commonly affect the spinal cord, causing transverse myelitis.[11]

Alterations in the immune response to viruses and intestinal helminths[12,13] have been reported during infection with schistosomiasis. The relationship between schistosomiasis and morbidity and mortality due to viral hepatitis remains controversial.

Diagnosis

Definitive diagnosis is made by identifying characteristic eggs in the stool or urine sample or by tissue biopsy.[14] Eggs of *S. japonicum* and *S. mekongi* are globular in shape without spines; *S. mansoni*, oval with a lateral spine; and *S. haematobium*, oval with a terminal spine. Concentration techniques should be employed for all urine and stool specimens, and multiple samples should be examined carefully before a negative report is given. The quantitative Kato-Katz (cellophane) thick fecal smear is a rapid, inexpensive method of detection of eggs in the stool. It has become a standard diagnostic tool in epidemiology for international comparison of data[1] and has largely replaced filtration and hatching techniques. Newer techniques, such as Visser filtration,[14] allow examination of larger amounts of stool and may be useful in documenting light infections. If eggs cannot be found in a chronic symptomatic case, rectal biopsy snips should be taken, pressed between two slides and examined by light microscopy for eggs.[15] Colposcopic biopsy with histologic examination may also be useful in such instances.

In urinary schistosomiasis, concentration and quantification of eggs in urine samples may be accomplished by centrifugation or a variety of filtration techniques. Since *S. haematobium* eggs are shed into the urine following a circadian rhythm, samples should be obtained between 10 A.M. and 2 P.M. Large volumes (>3 liters) of urine may need to be examined to detect eggs in light infections. In epidemiological studies, hematuria is often used as an indirect indicator of *S. haematobium* infection; however, the diagnostic value of hematuria at the individual level is limited by large variations in the predictive value of the test between different populations.[16]

The detection of antibodies against schistosomes may be helpful in documenting recent infection in visitors to endemic areas; however, the inability of such tests to distinguish between past and current infection limits their utility in endemic areas. More recently, a variety of schistosome antigen detection tests have been developed, of which serum circulating anodic antigen (CAA) and urine circulating cathodic antigen (CCA) are the best characterized.[17] Since antigen titers become positive early in infection and are correlated with the intensity of infection, serum CAA and urine CCA may be useful in the diagnosis of acute schistosomiasis and in assessing cure after chemotherapy.

Although abdominal ultrasonography is sometimes helpful diagnostically, findings may be nonspecific early in infection. Consequently, it is most useful in assessing morbidity and monitoring the response to treatment in patients with chronic disease.[7]

Treatment

The three drugs currently used to treat schistosomiasis in humans are praziquantel, oxamniquine, and metrifonate.[18] Praziquantel, a heterocyclic pyrazinoisoquinoline, is the drug of choice for all species of schistosomes, with cure rates from 60 to 98 percent in most series.[19] In patients with hepatosplenic involvement, periportal fibrosis may actually resolve with treatment.[20] The drug is well tolerated, with only mild transient side effects, including abdominal discomfort, nausea, diarrhea, headache, dizziness, drowsiness and pruritus. Three doses of 20 mg/kg given at 4-hour intervals are recommended for treatment of *S. japonicum* infections.[18] In most cases, a single dose of 40 mg/kg is sufficient for treatment of infection with other schistosome species.[18] Resistance to praziquantel has been induced in laboratory strains of *S. mansoni*,[21] but until recently had not been reported in a clinical isolate. Reports of decreased cure rates with praziquantel in an epidemic focus in Senegal,[22] coupled with the isolation of a resistant strain from an individual in this population,[23] suggest that drug resistance may soon become a problem in the treatment of schistosomiasis.

Oxamniquine, a tetrahydroquinoline, is active only against *S. mansoni*.[18] For the strain of South American origin, a single dose of 15 mg/kg is adequate for adults, and two doses of 10 mg/kg once daily are recommended for children. For the strain of African origin, a total dose of 30 to 60 mg/kg given over 2 to 3 consecutive days is required, depending upon the specific geographical origin of the infection. Oxamniquine resistance has been reported in a small number of South American patients with refractory infection,[24] but does not appear to be a widespread phenomenon. Side effects of oxamniquine therapy include mild drowsiness, dizziness, headache, and rarely, seizures.

Metrifonate, an organophosphorus ester, is active only against *S. haematobium*.[18] Three doses of 7.5 to 10 mg/kg given at 2-week intervals are required. It is generally well tolerated, but must be used cautiously in patients receiving neuromuscular blocking agents or exposed to high levels of organophosphorus insecticides, because of the possibility of potentiating the cholinergic effects of the drug.

Control and Prevention

Control and prevention of schistosomiasis are among the most complex problems in public health. Success in control depends on having a well-organized program based on a profound understanding of the epidemiology of the disease, the biology, ecology, and distribution of the parasite intermediate snail-host, and the geographic characteristics of the environment. It is also important to have sound knowledge of local socioeconomic conditions, support from health authorities, and cooperation of the communities.

The elimination of schistosomiasis through interruption of transmission has been attempted for the last four decades. It has been successful in certain countries, such as Japan and large parts of China, but has proved to be beyond the resources of many endemic areas.[1] Furthermore, ecological changes, both natural (e.g., drought) and artificial (e.g., water resource development projects, relocation of populations for political reasons), have led to recent outbreaks in some regions.[25] Overall, there has been no change in the global estimate of the prevalence of schistosomiasis in the last 20 years. As a result, a new program of schistosomiasis control, targeted at reducing the morbidity and prevalence of the disease implemented through a primary health care unit, has been recommended by the World Health Organization. The particular combination of measures is determined by local conditions and available resources.

Snail Control

Molluscicides provide a rapid and effective means of reducing the snail population and decreasing disease transmission;[26,27] however, their application must take into account the focal and seasonal patterns of disease transmission. A suitable molluscicide must be safe and nontoxic to mammals and aquatic organisms, stable in storage, and simple to apply. Niclosamide, a synthetic amide that has been used since the 1960s, fulfills most of these criteria and remains the molluscicide of choice. The major limitations to its widespread use are cost (as much as $100/kg in some areas of the world) and the high incidence of drug-associated fish mortality.[27] Natural molluscicides of plant origin provide the theoretical advantage of decreased cost, local production, and low toxicity, but to date have not been as effective as niclosamide in field trials. Newer agents, including *Millettia thonningii*, a natural molluscicide from a West African legume, are being developed and appear promising.

Long-lasting effects in the reduction of snail populations can be achieved by environmental modifications, such as the installation of overhead sprinklers and trickle-type irrigation systems, modification of canal design, alteration of water level, or lining of canals with cement. Simple methods, including weed control and drainage of unused standing water, can also reduce snail populations. Biological snail control methods are still in the experimental stages, and none has reached large-scale field trials. Preliminary studies using fish, insect, and molluscan competitors have met with only limited success.[26]

Chemotherapy

Chemotherapy not only decreases the morbidity and prevalence of disease but also reduces transmission. Three basic strategies have been advocated: mass treatment, selective population-based therapy of infected individuals, and therapy targeted to subpopulations of infected individuals (e.g., those with high intensity infection). The most appropriate treatment strategy depends on the endemicity of infection and the available resources. For example, in a highly endemic area, the cost of screening individuals for infection may exceed the cost of providing therapy for all persons living in the endemic area. Regardless of the strategy, reinfection generally occurs, especially in children where up to 40 percent may be reinfected 1 year after treatment,[28] and even a small residual egg output can sustain disease transmission if the snail population is not controlled. Thus, a continuing schedule of screening and retreatment is required. The long-term side effects (if any) of repeated drug treatment and the potential effects on drug resistance also need to be considered.

Education

Health education is an integral part of any successful schistosomiasis control program and has been shown in several studies to have an effect on human behaviour and ultimately on disease transmission and prevalence.[29,30] It is much more likely that people will minimize contact with infested water, avoid polluting water sources, and cooperate with community control programs if they understand the basic mechanism of disease transmission. Furthermore, simple and inexpensive water disinfection procedures, such as boiling, filtering, or storing for 24 hours, after which contaminating cercariae become noninfective, can be instituted. Finally, people who must have contact with contaminated water can be taught personal protection measures, including the use of repellents, rubber boots, and other barrier methods (e.g., wrapping the feet with cloth or puttees smeared with powdered *Thea oleosa* fruits[31]), which may provide partial protection against infection.

Sanitation and Water Supply

Although expensive, the provision of safe water and adequate sanitation is crucial to the long-term control of schistosomiasis. In St. Lucia, the installation of individual household water systems was associated with a 75 percent decrease in the incidence of new *S. mansoni* infections in children.[30] In theory, installation of latrines may protect snail-bearing waters from contamination with infectious human wastes; however, this has been less effective than provision of a safe water supply in decreasing transmission. The reason for this is likely multifactorial and includes accessibility and social issues limiting the use of latrines in many communities. Finally, since water resource development programs may spread schistosomiasis to previously uninfected areas, such programs should be planned by multidisciplinary teams, including epidemiologists, ecologists, biologists, engineers, and public health officials.

Successful short-term control has been achieved with an integrated approach in some endemic areas.[30,32] However, once prevalence has been reduced to the targeted level, a maintenance program is necessary to sustain it. This was highlighted by a recent study of community-based control of schistosomiasis in the Philippines, in which a marked increase in the incidence of hepatosplenomegaly was seen with suspension of antischistosomal chemotherapy for as little as 2 years.[32] The cost of such long-term, multifaceted control programs is not insignificant and may be as high as US$3 per "protected subject" per year (as compared to the less than US$5 per capita total expenditure for health in sub-Saharan Africa).[30] Although integration of schistosomiasis control programs with other local health programs has been successful in decreasing costs and increasing efficacy in some countries,[1,30] additional inexpensive and effective alternatives (such as a vaccine) are clearly needed.

The immune response to schistosome infection is extremely complex. Nevertheless, epidemiological studies in schistosomiasis-endemic areas suggest that acquired resistance to reinfection occurs with age. Furthermore, although vaccination of experimental animals (including nonhuman primates) with live attenuated schistosomes provides only partial immunity to reinfection (70 to 90 percent reduction in worm burden),[33] such levels of immunity could have a significant effect on morbidity by reducing the prevalence of high-intensity infections and potentially reduce transmission. Since the use of a live vaccine would be unethical in humans, recent attention has focused on recombinant or synthetic peptides as potential vaccine candidates,[33] and on the use of novel delivery systems (e.g., Bacillus Calmette-Guérin (BCG)[34]) and adjuvants (e.g., interleukin-12 (IL-12)[35]) to enhance their immunogenicity. Although several antigens have been shown to confer partial protection in animal challenge studies, none has reached the stage of human trials. Consequently, it seems unlikely that a safe and effective vaccine against human schistosomiasis will be available for use in the near future.

Staphylococcal Toxic Shock Syndrome

Arthur L. Reingold

Staphylococcal toxic shock syndrome (TSS) is an acute multisystem illness due to infection with *Staphylococcus aureus*. Although TSS has occurred in association with a wide variety of different kinds of *S. aureus* infections, most reported cases have occurred in previously healthy young women who were menstruating and using tampons at the time of onset of illness. TSS has been categorized into menstrual and nonmenstrual cases for epidemiological purposes, but the clinical picture, microbiologic findings, and treatment are similar in these groups.

Clinical Findings

Symptoms of TSS include fever, chills, vomiting, myalgias, dizziness, and diarrhea. Typically, onset is abrupt. On physical examination, patients have fever, hypotension, and rash. The rash has been described as a diffuse, sunburnlike erythroderma of the face and trunk. Oropharyngeal erythema, conjunctival infection, vaginal hyperemia, and muscle tenderness are common findings, and vaginal ulceration and discharge may also be present. Desquamation usually occurs 1 to 3 weeks after the acute illness and can be generalized or localized to the face or palms and soles, particularly around nail beds. In nonmenstrual cases associated with *S. aureus* surgical wound infections, the wound frequently does not display local signs of infection such as redness, tenderness, or drainage. Laboratory findings in patients with TSS may include leukocytosis, lymphocytopenia, thrombocytopenia, abnormal liver and renal function tests, hypocalcemia, hypophosphatemia, sterile pyuria, and proteinuria. The case-fatality rate for TSS is in the range of 1 to 2 percent. When death occurs, it is usually due to respiratory failure or irreversible hypotension.

The diagnosis of TSS is based on clinical criteria because a sensitive and specific laboratory test is not available. According to the accepted case definition, the criteria for a definite case include high fever, a characteristic rash, evidence of hypotension, and subsequent desquamation of the rash.[1] In addition, there must be evidence of involvement of at least three organ systems. If tests for other illness such as Rocky Mountain spotted fever, leptospirosis, or rubeola are performed, the results must be negative. If group A streptococci are recovered from a clinical specimen or there is other laboratory evidence of streptococcal infection, streptococcal TSS should be considered. Because the criteria for inclusion as a case are strict, confusion of TSS with diseases that resemble it is unlikely. Patients whose illnesses meet the current case definition are usually severely ill and generally require hospitalization. It is clear that a much wider spectrum of clinical presentations of TSS exists, however, and that milder cases occur; their identification and characterization is difficult in the absence of a diagnostic laboratory test.

History

TSS is believed to be the same clinical entity as staphylococcal scarlet fever, cases of which have been reported in the medical literature since 1927.[2] Todd and associates introduced the name TSS in 1978 when they reported a series of seven children, age 8 to 17 years, with high fever, erythroderma, hypotension, and renal and hepatic abnormalities, associated with infection with phage group I *S. aureus*.[3] TSS rose from being a disease of relative obscurity to one of notoriety when, in late 1979 and early 1980, an increasing number of cases were reported and it was recognized that most of these cases were occurring in young menstruating women.

A number of epidemiological studies performed in 1980 and 1981 showed that the use of tampons was associated with an increased risk of developing menstrual TSS.[4-8] In addition, four studies showed that a particular brand of tampons, when compared with other tampons, was associated with the highest risk of developing tampon-associated menstrual TSS,[4-6,9] and one study showed that the risk of developing tampon-associated menstrual TSS was related to the absorbency and chemical composition of tampons.[6] As a result, in September 1980 the manufacturer of the tampon brand that was particularly implicated voluntarily withdrew this product from the market. Later studies suggested that the increased risk of menstrual TSS among tampon users persisted and was associated with higher absorbency tampons.[10,11] As a result, the manufacturers of other brands began altering the chemical composition and reducing the absorbency of the tampons they produced. The absorbency of currently available tampons is approximately half that of tampons sold from 1980 to 1981,[12] and all currently available tampons are made exclusively of cotton and/or rayon. Although cases of TSS continue to occur (Fig. 16-2), the number of cases reported annually has dropped substantially and it is uncertain whether the use of currently available tampons is associated with an increased risk of TSS. Evidence from studies employing active surveillance or case detection methods suggests that the incidence of hospitalization for TSS associated with menstruation has, in fact, dropped substantially since 1980,[12,13] although it is also likely that the completeness of case reporting has lessened since the early 1980s.

Epidemiology

Between 1979 and 1995, 3,397 cases of TSS meeting the strict criteria were reported to the Centers for Disease Control and Prevention (CDC) as having occurred in the United States. Overall, 76 percent were known to have been associated with menstruation. The percentage of reported cases not associated with menstruation has increased from 7 percent in 1980, to 19, 28, 36, 40, and 54 percent in 1981–1982, 1983–1984, 1985–1986, 1987–1989, and 1990–1995, respectively. Of the reported menstrual cases, 98 to 99 percent have occurred in tampon users, whereas only 60 to 70 percent of menstruating women in the United States use tampons. The incidence of menstrual TSS in 1980 was estimated to be approximately 5 to 10 cases per 100,000 menstruating women per year.[7] Studies from several areas in the United States suggested that the incidence of menstrual TSS in the late 1980s was in the range of 1 to 1½ cases per 100,000 menstruating women.[12,14] More recent reliable incidence data for TSS are not available. Patients with menstrual TSS have ranged from 11 to 60 years of age, but almost 60 percent have been between the ages of 15 and 24; 97 percent have been white.

Patients with TSS not associated with menstruation have ranged from younger than 1 to over 80 years of age. Although reported menstrual cases have been primarily in whites, the racial distribution of patients with nonmenstrual TSS more closely reflects the racial distribution of the U.S. population. Of the nonmenstrual cases, 35 percent have occurred in men and boys. When the postpartum and nonmenstrual vaginal cases are excluded, there is only a slight female predominance.

The large proportion of nonmenstrual cases, about one-third, have occurred in association with nonsurgical cutaneous and subcutaneous *S. aureus* infections, such as abscesses, furuncles, infected burns, and insect bites. In addition, TSS cases have occurred in postpartum women, associated with either vaginal infection, mastitis, or infection of cesarean-section site, and in postoperative patients, associated

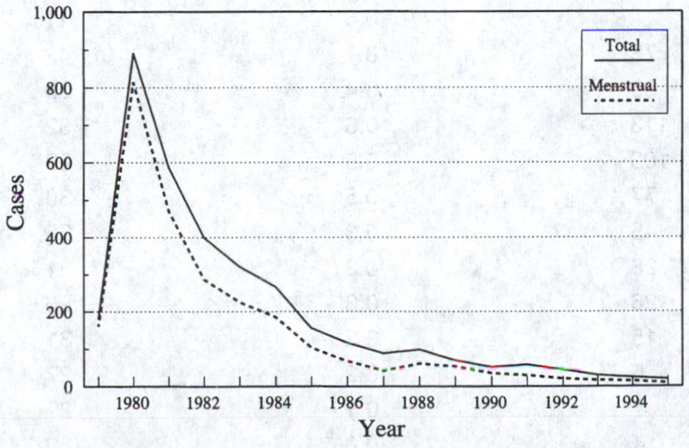

Figure 16-2. Reported cases of toxic-shock syndrome, by year, United States, 1979 to 1995.

with *S. aureus* surgical wound infections. Nonmenstrual TSS also has occurred in association with *S. aureus* infections at various body sites, and cases have been reported to develop coincident with or following diaphragm and contraceptive sponge use.

In the United States, cases have occurred in all states. While a disproportionate percentage of the cases reported in 1980 and 1981 were from a small number of states (Wisconsin, Minnesota, Utah, Colorado, and California), it is unknown to what extent this pattern reflected true geographic differences in incidence as opposed to increased surveillance activity in these states. However, studies employing active surveillance or review of hospital discharge records suggested that regional variation in the incidence of TSS at that time was not entirely due to differences in diagnosis and reporting of cases.[14,15] Cases outside the United States have occurred in Canada, Europe, Israel, South Africa, Australia, New Zealand, Japan, and elsewhere. While many of the cases reported from outside the United States also have occurred in young menstruating women who were using tampons, the association of TSS and tampons has been less prominent outside the United States.

Possible risk factors for menstrual TSS, other than factors related to tampon use, have been evaluated in several epidemiological studies. None of the other factors examined, including sexual activity, duration and quantity of menstrual flow, bathing or physical activity during menstruation, douching, or use of vaginal deodorants, were found to be associated with an increased risk of menstrual TSS. An early finding that use of oral contraceptives may decrease the risk of menstrual TSS was not substantiated in a later study.[11]

Bacteriology and Pathogenesis

Much research has been directed at characterizing TSS-associated *S. aureus* strains. Most *S. aureus* strains isolated from TSS patients are phage group I, with phage types 29 and 52 predominating.[16]

Because the clinical features of TSS, particularly the lack of bacteremia in most cases, suggested a toxin-mediated mechanism, attempts were made to identify one or more toxins responsible for TSS. It is now clear that toxic shock syndrome toxin-1 (TSST-1), an extracellular protein produced by *S. aureus*, can produce many, if not all, the signs and symptoms of TSS. Of the many *S. aureus* strains from women with menstrual TSS studied, 90 to 100 percent make TSST-1, compared with only 10 to 30 percent of non-TSS associated strains.[17] Purified TSST-1 has been shown to have a variety of biological properties, many mediated by interleukin-1. In vivo animal studies have shown that it can produce a TSS-like illness in rabbits.[18,19] However, only 60 to 70 percent of *S. aureus* strains recovered from normally sterile sites in patients with nonmenstrual TSS make TSST-1, strongly suggesting that one or more other staphylococcal products can produce a similar or identical clinical illness.[20] Staphylococcal enterotoxin B has been proposed as the responsible toxin in many of these cases.[21–23]

In addition to characteristics of *S. aureus* strains, host factors and interactions between tampons and *S. aureus* have been studied. There is evidence that patients with TSS lack preexisting antibody to TSST-1, suggesting that host susceptibility may be important. In menstrual TSS the role of the materials used in the manufacture of tampons has been investigated both in the laboratory and in epidemiological studies. The epidemiological studies suggest that the chemical composition of tampons has an effect on the risk of developing menstrual TSS that is independent of the tampon's absorbency.[10] At the same time, laboratory studies have produced conflicting results about the extent to which various tampons and their constituents affect the production of TSST-1 by *S. aureus* in vitro.[24–28]

Therapy and Prevention

Therapy for TSS should be directed at correcting hemodynamic, electrolyte, and acid-base abnormalities. Correction of hypovolemia with intravenous fluids and, when necessary, maintenance of blood pressure with vasopressors are the mainstays of treatment. Supportive measures for complications such as renal failure or adult respiratory distress syndrome are also required in some cases. Antimicrobial therapy directed against *S. aureus*, such as a β-lactamase-resistant penicillin, cephalosporin, or vancomycin, is recommended. Although there is no evidence that antimicrobial therapy shortens or ameliorates the acute illness, there is evidence that antimicrobial therapy prevents recurrences. High-dose corticosteroids and calcium replacement may be of benefit in severe cases of TSS, although data supporting their use are largely anecdotal.

Although an assay that measures antibody to TSST-1 has been developed, its use in screening individuals for susceptibility to TSS cannot be recommended. Similarly, routine vaginal cultures in healthy women are of no benefit in determining who is at risk of developing TSS. Women who have had menstrual TSS should be advised to discontinue tampon use. Women who have not had TSS can minimize their already small risk of developing menstrual TSS by not using tampons.

Reye's Syndrome

Robert B. Wallace

What is now known as Reye's syndrome was first described in Australia in 1963,[1,2] and shortly thereafter a series of similar cases was published in the United States.[3] It is unclear whether cases occurred in prior eras. The syndrome was characterized by an acute encephalopathic clinical picture and fatty liver in children, with major neurological and metabolic manifestations often leading to death.[4] Epidemiological, clinical, and metabolic studies have added considerable information on the nature of the condition, but it remains a syndrome that is likely comprised of diverse causes and pathogenetic mechanisms.

Case Definition and Surveillance

Rates of occurrence of Reye's syndrome depend in part on the skill in clinical case recognition, the rigor of surveillance, and case definition. Clearly some definitions and criteria are much more encompassing than others. The epidemiological case definition used by the U.S. Centers for Disease Control[5] includes

1. Acute noninflammatory encephalopathy with
   a. Microvascular fatty metamorphosis of the liver confirmed by biopsy or autopsy, or
   b. A serum alanine aminotransferase (ALT or SGPT), a serum ammonia greater than three times normal
2. If cerebrospinal fluid is obtained, leukocyte count must be ≤8/mm³.
3. In addition, there should be no other more reasonable explanations for the neurological or hepatic abnormalities.

Cases have been reported in the neonatal period and in adults, although most occur in infants and children. The syndrome has been clinically staged according to the level of consciousness and corresponding physical signs.[6]

Other definitions have been more specific,[7] but none will be wholly satisfactory until a "gold standard" for the diagnosis appears. Recent evidence suggests, for example, that at least some cases originally labeled as being the syndrome were associated with known inborn errors of metabolism.[7] Diagnosis rates may also vary according to the frequency of biopsy and autopsy, although the specificity of histopathological changes has been disputed. In fact, as more metabolic diseases are discovered that have a Reye's syndrome–like clinical picture, the clinical pattern of remaining cases may be changing over time.[8] Continuous surveillance of Reye's syndrome began in 1976 in the United States, and the incidence of the syndrome has clearly decreased since. There were as many as 555 cases reported in a single year. Table 16-1 shows the distribution of cases in a peak year—1980. However, in recent years the number of reported cases has been much

TABLE 16-1. PREDOMINANT INFLUENZA STRAINS, REPORTED CASES OF REYE'S SYNDROME [RS] AND VARICELLA-ASSOCIATED RS, RS INCIDENCE, AND RS FATALITY RATE, UNITED STATES, 1974 AND FROM 1977 TO 1988[a]

Year[a]	*Predominant Influenza Strains [Jan–May]*	*Total*	*Varicella-associated*	*Incidence of RS[b]*	*Case Fatality Rate [%]*
1974	B	379		0.6	41
1977	B	454	73	0.7	42
1978	A(H3N2)	236	69	0.4	29
1979	A(H1N1)	389	113	0.6	32
1980	B	555	103	0.9	23
1981	A(H3N2)	297	77	0.5	30
1982	B	213	45	0.3	35
1983	A(H3N2)	198	28	0.3	31
1984	A(H1N1)+B	204	26	0.3	26
1985	A(H3N2)	93	15	0.2	31
1986	B	101	5	0.2	27
1987	A(H1N1)	36	7	0.1	29
1988	A(H3N2)	20	4	0.0	30

[a]Continuous RS surveillance began in December 1976. Data for 1988 are provisional. RS reporting year begins December 1 of previous year.
[b]Per 100,000 U.S. population <18 years of age [U.S. Bureau of the Census data].

smaller. Despite this, the surveillance effort remains active, and reporting is encouraged.

There have also been differences in occurrence patterns among countries. For example, in Australia, occurrences are nonseasonal and children with Reye's syndrome have tended to be younger, generally less than 5 years of age. Cases in the United States occur predominantly in the fall and winter seasons, with a modal age distribution of 5 to 15 years. Further, the decline in the U.S. incidence rate for Reye's syndrome in the 1980s was initially more prominent in children under 10 years of age, although more recently all age groups have enjoyed some decrease. All of this suggests the possibility of age- and geography-related heterogeneity in the nature and causes of the syndrome.

Causes and Control of Reye's Syndrome

The causes of Reye's syndrome, including pathogenetic mechanisms, remain enigmatic. Sullivan-Bolyai and Corey have reviewed this area thoroughly.[9] Hypotheses include genetic predisposition, possibly related to selected inborn errors of metabolism; exposure to environmental toxins such as various chemicals, pesticides, and mycotoxins; and use of medications such as salicylates and antiemetics. Also, at least in the United States, most cases are preceded by an acute viral infection, usually beginning 7 to 10 days prior to syndrome onset. Instances of infection with many categories of viruses have been documented, but the two most prominent are varicella and influenza B. Table 16-1 shows that 5 to 30 percent of reported cases were varicella associated and explores the relation of case rates to the prevalent influenza strain.[6] The synergistic effect of a second or dual viral infection in causing the syndrome has been postulated. Other viruses have been the subject of speculation but have not been rigorously evaluated.

The 1980s were characterized by the epidemiological assessment as to whether salicylates, particularly aspirin, have a causal role in the syndrome. After some anecdotal reports and case series, several case-control studies were performed in the United States. Although some of these were criticized on methodological grounds, in aggregate they suggested that the syndrome was at least in part related to the use of aspirin as treatment for the febrile illness preceding or during syndrome onset.[10] No evidence was found for acetaminophen or other medications. In fact, the decline in Reye's syndrome incidence noted above has been related to public education and the subsequent decline in the use of aspirin for febrile conditions in children.[11] However, aspirin does not likely explain all cases of the syndrome, and other forces, yet unidentified, may be at work. In other countries such as Australia, aspirin was not related to the syndrome, particularly in children under 5 years of age,[12] and some of these cases are turning out to be other defined metabolic disorders. Several other chemical agents and drugs have been suggested to be related to the syndrome, but conclusive evidence is generally lacking.[13]

Summary

Reye's syndrome appears to be an important and at least partially preventable entity, even if not fully characterized or etiologically explained. However, modern biology continues to suggest pathogenetic mechanisms.[14] Continued surveillance is necessary to assess its public health impact, search for additional causes, and detect any important increases in incidence.

▶ REFERENCES

Dermatophytoses

1. Ajello L: Geographic distribution and prevalence of the dermatophytes. Ann N Y Acad Sci 89:30, 1960
2. Allen AM, et al: Griseofulvin in the prevention of experimental human dermatophytosis. Arch Dermatol 108:233–236, 1973
3. Elewski BE, Hay RJ: Update on the management of onychomycosis. Highlights of the Third International Summit on Cutaneous Antifungal Therapy. Clin Infect Dis 23:305–313, 1996
4. Elewski BE: Mechanisms of action of systemic antifungal agents. J Am Acad Dermatol 28 (5pt 1):328–534, 1993
5. English MP: The epidemiology of animal ringworm in man. Br J Dermatol 86(suppl 8):78, 1972
6. English MP, Gibson MD: Studies in the epidemiology of tinea pedis. I. Tinea pedis in school children. II. Dermatophytes on the floors of swimming-baths. Br Med J 1442–1448, 1959
7. Faergemann J, Zebender H, Millerioux L: Levels of terbinafine in plasma, stratus corneum, dermis-epidermis (without stratum corneum), sebum, hair and nails during and after 250 mg terbinafine orally once daily for 7 and 14 days. Clin Exp Dermatol 19:21–126, 1994
8. Georg L: Epidemiology of the dermatophytes. Sources of infection, modes of transmission and endemicity. Ann N Y Acad Sci 89, 1960
9. Grappel SF, Bishop CT, Blank F: Immunology of dermatophytes and dermatophytosis. Bacteriol Rev 38:222–250, June 1974
10. Gupta AK, Sauder DN, Shear NA: Antifungal agents: an overview (pt 2). J Am Acad Dermatol 30:911–933, 1994
11. Head ES, Henry JC, Macdonald EM: The cotton swab technique for the culture of dermatophyte infections—its efficacy and merit. J Am Acad Dermatol 11:797–801, 1984
12. Mitchell PC, Clayton YM: Some observations on fungal infections in tropical climates. Proc R Soc Med 55:559–561, 1962
13. Summerbell RC, Kane J, Krajden S: Onychomycosis, tinea pedis and tinea manuum caused by non-dermatophytic filamentous fungi. Mycoses. 32(8):609–619, 1989

Hookworm Disease: Ancyclostomiasis, Necatoriasis, Uncinariasis

1. Warren, KS: Selective primary health care and parasitic diseases. In McAdam KPWJ (ed): Frontiers of Infectious Diseases: New Strategies in Parasitology. Edinburgh: Churchill Livingstone, 1989, pp 217–231
2. Schad GA, Banwell JG: Hookworms. In Warren KS, Mahmoud AAF (eds): Tropical and Geographic Medicine. New York: McGraw-Hill, 1990, pp 379–393
3. Kappus KD, Lundgren RG, Juranek DD, Roberts JM, Spencer HC: Intestinal parasitism in the United States: update on a continuing problem. Am J Trop Med Hyg 50 (6):705–713, 1994
4. Crompton DWT, McKean PG, Schad GA: Hookworm disease: current status and new directions. Parasitol Today 5:1–2, 1989
5. Ju JS, Huang WI, Ryu TG, Oh SH: Protein absorption in intestinal parasite bearing adult man. Korean J Biochem 13(2):45–56, 1981
6. Prociv P, Croese J: Human eosinophilic enteritis caused by dog hookworm *Ancylostoma caninum*. Lancet (North American Edition) 335(8701):1299–1302, 1990
7. Croese J, Loukas A, Opdebeeck J, Prociv P: Occult enteric infection by *Ancylostoma caninum*: a previously unrecognized zoonosis. Gastroenterology 106(1):3–12, 1994
8. Croese J, Loukas A, Opdebeeck J, Fairley S, Prociv P: Human enteric infection with canine hookworms. Ann Intern Med 120(5): 369–374, 1994
9. Loukas A, Opdebeeck J, Croese J, Prociv P: Immunological incrimination of *Ancylostoma caninum* as a human enteric pathogen. Am J Trop Med Hyg 50(1):69–77, 1994
10. Chandler AC: Hookworm Disease: Its Distribution, Biology, Epidemiology, Pathology, Diagnosis, Treatment and Control. New York: Macmillan, 1929
11. Matsusaki G: Hookworm diseases and prevention. In Morishita K et al (eds): Progress of Medical Parasitology in Japan. Tokyo: Meguro Parasitological Museum 1966, vol 3, pp 187–282
12. Pritchard DL, McKean PG, Schad GA: An immunological and biochemical comparison of hookworm species. Parasitol Today 6:154–156, 1990
13. Hoagland KE, Schad GA: *Necator americanus* and *Ancylostoma duodenale* life history parameters and epidemiological implications of two sympatric hookworms of humans. Exp Parasitol 44:36–49, 1978

14. Beaver PC, Jung RC, Cupp EW: Clinical Parasitology. 9th ed. Baltimore: Lea & Febiger, 1984, p 270
15. Komiya Y, Yasuraoka K: The biology of hookworms. In Morishita K et al (eds): Progress of Medical Parasitology in Japan. Tokyo: Meguro Parasitological Museum 1966, vol 2, pp 5–114
16. Okamoto K: An experimental study of the migration route and development of *Ancylostoma duodenale* in pups after oral infection. J Kyoto Pref Med Univ 70:145–152, 1961
17. Yu SH, Jiang ZX, Xu LQ: Infantile hookworm disease in China: a review. Acta Trop 59(4):265–270, 1995
18. Wang MP, Yu YF, Peng JM, Wu DL, Yao SY: Persistent migration of *Ancylostoma duodenale* larvae in human infection. Chin Med J (Engl) 97(2):147–149, 1984
19. Soh CT: The distribution and persistence of hookworm larvae in the tissues of mice in relation to species and to routes of inoculation. J Parasitol 44:515–519, 1958
20. Harada Y: Wakana disease and hookworm allergy. Yonago Acta Med 6:109–118, 1962
21. Roche M, Layrisse M: The nature and causes of "hookworm anemia." Am J Trop Med Hyg 15(6)(part 2): 1966
22. Kalkofen UP: Intestinal trauma resulting from feeding activities of *Ancylostoma caninum.* Am J Trop Med Hyg 23:1046–1053, 1974
23. Carroll SM, Howse DJ, Grove DL: The anticoagulant effects of the hookworm, *Ancylostoma caninum.* Thromb Haemost 51:222–227, 1984
24. Cappello M, Vlasuk GP, Bergum PW, Huang S, Hotez PJ: *Ancylostoma caninum* anticoagulant peptide: a hookworm-derived inhibitor of human coagulation factor Xa. Proc Natl Acad Sci USA 92(13): 612–616, 1995
25. Moyle M, Foster DL, Magrath DE, Brown SM, Laroche Y, De Meutter J, Stanssens P, Bogowitz CA, Fried VA, Ely JA, Soule HR, Vlasuk GP: A hookworm glycoprotein that inhibits neutrophil function is a ligand of the integrin CD11b-CD18. J Biol Chem 269(13): 10008–10015, 1994
26. Rieu P, Ueda T, Haruta I, Sharma CP, Arnaout MA: The A-domain of beta-2 integrin CR3 (CD11b-CD18) is a receptor for the hookworm-derived neutrophil adhesion inhibitor NIF. J Cell Biol 127 (6 part 2):2081–2091, 1994
27. Nontasut P, Changbumrung S, Muennoo C, Hongthong K, Vudhivai N, Sanguankiat S, Yaemput S: Vitamin B_1, B_2 and B_6 deficiency in primary school children infected with hookworm. Southeast Asian J Trop Med Public Health 27(1):47–50, 1996
28. Variyam EP, Banwell JG: Nutrition implications of hookworm infection. Rev Infect Dis 4:830–835, 1982
29. Andy JJ: Helminthiasis the hyper eosinophilic syndrome and endomyocardial fibrosis: some observations and an hypothesis. Afr J Med Med Sci 12(3–4):155–164, 1983
30. Van Der Gaag R, Abdillahai H, Stilma JS, Vetter JCM: Circulating antibodies against corneal epithelium and hookworm in patients with Moorens ulcer from Sierra-Leone. Br J Ophthalmol 67(9):623–628, 1983
31. Ganguly NK, Mahajan RC, Sehgal R, Shetty P, Dilawari JB: Role of specific immunoglobulin E to excretory-secretory antigen in diagnosis and prognosis of hookworm infection. J Clin Microbiol 26(4): 739–742, 1988
32. Dipeolu OO: Laboratory investigations into the role of *Musca vicina* and *Musca domestica* in the transmission of parasitic helminth eggs and larvae. Int J Zoonoses 9(1):57–61, 1982
33. Sulaiman S, Sohadi AR, Yunus H, Iberahim R: The role of some Cyclorrhaphan flies as carriers of human helminths in Malaysia. Med Vet Entomol 2(1):1–6, 1988
34. Behnke JM: Do hookworms elicit protective immunity in man? Parasitol Today 3:200–206, 1987
35. Upatham ES, Viyanant V, Brockelman WY, Kurathong S, Ardsungnoen P, Chindaphol U: Predisposition to reinfection by intestinal helminths after chemotherapy in South Thailand. Int J Parasitol 22(6):801–806, 1992
36. Hominick WM, Dean CG, Shad GA: Population biology of hookworms in west Bengal: analysis of numbers of infective larvae recovered from damp pads applied to the soil surface at defaecation sites. Trans R Soc Trop Med Hyg 81:978–986, 1987
37. Kan S: Soil-transmitted helminthiases among inhabitants of an oilpalm plantation in West Malaysia. J Trop Med Hyg 92:263–269, 1989
38. Quinnell RJ, Slater AFG, Tighe P, Walsh EA, Keymer AE, Pritchard DI: Reinfection with hookworm after chemotherapy in Papua New Guinea. Parasitology 106(4):379–385, 1993

Other Intestinal Nematodes

Strongyloidiasis

Archibald LK, et al: Correspondence: albendazole is effective treatment for chronic strongyloidiasis. JAMA 270:2921, 1993
Braun TI, Fekete T, Lynch A: Strongyloidiasis in an institution for mentally retarded adults. Arch Intern Med 148:634–636, 1988
Gann PH, Neva FA, Gam AA: A randomized trial of single- and two-dose ivermectin versus thiabendazole for treatment of strongyloidiasis. J Infect Dis 169:1076–1079, 1994
Genta RM: Global prevalence of strongyloidiasis: critical review with epidemiologic insights into the prevention of disseminated disease. Rev Infect Dis 11:755–766, 1989
Lindo JF, Conway DJ, Atkins NS, Bianco AE, Robinson RD, Bundy DAP: Prospective evaluation of enzyme-linked immunosorbent assay and immunoblot methods for the diagnosis of endemic *Strongyloides stercoralis* infection. Am J Trop Med Hyg 51:175–179, 1994
Liu LX, Weller PF: Strongyloidiasis and other intestinal nematode infections. Infect Dis Clin North Am 7:655–682, 1993
Mahmoud AAF: Strongyloidiasis. Clin Infect Dis 23:949–953, 1996
Milder JE, Walzer PD, Kilgore G, Rutherford I, Klein M: Clinical features of *Strongyloides stercoralis* infection in an endemic area of the United States. Gastroenterology 80:1481–1488, 1981
Pelletier LL, Baker CB, Gam AA, Nutman TB, Neva FA: Diagnosis and evaluation of treatment of chronic strongyloidiasis in ex-prisoners of war. J Infect Dis 157:573–576, 1988
Woodring JH, Halfhill H, Berger R, Reed JC, Moser N: Clinical and imaging features of pulmonary strongyloidiasis. South Med J 89: 10–19, 1996

Ascariasis

Anonymous: Ascariasis: indiscriminate or selective mass chemotherapy? Lancet 339:1253, 1264, 1992
Villamizar E, Mendez M, Bonilla E, Varon H, de Onatra S: *Ascaris lumbricoides* infestation as a cause of intestinal obstruction in children: experience with 87 cases. J Pediatr Surg 31:201–205, 1996

Trichuriasis

Albonico M, Smith PG, Hall A, Chwaya HM, Alawi KS, Saviola L: A randomized controlled trial comparing mebendazole and albendazole against *Ascaris, Trichuris* and hookworm infections. Trans R Soc Trop Med Hyg 88:585–589, 1994
Cooper ES, Duff EMW, Howell S, Bundy DAP: 'Catch-up' growth velocities after treatment for *Trichuris* dysentery syndrome. Trans R Soc Trop Med Hyg 89:653, 1995
Pearson RD, Schwartzman JD: Nematodes limited to the intestinal tract. In Strickland GT (ed): Hunter's Tropical Medicine. 7th ed. Philadelphia: WB Saunders, 1991

Capillariasis

Cross JH: Intestinal capillariasis. Clin Micro Rev 5:120–129, 1992
Kang G, Mathan M, Ramakrishan BS, Mathai E, Sarada V: Human intestinal capillariasis: first report from India. Trans R Soc Trop Med Hyg 88:204, 1994

Enterobiasis

Cook GC: *Enterobius vermicularis* infection. Gut 35:1159–1162, 1994

Liu LX, Chi J, Upton MP, Ash LR: Eosinophilic colitis associated with larvae of the pinworm *Enterobius vermicularis*. Lancet 346: 410–412, 1995

Treatment

Drugs for parasitic infections. Med Lett 37:99–104, 1995

Schistosomiasis

1. Sturrock RF: The parasites and their life cycles. In: Human Schistosomiasis. Oxon: CAB International, 1993, pp 1–22
2. Arnon R: Life span of parasite in schistosomiasis patients [edit; comment]. Israel J Med Sci 26:404–405, 1990
3. Sturrock RF: The intermediate hosts and host-parasite relationship. In: Human Schistosomiasis. Oxon: CAB International, 1993, pp 33–85
4. Mao SP, Shao BR: Schistosomiasis control in the People's Republic of China. Am J Trop Med Hyg 31:92–99, 1982
5. Jordan P, Webbe G: Epidemiology. In: Human Schistosomiasis. Oxon: CAB International, 1993, pp 87–158
6. Hoeffler DF: Cercarial dermatitis: its etiology, epidemiology and clinical aspects. Arch Environ Health 29:225–229, 1974
7. Wiest PM: The epidemiology and morbidity of schistosomiasis. Parasitol Today 12:215–220, 1996
8. Rocha H, Kirk JW, Hearey CDJ: Prolonged *Salmonella* bacteremia in patients with *Schistosoma mansoni* infection. Arch Intern Med 128:254–257, 1971
9. Andrade ZA, Van Marck EAE: Schistosomal glomerular disease. A review. Mem Inst Oswaldo Cruz 79:499–506, 1984
10. Scrimgeour EM, Gadjusek DC: Involvement of the central nervous system in *Schistosoma mansoni* and *S. haematobium* infection: a review. Brain 108:1023–1038, 1985
11. Cohen J, Capildo R, Rose FC, et al.: Schistosomal myelopathy. Br Med J 1:1258, 1977
12. Actor JK, Shirai M, Kullberg MC, et al: Helminth infection results in decreased virus-specific CD8+ cytotoxic T-cell and Th1 cytokine responses as well as delayed virus clearance. Proc Natl Acad Sci USA 90:948–952, 1993
13. Chieffi PP: Interrelationship between schistosomiasis and concomitant disease [Review]. Mem Inst Oswaldo Cruz 87 (Suppl 4):291–296, 1992
14. Schutte CH, Pienaar R, Becker PJ, et al.: Observations on the techniques used in the qualitative and quantitative diagnosis of schistosomiasis. Ann Trop Med Parasitol 88:305–316, 1994
15. Rabello AL: Parasitological diagnosis of *Schistosoma mansoni*; fecal examination and rectal biopsy. Mem Inst Oswaldo Cruz 87 (Suppl 4):325–331, 1992
16. Mott KE, Dixon H, Osei-Tutu E, et al: Evaluation of reagent strips in urine tests for detection of *Schistosoma haematobium* infection: a comparative study in Zambia and Ghana. Bull WHO 63:125–133, 1985
17. De Jonge N, Rabello ALT, Krijger FW, et al: Levels of the schistosome circulating anodic and cathodic antigens in serum of schistosomiasis patients from Brazil. Trans R Soc Trop Med Hyg 85: 756–759, 1991
18. Drugs for parasitic infections. Med Lett Drugs Ther 37:99–108, 1995
19. Pearson RP, Guerrant RC: Praziquantel: a major advance in anti-helminthic therapy. Ann Intern Med 99:195–198, 1983
20. Homeida MA, el Tom I, Nash T, et al: Association of the therapeutic activity of praziquantel with the reversal of Symmers' fibrosis induced by *Schistosoma mansoni*. Am J Trop Med Hyg 45:360–365, 1991
21. Fallon PG, Doenhoff MJ: Drug-resistant schistosomiasis: resistance to praziquantel and oxamniquine induced in *Schistosoma mansoni* in mice is drug specific. Am J Trop Med Hyg 51:83–88, 1994
22. Stelma FF, Talla I, Sow S, et al: Efficacy and side effects of praziquantel in an epidemic focus of *Schistosoma mansoni*. Am J Trop Med Hyg 53:167–170, 1995
23. Fallon PG, Sturrock RF, Capron A, et al: Short report: diminished susceptibility to praziquantel in a Senegal isolate of *Schistosoma mansoni*. Am J Trop Med Hyg 53:61–62, 1995
24. Cioli D, Pica-Mattoccia L, Archer S: Drug resistance in schistosomes. Parasitol Today 9:162–166, 1993
25. Talla I, Kongs A, Verle P, et al: Outbreak of intestinal schistosomiasis in the Senegal river basin. Ann Soc Belg Med Trop 70:173–180, 1990
26. Sturrock RF: Current concepts of snail control. Mem Inst Oswaldo Cruz 90:241–243, 1995
27. Perrett S, Whitfield PJ: Currently available molluscicides. Parasitol Today 12:156–159, 1996
28. Polderman AM, Manshande JP: Failure of targeted mass treatment to control schistosomiasis. Lancet i:217–218, 1981
29. Bausch D, Cline BL: The impact of control measures on urinary schistosomiasis in primary school children in northern Cameroon: a unique opportunity for controlled observations. Am J Trop Med Hyg 53:577–580, 1995
30. Webbe G, Jordan P: Control. In: Human schistosomiasis. Oxon: CAB International, 1993, pp 405–451
31. Hsu HF, Hsu SYL: Schistosomiasis in the Shanghai area. In: China Medicine As We Saw It. Bethesda, MD: National Institutes of Health, 1974, pp 345–363
32. Olveda RM, Daniel BL, Ramirez BDL, et al: *Schistosomiasis japonica* in the Philippines: the long-term impact of population-based chemotherapy on infection, transmission and morbidity. J Infect Dis 174:163–172, 1996
33. Dunne DW, Hagan P, Abath FGC: Prospects for immunological control of schistosomiasis. Lancet 345:1488–1492, 1995
34. Kremer L, Riveau G, Baulard A, et al: Neutralizing antibody responses elicited in mice immunized with recombinant Bacille Calmette-Guérin producing the *Schistosoma mansoni* glutathione-*S*-transferase. J Immunol 156:4309–4317, 1996
35. Wynn TA, Reynolds A, James S, et al: IL-12 enhances vaccine-induced immunity to schistosomes by augmenting both humoral and cell-mediated immune responses against the parasite. J Immunol 157:4068–4078, 1996

Staphylococcal Toxic Shock Syndrome

1. Reingold AI, et al: Toxic shock syndrome surveillance in the United States, 1980 to 1981. Ann Intern Med 967:875–880, 1982
2. Stevens FR: The occurrence of *Staphylococcus aureus* infection with a scarlatiniform rash. JAMA 88:1957–1958, 1927
3. Todd J, Fishaut M, Kapral F, Welch T: Toxic-shock syndrome associated with phage group I staphylococci. Lancet 2:1116–1118, 1978
4. Schlech WF, Shands KN, Reingold AL, et al: Risk factors for the development of toxic-shock syndrome: association with a tampon brand. JAMA 248:834–839, 1982
5. Kehrberg MW, Latham RH, Haslam BT, et al: Risk factors for staphylococcal toxic-shock syndrome. Am J Epidemiol 114:873–879, 1981
6. Osterholm MT, Davis JP, Gibson RW, et al: Tri-state toxic-shock syndrome study: I. Epidemiologic findings. J Infect Dis 145:431–440, 1982
7. Davis JP, Chesney PJ, Wand PJ, LaVenture M, the Investigation and Laboratory Team: Toxic-shock syndrome: epidemiologic features, recurrence, risk factors, and prevention. N Engl J Med 303:1429–1435, 1980
8. Shands KN, Schmid GP, Dan BB, et al: Toxic-shock syndrome in menstruating women: its association with tampon use and *Staphylococcus aureus* and the clinical features in 52 cases. N Engl J Med 303:1436–1442, 1980
9. Helgerson SD, Foster LR: Toxic shock syndrome in Oregon: epidemiologic findings. Ann Intern Med 96:909–911, 1982

10. Berkley SF et al: The relationship of tampon characteristics to menstrual toxic shock syndrome. JAMA 258:917–920, 1987
11. Reingold AL et al: Risk factors for menstrual toxic shock syndrome: results of a multistate case-control study. Rev Infect Dis 11:S35–S42, 1989
12. Petitti DB et al: Update through 1985 on the incidence of toxic shock syndrome among members of a prepaid health plan. Rev Infect Dis 11:S22–S27, 1989
13. Todd JK et al: Toxic shock syndrome. II. Estimated occurrence in Colorado as influenced by case ascertainment methods. Am J Epidemiol 122:857–867, 1985
14. Gaventa S et al: Active surveillance for toxic shock syndrome in the United States, 1986. Rev Infect Dis 11:S28–S35, 1989
15. Markowitz LE et al: Toxic shock syndrome: evaluation of national surveillance data using a hospital discharge survey. JAMA 258:75–78, 1987
16. Altemeier WA et al: *Staphylococcus aureus* associated with the toxic-shock syndrome: phage typing and toxin capability testing. Ann Intern Med 96(part 2):978–982, 1982
17. Schlievert PM et al: Identification and characterization of an exotoxin from *Staphylococcus aureus* associated with toxic-shock syndrome. J Infect Dis 143:509–516, 1981
18. Parsonnet J: Mediators in the pathogenesis of toxic shock syndrome: overview. Rev Infect Dis 11:S263–S269, 1989
19. Melish ME et al: Endotoxin is not an essential mediator in toxic shock syndrome. Rev Infect Dis 11:S219–S230, 1989
20. Garbe PL et al: *Staphylococcus aureus* isolated from patients with nonmenstrual toxic shock syndrome: evidence for additional toxins. JAMA 253:2538–2542, 1985
21. Schlievert PM: Staphylococcal enterotoxin B and toxic shock syndrome toxin-1 are significantly associated with non-menstrual TSS. Lancet 1:1149–1150, 1986
22. Lee VTP, Chang AH, Chow AW: Detection of staphylococcal enterotoxin B among toxic shock syndrome (TSS)—non-TSS-associated *Staphylococcus aureus* isolates. J Infec Dis 166:911–915, 1992
23. Marples RR, Wieneke AA: Enterotoxins and toxic-shock syndrome toxin-1 in non-enteric staphylococcal disease. Epidemiol Infect 110:477–488, 1993
24. Lee AC et al: Investigation by syringe method of effect of tampons on production in vitro of toxic shock syndrome toxin-1 by *Staphylococcus aureus*. J Clin Microbiol 25:87–90, 1987
25. Schlievert PM, Deringer JR, Kim MH, Projan SJ, Novick RP: Effect of glycerol monolaurate on bacterial growth and toxin production. Antimicrob Agents Chemother 36:626–631, 1992
26. Projan SJ, Brown-Skrobot S, Schlievert PM, Vandenesch F, Novick RP: Glycerol monolaurate inhibits the production of β-lactamase, toxic shock syndrome toxin-1, and other staphylococcal exoproteins by interfering with signal transduction. J Bacteriol 176:4204–4209, 1994
27. Schlievert PM: Comparison of cotton and cotton/rayon tampons for effect on production of toxic shock syndrome toxin. J Infec Dis 172:1112–1114, 1995
28. Parsonnet J, Modern PA, Giacobbe KD: Effect of tampon composition on production of toxic shock syndrome toxin-1 by *Staphylococcus aureus* in vitro. J Infec Dis 173:98–103, 1996

Reye's Syndrome

1. Anderson RMcD: Encephalitis in childhood: pathologic aspects. Med J Aust 1:573–575, 1963
2. Reye RDK, Morgan G, Baral J: Encephalopathy and fatty degeneration of the viscera: a disease entity in childhood. Lancet 2:749–752, 1963
3. Johnson GM, Scurletis TD, Carroll NB: A study of sixteen fatal cases of encephalitis-like disease in North Carolina children. N C Med J 24:463–473, 1963
4. Glasgow JFT, Moore R: Current concepts in Reye's syndrome. Br J Hosp Med 50:599–604, 1993
5. Centers for Disease Control: Follow-up on Reye syndrome—United States, 1987 and 1988. MMWR 29:321–322, 1980
6. Centers for Disease Control: Reye syndrome surveillance—United States, 1987 and 1988. MMWR 38:325–327, 1989
7. Gauthier M, Guay J, LaCroix J, Lortie A: Reye's syndrome. A reappraisal of diagnosis in 49 presumptive cases. Am J Dis Child 143:1181–1185, 1989
8. Hardie RM, Newton LH, Bruce JC, Glasgow JFT, Mowat AP, Stephenson JBP, Hall SM: The changing clinical pattern of Reye's syndrome. 1982–1990
9. Sullivan-Bolyai JZ, Corey L: Epidemiology of Reye syndrome. Epidemiol Rev 3:1–26, 1981
10. Hurwitz ES: Reye's syndrome. Epidemiol Rev 11:249–253, 1989
11. Arrowsmith JB, Kennedy DL, Kuritsky JN, Faich GA: National patterns of aspirin use and Reye syndrome reporting, United States, 1980 to 1985. Pediatrics 79:858–863, 1987
12. Orlowski JP, Campbell P, Goldstein S: Reye's syndrome: a case control study of medication use and associated viruses in Australia. Cleve Clin J Med 57:323–329, 1990
13. Visentin M, Salmona M, Tacconi MT: Reye's and Reye-like syndromes, drug-related diseases? (causative agents, etiology, pathogenesis, and therapeutic approaches. Drug Metab Rev 27:517–539, 1995
14. Trost LC, Lemasters JJ: The mitochondrial permiability transition: a new pathophysiologic mechanism for Reye's syndrome and toxic liver injury. J Pharmacol Exp Ther 278:1000–1005, 1996.

III

Environmental Health

Edited by Arnold J. Schecter

17

The Status of Environmental Health

Arthur L. Frank

Environmental health concerns continue to be central to the modern practice of public health. Workplace and ambient exposures in air, water, and soil continue to meld, and individuals, communities, and even the "whole earth" now claim our attention. Traditional clinical, epidemiologic, and preventive activities all have a role in helping us understand and reduce environmentally induced problems.

One major focus for environmental health is the occupational setting where clinical activities include pre-employment examinations, injury evaluation, and screening for disease. Screening may be specifically related to workplace exposures to chemicals, noise, or other potentially hazardous agents or may be used for general population screening examinations such as for hypertension and diabetes. Workplaces often prove a suitable setting for intervention programs for stress and weight reduction, smoking cessation, and similar programs.

This section of the book reflects both traditional as well as newer concerns in the area of environmental and occupational health. A review of similar sections of prior editions highlights how much more significant is the role of environmental health among the overall array of topics relevant to public health. This section has grown over time and now represents a major portion of this book. Reviewed in this section are basic toxicological principles, the hazards of exposure to chemical and physical agents, and global issues concerning water, waste, and food. There is material on regulatory issues, problems of special groups, preventive strategies, and generic issues such as global warming.

While changes have occurred and some issues are better understood since the previous edition, some matters continue to be problematic. The response within the legal community has altered some of the ways in which litigation can be carried out relevant to environmental and occupational issues. Amounts and types of recovery are being limited in some settings. The growing body of evidence within the legal community, joining long-standing medical concerns of the hazards of smoking, may well have repercussions regarding workplace and environmental exposure issues. Congressional actions in the United States have attempted to prevent the collection of some necessary research data to plan appropriate response and intervention strategies in such areas as ergonomics—demonstrating how lawmakers' personal pique may interfere with societal needs.

Unchanged is the continuing significant shortage of appropriately trained professional personnel needed to work in occupational medicine settings, industrial hygiene, and similar occupations. Medical students and primary care physicians continue to receive too little training on occupational and environmental health topics. With some exceptions, funding support for such training, both for specialists and the education of others, remains weak. Worker education has not expanded significantly. The pace at which new programs have been created has slowed.

One new funded governmental initiative in recent years has been the creation and support for eight National Institute for Occupational Safety and Health agricultural safety and health centers strategically placed to cover all of the United States. In America less than 2 percent of the total population now work in agriculture, feeding much of the United States as well as other parts of the world. This small percentage of workers in agriculture is characteristic of industrialized countries; over 70 percent of the world's working population remains in agricultural pursuits. Regrettably, much of the research about agricultural safety and health addresses problems common in the mechanized and chemically dependent agriculture of the industrialized countries and may have little generalizability to the majority of agricultural workers in developing economies. Migrant and seasonal farm worker issues are also receiving increased attention.

This disparity between developed and developing countries highlights another significant shift in issues of worker safety and environmental health. Increasingly, potentially hazardous exposures are being reduced or eliminated in some countries, with the subsequent transfer of hazard, along with the transfer of jobs and technology, to developing nations. This pattern of shift, once seen in the United States between states when there were few federal regulations, is now being seen between nations. Tobacco profits now come predominantly from cigarette sales outside of the United States, and chemicals, such as dibromochloropropane, an agent causing male sterility in humans, is banned for use in the United States but can still be manufactured for export and use elsewhere, often resulting in unwitting "reimportation" after it has been used on agricultural products. Such globalization of environmental health hazards is a disturbing trend.

For medical professionals the continuing key to dealing with environmental health issues is obtaining an appropriate exposure history. Routine medical records are a notoriously poor source of exposure data, either for individual assessment of patients or for epidemiologic studies. Increasingly one reads of studies that use surrogates such as spouses or coworkers for exposure assessment, but these studies appear more to highlight their inadequacy than demonstrate their usefulness for research purposes. Table 17-1 provides a useful format for obtaining the essential features of an environmental and occupational exposure history. While not suitable for all settings, it is adequate for most, and when the information obtained is coupled with appropriate resources of information regarding hazardous exposures, such as this volume provides, one can be better prepared to deal with these issues.

TABLE 17-1. ENVIRONMENTAL AND OCCUPATIONAL EXPOSURE HISTORY

Current work: ______

How long at this job? ______

Description of work: ______

______

Any contact with dust, fumes, chemicals, radiation, noise, etc.?

______ Yes ______ No If yes, describe: ______

______

Describe any adverse effects noted: ______

Are any fellow workers ill? ______ Yes ______ No

If yes, describe: ______

Do you use any protective equipment at work?

______ Yes ______ No

Previous job history	*From*	*To*	*Exposures*
First regular job	______	______	______
Next job	______	______	______
Next job	______	______	______
Vacation or temporary job	______	______	______
Vacation or temporary job	______	______	______

Military service or related exposures: ______

______

Have you lived near an industrial facility or has a family member worked in a setting where hazardous materials have been brought home? ______ Yes ______ No

If yes, describe: ______

Hobby history: ______

Smoking history: ______

Alcohol and drug use history: ______

Comments: ______

The traditional differences between occupational and environmental exposure are continuing to diminish. This is reflected in many ways. Research initiatives that have traditionally focused on workers, such as pesticide exposures, are now being addressed as to the possible role of such substances in the development of breast cancer in women. Complex exposures related to wartime activities have been receiving special attention and involve chemicals including nerve gas weapons, vaccines, and potential antidotes. Even professional organizations and journal titles are reflecting this change with the addition of "environmental" to many long-standing names. The material in this section of the book should be looked upon as a resource for all who may be exposed, no matter under what circumstances.

18

Toxicology

Principles of Toxicology

Michael Gochfeld

Toxicology is the study of the harmful effects of chemicals, including drugs, on living organisms. Many books (see General References), and particularly *Toxicologic Profiles* published by the Agency for Toxic Substances and Disease Research, cover in detail the toxicology of individual substances. This chapter focuses on generic and conceptual issues relating to properties of toxic substances in general, how they enter and move through the body, and the kinds of pathophysiologic effects that they exert on various targets within the body that ultimately lead to the health effects.

Historians[1] trace the history of toxicology back to Paracelsus (1493–1541), who recognized that a substance that was physiologically ineffective at very low dose might be toxic at high dose and therapeutic at intermediate dose. Gallo[2] identified human use of natural venoms in antiquity with a number described in the famed "Ebers Papyrus" (ca 1500 B.C.). Modern toxicology developed under the combined impetus of a quest for therapeutic agents and concern over adulterated foods. In 1906 the United States enacted the Food and Drug Act, perhaps stimulated more by writings such as Upton Sinclair's *The Jungle*[3] than by toxicologists.[2]

Toxic chemicals (*a*) enter and move through the environment (air, water, soil, food) at various concentrations until they (*b*) come into contact with a target individual; (*c*) are taken up by inhalation, ingestion, or though the skin (exposure); (*d*) are absorbed into the bloodstream (uptake) reaching a certain concentration (dose); (*e*) undergo complex toxicokinetics involving metabolism, conjugation, excretion, storage, as well as (*f*) delivery to target organs (internal dose), where (*g*) they affect some molecular, biochemical, cellular, or physiologic target to produce their adverse effect.

Internal distribution and the dose reaching a target organ, tissue, or cell are constantly modified by binding to carrier molecules, metabolic activation (or inactivation), storage in various tissues (e.g., fat), and by excretion.[4] The relationship among these processes are demonstrated in Figure 18-1. This chapter covers the classification of toxic chemicals, the manner in which exposure occurs and how it can be measured, the absorption and distribution of chemicals within the body, and finally the kinds of toxic effects that are produced.

▸ BRANCHES OF TOXICOLOGY

Toxicology is a broad discipline embracing such traditionally medical areas as pathology, pharmacology and clinical toxicology on the one hand, and molecular biology and biochemistry on the other. Historically toxicology was linked with pharmacology and focused on the toxic effects of pharmaceuticals. Industrial toxicology emerged to investigate the toxic effects of raw materials, intermediates, products, and wastes produced by commerce. Toxicology has subdisciplines linked to behavior, nutrition, biochemistry, and genetics (including the Human Genome Project), which have opened new research horizons.

Toxicology is concerned with both lethal and sublethal effects. A decade ago molecular toxicology was a new frontier with an emphasis on the discovery of biomarkers.[2,5] Increasingly toxicologists have focused on the cellular, biochemical, and molecular interactions and changes wrought by foreign chemicals, thereby elucidating their mechanisms of action. Toxicological data is a major basis for environmental risk assessments, which in turn are increasingly used by regulatory agencies to assess chemical hazards, prioritize hazardous waste site cleanups, establish governmental policies, and set levels of allowable exposure. Such risk assessments produce quantitative or qualitative estimates of the magnitude of the risk of some adverse endpoint associated with a particular dose or exposure of a target population to a particular chemical, physical, or biological agent.

▸ TYPES OF STRESSORS

The stressors that potentially harm the body can be broadly classified as physical (noise, temperature, radiation), biological (infectious, immunologic), chemical, and psychosocial. Toxicologists focus mainly on chemicals, both synthetic and those of natural biologic origin, and on physical agents such as radiation. There are interactions among classes of stressors. Thus radiation, infection, or psychologic stress may modify the effects of toxic chemicals, and vice versa, and there is increasing attention to the effects of two or more chemicals administered together where synergistic or antagonistic effects may occur (see below).

The following definitions are important. *Toxicity* is the intrinsic ability of a substance to harm living things. A *xenobiotic* is any substance foreign to the body, including all synthetic chemicals as well as many natural substances. *Susceptibility* refers to the ability of a living thing to be harmed by an agent. It is influenced by genotype, by age and gender, and by environmental factors such as nutrition, prior exposure, and underlying state of health (for example, immune status). *Bioavailability* is the ability of a substance that enters the body to be liberated from its environmental matrix (air, water, soil, food) and to enter the circulation. *Biotransformation*, or *intermediary me-*

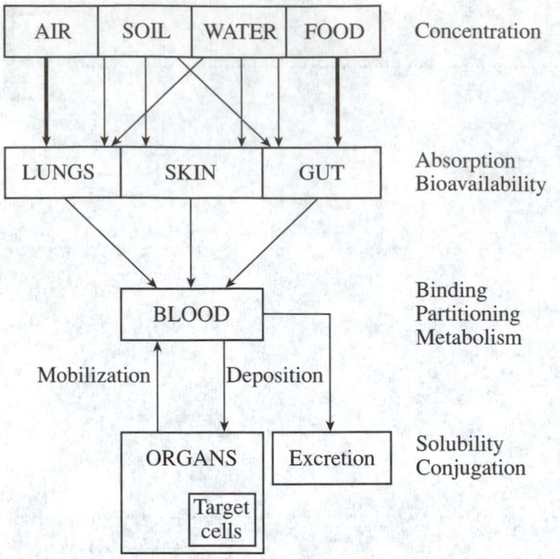

Figure 18-1. A multicompartment model of toxicant distribution.

tabolism, are the biochemical change(s) a chemical undergoes once it reaches the cells of the body. This may lessen its toxicity (*detoxification*) or enhance it (*activation*) and may facilitate excretion. *Mechanism* refers to the way in which the toxic substance acts on a cellular or subcellular level to disrupt the living organism. Some toxic agents are metabolic poisons, others disrupt cell membranes, interfere with chemical reactions, or bind to nucleic acids. *Threshold* is the lowest dose of a chemical that has a detectable effect.

► CLASSIFICATION OR TAXONOMY OF TOXIC AGENTS

One can organize knowledge in toxicology in terms of chemical agents or types of effect. Chemicals can be classified based on their structure, source, economic role, mechanism of action, or on their target organ. The lists below are not intended to be exhaustive.

Classification by Structure

Organic Chemicals	**Inorganic Chemicals**
Aromatics (e.g., phenols, benzene derivatives)	Acids and bases
Aliphatics (e.g., ethanes, ethenes)	Anions and cations
Polyaromatic hydrocarbons (PAHs)	Heavy metals
Chlorinated polyaromatics (e.g., dioxins, furans, polychlorinated biphenyls (PCBs))	Metalloids (e.g., selenium)
Chlorinated hydrocarbons (chlorinated alkanes and alkenes)	Salts
Amines	
Nitriles	
Ethers, ketones, aldehydes, alcohols	

Classification by Source

Many plants and animals secrete chemicals designed to keep them from being eaten. Butterflies, such as the monarch, may incorporate plant alkaloids in their own tissues, rendering themselves inedible. Beetles may squirt cyanide compounds to deter predators. Plants that have been partially eaten by herbivores may load increased levels of distasteful alkaloid compounds in newly regenerated leaves. Similarly, many fungi may secrete chemicals that inhibit bacterial growth. A wide variety of these naturally occurring bioactive substances or "toxins" have been adapted into some of our most familiar pharmaceuticals, for example antibiotics.

Natural or Biologic Compounds "Toxins"	**Synthetics**
Plant	Industrial reagent, by-product or product
Bacterial	Pharmaceutical
Invertebrate	
Vertebrate	

Environmental toxicology and risk assessment have focused mainly on synthetic chemicals, yet natural toxic compounds, called toxins or venoms, are widespread and include some of the most toxic agents known. Invertebrate toxins occasionally cause epidemic outbreaks of food-borne disease and have proven valuable research tools because of their highly specific modes of action. Many have very complex structures, for example, the chain of 13 heterocyclic 5- to 7-membered rings that make up the backbone of ciguatoxin. These plant and animal toxins have evolved specifically to damage either predators or prey. A review of their toxicology is beyond the scope of this chapter.[6]

Classification by Use

Very often in clinical toxicology, the first thing one learns about a chemical exposure is the type of compound. Thus a would-be suicide may be brought in with "an overdose of sleeping pills," or a worker may have been overcome while "using a solvent," or a homeowner may report "some pesticide spray" making them ill. Examples of common use classes of materials that may have toxic effects include:

Solvents	Pharmaceutical agents
Paints, dyes, coatings	Detergents, cleansers
Pesticides	Acids, bases

Pharmaceuticals and Abused Substances. These are grouped together because of the tendency for very high concentrations of bioactive agents to be deliberately introduced into the body. In fact, many abused substances that were originally developed as pharmaceuticals (e.g., amphetamines, barbiturates, and narcotics) have profound toxic effects, quite apart from their addictive properties. By whatever route, and whether legal or illicit, these chemicals are used because of their high level of bioactivity. Even when the dosage used is in the therapeutic range, there may be undesired side effects, which are manifestations of toxicity. These may occur in most users (e.g., soporific effects of diphenhydramine) or rarely (anaphylaxis from penicillin). Certainly the most widespread toxic exposures involve the chronic inhalation of tobacco smoke by the smoker and the chronic consumption of ethanol.

Classification by Mechanism of Action

Much exciting research in modern toxicology focuses on the mechanism by which a bioactive substance interacts with and alters its targets to produce its unwanted effects, for example:

Enzyme inhibition	Formation of free radicals/ active oxygen
Enzyme induction	Redox reactions
Metabolic poisons	Interference with signal transduction
Macromolecular binding (e.g., DNA, protein)	Interference with hormone activity
Cell membrane disruption including lipid peroxidation	Sensitizers
Competitive binding of active sites or receptors	Irritants

Classification by Target Organ

Toxins can act on any organ system in the body. The effects on these target organs are discussed in other chapters in this section. Standard textbooks of toxicology[7] are organized by organ system, and several of the general readings deal with organ systems. The next chapter deals specifically with neurobehavioral toxicology.

Neurotoxin	Pulmonary toxin	Genotoxin (including mutagens)
Hematotoxin	Metabolic toxin	Carcinogen (including initiators and promoters)
Nephrotoxin	Endocrine toxin	Teratogens
Hepatotoxin	Dermatotoxin	
Cardiotoxin	Reproductive toxin	

The liver is of particular importance since many substances, particularly ingested xenobiotics, are transported directly to the liver, where they undergo metabolism, which may either detoxify or activate them. The liver may conjugate substances to facilitate their excretion in the urine or may secrete some substances into the bile. Liver cells are particularly vulnerable to toxins, and toxic hepatitis, manifest often by abnormalities in liver function tests, is a common occurrence.

▶ CHEMICAL STRUCTURE AND TOXICOLOGY

Several chemical principles play important roles in toxicology. They influence how the chemical behaves in its environmental matrix, how it is absorbed into, metabolized by, distributed through, and excreted from the body and how it exerts its toxic effect.

Chemical Species

Although a rose may be a rose, a chemical may not always be what it appears to be. Thus toxicologists have demonstrated that slight modifications in a chemical may drastically alter its effect.[8] This is particularly true for the effects of certain metals, which, when in an organic complex, may have drastically different and more serious effects than their elemental or ionic form, for example, methyl mercury and orgonotin tin compared to inorganic mercury or tin compounds. The organic species have been incorporated in biocides such as fungicidal seed dressing and in marine paints to thwart the growth of barnacles. However, human exposure occurs through the food chain. Both methyl mercury and alkyltin compounds are potent neurotoxins.[9,10] Conversely organic arsenicals are generally less toxic to humans than inorganic arsenic compounds.

A chemical variant of a metal is called a "species." This may also refer to valence state; thus trivalent and hexavalent chromium are species of chromium,[11] and because CrIII is an essential nutrient while CrVI is a potent lung carcinogen,[12] the difficulty in reliably analyzing the concentrations of CrIII and CrVI in an environmental sample impedes our ability to protect potentially exposed people.

Isomers and Congeners

Two chemical compounds that have the same chemical formula but differ in structure are called *isomers*. Thus butane, a four-carbon chain can appear as either normal (linear) butane or branched isobutane. *Congeners* have the same basic structure, but different numbers of atoms. For instance, dichlorophenol and trichlorophenol would be congeners while 2,4-dichlorophenol and 2,5-dichlorophenol would be isomers. The behavior in the body and the toxicity may vary greatly among isomers and congeners. Thus different chlorinated dibenzodioxins vary by orders of magnitude in their toxicity.[13] Each compound can be assigned a toxicity potency (toxic equivalency factor) relative to 2,3,7,8-tetrachlorodibenzo-*p*-dioxin (TCDD).

Structure Activity Relationships

The converse of the variation in toxicity between isomers and congeners is that chemicals that are structurally similar may have similar types of toxic effects on the body, although the effects may be modulated in intensity by adjacent atoms. This forms the basis for much pharmaceutical research, the quest for agents that have a desired effect without undesired side effects. Understanding structure activity relationships (SARs) is important in toxicology since one can often infer the effects of a chemical by knowing the effects of related compounds. Thus many short-chain chlorinated hydrocarbons have a common general anesthesia effect, even though their potency varies with their structure. Similarly many metal ions are nephrotoxic to the proximal kidney tubule,[14] and many hallucinogenic compounds share a common active group. SARs have proven predictive of carcinogenicity identified by long-term animal bioassays.[15]

▶ CHEMICALS IN THE ENVIRONMENT

Environmental toxicology is generally concerned with chemicals in air, water, soil, and food we encounter in our home, community, and workplace environments. Our behavior greatly influences the microenvironment we frequent, the exposures we experience, and the way that chemicals enter our body via ingestion, inhalation, and percutaneous absorption. Table 18-1 indicates the factors that influence the uptake and toxicity of a material and the susceptibility of the host. Uptake varies by route of exposure and bioavailability. A given chemical may be readily absorbed from the lungs but may have negligible uptake through the skin or intestinal tract.

Chemicals in Air

Air pollution remains a major public health concern. Ozone is a major air pollutant of concern. Probably the main substrate for excess ozone formation are oxides of nitrogen (the term for the family of NO_x) emitted in automobile exhaust. Another substance of concern is sulfur dioxide, which forms an irritating acid mist. Both ozone and sulfur dioxide are irritating to the respiratory system. Recent research has focused attention on particulates less than 10 μm (PM-10 fraction), which are associated with increased rates of respiratory disease. Air pollution indoors has become a major concern since the fuel crisis of the early 1970s,[16] and new regulations proposed in November 1996 specifically use the PM-10 data.

Recently constructed office buildings tend to be relatively airtight, and fuel conservation programs greatly reduce the amount of fresh air (makeup air) added to air conditioning. Many homes have unsuspected air pollutants that are hazardous to health. Radon, a breakdown product from naturally occurring radioactive materials in soil, occurs in gaseous form and emits alpha particles which cause lung cancer. It occurs in many parts of the United States and may

TABLE 18-1. FACTORS THAT MODIFY TOXICITY

■ ***HOST***
Species, strain, genotype
Age
Gender
Infectious/immunologic history
Behavioral stress history
Activity level/fitness
Nutritional status
Toxicant exposure history

■ ***ENVIRONMENT***
Temperature
Light: cycle, intensity, spectral distribution
Air: flow rate, ion content, humidity

■ ***TOXICANT***
Matrix/bioavailability
Physical form
Chemical form

occur in relatively high concentrations in certain homes. A more common but less dreaded pollutant is nitrogen dioxide, which is formed by combustion in a gas cooking range. Elevated levels of this irritant can be measured in a kitchen while cooking is in progress. Children living in homes with gas ranges may experience an excess of respiratory symptoms.[17]

Air is the major route of exposure for industrial workers. Many processes emit vapors, smokes, or mists, which can be inhaled. Most of the standards regarding industrial exposure refer to airborne concentrations, above which inhalation could lead to adverse health effects.[18] See Chapter 35 on occupational exposures.

Chemicals in Water

Both surface and ground water are used as community water sources. Many industrial and municipal wastes, both treated and untreated, are discharged directly to surface waters, and discharge permits allow certain quantities of toxic chemicals to be piped into streams, lakes, rivers, canals, and the ocean. Ground water contamination occurs as contaminants leach downward through soil. The solubility in water is the primary factor determining the behavior of chemicals in water. Many metal salts dissolve readily, while most larger organic molecules do not. Drinking water sources are regulated with regard to several pollutants. Although ingestion is the major pathway for water contaminants, volatile compounds in water escape during cooking and showering, offering a significant potential for inhalation exposure.

Chemicals in Soil

Soils have complex physical structures and compositions that vary greatly. The physical texture and water and organic content determine how chemicals will move through soil and influences their bioavailability. Some soils are naturally rich in toxic elements, such as the nickel-rich soils of New Caledonia, to which a unique group of plant species has become adapted. However, human activities have resulted in soil contamination via fallout of air pollutants, discharge of liquid industrial or agricultural waste, or dumping of solid waste. Once a chemical is deposited on soil it may remain in place, may be washed away by water flowing over the surface (runoff), or may percolate down through the soil (leaching).

Some chemicals may be readily leached from the upper layers of soil and carried down or away by water. Others may undergo biodegradation or photodegradation with the aid of microorganisms or sunlight. Some chemicals are persistent; for example, the chlorinated hydrocarbon pesticides and PCBs tend to remain unchanged in the soil for many years.

Soil particles that form fine dusts can become airborne and can be inhaled. Particles less than 5 μm in diameter are likely to reach the alveoli. Other particles may settle on food or water and be ingested. People may also ingest particles of soil that get on their fingers or under their nails or that are on the outer surface of vegetables. The ingestion of contaminated soil by toddlers is a major route of exposure and is often the major pathway in a risk assessment.

Food

Food may contain toxic chemicals from a variety of sources. Although regulations governing pesticide application (for example, the minimum number of days between spraying and harvest) are designed to minimize residual pesticides in food, many vegetables still contain some pesticide residues. Some residues may be surface sprays that adhere to plant tissue, while others are systemic substances taken up through the roots and incorporated in the tissue. Hormones and antibiotics used in promoting animal growth can also be detected in certain foods as can food additives used to prolong shelf life or enhance flavor, texture, or color. Some of these compounds have been demonstrated to have toxic effects in long-term low-level exposure experiments (see Chapter 26).

Biological Amplification in the Food Chain. Among the phenomena that influence the movements of chemicals in the environment is the process of biological amplification. This phenomenon has been demonstrated in a variety of ecosystems and has implications for human exposure. Most examples of bioamplification concern lipophilic chemicals such as polyaromatic hydrocarbons or organometals such as methyl mercury. These substances may be present in water or soil at the parts per million level. When taken up by planktonic organisms, they tend to concentrate in the lipids of these organisms and only a small fraction of the uptake is excreted. At each step up the food chain (what ecologists call trophic levels), the organism retains more than it excretes and incorporates an ever-increasing amount of contaminant in its fat.

If the concentration factor were 10 for each level, then the plankton swimming in water with a 1 ppm concentration, would contain 10 ppm, the fish larvae 100 ppm, the small fish 1,000 ppm, and the large fish 10,000 ppm. This example leaves the hapless human consuming a huge dose of the amplified toxic material. A high lipid-water partition coefficient enhances bioamplification. However, some nonlipophilic materials may also undergo bioamplification if they concentrate in some other tissue (i.e., the thyroid) or bind to macromolecules.

▸ EXPOSURE TO TOXIC SUBSTANCES

Understanding human exposure is the unique feature of environmental medicine. Traditional approaches such as taking a history remain important, but much more sophisticated approaches are required to understand exposure which takes place in the home, community, and workplace.

Exposure Assessment

Exposure assessment has emerged as a discipline that combines chemical analysis, biomarkers, behavioral studies, and mathematical modeling to estimate the dose received by an individual.[19] It is necessary to investigate exposure formally as a system of coupled events.[20] Exposure pathways involve contaminated air, water, soil, or food entering through the lungs, gastrointestinal tract, or skin, each combination of which is a potential pathway as shown in Table 18.2 and Figure 18-1.

When a human comes in contact with a contaminated medium, there is always the question about how much enters the body, is absorbed into the bloodstream, and reaches the target tissue. The bioavailability of a material in a particular matrix and the absorptive capability through the skin, intestinal mucosa, or alveoli can vary greatly and are difficult to measure directly. Likewise, the actual exposure of the target cells, tissues, or organs, the internal dose,[19] is seldom known. Absorption varies with species, age, the vehicle or solvent, as well as the presence of carrier molecules. Children absorb some compounds such as lead more efficiently than do adults. Since they are also more likely to ingest soil and are more vulnerable to its effects, they are in triple jeopardy. Children who are undernourished are both more vulnerable and at the same time more likely to eat soil (pica) and more efficient at absorbing lead from a diet deficient in iron or calcium. Children consume about 0.1 g of soil per day.[21]

For a given contaminant, different pathways may be important for different species. For example, organic mercury is primarily taken up by ingesting contaminated seafood, while inorganic mercury usually enters by inhalation.

Advances in instrumentation and analytic chemistry have supported great strides in direct measurement of environmental exposure. This is not without cost, because as our ability to analyze vanishingly small quantities of an agent improves, our ability to deal environmentally and sociopolitically with such exposures has not kept pace. Analytic techniques that would formerly have yielded concentrations of "zero" or "nondetectable", now provide results at parts per quadrillion (e.g., femtograms/gram). This has been referred to as the "vanishing zero."[22]

The discipline of industrial hygiene is particularly concerned with estimating and preventing exposure to workplace hazards.[23] For

TABLE 18-2. EXAMPLES OF BIOMARKERS

■ ***BIOMARKERS OF EXPOSURE***
Specific chemical agents[a]
Metabolites
■ ***BIOMARKERS OF EFFECT***
Male reproduction
Sperm motility
Semen quality
Müllerian-inhibiting factor
Chromosomal aberrations
DNA adducts in sperm
Female reproduction
Chorionic gonadotropin assay
Urinary progesterone metabolites
Pulmonary
Pulmonary function testing
Airway reactivity (challenge tests)
Pulmonary cytology
Immunology
Immunoglobulin levels
Lymphocyte ratios
Lymphocyte functional assays
T-cell dependent antibody response
Plaque-forming assays
Lymphocyte proliferation tests
Interleukin-2 activity
Specific receptor expression assays
Macrophage/leukocyte respiratory burst response
Lead poisoning
Zinc or erythrocyte protoporphyrin
δ-amino levulinic acid in urine
δ-amino levulinic acid dehydratase activity
bone lead

[a] The American Conference of Governmental Industrial Hygienists has established Biological Exposure Indices (BEIs), which involve the measurement of a specific chemical in blood, urine, or exhaled air.

airborne hazards, industrial hygienists use a variety of pumps and collection media to capture pollutants in a known volume of air. These are then quantified in the laboratory and extrapolated to determine how much of the material a person is exposed to in an 8-hour period. Where particulates are involved it is necessary to establish a size distribution to determine the portion that is of respirable size (usually less than 5 μm in diameter). Because exposures are not constant throughout the day, measurements must be made either at several times during the day or over several 8-hour work shifts. Exposures are expressed in terms of a time-weighted average (TWA) corrected to an 8-hour exposure.[18]

Bioavailability

An important aspect of exposure alluded to above is bioavailability.[24] How readily is a toxicant released from its environmental matrix? In the case of ethanol dissolved in water, there is virtually 100 percent uptake of the alcohol into the bloodstream. In the case of a metal bound to protein in our food, the uptake may depend on the efficiency of protein digestion. In the case of substances bound to soil, bioavailability may vary greatly. Bioavailability of 2,3,7,8-tetrachlorodibenzodioxin ("dioxin") was low in soil from Newark, New Jersey, probably due to a high degree of organic compounds in the soil, while dioxin from the sandy soil at Times Beach, Missouri, had much higher bioavailability.[24]

Bioavailability is also important for plants and consequently for humans that consume the plants. Certain pollutants in soil may be taken up by a plant and translocated to the leaves or fruits, which are subsequently harvested for human consumption. Depending upon the chemical species, concentration, pH, competing ions, etc. the plant may take up a large amount of the pollutant or none at all. If the pollutant is taken up it is likely to be translocated and subsequently consumed by humans.

▶ ACUTE AND CHRONIC EXPOSURE AND TOXICITY

The terms "acute" and "chronic" can refer either to conditions of exposure or to the resultant health effects. A single "acute" exposure to a toxic chemical may be sufficient to induce health effects that in turn may be either acute (followed by recovery), subacute, or chronic. Long-term or chronic exposure may be followed by no adverse health effects (if the dose is low), or by acute effects (which may occur when a sufficient dose is accumulated), or by chronic effects. In addition to having a long duration, chronic effects tend to be nonreversible.

More specifically with respect to toxicological studies on animals, acute toxicity can be defined as adverse effects usually occurring within 24 hours after a single dose. Subchronic effects usually occur after repeated dosing over up to 10 percent of the life span.[25] Chronic exposure refers to dosing animals for more than 10 percent of their life span.[26]

▶ CHEMICALS IN THE BODY

Toxicokinetics

Toxicokinetics is the totality of reactions that govern the distribution of a toxic substance and its metabolites throughout the body. It is based on the different rate constants that exist for metabolic processes in different tissues under different circumstances and on different partitioning coefficients, binding properties, etc. These reactions are competitive, such that the amount of material available for metabolism depends on the amount that has been sequestered in fat, bound to protein, or excreted in the urine.

The fate and effect of every substance that enters the body depend upon its absorption, transport, metabolism, storage, and excretion. Metabolism, for example, alters the binding properties and solubility of the original chemical and influences its activity and whether it will be stored or excreted. Dynamic equilibria exist for all of these processes, and one can refer to Figure 18-1 for the various state changes that influence the effects of a substance.

Two factors that influence the entry of chemicals into cells include the perfusion rate of the organ and the diffusion rate of the substance across the membrane. Fick's law describes the passage of a xenobiotic across a membrane as proportional to the concentration gradient, the membrane surface area, and a compound-specific permeability coefficient. The latter in turn depends upon the condition of the membrane and the lipid-aqueous partitioning of the compound. This is often measured as the solubility in octanol divided by the solubility in water. Excretion via urine, feces, exhaled air, or sweat is in turn determined by the relative solubility of the compound and its delivery to the kidney, liver, lungs, or skin. In general, compounds that are water soluble or conjugated are excreted via urine, while lipid-soluble compounds are secreted via the bile into the intestine.

Metabolic Activation versus Detoxification

An important feature of metabolism is its ability to both reduce and enhance toxicity. Although it was formerly taught that the liver was the major site for detoxification of xenobiotics, many toxics do not exert activity until they reach the liver and are metabolically activated, usually through an oxidative reaction. This forms more highly reactive intermediate compounds that can interfere with other metabolic reactions or "attack" membranes, organelles, or macromolecules.

Phase I reactions involve oxidation or reduction resulting in hydrolysis or hydroxylation, the formation and hydrolysis of epoxides, and various other reactions. The P-450 cytochrome-dependent enzyme system (see below) plays a major role. Phase II involves linking the substance to a glucuronide or adding acetyl or methyl radicals or conjugating it with amino acids or glutathione. Phase II reactions usually increase the hydrophilic nature of the substance, facilitating its excretion in urine.

The liver is the main organ of metabolism, but the metabolic enzymes occur in most tissues. Within cells they are found mainly in the microsomal component of the endoplasmic reticulum, but also in the cytosol and other organelles. Certain xenobiotic compounds are metabolized by the intestinal flora. Recent studies[27] show that there are active P-450, glutathione-*S*-transferase, and other metabolic enzymes in the nasal mucosa that modify inhaled xenobiotics.

As an example, 1-methyl-4-phenyl-1,2,5,6-tetrahydropyridine (MPTP) was produced accidentally in an attempt to synthesize a narcotic analog. MPTP is oxidized to the neurotoxic metabolite MPP+ by monoamine oxidase B,[28] which in turn is transported by the dopamine transporter and concentrates in dopaminergic neurons where it inhibits cellular respiration, causing cell death. The deliberate consumption of this by-product by substance abusers produced parkinsonism in a large number of young people, and MPTP has now become a model drug for parkinsonism research. Monoanime oxidase inhibitors block the toxicity of MPTP.

The common analgesic, acetaminophen, undergoes metabolism by P-450 to a quinone, which interacts with liver proteins, causing centrilobular necrosis. It also undergoes activation through the prostaglandin H synthase (PHS) system in the kidney to produce a nephrotoxic free radical. The bladder epithelium is also relatively rich in PHS, which can metabolize certain aromatic amines into genotoxic metabolites which cause bladder cancer in humans and dogs. In rats the predominant pathway is *N*-hydroxylation in the liver, such that the same amines cause liver tumors rather than bladder tumors.[29]

Cytochrome P-450

This system of enzymes is very diverse.[30] An entire subdiscipline has developed around understanding the species, tissue, substrate, and reaction specificity (or lack thereof) of the many P-450s found in various organisms. P-450s have also been called the liver microsomal oxidase system since the highest concentration is found in the microsomes (endoplasmic reticulum) of hepatocytes, but P-450s are found in virtually all tissues. They are heme-containing proteins, which have peak absorption at 450 nm when complexed with carbon monoxide. This is a family of monooxygenase enzymes that catalyze a variety of reactions, many of which add oxygen to the substrate. These oxidation reactions can result in hydroxylation, the formation of epoxides from carbon=carbon double bonds, the cleavage of esters, dehalogenation, and other reactions.[31] Many new isoforms of P-450 are being discovered, and they are assigned to several families. Thus the P-450 that metabolizes caffeine is referred to as P-450 1A2 and is often abbreviated CYP1A2. Other examples of specific P-450 reactions are the hydroxylation of testosterone at position 6 by CYP3A4, and of coumarin at position 7 by CYP2A6. Many of the discrete P-450s have been detected in studies of drug metabolism, and their natural substrates have not always been identified. Many of the P-450s are inducible rather than constitutive enzymes. That is, the amount of P-450 activity is often low until a particular substrate is present which activates the gene that turns on the expression of a particular P-450. A particular substrate may be metabolized by more than one P-450, while conversely, a single P-450 may catalyze more than one reaction. Thus CYP3A4 can hydroxylate testosterone at several positions and also dehydrogenate it to 6-dehydrotestosterone.[29]

Current interest in P-450 focuses on heritable deficiencies or polymorphisms that influence individual susceptibility to xenobiotics.[32,33] A mutation in the gene for CYP2D6 interferes with metabolism of the drug debrisoquine, and about 5 to 10 percent of Caucasians but less than 1 percent of Japanese are "poor metabolizers." Conversely 20 percent of Japanese are poor metabolizers of the anticonvulsant *S*-mephenytoin due to deficiency of CYP2C19. Since these P-450s are not substrate specific, these deficient individuals may be intolerant of certain other xenobiotics, whether environmental or pharmacologic.

Tissue Specificity. CYP1A2 is expressed in liver cells but not in other tissues, while CYP1A1 is low in liver (of most mammals, but not guinea pigs or rhesus monkeys), but high in other tissues. Both are induced by polyaromatic hydrocarbons and indoles. Since the two catalyze different reactions, a single substrate may follow different metabolic pathways in different tissues. This is a rapidly evolving area of research with important applications on pharmacology and toxicology.[34]

Induction. It has long been known that certain xenobiotics induce the formation of metabolic enzymes.[35] CYP1A2 is induced by a variety of polyaromatic hydrocarbons and indoles. CYP3A4 is induced by barbiturates, while CYP2D6, which metabolizes many different drugs, is constitutive rather than inducible. CYP2D6-deficient individuals are hyperresponsive to certain drugs. However, they are likewise protected from certain environmentally caused cancers such as lung, bladder, and liver cancer, because of their failure to activate certain pro-carcinogens. Whether this is a direct effect of CYP2D6 deficiency remains to be determined. There is a 10-fold variation in the liver content of CYP3A4.[36,37,38] This may add credence to the use of a $10 \times$ uncertainty factor to protect the most susceptible individual.

Flavin-Containing Monooxygenases

Flavin-containing monooxygenases are another family of microsomal enzymes that require NADPH and oxygen to catlyze the metabolism of various xenobiotics that contain nitrogen (e.g., amines), sulfur (e.g., thiols), and phosphorus (e.g., organophosphates). There are several forms of these oxygenases, which have different distributions in various organs and species. Thus mouse and human liver have a high concentration of FMO3 and low concentration of FMO1 and the reverse is true in the rat, but both are present in high concentrations in the kidneys of all three species. Hepatocytes in female mice have higher expression of FMO1 and FMO3 than do male mice.[39]

Phase II Reactions

These include several important conjugation reactions, some of which accelerate the elimination of xenobiotics.

Glucuronidation. A series of enzymes called uridine diphosphate glucuronosyltransferases, found in various tissues of mammals other than felines, catalyze the conjugation of xenobiotics with glucuronides, which are usually water soluble, allowing excretion in the urine (low molecular weight forms) or in the bile.

Glutathione Conjugation. Many xenobiotics are electrophilic and will react with glutathione (GSH). The conjugation is accelerated by cytosolic glutathione-*S*-transferase (GST) enzymes. Glutathione conjugates can be excreted in the bile or can be transformed to water-soluble metabolites in the kidney and excreted in the urine. Polymorphisms at the GST loci result in variable efficiencies of the conjugation reaction. Divalent cations readily bind with sulfhydryl groups, including GSH, and indeed, treatment with mercury increases the activity of several enzymes involved in the synthesis of GSH and the reduction of glutathione disulfide (GSSG).[40] Conversely acetaminophen depletes GSH levels in liver; both the depletion and the subsequent hepatotoxicity are inhibited by diallyl sulfone, a metabolite of garlic,[41] which inhibits CYP2E1 which activates acetaminophen.

Other Reactions. Sulfation results in the formation of a water-soluble ester due to the transfer of the SO_3 moiety. Methylation and amino acid conjugation are minor pathways. *N*-Acetylation is a major pathway for aromatic amines or hydrazines. It is catalyzed by *N*-acetyltransferases (NAT). These are cytosolic enzymes found in most mammals, except canines. There are at least three forms of NAT, and a deficiency in either activity or structure of NAT2 results in slow acetylation of certain drugs (for example, the antituberculosis drug, isoniazid). This deficiency occurs in about 70 percent of the Middle East population, in 50 percent of Europeans, and in 20 percent of Asians. Sulfur transferases have been found to have a wide role; for example, the enzyme 3-mercaptopyruvate sulfurtransferase is capable of detoxifying cyanide by transfering a sulfur, forming the less toxic thiocyanate.

Sequestration of Xenobiotics. The amount of a substance available to affect a target organ or excrete depends on how much has been stored or bound. Sequestration of an agent in an organ need not be permanent. Stored substances may be slowly or quickly released from such relatively inactive depots as bone or fat. Lipophilic substances such as chlorinated hydrocarbons and organometals are generally found in fatty tissues or in lipid components of cells and membranes. They may be released in large concentrations from fat during starvation or illness. Metal ions such as strontium and lead compete with calcium for deposition in bone, and bone therefore provides a long-term storage depot for these ions.

Routes of Excretion

Xenobiotics and their metabolites are excreted mainly through the urine and feces, but also through the lungs, sweat, milk, and through the sloughing of skin and hair. Renal clearance is greatest for substances that are water soluble or that are conjugated into hydrophilic complexes. Fecal excretion usually occurs for substances that are lipophilic or can be conjugated into lipophilic complexes. Enterohepatic cycles may exist to interfere with excretion. A substance that is lipophilic can be secreted into the intestine, from which it is immediately reabsorbed, redistributed to the liver, conjugated with bile, and returned to the gut.

Volatile compounds are excreted through the lungs. At any moment the concentration of volatiles in expired air depends on how much has just been inspired (but not absorbed) as well as how much is released to the lungs from the bloodstream. Measurement of volatiles in expired air is gaining increasing utility as a means of monitoring exposure.

Short-chain chlorinated hydrocarbons are highly volatile, and whether consumed in water or inhaled, they are excreted via the lungs. Once they reach the liver they are oxidatively metabolized into polar metabolites, which are water soluble and are not excreted in the air.

Biological Half-Lives. The concept of a radiologic half-life, whereby a the radioactive decay of a compound can be predicted, is mirrored by the biological half-life, the time it takes for half of a dose of a xenobiotic to be eliminated. However, as elimination may follow a 2- or 3-phase decay curve, the half-life is only an approximation, and estimates of half-lives vary among studies, and among individuals as well. The individual variation in half-life of cadmium in the kidney has been estimated to range from a few years to a century.[42]

▸ TOXICOLOGIC EFFECTS

Endpoints or Response

A toxicologic effect may be manifest at the molecular, cellular, tissue, organ, individual, or population level. Some effects such as death, acute respiratory illness, skin rashes, and toxic hepatitis may be readily apparent, while others may be subtle, requiring sophisticated testing for identification. Endpoints depend on the toxic properties of a chemical and what the researcher chooses to study. A chemical may be highly specific, such as the effect of benzene on the bone marrow causing myelogenous leukemia, or nonspecific. Endpoints may be sought in any organ system or any tissue type. They need not be clinically significant.

Recently, attention has focused on subcellular and molecular targets of poisons and on biomarkers. Toxicology is concerned with all of these forms and levels of injury.

Dose-Response Curve

Although many toxicological studies simply report the presence or absence of a particular effect, the hallmark of toxicology is the dose-response curve. This is predicated on the fact that a high dose of a substance usually has a greater effect on any endpoint than does a low dose. The dose-response curve (Fig. 18-2) plots the dose along the x axis and the endpoint response indicated along the y axis. Often the response is measured as the percent of exposed animals that show a particular effect (*population curve*). The response could also reflect severity of effect experienced by an individual or the concentration of a biomarker (*individual curve*). The typical dose-response curve has the sigmoid shape illustrated. It is a cumulative percent response curve.

It is customary to measure dose in terms of the amount of the agent divided by the body weight of the organism, for example, milligrams of chemical per kilogram of body weight. In some cases, for example, acute toxic effects or sensitization of the skin, eye, or respiratory tree, the toxicant is not distributed throughout the body, and the dose per body weight is therefore not a good predictor of effect. In such cases different units must be used, such as concentration in a volume of air or on an area of skin.

In interpreting dose-response data from animal studies, it is necessary to know the species, strain, age, and sex of the test animals, the conditions of exposure, as well as the dose. Endpoints include death, presence of lesion (e.g., tumor), number of lesions, and anatomic, physiologic, biochemical, molecular, or behavioral changes. Thus if one were concerned with neurotoxic, nephrotoxic, and lethal characteristics of a particular chemical, one would draw three dose-response curves, graphing the severity of each effect against dose. Figure 18-3 shows different clinical consequences occurring as a percent of the population with different levels of organomercury exposure. Thus difficulty in speech occurred at a much lower dose than coma and death.

The common features of most dose-response curves are shown in Figure 18-2. Initially there is a flat subthreshold portion where an increase in dose produces no detectable effect. The threshold is the lowest dose that produces an observable effect. Beyond that point the curve tends to rise steeply and often enters a linear phase where the increase in response is proportional to the increase in dose. Eventually a maximal response is reached, and the curve flattens out. This usually means that all the exposed individuals, or at least all the susceptible individuals, have shown the effect.

Various endpoints have been used to reflect toxicity. Traditionally toxicologists were interested in the LD_{50}, which killed half of the exposed animals. Various chemicals could be ranked in terms of their LD_{50}. This proved to be a very narrow indication of toxicity. In recent

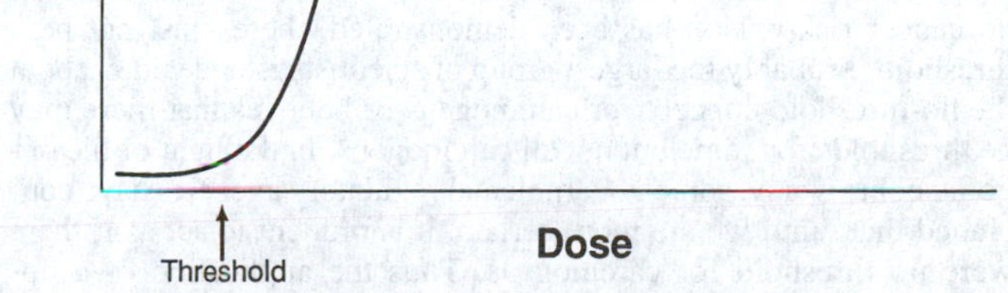

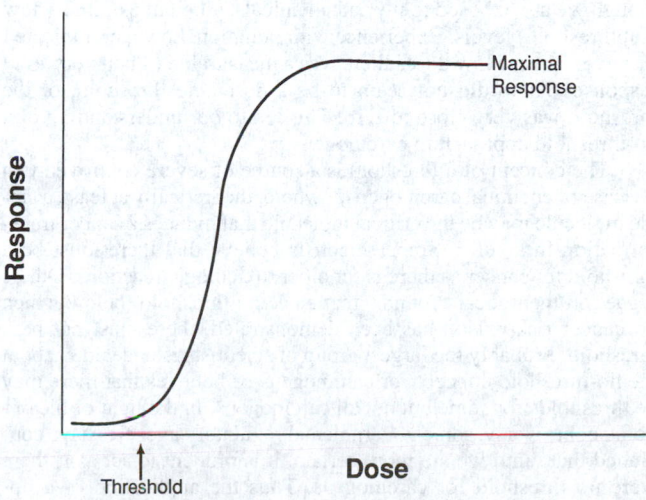

Figure 18-2. The dose-response curve.

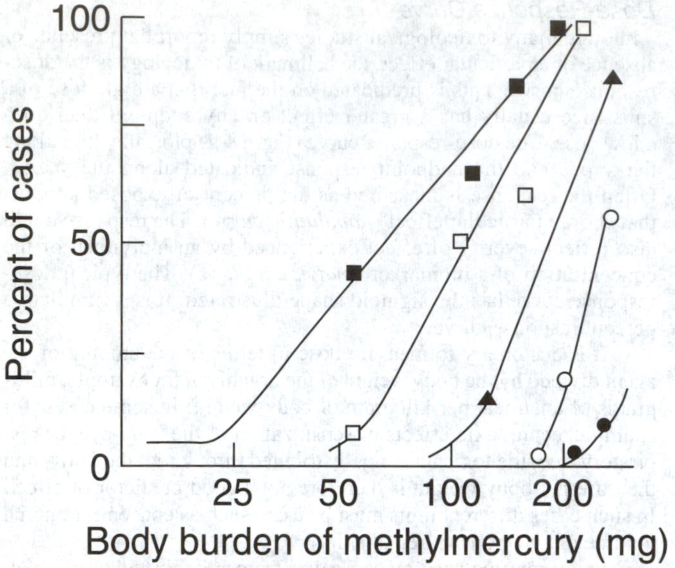

Figure 18-3. Dose-response curves for different clinical manifestations of organomercury poisoning based on the epidemic in Iraq, showing the relative progression in thresholds from relatively minor sign of paresthesias to lethality, estimated at the time exposure ceased. *Solid triangles* = paresthesias, *open squares* = ataxia, *solid squares* = dysarthria; *open circles* = deafness; *solid circles* = death. (Modified from Takizawa Y: Epidemiology of mercury poisoning. In Nriagu J, ed: *The biogeochemistry of mercury in the environment*, Amsterdam, 1979, Elsevier-North Holland.)

years a variety of other responses such as physiologic and behavioral responses are defined, but one can still speak of the response dose, or RD_{50}, or the effective dose, or ED_{50}. These doses can be calculated from data generated in animal studies using various computer programs.[43]

Hormesis. Many substances that are essential elements or nutrients at low doses, for example, iron and chromium, become toxic at high doses. Whether certain other nonessential, toxic chemicals also have a beneficial dose range (*hormesis*) is controversial.

Thresholds. Thresholds (Fig. 18-2) are a familiar concept to physiologists and biochemists. A particular response may not occur at a very low dose or intensity of stimulus. Thresholds probably exist for most toxicologic exposures. Thus we can live normal lives even though we are exposed to myriad chemicals, albeit at extremely low (subthreshold) levels. Experience with radiation, however, indicated that even at very low doses there was a measurable (albeit very low) response. There did not seem to be a definable threshold, or the threshold was very close to zero. This led to our understanding of a no-threshold approach to carcinogens.[44]

The concept of a threshold is a source of severe controversy in the case of chemical carcinogens,[45] where, theoretically at least, a single molecule may be the critical molecule that induces a cancer transformation in a cell.[46] Some scientists believe that there must be a threshold for cancer as there is for other toxicologic reactions. Others argue, on theoretical grounds, that since no threshold (below which no cancer risk exists) has been demonstrated, there must not be a threshold. Probably the largest group of scientists is undecided about the no-threshold concept for carcinogens or believes that there may be thresholds for some but not all carcinogens. In the light of the ongoing controversy, some governmental regulatory agencies have concluded that, until we are more certain, it is prudent to act as if there were no threshold for carcinogens. Thus the application of a no-threshold approach to carcinogens can be viewed as a policy decision rather than a scientific decision.[47]

Latency

Latency is the time between a stimulus and a response or, in toxicology, the time between an exposure and an effect. In some cases (for example, acute exposure to hydrogen sulfide), the effect is felt in seconds, and the latency is therefore measured in seconds. In the case of asbestos-induced mesothelioma, a cancer of the lining of the chest or abdomen, the latency is on the order of 40 years, that is, the cancer may not develop until 40 years after the first exposure occurred.[48]

If the latency is very short, as with acute effects, it is usually easy to establish a cause-effect relationship. When the latency is much longer, the cause may be long-forgotten before the outcome is realized. Accordingly, only sophisticated epidemiologic studies can identify cause-effect relationships with long latencies. In some cases there is a dose-response relationship for latency, i.e., at higher doses latency is reduced.

Interactions

When two chemicals are administered together or when an individual is exposed to a mixture of chemicals, there may be various interactions identified as follows: (*a*) *independence* or *additivity*: each substance produces its own effect appropriate for its dose; (*b*) *synergism*: the combined effect is greater than either substance would produce alone or additively, i.e., it is multiplicative; and (*c*) *antagonism*: the combined effect is less than one would have expected from one or both chemicals administered alone. A classic example of synergism is the case of asbestos and smoking.[49] Asbestos exposure increases the risk of lung cancer 5-fold over the risk of the unexposed person, while smoking increases the risk of lung cancer about 10-fold over the nonsmoker's risk. The asbestos worker who smokes has a risk about 50 times greater than the person with neither exposure. Synergism may occur when substance A enhances the effect of B, promotes its activation, or interferes with its degradation and excretion. Antagonism occurs when A interferes with the uptake of B, competes with it for metabolic enzymes or substrates, or enhances its degradation or excretion.

There is a synergistic interaction between aflatoxin B1 (itself a potent hepatocarcinogen) and hepatitis B. Hepatitis patients exposed to aflatoxin B are at greatly increased risk compared with normal subjects.[50] Many xenobiotics, such as the PCBs and dioxins, induce enzymes (for example the P-450s), which in turn alters the metabolism of endogenous chemicals and drugs.[51] The oxidation of toluene, for example, is greatly increased by prior exposure to PCBs.

Reversibility

Since most individuals recover from most toxic exposures, it is clear that many toxic effects are reversible. Inhibition of a biochemical pathway may be reversed if a competing agent is introduced to bind up the xenobiotic. If a cell is killed, that process is not reversible, but in almost all organs, regeneration of new cells occurs to take over the role of the damaged cells. In the case of genetic damage to the nucleic acid molecules, sophisticated biochemical reactions called "DNA repair" mechanisms are brought into play and eliminate, in various ways, the damaged DNA. Our DNA repair mechanism(s) become less efficient as we age, and this is believed to be one of the factors associated with the increased incidence of cancer in older people.

▸ SUSCEPTIBILITY

Although it is well known that individual humans vary in their susceptibility to different stressors, and although some of the factors modifying susceptibility are well known, there is a great need for research on susceptibility. In experimental animal species, strain, gender, and age influence susceptibility. Indeed some rodent strains are bred for enhanced susceptibility to certain diseases. If a population of organisms were exposed to a fixed dose of a chemical, one could graph the responses with a histogram—how many individuals had no, low, medium, or high response. If response is quantitative, a smoothed histogram could be drawn. This might take the form of a normal, log-normal distribution (Fig. 18-3), or some other distribution. If only one gender were susceptible the curve would be skewed. Or if only very young and very old individuals were susceptible the curve would be bimodal.

▶ MECHANISMS OF TOXICITY

Understanding how a chemical causes its adverse effect is important in directing research or influencing risk assessments. New advances in biology including understanding of gene regulation, transcription factors, polymorphisms, receptors, cytokines, oncogenes, cell cycling, DNA repair, and apoptosis have greatly expanded the horizons of toxicology in the past 5 years. Several of these advances are discussed briefly in this chapter.

Metabolic Poisons

These include substances that disrupt metabolic pathways, for example, cyanide compounds, which inhibit cellular respiration. Binding to an enzyme and altering its tertiary structure and its active site is a common mechanism. Some substances act within cells to alter the structure or function of internal membranes, such as endoplasmic reticulum, or organelles, such as mitochondria. Many chemicals act on mitochondria, interfering with their energetic function and resulting in swelling and loss of detail on electron micrographs.

Macromolecular Binding

Chemicals may bind to various macromolecules such as proteins, hemoglobin, and nucleic acids. These adducts may interfere with function or may be silent. Some are reversible, being repaired within hours, while others persist and may presage future cancer. The presence of DNA adducts may reflect genotoxic or carcinogenic properties, and the quest for these molecular markers of exposure is an important frontier in toxicologic research.

Cellular Poisons

Cellular poisons are substances that damage cells or cell membranes, causing necrosis or lysis. Membranes are functional as well as structural entities, and chemicals that interfere with membrane transport systems may have major consequences. Toxic agents may react with either the protein or lipid component of the membrane. Many naturally occurring toxins cause lysis of cells, for example, the hemolysins in certain plants and snake venoms. Some heavy metals act directly on the cell membrane, interfering with the sulfhydryl binding responsible for membrane integrity and altering membrane fluidity.[52]

Enzyme Induction

Because of the specificity of enzymes, the body cannot at all times maintain a full supply of all the enzymes that may be needed for every situation. Accordingly, many substances induce the synthesis of the enzymes that will act on them, and within 12 or 24 hours, the amount of enzyme present within a cell may increase by several orders of magnitude. Some enzyme systems are highly specific and act only on a single substrate, others are nonspecific and catalyze classes of reactions on a wide range of substrates. The substrates vary in their potency at inducing enzymes. Enzyme induction plays an important role in metabolizing xenobiotics, either enhancing their toxicity or reducing it. However, sometimes the most important consequence of the enzyme induction is the greatly accelerated metabolism of endogenous bioactive compounds.

Receptors

Advances in biochemistry include recognizing the role of receptors and their regulation as an important part of toxic interactions. Although some toxic interactions take place in solution, toxicologists have increasingly recognized that toxic effects usually involve binding of the toxicant to some active receptor site on an enzyme or membrane. A familiar example is the binding of neuroinhibitory substances to the receptors on the most synaptic membrane or the myoneural junction. Receptors are important components of normal cellular function and account for the remarkable specificity of many cell processes. Most familiar are the receptors on the postsynaptic membrane, which initiate a nerve impulse when binding acetylcholine. It is now realized that many hormone effects are mediated by hormone-specific receptors in particular target tissues. Some toxic effects occur because a xenobiotic is capable of binding to a hormone receptor or a neuroreceptor and interfering with the normal action of the endogenous chemical.

The compound 2,3,7,8-TCDD, often known simply as dioxin, has proven a valuable tool for toxicologic research.[53] Its effects are in part mediated by binding to the Ah (aromatic hydrocarbon) receptor.[54] Related substances that bind to the Ah receptor have effects similar to TCDD, but with vastly different dose-response curves related to their binding affinity.

A normal feature of receptor models is that they are reversible, allowing the same biologic function to be rapidly repeated. Toxic effects involving receptors often are much less reversible (for instance, the binding of carbon monoxide to hemoglobin or the inhibition of cholinesterase by organophosphate pesticides). This leads among other things to competitive inhibition between the xenobiotic and the endogenous compound.

By binding to estrogen-like receptors that might normally be activated by estrogens, dioxin may inhibit the proliferation of breast cancers. This is based on animal research. However, a study of the dioxin-exposed communities around the Seveso plant (in Italy) which exploded, releasing a cloud of dioxin, showed, as expected, a deficit of breast cancer, although other cancers were elevated.[55]

Immunotoxins

Immunotoxins act by suppressing or activating the immune system. Some alter the formation of immunoglobulins, while others affect the lymphocytes. Some agents interfere with the production or function or lifespan of the T and B lymphocytes. T cells mature in the thymus and are the main factor in cell-mediated immunity. B cells control antibody-mediated or humoral immunity. T cells are classified on the basis of surface antigens, and it is now possible to quantify a variety of T-cell populations and determine which functions have been inhibited. Many studies of T-cell function changes have provided conflicting results, but the recognition of variable phenotypes of the different types of lymphocytes offers the opportunity to clarify cell-mediated immunotoxicity.[56]

Substances known to interfere with the immune system include polyhalogenated aromatic compounds (e.g., 2,3,7,8-TCDD), metals (e.g, lead and cadmium), pesticides, and even air pollutants (e.g., NO_2, SO_2, tobacco smoke). Mercury, for example, causes autoimmune changes and glomerulonephritis in the brown Norway rat strain but none in the Lewis strain. This appears related to a depletion of the $RT6^+$ subpopulation of T-lymphocytes in the former but not in the latter.[57]

Sensitizers. Sensitizers are substances that act through the immune system to induce an increased immune response. These can be complete allergens or haptenes. The main target organs are the skin itself and the respiratory system. Nickel and poison ivy (*Rhus*) contact dermatitis are common examples of such skin sensitization. Occupational asthmas reflect sensitization of the lung and airways to aerosols.

Genotoxicity

Radiation and various chemicals are capable of damaging DNA, the genetic material, or interfering with the processes involved in chromosomal replication and cell division. Damage occurring in the germ cells may be heritable, while those occurring in somatic cells are not.

Mutagenesis. Some substances interact with genetic material, causing either point mutations, chromosomal damage, or interference with meiosis, mitosis, or cell division. A variety of tests can measure these effects including chromosomal aberrations, aneuploidy, sister chromatid exchange, translocation assays, micronucleus formation, glycophorin A assay, and T-cell receptor genes. New genetic techniques allow sequencing of genes and detection of changes at specific codons.

Mutation Spectrum. Genetic analysis can reveal a pattern of GC or AT base pair substitutions, deletions, or duplications at a single gene locus in individuals with a particular exposure. The relative frequency of the different mutations—the spectrum—may differ depending on the nature of the exposure. For example, somatic mutations at the X-linked hypoxanthine phosphoribosyltransferase (*hprt*) gene are mainly deletions (49 percent) or base pair substitutions (44 percent). Although GC substitutions are commoner in nonsmokers, there was a slight increase in AT substitutions in smokers.[58] However, after radiotherapy there was a substantial increase in rearrangements and deletions, which persisted for at least several years.[59]

ras Oncogenes. Genotoxic chemicals may cause mutation in proteins called proto-oncogenes producing the mutant oncogene that encodes for a modification of the natural protein product. Some changes such as that in the *ras* proto-oncogene increase cell susceptibility to cancer. The 21-kDa protein (*p*21) binds with a receptor on the inner cell membrane and mediates responses to growth factors. Mutation at codon 13 "locks" the protein into the active form such that it no longer responds to other cell signals. With signal transduction impaired, this permanent activation is associated with malignant transformation and proliferation.[60]

Tumor Suppressor Genes (p53). Certain proteins inhibit cell division cycles. If the genes that encode these control proteins mutate, the resulting gene product may lack the inhibitory effect, allowing unbridled cell proliferation. One of these, the *p*53 gene, encodes a 53-kDa protein, which among other functions inhibits cell growth, slowing the process of neoplastic transformation. Transgenic mice that lack *p*53 develop cancer at an early age.[61] There is an association between a change in the 249th codon of the *p*53 product in people exposed to aflatoxin B_1 and in people with hepatocellular carcinoma, suggesting that the toxin may cause cancer by this highly specific mutation.[62]

Reproductive Effects

The processes of gametogenesis, fertilization, implantation, embryogenesis, organogenesis, and birth are complex and subject to many errors. Major errors incompatible with life generally result in abortion, which can be viewed as a quality control procedure. Adverse reproductive consequences include failure to form gametes (e.g., azoospermia) and formation of abnormal gametes. Once gametes are formed, several factors may intervene to prevent the initiation of embryogenesis. There is concern that many synthetic chemicals, particularly those that bind to hormone receptors, may interfere with one or more of these steps. A notable case is dibromochloropropane (DBCP), a nematocide, which induced azoospermia in the men who manufactured and packaged DBCP. Some of these never recovered normal spermatogenesis after cessation of exposure. Lead also interferes with spermatogenesis. A long list of chemicals has been implicated in toxicity to the male reproductive system (including interfering with spermatogenesis, semen quality, erection, and libido). The list of chemicals affecting females includes cancer chemotherapeutic agents, other pharmaceuticals, metals, insecticides, and various industrial chemicals. (See Reference 63 for further details.)

Teratogenesis

From conception through birth and maturation, the organism undergoes a bewildering series of carefully timed events that require the formation and replacement of tissues. Some substances interfere with the complex processes of morphogenesis. Depending on the stage of embryogenesis and fetogenesis, they may affect different organ systems, leading to embryonic death, major structural birth defects, slowed maturation, or even postnatal effects such as learning difficulties.[64] In general, exposure prior to implantation is likely to be lethal. Exposure during organogenesis begets birth defects or embryolethality. Later in fetal life one sees intrauterine growth retardation or fetal death or functional changes that interfere with birth or postnatal development. Approximately 3 percent of live births have detectable congenital abnormalities, and additional congenital defects may become apparent later in life. Some of the defects are genetic or chromosomal in origin, but some are due to chemical exposures (including drugs taken by the mother).

The recently recognized field of behavioral teratology involves study of some of these affects, such as the impact of lead exposure on psychomotor development and learning. The fetal alcohol syndrome reflects the specific toxicity of ethanol ingested by the mother on the development and behavior of the newborn.

Endocrine Disruptors

This rubric applies to a wide range of substances and a wide range of effects and is an area of major controversy highlighted by Theo Colburn's book, *Our Stolen Future*.[65] The ability of DDT to influence estrogen metabolism through enzyme induction has been established since the early 1970s,[51] but recent research has shown a wide range of effects in various animal species of compounds that resemble hormones or that interact with hormone receptors to enhance or inhibit normal endocrinologic function particularly related to development, maturation, and reproduction.[66]

Many of these compounds occur naturally in vegetables and have been called "phytoestrogens." These include a group of isoflavonoid and lignin polycyclic compounds. At the same time that concern is voiced regarding interference with reproduction and development, their beneficial features are being exploited. One isoflavenoid, coumesterol, anatgonizes estrogen during embryonic development, leading to reproductive abnormalities in behavior and hormone function. Others, such as genistein, protect against certain hormone-dependent breast cancers by competing with estrogens, or against other cancers by inhibiting proliferation, differentiation, or the vascular supply.[67] Research on the adverse developmental effects of genistein is in its infancy.

Research is proceeding on many fronts, including using the bioengineered yeast estrogen screen, in which the human estrogen receptor and estrogen response elements are expressed to screen for the action of various xenobiotics. The potency of these compounds is influenced by environmental persistence and bioamplification, bioavailability, and binding affinities.[68]

Oxidative Stress and Free Radicals

In addition to its critical role in supporting cellular respiration and oxidation-reduction reactions throughout the body, oxygen plays a more sinister role in toxicity. Normally there is a balance between oxidative and antioxidant reactions. However, the oxidative reactions, so necessary for life, are now believed to play important roles in inflammation, aging, carcinogenesis, and toxicity.[69] Current research is increasing the number of toxicants for which oxidative stress is an important mechanism. Thus chromium increases the formation of superoxide anion and nitric oxide in cells and enhances DNA single-strand breaks.[70] Glucose-6-phosphate dehydrogenase (G6PDH) is essential in cells facing oxidative stress, which in turn increases the amount of G6PDH in exposed cells.

Toxicologists speak of reactive oxygen species, some of which are free radicals. Oxygen can receive an electron and form a superoxide anion radical, which can in turn react with hydrogen to form hydrogen peroxide, which reacts with free electrons and hydrogen ion to form water and a highly reactive hydroxide radical.

$$\text{O-O} + c^- \rightarrow \text{O-O}^{\cdot}$$

$$\text{O-O}^{\bullet} + c^- + 2\text{H}^+ \rightarrow \text{H-O-O-H}$$

$$\text{H-O-O-H} + c^- + \text{H}^+ \rightarrow \text{H}_2\text{O} + {}^{\bullet}\text{OH}$$

In the course of these reactions the highly reactive free radicals, particularly the hydroxy radical, are available to attack macromolecules, initiating a variety of toxic effects. The superoxide anion radical is formed in many oxidation reactions, where oxygen acts as an electron receptor.

In response to the potential harm that these reactive oxygen species may cause, the body has evolved antioxidant defenses. (See Reference 69 for more detailed description.) The defenses include water-soluble vitamin C and lipid-soluble vitamin E and vitamin A. Superoxide dismutase, a metalloprotein, and glutathione-dependent peroxidases, in association with glutathione reductase, serve to scavenge free radicals. One of the consequences of free radical formation is reaction with lipids, including those in cell and organelle membranes, to form lipid peroxides, which in turn lead to cell damage and dysfunction.

Lipid Peroxidation

Some cytotoxicity of chlorinated hydrocarbons such as carbon tetrachloride are mediated by peroxidation of membrane lipids, which can be caused by a variety of reactive oxygen species.[71] An active area of research involves identifying naturally occurring and synthetic compounds that interfere with lipid peroxidation.[72]

Nitric Oxide

A major new development has been recognition of the complex roles that nitric oxide (NO) plays in the cell as an intracellular messenger. This occurs in the nervous system, lung, and liver, where synthesis is altered by xenobiotics.[73] L-Arginine is converted to nitric oxide by a calcium-dependent, NADPH-dependent cytosolic enzyme, nitric oxide synthase (NOS).[74] This formation is coupled to activation of glutamate receptors.[75] Excess NO production increases intracellular free radicals enhancing neuronal degradation.[76]

▶ CARCINOGENESIS: INITIATION AND PROMOTION

Cancer is not a single disease, but includes a great many diseases that share a common property of uncontrolled cell proliferation. Normally cell proliferation proceeds in controlled fashion ensuring an adequate number of new cells for any given physiologic task. It is customary to divide carcinogenesis into stages: *initiation, promotion, proliferation*, and clinically apparent *disease*. Initiation is the process by which the genetic material of the cell is altered, predisposing it to cancer.[77] Such genetic abnormalities are often repaired, or initiated cells may be destroyed as part of the body's defense against cancer. However, we are exposed to initiating events throughout our lives. Initiated cells may survive but remain dormant, perhaps controlled by the immune system. In the presence of certain substances, *promoters*, initiated or mutated cells have a selective growth and division advantage over normal cells. Promotion is the process by which initiated cells are stimulated or allowed to become cancerous,[78] and proliferation is the stage of clonal expansion. At each of these stages, defenses may reverse or retard the process.[79]

Effects on Signal Transduction

Cell cycles are regulated by molecules that serve as signals to activate certain receptors that transduce signal (change the form of the signal) to influence genes. Signal transduction pathways typically alter gene expression or modify gene products, either enhancing or inhibiting their function. Many endogenous signal chemicals (such as hormones) as well as xenobiotics can alter gene expression by activating transcription factors, which in turn promote the transcription of certain genes.

Apoptosis

Programmed cell death is a necessary part of the life history of a cell. Gene activation leads to proteins that prepare the cell for apoptosis, which ends with phagocytosis of cell fragments, without concomitant inflammation.[80] This is an essential feature during development, allowing the remodeling of tissues. Apoptosis selectively eliminates cells with damaged DNA and also counters the clonal expansion of neoplastic cells. Inhibition of apoptosis, for example, by estrogens, allows mutations to accumulate and tumor proliferation to occur. Hormone-dependent tumors expand when the hormone inhibits apoptosis, while an antiestrogenic drug, such as tamoxifen, allows apoptosis to occur. Conversely, the tumor-promotor, phenobarbital, inhibits apoptosis.[81] Some chemicals appear to inhibit apoptosis, thus enhancing the proliferative phase of carcinogenesis.[82] New cancer treatment approaches focus on harnessing apoptosis to destroy tumor cells.[83]

▶ CLINICAL EVALUATION OF TOXICITY

Clinical toxicology usually refers to the emergency diagnosis and treatment of episodes of acute poisoning. Yet clinicians play an important role in the understanding of chronic poisonings as well. This requires an accurate identification of possible hazards and an estimation of the magnitude and circumstances of exposure, as well as delineation of toxic effects. The clinician obtains a detailed medical, social, environmental, and occupational history (see Chapter 17), performs a physical examination, and uses a variety of clinical and laboratory tests, including the assessment of biomarkers of exposure and effect.

Evaluation of pulmonary damage may be apparent on chest x-rays, pulmonary function tests, or by alterations in the cells obtained by bronchoalveolar lavage. Or pulmonary white cells may be used in a lymphocyte proliferation test to identify specific sensitivities, for example, to beryllium.[84] Damage to liver can often be detected by disturbances in the pattern of various enzymes that serve as markers of liver cell damage. Similarly severe kidney damage may be reflected in the excretion of large proteins such as albumin, while low molecular weight proteins may provide signs of earlier damage.[85]

▶ BIOMARKERS

The past decade has seen a tremendous emphasis on *biomarkers* in understanding toxic effects on humans[86,87] and other organisms.[88] In the broadest sense, anything that can be measured (for example, blood pressure and historical information) could be included under the rubric of "biomarker," for there is no clear distinction between these clinical measures and those identified through molecular biology, biochemistry, or analytic chemistry.

It has been convenient to divide biomarkers into three categories: markers of susceptibility, markers of exposure, and markers of effect. However, the distinction is blurred in practice. For example, when a xenobiotic (such as benzo[*a*]pyrene) forms an adduct with DNA, that can be considered an effect, a marker for exposure, or (if it increases the risk of cancer), a marker of susceptibility.

Familiar biomarkers include blood lead (a biomarker of exposure) and zinc protoporphyrin (a biomarker of effect from lead exposure). The study of biomarkers in various human populations has been labeled *molecular epidemiology*.[86]

The National Research Council's Board on Environmental Studies and Toxicology has a Committee on Biologic Markers, which has published monographs on markers in pulmonary toxicology,[89] reproductive toxicology,[90] and immunotoxicology.[91] The potential application of biomarkers are boundless. They can be used to estimate exposure, internal dose, and dose to target cells. They can be the endpoint in dose-response assessments. They can be used to distinguish exposed from unexposed populations for epidemologic studies. Biomarkers of susceptibility will greatly enhance the utility of risk assessments.

Adducts

Adducts are formed when a chemical or its metabolite binds with macromolecules, particularly nucleic acids, but also proteins such as hemoglobin. Smokers, for example, have higher levels of benzo(*a*)-

pyrene adducts to DNA than do nonsmokers.[92] Some adducts are repaired within hours, while others persist. A variety of techniques have been used to assess adduct formation, including the ^{32}P post-labeling (Randerath) technique based on differential mobility of DNA bases involved in adduct formation. This method has yet to prove useful in screening other populations. DNA-protein cross-linking is promoted by a variety of genotoxic chemicals including hexavalent chromium.[93] However, new techniques may greatly improve the sensitivity and utility of adducts.

Radiation Damage and Chromosomes

The main body of information on the genetic effects of ionizing radiation derives from the 50-year follow-up of atom bomb victims of Hiroshima and Nagasaki conducted cooperatively by the United States and Japan through the Radiation Effects Research Foundation. The chromosomal damage in 2,300 survivors shows a clear dose-response relationshp that parallels the incidence of leukemia in the same population.[94]

▸ CAUSALITY: ENVIRONMENTAL CHEMICAL EXPOSURE AND HEALTH EFFECTS

In the laboratory, establishing causality between a chemical exposure and a health effect depends upon sound experimental design with careful attention to alternative hypotheses. It may or may not involve careful definition of the mechanism by which the effect is achieved. In the community, determination of cause and effect is much more difficult. Under these "natural" conditions the hazardous substance is not always identified or may be present in mixtures, and the dose and the conditions and time frame of exposure are seldom known. It may be difficult to ascertain who is exposed as well as to what. Often there is a bewildering array of symptoms and signs suspected or attributed to the putative cause. Simply defining relevant health effects may be a costly and frustrating venture, while linking them to specific exposures may be impossible.[95]

Scientists and clinicians may not appreciate that the courts impose entirely different standards for establishing causation. Moreover, standards of causation differ under different bodies of law. Thus in some jurisdictions one may have to establish a "reasonable probability," in other cases it must be "more likely than not," or "without this event the outcome probably would not have occurred." In some circumstances one must establish an attributable risk, how much of the outcome can be related to the particular exposure. In other cases, the causation is assumed unless proven otherwise. For example, the U.S. Congress required the Veterans Administration to give veterans the benefit of the doubt in cases involving herbicide exposure, and certain diseases in exposed veterans are now presumed to be related to herbicide exposure and qualify for compensation.

▸ TOXICITY TESTING

Toxicologists employ a wide variety of systems and paradigms to test chemicals in order to predict their effects on human health or the environment. The factors that affect toxicity in humans (Table 18-2) must be considered in designing the experiments. One must choose the appropriate animal model or in vitro test system. If using animals the genetic strain, gender, and age of the animal must be selected. The dosage schedule, single or multiple, and acute, subchronic, chronic, as well as appropriate dose levels must be chosen. The route of administration should be relevant to natural conditions of exposure. The experiment should last long enough to fully encompass any effects that have a long latency. And naturally appropriate controls must be selected. In addition to these design features, there are standards for good laboratory practices which indicate how animals must be cared for and how data must be recorded. This provides for appropriate quality assurance methodology. Increasingly a variety of in vitro test systems are replacing many studies traditionally done in animals.

Bioassays of the National Toxicology Program

The National Toxicology Program (NTP), operated by the National Institute for Environmental Health Sciences, sponsors long-term rodent studies to detect the carcinogenic or other toxic properties of chemicals.[96] Chemicals are selected depending on the data needs of governmental agencies and in response to public concerns. The standard protocol is two species (rat, mouse), both sexes, and a minimum of 50 individuals for each category, with oral dosing over a 2-year "life span." These 2-year bioassays can provide information on metabolism and genetic, reproductive, and developmental toxicity as well as on toxic effects on various organ systems. The NTP bioassays serve an important role in screening new chemicals for carcinogenic activity and classifying them with respect to human carcinogenicity. However, the main application has been the use of the tumor incidence data in risk assessment.

Transgenic and Knockout Mice

For decades toxicologists have taken advantage of rodent strains inbred for specific metabolic or susceptibility characteristics that rendered a particular strain suitable for a particular test. Genetic engineering has produced mice with highly specific defects that might not have arisen by chance, thereby offering a new array of "tools" for toxicologic research. Thus a mouse can be designed to express a particular protein or lack of a protein, and traits can be combined in the same animal such as the severe combined immunodeficiency (SCID) mouse. The study of environmental carcinogenesis has been advanced by the availability of an otherwise normal mouse deficient at the *p*53 locus.[97,98]

▸ PRODUCT SUBSTITUTION

Both environmental and industrial toxicology have focused on the development of substitutes for widely used, but unacceptably toxic, chemicals that for various reasons are no longer acceptable. The chlorofluorocarbons (CFCs), used as refrigerants and propellants, have global effects catalyzing the destruction of atmospheric ozone, which resulted in an international agreement to phase out their use. The development of compounds that share their desirable properties and are also nontoxic and environmentally friendly is a major area of research. Likewise, the widely used dry-cleaning fluid tetrachloroethylene is a possible human carcinogen. This has prompted a quest for alternatives, including the use of liquid carbon dioxide.[99]

Chlorine. A highly charged issue is the recommendation that chlorine-containing products be banned. Many of the chlorinated solvents are classified as known or probable human carcinogens. Exposure to chlorination products in drinking water has been linked to small birth weight and head circumference,[100] and to intestinal cancer,[101] although the potency is low and causality is in question.

Organomanganese in Gasoline. The removal of organic lead from gasoline was a major success in applied toxicology. However, its proposed replacement, methylcyclopentadienyl manganese tricarbonyl (MMT) may greatly increase exposure to manganese, itself a potent neurotoxin, that causes a parkinsonian-like syndrome. MMT has been used in Canada since 1977, and urban pigeons have higher levels of manganese than do rural ones, consistent with traffic-related contamination.[102] Widespread use of this compound in gasoline seems bound to repeat the lead-in-gasoline tragedy of the midtwentieth century. In 1997, Canada terminated the use of MMT.

▸ ANIMAL WELFARE AND ANIMAL RIGHTS

Toxicologists have become increasingly attentive to the animal welfare/animal rights movements. Proponents of animal rights argue that animals have intrinsic rights that, in the extreme, should protect them from any and all use in experimental research. Whether "animal rights" are guaranteed by either human or divine "law," is beyond the scope of this chapter. However, animal welfare is clearly an important issue for toxicologists. The Animal Welfare Act (AWA) is administered by the Animal and Plant Health Inspection Service of the U.S. Department of Agriculture. Currently it applies only to mammals, exclusive of mice and rats.

Experimental animals should be spared unnecessary stress, discomfort, or pain. The AWA requires that alternatives to painful procedures be considered. Increasingly, researchers have sought alternative models that do not require whole animals. At the same time, animal research has been redesigned to use fewer animals and to minimize pain and discomfort. The National Science Foundation and National Institutes of Health have recognized the importance of animal welfare not only from a humane perspective but because stressed animals cannot provide an unbiassed response in experimental situations. Accordingly researchers using animals must take into account animal care guidelines, which stipulate the conditions under which animals must be kept and the availability of veterinary care. Research protocols must be reviewed by institutional animal care committees.

The concern over animal welfare reaches its peak when primates are used. Primates are expensive to acquire and maintain, and most studies of primates can afford only a few animals who often live under unnatural and extremely stressful conditions. In addition, since extrapolation from primates to humans is not always more appropriate than extrapolation from other animal models, most toxicology research does not involve primates. Molecular studies are showing significant differences between humans and other primates in the distribution of P-450 enzymes and in their response to xenobiotics.

▸ REGULATING TOXIC EXPOSURES

The past three decades have seen emergence of a complex governmental regulatory framework for toxic chemicals in the environment. Each agency has distinct jurisdiction, and unfortunately there is not always consistency among agencies. Among these agencies and programs are the following:

Food and Drug Administration

This agency is responsible for protecting the integrity of food, drugs, and cosmetics (see Chapter 36) and ensuring that harmful levels of xenobiotics, additives, and adulterants are not present. It sets allowable daily intakes (ADIs) for various chemicals. A major change in the Food Quality Protection Act of 1996 was to increase its coverage of chemicals while setting aside the Delaney Amendment, which forbid any residue of any animal carcinogen in food.

Occupational Safety and Health Administration

Established in 1970 by the Occupational Safety and Health Act, this branch of the U.S. Department of Labor is required to set standards that will protect workers from adverse health consequences (see Chapter 35). The Occupational Safety and Health Administration (OSHA) establishes permissible exposure limits (PELs), to which a worker could be exposed 40 hours a week for a 40-year working lifetime, and short-term exposure limits (STELs), the latter being ceiling values that cannot be exceeded for more than 15 minutes.

Environmental Protection Agency

The Environmental Protection Agency (EPA) has far-flung responsibility for protecting the environment. EPA sets and enforces regulations regarding amount of tolerable pollution and levels of contamination in soil, air, and water. It implements the Federal Insecticide, Fungicide and Rodenticide Act (FIFRA), originally passed in 1947, and the Toxic Substances Control Act (TSCA), originally passed in 1976, as well as Clean Air and Clean Water Acts, and many others. One of the latter acts established the National Toxicology Program and requires EPA to evaluate data on any new chemicals proposed for manufacture and importation.

Department of Transportation

The Transportation Act governs the labeling and handling of hazardous chemicals shipped in interstate commerce. It requires classification and testing of chemicals to determine the type and extent of hazard they might pose in the event of a spill.

Neurobehavioral Toxicity

Nancy Fiedler • Joanna Burger • Michael Gochfeld

The nervous system is a prominent target for many poisons that can cause morphological or functional damage.[1] Classical neurotoxic effects include the depression of central nervous function by anesthetic-like solvents, the weakness from anticholinesterase pesticides, the tremor of chronic mercurialism, or the peripheral neuropathy of lead poisoning. Recent attention has focused on dementia attributed to chronic solvent exposure and on neurodevelopmental disruption and cognitive impairment caused by prenatal exposure to lead and polychlorinated biphenyl (PCBs). Whereas evaluation of nervous system function was formerly the domain of the neurologist and electrophysiologist, neurobehavioral testing offers another dimension of evaluation that is important for several reasons. First, neurobehavioral tests are sensitive to subtle behavioral changes that may occur at doses lower than those required to cause anatomical or physiologic changes or even symptoms that can be observed by the clinician.[2-5] Second, because neurobehavioral toxins can affect the higher levels of function and functional integration essential for complex cognitive processes, neurobehavioral tests offer standardized methods to evaluate these critical and somewhat unique aspects of human behavior.

Although acute effects are often dramatic, the discipline has become increasingly concerned with chronic effects such as impaired learning, memory, vigilance, and depressed psychomotor performance. Persistent behavioral effects can occur as a consequence of acute poisoning or from prolonged exposure to low levels.[6] Neurobehavioral evaluations of exposed individuals or groups provide an opportunity to objectively evaluate the many nonspecific symptoms such as weakness, dizziness, irritability, listlessness, anorexia, depression, disorientation, incoordination, difficulty concentrating, or personality changes, which are sometimes attributed to environmental exposures.

Ultimately toxicity occurs through the interaction of a chemical and a molecular target,[7] yet in neurobehavioral toxicology we often treat the nervous system as a "black box."[1] Lotti[1] notes the frustrating search for morphologic correlates or markers of functional toxicity. In some instances, the molecular approach has been rewarding, although many mechanisms remain elusive. For example, neuropathy target esterase (NTE) was identified as the target for the delayed polyneuropathy associated with organophosphate (OP).[8] However, its physiological function remains unknown, and although the reaction of OPs with NTE is understood, the subsequent cascade leading to the polyneuropathy is unknown.[1] Moreover, the known function of NTE (which allows measurement of its activity) is not related to the likelihood of developing the polyneuropathy.

Similarly, lead alters the sensitivity of the *N*-methyl-D-aspartate (NMDA) receptor complex. Several areas of the brain are rich in NMDA receptors, and the density of receptors varies with time during development. Antagonists of NMDA receptors impair learning in several study designs.[9–11] For example, in birds, NMDA antagonists block the learning of song.[12] The ramifications of this change on imprinting, learning, and memory, which are influenced by the NMDA receptor in certain parts of the brain, are an active area of neurobehavioral research.[13]

While researchers continue the search for mechanisms to explain toxicity at the molecular level, behavioral methods to detect and quantify changes in function from acute and chronic exposure has developed in parallel. For example, in 1973 the National Institute for Occupational Safety and Health (NIOSH) convened a Behavioral Toxicology Workshop for Early Detection of Occupational Hazards,[3] which reviewed research findings on many substances in various organisms and considered the tools that could be applied for evaluation of behavioral toxicity.[2] During the past 15 years, the field has grown rapidly with a variety of experimental paradigms and clinical approaches for detecting behavioral manifestations of neurotoxicity.[14,15] There have been extensive reviews of experimental and clinical findings (see general references) and an entire journal, first published in 1979, is devoted to the field.

In this chapter we review the target components of the nervous system, examples of neurotoxicants, the kinds of behavioral abnormalities seen, and some of the neurobehavioral tests currently used for evaluating such abnormalities.

▶ TARGET COMPONENTS OF THE NERVOUS SYSTEM

Autonomic Nervous System

Toxins structurally similar to neurotransmitters may enhance (agonist) or inhibit (antagonist) the normal function of either the parasympathetic or sympathetic systems. Many widely used drugs have primary or side effects on the autonomic system, and organophosphates interfere with parasympathetic function.

Peripheral Nervous System

Peripheral neuropathies may occur when a xenobiotic kills nerve cells, destroys the axon, or causes myelinopathies. Even subtle damage to the myelin can be detected by nerve conduction velocity studies. Axonopathies involve a dying back of the axon itself (for example, that caused by *n*-hexane). These defects can be detected by electrophysiologists or neuropathologists. Peripheral neuropathies may affect either sensory nerves, motor nerves, or both; usually sensory nerve fibers are most susceptible.[16]

Central Nervous System

The central nervous system (CNS) is the primary domain of neurobehavioral toxicology. Neurotoxic effects in the brain are often complex, with elusive pathologic changes that affect associations among neuronal pathways. Improved histochemical approaches allow pathologists to detect changes in dendritic patterns and interconnections, for example, between two nuclei in the brain as well as the localized destruction of specific types of nerve cells. Many neurobehavioral effects are due to agonistic or antagonistic actions on neurotransmission in the CNS. At the subcellular level, the differential impact of organic and inorganic lead on microtubule assembly suggests an additional mechanism subject to disruption by certain toxins.

Our understanding of how the brain achieves the so-called higher functions (learning, memory, creativity, cognition, etc.) remains primitive. Ablation studies (opportunistic or deliberate) and computer analogy are examples of approaches to understanding brain function. In addition, with the advent of single-photon emission computed tomography (SPECT) and positron emission tomography (PET), functional imaging has revealed the brain structures involved in the performance of various cognitive functions.[17] For example, PET scanning has been used to document encephalopathy due to solvent exposure.[18] There is also a need for fusion among disciplines since, for example, the extensive literature on the neurobehavioral effects of alcohol and hallucinogens could provide important insights applicable to neurobehavioral toxicology.

▶ SELECTED NEUROBEHAVIORAL TOXINS

This section provides a brief overview of neurobehavioral toxicants. (For more detail, see General References.) Many commonly occurring chemicals are neurotoxic. Table 18-3 indicates the variability in effects produced by some common neurotoxicants. For example, carbon monoxide at relatively low levels (equivalent to Carboxy hemoglobin (COHb) < 10 percent) impairs vigilance, tracking, and ability to drive.[19,20]

Virtually all solvents, whether aliphatic or aromatic, chlorinated or not, have acute depressant effects on the nervous system, many of them sharing common anesthetic properties. It is also apparent that there are important chronic effects from solvent exposure apparent both in animals and workers, particularly based on research in Scandinavia.[21–23] Nerve conduction remains altered for many years following cessation of solvent exposure, while memory and learning, mood, impulse control, and motivation are impaired.[24] Long-term exposure causes a toxic encephalopathy with memory and motor deficits. Rats chronically exposed to toluene show permanent deple-

TABLE 18-3. EXAMPLE OF BEHAVIORAL IMPAIRMENTS ASSOCIATED WITH VARIOUS TOXIC SUBSTANCES

Impairments	*Pb*	*As*	*Mn*	*Hg*	*CS_2*	*Solv*	*OPP*
Acute psychosis			+		+		
Emotional lability			+	+	+		
Memory impairment	+	+	+		+		
Psychomotor impairment	+			+	+	+	+
Neurasthenia	+	+	+	+		+	
Extrapyramidal impairment			+		+		
Neuropathy	+	+					
Tremor			+	+	+		

Abbreviations: Pb, lead; As, arsenic; Mn, manganese; Hg, mercury; CS_2, carbon disulfide; Solv, solvents; OPP, organophosphate pesticides.

tion (approximately 16 percent) of neurons in the inferior regions of the hippocampus.[25] Styrene effects have been studied in several occupational groups[26,27] with both specific changes (impaired reaction time and color vision) and more general mood alterations.

Carbon disulfide effects are manifest in almost all components of the central and peripheral nervous systems in humans.[28] Evidence of peripheral neuropathy (paresthesia, numbness), cranial neuropathy, dementia (confusion), parkinsonism, acute psychoses, irritability, and memory loss have been attributed to this compound.[29,30]

Many metals, for example, lead, mercury, manganese, and arsenic, are also neurotoxic, but these tend to have discrete nervous system effects (Table 18-4). The species of metal influences its impact. Thus organic tin compounds cause weakness and paralysis as well as central disturbances. Organic arsenic affects the optic nerve and retina, while inorganic arsenic produces polyneuritis and weakness. Tremors, and in severe cases ataxia, occur with either inorganic or organic mercury poisoning; however, organic mercury also produces visual field changes, while inorganic mercury produces personality disturbances characterized as "erethism." This syndrome involves irritability, labile temper, pathologic shyness (avoiding close friends), depression, loss of sleep, fatigue, and blushing. In some cases there is even a dose-response curve between the occurrence of symptoms and the concentration of mercury in urine. Methyl mercury disrupts both the mature and the developing central nervous system, interfering with visual, auditory, and somatosensory function.[31] Exposed rats developed specific antibodies to neurotypic and gliotypic proteins and had reduced glial fibrillary acid protein in their cortex. Pathologic changes include neuronal degeneration and demyelination and an increase in astroglia with accumulation of methyl mercury.[32]

A more esoteric compound is MPTP (1-methyl-4-phenyl-1,2,3,6-tetrahydropyridine), a synthetic substance produced accidentally in the attempted synthesis of meperidine analogs by substance abusers. A metabolite of MPTP damages the dopaminergic cells of the substantia nigra, leading to irreversible parkinsonian symptoms.[33] This discovery is considered "one of the most important achievements in neurotoxicology of the last twenty years."[1] In addition many psychoactive chemicals both licit and illicit, including ethanol and hallucinogens, have their primary effects on neurobehavioral performance.

Lead has been the most extensively studied.[34,35] It is universally deleterious to the developing nervous system. Ultrastructural studies show altered axonal development and dendritic deployment with fewer neural connections, leading among other things to impaired cognition and concentration. This is associated with deficiency in expression of a specific nerve growth-associated protein (GAP-43). Perinatal and postnatal exposure to lead resulted in depressed mRNA levels for GAP-43 in rats.[36]

In several studies prenatal exposure to certain PCB isomers has been implicated in causing impaired neurobehavioral and cognitive development in babies and young children. Despite controversy, the evidence appears to be consistent using several populations and evaluation techniques[37–39] (see Behavioral Teratology below).

▶ BIOCHEMICAL MECHANISMS

The "black box," or phenomenological, approach to neurobehavioral toxicology has its limitations.

New advances in molecular and cell biology and biochemistry are elucidating many aspects of brain function that will facilitate making predictions and designing of new tests. An important benefit is to enhance interpretation of behavioral toxicology studies. Advances in molecular biology will suggest new populations to study and will provide new biomarkers to validate exposures.

Neurotransmitters

Neurobehavioral toxicology is intimately dependent on advances in understanding neurotransmitter function, which go beyond the role of transducing nerve impulses. The behavioral abnormalities attributed to low-level lead exposure may involve, in part, alterations in dopaminergic transmission,[40–42] while learning deficits from lead are related to glutamic transmitters.[43] Also, lead may have a more global effect on the release of several neurotransmitters by altering calcium homeostasis.[44]

Nitric oxide, an intracellular messenger, is formed from L-arginine by the enzyme nitric oxide synthase (NOS), found in many tissues including brain, where it is constitutive rather than inducible. It modulates the secretion of hormones such as adrenocorticotropic hormone (ACTH) and is in turn regulated by estrogen, which enhances the expression of mRNA for NOS in parts of the brain (e.g., ventromedial nucleus of the hypothalamus) rich in estrogen receptors.[45] This may be one of several mechanisms by which hormones modulate behavior.

5-Hydroxytryptamine (serotonin) research covers very broad areas directly central to neurobehavioral toxicology. Various receptor systems such as opioid receptor antagonists and agonists are under investigation for their control of serotonin synthesis and release.[46] This is known to be important in influencing mood.

Neuropeptides

An exciting area of neurobiology is the study of neuropeptides such as substance P, neurokinin A, thyrotropin-releasing hormone,

TABLE 18-4. AVAILABILITY OF NORMATIVE DATA (VALIDATED ON LARGE NORMAL AND NONNORMAL POPULATIONS) FOR VARIOUS NEUROBEHAVIORAL TESTS

Test	*Function*	*Validation Status*
Visual reaction time	Psychomotor	
Auditory reaction time	Psychomotor	
Santa Ana	Psychomotor	
Grooved pegboard	Psychomotor	
WAIS subtests		
Digit-Symbol	Perception/encoding	
Digit Span, Auditory	Memory	
Vocabulary and Comprehension	Cognitive verbal	
Block Design	Cognitive nonverbal	
California Verbal Learning Test	Cognitive verbal	
Benton Retention Test	Memory	
Embedded figures	Perception profile of mood states	
Mood/affect		
SCL-90	Mood affect	

and neuropeptide Y. Their functions, distribution, and control of synthesis and breakdown are an active area of research. For example, neuropeptide Y is a vasoconstrictor peptide found in sympathetic nerve terminals and the adrenal medulla as well as in the plasma.[47] A variety of stressors, including possibly xenobiotics, may influence its levels; its role in modulating behavior requires study.

Receptor Biology

Although the understanding of specific receptors for bioactive agents is not new, there have been great technical advances in ability to probe for the presence and upregulation or downregulation of specific receptors on various cell populations. Estrogen receptor studies illustrate how hormones can regulate neurotransmitters in the brain.[45] A family of receptors responsive to endogenous and exogenous opioids have been detected. They are coupled to a protein (G-protein), use adenylate cyclase as a second messenger, and regulate neurobehavioral function by altering electrolyte fluxes. Among these receptors the μ and δ receptors open potassium channels, while activation of K receptors close calcium channels.[48]

Thyrotropin-Releasing Hormone

Certain cells of the hypothalamus contain thyroid hormone receptors that, when activated, regulate gene expression of various proteins that mediate the hormone effect on the nervous system development.[49] These may play a role in behavioral teratology.

Nerve Growth Factors

In 1986 Montacalcini and Cohen received the Nobel Price for discovering growth factors that influence the differentiation of nerve cells. The mechanism by which growth factors are regulated and how they in turn "control" cell differentiation and ultimately behavior are being investigated using transgenic animals that lack particular receptors.[50] This is becoming an important tool in neurotoxicology and will provide new models for studying behavior.

► ANIMAL MODELS IN NEUROBEHAVIORAL TOXICITY

Animal research contributes significantly to our understanding of neurotoxicity and neurobehavioral changes. No animal model adequately mimics the complex neurobehavioral performance of humans, particularly in the intellectual domain. Although gorillas and chimpanzees appear to behave similarly to humans in some respects and are genetically very close to humans, our evolutionary divergence is particularly apparent in those functions that are the domain of the neurobehaviorist. Several researchers have employed primates to provide insights into human behavioral toxicology,[31,41,51] but primate research is extremely expensive, and many of the species used in research are threatened or endangered in the wild. Moreover, for wide-ranging, highly social species such as primates, captivity, and particularly restraint, may produce a chronic level of stress, which itself interferes with all aspects of behavior.

Many important advances in understanding brain function have been derived from studies on avian and rodent models. Rodent studies allow large sample sizes to be employed, while avian studies take advantage of the fact that, like humans, birds rely primarily on visual and acoustic rather than olfactory or tactile communication. The fact that a chemical produces the same effect on learning, for example, in a wide variety of animal species is important validation of its role in humans. Eye-limb coordination, cerebellar function, and even learning are common to all vertebrates, and even cognition may be identified in many so-called "lower" organisms.[52] In recognition of the important contribution of animal behavior studies to shaping our understanding of human behavior,[53] three pioneers of animal behavior research, Konrad Lorenz, Niko Tinbergen, and Karl von Frisch were awarded the Nobel Prize in biology and medicine in 1973.

Animal experimentation also provides the opportunity to assess exposures and effects that cannot be studied in humans. Developing species-appropriate test batteries is an exciting challenge for behavioral toxicologists.[54–56] Animal studies have focused on discrimination of stimuli, learning deficits, disturbance of locomotion or balance, decreased performance of previously learned tasks, memory deficits, altered activity patterns, and changes in normal behavior patterns related to reproduction or maintenance. A wide variety of paradigms have been employed to understand the effects of stresses on the nervous system, and many of these can be applied to humans. In addition, some research has examined how the neurobehavioral effects of a toxic chemical or physical stressors can be exhibited in offspring of the exposed individual.

Learning Tasks

Experimental intervention allows specific probes of behavior and performance. Early testing employed Y mazes and other learned visual discrimination tasks. Experiments with rats and mice examined how toxins affect the speed of learning a maze after a reward or punishment was offered in one or the other arms.[57,58] Learning impairment offers an valuable paradigm. Animals are treated with drugs or other chemicals before or after a learning situation or conditioning stimulus to see whether subsequent performance is enhanced or impaired. Injection of glucose enhances, and injection of insulin impairs, learning of foot-shock avoidance tasks.[59]

Memory

Passive avoidance training allows investigation of substances that effect a calcium-calmodulin–dependent protein kinase in the same forebrain nuclei. Kinase activity increases within 10 minutes after training. Antagonistic drugs cause amnesia.[60]

Imprinting

Many young animals form an attachment to a parent or other individual whom they see, hear, or smell shortly after birth. This "imprinting" behavior is pronounced in a variety of birds, and the ability of various chemicals to impair the imprinting behavior has been studied. Imprinting depends on *N*-methyl-D-aspartate receptors in the forebrain, where antagonistic drugs reduce imprinting behavior.[61] NMDA antagonists block olfactory imprinting in rats.[62]

Parental Recognition

An important function of imprinting is the ability to recognize parents and relatives to gain food or protection and avoid aggression from strangers. Since this behavior has direct survival value, it can be used to test the relevance of effects of neurotoxic chemicals. Lead-exposed herring gull chicks have poor discrimination and longer latency for choosing between a parental surrogate and a stranger[63] and these effects differ depending on the stage of exposure.

Conditioning Studies

In studies involving conditioning of psychomotor performance, animals are trained to perform tasks in response to certain stimuli. They are then exposed to a substance, and the disruption of performance is quantified.[54,64] With time, the behavioral tests have become more sophisticated and now include such paradigms as nonspatial and spatial delayed matching to a sample, serial position sequences, and multiple fixed-interval reinforcement tests in animals previously trained with operant conditioning.[51,54,65–67] These studies examined learned behavior and relied on the production of the desired behavior, followed by measurement of its sensitivity to environmental stimuli.[54] Alterations in visual performance can be useful endpoints in conditioned animals.[68] The great advantage of these methods is that they can detect subtle differences in behavior of animals that otherwise appear normal; however, they do require experience in the operant conditioning techniques.

Discrimination Conditioning

Animals can be conditioned to respond differentially to a variety of stimuli and the effects of various substances on this ability offers a sensitive test. This conditioning has been expanded to more relevant neurotransmitters, and animals can be trained to discriminate these from saline.[13]

Intracerebral Injection

In combination with stereotactic techniques and histochemical studies of the brain, the localized injection of agonist and antagonistic chemicals into specific regions of the brain is contributing to the understanding of localization of behavioral functions, and conversely, as functions are localized, it becomes feasible to test many new substances for specific agonist or antagonist activity. For example, serotonin inhibits the premating lordosis behavior of female rodents by acting on 5-hydroxytryptamine 1A receptors, but it enhances the same behavior at 2A/2C receptors. The relative activity of these receptor classes varies during the estrous cycle.[69]

Naturalistic Studies

Naturalistic observations of behavior conducted in the laboratory and in the field employ behaviors that occur naturally in the organisms (for example, locomotion, balance, or predator defense).[55,70] In many of these studies the toxic agent, such as lead, interferes with learning or learning-retention and the subsequent performance of learned tasks.

Under natural conditions, animals have somewhat predictable or stereotyped ways of behaving that can be quantified. Such behaviors may be directly relevant to their survival and successful reproduction. Toxics that affect such behavior can have far-reaching effects on fitness. Some behaviors examined including pecking accuracy and pecking rate of pigeons,[71] activity rates in mice,[72,73] nest site defense in falcons,[74] monkey behavior,[75] dove courtship sequences,[76] begging behavior and food manipulation in terns,[55] and web-weaving in spiders.[77] In most of these studies the effect was clearly demonstrable by directly observing individuals.

The advantage of the naturalistic behaviors is that the behaviors are important for fitness and have been shaped and perhaps optimized by evolution. Thus predator avoidance is a natural part of an animal's behavioral repertoire while pushing a button may not be. Conversely, operant conditioning paradigms afford tighter control of experimental situations. Yet natural behaviors such as locomotion,[56] exploration, righting ability, depth perception, thermoregulation, aggression, avoidance,[55] learning, and parental recognition are all amenable to laboratory and field experimentation where variables can be controlled.[55,78] Such naturalistic experiments with herring gulls injected with lead in the wild indicated that the effects that were observed were similar and as severe as results in the laboratory. Recovery was quicker and parental behavior partially ameliorated behavioral deficits to allow the chicks partial recovery of cognitive function.[70]

While most neurotoxicology studies on animals examine the direct effect of exposure, some multigeneration studies have yielded important results,[79,80] showing that the offspring and even grandchildren of treated animals may manifest behavioral deficits. Exposure of one or both parents can affect behavior in offspring. If both parents are exposed, the impact is greater than if either one is exposed alone.[79]

It seems reasonable to conclude that animal behavioral models will continue to be useful for understanding many aspects of behavioral toxicology, for developing useful questions and approaches for clinical application, and for validating generalizations developed in humans. Conversely, for some of the higher functions, humans will remain the primary test subjects and improved epidemiologic studies employing both old and new psychometric approaches will be fruitful. These must be opportunistic, recognizing exposures that have already occurred, while the animal models will allow the use of controlled exposures and testing of new paradigms.

► SYSTEMATIC EVALUATION OF THE NERVOUS SYSTEM

Sensory Systems

Earlier literature evaluating the effects of neurotoxicants on human behavior focused mainly on aspects of higher cognitive function. However, more recently, behavioral tests of sensory systems have been included as indicators sensitive to subtle neurologic effects.[81] The following discussion offers an overview of these sensory systems and tests to evaluate the effects of neurotoxicants.

Vision

Neuroophthalmologists, neurologists, and ophthalmologists examine the eyes and visual system for evidence of damage. Visual evoked potentials use electroencephalographic techniques to measure brain wave responses to light. Neurobehaviorists test such functions as visual perception, color vision, and eye-hand coordination. Direct perceptual changes include loss of visual acuity, alteration of visual fields, changes in color sensitivity, contrast sensitivity, and critical flicker fusion. For example, Mergler and colleagues reported loss of color vision and contrast sensitivity among workers exposed chronically to organic solvent mixtures.[82,83] Neuro-optic pathways are vulnerable to the effects of styrene which impair color discrimination. Although the current threshold limit value for styrene is 50 ppm, visual impairment can be detected at only 4 ppm (with the 95 percent confidence limit at 26 ppm).[27] This color vision loss is dose-dependent.[84] Loss begins with the distal retinal layers and progresses to the proximal layers and then the optic nerve.[85]

Reduced fusion threshold on critical flicker fusion was observed among lead-exposed workers.[86] Valciukas and Singer[87] emphasized the utility of testing complex perceptual tasks using the embedded figures, a task in which familiar objects are embedded in a confusing background. These different approaches thus evaluate the ability to direct the eyes, the receptive capability of the eye itself, and ultimately the ability of the brain to process and respond to information transmitted from the eye.

Hearing

Hearing evaluation is a necessary precursor to neurobehavioral testing since many tests rely on hearing for accurate performance. As with the eye, some tests evaluate the external receptor, while others determine the response of the brain to sound. Certain neurotoxic chemicals, for instance the antibiotics streptomycin and kanamycin, damage the auditory nerve pathway. More subtle changes in our ability to detect loudness, pitch, and timbre are the domain of the psychoacoustician and in special cases can be evaluated as part of a neurobehavioral assessment.

The working environment of those who are routinely exposed to neurotoxicants often includes exposure to noise, which may result in damage to the sensory cells of the inner ear. Also, neurotoxicants may directly interfere with hearing through effects on the central or peripheral nervous system. Morata et al.[88] suggested that noise and organic solvents such as carbon disulfide, toluene, and trichloroethylene may interact to produce hearing loss and perceptual impairments.

Olfaction

Unlike virtually all other mammals, humans rely relatively little on olfaction to find their food or detect danger. Unlike moths, which can locate a potential mate from a few molecules of a pheromone emitted a kilometer away, humans rely primarily on sight and sound for communication with mates. Nonetheless, olfaction has been shown to influence human appetite and sexual development,[89] and we are capable of distinguishing the odor of our mates from those of other individuals. Disruption in the olfactory sense either due to loss of olfaction (hyposmia or anosmia), hypersensitivity to odors, or persistent bad odors (cacosmia) has been associated with exposure to neurotoxicants.

For example, two studies of solvent-exposed workers showed discrepant results. One study of paint-manufacturing workers[90] documented decrements in the sense of smell following exposure to solvents, while the other study of clinic patients who attributed symptoms to solvents found heightened sensitivity and increased symptoms.[91] This apparent discrepancy may be accounted for by the different methodologies used to assess sensory changes. The first study tested odor discrimination objectively with the University of Pennsylvania Smell Identification Test (UPSIT),[92] while the second used self-report of hypersensitivity to assess sensory changes. The UPSIT, a multiple choice scratch and sniff test, evaluates the ability to correctly identify odors as a screen for normosmia.[92] Odor threshold testing has also been used to test unusual sensitivities to odors among patients reporting enhanced ability to detect chemical odors.[93] Exposure to metals, for example cadmium, also raises olfactory thresholds (decreases sensitivity).[94]

Taste

Although the food industry conducts extensive subjective research on tastes, there is little objective literature on the impact of chemicals on taste sensitivity. Many chemicals have specific "tastes," while others seem to induce abnormal tastes such as the metallic taste that characterizes lead poisoning (but is not a lead taste) and the garliclike taste that occurs with selenium but is not a selenium taste. There is a close linkage between olfaction and taste, albeit different peripheral receptors, and diminished olfactory sensitivity or discrimination will interfere with taste. Taste actually lends itself to objective study more readily than olfaction since one can control and determine the concentration of a substance in solution more easily than in air.

Touch

Physical examination of light touch and pain sensation and of temperature and two-point discrimination can be elaborate and time consuming, but in the hands of an experienced neurologist can detect subtle nervous system malfunction. However, evaluation of touch is actually quite complex. In addition to skin receptors, there are receptors in underlying tissues and muscle. Other tests are described in standard physical diagnosis textbooks and are a part of the sensory perceptual examination performed by a trained neuropsychologist.[95]

Vibration

Vibratory sensation appears to be quite sensitive to peripheral nerve damage.[96] Recent attempts to quantify vibratory sensation with a variety of devices have had substantial success in several workplace settings.[97,98] The subject presses a fingertip or toe against the detector and indicates when a vibration is felt. The amplitude and frequency of the vibration can be adjusted to determine the subject's threshold. The pressure applied by the patient potentially confounds the measurement, however, and use of a physical device to control the pressure applied compensates for this. Specific protocols for evaluating vibration thresholds are available through the manual from the Agency for Toxic Substances and Disease Registry (ATSDR).[81]

Temperature

Ability to discriminate slight changes in temperature is also affected by chemical exposure. Devices that provide objective control of temperature, combined with a forced-choice paradigm, allow the clinician or researcher to evaluate this modality.[97]

Position Sense

The dorsal columns of the spinal cord carry information on position to the brain and the sensorimotor system compensates by adjusting tone. Tests for sway,[99] straight-line walking, and the Romberg tests are traditional ways of measuring the performance of these tasks. In addition to testing position sense, these test are dependent on intact motor and vestibular functions.

Motor Function

Neuromuscular function provides the organism with its main modes of manipulating its environment or manipulating itself within its environment. Motor deficits may be due to muscle disease, disorders of the motor cortex or pathways, changes in the reflex pathways controlling tone, or central disorders (cerebellum, basal ganglia), which interfere with both volition, fine tuning, and coordination of motor function.

A physical examination can detect changes in muscle mass (particularly asymmetry) and physical weakness. Behavioral tests focus on the motor system as a manifestation of central function, for example, in terms of reaction time (see below), rapid alternating movements, and fine muscle control. Many compounds that produce acute intoxication (i.e., alcohol) affect sensory-motor function, producing alterations of gait and posture. Some neurotoxicants affect motor nerves, leading to reduced strength, coordination, and fine muscle control. Loss of ability to perform previously learned motor sequences, apraxias, may be an indication of neurotoxicity, and some of the animal paradigms appear directly analogous to this deficit.

Vestibular Function

The labyrinth and vestibular apparatus provides for maintenance of equilibrium and awareness of position. It senses the position of the eyes and head and reflexly controls tone in the limbs and body. Its function depends on the saccular and utricular macules that sense linear acceleration of the head and the semicircular canals, which sense angular acceleration. Visual and proprioceptive impulses also feed this system. Disruption of either the sensory components or the central vestibular function can cause dizziness and vertigo. Certain neurotoxicants such as ethanol and organic solvents[100] can have a specific impact on this system. Postural sway was impaired among workers exposed to formaldehyde.[101] A sway test is a gross procedure that evaluates the intactness of vestibular function as well as the proprioceptive inputs.

Basal Ganglia

The basal ganglia and cerebellum constitute the extrapyramidal motor system, often a target of toxic chemicals. The functional relationships of the basal ganglia to the striatum and cerebral cortex are described in standard texts. Damage to these ganglia or the cortico-striatal-pallidal-thalamic-cortical loop are associated with a variety of disorders including ataxias, tremors, akinesia or dyskinesia, athetosis, dystonia, and myoclonus. This system is characterized by the variety of neurotransmitters (e.g., γ-aminobutyric acid (GABA), dopamine) associated with particular functional components. Toxic damage by MPTP to the substantia nigra, for example, is known to produce parkinsonism.[33] Selected neurobehavioral tests of fine motor function may detect early damage to this system.

Cerebellar Function

The cerebellum refines motor function and contributes to balance, posture and tone, repetitive movement, coordination, and spatial location. Gross cerebellar dysfunction is manifest as staggering gait, swaying or stumbling, ataxias involving movements of specific limbs in which the timing of contraction of antagonistic muscle groups is disrupted, and loss of controlled rapid alternating movements, dysdiadochokinesia.

Personality, Mood, and Affect

A number of epidemiologic studies indicate that overall personality changes may be important manifestations of neurobehavioral toxicity. Erethism attributable to inorganic mercury (see above) is probably the classic example of this. Mood changes associated with solvents[102,103] and classroom behavior attributed to lead[104] are additional examples where mood and personality in general may be altered, without necessarily showing specific focal changes.

Cognitive Evaluation

Complete neurobehavioral examination is an interdisciplinary endeavor requiring the participation of the physician, psychologist, and electrophysiologist. A complete examination will include an interview, a physical examination, and one or more neurobehavioral tests, supplemented where necessary by electrophysiology.

Interview

The interview provides the examiner with an important opportunity to observe the mood, affect, and behavior of the individual. This can be supplemented by a structured psychiatric interview such as the Diagnostic Interview Survey or the Structured Clinical Interview for the DSM and mental status examination.[105] The interview allows one to explore the contribution of "organic" and "psychologic" pathology and to detect anxiety, depression, changes in intellectual function, and other performance.

Neurobehavioral Testing

In the presence of uncertainty, a major rationale for neurobehavioral testing is the prevailing assumption that subtle behavioral changes in cognitive function may be the most sensitive indicator of exposure to toxics.[4] Moreover, there is the increasing recognition that levels of exposure formerly thought safe or unlikely to produce health effects are now known to have far-reaching consequences on important behavioral functions. Most evident among these is the impact of low-level lead exposure on hyperactivity and intellectual development in children.[106]

Just as liver function tests can measure cell damage, conjugation, or metabolic ability, so neurobehavioral tests have distinct target functions. These include vigilance, time and accuracy of perception and task performance, simple and complex reaction times, visual-motor coordination, and intellectual function such as vocabulary and arithmetic skills, attention/concentration, memory, learning, and abstract thinking processes.

Psychometric Tests in Neurobehavioral Evaluation

Although an interview and a mental status examination can detect many gross changes, psychometric tests are useful to extend the sensitivity of the examination by detecting and quantifying subclinical effects. Psychometric tests for which there is a long history of validation and a database of normative data can be particularly useful in evaluating an individual. Many new tests, lacking such normative data, may be difficult to interpret on an individual basis, but may be useful in large-scale screenings or epidemiologic studies.

The following is a discussion of the core functions that potentially need to be assessed if a patient is exposed to neurotoxicants. There are many tests in the literature. Those cited as illustrative of various functions are those that have normative data to allow interpretation of an individual's performance. Unlike statistical group comparisons in a research context, individual assessment of dysfunction is dependent upon having a standard against which an individual's performance can be compared, either an individual baseline or group norms. For example, if an individual's performance on a test of a particular function is markedly lower (e.g., two or more standard deviations below the mean) than that of comparable peers (e.g., similar age, sex, race, and socioeconomic status), the clinician may suspect deficits due to exposure. Confronted by a poor test performance, the clinician must ascertain that the standard against which the individual is being compared is reasonably similar to the individual patient's demographic profile. It is particularly necessary to be alert to cultural and language biases of these tests.

A number of investigators and clinicians have developed neurobehavioral test batteries.[81,106,107] In general, these batteries include tests representative of several basic functions necessary for higher-order cognitive functioning. While the specific tests to assess each area may differ, the basic areas to be covered are consistent. In an effort to standardize assessment of neurobehavioral function internationally, the World Health Organization has recommended a core battery of functions and tests. These core functions include psychomotor, cognitive nonverbal, cognitive verbal, memory/learning, perceptual speed, and mood.[108] Tests are categorized as representative of a particular function, but a given test often involves more than one function. For example, reaction time is a basic skill that underlies performance on more complex tests. Thus, if a patient's reaction time is slowed, this will interfere with the ability to perceive and respond to more complex tests involving memory or construction of complex figures.[95]

Overall Intellectual Ability

Tests of cognitive verbal ability are generally more familiar to the patient and include such tests as vocabulary and comprehension (e.g., revised Wechsler Adult Intelligence Scale (WAIS-R)[109]). These tests are regarded as most resistant to the effects of neurotoxicants since they reflect abilities that are well-rehearsed and long-standing.[110] If an individual's verbal abilities have declined significantly, this usually reflects serious or chronic damage. Such deficits can occur with significant head injury or stroke but generally not with exposure to neurotoxicants unless the latter has occurred over a number of years at significant levels[111] producing a well-defined dementia such as "painter's syndrome."[108] Thus, the patient's performance on a vocabulary test is frequently used in the absence of information about premorbid function, as an estimate of premorbid ability. While this is a standard in the literature, a recent investigation directly comparing actual premorbid and current vocabulary scores revealed that exposures to neurotoxicants may have a more significant impact on tests of highly practical skills (e.g., vocabulary) than previously assumed.[112] Tests of cognitive nonverbal functions are generally more complex and reflect ability not related to verbal skills such as the Raven's Progressive Matrices.[113] These tests are useful in situations where estimates of ability, unbiased by verbal skills, are needed.

Psychomotor Functions

Psychomotor function requires integration of sensory perceptual processes, such as vision or hearing, with motor responses. For example, a test of simple reaction time in response to a visual or auditory cue provides the simplest method for assessing psychomotor function. The patient is instructed to press a button (motor response) as quickly as possible following the presentation of a visual or an auditory stimulus. The time between presentation of the stimuli is varied and may affect performance. At a more complex level, a patient may be asked to place pegs into holes as quickly as possible,[114] a task requiring more motor skill than reaction time. Tests of psychomotor function have consistently been among the most sensitive indicators of deficits due to neurotoxicants.[110] A test frequently shown to be sensitive to the effects of neurotoxicants is the Digit Symbol subtest of the WAIS-R.[109] The patient records symbols with their corresponding number according to a key while being timed. While memory substantially aids performance, it is not necessary since the key is always present. Studies of neurotoxicants such as solvents and lead have shown significantly reduced performance on this test.[115]

Attention/Concentration

A precursor to performance on neurobehavioral tasks is the ability to scan the environment, orient to the appropriate stimulus, and sustain attention to a task, with more complex tasks requiring relatively greater levels of sustained attention. Neurotoxicants can disrupt this ability as demonstrated with such tests as Digit Span of the WAIS-R in which the individual is asked to repeat an increasing string of digits (Digits Forward) or to reverse the digits (Digits Backward) immediately following their verbal presentation.[113] Trials A and B, in which the individual connects numbers or numbers and letters in sequence, tests psychomotor skills, visual attentiveness, and the ability to shift sets under time pressure. Simple reaction time also measures attention and is highly sensitive to the effects of neurotoxicants.[110]

Tests of vigilance require sustained attention over relatively longer periods of time such as for continuous performance tests in which the individual responds to a specific target flashed among similar nontarget stimuli. Vigilance tasks are sensitive to low-level effects of alcohol[116,117] and to the interaction of neurotoxicants, fatigue, and variation in the interstimulus interval.

Memory and Learning

Tests of memory/learning assess a patient's short-term memory by presenting stimuli (e.g., words, digits, pictures) visually or auditorially and asking the patient either to recall or recognize these stimuli immediately or after 30 minutes. The California Verbal Learning Test involves the presentation of a string of words that the patient is asked to recall.[118] For other memory tests, pictures of abstract drawings or actual objects are presented to the subject, who must then reproduce these drawings from memory (e.g., Benton Retention Test[119]). Short-term memory loss is one of the most frequent clinical complaints of patients exposed to neurotoxicants,[99] and it has frequently been substantiated in studies of neurobehavioral deficits due to solvents, lead, mercury, and pesticides.[113] If a patient's performance on a short-term memory task is well below his or her general ability as assessed by a vocabulary test, then complaints of memory problems may be substantiated.

Mood and Affect

Patients exposed to neurotoxicants often complain of mood changes including being depressed, anxious, and irritable. While a number of instruments document these complaints and compare an individual patient's level to a normative group, the cause of these symptoms cannot be ascertained. That is, such symptoms may be secondary to other cognitive deficits or may be a primary effect of exposure to neurotoxicants. The Profile of Mood States[120] and the Symptom Checklist-90[121] both document levels of mood disturbance. The factors to which these symptoms can be attributed requires a clinical assessment of other potential agents and/or stressors in an individual's life that could be causing mood disturbance.

Temporal Properties of Performance

One of the most subtle measures of neurobehavioral deficits is a slowing in function. While peripheral neuropathies are characterized by slowing of nerve impulse conduction, it is the slowing of central functions that are evaluated in neurobehavioral testing. Whether this can be thought of as an "increased resistance" in the central nervous system, or the need for adaptation wherein alternative pathways are sought for particular functions, is a subject for future research. It is not known whether cells die, interconnections shrink or wither, or biochemical communication is inhibited, but probably all of these mechanisms apply.

Computerized Test Batteries

In the late 1970s, researchers recognized the potential of computers to challenge the nervous system in a repeatable, objective fashion and to score performance in real time. The emergence of neurobehavioral toxicology has coincided with the ascendancy of the microcomputer, and it is no surprise that some of the early developments in neurobehavioral testing have relied heavily on the computer.[15] Many traditional psychometric tests have been adapted for computer application. The advantages of the computer are (*a*) consistency of application, (*b*) reduced need for highly trained testors, and (*c*) automatic recording of data in real time. Disadvantages have been (*a*) logistic considerations such as unreliable hardware and software and capital costs for purchasing several computers, (*b*) many target populations not being computer literate, (*c*) lack of motivation and stimulation provided by a live examiner and loss of opportunity to observe performance, and (*d*) lack of normative data.

▶ BEHAVIORAL TERATOLOGY

The developing nervous system undergoes dramatic growth and expansion of function, not only prior to birth, but throughout the first decade of life. Anatomical changes such as increasing myelinization occur during the first years of life, and associations are formed that make possible complex motor patterns, fine-tuning of coordination, concept formation, pattern recognition, and more highly learned tasks such as speech and communication. For some tasks such as learning language there appear to be "critical periods" during which learning proceeds more rapidly and effectively. Animals or humans that are isolated from speakers during the critical period may find it difficult or impossible to learn speech at a later time. There may be critical periods for development of other functions as well.[122] As organisms mature, their locomotory ability, learning, and knowledge should increase appropriately for their age. There is increasing evidence that even low-level chemical exposure may have profound impact on the orderly acquisition of nervous system function. The magnitude of such changes is not fully appreciated, and the field of behavioral teratology is in a rapid growth phase.

Lead and Child Development

Probably the best documented behavioral teratology is associated with lead. At blood lead levels formerly thought innocuous (i.e., below 25 μg/dL), children may still show depressed intellectual development,[123] and more subtle effects may occur at levels below 15 μg/dL. Elementary school children with higher body burdens of lead were rated by their teachers as being more easily distracted, less persistent, less independent and organized, more hyperactive and impulsive, more easily frustrated, and showing poorer overall functioning, compared with children in the lower lead groups.[104] Needleman et al.'s study shows remarkable dose-response relationships between dentine-lead levels and poor school ratings. Children with higher lead did more poorly on verbal and digit span components of IQ tests.[104]

Animal Studies of PCBs

It has long been known that PCBs interfere with locomotion and learning in rodents[124] and with learning and cognition in monkeys.[125] Interference with cellular metabolism, neurotransmitters, and thyroid hormone also have been proposed.[126,127]

Epidemiologic Studies of PCBs

Several epidemiologic studies have assessed neurobehavioral deficits in populations exposed to PCBs and related compounds.[128] There is evidence of developmental neurotoxicity including low IQ, from the Japanese Yusho Incident, involving prenatal exposure to PCBs and furans.[129] Several years later a similar event, the Yu-Cheng Incident in Taiwan, resulted in heavy PCB exposure (exceeding 1 g in some cases). Children born to exposed mothers had multiple defects at birth and showed developmental delays and lowered performance on neurological examination and standard tests of cognition. The fact that these abnormalities did not correlate well with measures of postbirth maternal exposure[130] illustrates the importance of measuring fetal exposure in determining neurodevelopmental defects. Linkage to a persistent chemical is evidenced by the poor performance of children born to exposed mothers more than 6 years after the exposure.[131]

Jacobson and colleagues studied babies born to women who ate PCB-contaminated fish from the Great Lakes. Some of these women had elevated serum and milk PCB levels, and their babies showed impaired neurobehavioral development,[132] which has persisted for several years. Some of the abnormalities are predicted by cord serum PCB levels.[133] Rogan and Gladen studied 931 children of mothers who did not, as a group, have unusually high PCB exposure. Children with higher prenatal PCB exposure at birth were more likely to be hypotonic and hyporeflexic and showed poorer psychomotor performance on the Bayley Scales. These changes were not related to postnatal PCB exposure.[134] These differences did not persist after age 5.[135]

The Oswego Newborn and Infant Development project examined the behavioral effects in human newborns, infants, and children of mothers who had consumed fish from Lake Ontario.[136] Fish from this lake are contaminated with a wide range of toxic chemicals, including PCBs, dioxin, dieldrin, lindane, chlordane, cadmium, mercury, and mirex. Newborns were classified into high, medium, and low maternal exposure groups and were tested on the Neonatal Behavioral Assessment Scale in their 1st and 2nd day after birth. The groups did not differ demographically, but after many confounders were eliminated, the high-exposure babies showed a greater number of abnormal reflexes and less mature autonomic responses than babies in the other groups. This confirms Jacobson et al.'s original findings.[132] This study also found a dose-response relationship between fish consumption and decreased habituation to mildly aversive stimuli and is similar to results found in laboratory rats fed Lake Ontario salmon.[137]

▸ CONFOUNDERS OF BEHAVIORAL PERFORMANCE

Neurobehavioral evaluation requires the concentration and cooperation of the subject, yet these behaviors too may be diminished in chemical-exposed individuals. Interpretation of test results in the individual must take into account a variety of confounders that are only briefly mentioned here. Many of the confounders have a *global* effect, that is, they interfere with all aspects of performance rather than with particular subtests. Subjects who have a high level of anxiety may find it difficult to concentrate on complex tasks, particularly on tests of vigilance. Lack of familiarity with the test context or with the expectations, particularly if the testing is not conducted in one's first language, will certainly interfere with performance. Subjects who believe they are being evaluated for poisoning may be hesitant about participating in so many "psychologic" tests that may suggest that the examiners don't believe their complaints are "real."

Physical Condition

Lack of sleep, drowsiness, a recent full meal, or recent use of drugs, alcohol, or tobacco may also have global effects on performance. Examiners should elicit subjective evaluations of wakefulness and should carefully observe the subject. A pretest questionnaire should determine the time at which alcohol, cigarettes, or specific medications were used. Unrelated illnesses may affect performance. Diabetes or other metabolic states may interfere with alertness. Dementias due to other causes such as head injuries will complicate interpretation of test results.

Learning and Experience

Learning poses an additional confounding problem in interpreting neurobehavioral tests, particularly when tests are to be repeated in a prospective study. The time interval between testing, the individual subject's learning ability, and the test's complexity will alter the learning curve or practice effect of repeat testing. This phenomenon needs to be quantified to interpret accurately changes in test performance over time. One method to deal with practice effects is to provide practice sessions for all tests to reduce the impact of a learning curve. Familiarity with computers enhances performance on the computerized batteries.

Language and Culture

Perhaps the most important problems are the inherent intellectual and cultural biases of many of the tests. Designed for white, English-speaking, educated, middle-class patients, the tests may require major modifications before being applied to less educated and/or non-English speaking cohorts, much less to worker populations from distant cultures. Studying cultural impacts on performance should be viewed as a challenge for the coming decade.

Aging

Many neurobehavioral functions decline steadily with age.[14,138] In addition to well-known effects on short-term memory, aging produces alterations in cognitive function as well, although this varies greatly among individuals, from frank dementia as in Alzheimer's disease to very subtle changes. Reaction time increases and performance on psychomotor tasks decreases with age. In rats, age may also indirectly impair performance by enhancing the negative effects of stress.[139] The dopaminergic neurons also degenerate with age, resulting in some cases of late-onset parkinsonism. Oxidation of dopamine produces reactive oxygen species, which may enhance the degeneration of these neurons. Glutathione blocks the dopamine-induced apoptosis.

▸ FUTURE DIRECTIONS

Building on the foundation of clinical psychology and neurobiology, behavioral toxicologists have assembled a variety of test approaches that yield important information about nervous system response to toxic chemicals. In many cases the mechanisms are uncertain and the pathologic lesion unrecognized. The molecular, biochemical, and microanatomic changes are being revealed. New ways of probing receptors and new breeds of transgenic or "knockout" animals that lack a particular gene offer the opportunity to identify specific mechanisms.

A neurotoxicant may act on a discrete target such as the basal ganglia or may disrupt associations between different parts of the brain, interfering with intellectual functions such as cognition and memory. These all provide an active domain for research in a variety of disciplines using a variety of models. New test equipment requires validation on a variety of populations and interpretation depends on improving exposure assessment as well. As the field of neurobehavioral testing matures and tests become validated on increasing numbers of "normal" individuals, one may achieve greater certainty in evaluating subtle abnormalities.

Neuronal peptides and nervous system development were two research needs underserved in 1980 and still central today. The interaction of xenobiotics with cytokines, genes, gene products, cell differentiation, apoptosis, cell assembly, and neuronal connections during development is basic to improving the understanding of neurobehavioral development and behavioral teratology.

Environmental and Ecological Risk Assessment

Michael Gochfeld • Joanna Burger

Risk assessment is a formalized process for characterizing and estimating the magnitude of harm resulting from some condition—usually exposure to one or more hazardous substances in the environment. "Environmental risk assessment" usually refers to human health consequences, while "ecological risk assessment" refers to damage to natural or artificial ecosystems. Risk assessments are intended to provide objective information to inform public policy decisions.[1]

Increasingly governments and the public have realized that it is critical to protect the health and well-being of ecological systems, both for their own value as well as for the ecological services that they provide for humans. Intact, functioning ecosystems provide a wealth of services including fertile land for agriculture, unpolluted waters for fisheries, safe drinking water, clean air, stabilization of coastal environments, and places for recreation and other aesthetic pursuits so important to people.[2,3] Moreover, changes in ecosystem health can have direct effects on human health by changing human exposure to disease organisms.[4]

Risk assessment is primarily a scientific endeavor, while risk management refers to those actions taken by society to ameliorate risks. Risk management takes into account human values and fiscal concerns and determines what risk assessments need to be done and how they are to be used, but the methods and outcomes of risk assessment should not be biased by these concerns.[5] Risk management may involve policy decisions that set particular standards for contaminants in air, water, soil, or food, or they may reflect particular decisions on whether and how much to remediate a hazardous waste site. There is ongoing controversy as to whether risk assessment can remain value-free or whether that is an illusion.

Protecting human health does not necessarily protect ecosystems and their component communities and organisms from harm.[6] Humans may be less or more susceptible to certain chemicals than either wild or experimental animals. Also the process of remediating contaminated soil may seriously disrupt fragile ecosystems, while conversely, the establishment of new wetland ecosystems is being used as an approach to preventing environmental contamination.[7]

Risk assessment involves *target populations*, either real or hypothetical, and the question of how much increased risk will occur if a group of people or a natural ecosystem is exposed to a certain amount of a hazardous substance or condition over a certain period of time. Major descriptions of the risk assessment process[5,8] and its role in policy[1] have been published, and various refinements are added to take into account the great uncertainties attached to risk estimation.

▸ APPLICATIONS OF RISK ASSESSMENT

There is a rapidly growing literature on specific applications of risk assessment,[9,10] and an entire journal, *Risk Analysis*, is devoted to the subject. The social implications of the risk assessment process have been discussed by many authors including Lowrance,[11] Imperato and Mitchell,[12] and Jasanoff[13] among others.

The U.S. National Academy of Science's National Research Council has several committees investigating various aspects of risk assessment to enhance its scientific quality and its effectiveness in informing public policy on the environment and health. Several important volumes have been published recently including the Committee on Risk Assessment Methodology volume on *Issues in Risk Assessment*[14] and the Committee on Risk Characterization's *Understanding Risk*,[1] the latter focusing specifically on the transfer of risk information to policy.

In its broadest sense[15] environmental risk assessment covers a wide variety of natural hazards including earthquakes, floods, and hurricanes. However, this chapter focuses on the narrower application to hazardous chemical and physical agents and their impact on human health and ecosystems.

There are several ways of applying environmental risk assessment in making policy decisions. One can estimate risks associated with a variety of hazards (for example, different hazardous waste sites) and use them to prioritize remediation, starting first with those sites that pose the greatest risk to the greatest number. One can compare an estimated risk with a level of so-called *acceptable risk* (see below) and decide whether or not to take an action. One can treat the reduction of risk as a benefit and perform a cost-benefit analysis for any proposed solution, recognizing that benefit in terms of lives, health, or environmental quality is not easily compared with monetary costs. In another mode, one can contrast the risks from two or more alternative decisions (e.g., to clean up or not to clean up or to ban or not to ban) and may choose the path with the lowest risk. This is called risk-risk balancing.

▸ ACCEPTABLE RISK

One common goal of environmental risk assessment is to identify whether a particular exposure scenario or environmental level of an agent is "acceptable" or whether a target population can continue to be exposed to a current level without unacceptably high consequences. This requires society to identify levels of harm that it considers "acceptable"[9] and to recognize that what may seem acceptable to a risk manager or regulator may not seem "acceptable" to a target population. What constitutes unacceptably high risk to one person (e.g., sky diving) may be a provocative challenge to another. The risk estimate can be used to establish an appropriate regulatory approach or policy that will protect the public from greater exposure.[16]

The process of establishing "acceptable risk" is a human values and social decision, not a biomedical one. For cancer, it has become traditional to state that an exposure to a hazard is acceptable if it does not cause an elevation in death rate of cancer greater than 1 in a million exposed people. If we accept for sake of argument that approximately 20 percent of people die of cancer, a 1 in a million or 10^{-6} elevation of risk means that instead of 200,000 of a million people dying of cancer, the level will be 200,001. Clearly this immeasurably small elevation of risk cannot be identified by any current or projected epidemiologic methods. By contrast, regulations regarding occupational exposures tolerate a much higher risk (on the order of 10^{-4}), but this too is immeasurably small. Most epidemiologists are content if they can identify as real a 50 percent increase in risk.

Before one determines whether a risk is acceptable or not, it is necessary to define an endpoint. Table 18-5 provides a spectrum of endpoints ranging from those like early death from cancer to emotional disturbances. There is a tendency to treat the first entries as the most consequential, and indeed risk assessment has been preoccupied with cancer. Yet some people are disabled by their emotional reactions to hazardous exposures. Society must determine how safe it wants to be[17] and how much it is prepared to sacrifice for that level of security.

Unfortunately, the persons who most often decide whether or not to invest in environmental safety are usually not those most at risk. For those, like the Environmental Protection Agency (EPA), who define acceptable risk as a lower than 10^{-6} excess, the exposure level at which the population is estimated to experience a 10^{-6} increase represents the cutoff between acceptable and unacceptable. Some persons argue that this is an unrealistically small level since most of the risks that most people willingly face (e.g., driving an automobile) are much higher. Indeed, the cancer risk of living in a home with 4 pCi of radon per cubic meter has been estimated on the

TABLE 18-5. SPECTRUM OF ADVERSE CONSEQUENCES CONSIDERED BY RISK ASSESSORS[a]

Shortening of life (mortality)
Cancer versus other causes
Illness or injury leading to disability
Acute versus chronic
Permanent versus temporary disability
Serious versus minor disability
Illness or injury with temporary disability followed by recovery
Chronic versus acute
Serious versus minor disability
Physical discomfort without disability
Psychological disorder with behavioral consequences
Posttraumatic stress disorder
Anxiety reaction
Stress reaction
Chronic frustration and anger
Emotional discomfort

[a] Each of these categories is weighted by the number of individuals involved.

order of 10^{-2} or 10^{-3}, but many people choose not to test their homes or remediate the elevated level.[18]

Once a risk estimate has been calculated, it becomes a major problem to communicate the risk to responsible officials and potentially at-risk individuals, for the manner in which individuals perceive risk often bears little resemblance to the actual magnitude of their risk.[19]

Environmental Equity

Although it has long been known that the most hazardous workplace or community exposures are not uniformly distributed, and that persons in lower socioeconomic groups are most likely to enounter such hazards in their work or home, only in the past decade has attention focused on "environmental justice" or "equity." This inequity is not universal, for depending on the economic history of a community, some industrialized counties are also quite affluent.[20] Only 20 years ago, companies wishing to site potentially hazardous facilities investigated what kind of remuneration would be necessary to encourage a community to accept a facility, with the consequence that the most disadvantaged communities would be most likely to accept an unpleasant facility.[21]

Attention is now focusing on how to rectify the unequal population risks fostered by the practice of siting hazardous facilities in lower socioeconomic (and often ethnic minority) communities. In many cases, communities grew up around the industrial facilities that employed people, with the result that industrialized areas often found themselves in close proximity to residential areas.

Risk Assessment versus Risk Management

One of the historical problems with risk assessment is the confusion between analyzing a level of risk and controlling that risk. Early risk estimates were often modified by the concerns over what it would take to manage the risk, and some policymakers considered risk management an integral part of risk assessment.[22] Accordingly the term *risk analysis* was introduced to refer to a value-free process of estimating risk, independent of any management or economic considerations. May[23] has criticized some blatant uses of cost-benefit analysis in evaluating risk data, wherein a company may choose to accept and pay for a certain level of risk rather than re-engineering to make a safer product.

Risk assessment is or can be used in applications for siting permits for hazardous facilities such as nuclear plants, liquified natural gas depots, municipal solid waste incinerators, and hazardous waste sites.[24] Because of the wide latitude or confidence limits around many risk estimates (*uncertainty*) and the controversies over how to do risk assessments, many management applications of risk analyses may be premature. Nonetheless risk analysis has played an important role in many governmental decisions, such as management of dioxin-contaminated soil[25] and the setting of safe drinking water standards.[26]

The dangers of allowing risk management to intrude on risk assessment are highlighted by the Office of Management and Budget's (OMB) attack on the Occupational Safety and Health Administration's risk-based cadmium standard. Not only did OMB display "a fundamental lack of understanding" about risk assessment, but it used a flawed approach to try to second-guess the risk assessment.[27]

▸ ENVIRONMENTAL RISK ASSESSMENT PARADIGM FOR CARCINOGENS

The basic four-step approach to environmental risk assessment for carcinogens as outlined below was codified by the National Research Council in 1983.[5] In the late 1970s there was heavy emphasis on improving dose-response information; by the early 1980s the research emphasis had shifted to improving understanding of the appropriate mathematical models for low-dose extrapolation. By the late 1980s it was realized that the exposure assessment phase required much research attention. In the 1990s attention is focusing on understanding the mechanisms by which agents produce disease and modifying the generic risk assessment process accordingly.[28]

Hazard Identification

The first step is to define the hazard and establish the endpoint that will be used in the risk assessment (Table 18-5). This means identifying a toxic substance or mixture and naming one or more endpoints (e.g., lung cancer, neurotoxicity) which are of concern.

Dose-Response Assessment

This usually involves extensive review of the toxicologic and/or epidemiologic literature to ascertain whether dose-response curves can be constructed for the endpoints of concern or whether specific thresholds have been determined. The goal is to construct a dose-response curve from the existing studies. The Carcinogen Assessment Group of the EPA has prepared cancer potency estimates for a number of common carcinogens.[28] These and other valuable data are available in EPA's *IRIS* database.

Exposure Assessment

Estimating exposure to the target population is essential.[29] This combines direct measurements of agents in environmental media (air, water, soil, food), coupled with exposure assessments, and often with mathematical models or projections of exposure under different scenarios. Exposure assessment must take into account the measured or estimated concentration of a substance (air, water, food, soil) and all applicable routes of exposure (inhalation, ingestion, skin absorption). This requires knowing how individuals behave: where they spend their time, what they eat, how much they drink. It must incorporate estimates of bioavailability and increasingly relies on physiologically based pharmacokinetic models to provide estimates of the internal dose, the dose actually delivered to the target site.

Risk Analysis, or Risk Characterization

This involves a quantitative estimate of the exposure level at which a particular level of excess risk exists. In the case of cancer, one constructs a dose-response curve based on animal studies of cancer and performs a low-dose extrapolation to estimate the dose that would produce a particular excess of cancer (usually a 10^{-6} increase). The toxicologic data used may involve the presence of tumors, the number of tumors per animal, or the time-to-tumor from initial dosing. A variety of biological models of carcinogenesis have been advocated, each leading to selection of different mathematical extrapolations. Among these are the linear no-threshold model,[30] the Armitage-Doll multistage model,[31] and more recently the Moolgavkar-Vernon-Knudsen model, which emphasizes mutational events[32] involved in initiation rather than in promotion.

Cancer is not a single disease, and no single model will explain all cancer-causing processes. Risk assessment texts provide details on the various mathematical models in use.[33,34] The linear non-threshold model assumes that chemical carcinogens behave like radiation such that no threshold exists (an infinitesimally small dose results in an increased risk).[30] The linearized multistage model is probably the most widely accepted and takes into account multistage models of carcinogenesis.[35] Other models such as dose-distribution models give higher estimates of dose and are considered less protective of the public health, although future research may validate their use for some substances. It is likely that, where several models give similar estimates of risk for a substance, and one model gives a very divergent estimate of risk, one can safely rely on the evidence of the concordant estimates.

The Maximally Tolerated Dose

Critics of risk assessment point to the reliance on the maximally tolerated dose (MTD) as leading inevitably to overestimates of risk. The MTD is the highest dose "that does not alter the animals' longevity or well-being" from unrelated effects.[14] The National Research Council's Committee on Risk Assessment Methodology (CRAM) concluded that the MTD is useful mainly for qualitatively identifying carcinogens and was not intended to be the only data used for quantitatively estimating risk.[14]

Low-Dose Extrapolation

Even below the MTD, many of the doses used in toxicologic research have been orders of magnitude greater than the doses encountered in the home, community, or workplace. Moreover a single study usually involves only two or three different doses, plus the no-dose control. How can one ascertain the risk facing humans at a low dose from the outcome in animals exposed at a high dose? Depending on what biological model one believes appropriate for a particular chemical, one selects from a variety of mathematical models, each purporting to describe a realistic biological concept. For example, if the risk assessor believes that the dose-response curve is linear and has no threshold (a common belief for carcinogens), one may employ the "linear no-threshold model."

▸ RISK ASSESSMENT FOR NONCANCER ENDPOINTS

Risk analyses for noncancer endpoints use a variety of approaches usually based on the highest dose known to produce no effect (no observed adverse effect level (NOAEL) or the lowest dose known to produce an effect (lowest observed adverse effect level (LOAEL)).[36] Ideally one would use data from epidemiologic studies including the most sensitive human subpopulations, where there has been a lifetime of adequate exposure by appropriate routes as well as a lifetime of follow-up (to ensure that events with long latency are not missed). This condition is virtually never met. One must rely either on incomplete epidemiologic studies or more frequently on animal studies. Since most published animal studies were not designed for risk assessment, one must be selective. Studies with very short-term exposure or with short-term follow-up are usually not incorporated in risk assessments.

Several terms need to be understood.

Benchmark Dose. An alternative to relying on a NOAEL, the benchmark dose is the lower confidence limit on a dose which produces an effect in some percent of test animals (usually set at 1, 5, or 10 percent). It is derived from modeling.

NOEL and NOAEL. In toxicologic studies these are the no observable effect level or no observed adverse effect level, respectively. The NOAEL is the dose at which there was no biological or statistically significant adverse effect. Often there may be measurable effects that are not known to have adverse consequences (hence the term NOEL). It is sensitive to the doses chosen for the study.

LOAEL. Lowest observed adverse effect level. In some studies even the lowest dose induced a significant adverse effect. Rather than throw out such studies, there has been a tendency to use these data, but to treat the LOAEL differently from a NOAEL. Since most toxicologic data used in risk assessment were not collected with risk assessment in mind, one is often confronted with LOAELs rather than NOAELs.

Reference Dose (RfD), or Acceptable Daily Intake (ADI). The RfD is established by the Environmental Protection Agency based on risk assessments for noncancer and nongenetic endpoints.[37] This is a daily dose expressed usually in µg/kg/day, that one could take every day without experiencing any adverse effect.

Safety Factor (SF), or Uncertainty Factor (UF). A margin of safety (often arbitrary) introduced into the regulatory process to account for uncertainties in the biomedical database. Since they do not necessarily ensure *safety*, most authors prefer to label them uncertainty factors. Various UFs are used to calculate an RfD from a NOAEL or LOAEL. The most common of these are:

To use animal data to protect humans[38] (UF 10);
To protect the most sensitive human individuals (UF 10);
To calculate a chronic or lifetime RfD from a study using only a subacute or acute exposure (UF 10);
If the RfD is based on a LOAEL rather than a NOAEL (UF 10).

Although the choice of these values of 10 may be arbitrary, subsequent data analyses has tended to support their utility.[34] However, if all four conditions hold, then the combined UF equals 10,000, resulting in a RfD that is four orders of magnitude lower than the LOAEL. Some authors believe that this is overly and unreasonably protective.

Making the Calculations

In using these levels one selects the highest NOAEL or the lowest LOAEL reported in the literature as the starting point for calculations. One also makes certain assumptions about exposure. The standard human target is the 70-kg adult male. However, if susceptible subpopulations include children, females, or ethnic groups, a more appropriate mass should be chosen. Exposure is assumed to occur over a 70-year life span, but in many cases involving childhood exposure a different critical period is selected.

The human daily dose can be calculated as

$$\text{Dose} = \frac{\begin{matrix}\text{Concentration} \\ \text{of agent in media}\end{matrix} \times \begin{matrix}\text{Estimated} \\ \text{intake of media}\end{matrix}}{\text{body weight}}$$

The acceptable daily intake, or reference dose, is calculated by the NOAEL/ΓUF, where Γ is the product of all applicable uncertainty factors. Examples of applications of this approach with much additional detail are provided by Hallenbeck.[34]

Physiologically Based, Pharmacokinetic Models (PBPK)

The above methodology has been criticized as being overconservative, introducing too many arbitrarily derived UFs. Since the value of "10" is a default value, critics seek more "realistic" estimates. The use of pharmacokinetic models may offer a way of avoiding reliance on the default values.[39] For example, using the concentration of tetrachloroethylene in the air in a shower, a PBPK can predict the concentration delivered to the brain after both inhalation and dermal exposure. Instead of relying on a RfD (daily intake), one can calculate a reference target tissue level (RTTL).[40]

Receptor Kinetics

Recent advances in molecular and cell biology point to the role of receptor-mediated gene expression in cells as part of toxicologic responses. Xenobiotics may bind to (or inhibit) receptors intended for naturally occurring mechanisms. Increasing knowledge of these mechanisms and modeling will improve understanding of the shape of the dose-response curve.[41]

Cancer Risk Assessment

Much of the literature on risk assessment has been concerned with cancer. This is partly because community concerns about cancer from long-term low-level exposures were frequently encountered by the EPA and provided the main stimulus for risk assessment. The basic process of risk assessment begins with a review of the literature on toxicological studies of a particular chemical. Then one can either analyze the number of animals at each dosage group that developed cancer, the number of cancers per animal, or the time to develop the tumor.

A variety of mathematical models have been used for low-dose extrapolation of cancer risks. In general the one-hit linear, no-threshold model produces the highest estimate of risk (or conversely the lowest allowable dose), while the logit and probit models are at the opposite end of the spectrum.[33] The one-hit model assumes a linear relationship between dose and outcome, with the slope of the line determined from the available studies. It assumes no threshold and is basically drawn from our understanding of radiation and cancer. Multistage models take into account our understanding of chemical carcinogenesis as a process involving initiation and promotion. Crump[35] proposed a linearized multistage model, now widely used.

Interspecies Extrapolations

One of the controversial aspects of risk assessment is comparing effects among species. It is important to realize that such basic phenomena as the presence of enzymes and consequent metabolism vary not only among species, but among strains of a species, between sexes, and even with age. The response of experimental animals (or of human subjects) may vary with many factors. In some cases the fact that a toxic substance produces the same effect (e.g., bladder cancer or leukemia) in several species of animals makes one confident that interspecies extrapolation is valid. A carcinogen produces cancer in many species, but in each case involving a different organ system. Extrapolation is more uncertain. Finally a substance may be a carcinogen in one species, but not in another.

Where data are available to estimate cancer potency for a single chemical from both animal studies and human epidemiologic studies there is a high correlation,[42] validating the use of animal toxicologic data. The basic problem is that one does not know whether the human is more or less susceptible to the agent than the experimental animal used in a study. Incorporating a safety factor of 10 assumes that humans are no more than 10-fold more sensitive. However, humans are just as likely to be less sensitive than more sensitive, and in many cases the sensitivity is not known. Thus in the case of 2, 3, 7, 8-TCDD dioxin, guinea pigs are about 1,000 times more sensitive than rats are, while it is not clear whether humans are closer to guinea pigs, to rats, or perhaps even less sensitive than either.

Interpreting the Model

Before selecting a model one establishes a level of acceptable risk.[11,17] For example, what dose of chemical would increase the cancer risk by 1 case in a million. The mathematical model allows one to extrapolate downward until one reaches that very low dose associated with 1 in a million excess risk.

If one uses the linear nonthreshold model, this dose will be much lower than if one uses the probit model. Environmentalists seeking to prevent any unnecessary exposure to carcinogens will tend to favor the model giving the lowest allowable dose, while an industrialist responsible for controlling exposures in and around his or her factory, will feel more comfortable if a probit model is used, thus relaxing his or her burden somewhat. Unfortunately much of the debate over which model to use has focused on the political consequences of the choice rather than on the scientific basis. This is perhaps inevitable since there has been only slow progress toward determining the biological basis for model selection for specific chemicals. This is an important rationale for understanding the mechanisms by which toxic substances produce their effects at the molecular and cellular level.

In addition to estimating a critical dose, one can calculate the 95 percent confidence limits around an estimate. To ensure protectiveness of public health, one reports the upper 95 percent confidence limit as the "upper bound" of the risk estimate. In addition, one can establish a science-policy decision of using a no-threshold model in cancer risk assessment.[30] In other countries a no-threshold model is used for genotoxic carcinogens, but not necessarily for other carcinogens such as promoters.[43]

One compromise solution is the linearized multistage model.[35] This takes into account the two-stage process of carcinogenesis, recognizing that a single hit may not be sufficient to cause a cancer. The dose estimated by the linearized multistage model is intermediate between the doses generated by the other two models. The EPA has also selected a "one in a million excess risk," often indicated as a 10^{-6} excess risk as the point at which it will make decisions to regulate exposures.

Modeling Endpoints Other than Cancer

Although the method described above under Risk Assessment for Noncancer Endpoints is still prevalent, there are attempts to bring dose-response extrapolation to bear on other endpoints. A model for developmental toxicology incorporates many parameters to estimate cell kinetic rates, and the population of cells with normal and abnormal kinetics, from which developmental abnormalities can be inferred.[44]

Limitations of Risk Assessment

Although risk assessment is becoming increasingly important to policymakers it is essential to understand its limitations: (*a*) for the most part it has been and will continue to be based on published animal research. However, until recently, toxicological research on animals was not designed with quantitative risk assessment in mind, hence the choice of doses and number of animals used may have been appropriate for descriptive purposes, but not for the low-dose extrapolations used in risk assessment. (*b*) Many of the endpoints of concern in humans have not been adequately studied in animal models. (*c*) The uncertainties inherent in extrapolating from animals to humans have engendered controversy. (*d*) Human epidemiologic studies of adequate power are usually too sparse to contribute to risk assessment, hence the continued necessity of relying on animal models. (*e*) Human exposure data are often inadequate. (*f*) In cancer risk assessments, there are dramatic differences depending on which mathematical model is used. (*g*) Risk estimates based on collective exposure are not easily translated into individual risk. (*h*) There is the continuing debate over what constitutes an acceptable level, which often overrides biomedical estimate of risk.

Although these concerns interfere with performance and application of risk assessments, the process has become increasingly robust, so that it does serve useful functions in ordering priorities, in comparing the risks of different solutions, and in providing some data for establishment of policy.

Uncertainty

Uncertainty permeates the risk assessment process. Even when the mechanism by which an agent produces disease is well understood, uncertainty is introduced in the dose-response data from animal studies, the exposure assessment, and the risk estimation process. These uncertainties may be multiplicative, leading to orders of magnitude differences in estimate depending on the assumptions one uses. Is is important to distinguish between uncertainty introduced by inadequate data or choice of methodology from the inherent variability among individuals.[45] Thus in a population for which an average exposure assessment can be estimated, some will behave in a way that minimizes, while others maximize, their potential exposures. Similarly individuals vary in their susceptibility to different hazards. A variety of approaches is being suggested to reduce the uncertainty in risk assessments. Monte Carlo (randomization) simulations have been used to produce a distribution of estimates.[46] However, formal uncertainty analysis is probably less important than efforts to reduce the uncertainties through toxicologic and epidemiologic research enhanced by the increasing availability of biomarkers and through careful site-specific studies of exposure.

Susceptibility

The past 5 years have seen awakened interest in individual variability in susceptibility to hazardous agents. This variability can be genetic or acquired. Age, gender, and race influence susceptibility. Acquired variability may reflect overall health status, concurrent exposures, diet, and lifestyle. Major research breakthroughs are being made in understanding the contribution of genetic variability, particularly in the P-450 enzyme system on susceptibility.

Individual versus Collective Risk

The process of risk assessment is concerned with collective risks facing a target population rather than an individual. Policymakers, likewise, are concerned with protecting groups from unacceptable exposures and risks. However, many decisions regarding risks are made at the individual level. And even when a group is exposed, its members try to interpret and respond to the risk as individuals. It seems reasonable to assume that, once a risk has been estimated for a group, any individual within that group will face the average risk. However, within a population the risk is distributed unevenly, depending on variation in exposure and susceptibility, such that any individual may have a risk much lower or higher than the estimate.

Risk Perception

Some individuals engage in extremely risky behavior on a regular basis as part of their job and may receive hazardous duty pay in recognition of this risk. Others engage in risks for recreational purposes or thrill. At the opposite pole of such risk-taking behavior are risk-aversive individuals. One might predict that a risk-taking individual, such as a skydiver or a mercenary soldier, would willingly undertake other risks such as smoking, driving without a seat belt, tolerating radon in their homes, or living next to a hazardous waste dump, while risk-aversive individuals take public transportation to a 9-to-5 job, frequently check their homes for radon, have their car undergo frequent safety inspections, and shun all activities or exposures that enhance their risk of becoming ill or injured.

However, risk perception is not that simple. Some individuals who willingly take great risks fear having their drinking water contaminated even at immeasurably low levels. The fact that, in general, individuals tend to overestimate negligible risks and underestimate severe ones is a source of frustration to risk analysts and policymakers alike, and this has engendered the rapidly growing field of "risk perception research."[47]

Unfortunately, many studies of *risk perception and risk communication* are aimed at marketing a particular viewpoint—that is, trying to convince people to accept a particular level of risk that is politically or economically expedient. Although not usually recognized, the field has its roots in the study of "marketing," which emerged in the 1950s and 1960s to understand factors motivating human purchasing decisions. Although the risk perception literature rarely references its parent discipline, many common principles can be recognized. Nonetheless, important advances and generalizations have been developed.[48]

Lowrance[11] is credited with popularizing the understanding of risk perception and what constitutes acceptable risk. He elaborated a series of "dichotomies," originally proposed by Fischoff, which influence human perception of risk. Some of these are shown in Table 18-6.

The goal of risk perception research is to understand how individuals appreciate risks, how they make their risk-taking and risk-avoiding decisions, and how to bring their understanding of specific risks into congruence with the actual levels of risk. This will reduce the anxiety levels where risk is overestimated and may influence behavior, preventing significant exposure where risk is underestimated. All too often, risk managers have the goal of reducing anxiety and encouraging people to accept exposures, particularly those that would be costly to mitigate. However, examples of the need to enhance awareness and response to underestimated exposures include convincing people to have their homes tested for radon and to have exposure mitigated if the radon level is high and educating people regarding the hazards of smoking tobacco.

Although people in different parts of the world and at different socioeconomic levels face different kinds of risks and make risk decisions driven by different factors, there are some universal features to risk perception. For example, Hinman et al.[49] showed a remarkable concordance between U.S. and Japanese respondents regarding the things they dread (with nuclear accidents, radiation waste, and nuclear war at the high end for both countries); however, there was less concordance between countries in the knowledge about the 30 hazards tested.

TABLE 18-6. RISK PERCEPTION DICHOTOMIES

Acceptable, or Reduces Apparent Riskiness	*Unacceptable, or Increases Apparent Riskiness*
Assumed voluntarily or self-imposed	Borne involuntarily or imposed by others
Adverse effect immediate	Outcome delayed
Alternatives not available a necessity	Alternatives available a luxury
Risk certain	Risk uncertain
Occupational exposure	Community exposure
Familiar hazard	Feared or "dread" hazard
Consequences reversible	Consequences irreversible
Some benefit gained from assuming risk	No apparent benefit to persons at risk
Hazard associated with perceived good	Someone else profits at "my expense"

Modified from Lowrance WW: Of Acceptable Risk. Los Altos, CA: William Kaufmann, 1976, p 87

Among scientists, those in the life sciences and those in academia tend to perceive greater risks from nuclear waste than do physical scientists or those in industry or government.[50] The latter are also more willing to impose risks on others. Not surprisingly, employees of a nuclear plant perceived a lower risk of accidents than did the general public.[51]

Demographic factors influence perception in complex ways. In some studies more educated people who may have a better understanding of science and technology are more accepting of technological hazards,[52] but the fact that people of lower socioeconomic status and education fear such developments relates in part to their perception that they personally are at greater risk.[53] Perceived risks for any hazard correlates with one's perception of personal risk from that hazard, but is tempered by any benefits from that hazard.[54]

Risk Communication

Like risk perception there is a growing field of research surrounding the methods that can be used to impart risk information to the public. The landmark book *Improving Dialogue with Communities: A Risk Communication Manual for Government* identified the challenges that government officials face when bringing news (particularly unpleasant news) about a local environmental hazard to communities.[55] Public utilities and corporations have also invested in improving their communication with their neighboring communities, both to comply with Superfund Ammendment Reauthorization Act (SARA) title 3 and with community right-to-know laws in some states and to create channels of communication in case of an accident.

Models of Risk Communication

In many circumstances risk communication has been a one-way path between the "expert" and the "public" following a *source-receiver model* in which the recipient is passive and is expected to respond to the message in a predicted manner. Very frequently the anticipated response does not materialize. Two-way communication (sometimes called a *convergence model*),[56] is necessary so that the receiver can inform the sender what parts of the problem are important, thereby shaping the message they receive.

Risk Comparisons

Risk assessors, not realizing that individuals must put risk into very personal contexts, often lament that the public reacts irrationally to risks. Risk comparison is an approach to communicating risk by contrasting unfamiliar risks with familiar ones. Common reference points include the risk of driving so many miles in a car, the radiation risk of a transcontinental air flight, and the lung cancer risk from smoking a pack of cigarettes per day. The implication is that a risk lower than these should be acceptable. Yet individuals may rationally accept the necessary risk of transcontinental flight, while shunning the perceived risk of having a communication tower constructed in their community. The concept of risk comparison thus makes more sense to the communicator than to the communicatee. The dichotomies shown in Table 18-6 help us understand this apparent paradox.

Temporal Characterization of Risk

As an alternative to risk comparison, very low lifetime risks can be transformed into a time frame that may help some people grasp their significance. Thus a 1 in 100,000 risk in a town of 2,000 people translates into 1 death in 3,500 years (50 × 70 yr lifetimes).[57]

Media Coverage of Risk

One often gains the impression that newspaper and television coverage exaggerates the hazards of everyday life, with stories that bear little relationship to the actual magnitude of public health hazard.[58] Nonetheless the media are an important source of hazard and risk information for many people, and the media therefore could play a crucial role in providing a balanced perspective on risk. Although many toxicologists shun journalists for fear of being misquoted, there is a substantial basis for believing that environmental news coverage can be improved if a dialogue between toxicologists, risk assessors, and reporters can be developed.[59]

Stakeholders and Citizens' Advisory Boards (CABs)

Various agencies, including large corporations and the Department of Energy, form advisory boards representing various types of stakeholders. These can voice concerns to which the company can respond proactively. CABs can focus attention on the risks that they view as significant and can identify acceptable alternatives or programs. At some factories they actually participate in fence-line monitoring programs. Their actual contribution to policy outcomes, however, is variable.[60]

Improving the involvement and usefulness of communities, particularly minority communities, in agency decisions, as well as a need to evaluate risk communication methodologies have been identified as high priorities for risk communication research.[61]

▸ ECOLOGICAL RISK ASSESSMENT

Ecological Risk Assessment has emerged as the discipline to evaluate the risk of stressors to ecological systems (including their component organisms), and it has borrowed heavily from the human risk assessment four-step paradigm[7,14,62]: hazard identification, dose-response, exposure assessment, and risk characterization. However, evaluating risk to ecological systems is far more difficult than is human health risk assessment because of the complexities of ecosystems. Ecosystems include both the abiotic (soil, air, water) and biotic components, and the latter includes a wide range of species with different life spans (from minutes to hundreds of years), different life history strategies (some have few offspring, others lay millions of eggs), different life stages (e.g., egg, larvae, adult), and vastly different susceptibilities to stressors. It is for this reason that ecological risk assessment must be conducted with a particular objective in mind, with a particular range of species of concern.

The hazard identification phase of ecological risk assessment therefore requires input from risk managers and the general public.[1,63] All of these stakeholders must work in an iterative framework to provide the background, scope, and objectives for an ecological risk assessment. Most of the federal agencies involved in ecological risk assessment have acknowledged the importance of this initial phase and of including stakeholders. Moreover, because of the complexities within ecosystems, the endpoints or measures of risk must be carefully defined and selected. This is not a trivial aspect. In human risk assessments one has to worry about only one species; in ecological assessments the structure and function of the system as well as the survival of component species are of concern.

Selecting the target endpoint is challenging. Is it a particular ecosystem function such as productivity, or the amount of energy or matter channeled through the system, or is it a size of a component population? One critical difference between human and ecological risk assessment is that, whereas the health and well-being of each individual human being is important, for ecological systems (except for endangered species) it is the population that is of concern.

At this stage there is still a lack of dose-response data and exposure data for plants and animals in most ecosystems. Most estimates of exposures come from measuring the levels of chemicals in various tissues. There are few monitors available for wild animals, and the cost would be prohibitive for obtaining either large sample sizes or data on many different species. Replicating ecosystems on a scale suitable for research has required aquarium-level (microcosm) and pond-level (mesocosm) models,[64] the latter still restricted to a few research stations.

A new phase in ecological risk assessment is to focus on a large area scale, a so-called *landscape* approach.[65] The problems that ecological systems face often can be examined only on a regional basis where the health and well-being of populations can be assessed. In addition, researchers are trying to estimate the resiliency of ecosystems or the time required for them to recover from a disturbance or contamination.[66] As with human health risk assessment, it is often challenging to determine whether a risk assessment has achieved its purpose since long-term studies are required to determine whether predictions have been borne out.[5]

Risk Characterization

Ellen K. Silbergeld

Risk characterization, risk assessment, and risk management are terms for methods of analyzing health and environmental issues. At one level, almost any decision requires individuals or institutions to gather and evaluate information for use in deciding whether or not to take actions to manage risk, which may range from individual choices (for instance, which medicine to prescribe) to complex regulations with major legal and economic consequences for society. While the elements of risk characterization and risk management are similar at most levels of organization, the processes of decision-making by government and other institutions are considerably more complicated and often controversial. The public demands a high degree of accountability and justification for these choices, since their costs and benefits may be felt widely, if not universally.

Risk characterization is usually defined as the linked analysis of risk assessment and exposure assessment, which is then divided into three steps: hazard identification, dose-response analysis, and exposure assessment.[1] Risk management utilizes these analyses, as shown in Figure 18-4, along with other factors—economic constraints, social values, legal mandates, technological capacity, and politics—that influence the use of a risk characterization in decision-making. While schematics such as Figure 18-4 separate these elements, in fact it is often difficult to distinguish the "science" of risk characterization from the "values" of risk management, as is now recognized.[2–4] It is essential to realize that risk management goals—such as how much risk of cancer is allowable from exposure to pesticide residues in food, or what level of incidence of lead poisoning is socially tolerable—are set not by science but by the politics of consensus and contention.

Risk characterization and its elements have become important steps in public policy-making, particularly in environmental health policy. Because environmental policy is often controversial, highly codified guidelines for risk characterization have been published at several points from 1979 onwards by the U.S. Environmental Protection Agency (EPA). These statements of increasingly detailed methods on the selection, evaluation, and analysis of scientific data and on using nonhuman toxicity data in estimating human health risks are intended to provide an explicit "road map" to policy and are also designed to explain how policymakers reach rational decisions when data are incomplete.

Risk characterization involves elements of biological and epidemiological information, and judgment, to guide policymakers in reaching sound decisions. This is not dissimilar to the demands of clinical judgment that physicians and health care providers have been trained to make. However, often the risk management questions that arise in environmental health are extremely complex, controversial, and costly. Frequently, there is insufficient information on human risk and exposures. This chapter outlines the general principles and sources of information that are used in the steps of risk characterization, to acquaint the reader with the challenges of making policy to protect human health from environmental risks. The process of risk characterization and risk management will always involve the combination of science and judgment.[5] While physicians participate in social decisions along with other citizens, they are often called upon to explain risk assessments to the public, particularly when local issues are involved.

▶ USES OF RISK ASSESSMENT

Risk assessment was developed primarily by regulatory agencies to provide a rationale for setting enforceable standards for toxic chemicals in air, water, food, soils, consumer products, and wastes, including cleanup of hazardous waste sites. It is now used to set priorities, to compare risks, to identify research needs, and to generate information for cost-benefit analysis. Determining priorities for action is the first step in policy-making since policy options or issues given low priority become decisions to accept the status quo. Comparative risk assessment is part of prioritization, but it has also become mandated by the 1990 amendments to the Clean Air Act, which direct the EPA to allow a regulated industry to "trade" among various risks as an alternative to reducing the risks of one chemical. Risk-risk analysis is promoted by those who are concerned that the consequences of strict regulation may be loss of jobs, which in itself can affect health. Risk assessment is also proposed as a useful method to identify critical research needs, both for specific chemicals as well a for more general validation of models.[6] Risk assessment is increasingly used to generate the benefits (reduced risks) for cost-benefit analyses of regulations. This use of risk assessment is provocative when benefits are expressed as lives saved and a monetized value is placed upon human life. Concerns have been raised as to the reality of "risks" in these calculations. Also, the valuation of health effects other than death has been difficult to determine.

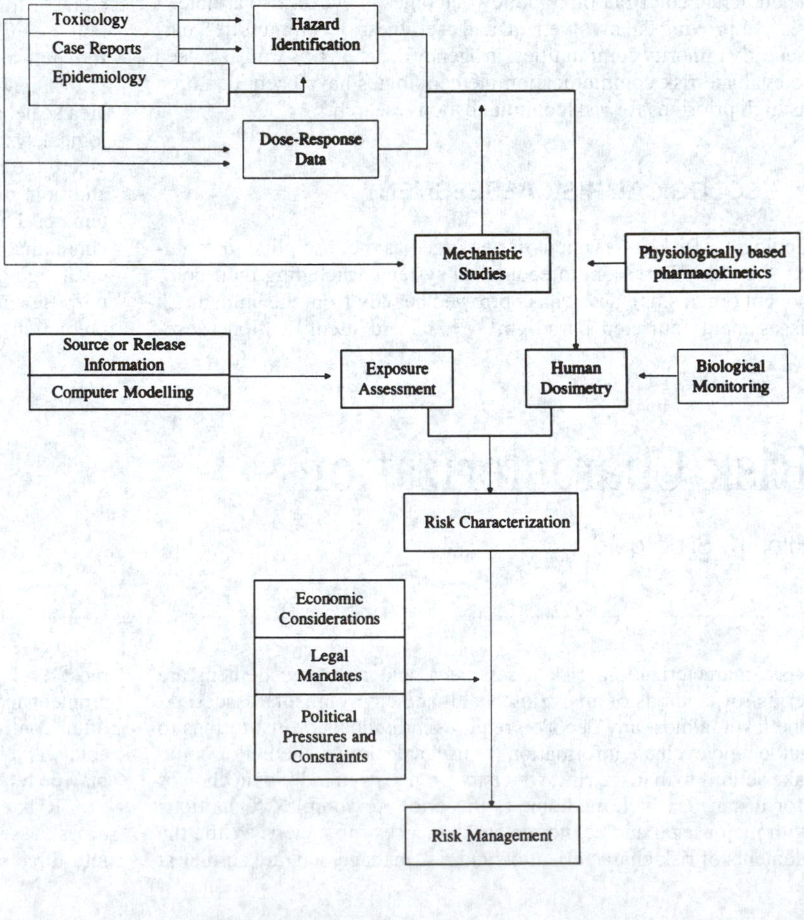

Figure 18-4. The role of risk characterization in understanding and managing risks.

▶ GENERAL PRINCIPLES OF RISK ASSESSMENT

From 1979 onwards, EPA has issued guidelines for the assessment and characterization of toxic chemicals that cause cancer or affect the nervous system, development, and reproduction. In the first statement of risk assessment or characterization principles in 1979, the Federal Government laid out some general guidelines that have remained policy principles in the United States. These are:

- Animal data are valid and relevant for both the identification and quantitative estimation of human health risk.
- Biologically based or mechanistic models are appropriate for estimating low-dose risk at levels of exposure where no increases in tumors or mortality can be detected in either animals or human populations.
- In assessing exposure, it is appropriate to assume that individuals or groups may be maximally exposed for a lifetime, unless more detailed information is available.
- The estimation of population risk is equivalent to individual risk times the number of people in the exposed population.
- No interactions other than simple addition occur in cases of multiple exposures.
- In cases of uncertainty (such as how to convert animal dose to human exposure), conservative assumptions as to risk should be employed.

The legal importance of risk assessment guidelines became clear in 1980 when the Supreme Court struck down the Occupational Safety and Health Administration's (OSHA's) regulations of benzene, a human leukemogen, on the grounds that OSHA had neither quantitated the risks of then-current benzene exposures in the workplace nor did it calculate the reduction in risk expected to be achieved by the proposed reduction in occupational exposures. Legislation since 1980 has encouraged or required the use of quantitative risk assessment. With increasing attention to the costs of regulation and other health policies, the importance of risk assessment has increased, since the risks to be reduced by government intervention or voluntary action are the "benefits" in a cost-benefit analysis framework.

▶ RISK CHARACTERIZATION METHODS

Most risk assessment methodologies incorporate the same general principles stated in the 1979 cancer guidelines, although there are some important differences specific to each endpoint, or risk. Underlying these differences are different fundamental assumptions about the nature of risk and the biological events in disease. Cancer risks are stochastic, that is, cancer either occurs or it does not occur. Thus the probability of cancer increases with increasing exposure, or dose. This can be compared to weather forecasting, in which the predicted occurrence of "rain" is expressed as a probability. In contrast, noncancer diseases, such as hypertensive heart disease, peripheral neuropathy, lead poisoning, or toxic hepatitis, are by nature nonstochastic. Their severity, rather than their likelihood or probability, increases with exposure, or dose. The expression of risk is therefore more complicated than a probability estimate. The basic biological model for assessing cancer risks has been based upon the hypothesis that all cancers involve the same initial and necessary molecular event of DNA damage.[7] Because a change (mutation or deletion) of even 1 base pair may be associated with cancer (as recent evidence suggests for mutations in the *p*53 gene),[8] then the risks of cancer can be increased by some very small but finite amount even at very low cellular concentrations. At these low levels, the incremental risk is considered to be linear with dose. Based on these assumptions, models for cancer risk assessment usually extend the curve fitted to data on dose and response well below the range of actual observation, using linear or nonlinear extrapolation. This extrapolation is necessary because the "acceptable" level of exposure, determined by a risk management goal mandated by statute or otherwise agreed upon, is well below the range detectable in actual toxicological or experimental studies. If the "acceptable" level of risk is set at 1 : 100,000 then the exposure associated with this risk level can be determined graphically only from the equation of the curve fitted and extrapolated.

In contrast, for noncarcinogens, there is no single unifying theory of toxic action even for one set of endpoints, such as neurotoxicity. Generally, it has been assumed that noncancer toxicity, or target organ toxicity, occurs only at some dose well above zero, at which functional reserves such as cell replacement, detoxifying enzymes, or sequestering proteins are unable to prevent biologically significant adverse or toxic effects at the site(s) of action. For example, it is known that the conduction velocity decrements observed in many types of peripheral neuropathy occur only when many nerve fibers within a specific nerve are damaged. Unless this amount of damage is induced, no measurable deficits in conduction velocity, grip strength, or other function is observed. The level at which detectable damage is induced by a toxicant is termed the threshold; below this level, there is no toxicity. Of course, much depends upon the definition of an adverse effect and the sensitivity of measurement. However, even with ideally sensitive measurement of effect, it is assumed that, as a consequence of mechanism, there are still thresholds for noncarcinogens.

Risk characterizations for cancer risk are expressed as a probability of cancer, in one of three ways: the probability at a specific dose (sometimes called "unit risk"); the benchmark dose[9] or the dose or exposure associated with a specific risk (sometimes related to a risk management goal, such as the 1 in 100,000 or 1 in 1,000,000 risk level); or even as the slope of the linear relationship between risk and dose (sometimes called Q* or potency). Risk characterizations for noncancer endpoints are usually expressed as an "acceptable" dose: this is determined by taking the exposure or dose associated with a defined effect in either animal studies or epidemiological studies and dividing this number by one or several so-called "safety" or "uncertainty" factors (each one usually valued at 10).[10] These factors represent such uncertainties or datagaps as: the true NOEL, or highest dose at which no adverse effect occurs, or true LOEL, or lowest dose at which an adverse effect occurs (which may not be discernible in the available data); differences in response between humans and animals, and among humans; and sometimes the severity of the observed effect. For instance, as shown below, if the data available indicate that mirex (an insecticide) causes early vaginal opening in rats, then the following calculation may be done:

where D = dose at which vaginal opening in rats is significantly affected

D_H = human equivalent dose (converted on a mg/kg or surface area basis)

Then AD = acceptable dose = $D_H/[(A)(B)(C)] = D_H \times 10^{-3}$

Where A = 10, animal to human safety or uncertainty factor, since no human data exist

B = 10, lack of **no** observed effect level data, since only data on the **lowest** observed effect dose are available

C = 10, severity of effect, since no information is available on more sensitive endpoints(s) in the development of the reproductive system.

These distinctions between cancer and noncancer risk have been challenged. Some have suggested that not all carcinogens involve point mutation (or "single hit") mechanisms, and thus the low dose-response relationship may not be linear.[11] Some carcinogens are nonmutagenic, and increased tumorigenesis has been observed only in experimental animals treated at doses that induce detectable target organ toxicity.[12] Accordingly, these mechanisms are likely to involve thresholds, like other target organ toxicities. Others have suggested that some noncancer endpoints, and nonmutagenic carcinogens, may induce adverse effects at the molecular level linear or near linear with dose at very low levels. This has been advocated for some types of neurotoxins and for receptor mediated carcinogens, such as the dioxins.

These debates are fiercely fought because much is at stake. The difference between assuming a linear or a threshold relationship between dose and effect at low dose can mean substantial differences in "allowable" exposures, and hence in the costs and other investments required to meet a regulatory standard. Research is unlikely to answer all the questions involved. Epidemiology is inadequately sensitive to detect increases in disease at the levels of increased risk deemed unacceptable by the political process; epidemiologists routinely argue about the meaning of an observed relative risk greater than 1 but less than 2. Toxicology may extend the sensitivity of the dose-effect relationship substantially, but even with large numbers of animals, it has proven impossible to resolve with statistical certainty the dose at which a known carcinogen increases risks of tumors by 10 percent, a level of risk that is politically unacceptable for environmental and occupational health standards in the United States. Molecular methods, such as the measurement of DNA adducts (carcinogenic chemicals bound to DNA bases), may increase sensitivity, but the meaning of an increase in DNA adducts in terms of ultimate disease risk is unknown.

▸ INFORMATION USED IN RISK CHARACTERIZATION

Epidemiology and experimental toxicology provide information for risk assessment. Epidemiological studies concern the appropriate species, humans, but they are often limited by uncertainties as to exposure and lack of power to detect small increases in risk. It is difficult to detect with statistical confidence an increase in risk (incidence of disease or death) unless it exceeds by more than 100 percent that which occurs in a reference or control group, and the use of methods such as meta-analysis to increase power is often controversial.[13] Toxicological studies have the advantage usually in terms of accuracy of exposure and dose measurements, but in many cases there are uncertainties on converting animal doses to human exposures and sometimes it is hard to define the relevance of an observed effect for predicting human disease or disability. For instance, while butadiene can induce bladder cancer in both mice and humans, we cannot tell if lead causes lowered IQ in young mice, although we can measure learning behavior in rodents exposed to lead.

Most risk assessments must rely upon toxicological data, for two reasons. First, since the stated purpose of our environmental and occupational health laws is to prevent disease and mortality, then risk management should be done before sufficient human exposure has occurred to increase disease/mortality incidence or prevalence such that it can be detected by clinical or epidemiological surveillance. Second, the lack of epidemiologic studies that are not compromised by uncertainties in human exposure assessment means that the effects of very few chemicals have been studied in human populations. Information is available from several sources, databases run by: the National Library of Medicine (TOXLINE, CANCERLINE), the EPA (IRIS), OSHA (RTECS), the World Health Organization (IRPTC), and private sources (such as the Reproductive Toxicology Center at George Washington University Medical School).

For clinicians and epidemiologists, it is important to recognize that "risk" calculated in a risk assessment is not the same as "risk" calculated in an epidemiological study as an odds ratio or relative risk calculation. An epidemiological risk is always based upon a study population, in which characteristics such as distribution of age, gender, and other factors are very important. A risk assessment risk is independent of these factors; as noted above, risk assessment equates population risk with individual risk multiplied by the size of the population. Also, risk assessment usually considers lifetime risk, rather than risk observed at some point in time, so it is a summation of expected events.

As discussed above, risk management goals almost always require that risks are estimated below the range of actual dose-response or dose-effect data. These estimations are done using biologically based or mechanistic information, which is obtained from toxicologic studies or other research using defined animal models or cell systems. This information may in some cases be directly useful in low dose-effect modeling, or it may be cited as reason to modify inferences of risk across species. For instance, it has been claimed that many rodent bladder carcinogens are not predictive of human tumorigenicity since they involve induction of a rodent-specific protein, β-microglobulin, which mediates specific damage to the kidney. Considerably more research is needed on mechanisms of carcinogenesis and target organ toxicity in order to develop more biologically based methods; in the meanwhile, it will remain necessary to use the general approaches described above (often called default models[5]).

The final step of the risk assessment phase is to express dose in human exposure terms. This involves both quantitative conversion of animal dose to human dose, which is usually done on simple metrics of body size (weight and/or surface area). Increasingly, this is supplemented by information on toxicokinetics, or the handling of the chemical by humans or animals. Toxicokinetic differences between sexes, ages, and species may complicate interpretation.[14] Nevertheless, there is growing support for the incorporation of what are called physiological-based pharmacokinetic (PBPK) models into the exposure assessment part of risk characterization, particularly as this information may modify relatively simplistic dosimetric conversions from rodents to humans.[15]

Risk assessment is then combined with exposure assessment to derive a risk characterization (Fig. 18-4). Exposure assessment is often neglected in the risk characterization process, but it is equally important in reaching sound risk management decisions. Exposure assessments include the following elements: sources of chemicals in the human environment; concentrations of chemicals in media such as ambient and indoor air, drinking water, and food; rates of consumption or intake of air, water, and food; absorption and retention; metabolism; and fraction of the lifetime in which exposures may occur. These data are mostly unavailable so that exposure is often assessed by modeling human exposures based upon general principles that link sources to receptors. Because of the enormous expense in human monitoring, most exposure assessments are based upon models of how chemicals move from a source, such as a smokestack or a consumer product, to portals of entry in individuals (inhalation, ingestion, skin absorption). EPA has developed a model for computing children's exposure to lead in dusts and soils (the Integrated Uptake Biokinetic Model (IUBK)), which will generate a prediction of individual or population blood lead levels based upon information related to lead concentrations in soils and dusts, age of children, and time spent in specified environments. Some studies have been conducted to characterize human exposures by personal monitoring, either by air samplers carried by individuals or by analyzing samples of human blood, fat tissue, or breast milk. There is always a question as to how representative the sample of persons monitored is and the extent to which the sample encompasses persons who for a variety of reasons (behavior, genetics, diet, activity patterns) may have considerably higher or lower exposures than the median or average. For instance, it is recognized that young children ingest substantially more dusts and surface soils through normal hand-to-mouth activities than do adults. Variations in food consumption patterns in the U.S. population can result in substantial differences in exposure, as shown for children[16] and for persons consuming large amounts of freshwater fish from contaminated ecoysystems such as the Great Lakes. Careful data gathering on exposure is particularly important for assessing risk in specific populations, such as communities living near a hazardous waste site.

▸ EXAMPLES OF RISK CHARACTERIZATIONS

Two examples of risk characterizations are presented: for a carcinogen and a noncarcinogen. It is important to note how risk characterization (hazard and exposure assessments) are interwoven with risk management (goals for public health protection). Physicians and others involved in advising individuals and communities need to recognize this interplay.

TABLE 18-7. ESTIMATED PERCENTAGE OF CHILDREN WITH BLOOD LEAD (PbB) LEVELS AT OR ABOVE 10 μg/DL FOR A RANGE OF DUST LEAD STANDARDS (μg/SQ FT) FOR VARIOUS SURFACES, ADJUSTED FOR OTHER COVARIATES

Dust Lead Standard	*% with PbB ≥10 μg/dL*	*95% CI*
■ ***CARPETED FLOORS***		
5	3.8	0.3, 7.4
10	9.9	5.2, 14.5
15	14.7	9.7, 19.7
20	16.6	11.5, 21.7
25	17.5	12.4, 22.6
30	18.1	13.0, 23.2
35	19.2	14.0, 24.4
40	19.8	14.5, 25.0
■ ***NONCARPETED FLOORS***		
5	4.3	0.5, 8.2
10	10.2	4.9, 15.6
15	13.5	8.0, 19.1
20	14.9	9.7, 20.2
25	17.0	12.0, 22.1
30	18.0	13.0, 23.1
35	18.9	14.0, 24.0
40	19.7	14.6, 24.9

Example 1: Habitability of a Community with Dioxin Contamination

This issue deals with the public health decision whether to relocate a community where hazardous waste has been discovered in the surface soils in public areas, including backyards, school grounds, and streets.[17] Among the chemicals present is 2,3,7,8-tetrachlorodibenzo-D-dioxin (TCDD), the most toxic of the chlorinated dibenzodioxins. This chemical is considered a human carcinogen (that is, there is definitive evidence that TCDD causes cancers in laboratory animals and strong evidence of carcinogenicity in some human populations exposed to TCDD). The risk to be assessed is cancer. The route of exposure is via inhalation and ingestion of soil. Scientists at CDC calculated the relationship between TCDD in soil and estimated excess cancer risk in two steps: first they evaluated the dose-response relationship for TCDD and cancer in rats and mice and converted the dose to a human exposure; then they estimated the exposures resulting from a lifetime of opportunity to contact soil. The highest exposures are associated with ingestion of soil by a young child, assuming 100 percent absorption of TCDD in soil. These calculations provide a graphical relationship between TCDD in soil and risk. Based upon the risk management goal (what level of excess risk is acceptable), a guideline for acceptable soil concentrations can be established and actions taken based on the extent to which soil concentrations in the community exceed this level.

Example 2: Clean Up Standards for Lead in House Dust

This issue deals with the public health decision as to how to deal with lead-based paint in a home. It is recognized that much of the risk of lead-based paint, for young children, comes from small particles of paint in house dust.[18] Moreover, when lead-based paint is removed, lead dust can be generated, and cleanup is an important part of preventing childhood lead exposure.[19] Many studies have documented the relationship between blood lead levels and decrements in children's learning and behavior. These studies suggest that, as blood lead levels increase by 10 μg/dL, then IQ performance decreases by 4–8 points.[20] In addition, studies have demonstrated a relationship between lead in house dust and blood lead levels in young children.[21] Based upon a risk management goal of preventing lead-induced neurotoxicity by keeping blood lead levels below 10 μg/dL, it can be seen from Table 18-7 that a dust level of below 10 to 20 μg/sq ft lead will be predicted to keep 90 percent of children below this level of toxicity. However, many studies have indicated that achieving this goal is very expensive and may prevent extensive lead paint abatement, particularly in low income housing. Moreover, enforcing a similar standard for surface soils would require massive cleanup of many urban neighborhoods, where decades of traffic have resulted in substantial contamination from leaded gasoline. For that reason, guidelines for acceptable levels in house dust and surface soils have generally embodied both a health goal and a feasibility standard.

Biomarkers

Paul W. Brandt-Rauf

The term biological marker or biomarker encompasses broad categories of indicators or signals of events in biologic systems, including those that are biochemical, molecular, genetic, immunologic, and physiologic. The use of biomarkers so broadly defined is clearly not new in preventive medicine or in the area of environmental health. In recent years, the tremendous increase in knowledge of the molecular mechanisms of disease processes has spurred a concomitant increased interest in specific molecular biomarkers. In environmental health, this interest has focused on molecular biomarkers that track the continuum from contact with exogenous toxins (biomarkers of exposure) to measurable toxic effects (biomarkers of response), as modified by interindividual variability (biomarkers of susceptibility).

Traditionally, exposure of individuals to toxins has been estimated based on monitoring of the ambient environment. For example, in the case of respirable toxins, exposure could be estimated from the amount in the air at the individual's breathing zone. However, this type of measure may not accurately reflect the amount of toxin that gets into the body (internal dose). The internal dose of many toxins can be measured in various body tissues and fluids by routine analytic methodologies (e.g., blood lead levels, urinary arsenic levels, salivary cotinine levels, dioxin fat levels) and are well established in environmental health. Increasingly sophisticated techniques have made possible such measurements at concentrations as low as the picomolar, femtomolar, and examolar (1 part in 10^{18}) levels, although the biological significance of such levels is unknown. In addition, biomarkers of internal dose may not necessarily correlate with the amount of toxin (or its active metabolite) that has interacted with the target molecule critical for the production of pathogenic changes (biologically effective dose). For example, certain carcinogens must form DNA adducts to produce the mutations that will cause cancer. The biologically effective dose of such carcinogens is thus the amount of DNA adducts that they produce. The presence of

DNA adducts can be detected using ^{32}P-postlabeling of DNA extracted from target tissue (or surrogate sites such as white blood cells) with good sensitivity (one adduct per 10^9 to 10^{10} bases). Specific identification of DNA adducts can be accomplished by various methods. In experimental situations, accelerator mass spectrometry with radiolabeled compounds is very sensitive (one adduct in 10^{14} DNA bases, or less than one adduct per cell). For practical applications, high pressure liquid chromatography coupled with mass spectrometry or fluorimetry and immunochemical methods such as radioimmunoassays and enzyme linked immunosorbent assays (ELISA), based on monoclonal antibody technology, are being employed to study exposed workers, cigarette smokers, or groups with environmental exposures. Although current monoclonal antibody techniques have sensitivities of an adduct in 10^8 DNA bases, new developments (such as immuno–polymerase chain reaction (PCR)) may increase this by orders of magnitude in the future.

Since biomarkers of exposure may not be able to establish that a disease process has actually been initiated by a given dose, they may not be as specific indicators of pathogenesis as indicators of altered structure or function of the cellular components that control the disease process (biomarkers of response). Many biomarkers of response are well-known in environmental health (e.g., degree of inhibition of blood acetylcholinesterase from organophosphate pesticide exposure, levels of blood liver isoenzynes from hepatotoxin exposure, levels of urinary enzymes or proteins from renal toxin exposure). Recent advances in molecular biology have stimulated greatly increased interest in potential biomarkers of response to the effects of genotoxins. DNA amplification techniques, such as polymerase chain reaction, and DNA sequencing techniques have made possible the identification of specific point mutations in the genes that are presumed to be causally related to carcinogenesis. Thus, in certain cases, there is now the potential to link specific types of mutations in cancer-related genes with specific genotoxic exposures (mutational spectrum). For example, tentative associations have been made between specific alterations in oncogenes or tumor suppressor genes from environmental carcinogens and the resultant cancers, such as ultraviolet radiation and skin cancer, aflatoxin B and hepatocellular carcinoma, polycyclic aromatic hydrocarbons (PAH) or radon and lung cancer, and vinyl chloride and angiosarcoma of the liver. Since alterations in DNA exert their effect through the expression of the encoded protein product, alternative biomarkers of response rely on the detection of altered expression of these proteins. This can be done in cellular samples using monoclonal antibodies specific for the proteins in immunohistochemical techniques or in biologic fluids such as serum or urine via Western blotting or ELISA.

Even with the same exposures, different individuals can exhibit different responses due to variations in susceptibility that are partly attributable to variations in metabolism. For example, people can inherit different alleles for the genes that encode metabolic enzymes (that will have different levels of activity), and this inherited genotype is further modifiable in its phenotypic expression by exposures themselves, since the expression of several of these genes is inducible. The genotype and phenotype of certain metabolic enzymes are thus potential biomarkers of susceptibility. Genotyping can be determined by DNA sequencing techniques, and phenotype can be determined by biochemical assays of enzyme activity. In several cases, associations have been made between certain genotypes and/or phenotypes and the resultant cancers in exposed populations, such as *N*-acetyltransferase and bladder cancer in those exposed to aromatic amines; glutathione-*S*-transferase or debrisoquine metabolism via P-450 2D6 or PAH metabolism via P-450 1A1 and lung cancer in cigarette smokers.

Although new biomarkers of exposure, response, and susceptibility provide many opportunities for the refinement of epidemiologic and toxicologic research, the improvement of risk assessment, and the prevention of environmental illnesses, many issues remain unanswered. For example, the successful utilization of the potential predictive value of biomarkers requires the existence or development of appropriate preventive interventions. Inappropriate access to the information concerning an individual's biomarker status may lead to adverse consequences concerning his or her employability or insurability. For biomarkers to be widely useful, these social concerns will need to be addressed as rigorously as the scientific concerns.

► REFERENCES

Principles of Toxicology

1. Oser BL: Toxicology then and now. Regul Toxicol Pharmacol 7:427–443, 1987
2. Gallo M: History and scope of toxicology. In Klaassen C (ed): Casarett and Doull's Toxicology. 5th ed. New York: McGraw-Hill, 1996, pp 3–12
3. Sinclair U: The Jungle. New York: Viking, 1946 (originally published 1905)
4. Rozman KK, Klaassen CD: Absorption, distribution, and excretion of toxicants. In Klaassen C (ed): Casarett and Doull's Toxicology. 5th ed. New York: McGraw-Hill, 1996, pp. 91–112
5. Mendelsohn ML: Can chemical carcinogenicity be predicted by short-term tests. Ann N Y Acad Sci 534:115–126, 1988
6. Singh BR, Tu AT (eds): Natural toxins 2: structure, mechanism of action and detection. Adv Exp Med Biol 391, 1996
7. Klaassen CD (ed): Casarett and Doull's Toxicology. 5th ed. New York: McGraw-Hill, 1996
8. Dawson JH: Probing structure-function relations in heme-containing oxygenases and peroxidases. Science 240:433–439, 1988
9. d'Itri, FM: Mercury contamination—what we have learned since Minamata. Environ Monitor Assess 19:165–182, 1991
10. Wenger GR, McMillan DE, Chang LW: Behavioral effects of trimethyltin in two strains of mice. Toxicol Appl Pharmacol 73: 78–88, 1984
11. Agency for Toxic Substances and Disease Registry: Toxicological Profile: Chromium. USPHS, ATSDR/TP-88/10. Atlanta: Centers for Disease Control, 1989
12. Nieboer E, Jusys AA: Biologic chemistry of chromium. In Nriagu JO, Nieboer E (eds): Chromium in the Natural and Human Environments. New York: John Wiley & Sons, 1988, pp 21–80
13. Davis D, Safe S: Immunosuppressive activities of polychlorinated dibenzorfuran congeners: quantitative structure-activity relationships and interactive effects. Toxicol Appl Pharmacol 94:141–149, 1988
14. Goldstein RS, Schnellmann RG: Toxic responses of the kidney. In Klaasen CD, Amdur MO, Doull J (eds): Casarett and Doull's Toxicology. McGraw-Hill, New York. 1996, pp 417–438
15. Ashby J, Tennant RW: Prediction of rodent carcinogenicity for 44 chemicals: results. Mutagenesis 9:7–15, 1994
16. Environmental Protection Agency: Introduction to Indoor Air Quality: A Reference Manual. EPA/400/3-91/003. Washington, DC: Environmental Protection Agency, 1991
17. Goldstein BD, Melia RJW, du V Florey C: Indoor nitrogen oxides. Bull N Y Acad Med 58:873–882, 1981
18. American Conference of Governmental Industrial Hygienists: Threshold Limit Values and Biological Exposure Indices for 1995–1996. Cincinnati: American Conference of Governmental Industrial Hygienists, 1995
19. Lioy P: Total human exposure analysis: a multidisciplinary science for reducing human contact with contaminants. Environ Sci Technol 24:938–945, 1990
20. Georgopoulos PG, Lioy PJ: Conceptual and theoretical aspect of human exposure and dose assessment. J Expo Anal Environ Epidemiol 4:253–285, 1994
21. Environmental Protection Agency: Estimating exposure to dioxin-like compounds. EPA/600/6-88/005Ca,Cb,Cc. Washington DC: Environmental Protection Agency, 1994

22. Zweig G: The vanishing zero: the evolution of pesticide analyses. Essays Toxicol 2:156–198, 1970
23. Plog B: Fundamentals of Industrial Hygiene. 3rd ed. Chicago: National Safety Council, 1988
24. Umbreit TH, Hesse EJ, Gallo MA: Bioavailability of dioxin in soil from a 2,4,5,-T manufacturing site. Science 232:497–499, 1986
25. Chan PK, O'Hara GP, Hayes AW: Principles and methods for acute and subchronic toxicity. In Hayes AW (ed): Principles and Methods of Toxicology. New York: Raven Press, 1982, pp 1–51
26. Stevens KP, Gallo MA: Practical considerations in the conduct of chronic toxicity studies. In Hayes AW (ed): Principles and Methods of Toxicology. New York: Raven Press, 1982, pp 53–77
27. Brittebo EB: Metabolism of xenobiotics in the nasal olfactory mucosa: implications for local toxicity. Pharmacol Toxicol 72(Suppl 3):50–52, 1993
28. Gerlach M, Riederer P, Przuntek H, Youdim MBH: MPTP mechanisms of neurotoxicity and their implications for Parkinson's disease. Eur J Pharmacol 208:273–286, 1991
29. Parkinson A: Biotransformation of xenobiotics. In Klaassen CD (ed): Casarett and Doull's Toxicology. 5th ed. New York: McGraw-Hill, 1996, pp 113–186
30. Guengerich FP: Mammalian Cytochrome P-450. Boca Raton, FL: CRC Press, 1987
31. Guengerich FP: Reactions and significance of cytochrome P-450 enzymes. J Biol Chem 66:10019–10022, 1991
32. Tucker GT: Clinical implications of genetic polymorphism in drug metabolism. J Pharm Pharmacol 46(Suppl 1): 417–424, 1994
33. Meyer UA: The molecular basis of genetic polymorphisms of drug metabolism. J Pharm Pharmacol 46(Suppl 1): 409–415, 1994
34. Guengerich FP: Catalytic selectivity of human cytochrome P-450 enzymes: relevance to drug metabolism and toxocity. Toxicol Lett 70:133–138, 1994
35. Conney AH: Pharmacological implications of microsomal enzyme induction. Pharmacol Rev 19:317–366, 1967
36. Wrighton SA, Stevens JC: The human hepatic cytochromes P-450 involved in drug metabolism. Crit Rev Toxicol 22:1–21, 1992
37. Shimada T, Yamazaki H, Mimura M, et al: Interindividual variations in human liver cytochrome P-450 enzymes involved in the oxidation of drugs, carcinogens and toxic chemicals: studies with liver microsomes of 30 Japanese and 30 Caucasians. J Pharmacol Exp Ther 270:414–423, 1994
38. Guengerich FP, Shimada TL: Oxidation of toxic and carcinogenic chemicals by human cytochrome P-450 enzymes. Chem Res Toxicol 4:391–407, 1991
39. Falls JG, Blake BL, Cao Y, Levi PE, Hodgson E: Gender differences in hepatic expression of flavin-containing monooxygenase isoforms (FMO1, FMO3, and FMO5) in mice. J Biochem Toxicol 10:171–177, 1995
40. Lash LH, Zalups RK: Alterations in renal cellular glutathione metabolism after in vivo administration of a subtoxic dose of mercuric chloride. J Biochem Toxicol 11:1–9, 1996
41. Lin MC, Wang EJ, Patten C, Lee MJ, Xiao F, Reuhl KR, Yang CS: Protective effect of diallyl sulfone against acetaminophen-induced hepatotoxicity in mice. J Biochem Toxicol 11:11–20, 1996
42. Sugita M, Tsuchiya K: Estimation of variation among individuals of biological half-time of cadmium calculated from accumulation data. Environ Res 68:31–38, 1995
43. Abou-Setta MM, Sorrell RW, Childers CC: A computer program in BASIC for determining probit and log-probit or Logit correlation for toxicology and biology. Bull Environ Contam Toxicol 36: 242–249, 1986
44. National Research Council: Drinking Water and Health. Washington DC: National Academy Press, 1986, vol 6
45. Schneiderman MA, DeCouflé P, Brown CC: Thresholds for environmental cancer: biological and statistical considerations. Ann N Y Acad Sci 329:92–130, 1979
46. Gots RE: Toxic Risks. Boca Raton, FL: Lewis Publications, 1993
47. Environmental Protection Agency: Proposed guidelines for carcinogen risk assessment. Federal Register 49:46294–46301, 1984
48. Bianchi C, Brollo A, Raman L, Zuch C: Asbestos-related mesothelioma in Monfalcone, Italy. Am J Ind Med 24:149–160, 1993
49. Selikoff, IJ, Seidman H: Asbestos-associated deaths among insulation workers in the United States and Canada, 1967–1987. Ann N Y Acad Sci 643:1–14, 1991
50. Ross RK, Yuan J-M, Yu MC, Wogan GN, Qian G-S, Tu J-T, Groopman JD, Gao Y-T, Henderson BE: Urinary aflatoxin biomarkers and risk of hepatocellular carcinoma. Lancet 339:943–946, April 1992
51. Conney AH, Burns JJ: Metabolic interactions among environmental chemicals and drugs. Science 178:576–586, 1972
52. Johnson DR: Role of renal cortical sulfhydryl groups in development of mercury-induced renal toxicity. J Toxicol Environ Health 9:119–126, 1982
53. Schecter A: Dioxins and Health. New York. Plenum, 1994
54. Lucier GW, Portier CJ, Gallo MA: Receptor mechanisms and dose-response models for the effects of dioxins. Environ Health Perspect 101:36–44, 1993
55. Bertazzi PA, Pesatori AC, Consonni D, Tironi A, Landi MT, Zocchett C: Cancer incidence in a population accidentally exposed to 2,3,7,8-tetrachlorodibenzo-para-dioxin. Epidemiology 4:398–406, 1993
56. Powrie F, Mason D: Phenotypic and functional heterogenity of $CD4^+$ T-cells. Immunol Today 9:274–277, 1988
57. Kosuda LL, Greiner DL, Bigazzi PE: Mercury-induced renal autoimmunity: changes in RT6+ T-lymphocytes of susceptible and resistant rats. Environ Health Perspect 101:178–185, 1993
58. Burkhart-Schultz K, Thomas CB, Thompson CL, Stout CL, Brinson E, Jones IM: Characterization of in vivo somatic mutations at the hypoxanthine phosphoribosyltransferase gene of a human control population. Environ Health Perspect 103:68–74, 1993
59. Nicklas JA, O'Neill JP, Hunter TC, Falta MT, Lippert MJ, Jacobson-Kram D, Williams JR, Albertini RJ: In vivo ionizing irradiations produce deletions in the *hprt* gene of human T-lymphocytes. Mutat Res 250:383–391, 1991
60. Brandt-Rauf P, Marion M-J, DeVivo I: Mutant p21 protein as a biomarker of chemical carcinogenesis in humans. In Mendelsohn ML, Peeters JP, Normandy MJ (eds): Biomarkers and Occupational Health. Washington DC: Joseph Henry Press, 1995, pp 163–173
61. Harris CC: *p53*: at the crossroads of molecular carcinogenesis and risk assessment. Science 262:1980–1981, 1993
62. Aguilar F, Hussain SP, Cerutti P: Aflatoxin B_1 induces the transversion of G $\rightarrow$ T in codon 249 of the *p53* tumor suppressor gene in human hepatocytes. Proc Natl Acad Sci U S A 90:8586–8590, 1993
63. Thomas JA: Toxic responses of the reproductive system. In Klaassen CD (ed): Casarett and Doull's Toxicology. 5th ed. New York: McGraw-Hill, 1996, pp 547–582
64. Needleman HL, Schell A, Bellinger D, Leviton A, Allred EN: The long-term effects of exposure to low doses of lead in childhood. N Engl J Med 322:83–88, 1990
65. Colburn T, Dumanoski D, Myers JP: Our Stolen Future. New York: Dutton, 1996
66. Guillette LJ Jr, Gross TS, Masson GR, Matter JM, Percival HF, Woodward AR: Developmental abnormalities of the gonad and abnormal sex hormone concentrations in juvenile alligators from contaminated and control lakes in Florida. Environ Health Perspect 102:680–688, 1994
67. Adlercreutz H: Phytoestrogens: epidemiology and a possible role in cancer protection. Environ Health Perspect Suppl 103(7):103–112, 1995
68. Arnold SF, Robinson MK, Notides AC, Guillette LJ Jr, McLachlan JA: A yeast estrogen screen for examining the relative exposure of

cells to natural and xenoestrogens. Environ Health Perspect 104: 544–548, 1996

69. Sies H: Oxidative stress: introductory remarks. In Sies H (ed): Oxidative Stress. New York, Academic Press, 1985, pp 1–10
70. Houssoun EA, Stohs SJ: Chromium-induced production of reactive oxygen species, DNA single-strand breaks, nitric oxide production, and lactate dehydrogenase leakage in J774A.1 cell cultures. J Biochem Toxicol 10:315–322, 1995
71. Tappel AL: Lipid peroxidation damage to cell components. Fed Proc 32:1870–1874, 1973
72. Melin AM, Perromat A, Clerc M: In vivo effect of diosmin on carrageenan and CCl_4-induced liver peroxidation in rat liver microsomes. J Biochem Toxicol 11:27–32, 1996
73. Laskin DL, Heck DE, Gardner CR, Fedor LS, Laskin JD: Distinct patterns of nitric oxide production in hepatic macrophages and endothelial cells following acute exposure of rats to endotoxin. J Leukoc Biol 56:751–758, 1994
74. Bredt DS, Snyder SH: Isolation of nitric oxide synthase, a calmodulin-requiring enzyme. Proc Natl Acad Sci U S A 87:682–685, 1990
75. Dawson TM, Dawson VL, Snyder SH: A novel neuronal messenger molecule in brain: the free radical, nitric oxide. Ann Neurol 32:297–311, 1992
76. Dawson VL, Dawson TM, Bartley DA, Uhl GR, Snyder SH: Mechanisms of nitric oxide-mediated neurotoxicity in primary brain cultures. J Neurosci 13:2651–2661, 1993
77. Armitage P: Multistage models of carcinogenesis. Environ Health Perspect 63:195–201, 1985
78. Report of the EPA Workshop on the Development of Risk Assessment Methodologies for Tumor Promoters. EPA/600/9-87/013. Washington, DC: Environmental Protection Agency, 1987
79. Cohen SM, Ellwein LB: Genetic errors, cell proliferation, and carcinogenesis. Cancer Res 51:6493–6505, 1991
80. Bursch W, Oberhammer F, Schulte-Herman R: Cell death by apoptosis and its protective role against disease. Trends Pharmacol Sci 13:245–251, 1992
81. Schulte-Herman R, Timmermann-Trosiener I, Barthel G, Bursch W: DNA synthesis, apoptosis, and phenotypic expression and determinants of growth of altered foci in rat liver during phenobarbital promotion. Cancer Res 50:5127–5135, 1990
82. Marsman DS, Barrett JC: Apoptosis and chemical carcinogenesis. Risk Anal 14:321–326, 1994
83. Thompson CB: Apoptosis in the pathogenesis and treatment of disease. Science 267:1456–1460, 1995
84. Newman LS: To Be^{2+} or not to Be^{2+}: immunogenetics and occupational exposure. Science 262:197–198, 1993
85. Lauwerys R, Bernard A: Preclinical detection of nephrotoxicity: description of the tests and appraisal of their health significance. Toxicol Lett 46:13–30, 1989
86. Schulte PA, Perera FP: Molecular Epidemiology: Principles and Practices. San Diego: Academic Press, 1993
87. Mendelsohn ML, Peeters JP, Normandy MJ (eds): Biomarkers and Occupational Health: Progress and Perspectives. Washington DC: Joseph Henry Press, 1995
88. Peakall D: Animal Biomarkers as Pollution Indicators. London: Chapman & Hall, 1992
89. National Research Council: Biomarkers in Pulmonary Toxicology. Washington, DC: National Academy Press, 1989
90. National Research Council: Biomarkers in Reproductive Toxicology. Washington, DC: National Academy Press, 1992
91. National Research Council: Biomarkers in Immunotoxicology. Washington, DC: National Academy Press, 1992
92. Santella RM, Grinberg-Funes RA, Young TL, Singh VN, Wang LW, Perera FP: Cigarette smoking related polycyclic aromatic hydrocarbon-DNA adducts in peripheral mononuclear cells. Carcinogenesis 13:2041–2045, 1992
93. Costa M, Zhitkovich A, Toniolo P: DNA-protein cross-links in welders: molecular implications. Cancer Res 53:460–465, 1991
94. Mendelsohn ML: The current applicability of large scale biomarker programs to monitor cleanup workers. In Mendelsohn ML, Peeters JP, Normandy MJ (eds): Biomarkers and Occupational Health. Washington, DC: Joseph Henry Press, 1995, pp 9–19
95. Kimbrough RD: Determining exposure and biochemical effects in human population studies. Environ Health Perspect 48:77–79, 1983
96. Rall D, Hogan MD, Huff JE, Schwetz BA, Tennant RW: Alternatives to using human experience in assessing health. Ann Rev Public Health 8:355–385, 1987
97. Donehower L, Harvey M, Slagle B, McArthur M, Montgomery C, Butel J, Bradley A: Mice deficient for p53 are developmentally normal but susceptible to spontaneous tumours. Nature 356:215–221, 1992
98. Jacks T, Remington L, Williams B, Schmitt E, Halachmi S, Bronson R, Weinberg R: Tumor spectrum analysis in p53-mutant mice. Curr Biol. 4:1–7, 1994
99. Black H: A cleaner bill of health. Environ Health Perspect 104: 488–490, 1996
100. Kanitz S, Franco Y, Patrone V, Caltabellotta M, Raffo E, Riggi C, Timitilli D, Ravera G: Association between drinking water disinfection and somatic parameters at birth. Environ Health Perpsect 104:516–521, 1996
101. Alavanja M, Goldstein I, Susser M: A case-control study of gastrointestinal and urinary tract cancer mortality and drinking water chlorination. In Jolley RL, Gorchev H, Hamilton DH Jr (eds): Water Chlorination: Environmental Impact and Health. Ann Arbor, MI: Ann Arbor Scientific Publishing, 1990
102. Loranger S, Demers G, Kennedy G, Forget E, Zayed J: The pigeon (*Columba livia*) as a monitor for manganese contamination from motor vehicles. Arch Environ Contam Toxicol 27:311–317, 1994

General References

Aldredge WN: Mechanisms and Concepts in Toxicology. London: Taylor and Francis, 1996

Arias IM, Jakoby WB, Popper H, Schacter D: The Liver: Biology and Pathobiology. 2nd ed. New York: Raven Press, 1988

Ballantyne B, Marrs T, Turner P: General and Applied Toxicology. London: Macmillan Press, Ltd, 1995

Davies KJA, Ursini F (eds): The Oxygen Paradox. CLEUP University Padova, Italy, 1995

Francis BM: Toxic Substances in the Environment. New York: John Wiley & Sons, 1994

Fun AM, Chang LW (eds): Toxicology and Risk Assessment: Principles, Methods, and Applications. New York: Marcel Dekker, 1996

Galli CL, Marinovich M, Goldberg AM (eds): Modulation of Cellular Responses in Toxicity. Berlin: Springer, 1995

Gallo MA, Hesse EJ, MacDonald GJ, Umbreit TH: Interactive effects of estradiol and 2,3,7,8-tetrachloro-dibenzo-*p*-dioxin on hepatic cytochrome P-450 and mouse uterus. Toxicol Lett 32:123–132, 1986

Gossel TA, Bricker JD: Principles of Clinical Toxicology. 3rd ed. New York: Raven Press, 1994

Hayes AW: Principles and Methods of Toxicology. New York: Raven Press, 1989

Hayes WJ, Laws ER Jr: Handbook of Pesticide Toxicology. New York: Academic Press, 1997, vols 1–3

Hughes WW: Essentials of environmental toxicology: the effects of environmentally hazardous substances on human health. Washington, DC: Taylor and Francis, 1996

Josephy PD: Molecular Toxicology. New York: Oxford University Press, 1997

Kiran R, Varma MN: Biochemical studies on endosulfan toxicity in different age groups of rats. Toxicol Lett 44:247–252, 1988

Klaasen CD (ed): Casarett and Doull's Toxicology: The Basic Science of Poisons. 5th ed. New York: McGraw-Hill, 1996

Loomis TA, Hayes AW: Loomis's Essentials of Toxicology. 4th ed. San Diego: Academic Press, 1996

Lu FC: Basic toxicology: fundamentals, target organs, and risk assessment. 3rd ed. Washington DC: Taylor and Francis, 1996

Malins DC, Ostrander GK (eds): Aquatic toxicology; molecular, biochemical, and cellular perspectives. Boca Raton, FL: Lewis Publishers, 1994

National Research Council: Toxicants Occurring Naturally in Food. Washington, DC: National Academy of Science, 1973

Parker MG: Nuclear hormone receptors: molecular mechanisms, cellular functions, clinical abnormalities. London: Academic Press, 1991

Salsburg DS: Statistics for Toxicologists. New York: Marcel Dekker, 1986

Schardein JL: Chemically induced birth defects. 2nd ed. New York: Marcel Dekker, 1993

Sipes IG, McQueen CA, Gandolfi AJ: Comprehensive Toxicology. New York: Pergamon 1997 (13 volumes)

Timbrell JA: Introduction to Toxicology. 2nd ed. London: Taylor and Francis, 1995

Walker CH, Hopkin SP, Sibly RM, et al: Principles of Ecotoxicology. London: Taylor and Francis, 1996

Wexler P: Information Resources in Toxicology. New York: Elsevier, 1988

Williams PL, Burson JL: Industrial Toxicology. New York: Van Nostrand, 1985

Exposure

Barrett JC: Prevention of environmentally related disease. Environ Health Perspect 102:812–813, 1994

Lioy PJ, Waldman JM, Greenberg A, Harkov R, Pietarinen C: The Total Human Environmental Exposure Study (THEES) to benzo(a)pyrene: comparison of the inhalation and food pathways. Arch Environ Health 43:304–312, 1988

Miller FJ, Graham JA: Research needs and advances in inhalation dosimetry identified through the use of mathematical dosimetry models of ozone. Toxicol Lett 44:231–246, 1988

Morris RD: Chlorination, chlorination by-products and cancer: a meta-analysis. Am J Public Health 82:955–962, 1992

Carcinogenesis

Dragani T, Manenti G, Gariboldi M, Falvella S, Pierotti M, Della Porta G: Genetics of hepatocarcinogenesis in mouse and man. In Zervos C (ed): Oncogene and Transgenics Correlates of Cancer Risk Assessments. New York: Plenum Press, 1992, pp 67–80

Drinkwater N, Bennett L: Genetic control of carcinogenesis in experimental animals. Prog Exp Tumor Res 33:1–20, 1991

Haseman J, Lockhart A: The relationship between use of the maximum tolerated dose and study sensitivity for detecting rodent carcinogenicity. Fund Appl Toxicol 22:382–391, 1994

Huff J: Chemicals and cancer in humans: first evidence in experimental animals. Environ Health Perspect 100:201–210, 1993

Huff J, Boyd J, Barrett JC: Cellular and molecular mechanisms of hormonal carcinogenesis: environmental influences. New York: John Wiley & Sons, 1996

Li JJ, Li SA, Gustafsson J-A, Niendi S, Sekely LI (eds): Hormonal carcinogenesis. New York: Springer Verlag, 1996, vols 1–2

Mixtures

Vick J, Joseph X, Whitehurst V, Herman E, Balazs T: Cardiotoxic effects of the combined use of caffeine and isoproterenol in the minipig. J Toxicol Environ Health 26:425–436, 1989

Specific Substances

Lee JS, White KL: A review of the health effects of cadmium. Am J Ind Med 1:307–317, 1980

Haseman JK, Lockhart A: Correlations between chemically related site-specific carcinogenic effects in long-term studies in rats and mice. Environ Health Perspect 101:50–55, 1993

Ashby J, Hilton J, Dearman RJ, Callander RD, Kimber I: Mechanistic relationship among mutagenicity, skin sensitization and skin carcinogenicity. Environ Health Perspect 101:62–67, 1993

Lucier GW, Portier CJ, Gallo MA: Receptor mechanisms and dose-response models for the effects of dioxins. Environ Health Perspect 101:36–44, 1993

Neurobehavioral Toxicology

1. Lotti M: Neurotoxicology: The cinderella of neuroscience. Neurotoxicology 17:313–322, 1996
2. Weiss B: Tools for the assessment of behavioral toxicity. In Xinteras C, Johnson BL, de Groot I (eds): Behavioral Toxicology: Early Detection of Occupational Hazards. Washington, DC: US Department of Health, Education and Welfare, National Institute of Occupational Safety and Health, 1974, pp 444–449
3. Xintaras C, Johnson BL, de Groot I: Behavioral Toxicology: Early Detection of Occupational Hazards. Washington DC: US Department of Health, Education and Welfare, 1974
4. Zenick H, Reiter LW: Behavioral toxicology, an emerging discipline. Research Triangle Park, NC: U.S. Environmental Protection Agency, 1977
5. Valciukas JA, Lilis R: Psychometric techniques in environmental research. Environ Res 21:275–297, 1980
6. Lotti M: Central neurotoxicity and behavioral effects of anticholinesterases. In Ballantyne B, Marrs TC (eds): Clinical and Experimental Toxicology of Organophosphates and Carbamates. London: Butterworth-Heinemann, 1992, pp 75–83
7. Aldridge WN: The biological basis and measurement of thresholds. Ann Rev Pharmacol Toxicol 26:39–58, 1986
8. Johnson MK: The delayed neuropathy caused by some organophosphorus esters: mechanism and challenge. CRC Crit Rev Toxicol 3:289–316, 1975
9. Cohn J, Cory-Slechta DA: Lead exposure potentiates the effects of NMDA on repeated learning. Neurotoxicol Teratol 16:455–465, 1994
10. Cohen SA, Muller WE: Age-related alterations of NMDA-receptor properties in the mouse forebrain: partial restoration by chronic phosphatidylserine treatment. Brain Res 584:174–180, 1992
11. France CP, Lu Y, Woods JH: Interactions between *N*-methyl-D-aspartate and CGS 19755 administered intramuscularly and intracerebroventricularly in pigeons. J Pharmacol Exp Ther 225:1271–1277, 1990
12. Aamodt SM, Nordeen EJ, Nordeen KW: Blockade of NMDA receptors during song model exposure impairs song development in juvenile zebra finches. Neurobiol Learn Mem 65:91–98, 1996
13. Cory-Slechta DA, Pokora MJ, Preston RA: The effects of dopamine agonists on fixed interval schedule-controlled behavior are selectively altered by low-level lead exposure. Neurotoxicol Teratol 18:565–575, 1996
14. Johnson BL, Anger WK: Behavioral toxicology. In Rom W (ed): Environmental and Occupational Medicine. Boston: Little, Brown, 1983, pp 329–350
15. Baker EL, Letz R, Fidler A: A computer-administered neurobehavioral evaluation system for occupational and environmental epidemiology. J Occup Med 27:206–212, 1985
16. Singer R, Valciukas JA, Lilis R: Lead exposure and nerve conduction velocity: the differential time course of sensory and motor nerve effects. Neurotoxicology 4:193–202, 1983
17. Gilman S: Medical progress: advances in neurology. N Engl J Med 326:1608–1616, 1992
18. Morrow LA, Callender T, Lottenberg S, Buchsbaum MS, Hodgson MJ, Robin N: PET and neurobehavioral evidence of tetra-

bromoethane encephalopathy. J Neuropsychiatry Clin Neurosci 2:431–435, 1990
19. Laties VG, Merigan WH: Behavioral effects of carbon monoxide on animals and man. Annu Rev Pharmacol Toxicol 19:357–392, 1979
20. O'Hanlon JF: Preliminary studies of the effects of carbon monoxide on vigilance in man. In Weiss B, Laties VG (eds): Behavioral Toxicology. New York: Plenum Press, 1975, pp 61–75
21. Seppalainen AM: Neurophysiological findings among workers exposed to organic solvents. Scand J Work Environ Health 7(Suppl 4):29–33, 1981
22. Lindstrom K, Martelin T: Personality and long term exposure to organic solvents. Neurobehav Toxicol 2:89–100, 1980
23. Flodin U, Edling C, Axelson O: Clinical studies of psychoorganic syndromes among workers with exposure to solvents. Am J Ind Med 5:287–295, 1984
24. National Institute for Occupational Safety and Health: Organic solvent neurotoxicity. NIOSH Curr Intelligence Bull 48:1–39, 1987
25. Korbo L, Ladeefoged O, Lam HR, Østergaard G, West MJ, Arlien-Søbert: Neuronal loss in hippocampus in rats exposed to toluene. Neurotoxicology 17:359–366, 1996
26. Cherry N, Waldron HA, Wells GG, Wilkinson RT, Wilson HK, Jones S: An investigation of the acute behavioural effects of styrene on factory workers. Br J Ind Med 37:234–240, 1980
27. Campagna D, Gobba F, Mergler D, Moreau T, Galassi C, Cavalleri A, Huel G: Color vision loss among styrene-exposed workers: neurotoxicological threshold assessment. Neurotoxicology 17:367–374, 1996
28. Cavanaugh JV: Peripheral neuropathy caused by chemical agents. CRC Crit Rev Toxicol 2:365–376, 1980
29. Teisinger J: New advances in the toxicology of carbon dislufide. Am Ind Hyg Assoc J 35:55, 1974
30. Vigilani EC: Carbon disulfide poisoning in viscose rayon factories. Br J Ind Med 11:235, 1954
31. Rice DC: Sensory and cognitive effects of developmental methyl mercury exposure in monkeys, and a comparison to effects in rodents. Neurotoxicology 17:139–154, 1996
32. El-Fawal HAN, Gong Z, Little AR, Evans HL: Exposure to methyl mercury results in serum autoantibodies to neurotypic and gliotypic proteins. Neurotoxicology 17:531–540, 1996
33. Langston JW, Ballard P, Tetrud JW, Irwin I: Chronic parkinsonism in humans due to a product of meperidine-analog synthesis. Science 219:979–980, 1983
34. Valciukas JA, Lilis R, Fischbein A, Selikoff IJ: Central nervous system dysfunction due to lead exposure. Science 201:465–467, 1978
35. Agency for Toxic Substances and Disease Registry (ATSDR): The nature and extent of lead poisoning in children in the United States: a report to Congress. Atlanta: U.S. Public Health Service, 1988
36. Schmitt TJ, Zawia N, Harry GJ: GAP-43 mRNA expression in the developing rat brain: alterations following lead-acetate exposure Neurotoxicology. 17:407–414, 1996
37. Rogan WJ, Gladen BC, McKinney JD, Carreras N, Hardy P, Thullen J, Tinglestad J, Tully M: Neonatal effects of transplacental exposure to PCBs and DDE. J Pediatr 109:335–341, 1986
38. Jacobson JL, Jacobson SW, Padgett RJ, Brumitt GA, Billings RL: Effects of prenatal PCB exposure on cognitive processing efficiency and sustained attention. Dev Psychobiol 28:297–306, 1992
39. Jacobson JL, Jacobson SW: Intellectual impairment in children exposed to polychlorinated biphenyls in utero. N Engl J Med 335:783–789, 1996
40. Silbergeld EK: Mechanisms of lead neurotoxicity, or looking beyond the lamppost. FASEB J 6:3201–3206, 1992
41. Cory-Slechta DA, Pokora MJ, Fox RAV, O'Mara DJ: Lead-induced changes in dopamine D_1 sensitivity: modulation by drug discrimination training. Neurotoxicology 17:445–458, 1996
42. Cory-Slechta DA, Pokora MJ, Johnson JL: Postweaning lead exposure enhances the stimulus properties of *N*-methyl-D-aspartate: possible dopaminergic involvement? Neurotoxicology 17:509–522, 1996
43. Cory-Slechta DA: Relationships between lead induced learning impairments and changes in dopaminergic, cholinergic, and glutaminergic neurotransmitter system functions. Annu Rev Pharmacol Toxicol 3:391–415, 1995
44. Simmons TJB: Lead-calcium interactions in cellular lead toxicity. Neurotoxicology 14:77–86, 1993
45. Ceccatelli S, Grandison L, Scott REM, Pfaff DW, Kow L-M: Estradiol regulation of nitric oxide synthase mRNAs in rat hypothalamus. Neuroendocrinology 64:357–363, 1996
46. Franck J, Nylander I, Rosén A: Met-enkephalin inhibits 5-hydroxytrypatmine release from the rat ventral spinal cord via δ opioid receptors. Neuropharmacology 35:743–748, 1996
47. Hauser GJ, Danchak MR, Colvin MP, Hopkins RA, Wocial B, Myers AK, Zukowska-Grojec Z: Circulating neuropeptide Y in humans: relation to changes in catecholamine levels and changes in hemodynamics. Neuropeptides 30:159–165, 1996
48. Haberstock H, Marotti T, Banfic H: Neutrophil signal transduction in Met-enkephalin modulated superoxide anion release. Neuropeptides 30:193–201, 1996
49. Ribeiro RCJ, Apriletti JW, West BL, Wagner RL, Fletterick RJ, Schaufele F, Baxter JDL: The molecular biology of thyroid hormone actin. Ann N Y Acad Sci: 758L:366–389, 1995
50. Li M, Sendtner M, Smith M: Essential function of LIF receptor in motor neurons. Nature 378:724–727, 1995
51. Rice DC, Gilbert SG, Willes RF: Neonatal low-level lead exposure in monkeys: locomotor activity, schedule-controlled behavior, and the effects of amphetamine. Toxicol Appl Pharmacol 51:503–513, 1979
52. Griffin DR: The Question of Animal Awareness: Evolutionary Continuity of Mental Experience. New York: Rockefeller University Press, 1976
53. Lorenz K: On Aggression. New York: Harcourt, Brace & World, 1966
54. Laties VG: How operant conditioning can contribute to behavioral toxicology. Environ Health Perspect 26:29–35, 1978
55. Burger J, Gochfeld M: Early postnatal lead exposure: behavioral effects in common tern chicks (*Sterna hirundo*). J Toxicol Environ Health 16:869–886, 1985
56. Reiter L: Use of activity measures in behavioral toxicology. Environ Health Perspect 26:9–20, 1978
57. Brown DR: Neonatal lead exposure in the rat: decreased learning as a function of age and blood lead concentration. Toxicol Applied Pharmacol 32:628–637, 1975
58. Ogilvie DM: Sublethal effects of lead acetate on the Y-maze performance of albino mice (*Mus musculus* L.). Can J Zoology 55:771–775, 1977
59. Kopf SR, Baratti CM: Memory modulation by post-training glucose or insulin remains evident at long retention intervals. Neurobiol Learn Mem 65:189–191, 1996
60. Zhao WQ, Bennett P, Rickard N, Sedman GL, Gibbs ME, Ng KT: The involvement of Ca^{2+}/calmodulin-dependent protein kinase in memory formation in day-old chicks. Neurobiol Learn Mem 66:24–35, 1996
61. Bock J, Wolf A, Braun K: Influence of the *N*-methyl-D-aspartate receptor antagonist DL-2-amino-5-phosphonovaleric acid on auditory filial imprinting in the domestic chick. Neurobiol Learn Mem 65:177–188, 1996
62. Lincoln J, Coopersmith R, Harris EW, Cotman CW, Leon M: NMDA receptor activation and early olfactory learning. Brain Res 467:309–312, 1988
63. Burger J, Gochfeld M: Lead and behavioral development: parental compensation for behaviorally impaired chicks. Pharmacol Biochem Behav 55:339–349, 1996
64. Cory-Slechta DA, Weiss B, Cox C: Delayed behavioral toxicity of lead with increasing exposure concentration. Toxicol Appl Pharmacol 71:342–352, 1983

65. Rice DC, Gilbert SG: Early chronic low-level methyl mercury poisoning in monkeys impairs spatial vision. Science 206:759–771, 1982
66. Rice DC: Behavioral deficit (delayed matching to sample) in monkeys exposed from birth to low levels of lead. Toxicol Appl Pharmacol 75:337–345, 1984
67. Dietz DD, McMillan DE, Mushak P: Effects of chronic lead administration on acquisition and performance of serial position sequences by pigeons. Toxicol Appl Pharmacol 47:377–384, 1979
68. Laties VG, Evans HL: Methyl mercury–induced changes in an operant discrimination in the pigeon. J Pharmacol Exp Ther 214:620–628, 1980
69. Uphouse L, Andrade M, Caldarola-Pastuszka M, Jackson A: 5-HT_{1A} receptor anatgonists and lordosis behavior. Neuropharmacology 35:489–495, 1996
70. Burger J, Gochfeld M: Behavioral impairments of lead-injected young herring gulls in nature. Fundam Appl Toxicol 23:553–561, 1994
71. Barthalamus GT, Leander JD, McMillan DE, Mushak P, Krigman MR: Chronic effects of lead on schedule-controlled pigeon behavior. Toxicol Appl Pharmacol 41:459–471, 1977
72. Crofton KM, Howard JL, Moster VC, Gill MW, Reiter LW, Tilson HA, MacPhail RC: Interlaboratory comparison of motor activity experiments: implications for neurotoxicological assessments. Neurotoxicol Teratol 13:599–609, 1991
73. Silbergeld E, Goldberg A: A lead-induced behavioral disorder. Life Sci 13:1275–1283, 1973
74. Fox GA, Donald T: Organochlorine pollutants, nest-defense behavior and reproductive success in merlins. Condor 82:81–84, 1980
75. Bushnell PJ, Bowman RE, Allen JR, Marlar RJ: Scotopic vision deficits in young monkeys exposed to lead. Science 196:333–335, 1977
76. McArthur MLB, Fox GA, Peakall DB, Philogene BJR: Ecological significance of behavioral and hormonal abnormalities in breeding ring doves fed an organochlorine chemical mixture. Arch Environ Contam Toxicol 12:343–353, 1983
77. Witt PN: Drugs alter web-building of spiders: a review and evaluation. Behav Sci 16:98–113, 1971
78. Laties V, Cory-Slechta DA: Some problems in interpreting the behavioral effects of lead and methyl mercury. Neurobehav Toxicol 1:129–135, 1979
79. Brady K, Herrera Y, Zenick H: Influence of parental lead exposure on subsequent learning ability of offspring. Pharmacol Biochem Behav 3:561–565, 1975
80. Dahlgren RB, Linder RL: Effects of dieldrin in penned pheasants through the third generation. J Wildlife Manag 39:320–330, 1974
81. Hutchinson LJ, Amler RW, Lybarger JA, Chappell W: Neurobehavioral test batteries for use in environmental health field study. Atlanta: U.S. Department of Health and Human Services, Agency for Toxic Substances and Disease Registry, 1992
82. Mergler D, Blain L: Assessing color vision loss among solvent-exposed workers. Am J Ind Med 12:195–203, 1987
83. Mergler D, Huel G, Bowler R, Frenette B, Cone J: Visual dysfunction among former microelectronics assembly workers. Arch Environ Health 46:326–334, 1991
84. Mergler D: Color vision loss: a sensitive indicator of the severity of optic neuropathy. In Johnson BL (ed): Advances in Neurobehavioral Toxicology: Applications in Environmental and Occupational Health. Chelsea, MI: Lewis Publishers, 1990, pp 175–182
85. Mergler D: Behavioral Neurophysiology: Quantitative Measures of Sensory Toxicity Neurotoxicology: Approaches and Methods. New York: Academic Press, 1995, pp 727–736
86. Williamson AM: The development of a neurobehavioral test battery for use in hazard evaluations in occupational settings. Neurotoxicol Teratol 12:509–514, 1990
87. Valciukas JA, Singer RM: An embedded figures test in environmental and occupational neurotoxicology. Environ Res 28:183–198, 1982
88. Morata TC, Dunn DE, Sieber WK: Occupational exposure to noise and ototoxic organic solvents. Arch Environ Health 49:359–365, 1994
89. Burger J, Gochfeld M: A hypothesis on the role of pheromones on age of menarche. Med Hypotheses 17:39–46, 1985
90. Schwartz BS, Ford P, Bolla KI, Agnew J, Rothman N, Bleecker ML: Solvent-associated decrements in olfactory function in paint manufacturing workers. Am J Ind Med 18:697–706, 1990
91. Ryan CM, Morrow LA, Hodgson M: Cacosmia and neurobehavioral dysfunction associated with occupational exposure to mixtures of organic solvents. Am J Psychiatry 145(11):1442–1445, 1988
92. Doty RL, Gregor T, Monroe C: Quantitative assessment of olfactory function in an industrial setting. J Occup Med 28:457–460, 1986
93. Doty RL, Deems DA, Frye RE, et al. Olfactory sensitivity, nasal resistance, and autonomic function in patients with multiple chemical sensitivities. Arch Otolaryngol Head Neck Surg 114:1422–1427, 1988
94. Rose CS, Heywood PG, Costanzo RM: Olfactoric impairment after chronic occupational cadmium exposure. J Occup Med 34:600–605, 1992
95. Lezak M: Neuropsychological Assessment. New York: Oxford University Press, 1995
96. McConnell R, Keifer M, Rosenstock L: Elevated quantitative vibrotactile threshold among workers previously poisoned with methamidophos and other organophosphate pesticides. Am J Ind Med 25:325–334, 1994
97. Bove F, Litwak MS, Arezzo JC, Baker EL: Quantitative sensory testing in occupational medicine. Semin Occup Med 1:185–188, 1986
98. Mergler D: Behavioral neurophysiology: quantitative measures of sensory toxicity. In Chang LW, Slikker W (eds), Neurotoxicology: Approaches and Methods. San Diego: Academic Press, 1995, pp 727–736
99. Kilburn KH, Warshaw RH, Hanscom B: Are hearing loss and balance dysfunction linked in construction iron workers? Br J Industr Med 49:138–141, 1992
100. Gyntelberg F, Vesterhauge S, Fog P, Isager H, Zillstorff K: Acquired intolerance to organic solvents and results of vestibular testing. Am J Ind Med 9:363–370, 1986
101. Kilburn KH, Warshaw R, Thornton JC: Formaldehyde impairs memory, equilibrium, and dexterity in histology technicians: effects which persist for days after exposure. Arch Environ Health 42: 117–120, 1987
102. Morrow LA, Ryan CM, Goldstein G, Hodgson MJ: A distinct pattern of personality disturbance following exposure to mixtures of organic solvents. J Occup Med 31:743–750, 1989
103. Kilburn KH, Seidman BC, Warshaw R: Neurobehavioral and respiratory symptoms of formaldehyde and xylene exposure in histology technicians. Arch Environ Health 40:229–233, 1985
104. Needleman H, Gunnoe C, Leviton A, Reed R, Peresie H, Maher C, Barrett P: Deficits in psychologic and classroom performance of children with elevated dentine lead levels. N Engl J Med 300: 689–695, 1979
105. Spitzer RL, Williams JBW, Gibbon M, et al: User's Guide for the Structured Clinical Interview for DSM-III-R. Washington, DC: American Psychiatric Press, 1990
106. Baker EL, Letz R: Solvent neurobehavioral testing in monitoring hazardous workplace exposures. J Occup Med 28:126–129, 1986
107. Hanninen H, Lindstrom K: Behavioral Test Battery for Toxicopsychological Studies. Helsinki: Institute of Occupational Health, 1979
108. World Health Organization: Organic Solvents and the Central Nervous System. Document 5, Copenhagen: World Health Organization, 1985
109. Wechsler D: WAIS-R Manual. New York: The Psychological Corporation, 1981

110. Gamberale F: Use of behavioral performance tests in the assessment of solvent toxicity. Scand J Work Environ Health 11:65–74, 1985
111. Hartman DE: Neuropsychological toxicology. New York: Pergamon Press, 1988
112. Michelsen H, Lundberg I: Neuropsychological verbal tests may lack "hold" properties in occupational studies of neurotoxic effects. Occup Environ Med 53:478–483, 1996
113. Dick RB: Neurobehavioral assessment of occupational relevant solvents and chemicals in humans. In Chang LW, Dyer RS, (eds): Handbook of Neurotoxicology. New York: Marcel Dekker, 1995, pp 217–322
114. Matthews CG, Klove H: Instruction manual for the Adult Neuropsychology Test Battery. Madison, WI: University of Wisconsin Medical School, 1964
115. Anger WK: Worksite behavioral research: results, sensitive methods, test batteries and the transition from laboratory data to human health. Neurotoxicology 11:629–720, 1990
116. Jansen AAI, deGier JJ, Slangen JL: Alcohol effects on signal detection performance. Neuropsychobiology 14:83–87, 1985
117. Gustafson R: Alcohol, reaction time, and vigilance settings: importance of length of intersignal interval. Percept Motor Skills 63:424–426, 1986
118. Delis D, Kramer J, Kaplan E, Ober B: California Verbal Learning Test Manual. San Antonio, TX: The Psychological Corporation, 1987
119. Benton A: Visual Retention Test Manual. San Antonio, TX: The Psychological Corporation, 1974
120. McNair D, Lorr M, Droppleman L: Profile of Mood States. In: Educational and Industrial Testing Service Manual, San Diego: 1981
121. Derogatis L: SCL-90-R Manual-II. Towson, MD: Clinical Psychometric Research, 1983
122. Burger J, Gochfeld M: Lead and behavioral development: effects of varying dosage and schedule on survival and performance of young common terns (*Sterna hirundo*). J Toxicol Environ Health 24:173–182, 1988
123. Needleman HL, Gatsonis CA: Low-level lead exposure and the IQ of children: a meta-analysis of modern studies. JAMA 263:673–678, 1990
124. Tilson HA, Davis GJ, MaLachlan JA, Lucier GW: The effects of polychlorinated biphenyls given prenatally on the neurobehavioral development of mice. Environ Res 18:466–474, 1979
125. Schantz SL, Levin ED, Bowman RE, Heironimus MP, Laughlin NK: Effects of perinatal PCB exposure on discrimination-reversal learning in monkeys. Neurotoxicol Teratol 1:243–250, 1989
126. Maier WE, Kodavanti PRS, Harry GJ, Tilson HA: Sensitivity of adenosine triphosphatases in different brain regions to polychlorinated biphenyl congeners. J Appl Toxicol 14:225–229, 1994
127. Kodavanti PRS, Ward TR, McKinney JD, Tilson HA: Increased [^{3}H]phorbol ester binding in rat cerebellar granule cells by polychlorinated biphenyl mixtures and congeners: structure-activity relationships. Toxicol Appl Pharmacol 130:140–148, 1995
128. Krasnegor NA, Otto DA, Bernstein JH, Burke R, Chappell W, Eckerman DA, Needleman HL, Oakley G, Rogan W, Terracciano G, Hutchinson L: Neurobehavioral test strategies for environmental exposures in pediatric populations. Neurotoxicol Teratol 16:499–509, 1994
129. Harada M: Intrauterine poisoning: clinical and epidemiologial studies and significance of the problem. Bull Inst Constit Medicine, Kumanoto Univ 25(suppl):1–69, 1976
130. Yu M, Hsu C, Gladen BC, Rogan WJ: In utero PCB/PCDF exposure: relation of developmental delay to dysmorphology and dose. Neurotoxicol Teratol 13:195–202, 1991
131. Chen YJ, Gue Y, Hsu C, Rogan WJ: Cognitive development of Yu-Cheng ("oil disease") children prenatally exposed to heat-degraded PCBs. JAMA 268:3213–3218, 1992
132. Jacobson SW, Fein GG, Jacobson JL, Schwartz PM, Dowler JK: The effect of intrauterine PCB exposure on visual recognition memory. Child Dev 56:853–860, 1985
133. Jacobson JL, Jacobson SW, Humphrey JB: Effects of in utero exposure to polychlorinated biphenyls and related contaminants on cognitive functioning in young children. J Pediatr 116:38–45, 1990
134. Rogan WJ, Gladen BC: PCBs, DDE, and child development at 18 and 24 months. Ann Epidemiol 1:407–413, 1991
135. Gladen BC, Rogan WJ: Effects of perinatal polychlorinated biphenyls and dichlorodiphenyl dichloroethene on later development. J Pediatr 119:58–63, 1991
136. Lonky J, Relhman J, Darvill T, Mather J Sr, Daly H: Neonatal behavioral assessment scale performance in humans influenced by maternal consumption of environmentally contaminated Lake Ontario fish. J Great Lakes Res 22:198–212, 1996
137. Daly HB: The evaluation of behavioral changes produced by consumption of environmentally contaminated fish. In Issacson RL, Jensen KR (eds): The Vulnerable Brain and Environmental Risks. Malnutrition and Hazard Assessment. New York: Plenum Press, 1992, vol 1, pp 151–171
138. Doty RL, Shaman PL, Applebaum SL, Giberson R, Siksorski L, Rosenberg L: Smell identification ability: changes with age. Science 226:1441–1443, 1984
139. Mabry TR, McCarty R, Gold PE, Foster TC: Age and stress history effects on spatial performance in a swim task in Fischer-344 rats. Neurobiol Learn Mem 66:1–10, 1996

General References

Anastasi A: Psychological Testing, New York: Macmillan, 1976
Annau Z: Neurobehavioral Toxicology. Baltimore: Johns Hopkins University Press, 1986
Belgrave BE, Bird KD, Chesher GB, Jackson DM, Lubbe KE, Starmer GA, Teo RKC: The effect of cannabidiol, alone and in combination with ethanol, on human performance. Psychopharmacology 64:243–246, 1979
Bender L: A visual motor gestalt test and its clinical use. New York: American Orthopsychiatric Association, 1938
Brown GG, Nison R: Exposure to polybrominated biphenyls: some effects on personality and cognitive functioning JAMA 242:523, 1979
Camhi JM: Neuroethology: Sunderland, MA: Sinauer Associates Press, 1984
Chang LW, Dyer RS: Handbook of Neurotoxicology. New York: Marcel Dekker, 1995
Chang LW, Slikker W Jr (eds): Neurotoxicology: Approaches and Methods. San Diego: Academic Press, 1995
Davis DD, Templer DI: Neurobehavioral functioning in children exposed to narcotics in utero. Addict Behav 13:275–283, 1988
Donovick PJ, Horowitz GP: On the choice of subject populations for research in neurobehavioral toxicology. J Toxicol Environ Health 10: 1–9, 1982
Dun NJ, Perlman RL (eds): Neurobiology of Acetylcholine. New York: Plenum Press, 1987
Feldman RG, Ricks NL, Baker EL: Neuropsychological effects of industrial toxins: a review. Am J Ind Med 1:211–227, 1980
Flodin U, Edling C, Axelson O: Clinical studies of psychoorganic syndromes among workers with exposure to solvents. Am J Ind Med 5:287–295, 1984
Gale A, Edwards JA (eds): Physiological Correlates of Human Behavior. New York: Academic Press, 1983, vols 1–3
Gamberale F: Use of behavioral performance tests in the assessment of solvent toxicity. Scand J Work Environ Health 11(1):65–74, 1985
Gilioli R, Cassitto MG, Foa V: Neurobehavioral Methods in Occupational Health. New York: Pergamon Press, 1982

Grandjean P: Symposium synthesis: application of neurobehavioral methods in environmental and occupational health. Environ Res 60: 57–61, 1993

Hanninen H: Behavioral effects of occupational exposure to mercury and lead. Acta Neurol Scand 66:(suppl) 92:167, 1982

Hartman DE: Neuropsychological toxicology. New York: Pergamon Press, 1988

Head H: The conception of nervous and mental energy: vigilance, a physiological state of the central nervous system. Br J Psychol 14:126–146, 1923

Hook GER, Lucier GW: Human developmental neurotoxicity. 102(suppl 2):115–161, 1994

Huber F, Markl H: Neuroethology and Behavioral Physiology. New York: Springer Verlag, 1983

Hunting KL, Matanoski GM, Larson M, Wolford R: Solvent exposure and the risk of slips, trips and falls among painters. Am J Industr Med 20:353–370, 1991

Johnson BL (ed): Prevention of Neurotoxic Illness in Working Populations. New York: John Wiley & Sons, 1987

Kilburn KH, Warshaw RH: Neurobehavioral testing of subjects exposed residentially to groundwater contaminated from an aluminum diecasting plant and local referents. J Toxicol Environ Health 39:483–496, 1993

Kilburn KH, Seidman BC, Warshaw R: Neurobehavioral and respiratory symptoms of formaldehyde and xylene exposure in histology technicians. Arch Environ Health 40:229–233, 1985

Lehner PN: Handbook of Ethological Methods. New York: Garland STPM Press, 1979

Lewis JA, Baddeley A, Banham KG, Lovitt D: Traffic pollution and mental efficiency. Nature 225:95–96, 1969

Lindstrom K, Harkonen H, Hernberg S: Disturbances in psychological functions of workers occupationally exposed to styrene. Scand J Work Environ Health 3:129–139, 1976

Lindstrom K, Martelin T: Personality and long term exposure to organic solvents. Neurobehav Toxicol 2:89–100, 1980

Marlow M, Stellern J, Errera J, Moon C: Main and interaction effects of metal pollutants on visual-motor performance. Arch Environ Health 40:221–224, 1985

Mutti A, Mazzucchi A, Rustichelli P, Frigeri G, Arfini G, Franchini I: Exposure-effect and exposure-response relationships between occupational exposure to styrene and neuropsychological functions. Am J Ind Med 5:275–281, 1984

Reiter L: An introduction to neurobehavioral toxicology. Environ Health Perspect 26:5–7, 1978

Seppalainen AN, Lindstrom K, Martelin T: Neurophysiological and psychological picture of solvent poisoning. Am J Ind Med 1:31–42, 1980

Tilson HA, Sparber SB: Neurotoxicants and Neurobiological Function. New York: John Wiley & Sons, 1987

Tilson HA, Cabe PA, Mitchell CL: Behavioral and neurological toxicity of polybrominated biphenyls in rats and mice. Environ Health Perspect 23:257–263, 1978

Tinbergen N: The Study of Instinct. New York: Oxford University Press, 1974

Valciukas JA: Foundations of Environmental and Occupational Neurotoxicology. New York: Van Nostrand Reinhold, 1991

Valciukas JA, Lilis R: Psychometric techniques in environmental research. Environ Res 21:275–297, 1980

Weiss B: Behavioral toxicology and environmental health science: opportunity and challenge for psychology. Am Psychol 38:1174, 1983

Weiss B: Experimental implications of behavior as a criterion of toxicity. In Weiss B, Laties VG (eds): Behavioral Pharmacology: The Current Status. New York: Alan R. Liss, 1985, pp 467–472

Weiss B, Laties VG: Behavioral Pharmacology: The Current Status. New York: Alan R. Liss, 1985

Winlow W, Vinogradova OS, Sakharov DA: Signal Molecules and Behavior. New York: Manchester University Press, 1991

Xintaras C, Johnson BL, de Groot I: Behavioral Toxicology: Early Detection of Occupational Hazards. DHEW (NIOSH) 74-126. NIOSH, Washington, DC: U.S. Department of Health, Education and Welfare, 1974

Yerkes RM: The mental life of monkeys and apes: a study of ideational behavior. Behav Monogr 3:1–145, 1916

Yerkes RM: The mind of a gorilla: memory. Comp Psychol Monogr 5(2):1–91, 1928

Yesavage JA, Dolhert N, Taylor JL: Flight simulator performance of younger and older aircraft pilots: effects of age and alcohol. J Am Geriatr Soc 42:577–582, 1994

Zenick H, Reiter LW: Behavioral toxicology, an emerging discipline. Research Triangle Park, NC: U.S. Environmental Protection Agency, 1977

Zbinden G, Cuomo V, Racagni G, Weiss B (eds): Application of Behavioral Pharmacology in Toxicology. New York: Raven Press, 1983

Neurobehavioral Effects of Lead

Bushnell PJ, Bowman RE: Persistence of impaired reversal learning in young monkeys exposed to low levels of dietary lead. J Toxicol Environ Health 5:1015–1023, 1979

Cory-Slechta DA, Weiss B, Cox, C: Delayed behavioral toxicity of lead with increasing exposure concentration. Toxicol Appl Pharmacol 71:342–352, 1983

David OJ, Hoffman SP, Sverd J, Clark J: Lead and hyperactivity: lead levels among hyperactive children. J Abnorm Child Psychol 5:405–417, 1977

Jason KM, Kellogg CK. Behavioral neurotoxicity of lead. In Singhal RL, Thomas JA (eds): Lead Toxicity. Baltimore Urban & Schwarzenberg, pp 241–271, 1980

Lucier GW (ed): Advances in lead research: implications for environmental health. Environ Health Perspect 89:3–239, 1990

McMichael AJ, Baghurst PA, Wigg NR, Vimpani GV: Port Pirie cohort study: environmental exposure to lead and children's abilities at four years. N Engl J Med 319:468–475, 1988

Needleman HL: Human Lead Exposure. Boca Raton, FL: CRC Press, 1992

Roderer G, Doenges KH: Influence of trimethyl lead and inorganic lead on the in vitro assembly of microtubules from mammalian brain. Neurotoxicology 4:171–180, 1983

Seeber A, Kiesswetter E, Neidhart B, Blaszkewicz M: Neurobehavioral effects of a long-term exposure to tetraalkyllead. Neurotoxicol Teratol 12:653–655, 1990

Singer R, Valciukas JA, Lilis R: Lead exposure and nerve conduction velocity: the diferential time course of sensory and motor nerve effects. Neurotoxicology 4:193–202, 1982

Smith M: Intellectual and behavioral consequences of low level lead exposure: a review of recent studies. Clin Endocrinol Metab 14:657–680, 1985

Yule W, Lansdown R, Millar IB, Urbanowicz M: The relationship between blood lead concentrations, intelligence and attainment in a school population: a pilot study. Dev Med Child Neurol 23:567–576, 1981

Environmental and Ecological Risk Assessment

1. National Research Council: Understanding Risk—Informing Decisions in a Democratic Society. Washington, DC: National Academy Press, 1996
2. Cairns J: Restoration ecology: a major opportunity for ecotoxicologists. Environ Toxicol Chem 10:429–432, 1991
3. Burger J, Gochfeld M: Ecological and human health risk assessment: a comparison. In DiGuilio RT, Monosson E (eds): Interconnections between human and ecosystem health. London: Chapman & Hall, 1996, pp 127–148
4. Morse SS: Factors in the emergence of infectious diseases. Emerg Infect Dis 1:7–15, 1995

5. National Research Council: Risk Assessment in the Federal Government. Washington DC: National Academy Press. 1983
6. Burger J: How should success be measured in ecological risk assessment? The importance of "predictive accuracy." Environ Health Toxicol 42:367–376, 1994
7. Mitsch WJ: Ecological engineering. Environ Sci Technol 27:438–445, 1993
8. United States Environmental Protection Agency: Risk Assessment Guidelines for Carcinogenicity, Mutagenicity, Complex Mixtures, Suspect Developmental Toxicants, and Estimating Exposures. Federal Register 51:33992–34054, 1986
9. Derby SL, Keeney RL: Risk analysis: understanding "how safe is safe enough?" Risk Anal 1:217–224, 1981
10. National Research Council: Report of the Commission on Risk Assessment and Risk Management. Washington DC: National Research Council, 1996
11. Lowrance WW: Of Acceptable Risk. Los Altos, CA: William Kaufmann, 1976
12. Imperato PJ, Mitchell G: Acceptable Risk. New York: Viking, 1985
13. Jasanoff S (ed): Learning from Disaster. Philadelphia: University of Pennsylvania Press, 1994
14. National Research Council: Committee on Risk Assessment Methodology: Issues in Risk Assessment. Washington, DC: National Academy Press, 1993
15. Whyte AV, Burton I: Environmental risk assessment. New York: John Wiley & Sons, 1980
16. Goldstein BD: Risk assessment/risk management is a three step process: in defense of EPA's risk assessment guidelines. J Am Coll Toxicol 7:543–549, 1988
17. Fischoff B, Slovic P, Lichtenstein S, Read S, Combs B: How safe is safe enough?: a psychometric study of attitudes towards technological risks and benefits. Policy Sci 8:127–152, 1978
18. Sandman PM: Hazard Versus Outrage: The Case of Radon. New Brunswick, NJ: Rutgers Environmental Communication Research Program, 1988
19. Kasperson RE, Renn O, Slovic P, Brown HS, Emel J, Goble R, Kasperson JX, Ratick S: The social amplification of risk: a conceptual framework. Risk Anal 8:177–187, 1988
20. Cutter SL, Holm D, Clark L: The role of geographic scale in monitoring environmental justice. Risk Anal 16:517–526, 1996
21. Greenberg M, Krueckeberg D, Kaltman M, Metz W, Wilhelm C: Local planning v national policy: urban growth near nuclear power stations in the United States. Town Plan Rev 57:225–238, 1986
22. Doderlein JM: Understanding risk management. Risk Anal 3:17–21, 1983
23. May WW: $s for lives: ethical considerations in the use of cost/benefit analysis by for-profit firms. Risk Anal 2:35–46, 1982
24. Greenberg MR, Anderson RF: Hazardous Waste Sites: The Credibility Gap. New Brunswick, NJ: Center for Urban Policy Research, 1984
25. Environmental Protection Agency: Office of Research and Development: Health Assessment Document for 2,3,7,8-tetrachlorodibenzo-*p*-dioxin (TCDD) and related compounds. Washington, DC: Environmental Protection Agency, 1994
26. National Research Council, Safe Drinking Water Committee: Drinking Water and Health. Selected Issues in Risk Assessment. Washington, DC: National Academy Press, 1989, vol 9
27. Crump KS, Gentry R: A response to OMB's comments regarding OSHA's approach to risk assessment in support of OSHA's final rule on cadmium. Risk Anal 13:487–489, 1993
28. Environmental Protection Agency: Intergrated Risk Information System (IRIS) database. Washington, DC. Environmental Protection Agency, 1996
29. Lioy P: Assessing total human exposure to contaminants. Environ Sci Technol 24:938–945, 1990
30. Environmental Protection Agency: Proposed Guidelines for Carcinogen Risk Assessment. Federal Register 49:46294–46301, 1984
31. Armitage P: Multistage models of carcinogenesis. Environ Health Perspect 63:195–201, 1985
32. Moolgavkar SH, AG Knudsen Jr: Mutation and cancer: a model for human carcinogenesis. J Nat Cancer Inst 66:1037–1052, 1981
33. Krewski D, Van Ryzin J: Dose response models for quantal response toxicity dates. In Csorgo M, Dawson D, Rao JNK, Saleh E (eds): Current Topics in Probability and Statistics. New York: North-Holland, 1981
34. Hallenbeck WH: Quantitative evaluation of human and animal studies. In Hallenbeck WH, Cunningham KM (eds): Quantitative Risk Assessment for Environmental and Occupational Health. Chelsea, Michigan: Lewis, 1987, pp 43–60
35. Crump KS, Howe RB: The multistage model with a time-dependent dose pattern: application to carcinogenic risk assessment. Risk Anal 4:163–176, 1984
36. Farland W, Dourson M: Noncancer health endpoints: approaches to quantitative risk assessment. In Cothern CR (ed): Comparative Environmental Risk Assessment. Boca Raton, FL: Lewis, 1993, pp 87–106
37. Barnes DG, Dourson M: Reference dose (Rfd): description and use in health risk assessments. Reg Toxicol Pharmacol 8:471–486, 1988
38. Environmental Protection Agency: IRIS: Integrated Risk Information System. Washington, DC: Environmental Protection Agency, 1992
39. Clewell HJ III, Jarnot BM: Incorporation of pharmacokinetics in noncancer risk assessment: example with chloropentafluorobenzene. Risk Anal 14:265–276, 1994
40. Rao HV, Brown DR: A physiologically-based pharmacokinetic assessment of tetrachloroethylene in groundwater for a bathing and showering determination. Risk Anal 13:37–50, 1993
41. Kohn MC, Portier CJ: Effects of the mechanisms of receptor-mediated gene expression on the shape of the dose-response curve. Risk Anal 13:565–572, 1993
42. Allen BC, Crump KS, Shipp AM: Correlation between carcinogenic potency of chemicals in animals and humans. Risk Anal 8:531–544, 1988
43. IARC: General principles for evaluating the carcinogenic risk of chemicals. In: IARC Monographs on the Evaluation of Carcinogenic Risk of Chemicals to Humans. Suppl 4. Lyon, France: International Agency for Research on Cancer, 1982
44. Leroux BG, Leisenring WM, Mollgavkar SH, Faustman EM. A biologically-based dose-response model for developmental toxicology. Risk Anal 16:449–458, 1996
45. Hattis D, Burmaster DE: Assessment of variability and uncertainty distributions for practical risk analyses. Risk Anal 14:713–730, 1994
46. Thompson KM, Burmaster DE, Crouch EAC: Monte Carol techniques for quantitative uncertainty analysis in public health risk assessments. Risk Anal 12:53-64, 1992
47. Slovic P, Fischoff B, Lichtenstein S: Why study risk perception. Risk Anal 2:83–94, 1982
48. Covello VT, Flamm WG, Rodricks JV, Tardiff RG (eds): The Analysis of Actual vs. Perceived Risks. New York: Plenum Press, 1983
49. Hinman GW, Rosa EA, Kleinhesselink RR, Lowinger TC: Perceptions of nuclear and other risks in Japan and the United States. Risk Anal 13:449–455, 1993
50. Barke RP, Jenkins-Smith HC: Politics and scientific expertise: scientists, risk perception and nuclear waste policy. Risk Anal 13:425–439, 1993
51. Kivimäki M, Kalimo R: Risk perception among nuclear power plant personnel: a survey. Risk Anal 13:421–424, 1993
52. Pilisuk M, Acredolo C: Fear of technological hazards: one concern or many? Soc Behav 3:17–24, 1988
53. Savage I: Demographic influences on risk perceptions. Risk Anal 13:413–420, 1993
54. Gregory R, Mendelsohn R: Perceived risk, dread, and benefits. Risk Anal 13:259–264, 1993

55. Hance BJ, Chess C, Sandman PM: Improving Dialogue with Communities: A Risk Communication Manual for Government. Trenton, NJ: NJ Department of Environmental Protection, 1988
56. Bradbury JA: Risk communication in environmental restoration programs. Risk Anal 14:357–363, 1994
57. Weinstein ND, Kolb K, Goldstein BD: Using time intervals between expected events to communicate risk magnitudes. Risk Anal 16:305–308, 1996
58. Greenberg MR, Sachsman DB, Sandman PM, Salomone KL: Network evening news coverage of environmental risk. Risk Anal 9:119–126, 1987
59. Sandman P, Sachsman D, Greenberg M, Gochfeld M: Environmental Risk and the Press. New Brunswick, NJ: Transaction Books, 1987
60. Lynn FM, Busenberg GJ: Citizen advisory committees and environmental policy: what we know, what's left to discover. Risk Anal 15:147–162, 1995
61. Chess C, Salomone KL, Hance BJ: Improving risk communication in government: research priorities. Risk Anal 15:127–136, 1995
62. Environmental Protection Agency: Risk Assessment and Management: Framework for Decision Making. Washington DC: Environmental Protection Agency, 1984
63. Norton SB, Rodier DR, Gentile JH, van der Schalie WH, Wood WP, Slimak MW: A framework for ecological risk assessment at the EPA. Environ Toxicol Chem 11:1663–1672, 1992
64. Bartell SM, Gardner RH, O'Neill, RV: Ecological Risk Estimation. Boca Raton, FL: Lewis Press, 1992
65. Graham RL, Hunsaker CT, O'Neill RV, Jackson BL: Ecological risk assessment at the regional scale. Ecol Applic 1:196–206, 1991
66. Gochfeld M, Burger J: Evolutionary consequences for ecological risk assessment and management. Environ Monitor Assess 28:161–168, 1993

General References on Risk Assessment

Bates DV: Environmental Health Risks and Public Policy. Seattle: University of Washington Press, 1994

Conway RA: Environmental Risk Analyses for Chemicals. New York: Van Nostrand, 1982

Environmental Protection Agency: Reducing Risk: Setting Priorities and Strategies for Environmental Protection. Washington, DC: Environmental Protection Agency, 1990

Environmental Protection Agency: Risk Assessment Guidance for Superfund. Washington, DC: Environmental Protection Agency, 1991

Environmental Protection Agency: Guidelines for Exposure Assessment. Federal Register 57 (May 29):22888–22938, 1992

Environmental Protection Agency: Health Effects Assessment Summary Tables. Washington, DC: Environmental Protection Agency, 1992

Environmental Protection Agency: Health Assessment Document for 2,3,7,8-Tetrachlorodibenzo-*p*-dioxin (TCDD) and Related Compounds. Washington, DC: Environmental Protection Agency, 1994, vols 1–3

Faustman EM, Omenn GS: Risk assessment. In Klaassen CD (ed): Casarett and Doull's Toxicology. New York: McGraw-Hill, 1996, pp. 75–88

Finkel AM, Golding D: Worst Things First? The Debate over Risk-Based National Environmental Priorities. Baltimore: Johns Hopkins University Press, 1994

Goldring D, Krimsky S: Theories of Risk. New York: Praeger, 1992

Goldsmith DF: Risk assessment applied to environmental medicine. In Brooks S, Gochfeld M, Herzstein J, Schenker M, Jackson R (eds): Environmental Medicine. St. Louis: CV Mosby, 1995, pp 30–36

Goldstein BD: The maximally exposed individual: an inappropriate basis for public health decisionmaking. Environ Forum November–December 13–16, 1989

Guzelian PS, Henry CJ, Olin SS: Similarities and Differences between Children and Adults: Implications for Risk Assessment. Washington, DC: International Life Sciences Institute, 1992

Hallenbeck WH, Cunningham KM: Quantitative risk assessment for environmental and occupational health. Chelsea, MI: Lewis Press, 1987

Hawkins NC, Graham JD: Expert scientific judgment and cancer risk assessment: a pilot study of pharmacokinetic data. Risk Anal 8:615–625, 1988. (Expert opinion is polarized on formaldehyde.)

Imperato PJ: On Acceptable Risk. Viking, New York, 1985

Kunreuther H, Gowda MVR (eds): Integrating Insurance and Risk Management for Hazardous Wastes. Boston: Kluwer, 1990

Long FA, Schweitzer GE: Risk assessment at hazardous waste sites. Am Chem Soc Symp 204, 1982

Lowrance WW: Of Acceptable Risk. Los Altos, CA: William Kaufmann, 1976

Lucier GW: Risk assessment: good science for good decisions. Environ Health Perspect 101:366, 1993

Oftedal P, Brogger A: Risk and Reason: Risk Assessment in Relation to Environmental Mutagens and Carcinogens. New York: Alan R. Liss, 1986

Olin S, Farland W, Park C, Rhomberg L, Scheuplein R, Starr T, Wilson J (eds): Low-dose Extrapolation of Cancer Risks. Washington, DC: International Life Sciences Institute Press, 1995

Presidential/Congressional Commission on Risk Assessment and Risk Management: Framework for Environmental Health Risk Management, Final Report. Washington, DC: The Commission, 1997

Risk Analysis: An International Journal of the Society for Risk Analysis. New York: Plenum Press, 1981 to present

Saxena J: Hazard assessment of chemicals. New York: Academic Press, vols 1–2, 1986

Sielken RL: Quantitative cancer risk assessment for TCDD. Food Chem Toxicol 25:257–267, 1987

Whyte AV, Burton I: Environmental Risk Assessment. New York: John Wiley & Sons, 1980

Nicholson WJ (ed): Management of Assessed Risk for Carcinogens. Ann NY Acad Sci 363:1–300, 1981

General References on Quantitative Risk Assessment

Allen BC, Crump KS, Shipp AM: Correlation between carcinogenic potency of chemicals in animals and humans. Risk Anal 8:531–544, 1988

Andersen ME, Clewell HI, Gargas ML, Smith FA, Reitz RH: Physiologically based pharmacokinetics and the risk assessment process for methylene chloride. Toxicol Appl Pharmacol 87:185–205, 1987

Armitage P: Multistage models of carcinogenesis. Environ Health Perspect 63:195–201, 1985

Crump KS: A critical analysis of a dose-response assessment for TCDD. Food Chem Toxicol 26:79–83, 1988

Finkel AM: Dioxin: are we safer now than before? Risk Anal 8:161–166, 1988

Gerrity TR, Henry CJ: Principles of Route-to-Route Extrapolation for Risk Assessment. Amsterdam: Elsevier, 1990

Knight FH: Risk, Uncertainty and Profit, New York: Harbor Torchbooks, 1921

Moolgavkar SH, Knudsen AG Jr: Mutation and cancer: a model for human carcinogenesis. J Nat Cancer Inst 66:1037–1052, 1981

National Research Council: Science and Judgment in Risk Assessment. Washington, DC: National Academy Press, 1994

Purchase IFH, Auton TR: Thresholds in chemical carcinogenesis. Reg Toxicol Pharmacol 22:199–205, 1995

Safe Drinking Water Committee, National Academy of Science: Drinking Water and Health. Washington, DC: National Academy Press, 1986, vol 6

Upton AC: The question of thresholds for radiation and chemical carcinogenesis. Cancer Invest 7:267–276, 1989

General References on Risk Perception and Risk Communication

Burger J, Gochfeld M: Fishing a superfund site: dissonance and risk perception of environmental hazards by fishermen in Puerto Rico. Risk Anal 11:269–277, 1991

Burger J, Gochfeld M: Ecological and human health risk assessment: a comparison. pp. 127–148 In Di Giulio RT, Monosson E (eds): Interconnections between Human and Ecosystem Health. London: Chapman & Hall, 1996
Covello VT, Flamm WG, Rodricks JV, Tardiff RG (eds): The analysis of actual vs. perceived risks. New York: Plenum Press, 1983
Davies JC, Covello VT, Allen FW (eds): Risk Communication: Proceedings of the National Conference on Risk Communication. Washington, DC: Conservation Foundation, 1986
Epple D, Slovic P: Taxonomic analysis of perceived risk: modeling individual and group perceptions within homogeneous hazard domains. Risk Anal 8:435–456, 1988
Johnson B, Covello V (eds): Social and Cultural Construction of Risk. Boston: Reidel, 1987
Kahneman D, Slovic P, Tversky A: Judgement under Uncertainty: Heuristics and Biases. New York: Cambridge University Press, 1982
National Research Council: Regulating Pesticides in Food: The Delaney Paradox. Washington, DC: National Academy Press, 1987
National Research Council: Improving Risk Communication. Washington, DC: National Academy Press, 1989
National Research Council: Issues in Risk Assessment. Washington, DC: National Academy Press, 1993
National Research Council: Pesticides in the Diets of Infants and Children. Washington, DC: National Academy Press, 1993
National Research Council: Building Consensus through Risk Assessment and Management of the Department of Energy's Environmental Remediation Program. Washington, DC: National Academy Press, 1994
National Research Council: Science and Judgement in Risk Assessment. Washington, DC: National Academy Press, 1994
Sandman P, Sachsman D, Greenberg M, Gochfeld M: Environmental Risk and the Press. New Brunswick, NJ: Transaction Books, 1987
Short JF Jr: Social dimensions of risk: the need for a sociological paradigm and policy research. Am Sociol 22:167–172, 1987
Slovic P: Informing and educating the public about risk. Risk Anal 6:403–415, 1986
Slovic P: Perception of risk. Science 236:28–290, 1987
Slovic P, Fischoff B, Lictenstein S: Facts versus fears: understanding perceived risk. In Kahneman D, Slovic P, Tversky A (eds): Judgement under Uncertainty: Heuristics and Biases. New York: Cambridge University Press, 1982
von Winterfeldt D, John RS, Borcherding K: Cognitive components of risk ratings. Risk Anal 1:277–288, 1981

General References on Applications of Risk Assessment

Carnegie Commission: Risk and the Environment: Improving Regulatory Decision Making. New York: Carnegie Commission, 1993
Denison RA, Silbergeld EK: Risks of municipal solid waste incineration: an environmental perspective. Risk Anal 8:343–357, 1988
Ditz DW: Hazardous waste incineration at sea. EPA decision making on risk. Risk Anal 8:499–508, 1988. (criticizes EPA for underestimating risk)
Gough M: Science policy choices and the estimation of cancer risk associated with exposure to TCDD. Risk Anal 8:337–342, 1988
Jasanoff S: Learning from disaster: risk management after Bhopal. Philadelphia: University of Pennsylvania Press, 1994
Kroes R: Contribution of toxicology toward risk assessment of carcinogens. Arch Toxicol 60:224–228, 1987 (Genotoxic carcinogens get no threshold model, others get threshold model.)
Kunreuther H, Lathrop JW: Siting hazardous facilities: lessons from LNG. Risk Anal 1:289–302, 1981
Kunreuther H, Slovic P: Decision making in hazard and resource management. In Kates RW, Burton I (eds): Geography, Resources and Environment. Chicago: University of Chicago Press, 1986, vol II, pp 153–187
National Research Council: Pesticides in the Diets of Infants and Children. Washington, DC: National Academy Press, 1993
Rycroft TW, Regens JL, Dietz T: Incorporating risk assessment and benefit-cost analysis in environmental management. Risk Anal 8:415–420, 1988

General References on Ecological Risk Assessment

Barnthouse LW: The role of models in ecological risk assessment: a 1990s perspective. Environ Toxicol Chem 11:1751–1760, 1992
Bartell SM, Gardner RH, O'Neill RV: Ecological Risk Estimation. Boca Raton, FL: Lewis Press, 1992
Burger J, Gochfeld M: Temporal scales in ecological risk assessment. Arch Environ Contam Toxicol 23:484–488, 1992
Cairns J, Niederlehner BR, Orvos DR (eds): Predicting Ecosystem Risk. Princeton Scientific Publishing, Princeton, 1992
Commission on Risk Assessment and Risk Management: Report of the Commission on Risk Assessment and Risk Management. Washington, DC: National Academy Press, 1996
Di Giulio RT, Monosson E: Interconnections between Human and Ecosystem Health. London: Chapman & Hall, 1996
Linthurst RA, Bourdeau P, Tardiff RC (eds): Methods to Assess the Effects of Chemicals on Ecosystems. SCOPE Monograph No. 53. New York: John Wiley & Sons, 1995
National Research Council: Risk Assessment in the Federal Government: Managing the Process. Washington, DC: National Academy Press, 1983
National Research Council: Ecological Knowledge and Environmental Problem Solving. Washington, DC: National Academy Press, 1986
National Research Council: Animals As Sentinels of Environmental Health Hazards. Washington, DC: National Academy Press, 1991
Norton SB, Rodier DR, Gentile JH: A framework for ecological risk assessment at the EPA. Environ Toxicol Chem 11:1663–1672, 1992
Peakall D: Animal Biomarkers as Pollution Indicators. London: Chapman & Hall, 1992
Römbke J, Moltmann JF: Applied Ecotoxicology. Boca Raton, FL: Lewis Publishers, 1996
Suter GW II: Endpoints for regional ecological risk assessment. Environ Manag 14:9–23, 1990
Suter GW II: Ecological Risk Assessment. Boca Raton, FL: Lewis Publishers, 1993
Travis CC, Morris JM: The emergence of ecological risk assessment. Risk Anal 12:167–169, 1992
National Research Council: Issues in Risk Assessment. Washington, DC: National Academy Press, 1993

Susceptibility

Alavanja M, Aron J, Brown C, Chandler J: From biochemical epidemiology to cancer risk assessment. J Natl Cancer Inst 78:633–643, 1987
Armitage P, Doll R: Age distribution of cancer. Bri J Cancer 8:1–12, 1954
Finkel AM: A quantitative estimate of the variations in human susceptibility to cancer and its implications for risk management. In Olin S, Farland W, Park C, Rhomberg L, Scheuplein R, Starr T, Wilson J (eds): Low-dose Extrapolation of Cancer Risks. Washington, DC: International Life Sciences Institute Press, 1995, pp 297–328
Fraumeni JF Jr (ed): Persons at High Risk of Cancer: An Approach to Cancer Etiology and Control. New York: Academic Press, 1975
Goodlett CR, Peterson SD: Sex differences in vulnerability to developmental spatial learning deficits induced by limited binge alcohol exposure in neonatal rats. Neurobiol Learn Mem 64:265–275, 1995
Greenberg GN, Dement JM: Exposure assessment and gender differences. J Occup Med 36:908–912, 1994
Harris CC: Interindividual variation among humans in carcinogen metabolism, DNA adduct formation, and DNA repair. Carcinogenesis 10:1563–1566, 1989

Mendelsohn ML, Mohr LC, Peeters JP: Biomarkers, the Genome and the Individual. Washington, DC: Joseph Henry Press, National Academy of Sciences, in press

Nebert D: Possible clinical importance of genetic differences in drug metabolism. Br Med J 283:537–542, 1981

Risk Characterization

1. National Research Council: Risk Assessment in the Federal Government: Managing the Process. Washington, DC: National Academy Press, 1983
2. Silbergeld EK: Risk assessment and risk management: an uneasy divorce. In: May D, Hollander R (eds): Acceptable Evidence: Science and Values in Risk Assessment. New York: Oxford University Press, 1991, pp 99–114
3. Finkel A: Is risk assessment really too conservative: revising the revisionists. Columbia J Environ Law 14:427–467, 1989
4. Slovic P: Perception of risk. Science 236:280–285, 1987
5. National Research Council, Committee on Risk Assessment of Hazardous Air Pollutants, Commission on Life Sciences: Science and Judgement in Risk Assessment. Washington, DC: National Academy Press, 1994
6. Office of Technology Assessment: Identifying and Regulating Carcinogens. Washington, DC: Government Printing Office, 1987
7. Barrett JC: Mechanisms of multistep carcinogenesis and carcinogen risk assessment. Environ Health Perspect 100:9–20, 1993
8. Harris CC, Hollstein M: Clinical implications of the p53 tumor suppressor gene. N Engl J Med 329:1318–1327, 1993
9. Barnes DG, Daston GP, Evans JS, et al: Benchmark dose workshop: criteria for use of a benchmark dose to estimate a reference dose. Regul Toxicol Pharmacol 21:296–306, 1995
10. Krewski D, Brown C, Murdoch D: Determining "safe" levels of exposure: safety factors of mathematical models. Fund Appl Toxicol 4: S383–394, 1984
11. Ames BN, Gold LS: Chemical carcinogenesis: too many rodent carcinogens. Proc Natl Acad Sci USA 87:7772–7776, 1990
12. Cohen SM, Ellwein LB: Cell proliferation and carcinogenesis. Science 249:1007–1011, 1990
13. Blair A, Burg J, Foran J, et al: Guidelines for application of meta-analysis in environmental epidemiology. Regul Toxicol Pharmacol 22:189–197, 1995
14. Harris CC: Interindividual variation among humans in carcinogen metabolism, DNA adduct formation and DNA repair. Carcinogenesis 10:1563–1566, 1989
15. Connolly RB, Andersen ME: Biologically based pharmacodynamic models: tools for toxicological research and risk assessment. Annu Rev Pharmacol Toxicol 31:503–523, 1991
16. National Research Council, Committee on Pesticides in the Diets of Infants and Children, Commission on Life Sciences: Pesticides in the Diets of Infants and Children. Washington, DC: National Academy Press, 1993a
17. Stehr PA, Stein G, Falk H, et al: A pilot epidemiologic study of possible health effects associated with 2,3,7,8-tetrachlorodibenzo-*p*-dioxin. Arch Environ Health 41:16–22, 1986
18. Lanphear BP, Weitzman M, Winter NL: Lead-contaminted house dust and urban children's blood lead levels. Am J Public Health 86(10):1416–1421, 1996
19. Farfel MR, Chisolm JJ: Health and environmental outcomes of traditional and modified practices for abatement of residential lead-based paint. Am J Public Health 80:1240–1245, 1990
20. Needleman HL, Gaszonis CA: Low-level lead exposure and the IQ of children. JAMA 263:673–678, 1990
21. Bornschein RL, Succop PA, Kraft KM, Clark CS, Peace B, Hammond PB: Exterior surface dust lead, interior house dust lead and childhood lead exposure in an urban environment. In: Hemphill DD (eds): Trace Substances in Environmental Health—XX: Proceedings of University of Missouri's 20th Annual Conference, June 1986. Columbia, MO: University of Missouri; 322–332, 1987

19

Asbestos and Other Fibers

Kaye H. Kilburn

▸ ASBESTOS

Asbestos-Associated Diseases

Prevention of asbestosis and reduction in lung cancer mortality in asbestos-exposed subjects has occurred in the last generation in the United States. Massive medical evidence compelled the primary industry to shut down as the use of asbestos was made excessively expensive as an uninsurable risk. This followed successive waves of court awards for liability and punitive damages and settlements negotiated to user workers, co-contaminated workers, and bystanders. Jury awards for mesotheliomas were frequently in the range of $1 million, and those for asbestosis ranged from thousands to hundreds of thousands of dollars. This was a novel but effective way to stem an epidemic. It is to be hoped that widespread substitution of human-made fibers in construction has not predestined a repeat performance. Seventy-five years ago, Dr. Cooke, who associated lung fibrosis with asbestos and named it asbestosis, thought its recognition would lead quickly to its prevention.

Clinical Recognition of Asbestosis

Asbestosis is defined as a fibrotic disease of the lung from asbestos exposure that occurs after a suitable latent period. Pathologic changes consisting of cellular infiltrates and fibrosis surround small bronchioles, limit forced expiratory flow, and thereby impair pulmonary function. Asbestosis is diagnosed from chest radiographs by diffuse, irregular opacities in the lung fields or by circumscribed or diffuse pleural thickening, which are defined by international criteria.[1]

Asbestos exposure produces *no acute symptoms*. The pathologic changes of fibrosis in lung or pleura are well advanced when the recognition of expiratory obstruction permits "early diagnosis" before the development of radiographic abnormality, *breathlessness on exertion*, or *cough productive of phlegm*. Usually asbestosis has been incubating for years, frequently two decades or more from the first exposure; this is called the "latent" period. Asbestos and cigarette smoking are *synergistic* in impairing function and producing fibrosis and carcinoma.

History

Although the first use of asbestos by humans is lost in antiquity, it is mentioned by Plinius, who referred to asbestos as *immun vivum*, "durable linen," and Roman slaves who worked in these mines grew breathless and died prematurely. Asbestos has properties of incombustibility, durability, and resistance to friction that have made it useful for insulation and heat protection in modern industrial society. H. Montague Murray,[2] a London physician, recognized a new disease in the badly scarred lungs of an asbestos worker, presumably from a textile factory, who died after a brief illness characterized by extreme breathlessness. Murray connected the workplace exposure to the scarring in testifying before an inquiry at the British Government Commission on Occupational Disability in 1907 and stated hopefully that with the recognition of the cause, he would predict few future cases. His singular finding was ignored until 1924, when Cooke[3] described pulmonary fibrosis in a woman who had worked for 20 years in an asbestos textile factory. The illness was widely regarded as a manifestation of tuberculosis, the plague of those times, and thus was largely ignored. Cooke[4] also introduced the name "pulmonary asbestosis" as a pneumoconiosis, one of the dust diseases (as named by Zenker 60 years earlier).

After further scattered reports of asbestosis in individual workers, an epidemiologic investigation was conducted by Merewether and Price[5] of the workers in British asbestos textile factories in 1930. They systematically associated factory dust containing asbestos with radiographic findings of asbestosis, as reported by Pancoast et al[6] in 1918. Their study related levels of dust and prevalence of asbestosis in the card rooms. Gloyne's autopsy studies of the workers' lungs[7] showed lesions of membranous and respiratory bronchioles. Later in the 1930s there were two supporting studies. One, for the Metropolitan Life Insurance Company by Lanza et al,[8] reported that two-thirds of the x-ray films of 126 persons "randomly selected" from those with 3 or more years of employment had asbestosis. In 1938, Dreessen et al[9] studied 511 employees of asbestos textile factories in North Carolina and found a low prevalence of abnormalities in the x-ray films in largely newly hired hands with short exposures. When several dozen workers who had been discharged from these factories were traced, of many of their x-ray films showed characteristic asbestosis.[10–12] Dreessen's study and the associated reports made it clear that asbestosis produced abnormalities in the chest x-ray and shortness of breath.

In the 1930s, additional reports of insulators, boilermakers, and men in other trades who manufactured or used asbestos showed that they had abnormal x-ray films, shortness of breath, and in some cases rales in the chest, clubbing of the digits, and cyanosis. However, World War II intervened before the prevalence was measured or exposure controlled. Thus knowledge of the pervasiveness of asbestosis was left until the 1960s and 1970s, when studies in the shipbuilding and construction trades showed chest x-rays were abnormal in many workers exposed to asbestos. Large studies of asbestos miners and millers[13] showed that airway obstruction and reductions in vital capacity and in diffusing capacity occurred before the chest x-ray abnormalities.

Lung Cancer

Lung cancer in individuals exposed to asbestos was reported in the 1930s, but the causal impact developed slowly. Merewether[14] reported in 1947 that 13.5 percent of the asbestos textile workers studied in 1931 had died of lung cancer within 16 years. Heuper[15] by 1942 concluded in his textbook that asbestos was a more important cause of lung cancer than was arsenic or radium. However, Richard Doll,[16] in a well-designed study of a textile factory cohort (a defined population), noted long latency of cancer and accounted for all causes of death. In 1955 occupational exposure to asbestos increased lung cancer deaths 10-fold above the expected rate. Mancuso and Coulter,[17] who confirmed Doll's findings in the United States, and Selikoff[18] first reported a large excess of lung cancer among major users of asbestos—insulators. The finding that users were in danger vastly increased the numbers of persons at risk for lung cancer and made control urgent. In their 20-year prospective study of mortality rates among almost 18,000 insulators begun in 1967, Selikoff and Seidman,[19] by 1979, found excessive death rates not only for lung cancer, mesothelioma, and asbestosis but also for cancers of the gastrointestinal tract, larynx, oropharynx, and kidney (Tables 19-1 and 19-2), and synergistic interactions between cigarette smoking and asbestos in these cancers. Age-standardized rates per 100,000 person-years are as follows: Individuals who neither worked with asbestos nor smoked cigarettes had a calculated death rate of 11.3; asbestos workers who did not smoke had a rate of 58.4. Smokers in general (not asbestos workers) showed a rate of 122.6, whereas those who had both types of exposure, cigarettes and asbestos, had a rate of 601.6.

Mesothelioma, a Twentieth-Century Tumor

Klemperer and Rabin[20] in 1931 described this rare tumor, characteristically spread on the pleural surface, and reasoned that the responsible carcinogen must penetrate to these inaccessible pleura and peritoneum surfaces. Reports of mesotheliomas in subjects exposed to asbestos were rare in the 1940s and 1950s until Wagner et al,[21] in 1960, reported 47 mesotheliomas in people who had worked in or lived near the crocidolite works in South Africa 15 years earlier. Such a clear association between a rare tumor and a causal agent was unprecedented, but it was quickly corroborated by other studies. Although Wagner's study lacked control subjects, the germinal observations were confirmed by population-based data. Consequently, the diagnosis of a mesothelioma now provokes a search for asbestos exposure that is seldom unfulfilled. Latent intervals of 30 to 40 years are characteristic, so many recent and current patients were exposed in U.S. shipyards that built and repaired a two-ocean navy and shipping fleet during World War II.

Asbestos Minerals

Fibers and Fibrils

"Asbestos" is a general name for naturally occurring fibrous minerals that include serpentine and amphibole fibers, but excludes fibrous forms of other minerals such as wollastonite, brucite, gypsum, and calcite. Chrysotile, the only serpentine asbestos, occurs in "cobs" about the size of a hand that are found in pockets, often within plate-like and nonfibrous silica deposits. The fibers can be seen with an optical microscope; the fibrils that compose them are of micrometer size, and therefore single fibrils isolated or in tissue are ordinarily visible only with an electron microscope. Fortunately there are crude associations among "dustiness" (the gravimetric measurement of the total airborne concentration), the visible fibers recognized with the optical microscope (particularly with the help of phase contrast or polarized light), and the concentrations of fibrils measured with the electron microscope. For industrial hygiene, the rough relationships between total dust measured gravimetrically from air samples and fibers visible with the light microscope have produced reasonable dose-response relationships in miners and millers of asbestos, asbestos textile workers, and workers producing asbestos (calcite) pipe. Estimates of maximal human exposure to fine fibers range widely from several hundred fibrils per cubic meter of air to several hundred millions of fibrils per cubic meter.

Sources

The commercially important asbestos fibers are chrysotile, amosite, and crocidolite. Chrysolite, or white asbestos, is mined mainly in Canada's Quebec province and in the Ural Mountains of the former Soviet Union. U.S. mines in Arizona and California produced small quantities. The three amphiboles are crocidolite, or blue asbestos, which is highly associated with mesothelioma; amosite (named for the Asbestos Mining Organization of South Africa), called brown asbestos because of its iron content; and anthophyllite, which is found in Finland. Actinolite, or fibrous tremolite, contaminates minerals. Examples include crocidolite and talc from many sources, particularly the Gouverneur district of New York State.

TABLE 19-1. DEATHS AMONG 17,800 ASBESTOS INSULATION WORKERS IN THE UNITED STATES AND CANADA, JANUARY 1, 1967–DECEMBER 31, 1986

		Observed		SMR Values[d]	
Underlying Cause of Death	***Expected Deaths***[a]	***DC***[b]	***BE***[c]	***DC***	***BE***[e]
Total deaths, all causes	3,453.50	4,951	4,951	143***	143***
Total cancer, all sites	761.41	2,127	2,295	279***	301***
Lung cancer	268.66	1,008	1,168	375***	435***
Pleural mesothelioma[f]	—	89	173	—	—
Peritoneal mesothelioma[f]	—	92	285	—	—
Gastrointestinal cancer[g]	135.69	188	189	139***	139***
Gastrointestinal cancer, extended[h]	191.66	324	269	169***	140***
Noninfectious pulmonary diseases, total	144.82	465	507	321***	350***
Asbestosis[f]	—	201	427	—	—
All other causes	2, 547.27	2,359	2,149	93***	84***

From Selikoff IJ, Seidman H: Asbestos associated deaths among insulation workers in the United States and Canada, 1967–1987. Ann NY Acad Sci 643:1–14, 1991.
[a] Expected deaths are based upon white male, age-specific death rates of the U.S. National Center for Health Statistics, 1967–1986.
[b] DC: Number of deaths as recorded from death certificate information only.
[c] BE: Best evidence. Number of deaths categorized after review of best available information (autopsy, surgical, clinical). Where no such data were available, the death certificate diagnosis was used.
[d] SMR: Standardized mortality ratio. Observed deaths/expected deaths × 100.
[e] Calculated for information only, since it utilized "best evidence" vs. "death certificate" diagnoses, which are not strictly comparable because of different ascertainment and verification.
[f] Rates are not available since these have been rare causes of death in the general population.
[g] Includes cancer of stomach, esophagus, and colon/rectum.
[h] Includes cancer of stomach, esophagus, colon/rectum, liver, gallbladder, and bile ducts.
Probability levels: * $P < 0.05$; ** $P < 0.01$; *** $P < 0.001$.

TABLE 19-2. LESS COMMON MALIGNANT NEOPLASMS: DEATHS AMONG 17,800 ASBESTOS INSULATION WORKERS IN THE UNITED STATES AND CANADA, JANUARY 1, 1967–DECEMBER 31, 1986

		Observed		Ratio o/e	
Site of Cancer Causing Death	*Expected Deaths*[a]	*DC*[b]	*BE*[c]	*DC*	*BE*[d]
Increased incidence at these sites:					
Larynx	10.57	17	18	1.61	1.70*
Oropharynx	22.02	38	48	1.73**	2.18***
Kidney	18.87	32	37	1.70**	1.96***
Pancreas	39.52	92	54	2.33***	1.37*
Esophagus	17.80	29	30	1.63*	1.68*
Stomach	29.36	34	38	1.16	1.29
Colon/rectum	88.49	125	121	1.41***	1.37**
Gall bladder/bile ducts	5.37	13	14	2.42**	2.61**
No increased incidence at these sites:					
Urinary bladder	20.77	17	22	0.82	1.06
Prostate	52.56	59	61	1.12	1.16
Liver	11.06	31	12	2.80***	1.08
Brain tumors (all)	26.35	40	33	1.52*	1.25
Cancer of brain	22.55	29	27	1.29	1.20
Leukemia	28.74	32	33	1.11	1.15
Lymphoma	43.24	33	39	0.76	0.90

From Selikoff IJ, Seidman H: Asbestos associated deaths among insulation workers in the United States and Canada, 1967–1987. Ann NY Acad Sci 643:1–14, 1991.
[a] Expected deaths are based upon white male, age-specific death rates of the U.S. National Center for Health Statistics, 1967–1986.
[b] DC: Number of deaths as recorded from death certificate information only.
[c] BE: Best evidence. Number of deaths categorized after review of best available information (autopsy, surgical, clinical). Where no such data were available, the death certificate diagnosis was used.
[d] Calculated for information only, since it utilized "best evidence" vs. "death certificate" diagnoses, which are not strictly comparable because of different ascertainment and verification.
Probability range: * $P < 0.05$; ** $P < 0.01$; *** $P < 0.001$.

Far fewer human subjects are exposed to the mining and milling of asbestos than to thermal insulation and construction materials: surfacing materials, preformed thermal insulating products, textiles, cementitious (concrete-like) products, paper products, roofing felts, asbestos-containing compounds, flooring tile and sheet goods, wall coverings, and paints and coatings. Dispersal of the fibrils into the air of "massive containers"—ships and industrial facilities such as aluminum refineries, copper smelters, glass and fiberglass factories, paper mills, and powerhouses—exposes all workers, well beyond those whose hands come in contact with asbestos products.

Use of Asbestos in Industry and Construction

The general uses of asbestos are in heat insulation, friction-resistant products, and construction.[22] As heat insulation, asbestos cloth is used in blankets, gloves, suits, and boiler packing and is combined with magnesia in pipe insulation. Asbestos combined with portland cement, or blue mud, was widely used to free-form insulation around pipes and boilers. Friction products included brake shoes and pads, clutch facings, and other woven products that must resist both friction and the heat it generates. The major tragedy of asbestos exposure since World War II was in workers in the construction trades, where, for reasons never stated but including availability, cheapness, and binding properties, asbestos has been used in drywall, in spray ceilings, paint, floor tile, ceiling tile, and as filler in many other products. Analogous to fine sand, as the inert material in paint, asbestos was added to products whether or not it conferred useful properties.

TABLE 19-3. PULMONARY PARENCHYMAL ASBESTOSIS OF PROFUSION 1/0 OR MORE INTERNATIONAL LABOR ORGANIZATION CRITERIA IN 419 MIDWESTERN INSULATORS BY HISTORY OF CIGARETTE SMOKING

Smoking Category	*Mean Age [Years]*	*Number with Asbestosis/ Number in Population*	*Percent*	*Risk Ratio*
Nonsmokers	40	7/97	7.2	
Exsmokers	44	29/131	22.1	3.1
Current smokers	48.2	37/191	19.4	2.7

Peak Use of Asbestos

The peak use of asbestos in the United States was probably in the early 1970s, although the yearly consumption rose steadily from 1890 to 1950, was virtually level at more than 7,000 metric tons per year from 1950 through 1969, and fell precipitously in the 1980s. The profile is similar for other developed nations of the world, where asbestos was widely used in construction.

Patterns of Use

Asbestos litigation and regulation since the mid-1970s have excluded asbestos from many consumer products, from building materials, and lastly from brakes and friction goods. Pioneering synthetic brake materials, Volvo Corporation in Sweden produced pads and shoes that, although twice as expensive, last three or four times as long as asbestos. Progress has been uneven. Asbestos insulating products continued to be installed in New Jersey schools (without the addition of warning labels) well into the early 1980s, and in 1986 an inventory of a U.S. Navy warehouse for ship fittings disclosed 130 products containing asbestos. Many of these were gaskets and other relatively low-exposure items, but others included thermal insulation and blankets. Because asbestos use accompanied the intense industrialization of the twentieth century, a key concern is whether developing countries will continue to let economic determinants take precedence over health. For example, in Israel, asbestos pipe containing crocidolite was manufactured through the 1970s, and asbestos remains in place in sugar mills and oil refineries in Mexico, Brazil, and China.

Removal of Asbestos

Fragmentation and degeneration due to heat and vibration increase the liberation of fibrils from asbestos during renovation, removal, or repair.[23] The highest doses for workers may be generated during the removal of asbestos unless proper procedures are followed, including wetting material down and restricting the area to properly suited, well-trained personnel using air-supply respirators.[22] If the asbestos is placed in plastic bags and buried, the hazard is minimized. These safeguards have been neglected in many asbestos-removal efforts, where levels of more than 100 fibers per millimeter have been measured.

Biological Effects of Asbestos

Molecular Effects

Asbestos fibrils in vitro hemolyze red blood cells. Chrysotile also mediates the uptake of exogenous DNA into monkey cells in such a way that the genes on the DNA are expressed.[24] In several cultured human cell lines chrysotile and amosite induce changes.[25–27] Rat alveolar macrophages are induced to form and release tissue necrosis factor-α by asbestos and human-made fibers.[28] Dose-response cytotoxic effects were found to amphiboles in a cultured line of macrophages, which caused hyperplasia and squamous cell metaplasia.[25] Chrysotile was more toxic than amosite in normal and transformed epithelial cell lines and in plasminogen activation.[28]

Cellular Effects

Heppleston[29,30] and Allison[31] two decades ago showed that important signals were generated by macrophages that had phagocytosed asbestos fibrils. Macrophages caused fibrosis in animal models[32,33] and in the human lung, where asbestos caused both recruitment and proliferation.[34] In contrast, quartz was disturbingly lethal for cells. Observations of cells in vitro and in permeable chambers implanted in the peritoneum of rats showed that macrophages produce peptides that stimulate fibroblasts (fibronectin and others) to replicate and produce collagen.[35,36]

Target Organ

Processing asbestos in the lung[38,39] evidently begins in airways, particularly the small airways where fibrils impinge. Short-term clearance depends on fiber size and type; chrysotile, for example, clears from guinea pig lungs faster than does amosite.[40] The probable scenario in airways is that fibrils pass between the epithelial cells, cross the basement membrane, and lodge in the connective tissue, attracting macrophages. Macrophages on the airway surfaces may phagocytose some fibrils, but many fibrils are simply carried away on the mucociliary escalator. Others, apparently a small minority, are coated with iron-rich protein and become asbestos (ferruginous) bodies (Fig. 19-1). Airway walls thicken beneath the epithelium, and cells are attracted to the alveolar side of membranous small airways. It appears likely that the next step is bridging, via the lymphatic vessels, between the peribronchiolar scars, linking them together in a laticelike network. It was assumed previously that this linked-up network "shrank" the lung, that is, reduced its volume; however, this hypothesis is no longer tenable. Volumes lost to shrunken zones are compensated for by areas of emphysema. Interstitial fibrosis is seen only with advanced asbestosis, particularly in subjects who have smoked cigarettes.

Transport of Fibrils

Fibrils are transported to other sites, via regional lymphatic vessels, and into the pleural space. Hillerdal[42] suggested that the fibrils, absorbed in small airways and alveoli, move via the lymphatic vessels or within cells to the pleural surface, cross the pleural "space," and impinge on the parietal pleura, where the macrophages are retained. Here they send signals to fibroblasts or perhaps also to mesothelial cells to undergo fibroblastic proliferation and to produce collagen.[43] Under this stimulation, characteristic hyaline plaques of the parietal pleura develop. When pleural effusion intercedes, there may be symphysis between the pleural layers, with dense adhesions. At this stage it appears that in some instances fibrosis invades the lung from pleural surfaces via the perivenous lymphatics. Retrograde flow may occur because symphysis obliterates the pleural space so that it is no longer accessible as a sump for the fibrils, which move into the peripheral lung. Fibrils remain in the perivenous lymphatics. Whatever the mechanism, such fibrous strands, as seen on cut surfaces of the lung or on high-resolution computer-augmented tomographs, are most dense at the pleura and attenuate progressively toward the hilum.

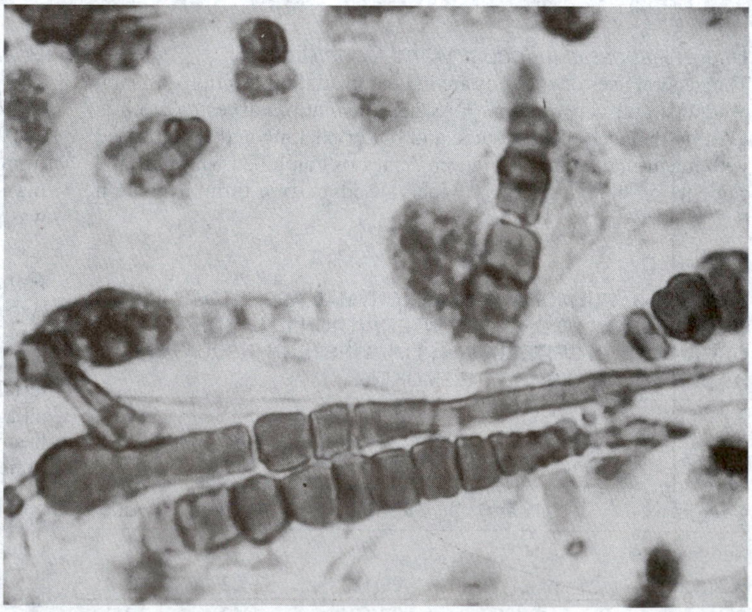

Figure 19-1. Asbestos (ferruginous) bodies in lung tissue consist of an asbestos core with an iron protein coat that make them appear tan or brown, (×600).

Immune Responses

Association of rheumatoid factor with asbestosis[44,45] has posed unresolved questions: first, whether those subjects who develop rheumatoid factor are more susceptible to the clinical manifestations of disease after asbestos exposure; second, whether immune globulin synthesis is stimulated by asbestos; and third, whether such elevations enhance the development of asbestosis. Alterations in populations of lymphatic T cells have also been associated with asbestos exposure and with asbestosis.[45,46] However, the meaning of these observations is uncertain and poses questions similar to those regarding the role of immune globulins.

Summary

Macrophages export peptides that stimulate fibroblasts to proliferate and to produce collagen in cell systems and diffusion chambers of plants and animals.[30,31] Fibronectin and at least one other fibroblast-stimulating factor can be stimulated by asbestos in cells.[47–49] Implantation of asbestos and human-made fibers in the pleural space of experimental animals, and refinements of this technique with milling and sizing of the fibrils, led Stanton and Wrench[50] to propose that the physical properties—the diameters and lengths of the fibers or fibrils—were responsible for mesothelioma. Intracellular asbestos fibrils interfere with chromosome aggregation in mitosis, although whether this interference is linked to neoplasia is unclear.[24] It appears that physical, surface, and chemical properties of the fibrils may be important in cell proliferation and in forming tumors.

Human Exposure

Workers

Contained air space into which asbestos has been dispersed, such as in a textile factory, ship, power station, factory, smelter, or refinery where there is heat conservation and protection concentrates the dose. Thus, when asbestos insulation was sprayed on the structural steel of high-rise buildings in New York City, sprayers were heavily exposed and asbestos was detected in ambient air as far away as Cape May, NJ. However, it is clear that the sprayers themselves, within the skeleton of the building, were at greatest risk to asbestos exposure. It is probable that, in mining and milling, moisture and nonasbestos rock bind fibers together and impair the discharge of fibrils into the air. In comparison, textile operations, in which the fibers are carded and spun, generate fibrils into the workplace air, similar to the spraying of asbestos insulation. Obviously, partially bound asbestos-containing materials are less hazardous than those that are friable and that readily release fibers or allow for the generation of fibrils into the air. Cleaning brake drums with compressed air disturbs many fine fibrils (Fig. 19-2), as does the removal of insulation that has been cooked on boilers or steam lines. If prevalence of asbestosis reflects cumulative exposures, insulators, sheet metal workers, boilermakers, and pipefitters are at high risk whereas electricians, carpenters, laborers, workers, and mechanics have had less exposure and less disease after 15 to 25 years. Ships with decks and hulls made of perforated plates are ideal for maintaining fibrils in the air space, similar to that in asbestos textile factories.[51] Thus in taking a patient's history, determining patient involvement in asbestos heat-conservation or heat-protection is essential. For example, asbestosis has been diagnosed in cafeteria and office workers employed in asbestos pipe plants where they had shared a single structure with production workers for 15 or 20 years.

Secondary Human Exposure

Family Members

Exposure to asbestos brought home by workers on their person and clothes was discovered in families of amosite factory workers[52] in Paterson, New Jersey. Fourty-eight percent of wives, 21 percent of daughters, and 42 percent of sons showed parenchymal or pleural evidence of asbestosis. Shifting to a less intense work exposure, that of shipyards, another family study showed that 11.3 percent of wives, 2.1 percent of daughters, and 7.6 percent of sons had signs of asbestosis.[53] Although consumer electrical goods such as irons, hair dryers, and fans have contained asbestos, to date there has been no evidence of disease resulting from exposure at the levels of fibrils released from electric irons, electric hair dryers, or even asbestos-containing artificial logs used in fireplaces. However, discontinuance of such exposure is the responsibility of the Consumer Products Safety Administration.

Schools and Other Buildings

Passive bystander asbestos exposure—as occurs to people in buildings with asbestos as heat insulation on steam pipes, boilers, and ducts leading to the rooms and sprayed on ceilings and walls or as construction materials—has been the subject of contentious discussion, rule making,

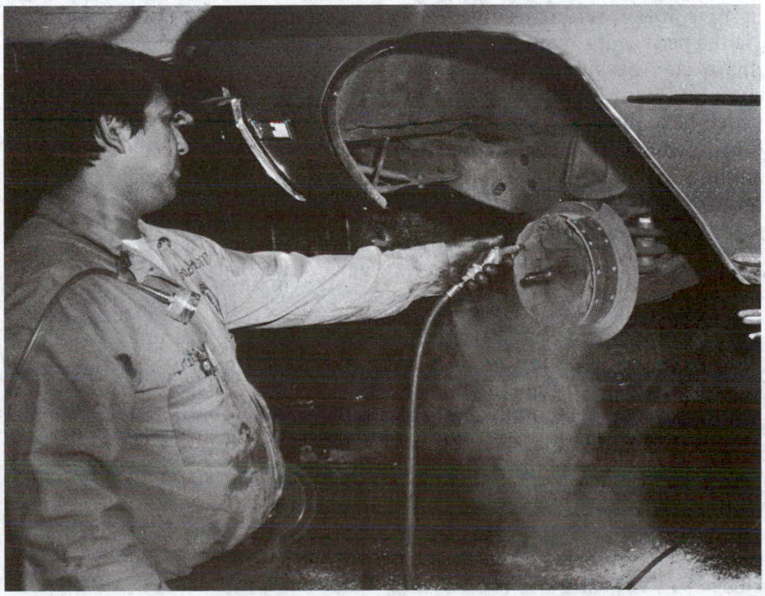

Figure 19-2. Removal of dust from brake drum and back plate using compressed air generates cloudy or fine fibers and dust.

and litigation in the past decade.[54,55] Surveys by the U.S. Environmental Protection Agency (EPA) in 1985 estimated that 31,000 schools and 733,000 public and commercial buildings contained friable, easily crumbled asbestos-containing material.[22] In a preliminary study of school custodians that was stimulated by the finding of mesotheliomas in three of this group, a Los Angeles study of 205 school maintenance workers and custodians with 10 years on the job showed 16 percent had pleural and 13 percent had parenchymal signs of asbestosis.[56] A similar prevalence was found in a study of New Jersey custodians (S Levine, personal communication). In neither of these studies were custodians with prior exposure to asbestos excluded nor was it possible to ascertain which ones were working on the maintenance of boilers and heat- and power-generating facilities. In Boston schools[57] 52 custodians showed signs of asbestosis. School custodial workers have asbestosis as a result of workplace exposure. Teachers and students sharing these air spaces may show signs as well, but neither has been studied. Many school boards have removed asbestos from the schools; some have issued bonds for this purpose, and some have sued the suppliers of asbestos-containing products to recover the costs. In response to pressure from consumer groups and legislatures, the EPA has recommended removal of such products when air levels of asbestos are 0.1 to 0.01 fiber/mL.[21] The problem can be solved if a society will make changes based on the known harmfulness of asbestos, without assessing morbidity and mortality rates for a particular exposure.[53,54]

Asbestosis

Diagnosis

The diagnosis of asbestosis requires, first, a history of exposure, usually occupational or as a bystander in a trade in which asbestos has been used. Second, a suitable period must have elapsed since the start of exposure (latent period). The third criterion is typical pulmonary or pleural abnormalities on the chest x-ray. The latent period, at the levels of exposure prevalent in developed countries in the past 30 years, is at least 10 years, with progressively higher prevalences of asbestosis at 20, 30, and 40 years. In most shipbuilding and construction trades, among workers who were virtually continuously exposed for 25 to 35 years, the prevalence of asbestosis, including pleural disease, is 25 to 35 percent. Full-size posteroanterior chest radiographs show irregular opacities in the lower half of the lung fields near the lateral pleural surfaces. Pleural signs are circumscribed or diffuse areas of pleural thickening, so-called hyaline plaques of the parietal pleura, which are seen best when located laterally or on the diaphragm but may also be located posteriorly or anteriorly and seen face on (en face) or in profile. Descriptions of the patterns of changes in chest radiographs as a result of asbestosis have been progressively enhanced and detailed by the International Labour Organization (ILO) working committees since 1919. The 1980 revision[1] included a set of standard radiographs with the major ILO categories portrayed (Fig. 19-3, *A* to *E*). Pleural changes are described by their location, thickness, and extent (Fig. 19-3*F*). Use of the ILO classification scheme has improved communication between investigators in various countries. Recent studies of several thousand exposed workers showed that the functional implications of pleural and pulmonary signs are similar: both impair expiratory flow and produce air trapping.[58–60] Furthermore, despite radiographic distinctions between circumscribed plaquelike and diffuse pleural thickening, there was no difference in physiological impairment except that greater impairment occurred when diffuse thickening surrounded the base of the lung.

Pathology

British pathologist Roodhouse Gloyne[7] described in the classic cellular aggregates and cell proliferation around the small airways, the terminal and respiratory bronchioles, a diagnostic gold standard. The primacy of this lesion was obscured in later descriptions of fibrosis throughout the lung, with dense aggregates of macrophages and asbestos bodies in the surviving alveoli and led to characterization of asbestosis as an interstitial fibrosis. However, in the past decade, descriptions of the human pathological changes and considerable animal experimentation have drawn attention to the membranous and respiratory bronchioles as the focus of fibrosis (Fig. 19-4). Subsequent bridging extends between the bronchioles, creating a latticework; additional interstitial fibrosis may develop at a more advanced stage.[41] A possible second and more distinctive lesion probably involves the perivenous lymphatics and has been visualized on extended-scale computer-assisted tomograms of subjects showing increased markings in the lung bases.[61,62] This lesion creates a distinct pattern on the extended-scale tomograms. Fibrosis is well visualized peripherally and attenuates as it extends toward the hilum. This is in contrast to ordinary vascular and bronchial markings, which attenuate toward the pleural surfaces. Accentuated secondary lobular septa occur at about 1-cm intervals along the lateral margins of the lung, where they are recognized as laddering on the chest radiograph.

A small percentage of asbestos-exposed subjects have their course complicated by pleural effusions. Healing of these effusions may obliterate the costophrenic angles and produce diffuse pleural scarring.[63,64]

Undoubtedly, fibrils migrate to the pleura from their locus of deposition in small airways or alveoli.[42] Whether they are translocated as free fibrils or within macrophages after phagocytosis is still unknown. In either case they must exit the lung to the pleural space and move with the lymph flow to the parietal pleural lymphatic vessels.[42] Here they apparently stimulate macrophages or stimulate the retention of the macrophages in the outer layers of the pleura and once again stimulate fibroblastic proliferation. Thus circumscribed thickening

Figure 19-3. The International Labor Organization (ILO) classification for pneumoconiosis has provided criteria for asbestosis on chest x-ray films since 1959, using a scheme that originated in 1916. Classification is based on a standard 14 × 17 = inch posteroanterior radiograph of a technical quality that distinguishes details in the lungs. In 1980, copies of radiographs were supplied for normal, 0/0, and for the three major categories of profusion of opacities for each size: s, t, and u. 1/1 slight opacities, notable in outer lung regions; 2/2 = moderate opacities, partly obscuring pulmonary vessels; and 3/3 = opacities so profuse as to obscure the pulmonary vessels. **A** shows the standard films for opacities 3 to 10 mm in diameter (u/u). **F** shows circumscribed plaque (UL), diffuse pleural plaques (UR), calcified diaphragmatic plaque (LR), and calcified wall (LL).
Technical quality. With modern x-ray equipment, dedicated technicians can produce nearly ideal maximally inflated chest radiographs in all instances except morbid obesity, severe infirmity, or distortion of the chest cage or internal organs. The common correctable error is underinflation, which is recognized when the right side of the diaphragm is above the ninth intercostal space. Such films must be repeated after the subject is instructed in holding a deep breath. Films of high quality can be ensured if a qualified reader repeats suboptimal films before the subject leaves the x-ray unit.
The 12-point scale. The profusion of opacities was classified into one of four major categories by comparison with standard radiographs and a number, 0 to 3, written to the left of the slash. If during this rating the major category above or below was seriously considered as an alternative, this was recorded on the right side of the slash, thus, "2/1" represents a profusion of major category 2 but with category 1 having been seriously considered. Profusion without serious doubt, in the middle of the major category, was recorded as 2/2. If the category above was seriously considered, profusion was recorded as 2/3.

A B C D E F

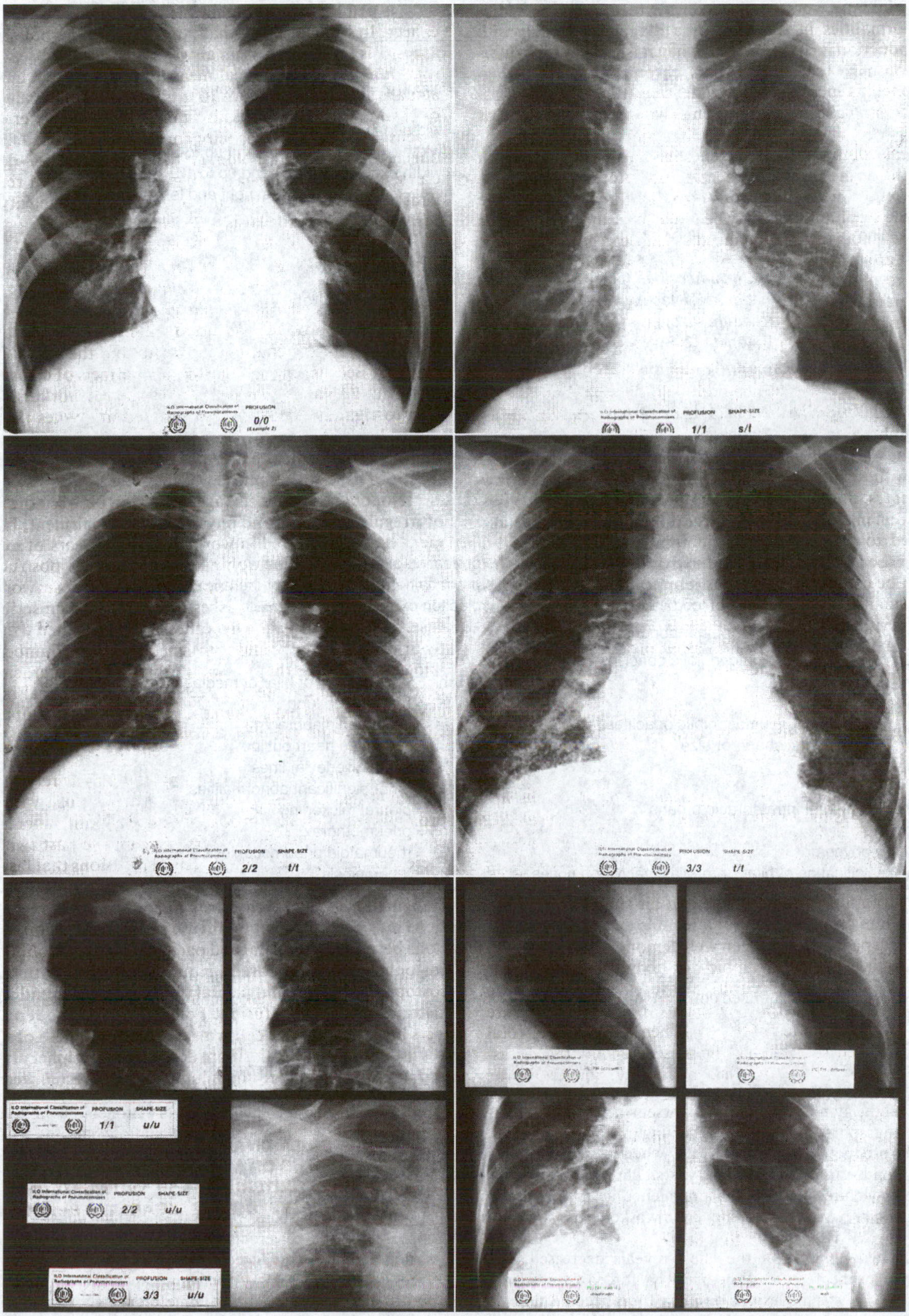

Figure 19-3. For legend see facing page. Figure table information appears on page 466.

Figure 19-3. Table information
ILO CLASSIFICATION OF CHEST RADIOGRAPHS FOR ASBESTOSIS

Small Opacities Irregular		***Short (1971) Classification***	***1980 Extended Classification***
Profusion		1, 2, 3	0/0, 0/1, 1/0, 1/1, 1/2, 2/1, 2/2, 2/3, 3/2, 3/3, 3/4
			1 = slight, 2 = moderate, 3 = advanced
Type		s, t, u	s, t, u
			s = width to about 1.5 mm
			t = width exceeding 1.5 mm and up to 3 mm
			u = width exceeding 3 mm and up to 10 mm
Extent		—	6 zones: right and left—upper, middle, and lower
Large opacities:	>10 mm		
Pleural thickening:			
Chest wall			
	■ ***Circumscribed*** (plaques)		
	Face-on (en face)		Right, left
	Width (a, b, c)		
	Extent (1, 2, 3)		
	■ ***Diffuse***		
	Face-on		
	Width (a, b, c)		
	Extent (1, 2, 3)		
	Diaphragm		Right, left
	Costophrenic angle obliteration		Right, left
	a = maximum width up to ≈ 5 mm		
	b = maximum width > ≈ 5 mm and up to ≈ 10 mm		
	c = maximum width > ≈ 10 mm		
	1 = total length up to one fourth (of the projection of the lateral chest wall)		
	2 = total length exceeding one fourth but not half of the projection of the lateral chest wall		
	3 = total length exceeding half of the projection of the lateral chest wall		

Additional symbols: classification of other abnormalities on the x-ray films.

ax = coalescence of small pneumoconiotic opacities	fr = fracture rib
bu = bullae	hi = enlargement of hilar or mediastinal lymph nodes
ca = cancer of lung or pleura	ho = honeycomb lung
cn = calcification of small pneumoconiotic opacities	id = ill-defined diaphragm
co = abnormality of cardiac shape or size	ih = ill-defined heart outline
cp = cor pulmonale	kl = septal (Kerley's) lines
cv = cavity	od = other significant abnormalities
di = marked distortion of intrathoracic organs	pi = pleural thickening
ef = effusion	px = pneumothorax
em = definite emphysema	rp = rheumatoid pneumoconiosis
es = eggshell calcification of hilar or mediastinal lymph nodes	tb = tuberculosis

(plaques) is found in the lower two-thirds of the lateral dorsal and ventral parietal pleura and on the dome of the diaphragm. Plaques are disks composed of dense hyalinized collagenous connective tissue up to several millimeters in thickness.

Clinical Features

The principal symptom is shortness of breath on exertion; onset is insidious, and the symptom gradually worsens before either recognition of radiograph abnormalities in the lung or a diagnosis. Cough with phlegm production is common and, when present for a duration of 3 months in 2 succeeding years, chronic bronchitis is diagnosed. Bronchitis increases in prevalence as the duration of asbestos exposure passes 20 years, even in workers who have never smoked.

Physical examination of the chest reveals decreased breath sounds as the prime feature. Wheezing on forced expiration increases in frequency as the lesions on x-ray films become more profuse. Fine crepitant rales may be heard after the radiographic changes are moderately advanced (ILO category 2/2 and greater) but are rare earlier. Peripheral cyanosis and clubbing of the phalanges, although described in advanced asbestosis, are such uncommon signs that their presence should arouse suspicion of other causes. Asbestos "warts," which occur from inoculation of asbestos fibers through the skin, once common in insulators who handled asbestos daily, are rare.

Physiological Impairment

The principal pathological lesions of asbestos in the lungs narrow and constrict membranous and respiratory bronchioles. These lesions, in turn, physically limit mid and terminal flow rates,[65,66] that is, obstruct expiratory air flow, which is the earliest physiological finding in asbestosis.[13,58] Over 1,700 workers who had never smoked cigarettes were studied to define the effects of asbestos alone.[13,58] Their small airways were obstructed before the irregular opacities of asbestosis appeared on the posteroanterior chest radiograph (Fig. 19-5). Such airflow limitation produced air trapping noted by an increased ratio of residual volume (RV) to total lung capacity (TLC ratio) (RV/TLC), and the increased residual volume reduced vital capacity. The reduced vital capacity led to the concept that asbestosis is a restrictive lung disease similar to idiopathic pulmonary fibrosis. However, vital capacity is a reliable measure of restrictive disease, which is defined solely by loss of lung volume, only in the *absence of obstruction*.[67]

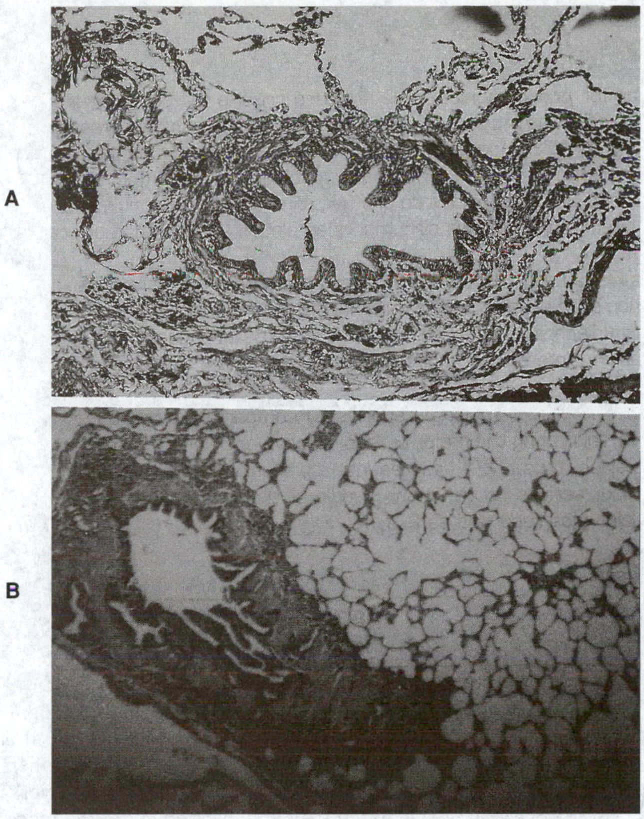

Figure 19-4. A, normal terminal bronchiole (small airway) has thin walls beneath the epithelial layer and is near to alveoli. **B,** An abnormal terminal bronchiole is surrounded by a thick cuff of connective tissue.

These effects are exaggerated by cigarette smoking (Fig. 19-6). Gas dilution using helium or nitrogen must ignore air trapping and does not measure total lung capacity, as happens in patients with emphysema. Thus radiographic[68] or body plethysmographic methods must be used for accurate measurement of total lung capacity.[67] In the former method, radiographs must be obtained when the lungs are fully inflated, while in the latter one, expiratory reserve volume must be measured carefully. Total lung capacity is slightly increased due to effects of cigarette smoking; 85 percent of workers exposed to asbestos also smoked cigarettes for many years.

When the profusion of irregular opacities on the chest radiograph is used to measure severity of asbestosis, to plot against key pulmonary function measurements, progressive impairment of airflow and air trapping occur with an increasing profusion of opacities on radiographs[59,60] (Figs. 19-5, *A* and *B*, and 19-6, *A* and *B*). Further limitation of expiratory flow from 25 to 75 percent of vital capacity (FEF_{25-75}) indicates increased airway obstruction, which has increased air trapping, within a normal total lung capacity. As flow (FEF_{25-75}) decreased, both forced expiratory volume, in 1 second, and vital capacity decreased; lung volume was maintained. Further evidence came from the 46 men with severe asbestosis as shown by ILO profusions of 2/3 and greater from 8,000 asbestos exposed workers. None had reduced thoracic gas volume. There were four additional subjects who appeared to have restrictive disease but each had had a lobe or more of lung removed for cancer. In summary, "a small, tight lung" does not characterize asbestosis. Rather it is an airway obstructive disease in which total lung volume, the measure of restrictive lung disease, has increased by 10 percent due to cigarette smoking. Gas transfer capacity—that is, the diffusing capacity for carbon monoxide, measured during a single breath-hold of 10 seconds—does not decrease until air trapping has reduced vital capacity; thus decreased diffusing capacity is not an early sign of asbestosis.

Cigarette Smoking Interaction

Men with asbestosis who smoked cigarettes have an increasing profusion of irregular opacities (Table 19-2).[69] Cigarette smoking produces obstructive lesions of the small airways and causes emphysema by departitioning the distal portion of the lung. Because of these well-known effects of cigarette smoke on the airways, obstruction in asbestos workers was attributed to cigarette smoke. However, recent studies of large numbers of workers who never smoked showed that airway obstruction is characteristic of asbestosis alone.[13,58-60]

Not only is there a strong correlation between the profusion of irregular opacities and physiological impairment, but impairment can be measured in workers after 15 years of exposure in the absence of radiographic lesions. Airway obstruction also characterizes the physiological pattern in those workers who show only pleural signs of asbestosis, either circumscribed or diffuse,[70] as hypothesized by Fridriksson et al[71] and confirmed by many physiological studies.

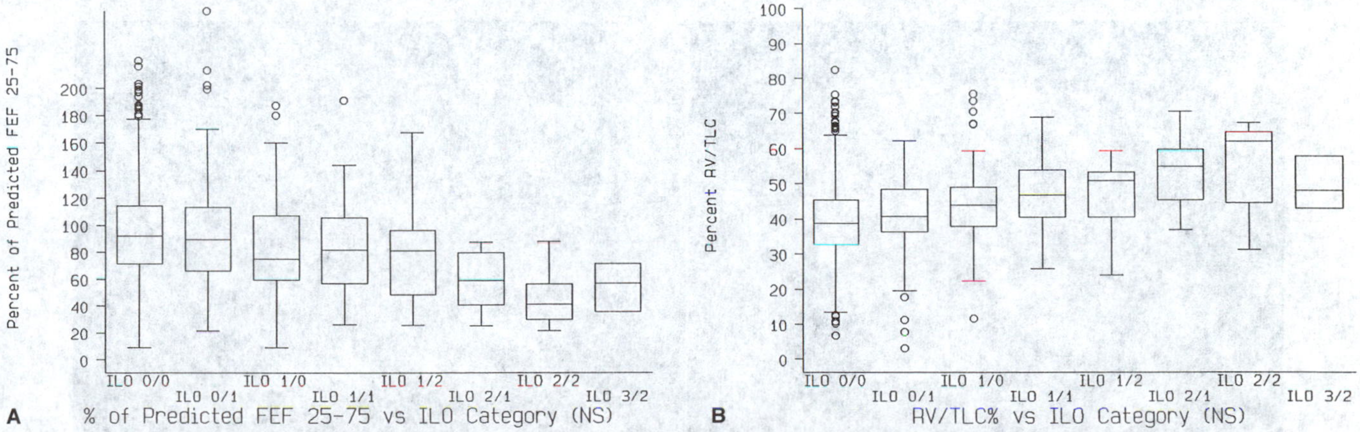

Figure 19-5. A, Mid flows (FEF25-75) in 1,777 men who were never smokers as a percentage of predicted (adjusted for height and age) are shown as box plots against ILO categories 0/0 to 3/3 with median line, 25 to 75 percent limits as the box bottoms and tops and whiskers equal to three halves of the interquartile range rolled back to where there are data. Regression equation for FEF25–75 percent predicted = 99.01 – 4.92 ILO category ($P < 0.0001$, R^2 = 2.4 percent). **B**, Residual volume/total lung capacity (RV/TLC) is plotted against ILO categories as in top. RV/TLC = 36.6 + 2.54 ILO category ($P < 0.0001$, R^2 = 6.7 percent).
(From Kilburn KH, Warshaw RH: Airways obstruction from asbestos exposure: effects of asbestosis and smoking. Chest 106:1061–1070, 1994.)

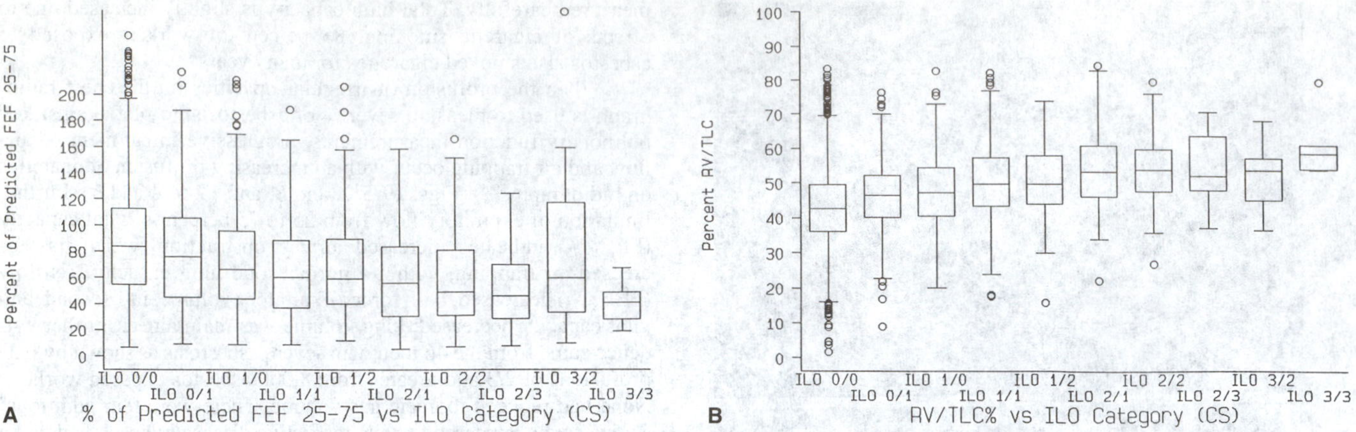

Figure 19-6. **A**, Mid flows (FEF25–75) in 4,550 men who were current smokers as percentage of predicted (adjusted for height, age, and duration of cigarette smoking) are plotted against ILO categories as in Figure 19-5. FEF25–75 percent predicted 89.4–4.93 ILO category ($P < 0.0001$, $R^2 = 3.5$ percent). **B**, Residual volume/total lung capacity (RV/TLC) is plotted against ILO categories for current smokers. RV/TLC = 41 2 + 2.04 ILO category ($P < 0.0001$, $R^2 = 7.9$ percent).
(From Kilburn KH, Warshaw RH: Airways obstruction from asbestos exposure: effects of asbestosis and smoking. Chest 106:1061–1070, 1994.)

Subjects with both pleural and parenchymal asbestosis are more impaired than those with either pleural or pulmonary changes alone.

Pleural Effusions and Their Sequelae

The recognition that pleural effusions occur in subjects with asbestosis without other proximate causes was probably delayed until tuberculosis became rare in American workers. During the past two decades, there have been reports[63,64] of pleural effusions that last weeks to months; are without bacterial flora, stigmata of tuberculosis, or malignant cells; and have a benign course. Such effusions may precede diffuse pleural thickening with adhesions between the visceral and parietal pleura and obliteration of costophrenic angles, as many workers with these signs have histories of pleural effusion. Follow-up of some reported subjects has been likewise confirmatory.[64] From these observations it is inferred that fibrosis, more dense in the periphery of the lung and attenuating toward the hilum, which is recognized with extended-scale, computer-augmented tomography[61,62] (Fig. 19-7), may be due to asbestosis pleural effusions. It is clear that these workers have more functional impairment than others with pleural asbestos disease.[70] The logical inference that these workers are the ones who develop thick pleural encasement of the lungs, which occasionally requires surgical removal (decortication) for relief of lung trapping, is not yet confirmed.

Mesothelioma

The pleura and peritoneum are lined with mesothelial cells. These cells are derived from mesoderm and may develop into connective tissue cells or epithelial cells. Asbestos is translocated to mesothelial cells and initiates tumors that grow rapidly, have an excellent blood supply, and thus rarely show necrosis. They invade nerves to cause and kill by interference with vital functions. Microscopic metastases

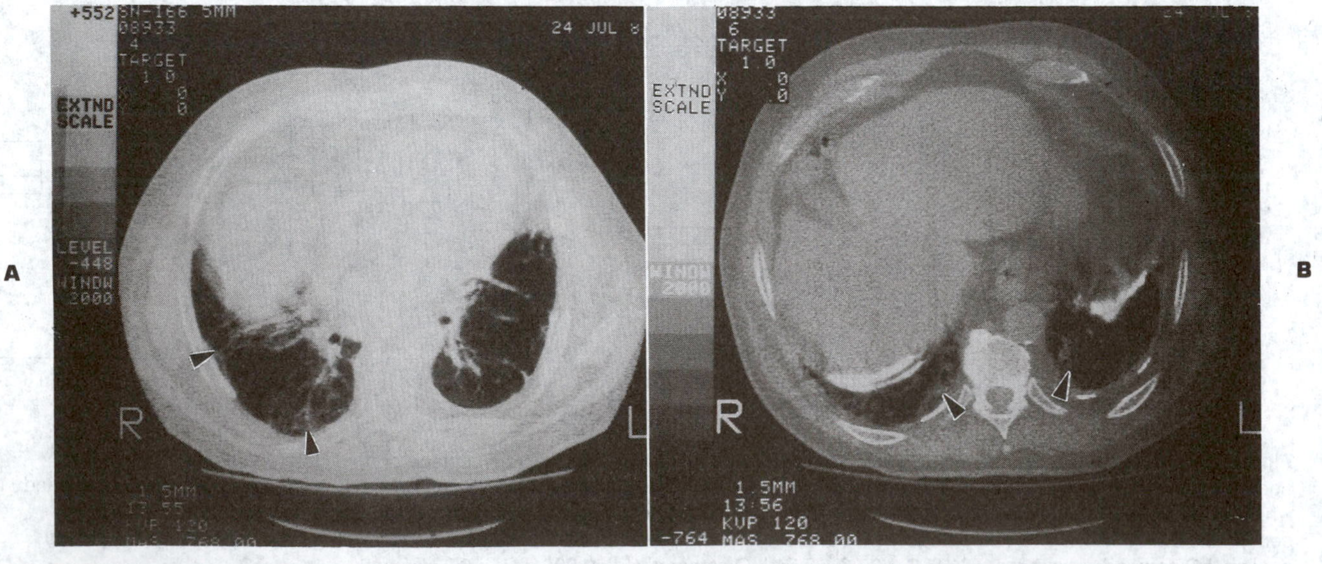

Figure 19-7. A, Extended-scale, computer-augmented scan shows pleura plaques *(white)* and networks of abnormal connective tissue (*arrows*) extended from mid-lung structures to the chest wall and to plaques on the right (*R*) side. **B,** Similar scan has gray-shaded area showing connective tissue.

are frequent but rarely clinically important. These tumors arise in response to asbestos fibers or fibrils that have either penetrated the lung to reach the pleural space or penetrated the bowel wall to reach the peritoneum. Mesotheliomas grow and spread rapidly and widely over the surfaces, displacing or engulfing vital organs rather than invading them (Fig. 19-8). In the peritoneum or pleura the bumpy growths are white or light yellow and vascular without necrosis. Histological sections show either a dense fibroblastic connective tissue, with stroma cells forming tubular structures resembling capillaries, or small vessels or glands, or a combination of fibroblastic and epithelial cell types.[72] It is sometimes difficult to distinguish from the tumors of metastatic adenocarcinoma from lung, pancreas, colon, or stomach tissue without ultrastructural and histochemical studies.[73]

Rare tumors such as these serve as sentinel or signal neoplasms, strongly suggesting specific exposures. Thus mesotheliomas are sentinels for asbestosis. Nasal sinus carcinomas connote exposure to nickel carbonyl or wood dust from certain tropical hardwood trees. Angiosarcoma of the liver in the United States suggests exposure to vinyl chloride monomer, but similar tumors of the liver in Africa indicate aflatoxin exposure. Historically the scrotal cancers in the chimney sweeps causally related to coal tar by Percival Pott were sentinels.

In the general population the incidence of mesothelioma varies between 1:1000 and 1:10,000 deaths or fewer, but in insulators heavily exposed throughout their careers, it caused 8 to 10 percent of deaths. Add to these the deaths from contamination of the home by asbestos brought into it by a worker in a shipyard or an asbestos factory and deaths of subjects who had exposures for only a year or so. Although the latency period averages 35 to 40 years, it may be as brief as 5 years. There is no relation to cigarette smoking, nor is there convincing evidence for a dose-response or an enhanced risk from intensive or prolonged exposure to asbestos although amphiboles may be more potent than is chrysotile. Thus in the shipbuilding trades the incidence of mesothelioma is related to the number of workers at risk in all of the trades, whereas the prevalence of asbestosis is much higher in more heavily exposed workers such as pipe coverers, pipefitters, and boilermakers.

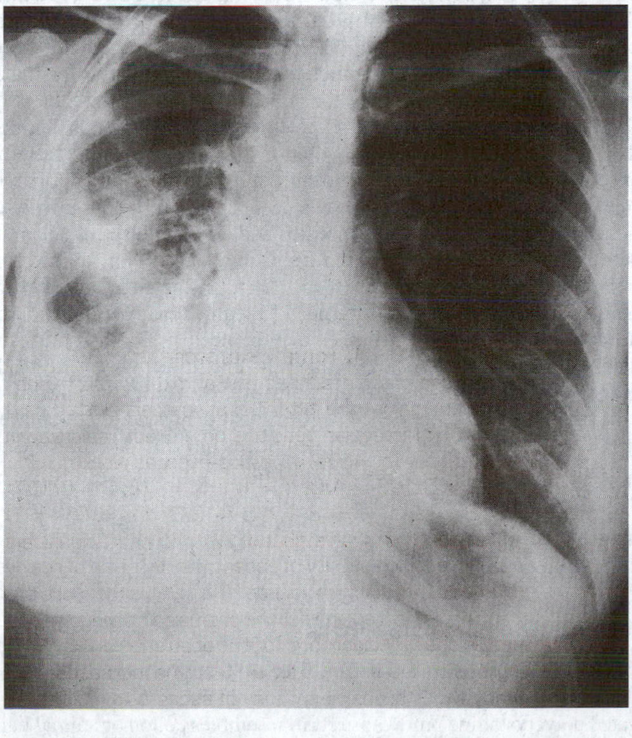

Figure 19-8. Pleural mesothelioma in a 35-year-old housewife. Her father, a shipyard employee, had brought dusty work clothes home from the shipyard to be cleaned. He died of lung cancer. Her mother died of pleural mesothelioma.

By experimental implanting of fibers of various types and sizes into the pleural space of rats and guinea pigs, Stanton and Wrench showed that fibrous glass, rock wool, palygorskite, and brucite caused mesothelioma.[50] In Turkey, erionite, a fibrous zeolite, has been associated with an extraordinary prevalence of mesotheliomas around Cappadocia.[74,75] Before zeolite can be accepted as a cause, however, it must be noted that fibrous tremolite has also been found in this area and is a contaminant of natural products used for building material. Thus fibrous tremolite, an amphibole, may be responsible for the mesotheliomas. The animal experiments caution against widespread adoption of human-made substitutes for asbestos. Carbon fibers, because of their size and shape, may share the potential for inducing mesothelioma, and they and vitreous fibers may also produce pulmonary fibrosis although they have not been tested.

Management of mesothelioma is discouraging to the patient and frustrating to the physician. Survival after diagnosis is usually 1 year. Patients rarely live 5 years. Used alone, radiotherapy, chemotherapy, and surgery offer no advantage to the natural course. Debulking of the tumor surgically, if possible, and multidrug hemotherapy, with doxorubicin (adriamycin), cyclophosphamide, and cisplatinate, increase the after-diagnosis life span about 1 year. Because mesotheliomas invade nerves, pain relief is the major concern.

Lung Cancer

The major public health concern and principal cause of death from asbestos in developed countries is lung cancer. In some groups of asbestos-exposed workers, the lung cancer mortality rate is as high as one in five. The cocausality with cigarette smoking is clear, and the relative risk may be 50 to 100 times as high in the asbestos-exposed smoker as in the non-asbestos–exposed subject who has never smoked.[19,76] Because 65 to 85 percent of workers exposed to asbestos have smoked and about 50 percent, in 1990, continued to do so,[77] their excessive risk of lung cancer calls for intervention to quit smoking. Although the smoking rate for males in the general population is now less than 30 percent and there is clear evidence that stopping smoking reduces the risk of cancer,[78] more than 50 percent of asbestos workers surveyed from 1987 to 1994 (69, 70, 77) in the construction, shipbuilding, and metal trades continued smoking. Thus there are workers with an extreme risk of cancer for whom there is only one practical approach: motivate them to discontinue smoking. Treatment of lung cancer has advanced but little in the past 30 years. Only 5 to 8 percent of patients survive 5 years after discovery of the cancer by symptoms or ordinary clinical detection. Although investigations with genetic markers and surface antigens suggest that we may be on the verge of earlier clinical recognition, the logistics of extending the present expensive and time-consuming methods to several million asbestos-exposed active and retired workers suggest that little immediate benefit can be expected from this avenue.

The latency for lung cancer in asbestos-exposed workers appears to be similar to that in non-asbestos–exposed workers, with a peak incidence in the early 60s.[19,76,79] Because of the demonstration of a rapidly decreasing risk with the cessation of smoking, serious and continuous efforts to induce asbestos-exposed persons to stop smoking are a public health priority. Similar risk reduction is postulated for the bystander and household-exposed groups, as well as for those persons who share lesser degrees of exposure in buildings containing asbestos. Although proof that the tumors are due to asbestos is at times difficult in the absence of radiographically demonstrated asbestosis, a recent study showed that almost all the lungs removed for cancer from asbestos-exposed individuals show microscopic fibrosis.[80] One lesson from history is clear: when asbestos exposure was sufficiently great that asbestosis was a principal cause of death, then the opportunity to survive long enough to develop lung cancer is diminished. This was illustrated in a German asbestos industry study centered in Dresden, which showed that one-fourth of the deaths after World War II in asbestos workers were due to asbestosis; less than 2 percent had lung cancer.[81] After the war, extensive industrial hygiene controls reduced the risk of fatal asbestosis in asbestos workers, and they lived longer only to die of lung cancer.

The dismal prospect for medical treatment of lung cancer and the large number of people exposed to asbestos who still smoke place the public health priority on cessation of smoking among blue collar workers who have been in proximity to airborne asbestos. Much of the smoking cessation effort has been directed to aid individuals who are already motivated to cease smoking. Relatively little has been written about motivation to quit. Workers can be motivated by a physician directing personal attention to effects of cigarette smoke such as signs of chronic bronchitis and emphysema and emphasizing the higher cancer risks when combined with asbestos exposure.[77] This strategy should be extended in the United States and most of the developed world, as during the past 20 years asbestos exposure has been progressively reduced. Millions of peoples' risk for lung cancer from exposure in the previous era can be substantially reduced if they cease smoking, thus also improving public health and decreasing medical and societal costs.

Other Asbestos-Related Neoplasms

Attribution of other neoplasms to asbestos is complex, meaning that large numbers of study subjects and a long time are required because many individuals in the study populations also smoke cigarettes, use alcohol, and are exposed to other occupational carcinogens. However, associations have been made between asbestos exposure and neoplasms of the pancreas and kidney, certain types of lymphoma, and neoplasms of the gastrointestinal tract, including the esophagus, mouth, and colon. The most extensive study, which serves to anchor the experience, is that of the heat and frost insulators, a cohort of 17,800 workers who have been studied by Selikoff and Seidman[19] since January 1967. In this group the ratio of observed to expected cancers of the esophagus, larynx, kidney, pharynx, and buccal mucosa was greater than 2; whereas the ratio for cancers of the stomach, colon, and rectum was greater than 1.5. Thus it appears that these common epithelial cancers are related to asbestos exposure, although the relationship of several are complex because of causal interaction with cigarette smoke and alcohol (Table 19-2).

The mortality rate from asbestos disease is elevated 2.6 times the expected rate, and that due to lung cancer is 9.1 times the expected rate.[76] Of British workers certified by medical panels as having asbestosis on the basis of sufficient exposure and the presence of two or four conditions (radiological (pulmonary) abnormality, pulmonary functional impairment, basal rales, and finger clubbing), 39 percent died of lung cancer; 9 percent, of mesothelioma; and 20 percent, of asbestosis. Selikoff and Seidman[19] studied all deaths in U.S. and Canadian insulators, found in the 1967 to 1987 interval an excess of deaths was 1.4 times the expected number, with deaths from cancer 3.0 times the expected number. Lung cancer accounted for 23.6 percent of deaths; mesothelioma, 9.3 percent; and asbestosis, 8.6 percent.

Societal Impact

Beginning slowly in the 1970s, workers' compensation and tort litigation were both undertaken for workers with mesothelioma, lung cancer, and asbestosis who were either threatened by death or showed impairment of function. In part because of 50 different laws in the states, there are no accurate figures on the numbers of plaintiffs who have successfully threaded through the legal maze of workers' compensation. This system was a social construct to avoid litigation and provide compensation without adversarial confrontation. It was focused on workplace injuries. The tradeoff for the worker (plaintiff) was to give up all legal redress for injury or illness. In practice, obtaining workers' compensation may be more difficult than pursuing third-party litigation. Thus society rather than industry has borne those costs after the workers' resources have been exhausted, employing public assistance, disability compensation, Social Security payments, Medicare, and Medicaid.

In the mid-1970s, civil actions (torts) began to be filed against major asbestos suppliers and manufacturers on behalf of patients with asbestos disease. More than a decade of such litigation has made the use of asbestos expensive because insurance is difficult or impossible to buy. Juries awarded large sums to a small fraction of plaintiffs with asbestos disease, particularly those with fatal neoplasms. Small awards or settlements were made for pulmonary impairment along with asbestosis in the lungs. The associated (nonpulmonary) neoplasms and pleural asbestosis have fared less well, with smaller jury awards and less frequent settlements. The co-responsibility of cigarette smoking has not been accepted by the tobacco companies, nor has litigation succeeded against them for their contribution to the lung cancer death toll. In 1978 the U.S. Congress asked for an appraisal of workers' compensation programs for occupationally related lung disease, which included asbestosis, byssinosis, and black lung, as the prelude to an omnibus bill. However, no omnibus bill has been passed. Although on paper the situation remains perhaps worse than it was in 1978, society has responded through the courts. The bankruptcy proceedings of Johns Mansville and several of the other asbestos firms affirm their loss of insurability and their large costs in fighting and settling asbestos cases. Meanwhile, installation and use of new asbestos have virtually ceased. More members of the exposed workforce know the hazards and hygiene of asbestos removal. Exposure has certainly decreased in developed countries. Currently the burden of asbestosis is on the individual who tries to obtain Social Security, county welfare, public assistance, disability compensation, or Medicare payments. The likelihood of obtaining such help apparently depends on luck.

Regulations to control exposure in the workplace were enacted in 1977; a temporary standard allowed workers to be employed in environments that contained up to 2 fibers/mL of air, or 2 million fibers/m^3.[82,83] The National Institute for Occupational Safety and Health (NIOSH) has recommended to the Occupational Safety and Health Administration (OSHA) a 0.1 fiber/mL industrial exposure in the United States, which was adopted in 1990 as a time-weighted average value. In view of the temporizing slowness of this approach, it is reassuring that the use of asbestos in the United States has steadily fallen since 1978, that it is or will be proscribed in most consumer products, that in California a home cannot be sold without an asbestos inspection and amelioration of any problems found, and that there is a public sense of asbestos avoidance. New asbestos products are not being installed because of EPA rulings regarding most new construction. The EPA expanded its asbestos ban to most uses in July 1989[84] but brake blocks, pipe, and shingles were not affected until 1996 after three phase-out stages. By 1990 only 10 percent of products were phased out but most exceeding the EPA requirements were not being produced by November 1993, including brake linings, friction materials, flooring felt, and tile. Disappearance of asbestosis will be slow because of its long latency and some exposure from asbestos that was in place. Although in many jurisdictions removal is done legally by specially trained workers in disposable suits and using air supply respirators, some fly-by-night removal companies use laborers who do not even know the dangers of asbestos and lack any instructions in its safe handling. Such avoidance of responsibility also characterized earlier eras in this industrial society. Such unconscionable disregard of human suffering underscores the need for tighter controls and genuine accountability. Criminal penalties may be needed. On the optimistic side, friction products such as brakes and clutch facings can be made free of asbestos materials, and although they cost more than the products replaced, early experience suggests that they need to be replaced less often. Asbestos use in the United States fell from 240,000 metric tons in 1984 to 85,000 metric tons in 1987.[84,85]

▶ NATURAL NONASBESTOS AND HUMAN-MADE FIBERS

Natural Nonasbestos Fibers

According to the Mine Safety and Health Administration, about 150 minerals occur in fibrous form or may contain fibers. A fiber is an elongated polycrystalline unit whose form resembles cotton or animal hair. Some mineralogists define fibers as particles with an aspect ratio (length to diameter) equal to or greater than 10 to 1. "Asbestiform" denotes a type of silicate fiber that has a high tensile strength, extreme aspect ratio (i.e., high length/diameter ratio), flexibility, heat resistance, and aggregation of fibrils into bundles. Chrysotile is a good example. The Occupational Safety and Health Administration has defined the asbestos fiber as being greater than 5 μm in length with an aspect ratio of 3 to 1 or greater.

The pulmonary toxicity of natural and human-made fibers is related to the dose delivered and to the dimensions and durability of the fiber. Fibers with long residence time because of high durability are more toxic than those with shorter residence time. Pleural or peritoneal injection of fibers such as amosite and crocidolite, chrysotile, anthophyllite, tremolite, attapulgite, erionite (zeolite), borosilicate glass, aluminum silicate glass, mineral wool, aluminum oxide, potassium titanate, silicon carbide, sodium aluminum carbonate, and wollastonite produce mesotheliomas in animal models.[86] It is clear that both in solution and in animal tissues, including lung tissue, the amphiboles are more durable than chrysotile.

Whether talc, a sheetlike silicate, is toxic to the lung is unclear because in most North America deposits it is significantly contaminated by tremolite, anthophyllite, and quartz.[87] Exposure to pure cosmetic talc, that is, talc with minimal fiber content, produces few if any toxic reactions. Thus it appears that the toxicity of talc is due to its fiber contamination, or perhaps to its free silica content.

Vermiculite, a family of hydrated magnesium-aluminum-iron silicates, is sheetlike. The mineral is expanded by heat after removal from the mines and used for insulation and for fillers in paint, plasters, rubber, and other materials. The health hazard from vermiculite is attributable to its contamination with fibrous tremolite.[88]

Zeolites, a group of crystalline and hydrated aluminum silicate minerals, consist of extremely fine tubes of mordenite or erionite. The tubes are 10 to 20 μm in length and less than 1 to 3 μm in diameter. Naturally occurring deposits of zeolites are distributed worldwide, but adverse health effects have been investigated near Karain, Turkey, in the central Anatolia.[89,90] Although mesotheliomas, pleural thickening, and plaques were attributed to exposure to erionite, it appears that it is contaminated with chrysotile and tremolite.[89] Airborne fibers in Karain, which average less than 0.01 fiber/m^3 and a peak level of 1.38 fibers/m^3, are significantly below the current standard for asbestos fibers. Either this is an unrecognized hazard from low-level airborne fiber exposure, or alternatively, low-level exposure to tremolite, in contrast to erionite, may be responsible for the adverse health effects.[87] Wollastonite deposits are scattered around the world. A study in Finland showed that workers from a limestone-wollastonite quarry had a high frequency of pleural thickening and pulmonary fibrosis. Fibrosis was observed in only 3 percent of a worker cohort in the United States, but these subjects' reductions in expiratory airflow were related to dust levels.[91] Further studies of effects of erionite and wollastonite on human populations are needed, but these materials should be handled with caution.

Human-Made Fibers

The physical characteristic of fibers made by humans, from slag, rock, glass, or ceramics, vary greatly with their manufacture.[92] This also applies to the most recent species, carbon fiber. Carbon fibers are used in making sailboat masts and aircraft components (as in the Stealth bomber). The same considerations of dose, dimensions, and durability that apply to natural fibers extend to human-made filaments.[93] These products have a wide range of diameters. It is clear that little human respiratory hazard should be predicted for fibers with diameters greater than 10 μm because there is no way for these fibers to be split into fragments that are respirable. However, numerous samples of current commercial fibrous glass are highly heterogeneous, with some fiber diameters of 1 μm or less. Both rotary spinning and flame attenuation produce fibers less than 1 μm (Fig. 19-9, *A* and *B*). Currently the National Institute for Occupational Safety and Health[94] recommends that fibrous glass exposure be limited to 3 fibers/m^3. These fibers are defined as less than 3.5 μm in diameter and equal to or greater than 10 μm in length. Rotary spinning, the process analogous to that for making cotton candy, requires less energy and is replacing flame attenuation for producing fine fibers. The thermal coefficient, a measure of insulating capacity, is increased as fiber diameters are reduced (Fig. 19-9*C*) where high thermal coefficients are needed with low weight, such as in aerospace applications. Uniformly fine fiberglass is preferred. Fine fiberglass is also found in refrigerator doors and in insulating industrial construction and homes because it is mixed

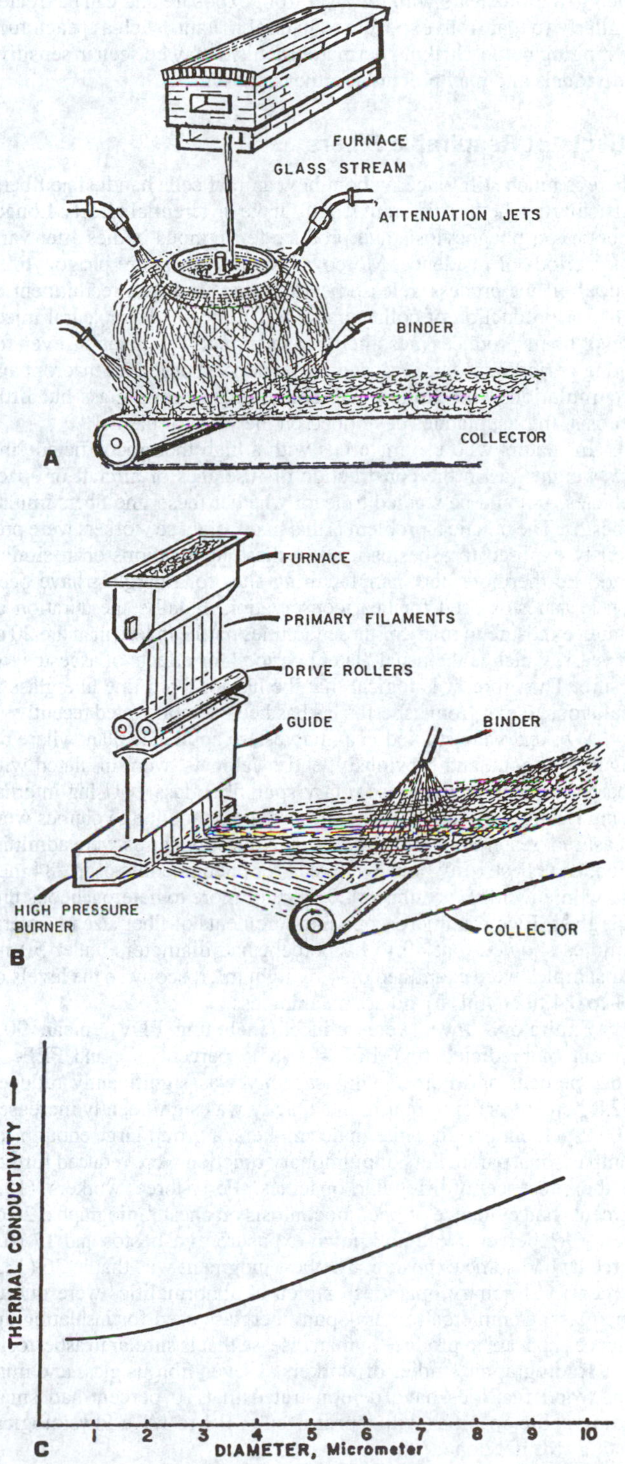

Figure 19-9. A, Rotary process of producing fine Fiberglass used both centrifugal force and air jets to attenuate the glass. Heterogeneous fiber diameters result. **B,** Flame attenuation provides heat and drive force to pull the fibers into smaller diameters. **C,** Insulating capacity, the reciprocal of thermal conductivity, is increased as fiber diameter is reduced.

heterogeneously with larger fibers. This usage exposes production and construction workers to some respirable airborne fibers.

Effects of Nonrespirable Fibers

Nonrespirable fibers irritate the skin, causing itching, burning, and irritation of the conjunctivae and the nasal and pharyngeal passages.[95] Such irritation clears with removal from exposure and can be treated similarly to that from exposure to natural irritants such as peach fuzz or stinging nettle. Striking dermatographism may be seen in sensitive individuals and may preclude further exposure.

Effects of Respirable Fibers

There is much still to learn about how animal cells handle fine fibers, particularly whether different lengths have differential effects. Longer fibers resist phagocytosis and produce ferruginous bodies after variable periods of residence. Moreover, shorter fibers are phagocytized and, after this process, release peptides that stimulate recruitment of cells for production of collagen and other fibers.[96] Intrapleural injection of fibers produces mesothelioma in animals.[85] Inhalation, even for a long period in rodents[97–99] and in monkeys,[98] produces macrophage accumulations and granulomas containing fibrous glass but little fibrosis. In rats, plaques developed on the visceral pleura.[98]

Insulators who use materials with a high thermocoefficient and low weight—as in the construction of fuselages of aircraft or space vehicles—should be studied to learn whether these fine fibers imitate asbestos. The practical problem is that many of these workers were previously exposed to asbestos used in these applications or in similar work. Furthermore, the manufacturing sites for fiberglass have been rich in asbestos used for heat conservation. Finally, the duration of human exposure in many of these facilities has been less than the 20 or 25 years, which is the usual "latent period" for effects of asbestos exposure. Therefore, it is logical that the hazard from fine fiberglass is analogous to that from asbestos, as has been demonstrated recently.

Workers were studied in a midwestern appliance plant where refrigerator doors, and previously, entire cabinets, were insulated with fiberglass sheeting and loose rotary-spun fiberglass.[100] Using International Labour Office 1980 criteria, spirometry and lung volumes were measured, respiratory and occupational questionnaires were administered, and chest x-ray films were read for pneumoconiosis in 284 men and women with exposures of 20 years or more to heterogeneous fine fiberglass. Electron microscope measurements of fiber size in several samples showed that 49 to 83 percent had diameters under 5 μm. Air samples were examined only by light microscopy so the levels of 0.1 to 0.4 fibers/mL found are meaningless.

Expiratory flows were reduced including FEV_1 (mean 90.3 percent of predicted (pr), FEF_{25-75} (85.5 percent pr), and FEF_{75-85} (76.2 percent pr). Forced vital capacity was significantly reduced (92.8 percent pr) and total lung capacity was significantly increased (109.2 percent pr). In white male smokers, a group large enough for comparisons, parameters of pulmonary function were reduced further in the presence of irregular opacities. Forty-three workers (15.1 percent) had evidence of pneumoconiosis on chest radiographs: 26 of these (9.1 percent) had no known exposure to asbestos and 17 (6.0 percent) had some exposure. The best judgment was that in 36 (13.0 percent) pulmonary opacities or pleural abnormalities were due to fiberglass. Commercial rotary-spun fiberglass used for insulating appliances appears to produce human disease that is similar to asbestosis.

Radiographic studies of workers at seven fibrous glass and mineral wood facilities have demonstrated that 10 percent had small radiographic opacities with a profusion of 0/1 to 1/1.[17] Physiological testing was not done.[99,101]

Mortality rates for fibrous glass workers have been studied without regard to the respirability (size) of the fibers; generally there have been no excess deaths from malignant or nonmalignant respiratory disease.[102] Two large studies include a 17-plant study in the United States under the auspices of the Thermal Insulation Manufacturers Association and a 72-plant seven-country European study by the European Insulation Manufacturers Association. In the United States, risks for lung cancer are above those of control populations, a 12 percent increase in glass wool workers and a 36 percent increase in those exposed to mineral wool.[102] Preliminary analyses of results have raised serious questions about the suitability of national versus regional versus area controls for tracking cancer mortality rates. The mortality rate question remains unsettled[103–105] because these problems are general, beyond merely understanding the effects of fiberglass. However, in societies whose members are contaminated by many chemicals, suitable comparison groups are difficult to locate. Human mesotheliomas from fiberglass have not been identified yet in construction workers installing loose fiberglass who had exposures of 7 fibers/mL.[104]

Public Health Considerations

Research

Because of the analogous dimensions and respirability of fine fibrous glass and other human-made fibers and a range of durability, additional studies are needed of health effects and mortality in populations that have been exposed for at least 20-year latent periods and without *exposure* to asbestos. If these studies confirm those reviewed above, they will guide choosing the best alternatives to asbestos in many applications. Meanwhile, the association of mesothelioma with siliceous filaments in sugar cane factory workers in India[106] raises the possibility of a "natural fiber" of plant origin mimicking asbestos exposure or that asbestos exposure has not been shown by the methods used. A better history of exposure, examination of lung tissue, and analysis of its fiber content with scanning electron microscopy and energy-dispersive analysis will help answer many questions of competing etiology as asbestos use is stopped.

Control Measures

It seems ironic that we are witnessing widespread adoption of fibrous glass and, despite the lessons of 75 years, facing this adoption without the key information needed to determine the human health risks.[93,94,103–105] Clearly, determination of the health hazards of fine human-made fibers is a high priority before widespread use in the production and application industries produces a problem for the next century that mimics the one we have experienced with asbestos. Meanwhile, it is prudent to regard materials that contain fibers of respirable dimension as needing the same precautions as does asbestos.[105]

▶ REFERENCES

1. International Labour Office: U/C International Classification of Radiographs of Pneumoconiosis in Occupational Safety and Health Series. Geneva: International Labour Office, 1980
2. Murray HM: Report of the Departmental Committee on Compensation for Industrial Disease. London: HM Stationery Office, 1907
3. Cooke WE: Fibrosis of the lungs due to the inhalation of asbestos dust. Br Med J 2:147, 1924
4. Cooke WE: Pulmonary asbestosis. Br Med J 2:1024–1026, 1927
5. Merewether ERA, Price CV: Report on effects of asbestos dust on the lungs and dust suppression in the asbestos industry. London: HM Stationery Office, 1930
6. Pancoast HK, Miller TG, Landish HRM: A roentgenologic study of the effects of dust inhalation upon the lungs. Am J Roentgenol (N.S.) 5:129–138, 1918
7. Gloyne SR: The morbid anatomy and histology of asbestosis. Tubercule (London) 14:445–451, 493–497, 550–559, 1933
8. Lanza AJ, McConnell WJ, Fehnel JW: Effects of the inhalation of asbestos dust on the lungs of asbestos workers. Public Health Rep 50:1–48, 1935
9. Dreessen WC, Dallavalle JM, Edwards TI, et al: A study of asbestosis in the asbestos textile industry. Public Health Bull 241:1–147, 1938
10. Donnelly J: Pulmonary asbestosis: incidence and prognosis. J Ind Hyg 18:222–228, 1936
11. Shull JR: Asbestosis: a roentgenologic review of 71 cases. Radiology 27:279–292, 1936

12. McPheeters SB: A survey of a group of employees exposed to asbestos dust. J Ind Hyg 18:229–239, 1936
13. Becklake MR, Fournier-Massey G, McDonald JC, Siemiatycki J, Rossiter CA: Lung function in relation to chest radiographic changes in Quebec asbestos workers. I. Methods, results and conclusions. Bull Physio Pathol Resp 6:637–659, 1970
14. Merewether ERA: Annual Report of the Chief Inspector of Factories. London: HM Stationery Office, 1947
15. Hueper WC: Occupational tumors and allied diseases. Springfield, IL: Charles C Thomas, 1942
16. Doll R: Mortality from lung cancer in asbestos workers. Br J Ind Med 12:81–86, 1955
17. Mancuso TF, Coulter EJ: Methodology in industrial health studies: the cohort approach, with special reference to an asbestos company. Arch Environ Health 6:210–222, 1963
18. Selikoff IJ: Asbestos disease in the United States, 1918–1975. Rev Fr Mal Resp 4:7–24, 1976
19. Selikoff IJ, Seidman H: Asbestos associated deaths among insulation workers in the United States and Canada, 1967–1987. Ann N Y Acad Sci 643:1–14, 1991
20. Klemperer P, Rabin CB: Primary neoplasms of the pleura: a report of five cases. Arch Pathol 11:385–412, 1931
21. Wagner JC, Sleggs CA, Marchand P: Diffuse pleural mesothelioma and asbestos exposure in the North Western Cape Province. Br J Ind Med 17:260–271, 1960
22. Guidance for Controlling Asbestos-containing Materials in Buildings. EPA 560/5-85-024. Washington, DC: U.S. Environmental Protection Agency, June 1985
23. Spurny KR: On the release of asbestos fibers from weathered and corroded asbestos cement products. Environ Res 48:100–116, 1989
24. Appel JD, Fasy TM, Kohtz DS, Kohtz JD, Johnson EM: Asbestos fibers mediate transformation of monkey cells by exogenous plasmid DNA. Proc Natl Acad Sci USA 85:7670–7674, 1988
25. Mossman BT, Craighead JE, MacPherson BV: Asbestos-induced epithelial changes in organ cultures of hamster trachea: inhibition by retinyl methyl ether. Science 207:311–313, 1980
26. Wade MJ, Lipsin LE, Tucker RW, Frank AL: Asbestos cytotoxicity in a long-term macrophage-like cell culture. Nature 264:444–446, 1976
27. Neugut AI, Eisenberg D, Silverstein M, Pulkribek P, Weinstein IB: Effects of asbestos epithelial cell lines. Environ Res 17:256–265, 1978
28. Ljungman AJ, Lindahl M, Tagnession C: Asbestos fibers and man-made mineral fibers: induction and release of tumor necrosis factor from rat alveolar macrophages. Occup Environ Med 15:777–783, 1994
29. Heppleston AG: Silica and asbestos: contrasts in tissue response. Ann NY Acad Sci 330:725–744, 1979
30. Heppleston AG: The fibrogenic action of silica. Br Med Bull 25:282–287, 1969
31. Allison AC: Pathogenic effects of inhaled particles and antigens. Ann NY Acad Sci 221:299–308, 1974
32. Davis JMG: The effects of chrysotile asbestos dust on lung macrophages maintained in organ culture. Br J Exp Pathol 48: 379–385, 1967
33. Davis JMG, Beckett ST, Bolton RE, Collings P, Middleton AP: Mass and number of fibres in the pathogenesis of asbestos-related lung disease in rats. Br J Cancer 37:673–688, 1978
34. Spurzem JR, Saltini C, Rom W, Winchester RJ, Crystal RG: Mechanisms of macrophage accumulation in the lungs of asbestos-exposed subjects. Am Rev Respir Dis 136:276–280, 1987
35. Wagner JC, Burns J, Munday DE, McGee J: Presence of fibronection in pneumoconiotic lesions. Thorax 37:54–56, 1982
36. Rom WN, Bitterman PB, Rennard SI, Catin A, Crystal RG: Characterization of the lower respiratory tract inflammation of nonsmoking individuals with interstitial lung disease associated with chronic inhalation of inorganic dusts. Am Rev Respir Dis 136:1429–1434, 1987
37. Davis HV, Reeves AL: Collagen biosynthesis in rat lungs during exposure to asbestos. Am Ind Hyg Assoc J 32:599–602, 1971
38. Wagner JC, Berry G, Skidmore JW, Timbrell V: The effects of the inhalation of asbestos in rats. Br J Cancer 29:252–269, 1974
39. Wagner JC: Asbestosis in experimental animals. Br J Ind Med 20:1–12, 1963
40. Churg A, Wright JL, Gilks B, DePaoli L: Rapid short-term clearance of chrysotile compared to amosite asbestos in the guinea pig. Am Rev Respir Dis 139:A214, 1989
41. Craighead JE, Abraham JL, Churg A, Green FHY, Kleinerman J, Pratt PC, Seemayer TA, Vallyathan V, Weill H: Asbestos-associated disease. Arch Pathol Lab Med 106:544–597, 1982
42. Hillerdal G: The pathogenesis of pleural plaques and pulmonary asbestosis: possibilities and impossibilities. Eur J Respir Dis 61: 129–138, 1980
43. Rennard SI, Jaurand M-C, Bignon J, Kawanami O, Ferrans VJ, Davidson J, Crystal RG: Role of pleural mesothelial cells in the production of the submesothelial connective tissue matrix of lung. Am Rev Respir Dis 130:267–274, 1984
44. Turner-Warwick M, Parkes WR: Circulating rheumatoid and anti-nuclear factors in asbestos workers. Br Med J 3:492–495, 1970
45. Kagan E, Solomon A, Cochrane JC, Kuba P, Rocks PH, Webster I: Immunological studies of patients with asbestosis. II. Studies of circulating lymphoid cell numbers and humoral immunity. Clin Exp Immunol 28:268–275, 1977
46. Kagan E, Solomon A, Cochrane JC, Beissner EI, Gluckman J, Rocks PH, Webster I: Immunological studies of patients with asbestosis. I. Studies of the cell-mediated immunity. Clin Exp Immunol 28: 261–267, 1977
47. Bitterman P, Rennard SI, Ozaki T, Adelberg S, Crystal RG: PGE_2: a potential regular of fibroblast replication in normal alveolar structures. Am Rev Respir Dis 127:271A, 1983
48. Rennard SI, Crystal RG: Fibronection in human bronchopulmonary lavage fluid elevation in patients with interstitial lung disease. J Clin Invest 69:113–122, 1981
49. Rennard SI, Bitterman PB, Crystal RG: Pathogenesis of granulomatous lung disease. IV. Mechanisms of fibrosis. Am Rev Respir Dis 30: 492–496, 1984
50. Stanton MF, Wrench C: Mechanisms of mesothelioma induction with asbestos and fibrous glass. J Natl Cancer Inst 48:797, 1972
51. Kilburn KH, Warshaw RH, Thornton JC: Asbestosis, pulmonary symptoms and functional impairment in shipyard workers. Chest 88:254–259, 1985
52. Anderson HA, Lilis R, Daum SM, Selikoff IJ: Asbestosis among household contacts of asbestos factory workers. Ann N Y Acad Sci 330:387–399, 1979
53. Kilburn KH, Lilis R, Anderson HA, Boylen CT, Einstein HE, Johnson SJS, Warshaw RH: Asbestos disease in family contacts of shipyard workers. Am J Public Health 75:615–617, 1985
54. Nicholson WJ, Swoszowski EJ Jr, Rohl AN, Todaro JD, Adams A: Asbestos contamination in United States schools from use of asbestos in surfacing materials. Ann N Y Acad Sci 330:587–596, 1979
55. Sawyer RN, Swoszowski EJ Jr: Asbestos abatement in schools: observations and experiences. Ann N Y Acad Sci 330:765–775, 1979
56. Balmes JR, Warshaw R, Chong S, Kilburn KH: Effects of occupational exposure to asbestos containing materials in public schools. Am Rev Respir Dis 129:A174, 1984
57. Oliver LC, Sprunce NL, Green RE: Asbestos-related disease in public school custodians. Am Rev Respir Dis 139:A211, 1989
58. Kilburn KH, Warshaw RH, Einstein K, Bernstein J: Airway disease in non-smoking asbestos workers. Arch Environ Health 40:293–295, 1985
59. Kilburn KH, Warshaw RH: Correlation of pulmonary functional impairment with radiographic asbestosis (ILO category). Am Rev Respir Dis 139:A210, 1989
60. Kilburn KH, Warshaw RH: Airways obstruction from asbestos exposure: effects of asbestosis and smoking. Chest 106:1061–1070, 1994
61. Wollmer P, Jakobsson K, Albin M, Albrechtsson U, Brauer K, Eriksson L, Johnson B, Skerfving S, Tylen U: Measurement of lung density by x-ray computed tomography. Chest 91:865–869, 1987

62. Aberle DR, Gamsu G, Ray CS: High-resolution CT of benign asbestos-related disease: clinical and radiographic correlation. Am J Radiol 151:883–891, 1988
63. Gaensler EA, Kaplan AI: Asbestos pleural effusion. Ann Intern Med 74:178–191, 1971
64. Epler GR, McLoud TC, Gaensler EA: Prevalence and incidence of benign asbestos pleural effusion in a working population. JAMA 247:617–622, 1982
65. Morris JF, Koski A, Johnson LC: Spirometric standards for healthy nonsmoking adults. Am Rev Respir Dis 103:57–67, 1971
66. Morris JF, Koski A, Breese JD: Normal values and evaluation of forced end-expiratory flow. Am Rev Respir Dis 111:755–762, 1975
67. Kilburn KH, Warshaw RH: Measuring lung volumes in advanced asbestosis: comparability of plethysmographic and radiographic versus helium rebreathing and single breath methods. Respir Med 87: 115–120, 1993
68. Kilburn KH, Warshaw RH: Total lung capacity in asbestosis: a comparison of radiographic and body plethsymographic methods. Am J Med Sci 305:84–87, 1993
69. Kilburn KH, Lilis R, Anderson HA, Miller A, Warshaw RH: Interaction of asbestos, age and cigarette smoking in producing radiographic evidence of diffuse pulmonary fibrosis. Am J Med 80: 377–381, 1986
70. Kilburn KH, Warshaw RH: Pulmonary functional consequences of pleural asbestos disease circumscribed and diffuse. Chest 98:965–972, 1990
71. Fridriksson HV, Hedenstrom H, Hillerdal G, Malmberg P: Increased lung stiffness in persons with pleural plaques. Eur J Respir Dis 62:412–424, 1981
72. Suzuki Y: Pathology of human malignant mesotheliomas. Semin Oncol 8:268–282, 1980
73. Suzuki Y, Churg J, Kannerstein M: Ultrastructure of human malignant mesothelioma. Am J Pathol 85:241–262, 1976
74. Baris YI, Sakin AA, Ozesmi M, Kerse I, Ozen E, Kolocan B, Altinors M, Ghoktepeli A: An outbreak of pleural mesothelioma and chronic fibrosing pleurisy in the village of Karain Urgup in Anatolia. Thorax 33:181–192, 1978
75. Lilis R: Fibrous zeolites and endemic mesothelioma in Cappadocia, Turkey. J Occup Med 23:548–558, 1981
76. Berry G: Mortality of workers certified by pneumoconiosis medical panels as having asbestosis. Br J Ind Med 38:130–137, 1981
77. Kilburn KH, Warshaw RH: Effects of individually motivated smoking cessation on male blue collar workers. Am J Public Health 80:1334–1337, 1990
78. Hammond EC, Selikoff IJ, Seidman H: Asbestos exposure, cigarette smoking and death rates. Ann N Y Acad Sci 330:473–490, 1979
79. Selikoff IJ, Seidman H, Hammond EC: Mortality effects of cigarette smoking among amosite asbestos factory workers. J Natl Cancer Inst 65:507–513, 1980
80. Kipen HM, Lilis R, Suzuki Y, Valciukas JA, Selikoff IS: Pulmonary fibrosis in asbestos insulation workers with lung cancer: a radiological and histopathological evaluation. Br J Ind Med 44:96–100, 1987
81. Jacob G, Anspach M: Pulmonary neoplasia among Dresden asbestos workers. Ann N Y Acad Sci 132:536–548, 1965
82. Peto J: Dose-response relationships for asbestos-related disease: implications for hygiene standards. II. Mortality. Ann NY Acad Sci 330:195–203, 1979
83. Berry G, Lewinsohn HC: Dose-response relationships for asbestos-related disease: implications for hygiene standards. I. Morbidity. Ann N Y Acad Sci 330:184–194, 1979
84. EPA announces final regulation to ban new asbestos products. Washington, DC: US Environmental Protection Agency, Office of Public Affairs (A107), 1989
85. EPA orders more bans on asbestos. Salt Lake Tribune, July 7, 1989
86. Stanton MF, Wrench C: Mechanisms of mesothelioma induction with asbestos and fibrous glass. J Natl Cancer Inst 48:797–821, 1972
87. Lockey JE, Moatamed F: Health implications of non-asbestos fibers. In Gee B (ed): Occupational Lung Diseases. New York: Churchill Livingstone, 1984, pp 75–98
88. Hassell PA, Sluis-Cremer GK: X-ray findings, lung function and respiratory symptoms in black South African vermiculate workers. Am J Ind Med 15:21–29, 1989
89. Baris YI, Sakin AA, Ozesmi M, Kerse I, Ozen E, Kolocan B, Altinors M, Goktepeli A: An outbreak of pleural mesothelioma and chronic fibrosing pleurisy in the village of Karain Urgup in Anatolia. Thorax 33:181–192, 1978
90. Lilis R: Fibrous zeolites and endemic mesothelioma in Cappadocia, Turkey. J Occup Med 23:548–553, 1981
91. Hanke W, Sepulveda M-J, Watson A, Jankovic J: Respiratory morbidity in wollastonite workers. Br J Ind Med 41:474–479, 1984
92. Kilburn KH: Flame-attenuated fiberglass: Another asbestos? Am J Ind Med 3:121–125, 1982
93. Stanton MF: Fiber carcinogenesis: is asbestos the only hazard? J Natl Cancer Inst 52:633–634, 1974
94. National Institute for Occupational Safety and Health: Criteria for a Recommended Standard Occupational Exposure to Fibrous Glass. Publication No. DHEW (NIOSH) 77-152. US Public Health Service, Department of Health, Education, and Welfare, 1977
95. Bjornberg A: Glass fiber dermatitis. Am J Ind Med 8:395–400, 1985
96. Maroudas NG, O'Neill CH, Stanton MF: Fibroblast anchorage in carcinogenesis by fibres. Lancet 1:807–809, 1973
97. Gross P, Kaschak M, Tolker EB, Babyak MA, de Treville RTP: The pulmonary reaction to high concentrations of fibrous glass dust. Arch Environ Health 20:696–704, 1970
98. Mitchell RI, Donofrio DJ, Moorman WJ: Chronic inhalation toxicity of fibrous glass in rats and monkeys. J Am Coll Toxicol 5:545–574, 1986
99. Smith DM, Ortiz LW, Archuleta RF, Johnson NF: Long-term health effects in hamsters and rats exposed chronically to man-made vitreous fibres. Ann Occup Hyg 31:731–754, 1987
100. Enterline PE, Marsh GM, Esmen NA: Respiratory disease among workers exposed to man-made fibers. Am Rev Respir Dis 128:1–7, 1983
101. Kilburn KH, Powers, B, Warshaw RH: Pulmonary effects of exposure to fine fibreglass: irregular opacities and small airway obstruction. Br J Ind Med 49:714–720, 1992
102. Nasr AN, Ditchek T, Scholtens PA: The Prevalence of Radiographic Abnormalities in the Chests of Fiber Glass Workers: Occupational Exposure to Fibrous Glass. Publication No. USPHS NIOSH 76-151. US Department of Health, Education, and Welfare, 1976
103. Enterline PE, Marsh GM, Stone RA, Henderson VL: Mortality among a cohort of U.S. man-made fiber workers. J Occup Med 32:594–604, 1990
104. Doll R: Overview and conclusions. Symposium on Man-made Mineral Fibers, Copenhagen, October 1986. Ann Occup Hyg 31: 805–819, 1987
105. Simonato L, Fletcher AC, Cherrie JW, et al: International Agency for Research on Cancer. Historical cohort study of MMMF production workers in seven European countries: extension of the follow-up. Ann Occup Hyg 31:603–623, 1987
106. Infante PF, Schuman LD, Dement J, Huff J: Fibrous glass and cancer: commentary. Am J Ind Med 26:559–584, 1994
107. Das PB, Fletcher AG Jr, Deodhare SG: Mesothelioma in an agricultural community of India: a clinicopathological study. Aust N Z J Surg 46:218–226, 1976
108. Hallin N: Report on Mineral Wool Dust in Construction Sites. Stockholm, Sweden: Bygghalsan, The Construction Industry's Organization for Working Environment, Safety and Health, 1981

20

Coal Workers' Lung Diseases

Gregory R. Wagner • Michael D. Attfield • James A. Merchant

Historical Perspective

Lung disease among underground coal miners has been a recognized occupational hazard since at least the mid-seventeenth century. Miners' black lung, now called coal workers' pneumoconiosis (CWP) was first documented among Scottish coal miners in 1836.[1] Although the disease was thought to be disappearing in Britain at the turn of this century, wider use of chest radiographs following World War I showed pneumoconiosis, similar to silicosis, among coal miners in South Wales. By 1934, British physicians were beginning to accept coal dust as an occupational exposure that could result in disability and death. In 1942, the Committee on Industrial Pulmonary Diseases of the Medical Research Council introduced the term "coal workers' pneumoconiosis."[2,3]

In marked contrast, appreciation of CWP as an occupational disease and public health problem occurred much later in the United States, as did legislation to prevent CWP or to compensate for CWP and associated respiratory disease. One reason for the relatively late recognition of CWP as a distinct disease entity in the United States was the early emphasis placed on the etiological role of silica in pneumoconiosis. The Hawk's Nest tragedy (1932 to 1934), in which more than 400 workers died of acute silicosis and tuberculosis after working on the tunnel at Gauley Bridge, West Virginia, reinforced the prevalent theory that silica content was the critical etiological agent in pneumoconiosis.

The first systematic study of U.S. coal miners was conducted by the Public Health Service between 1928 and 1931 in the anthracite coal fields in eastern Pennsylvania.[4] Because of the relatively high silica content and similarity to silicosis, the term "anthracosilicosis" was used to describe the pneumoconiosis found among those miners. Of 2,711 men studied, 23 percent were found to be affected. The prevalence of pneumoconiosis was related to the number of years underground, particles per cubic meter, and free silica content of the dust. "Pulmonary infection" was more frequent among miners with higher dust exposure and more than 15 years underground. Among miners over age 55, pulmonary tuberculosis was as much as 10 times more common than in the general population.[5]

Little additional progress was made in the United States until 1954, when the Public Health Service published a bibliography of American and British reports on respiratory disease among coal miners.[6] Following this, various clinical and epidemiologic studies by Levine and Hunter,[7] Lieben et al.,[8] and Stoeckle et al.[9] further documented the importance of coal workers' pneumoconiosis. At the direction of Congress, the Public Health Service began a comprehensive survey of the Appalachian coal fields in 1963. Of 2,549 working miners and 1,191 nonworking miners, 9 percent of the working and 18 percent of the nonworking miners were found to have radiographic evidence of pneumoconiosis.[10] This study, published in 1968, together with the disastrous November 20, 1968, Farmington, West Virginia, mine explosion that killed 78 miners, triggered increased pressure from miners, their union (the United Mine Workers of America), and public health advocates and led to passage of the Federal Coal Mine Health and Safety Act of 1969 (Public Law 1973).[11] This was the first American mining bill to recognize the importance of both health and safety hazards and provide a mandate for strong preventive measures.

Since that time, an awareness has grown indicating that CWP is not the only occupational pulmonary disease affecting coal miners. The results of the study by Rogan and colleagues[12] were the first to show a clear link between chronic airflow obstruction and dust exposure, independent of CWP status, while Rae et al.[13] demonstrated that respiratory symptom prevalence was related to level of dust exposure. Emphysema is increased in coal miners,[14] and related to both FEV_1, retained dust in the lung, and to cumulative dust exposure.[15,16]

Legislation

Although the Federal Coal Mine Health and Safety Act of 1969 was a landmark piece of legislation, it was by no means the first or last legislation to deal with occupational hazards of mining (Table 20-1). The 1969 act addressed several issues specifically and has served as a model for subsequent occupational safety and health legislation. The provisions included the following:[17]

- Mandatory health standards to be prescribed by the Secretary of Health and Human Services (HHS)
- Right of entry for inspection (Department of Interior) and investigation (HHS)
- Power to close mining operations, issue abatement orders, and penalize operators for noncompliance
- A respirable dust standard of 3 mg/m^3 to be reduced to 2 mg/m^3 3 years after passage of the act
- Medical surveillance of underground coal miners through entry and periodic medical examinations
- Rights of miners (transfer rights) with evidence of pneumoconiosis to work in a low-dust area (now <1 mg/m^3) with increased dust monitoring. If job transfer is necessary, there is no loss of pay (rate retention)
- Autopsies on deceased miners, administered by the National Institute for Occupational Safety and Health (NIOSH) through the National Coal Workers' Autopsy Study
- Compensation for miners with total disability and for dependents of miners who die of lung disease from coal mine employment
- Research and training

The medical surveillance provisions of the act were implemented through specifications developed by the NIOSH Appalachian Laboratory for Occupational Safety and Health in August 1970. Since that date, more than 350,000 examinations have been performed.

TABLE 20-1. COAL MINING HEALTH AND SAFETY LEGISLATION IN THE UNITED STATES

1865:	Bill is introduced to create Federal Mining Bureau. It is not passed.
1910:	Bureau of Mines is established but specifically denied right of inspection.
1941:	Bureau of Mines is granted authority to inspect, but it is not given authority to establish or enforce safety codes (Title I, Federal Coal Mine Safety Act).
1946:	Federal Mine Safety Code for Bituminous Coal and Lignite Mines is issued by the Director, Bureau of Mines (agreement between Secretary of the Interior and the United Mine Workers of America) and included in the 1946 (Krug-Lewis) UMWA Wage Agreement.
1947:	Congress requests coal mine operators and state agencies to report compliance with the Federal Mine Safety Code; 33 percent compliance is reported.
1952:	Title II of the Federal Coal Mine Safety Act is passed. All mines employing 15 or more persons underground must comply with the act. Enforcement is limited to issuing orders of withdrawal for imminent danger or for failure to abate violations within a reasonable time.
1966:	Amendments to 1952 law are passed. Mines employing under 15 employees are included under 1952 act; stronger regulatory powers are given to Bureau of Mines, such as the provision permitting the closing of a mine or section of a mine because of an unwarrantable failure to correct a dangerous condition.
1969:	Federal Coal Mine Health and Safety Act is passed. The hazards of pneumoconiosis are, for the first time, given prominence, in addition to those of accidents.
1972:	Black Lung Benefits Act of 1972 is passed. Several sections of the Title IV are amended, liberalizing the awarding of compensation benefits.
1977:	Federal Mine Safety and Health Act of 1977 is passed. It amends Coal Mine Health and Safety Act of 1969 largely by adding health and safety standard setting, inspections, and research provisions for metal and nonmetal miners, while leaving the 1969 act largely intact. This act also consolidates health and safety compliance activities for general industry (OSHA) and mining (MSHA) in the Department of Labor.
1977:	Black Lung Benefits Revenue Act of 1977 is passed. This provides for an excise tax on the sale of coal by the producer to establish trust funds to pay black lung benefits.
1977:	Black Lung Benefits Reform Act of 1977 is passed, to improve and further define provisions for awarding black lung benefits. Additionally, it establishes (a mandate) that a detailed study of occupational lung disease would be undertaken by the Department of Labor and NIOSH.

From Key MM, Kerr LE, Bundy M (eds): Pulmonary Reactions to Coal Dust. New York: Academic Press, 1971, with permission.

Subsequently, Title IV of the 1969 act has been amended twice by Congress, each time modifying requirements that qualify miners for benefits and making coal operators responsible for providing trust funds to pay these benefits. In 1977, the 1969 act was revised and largely incorporated into a new, comprehensive mining law—the Federal Mine Safety and Health Act of 1977, Public Law 91-173, amended by Public Law 95-164, 101[18]—which extended many of the provisions of the 1969 act to metal and nonmetal miners. Significant new responsibilities were given to the Department of Labor (Mine Safety and Health Administration) for establishing health standards and mine inspections and to HHS (NIOSH) for research and surveillance in noncoal mines.

Definition of CWP

CWP is a specific occupational lung disease arising from the prolonged inhalation of coal mine dust. Black lung is a generic term that has been used legislatively and popularly to mean any lung disease that may arise from coal mine employment. This includes both pathologically defined CWP and also obstructive airway disease among coal miners. CWP occurs in two forms: (*a*) simple (chronic) CWP and (*b*) complicated CWP, or progressive massive fibrosis (PMF). The characteristic lesion of simple CWP is the coal macule, which is a focal collection of dust-laden macrophages at the division of the respiratory bronchioles together with associated focal emphysema.[19] Micronodules and macronodules of simple CWP usually are smaller than 1 cm in diameter. Complicated CWP, or PMF, consists of solid, heavily pigmented masses generally greater than 2 cm in diameter, commonly located in the apical region of the lung and occurring on a background of simple CWP.

Environmental Exposures

Significant exposure to coal mine dust may occur not only underground but also in surface strip and auger mines, in coal preparation plants, and in coal-handling operations. U.S. coal reserves are extensive, covering some 400,000 square miles across the country (Fig. 20-1). Coal in the United States may be classified by four ranks: lignite, subbituminous, bituminous, and anthracite, reflecting the degree of metamorphosis of the coal. Anthracite deposits, which are mined on a limited basis only in northeastern Pennsylvania, are associated with the highest rates of pneumoconiosis. Bituminous coals, which are mined from central Pennsylvania westward to Utah are less fibrogenic than anthracite, there being a gradient in toxicity from low volatile bituminous (more fibrogenic) to subbituminous coal (less fibrogenic). Lignite, which also is mined on a limited basis, has not been adequately studied epidemiologically. Workers engaged in face work (coal cutting) and coal preparation often have the highest exposures to respirable coal dust and thus the highest rates of CWP. Drillers and other workers involved in tasks that generate free silica dust are also at risk of contracting silicosis.

Prior to 1970, dust concentrations in face jobs in underground mining were ranging from 6 to 10 mg/m^3. Subsequent to the 1969 act,[11] dust levels were limited first to 3 mg/m^3, and then to 2 mg/m^3. Overall, there is evidence that the regulations have brought about a marked reduction in dust exposures in coal mines,[20,21] although there has been continued concern that overexposure is still occurring.[22,23] The relatively new high-production technology of longwall mining poses a challenge to control engineers for maintenance of exposure levels within the compliance limit.[24]

Surface coal miners generally experience lower levels of dust exposure than do their counterparts underground.[25] Some surface mine jobs, however, can involve very high exposures to silica, especially if dust control measures are missing or ineffective. Drillers, in particular, are at risk of both acute and chronic silicosis, and severe cases have been reported.[26]

Pathophysiology

Pathologically defined simple CWP consists, at a minimum, of the characteristic coal macule lesion(s).[17,19] These may occur as microscopic manifestations of CWP associated with little or no functional impairment. With greater dust deposition in the lung, micronodules

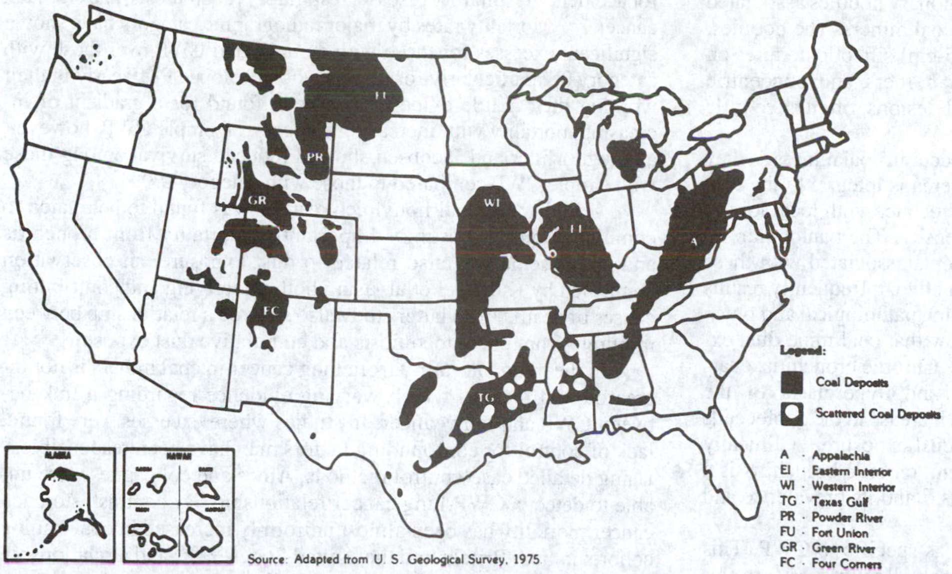

Figure 20-1. Coal deposits in the United States.

(less than 7 mm in diameter) and nodules (larger than 8 mm but less than about 1 cm) are found, predominantly in the upper lung zones (Fig. 20-2). These nodules consist of collagen in addition to a preponderance of reticulin. With increased profusion of nodular lesions in the lung comes greater functional abnormalities, but until marked, CWP often is not associated with significant respiratory symptoms or limiting impairment.

The presence of simple CWP is a significant risk factor for development of PMF; and its probability increases with the severity of simple CWP (Fig. 20-3).[27,28] PMF lesions usually occur in the posterior portion of the upper lobes and in the superior segment of the lower lobes. Unlike silicotic lesions, they cut easily and may have cavities containing inky fluid. The margins may be rounded or irregular, with fibrous strands extending into adjacent lung tissue.

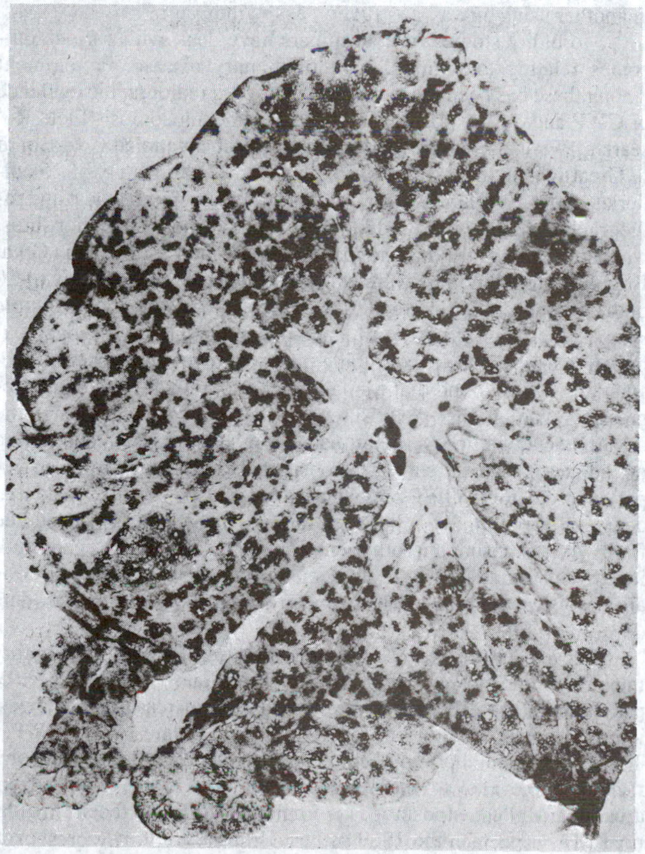

Figure 20-2. Whole lung section showing simple CWP with associated focal emphysema but otherwise preserved lung architecture.

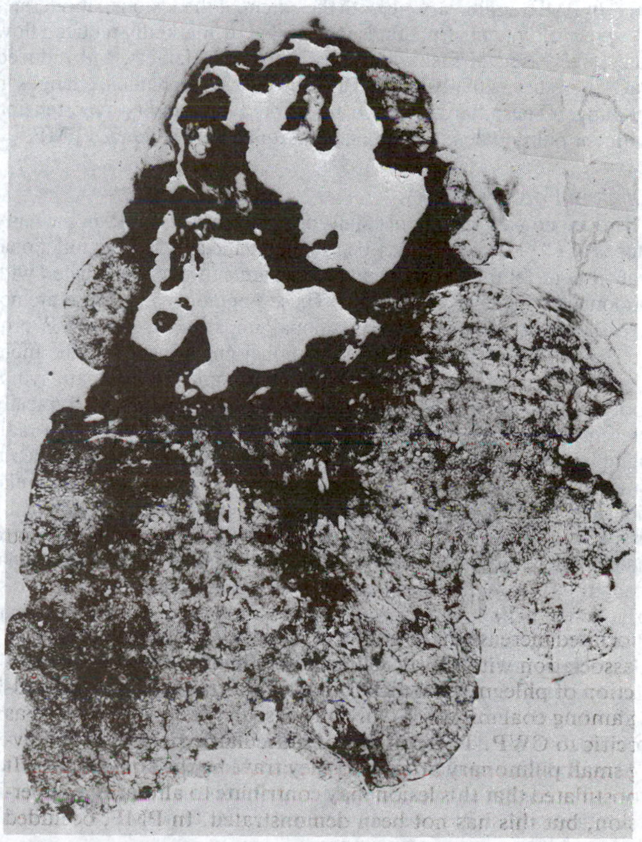

Figure 20-3. Whole lung section showing progressive massive fibrosis with cavitation involving the superior segments of the lung on a background of simple CWP and extensive emphysema.

Caplan's syndrome, consisting of pulmonary nodules associated with rheumatoid arthritis, occurs rarely in coal miners. The nodules, Caplan lesions, are similar to large (up to 5-cm) silicotic nodules on gross examination, usually have smooth borders and concentric internal laminations, and in contrast to PMF lesions, often have little dust contained with the lesion.[19]

Although other forms of emphysema occur in coal miners as they do in the general population, focal emphysema is integral to the coal macule (Fig. 20-2). Focal emphysema is associated with local loss of elastic fibers and alterations in capillary density. The panlobular, irregular, centrilobular, and bullous emphysema associated with these massive lesions is often extensive and destructive; it frequently results in marked pulmonary impairment.[19] Increasing pathological and physiological evidence has strengthened the view that coal mine dust exposure causes centrilobular emphysema.[29–31] Chronic bronchitis, characterized pathologically by hypertrophy and hyperplasia of the bronchial mucous glands with an associated increase in the goblet cells of the small airways, occurs as a result of dust exposure.[32] Clinically defined as the chronic production of phlegm, chronic bronchitis is a frequent clinical finding among coal miners,[33] and its prevalence and incidence are related to dust exposure.[13,34]

Only one vascular lesion is accepted as specific to CWP. This consists of muscular hypertrophy involving small pulmonary arteries as they traverse the coal macule. It is postulated that this lesion may contribute to alterations in perfusion, but this has not been demonstrated. In PMF, occluded and destroyed blood vessels are common and contribute to right ventricular hypertrophy or cor pulmonale, which is frequent among miners with severe CWP.[19] Physiologically, miners with simple CWP have been found to have increased residual volumes, decreased maximal expiratory flow rates, reduction in PaO_2, increased alveolar arterial oxygen differences, and slight hyperventilation, especially with exercise.[35,36] These findings may be nonexistent or slight in those in the earliest stages of CWP, but become progressively more significant with increasing extent of disease.

In PMF (again varying with the extent of the lesions), moderate-to-severe airway obstruction is manifested by markedly reduced flow rates, decreased diffusing capacity, perfusion defects, and reduced PaO_2, together with obstructive and restrictive mechanical changes in the lung.[35] These findings often are marked. Pulmonary hypertension with cor pulmonale is a frequent consequence of advanced PMF.

Clinical Features

There are no pathognomonic signs or symptoms of CWP. In the early stages of CWP, workers may be asymptomatic and without functional impairment. Chronic cough and phlegm are, however, associated with prolonged inhalation of coal dust. These symptoms per se also are not necessarily associated with functional impairment. As CWP progresses, shortness of breath and functional impairment become more common, yet some miners with advanced simple CWP remain symptom free. Those with PMF, especially those with large lesions, typically present with cough, phlegm, and shortness of breath. The chest radiograph is the standard method for detection of CWP. Although the radiographic examination is somewhat limited in sensitivity, the correlation between the profusion of CWP pathologically and radiographically is reasonably good.[37] An internationally developed and accepted method of radiograph classification distributed by the International Labour Office can be used to describe the extent, size, shape, and distribution of radiographic opacities and also to describe pulmonary, cardiac, pleural, and other thoracic abnormalities that may appear on a chest radiograph.[38] This classification divides simple pneumoconiosis into four major subcategories (0, 1, 2, and 3), each of which is subdivided into three categories (i.e., 1/0, 1/1, and 1/2), resulting in an approximation to a continuous scale. PMF is divided into three categories (A, B, and C), depending on lesion size. Although designed as a tool for public health surveillance and epidemiological investigation, this classification also has been adopted worldwide to describe CWP clinically and for compensation purposes.

Epidemiology

Mortality patterns among coal miners have been studied extensively and have generally shown increased standard mortality ratios (SMRs) for accidents, respiratory disease, respiratory tuberculosis, and stomach cancer.[39–43] Mortality rates by major radiographic category have shown significant excesses for those with complicated CWP over those with category 0,[44] particularly for miners who developed PMF early in their working life.[45] Little evidence has been found for a gradient of increasing mortality with increasing category of simple CWP, however, although Miller and Jacobsen showed reduced survival among those with simple CWP compared to those with category 0.[45]

Mortality from all nonviolent causes was found to be related to cumulative dust exposure.[45] Importantly, mortality from bronchitis and emphysema was also related to dust exposure, an observation confirmed by Kuempel et al. using both underlying and contributing causes of death.[46] The latter study also showed a relationship between mortality from pneumoconiosis and cumulative dust exposure.

In the main, mortality from lung cancer in coal miners is not increased, but there is widely varying evidence regarding a link between CWP and lung cancer. In studies where excesses were found, lack of control for confounding factors may have been responsible.[47] Using detailed case-control methods, Ames and colleagues were unable to detect a CWP-lung cancer relationship. By contrast, stomach cancer mortality has been almost uniformly increased in coal mining cohorts in both Britain and the United States,[39,40,43] and a relationship with dust exposure has been detected.[45] Ong and coworkers[48] have hypothesized, supported by laboratory mutagenesis data, that compounds in coal may undergo intragastric nitrosation or interaction with exogenous chemicals or both to form carcinogenic compounds that may with time cause stomach cancer. The Meyer hypothesis,[49] which posits that miners with good lung clearance are at increased risk of stomach cancer because of ingestion of cleared dust while those with impaired clearance get nonmalignant lung disease, has been invoked as one explanation of the increased mortality from stomach cancer in coal miners. This hypothesis was confirmed in one analysis using CWP as an indicator of impaired clearance,[50] but not in another using airway obstruction as the indicator.[51]

Morbidity studies of coal miners have dealt with various outcomes relating to nonmalignant pulmonary disease. Pre-eminent among these has been the association between radiographic evidence of CWP and dust exposure. In 1959, the Pneumoconiosis Field Research (PFR), a scientific study initiated by the National Coal Board of Great Britain, began a massive, long-term cohort study of 26 collieries. After 10 years of study, analysis of the respirable dust and radiographic findings provided clear dose-response relationships, which resulted in new dust standards in the United States and in Great Britain.[52] These findings were confirmed in a subsequent study of 10 of the original collieries (Fig. 20-4).[53] Free silica content in respirable samples was found not to influence pneumoconiosis risk, once cumulative exposure to mixed mine dust was taken into account. Despite this, it was found that a small number of miners with rapid progression had higher exposure to free silica, suggesting the development of silicosis rather than CWP.[54] Coal rank, in addition to mixed mine dust exposure, has consistently been found to be an important predictor of CWP prevalence and incidence.[55–57] A substantial degree of variation exists between mines which cannot be accounted for by dust exposure and other environmental factors.[58] Recent findings from similar studies in the United States conducted by NIOSH are consistent with the British pneumoconiosis field research data (Fig. 20-5).[56,59]

Because of the strong association between PMF and respiratory impairment and increased mortality, the attack rate of PMF has been of particular interest. The risk of developing PMF increases with increasing radiographic category of CWP[60] and with progression of CWP.[28] These studies are important because they provide the basis for recommending removal of a miner with radiographic evidence of CWP from areas of high-dust exposure, as is implemented in the federal regulations associated with the 1969 act.[11] It is important to note, however, that recent findings show the potential for PMF to develop in response to dust exposure directly from a background of category 0.[61] This indicates that the incidence of PMF cannot be controlled merely by the prevention of simple CWP. The attack rate of PMF does not appear to depend on presence of pulmonary tuberculosis, as once suspected.[17,19,62]

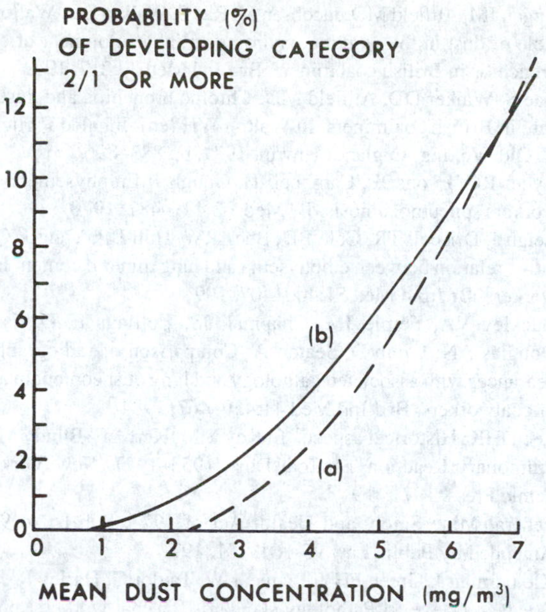

Figure 20-4. Lines (*a*) and (*b*) are estimates of probabilities of developing category 2 or 3 of simple pneumoconiosis over an approximately 35-year working life at the coalface, in relation to the mean dust concentration experienced during that period. (*a*) is based on 10 years of data, Interim Standards Study, Pneumoconiosis Field Research. (*b*) is update of (*a*), based on 20 years of data, Pneumoconiosis Field Research. (From Hurley JF, et al: Simple Pneumoconiosis and Exposure to Respirable Dust: Relationships from Twenty-five Years' Research at Ten British Coal Mines. Institute of Occupational Medicine, Report No. TM/79/13.)

Smoking has not been found to affect CWP development,[63] nor did bronchitis appear to play a role.[64] The exposure-response relationship for CWP and dust exposure is similar for current coal miners and ex-miners, although ex-miners had more disease owing to higher exposures.[65] Although rounded-type small radiographic opacities have been traditionally studied in connection with CWP, there is evidence that small irregular opacities also increase in prevalence with degree of dust exposure.[66,67] Small irregular opacities may be linked with lung function deficits.[68]

While radiographic evidence of CWP has been the major focus of epidemiological research on CWP, much attention has also been

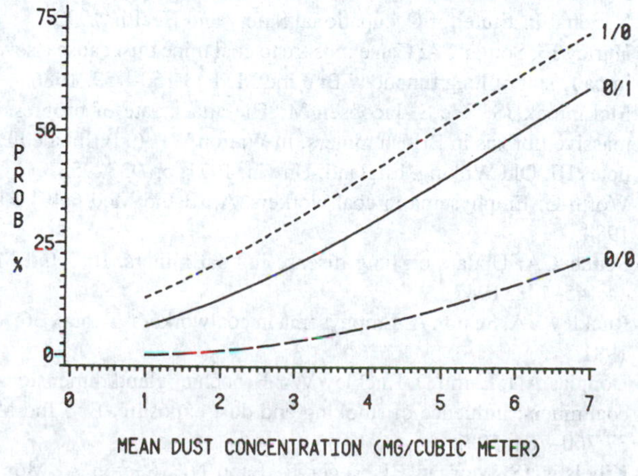

Figure 20-5. Ten-year predicted incidence and progression of CWP for various starting categories (From the Division of Respiratory Disease Studies/NIOSH.)

paid to coal dust exposure and other nonmalignant lung diseases (including bronchitis, obstructive airway disease, and emphysema). Unlike CWP, these diseases are known to be of multifactorial etiology, including a major influence of cigarette smoking among smokers. Hence their interpretation and significance in terms of occupational exposure has been associated with some controversy.

There is now overwhelming evidence of an exposure-response relationship for ventilatory function and cumulative dust exposure. This has been found in cross-sectional studies,[12,69–71] and in longitudinal studies.[72,73] Smoking was not found to potentiate the effect of dust exposure, nor was presence of CWP a prerequisite for ventilatory function loss. Although the average effect of dust exposure obtained from the exposure-response analyses may appear small, this appearance is misleading, and there is evidence that some miners suffer important deficits in ventilatory function from their work.[27,74] There is no epidemiologic evidence that the effect of smoking and dust exposure differ in nature.[75] Recent evidence suggests that new recruits to mining suffer large initial declines in ventilatory function; these then ameliorate.[34,76,77]

Respiratory symptoms associated with chronic bronchitis have been shown to be related to cumulative dust exposure and its surrogates, in both smokers and never smokers.[13,33,78] The presence of emphysema, as detected on the chest radiograph, is linked with extent of cumulative dust exposure.[79] This finding is consistent with the results of several pathologic studies, which indicate that emphysema is associated with both retained dust and cumulative exposure (or its surrogates) during life.[15,16,80]

Prevention

The key to preventing coal workers' pneumoconiosis is prevention of prolonged inhalation of significant concentrations of coal mine dust. This can be accomplished in two ways (*a*) by the control of respirable coal mine dust through proper ventilation, use of water spray dust suppression, and enclosure of mining operations, or (*b*) by removal of miners with early evidence of CWP to low-dust jobs. Of these two, dust control clearly is more effective. These two provisions were mandated by Congress in the Federal Coal Mine Health and Safety Act of 1969 and have been implemented successfully in underground operations of the U.S. coal industry. Since passage of the 1969 act, respirable dust levels have been reduced for most high-risk jobs to meet the 2.0 mg/mL standard. Although the vast majority of mining sections are in compliance with the standard, certain operations such as longwalls have proved difficult to control. Dust concentration in surface mines has averaged less than half that of underground mining; however, high exposure to coal dust and free silica may occur for those who drill, crush, and prepare coal for transport. NIOSH recently described several cases of acute or accelerated silicosis in young (<35 years old) drillers, and has recommended the use of wet drilling and exhaust ventilation as effective prevention measures.[26]

NIOSH CWP surveillance of U.S. miners has documented decreases in radiographic prevalence of CWP (category 1 or greater) over the period 1970 to 1991 from about 32 to about 20 percent in miners with 25 or more years in mining, and from 7 to about 3 percent in miners with 10 to 14 years in mining (Fig. 20-6). Although there was a sharp decline in prevalence from 1970 to 1980, rates since then have leveled off.

In response to this evidence of limitations in the effectiveness of current U.S. effort to fully control lung disease in coal miners, NIOSH produced new comprehensive recommendations for addressing this problem.[81] This criteria document makes the following recommendations:

- Control of respirable coal mine dust to 1 mg/m^3
- Improved engineering control and work practices
- Improved hazard surveillance
- Extension of health screening and surveillance to include tests of pulmonary function with all coal miners being eligible

Recently the U.S. Secretary of Labor empaneled an Advisory Committee on the Elimination of Pneumoconiosis Among Coal Mine

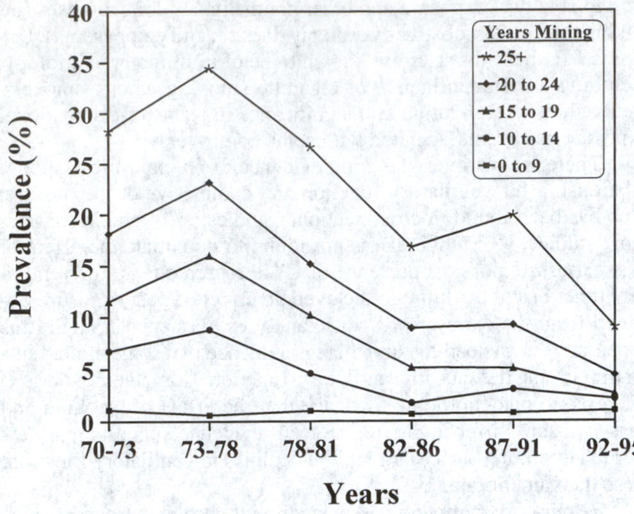

Figure 20–6. Radiographic prevalence of CWP in miners.

Workers.[82] This committee reviewed the scientific data on the causes of disease persistence and issued 20 recommendations. Those include recommendations for improved dust control, and inspection and enforcement of exposures to coal mine dust including silica dust. A strengthened program of medical screening and health surveillance was also endorsed.

Ultimately, improved prevention depends on adoption and application of these recommendations.

▶ REFERENCES

1. Thomson W: On black expectoration and deposition of black matter in the lungs. Med Chir Tr 20:230, 1836
2. Medical Research Council of Great Britain: Chronic pulmonary diseases in South Wales coal miners. Special Report Series 243. London: Medical Research Council of Great Britain, 1942
3. Medical Research Council of Great Britain: Chronic pulmonary diseases in South Wales coal miners. Special Report Series 244. London: Medical Research Council of Great Britain, 1943
4. Sayers RR, Bloomfield JJ, Dallavalle JM: Anthraco-Silicosis (Miners' Asthma): A Preliminary Report of a Study Made in the Anthracite Region of Pennsylvania. Spec. Bull. No. 41. Harrisburg, PA: Pennsylvania Department of Labor and Industry, 1934
5. Subcommittee of the Committee of Labor, House of Representatives: An Investigation Relating to Health Conditions of Workers Employed in Construction and Maintenance of Public Utilities. Washington, DC: 74th Congress, HJ Res. 449, 1936
6. Doyle HN, Noehren TH: Pulmonary Fibrosis in Soft Coal Miners: An Annotated Bibliography on the Entity Recently Described as Soft Coal Pneumoconiosis. US Public Health Service Bibliography, Ser 11. Washington, DC: US Public Health Service, 1954
7. Levine MD, Hunter MB: Clinical study of pneumoconiosis of coal workers in Ohio River Valley. JAMA 163:1–9, 1957
8. Lieben J, Pendergrass E, McBride WW: Pneumoconiosis study in central Pennsylvanian coal miners. J Occup Med 5:376–388, 1961
9. Stoeckle JD, Hardy HL, King WB, Nemiah JC: Respiratory disease in U.S. soft-coal miners: clinical and etiological considerations: A study of 30 cases. J Chron Dis 15:887–905, 1961
10. Lainhart WS, Felson B, Jacobson G, Pendergrass EP: Pneumoconiotic lesions in bituminous coal miners and metal miners. Arch Environ Health 16:207–210, 1968
11. Federal Coal Mine Health and Safety Act: Public Law 91-173, 2917, 1969
12. Rogan JM, Attfield MD, Jacobsen M, Rae S, Walker DD, Walton WH: Role of dust in the working environment in development of chronic bronchitis in British coal miners. Br J Ind Med 30:217, 1973
13. Rae S, Walker DD, Attfield MD: Chronic bronchitis and dust exposure in British coalminers. In Walton WH (ed): Inhaled Particles III, II. Old Woking, England: Unwin, 1971, pp 883–896
14. Ryder RC, Lyons JP, Campbell H, Gough J: Emphysema and coal workers' pneumoconiosis. Br Med J 3:481–487, 1970
15. Leigh J, Driscoll TR, Cole BD, Beck RW, Hull BP, Yang J: Quantitative relation between emphysema and lung mineral content in coalworkers. Br J Ind Med 51:400–407, 1994
16. Ruckley VA, Fernie JM, Chapman JS, Collings P, Davis JMG, Douglas AN, Lamb D, Seaton A: Comparison of radiographic appearances with associated pathology and lung dust content in a group of coalworkers. Br J Ind Med 41:459–467, 1984
17. Lee DHK: Historical aspects. In Key MM, Kerr LE, Bundy M (eds): Pulmonary Reactions to Coal Dust, 1953–1977. New York: Academic Press, 1971, p 9
18. Federal Mine Safety and Health Act of 1977: Pub L No 91-173. Amended by Public Law 95-164, 101, 1977
19. Kleinerman J, Green FHY, Laqueur W, Taylor G, Harley R, Pratt P, Wyatt S, Naeye R: Pathology standards for coal workers' pneumoconiosis. Arch Pathol Lab Med 103:375–432, 1979
20. Parobeck PS, Jankowski RA: Assessment of the respirable dust levels in the nation's underground and surface coal mining operations. Am Ind Hyg Assoc J 40:910–915, 1979
21. Watts WF: Respirable dust trends in coal mines with longwall or continuous miner sections. Proceedings of the VIIth International Pneumoconiosis Conference, August 1988, Pittsburgh. DHHS (NIOSH) Publication No. 90-108. Washington, DC: Department of Health and Human Services, 1990, pp 94–99
22. Boden LI, Gold M: The accuracy of self-reported regulatory data: the case of coal mine dust. Am J Ind Med 6:427–440, 1984
23. Mine Safety and Health Administration: Report of the Statistical Task Team of the Coal Mine Respirable Dust Task Group. Washington DC: US Department of Labor, 1993
24. Weeks JL: Characteristics of chronically dusty longwall mines in the U.S. Proceedings of the VIIth International Pneumoconiosis Conference, August 1988, Pittsburgh. DHHS (NIOSH) Publication No. 90-108. Washington, DC: Department of Health and Human Services, 1990, pp 76–80
25. Piacitelli GM, Amandus HA, Dieffenbach A: Respirable dust exposures in U.S. surface coal mines (1982–1986). Arch Environ Health 45:202–209, 1990
26. National Institute for Occupational Safety and Health: Request for Assistance in Preventing Silicosis and Deaths in Rock Drillers. NIOSH Alert DHHS (NIOSH) Publication No. 92-107. Cincinnati: National Institute for Occupational Safety and Health, 1992
27. Hurley JF, Soutar CA: Can exposure to coal mine dust cause a severe impairment of lung function? Br J Ind Med 43:150–157, 1986
28. McLintock JS, Rae S, Jacobsen M: The attack rate of progressive massive fibrosis in British miners. In Walton WH (ed): Inhaled Particles III. Old Woking, England: Unwin, 1971, pp 933–952
29. Worth G: Emphysema in coal workers. Am J Ind Med 6:401–403, 1984
30. Soutar CA: Update on lung disease in coal miners. Br J Ind Med 44:145–148, 1987
31. Ruckley VA, Seaton A: Emphysema in coalworkers. Thorax 36:716, 1981
32. Douglas AN, Lamb D, Ruckley VA: Bronchial gland dimensions in coalminers: influence of smoking and dust exposure. Br J Ind Med 37:760–764, 1982
33. Kibelstis JS, Morgan EJ, Reger R, Lapp NL, Seaton A, Morgan WKC: Prevalence of bronchitis and airway obstruction in American bituminous coal miners. Am Rev Respir Dis 108:886–893, 1973

34. Seixas NS, Robins TG, Attfield MD, Moulton LH: Exposure-response relationships for coal mine dust and obstructive lung disease following enactment of the Federal Coal Mine Health and Safety Act of 1969. Am J Ind Med 21:715–734, 1992
35. Lapp NL, Seaton A: Pulmonary function in coal workers' pneumoconiosis. In Key MM, Kew LE, Bundy M (eds): Pulmonary Reactions to Coal Dust. New York: Academic Press, 1971, pp 153–185
36. Rasmussen DL, Laqueur WA, Futterman HD: Pulmonary impairment in Southern West Virginia coal miners. Am Rev Respir Dis 98:658–667, 1968
37. Wagner GR, Attfield MD, Parker JE: Chest radiography in dust-exposed miners: Promise and problems, potential and imperfections. Occup Med 8(1):127–141, 1993
38. International Labour Office: International classification of radiographs of pneumoconiosis. Occupational Safety and Health Series No. 22 (rev 80). Geneva: International Labour Office, 1980
39. Stocks P: On the death rates from cancer of the stomach and respiratory diseases in 1949–53 among coal miners and other residents in counties of England and Wales. Br J Cancer 16:592–598, 1962
40. Enterline PE: Mortality rates among coal miners. Am J Public Health 54:758–768, 1964
41. Carpenter RG, Cochrane AL, Clarke WG, Jonathan G, Moore F: Death rates of miners and ex-miners with and without coalworkers' pneumoconiosis in South Wales. Br J Ind Med 50(7):577–585, 1993
42. Cochrane AL, Carpenter RG, Moore F, Thomas J: The mortality of miners and ex-miners in the Rhondda Fach. Br J Ind Med 21:38–45, 1964
43. Rockette H: Mortality among coal miners by the UMWA health and retirement funds. DHEW (NIOSH) Publication No. 77-155. Washington, DC: US Department of Health, Education, and Welfare, 1977
44. Ortmeyer CE, Costello J, Morgan WKC, Swecker S, Petersen MR: The mortality of Appalachian coal miners. Arch Environ Health 29:67–72, 1974
45. Miller BG, Jacobsen M: Dust exposure, pneumoconiosis, and mortality of coal miners Br J Ind Med 42:723–733, 1985
46. Kuempel ED, Stayner LT, Attfield MD, Buncher CR: Exposure-response analysis of mortality among coal miners in the United States. Am J Ind Med 28:167–184, 1995
47. Ames RG, Amandus H, Attfield M, Green FY, Vallyathan V: Does coal mine dust present a risk for lung cancer? A case-control study of U.S. coal miners. Arch Environ Health 38:331–333, 1983
48. Ong TM, Whong WZ, Ames RG: Gastric cancer in coal miners: an hypothesis of coal mine dust causation. Med Hypotheses 12:159–165, 1983
49. Meyer MB, Luk GD, Sotelo JM, Cohen BH, Menkes HA: Hypothesis: the role of the lung in stomach carcinogenesis. Am Rev Respir Dis 121:887–892, 1980
50. Swaen GMH, Meijers JMM, Slangen JJM: Risk of gastric cancer in pneumoconiotic coal miners and the effect of respiratory impairment. Occup Environ Med 52:606–610, 1995
51. Ames RG, Gamble JF: Lung cancer, stomach cancer, and smoking status among coal miners. Scand J Work Environ Health 9:443–448, 1983
52. Jacobsen M, Rae S, Walton WH, Rogan JM: The relation between pneumoconiosis and dust exposure in British coal mines. In Walton WH (ed): Inhaled Particles III. Old Woking, England: Unwin, 1971, pp 903–919
53. Hurley JF, Burns J, Copland L, Dodgson J, Jacobsen M: Coalworkers' simple pneumoconiosis and exposure to dust at 10 British coalmines. Br J Ind Med 39:120–127, 1982
54. Seaton A, Dodgson J, Dick JA, Jacobsen M: Quartz and pneumoconiosis in coalminers. Lancet 1272–1275, 1981
55. Walton WH, Dodgson J, Hadden GG, Jacobsen M: The effect of quartz and other non-coal dusts in coalworkers' pneumoconiosis. In Walton WH (ed): Inhaled Particles IV. Old Woking, England. Unwin, 1977, vol 2, pp 669–689
56. Attfield MD, Morring K: An investigation into the relationship between coal workers' pneumoconiosis and dust exposure in U.S. coal miners. Am Ind Hyg Assoc J 53:486–492, 1992
57. Reisner MTR, Robock K: Results of epidemiological, mineralogical, and cytotoxicological studies on the pathogenicity of coal-mine dusts. In Walton WH (ed): Inhaled Particles IV. Oxford: Pergamon Press, 1977, vol 2, pp 703–716
58. Crawford NP, Bodsworth FL, Dodgson J: A study of the apparent anomalies between dust levels and pneumoconiosis at several British collieries. Ann Occup Hyg 26:725–744, 1982
59. Attfield MD, Seixas NS. Prevalence of pneumoconiosis and its relationship to dust exposure in a cohort of U.S. bituminous coal miners and ex-miners. Am J Ind Med 27:137–151, 1995
60. Cochrane AL: The attack rate of progressive massive fibrosis. Br J Ind Med 19:52–64, 1962
61. Hurley JF, Maclaren WM: Dust-Related Risks of Radiological Changes in Coalminers over a 40-Year Working Life Report on Work Commissioned by NIOSH. TM/79/09: Edinburgh, Scotland Institute of Occupational Medicine, 1987
62. Dick JA: The role of pulmonary tuberculosis in the causation of progressive massive fibrosis in coal workers in Great Britain. Vth International Pneumoconiosis Conference, 29 October to 3 November 1978, Caracas, Venezuela. Bremerhaven: Wirtschaftverlag NW, 1985, pp 409–421
63. Jacobsen M, Burns J, Attfield MD: Smoking and coalworkers' simple pneumoconiosis. In Walton WH (ed): Inhaled Particles IV. Oxford Pergamon Press, 1977, pp 759–772
64. Muir DCF, Burns J, Jacobsen M, Walton WH: Pneumoconiosis and chronic bronchitis. Br J Ind Med 2:424–427, 1977
65. Soutar CA, Maclaren WM, Annis R, Melville AWT: Quantitative relations between exposure to respirable coalmine dust and coalworkers' simple pneumconiosis in men who have worked as miners but have left the industry. Br J Ind Med 43:29–36, 1986
66. Amandus HE, Lapp NL, Jacobson G, Reger RB: Significance of irregular small opacities in radiographs of coalminers in the USA. Br J Ind Med 33:13–17, 1976
67. Collins HPR, Dick JA, Bennett JG, Pern PO, Rickards MA, Thomas DJ, Washington JS, Jacobsen M: Irregularly shaped small shadows on chest radiographs, dust exposure, and lung function in coalworkers' pneumoconiosis. Br J Ind Med 45:43–55, 1988
68. Cockcroft AE, Wagner JC, Seal EME, Lyons JP, Campbell MJ: Irregular opacities in coalworkers' pneumoconiosis—correlation with pulmonary function and pathology. Ann Occup Hyg 26:767–787, 1982
69. Hankinson JL, Reger RB, Fairman RP, Lapp NL, Morgan WKC: Factors influencing expiratory flow rates in coal miners. In Walton WH (ed): Inhaled Particles IV. Oxford Pergamon Press, 1977, pp 737–755
70. Soutar CA, Hurley JF: Relation between dust exposure and lung function in miners and ex-miners. Br J Ind Med 43:307–320, 1986
71. Attfield MD, Hodous TK: Pulmonary function of U.S. coal miners related to dust exposure estimates. Am Rev Respir Dis 14:605–609, 1992
72. Love RG, Miller BG: Longitudinal study of lung function in coal miners. Thorax 37:193–197, 1982
73. Attfield MD: Longitudinal decline in FEV_1 in United States coalminers. Thorax 40:132–137, 1985
74. Marine WM, Gurr D, Jacobsen M: Clinically important respiratory effects of dust exposure and smoking in British coal miners. Am Rev Respir Dis 137:106–112, 1988
75. Attfield MD, Hodous TK: Does regression analysis of lung function data obtained from occupational epidemiologic studies lead to misleading inferences regarding the true effect of smoking? Am J Ind Med 27:281–291, 1995
76. Seixas NS, Robins TG, Attfield MD, Moulton LH: Longitudinal and cross sectional analyses of exposure to coal mine dust and pulmonary function in new miners. Br J Ind Med 50:929–937, 1993

77. Henneberger PK, Attfield MD: Coal mine dust exposure and spirometry in experienced miners. Am J Respir Crit Care Med 153:1560–1566, 1996
78. Leigh J, Wiles AN, Glick M: Total population study of factors affecting chronic bronchitis prevalence in the coal mining industry of New South Wales, Australia. Br J Ind Med 43:263–271, 1986
79. Wagner GR, Attfield MD: Radiographic appearances of emphysema in coal miners. Its relationship to pathologic abnormality and dust exposure [Abstract]. Epidemiology 6:S117, 1995
80. Leigh J, Outhred KG, McKenzie HI, Glick M, Wiles AN: Quantified pathology of emphysema, pneumoconiosis, and chronic bronchitis in coal workers. Br J Ind Med 40:258–263, 1983
81. National Institute for Occupational Safety and Health: Criteria for a Recommended Standard. Occupational Exposure to Coal Mine Dust. Washington, DC: National Institute for Occupational Safety and Health, 1995
82. US Department of Labor: Report of the Secretary of Labor's Advisory Committee on the Elimination of Pneumoconiosis among Coal Mine Workers. Washington, DC: US Department of Labor, 1996

21

Silicosis

Stephen M. Levin • Ruth Lilis

Silicosis is a fibrotic lung disease produced by the inhalation of dust containing free crystalline silicon dioxide (SiO_2). Free silica and silicates represent a large part of the earth's crust. Silicon and oxygen are the two most important elements in the crust; about 27.7 percent of its composition is silicon, and 46.6 percent is oxygen. Free silica, the most widespread naturally occurring substance known to have a fibrogenic effect on the lungs, occurs in crystalline and amorphous forms. The crystalline forms that are fibrogenic are quartz, tridymite, and cristobalite; cryptocrystalline forms (consisting of minute crystals) are flint, chert, opal, and chalcedony. There are numerous forms of amorphous silica.

At high temperatures (800 to 1000°C), quartz, the most common crystalline form of free silica, is converted into tridymite, and at even higher temperatures (1100 to 1400°C) it is transformed into cristobalite. Flint, chert, opal, chalcedony, and amorphous forms of free silica, including kaolin and diatomaceous earth, are also transformed into tridymite and cristobalite at these temperatures. This effect of high temperatures is of importance, since both tridymite and cristobalite are more potent than quartz in producing pulmonary fibrosis.

History

Silicosis undoubtedly originated in antiquity with the mining and processing of metals and building stone. Agricola, in his book *De Re Metallica* (1556), was probably the first to recognize the adverse effects of inhaled dust. The first monograph on miners' diseases, *Von der Bergsucht* by Paracelsus in 1567, included a classic description of "miners' phthisis." Van Diemerbroeck described how the lungs of stonecutters dying of "asthma" cut like masses of sand (*Anatomi Corporis Humani*, 1672). Bernardino Ramazzini included a description of diseases of stonemasons and miners in *De Morbis Artificium Diatriba* (1700). In England the disease ("phthisis") was described in flint knappers, needle pointers, knife grinders, fork sharpeners, and cutters of sandstone. John Scott Haldane (1923) described the cellular storage and retention of dust, including the long-term retention of silica, and recommended better ventilation of mines and factories. The distinction between tuberculosis and silicosis followed Koch's discovery of the tubercle bacillus in 1882. The earliest description of silicosis in the United States, in the nineteenth century, was of employees of a cutlery plant; the disease was then detected among miners. Tunnel work generated numerous cases of silicosis. The tunnel at Gauley Bridge in West Virginia, where many workers contracted both acute and chronic silicosis in the 1930s, attracted much public attention. This resulted in the initiation of dust suppression and respiratory protection methods, improved industrial hygiene, and the introduction of laws for compensation of silicosis victims.

Although the magnitude of the silicosis risk was gradually reduced in tunnel drilling and mining operations, significant silica exposure continued to occur in other industrial operations, such as foundries, the manufacture and use of silica flour, the production of detergent soaps with a high content of free silica, and sandblasting.

Work Exposures

Mines. The quartz content of the ores mined and the intensity of exposure to dusts determine the relative risks of working in the following situations: metal ore mines, especially gold, copper, tin, silver, nickel, tungsten, uranium, and platinum; coal mines (drilling through rock or work in areas with narrow seams); mines or quarries for silicates (talc, kaolin, bentonite, mica, clays, etc.), slate, graphite, and fluorspar and their processing; drilling for exploration; and crushing operations.

Quarries. Quarries of materials with high free crystalline silica content (quartz, sandstone, granite, slate, porphyry, etc.) and the processing of such materials place workers at risk for silicosis. Sandstone is almost pure silica; granite may have a variable silica content, 20 to 70 percent; and slate usually is approximately 40 percent silica. The cottage industry producing slate pencils in India has produced numerous cases of severe silicosis.[1]

Tunnels. Tunnel drilling and other excavations in rocks with high SiO_2 content may represent a severe hazard, especially since ventilation usually is poor. Among the earliest studies of silicosis in the United States were those of disease in subway and tunnel builders in New York City in the mid-1920s. Cases of silicosis also have been traced to the excavation of deep foundations in sandstone in Australia. In northeastern Brazil, a high incidence of silicosis in pit diggers was recently reported.[2]

Stonemasonry. Stonemasons may be subjected to significant and seldom well-controlled silica exposure. Sandstone and granite are the most important materials.

Foundry Work. A significant risk of silica exposure is associated with the mixture of sand and clays used for molds; the temperature of the molten metal poured into the molds fuses some sand to the surface of the castings and converts some quartz into tridymite or even cristobalite. Sometimes the molds are dusted with powders of high free-silica content, which adds a significant risk. The separation of castings from molds and cores, by shaking or knocking or automatically on vibrating tables, generates dangerous concentrations of dust. Fettling, the process by which the remnants of molds are removed from the castings by various abrading and polishing techniques, carries a substantial risk.

Grinding. Grinding and polishing with sandstone or other abrasive materials of high silica content have been replaced largely by less hazardous procedures, since these methods have resulted in numerous severe cases of silicosis. Nevertheless, grinding with such synthetic materials as Carborundum does not totally eliminate the risk, since remnants of the silica-containing mold are a source of airborne silica dust. Crushed sand, sandstone, and quartzite have been used for metal polishes and sandpaper.

Sandblasting. Sandblasting, used in foundries, in construction work, especially for the polishing of metal surfaces before painting and for cleaning building stone, and in the etching of glass and plastics, is an extremely hazardous occupation with high levels of exposure to very fine particles. Steel shot, iron garnet, and Carborundum are sometimes used instead of sand, but this has not universally eliminated the risk. Sandblasting of relatively small objects can be done in enclosed chambers operated from the outside. A hazardous exposure persists, however, for workers entering the sandblasting booths to remove the objects or clean the floors. Sandblasting in construction work or shipbuilding is much more difficult to enclose; hence adequate respiratory protection of all persons in the work area is essential. Sandblasting was banned in the United Kingdom in 1951 and in the European Economic Community in 1966 but is still widely used in the United States, where cases of rapidly progressing silicosis attributed to this type of exposure have been reported.[3]

Refractory Brick Manufacture. Manufacture of refractory brick and other refractory products (especially the acid refractories) carries a high risk of silicosis. Quartzite, sandstone, sands, or grits with a high quartz content are crushed, milled, shaped, dried, and fired at high temperatures, and a proportion of quartz is converted to tridymite and cristobalite.

Bricklaying. Bricklaying and dismantling or repair of refractory bricks in ovens, furnaces, kilns, and boilers carry a high risk of silicosis, especially because of the presence of cristobalite along with the quartz.

Pottery. The pottery industry may generate significant risks when the raw materials (mostly clays) contain free silica, even though use of powdered flint, which was a major source of silica in the pottery industry in Great Britain, has been discontinued. Glazes with variable contents of quartz also are used; firing at high temperatures (up to 1400°C) may create another source of significant silica exposure. In the United States, wollastonite, a calcium metasilicate, is used instead of flint, quartz, sand, and china clay, and therefore the health hazard in this industry is less than that reported in Great Britain in the past.

Glass. Glass industry workers, especially those grinding and polishing with fine quartz, and sandblasters of glass have considerable silica exposure.

Manufacture of Abrasive Soaps. The manufacture of soaps containing fine sand (silica flour) has in the past been a cause of rapidly progressing silicosis, "abrasive soap pneumoconiosis."

Fillers. Fillers used in the paint, rubber, plastic, and paper manufacturing industries may include silica flour, a finely ground, highly toxic quartz. It is sometimes incorrectly labeled as amorphous silica.[4] Rapidly progressing silicosis has resulted from the production of silica flour in Australia[5] and the United States.[6]

Enamel. Vitreous enameling, using mixtures of pulverized materials containing quartz at high temperatures, may present a significant risk. Enamel spraying is particularly hazardous.

Diatomaceous Earth. Calcined diatomaceous earth carries a significant risk, since part of the amorphous silica is transformed through calcination into cristobalite and tridymite. It is used in filters, absorbents, and abrasives and may generate significant exposure and risk of silicosis.

Ceramic Fiber Insulation. Ceramic fiber insulation is being used increasingly as a refractory lining for heat-treating and preheating furnaces in the iron and steel industry. Recent studies have shown that the fibers undergo partial conversion to cristobalite when exposed to high temperatures.[7]

In rural African women, cases of pneumoconiosis ("Transkei silicosis") recently were identified and attributed to silica inhalation during hand grinding of maize between rocks (sandstone). The criteria for diagnosis included rural domicile, radiographic and lung biopsy evidence of pneumoconiosis, no exposure to mining or industry, and no evidence of active tuberculosis.[8]

Occurrence

Accurate data on the occurrence of silicosis in various industries and in different parts of the world are difficult to obtain and hard to compare, in part because of different notification systems. Cross-sectional surveys of exposed populations, such as miners, indicate the prevalence of the disease. The attack rate or incidence of the disease is less well known. The incidence of silicosis undoubtedly increased in the majority of the industrialized countries until the 1950s. Methods of dust suppression and control that had been developed and applied mainly in large industrial facilities then led to a decrease in the incidence of silicosis. Dust control became more rigorous as the hazards were recognized, but smaller industries and new industrial processes continued to expose workers to dangerous levels of silica.

In industrialized countries with intensive mining, such as West Germany, silicosis is still one of the most important problems of occupational medicine; as many as 3,500 new cases and approximately 1,500 deaths due to silicosis occurred annually in the 1960s, five times more than the total number of fatal work accidents. France reported a similar incidence and mortality from silicosis.

In India, silicosis was diagnosed as soon as systematic examinations of miners were initiated in the 1950s and 1960s. In the Bihar mining area, 34 percent of those examined were found to have advanced silicosis. Similarly, in Japan a high prevalence of silicosis (63 percent) was found in some metal ore miners.

Much of the available information is based on compensation cases. Because the criteria for compensation differ from country to country, only general trends can be detected. In the United Kingdom, for example, 721 persons were awarded industrial injury compensation for silicosis in 1957; in 1969, only 162 new awards for silicosis were made. Mining, quarrying, and slate industries had not shown a significant downward trend, however.

In the United States, the incidence of silicosis has decreased in the Vermont granite quarries,[7] but metal mining is still an important cause of silicosis. A survey of more than 76 percent of the work force in 50 metal mines, conducted by the Public Health Service and the Bureau of Mines between 1958 and 1961, revealed a silicosis prevalence of 3.4 percent. In one-third of cases, complicated silicosis was present. Prevalence was related to silica content of the rock, occupation, and length of exposure. Trasko[9] estimated the total number of silicosis cases in 20 states to be about 6,000. Miners and foundry workers were each represented by more than 1,600 cases, but the number of cases was probably underestimated. In a British study of foundry workers,[10] the prevalence of simple pneumoconiosis was 34 percent among fettlers and 14 percent in foundry floor workers. Similar data for the United States are not available.

In 1971, milling of bentonite (sodium montmorillonite) was found to have produced severe silicosis in Wyoming;[11] a silicosis risk in this industry had not been suspected in the past.

In 1983, the National Institute of Occupational Safety and Health (NIOSH) estimated that approximately 3.2 million workers in 238,000 plants in the United States were potentially exposed to crystalline silica.

Watts et al.[12] analyzed respirable silica exposures in metal and nonmetal mines in the United States (41,502 samples taken from 1974 to 1981). Workers in sandstone, clay, shale, and various nonmetallic mineral mills had the highest exposures to silica dust. Crushing, grinding, sizing, and bagging operations and general labor had the highest exposures.

In 1984 the U.S. Mine Safety and Health Administration identified approximately 2,400 work sites in coal mines where the level of

5 percent silica in respirable dust had been exceeded, representing the work environment of 15,000 to 20,000 coal miners (about 10 percent of U.S. coal miners). Floor and roof samples were found to contain 18 to 82 percent quartz; coal itself contained only 1 to 4 percent.[13] Continuous mining machines, cutting of roof, floor, and inclusion rock bands, and roof bolting operations were the major sources of silica exposure.

Mean quartz content of respirable dust was found to range from 4.2 to 14 percent in Belgium, 0.8 to 9.3 percent in Germany, 1.59 to 10.3 percent in Great Britain, 0.4 to 12.5 percent in the former Soviet Union, and 2.1 to 12.7 percent in Bulgarian coal mines.[14]

The median silica content of respirable dust in 1,743 personal air samples collected by the U.S. Occupational Safety and Health Administration in U.S. foundries from 1974 to 1981 ranged from 7.3 to 12.0 percent. Of 10,850 samples collected in iron and steel foundries, 23 percent had concentrations in excess of 0.20 mg/m^3 respirable silica.

Reports on a high (37 percent) prevalence of silicosis in workers in silica flour mills, with a significant proportion of cases developing massive fibrosis,[6] and reports of acute silicosis in sandblasters in the Louisiana Gulf area[15] point to the fact that silicosis continues to be an important occupational health risk, although the number of individuals affected probably has been reduced substantially.

Effects on Health

Classic silicosis is a chronic and slowly progressive disease. Acute silicosis and silicoproteinosis (alveolar lipoproteinosis-like silicosis) occur in epidemic outbreaks under circumstances of heavy silica exposure. Sandblasting, abrasive soap manufacture, tunnel drilling, and refractory brick manufacture have been the major sources of such outbreaks.

Dust concentration, particle size (in the 2- to 0.1-µm range, which penetrate respiratory bronchioles and alveoli), and duration of dust exposure define the hazard. Thus high concentrations of fine dust overburden the limited direct clearance capacity of the distal zones of the lung, and longer exposures increase the risk of developing silicosis.

The interactions of concentration, particle size, and duration of exposure are the main determinants of the attack rate, latency period, incidence, rate of progression, and outcome of the disease.

In industrial processes in which silica-containing materials are heated at temperature exceeding 800°C so that transformation into tridymite and cristobalite occurs, the higher fibrogenic potency of these forms of SiO_2 results in a higher attack rate and more severe silicosis. In the superficial layers of refractory brick that have been repeatedly subject to contact with molten metal, cristobalite may reach a concentration of 94 percent. Fusicalcination of diatomaceous earth also results in high cristobalite concentrations (up to 35 percent).

In experimental studies and in an investigation of human subjects with silicosis, silica particles have been shown to initially produce an alveolitis, characterized by sustained increases in the total number of alveolar cells, including macrophages, lymphocytes, and neutrophils.

Recent studies in human subjects and on animal models have shown that alveolar macrophages that have engulfed silica particles maintain normal viability, including unaltered phagocytosis. In vitro and in vivo animal studies, as well as investigations in humans strongly support the role of macrophage products in the development and progression of silicosis. Such products include enzymes and reactive oxygen species, which may cause lung damage; cytokines, which recruit and/or activate polymorphonuclear leukocytes and thus result in further oxidant damage to the lung; and fibrogenic factors, which induce fibroblast proliferation and collagen synthesis.[16]

The alveolar macrophage (AM) plays a prominent role in lung inflammation via the production of oxygen radicals, enzymes, arachidonic acid metabolites and cytokines. Bronchoalveolar lavage in silicosis and coal workers' pneumoconiosis showed a large influx of mononuclear phagocytes, increased production of oxidants, fibronectin, neutrophil chemotactic factor, interleukin-6, and tumor necrosis factor-α (TNF-α).[17] Macrophage-derived growth-promoting activity factors were shown to have characteristics consistent with platelet-derived growth factor-like insuline-like growth factor 1-like and fibroblast growth factor-like molecules.[18]

Transforming growth factor-α (TGF-α). a cytokine with potent mitogenic activity for epithelial and mesenchymal cells, may play a role in the lung remodeling of silicosis. TGF-α may be critical in directing the proliferation of pneumocytes type II that characterize silicosis.[19] Transforming growth factor-β_1 was demonstrated in fibroblasts and macrophages located at the periphery of silicotic granulomas and in fibroblasts adjacent to hyperplastic type II pneumocytes.[20] Silica causes release of TNF from mononuclear phagocytes. Experimental studies indicate that silica can upregulate the TNF gene and thus increase TNF gene transcription in exposed cells.[21]

Inhalation of crystalline silica particles produces a rapid increase in the rate of synthesis and deposition of lung collagen. Silica-induced fibrosis is unique among all the animal models and most human fibrotic lung disease thus far examined in that the excess collagen deposited in the lung contains normal ratios of the two major collagen types of the lung, types I and II; nevertheless it is biochemically different from normal lung collagen. The difference seems to be due to altered intermolecular cross-links; there is an increased hydroxylysine content of collagen. Dysfunctional cross-links are more likely to be derived from hydroxylysine. Hydroxylysine replaces lysine in the primary structure of a specific collagen α-chain to form the altered cross-links.

In the alveolar spaces of rats exposed to very high concentrations of quartz or cristobalite, a material similar to that found in human alveolar lipoproteinosis together with a significant increase in the number of type II alveolar cells have been detected. This alveolar material is acellular and has a high phospholipid content with osmophilic bodies similar to those present as inclusions in type II alveolar cells. Phosphatidylcholine and phosphatidylglycerol are components of the increased amounts of surfactant found in the alveolar spaces under such circumstances.

Significant increases in surfactant production associated with type II epithelial cell hypertrophy and hyperplasia were shown to be associated with a proportional enhancement of surfactant proteins (SP-A and SP-B) and phospholipids.[22]

Thus it seems that two different types of reactions can occur as a result of the penetration of silica particles into alveolar spaces: triggering of a fibrogenic reaction by altered macrophages or production of excess phospholipids by type II alveolar cells. The rate at which silica particles accumulate in the alveoli is of great importance; exposure to high concentrations results in lipoproteinosis; exposure to relatively lower concentrations of silica, over longer periods of time, leads to the development of typical nodular fibrosis. Most silicosis cases are of the classic nodular type, characterized by the presence of collagenous and hyaline nodules.

Pathology

Silicotic nodules are readily felt in the lung and seen on the cut surface. Their size usually varies between 2 and 6 mm; they are hard, grayish, and more frequent in the apical and posterior parts of the lung. Sectioned nodules show a characteristic whorled pattern. The hilar lymph nodes most often are enlarged and also contain silicotic nodules.

Large fibrotic masses tend to be located mostly in the upper and posterior parts of the lungs; they are the result of coalescence of individual nodules when their profusion is high. Cavitation in large fibrotic masses can occur and most often is due to complicating tuberculous infection; cavitation due to ischemic necrosis is relatively rare in silicosis. Emphysema frequently is present when large fibrotic masses have developed. Enlargement of the right chambers of the heart and the pulmonary artery can be found in advanced silicosis.

In a classic example of nodular disease in gold miners, the quartz content of the lungs is 2.5 to 3 g of the total 7 to 10 g of dust content; in foundry workers it is between 1 and 2 g with approximately 10 g of total dust content. In contrast, in stellate or diffuse fibrosis in hematite miners, the total dust content may be 60 g with 3.5 g of quartz; and in coal miners, 40 to 55 g with 1 to 1.5 g of quartz.[23]

Silicotic nodules initially appear in the area of the respiratory bronchiole and around arterioles. The nodules consist of concentric layers of collagen; hyalinization of the collagen occurs with time and progresses from the center to the periphery of the nodule; reticulin fibers usually are present in the periphery. A cellular peripheral layer is characteristic of relatively early lesions; it consists mostly of fibroblasts and macrophages. Particles of silica can be found in the center of the nodules; polarized light is particularly useful to visualize the birefringent SiO_2 particles.

The alveoli around the silicotic nodule most often are normal, although scar emphysema occasionally can be observed; centrilobular emphysema is not a feature of silicosis.[24,25] Small pulmonary arterioles and venules are involved in the fibrotic process and are often obliterated. With continuous exposure the silicotic nodules grow and new nodules appear. Progression may continue even after exposure has been discontinued, especially when the dust is characterized by high silica concentration and small particle size.

Coalescence of nodules occurs when the profusion of silicotic nodules has increased beyond a critical level. Dense, hyalinized collagen masses develop in which individual nodules can still be identified, especially at the periphery. These lesions destroy the normal architecture of the lung; necrosis in the avascular center can occur even in the absence of tuberculous infection, although the latter is a frequent complication.

In *rapidly developing silicosis*, because of exposure to high concentrations of fine silica particles, the characteristic pathological features consist of the rapid development of numerous small nodules, together with areas of diffuse fibrosis and the rapid coalescence of nodules into large fibrotic masses.

Acute or hyperacute silicosis resembles idiopathic alveolar lipoproteinosis and has been associated with extremely high exposures to pure or almost pure free silica and very small particle sizes. The term *silicolipoproteinosis* has been proposed for this condition.[26] Exposures in the manufacture of abrasive soap, quartz milling, the grinding of quartzite and sandstone to produce silica flour, and sandblasting with quartzite have been associated with silicolipoproteinosis.

In this form of silicosis, the lungs are firm and edematous. A few silicotic nodules can be present; alveolar walls are infiltrated by mononuclear and plasma cells or thickened by fibrosis, and alveoli are filled with an eosinophilic periodic acid-Schiff (PAS)-positive lipid and proteinaceous fluid with numerous fine granules and desquamated cells. The latter are mostly type II alveolar cells, containing osmiophilic lamellar bodies. Diffuse interstitial pulmonary fibrosis is present, but silicotic nodules are rare or absent. These lesions have been reproduced in experimental animals exposed to inhalation of high concentrations of fine quartz particles.[27,28]

Proteinuria and renal failure have been associated with silica exposure from sandblasting or refractory bricks.[29,30] This appears to represent the effect of high levels of renal silicon dioxide crystals transferred to the kidney after pulmonary deposition.

Clinical Features

Classic nodular silicosis sometimes can be completely asymptomatic, although relatively numerous silicotic nodules can be present on the chest x-ray film. In most such cases, no abnormalities can be detected on physical examination. As the disease progresses, cough, sputum production, and dyspnea on exertion gradually develop in most cases. In some there is only a dry cough; in others small amounts of mucoid sputum are produced. An increased susceptibility to repeated respiratory infections develops in many patients and can result in larger amounts of mucopurulent sputum.

In the advanced stages of silicosis, distortion of the normal architecture of the bronchi develops, especially when coalescence into massive fibrosis has taken place. Rhonchi and wheezes can be detected in such cases and paroxysms of coughing can occur. Shortness of breath develops gradually as the disease progresses; initially it is limited to heavy exercise, but later it manifests itself with moderate or even minor effort. Physical signs are practically absent in the initial stages of silicosis. With the development of massive fibrosis or of a major infectious complication such as tuberculosis, abnormalities on percussion and auscultation (rales, rhonci, areas of reduced or increased resonance) and cyanosis can develop.

Cor pulmonale is the most frequent complication of silicosis in industrialized countries. Pulmonary hypertension with a loud second pulmonic sound and corresponding electrocardiographic signs can be detected; overt congestive heart failure with hepatomegaly and peripheral edema is less frequent and is thought to occur mainly in cases with significant associated emphysema or marked chronic bronchitis.

In patients with "acute" silicosis similar to idiopathic alveolar lipoproteinosis, symptoms develop rapidly over a period of several weeks or months; time from onset of exposure to first symptoms can vary from less than 1 year to a few years. Fatigue, cough, sputum production (mostly mucoid), chest pain of a pleuritic type, rapidly progressive shortness of breath, weight loss, and rapid deterioration are characteristic for such cases. Shortness of breath at rest, cyanosis, and abnormalities on percussion and auscultation with presence of crepitations are noted frequently. The rapid and fatal course of the disease leads to death in hypoxic respiratory failure.[31]

Radiographic Findings

The radiographic changes in silicosis are essential for the diagnosis and classification of the disease, for the evaluation of its progression, and for the detection of important complications, such as tuberculosis, emphysema, and cor pulmonale. Nevertheless, it should be emphasized that pathological changes precede, often by several years, the appearance of the earliest radiographic changes, since to be detected on the standard posteroanterior chest film the pathological changes (silicotic nodules) have to reach a certain size, profusion, and radiological density. Because of this radiological latency period of silicosis, a normal chest x-ray film does not exclude the existence of the pathological process of silicosis in a person with significant exposure. Nevertheless, the disease seldom is symptomatic in this stage of radiological latency, with the notable exceptions of "acute silicosis," alveolar lipoproteinosis, and chronic bronchitis due to silica.

The earliest radiographic changes consist of fine linear-reticular opacities, often described as "lacelike," in the upper and middle lung fields and extending to the periphery. These linear reticular opacities increase in thickness with time.

The most characteristic radiographic abnormalities are silicotic nodules (Fig. 21-1), which usually appear initially in the middle and upper right lung fields. The earliest discrete round opacities are small, with a diameter of 1 to 3 mm and of low radiopacity. The diameter of silicotic nodules increases with time, as does their profusion and radiopacity, and they become more visible in most of the lung fields, with the exception of the lower lateral areas. The International Labor Office's Classification of Radiographs of Pneumoconioses (1980) grades simple silicosis according to the profusion of the opacities, from 1/0 to 3/+, and to the size of most of the nodules, p for less than 1.5 mm, 4 for between 1.5 and 3 mm, and r for opacities with a diameter of more than 3 mm but less than 10 mm. The nodules often are seen against a background of a linear-reticular pattern.

As the number of rounded opacities increases, the profusion progresses, and eventually coalescence of nodules, initially in small limited areas in the upper lateral parts of the lung fields, becomes apparent. At this stage when coalescence into large opacities is suspected (and their size is relatively small, less than 5 cm in diameter), they are classified as Ax. This marks the point at which simple silicosis progresses to complicated silicosis.

As the large opacity becomes definite, it is classified according to size into category A (less than 5 cm), B (one or more opacities with a diameter of more than 5 cm but with a combined area of less than the equivalent of the right upper zone), and C (one or more opacities whose combined area exceeds the equivalent of the right upper zone). The large opacities in silicosis usually are bilateral and most often located in the upper, but also in the middle, lung fields (Figs. 21-2 and 21-3). When the opacities are observed over time, contraction may be

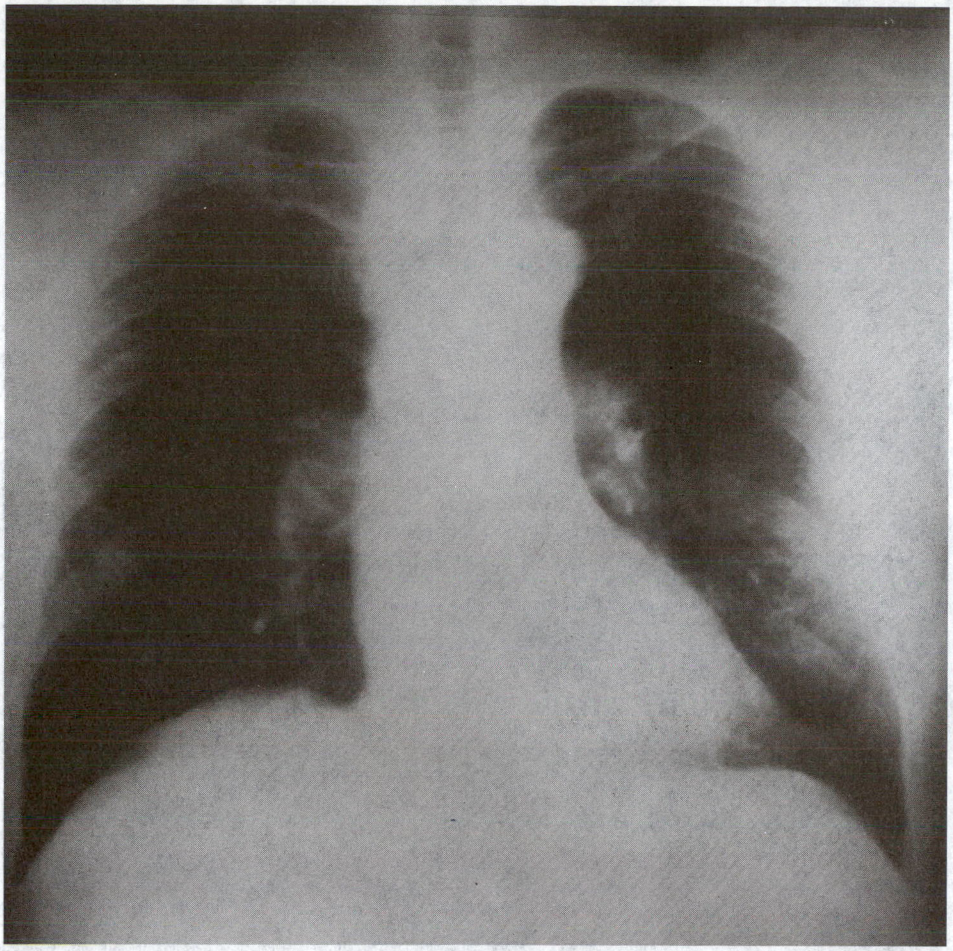

Figure 21-1. Simple silicosis. Small, rounded opacities (q-diameter, approximately 3 mm) in upper lung fields, bilaterally.

noted, and migration to the enlarged hilar opacities is not unusual. Distortion of the pulmonary and mediastinal structures is frequent in this stage, as are emphysematous changes, including bullae, in the rest of the lung. Hilar lymph node enlargement is observed consistently in silicosis; calcification of the periphery of the lymph nodes, "eggshell" calcification, may be present occasionally. Pleural adhesions also may be found; quite characteristic are the longitudinal pleural plicatures extending from the diaphragmatic pleura along the interlobar fissures.

In rapidly progressive silicosis the radiological latency period, a few months to 2 years, is much shorter than in classic silicosis. The radiological abnormalities are different from those of classic (nodular) silicosis, a fact that may have contributed to the underestimation of the incidence of this form of silicosis. Early changes consist of a diffuse haziness of reticular, irregular opacities in the middle and lower lung fields. Rounded and linear opacities develop rapidly over the entire lung fields. Occasionally, very small opacities are the main feature. The hilar shadows are only moderately enlarged. Rapid coalescence and large opacities, sometimes involving an entire lobe, can be observed in some cases; in others the numerous small, rounded opacities do not coalesce, and death ensues rapidly.

Alveolar lipoproteinosis is characterized by diffuse, hazy infiltrates found most often in the lower lung fields, particularly above the diaphragm. Changes similar to those characteristic for pulmonary edema are present sometimes; in other cases, small rounded opacities indicating alveolar filling can be observed.

Pulmonary Function

With classic silicosis the typical change in pulmonary function is a gradual reduction in lung volume, beginning with reduction in vital capacity. The functional changes are less than would be predicted from the radiographic evidence. Airway obstruction, however, often is present because chronic bronchitis frequently coexists, especially in foundry workers, brickworkers, hematite miners, and workers in user industries. The diffusing capacity is normal until relatively late in the course of the disease. Thus in classic silicosis there is a decrease in total lung capacity, vital capacity, and residual volume, with arterial blood oxygen tension normal or slightly decreased. A mixed pattern of restrictive and obstructive ventilatory dysfunction is found most often in advanced, complicated silicosis.

Imbalance of ventilation-perfusion occurs in the more advanced stages of the disease. Impairment of gas exchange and signs of cor pulmonale can develop. The coexistence of chronic bronchitis with airway obstruction results in reduced forced expiratory volume in 1 second (FEV_1), reduced flow at 25 to 75 percent of vital capacity (FEF_{25-75}), and in increased airway resistance. With severe obstruction arterial blood oxygen tension is reduced and carbon dioxide tension increased. Acute silicolipoproteinosis almost always causes marked restrictive dysfunction with reduced diffusing capacity and arterial desaturation.

Complications

The complications of silicosis include tuberculosis, cor pulmonale, and Caplan's syndrome.

Tuberculosis has been the most persistent problem over the past 150 years. There is no doubt that involvement of the lungs by silicosis increases the susceptibility for tuberculosis infection. In contrast, there is no added risk of tuberculosis after exposure to asbestos or other nonsilica dusts. Thus patients with silicosis in whom tuberculosis is suspected on the basis of a positive tuberculin test and a suggestive x-ray film should be treated with antituberculous chemotherapy because demonstration of mycobacteria by smear or culture is

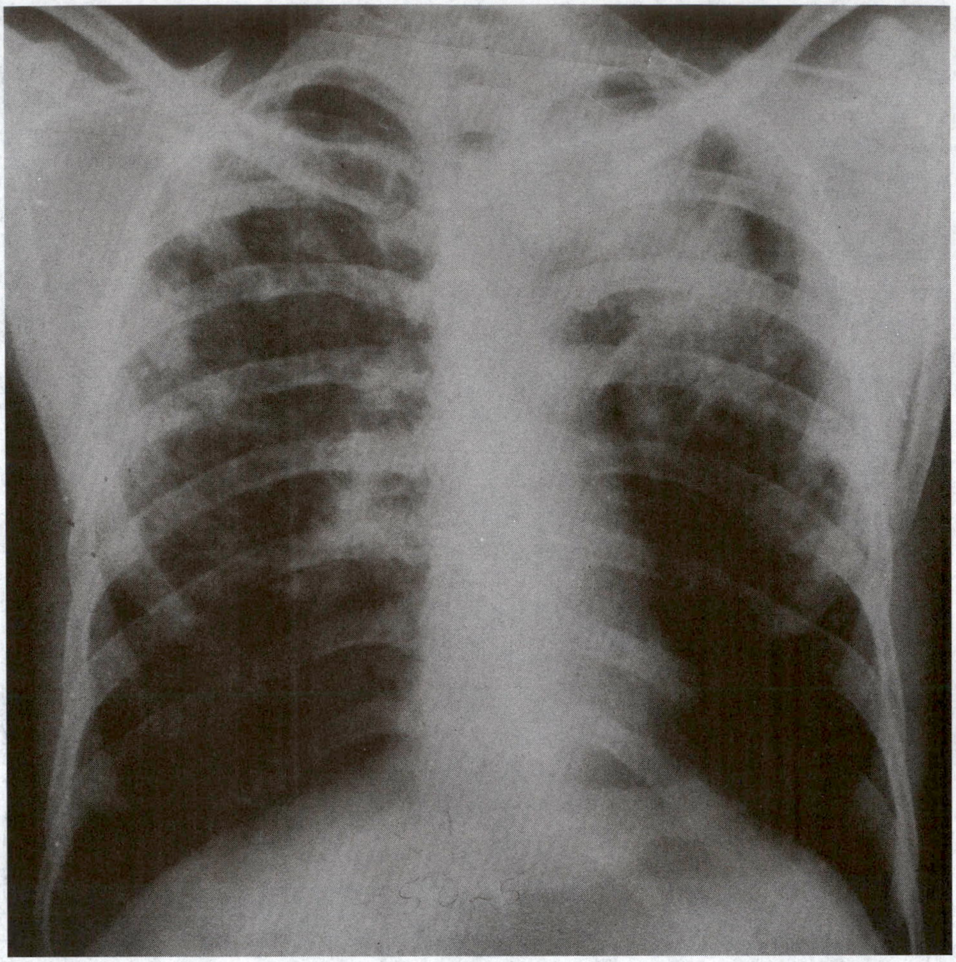

Figure 21-2. Small, rounded opacities (r-diameter, approximately 3 to 10 mm) predominantly in upper and middle lung fields; large opacity due to coalescence of nodules in left upper lung field (size B, according to International Classification of Radiographs of Pneumoconioses).

difficult in silicotuberculosis, and the disease sometimes advances rapidly.

The high risk of tuberculosis in subjects with silicosis has recently been quantified in a cohort study of 1,153 gold miners with and without silicosis, followed for 7 years. The annual incidence of tuberculosis was 981/100,000 in the 335 men without silicosis and 2,707/100,000 in the 818 men with silicosis.[32]

Chronic bronchitis is not infrequent in some occupational groups exposed to silica dust, such as foundrymen.[10] Bronchitis due to acute or subacute infections of the distorted bronchi associated with advanced silicosis has been well characterized.

Emphysema is considered a side effect in the silicotic process. Small areas of scar emphysema can be found around nodules; coalescence of nodules into fibrotic masses often produces larger areas of emphysema, often bullous, mostly in the lower lung fields. In a group of 1553 South African gold miners who had undergone autopsy examination between 1974 and 1987 it was found that a miner with 20 years in high-dust occupations had 3.5 times higher odds of significant emphysema at autopsy than a miner not in a dusty occupation.[33] In a study of 207 workers evaluated for possible pneumoconiosis using high-resolution CT scans for detection, typing, and grading of emphysema, a significant excess of emphysema was found in those with pneumoconiosis and in smokers with silica exposure (as compared to those with asbestos exposure). Thus silica exposure was shown to be a significant contributing factor to the development of emphysema.[34]

Cor pulmonale is a well-recognized complication of silicosis; the massive involvement of the pulmonary vasculature in the fibrotic process with obliteration of numerous arterioles eventually results in a marked increase in resistance and consequently in pulmonary artery pressure. Right ventricular heart failure with overt clinical signs is seen less frequently, although it is not unusual. In such cases death due to congestive heart failure can occur. In cases with coexistent emphysema and chronic bronchitis with marked airflow obstruction or complicating tuberculosis, right ventricular heart failure is encountered more frequently.

The presence of cor pulmonale at death was analyzed in a study of 732 South African gold miners. Marked emphysema was the highest risk factor, with an odds ratio of 21.32 (95 percent C.I. 5.02 to 90.7), followed by extensive silicosis (odds ratio 4.95, 95 percent C.I. 2.92 to 8.38).[35]

Progressive systemic sclerosis (scleroderma) has been reported by some investigators to be associated with silicosis with a frequency greater than would be expected in the population at large. It is not clear in these cases whether the association was merely due to coincidence.

Caplan's syndrome, the association between rheumatoid arthritis and silicosis, is rare. It is characterized by the appearance of large nodules (more than 1 cm in diameter) on a background of preexisting silicotic nodules. The larger nodules of Caplan's syndrome occasionally cavitate.

Renal lesions have been described in cases in which heavy occupational exposure to free silica has led to silico-lipoproteinosis. Glomerular and tubular lesions have been described. Proteinuria and hypertension were associated with these renal lesions.[24] The silica content of the kidney was found to be high in such cases.

In recent years the problem of a possible *carcinogenic effect of silica* has received considerable attention. Experimental studies on the possible carcinogenic effect of crystalline silica have been conducted on rats, mice, and hamsters, using various routes of administration: inhalation, intratracheal instillation, and intrapleural and intraperitoneal injection.

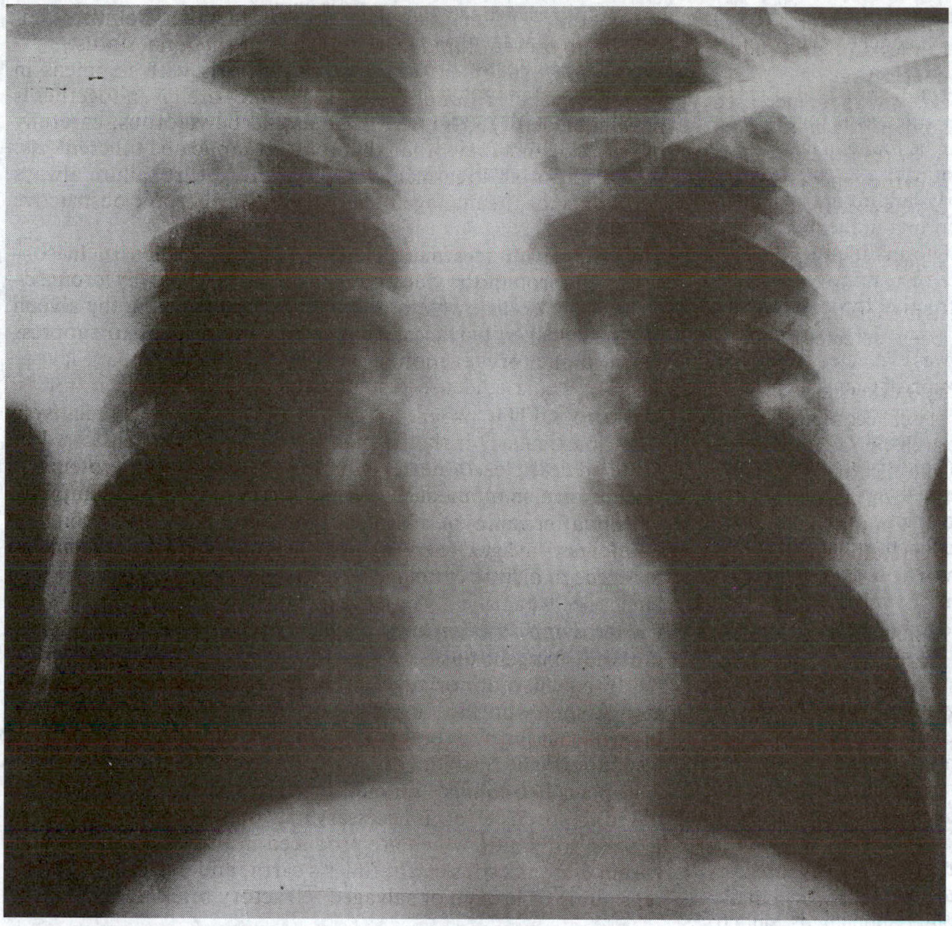

Figure 21-3. Rounded opacities (r/q) in upper and middle lung fields; bilateral multiple large opacities due to coalescence of nodules.

Findings from these studies were negative in mice and hamsters. In rats the incidence of adenocarcinoma of the lung and squamous cell carcinoma was significantly increased, and the intraperitoneal injections caused malignant lymphomas.

Epidemiological studies have been conducted on numerous silica-exposed groups, such as metal ore miners, coal miners, and workers in the granite and stone industry, the ceramics, glass, and related industries, foundries, and in persons diagnosed as having silicosis. There were methodologic difficulties with many of these studies; confounding by cigarette smoking and insufficient information on exposure to other carcinogens, such as radon (mostly in mining and quarrying operations), polycyclic aromatic hydrocarbons (mostly in foundries), and arsenic (in metal ore mining and possibly in the ceramics and glass industries) were the most important issues of concern.

Metal ore mining has not been associated with an increased incidence of respiratory cancer in some studies;[36,37] in other cohorts of metal ore miners, mortality rates for respiratory cancer were found to be 20 to 50 percent above levels in the general population.[38,39] In most studies of coal miners, no increased incidence of lung cancer has been detected.

Studies of granite workers generally have yielded negative findings also.[40,41]

In the ceramics and pottery industry a moderately increased mortality from respiratory cancer has been detected in some studies.[42,43]

A number of recent reports on foundry workers have pointed to slightly to moderately increased respiratory cancer mortality.[44–46]

The International Agency for Research on Cancer monograph on the evaluation of the carcinogenic risk of silica in 1987 concluded that "there is sufficient evidence for carcinogenicity of crystalline silica to experimental animals [and that] there is limited evidence for the carcinogenicity of crystalline silica to humans."

A mortality study of 716 cases of silicosis, diagnosed from 1940 through 1983, was undertaken as part of the North Carolina pneumoconiosis surveillance program for dusty trades workers. Five hundred forty-six death certificates were obtained among 550 deceased. Mortality for lung cancer was increased among whites (standard mortality ratio (SMR) 2.6; the SMR was 2.3 in those without other exposure to known carcinogens. Age- and smoking-adjusted rates in silicotic metal miners were 3.9 times higher than in nonsilicotic metal miners.[47]

The association between silicosis and lung cancer mortality was studied in 9,912 (369 silicotic and 9,543 nonsilicotic) white metal miners examined by the U.S. Public Health Service from 1959 to 1961 and followed through 1975. The SMR for lung cancer was 1.73 (95 percent, C.I. 0.94 to 2.90) in silicotic metal miners and 1.18 (C.I. 0.98 to 1.42) in nonsilicotic metal miners. Confounding from exposure to radon or other carcinogens, such as arsenic, could not be ruled out.[48] A mortality study of 3,328 gold miners in South Dakota found an SMR for lung cancer of 1.13 (C.I. 0.94 to 1.36). No positive exposure-response trend was evident with cumulative exposure. Silicosis and tuberculosis were significantly increased (SMRs of 3.44 and 2.61, respectively).[49]

DNA binding to crystalline silica surfaces may be important in silica carcinogenesis by anchoring DNA and its target nucleotides to within a few angstroms of sites of oxygen radical production on the silica surface.[50]

As recently summarized by the American Thoracic Society, "The balance of evidence indicates that silicotic patients have increased risk for lung cancer. It is less clear whether silica exposure in the absence of silicosis carries increased risk for lung cancer."[51]

Diagnosis

A history of exposure to free silica is important for the diagnosis of silicosis. A detailed work history is necessary, with appropriate attention to occupations held in the past, since the latency period for the appearance of characteristic chest x-ray abnormalities is often decades, especially with relatively low silica concentrations in the airborne dust.

The other essential element for a correct diagnosis of silicosis is a good quality chest x-ray film. Nodular silicosis is not difficult to recognize, although nodular opacities can be found in many other diseases. Enlarged hilar opacities are characteristic for silicosis. Pulmonary function tests are not particularly helpful in the diagnosis of silicosis since they can be entirely normal in the presence of well-developed nodular opacities. When abnormalities are present, they are most often of a mixed, obstructive-restrictive type, although cases with only restrictive or obstructive dysfunction also can be found.

The sensitivity of the chest radiograph was evaluated in 557 gold miners in South Africa by comparing profusion of rounded opacities with pathological findings (average 2.7 years between chest x-ray and pathological examination). The sensitivity of the chest x-ray (using ILO category 1/1 or greater as a positive diagnosis of silicosis) was found to be 0.393, 0.371, and 0.236 (for three independent readers). A large proportion of those with moderate silicosis were not diagnosed radiologically. The authors concluded that the sensitivity of the chest radiograph could be improved by using 1/0 as a cutoff point for a positive diagnosis of silicosis (for exposure to relatively low dust concentrations) and 0/1 for workers exposed to high average concentrations of silica dust.[52]

Computed tomography scanning in the early detection of silicosis was shown to be significantly more informative than the chest radiograph. Thirteen of 32 subjects classified as normal on standard chest x-rays were found to be abnormal on CT scanning using conventional and high-resolution techniques, as were 4 of 6 subjects classified as "indeterminate" on the standard chest radiograph. In addition, the CT scans added 6 cases of confluence of small opacities to the 3 cases detected with standard chest x-rays.[53]

The differential diagnosis has to exclude conditions such as sarcoidosis, miliary tuberculosis, carcinomatous lymphangitis, pulmonary hemosiderosis, rheumatoid lung, fibrosing alveolitis, alveolar microlithiasis, and histoplasmosis.

Massive fibrosis seldom presents difficulties in diagnosis, although early in its development, when a single large opacity is detected, differential diagnosis with lung cancer can be a problem. The presence of nodular opacities around the large opacity most often facilitates the correct diagnosis of silicosis with coalescent, massive fibrosis.

The diagnosis of tuberculosis in the presence of silicosis is difficult; this complication should always be considered, and frequent sputum cultures are indicated.

The diagnosis of acute silicosis is more difficult than that of classic nodular silicosis because the radiographic changes are less characteristic and the clinical course more rapid. Idiopathic alveolar proteinosis, acute allergic alveolitis, and tuberculosis have to be considered in the differential diagnosis. A careful occupational history with evidence of exposure to high silica dust levels is extremely important for the diagnosis of this form of silicosis.

Treatment

Although poly-2-vinyl-pyridine-1-oxide and polybetaine prevent silicosis in experimental animals, possibly by altering the surface charge on silica particles, the results of clinical trials have been unrewarding. Treatment of patients with silicosis by the inhalation of powdered aluminum was undertaken in the 1950s, but aluminum itself carries the risk of diffuse interstitial fibrosis. Thus neither of these forms of prophylactic treatment can be recommended.

There is no specific treatment for established silicosis; therapy of complications, such as bronchitis and pneumonitis, is important to prevent rapid deterioration of functional status.

Prompt treatment of silicotuberculosis with regimens in which isoniazid, rifampin, and ethambutol are given together is most satisfactory. The treatment should be vigorous, carefully monitored, and longer than that for uncomplicated tuberculosis.

Appropriate treatment for congestive heart failure always has to include the management of coexisting chronic obstructive bronchitis.

No specific treatment is useful for rapidly progressive silicosis. In contrast, lipoproteinosis due to silica can be treated by bronchopulmonary lavage, which may be helpful in clearing the alveoli of the deposited particles,[54] and by steroid therapy to suppress the inflammatory reaction.

Prognosis

The prognosis for nodular silicosis is relatively good, particularly if the progression of the disease is slow. For rapidly progressing silicosis, early death is almost the rule. Lipoproteinosis may resolve spontaneously without treatment or may improve rapidly after removal of free silica from the lung by bronchopulmonary lavage. There is some evidence that lipoproteinosis proceeds to diffuse fibrosis if left untreated.[55]

Control and Prevention

The recognition of the silicosis hazard and stringent dust control engineering measures are essential. Frequent monitoring of airborne dust levels is needed to ensure a safe working environment. The effectiveness of dust control measures in preventing silicosis has been emphasized dramatically by the reduction in silicosis in Great Britain and the European Economic Community since sandblasting was outlawed. A special effort is necessary to avoid exposure to cristobalite and tridymite, which are produced in the calcining of silica within diatomaceous earth, fuller's earth, and particularly in the regrinding of broken or salvaged refractory brick, in the scaling of boilers, and in steel foundries.

Reduction of exposure to quartz above the threshold limit value of

$$\frac{10 \text{ mg/m}^3}{\%SiO_2 + 2}$$

would reduce the silicosis attack rate considerably. NIOSH has proposed a further reduction of the time-weighted average silica exposure to 50 $\mu g/m^3$. The effects of dust levels on other workers in the area must be considered because, even if sandblasters or brick grinders are protected by appropriate respirators, workers in other trades within the same area may be affected. Failure to apply occupational standards to workplaces employing five or fewer workers also has resulted in cases of silicosis. In addition, it appears essential to regard silica in quantities of 5 percent or less within other rock, such as limestone, kaolin, gypsum, graphite, or portland cement, as important and capable of producing disease if total dust concentrations are as high as they often are in mining or other operations. The problem of silica exposure in foundries is well known and may require changes in technology to bring it under control. Personal respiratory protection is valuable when it is otherwise impossible to control environmental dust levels.

▶ REFERENCES

1. Jain SM, Sepha GC, Khare KC, Dubey VS: Silicosis in slate pencil workers. Chest 71:423–426, 1977
2. Holand MA, Holanda MA, Martins MP, Felismino PH, Pinheiro VG: Silicosis in Brazilian pit diggers: relationship between dust exposure and radiologic findings. Am J Ind Med 27:367–378, 1995
3. Buechner HA, Ansari A: Acute silico-proteinosis, a new pathologic variant of acute silicosis in sandblasters, characterized by histologic features resembling alveolar proteinosis. Dis Chest 55:274–284, 1969
4. Banks DE, Morring KL, Boehlecke BE: Silicosis in the 1980's. Am Ind Hyg Assoc J 42:77–79, 1981
5. Zimmerman PV, Sinclair RA: Rapidly progressive fatal silicosis in a young man. Med J Aust 2:704–706, 1981

6. Banks DE, Morring KI, Boehlecke BE: Silicosis in silica flour workers. Am Rev Respir Dis 124:445–450, 1981
7. Ashe HB, Bergstrom DE: Twenty six years' experience with dust control in the Vermont granite industry. Ind Med Surg 33:973–978, 1964
8. Grobbelaar JP, Bateman ED: Hut lung: a domestically acquired pneumoconiosis of mixed aetiology in rural women. Thorax 46: 334–340, 1991
9. Trasko VM: Some facts on the prevalence of silicosis in the United States. Arch Ind Health 14:379–386, 1956
10. Lloyd-Davies TAL: Respiratory Disease in Foundry Men. London: Her Majesty's Stationary Office, 1971
11. Phibbs BP, Sundin RE, Mitchell RS: Silicosis in Wyoming bentonite workers. Am Rev Respir Dis 103:1–17, 1971
12. Watts WF, Parker DR, Johnson RL, Jensen KL: Analysis of Data on Respirable Quartz Dust Samples Collected in Metal and Nonmetal Mines and Mills. Information Circular 8967. Washington, DC: Bureau of Mines, U.S. Department of the Interior, 1984
13. Jankosvski RA, Nesbit RE, Kissel FN: Concepts for controlling quartz dust exposure of coal mine workers. In Peng SS (ed): Coal Mine Dust Conference Proceedings. Cincinnati: American Conference of Governmental Industrial Hygienists, 1984, pp 126–136
14. Silica and some silicates. In: Evaluation of the Carcinogenic Risk of Chemicals to Humans. International Agency for Research on Cancer, Lyons, France, 1987, vol 42, pp 39–143
15. Hughes JM, Jones RN, Gilson JC, et al: Determinants of progression in sandblasters' silicosis. In Walton WH (ed): Inhaled Particles V. Oxford: Pergamon Press, 1983, p 701
16. Lapp NL, Castranova V: How silicosis and coal-workers' pneumoconiosis develop—a cellular assessment. Occup Med 8:35–56, 1993
17. Vanhee D, Gosset P, Boitelle A, Wallaert B, Tonnel AB: Cytokines and cytokine network in silicosis and coal workers' pneumoconiosis. Eur Respir J 8:834–842, 1995
18. Melloni B, Lesur O, Bouhadiba T, Cantin A, Begin R: Partial characterization of the proliferative activity for fetal lung epithelial cells produced by silica-exposed alveolar macrophages. J Leukoc Biol 55:574–580, 1994
19. Absher M, Sjostrand M, Baldor LC, Hemenway DR, Kelley J: Patterns of secretion of transforming growth factor-alpha (TGF-alpha) in experimental silicosis. Acute and subacute effects of cristobalite exposure in the rat. Reg Immunol 5:225–231, 1993
20. Williams AO, Flanders KC, Saffiotti U: Immunohistochemical localization of transforming growth factor-beta 1 in rats with experimental silicosis, alveolar type II hyperplasia, and lung cancer. Am J Pathol 142:1831–1840, 1993
21. Savici D, He B, Geist LJ, Monick MM, Hunninghake GW: Silica increases tumor necrosis factor (TNF) production, in part, by upregulating the TNF promoter. Exp Lung Res 20:613–625, 1994
22. Lesur O, Veldhuizen RA, Whitsett JA, Hull WM, Passmayer F, Cantin A, Begin R: Surfactant-associated proteins (SP-A, SP-B) are increased proportionally to alveolar phospholipids in sheep silicosis. Lung 17:63–74, 1993
23. Nagelschmidt G: The relationship between lung dust and lung pathology in pneumoconiosis. Br J Ind Med 17:247–259, 1960
24. Gardner LV: Pathology of so-called acute silicosis. Am J Public Health 23:1240–1249, 1930
25. Heppleston AG: The fibrogenic action of silica. Br Med Bull 25:282–287, 1969
26. Parkes WR: Diseases due to free silica. In: Occupational Lung Disorders. 2nd ed. London: Butterworth, 1982, pp 134–174
27. Gross P, deTreville RTP: Alveolar proteinosis: its experimental production in rodents. Arch Pathol 86:255–261, 1968
28. Heppleston AG: A typical reaction to inhaled silica. Nature 213:199–200, 1967
29. Saldanha LF, Rosen VJ: Silicon nephropathy. Am J Med 59:95–103, 1975
30. Giles RD, Sturgill BC, Suratt PM, Bolton WK: Massive proteinuria and acute renal failure in a patient with acute silico-proteinosis. Am J Med 64:336–342, 1978
31. Ruttner JR, Heer HR: Silikose and Lungenkarzinom. Schweiz Med Wochenschr 99:245–249, 1969
32. Cowie RL: The epidemiology of tuberculosis in gold miners with silicosis. Am J Respir Crit Care Med 150:1460–1462, 1994
33. Hnizdo E, Sluis-Cremer GK, Abramowitz JA: Emphysema type in relation to silica dust ezposure in South African gold miners. Am Rev Respir Dis 143:1241–1247, 1991
34. Begin R, Filion R, Ostiguy G: Emphysema in silica- and asbestos-exposed workers seeking compensation. A CT scan study. Chest 108:647–655, 1995
35. Murray J, Reid, G, Kielkowski D, de-Beer M: Cor pulmonale and silicosis: a necropsy-based case-control study. Br J Ind Med 50: 544–548, 1993
36. Brown DP, Kalplan SD, Zumwalde RD, Kaplowitz M, Archer VE: Retrospective cohort mortality study of underground gold mine workers. In Goldsmith DF, Winn DM, Shy CM (eds): Silica, Silicosis, and Cancer. Controversy in Occupational Medicine. New York: Praeger, 1986, pp 335–350
37. Lawler AB, Mandel JS, Scuman LM, Lubin JH: Mortality study of Minnesota iron ore miners: Preliminary results. In Wagner WL, Rom WN, Merchant JA (eds): Health Issues Related to Metal and Nonmetallic Mining. Boston: Butterworth, 1983, pp 211–226
38. Muller J, Wheeler WC, Gentleman JF, Suranyi G, Kusiak RA: Study of Mortality of Ontario Miners, 1955–1977. Part I. 1. Toronto: Ontario Ministry of Labour/Ontario Workers' Compensation Board/ Atomic Energy Control Board of Canada, 1983
39. Costello J: Mortality of metal miners. A retrospective cohort and case-control study. In Proceedings of an Environmental Health Conference, April 6–9 1982, Park City, UT. Morgantown, WV: National Institute of Occupational Safety and Health, 1982
40. Davis LK, Wegman DH, Monson RR, Froines J: Mortality experience of Vermont granite miners. Am J Ind Med 4:705–723, 1983
41. Costello J, Graham WGB: Vermont granite workers' mortality study. In Goldsmith DF, Winn DM, Shy CM (eds): Silica, Silicosis, and Cancer. Controversy in Occupational Medicine, New York: Praeger, 1986, pp 437–440
42. Thomas TL: A preliminary investigation of mortality among workers in the pottery industry. Int J Epidemiol 27:175–180, 1982
43. Forastiere F, Lagorio S, Michelozzi P, Cavariani F, Arca M, Borgia P, Perucci C, Axelson O: Silica, silicosis, and lung cancer among ceramic workers: a case-referent study. Am J Ind Med 10:363–370, 1986
44. Sherson D, Iversen E: Mortality among foundry workers in Denmark due to cancer and respiratory and cardiovascular disease. In Goldsmith DF, Winn DM, Shy CM (eds): Silica, Silicosis, and Cancer. Controversy in Occupational Medicine, New York: Praeger, 1986, pp 403–414
45. Fletcher AC: The mortality of foundry workers in the United Kingdom. In Goldsmith DF, Winn DM, Shy CM (eds): Silica, Silicosis, and Cancer. Controversy in Occupational Medicine. New York: Praeger, 1986, pp 385–401
46. Silverstein M, Maizlish N, Park R, Silverstein B, Brodsky L, Mirer F: Mortality among ferrous foundry workers. Am J Ind Med 10:27–43, 1986
47. Amandus HE, Shy C, Wing S, Blair A, Heineman EF: Silicosis and lung cancer in North Carolina dusty trades workers. Am J Ind Med 20:57–70, 1991
48. Amandus HE, Costello J: Silicosis and lung cancer in U.S. metal miners. Arch Environ Health 46:82–89, 1991
49. Steenland K, Brown D: Mortality study of gold miners exposed to silica and nonasbestiform amphibole minerals: an update with 14 more years of follow-up. Am J Ind Med 27:217–229, 1995

50. Saffiotti U, Daniel LN, Mao Y, Shi X, Williams AO, Kaighn ME: Mechanisms of carcinogenesis by crystalline silica in relation to oxygen radicals. Environ Health Perspect 102(Suppl 10): 159–163, 1994
51. Report of the ATS Committee on Adverse Effects of Crystalline Silica Exposure. Beckett WS (Chair), 1996, p 12
52. Hnizdo E, Murray J, Sluis-Cremer GK, Thomas RG: Correlation between radiological and pathological diagnosis of silicosis: an autopsy population based study. Am J Ind Med 24:427–445, 1993
53. Begin R, Ostiguy G, Fillion R, Colman N: Computed tomography scan in the early detection of silicosis. Am Rev Respir Dis 144: 697–705, 1991
54. Ramieriz RJ, Keiffer RE, Ball WC: Bronchopulmonary lavage in man. Ann Intern Med 63:819–828, 1965
55. Hudson AR, Halprine GM, Miller JA, Kilburn KH: Pulmonary interstitial fibrosis following alveolar proteinosis. Chest 65:700–702, 1974

22

Health Significance of Metal Exposures

Philippe Grandjean

The term metal has important meanings in physics and chemistry. In environmental medicine, arsenic and selenium are often considered along with the group of metals. Nutritionists often refer to trace metals as those constituting less than 1 g of the human body, an arbitrary limit which would exclude iron. Although toxic metals is a common term, all metals may actually exert toxic effects, and the dose determines whether or not toxicity ensues. Frequently, heavy metals (with a gravity of 4 g/cm^3 and above) are considered most important with regard to adverse health effects. This belief is related to the observation that the toxicity of the metals tends to increase toward the right and downward in the periodic system. However, gravity as such is of little medical significance and would not account for the toxic potential of beryllium. Rather, the relative toxicity on a molar basis would seem to be related to the affinity to various ligands and the resulting biochemical activity. On the basis of such considerations, the metals may be separated into soft metals (class B), with a higher affinity toward sulfur and nitrogen than toward oxygen, and the hard metals (class A), where the opposite is the case.[1]

Among the metals considered in this chapter, aluminum, barium, beryllium, magnesium, and lanthanum (rare earths) belong to the less toxic class A, while the other metals are either borderline or class B metals.

In contrast to organic compounds, which may be broken down by detoxification processes, metals will remain metals. However, some changes may occur due to oxidation/reduction, as with mercury vapor and chromate, and most metals will be bound to organic compounds, notably proteins such as metallothionein. Some metals form rather stable organometal compounds with a covalent bond between carbon and the metal. Some organic compounds, such as tetraalkyl lead, are dealkylated in the body. On the other hand, methylation in the liver is an important part of arsenic and selenium kinetics. These metabolic processes affect the toxicity and may vary between individuals.

When present as airborne particles, retention in the airways is governed by physical principles related to the aerodynamic diameter of the particles. Some metal compounds are corrosive and exert their effect on the mucous membranes. Such is the case with osmium tetroxide and zinc chloride. In other situations, systemic effects, whether mediated by oral or respiratory intake, are most important and will then depend on the amount absorbed. Solubility of metal compounds is of major significance. In the gut, some interaction between metals may occur. Thus, zinc and copper tend to mutually inhibit the absorption of the other metal. The same appears to be true for iron and cobalt, but the absorption of both is increased in iron deficiency. In addition, phosphate and other components may decrease the absorption due to formation of insoluble compounds. The variability is illustrated by the fact that gastrointestinal absorption of lead sulfide is barely detectable, while a soluble compound ingested during a fasting period may result in a 50 percent absorption.

Exposure potentials have increased considerably due to the development of metallurgy and associated processes and due to the contamination from energy production. Chemical elements that are rare in the earth's crust may now result in heavy exposures of workers, neighbors, and consumers. In comparison with atmospheric emissions from natural sources, air pollution with lead from human activities is more than 10-fold greater, and the amounts of cadmium, zinc, and other metals in anthropogenic air pollution are also comparatively large. Table 22–1 shows an arbitrary grouping of some metals according to their abundance and the annual production rate. Although only major tendencies would appear from such crude grouping, the rarer metals seem to cause much less prevalent exposures than do the metals that are common in the earth's crust. However, production figures tend to increase, in particular for aluminum, molybdenum, nickel, and rare earths.

The metals have all occurred in the biosphere since primeval times, though mostly in lower concentrations than today; some of the common metals were used in metabolic processes and became essential nutrients (Table 22–1). When the intake of essential metals is insufficient, signs of deficiency may develop. Many of such cases have occurred as part of multiple nutrient deficiencies or as a result of long-term parenteral nutrition. Low environmental levels may locally cause a risk of certain deficiencies, while refined food in general tends to be an insufficient source of essential minerals.

When toxicity is compared, the rarer metals appear to be more toxic than elements that are more common components of the earth's crust and the "natural" environment. In Table 22–1, the molar limits for occupational exposure have been used for classifying metals into three groups with different toxicities. LD_{50} values from animal experiments could have been used as well and would yield almost the same result.

In preventive medicine, the target organ is of special importance. The earliest effects of metal toxicity are said to originate from the target organ, sometimes referred to as the critical organ. As a consequence, if effects in the target organ can be prevented, no other toxicity should be expected. However, prevention becomes somewhat more difficult when considering that the critical effect of respiratory exposure to some chromate or nickel compounds is respiratory cancer; such stochastic effects may be totally prevented only if exposures are effectively eliminated. Other complex problems relate to the prevention of contact dermatitis in individuals who have developed metal allergies; even oral intake of the offending metal can induce or worsen the hand eczema in these patients. Individual susceptibility must therefore be taken into account. In this regard, interactions between metals are also of importance. Thus, zinc supplements may

TABLE 22-1. NATURAL OCCURRENCE, PRODUCTION, AND HEALTH SIGNIFICANCE OF METALS, AS INDICATED BY ARBITRARY GROUPING OF RELEVANT PARAMETERS

Abundance in Earth's Crust	*Annual Production*	*Occupational Exposure Limit*	*Significance of Daily Oral Intake*
I. Common ($>10^{-2}$ mol/kg) Al, Fe, Mg, Mn, Ti	I. Large ($>10^{11}$ mol/yr) Al, Cu, Fe, Mg, Mn, Zn	I. High ($>10^{-4}$ mol/m^3) Al, Fe, Mg, Ti, Zn	I. Deficiency recorded Cr, Cu, Fe, Mg, Se, Zn
II. Medium (10^{-4}–10^{-2} mol/kg) Ba, Be, Co, Cr, Cu, Ni, V, Zn, Zr	II. Medium (10^{9}–10^{11} mol/yr) Ba, Cr, Mo, Ni, Pb, Sb, Sn, Ti, Zr	II. Medium (10^{-6}–10^{-4} mol/m^3) As, Ba, Be, Cd, Co, Cr, Cu, Mn, Mo, Ni, Sb, Se, Sn, Ta, V, W, Zr, rare earths	II. Unknown or no significance Ag, Al, Be, Mn, Mo, Ni, Os, Pt, Sb, Sn, Ta, Te, Ti, Tl, V, W, Zr, rare earths
III. Rare ($<10^{-4}$ mol/kg) Ag, As, Cd, Hg, Mo, Os, Pb, Pt, Sb, Se, Sn, Ta, Te, Tl, U, W, rare earths	III. Low ($<10^{9}$ mol/yr) Ag, As, Be, Cd, Co, Hg, Os, Pt, Se, Ta, Te, Tl, U, V, W, rare earths	III. Low ($<10^{-6}$ mol/m^3) Ag, Hg, Os, Pb, Pt, Te, Tl, U	III. Environmental toxicity recorded As, Ba, Cd, Co, Hg, Pb, U

prevent cadmium toxicity in experimental animals, and selenium may to some degree protect against mercury toxicity.

As preventive efforts become more efficient, the patterns of adverse effects change and, in fact, become more difficult to recognize. Most metals accumulate in the body, and storage depots or "slow compartments" may slowly release metals to the blood or may actually be the site of delayed toxicity. The resulting insidious, delayed effects are often hard to detect, also for the patient. In the absence of pathognomonic symptoms and a history of a recent hazardous exposure, an etiologic diagnosis may be almost impossible to verify.

The diagnosis of metal poisoning has been frequently supported by the detection of increased or toxic levels of the metal in blood or urine. Methods have now been further refined and become routine parameters for biological monitoring of metal exposures.[2] Recent developments have included more sensitive analyses and methods for in vivo detection of cadmium and mercury in kidney and liver, for measurement of lead levels in calcified tissues, and for assessment of various biochemical abnormalities which indicate early biological effects of metal exposures. Biological monitoring will become an essential part of future preventive activities with regard to environmental and occupational metal exposures. However, because metals are ubiquitous and often disseminated through a multitude of pathways, the sources of human exposures must be known before a preventive strategy can be planned.

In the following pages, individual metals are dealt with in alphabetical order. The general outline includes: environmental occurrence, uses, exposure sources; absorption and fate in the human organism; essential functions and toxic effects in humans; preventive measures; and limits applicable. Relevant publications from the International Programme on Chemical Safety and from the International Agency for Research on Cancer are mentioned, but otherwise references have been limited to a few recent key studies or reports. For more detailed information and reference to additional literature sources, some recent handbooks should be consulted.[3–5]

▸ ALUMINUM

Exposures

Aluminum is a light metal with a high resistance against corrosion and is used in light metal alloys, in particular with magnesium. Kitchenware, aluminum foil, and automobile bodies are important uses, and the aircraft industry is one of the major consumers. The most intense occupational exposures occur in the aluminum refineries, where the metal is produced by electrolysis of aluminum oxide dissolved in molten cryolite. Refinery and foundry workers, welders, and grinders working with aluminum or its alloys may be exposed to high levels of aluminum fumes or particles. Aluminum chloride is used in petroleum processing and in the rubber industry, and alkyl compounds are used as catalysts in the production of polyethylene. Other aluminum compounds are also widely used, notably for flocculation of drinking water.

Aluminum compounds in soil are soluble at low pH values (below 6), e.g., caused by acidification. Soft drinking water may also dissolve traces of aluminum flocculants used in municipal water treatment. In such cases, the aluminum concentration may occasionally exceed 1 mg/L, but otherwise the concentrations in water are usually well below 100 μg/L. Among food items, meat products and vegetables may exhibit relatively high levels; the total daily intake through food and beverages are generally about 10 mg. Sources of excess exposures include aluminum silicate used as an anticaking agent and aluminum powder used for decorating pastry. Small amounts may be released from aluminum pots and pans at low pH levels, especially when acid foods are stored. Ulcer patients may ingest several grams of aluminum hydroxide every day in their antacid medicine.

Aluminum is barely absorbed from the gastrointestinal tract, probably because sparingly soluble aluminum phosphate is formed. Patients who ingest aluminum-containing antacids appear to absorb about 0.1 percent of the amount ingested. Concurrent intake of fruit juices may substantially increase the absorption. Inhalation of fine aluminum dust can lead to retention in the alveoli, and the concentration of this metal in the lungs increases with advancing age. When released to the blood, aluminum appears to effectively excreted, almost entirely in the urine.

Effects

Salts of aluminum are irritants because acid is liberated on hydrolysis. Thus, conjunctivitis, eczema, and upper airway irritation may result, and even local necrosis of the cornea has been recorded. A form of pneumoconiosis, sometimes called aluminum lung or aluminosis, is associated with severe exposures to aluminum oxide; the most frequent symptoms are dyspnea and dry cough. Unilateral pneumothorax has been seen more often than expected in workers exposed to aluminum dust.

Aluminum exposure may cause neurotoxicity, particularly in patients undergoing dialysis.[6,7] Due to the deficient excretion of aluminum in the urine of these patients, accumulation in the body occurs from small amounts from the dialysis water and if aluminum hydroxide gels are used to decrease phosphate absorption in the gut. In particular, aluminum accumulates under those circumstances in the brain and seems to be at least a partial cause of dialysis dementia. The early symptoms are speech impairment and dysphasia, followed by myoclonic movements, seizures, and progressive global dementia with prominent symptoms from the parietal lobe. This disease appears to be irreversible, and survival beyond a few years is uncommon.

In addition, aluminum seems to accumulate, although to a much lesser extent, in the brain of patients with Alzheimer's disease. This accumulation seems to be a phenomenon secondary to the disease development, and the possible causative role of aluminum has not yet been determined. A different type of encephalopathy may develop as an apparent result of heavy occupational aluminum exposure. Thus, aluminum is undoubtedly neurotoxic, but the extent to which this occurs in individuals with normal kidney function still has to be clarified.

Dialysis osteomalacia is a complication that occurs rarely in patients undergoing long-term dialysis treatment; it causes development of sclerosis and osteoporosis, leading to skeletal pains and multiple fractures.[6,7] The occurrence of this disease is closely associated with long-term aluminum accumulation. Bone toxicity has also been described in patients receiving chronic parenteral nutrition containing aluminum-contaminated casein hydrolysate and in patients who had ingested large doses of aluminum-containing antacids for extended periods.

Prevention

Aluminum measurements of serum are extensively used in the monitoring of patients undergoing dialysis treatment. Although high levels of aluminum may be accurately estimated by most laboratories, reference levels have decreased significantly, indicating an improved contamination control in the laboratories. Serum levels below 10 μg/L (0.37 μmol/L) are usually considered normal. Dialysis patients may have serum levels of 50 μg/L (1.85 μmol/L) and above, and the risk of adverse effects of aluminum is much increased if the serum level exceeds 100 μg/L (3.7 μmol/L). Aluminum has a short biological half-life in the blood of individuals with normal kidney function, thus rendering aluminum measurements of serum samples of limited value in occupational health practice. However, urinary excretion of aluminum reflects short-term exposures, while a better indication of the chronic accumulation is the excretion after an exposure-free interval of several days. A measure of the body burden is the concentration in a bone biopsy from the iliac crest.

Aluminum toxicity in dialysis patients should be prevented by using dialysis water with an aluminum concentration below 10 μg/L (0.37 μmol/L) after reverse osmosis or other effective treatment. Also, restriction or substitution of oral aluminum-containing phosphate binders should be instituted. Solutions used for parenteral nutrition should be examined for aluminum contents, and low-level products should be preferred. Desferrioxamine has a limited therapeutic use as an aluminum chelator.

In the United States aluminum is regulated as an inert dust, with an exposure limit of 15 mg/m^3 for dust and 5 mg/m^3 for respirable particles. This limit may not entirely protect against adverse effects. The limits recommended by the American Conference of Governmental Industrial Hygienists (ACGIH) are: 10 mg/m^3 for aluminum metal and oxide, 5 mg/m^3 for aluminum pyro-powders and welding fumes, and 2 mg/m^3 for soluble aluminum salts and for (unstable) aluminum alkyls.

▶ ANTIMONY

Antimony is used for various alloys with lead and other metals, for semiconductors, and for thermoelectric devices, and antimony compounds are widely employed, especially as pigments. Occupational antimony exposures occur in the mining and refining of the metal and in the production of pewter, solder, storage battery plates, and babbitt metal. Exposure to antimony compounds has been reported in the glass industry and from the production of abrasives, textile dyeing, and handling of pigments and catalysts. Antimony-containing pharmaceuticals (e.g., against leishmaniasis and schistosomiasis) are still in wide use in certain parts of the world.

The medical literature on antimony mainly deals with the use of organic compounds as therapeutic agents, and much less information is available on the significance of environmental and occupational exposures.[8] Adverse health effects seen in relation to occupational antimony exposures are difficult to evaluate, because concomitant exposures to arsenic may have occurred. While cardiotoxicity has been documented as a side effect in antimony pharmaceuticals, electrocardiogram changes related to occupational exposures have only occasionally been reported. More commonly, antimony compounds have given rise to irritation of the mucous membranes, irritant eczema, and even chemical burns and perforation of the nasal septum. In particular, antimony trioxide frequently causes the so-called antimony spots, i.e., small, erythematous papules that develop under intense itching on exposed, moist skin areas in hot environments; they are fortunately short lasting. A benign pneumoconiosis is related to antimony exposures. The lung cancer risk may be increased by exposures to this metal, and a relation to increased frequency of abortions has been reported in one study.

In the presence of strong acid, stibine (SbH_3) may be formed. Storage battery workers and metal etchers may be exposed to this hazard. This gas is very toxic and causes severe hemolysis, shock, central nervous system (CNS) symptoms, and even death due to anuria.

Most antimony absorbed is rather rapidly excreted, Sb(V) mostly in the urine, Sb(III) mostly via the gastrointestinal tract. A slow compartment seems to exists, probably mainly due to accumulation in liver and kidneys. Severe toxicity has not been documented at urine levels below 1 mg/L (8.2 μmol/L), but biological monitoring of antimony levels in blood and urine has so far been used only rarely. The limit for occupational antimony exposures is 0.5 mg/m^3; for stibine this level corresponds to 0.1 ppm.

▶ ARSENIC

Exposures

Arsenic occurs widely in the environment. Major sources of environmental pollution are primary metal smelters and coal burning. Well water may be severely contaminated, especially in certain parts of South America, West Bengal, and Taiwan. Some crustaceans may contain as much as 100 mg/kg, but most arsenic in seafood occurs as organic complexes. Other food items contain little arsenic. Fowler's solution (sodium arsenite) was used in the past to treat leukemia, psoriasis, and other diseases, and arsenic may still be employed for therapeutic purposes in some parts of the world.

Occupational exposure to arsenic occurs in the following branches of industry: metal smelting, where arsenic occurs as a contaminant or by-product; production and use of various alloys, especially with lead and copper; semiconductor industry; production and use of pesticides (e.g., calcium and lead arsenate); production of opal glass; certain kinds of enameling; production of pharmaceuticals; production of paints and coatings; leather tanning and the taxidermist industry; and the production, handling, analysis, etc. of arsenic and arsenic compounds. When arsenic-containing ores are heated, arsenic trioxide (As_2O_3, white arsenic) is formed, and this compound constitutes the main product for the arsenic-consuming industry. Experimental studies suggest that this As(III) is more toxic than the As(V), which occurs in arsenate compounds, e.g., wood treatment products. Arsine (AsH_3) is particularly toxic. However, little is known about the speciation of arsenic in occupational exposures.

Easily soluble arsenic compounds may be absorbed rather efficiently through the respiratory and gastrointestinal tracts; absorption through the skin has also been documented. As(V) seems to be partially converted to As(III). Methylation occurs in the liver, and the methylated arsenic species usually constitute the main part of the urinary arsenic excretion after exposure to inorganic arsenic compounds. Arsenobetaine and arsenocholine almost entirely account for the arsenic content of fish and crustacea. These compounds are relatively rapidly excreted unchanged in the urine. The biological half-life for inorganic arsenic in the blood is about 1 to 2 days; after an acute exposure to inorganic arsenic, the arsenic excretion in urine is therefore increased for a week or more. An additional, somewhat slower excretion occurs through hairs, nails, and skin cells. Both skin and lungs may constitute a "slow" arsenic compartment with a long biological half-time.

Effects

Acute intoxication due to ingestion of arsenic trioxide or lead arsenate first causes vomiting, colics, and diarrhea, then follows fever, cardiotoxicity, peripheral edema, and shock, which can lead to death within 12 to 48 hours. Patients who survive an acute intoxication usually exhibit anemia and leukopenia and may experience peripheral nervous damage 1 to 2 weeks later. Late effects include loss of hair and nail deformities. Recovery from peripheral neurotoxicity is slow and may take several months.

Another kind of acute poisoning may occur following inhalation of the extremely toxic arsine (AsH_3), which smells like garlic. This compound is formed when arsenic (frequently as an impurity) comes into contact with strong acid, and prolonged inhalation of 10 ppm or more of arsine is lethal. The patient first suffers dizziness, headache, pains in the stomach, arms, and legs and subsequently hemolysis, janudice, and kidney damage, which may lead to death.

Under chronic exposure conditions, the critical effect is the neuropathy, which is usually of the sensorimotor type causing paresthesias in the extremities, muscle weakness, especially in the fingers, motor incoordination, and neuralgic pains. It may occur as a late result of an acute exposure or it may be the only lasting result of a long-term exposure to arsenic, although chronic skin symptoms often occur at the same time. A subclinical neuropathy, detectable by neurophysiological methods, has been described in relation to relatively low arsenic exposures. Long-term exposure to inorganic arsenic compounds can cause chronic eczema, hyperpigmentation of the skin, and hyperkeratosis, especially on footsoles and palms. Development of skin cancer may be seen at a later time: squamous cell carcinomas mostly at the hyperkeratoses on the extremities, basal cell carcinomas in any region. Vascular effects may result in Raynaud's syndrome, acrocyanosis, and necroses ("blackfoot disease"). Epidemiological studies of pesticide production workers, sprayers, smelter workers, residents near polluting industries, and patients treated with arsenicals convincingly indicate that respiratory exposure to arsenic results in an increased risk of lung cancer. The incidence of other cancer forms may be increased as well, though this evidence is less certain.[9] In most studies, the exposures were mixed, and the effects of As(III) and As(V) cannot be separated. Arsenic may act synergistically with tobacco smoke. Teratogenic effects have also been reported.

Prevention

Biological monitoring of arsenic levels in blood is of limited interest, because arsenic is rapidly cleared from the blood. Hair analysis has been employed in forensic medicine, but the significance of external contamination excludes the use of this method in the surveillance of dust exposures in industry. Measurement of arsenic levels in urine may be used for the evaluation of current exposures, because a major part, about 60 percent at steady-state, of the absorbed arsenic is excreted in the urine. However, due to the somewhat variable proportion excreted by this route, the daily variations related to the short biological half-life, and the contribution of arsenic compounds from food items, urine tests for total arsenic are useful only on a group basis. If the excretion is above 1 mg/L (13 μmol/L), the result can be used as an indication of arsenic intoxication. Normally the arsenic content in urine is below 100 μg/L (1.3 μmol/L), but levels more than twice that high may be seen after a good seafood meal. After exposure to inorganic arsenic compounds, the urinary arsenic consists of no more than 25 percent inorganic arsenic, one-third of the rest being monomethylarsonate, and two-thirds being dimethylarsinate (cacodylate). Background levels of these compounds would probably be below 20 μg/L (0.27 μmol/L), unless exposures from contaminated wells were prevalent. The organoarsenicals from seafood do not affect the urinary excretion of the methylated compounds.

The limit for airborne arsenic and inorganic arsenic compounds is 0.01 mg/m^3; for organic compounds, 0.5 mg/m^3; and for arsine the limit is 0.05 ppm, which corresponds to 0.2 mg/m^3. However, on the basis of the carcinogenic effects, the National Institute of Occupational Safety and Health (NIOSH) has recommended a limit of 0.002 mg/m^3 for all arsenic compounds; exposures below this limit would result in minor or undetectable increases of arsenic levels in urine. A WHO/FAO expert group has suggested a limit for daily intake of inorganic arsenic of 0.002 mg/kg body weight.

▶ BARIUM

Barium is used in drilling muds, in glass and ceramic glazes, paper coating, pesticides, and as a plastic stabilizer. Sparingly, soluble barium salts cause negligible gastrointestinal absorption. Thus the use of barium sulfate as x-ray contrast material is generally safe. If absorbed, barium mainly accumulates in the skeleton. Inhalation of insoluble barium compounds has resulted in the development of a benign pneumoconiosis, baritosis. Soluble barium salts cause a movement of potassium into the cells and subsequently hypokalemia. In barium poisoning, the first symptom is smooth muscle stimulation (vomiting, colic, diarrhea), followed by general muscle stimulation; in severe cases, paralysis then develops.[10] In the Szechuan province of China, an endemic occurrence of a periodic, familial paralysis was traced to the table salt produced from a mine with a very high barium content. The occupational exposure limit for soluble barium compounds is 0.5 mg/m^3, but the sulfate is regulated as an inert dust.

▶ BERYLLIUM

Beryllium, the fourth lightest element, is extracted from beryl ore. Most cases of beryllium-induced disease have been the result of past exposures in connection with the production of fluorescent lamps. Beryllium is used for coating of cathode-ray tubes, e.g., for radar equipment, in electrical or electronic instruments, and in nuclear reactors. Moreover, beryllium is used in many light metal alloys for the space and aircraft industry. Most of the environmental pollution is due to combustion of fossil fuels.[11]

Most beryllium salts are practically insoluble at neutral pH, and absorption after oral intake is therefore limited. Skin contact may result in allergic dermatitis. Inhalation of beryllium dusts is the major hazard. Once absorbed, excretion is slow. An acute, severe exposure to airborne beryllium may result in an inflammation of mucous membranes and in a chemical pneumonia. Inhalation of as little as 45 μg of this metal is sufficient to cause acute disease.

Chronic beryllium disease (sometimes called berylliosis) has similarities to sarcoidosis.[11] This pulmonary granulomatosis can evolve following an acute phase by a long but variable latency period. Often the diagnosis is made several years after cessation of exposure. Cases have occurred in several household contacts. The most frequent symptom is dyspnea at exertion. The chest x-ray usually reveals a mixture of small, rounded, and irregular opacities. Pulmonary function tests show decreased diffusion, later followed by more generalized pulmonary impairment. Granulomas may also occur in the liver and other organs, but the Kveim test for sarcoidosis is negative, while the lymphocyte blast transformation test is positive for beryllium. The course of the disease is irregular, and some form of predisposition seems to affect the pathogenesis. Although steroid treatment is beneficial, no complete recovery has been recorded. The beryllium case registry at NIOSH has recorded almost 1,000 cases, though almost none recently.

Experimental evidence suggests that beryllium is a carcinogen. Epidemiological evidence from refining, machining, and production of beryllium metal and alloys confirms that beryllium-exposed individuals suffer lung cancer more frequently than expected.[12]

Biological monitoring is of limited interest and plays no role in the prevention of excess beryllium exposures. The limit for occupational beryllium exposure is 0.002 mg/m^3, with a peak value of 0.025 mg/m^3 for short exposures.

▶ CADMIUM

Exposures

Cadmium concentration in agricultural soils is increasing because of the deposition of airborne cadmium particles and because of the cadmium content of phosphate fertilizers and sewage sludge used for fertilization. Cadmium is a relatively mobile metal in soils, and many crops retain relatively high cadmium levels. In particular, tobacco leaves are high in cadmium.[13] The total daily intake of cadmium via food varies according to dietary habits, but averages range from less than 10 to more than 50 μg/day. Cereals, molluscs and crustaceans, wild mushrooms, and beef kidney are main sources of increased dietary cadmium exposure.[14]

The most important application of this metal is cadmium plating for corrosion treatment of metals, especially iron and steel. Brazing is still carried out with solders containing cadmium. Rechargeable nickel-cadmium batteries are increasingly used in modern-day electronic products. To a limited degree cadmium is also used in certain copper alloys and in bearing metal. Cadmium rods are used in nuclear power plants. Cadmium sulfide and selenide are used as pigments in enamel, ceramics, glass, plastic, and leather. Many of these uses are now being restricted. However, considerable occupational cadmium exposure may still be a result of various work processes, such as welding or cutting of metals with cadmium-containing coatings, spray-painting with cadmium pigments, or primary production of copper and zinc from cadmium-containing ores. Raw phosphate often contains significant amounts of cadmium, and exposures may occur during the production of phosphate fertilizers. This metal has a melting point of 320°C, and dangerous fumes are generated by rather low temperatures.

Pulmonary absorption depends on particle size and solubility, while 2 to 10 percent of oral intake is transferred to the bloodstream. Uptake by the liver induces the synthesis of metallothionein, which binds cadmium. When released to the blood, the complex is subsequently excreted through the kidney glomeruli; most is again reabsorbed by the tubulus cells, and an accumulation in the kidney cortex takes place. In general, about one-half of the human body burden of cadmium is located in liver and kidneys. The liver is the main storage organ for cadmium in the body, but the highest concentration is eventually reached in the kidneys. The biological half-life is 10 to 20 years, and cadmium accumulation in the body therefore seems to occur during the major part of a lifetime.

Effects

Acute cadmium poisoning most frequently occurs after inhalation of cadmium fume, e.g., cutting cadmium-plated steel with an oxyacetylene torch. After a latency of a few hours, the first symptoms may suggest metal fume fever, but a toxic pneumonitis then develops. Recovery is often slow and may take months; several years after acute cadmium pneumonitis, progressive pulmonary fibrosis has been observed. Oral cadmium exposure may cause acute poisoning, e.g., when large amounts of the metal is released from solder materials in soft-drink machines or from ceramic glazes of kitchenware.

The chronic form of cadmium poisoning is a result of long-term accumulation in the body, where the kidneys constitute the target organ. The toxic damage mostly seems to occur in the proximal tubuli, but glomerular changes often appear at a later state and may even in some cases be the first indication of cadmium-induced nephropathy. The first sign of kidney dysfunction is usually an increased excretion of low-molecular proteins in the urine, notably β_2-microglobulin. In case of glomerular dysfunction, larger proteins also occur in the urine. Subsequent losses of protein and minerals may lead to skeletal changes, as seen in Japan where a large number of cadmium-exposed patients suffered osteomalacia with skeletal pains and pseudofractures, the so-called Itai-Itai disease. Low-level environmental exposure to cadmium in women over 60 years of age has been related to increased urinary leakage of small proteins; patients with diabetes also seem to be at an increased risk of cadmium nephrotoxicity.[14] Thus, environmental cadmium pollution may accelerate age-related declines of renal function.

Long-term inhalation of cadmium can lead to emphysema. This disease has been linked to cadmium retention in the lungs in smokers. Experimental animal studies show that pulmonary exposure to cadmium compounds may cause lung cancer. Epidemiological evidence has suggested a similar link, and cadmium should therefore be regarded a carcinogenic metal.[12] Additional animal experiments suggest that this metal may be a teratogen.

Prevention

The cadmium level in the blood is an indication of the current exposure (during the last few months) and is frequently used for biological monitoring. Levels up to 10 μg/L (89 nmol/L) may occur in heavy smokers, while never-smokers usually show levels below 1 μg/L (9 nmol/L). For industrial exposures, a recommended limit for blood cadmium is 5 μg/100 mL (44 nmol/L), but this limit may not protect against kidney damage under long-term exposure conditions. Urinary excretion of cadmium is limited in the beginning, and immediate increases occur only under rather heavy exposures. Higher urinary cadmium levels are more frequently found when the kidneys over a long period have accumulated rather large amounts of cadmium, which then start to leak, and an upper normal level of 3 μg/L (26 nmol/L) is then exceeded. If the exposure continues, tubular and perhaps glomerular dysfunction develops, and relatively large amounts of cadmium are then excreted in the urine, thus decreasing the kidney burden of the metal. Considerable evidence suggests that the threshold for development of nephrotoxicity may be exceeded when the cadmium concentration in the kidney cortex reaches about 200 μg/g, a level that would correspond to a urinary cadmium excretion of 10 μg/L (89 nmol/L), and a daily absorption of 10 to 15 μg over a lifetime. β_2-Microglobulin may be assessed in urinary samples, but excess levels are found only in case of early or imminent kidney damage, i.e., when preventive efforts have failed.

The exposure limit in the United States is 0.005 mg/m^3 due to the carcinogenic risk. This limit will protect against nephrotoxicity.[15] Many countries have adopted regulations concerning cadmium release from ceramic glazes and other materials that may leach cadmium to food and beverages. The International Standards Organization (ISO) has adopted a limit for cadmium release from ceramic flatware of 0.17 mg/dm^2, with higher limits for hollowware. With regard to dietary intake of cadmium, a WHO/FAO expert group several years ago suggested a Provisional Tolerable Weekly Intake (PTWI) limit of 0.4 to 0.5 mg/week. Since then, kidney function in the elderly and diabetes patients has turned out to be more vulnerable than expected, and lifelong cadmium accumulation from environmental exposures would seem to eventually cause adverse effects, perhaps even below the PTWI. However, even the current PTWI seems already to be exceeded by some population groups, and prevention of cadmium pollution from all sources would seem to be a major environmental priority.

▶ CHROMIUM

Exposures

Chromium most commonly occurs as trivalent compounds. Divalent compounds are rather unstable, and hexavalent chromates are reduced to trivalent compounds in the presence of oxidizable substances. Only scattered information is available on environmental exposures to chromium. In the United States, daily intake through food is usually below 100 μg, but higher intake occurs in northern Europe.

However, the chemical form of chromium present in food and drinking water is largely unknown.

Occupational exposures to chromium occur in several branches of industry: production of chromium and chromium compounds, stainless steel, and other metal alloys; chromium plating of metals; production of heat-resistant bricks with chromate additives; use of chromates as pigments and bichromates for tanning; welding of chromium-plated metals and chromium-containing alloys; development of photographic emulsions; and production and usage of wood preservatives. The main consumption of chromium is in the steel industry, and stainless steel usually contains between 8 and 18 percent chromium. In addition, chromate present in cement results in considerable cutaneous exposures.

The gastrointestinal uptake of Cr(VI) is a few percent, while the absorption of Cr(III) is much less; organic complexes of chromium may be more easily absorbed. The fate of inhaled chromium particles and the transfer within the body depends on the solubility of the compounds. Excretion is mainly via the urine.

Effects

Chromium is an essential trace metal (as glucose tolerance factor) for several species, including humans. Glucose intolerance, weight loss, and peripheral neuropathy in patients undergoing long-term intravenous nutrition may be cured by Cr(III) supplements. Chromium deficiency in humans is otherwise unknown, and the daily chromium need is unclear.

The toxicity of the various chromium compounds varies, partly in relation to the different solubilities.[16] In general, hexavalent compounds are more easily soluble than the trivalent compounds. The chromate ion is strongly oxidizing and is capable of passing through biological membranes. Trivalent chromium is less toxic, apparently due to the lower solubility and lower biological mobility. However, Cr(III) may be the ultimate toxicant in relation to some of the Cr(VI)-associated effects. The major effects include corrosion of skin and mucous membranes, allergic responses, and carcinogenicity.

Long-term inhalation of Cr(VI) compounds in chromium-plating workshops has in the past caused severe corrosion of the nasal mucous membranes with defects in the nasal septum. These effects are now seen more rarely. Chromate may cause circumscribed ulcers (chrome holes) at the knuckles, nail roots, or other exposed skin areas. Even though they may be quite deep, they are almost painless. Healing often takes several weeks and leaves a depressed scar, but the ulcers are apparently not related to development of skin cancer.

Chromium is one of the best known allergens in the occupational environment, and chromate is frequently the most common cause of allergic contact dermatitis among males. Cement eczema is a common occupational disease in construction workers, and chromate allergy is the most frequent allergen. This disease also occurs in tanners, furriers, and workers exposed to chromates in photographic laboratories and in relation to wood treatment. Although Cr(VI) may be the primary sensitizer, subsequent allergic responses have allegedly also been elicited by Cr(III). In a few cases, chromate has also been identified as a cause of asthma, probably mediated by a type I allergic reaction. Chromite mining has apparently caused several cases of a benign pneumoconiosis.

Chromium is a well-documented human carcinogen, and occupational exposures resulting from the production of ferrochrome and of chromates have caused an increased frequency of cancer in the respiratory tract.[17] An increased occurrence of lung cancer in welders may be due to the content of insoluble chromates in welding fumes from stainless steel. Although trivalent chromium compounds may constitute the ultimate carcinogen, exposures to such compounds have not been shown in epidemiological studies to cause cancer.

Prevention

Biological monitoring of chromium levels in the urine is useful to follow the exposure to soluble, hexavalent chromium compounds. The biological half-time in plasma is a few days. When external contamination of the sample has been avoided, the upper reference level is usually about 0.5 µg/L (10 nmol/L). Plasma chromium levels parallel the urinary excretion, but chromium concentrations in erythrocytes or whole blood reflect longer-term chromate exposures. Exposure to trivalent compounds or sparingly soluble chromates will not result in detectable changes in body fluids available for biological monitoring.

The exposure limit for airborne chromate and chromium acid is a ceiling value of 0.1 mg/m^3; for soluble chromic and chromous salts, the limit is 0.5 mg/m^3; and for chromium metal and insoluble chromium salts, 1 mg/m^3. Cr(VI) compounds are regarded as carcinogenic, and a permissible exposure limit of 0.001 mg/m^3 has been suggested by NIOSH. Skin contact with Cr(VI) compounds should be avoided, and any skin contamination should be immediately removed with soap and water. This problem is even more important for patients with chromate allergy who may have to avoid contact with leather products and plastic articles with leachable chromate pigments. The sulfur on matches contains chromate as well. On the other hand, chromium alloys release only insignificant amounts, because of oxide formation in the surface layer. In some countries the addition of 0.4 percent of ferrous sulfate to the cement is required by law, because it effectively reduces the chromate to insoluble Cr(III) compounds.

► COBALT

Human cobalt exposures from natural sources are very limited, and daily intake through food has usually been estimated at somewhat below 50 µg. Cobalt levels in drinking water are usually low and of little concern, and atmospheric levels are frequently undetectable.

Occupational exposures have become prevalent.[18] The most important use is "hard metal," which consists of various metal carbides (mainly tungsten) cemented by a cobalt binder. Cobalt has also found considerable use in alloys, to which it adds a high melting point, tensile strength, and resistance to corrosion. Cobalt compounds are increasingly used as catalysts, including desiccators in paints. Cobalt pigments are used in ceramic and glass products. The alloys are extensively used in the electrical, automobile, and aircraft industries, and cobalt is also used for electroplating.

Absorption in the gastrointestinal tract varies, but probably averages about 25 percent for soluble compounds, unless cobalt is ingested in the form of vitamin B_{12}, and in iron deficiency, which increased the absorption of cobalt. Cobalt induces hematopoiesis and has a therapeutic application in patients with refractory anemia. Ingestion of excessive amounts of cobalt will induce vomiting and diarrhea.

Cobalt is an essential micronutrient and has important actions as an enzyme activator and as a component of vitamin B_{12}. However, cobalt deficiency has not been documented in humans, but enzootic deficiency may be a problem in certain regions of the United States, Australia, Scotland, and other parts of the world. Thus, cobalt is added to cattle feed and sometimes to fertilizers.

Respiratory exposure to cobalt dust may lead to airway irritation, asthma, and measurable systemic absorption. Cemented carbide production workers may develop a pneumoconiosis called hard metal lung, frequently following long-term exposures of more than 10 years. The pathogenesis of cobalt-induced pulmonary disease is not known in detail, but some individual hypersensitivity may predispose to the pulmonary reactions. Some studies suggest that cobalt exposure may lead to an increased risk of lung cancer.

Cutaneous exposures to cobalt are common. Small concentrations of this metal are present in cement, and cobalt may contaminate cutting oils and may leach from metal objects. In fact, cobalt allergy is frequent, but occurs frequently in connection with allergy toward nickel or chromate. Hand eczemas in patients with such cross-reactions have a relatively poor prognosis.

An outbreak of cardiomyopathy, sometimes complicated by pericardial effusion, was reported in Quebec City 25 years ago.[19] This disease occurred exclusively in beer drinkers, and subsequent investigations showed that the local brewery added cobalt sulfate to the beer. The same practice was discovered in Omaha, Minneapolis, and in Brussels, where similar epidemics occurred. Although probably not solely due to the addition of about 1 mg of cobalt to each liter of beer, the epidemics faded after discontinuation of the addition of cobalt. Several similar cases have been linked to industrial cobalt exposures.

Biological monitoring may be of some use. The kinetics of cobalt in the organism show the existence of two fast compartments with half-lives of up to 2 days, while about 10 percent of absorbed cobalt is excreted much more slowly. Urinary cobalt excretion levels are normally below 2 μg/L (30 nmol/L), unless the individual takes a mineral supplement. Following occupational exposures, urinary excretion levels may be 100-fold the normal upper limit, but the levels may change rapidly due to the short half-life. Thus more information may be obtained on the average long-term exposure by measuring the cobalt level in urine or blood on Monday morning after an exposure-free period.

Occupational exposures to cobalt metal fume and dust should be limited as much as possible and also respect the current exposure limit of 0.1 mg/m^3. Due to the increasing awareness concerning hard metal disease, a limit of 0.05 mg/m^3 for cobalt metal, dust, and fume has been proposed by ACGIH. Even this limit may not sufficiently protect a worker with pulmonary hypersensitivity, however.

▸ COPPER

Copper is a widely used metal that has both beneficial and adverse health effects. This metal is used in electrical equipment, in alloys, and in plumbing and heating systems. The daily intake through food averages about 1 mg or more. Copper is an essential element that is necessary for various metalloenzymes, and possible signs of copper deficiency in humans have been documented in depletion experiments. Accidental intake of large amounts of this metal results in acute gastrointestinal symptoms. Copper sulfate has therefore been used as an emetic, but the potential absorption of toxic quantities of the metal limits its usefulness. Occupational exposures to copper fume and fine dust may cause metal fume fever, and copper dust is a respiratory irritant. Patients with Wilson's disease (hepatolenticular fibrosis) accumulate copper in the liver related to insufficient formation of the copper-binding ceruloplasmin; these patients and the heterozygous carriers may be particularly sensitive to excess copper exposures. Serum concentrations are affected by ceruloplasmin levels and increase during pregnancy and during anticonceptive hormone treatment. Excretion is mainly via the bile. The exposure limit for copper dusts or mists is 1 mg/m^3; and for copper fume, 0.1 mg/m^3, although ACGIH has suggested 0.2 mg/m^3 for fumes. Copper is included in the list of essential minerals with a recommended daily dietary intake of 2.3 mg for adults.

▸ IRON

Iron is necessary for life but may also cause toxicity at excess exposures. Iron deficiency is the most prevalent metal deficiency syndrome in humans, especially among women of the reproductive age groups and certain groups of small children. Several nutrients interfere with iron absorption, but it is always increased in case of deficiency. Ingestion of iron supplements in considerable excess may cause acute gastrointestinal lesions followed by metabolic acidosis, toxic hepatitis, and shock. Chronic iron overload, as in hereditary hemochromatosis, leads to hemosiderosis, liver cirrhosis, and increased cancer risk. Foundry workers, grinders, and welders are exposed to considerable quantities of iron oxide fume, which accumulates in the lungs and may result in siderosis, a benign pneumoconiosis. Hematite miners have exhibited an excess incidence of lung cancer; although iron may not be the primary cause, an interaction between the iron dust and other factors, such as radon and asbestos, is possible. The exposure limit for iron oxide fume is 10 mg/m^3, but ACGIH has recommended a limit of half as much and 1 mg/m^3 for soluble iron salts. Recommendations for daily iron intakes suggest that iron supplements are necessary for large population groups, but the supplement should always be stored in child-proof containers.

Iron pentacarbonyl may be formed when carbon monoxide comes in contact with iron at high partial pressures. This liquid is extremely toxic and, when the vapor is inhaled, results in almost immediate headache, dyspnea, and dizziness. The symptoms then fade, only to return after several hours when pulmonary consolidation and cerebral degeneration are progressing. The ACGIH exposure limit is 0.1 ppm.

▸ LEAD

Exposures

Lead has a wide spectrum of applications. Metallic lead is used in various alloys, and several inorganic compounds have important uses. Almost 10 percent of the production is used for organolead compounds, tetraethyl lead and tetramethyl lead, which are added to gasoline as octane boosters. These compounds are dealt with separately. The extensive use of lead resulted in considerable redistributions in the biosphere, particularly as a result of the air pollution, which reached a maximum of about 1,000 tons/day in the late 1970s. Most was emitted in the northern hemisphere, but pollution levels in the southern hemisphere are still increasing.[20] Calculations of natural lead exposures, supplemented by measurements of lead retention levels in archeological samples of bones and teeth, suggest that environmental lead exposures averaged about 100-fold above typical exposure levels in premetallurgical times. Dietary lead intakes have decreased considerably in many countries as a result of the decreased use of lead additives to gasoline, and the daily oral intake of lead is mostly below 100 μg for adults. The major sources of environmental lead exposure include: gasoline additives, lead-based paint, lead-soldered food cans, ceramic glazes, and industrial pollution. Drinking water levels may be of particular concern in soft water areas; where lead pipes are used, the highest lead concentrations occur in the "first draw" water in the morning.

The melting point for lead is 327°C, and hazardous evaporation results when the temperature exceeds about 500°C. This fact is of importance where lead is melted or molded in factories and workshops. Various inorganic compounds are used as pigments and desiccators, for corrosion treatment and enameling, and as an additive to glass and a stabilizer in polyvinyl chloride (PVC) plastic. Lead compounds that are used in ceramic glazes are usually fritted, i.e., aggregated as larger particles by preheating.

Occupational lead exposure occurs in particular in the following processes: primary production of lead from lead ores; secondary lead production from used automobile batteries and scrap metal; production of batteries; welding and flame cutting of lead-containing or minium-treated alloys; molding of lead-containing alloys in foundries; soldering with lead solder, if the temperature is too high; production of and spray painting with paints containing lead pigments and dessicators; addition of lead stearate as stabilizer in PVC plastic; batch mixing with lead compounds for the production of crystal glass; and grinding and sandblasting of lead alloys and coatings. High exposures have also been documented in instructors from indoor shooting ranges, in workers producing leaded panes, and in gunsmiths.

Inorganic lead compounds are absorbed only to a minor degree in the gastrointestinal tract of adults, usually about 10 percent or slightly less, somewhat higher during fasting, and somewhat lower when excess calcium, phosphate, and phytate are present. However, the immature gastrointestinal tract is relatively permeable to lead, and balance studies in small children have suggested that oral intake may result in absorption rates of 30 to 50 percent.

Almost all lead in the blood is bound to the erythrocytes, and the lead content of serum or plasma is so low that it cannot be reliably measured by conventional analytical methods. Measurements therefore refer to the lead content of whole blood (or erythrocytes). Due to the low solubility of lead phosphate, lead accumulates in calcified tissues. About 95 percent of the lead burden of an adult person is located in the skeleton, with a very long biological half-life related to the slow tissue remodeling rate. Skeletal lead is more mobile in children. Much less lead is present in the soft tissues, and the half-life is generally about 2 months. The brain probably constitutes an exception: lead that has passed through the blood-brain barrier has a biological half-life of more than a year. The placenta does not constitute any major barrier to lead passage, and the fetus is therefore exposed to lead through the mother. Some lead is excreted into the gastrointestinal tract, but the major excretion is via the urine. Only low concentrations of lead have been detected in human milk.

Effects

Lead is an important enzyme inhibitor. Of major clinical importance are the chronic effects on blood cells and the nervous system. Anemia is a typical symptom in classic lead poisoning. Lead inhibits the Na-K-ATPase in the cell membranes of the erythrocytes and thereby makes them less stable, with a shortened life span as a result. Of quantitatively less importance is the interference with hemoglobin synthesis, several steps of the heme formation being inhibited by lead. Most sensitive is the enzyme amino-levulinic acid dehydratase (ALAD), which is inhibited already at low lead concentrations in the blood at 50 μg/L (0.25 nmol/L) and above. The erythrocyte ALAD activity correlates very closely with the lead content in the blood, but in occupational lead exposure, the activity of this enzyme may become very low. Less sensitive to lead is the incorporation of ferrous ion into protoporphyrin IX to form heme. When this reaction is inhibited, zinc substitutes for iron and the resulting zinc protoporphyrin (ZPP) binds instead of heme to the hemoglobin molecule, thereby rendering it unable to carry oxygen. Each erythrocyte in the blood contains a ZPP amount as a message of the lead exposure at the time when the cell was formed. A blood sample containing erythrocytes that have been formed within the last 4 months or so, and the ZPP concentration in the blood, is therefore an indication of the average lead exposure within this time interval. The measurement may be carried out by a portable fluorometer in a few seconds. In adult men, the ZPP concentration increases significantly when the blood-lead concentration averages above 250 μg/L (1.25 nmol/L). In women, the threshold is somewhat lower because of the increased sensitivity related to lower iron stores in the body. In children, the threshold for ZPP increase seems to be about 150 μg/L (0.75 nmol/L). An increased amount of ZPP in the blood can also be caused by iron deficiency alone, but iron deficiency may at the same time make the patient more sensitive to the toxic effects of lead.

Lead affects both the central and the peripheral nervous system. Cases of encephalopathy in adults have been caused by consumption of moonshine whiskey distilled in old car radiators. More insidiously, a chronic toxic encephalopathy may develop. Typically, the lead-poisoned worker is taken to the doctor or the hospital by the wife who is worried about by his failing health and his unbearable irritability. Clinical examination and neuropsychological testing frequently show that attention, concentration, memory, and abstraction are affected. Early effects, detectable by psychological tests, may develop when blood lead concentrations exceed 400 μg/L (2.0 nmol/L) for extensive periods. Prospective studies suggest that decreasing performance may occur in men when a lead level of 300 μg/L (1.5 nmol/L) is exceeded.

Children are more susceptible to the central nervous effects, and severe cases of encephalopathy with seizures still occur, sometimes as a result of ingesting of lead-containing paint flakes from peeling walls. More commonly, effects are detected in children with elevated levels of lead in the blood in the absence of any past history of acute lead toxicity. The studies suggest that attention and vigilance are sensitive measures of lead toxicity, and decreased performance may be detected in IQ tests. Several other factors may influence the performance of small children in such tests, and the contribution of lead to decreased functioning of children has raised considerable controversy. The relative contribution by prenatal and postnatal exposures is still unclear. When carefully evaluated, however, the studies in concert suggest that even low lead levels may contribute to decreased intellectual performance of children.[21] The threshold for such effects of course depends on the sensitivity of the methods employed, the sample size, and the validity of the study, but the general impression is that levels only slightly above 100 μg/L (0.5 nmol/L) may cause measurable deficits.

The adult patient with an acute lead poisoning has a weak handshake and a decreased function of the extensor muscles of the forearm ("lead palsy," Teleky's sign). Decreased nerve conduction velocity has been documented in chronically exposed workers. Related subjective symptoms may include muscle weakness, fatigue, pains in the extremities, and sometimes even tremor. The earliest detectable effects on nerve conduction velocity appear to occur when blood lead levels exceed 400 μg/L (2.0 nmol/L). Children may be somewhat more sensitive with regard to the peripheral nervous system effects, but less information is available in this regard.

Acute lead exposure may also affect the kidney function, but this effect appears to be reversible. Symptoms from the gastrointestinal tract include anorexia, dysphagia, constipation, or in some cases diarrhea and occur as a result of chronic exposures as well as acute intoxication. In severe poisoning, colicky pains occur, and several such patients have been subject to surgery for a suspected appendicitis or ulcer. Under chronic exposure conditions and bad oral hygiene, the accumulation of lead sulfide can cause a formation of a blue-grey seam of the gingival edge, the so-called lead seam.

Some studies have suggested that severe lead exposure may result in a decreased life span, in particular due to an increased incidence of stroke. A similar tendency has also been postulated in relation to kidney disease, and kidney cancer has been suggested by animal studies. Although lead may be a weak cancer promotor and augment the development of other disease, current lead exposure levels would probably not cause a detectable increase in cause-specific mortality, although the influence on individual health could be considerable. Teratogenic effects are well documented, and some reports have indicated toxic effects on spermatozoa.

Prevention

The current lead exposure of an individual is best reflected in the lead concentration of whole blood. Prevention of adverse health effects requires that blood lead levels be maintained below 400 μg/L (2.0 nmol/L). Furthermore, the Occupational Safety and Health Administration (OSHA) lead standard includes the provision that blood lead concentrations should be kept below 300 μg/L (1.5 nmol/L) in male and female workers who intend to have children. The long-term exposure may be evaluated by measuring the ZPP level in the blood, and this test can efficiently be used for screening purposes. Medical surveillance is required as an additional safeguard and must be made available to all employees exposed above the action level of 30 $\mu g/m^3$ for more than 30 days a year. Blood lead examination must be carried out at least every 6 months, every 2 months if the blood lead level exceeds 400 μg/L (2.0 nmol/L). The removal protection provision means that workers with a blood lead level above 500 μg/L (2.5 nmol/L), or if otherwise indicated by the medical surveillance, should be removed without losing wage or benefits, until the level has returned to 400 μg/L (2.0 nmol/L) or below that level. If the air lead level cannot be kept below 50 $\mu g/m^3$, engineering control measures must be initiated. Regular air monitoring is required if levels exceed the action limit of 30 $\mu g/m^3$. The standard also includes provision for employee information and respirator use.

The goal for the U.S. Centers for Disease Control and Prevention is to reduce children's blood lead concentrations below 100 μg/L (0.5 nmol/L).[22] If many children exceed this level in a local area, communitywide interventions (primary prevention) should be considered. Interventions for individual children should begin at blood lead concentrations of 150 μg/L (0.75 nmol/L).

An FAO/WHO expert group has recommended that the weekly oral intake of lead should be below 3 mg. This limit may protect most adults against adverse effects of lead, but a special limit for children at half that level when adjusted for body weight is clearly insufficient to protect children.

The action level set by the U.S. Environmental Protection Agency for lead in drinking water is 15 μg/L, a limit that must be respected in at least 90 percent of the homes. Some countries have adopted a limit for lead in wine (250 μg/L); milligram quantities may occur in a vintage bottle if the lead cap has been eroded. Lead caps are no longer used. Also, specific limits may apply to ceramic glazes. The lead release is usually measured by means of a 5 percent dilute acetic acid test, and the release is measured during boiling for three times 30 minutes. Exposures are also limited by setting standards for lead contents of paints. Major efforts have been initiated to remove old, peeling lead paint as part of restoration of houses with a lead hazard.

Organolead Compounds

Organolead compounds have a covalent bond between lead and carbon, and this results in chemical and toxic properties that differ from those of inorganic lead.[23] Tetraethyl lead has been used since 1924, and tetramethyl lead since 1960, as octane boosters of gasoline. Although the formation of methylated lead compounds in aquatic sediments may be possible, pollution with organolead compounds in cities is entirely due to gasoline lead. Evaporation from the carburetor and gasoline tank is a problem of older automobiles, and filling stations also contribute significant amounts of organolead vapors. In addition, uncombusted organolead compounds may be present in considerable quantities in the exhaust gases during cold starts.

Organolead compounds are still produced at several facilities in the United States and in Europe. Occupational exposures may occur during the production, transportation, and blending procedures with raw gasoline. Particularly hazardous procedures include the cleaning of large storage tanks, where the inside organolead levels have been extremely high and caused a large number of fatal intoxications. Organolead compounds may pass through the skin, but apparently only in minor quantities when diluted in gasoline.

Due to the lipid solubility, organolead compounds may pass membranes, including the blood-brain barrier. In the body, they are dealkylated to the trialkyl lead compounds, which are responsible for the toxic actions. The symptoms of acute poisoning include sleepiness, dizziness, fatigue, and at higher exposure levels, insomnia, hallucinations, and a toxic psychosis may ensue. Symptoms of chronic intoxication are mild and may resemble the nonspecific symptoms of the prodromal period. The measurement of blood lead levels is of limited use, but lead excretion in the urine may provide important information.

Gasoline sniffing has been reported in several ethnic groups in different parts of the world, but gasoline sniffers are most frequently teenagers from traditional societies under severe pressures. A euphoric state with hallucinations results from inhalation of gasoline fumes, and subsequent effects including nausea, vomiting, agitation, and anxiety could be partly due to organolead toxicity. The ataxia, tremor, confusion, and other neurological symptoms seen in habitual gasoline sniffers are probably produced by organolead compounds.

The occupational exposure limit for the two tetraalkyl lead compounds is 0.075 mg/m^3. This situation may be somewhat difficult to understand, since inorganic lead, to which the organolead compounds are detoxified, has a lower exposure limit. Environmental pollution with organolead compounds will decrease, as the use of these octane boosters are phased out, and as older car models are scrapped. In Japan and some European countries, all gasoline consumed is now unleaded. The production of these compounds is now increasingly exported to developing countries.

▶ MAGNESIUM

Magnesium is required as an activator for at least 300 enzymes, and a daily intake of 0.6 g for an adult individual has been recommended. Deficiency states may be caused by insufficient intake, decreased absorption, and increased loss; alcoholism, parenteral nutrition, certain drugs, and various diseases are major causes of magnesium deficiency. A high body store of magnesium seems to decrease the mortality in patients with recent myocardial infarction, perhaps by preventing arrythmias, and magnesium deficiency may therefore be more widespread than previously thought.[24] Occupational exposures to magnesium oxide result in eye and upper airway irritation, and controlled exposure with magnesium oxide fumes have demonstrated that metal fume fever may be induced in humans. Magnesium metal silvers implanted in the skin cause a slow-healing burn with ulceration. About one-half of the magnesium in the body is retained in the skeleton, and a similar amount is contained intracellularly, while only about 1 percent is found in the serum. However, measurement of serum and urine magnesium levels are frequently useful. The current standard for occupational magnesium oxide exposure is 15 mg/m^3, while ACGIH has recommended a threshold limit value of 10 mg/m^3. The daily requirement for this essential element in food is about 0.3 to 0.4 g.

▶ MANGANESE

Manganese has a wide range of applications, ferromanganese being the main product, with 90 percent of this production used in various metal alloys, including welding rods. Other applications include dry batteries (manganese dioxide) and pigments for the glass and ceramics industry. Methylcyclopentadienyl manganese tricarbonyl (MMT) is used as an octane-boosting additive to gasoline. Occupational exposures to manganese may occur in the primary production and in the various user industries, especially when manganese-containing alloys are welded. Daily intakes through food usually average about 2 to 3 mg, but may vary considerably, depending on the intake of cereals and rice, which are high in manganese. High levels in drinking water occur in some regions, although low limits are set for technical reasons. Increasing use of MMT in gasoline may cause atmospheric manganese levels above 1 μg/m^3 in cities, and similar levels may be encountered near ferromanganese plants.

The gastrointestinal absorption of manganese appears to be below 5 percent of that ingested, although higher at lower intakes and in case of iron deficiency; a considerable excretion occurs through the bile, some of which is reabsorbed. Manganese is an essential element in metalloenzymes and as enzyme activator, but deficiency states are unlikely to occur under normal circumstances.

Characteristic, manganese-related diseases appear to be relatively rare. Two different pictures may emerge: pulmonary and neurological pathologies. In acute respiratory exposure to manganese, a chemical pneumonitis may develop with cough, phlegm, fever, and changes on the chest x-ray. Also, manganese aerosols may cause metal fume fever (as described under Zinc). However, pulmonary effects are unlikely to occur at manganese exposures below 0.3 mg/m^3.

Manganism is a central nervous system disease with clinical manifestations somewhat similar to those of parkinsonism. This chronic intoxication has primarily been described in miners and workers in ore processing plants. The onset is delayed and sometimes occurs after the exposure has ceased. The first symptoms are nonspecific, such as asthenia, fatigue, headache, irritability, and memory difficulties. The more characteristics signs then develop insidiously: stiff movements, hoarse and low voice, stiffened facial expression, muscular hypertonia, and tremor. At least partial, and temporary, recovery may be obtained by treatment with L-dopa. The severe manganism appears to effect only a small number of the exposed individuals, and individual vulnerability may therefore be of importance. Recent studies have suggested that the early, nonspecific symptoms occur at an increased frequency in welders and other workers with increased exposures to manganese. In patients with compromised liver function, manganese may be less effectively excreted, and accumulation in the basal ganglia has been demonstrated. Although occupational manganese exposure had not occurred in these patients, it was suggested that manganese could contribute to the development of the encephalopathy seen in severe liver disease.[25]

Biological monitoring for manganese is of some interest and needs further exploration. In the blood, some of the manganese has a half-life of about 1 month. Urine analyses are not useful, except perhaps in case of MMT exposure, but analysis of hair samples has occasionally been used for screening purposes.

The limit for occupational exposures is currently 5 mg/m^3, although NIOSH has suggested a limit of 1 mg/m^3. Due to the possible subclinical effects on the central nervous system, a WHO working group recommended a limit of 0.3 mg/m^3.[15] Although only few countries have adopted a limit of this magnitude, the exposure limits for manganese have tended to decrease. In the surveillance of workers exposed to manganese above the WHO recommendation, neurological tests should be included so that the exposure can be stopped if early neurotoxic effects develop. Due to beneficial effects of trace amounts of manganese, a daily intake of about 2.5 to 5 mg of this metal in the diet has been recommended.

▸ MERCURY

Exposures

The toxicity of mercury has been known since antiquity, but its therapeutic effects were also used in a variety of drugs. In particular, mercury became an important drug from the sixteenth century when syphilis patients were treated with mercurous chloride (calomel). Such treatments invariably caused numerous intoxications. Occupational mercury poisoning has been vividly described in the past, for example, by Ramazzini, who 300 years ago noted about the mirror makers: "At Venice on the island called Murano where huge mirrors are made, you may see these workmen gazing with reluctance and scowling at the reflection of their own sufferings in their mirrors and cursing the trade they have adopted."

Natural evaporation of mercury is the major source of atmospheric pollution. Cinnabar, i.e., mercury sulfide, has been used since ancient times as a pigment and constitutes the most important mercury ore. Inorganic mercury in the aquatic environment tends to sediment, where certain microorganisms are able to methylate mercury, possibly as a means of detoxication. The methylmercury generated then accumulates in fish, particularly in fatty species at the higher trophic levels. Particularly high methylmercury concentrations are reached by marine carnivores. Increased human exposures therefore occur in individuals frequently eating fish; the highest exposures are seen in the arctic where meat from marine carnivores are included in the diet.[26]

Mercury is used for a variety of instruments, including thermometers, manometers, polarographs, and electrical equipment. Mercury is also used for the production of fluorescent light tubes, as a catalyst in chemical industry, including the production of chlorine, and in amalgams for dentistry practice. Mercury may evaporate at room temperature, and the rate depends on the surface area, temperature, and the ventilation. Thus increased amounts will evaporate if mercury is scattered on the floor as small droplets. The amount that evaporates at 40°C is four times the amount that evaporates at 20°C. At saturation, the air at 20°C contains 15 mg/m^3, which is more than 100 times the occupational exposure limit.

Inorganic mercury compounds are used for the production of certain pharmaceuticals, including mercurous bromide, certain inorganic pesticides, and antifouling agents for marine paints, and various other purposes, such as treatment of felt for hats.

Organomercury compounds contain a covalent bond between mercury and carbon, and the organic part of the molecule is often an alkyl group or an alkoxialkyl group. The former compounds are more toxic, because they are more easily absorbed and more slowly metabolized. Organomercury compounds are used as a fungicide on seed grain. Methyl mercury was extensively used for this purpose in the past, until environmental effects were discovered, and now methoxymethyl mercury is the compound preferred. The paper and pulp industry has previously used these compounds as antislime agents.

The various uses of mercury and mercury compounds result in occupational exposures in a range of occupations. Also, the industrial use of mercury may lead to releases to the environment, in particular through sewage water.[27] Localized problems relating to contamination of river systems and bays have been caused by such contamination from chloralkaline plants, paper and pulp industries, and pesticide factories. In Japan, Minamata Bay became severely contaminated from a factory that used methyl mercury as a catalyst in the production of vinyl chloride.

Inhalation of metallic mercury results in an almost complete absorption of the vapors in the alveoli. Small amounts are released from dental amalgam fillings, especially from those in the molar teeth that are subjected to the highest pressures during chewing. However, only negligible absorption of the metal takes place in the gastrointestinal tract, unless some is retained, e.g., in diverticula or appendix.

Inorganic mercury compounds from aerosols may be absorbed through the lungs as well, and some absorption (about 5 to 10 percent) also takes place in the gastrointestinal tract. A higher absorption rate has been demonstrated in newborn rats, but data on humans is lacking. The organomercury compounds are also absorbed when taken in by this route, methyl mercury almost completely.[26] Occupational exposures are frequently of a mixed type, and absorption patterns may therefore vary.

In the blood, inorganic mercury is almost evenly distributed between plasma and erythrocytes, while about 90 percent of organomercury compounds are bound to the cells. Mercury vapor and methyl mercury are lipophilic and may pass biological membranes, including the blood-brain barrier and placenta, and result in considerable deposition in the central nervous system and the fetus, respectively. The vapor dissolved in the blood and tissues rapidly becomes oxidized. Mercuric ions become bound to some extent to metallothionein and accumulate in the kidneys. Excretion takes place mainly through feces and urine, but significant amounts may be eliminated in sweat. The presence of ethanol in the blood influences the equilibrium between dissolved mercury vapor and mercury ions. Thus, after ethanol ingestion, mercury vapor may be detected in the expired air in individuals with high levels of mercuric ions in the blood. When selenium is present in the blood, a complex is formed that results in a longer half-life but also decreased toxicity, as judged from animal experiments. Methyl mercury is slowly metabolized in the liver and is excreted partly as inorganic mercury in the feces.

Effects

Acute poisoning with mercury vapor may cause a severe airway irritation, chemical pneumonitis, and pulmonary edema in severe cases. Ingestion of inorganic compounds results in symptoms of gastrointestinal corrosion and irritation, such as vomiting, bloody diarrhea, and stomach pains. Subsequently, shock and acute kidney dysfunction with uremia may ensue. Cutaneous exposure to mercury compounds may result in local irritation, and mercury compounds are among the most common allergens in patients with contact dermatitis.

Chronic intoxication may develop a few weeks after the onset of a mercury exposure, more commonly if the exposure has lasted for several months or years. The symptoms depend on the degree of exposure and the kind of mercury in question. The symptoms may involve the oral cavity, the nervous system, and the kidneys.

Severe exposure to inorganic mercury causes an inflammation of gingiva and oral mucosa, which become tender and bleed easily. Salivation is increased, most obviously so in subacute cases. Often the patient complains of a metallic taste in the mouth. Especially when oral hygiene is bad, a grey border is formed on the gingival edges.

Mercury may damage both the peripheral and the central nervous system. In exposures to mercury vapor, the central nervous system is the critical organ, and the classic triad of symptoms includes erethism, intention tremor, and the gingivitis described above. The fine intention tremor of fingers, eyelids, lips, and tongue may progress to spasms of arms and legs. A jerky micrographia is typical as well. The changes in the central nervous system result in psychological effects known as erethism: restlessness, irritability, insomnia, concentration difficulties, decreased memory, and depression, sometimes in combination with shyness, unusual psychological vulnerability, anxiety, and total neglect concerning economic problems and daily needs. Newer studies suggest that early stages of erethism may occur, and this psychoasthenic-vegetative syndrome has been dubbed "micromercurialism" by Russian authors. The main problem here appears to be decreased memory, and headache, dizziness, and irritability may also be part of the picture. Similar nonspecific symptoms are described by patients who attribute their ill health to mercury from their dental fillings. Although slight adverse effects are difficult to rule out in susceptible subjects, little evidence is available to support this notion.[28]

Nephrotoxic effects include proximal tubular damage, as indicated by an increased excretion of small proteins in the urine, e.g., β_2-microglobulin. Glomerular damage seems to be caused by an autoimmune reaction to mercury complexes in the basal membrane, and mercury-related cases of nephrotic syndrome have been traced to this pathogenesis.

In children, a different syndrome is seen, the so-called "pink-disease" or acrodynia, diagnosed most frequently in children treated with teething powders that contained calomel and also occasionally seen in children who had inhaled mercury vapor, e.g., from broken thermometers.[29] A generalized eruption develops, and the hands and feet show a characteristic, scaly, reddish appearance. In addition, the children are irritable, sleep badly, fail to thrive, sweat profusely, and have photophobia. This condition was extremely common until 30 years ago, when the etiology was finally found and teething powders were phased out.

Intoxications with alkoxialkyl or aryl compounds are similar to intoxications with inorganic mercury compounds, because these organomercurials are relatively unstable. Alkyl mercury compounds, such as methyl mercury, result in a different syndrome. The earliest symptoms in adults are paresthesias in the fingers, the tongue, and the face, particularly around the mouth. Later on, disturbances occur in the motor functions, resulting in ataxia and dysphasia. The visual field is decreased, and in severe cases the result may be total blindness. Similarly impaired hearing may progress to complete deafness. This syndrome has been caused by methyl mercury–contaminated fish in Japan and by methyl mercury–treated grain used for baking or animal feed in Iraq and elsewhere. Children are more susceptible to the toxic effects of methyl mercury than are adults, and congenital methyl mercury poisoning may result in a cerebral palsy syndrome, even though the mother remains healthy or suffers only minor symptoms due to the exposure.[30] In various populations with a high consumption of large marine fish or marine mammals, methyl mercury intakes may approach the levels that resulted in such serious disease in Japan and Iraq. While, no clear-cut cases of intoxication have been reported in these populations, delays in cognitive development in children may occur.

Sufficient evidence exists that methyl mercury chloride is carcinogenic to experimental animals. In the absence of comprehensive epidemiological data, methyl mercury is considered a possible human carcinogen (class 2B).[12]

Prevention

Biological monitoring is useful in the diagnosis of mercury exposure and in the control of occupational exposure levels. In the blood, inorganic mercury has a half-life of about 30 days, and methyl mercury has a half-life of about twice as long. Unfortunately, blood levels do not reflect mercury retained in the brain where mercury after vapor inhalation has a half-life of several years. Urine levels are usually preferred as an indicator of occupational exposures. Long-term mercury vapor exposures should respect a time-weighted average limit of 25 μg/m^3 and a corresponding urinary mercury excretion limit of 50 μg/g creatinine (28 μmol/mol creatinine). Induction of minimal tremor by mercury vapor has been reported at urinary excretion levels of 50 μg/L (0.25 μmol/L) and above. With regard to methyl mercury, the earliest effects, such as paresthesias, appear to occur when blood concentrations are above 200 μg/L (1 μmol/L), but an uncertainty factor of perhaps 10 should be applied to take into account possible individual susceptibility and the increased vulnerability of the fetus. Methyl mercury is incorporated in hair, and hair mercury analyses have proved useful for screening and reliable as indicators of individual exposures. Methyl mercury toxicity has been seen at hair levels above 50 μg/g (0.25 μmol/g). WHO recommends that hair mercury concentrations be kept below 10 to 20 ppm (0.05 to 0.10 μmol/g) to protect the fetus. Using an uncertainty factor of 10, the U.S. EPA recommends a Reference Dose corresponding to 1.1 ppm.

Preventive measures should include the limitation of mercury released from industrial operations to the environment. Important nonindustrial sources are discarded batteries (for cameras and watches) and thermometers. Some countries have instituted a practice of collecting and recycling the mercury from such consumer products. If mercury is used for fungicidal treatment of grain, the grain should be dyed red to indicate that it is unsuitable for human consumption. Mercury exposures from dental amalgam fillings should be minimized, but alternative restorative materials should be used only if their safety and durability are known to be superior to amalgam. Concentration limits have been proposed for various fish products, especially for tuna, swordfish, and shark. A level of 0.5 or 1.0 mg/kg is frequently used. A PTWI level has been recommended at 0.3 mg/week, of which no more than 0.2 mg/week may be methylmercury. The EPA Reference Dose is 0.1 μg/kg body weight per day.

The current occupational exposure limits are 0.1 mg/m^3 as a ceiling value for inorganic mercury and 0.01 mg/m^3 for organic (alkyl) mercury. NIOSH has recommended a time-weighted average limit for inorganic mercury at 0.05 mg/m^3.

▸ MOLYBDENUM

The largest deposit of molybdenite, the major molybdenum ore, is in Climax, Colorado. Most of the molybdenum consumption is used in alloys, but various compounds are also employed as catalyst and pigments. Considerable experimental evidence is available on the essential functions of molybdenum, but little information has been gathered on the toxic potentials. The human intake of this metal appears to be below 0.2 mg per day, unless significant contamination occurs. Absorption of molybdenum in food may be about 25 to 50 percent in humans, and excretion is mainly through the urine; the biological half-life in the blood is probably only a few hours, although some molybdenum may be retained in the liver and other tissues for a longer time. Molybdenum serves a constituent of three oxidases, including xanthine oxidase, but deficiency states have not been reported in humans. Molybdenum poisoning in livestock may produce "teart disease" with anemia, growth retardation, and bone abnormalities, especially if the copper intake is low. In humans, the frequent occurrence of arthralgias in some Armenian villages has been linked to the high intake of molybdenum, possibly via abnormalities of uric acid metabolism. Pulmonary fibrosis has been reported in experimental animals, and a few cases of pneumoconiosis have been seen in workers exposed to sparingly soluble forms of molybdenum. The current exposure limits are 5 mg/m^3 for soluble compounds and 15 mg/m^3 for insoluble molybdenum compounds, while the ACGIH limits are 5 mg/m^3 and 10 mg/m^3, respectively. A dietary intake of 0.15 to 0.5 mg of this metal per day has been recommended as safe and adequate for adults.

▸ NICKEL

Exposures

Nickel ores of sufficient quality occur only at a few places, notably at Sudbury, Ontario. Nickel is particularly used for alloys but also for surface treatment of metals, as a catalyst, in the electronics industry, and in the production of nickel-cadmium batteries. Nickel exposures occur in the production trades and the various user industries, e.g., when welding stainless steel. The nickel intake through food may average about 0.1 to 0.2 mg per day, but it varies considerably because high contents may be encountered in legumes, cereals, nuts, and chocolate. Nickel may leach to food and beverages from nickel-plated or nickel-containing kitchen utensils. Gastrointestinal absorption of nickel from food is about 1 percent, but absorption from an aqueous solution taken on an empty stomach may be about 25 percent.[31] Internal exposures may result from implantation of orthopedic prostheses and from intravenous infusion of nickel-contaminated solutions.

Effects

Nickel apparently has limited acute toxicity in humans, including airway irritation, and the important adverse effects relate to allergic eczema and respiratory cancers.[32] Nickel carbonyl may cause acute pulmonary disease and systemic toxicity.

Respiratory exposure to nickel compounds in nickel production plants results in an increased risk of nasal and respiratory cancer.[17] An increased respiratory cancer risk has also been seen in welders, but the contribution by nickel in welding fumes is unclear. Most respiratory cancers in refinery workers have been primary carcinoma of the lung, but nasal cancers may be 100-fold as frequent as otherwise expected.

Nickel allergy is the most frequent cause of contact eczema in women. The development of allergy is frequently provoked by earrings, but metal buttons, bracelets, and watches are frequent causes as well. More rarely, the primary allergy develops due to an occupational exposure. However, hand eczema often results as a consequence of exposures at work if nickel allergy is already present, as indicated, e.g., by earlobe dermatitis in the past. Some studies suggest that about 10 to 15 percent of women become allergic to nickel, and that almost half of them at some point develop hand eczema, in some cases so severe that the patient has to give up working. A much smaller proportion of the male population appears to be allergic to nickel. Nickel allergy is probably increasing worldwide in prevalence, and it most frequently develops during the teenage years. The hand eczema in a nickel-allergic patient may develop or progress as a result of increased nickel intake through food and beverages.[33] In addition, inhalation allergy has resulted in asthmatic symptoms in a few recorded cases.

Nickel carbonyl ($Ni(CO)_4$) is a liquid that can evaporate at room temperature. Nickel carbonyl is produced in the Mond refining process of nickel. In addition, it may be formed or used in other branches of industry, such as electronics, oil refining, and plastics. After an acute exposure, dyspnea, headache, dizziness, vomiting, and substernal and hypogastric pain may occur, followed by a virtually symptom-free interval of 12 to 36 hours. Severe pulmonary symptoms then develop, and physical examination suggests pneumonia. The intoxication can lead to cerebral toxicity and death within 3 to 10 days. Pulmonary cancer has been reported in animal experiments, but the epidemiological evidence is uncertain on this point.

Prevention

Exposure to soluble nickel compounds and nickel carbonyl, which is metabolized to form nickel ions and carbon monoxide, may be evaluated by analysis of nickel concentrations in plasma and urine. The biological half-life in the body and the release from particles retained in the lungs will depend on the solubility of the nickel compounds concerned. Nickel present in the blood seems to be cleared relatively rapidly by the kidneys, and animal experiments suggest a half-life of a few days. Limits for plasma levels must therefore depend on the nickel speciation in the exposure. Nickel levels in plasma are usually below 1 μg/L (17 nmol/L) in individuals without occupational exposures, at least when analysis of uncontaminated samples has been carried out by an experienced laboratory.

Limits for occupational exposure are 1 mg/m^3 for nickel metal and soluble nickel compounds, and 0.001 ppm for nickel carbonyl. The ACGIH limits are: 1 mg/m^3 for nickel metal, nickel sulfide roasting, fumes, and dust; 0.1 mg/m^3 for soluble compounds; and 0.05 ppm for nickel carbonyl. NIOSH has recommended that the permissible exposure limit for nickel be reduced to 0.015 mg/m^3.

Specific preventive measures apply with regard to nickel-induced contact dermatitis. Primary prevention would mean that nickel-containing or nickel-plated metals should not be used in products that come into contact with the skin. Unfortunately, current fashions and the usefulness of nickel in cheap alloys (including coinage metal) seem to strongly oppose such measures. Contact with such products should be limited, if not totally avoided, in patients who have already developed allergy toward nickel. Many dermatologists have experienced some success in advising their patients to refrain from eating oatmeal, legumes, nuts, and chocolate and from using nickel-plated kitchen utensils. Beverages should not be ingested on an empty stomach. Some countries have enacted legislation concerning the acceptable degree of nickel release from metal objects that may come into contact with the skin. The degree of nickel leaching from white metal objects may be determined by Fisher's test (dimethylglyoxime and ammonium hydroxide), which enables the allergic patient to identify and discard objects that could provoke an outbreak of dermatitis.

► OSMIUM

Environmental exposures are of limited significance, but the information on kinetics in the human body is incomplete. Of main interest is osmium tetroxide (osmic acid), which is used for various laboratory purposes, mainly as a fixative for tissue sections. The highly volatile osmium tetroxide may also be formed by oxidation of the finely divided metal. Inhalation of osmium tetroxide causes immediate irritation of the mucous membranes with cough and shortness of breath. These symptoms may last for several hours after a short exposure. Osmium tetroxide also has corrosive effects on the eyes, as indicated by severe irritation and lacrimation. After these symptoms have ceased, the patient may see large halos around lights until the tissue damage has been completely repaired. Skin contact results in irritant dermatitis. Repeated respiratory exposures have allegedly caused headache, insomnia, chronic airway irritation, and gastrointestinal disturbance. The permissible limit for occupational exposures to osmium tetroxide is 0.002 mg/m^3.

► PLATINUM

Platinum is used in jewelry, in dentistry, and in chemical and electrical industries. Platinum compounds are employed in electroplating, in photography, and as a catalyst in the petroleum and pharmaceutical industries. Exposures to hexachloroplatinic acid and platinum tetrachloride are most frequent. When inhaled, the platinum compounds may cause upper airway irritation with violent sneezing, dyspnea, wheezing, and even cyanosis. Platinum rhinorrhea and platinum asthma are more typical clinical pictures that fade away shortly after the worker has left work for the day, and skin contact with chlorinated platinum salts may result in a scaly erythema, sometimes urticaria, and mostly only on hands and forearms.[34] These allergic manifestations have been called platinosis. Long-term effects, such as lung fibrosis, are unlikely, but a worker with a past history of platinosis may not be able to work with platinum again without suffering a severe reaction to minute amounts of platinum salts in the atmosphere. Some platinum compounds, notably *cis*-diamino-dichloroplatinum (*cis*-platin), inhibit cell growth in tumors and have therefore been used as cytostatic agents, especially for testicular cancer. Environmental exposures result from industrial emissions and from the use of catalytic converters on automobile exhaust systems. Platinum is employed as a catalyst in catalytic converters on cars, and about 1 μg of the metal is lost per kilometer of driving with a pellet-type catalyst; much lower losses have been measured from the newer monolith-type catalysts. The limit for occupational exposures is 0.002 mg/m^3 for soluble platinum salts, and ACGIH has adopted a limit of 1 mg/m^3 for platinum metal. Limited information exists concerning biological monitoring, but platinum allergy can be diagnosed by specific IgE antibodies.

► RARE EARTHS

The rare earths or lanthanons constitute a group of metals that include lanthanum and the following 14 elements of the periodic system.

Most extensively used are cerium and lanthanum. Major uses include steel alloys, lighter flints, catalysts, and additives in glass manufacture. Mischmetal is an unseparated mixture of rate earths and yttrium. Various prognoses suggest that these metals will experience a rapidly increasing demand, particularly for production of alloys. Thus exposure potentials may change in the future. So far, few problems have been discovered as a result of occupational exposure. A small number of reports have described cases of benign pneumoconiosis related to rare earth exposures, and similar conditions have been produced in animal experiments. Subcutaneous implantation of some rare earths have caused granulomas. Gastrointestinal absorption is limited and possibly negligible. Experiments with laboratory animals have documented toxic effects on several organ systems, especially fatty liver degeneration, blocking of the reticuloendothelial system, and interference with calcium metabolism. Due to the pyrophoric effects, rare earths may cause thermal burns and eye injuries. Although the limited information available suggests that these metals belong among the relatively less toxic ones, the increasing use and the scarcity of data should inspire additional studies and considerable caution in the handling of rare earth. Yttrium, which is often dealt with as a rare earths, has an exposure limit of 1 mg/m^3.

► SELENIUM

Selenium is often referred to as a metalloid, although it shares some chemical properties with sulfur. Selenium is usually a by-product obtained from primary copper production. This element has found considerable use in semiconductor technology and other electronic applications, in photocopy machines, as pigments in paints and glass, as an ingredient in certain alloys, in antidandruff shampoos, and several other applications. Perhaps the most intensive exposures occur in sulfide ore refineries, but harmful exposures may also result when selenium-containing rectifiers are overloaded or when scrap metal is melted. Environmental selenium exposures vary geographically, with average daily intakes through the diet varying from a low 30 to 50 μg in Scandinavia, Egypt, and New Zealand to a high of about 300 μg in Venezuela. Increased levels may occur due to emissions from coal combustion and manufacturing industries, but geological factors are generally most important. Some plants concentrate selenium and may contain concentrations up to several thousand parts per million.

Effects of selenium used to be a concern mainly with regard to domestic animals. Acute poisoning ("blind staggers") and chronic toxicity ("alkali disease") have been known in livestock for over 50 years. Later, selenium deficiency was discovered as the cause of white muscle disease in ruminants, hepatosis diatetica in swine, and exudative diathesis in chickens.

Soluble selenium compounds are almost completely absorbed from the gastrointestinal tract. Absorption through the skin may occur as well. The selenium concentrations in blood and urine seem to reflect recent absorption. Part of the selenium in the blood is associated with a glutathione peroxidase, and the activity of this enzyme is associated with the selenium levels. Selenium compounds are metabolized in the liver, in part by reduction and methylation. Dimethylselenide is an intermediary metabolite that is exhaled when the formation of this compound at high exposures exceeds the further formation of trimethylselenonium ions, which are excreted in the urine. The kinetics depend on the absorption level and perhaps on individual differences and on interfering substances, such as arsenic, cadmium, and mercury.

Inhalation of selenium results in mucous membrane irritation, gastrointestinal symptoms, increased body temperature, headache, and malaise. Garlicky breath from dimethylselenide is frequently present. This symptom was already noted by the housekeeper of Berzelius, who discovered this element. In fact most of the systemic toxicity may be due to the liberation of this metabolite from the liver. Selenium dioxide forms caustic selenous acid in contact with water and is therefore highly irritant and may produce burns and pulmonary edema. The nail beds become tender, deformed nails develop, and skin, teeth, and hair may be dyed red from precipitation of amorphous selenium. Hydrogen selenide is more toxic than hydrogen sulfide; immediate symptoms are related to the irritant properties. Seleniferous food has been related to vague symptoms, but lack of proper reference groups and other deficiencies hamper the interpretation of the data.

Selenium deficiency is of increasing relevance. Keshan disease, an endemic, juvenile cardiomyopathy in China, occurs in selenium-low areas, and successful treatment of a large number of patients has apparently been achieved by selenium supplements. Low selenium intakes may predispose to the development of cancer and arteriosclerosis. In addition, clinical improvement has been recorded in other groups of patients, including some on parenteral nutrition and some with lipidoses of the central nervous system. However, much needs to be discovered in these areas before conclusions concerning minimal daily intakes can be made, although a daily intake of 0.05 to 0.2 mg is currently recommended.

Monitoring of urine levels, which should be kept below 0.1 mg/L, and perhaps analysis of exhaled air for dimethylselenide, could be considered. The occupational exposure limit is 0.2 mg/m^3 for selenium and its inorganic compounds and 0.05 ppm for selenium hexafluoride, an airway irritant. In Finland, where the dietary intake of selenium was among the lowest in the world, selenium is now added to fertilizers to increase the selenium concentration of agricultural products.

► SILVER

Major uses of silver in the past, such as jewelry, silverware, and photographic emulsions, still continue to be important, but a range of other applications have increased the demand due to developments in coatings and alloy technology. Silver solder is also in use, although the adverse effects related to the cadmium content have necessitated a change of ingredients. Argyria is a bluish discoloration of the skin due to deposition of silver metal particles. A localized form is due to penetration of particles through the stratum corneum, but generalized argyria is due to absorption of silver compounds into the body. Argyrosis of the respiratory tract has been diagnosed by bronchoscopy, but ocular argyrosis, especially as evidenced by conjunctival discoloration, may be more easily detected. These signs occur as a result of occupational exposures but may also be caused by oral or dermal pharmaceuticals containing silver; they appear to be relatively benign. The current exposure limit is 0.01 mg/m^3 for silver metal and soluble silver compounds, but ACGIH has recommended a limit of 0.1 mg/m^3 for silver metal.

► TANTALUM

Tantalum is increasingly used in alloys for electronic equipment and applications in the nuclear and aerospace industries. Additional uses include surgical prostheses and additives in glass manufacture. This metal has caused few health problems due to occupational exposures. To date, animal experiments suggest that airway irritation and pneumonitis may result from inhalation of tantalum dusts, and sequelae in the form of emphysema, slight fibrosis, and epithelial hyperplasia have been recorded. The current occupational exposure limit is 5 mg/m^3.

► TELLURIUM

This element is similar to selenium and occurs as an impurity of various metal ores. It is used in various alloys and for rubber compounding. Tellurium causes garlicky breath at a lower exposure level than does selenium. Not surprisingly, some workers from an electronic company were referred to the late Dr. Harriet L. Hardy with the chief complaint that their wives refused to kiss them. This symptom disappears in about a week after selenium exposure but is longer lasting when due to tellurium. In addition, the latter also causes dry mouth and inhibits sweating. The exposure limit is 0.1 mg/m^3, but for the irritant tellurium hexafluoride, it is 0.02 ppm or 0.2 mg/m^3.

▸ THALLIUM

Past uses included thallium as a therapeutic agent against syphilis, dysentery, and other diseases, as well as a depilatory agent, and as a rodenticide or insecticide. Thallium has important uses in various industrial processes, including the fabrication of phosphorescent pigments and glassware, and as a catalyst in organic synthesis. Environmental thallium pollution occurs near mines and refineries because zinc, cadmium, and copper ores usually contain thallium. Cement production and coal burning also cause thallium emissions. Most environmental effects have been due to extensive application of thallium rodenticides in the past.[35]

Thallium compounds are without taste and odor, and lethal doses may be less than 1 g. Absorption through the skin has led to several cases of intoxication, and gastrointestinal absorption is almost complete. Many poisonings were related to the easy access in the past to thallium pesticides. The acute gastrointestinal effects are followed, within a few days, by peripheral neuropathy with muscle weakness and "burning feet syndrome." The associated mental disturbances include irritability, concentration difficulties, and somnolence. Hair loss (alopecia) occurs about 1 to 3 weeks after the acute exposure. Thus, the characteristic triad, gastroenteritis, polyneuropathy, and hair loss, is seen only at a rather late stage of the intoxication. In survivors of severe poisoning, some nervous system damage may remain after recovery. Inhalation of thallium-containing dust at work over longer time periods may be associated with vague symptoms of joint pains, anorexia, fatigue, trembling, and with partial hair loss and polyneuropathy.

Excretion is mainly via the gastrointestinal tract and the kidney. Urine levels of thallium may remain high for several weeks, although plasma concentrations have decreased. A biological half-life of a couple of weeks seems to apply to humans. A slow excretion takes place through hair and nails, which may provide a profile of recent thallium levels in the body. The limit for occupational exposure to soluble thallium compounds is 0.1 mg/m^3.

▸ TIN

Tin has been used for many centuries in brass and pewter, and current uses also include tin plating, which consumes about half of the total tin production, tin foil, collapsible tubes, and pipes. Cans for food products are often plated with tin on the inner side, and leaching may be considerable to acid contents, especially if the can is left open for a few days. The dietary intake of tin is variable, although mostly about 1 to 4 mg per day. A large number of organotin compounds are in use, e.g., dioctyltin as a stabilizer in PVC, triorganotins as pesticides, in particular fungicides and antifouling agents, and in various compounds as catalysts.

Ingestion of 50 mg of tin results in vomiting, but gastrointestinal absorption in only a few percent. Organotin compounds are more easily absorbed, also through the skin. Tin may be an essential element in some species, perhaps including humans. Inhalation of tin dust is usually not a matter of major concern. However, a benign pneumoconiosis, called stannosis, has been described, where pulmonary function abnormalities are minor, if detectable at all.

The organotin compounds, including dialkyl and trialkyl compounds, are strong skin irritants. The systemic toxicity in experimental animals has been studied in some detail; the neurotoxic potential is higher in trialkyltins than in dialkyltins, and it decreases with the length of the alkyl chains. Some compounds may be immunotoxic, and endocrine disruption in some marine organisms has been related to organotin pollution levels. More than 200 human cases of poisoning, half of them fatal, were described after the application of an ointment containing organotin compounds (mainly diethyltin) against staphylococcal infections. The symptoms included headache, vomiting, dizziness, visual disturbances, convulsions, and paresis.

The limit for occupational exposure is 2 mg/m^3, and for organotin compounds is 0.1 mg/m^3. Biological monitoring seems to be of limited use, although urinary tin excretion may be worth studying more closely. In the preventive measures, eye protection and prevention of skin contact with organotin compounds should be included.

▸ TITANIUM

Titanium dioxide pigment constitutes the major part of titanium uses. It is used in paints, paper coatings, pharmaceuticals, bread flour, etc., due to its extreme whiteness and high index for refraction. Titanium tetrachloride may be encountered as an intermediate and as a catalyst, the carbide is a component of "hard metal," and titanium metal is alloyed with other metals. The daily intake, mainly through food, may be up to a few milligrams, depending on local point sources and the content of titanium dioxide additives in food items, such as bread and cheese. Occupational exposures mainly concern the metal and the dioxide, which appear to be rather nontoxic.[36] Findings of obstructive lung disease, pulmonary fibrosis, and airway irritation in titanium-exposed workers deserve to be further explored. Titanium tetrachloride is strongly irritant, because acid is liberated in contact with water, and pulmonary edema may result. Systemic toxicity is known from experimental toxicology but is probably of little significance in environmental health, because titanium is poorly absorbed from the gastrointestinal tract. Titanocene, an organotitanium compound, has been found carcinogenic when injected into rodents. Also, titanium phosphate, a fibrous material, may possess important biological activities. The consumption of this metal is rapidly increasing, and additional studies of its health significance would be warranted. Titanium dioxide is regarded a nuisance dust with an exposure limit of 15 mg/m^3, while ACGIH has adopted a limit of 10 mg/m^3. NIOSH regards this compound as a potential carcinogen, although the International Agency for Research on Cancer (IARC) was unable to classify it.[36]

▸ TUNGSTEN

Tungsten (or wolfram) is present in the environment in small quantities. Major exposures are associated with the primary production of tungsten and with the manufacture of tungsten carbide for hard metal products. Although a considerable fraction of soluble tungsten compounds are absorbed in the gut, urinary excretion is rapid. Systemic toxicity has been produced in laboratory animal experiments but appears to be of little relevance to human exposure situations. Pulmonary disease has been documented from the manufacture of cemented carbide tools, but the adverse effects are probably caused by cobalt, and any contribution from tungsten exposures is difficult to assess. The ACGIH limits are 1 mg/m^3 for tungsten and soluble compounds and 5 mg/m^3 for insoluble compounds. NIOSH has recommended similar limits.

▸ URANIUM

Uranium is a radioactive metal that may cause serious chemical toxicity. Most natural uranium is ^{238}U, which has a half-life of almost 5 billion years. It is extracted from ores that may contain less than 1 percent of the metal. The main use is as fuel in nuclear power plants, but small amounts are used as pigments and catalysts. Gastrointestinal absorption varies with solubility, and human studies would suggest that perhaps 20 percent of uranium from food is absorbed. Tetravalent uranium is oxidized in the organism to hexavalent ions, which are excreted through the glomeruli. At low pH, uranyl ions (UO_2^{2+}) will be reabsorbed in the tubuli, where they may cause cell damage or necrosis. Less-soluble uranium compounds from respiratory exposures will tend to accumulate in the lungs. Such accumulation, especially if the uranium is enriched with ^{235}U, would tend to cause health effects associated with the alpha-radiation. However, the excess cancer risk in uranium miners seems to be mainly due to radon gas and radon progeny. Uranium may sometimes occur in drinking water, and such contamination has been linked to excess excretion of β_2-microglobulin in the urine as an indication of early tubulus dysfunction. The drinking-water standard is 5 mg/L. The standard for occupational exposure to uranium and insoluble compounds is 0.25 mg/m^3, and for soluble compounds is 0.05 mg/m^3, while ACGIH has recommended 0.2 mg/m^3 for all uranium.

▶ VANADIUM

Vanadium is frequently used in various alloys, frequently in the form of ferrovanadium, which accounts for the majority of vanadium consumption. Vanadium oxides are important catalysts in the inorganic and organic chemical industries, and other vanadium compounds are used in the electronics, ceramics, glass, and pigment industries. Occupational exposure to vanadium may also occur at primary production of other metals when the ores contain considerable amounts of vanadium; certain qualities of oil contain much vanadium, and unexpected exposures may occur when servicing burners and filters.

The daily intake through food is frequently below 0.1 mg, and gastrointestinal absorption may be less than 1 percent. Vanadium is an essential element for chickens and rats, but the possible essentiality to humans has not been determined. Environmental exposures have not been reported to cause significant toxicity.

Pentavalent vanadium compounds are more toxic than are the tetravalent compounds. Vanadium pentoxide (V_2O_5) dust and fume result in conjunctivitis, rhinitis, and other irritation of the mucous membranes, and in severe cases, in dyspnea and chemical pneumonitis. Some workers may become particularly sensitive to these actions, while others seem to show some adaptation. Vanadium-induced cough may be particularly bothersome, since it lasts for several days. Chronic bronchitis has been recorded as an apparent long-lasting effect following long-term exposures. Animal studies have indicated that vanadium could induce systemic effects, such as fatty degeneration of liver and kidneys, polycythemia, and cardiotoxicity at high doses. In humans, a lowering of serum cholesterol levels has been demonstrated as well as a reduction of cystine incorporation in fingernails. After oral intake of vanadium, records indicate that the tongue may be covered by a green layer.

Vanadium is efficiently excreted via the urine, and about one-half of the absorbed amount is excreted within the first 1 to 2 days, but the existence of a slower compartment with a half-life of about several weeks has been suggested. Analysis of urine samples for vanadium may be useful to indicate the acute exposure levels, and levels below 0.5 mg/L (10 nmol/L) are believed to reflect safe exposures. The ceiling limits for occupational exposures to vanadium pentoxide are 0.5 mg/m^3 for dust and 0.1 mg/m^3 for fume, while NIOSH has recommended a limit of 0.05 mg/m^3 for both.

▶ ZINC

Zinc is a common and essential metal with a low toxic potential. This metal is added to bronze, brass, and various other alloys to add corrosion resistance, and it is used for galvanizing steel and other iron products. In the presence of carbon dioxide and humidity, a surface film of alkaline zinc carbonate is formed, which protects against corrosion. Various zinc compounds are used in the chemical, ceramic, pigment, plastic, rubber, and fertilizer industries, and most frequently used are zinc oxide, carbonate, sulfate, chloride, and some organic compounds. The most significant occupational exposures occur during alloy founding, galvanizing, zinc smelting, and welding, especially of galvanized metals.

The daily intake of zinc varies considerably, seafood and meat being high in zinc, but typically ranges from 10 to 15 mg. Also, soft drinking water may contain high concentrations of zinc leached from the water pipes. The average oral intake is several milligrams. The gastrointestinal absorption is difficult to evaluate, because the major excretion route is via the gut. Also, the absorption of zinc may vary with the speciation and the presence of phytate, calcium, phosphate, and vitamin D. Under normal circumstances, the absorption is probably about 25 to 50 percent while under zinc deficiency the absorption may approach 100 percent.

Zinc is an essential metal, and more than 20 zinc-dependent enzymes have been identified. Zinc deficiency in children has resulted in endocrine disturbances with retarded growth and delayed puberty. This condition may be completely cured when zinc therapy is instituted. Acrodermatitis enterohepatica, a rare familial skin disease, has been found to be related to deficient zinc absorption. In addition, recent research has suggested that zinc supplements may be beneficial in certain dermatological conditions and in accelerating wound healing in surgical patients. Zinc also seems to somewhat protect against cadmium toxicity. However, in the occupational setting, the latter metal is a frequent impurity in zinc and may result in serious adverse effects.

Oral zinc poisoning has occurred in a few instances due to zinc release from galvanized food containers. Symptoms included nausea, vomiting, stomach pains, and diarrhea.

Inhalation of high concentrations of zinc oxide may cause metal fume fever, a condition that may also be caused by freshly formed oxides of several other metals, including copper, magnesium, manganese, and nickel. This condition is also referred to by other names, such as metal shakes or zinc chills. The metal oxide particles tend to aggregate after their formation and would then be unable to pass through to the lungs as easily; therefore only the freshly formed particles cause the disease. A few hours after the exposure, the first symptoms may be slight feeling of malaise, dry cough and sore throat, and a sweetish, metallic taste in the mouth. Six to 8 hours later, the patient develops an influenza-like syndrome with chills, muscle pains, headache, and medium-grade fever, then follows sweating and recovery. Blood tests show leukocytosis, increased sedimentation rate, and lactate dehydrogenase. Depending on the extent of the exposure, the total attack usually lasts less than 24 hours, and the patient usually returns to work the next morning. Many workers have experienced repeated, almost weekly spells of metal fume fever, and chronic damage could conceivably occur. However, this question is difficult to address, and no evidence currently suggests that repeated attacks of metal fume fever leave sequelae. In fact the patient develops a temporary resistance after each spell, and metal fume fever is therefore most seen on Mondays, which accounts for the name, Monday morning fever.

Zinc chloride has been in extensive use as a flux in soldering. In contact with water, hydrochloric acid is liberated, and the result is painful burns. Zinc chloride is also used in smoke bombs, and inhalation of the fume has caused corrosive effects in the airways with pulmonary edema and, in the survivors, bronchopneumonia.

Biological monitoring is yet of dubious value, since the serum zinc concentrations seem well regulated, and the urine represents only a minor part of the total amount excreted.

Metal fume fever seems to be caused by zinc fume levels of 15 mg/m^3, but insufficient information is available on exposures below that level. The exposure limit for zinc oxide is 5 mg/m^3, but NIOSH has recommended an additional ceiling limit of 15 mg/m^3 be respected. The standard for zinc chloride fume is 1 mg/m^3. With regard to the beneficial effects, recommended values for daily requirements are 15 mg for adults, 20 mg for pregnant women, and 25 mg for lactating women.

▶ ZIRCONIUM

Zirconium uses are rather limited, with major consumptions being glass and ceramics production, shielding materials for nuclear power plants, and some alloys. The meager evidence contains no well-documented case of zirconium toxicity in industry. However, use of deodorants containing this metal have induced subcutaneous granulomata, possibly due to hypersensitivity. The exposure limit is 5 mg/m^3.

▶ REFERENCES

1. Nieboer E, Richardson DHS. The replacement of the nondescript term "heavy metals" by a biological and chemically significant classification of metal ions. Environ Pollut (Ser B) 1:3–26, 1980
2. Elinder C-G, Friberg L, Kjellström T, Nordberg G, Oeberdoerster G. Biological monitoring of metals. Geneva: World Health Organization, 1994 (May be obtained free of charge from Office of Global and Integrated Environmental Health, World Health Organization, 1211 Geneva 27, Switzerland.)
3. Berton G (ed): Handbook of Metal-Ligand Interactions in Biological Fluids. Bioinorganic Medicine. New York: Marcel Dekker, 1995, vols 1–2
4. Clarkson TW, Friberg L, Nordberg GF, Sager PR (eds): Biological Monitoring of Toxic Metals. New York: Plenum Press, 1988
5. Friberg L, Nordberg GF, Vouk VB: Handbook on the Toxicology of Metals. 2nd ed. Amsterdam: Elsevier, 1996
6. de Broe ME, Coburn JW (eds): Aluminum and Renal Failure. Dordrecht: Kluwer, 1990
7. Wills MR, Savory J: Aluminum poisoning: dialysis encephalopathy, osteomalacia, and anaemia. Lancet 2:29–34, 1983
8. Criteria for Recommended Standard: Occupational Exposure to Antimony. DHEW (NIOSH) Publication No. 78-216. Cincinnati: National Institute for Occupational Safety and Health, 1978
9. Bates MN, Smith AH, Hopenhayn-Rich C: Arsenic ingestion and internal cancers: a review. Am J Epidemiol 135:462–476, 1992
10. International Programme on Chemical Safety: Barium. Environmental Health Criteria 107. Geneva: World Health Organization, 1990
11. International Programme on Chemical Safety: Beryllium. Environmental Health Criteria 106. Geneva: World Health Organization, 1990
12. International Agency for Research on Cancer: Beryllium, cadmium, mercury, and exposures in the glass manufacturing industry. Monographs on the Evaluation of Carcinogenic Risks to Humans. Lyon: Agency for Research on Cancer, 1993, vol 38
13. International Programme on Chemical Safety: Cadmium. Environmental Health Criteria 134. Geneva: World Health Organization, 1992
14. Buchet J-P, Lauwerys R, Roels H, Bernard A, Bruaux P, Claeys F, et al. Renal effects of cadmium body burden of the general population. Lancet 336:699–702, 1990
15. WHO Study Group: Recommended Health-Based Limits in Occupational Exposure to Heavy Metals. Technical Report Series 647. Geneva: World Health Organization, 1980
16. Langård S (ed): Biological and Environmental Aspects of Chromium. Amsterdam: Elsevier Biomedical, 1982
17. International Agency for Research on Cancer: Chromium, nickel and welding. Monographs on the Evaluation of Carcinogenic Risks to Humans. Lyon: Agency for Research on Cancer, 1988, vol 47
18. Criteria for controlling occupational exposure to cobalt. DHHS (NIOSH) Publication No. 82-107. Cincinnati: National Institute for Occupational Safety and Health, 1982
19. Alexander CS: Cobalt-beer cardiomyopathy. Am J Med 53:395–417, 1972
20. International Programme on Chemical Safety: Inorganic Lead. Environmental Health Criteria 165. Geneva: World Health Organization, 1995
21. Needleman HL, Gatsonis CA: Low-level lead exposure and the IQ of children. JAMA 263:673–678, 1990
22. Preventing Lead Poisoning in Young Children. A Statement by the Centers for Disease Control. Atlanta: U.S. Department of Health and Human Services, 1991
23. Grandjean P (ed): Biological Effects of Organolead Compounds. Boca Raton, FL: CRC Press, 1984
24. Durlach J, Durlach V, Bac P, Bara M, Guiet-Bara A: Magnesium and therapeutics. Magnes Res 7:313–328, 1994
25. Krieger D, Krieger S, Jansen O, Gass P, Theilmann L, Lichtnecker H: Manganese and chronic hepatic encephalopathy. Lancet 346:270–274, 1995
26. International Programme on Chemical Safety: Methylmercury. Environmental Health Criteria 101. Geneva: World Health Organization, 1990
27. International Programme on Chemical Safety: Inorganic Mercury. Environmental Health Criteria 118. Geneva: World Health Organization, 1991
28. Friberg LT, Schrauzer GN (eds): Status quo and perspectives of amalgam and other dental materials. Stuttgart: Georg Thieme, 1995
29. Agocs MM, Etzel RA, Parrish RG, Paschal DC, Campagna PR, Cohen DS, Kilbourne EM, Hesse JL: Mercury exposure from interior latex paint. N Engl J Med 323:1096–1101, 1990
30. Davis LE, Kornfeld M, Mooney HS, et al: Methylmercury poisoning: long-term clinical, radiological, toxicological, and pathological studies of an affected family. Ann Neurol 35:680–688, 1994
31. Sunderman FW Jr, Hopfer SM, Sweeney KR, Marcus AH, Most BM, Creason J: Nickel absorption and kinetics in human volunteers. Proc Soc Exp Biol Med 191:5–11, 1989
32. International Programme on Chemical Safety: Nickel. Environmental Health Criteria 108. Geneva: World Health Organization, 1991
33. Nielsen GD, Jepsen LV, Jørgensen PJ, Grandjean P, Brandrup F: Nickel-sensitive patients with vesicular hand eczema: oral challenge with a diet naturally high in nickel. Br J Dermatol 122:299–308, 1990
34. International Programme on Chemical Safety: Platinum. Environmental Health Criteria 125. Geneva: World Health Organization, 1991
35. International Programme on Chemical Safety: Thallium. Environmental Health Criteria 182. Geneva: World Health Organization, 1996
36. International Agency for Research on Cancer: Some Organic Solvents, Resin Monomers and Related Compounds, Pigments and Occupational Exposures in Paint Manufacture and Painting. Monographs on the Evaluation of Carcinogenic Risks to Humans. Lyon: Agency for Research on Cancer, 1989, vol 47

23

Diseases Associated with Exposure to Chemical Substances

Organic Compounds

Stephen M. Levin • Ruth Lilis

▶ ORGANIC SOLVENTS

Organic solvents are comprised of a large group of compounds (alcohols, ketones, ethers, esters, glycols, aldehydes, aliphatic and aromatic saturated and nonsaturated hydrocarbons, halogenated hydrocarbons, carbon disulfide, etc.) with a variety of chemical structures. Their common characteristic, related to their widespread use in many industrial processes, is the ability to dissolve and readily disperse fats, oils, waxes, paints, pigments, varnishes, rubber, and many other materials.[1,2]

Solvent exposure affects many persons outside industrial and occupational settings. The use of solvents in household products and in arts, crafts, and hobbies has significantly increased the population that may be affected by repeated exposure. Moreover, the deliberate inhalation of solvents as a form of addiction ("sniffing") occurs, especially in younger population groups.

Some solvents are well known for their specific toxic effects on the liver, kidney, and bone marrow,[3] and a few organic solvents have specific toxicity for the nervous system. Carbon disulfide may induce a severe toxic encephalopathy with acute psychosis;[3] methyl alcohol may induce optic neuritis and atrophy; methyl chloride and methyl bromide may cause severe acute, even fatal, toxic encephalopathy. Exposures to *n*-hexane, methyl-*n*-butyl ketone,[4–6] and carbon disulfide have produced peripheral neuropathy.

Most organic solvents share some common nonspecific toxic effects, the most important of which are those on the central nervous system (CNS). The depressant narcotic effects of organic solvents have long been recognized; numerous members of this heterogeneous group of chemical compounds have been used as inhalation anesthetics (chloroform, ethyl ether, trichloroethylene, etc.).

The sequence of stages of anesthesia achieved with volatile solvents is of interest: the cerebral cortex is affected first, the lower centers of reflex activity in the brainstem and medulla oblongata, which control vital cardiovascular and respiratory functions, are the last to be depressed. This characteristic sequence makes it possible to use volatile anesthetic compounds for medical purposes. The earliest manifestations of the anesthetic effects of solvents are slight disturbances in psychomotor coordination. These may progress to more pronounced incoordination and, if exposure continues, through an excitation stage of longer or shorter duration, to loss of consciousness.

Occupational exposure to solvents may reproduce the entire sequence of medical anesthesia, up to loss of consciousness and even death through paralysis of vital cardiovascular and respiratory centers. While such severe cases of occupational solvent poisoning are relatively uncommon under normal conditions, they may occur with unexpected accidental overexposure.

The initial manifestations of CNS depression are frequent in workers handling solvents or mixtures of solvents in various industrial processes. A low boiling point, with generation of significant airborne concentrations of vapor, large surfaces from which evaporation may take place, lack of appropriate enclosure and/or exhaust ventilation systems, relatively high temperature of the work environment, and physical exercise required by the actual work performed (increasing the ventilatory volume per minute and thus the amount of solvent vapor absorbed) may all contribute to uptake of sufficient solvent to induce prenarcotic CNS symptoms.

Early prenarcotic effects are dizziness, nausea, headache, slight incoordination, paresthesia, increased perspiration, tachycardia, and hot flushes. These symptoms are mostly subjective and transitory, and their causal relationship with solvent exposure has therefore often been overlooked. The transitory nature of prenarcotic symptoms is due to the common characteristics of the metabolic model for solvents: once exposure ceases after the end of the work shift, the body burden of solvents is usually rapidly depleted, mostly eliminated through exhalation. The prenarcotic symptoms subside as the concentration of solvent in blood and in the CNS decreases.

With exposure to higher concentrations or with longer exposure, more marked incoordination and a subjective feeling of drunkenness may occur. The risk of accidents is increased, even with early prenarcotic symptoms and more so with more pronounced symptoms.

While acute overexposure of higher magnitude with loss of consciousness is generally accepted as a serious condition (with possible persistent aftereffects, including neurological deficit), the long-term effect of repeated episodes of slight prenarcotic symptoms has remained unexplored until relatively recently, although it had been recognized that such symptoms are an expression of functional changes in some cortical neurons.

It had been suspected for some time that repeated functional change may lead to permanent impairment of neuronal functions, and various possible mechanisms had been considered, including interference with cell membrane or neurotransmitter functions or even neuronal loss. Since no regeneration of neurons occurs, neuronal loss can result in permanent, irreversible neurological damage. The diffuse nature of such effects and the lack of major, well-localized neurological deficits have contributed to the relatively slow recognition of chronic, irreversible solvent-induced neurological impairment.

Repeated exposure to organic solvents may result in the gradual development of persistent symptoms, such as headache, tiredness, fatigue, irritability, memory impairment, diminished intellectual capacity, difficulty in concentration, emotional instability, depression, sleep disturbances, alcohol intolerance, loss of libido and/or potency. These symptoms, often reported by workers with repeated solvent exposure and mentioned in many studies on chronic effects of solvents, had received relatively little attention until relatively recently, probably because of their nonspecific nature. Nevertheless, the term *toxic encephalosis* was proposed as early as 1947.[7] More recently, the term *psycho-organic syndrome* has been used for this cluster of symptoms related to long-term solvent exposure. Effects on the CNS, including the diencephalic centers of the autonomic system with their interrelationships with endocrine functions, are probably important components in the development of the syndrome.

Over the last two decades, chronic neurotoxicity of solvents related to long-term exposure has received increasing attention. Research has been particularly active in the Scandinavian countries. Epidemiological studies of exposed workers and control groups have significantly contributed to recognition of the association between the psycho-organic syndrome and exposure to solvents; neurobehavioral and electrophysiologic methods, including electroencephalographic, visual evoked potential, and nystagmographic investigations, have added objective, quantitative measures for the assessment of CNS functions.

In case-control studies,[8] neuropsychiatric disease has been found to occur more frequently among solvent-exposed workers than in age-matched controls. In a large study in Denmark, in which solvent-exposed painters were compared with nonexposed bricklayers,[9] the painters had a relative risk of 3.5 for disability due to cryptogenic presenile dementia. With modern methods of investigation and brain imaging, including computed tomographic (CT) scan magnetic resonance imaging (MRI), and cerebral blood flow studies, diffuse cerebral cortical atrophy has been demonstrated in cases of chronic solvent poisoning.[10–12]

Thus recent studies converge to indicate that long-term exposure to solvents may lead to chronic, irreversible brain damage. The clinical expression is that of intellectual impairment and decrements in performance, which can be detected by means of neurobehavioral testing; electroencephalographic abnormalities are frequent and characterized mostly by a diffuse low wave pattern. The underlying pathological changes are represented by cortical atrophy; these changes can be of varying severity, with extreme cases of severe diffuse cerebral and cerebellar cortex atrophy in chronic poisoning due to solvent sniffing addiction.[11,13]

The axons and myelin sheaths may also be affected by organic solvents. This is well known for peripheral nerves, and peripheral neuropathy has been well documented with exposure to such solvents as carbon disulfide, methyl-*n*-butyl ketone, and *n*-hexane. Specific CNS effects are also known to occur with carbon disulfide. Other solvents capable of producing peripheral neuropathy such as *n*-hexane and methyl-*n*-butyl ketone have an effect on both long and short axons, and axonal degeneration of fibers in the anterior and lateral columns of the spinal cord, cerebellar vermix, spinocerebellar tracts, optic tracts, and tracts in the hypothalamus can also occur.[6]

▶ ALIPHATIC HYDROCARBONS

Aliphatic hydrocarbons are mostly derived from petroleum by distillation or cracking; their chemical structure is relatively simple, since they are linear carbon chains of various lengths with a certain number of hydrogen atoms attached. They are either saturated (alkanes or paraffins) or unsaturated (alkenes or olefins, with one or several double bonds) and alkynes or acetylenes, with one or more triple bonds.

The aliphatic hydrocarbons occur in mixtures that have numerous industrial uses: natural gas; heating fuel; jet fuel; gasoline; solvents for a variety of materials such as pigments, dyes, inks, pesticides, herbicides, resins, and plastic materials; in degreasing and cleaning; in the extraction of natural oils from seeds; and increasingly as raw material for the synthesis of numerous compounds in the chemical industry.

Compounds with a low number of carbon atoms are gases (methane, ethane, propane, butane). Compounds with a higher number of carbon atoms (up to eight) are highly volatile liquids at room temperature, whereas those with longer carbon chains have higher boiling temperatures and usually do not generate dangerous air concentrations. Compounds with more than 16 carbon atoms are solids. The only adverse effect attributed to the lower members of the group is the indirect one they might exert when present in high concentrations, displacing oxygen.

Toxic effects of *paraffins* (alkanes) are significant for the highly volatile liquid compounds from pentane through octane. These compounds are potent depressants of the CNS, and overexposure may result in deep anesthesia with loss of consciousness, convulsions, and death. Such high levels of exposure are infrequent under usual circumstances, but they may occur accidentally. Moderate irritation of mucous membranes of the airways and conjunctivae is a common but less severe effect; defatting of the skin might contribute to dermatitis, with repeated contact. Aspiration of liquid mixtures of aliphatic hydrocarbons into the airways or accidental ingestion of such liquids usually results in chemical pneumonitis, often severe and necrotizing.

n-Hexane exposure may result in toxic peripheral neuropathy, affecting both the sensory and motor components of peripheral nerves, initially in the lower extremities, but eventually, with longer exposure, also in the upper extremities. Paresthesia, numbness, and tingling progressing from distal to proximal, distal hypoesthesia (touch, pain), followed by muscle weakness due to motor deficit, with difficulty in walking and eventual muscular atrophy, and diminished or absent deep tendon reflexes are the characteristic clinical findings. Electromyographic abnormalities indicating peripheral nerve lesions, including abnormal fibrillation patterns and significant decreases in nerve conduction velocities (sensory and motor) are usually detected. Axonal degeneration and secondary demyelination have been found to be the underlying pathological abnormalities. Abnormalities in visual, auditory, and somatosensory evoked potentials have been reported after experimental *n*-hexane exposure; longer latencies and central conduction times were interpreted as reflecting neurotoxic effects at the level of the cerebrum, brainstem, and spinal cord.[14]

n-Hexane peripheral neuropathy, first described by Japanese investigators[15] in 1969, has since been repeatedly reported from various European countries and the United States. It has also been reproduced in animal experiments at concentrations as low as 250 ppm. Outbreaks of toxic peripheral neuropathy due to *n*-hexane have continued to be reported. Such cases have occurred in press proofing workers in Taiwan, associated with exposure to a solvent mixture with a high (60 percent) *n*-hexane content. The outbreak of peripheral neuropathy cases had been preceded by a gradual change (to a high *n*-hexane content) in the solvent mixture used to clean rollers of press proofing machines.[16] In an offset printing plant with 56 workers, 20 (36 percent) developed symptomatic peripheral neuropathy due to exposure to *n*-hexane. Optic neuropathy and CNS involvement were uncommon and autonomic neuropathy was not encountered.[17]

Cases of *n*-hexane subacute, predominantly motor, peripheral neuropathy have also been reported in young adults and in children after several months of glue sniffing. Although functional improvement after discontinuation of toxic exposure has been reported, in some cases full recovery has not been observed, even after long-term (16 years) follow-up.[18–20] Experiments involving exposure of rats to high concentrations of *n*-hexane have revealed adverse effects on the seminiferous epithelium; repeated exposures resulted in severe, irreversible testicular lesions.[21] The main *n*-hexane metabolites are 2-hexanol and 2,5-hexanedione. *n*-Hexane is metabolized to the γ-diketone 2,5-hexanedione (2,5-HD), a derivative that covalently binds to lysine residues in neurofilament proteins (NF) to yield 2,5-dimethylpyrrole adducts. Pyrrolylation is an absolute requirement in neuropathogenesis.[22] Effects of chronic exposure to *n*-hexane on some nerve-specific marker proteins in rats' central and peripheral nervous systems were studied after high exposure (2,000 ppm *n*-hexane for 24 weeks). The level of neuron-specific enolase (NSE), creatine kinase-B (CK-B), and beta-S100 protein decreased significantly in the distal sciatic nerve, while the markers remained unchanged in the CNS.[23] *n*-Hexane accumulates in adipose tissue, where it persists longer (estimated half-life, 64 hours); complete elimination from fat tissue after cessation of exposure has been estimated to require at least 10 days.[24]

In humans chronically exposed to a mixture of hexane isomers with concentrations ranging from 10 to 140 ppm, the urinary 2,5-hexanedione excretion ranged from 0.4 to 21.7 mg/L.[25] Urinary concentrations of 2,5-hexanedione in subjects not exposed to *n*-hexane or related hydrocarbons were found to range from 0.12 to 0.78 mg/L.[26] The urinary 2,5-hexanedione excretion reaches its highest level 4 to 7 hours after the end of exposure.[27] Biological monitoring to assess worker exposure to toxic chemicals has gained increasing recognition, especially for occupations characterized by highly variable exposure levels. The American Conference of Government Industrial Hygenists has recommended biological exposure indices (BEIs—levels of a biological indicator after an 8-hour exposure to the current threshold limit value) for a limited number of widely used chemicals; *n*-hexane is one of these. 2,5-Hexanedione was found to be significantly correlated with a score of electroneuromyographic abnormalities. There is general agreement that, for practical purposes, the urinary concentrations of 2,5-hexanedione can predict the likelihood of subclinical peripheral neuropathy in persons exposed to *n*-hexane.[28] 4,5-Dihydroxy-2-hexanone as a metabolite of *n*-hexane has recently been identified in rats and in humans; it is excreted in amounts that at times exceed those of 2,5-hexanedione. It has been suggested that this metabolite indicates a route of detoxification.[29] While there is no definitive evidence that other aliphatic hydrocarbons, such as pentane, heptane, or octane, have similar effects, some case reports suggest an association. In inhalation exposure of rats to *n*-hexane vapors at 900, 3,000, and 9,000 ppm, reproductive parameters were unaffected over two generations.[30] The potential of commercial hexane to produce chromosome aberrations was evaluated in vitro and in vivo. No increase in chromosome aberrations was observed in either test system.[31]

Commercial hexane that had been used in industrial processes where workers had peripheral neuropathy was found to contain 2-methyl pentane, 3-methyl pentane, and methyl cyclopentane, in addition to *n*-hexane. The neurotoxicity of these compounds has been tested in rats, and significant effects on peripheral nerves of a similar type but of lesser magnitude than those of *n*-hexane were detected. The order of neurotoxicity was found to be *n*-hexane > methyl cyclopentane > 2-methyl pentane = 3-methyl pentane.[32]

Other solvent mixtures, such as one containing 80 percent pentane, 5 percent hexane, and 14 percent heptane, have produced cases of peripheral neuropathy in humans. White spirit mixtures containing more than 10 percent *n*-nonane have been shown by neurophysiological and morphological criteria to produce axonopathy in rats after 6 weeks of daily exposure. Since the various members of the group are most often used in mixtures, a time-weighted average (TWA) of 100 ppm (350 mg/m^3) has been proposed.[3]

Peripheral neuropathy similar to that associated with hexane has been found to result from exposure to methyl *n*-butyl ketone. DiVincenzo et al.[33] identified the metabolites of *n*-hexane and of methyl *n*-butyl ketone; the similarity of chemical structure between the metabolites of these two neurotoxic agents suggested the possibility of a common mechanism in the very similar peripheral neuropathy.

n-hexane	methyl *n*-butyl ketone
↓	↓
2-hexanol	5-hydroxy-2-hexanone
↓	↓
2,5-hexanediol	2,5-hexanedione

It is now well established that 2,5-hexanedione is the most toxic metabolite. The biochemical mechanism of 2,5-hexanedione neurotoxicity is related to its covalent binding to lysine residues in neurofilament protein and cyclization to pyrroles. Pyrrole oxidation and subsequent protein cross-linking then lead to the accumulation of neurofilaments in axonal swellings, the histopathologic earmark of γ-diketone peripheral neuropathy. Massive accumulation of neurofilaments has been shown to occur within the axoplasm of peripheral and some central nervous system fibers.[34]

Ethyl-*n*-butyl ketone (EBK, 3-heptanone) administered in relatively high doses for 14 weeks by gavage produced a typical central peripheral distal axonopathy in rats, with giant axonal swelling and hyperplasia of neurofilaments. Methyl-ethyl ketone (MEK) potentiated the neurotoxicity of EBK and increased the urinary excretion of two neurotoxic γ-diketones, 2,5-heptanedione and 2,5-hexanedione. The neurotoxicity of EBK seems to be due to its metabolites, 2,5-heptanedione and 2,5-hexanedione.

Methyl-ethyl ketone is a widely used industrial solvent to which there is considerable human exposure. The potential to cause developmental toxicity was tested in mice. Mild developmental toxicity was observed after exposure to 3,000 ppm, which resulted in reduction of fetal body weight. There was no significant increase in the incidence of any single malformation, but several malformations not observed in the concurrent control group were found at a low incidence: cleft palate, fused ribs, missing vertebrae, and syndactyly.[35] MEK potentiates EBK neurotoxicity by inducing the metabolism of EBK to its neurotoxic metabolites.

Commercial-grade methyl-heptyl ketone (MHK, 5-methyl-2-octanone) also produced toxic neuropathy in rats, clinically and morphologically identical to that resulting from *n*-hexane, methyl-*n*-butyl ketone (MBK), and 2,5-hexanedione. The MHK mixture was found by gas chromatography-mass spectrometry to contain 5-nonanone (12 percent), MBK (0.8 percent) and C_7-C_{10} ketones and alkanes (15 percent), besides 5-methyl-2-octanone. Purified 5-nonanone produced clinical neuropathy, whereas purified 5-methyl-2-octanone was not neurotoxic; given together with 5-nonanone, it potentiated the neurotoxic effect. In vivo conversion of 5-nonanone to 2,5-nonanedione was demonstrated.[36] The toxicity of 5-nonanone was shown to be enhanced by simultaneous exposure to MEK. This effect is attributed to the microsomal enzyme-inducing properties of MEK. The neurotoxicity of methyl-*n*-butyl ketone has been shown to be enhanced by other aliphatic monoketones, such as methyl-ethyl ketone, methyl-*n*-propyl ketone, methyl-*n*-amyl ketone, and methyl-*n*-hexyl ketone; the longer the carbon chain of the aliphatic monoketone, the stronger the potentiating effect on methyl-*n*-butyl ketone neurotoxicity.[37]

Neuropathological studies have shown that the susceptibility of nerve fibers to linear aliphatic hydrocarbons and ketones is proportional to fiber length and the diameter of the axon. Fibers in the peripheral and central nervous systems undergo axonal degeneration, with shorter and smaller fibers generally being affected later. The long ascending and descending tracts of the spinal cord and the spinocerebellar and the optic tracts can be affected. Giant axonal swelling, axonal transport malfunction, and secondary demyelination are characteristic features of this central peripheral distal axonopathy.

The unsaturated *olefins* (with one or more double bonds), such as ethylene, propylene, and butylene, and the diolefins, such as 1,3-butadiene and 2-methyl-1,3-butadiene, mainly obtained through cracking of crude oil, are of importance as raw materials for the manufacture of polymers, resins, plastic materials, and synthetic rubber. Their narcotic effect is more potent than that of the corresponding saturated linear hydrocarbons, and they have moderate irritant effects.

1,3-Butadiene, a colorless, flammable gas, is a by-product of the manufacture of ethylene; it can also be produced by dehydrogenation of *n*-butane and *n*-butene. Major uses of 1,3-butadiene are in the manufacture of styrene-butadiene rubber, polybutadiene rubber, and neoprene rubber; acrylonitrile-butadiene-styrene resins; methyl methacrylate-butadiene-styrene resins; and other copolymers and resins. It is also used in the production of rocket fuel. In studies of chronic 1,3-butadiene inhalation, malignant tumors developed at multiple sites in rats and mice, including mammary carcinomas and uterine sarcomas in rats and hemangiosarcomas, malignant lymphomas, and carcinomas of the lung in mice.[38] Other important effects were atrophy of the ovaries and testes. Ovarian lesions produced in mice exposed by inhalation to 1,3-butadiene included loss of follicles, atrophy, and tumors (predominantly benign, but also malignant granulosa cell tumors).[39] A macrocytic megaloblastic anemia, indicating bone marrow toxicity, was also found in inhalation experiments on mice.[40]

Epidemiological studies on occupational groups exposed to 1,3-butadiene in the manufacture of styrene-butadiene rubber were conducted. The results in some studies were inconclusive, most probably because of the relatively short period of observation from onset of exposure and the relatively small number of workers in the cohorts. The standardized mortality ratio for non-Hodgkin's lymphoma was found to be increased in a large cohort of employees at a butadiene-production facility. There were, nevertheless, no clear exposure group or latency period relationships.[41] 1,3-Butadiene is metabolized to 1,2-epoxy-3-butene. This metabolite has been shown to be carcinogenic in skin-painting experiments on mice. 1,3-Butadiene has been found to be mutagenic in in vitro tests on *Salmonella* and genotoxic to mouse bone marrow in vitro in the sister chromatid exchange test. A second metabolite of 1,3-butadiene is 1,2,3,4-diepoxybutane, also shown to be genotoxic in various test systems in vitro.[42] Binding of ^{14}C-labeled 1,3-butadiene to liver DNA was demonstrated in mice and rats.[43] The International Agency for Research on Cancer concluded in 1986 that the evidence of a carcinogenic effect of 1,3-butadiene in humans is inadequate, but that there is sufficient evidence of carcinogenic potential in experimental animals to consider a carcinogenic risk in humans.[44]

The National Institute for Occupational Safety and Health (NIOSH) has recommended that the present Occupational Safety and Health Administration (OSHA) standard of 1,000 ppm TWA for 1,3-butadiene be reexamined, since carcinogenic effects in rodents (mice) have been observed at exposure levels of 650 ppm. To minimize the carcinogenic risk for humans, it was recommended that exposures be reduced to the lowest possible level.

Isoprene (2-methyl-1,3-butadiene), a naturally occurring volatile compound and close chemical relative of 1,3-butadiene, has been studied in inhalation experiments on rats. A mutagenic metabolite, isoprene diepoxide, was tentatively identified in all tissues examined.[45]

The principal member of the series of aliphatic hydrocarbons with triple bonds—*alkynes*—is acetylene (HCCH), a gas at normal temperature. Acetylene is widely used for welding, brazing, metal buffing, metallizing, and other similar processes in metallurgy. It is also a very important raw material for the chemical synthesis of plastic materials, synthetic rubber, vinyl chloride, vinyl acetate, vinyl ether, acrylonitrile, acrylates, trichloroethylene, acetone, acetaldehyde, and many others.

While the narcotic effect of acetylene is relatively low and becomes manifest only at high concentrations (15 percent) not found under normal circumstances, the frequent presence of impurities in acetylene represents the major hazard. Phosphine is the most common impurity in acetylene, but arsine and hydrogen sulfide may also be present. The hazard is especially significant in acetylene-producing facilities or when acetylene is used in confined, poorly ventilated areas.

▶ ALICYCLIC HYDROCARBONS

Alicyclic hydrocarbons are saturated (cycloalkanes, cycloparaffins, or naphthenes) or unsaturated cyclic hydrocarbons, with one or more double bonds (cycloalkenes or cycloolefins). The most important members of the group are cyclopropane, cyclopentane, methylcyclopentane, cyclohexane, methylcyclohexane ethylcyclohexane, cyclohexene, cyclopentadiene, and cyclohexadiene. These compounds are present in crude oil and its distillation products.

Cyclopropane is used as an anesthetic. Most of the members of the group are used as solvents and, in the chemical industry, in the manufacture of a variety of other organic compounds, including adipic, maleic, and other organic acids; methylcyclohexane is a good solvent for cellulose ethers. Their toxic effects are similar to those of their linear counterparts, the aliphatic hydrocarbons, but they have more marked narcotic effects; the irritant effect on skin and mucosae is similar.

▶ COMMERCIAL MIXTURES OF PETROLEUM SOLVENTS

Mixtures of hydrocarbons obtained through distillation and cracking of crude oil are gasoline, petroleum ether, rubber solvent, petroleum naphtha, mineral spirits, Stoddart solvent, kerosene, and jet fuels. These are all widely used commercial products.

The composition of these mixtures is variable: all contain aliphatic saturated and nonsaturated hydrocarbons, alicyclic saturated and nonsaturated hydrocarbons, and smaller amounts of aromatic hydrocarbons such as benzene, toluene, xylene, and polycyclic hydrocarbons; the proportion of these components varies. The boiling temperature varies from 30 to 60°C for petroleum ether to 175 to 325°C for kerosene; the hazard of overexposure is higher with the more volatile mixtures with lower boiling temperatures.

The toxic effects of these commercial mixtures of hydrocarbons are similar to those of the individual hydrocarbons: the higher the proportion of volatile hydrocarbons in the mixture, the greater the hazard of acute CNS depression, with possible loss of consciousness, coma, and death resulting from acute overexposure. Exposure to high concentrations, when not lethal, is usually followed by complete recovery. Nevertheless, irreversible brain damage may occur, especially after prolonged coma. The underlying pathologic change is represented by focal microhemorrhages. The irritant effects on the respiratory and conjunctival mucosae are generally moderate.

Exposure to lower concentrations over longer periods is common; the potential effects of aromatic hydrocarbons, especially benzene, have to be considered under such circumstances. Bone marrow depression with resulting low red blood cell counts and leukopenia with neutropenia and/or low platelet counts can develop, and medical surveillance should include periodic blood counts for the early detection of such effects; cessation of exposure to mixtures containing aromatic hydrocarbons is necessary when such abnormalities occur. Long-term effects of benzene exposure include increased risk of leukemia; therefore, exposure should be carefully monitored and controlled so that the recommended standard for benzene not be exceeded.

Chronic effects on the central and peripheral nervous systems with exposure to commercial mixtures of hydrocarbons have received more attention only in recent years. Since some of the common components of such mixtures have been shown to produce peripheral neuropathy and to induce similar degenerative changes of axons in the CNS, such effects might also result from exposure to mixtures of hydrocarbons. Long-term exposure to solvents, including commercial mixtures of hydrocarbons, has been associated, in some cases, with chronic, possibly irreversible CNS impairment. Such effects have been documented by clinical, electrophysiological, neurobehavioral, and brain-imaging techniques.

Accidental ingestion and aspiration of gasoline or other mixtures of hydrocarbons can occur, mainly during siphoning, and result in severe chemical pneumonitis, with pulmonary edema, hemorrhage, and necrosis.

Gasoline and other hydrocarbon mixtures used as engine fuel have a variety of additives to enhance desired characteristics. Lead tetraethyl probably has the highest toxicity. Workers employed in the manufacture of this additive and in mixing it with gasoline have the highest risk of exposure, and their protection has to be extremely thorough. Ethylene dibromide (EDB) is another additive with important toxicological effects which has received increased attention recently.

Skin irritation, related to the defatting properties of these solvents, and consequent increased susceptibility to infections, is frequent when there is repeated contact with such mixtures of hydrocarbons or with individual compounds. Chronic dermatitis is a common finding in exposed workers; protective equipment and appropriate work practices are essential in its prevention.

Prevention and Surveillance

Exposure to airborne aliphatic hydrocarbons should be controlled to not exceed a concentration of 350 mg/m^3 as a time-weighted average. This concentration is equivalent to 120 ppm pentane, 100 ppm hexane, and 85 ppm heptane. For the commercial mixtures, a similar TWA has been recommended, except for petroleum ether (the most volatile mixture) for which a TWA of 200 mg/m^3 is recommended.[3] Exposure to benzene should not exceed the recommended standard of 1 ppm (3.2 mg/m^3), given the marked myelotoxicity of benzene and the increased incidence of leukemia. There is a definite need to monitor for the presence and amount of aromatic hydrocarbons in mixtures of petroleum solvents.

Medical surveillance programs should aim at the early detection of such adverse effects as toxic peripheral neuropathy, chronic CNS dysfunction, hematological effects, and dermatitis. Since accidental overexposure may result in rapid loss of consciousness and death (CNS depression), adequate and prompt therapy for such cases is urgent. Education of employees and supervisory personnel concerning potential health hazards, safe working practices (including respirator use when necessary), and first-aid procedures is essential.

▶ AROMATIC HYDROCARBONS

Aromatic hydrocarbons are characterized by a benzene ring in which the six carbon atoms are arranged as a hexagon, with a hydrogen atom attached to each carbon $-C_6H_6$. According to the number of benzene rings and their binding, the aromatic hydrocarbons are classified into three main groups:

1. Benzene and its derivatives: toluene, xylene, styrene, etc.
2. Polyphenyls: two or more noncondensed benzene rings—diphenyls, triphenyls
3. Polynuclear aromatic hydrocarbons: two or more condensed benzene rings—naphthalene, anthracene, phenanthrene, and the carcinogenic polycyclic hydrocarbons (benz[*a*]pyrene, methylcholanthrene, etc.)

Distillation of coal in the coking process was the original source of aromatic hydrocarbons; an increasing proportion is now derived from petroleum through distillation, dehydrogenation of cycloparaffins, and catalytic cyclization of paraffins.

Benzene

Benzene is a clear, colorless, volatile liquid with a characteristic odor; the relatively low boiling temperature (80°C) is related to the high volatility and the potential for rapidly increasing air concentrations.

Commercial-grade benzene contains variable amounts—up to 50 percent—of toluene, xylene, and other constituents that distill below 120°C. More important is that commercial grades of other aromatic hydrocarbons, toluene and xylene, also contain significant proportions of benzene (up to 15 percent for toluene); this also applies to commercial mixtures of petroleum distillates, such as gasoline and aromatic petroleum naphthas, where the proportion of benzene may reach 16 percent. Benzene exposure is therefore a more widespread problem than would be suggested by the number of employees categorized as handling benzene as such. Many others exposed to mixtures of hydrocarbons or commercial grades of toluene and xylene may also be exposed to significant concentrations of benzene.

Exposure to benzene may occur in the distillation of coal in the coking process; in oil refineries; and in the chemical, pharmaceutical, and pesticides industries, where benzene is widely used as a raw material for the synthesis of products. Exposure may also occur with its numerous uses as a solvent, in paints, lacquers, and glues; in the linoleum industry; for adhesives; in the extraction of alkaloids; in degreasing of natural and synthetic fibers and of metal parts; in the application and impregnation of insulating material; in rotogravure printing; in the spray application of lacquers and paints; and in laboratory extractions and chromatographic separations. An important use of benzene in some parts of the world is as an additive in motor fuel, including gasoline. In Europe, gasolines have been found to contain up to 5 percent benzene; in the United States levels up to 2 percent have been reported. Environmental levels of benzene in areas with intense automotive traffic have been found to range from 1 to 100 ppb. The largest amounts of benzene are used for the synthesis of other organic compounds, mostly in enclosed systems, where exposure is generally limited to equipment leakage, liquid transfer, and repair and maintenance operations. Exposures with the use of benzene as a solvent or solvent component present a more difficult problem, since enclosure of such processes and adequate control of airborne concentrations have not been easily achieved.

Production has continuously expanded. It is estimated that more than 2 million workers are exposed to benzene in the United States.[3] In recent years there has been increasing concern with respect to benzene in hazardous waste-disposal sites. Benzene has been found in almost one-third of the 1,177 National Priorities List hazardous waste sites. Other environmental sources of exposure include gasoline filling stations, vehicle exhaust fumes, underground gasoline storage tanks that leak, wastewater from industries that use benzene, and ground water next to landfills that contain benzene. Consumer products that contain benzene include glues, adhesives, some household cleaning products, paint strippers, some art supplies, and gasoline.

Inhalation of the vapor is the main route of absorption; skin penetration is of minor significance. Benzene retention is highest in lipid-rich organs. In adipose tissue and bone marrow, benzene concentrations may reach a level 20 times higher than the blood concentration; its persistence in these tissues is also much longer. Elimination is through the respiratory route (45 to 70 percent of the amount inhaled); the rest is excreted as urinary metabolites.

Benzene is metabolized in the liver by the mixed-function microsomal oxidases; the first intermediate in its biotransformation, benzene epoxide, is possibly the active substance responsible for the carcinogenic effect of benzene. The metabolites of benzene include phenol, catechol, hydroquinone, *p*-benzo-quinone, and *trans-trans*-mucondialdehyde. It has been shown that deoxyribonucleic acid (DNA) adducts (guanine nucleoside adducts) are formed by incubation of rabbit bone marrow with ^{14}C-labeled benzene; *p*-benzoquinone, phenol, hydroquinone, and 1,2,4-benzenetriol also form adducts with guanine.[46] The stromal macrophage that produces interleukin-1 (IL-1), a cytokine essential for hematopoiesis, is a target of benzene toxicity. Hydroquinone, a bone marrow toxin, inhibits the processing of pre-interleukin-1α (IL-1α) to the mature cytokine in bone marrow macrophages.[47]

The aromatic hydrocarbons (benzene, toluene, styrene, xylene, ethyl benzene) have been shown to inhibit the ATPase activities of (Na^+, K^+)-ATPase and Mg^{2+}-ATPase according to their lipid solubilities. This effect is probably important for the neurotoxic effects of these solvents.[48]

Benzene is metabolized to a series of phenolic and ring-opened products and their conjugates. Differences in measured hepatic P-450 (CYP) 2E1 activity may be an important factor in both interindividual and interspecies variations in hepatic metabolism of benzene. Both hydroquinone and catechol formation were found to be directly correlated to CYP 2E1 activity.[49] The mechanism of aplastic anemia appears to involve the concerted action of several metabolites acting together on early stem and progenitor cells, as well as on early blast cells, to inhibit maturation and amplification. Benzene and its metabolites do not function well as mutagens, but are highly clastogenic, producing chromosome aberrations, sister chromatid exchange, and micronuclei.[50]

Trans, trans-muconaldehyde (MUC), a six-carbon-diene-dialdehyde, is a microsomal, hematotoxic ring-opened metabolite of benzene. MUC is metabolized to compounds formed by oxidation and reduction of the aldehyde group(s). MUC and its aldehydic metabolites 6-hydroxy-*trans, trans*-2,4-hexadienal and 6-oxo-*trans, trans*-dexadienoic acid are mutagenic in that order of potency. The order of mutagenic activity correlates with reactivity toward glutathione, suggesting that alkylating potential is important in the genotoxicity of these compounds.[51]

The triphenolic metabolite of benzene 1,2,4-benzenetriol (BT) is readily oxidized to its corresponding quinone. During this process active oxygen species are formed that may damage DNA and other macromolecules. BT increases the frequency of micronuclei formation. BT also increases the level of 8-hydroxy-2′-deoxyguanosine (8-OH-dG), a marker of active oxygen-induced DNA damage. Thus BT can cause structural chromosomal changes and point mutations indirectly by generating oxygen radicals. BT may therefore play an important role in benzene-induced leukemia.[52] Catechol and hydroquinone were found to be highly potent in inducing sister chromatic exchange and delaying cell division; these effects were much more marked than those of benzene and phenol.[53]

Cytogenetic damage induced by benzene in mice was evaluated by determining the frequencies of chromosomal aberrations in bone marrow and spermatogonial cells. The clastogenic effect was dose-dependent in both cell types. The damage was greater in bone marrow than in spermatogonial cells.[54]

Exposure to high airborne concentrations of benzene results in CNS depression with acute, nonspecific, narcotic effects. With very high exposure (thousands of parts per million), loss of consciousness and depression of the respiratory center or myocardial sensitization to endogenous epinephrine with ventricular fibrillation may result in death. Recovery from acute benzene poisoning is usually complete if removal from exposure is prompt; in cases of prolonged coma (after longer exposure to high concentrations), diffuse or focal electroencephalographic (EEG) abnormalities have been observed for several months after recovery, together with such symptoms as dizziness, headache, fatigue, and sleep disturbances.

Chronic benzene poisoning is a more important risk, since it can occur with much lower exposure levels. It can develop insidiously over months or years, often without premonitory warning symptoms, and result in severe bone marrow depression. Benzene is a potent myelotoxic agent. Red blood cell, white blood cell, and platelet counts may initially increase, but more often anemia, leukopenia, and/or thrombocytopenia are found. The three cell lines are not necessarily affected to the same degree, and all possible combinations of hematological changes have been found in cases of chronic benzene poisoning. In some older reports, the earliest abnormalities have been described as reduction in the number of white blood cells (WBCs) and relative neutropenia; in later studies, lower than normal red blood cell (RBC) counts and macrocytosis with hyperchromic anemia have been found more often to be the initial hematologic abnormalities.[55,56] Thrombocytopenia has also been frequently reported.[57] The bone marrow may be hyperplastic or hypoplastic; in extreme cases, bone marrow failure with aplastic anemia may be seen.

Hematologic abnormalities detected in the peripheral blood do not always correlate with the pattern of bone marrow changes. Relatively minor deviations from normal in the blood count (RBCs, WBCs, or platelets) may coexist with marked bone marrow changes (hyperplastic or hypoplastic), and abnormalities are sometimes first found after cessation of exposure. Benzene-induced aplastic anemia can be fatal, with hemorrhage secondary to the marked thrombocytopenia and increased susceptibility to infections due to neutropenia. The number of reported cases of severe chronic benzene poisoning with aplastic anemia gradually decreased after World War II, because of better engineering controls, progressive reduction of the permissible exposure limits, and efforts to substitute less toxic solvents for benzene in numerous industrial processes. Suppression of cell growth and function in the lymphocytic line have also been shown to result from benzene exposure and to be correlated with the concentrations of benzene metabolites. The possibility that depressed immune system function might contribute to carcinogenesis has been raised.

Leukemia secondary to benzene exposure has been repeatedly reported since the 1930s. All types of leukemia have been found; myelogenous leukemia (chronic and acute) and erythroleukemia (Di Guglielmo's disease) apparently more frequently, but acute and chronic lymphocytic or lymphoblastic leukemia is represented as well. Malignant transformation of the bone marrow has been noted years after cessation of exposure, an added difficulty in the few epidemiological studies on long-term effects of benzene exposure. In Italy, with a large shoe-manufacturing industry, where benzene-based glues had been used for many years, at least 150 cases of benzene-related leukemia were known by 1976.[58] In Turkey more than 50 cases of aplastic anemia and 34 cases of leukemia have been reported from the shoe-manufacturing industry.[59] Epidemiological studies in the U.S. rubber industry have indicated a more than 3-fold increase in leukemia deaths; occupations with known solvent exposure (benzene widely used in the past and still a contaminant of solvents used) showed a significantly higher leukemia mortality than other occupations. Lymphatic leukemia showed the highest excess mortality. The risk of leukemia was much higher in workers exposed 5 years or more (standard mortality ratio (SMR) of 2100). Four additional cases of leukemia occurred among employees not encompassed by the definition of the cohort.[60] In Japan the incidence of leukemia among Hiroshima and Nagasaki survivors was found to be significantly increased by occupational benzene exposure in the years subsequent to the bomb.[61]

Chromosomal aberrations in lymphocytes of benzene-exposed workers have been well documented;[62] they were shown to persist even years after cessation of toxic exposure. The "stable" aberrations are more persistent and have been considered to be the origin of leukemic clones. Cytogenetic effects of benzene have been reproduced in animal models. In rats exposed to 1,000 and 100 ppm, a significant increase in the proportion of cells with chromosomal abnormalities was detected; exposure to 10 and 1 ppm resulted in elevated levels of cells with chromosomal abnormalities that showed evidence of being dose-related, although they were not statistically significant.[63] A significant increase in sister chromatic exchanges in bone marrow cells of mice exposed to 28 ppm benzene for 4 hours was also reported.[64]

Benzene is an established animal and human carcinogen. The modified base 8-hydroxydeoxyguanosine (8-OH-dG) is a sensitive marker of DNA damage due to hydroxyl radical attack at the C8 guanine. A biomonitoring study of 65 filling station attendants in Rome, Italy, found the urinary concentration of 8-OH-dG to be significantly correlated with benzene exposure calculated on the basis of repeated personal samples collected during 1 year.[65]

Toxic effects on reproductive organs have received increased attention. In subchronic inhalation studies, histopathological changes in the ovaries (characterized by bilateral cyst formation) and in the testes (atrophy and degenerative changes, including a decrease in the number of spermatozoa and an increase in abnormal sperm forms) have been reported.[66] Benzene was shown to be a transplacental genotoxicant in mice, where it was found to significantly increase micronuclei and sister chromatic exchange in fetal liver when administered at a high dose (1,318 mg/kg) to mice on days 14 and 15 of gestation.[67]

Experimental studies have demonstrated carcinogenic effects of benzene in experimental animals; in addition to leukemias,[68] benzene has produced in rodents significant increases in the incidence of Zymbal gland carcinomas, cancer of the oral cavity, hepatocarcinomas, and possibly mammary carcinomas and lymphoreticular neoplasias.[69] In experimental studies on mice, in addition to a high increase in leukemias, a significant increase in lymphomas was found.[70] The National Toxicology Program (NTP) conducted an oral administration experimental study in which malignant lymphoma and carcinomas in various organs, including skin, oral cavity, alveoli/bronchioli, and mammary gland in mice, and carcinomas of the skin, oral cavity, alveoli/bronchioli, and mammary gland in mice, and carcinomas of the skin, oral cavity, and Zymbal gland in rats were found with significantly increased incidence. Thus NTP concluded that there was clear evidence of carcinogenicity of benzene in rats and mice.[71] The Environmental Protection Agency (EPA) has come to the same conclusion.

The International Agency for Research on Cancer (IARC) has acknowledged the existence of limited evidence for chronic myeloid and chronic lymphocytic leukemia. In addition, it was noted that studies had suggested an increased risk of multiple myeloma,[72] while others indicate a dose-related increase in total lymphatic and hematopoietic neoplasms.

There is little information on developmental toxicity of benzene in humans. Case reports have documented that normal infants without chromosomal aberrations can be born to mothers with an increased number of chromosomal aberrations;[73] other investigators have reported increases in the frequency of sister chromatid exchanges and chromatid breaks in children of women exposed to benzene and other solvents during pregnancy. In animal experiments in vivo, benzene has not been found to be teratogenic; a decrease in fetal weight and an increase in skeletal variants have been associated with maternal toxicity.

The embryotoxicity of toluene, xylene, benzene, and styrene and its metabolite, styrene oxide, was evaluated using the in vitro culture of postimplantation rat embryos. Toluene, xylene, benzene, and styrene all have a concentration-dependent embryotoxic effect on the developing rat embryo in vitro at concentrations ranging from 1.00 μmol/mL for styrene, 1.56 μmol/mL for benzene, and 2.25 μmol/mL for toluene. There was no evidence of synergistic interaction among the solvents.[74]

Prevention and Control

Prevention of benzene poisoning and of malignant transformation of the bone marrow is based on engineering control of exposure. The threshold limit value (TLV) for benzene has been repeatedly reduced in the last several decades.[2,3] In 1987 the OSHA occupational exposure standard for benzene was revised to 1 ppm TWA, with a 5 ppm short-term exposure limit (STEL). NIOSH has recommended that the standard be revised to a TWA of 0.1 ppm, with a 15-minute ceiling value of 1 ppm.

Biological monitoring through measurements of urinary metabolites of benzene is useful as a complement to air sampling for the measurement of benzene concentrations. Elevation in the total urinary phenols (normal range 20 to 30 mg/L) indicates excessive benzene exposure, and 50 mg/L should not be exceeded. The urinary inorganic/total sulfate ratio may also be monitored. Biological monitoring is recommended at least quarterly but should be more frequent when exposure levels are equal to or higher than the TWA. Current methods of biological monitoring lack sensitivity at levels corresponding to inhalation exposures below 10 ppm. A urinary phenol level of 75 mg/L was found in one study to correspond to a TWA exposure to 10 ppm; in other studies the urinary phenol level corresponding to 10 ppm benzene was 45 to 50 mg/L.

Animal studies indicate that muconic acid is a metabolite of benzene that is excreted in urine as an increasing fraction of the total benzene metabolite with decreasing dose of benzene. Thus urinary muconic acid is potentially useful as a monitor for low levels of exposure to benzene. A gas chromatography-mass spectrometry assay was developed that detects muconic acid in urine of exposed workers at levels greater than 10 ng/mL.

Preplacement and periodic examinations should include a history of exposure to other myelotoxic chemical or physical agents or medications and of other hematologic conditions. A complete blood count, a mean corpuscular volume determination, reticulocyte and platelet counts, and the urinary phenol test are basic laboratory tests. The frequency of these examinations and tests should be related to the level of exposure.[3] Possible neurological and dermatological effects should also be considered in comprehensive periodic examinations. Adequate respirators should be available and should be used when spills, leakage, or other incidents of higher exposure occur.

In recent years the possibility of excessive benzene ingestion from contaminated water has received increasing attention. Benzene concentrations in water have been found to range from 0.005 ppb (in the Gulf of Mexico) to 330 ppb in contaminated well water in New York, New Jersey, and Connecticut. In 1985 the EPA proposed a maximum contamination level (MCL) for benzene in drinking water at 0.005 mg/L; this standard was promulgated in 1987.

Toluene

Toluene (methylbenzene, $C_6H_5CH_3$) is a clear, colorless liquid, with a higher boiling point (110°C) than benzene and therefore lower volatility. The production of toluene has increased markedly over the last several decades because of its use in numerous chemical synthesis processes, such as those of toluene diisocyanate, phenol, benzyl, and benzoyl derivatives, benzoic acid, toluene sulfonates, nitrotoluenes, vinyl toluene, and saccharin. Toluene is also used as a solvent, mostly for paints and coatings, and is often a component of mixtures of solvents. Technical grades of toluene contain benzene in variable proportions, reaching 25 percent in some products.

Hematological effects in workers exposed to toluene have been reported in the past.[1,2] Such effects were most probably due to the benzene content of toluene or to prior benzene exposure. Animal experiments indicate that pure toluene has no myelotoxic effects. Toluene has been shown to induce microsomal cytochrome P-450 and mixed-function oxidases in the liver. Toluene exposure induces P-450 isoenzymes CYP1A1/2, CYP2B1/2, CYP2E1, and CYP3A1, but decreases CYP2C11/6 and CYP2A1 in adult male rats. The inductive effect is more prominent in younger than in older animals and in males more than in females. Exposure to toluene does not influence pulmonary or renal microsomal P-450–related enzyme activity in rats.[75]

Exposure to toluene concentrations higher than 100 ppm results in CNS depression, with prenarcotic symptoms, and in moderate eye, throat, airway, and skin irritation. These effects are more pronounced with higher concentrations.

Volatile substance abuse has now been reported from most parts of the world, mainly among adolescents, individuals living in isolated communities, and in those who have ready access to such substances. Solvents from contact adhesives, cigarette lighter refills, aerosol propellants, gasoline, and fire extinguishers containing mostly halogenated hydrocarbons may be abused by sniffing. Euphoria, behavioral changes similar to those produced by ethanol, and hallucinations and delusions are the most frequent acute effects. Higher doses can result in convulsions and coma. Cardiac or central nervous system toxicity can lead to death. Chronic abuse of solvents can produce severe organ toxicity, mostly of the liver, kidney, and brain.[76]

Numerous reports on toluene addiction (sniffing) have indicated that irreversible neurological effects are possible. Severe multifocal CNS damage[77–79] with impairment in cognitive, cerebellar, brainstem, auditory, and pyramidal tract function has been well documented in glue sniffers. Diffuse electroencephalographic abnormalities are usually present. Cerebral and cerebellar atrophy have been demonstrated by CT scans of the brain; brainstem atrophy has also been reported.[79] Toluene exposure in rats (2,200 ppm 8 hours/day; 4,400 ppm, 30 minutes each hour, 8 hours/day; or 6,200 ppm, 15 minutes each hour, 8 hours/day) for 11 weeks, resulted in a persisting motor syndrome, with shortened and widened gait and widened landing foot splay, and hearing impairment. This motor syndrome resembles the syndrome (e.g., wide-based, ataxic gait) seen in some heavy abusers of toluene-containing products.[80]

Subchronic exposure of rats to toluene in low concentrations (80 ppm, for 4 weeks, 5 days/week, 6 hours/day) causes a slight but persistent deficit in spatial learning and memory, a persistent decrease in dopamine-mediated locomotor activity, and an increase in the number of dopamine D2 receptors.[81] Toluene exposure of rats to concentrations of 100, 300, and 1,000 ppm was found to produce a significant increase in three glial cell marker proteins (α-enolase, creatine kinase-B, and β-S100 protein) in the cerebellum. β-S100 protein also increased in a dose-dependent manner in the brainstem and spinal cord. The two neuronal cell markers did not show a quantitative decrease in the CNS. This indicates that the development of gliosis, rather than neurone death, is induced by chronic exposure to toluene.[82]

Progressive optic neuropathy and sensory hearing loss developed in some cases. Toluene causes midfrequency auditory damage; a morphological study in rats and mice showed the cochlear outer hair cells to be mainly affected. Noise exposure enhanced the loss in auditory sensitivity due to toluene. Toluene exposure was also shown to accelerate age-related hereditary hearing loss in one genotype of mice.[83] Peripheral neuropathy associated with severe CNS damage has been reported.

Hepatotoxic and nephrotoxic effects have also been found in cases of toluene addiction; the possibility that other toxic agents might have contributed cannot be excluded. Sudden death in toluene sniffers has been reported and is thought to be due to arrhythmia secondary to myocardial sensitization to endogenous catecholamines,[84] a mechanism of sudden death similar to that reported with trichloroethylene and other halogenated hydrocarbons.

Adverse developmental effects in offspring of women who are solvent sniffers have been reported. These include CNS dysfunction, microcephaly, minor craniofacial and limb abnormalities,[85] and growth retardation. Developmental disability, intrauterine growth retardation, renal anomalies, and dysmorphic features have been described in offspring of women who abuse toluene during pregnancy. Experimental results[86] confirm adverse developmental effects: skeletal abnormalities and low fetal weight were observed in several animal species (mice, rabbits).

Adverse reproductive effects have not been detected in other human or experimental studies. In an experimental study on rats receiving toluene by gavage (520 mg/kg body weight during days 6 to 19 of gestation), no major congenital malformations or neuropathologic changes were found; the number of implantations and stillbirths were not affected. The weight of fetuses and placental weights were reduced, as were the weights of most organs. Prenatal toluene exposure produced a generalized growth retardation.[87] Toluene was not embrotoxic, fetotoxic, or teratogenic for rabbits exposed during the period of organogenesis. The highest concentration tested was 500 ppm.[88]

Toluene has been found to be nonmutagenic and nongenotoxic. There are no indications, from human observations, that toluene has carcinogenic effects; long-term experimental studies on several animal species have been consistently negative.

Prevention and Control

The recommended TWA for toluene is 100 ppm. It is important to monitor the benzene content of technical grades of toluene and to control exposures so that the TWA of 1 ppm for benzene is not exceeded. Engineering controls, such as enclosure and exhaust ventilation, are essential for the prevention of excessive exposure; adequate respirators should be provided for unusual situations, when higher exposures might be expected.[3]

Biological monitoring of exposure can be achieved by measuring urinary hippuric acid, the main urinary metabolite of toluene. Excretion of hippuric acid in excess of 3 g/L indicates an exposure in excess of 100 ppm. A second important urinary metabolite of toluene is *o*-cresol; as for hippuric acid, the excretion of *o*-cresol reaches its peak at the end of the exposure period (work shift). Interindividual differences in the pattern of toluene metabolism have been found, resulting in variable ratios between urinary hippuric acid and *o*-cresol. For these reasons, biological monitoring should include measurements of both urinary metabolites. Simultaneous exposure by inhalation to toluene and xylene resulted in lower amounts of excreted hippuric acid and methylhippuric acid in urine, while concentrations of solvents in blood and brain were found during the immediate post-exposure period. These results strongly suggest mutual metabolic inhibition between toluene and xylene.[89]

Preemployment and periodic medical examinations should encompass possible neurological, hematological, hepatic, renal, and dermatological effects. Hematological tests, as indicated for benzene, have to be used because, as noted, variable amounts of benzene may be present in commercial grades of toluene.

Potential environmental toluene exposure is currently also of concern. The largest source of environmental toluene release is the production, transport, and use of gasoline, which contains 5 to 7 percent toluene by weight. Toluene in the atmosphere reacts with hydroxyl radicals; the half-time is about 13 hours. Toluene in soil or water volatilizes to air; the remaining amounts undergo microbial degradation. There is no tendency toward environmental buildup of toluene. Toluene is a very common contaminant in the vicinity of waste-disposal sites, where average concentrations in water have been found to be 7 to 20 μg/L; and average concentrations in soil, 70 μg/L. The EPA, in a 1988 survey, found toluene in ground water, surface water, and soil at 29 percent of the hazardous waste sites tested. Toluene is not a widespread contaminant of drinking water; it was present in only approximately 1 percent of ground-water sources, in concentrations lower than 2 ppb.

Biodegradation of trichloroethylene and aromatic compounds by microbial consortia enriched from contaminated subsurface sediments has been extensively studied. The consortia were capable of utilizing methane (15 percent) and propane (3 percent) as sources of carbon and energy. Two continuously recycled expanded-bed bioreactors were inoculated with (*a*) the subsurface consortium and (*b*) *Pseudomonas fluorescence, Pseudomonas putida*, and *Methylosinus trichosporium*. Greater than 97 percent degradation of trichloroethylene was observed over a period of 12 days. More than 99 percent of benzene, toluene, and xylene were degraded within the first 7 days.[90]

Xylene

Xylene (dimethylbenzene, $C_6H_4(CH_3)_2$) has three isomeric forms: *ortho-*, *meta-*, and *para*-xylene. Commercial xylene is a mixture of these but may also contain benzene, ethylbenzene, toluene, and other impurities. With a boiling temperature of 144°C, xylene is less volatile than benzene and toluene. It is used as a solvent and as the starting material for the synthesis of xylidines, benzoic acid, phthalic anhydride, and phthalic and terephthalic acids and their esters. Other uses are in the manufacture of quartz crystal oscillators, epoxy resins, and pharmaceuticals. In a study of two paint manufacturing plants and 22 spray painting operations (car painting, aircraft painting, trailer painting, and video terminal painting), the main constituents of the mixtures of solvents used were xylene and toluene, with average contents of 46 and 29 percent, on a weight basis, of 67 air samples.[91] It is estimated that 140,000 workers are potentially exposed to xylene in the United States. As with toluene, early reports on adverse effects of xylene have to be evaluated in light of the frequent presence of considerable proportions of benzene in the mixture.[2,3]

Xylene has been shown to induce liver microsomal mixed function oxidases and cytochrome P-450 in a dose-dependent manner.[92] *m*-Xylene treatment led to elevated P-450 2B1/2B2 without significantly depressing P-450 2C11 and produced significant increases in activities efficiently catalyzed by both isozymes.[93] The metabolism of *n*-hexane to its highly neurotoxic metabolite 2,5-hexanedione was shown to be markedly enhanced in rats pretreated with xylene.[124] Xylene also increases the metabolism of benzene and toluene. Thus, when present in mixtures with other solvents, xylene can increase the adverse effects of those compounds, which exert their toxicity mainly through more toxic metabolites.

Xylene was also found to facilitate the biotransformation of progesterone and 17, β-estradiol in pregnant rats by inducing hepatic microsomal mixed-function oxidases. Decreased blood levels of these hormones were thought to result in reduced weight of the fetuses.[94] Xylene exposure (500 ppm) of pregnant rats on gestation days 7 to 20 resulted in a lower absolute brain weight and impaired performance in behavioral tests of neuromotor abilities and for learning and memory.[95] The effects of lacquer thinner and its main components, toluene, xylene, methanol, and ethyl acetate, on reproductive and accessory reproductive organs in rats were studied; the vapor from the solvents was inhaled twice a day for 7 days. Both xylene and ethyl acetate caused a decrease in the weights of testes and prostate and reduced plasma testosterone. Spermatozoa levels in the epididymis were decreased. In contrast, toluene and methanol had no effects on organ weights and circulating testosterone levels.[96]

Acute effects of xylene exposure are depression of the CNS (prenarcotic and narcotic with high concentrations) and irritation of eyes, nose, throat, and skin. Acute effects of *m*-xylene were studied in 9 volunteers exposed at rest or while exercising to concentrations of 200 ppm (TWA), with short-term peak concentrations of 400 ppm or less. Exposure increased the dominant alpha frequency and alpha percentage in the EEG during the early phase of exposure. The effects of short-term *m*-xylene exposure on EEG were minor, and no persistent deleterious effects were noted.[97] Liquid xylene is irritant to the skin, and repeated exposure may result in dermatitis. Hepatotoxic and nephrotoxic effects have been found in isolated cases of excessive exposure. Myelotoxic effects and hematologic changes have not been documented for pure xylene; the possibility of benzene admixture to technical-grade xylene has to be emphasized.

The TWA for xylene exposure is 100 ppm. The metabolites of *ortho-*, *meta-*, and *para*-xylene are the corresponding methyl hippuric acids. A concentration of 2.05 g *m*-methyl hippuric acid corresponds to 100 ppm (TLV) exposure to *m*-xylene. Prevention, control, and medical surveillance are similar to those indicated for toluene and benzene. Complete blood counts, urinalysis, and liver function tests should be part of the periodic medical examinations.

Styrene

Styrene (vinyl benzene, $C_6H_5CH{=}CH_2$), a colorless or yellowish liquid, is used in the manufacture of polystyrene (styrene is the monomer; at temperatures of 200°C, polymerization to polystyrene occurs) and of copolymers with 1,3-butadiene (butadiene-styrene rubber) and acrylonitrile (acrylonitrile-butadiene-styrene (ABS)). The most important exposures to styrene occur when it is used as a solvent-reactant in the manufacture of polyester products in the reinforced plastics industry. TWA exposures can be as high as 150 to 300 ppm, with excursions into the 1,000 to 1,500 ppm range.

The metabolic transformation of styrene is characterized by its conversion to styrene-7,8-oxide by the mixed function oxidases and cytochrome P-450 enzyme complex. Styrene-7,8-oxide is mutagenic in several prokaryotic and eukaryotic test systems. It has been shown to produce single-strand breaks in DNA of various organs in mice: kidney, liver, lung, testes, and brain.[98] Styrene-7,8-oxide is an alkylating agent and reacts mostly with deoxyguanosine, producing 7-alkylguanine, and with deoxycytidine, producing *N*-3-alkylcytosine. Chromosome aberrations and sister chromatic exchanges were reported to be significantly increased in several studies of styrene-exposed workers. Styrene-7,8-oxide is a potent carcinogen in rodents.

Mandelic acid (MA) and phenyl glyoxylic acid (PGA) are the main urinary metabolites of styrene.

Styrene has an irritant effect on mucous membranes (eyes, nose, throat, airways) and skin. Inhalation of high concentrations may result in transitory CNS depression, with prenarcotic symptoms. Chronic neurotoxic effects have been reported with repeated exposure to relatively high levels in the boat-construction industry, mostly in Scandinavian countries, where styrene is widely used by brush application on large surfaces. Electroencephalographic changes, performance test abnormalities, and peripheral nerve conduction velocity changes have been reported.[99] There is no indication from epidemiological studies that styrene is carcinogenic in humans.

Contact allergy to styrene has been reported. Cross-reactivity on patch testing with 2-, 3-, and 4-vinyl toluene (methyl styrene) and with the metabolites styrene epoxide and 4-vinyl phenol has been found.

Prevention

In view of reports of persistent neurological effects with long-term exposure, the present federal standard for a styrene TWA of 100 ppm appears to be too high, and reduction has been suggested. NIOSH has proposed a TWA of 50 ppm. Biological limits of exposure have been proposed corresponding to a TLV of 50 ppm styrene. At the end of the shift, urinary MA should not exceed 800 mg/g creatinine and the sum of MA and PGA should not be more than 1,000 mg/g creatinine. In the morning, before the start of work, the values should not exceed 150 and 300 mg/g creatinine, respectively. Preemployment and periodic medical examinations should assess neurological status, liver and kidney function, and hematological parameters.

▸ HALOGENATED HYDROCARBONS

The compounds in this group result from the substitution of one or more hydrogen atoms of a simple hydrocarbon by halogens, most often chlorine. Simple chlorinated hydrocarbons are used in a wide variety of industrial processes. The majority are excellent solvents for oils, waxes, fats, rubber, pigments, paints, varnishes, etc. In the chemical industry these compounds are used for chlorination in the manufacture of such products as plastics, pesticides, and other complex halogenated compounds.[1,2] Most are nonflammable; some, such as carbon tetrachloride, have been used as fire extinguishers. (This use has been stopped because of the marked toxicity of carbon tetrachloride and the formation of highly irritant combustion products.) The most widely used simple chlorinated hydrocarbons are as follows:

Monochloromethane (methyl chloride)	CH_3Cl
Dichloromethane (methylene chloride)	CH_2Cl_2
Trichloromethane (chloroform)	$CHCl_3$
Tetrachloromethane (carbon tetrachloride)	CCl_4
1,2-Dichloroethane (ethylene chloride)	CH_2ClCH_2Cl
1,1-Dichloroethane	$CHCl_2CH_3$
1,1,2-Trichloroethane	$CH_2ClCHCl_2$
1,1,1-Trichloroethane (methyl chloroform)	CH_3CCl_3
1,1,2,2-Tetrachloroethane	$CHCl_2CHCl_2$
Monochloroethylene (vinyl chloride)	$CHCl{=}CH_2$
1,2-Dichloroethylene (*cis* and *trans*)	$CHCl{=}CHCl$
Trichloroethylene	$CHCl{=}CCl_2$
Tetrachloroethylene	$CCl_2{=}CCl_2$

Many of the members of this series of compounds have a low boiling point and are highly volatile at room temperature; hazardous exposure levels may develop in a very short time. The application of heat is common in numerous industrial processes; air concentrations of halogenated hydrocarbons increase sharply under such circumstances.

Many industrial solvents are sold as mixtures. These may sometimes contain highly toxic products, and hazardous exposure may occur without the exposed person's knowledge of the specific chemical composition of the solvent mixture used. Carbon tetrachloride has been generally accepted as the prototype for a hepatotoxic agent; other members of the group have similar or lesser hepatotoxicity.

The majority of the compounds have a narcotic effect on the central nervous system; in this respect they are more potent than the hydrocarbons from which they are derived. Some (chloroform, trichloroethylene) were used as anesthetics until their marked toxicity was recognized. Moderate irritation of mucous membranes (conjunctivae, upper and lower airways) is also a common effect of halogenated hydrocarbons.

With acute overexposure or repeated exposures of a lesser degree, toxic damage to the liver and kidney is common; the severity of these effects is largely dependent on the specific compound and on the level and pattern of exposure. Individual susceptibility may also contribute but is of lesser importance. Halogenated hydrocarbons may produce liver injury and centrilobular necrosis with or without steatosis. They also have marked nephrotoxicity; tubular cellular necrosis is the specific lesion that may lead to anuria and acute renal failure. Many of the fatalities due to acute overexposure to halogenated hydrocarbons have been attributed to this effect, although concomitant liver injury was always present.[1,2]

The toxicity of many halogenated solvents is associated with their biotransformation to reactive electrophilic metabolites, which can alkylate macromolecules and thus produce organ injury. The microsomal mixed function oxidases and cytochrome P-450 complex of enzymes are effective in the biotransformation of halogenated solvents. The role of human microsomal cytochrome P-450 IIE1 in the oxidation of a number of chemical compounds has been established. P-450 IIE1 is a major catalyst of the oxydation of benzene, styrene, CCl_4, $CHCl_3$, CH_2Cl_2, CH_3Cl, CH_3CCl_3, 1,2-dichloropropane, ethylene dichloride, ethylene dibromide, vinyl chloride, vinyl bromide, acrylonitrile, and trichloroethylene. Levels of P-450 IIE1 can vary considerably among individuals.[100] The P-450 enzyme is highly inducible by ethanol.[101] Chloroethanes (1,2-dichloroethane, 1,1,1-trichloroethane, and 1,1,2,2-tetrachloroethane) have also been shown to be metabolized by hepatic cytochrome P-450.

Food deprivation, more specifically a low intake of carbohydrates, and alcohol consumption enhance the metabolic transformation of the halogenated hydrocarbon solvents chloroform, carbon tetrachloride, 1,2-dichloroethane, 1,1-dichloroethylene, and trichloroethylene. Carbon tetrachloride rapidly promotes lipid peroxidation and inhibits calcium sequestration, glucose-6-phosphatase activity, and cytochrome P-450. The urinary excretion of the lipid metabolites formaldehyde, malondialdehyde, acetaldehyde, and acetone was increased after administration of CCl_4. The increased excretion of these lipid metabolites may serve as noninvasive markers of xenobiotic-induced lipid peroxidation.[102]

Pretreatment of rats with large doses of vitamin A potentiates the hepatotoxicity of CCl_4. Vitamin A enhances CCl_4-induced lipid peroxidation and release of active oxygen species from Kupffer cells and possibly other macrophages activated by vitamin A.[103] The in vivo formation of PGF_2-like compounds (F2-isoprostanes) derived from free radical-catalyzed nonenzymatic peroxidation of arachidonic acid has been found to be considerably increased (up to 50-fold) in rats administered CCl_4. F2-isoprostanes are esterified to lipids in various organs and plasma. The measurement of F2-isoprostanes may facilitate the investigation of the role of lipid peroxidation in human disease.[104]

Considerable indirect evidence suggests that the cytokine tumor necrosis factor contributes to the hepatocellular damage resulting from toxic liver injury. By administering a soluble tumor necrosis factor receptor, the mortality from CCl_4 was lowered from 60 to 16 percent in an experimental study. The degree of liver injury was reduced, as measured by levels of serum enzymes. There was no detrimental effect on liver regeneration. These results suggest that soluble tumor necrosis factor receptor may be of benefit in the treatment of toxic human liver disease.[105]

Cellular phosphatidylcholine hydroperoxide (PCOOH) and phosphatidylethanolamine hydroperoxide (PEOOH) were increased more than four times by exposure of cultured hepatocytes to CCl_4, 1,1,1-trichloroethane, tetrachloroethylene, and 1,3-dichloropropene in a concentration of 10 mM. Peroxidative degradation of membrane phospholipids may play an important role in the cytotoxicity of some chlorinated hydrocarbons.[106]

It has been proposed that the nephrotoxicity of some compounds in this group is due to metabolic transformation in the kidney of the glutathione conjugates into the corresponding cysteine conjugates. The cysteine conjugates may be directly nephrotoxic or they may be further transformed in the kidney by renal cysteine conjugate β-lyase into reactive alkenyl mercaptans.

Another toxic effect, more recently identified, is related to the arrhythmogenic properties of halogenated hydrocarbons. These were first reported with chloroform and trichloroethylene used as anesthetics; they have also been found to occur with occupational exposure and, more recently, in persons addicted to the euphoric effects of short-term exposure (solvent sniffers).[3] Ventricular fibrillation secondary to myocardial sensitization to endogenous epinephrine and norepinephrine has been postulated as the mechanism underlying the arrhythmias and sudden deaths. Incorporation of halocarbons in the membrane of cardiac myocytes may block intercellular communication through modification of the immediate environment of the gap junctions. Inhibition of gap junctional communication is possibly a factor in the arrhythmogenic effects of acute halogenated hydrocarbon exposure.[107]

The hepatotoxicity of carbon tetrachloride has been studied extensively, both clinically and in various experimental models. The mechanisms of toxic liver injury, the underlying biochemical and enzymatic disruptions, and the corresponding ultrastructural changes have been progressively defined. Hepatic cirrhosis may follow repeated exposure to carbon tetrachloride. Hepatic perisinusoidal cells (PSCs) proliferate and are thought to be the principal source of extracellular matrix proteins during the development of liver fibrosis. The PSCs have been shown to be modulated into a synthetically active and contractile myofibroblast in the course of liver fibrosis.[108]

Simultaneous administration of trichloroethylene (TCE) and carbon tetrachloride (0.05 mL/kg) resulted in a marked potentiation of liver injury caused by CCl_4. Hepatic glutathione levels were depressed only in rats given both TCE and CCl_4. The regenerative activity in the liver appeared to be delayed by TCE.[109] Acetone (A), MEK, and methyl isobutyl ketone (MiBK) markedly potentiate CCl_4 hepatotoxicity and chloroform ($CHCl_3$) nephrotoxicity. The potency ranking for this potentiating effect is MiBK > A > MEK for hepatotoxicity and A > MEK ≥ MiBK for nephrotoxicity.[110] An unusual type of fibrosis of the liver and spleen, including subcapsular fibrosis, and the development of portal hypertension can result from vinyl chloride exposure.

Liver carcinogenicity has been documented for several compounds of this series. Hepatocellular carcinoma developing several years after acute carbon tetrachloride poisoning has been reported.[111] In other cases long-term exposure, even without overt acute toxicity, may lead to the same end result. In animal studies, carbon tetrachloride has proved a potent hepatocarcinogen. Chloroform and trichloroethylene have been shown to be hepatocarcinogens in animals.[112] Human data are not available; no long-term epidemiological study has been reported, and the possibility exists that instances of hepatocellular carcinoma may have occurred in workers exposed to these substances without recognition of the etiological link between exposure and malignancy. That this is a possibility has been illustrated by the example of vinyl chloride. Hemangiosarcoma of the liver was identified as one of the possible effects of vinyl chloride exposure in 1974, and many cases have since been reported from various industrial countries. Some of these cases had occurred in prior years, but at that time the link between toxic exposure and malignancy had not been suggested. Only after the etiological association was established, both by the first human cases reported and by results of animal experiments,[113] was information on many other cases published. There are indications that vinyl chloride may induce hepatoma as well as hemangiosarcoma. Vinylidene chloride has also come under close scrutiny, since animal data seem to indicate a carcinogenic effect. Chemical enhancement of viral transformation of Syrian hamster embryo cells has been demonstrated for 1,1,1-trichloroethane, 1,2-dichloroethane, 1,1-dichloroethane, chloromethane, and vinyl chloride; other chlorinated methanes and ethanes did not show such an effect.[114]

Exposure to halogenated hydrocarbons and other volatile organic compounds in the general environment, from various sources including contaminated water and toxic waste-disposal sites, has received increasing attention during recent years. Methods have been developed to determine individual exposures with personal monitors to determine ambient air levels and special equipment for the collection of expired air samples in field settings; gas chromatography-mass spectroscopy analysis has permitted adequate detection and has clarified patterns of relationships between breathing zone concentrations and results of breath analysis.

In a study on students in Texas and North Carolina, air has been found to be the major source of absorption, except for two trihalomethanes, chloroform and bromodichloromethane. Estimated total daily intake from air and water ranged from 0.3 to 12.6 mg, with 1,1,1-trichloroethane at the highest concentrations.[115] Monitoring of airborne levels of mutagens and suspected carcinogens, including linear and cyclic halogenated hydrocarbons, has been undertaken in many urban centers of the United States. Average concentration levels for halogenated hydrocarbons were in the 0 to 1 ppb range. Similar efforts have been undertaken regarding the monitoring of water contamination with halogenated hydrocarbons. Rivers, lakes, and drinking water from various sources have been tested. Analytical methods have been developed for the detection of volatile organic compounds, including chlorinated hydrocarbons, in fish and shellfish. Regional data from Germany indicate that approximately 25 percent of the ground-water samples contained more than 1 μg/L of a single solvent, most prominent being trichloroethene, tetrachloroethane, 1,1,1-trichloroethane, and dichloromethane, but also chloroform. Since the long-term effects of low-level exposure to halogenated hydrocarbon solvents, especially with regard to carcinogenicity and mutagenicity, are not known, it is necessary to monitor current exposures from all possible sources and to reduce such exposures to a minimum to protect the health of the general population.

Carbon Tetrachloride

The production of carbon tetrachloride in the United States has varied from 250 to 400 million kg in recent years. It is currently used mainly in the synthesis of dichlorofluoromethane (fluorocarbon 12) and trichlorofluoromethane (fluorocarbon 11); a small proportion is still applied as a fumigant and pesticide for certain crops (barley, corn, rice, rye, wheat) and for agricultural facilities, such as grain bins and granaries.

Airborne concentrations of carbon tetrachloride in the general environment have been found to vary from 0.05 to 18 ppb. In rural areas, levels of CCl_4 were lower, in the range of 80 to 120 ppt. The photodecomposition of tetrachloroethylene results in the formation of about 8 percent (by weight) carbon tetrachloride[116] and is thought to be possibly responsible for a significant proportion of atmospheric carbon tetrachloride.

Carbon tetrachloride has also been found in rivers, lakes, and drinking water. Through 1983, about 95 percent of all surface water supplies contained less than 0.5 μg/L; in drinking water, detectable levels (>0.2 μg/L) were present in 3 percent of 945 samples tested.

The toxicity of carbon tetrachloride (CCl_4) is enhanced by its metabolic transformation in the liver. Induction of mixed function microsomal enzymes significantly increases CCl_4 toxicity, while inhibition of the enzymatic system decreases its toxicity.

Carbon tetrachloride can produce disruption of all elements of the hepatocyte—plasma membrane, endoplasmic reticulum, mitochondria, lysosomes, and nucleus. The resulting cellular destruction is reflected in zonal (centrilobular) necrosis, which can be accompanied by steatosis. The corresponding clinical manifestation is hepatocellular jaundice; in severe cases hepatic failure and death may occur. With lesser exposure, less extensive subclinical pathologic changes may result; nonspecific symptoms, such as fatigability, loss of appetite, and nausea, may be present without jaundice. Elevated serum enzymes (SGOT, SGPT, LDH), bilirubin, and sometimes alkaline phosphatase, a rise in bromsulphalein retention, reduction of prothrombin, and increased urinary urobilin excretion may nevertheless be detected. Repeated toxic insults may lead to the development of postnecrotic cirrhosis.

The toxic effect of carbon tetrachloride is due to a metabolite, a free radical (CCl_3) that appears to produce peroxidation of the unsaturated lipids of cellular membranes. Metabolism of CCl_4 to the more toxic metabolite (free radical) is thought to occur in the endoplasmic reticulum. Cytochrome P-450 is destroyed in the process. As the metabolite accumulates, membranes of lysosomes and mitochondria are also injured, and necrosis results.

Individual variation in the response to CCl_4 is now better understood. Carbon tetrachloride hepatotoxicity was found to be much less severe in old rats than in young adult rats, as assessed by serum hepatic enzymes and disappearance of hepatic microsomal cytochrome P-450.[117] Previous mixed-function microsomal enzyme induction has been shown to enhance CCl_4 toxicity through enhanced metabolic transformation to the active intermediate free radical. Alcohols, ketones, and some other chemical compounds enhance carbon tetrachloride toxicity: ethanol, isopropyl alcohol, butanol, acetone, PCBs and PBBs, chlordecone, and trichloroethylene have all been shown to potentiate CCl_4 toxicity, mostly by hepatic enzyme induction. These observations are important for the assessment of potential toxicity of chemical mixtures, including those from waste-disposal sites, that could be or are found to contaminate drinking water.

Carbon tetrachloride metabolites form irreversible covalent bonds to hepatic macromolecules, and binding of radiolabeled CCl_4 to DNA also occurs:[118] Experimental evidence of carcinogenicity in mice and rats has accumulated. Liver tumors, including hepatocellular carcinomas, developed in various strains of mice, and benign and malignant liver tumors developed in rats.[119]

Prevention and Control

The federal OSHA standard for a permissible exposure limit (PEL) for carbon tetrachloride exposure is 2 ppm. Replacement by less toxic substances, engineering controls, and enclosed processes are necessary. Respiratory protection should be available for emergency situations. Medical surveillance must include careful evaluation of liver and kidney function, central and peripheral nervous system function, and the skin. The World Health Organization has adopted a guideline for permissible CCl_4 concentration of 0.003 mg/L in drinking water.

Chloroform

Chloroform is a colorless, very volatile liquid, with a boiling point of 61°C. Most of the more than 300 million pounds produced annually in the United States is used in the manufacture of fluorocarbons. Chloroform has also been used in cosmetics and numerous products of the pharmaceutical industry; the FDA banned these uses in 1976. Another application of chloroform has been as an insecticidal fumigant for certain crops, including corn, rice, and wheat. Chloroform residues have been detected in cereals for weeks after fumigation. They have also been found in food products, such as dairy produce, meat, oils and fats, fruits, and vegetables, in amounts ranging from 1 to more than 30 mg/kg.

The presence of chloroform in the water of rivers and lakes, in ground water, and in sewage treatment plant effluents has been documented at various locations. In drinking water, concentrations of 5 to 90 μg/L have been detected. Chlorination of water is thought to be responsible for the presence of chloroform in water.

Chloroform has toxic effects similar to those of carbon tetrachloride, but fewer severe cases have been reported after industrial exposure. Chloroform undergoes metabolic transformation; one of the metabolites has been shown to be phosgene ($COCl_2$). Microsomal cytochrome P-450 is active in the metabolism of chloroform; induction of cytochrome P-450 results in increased chloroform hepatotoxicity. Methyl-*n*-butyl ketone (MBK) and 2,5-hexanedione, the common metabolite of MBK, and *n*-hexane enhance chloroform hepatotoxicity by induction of cytochrome P-450. Extensive covalent binding to liver and kidney proteins has been found, in direct relationship with the extent of hepatic centrilobular and renal proximal tubular necrosis. Neither chloroform nor its metabolites are directly DNA reactive; the carcinogenicity of chloroform is secondary to induced cytolethality and regenerative cell proliferation.[120]

The National Cancer Institute report on the carcinogenic effect of chloroform in animals (hepatocellular carcinomas in mice and renal tumors in rats) draws attention again to the lack of long-term epidemiologic observations. As with other carcinogens, industrial exposure must not exceed the limit of detection, and appropriate engineering methods must be used to protect the health of employees. NIOSH recommended a ceiling of 2 ppm. Environmental exposure of the general population to chloroform in water and food also has to be reduced to a minimum, given that sufficient experimental evidence for the carcinogenicity of chloroform has accumulated.

Trichloroethylene

Trichloroethylene (TCE) is a colorless, volatile liquid with a boiling point of 87°C. Trichloroethylene was thought to be much less toxic than carbon tetrachloride and was used, to a large extent, to replace CCl_4 in many industrial processes. It is one of the most important chlorinated solvents. Its main applications have been as a dry-cleaning agent and a metal degreaser. In smaller amounts, it is used in extraction of fats and other natural products, in the manufacture of adhesives and industrial paints, and in the chemical industry, mainly in the production of fluorocarbons.

NIOSH has estimated that 3.5 million workers in the United States are occupationally exposed to trichloroethylene; about 100,000 are exposed full-time.

Trichloroethylene is absorbed rapidly through the respiratory route, and only a relatively small fraction of the amount inhaled is eliminated unchanged in the exhaled air. The metabolic transformation of trichloroethylene has been shown to proceed through formation of a complex with cytochrome P-450; several pathways can then follow:

- Destruction of heme
- Formation of chloral, which can be reduced to trichloroethanol or oxidized to trichloroacetic acid
- Formation of trichloroethylene oxide, which then decomposes into carbon monoxide and glyoxylate
- Formation of metabolites that bind irreversibly to protein, RNA, and DNA

The relative proportion of these four different metabolic pathways can vary. Species differences in TCE metabolism have been demonstrated. Following a single oral dose of TCE of 1.5 to 23 mmol/kg, peak blood concentrations of trichloroethylene, trichloroacetate, and trichloroethanol were much greater in mice than in rats.[121] Dichloroacetate, an inducer of hepatic tumors in mice, has been found to be an important metabolite of TCE in the mouse.[122]

The levels of protein and DNA adducts vary from species to species and may contribute to species differences found in carcinogenicity bioassays. In some studies in rodents, no direct evidence of formation of liver DNA adducts could be detected. In other studies, covalent binding to liver and kidney RNA and to DNA in kidney, testes, lung, pancreas, and spleen was found. Dichlorovinylcysteine, a metabolite of TCE thought to be responsible for the nephrocarcinogenicity of trichloroethylene, has been found to induce DNA double-strand breaks followed by increased poly(ADP-ribosyl)ation of nuclear proteins in cultured renal cells in male Wistar rats.[123]

In humans, most trichloroethylene is metabolized to trichloroacetic acid and trichloroethanol. The urinary excretion of these metabolites can be used for biologic monitoring of trichloroethylene exposure; trichloroethanol excretion reaches its peak 24 hours after exposure, while trichloroacetic acid reaches its highest urinary level 3 days after exposure. Trichloroethylene has a depressant effect on the CNS; prenarcotic and narcotic symptoms can develop in rapid sequence with high concentrations of vapor. TCE is also an irritant to the skin, conjunctivae, and airways.

Hepatotoxicity and nephrotoxicity of trichloroethylene are much lower than those of carbon tetrachloride; there are few reports of acute fatal toxic hepatitis and only isolated reports of acute renal failure due to TCE. Trichloroethylene can enhance the hepatotoxicity of carbon tetrachloride, possibly potentiating lipid peroxidation. Hepatotoxicity with moderate, long-term exposure has not been found in humans. Cardiac arrest[124] and sudden deaths in young workers exposed to TCE have been reported repeatedly and have been attributed to ventricular fibrillation, through myocardial sensitization to increased levels of epinephrine. Recent studies have demonstrated the capacity of TCE to inhibit Ca^{2+} dynamics in cardiomyocytes.[125]

Chronic effects on the central and peripheral nervous system have been described in TCE-exposed workers.[126] TCE has been shown to alter the fatty acid composition of mitochondria in neural cells in the rat.[127] Visual evoked potential (VEP) amplitudes were significantly decreased in rabbits exposed to TCE via inhalation compared with VEPs obtained prior to exposure; a significant increase in VEP amplitude followed exposure at 700 ppm.[128] Persistent midfrequency hearing loss has been demonstrated in rats following a 5-day inhalation exposure to TCE, noted especially at 8 and 16 kHz.[129] Brainstem auditory evoked potentials were depressed in TCE-exposed rats, with high-frequency hearing loss predominating.[130]

Trichloroethylene has been reported to be a hepatocarcinogen in experimental animals. An increased incidence of hepatocellular carcinomas was found in mice, but this effect was not observed in rats. Kidney adenocarcinomas, testicular Leydig cell tumors, and possibly leukemia were found to be significantly increased in some experimental studies in rats.

Epidemiological data have accumulated which suggest that TCE may be carcinogenic in humans. In a study of cancer incidence among 2,050 male and 1,924 female workers in Finland, those who were exposed to TCE had an increased overall cancer incidence when compared with that of the Finnish general population. Excesses of cancer of the stomach, liver, prostate, and lymphohematopoietic tissues was found.[131] Among workers exposed for at least 1 year to TCE, renal cell/urothelial cancers occurred in excess. Associations of astrocytic brain tumors with trichloroethylene exposure among workers have been reported.[132] A study of cancer mortality and morbidity among 1,421 men exposed to TCE found no significant increase in cancer incidence or mortality at any site, but for a doubling of the incidence of nonmelanocytic skin cancer without correlation with exposure categories.[133]

Trichloroethylene has been shown to induce congenital cardiac malformations in Sprague-Dawley rats when females were given TCE in drinking water before and during pregnancy.[134] Trichloroethylene had no effect on reproductive function in mice at doses up to 1/10 of the oral LD_{50}.[135] TCE exposure does not produce dominant lethal mutations in mice. An increased proportion of morphologically abnormal spermatozoa was found in mice exposed to TCE by inhalation. Trichloroethylene oxide, an intermediate metabolite of TCE formed by mixed function oxidase metabolism, has been reported to be highly embryotoxic in the Frog Embryo Teratogenesis Assay.[136]

Medical surveillance of populations currently exposed or exposed in the past is necessary, with special attention to long-term and potential carcinogenic effects, neurological effects, and liver and kidney function abnormalities.

The present federal standard for a permissible level of occupational TCE exposure is 50 ppm. A lower exposure limit has been proposed in view of information on carcinogenicity in animals. Exposure of the general population to TCE has received increasing attention. In 1977 the FDA proposed a regulation prohibiting the use of TCE as a food additive; this included the use of TCE in extraction processes in the manufacture of decaffeinated coffee and of spice oleoresins.

Trichloroethylene has been found in at least 460 of 1,179 hazardous waste sites on the National Priorities List. Federal and state surveys have shown that between 9 and 34 percent of water supply sources in the United States are contaminated with TCE; the concentrations are, on the average, 1 to 2 ppb or less. Higher levels have been found in the vicinity of toxic waste-disposal sites; under such circumstances, concentrations of several hundred up to 27,000 ppb have been detected. In 1989 the EPA established a drinking water standard of 5 ppb.

In a recent study, birth outcome status and maternal risk factor information for 80,938 live births and 594 fetal deaths were obtained from vital records and the New Jersey Birth Defects Registry. Tap water sample data were used to estimate exposure to TCE during pregnancy. A relationship between trichloroethylene exposure during pregnancy and central nervous system defects, neural tube defects, and oral cleft defects was found (odds ratio, 1.50 or more).[137] Long-term, low-level exposure to a mixture of common organic ground-water contaminants (benzene, chloroform, phenol, and trichloroethylene) was shown to induce significant increases in hepatocellular proliferation in F344 rats, in the absence of histopathological lesions or an increase in liver enzyme levels in serum.[138] Synergy between TCE and CCl_4 when administered in drinking water has been demonstrated in the rat.[139]

Considerable effort has been directed toward the development of microbial systems for the detoxification of TCE-contaminated sites. Most systems have employed obligate methane-oxidizing bacteria (methanotrophs) altered by molecular genetic techniques.[140]

Perchloroethylene

Perchloroethylene (PCE, tetrachloroethylene) is used in the textile industry for dry cleaning, processing, and finishing. More than 70 percent of all dry-cleaning operations in the United States use perchloroethylene. Another important use is in metal cleaning and degreasing. Perchloroethylene is also a raw material for the synthesis of fluorocarbons.

Perchloroethylene is similar in most respects to trichloroethylene. Its hepatotoxicity, initially thought to be very low, has been well documented, with abnormal levels of liver enzymes after exposure and persistence of elevated urinary urobilinogen and serum bilirubin in asymptomatic persons.

An arrhythmogenic effect of perchloroethylene has also been well documented in humans; premature ventricular contractions in young adults were frequent with high blood levels of perchloroethylene and disappeared completely after removal from exposure. Alteration of Ca^{2+} dynamics in cardiomyocytes is a common mechanism of cardiotoxic halogenated hydrocarbons' action.[141]

In a collaborative European study, renal effects of perchloroethylene exposure in dry cleaners were assessed by a battery of tests, and the findings compared with those of matched controls. Increased high–molecular weight protein in urine was frequently associated with tubular alterations, including changes consistent with diffuse abnormalities along the nephron, in workers exposed to low levels of PCE (median 15 ppm). Generalized membrane disturbances were thought to account for the increased release of laminin fragments, fibronectin and glycosaminoglycans, for high–molecular weight proteinuria, and for increased shedding of epithelial membrane components from tubular cells at different locations along the nephron (brush-border antigens and Tamm-Horsfall glycoprotein). These findings of early renal changes indicate that dry cleaners need to be monitored for chronic renal changes.[142]

Deaths due to massive perchloroethylene overexposure have occurred, especially in small dry-cleaning establishments. Increases in the brain content of an astroglial protein (S-100) and of glutamine synthetase, a biomarker for astroglial hypertrophy, provide biochemical evidence of astroglial proliferation secondary to neuronal damage.

The metabolism of perchloroethylene is characterized by a cytochrome P-450–catalyzed oxidative reaction; an epoxide intermediate has been postulated, but current technology has not yet allowed its isolation. For biological monitoring of exposure to perchloroethylene, measurements of urinary trichloroacetic acid and blood levels of perchloroethylene can be used. A blood level of 1 mg/L found 16 hours after exposure corresponds to a TWA exposure of less than 50 ppm. Such an exposure was found to result in no adverse effects on the CNS, liver, or kidney. The excretion of urinary trichloroacetic acid is slow and therefore not very useful for biological monitoring. Concentrations of PCE in exhaled air may prove useful after recent exposure.

In chronic inhalation studies, perchloroethylene increased the incidence of leukemia in rats and hepatocellular adenomas and carcinomas in mice. Epidemiological studies on workers exposed to perchloroethylene are considered inconclusive. Liver cancer and leukemia, of a priori concern because of results in experimental animals, have not been found with increased frequency in dry-cleaning personnel. Rates for esophageal cancer and bladder cancer were elevated by a factor of two. The confounding effect of alcohol and cigarette smoking is to be considered, and other solvents may have played a role in bladder cancer incidence.[143] The International Agency for Research on Cancer (IARC) and the EPA have classified perchloroethylene as a category 2B carcinogen. NIOSH has designated perchloroethylene as a carcinogen and has recommended that occupational exposure be limited to the lowest feasible limit. In 1986 the American Conference of Government Industrial Hygienists (ACGIH) recommended a TLV-TWA of 50 ppm.

Mutagenicity tests with perchloroethylene have been negative. No increase in the rate of chromosomal aberrations or sister chromatic exchange has been found in workers occupationally exposed to perchloroethylene. In rats treated by gavage, malformations suggestive of teratogenicity were represented by microophthalmia (TCE, PCE); full litter resorption and delayed parturition were caused by PCE.[144]

Contamination of the general environment with perchloroethylene has been documented. Perchloroethylene exposure in 28 dry-cleaning establishments and in 25 homes occupied by dry-cleaners in Modena, Italy, showed wide variations in PCE concentrations from establishment to establishment (2.6 to 221.5 mg/m^3, 8-hour TWA personal sampling values). PCE inside the homes were significantly higher than in 29 houses selected as controls; alveolar air samples collected at home suggest that nonoccupational exposure to PCE exists for family members.[145] Perchloroethylene may be formed in small amounts through chlorination of water. It has been found in drinking water in concentrations of 0.5 to 5 μg/L. In trace amounts, it has also been detected in foodstuffs. The EPA has recommended that perchloroethylene in drinking water not exceed 0.5 mg/L.

Methyl Chloroform

Methyl chloroform (1,1,1-trichloroethane) has recently gained widespread use because of its relatively low toxicity. It is mostly used as a dry-cleaning agent, vapor degreaser, and aerosol vehicle and in the manufacture of vinylidene chloride. Hepatotoxicity and nephrotoxicity are low, but narcotic effects and even fatal respiratory depression have been reported. Cardiac arrhythmias due to myocardial sensitization to epinephrine have sometimes led to fatal outcomes. Methyl chloroform, rather than its metabolites, produces the arrhythmias.

Fatal cases of 1,1,1-trichloroethane poisoning have occurred. Intentional inhalation of typewriter correction fluid has resulted in deaths. 1,1,1-Trichloroethane and trichloroethylene are the components of this commercial product. Decrease in the availability of toluene-based glues, because of measures to combat glue sniffing, has resulted in abuse of more accessible solvents, such as 1,1,1-trichloroethane. In subchronic inhalation experiments, 1,1,1-trichloroethane was shown to lead to a decrease in DNA concentration in several brain areas of Mongolian gerbils. These results were interpreted as indicating decreased cell density in sensitive brain areas.[146]

Technical-grade methyl chloroform often contains vinylidene chloride; elimination of this contaminant seems desirable in view of its potential carcinogenic and mutagenic risk.

Vinyl Trichloride

Vinyl trichloride (1,1,2-trichloroethane) is a more potent narcotic and is a potent hepatotoxic and nephrotoxic agent. Significant increases in hepatocellular carcinomas and adrenal pheochromocytomas have been found in mice, but not in rats. DNA adduct formation in vivo was found to occur to a greater extent in mouse liver than in rat liver.[147] The IARC (1987) has classified 1,1,2-trichloroethane in group 3 (not classifiable as to its carcinogenicity in humans). The EPA (1988) has included 1,1,2-trichloroethane in category C (possible human carcinogen). The permissible level for occupational exposure to 1,1,2-trichloroethane is 10 ppm. The EPA (1987) has recommended that the concentration in drinking water not exceed 3 μg/L.

Tetrachloroethane

Tetrachloroethane (1,1,2,2,-tetrachloroethane) is the most toxic of the chlorinated hydrocarbons. It is an excellent solvent and has been widely used in the past in the airplane industry, from which numerous cases of severe and even fatal toxic liver injury have been reported. This has prompted its replacement by other, less toxic solvents in most industrial processes. Toxic liver damage due to tetrachloroethane is known to have been associated with the development of cirrhosis of the liver.

1,1,2,2-Tetrachloroethane has produced hepatocellular carcinomas in mice. In rats, no significant increase in hepatocellular carcinomas was found. It has been recommended by NIOSH that occupational exposure to 1,1,2,2-tetrachloroethane not exceed 1 ppm.

Vinyl Chloride

Vinyl chloride, an unsaturated, asymmetrical chlorinated hydrocarbon, has found widespread use in the production of the polymer polyvinyl chloride. Although its industrial use had expanded in the 1940s and 1950s, it was not until 1973 that its hepatotoxicity and carcinogenicity[148] were recognized. The acute narcotic effects had long been known: some rather unusual chronic effects had been reported in the 1960s, their main feature being Raynaud's syndrome involving the fingers and hands, skin changes described as similar to those of scleroderma, and bone abnormalities with resorption and spontaneous fractures of the distal phalanges. This syndrome was reported under the name vinyl chloride acroosteolysis.

In 1973 unusual hepatosplenic changes were described in vinyl chloride–exposed workers in Germany. Soon thereafter, the first cases of hemangiosarcoma of the liver were reported in workers of one vinyl chloride-polyvinyl chloride polymerization plant in the United States,[148] and the search for similar cases elsewhere led to the identification of some 90 such otherwise rare tumors in workers of this industry in many industrialized countries. The first case of vinyl chloride-related hepatic angiosarcoma in Australia has recently been reported: a 57-year-old former polyvinyl chloride autoclave cleaner developed angiosarcoma of the liver 15 years after his last exposure.[149]

The nonmalignant pathological changes in the liver are characterized by activation of hepatocytes, smooth endoplasmic reticulum proliferation, activation of sinusoidal cells including lipocytes, nodular hyperplasia of hepatocytes and sinusoidal cells, dilation of sinusoidal spaces, networklike collagen transformation of the sinusoidal walls, moderate portal fibrosis, and subcapsular fibrosis.

Portal hypertension has been the prominent feature in some cases of nonmalignant vinyl chloride liver disease; esophageal varices and bleeding have occurred. Fatty degenerative changes in the hepatocytes and focal necrosis have sometimes been observed and are thought to be more pronounced in cases studied shortly after cessation of toxic exposure.

The dilation of sinusoidal spaces and the proliferative changes of sinusoidal cells are precursors of the malignant transformation and the appearance of angiosarcomas. While the pathological characteristics of hemangiosarcomas may differ, and several types (sinusoidal, papillar, cavernous, and anaplastic) have been described, the biological characteristics are similar, with rapid growth and a downhill clinical course. No effective therapeutic approach has been identified.

Hemangiosarcoma of the liver is a very rare tumor, and therefore the identification of vinyl chloride as the etiologic carcinogen was facilitated. Excess lung cancers, lymphomas, and brain tumors have also been reported in some epidemiological studies. A significant mortality excess in angiosarcoma (15 cases), and cancer of the liver and biliary tract was found in a cohort of 10,173 men who had worked for at least 1 year in jobs with vinyl chloride exposure. The SMR for cancer of the brain was 180.[150]

In experimental animals exposed to vinyl chloride, carcinomas of the liver (hepatomas) also occur; sometimes both hemangiosarcoma and hepatoma have been found in the same animal. Malignant tumors of kidney, lung, and brain have also been found with increased incidence. Vinyl chloride is a transplacental carcinogen in the rat.

Vinyl chloride is metabolically activated by liver microsomal enzymes to intermediates that bind covalently to proteins and nucleic acids.

The toxic active metabolite of vinyl chloride is, according to several groups of investigators, most probably the epoxide chloroethylene oxide:

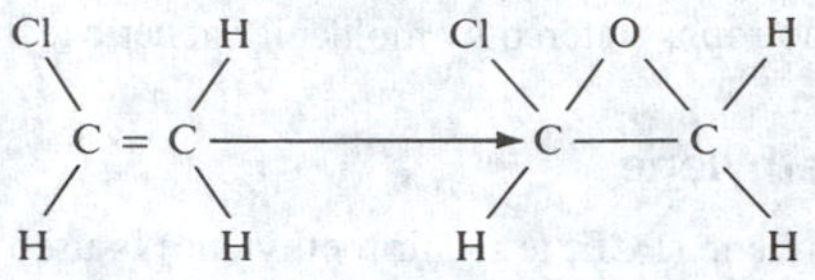

The electrophilic epoxide may react with cellular macromolecules, including nucleic acids; covalent and noncovalent binding occurs. The vinyl chloride epoxide metabolite appears to represent an optimal balance between stability that allows it to reach the DNA target and reactivity that leads to DNA binding and thus to the carcinogenic effect. Proven sites of alkylation are adenine, cytosine, and guanine moieties of nucleic acids and sulfhydryl groups of protein. Covalent binding with hepatocellular proteins can lead to liver necrosis; it has been observed that after microsomal enzyme induction, high doses of vinyl chloride may result in acute necrosis of the liver.

Binding to DNA is considered potentially important for mutagenicity and carcinogenicity. Ethenocytosine (epsilon C) is a highly mutagenic exocyclic DNA lesion induced by the carcinogen vinyl chloride. 3,*N*4-Ethano-2′-deoxycytidine, 3-(hydroxyethyl)-2′-deoxyuridine and 3,*N*4-etheno-2′-deoxycytidine are also formed in cells treated with vinyl chloride.[151] 1-*N*6-Ethenodeoxyadenosine (edA) and 3,-*N*4-ethenodeoxycytidine (edC) are two mutagenic adducts associated with exposure to vinyl chloride. Sensitive methods for determining the molecular dose of adducts in cellular DNA have recently been developed.[152] Four cyclic theno adducts—1,*N*6-ethenodeoxyadenine (epsilon A), 3,*N*4-ethenocytosine (epsilon C), *N*2,3-ethenoguanine (*N*2,3-epsilon G), and 1,*N*2-ethenoguanine (1,*N*2-epsilon G)—have been reported from human cells and tissues treated with the vinyl chloride metabolite chloroacetaldehyde.[153] Epsilon G,*N*2,3-ethenoguanine, a cyclic base derivative in DNA, was shown to specifically induce G → A transitions during DNA replication in *Escherichia coli*.[154] Under normal circumstances, altered DNA molecules are eliminated through physiological enzymatic systems. With defective function of repair mechanisms, cell populations modified by the toxic metabolite develop, with increasing metabolic autonomy and eventual malignant growth.

The p53 tumor suppressor gene is often mutated in a wide variety of cancers, including angiosarcoma of the liver. Anti-p53 antibodies have been detectected in sera of patients with a variety of cancers and can predate diagnosis of certain tumors such as angiosarcoma, making possible the identification of individuals at high cancer risk among the vinyl chloride-exposed workers.[155]

Activation of the Ki-ras 2 gene by GC → AT transition at the second base of codon 13 in human liver angiosarcoma associated with exposure to vinyl chloride has been recently reported. Experiments in rats exposed to vinyl chloride and developing liver angiosarcomas and hepatocellular carcinomas showed other sites of mutations affecting the Ha-ras gene in the hepatocellular carcinomas and the N-ras A gene in angiosarcomas. The nature of the ras gene affected by a given carcinogen depends on host factors specific to cell types. The molecular pathways leading to tumors in humans and rats are different, and differences are detected within a given species between different cell types.[156] Mutations of ras oncogenes and expression of their encoded p21 protein products are thought to have an important role in carcinogenesis. In 5 patients with angiosarcoma of the liver and heavy past exposure to vinyl chloride, four were found to have the mutation (Asp 13 c-Ki-ras) and to express the corresponding mutant protein in their tumor tissue and serum. In 45 vinyl chloride–exposed workers with no evidence of liver neoplasia, 49 percent were positive for the mutant p21 in their serum. In 28 age-, gender-, and race-matched, unexposed controls, results were all negative.[157]

Active research on the metabolic transformations of vinyl chloride has also resulted in a better understanding of the metabolic transformations of other chlorinated hydrocarbons, identification of reactive intermediate products (epoxides), and structural reasons for higher or lower reactivity.

Tetrachloroethylene, 1,2-*trans*-dichloroethylene, and 1,2-*cis*-dichloroethylene have been found not to be mutagenic, while trichloroethylene, 1,1-dichloroethylene, and vinyl chloride are mutagenic. The respective epoxides have been found to be symmetrical and relatively stable for the first group but asymmetrical, unstable, and highly reactive for the second.

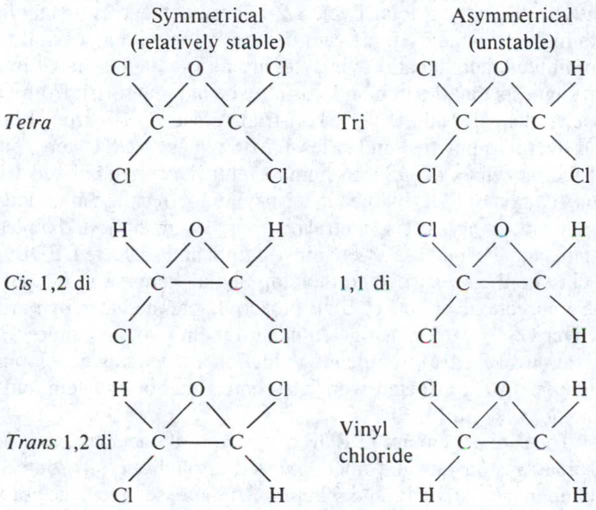

Mutagenicity of vinyl chloride has been demonstrated in a variety of test systems. Cytogenetic studies have indicated that vinyl chloride produces chromosomal aberrations.[158] The federal standard for exposure to vinyl chloride is 1 ppm for an 8-hour period; the ceiling of 5 ppm should never be exceeded for more than 15 minutes. Air-supplied respirators should be available and are required when exposure levels exceed these limits.

Vinyl Bromide

Production of vinyl bromide in the United States has expanded recently. It is used in the chemical, plastic, rubber, and leather industries. Experimental studies have shown that vinyl bromide has produced angiosarcoma of the liver, lymph node angiosarcoma, lymphosarcoma, and bronchioloalveolar carcinoma in rats exposed to 50 and 25 ppm by inhalation. Mutagenicity of vinyl bromide has also been reported.[159] On the basis of these data, NIOSH and OSHA jointly recommended that vinyl bromide be considered a potential carcinogen for humans and be controlled in a way similar to vinyl chloride, with a recommended exposure standard of 1 ppm.

Vinylidene Chloride

Vinylidene chloride (1,1-dichloroethylene (DCE)), like other vinyl halides, is used mainly in the plastics industry; it is easily polymerized and copolymerized to form plastic materials and resins with valuable properties.

Vinylidene chloride produces proximal tubular damage in mice. DCE undergoes biotransformation by NADPH-cytochrome P-450 to several reactive species that conjugate with glutathione (GSH). Further activation of these conjugates occurs in renal tubular cells.[160] DCE requires cytochrome P-450–catalyzed bioactivation to electrophylic metabolites (1,1-dichloroethylene oxide, 2-chloroacetyl chloride, and 2,2-dichloroacetaldehyde) to exert toxic effects. Conjugation of GSH with 1,1-dichloroethylene oxide leads to formation of monoglutathione and diglutathione adducts. Species differences were detected; microsomes from mice were 6-fold more active than those from rats. The epoxide is the major metabolite of DCE that is responsible for GSH depletion, suggesting that it may be involved in hepatotoxicity of DCE; mice are more susceptible than rats.[161]

In experimental studies, vinylidene chloride has been found to be carcinogenic in rats and mice: angiosarcoma of the liver, adenocarcinoma of the kidney, and other malignant tumors have been produced in inhalation experiments. In a recent study, DCE caused renal tumors in male mice after inhalation. Renal tumors were not observed in female mice or in rats of either sex. Kidney microsomes from male mice biotransformed DCE to chloroacetic acid. Cytochrome P-450 2E1 was detected in male mouse kidney microsomes; the expression of this protein was regulated by testosterone and correlated well with the ability to oxidize *p*-nitrophenol, a specific substrate for cytochrome P-450 2E1. In kidney microsomes from rats of both sexes and in six samples of human kidney (male donors), no *p*-nitrophenol oxidase was detected. The data suggest that cytochrome P-450 2E1 or a P-450 enzyme with very similar molecular weight and substrate specificities is expressed only in male mouse kidney and bioactivates DCE.[162]

Workers occupationally exposed to vinylidene chloride have not been shown to have excessively high cancer mortality; nevertheless, the possibility of a carcinogenic risk for humans exposed to vinylidene chloride cannot yet be excluded. Vinylidene chloride has been shown to be mutagenic in several assay systems. Embryotoxicity and fetal malformations have been observed in rats and rabbits after inhalation exposure to maternally toxic concentrations. In studies using a chick model, significantly more embryonic deaths occurred in the DCE-treated group than in controls.[163] Vinylidene chloride has not been shown to produce chromosomal aberrations or sister chromatic exchanges. In some experiments, vinylidene chloride has induced unscheduled DNA synthesis in rat hepatocytes and has alkylated DNA and induced DNA repair in mouse liver and kidney; the validity of these results has been questioned. The IARC has concluded that no evaluation of the carcinogenic risk of vinylidene chloride in humans could be made. The recommended exposure standard for vinylidene chloride is 1 ppm.

Ethylene Dichloride

Ethylene dichloride (1,2-dichloroethane, $ClCH_2-CH_2Cl$) is a colorless liquid at room temperature; with a boiling temperature of 83.4°C, it is highly volatile. Ethylene dichloride has a rapidly increasing volume of annual production; approximately 10 to 13 billion pounds were manufactured in the United States in recent years. Most of it (approximately 75 percent) is used in the production of vinyl chloride; it has also found applications in the manufacture of trichloroethylene, perchloroethylene, vinylidene chloride, ethylene amines, and ethylene glycol. It is a frequent constituent of antiknock mixtures of leaded gasoline and a component of fumigant insecticides. Other uses are as an extractor solvent, as a dispersant for nylon, viscose rayon, styrene-butadiene rubber, and other plastics, as a decreasing agent, as a component of paint and varnish removers, and in adhesives, soaps, and scouring compounds.

The main route of absorption is by inhalation; absorption through the skin is also possible. Ethylene dichloride is metabolized by cytochrome P-450; chloroacetoaldehyde and chloroacetic acid are the resulting metabolites. Microsomal cytochrome P-450 and nuclear cytochrome P-450 have been shown to metabolize ethylene dichloride. The possibility that the metabolic transformation of ethylene dichloride by nuclear cytochrome P-450 may in part mediate its mutagenicity, and carcinogenicity has been considered. Covalent alkylation of DNA by ethylene dichloride has been demonstrated.

Narcotic and irritant effects occur during or soon after acute overexposure; hepatotoxic and nephrotoxic effects become apparent several hours later and can be severe, with centrilobular hepatic necrosis, jaundice, or proximal renal convoluted tubular necrosis and anuria; fatalities with high exposure levels have been reported.[2,3] A hemorrhagic tendency in acute ethylene dichloride poisoning has also been reported; disseminated intravascular coagulopathy and hyperfibrinolysis have been found in several cases. Experiments on rats and mice fed ethylene dichloride in corn oil revealed a statistically significant excess of malignant and benign tumors. Glutathione conjugation is important in the metabolic transformation of 1,2-dichloroethane.

The metabolic pathways for 1,2-dichloroethane biotransformation are saturable; saturation occurs earlier after ingestion than after inhalation. Such differences in metabolic transformation have been thought to explain differences in results of experimental carcinogenicity studies, positive after oral administration but negative in inhalation experiments. A statistically significant increase in sister chromatic exchanges was detected in bone marrow cells of mice after acute 1,2-dichloroethane exposure.

Ethylene dichloride has been found to be mutagenic in a variety of bacterial systems and to enhance the viral transformation of Syrian hamster embryo cells. Testing for teratogenic effects and dominant lethal effects in mice was negative.[164]

Environmental surveys conducted by the EPA have detected 1,2-dichloroethane in ground-water sources in the vicinity of contaminated sites in concentrations of about 175 ppb (geometric mean). In a survey of 14 river basins in heavily industrialized areas in the United States, 1,2-dichloroethane was present in 53 percent of more than 200 surface-water samples. In drinking water the compound has been detected at concentrations ranging from 1 to 64 μg/L.[165] The OSHA permissible exposure limit for occupational exposure is 1 ppm. The MCL for drinking water has been regulated by the EPA at 0.005 mg/L. The EPA has classified 1,2-dichloroethane for its carcinogenic potential in group 2B.

Ethylene Dibromide

Ethylene dibromide (1,2-dibromoethane, $BrCH_2CH_2Br$) (EDB) is a colorless liquid with a boiling point of 131°C. One of the most important uses is in antiknock compounds added to gasoline to prevent the deposition of lead on the engine cylinder. It has also been used as a fumigant for grains, fruit, and vegetables, as a soil fumigant, as a special solvent, and in organic synthesis.

EDB has an irritant effect on the skin, with possible development of erythema, blistering, and ulceration after prolonged contact. It is also a potent eye and respiratory mucosal irritant. Systemic effects include CNS depression; after accidental ingestion, hepatocellular necrosis and renal proximal tubular epithelium necrosis have been reported. Cases of fatal ethylene dibromide poisoning have been reported. In experimental studies, hepatotoxicity and nephrotoxicity have been found at exposure levels of 50 ppm in all animals tested (rats, guinea pigs, rabbits, and monkeys).

EDB has been shown to produce significant decreases in cytochrome P-450 levels in liver, kidney, testes, lung, and small intestine microsomes. Hepatic microsomal mixed-function oxidase activities decreased in parallel with the cytochrome P-450 content. Dibromoalkane cytotoxicity is due to lipid peroxidation as well as cytochrome P-450–dependent formation of toxic bromoaldehydic metabolites, which can bind with cellular macromolecules. Dibromoethane-GSH conjugates also contribute to EDB cytotoxicity.[166]

The liver toxicity of several halogen compound mixtures has been studied. Carbon tetrachloride (CT) and trichlorobromomethane (TCBM) undergo dehalogenation via the P-450–dependent enzyme system. DCE and EDB are mainly conjugated with the cytosolic GSH by means of GSH-*S*-transferase. The mixture TCBM and DBE shows a more than additive action on lipid peroxidation and liver necrosis. TCBM, like CT, reduces hepatic levels of GSH-*S*-transferase, increasing the amount of EDB available for P-450–dependent metabolism, with the production of toxic metabolites. The toxicity of mixtures of halogen compounds can be partly predicted. When their metabolism is quite different, a synergistic toxicity can occur if one pathway interferes with a detoxification mechanism of the other compound.[167]

EDB exerts a toxic effect on spermatogenesis in bulls, rams, and rats, with oligospermia and degenerative changes in spermatozoa. Effects of ethylene dibromide on spermatogenesis have been studied in 46 men employed in papaya fumigation; the highest measured exposure was 262 ppb, and the geometric mean was 88 ppb. When compared with a nonexposed reference group, there were statistically significant decreases in sperm count, in percentage of viable and mobile sperm, and in the proportion of sperm with specific morphologic abnormalities.[168]

Mutagenic effects of EDB have been detected in several test systems.

A teratogenic effect is suspected; in rats and mice an increased incidence of CNS and skeletal malformations was found to be related to ethylene dibromide exposure. GSH-*S*-transferase occurs abundantly in the human fetal liver. 1,2-Dibromoethane is metabolized with high efficiency. Significant bioactivation with a possibility of only limited detoxification via cytochrome P-450–dependent oxidation suggests that the human fetus may be at greater risk from DBE toxicity than the adult.[169] GSH-*S*-transferase (GST) from human fetal liver was purified and at least 5 isozymes of GST were found. All the isozymes of GST in human fetal liver metabolized EDB. Bioactivation of EDB by the GST isozyme P-3 resulted in toxicity to cultured rat embryos. The central nervous system, optic and olfactory system, and the hind limb were most significantly affected. EDB may be classified as a suspected developmental toxicant in humans.[170] The embryotoxic effects of EDB bioactivation, mediated by purified rat liver GST, were investigated using rat embryos in culture. EDB activation caused a significant reduction in general development structures. Most affected were the central nervous system and the olfactory system.[171]

The carcinogenicity of EDB has been well documented in several bioassays on rats and mice exposed through various routes, including inhalation of 10 and 40 ppm. An increased incidence of various malignant tumors occurred in one or both sexes of one or both species tested. Among these were tumors of the mammary gland and nasal cavity, alveolar bronchiolar carcinomas, hemangiosarcomas, and tumors of the adrenal cortex and kidney.

An epidemiological study[3,172] of a relatively small group of EDB-exposed workers suggests an increase in total mortality and total deaths from malignant diseases in the population with higher exposure.

EDB is considered to be a bifunctional alkylating agent because of the two replaceable bromine atoms. It may form covalent bonds with cellular constituents; the reaction with DNA is thought to be especially important, with possible covalent cross-links between DNA strands. Irreversible binding of EDB to DNA and RNA has been demonstrated. A complex between reduced glutathione and ethylene dibromide seems to be implicated in the covalent binding of EDB to DNA; this is unusual in that glutathione seems to play a role in the bioactivation of the carcinogen, as opposed to its more typical detoxification reactions. The major DNA adduct (greater than 95 percent of the total) resulting from the bioactivation of ethylene dibromide by conjugation with GSH is *S*-(2-(*N*7-guanyl)ethyl)GSH. Other adducts are present at much lower levels.[173]

Environmental exposure of the general population to EDB has recently received increased attention. Several uses of EDB—as an antiknock additive in leaded gasoline, for soil fumigation, fumigation of citrus and other fruit to prevent insect infestation, and treatment of grain-milling equipment—have resulted in contamination of air, water, fruit, grain, and derived products.

EDB has been found in ground water in areas where it had been extensively used for soil fumigation. In the air of major cities, levels of EDB ranging from 16 to 59 ppt have been detected. Citrus fruits that had been fumigated were found to contain amounts of EDB of several hundred parts per billion; in lychee fruit (imported to Japan from Taiwan) levels varying from 0.14 to 2.18 ppm were detected.[174] An important and rather widespread contamination problem is that of EDB residues in commercial flour; levels from 8 ppb to 4 ppm were detected. In some ready-to-eat food products, levels up to 260 ppb were found.

In 1983 the EPA introduced regulations to discontinue the use of EDB for soil fumigation, grain fumigation, treatment of grain-milling equipment, and postharvest fruit fumigation. In 1984 the EPA recommended guidelines for acceptable levels of the chemical in food for human consumption, based on samplings of grain stocks and packaged foods in markets. It was recommended that EDB concentrations in grain intended for human consumption not exceed 90 ppb; for flour the residue level should not be higher than 150 ppb, and for ready-to-eat products it should not be more than 30 ppb. These guidelines have been critically reviewed and requests for even lower acceptable levels have been made. The proposed OSHA TWA standard for ethylene dibromide exposure is 100 ppb. NIOSH has recommended 45 ppb.

Methyl Chloride and Methyl Bromide

Methyl chloride and methyl bromide are gases at normal temperatures. Methyl chloride (CH_3Cl) is used in the chemical industry as a chlorinating agent but mainly as a methylating agent; it is also used in oil refineries for the extraction of greases and resins, as a solvent in the synthetic rubber industry, and as an expanding agent in the production of polystyrene foam. In recent years methyl chloride has been used primarily in the production of methyl silicone polymers and resins and organic lead additives for gasoline. Methyl bromide (CH_3Br) is used as a fumigant for soil, grain, warehouses, and ships. Other important uses are as a methylating agent, a herbicide, a fire-extinguishing agent, a degreaser, in the extraction of oils, and as a solvent in aniline dye manufacture. Currently most of the methyl bromide produced in the United States is used to manufacture pesticides.

Methyl chloride and methyl bromide are irritants; exposure to high concentrations may result in toxic pulmonary edema. They are potent depressants of the CNS; with high exposure, toxic encephalopathy with visual disturbances, tremor, delirium, convulsions, and coma may occur and may be fatal. Permanent neurological deficits have been reported after recovery from acute toxic encephalopathy caused by methyl chloride and methyl bromide. Hepatotoxic and nephrotoxic effects may also occur.

Fatal poisonings after accidental exposure to high concentrations of methyl bromide, used as a fumigant, have occurred. In California in recent years, the most frequent cause of methyl bromide-related fatalities has been unauthorized entry into structures under fumigation. Toxic acute pulmonary edema, with hemorrhage, has been the most frequently reported lesion in such cases.[175]

Systemic methyl bromide poisoning developed in nine greenhouse workers after acute inhalational exposure on 2 consecutive days. Measurements of CH_3Br at the site within hours after the accident suggested that exposure on the second day may have been in excess of 200 ppm (800 mg/m^3). Two patients needed intensive care for several weeks because of severe myoclonus and tonic-clonic generalized convulsions, which could be suppressed effectively only by thiopental. Prior, subchronic exposure to methyl bromide and high serum bromide (Br^-) concentrations are likely to have contributed to the severity of the symptoms.[176] A case of preventable fatality as a result of methyl bromide fumigation of a restaurant has been reported. Worker and community notification of the hazard whenever fumigation takes place are absolutely necessary.[177]

Methyl chloride, methyl bromide, and methyl iodide are alkylating agents; all three are direct mutagens in in vitro tests. Monohalogenated methanes (methyl chloride, methyl bromide, and methyl iodide) produced DNA adducts 7-methylguanine and *O*6-methylguanine in exposed rats.[178]

^{14}C-Methyl bromide was administered to rats orally or by inhalation. DNA adducts were detected in the liver, lung, and stomach. ^{14}C-3-methyladenine, ^{14}C-7-methylguanine, and ^{14}C-*O*6-methylguanine were identified. A systemic DNA-alkylating potential of methyl bromide was thus demonstrated.[179]

Sister chromatid exchange (SCE) was determined in the lymphocytes of methyl bromide fumigators as an additional biomonitoring parameter. The new method for determination of blood protein adducts can be applied for evaluation of environmental exposure.[180]

A hitherto unknown glutathione-*S*-transferase in human erythrocytes displays polymorphism: three quarters of the population ("conjugators") possess, whereas one-quarter ("nonconjugators") lack this specific activity. A standard method for identification of conjugators and nonconjugators with the use of methyl bromide and gas chromatography (head space technique) has been developed. Methyl bromide, ethylene oxide and dichloromethane (methylene chloride) were incubated in vitro with whole blood samples of conjugators and nonconjugators. All three substances led to a marked increase of SCEs in the lymphocytes of nonconjugators. A protective effect of the glutathione-*S*-transferase activity in human erythrocytes for the cytogenetic toxicity of these chemicals in vitro is thus confirmed.[181]

The formation of formaldehyde from dichloromethane (methylene chloride) is influenced by the polymorphism of GST theta, in the same way as the metabolism of methyl bromide, methyl chloride, methyl iodide, and ethylene oxide. Carcinogenicity of dichloromethane in long-term inhalation exposure of rodents has been attributed to metabolism of the compound via the GST-dependent pathway. Extrapolation of the results to humans for risk assessment should consider the newly discovered polymorthic enzyme activity of GST theta.[182]

Methyl chloride has produced a teratogenic effect (heart malformation) in offspring of pregnant mice exposed by inhalation. Methyl chloride and methyl bromide have been shown to produce testicular degeneration.

The hemoglobin adduct methyl cysteine has been proposed as a biological indicator of methyl bromide exposure. The NIOSH recommends that methyl chloride and methyl bromide be considered as potential occupational carcinogens. The IARC (1986) found the evidence of carcinogenicity in humans and animals inconclusive. The 1987 TLV for methyl chloride is 50 ppm; for methyl bromide, it is 5 ppm.

Chloroprene

Chloroprene (2-chloro-1,3-butadiene, $H_2C{=}CCl{-}CH{=}CH_2$) is a colorless, flammable liquid with a low boiling point of 59.4°C. The major use is as a monomer in the manufacture of synthetic rubber, neoprene, since it can polymerize spontaneously at room temperature. The annual neoprene production in the United States is approximately 400 million pounds.

Inhalation of vapor and skin absorption are the routes of absorption. Chloroprene is an irritant of skin and mucosae (eyes, respiratory tract); it is a potent CNS depressant and has definite liver and kidney toxicity. Hair loss has also been associated with chloroprene exposure.

There are very few epidemiological studies on long-term effects of chloroprene. An excess of lung cancer and skin cancer has been reported by Russian investigators; the mean age of chloroprene-exposed workers with cancer was significantly younger than that in other groups.[183] The methodological limitations of these studies preclude firm conclusions on the carcinogenicity of chloroprene. A cohort study of chloroprene production and polymerization workers[184] gave negative results with regard to lung cancer but raised the possibility of an increased incidence of gastrointestinal cancer and hematopoietic and lymphatic cancer. Methodological difficulties of this latter study make it impossible to reach definitive conclusions.

Experimental studies on the carcinogenicity of chloroprene have been assessed by the International Agency for Research on Cancer and found to be inconclusive.

An immunosuppressive effect of chloroprene is suspected. Chloroprene produces degenerative changes in male reproductive organs. Reproductive capacity in male mice and rats was affected after inhalation of chloroprene in concentrations of 12 to 150 ppm. Reduction in the number and mobility of sperm and testicular atrophy have been observed in rats after chloroprene exposure. In experiments on rats and mice, it was also found to be embryotoxic.

Although chloroprene has been shown to be mutagenic in several test systems, the genotoxicity of 2-chloro-1,3-butadiene is controversial. A recent mutagenicity study detected a mutagenic effect that occurred linearly with increasing age of chloroprene. Major by-products of chloroprene, probably responsible for mutagenic properties of aged chloroprene, were identified as cyclic chloroprene dimers.[185] Chromosome aberrations have been reported in bone marrow cells of exposed rats. In several groups of chloroprene-exposed workers, an increased incidence of chromosome aberrations in peripheral blood lymphocytes was noted.

Prevention

Occupational exposure to chloroprene should be limited to a maximum concentration of 1 ppm. Protective equipment to exclude the possibility of skin absorption, safety goggles, and air-supplied respirators are necessary to minimize exposure. Medical surveillance must be aimed not only at detection of short-term toxic and irritant effects but also at long-term effects on the CNS, liver and kidney function, reproductive abnormalities, and cancer risk.

Fluorocarbons

Fluorocarbons are hydrocarbons with fluorine, often with additional chlorine or bromine substitution of hydrogen atoms in their molecules. Most of them are nonflammable gases, and some are liquids at room temperature. Contact with open flame or heated metallic objects results in decomposition products, some of which are highly irritant, especially with chlorofluorocarbons (hydrogen fluoride, hydrogen chloride, phosgene, chlorine).

The fluorocarbons are used as refrigerants (Freon is one of the most widely used trademarks), as aerosol propellants, in fire extinguishers, for degreasing of electronic equipment, in the production of polymers, and as expanding agents in the manufacture of plastic foam.

Exposure to fluorocarbons in chemical plant operations and production is generally low but highly variable; high exposures can occur in areas without proper ventilation, during tank farm operations, tank and drum filling, and cylinder packing and shipping. Exposure to fluorocarbons can also occur during manufacturing, servicing, or leakage of refrigeration equipment.

The use of fluorocarbons as solvents in the electrical and electronic industry can generate higher exposures, especially when open containers are used. Emissions of fluorocarbons from plastic foams, where they have been entrapped during foam blowing, is another source of exposure. Use of fluorocarbons in sterilization procedures for reusable medical equipment, mostly with ethylene oxide, does not usually generate major exposures.

Fluorocarbons, especially trichlorofluoromethane (FC 11), have been used in the administration of certain drugs by inhalation, mostly sympathomimetics and corticosteroids for the treatment of asthma.

Fluorocarbons with the widest use are the following:

Bromotrifluoromethane
Dibromodifluoromethane
Dichlorodifluoromethane
Dichloromonofluoromethane
Dichlorotetrafluoroethane
Fluorotrichloromethane
1,1,1,2-Tetrachloro-2,2-difluoroethane
1,1,2,2-Tetrachloro-1,2-difluoroethane
1,1,2-Trichloro-1,2,2-trifluoroethane
Bromochlorotrifluoroethane
Chlorodifluoromethane
Chloropentafluoroethane
Chlorotrifluoroethylene
Chlorotrifluoromethane
Difluoroethylene
Fluoroethylene
Hexafluoropropylene
Octafluorocyclobutane
Tetrafluoroethylene

Irritative effects of fluorocarbons are mild; after exposure to decomposition products, such effects may be severe. A bronchoconstrictive effect after inhalation of fluorocarbons has been demonstrated to occur at concentrations higher than 1000 ppm.

Narcotic effects occur at high concentrations. Liver and kidney toxicity have been reported with fluoroalkenes, thought to be more toxic than fluoroalkanes. Fatalities have been reported after acute overexposure to high concentrations of fluorocarbons used as refrigerants; in some of these cases simultaneous exposure to methyl chloride or to phosgene (a decomposition product of fluorocarbons) made it difficult to assess the contribution of fluorocarbon exposure to the lethal outcome.

A significant increase in the number of deaths from bronchial asthma was observed in Great Britain and found to coincide in time with the introduction and use of bronchodilator aerosols with fluorocarbon propellants. After withdrawal of these products from over-the-counter sale, the number of deaths from bronchial asthma decreased significantly.[186] Numerous deaths due to inhalation of fluorocarbon FC 11 (trichlorofluoromethane) have occurred. Addiction to fluorocarbon propellants in bronchodilator aerosols has been reported.[187]

Experimental evidence from studies on various animal species, documenting the arrhythmogenic properties of fluorocarbons, has established that sudden deaths due to cardiac arrhythmias, most probably through a mechanism similar to that identified for many chlorinated hydrocarbons, can occur with exposure to fluorocarbons. This prompted a reassessment of the permissible exposure levels.

Mutagenicity tests were conducted on a series of fluorocarbons in two in vitro systems. Chlorodifluoromethane (FC 22), chlorofluoromethane (FC 31), chlorodifluoroethane (FC 142b), and trifluoroethane (FC 143a) gave positive results in one or two of the tests. Potential carcinogenicity was considered, and limited carcinogenicity bioassays have indicated that FC 31 and FC 133 were potent carcinogens.[188]

Fluorocarbons that are lighter than air accumulate at high altitudes, where they may interact with and degrade the ozone layer, leading to penetration to the earth's surface of greater amounts of ultraviolet light. The problem of the ozone layer depletion is thought to be more specifically related to the fully halogenated, nonhydrogenated fluorocarbons, which produce free-radical reactions with ozone by photodissociation in the upper atmosphere. Regulatory action has been taken to eliminate the use of fluorocarbon aerosol products in the United States. Other aspects of fluorocarbon use are still under consideration.

▸ ALCOHOLS AND GLYCOLS

Alcohols are characterized by the substitution of one hydrogen atom of hydrocarbons by a hydroxyl (—OH) group; glycols are compounds with two such hydroxyl groups. Both are used extensively as solvents. Under usual industrial exposure conditions, alcohols and glycols do not represent major acute health hazards, mostly because their volatility is much lower than that of most other solvents.

Cases of severe poisoning with methyl alcohol or ethylene glycol are usually caused by accidental ingestion. They have an irritative effect on mucous membranes; the narcotic effect is much less prominent than with the corresponding hydrocarbons or halogenated hydrocarbons.

Glycols are liquids with low volatility; the low vapor pressure prevents significant air concentrations, except when the compounds are heated or sprayed. Inhalation or skin contact does not usually result in absorption of toxic amounts; accidental ingestion accounts for the majority of poisoning cases. Glycols are used mainly as solvents and, because of their low freezing point, in antifreeze mixtures.

Methyl Alcohol

Methyl alcohol (methanol, wood alcohol, CH_3OH) is used in the chemical industry in the manufacture of formaldehyde, methacrylates, ethylene glycol, and a variety of other compounds such as plastics, celluloid, and photographic film.[2,3] It is also used as a solvent for lacquers, adhesives, industrial coatings, inks, and dyes and in paint and varnish removers. It is used in antifreeze mixtures, as an additive to gasoline, and as an antidetonant additive for aircraft fuel. Increases in the use of methanol as a transportation fuel would result in greater potential for inhalation exposures.[189] Methanol will be present as a new air pollutant when methanol-powered vehicles are introduced in the United States. Twenty-six human volunteers were exposed for 4 hours to 200 ppm methanol vapor in a randomized, double blind study using a whole-body exposure chamber. No significant differences in serum formate concentrations between exposed and control groups were detected. It was concluded that, at 200 ppm, methanol exposure does not contribute substantially to endogenous formate quantities.[190]

Methyl alcohol is a moderate irritant and depressant of the CNS. Systemic toxicity due to inhalation and skin absorption of methyl alcohol has been reported with very high exposure levels because of large amounts being handled in enclosed spaces. Accidental ingestion of methyl alcohol can be fatal; after a latency period of several hours (longer with smaller amounts), neurological abnormalities, visual disturbances, nausea, vomiting, abdominal pain, metabolic acidosis, and coma may occur in rapid sequence.

Toxic optic retrobulbar neuritis is a specific effect of methyl alcohol and may result in permanent blindness due to optic atrophy. Bilateral putaminal necrosis is often recognized radiologically in severe methanol toxicity. A case of bilateral putaminal and cerebellar cortical lesions demonstrable on CT and MRI has been reported.[191] Nephrotoxic effects and toxic pancreatitis have also been reported. Methyl alcohol is slowly metabolized to formaldehyde and formic acid; the extent to which these metabolites are responsible for the specific toxic effects has not been completely clarified. Formate metabolism to CO_2 is governed by tissue H_4folate and 10-formyltetrahydrofolate dehydrogenase (10-FTHFDH) levels. 10-FTHFDH was found to be present in rat retina, optic nerve, and brain. It was concluded that, in rats, target tissues possess the capacity to metabolize formate to CO_2 and may be protected from formate toxicity through this folate-dependent system.[192]

Nonprimate laboratory animals do not develop the characteristic human methanol toxicities even after a lethal dose.[193] In humans, methanol causes systemic and ocular toxicity after acute exposure. The folate-reduced (FR) rat is an excellent animal model that mimics characteristic human methanol toxicity. Blood methanol levels were not significantly different in FR rats compared with folate-sufficient rats. FR rats, however, had elevated blood and vitreous humor formate and abnormal electroretinograms at 48 hours postdose, suggesting that formate is the toxic metabolite in methanol-induced retinal toxicity.[194]

Control of acidosis is very important in methyl alcohol poisoning, and intravenous bicarbonate has been beneficial. Since methanol is metabolized by alcohol dehydrogenase, and its metabolites were considered more toxic than methanol itself, ethanol was thought to be helpful through competition for the metabolizing enzyme. The median half-life of methanol in patients treated with ethanol was found to be 43.1 hours. Because of the significant risk of toxicity and complications during methanol monotherapy with ethanol, hemodialysis should be considered in patients who are treated with ethanol infusion.[195] Hemodialysis has markedly improved the outlook in accidental methanol poisoning, as has the adequate management of metabolic acidosis.

Prevention

The federal standard for methanol exposure is 200 ppm.[3] Warning signs must be posted wherever methyl alcohol is stored or can be present in the working environment, with emphasis on the extreme danger of blindness if swallowed. Employees' education and training must be thorough. Medical surveillance with attention to visual, neurological, hepatic, and renal functions is necessary. Formic acid in urine and methyl alcohol in blood can be used for the assessment of excessive exposure.

Significant toxicity can result from *intentional* methanol inhalation. Several cases of intentional inhalation of a carburetor cleaner containing toluene 43.8 percent, methanol 23.2 percent, methylene chloride 20.5 percent, and propane 12.5 percent were recently reported. Patients arrived at the emergency department with central nervous system depression, nausea, vomiting, shortness of breath, photophobia, and/or decreased visual acuity. Treatment included correction of acidosis, folic acid, ethanol infusions, and supportive care. Hemodialysis was necessary in three cases. Methanol in blood ranged from 50.4 to 128.6 mg/dL. Blood formic acid ranged from 120 to 480 µg/mL. Ophthalmic examination revealed hyperemic discs and decreased visual acuity in one patient. One individual was found pulseless, and attempts at revival were unsuccessful.[196]

Allyl Alcohol

Allyl alcohol ($H_2C{=}CHCH_2OH$) is a liquid with a boiling point of 96.0°C. It is used in the manufacture of allyl esters and of monomers for synthetic resins and plastics, in the synthesis of a variety of organic compounds, in the pharmaceutical industry, and as a herbicide and fungicide.

Absorption occurs through inhalation and percutaneous penetration. Allyl alcohol is a potent irritant for the eyes, the respiratory system, and the skin. Muscle pain underlying the site of skin absorption, lacrimation, photophobia, blurring of vision, and corneal lesions have been reported.[2] The marked irritant properties probably prevent greater exposure, which would result in liver and kidney toxicity, effects found in experimental animals but not reported in humans.

Prevention

The federal standard for permissible exposure limit to allyl alcohol is 2 ppm. Protective equipment is very important, given the possible skin absorption; the material of choice is neoprene.

Isopropyl Alcohol

Isopropyl alcohol ($CH_3CHOHCH_3$, isopropanol) is a colorless liquid with a boiling point of 82.3°C and high volatility. It is used in the production of acetone and isopropyl derivatives. Other important uses are as a solvent for oils, synthetic resins, plastics, perfumes, dyes, and nitrocellulose lacquers and in the extraction of sulfonic acid from petroleum products. Isopropyl alcohol has many applications in the pharmaceutical industry, in liniments, skin lotions, mouthwashes, cosmetics, rubbing alcohol, etc.

Isopropyl alcohol absorption takes place mainly by inhalation, although skin absorption is also possible. The irritant effects are slight; dermatitis has seldom been reported. Depressant (narcotic) effects have been observed in cases of accidental or intentional isopropyl alcohol ingestion. Coma and renal tubular degenerative changes have occasionally resulted in death. Acetone has been found in the exhaled air and in urine; isopropyl alcohol concentrations in blood can be measured.

In the early 1940s an unusual clustering of neoplasms of the respiratory tract—malignant tumors of the paranasal sinuses, lung, and larynx—was reported in workers in isopropyl alcohol manufacturing. It was thought that the carcinogenic compounds were associated with the "strong acid process" and especially with heavier hydrocarbon oils (tars) containing polyaromatic compounds.

In the more modern direct catalytic hydration (weak acid process) of propylene, the isopropyl oil seems to contain compounds with lower molecular weight, although the precise composition is not known. Attempts to identify the carcinogen(s) in experimental studies have not been successful,[3] and the question of a carcinogen present in the manufacture of isopropyl alcohol is still open.

Prevention

The federal standard for a permissible level of isopropyl alcohol exposure is at present 400 ppm.

Ethylene Chlorhydrin

Ethylene chlorhydrin (CH_2ClCH_2OH)—synonyms: glycol chlorohydrin, 2-chloroethanol, β-chloroethyl alcohol—is a very toxic compound.[2] It is used in the synthesis of ethylene glycol and ethylene oxide and in a variety of other reactions, especially when the hydroxyethyl group ($-CH_2CH_2OH$) has to be incorporated in molecules. Other uses are as a special solvent, for cellulose acetate and esters, resins, waxes, and for the separation of butadiene from hydrocarbon mixtures. Agricultural applications include seed treatment and application to accelerate the sprouting of potatoes.

Ethylene chlorhydrin is absorbed through inhalation and readily through the skin. It is irritant to the eyes, airways, and skin. Exposure to high concentrations may result in toxic pulmonary edema. Systemic effects are marked: depression of the CNS, hypotension, visual disturbances, delirium, coma and convulsions, hepatotoxic and nephrotoxic effects with nausea, vomiting, hematuria, and proteinuria. Death may occur as a result of pulmonary edema or cerebral edema. Even cases with slight or moderate initial symptoms may be fatal.

Prevention

The federal standard for the limit of permissible exposure is 5 ppm. The use of ethylene chlorhydrin other than in enclosed systems should be completely eliminated. Protective clothing should use materials impervious to this compound; rubber is readily penetrated and has to be excluded. Protective clothing must be changed regularly so that no deterioration will jeopardize its effectiveness.

Ethylene Glycol

Ethylene glycol ($OHCH_2CH_2OH$) is a viscous colorless liquid, used mainly in antifreeze and hydraulic fluids but also in the manufacture of glycol esters, resins, and other derivatives, and as a solvent.

CNS depression, nausea, vomiting, abdominal pain, respiratory failure, and renal failure with oliguria, proteinuria, and oxalate crystals in the urinary sediment are manifestations of ethylene glycol poisoning.[2] Glycolic acid is the metabolite that is found in the highest concentrations in blood; serum and urine levels of glycolic acid correlate with clinical symptoms.[197] The active enzyme is alcohol dehydrogenase. It is estimated that 50 deaths occur annually in the United States from accidental ingestion of ethylene glycol. Hemodialysis has been successfully used in the treatment of accidental ethylene glycol poisoning by ingestion. The therapeutic use of 4-methyl pyrazole, an alcohol dehydrogenase inhibitor, has been recommended for the management of accidental or suicidal ethylene glycol poisoning.

Prevention

No federal standard for ethylene glycol exposure has been established. The American Conference of Industrial Hygienists recommended a threshold limit value of 100 ppm. The most important preventive action is to alert employees to the extreme hazard of ingestion. Adequate respiratory protection should be provided wherever the compound is heated or sprayed.

Increasing use of glycols as deicing agents for aircraft and airfield runways has generated concern about surface-water contamination that may result from runoff. Degradation of ethylene glycol in river water is complete within 3 to 7 days (depending on temperature); degradation of diethylene glycol is somewhat slower. At low temperatures (8°C or less), both glycols degrade at a minimal rate.[198]

Diethylene Glycol

Diethylene glycol is similar in its effects to ethylene glycol; its importance is mainly historical, since more than 100 deaths occurred in the United States when it was used in the manufacture of an elixir of sulfanilamide. Fatal cases were caused by renal proximal tubular necrosis and renal failure.[2]

▸ ETHYLENE GLYCOL ETHERS AND DERIVATIVES

The most important alkyl glycol derivatives are ethylene glycol monoethyl ether (ethoxyethanol, cellosolve) ($CH_3CH_2OCHCH_2OH$) and its acetate; ethylene glycol monomethyl ether (methoxyethanol, methyl cellosolve, EGME) ($CH_3OCH_2CH_2OH$) and its acetate; and ethylene glycol monobutyl ether (butoxyethanol, butyl cellosolve) ($CH_3CH_2CH_2CH_2OCH_2CH_2OH$).[2] These compounds are colorless liquids with wide applications as solvents for resins, lacquers, paints, varnishes, coatings (including epoxy resin coatings), dyes, inks, adhesives, and plastics. They are also used in hydraulic fluids, as anti-icing additives, in brake fluids, and in aviation fuels. Ethylene glycol monoethyl ether is used in the formulation of adhesives, detergents, pesticides, cosmetics, and pharmaceuticals.

Inhalation, transcutaneous absorption, and gastrointestinal absorption are all possible. These derivatives are irritants for the mucous membranes and skin. The acetates are more potent irritants. Corneal clouding, usually transitory, may occur. Acute overexposure may result in marked narcotic effects and encephalopathy; pulmonary edema and severe kidney and liver toxicity are also possible. At lower levels of exposure, CNS effects result in such symptoms as fatigue, headache, tremor, slurred speech, gait abnormalities, blurred vision, and personality changes.

Anemia is another possible effect; macrocytosis and immature forms of leukocytes can be found. Exposure to ethylene glycol monomethyl ether has also been associated with pancytopenia. In animal experiments, butyl cellosolve has been shown to produce hemolytic anemia; this has not been reported in humans.

Exposure to ethylene glycol monomethyl ether and to ethylene glycol monoethyl ether has been shown to result in adverse reproductive effects in mice, rats, and rabbits. These effects include testicular atrophy, degenerative testicular changes,[199] abnormal sperm head morphology, and infertility in males. Glycol ethers produce hematotoxicity and testicular toxicity in animals, which are dependent on both the alkyl chain length and the animal species used. Ethylene glycol monobutyl ether (2-butoxyethanol, BE) causes hemolytic anemia in rats but not in guinea pigs (or in humans).

2-Methoxyethanol (ME) produces testicular lesions in rats, characterized primarily by degeneration of spermatocytes undergoing meiotic division, with minimal or no hemolytic changes. In guinea pigs, a single dose or multiple (3 daily) doses of 200 mg ME/kg were given, and animals were examined 4 days after the start of treatment. In guinea pigs, spermatocyte degeneration was observed in stage III/IV tubules, but was much less severe than in rats.[200] The stage-specific effect of a single oral dose (500 mg/kg body weight) of ethylene glycol monomethyl ether was characterized during one cycle of seminiferous epithelium in rats. Maximum peritubular membrane damage and germinal epithelium distortion were observed in stages IX–XII. Cell death occurred during conversion of zygotene to pachytene spermatocytes (stage XIII) and between dividing spermatocytes and step I spermatids (stage late XIII–XIV).[201]

Exposure of pregnant animals resulted in increased rates of embryonic deaths and in various congenital malformations. The acetate esters of ethylene glycol monomethyl ether and of ethylene glycol monoethyl ether have produced similar adverse male reproductive effects.

Ethylene glycol monomethyl ether is metabolized to the active compound methoxy-acetic acid, which readily crosses the placenta and impairs fetal development. Pregnant mice exposed to EGME from gestational days 10 to 17 and offspring were examined on gestational day 18. Significant thymic atrophy and cellular depletion were found in EGME-exposed fetal mice, with decreased CD4+8+ thymocytes and increased percentages of CD4–8– thymocytes. In addition, fetal liver prolymphocytes were also sensitive targets of EGME exposure.[202]

Methoxyacetic acid (MAA), a teratogenic toxin, is the major metabolite of EGME. Electron paramagnetic resonance (EPR) spin-labeling techniques were used to gain insight into the mechanism of MAA toxicity. The results suggested that MAA may lead to teratological toxicity by interacting with certain protein components, i.e., transport proteins, cytoskeleton proteins, or neurotransmitter receptors.[203]

A cross-sectional study of 97 workers exposed to ethylene glycol monomethyl ether, with semen analysis in 15, did not reveal abnormalities other than possibly smaller testicular size.[204] The occurrence of adverse male reproductive effects in humans cannot be excluded on the basis of this study.

Ethylene glycol monomethyl ether, ethylene glycol monoethyl ether, ethylene glycol *n*-butyl ether and their aldehyde and acid derivatives were tested for mutagenicity with the Ames test, with and without the rat S9 mix. Ethylene glycol *n*-butyl ether and the aldehyde metabolite of ethylene glycol monomethyl ether, methoxyacetaldehyde, were found to be mutagenic in strain *Salmonella typhimurium* 97a, with and without S9 mix.[205] Administration of EGME and its metabolite methoxyacetaldehyde (MALD), in concentrations of 35 to 2500 mg/kg for EGME and 25 to 1,000 mg/kg for MALD, did not cause any chromosomal aberrations in mice after acute or subchronic exposure by the oral route.[206]

Prevention

Federal standards for permissible exposure limits are ethylene glycol monoethyl ether, 200 ppm; ethylene glycol monoethyl ether acetate, 100 ppm; ethylene glycol monomethyl ether, 25 ppm; ethylene glycol monomethyl ether acetate, 25 ppm; and ethylene glycol monobutyl ether, 50 ppm.

The American Conference of Governmental Industrial Hygienists has recommended a TLV of 25 ppm for ethylene glycol monomethyl ether and 100 ppm for ethylene glycol monoethyl ether; this later TLV was lowered in 1981 to 50 ppm. In 1982 it was proposed that the time-weighted average exposure limits for both these compounds and their acetates be reduced to 5 ppm in view of the testicular effects observed in recent animal studies.

▶ ORGANIC ACIDS, ANHYDRIDES, LACTONES, AND AMIDES

These compounds have numerous industrial applications. Their common clinical characteristic is an irritant effect on eyes, nose, throat, and the respiratory tract. Skin irritation can be severe, and some of the acids (formic, acetic, oxalic, and others) can produce chemical burns. Accidental eye penetration may result in severe corneal injury and consequent opacities. Toxic pulmonary edema can occur after acute overexposure to high concentrations.

Phthalic Anhydride

Phthalic anhydride ($C_6H_4(CO)_2O$) is a crystalline, needlelike white solid. It is used in the manufacture of benzoic and phthalic acids, as a plasticizer for vinyl resins, alkyd, and polyester resins, in the production of diethyl and dimethyl phthalate, phenolphthalein, phthalamide, methyl aniline, and other compounds.

Phthalic anhydride as dust, fumes, or vapor is a potent irritant for the eyes, respiratory system, and skin; with prolonged skin contact, chemical burns are possible. Repeated exposure may result in chronic industrial bronchitis. Phthalic anhydride is also a potent sensitizing substance: occupational asthma can be severe and hypersensitivity pneumonitis has been reported. Skin sensitization may result in eczematiform dermatitis.

Prevention

The federal standard for phthalic anhydride is a TLV of 1 ppm. Enclosure of technological processes where phthalic anhydride is used and protective clothing, including gloves and goggles, are necessary; respiratory protection must be available. Periodic examinations should focus on possible sensitization and chronic effects, such as bronchitis and dermatitis.

Maleic Anhydride

Maleic anhydride (O *CO CH*=*CO*) is used mainly in the production of alkyd and polyester resins; it has also found applications for siccatives. Maleic anhydride can produce severe chemical burns of the skin and eyes. It is also a sensitizing substance and can lead to clinical manifestations similar to those described for phthalic anhydride. The 1987 TLV is 0.25 ppm.

Trimellitic Anhydride

Trimellitic anhydride (1,2,4-benzenetricarboxylic acid, cyclic 1,2-anhydride, $C_9H_4O_5$) is used as a curing agent for epoxy resins and other resins, in vinyl plasticizers, polyesters, dyes and pigments, paints and coatings, agricultural chemicals, surface-active compounds, pharmaceuticals, etc. Chemical pneumonitis has been reported after an epoxy resin containing trimellitic anhydride was sprayed on heated pipes. Respiratory irritation after exposure to high concentrations of trimellitic anhydride was reported in workers engaged in the synthesis of this compound. It was also found that in some cases sensitization occurs after variable periods following onset of exposure (sometimes years); allergic rhinitis, occupational asthma, and hypersensitivity pneumonitis can be manifestations of sensitization. Trimellitic anhydride as the etiologic agent in cases of sensitization was confirmed by inhalation challenge tests.[207]

Prevention

The NIOSH recommended in 1978 that trimellitic anhydride be considered an extremely toxic agent, since it can produce severe irritation of the respiratory tract, including pulmonary edema and chemical pneumonitis; sensitization, with occupational asthma or hypersensitivity pneumonitis, can occur at lower levels. Guidelines for engineering controls and protective equipment have been outlined by NIOSH.[3] The current OSHA TLV standard is 0.04 mg/m^3.

β-Propiolactone

β-Propiolactone ($OCH_2CH2C{=}O$) is a colorless liquid with important applications in the synthesis of acrylate plastics; it is also used as a disinfectant and as a sterilizing agent against viruses. It is easily absorbed through the skin; inhalation is also important.

β-Propiolactone is a very potent irritant. In animal experiments it has been found to produce hepatocellular necrosis, renal tubular necrosis, convulsions, and circulatory collapse. In several animal studies it has also been shown to be carcinogenic; skin cancer, hepatoma, and gastric cancer have been induced. Reports on systemic or carcinogenic effects in humans are not available.

β-Propiolactone is included in the federal standard for carcinogens; no exposure should be allowed to occur. Protective equipment designed to prevent all skin contact or inhalation is necessary; this includes full-body protective clothing and full-face air-supplied respirators. Showers at the end of the shift are absolutely necessary. The 1987 TLV is 0.05 ppm.

N,N-Dimethylformamide

N,N-Dimethylformamide, $HCON(CH_3)_2$, is a colorless liquid with a boiling point of 153°C. It is miscible with water and organic solvents at 25°C. It has excellent solvent properties for numerous organic compounds and is used in processes where solvents with low volatility are necessary. Its major applications are in the manufacture of synthetic fibers and resins, mainly polyacrylic fibers and butadiene. It is absorbed through inhalation and through the skin and is irritating to the eyes, mucous membranes, and skin.[2] Adverse effects of absorption include loss of appetite, nausea, vomiting, abdominal pain, hepatomegaly, and other indications of liver injury. Recently clusters of testicular germ cell tumors have been reported among airplane manufacturing employees and tannery workers.[208,209] An increased incidence of cancer (oropharyngeal and melanoma) was reported in a cohort of formamide-exposed workers.[210]

Dimethylformamide (DMF) administered to mice and rats 5 days/week for 18 months did not produce effects on the estrous cycle. Compound-related morphological changes were observed only in the liver. Centrilobular hepatocellular hypertrophy and centrilobular single cell necrosis were found in rats and mice. DMF was not oncogenic under these experimental conditions.[211] Diemethylformamide exposure did not result in adverse effects on semen or menstrual cycle in cynomolgus monkeys, exposed for 13 weeks to concentrations up to 500 ppm.[212]

The federal standard for a permissible exposure limit is 10 ppm (30 mg/m^3).

N,N^1-Dimethylacetamide

N,N^1-Dimethylacetamide ($CH_3CON(CH_3)_2$) is a colorless liquid that is easily absorbed through the skin. Inhalation is a less important route of absorption, since the volatility is low. *N,N^1*-Dimethylacetamide is used as a solvent in a variety of industrial processes.

Hepatotoxicity is the most severe adverse effect; hepatocellular degenerative changes and jaundice have been reported in exposed workers. Experimental studies have also indicated hepatotoxicity as the prominent effect in rats and dogs. With high exposure, depressant neurotoxic effects become evident. Dimethylacetamide has been shown, in experiments on rodents, to produce testicular changes in rabbits and rats. Its hepatotoxicity was comparable to and possibly higher than that of dimethylformamide.[213]

The federal standard for a PEL is 10 ppm (35 mg/m^3). Protective equipment to exclude percutaneous absorption is necessary, as are eye and respiratory protection if high vapor concentrations are possible.

Acrylamide

Acrylamide ($CH_2{=}CHCONH_2$) is a white crystalline material with a melting point of 84.5°C and a tendency to sublime; it is readily soluble in water and in some other common polar solvents. Large-scale production started in the early 1950s; the major industrial applications are as a vinyl monomer in the production of high-molecular polymers such as polyacrylamides. These have many applications, including the clarification and treatment of municipal and industrial effluents and potable water; in the oil industry (for fracturing and flooding of oil-bearing strata); as flocculants in the production of ores, metals, and coal; as strengtheners in the paper industry; for textile treatment, etc. Acrylamide is of major concern because of its extensive use in molecular biology laboratories, where, in the United States, 100,000 to 200,000 persons are potentially exposed in chromatography, electrophoresis, and electron microscopy.[214]

Although the pure polyacrylamide polymers are nontoxic, the problem of residual unreacted acrylamide exists, since up to 2 percent residual monomer is acceptable for some industrial applications. The Food and Drug Administration (FDA) has established a maximum 0.05 percent residual monomer level for polymers used in paper or cardboard in contact with food; similar levels are accepted for polymers used in clarification of potable water. Since acrylamide has cumulative toxic effects, it has been recommended that the general population not be exposed to daily levels in excess of 0.0005 mg/kg.

The initial indication of a marked neurotoxic effect of acrylamide came when a recently introduced acrylamide production method (from acrylonitrile) was first used in 1953; several workers experienced weakness in their extremities, with numbness and tingling, strongly suggestive of toxic peripheral neuropathy. Cases of acrylamide neuropathy have since been reported from Japan, France, Canada, and Great Britain.

Acrylamide is readily absorbed through the skin, which is considered an important route of absorption. Respiratory absorption and ingestion of acrylamide are also important; severe cases of acrylamide poisoning have resulted from ingestion of contaminated water in Japan.

Acrylamide is metabolized to the epoxide glycidamide, whose adducts to hemoglobin and to DNA have been identified in animals and humans. This metabolite may be involved in the reproductive and carcinogenic effects of acrylamide. The neurotoxicity of acrylamide and glycidamide were shown to differ in rats, suggesting that acrylamide itself is primarily responsible for peripheral neurotoxicity.[215]

Acrylamide poisoning in occupationally exposed workers has occurred after relatively short periods of exposure (several months to a year). Erythema and peeling of skin, mainly in the palms but also on the soles, usually precede neurologic symptoms; excessive fatigue, weight loss, and somnolence are followed by a slowly progressive symmetrical peripheral neuropathy. The characteristic symptoms include muscle weakness, unsteadiness, paresthesia, signs of sympathetic nervous system involvement (cold, blue hands and feet, excessive sweating), impairment of superficial sensation (touch, pain, temperature) and position sense, diminished or absent deep tendon reflexes in legs and arms, and the presence of Romberg's sign. Considerable loss of muscle strength may occur, and muscular atrophy, usually starting with the small muscles of the hands, has been reported. This toxic neuropathy has a distal to proximal evolution; the earliest and most severe changes are in the distal segments of the lower and upper extremities, and progression occurs with involvement of more proximal segments ("stocking and glove" distribution). Signs indicating CNS involvement are somnolence, vertigo, ataxic gait, and occasionally slight organic mental syndrome. EEG abnormalities have also been described.

Sensory nerve conduction velocities have been found to be more affected than motor nerve conduction velocities; potentials with markedly prolonged distal latencies are described. Recovery after cessation of exposure is slow; it may take several months to 2 years. Experimental acrylamide neuropathy has been produced in all mammals studied; medium- to large-diameter fibers and long fibers are more susceptible to the primary giant axonal degeneration and secondary demyelination characteristic of acrylamide neuropathy. CNS pathology consists of degenerating fibers in the anterior and lateral columns of the spinal cord, gracile nucleus, cerebellar vermis, spinocerebellar tracts, CNS optic nerve tracts, and tracts in the hypothalamus.

Changes in somatosensory evoked potentials have been found to be useful in the early detection of acrylamide neurotoxicity. They precede abnormalities of peripheral nerve conduction and behavioral signs of intoxication. Deterioration of visual capacity, with an increased threshold for visual acuity and flicker fusion and prolonged latency in visual evoked potentials, was reported in monkeys. These abnormalities were detected before overt signs of toxicity became apparent. Acrylamide preferentially damages P retinal ganglion cells in macaques, with marked effects on visual acuity, contrast discrimination, and shape discrimination.[216]

An underlying mechanism of acrylamide peripheral neuropathy has been found to be impaired retrograde transport of material from the more distal parts of the peripheral nerve. The buildup of retrogradely transported material has been shown to be dose-related. Changes in retrograde axonal transport are thought to play an initial and important role in the development of toxic axonopathies, possibly the primary biochemical event in acrylamide neuropathy.

Local disorganization of the smooth endoplasmic reticulum, forming a complex network of tubules intermingled with vesicles and mitochondria, is thought to be responsible for the focal stasis of fast-transported proteins. These seem to be the earliest changes detectable in axons damaged by acrylamide.

Acrylamide reduced microtubule-associated proteins (MAP1 and MAP2) in the rat extrapyramidal system. The effect was more marked in the caudate-putamen than in other components of the extrapyramidal system. The loss of MAPs occurs first in dendrites and proceeds towards the perikarya. The depletion of microtubule-associated proteins in the extrapyramidal system appears to be an early biochemical event preceding peripheral neuropathy.[217] In addition, acrylamide also produces necrosis of cerebellar Purkinje cells after high dose (50 mg/kg) administration in rats.[218] Acrylamide has been found to depress fast anterograde transport of protein, resulting in reduction in delivery of protein to the axon and distal nerve degeneration.[219]

Acrylamide has been reported to produce effects on neurotransmitter and neuropeptide levels in various areas of the brain. Elevated levels of 5-hydroxyindolacetic acid in all regions of the rat brain were interpreted as being the result of an increased serotonin turnover. Changes in the affinity and number of dopamine receptor sites have also been found. Elevated levels of some neuropeptides were detected mainly in the hypothalamus. Significant decreases in plasma levels of testosterone and prolactin were found after repeated acrylamide administration.

Experimental neurotoxicity studies of 14 acrylamide analogs were undertaken; 5 produced neuropathy. The order of neurotoxicity was acrylamide > *N*-isopropylacrylamide > *N*-methylacrylamide = methacrylamide > *N*-hydroxymethylacrylamide. All these compounds also produced testicular atrophy, with degenerative changes in the epithelial cells of seminiferous tubules.

Acrylamide produces chromosomal aberrations in mouse bone marrow cells. The micronucleus test was also positive.[220] Acrylamide treatment produced significant increases in chromosomal structural aberrations in late spermatids-spermatozoa of mice. Chromosomal damage was consistent with alkylation of DNA-associated protamines. A dose-dependent depletion of mature spermatids after treatment of spermatogonia and a toxic effect upon primary spermatocytes were also detected.[221] Acrylamide (IP) produced a meiotic delay in spermatocytes of mice. This was predominately due to prolongation of interkinesis. The disturbances in cell division caused by acrylamide suggest that acrylamide might induce aneuploidy by interfering with proper functioning of the spindle; errors in chromosome segregation may also occur.[222] Genotoxic effects of acrylamide and glycidamide have also been detected in several in vitro and/or in vivo unscheduled DNA synthesis assays.[223] Acrylamide is highly effective in breaking chromosomes in germ cells of male mice, resulting both in early death of conceptuses and in the transmission of reciprocal translocation to live-born progeny. This effect has been demonstrated after topical application and absorption through the skin.[224] Oncogenicity studies on rats treated with acrylamide in drinking water for 2 years have been positive for a number of tumors (central nervous system, thyroid, mammary gland, uterus in females, and scrotal mesothelioma in males).

In a mortality study involving a cohort of 371 employees exposed to acrylamide, an excess in total cancer deaths was due to excess in digestive and respiratory cancer in a subgroup that had had previous exposure to organic dyes.[225]

Control and Prevention

Engineering designs that prevent the escape of both vapor and dust into the environment are necessary; enclosure, exhaust ventilation, and automated systems must be used to minimize exposure. Prevention of skin and eye contact is especially important in handling of aqueous solutions, and closed systems are to be preferred.

Measurements of hemoglobin adducts were developed as a way to monitor exposure to acrylamide and have been successfully applied in a field study of occupationally exposed workers.[226] A study of 41 workers heavily exposed to acrylamide and acrylonitrile in Xinxiang, China, was undertaken because of frequent signs and symptoms indicating neuropathy. Hemoglobin adducts of acrylamide were significantly correlated with a "neurotoxicity index" based on signs and symptoms of peripheral neuropathy, vibration thresholds, and electroneuromyography measurements.[227]

The present recommended TWA for acrylamide exposure is 0.3 mg/m^3. Skin exposure has to be carefully avoided by the use of appropriate protective clothing and work practices. Showers and eyewash fountains should be available for immediate use if contamination occurs. Pre-employment and periodic medical examinations with special attention to skin, eyes, and nervous system are necessary. It is essential that employees be warned of the potential health hazards and the importance of personal hygiene and careful work practices. Frequent inspection of fingers and hands by medical or paramedical personnel is useful in detecting peeling of skin, which usually precedes clinical neuropathy.

▶ ALDEHYDES

Aldehydes are aliphatic or aromatic compounds with the general structure:

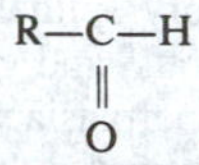

The aldehydes are highly reactive substances and are used extensively throughout the chemical industry. Formaldehyde is a gas that is readily soluble in water; the other aldehydes are liquids.

The common characteristic of aldehydes is their strong irritative effect on the skin, eyes, and respiratory system. Acute overexposure may result in toxic pulmonary edema. Sensitization to aldehydes is possible, and allergic dermatitis and occupational asthma can occur.

Formaldehyde

Formaldehyde (HCHO) is a colorless gas with a strong odor and is readily soluble in water; the commercial solutions may contain up to 15 percent methanol to prevent polymerization. It has numerous industrial applications in the manufacture of textiles, cellulose esters, dyes, inks, latex, phenol, urea, melamine, pentaerythrol, hexamethylenetetramine, thiourea, resins, and explosives, and as a fungicide, disinfectant, and preservative. More than half of formaldehyde is used in the United States in the manufacture of plastics and resins: urea-formaldehyde resins and phenolic, polyacetal, and melamine resins. Among the many other uses is in the manufacture of 4,4′-methylene dianiline and 4,4′-methylene diphenyl diisocyanate. Some relatively small-volume uses of formaldehyde are in agriculture, for seed treatment and as a soil disinfectant, in cosmetics, deodorants, in photography, and in histopathology.

Formaldehyde has been found to be a relatively common contaminant of indoor air; it originates in urea-formaldehyde resins used in the production of particle board or in urea-formaldehyde foam used for insulation. Such insulation was applied in the United States in approximately 500,000 houses during the period 1975 to 1980. Concentrations of formaldehyde in residential indoor air have varied from 0.01 to 31.7 ppm.

Significant concentrations of formaldehyde have been found in industrial effluents, mainly from the production of urea-, melamine- and phenol-formaldehyde resins, and also from users of such resins (e.g., plywood manufacturers). In water, formaldehyde undergoes rapid degradation and therefore does not represent a major source of absorption. Formaldehyde is also readily degraded in soil. Bioaccumulation does not occur.

Other sources of formaldehyde exposure for the general population are from cigarette smoke (37 to 73 μg/cigarette) and from small amounts in food, especially after the use of hexamethylenetetramine as a food additive.

Formaldehyde resins applied to permanent-press textiles can emit formaldehyde when stored. Fingernail hardeners containing formaldehyde are a relatively recent addition to the potential sources of formaldehyde exposure.

Absorption occurs through inhalation. Skin and eye contact may result in chemical burns. Guinea pigs exposed by inhalation to formaldehyde (1 ppm for 8 hours) developed increased airway resistance and enhanced bronchial reactivity to acetylcholine, mediated through leukotriene biosynthesis.[228] Smooth muscle reactivity in the airways was altered, despite absence of epithelial damage or inflammation histologically.[229] Acute overexposure to very high concentrations may result in pulmonary edema. Sensitization resulting in allergic dermatitis is not uncommon; occupational asthma is also possible.

Formaldehyde carcinogenicity assays have revealed that inhalation exposure to concentrations of 14.3 ppm resulted in a significantly increased incidence of nasal squamous cell carcinomas in rats of both sexes. Induction of nasal carcinomas in rats exhibited a nonlinear relationship with formaldehyde dose, the rates increasing rapidly with increasing exposure concentrations.[230]

In mice only a very small number of squamous cell carcinomas developed, and the incidence was not statistically significant. Dysplasia and squamous metaplasia of the respiratory epithelium, rhinitis, and atrophy of the olfactory epithelium were observed in mice; similar lesions were seen in rats, and goblet cell hyperplasia, squamous atypia, and papillary hyperplasia were also found. A 2-year experimental study on rats investigated the effects of formaldehyde in drinking water. Although pathologic changes in the gastric mucosa were found in the high-dose rats, no gastric tumors or tumors at other sites were detected.[231]

Mortality studies on human populations exposed to formaldehyde only are rare. A study of pathologists and laboratory technicians in Great Britain was negative. Among morticians practicing embalming in New York State, an excess of skin cancer, kidney cancer, and brain cancer was found, although the small numbers preclude definitive conclusions. There were no cancers of the nose or nasal sinuses and no excess of respiratory cancer. A cohort study of 2,490 employees in a chemical plant manufacturing and using formaldehyde was also conducted. An elevated proportional mortality for digestive tract cancer in white males was found; the small numbers make it difficult to draw conclusions. No deaths from cancers of the nose or nasal sinuses had occurred. The duration of employment was relatively short. The studies had a very limited power to detect excess mortality from nasal cancer. In a large retrospective cohort mortality study of more than 11,000 workers exposed to formaldehyde in the garment industry, significant excess mortality from cancer of the buccal cavity and connective tissue was found. The incidence of such cancers as leukemia and lymphoma was higher than expected, without reaching the level of statistical significance.

Formaldehyde is mutagenic to bacteria, yeast, and *Drosophila*. Recently, formaldehyde-induced mutagenesis has been demonstrated in Chinese hamster ovary cells, primarily point mutations with single-base transversions.[232] Formaldehyde is metabolized to carbon dioxide and formate. Studies using ^{14}C-formaldehyde have demonstrated the presence of ^{14}C-labeled cellular macromolecules.

Formaldehyde has been reported to react with nucleic acids and has been found to be among the most potent of DNA-protein cross-link inducers, compared with aldehydes with greater carbon chain length.[233] DNA-protein cross-links were induced, along with cell proliferation, squamous metaplasia, and squamous cell carcinomas, in the nasal lateral meatus (a high tumor site in bioassays) of F344 rats exposed to formaldehyde.[234]

Sister chromatid exchanges in lymphocytes of formaldehyde-exposed anatomy students showed a small but statistically significant increase when compared with pre-exposure findings in the same persons.[235] Nasal respiratory cell samples collected from formaldehyde-exposed sawmill and shearing press workers showed a significantly higher frequency of micronucleated cells than found among unexposed control subjects.[236] DNA-protein cross-links were found with significantly greater frequency in the white blood cells of 12 formaldehyde-exposed workers than in the white blood cells of 8 unexposed control subjects.[237]

Evidence has acculumated that indicates that formaldehyde is an important metabolite of a number of halogenated hydrocarbons, mediated through glutathione-*S*-transferase theta activity, including dichloromethane, methyl bromide, methyl chloride, and carbon tetrachloride.[238,239]

Formaldehyde administered to male rats at 10 mg/kg body weight/day for 30 days caused a significant fall in sperm motility, viability, and count.[240]

The federal standard for formaldehyde is 1 ppm (1.2 mg/m^3). Engineering controls are essential to control exposure. Protective equipment to prevent skin contact, adequate respirators for situations in which higher exposure could result, proper work practices, and continuous education programs for employees are necessary. The Environmental Protection Agency and the Occupational Health and Safety Administration, in their consideration of available epidemiological and toxicological studies, now regard formaldehyde as a possible human carcinogen, although the evidence in humans is limited and controversial.

Acrolein

Acrolein ($H_2C{=}CHCHO$), a clear liquid, is used in the production of plastics, plasticizers, acrylates, synthetic fibers, and methionine; it is produced when oils and fats containing glycerol are heated. It is one of the strongest irritants. Skin burns and severe irritation of eyes and respiratory tract, including toxic pulmonary edema, are possible.

Inhalation of smoke containing acrolein, the most common toxin in urban fires after carbon monoxide, causes vascular injury with noncardiogenic pulmonary edema containing edematogenic eicosanoids such as thromboxane, leukotriene B_4, and the sulfidopeptide leukotrienes. Thromboxane is probably responsible for the pulmonary hypertension that occurs after the inhalation of acrolein smoke.[241] Acrolein acts as a strong peroxidizing agent.[242]

Acrolein is embryotoxic and teratogenic in rats and chick embryos after intra-amniotic administration. Acrolein is genotoxic and causes DNA single-strand breaks and DNA cross-links in human bronchial epithelial cells. Acrolein is a much more potent DNA-protein cross-linking agent, 500-fold more potent than propionaldehyde.[243] Acrolein forms cyclic deoxyguanosine adducts when it reacts with DNA in vitro and in *S. typhimurium* cultures.

2-Chloroacrolein and 2-bromoacrolein are very potent direct mutagens not requiring metabolic activation in *S. typhimurium* strains.[244] Acrolein was not found to be a developmental toxicant or teratogen at doses not toxic to the does, when administered via stomach tube to pregnant white rabbits (0.1, 0.75, and 2.0 mg/kg/day).[245] Acrolein is not a selective reproductive toxin in the rat.[246]

The federal standard for a permissible exposure limit for acrolein is 0.1 ppm.

Environmentally relevant concentrations of aldehydes acrolein and formaldehyde can induce bronchial hyperactivity in guinea pigs through a mechanism involving injury to cells present in the airways. There is evidence that this response is dependent on leukotriene biosynthesis.[228,247]

Other widely used aldehydes are acetaldehyde and furfural. They have irritant effects but are less potent in this respect than formaldehyde and acrolein. Evidence for carcinogenic potential in experimental animals is convincing for formaldehyde and acetaldehyde, limited for crotonaldehyde, furfural, and glycidaldehyde, and very weak for acrolein.[248]

▶ ESTERS

Esters are organic compounds that result from the substitution of a hydrogen atom of an acid (organic or inorganic) with an organic group. They constitute a very large group of substances with a variety of industrial uses in plastics and resins, as solvents, and in the pharmaceutical, surface coating, textile, and food-processing industries.

Narcotic CNS effects and irritative effects (especially with the halogenated esters such as ethyl chloroformate, ethyl chloroacetate, and the corresponding bromo- and iodo- compounds) are common to most esters. Sensitization has been reported with some of the aliphatic monocarboxylic halogenated esters. Some of the esters of inorganic acids have specific, potentially severe toxicity. For a discussion of phosphate esters, see Chapter 26.

Dimethyl Sulfate

Dimethyl sulfate, $(CH_3)_2SO_4$, is an oily fluid. It is used mainly for its methylating capacity; another use is as a solvent in the separation of mineral oils. Absorption is mainly through inhalation, but skin penetration is also possible.

Toxic effects are complex and severe; many fatalities have occurred. After a latency period of several hours, the irritant effects on the skin, eyes, and respiratory system become manifest; toxic pulmonary edema is not unusual. Vesication of the skin and ulceration can occur. Eye irritation usually results in conjunctivitis, keratitis, photophobia, palpebral edema, and blepharospasm. Irritation of the upper airways may also be severe, with dysphagia and sometimes edema of the glottis. Dyspnea, cough, and shallow breathing are the signs of toxic pulmonary edema. If the patient survives this critical period, 48 hours later the signs and symptoms of hepatocellular necrosis and renal tubular necrosis may become manifest.

At very high levels of exposure, neurotoxic effects are prominent, with somnolence, delirium, convulsions, temporary blindness, and coma.

Dimethyl sulfate is an alkylating agent. In experimental studies on rats it has been shown to be carcinogenic. Prenatal exposure has also produced tumors of the nervous system in offspring. The IARC has concluded that there is sufficient evidence of dimethyl sulfate carcinogenicity in animals and that it has to be assumed to be a potential human carcinogen. In inhalation experiments on rodents, embryotoxic and teratogenic effects have also been observed.

The federal standard for a permissible level of dimethyl sulfate exposure is 0.1 ppm.

Diethyl sulfate, methylchlorosulfonate, ethylchlorosulfonate, and methyl-*p*-toluene sulfonate have effects similar to those of dimethyl sulfate, and the same extreme precautions in their handling are necessary. The skin, eyes, and respiratory tract should be protected continuously when there may be exposure to dimethyl sulfate or the other esters that have similar effects. Contaminated areas should be entered only by trained personnel with impervious protective clothing and air-supplied respirators.[2]

▶ KETONES

The chemical characteristic of this series of compounds known as ketones is the presence of the carbonyl group. Their general structure is

$$R{-}\underset{\underset{\displaystyle O}{\|}}{C}{-}R'$$

Ketones are excellent solvents for oils, fats, collodion, cellulose acetate, nitrocellulose, cellulose esters, epoxy resins, pigments, dyes, natural and synthetic resins (especially vinyl polymers and copolymers), and acrylic coatings. They are also used in the manufacture of paints, lacquers, and varnishes and in the celluloid, rubber, artificial leather, synthetic rubber, lubricating oil, and explosives industries. Other uses are in metal cleaning, rapidly drying inks, airplane dopes, as paint removers and dewaxers, and in hydraulic fluids.

The most important members of the ketone group, because of extensive use, are as follows:

Acetone	CH_3COCH_3
Methyl-ethyl-ketone	$CH_3COCH_2CH_3$
Methyl-*n*-propyl ketone	$CH_3(CH_2)_2COCH_3$
Methyl-*n*-butyl ketone	$CH_3CO(CH_2)_3CH_3$
Methyl isobutyl ketone	$CH_3COCH_2CH(CH_3)_2$
Methyl-*n*-amyl ketone	$CH_3CO(CH_2)_4CH_3$
Methyl isoamyl ketone	$CH_3CO(CH_2)_2CH(CH_3)_2$
Diisobutyl ketone	$(CH_3)_2CHCH_2COCH_2CH(CH_3)_2$
Cyclohexane	$C_6H_{10}O$
Mesityl oxide	$CH_3COCH{=}C(CH_3)_2$
Isophorone (3,5,5-trimethyl-2-cyclohexen-1-one)	$C_{10}H_{14}O$

Methyl isobutyl ketone is used in the recovery of uranium from fission products. It has also found applications as a vehicle for herbicides, such as 2,4,5-T, and insecticides. Many of the ketones are valuable raw materials or intermediates in the chemical synthesis of other compounds. For example, approximately 90 percent of the 2 billion pounds of acetone produced each year is used by the chemical industry for the production of methacetylates and higher ketones.

The major route of absorption is through inhalation of vapor; with some of the ketones, such as methyl-ethyl ketone (MEK) and methyl-butyl ketone (MBK), skin absorption may contribute significantly to the total amount absorbed if work practices allow for extensive contact (immersion of hands, washing with the solvents).

All the ketones are moderate mucous membrane irritants (eyes and upper airways); at higher concentrations, CNS depression with prenarcotic symptoms progressing to narcosis may occur.

A specific neurotoxic effect of MBK, peripheral neuropathy, was reported in 1975 in workers exposed in the plastic coatings industry.[249] In 1976 similar cases were identified among spray painters. Cases of peripheral neuropathy were also found in furniture finishers exposed to methyl-*n*-butyl ketone (MnBK) and in workers employed in a dewaxing unit in a refinery, where the exposure was reported to be to MEK.

The toxic sensorimotor peripheral neuropathy caused by MnBK exposure is very similar to that caused by other neurotoxic substances such as acrylamide and *n*-hexane. Typically, sensory dysfunctions (touch, pain, temperature, vibration, and position) are the initial changes, affecting the hands and feet. Distal sensory neuropathy can be the only finding in some affected persons; in more severe cases motor impairment (muscle weakness, diminished or abolished deep tendon reflexes) in the distal parts of the lower and then the upper extremities becomes manifest. With progression, and in more severe cases, both the sensory and motor deficits may also affect the more proximal segments of the extremities; muscle wasting may be present in severe cases. Electromyographic abnormalities and slowing of nerve conduction velocity can be detected in the vast majority of cases; these electrophysiological abnormalities are useful for early detection, since they most often precede clinical manifestations. The clinical course is protracted, and cessation of toxic exposure does not result in recovery in all cases; progressive dysfunction was observed to occur for several months after exposure had been eliminated.

Animal experiments have demonstrated that exposure to methyl-*n*-butyl ketone (MnBK) results in peripheral neuropathy in all tested species; moreover, mixed exposure to MEK and MnBK (in a 5 : 1 ratio) resulted in a more rapid development of peripheral neuropathy in rats than exposure to MnBK alone, indicating a potentiating effect of MEK. These experimental data are of importance for human exposure, since mixtures of solvents are often used.

MnBK produces primary axonal degeneration, with marked increase in the number of neurofilaments, reduction of neurotubules, axonal swelling, and secondary thinning of the myelin sheath. Spencer and Schaumberg[250] have identified similar changes in certain tracts of the CNS, the distal regions of long ascending and descending pathways in the spinal cord and medulla oblongata, and preterminal and terminal axons in the gray matter. For this reason, they have proposed central-peripheral distal axonopathy as a more appropriate term for this type of neurotoxic effect. The "dying back" axonal disease therefore seems not to be limited to the peripheral nerves but to be quite widespread in the CNS. Recovery from peripheral neuropathy is slow; it is thought that recovery of similar lesions within the CNS is unlikely to occur and might result in permanent deficit, such as ataxia or spasticity.

The predominant metabolite of MnBK identified by DiVincenzo et al[33] is 2,5-hexanedione. A similar type of giant axonal neuropathy was reproduced in animals exposed to this metabolite. 2,5-Hexanedione is also the main metabolite of *n*-hexane, another solvent with marked similar neurotoxicity. Other metabolites of MnBK are 5-hydroxy-2-hexanone, 2-hexanol, and 2,5-hexanediol; all have been shown to produce typical giant axonal neuropathy in experiments on rats.[3] The transformation of MnBK to its toxic metabolites is mediated by the liver mixed-function oxidase system.[33] MEK potentiates the neurotoxicity of MnBK by induction of the microsomal mixed-function enzyme system.

It is generally accepted that 2,5-hexanedione, the γ-diketone metabolite of MnBK, has the most marked neurotoxic effect of all MnBK metabolites. Another ketone, ethyl-*n*-butyl ketone (EnBK, 3-heptanone) has also been reported to produce typical central-peripheral distal axonopathy in rats. MEK potentiated EnBK neurotoxicity; the excretion of two neurotoxic γ-diketones—2,5-heptanedione and 2,5-hexanedione—was increased.

Technical-grade methyl-heptyl ketone (MHK) was also found to produce toxic neuropathy in rats; the effect was shown to be due to 5-nonanone. Metabolic studies have demonstrated the conversion of 5-nonanone to 2,5-nonanedione, MnBK, and 2,5-hexanedione.[36] Other γ-diketones—2,5-heptanedione and 3,6-octanedione—have also produced neuropathy.

Nephrotoxic (degenerative changes in proximal convoluted tubular cells) and hepatotoxic effects have been detected in experimental exposure of several animal species to the following ketones: isophorone (at 50 ppm), mesityl oxide (at 100 ppm), mesityl isobutyl ketone (at 100 ppm), cyclohexanone (at 190 ppm), and diisobutylketone (at 250 ppm).

The potential for methyl ethyl ketone to cause developmental toxicity was tested in mice. Mild developmental toxicity was observed after exposure to 3,000 ppm, which resulted in reduction of fetal body weight. There was no significant increase in the incidence of any single malformation, but several malformations not observed in the concurrent control group were found at a low incidence—cleft palate, fused ribs, missing vertebrae, and syndactyly.[251]

Prevention

Appropriate engineering, mainly enclosure and exhaust ventilation, and adequate work practices preventing spillage and vapor generation are essential to maintain exposure to ketones below the exposure limits. Adequate respiratory protection is recommended for situations in which excessive concentrations are possible (maintenance and repair, emergencies, installation of engineering controls, etc.). Appropriate protective clothing is necessary, and skin contact must be avoided.

All ketones are flammable or combustible, and employees should be informed of this risk as well as of the specific health hazards. Warning signs in the work areas and on vessels and special educational programs for employees, especially new employees, are necessary as part of a comprehensive prevention program.

The NIOSH recommends that occupational exposure to ketones be controlled so that the TWA concentration does not exceed the following exposure limits:

MnBK	1 ppm
Isophorone	4 ppm
Mesithyl oxide	10 ppm
Cyclohexanone	25 ppm
Diisobutyl ketone	25 ppm
Methyl isobutyl ketone	50 ppm
Methyl isoamyl ketone	50 ppm
Methyl *n*-amyl ketone	100 ppm
Methyl *n*-propyl ketone	150 ppm
MEK	200 ppm
Acetone	250 ppm

The marked neurotoxicity of at least one member of this group (MnBK), the slow recovery in cases of distal axonal degeneration, and the possibility that irreversible damage may occur, possibly also in the central nervous system, indicate the need for appropriate protection and medical surveillance.[3] Neurophysiological methods—electromyography and nerve conduction velocity measurements—are indicated wherever MnBK, mixtures of MEK and MnBK, or other neurotoxic ketones are used. Liver-function tests and indicators of renal function should be included in the periodic medical examination along with the physical examination and medical history.

ETHERS

Ethers are organic compounds characterized by the presence of a $-C-O-C-$ group. They are volatile liquids, used as solvents and in the chemical industry in the manufacture of a variety of compounds. Some of the halogenated ethers are potent carcinogens (see Halogenated Ethers). While all ethers have irritant and narcotic properties, dioxane ($O-CH_2-CH_2-O-CH_2-CH_2$) has marked specific toxicity.

Diethylene Dioxide (Dioxane)

Dioxane is a colorless liquid with a boiling temperature of 101.5°C. It has applications as a solvent similar to those indicated for the ethylene glycol ethers; it is also a good solvent for rubber, cellulose acetate and other cellulose derivatives, and polyvinyl polymers. Dioxane has been used in the preparation of histologic slides as a dehydrating agent.

Absorption is mainly through inhalation but also through the skin. Dioxane is slightly narcotic and moderately irritant. The major toxic effect is kidney injury, with acute renal failure due to tubular necrosis; in some cases, renal cortical necrosis was reported. Centrilobular hepatocellular necrosis is also possible.

1,4-Dioxane was not genotoxic in vitro, but was an inducer of micronuclei in the bone marrow of rats and a carcinogen for both rats and mice. Together with the previously reported in vivo induction of DNA strand breaks in the rat liver, these data raise the possibility of a genotoxic action for 1,4-dioxane.[252] Dioxane has been shown to be carcinogenic (by oral administration) in rats and guinea pigs. Several long-term studies with 1,4-dioxane have shown it to induce liver tumors in mice, and nasal and liver tumors in rats when administered in amounts from 0.5 to 1.8 percent in drinking water.[253]

Prevention

The federal standard for the permissible exposure limit is 100 ppm; because of the high toxicity, the ACGIH recommended 50 ppm. Protective equipment, appropriate work practices, and medical surveillance are similar to those indicated for the ethylene glycol ethers.

Carbon Disulfide

Carbon disulfide (CS_2) is a colorless, very volatile liquid (boiling temperature, 46°C). It is used in the production of viscose rayon and cellophane.[3] Another important application is in the manufacture of carbon tetrachloride. Other uses are in the manufacture of the neoprene cement and rubber accelerators, the fumigation of grain, various extraction processes, as a solvent for sulfur, iodine, bromine, phosphorus, and selenium, in paints, varnishes, paint and varnish removers, and in rocket fuel. Absorption is mainly through inhalation; skin absorption has been demonstrated but is practically negligible.

After inhalation, at least 40 to 50 percent of carbon disulfide is retained, while 10 to 30 percent is exhaled; less than 1 percent is excreted unchanged in the urine.

Oxidative metabolic transformation of carbon disulfide is mediated by microsomal mixed-function oxidase enzymes. The monoxygenated intermediate is carbonyl sulfide (COS); the end product of this metabolic pathway is CO_2, with generation of atomic sulfur. Atomic sulfur is able to form covalent bonds.

Carbon disulfide is a very volatile liquid, and high airborne vapor concentrations can easily occur; under such circumstances, specific toxic effects on the central nervous system are prominent and may result in severe acute or subacute encephalopathy. The clinical symptoms includes headache, dizziness, fatigue, excitement, depression, memory deficit, indifference, apathy, delusions, hallucinations, suicidal tendencies, delirium, acute mania, and coma. The outcome may be fatal; in less severe cases, incomplete recovery may occur with persistent psychiatric symptoms, indicating irreversible CNS damage. Many such severe cases of carbon disulfide poisoning have occurred in the past, during the second half of the nineteenth century in the rubber industry in France and Germany; as early as 1892 the first cases in the rubber industry were reported from the United States. Acute mania often led to admission to hospitals for the insane. With the rapid development of the viscose rayon industry, cases of carbon disulfide poisoning became more frequent, and Alice Hamilton repeatedly called attention to this health hazard in the rubber and rayon viscose industries.[254] The first exposure standard for carbon disulfide in the United States was adopted in 1941. As late as 1946, cases of carbon disulfide psychosis were reported as still being admitted to state institutions for the mentally ill,[2] often without any mention of carbon disulfide as the etiological agent. Chronic effects of carbon disulfide exposure were recognized later, when the massive overexposures leading to acute psychotic effects had been largely eliminated.

Peripheral neuropathy of the sensorimotor type, initially involving the lower extremities but often also the upper extremities, with distal to proximal progression, can lead in severe forms to marked sensory loss, muscle atrophy, and diminished or abolished deep tendon reflexes. CNS effects can also often be detected in cases of toxic carbon disulfide peripheral neuropathy; fatigue, headache, irritability, somnolence, memory deficit, and changes in personality are the most frequent symptoms.[2,255] Optic neuritis has often been reported. Constriction of visual fields has been found in less severe cases.

Electromyographic changes and reduced nerve conduction velocity have been useful in the early detection of carbon disulfide peripheral neuropathy.[255] Behavioral performance tests have been successfully applied for the early detection of CNS impairment. In rats exposed to CS_2 inhalation (200 and 800 ppm for 15 weeks), auditory brainstem responses were found to be delayed, suggesting a conduction dysfunction in the brainstem.[256] In CS_2-exposed rats, visual evoked potentials (flash and pattern reversal) were shown to be decreased in amplitude with an increase in latency. Repeated exposures had a more marked effect than acute exposure.[257]

With the recognition of carbon disulfide peripheral neuropathy, efforts to further reduce the exposure limits were made. As the incidence of carbon disulfide peripheral neuropathy decreased, previously unsuspected cardiovascular effects of long-term carbon disulfide exposure, even at lower levels, became apparent. Initially cerebrovascular changes, with clinical syndromes including pyramidal, extrapyramidal, and pseudobulbar manifestations, were reported with markedly increased incidence and at relatively young ages in workers exposed to carbon disulfide. A significant increase in deaths due to coronary heart disease was documented in workers with long-term carbon disulfide exposure at relatively low levels, and this led to the lowering of the TLV to 10 ppm in Finland in 1972.

A higher prevalence of hypertension and higher cholesterol and lipoprotein levels have also been found in workers exposed to carbon disulfide and most probably contribute to the higher incidence of atherosclerotic cerebral, coronary, and renal disease. A high prevalence of retinal microaneurysms was found in Japanese and Yugoslavian workers exposed to carbon disulfide; retinal microangiopathy was more frequent with longer carbon disulfide exposure.

Adverse effects of carbon disulfide exposure on reproductive function and more specifically on spermatogenesis have been reported in exposed workers, with significantly lower sperm counts and more abnormal spermatozoa than in nonexposed subjects. This toxic effect on spermatogenesis was confirmed in experiments on rats, where marked degenerative changes in the seminiferous tubules and degenerative changes in the Leydig cells, with almost complete disappearance of spermatogonia, were found.

Carbon disulfide has a high affinity for nucleophilic groups, such as sulfhydryl, amino, and hydroxy. It binds with amino groups of amino acids and proteins and forms thiocarbamates; these tend to undergo cyclic transformation, and the resulting thiazolidines have been shown to chelate zinc and copper (and possibly other trace metals), essential for the normal function of many important enzymes. The high affinity for sulfhydryl groups can also result in interference with enzymatic activities.

Effects of carbon disulfide on catecholamine metabolism have been reported. The concentration of norepinephrine in the brain decreased in rats exposed to carbon disulfide, while dopamine levels increased in both the brain and the adrenal glands. The possibility that carbon disulfide might interfere with the conversion of dopamine to norepinephrine has been considered; the converting enzyme dopamine-β-hydroxylase contains copper, and the copper-chelating effect of carbon disulfide probably results in its inhibition.

Carbon disulfide interference with vitamin B_6 metabolism has also been considered as a possible mechanism contributing to its neurotoxicity. Carbon disulfide reacts with pyridoxamine in vitro, with formation of a salt of pyridoxamine dithiocarbonic acid.

Carbon disulfide has been shown to produce a loss of cytochrome P-450 and to affect liver microsomal enzymes. This effect is thought to be related to the highly reactive sulfur (resulting from the oxidative desulfuration of carbon disulfide), which binds covalently to microsomal proteins.

Carbon disulfide peripheral neuropathy is characterized by axonal degeneration, with multifocal paranodal and internodal areas of swelling, accumulation of neurofilaments, abnormal mitochondria, and eventually thinning and retraction of myelin sheaths. Such axonal degeneration has been detected also in the central nervous system, mostly in long-fiber tracts. A marked reduction in metenkephalin immunostaining in the central amygdaloid nuclei and the globus pallidus has been measured, with a parallel elevation in the lateral septal nucleus and the parietal cortex. These findings suggest that the enkephalinergic neuromodulatory system could play a role in CS_2 neurotoxicity.[258]

Thus carbon disulfide neuropathy is of the type described as central peripheral distal axonopathy, very similar to those produced by *n*-hexane and methyl-*n*-butyl ketone. Covalent binding of the highly reactive sulfur to enzymes and proteins essential for the normal function of axonal transport is thought to be the mechanism of axonal degeneration leading to carbon disulfide peripheral neuropathy. Covalent cross-linking of proteins by CS_2 has been demonstrated in vitro. Intraperitoneal injection of CS_2 in rats produced several high–molecular weight proteins eluted from erythrocyte membranes which were not present in control animals. The high–molecular weight proteins were shown to be α, β heterodimers. The production of multiple heterodimers was consistent with the existence of several preferred sites for cross-linking. Dimer formation showed a cumulative dose-response in CS_2-treated rats.[259] CS_2 has been shown to produce intermolecular and intramolecular cross-linking of the low–molecular weight component of the neurofilament triplet proteins.[260]

CS_2 is a member of the class of neuropathy-inducing xenobiotics known as "neurofilament neurotoxicants." Current hypotheses propose direct reaction of CS_2 with neurofilament lysine epsilon-amine moieties as a step in the mechanism of this neuropathy. A lysine-containing dipeptide and bovine serum albumin, when incubated with $^{14}CS_2$, exhibited stable incorporation of radioactivity. A specific intramolecular cross-link was also detected.[261]

Approximately 70 percent to 90 percent of absorbed carbon disulfide is metabolized. Several metabolites are excreted in the urine. Among these, thiocarbamide and mercaptothiazolinone have been identified.

The urinary metabolites of carbon disulfide have been found to catalyze the iodine-azide reaction (i.e., the reduction of iodine by sodium azide). The speed of the reaction is accelerated in the presence of carbon disulfide metabolites, and this is indicated by the time necessary for the disappearance of the iodine color. A useful biological monitoring test has been developed[262] from these observations; departures from normal are found with exposures exceeding 16 ppm. It has been recommended that workers with an abnormal iodine-azide test reaction at the end of a shift, in whom there is no recovery overnight, should be removed (temporarily) from carbon disulfide exposure.

Prevention

The present federal standard for a permissible level of carbon disulfide exposure is 10 ppm. Prevention of exposure should rely on engineering controls, and mostly on enclosed processes and exhaust ventilation. When unexpected overexposure can occur, appropriate[3] respiratory protection must be available and used. Skin contact should be avoided, and protective equipment should be provided; adequate shower facilities and strict personal hygiene practices are necessary. Worker education on health hazards of carbon disulfide exposure and the importance of adequate work practices and personal hygiene must be part of a comprehensive preventive medicine program. Medical surveillance should encompass neurologic (behavioral and neurophysiological), cardiovascular (electrocardiogram and ophthalmoscopic examination), renal function, and reproductive function assessment. The iodine-azide test is useful for biological monitoring: it is an integrative index of daily exposure.

► AROMATIC NITRO- AND AMINO-COMPOUNDS

Aromatic nitro- and amino- compounds make up a large group of substances characterized by the substitution of one or more hydrogen atoms of the benzene ring by the nitro-($-NO_2$) or amino-($-NH_2$) radicals; some of the compounds have halogens (mainly chlorine and bromine) or alkyl radicals (CH_3, C_2H_5, etc.). Substances of this group have numerous industrial uses in the manufacture of dyes, pharmaceuticals, rubber additives (antioxidants and accelerators), explosives, plastic materials, synthetic resins, insecticides, and fungicides. New industrial uses are continuously found in the chemical synthesis of new products.[2] The physical properties of the aromatic nitro- and amino- compounds influence the dimension of the hazards they may generate. Some are solid, and some are fluids with low volatility; most are readily absorbed through the skin, and dangerous toxic levels can easily be reached in persons thus exposed.

A common toxic effect of most of these compounds is the production of methemoglobin and thus interference with normal oxygen transport to the tissues. This effect is thought to result not through a direct action of the chemical on hemoglobin but through the effect of intermediate metabolic products, such as paraaminophenol, phenylhydroxyl-1-amine, and nitrosobenzene. The microsomal mixed-function oxidase system is directly involved in these metabolic transformations.

Methemoglobin (metHb) results from the oxidation of bivalent Fe^{2+} in hemoglobin to trivalent Fe^{3+}. Methemoglobin is a ferrihemoglobin (Hgb $Fe^{3+}OH$) as opposed to hemoglobin, which is a ferrohemoglobin. Methemoglobin cannot serve in oxygen transport, since oxygen is bound (as $-OH$) in a strong bond and cannot easily be detached. The transformation of hemoglobin into methemoglobin is reversible; reducing agents, such as methylene blue, favor the reconversion. In humans methemoglobin is normally present in low concentrations, not exceeding 0.5 g/100 mL whole blood. An equilibrium exists between hemoglobin and methemoglobin, the latter being continuously reduced by intracellular mechanisms in which a methemoglobin reductase-diaphorase has a central place.

The production of methemoglobin after exposure to and absorption of nitro- and amino-aromatic compounds results in hypoxia, especially when higher concentrations of metHb (in excess of 20 to 25 percent of total hemoglobin) are reached. The most prominent and distinctive symptom is cyanosis (apparent when metHb exceeds 1.5 g/100 mL); most of the other symptoms and signs are due to the effects of hypoxia on the central nervous and cardiovascular systems. With high levels of methemoglobinemia, coma, arrhythmias, and death may occur. After cessation of exposure, recovery is usually uneventful, taking place in a matter of hours or days, depending on the specific compound. Methemoglobinemia develops more rapidly with aromatic amines, such as aniline, than with nitro-aromatic compounds; with the latter, the reconversion of methemoglobin into hemoglobin is slower (several days).

While the methemoglobin-forming effect is of an acute type, several significant chronic toxic effects have resulted from exposure to some of the members of this group. Liver toxicity, with hepatocellular necrosis, can be prominent, especially for polynitroaromatic derivatives. Aplastic anemia is another severe effect, sometimes associated with the hepatotoxic effect, especially with trinitrotoluene.

The major nitro- and amino-aromatic compounds are as follows:

Aniline	$C_6H_5NH_2$
Nitrobenzene	$C_6H_5NO_2$
Dinitrobenzene	$C_6H_4(NO_2)_2$
Trinitrobenzene	$C_6H_3(NO_2)_3$
Dinitrotoluene	$C_6H_3CH_3(NO_2)_2$
Trinitrotoluene	$C_6H_2CH_3(NO_2)_3$
Nitrophenol	$C_6H_4OHNO_2$
Dinitrophenol	$C_6H_3OH(NO_2)_2$
Tetranitromethylaniline (tetryl)	$C_6H_2(NO_2)_3N(CH_3)NO_2$
Toluylenediamine	$C_6H_3CH_3(NH_2)_2$
Xylidine	$C_6H_3(CH_3)_2NH_2$
Phenylenediamine	$C_6H_4(NH_2)_2$
4,4′-Diaminodiphenyl methane (methylene dianiline)	$NH_2(C_4H_4)CH_2(C_4H_4)NH_2$

Diazo-positive metabolites (DPM) have been proposed as biological indicators of aromatic nitro- and amino- compound absorption, including that of trinitrotoluene.

Nitrobenzene

Nitrobenzene, easily absorbed through the skin and the respiratory route, is known to have resulted in numerous cases of industrial poisoning. Its toxicity is higher than that of aniline, and liver and kidney damage are not unusual, although most often these are transitory. Anemia of moderate degree and Heinz bodies in the red blood cells may also be found.

Dinitrobenzene

Dinitrobenzene, especially the meta-isomer, is more toxic than both aniline and nitrobenzene. Liver injury, sometimes severe, may even result in hepatocellular necrosis.

Dinitrotoluene

Dinitrotoluene is another compound that may produce toxic hepatitis.

Trinitrotoluene

Trinitrotoluene (TNT) has produced thousands of cases of industrial poisoning. The first reported cases occurred during World War I, and several hundred fatalities were reported from the ammunition industry in Great Britain and the United States. During World War II, there were another several hundred cases and a smaller number of fatalities in both countries.[2]

Absorption takes place through the skin and also through the respiratory and gastrointestinal routes.

Functional disturbances of the gastrointestinal, central nervous, and cardiovascular systems, and skin irritation or eczematous lesions may precede the development and clinical manifestations of toxic liver injury or aplastic anemia. Abdominal pain, loss of appetite, nausea, and hepatomegaly may be the first indications of toxic hepatitis. Clinically recognizable jaundice can be preceded by moderate elevations in bilirubin levels and a decrease in total plasma protein levels.

According to available records, toxic hepatitis developed in approximately 1 of 500 workers exposed, but the fatality rate was around 30 percent and higher in some reported series. High urinary coproporphyrin levels are a feature of TNT-induced toxic hepatitis. Acute liver failure may develop rapidly and may be fatal. Massive subacute hepatocellular necrosis has been found in fatal cases. A chronic, protracted course with development of cirrhosis was observed in other cases. Postnecrotic cirrhosis, becoming clinically evident as long as 10 years after apparent recovery from TNT-induced acute toxic hepatitis, has also been reported.

The number of nonfatal cases of TNT poisoning during World War II is unknown, since only fatalities due to hepatocellular necrosis or to aplastic anemia were reported. It is almost certain that many cases of toxic hepatitis were never diagnosed during exposure, and the number of such cases eventually resulting in chronic liver disease—postnecrotic cirrhosis—is unknown. Acute hemolytic anemia has been reported after TNT exposure of workers with glucose-6-phosphate dehydrogenase deficiency. Early equatorial cataracts were described in workers exposed to TNT.

Urinary metabolites of trinitrotoluene are 4-aminodinitrotoluene and 2-aminodinitrotoluene; they can be used for biological monitoring of exposed workers. Complete blood counts, bilirubin, prothrombin, liver enzyme (SGOT, SGPT, etc.) levels, and urinary coproporphyrins have been recommended in the medical surveillance of exposed workers.

Toluylenediamine

Toluylenediamine can produce severe toxic liver damage, with massive hepatic necrosis.

Xylidine

Xylidine has been shown to produce severe toxic hepatitis; postnecrotic cirrhosis has developed in experimental animals.

4,4′-Diaminodiphenylmethane

More than 200 million pounds of 4,4′-diaminodiphenylmethane (methylene dianiline, MDA) are manufactured each year in the United States. It is widely used in the production of isocyanates and polyisocyanates, which are the basis for polyurethane foams. Other uses are as an epoxy hardener, as a curing agent for neoprene in the rubber industry, and as a raw material in the production of nylon and polyamideimide resins.

4,4′-Diaminodiphenylmethane was the cause of an epidemic outbreak (84 cases) of toxic hepatitis with jaundice in Epping, England, in 1965 (an episode since known as "Epping jaundice"). The accidental spillage of the chemical from a plastic container and contamination of flour used for bread was the cause of this epidemic. Both the contaminated bread and the pure aromatic amine produced similar lesions in mice.

In 1974 the first industrial outbreak of 13 cases of toxic hepatitis caused by 4,4′-diaminodiphenylmethane was reported. The aromatic amine had been used as an epoxy resin hardener for the manufacture of insulating material. The pattern of illness was similar to that described for the Epping epidemic, with abrupt onset, epigastric or right upper quadrant pain, fever, and jaundice. The duration of the illness ranged from 1 to 7 weeks. Skin absorption had been important in some of the cases.

Another small outbreak of methylene dianiline poisoning occurred when 6 of approximately 300 men who applied epoxy resins as a surface coat for concrete walls at the construction site of a nuclear power electric generating plant contracted toxic hepatitis 2 days to 2 weeks after starting work. The clinical picture was similar to the cases previously described. Methylene dianiline has been shown to produce hepatocellular necrosis in all animals tested, although there are species differences. Cirrhosis has developed in rats and dogs in several experimental series.

MDA exhibits all the characteristics of a direct or predictable hepatotoxin, such as dose dependency, short latent period, and effect on animal models. Nephrotoxicity has also been demonstrated in animal experiments. In recent years 4,4-diaminodiphenylmethane has been the etiologic agent of an increasing number of cases of contact allergies.

Limited data suggest that workers in the textile, dye, and rubber industries experience a higher incidence of gallbladder and biliary tract cancer than control groups.[3] In view of the very large number of chemicals used, however, direct association with MDA has not been established. Long-term observations on workers exposed only to chemicals of this group are almost nonexistent, and therefore no firm conclusions can be drawn.

In a chronic feeding experiment on rats and mice, MDA was found to produce thyroid carcinoma, hepatocellular carcinoma, lymphomas, and pheochromocytomas. The NIOSH recommended that MDA be considered a potential human carcinogen and that exposures be controlled to the lowest feasible limit. The IARC concluded that there is sufficient evidence for carcinogenic effect of 4,4-methylenedianiline in experimental animals to consider a carcinogenic risk to humans.

Dinitrochlorobenzenes

Dinitrochlorobenzenes are strong skin sensitizers.[2]

Paraphenylenediamine and Paraaminophenol

Paraphenylenediamine and paraaminophenol are dye intermediates and are used mostly in the fur industry. They are potent skin and respiratory sensitizers. Severe occupational asthma is not unusual in exposed workers.[2] Paraphenylenediamine was shown to induce sister chromatic exchanges in ovary cells of Chinese hamsters.

4,4′-Methylene-Bis-Ortho-Chloroaniline

4,4′-Methylene-bis-ortho-chloroaniline (MOCA) is used mainly in the production of solid elastomeric parts, as a curing agent for epoxy resins, and in the manufacture of polyurethane foam. Absorption through inhalation and skin contact is possible. In rats, liver and lung cancer have followed the feeding of MOCA. MOCA is included in the federal standard for carcinogens; all contact must be avoided.

Tetranitromethylaniline (Tetryl)

Tetryl is a yellow solid used in explosives and as a chemical indicator.[2] It can be absorbed through inhalation and skin absorption. It is a potent irritant and sensitizer; allergic dermatitis can be extensive and severe. Anemia with hypoplastic bone marrow has occurred. In animal experiments, hepatotoxic and nephrotoxic effects have been detected.

Prevention and Control

Adequate protective clothing and strict personal hygiene with careful cleaning of the entire body, including hair and scalp, are essential to minimize skin absorption, which is particularly hazardous with this group of substances. Clean work clothes should be supplied at the beginning of every shift. Soiled protective equipment must be immediately discarded. Adequate shower facilities and a mandatory shower at the end of the shift, as well as immediately after accidental spillage, are necessary. Respirators must be available for unexpected accidental overexposure.

Medical surveillance should comprise dermatological examination and hematological, liver, and kidney function evaluation. Workers must be informed of the health hazards and educated and trained to use appropriate work practices and first-aid procedures for emergency situations.

► ALIPHATIC AMINES

Aliphatic and alicyclic amines are derivatives of ammonia (NH_3) in which one atom (primary amine) or more hydrogen atoms (secondary or tertiary amines) are substituted by alkyl, alicyclic, or alkanol radicals (ethanolamines). They have a characteristic fishlike odor; most are gases or volatile liquids. They are widely used in industry; one of the most important applications is as "hardeners" (cross-linking agents) and catalysts for epoxy resins. Other uses are in the manufacture of pharmaceutical products, dyes, rubber, pesticides, fungicides, herbicides, emulsifying agents, and corrosion inhibitors.

The amines form strongly alkaline solutions that can be very irritating to the skin and mucosae. Chemical burns of the skin can occur. Skin sensitization and allergic dermatitis have been reported.[2] Some of the amines can produce bronchospasm, and cases of amine asthma have been documented.[2] Corneal lesions may result from accidental contact with liquid amines or solutions of amines.

Prevention

Appropriate engineering controls, protective clothing, eye protection (goggles), and air-supplied respirators when concentrations exceeding the federal standard for exposure limits (from 3 to 10 ppm for various amines) are expected, and training programs for employees are necessary to prevent adverse effects due to exposure to these compounds.

► ORGANIC NITROSO-COMPOUNDS

The organic nitroso- compounds compose nitrosamines and nitrosamides, in which the nitroso- groups (−N=0) are attached to nitrogen atoms,

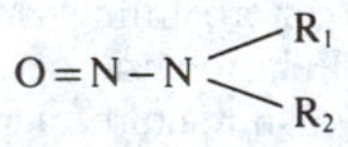

and C-nitroso-compounds, in which the nitroso-groups are attached to carbon atoms. Nitrosamines are readily formed by the reaction of secondary amines with nitrous acid (nitrite in an acid medium).

A large number of *N*-nitroso-compounds are known; several examples of dialkyl, heterocyclic, and aryl alkylnitrosamines with marked toxic activity are shown below, together with two *N*-nitrosamides, *N*-nitrosomethyl urea and *N*-nitro-*N*′-nitro-*N*-methyl guanidine. The nitrosamines are more unstable in an alkaline medium, yielding the corresponding dialkanes; they are extensively used in synthetic organic chemistry for alkylating reactions.

Interest in the toxicity of *N*-nitroso-compounds was first aroused in 1954, when Barnes and Magee[263] reported on the hepatotoxicity of dimethylnitrosamine. This compound had recently been introduced into a laboratory as a solvent, and two cases of clinically overt liver damage were etiologically linked to it. A search of the literature at that time revealed only a single short report of the toxic properties of dimethylnitrosamine (DMN). Hamilton and Hardy had reported in 1949 that the use of DMN in an automobile factory had been followed by illness in some of the exposed workers. Experiments on dogs showed DMN to be capable of producing severe liver injury.

N-nitrosodimethylamine (dimethylnitrosamine)

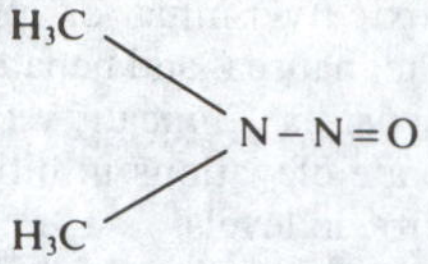

N-nitrosodibutylamine (dibutylnitrosamine)

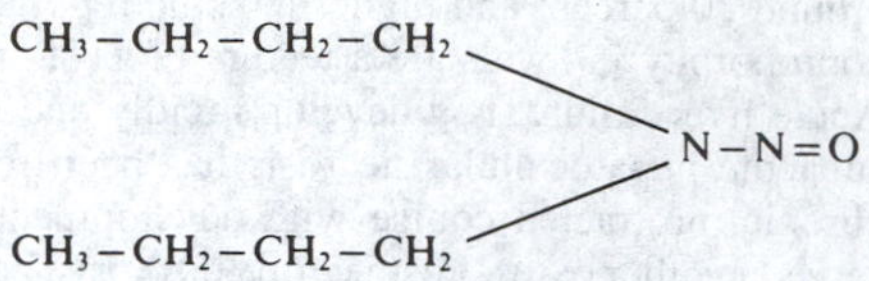

N-nitrosopyrolidine

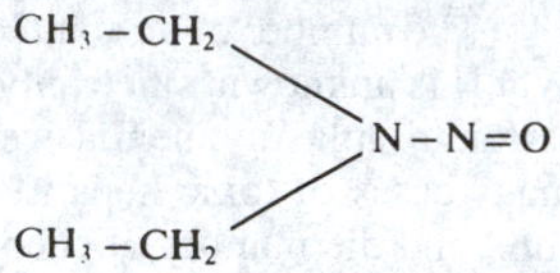

N-nitrosomethylaniline

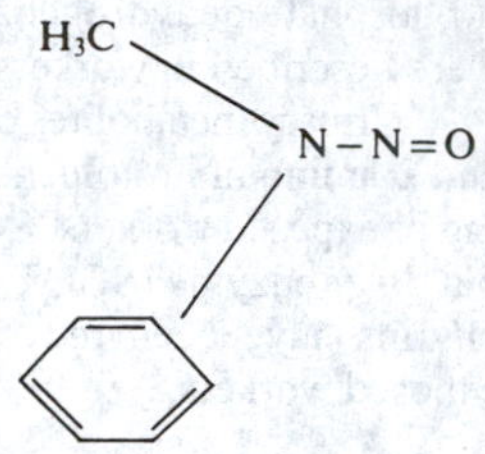

N-nitrosomethyl urea

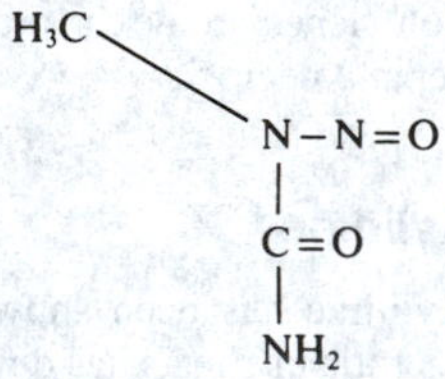

N-nitroso-*N*′-nitro-*N*-methyl guanidine

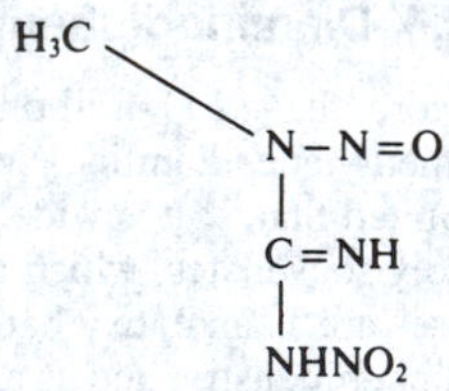

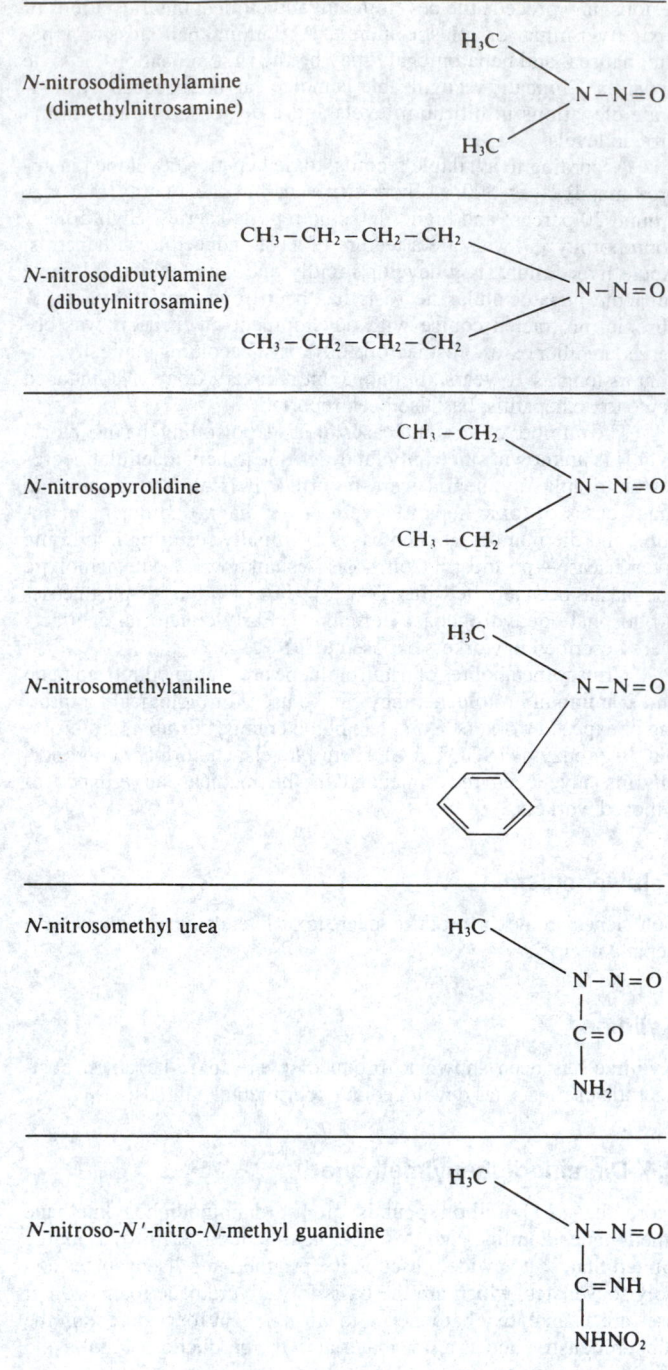

As a solvent, DMN is highly toxic and dangerous to handle, although its volatility is relatively low. The absence of a specific odor or irritant properties may favor the absorption of toxic amounts without any warning; contamination of skin and clothes may pass unnoticed.

Information on the industrial uses of nitrosamines is incomplete. A relatively large patent literature indicates many potential applications. The manufacture of rubber, dyes, lubricating oils, explosives, insecticides and fungicides, the electrical industry, and the industrial applications of hydrazine chemistry appear to be the main uses for nitrosamines.

The use of DMN as an intermediate in the manufacture of 1,1-dimethylhydrazine is well known. *N*-Nitrosodiphenylamine is used in the rubber industry as a vulcanizing retarder, and dinitrosopentamethylene-tetramine is used as a blowing agent in the production of microcellular rubber.

Experiments conducted by Barnes and Magee[263] indicated that DMN readily produced severe liver injury in rats, rabbits, mice, guinea pigs, and dogs. Centrilobular and midzonal necrosis, depletion of glycogen and fat deposition, and dilation of sinusoidal spaces were the prominent changes in the acute stage. Hemorrhagic peritoneal exudate and bleeding into the lumen of the gut were striking features; such changes are not encountered in liver injury caused by carbon tetrachloride, phosphorus, or beryllium. Repeated doses were found to result in fibrosis of the liver. These experimental observations pointed to the conclusion that DMN, shown to produce severe liver injury in a variety of experimental animals, had been the etiological agent in the development of cirrhosis of the liver in the two laboratory technicians handling the solvent.

In 1956 Magee and Barnes[264] reported on the hepatocarcinogenicity of DMN. The metabolic degradation of DMN in the liver proceeds through enzymatic oxidative demethylation; the resulting monomethyl nitrosamine is then decomposed, and diazomethane was thought by Magee to be the alkylating agent with carcinogenic potential.

In 1962 Magee and Farber,[265] by administering ^{14}C-DMN to rats, were able to demonstrate the methylation of nucleic acids in the liver, especially at the N7 site of guanidine. Thus an alteration of the genetic information in the hepatocyte was detected and was considered the basis for the carcinogenic effect. This was the first experimental proof of such a molecular alteration of DNA by a carcinogen. The discovery of the role of drug-metabolizing microsomal enzymes in the biotransformation of DMN into a carcinogen opened an important field of investigation. Similar pathways were found to be effective for another compound of this group, diethylnitrosamine.[266]

The acute hepatotoxic effect on *N*-nitroso- compounds is also caused by the alkylating intermediate metabolites. The acute toxicity is due to alkylation of proteins and enzymes, while the carcinogenic effect is related to alkylation of nucleic acids. Several fundamentally important observations were also made by Druckrey and coworkers.[266]

1. A carcinogenic effect of a single dose of some of these compounds was demonstrated (tumors developed after various latency periods), and the kidney, liver, esophagus, stomach, and CNS were the main organs in which the primary tumors were detected.
2. The site of the primary malignant tumor was found to be, for certain compounds, in a clear relationship with the administered dose.
3. DMN was shown to be a more potent carcinogen than diethylnitrosamine.
4. The transplacental carcinogenicity of DMN was demonstrated; hepatocarcinogenicity was detected in offspring of treated pregnant rats.
5. Di-*n*-butyl-nitrosamine induced hepatocellular carcinoma and cirrhosis of the liver when administered orally in relatively high amounts. With the gradual decrease of the dose, fewer hepatocellular carcinomas and more cancers of the esophagus and the urinary bladder were found. Diamylnitrosamine resulted in hepatocellular carcinoma when given in high doses. Subcutaneous injections resulted in squamous cell and alveolar cell carcinoma of the lung, in addition to relatively few hepatocellular carcinomas. This finding was thought to be important since it indicated that lung cancer can develop not only after inhalation of carcinogens but also as a result of absorption of carcinogens through other routes.

Cyclic *N*-nitroso- compounds (*N*-nitrosopyrrolidine, *N*-nitrosomorpholine, *N*-nitrosocarbethoxypiperazine) were also found to produce hepatocellular carcinomas. Heterocyclic nitrosamines (*N*-nitrosoazetidine, *N*-nitrosohexamethyleneimine, *N*-nitrosomorpholine, *N*-nitrosopyrrolidine, and *N*-nitrosopiperidine) result in characteristic hepatic centrilobular necrosis; they have also been shown to produce a high incidence of tumors of the liver and other organs. The earliest change in the liver is the development of foci of altered hepatocytes (FAH), demonstrated histochemically by changes in the activities of glucose-6-phosphate dehydrogenase and glycogen phosphorylase and in the glycogen content. Proliferating cells have been detected by immunohistochemical reaction for proliferating cell nuclear antigen. The number and size of foci of altered hepatocytes increased in a time- and dose-related manner.[267]

Pancreatic cancer developed in Syrian hamsters after subcutaneous administration of three nitrosamines, including *N*-nitro-2,6-dimethylmorpholine. *Ras*-oncogene activation was investigated in bladder tumors of male rats given *N*-butyl-*N*-(4-hydroxybutyl) nitrosamine. Enhanced expression of p21 was detected in all tumors. The tobacco-specific nitrosamine 4-(methylnitrosamine)-1-(3-pyridyl)-1-butanone (NNK) is a potent carcinogen in laboratory animals. Analysis of DNA for K-ras mutation showed G → A transition of codon 12 of the K-ras oncogene in tumor cells derived from pancreatic duct cells treated with NNK.[268]

In human esophageal cancers, no ras gene mutations, but a relatively high prevalence of p53 gene mutations, have been reported. A high prevalence of point mutations in Ha-ras and p53 genes was found in *N*-nitrosomethylbenzylamine (NMBA)-induced esophageal tumors in rats. The prevalent mutations were G → A.[269] The carcinogenic properties of *N*-nitroso- compounds are associated with their ability to alkylate DNA, in particular to form *O*6-alkylguanine and *O*4-alkylthymine.[270]

DMN was shown to induce, besides typical centrilobular necrosis, veno-occlusive lesions in the liver in animals followed for longer periods after a high, nearly lethal dose. Prolonged oral administration of relatively low doses of dimethylnitrosamine resulted in gross, nodular cirrhosis of the liver; with lower doses, longer survival of the animals was achieved, and several malignant liver-cell–type tumors occurred.

The dialkylnitrosamines, stable compounds, are decomposed only by enzymatic action and result in cell damage after having undergone an enzymatic activation process in organs that have adequate enzymatic systems. The toxic, mutagenic, teratogenic, and carcinogenic effects of nitroso- compounds all depend on this biologic activation by enzymatic reactions. Inhibition of hepatic microsomal enzymatic systems by a protein-deficient diet has been shown to result in a decrease in dimethylnitrosamine toxicity, confirming that the hepatotoxic effect is dependent on microsomal enzymatic activation.

The predominant effect of the dialkylnitrosamines is liver injury, the characteristic lesion being a hemorrhagic type of centrilobular necrosis. This specificity of action is related to the fact that these compounds require metabolic transformation-activation for their toxic effect. The enzymatic systems effective for these metabolic transformations are present in highest amounts in the microsomal fraction of the liver, but also in the kidney, lung, and esophagus. Species differences have been documented; these metabolic differences parallel differences in the main site of effects—toxic, carcinogenic, or both.

In contrast to the relative chemical stability of nitrosamines, the nitrosamides show varying degrees of instability. Many of these compounds yield diazoalkanes when treated with alkali, and they are extensively used in the synthetic chemical industry.

The nitrosamides differ in their effects from the nitrosamines; they have a local irritation effect at the site of administration; some have marked local cytopathic action, sometimes resulting in severe tissue necrosis. *N*-methyl-*N*-nitrosomethane causes severe necrotic lesions of the gastric mucosa and also periportal liver necrosis. In addition to their local action, some of the nitrosamides have a radiomimetic effect on organs with rapid cell turnover, with the bone marrow, lymphoid tissue, and small intestine being injured most. Several substances of the nitrosamide group are known to induce cancer at the site of chronic application.

Morpholine is widely used in industry as a solvent for waxes, dyes, pigments, and casein; it has also found applications in the rubber industry.

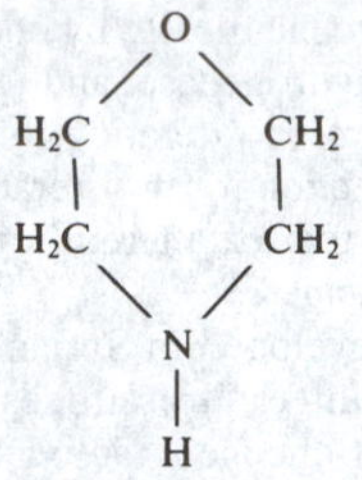

As an anticorrosive agent and as an emulsifier (after reaction with fatty acids), morpholine is used in the manufacture of cleaning products. Long considered a relatively nontoxic substance, morpholine was also used in the food industry, in the coating of fresh fruit and vegetables (fatty acid salts of morpholine), and for anticorrosive treatment of metals (including those to be used in the food industry). Industrial occupational exposure and household exposure are therefore quite frequent. Absorption of morpholine through the oral route may, in the presence of nitrites from alimentary sources, result in the production of hazardous gastric levels of nitrosamine. In the rubber industry, efforts have been made to replace amino- compounds that can generate *N*-nitrosamines in accelerators with "safe" amino components. Derivatives of the dithiocarbamate and sulfenamide class were synthesized and found to be suitable for industrial application.

The organic *N*-nitroso- compounds are characterized by marked acute liver toxicity; chronic absorption of smaller amounts has been shown to result in cirrhosis in experimental animals. Initial reports of human cases of postnecrotic cirrhosis, however, have not been followed by other reports on human effects. Suitable epidemiological data are not yet available on the real incidence of toxic liver damage, cirrhosis of the liver, hepatocellular carcinoma, and other malignant tumors in industrially exposed populations.

The presence of nitrosamines in cutting oils has been reported.[1] The formation of nitrosamines had been suspected, since nitrites and aliphatic amines are known constituents of some cutting fluids. Concentrations of nitrosamines up to 3 percent have been found in randomly selected cutting oils; metal machining operators using cutting oils may therefore be significantly exposed to nitrosamines. Semisynthetic cutting oils and the synthetic cutting fluids most often contain amines as a soluble base and nitrites as additives. NIOSH estimated that almost 800,000 persons are occupationally exposed in the manufacture and use of cutting fluids and issued guidelines for industrial hygiene practices in an effort to minimize skin and respiratory exposure.

Environmental Nitrosamines

The possibility that exposure to compounds of the nitrosamine group may occur in situations other than the industrial environment was revealed by an outbreak of severe liver disease in sheep in Norway in 1960. Severe necrosis of the liver was the main pathologic feature. The sheep had been fed fish meal preserved with nitrite. This suggested that nitrosamines may have resulted from the reaction between secondary and tertiary amines present in the fish meal and the nitrites added as a preservative. The presence of dimethylnitrosamine at levels of 30 to 100 ppm was detected. Subsequently, the presence of nitrosamines in small amounts in food for human consumption has been documented. Smoked fish, smoked sausage, ham and bacon, mushrooms, some fruits, and alcoholic beverages (from areas in Africa with a high incidence of esophageal cancer) have been shown to contain various amounts of nitrosamines (0.5 to 40 μg/kg).

Nitrosamines can be formed in the human stomach from secondary amines and nitrites. The methylation of nucleic acids of the stomach, liver, and small intestine in rats given ^{14}C-methyl urea and sodium nitrite simultaneously was also demonstrated, and malignant liver and esophageal tumors in rats have resulted from simultaneous feeding of morpholine or *N*-methylbenzylamine and sodium nitrite. Several bacterial species—*Escherichia coli, Enterococcus dispar, Proteus vulgaris*, and *Serratia marcescens*—can form nitrosamines from secondary amines. The bacterial reduction of nitrate to nitrite in the human stomach has been shown.

Tobacco-specific nitrosamines have been identified and have received considerable attention. Nicotine and the minor tobacco alkaloids give rise to tobacco-specific *N*-nitrosamines (TSNAs) during tobacco processing and during smoking (≤25 μg/g) and in mainstream smoke of cigarettes (1.3 TSNA/cigarette). In mice, rats, and hamsters, three TSNAs, *N*′-nitrosonornicotine (NNN), 4-(methylnitrosamino)-1-(3 pyridyl)-1-butanone (NNK), and 4-(methylnitrosamino)-1-(3 pyridyl)-1-butanol (NNAL), are powerful carcinogens; two TSNAs are moderately active carcinogens and two TSNAs appear not to be carcinogenic. The TSNAs are procarcinogens that require metabolic activation. The active forms react with cellular components, including DNA, and with hemoglobin. The Hb adducts serve as biomarkers in smokers or tobacco chewers, and the urinary excretion of NNAL is an indicator of TSNA uptake. The TSNAs contribute to the increased risk of upper digestive tract cancer in tobacco chewers and lung cancer in smokers. The high incidence of cancer of the upper digestive tract in the Indian subcontinent has been casually associated with chewing of betel quid mixed with tobacco. Betel quid is the source of four *N*-nitrosamines from the Areca alkaloids; two of these are carcinogenic.[271]

TSNAs NNN and NNK are metabolites of nicotine and are the major carcinogens in cigarette smoke. In fetal human lung cells exposed to NNN and NNK, a dose-dependent increase in DNA single-strand breaks was observed. In combination with enzymatically generated oxygen radicals, strand breakage increased by approximately 50 percent for both NNN and NNK.[272] Tobacco-specific nitrosamine NNK produces DNA single-strand breaks (SSB) in hamster and rat liver. DNA SSB reached a maximum at 12 hours after treatment and persisted 2 to 3 weeks, reflecting deficient repair of some DNA lesions.[273] NNK injected subcutaneously or instilled intratracheally into pregnant hamsters resulted in high incidence of respiratory tract tumors in offspring; target organs included the adrenal glands and the pancreas. The results suggested that NNK, at doses comparable to the cumulative exposure during a 9-month period in women, is a potent transplacental carcinogen in hamsters.[274]

Evidence of nitrosamine-induced DNA damage was found in the increased levels of 8-oxodeoxyguanosine and 8-hydroxydeoxyguanosine (8-OH-dG) in tissue DNA of mice and rats treated with the tobacco-specific nitrosamine NNK. These lesions were detected in lung DNA and liver DNA, but not in rat kidney (a nontarget tissue). These findings support the role of oxidative DNA damage in NNK lung tumorigenesis.[275] NNK produced pulmonary tumors in adult mice treated with a single dose (100 mg/kg IP). Progression of pulmonary lesions was noted from hyperplasia through adenomas to carcinomas (to 54 weeks). DNA was isolated from 20 hyperplasias and activation of the K-ras gene was found in 17 lesions, 85 percent of the mutations involving a GC → AT transition within codon 12, a mutation consistent with base mispairing produced by the formation of the *O*6-methylguanine adduct.[276] NNK is a potent carcinogen in adult rodents and variably effective transplacentally, depending on species. NNK was tested in infant mice; at 13 to 15 months, 57 percent of NNK-exposed male offspring had hepatocellular tumors; a lower occurrence (14 percent) was found in female offspring. In addition, primary lung tumors were also found in 57 percent of males and 37 percent of females. These results call attention to the possibility that human infants may be especially vulnerable for tumor initiation by tobacco smoke constituents.[277]

The number of lung tumors and fore-stomach tumors in mice given 6.8 ppm *N*-nitrosodiethylamine was considerably increased when ethanol 10 percent was also added. Ethanol increased lung tumor multiplicity 5.5-fold when *N*-nitrosopyrrolidine was given. It is thought that coadministered ethanol increases the tumorigenicity of nitrosamines by blocking hepatic first-pass clearance.[278]

Numerous epidemiological studies have established that asbestos causes occupational lung cancer and mesothelioma; a cocarcinogenic effect of cigarette smoking on the incidence of lung cancer in asbestos workers has been well documented. In an experimental study on rats, chrysotile asbestos was administered intratracheally, *N*-bis(hydryoxypropyl)nitrosamine (DHPN) was injected intraperitoneally, and the animals were exposed to smoke from 10 cigarettes/day for their entire life span. Lung tumors were detected in one of 31 rats receiving only asbestos; they occurred in 22 percent of rats receiving DPNH alone and in 60 percent of the rats receiving DPNH and asbestos. Thus the cocarcinogenic effect of tobacco-specific nitrosamines was clearly demonstrated.[279]

The Areca-derived 3-(methylnitrosamino)propionitrile (MNPN) when tested on mouse skin produced multiple distant tumors in the lungs. When applied by swabbing the oral cavity, strong organ-specific carcinogenicity resulted in nasal tumors, lung adenomas, liver tumors, and papillomas of the esophagus, with relatively few oral tumors.[280]

Certain environmentally relevant nitrosamines specifically induce malignant tumors in the urinary bladder in several animal species. Butyl-3-carboxypropylnitrosamine, methyl-3-carboxypropylnitrosamine, and methyl-5-carboxypropylnitrosamine were found to be β-oxidized by mitochondrial fractions to butyl-2-oxopropylnitrosamine or methyl-2-oxopropylnitrosamine. By this reaction, water-soluble carboxylated nitrosamines of low genotoxic potential are converted into rather lipophilic 2-oxopropyl metabolites, with high genotoxic and carcinogenic potency.[281]

In northeast Thailand the consumption of raw freshwater and salt-fermented fish results in repeated exposure to liver fluke (*Opisthorchis viverrini*) infection and ingestion of nitrosamine-contaminated food. A high prevalence of cholangiocarcinoma is known to exist in this region. The Syrian golden hamster receiving subcarcinogenic doses of dimethylnitrosamine (DMN) and infection with flukes developed cholangiocarcinomas. Nitrosamines are considered to be genotoxicants, while liver flukes are assumed to play an epigenetic role.[282] Samples of food frequently consumed in Kashmir, a high-risk area for esophageal cancer, revealed high levels of *N*-nitrosodimethylamine, *N*-nitrosopiperidine, and *N*-nitrosopyrrolidine in smoked fish, sun-dried spinach, dried mixed vegetables, and dried pumpkin.[283]

A reduction of the high exposures to *N*-nitrosamines in the rubber and tire industry is possible by using vulcanization accelerators that contain amine moieties that are both difficult to nitrosate, and, on nitrosation, yield noncarcinogenic *N*-nitroso- compounds. The toxicological and technological properties of some 50 benzothiazole sulfenamides derived from such amines have been evaluated.[284]

Laboratory research conducted over the last 20 years has identified the organic nitroso- compounds as some of the most potent carcinogens, mutagens, and teratogens for a variety of animal species. The possibility of nitrosamine formation from nitrites (or nitrates) and secondary or tertiary amines in the stomach and the possibility of a similar effect attributable to microorganisms normally present in the gut and frequently in the urinary tract suggest a potential hazard for the population at large.

The identification of tobacco-specific nitrosamines and of nitrosamines in betel and in foodstuffs in areas with high cancer incidence emphasizes the growing importance of this group of chemical carcinogens.

▸ EPOXY COMPOUNDS

Epoxy compounds are cyclic ethers characterized by the presence of an epoxide ring.

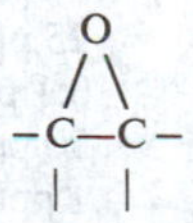

These ethers, with an oxygen attached to two adjacent carbons, readily react with amino, hydroxyl, and carboxyl groups and also with inorganic acids to form relatively stable compounds. The epoxide group is very reactive and can form covalent bonds with biologically important molecules.

Industrial applications have expanded rapidly in the manufacture of epoxy resins, plasticizers, surface-active agents, solvents, etc.

Most epoxy resins are prepared by reacting epichlorhydrin with a polyhydroxy compound, most frequently bisphenol A, in the presence of a curing agent (cross-linking agents—"hardeners," mainly polyamines or anhydrides of polybasic acids, such as phthalic anhydride). Catalysts include polyamides and tertiary amines; diluents such as glycidyl ethers, styrene, styrene oxide, or other epoxides are sometimes used to achieve lower viscosity of uncured epoxy resin systems.

Epoxy compounds can adversely affect the skin, mucosae, airways, and lungs; some have hepatotoxic and neurotoxic effects. Most epoxy compounds are very potent irritants (to eyes, airways, skin), and they can produce pulmonary edema. Skin lesions can be due to the irritant effect or to sensitization. Respiratory sensitization can also occur. Carcinogenic effects in experimental models have been demonstrated for several epoxy compounds.

Epichlorhydrin

Epichlorhydrin (1-chloro-2,3,-epoxypropane, $CH_2OCH\text{-}CH_2Cl$) is a colorless liquid with a boiling point of 116.4°C. The most important uses are for the manufacture of epoxy resins, surface-active agents, insecticides and other agricultural chemicals, coatings, adhesives, plasticizers, glycidyl ethers, cellulose esters and ethers, paints, varnishes, and lacquers.[2,3]

Absorption through inhalation and skin is of practical importance. Epichlorhydrin is a strong irritant of the eyes, respiratory tract, and skin. Skin contact may result in dermatitis, occasionally with marked erythema and blistering. Skin sensitization with allergic dermatitis has also been reported. Severe systemic effects have been reported in a few cases of human overexposure: these included nausea, vomiting, dyspnea, abdominal pain, hepatomegaly, jaundice, and abnormal liver function tests.

In experimental studies, nephrotoxic effects have been found; an adverse effect on liver mixed-function microsomal enzymes has also been reported. In experiments on rats, epiochlorhydrin was found to significantly decrease the content in cytochrome P-450 of microsomes isolated from the liver, kidney, testes, lung, and small intestine mucosa.

In experimental studies on rats, it was found that the incidence of squamous cell nasal carcinoma was significantly higher than in control animals. Limited epidemiological data have produced equivocal results. The carcinogenic risk to humans cannot be considered as having been fully assessed because of insufficient follow-up periods and relatively small cohorts. The IARC has concluded that there is sufficient evidence of carcinogenicity in animals but as yet inadequate evidence in humans.

Chromosomal aberrations have been found in exposed workers. Several experimental studies suggest that interference with male reproductive function can result from epichlorhydrin exposure. In rats, epichlorhydrin was found to produce progressive testicular atrophy, reduction of sperm concentration, and an increase in the number of morphologically abnormal spermatozoa. Testicular function was studied in epichlorhydrin-exposed workers; no effects were demonstrated. Epichlorhydrin did not produce teratogenic effects in rats, rabbits, or mice.

Epichlorhydrin is considered a bifunctional alkylating agent; it reacts with nucleophilic molecules by forming covalent bonds; cross-linking bonds may also be formed. These chemical characteristics are believed to be of importance for their carcinogenic, mutagenic, and reproductive effects.

Prevention

The recommended standard[3] for exposure to epichlorhydin is 2 mg/m^3 (0.5 ppm), with a ceiling of 19 mg/m^3 (5 ppm) not to exceed

15 minutes. In 1978, when data on a potential carcinogenic effect in humans became available, additional emphasis was given to the importance of minimizing occupational exposure to epichlorhydrin by engineering and work practice controls.

Ethylene Oxide

Ethylene oxide (1,2-epoxyethane, H_2COCH_2), is a colorless gas used in the organic synthesis of ethylene glycol and glycol derivatives, ethanolamines, acrylontrile, polyester fibers, and film and surface-active agents; it has been used as a pesticide fumigant and for sterilization of surgical equipment. Ethylene oxide is highly reactive and potentially explosive; it is relatively stable in aqueous solutions or when diluted with halogenated hydrocarbons or carbon dioxide.

Ethylene oxide is a high-volume production chemical; production capacity in the United States was 6.1 billion pounds a year in 1981. Exposure to ethylene oxide is very limited in chemical plants, where it is produced and used for intermediates, mostly in closed systems. Maintenance and repair work, sampling, loading and unloading, and accidental leaks can generate exposure.

Although only a small proportion of ethylene oxide is used in health care and medical equipment manufacturing industries, and even less for sterilization of equipment in medical care facilities, NIOSH has estimated that more than 75,000 employees in sterilization areas have been exposed; concentrations as high as hundreds of parts per million were found on occasion, mostly in the vicinity of malfunctioning or inadequate equipment.

Absorption occurs through inhalation. Ethylene oxide is a strong irritant, especially in aqueous solutions. Severe dermatitis and even chemical burns, marked eye irritation, and toxic pulmonary edema have occurred with high concentrations. The presence of lens opacities in combination with loss of visual acuity was found to be significantly increased among sterilization workers exposed to ethylene oxide, when compared with unexposed controls.[285] Allergic dermatitis may develop. With high levels of exposure, CNS depression with drowsiness, headaches, and even loss of consciousness have occurred. A number of cases of sensory motor peripheral neuropathy have been reported in personnel performing sterilization with ethylene oxide. Removal from exposure resulted in gradual improvement over several months. The distal axonal degenerative changes have been reproduced in rats exposed to 500 ppm for 13 weeks. In rats chronically exposed to ethylene oxide (500 ppm for 6 hours/day, 3 days/week for 15 weeks), the distal portions of the sural nerve showed degenerational changes in myelinated fibers and fewer large myelinated fibers in the distal peroneal nerve, with a decrease in the velocity of anterograde axonal transport.[286]

Ethylene oxide has been shown to be mutagenic in several assay systems including human fibroblasts.[287] Covalent binding to DNA has been demonstrated.

Sterilization plant workers have been shown to exhibit evidence of DNA damage. DNA strand breaks, alkali-labile sites of DNA, and DNA cross-links were seen in excess in peripheral mononuclear blood cells, compared with findings in unexposed controls.[288] The frequency of hemoglobin adducts and SCEs in peripheral blood cells increased with cumulative exposure to ethylene oxide among hospital workers.[289] Increased frequencies of hypoxanthine-quanine phosphonbosyl transferase (HPRT) mutants, chromosomal aberrations, micronuclei, and sister chromatid exchanges have been reported among sterilization plant workers.[290] Chromosomal aberrations and sister chromatic exchange have been found to occur with significantly increased frequency in workers exposed to ethylene oxide at concentrations not exceeding a time-weighted average of 50 ppm (but with occasional excursions to 75 ppm). More recently, exposures near or below 1 ppm among workers in a hospital sterilization unit were associated with increased hemoglobin adduct formation and SCEs, independent of smoking history.[291]

Adverse reproductive effects (reduced numbers of pups per litter, fewer implantation sites, and a reduced ratio of fetuses to number of implantation sites) were observed in rats exposed to 100 ppm ethylene oxide. An increased proportion of congenital malformations (mostly skeletal) was also reported. The effect occurred predominately when exposure occurred during the zygotic period rather than during organogenesis.[292] Genotoxic effects on male germ cells in postmeiotic stages have been demonstrated in both *Drosophila* and the mouse.[293] Testicular damage following ethylene oxide exposure in rats has been reported, with specific but reversible injury to Sertoli cells.[294] Women hospital employees exposed to ethylene oxide were found to have a higher incidence of miscarriages than a comparison group.

In 1981, the NIOSH recommended that ethylene oxide be regarded in the workplace as a potential carcinogen and that appropriate controls be used to reduce exposure. This recommendation was based on the results of a carcinogenicity assay, clearly indicating that ethylene oxide can produce malignant tumors in experimental animals. In a chronic inhalation study, mononuclear cell leukemias and peritoneal mesotheliomas were found to be significantly increased in ethylene oxide-exposed rats; both were dose-related and occurred at concentrations of 33 ppm.

A mortality study of workers in a Swedish ethylene oxide plant[295] showed an increased incidence of total cancer deaths, with leukemia and stomach cancer accounting for most of these excess cancer deaths. Other chemical exposures (including some well-known carcinogens) had also been possible in that plant. An excess of leukemia was also found in another plant in which 50 percent ethylene oxide and 50 percent methyl formate were used for sterilization of hospital equipment.[296] The small number of observed deaths and the complex chemical exposures[295] do not allow definitive conclusions regarding the human evidence of ethylene oxide carcinogenicity, although it is entirely consistent with the experimental data. A more recent study of the mortality experience among 18,254 U.S. sterilization plant workers (4.9 years average exposure duration and 16 years of follow-up), with 8-hour TWAs averaging 4.3 ppm, reported a significant trend toward increased mortality with increasing length of time since first exposure for all hematopoietic cancers; among men, but not women, there was a significant increase in mortality from hematopoietic cancers.[297]

The current (1987) TLV for ethylene oxide is 1 ppm.

Glycidyl Ethers

Glycidyl ethers are characterized by the group:

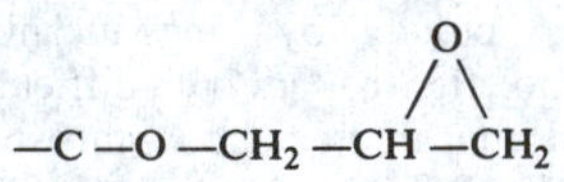

Their most important use is for epoxy resins; diglycidyl ether of bisphenol A is one of the basic ingredients used to react with epichlorhydrin.[97] Glycidyl ethers are also used as diluents, to reduce the viscosity of uncured epoxy resin systems. These find applications in protective coatings, bonding materials, reinforced plastics, etc. The NIOSH estimates that about 1 million workers are exposed to epoxy resins; it is difficult to reach an accurate estimate of the number exposed to glycidyl ethers, but it is probably around 100,000 workers.

Glycidyl ethers are irritants for the skin and mucosae; dermatitis and sensitization have been reported. In experimental studies, an adverse effect on spermatogenesis and testicular atrophy have been the result of glycidyl ether exposure of several species (rats, mice, rabbits) to concentrations as low as 2 to 3 ppm. A potent effect on lymphoid tissue, including atrophy of the thymus and of lymph nodes, low white blood cell counts, or bone marrow toxicity have also been reported in rats, rabbits, and dogs. Information on immunosuppressive or myelotoxic effects in humans is not available, and the possibility that such effects have not been detected in the past cannot be excluded. The present federal standard for permissible exposure limits are listed below:

Allyl glycidyl ether	5 ppm
n-Butyl glycidyl ether	25 ppm
Diglycidyl ether	0.1 ppm
Isopropyl glycidyl ether	50 ppm
Phenyl glycidyl ether	1 ppm

Carcinogenicity Results in Animals Predict Cancer Risks to Humans

James Huff

> Hee is a better physician
> that keeps diseases off us,
> than hee that cures them being on us.
> Prevention is so much better than healing,
> because it saves us the labor of being sick.
>
> —Thomas Adams (seventeenth century)

▸ PERSPECTIVE

Cancers are the second leading cause of death in the United States, with heart diseases being number one and cerebrovascular diseases at number three. As cardiovascular diseases are conquered, cancers are predicted to become the primary killer of Americans in the early twenty-first century. The organs or systems associated with the leading sites of cancer morbidity and mortality include lung, colon and rectum, breast, and prostate gland. Logical grouping of sites leads to these rankings: genital organs, digestive organs, respiratory system, breast, and urinary organs (Fig. 23-1).

In the United States alone, estimates of the number of new cancer cases for the year 1997 indicate that 1,382,400 individuals (785,800 males; 596,600 females) will be diagnosed with cancer (Fig. 23-1) and that 560,000 cancer-associated deaths (294,100 males; 265,900 females) will occur, with both figures almost equally divided among males and females. Estimated numbers of new cancer cases by state are shown on the map of the United States (Fig. 23-2). These figures do not include carcinoma in situ or basal and squamous cell cancers of the skin, which will afflict an additional 900,000 people annually. Many of these cancers are preventable—more than 1 million easily eliminated cancers are those induced by alcoholic beverages (19,000), tobacco smoke (174,000), and solar exposure (900,000).

Even though much is known about certain causes of cancer (e.g., occupational and cancer chemotherapeutic agents), the etiologies of

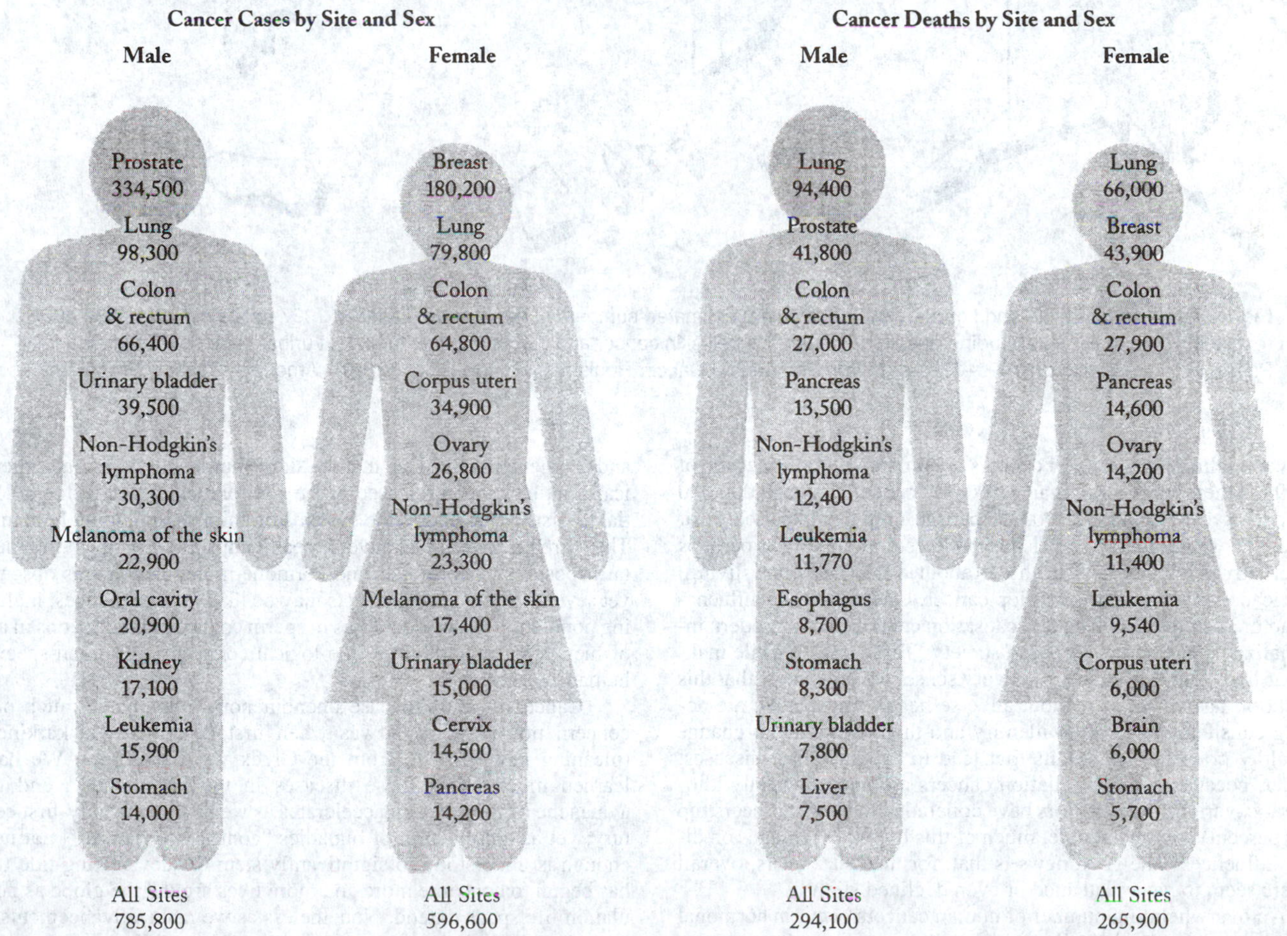

Figure 23-1. Leading sites of new cancer cases and deaths, 1997 estimates. Data exclude basal and squamous cell skin cancer and in situ carcinomas except urinary bladder. (From American Cancer Society Surveillance Research, 1997, American Cancer Society, Cancer Facts and Figures, Atlanta, GA, p 9, 1997.)

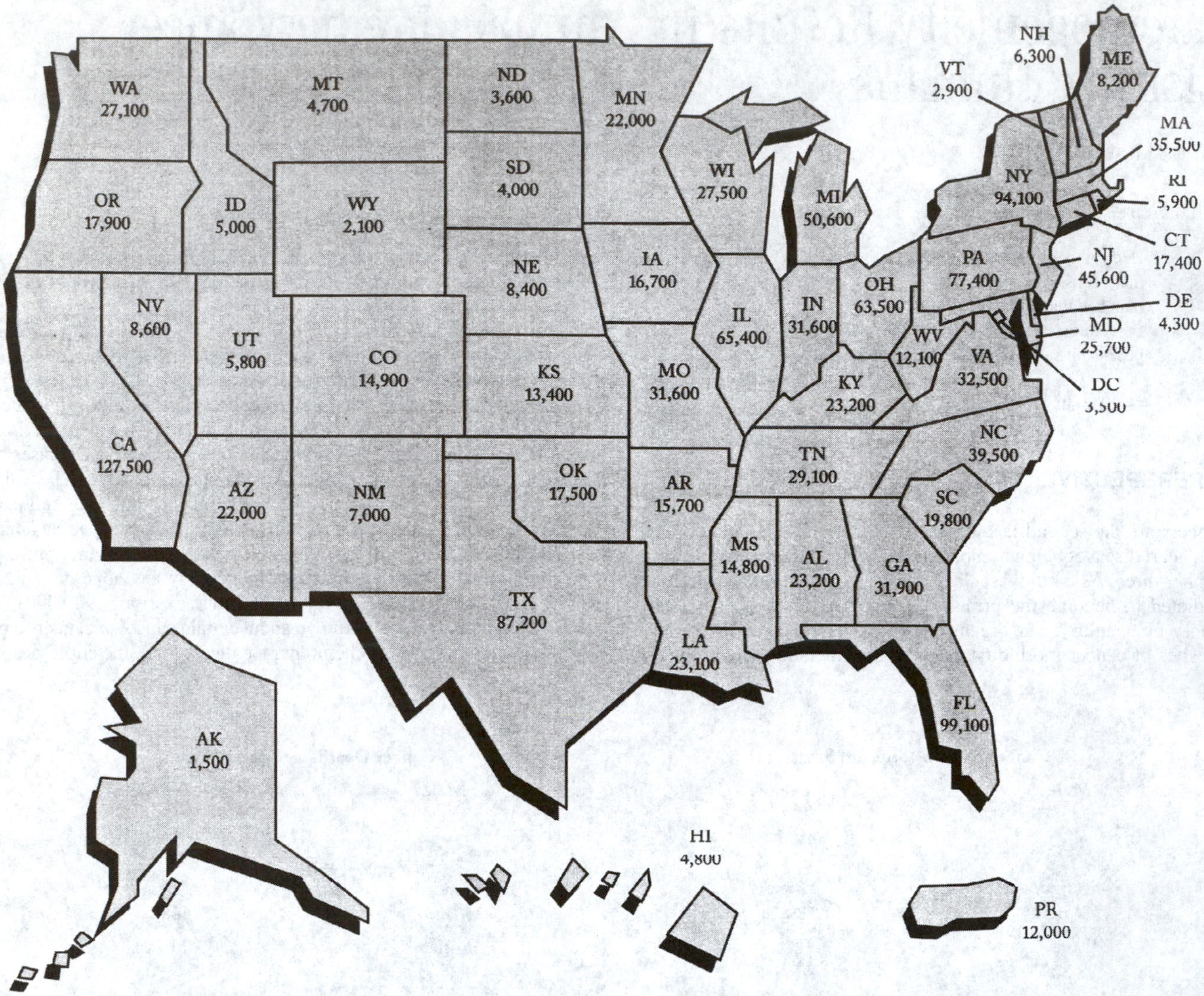

Figure 23-2. Cancer facts and figures, 1997. Shown are estimated numbers of new cancer cases in 1997 by state: total, 1,382,400 (excluding Puerto Rico), excluding basal and squamous cell skin cancer and carcinoma in situ except urinary bladder. Estimates for Puerto Rico are based on 1990–1991 data from the Central Cancer Registry of Puerto Rico. (©1997, American Cancer Society, Inc.)

the overwhelming majority of cancers are unknown. In the decade of the 1980s there were more than 4,500,000 cancer deaths, 9,000,000 new cancer cases, and 12,000,000 people under medical care for cancer. These numbers keep rising, and predictions (albeit perhaps conservative) indicate one in three (about 85,000,000 now living) Americans will eventually develop cancer. One consensus influencing factor associated with cancer causation centers on our modern industrialized and chemically based society (Table 23-1). While making our lives longer and better in every sense, we now know that this revolution has not been without adverse health impact. We are devoting considerable effort to identify and then overcome or change unhealthy practices and habits that lead to or exacerbate diseases. Further, because many population cancers are geographically idiosyncratic, various investigators have concluded that most cancers (up to 90 percent) are preventable; much of this hypothesis hinges on dietary influences. The good news is that, for the last 2 years, overall cancers seem to have plateaued or even declined slightly.

An overwhelming number of human cancers occur in hormonal organs or are mechanistically linked to hormone-associated etiologies,[1] which can be endogenous or exogenous in origin, or both. The extent to which environmental estrogens or "endocrine disruptors" contribute to these cancers remains to be determined. To illustrate possible exogenous causes of hormonally related cancers, Colborn and Clement[2] emphasized that the "large number of man-made chemicals that have been released in the environment . . . have the potential to disrupt the endocrine systems of animals, including humans." The current and eventual adverse health impacts of these environmental exposures to hormones and hormone-mimetics remains obscure, yet several recent global effects may be likely consequences, including population-based decreases in sperm counts and reductions in age of menarche, in addition to the logical connection to organ-specific human cancers.

Cancer—a multidisease phenomenon—remains as much of a concern nowadays as it was when first described as "karkinos" (meaning new growth, from the Greek word for crab). We have learned much about these diseases in the last century, and the avalanche of information accelerates as we near the twenty-first century; yet as a collection of maladies "contrary to nature,"[3] not near enough is understood to significantly stem the devastating tide that has begun to consume more and more lives around the globe as population life spans extend. Nonetheless as we make advancements to extend our knowledge and understanding of these diseases, many believe intervention strategies and better treatment regimens are imminent. Meanwhile, implementation of known prevention action plans (e.g., for tobacco and lung cancers) could easily reduce existing cancer trends and societal burdens. Reducing or eliminating exposures to

TABLE 23-1. BACKGROUND TO THE PROBLEM

1. CHEMICALS

A. 11,000,000 synthesized or characterized and part of CAS registry
B. 65,000–85,000 in common and/or commercial use
C. 1500(+/–?) have been tested adequately for carcinogenicity
D. Thousands to millions of combinations and mixtures and consumer products containing chemicals
E. Synthetic organic chemicals produced in the United States for 1992, 177,800,000,000 kg or 391,200,000,000 lb
F. Top 50 US chemical production: 650,000,000 lb (64% inorganics; 36% organics)
G. Uncharacterized, unidentified, and unpredictable exposures:
   I. Occupational
   II. "Pollution" of air, water, soil
   III. Waste sites and facilities
   IV. "Local" unique exposures
      e.g., arsenic smelter
      e.g., refineries, chemical plants
      e.g., accidents/spills (dioxin, MIC, methylisocyanate)
   V. Individual multiplicity: workplace, drugs, tobacco smoke, alcohol, lifestyle, social, pesticides, Cl and F water, smog, diet, acid rain, "home" (e.g., insulation, HCHO, formaldehyde) comestics, fuel exhausts, nature, hobbies, pollution burdens, work, etc.

2. CANCER FACTS AND FIGURES

A. In 1997
   I. 1,382,400 humans will be newly diagnosed with cancer (158 persons/hr) (another 900,000 people with skin cancer)
   II. 560,000 humans will die from cancer (64/hr or 1534/day)
   III. "Equally" divided among genders
B. During the 1980s
   I. 4,500,000 cancer deaths
   II. 9,000,000 new cancer cases
   III. 12,000,000 under medical care
C. Living Americans
   I. 1 in 3 will develop cancer
   II. 85,000,000 will get cancer
D. Since 1957–1959 to 1987–89 (each per 100,000 population)
   I. Deaths, males: 180–216; +20%
   II. Deaths, females: 138–140; +1%
E. National cancer death rates (age-adjusted compared with 1930; /100,000) 1930: 143, base; 1940: 152 +6%; 1970: 163 +14% 1990: 175+22%

cancer-causing agents could have a dramatic effect on cancer morbidity, mortality, and attendant sequelae.

▶ INTRODUCTION

Primary prevention strategies are designed and implemented to reduce or eliminate the occurrences, disabilities, and mortalities from diseases. Basic and applied research using laboratory animals is fundamental for the discovery of new drugs and other beneficial chemical substances, for the development of medical procedures and other lifesaving technologies, and for the betterment of both animal and human health. Likewise, toxicological characterization of chemicals, mixtures of chemicals, and various exposure circumstances remains essential to the identification and prevention of potential hazards or of adverse effects that these agents or situations may impose on public and environmental health. Prevention and intervention better reduce or eliminate diseases in general, and illnesses associated with chemical exposures in particular, than do treatment and other after-the-fact remediation.[4,5]

Of the nearly 500,000 deaths from cancer in the United States each year, at least 4 percent [20,000 people] are thought to be related to occupation and workplace exposure circumstances. This percentage is likely to be higher, given the difficulties of describing attributable risks and in identifying causes of death. Fortunately, and largely due to agencies such as the National Institute of Occupational Safety and Health (NIOSH) and the Occupational Safety and Health Administration (OSHA), overt exposures to many identified occupational carcinogens have been reduced or eliminated. Nonetheless, workers—as well as the general population—continue to be exposed unnecessarily to carcinogens, mixtures of carcinogens, and myriad hazardous exposure circumstances (Tables 23-1 and 23-2).

Estimates indicate that about 10 percent of lung cancers, 21 to 27 percent of urinary bladder cancers, and close to 100 percent of mesotheliomas in the general population are related to occupational exposures to known human and animal carcinogens. Regarding exposures to specific carcinogens, the occurrence of site-specific cancers attributed to a particular exposure approaches 50 percent for asbestos and lung cancer and 100 percent for vinyl chloride and angiosarcoma of the liver.[6] Other site-specific carcinogens discovered in animals could and did lead to causative cancers in humans, for example, butadiene and lymphohematopoietic cancers; trichloroethylene and kidney cancer; dioxins and multiple cancers; and benzene and lung cancer. Nearly one-third of those agents considered to cause cancer in humans had been first discovered in experimental animals.

Carcinogenesis bioassays using laboratory animals have a solid history for identifying (*a*) natural and synthetic chemicals, (*b*) mixtures of chemicals, (*c*) drugs, and (*d*) commercial products as being most likely or predictive to be carcinogenic to humans.[7–14] Nearly 30 agents causing cancer in humans were first found to induce cancer in laboratory animals.[15] Hurtfully, however, these findings were and are largely ignored in protecting human health. Rather than waiting for epidemiologic data, the bare implications of this knowledge must be better used to prevent future cancers.[4]

Some have adopted a newer strategy to discount bioassay data: opining that mechanisms of "rodent-specific, organ-site" carcinogenesis has little to do with human risks or prevention reality. We have yet to adjudicate a complete step-by-step or stage-by-stage illustration of a chemical-induced mechanism of carcinogenic action. It is not certain that a "mechanism of carcinogenesis" in rodents (mammals) is or will be different than that predicted to occur in humans (mammals). Several examples include urinary bladder tumors and calculi; tumors of the thyroid gland and goiter; tumors of the kidney and α-2u-globulin; and in general tumors of the liver in mice. From the perspective of protecting public health, one should not be too quick to discount warnings from long-term bioassays in animals, especially given the long history of correlations between biologic feasibility of extrapolations among mammalian species, together with the findings that 100 percent of the agents known to cause cancer in humans likewise cause cancer in laboratory animals.

TABLE 23-2. NUMBERS OF CHEMICALS, GROUPS OF CHEMICALS, AND EXPOSURE CIRCUMSTANCES EVALUATED FOR CARCINOGENICITY BY THE IARC AND THE NTP

Number of chemicals studied for carcinogenicity	±1500
IARC Evaluations	825
Group 1: Carcinogenic to humans	72[a]
Group 2A: Probably carcinogenic	57[b]
Group 2B: Possibly carcinogenic	225[c]
Group 3: Not classifiable	470[d]
Group 4: Probably not carcinogenic	1
NTP evaluations	
Annual report on carcinogens	±700[e]
Known to be carcinogenic to humans	29
Reasonably anticipated to be carcinogenic	169

[a] 38 agents; 9 viruses/infections with; 12 mixtures; 13 exposure circumstances.
[b] 45 agents; 3 viruses/infections with; 5 mixtures; exposure circumstances.
[c] 208 agents; 13 mixtures; 4 exposure circumstances.
[d] 451 agents; 12 mixtures; 7 exposure circumstances.
[e] Estimated number of agents evaluated for listing.

TABLE 23-3. SOURCES AND STRATEGIES FOR IDENTIFYING CHEMICAL CARCINOGENS ASSOCIATED WITH CANCER HAZARDS TO HUMANS

1. Epidemiologic studies
2. Long-term bioassays
3. Midterm in vivo assays
4. Short-term in vivo and in vitro assays
5. Artificial intelligence; structure-biological-activity
6. Mechanism-based inference

Unfortunately, however, carcinogenesis bioassays have not been nor typically can they be used to evaluate or discover industrial processes or occupational exposure circumstances that cause or might cause cancer in humans, for example, (*a*) the rubber industry: urinary bladder cancer and leukemia; (*b*) painters: lung cancer; (*c*) furniture making: nasal cancers; (*d*) aluminum production, iron and steel founding, and coke production industries: lung cancer.[7,14] Equally difficult to test for carcinogenesis are environmental mixtures, diets and dietary factors, and actual (or simulating) human exposures to myriad chemicals, coupled with varied lifestyles and socioeconomic situations.[11,16–19,19a]

Despite these obstacles, all chemicals known to cause cancer in humans that could be properly tested in animals are likewise carcinogenic[11]—a remarkable correlation. Does this imply that any chemical that causes cancer in animals will be carcinogenic in humans? No. In fact, using a multifactorial matrix approach including mechanistic information, structure-activity relationships, exposure circumstances, levels and potency of carcinogenic responses, and human experience, we have predicted that fewer than 5 to 10 percent of all chemicals would eventually be considered reasonably anticipated to cause cancer in humans.[9] Importantly, most agents tested in animals do not cause cancer.[15,16,20] Nonetheless, we must remain equally mindful that a "negative" bioassay does not mean that a particular chemical will be absolutely devoid of any potential carcinogenic activity. In any event, a further benefit of these carcinogenic activity tests allows identification of possible anticarcinogens in routine bioassays.[21–23]

Prudent public health policy requires us to continue with the rational strategy of reducing or eliminating exposures to chemical carcinogens, to chemicals in general, and to unhealthy or improvable workplace circumstances. Additionally, we need to persevere in our efforts to reduce or eliminate unnecessary industrial emissions and chemical contaminations of our air; domestic and feral animals, and plant life; lands and food crops; and waters, fishes, and

TABLE 23-4. METHODS FOR IDENTIFYING CANCER RISKS: ADVANTAGES AND DISADVANTAGES

1. Epidemiological Studies

Advantages
1. Humans are ultimate indicators of disease
2. Evaluate sensitive populations
3. Occupational exposure cohorts
4. Environmental sentinel alerts

Disadvantages
1. Generally retrospective (death certificates, recall biases, etc.)
2. Insensitive, costly, lengthy
3. Reliable exposure data not available or difficult to obtain
4. Combined, multiple, and complex exposures; lack of appropriate cohorts
5. Experiments on humans not done
6. Cancer detection not prevention

2. Long-term Chemical Carcinogenesis Bioassays

Advantages
1. Prospective and retrospective (validation) evaluations
2. Excellent correlation with identified human carcinogens
3. Exposure levels and conditions known
4. Identifies chemical toxicity and carcinogenicity effects
5. Results obtained relatively quickly
6. Qualitative comparisons among chemical classes
7. Integrative and interactive biologic systems related closely to humans

Disadvantages
1. Rarely replicated
2. Resource intensive (staff, money, facilities)
3. Shortage of adequate facilities, scientific expertise, and experience, or research interest
4. Debate regarding relevancy of results (rodents are not humans, routes of exposure, too sensitive)
5. Studies at exposure levels often in excess of those anticipated for humans
6. Single chemical bioassays do not mimic human exposure circumstances

3 and 4. Midterm in Vivo Bioassays and Short-term in Vivo and in Vitro Assays

Advantages
1. More rapid and less expensive
2. Large samples and easily replicated
3. Biologically valuable endpoints measured (e.g., mutations, preneoplasia)
4. Assays easily manipulated (e.g., two-stage models; organ systems: liver, urinary bladder)
5. Single or multiple chemicals, simple or complex mixtures, environmental or occupational samples
6. Screening assays to select chemicals for subsequent bioassay and mechanistic studies

Disadvantages
1. In vitro not fully predictive for in vivo
2. In vivo measures purported preneoplastic lesions
3. Not generally predictive for toxicity or carcinogenicity
4. Usually organism- or organ-specific
5. Systems manipulated toward select and sensitive endpoints
6. Not reliable surrogates for whole animals, long-term bioassays, or for humans
7. Potencies not comparable to whole animals or humans

5. Artificial Intelligence; Chemical Structure–Biological Activities Associations

Advantages
1. Relatively easy, rapid, and inexpensive
2. Reliable for certain chemical classes (e.g., nitrosamines, antibiotics, anthraquinones, benzidine dyes)
3. Developed using biological information, yet not dependent on animal or human data
4. Computer adaptable and compatible

Disadvantages
1. Not "biological"
2. Many exceptions to formulated rules
3. False positives and false negatives
4. Disparate theoretical systems and versions available with conflicting predictions
5. Retrospective and rarely (but becoming) prospective

6. Mechanism-Based Inferences

Advantages
1. Reasonably accurate for classes of chemicals; or known mechanisms for different chemicals
2. Permits evaluations of chemicals without doing long-term bioassays
3. Can "test" more chemicals and classes of chemicals
4. Allows refinements and further hypotheses
5. Can adjust or orient risk assessments to sensitive populations (genetic susceptibility)
6. Strengthen risk assessments (low dose and species extrapolation)

Disadvantages
1. Mechanisms of chemical carcinogenesis undefined, multiple, and likely chemical-class-specific
2. Exceptions to posed mechanisms: DNA interactions; adduct formation; stones; irritation; cell proliferation; receptor-mediated; toxicity; genotoxic/nongenotoxic; α-2u-globulin-induced nephropathy; structural alerts; epoxides; etc.
3. Nonconfirmation of purported mechanisms or nonreproducible
4. Flaws lead to faulty risk assessments (under- and overestimates)

TABLE 23-5. BASIC DESIGN PROTOCOL FOR LONG-TERM CHEMICAL CARCINOGENESIS STUDIES

1. *Purpose:* Identify chronic toxicity (nonneoplastic) and carcinogenic (neoplastic) effects of chemicals
2. *Animals:* Fischer 344 hybrid rats or other strains
   B6C3F1 inbred mice (C3H × C57Bl/6) or other strains
3. *Groups and group sizes:*
   Males and females of each species
   50–60+ animals/sex/species groups
   Concurrent controls plus 2–4 experimental exposure groups
4. *Exposure levels:* Chosen to show some minimal yet obvious chemical-associated effects of a degree not to compromise normal well-being or growth and survival
5. *Exposure duration:* 24 months (typically ⅔ lifespan); 30 months
6. *Routes of exposure:* Priority to human exposure. Historically, in NTP, via feed (60%), oral intubation (27%), inhalation (5%), skin (3%), IP injection (3%), drinking water (2%)
7. *Pathology:* All animals, complete gross and histologic examination

shellfish. Otherwise the increasing pollution-burden continues to add to the disease quotient.

In this chapter, primary emphasis centers on the usefulness, value, and relevance of the long-term carcinogenesis bioassay toward avoiding, reducing, and preventing carcinogenic risk to humans. Particular topics covered include: (*a*) methods for identifying carcinogens, (*b*) value and validity of experimental carcinogenesis, (*c*) correspondence of laboratory and human evidence, and (*d*) cumulative importance and worth of experimental findings. Other relevant topics can be discovered in the appended reference and background reading lists.

Identifying Carcinogens

The major efforts being used today for identifying existing or predicted cancer causes in humans are detailed in Table 23-3. These six methods are given together with key advantages and disadvantages for each (Table 23-4). Much as we would like to reduce our reliance on long-term carcinogenesis bioassays, and perhaps use other methods including shorter term assays, transgenic models, and prospective predictive techniques,[13,24] no proposed paradigm has been proven to be a better indicator of potential human cancer risks than have long-term carcinogenesis bioassays.[10,16]

Clinical and epidemiologic studies, which frequently involve the observation and evaluation of human experience with exposure to possibly hazardous agents, obviously offer the most direct means of assessing human health risks associated with such exposures.[25] However, for chronic diseases such as cancer, the long time interval or latency period that often occurs between the initial exposure to the hazardous agent and the onset of clinically recognizable disease may mean that there will not yet be sufficient human experience with the agent to determine its full toxicologic potential. In other instances, an agent may have been present in the human environment long enough for its toxicologic effects to be apparent, but lack of adequate historical exposure data on individuals whose initial exposures occurred one or more decades in the past may inhibit the use of available epidemiologic information in the quantitative estimation of potential adverse health effects. As a result, data generated from laboratory experiments most often form the primary basis for the identification and evaluation of possible human health risks, including cancer.[7,14,26,27]

Long-Term Carcinogenesis Bioassay

A typical bioassay involves anywhere from a single sex of a particular strain and species to both genders of two species; from single exposure regimens to multiple levels of exposure; from 18 months to lifetime durations; and from compiling tumor findings to mechanistic and other additional studies together with neoplastic responses. A starting-point design used by the National Toxicology Program[10,16,28] is described in Table 23-5. Frequent options for flexibility are given in Table 23-6.

Results

Since the middle 1970s when the National Cancer Institute (NCI) issued its first chemical carcinogenicity technical report, which was on trichloroethylene, more than 450 studies have been completed, evaluated in public sessions, and reported. The complete listing—with chemical names and summary results on each of the chemicals—has been published[29] and is available upon request.

An overall summary of the results indicates that more than half the chemicals tested show some evidence of carcinogenic activity (Table 23-7A). This figure is misleading and often misused because a chemical is considered "positive" regardless of the overall qualitative strength of the evidence; that is, a chemical causing cancer in one organ of one sex of one strain of one species at one exposure level is placed in the same context of positivity as a chemical that induces dose-related cancers in multiple organs in both sexes of multiple strains of multiple species. Dividing the carcinogenicity findings by some of these parameters (i.e., by sex/strain/species) leads to a different and perhaps more relevant comparative stratification (Table 23-7B). These

TABLE 23-6. ALTERNATIVE DESIGN CONSIDERATIONS FOR LONG-TERM BIOASSAYS

1. *Animals:* Chemical and target site specific, e.g., for a potential leukemogen or testicular carcinogen *do not use* Fischer 344 rats (high background rates for this cancer); for a possible mammary carcinogen *do not use* Sprague-Dawley rats (high background); for skin carcinogens *do not use* insensitive B6C3F1 mice; for lung carcinogens *do not use* hamsters.
2. *Sex/species:* Consider a single sex of two species, e.g., male rats and female mice. For chlorinated solvents use two strains of mice (rats appear "resistant" to these solvents).
3. *Groups and groups sizes:* At least 100 per group, with up to 1,000 per group for a predictably "weak" environmental carcinogen (e.g., electromagnetic fields), or a chemical with extensive population exposure (e.g., fluoride or aspartame).
4. *Exposures:* Highest concentration at the MTE (minimal toxic exposure; often called MTD or maximum tolerated dose); lower levels at "metabolic saturation point" or at "pharmacokinetic inflection point" or at human (drugs) or environmental exposure levels. Consider intermittent exposure regimens (e.g. 2–3 days on and 2–3 days off).
5. *Routes:* Mimic main route of human exposure. Use multiple routes when relevant, e.g., chemical(s) could be given simultaneously by inhalation and in drinking water and by skin painting and by gavage where appropriate (e.g., solvents; water supply contaminants as trihalomethanes; and added chemicals such as fluoride).
6. *Duration:* Flexible, (*a*) at least 2 years for "unknowns"; (*b*) longer periods for metals (e.g., cadmium carcinogenesis not apparent before 30 months) and most other chemicals; (*c*) supplemental routine shorter exposure groups (e.g., 13 weeks) to determine tumor progression/regression; (*d*) preconception, gestation, lactation, and F1 exposures for 30–36 months if large human populations (e.g., fluoride, food additives, electromagnetic fields (EMF); aspartame), intermittent exposures for solvents.
7. *Chemicals:* Multiple exposures and mixtures more closely to human exposure patterns, e.g., oxazapam by gavage, fluoride by drinking water, pesticides by feed, solvents by skin.
8. *Pathology:* More selective; reduce general histopathology; use routine multiple sections for predicted or grossly observed target organs (e.g., solvents and kidney; hormones and glands; aniline dyes and spleen, halogenated hydrocarbons and liver; "site-of-application" as lung and inhalation, stomach and gavage, oral and water).

TABLE 23-7. SUMMARY OF NCI AND NTP LONG-TERM CARCINOGENESIS BIOASSAY RESULTS

A. CARCINOGENESIS BIOASSAY RESULTS ON 457 CHEMICALS	
Evidence of carcinogenicity	238 (52%)
No evidence of carcinogenicity	147 (32%)
Marginal/equivocal evidence	64 (14%)
Experiments inadequate for evaluation	8 (2%)
B. CARCINOGENICITY RESULTS ON 367 CHEMICALS BY NUMBER OF EXPERIMENTS PER BIOASSAY	
"Positive" Results in Sex/Species Groups	***Number in Category***
4/4	54 (14.7%)
3/4	29 (7.9%)
2/4	67 (18.3%)
1/4	45 (12.3%)
0/4	172 (46.9%)

Note: for these 367 bioassays, four experimental groups were used for each chemical: male rats, female rats, male mice, female mice; the left colume indicates a qualitative level of "potency" whereby a chemical in the 4/4 category shows that chemical-associated cancer(s) were induced in each of the four groups; 0/4 shows no cancers related to chemicals were induced.

data clearly indicate that less than 25 percent of the chemicals tested by the NCI/NTP would meet the two-species entry criteria to be even considered as being "anticipated to be carcinogenic to humans."[30]

Moreover, Fung et al.[9] evaluated the carcinogenicity findings based on the rationale for selecting and testing the chemicals in the first place. Dividing the 400 chemicals into (*a*) those that were selected with a strong suspicion of causing cancer in animals and (*b*) those that were selected primarily on the basis of production volume and numbers of people exposed led to the dramatic finding that while 64 percent of the suspected chemicals showed evidence of carcinogenicity, only 22 percent of the large volume chemicals gave some positive responses (Table 23-8). Based on these observations and extrapolating to the universe of chemicals, Fung et al[9] posed that only 5 to 10 percent of all chemicals if tested would be likely to represent potential carcinogenic risks to humans.

Likewise, if one examines the list of chemicals evaluated for carcinogenicity by the International Agency for Research on Cancer (IARC), only 72 (8.7 percent) of the 825 agents or exposure circumstances studied and interpreted were considered to be "carcinogenic to humans."[14] Of course if one adds the 57 agents or groups of agents considered "probably carcinogenic to humans," then the figure nearly doubles to 15.6 percent (129/825). Table 23-2 summarizes the IARC conclusions, Table 23-9A lists the agents in Group 1 ("carcinogenic to humans"), and Table 23-9B categorizes those in Group 2A ("probably carcinogenic to humans").

Since testing chemicals for carcinogenicity began, somewhere between 1,200 and 1,500 agents have been tested adequately; others such as pesticides, food additives, and drugs have been tested for regulatory purposes but the results have often not been published. In some cases a single agent has been tested over and over again, often to evaluate other species responses (urethane),[31] to explore mechanisms (dioxin),[32,33] or to simply "do it right" with more modern protocols for chemicals previously tested but whose tests were considered inadequate for evaluation (benzene).[34,35] Further, some chemicals that have been tested and found limited need additional testing because of large population-based exposures (aspartame),[36] because the agent is carcinogenic to humans and had not been found convincingly to cause cancer in laboratory animals (benzene;[34,37,38] arsenic[39]) or because certain agents shown to be carcinogenic to humans have not been tested (treosulfan).[11,16,39,40]

Obviously the majority of chemicals in commerce and in daily use have not been tested in vivo for carcinogenicity using standard and current protocols.[8,10,16,26,30] Our quest for shorter term in vivo and in vitro tests has not yet been successful to adequately replace or even reduce the need for 2-year bioassays. The latest on the scene is the use of transgenic models.[41]

Other techniques being explored or revisited include "predictive toxicology"[24] using structure-activity relations, machine learning, or "experience."[13] Certainly the era of short-term tests continues with a spat of tests and test systems; these are introduced with much less fanfare than in the past, whereby the initial optimism gave way to realism or even pessimism.[42]

However, the quest does and should continue. For example, medium term models developed by Ito need to be studied by others for validation and for species comparisons.[43] And the neonatal model created by Vesselinovitch should be revived.[44] Several other in vivo models have been tried with limited success (Table 23-10).

Thus at the present time, these other test methods as well as the current popular trend to use computer-assisted predictions to guess whether a chemical would eventually induce cancer in experimental animals and hence represent a carcinogenic hazard to humans are fraught with considerable uncertainty, uncertainty that can be relieved only by long-term testing in animals or by conducting an epidemiological investigation of exposed individuals or groups. Nonetheless, the day may come when our predictive acumen or short-term test barrage will be upgraded to such an extent that we might eventually obviate cancer testing. Until then, and in the best interests of public health, however, we urge long-term testing of chemicals be continued, at increased pace.

Mechanistic Considerations for Identifying Carcinogens

The quest to use what we know or think we know regarding purported mechanisms of chemical carcinogenesis often overshadows reality. Momentum has grown over the last decade in particular. However, we can no longer approach this conundrum by searching for a "silver bullet" mechanism of cancer. We now know that "there are more than 100 types of human cancers, and, thus, likely to be at a minimum 100 different sequences of mutational events that occur during the creation of these tumors. Each of these sequences would represent the life history of a particular type of tumor cell. Yet, with the single exception of colorectal cancer . . . we know almost nothing about the genetic biographies of human tumors, that is, the succession of mutational events that is responsible for creating them."[45]

Despite the long and costly (albeit worthy) investment in identifying chemical mutagens as posed mechanisms of chemical carcinogenesis, "most of the agents and stimuli that are responsible for inducing human cancer may not act through their ability to damage DNA."[11] Indeed, almost half a century after its description, the precise mechanism of action of the best-studied of tumor promoters—phorbol ester used by Berenblum—remains unclear,[11] Nongenotoxic promoting agents . . . may be vital forces driving human cancer patho-

TABLE 23-8. STATISTICS ON SELECTION RATIONALE FOR 400 CHEMICALS/CHEMICAL MIXTURES

		Number of Chemicals with	
Selection Basis	***Number of Chemicals (%)***	***Positive Results (%)***	***Negative Results (%)***
Completed bioassays	400	210 (52)	190 (48)
Suspicion of carcinogenicity	267 (67)	181 (68)	88 (32)
Large production volumes and/or widespread occupation/ population exposures	133 (33)	29 (22)	104 (78)

TABLE 23-9. AGENTS, MIXTURES, AND EXPOSURE CIRCUMSTANCES CONSIDERED CARCINOGENIC TO HUMANS OR PROBABLY CARCINOGENIC TO HUMANS (*IARC MONOGRAPHS* VOLUMES 1–69; 1972–1997)

A. GROUP 1—CARCINOGENIC TO HUMANS

Agents and Groups of Agents

- Aflatoxins, naturally occurring
- 4-Aminobiphenyl
- Arsenic and arsenic compounds[a]
- Asbestos
- Azathioprine
- Benzene
- Benzidine
- Beryllium and beryllium compounds[b]
- *N,N*-Bis(2-chloroethyl)-2-naphthylamine (Chlornaphazine)
- Bis(chloromethyl)ether and chloromethyl methyl ether (technical-grade)
- 1,4-Butanediol dimethanesulfonate (Busulphan; Myleran)
- Cadmium and cadmium compounds[b]
- Chlorambucil
- 1-(2-Chloroethyl)-3-(4-methylcyclohexyl)-1-nitrosourea (methyl-CCNU; Semustine)
- Chromium[VI] compounds[b]
- Cyclosporine
- Cyclophosphamide
- Diethylstilbestrol
- Erionite
- Estrogen replacement therapy
- Estrogens, nonsteroidal[a]
- Estrogens, steroidal[a]
- Ethylene oxide[c]
- *Helicobacter pylori* (infection with)
- Hepatitis B virus (chronic infection with)
- Hepatitis C virus (chronic infection with)
- Human immunodeficiency virus type 1 (infection with)
- Human papillomavirus type 16
- Human papillomavirus type 18
- Human T-cell lymphotropic virus type I
- Melphalan
- 8-Methoxypsoralen (Methoxsalen) plus ultraviolet A radiation
- MOPP and other combined chemotherapy including alkylating agents. MOPP = procarbazine, nitrogen mustard, vincristine, prednisone
- Mustard gas (Sulfur mustard)
- 2-Naphthylamine
- Nickel compounds[b]
- *Opisthorchis viverrini* (infection with)
- Oral contraceptives, combined[d]
- Oral contraceptives, sequential
- Radon and its decay products
- *Schistosoma haematobium* (infection with)
- Silica, crystalline
- Solar radiation
- Talc containing asbestiform fibers
- Tamoxifen[e]
- 2,3,7,8-Tetrachloro-para-dioxin[c]
- Thiotepa
- Treosulfan
- Vinyl chloride

Mixtures

- Alcoholic beverages
- Analgesic mixtures containing phenacetin
- Betel quid with tobacco
- Coal-tar pitches
- Coal-tars
- Mineral oils, untreated and mildly treated
- Salted fish (Chinese-style)
- Shale-oils
- Soots
- Tobacco products, smokeless
- Tobacco smoke
- Wood dust

Exposure Circumstances

- Aluminium production
- Auramine, manufacture of
- Boot and shoe manufacture and repair
- Coal gasification
- Coke production
- Furniture and cabinet making
- Hematite mining (underground) with exposure to radon
- Iron and steel founding
- Isopropanol manufacture (strong-acid process)
- Magenta, manufacture of
- Painter (occupational exposure as a)
- Rubber industry
- Strong-inorganic-acid mists containing sulfuric acid (occupational exposure to)

B. GROUP 2A—PROBABLY CARCINOGENIC TO HUMANS

Agents and Groups of Agents

- Acrylamide[f]
- Acrylonitrile
- Adriamycin[f]
- Androgenic (anabolic) steroids
- Azacitidine[f]
- Benz(*a*)anthracene[f]
- Benzidine-based dyes[f]
- Benzo[*a*]pyrene[f]
- Bischloroethyl nitrosourea (BCNU)
- 1,3-Butadiene
- Captafol[f]
- Chloramphenicol[f]
- 1-(2-Chloroethyl)-3-cyclohexyl-1-nitrosourea (CCNU)[f]
- *para*-Chloro-*ortho*-toluidine and its strong acid salts[b]
- Chlorozotocin[f]
- Cisplatin[f]
- *Clonorchis sinensis* (infection with)[f]
- Dibenz[*a,h*]anthracene[f]
- Diethyl sulfate
- Dimethylcarbamoyl chloride[f]
- Dimethyl sulfate[f]
- Epichlorohydrin[f]
- Ethylene dibromide[f]
- *N*-Ethyl-*N*-nitrosourea[f]
- Formaldehyde
- Human papillomavirus type 31
- Human papillomavirus type 33
- IQ[f] (2-Amino-3-methylimidazo [4,5-*f*]quinoline)
- 5-Methoxypsoralen[f]
- 4,4′-Methylene bis(2-chloroaniline) (MOCA)[f]
- *N*-Methyl-*N*′-nitro-*N*-nitrosoguanidine (MNNG)[f]
- *N*-Methyl-*N*-nitrosourea[f]
- Nitrogen mustard
- *N*-Nitrosodiethylamine[f]
- *N*-Nitrosodimethylamine[f]
- Phenacetin
- Procarbazine hydrochloride[f]
- Styrene-7,8-oxide[f]
- Tetrachloroethylene
- Trichloroethylene
- 1,2,3-Trichloropropane
- Tris(2,3-dibromopropyl)phosphate[f]
- Ultraviolet radiation A[f]
- Ultraviolet radiation B[f]
- Ultraviolet radiation C[f]
- Vinyl bromide[f]
- Vinyl fluoride

Mixtures

- Creosotes
- Diesel engine exhaust
- Hot mate
- Nonarsenical insecticides (occupational exposures in spraying and application of)
- Polychlorinated biphenyls

Exposure Circumstances

- Art glass, glass containers, and pressed ware (manufacture of)
- Hairdresser or barber (occupational exposure as a)
- Petroleum refining (occupational exposures in)
- Sunlamps and sunbeds (use of)

[a] This evaluation applies to the group of chemicals as a whole and not necessarily to all individual chemicals within the group.
[b] Evaluated as a group.
[c] Overall evaluation upgraded from 2A to 1 with supporting evidence from other data relevant to the evaluation of carcinogenicity and its mechanisms.
[d] There is also conclusive evidence that these agents have a protective effect against cancers of the ovary and endometrium.
[e] There is also conclusive evidence that this agent (tamoxifen) reduces the risk of contralateral breast cancer.
[f] Overall evaluation upgraded from 2B to 2A with supporting evidence from other data relevant to the evaluation of carcinogenicity and its mechanisms.
Source: IARC monographs (see reference 14).

TABLE 23-10. POSSIBLE IN VIVO ALTERNATIVES TO THE LONG-TERM CARCINOGENESIS BIOASSAY

1. Skin painting (mouse): multiple exposures: 26–78 wks; skin
2. A/J mouse lung: IP injection [3/wk/8 wks]; 24 wks; lung
3. Subcutaneous (mouse): single/multiple; 13–52 wks
4. Neonatal mouse: single exposure; IP injection or gavage; ≤1 yr, liver
5. "Pitot" 2-stage liver: partial hepatectomy; initiator; chemical in feed; 10–26–52 wks; liver (foci, tumor)
6. "Ito" midterm:
   a. initiator; chemical in feed; partial hepatectomy; 8 wks; liver
   b. initiators; chemical in feed; partial hepatectomy; 12–20 wks; liver, kidney, +others
7. Fish: medaka; guppy: environmental conditions; evaluate mixtures, chemical combinations; multi-generational; flexible duration
8. Transgenics
9. a. *Toad:* SC; skin; or gavage; 13 wks
   b. *Hamster cheek pouch:* 3 times/wk; painted; 30 wks; local tumors
   c. *Rat mammary:* initiator; chemical; 32 wks
   d. *Urinary bladder:* initiator; drinkng water 4 wks; chemical 32 wks
   e. *Stomach:* methylnitrosonitroguanidine; chemical; 16–20 wks
   f. *Others:* kidney; lung; thyroid; pancreas

In Vivo Alternatives—Comments and Conclusions

+1. Typically quicker; less expensive; reasonably reliable (especially positives)
+2. Fewer animals; smaller facilities; less resources
+3. Chemicals: classes; mixtures; combinations; test/alternative variables (e.g., diet, duration, single/multiple routes)
+4. Screen: select chemicals for 2-yr bioassay (negatives) and to study/explore mechanism (positive)
–5. Diminished sensitivity: "single" target site; reduced sex/species correlations and strength of evidence
–6. Nontumor endpoints: biomarkers, enzymes, foci, and toxic or preneoplastic lesions
–7. Screen: notably for nonconclusive results—"no" or "equivocal" evidence (false negatives?)
–8. Not "validated" and often not standardized

Note: items 1–4 are positive aspects; items 5–8 are negative aspects

genesis, more important than those substances classified as clear mutagens. But in general, we know rather little about their identities."[45] Again, the best and perhaps only established method to identify nongenotoxic carcinogens is the long-term bioassay.[10,26,28]

A "mechanistic trend" seems to be developing to discount or modulate certain chemically induced carcinogenic responses in laboratory animals as being "rodent specific," and thus not relevant to humans. This is premature at best, and, at worse, antithetical to public health.

So far, the list of tumors with their assigned "mechanism" considered irrelevant includes

- Male rat kidney tumors when/if associated with α-2u-globulin–induced nephropathy;
- Forestomach tumors with local hyperplasia;
- Male rat urinary bladder tumors with reactive hyperplasia from cytotoxic precipitated chemicals;
- Lung tumors with overwhelming of clearance mechanisms;
- Thyroid gland tumors with sustained excessive hormonal stimulation.

First, these tumors and the posed tumor "mechanisms" are not mechanisms in the classic sense because they are simply histological observations made after a bioassay has been completed. That is, if a male rat has a tumor of the urinary bladder, and that same bladder contains calculi or a stone, then a claim is made that there is an association. Likewise for the rest mentioned above. These do not represent scientific proof.[46]

Second, these associations have not been proven experimentally. Again, there are select data to show that certain chemicals that induce male rat kidney tumors also have α-2u-globulin–induced nephropathy. However, there are chemicals that also induce this same nephropathy that do not cause male rat kidney tumors.[47] Thus, how does one "selectively" assign a mechanism of irrelevancy?

Third, these "mechanistic associations" are inconsistently allied with a "cause and effect" paradigm. In many long-term bioassays, animals frequently exhibit these "mechanisms" (be they local or regenerative hyperplasia, goiter, stones, α-2u-globulin–induced nephropathy) and yet do not develop tumors.

Fourth, in almost all bioassays these tumors/mechanisms are not the only carcinogenic responses induced by a particular chemical. Does this mean that chemicals elicit multiple mechanisms? Probably. Does this mean that tumor A is not relevant to humans but tumor B or C is relevant? What would one decide if each of the above five tumor sites were induced by a single chemical? Are these effects considered not relevant to humans only if the chemicals are nongenotoxic?

Contrary to these isolated chemical "mechanistic associations," large collections of evaluated empirical data do not support these relationships.[46–49] That is not to say that these "associative mechanisms"never do or cannot influence a particular site-specific tumor pathogenesis by some cocarcinogenic consequence. However, before altering public health policy by using mechanistic evidence, the mechanism should meet exhaustive scientific scrutiny and should be operative all the time.[47] That is, for example, if α-2u-globulin–induced nephropathy is observed in male rats, and as this is posed as a mechanism for inducing kidney tumors, then tumors of the kidney should be induced by all chemicals that incite this nephrotic syndrome. This does not happen consistently, and thus I believe that α-2u-globulin–induced nephropathy cannot be considered as a mechanism of tumorigenicity, nor as being irrelevant to human cancer risk.

Similar findings are available for each of the other four posed rodent-specific mechanisms. These are not recitated here.[33,46,47,50,51]

Obversely, mechanisms have been used to declare chemicals as being human carcinogens in the absence of overwhelming or scientifically convincing epidemiological evidence; that is, associations with cancer in humans have been made, but were not of the strength to declare that agent or exposure circumstance a human carcinogen based solely on epidemiologic information. The International Agency for Research on Cancer has upgraded two chemicals from the category "probably carcinogenic to humans" (Category 2A) to "carcinogenic to humans" (Category 1) based on solid mechanistic information. These are ethylene oxide and 2,3,7,8-tetrachlorodibenzodioxin ("dioxin"). Likewise, because benzidine is a "human carcinogen" and benzidine-based dyes are all carcinogenic to laboratory animals and are usually more potent than the parent compound and metabolic forms of benzidine in vivo, one could propose that all benzidine-based dyes should be upgraded to the category "carcinogenic to humans." Other classes of chemicals would similarly fit this situation.

Conclusions

> "Students of the history of medicine have long known that diseases can be prevented or effectively treated long before causative mechanisms and therapeutic activity are understood."[52]
>
> Wynder, 1994

To make public health policy in cancer reduction and prevention, in the absence of reliable or unequivocal epidemiological data, one must continue to rely on results from long-term carcinogenesis bioassays. Utilization of experimental carcinogenicity data has been proven over several decades to be the most appropriate thing to do. This at times may be undergirded using current knowledge of mechanisms, yet this knowledge most often is not yet understood completely enough to discount bioassay experimental findings. Thus, where mechanisms of carcinogenesis are valuable for gaining insights into causation of cancer in rodents and in humans, more needs to be learned about these before uniform adoption and before making public health policy decisions.

Polychlorinated Biphenyls (PCBs) and Polybrominated Biphenyls (PBBs)

Alf Fischbein • Mary S. Wolff • George Bekesi

▶ POLYCHLORINATED BIPHENYLS (PCBs)

Polychlorinated biphenyls (PCBs) are a group of complex synthetic organic chemicals belonging to the class of chlorinated aromatic hydrocarbons. Because of their chemical and thermal stability, they have been widely used in industry. They are useful as components of dielectric fluid in transformers, capacitors, and other electrical equipment due to their excellent dielectric or nonconductor (insulating) properties. PCBs are present in these items in conjunction with other insulating chemicals, including chlorinated benzenes and epoxy compounds. PCBs have also been used as additives in paints and surface coatings, inks, adhesives, and as components in hydraulic fluid, metal presses, elevators, forklifts, and heat exchangers. They are used for microencapsulation of dyes in carbonless copying paper, and in immersion oil for microscopic analysis. Although most principal uses are in enclosed systems, some uses allow direct entry of these chemicals into the environment.

PCBs have attracted much public health concern; attention to these chemicals is widespread, especially in connection with detection of PCBs in waterways and toxic waste sites and in association with accidental spills and fires involving transformers and other equipment containing PCBs. It is the only group of chemicals in the United States regulated by an act of Congress, with specific policies for control of their spread in the environment.[1] Chronic health effects in humans as a result of environmental or occupational exposures to PCBs have not been well documented.[2,3] However, because of their chemical stability and low degree of biodegradation, they are very persistent and their ubiquity in the environment has resulted in the accumulation of these substances in the biota and human tissues.

The manufacturing of PCBs, which began in the 1920s, was discontinued in the United States in 1977, and their use has been restricted to enclosed systems. The regulatory framework concerning disposal of PCBs and the minimizing of reentry into the human environment is extensive in the United States.[4,5] The National Institute for Occupational Safety and Health (NIOSH) recommends an exposure limit to all PCBs of 1.0 mg/m^3, determined as a time-weighted average (TWA) concentration for up to a 10-hour workday or a 40-hour workweek. The Occupational Safety and Health Administration's (OSHA) permissible occupational exposure limits are 0.5 mg/m^3 for mixtures with 54 percent chlorine content and 1 mg/m^3 for 42 percent chlorine mixtures for an 8-hour workday. It is estimated that more than 750 million pounds of PCBs are distributed throughout the United States in more than 900 million items of equipment. Certain occupational groups may, therefore, continue to be at risk of possible exposure, including utility workers handling transformers and capacitors, electricians, appliance service persons, and clean-up workers involved in decontaminations of hazardous spills.[6,7]

When evaluating human risk of PCB exposure, consideration must be given to other chemically related compounds present in environments along with PCBs. Accidents, especially fires involving transformers containing PCBs and other chlorinated compounds, have focused attention on potential health effects to firefighters and emergency crew workers. In this context, heating or pyrolysis of materials containing PCBs and chlorinated benzenes can, under some circumstances, generate chemically related and toxic polychlorinated dibenzofurans (PCDFs) and polychlorinated dibenzodioxins (PCDDs), respectively.[8] It is unclear the degree to which these chemicals are causally related to health effects in situations in which PCBs are present in the exposure source. It appears, however, that PCDFs, often referred to as "contaminants," have played a role in the cause of clinical signs and symptoms connected with two major outbreaks of accidental poisonings in Japan and Taiwan. In these episodes, persons ingested rice oil that had become contaminated with heat-exchange fluid. This fluid was initially thought to contain PCBs, but was subsequently found to contain both PCDFs and other polychlorinated compounds such as polychlorinated quarterphenyls (PCQs) as well. These chemicals were also identified in the blood of patients who had consumed the contaminated oil.[9] Exposure to these chemicals will likely become of greater health concern in the future, especially among firefighters and clean-up operaters.

It is now known that mono-ortho substituted and coplanar PCBs contribute to dioxin toxic equivalents and that dioxinlike PCBs must be measured with dioxins and dibenzofurans to accurately assess total dioxin-like toxicity.[10]

Chemistry and General Toxicity

PCBs are produced by the chlorination of biphenyl hydrocarbons at elevated temperatures in the presence of anhydrous chlorine and a catalyst, such as iron or ferric chloride. The chlorination results in a biphenyl nucleus in which one to 10 chlorine atoms are substituted on either or both aromatic rings. Substitution of ring positions by chlorine ranges from dichloroisomers (two substitutions) to decachloroderivatives (10 substitutions). Commercial PCB mixtures contain 60 to 100 congeners from among 209 possible structures.

PCBs appear as colorless crystals when isolated in pure form. Most commercial products are liquid with low solubility in water, ranging from 0.007 to 5.9 mg/L for the most commonly occurring isomers. They are also soluble in oils and organic solvents.[11]

PCBs were manufactured in the United States under the name Aroclor. Most of these commercial mixtures are numerically described according to their chlorine content; for example, Aroclor 1254 and Aroclor 1260 refer to 54 and 60 percent chlorine content, respectively. The degree of chlorination and the chlorine substitution pattern are related to biological activity and environmental persistence. Generally, more highly chlorinated PCBs tend to be less readily metabolized than those with lower chlorine content. PCBs are lipophilic compounds and readily accumulate in adipose tissue. In various studies, as many as 70 individual congeners have been detected in human tissues. PCBs have low acute toxicity; of greater public health concern is the potential risk of chronic or delayed effects resulting from residues in the body.

Environmental Contamination

During widescale industrial manufacturing of PCBs from the 1920s to the early 1970s, there was ample opportunity for PCBs to enter the human environment, since there were no restrictions regarding their use or disposal. Only in 1966 were PCBs identified as a major environmental pollutant. This was determined only after a survey of wildlife and vegetation in Stockholm, Sweden, provided evidence of the presence of PCBs in many tissue and plant samples.[12] Similar findings were subsequently made by analysis of samples taken from areas remote from industrial activity, and soon after, scientists detected PCBs in several international locations. There is no evidence that PCBs are formed in the environment from natural sources; thus, environmental contamination is a reflection of contamination associated with human-made production and long-term industrial use of

PCBs. Despite recent regulations concerning their use and disposal, there are significant reservoirs of PCBs in the environment that constitute a potential source of future exposure to humans.

The principal sources of PCBs contributing to environmental contamination include industrial and municipal effluents and paper recycling. The latter is related to the use of PCBs in carbonless copy paper and contamination from migration to food products through packaging materials. Incineration of paper and other PCB-containing products under conditions that do not destroy PCBs is another potential source of exposure, along with release of PCBs into soil, primarily from disposal sites. It is uncertain whether such exposure is associated with increased absorption among persons living in the vicinity of waste sites.[13]

Accumulation of PCBs in fresh water biota has been a particular concern; fish is a major source of PCB exposure to humans via the food chain. Past surveys in the United States have revealed that fish from some industrially polluted waters known to be contaminated with PCBs had exceeded the Food and Drug Administrations tolerance level of 2 mg/kg. Such water sources include Lake Michigan, the Fox River in Wisconsin, and the Hudson River in New York State.

Because of the ubiquity of PCBs in the environment and magnification through the food chain, PCBs are present in humans. In the United States, serum PCB levels ranging from 0 to 10 ppb are frequently found among persons of the general population with no specific history of occupational or environmental exposure. Polychlorinated biphenyls have also been detected in human breast milk. Significant correlation between consumption of fish from PCB-contaminated waters and serum levels of PCBs has been reported.

Experimental Laboratory Studies

The toxicity of PCBs has been evaluated extensively in numerous experimental animal studies demonstrating a wide spectrum of toxic effects on the skin, liver, lipid metabolism, and the immune, endocrine, and reproductive systems.[14,15]

One of the principal biochemical effects of PCBs is their ability to induce phase I and II enzymes in liver and other tissues. The induction of these systems has the potential for both activation and detoxification of a wide variety of drugs and other substances. Structure-activity relationships exist between PCB congener subgroups and their ability to induce specific cytochrome P-450 isozymes.[15] The most widely studied response is toxicity associated with CYP1A1 induction through the Ah receptor. These dioxin-(TCDD) or methylcholanthrene-like effects include immunotoxicity and are structure-specific. CYP1A1 and CYP1A2 are induced by the dioxinlike, non-ortho–substituted coplanar PCBs, whereas other genes are more responsive to PCBs with orthochlorine substituents. Effects have been identified for P-450 enzymes governed by the CYP1A, CYP2A, CYP2B, CYP3B, and CYP4A genes. In addition, phase II enzymes including glutathione-*S*-transferase are also upregulated by PCBs. Since both endogenous and exogenous substances are metabolized by these enzyme systems, many such compounds are more rapidly metabolized by animals and humans with excessive exposure to PCBs. For example, PCBs have been shown to increase the metabolism of polycyclic aromatic hydrocarbons, drugs, and hormones (testosterone, progesterone, estrogen) by their ability to induce liver microsomal enzymes.

Dermatological abnormalities are frequently found in PCB-exposed animals; the pilosebaceous unit of the skin appears to be the most commonly affected organ. In laboratory studies acneiform lesions are considered typical sequelae of exposure to PCBs and related substances. Enlargement of the meibonian glands and swelling of the upper eyelids are also manifestations of experimental animal PCB poisoning.

Animal studies have also revealed a neurotoxic action of certain PCB congeners. Exposure to PCBs in utero has shown alterations in activity levels and impaired learning in offspring. Although it is difficult to extrapolate PCB-related effects from animal studies directly to humans, there appears to be a significantly high degree of similarity among species with regard to neurotoxic effects.[16]

Certain types of PCBs administered in high doses have been found to produce hepatomas and hepatocellular carcinomas in mice and rats.[14,17] Similar to many other toxic effects, a wide range of biological responses have been noted among various species. Therefore, in terms of risk assessment, it is difficult to determine which animal model is the most appropriate predictor of the carcinogenic risk of long-term exposure for humans.

Human Health Effects

Despite the widespread industrial use of PCBs since the 1930s, it was not until 1966, as mentioned, that PCBs were first recognized as a major environmental pollutant.[12] Adverse effects of excessive exposure to chlorinated naphthalenes, PCBs, and related substances were initially reported in the 1930s and 1940s.[18,19] These reports described multiple skin lesions characterized by chloracne and, occasionally, systemic health effects among workers who either manufactured these chemicals or handled products containing mixtures of them. In one investigation of an insulation material known as Halowax, the rate of skin symptoms from contact ("cable rash") was found to be very high. Chlorinated naphthalenes, a principal ingredient of Halowax, is a known cause of chloracne and liver dysfunction; Halowax contained a biphenyl compound as a minor ingredient.

In most instances, in which adverse effects have been attributed to exposure to PCBs, concomitant exposure to other halogenated hydrocarbons, including polychlorinated naphthalenes, styrene chloride, and polychlorinated dibenzofurans, has occurred. A report from 1954 described chloracne among workers with exposure to an Aroclor compound in a heat-exchanger system. Whether contaminants were present in the heated oil was not reported.[20]

Attributing adverse health effects in humans to singular PCB exposure has been a difficult problem, since several major exposure incidents have usually involved toxic contaminants in the PCBs. Two major epidemic outbreaks of disease (yusho and yu-cheng), were initially thought to have been caused by the consumption of vegetable oil accidentally contaminated with PCBs, but the disease was later found to have been associated with other toxic compounds in the oil, especially the PCDFs.[21,22] This became known only after subsequent improvements were made in the analytical methods for the determination of the chemicals involved. Similarly, industrial accidents that involve heating of PCBs also have produced similar contaminants.

Yusho and Yu-cheng

During the summer of 1968 in Japan, a large number of people from one area sought medical attention because of a variety of skin symptoms.[21,22] Chloracne was diagnosed in the majority of affected persons with characteristic signs, such as comedones, pustules, and straw-colored cysts. Other abnormalities on the skin and mucous membranes, including hyperpigmentation, swelling of the eyelids, eye discharge (caused by hypersecretion of the Meibomian glands), and hyperemia of the conjunctiva were noted. Approximately 80 percent of the first group of patients manifested skin symptoms. Skin abnormalities, particularly dark brown pigmentation and facial edema, were also noted among newborn infants who were also found to exhibit low–birth weight, pigmented nails, and dental abnormalities.[21,22]

Epidemiological investigation demonstrated that affected persons had consumed food prepared in a rice cooking oil, which had been produced or distributed on 2 consecutive days from a certain company. It was initially estimated from a chlorine analysis of the oil that the PCB concentration was approximately 2,000 to 3,000 ppm. When improved analytical methods were subsequently applied, other chlorinated compounds were found in the oil including PCQs and PCDFs. More than 40 different isomers were identified among the latter group of chemicals.

The clinical findings of this investigation became known as "PCB poisoning" or "yusho" (in Japanese, literally, "oil disease").

Observations similar to those made in patients with yusho were reported in a second outbreak of intoxication that occurred in Taiwan in 1979. The oil consumed in that incident contained 100 ppm PCBs and 0.1 PCDFs. The clinical syndrome resulting from this episode was named yu-cheng (in Chinese, "oil disease").[21,22]

In addition to the dermatological abnormalities mentioned above, there were effects on other organ systems noted in both epidemics. A prominent clinical-biochemical finding in patients with yusho and yu-cheng was elevated levels of serum triglycerides. Abnormal results for liver function tests were also found in some of the severely affected persons. Neurophysiological examinations revealed sensory neuropathy, and abnormal measurements of velocity of motor nerve conduction were reported, particularly in yu-cheng patients. Also reported were nonspecific symptoms including fatigue, anorexia, and weight loss and effects on the respiratory and immune systems.

In the outbreak in Taiwan, transplacental exposure and possible exposure through breast milk from exposed mothers resulted in signs of poisoning such as skin and mucous membrane abnormalities, with developmental effects also being noted.[23]

These observations represent an unusual description of effects in offspring associated with this type of exposure. Long-term follow-up of Taiwanese children with prenatal exposure to PCBs and other related polychlorinated contaminants consequent to heating of the cooking oil appear to reinforce initial observations of slight impairment of cognitive development.[24] In a subsequent study, assessment of developmental and behavioral parameters in children born 7 to 12 years after their mother's intoxication has also demonstrated delayed gonadal development.[25]

Carcinogenic effects on survivors of the yusho and yu-cheng episodes are as yet preliminary; epidemiological surveillance after a sufficient latency period is necessary for a detailed assessment, and findings until now have revealed very few observations.

There is a general consensus that the contaminants PCDFs, PCQs, and perhaps others have contributed to the development of the clinical and biochemical effects observed in yusho and yu-cheng.

Occupational Exposure to PCBs and Their Contaminants

Recent investigations of occupationally overexposed workers have not demonstrated clinical abnormalities of the severity found in patients with yusho and yu-cheng. Except for early reports, mentioned above, of skin and liver abnormalities from exposure to chlorinated compounds mixed with PCBs (e.g., chlorinated naphthalenes), overt clinical findings have been rare.

Abnormal liver function tests and various dermatological abnormalities, including some cases suggestive of chloracne, have been reported.[3,14,26] However, the majority of studies have not identified clinically noticeable effects in workers, despite long-term exposure and high serum concentrations of PCBs, i.e., even several times the amount typically found in the general population. Significant correlations between serum levels of PCBs and liver function tests have been reported, but liver function tests have mostly been within the normal range as compared with those of nonexposed workers.

Other clinical-biochemical parameters, such as plasma triglyceride levels, have been significantly correlated with serum levels of PCBs.[27] It is unclear whether there is a direct cause-effect relationship between serum lipids and PCBs. This observation could be a consequence of the lipophilic properties of PCBs. Thus a positive association between PCBs and serum lipids could be related to the increased solubility of PCBs in serum with higher lipid concentrations.[28]

Adverse reproductive effects, immunosuppression, respiratory symptoms, neurological abnormalities, effects on the endocrine system and other health consequences attributed to PCBs and their contaminants (such as those described among patients with yusho and yu-cheng), have not been well documented in occupationally exposed subjects. Dose-response relationships have also been poorly defined in studies of human populations.

Mortality studies of occupationally exposed populations have not demonstrated conclusive evidence that exposure to PCBs increases the risk of cancer or other chronic disease. Most of the existing reports use historical measures of exposure such as duration of employment rather than more accurate individual exposure assessments.

An early mortality study of employees potentially exposed to PCBs during a 10-year period in a refinery plant reported an excess mortality rate due to melanoma and cancer of the pancreas. Association with PCBs is uncertain because there was exposure to several other chemicals as well during the same period and the population was small.[29] Melanoma was also reported in a later study of capacitor manufacturing workers.[30]

Studies of workers employed in capacitor manufacturing plants have provided limited information.[31] The number of deaths is small, and meaningful interpretations are often difficult to make. However, a high rate of deaths due to cancer of the liver and rectum were found in two studies, but the risk with regard to specific organs has not been clearly determined.[32] Deaths due to cancer of the liver, gallbladder, and the biliary tract are of particular interest in view of experimental study results.[31] Other investigations demonstrated different mortality patterns and were inconclusive. However, evidence of increased mortality risk from malignant melanoma and brain cancer was apparent in one study of capacitor manufacturing workers.

Recently, findings of higher concentrations of specific PCB congeners in patients with non-Hodgkin's lymphoma as compared with comparison subjects without malignant disease have been reported. None examined in this study had a risk of occupational exposure to PCBs.[33] The number of study subjects was small, however, and the findings need confirmation in larger populations. Similar observations have also been made by the same researchers with regard to chlordane, a pesticide.[34]

Low-Level Environmental Exposure

Health effects of levels of exposure commonly encountered in the general environment and associated with serum concentrations of PCBs considered to be within the general population range (0 to 10 ppb total PCBs) have not been reported. Blood pressure and serum levels of PCBs were associated in one study of a community in the southern United States.[35] Other concomitant exposures and significant associations with blood pressure were also recognized in that study. A follow-up study addressing the issue of blood pressure and exposures experienced by patients with yusho did not report a similar association.[36]

While the yusho and yu-cheng incidents have elicited clinically apparent neurotoxicity, lower levels of environmental exposure to PCBs in utero appear to be associated with subclinical neurologic changes. An association between prenatal PCB exposures and small deficits in motor-sensory and intellectual function has now been seen among infants and young children in several independent studies. For example, children whose mothers had potentially been exposed to PCB-laden fish from Lake Michigan had lower scores on verbal IQ and reading comprehension and adverse effects on memory and attention at 11 years of age. Deficits were believed to be related to transplacental exposure and not to breast-feeding, suggesting higher vulnerability of the developing nervous system in utero.[37] Exposures were not excessively high; levels in the mothers at the time of delivery were at the upper range of normal as compared with levels usually found in the general population without a specific exposure source, such as consumption of PCB-contaminated fish. Similar findings have been reported by other investigations in North Carolina and Europe.[38]

Patients often voice concern to their clinicians over potential adverse health effects of exposures to various materials containing PCBs. Typical situations include brief contact with contaminated soil (e.g., from a leaking transformer or similar equipment) or being present in the vicinity of an accidental fire involving electrical instruments containing dielectric fluids. Evidence of significantly increased absorption of PCBs or of adverse health effects has rarely been reported from such exposures.

Disposal and Destruction

The Toxic Substances Control Act has prescribed strict regulations for the disposal of PCBs. Among the types of disposal methods approved by the U.S. Environmental Protection Agency are landfill disposal, high-temperature incineration, and chemical dechlorination. The various disposal methods are aimed at the destruction of specific items and wastes containing PCBs. For example, nonliquid PCB-containing materials are most frequently disposed of in landfills, while the disposal of free fluids is not permitted in a landfill, unless prior to pre-treatment dilution, the fluid contained 500 ppm PCBs or less. For liquids with a PCB concentration of 500 ppm or higher, incineration is the preferred method of disposal.[1] To avoid the formation of PCDFs and PCDDs, incineration must take place at temperatures in the range of 1500°C.[39]

Dechlorination and other chemical modification are the techniques most often applied to PCBs in mineral oil. Some methods make possible recycling of the purified mineral oil for reuse in transformers. Degradation of PCBs also occurs in nature by bacterial action.[40] Major international efforts are currently being made to dispose of PCBs and related chemicals, and international coordination is desirable.[41]

Exposure Tests and Clinical Evaluation

Clinical evaluation is usually limited to those with previous employment in environments with exposure to PCBs and related substances. Another group frequently undergoing examination consists of maintenance personnel in industrial facilities where transformers and similar electrical equipment are still in use.

Several laboratories throughout the United States perform analysis of PCBs in serum. The serum concentration of PCBs is a good indicator of exposure and absorption, which primarily occurs via the lungs or the skin. Adipose measurements are useful when a lower limit of detection is desired. The levels measured in an individual or a group of workers are best evaluated in comparison with those found in nonoccupationally exposed controls. Typical serum levels of PCBs in the U.S. adult population are now less than 10 ng/mL (ppb). Because of great variations in laboratory techniques, the same laboratory should perform the analyses in sequential measurements. Routine measurement of PCDFs and other contaminants is not widely performed by clinical biochemistry laboratories; analyses are done by specialized laboratories, usually on a research basis, since costs are high. The identification of individual PCB congeners and related compounds in serum, milk, or adipose tissue is essential to link exposure with occupational or environmental circumstances, such as in firefighters and workers engaged in decontamination following fires where equipment contains chlorinated substances mixed with PCBs.

Clinical examination should include the skin, with attention to the presence of comedones, papules, pustules, and straw-colored cysts consistent with chloracne. The location of acne lesions associated with chlorinated substances differs from that seen in acne vulgaris (youth acne), but the diagnosis must often be made by an experienced occupational dermatologist. The occurrence of typical chloracne after occupational exposure to pure or unheated PCBs is rare.

Liver function tests are also an essential part of the medical examination. Despite the nonspecific and insensitive nature of such clinical biochemistry tests (γ-GTP, AST (SGOT), ALT (SGPT), alkaline phosphatase, and bilirubin), they are frequently used both for screening purposes and in the evaluation of individual patients. History of alcohol and drug use should be considered when evaluating the results of liver function tests. The usefulness of these tests is usually increased when the individual worker serves as his or her own control in serial tests, performed in relation to specific exposure situations.

Measurements of serum cholesterol and triglyceride levels are useful procedures in general health maintenance and may be of additional significance among persons with a history of significant exposure to PCBs. Fractionation of serum lipids into high- and low-density lipoproteins has also been suggested in evaluation of occupationally exposed groups. It is uncertain whether associations between serum lipids and serum or plasma levels of PCBs are a reflection of the solubility of PCBs in lipids or whether there is a direct cause-and-effect relationship between these two variables.

Evaluation of the endocrine and nervous system (neurophysiological studies and testing of the immune status) are usually not considered part of the routine laboratory tests in the evaluation of PCB-exposed workers, but, if indicated, should be performed in accordance with presenting symptoms and the clinical judgment of the examiner. Although abnormalities in these organ systems were reported in yusho and yu-cheng, these are usually not associated with a history of occupational or environmental exposure to PCBs alone.

▶ POLYBROMINATED BIPHENYLS (PBBs)

Polybrominated biphenyls (PBBs) have a chemical structure similar to that of PCBs and are a mixture of brominated biphenyls which are industrially produced by perbromination of the biphenyl ring. Although PBBs are no longer produced in the United States, their principal use has been as fire retardants in thermoplastic resins, lacquers, and polyurethane foam.[1] Like other halogenated hydrocarbons, PBBs are lipophilic and are resistant to chemical and metabolic degradation. While there is potential for accumulation of these compounds in biota and along the food chain, use of PBBs has been relatively limited. Worldwide environmental contamination by PBBs similar to that by PCBs has not occurred; however, a unique situation involving accidental exposure to PBBs did take place in Michigan in 1974. This unfortunate episode led to the discovery of a wide spectrum of toxic effects in exposed animals and humans. Longitudinal investigations of immunological effects in exposed populations have provided information about biochemical markers of exposure which may be important for future epidemiological surveillance.

PBB Exposure in Michigan

Health effects of exposure to PBBs were essentially unknown prior to the major outbreak of PBB poisoning in Michigan in 1974, when approximately 1000 kg of a commercial preparation containing PBBs was inadvertently substituted for a dairy cattle feed supplement (i.e., magnesium oxide) in a manufacturing process.[2] The contaminating agent was a mixture of brominated biphenyls which consisted of mainly penta-, hexa-, and octabromo biphenyls. It is estimated that the PBB concentration in the contaminated feed supplement was between 4,000 and 13,500 ppm. It was also reported that small amounts of brominated naphthalene and brominated methylfuran were present in the mixture.[3]

This outbreak was initially epizootic. It was estimated that cattle on approximately 25 farms had consumed as much as 200 g of PBBs per head. Because of widespread contamination of livestock, the episode subsequently had implications for human health. Large scale investigations of the toxicity of PBBs and their potential acute and chronic health effects on residents in Michigan were undertaken. Adverse effects of PBBs that were first described in lactating cows in 1974 included anorexia, weight loss, decreased milk production, abnormal hoof growth, hyperkeratosis, alopecia, and severe infections of the joints.[4] In numerous cases, cachexia and death followed within months after ingestion of the PBB-containing compound. Subsequently, more than 500 dairy and poultry farms were quarantined during 1974. Some 30,000 head of cattle and 1.5 million chickens died or were destroyed, and 5 million eggs were destroyed. Despite the quarantines, exposure to PBBs was widespread among the general population of Michigan. The exposure was especially high in persons who had consumed products from their own highly contaminated farms. In a study of postmortem tissue specimens from a series of autopsies from the Grand Rapids area in Michigan (considered one of the most highly exposed regions), PBBs were detected in 192 of 196 samples 10 years after the accident. The chemicals were primarily distributed in perirenal adipose tissue, adrenals, and thymus.[5] Ninety-six percent of farmers with a history of high exposure had detectable levels of PBBs (i.e., more than 0.5 ppm) in their serum, and persons living on or consuming products from quarantined farms had significantly higher PBB levels than those living on nonquarantined farms. Furthermore, it was estimated that the elimination half-time of PBBs in adipose tissue is at least 72 years and that PBBs are likely to persist in tissues of contaminated persons throughout their lifetimes.[6,7] A follow-up study of a cohort of PBB-exposed Michigan residents suggested an estimated half-life of about 11 years in human serum.[8]

Animal Experimentation Data

Toxicological data derived from animal experiments indicate that PBBs are fat-soluble substances and are stored especially in the thymus, liver, brain, and adipose tissues, where they persist for a long time. Polybrominated biphenyls have been shown to pass through the placenta and are excreted also in milk.[9] A wide spectrum of toxic effects on the liver, thyroid, thymus, and lymph nodes have been described; these include intrahepatic bile duct hyperplasia, thyroid gland hyperplasia, and the induction of hypocellular lymph nodes with a depleted T-cell–dependent area.[10] Significant thymic atrophy and chronic injury to the lymphatic tissues were also described in the "toxic PBB syndrome."

PBBs possess tumor-promoting activity[11] and induce hepatocellular carcinomas in rats[12] and tracheal papillomas in hamsters.[13]

Health Effects

Concomitant with the reporting of toxic effects in animals, investigations about potential health effects were performed. In one study, a high prevalence of clinical symptoms was reported among Michigan dairy farmers and members of their families. Four major categories of symptoms were recognized: neurological, musculoskeletal, dermatological, and gastrointestinal. The neurological symptoms were the most prominent and included headaches, dizziness, irritability, decreased capacity for physical and intellectual work, and memory impairment. The musculoskeletal symptoms consisted of arthritis-like abnormalities with pain and swelling of the joints, joint deformity, and various degrees of impaired movement. Knees and ankles mostly were affected. Individuals often reported multiple symptoms from several organ systems. The neurological and musculoskeletal symptoms, however, were the most prevalent. The existence of a "human toxic PBB syndrome" was suggested.[14]

PBB-Induced Immune Dysfunction

The clinical studies were accompanied by investigations of the potential immunotoxic effects by PBBs in Michigan dairy farmers and other residents of the state. The interest in studying the immunobiological aspects of PBB exposure was stimulated by the observed effects of PBBs on the thymus and lymphoid tissues in affected cattle and in experimental animals. That the immune system was a potential target organ for PBB-related toxicity was supported by the binding of a higher concentration of the most abundant hexa-isomers (HBB) on the surface membrane of white blood cells of Michigan dairy farm residents as compared with surface membranes' erythrocytes and plasma components.[15]

Initial studies[16,17] included 332 adult dairy farmers from Michigan, 156 persons from the general population of the state, and 29 chemical plant workers who had been engaged in the manufacture of PBBs. Significant deviation from normal in both percentage and absolute number of T lymphocytes was observed in the PBB-exposed farmers and PBB-manufacturing chemical workers with a reduction of T cells and increase in lymphocytes without detectable surface markers.

Moreover, both direct occupational and indirect exposure to PBBs were associated with abnormalities in cell-mediated immunity (CMI) assessed by delayed cutaneous hypersensitivity to PPD, mumps, *Candida*, Varidase, and dermatophytin. Whereas 43 of 46 tested persons of a control group responded to at least one recall antigen, 18 percent of the Michigan dairy farmers were completely anergic to each of the recall antigens. The functional integrity of peripheral blood lymphocytes of PBB-exposed persons was also adversely affected. Marked decreases were observed in lymphocyte responses to T cell–specific mitogens as well as in the proliferative T-lymphocyte responses in the mixed lymphocyte culture reaction.

Effects on the humoral immune system have also been observed and associated with PBB exposure. A dose-response relationship was suggested between PBBs and immunoglobulins (IgG, IgM, and IgA). Associations between cellular abnormalities, such as polyclonal hypergammaglobulinemia, reduced number of T cells, and heightened in vivo response to recall antigens were also suggested, as well as neurological and musculoskeletal symptoms.

Despite such observations, no apparent relationship between serum or adipose levels of PBBs and clinical symptoms or immune dysfunction was detected. However, family clustering of the observed abnormalities was noted, suggesting a common dietary source as the origin of exposure rather than genetic predisposition.

Five-year follow-up examination of farm residents originally examined in 1976 and of dairy farmers from another state[18,19] provided results similar to those obtained in 1976, with high correlations between the two examinations for both T-cell and B-cell functions ($r = 0.87$ and $r = 0.85$, respectively) suggesting persistence of the immunological abnormalities. This finding, coupled with the long half-life of PBBs in human tissues, warrants long-term epidemiological surveillance of the exposed populations. A carcinogenic effect of the PBBs in humans has not been demonstrated conclusively; however, the observation period since initial exposure is relatively short, assuming the latency period for PBB-related carcinogenic effects follows the pattern characteristic for occupational and environmental exposures. In a nested case-control study to examine the association between breast cancer and serum levels of PBBs, women who developed breast cancer were matched to control subjects. Women with serum PBB concentrations of 2 to 3 ppb, 4 ppb, or greater had a higher estimated risk for the disease than women with less than 2 ppb. The odds ratios were unchanged when adjusted for other known risk factors.[20] Future epidemiological surveillance of large PBB-exposed populations is necessary.

DEVELOPMENTAL TOXICITY

There is also data showing that PBBs are transmitted to nursing infants via mother's milk.[21] One investigation of 285 serum samples from 4-year-old children in Michigan demonstrated that PBBs were detected in 13 to 21 percent of the samples.[22] Fetal toxicity has been shown to accompany maternal toxicity in experimental animals.[23] Lower survival rates from birth to weaning and increased mortality rate after 2 years, including the development of hepatocellular carcinoma, have been reported in offspring of rats fed PBBs during pregnancy.[24] Growth retardation and neurobehavioral toxicity have also been shown at concentrations of PBBs in adipose tissue of offspring, similar to concentration levels reported for highly exposed humans with neurological abnormalities.[25]

Evaluation of PBB-related effects in developing children have not yet been performed on a large-scale basis, but this matter also requires future epidemiological surveillance. Although the present concentrations of brominated fire retardants do not yet appear to pose a significant environmental health risk, the replacement of PBBs by safer alternative substances is warranted. There is also a possibility that debromination of the commercial polybrominated compound, which caused the public health problem in Michigan, can sometimes occur by anaerobic microorganisms, contributing to biodegradation of the environmental burden of PBBs.[26]

Polychlorinated Dioxins and Polychlorinated Dibenzofurans

Yoshito Masuda • Arnold J. Schecter

Polychlorinated dioxins have been described as the most toxic man-made chemicals known. They are synthetic, lipophilic, and very persistent. They are also relatively controversial. Dioxin animal toxicology studies demonstrate dose–dependent toxic responses to the dioxins and related chemicals such as the polychlorinated dibenzofurans, which frequently accompany dioxins and polychlorinated biphenyls (PCBs). (Both dibenzofurans and PCBs are chemically and biologically similar to dioxins.) However, the findings from human studies, at least until recently, have been less consistent.

The animal health effects include but are not limited to: death several weeks after dosing, usually accompanied by a "wasting" or loss of weight syndrome; increase in cancers (found in all animal cancer studies); increased reproductive and developmental disorders including fetal death in utero, malformations, and, in offspring dosed in utero, endocrine disruption with altered thyroid and sex hormone blood levels; immune deficiency sometimes leading to death of newborn rodents, especially following dosing with infectious agents; liver damage including transient increase in serum liver enzymes as well as the characteristic lesions of hepatocytes to chlorinated organics, enlarged cells, intracytoplasmic lipid droplets, increase in endoplasmic reticulum, enlarged and pleomorphic mitochondria with altered structure of the cristae mitochondriales and enlarged dense intramitochondrial granules; central nervous system and peripheral nervous system changes including altered behavior and change in nerve conduction velocity; altered lipid metabolism with increase in serum lipids; and skin disorders including rash and chloracne (acne caused by chlorinated organic chemicals). Some effects are species specific. Other findings have been reported but with less frequency or consistency.[1]

Findings reported in some human studies are similar to those from animal studies. These include an increase in cancers of certain types, including soft tissue sarcomas, Hodgkin's lymphoma, non-Hodgkin's lymphoma, lung cancer, and liver cancer; adverse reproductive and developmental effects following intrauterine and nursing exposure such as lower birth weight and smaller head circumference for gestational age, decreased cognitive abilities, behavioral impairment, and endocrine disruptions including altered thyroid hormone levels; immune deficiency; liver damage; altered lipid metabolism with increase in serum lipids; altered nerve conduction velocity; altered sex ratio in children born to dioxin-exposed women (more females than males); increase in diabetes or altered glucose metabolism in exposed chemical workers and sprayers of dioxin-contaminated Agent Orange herbicide; and behavioral changes including anxiety, difficulty sleeping, and decrease in sexual ability in males.[1–10] Some of the human health effects are subtle such as those reported in the Dutch studies. These effects are not likely to be detected by the clinician on individual patients but only in a larger population-based study. Skin disorders including rash and chloracne are also observed in some exposed persons.

Dioxins and dibenzofurans are not manufactured as such, but are usually found as unwanted contaminants of other synthetic chemicals or as products of incineration of chlorinated organics. Dioxins consist of two benzene rings connected by a third middle ring containing two oxygens in the para position. Dibenzofurans have a similar structure but the middle connecting ring contains only a single oxygen atom. PCBs consist of two connected biphenyl rings with no oxygen (Fig. 23-3). When chlorine atoms are in the 2, 3, 7, and 8 positions, dioxins and dibenzofurans are extremely toxic. The most toxic congener is 2,3,7,8-tetrachlorodibenzo-*p*-dioxin (2,3,7,8-TCDD). It is defined as having a "dioxin toxic equivalency factor" (TEF) of 1.0; other toxic dioxins have TEFs as small as 0.001. Dioxins and dibenzofurans without chlorines in the 2, 3, 7, and 8 positions are devoid of dioxinlike tox-icity. Some PCBs also have dioxinlike toxicity. The dioxin toxic equivalency (TEQ) approximates the toxicity of the total mixture. The TEQ is determined by multiplying the measured level of each congener by the congener's TEF and then adding the products. The total dioxin toxicity of a mixture is the sum of the TEQs from the dioxins, the dibenzofurans, and the dioxinlike PCBs. There are characteristic levels and patterns of dioxin and dibenzofuran congeners found in human tissues which correspond to levels of industrialization and contamination in a given country. At the present time seven toxic dioxin and 10 toxic dibenzofuran congeners as well as many PCBs can usually be identified in human tissue in persons living in more industrialized countries (Fig. 23-3). The measurement of the individual congeners is done by capillary column gas chromatography coupled to high-resolution mass spectrometry. Extraction, chemical cleanup, and the use of known chemical standards has markedly improved specificity and sensitivity of such measurements in recent years.

Intake of 1 to 6 pg/kg body weight (BW)/day of TEQ of dioxin-like chemicals (dioxins, dibenzofurans, and PCBs) is characteristic of adult daily intake in the United States at the present time.[11] Intake of TEQ is mostly from food, especially meat, fish, and dairy products. Fruits and vegetables have very low levels of dioxins, which are from surface deposition. Air and water contain very low levels of the fat-soluble dioxins and are believed to usually contribute little to human intake, as food intake has been demonstrated in several studies to result in more than 90 percent of human exposure. Nursing infants in the United States consume approximately 35 to 65 pg/kg BW/day of TEQ during the first year of life. The U.S. Environmental Protection Agency (EPA) has used a value of 0.006 pg/kg BW/day of TEQ over a 70-year lifetime as a dose believed to possibly lead to an excess of one cancer per 1 million population. The current EPA Dioxin Reassessment draft document is considering a change from 0.006 to 0.01 pg/kg BW/day of TEQ as a cancer reference dose. Some European countries use values between 1 and 10 pg/kg BW/day of TEQ as their reference value or acceptable daily intake (ADI). These different values are all based on review of the same published animal and human literature and each involves certain assumptions and safety factor considerations including extrapolation between animal species and from animals to humans. From a public health perspective, however, it is noteworthy that the U.S. daily intake of dioxins, especially in the presumably more sensitive nursing infant, exceeds reference values.[12–14]

The PCBs, which, unlike dioxins and dibenzofurans, were deliberately manufactured, are also found in most countries as environmental contaminants in humans, wildlife, and environmental samples. They were used as electrical and thermal insulating fluids for electrical transformers and capacitors, as hydraulic fluids, in carbonless copying paper, and in microscope oil. Higher levels are found in more industrialized countries. One of the most well-known PCB and dibenzofuran contaminations is the rice oil poisoning (the 1968 yusho incident) in Japan where PCBs and dibenzofurans contaminated rice oil used for cooking. We describe this incident in detail later because it clearly documented the human toxicity of dioxinlike

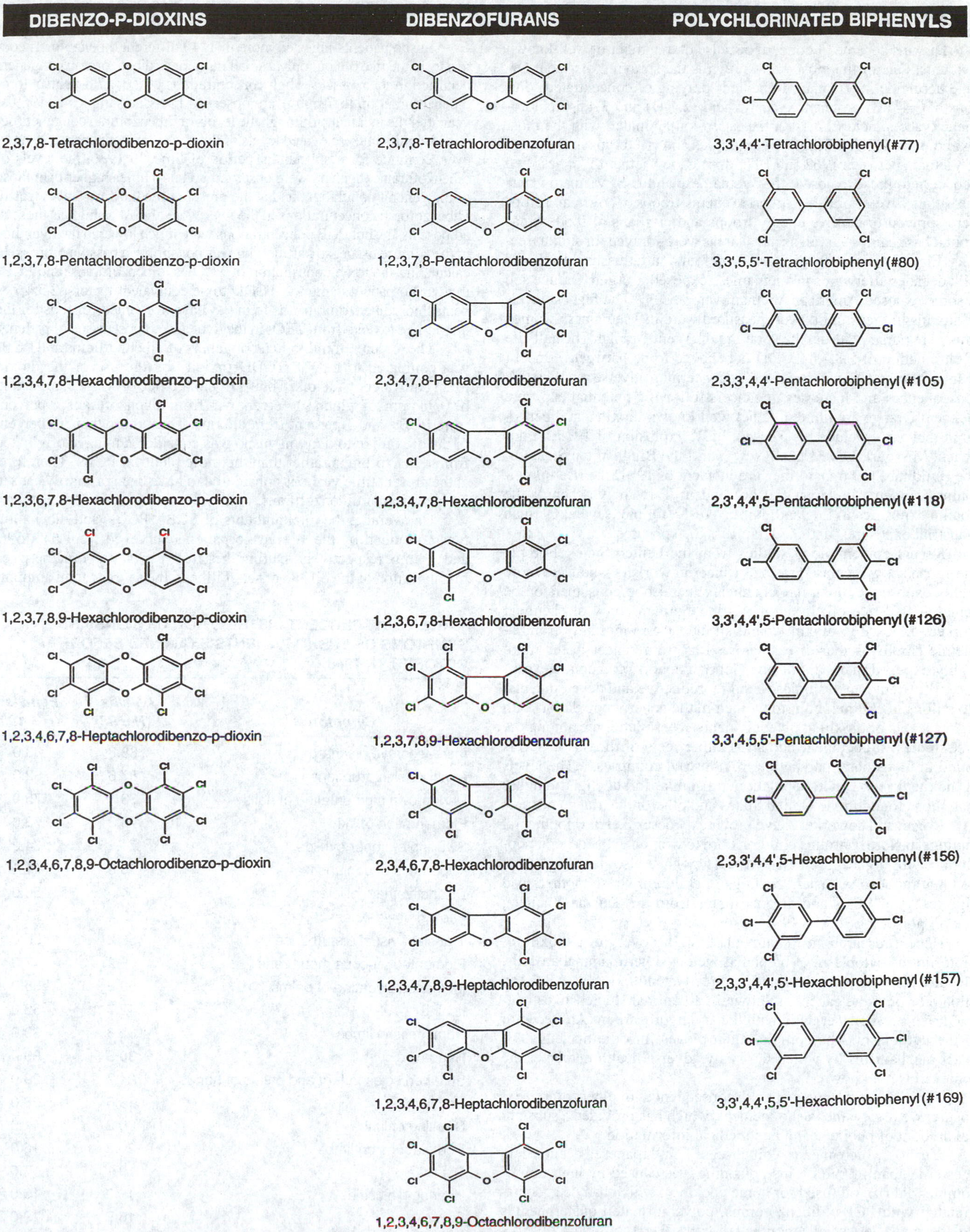
DIBENZO-P-DIOXINS
DIBENZOFURANS
POLYCHLORINATED BIPHENYLS
2,3,7,8-Tetrachlorodibenzo-p-dioxin
1,2,3,7,8-Pentachlorodibenzo-p-dioxin
1,2,3,4,7,8-Hexachlorodibenzo-p-dioxin
1,2,3,6,7,8-Hexachlorodibenzo-p-dioxin
1,2,3,7,8,9-Hexachlorodibenzo-p-dioxin
1,2,3,4,6,7,8-Heptachlorodibenzo-p-dioxin
1,2,3,4,6,7,8,9-Octachlorodibenzo-p-dioxin
2,3,7,8-Tetrachlorodibenzofuran
1,2,3,7,8-Pentachlorodibenzofuran
2,3,4,7,8-Pentachlorodibenzofuran
1,2,3,4,7,8-Hexachlorodibenzofuran
1,2,3,6,7,8-Hexachlorodibenzofuran
1,2,3,7,8,9-Hexachlorodibenzofuran
2,3,4,6,7,8-Hexachlorodibenzofuran
1,2,3,4,7,8,9-Heptachlorodibenzofuran
1,2,3,4,6,7,8-Heptachlorodibenzofuran
1,2,3,4,6,7,8,9-Octachlorodibenzofuran
3,3',4,4'-Tetrachlorobiphenyl (#77)
3,3',5,5'-Tetrachlorobiphenyl (#80)
2,3,3',4,4'-Pentachlorobiphenyl (#105)
2,3',4,4',5-Pentachlorobiphenyl (#118)
3,3',4,4',5-Pentachlorobiphenyl (#126)
3,3',4,5,5'-Pentachlorobiphenyl (#127)
2,3,3',4,4',5-Hexachlorobiphenyl (#156)
2,3,3',4,4',5'-Hexachlorobiphenyl (#157)
3,3',4,4',5,5'-Hexachlorobiphenyl (#169)

Figure 23-3. Chemical structures of selected polychlorinated dioxins, dibenzofurans, and biphenyls.

chemicals as early as 1968. An almost identical incident, known as yu-cheng, occurred in Taiwan in 1979.

Dioxins became of concern because of a number of well-known incidents. One of the most well-known is the spraying of Agent Orange herbicide in Vietnam. Repeated spraying of concentrated solutions of 2,4-dichlorophenoxyacetic acid (2,4-D) and 2,4,5-trichlorophenoxyacetic acid (2,4,5-T), the latter contaminated with the most toxic dioxin, 2,3,7,8-TCDD, over jungles and rice crops in the south of Vietnam between 1962 and 1971 during the Vietnam War has been a concern to those exposed: the Vietnamese and U.S. Vietnam veterans. Jungles were sprayed to deprive enemy troops of cover, and crops were sprayed to deprive enemy troops and civilians of food. Areas around base camps as well as naval areas were sprayed for similar reasons. Elevated dioxin levels have been found in fat tissue, blood, and milk decades afterwards in Vietnamese exposed to Agent Orange and in some exposed American Vietnam veterans.[15,16] The highest levels of dioxins in breast milk ever measured were in Vietnamese women who were nursing during the spraying of Agent Orange. The half-life of elimination of 2,3,7,8-TCDD is believed to be between 7 and 11 years in humans. Vietnamese studies concerning adverse reproductive consequences and increases in cancers following potential exposure to Agent Orange are limited. Other well-known dioxin and dibenzofuran incidents include the Seveso, Italy, explosion of 1976; Times Beach, Missouri; Love Canal, New York; the Binghamton State Office Building PCB transformer fire incident of 1981; the rice oil poisoning incidents in Japan (yusho) and in Taiwan (yu-cheng); the Coalite exposures in England; Nitro, West Virginia; several German industrial exposures; and the Ufa, Russia, exposures.[1]

Recent epidemiology studies from the United States, Europe, and Japan show increased rates of cancer in workers who were more highly exposed to dioxinlike chemicals and also in consumers of the contaminated rice oil. In addition, one German study of chemical workers exposed to dioxins found an increase in mortality from ischemic cardiovascular disease as well as from cancer in the more highly exposed members of one German cohort of chemical workers.[17–21] Recent Dutch studies found reproductive and developmental alterations in children born to women in the general population with higher levels of dioxin toxic equivalents. These latter are among the first studies to document human health effects of dioxins at levels found in the general population in industrial countries.[4,6] The levels of dioxins in the Dutch population are similar to but slightly higher than those found in the United States and other industrial countries.

Rogan and coworkers have previously described developmental findings in North Carolina children born to women in the general population with higher levels of PCBs. They have also described more striking and also persistent findings in children whose mothers had high levels of PCBs and dibenzofurans from the Taiwan Yucheng rice oil poisoning.[22–26]

Recent research has documented the discovery of a dioxin receptor in the cytoplasm of human as well as other mammalian cells. The dioxins, which appear not to be directly genotoxic, but which can initiate or promote cancer as shown in all animal studies investigating dioxins and cancer, bind with the aryl hydrocarbon (Ah) receptor in the cytoplasm. The complex then moves into the nucleus. The exact mechanisms by which the many adverse health outcomes are achieved is not known.[27]

To illustrate the human health consequences of dibenzofuran exposure, we review the yusho incident, which has provided a substantial amount of public health and medical information.

Yusho, which means "oil disease" in Japanese, occurred in Western Japan in 1968. This poisoning was caused by ingestion of commercial rice oil (used for home cooking), which had been contaminated with PCBs, dibenzofurans, polychlorinated quaterphenyls (PCQs) and a very small amount of dioxins. Two thousand people became ill and sought medical care. The marked increase of dibenzofurans in the rice oil is believed to have occurred in the following way. Although PCBs are usually contaminated with small amounts of dibenzofurans, the commercial PCBs used as a heat-transfer medium for deodorizing rice oil were heated above 200°C and the PCBs were gradually converted into dibenzofurans. The PCBs with increased dibenzofuran concentration leaked into the rice oil through holes formed in a heating pipe because of inadequate welding.

Yusho patients ingested more than 40 different dibenzofuran congeners in the rice oil, but only a small number of dibenzofuran congeners persisted in their tissues. High concentrations of 2,3,4,7,8-pentachlorodibenzofuran, up to 7 ppb, were observed in tissue samples in 1969, a year after the incident. Although the levels of dibenzofuran congeners declined significantly, elevated levels of dibenzofuran congeners did, however, continue for a substantial period of time. In 1986, the levels of dibenzofuran congeners were observed up to 40 times higher than those of the general population, and at the present time they are still elevated. Dibenzofuran concentrations in the liver were almost as high as those in adipose tissue, but PCB concentrations were much lower in the liver than in the adipose tissue, so partitioning was not simply a passive process. In calculating the toxic contribution of PCDDs, dibenzofurans, and PCBs in a yusho patient using the TCDD toxic equivalent factors, 2,3,4,7,8-pentachlorodibenzofuran was found to have accounted for most of the dioxin-like toxicity from TEQs in the liver and adipose tissue of patients.

The toxicity of individual congeners of dibenzofurans and PCBs was compared to 2,3,7,8-TCDD toxicity by the use of the dioxin toxin equivalency factors. Total TEQ in the rice oil was calculated to be 0.98 ppm, of which 91 percent was from dibenzofurans, 8 percent from PCBs, and 1 percent from dioxins. Thus, more than 90 percent of the dioxinlike toxicity in yusho was considered to have originated from dibenzofurans rather than the more plentiful PCBs. Therefore, at the present time yusho is considered to have been primarily caused by ingestion of dibenzofurans.

On average, the total amounts of PCBs, PCQs, and dibenzofurans consumed by the 141 yusho patients surveyed were 633, 596, and 3.4 mg, respectively. During the latent period, the time between first ingestion of the oil and onset of illness, the average total amounts

TABLE 23-11. PERCENT DISTRIBUTION OF SIGNS AND SYMPTOMS OF YUSHO PATIENTS EXAMINED BEFORE OCTOBER 31, 1968

Symptoms	*Males (N = 98)*	*Females (N = 100)*
Increased eye discharge	88.8	83.0
Acnelike skin eruptions	87.6	82.0
Dark brown pigmentation of nails	83.1	75.0
Pigmentation of skin	75.3	72.0
Swelling of upper eyelids	71.9	74.0
Hyperemia of conjunctiva	70.8	71.0
Distinctive hair follicles	64.0	56.0
Feeling of weakness	58.4	52.0
Transient visual disturbance	56.2	55.0
Pigmented mucous membrane	56.2	47.0
Increased sweating of palms	50.6	55.0
Itching	42.7	52.0
Numbness in limbs	32.6	39.0
Headache	30.3	39.0
Stiffened soles in feet and palms of hands	24.7	29.0
Vomiting	23.6	28.0
Swelling of limbs	20.2	41.0
Red plaques on limbs	20.2	16.0
Diarrhea	19.1	17.0
Hearing difficulties	18.0	19.0
Fever	16.9	19.0
Jaundice	11.2	11.0
Spasm of limbs	7.9	8.0

Kuratsune M. Yoshimura, T, Matsukzaka J, Yamaguchi A: Epidemiologic study on yusho, a poisoning caused by ingestion of rice oil contaminated with a commercial brand of polychlorinated biphenyls. Environ Health Perspect 1:119–128, 1972

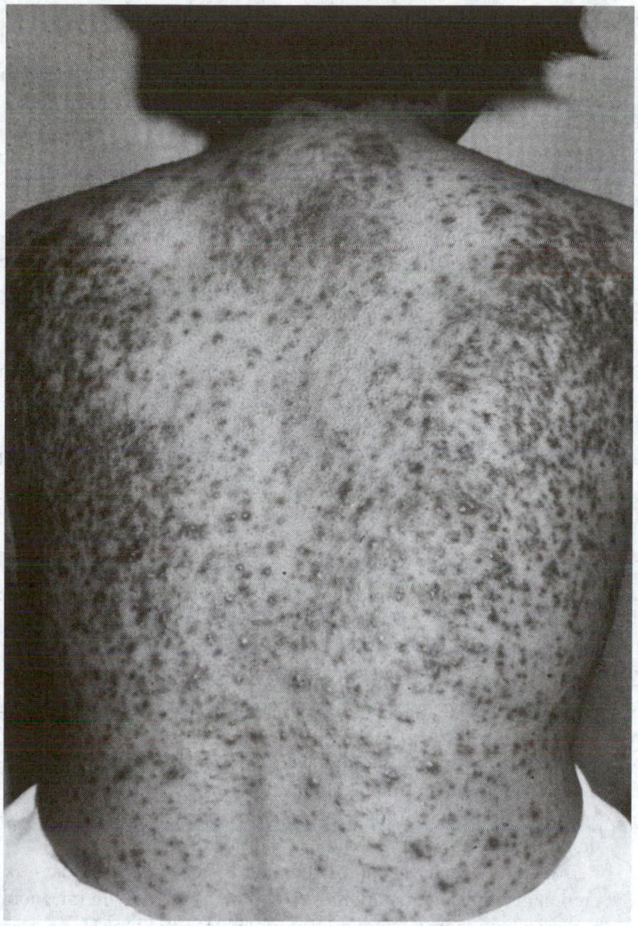

Figure 23-4. Acneform eruption on the back of a yusho patient (female, age 33, photographed in December, 1968).

consumed were 466, 439, and 2.5 mg of PCBs, PCQs, and dibenzofurans, respectively. The smallest amounts consumed which caused yusho were 111, 105, and 0.6 mg of PCBs, PCQs, and dibenzofurans, respectively. In yusho, it took on average about 3 months for clinical effects to be readily detected.

Most patients were affected within the 9-month period beginning February 1968, when the contaminated rice oil was shipped to the market from the Kanemi rice oil producing company, to October 1968, when the epidemic of yusho was reported to the public. Prominent signs and symptoms of yusho are summarized in Table 23-11. Pigmentation of nail, skin, and mucous membranes; distinctive follicles; acneform eruptions; increased eye discharge; and increased sweating of the palms were frequently noted. Common symptoms included pruritus and a feeling of weakness or fatigue.

The most notable initial signs of yusho were dermal lesions such as follicular keratosis, dry skin, marked enlargement and elevation of the follicular orifice, comedo formation, and acneform eruption (Fig. 23-4). Acneform eruptions developed in the face, cheek, jaw, back, axilla, trunk, external genitalia, and elsewhere. Dark pigmentation of the corneal limbus, conjunctivae, gingivae, lips, oral mucosa, and nails was a specific finding of yusho. Severity of the dermal lesions was proportional to the concentrations of PCBs and dibenzofurans in the blood and adipose tissue. The skin symptoms diminished gradually in the 10 years after the onset, probably related to the decreasing dibenzofuran concentrations in the body, while continual subcutaneous cyst formation with secondary infection persisted in a relatively small number of the most severely affected patients.

The most prominent ocular signs immediately after onset were hypersecretion of the meibomian glands and abnormal pigmentation of the conjunctiva. Cystic swelling of the meibomian glands filled with yellow infarctlike contents was observed in typical cases (Fig. 23-5). These signs markedly subsided in the 10 years after the onset of yusho. Eye discharge was a persistent complaint in many patients.

A brownish pigmentation of the oral mucosa was one of the characteristic signs of yusho. Pigmentation of the gingivae and lips was observed in many victims during 1968 and 1969. This pigmentation persisted for a considerable period of time and was still observed in most patients in 1982. Radiographic examination of the mouth of yusho patients demonstrated anomalies in the number of teeth and in the shape of the roots and marginal bone resorption at the roots.

Irregular menstrual cycles were observed in 58 percent of female patients in 1970. This was not related to elevation of yusho tissue levels. Urinary excretion of estrogen, pregnanediol, and pregnanetriol tended to be low in yusho patients. Thyroid function was investigated in 1984, 16 years after onset. The serum triiodothyronine and thyroxine levels were significantly higher than those of the general population, while thyroid-stimulating hormone levels were normal. Marked elevation of serum triglycerides was one of the abnormal laboratory findings peculiar to yusho in its early stages. Significant positive correlation was observed between serum triglyceride levels and blood PCB concentrations in 1973. Significantly elevated levels of triglycerides persisted in yusho patients for 15 to 20 years after exposure to PCBs and dibenzofurans.

A statistically significant excess mortality was observed for malignant neoplasm of all sites. This was also the case for cancer of the liver in males. However, excess mortality for such cancer was not statistically significant in females. It is still too early to draw any firm conclusion from this mortality study. However, the yusho rice oil poisoning incident was one of the first to demonstrate human health effects caused by the dioxinlike dibenzofurans and PCBs. These effects are similar to those noted in laboratory animals and wildlife from dioxin, dibenzofuran, or PCB exposure.[10,28]

Reduction of dioxins, dibenzofurans, and related chemicals in the environment can be and has been addressed in a variety of ways. One way is preventing the manufacture of certain chemicals such as PCBs. Another is banning the use of certain phenoxyherbicides such as 2,4,5-T, which is contaminated with the most toxic dioxin, 2,3,7,8-TCDD. Improved municipal, toxic waste, and hospital incinerators that produce less dioxin is another approach, as is not burning certain chlorine-containing compounds, such as the very common polyvinyl chlorides (PVCs). The use of unleaded gasoline avoids chlorinated scavengers found in leaded gasoline, which may facilitate formation

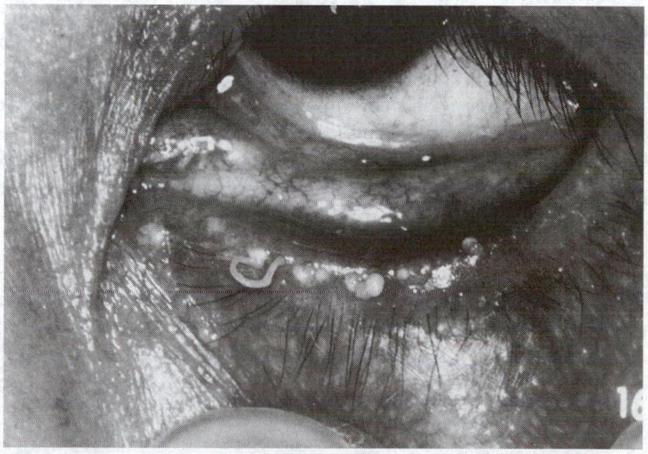

Figure 23-5. The lower eyelid of a 64-year-old yusho patient, 13 years after onset. White cheesy secretions were noted from the ducts of the meibomian glands when the eyelid was manually squeezed. (From Masuda Y: Causal agents of yusho, In: Kuratsune M, et al (eds): Yusho: A Human Disaster Caused by PCBs and Related Compounds. Fukuoka, Japan: Kyushu University Press, 1996, pp 47–80.)

of dioxins. Cigarette smoke contains a small amount of dioxins. Cessation of smoking and provision of smoke-free workplaces, eating establishments, airports, etc. helps prevent dioxin formation and exposure. In Europe over the past decade dioxin and dibenzofuran levels appear to be declining in human tissue, including breast milk and blood. This decline coincides in time with regulations and enforcement of regulations designed to decrease dioxin and dibenzofuran formation, especially with respect to incineration. Since intrauterine exposure cannot be prevented on an individual basis, and breast-feeding, which involves substantial dioxin transfer to the child, is otherwise desirable, worldwide environmental regulations with strong enforcement are clearly indicated as a preventive public health measure.

▶ REFERENCES

Organic Compounds

1. Browning E: Toxicity and Metabolism of Industrial Solvents. Amsterdam: Elsevier, 1965
2. Finkel AJ: Hamilton and Hardy's Industrial Toxicology, 4th ed. Boston: John Wright, 1983
3. National Institute for Occupational Safety and Health: Criteria for a Recommended Standard—Occupational Exposure to: Trichloroethylene, 1978; Benzene, 1974; Carbon Tetrachloride, 1976; Carbon Disulfide, 1977; Alkanes (C5-C8), 1977; Refined Petroleum Solvents, 1977; Ketones, 1978; Toluene, 1973; Xylene, 1975; Trichloroethylene, 1978; Chloroform, 1974; Epichlorhydrin, 1976; Ethylene Dichloride (1,2, dichloroethane), 1978 (revised); Ethylene Dichloride (1,2 dichloroethane), 1976; Ethylene Dibromide, 1977; Methyl Alcohol, 1976; Isopropyl Alcohol, 1976; Acrylamide, 1976; Formaldehyde, 1977. Washington, DC: U.S. Government Printing Office
4. Cavanagh JB: Peripheral neuropathy caused by chemical agents. CRC Crit Rev Toxicol 2:365–417, 1973
5. Spencer PS, Schaumburg HH: A review of acrylamide neurotoxicity. II. Experimental animal neurotoxicity and pathologic mechanisms. Can J Neurol Sci, August 1974, pp 152–169
6. Spencer PS, Schaumburg HH: Experimental neuropathy produced by 2,5-hexanedione—a major metabolite of the neurotoxic industrial solvent methyl *n*-butyl ketone. J Neurol Neurosurg Psychiatry 38(8):771–775, 1975
7. Borbely F: Erkennung und Behandlung der organischen Losungs mittel-vergiftungen. Bern: Medizinischer Verlag Hans Huber, 1947
8. Olsen J, Sabroe S: A case-reference study of neuropsychiatric disorders among workers exposed to solvents in the Danish wood and furniture industry. Scand J Soc Med 16:44–49, 1980
9. Mikkelson S: A cohort study of disability pension and death among painters with special regard to disabling presenile dementia as an occupational disease. Scand J Soc Med 16:34–43, 1980
10. Juntunen J, Hupli V, Hernberg S, Luisto M: Neurological picture of organic solvent poisoning in industry: a retrospective clinical study of 37 patients. Int Arch Occup Environ Health 46(3):219–231, 1980
11. Escobar A, Aruffo C: Chronic thinner intoxication: clinico-pathologic report of a human case. J Neurol Neurosurg Psychiatry 43(11): 986–994, 1980
12. Arlien-Sborg P, Henriksen L, Gade A, Gyldensted C, Paulson OB: Cerebral blood flow in chronic toxic encephalopathy in house painters exposed to organic solvents. Acta Neurol Scand 66(1): 3441, 1982
13. Sasa M, Igarashi S, Miyazaki T, et al: Equilibrium disorders with diffuse brain atrophy in long-term toluene sniffing. Arch Otorhinolaryngol 221(3):163–169, 1978
14. Chang YC: Neurotoxic effects of *n*-hexane on the human central nervous system: evoked potential abnormalities in *n*-hexane polyneuropathy. J Neurol Neurosurg Psychiatry 50(3):269–274, 1987
15. Yamamura Y: *N*-hexane polyneuropathy. Folia Psychiatr Neurol Jpn 23:45–57, 1969
16. Aksoy M, Erdem S, Dincol G: Types of leukemia in chronic benzene poisoning: a study in thirty-four patients. Acta Haematol 55: 65–72, 1976
17. Chang CM, Yu CW, Fong KY, Leung SY, Tsin TW, Yu YL, Cheung TF, Chan SY: N-hexane neuropathy in offset printers. J Neurol Neurosurg Psychiatry 56(5):538–542, 1994
18. Kurihara K, Kita K, Hattori T, Hirayama K: N-hexane polyneuropathy due to sniffing bond G10: clinical and electron microscope findings. No To Shinkei 38(11):1011–1017, 1986
19. Hall D MB, Ramsey J, Schwartz MS, Dookun D: Neuropathy in a petrol sniffer. Arch Dis Child 61(9):900–901, 1986
20. Oryshkevich RS, Wilcox R, Jhee WH: Polyneuropathy due to glue exposure: case report and 16-year follow-up. Arch Phys Med Rehabil 67(11):827–828, 1986
21. De Martino C, Malorni W, Amantini MC, Barcellona PS, Frontali N: Effects of respiratory treatment with *n*-hexane on rat testis morphology. I. A light microscopic study. Exp Mol Pathol 46(2):199–216, 1987
22. Zhu M, Spink DC, Yan B, Bank S, DeCaprio AP: Inhibition of 2,5-hexanedione-induced protein cross-linking by biological thiols: chemical mechanisms and toxicological implications. Chem Res Toxicol 8(5):764–771, 1995
23. Huang J, Kato K, Shibata E, Asaeda N, Takeuchi Y: Nerve-specific marker proteins as indicators of organic solvent neurotoxicity. Environ Res 63(1):82–87, 1993
24. Perbellini L, Mozzo P, Brugnone F, Zedde A: Physiologico-mathematical model for studying human exposure to organic solvents: kinetics of blood/tissue *n*-hexane concentrations and of 2,5-hexanedione in urine. Br J Ind Med 43(11):760–768, 1986
25. Perbellini L, Amantini MC, Brugnone F, Frontali N: Urinary excretion of *n*-hexane metabolites: a comparative study in rat, rabbit and monkey. Arch Toxicol 50(3–4):203–215, 1982
26. Fedtke N, Bolt HM: Detection of 2,5-hexanedione in the urine of persons not exposed to *n*-hexane. Int Arch Occup Environ Health 57(2):143–148, 1986
27. Ahonen I, Schimberg RW: 2,5-Hexanedione excretion after occupational exposure to *n*-hexane. Br J Ind Med 45(2):133–136, 1988
28. Governa M, Calisti R, Coppa G, Tagliavento G, Colombi A, Troni W: Urinary excretion of 2,5-hexanedione and peripheral polyneuropathies in workers exposed to hexane. J Toxicol Environ Health 20(3):219–228, 1987
29. Fedtke N, Bolt HM: The relevance of 4,5-dihydroxy-2-hexanone in the excretion kinetics of *n*-hexane metabolites in rat and man. Arch Toxicol 61(2):131–137, 1987
30. Daughtrey WC, Neeper-Bradley T, Duffy J, Haddock L, Keenan T, Kirwin C, Soiefer A: Two-generation reproduction study on commercial hexane solvent. J Appl Toxicol 14(5):387–393, 1994
31. Daughtrey WC, Putman DL, Duffy J, Sopiefer AI, Kirwin CJ, Curcio LN, Keenan TH: Cytogenetic studies on commercial hexane solvent. J Appl Toxicol 14(3):161–165, 1994
32. Takeuchi Y, Ono Y, Hisanaga N: An experimental study on the combined effects of *n*-hexane and toluene on the peripheral nerve of the rat. Br J Ind Med 38(1):14–19, 1981
33. DiVincenzo GD, Kaplan CJ, Dedinas J: Characterization of the metabolites of methyl *n*-butyl ketone, methyl iso-butyl ketone, methyl ethyl ketone in guinea pigs and their clearance. Toxicol Appl Pharmacol 36:511–522, 1976
34. DeCaprio AP: Molecular mechanisms of diketone neurotoxicity. Chem Biol Interact 54(3):257–270, 1985
35. Schwetz BA, Mast TJ, Weigel RJ, Dill JA, Morrisey RE: Developmental toxicity of inhaled methyl ethyl ketone in Swiss mice. Fundam Appl Toxicol 16(4):742–748, 1991
36. O'Donoghue JL, Krasavage WJ, DiVincenzo GD, Ziegler PA: Commercial grade methyl heptyl ketone (5-methyl-2-octonone)

neurotoxicity: contribution of 5-nonanone. Toxicol Appl Pharmacol 62(6):307–316, 1982
37. Misvmi J, Nagano M: Experimental study on the enhancement of the neurotoxicity of methyl *n*-butyl ketone by non-neurotoxic aliphatic monoketones. Br J Ind Med 42(3):155–161, 1985
38. National Institute for Occupational Safety and Health: 1,3 Butadiene. NIOSH Current Intelligence Bulletin 41. Washington, DC: National Institute for Occupational Safety and Health, 1984
39. Maronpot RR: Ovarian toxicity and carcinogenicity in eight recent national toxicology program studies. Environ Health Perspect 73: 125–130, 1987
40. Irons RD, Smith CN, Stillman WS, Shah RS, Steinhagen WH, Leiderman LJ: Macrocytic-megaloblastic anemia in male NIH Swiss mice following repeated exposure to 1,3-butadiene. Toxicol Appl Pharmacol 85(3):450–455, 1986
41. Downs TD, Crane MM, Kim KW: Mortality among workers at a butadiene facility. Am J Ind Med 12(3):311–329, 1987
42. Norppa H, Sorsa M: Genetic toxicity of 1,3-butadiene and styrene. IARC Sci Publ 127:185–193, 1993
43. deMeester C: Genotoxic properties of 1,3-butadiene. Mutat Res 195(1–4):273–281, 1988
44. Some chemicals used in plastics and elastomers. In: IARC Monographs on the Evaluation of the Carcinogenic Risk of Chemicals to Humans. Vol 39. Lyon, France: International Agency for Research on Cancer, 1986, pp 155–179
45. Dahl AR, Birnbaum LS, Bond JA, Gervasi PG, Henederson RF: The fate of isoprene inhaled by rats: comparison to butadiene. Toxicol Appl Pharmacol 89(2):237–248, 1987
46. Rushmore T, Snyder R, Kalf G: Covalent binding of benzene and its metabolites to DNA in rabbit bone marrow mitochondria in vitro. Chem Biol Interact 49(1–2):133–154, 1984
47. Renz JF, Kalf GF: Role for interleukin-1 (IL-1) in benzene-induced hematotoxicity: inhibition of conversion of pre-IL-1 alpha to mature cytokine in murine macrophages by hydroquinone and prevention of benzene-induced hematotoxicity in mice by IL-1 alpha. Blood 78(4):938–944, 1991
48. Vaalavirta L, Tahti H: Effects of selected organic solvents on the astrocyte membrane ATPase in vitro. Clin Exp Pharmacol Physiol 22(4):293–294, 1995
49. Seaton MJ, Schlosser PM, Bond JA, Medinsky MA: Benzene metabolism by human live microsomes in relation to cytochrome P-450 2E1 activity. Carcinogenesis 15(9):1799–1806, 1994
50. Snyder R, Witz G, Goldstein BD: The toxicology of benzene. Environ Health Perspect 100:293–306, 1993
51. Chang RL, Wong CQ, Kline SA, Conney AH, Goldstein BD, Witz G: Mutagenicity of *trans, trans*-muconaldehyde and its metabolites in V79 cells. Environ Mol Mutagen 24(2):112–115, 1994
52. Zhang L, Robertson ML, Kolachana P, Davison AJ, Smith MT: Benzene metabolite, 1,2,4-benzenetriol, induces micronuclei and oxidative DNA damage in human lymphocytes and HL60 cells. Environ Mol Mutagen 21(4):339–348, 1993
53. Morimoto K, Wolff S: Increase in sister chromatic exchanges and perturbations of cell division kinetics in human lymphocytes by benzene metabolites. Cancer Res 40(4):1189–1193, 1980
54. Ciranni R, Barale R, Adler ID: Dose-related clastogenic effects induced by benzene in bone marrow cells and in differentiating spermatogonia of Swiss CD1 mice. Mutagenesis 6(5):417–421, 1991
55. Greenburg L: Benzol poisoning as an industrial hazard. Vll. Results of medical examination and clinical tests made to discover early signs of benzol poisoning in exposed workers. Public Health Rep 41:1526–1539, 1926
56. Greenburg L, Mayers MR, Goldwater L, Smith AR: Benzene (benzol) poisoning in the rotogravure printing industry in New York City. J Ind Hyg Toxicol 21:295–420, 1939
57. Savilahti M: More than 100 cases of benzene poisoning in a shoe factory. Arch Gewerbepathol Gewerbebyg 15:147–157, 1956
58. Vigliani EC: Leukemia associated with benzene exposure. Ann NY Acad Sci 271:143–151, 1976
59. Aksoy M, Erdem S, Dincol G: Types of leukemia in chronic benzene poisoning: a study in thirty-four patients. Acta Haematol 55:65–72, 1976
60. Rinsky RA, Young RJ, Smith AB: Leukemia in benzene workers. Am J Ind Med 2(3):217–245, 1981
61. Ishimaru T, Okada H, Tomiyasu T, et al: Occupational factors in the epidemiology of leukemia in Hiroshima and Nagasaki. Am J Epidemiol 93:157–165, 1971
62. Forni A, Cappellini A, Pacifico E, Vigliani EC: Chromosome changes and their evolution in subjects with past exposure to benzene. Arch Environ Health 23:285–391, 1971
63. Styles J, Richardson CR: Cytogenetic effects of benzene: dosimetric studies on rats exposed to benzene vapour. Mutat Res 135(3): 203–209, 1984
64. Tice RR, Vogt TF, Costa DL: Cytogenetic effects of inhaled benzene in murine bone marrow. Environ Sci Res 25:257–275, 1982
65. Lagorio S, Tagesson C, Forastiere F, Iavarone I, Axelson O, Carere A: Exposure to benzene and urinary concentrations of 8-hydroxydeoxyguanosine, a biological marker of oxidative damage to DNA. Occup Environ Med 51(11):739–743, 1994
66. Ward CO, Kuna RA, Snyder NK, Alsaker RD, Coate WB, Craig PH: Subchronic inhalation toxicity of benzene in rats and mice. Am J Ind Med 7:457–473, 1985
67. Xing SG, Shi X, Wu ZL, Chen JK, Wallace W, Whong WZ, Ong T: Transplacental genotoxicity of triethylenemelamine, benzene, and vinblastine in mice. Teratog Carcinog Mutagen 12(5):223–230, 1992
68. Snyder CA, Goldstein BD, Sellakumar AR, Albert RE: Evidence for hematotoxicity and tumorigenesis in rats exposed to 100 ppm benzene. Am J Ind Med 5(6):429–434, 1984
69. Maltoni C, Conti B, Cotti G: Benzene: a multipotential carcinogen; results of long-term bioassays performed at the Bologna Institute of Oncology. Am J Ind Med 4(5):589–630, 1983
70. Cronkite EP: Benzene hematotoxicity and leukemogenesis. Blood Cells 12:129–137, 1986
71. National Toxicology Program: Toxicology and Carcinogenesis Studies of Benzene. Research Triangle Park, NC: National Toxicology Program, 1986
72. Rinsky RA, Alexander B, Smith MD, et al: Benzene and leukemia: an epidemiological risk assessment. N Engl J Med 316:1044–1050, 1987
73. Messerschmitt J: Bone-marrow aplasias during pregnancy. Nouv Rev Fr Hematol 12:115–128, 1972
74. Brown-Woodman PD, Webster WS, Picker K, Huq F: In vitro assessment of individual and interactive effects of aromatic hydrocarbons on embryonic development of the rat. Reprod Toxicol 8(2):121–135, 1994
75. Nakajima T, Wang RS: Induction of cytochrome P450 by toluene. Int J Biochem 26(12):1333–1340, 1994
76. Flanagan RJ, Ives RJ: Volatile substance abuse. Bull Narc 46(2):49–78, 1994
77. Knox JW, Nelson JR: Permanent encephalopathy from toluene inhalation. N Engl J Med 275:1494–1496, 1966
78. Fornazzari L, Wilkonson DA, Kapur BM, Carlen PL: Cerebellar, cortical and functional impairment in toluene abusers. Acta Neurol Scand 67(6):319–329, 1983
79. Streicher HA, Gabow PA, Moss AH, Kano D, Kaehny WD: Syndromes of toluene sniffing in adults. Ann Intern Med 94(6):758–762, 1981
80. Pryor GT: A toluene-induced motor syndrome in rats resembling that seen in some human solvent abusers. Neurotoxicol Teratol 13(4):387–400, 1991
81. von Euler G, Ogren SO, Li XM, Fuxe K, Gustafsson JA: Persistent effects of subchronic toluene exposure on spatial learning and

memory, dopamine-mediated locomotor activity and dopamine D2 agonist binding in the rat. Toxicology 77(3):223–232, 1993
82. Huang J, Asaeda N, Takeuchi Y, Shibata E, Hisanaga N, Ono Y, Kato K: Dose dependent effects of chronic exposure to toluene on neuronal and glial cell marker proteins in the central nervous system of rats. Br J Ind Med 49(4):282–286, 1992
83. Johnson AC: The ototoxic effect of toluene and the influence of noise, acetyl salicylic acid, or genotype. A study in rats and mice. Scand Audiol Suppl 39:1–40, 1993
84. Reinhardt DF, Azar A, Maxfield ME, Smith PE, Mullin LS: Cardiac arrhythmias and aerosol "sniffing." Arch Environ Health 22:265, 1971
85. Hersh JH, Podruch PE, Rogers G, et al: Toluene embryopathy. J Pediatr 106:922–927, 1985
86. Courtney KD, Andrews JE, Springer J, et al: A perinatal study of toluene in CD-1 mice. Fundam Appl Toxicol 6:145–154, 1986
87. Gospe SM Jr, Saeed DB, Zhou SS, Zeman FJ: The effects of high-dose toluene on embryonic development in the rat. Pediatr Res 36(6):811–815, 1994
88. Klimisch HJ, Hellwig J, Hofmann A: Studies on the prenatal toxicity of toluene in rabbits following inhalation exposure and proposal of a pregnancy guidance value. Arch Toxicol 66(6):373–381, 1992
89. Tardif R, Plaa GL, Brodeur J: Influence of various mixtures of inhaled toluene and xylene on the biological monitoring of exposure to these solvents in rats. Can J Physiol Pharmacol 70(3):385–393, 1992
90. Korde VM, Phelps TJ, Bienkowski PR, White DC: Biodegradation of chlorinated aliphatics and aromatic compounds in total-recycle expanded-bed biofilm reactors. Appl Biochem Biotechnol 39–40: 631–641, 1993
91. Chen JD, Wang JD, Jang JP, Chen YY: Exposure to mixtures of solvents among paint workers and biochemical alterations of liver function. Br J Ind Med 48(10):696–701, 1991
92. Toftgard R, Halpert J, Gustafsson JA: Xylene induces a cytochrome P-450 isozyme in rat liver similar to the major isozyme induced by phenobarbital. Mol Pharmacol 23(1):265–271, 1983
93. Backes WL, Sequeira DJ, Cawley GF, Eyer CS: Relationship between hydrocarbon structure and induction of P450: effects on protein levels and enzyme activities. Xenobiotica 23(12):1353–1366, 1993
94. Unguary G, Varga B, Horvath E, Tatrai E, Folly C: Study on the role of maternal sex steroid production and metabolism in the embryotoxicity of *para*-xylene. Toxicology 19(3):263–268, 1981
95. Hass U, Lund SP, Simonsen L, Fries AS: Effects of prenatal exposure to xylene on postnatal development and behavior in rats. Neurotoxicol Teratol 17(3):341–349, 1995
96. Yamada K: Influence of lacquer thinner and some organic solvents on reproductive and accessory reproductive organs in the male rat. Biol Pharm Bull 16(4):425–427, 1993
97. Seppalainen AM, Laine A, Salmi T, Verkkala E, Hiihimaki V, Luukkonen R: Electroencephalographic findings during experimental human exposure to m-xylene. Arch Environ Health 46(1): 16–24, 1991
98. Solveig-Walles SA, Orsen I: Single-strand breaks in DNA of various organs of mice induced by styrene and styrene oxide. Cancer Lett 21(1):9–15, 1983
99. Harkonen H, Lindstrom K, Seppalainen AM, et al: Exposure-response relationship between styrene exposure and central nervous functions. Scand J Work Environ Health 4:53–59, 1978
100. Guengerich FP, Kim DH, Iwasaki M: Role of human cytochrome P-450 IIE1 (P-450 IIE1) in the oxidation of many low molecular weight cancer suspects. Chem Res Toxicol 4(2):168–179, 1991
101. Raucy JL, Kraner JC, Lasker JM: Bioactivation of halogenated hydrocarbons by cytochrome P450 2E1. Crit Rev Toxicol 23(1):1–20, 1993
102. Bagchi D, Bagchi M, Hassoun E, Stohs SJ: Carbon tetrachloride-induced urinary excretion of formaldehyde, malondialdehyde, acetaldehyde and acetone in rats. Pharmacology 47(3):209–216, 1993
103. elSisi AE, Earnest DL, Sipes IG: Vitamin A potentiation of carbon tetrachloride hepatotoxicity: role of liver macrophages and active oxygen species. Toxicol Appl Pharmacol 119(2):295–301, 1993
104. Morrow JD, Awad JA, Kato T, Takahashi K, Badr KF, Roberts LJ 2d, Burk RF: Formation of novel non-cyclooxygenase-derived prostanoids (F2-isoprostanes) in carbon tetrachloride hepatotoxicity. An animal model of lipid peroxidation. J Clin Invest 90(6): 2502–2507, 1992
105. Czaja MJ, Xu J, Alt E: Prevention of carbon tetrachloride-induced rat liver injury by soluble tumor necrosis factor receptor. Gastroenterology 108(6):1849–1854, 1995
106. Suzuki T, Nezu K, Sasaki H, Miyazawa T, Isono H: Cytotoxicity of chlorinated hydrocarbons and lipid peroxidation in isolated rat hepatocytes. Biol Pharm Bull 17(1):82–86, 1994
107. Toraason M, Breitenstein MJ, Wey HE: Reversible inhibition of intercellular communication among cardiac myocytes by halogenated hydrocarbons. Fundam Appl Toxicol 18(1):59–65, 1992
108. Schmitt-Graff A, Chakroun G, Gabbiani G: Modulation of perisinusoidal cell cytoskeletal features during experimental hepatic fibrosis. Virchows Arch A Pathol Anat Histopathol 422(2):99–107, 1993
109. Steup DR, Hall P, McMillan DA, Sipes IG: Time course of hepatic injury and recovery following coadministration of carbon tetrachloride and trichloroethylene in Fischer-344 rats. Toxicol Pathol 21 (3):327–334, 1993
110. Raymond P, Plaa GL: Ketone potentiation of haloalkane-induced hepato- and nephrotoxicity. I. Dose-response relationships. J Toxicol Environ Health 45(4):465–480, 1995
111. Tracey JP, Sherlock P: Hepatoma following carbon tetrachloride poisoning. NY State J Med 68:2202–2204, 1968
112. National Institute for Occupational Safety and Health: Current Intelligence Bulletin. Bull. 2, Trichloroethylene, June 6, 1975; Trichloroethylene, February 28, 1978; Bull. 28, Vinyl Halides Carcinogenicity, September 21, 1978; Bull. 25, Ethylene Dichloride, April 19, 1978; Bull. 1, Chloroprene, January 20, 1975; Bull. 9, Chloroform, March 15, 1976; Bull. 21, Trimellitic Anhydride (TMA), February 3, 1978; Bull. 8, 4,4-Diaminodiphenyl-methane (DDM), January 30, 1976; Bull. 15, Nitrosamines in Cutting Fluids, October 6, 1976; Bull. 30, Epichlorhydrin, October 12, 1978. Washington, DC: U.S. Government Printing Office
113. Maltoni C: Predictive value of carcinogenesis bioassays. Ann NY Acad Sci 271:431–447, 1976
114. Hatch GG, Mamay PD, Ayer ML, Castro BC, Nesnow S: Chemical enhancement of viral transformation in Syrian hamster embryo cells by gaseous and volatile chlorinated methanes and ethanes. Cancer Res 43(5):1945–1950, 1983
115. Wallace L, Zweidinger R, Erikson M, et al: Monitoring individual exposure: measurements of volatile organic compounds in breathing zone air, drinking water, and exhaled breath. Environ Int 8(16):269–282, 1982
116. Singh BH, Lillian D, Appleby A, Lobban L: Atmospheric formation of carbon tetrachloride from tetrachloroethylene. Environ Lett 10:253–256, 1975
117. Rikans LE, Hornbrook KR, Cai Y: Carbon tetrachloride hepatotoxicity as a function of age in female Fischer 344 rats. Mech Ageing Dev 76(2–3):89–99, 1994
118. Dias Gomez MI, Castro JA: Covalent binding of carbon tetrachloride metabolites to liver nuclear DNA, proteins, and lipids. Abstract No. 223. Toxicol Appl Pharmacol 45:315, 1970
119. Some Halogenated Hydrocarbons. In: Monographs on the Evaluation of the Carcinogenic Risk of Chemicals to Humans. vol. 20. Lyon, France: International Association of Research on Cancer, 1979

120. Larson JL, Sprankle CS, Butterworth BE: lack of chloroform-induced DNA repair in vitro and in vivo in hepatocytes of female B6C3F1 mice. Environ Mol Mutagen 23(2):132–136, 1994
121. Larson JL, Bull RJ: Species differences in the metabolism of trichloroethylene to the carcinogenic metabolites trechloroacetate and dichloroacetate. Toxicol Appl Pharmacol 115(2):278–285, 1992
122. Templin MV, Parker JC, Bull RJ: Relative formation of dichloroacetate and trichloroacetate from trichloroethylene in male B6C3F1 mice. Toxicol Appl Pharmacol 123(1):1–8, 1993
123. McLaren J, Boulikas T, Vanvakas S: Induction of poly(ADP-ribosyl)ation in the kidney after in vivo application of renal carcinogens. Toxicology 88(1–3):101–112, 1994
124. Wernisch M, Paya K, Palasser A: [Cardiovascular arrest after inhalation of leather glue.] Wien Med Wochenschr 141(3):71–74, 1991
125. Hoffmann P, Heinroth K, Richards D, Plews P, Toraason M: Depression of calcium dynamics in cardiac myocytes—a common mechanism of halogenated hydrocarbon anesthetics and solvents. J Mol Cell Cardiol 26(5):579–589, 1994
126. Rasmussen K, Jeppesen HJ, Sabroe S: Solvent-induced chronic toxic encephalopathy. Am J Ind Med 23(5):779–792, 1993
127. Okamoto T, Shiwaku K: Fatty acid composition in liver, serum and brain of rat inhalated with trichloroethylene. Exp Toxicol Pathol 46(2):133–141, 1994
128. Blain L, Lachapelle P, Molotchnikoff S: Evoked potentials are modified by long term exposure to trichloroethylene. Neurotoxicology 13(1):203–206, 1992
129. Crofton KM, Zhao X: Mid-frequency hearing loss in rats following inhalation exposure to trichloroethylene: evidence from reflex modification audiometry. Neurotoxicol Teratol 15(6):413–423, 1993
130. Rebert CS, Day VL, Matteucci MJ, Pryor GT: Sensory-evoked potentials in rats chronically exposed to trichloroethylene: predominant auditory dysfunction. Neurotoxicol Teratol 13(1):83–90, 1991
131. Anttila A, Pukkala E, Sallmen M, Hernberg S, Hemminki K: Cancer incidence among Finnish workers exposed to halogenated hydrocarbons. J Occup Environ Med 37(7):797–806, 1995
132. Heineman EF, Cocco P, Gomez MR, Dosemeci M, Stewart PA, Hayes RB, Zahm SH, Thomas TL, Blair A: Occupational exposure to chorinated aliphatic hydrocarbons and risk of astrocytc brain cancer. Am J Ind Med 26(2):155–169, 1994
133. Axelson O, Selden A, Andersson K, Hogstedt C: Updated and expanded Swedish cohort study on trichloroethylene and cancer risk. J Occup Med 36(5):556–562, 1994
134. Dawson BV, Johnson PD, Goldberg SJ, Ulreich JB: Cardiac teratogenesis of halogenated hydrocarbon-contaminated drinking water. J Am Coll Cardiol 21(6):1466–1472, 1993
135. Cosby NC, Dukelow WR: Toxicology of maternally ingested trichloroethylene (TCE) on embryonal and fetal development in mice and of TCE metabolites on in vitro fertilization. Fundam Appl Toxicol 19(2):268–274, 1992
136. Fort DJ, Stover EL, Rayburn JR, Hull M, Bantle JA: Evaluation of the developmental toxicity of trichloroethylene and detoxification metabolites using Xenopus. Teratog Carcinog Mutagen 13(1):35–45, 1993
137. Bove FJ, Fulcomer MC, Klotz JB, Esmart J, Dufficy EM, Savrin JE: Public drinking water contamination and birth outcomes. Am J Epidemiol 141(9):850–862, 1995
138. Constan AA, Yang RS, Baker DC, Benjamin SA: A unique pattern of hepatocyte proliferation in F344 rats following long-term exposures to low levels of a chemical mixture of groundwater contaminants. Carcinogenesis 16(2):303–310, 1995
139. Steup DR, Wiersma D, McMillan DA, Sipes IG: Pretreatment with drinking water solutions containing trichloroethylene or chloroform enhances the hepatotoxicity of carbon tetrachloride in Fischer 344 rats. Fundam Appl Toxicol 16(4):798–809, 1991
140. Murrell JC: Genetics and molecular biology of methanotrophs. FEMS Microbiol Rev 8(3–4):233–248, 1992
141. Hoffmann P, Heinroth K, Richards D, Plews P, Toraason M: Depression of calcium dynamics in cardiac myocytes—a common mechanism of halogenated hydrocarbon anesthetics and solvents. J Mol Cell Cardiol 26(5):579–589, 1994
142. Mutti A, Alinovi R, Bergamaschi E, Giagini C, Cavazzini S, Franchini I, Lauwreys RR, Bernard AM, Roels H, Gelpi E, et al: Nephropathies and exposure to perchloroethylene in dry-cleaners. Lancet 340(8813):189–193, 1992
143. Weiss NS: Cancer in relation to occupational exposure to perchloroethylene. Cancer Causes Control 6(3):257–266, 1995
144. Narotsky MG, Kavlock RJ: A multidisciplinary approach to toxicological screening: II. Developmental toxicity. J Toxicol Environ Health 45(2):145–171, 1995
145. Aggazzotti G, Fantuzzi G, Righi E, Predieri G, Gobba FM, Paltrinieri M, Cavalleri A: Occupational and environmental exposure to perchloroethylene (PCE) in dry cleaners and their family members. Arch Environ Health 49(6):487–493, 1994
146. Karlsson JE, Rosengren LE, Kjellstrand P, Haglid KG: Effects of low-dose inhalation of three chlorinated aliphatic organic solvents on deoxyribonucleic acid in gerbil brain. Scand J Work Environ Health 13(5):453–458, 1987
147. Mazzullo M, Colacci A, Grilli S, et al: 1,1,2-Trichloroethane: evidence of genotoxicity from short-term tests. Jpn J Cancer Res 77: 532–539, 1986
148. Creech JL Jr, Johnson MN: Angiosarcoma of liver in the manufacture of polyvinyl chloride. J Occup Med 16:150, 1974
149. Riordan SM, Loo CK, Haber RW, Thomas MC: Vinyl chloride related hepatic angiosarcoma in a polyvinyl chloride autoclave cleaner in Australia. Med J Aust 155(2):125–128, 1991
150. Wong O, Whorton MD, Foliart DE, Ragland D: An industry-wide epidemiologic study of vinyl chloride workers, 1942–1982. Am J Ind Med 20(3):317–334, 1991
151. Nair J, Barbin A, Guichard Y, Bartsch H: 1,N6-ethenodeoxyadenosine and 3,N4-ethenodeoxycytine in liver DNA from humans and untreated rodents detected by immunoaffinity/32P-postlabeling. Carcinogenesis 16(3):613–617, 1995
152. Misra RR, Chiang SY, Swenberg JA: A comparison of two ultrasensitive methods for measuring 1,N6-etheno-2′-deoxyadenosine and 3,N4-etheno-2′-deoxycytidine in cellular DNA. Carcinogenesis 15(8):1647–1652, 1994
153. Dosanjh MD, Chenna A, Kim E, Fraenkel-Condrat H, Samson L, Singer B: All four known cyclic adducts formed in DNA by the vinylochloride metabolite chloroacetaldehyde are released by a human DNA glycosylase. Proc Natl Acad Sci USA 91(3):1024–1028, 1994
154. Cheng KC, Preston BD, Cahill DS, Dosanjh MK, Singer B, Loeb LA: Proc Natl Acad Sci USA 88(22):9974–9978, 1991
155. Trivers GE, Cawley HI, DeBenedetti VM, Hosstein M, Marion MJ, Bennett WP, Hoover ML, Prives CC, Tamburro CC, Harris CC: Anti-p53 antibodies in sera of workers occupationally exposed to vinyl chloride. J Natl Cancer Inst 87(18):1400–1407, 1995
156. Froment O, Boivin S, Barbin A, Bancel B, Trepo C, Marion MJ: Mutagenesis of ras proto-oncogenes in rat liver tumors induced by vinyl chloride. Cancer Res 54(20):5340–5345, 1994
157. DeVivo I, Marion MJ, Smith SJ, Carney WP, Brandt-Rauf PW: Mutant c-Ki-ras p21 protein in chemical carcinogenesis in humans exposed to vinyl chloride. Cancer Causes Control 5(3):273–278, 1994
158. Heath CW Jr, Dumont CR, Gamble J, Waxweiler RJ: Chromosomal damage in men occupationally exposed to vinyl chloride monomer and other chemicals. Environ Res 14:68–72, 1977
159. Bartsch H, Malaveille C, Barbin A, et al: Alkylating and mutagenic metabolites of halogenated olefins produced by human and animal tissues. Proc Am Assoc Cancer Res 17:17, 1976

160. Ban M, Hettich D, Huguet N, Cavelier L: Nephrotoxicity mechanism of 1,1-dichloroethylene in mice. Toxicol Lett 78(2):87–92, 1995
161. Dowsley TF, Forkert PG, Benesch LA, Bolton JL: Reaction of glutathione with the electrophilic metabolites of 1,1-dichloroethylene. Chem Biol Interact 95(3):227–244, 1995
162. Speerschneider P, Dekant W: Renal tumorigenicity of 1,1-dichloroethene in mice: the role of male-specific expression of cytochrome p450 2E1 in the renal bioactivation of 1,1-dichloroethene. Toxicol Appl Pharmacol 130(1):48–56, 1995
163. Goldberg SJ, Dawson BV, Johnson PD, Hoyme HE, Ulreich JB: Cardiac teratogenicity of dichloroethylene in a chick model. Pediatr Res 32(1):23–26, 1992
164. Lane BW, Riddle BL, Borzelleca JF: Effects of 1,2-dichloroethane and 1,1,1-trichloroethane in drinking water on reproduction and development in mice. Toxicol Appl Pharmacol 63(3):409–421, 1982
165. Toxicological Profile for 1,2-Dichloroethane. Agency for Toxic Substances and Disease Registry, U.S. Public Health Service, 1989
166. Khan S, Sood C, O'Brien PJ: Molecular mechanisms of dibromoalkane cytotoxicity in isolated rat hepatocytes. Biochem Pharmacol 45(2):439–447, 1993
167. Danni O, Aragno M, Tamagno E, Ugazio G: In vivo studies on halogen compound interactions. IV. Interaction among different halogen derivatives with and without synergistic action on liver toxicity. Res Commun Chem Pathol Pharmacol 76(3):355–366, 1992
168. Ratcliffe JM, Schrader SM, Steenland K, Clapp DE, Turner T, Hornung RW: Semen quality in papaya workers with long term exposure to ethylene dibromide. Br J Ind Med 44(5):317–326, 1987
169. Kulkarni AP, Edwards J, Richards IS: Metabolism of 1,2-dibromoethane in the human fetal liver. Gen Pharmacol 23(1):1–5, 1992
170. Mitra A, Hilbelink DR, Dwornik JJ, Kulkarni A: A novel model to assess developmental toxicity of dihaloalkanes in humans: bioactivation of 1,2-dibromoethane by the isozymes of human fetal liver glutathione S-transferase. Teratog Carcinog Mutagen 12(3):113–127, 1992
171. Mitra A, Hilbelink DR, Dwornik JJ, Kulkarni A: Rat hepatic glutathione S-transferase-mediated embryotoxic bioactivation of ethylene dibromide. Teratology 46(5):439–446, 1992
172. Ott MG, Scharnweber HC, Langner RR: The mortality experience of 161 employees exposed to ethylene dibromide in two production units. Report submitted to NIOSH by the Dow Chemical Co., Midland, MI, March 1977
173. Cmarik JL, Humphreys WG, Bruner KL, Lloyd RS, Tibbetts C, Guengerich FP: Mutation spectrum and sequence alkylation selectivity resulting from modification of bacteriophage M13mp18DNA with *S*-(2-chloroethyl)glutathione. Evidence for a role of *S*-(2-N7-guanyl)ethyl)glutathione as a mutagenic lesion formed from ethylene dibromide. J Biol Chem 267(10):6672–6679, 1992
174. Sekita H, Takeda M, Uchiyama M: Analysis of pesticide residues in foods: 33. Determination of ethylene dibromide residues in litchi (lychee) fruits imported from Formosa. Eisei Shikenjo Hokoku 99:130–132, 1981
175. Yang RS, Witt KL, Alden CJ, Cockerham LG: Toxicology of methyl bromide. Rev Environ Contam Toxicol 142:65–85, 1995
176. Hustinx WN, van de Laar RT, van Huffelen AC, Verwey JC, Meulenbelt J, Savelkoul TJ: Systemic effects of inhalational methyl bromide poisoning: a study of nine cases occupationally exposed to inadvertent spread during fumigation. Br J Ind Med 50(2):155–159, 1993
177. Fuortes LJ: A case of fatal methyl bromide poisoning. Vet Hum Toxicol 34(3):240–241, 1992
178. Xu DG, He HZ, Zhang GG, Gansewendt B, Peter H, Bolt HM: DNA methylation of monohalogenated methanes of F344 rats. J Tongjii Med Univ 13(2):100–104, 1993
179. Gansewendt B, Foest U, Xu D, Hallier E, Bolt HM, Peter H: Formation of DNA adducts in F-344 rats after oral administration or inhalation of [^{14}C]methyl bromide. Food Chem Toxicol 29(8):557–563, 1991
180. Goergens HW, Hallier E, Muller A, Bolt HM: Macromolecular adducts in the use of methyl bromide as a fumigant. Toxicol Lett 72(1–3):199–203, 1994
181. Hallier E, Langhof T, Dannappel D, Leutbecher M, Schroder K, Goergens HW, Muller A, Bolt HM: Polymorphism of glutathione conjugation of methyl bromide, ethylene oxide and dichloromethane in human blood: influence on the induction of sister chromatid exchanges (SCE) in lymphocytes. Arch Toxicol 67(3):173–178, 1993
182. Hallier E, Schroder KR, Asmuth K, Dommermuth A, Aust B, Goergens HW: Metabolism of dichloromethane (methylene chloride) to formaldehyde in human erythrocytes: influence of polymorphism of glutathione transferase theta (GST T1-1). Arch Toxicol 68(7): 423–427, 1994
183. Khachatryan EA: The occurrence of lung cancer among people working with chloroprene. Probl Oncol 18:85, 1972
184. Pell S: Mortality of workers exposed to chloroprene. J Occup Med 20:21–29, 1978
185. Westphal GA, Blaszkewicz M, Leutbecher M, Muller A, Hallier E, Boldt HM: Bacterial mutagenicity of 2-chloro-1,3-butadiene (chloroprene) caused by decomposition products. Arch Toxicol 68(2): 79–84, 1994
186. Toxicology. In: Clayton GD, Clayton FE (eds): Patty's Industrial Hygiene and Toxicology. 3rd ed. vol. 2B. New York: John Wiley, 1981
187. Brennon PD: Addiction to aerosol treatment. Br Med J 287:1877, 1983
188. Longstaff E, Robinson M, Bradbrook C, Styles JA, Purchase IF: Genotoxicity and carcinogenicity of fluorocarbons: assessment by short-term in vitro tests and chronic exposure in rats. Toxicol Appl Pharmacol 72(1):15–31, 1984
189. Simmons JE, McDonald A, Seely JC, Sey YM: Potentiation of carbon tetrachloride hepatotoxicity by inhaled methanol: time course of injury and recovery. J Toxicol Environ Health 46(2):203–216, 1995
190. d'Alessandro A, Osterloh JD, Chuwers P, Quinlan PJ, Kelly TJ, Becker CE: Formate in serum and urine after controlled methanol exposure at the threshold limit value. Environ Health Perspect 102(2): 178–181, 1994
191. Chen JC, Schneiderman JF, Wortzman G: Methanol poisoning: bilateral putaminal and cerebellar cortical lesions on CT and MR. J Comput Assist Tomogr 15(3):522–524, 1991
192. Neymeyer VR, Tephly TR: Detection and quantification of 10-formyltetrahydrofolate dehydrogenase (10-FTHFDH) in rat retina, optic nerve, and brain. Life Sci 54(22):PL395–399, 1994
193. Lee EW, Garner CD, Terzo TS: A rat model manifesting methanol-induced visual dysfunction suitable for both acute and long-term exposure studies. Toxicol Appl Pharmacol 128(2):199–206, 1994
194. Garner CD, Lee EW, Terzo TS, Louis-Ferdinand RT: Role of retinal metabolism in methanol-induced retinal toxicity. J Toxicol Environ Health 44(1):43–56, 1995
195. Palatnick W, Redman LW, Sitar DS, Tenegein M: Methanol half-life during ethanol administration: implications for management of methanol poisoning. Ann Emerg Med 26(2):202–207, 1995
196. Frenia ML, Schauben JL: Methanol inhalation toxicity. Ann Emerg Med 22(12):1919–1923, 1993
197. Hewlett TP, McMartin KE, Lauro AJ, Ragan FA Jr: Ethylene glycol poisoning: the value of glycolic acid determinations for diagnosis and treatment. J Toxicol Clin Toxicol 24(5):389–402, 1986
198. Evans W, David EJ: Biodegradation of mono-, di-, and triethylene glycols in river waters under controlled laboratory conditions. Water Res 8(2):97–100, 1974
199. Miller ER, Ayres JA, Young JT, McKenna MJ: Ethylene glycol monomethyl ether. I. Subchronic vapor inhalation study in rats and rabbits. Fundam Appl Toxicol 3(1):49–54, 1983

200. Ku WW, Ghanayem BI, Chapin RE, Wine RN: Comparison of the testicular effects of 2-methoxyethanol (ME) in rats and guinea pigs. Exp Mol Pathol 61(2):119–133, 1994
201. Vachhrajani KD, Dutta KK: Stage specific effect during one seminiferous epithelial cycle following ethylene glycol monomethyl ether exposure in rats. Indian J Exp Biol 30(10):892–896, 1992
202. Holladay SD, Comment CE, Kwon J, Luster MI: Fetal hematopoietic alterations after maternal exposure to ethylene glycol monomethyl ether: prolymphoid cell targeting. Toxicol Appl Pharmacol 129(1):53–60, 1994
203. Lee J, Trad CH, Butterfield DA: Electron paramagnetic resonance studies of the effects of methoxyacetic acid, a teratologic toxin, on human erythrocyte membranes. Toxicology 83(1–3):131–148, 1993
204. Cook RR, Bodner KM, Kolesar RC, et al: A cross-sectional study of ethylene glycol monomethyl ether process employees. Arch Environ Health 37(6):346–351, 1982
205. Hoflack JC, Lambolez L, Elias Z, Vasseur P: Mutagenicity of ethylene glycol ethers and of their metabolites in *Salmonella typhimurium* his-. Mutat Res 341(4):281–287, 1995
206. Au WW, Morris DL, Legator MS: Evaluation of the clastogenic effects of 2-methoxyethanol in mice. Mutat Res 300(3–4):273–279, 1993
207. Leach CL, Hatoum NS, Ratajczak HV, Zeiss CR, Garvin PJ: Evidence of immunologic control of lung injury induced by trimellitic anhydride. Am Rev Respir Dis 137(1):186–190, 1988
208. Ducatman AM, Conwill DE, Crawl J: Germ cell tumors of the testicles among aircraft repairmen. J Urol 136(4):834–836, 1986
209. Levin SM, Baker DB, Landrigan PJ, Monaghan SV, Frumin E, Braithwaite M: Testicular cancer in leather tanners exposed to dimethylformamide. Lancet 2(8568):1153, 1987
210. Chen JL, Fayerweather WE, Pell S: Cancer incidence of workers exposed to dimethylformamide and/or acrylonitrile. J Occup Med 30(10):813–818, 1988
211. Malley LA, Slone TW Jr, Van-Pelt C, Elliott GS, Ross PE, Stadler JC, Kennedy GL Jr: Chronic toxicity/oncogenicity of dimethylformamide in rats and mice following inhalation exposure. Fundam Appl Toxicol 23(2):268–279, 1994
212. Hurtt ME, Placke ME, Killinger JM, Singer AW, Kennedy GL Jr: 13-week inhalation toxicity study of dimethylformamide (DMF) in cynomolgus monkeys. Fundam Appl Toxicol 18(4):596–601, 1992
213. Kennedy GL Jr, Sherman H: Acute and subchronic toxicity of dimethylformamide and dimethylacetamide following various routes of administration. Drug Chem Toxicol 9(2):147–170, 1986
214. Costa LG, Deng H, Gregotti C, Manzo L, Faustman EM, Bergmark E, Calleman CJ: Comparative studies on the neuro- and reproductive toxicity of acrylamide and its epoxide metabolite glycidamide in the rat. Neurotoxicology 13(1):219–224, 1992
215. Costa LG, Deng H, Calleman CJ, Bergmark E: Evaluation of the neurotoxicity of glycidamide, an epoxide metabolite of acrylamide: behavioral, neurochemical and morphological studies. Toxicology 98(1–3):151–161, 1995
216. Lynch JJ 3d, Silveira LC, Perry VH, Merigan WH: Visual effects of damage to P ganglion cells in macaques. Vis Neurosci 8(6):575–583, 1992
217. Chauhan NB, Spencer PS, Sabri MI: Acrylamide-induced depletion of microtubule-associated proteins (MAP1 and MAP2) in the rat extrapyramidal system. Brain Res 602(1):111–118, 1993
218. Jortner BS, Ehrich M: Comparison of toxicities of acrylamide and 2,5-hexanedione in hens and rats on 3-week dosing regimens. J Toxicol Environ Health 39(4):417–428, 1993
219. Sickles DW: Toxic neurofilamentous axonopathies and fast anterograde axonal transport. III. Recovery from single injections and multiple dosing effects of acrylamide and 2,5-hexanedione. Toxicol Appl Pharmacol 108(3):390–396, 1991
220. Adler ID, Ingwersen I, Kliesch U, el Tarras A: Clastogenic effects of acrylamide in mouse bone marrow cells. Mutat Res 206(3):379–385, 1988
221. Pacchierotti F, Tiveron C, D'Archivio M, Bassani B, Cordelli E, Leter G, Spano M: Acrylamide-induced chromosomal damage in male mouse germ cells detected by cytogenetic analysis of one-cell zygotes. Mutat Res 309(2):273–284, 1994
222. Adler ID, Zouh R, Schmid E: Perturbation of cell division by acrylamide in vitro and in vivo. Mutat Res 301(4):249–254, 1993
223. Butterworth BE, Eldridge SR, Sprankle CS, Working PK, Bentley KS, Hurtt ME: Tissue-specific genotoxic effects of acrylamide and acrylonitrile. Environ Mol Mutagen 20(3):148–155, 1992
224. Gutierrez-Espeleta GA, Hughes LA, Piegorsch WW, Shelby MD, Generoso WM: Acrylamide: dermal exposure produces genetic damage in male mouse germ cells. Fundam Appl Toxicol 18(2): 189–192, 1992
225. Sobel W, Bond GG, Parsons TW, Brenner FE: Acrylamide cohort mortality study. Br J Ind Med 43(11):785–788, 1986
226. Costa LG, Manzo L: Biochemical markers of neurotoxicity: research strategies and epidemiological applications. Toxicol Lett 77(1–3):137–144, 1995
227. Calleman CJ, Wu Y, He F, Tian G, Bergmark E, Zhang S, Deng H, Wang Y, Crofton KM, Fennell T, et al: Relationships between biomarkers of exposure and neurological effects in a group of workers exposed to acrylamide. Toxicol Appl Pharmacol 126(2):361–371, 1994
228. Leikauf GD: Mechanisms of aldehyde-induced bronchial reactivity: role of airway epithelium. Res Rep Health Eff Inst 49(1):1–35, 1992
229. Swiecichowski AL, Long KJ, Miller ML, Leikauf GD: Formaldehyde-induced airway hyperreactivity in vivo and ex vivo in guinea pigs. Environ Res 61(2):185–199, 1993
230. Monticello TM, Swenberg JA, Gross EA, Leininger JR, Kimbell JS, Seilkop S, Starr TB, Gibson JE, Morgan KT: Correlation of regional and nonlinear formaldehyde-induced nasal cancer with proliferating populations of cells. Cancer Res 56(5):1012–1022, 1996
231. Til HP, Woutersen RA, Feron VJ, Hollanders VH, Falke HE, Clary JJ: Two-year drinking water study of formaldehyde in rats. Food Chem Toxicol 27(2):77–87, 1989
232. Graves RJ, Trueman P, Jones S, Green T: DNA sequence analysis of methylene chloride-induced HPRT mutations in Chinese hamster ovary cells: comparison with the mutation spectrum obtained for 1,2-dibromoethane and formaldehyde. Mutagenesis 11(3):229–233, 1996
233. Kuykendall JR, Bogdanffy MS: Efficiency of DNA-histone crosslinking induced by saturated and unsaturated aldehydes in vitro. Mutat Res 283(2):131–136, 1992
234. Casanova M, Morgan KT, Gross EA, Moss OR, Heck HA: DNA-protein cross-links and cell replication at specific sites in the nose of F344 rats exposed subchronically to formaldehyde. Fundam Appl Toxicol 23(4):525–536, 1994
235. Yager JW, Cohn KL, Spear RC, Fisher JM, Morse L: Sister chromatid exchanges in lymphocytes of anatomy students exposed to formaldehyde-embalming solution. Mutat Res 174(2):135–139, 1986
236. Ballarin C, Sarto G, Giacomelli L, Bartolucci GB, Clonfero E: Micronucleated cells in nasal mucosa of formaldehyde-exposed workers. Mutat Res 280(1):1–7, 1992
237. Shaham J, Bomstein Y, Meltzer A, Kaufman Z, Palma E, Ribak J: DNA-protein crosslinks, a biomarker of exposure to formaldehyde—in vitro. Carcinogenesis 17(1):121–125, 1996
238. Hallier E, Schroder KR, Asmuth K, Dommermuth A, Aust B, Goergens HW: Metabolism of dichloromethane (methylene chloride) to formaldehyde in human erythrocytes: influence of polymorphism on glutathione transferase theta (GST T1-1). Arch Toxicol 68(7): 423–427, 1994

239. Dennis KJ, Ichinose T, Miller M, Shibamoto T: Gas chromatographic determination of vapor-phase biomarkers formed from rats dosed with CCl_4. J Appl Toxicol 13(4):301–303, 1993
240. Majumder PK, Kumar VL: Inhibitory effects of formaldehyde on the reproductive system of male rats. Indian J Physiol Pharmacol 39(1):80–82, 1995
241. Janssens SP, Musto SW, Hutchison WG, Spence C, Witten M, Jung W, Hales CA: Cyclooxygenase and lipoxygenase inhibition by BW-755C reduces acrolein smoke-induced acute lung injury. J Appl Physiol 77(2):888–895, 1994
242. Awasthi S, Boor PJ: Lipid peroxidation and oxidative stress during acute allylamine-induced cardiovascular toxicity. J Vasc Res 31(1):33–41, 1994
243. Kuykendall JR, Bogdanffy MS: Efficiency of DNA-histone cross-linking induced by saturated and unsaturated aldehydes in vitro. Mutat Res 283(2):131–136, 1992
244. Eder E, Deininger C, Deininger D, Weinfurtner E: Genotoxicity of 2-halosubstituted enals and 2-chloroacrylonitrile in the Ames test and the SOS-chromotest. Mutat Res 322(4):321–328, 1994
245. Parent RA, Caravello HE, Christian MS, Hoberman AM: Developmental toxicity of acrolein in New Zealand white rabbits. Fundam Appl Toxicol 20(2):248–256, 1993
246. Parent RA, Caravello HE, Hoberman AM: Reproductive study of acrolein on two generations of rats. Fundam Appl Toxicol 19(2): 228–237, 1992
247. Leikauf GD: Mechanisms of aldehyde-induced bronchial reactivity: role of airway epithelium. Res Rep Health Eff Inst 49:1–35, 1992
248. Feron VJ, Til HP, de-Vrijer F, Woutersen RA, Cassec FR, van-Bladeren PJ: Aldehydes: occurrence, carcinogenic potential, mechanism of action and risk assessment. Mutat Res 259(3–4):363–385, 1991
249. Allen N, Mendell JR, Billmaier DJ, et al: Toxic polyneuropathy due to methyl *n*-butyl ketone. Arch Neurol 32:209–218, 1975
250. Spencer PS, Schaumburg HH: Ultrastructural studies of the dying-back process. IV. Differential vulnerability of PNS and CNS fibers in experimental central-peripheral distal axonopathies. J Neuropathol Exp Neurol 36:300–320, 1977
251. Schwetz BA, Mast TJ, Weigel RJ, Dill JA, Morrissey RE: Developmental toxicity of inhaled methyl ethyl ketone in Swiss mice. Fundam Appl Toxicol 16(4):742–748, 1991
252. Rosenkranz HS, Klopman G: 1,4-Dioxane: prediction of in vivo clastogenicity. Mutat Res 280(4):245–251, 1992
253. Goldsworthy TL, Monticello TM, Morgan KT, Bermudez E, Wilson DM, Jackh R, Butterworth BE: Examination of potential mechanisms of carcinogenicity of 1,4-dioxane in rat nasal epithelial cells and hepatocytes. Arch Toxicol 65(1):1–9, 1991
254. Hamilton A: The making of artificial silk in the United States and some of the dangers attending it. In U.S. Department of Labor, Division of Labor Standards: Discussion of Industrial Accidents and Diseases. Bulletin No. 10. Washington, DC: Government Printing Office, 1937, pp 151–160
255. Lilis R: Behavioral effects of occupational carbon disulfide exposure. In Xintaras C, Johnson BL, de Groot I (eds): Behavioral Toxicology, Early Detection of Occupational Hazards. Washington, DC: National Institute for Occupational Safety and Health, 1974, pp 51–59
256. Hirata M, Ogawa Y, Okayama A, Goto S: Changes in auditory brainstem response in rats chronically exposed to carbon disulfide. Arch Toxicol 66(5):334–338, 1992
257. Herr DW, Boyes WK, Dyer RS: Alterations in rat flash and pattern reversal evoked potentials after acute or repeated administration of carbon disulfide (CS2). Fundam Appl Toxicol 18(3):328–342, 1992
258. de Gandarias JM, Echevarria E, Mugica J, Serrano R, Casis L: Changes in brain enkephalin immunostaining after acute carbon disulfide exposure in rats. J Biochem Toxicol 9(2):59–62, 1994
259. Valentine WM, Graham DG, Anthony DC: Covalent cross-linking of erythrocyte spectrin by carbon disulfide in vivo. Toxicol Appl Pharmacol 121(1):71–77, 1993
260. Valentine WM, Amarnath V, Amarnath K, Rimmele F, Graham DG: Carbon disulfide mediated protein cross-linking by *N,N*-diethyldithiocarbamate. Chem Res Toxicol 8(1):96–102, 1995
261. DeCarpio AP, Spink DC, Chen X, Fowke JH, Zhu M, Bank S: Characterization of isothiocyanates, thioureas, and other lysine adduction products in carbon disulfide-treated peptides and protein. Chem Res Toxicol 5(4):496–504, 1992
262. Djuric D, Surducki N, Berkes I: Iodine-azide test on urine of persons exposed to carbon disulfide. Br J Ind Med 22:321–323, 1965
263. Barnes JM, Magee PN: Some toxic properties of dimethylnitrosamine. Br J Ind Med 11:167, 1954
264. Magee PN, Barnes JM: Carcinogenic nitroso compounds. Adv Cancer Res 10:163, 1956
265. Magee PN, Farber E: Toxic liver injury and carcinogenesis: methylation of rat-liver nucleic acids by dimethylnitrosamine in vivo. Biochem J 83:114, 1962
266. Druckrey H, Preussman R, Ivankovic S, Schmahl D: Organotrope carcinogene Wirkungen bei 65 verschiedenen *N*-Nitroso-Verbindungen an BD-Ratten. Z Krebsforsch 69:103–201, 1967
267. Enzmann H, Zerban H, Kopp-Schneider A, Loser E, Bannach P: Effects of low doses of *N*-nitrosomorpholine on the development of early stages of hepatocarcinogenesis. Carcinogenesis 16(7):1513–1518, 1995
268. Baskaran K, Laconi S, Reddy MK: Transformation of hamster pancreatic duct cells by 4-(methylnitrosamino)-1-butanone (NNK), in vitro. Carcinogenesis 15(11):2461–2466, 1994
269. Lozano JC, Nakazawa H, Cros MP, Cabral R, Yamasaki H: G → A mutations in p53 and Ha-ras genes in esophageal papillomas induced by *N*-nitrosomethylbenzylamine in two strains of rats. Mol Carcinog 9(1):33–39, 1994
270. Georgiadis P, Xu YZ, Swann PF: Nitrosamine-induced cancer: *O*4-alkylthymine produces sites of DNA hyperflexibility. Biochemistry 30(50):11725–11732, 1991
271. Hoffmann D, Brunnemann KD, Prokopczyk B, Djordjevic MV: Tobacco-specific *N*-nitrosamines and Areca-derived *N*-nitrosamines: chemistry, biochemistry, carcinogenicity, and relevance to humans. J Toxicol Environ Health 41(1):1–52, 1994
272. Weitberg AB, Corvese D: Oxygen radicals potentiate the genetic toxicity of tobacco-specific nitrosamines. Clin Genet 43(2):88–91, 1993
273. Jorquera R, Castonguay A, Schuller HM: DNA single-strand breaks and toxicity induced by 4-(methyl-nitrosamino)-1-(3-pyridyl)-1-butanone or *N*-nitrosodimethylamine in hamster and rat liver. Carcinogenesis 15(2):389–394, 1994
274. Schuller HM, Jorquera R, Lu X, Riechert A, Castonguay A: Transplacental carcinogenicity of low doses of 4-(methylnitrosamino)-1-(3-pyridyl)-1-butanone administered subcutaneously or intratracheally to hamsters. J Cancer Res Clin Oncol 120(4): 200–203, 1994
275. Chung FL, Xu Y: Increased 8-oxodeoxyguanosine levels in lung DNA of A/J mice and F344 rats treated with the tobacco-specific nitrosamine 4-(methylnitrosamino)-1-(3-pyridyl)-1-butanone. Carcinogenesis 13(7):1269–1272, 1992
276. Belinsky SA, Devereux TR, Foley JF, Maronpot RR, Anderson MW: Role of the alveolar type II cell in the development and progression of pulmonary tumors induced by 4-(methylnitrosamino)-1-(3-pyridyl)-1-butanone in the A/J mouse. Cancer Res 52(11): 3164–3173, 1992
277. Tumorigenicity of the tobacco-specific carcinogen 4-(methylnitrosamino)-1-(3 pyridyl)-1-butanone in infant mice. Cancer Lett 58(3):177–181, 1991
278. Anderson LM, Carter JP, Driver CL, Logsdon DL, Kovatch RM, Giner-Sorolla A: Enhancement of tumorigenesis by *N*-nitrosodi-

ethylamine, *N*-nitrosopyrrolidine and *N*6-(methylnitroso)-adenosine by ethanol. Cancer Lett 68(1):61–66, 1993
279. Yoshimura H, Takemoto K: Effect of cigarette smoking and/or *N*-bis(2-hydroxypropyl)nitrosamine (DHPN) on the development of lung and pleural tumors in rats induced by administration of asbestos. Sangyo Igaku 33(2):81–93, 1991
280. Prokopczyk B, Rivenson A, Hoffmann D: A study of betel quid carcinogenesis. IX. Comparative carcinogenicity of 3-(methylnitrosamino)propionitrile and 4-(methylnitrosamino)-1-(3-pyridyl)-1-butanone upon local application to mouse skin and rat oral mucosa. Cancer Lett 60(2):153–157, 1991
281. Janzowski C, Landsiedel R, Golzer P, Eisenbrand G: Mitochondrial formation of beta-oxopropyl metabolites from bladder carcinogenic omega-carboxyalkylnitrosamines. Chem Biol Interact 90(1):23–33, 1994
282. Pairojkul C, Shirai T, Hirohashi S, Tharnavit W, Bhudisawat W, Utaravicien T, Itoh M, Itoh N: Multistage carcinogenesis of liver-fluke-associated cholangiocarcinoma in Thailand. Princess Takamatsu Symp 22:77–86, 1991
283. Siddiqi MA, Tricker AR, Kumar R, Fazili Z, Preussmann R: Dietary sources of *N*-nitrosamines in a high-risk area for oesophageal cancer—Kashmir, India. IARC Sci Publ 1991(105):210–213
284. Wacker DC, Spiegelhalder B, Preussmann R: New sulfenamide accelerators derived from 'safe' amines for the rubber and tyre industry. IARC Sci Publ 1991(105):592–594
285. Deschamps D, Leport M, Cordier S, Laurent AM, Festy B, Hamard H, Renard G, Pouliquen Y, Conso F: Toxicity of ethylene oxide on the crystalline lens in an occupational milieu. Difficulty of epidemiologic surveys of cataract. J Fr Ophthalmol 13(4):189–197, 1990
286. Nagata H, Ohkoshi N, Kanazawa I, Oka N, Ohnishi A: Rapid axonal transport velocity is reduced in experimental ethylene oxide neuropathy. Mol Chem Neuropathol 17(3):209–217, 1992
287. Kolman A, Bohusova T, Lambert B, Simons JW: Induction of 6-thioguanine-resistant mutants in human diploid fibroblasts in vitro with ethylene oxide. Environ Mol Mutagen 19(2):93–97, 1992
288. Oesch F, Hengstler JG, Arand M, Fuchs J: Detection of primary DNA damage: applicability to biomonitoring of genotoxic occupational exposure and in clinical therapy. Pharmacogenetics 5: S118–S122, 1995
289. Schulte PA, Boeniger M, Walker JT, Schober SE, Pereira MA, Gulati DK, Wojciechowski JP, Garza A, Froelich R, Strauss G, et al: Biologic markers in hospital workers exposed to low levels of ethylene oxide. Mutat Res 278(4):237–251, 1992
290. Tates AD, Grummt T, Tornqvist M, Farmer PB, van Dam FJ, van Mossel H, Schoemaker HM, Osterman-Golkar S, Uebel C, Tang YS, et al: Biological and chemical monitoring of occupational exposure to ethylene oxide. Mutat Res 250(1–2):483–497, 1991
291. Mayer J, Warburton D, Jeffrey AM, Pero R, Walles S, Andrews L, Toor M, Latriano L, Wazneh L, Tang D, et al: Biological markers in ethylene oxide-exposed workers and controls. Mutat Res 248(1): 163–176, 1991
292. Polifka JE, Rutledge JC, Kimmel GL, Dellarco V, Generoso WM: Exposure to ethylene oxide during the early zygotic period induces skeletal anomalies in mouse fetuses. Teratology 53(1):1–9, 1996
293. Vogel EW, Natarajan AT: DNA damage and repair in somatic and germ cells in vivo. Mutat Res 330(1–2):183–208, 1995
294. Kaido M, Mori K, Koide O: Testicular damage caused by inhalation of ethylene oxide in rats: light and electron microscopic studies. Toxicol Pathol 20(1):32–43, 1992
295. Hogstedt C, Rohlen BS, Berndtsson O, Axelson O, Ehrenberg L: A cohort study of mortality and cancer incidence in ethylene oxide production workers. Br J Ind Med 36:276–280, 1979
296. Hogstedt C, Malmquist N, Wadman B: Leukemia in workers exposed to ethylene oxide. JAMA 241:1132–1133, 1979
297. Steenland K, Stayner L, Greife A, Halperin W, Hayes R, Hornun R, Nowlin S: Mortality among workers exposed to ethylene oxide. N Engl J Med 324(20):1402–1407, 1991

Carcinogenicity Results in Animals Predict Cancer Risks to Humans

1. Huff JE, Boyd JA, Barrett JC (eds): Cellular and Molecular Mechanisms of Hormonal Carcinogenesis: Environmental Influences. New York: Wiley-Liss, 1996
2. Colborn T, Clement C (eds): Chemically-induced alterations in sexual and functional development: the wildlife/human connection. Adv Mod Environ Toxicol 21:1–403. Princeton, NJ: Princeton Scientific Pub Co., 1992
3. Shimkin MB: Contrary to nature. DHEW Pub No [NIH] 79-720. National Institutes of Health, Bethesda, MD, 1977, 498 pp
4. Tomatis L, Huff JE, Hertz-Picciotto I, Sandler DP, Bucher J, Boffetta P, Axelson O, Blair A, Taylor J, Stayner L, Barrett JC: Avoided and avoidable risks in cancer. Carcinogenesis 18:97–105, 1997
5. Goldenhar LM, Connally LB, Schulte PA (eds): Intervention research in occupational health and safety: science, skills, and strategies. Am J Ind Med 29:285–434, 1996
6. NIOSH: National Occupational Research Agenda. National Institute for Occupational Safety and Health, Cincinnati, 1996, 75 pp
7. Tomatis L, Aitio A, Wilbourn J, Shuker L: Human carcinogens identified so far. Jpn J Cancer Res 80:795–807, 1989
8. Fung VA, Huff JE, Weisburger E, Hoel DG: Predictive strategies for selecting 379 NCI/NTP chemicals evaluated for carcinogenic potential: scientific and public health impact. Fund. Appl. Toxicol. 20:413–436, 1993
9. Fung VA, Barrett JC, Huff JE: The carcinogenesis bioassay in perspective: application in identifying human cancer hazards. Environ Health Perspect 103:680–683, 1995
10. Huff JE, Haseman JK: Long-term chemical carcinogenesis experiments for identifying potential human cancer hazards. Collective data base of the National Cancer Institute & National Toxicology Program (1976–1991). Environ Health Perspect 96:23–31, 1991
11. Huff JE: Chemicals causally associated with cancers in humans and in laboratory animals: a perfect concordance. In Waalkes MP, Ward JM (eds): Carcinogenesis. New York: Raven Press, 1994, pp 25–37
12. Huff JE: Carcinogenic hazards from eating fish & shellfish contaminated with disparate and complex chemical mixtures. Chapter 9: 157–194. In: Yang RSH [ed]. Toxicology of chemical mixtures: from real life examples to mechanisms of toxicological interactions. Academic Press, New York, 1994
13. Huff JE, Weisburger E, Fung VA: Multicomponent criteria for predicting carcinogenicity: dataset of 30 NTP chemicals. Environ Health Perspect 104(Suppl 5):1105–1112, 1996
14. IARC: IARC Monographs on the Evaluation of carcinogenic Risk to Humans. Vol 1–69. International Agency for Research on Cancer, Lyon, 1997
15. Huff JE: Chemicals and cancer in humans: first evidence in experimental animals. Environ Health Perspect 100:201–210, 1993
16. Huff JE, Haseman JK, Rall DP: Scientific concepts, value, and significance of chemical carcinogenesis studies. Annu Rev Pharmacol Toxicol 31:621–652, 1991
17. Tomatis L: Ethical aspects of prevention. Scand J Work Environ Health 212:245–251, 1995
18. Tomatis L: Socioeconomic factors and human cancer. Int J Cancer 62:121–125, 1995
19. Huff JE, Bucher JR, Yang RSH: Carcinogenesis studies in rodents for evaluating risks associated with chemical carcinogens in aquatic food animals. Environ. Health Perspect. 90:127–132, 1991
19a. Huff JE: Carcinogenic hazards from eating fish & shellfish contaminated with disparate and complex chemical mixtures. Chapter 9:157–194. In: Yang RSH [ed]. Toxicology of chemical mixtures: from real life examples to mechanisms of toxicological interactions. Academic Press, New York, 1994

20. Huff JE, Hoel DG: Perspective and overview of the concepts and value of hazard identification as the initial phase of risk assessment for cancer and human health. Scand J Work Environ Health 18(Suppl 1):83–89, 1992
21. Douglas JF, Huff JE, Peters AC: No evidence of carcinogenicity for L-ascorbic acid (vitamin C) in rodents. J Toxicol Environ Health 15:605–609, 1984
22. Chhabra RS, Huff JE, Haseman JK, Hall A, Baskin G, Cowan M: Inhibition of some spontaneous tumors by 4-hexylresorcinol in F344/N rats and B6C3F1 mice. Fundam Appl Toxicol 11:685–690, 1988
23. Haseman JK, Johnson FM: Analysis of National Toxicology Program rodent bioassay data for anticarcinogenic effects. Mut Res 350:131–141, 1996
24. Bristol DW, Wachsman JT, Greenwell A: The NIEHS Predictive-toxicology evaluation project. Environ Health Perspect 104(Suppl 5):1001–1010, 1996
25. Rall DP, Hogan MD, Huff JE, Schwetz BA, Tennant TW: Alternatives to using human experience in assessing health risks. Annu Rev Public Health 8:355–385, 1987
26. Huff JE, McConnell EE, Haseman JK, Boorman GA, Eustis SL, Schwetz BA, Rao GN, Jameson CW, Hart LG, Rall DP: Carcinogenesis studies: results from 398 experiments on 104 chemicals from the U.S. National Toxicology Program. Ann NY Acad Sci 534:1–30, 1988
27. Lijinsky W: In vivo testing for carcinogenicity. Chapter 6:180–209. In: Cooper CS, Grover PL (eds). Handbook of experimental pharmacology. Springer-Verlag, New York, 1990
28. Chhabra RS, Huff JE, Schwetz BS, Selkirk J: An overview of prechronic and chronic toxicity/carcinogenicity experimental study designs and criteria used by the National Toxicology Program. Environ Health Perspect 86:313–321, 1990
29. Huff JE: Value, validity, and historical development of carcinogenesis studies for predicting and confirming carcinogenic risks to humans. In Kitchen K (ed): Testing, Predicting, Interpreting Chemical Carcinogenicity. New York: Marcel Dekker, in press
30. NTP: NTP Report on Carcinogens 1998. National Toxicology Program, Research Triangle Park, NC [in press].
31. Salmon AG, Zeise L: Risks of carcinogenesis from urethane exposure. CRC Press, Boca Raton, 1991, 231 pp
32. Huff JE, Lucier G, Tritscher A: Carcinogenicity of TCDD: experimental, mechanistic, and epidemiologic evidence. Ann Rev Pharmacol Toxicol 34:343–372, 1994
33. Huff JE: Dioxins and mammalian carcinogenesis. Chapter 12: 389–407. In: Shechter A [ed]. Dioxins and Health. Plenum Press, NY, 1994, 710 pp
34. Maltoni C, Ciliberti A, Cotti G, Conti B, Belpoggi F: Benzene, an experimental multipotential carcinogen: results of the long-term bioassays performed at the Bologna Institute of Oncology. Environ Health Perpospect. 82:109–124, 1989
35. Huff JE, Haseman JK, DeMarini DM, Eustis S, Maronpot RR, Peters AC, Persing RL, Chrisp CE, Jacobs AC: Multiple-site carcinogenicity of benzene in Fischer rats and B6C3F1 mice. Environ. Health Perspect. 82:125–163, 1989
36. Olney JW, Farber NB, Spitznagel E, Robins LN: Increasing brain cancer rates: is there a link to asparatame? J Neuropathol Exp Neurol 55:1115–1123, 1996
37. Huff JE: Applicability to humans of rodent-specific sites of chemical carcinogenicity: tumors of the forestomach and of the harderian, preputial, and zymbal glands induced by benzene. J Occup Med Toxicol 1:109–141, 1992
38. Tsutsui T, Hayashi N, Maizumi H, Huff JE, Barett JC: Benzene-, catechol-, hydroquinone-, and phenol-induced cell transformation, gene mutations, chromosome aberrations, aneuploidy, sister chromatid exchanges, and unscheduled DNA synthesis in Syrian hamster embryo cells. Mutat Res 373:113–123, 1997
39. IARC: Overall evaluations of carcinogenicity: an updating of IARC Monographs 1 to 42. Suppl 7:363. IARC Monographs on the evaluation of carcinogenic risks to humans. International Agency for Research on Cancer, Lyon, 1987, 440 pp
40. Huff JE, Cirvello J, Haseman JK, Bucher JR: Chemicals associated with site-specific neoplasia in 1394 long-term carcinogenesis experiments in laboratory rodents. Environ Health Perspect 93:247–271, 1991
41. Tennant RW, Spalding J, French J: Evaluation of transgenic mouse bioassays for identifying carcinogens and non carcinogens. Mut Res 365:119–127, 1996
42. Tennant RW, Margolin BH, Shelby MD, Zeiger E, Haseman JK, Spalding J, Caspary W, Resnick M, Stasiewicz S, Anderson B, Minor R: Prediction of chemical carcinogenicity in rodents from in vitro genetic toxicity assays. Science 236:933–941, 1987
43. Ito N, Shirai T, Hasegawa R: Medium-term bioassays for carcinogens. In: Vainio H, Magee P, McGregor D & McMichael A [eds]. Mechanisms of Carcinogenesis in Risk Identification. IARC Sci. Pub. 116:353–388. International Agency for Research on Cancer, Lyon, France, 1992, 615 pp
44. Vesselinovitch SD, Rao KVN, Mihailovich N: Neoplastic response or mouse tissues during prenatal age periods and its significance to chemical carcinogenesis. Natl Cancer Inst Monogr 51:239–250, 1979
45. Weinberg RA: Two decades of progress. In: Fortner JG, Sharp PA (eds): Accomplishments in Cancer Research. Philadelphia: Lippincott-Raven, 1995, pp 214–222
46. Huff JE: Chemical toxicity and chemical carcinogenesis. Is there a causal connection? A comparative morphological evaluation of 1500 experiments. In Vainio H, Magee P, McGregor D, McMichael A (eds): Mechanisms of Carcinogenesis in Risk Identification. IARC Scientific Publication 116. Lyon, France: International Agency for Research on Cancer, 1992, 437–475
47. Huff JE: α2μ-Globulin nephropathy, posed mechanisms, and white ravens. Environ Health Perspect 104:1264–1267, 1996
48. Hoel DG, Haseman JK, Hogan MD, Huff JE, McConnell EE: The impact of toxicity on carcinogenicity studies: Implications for risk assessment. Carcinogenesis 9:2045–2052, 1988
49. Tennant RW, Elwell R, Spaulding JW, Greisemer RA: Evidence that toxic injury is not always associated with induction of chemical carcinogenesis. Mole Carc 4:420–440, 1991
50. Melnick RL, Kohn MC, Huff JE: Weight of evidence versus weight of speculation to evaluate the α2u-globulin hypothesis. Environ Health Perspect. 105:904–906
51. Huff JE: Issues and controversies surrounding qualitative strategies for identifying and forecasting cancer causing agents in the human environment. Pharmacol Toxicol 72 (Suppl 1):12–27, 1993
52. Wynder: Studies in mechanism and prevention. Striking a proper balance. Am J Epidemiol 139:547–549, 1994

General References

DeMarini DM, Huff JE: Genetic toxicity assessment: toxicology test methods. Chapter 33:43–45. In: Stellman JM (ed.) ILO Encyclopaedia of Occupational Health and Safety, 4th ed. Geneva: International Labour Office, 1998

Dunnick JK, Elwell MR, Huff JE, Barrett JC: Chemically induced mammary gland cancer in the National Toxicology Program's carcinogenesis bioassy. Carcinogenesis 16:173–179, 1995

Haseman JK, Huff JE: Species correlation in long-term carcinogenicity studies. Cancer Lett 37:125–132, 1987

Haseman JK, Huff JE: Arguments that discredit animal studies lack scientific support. Chem Engineer News 69:49–51, 1991

Haseman JK, Huff JE, Rao GN, Arnold JE, Boorman GA, McConnell EE: Neoplasms observed in untreated and corn oil gavage control groups of F344/N rats and (C57Bl/6N × C3H/HeN)F1 (B6C3F1) mice. J Natl Cancer Inst 75:975–984, 1985

Haseman JK, Huff JE, Rao GN, Eustis SL: Sources of variability in rodent carcinogenicity studies. Fundam Appl Toxicol 12:793–804, 1989

Haseman JK, Huff JE, Zeige E, McConnell EE: Comparative results of 327 chemical carcinogenicity studies. Environ Health Perspect 74: 229–235, 1987

Hoel DG, Haseman JK, Hogan MD, Huff JE, McConnell EE: The impact of toxicity on carcinogenicity studies: implications for risk assessment. Carcinogenesis 9:2045–2052, 1988

Huff JE: The value of in-life and retrospective data audits. In Hoover BK, Baldwin JK, Uelner AF, Whitmire CE, Davies CL, Bristol DW (eds): Managing Conduct and Data Quality of Toxicology Studies. Princeton, NJ: Princeton Scientific, 1986, pp 99–104

Huff JE, Eustis SL, Haseman JK: Occurrence and relevance of chemically induced benign neoplasms in long-term carcinogenicity studies. Cancer Metastasis Rev 8:1–21, 1989

Huff JE: Design strategies, results, and evaluations of long-term chemical carcinogenesis studies. Scand J Work Environ Health 18(Suppl 1): 31–37, 1992

Huff JE: A historical perspective of the classification developed and used for chemical carcinogens by the National Toxicology Program during 1983–1992. Scand J Work Environ Health 18(Suppl 1):74–82, 1992

Huff JE: Absence of morphologic correlation between chemical toxicity and chemical carcinogenesis. Environ Health Perspect 101(Suppl 5): 45–54, 1993

Huff JE, Bucher JR, Yang RSH: Carcinogenesis studies in rodents for evaluating risks associated with chemical carcinogens in aquatic food animals. Environ Health Perspect 90:127–132, 1991

Huff JE, Haseman JK: Exposure to certain pesticides may pose real carcinogenic risk. Chem Engineer News 69:33–37, 1991[Reprinted in J Pest Reform 11:10–14, 1991; Pesticides News 12:7–10, 1991]

Huff JE, Rall DP: Relevance to humans of carcinogenesis results from laboratory animal toxicology studies, 433–440 & 453–457. In Last JM, Wallace RB (eds): Maxcy-Rosenau-Last Public Health & Preventive Medicine. 13th ed. Norwalk, CT: Appleton & Lange, 1992, pp 433–440, 453–457

Huff JE: Mechanisms, chemical carcinogenesis, and risk assessment: cell proliferation and cancer. Am J Ind Med 27:293–300, 1995

Huff JE: Chemically induced cancers in hormonal organs of laboratory animals and of humans. In Huff JE, Boyd JA, Barrett JC (eds): Cellular and Molecular Mechanisms of Hormonal Carcinogenesis: Environmental Influences. New York: Wiley-Liss, 1996, pp 77–102

MacGregor JT, Shane BS, Spalding J, Huff JE: Carcinogenicity and genotoxicity assays for cancer risk to humans. In: Screening and Testing Chemicals in Commerce. OTA-BP-ENV-166. Workshop Proceedings on Genotoxic & Carcinogenic Assays for Identifying Carcinogens. Washington, DC: Office of Technology Assessment, 1995, pp 11–28

Maronpot RR, Haseman JK, Boorman G, Eustis S, Rao GN, Huff JE: Liver lesions in B6C3F1 mice: The National Toxicology Program experience and position. Arch Toxicol Suppl 10:10–26, 1987

Melnick RL, Barrett JC, Huff JE (eds): Cell proliferation and chemical carcinogenesis: proceedings. Environ Health Perspect 101(Suppl 5): 1–285, 1993

Rao G, Huff JE: Refinement of long-term toxicity & carcinogenesis studies. Fundam Appl Toxicol 15:33–43, 1990

Waalkes MP, Infante P, Huff JE: The scientific fallacy of route specificity of carcinogenesis with particular reference to cadmium. Regul Toxicol Pharmacol 20:119–121, 1994

Wolff M, Coleman G, Barrett JC, Huff JE: Breast cancer and environmental risk factors: epidemiological and experimental findings. Annu Rev Pharmacol Toxicol 36:573–596, 1996

Polychlorinated Biphenyls (PCBs)

1. Woodyard JP, King JJ: PCB Management Under TSCA. The Hazardous Waste Management Handbook Series. New York: Executive Enterprises, 1989
2. Kimbrough RD: Polychlorinated biphenyls (PCBs) and human health: an update. Crit Rev Toxicol 25:133–163, 1995
3. Swanson GM, Ratcliffe HE, Fischer LJ: Human exposure to polychlorinated biphenyls (PCBs): a critical assessment of the evidence for adverse health effects. Regul Toxicol Pharmacol 21(1):136–150, 1995
4. U.S. Environmental Protection Agency: Polychlorinated biphenyls (PCBs); manufacturing, processing, distribution in commerce and use prohibition; use in closed and controlled waste manufacturing processes. Federal Register 47(204):46980–46996, 1982
5. Polychlorinated biphenyls spill cleanup policy. Federal Register 52(63):10688, 1987
6. Letz G: The toxicology of PCBs—an overview for clinicians. West J Med 138:534–540, 1983
7. Mosley CL, Geraci CL, Burg J: Polychlorinated biphenyl exposure in transformer maintenance operations. Am Ind Hyg Assoc J 43: 170–174, 1982
8. Hutzinger O, Blumich MJ, von den Berg M, Olie K: Sources and fate of PCDDs and PCDFs: an overview. Chemosphere 14:581–600, 1985
9. Kashimoto T, Miyata H, Shigehiko F, Kunita N, Ohi G, Tung TC: PCBs, PCQs and PCDFs in blood of yusho and yu-cheng patients. Environ Health Perspect 59:73–78, 1985
10. Schecter A, Stanley J, Boggess K, Masuda Y, Mes J, Wolff M, Furst P, Furst C, Wilson-Yang K, Chisholm B: Polychlorinated biphenyl levels in the tissues of exposed and nonexposed humans. Environ Health Perspect 102(Suppl 1):149–158, 1994
11. Waid JS (ed): PCBs and the Environment. vol 1. Boca Raton, FL: CRC Press, 1987
12. Jensen S: The PCB story. Ambio 1:123–131, 1972
13. Stehr-Green PA, Burse VW, Welty E: Human exposure to polychlorinated biphenyls at toxic waste sites: investigations in the United States. Arch Environ Health 43:6:420–424, 1988
14. Toxicological profile for selected PCBs (aroclor-1260, -1254, -1248, -1232, -1221 and -1016). Agency for Toxic Substances and Disease Registry (ATSDR). ATSDR/TP-88/21. Washington, DC: U.S. Public Health Service, 1989
15. Alvares AP, Bickers DR, Kappas A: Polychlorinated biphenyls: new type of inducer of cytochrome P-448 in the liver. Proc Natl Acad Sci USA 70:1321–1325, 1973
16. Tilson HA, Jacobson JL, Rogan WJ: Polychlorinated biphenyls and the developing nervous system: cross species comparisons. Neurotoxicol Teratol 12(3):239–248, 1990
17. Kimbrough RD, Squire R, Linder RE, et al: Induction of liver tumors in Sherman strain female rats by polychlorinated biphenyl (Aroclor 1260). J Natl Cancer Inst 55:1453–1459, 1975
18. Jones JW, Alden HS: An acneform dermatergosis. Arch Dermatol Syphilol 33:1022–1034, 1936
19. Schwartz L: An outbreak of halowax acne ("cable rash") among electricians. JAMA 122:158–161, 1943
20. Meigs JW, Albom JJ, Siyali DS: Chloracne from an unusual exposure to Arochlor. JAMA 154:1417–1418, 1954
21. PCB Poisoning in Japan and Taiwan. In Kuratsune M, Shapiro RE (eds): Progress in Clinical and Biological Research. vol 137. New York: Alan R. Liss, 1984
22. Environmental Health Perspectives. vol 59. Washington, DC: National Institute of Environmental Health Sciences, 1985
23. Rogan WJ, Gladen BC, Hung KL, Koong SL, Shih LY, Taylor JS, Wu YC, Yang D, Regan NB, Hsu CC: Congenital poisoning by polychlorinated biphenyls and their contaminants in Taiwan. Science 241:334–336, 1988
24. Chen YC, Guo YL, Hsu CC, Rogen WJ: Cognitive development of Yu-Cheng ("oil disease") children prenatally exposed to heat degraded PCBs. JAMA 268(22):3213–3218, 1992
25. Guo YL, Chen YC, Yu ML, Hsu CC: Early development of Yu-Cheng children born seven to twelve years after the Taiwan PCB outbreak. Chemosphere 29(9–11):2395–2404, 1994

26. Acquavella JF, Hanis NM, Nicolich MJ, Phillips SC: Assessment of clinical, metabolic, dietary and occupational correlations with serum polychlorinated biphenyl levels among employees at an electrical capacitor manufacturing plant. J Occup Med 28:1177–1180, 1986
27. Smith AB, Schloemer J, Lowry LK, Smallwood AW, Ligo RN, Tanaka S, Stringer W, Jones M, Hervin R, Glueck CJ: Metabolic and health consequences of occupational exposure to polychlorinated biphenyls. Br J Ind Med 39:361–369, 1982
28. Lawton RW, Ross MR, Feingold J, Brown JF Jr: Effects of PCB exposure on biochemical and hematological findings in capacitor workers. Environ Health Perspect 60:165–184, 1985
29. Bahn AK, Rosenwaike I, Herrman N, Grover P, Stellman J, O'Leary K: Melanoma after exposure to PCB. N Engl J Med 295:450, 1976
30. Sinks T, Steele G, Smith AB, Watkins K, Shults RA: Mortality among workers exposed to polychlorinated biphenyls. Am J Epidemiol 136(4):389–398, 1992
31. Brown DP: Mortality of workers exposed to polychlorinated biphenyls—and update. Arch Environ Health 42:333–339, 1987
32. Bertazzi PA, Riboldi L, Pesatori A, Radice L, Zocchetti C: Cancer mortality of capacitor manufacturing workers. Am J Indust Med 11:165–176, 1987
33. Hardell L, Van Bavel B, Lindström G, Fredrikson M, Hagberg H, Liljegren G, Nordström M, Johansson B: Higher concentrations of specific polychlorinated biphenyl congeners in adipose tissue from non-Hodgkin's lymphoma patients compared with controls without a malignant disease. Int J Oncol 9:603–608, 1996
34. Hardell L, Liljegren G, Lindström G, Van Bavel B, Broman K, Fredrikson M, Hagberg H, Nordström M, Johansson B: Increased concentrations of chlordane in adipose tissue from non-Hodgkin's lymphoma patients compared with controls without a malignant disease. Int J Oncol 9:1139–1142, 1996
35. Kreiss K, Zack MM, Kimbrough RD, Needham LL, Smrek AL, Jones BT: Association of blood pressure and polychlorinated biphenyls. JAMA 245:2505–2509, 1981
36. Akagi K, Okumura M: Association of blood pressure and PCB level in yusho patients. Environ Health Perspect 59:37–39, 1985
37. Jacobsen JL, Jacobsen SW: Intellectual impairment in children exposed to polychlorinated biphenyls in utero. N Engl J Med 335(11): 783–789, 1996
38. Rogan WJ, Gladen BC: Neurotoxicology of PCBs and related compounds. Neurotoxicology 13(1):27–35, 1992
39. Piver WT, Lindstrom FT: Waste disposal technologies for polychlorinated biphenyls. Environ Health Perspect 59:163–177, 1985
40. Furukawa K: Microbial degradation of polychlorinated biphenyls (PCBs). In Chakrabarty AM (ed): Biodegradation and Detoxification of Environmental Pollutants. Boca Raton, FL: CRC Press, 1982, pp 33–37
41. Jones GRN: Polychlorinated biphenyls: where do we stand now? Lancet 2:791–794, 1989

Polybrominated Biphenyls (PBBs)

1. Pijnenburg AM, Everts JW, de Boer J, Boon JP: Polybrominated biphenyl and diphenylether flame retardants: analysis, toxicity, and environmental occurrence. Rev Environ Contam Toxicol 141:1–26, 1995
2. Carter LT: Michigan's PBB incident: chemical mix-up leads to disaster. Science 192:240–243, 1976
3. Kay K: Polybrominated biphenyls (PBB) environmental contamination in Michigan, 1973–1976. Environ Res 13:74–93, 1977
4. Jackson TF, Halbert FL: A toxic substance associated with the feeding of polybrominated biphenyls-contaminated concentrate to dairy cattle. J Am Vet Med Assoc 165:437–439, 1974
5. Miceli JN, Nolan DC, Marks B, Hariharan M: Persistence of polybrominated biphenyls (PBB) in human post-mortem tissue. Environ Health Perspect 60:399–403, 1985
6. Wolff MS, Aubrey B, Camper F, Haymes N: Relation of DDE and PBB serum levels in farm residents, consumers, and Michigan Chemical Corporation employees. Environ Health Perspect 23:177–181, 1978
7. Wolff MS, Anderson HA, Selikoff IJ: Human tissue burdens of halogenated aromatic chemicals in Michigan. JAMA 247:2112–2116, 1982
8. Rosen DH, Flanders WD, Friede A, Humphrey HE, Sinks TH: Half-life of polybrominated biphenyl in human sera. Environ Health Perspect 103(3):272–274, 1995
9. Gutermann WH, Lisk DJ: Tissue storage and excretion in milk of polybrominated biphenyls in ruminants. J Agric Food Chem 23: 1005–1007, 1975
10. Farber T, Kasza L, Giovetti A, et al: Effect of polybrominated biphenyls (Firemaster BP) on the immunologic system of the beagle dog. Toxicol Appl Pharmacol 45:343–344, 1978
11. Rangga-Tabbu C, Sleight SD: Development of preneoplastic lesions in the liver and nasal epithelium of rats initiated with *N*-nitrosodimethylamine or *N*-nitrosopyrrolidine and promoted with polybrominated biphenyls. Food Chem Toxicol 30(11):921–926, 1992
12. Tsushimoto G, Trosko JE, Chang CC, Aust SD: Inhibition of metabolic cooperation in Chinese hamster V79 cells in culture by various polybrominated biphenyl (PBB) congeners. Carcinogenesis 3:181–186, 1982
13. Wasito L, Sleight SD: Promoting effect of polybrominated biphenyls on tracheal papillomas in Syrian golden hamsters. J Toxicol Environ Health 27:173–187, 1989
14. Anderson HA, Lilis R, Selikoff LJ, et al: Unanticipated prevalence of symptoms among dairy farmers in Michigan and Wisconsin. Environ Health Perspect 23:217–266, 1978
15. Roboz J, Suzuki RK, Bekesi JG, et al: Mass spectral identification and quantification of polybrominated biphenyl in blood compartments of exposed Michigan chemical workers. J Envir Pathol Toxicol 3:363–378, 1979
16. Bekesi JG, Holland JF, Anderson HA, et al: Lymphocyte function of Michigan dairy farmers exposed to polybrominated biphenyls. Science 199:1207–1209, 1978
17. Bekesi JG, Roboz JP, Solomon S, et al: Altered immune function in Michigan residents exposed to polybrominated biphenyls. In Gibson GG, Hubbard R, Parke DV (eds): Immunotoxicology. New York: Academic Press, 1983, pp 181–191
18. Bekesi JG, Roboz J, Fischbein A, Mason P: Immunotoxicology: environmental contamination by polybrominated biphenyls and immune dysfunction among residents of the state of Michigan. Cancer Detect Prev 1(Suppl):29–37, 1987
19. Bekesi JG, Roboz J, Fischbein A, Roboz JP, Solomon S, Greaves J: Immunological, biochemical and clinical consequences of exposure to polybrominated biphenyls. In Dean JH, Luster MI, Munson AE, Amos H (eds): Immunotoxicology and Immunopharmacology: New York: Raven Press, 1985, 393–405
20. Henderson AK, Rosen D, Miller GL, Piggs LW, Zahm SH, Sieber SM, Humphrey HE, Sinks T: Breast cancer among women exposed to polybrominated biphenyls. Epidemiology 6(5):544–546, 1995
21. Brilliant LB, Van Amburg GA, Isbister J, Humphrey H, Wilcox K, Eyster J, et al: Breast-milk monitoring to measure Michigan's contamination with polybrominated biphenyls. Lancet 2:643–646, 1978
22. Jacobson JL, Humphrey HE, Jacobson SW, Schantz SL, Mullin MD, Welch R: Determinants of polychlorinated biphenyls (PCBs), polybrominated biphenyls (PBBs) and dichlorodiphenyl trichloroethane (DDT) levels in the sera of young children. Am J Public Health 79:1401–1404, 1989
23. Breslin WJ, Kirk HD, Zimmer MA: Teratogenic evaluation of a polybromodiphenyl oxide mixture in New Zealand white rabbits following oral exposure. Fundam Appl Toxicol 12:151–157, 1989

24. Groce DF, Kimbrough RD: Stunted growth, increased mortality and liver tumors in offspring of polybrominated biphenyl (PBB) dosed Sherman rats. J Toxicol Environ Health 14:695–706, 1984
25. Henck JW, Mattsson JL, Rezabek DH, Carlson CL, Rech RH: Developmental neurotoxicity of polybrominated biphenyls. Neurotoxicol Teratol 16(4):391–399, 1994
26. Morris PJ, Quensen JF 3rd, Riedje JM, Boyd SA: Reductive debromination of the commercial polybrominated biphenyl mixture firemaster BP6 by anaerobic microorganisms from sediments. Appl Environ Microbiol 58(10):3249–3256, 1992

Polychlorinated Dioxins and Polychlorinated Dibenzofurans

1. Schecter A (ed): Dioxins and Health. New York: Plenum Press, 1994
2. Institute of Medicine: Veterans and Agent Orange: Health Effects of Herbicides Used in Vietnam. Washington, DC: National Academy Press, 1994
3. Institute of Medicine: Veterans and Agent Orange: Update 1996. Washington, DC: National Academy Press, 1996
4. Huisman M, Koopman-Esseboom C, Fidler V, et al: Perinatal exposure to polychlorinated biphenyls and dioxins and its effect on neonatal neurological development. Early Hum Dev 41:111–127, 1995
5. Koope JG, Pluim HJ, Olie K: Breast milk, dioxins and the possible effects on health of newborn infants. Sci Total Environ 106:33–41, 1991
6. Koopman-Esseboom C, Morse DC, Weisglas-Kuperus N, et al: Effects of dioxins and polychlorinated biphenyls on thyroid hormone status of pregnant women and their infants. Pediatr Res 36:468–473, 1994
7. Henriksen GL, Ketchum NS, Michalek JE, Swaby JA: Serum dioxins and diabetes mellitus in veterans of operation ranch hand. Epidemiology, 8(3):252–258, 1997
8. Sweeney MH, Hornung RW, Wall DK, Fingerhut MA, Halperin WE: Prevalence of diabetes and elevated serum glucose levels in workers exposed to 2,3,7,8-tetrachlorodibenzo-*p*-dioxin (TCDD). Organohalogen Compds 10:225–226, 1992
9. Mocarelli P, Brambilla P, Gerthoux PM: Change in sex ratio with exposure to dioxin. Lancet 348:409, 1996
10. Masuda Y: Causal agents of Yusho. In Kuratsune M, Yoshimura H, Hori Y, Okumura M, Masuda Y (eds): Yusho: A Human Disaster Caused by PCBs and Related Compounds. Fukuoka, Japan: Kyushu University Press, 1996, pp 47–80
11. Schecter A, Startin J, Wright C, et al: Congener-specific levels of dioxins and dibenzofurans in U.S. food and estimated daily dioxin toxic equivalent intake. Environ Health Perspect 102(11):962–966, 1994
12. U.S. Environmental Protection Agency: Exposure Factors Handbook. EPA/600/8-89/043. Washington, DC: U.S. Environmental Protection Agency, Office of Health and Environmental Assessment, 1989
13. U.S. Environmental Protection Agency: Estimating Exposure to Dioxin-Like Compounds (Review Draft). Washington, DC: U.S. Environmental Protection Agency, Office of Health and Environmental Assessment, 1994
14. U.S. Environmental Protection Agency: Health Assessment Document for 2,3,7,8-Tetrachlorodibenzo-*p*-Dioxin (TCDD) and Related Compounds (Review Draft). Washington, DC: U.S. Environmental Protection Agency, Office of Health and Environmental Assessment, 1994
15. Schecter A, Dai LC, Thuy LTB, et al: Agent Orange and the Vietnamese: the persistence of elevated dioxin levels in human tissue. Am J Public Health 85(4):516–522, 1995
16. Schecter A, McGee H, Stanley J, Boggess K, Brandt-Rauf P: Dioxins and dioxin-like chemicals in blood and semen of American Vietnam veterans from the state of Michigan. Am J Ind Med 30(6):647–654, 1996
17. Fingerhut MA, Halperin WE, Marlow DA, et al: Cancer mortality in workers exposed to 2,3,7,8-tetrachlorodibenzo-p-dioxin. N Engl J Med 324:212–218, 1991
18. Flesch-Janys D, Berger J, Gurn P, et al: Exposure to polychlorinated dioxins and furans (PCDD/F) and mortality in a cohort of workers from a herbicide-producing plant in Hamburg, Federal Republic of Germany. Am J Epidemiol 142(11):1165–1175, 1995
19. Manz A, Berger J, Dwyer JH, et al: Cancer mortality among workers in chemical plant contaminated with dioxin. Lancet 338:959–964, 1991
20. Saracci R, Kogevinas M, Bertazzi PA, et al: Cancer mortality in workers exposed to chlorophenoxy herbicides and chlorophenols. Lancet 338:1027–1032, 1991
21. Zober A, Messerer P, Huber P: Thirty-four-year mortality follow-up of BASF employees exposed to 2,3,7,8-TCDD after the 1953 accident. Int Arch Occup Environ Health 62:139–157, 1990
22. Rogan WJ, Gladen BC, McKinney JD, et al: Neonatal effects of transplacental exposure to PCBs and DDE. J Pediatr 109:335–341, 1986
23. Rogan WJ, Gladen BC, McKinney JD, et al: Polychlorinated biphenyls (PCBs) and dichlorodiphenyl dichloroethene (DDE) in human milk: effects on growth, morbidity, and duration of lactation. Am J Public Health 77:1294–1297, 1987
24. Rogan WJ, Gladen BC: PCBs, DDE, and child development at 18 and 24 months. Ann Epidemiol 1:407–413, 1991
25. Gladen BC, Rogan WJ: Effects of perinatal polychlorinated biphenyls and dichlorodiphenyl dichloroethene on later development. J Pediatr 119:58–63, 1991
26. Hsu C-C, Yu M-L M, Chen Y-C J, Guo Y-L L, Rogan WJ: The Yucheng rice oil poisoning incident. In Schecter A (ed): Dioxins and Health. New York: Plenum Press; 1994, pp 661–684
27. DeVito MJ, Birnbaum LS: Toxicology of dioxins and related chemicals. In Schecter A (ed): Dioxins and Health. New York: Plenum Press, 1994, pp 139–162
28. Masuda Y: The Yusho rice oil poisoning incident. In Schecter A (ed): Dioxins and Health. New York: Plenum Press, 1994, pp 633–659

24

Multiple Chemical Sensitivities

Mark R. Cullen

During the 1980s a curious clinical syndrome emerged in occupational and environmental health practice, characterized by apparent intolerance to low levels of human-made chemicals. Although still lacking a widely agreed upon definition or designation, the disorder idiosyncratically occurs in individuals who have experienced a single episode or recurring episodes of a typical chemical intoxication or injury such as solvent or pesticide poisoning. Subsequently, an expansive array of divergent environmental contaminants in air, food, or water may elicit a wide range of symptoms at doses far below those that typically produce toxic reactions. Although these symptoms are not associated with objective impairment of the organs to which they are referable, the complaints may be impressive, causing considerable dysfunction and disability.

Although such reactions to chemicals are not new, there is an unmistakable impression that multiple chemical sensitivities, or MCS, as the syndrome is now most frequently called, is occurring and presenting to medical attention far more commonly than in the past. Although little is known about its epidemiology (see below), it has become prevalent enough to have attracted its own group of specialists—clinical ecologists or environmental physicians—and substantial public controversy. Unfortunately, despite widespread debate over who should treat patients suffering with the disorder and who should pay for it, little compelling research has yet emerged to elucidate virtually any important scientific question. The cause, pathogenesis, treatment, and prevention of MCS remain entirely unknown.

This state of affairs notwithstanding, MCS is clearly occurring and causing significant morbidity in the workforce and general populations. It is the goal that this chapter elucidate what is known about the disorder in the hope of improving recognition and management in the face of uncertainty and stimulating constructive scientific engagement of this timely problem.

▸ DEFINITION AND DIAGNOSIS

Although, as noted, there has yet to be general consensus on a single definition of MCS, certain features can be described that allow differentiation from other well-characterized entities.[1] These include

1. Symptoms appear to begin after the occurrence of a more typical occupational or environmental disease such as an intoxication or chemical insult. This "initiating" problem may be one episode, such as a smoke inhalation, or repeated episodes, as in solvent intoxication. Often the preceding events are mild and may blur almost imperceptibly into the syndrome that follows.
2. Symptoms, often initially very similar to those of the initiating illness, begin to occur after re-exposures to lower levels of the same or related compounds, in environments previously well tolerated, such as the home, stores, etc.
3. Generalization of symptoms occurs such that multiorgan-system complaints are involved. Invariably these include symptoms referable to the central nervous system such as fatigue, confusion, headache, etc.
4. Generalization of precipitants occurs such that low levels of chemically diverse agents become capable of eliciting the responses, often at levels orders of magnitude below accepted threshold limit values (TLVs) or guidelines.
5. Workup of complaints fails to reveal impairment of organs which would explain the pattern or intensity of complaints.
6. Psychosis or systemic illness, which might explain the multiorgan symptoms, is absent.

While not every patient will fit this description precisely, it is important to consider each point before "labeling" a patient with MCS or including them in any study population. Each of the criteria serves to rule out other disorders with which MCS may be confused: typical somatization disorder, classic sensitization to environmental antigens (e.g., occupational asthma), pathologic sequelae of organ system damage (e.g., reactive airways dysfunction syndrome after a toxic inhalation) or a masquerading systemic disease (e.g., cancer with paraneoplastic phenomena). On the other hand, it is important to recognize that MCS is not a diagnosis of exclusion, nor should exhaustive and therapeutically disruptive (see below) tests be required in most cases. While many variations will be encountered, MCS has an unmistakable character that should allow prompt recognition in most cases.

In practice, the most difficult diagnostic problems with MCS fall into two categories. The first occurs with patients early in their course in whom it is often challenging to separate MCS from the more classic occupational or environmental health problem that generally precedes it. For example, patients who have experienced untoward reactions around organic solvents may find that their reactions are persisting even when they have been removed from high exposure areas or after the exposures have been properly abated; clinicians may assume that high exposures that could be remedied are still occurring and direct attention to that, an admirable but unhelpful error. This is especially troublesome in the office setting where MCS may be seen as a complication of typical sick building syndrome. Whereas the typical office worker will respond promptly to steps that improve indoor air quality, the patient who has acquired MCS typically will continue to experience symptoms despite the far lower exposures involved. Again, attempts to improve the air quality further may be frustrating to patient and employer alike.

Later in the disorder, confusion often is created by patient reactions to chronic illness. The MCS patient who has been symptomatic for many months is often depressed and anxious, as are most medical patients with new chronic diseases to which they have not adapted. This may lead to a focus exclusively on psychiatric aspects of which the chemically stimulated symptoms are viewed as a part. Without questioning the importance of recognizing and treating these complications of MCS, nor the possibility that MCS itself has psychological origins, the underlying pattern of MCS must be recognized to facilitate appropriate management. Focusing exclusively on psychological aspects, while ignoring the patient's perception of clinical response to chemical exposures, is therapeutically counterproductive.

▶ PATHOGENESIS

The sequence of events that leads in some individuals from a self-limited episode or episodes of occupational or environmental illness to the development of potentially disabling symptomatic responses to very low levels of ubiquitous chemicals is presently unknown. Several theories have been offered, including the following:

1. The clinical ecologists and their adherents initially attributed the illness to immune dysfunction caused by excessive cumulative burden of xenobiotic material in susceptible hosts.[2–4] According to this view, such factors may include relative or absolute nutritional deficiencies (vitamins, antioxidants, essential fatty acids, etc.) or the presence of subclinical infections, such as *Candida* or other yeasts, or other life stresses. In this view the role of the "initiating" illness is important only insofar as it may contribute heavily to this overload.
2. Critics of clinical ecology have invoked a primarily psychological view of the disorder, characterizing it in the spectrum of somatoform illnesses.[5–7] Variations of this view include the concept that MCS is a variant of classic posttraumatic stress disorder or a conditioned response to an unpleasant experience. In these views the initiating illness plays an obviously more central role in the pathogenesis of the disorder. Host factors may also be important, especially the predisposition to somaticize.
3. More recently several theories have emerged that invoke a synthesis of biologic and neuropsychologic mechanisms. Central in these theories is the role of altered chemoreception of odor and irritation stimuli in the nose,[8,9] resulting in altered CNS responses to otherwise minimally noxious stimuli. A model of sensitization or "kindling" of limbic pathways, analogous to mechanisms postulated to explain drug addictions and other CNS adaptations, has also been proposed.[10] The rich network of neural connections between the nasal epithelium and the CNS provide an intriguing theoretical basis for these hypotheses.

Unfortunately, despite considerable literature generated on the subject, especially by the clinical ecologist group, little compelling clinical or experimental science has been published to conclusively prove any of these views. Limitations of published clinical studies include failure to define rigorously the population on which tests have been performed and problems with identifying appropriately matched groups of referent subjects for comparison. Neither subjects of research nor observers have been blind to subjects' status or research hypotheses. In the end, almost all existing data must be characterized as anecdotal.

Most unfortunate of all, the legitimate debate over the etiologic basis of the disorder has been heavily clouded by dogma. Since major economic decisions may hinge on the terms in which an individual case or cases generally are viewed (e.g., patient benefit entitlements, physician reimbursement acceptance), many patients as well as their physicians may have very strong views of the illness which have inhibited scientific progress as well as patient care. It is essential to an understanding of MCS itself that the above theories are extant and often well known to patients who often have very strong views themselves. As such, MCS differs markedly from other environmentally related disorders, like progressive massive fibrosis in miners, in which uncertainty about pathogenesis has not interfered with efforts to study the problem or manage its victims.

▶ EPIDEMIOLOGY

Given the absence of a clear case definition, it is not surprising that detailed knowledge about the occurrence of MCS is lacking. Although estimates of its prevalence in the population range as high as several percent, the scientific basis of these remains obscure.[11] Almost all available data derive from anecdotal reports of practitioners who have treated patients with the disorder.

The limitations of this database notwithstanding, some general observations merit mention.[12] Compared to other occupational disorders, MCS appears to occur more commonly in younger (especially fourth and fifth decades) workers and among those of higher socioeconomic status. Economically disadvantaged and non-whites seem underrepresented in most reports, although this may be an artifact of differential access, disease perception, or diagnostic bias. Women seem to be more frequently affected than men. Importantly, epidemiologic evidence strongly suggests host idiosyncrasy as a factor, since more than isolated cases have uncommonly occurred after outbreaks of acute occupational or environmental disease, which predispose.

In addition to these demographic features, some insights may be gleaned about the settings in which the illness occurs. Although many develop after nonoccupational exposures, e.g., in cars, homes etc., several groups of chemicals appear to account overwhelmingly for the majority of initiating events—organic solvents, pesticides, and respiratory irritants. While this may be a function of the broad usage of these materials in our workplaces and general environment, the impression is that they are overrepresented. The other special setting in which many cases occur is in the so-called tight building, with victims of the typical "sick building syndrome" occasionally evolving into classic MCS pictures. Although the two illnesses have a great deal in common, their epidemiologic features readily distinguish them. Sick building syndrome typically affects most individuals sharing a common ("sick") environment and responds characteristically to environmental improvement; MCS occurs in isolation and does not abruptly respond to quantitative modifications of the environment.

A final issue of considerable interest is whether MCS is, in fact, a truly new disorder or whether it has only recently come to attention because of widespread interest in the environment as a source of human disease. Views on this are split, largely along the same lines as opinion regarding the pathogenesis of the disorder. Those, including the clinical ecologists, who suspect a primarily biologic role for environmental agents would argue that MCS is uniquely a twentieth century disease with rapidly rising incidence because of increased chemical contamination of the environment.[2–4] Contrarily, those who invoke primarily psychological mechanisms have argued that only the societal context of the disease is in any sense new.[13] According to this view, the social perception of the environment as a hostile agent has resulted in the evolution of new symbolic content to the age-old problem of psychosomatic disease, changing the perception of patient and doctor but not the fundamental disease mechanism.[14]

▶ NATURAL HISTORY

Although MCS has yet to be subjected to careful clinical study sufficient to delineate its course or outcome, anecdotal experience with large numbers of patients has shed some preliminary light on this issue, which may be of great importance in appropriate management. Based on this information, the general pattern of illness appears to be one of initial progression as the process of generalization evolves, followed by cyclical periods of gradual improvements and exacerbations. While these cycles are generally perceived by the patient to be related to improvement or contamination of his or her environment, the pattern seems to have some life of its own as well, although the basis for it is far from clear.

Two important corollaries follow from this observation. Other than during the early stages in which the process initially emerges, there is little evidence to suggest that the disease is in any sense progressive.[15] Patients do not tend to deteriorate from year to year, nor have obvious complications such as infections or organ system failure, resulted. There is no evidence of mortality from MCS, although many patients become convinced that progression and death are inevitable based on the profound change in perception of health which the disorder engenders.

While this observation may provide the basis for a sanguine prognosis and reassurance, it has been equally clear from described clinical experience that true remission of symptoms is also highly improbable. While various good outcomes have been described, these are invariably based on improved patient function and sense of well-being. The underlying tendency to react adversely to chemical exposures continues, although symptoms may become sufficiently tolerable to allow return to a near-normal lifestyle.

In sum, MCS would appear to be a disorder with well-defined upper and lower bounds in outcome. While neither limit has been confirmed by large, well-characterized series, it is probably not premature to include this assumption in planning treatment and assisting in vocational rehabilitation.

▸ CLINICAL MANAGEMENT

Very little is known about treatment of MCS. Although a vast array of modalities have been proposed and tried, none has been subjected to the usual scientific standards to determine efficacy. As with other aspects, theories of treatment follow closely the theories of pathogenesis. Clinical ecologists, convinced that MCS represents immune dysfunction caused by excessive body burdens of xenobiotics, focus much of their attention on reducing burden by strict avoidance of chemicals; some have advocated extreme steps resulting in complete alterations in patient lifestyle. This approach is often accompanied by efforts to determine "specific" sensitivities by various forms of skin and blood testing—none as yet validated by acceptable standards—and using therapies akin to desensitization with a goal of inducing "tolerance." Coupled with this are a variety of strategies to bolster underlying immunity with dietary supplementation, eradication of "infections," such as *Candida*, and other metabolic supports. A most radical approach involves efforts to eliminate toxins from the body by chelation or accelerated turnover of fat (where some presumed causal agents are stored).

Those inclined to a more psychological view of the disorder have explored alternative approaches consistent with their theories. Supportive individual or group therapies and more classic behavioral methods have been described.[16] However, as with the more biological theories, the efficacy of these approaches remains conjectural.

Although none of these modalities is likely to be directly dangerous, limitations to present knowledge would suggest that they would best be reserved for settings in which well-controlled trials are being undertaken. In the meantime, certain treatment principles have emerged that can be justified based on present knowledge and experience. These include

1. Taking steps to limit to the extent possible the search for the mysterious "cause" of the disease is an important first aspect of treatment. Many patients will have had considerable workup by the time MCS is considered and will equate, not irrationally, extensive testing with extensive pathology. Uncertainty feeds this cycle as well as the patient's common underlying fear that they have been irrevocably poisoned.
2. Whatever the theoretical proclivity of the clinician, it is crucial that the existing knowledge and uncertainty about MCS be explained to the patient, including specifically that the cause is unknown. The patient must be reassured that the possibility of a psychological basis does not make the illness less real, less serious, or less worthy of treatment. Further reassurance that the disease will not lead to death is also valuable, coupled with caution that total cure is unrealistic.
3. Steps to remove the patient from the most obviously offensive aspects of his or her environment are almost always necessary, especially if the patient still lives or works in the same environment where the initiating illness occurred. While radical avoidance is probably counterproductive, given the goal of improving function, protection from daily misery is important in establishment of a strong therapeutic relationship, which the patient needs. In general, this means a vocational change, which will also require attention to sufficient benefits to make this choice viable for the patient. For cases that occur as a consequence of an occupational illness, however mild, workers' compensation may be available; most jurisdictions do not require detailed understanding of disease pathogenesis if MCS can be demonstrated to be a complication of a disorder that is accepted by local convention as work related.
4. Having established this foundation of support, the goal of all subsequent therapy should be development of improved function. Obviously psychological problems, like adjustment difficulties, anxiety, or depression should be treated, as should coexistent pathology, such as usual allergic manifestations. Unfortunately, since MCS patients do not tolerate chemicals readily, nonpharmacologic approaches may be necessary. Beyond these measures, patients need direction, counseling, and reassurance to begin the challenging process of adjusting to an illness without established treatment. To the extent consistent with tolerable symptoms, patients should be encouraged to expand the range of their activities and should be discouraged from passivity, dependence, or resignation, which intermittently recur throughout the course of the illness. It is worth emphasizing that there is no evidence to suggest that chemical exposures that induce symptoms otherwise adversely modify the future course of the illness.
5. Although it is appropriate to provide patients with all available factual information about MCS, as well as fairly representing the view of the clinician, it must be recognized that many patients will get desperate and will try available alternative treatment modalities, sometimes several at once or in sequence. It is probably not reasonable to strongly resist such efforts or to undermine a therapeutic relationship on this account, but rather to hold steadily to a single coherent perspective, treating such "treatments" as yet another troublesome aspect of a troublesome condition.

▸ PREVENTION

It goes without saying that primary prevention cannot be seriously considered given present knowledge of the pathogenesis of the disorder or the host factors that render certain individuals susceptible to it. At this time the most reasonable approach is to reduce the opportunities in the workplace and ambient environment for the kinds of acute exposures, especially solvents and pesticides, that would appear to precipitate MCS in some hosts. Reduction in the proportion of poorly ventilated offices would also appear likely to help.

Secondary prevention appears to offer some greater control opportunity, although no intervention has been studied. On the possibility that psychological factors may play a role in victims of environmental mishaps, careful early management of such individuals would seem advisable, even if the prognosis from a biologic perspective is good. For example, patients seen in clinics or emergency rooms after acute exposures should have some exploration of their reactions to the events and should probably receive very close follow-up where undue fears of long-term effects or recurrence are expressed. Equally important, efforts must be made on behalf of such patients to ensure that preventable recurrences do not occur, since this may be an important pathway leading to MCS by whichever mechanism is truly responsible.

► REFERENCES

1. Cullen MR: The worker with multiple chemical sensitivities: an overview. Occup Med 2:655–661, 1987
2. Bell IR: Clinical Ecology. Colinas, CA: Common Knowledge Press, 1982
3. Levine AS, Byers VS: Environmental illness: A disorder of immune regulation. Occup Med 2:669–682, 1987
4. Asford NA, Miller CS: Chemical Exposures: Low Levels and High Stakes. New York: Van Nostrand Reinhold, 1991
5. Brodsky CM: Psychological factors contributing to somatoform diseases attributed to the workplace. The case of intoxication. J Occup Med 25:459–464, 1983
6. Black DW, Rathe A, Goldstein RB: Environmental illness: a controlled study of 26 subjects with 20th century disease. JAMA 264:3166–3170, 1990
7. Bolle-Wilson K, Wilson RJ, Bleecker ML: Conditioning of physical symptoms after neurotoxic exposure. J Occup Med 30:684–686, 1988
8. Doty R, Deems DA, Frye RE, Pelberg R, Shapiro A: Olfactory sensitivity, nasal resistance and autonomic function in patients with multiple chemical sensitivities. Arch Otolaryngol Head Neck Surg 114:1422–1427, 1988
9. Meggs WJ, Cleveland CH: Rhinolaryngoscopic examination of patients with the multiple chemical sensitivity syndrome. Arch Environ Health 48:14–18, 1993
10. Bell IR, Miller CS, Schwartz GE: An olfactory-limbic model of multiple chemical sensitivity syndrome: possible relationships to kindling and affective spectrum disorders. Biol Psychiatry 32:218–242, 1992
11. Mooser SB: The epidemiology of multiple chemical sensitivities. Occup Med 2:663–668, 1987
12. Cullen MR: Multiple chemical sensitivities: development of public policy in the face of scientific uncertainty. New Solutions Fall:16–24, 1991
13. Brodsky CM: Multiple chemical sensitivities and other “environmental illnesses”: a psychiatrist’s view. Occup Med 2:695–704, 1987
14. Shorter E: From paralysis to fatigue: a history of psychosomatic illness in the modern era. New York: Macmillan, 1992, pp 233–323
15. Cullen MR, Pace PE, Redlich CA: The experience of the Yale occupational and environmental medicine clinic with MCS 1986–91. In Mitchell FL (ed): Multiple Chemical Sensitivity: A Scientific Overview. Princeton: Princeton Scientific, 1995, pp 15–20
16. Lewis BM: Workers with multiple chemical sensitivities: psychosocial interventions. Occup Med 2:791–800, 1987

25

Pulmonary Responses to Gases and Particles

Kaye H. Kilburn

This chapter defines the functional zones of human lung, describes responses to occupationally polluted air, reviews the adverse health effects caused by environmental air pollution, and considers indoor air pollution.

▸ FUNCTIONAL ZONES OF HUMAN LUNG

The lung has two regions: the conducting airways and the gas-exchanging alveolar zone. In the former, a mucociliary escalator removes deposited particles. The alveolar zone, which includes alveolarized respiratory bronchioles and alveolar ducts, lacks this ability[1] (Fig. 25-1). The two zones have vastly different defenses and susceptibilities to damage. For example, water-soluble gases such as sulfur dioxide and ammonia adsorb to proximal conducting airways, while relatively insoluble ozone and nitrogen dioxide damage the nonmucous-covered alveolar zone (Table 25-1). The airways selectively filter particles from the nose to the alveolar ducts. Thus large particles (50 μm in diameter) lodge in the nose or pharynx, but particles must be less than 10 μm (and usually less than 5 μm) to reach the alveolar zone.[2] Fungal spores with diameters of 17 to 20 μm affect only proximal conducting airways (Fig. 25-2), while the 1 μm diameter spores of *Micropolyspora faeni* affect alveoli as well (Fig. 25-3). As a first approximation, reactions to particles can be predicted from their size, which is best defined by the mean median diameter, and from solubility in water. Where fibers and fibrils lodge is predicted from aerodynamic diameter, not from length.

▸ OCCUPATIONAL POLLUTED AIR

Acute Alveolar Reactions

Asphyxiant Gases

Asphyxiant gases, which include carbon dioxide, carbon monoxide, hydrogen cyanide, hydrogen sulfide, methane, and the fluorocarbons, essentially displace oxygen from alveoli and cause death. Their properties, exposure sources, toxicity, and applicable standards for occupational exposure in the United States are listed in Table 25-1. Carbon dioxide stimulates respiration at concentrations less than 10 percent but depresses breathing at higher concentrations and is anesthetic. The occupational hazard generally occurs in people going into poorly ventilated chambers, often underground. For example, carbon dioxide, methane, and hydrogen sulfide are generated from manure collected from cattle feeding lots or from sewage and in wells, pits, silos, holds of ships, or abandoned mine shafts. Workers entering these areas collapse after a few breaths. Tragically, the first attempted rescuer often dies of asphyxiation before it is realized that the exposure is lethal.

Arc welding is a particular hazard in small compartments, since it does not require oxygen but burns organic material with oxygen to produce carbon monoxide; if ventilation is restricted, lethal quantities of carbon monoxide may accumulate in the compartment. Methane, as coal damp, is an asphyxiant and an explosion hazard for miners. Community contamination with hydrogen sulfide has occurred from coal seams in Gillette, Wyoming, from evaporative (salt crystallization) chemistry in Trona, California, and from hydrocarbon petroleum refining in Ponca City, Oklahoma, and Nipoma, California. However, the most serious incident of this type was the Bhopal, India, disaster of 1984. Methyl isocyanate (used in manufacturing the insecticide carbaryl (Sevin)) escaped from a 21-ton liquid storage tank, killing more than 2,300 people and injuring more than 30,000.

Hydrogen sulfide inhalation produced nausea, headache, shortness of breath, sleep disturbances, and throat and eye irritation at concentrations of 0.003 to 11 mg/m^3 during a series of intermittent air pollution episodes over a 2-month period. Hydrogen sulfide at concentrations of about 150 ppm quickly paralyzes the sense of smell, so that victims may be unaware of danger. Instantaneous death has occurred at levels of 1,400 mg/m^3 (1,000 ppm) to 17,000 mg/m^3 (12,000 ppm). As the level of hydrogen sulfide increases in the ambient environment, symptoms vary from headache, loss of appetite, burning eyes, and dizziness at low concentrations, to low blood pressure, arm cramps, and unconsciousness at moderate concentrations, to pulmonary edema, coma, and death at higher concentrations. The recommended occupational standard for carbon dioxide is 0.5 percent, but for carbon monoxide it is 50 ppm for an 8-hour workday, with a single exposure to 200 ppm considered dangerous for chronic as well as acute impairment of the central nervous system (CNS). Since hydrogen sulfide is highly toxic even at low concentrations, the Occupational Safety and Health Administration (OSHA) has not set a time-weighted average for an 8-hour day. Instead, 20 ppm has been set as a maximum 15-minute exposure.

Oxidant Gases

A potent oxidizing agent, ozone is a bluish pungent gas generated by electrical storms, arcs, and ultraviolet light. Ozone and nitrogen oxides are important in environmental air pollution. At high altitudes the ozone shield protects against solar radiation. Excess ozone is found aboard high-flying long-distance aircraft, particularly over the Poles if adequate adsorption is absent. Otherwise exposure to ozone,

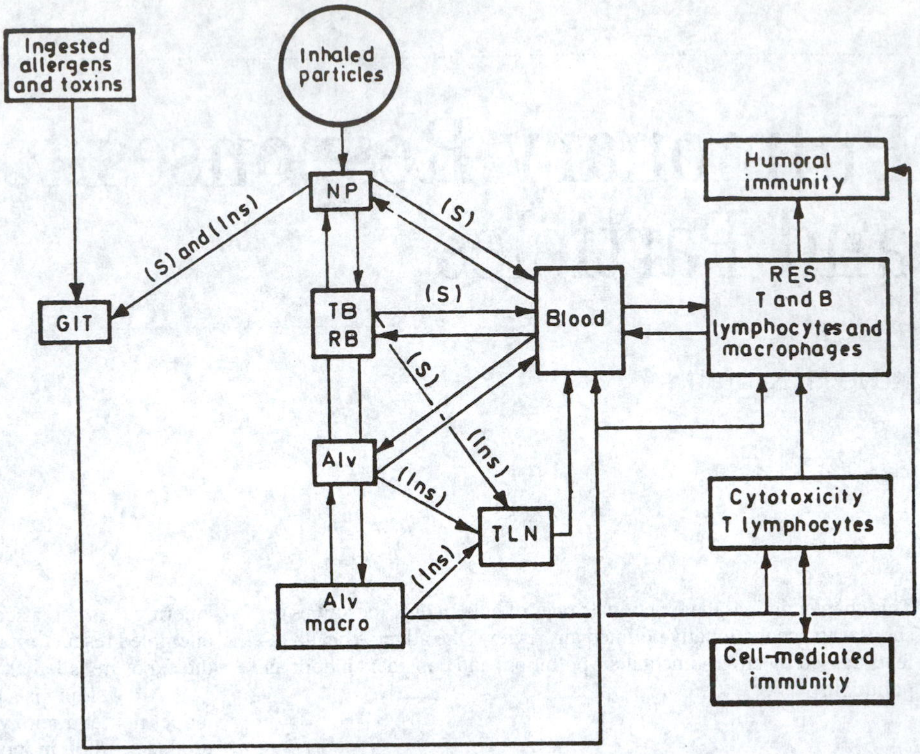

Figure 25-1. Diagram showing the possible fates and influence of inhaled aerosols and ingested materials. *Alv,* alveolus; *Alv macro,* alveolar macrophages; *GIT,* gastrointestinal tract; *Ins,* insoluble particles; *NP,* nasopharynx; *RB,* red blood cell; *RES,* reticuloendothelial system; *S,* soluble particles; *TB,* terminal bronchioles; *TLN,* thoracic lymph nodes. (Adapted from Kilburn KH: A hypothesis for pulmonary clearance and its implications. Am Rev Respir Dis 98:449–463, 1968. Courtesy of the Editor of *American Review of Respiratory Diseases.*)

nitrogen dioxide, and other oxidant gases is found mainly in welding, near electric generation, and in the chemical industry (Table 25-1). Nitrogen dioxide has a pungent odor most remarkable in fuming nitric acid, silos containing alfalfa, and manufacture of feeds, fertilizers, and explosions. Although ozone and nitrogen dioxide irritate mucous membranes and the eyes, they exert their effects in the distal zone of the lung, the respiratory bronchioles, and alveoli ducts. These gases enter alveolar epithelial cells, produce swelling, and secondarily affect the capillary endothelial cells. The thin alveolar membranes are then rendered permeable to plasma fluids and proteins, which leads to pulmonary edema after exposure to large concentrations. Exposure to nitrogen oxides, principally nitrogen dioxide generated in silos by silage, in animal feed processing, and in nitrocellulose film fires in movie theaters, caused subacute necrotizing bronchiolitis in survivors of acute pulmonary edema. Sulfur dioxide may also cause alveolar edema but is extremely irritating; unless doses are unbearably high, the nose and upper airways absorb enough to reduce the amount reaching the alveoli.

Irritant Gases

The irritant gases include several halogens (fluorine, bromine, and chlorine), hydrochloric acid, hydrogen fluoride, phosgene (and chlorine, which were poison gases used in World War I), sulfur dioxide, ammonia, and dimethyl sulfate. Oxides of vanadium, oxmium, cadmium and platinum as finely divided fumes act like gases. The sources are generally industrial processing, although inadvertent production may occur. In addition, bromine and chlorine are injected to sterilize municipal water supplies, so that large amounts of concentrated gas are stored in heavily populated cities. One desulfurization processes for petroleum uses vanadium pentoxide as a catalyst for hydrogen sulfide, and although portions of this are regenerated, workplace and environmental exposures have occurred. When ammonia is injected into soil as liquid ammonia for agricultural or industrial purposes, workers may be exposed to large quantities.

The so-called irritant gases in large quantities damage alveolar lining cells and capillary endothelial cells, causing alveolotoxic pulmonary edema. They may also severely damage the epithelial surface of airways. The mechanism of pulmonary edema is destruction of both alveolar epithelial cells and the capillary endothelium, such that fluid and protein beyond what the lymphatic system can remove overflow into alveoli. The fluid moves up into the terminal bronchioles and hence into the conducting airways, to be heard as rales on examination.

Recent observations show that the brain is the target of several of these gases including chlorine, hydrochloric acid, ammonia, formaldehyde, and hydrogen sulfide. Sensitive measurements show impaired balance, reaction time, visual fields, recall, problem solving, and decision-making and high frequencies of headache, memory loss, dizziness, and other symptoms.[3]

Particles

Particles causing alveolar edema include small fungal spores such as *M. faeni*, bacterial endotoxins, and metal fumes (particles), particularly vanadium pentoxide, osmium, platinum, cadmium, and cobalt. Particles may be generated from vegetable crops used as food, fiber, or forage; as aerosols from sewage or animal fertilizer; or from petroleum desulfurization in large enough amounts that acute inhalation produces pulmonary edema. Onset may range from minutes to hours.

Mixtures

Mixtures created by combustion of fuel, such as diesel exhaust in mines and welding fumes, particularly in compartments with limited ventilation, may reach edemagenic levels due to concentrations of ozone, nitrogen dioxide, formaldehyde, and acrolein. Again, if combustion or arcing takes place in a limited air space without adequate ventilation, pulmonary edema or acute airways obstruction is likely.

Therapy

Afflicted individuals require oxygen delivered under positive pressure by mask. This restores oxygen to alveoli blocked by foaming of edema fluid and rapidly improves systemic oxygenation. Morphine (which is a respiratory depressant), diuretics, fluid restriction, or adrenal corticosteroids are secondary measures. Speed is crucial. If

TABLE 25-1. PROPERTIES, SOURCES, AND TOXICITY OF COMMON GASES

Name	Formula	Color and Odor	Sources of Exposure	Health Effects: Acute	Health Effects: Chronic	OSHA [TWA][a] (ppm)	IDLH[b] (ppm)
■ ***ASPHYXIANT GASES***							
Carbon dioxide	CO_2	c, ol	M, We, FC	A, H, D, Ch		5,000	50,000
Carbon monoxide	CO	c, ol	CS, T, FC	A, H, Cv, Co		50	1,500
Carbon disulfide	CS_2	c, so	CM	H, D	Np	20	500
Hydrogen sulfide	H_2S	c, re	Ae, D, Ng, P	A, Pe, D, H, Co	Np	(20) ceiling	300
Methane	CH_4	c, ol, f	Ng, D	A			
■ ***OXIDANT GASES***							
Ozone	O_3	c, po	S, EA, W, AC	T, Pe, Mm, Tp	AO	0.1	10
Nitrogen oxides	NO	rb, po	W	T, Mm, Pe, Tp		25	100
	$NO_2(N_2O_4)$	rb, po	CS, W, FC	Ch	AO	5	50
■ ***IRRITANT GASES***							
Sulfur dioxide	SO_2	c, po	P	T, Mm, Tp, Pe, Ch		5	100
Ammonia	NH_3	c, po	Ae, Af, Cm	A, Pe, Mm, Tp, T, Ch	Np	50	500
Formaldehyde	$HCHO$	c, po, p	CS, CM	T, Mm, Ch, Tp	AO, Ca, Np		
Acetaldehyde	CH_3CHO	c, po, p	CS, CM	T, Mm, Ch, Tp	AO, N	2	100
Acrolein		c, po, p	CS, CM	T, Mm, Ch, Tp	AO, Np	0.1	5
Chlorine		gy, po	CM	Pe, Mm, Ch, T, H, D, L	AO, Np	1	25
Bromine		rb, po	CM	Pe	AO	1	10
Fluorine		y, po	CM	Pe	AO	0.1	25
Hydrogen fluoride	HF	c, po	CM	Pe, T, Mm, B	AO	3	20
Hydrogen bromide	HB_r	c, po	CM	Pe, T, Mm, B	AO	3	50
Hydrogen chloride	HCl	c, po	CM	Pe, T, Mm, B	AO, Np	5	100
Phosgene	$COCl_2$	c, ol-po	CM	Pe, T, Mm, Ch Tp, B	AO	0.1	2
Carbon tetrachloride	CCl_4	c, so		H, D, Pe	L, Np	10	300
Chloroform	$CHCl_3$	c, so	CM	H, D, Pe, Co	L, Np	50	1,000
Vinyl chloride	$CH_2 = CHCL$	c, so, p	CM	H, D, Mm	Ca, AOL, Np	1	5
Vinylidene chloride	$CH_2 = CCl_2$	c, so, p	CM	B, Mm	Ca	10	50

Color and Odor: c, colorless; f, flammable; gy, green, yellow; o, odorless; p, polymerizes; po, pungent; rb, red-brown; re, rotten eggs; so, sweet.
Sources: AC, aircrew; Ae, animal excreta; Af, agrifertilizer; CM, chemical manufacture; CS, cigarette smoke; D, dumps; EA, electric arcs; FC, fuel combustion; M, mining; Ng, natural gas; P, petroleum drilling, refining; S, stratosphere; T, tunnels; W, welding; We, wells.
Health Effects: A, asphyxiant; AO, airways obstruction; AOL, acroosteolysis; B, burns, skin; Ca, cancer; Ch, cough; Co, coma; Cv, depressed heart rate; D, dizziness; H, headache; L, liver; Mm, mucous membrane irritation; Np, neuropsychological toxin; Pe, pulmonary edema; T, tearing; Tp, tracheal pain.
[a] TWA, time-weighted average.
[b] IDLH, level of immediate danger to life or health.

breathing is impaired or the patient is unconscious, intubation and artificial ventilation may be required.

Control

Control and surveillance include avoiding areas where harmful gases may collect. Personnel must don self-contained breathing apparatus or air supply respirators before entering such areas and work in such areas only with adequate provision for air exchange. All rescuers of afflicted individuals should wear an individual air or oxygen supply and be attached to a safety harness by which they can be retrieved safely by fellow workers. Appropriate and specific rules should be devised and posted for personnel.

Prevention

Opportunities for gas leakage and accumulation should be minimized by industrial hygiene surveillance; the above advice postulates that every effort has been made to minimize leakage and maximize avoidance.

Chronic Alveolar Disease

Extrinsic allergic alveolitis, lipoproteinosis, and granulomatous alveolitis are disorders of the alveolar cells or alveolar spaces that are caused by inhalation of chemically active particles. They are described briefly below.

Nongranulomatous Alveolitis, Allergic Pneumonitis

The original description of extrinsic allergic alveolitis, or farmer's lung, implicated inhalation of fungal spores and vegetable material from hay or grain dust,[4] which recruited cells to alveoli. Some exposed farmers developed shortness of breath. Frequently, precipitating antibodies to crude preparations of fungi were found in their serum. However, antibodies were also found in asymptomatic farmers. Farmer's lung occurred in areas where animal feeds were stored wet, with the consequent enhanced generation of fungal spores. Classic descriptions came from Northwest England,[5] Scotland, and the north-central U.S. dairy states.[6] Both the size of the spores, less than 7 μm to be respirable but less than 3 μm to reach alveoli, and their solubility influence the disorder. Their toxins, including endotoxins, are important in the pathogenesis of farmer's lung, and hypersensitivity may be responsible for part of the pathological picture. Whether this is type IV allergy or also type III is not clear. Initial high-dose exposure to spores frequently produces both airway narrowing and acute pulmonary edema[7] (Fig. 25-3). Hospitalization with oxygen therapy has been required. After repeated exposure and development of precipitating antibodies, many cells may be recruited into alveoli. This pneumonitis can be lethal with repeated heavy exposure. On the other hand, the reaction may clear completely during absence from exposure. Adrenal corticosteroids frequently help resolve the acute phase but do not affect the chronic fibrotic stage.

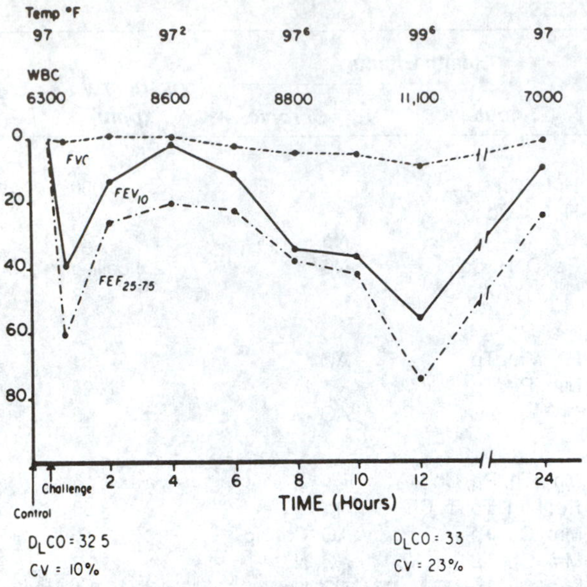

Figure 25-2. Effects of exposure to aspergilli.

Berylliosis

Beryllium, a dense, corrosion-resistant metal, produces fulminant chemical pneumonia when inhaled as a soluble salt in large doses. Inhalation of fumes or fine particles leads to chronic granulomatous alveolitis. Originally beryllium disease was interpreted as an accelerated sarcoidosis.[8] First recognized in workers making phosphores for fluorescent lamps, berylliosis is recognized pathologically by noncaseating granuloma with giant cells and the absence of necrosis. Specific helper-inducer T cells accumulate in the lung, leading to the identification of berylliosis as a hypersensitivity disease.[9] Insidious shortness of breath was accompanied by characteristic x-ray changes, which led to hospitalization in a tuberculosis sanitarium. Patients with accelerated sarcoidosis were brought to the attention of Dr. Harriet Hardy, who isolated the cause as beryllium from 42 materials used at work by the original patients.[8] Subsequently, the problem was recognized in workers from other electrical factories using beryllium nitrate phosphores. Some of the patients with advanced disease died. Those with less advanced berylliosis gradually improved but were left with residual interstitial fibrosis.[10] Because beryllium is irreplacable in nuclear reactors and in exotic alloys for spacecraft, exposure to beryllium fumes continues to be a problem for both engineers and skilled workers. Beryllium must be handled in a protective enclosure.

Lipoproteinosis

In this disorder alveolar spaces are filled with a combination of neutral lipids resembling pulmonary surfactant and proteins similar to the apoproteins of surfactant.[11] Inorganic particles and *Myobacterium tuberculosis* have been causally associated most frequently.[12] Thus areas of lipoproteinosis are frequently found in lung biopsies or in lungs at autopsy from workers exposed to silica.[13] Many other particles have been associated with occupational exposures. Diagnosis is usually made by sampling alveolar fluids by minibronchial lavage through the fiberoptic bronchoscope or by lung biopsy. Treatment is by lung lavage.

Both granulomatous and nongranulomatous alveolitis may be seen in a person exposed to moldy plant debris. Animal experiments suggest that granulomas may be due to poorly digestible complex chitins, which are complex carbohydrates forming the walls of spores and of plant cells.[14] Pulmonary fibrosis may result from chronic farmer's lung and lipoproteinosis[15] and appear to depend on particle composition, the host's immune status, and other factors.

Fibrosis

Chronic interstitial fibrosis has been observed after exposure to hard metal (tungsten carbide), silicon carbide, rare earths, copper (as sulfate in vineyard sprayer's lung), aluminum, beryllium, and cadmium. As mentioned above in berylliosis, fibrosis follows the granulomatous sarcoidlike response. Aluminum has been associated with fibrosis in workers making powdered aluminum for paints,[16] but is infrequent and must be differentiated radiographically or by lung biopsy from asbestosis and silicosis.

To make hard metal, powdered tungsten and carbon are fluxed with cobalt. Animals exposed to cobalt alone show the same lesions seen in workers,[17] namely, proliferation of alveolar and airway cells.[18] One similarity to the beryllium reaction is that removing the worker from exposure leads to prompt improvement; reexposure causes exacerbation. Its similarity to farmer's lung or alveolar lipoproteinosis suggests that lung lavage may be helpful. Adrenal corticosteroids help reverse the airways obstruction. Cadmium has the unusual distinction of producing both pulmonary edema (acute respiratory distress syndrome), particularly when fumes are generated from silver (cadmium) soldering, and pulmonary fibrosis, which is fine and non nodular in cadmium refinery workers.[19] Because of the frequency of asbestos exposure and asbestosis among metal smelting and refinery workers,[20] caution is advised in attributing pulmonary fibrosis to cadmium alone. Nodular infiltrates resembling those of berylliosis, hard metal disease, and silicosis have been reported among dental technicians and workers machining alloys of exotic metals. Because these illnesses occur infrequently among exposed workers (e.g., only 12.8 percent of 425 workers exposed to hard metal had radiographic evidence of disease),[21] individual immune response or susceptibility factors appear to be important.

Asthma, Acute Airway Reactivity

Acute airway narrowing, or asthma, is defined by shortness of breath or impaired breathing usually accompanied by wheezing that is relieved spontaneously or with therapy. Within this physiological definition of asthma are acute responses that develop within a few minutes of exposure in a sensitized individual as well as responses that may require several hours to reach their peak after beginning exposure, as with cotton dust.[22] Asthma has the fastest increasing incidence of the lung diseases as the twenty-first century approaches. Although the causes of the increase are not agreed upon, chemicals are important at work and at home. It is estimated that asthma increased by 60 percent in the 1980s.[23] Asthma currently affects 5 to 10 percent of children in the United States and 5 to 10 percent of

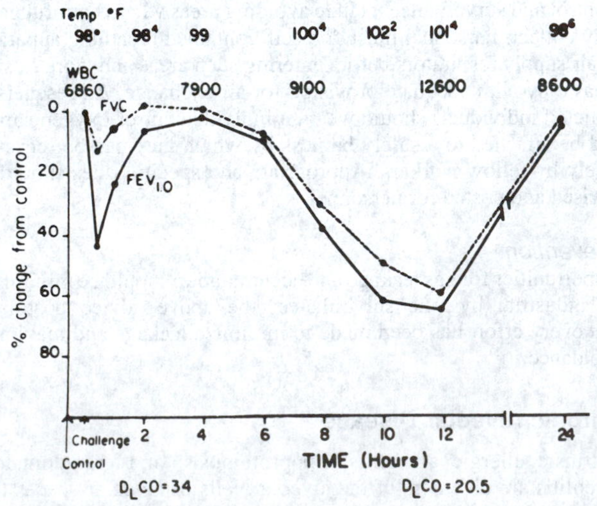

Figure 25-3. Effects of exposure to thermophiles.

adults.[24] African Americans are three times more likely to die of asthma than are whites.[23] They are also frequent victims of environmental inequality, meaning living in chemical "soups." Asthma is a disease of increasing mortality in the United States and across the world, particularly in developed countries such as Sweden, Denmark, and New Zealand. In 1979 the mortality in the United States was 1.2 per 100,000 and it had risen to 1.5 in 1983–1984.[25] In African Americans the corresponding figures are 1.8 in 1979 and 2.5 in 1984. Possible causes of this startling increase in asthma were not identified nor was it speculated why this disease has become epidemic. Many authors[23] have elaborated on the mechanisms, as if dismissing the evident multiplicity and complexity of causes. This chapter develops the view that the synthetic chemical triggers for asthma have increased manyfold in the past 50 years, and meanwhile buildings and homes have become tighter containers for these triggering chemicals. It will be argued that prevention of asthma, which is the most effective control measure, depends on stopping or at least reducing exposures to the chemical causes.

Prevalence

The prevalence of occupational asthma has been estimated for only a few situations. Although the total number of workers at risk is known in the United States by using data compiled by the National Institute of Occupational Safety and Health, the prevalence of asthma is known only within wide limits for portions of this population. For example, in 1973 the prevalence of byssinosis varied from 5 to 60 percent among the 700,000 U.S. textile workers. Estimates of disability from byssinosis were as high as 35,000 workers, although most of these individuals had already retired from the workforce. Based on the shift of cotton carding, spinning, and weaving to developing countries, world exposure to cotton dust may be 10 times the U.S. estimate. Although in the United States effective dust control in textile mills mandated by National Occupational Safety and Health Standards has reduced the prevalence of byssinosis to 5 percent or less, no dust controls exist in many countries.

Because the processing of common materials, for example cereal grains and flour, maximizes opportunities for exposure, farmers, grain handlers, millers, and bakers probably constitute the largest worldwide group with reactive airways disease.[26,27] Fortunately, exposures that produce the highest prevalence of airways reactivity, such as exposure to diisocyanates and cotton dust, have been controlled in the United States or the amounts used reduced.[28] An estimated 8 million workers in the world are exposed to welding gases and fumes. Such exposure produces symptoms but practically no acute airway response and relatively mild impairment of function. This is detectable 10 or 11 years after beginning exposure and is greater in cigarette smokers.[29]

Diagnosis

Acute or reactive airway response is recognized by an increased resistance to expiratory flow from either contraction of airway smooth muscle or swelling of airway walls. Tightness in the chest, shortness of breath, and wheezing develop quickly or insidiously. Nonproductive cough occurs with increasing frequency, but as mucus secretion is stimulated, the cough becomes productive. Generalized wheezing is heard low and posterior as the lung empties during forced expiration. Alternatively, scattered localized wheezing may be heard. The chest x-ray film is usually negative. Abnormalities seen are often due to preexisting disease. One exception is occasionally hyperinflation with increased radiolucency and even a low and flattened diaphragm, suggesting emphysema. A second exception is accentuated venous markings and a prominent minor lung fissure, suggesting pulmonary edema. Symptoms occur within a few hours of beginning work, are more frequent on Monday or the first day back after a holiday, and gradually increase during the work shift.[22] The diagnosis is confirmed by finding decreases in expiratory flow when comparing measurements at the middle or end of the shift with those made before entry to the workplace. The workplace is convenient to find cross-shift decrements, but if specific agent testing is needed, a laboratory exposure challenge may be required.[4,7] Workers' exposure must be long enough to stimulate workplace conditions. With management's cooperation, exposures can be measured during the work shift and dose-response curves constructed.

Mechanisms

Acute airway responses may be nociceptive, inflammatory, or immune. The reactive segment of a workforce includes but is not limited to atopic individuals, those with IgE antibodies. In the instance of toluene diisocyanate (TDI), which has been well studied, reactivity to low doses does not appear to correlate with atopic status.[30] Etiologies of many workplace exposures are imperfectly understood because cotton dust, grain dust, flour, coal dust, and foundry dust are complex mixtures. Only a few chemical agents can be singled out as specific causes. Included are metal fumes from zinc, copper, magnesium, aluminum, osmium, and platinum. Clearly endotoxin from Gram-negative bacteria and possibly from fungi is an important one. Many organic, naturally occurring food, fodder, and fiber plant products are enriched with endotoxin. Endotoxin concentrations increase with senescence of plants and thus are maximal at harvest time, as with cotton.

Causal Agents

To cover comprehensively the occupational exposures of importance is an encyclopedic job. However, Table 25-2 provides an index of the categories of materials and types of reactions. Causative agents are logically grouped so the reader can add new materials and reactions to them.

Control, Surveillance, and Prevention

The first principle of control and prevention is to reduce exposure for all workers by improved industrial hygiene. This has been demonstrated in the control of byssinosis (cotton dust disease) in the United States. Since 1973, dust has gradually been reduced in cotton textile mills. Abatement was so successful that after 15 years there was debate on whether byssinosis had existed. However, it continues to be a problem in the waste cotton industry[31] and in developing countries[32] lacking adequate engineering controls. The second principle of control and prevention is to remove reactive individuals from exposure. Reactivity is judged from symptoms or objectively from impaired function. Often individuals who react sharply to inhaled agents select themselves out of work. Because removing impaired workers from cotton textile mills did not improve their function, at least in the short term, it appears that byssinosis is a disease for which surveillance should be longitudinal as well as across the acute shift exposure so that workers whose function deteriorates at an accelerated rate can be removed from exposure before they have suffered enough impairment to interfere with their ability to work. This can be determined after measurements at 6- and 12-month intervals after the baseline measurement. Annual and semiannual surveillance by pulmonary function testing was mandated by the cotton dust standards invoked in 1978[24] under the 1970 amendments to the Occupational Health and Safety Act (OSHA).

Chronic Airway Disease: Chronic Bronchitis

Definition

Chronic bronchitis is defined by the presence of phlegm or sputum production for more than 3 months of 2 succeeding years. Cough is generally the presenting symptom. It is probably the most common respiratory disease in the world.[33]

Effects of Cigarette Smoking

The prevalence of chronic bronchitis is related mainly to the widespread smoking of cigarettes, a plague of this century largely since World War I. Although the habit is on the wane in the United States, it appears to be entrenched in Europe and to have taken developing

TABLE 25-2. PARTICLES AFFECTING HUMAN LUNGS: CLASSES AND EXAMPLES

Source	Persons Affected	Airways	Alveoli	Reference
■ ***BACTERIA***				
Aerobacter cloaceae *Phialophora species*	Air conditioner, humidifier workers		+	Friend JAR: Lancet 1:297, 1977
Escherichia coli endotoxin	Textile workers (mill fever)	+	+	Pernis B, et al: Br J Ind Med 18:120, 1961
Pseudomonas sp.	Sewer workers	+	+	Rylander R: Schweiz Med Wochenschr 107:182, 1977
■ ***FUNGI***				
Aspergillus sp. *Micropolyspora faeni*	Farmers	+		Emanuel DA, et al: Am J Med 37:392, 1964
Aspergillus clavatus	Malt workers	+		Channell S, et al: Q J Med 38:351, 1969
Cladosporium sp.	Combine operators	+	+	Darke CS, et al: Thorax 31: 294–302, 1976
Verticillium sp. *Alternaria* sp. *Micropolyspora faeni*	Mushroom workers	+	+	Lockey SD: Ann Allergy 33:282, 1974
Penicillium casei	Cheese washers	+		Minnig H, deWeck: AL Schweiz Med Wochenschr 102:1205, 1972
Penicillium frequentans	Cork workers [suberosis]	+		Arila R, Villar TG: Lancet 1:620, 1968
Thermoactinomyces (vulgaris) sacchari	Sugar cane workers [bagassosis]	+	+	Seabury J, et al: Proc Soc Exp Biol Med 129:351, 1968
■ ***AMOEBA***				
Acanthamoeba castellani *Acanthamoeba polyphaga* *Naegleria gruberi*	Air conditioning, humidifier workers	+	+	Edwards JH, et al: Nature 264:438, 1976
■ ***VEGETABLE ORIGIN***				
Barley dust	Farmers	+		McCarthy PE, et al: Br J Ind Med 42:106–110, 1985
Carbon black	Production workers	+		Crosbie WA: Arch Environ Health 41:346–353, 1986
Castor bean [ricin]	Oil mill workers	+		Panzani R: Int Arch Allergy 11:224–236, 1957
Cinnamon	Cinnamon workers	+		Uragada CG: Br J Ind Med 41:224–227, 1984
Coffee bean	Roasters	+		Freedman SD, et al: Nature 192:241, 1961
				Van Toorn DW: Thorax 25:399–405, 1970
Cotton, hemp, flax, jute, kapok	Textile workers	+		Roach SA, Schilling RSF: Br J Ind Med 17:1, 1960
				Jamison JP, et al: Br J Ind Med 43:809–813, 1986
				Buck MG, et al: Br J Ind Med 43:220–226, 1986
Flour dust	Millers	+		Tse KS, et al: Arch Environ Health 27:74, 1973
Grain dust	Farmers	+		Warren P, et al: J Allergy Clin Immunol 53:139, 1974
				Awad el Karim MA, et al: Arch Environ Health 41:297–301, 1986
Gum arabic, gum	Printers	+		Gelfand HH: J Allergy 14:208, 1954
Papain	Preparation workers		+	Flindt MLH: Lancet 1:430, 1978
Proteolytic enzymes—*Bacillus subtilis* [subtilisin, alcalase]	Detergent workers		+	Pepys J, et al: Lancet 1:1181, 1969
Soft paper	Paper mill workers	+		Enarson DA, et al: Arch Environ Health 39:325–330, 1984
				Thoren K, et al: Br J Ind Med 46:192–195, 1989

TABLE 25-2. PARTICLES AFFECTING HUMAN LUNGS: CLASSES AND EXAMPLES (Continued)

Source	Persons Affected	Airways	Alveoli	Reference
■ ***VEGETABLE ORIGIN*** (cont'd)				
Tamarind seed powder	Weavers	+		Murray R, et al: Br J Ind Med 14:105, 1957
Tea	Tea workers	+		Zuskin ES, Kuric Z: Br J Ind Med 41:88–93, 1984
Tobacco dust	Cigarette, cheroot factory workers	+		Viegi G, et al: Br J Ind Med 43: 802–808, 1986 Huuskonen MS, et al: Br J Ind Med 41:77–83, 1984
Wood dust	Those who work with Canadian red cedar, South African box-wood, rosewood (*Dalbergia* sp.)	+		Chan-Yeung M, et al: Am Rev Respir Dis 108:1094–1102, 1973 Carosso A, et al: Br J Ind Med 44:53–56, 1987 Vedal S, et al: Arch Environ Health 41:179–183, 1986
	Furniture workers		+	Gerhardsson MR, et al: Br J Ind Med 42:403–405, 1985
■ ***ANIMAL ORIGIN***				
Ascaris lumbricoides	Zoologists	+		Hansen K: Occupational Allergy. Springfield, IL: Charles C Thomas, 1958
Ascidiacea	Oyster culture workers	+		Nakashima T: Hiroshima J Med Sci 18:141, 1969
Dander	Farmers, fur workers, grooms	+		Squire JR: Clin Sci 9:127, 1950
Egg protein	Turkey and chicken farmers	+		Smith AB, et al: Am J Ind Med 12:205–218, 1987
Feathers	Poultry workers	+		Boyer RS, et al: Am Rev Respir Dis 109:630–635, 1974
Furs	Furriers			Zuskin E, et al: Am J Ind Med 14:189–196, 1988
Insect chitin [*Sitophilus granarius*]	Flour	+		Lunn JA, Hughes DTD: Br J Ind Med 24:158, 1967
Mayfly	Outdoor enthusiasts	+		Figley KD: J Allergy 11:376, 1940
Screwfly	Screwworm controllers	+		Gibbons HL, et al: Arch Environ Health 10:424–430, 1965
King crab	Processors	+		Orford RR, Wilson JT: Am J Ind Med 7:155–169, 1985
Pancreatic enzymes	Preparation workers	+	+	Colten HR, et al: N Engl J Med 292:1050–1053, 1975 Flood DFS, et al: Br J Ind Med 42:43–50, 1985
Rat serum and urine	Laboratory workers	+	+	Taylor AN, et al: Lancet 2:847, 1977 Agrup G, et al: Br J Ind Med 43:192–198, 1986
Swine confinement	Farm workers	+		Donham KJ: Am J Ind Med 5: 367–375, 1984
■ ***CHEMICALS***				
Inorganic				
Beryllium	Metal workers		+	Saltini C, et al: N Engl J Med 320:1103–1109, 1989
Calcium hydroxidetricalium silicate	Cement workers	+		Eid AH, El-Sewefy AZ: J Egypt Med Assoc 52:400, 1969
Chromium	Casters	+		Dodson VN, Rosenblatt EC: J Occup Med 8:326, 1966
Copper sulfate and lime	Vineyard sprayers		+	Pimental JC, Marques F: Thorax 24:678–688, 1969
Hard metal	Sintering and finishing workers	+	+	Meyer-Bisch C, et al: Br J Ind Med 46:302–309, 1989

(Continued)

TABLE 25-2. PARTICLES AFFECTING HUMAN LUNGS: CLASSES AND EXAMPLES (Continued)

Source	Persons Affected	Airways	Alveoli	Reference
■ ***CHEMICALS*** (cont'd)				
Vanadium pentoxide	Refinery workers	+		Zenz C, et al: Arch Environ Health 5:542, 1962
Nickel sulfate	Platers	+		McConnell LH, et al: Ann Intern Med 78:888, 1973
Platinum chloroplatinate	Photographers	+		Pepys J, et al: Clin Allergy 2: 391, 1972
Titanium chloride	Pigment workers		+	Redline S, et al: Br J Ind Med 43:652–656, 1986
Titanium oxide	Paint factory			Oleru UG: Am J Ind Med 12: 173–180, 1987
Tungsten carbide (cobalt); hard metal	Hard metal workers	+	+	Coates EO, Watson JHL: Ann Intern Med 75:709, 1971
Zinc, copper, magnesium fumes	Welders, bronze workers [metal fume fever]	+		Gleason RP: Am Ind Hyg Assoc J 29:461, 1968
Iron, chromium, nickel [oxides]	Welders	+		Kilburn KH: Am J Indust Med 87:62–69, 1989
Organic				
Aminoethyl ethanolamine	Solderers			McCann JK: Lancet 1:445, 1964
Ayodicarbonemide	Plastic injection molders	+		Whitehead LW, et al: Am J Ind Med 11:83–92, 1987
Chlorinated biphenyls	Transformer manufacturers		+	Shigematsu N, et al: PCB's Environ Res 1978
Colophony (pine resin)	Solderers	+		Fawcett IW, et al: Clin Allergy 6(4)577, 1976
Diazonium salts	Chemical workers	+		Perry KMA: Occupational Lung Diseases. In Perry KMA, Sellers TH (eds): Chest Diseases. London: Butterworth, 1963, p 518
Diisocyanates—toluene, diphenylmethane	Production workers, foundry workers	+		Brugsch HG, Elkins HG: N Engl J Med 268:353–357, 1963 Zammit-Tabona M, et al: Am Rev Respir Dis 128: 226–230, 1983
Formaldehyde (Permapress, urethane foam)	Histology technicians, office workers	+		Popa V, et al: Dis Chest 56: 395; 1969; Alexandersson R, et al: Arch Environ Health 43:222, 1988
Paraphenylenediamine	Solderers	+		Perry KMA: Occupational lung diseases. In Perry KMA, Sellers TH (eds): Chest Diseases. London: Butterworth, 1963, p 518; Dally KA, et al: Arch Environ Health 36:277–284, 1981
Paraquat	Sprayers	+	+	Bainova A, et al: Khig-i zdravespazane 15:25, 1972
Penicillin, ampicillin	Production workers, nurses	+		Davies RJ, et al: Clin Allergy 4: 227, 1974
Parathion	Sprayers	+		Ganelin RS, et al: JAMA 188: 108, 1964
Piperazine	Chemists	+		Pepys J: Clin Allergy 2:189, 1972
Polymer fumes (polytetrafluoroethylene)	Teflon manufacturers, users	+	+	Harris DK: Lancet 2:1008, 1951 Lewis CE, Kirby GR: JAMA 191:103, 1965
Polyvinyl chloride	Fabrication workers	+		Ernst P, et al: Am J Ind Med 14:273–279, 1988
■ ***SYNTHETIC FIBERS***				
Nylon, polyesters, Dacron	Textile workers		+	Pimental JC, et al: Thorax 30: 204, 1975
Rubber (neoprene)	Injection press operators	+		Thomas RJ, et al: Am J Ind Med 9:551–559, 1986

TABLE 25-2. PARTICLES AFFECTING HUMAN LUNGS: CLASSES AND EXAMPLES (Continued)

Source	*Persons Affected*	*Airways*	*Alveoli*	*Reference*
Tetralzene	Detonators	+		Burge SB, et al: Thorax 39: 470, 1984
Vinyl chloride [phosgene, hydrogen chloride]	Meat wrappers [asthma]	+		Sokol WN, et al: JAMA 226: 639, 1973
	Firefighters		+	Dyer RE, Esch VH: JAMA 235: 393, 1976
	Polymerization plant workers		+	Arnard A, et al: Thorax 33:19, 1978

nations by storm, where the peak prevalence of cigarette smoking may not yet have been reached. Certainly there is no evidence that quitting has become the more accepted social behavior, as it has in the United States. Chronic bronchitis has such a high prevalence in cigarette smokers, particularly 20 years or more after they start smoking, that it often takes careful analysis to find occupational chronic bronchitis. This is because blue collar workers are more frequently cigarette smokers than others in the population.[34]

Occupational effects can be assessed most securely by studying large populations of individuals who have never smoked.[35] Alternately, effects of cigarette smoking and occupational exposure can be partitioned by adjusting predicted function values for expiratory flows for duration of smoking using standard regression coefficients.[36] Similarly, accelerated functional deterioration or increased prevalence of symptoms across years of occupational exposure after adjusting for the cumulative effects of smoking may show the effects of occupational exposure. Based on interactive effects of cigarette smoking with occupational dusts and fumes and with atmospheric air pollution in many studies, if the age decrement for forced expiratory volume (FEV_1) in a person who has never smoked exceeds 21 to 25 mL/year, this represents an excessive decrement. Cigarette smoking alone in men increases the age-associated decrement by 9 mL/year, an almost 40 percent increase. Women show no such effect, probably because they smoke fewer cigarettes daily but still show increased lung cancers. In groups of men, decrements in FEV_1 of more than than 30 mL/year would be attributable to occupational or environmental exposures. Airborne particle burdens increase age-related decrements.

Occupational Exposures

Many dusts of occupational exposure, including those containing silica, coal, asbestos, and cotton (including flax and hemp) dust, and exposures during coking, foundry work, welding, and papermaking increase the prevalence or lower the age of appearance of chronic bronchitis. Although it is clear that high exposures to silica and asbestos produce pneumoconiosis, lower doses cause airways obstruction. Symptoms and later airways obstruction from cotton and other vegetable dusts have been well studied since recognition more than a century ago.[37] In the 1960s studies in British textile mills (using American-grown cotton), the severity of this Monday-morning asthma (byssinosis) and of shortness of breath and tightness in the chest were correlated with concentrations of respirable cotton dust.[38] Similarly, exposure to welding gases and fumes has been associated with accelerated reductions in expiratory flows.[29] It is noteworthy that the trades of shipbuilding and construction work, so frequently associated with asbestosis and to a lesser extent with silicosis, are also strongly correlated with chronic bronchitis, as are coal mining[39,40] and work in foundries.[41] The common thread is inhalation of respirable particles with inflammation stimulated by one or more chemically active species contained or absorbed. Clinical signs are cough with mucus production due to goblet cell hyperplasia in small airways and to hyperplasia of mucous glands in large bronchi and exertional dyspnea due to small airways obstruction.[42]

Inhalation of 200 to 400 ppm of sulfur dioxide by rats or guinea pigs produces a useful model of chronic bronchitis. However, the levels exceed, by 2 orders of magnitude, levels found in usual smelting or metal roasting operations to which workers are exposed or by 3 orders of magnitudes the most ambient air pollution exposures. However, human exposures are almost always accompanied by quantities of respirable particles. Similarly, exposure to chlorine, fluorine, bromine, phosgene, and vapors of hydrogen fluoride and hydrogen chloride produce bronchitic reactions, but because exposure is seldom continuous, these pulses of damage tend to produce cycles of injury and repair rather than chronic bronchitis.

Gases are adsorbed on particles in many occupational exposures. Examples include welding, metal roasting, and smelting operations, as well as situations in foundries or where compressed air jets are used for cleaning. Gas molecules adsorbed on particles deposit in small airways.[2] This deposition is studied in animal models with gases and pure carbon. Carbon, by itself an innocuous particle, adsorbs gas molecules and creates a nidus of damage because the particle is difficult to remove and the adsorbed gas molecules leach into cells.[43] Perhaps the best examples are the adsorption of ozone, nitrogen dioxide, and hydrocarbons on respirable particles[35] in Los Angeles, Mexico City, Athens, and other cities where large amounts of fossil fuel are combusted with limited atmospheric exchanges because of mountains, prevailing winds, and weather conditions.

The prevalence of occupational chronic bronchitis has declined in the postindustrial era in the United States, Great Britain, and Northern Europe. Byssinosis and chronic bronchitis from cotton dust have been on the wane since the early 1970s.[44,45] A similar decline in prevalence in workers in foundries, coke ovens, welding, and other dusty trades is attributed to better awareness of the health hazards and improved air hygiene often dictated by economic or processing imperatives.[39,41,46] Workers in Eastern Europe and emerging economies in China, India, Southeast Asia, and South America are now plagued by these "solved" problems.

Natural History

The natural history of chronic bronchitis in urban dwellers has been investigated since the early nineteenth century.[47] Chronic inhalation of polluted air stimulates mucus production, recognized by cough and phlegm, which define chronic bronchitis epidemiologically.[48] Chronic bronchitis identified by the symptoms of cough and sputum was studied in more than 1,000 English civil servants and transport workers over a decade.[48,49] Approximately the same proportion were symptomatic at the end of the decade as at the beginning, although some individuals had left and others had entered the symptomatic group over the interval.[49]

Clearly, the prevalence of chronic bronchitis increases with age in both females and males. The male predominance may be entirely due to cigarette smoking. The latent period before deterioration of expiratory airflow may be long if chronic bronchitis begins in childhood or early adulthood but short if it begins in late middle age.[49,50]

Chronic bronchitis has another course, that with an abrupt onset of bronchitis, which is not associated with cigarette smoking or occupational exposure.[50] It is more common in women and is generally preceded by a viral or chemical respiratory illness, after which there is chronic phlegm production and more rapid than expected airflow limitation with deterioration of pulmonary function. When shortness of breath accompanies the cardinal symptoms, airflow limitation is generally present, and the yearly decrements in function are usually twice as large as predicted. For many individuals who smoke and have had an insidious onset of shortness of breath, expiratory airflow declines more steeply after age 50.[49]

Epidemiology

Since the early 1960s, atmospheric air pollution has been recognized as an important cause of chronic bronchitis.[51] Studies in Groningen, The Netherlands,[52] Cracow, Poland,[53] and London[49] firmly established that episodic severe pollution increased mortality and that chronic levels of atmospheric air pollution were associated with increased prevalence and morbidity from chronic bronchitis. Mortality from asthma and chronic bronchitis fell in Japan when sulfur dioxide air pollution decreased.[54] In 1986, restudy of Italian schoolchildren showed that previously reduced expiratory flows rose to levels of controls when air pollution decreased.[55]

Control Measures

Control measures for chronic bronchitis depend on avoiding exposure—to cigarette smoke, to contaminated respirable particles in coal mines, smelters, and foundries, and to air pollution from fossil fuel combustion. Socioeconomic level is also important since, as the standard of living rises, the prevalence of chronic bronchitis falls. Probably the factor is residence near fuel combustion effluents. Control ultimately depends on improving the population's general health and curtailing its exposure to respirable particles.

Surveillance

Effects of a personal, occupational, or atmospheric air pollution control program are best assessed by surveying symptoms and pulmonary functional performance of a random sample of the affected population. Most essential data—the prevalence of chronic bronchitis and measurement of expiratory airflow—are easily obtained and can be appraised frequently. Measures that decrease exposure should reduce the prevalence of cough and phlegm and the rate of deterioration of expiratory airflow.

Prevention

The prevention of chronic bronchitis essentially centers on avoiding generation of respirable particles into the human air supply. Cigarette smoking cannot be condoned. Air filtration helps if particle generation is not avoidable, as in cotton textile mills. Socioeconomic measures include cleaner combustion of fossil fuels, reduction of human crowding, provisions for central heating, and improvements in the standard of living. Patients with acute bronchitis should be treated with a broad-spectrum antibiotic to reduce chronic bronchitis of abrupt onset.

Neoplastic Disease of Airways

Lung cancer from occupational exposure to uranium, asbestos, chromate pigments, and arsenic was described before the worldwide epidemic of lung cancer from cigarette smoking. Unfortunately, early reports often failed to mention cigarette smoking, so that secure attribution of cause was delayed until large studies had sufficient numbers of individuals who had never smoked. Certainly with asbestosis, there is firm data on which to establish the causal linkage of asbestos to lung cancer without smoking. The histological types of cancer are those seen in the general population, including adenocarcinoma, squamous cell, undifferentiated, and small-cell or oat cell carcinoma. One sentinel disorder has been described, small-cell carcinoma, after exposure to chloromethyl ethers.

The association of lung cancer with exposure to polycyclic aromatic hydrocarbons in coke oven workers and roofers has been clearly established and follows Percival Pott's attribution of the scrotal skin cancers in chimney sweeps to coal tar in London, over 200 years ago. Similarly, the occupational exposures to radon, radium, and uranium in mining and metalworking cause lung cancers. A recent example is uranium-mining Navaho Indians on the Colorado Plateau, who, despite a low prevalence of smoking and a low consumption of cigarettes among those who smoked, had a 10-fold increase (observed over expected) in lung cancer.[56] Sentinel nasal sinus cancers and excessive lung cancers have resulted from exposure to the nickel refining in calcination of impure nickel and copper sulfide to nickel oxide or in the carbonyl process.

Lung cancer may be caused by other exposures to nickel, to chromium, and to arsenic, but the data are less convincing than the foregoing examples.[57] Thus, another agent or agents may be responsible for the cancer mortality from lung cancer in smelter workers. That this additional factor may be asbestos was suggested in recent studies of copper smelter workers and aluminum refinery workers, whose prevalences of asbestosis were between 8 and 25 percent using the International Labor Organization (ILO) criteria for x-ray diagnosis.[20]

It appears that the common denominator for the higher pulmonary disease prevalence and lung cancer mortality among metal smelter workers may be asbestos. In these work sites, asbestos has been used for heat insulation; for patching of calciners, retorts, and roasters; and for heat protection for personnel. In a way reminiscent of the studies before the contribution of cigarette smoking was recognized, it appears that the contribution of asbestos must be taken into account before attributing cancer or irregular opacities in the lung to the useful metals.

▸ ENVIRONMENTAL AIR POLLUTION

History

The famous fogs along the Thames in the City of London chronicled by Sir Arthur Conan Doyle in the Sherlock Holmes stories 100 years ago underscored a problem first noted in the early seventeenth century, at the beginning of the Industrial Revolution with John Evelyn's description in 1621. That such exposure could produce death was first recognized in the Meuse Valley of Belgium during a thermal inversion in December 1930.[51] Sixty people died. In Donora, Pennsylvania, a town of about 14,000 people along the Monongahela River with steel mills, coke ovens, a zinc production plant, and a chemical plant manufacturing sulfuric acid, a continuous temperature inversion created a particularly malignant fog that caused many illnesses and 20 deaths in October 1948. Deaths occurred the third day after onset. In December 1952, a particularly vicious episode produced excessive mortality in London among infants, young children, and elderly persons with cardiorespiratory disease. High values reported were 4.5 mg/m^3 for smoke and 3.75 mg/m^3 for sulfur dioxide. A 1953 episode in New York City called further attention to this twentieth century plague. Other episodes described in Tokyo, Yokohama, New Orleans, and Los Angeles led to investigation of the health effects of environmental air pollution in the 1960s and early 1970s.

A singular air pollution episode swept across the Northern Hemisphere between November 27 and December 10, 1962. Excessive respiratory symptoms were observed in Washington, D.C., New York City, Cincinnati, and Philadelphia. London had 700 excess deaths due to high sulfur dioxide levels, and in Rotterdam, sickness, absenteeism, and increased hospital admissions occurred, with a 5-fold increase in sulfur oxides. Hamburg, West Germany, reported increased sulfur dioxide and dust and increased heart disease mortality. In Osaka 60 excess deaths were linked to high pollution levels.

Currently, several cities stand out as worst cases of air pollution. Mexico City, with extreme levels of pollution and an altitude of 7,000 feet in an enclosed valley with over 20 million people, is the world's capital of air pollution. Athens, located like Los Angeles with a mountain backdrop to prevailing westerly winds, has experienced such serious pollution as to jeopardize some of its monuments of antiquity. Adverse health effects from air pollution have been observed in São Paulo and Cubatao, Brazil, which have many diesel vehicles, a heavy petrochemical industry, and fertilizer plants. Brazil is experimenting with methyl alcohol as fuel for internal combustion engines. As more developing countries industrialize, the lessons that should have been learned from Donora, London, and New York continue to be ignored.

Sources

The major source of modern environmental air pollution is combustion of fossil fuels.[58] During this century, oil (gasoline)-based transportation has become the predominant contributor, with a shift from coal for space heating and industrial production. In fact, the internal combustion automobile engine is now the major source of both particles and gases, including hydrocarbons. The interaction of atmospheric gases with hydrocarbons under sunlight (photocatalysis) produces ozone and nitrogen dioxide. Adding these to the direct products of combustion in air produces the irritating acrid smoke and smog, a word coined to describe the mixture of smoke and fog. Thus, the horizon of many cities shows a burnished copper glow from nitrogen oxides. The smog in Los Angeles has remained practically static for 30 years; efforts to ameliorate the problem have simply kept pace with the additional population and its motor vehicle exhaust.[59,60]

In certain areas, such as the Northeastern United States, industrial processing, coking, steel production, as well as paper mills and oil refineries contribute their selective and somewhat specific flavor to the problem.[61] In occupational exposures, the particles are of respirable size and gases adsorb on them. Fly ash, from the combustion of coal in power stations, from space heating, and in industry, consists of fused glass spheres with adsorbed metals and acidic gases.[62] Adsorbed chemicals increase particle toxicity and determine the zones of injury in the lung.

Waste incineration has increased the burden in the air, and greater population has nearly exhausted available canyons and open spaces for landfills for garbage around major cities. Although it appears that selective incineration under properly controlled conditions may help solve the solid waste problem, it increases the burden of particles and gases in the atmosphere unless carefully controlled. Moreover, nature may be responsible for freak episodes of air pollution. In 1986, release of carbon dioxide from Lake Nyos in West Africa killed 1,700 people as they slept, and already the lake may be partly recharged.[63]

Regulated Pollutants

Since 1970 in the United States, carbon monoxide, hydrocarbons, sulfur dioxide, nitrogen oxides, and ozone have been regulated by the Environmental Protection Agency (EPA). In various urban areas, ozone and oxidant concentrations have been defined above which occupants are alerted to limit physical activity. Although the respirable particles, particularly flyash, hydrocarbons, and coated carbon particles from diesel engines, provide the principal components that make up the visible pollution, recently considerable attention has focused on acids and chlorofluorocarbons.

Chlorofluorocarbons manufactured as refrigerants and also used to power convenience aerosols liberate chlorine into the stratosphere, where it combines with ozone to reduce the shield against ultraviolet radiation.[64,65] The combination of loss of the ozone shield and increase in carbon dioxide from combustion of fuel and destruction of tropical rain forests, among other causes, has increased atmospheric carbon dioxide, leading to global warming, the so-called greenhouse effect.[66] This constitutes an entirely different but potentially very serious complication of environmental air pollution. Northern Europeans, particularly in Sweden, Norway, and the city of Cologne, West Germany, have been greatly concerned with the problem of acid rain, which is precipitation of large amounts of acid from acidic gases combined with water.[67] The acidity of these solutions has been sufficient to etch limestone buildings and to acidify lakes and reservoirs, killing aquatic life and changing natural habitats. Ozone loss (which increases the risk of cancer),[68] acid rain, and global warming are likely to produce future human health problems.

Modifiers

The effects of particles and gases in the atmosphere are lessened by wind and rain dilution and made worse by thermal inversion. Studies in Tokyo showed that the heat worked with ozone to produce respiratory symptoms in schoolchildren.[69] There have been enough spontaneous experiments to show that stopping automotive transportation in a city such as New York, for a day or two, is sufficient to ameliorate problems from rising levels of air pollutants. Thus it appears obvious that a solution to transportation in urban areas would greatly relieve air pollution. Because combustion of diesel fuel and gasoline in automobiles and trucks is the major problem, it appears that designing cleaner engines is fundamental to improving air quality. Alternate fuels emphasizing methanol and ethanol alone or mixed with gasoline may be important and are included in the EPA plans for clearer air for the United States in the next decade. One additive methyl-*n*-butyl ether has increased respiratory illnesses in winter and asthma. Almost 20 years of retrofit (regressive) engineering, the installation of catalytic converters, has been less satisfactory. Although it has kept levels of air pollution from increasing in Los Angeles, it is unclear whether this technology would help in Mexico City, Athens, or São Paulo.

Effects

Toxicity is determined by particle size, adsorption, and respiratory deposition profiles.[70] Respirable particles are those capable of depositing beyond the ciliated conducting airways of the human lung.[1,2] The effects of air pollution can be classified as symptoms, impaired pulmonary function, respiratory diseases, and mortality. Acute symptoms, including eye irritation, nasal congestion, and chest tightness, appear to be due to the oxidant gases, aldehydes, and hydrocarbons largely in the gaseous phase, including peroxyacetyl nitrate.[71] In the most sensitive 7 to 10 percent of the population, exposure to these same gases may limit expiratory air flow, with wheezing and cough. Symptoms increase with exercise and are usually relieved within a few hours of removal from exposure.

Large studies of European populations exposed to air pollution have shown that airways obstruction varied on days of greater or lesser levels of sulfur dioxide and particles.[52,55] However, the question of reversibility is unanswered. Whether or how quickly airflow limitation is relieved by removal from exposure has not been tested. Meanwhile, to assume that the situation resembles that of cigarette smoking, in that airways obstruction is irreversible, is justified.

The prevalence of chronic bronchitis in the exposed population is one of the most reliable indicators of exposure to the gases and particles of atmospheric air pollution.[71] A number of classic studies—Grotingen, The Netherlands; Cracow; Poland; London; Tokyo; and Los Angeles—have shown that prevalence of chronic bronchitis rises with level and duration of air pollution.[72] Obviously, this is best studied in individuals who have never smoked and in children. The production of enough mucus to necessitate coughing for its removal appears to be essentially a protective mechanism for the respiratory tract. Both clinical and experimental data show goblet cell metaplasia in small airways[42] and goblet cell and mucous gland hyperplasia in large conducting airways. This latter finding is the consistent pathological accompaniment of chronic bronchitis in autopsies from exposed populations.[73]

Deaths from the air pollution disasters, and from current levels of air pollution, have largely occurred in infants who have died of pneumonia and in adults with cardiorespiratory disease, particularly chronic bronchitis and emphysema. Those with precarious respiratory function are highly susceptible to additional insult and by analogy constitute, in the picturesque lumberjack terms, "standing dead timber," susceptible to the "strong wind" provided by a prolonged period of increased air pollution.

Other results of severe air pollution include the retardation of children's mental development from airborne lead,[74] which constituted the principal reason for first reducing lead tetraethyl and similar additives and finally removing them from gasoline and motor fuel in the United States during the 1970s. The clear inverse relationship between lead and population intelligence is being verified again in Mexico City.[75]

▸ INDOOR AIR POLLUTION

Living Agents

Illness and excessive symptoms from indoor exposures to sick buildings have increased rapidly in a generation. Illness associated with exposure indoors has been observed repeatedly[76,77] and reviewed at length.[78,79] Episodes such as in Pontiac, Michigan, have stimulated investigations into bacterial and fungal contamination with some fruitful results. For example. Legionnaire's disease was discovered from an investigation of illnesses occurring at a convention of the American Legion at the Bellvue Stratford Hotel in Philadelphia. Its etiology was a bacterium since named *Legionella pneumophila*.[80] Episodes of the tight building syndrome became more frequent with the energy crisis of 1973. These many investigations failed to find a bacterial or fungal source and engendered a search for chemical contamination.

Sources of Chemicals

Indoor air receives gases, vapors, and some particles generated by the activities therein (Table 25-3). Their concentrations reflect the amounts generated or released in the volume, the number of air exchanges, and the purity of makeup air. Thus, human effluents, chiefly carbon dioxide and mercaptans, combine with products of space heating and cooking, cigarette smoke, and contributions from air-conditioning systems. Added to these are outgassing of building construction, adhesive, and decorating materials to make a potent witches' brew. If the building has a sufficient number of air exchanges, the concentration gradient may be reversed and the building atmosphere made hospitable. On the other hand, reducing the air exchanges to conserve heat or cold can lead to buildup of noxious odors, vapors, and gases. Location of air intakes, types of filtration, and refrigeration and heating systems all decrease the quality of indoor air and increase volatile organic chemicals (VOCs). New evidence shows that pesticides such as chlordane and organophosphates such as chlorprifos, sprayed indoors in xylene-water, appear responsible for excessive neurobehavioral symptoms and measurable brain injury.[3]

A causal analytical approach to personal factors and indoor air quality in Sweden found that total hydrocarbon concentrations were significantly correlated with eye, skin, and upper airway irritation, headache, and fatigue.[81] Smoking, psychosocial factors, and static electricity were also contributory. Hyperactivity, as well as sick leave due to airway diseases, were important chronic effects in this study. Neither atopy, age, nor sex were correlated with symptoms. The studies were extended to 129 teaching and maintenance personnel of six primary schools in Uppsala,[82] a Swedish city 50 km from Stockholm. All buildings had elevated carbon dioxide levels of more than 800 ppm, indicating a poor air supply. Mean indoor VOCs ranged from 70 to 180 μg/m^3. Arithmetic mean was 130 μg/m^3, aromatics mean was 39 μg/m^3, while formaldehyde was below the detection limit of 10 μg/m^3. Chronic sick building symptoms were not related to carbon dioxide levels, but instead were correlated with VOCs, as well as wall-to-wall carpeting, hyperactivity, and psychosocial factors.

Formaldehyde. Because many building materials are bonded with resins that use formaldehyde, this gas, which also is a constituent of

TABLE 25-3. SELECTED GUIDELINES FOR AIR CONTAMINANTS OF INDOOR ORIGIN

Contaminant[a]	*Concentration*	*Exposure Time*	*Comments*
Acetone—O	—	—	—
Ammonia—O	—	—	—
Asbestos	—	—	Known human carcinogen; best available control technology
Benzene—O	—	—	Known human carcinogen; best available control technology
Carbon dioxide	4.5 g/m^3	Continuous	—
Chlordane—O	5 μg/m^3	Continuous	—
Chlorine	—	—	—
Cresol—O	—	—	—
Dichloromethane—O	—	—	—
Formaldehyde—O	120 μg/m^3	Continuous	West German and Dutch guidelines
Hydrocarbons, aliphatic—O	—	—	—
Hydrocarbons, aromatic—O	—	—	—
Mercury	—	—	—
Ozone—O	100 μg/m^3	Continuous	—
Phenol—O	—	—	—
Radon	0.01 working level	Annual average	Background 0.002–0.004 working level
Tetrachloroethylene—O	—	—	—
Trichloroethane—O	—	—	—
Turpentine—O	—	—	—
Vinyl chloride—O	—	—	Known human carcinogen; best available control technology

Reprinted with permission from American National Standards Institute/American Society of Heating, Refrigeration, Air-Conditioning Engineers: Standard 62-1981—Ventilation for Acceptable Indoor Air Quality. New York: The Society, 1981, 48 pp which states: "If the air is thought to contain any contaminant not listed (in various tables), guidance on acceptable exposure . . . should be obtained by reference to the standards of the Occupational Safety and Health Administration. For application to the general population the concentration of these contaminants should not exceed 1/10 of the limits that are used in industry. . . . In some cases, this procedure may result in unreasonable limits. Expert consultation may then be required. . . . These substances are ones for which indoor exposure standards are not yet available."

[a] Contaminants marked "O" have odors at concentrations sometimes found in indoor air. The tabulated concentrations do not necessarily result in odorless conditions.

cigarette smoke and is used in permanent press fabrics, has been consistently found in indoor air.[83] Most studies have found major contamination from cigarette smoking. Thus, prohibition of smoking indoors makes air more pleasant. Cooking, particularly with natural gas, generates nitrogen oxides that rival formaldehyde in their capacity to irritate.

Asbestos. During the late 1970s and early 1980s, concern for release of asbestos from construction materials into indoor air stimulated measurement of fiber levels.[84] Generally these have been well below occupational levels, usually between 0.01 and 0.0001 fibers/mL. However, during repair or renovation of heating systems, with maximal conservation of air, levels may reach 0.2 to 1.0 fibers/mL. The experience with asbestos has raised concerns about fibrous glass, which has been widely used in insulation. Even less is known of its possible effects on health from bystander exposure.

Freon and Chlorofluorocarbons. The leakage of freon, a refrigerant used in air-conditioning systems, is particularly noxious because phosgene is generated at ignition points such as electric arcs, burning cigarettes, and open flames. This problem was first identified aboard nuclear submarines, which remained submerged for long periods. Paint solvents contributed most to indoor pollution on board these vessels. Regulations now prohibit painting less than 30 days before putting to sea.

Radon. Another concern indoors is radon and daughter products, which may concentrate in indoor air due to building location (e.g., the granite deposits of Reading Prong in Pennsylvania, New York, and New Jersey) or be released from concrete and other building materials.[85] As with asbestos, the human health hazard of large exposures to radon and daughter products is well known from the miners of Schneeberg, Germany, and Jacymov, Czechoslovakia. The long-term health impact of low doses of radon products from basements, particularly from building materials or the substrata of rock, is poorly demonstrated.[86] Related decisions are difficult both for individuals and from a public health perspective, and thus both legislation and rule making have wavered in the breezes of indecision.

In summary, living organisms do cause disease in buildings spread by heating and air-conditioning systems. It is unknown if materials such as trichloroethylene, which appears in culinary water that is dispersed into the air by showering and other water use, make chronic exposure dangerous. Such low-level exposure appears to produce harmful effects after 20 or 25 years.[72]

Effects

Symptoms. The major ill effects from indoor exposure begin several minutes to several hours after exposure and disappear in a few hours or overnight after individuals exit the building. They recur on reentry. Symptoms include fatigue, feeling of exhaustion, headache, and sometimes anorexia, nausea, lack of concentration, and lightheadedness. As occupants talk about their problems, irritability and recent memory loss may be noted along with the irritation of eyes and throat. Attempts to demonstrate physiological changes are beset by difficulties in measuring slight changes and interpreting findings. This has led to concerns over possible mass hysteria, or "crowd syndrome." The methods for proving these diagnoses are frequently poorly grounded and there is as yet no standard investigational method for these problems. However, the following are suggested.

Investigation. Use a standard inventory of symptoms and obtain information on as many occupants of a structure as possible. Affective disorder inventories such as the profile of mood states are useful. This information should be accompanied by mapping of affected and unaffected subjects' work areas and their locations in the building. Air sampling should aim at recognizing chemical groups such as aldehydes, solvents, mercaptans, oxidant gases, chlorofluorocarbons (freons), carbon monoxide, and pesticides (organochlorines and organophosphates). The decision to use physiological tests for pulmonary or neurological function should be made after reviewing the exposure and the symptom inventories.

Control and Prevention

Provision for adequate air exchange with entrainment of fresh air not contaminated by motor vehicle exhaust or effluents from surrounding industrial activities is the most prudent control and preventive measure. Removal of sources of contaminated air should be by hoods with back- or down-draft suction for welding, painting, and similar operations. Internal filtration of air removes particles in cotton textile mills and metal machining operations but is rarely useful in indoor pollution, where total particle burdens are rarely more than 0.2 or 0.3 mg/m^3 and VOCs are incriminated. On high-altitude aircraft, activated charcoal absorbers for ozone are workable, as they are on submarines. However, the cost of these for buildings, compared with cost for air exchanges, is prohibitively high. Freon, formaldehyde, solvents, and asbestos should be controlled to as low levels as possible in the indoor environment. These concerns will be pushed by needs for energy conservation. The problems of indoor air pollution in "sick buildings," especially neurobehavioral impairment associated with VOCs and pesticides, demand attention as workers are forced to retire early for neurobehavioral disability.

▸ REFERENCES

1. Kilburn KH: A hypothesis for pulmonary clearance and its implications. Am Rev Respir Dis 98:449–463, 1968
2. Kilburn KH: Particles causing lung disease. Environ Health Perspect 55:97–109, 1984
3. Kilburn KH: Chemical brain injury. New York: John Wiley, 1979
4. Pepys J: Hypersensitivity disease of the lungs due to fungi and organic dusts. In Kolos A (ed): Monograph in Allergy. New York: Karger, 1969, vol 4, pp 1–147
5. Morgan DC, Smyth JT, Lister RW, et al: Chest symptoms in farming communities with special reference to farmer's lung. Br J Ind Med 32:228–234, 1975
6. Roberts RC, Wenzel FJ, Emanuel DA: Precipitating antibodies in a midwest dairy farming population toward the antigens associated with farmer's lung disease. J Allergy Clin Immunol 57:518–524, 1976
7. Schlueter DP: Response of the lung to inhaled antigens. Am J Med 57:476–492, 1974
8. Hardy HL, Tabershaw IR: Delayed chemical pneumonitis in workers exposed to beryllium compounds. J Ind Hyg Toxicol 28:197–211, 1946
9. Saltini C, Winestock K, Kirby M, Pinkston P, Crystal RG: Maintenance of alveolitis in patients with chronic beryllium disease by beryllium-specific helper T cells. N Engl J Med 320:1103–1109, 1989
10. Hardy HL: Beryllium poisoning—lessons in control of man-made disease. N Engl J Med 273:1188–1199, 1965
11. Passero MA, Tye RW, Kilburn KH, Lynn WS: Isolation characterization of two glycoproteins from patients with alveolar proteinosis. Proc Natl Acad Sci USA 70:973–976, 1973
12. Davidson JM, MacLeod WM: Pulmonary alveolar proteinosis. Br J Dis Chest 63:13–28, 1969
13. Heppleston AG, Wright NA, Stewart JA: Experimental alveolar lipoproteinosis following the inhalation of silica. J Pathol 101:293–307, 1970
14. Smetana HF, Tandon HG, Viswanataan R, Venkitasubrunarian TA, Chandrasekhary S, Randhawa HS: Experimental bagasse disease of the lung. Lab Invest 11:868–884, 1962
15. Seal RME, Hapke EJ, Thomas GO, Meck JC, Hayes M: The pathology of the acute and chronic stages of farmer's lung. Thorax 23: 469–489, 1968

16. Mitchell J, Mann GB, Molyneux M, Lane RE: Pulmonary fibrosis in workers exposed to finely powdered aluminum. Br J Ind Med 18: 10–20, 1961
17. Coates EO, Watson JHL: Diffuse interstitial lung disease in tungsten carbide workers. Ann Intern Med 75:709–716, 1971
18. Schepers GWEH: The biological action of particulate cobalt metal. AMA Arch Ind Health 12:127–133, 1955
19. Smith TJ, Petty TL, Reading JC, Lakshminarayans: Pulmonary effects of chronic exposure to airborne cadmium. Am Rev Respir Dis 114:161–169, 1976
20. Kilburn KH: Re-examination of longitudinal studies of workers. Arch Environ Health 44:132–133, 1989
21. Meyer-Bisch C, Pham QT, Mur JM, Massin N, Moulin JJ, Teculescu D, Carton B, Pierre F, Baruthio F: Respiratory hazards in hard-metal workers: a cross sectional study. Br J Ind Med 46: 302–309, 1989
22. Merchant JA, Lumsden JC, Kilburn KH, et al: Dose response studies in cotton textile workers. J Occup Med 15:222–230, 1973
23. Lichtenstein LM: Allergy and the immune system. Sci Am 269: 116–124, 1993
24. Knicker WT: Deciding the future for the practice of allergy and immunology. Ann Allergy 55:106–113, 1985
25. Sly RM: Mortality from asthma 1979–1984. J Allergy Clin Immunol 82:705–717, 1988
26. Manfreda J, Cheang M, Warren CPW: Chronic respiratory disorders related to farming and exposure to grain dust in rural adult community. Am J Ind Med 15:7–19, 1989
27. Anto JM, Sunyer J, Rodriguez-Roisin R, Suarez-Cervera M, Vasquez L: Community outbreaks of asthma associated with inhalation of soybean dust. N Engl J Med 320:1097–1102, 1989
28. Musk AW, Peters JM, Wegman DH: Isocyantes and respiratory disease: current status. Am J Ind Med 13:331–349, 1988
29. Kilburn KH, Warshaw RH: Pulmonary function impairment from years of arc welding. Am J Med 87:62–69, 1989
30. Diem JE, Jones RN, Hendrich DJ, et al: Five-year longitudinal study of workers employed in a new toluene diisocyanate manufacturing plant. Am Rev Respir Dis 126:420–428, 1982
31. Engelberg AL, Piacitelli GM, Petersen M, Zey J, Piccirillo R, Morey PR, Carlson ML, Merchant JA: Medical and industrial hygiene characterization of the cotton waste utilization industry. Am J Ind Med 7:93–108, 1985
32. Pei-lian L, Christiani DC, Ting-ting Y, Nai-yi S, Zhi-Chu G, He-lian D, Wei-de Z, Jun-Wei H, Mu-Zhen L: The study of byssinosis in China: a comprehensive report. Am J Ind Med 12:743–753, 1987
33. Ciba Guest Symposium: Terminology, definitions and classification of chronic pulmonary emphysema and related conditions. Thorax 14:286, 1959
34. Kilburn KH, Warshaw RH: Effects of individually motivating smoking cessation on male blue collar workers. Am J Public Health 80:1334–1337, 1990
35. Hodgkin JE, Abbey DE, Euler GL, Magie AR: COPD prevalence in non-smokers in high and low photochemical air pollution areas. Chest 86:830–838, 1984
36. Miller A, Thornton JC, Warshaw RH, Bernstein J, Selikoff IJ, Teirstein AS: Mean and instantaneous expiratory flows, FVC and FEV_1: prediction equations from a probability sample of Michigan, a large industrial state. Bull Eur Physiopathol Respir 22:589–597, 1986
37. Schilling RSF, Hughes JPW, Dingwall-Fordyce I, Gilson JC: An epidemiological study of byssinosis among Lancashire cotton workers. Br J Ind Med 12:217–226, 1955
38. McKerrow CB, McDermott M, Gilson JC, Schilling RSF: Respiratory function during the day in cotton workers: a study in byssinosis. Br J Ind Med 15:75–83, 1958
39. Lowe CR, Khosla T: Chronic bronchitis in ex-coal miners working in the steel industry. Br J Ind Med 29:45–49, 1972
40. Sluis-Cremer GK, Walters LG, Sichel HS: Ventilatory function in relation to mining experience and smoking in a random sample of miners and non-miners in a Witwatersrand Town. Br J Ind Med 24:13–25, 1967
41. Davies TAL: A survey of respiratory disease in foundrymen. London: HM Stationery Office, 1971
42. Karpick RJ, Pratt PC, Asmundsson T, Kilburn KH: Pathological findings in respiratory failure. Ann Intern Med 72:189–197, 1970
43. Boren HG, Lake S: Carbon as a carrier mechanism for irritant gases. Arch Environ Health 8:119–124, 1964
44. Merchant JA, Lumsden JC, Kilburn KH, et al: An industrial study of the biological effects of cotton dust and cigarette smoke exposure. J Occup Med 15:212–221, 1973
45. Kilburn KH: Byssinosis 1981. Am J Ind Med 2:81–88, 1981
46. Higgins ITT, Cochrane AL, Gilson JC, Wood CH: Population studies of chronic respiratory disease. Br J Ind Med 16:255–268, 1959
47. Oswald NC, Harold JT, Martin WJ: Clinical pattern of chronic bronchitis. Lancet 2:639–643, 1953
48. Fletcher CM: Chronic bronchitis, its prevalence, nature and pathogenesis. Am Rev Respir Dis 80:483–494, 1959
49. Fletcher CM, Peto R, Tinker C, Speizer FE: The natural history of chronic bronchitis and emphysema. Oxford: Oxford University Press, 1976
50. Gregory J: A study of 340 cases of chronic bronchitis. Arch Environ Health 22:428–439, 1971
51. Goldsmith JR: Effects of air pollution on human health. In Stern AC (ed): Air Pollution. 2nd ed. New York: Academic Press, 1968, pp 547–615
52. Van der Lende R, Kok T, Peset R, Quanjer PhH, Schouten JP, Orie NGM: Longterm exposure to air pollution and decline in VC and FEV_1. Chest 80:23S–26S, 1981
53. Kryzyanowski M, Jedrychowski W, Wysocki M: Factors associated with the change in ventilatory function and the development of chronic obstructive pulmonary disease in the 13 year follow-up of the Cracow study. Am Rev Respir Dis 134:1011–1090, 1986
54. Imai M, Yoshida K, Kitabtake M: Mortality from asthma and chronic bronchitis associated with changes in sulfur oxides air pollution. Arch Environ Health 41:29–35, 1986
55. Arossa W, Pinaci SS, Bugiani M, Natale P, Bucca C, de Candussio G: Changes in lung function of children after an air pollution decrease. Arch Environ Health 42:170–174, 1987
56. Samet JM, Kutvirb DM, Waxweiler RJ, Kay CR: Uranium mining and lung cancer in Navajo men. N Engl J Med 310:1481–1484, 1984
57. Sunderman FW Jr: Recent progress in nickel carcinogenesis. Toxicol Environ Chem 8:235–252, 1984
58. Comar CL, Nelson N: Health effects of fossil fuel combustion products: report of a workshop. Environ Health Perspect 12:149–170, 1975
59. Health and Welfare Effects Staff Report: Ambient air quality standard for ozone. Sacramento: Research Division Air Resources Board, 1987
60. South Coast Air Quality Management District: Seasonal and diurnal variation in air quality in California's south coast air basin. El Monte, CA, 1987
61. Rahn KA, Lowenthal DH: Pollution aerosol in the Northeast: Northeastern-Midwestern contributions. Science 228:275–284, 1985
62. Fisher GL, Chang DPY, Brummer M: Fly ash collected from electrostatic precipitators: Microcrystalline structures and the mystery of the spheres. Science 192:553–555, 1976
63. Kerr RA: Nyos, the Killer Lake, may be coming back. Science 244:1541–1542, 1989
64. Hively W: How bleak is the outlook for ozone? Am Sci 77:219–224, 1989
65. Rowland SF: Chlorofluorocarbons and the depletion of stratospheric ozone. Am Sci 77:36–45, 1989

66. Houghton RA, Woodwell GM: Global climate change. Sci Am 260: 36–44, 1989
67. La Bastille A: Acid rain—how great a menace? National Geographic 160:652–680, 1981
68. Jones RR: Ozone depletion and cancer risk. Lancet 2:443–446, 1987
69. Kagawa J, Toyama T, Nakaza M: Pulmonary function test in children exposed to air pollution. In Finkel AJ, Duel WC (eds). Clinical Implications of Air Pollution Research. Acton, MA: Publishing Sciences Group, 1976
70. Natusch FS, Wallace JR: Urban aerosol toxicity: the influence of particle size. Science 186:695–699, 1974
71. World Health Organization Regional Office for Europe, Copenhagen: Air quality guidelines for Europe. Geneva: WHO Regional Publications, European series, No. 23, 1987
72. National Research Council: Epidemiology and air pollution. Washington, DC: National Academy Press, 1985
73. Reid L: Measurement of the bronchial mucous gland layer: a diagnostic yardstick in chronic bronchitis. Thorax 15:132–141, 1960
74. Needleman HL, Gunnoe C, Leviton A, Reed R, Peresie H, Maher C, Barrett P: Deficits in psychologic and classroom performance of children with elevated dentine lead levels. N Engl J Med 300:689–695, 1979
75. Grove N: Air—an atmosphere of uncertainty. National Geographic 171:502–537, 1987
76. Arnow PM, Fink JN, Schlueter DP, Barboriak JJ, Mallison G, Said SI, Martin S, Unger GF, Scanlan GT, Kurup VP: Early detection of hypersensitivity pneumonitis in office workers. Am J Med 64:236–242, 1978
77. Hodgson MJ, Morey PR, Attfied M, Sorenson W, Fink JN, Rhodes WW, Visvesvara GS: Pulmonary disease associated with cafeteria flooding. Arch Environ Health 40:96–101, 1985
78. National Academy Press: Indoor Pollutants. Washington, DC: The Press, 1981
79. Spengler JD, Sexton K: Indoor air pollution: a public health perspective. Science 221:9–17, 1983
80. Morey PR: Microbial agents associated with building HVAC systems. Presented at The California Council—American Institute of Architects' National Symposium on Indoor Pollution: The Architect's Response. San Francisco, Nov. 9, 1984
81. Norback D, Michel I, Widstroem J: Indoor air quality and personal factors related to sick building syndrome. Scand J Work Environ Health 16:121–128, 1990
82. Norbach D, Torgen M, Ealing C: Volatile organic compounds, respirable dust and personal factors related to the prevalence and incidence of sick building syndrome in primary schools. Br J Ind Med 47:733–741, 1990
83. Konopinski VJ: Formaldehyde in office and commercial environments. Am Ind Hyg Assoc J 44:205–208, 1983
84. Board on Toxicology and Environmental Health Hazards, Commission on Life Sciences, National Research Council: Asbestiform Fibers: Nonoccupational Health Risks. Washington, DC: National Academy Press, 1984
85. Archer VE: Association of lung cancer mortality with Precambrian granite. Arch Environ Health 42:87–91, 1987
86. Stebbings JH, Dignam JJ: Contamination of individuals by radon daughters: a preliminary study. Arch Environ Health 43:149–154, 1988

26

Pesticides

Marion Moses

Pesticides are among the few toxic substances deliberately added to our environment. They are, by definition, toxic and biocidal, since their purpose is to kill or harm living things. Pesticides are ubiquitous global contaminants found in air, rain, snow, soil, surface and ground water, fog, even the Arctic ice pack. All living creatures tested throughout the world are contaminated with pesticides—birds, fish, wildlife, domestic animals, livestock, and human beings, including newborn babies.

The federal law regulating pesticides defines them as "Any substance or mixture of substances intended for preventing, destroying, repelling or mitigating any insects, rodents, nematodes, fungi, or weeds, or any other forms of life declared to be pests; . . . or for use as a plant regulator, defoliant, or desiccant." The term *pesticide* is generic and different classes are named for the pest they control: insecticides (e.g., ants, aphids, beetles, bugs, caterpillars, cockroaches, mites, mosquitoes, termites), herbicides (e.g., weeds, grasses, algae, woody plants), fungicides (e.g., mildew, molds, rot, plant diseases), acaricides (mites, ticks), rodenticides (rats, gophers, vertebrates), picisides (fish), avicides (birds), and nematocides (nematodes).

▸ HISTORY

Use of sulfur and arsenic as pesticides dates back to ancient times. Botanicals such as nicotine (tobacco extract) date from the sixteenth century, and pyrethrum (from a type of chrysanthemum) since the nineteenth century. In the United States, Paris green (copper-aceto-arsenite) was first used in 1867 to control the Colorado potato beetle. Lead arsenate and other metallic salts were the dominant pest control agents until the 1940s.[1]

Widespread use of petrochemical-based synthetic pesticides began in the middle to late 1940s. In 1939, Swiss chemist Paul Mueller discovered the insecticidal properties of dichlorodiphenyltrichloroethane (DDT). DDT's first uses were military; it was marketed for commercial use in the United States in 1945. German scientists experimenting with nerve gas during World War II synthesized the first organophosphate insecticide, parathion, marketed in 1943. The phenoxy herbicides 2,4-dichlorophenoxy acetic acid (2,4-D) and 2,4,5-trichlorophenoxy acetic acid (2,4,5-T) were introduced in the 1940s, *N*-methyl carbamate insecticides in the 1950s, and the synthetic pyrethroid insecticides in the 1960s.

During World War II, DDT dusting of allied troops in Italy to kill body lice averted a typhus epidemic, making it the first war in history in which more soldiers died of wounds than of disease. By the 1950s, synthetic chemical pesticides were major pest control agents in agriculture in the United States. In developing countries, use was primarily for vector control in malaria and other tropical diseases.

The first serious challenge to synthetic pesticides was the 1962 publication of *Silent Spring* by wildlife biologist Rachel Carson.[2] Her book was a powerful indictment of DDT and related chlorinated hydrocarbon insecticides. Carson documented their environmental persistence, bioaccumulation in human and animal tissues, severe toxic effects on birds, fish, and other nontarget species, and potentially devastating ecological and human health effects.

In 1972, authority for administration and enforcement of the federal pesticide law was transferred from the U.S. Department of Agriculture to the Environmental Protection Agency (EPA), created in 1970.

▸ PRODUCTION AND USE

In 1939 there were 32 pesticide products registered in the United States. In 1996 there were 620 active ingredient pesticides formulated into 20,000 commercial products registered with the EPA. There are 20 major basic producers of pesticides in the United States, 100 smaller producers, 200 major formulators, 2,000 small formulators, 350 major distributors, and 16,900 small dealers.[3] Twenty-four new pesticide active ingredients were registered in 1996.[4]

In 1993, the United States produced 1.3 billion pounds of conventional pesticides (herbicides, insecticides, fungicides, rodenticides, and fumigants). There were 440 million pound of exports and 210 million pounds of imports. Total sales were $8.25 billion, including exports of $2.48 billion, and imports of $2.16 billion.

The top 15 pesticides used were: atrazine, metolachlor, sulfur, alachlor, methyl bromide, cyanazine, dichloropropene, 2,4-D, metam-sodium, trifluralin, petroleum oil, pendimethalin, glyphosate, ethyl dipropylthiocarbamate (EPTC), and chlorpyrifos.

Over four billion pounds of other chemicals regulated as pesticides by the EPA were also used in 1993—approximately 2.5 billion pounds of chlorine compounds, 830 million pounds of wood preservatives, and 320 million pounds of disinfectants.[3]

The United States is the world's largest pesticide user, accounting for 20 percent of the estimated six billion pounds used worldwide. California, which accounts for 25 percent of U.S. pesticide use, mandates reporting of all agricultural and commercial use. In 1994 there were 199.5 million pounds reported. Sulfur alone accounted for 35 percent (70.5 million pounds); its major use is as a fungicide in grape production. Of the remaining 129 million pounds reported, 24 percent were fumigants; 19 percent, herbicides; 18 percent, petroleum oil and related products; 12 percent, insecticides; and 5 percent, fungicides (other than sulfur). Pesticides for which one million or more pounds were used in 1994 were: sulfur, petroleum oils and distillates, methyl bromide, glyphosate, propargite, sulfuryl fluoride, molinate, diazinon, trifluralin, maneb, and ziram. These figures do not include individual householder use.[5]

Agricultural Use

Seventy-five percent of conventional pesticide use in the United States is in agriculture, of which 75 percent is for three crops—corn, soybeans, and cotton. Of the estimated 811 million pounds used in agriculture in 1993, almost 60 percent were herbicides. Insecticides were 21 percent of total use and fungicides and other types were 20 percent. In California about 80 percent of reported use is in agriculture.

Agricultural pesticide use in Canada and Western Europe is similar to that of the United States. Patterns in Latin America, the Asia-Pacific region, and Africa are similar to those of the 1950s United States, with insecticides accounting for 60–80 percent of use and herbicides being 10–15 percent.

Nonagricultural Use

Major nonagricultural uses of pesticides include: wood preservation, lawn and turf treatment, landscape and right-of-way maintenance, and structural, industrial, public health, and home and garden use. There are 40,000 commercial pest control firms in the United States. The most commonly used nonagricultural pesticides in 1993 were: 2,4-D, chlorpyrifos, diazinon, glyphosate, malathion, dicamba, diuron, naled, methyl chlorophenoxy propionate (MCPP) and carbaryl.[3]

Wood Preservatives

Over one billion pounds of wood preservatives are used annually in the United States. The largest single use is creosote on railroad ties. Pentachlorophenol and copper-chromium-arsenate are used for preservation of utility poles, dock pilings, and lumber for construction purposes.

Lawn, Turf, Golf Courses

If home lawns were a single crop, it would be the largest one in the United States, covering some 50,000 square miles (the size of Pennsylvania). About $30 billion is spent annually for lawn care.[6] The use of lawn and turf pesticides is widespread and increasing according to EPA surveys. About 40 percent of lawns are treated, with 32 million pounds applied by householders themselves, and an additional 38 million pounds by commercial firms. Herbicides account for 70 percent of use; insecticides, 32 percent; and fungicides, 8 percent.[3]

There are 14,000 golf courses in the United States and most are intensively chemically managed. In some areas it is common practice to apply chemical treatments on a daily basis. Herbicides and fungicides are the most extensively used.

Maintenance of Right-of-Way

Herbicides are extensively used for maintenance of right-of-way along highways, power transmission lines, and railroads. County and state agencies can be major users. The California Transportation Agency (CalTrans) is the largest single pesticide user in the state, treating 25,000 miles of highway with herbicides annually.

Structural Use

Use of pesticides in homes, apartments, offices, retail stores, commercial buildings, sports arenas, and other structures is a major nonagricultural use of pesticides. Common practice is to contract for regular spraying for cockroaches, ants, and other indoor pests. Subterranean and dry-wood termites are major structural pests. Estimates are that 1 million termite treatments of 500,000 households occur annually in the United States. Twenty percent of all termite jobs are in Texas alone where estimates are that consumers spend more than $1 billion annually for pest control services. About 30 million homes were treated with chlordane for subterranean termites before it was banned in 1988; chlorpyrifos has largely replaced it. Tenting structures and fumigating with methyl bromide or sulfuryl fluoride (Vikane®) is the usual treatment for dry-wood termites.

Over-the-Counter Products

About 71 million pounds of pesticides were sold directly to the consumer as aerosols, foggers, pest strips, baits, pet products, and lawn and garden chemicals in 1993.[3] With few exceptions, most of the pesticides in home and garden products are different formulations of agricultural pesticides. Surveys in San Francisco, and Sarasota, Florida, summarize information on brand name products sold for home, lawn, human, and pet use.[7]

Home use pesticides include the herbicides 2,4-D, glyphosate (Roundup®), and simazine; home use insecticides include diazinon, chlorpyrifos (Dursban®), carbaryl (Sevin®), dichlorvos (DDVP), methoxychlor, malathion, pyrethrins, pyrethroids, and propoxur (Baygon), and the fungicides, maneb, Captan, benomyl, and chlorothalonil (Daconil®).

Industrial Use

Fungicides are widely used as mildewcides; preservatives and antifoulants in paints, glues, pastes, and metalworking fluids; and in fabrics for tents, tarpaulins, sails, tennis nets, and exercise mats. Carpets are routinely treated with insecticides for protection against insects and moths. Pesticides are used in many consumer products including cosmetics, shampoos, soaps, household disinfectants, cardboard and other food packaging materials, and in many paper products. The pulp and paper products industry uses large amounts of slimicides. Water for industrial purposes and in cooling towers is treated with herbicides and algicides to prevent growth of weeds, algae, fungi, and bacteria. Canals, ditches, reservoirs, sewer lines, and other water channels are similarly treated.

Public Health Use

The major public health use of pesticides in the United States is the treatment of drinking water and sewage, primarily with chlorine compounds. Other uses are in rodent and vector control, especially mosquitoes. Worldwide the biggest public health use is in malaria control, where DDT is still widely used in developing countries.

Aircraft Use

Cargo holds, passenger cabins, and other areas of aircraft are sprayed with a wide variety of insecticides. A controversial policy is the spraying of occupied cabins with aerosol insecticides, usually synthetic pyrethroids. U.S. airlines have abandoned this practice within U.S. borders, but spray them on international flights to countries that require it by law, including Australia and the Caribbean.

▶ PESTICIDE FORMULATIONS

Pesticide products are mixtures of active and inert ingredients, and can contain toxic contaminants and metabolites. All must be considered in the potential for adverse effects on human health.

Pesticide products are formulations of the active pesticide(s) mixed with solvents, oils, surfactants, detergents, adjuvants, spreaders, stickers, and a variety of other "inert" ingredients. Typical solvents are light aromatics such as xylene, chlorinated organics such as 1,1,1-trichloroethane, and mineral spirits. There are four basic types: (*a*) foggers, bombs, and aerosols, (*b*) liquids and sprays, (*c*) powders, dusts, and granules, and (*d*) baits and traps.

Aerosols are mixed with solvents and a propellant; baits, with palatable grains, pastes, or other food attractive to the pest; emulsifiable concentrates, with a solvent and emulsifier (the solvent dissolves the pesticide and the emulsifier allows it to be mixed with water); dusts, with finely ground clay, talc or volcanic ash; granules, with clay or sand particles much larger than dusts; wettable powders, a distribution in dry powderlike particles for mixture with water before application.

Active Ingredients. The active ingredient is the pesticidal chemical in the product that is responsible for the specific toxic effect. There are 620 active ingredient pesticide chemicals registered with the EPA, formulated into 20,000 commercial products.[3] Table 26–1 lists the major classes and types of chemicals used as pesticides in the United States.

Inert Ingredients. Inert ingredients are so-called because they are not active as pesticides. The term is a misnomer since most inert ingredients are chemically and biologically active and can be equally as toxic or even more toxic than the active ingredient pesticide(s). There are 1,200 inert ingredients registered with the EPA including solvents, propellants, adjuvants (stickers, spreaders, surfactants), and other chemicals. Typical solvents include xylene, deodorized kerosene, 1,1,1-trichloroethane, methylene chloride, and mineral spirits. Over-the-counter aerosol pesticide products may contain carcinogenic solvents such as trichlorethylene and methylene chloride as "inert" ingredients.

Contaminants. Many technical pesticide products contain varying amounts of metabolites and process contaminants. Pesticides manufactured from chlorinated phenols contain dibenzodioxins and dibenzofurans (e.g., 2,4-D, 2,4,5-T, pentachlorophenol). Hexachlorobenzene contaminates the fungicides chlorothalonil, dacthal, pentachloronitrobenzene (PCNB), and pentachlorophenol; DDT is a contaminant of the miticide dicofol (Kelthane). Many pesticides are contaminated with nitrosoamines, including trifluralin, glyphosate, and carbaryl. The ethylenebisdithiocarbmate fungicides contain the metabolite ethylene thiourea (ETU), and carbon disulfide is a biodegradation product. Lengthy storage can also increase the toxicity of contaminants and metabolites in pesticide formulations, including sulfotepp in diazinon, and isopropylmalathion and *O,O,S*-trimethylphosphorothioate in malathion.

Intermediates. Pesticide intermediates can be highly toxic. Methylisocyanate (MIC), the chemical that poisoned and killed thousands of people in Bhopal, India, in 1984, is an intermediate in the manufacture of the *N*-methyl carbamate insecticides aldicarb (Temik®) and carbaryl (Sevin®).

TABLE 26-1. SELECTED PESTICIDES IN CURRENT USE IN THE UNITED STATES BY CATEGORY OF USE AND CHEMICAL CLASS

■ ***INSECTICIDES***

- Chlorinated hydrocarbons
  - dicofol (Kelthane)
  - dienochlor (Pentac®)
  - endosulfan (thiodan)
  - lindane (γ-HCH, Kwell®)
  - methoxychlor
- *N*-methyl carbamates
  - aldicarb (Temik®)
  - bendiocarb (Ficam®)
  - carbaryl (Sevin®)
  - carbofuran (Furadan®)
  - methomyl (Lannate®)
  - propoxur (Baygon®)
- Organophosphates
  - acephate (Orthene®)
  - azinphos-methyl (Guthion®)
  - chlorpyrifos (Dursban®)
  - diazinon, dichlorvos (DDVP)
  - dimethoate, malathion
  - methidathion (Supracide®)
  - methimidophos (Monitor®)
  - parathion/methyl parathion
  - tetrachlorvinphos
- Pyrethrins
- Pyrethrums
- Sulfite esters
  - porpargite (Omite®)
- Synthetic pyrethroids
  - cyfluthrin (Tempo®)
  - λ-cyhalothrin (Karate®)
  - cypermethrin (Demon®)
  - deltamethrin, fenvalerate
  - permethrin (Dragnet®)
  - phenothrin, resmethrin

■ ***RODENTICIDES***

- Anticoagulants
  - brodifacoum, bromadiolone
  - chloro/diphacinone, warfarin
- Phosphine gas releasers
  - aluminum/zinc phosphide

■ ***HERBICIDES***

- Acetanilides
  - alachlor (Lasso®)
- Amides
  - propachlor, propanil
- Arsenicals
  - cacodylic acid
- Bipyridyls
  - paraquat, diquat
- Carbamates/thiocarbamates
  - cycloate, EPTC, molinate
  - pebulate
- Dinitroanilines
  - trifluralin (Treflan®)
  - pendimethalin (Prowl®)
- Diphenyl ethers
  - oxyflurofen (Goal®)
- Organophosphates
  - DEF, merphos
- Phenoxyaliphatic acids
  - 2,4-D, dicamba, MCPA
- Phosphonates
  - glyphosate (Roundup®)
  - fosamine (Krenite®)
- Phthalates
  - dacthal, endothall
  - thiobencarb
- Substituted ureas
  - diuron, monuron
- Sulfanilimides
  - oryzalin (Surflan®)
- Sulfonylureas
  - chlorsulfuron (Glean®)
  - sulfometuron (Oust®)
- Substituted phenols
  - dinocap, dintriophenol
  - pentchlorophenol
- Triazines
  - atrazine, cyanazine, simazine
- Triazoles
  - amitrole

■ ***FUNGICIDES***

- Carboximides
  - captan, iprodione (Rovral®)
  - vinclozolin (Ronilan®)
- Dithio/thiocarbamates
  - maneb, mancozeb,
  - nabam, zineb, ferbam
  - thiram, ziram
- Heterocyclic nitrogens
  - benomyl (Benlate®), thiabendazole, thiophanate-methyl
- Organotins
  - triphenyl/tributyl tins
- Substituted benzenes
  - chlorothalonil (Daconil®), chloroneb, hexachlorobenzene, pentachloronitrobenzene
- Triazines
  - anilazine (Dyrene®)
- Triazoles
  - triadimefon (Bayleton®)

■ ***FUMIGANTS***

- Halogenated hydrocarbons
  - dichloropropene (Telone-II®)
  - methyl bromide, naphthalene, *para*-dichlorobenzene
- Oxides/aldehydes
  - ethylene oxide, formaldehyde
- Sulfur compounds
  - sulfur dioxide, sulfuryl fluoride (Vikane®)
- Thiocarbamates
  - metam-sodium (Vapam®)

■ ***WOOD PRESERVATIVES***

- arsenic, copper, creosote, boric acid/polyborates, copper/zinc naphthenate, pentachlorophenol

► EXPOSURE TO PESTICIDES

Occupational Exposure to Pesticides

The EPA estimates that there are 351,600 professionals certified to apply pesticides commercially (pest control operators/exterminators), and 965,692 certified private applicators (primarily individual farmers).[3] Pesticide law allows noncertified applicators to work "under the supervision of" certified applicators. Thus, there are thousands more noncertified applicators working with commercial pest control firms and on farms. There is no estimation of their actual numbers, nor of their qualifications and training.

Those with the greatest exposure handle concentrated formulations—including farm workers, exterminators, and lawn, landscape, golf course, highway maintenance, and other workers in agriculture and forestry who mix, load, and apply pesticides. Exposures tend to be lower in pesticide manufacturing since batch processing requires little direct contact.

Farm workers who cultivate and harvest crops are exposed to dislodgeable pesticide residues on leaf surfaces, on the crop itself, in the soil, or duff (decaying plant and organic material that collects under vines and trees). Field workers are exposed to overspray from crop dusting aircraft and drift from airblast and other ground rig sprayers. Farm worker children are at high risk of exposure because they work in the fields or may be taken to the fields by their parents since child care is rarely available. Farm worker families, especially migrant workers, often live in camps surrounded by fields that are sprayed.

Drift

Drift is the movement of pesticides away from the site of application. Approximately 85 to 90 percent of pesticides applied as broadcast sprays drift off target and can affect birds, bees, fish, and other species, including human beings. Significant concentrations can drift a mile or more; lower concentrations can drift many miles depending on droplet size, wind conditions, ambient temperature, and humidity.

Nonoccupational exposures to bystanders and community residents from drift are increasing with the building of residential housing adjacent to agricultural fields and golf courses. Off-gassing from fields where fumigants such as methyl bromide have been injected into the soil is another source of exposure and has resulted in evacuation of community residents.[9] Problems are increasing in urban areas with increasing chemical treatment of lawns, sports playing areas, and parks and recreation areas.

Children's Exposures

Children's exposures to pesticides are magnified by their greater likelihood of direct exposure from skin contact with contaminated floors, carpets, lawns, and other surfaces due to their crawling, toddling, and exploring activities. They can swallow significant amounts from ingesting contaminated house dust, and mouthing and chewing pesticide-contaminated objects. Their higher respiratory rate, larger skin surface for their size, and less mature immune and detoxifying systems put them at greater risk than are adults at comparable exposure levels.[10,11]

Absorption of Pesticides

Pesticides are readily absorbed through the skin, the respiratory tract (inhalation), and the gastrointestinal tract (ingestion). The eyes can be a significant route of exposure in splashes and spills. The rate of absorption of pesticides into the body is product specific and depends on the properties of the active ingredient pesticide and the inert ingredients in a particular formulation.

The skin, not the respiratory system as is commonly believed, is the chief route of absorption. Fumigants, which are in the form of gases are a notable exception, which accounts in part for their greater toxicity. Inhalation can be an important route of exposure in the home from the use of aerosols, foggers, bug bombs, and moth control products,[7] but the dermal route is still the most important route, especially in children.[10,11]

► TOXICOLOGY

The U.S. EPA ranks pesticides into four categories based on acute toxicity (Table 26–2). Most of the rest of the world uses the World Health Organization (WHO) classification (Table 26–3).

Poisoning and Death

The total number of pesticide poisonings in the United States is not known. The American Association of Poison Control Centers compiles an annual report called Toxic Exposure Surveillance System (TESS). In 1995, there were 84,346 pesticide-related incidents, 4.2 percent of the total. Of these incidents, 44,150 (52 percent) were in children less than 6 years old. There were 14 fatalities, including seven suicides. A 34-year-old man died within hours of repeated dermal application of the insect repellent, deet. Organophosphate insecticides accounted for 19,866 reports. (An EPA review showed that clorpyrifos was responsible for the greatest number.) There were 13,972 incidents related to pyrethrins/pyrethroids.[12]

The World Health Organization estimates that the total number of acute unintentional poisonings annually throughout the world is between 3.5 to 5 million cases, of which 3 million are severe poisonings resulting in 20,000 deaths. WHO estimates that intentional poisonings number 2 million with 200,000 resulting in death by suicide. Developing countries account for 25 percent of pesticide use, but 50 percent of acute poisonings, and 75 percent of deaths.[13]

In California, which mandates physician reporting of pesticide-related illness, 2,111 reports were received in 1993, and 1,995 were filed in 1994. Of the 1,435 classified as "definitely, probably, or possibly" related to pesticide exposure in 1993, 1,307 were occupational; and 448 of 1,332 in 1994.[14,15]

Most of the systemic poisonings in California were caused by organophosphate pesticides, primarily mevinphos (Phosdrin) and parathion.[16,17] A farm worker in a crew spraying almond groves died from parathion poisoning in 1989.[18]

In Washington state from June to August, 1993, there were 26 reports of severe poisoning in workers applying phosdrin in 19 different apple orchards.[19] Washington state banned the pesticide in 1993, and the federal EPA banned it in 1995 (Table 26–4).

Severe poisonings have occurred from wearing laundered uniforms previously contaminated with parathion.[20]

Reentry Poisoning

Dermal absorption of dislodgeable residues on crops they are harvesting has caused systemic poisoning of thousands of farm workers. Since California is the only state that enforces mandatory reporting of pesticide illness, most information on reentry poisonings is from that state. In the 1960s and 1970s many incidents of poisonings were reported in crops with high foliar contact such as grapes, peaches, and citrus, that had been sprayed with organophosphates such as parathion, phosdrin, and azinphos-methyl (Guthion®).

In the early 1970s, waiting periods before workers could be sent into the fields, called reentry intervals (REIs), were established to deal with this problem. Most intervals were 1 to 2 days, but for parathion could be up to 45. In California, the number of farm workers affected by pesticide residues in the fields decreased to 117 in 1993, compared to an average of 168 from 1989 through 1992. Prior to 1989, the average number of field residue cases per year had been 279.[14]

One of the largest outbreaks of pesticide-related dermatitis in California occurred in May, 1986, when 198 farm workers were sent to pick oranges after the groves had been sprayed with propargite (Omite-CR®). Fifty-two percent of the workers (114) sustained severe chemical burns. No violations of reentry intervals or application rates was found. A new inert ingredient that prolonged residue degradation had been added to the formulation.[21] Subsequent studies showed that the proper reentry interval should have been 42 days, not 7. Omite-CR® was banned for any use in California but is still used in other states.

TABLE 26-2. ENVIRONMENTAL PROTECTION AGENCY PESTICIDE TOXICITY CATEGORIES BY MEDIAN LETHAL DOSE (LD_{50}) IN MG/KG BODY WEIGHT IN THE RAT[a]

Toxicity Class and Signal Word	*Oral Required on Label*	*Dermal (mg/kg)*	*Inhalation (mg/kg)*	**Effects** *(mg/L)*	*Eye Skin*
I Highly toxic *DANGER*	<50	<200	<0.2	Corneal opacity (irreversible)	Corrosive
II Moderately toxic *WARNING*	50–500	200–2,000	0.2–2	Corneal opacity (reversible 7 days)	Severe irritation
III Minimally toxic *CAUTION*	500–5,000	2,000–20,000	2–20	Irritation	Moderate irritation
IV Least toxic *CAUTION*	>5,000	>20,000	>20	No irritation	Mild irritation

[a] The median lethal dose (LD_{50}) is the amount that will kill 50 percent of the exposed animals. The lower the median lethal dose, the more hazardous the chemical.

In Florida in 1989, 185 farm workers were severely poisoned when sent to work in a cauliflower field 12 hours after it had been sprayed with Phosdrin. The legal reentry interval was 4 days.

Organophosphates

Organophosphates are responsible for the majority of occupational poisonings and deaths from pesticides in the United States and throughout the world. There are many reports of severe poisoning and fatalities from accidental and suicidal ingestion of these compounds.[22–25] Even organophosphates thought to be "safe" can be deadly. In 1975, malathion caused five deaths and 2,800 poisonings in Pakistan during spraying for malaria control. The deaths were due to the contaminant isomalathion, a toxic isomerization product found in one country's product.[26]

Signs and symptoms of poisoning occur soon after exposure, from minutes to hours. Mild poisoning results in fatigue, headache, dizziness, nausea, vomiting, chest tightness, excess sweating, salivation, abdominal pain, and cramping. In moderate poisoning the victim usually cannot walk, has generalized weakness, difficulty speaking, muscular fasciculations, and miosis. Central nervous system effects also occur, including restlessness, anxiety, tremulousness, insomnia, excessive dreaming, nightmares, slurring of speech, confusion, and difficulty concentrating. Coma and convulsions accompany severe poisoning, which can result in death without proper treatment.[22,27]

The organophosphates are readily metabolized and excreted, and with early and proper treatment most poisoned workers will recover. In accidental or suicidal ingestion, recovery depends on the amount ingested, the interval before emergency resuscitation, and the appropriateness of treatment. While recovery appears to be complete, long-term neurological effects can occur (vide infra).

Organophosphates are similar to nerve gas and exert their toxic action by inhibition of the enzyme acetylcholinesterase at synaptic sites in muscles, glands, autonomic ganglia, and the brain. The signs and symptoms of poisoning result from the subsequent build-up of the neurotransmitter acetylcholine. Enzymes that hydrolyze choline esters in humans are found in red blood cells (RBCs) ("true" or RBC cholinesterase) and plasma ("pseudocholinesterase"). Decreased activity of RBCs and plasma cholinesterase is an indicator of excess absorption or poisoning by organophosphates. Testing for cholinesterase activity levels is thus an excellent tool for diagnosing pesticide poisoning and for monitoring worker exposure.

A 10 to 40 percent reduction in cholinesterase activity usually results in latent poisoning without clinical manifestations. A 50 to 60 percent reduction usually results in mild poisoning. A reduction of 70 to 80 percent results in moderate poisoning and 90 percent or more indicates severe poisoning that can be fatal without treatment.

The *rate* of reduction in activity of cholinesterase is an important determinant of poisoning. A rapid reduction over a few minutes or hours can produce marked signs and symptoms. A gradual drop of the same magnitude over of period of days or weeks may cause only minimal signs and symptoms. In worker monitoring programs, a reduction in RBC enzyme activity of 25 percent or more, or in plasma cholinesterase of 40 percent or more from a preexposure or "baseline" level, is evidence of excess absorption. The workers should be removed from further exposure until recovery of activity to at least 80 percent of baseline.

Atropine, which blocks the effects of acetylcholine, is the antidote for organophosphate (OP) pesticide poisoning. Pralidoxime (2-PAM), if given within 24 to 48 hours of exposure, can reactivate cholinesterase and restore enzyme function. After this time, "aging" of the enzyme-pesticide complex occurs, making it refractory to reactivation.

Alkylphosphate metabolites of the most widely used organophosphates are excreted in the urine. As a measure of recent absorption, they can be useful in biomonitoring workers, and in exposure assessment.[28,29] Levels peak within 24 hours of exposure and usually cannot be detected 48 hours or more after exposures ceases.

TABLE 26-3. WORLD HEALTH ORGANIZATION RECOMMENDED CLASSIFICATION OF PESTICIDES BY HAZARD BY MEDIAN LETHAL DOSE (LD_{50}) IN MG/KG BODY WEIGHT IN THE RAT[a]

	Oral		**Dermal**	
Hazard Class	*Solids*	*Liquids*	*Solids*	*Liquids*
IA Extremely hazardous	≤5	≤20	≤10	≤40
IB Highly hazardous	5–50	20–200	10–100	40–400
II Moderately hazardous	50–500	200–2,000	100–1,000	400–4,000
III Slightly hazardous	>500	>2,000	>1,000	>4,000

[a] The median lethal dose (LD_{50}) is the amount that will kill 50 percent of the exposed animals. The lower the median lethal dose, the more hazardous the chemical.

TABLE 26-4. PESTICIDES BANNED, SUSPENDED, OR SEVERELY RESTRICTED IN THE UNITED STATES

Pesticide	*Action*	*Year*
Aldrin	All uses canceled except termite control	1974
Amitrole	Voluntary cancellation, liquid formulation	1996
	Cancellation ornamental plant nursery stock use	1996
Bacillus popilliae	Voluntary cancellation, all uses	1996
BHC	All uses canceled	1978
Chlordane	Cancellation, most uses, except termite control	1978
	All uses canceled	1988
Chlordimeform	Registration voluntarily withdrawn	1989
Cloprop	Voluntary cancellation, all uses	1996
Cyanazine	Voluntary phase out of all use by 1999	1995
Daminozide (Alar)	All food uses canceled	1990
DBCP	All uses canceled except for pineapple in Hawaii	1979
	Use on pineapple canceled	1985
DDT	All agricultural use canceled	1972
	Use only for public health emergencies	
Diazinon	Use on golf courses, sod farms canceled	1986
Dieldrin	Cancellation, most uses	1974
Dinoseb	Emergency suspended and registration canceled	1986
EDB	All uses canceled	1984
Endrin	Voluntary cancellation	1985
EPN	Use as mosquito larvacide canceled	1983
Heptachlor	All uses canceled except seed treatment	1978
	Seed treatment use canceled	1989
Kepone	All uses canceled	1976
Lindane	Indoor smoke fumigation use canceled	1986
Maleic hydrazide	All use suspended	1981
Methyl bromide	To be phased out by 2001 (ozone depleter)	1993
Mirex	All uses canceled except pineapple in Hawaii	1977
Nitrofen (TOK)	Voluntary cancellation, all uses	1983
Oil of Pennyroyal	Voluntary cancellation	1996
Phosdrin	Voluntary cancellation, all uses	1994
Phosdrin	Cancellation delayed for 1 year	1995
Phosphamidon	Voluntary cancellation, all uses	1996
2,4,5-T/Silvex	Emergency suspended	1979
	All uses canceled	1985
Simazine	Cancellation algicide swimming pools/hot tubs	1994
Toxaphene	All uses canceled except sheep/cattle dip and bananas/pineapple in Puerto Rico, Virgin Islands	1982

N-Methyl-Carbamate Insecticides

The *N*-methyl-carbamate insecticides are similar to the organophosphates in their acute toxic effects and mechanism of action. However, the inhibition of acetylcholinesterase is readily reversible. Signs and symptoms appear earlier, and workers are more likely to remove themselves from excess exposure. Except for an aldicarb (Temik®)-related tractor accident death of a farm worker reported in 1984, no deaths from occupational exposure have been reported in the United States.

Atropine is also the antidote for *N*-methyl-carbamate poisoning. 2-PAM is not recommended unless there is concomitant exposure to an organophosphate.[27,30] Testing RBC and plasma cholinesterase activity is less useful in poisoning with the carbamates. Carbamylation of the enzyme, unlike phosphorylation, is readily reversible, and can occur in vitro during transport of the specimen to the laboratory. Poisoning of grape girdlers in California with prolonged exposure to methomyl (Lannate®) was unusual in the occurrence of significant depression of cholinesterase activity in the workers.

Chlorinated Hydrocarbon Insecticides

The chlorinated hydrocarbons are less acutely toxic than the organophosphates and *N*-methyl carbamate. They are central nervous system stimulants, and in toxic doses cause anxiety, tremor, hyperexcitability, confusion, agitation, generalized seizures, and coma that can result in death. Convulsions or abnormal electroencephalograms can occur without overt signs or symptoms of clinical toxicity. The exact mechanism of neurotoxicity is unknown.[31]

Most organochlorine insecticides are no longer used in the United States, including DDT, aldrin, endrin, dieldrin, chlordane, heptachlor, and toxaphene (Table 26–4). The currently registered chlorinated hydrocarbon insecticides dienochlor, endosulfan (thiodan), and methyoxychlor biodegrade and are readily excreted and do not persist in the environment. The acaricide dicofol (Kelthane) is contaminated with DDT.

Lindane

The only persistent chlorinated hydrocarbon insecticide on the market in the United States is lindane (γ-hexachlorocyclohexane, γ-HCH, Kwell®). The 1 percent shampoo or lotion is available by prescription only for use as a pediculicide and scabicide. Generalized seizures have been reported in children[32] and adults[33] from dermal application for lice and scabies. A 20 percent formulation is available over-the-counter for control of lawn, turf, and tree insects.[7]

Kepone

The most serious outbreak of chlorinated hydrocarbon poisoning in the United States occurred at a plant manufacturing chlordecone (Kepone®) in Hopewell, Virginia, in 1974–1975. Workers manifested nervousness, apprehension, tremor, head bobbing, opsoclonus, ataxia, and vision and speech disturbances. Toxic psychosis occurred in the most severely affected worker. Generalized seizures, characteristic of poisoning with these compounds, did not occur. Sperm abnormalities and oligospermia were also found.[34] The State of Virginia closed the plant in 1975. The EPA canceled Kepone®'s registration in 1976.

Hexachlorobenzene

More than 3,000 cases of acquired porphyria cutanea tarda occurred in Turkey from 1956 to 1959. Those affected had eaten hexachlorobenzene-treated seed wheat illegally sold for food use in several villages. The mortality rate of about 10 percent occurred largely in infants who nursed from mothers with porphyria and in children who had eaten bread made from the contaminated wheat.[35] Turkey banned hexachlorobenzene in 1959. The United States still allows its use for seed treatment.

Hexachlorobenzene is a contaminant of the herbicide Dacthal, and the fungicides, chlorothalonil (Daconil), PCNB, and pentachlorophenol. It is a widespread environmental contaminant as a by-product of perchlorethylene manufacture and an ubiquitous contaminant of human breast milk.

Pyrethrums/Pyrethrins/Synthetic Pyrethroid Insecticides

Pyrethrums are crushed petals of a type of chrysanthemum that contains insecticidal chemicals called pyrethrins. Pyrethrins are much more concentrated formulations in which the active pyrethins have been solvent extracted from the flowers. They are more acutely toxic than pyrethrums. Pyrethroids are synthetic analogs of natural pyrethrins. The synergist piperonyl butoxide is added to most pyrethrin and pyrethroid formulations to prolong their residual action.

The pyrethrins and pyrethroids are readily metabolized and excreted and do not bioaccumulate in humans or the environment. They are less acutely toxic than most organophosphate insecticides; most are in toxicity categories III and IV (Table 26–2). Many household aerosols and pet care products contain pyrethrins and synthetic pyrethroids.[7] Exterminators use them extensively for structural treatments of homes and buildings.

Characteristic symptoms of exposure to synthetic pyrethroids are transient facial and skin sensations such as burning, itching, tingling sensations, not associated with dermatoses. These cutaneous paresthesias and dysesthesias disappear soon after exposure ceases and are often exacerbated by sweating and washing with warm water.

Signs and symptoms of mild to moderate poisoning include dizziness, headache, nausea, anorexia, and fatigue. Severe poisoning results in coarse muscular fasciculations in large muscles of the extremities and generalized seizures.[36] Recovery is usually rapid after exposure ceases. There are no specific antidotes to poisoning, and treatment is supportive.

Pyrethrins cross-react with ragweed and other pollens. Members of this class of chemicals, including the synthetic pyrethroids, are potential allergens and skin sensitizers.

Pyrethrins and pyrethroids slow the closing of the sodium activation gate in nerve cells. Pyrethroids with the α-cyano moiety (cyfluthrin, λ-cyhalothrin, cyphenothrin, cypermethrin, esfenvalerate, fenvalerate, fenpropathrin, fluvalinate, tralomethrin) are more toxic than those without this functional group (permethrin, *d*-phenothrin, resmethrin).

Phenolic and Cresolic Pesticides

These highly toxic pesticides include pentachlorophenol, dinoseb (dinitrophenol), 4,6-dinitro-ortho-cresol (DNOC), and dinocap. They are uncouplers of oxidative phosphorylation, and poisoning results in a severe hypermetabolic state. Clinical manifestations include anorexia, flushing, severe thirst, weakness, profuse diaphoresis, and hyperthermia, which can progress to coma and death. Aspirin is contraindicated in treatment.

Many occupational deaths have occurred from these compounds, as well as deaths in infants in a newborn nursery where sodium pentachlorophenate was mistakenly used to wash diapers. Dinoseb, DNOC, and related compounds stain the skin yellow on contact, which must be differentiated from diffuse jaundice of the skin and sclerae, a sign of hepatotoxicity and indicator of serious poisoning.

Phenoxy Herbicides

2,4-D is the most widely used of this group of chemicals, which also includes: 2,4-dichlorophenoxy propionic acid (2,4-DP), 2,4-dichlorophenoxy butyric acid (2,4-DB), 2-methyl-4-chlorophenoxy acetic acid (MCPA), 2-(2-methyl-4-chlorophenoxy) propionate (MCPP), and dicamba (2-methyl-3,5-dichlorobenzoic acid). The acute toxicity of these compounds is relatively low and they are readily metabolized and excreted. However, since they are made from chlorinated phenols, they can be contaminated with dibenzodioxins.

Agent Orange, used as a defoliant during the war in Vietnam from 1962 to 1971, was a 50/50 combination of the *n*-butyl esters of 2,4-D and 2,4,5-T. 2,4,5-T, which was banned in 1979 for most uses, is contaminated with 2,3,7,8-tetrachlorodibenzodioxin (TCDD), the most toxic of the 75 different dioxin isomers.

Chloracne is the most easily observed effect of exposure to dibenzodioxins. Adverse health effects in chemical workers with severe dioxin poisoning include: hyperirritability, sleep disturbances, decreased libido, impotence, toxic hepatitis, abnormalities in liver enzymes, elevated blood lipids, sensory-motor peripheral neuropathy, acquired porphyria cutanea tarda, increase in cancer mortality, and possible increase in adult onset diabetes mellitus. Additional health effects are described in the section on dioxins and dibenzofurans.

Bipyridyl Herbicides

Paraquat (Gramoxone) used to be one of the most widely used herbicides in the world. Many fatalities are related to its accidental or suicidal ingestion. Diquat, a related compound, is mainly used for aquatic weed control and is much less toxic.

Paraquat is an epithelial toxin and a powerful irritant that can cause severe injury to the eyes, skin, nose, and throat, resulting in ulceration, epistaxis, and severe dystrophy or complete loss of the fingernails. Acute poisoning can result in hepatic and renal failure; the patient may recover only to die of asphyxiation due to a relentlessly progressive pulmonary fibrosis. Death occurs most often 1 to 3 weeks after ingestion, depending on the dose and treatment. Dermal exposure to paraquat has also caused fatal pulmonary fibrosis. Deaths have been reported in farmers and landscape maintenance workers and from application to the skin for treatment of lice and scabies.

The toxic action is most likely due to lipid peroxidation from reaction with molecular oxygen to form superoxide ion. There is no antidote to paraquat poisoning and most patients who absorb or ingest an amount sufficient to cause severe organ toxicity do not survive.[37]

Other Pesticides

Most widely used herbicides and fungicides are not highly acutely toxic. Because they do not cause immediate or apparent illness, or are seen as minor skin or eye irritants, a false sense of security surrounds their use. Many of these product may have potential long-term effects or contain toxic inert ingredients.

Glyphosate (Roundup®) is much less toxic than paraquat, the herbicide it primarily replaced. Occupational illness reports involving glyphosate products are among the most frequently reported in agricultural and landscape maintenance workers in California.[38] A toxic inert ingredient in Roundup®, polyoxyethylenamine (POEA), is linked to fatalities from accidental or suicidal ingestion of the product.

Atrazine, the most widely used herbicide in the country, primarily on corn, is also not highly acutely toxic. It is also sold over-the-counter in some states and used by pest control companies for lawn and turf management.[7] It is persistent in soil, is a widespread groundwater contaminant, and causes mammary cancer and other tumors in rodents. Atrazine is under review by the EPA.

Most of the widely used fungicides are in toxicity category IV, the least acutely toxic. Many cause contact dermatitis and can be potent allergens and sensitizers (vide infra). Many are also known or suspect carcinogens—including benomyl, captan, chlorothalonil, maneb, and mancozeb (Table 26–5).

Insect Repellents

N,N-diethyl-*m*-toluamide (deet, OFF®, Skintastic®) first marketed in 1954, is a widely used insect repellent applied directly to the skin. Its use has been increasing, especially among children, because of concerns regarding ticks that carry Lyme disease. It is extensively used by the military for troops in the field. Concerns have been raised by the combination of its use with permethrin-impregnated uniforms in the etiology of "Gulf War syndrome."

Deet is neurotoxic, and signs and symptoms of mild poisoning include headache, restlessness, irritability, crying spells in children, and other changes in behavior. Severe poisoning is one of toxic encephalopathy, with slurring of speech, tremor, generalized seizures, and coma.[39] There are reports of generalized seizures in children when used according to label directions. Fatalities have been reported in children and adults within hours of repeated dermal exposure. Anaphylactic shock, though rare, has also been reported.

Fumigants

Fumigants are among the most highly toxic pesticide products. Since they are gases, they are rapidly absorbed through the lungs and distributed throughout the body. Most are alkylating agents, mutagens, and carcinogens and are neurotoxic and hepatotoxic. They, especially methyl bromide, are responsible for many deaths.[40] The central nervous system, lungs, liver, and kidneys can be severely affected. Pulmonary edema can occur and is a frequent cause of death.

Severe neurotoxic and behavioral effects, including toxic psychosis, can result from poisoning with methyl bromide. Mental and behavioral changes can occur after acute overexposures or from low-level chronic exposure. There are many reports of permanent sequelae after recovery from acute methyl bromide poisoning. Anxiety, difficulties in concentration, memory deficits, changes in personality, and other behavioral effects occur and can be progressive and irreversible.[41]

Methyl bromide is a potent ozone depleter. The United States is a signatory to the Montreal Protocol, an international agreement to phase out all use of the fumigant by 2001.

TABLE 26-5. SELECTED PESTICIDES BY EPA CARCINOGENICITY CATEGORY

A	Metiram	Dichlobenil	Phosphamidon
Arsenic acid	Orthophenylphenol	Diclofop	Prochloraz
Arsenic pentoxide	PCNB	Dicofol	Prodiamine
Chromic acid[a]	Pentachlorophenol	Dimethipin	Pronamide
B1	Procymidone	Dimethoate	Propazine
Cadmium chloride[a]	Propargite	Dinoseb[a]	Propiconazole
Ethylene oxide	Propoxur	Ethophenprox	Quinclorac
B2	Terrazole	Fomesafen	Simazine
Aciflurofen	Toxaphene[a]	Fosetyl-al	Terbutryn
Alachlor	Zineb	Hexaconazole	Tetrachlorvinphos
Amitrole	***B2/C***	Hexakis	Tetramethrin
Captafol[a]	Haloxyfop-methyl	Hexazinone	Thiodicarb
Captan	Lindane	Hexythiazox	Thiophanate-methyl
Chlordane[a]	Paradichlorobenzene	Hydramethylnon	Triadimefon
Chlorothalonil	***C***	Isoxaben	Triadimenol
Creosote	Acephate	Linuron	Triallate
Daminozide	Acrolein	Methidathion	Tribenuron methyl
1,3-dichloropropene	Amitraz	Methomyl	Tridiphane
Dichlorvos	Asulam	Methyl parathion	Trifluralin
ETU[b]	Atrazine	Metolachlor	Uniconazole
EDB[a,c]	Benomyl	Norfluazon	***D***
Folpet[a]	Bifenthrin	Oryzalin	Aldicarb
Heptachlor[a]	Bromacil	Oxadiazon	Azinphos-methyl
Hexachlorobenzene	Bromoxynil	Oxadixyl	2,4-D
Lactofen	Clofentizine	Oxyfluofen	Fenarimol
Mancozeb	Cyanazine	Parathion	Glyphosate
Maneb	Cypermethrin	Pendamethalin	Malathion
Methylene chloride	Cyproconazole	Permethrin	Phorate
		Phosmet	

Category: A, human carcinogen; B1, probable human carcinogen based on animal data and human epidemiology; B2, probable human carcinogen based on animal data; C, possible human carcinogen; D, not classifiable as to human carcinogenicity.

[a] No longer registered for use in the United States.

[b] Ethylene thiourea, found in dithio/thiocarbamate fungicides (Table 26–1).

[c] Ethylene dibromide.

▶ HEALTH EFFECTS

Epidemiological studies in populations with occupational and environmental exposure to pesticides show increased risk of cancer, birth defects, adverse effects on reproduction and fertility, and neurological damage. The increased risk can occur without any evidence of past acute health effects or poisoning and from long-term exposure to low levels not considered toxicologically significant.

Constraints in chronic disease epidemiology of pesticides include: difficulty in assessing and documenting exposure; simultaneous exposure to other pesticides (and inert ingredients); the changing nature of exposures over time; and potential additive and synergistic effects from multiple exposures, especially in exposures to the fetus, infants, and children at critical periods in development.

Asthma and Allergies

Asthmatics are extremely susceptible to adverse health effects from pesticides; they can experience severe symptoms at levels of exposure considered "safe" or trivial. Organophosphates can trigger or exacerbate an attack and prolong recovery.[42] While organophosphates and pyrethrins/pyrethroids are most frequently implicated, any pesticide or inert ingredient can be a hazard. Children are at risk from pesticides used inside and outside the home (including the neighbor's use); from use on carpets and on pets; and from sprays used in schools, parks, play, and other recreation areas. An increase in number and or severity of asthma attacks in children is often the first clue to pesticide exposures from drift.

People with allergies and multiple chemical sensitivities can experience adverse effect from low levels of exposure that would not affect those without these conditions.

Any pesticide or inert ingredient can potentially be an allergen or sensitizer. But most skin reactions are due to an irritant contact dermatitis; allergic dermatitis is much less common. Fungicides as a group are the most likely to cause allergic dermatitis and sensitization. Pesticides that are potential allergens and sensitizers include anilazine, chlorothalonil (Daconil), deet, diazinon, dicofol, maneb, and PCNB.

Chronic Effects on the Brain and Nervous System

Although there is a dearth of data on chronic neuropathological and neurobehavioral effects of pesticides, available studies show adverse effects in two areas: long-term sequelae of acute poisoning and organophosphate-induced delayed neuropathy.

Long-term Sequelae of Acute Poisoning

The percentage of acutely poisoned individuals who develop clinically significant sequelae is not known. Early reports document that organophosphate pesticides can cause profound mental and psychological changes.[44]

Follow-up studies in persons poisoned by organophosphates suggest that long-term neurological sequelae occur even though recovery appeared to be complete. Even single episodes of severe poisoning may be associated with a persistent decrement in function. Neuropsychological status of 100 persons poisoned by organophosphate pesticides (mainly parathion), an average of 9 years prior, was significantly different from that in control subjects in measures of memory, abstraction, and mood. Twice as many had scores consistent with cerebral damage or dysfunction, and personality scores showed greater distress and complaints of disability.[45]

Other studies find that auditory attention, visual memory, visual-motor speed, sequencing, problem solving, motor steadiness, reaction time, and dexterity are significantly poorer among the poisoned cohort. Complaints of visual disturbances were found in 10 of 117 individuals 3 years after occupational organophosphate poisoning (mainly from parathion and phosdrin). One-fourth of workers poisoned 10 to 24 months after hospitalization for acute organophosphate poisoning had abnormal vibrotactile thresholds.

Pesticide-Induced Delayed Neuropathy

Certain organophosphate pesticides can cause delayed neuropathy. Demyelination of long and large-diameter fibers in the spinal cord and peripheral nervous system results in muscle weakness that may progress to paralysis. Onset is usually 2 to 4 weeks after an acute exposure.[46]

The first reported human case of organophosphate pesticide–induced delayed neuropathy (OPIDN) was in 1953 in a research chemist experimenting with the insecticide Mipafox. In 1979 a cluster of 12 cases at a plant in Texas manufacturing leptophos (Phosvel) for export was determined by NIOSH to be work-related. Affected workers were initially diagnosed with multiple sclerosis, psychiatric disorders, and encephalitis. More recent reports link OPIDN in humans to methamidophos (Monitor®), chlorpyrifos (Dursban®, Lorsban®), and perhaps fenthion.

The mechanism involved in OPIDN probably requires the inhibition and subsequent aging of a poorly characterized esterase known as "neuropathy target esterase" or "neurotoxic esterase" (NTE), which is distinct from acetylcholinesterase. In a patient poisoned with chlorpyrifos, the inhibition and aging of NTE in human lymphocytes were shown to predict the onset of OPIDN. The hen brain inhibition bioassay is required by the EPA for screening new organophosphate insecticides for delayed neuropathic effects.

Other Neurological Disease

There are reports of severe psychological disturbances, including toxic psychosis, related to poisoning from organophosphates, chlordecone (Kepone®), methyl bromide, and other pesticides. There are rare reports of Guillain-Barré syndrome following acute overexposure or poisoning with pesticides.

Parkinson's Disease

An association between organophosphate pesticide exposure and Parkinson's disease was first suggested in 1978, and with choreoathetosis in 1984. Recent reports suggest a higher prevalence of Parkinson's disease in agricultural areas and increased risk in herbicide applicators and in pesticide exposures, especially in those who develop the disease at age 50 or younger.[47] Studies in Canada and Germany found elevated risk for Parkinson's disease with occupational exposures to herbicides and wood preservatives, respectively. There is a case report of two young agricultural workers with a parkinsonian syndrome who were exposed to the magnesium-containing fungicide maneb.

Pesticides and Cancer

A large number of pesticide active ingredients are known or suspect animal carcinogens. Based on the evidence for cancer in humans, the EPA classifies pesticides into five categories: A, human carcinogen; B, probable human carcinogen; C, possible human carcinogen; D, not classifiable as to human carcinogenicity; and E, no evidence of carcinogenic risks to humans (Table 26–5). Epidemiological studies done in the United States and other countries report significant increased risk of certain cancers with occupational pesticide exposure.[48]

Farmers

In the United States, statistically significant increased risks were found for non-Hodgkin's lymphoma, leukemia, multiple myeloma, and cancer of the prostate, testis, pancreas, colon, and liver. Several studies report a nonsignificant increase in risk of brain cancer. Studies of farmers in Canada, China, France, Germany, Italy, Japan, New

Zealand, and Sweden report increased risk for non-Hodgkin's lymphoma, multiple myeloma, and cancer of the brain, prostate, and pancreas.[49–51]

Other Agricultural Exposures

Agricultural extension agents[52] and soil conservation agents[53] were at significantly increased risk of non-Hodgkin's lymphoma, leukemia, multiple myeloma, and cancer of the brain, prostate, and colon.

Exterminators

A Florida study found significant increased risk for brain cancer and leukemia in licensed exterminators.[54] Urban applicators in Rome were at significantly increased risk of brain cancer.[55]

Pesticide Manufacturing Workers

Studies of U.S. pesticide workers show significant increased risk of non-Hodgkin's lymphoma, leukemia, and hepatobiliary and testicular cancer.[56] Long-term follow-up of DDT workers found significant increased risk for pancreatic cancer.[57]

Golf Course Superintendents

A nationwide mortality study found significant risk for non-Hodgkin's lymphoma and cancer of the prostate, brain, and colon. Nonsignificant increased risk was found for leukemia and cancer of the liver, pancreas, and bone.[58]

Cancer in Children

Children's exposure to pesticides depends on the actions and occupations of their parents. Studies in the United States and other countries show an association between cancer in children and use of home, yard, and garden pesticides and parents' occupation in agriculture.[59]

Statistically significant increased risk for brain cancer has been associated with home use of aerosol bombs/foggers, pest strips, pet flea collars, home extermination, and lice treatment with lindane,[60,61] and with parental occupation in agriculture.[62]

Significant increased risk for leukemia, lymphoma, and soft tissue sarcoma have been associated with home, yard, and garden pesticide use.[61,63] Studies of parental occupation in agriculture found significant risk for Wilms' tumor[64,65] and osteosarcoma.[66]

Aplastic Anemia

There are fewer reports of pesticide-related aplastic anemia since the banning of DDT, dieldrin, and other persistent chlorinated hydrocarbons. Cases associated with lindane (γ-hexachlorocyclohexane, Kwell®) are still being reported. A recent report links pentachlorophenol exposure as well.[67]

Breast Cancer

Recent studies in the United States found that women with breast cancer had higher levels of the DDT metabolite DDE in their breast tissue and blood (serum) than did a comparison group of women without breast cancer.[68–70]

Reproductive Effects

Maternal and paternal pesticide exposure has been found to be a risk factor for infertility, sterility, spontaneous abortion, stillbirth, and birth defects.[71]

Sterility and Pesticide Exposure

In 1977 the soil fumigant 1,2-dibromo-3-chloropropane (DBCP) was found to cause sterility (azoospermia) and decreased fertility (oligospermia) in workers in California. Two of the sterile workers had had no exposure to DBCP for 9 and 13 years, respectively, and both had fathered children before their exposure. A follow-up found that some had recovered, but in others, damage to their testes was permanent. The EPA banned DBCP in 1979 (1989 in Hawaii). DBCP, the most frequently found contaminant of groundwater in California, is still leaching into groundwater 20 years after all use stopped.

Studies of workers exposed to a related soil fumigant, ethylene dibromide (EDB) found lowered sperm counts and impaired fertility. EDB, which replaced DBCP in 1979, was banned in 1984 due to concerns about carcinogenicity. Both DBCP and EDB are potent animal carcinogens.

Danish organic farmers, who did not use synthetic chemical pesticides or fertilizers, had significantly higher sperm counts than conventional farmers.[72]

Birth Defects and Pesticide Exposure

There are few studies of birth defects and pesticide exposure. U.S. studies found significantly increased risk of limb reduction defects in infants of agricultural workers. A Finnish study of maternal agricultural work during the first trimester found increased pooled risk for several defects that was significant only for orofacial clefts. Risk of craniosynostosis was found to be increased but not significant for parental agricultural/forestry occupation. There is a case report of a farm worker poisoned by Metasystox-R, a known animal teratogen, who delivered a chromosomally normal child with multiple severe defects that died 2 weeks later.

Studies in Arkansas, New Zealand, and Hungary of parental environmental or occupational exposures to the phenoxy herbicides 2,4,5-T and 2,4-D found no association between exposure to these herbicides and major structural defects in the offspring of exposed parents.

Vietnam veterans raised concerns about their exposure to Agent Orange. Earlier case-control studies in Atlanta and Australia found no relationship between service in Vietnam and fathering a child with a birth defect. In a follow-up of the Ranch Hands (Air Force pilots who flew the herbicide missions) an increase in neural tube defects was found with increasing paternal dioxin levels.[73]

The failure to find a high rate of birth defects associated with pesticide exposures may be due to the embryotoxicity or fetotoxicity of the pesticide, resulting in early spontaneous abortion. A U.S. study of maternal occupation and fetal death found farm worker women to be at increased risk for spontaneous abortion. A study in India found increased rates of spontaneous abortion, stillbirth, and sterility in vineyard workers. A large study in Montreal found women in agricultural and horticultural occupations to be at significantly increased risk for stillbirth.[74]

Endocrine Disruptors

Rachel Carson was the most eloquent spokesperson for wildlife as harbingers of potential health hazards to humans from toxic chemicals.[2] DDT and other persistent chlorinated hydrocarbons, which devastated bird populations, are known to act hormonally as xenoestrogens—foreign compounds not found in nature that can mimic or act like female hormones.[75]

Wildlife biologists continue to document severe disruptions in wildlife that are thought to be due to pesticides, PCBs, dioxins, plasticizers, and other environmental toxins. The findings include: abnormal thyroid function; decreased fertility; decreased hatching success in birds, fish, turtles, and mammals; demasculinazation and defeminization in fish and birds; and alterations in immune function in birds and mammals.[76]

The normal function of all organ systems is regulated by the endocrine system. Small disturbances in hormonal function (e.g., pituitary, adrenal, thyroid, testes, ovaries) especially during critical phases of development and growth, can lead to profound and lasting effects.

Questions have been raised about the relevance of the findings in wildlife to human populations, whether possible decreasing quantity and quality of human sperm, increasing incidence of breast and prostate cancer in industrialized countries, and increasing incidence of cryptorchidism and ectopic pregnancies could be related to endocrine-disrupting environmental contaminants.[77]

Pesticides that are known endocrine disruptors include: DDT, Kepone®, heptachlor, dieldrin, chlordane, toxaphene, lindane, endosulfan, methyxychlor (all chlorinated hydrocarbons) and atrazine, simazine, and cyanazine (triazine herbicides). The fungicide vinclozin can act as an antiandrogen,[78] the synthetic pyrethroids can affect levels of sex hormone binding globulin,[79] and the dithiocarbamate fungicides contain ethylene thiourea (ETU), which affects thryroid function. As discussed earlier, simultaneous exposure to a combination of pesticides at a dose that is toxicologically insignificant for any single chemical can increase toxicity 150 to 1,600 times.[43]

Endocrine effects on the developing fetus can be mediated by very low levels of exposure during critical periods of organogenesis, which may not be manifested until adulthood. Can exposure of the mother (or father) at any time during life before producing offspring result in transgenerational exposures? These and other questions are discussed in a book written for the general public on these issues.[80]

The U.S. Congress has passed a law mandating the EPA to devise a screening and testing program for pesticides and other chemicals to determine if they are endocrine disruptors.

▶ REGULATION AND CONTROLS

Legislation

The Federal Insecticide Act of 1910, primarily a labeling law to prevent adulteration, was repealed by the Federal Insecticide Fungicide and Rodenticide Act (FIFRA) of 1947. FIFRA was administered by the U.S. Department of Agriculture (USDA) until 1972, when control passed to the Environmental Protection Agency. Most pesticides now on the market were approved by the USDA in the 1940s through the early 1970s, without the chronic toxicity, health, and environmental fate data required by current law.

Pesticides must be registered with the EPA before they can be sold. Registration is contingent upon submission, by the registrant (manufacturer), of scientific evidence that when used as directed the pesticide will effectively control the indicated pest(s); that it will not injure humans, crops, livestock, wildlife, or the environment; and that it will not result in illegal residues in food and feed.

In 1972 Congress passed extensive amendments to FIFRA, including requirements that all pesticides be reregistered by 1975 to meet current health and safety standards. Toxicity testing required was: oncogenicity/carcinogenicity, chronic toxicity, reproductive toxicity, teratogenicity, gene mutation, chromosomal aberrations, DNA damage, and delayed neurotoxicity. As of 1986, only one of the 1,200 registered pesticide active ingredients had met the new standards.

In 1988, Congress again amended FIFRA, requiring the EPA to undertake a comprehensive reregistration review of the 1,138 active-ingredient pesticides first registered before November, 1984. Registration Eligibility Decisions (REDs) summarize the reviews of these older chemicals. As of 1996, 61 percent have yet to be reviewed. There were a large number of voluntarily cancellations due to the review process.[3]

All pesticides are classified as either general or restricted use. Restricted use pesticides must be applied by a state-certified applicator or under the supervision of a certified applicator. The states vary enormously in the quality of their education and training programs for pesticide applicators. Usually one person on each farm or in each company is certified, most often a supervisor or manager. In actual practice, most pesticide applications are done by persons "under the supervision of a certified applicator." The majority of the workers applying pesticides are not certified. Many are not even minimally trained, and turnover is high.

Worker Protection Standards

Chemical workers who manufacture and formulate pesticides are covered by the Occupational Safety and Health Act (OSHA) passed in 1970. Agricultural workers were specifically excluded from the law, including the Hazard Communication Standard (Right-to-Know).

It was not until 1992 that the EPA issued Worker Protection Standards (WPS) under section 170 of FIFRA, with full implementation by October 1995. The EPA estimates that about four million workers on farms, and in nurseries, greenhouses, and forestry are covered by the rules.

The regulations require restricted entry intervals (REIs) for all pesticides: 48 hours for all toxicity category I products, which can be extended up to 72 hours for organophosphates applied outdoors in arid areas; 24 hours for toxicity category II products; and 12 hours for all other products, later amended to exempt cut-rose workers. The rules require posting of warning signs for certain applications, worker education and training, and providing pesticide-specific materials upon request.

The WPS are based on acute toxicity only, and there are no rules that specifically address the exposures to pesticides that are known or suspect carcinogens and teratogens. The rules apply to adult workers, without any modifications or consideration of exposures to children and pregnant women.

Federal and State Administration and Enforcement

The EPA delegates administration and enforcement of FIFRA to the states through working agreements. In most states, enforcement authority is in the state department of agriculture.

The pesticide label is the keystone of FIFRA enforcement, and any use inconsistent with the label is illegal. The label must contain: brand name, chemical name, percentage active ingredient(s) and inert ingredient(s); directions for use; pests that it is effective against; crops, animals, or sites to be treated; dosage, time, and method of application; reentry interval, preharvest interval; protective clothing and equipment required for application; first aid and emergency treatment; name and address of the manufacturer; and toxicity category. The toxicity category and associated signal word (Table 26–2) must also be on the label.

Action on Chlorpyrifos

Chlorpyrifos is the common name for the most widely used organophosphate in the United States. First marketed in 1975, its use has increased 26 times. Almost 1,000 registered pesticide products contain this chemical, most with names other than Dursban® and Lorsban®, their common trade names. In April 1995, the EPA fined the basic manufacturer, DowElanco, $732,000,000, for failing to report to the agency adverse health effects known to the company over the past decade. The bulk of the information arose from personal injury claims filed against the company relating to chlorpyrifos, primarily for peripheral neuropathy and other chronic neurological effects, as well as asthma and birth defects.

The EPA recently completed a review of chlorpyrifos in addition to the regular review for reregistration. Concerns were expressed about potential chronic neurological disease from long-term exposure from household use. The EPA is working on an agreement that would withdraw chlorpyrifos from the indoor broadcast flea control market; the indoor total release fogger market; the paint additive market; and the direct application pet care products market (shampoos, dips, sprays). These actions are part of measures that will apply not only to chlorpyrifos, but to other household products.[81]

Inert Ingredients

A U.S. federal district court ruled on October 11, 1996, that pesticide companies must disclose information about inert ingredients in six pesticide products under the Freedom of Information Act. Environmental groups had filed a lawsuit against the EPA in 1994, demanding public disclosure of the inert ingredients. The products involved are: Aatrex 80W (atrazine), Weedone LV4 (2,4-D), Roundup® (glyphosate), Velpar (hexazinone), Garlon 3A (triclopyr), and Tordon 101 (picloram and 2,4-D). The EPA routinely withholds this information from the public because of industry claims that inert ingredients are subject to the trade secret provisions of FIFRA and are therefore confidential.

Action on Glyphosate

In 1991, New York State's Office of the Attorney General charged the Monsanto Chemical Company with deceptive and misleading advertising. The state challenged unsubstantiated safety and health claims for Roundup® and other products containing glyphosate. In 1996 the company agreed to discontinue the use of terms such as "biodegradable" and "environmentally friendly" and to pay $50,000 toward the costs of pursuing the case.

Other Agencies

Other Federal agencies with responsibilities for enforcement of pesticide regulations include the Food and Drug Administration (FDA), the USDA, and the Federal Trade Commission (FTC). The EPA sets the maximum legal residues of pesticides (called tolerances) allowed to be on food at the time of retail sale, but does not enforce them. The FDA is responsible for enforcement of tolerances in fruits, vegetables, grains, feed, and fiber; and the USDA, for meat, poultry, and fish.

The Food Quality Protection Act, passed in 1996, amends Federal Food Drug and Cosmetic Act (FFDCA) to establish a single, health-based standard for pesticide residues in all types of foods, replacing the Delaney clause as it applied to some residues in ready-to-eat processed foods.

The FTC protects consumers against false and deceptive advertising claims by pesticide distributors and professional applicators—the FTC has brought only three actions in the past 10 years.

Banned, Suspended, and Severely Restricted Pesticides

Table 22–4 lists selected pesticides that have been banned, suspended, or severely restricted for use in the United States. Many pesticides that are banned or severely restricted in the United States, Canada, and Western Europe are widely used in developing countries. The impact of the North American Free Trade Agreement (NAFTA) is yet unknown; but is expected to increase both pesticide use and exposures to workers and children.

The Pesticide Action Network (PAN), a coalition of over 300 non-government organizations from 50 countries, has called for the world-wide ban of a group of pesticides called "The Dirty Dozen." These pesticides are: aldicarb (Temik), chlordane/heptachlor, chlordimeform, DBCP/EDB, DDT, Aldrin/Dieldrin/Endrin, BHC/Lindane, Paraquat, Parathion (ethyl and methyl), pentachlorophenol 2,4 -D, and 2,4,5-T.

An Executive Order signed in 1979 requires agencies such as the Agency for International Development to file Environmental Impact Statements before beginning projects in foreign countries. Another Executive Order requires the United States to inform third world countries if an exported pesticide is banned in the United States and to obtain official approval before it can be exported.

▸ REFERENCES

1. Whorton J: Pesticide Use in Pre-DDT America. NJ: Princeton University Press, Princeton, 1974
2. Carson R: Silent Spring. Boston: Houghton Mifflin, 1962
3. Aspelin AL: Pesticides Industry Sales and Usage: 1992 and 1993 Market Estimates. Environmental Protection Agency, Office of Pesticide Programs, US 733-K-94-001. Washington, DC: 1994
4. Environmental Protection Agency: Office of Pesticide Programs Annual Report for 1996. 735R6001. Washington, DC: US Environmental Protection Agency: 1996
5. California Environmental Protection Agency: Annual Report of Pesticide Use in 1994 by Chemical and by Commodity. Sacramento: Department of Pesticide Regulation, 1996
6. Graham W: The Grassman. The New Yorker, August 19:34–37, 1996
7. Moses M: Designer Poisons: How to Protect Your Health and Home from Toxic Pesticides. San Francisco: Pesticide Education Center, 1995
8. Moses M, Johnson ES, Anger WK, et al: Environmental equity and pesticide exposure. Toxicol Ind Health 9(5):913–959, 1993
9. Goldman LR, Mengle D, Epstein DM: Acute symptoms in persons residing near a field treated with the soil fumigants methyl bromide and chloropicrin. West J Med 147:95–98, 1987
10. Fenske RA, Black KG, Elkner KP, et al: Potential exposure and health risks of infants following indoor residential pesticide applications. Am J Public Health 80(6):689–693, 1990
11. Lewis RG, Fortmann RC, Camann DE: Evaluation of methods for monitoring the potential exposure of small children to pesticides in the residential environment. Arch Environ Contam Toxicol 26(1): 37–46, 1994
12. Litovitz TL, Felberg L, White SW, et al: 1995 Annual Report of the American Association of Poison Control Centers Toxic Exposure Surveillance System. Am J Emerg Med 14(5):487, 1996
13. World Health Organization: Public Health Impact of Pesticides Used in Agriculture. Report of a WHO/UNEP Working Group. Geneva: World Health Organization, 1989
14. State of California: The California Pesticide Illness Surveillance Program—1993. Sacramento: Department of Pesticide Regulation, 1994
15. State of California: The California Pesticide Illness Surveillance Program—1994. Sacramento: Department of Pesticide Regulation, 1995
16. O'Malley M: Systemic illness associated with exposure to parathion in California 1982–1989. Report HS-1625. Sacramento: Department of Pesticide Regulation, Worker Health and Safety Branch, 1992
17. O'Malley M: Systemic illness associated with exposure to mevinphos in California 1982–1989. Report HS-1626. Sacramento: Department of Pesticide Regulation, Worker Health and Safety Branch, 1992
18. Osorio AM, Ames R: Investigation of a fatality among parathion applicators: Kern County, California. Berkeley: Department of Health Services, HESIS and Pesticide Unit, 1990
19. Centers for Disease Control and Prevention: Occupational pesticide poisoning in apple orchards—Washington, 1993. MMWR 42(51–52): 993–995, 1994
20. Clifford NJ, Nies AS: Organophosphate poisoning from wearing a laundered uniform previously contaminated with parathion. JAMA 262(21):3035–3036, 1989
21. Saunders LD, Ames RG, Knaak JB, et al: Outbreak of Omite-CR-induced dermatitis among orange pickers in Tulare County, California. J Occup Med 29(5):409–413, 1987
22. Tafuri J, Roberts J: Organophosphate poisoning. Ann Emerg Med 16(2):193–202, 1987
23. Mortensen ML: Management of acute childhood poisonings caused by selected insecticides and herbicides. Pediatr Clin North Am 33(2):421–445, 1986
24. Zwiener RJ, Ginsburg CM: Organophosphate and carbamate poisoning in infants and children [published erratum in Pediatrics 81(5):683]. Pediatrics 81(1):121–126, 1988
25. Hayes WJ Jr, Law E: Handbook of Pesticide Toxicology. San Diego: Academic Press, 1991
26. Baker EL, Zack M, Miles JW, et al: Epidemic malathion poisoning in Pakistan malaria workers. Lancet 1:31–34, 1978
27. Morgan DP: Recognition and Management of Pesticide Poisoning. 4th ed. EPA-540/9-88-001. Washington, DC: US Environmental Protection Agency, 1989
28. Rees H: Exposure to sheep dip and the incidence of acute symptoms in a group of Welsh sheep farmers. Occup Environ Med 53(4):258–263, 1996
29. Richter ED, Kowalski M, Leventhal A, et al: Illness and excretion of organophosphate metabolites four months after household pest extermination. Arch Environ Health 47(2):135–138, 1992
30. Lifshitz M, Rotenberg M, Sofer S, et al: Carbamate poisoning and oxime treatment in children: a clinical and laboratory study. Pediatrics 93(4):652–655, 1994
31. Ecobichon DJ, Davies J, Doull J, et al: Neurotoxic Effects of Pesticides. In Baker S (ed): Effects of Pesticides on Human Health. New Jersey. Princeton Scientific Publishing Co., Princeton, 1990, pp 131–199

32. Solomon LM, Fahrner L, West DP: Gamma benzene hexachloride toxicity: a review. Arch Dermatol 113:353–357, 1977
33. Fischer TF: Lindane toxicity in a 24-year-old woman. Ann Emerg Med 24(5):972–974, 1994
34. Taylor JR, Selhorst, JB, Houff SA, et al: Chlordecone intoxication in man. I. Clinical observations. Neurology 28:626–630, 1978
35. Cripps DJ, Goemen A, Peters HA: Porphyria turcica, twenty years after hexachlorobenzene intoxication. Arch Dermatol 116:46–50, 1980
36. He F, Wang S, Liu L, et al: Clinical manifestations and diagnosis of acute pyrethroid poisoning. Arch Toxicol 63(1):54–58, 1989
37. Lheureux P, Leduc D, Vanbinst R, et al: Survival in a case of massive paraquat ingestion. Chest 107(1):285–289, 1995
38. Pease WS, Morello-Frosch RA, Albright DS, et al: Preventing Pesticide-Related Illness in California Agriculture. California Policy Seminar. Berkeley: University of California, 1993
39. Roland EH, Jan JE, Riggs JM: Toxic encephalopathy in a child after brief exposure to insect repellents. Can Med Assoc J 132:155–156, 1985
40. Centers for Disease Control and Prevention: Deaths associated with exposure to fumigants in railroad cars—United States. MMWR 43(27):489–491, 1994
41. Bishop CM: A case of methyl bromide poisoning. Occup Med 42(2): 107–109, 1992
42. Deschamps D, Questel F, Baud FJ, et al: Persistent asthma after acute inhalation of organophosphate insecticide. Lancet 344:1712, 1994
43. Arnold SF, Klotz DM, Collins B, et al: Synergistic activation of estrogen receptor with combinations of environmental chemicals. Science 272:1489–1492, 1996
44. Sharp DS, Eskenazi B, Harrison R, et al: Delayed hazards of pesticide exposure. Ann Rev Public Health 7:441–471, 1986
45. Savage EP, Keefe TJ, Mounce LM, et al: Chronic neurological sequelae of acute organophosphate poisoning. Arch Environ Health 43:38–45, 1988
46. Richardson RJ: Assessment of the neurotoxic potential of chlorpyrifos relative to other organophosphorus compounds: a critical review of the literature. J Toxicol Environ Health 44(2):135–165, 1995
47. Butterfield PG, Valanis BG, Spencer PS, et al: Environmental antecedents of young-onset Parkinson's disease. Neurology 43:1150–1158, 1993
48. Moses M: Occupational Exposure to Pesticides and Cancer in Humans, Summary of Selected Studies. San Francisco: Pesticide Education Center, 1996
49. Blair A, Zahm SH, Pearce NE, et al: Clues to cancer etiology from studies of farmers. Scand J Work Environ Health 18:209–215, 1992
50. Blair A, Dosemeci M, Heineman EF: Cancer and other causes of death among male and female farmers from twenty-three states. Am J Ind Med 23(5):729–742, 1993
51. Kristensen P, Andersen A, Irgens LM, et al: Incidence and risk factors of cancer among men and women in Norwegian agriculture. Scand J Work Environ Health 22:14–26, 1996
52. Alavanja MCR, Blair A, Merkele S, et al: Mortality among agricultural extension agents. Am J Ind Med 14:167–176, 1988
53. Alavanja MCR, Blair A, Merkle S, et al: Mortality among forest and soil conservationists. Arch Environ Health 44:94–101, 1989
54. Blair A, Grauman DJ, Lubin JH: Lung cancer and other causes of death among licensed pesticide applicators [Abstract]. J Nat Cancer Inst 71(1):31–37, 1983
55. Figa-Talamanca I, Mearelli I, Valente P, et al: Mortality in a cohort of pesticide applicators in an urban setting. Int J Epidemiol 22(4): 674–675, 1993
56. Leet T, Acquavella J, Lynch C, et al: Cancer incidence among alachlor manufacturing workers. Am J Ind Med 30(3):300–306, 1996
57. Garabrant DH, Held J, Langholz B, et al: DDT and related compounds and risk of pancreatic cancer. J Nat Cancer Inst 84:764–771, 1992
58. Kross BC, Burmeister LF, Ogilvie LK, et al: Proportionate mortality study of golf course superintendents. Am J Ind Med 29(5):501–506, 1996
59. Moses M: Pesticide Exposure and Cancer in Children, Summary of Selected Studies. San Francisco: Pesticide Education Center, 1996
60. Davis JR, Brownson RC, Garcia R, et al: Family pesticide use and childhood brain cancer. Arch Environ Contam Toxicol 24:87–92, 1993
61. Leiss JK, Savitz DA: Home pesticide use and childhood cancer: a case-control study. Am J Public Health 85(2):249–252, 1995
62. Kristensen P, Andersen A, Irgens LM, et al: Cancer in offspring of parents engaged in agricultural activities in Norway: incidence and risk factors in the farm environment. Int J Cancer 65(1):39–50, 1996
63. Lowengart RA, Peters JM, Cicioni C, et al: Childhood leukemia and parents' occupational and home exposures. J Natl Cancer Inst 79(1):39–46, 1987
64. Olshan AF, Breslow NE, Falletta JM, et al: Risk Factors for Wilms tumor: Report from the National Wilms Tumor Study. Cancer 72(3–4):938–944, 1993
65. Sharpe CR, Franco EL, deCamargo B, et al: Parental exposures to pesticides and risk of Wilms' tumor in Brazil. Am J Epidemiol 141(3):210–217, 1995
66. Holly EA, Aston DP, Ahn PKA, et al. Ewing's bone sarcoma, parental occupational exposures and other factors. American Journal Epidemiology 135 (2):122–129, 1992
67. Rugman FP, Cosstick R: Aplastic anaemia associated with organochlorine pesticide: case reports and review of evidence. J Clin Pathol 43(2):98–101, 1990
68. Falck F Jr, Andrew R Jr, Wolff MS, et al: Pesticides and polychlorinated biphenyl residues in human breast lipids and their relation to breast cancer. Arch Environ Health 47:143–146, 1992
69. Kreiger N, Wolff MS, Hiatt RA, et al: Breast cancer and serum organochlorines: a prospective study among white, black, and Asian women. J Natl Cancer Inst 86(8):589–599, 1994
70. Wolff MS, Toniolo PG, Lee EW, et al: Blood levels of organochlorine residues and risk of breast cancer. J Natl Cancer Inst 85(8): 648–652, 1993
71. Moses M: Pesticides. In Paul M (ed): Occupational and Environmental Reproductive Hazards: A Guide for Clinicians. Baltimore: Williams & Wilkins, 1993, pp 296–309
72. Abell A, Ernst E, Bonde JP: High sperm density among members of an organic farmers' association. Lancet 343:1498, 1994
73. Wolfe WH, Michalek JE, Miner JC, et al: Paternal serum dioxin and reproductive outcomes among veterans of Operation Ranch Hand. Epidemiology 6:17–22, 1995
74. McDonald AD, McDonald JC, Armstrong B, et al: Occupation and pregnancy outcome. Br J Ind Med 44(8):521–526, 1987
75. Soto AM, Chung KL, Sonnenschein C: The pesticides endosulfan, toxaphene, and dieldrin have estrogenic effects on human estrogen-sensitive cells. Environ Health Perspect 102(4):380–383, 1994
76. Colborn T, Vom Saal FS, Soto AM: Developmental effects of endocrine-disrupting chemicals in wildlife and humans. Environ Health Perspect 101(5):378–384, 1993
77. Kavlock RJ, Daston GP, DeRosa C, et al: Research needs for the risk assessment of health and environmental effects of endocrine disruptors: A report of the U.S. EPA-sponsored workshop. Environ Health Perspect 104(Suppl 4):1–26, 1966
78. Gray LE Jr, Ostby JS, Kelce WR: Developmental effects of an environmental antiandrogen: the fungicide vinclozolin alters sex differentiation of the male rat. Toxicol Appl Pharmacol 129(1):46–52, 1994
79. Eil C, Nisula BC: The binding properties of pyrethroids to human skin fibroblast androgen receptors and to sex hormone binding globulin. J Steroid Biochem 35(3–4):409–414, 1990
80. Colburn T, Dumanowski D, Myers JP: Our Stolen Future. New York: Dutton, 1996
81. U.S. Environmental Protection Agency. Letter from Lynn R. Goldman, M.D. to Mr. John Hagaman. Washington, DC: Office of Prevention, Pesticides, and Toxic Substances, January 14, 1997

27

Illness Due to Thermal Extremes

Edwin M. Kilbourne

▸ THERMOREGULATION

Humans are a homeothermic (warm-blooded) species and must maintain a relatively constant deep body (core) temperature. The temperatures of the extremities and superficial body parts may vary, but only within limits. Substantial deviations from "normal" body temperatures can result in adverse effects that range in severity from minor annoyance to life-threatening illness.

Body temperature is affected by four fundamental physical processes. They are (*a*) biochemical heat production—metabolic heat must constantly be dissipated; (*b*) heat loss by evaporation of moisture from skin and respiratory passages; (*c*) heat transfer to or from matter with which the body may be in contact, whether solid (conduction) or fluid (convection, i.e., to a medium such as air or water); and (*d*) heat gain or loss due to thermal radiation (e.g., heat gain from direct sun exposure or proximity to a hot object).[1]

▸ ADVERSE EFFECTS OF HEAT

Heat Stress

Heat stress may result from alteration of any of the physical processes involved in determining body temperature. A runner in a long-distance race or a soldier on strenuous military maneuvers may suffer heat stress as a result of increased metabolic heat production caused by physical activity. A steel worker may experience heat stress because of the radiant heat emitted from a furnace at the workplace. At a hazardous waste site, a worker who must wear a heavy, impermeable suit may develop heat stress as the air in the suit becomes humid (decreasing evaporative cooling) and warm (limiting heat loss by convection).

People seek to relieve heat stress by altering one or more of the processes by which the body gains or loses heat. They may rest (lowering metabolic heat production), move to the shade (avoiding radiant solar heat), sit in front of a fan (increasing convective and evaporative heat loss), or swim (facilitating heat loss by conduction/convection through water).

The acute physiological response to heat stress includes perspiration and peripheral vasodilation. Perspiration increases cutaneous moisture, allowing greater evaporative cooling. Peripheral vasodilation tends to reroute blood flow, enhancing transmission of heat from the body's core to peripheral body parts, from which it can be more readily lost.[2,3]

With continuing exposure to heat stress, a process of physiological adaptation takes place. Although maximal adaptation may take weeks, significant acclimatization occurs within a few days of the first exposure.[4,5]

Indices of Heat Stress

In most circumstances, there are four principal environmental determinants of heat stress. They are ambient (dry-bulb) temperature, humidity, air speed, and thermal radiation. A number of heat indices have been developed to attempt to combine some or all of these separate factors into a single number indicating how hot "it feels" and, by implication, attempting to quantify the net pathophysiological significance of a given set of environmental conditions.

The original "effective temperature" (ET) index is determined from a nomogram reflecting dry-bulb and wet-bulb temperatures and air speed. ET was derived empirically, based on subjective reports of thermal sensations of subjects placed in a wide variety of conditions of temperature, humidity, and air movement. As originally conceived, ET aimed to quantify the dry-bulb temperature of still, saturated air that would produce the same subjective thermal effect as the conditions being evaluated.[6] A revision of ET, the corrected effective temperature (CET), was developed to take radiant heat into account and substitutes globe thermometer temperature for dry-bulb temperature. (The globe thermometer is a dry-bulb thermometer with the bulb located at the center of a 6-inch diameter thin copper sphere, the outside of which is painted matte black.) Because of concern that the original ET is too sensitive to the effect of humidity at low temperatures and not sensitive enough to humidity at high temperatures, a reformulated version of ET has been published.[7,8]

The wet-bulb globe temperature (WBGT) is a heat stress index calculated as a weighted average of wet-bulb, globe, and dry-bulb thermometer temperatures:

$$\text{Outdoors: } \quad WBGT = 0.7T_{wb} + 0.2T_g + 0.1T_{db}$$
$$\text{Indoors: } \quad WBGT = 0.7T_{wb} + 0.3T_g$$

where T_{wb} is the temperature read by a naturally convected wet-bulb thermometer, T_g is the globe thermometer temperature, and T_{db} is the dry-bulb temperature. Its formulae were chosen to yield values close to those of the ET for the same conditions.[9] The WBGT has been used to assess the danger of heatstroke or heat exhaustion occurring in persons exercising in hot environments. Curtailing certain types of activities when the WBGT is high decreases the incidence of serious heat-related illness among military recruits.[10] Current standards and recommendations for limiting heat stress in the workplace are frequently expressed in terms of WBGT, although a person's degree of acclimatization, the energy expenditure required, and the amount of time spent performing the stressful task are often factored in as well.[11]

The "Botsball" (BB) or wet-globe thermometer consists of a thermal probe within a black sphere 6 cm in diameter, the surface of which is covered with black cloth kept wet by water in a reservoir. The BB is smaller and lighter than the equipment required to take WBGT readings and has a shorter stabilization time. These attributes facilitate its use to measure conditions in an employee's personal workspace. BB readings approximate those of WBGT according to the formula:[12]

$$\text{WBGT} = (1.01 \times \text{BB}) + 2.6$$

Steadman's scheme of apparent temperature (AT) is favored by many U.S. meteorologists and climatologists as a measure of the heat stress associated with a given set of meteorological conditions (Table 27-1). For conditions of high temperature, the dry-bulb temperature and humidity components of AT are frequently used alone and referred to as "heat index." Unlike effective temperature, which was derived empirically, AT is the product of mathematical modeling based on principles of physics and physiology. The AT for a given set of conditions of temperature, humidity, air speed, and radiant heat energy is equal to the dry-bulb temperature with the same predicted thermal impact on an adult walking in calm air of "moderate" humidity with surrounding objects at the same temperature as ambient air (no "extra" radiation).[13]

There are other heat-stress indices, and no attempt is made here to present an exhaustive list. For public health purposes, heat stress indices may be helpful in assessing the danger posed by particular weather conditions, but they are limited by underlying assumptions regarding metabolic heat production, clothing, body shape and size, and other factors. Moreover, indices yield instantaneous values that do not reflect the time course of a community's heat exposure, which may be critical to occurrence (or not) of adverse health effects.

Heatstroke

The most serious illness caused by elevated temperature is heatstroke. Its hallmark is a core body temperature elevated to more than 105°F (40.6°C). Temperature elevations to 110°F (43.3°C) or higher are not uncommon. Mental status is altered, and initial lethargy proceeds to confusion, stupor, and finally unconsciousness. Classically, sweating is said to be absent or diminished, but many victims of clear-cut heatstroke perspire profusely. The outcome is often fatal, even when patients are brought quickly to medical attention. Death-to-case ratios of 40 percent or more have been reported.[14–16]

Heatstroke is a medical emergency requiring immediate steps to lower core body temperature. A patient can be cooled with an ice-water bath, ice massage, or specialized evaporative cooling procedures. Further treatment is supportive and directed toward potential complications of hyperthermia, including fluid and electrolyte abnormalities, rhabdomyolysis, and bleeding diathesis. Maximal recovery may occur quickly or may not occur for a period of days or weeks, and there may be permanent neurological residua.[14,16]

Heat Exhaustion

Heat exhaustion is a milder illness than heatstroke, due primarily to the unbalanced or inadequate replacement of water and salts lost in perspiration. It typically occurs after several days of heat stress. Body temperature is normal to moderately elevated; it rarely exceeds 102°F (38.9°C). The symptoms, primarily dizziness, weakness, and fatigue, are those of circulatory distress. Treatment is supportive and directed toward normalizing fluid and electrolyte balance.[15,16]

Heat Syncope and Heat Cramps

Heat syncope and heat cramps occur principally in persons exercising in the heat. Heat syncope is a transient fall in blood pressure with an associated loss of consciousness. Consciousness generally returns promptly in the recumbent posture. The disorder is thought to arise from circulatory instability due to cutaneous vasodilation in response to heat stress. Prevention is accomplished by avoiding strenuous exercise in the heat, unless one is well trained and acclimatized.[17]

Heat cramps are muscle cramps, particularly in the legs, that occur during or shortly after exercise in a hot environment. They are thought to arise as a result of transient fluid and electrolyte abnormalities. Heat cramps decrease in frequency with athletic training and acclimatization to hot weather. They may be treated by increasing salt intake.[15]

TABLE 27-1. APPARENT TEMPERATURE IN DEGREES CELSIUS SHOWING EFFECT OF HUMIDITY AT HIGHER TEMPERATURE (WIND AND RADIATION COMPONENTS NOT SHOWN)

Dry-Bulb Temperature (°C)	**Relative Humidity (%)**										
	0	*10*	*20*	*30*	*40*	*50*	*60*	*70*	*80*	*90*	*100*
20	17.1	17.5	17.9	18.4	18.8	19.2	19.6	20.0	20.4	20.8	21.2
22	19.1	19.6	20.1	20.6	21.1	21.5	22.0	22.4	22.8	23.2	23.5
24	21.3	21.9	22.4	22.9	23.3	23.8	24.2	24.6	25.2	25.8	26.4
26	23.6	24.2	24.7	25.1	25.6	26.1	26.7	27.3	28.0	28.9	29.8
28	25.4	25.9	26.5	27.1	27.8	28.6	29.4	30.4	31.7	32.8	34.3
30	27.1	27.7	28.4	29.2	30.1	31.1	32.3	33.7	35.3	37.2	39.6
32	28.7	29.5	30.4	31.4	32.8	34.0	35.7	37.6	40.1	43.0	
34	30.3	31.3	32.5	33.8	35.0	37.4	39.6	42.7	46.0		
36	31.9	33.1	34.6	35.5	37.3	40.0	43.0	48.3			
38	33.4	35.0	36.8	39.0	41.8	45.3	49.7				
	Relative Humidity (%)										
	0	*5*	*10*	*15*	*20*	*25*	*30*	*35*	*40*	*45*	*50*
40	35.0	35.9	36.9	38.0	39.2	40.6	42.0	43.9	45.8	48.2	50.6
42	36.6	37.4	38.2	39.6	40.9	42.9	45.0	46.7	48.6		
44	38.1	39.4	40.8	42.4	44.4	46.5	49.0	51.8	54.1		
46	39.7	41.2	43.0	45.0	47.4	50.1	53.3				
48	41.2	43.1	44.5	46.8	49.6	52.8					
50	42.8	45.0	47.5	50.5	54.0	58.1					

Used with permission from Steadman RG: A universal scale of apparent temperature. J Climate Appl Meteorol 23:1674–1687, 1984.

Reproductive Effects

Among men, frequent or prolonged exposure to heat can result in elevated intrascrotal temperatures, causing a substantial decrease in sperm count.[18] Occupational exposure to heat has been associated with delayed conception.[19] Maternal hyperthermia has been implicated in the genesis of neural tube defects.[20,21]

▸ EPIDEMIOLOGY OF HEAT-RELATED ILLNESS

Heat Waves

Prolonged spells of unusually hot weather can cause dramatic increases in mortality, particularly in the urban areas of temperate regions. During the heat wave of 1980 in St. Louis, Missouri, some 300 more persons died than would have been expected on the basis of death rates observed before and after the heat wave (Fig. 27-1).[22] More recently, in the summer of 1995, record-breaking heat resulted in the loss of more than 700 lives in Chicago, largely in the course of a single week.[23] In fact, more than 150 excess deaths occurred in a single day.[24]

A surprisingly small proportion of heat wave-related mortality is identified as being caused by or precipitated by the heat. In general, recognized heat-related deaths compose from none to fewer than two-thirds of the heat-wave mortality increase.[25]

The connection of heat with many heat wave-related deaths is simply unrecognizable. Retrospective reviews of death certificates and clinical records have shown that increases in three categories of deaths largely account for the heat-related increase: Cardiovascular, cerebrovascular, and respiratory deaths are among the most common causes of death.[25] As a practical matter, it may be difficult or impossible for a physician to distinguish a case of myocardial infarction or stroke that occurred because of the heat from a case that he or she would have seen whether or not hot weather occurred.

Frequently, the overall health effects of the heat are most evident in the office of the medical examiner or coroner, where elevated mortality due to the heat presents as an abrupt increase in the number of sudden unattended deaths. Such cases are generally referred to the medical examiner or coroner. However, the sheer volume of cases may preclude in-depth investigation of each one, further complicating the task of distinguishing those that are heat-related. Moreover, procedures for determining whether a case is heat-related are at the discretion of individual medical examiners and are not standardized.

Nevertheless, the increased numbers of deaths apparently due to cerebrovascular disease (largely stroke) and cardiovascular disease (principally ischemic heart disease) are biologically plausible. Some studies have indicated that heat stress may induce some degree of blood hypercoagulability.[26,27] Heat stress may therefore favor the development of thrombi and emboli and may cause an increase in fatal strokes and myocardial infarctions.

The increase in mortality during heat waves is paralleled by an increase in nonspecific measures of morbidity. During hot weather, the numbers of hospital admissions and emergency room visits increase.[22,28]

Excess mortality due to heat waves occurs primarily in urban areas. Suburban and rural areas are at far less risk.[22,28] The urban predominance of adverse health consequences of the heat may be explained, in part, by the phenomenon of the urban "heat island."[29] The masses of stone, brick, concrete, asphalt, and cement that are typical of modern urban architecture absorb much of the sun's radiant energy, functioning as heat reservoirs and reradiating heat during nights that would otherwise be cooler. In many urban areas there are few trees to provide shading. In addition, tall buildings may effectively decrease wind velocity, decreasing in turn the cooling convective and evaporative effects of moving air. Other factors contributing to the severity of heat-related health effects in cities include the relative poverty of some urban areas.[22,28] Poor people are less able to afford cooling devices such as air conditioners and the energy needed to run them.

Impact on the Elderly

The elderly are at particularly high risk of severe, heat-related health effects. Except for infancy and early childhood, the risk of death due to heat increases throughout life as a function of age (Fig. 27-2). In

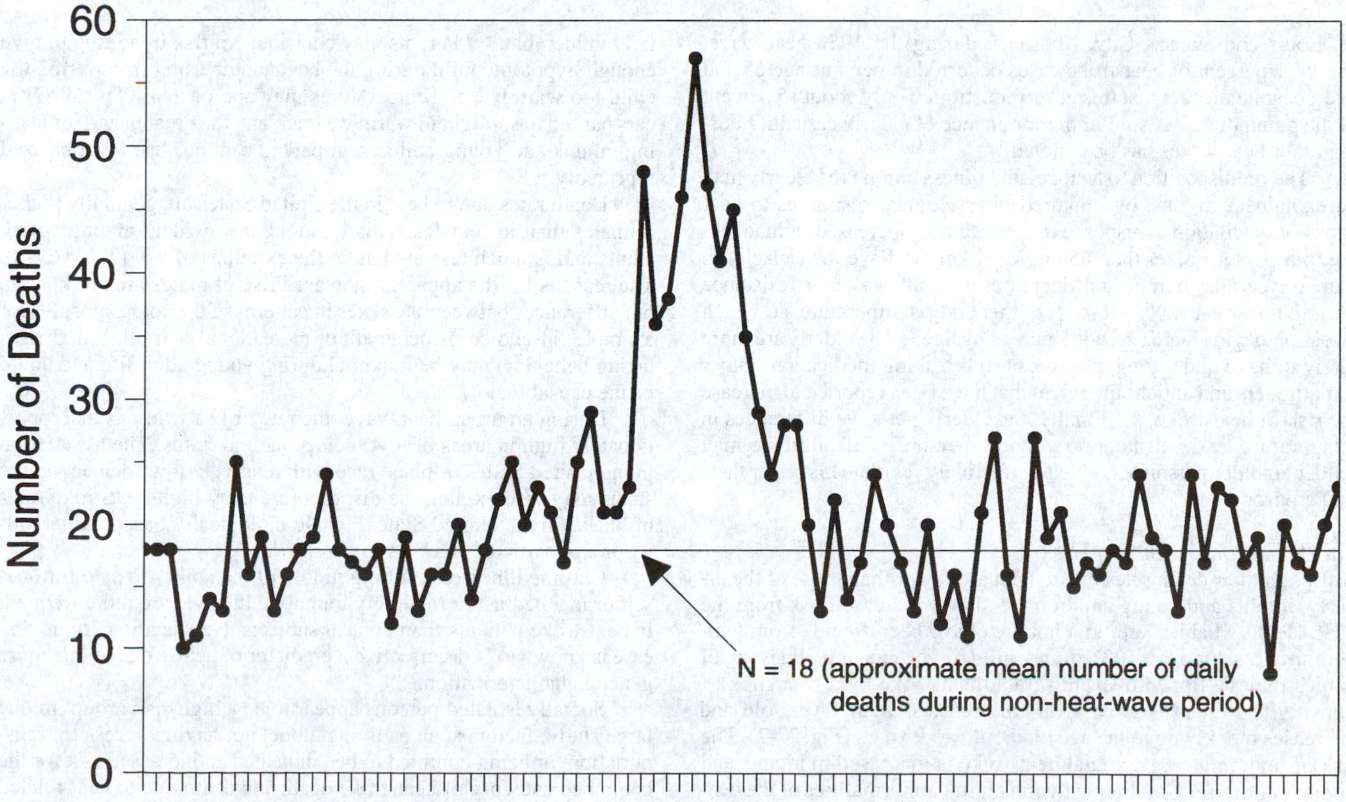

Figure 27-1. Plot of deaths by day, residents of St. Louis, Missouri, June–August, 1980.

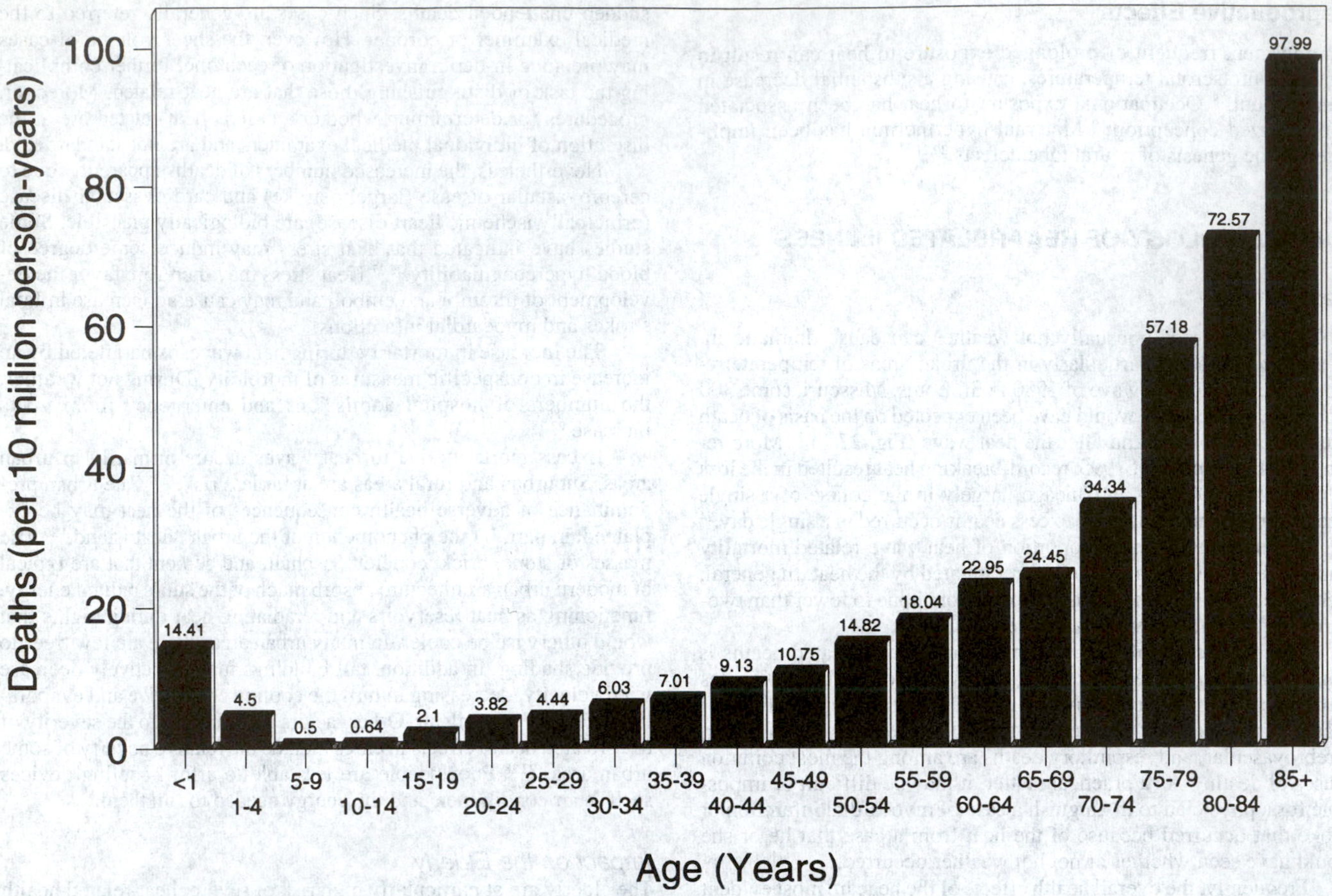

Figure 27-2. Rates of death caused by heat (International Classification of Diseases. 8th and 9th revs. Code E900) by age, United States, 1983–1993.

St. Louis and Kansas City, Missouri, during the 1980 heat wave, about 71 percent of heatstroke cases occurred in persons age 65 and over, despite the fact that this group constituted only about 15 percent of the population.[22] A similar predominance of elderly casualties during other heat waves has been noted.[30]

The predisposition to heat-related illness among the elderly may be explained, in part, by impaired physiological responses to heat stress. Vasodilation in response to heat requires increased cardiac output, but persons older than 65 are less likely to have the capacity to increase cardiac output and decrease systemic vascular resistance during hot weather.[31] Moreover, the body temperature at which sweating begins increases with increasing age.[32] The elderly are more likely to have underlying diseases or to be taking medication (major tranquilizers and anticholinergics) that have been reported to increase the risk of heatstroke.[33–36] Finally, the elderly perceive differences in temperature less well than do younger persons. This attribute may render an older person less able to effectively regulate his or her thermal environment.[37]

Other Factors Affecting Risk

Although their death rates due to heat are lower than those of the elderly, infants and young children are also at increased risk from the heat. Healthy babies kept in a hot area have been found to run temperatures as high as 103°F, and mild fever-causing illnesses of babies may be tipped over into frank heatstroke by a heat stress.[38] Sensitivity to heat is greatest in children less than 1 year old and decreases quickly up to the age of about 5 to 9 years (Fig. 27-2). The risk of both fatal and nonfatal heatstroke is increased in infants and young children.[39] Children with congenital abnormalities of the central nervous system and with diarrheal illness appear to be particularly vulnerable.[38,39] Parents may contribute to risk by failing to give enough hypotonic fluid during the heat and dressing or covering the child too warmly.[39,40] Temperatures may approach 140°F (60°C) in cars parked in sunlight in warm weather, and the great hazard of leaving infants and young children in parked cars has been emphasized repeatedly.[41,42]

Death rates due to heat in the United States are generally higher in males than in females. This trend is most evident among young adults and is much less evident at the extremes of age (Table 27-2). The reasons for the apparent increased risk of males are not known, but differences between the sexes in patterns of thermal exposure (for example, in choice of occupation, recreational activities, and risk-taking behavior) may be maximal during young adult life and could be the causal factor.

During an urban heat wave, the rate of heatstroke is disproportionately high in areas of low socioeconomic status. The association in the United States of black race with relatively low socioeconomic status may well explain the disproportionately high heatstroke rates of blacks in the United States.[22,28] No biologically based vulnerability of any particular race has been shown.

Chronic illnesses resulting in loss of the ability to care for oneself or in a bedfast or relatively immobile lifestyle are more frequent in heatstroke patients than control subjects. No specific chronic disease is known to be as effective a predictor of heatstroke as this more general characterization.[23,33]

Socially isolated persons appear to be a high-risk group. In one large study, factors such as living alone, not having access to transportation, or being confined to bed indicated an increased risk for the combined category of heatstroke death and death due to heat-related exacerbation of underlying cardiovascular disease.[23]

TABLE 27-2. RATES OF DEATH DUE TO HEAT AND COLD BY SEX AND AGE WITH RATE RATIOS, U.S. RESIDENTS, 1983–1993

	Heat (ICD E900)[a]			Cold (ICD E901)[a]		
Age Group	*Male*	*Female*	*RR*[b]	*Male*	*Female*	*RR*[b]
<1	15.48	13.3	1.16	12.71	8.67	1.47
1–4	4.93	4.06	1.21	1.41	0.74	1.91
5–9	0.49	0.51	0.95	1.57	0.62	2.54
10–14	0.93	0.33	2.86	3.21	0.33	9.84
15–19	3.4	0.74	4.62	13.48	2.63	5.13
20–24	6.39	1.17	5.47	14.75	2.53	5.83
25–29	7.65	1.2	6.38	17.68	3.85	4.59
30–34	10.28	1.82	5.65	20.06	4.05	4.95
35–39	12.3	1.81	6.81	28.09	5.24	5.36
40–44	15.48	2.95	5.24	37.86	7.64	4.96
45–49	16.69	5.02	3.32	47.65	8.62	5.53
50–54	22.09	7.94	2.78	79.13	14.33	5.52
55–59	26.73	10.09	2.65	87.4	15.21	5.74
60–64	31.97	15.07	2.12	110.26	23.57	4.68
65–69	32.29	18.09	1.79	107.31	29	3.7
70–74	42.93	27.95	1.54	123.99	46.59	2.66
75–79	64.02	52.76	1.21	198.5	81.1	2.45
80–84	91.83	62.31	1.47	273.51	126.4	2.16
85+	142.03	80.99	1.75	489.68	240.93	2.03

[a] International Classification of Diseases code for cause of death.
[b] Rate ratio male-female.

Persons with a history of prior heatstroke maintained thermal homeostasis in a hot environment less well than comparable volunteers who have never suffered heatstroke.[43] Whether heatstroke causes damage to the body's ability to regulate its temperature or thermoregulative abnormalities antedate the first heatstroke is not known.

Frequently referred to as a risk factor, the role of obesity in heatstroke risk is unclear. Obese subjects exercising in a hot environment showed a greater increase in rectal temperature and heart rate than did lean subjects.[44,45] Soldiers in the U.S. Army who died of exertional heatstroke during basic training in World War II were more likely to be obese than their peers.[46] However, studies of heatstroke and fatal cardiovascular disease among the relatively sedentary older persons principally at risk during urban summer heat waves have failed to demonstrate high body mass index as a risk factor.[23,33]

Neuroleptic ("major tranquilizing") drugs have been strongly implicated in increasing risk from the heat in both animal and human studies.[33,34,36,47] Neuroleptics appear to impair thermoregulatory function in both directions, sensitizing to cold as well as to heat.[56]

Anticholinergics decreased heat tolerance in laboratory tests of human volunteers. Persons treated with anticholinergics while exposed to heat had a decrease or cessation of sweating and a rise in rectal temperature.[35] Many commonly used prescription drugs (e.g., tricyclic antidepressants, some antiparkinsonian agents) and nonprescription drugs (e.g., antihistamines, sleeping pills) have prominent anticholinergic effects, and in one study the use of such drugs was more common in heatstroke victims than in control subjects.[33]

▸ PREVENTION OF HEAT-RELATED ILLNESS

In most parts of the United States, heat waves severe enough to threaten health do not occur every year. Several relatively mild summers may intervene between major heat waves. The erratic occurrence of heat waves hinders prevention planning. It is administratively difficult to plan for adequate resources to be available if needed, but not wasted if not needed.

Programs to prevent heat-related illness should concentrate on measures the efficacy of which is supported by empirical data. Many heatstroke prevention efforts for the community at large have been based on the distribution of electric fans to persons at risk. Nevertheless, systematic studies of urban heat waves failed to demonstrate any protective effect of electric fans.[23,33] Indices of heat stress predict a diminished cooling effect of air movement as dry-bulb temperature increases.[6,13] Physiologic experimentation confirms the inability of increasing air movement to increase heat tolerance at high temperatures.[45] Fans thus appear unlikely to offer protection from heat under the conditions of very high ambient temperature at which heat-related health effects are most likely to occur. Accordingly, the distribution of free fans during heat waves as a public health measure should be abandoned.

Air conditioning, on the other hand, is the single most effective intervention for prevention of heatstroke. In separate studies, the availability of home air conditioning was associated with a 70 percent decrease in fatality from the combined endpoint of either heatstroke or cardiovascular disease[23] and a 98 percent decrease in fatal heatstroke.[33] Moreover, both studies showed additional major reductions in risk (50 and 75 percent, respectively) from simply spending more time in air conditioned places.[23,33] Thus, such strategies as setting up air-conditioned heat wave shelters and air conditioning the lobbies of apartment buildings of lower socio-economic status tenants may be effective in preventing heat wave-related illness and death. Even when shelters cannot be provided, elderly and other persons at high risk can be encouraged to spend a few hours each day at public air conditioned places, such as movie theaters and shopping malls.

Heatstroke is an occupational risk for an estimated 6 million Americans who work in "hot" industries (e.g., foundries, glassworks, and mines). To prevent heat-related illness among the occupationally exposed, the U.S. National Institute for Occupational Safety and Health (NIOSH) recommends acclimatizing new workers and those returning from leave, arranging frequent rest periods in a cool environment, scheduling hot operations for the coolest part of the day, making drinking water readily available, conducting preemployment and periodic medical examinations, and instructing workers and supervisors about preventive measures and early recognition of heat-related illnesses.[11]

▸ COLD WEATHER

Seasonal Trends in Mortality

Human mortality is highly seasonal. In the United States, the death rate is greatest in late winter (usually February) and lowest in the late summer (August) (Fig. 27-3). A similar seasonal pattern of mortality occurs in other countries in the temperate zones of both the Northern and Southern Hemispheres, although the mortality curves of the two hemispheres are 6 months out of phase.[1]

The wintertime increase in the death rate is most marked in the elderly and becomes increasingly prominent with advancing age. For persons age 45 and younger, however, the pattern is reversed; the death rate is smallest in the winter and is greater in the summer.[48]

The extent of seasonal variation in mortality varies greatly by cause of death. The death rates for diseases of the heart, cerebrovascular disease, pneumonia, influenza, and chronic obstructive pulmonary disease show substantial increases in the winter. In contrast, the occurrence of death due to malignant neoplasms remains virtually constant throughout the year.[48,49]

Some of the seasonal winter increase in deaths due to major chronic diseases such as stroke and myocardial infarction may reflect seasonal changes in underlying risk factors for vascular diseases. For example, it is well documented that blood pressure in humans is seasonal and is higher in the winter.[50] Cold stress can physiologically potentiate the coagulation of blood, possibly contributing to the winter excess of deaths due to stroke and ischemic heart disease.[51] In addition, many types of exercise are practiced seasonally, with sedentary periods tending to occur in winter.[52]

The winter death increase cannot be attributed entirely to the direct effect of cold exposure. The increase occurs even in states noted for their relatively mild winter climates (e.g., Florida and Hawaii) and is of approximately the same order of magnitude as in colder states (e.g., Minnesota and Montana).[48] Low winter humidity may contribute to the winter death excess, since it favors the transmission of certain infectious agents, notably influenza.[53] In addition, winter increases in deaths due to certain unintentional injuries may reflect seasonal increases in certain behaviors. For example, deaths due to fire are more common in the winter, perhaps a result of the use of fireplaces and heating devices. Finally, the peaks and valleys in the U.S. death rate have not always come in mid to late winter and late summer, respectively, as they usually do now. In the early part of this century, the peak was usually in February or March and the nadir in June rather than August.[49] This change in seasonal pattern is further evidence that temperature is not necessarily the most important immediate determinant of seasonality in mortality.

Cold Stress and Its Indices

The two most important adaptive physiological responses to the cold are vasoconstriction and shivering. Peripheral vasoconstriction causes a rerouting of some blood away from cutaneous and other superficial vascular beds toward deeper tissues where the blood's heat is less easily lost. In addition, blood is rerouted from the superficial veins of the limbs to the venae comitantes of the major arteries. Such rerouting activates a "countercurrent" mechanism by which arterial blood warms venous blood before the venous blood returns to the core. Conversely, venous blood cools arterial blood so that it gives up less heat when it reaches the periphery. The result is a fall in the temperature of superficial body parts in defense of core temperature.[1,54]

Humidity and radiant heat energy are less important in the evaluation of cold environments than of hot. Thus the popular "wind chill" index of Siple expresses the intensity of cooling expected from a cold environment as a function only of ambient temperature and wind speed:

$$H = (10.45 + 10s^{1/2} - s)(33 - t)$$

where H is the wind chill expressed in kcal m^{-2} hr^{-1}, s is the wind speed in $msec^{-1}$, and t is the ambient temperature in degrees Celsius.[55] The value of H permits comparison of the cooling effect of various

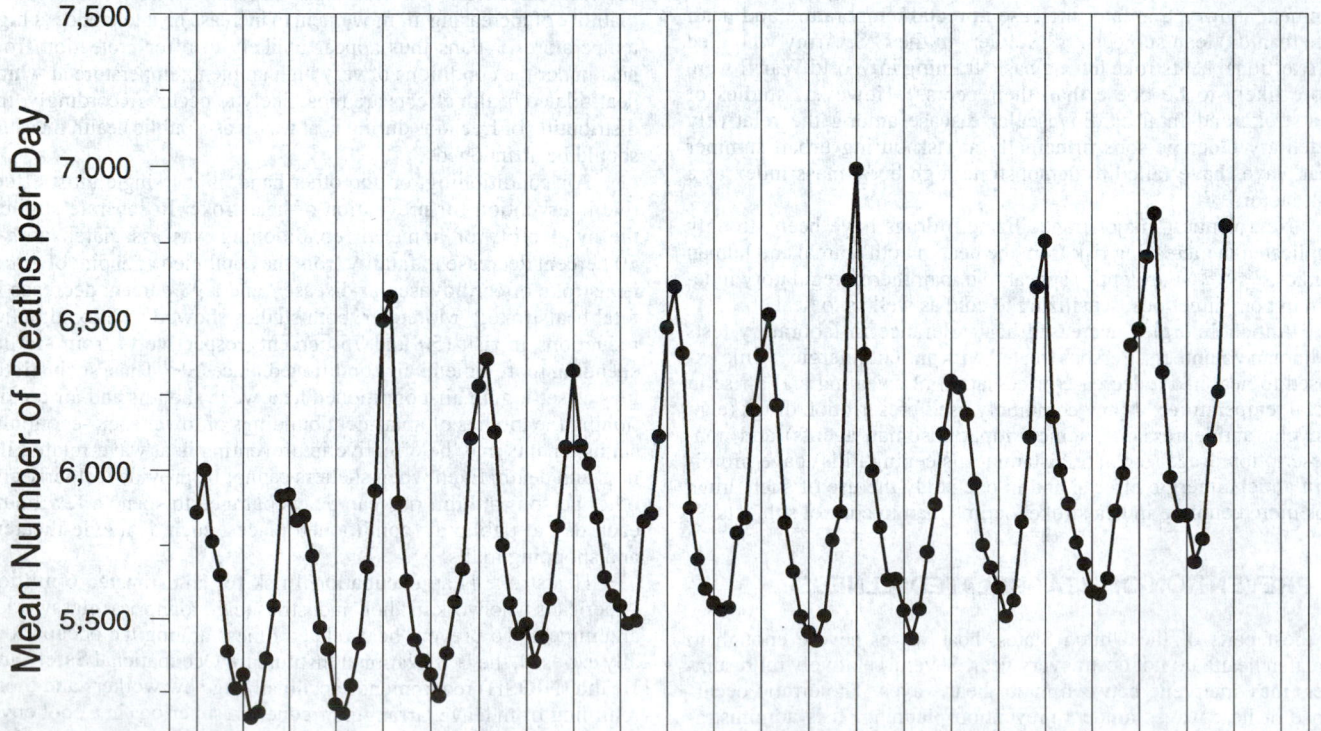

Figure 27-3. Mean daily number of deaths from all causes by month, United States, January 1983–December 1993.

temperature and wind speed combinations. The subjective thermal perception associated with any given value of H is influenced greatly by one's level of activity and the type and amount of clothing worn.

Often, the wind-chill effect is described in terms of a wind-chill equivalent temperature. This is the temperature that would produce the same intensity of cooling as the temperature-wind speed combination under consideration if the wind speed were some relatively low reference value.[56] A wind-chill equivalent temperature can be calculated from a modification of the Siple formula:

$$t_{eq} = 33 - \frac{(10.45 + 10s^{1/2} - s)(33 - t)}{(10.45 + 10s_{ref}^{1/2} - s_{ref})}$$

where t_{eq} and t are the wind-chill equivalent and ambient temperatures in degrees Celsius, and s and s_{ref} are the actual and reference wind speeds in $msec^{-1}$. Wind-chill equivalent temperatures in degrees Fahrenheit for a reference wind speed of 4 mph (1.79 $msec^{-1}$) are listed in Table 27-3.

The wind-chill formula of Siple has been criticized as being too sensitive to changes in wind speed when wind speed is low, and not sensitive enough to changes in wind speed at higher velocities.[56] The formula is clearly only an approximation since, for any temperature, H, the wind chill, is maximal at winds of 25 $msec^{-1}$ (56 mph) and actually *decreases* as wind speed goes even higher, a physical impossibility.

▸ ILLNESSES CAUSED BY COLD

Hypothermia

Hypothermia refers to a decrease in core body temperature below 35°C (95°F). Hypothermia may be purposefully induced (e.g., to decrease oxygen consumption during surgery). However, hypothermia also occurs unintentionally (so-called accidental hypothermia) as a result of exposure to cold environmental conditions. Unintentional hypothermia is a problem of considerable public health importance and is the only type of hypothermia considered further.

As body temperature drops, consciousness becomes clouded, and the patient appears confused or disoriented. Intense vasoconstriction causes pallor. Shivering is maximal in the higher range of hypothermic core temperatures, but decreases markedly in intensity as body temperature falls further and hypothermia itself impairs thermoregulation. In severe hypothermia (body temperature below about 86°F or 30°C), consciousness is lost, respirations may become imperceptibly shallow, and the pulse may not be palpable.[1]

At such low temperatures, the myocardium becomes irritable and ventricular fibrillation is common. The patient may appear dead even though he or she may yet be revived with proper treatment. Persons found apparently dead in circumstances suggesting that they may have suffered hypothermia should be treated for hypothermia until death can be confirmed. In particular, the potential for recovery of cold-water drowning victims should not be underestimated, since there have been reports of virtually complete recovery in patients who were without an effective heartbeat for periods as long as 2½ hours.[57]

Hypothermia occurs both as a direct consequence of overexposure to the cold (primary hypothermia) and as the apparent result of thermoregulatory failure due principally to other severe illness (e.g., sepsis, myocardial infarction, central nervous system damage, metabolic derangements), although cold exposure may also contribute to such secondary hypothermia. Primary hypothermia has a better prognosis than hypothermia that occurs as a result of concomitant illness.[58] Death is also more likely in patients who present with particularly low body temperatures.[59]

There is considerable debate in the medical literature regarding the optimal method of rewarming hypothermic patients. However, a consensus is emerging that treatment must vary according to the severity of the illness. Noninvasive, external rewarming is appropriate for mildly hypothermic patients who have a perfusing cardiac rhythm. On the other hand, cardiopulmonary bypass with extracorporeal rewarming of the blood may be required in patients with severe hypothermia and no effective cardiac function.[60,61] In addition, all but very mild hypothermia cases require additional intensive supportive medical care.[61]

Frostbite

Local tissue injury as a result of exposure to cold may be seen in hypothermia cases but often occurs independently from it. Frostbite involves actual freezing of tissue. It affects primarily acral body parts (e.g., distal extremities, ears, and nose) and can occur over a period of minutes to hours in severe cold. Severe frostbite may result in a loss of tissue viability that may require amputation. Such injuries may be frequent during a spell of unusually cold weather.[62]

Nonfreezing Local Tissue Injury

Perniosis (chilblains) is characterized by tender and/or pruritic, erythematous or violaceous papules occurring in the skin of acral body parts, particularly the hands. When severe, the lesions may blister or

TABLE 27-3. WIND CHILL EQUIVALENT TEMPERATURES IN DEGREES FAHRENHEIT FOR A REFERENCE WIND SPEED OF 4 MPH

	Actual Wind Speed (mph)						
Temperature (°F)	*4*	*5*	*10*	*20*	*30*	*40*	*50*
40	40	37	28	18	13	10	9
35	35	32	22	11	5	2	1
30	30	27	16	4	−2	−6	−7
25	25	22	10	−3	−10	−14	−15
20	20	16	4	−10	−18	−22	−23
15	15	11	−3	−18	−25	−29	−31
10	10	6	−9	−25	−33	−37	−39
5	5	1	−15	−32	−41	−45	−47
0	0	−5	−21	−39	−48	−53	−55
−5	−5	−10	−27	−46	−56	−61	−63
−10	−10	−15	−33	−53	−64	−69	−71
−15	−15	−20	−40	−60	−71	−77	−79
−20	−20	−26	−46	−67	−79	−85	−87

ulcerate. The condition is typically present only during the colder months of the year, and women are afflicted more frequently than men are.[63] The underlying pathophysiology may involve cold-induced ischemia of involved areas or a cold-mediated inflammatory reaction. Vasodilators (for example, nifedipine) may be useful both in treatment of the lesions and in the prevention of recurrences.[64]

A condition known as "cold water immersion injury" or "trench foot" (when it affects the lower extremity) results from the continuous exposure of parts of the body (typically, the lower extremities) to wet and above-freezing cold conditions for a period of days to weeks. Local tissue injury occurs, possibly from reduced blood flow due to prolonged vasoconstriction. When affected extremities are warmed, they are swollen and numb at first. Later, a painful hyperemic phase develops. Still, later, muscle weakness and atrophy and fibrosis may develop, and there may be other long-lasting sequelae, including persistent pain, hypesthesia, or increased sensitivity to the cold.[65] Anyone with prolonged continuous exposure to cold water and/or cold wet clothing is at risk. The condition is prevented by fully rewarming and drying the body at frequent intervals.

▶ EPIDEMIOLOGY OF COLD INJURY

Hypothermia in the Elderly

The extent to which indoor cold causes clinically significant hypothermia has been increasingly appreciated in recent years. In particular, the special vulnerability of elderly persons to this condition has been recognized. After the first year or so of life, the rate of death due to effects of the cold increases steadily with advancing age (Fig. 27–4). In the United States, approximately 700 to 1,000 deaths due to cold exposure occur each year. More than half of these cases occur in persons aged 60 years or older,[66] although persons in this age group comprise less than 17 percent of the population.[67]

The extent of hypothermia morbidity is difficult to measure. A nationwide study of hypothermia in New Zealand found an incidence of hypothermia hospital admissions that was 12 times the hypothermia death rate. However, hypothermia hospitalizations primarily involved infants, whereas hypothermia deaths occurred primarily among the elderly and among males 13 to 65 years old.[68]

A wintertime survey conducted in Great Britain of 1,020 persons age 65 and over revealed that relatively few (0.58 percent) persons surveyed had hypothermic morning deep-body temperatures (≤35°C) and none had hypothermic evening temperatures. Nevertheless, a substantial number (10 percent) had near-hypothermic temperatures (≤35.5°C but >35°C).[69] In contrast, 3.6 percent of 467 patients more than 65 years old admitted to London hospitals in late winter and early spring were hypothermic.[70] That hypothermia is relatively common among elderly persons admitted to hospitals, although virtually absent in the community, has been interpreted as showing that most elderly Britons with hypothermia are quickly hospitalized.

The apparent cold sensitivity of the elderly may be due to physiological factors. Collins and others found that a high proportion of persons age 65 and older failed to develop physiologically significant vasoconstriction in response to a controlled cold environment and that the proportion of such persons increased with the age of the cohort examined. These elderly subjects with abnormal vasoconstriction tended to have relatively low core temperatures.[71] The basal metabolic rate (BMR) declines substantially with age, requiring elderly people to battle cold stress from a relatively low level of basal thermogenesis.[72] Shivering, a mechanism by which metabolic thermogenesis can be increased, may be impaired in some older persons.[73] Voluntary muscular activity also releases heat, but the elderly

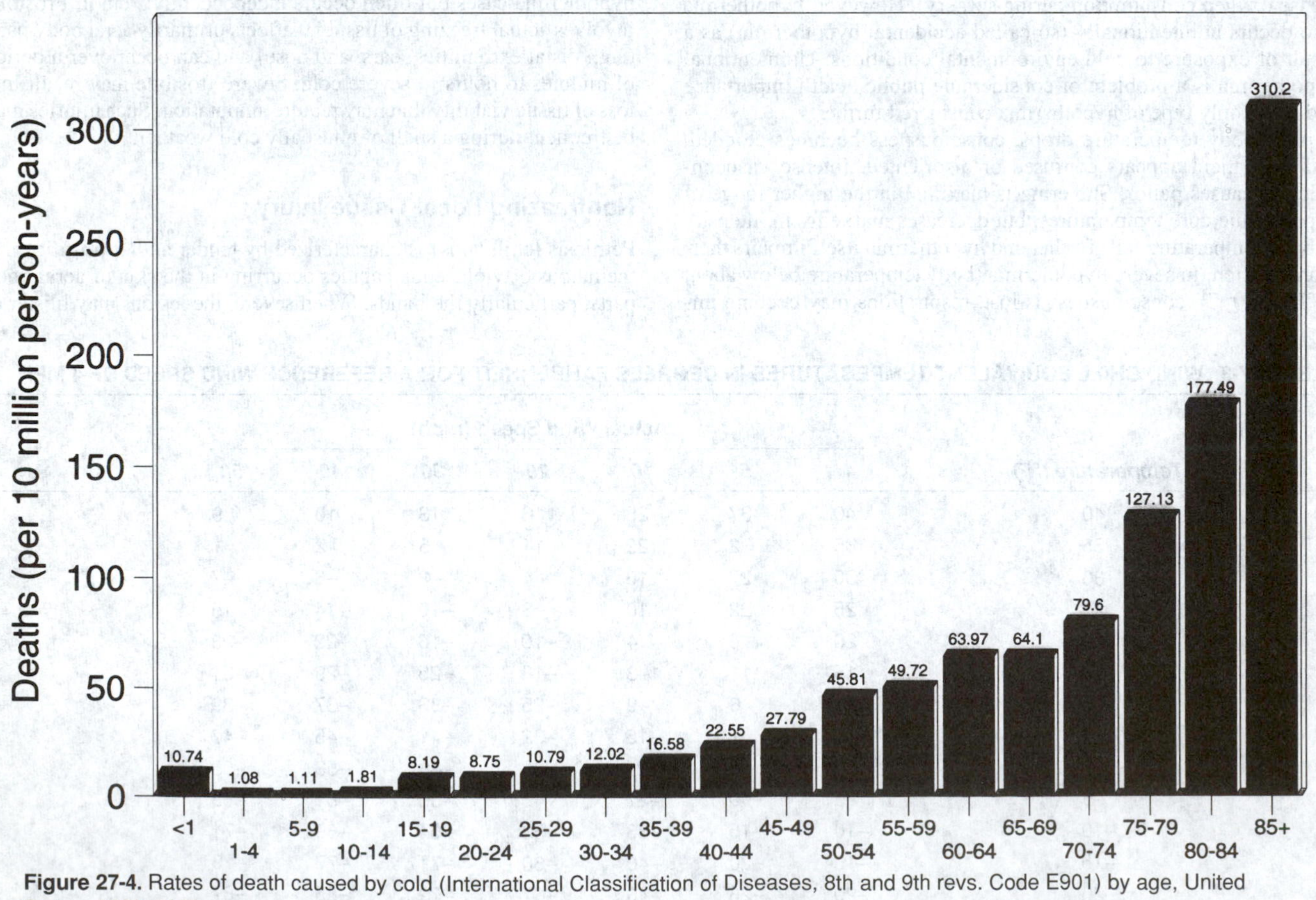

Figure 27-4. Rates of death caused by cold (International Classification of Diseases, 8th and 9th revs. Code E901) by age, United States, 1983–1993.

are more prone than others to debilitating chronic illnesses that limit mobility. Metabolic heat produced through the oxidation of brown fat is less available to the elderly, in whom this type of adipose tissue is less abundant than in children and younger adults.[74]

Elderly persons appear to perceive cold less well than younger persons and may voluntarily set thermostats to relatively low temperatures.[13,75] In addition, the high cost of energy, together with the relative poverty of some elderly people, may discourage their setting thermostats high enough to maintain comfortable warmth.[76]

Drugs Predisposing to Hypothermia

Ethanol ingestion is an important predisposing factor for hypothermia. The great majority of patients in many hypothermia case series are middle-aged alcoholic men.[77,78] Ethanol produces vasodilation, interfering with the peripheral vasoconstriction that is an important physiological defense against the cold.[54] Although ethanol-containing beverages are sometimes taken in cold surroundings for the subjective sense of warmth they produce, this practice is dangerous. Ethanol also predisposes to hypothermia indirectly, by inhibiting hepatic gluconeogenesis, and thus producing hypoglycemia in carboydrate-depleted persons (e.g., many chronic alcoholics). Ethanol-induced hypoglycemia has been clearly shown to produce hypothermia in healthy volunteers.[79]

Treatment with the neuroleptic drugs (phenothiazines, butyrophenones, and thioxanthenes) also predisposes to hypothermia. Chlorpromazine, the prototype drug of this group, has been used to induce hypothermia pharmacologically.[1,80] Chlorpromazine suppresses shivering, probably by a central mechanism, and causes vasodilation.[47] The hypothermic action of drugs of this class becomes more pronounced with decreasing ambient temperature.[81]

Other Hypothermia Risk Factors

Infants under 1 year of age have a higher rate of death due to cold than do older children (Fig. 27-4). Neonates, especially premature or small-for-gestational-age babies, are at particularly high risk. Although the mechanisms for maintaining thermal homeostasis (vasoconstriction and thermogenesis by shivering) are present at birth, they seem to function less effectively than in older children. Infants have a relatively large ratio of heat-losing surface to heat-generating volume, and the layer of insulating subcutaneous fat is relatively thin. Perhaps most importantly, a baby is unable to control his or her own environment. Babies are totally dependent on others to keep them warm, and if sufficient warmth is not provided, hypothermia results.[54]

Hypothermia in infants can be a substantial public health problem in areas with severe winter weather. During December and January of the winters of 1961–1962 and 1962–1963, 110 hypothermic (T < 90°F, 32.2°C) babies were admitted to hospitals in Glasgow, Scotland. Mortality in this group was 46 percent.[82] Hypothermia, however, is not a problem only in cold climates. In tropical climates, hypothermia among babies and young children can also be a problem in winter. Children and infants suffering from protein-calorie malnutrition are particularly susceptible.[83]

In older children and young adults, lethal hypothermia is relatively infrequent (Fig. 27-4). However, persons in this age group are still susceptible to an overwhelming cold stress.

Unintentional immersion in very cold water can lead rapidly to hypothermia.[84] Cold and wet weather may be especially dangerous, because the insulating properties of clothing are markedly reduced by moisture.[85]

The rate of death due to cold is greater in males than in females in all age groups (Table 27-2). Behavioral differences (for example, in choice of occupation and recreational activities) resulting in increased frequency of in exposure to cold may account for the particularly great relative risk of males during the teenage years through late middle age but do not fully explain the apparent difference between the sexes in susceptibility.

Homelessness is an important hypothermia risk factor. Substantial proportions of hypothermia case series involve persons without a fixed address.[77,86,87]

Epidemiology of Frostbite

Serious frostbite injury occurs predominantly among males and is less frequent among babies, young children, and the elderly than among other age groups. Alcohol intoxication plays a role in about of half of each of several case series. Other factors frequently contributing to frostbite injury are psychiatric illness, vehicular failure or crash, and drug use. Hypothermia is frequently present. In one case series, 12 percent of frostbite patients had hypothermia (temperature less than 32°C).[88] Finnish conscripts were found to be at increased risk of frostbite if they did not wear scarves or headgear with earflaps or if they did wear supposedly protective ointments.[89]

▸ PREVENTION OF COLD-RELATED ILLNESS

Hypothermia is best prevented by limiting the cold stress of susceptible populations. Thus, programs to help the elderly poor receive financial assistance in paying heating bills may be helpful. Both government agencies and utility companies have been involved in establishing programs that either provide direct financial aid toward the payment of elderly people's energy bills or allow deferred payment.

Awareness of the problem of neonatal hypothermia by pediatricians and communication of this concern to new parents may help prevent hypothermia in infants.

Children and young adults who are at low risk from the cold should nevertheless take appropriate precautions when they go into a cold environment. The clothing chosen should provide sufficient insulation, and care should be taken that it not get wet. One should especially guard against the possibility of immersion in cold water.

To prevent frostbite when venturing into below-freezing temperatures, care should be taken to minimize the area of exposed skin.

▸ REFERENCES

1. Collins KJ: Hypothermia: The Facts. New York: Oxford University Press, 1983
2. Rowell LB: Human adjustments and adaptations to heat stress. Where and how? In Folinsbee LJ, Wagner JA, Borgia JF, et al (eds): Environmental Heat Stress: Individual Human Adaptations. New York: Academic Press, 1978, pp 3–27
3. Nadel ER, Roberts MF, Wenger CB: Thermoregulatory adaptations to heat and exercise: comparative responses of men and women. In Folinsbee LJ, Wagner JA, Borgia JF, et al (eds): Environmental Heat Stress: Individual Human Adaptations. New York: Academic Press, 1978, pp 29–38
4. Bonner RM, Harrison MH, Hall CJ, Edwards RJ: Effect of heat acclimatization on intravascular responses to acute heat stress in man. J Appl Physiol 41:708–713, 1976
5. Wyndham CH, Rogers GG, Senay LC, Mitchell D: Acclimatization in a hot, humid environment: cardiovascular adjustments. J Appl Physiol 40:779–785, 1976
6. Yaglou CP: Temperature, humidity, and air movement in industries: the effective temperature index. J Ind Hyg 9:297–309, 1927
7. American Society of Heating, Refrigerating, and Air Conditioning Engineers (ASHRAE): Handbook of Fundamentals. Atlanta: ASHRAE, 1981
8. American Society of Heating, Refrigerating, and Air Conditioning Engineers (ASHRAE): 1989 ASHRAE Handbook: Fundamentals (I-P ed.). Atlanta: ASHRAE, 1989

9. Lee DHK: Seventy-five years of searching for a heat index. Environ Res 22:331–356, 1980
10. Minard D, Belding HS, Kingston JR: Prevention of heat casualties. JAMA 1655:1813–1818, 1957
11. National Institute for Occupational Safety and Health: Criteria for a Recommended Standard: Occupational Exposure to Hot Environments. Revised Criteria 1986. Washington, DC: Government Printing Office, 1986
12. Beshir MY, Ramsey JD, Burford CL: Threshold values for the Botsball: a field study of occupational heat. Ergonomics 25:247–254, 1982
13. Steadman RG: A universal scale of apparent temperature. J Climate Appl Meteorol 23:1674–1687, 1984
14. Hart GR, Anderson RJ, Crumpler CP, et al: Epidemic classical heat stroke: clinical characteristics and course of 28 patients. Medicine 61:189–197, 1982
15. Knochel JP: Environmental heat illness: an eclectic review. Arch Intern Med 133:841–864, 1974
16. Knochel JP: Heat stroke and related heat stress disorders. Dis Mon 35:301–377, 1989
17. National Institute for Occupational Safety and Health: Criteria for a Recommended Standard: Occupational Exposure to Hot Environments. Washington, DC: U.S. Department of Health, Education and Welfare, 1972
18. Levine RJ: Male fertility in hot environments [Letter]. JAMA 252:3250–3251, 1984
19. Rachootin P, Olsen J: The risk of infertility and delayed conception associated with exposures in the Danish workplace. J Occup Med 25:394–402, 1983
20. Miller P, Smith DW, Shepard TH: Maternal hyperthermia as a possible cause of anencephaly. Lancet 1:519–521, 1978
21. Layde PM, Edmonds LD, Erickson JD: Maternal fever and neural tube defects. Teratology 21:105–108, 1980
22. Jones TS, Liang AP, Kilbourne EM, et al: Morbidity and mortality associated with the July 1980 heat wave in St. Louis and Kansas City, Missouri. JAMA 247:3327–3331, 1982
23. Semenza JC, Rubin CH, Falter KH, Selanikio JD, Flanders D, Howe HL, Wilhelm JL: Heat-related deaths during the July 1995 heat wave in Chicago. N Engl J Med 335:84–90, 1996
24. Centers for Disease Control and Prevention: Heat-related mortality—Chicago, July 1995. MMWR 44:577–580, 1995
25. Kilbourne EM: Heat waves and hot environments. In Noji E (ed): The Public Health Consequences of Disasters. New York: Oxford University Press, pp 245–269
26. Keatinge WR, Coleshaw SRK, Easton JC, Cotter F, Mattock MB, Chelliah R: Increased platelet and red cell counts, blood viscosity, and plasma cholesterol levels during heat stress, and mortality from coronary and cerebral thrombosis. Am J Med 81:795–800, 1986
27. Strother SV, Bull JMC, Branham SA: Activation of coagulation during therapeutic whole body hyperthermia. Thromb Res 43:353–360, 1986
28. Applegate WB, Runyan JW Jr, et al: Analysis of the 1980 heat wave in Memphis. J Geriatr Soc 29:337–342, 1981
29. Clarke JF: Some effects of the urban structure on heat mortality. Environ Res 5:93–104, 1972
30. Austin MG, Berry JW: Observations on one hundred cases of heatstroke. JAMA 161:1525–1529, 1956
31. Sprung CL: Hemodynamic alterations of heat stroke in the elderly. Chest 75:362–366, 1979
32. Crowe JP, Moore RE: Physiological and behavioral responses of aged men to passive heating. J Physiol 236:43P–45P, 1973
33. Kilbourne EM, Choi K, Jones TS, et al: Risk factors for heatstroke. A case-control study. JAMA 247:3332–3336, 1982
34. Wise TN: Heatstroke in three chronic schizophrenics: case reports and clinical considerations. Compr Phsychiatry 14:263–267, 1973
35. Littman RE: Heat sensitivity due to autonomic drugs. JAMA 149: 635–636, 1952
36. Adams BE, Manoguerra AS, Lilja GP, Long RS, Ruiz E: Heatstroke: associated with medications having anticholinergic effects. Minn Med 60:103–106, 1977
37. Collins KJ, Exton-Smith AN, Dore C: Urban hypothermia: preferred temperature and thermal perception in old age. Br Med J 282:175–177, 1981
38. Cardullo HM: Sustained summer heat and fever in infants. J Pediatr 35:24–42, 1949
39. Danks DM, Webb DW, Allen J: Heat illness in infants and young children. A study of 47 cases. Br Med J 2:287–293, 1962
40. Bacon C, Scott D, Jones P: Heatstroke in well-wrapped infants. Lancet 1:422–425, 1979
41. Gibbs LI, Lawrence DW, Kohn MA: Heat exposure in an enclosed automobile. J La State Med Soc 147:545–546, 1995
42. Centers for Disease Control and Prevention: Heat-related illnesses and deaths—United States, 1994–1995. MMWR 44:465–468, 1995
43. Shapiro Y, Magazanik A, Udassin R, et al: Heat intolerance in former heatstroke patients. Ann Intern Med 90:913–916, 1979
44. Bar-Or O, Lundegren HM, Buskirk ER: Heat tolerance of exercising obese and lean women. J Appl Physiol 26:403–409, 1969
45. Haymes EM, McCormick RJ, Buskirk ER: Heat tolerance of exercising lean and obese prepubertal boys. J Appl Physiol 39:457–461, 1975
46. Schickele E: Environment and fatal heat stroke: an analysis of 157 cases occurring in the army in the U.S. during World War II. Mil Surg 98:235–256, 1947
47. Kollias J, Ballard RW: The influence of chlorpromazine on physical and chemical mechanisms of temperature regulation in the rat. J Pharmacol Exp Ther 145:373–381, 1964
48. Feinlieb M: Statement of Manning Feinleib. In: Deadly Cold: Health Hazards due to Cold Weather. Washington, DC: Government Printing Office, 1984, pp 85–125
49. Rosenwaike I: Seasonal variation of deaths in the United States, 1951–1960. J Am Stat Assoc 61:706–719, 1966
50. Giaconi S, Ghione S, Palombo C, Genovesi-Ebert A, Marabotti C, Fommei E, Donato L: Seasonal influences on blood pressure in high normal to mild hypertensive range. Hypertension 14:22–27, 1989
51. Keatinge WR, Coleshaw SRK, Cotter F, Mattock M, Murphy M, Chelliah R: Increases in platelet and red cell counts, blood viscosity and arterial pressure during mild surface cooling: factors in mortality from coronary and cerebral thrombosis in winter. Br Med J 289: 1405–1408, 1984
52. Dannenberg AL, Keller JB, Wilson PWF, Castelli WP: Leisure time physical activity in the Framingham offspring study. Am J Epidemiol 129:76–88, 1989
53. Schulman JL, Kilbourne ED: Experimental transmission of influenza virus in mice: II. Some factors affecting incidence of transmitted infection. J Exp Med 118:267–275, 1963
54. Maclean D, Emslie-Smith D: Accidental Hypothermia. Oxford: Blackwell Scientific Publications, 1977
55. Siple PA, Passel CF: Measurement of dry atmospheric cooling in subfreezing temperatures. Proc Am Philos Soc 89:177–199, 1945
56. Steadman RG: Indices of wind chill of clothed persons. J Appl Meteorol 10:674–683, 1971
57. Young RSK, Zaineratis EL, Dooling EC: Neurological outcome in cold water drowning. JAMA 244:1233–1235, 1980
58. Miller JW, Danzl DF, Thomas DM: Urban accidental hypothermia: 135 cases. Ann Emerg Med 9:456–460, 1980
59. Danzl DF, Pozos RS, Auerbach PS, et al: Multicenter hypothermia survey. Ann Emerg Med 16:1042–1055, 1987
60. Danzl DF, Pozos RS: Accidental hypothermia. N Engl J Med 331: 1756–1760, 1994
61. Anonymous: Treatment of hypothermia. Med Let Drugs Ther 36: 116–117, 1994

62. Bishop HM, Collin J, Wood RAM, Morris PJ: Frostbite in Oxfordshire: the impact of a severe winter on an unprepared civilian population. Injury 15:379–380, 1984
63. Goette DK: Chillblains (perniosis). J Am Acad Dermatol 23:257–262, 1990
64. Rustin MHA, Newton JA, Smith NP, Dowd PM: The treatment of chilblains with nifedipine: the results of a pilot study, a double-blind placebo-controlled randomized study and a long-term open trial. Br J Dermatol 120:267–275, 1989
65. Mills WJ Jr, Mills WJ III: Peripheral non-freezing cold injury: immersion injury. Alaska Med 35:117–128, 1993
66. National Center for Health Statistics: Public use mortality data tapes for the years 1983–1993. Hyattsville, MD:
67. U.S. Bureau of the Census: Decennial Census for 1990
68. Taylor NAS, Griffiths RF, Cotter JD: Epidemiology of hypothermia: fatalities and hospitalisations in New Zealand. Aust N Z J Med 24:705–710, 1994
69. Fox RH, Woodward PM, Exton-Smith An, et al: Body temperatures in the elderly: a national study of physiological, social, and environmental conditions. Br Med J 1:200–206, 1973
70. Goldman A, Exton-Smith AN, Francis G, O'Brien A: A pilot study of low body temperatures in old people admitted to hospital. J R Coll Physicians Lond 11:291–306, 1977
71. Collins KJ, Dore C, Exton-Smith AN, et al: Accidental hypothermia and impaired temperature homeostasis in the elderly. Br Med J 1:353–356, 1977
72. Shock NW, Watkin DM, Yiengst MJ, et al: Age differences in the water content of the body as related to basal oxygen consumption in males. J Gerontol 18:1–8, 1963
73. Collins KJ, Easton JC, Exton-Smith AN: Shivering thermogenesis and vasomotor responses with convective cooling in the elderly. J Physiol 320:76P, 1981
74. Heat J: The distribution of brown adipose tissue in the human. J Anat 112:35–39, 1972
75. Watts AJ: Hypothermia in the aged: a study of the role of cold-sensitivity. Environ Res 5:119–126, 1971
76. Morgan R, King D, Blair A: Urban hypothermia. Many elderly people cannot keep warm in winter without financial hardship (Letter). Br Med J 312:124, 1996
77. Centers for Disease Control: Exposure-related hypothermia deaths—District of Columbia, 1972–1982. MMWR 31:669–671, 1982
78. Weyman AE, Greenbaum DM, Grace WJ: Accidental hypothermia in an alcoholic population. Am J Med 56:13–21, 1974
79. Haight JSJ, Keatinge WR: Failure of thermoregulation in the cold during hypoglycemia induced by exercise and ethanol. J Physiol 229: 87–97, 1973
80. Courvoisier S, Fournel J, Ducrot R, Kolsky M, Koetschet P: Proprietes pharmacodynamiques du chlorhydrate de chloro-3 (dimethyl-amino-3′ propyl)-10 phenothiazine (4.560 R.P.). Arch Int Pharmacodyn Ther 92:305–361, 1953
81. Higgins EA, Iampietro PF, Adams T, Holmes DD: Effects of a tranquilizer on body temperature. Proc Soc Exp Biol Med 115:1017–1019, 1964
82. Arneil GC, Kerr MM: Severe hypothermia in Glasgow infants in winter. Lancet 2:756–759, 1963
83. Cutting WAM, Samuel GA: Hypothermia in a tropical winter climate. Indian Pediatr 8:752–757, 1971
84. Bullard RW, Rapp GM: Problems of body heat loss in water immersion. Aerospace Med 41:1269–1277, 1970
85. Pugh LGC: Clothing insulation and accidental hypothermia in youth. Nature 209:1281–1286, 1966
86. Centers for Disease Control and Prevention: Hypothermia-related deaths—Cook County, Illinois, November 1992–March 1993. MMWR 42:917–919, 1993
87. Centers for Disease Control and Prevention: Hypothermia-related deaths—New Mexico, October 1993–March 1994. MMWR 44:933–935, 1995
88. Valnicek SM, Chasmar LR, Clapson JB: Frostbite in the prairies. A 12-year review. Plast Reconstr Surg 92:633–641, 1993
89. Lehmuskallio E, Lindholm H, Koskenvuo K, Sarna S, Friberg O, Viljanen A: Frostbite of the face and ears: epidemiological study of risk factors in Finnish conscripts. Br Med J 311:1661–1663, 1995

28

Ionizing Radiation

Arthur C. Upton

Since the discovery of the x-ray, in 1895, studies of the health effects of ionizing radiation have received continuing impetus from the expanding uses of radiation in medicine, science, and industry, as well as from the peaceful and military applications of atomic energy.[1] The extensive knowledge of the effects of ionizing radiation generated by these studies has prompted strategies for protection against radiation that have been influential in shaping measures for protection against other hazardous physical and chemical agents as well.

▶ PHYSICAL PROPERTIES OF IONIZING RADIATION

Ionizing radiations differ from other forms of radiant energy in being able to disrupt atoms and molecules on which they impinge, giving rise to ions and free radicals in the process. Ionizing radiations include: (*a*) electromagnetic radiations of short wave length and high energy (e.g., x-rays and gamma rays) and (*b*) particulate radiations, which vary in mass and charge (e.g., electrons, protons, neutrons, alpha particles, and other atomic particles).

Ionizing radiation, impinging on a living cell, collides randomly with atoms and molecules in its path, giving rise to ions and free radicals, and depositing enough localized energy to damage genes, chromosomes, or other vital macromolecules. The distribution of such events along the path of the radiation (i.e., the "linear energy transfer" of the radiation) varies with the energy and charge of the radiation, as well as the density of the absorbing medium. Along the path of an alpha particle, for example, the collisions occur so close together that the radiation typically loses all of its energy in traversing only a few cells, whereas along the path of an x-ray the collisions are far enough apart so that the radiation may be able to traverse the entire body (Fig. 28-1).

Because the biological effects of ionizing radiation result from the deposition of energy in exposed cells, doses of ionizing radation are customarily expressed in terms of energy deposition (Table 28-1). On traversing a cell, however, a densely ionizing radiation (e.g., an alpha particle) is more likely than a sparsely ionizing radiation (e.g., an x-ray) to deposit enough energy in a critical site, such as a gene or chromosome, to injure the cell.[3] Hence an additional dose unit (the *equivalent dose*) is used in radiation protection to enable different types of radiation to be normalized in terms of relative biological effectiveness (RBE). The equivalent dose (expressed in sievert (Sv)) is the dose in gray (Gy) multiplied by an appropriate weighting factor to adjust for differences in RBE; i.e., 1 Sv of alpha radiation is that dose (in gray) of alpha radiation that is roughly equivalent in biological effectiveness to 1 Gy of gamma rays (Table 28-1).

The uptake, distribution, and retention of internally deposited radionuclides vary, depending on their physical and chemical properties. Once deposited, the amount of radioactivity remaining in situ decreases with time as a result of both physical decay and biological removal. The physical half-lives of the different radionuclides vary, from less than a second in some to billions of years in others. Biological half-lives also vary, tending to be longer with radionuclides that localize in bone (e.g., radium, strontium, plutonium) than with those that are deposited predominantly in soft tissue (e.g., iodine, cesium, tritium).[4]

▶ SOURCES AND LEVELS OF IONIZING RADIATION IN THE ENVIRONMENT

Life has evolved in the continuous presence of natural background radiation. The major sources of natural background radiation to which the human population is exposed are (*a*) cosmic rays, which originate in outer space; (*b*) terrestrial radiations, which emanate from the thorium, uranium, radium, and other radioactive constituents of the earth's crust; (*c*) internal radiation, which is emitted by the potassium-40, carbon-14, radium, and other radionuclides normally present in living cells, and (*d*) radon and its daughter elements, which are inhaled in indoor air (Table 28-2). The dose from cosmic rays varies appreciably with altitude, being higher by a factor of 2 in the mountains than at sea level and being higher by orders of magnitude at jet aircraft altitudes.[6] Likewise, the dose from internally deposited radium may be higher by a factor of 2 or more in geographic regions where the earth's crust is rich in this element.[6] The dose to the bronchial epithelium from radon also may vary by an order of magnitude or more, depending on the concentration of radon in indoor air, and it typically exceeds by far the dose from all other sources combined.[6] In cigarette smokers, moreover, portions of the bronchial epithelium may receive additionally as much as 0.2 Sv (20 rem) per year from the polonium that is normally present in cigarette smoke.[6]

In addition to natural background radiation, populations in the modern world are exposed to radiation from various artificial sources as well. The largest such source is the use of x-rays in medical diagnosis (Table 28-2). Lesser sources include (*a*) radioactive minerals in building materials, phosphate fertilizers, and crushed rock; (*b*) radiation-emitting components of TV sets, video display terminals, smoke detectors, and other consumer products; (*c*) radioactive fallout from nuclear weapons and nuclear accidents; and (*d*) radionuclides released in the production of nuclear power (Table 28-2).

Additional doses of radiation are received by workers in various occupations, depending on their particular work assignments and working conditions. The average annual effective dose received occupationally by monitored workers in the United States is lower than the dose from natural background radiation, and in any given year less than 1 percent of such workers receive a dose that approaches the maximum permissible yearly limit of 50 mSv (5 rem).[7]

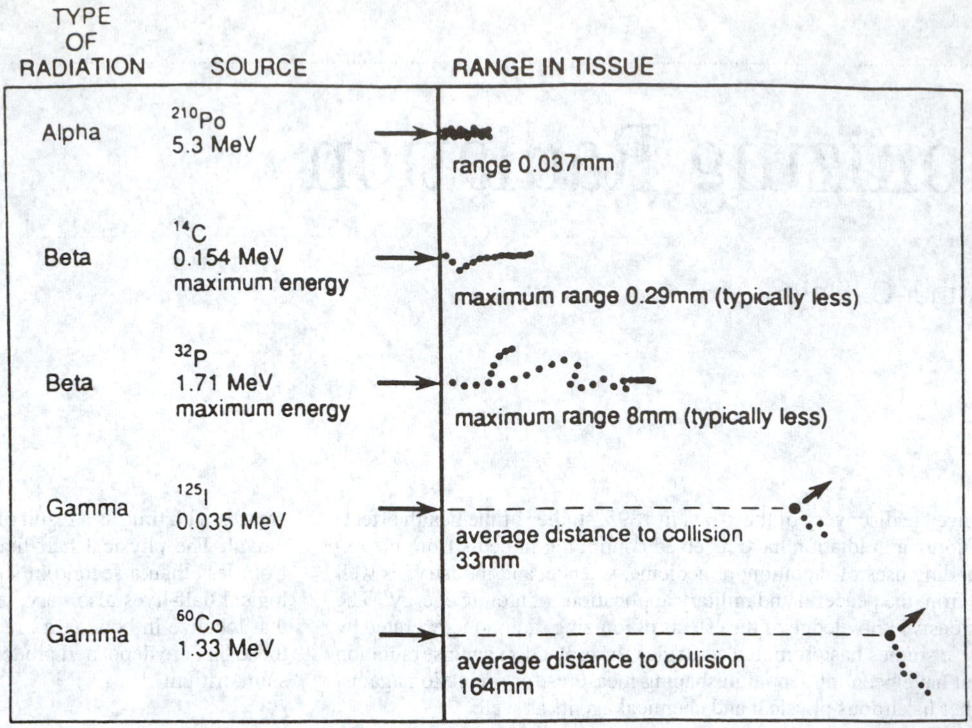

Figure 28-1. Differences among various types of ionizing radiation in penetrating power in tissue. (Reprinted by permission of the publisher from RADIATION PROTECTION: A GUIDE FOR SCIENTISTS AND PHYSICIANS, Third Edition, by Jacob Shapiro, Cambridge, Mass: Harvard University Press, Copyright © 1972, 1981, 1990 by the President and Fellows of Harvard College.)

Radiation accidents have been another source of exposure for workers and members of the public.[8,9,10] In spite of elaborate precautions, some 285 nuclear reactor accidents (excluding the Chernobyl accident) were reported in various countries between 1945 and 1987, resulting in the exposure of more than 1,350 persons and 33 fatalities.[8] In the Chernobyl accident alone, enough radioactivity was released to require the evacuation of tens of thousands of people and farm animals from the surrounding area and to result in a collective committed effective dose to the Northern Hemisphere of 600,000 person-Sv (60,000,000 person-rem).[9,10] The large amounts of radioactive iodine (>600 PBq) that were released in the accident[10] have since been implicated in an increase in the incidence of thyroid cancer in Byelorussia and the Ukraine, as noted below. More numerous than reactor accidents, although less catastrophic, are accidents involving medical and industrial sources.[10] In 1987, for example, a cesium-137 radiotherapy source that was inadvertently dismantled by junk dealers severely contaminated parts of Goiania, Brazil, exposing more than 120 persons, 54 of whom required hospitalization and four of whom were injured fatally as a result.[10]

▶ RADIATION EFFECTS

Types of Effects

In radiation protection, it is customary to distinguish between effects for which there are dose thresholds and effects for which there may be no dose thresholds. The former—so-called *nonstochastic* (or *deterministic*) effects—include various tissue reactions that are elicited only by doses large enough to kill many cells in the affected organs. The latter, by contrast—which include the mutagenic and carcinogenic effects of radiation—are viewed as *stochastic* (or *probabilistic*) phenomena of a type that may be produced by a subtle change within a single cell in an affected organ and which may be expected to increase in frequency as a linear-nonthreshold function of the dose of radiation.[3]

Effects on Genes and Chromosomes

Any molecule in the cell may be damaged by ionizing radiation, but damage to a single gene, unless properly repaired, may permanently alter or kill the cell. A dose large enough to kill the average dividing

TABLE 28-1. QUANTITIES AND DOSE UNITS OF IONIZING RADIATION

Quantity Being Measured	*Definition*	*Dose Unit[a]*
Absorbed dose	Energy deposited in tissue (1 J/kg)	Gray (Gy)
Equivalent dose	Absorbed dose weighted for the relative biological effectiveness of the radiation	Sievert (Sv)
Effective dose	Equivalent dose weighted for the sensitivity of the exposed organ(s)	Sievert (Sv)
Collective effective dose	Effective dose applied to a population	Person-Sv
Committed effective dose	Cumulative effective dose to be received from a given intake of radioactivity	Sievert (Sv)
Radioactivity	One disintegration per second	Becquerel (Bq)

[a] The units of measure listed are those of the International System, introduced in the 1970s to standardize usage throughout the world.[3] They have largely supplanted the earlier units; namely, the rad (1 rad = 100 ergs per gm = 0.01 Gy), the rem (1 rem = 0.01 Sv), and the curie (1 Ci = 3.7 × 10^{10} disintegrations per second = 3.7 × 10^{10} Bq).

TABLE 28-2. AVERAGE AMOUNTS OF IONIZING RADIATION RECEIVED ANNUALLY FROM DIFFERENT SOURCES BY A MEMBER OF THE U.S. POPULATION

	Dose[a]		
Source	***(mSv)***	***(mrem)***	***(%)***
Natural			
Radon[b]	2.0	200	55
Cosmic	0.27	27	8
Terrestrial	0.28	28	8
Internal	0.39	39	11
Total natural	2.94	294	82
Artificial			
X-ray diagnosis	0.39	39	11
Nuclear medicine	0.14	14	4
Consumer products	0.10	10	3
Occupational	<0.01	<1.0	<0.3
Nuclear fuel cycle	<0.01	<1.0	<0.03
Nuclear fallout	<0.01	<1.0	<0.03
Miscellaneous[c]	<0.01	<1.0	<0.03
Total artificial	0.63	63	18
Total natural and artificial	3.57	357	100

Adapted from National Council on Radiation Protection and Measurements: Ionizing Radiation Exposure of the Population of the United States. (NCRP) Report 93. Bethesda, MD: National Council on Radiation Protection and Measurements, 1987 and National Academy of Sciences Advisory Committee on the Biological Effects of Ionizing Radiation: The Effects on Populations of Exposure to Low Levels of Ionizing Radiation (BEIR V). Washington, DC: National Academy of Sciences, 1990.

[a] Average effective dose to soft tissues, excluding bronchial epithelium.

[b] Average effective dose to bronchial epithelium alone.

[c] Department of Energy facilities, smelters, transportation, etc.

cell (1 to 2 Sv) suffices to cause dozens of lesions in its DNA. Most such lesions tend to be reparable, depending on the effectiveness of the cell's repair processes, but residual damage, expressed in the form of mutations, appears to increase as a linear-nonthreshold function of the dose in human somatic cells and the cells of other organisms. The frequency of mutations approximates 10^{-5} to 10^{-6} per locus per Sv, depending on the genetic locus and conditions of irradiation.[3–5,9]

Chromosomal aberrations also increase in frequency with the dose of ionizing radiation, approximating 0.1 aberration per cell per Sv in the low-to-intermediate dose range (Fig. 28-2). The dose-dependent increase in the frequency of such aberrations, which has been reported to be detectable in radiation workers and persons residing in areas of elevated natural background radiation levels, may be of use as a biological dosimeter in radiation accident victims.[12]

Evidence that there may be no threshold in the dose-response relationship for mutations and for chromosomal aberrations has prompted efforts to estimate the risks of harm to future human generations that might result from radiation-induced damage to the germ cells of those living today. Although extensive studies of the children of the A-bomb survivors have been largely negative thus far, the findings are not incompatible statistically with the results of experiments on laboratory animals in which mutagenic effects of radiation have been well documented.[5,9] Hence on the basis of the available data, it is estimated that a dose in excess of 1.0 Sv would be required to double the frequency of heritable mutations in the human species, and that less than 1 percent of all genetically related human diseases is, therefore, attributable to natural background radiation (Table 28-3).

Cytotoxic Effects

As noted early in this century by Bergonie and Tribondeau, cells generally vary in radiosensitivity in proportion to their rate of proliferation and inversely in relation to their degree of differentiation. Cells of only few types (e.g., lymphocytes and oocytes) are radiosensitive in a nonproliferative state. The percentage of clonogenic human cells retaining the ability to proliferate decreases exponentially with increasing dose, acute exposure to 1 to 2 Sv typically sufficing to reduce the surviving population by 50 percent. Successive exposures tend to be less than fully additive in their cytotoxicity if they are sufficiently separated in time, owing to repair of radiation damage during the interim.[5,13]

Through cytotoxic effects on dividing cells, intensive irradiation can give rise to a wide variety of acute and chronic tissue reactions, depending on the tissue or organ irradiated, the dose, and the conditions of exposure.[4] In such reactions—exemplified by erythema of the skin, depression of the blood count, impairment of fertility, and cataract of the lens—interference with normal cell replacement in the exposed area leads to hypoplasia, functional disturbances, and atrophy of the affected part. If enough stem cells remain viable to repopulate the tissue in question, regeneration may ensue within days or weeks; however, a second wave of degenerative changes may occur months or years later, as a result of gradually progressive radiation-induced fibrosis of the exposed connective tissue and vasculature.[4]

► THE ACUTE RADIATION SYNDROME

Intensive irradiation of the hemopoietic system, gastrointestinal tract, lungs, or brain can cause the *acute radiation syndrome*. The syndrome may take one of several forms, depending on the size and anatomical distribution of the dose (Table 28-4). In each of the forms, anorexia, nausea, and vomiting typically occur within minutes or hours after irradiation, to be followed by a symptom-free interval that lasts until the onset of the main phase of the illness.

In the cerebral form of the syndrome, the main phase of the illness is characterized by headache, disorientation, ataxia, loss of conciousness, and convulsions, which develop within minutes or hours after irradiation and terminate fatally in 1 to 2 days (Table 28-4).

In the intestinal form, the main phase of the illness typically begins 2 to 3 days after irradiation, with abdominal pain, fever,

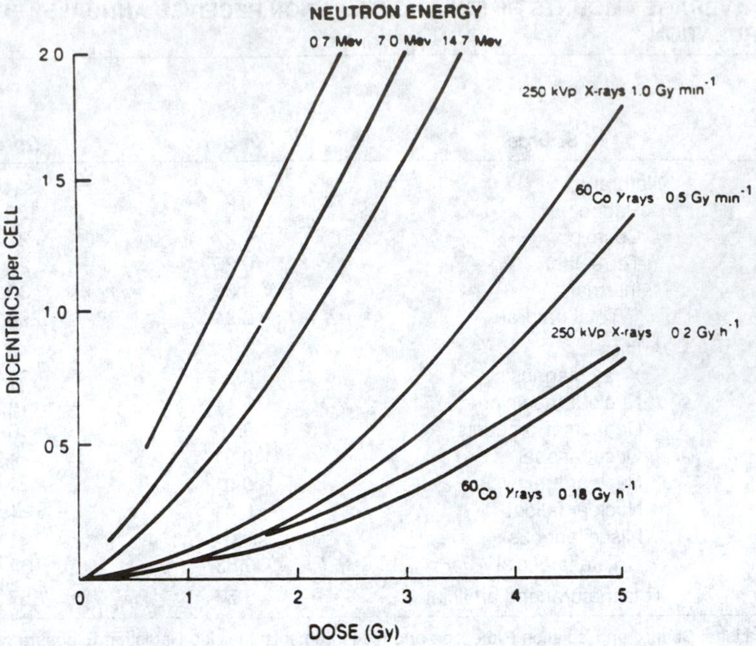

Figure 28-2. Frequency of dicentric chromosome aberrations in human lymphocytes in relation to dose, dose rate, and quality of irradiation in vitro. (From Lloyd DC, Purrott RJ: Chromosome aberration analysis in radiological protection dosimetry. Radiat Protect Dosim 1:19-28, 1981.)

increasingly severe diarrhea, dehydration, prostration, and toxemia, which progress rapidly to a fatal shocklike state within several days (Table 28-4).

In the hemopoietic form, the main phase of the illness is referable primarily to leukopenia and thrombocytopenia, effects that typically do not become severe enough to produce symptoms (e.g., malaise, fever, infection, hemorrhage) until the second or third week after irradiation. If sufficiently severe, injury of the bone marrow is likely to cause death from infection and/or hemorrhage between the fourth and the sixth week after irradiation (Table 28-4).

In the pulmonary form, an acute inflammatory process develops within 30 to 90 days after irradiation in lung tissue exposed to a dose of 6 to 10 Sv (Table 28-4). If the process is sufficiently extensive, it may terminate within weeks in respiratory failure, or it may develop into pulmonary fibrosis and cor pumonale months or years later.[10]

► CARCINOGENIC EFFECTS

Cancers of various types have been observed to increase in frequency with the dose of ionizing radiation in atomic bomb survivors, radiotherapy patients, early radiologists, radium dial painters, uranium miners, and other irradiated human populations.[1,4,5,9] Such growths have not appeared until years or decades after irradiation, and none has exhibited features identifying it as having been produced specifically by radiation, as opposed to some other cause. The causal connection between these cancers and previous irradiation can, therefore, be inferred only from appropriate epidemiological analysis of the dose-incidence relationship.[5]

The most extensive source of dose-reponse data thus far has been the study of atomic bomb survivors, in whom the overall incidence of cancer has increased roughly in proportion with the radia-

TABLE 28-3. ESTIMATED FREQUENCIES OF HERITABLE DISORDERS ATTRIBUTABLE TO NATURAL BACKGROUND IONIZING IRRADIATION

		Contribution from Natural Background Radiation[a] (per million live births)[b]	
Type of Disorder	***Natural Prevalence (per million live births)***	***First Generation***	***Equilibrium Generations[c]***
Autosomal dominant	180,000	20–100	300
X-linked	400	<1	<15
Recessive	2,500	<1	Very slow increase
Chromosomal	4,400	<20	Very slow increase
Congenital defects	20,000–30,000	30	30–300
Other disorders of complex etiology			
Heart disease	600,000	Not estimated[d]	Not estimated[d]
Cancer	300,000	Not estimated[d]	Not estimated[d]
Selected others	300,000	Not estimated[d]	Not estimated[d]

Based on National Academy of Sciences Advisory Committee on the Biological Effects of Ionizing Radiation: The Effects on Populations of Exposure to Low Levels of Ionizing Radiation (BEIR V). Washington, DC: National Academy of Sciences, 1990.

[a] Equivalent to ~1 mSv (100 mrem) per year (Table 28.2) or ~30 mSv (3 rem) per generation (30 years).

[b] Values rounded.

[c] After hundreds of generations, the addition of unfavorable radiation-induced mutations eventually becomes balanced by their loss from the population, resulting in a genetic "equilibrium."

[d] Quantitative risk estimates are lacking because of uncertainty about the mutational component of the disease(s) indicated.

TABLE 28-4. MAJOR FORMS AND FEATURES OF THE ACUTE RADIATION SYNDROME

Time after Irradiation	*Cerebral Form (>50 Sv)*	*Gastrointestinal Form (10–20 Sv)*	*Hemopoietic Form (2–10 Sv)*	*Pulmonary Form (>6 Sv to Lungs)*
First day	Nausea Vomiting Diarrhea Headache Disorientation Ataxia Coma Convulsions Death	Nausea Vomiting Diarrhea	Nausea Vomiting Diarrhea	Nausea Vomiting
Second week		Nausea Vomiting Diarrhea Fever Erythema Prostration Death		
Third to sixth weeks			Weakness Fatigue Anorexia Fever Hemorrhage Epilation Recovery (?) Death (?)	
Second to eighth months				Cough Dyspnea Fever Chest pain Respiratory failure (?)

Modified from United Nations Scientific Committee on the Effects of Atomic Radiation (UNSCEAR): *Souces, Effects, and Risks of Ionizing Radiation, Report to the General Assembly, with Annexes*. New York: United Nations, 1988.

tion dose (Fig. 28-3). The magnitude of the dose-dependent increase varies, however, from one type of cancer to another, and not all types of cancer appear to have been affected (Fig. 28-4). The most extensive data available to date concerning dose-response relationships for individual types of cancer pertain to leukemia, cancer of the female breast, and cancer of the thyroid gland.

Leukemia. All major types of leukemia except chronic lymphocytic leukemia have been observed to increase with dose after exposure of the whole body or a major part of the hemopoietic system. In A-bomb survivors and other irradiated populations, the increase has appeared within 2 to 5 years after exposure; has been dose-dependent, averaging approximately 1 to 3 cases per 10,000 persons per year per Sv to the bone marrow over the first 25 years after irradiation; and has persisted for 15 years or longer, depending on the type of leukemia, age at irradiation, and other variables.[3–5,9,15] A comparable excess has been reported in radiation workers, based on combined analyses of different occupational cohorts.[16] While the data do not suffice to define precisely the shape of the dose-incidence relationship, they are most consistent with a linear-quadratic function.[3–5,13,15]

Leukemia has also been observed to be increased in frequency in children who were x-irradiated prenatally through maternal abdominal radiography, the increase approximating 25 cases per 10,000 per Sv per year during the first 10 years of life.[4,5,9,15] Although no such increase was evident in prenatally exposed A-bomb survivors, the difference is not statistically significant in view of the limited numbers involved.[4,5,9,15]

Preconceptional irradiation of maternal or paternal germ cells also has been tentatively implicated to account for the excesses of childhood leukemia noted in some epidemiological studies; however, the prevailing evidence is interpreted to argue against this hypothesis.[17]

Breast Cancer. The incidence of breast cancer has appeared to increase in proportion to the radiation dose in women surviving A-bomb irradiation, women given radiotherapy to the breast for acute postpartum mastitis, women fluoroscoped repeatedly in the treatment of pulmonary tuberculosis with artificial pneumothorax, and women

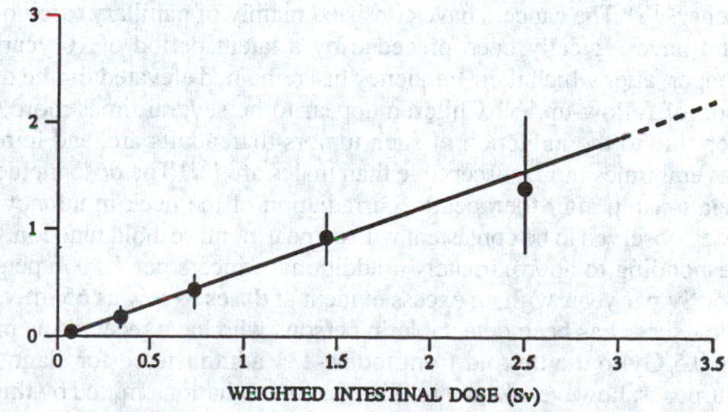

Figure 28-3. Dose-response relationship for total incidence of cancer, all types excluding leukemia, in atomic bomb survivors, 1958–1987. (From Thompson DE, Mabuchi K, Ron E, Soda M, Tokinaga M, Ochkubo S, Sugimoto S, Ikeda T, Terasaki M, Izumi S, Preston DL: Cancer incidence in atomic bomb survivors. Part II: Solid tumors, 1958–1987. Radiat Res 137:S17–S67, 1994.)

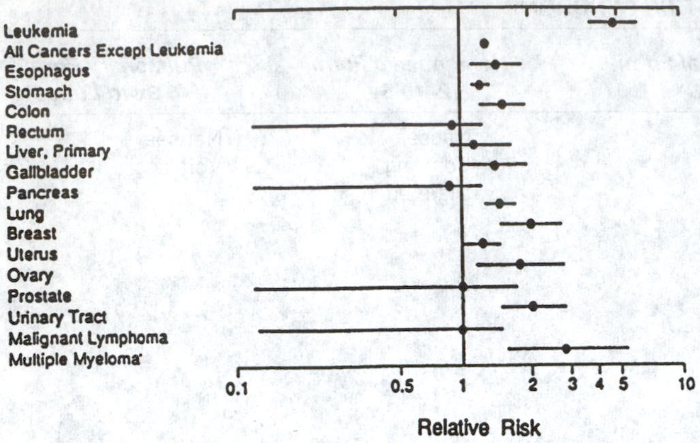

Figure 28-4. Relative risks of different types of cancer in atomic bomb survivors at 1-Gy exposure (shielded kerma), 1950–1985, with 90 percent confident intervals. (Modified from Shimizu Y, Kato H, Schull WJ: Studies of the mortality of A-bomb survivors. Mortality 1950–1985: Part 2. Cancer mortality based on the recently revised doses (DS 86). Radiat Res 121:120–141, 1990.)

employed as radium dial painters.[4,5,9,15] In all four groups, the excess did not become evident until at least 5 to 10 years after irradiation, depending on age at the time of exposure, and it has persisted for the duration of follow-up. The excess, averaged over all ages, has also been of similar magnitude in each group, in spite of marked differences among the groups in the rapidity with which the total doses of radiation were received, implying that successive small doses were additive in their cumulative carcinogenic effects.[4,5,9,15]

Susceptibility decreases markedly with increasing age at the time of irradiation, little excess being detectable in women exposed beyond the age of 40.[4,5,18] Following irradiation in childhood, moreover, the resulting cancers are similar in age distribution to those occurring in the general population, implying that expression of the carcinogenic effects of radiation on the breast depends on the hormonal stimulation associated with sexual maturation.[18] In A-bomb survivors who were the first to develop tumors, the excess was disproportionately large, suggesting that such women may have represented a genetically susceptible subgroup.[19]

Thyroid Gland. Dose-dependent excesses of thyroid cancer have been observed in A-bomb survivors, patients treated with x-rays for various benign conditions in childhood, Marshall Islanders and others exposed during childhood to radioactive fallout from nuclear weapons tests, and children exposed to radionuclides from the Chernobyl accident.[4,5,15,20] The cancers have consisted mainly of papillary carcinomas and have typically been preceded by a latent period of 10 years or longer, after which their frequency has remained elevated for the duration of follow-up.[4,5,15] Children appear to be several times more susceptible to the induction of such tumors than adults are, and females several times more susceptible than males are.[4,5,15] The dose-incidence relationship after therapeutic x-irradiation of the neck in infancy has been observed to be consistent with a linear-nonthreshold function, corresponding to approximately 4 additional cancers per 10,000 persons per Sv per year, with an excess evident at doses as low as 65 mSv.[4,5,15] No excess has been detectable in persons who have received as much as 0.5 Gy to the thyroid from iodine-131 administered for diagnostic purposes, however, which implies that the radiation emitted by this radionuclide is appreciably less carcinogenic to the thyroid than external x- or gamma radiation, possibly because of spatial and temporal differences in the distribution of the radiation within the gland.[4,5,15]

Assessment of the Risks from Low-Level Exposure. Although existing evidence does not suffice to define precisely the dose-incidence relationship for the carcinogenic effects of low-level radiation or to exclude the possibility that a threshold for such effects may exist in the millisievert dose range, the available epidemiologic and experimental data argue against the likelihood of a threshold for all types of cancer.[4,5,15] Attempts to estimate the risks of radiation-induced cancers from low doses have, therefore, generally been based on the assumption that the overall incidence of cancer varies as a linear, nonthreshold function of the dose, in spite of evidence for the existence of reparative processes affording cells some capacity to adapt to low-level radiation.[3,5,15]

Extrapolations based on the linear-nonthreshold dose-response model have yielded risk estimates for cancers of different organs (Table 28-5). These estimates imply that less than 3 percent of all cancers in the general population are attributable to natural background radiation, although a larger percentage—perhaps up to 10 percent—of lung cancers may be attributable to inhalation of indoor radon.[3–5,15]

The extent to which a cancer arizing in a previously irradiated individual can be attributed to the radiation that he or she may have received cannot be determined with certainty; however, it may be assumed to increase with the radiation dose in question, all other things being equal.[22] On the basis of this assumption, one may arrive at a crude estimate of the probability of causation, given sufficient knowledge of the dose, when the dose was received, and the extent to which other causal factors also may have been involved.[22]

▶ EFFECTS OF PRENATAL IRRADIATION

Apart from the relatively high susceptibility of the unborn child to the carcinogenic effects of ionizing radiation, noted above, the embryo is also highly susceptible to the teratogenic effects of radiation. Thus although the latter are generally considered to be nonstochastic in nature, exposure to as little as 0.25 Sv during critical stages of organogenesis has sufficed to cause malformations of many types in laboratory animals,[23,24] and similar developmental disturbances have been reported to follow intensive prenatal irradiation in humans.[4,10,23,24] Noteworthy examples of the latter include the dose-

TABLE 28-5. ESTIMATED LIFETIME RISKS OF CANCER ATTRIBUTABLE TO 0.1 Sv (10 REM) RAPID IRRADIATION

	Excess Cancer Deaths per 100,000	
Type or Site of Cancer	***(No.)***	***(%)[a]***
Stomach	110	17
Lung	85	2
Colon	85	7
Leukemia (excluding chronic lymphocytic leukemia)	50	14
Urinary bladder	30	12
Esophagus	30	8
Breast	20	2
Liver	15	8
Gonads	10	3
Thyroid	8	40
Osteosarcoma	5	12
Skin	2	30
Remainder	50	1
Total	500	3

Modified from International Commission on Radiological Protection: 1990 Recommendations of the International Commission on Radiological Protection. ICRP Publication 60. Ann. ICRP 21, No. 1–3. Oxford: Pergamon Press, 1991 and Puskin JS, Nelson CB: Estimates of radiogenic cancer risks. Health Phys 69:93–101, 1995.

[a] Percentage of the "spontaneous," baseline rate in the general population.

TABLE 28-6. RECOMMENDED LIMITS OF EXPOSURE TO IONIZING RADIATION FOR RADIATION WORKERS AND THE PUBLIC[a]

Type of Exposure	*Maximum Permissible Dose (mSv)*
A. Occupational exposures	
1. For protection against stochastic effects	
a. Annual (effective dose)	50
b. Cumulative (effective dose)	age × 10
2. For protection against nonstochastic effects in individual organs	
a. Lens of the eye (annual effective dose)	150
b. All other organs (annual effective dose)	500
3. Planned special exposure (effective dose)[b]	100
4. Emergency exposure	—[c]
B. Public exposures	
1. Continuous or frequent exposure (effective dose/year)	1
2. Infrequent exposure (effective dose/year)	5
3. Remedial action recommended when:	
a. Effective dose	>5
b. Exposure to radon and its decay products	>0.007 Jhm^{-1}
C. Education and training exposures[d]	
1. Effective dose (annual)	1
2. Equivalent dose (lens of eye, skin, extremities) (annual)	50
D. Exposure of the embryo-fetus	
1. Total equivalent dose	5
2. Equivalent dose in any 1 month	0.5

From National Council on Radiation Protection and Measurements: Limitation of Exposure to Ionizing Radiation. (NCRP) Report No. 116, Bethesda, MD: National Council on Radiation Protection and Measurements, 1993.

[a] Including natural background radiation exclusive of that from internally deposited radionuclides.

[b] Sum of internal and external exposures, excluding medical irradiation.

[c] Effective dose in any one planned event or cumulative effective dose in planned special exposures over a working lifetime should not exceed 100 mSv (10 rem).

[d] Short-term exposure to more than 100 mSv (10 rem) is justified only in lifesaving, emergency situations.

dependent increase in the frequency of severe mental retardation and the dose-dependent decreases in IQ and school performance scores observed in prenatally irradiated A-bomb survivors who were exposed between the 8th and 15th weeks (and to a lesser extent the 16th and 25th weeks) after conception.[4,5,10,24]

Furthermore, unlike mutagenic and carcinogenic effects, which are expressed in only a small percentage of exposed individuals, some disturbance of growth and development may be projected to affect all who are exposed at a vulnerable stage during prenatal life to a dose that exceeds the relevant threshold. Thus, while only a small percentage of the individuals who were exposed prenatally to atomic bomb radiation at a critical stage in brain development (i.e., 8 to 26 weeks after conception) exhibited severe mental retardation, a larger percentage exhibited less marked decrements in intelligence and school performance, implying that there was a dose-dependent downward shift in the distribution of intelligence levels within the entire cohort.[5,10]

▶ RADIATION PROTECTION

With the abandonment of the threshold dose-response hypothesis for the mutagenic and carcinogenic effects of radiation, the goal of minimizing the risks of such effects has become pre-eminent in radiation protection. In pursuit of this goal, the following guidelines have been recommended for any activity involving exposure to ionizing radiation: (*a*) *justification*, i.e., the activity should not be considered justifiable unless it produces a sufficient benefit to those who are exposed, or to society at large, to offset any harm it may cause; (*b*) *optimization*, i.e., the dose and/or likelihood of exposure should be kept as low as is reasonably achievable (ALARA), all relevant economic and social factors considered; and (*c*) *dose limits*, i.e., the likelihood of exposure and the resulting dose to any individual should be subject to control by operating limits.[3]

The dose limits that have been recommended (Table 28-6) are intended to restrict exposures sufficiently to completely prevent nonstochastic effects in any organ of the body, even in the most sensitive members of the population.[3] Although the limits are not expected to protect completely against the mutagenic and carcinogenic effects of radiation, since there may be no thresholds for such effects, the limits are judged to be low enough to prevent the risks of mutagenic and carcinogenic effects from reaching levels that are socially unacceptable.[3]

Implicit in the above guidelines are requirements that any facility dealing with ionizing radiation (*a*) be properly designed; (*b*) carefully plan and oversee its operating procedures, including dose calibration; (*c*) have in place a well-conceived radiation protection program; (*d*) ensure that its workers are adequately trained and supervised, and (*e*) maintain a well-developed and well-rehearsed emergency preparedness plan, to be able to respond promptly and effectively in the event of a malfunction, spill, or other type of radiation accident.[2]

Since the doses received from medical radiographic examinations and from indoor radon constitute the most important controllable sources of exposure to ionizing radiation for members of the general public, measures to limit these exposures are also called for.[3] Other potential sources of exposure against which protection is warranted are those posed by the millions of cubic feet of radioactive and mixed wastes (mine and mill tailings, spent nuclear fuel, waste from the decommissioning of nuclear power plants, dismantled industrial and medical radiation sources, radioactive pharmaceuticals and reagents, heavy metals, polyaromatic hydrocarbons, and other contaminants), which tax increasingly severely the existing storage capacities at numerous waste sites.[26,27]

▶ SUMMARY

The health effects of ionizing radiation are widely diverse, ranging from rapidly fatal injuries to cancers, birth defects, and hereditary disorders appearing months, years, or decades later. The nature, frequency, and severity of the effects depend on the quality of the radiation in question, as well as on the dose and conditions of exposure. For most effects, radiosensitivity varies with the rate of proliferation and inversely with the degree of differentiation of the exposed cells; as a result, the embryo and growing child are especially vulnerable to radiation injury. Although many types of effects require relatively high levels of exposure, the genotoxic and carcinogenic effects of ionizing radiation appear to increase in frequency as linear-nonthreshold functions of the dose. Therefore, to minimize the risks of the latter, exposures to ionizing radiation need to be limited accordingly.

▶ REFERENCES

1. Upton AC: Historical perspective on radiation carcinogenesis. In Upton AC, Albert RE, Burns FJ, Shore RE (eds): Radiation Carcinogenesis. New York: Elsevier Science Publishing; 1986, pp 1–10
2. Shapiro J: Radiation Protection: A Guide for Scientists and Physicians, 3rd ed. Cambridge, MA: Harvard University Press, 1972
3. International Commission on Radiological Protection: 1990 Recommendations of the International Commission on Radiological Protection. ICRP Publication 60. Ann. ICRP 21, No. 1–3. Oxford; Pergamon Press, 1991
4. Mettler FA Jr, Upton AC: Medical Effects of Ionizing Radiation. New York: WB Saunders, 1995
5. National Academy of Sciences Advisory Committee on the Biological Effects of Ionizing Radiation: The Effects on Populations of Exposure to Low Levels of Ionizing Radiation (BEIR V). Washington, DC: National Academy of Sciences, 1990
6. National Council on Radiation Protection and Measurements: Ionizing Radiation Exposure of the Population of the United States. (NCRP) Report 93: Bethesda, MD: National Council on Radiation Protection and Measurements, 1987
7. National Council on Radiation Protection and Measurements: Exposure of the U.S. Population from Occupational Radiation. (NCRP) Report 101. Bethesda, MD: National Council on Radiation Protection and Measurements, 1989
8. Lushbaugh CC, Fry SA, Ricks RC: Nuclear radiation accidents: preparedness and consequences. Br J Radiol 60:1159–1183, 1987
9. United Nations Scientific Committee on the Effects of Atomic Radiation (UNSCEAR): Sources, Effects, and Risks of Ionizing Radiation. Report to the General Assembly, with Annexes. New York: United Nations, 1988
10. United Nations Scientific Committee on the Effects of Atomic Radiation (UNSCEAR): Sources and Effects of Ionizing Radiation. UNSCEAR 1993 Report to the General Assembly, with Annexes. New York: United Nations, 1993
11. Lloyd DC, Purrott RJ: Chromosome aberration analysis in radiological protection dosimetry. Radiat Protect Dosim 1:19–28, 1981
12. International Atomic Energy Agency (IAEA): Biological Dosimetry: Chromosomal Aberration Analysis for Dose Assessment. Technical Report No. 260. Vienna: International Atomic Energy Agency, 1986
13. Thompson DE, Mabuchi K, Ron E, Soda M, Tokinaga M, Ochkubo S, Sugimoto S, Ikeda T, Terasaki M, Izumi S, Preston DL: Cancer incidence in atomic bomb survivors. Part II: Solid tumors, 1958–1987. Radiat Res 137:S17–S67, 1994
14. Shimizu Y, Kato H, Schull WJ: Studies of the mortality of A-bomb survivors. Mortality 1950–1985: Part 2. Cancer mortality based on the recently revised doses (DS 86). Radiat Res 121:120–141, 1990
15. United Nations Scientific Committee on the Effects of Atomic Radiation (UNSCEAR): Sources and Effects of Ionizing Radiation. UNSCEAR 1994 Report to the General Assembly, with Annexes. New York: United Nations, 1994
16. Cardis E, Gilbert ES, Carpenter L, Howe G, Kato I, Armstrong BK, Beral V, Cowper G, Douglas A, Fix J, Fry SA, Kaldor J, Lave C, Salmon L, Smith PG, Voelz GL, Wiggs LD: Effects of low doses and low dose rates of external ionizing radiation: cancer mortality among nuclear industry workers in three countries. Radiat Res 142:117–132, 1995
17. Wakeford, R: The risk of childhood cancer from intrauterine and preconceptional exposure to ionizing radiation. Environ Health Perspect 103:1018–1025, 1995
18. Mettler FA, Upton AC, Kelsey CA, Ashby RN, Rosenberg RD, Linver MIN: Benefits versus risks from mammography. A critical reassessment. Cancer 77:903–909, 1996
19. Tokunaga M, Land C, Tukapa S, Nishimori I, Soda M, Akiba S: Incidence of female breast cancer in atomic bomb survivors, 1950–1985. Radiat Res 138:209–223, 1994
20. Kreisel W: International program on the health effects of the Chernobyl accident. Stem Cells 13(Suppl 1):33–39, 1995
21. Puskin JS, Nelson CB: Estimates of radiogenic cancer risks. Health Phys 69:93–101, 1995
22. Rall JE, Beebe GW, Hoel DG, Jablon S, Land CE, Nygaard OF, Upton AC, Yalow RS, and Zeve VH: Report of the National Institutes of Health Ad Hoc Working Group to Develop Radioepidemiological Tables. NIH Publication No. 85-2748. Washington, DC: Government Printing Office, 1985
23. United Nations Scientific Committee on the Effects of Atomic Radiation (UNSCEAR): Ionizing Radiation: Sources and Biological Effects. 1982 Report to the General Assembly, with Annexes. New York: United Nations, 1982
24. United Nations Scientific Committee on the Effects of Atomic Radiation (UNSCEAR): Genetic and Somatic Effects of Ionizing Radiation, Report to the General Assembly, with Annexes. New York: United Nations, 1986
25. National Council on Radiation Protection and Measurements: Limitation of Exposure to Ionizing Radiation. (NCRP) Report No. 116, Bethesda, MD: National Council on Radiation Protection and Measurements, 1993
26. National Academy of Sciences/National Research Council: The Nuclear Weapons Complex. Washington, DC: National Academy Press, 1989
27. U.S. Department of Energy (USDOE): U.S. Department of Energy Interim Mixed Waste Inventory Report: Waste Streams, Treatment Capacities, and Technologies. DOE/NBM-1100, Washington, DC: Government Printing Office, 1993

29

Nonionizing Radiation

Arthur L. Frank • Louis Slesin

The term *nonionizing radiation* refers to several forms of electromagnetic radiation of wavelengths longer than those of ionizing radiation. As wavelength lengthens, the energy value of electromagnetic radiation decreases, and all nonionizing forms of radiation have less energy than cosmic, gamma, and x-radiation. In order of increasing wavelength, nonionizing radiation includes ultraviolet (UV) radiation, visible light, infrared radiation, microwave radiation, and radiofrequency radiation. The latter two are often treated as a single category. The energy, frequency, and wavelength range for electromagnetic forces are shown in Table 29-1. All forms of electromagnetic radiation have the same velocity of 3×10^{10} cm/s in a vacuum.

Radiation is emitted continuously from the sun over a wide range from 290 nm in the ultraviolet range to more than 2,000 nm in the infrared range with a maximum intensity at about 480 nm in the visible range. The radiation from the sun is modified as it passes through the earth's atmosphere. Ozone, which is found in the upper atmosphere, absorbs the highest energy ultraviolet radiation. Infrared radiation is absorbed by water vapor, and other wavelengths are altered by passage through smoke, dust, and gas molecules.

All objects above absolute zero temperature emit radiation, much of it as infrared radiation. At low temperatures, only long wavelength radiation is emitted, but as the temperature of the object increases, shorter wavelength radiation is emitted. Heated metal gives off a red glow; if heating continues, the metal becomes "white hot" as energy throughout the whole visible spectrum is given off. Heated gases may give off wavelengths in the ultraviolet, visible, or infrared regions. Ultraviolet radiation is given off with the use of extremely high-temperature welding equipment such as carbon or electric arcs.

The biological effect of radiation exposure depends on the type and duration of exposure and on the amount of absorption by the organism. The carcinogenic and other effects of ionizing radiation are discussed in Chapter 28.

▸ ULTRAVIOLET RADIATION

The sun is the major source of ultraviolet radiation. There are some artificial sources such as electric arc lights, welding arcs, plasma jets, and special ultraviolet bulbs. The amount of ultraviolet radiation reaching the earth from the sun varies with season, time of day, latitude, altitude, and specific atmospheric conditions. Intensity is greatest at midday and is greater in summer than in winter. In a summer month, about as much ultraviolet radiation reaches the earth's surface as in the entire period from autumn to spring equinoxes. Total ultraviolet exposure is greater on a cloudy day due to reflection, and snow reflects about 75 percent of ultraviolet radiation. Therefore, sunburn may be more severe on a cloudy than a clear day and may be especially severe in those spending a great deal of time on snow. Window glass and light clothing filter out ultraviolet radiation efficiently.

There is a wide range of potential occupational exposures[1,2] to ultraviolet radiation in both outdoor work and industrial settings (Table 29-2).

Biological Effects

Since ultraviolet radiation has little ability to penetrate, the organs primarily affected are the skin and eyes. Ultraviolet radiation is strongly absorbed by nucleic acids and proteins, and the effects in humans are largely chemical rather than thermal. Mutations resulting from ultraviolet exposure occur in organisms such as plants and flies but not in humans, because of the low penetration.

Short-term effects on humans include acute changes in the skin. These are of four types: (*a*) darkening of pigment, (*b*) erythema (sunburn), (*c*) increase in pigmentation (tanning), and (*d*) changes in cell growth. Ultraviolet radiation does not penetrate through the subcutaneous tissue. The corneum, or outermost layer of skin, which is about 0.03 mm thick, absorbs the shortest wavelength ultraviolet radiation. The longer the wavelength, the deeper the radiation penetrates; the longest ultraviolet radiation passes through the corneum and corium into the malpighian layer. The darkening of preformed pigment occurs immediately and is particularly noted at wavelengths between 300 and 400 nm. The erythema (sunburn) does not begin for at least one-half hour, and there are several peaks within the ultraviolet spectrum with variable times of maximum effect, ranging from 12 hours for radiation at 254 nm to 48 hours for radiation at 297 nm. Darker skin has a protective effect, and estimates for the darkest skin shades suggest a 2- to 10-fold threshold value for erythema production. Subsequent exposure reduces the threshold value for erythema production. The increase in pigmentation (tanning) results from a migration of melanin pigment into more superficial skin cells and also from an increased production of melanin pigment. Ultraviolet radiation works as a catalyst to oxidize tyrosine to dihydroxyphenol 1-alanine, which is a precursor of melanin. Changes in skin cell growth follow exposure to ultraviolet radiation. First, there occurs a cessation of cell growth followed after 24 hours by an increase in cell division. At this time there is an intracellular and intercellular edema that thickens the skin. Eventually there is shedding of cells by scaling. Severe reactions can be seen with blistering, desquamation, or even ulceration of the skin.

Ultraviolet radiation also causes acute effects on tissues of the eye. Exposure can lead to keratitis, inflammation of the cornea, and conjunctivitis. The keratitis may develop after a latent period of several hours and returns to normal in a few days. Since the cornea possesses a large number of nerve endings, even a small amount of inflammation can be painful. The effect in the eye is independent of skin color, and there appears to be no development of protection of the eye with repeated exposures.

Long-term effects of ultraviolet exposure include an increase in the rate of aging of skin with degeneration of skin tissue and a de-

TABLE 29-1. ENERGY, FREQUENCY, AND WAVELENGTH RANGE FOR ELECTROMAGNETIC FORCES

Type of Radiation	Energy Range	Frequency Range	Wavelength Range
Ionizing (includes cosmic, gamma, and x-ray)	>12.4 eV	>3000 THz	<100 nm
Ultraviolet	6.2–3.1 eV	1500–750 THz	200–400 nm
Visible	.3.1–1.8 eV	750–429 THz	400–700 nm
Violet			400–424
Blue			424–491
Green			491–575
Yellow			575–585
Orange			585–647
Red			647–700
Infrared	1.8 eV–1.2 meV	429 THz–300 GHz	700 nm–1 mm
Microwave	1.2 meV–1.2 μeV	300 GHz–300 MHz	1 mm–1 m
Radiofrequency	1.2 μeV–1.2 neV	300 MHz–300 kHz	1 m–1 km

Adapted from NIOSH Technical Report—Ionizing Radiation. Washington, DC: NIOSH Publication No. 78-142, 1978.

crease in elasticity. Late effects of ultraviolet radiation on the eye include the development of cataracts. The most serious chronic effect of ultraviolet exposure is skin cancer.

More than 90 percent of skin cancers occur on parts of the body exposed to sunlight. Approximately 40 percent of all cancers in the United States are skin cancers, and in general they are the most common malignancy in light-skinned populations. Rates for skin cancer vary from less than 2 cases per 100,000 in dark-skinned populations to more than 100 per 100,000 in South African whites and Australians.[3] The incidence of skin cancer on a worldwide basis correlates with decreasing latitude. Skin cancer occurs in great excess in those with outdoor occupations such as agricultural, forestry, and marine workers. Most skin cancers in humans are of epithelial cell origin; most commonly noted are basal cell carcinomas followed in frequency by squamous cell carcinomas followed in frequency by squamous cell melanomas.

Some individuals, for example, those with xeroderma pigmentosum, have particular sensitivity to ultraviolet radiation and are at increased risk for developing disease on exposure. Photosensitivity reactions occur after exposure to a variety of chemicals and drugs, including dyes, phenothiazine, sulfonamide, and sulfonylurea.

Ultraviolet radiation has an important role in the prevention of rickets. Vitamin D is produced by the action of ultraviolet radiation on 7-dehydrocholesterol or related steroidal compounds.

Protection

Protective measures include administrative controls, equipment design, and personal protection. Administrative actions include education and instruction of individuals who will be exposed, posting of notices, limiting access in the workplace, and regulation of exposure time. Equipment design includes placement of ultraviolet glass shields. Personal protection includes the use of shields, goggles, and appropriate clothing. Polyvinyl chloride can be used for gloves, and the use of barrier creams is also possible. Exposure during recreation, such as winter sports and sunbathing, including the use of tanning beds, should be done in moderation, especially by fair-skinned persons.

TABLE 29-2. OCCUPATIONAL EXPOSURE TO ULTRAVIOLET RADIATION

Aircraft workers	Glassblowers
Barbers	Metal casting inspectors
Bath attendants	Oil field workers
Construction workers	Railroad tract workers
Drug makers	Ranchers
Electricians	Seaman
Farmers	Steel mill workers
Fishermen	Tobacco irradiators
Food irradiators	Vitamin D makers
Foundry workers	Welders

Recommended Values for Protection against Ultraviolet Radiation. Based on regulations adopted from the American Conference of Governmental and Industrial Hygienists in 1976, the federal limits in the United States are as follows:

1. For the near ultraviolet spectral region (320 to 400 nm), total irradiance incident upon the unprotected skin or eye should not exceed 1 mW/cm^2 for periods greater than 10^3 seconds (approximately 16 minutes) and for exposure times less than 10^3 seconds should not exceed 1 J/cm^2.
2. For the actinic ultraviolet spectral region (200 to 315 nm), radiant exposure incident upon the unprotected skin or eye should not exceed the values given in Table 29-3 within an 8-hour period.

TABLE 29-3. THRESHOLD LIMIT VALUES (TLV) FOR ULTRAVIOLET RADIATION

Wavelength [nm]	TLV [mJ/cm^2]	Relative Spectral Effectiveness [S_γ]
200	100.0	0.03
210	40.0	0.075
220	25.0	0.12
230	16.0	0.19
240	10.0	0.30
250	7.0	0.43
254	6.0	0.5
260	4.6	0.65
270	3.0	1.0
280	3.4	0.88
290	4.7	0.64
300	10.0	0.30
305	50.0	0.06
310	200.0	0.015
315	1000.0	0.003

3. To determine the effective irradiance of a broadband source weighted against the peak of the spectral effectiveness curve (270 nm), the following weighting formula should be used:

$$E_{eff} = \Sigma E_{\lambda} S_{\lambda} \Delta_{\lambda}$$

where

E_{eff} = effective irradiance relative a E_{λ}
E_{λ} = monochromatic source at 270 nm spectral irradiance in W/cm²/nm
S_{λ} = relative spectral effectiveness (unitless)
Δ_{λ} = band width in nanometers

4. Permissible exposure time in seconds for exposure to actinic ultraviolet radiation incident upon the unprotected skin or eye may be computed by dividing 0.003 J/cm by E_{eh} in W/cm². The exposure time may also be determined using Table 29-4, which provides exposure times corresponding to effective irradiances in μW/cm².

▶ VISIBLE LIGHT

Visible light[4,5] is radiation with a wavelength between 400 and 700 nm. The sun is the major source of visible light, but it can also be produced by heating tungsten or other filaments and by electrical discharge in a gas such as mercury or neon. Any ultraviolet radiation given off is largely absorbed by the glass enclosing the bulb.

The abnormal biological effects of visible radiation are generally not serious. A flash of light will bleach visual pigments, causing "spots" in the visual field. Intense visible light, such as one may experience by staring directly into the sun for extended periods, may cause coagulation of the retina, and the scotoma that results may be permanent. Snow blindness results from overexposure to sunlight and is characterized by conjunctivitis and keratitis accompanied by photophobia. Use of appropriate lenses will protect against the above effects.

Of potentially greater seriousness are injuries caused by lasers. Laser stands for *l*ight *a*mplification of *s*timulated *e*mission of *r*adiation. Lasers are used in industry, communications, surveying, construction, medicine, and electronics. There are many types of laser apparatus, but all are characterized by their ability to produce an intense, monochromatic, coherent beam in which all waves are parallel and all are in phase. There are three types of lasers: (*a*) continuous, (*b*) pulsed, and (*c*) Q-switched, which are pulsed, but the beam is turned on and off at a rapid rate to produce a beam with higher peak power of shorter duration than the pulsed variety.

TABLE 29-4. THRESHOLD LIMIT VALUES FOR ULTRAVIOLET RADIATION

Duration of Exposure per Day	*Effective Irradiance, E_{eff} [μW/cm²]*
8 h	0.1
4 h	0.2
2 h	0.4
1 h	0.8
30 min	1.7
15 min	3.3
10 min	5.0
5 min	10.0
1 min	50.0
30 s	100.0
10 s	300.0
1 s	3,000.0
0.5 s	6,000.0
0.1 s	30,000.0

Because the laser is a light beam, it follows all the laws of optics and can be manipulated like other light beams. When focused on a spot, a laser can produce enormous heat for drilling and related purposes.

Burns may occur with exposure to lasers, either to the skin or to the eye, if the laser beam hits the retina. This can cause blindness. Lasers also emit ultraviolet radiation, which can cause corneal damage, and infrared radiation, which can cause opacification of the lens.

Threshold values have been proposed for a wide variety of laser equipment.

▶ ILLUMINATION

Units for Expressing Amount of Light

The amount of visible radiation (light) emitted by a luminous object, such as an electric light bulb, is measured in terms of candle power, based on a standard international candle. The amount of illumination that falls on a surface from a light source is expressed in terms of foot-candles. One foot-candle of illumination is the intensity of illumination at any point on a surface 1 foot away from a light source of 1 candle power. The illumination falling on a surface varies inversely as the square of the distance from the light source. The total amount of light that falls on 1 square foot of surface, all points of which are 1 foot from a light source of 1 standard candle, is called 1 lumen, lumen being the term used to measure light flux. The brightness of the light source or of an object reflecting light is usually expressed in terms of foot-lamberts or candles per square inch. One foot-lambert is equivalent to 1 lumen emitted per square foot of the light source. One candle per square inch is the candle power emitted per square inch of light source and is equivalent to 452 foot-lamberts.

General Principles of Illumination

Intensity of Illumination. Sufficient illumination is essential for visual acuity, maximum speed of seeing, prevention of eye fatigue and eye strain, and thus for efficient work and prevention of accidents. Definite proof that poor illumination leads to permanent eye injury is lacking, but the character of the illumination may affect psychological reactions. Most authorities agree that high levels of illumination, except under such unusual circumstances as direct viewing of the sun, do not produce harmful effects on the eye. The human eye is adapted for vision outdoors where foot-candle levels may range from 1,000 in the shade to 10,000 in the sun.

Standards of illumination usually are set in terms of the amount of illumination that falls on the work area. Since vision depends on the light reaching the eye, however, the important consideration is not the amount of illumination on the desk or workbench but the amount of light reflected to the eye. For example, if there are 50 foot-candles of illumination falling on a white object, which reflects about 80 percent of the visible light, then 40 foot-candles of illumination are reflected toward the eye. If the same amount of light falls on a dark object, which reflects 20 percent of the light, only 10 foot-candles of illumination are reflected to the eye. Hence it is necessary to specify different standards of illumination for different circumstances, depending on the amount of light reflected from each work area.

Authorities differ on the amount of illumination essential for vision. Visual acuity and speed of vision increase markedly with an increase in illumination up to about 10 foot-candles, and then increase more slowly up to about 20 foot-candles. Hence 15 to 20 foot-candles can be accepted as a bare minimum level of illumination for vision under the most optimum conditions. When the reflection factor is reduced, as in work on dark colors or when the contrast in color between the object and its background is reduced, higher levels of illumination are necessary for good visual acuity and speed of vision. Higher levels are required also for continuous and fine eye work. Persons with poor vision or eye defects require more illumination than those with normal eyesight. Generally it is recommended that when the contrast in color and brightness between the object and the immediate background is good and when the object being viewed is the size of normal print, the lighting for continuous eye work should supply a minimum of 30 foot-candles on the object. Where poor contrast exists or the size of the object is small, the minimum illumination requirement should be set at 50 foot-candles. Higher levels are necessary under certain conditions. In 1965, the American National Standards Institute (ANSI) in cooperation with the Illuminating Engineering Society published an American Standard Practice for Industrial Lighting, including a list of the current recommended practice foot-candles in service applicable to many types of industrial operations. More recently, the Illuminating Engineers and some other authorities have recommended much higher levels of illumination, but the 1965 standards were reconfirmed in 1970 by the American National Standards Institute and adopted by the United States Department of Labor as the standards to be used under the 1971 Occupational Safety and Health Act.

Brightness and Glare. The amount of light reaching the eye from a light source or by reflection from an object is commonly designated as the brightness of the source or object and is usually expressed in foot-lamberts. Although the eye can adapt to very high levels of brightness, such as daylight outdoors, it cannot tolerate great contrasts in brightness between the central field of vision and the surrounding area. Such contrasts interfere with vision and may produce an uncomfortable sensation. In viewing an object against its surroundings, the visual acuity is greatest when the surrounding area has the same brightness as the central field of vision. The brightness of this central field should never be less than that of the surroundings.

Brightness contrasts are produced also when bright light sources are in the field of view. If the eye is adapted to a high level of illumination and the contrast is not great, a bright light in the field of vision does not produce discomfort. The degree of the glare sensation depends on the distance of the eye from the light source, the brightness of the light source in relation to that of its surroundings, and the position of the light source in the field of vision in relation to that of the object on which the eye is focused. Excessive reflection from shiny surfaces, so-called reflected glare, produces an uncomfortable sensation and may completely obliterate the outline of an object. The effect of glare on vision increases sharply in older age groups; bare light bulbs should never be permitted in the field of vision.

Differences in Illumination. Great differences in illumination between one work space and another or between a work area and a hallway are dangerous if people are required to move from one space to the other. When passing from a brightly lighted area to one with a low level of illumination, the visual acuity is markedly decreased until dark adaptation has occurred. Although some adaptation occurs fairly rapidly, it requires at least one-half hour for adequate readjustment of vision to dim light. The greater the light adaptation, the slower the dark adaptation that follows. During the readjustment period, the ability of the eye to see clearly is so reduced that the danger of accidents is increased. Adaptation requires only a few minutes when passing from a dimly lighted space to one at a high level of illumination.

Color of Light and Surroundings and Surface Finish

A contrast in color between the object and its immediate background is important; the more definite the color contrast, the greater the visual acuity and speed of vision. The value of color contrast is due partly to the dissimilarity in color and partly to differences in the amount of light reflected by the different colors. Recognition of an object becomes most difficult when a black object is viewed against a black background. Here, differences in texture and shadows are necessary for vision. Higher levels of illumination are required where the color contrast is reduced. The color and finish of the walls, ceiling, furniture, and machinery are of great importance in illumination because the amount of light reflected is determined chiefly by the color.

Recommendations: Artificial and Natural Lighting

Artificial Illumination. It is evident from the above discussion that a basic amount of general illumination must be supplied to all areas of a room to prevent great contrasts in brightness. Local or supplemental lighting, in addition to general lighting, is necessary when very high levels of illumination are required, when illumination is needed in specific areas not accessible to general lighting, where the light must come from a particular angle, where hand readjustments are needed, where shadows are required for the prevention of reflected glare, and in various other circumstances. Supplementary lighting sources should be arranged so that other persons in the vicinity are not exposed to excessively bright spots of light.

Lighting fixtures fall into four types:

1. Totally indirect units give diffuse illumination with no shadows or glare, but they are uneconomical and accumulate dirt. Good reflection from the ceiling is necessary, but excessive brightness of the ceiling must be avoided.
2. Direct units are economical but cause shadows, produce glare, and give spot rather than diffuse illumination. They are used chiefly with high ceilings or for local lighting.
3. Semi-indirect units are satisfactory when equipped with diffusers, when ceiling reflection is adequate, and when they are properly placed to avoid too much brightness in the field of view.
4. Large units having a lower candle power per square inch, for example, long tabular fluorescent lights give less concentrated lighting than round tungsten-filament bulbs, which have a higher brightness per unit area (Table 29–5). Large units with moderate brightness also may cause discomfort if placed directly in the field of view.

Natural Illumination. Daylight, if properly arranged, may be a very effective source of good illumination in a room. Much more difficulty is encountered in designing for daylighting than for artificial lighting, however. The amount of daylight reaching a room varies with the location and orientation of the building, with the presence of surrounding buildings, and with the time of day, season, weather, and degree of atmospheric pollution. Furthermore, while artificial lighting can be evenly spaced throughout a room and directed as desired, daylight is available only from certain areas, and its distribution is more difficult to control. Because of these variable factors, only a few general recommendations for providing daylight illumination can be given.

Windows facing south give maximum heat in cold climates but considerable glare; those facing north are advised for buildings in warm climates. The glass area should be at least 20 percent of the floor area of the room. The tops of the windows should be as near the ceiling as possible, since the higher the windows, the more effectively the light reaches the opposite side of the room. An increase in the height of a window produces a much greater increase in illumination than a proportional increase in the width. Windows on two sides of the room are desirable, but where windows are only on one side of a room, the glass area should extend the full length of the room if possible. It is recommended that windows should not be in the field of view for normal working conditions. The size and position of monitors and skylights also must be related to the size of the building. Since direct sunlight often produces excessive brightness, it is necessary to provide some means of sunlight control, such as venetian blinds, shades, louvers, outside projectors, and glass block.

A complete discussion of recommended practices for daylighting in schools, factories, offices, and homes has been published by the Committee on Daylighting of the Illuminating Engineering Society.

TABLE 29-5. BRIGHTNESS OF NATURAL AND ARTIFICIAL LIGHT SOURCES

Light Source	Brightness	
	Foot-lamberts	Candles per Square Inch
Sun as observed at earth's surface	450,000,000	1,000,000.0
Full moon, clear sky	1,500	3.3
1000 W type H-6 mercury lamp	104,000,000	230,000.0
400 W type H-1 mercury lamp	443,000	980.0
Brightest spot on bulb of:		
500 W tungsten-filament lamp	131,000	290.0
100 W tungsten-filament lamp	58,800	130.0
40 W tungsten-filament lamp	24,800	55.0
30 W fluorescent, 1-inch tube [white]	2,400	5.3
40 W white fluorescent, 1½ in tube	1,750	3.9
100 W white fluorescent, 2⅛ in tube	2,180	4.8

From Taylor: Illum Engin 37, 19, 1947, with permission.

▶ INFRARED RADIATION

Infrared radiation, of longer wavelength than visible light, ranges in wavelength from 700 nm to 1 mm. All objects above absolute zero radiate some infrared radiation. Objects of higher temperature radiate to objects of lower temperature; the sensation of a hot stove results from this. Infrared radiation is the most important part of the spectrum for the production of heat.

Infrared radiation causes dilation of the capillary bed of the skin and if strong enough can cause a burn. Infrared radiation can cause damage to the eye and is a cause of cataract development among glassblowers and others. Occupations exposed to infrared radiation are listed in Table 29-6.

▶ EXTREMELY LOW FREQUENCY ELECTROMAGNETIC FIELDS

Electromagnetic fields (EMFs) in the extremely low frequency (ELF) range encompass the 0- to 300-Hz frequency band of the electromagnetic spectrum. Transmission and distribution power lines, which operate at 60 Hz in the United States and at 50 Hz in Europe, are the most common sources of ELF EMF exposures. The strength of the magnetic field is a function of the *current* flowing in the power line, not the *voltage*. The electric field is a function of the voltage on the line. The only reliable way to gauge magnetic fields is with a gaussmeter, a device that is marketed by a number of companies; the cost varies widely, but some units are available for several hundred dollars. The price for 3-axis meters has dropped dramatically in recent years.

Although the primary source of the public's chronic exposure to EMFs comes from power lines, surveys show that more than 75 percent of American homes have ELF fields of less than 1 mG.[6] All electric appliances also emit EMFs—the greater the current draw, the higher the fields. Appliances give off more intense fields than power lines, particularly up close. But fields from appliances diminish quickly with distance.

TABLE 29-6. OCCUPATIONAL EXPOSURE TO INFRARED RADIATION

Bakers	Foundry workers
Blacksmiths	Glass workers
Chemists	Solderers
Cooks	Steel mill workers
Electricians	Welders

Possible health effects of EMFs—principally the promotion of cancer—remain a controversial subject with no resolution in sight. As one observer commented:

> We are here faced with a situation familiar to the clinician looking at two X-ray views, one showing a suspicious lesion and another not. Is the difference due to artifact, masking of the lesion or quality of the film?[7]

The lack of consensus is illustrated by the startlingly opposite conclusions reached by expert panels. A draft Environmental Protection Agency (EPA) report released in 1990 stated that epidemiological studies of ELF exposures and leukemia, lymphoma, and cancers of the nervous system among children and workers "show a consistent pattern of response which suggests a causal link."[8] In contrast, a review commissioned by the White House Office of Science and Technology Policy found that there is "no conclusive evidence in the published literature" to support the possibility that exposures to ELF EMFs are "demonstrable health hazards."[9]

Five years later, agreement remained elusive. In the summer of 1995, a draft report of a committee of the National Council on Radiation Protection and Measurements urged strong action to limit public exposures to EMFs. The draft report generally endorsed a 2-mG exposure limit for new day care centers, schools, and playgrounds.[10] The following year, a panel convened by the National Research Council (NRC) of the National Academy of Sciences found that there was "no conclusive and consistent evidence" that residential exposures to EMFs present a human health hazard.[11]

Epidemiological Studies

The bulk of the evidence implicating EMFs in the development of cancer comes from epidemiological studies. In 1979, Wertheimer and Leeper first identified a link between childhood cancer and living near high-current power lines.[12] This study was repeated under the auspices of the New York Power Line Project by a team headed by Savitz, who essentially replicated the original findings.[13] The scientists who ran the New York project concluded that if the association between EMFs and cancer was causal, "10–15 percent of all childhood cancers are attributable to magnetic fields."[14]

In general, the association between cancer and present-day measurements of EMF levels has been weaker than that observed between cancer and the presence of high-current power lines. In some ways, this should not be surprising—it is similar to testing lead levels in the home years or even decades after a child develops lead poisoning. A landmark study by Swedish researchers gave strong support for the EMF-childhood cancer link using detailed power company records to estimate *past* EMF exposures. But Feychting and Ahlbom found a statistically reliable association with the calculated historical fields at or around the time of diagnosis. The risk of childhood cancer rose with exposures above 1 mG and there was a dose-response relationship.[15]

The Swedish childhood cancer study is limited by the small number of cases. A subsequent combined analysis of the Swedish study with similar studies from Denmark and Finland reaffirmed the link.[16] Also, a meta-analysis of 13 studies found statistically significant increases in leukemia and nervous system tumors.[17] Indeed, the 1996 NRC study featured its own meta-analysis of the residential EMF studies and estimated that children living near high-current wire power lines had a 50 percent higher rate of leukemia, a statistically significant association.[11] However, the NRC panel declined to implicate EMFs as a possible carcinogen, although it could not point to any other credible risk factors.

The status of the adult residential studies is much less clear. While some have documented a link for adults, others have not. A 1996 review found that, "[I]t seems that the evidence is not strong enough to support the putative causal relation between residential exposure to magnetic fields and adult leukemia or breast cancer."[18]

Over 100 occupational studies—of varying quality—have been published, and many show links between EMFs and leukemia, brain cancer, or both. In the mid-1990s, a number of research teams collected detailed magnetic field measurements in their epidemiological investigations, and, while showing a cancer risk, they have not been consistent. For instance, a Canadian-French effort found an association between EMFs and leukemia among utility workers.[19] But a similar study in the United States pointed instead to a brain tumor risk.[20] In another large study, Sweden's Floderus found higher rates of leukemia and brain cancer among EMF-exposed workers, though in her case, the link was stronger for leukemia.[21] This lack of consistency has clouded the ability to draw firm conclusions of an EMF-cancer link.

A meta-analysis of 29 occupational studies, sponsored by the Electric Power Research Institute found a "small but significant" increase in the risk of brain cancer among workers exposed to EMFs.[22]

In the 1990s, a number of investigators have implicated EMFs in the development of breast cancer. The first reports found that men in jobs with EMF exposures had unexpectedly high rates of breast cancer—a very rare disease among males with only approximately 900 cases a year in the United States. Attention soon turned to female breast cancer and the first studies have had mixed results. Loomis[23] and Coogan[24] found an association, while Canton[25] did not. At least four major breast cancer epidemiological studies are now under way in the United States and Sweden.

A contentious issues in the EMF controversy is the possible mechanism of interaction. One hypothesis centers on the hormone melatonin, which is a known oncostatic agent. Sunlight can inhibit the flow of melatonin and there are indications that ELF EMFs can do so as well.[26] Lower levels of melatonin, according to the theory, could lead to a general increase in various types of cancer—not necessarily in one specific site. Still in its infancy, this hypothesis could explain much of the variation in epidemiological findings.

In addition, if EMFs are cancer promoters, exposures to cancer-initiating agents (such as chemical carcinogens and ionizing radiation) could be an important factor in determining which types of cancer develop.

In the mid-1990s, Sobel opened a new area of research when he reported a link between occupational EMF exposure and Alzheimer's disease. In four separate groups of subjects in the United States and Finland, he and his coworkers found that those who had worked in jobs with medium-to-high EMF exposures were three to four times more likely to develop Alzheimer's disease.[27,28] Sobel has also proposed a biological mechanism to explain the role of EMFs in the development of Alzheimer's disease.[29]

Animal and Cellular Studies

Research on in vivo and in vitro effects is much less developed than the epidemiological studies. A number of large-scale animal studies are in progress in various countries around the world. But at present no reliable animal model for EMF effects is available.

A German group led by Dr. Wolfgang Löscher of the School of Veterinary Medicine in Hannover has carried out a series of studies that clearly show that magnetic fields can promote breast cancer in animals.[30,31] The effect follows a clear dose-response relationship. Replication studies are under way in the United States.

Cellular studies have not produced definitive results. Much of the in vitro work focuses on the possible impact of EMFs on gene expression, since this could explain the elevated risks observed in the epidemiological studies. Experiments by Goodman and Henderson[32,33] indicating than EMFs can alter the course of protein synthesis have led many others to try to replicate their work—some without success.[34] A congressionally mandated research project, known as EMF RAPID (Research and Public Information Dissemination), has sponsored a host of experimental work on gene expression, and these results, which are due over the next few years, should clarify the status of this possible EMF effect.

What Is the Right Index of Exposure?

One of the problems that has plagued an understanding of EMF health effects is the definition of dose. EMF research began in the 1970s with an emphasis on electric fields. In the mid-1980s, partially due to the confirmation of the Wertheimer-Leeper[12] study by Savitz,[13] the focus moved to magnetic fields. But, in the mid-1990s, there has been renewed interest on the role of electric fields acting in concert with magnetic fields. For instance, a combined analysis of electric and magnetic field exposures by Miller[35] found leukemia risks that were greater than 10 times that expected—a risk that was some three times larger than that seen when only considering magnetic fields.

A group led by Henshaw[36] in Bristol, United Kingdom, has argued that electric fields can concentrate radon daughter particles and that this mechanism could explain the observed increases in cancer rates.

But there are many other exposure variables that might be responsible for EMF health effects. These include: frequency, harmonic content, high-frequency transients, and polarization, as well as whether the exposure is continuous or intermittent. In addition, the magnitude and direction of the earth's magnetic field may be important.

A set of animal studies carried out in Sweden showed that mice exposed to *intermittent* 50-Hz magnetic fields had significantly more skin tumors than those exposed to *continuous* 50-Hz fields.[37] It is not yet clear whether the difference was due to the fact that fields were not on all the time (intermittency) or from high-frequency transients created in the course of turning the field on and off.

While measuring 60-Hz magnetic fields is relatively easy and cheap, measuring more complex EMFs, such as transients, is more difficult and more expensive.

EMF Standards

There are no federal standards governing human exposures to ELF EMFs in the United States. The states of Florida and New York have set interim standards for magnetic fields—in the range of 150 to 200 mG—but these are designed to ensure that current exposure levels do not increase rather than to protect against known health hazards.

The International Non-Ionizing Radiation Committee of the International Radiation Protection Association (which has become the International Commission on Non-Ionizing Radiation Protection) has a set of exposure 50/60-Hz guidelines for the general public and for workers. These recommend maximum exposures of 1,000 mG and 5 kV/m for the public and 5,000 mG and 10 kV/m for workers.[38] These limits are based on "established or immediate health effects," such as shocks and burns, and not on a possible cancer risk.

In the absence of standards that address the contentious data on cancer, many standard-setting bodies have opted for a policy of "prudent avoidance," as first proposed by an influential report from the now-disbanded Office of Technology Assessment.[39] Prudent avoidance may be defined in many ways, but the OTA report suggested that it would prompt lower exposures by rerouting power lines and redesigning electrical systems and appliances when these actions entail "modest costs." Prudent avoidance is a variation on the ALARA (as low as reasonably achievable) strategy, which was developed to limit exposures to ionizing radiation.

▶ VIDEO DISPLAY TERMINALS

Video display terminals (VDTs) have become a permanent fixture of the modern office and are nearly as common in American homes. As early as 1980, VDT operators were concerned about possible miscarriages and birth defects from working at the units. These fears were fueled by many reports of "clusters" of problem pregnancies. In 1988, Goldhaber and coworkers at Kaiser Permanente in Oakland, California, appeared to legitimize these concerns with a report that women who used VDTs more than 20 hours a week had twice as many miscarriages as non-VDT workers. No measurements were made on radiation emissions from the terminals.[40]

An epidemiological study by a team at the National Institute for Occupational Safety and Health (NIOSH)[41] failed to find any miscarriage risk. After the pregnancy questionnaires had been completed, NIOSH hired a consultant to measure the radiation levels from the type of VDTs used by the women who had participated in the study. Surprisingly, the survey showed that both cases and controls were exposed to similar levels of ELF EMFs, thus precluding any firm conclusions about potential radiation effects.[42]

The following year, a Finnish group reported a more than tripling of the miscarriage risk among VDT operators who used units with high ELF magnetic field emissions—defined as entailing average exposures of more than 3 mG. This study, the first to categorize VDT operators by their actual EMF exposure rather than the more imprecise number of hours at a terminal, has not been repeated, leaving the nature and extent of the possible pregnancy risk unsettled.[43]

Meanwhile, most new VDTs are now shielded to reduce EMF emissions. In 1990, standards were developed by a group of international experts working under the auspices of a Swedish organization now known as SWEDAC, then called MPR. The standards, known as MPR2, limit operator exposures to ELF EMFs to 2.5 mG at a distance of 50 cm from the set. Most terminals now on the market meet the MPR2 limits.[44] The Swedish white collar union, known as TCO, has developed even tougher exposure limits (2 mG at a distance of 30 cm from the front of the terminal) and a growing number of VDT manufacturers have met these limits. It is important to note that these standards are based on what is technologically achievable, not on documented health impacts.

With the introduction of low-emission VDTs, most of the attention on adverse health impacts due to working at a computer is now on ergonomic issues, specifically the threat of repetitive strain injuries such as carpal tunnel syndrome.

▶ RADIOFREQUENCY AND MICROWAVE RADIATION

Radiofrequency and microwave (RF/MW) radiation refers to electromagnetic radiation in the frequency band between 3 MHz and 300 GHz. The major sources of exposure to RF/MW radiation are: radio and television broadcasting, cellular phones and towers, radar, uplink satellite dishes, and industrial heating machines. Microwaves are also used in hyperthermia units for the treatment of cancer.

For many years, the only accepted mechanism for health effects from RF/MW exposure was from heating of tissue. Indeed, all current health standards are still based on heating. However, a growing number of researchers have come to believe that there are so-called nonthermal or athermal biological effects.

The specific absorption rate (SAR) is the unit of measurement often used to define the amount of energy absorbed by a biological system. SARs are measured in terms of watts per kilogram (W/kg). For humans an SAR of 4 W/kg is approximately equivalent to a power density of 10 mW/cm^2 at frequencies of 30 to 300 MHz. SARs are much more difficult to measure than power densities. A number of meters are available to measure RF/MW radiation exposures.

Epidemiological Studies

There are very few epidemiological studies of RF/MW exposed populations and those that have been carried out suffer from very poor exposure assessment.

Szmigielski of the Center for Radiobiology and Radiation Safety in Warsaw has been studying Polish military personnel exposed to RF/MW radiation for many years. In 1996, he published a detailed analysis that showed that such soldiers had significantly higher rates of leukemia and lymphoma. For younger soldiers, the risk of developing these cancers was more than eight times the expected rate.[45]

With the proliferation of wireless communications, especially cellular telephones and personal communication services, there are growing concerns over the possible effects of RF/MW towers. The power outputs of these towers are relatively low compared with conventional radio and television transmitters. For these latter sources, however, there are some preliminary reports indicating higher cancer rates among those living in the shadow of broadcast towers.

In Australia, Hocking has shown that children living near a television tower in Sydney had approximately double the rate of leukemia than those living further away.[46] And in 1997, Dolk reported a similar pattern among adults living near a television and FM radio tower in Birmingham, England.[47] A second study by Dolk was less clear.

Animal and Cellular Studies

The first chronic animal study of RF/MW exposures, by Guy and coworkers at the University of Washington, Seattle, indicated that pulsed 2,450-MHz radiation caused a statistically significant increase in total malignant tumors among rats. This experiment is considered quite controversial, as the sponsoring agency, the U.S. Air Force, has tried to dismiss this finding. Although completed in 1984, the study was not published until 1992.[48]

A more recent—and still unpublished—effort by Adey to investigate the possible long-term consequences of digital cellular phone radiation indicated a possible "protective effect." The exposed animals, which had been initiated by a chemical carcinogen, had *fewer* brain tumors than those who were unexposed.[49] Interestingly, a parallel study using frequency-modulated signals simulating analog phone radiation had no such effect. Adey has speculated that the pulsed radiation may enhance DNA repair mechanisms. Adey's results would, however, indicate that nonthermal levels of RF/MW radiation can have an effect on living systems, which might be beneficial or deleterious.

In another much discussed experiment, Lai and Singh of the University of Washington, Seattle, have shown that a single 2-hour exposure of low-level RF/MW radiation can increase the number of breaks in the DNA of the brains of live rats.[50] Like Adey, Lai and Singh have suggested that the radiation can alter DNA repair processes, though in this case negatively.

One of the most widely discussed cellular effects of RF/MW radiation is the finding by Cleary of the Medical College of Virginia that human brain tumor cells continued to proliferate at an abnormally high rate 5 days after a 2-hour exposure at levels of 5 or 24 W/kg.[51]

Given the worldwide explosion in the use of hand-held phones—over 100 million will be in use by the year 2000, according to current projections—there are initiatives all over the world to sponsor more studies on RF/MW radiation and specifically to look at the possible effects on brain biochemistry.

RF/MW Exposure Standards

The two most cited exposure standards for RF/MW radiation are those recommended by the National Council on Radiation Protection and Measurement (NCRP) in 1986[52] and those of the Institute of Electrical and Electronics Engineers, which were adopted by the American National Standards Institute (ANSI/IEEE) in 1992.[53] While the NCRP adopted the traditional distinction between occupational and general population RF/MW exposures (the latter being five times more stringent than the on-the-job limits), the ANSI/IEEE favored separate limits for "controlled" and "uncontrolled" environments. Here again, limits for uncontrolled exposures are stricter by a factor of five, but for some situations—such as the use of hand-held phones—it is not always clear which limits apply.

Both the NCRP and the ANSI/IEEE guidelines are based on thermal hazards and do not take into account possible health risks due to long-term exposures at low levels. The two sets of limits are based on the conclusion that there are no deleterious effects at exposures below 4 W/kg, with a safety factor of 10 added. Thus, exposure standards are based on SARs of 0.4 W/kg. They are therefore quite similar, except at the low and high frequencies. At frequencies below 100 MHz, the ANSI/IEEE guidelines take into account induced and contact currents. And at the high frequencies, above approximately 1 GHz, the ANSI/IEEE are twice the levels recommended by the NCRP. The logic for this loosening has been challenged by the EPA.

Neither standard limits exposures from specific peak pulses of energy from radar.

There are no enforceable federal standards for workers or the general public. The EPA was about to set safety limits in the mid-1980s, but backed off in face of intense pressure from industry.

The NCRP is in the process of revising its 1986 limits, but this will take many years and a report is not expected until sometime after the year 2000.

Essentially all ongoing health research at these frequencies is sponsored by the military and by industry, primarily by the wireless communications industry.

▸ REFERENCES

1. Hughes D: Hazards of Occupational Exposure to Ultraviolet Radiation. Occupational Hygiene Monograph No. 1. Leeds, England: University of Leeds Industrial Services, 1978
2. Occupational Exposure to Ultraviolet Radiation: NIOSH Criteria Document. Washington, DC. US Department of HEW, NIOSH Publication No. 73-11009, 1973, p 108
3. Urbach F: Geographic distribution of skin cancer. J Surg Oncol 3:219–234, 1971
4. American National Standards Institute: Practice of Industrial Lighting A 11.1, 1965 (reaffirmed 1970). Practice for Office Lighting A 132. 1, 1966. Guide for School Lighting A 23.1, 1962 (reaffirmed 1970). New York: The Institute
5. Illuminating Engineering Society, Committee on Daylighting: Recommended Practice of Daylighting. Baltimore: The Society, 1950
6. Zaffanella LE: Survey of Residential Magnetic Field Sources. Goals, Results and Conclusions, Report No. TR-102759-V1. Palo Alto, CA: Electric Power Research Institute, 1993
7. Ozonoff DM: Fields of controversy. The Lancet 349:74, 1997
8. Environmental Protection Agency (EPA): Evaluation of the Potential Carcinogenicity of Electromagnetic Fields. Washington, DC: Environmental Protection Agency, 1990
9. Oak Ridge Associated Universities: Health Effects of Low-Frequency Electric and Magnetic Fields. Washington, DC: Government Printing Office, 1992
10. National Council on Radiation Protection and Measurements (NCRP): Extremely Low Frequency Electric and Magnetic Fields, Draft Report, 1995. Conclusions and Recommendations. Microwave News 15(4):12–14, 1995
11. National Research Council: Possible Health Effects of Exposure to Residential Electric and Magnetic Fields. Washington, DC: National Research Council, 1996
12. Wertheimer N, Leeper E: Electrical wiring configurations and childhood cancer. Am J Epidemiol 109:273–284, 1979
13. Savitz D et al: Case control study of childhood cancer and exposure to 60 Hz magnetic fields. Am J Epidemiol 128:21–38, 1988
14. Ahlbom A et al: Biological Effects of Power Line Fields. Final Report of the New York State Power Line Project. Albany, New York: Department of Health, 1987
15. Feychting M, Ahlbom A: Magnetic fields and cancer in children residing near Swedish High-Voltage Power Lines. Am J Epidemiol 138:467–481, 1993
16. Ahlbom A et al: Electromagnetic fields and childhood cancer. The Lancet 342:1295–1296, 1993
17. Washburn EP et al: Residential proximity to electricity transmission and distribution equipment and risk of childhood leukemia, childhood lymphoma and childhood nervous system tumors: systematic review, evaluation and meta-analysis. Cancer Causes Control 5:299–309, 1994
18. Li C-Y, Thériault G, Lin RS: Epidemiological appraisal of studies of residential exposure to power frequency magnetic fields and adult cancers. Occup Environ Med 53:505–510, 1996
19. Thériault G et al: Cancer risks associated with occupational exposure to magnetic fields among electric utility workers in Ontario and Quebec, Canada, and France: 1979–1989. Am J Epidemiol 139:550–572, 1994
20. Savitz DA, Loomis DP: Magnetic field exposure in relation to leukemia and brain cancer mortality among electric utility workers. Am J Epidemiol 141:123–134, 1995
21. Floderus B et al: Occupational exposure to electromagnetic fields in relation to leukemia and brain tumors: a case-control study in Sweden. Cancer Causes Control 4:464–476, 1993
22. Kheifets LI et al: Occupational electric and magnetic field exposure and brain cancer: a meta-analysis, J Occup Environ Med 137: 1327–1341, 1995
23. Loomis DP, Savitz DA, Ananth CV: Breast cancer mortality among female electrical workers in the United States. J Nat Cancer Inst 86:921–925, 1994
24. Coogan PF et al: Occupational exposure to 60 Hz magnetic fields and risk of breast cancer in women. Epidemiology 7:459–464, 1996
25. Cantor KP et al: Occupational exposures and female breast cancer mortality in the United States. J Occup Environ Med 37:336–348, 1995
26. Reiter RJ: Static and extremely low frequency electromagnetic field exposure: reported effects on the circadian production of melatonin. J Cell Biochem 51:394–403, 1993
27. Sobel E et al: Occupations with exposure to electromagnetic fields: a possible risk factor with Alzheimer's disease. Am J Epidemiol 142:515–524, 1995
28. Sobel E et al: Elevated risk of Alzheimer's disease among workers with likely electromagnetic field exposure. Neurology 47:1477–1481, 1996
29. Sobel E, Davanipour Z: Electromagnetic field exposure may cause increased production of amyloid beat and eventually lead to Alzheimer's disease. 47:1594–1600, 1996
30. Löscher W, Mevissen M: Linear relationship between flux density and tumor co-promoting effect of prolonged magnetic field exposure in a breast cancer model. Cancer Lett 96:175–180, 1995
31. Mevissen M et al: Exposure of DMBA-treated female mice in a 50 Hz, 50 μTesla magnetic field: effects on mammary tumor growth, melatonin levels and T-lymphocyte activation. Carcinogenesis 17:903–910, 1996
32. Goodman R, Henderson AS: Exposure to salivary gland cells to low-frequency electromagnetic fields alters polypeptide synthesis. Proc Nat Acad Sci USA 85:3928–3932, 1988
33. Goodman R, Henderson AS: Transcription and translation in cells exposed to extremely low frequency electromagnetic fields. Bioelectrochem Bioenerg 25:335–355, 1991
34. Saffer JD, Thurston SJ: Short exposures to 60 Hz magnetic fields do not alter MYC expression in HL60 or Daudi cells. Radiat Res 144:18–25, 1995

35. Miller A et al: Leukemia following occupational exposure to 60 Hz electric and magnetic fields among Ontario electric utility workers. Am J Epidemiol 144:150–160, 1996
36. Henshaw DL et al: Enhanced deposition of radon daughter nuclei in the vicinity of power frequency electromagnetic fields. Int J Radiat Biol 69:25–38, 1996
37. Rannug A et al: Intermittent 50 Hz magnetic fields and skin tumor promotion in SENCAR mice. Carcinogenesis 15:153–157, 1994
38. International Non-Ionizing Radiation Committee, International Radiation Protection Association: Interim guidelines on limits of exposure to 50/60 Hz electric and magnetic fields. Health Phys 58:113–122, 1990
39. Office of Technology Assessment: Biological Effects of Power Frequency Electric and Magnetic Fields—Background Paper, No. OTA-BP-E-53, Washington, DC: Government Printing Office, 1989
40. Goldhaber MK, Polen MR, Hiatt RA: The risk of miscarriage and birth defects among women who use video display terminals during pregnancy. Am J Ind Med 13:695–706, 1988
41. Schnorr TM et al: Video display terminals and the risk of spontaneous abortion. N Engl J Med 324:727–733, 1991
42. Slesin L, Connelly M: Video display terminals and spontaneous abortions. N Engl J Med 325:811–812, 1991
43. Lindbohm M-L et al: Magnetic fields of video display terminals and spontaneous abortion. Am J Epidemiol 136:1041–1051, 1992
44. SWEDAC, Test Methods for Visual Display Units (MPR 1990:8) and User's Handbook for Evaluating Visual Display Units (MPR 1990:10). Borås, Sweden: SWEDAC, 1990
45. Szmigielski S: Cancer morbidity in subjects occupationally exposed to high frequency (radiofrequency and microwave) electromagnetic radiation. Sci Total Environ 180:9–17, 1996
46. Hocking B et al: Cancer incidence and mortality and proximity to TV towers. Med J Aust 165:601–605, 1996
47. Dolk H et al: Cancer incidence near radio and television transmitters in Great Britain. I: Sutton Coldfield Transmitter and II: All High Power Transmitters. Am J Epidemiol 145:1–9, 10–17, 1997
48. Chou CK et al: Long-term, low-level microwave irradiation of rats. Bioelectromagnetics 13:469–496, 1992
49. Adey WR et al: Brain tumor incidence in rats chronically exposed to digital cellular telephone fields in an initiation—promotion model. Abstract A-7-3. 18th Annual Meeting of the Bioelectromagnetics Society, Victoria, Canada, 1996
50. Lai H, Singh NP: Single- and double-strand DNA breaks in rat brain cells after acute exposure to radiofrequency electromagnetic radiation. Int J Radiat Biol 69:513–521, 1996
51. Cleary SE, Liu L-M, Merchant RE: Glioma proliferation modulated in vitro by isothermal radiofrequency radiation exposure. Radiat Res 121:38–45, 1990
52. National Council on Radiation Protection and Measurements (NCRP): Biological Effects and Exposure Criteria for Radiofrequency Electromagnetic Fields. Report No. 86. Bethesda, MD: National Council on Radiation Protection and Measurements, 1986
53. American National Standards Institute (ANSI): IEEE Standard for Safety Levels with Respect to Human Exposure to Radiofrequency Electromagnetic Fields, 3 kHz to 300 GHz (C95.1-1992). New York: American National Standards Institute, 1992

General References

Ahlbom A: A review of the epidemiologic literatures on magnetic fields and cancer. Scand J Work Environ Health 14:337–343, 1988

Archimbaud E et al: Acute myelogenous leukemia following exposure to microwaves. Br J Haematol 73:272–273, 1989

Armstrong B et al: Association between exposure to pulsed electromagnetic fields and cancer in electric utility workers in Quebec, Canada, and France. Am J Epidemiol 140:805–820, 1994

Becker RO, Selden G: The Body Electric. New York: William Morrow, 1985

Brodeur P: Currents of Death. New York: Simon and Schuster, 1989

Brown HD, Chattopadhyay SK: Electromagnetic field exposure and cancer. Cancer Biochem Biophys 9:295–342, 1988

Carpenter DO, Ayrapetyan S (eds): Biological Effects of Electric and Magnetic Fields. Sources and Mechanisms. Beneficial and Harmful Effects. San Diego, CA: Academic Press, 1994, vols 1 and 2

Feychting M, Ahlbom A: Childhood leukemia and residential exposure to weak extremely low frequency magnetic fields. Environ Health Perspect 103(Suppl 2):59–62, 1995

Florig HK: Containing the cost of the EMF problem. Science 257: 468–469, 488–492, 1992

Grandjean E: Ergonomics in Computerized Offices. Philadelphia: Taylor & Francis, 1987

Hendee WR, Boteler JC: The question of health effects from exposure to electromagnetic fields. Health Phys 66:127–136, 1994

Holmberg B: Magnetic fields and cancer. Animal and cellular evidence—an overview. Environ Health Perspect 103(Suppl 2):63–67, 1995

Horton WH, Goldberg S: Power Frequency Magnetic Fields and Public Health. Boca Raton, FL: CRC Press, 1995

Kuster N, Balzano Q, Lin JC: Mobile Communications Safety. London: Chapman & Hall, 1997

National Council on Radiation Protection and Measurements (NCRP): Biological Effects and Exposure Criteria for Electromagnetic Fields. Bethesda, MD: National Council on Radiation Protection and Measurement, 1986

National Institute of Child Health and Development. Proceedings of the NICHD Workshop on the Reproductive Effects of VDT Use. Reprod Toxicol 4:39–69, 1990

Okuno T: Thermal effect of visible light and infra-red radiation on the eye: a study of infra-red cataract based on a model. Ann Occup Hyg 38:351–359, 1994

Polk C, Postow E: Handbook of Biological Effects of Electromagnetic Fields. 2nd ed. Boca Raton, FL: CRC Press, 1996

Reiter RJ, Robinson J: Melatonin: Your Body's Natural Wonder Drug. New York: Bantam Books, 1995

Reilly JP: Electrical Stimulation and Electropathology. New York: Cambridge University Press, 1992

Salzinger K et al: Altered operant behavior of adult rats after perinatal exposure to a 60 Hz electromagnetic field. Bioelectromagnetics 11:105–116, 1990

Savitz D: Overview of occupational exposure to electric and magnetic fields and cancer: advancements in exposure assessment. Environ Health Perspect 103(Suppl 2):69–74, 1995

Savitz D, Calle E: Leukemia and occupational exposure to electromagnetic fields: review of epidemiologic surveys. J Occup Med 29:47–51, 1987

Sellers D: Zap! How Your Computer Can Hurt You—and What You Can Do About It. Berkeley, CA: Peachpit Press, 1994

Speers M, Dobbins J, Miller V: Occupational exposures and brain cancer: a preliminary study of East Texas residents. Am J Ind Med 13: 629–639, 1988

Stevens R et al (eds): The Melatonin Hypothesis: Breast Cancer and Use of Electric Power. Columbus, OH: Battelle Press, 1997

Thomas T et al: Brain tumor mortality risk among men with electrical and electronics jobs: a case-control study. Natl Conser Dist 79:233–238, 1987

Wilson B, Stevens R, Anderson L: Extremely Low Frequency Electromagnetic Fields. Columbus, OH: Battelle Press, 1990

30

Effects of the Physical Environment: Noise As a Health Hazard

Aage R. Møller

Noise is mainly hazardous to health because it can damage the ear, but it may also influence a number of other bodily functions. A temporary or permanent decrease in hearing acuity, such as that from noise exposure, may impair speech communication. Noise can also mask warning signals and thus poses a risk to safety and to the general health of workers.

The most apparent and best-known health risk from noise is damage to the ear, so this will be addressed first. The other effects of noise are dealt with later in the chapter.

▸ EFFECT OF NOISE ON HEARING

"Noise" is commonly used to describe sounds that are unwanted or unpleasant, in contrast to music or speech. Several textbooks, in fact, define noise as sound that is discordant and nonperiodic, probably because such sound often has unpleasant qualities. The potential of noise to damage hearing, however, is entirely related to its physical properties. In this chapter, we use the word *noise* to describe sound that may be damaging to the ear, because this word has traditionally had negative connotations and thus will be identified more readily with health hazards.

Noise that has a sufficient intensity and duration to cause hearing impairment is usually associated with industry. Since it is the physical characteristics of the sound that determines its potential for causing hearing loss, the origin of the sound, by itself, has no influence upon the degree of risk it presents for hearing damage. Sounds to which people are exposed during recreational activities may pose as great a risk to hearing as noise that is associated with work activities (including military activities, where gunshot noise in particular poses a high degree of risk to hearing).

There is great variation in an individual person's susceptibility to noise-induced hearing loss. Thus only the *average* probability for acquiring a hearing loss can be predicted on the basis of knowledge about the physical characteristics of noise and time of exposure to noise to which a person is exposed. The average risk of acquiring noise-induced hearing loss is in proportion to the intensity and duration of the noise exposure. The character of the noise—whether it is continuous or transient (such as gunshots)—also plays a role. Thus different types of noise pose different degrees of risk to hearing, even though the overall intensity of the noises is the same; impulsive sounds such as gunshots generally pose a greater risk than continuous noise.[1]

The risk of hearing loss also depends on the spectral composition of the noise and the pattern of exposure (constant intensity versus fluctuating intensity or noise interspersed with intervals of relative silence). Low-frequency sounds are considered to be less damaging than high-frequency sounds of the same physical intensity. For this reason, when noise intensity is measured with a sound-level meter for predicting its effect on hearing, a frequency weighing is used, where energy at low frequencies has less weight than energy at high frequencies (A-weighing). The importance of the temporal pattern is more difficult to represent in standard measurement of noise level.

Temporal Threshold Shift and Permanent Threshold Shift

The first effect of exposing an ear to noise above a certain intensity for a certain period of time is a reduction in the ear's sensitivity (an elevated auditory threshold). This reduction in hearing is greatest immediately after the exposure and decreases gradually. If the noise has not been too loud or the exposure too long, hearing will gradually return to its original level. This type of hearing loss is known as a *temporary threshold shift* (TTS) (Fig. 30-1). If the noise is more intense than a certain value and/or the exposure time longer than a certain time, the resulting hearing threshold never returns to its original value and a *permanent threshold shift* (PTS) has occurred. PTS is the stable threshold shift that is experienced after the temporary threshold shift has vanished (Fig. 30-1). For people who have been exposed to common industrial noise exposure for many years, it is the PTS that is most noticeable and the TTS component is small. TTS is experienced in uncommon situations, such as in explosions and from gunfire. There is a considerable individual variation in susceptibility to noise-induced hearing loss. Therefore, the curves in Figure 30-1 represent the *average* course of hearing loss.

While a temporary threshold shift probably results from temporary impairment of the function of the sensory cells in the cochlea (which is a part of the inner ear), a permanent threshold shift is associated with irreversible damage to these cells. This damage can be seen when the cells are examined histologically under high-power magnification (Fig. 30-2). The basilar membrane of the cochlea, along which the sensory cells are located, is a complex and intricate organ that performs spectral analysis of sounds so that specific groups of sensory cells become activated in accordance with the spectrum of a sound. There are two types of hair cells, inner and outer hair cells (Fig. 30-2). Although they are similar in appearance, they have totally different functions. The inner hair cells convert sounds into a neural

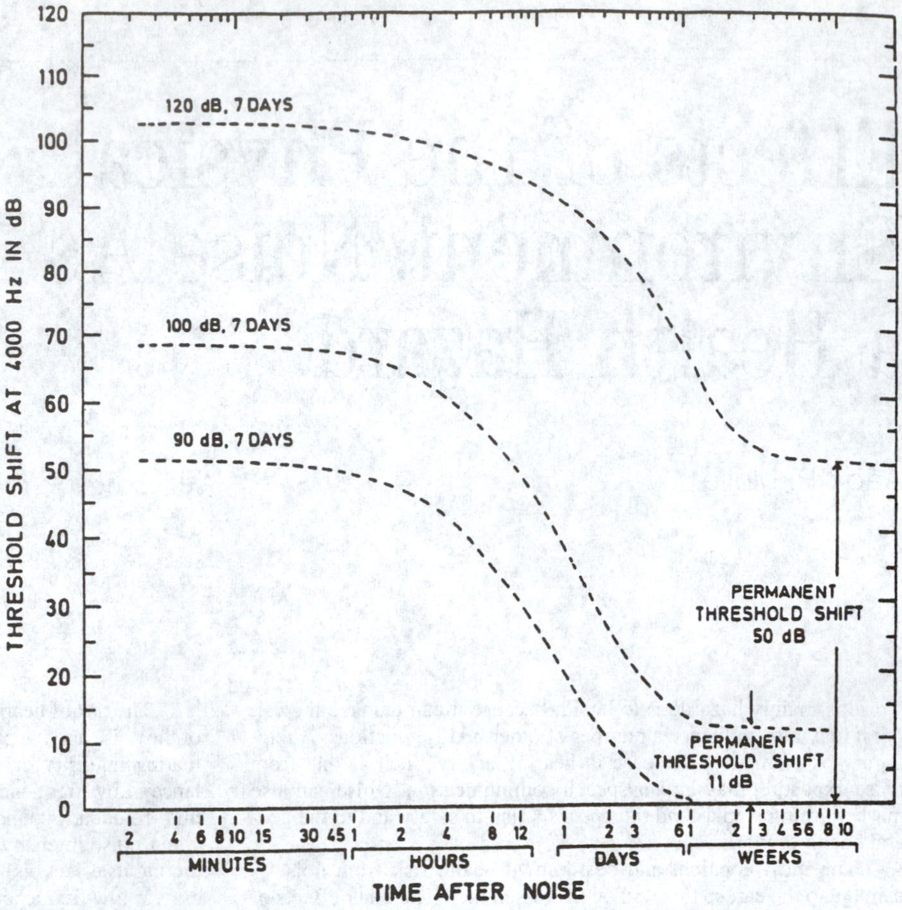

Figure 30-1. Schematic diagram illustrating how noise can affect hearing. The graph shows the hearing loss (*threshold shift*) at 4000 Hz a certain time (*horizontal axis*) after noise exposure. Noise with an intensity below a certain value is expected to give rise to a temporary threshold shift (*90 dB, 7 days curve*), while a louder noise (*100 dB, 7 days*) results in a permanent threshold shift. A very intense noise (*120 dB, 7 days*) gives rise to a considerable permanent shift in threshold. (Modified from Miller J: J Acoust Soc Am 56:3, 1974, with permission.)

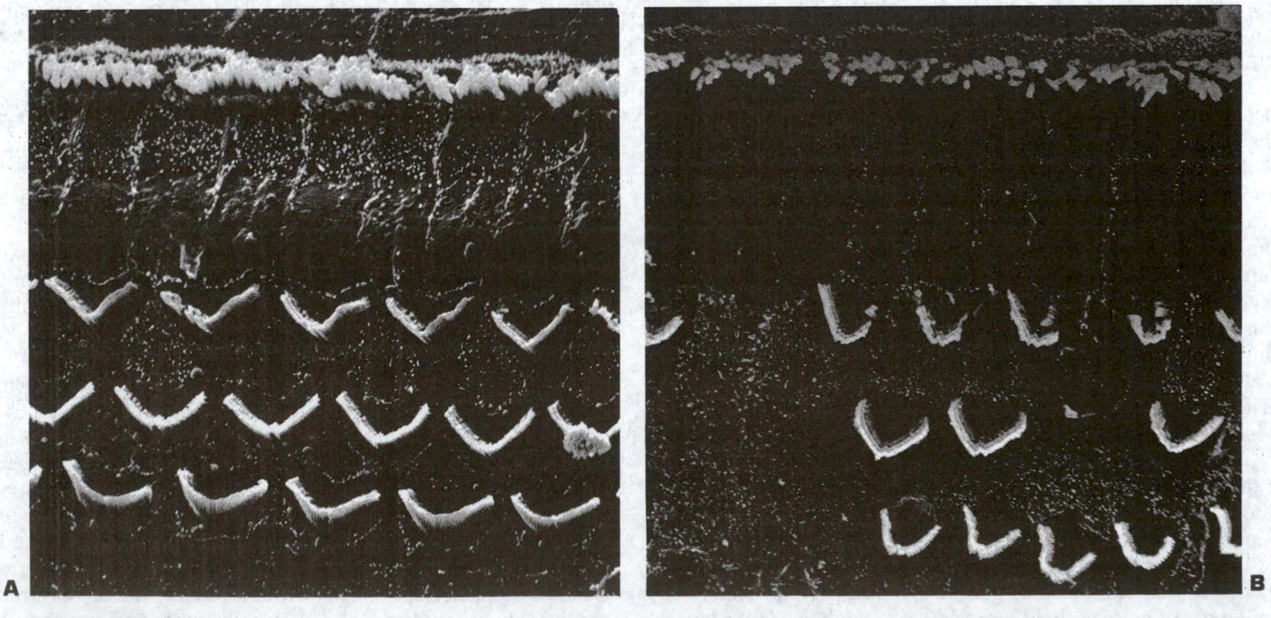

Figure 30-2. Scanning electron micrographs of sensory cells (hair cells) from a small segment of the basilar membrane of a monkey. *A*, normal hair cells. *B*, hair cells after noise exposure (gunshots). (Courtesy of Professor Hans Engstrom, Uppsala, Sweden.)

code in the individual fibers of the auditory nerve, but the outer hair cells' function is mechanical; they act as "motors" that amplify the motion of the basilar membrane and thereby increase the sensitivity of the ear. It is the outer hair cells that are damaged first by noise exposure. As a result of noise capable of producing hearing loss, destruction of outer hair cells is more frequent and more extensive than destruction of inner hair cells.[2,3] Destruction of outer hair cells reduces the sensitivity of the ear because the "cochlear amplifiers" have been destroyed. There is no way to restore hearing to normal in people with damaged hair cells. Noise exposure may also cause damage to the auditory nervous system, but the exact nature and extent of such damage is poorly understood.

► NATURE OF NOISE-INDUCED HEARING LOSS

Hearing loss is measured in decibels (dB)[a] relative to a normative average hearing threshold obtained by measuring the hearing thresholds of young people who have had no known exposure to noise. Slightly different standards for "normal" hearing are used in different parts of the world.[4,5] The difference between the hearing threshold of an individual and the "standard" hearing threshold is known as the "hearing level" (HL) and is measured in decibels. When the hearing level is plotted on the vertical axis as a function of the frequency tested, a graph results that is known as an audiogram. (Usually, the hearing thresholds are determined only in the frequency range of 125 to 8,000 Hz (8 kHz), despite the fact that a person with normal hearing can hear sounds in the frequency range of about 18 Hz to 20 kHz.)

Predicted Hearing Loss from Noise Exposure

Median predicted hearing loss determined by the International Organization for Standardization (ISO)[5] (Fig. 30-3) shows that the resulting hearing loss is greatest in a restricted frequency range around 4 kHz. When the exposure time to noise is increased, or the level of the noise is increased (100 versus 90 dB), the magnitude of the hearing loss increases and the frequency range of the hearing loss widens. Most of the hearing loss that is expected after 40 years of noise exposure is already acquired during the first 10 years of the exposure (Fig. 30-3).

The results shown in Figure 30-3 are typical for those exposed to noise in various manufacturing industries, where the noise tends to be of a broad spectrum and continuous in nature. However, it is a consistent finding that the greatest hearing loss occurs around 4 kHz. The frequency distribution of hearing loss as a result of noise exposure depends to some extent on the spectrum of the noise, but even noise with widely different spectra seems to produce its greatest effect in the 4-kHz range. The reason for this is not known with certainty. Hearing loss caused by exposure to pure tones, or a noise of which the energy is limited to a narrow range of frequencies, is largest in a frequency range that is about one-half octave above that at which the noise has its highest energy.

Individual Variation in Noise Susceptibility

There is a great degree of individual variation in the susceptibility to noise-induced hearing loss: people who are exposed to exactly the same noise for exactly the same period of time may suffer rather different degrees of hearing loss. Data such as those shown in Figure 30-3 thus do not predict the extent of hearing loss that an individual person will acquire when exposed to a certain noise. Some people can tolerate high-intensity noise for a lifetime and not suffer any noticeable degree of hearing loss. Other people may acquire a substantial

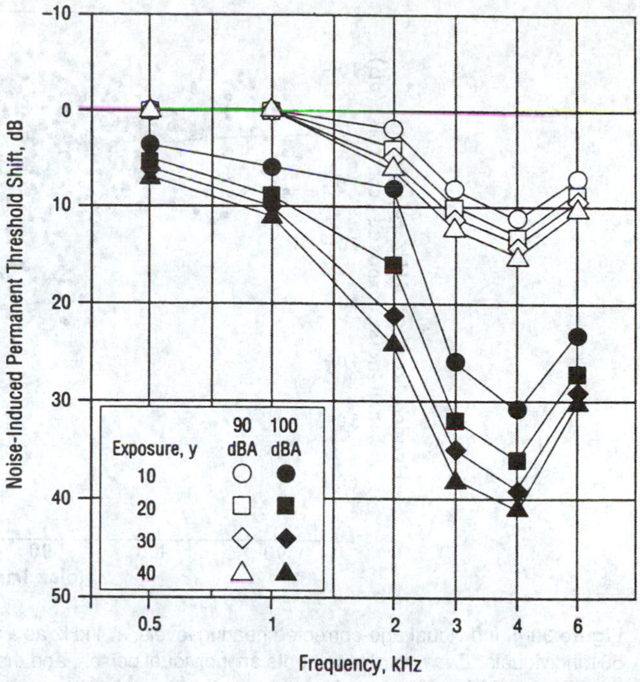

Figure 30-3. Median estimated noise-induced permanent threshold shift plotted as a function of frequency for two exposure levels (assuming 8-hour daily exposure) and four durations of exposure. (Reproduced from Dobie RA: Prevention of noise-induced hearing loss. Arch Otolaryngol Head Neck Surg 121:385–391, 1995; after ISO-1999, Annex E.)

hearing loss from exposure to much less intense noise. The individual variation in hearing loss as a function of noise exposure is illustrated in Figure 30-4, which shows hearing losses at 4 kHz for a number of people as a function of the *noise immission level*.[6] The *noise immission level* combines the two characteristics of noise—duration and intensity—which are assumed to be of the greatest importance in defining its potential for harm. The graph thus shows that the *average* hearing loss as a result of exposure to continuous noise with a sound intensity of 85 dB(A) for 20 years is less than 5 dB at 4,000 Hz, but that a number of people experience a 30- to 40-dB hearing loss (threshold shift).

A wide variety of factors that could influence the individual susceptibility to noise exposure have been suggested, including individual variations in blood supply to the cochlea, differences in the nervous system, and many more. Although solid evidence is lacking, it has also been suggested that environmental factors and differences in lifestyle, such as smoking cigarettes, physical activity, etc, could affect susceptibility to noise exposure.

Studies in animals have pointed toward some factors that may predispose to noise-induced hearing loss. For example, studies in rats showed that rats that were genetically predisposed to high blood pressure acquired a higher degree of hearing loss from noise exposure than normal rats when both groups were exposed to noise for their entire lifetimes.[7,8] Although these findings have not been duplicated in humans, the results of some studies in humans support a relationship between high blood pressure and hearing loss from noise exposure.[9] Alterations in cochlear blood flow may also affect susceptibility to noise-induced hearing loss.[10] (For a review see Borg et al.).[2] Research along these lines has provided important knowledge. To date, however, it has not resulted in the development of efficient ways to assess an individual's susceptibility to noise-induced hearing loss or to effectively decrease a person's susceptibility to noise-induced hearing loss.

Attempts have been made to estimate an individual's susceptibility to PTS by the degree of TTS evidenced on exposure to a test

---

[a] *dB is an abbreviation of decibel and is a logarithmic measure, used here as a measure of sound pressure. 1 dB is one-tenth of a logarithmic unit (a ratio of 1:10). The reason for using a logarithmic measure of sound pressure to measure hearing thresholds is that the subjective sensation of sound intensity is approximately related to the logarithm of the sound pressure.*

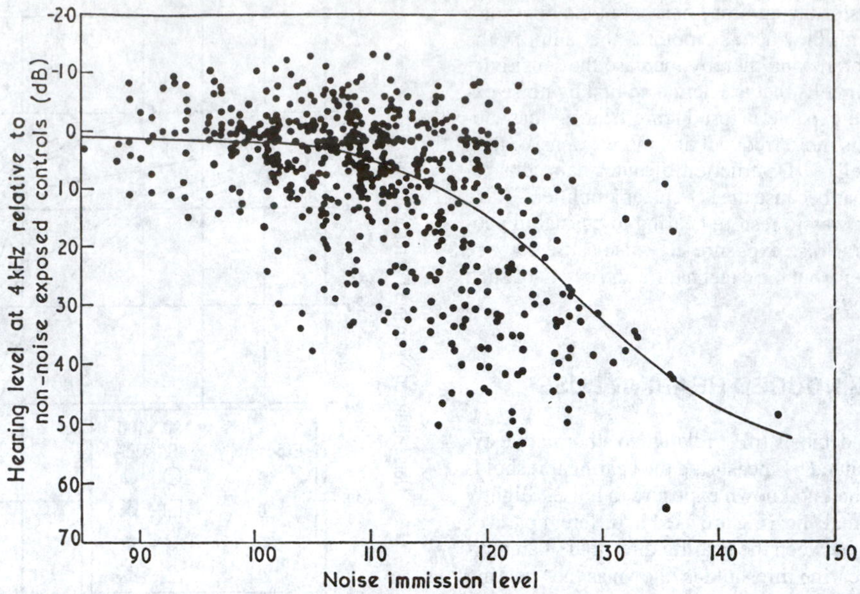

Figure 30-4. Individual age-corrected hearing levels, at 4 kHz as a function of the total amount of noise exposure (immission level), for 581 individuals. *Each point* represents an individual person, and the *solid lines* are the mean values of the threshold. The noise immission level E = L + 10 log(T), where L represents the sound level (measured with A-weighting) that is exceeded during 2 percent of the exposure time, T, in months. For example, exposure to 85-dB noise during 20 years of work corresponds to 85 + 10 log(20 * 12) = 85 + 10 log 240 = 85 + 24 = 109. For continuous noise, L deviates only slightly from the A-weighted sound intensity, but for noise that contains transient or intermittent noises (i.e., noises that vary considerably in intensity) the difference between these two values is great. (From Burns W, Robinson DW: Hearing and Noise in Industry. London: Her Majesty's Stationery Office, 1970, p 158.)

sound that is not loud enough to cause permanent hearing loss, but the results have been discouraging. It appears that there is only a weak correlation between susceptibility to PTS and the degree of TTS in any individual person. At the present time the only way to determine an individual's susceptibility to noise-induced hearing loss is to test, at frequent intervals, the hearing of those who were exposed to loud noise. It is interesting that the effect on hearing from noise exposure can be altered (decreased) by exposure to a sound of a lower intensity prior to the exposure to noise. Animal studies have disclosed that activation of a particular neural circuit in the brainstem (the olivocochlear bundle) may protect the ear from noise-induced hearing loss.[11] Pre-exposure to sound seems also to "harden" the ear against damage from noise exposure.[2,12]

Subjective Signs of Hearing Loss

Since hearing loss induced by industrial noise usually first affects the hearing threshold at frequencies around 4 kHz (and thus above the 300 Hz to 3 kHz range that is essential for perception of speech), a person who suffers from noise-induced hearing loss often does not notice the loss before it has reached a relatively severe level. Nevertheless, hearing tests can easily reveal hearing loss before it affects the ability to discriminate speech. Since a beginning hearing loss may indicate that the person in question is particularly susceptible to noise-induced hearing loss, it is important to do frequent hearing tests in workers who are exposed to noise. This testing is part of modern hearing conservation programs.

People who have noise-induced hearing loss often have difficulties in understanding speech, even when the sound has been amplified properly. This aspect of noise-induced hearing loss is more noticeable when in a noisy environment or in a place in which several people are speaking at the same time. Recent developments of "intelligent" hearing aids have, however, improved the situation for many hearing-impaired individuals. Measurement of speech perception is not standardized and the outcome depends on whether the tests are done in quiet or with a background of noise.[13] Also, there is a great individual variation in the relation between the tone audiogram and the ability to understand speech. Other effects of noise exposure on people with noise-induced hearing loss may include ringing in the ears (tinnitus) and headaches.

▶ NOISE STANDARDS

To reduce the risk of noise-induced hearing loss, a number of recommendations of acceptable noise levels have been established and appear in the form of "noise standards." Different countries have adopted slightly different standards, and the ways in which the standards are enforced also differ. All presently accepted standards use a single-value that is a combination of noise level and the duration of the exposure to calculate the risk of noise-induced permanent hearing loss. Some of these standards include correction factors regarding the nature of the sound (for instance, impulsive versus continuous sounds). Some standards take normal age-related hearing loss (presbycusis) into account while others do not.

Establishing Noise Standards and Damage Risk Criteria

The maximal noise level and duration accepted in most industrial countries is either 85 or 90-dB(A),[b] for 8 hours a day, 5 days a week. In Europe the 85-dB(A) level is more common. In the United States 90 dB(A) is the accepted level stated by the Occupational Safety and Health Administration (OSHA), although certain measures have to be taken if workers are exposed to noise levels above 85 db(A). (For a review of noise standards see Suter.)[14]

Because the great individual variation in susceptibility to noise-induced hearing loss makes it impossible to predict what hearing loss an individual will acquire when exposed to a certain noise, noise stan-

[b] *The (A) after dB indicates that the noise spectrum has been weighted to place less emphasis on low frequencies than on high frequencies. This is done because low-frequency sounds generally possess less risk for causing hearing loss than do high-frequency sounds.*

dards at best merely predict the percentage of people in a population with normal hearing who will acquire less than a certain specified (acceptable) hearing loss when exposed to noise no louder than a certain value.[15,16] The standards thus allow that a certain (small) percentage of a normal-hearing population will acquire a permanent hearing loss (threshold elevation) that is greater than a certain value.

Noise Level and Exposure Time

Noise standards are based on exposure for 8 hours per day. If the exposure time is shorter, a higher level of noise can be tolerated. To estimate how much higher level of noise can be tolerated when the duration of the exposure to noise is less than 8 hours per day, a conversion factor is used, which is different in the United States and Europe. Europe uses a 3-dB "doubling factor" while the United States uses a 5-dB doubling factor. A 3-dB doubling factor implies that, given a reduction of the exposure time by a factor of 2 (e.g., from 8 to 4 hours), a 3-dB higher sound level can be accepted. Thus 88 dB(A) for 4 hours is assumed to have the same effect on hearing as 85 dB(A) for 8 hours. If the exposure time to noise is 2 hours per day, a 6-dB higher sound level is assumed to be acceptable, and so on. This way of calculating an acceptable noise level reflects "the equal energy principle," which assumes that it is the total energy of the noise that determines the risk for permanent hearing loss. The acceptance of a 5-dB doubling factor assumes that the noise level may be increased by 5 dB when the exposure time is shortened by a factor of 2 without increasing the risk of hearing loss. Thus a noise level of 90 dB(A) for 8 hours is assumed to have the same risk as exposure to noise at 95 dB(A) for 4 hours, which again is considered to be equally hazardous as 2 hours of exposure to 100 dB(A), 1 hour of exposure to 105 dB(A), 30 minutes of exposure to 110 dB(A), and 15 minutes of exposure to 115 dB(A), and so on.

Research indicates that a doubling factor of 5 dB may be adequate for relatively low noise levels, but that a smaller doubling factor (3 dB, i.e., equal energy) more correctly reflects the hazards presented by noise of a high level. There are thus indications that a doubling factor of less than 5 dB should be applied for high noise levels. In the United States, standards have been tightened accordingly by stating that no worker should be exposed to continuous noise above 115 dB(A) or impulsive noise above 140 dB(A). This action sets a ceiling for acceptable combination of noise intensity and exposure time.

Because the level of noise exposure usually varies during a work day, noise exposure is often described by its *equivalent level* (L_{Eq}), which is defined as the level of a noise that has the same *average* energy as the noise that is measured during a work day. The equivalent level is measured by summing the total noise energy to which a person is exposed and dividing it by the duration of exposure. The calculation of this equivalent level assumes that the equal energy principle discussed above is valid.

▶ MEASUREMENT OF NOISE

The fact that the present noise standards are based on a simplified measure of noise, namely the A-weighted measure dB(A), adds to the uncertainty in predicting the risk of acquiring a hearing loss that may result from exposure to a certain noise. The dB(A) measure does not take into account the spectrum of the noise, nor does it take into account whether or not the noise contains sharp transient sounds or sounds with other characteristics important in hearing loss.

Measurements of sound levels are usually made at a location where people work, but sound level at the entrance of the ear canal of a person in that location will be different because the head and the pinna amplify sounds within frequencies between 2 and 5 kHz by as much as 10 to 15 dB. If the noise contains much energy in that frequency range, the sound that actually reaches the ear may be as much as 10 to 15 dB higher than the actual reading on a sound-level meter placed in the person's location when the person is not present. Because the noise level is often different at different locations and when a person walks around, the exposure varies and it becomes difficult to estimate the average exposure. Noise dosimeters have been developed to improve the accuracy of determination of the average noise exposure. These devices, worn by the person, function similarly to radiation monitors. They register the sound level near the ear or, sometimes, at other locations on the body and integrate the energy over an entire working day.

Impulsive Noise. Determination of the risk from noise that is impulsive in nature poses particular problems. Since the ear requires 100 ms (0.1 sec) to integrate a sound in order to perceive its loudness, noise-level meters in earlier times were designed to integrate sound over about 100 ms to provide a reading that was in accordance with the perceived loudness of sounds. This is appropriate when the purpose is to assess the subjective intensity (or annoyance) of sound. It is not appropriate when noise levels are measured for the purpose of assessing the risk they pose to hearing. The ear (cochlea) has a much shorter integration time than the brain, and since the injury from noise exposure occurs in the cochlea, a sound-level meter, the reading of which should reflect the potential of a sound to injure the ear, should have a much shorter integration time. The cochlea, where the damage for noise exposure occurs, integrates sound energy over a few milliseconds. The presently available sound-level meters (so-called impulse sound–level meters) have an integration time of 35 ms. It is not known how that value, which does not have any physiologic relevance, was derived. A noise-level meter that has an integration time of 35 ms will underestimate the peak intensities of impulsive sounds and thus the potential of such sounds to cause injury to the cochlea.[17]

What Degree of Hearing Loss Is Acceptable? In the beginning of the era in which efforts were made to reduce (or prevent) noise-induced hearing loss, the "acceptable hearing loss" was defined as the level of hearing loss at which an individual begins to experience difficulty in understanding everyday speech in a quiet environment. This definition was based on the American Academy of Ophthalmology and Otolaryngology (AAOO) guidelines for evaluation of hearing impairment (revised in 1979, from 1959 and 1973)[18] which state that the ability to understand normal everyday speech at a distance of about 1.5 m (5 ft) does not noticeably deteriorate as long as the hearing loss does not exceed an average value of 25 dB at frequencies H 500 Hz, 1 kHz and 2 kHz, and that hearing loss was regarded as a just-noticeable handicap for which a worker in the United States was entitled to receive worker's compensation for loss of earning power. It is puzzling that this degree of hearing loss was later designated as acceptable.

The NIOSH Criteria Document[19] states that the ability to hear sounds at 25 dB below normal at H 500 Hz, 1 kHz and 2 kHz is not good enough to ensure that speech will be understood under normal conditions. It has been advocated that, instead, the average hearing loss at 1, 2, and 3 kHz be used as a basis for evaluating the effects of noise exposure. The inclusion of the hearing level at 3 kHz seems justified, because hearing at 3 kHz is important for speech perception. It has also been suggested that the average hearing level of 25 dB be replaced by 22 dB, while keeping the same frequencies defined by the EPA (1, 2, and 4 kHz).[20] The reasoning behind this suggestion was endorsed by the AAOO, which, however, maintained that a "low fence" of 25 dB was acceptable.[18]

Effect of Age-Related Hearing Loss. Hearing loss from causes other than noise interacts with noise-induced hearing loss in a complex way. For instance, the "normal" progressive hearing loss that occurs with age (presbycusis) is not directly additive to hearing loss from noise (Fig. 30-5). If one would attempt to determine the hearing loss from noise alone by subtracting the hearing loss from aging, a paradoxical result will in many cases become evident, namely, that the noise-induced hearing loss will *decrease* with age and with the duration of the exposure to noise. This has caused much controversy because some investigators have proposed that the hearing loss from presbycusis should be subtracted from the total hearing to get a "clean" measure of noise-induced hearing loss. The reasons for the

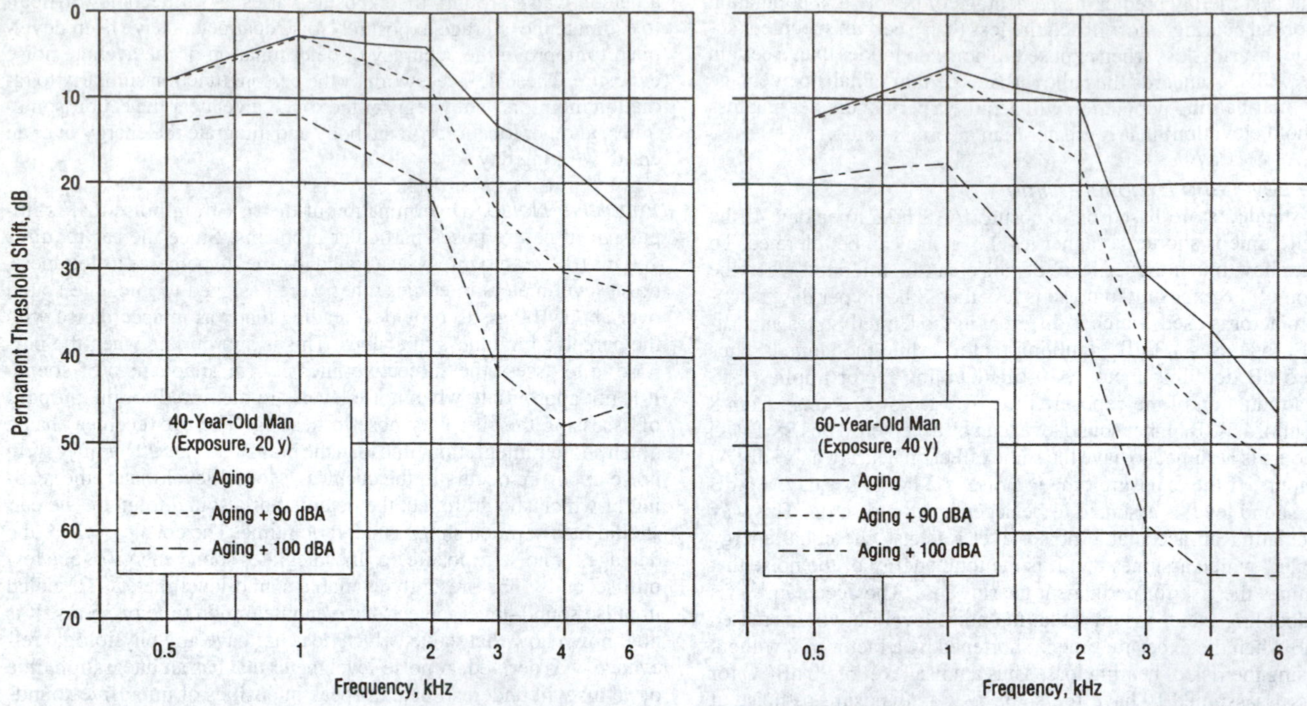

Figure 30-5. Median age-related permanent threshold shifts plotted alone (*solid lines*) and after addition of noise-induced permanent threshold shifts by the methods of ISO-1999 (*dashed lines*) assuming daily exposures of 90 or 100 dB(A). (From Dobie RA: Prevention of noise-induced hearing loss. Arch Otolaryngol Head Neck Surg 121:385–391, 1995.)

paradoxical findings is that subtracting presbycusis from the total hearing loss to get the PTS assumes that these two factors add in a linear way, which they do not. Presbycusis also varies very much from individual to individual, which adds to the uncertainty in predictions of an individual person's hearing loss.

Present Noise Standards

In the United States, legislation that covers noise includes the Federal Aviation Act of 1958, the 1969 Amendment of the Walsh-Healy Public Contracts Act, the Occupational Safety and Health Act of 1970, the Noise Control Act of 1972, and the Mine Safety and Health Act of 1978. These acts require certain agencies to regulate noise. In Europe, legislation in various countries regarding the limitations on industrial noise has largely been guided by recommendations made by the International Organization for Standardization (ISO). These recommendations have generally set an upper limit of acceptable noise exposure at 85 dB(A) for 8 hours a day, 5 days per week, while in the United States 90 dB(A) has been the standard.

The ISO recommendation is based on the probabilities of acquiring a hearing loss of 25 dB, averaged for 500 Hz, 1 kHz, and 2 kHz, with exposure to noises of different intensities for different lengths of time. According to ISO recommendations,[5] as much as 10 percent of a population with initially normal hearing will acquire a hearing loss of 25 dB or more averaged over frequencies 500 Hz, 1 kHz, and 2 kHz after 40 years of exposure to noise at a level of 85 dB(A). For 90 dB(A), the figure is 21 percent. These values are based on studies of workers in the weaving industry, and research indicates that the number of people with noise-induced hearing losses may be higher in other industries. The difference between 85 and 90 dB(A) daily average exposure is, however, that the risk of hearing impairment doubles, regardless of which data are used as a basis (see Suter[14]). In this connection, it deserves to be mentioned that the Environmental Protection Agency in the United States has regulated exposure to noise of the general population, deciding that no more than 5 dB hearing loss can be allowed at 4 kHz as a result of environmental noise.[21]

Models of Noise-Induced Hearing Loss. Elaborate models of noise-induced hearing loss have been developed, and there are formulae that claim to make it possible to predict the noise-induced hearing loss that a certain noise exposure will cause. One of the earliest such formulae was proposed by Robinson, and several subsequent models or formulae have been proposed (ISO). Such models are mainly used for prediction of hearing loss from noise exposure, but some models have also been used to predict previous exposure on the basis of hearing loss.[22] The latter are mainly of interest for medicolegal purposes. While such models may provide valid predictive values of the *average* hearing loss or average noise exposure, the large individual variation makes the accuracy of such predictions low when used for individual people. It is therefore questionable to use such models for prediction of the hearing loss that an individual will acquire, or for predicting what noise exposure a person has had on the basis of his or her hearing loss.

▶ PREVENTION OF NOISE-INDUCED HEARING LOSS

It has been advocated that noise standards be modified to reduce the number of people who acquire a hearing loss that can be regarded as a social handicap. The maximal tolerable noise level for an 8-hour exposure is around 75 dB(A) if significant noise-induced hearing loss is to be eliminated.[23] The main obstacles in adopting a lower noise level are economic: the cost of having all workplaces comply with such regulations have been considered prohibitive. However, a much less expensive alternative, having all *new* equipment comply with regulations, was not even considered.

Reduction of Noise at the Source

To lower the risk of noise-induced hearing loss, the standard in the United States from the earlier 90 dB(A) to 85 dB(A)[24] and the OSHA Hearing Conservation Amendment state that a noise monitoring program (hearing conservation program) is mandatory in environments where the daily average noise level is 85 dB(A) or higher.[25,26]

Lowering noise exposure has often been disputed because of its heavy economic implications; however, when implemented on new equipment only, the economic consequences are small. For example, when a fast paper-making machine was constructed in a very noisy industry it was possible to reduce the noise level to 85 dB(A) by using known technology. The old machinery that it replaced had a noise level of more than 110 dB(A).[27] The total cost of reducing noise was only 1.1 percent of the cost of the plant. This anecdotal example of noise control shows how implementation of state-of-the-art engineering can reduce noise without excessive economic consequences. Undeniably, there are several industries in which the cost of noise reduction is greater than in the example given, but in many instances the cost is less, and there may even be cases in which the cost would be negligible. In this connection it needs to be pointed out that it is not the noise level that machinery emits that is important, but rather the noise level to which workers are exposed. Moving people to less noisy locations can reduce the exposure levels, which means that changes in operating machinery can, in fact, lead to reduction in the risk of noise-induced hearing loss.

Personal Protection

Two types of personal protection are in common use: earmuffs, which are attached to a helmet or worn on a headband, and earplugs. Earmuffs can be removed more easily than earplugs and are therefore better suited for intermittent use as in situations when people are walking in and out of noisy areas (such as airports). On the other hand, earplugs are more practical for people who spend long periods of time in noisy environments. The sound attenuation of different types of earplugs and earmuffs depends on the type of device and how well it fits the individual person. When measured in the laboratory, earmuffs are found to attenuate sound more than earplugs.[28] But when hearing loss is assessed in people using these two types of ear protectors, earmuffs are usually shown to be less efficient than earplugs, even though earmuffs attenuate sound more.[28,29] The gain that is achieved in practice from wearing ear protection may be less than anticipated. The efficacy of ear protectors depends not only on their sound attenuation determined in the laboratory but also on compliance with the use of ear protectors, which is difficult to control and poorly documented. For ethical reasons, it is not possible to do studies making use of a controlled situation where participants who wear ear protectors are randomized with control participants who do not wear ear protectors. Nilsson and Lindgren's study in which the hearing loss in groups of people wearing ear protectors was compared with the hearing loss in people not wearing ear protectors[29] found that people who did not wear ear protectors were almost twice as likely to acquire a hearing threshold shift of 15 dB or more than those who used earmuffs. Other studies showed similar results.[26] This controversy may be due to the way sound attenuation is measured, or it may be psychological in nature: earmuffs are easier to remove and may not always be worn when indicated.[29] Earmuffs tend to lose some of their sound attenuating power over time. When the efficacy of ear protectors was studied in shipyards, in combination with intense continuous noise and superimposed impulsive noise, thus presenting an extreme hazard to hearing,[29] those who were exposed to low-intensity noise suffered more hearing loss than did those in the high-intensity noise group. This surprising result is likely due to workers' different habits of wearing ear protectors: many more workers exposed to high-intensity noise rather than low-intensity noise wore ear protectors.[29]

Solving the problem of noise-induced hearing loss by the use of personal protection devices has substantial drawbacks. Wearing ear protectors for long periods may be hot and inconvenient, and ear protectors impair speech communication, which makes it more difficult for people to hear alarm signals or other acoustic signs of danger. Nevertheless, there are situations where ear protectors are appropriate.

▶ HEARING CONSERVATION PROGRAMS

Regulations on noise-induced hearing loss[19,25] state that hearing conservation programs must be designed so that people who are exposed to noise levels of 85 dB(A) (8-hour weighted average) or more can be identified and that measures must be taken to reduce the noise. If these measures do not result in a reduction of the noise level to 90 dB(A) or lower, workers must participate in a hearing conservation program, and employers must make personal hearing protection devices (ear protectors) available to such workers and perform hearing tests at specified intervals during employment. If a hearing loss of 10 dB average over frequencies 2, 3, and 4 kHz is detected, then the person must be referred for further evaluation and action must be taken to avoid further deterioration of hearing. The progress of hearing deterioration can usually be halted by moving to a less noisy environment, thus preventing the progress of the hearing loss before it becomes a social handicap.

▶ EFFECTS OF NOISE ON OTHER BODILY FUNCTIONS

The effects of noise on bodily functions other than hearing are poorly understood. It is reported that noise exposure can cause an increase in blood pressure and changes in other important bodily functions such as change (usually increases) in the secretion of pituitary hormones.

It has been known for a long time that workers in noisy industries have a higher incidence of peripheral circulatory problems and heart problems than do those who are not exposed to such high levels of noise. However, there is evidence that individuals with a predisposition for circulatory diseases acquire more PTS when exposed to noise than people in general. The observed correlation between PTS and elevated blood pressure may thus be the result of a higher susceptibility of people with hypertension. Rats with hereditary predisposition for hypertension developed considerably greater degrees of hearing loss from exposure to noise than did rats without this hereditary predisposition to high blood pressure.[2,7,30,31]

Some retrospective studies (i.e., Jonsson and Hansson[9]) of the effects of exposure to noise on the blood pressures of industrial workers found that workers who were exposed to industrial noise had higher systolic and diastolic blood pressures, while other studies (i.e., Sanden and Axelsson[32]) found no relationship between noise-induced hearing loss and blood pressure in shipyard workers. If the results of these experiments in spontaneously hypertensive rats[7,33] can be applied to humans, then the results of the study of hypertension reported by Jonsson and Hansson[9] may have to be reevaluated. By using hearing loss as the criterion for degree of noise exposure, they may inadvertently have selected workers who were predisposed to hearing loss because of their hypertension and not vice versa, as was intended.

▶ EFFECTS OF SOUNDS ABOVE AND BELOW THE AUDIBLE FREQUENCY RANGE (ULTRASOUND AND INFRASOUND)

Sounds that are not audible to humans because their frequencies are above or below our audible frequency range are known as ultrasound and infrasound, respectively. There is no evidence to indicate that exposure to sounds that are not audible can damage the ear, and there is little evidence that such sounds could have other untoward effects.

Ultrasounds are rapidly attenuated when transmitted in air and therefore decrease rapidly in intensity with distance from the source. Although very high intensities of ultrasound can kill furred animals such as mice, rats, and guinea pigs because of the buildup of heat by sound absorption in the fur, such an effect could not occur in humans because bare skin cannot absorb enough energy to cause damage.

Exposure to low-frequency sounds (infrasound) of high intensity has been reported to cause various diffuse symptoms such as headache, nausea, and fatigue. Although very few controlled studies have been conducted, it is possible that exposure to such sounds may have some effect on general bodily functions. The results of some experiments indicate that infrasounds may give rise to a *decrease* in blood pressure, possibly mediated through stimulation of the vestibular part of the inner ear. However, there is no evidence that such sounds can be hazardous to hearing.

▶ REFERENCES

1. Price GR, Kim HN, Lim DJ, Dunn D: Hazard from weapons impulses: histological and electrophysiological evidence. J Acoust Soc Am 85:1245–1254, 1989
2. Borg E, Canlon B, Engstrom B: Noise-induced hearing loss. Literature review and experiments in rabbits. Scand Audiol 24(Suppl 40): 1–147, 1995
3. Borg E, Engstrom B: Noise level, inner-hair cell damage audiometric features and equal-energy hypothesis. J Acoust Soc Am 86: 1776–1782, 1989
4. American National Standard Institute (ANSI): Standard for Audiometrics, S3:6, 1969
5. International Organization for Standardization (ISO): Acoustics: Determination of Occupational Noise Exposure and Estimation of Noise-Induced Hearing Impairment. ISO-1999. Geneva: International Organization for Standardization, 1990
6. Burns W, Robinson DW: Hearing and Noise in Industry London: Her Majesty's Stationery Office, 1970
7. Borg E, Møller AR: Noise and blood pressure: effects of lifelong exposure in the rat. Acta Physiol Scand (Stockh) 103:340–342, 1978
8. Borg E: Noise, hearing, and hypertension. Scand Audiol 10:125–126, 1981
9. Jonsson A, Hansson L: Prolonged exposure to a stressful stimulus (noise) as a cause of raised blood-pressure in man. Lancet 1:86–87, 1977
10. Axelsson A, Borg E, Hornstrand C: Noise effects on the cochlear vasculature in normotensive and spontaneously hypertensive rats. Acta Otolaryngol (Stockh) 96:215–225, 1983
11. Rajan R, Johnstone BM: Contralateral cochlear destruction mediates protection from monaural loud sound exposures through the crossed olivocochlear bundle. Hear Res 39:263–278, 1989
12. Canlon B, Borg E, Flock A: Protection against noise trauma by preexposure to low level acoustic stimulus. Hear Res 34:197–200, 1988
13. Smoorenburg GF: Speech reception in quiet and in noisy conditions by individuals with noise-induced hearing loss in relation to their tone audiogram, J Acoust Soc Am 91:421–437, 1992
14. Suter AH: The development of federal noise standards and damage risk criteria. In Lipscomb DM (ed): Hearing Conservation in Industry, Schools, and the Military. London: Taylor & Francis, 1988, pp 45–66
15. Kryter KD: Impairment to hearing from exposure to noise. J Acoust Soc Am 53:1211–1234, 1973
16. Møller AR: Noise as a health hazard. Ambio 4:6–13, 1975
17. Bruel PV: Noise: Do We Measure It Correctly? Bruel and Kjaer, Denmark: Naerum, 1975, p 40
18. American Academy of Ophthalmology and Otolaryngology (AAOO), Committee on Hearing and Equilibrium and the American Council of Otolaryngology, Committee on Medical Aspects of Noise: Guide for evaluation of hearing handicap. Am J Med Assoc 241: 2055–2059, 1979
19. National Institute for Occupational Safety and Health (NIOSH): Criteria for a Recommended Standard: Occupational Exposure to Noise. Publication No. HSM 73-11001. Cincinnati: National Institute for Occupational Safety and Health, 1972
20. Suter AH: The ability of mildly hearing impaired individuals to discriminate speech in noise. US Environmental Protection Agency (EPA 550/9-78-100) and US Air Force (AMRL-TR-78-4) Reports. Washington, DC: Government Printing Office, 1978
21. Environmental Protection Agency (EPA), Office of Noise Abatement and Control Information on Levels of Environmental Noise. Requisite to Protect Public Health and Welfare with Adequate Margin of Safety. Washington, DC EPA 550/9-74-004 1974
22. Dobie RA: Medical-Legal Evaluation of Hearing Loss. New York: van Nostrand Reinhold, 1993
23. von Gierke HE, Johnson DL: Summary of present damage risk criteria. In Henderson D, Hamernik RP, Dosaujh DS, Mills JHM (eds): Effects of Noise on Hearing. New York: Raven Press, 1976, pp 547–560
24. Suter A: Essentials of noise regulations. Otolaryngol Clin North Am 21(3):551–562, 1979
25. Occupational Safety and Health Administration (OSHA): Occupational Noise Exposure. Hearing Conservation Amendment, Final Rule. Federal Register 48:9738–9785, 1983
26. Dobie RA: Prevention of noise-induced hearing loss. Arch Otolaryngol Head Neck Surg 121:385–391, 1995
27. Møller AR: Noise as a health hazard. Scand J Work Environ Health 3:73–79, 1977
28. Erlandsson B, Hakanson H, Ivarsson A, Nilsson P: The difference in protection efficiency between earplugs and earmuffs. Scand Audiol (Stockh) 9:215–221, 1980
29. Nilsson R, Lindgren F: The effect of long term use of hearing protectors in industrial noise. Scand Audiol Suppl 12:204–211, 1980
30. Nilsson R, Liden G, Sanden A: Noise exposure and hearing impairment in the shipbuilding industry. Scand Audiol 6:59–68, 1977
31. Borg E: Physiological and pathogenic effects of sound. Acta Otolaryngol Suppl (Stockh) 381:1–68, 1981
32. Sanden A, Axelsson A: Comparison of cardiovascular responses in noise-resistant and noise-sensitive workers. Acta Otolaryngol Suppl (Stockh) 377:75–100, 1981
33. Borg E: Noise-induced hearing loss in normotensive and spontaneously hypertensive rats. Hear Res 8:117–130, 1982

General References

Burns W, Robinson DW (eds): Hearing and Noise in Industry. London: Her Majesty's Stationery Office, 1970

Dobie RA: Medical-Legal Evaluation of Hearing Loss. New York: van Nostrand Reinhold, 1993

Hamernik RP, Henderson D, Salvi R (eds): New Perspectives on Noise-Induced Hearing Loss. New York: Raven Press, 1982

Kryter KD: The Effects of Noise on Man. 2nd ed. New York: Academic Press, 1985

Lipscomb DM (ed): Hearing Conservation in Industry, Schools, and the Military. Boston: Little, Brown, 1988

Pickles JO: Physiology of the Ear. 2nd ed. New York: Academic Press, 1988

Salvi RJ, Henderson D, Hamernik RP, Colletti V: Basic and Applied Aspects on Noise-Induced Hearing Loss. New York: Plenum Press, 1985

31

Ergonomics and Work-Related Musculoskeletal Disorders

W. Monroe Keyserling • Thomas J. Armstrong

Ergonomics is the study of humans at work in order to understand the complex relationships among people, machines, job demands, and work methods. All work, regardless of its nature, places both physical and mental stresses on the worker. As long as these stresses are kept within reasonable limits, work performance will be satisfactory and the worker's health and well-being will be maintained. However, if stresses are excessive, undesirable outcomes may occur in the form of errors, accidents, injuries, and/or a decrement in health.

Ergonomists are concerned with evaluating the stresses that occur in the work environment and the ability of people to cope with these stresses. The goal of ergonomics is to design facilities (e.g., factories and offices), furniture, equipment, tools, and job demands to be compatible with human dimensions, capabilities, and expectations. Ergonomics is a multidisciplinary science with four major areas of specialization:

- *Cognitive ergonomics* (sometimes called engineering psychology) is concerned with the information-processing requirements of work. Major applications include designing displays (e.g., gauges, warning buzzers, signs, instructions), controls (e.g., knobs, buttons, joysticks, steering wheels), and software to enhance human performance while minimizing the likelihood of error.[1–3]
- *Anthropometry* is concerned with the measurement and statistical characterization of body size. Anthropometric data provide important information to the designers of clothing, furniture, machines, tools and work stations.[4–6]
- *Work physiology* is concerned with the responses of the cardiovascular system, pulmonary system, and skeletal muscles to the metabolic demands of work. This discipline is concerned with the prevention of whole body and/or localized fatigue that results from a mismatch between job demands and worker capacities.[7]
- *Biomechanics* is concerned with the mechanical properties of human tissue, particularly the responses of tissue to mechanical stresses.[8] Many mechanical stresses can cause *overt* injuries (e.g., a concussion when a worker is struck in the head by a dropped object). In most cases, overt injury hazards are readily recognized and can be controlled through safety engineering techniques such as machine guarding and personal protective equipment.[9] Other stresses are more subtle and can cause chronic or cumulative injuries and disorders. These stresses may be external (e.g., a vibrating tool that causes white finger syndrome) or internal (e.g., tension in a tendon when the attached muscle contracts).

The primary emphasis of this chapter is the prevention of work-related musculoskeletal injuries, disorders, and syndromes that result from excessive physical demands in the work environment. Typical examples include:

- A poultry worker develops numbness and tingling in the hand and fingers due to the repetitive hand motions associated with dismembering chickens;
- A farm worker experiences pain in the lower back attributed to the awkward stooping posture required to harvest vegetables;
- A nurse's aide suffers a back strain when transferring a patient from a hospital bed to a wheelchair.

It is important to note that the health problems described above typically are not the result of an accident. (An *accident* is defined as an unanticipated, sudden, and discrete event that results in an undesired outcome such as property damage, injury, or death.[9]) Instead, they can be generally classified as overexertion or overuse disorders and syndromes that are caused by performing work tasks that are regular and predictable requirements of the job.

Anthropometry, work physiology, and biomechanics are the ergonomic disciplines that are most relevant to the development of programs for ameliorating overexertion injuries and chronic musculoskeletal disorders and are emphasized in the following sections. Readers who desire additional information pertaining to cognitive ergonomics are directed to the References for a short list of general survey texts.[1–3]

▸ ANTHROPOMETRY

Anthropometry is concerned with measuring the size of the human body and using this information to design facilities, equipment, tools, and personal protective equipment (e.g., gloves, respirators, etc.) to accommodate the physical dimensions of the user. As illustrated in Figure 31-1, most anthropometric design problems are nontrivial due the large variation in body dimensions within the working population. In this example, a designer must specify the height of an overhead conveyor used to transport parts between two areas of a plant. If the conveyor is too high, short workers would not be able to load or unload parts without elevating the shoulder to an extended reach posture. On the other hand, if the conveyor is too low, tall workers could sustain head injuries from collisions with hung parts.

Suppose that the designer's primary goal is to avoid head injuries to tall workers. To accomplish this, he or she decides to

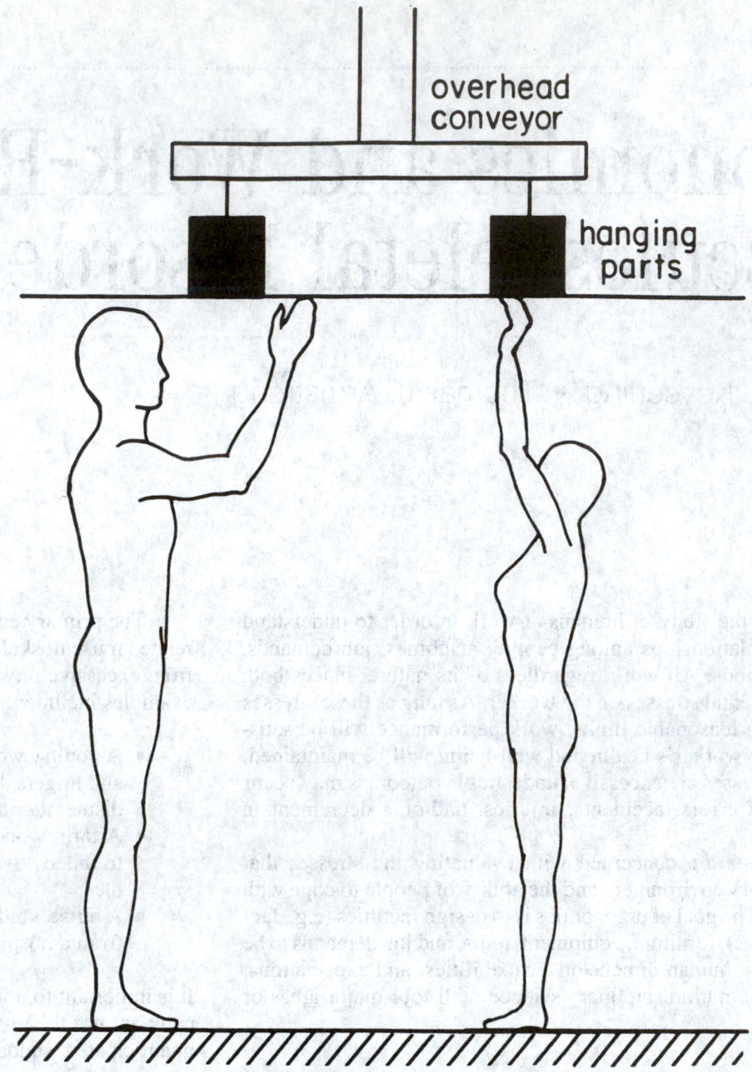

Figure 31-1. For safety reasons, an overhead conveyor should be higher than the stature of a tall worker (95th percentile male illustrated). This can create a difficult reach for a short worker (5th percentile female illustrated).

provide sufficient overhead clearance to accommodate 95 percent of the U.S. male population by positioning the conveyor so that the lowest point of the hung parts is 189.4 cm (74.6 inches) above the floor. (Note: This dimension is computed using nude stature data for a 95th percentile male from Table 31-1 and adding 2.5 cm (1 inch) as an adjustment for shoes.[5,10] With this design, a short worker (a 5th percentile female is illustrated) can reach the parts only by raising the shoulder into an elevated, awkward position, which may cause fatigue and/or musculoskeletal injury in the shoulder region.[11] In this situation, there is no simple solution that will simultaneously satisfy the needs of persons who are very tall or very short.

The characterization of body size must consider the large variations in dimensions from person to person and from population to population. Consequently, statistical methods are used to analyze body dimensions and the results are typically reported as means and standard deviations for various body segments.[12] Extensive tables of these statistics are available in reference texts.[4–6,10,12] By assuming that dimensions follow the "normal" or "log-normal" distribution, statistical procedures can be used to compute dimensions for various percentiles of the population of interest. Table 31-1 and Figure 31-2 present a summary of useful body dimensions for anthropometric applications.

In the following sections, several examples are presented that illustrate how awkward postures can contribute to the onset of fatigue and musculoskeletal and nerve disorders. Body posture is frequently determined by the physical dimensions of a work station and the location and orientation of equipment and tools. Anthropometric methods can be used during the design of work stations to avoid situations that require the use of awkward working postures.

▶ FATIGUE

Repeated or sustained exertions are associated with a constellation of performance impairments and symptoms that are collectively referred to as fatigue. Fatigue is typically characterized as "whole body" or "localized." Whole body fatigue is associated with activities where the work load is distributed over many parts of the body (e.g., legs, torso, and arms) concurrently, causing high rates of energy expenditure, such as when walking briskly, shoveling snow, or stacking containers. Localized fatigue is associated with tasks in which one segment of the body performs repeated or sustained work, e.g., forearm fatigue when using a hand tool, shoulder fatigue associated with overhead work, or back fatigue resulting from sustained trunk flexion.

Fatigue not only affects how workers feel; it also affects their ability to manipulate parts and tools precisely and may increase their risk of an accident. Symptoms of localized fatigue include localized discomfort, a sense of tiredness, reduced strength, reduced motor control, and tremor. In addition, there are circulatory, biochemical, and electrical changes within the muscle tissue.

TABLE 31-1. BODY DIMENSIONS FOR 5TH, 50TH, AND 95TH PERCENTILES OF THE U.S. CIVILIAN POPULATION

	U. S. Civilian Females			U. S. Civilian Males		
Dimension	***5th Percentile***	***50th Percentile***	***95th Percentile***	***5th Percentile***	***50th Percentile***	***95th Percentile***
Stature (cm)	151.1	161.5	172.2	163.6	175.3	186.9
Floor-knee	43.1	46.0	49.1	46.6	50.0	53.3
Floor-hip	80.1	85.6	91.3	86.7	92.9	99.1
Floor-elbow	95.2	101.7	108.5	103.1	110.4	117.7
Floor-shoulder	123.6	132.1	140.9	133.8	143.4	152.9
Floor-eye	141.4	151.2	161.2	153.1	164.1	174.9
Floor-finger	57.0	60.9	64.9	61.7	66.1	70.5
Floor-wrist	73.3	78.3	83.5	79.3	85.0	90.6
Sagittal plane-shoulder	19.5	20.8	22.2	21.1	22.6	24.1
Shoulder-elbow	28.1	30.0	32.0	30.4	32.6	34.8
Elbow-wrist	22.1	23.6	25.1	23.9	25.6	27.3
Wrist-finger	16.3	17.4	18.6	17.7	18.9	20.2
Foot length	23.0	24.5	26.2	24.9	26.6	28.4
Foot breadth	8.5	9.0	9.6	9.2	9.8	10.5

Stature from NASA[10] and link lengths from Drillis and Contini.[13]

Localized fatigue entails physiological and biomechanical processes.[14,15] Muscle contraction results in consumption of substrates and accumulation of by-products. At low-level exertions, blood flow increases and these concentrations are maintained at work levels. At high exertion levels, increased muscle pressure and deformation of the vascular bed impede circulation, and concentrations of substrates and metabolites become excessive. In addition to increased muscle pressure, there also is deformation of connective tissues that causes pain and may be a precursor to chronic soft tissue injuries.

Localized fatigue can develop over periods as short as several seconds or as long as several hours. Similarly, recovery occurs within periods of seconds, minutes, or hours and should be complete after a night of rest, or in extreme cases, after a few days. Altering the work activity will generally provide prompt relief of fatigue symptoms. For

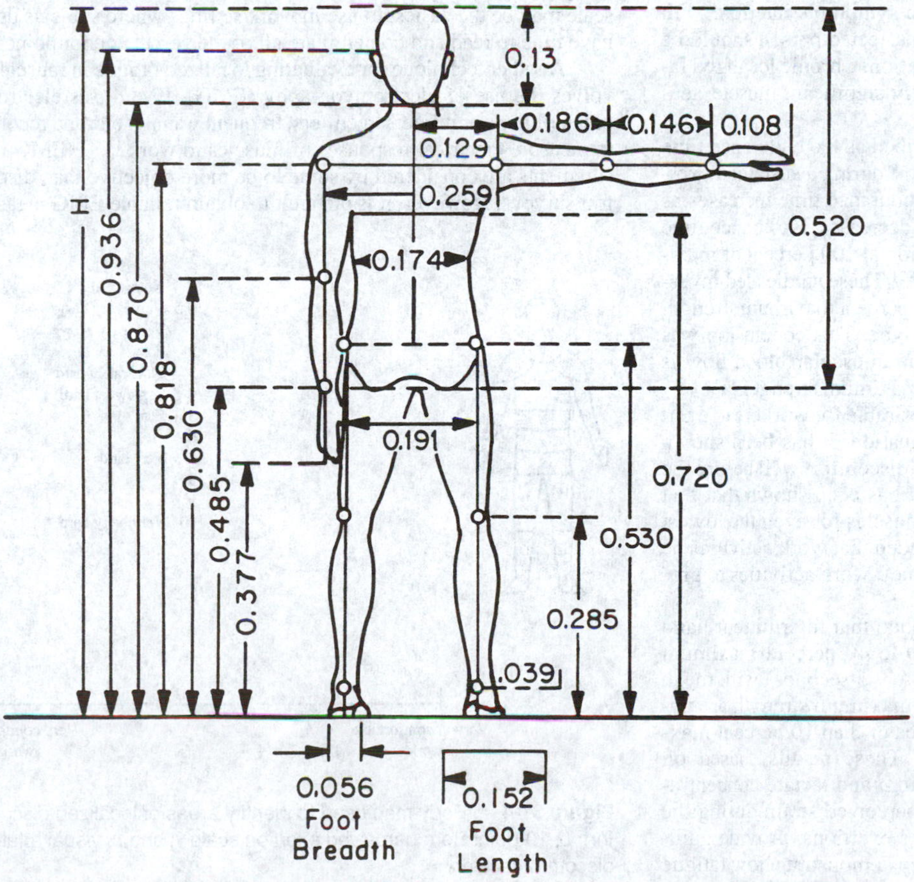

Figure 31-2. Link lengths of body segments expressed as a proportion of stature. (From Drillis R, Contini R: Body Segment Parameters. Department of Health, Education and Welfare, Office of Vocational Rehabilitation, Report No 1166-03. New York: New York University School of Engineering and Science, 1966.)

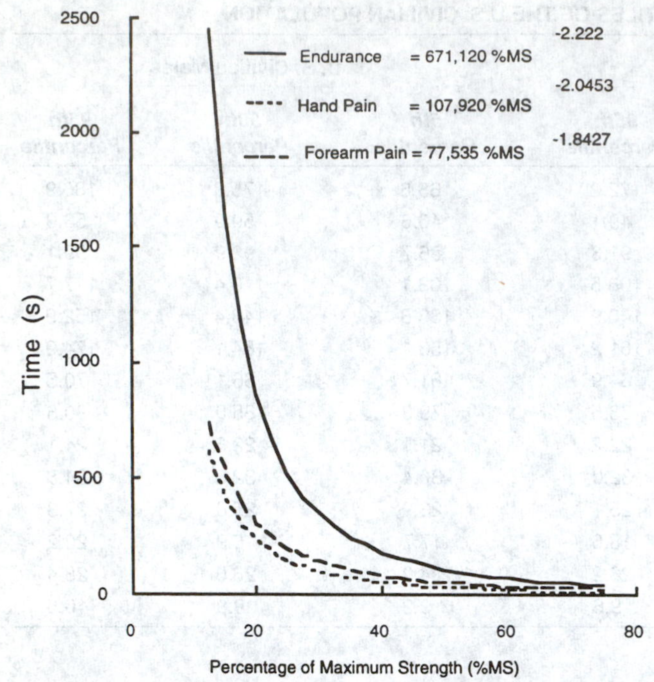

Figure 31-3. Average work endurance, time to hand pain, and time to forearm pain are shown plotted as functions of percentage of maximum strength for two college females and two college males. (From Armstrong TJ: Circulatory and Local Muscle Responses to Static Manual Work. Ann Arbor, MI: University of Michigan, 1976.)

example, a seated operator usually gets relief from stretching, changing seat position, standing up, or from a night of rest. If altering the work activity or posture does not provide prompt relief, if symptoms persist from one day to the next, or if the symptoms interfere with activities of work or daily living, then the affected person should be referred to a health care provider for evaluation. Chronic localized fatigue may be a harbinger of more clinically significant muscle, tendon, and nerve disorders.[16–18]

Localized fatigue has also been described as the endurance time prior to the onset of objectionable discomfort during a sustained exertion. Numerous studies have shown that endurance time increases as the intensity (forcefulness of the exertion) decreases. Endurance time is only a few seconds for a sustained exertion at 100 percent of maximum strength as shown in Figure 31-3.[15,19–21] These studies led investigators to conclude that exertions below 15 percent maximum strength could be sustained indefinitely without fatigue. This conclusion was also supported by studies showing that intramuscular blood flow is unimpeded in exertions below 15 percent maximum strength.[15,22]

Under most circumstances, it is not desirable for workers to exert themselves to the point of complete exhaustion. It has been shown that workers will experience objectionable discomfort well before the point of exhaustion[20,23–25] (Figure 31-3). It has been shown that that significant fatigue occurs within parts of muscles for even the lowest levels of exertion.[16–28] Thus it is recommended that work activities be designed so that workers can rest or alter their work activities to provide periods of rest as needed.

Bystrom and Fransson-Hall[29] concluded that intermittent hand exertions (5 seconds of static work at 10 to 40 percent maximum strength alternating with rest periods of 3 to 7.5 seconds) with mean contraction forces greater than 17 percent maximum strength are unacceptable, while continuous exertions greater than 10 percent maximum strength were also unacceptable. These results, based on strength, electromyography, blood potassium and lactate concentrations, muscle blood flow, heart rate, and perceived strain during the exertions and up to 24 hours following the exertions, provide guidance for design of work activities. They also demonstrate how fatigue is a complex process involving multiple physiological and biomechanical mechanisms, which are dependent on the intensity and temporal qualities of exertion.

Thus fatigue can be assessed through the intensity, location, and consistency of discomfort.[24–26] Advantages of using discomfort for assessing fatigue are: (*a*) it is relevant to how workers feel, (*b*) it provides information about many tissues and parts of the body, and (*c*) it requires minimum equipment. Disadvantages are: (*a*) it requires worker cooperation, (*b*) it can be hard to separate the symptoms of work-related fatigue from other causes, and (*c*) it is necessary to study multiple workers to control intrasubject and intersubject variability.

In its simplest form, assessment of effort or discomfort entails asking workers how they feel; however, it is important to ask the question in a way that does not suggest that they should be experiencing discomfort or pain. It also is important to ask the question so that the actual areas of discomfort can be identified. Several scales and procedures have been suggested and used for this purpose. The Borg scale on which 10 verbal anchor points are arranged in a geometric progression on a 14-point scale is widely used for assessing the intensity of fatigue.[30] The original scale (which ranged from 6 to 20 with verbal anchor points on a geometric progression) showed a high correlation with heart rate among subjects running on a treadmill. The Borg scale was later modified to use a 0 to 10 scale with the same anchor points. The modified version, shown in Figure 31-4, is used most widely today. It can be argued that perceived exertion data should be treated as ordinal data and analyzed using nonparametric statistics, but many investigators use parametric analyses. Borg characterized these scales as categorical with analog properties.[30]

Another way to query a worker is with a visual analog scale. Visual analog scales are lines with verbal anchor points at various locations.[26,31] The subjects place a check at the location on the line that corresponds to the level of their perceived discomfort or effort (Figure 31- 4). Studies by Harms-Ringdahl[26] found that subject ratings of elbow pain using the 10-point Borg scale and a visual analog scale agreed favorably; Ulin et al.[31] reported similar findings for subjects using powered hand tools. As a practical matter, the visual analog scale may be the easiest to use in work settings where subjects do not have time to read and contemplate all of the verbal anchor points.

Another technique for evaluating localized fatigue in muscles involves the use of electromyography (EMG). EMG uses electrodes, preamplifiers, amplifiers, rectifiers, frequency analyzers, and recorders to measure electrical responses of muscles to work.[14,23,32] EMG measurements are considered by some to be more objective than discomfort surveys. However, it is difficult to obtain reliable EMG measure-

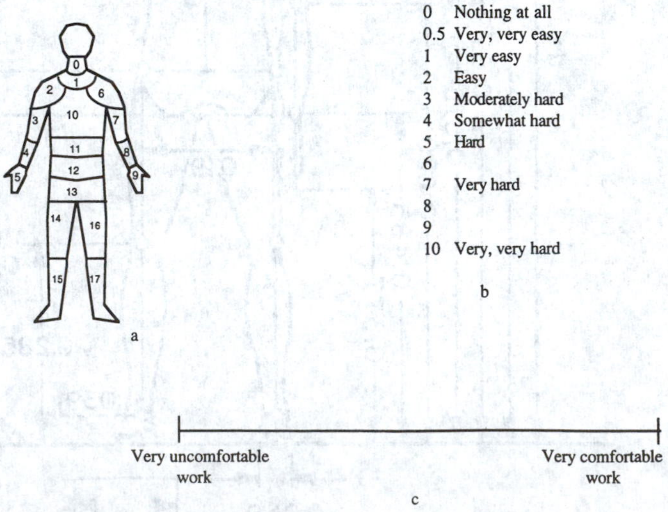

Figure 31-4. *a*, Body map used to identify areas of localized discomfort; *b*, 10-point Borg perceived exertion scale[30]; and *c*, visual analog discomfort scale.

ments on some subjects and in certain work environments; and the intrasubject and intersubject variability of those measurements may be quite high. EMG responses are most useful after the affected muscles have been identified using discomfort surveys or other methods. Use of EMG is beyond the scope of this discussion.

To summarize, localized fatigue is characterized as discomfort and/or performance decrement caused by repeated or sustained exertions. The development of and recovery from localized fatigue can occur in seconds, minutes, or hours. Failure to control localized fatigue through the design of work equipment and/or the effective management of work activities may lead to more severe, long-lasting pain or recognized medical conditions. Workers who experience persistent symptoms should be referred to a qualified health care provider.

▶ CHRONIC WORK-RELATED MUSCULOSKELETAL DISORDERS

Musculoskeletal disorders are a leading cause of worker impairment, lost work, and compensation. There is strong evidence that both personal and work-related factors are important in the pathogenesis of these disorders. The World Health Organization uses the term "work related" to characterize disorders that involve both personal and work-related factors and distinguishes them from occupational diseases where the entire cause is attributed to work exposures.[17,33,34] Frequently cited personal factors associated with chronic musculoskeletal disorders include history of certain injuries or illnesses, age, vitamin deficiencies, gender, and obesity. Work factors include repeated or sustained exertions, high forces, certain postures, mechanical contact stresses, low temperature, and vibration. Personal factors are important and should be considered during clinical assessments of patients and controlled in studies of the causes and amelioration of work-related musculoskeletal disorders.

Other terms such as cumulative trauma disorders, repetitive strain injuries, and overexertion injuries and overuse syndromes are sometimes used in place of the term "work-related musculoskeletal disorders" (WMSDs).[17,34] These terms are not intended to be used in place of specific diagnoses such as tendinitis, epicondylitis, bursitis, fibromyalgia, or carpal tunnel syndrome for the upper extremity; or sciatica, spondylosis, or osteoarthrosis for the lower back. WMSDs refer to a group of disorders that possess work activities as a common factor. Some important characteristic of WMSDs include:

1. Their pathogenesis involves both mechanical and physiological processes;
2. Weeks, months, and years may be required for them to develop;
3. Weeks, months, and years may be required for recovery, and in extreme cases, recovery may never be complete;
4. Their symptoms are often nonspecific, poorly localized, and episodic;
5. They often go unreported.

Mechanical processes refer to the deformation and, in some cases, damage that results from exertions and movements of the body. Physiological processes refer to pain and metabolic, repair, and adaptive responses that result from deformation of tissue.

The symptoms of WMSDs set them apart from acute injures such as lacerations or fractures where there is a conspicuous event and conspicuous effect that can be observed by a health care provider, supervisor, or coworker. Work factors associated with WMSDs are often overlooked, and the symptoms may not be observable by a third party. Workers themselves may not recognize an association between what they do at work and how they feel. This may explain why WMSDs are often under reported. Even when workers do suspect an association with their job, they may be reluctant to report their condition to an employer for fear of loosing their job. These factors contribute to the great reporting differences of WMSDs that sometimes occur between one site and another.

WMSDs are observed most frequently in the upper extremity and the lower back, as discussed in the following sections.

▶ WORK-RELATED MUSCULOSKELETAL DISORDERS OF THE UPPER EXTREMITY

Morbidity

One of the earliest references to these disorders is that of Bernardino Ramazzini[35] who in 1713 attributed "diseases reaped by certain workers" to "violent and irregular motions and unnatural postures." Gray[36] in 1893 described "washer-women's sprain," which is commonly referred to as de Quervain's disease, or tendinitis of the extrinsic abductor and extensor muscles of the thumb near the radial styloid process.[37]

Reports of insurance claims due to tendinitis were recorded in the early twentieth century. For example, from Swiss insurance records in 1927 Zollinger[38] reported 929 cases of crepitant tenosynovitis attributed to repeated strain. The work-relatedness and compensability of musculoskeletal disorders has been surrounded with controversy starting with the implementation of workers' compensation laws in the early part of this century. Conn reported that the state of Ohio, following 12 years of debate in the state legislature, amended its state workers' compensation rules in 1931 to include musculoskeletal disorders.[39]

The controversy centers on how causation is divided between personal and work-related factors. Work-related musculoskeletal disorders are now compensable in most states of the United States; however, the rules and reporting behavior may vary considerably from one state to another. In most cases, workers must initiate a claim against their employer to receive compensation. This may create an adversarial relationship, which may inhibit some workers from taking action. While workers compensation claims provide valuable documentation of the severity of work-related musculoskeletal disorders, only in a few cases have investigators been able to develop meaningful generalizations from compensation data.[40,41]

The reporting of work-related musculoskeletal disorders has increased substantially since the passage of the 1970 Occupational Safety and Health Act.[42] This law created the regulations that require the reporting of work-related musculoskeletal disorders and established the Occupational Safety and Health Administration (OSHA) to enforce those regulations. Under OSHA regulations, employers are required to maintain a record of all work-related musculoskeletal disorders or

> disorders associated with repeated trauma. Examples include: . . . synovitis, tenosynovitis, and bursitis; Raynaud's phenomena; and other conditions due to repeated motion, vibration, and pressure.[43]

The Department of Labor uses such records for determining if employers are in compliance with the General Duty Clause of the Occupational Safety and Health Act[42] which requires that

> Each employer shall furnish to each of his employees employment and a place of employment which are free from recognized hazards that are likely to cause death or serious physical harm to his employees.

Employers are expected to monitor WMSDs and intervene when new cases or high-risk jobs are identified. Like workers' compensation reports, the incidence of musculoskeletal disorders based on OSHA reports will vary considerably from site to site.[40]

In summary, the overall prevalence, incidence, and severity of various WMSDs of the upper extremity in the United States are not yet available. The data that are available suggest that, while there is significant underreporting, these disorders are a major cause of impairment and work disability.

Individual and Work-Related Risk Factors

Commonly cited individual risk factors include age, female gender, acute trauma, rheumatoid arthritis, diabetes mellitus, hormonal factors, wrist size or shape, and vitamin deficiency.[34] These factors

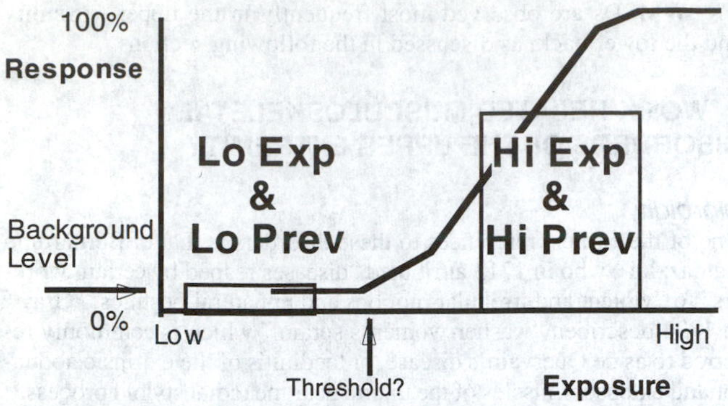

Figure 31-5. Exposure-response relationship between WMSDs and work factors.

should be evaluated as possible causes in each reported case; however, the sensitivity and specificity of these factors is not sufficient for use as a screening test at the time of employment to identify workers at risk. Even if such tests were available, affirmative action regulations would require employers to show that workplace modifications to accommodate "at-risk" workers are unfeasible before those workers could be denied employment. Attempts to use individual risk factors for worker selection or screening should be regarded as experimental and must include appropriate safeguards for risks and rights. It may be advisable to monitor workers with recognized personal risk factors and to counsel these individuals in regard to the potential risks of certain types of work.

Work-related factors include repeated and sustained exertions, forceful exertions, certain postures, mechanical contact stress, vibration, low temperatures, and work organization.[17,34,44] It has been shown that the prevalence of WMSDs increases with exposure to certain risk factors; however, it is not known at what level the risk becomes significantly elevated for a single factor or combination of work factors (Fig. 31-5). While it is not yet possible to state specific design standards for equipment and work procedures, it is possible to identify some of the most conspicuous risk factors, to identify possible work-related causes when new cases are reported, and to modify jobs to accommodate affected workers and prevent future cases.

Control of Upper Extremity WMSDs

A process for controlling WMSDs, presently under consideration as a voluntary standard/guideline in the United States, is shown in Figure 31-6.[45] It includes surveillance for identification of new cases, ongoing analysis of available health data, and proactive inspections of workplaces and jobs for possible risk factors. It also includes evaluation, treatment, and follow-up of new cases, and analysis, design, and evaluation of new or significantly changed jobs. Finally, it includes management commitment, education of company personnel and health care providers, and worker involvement. The process is intended as a general model that can be tailored to the needs of each organization and be integrated into existing programs rather than duplicate them. It is recognized that the needs of a large manufacturing organization will be different than those of a small office. Employers are referred to their

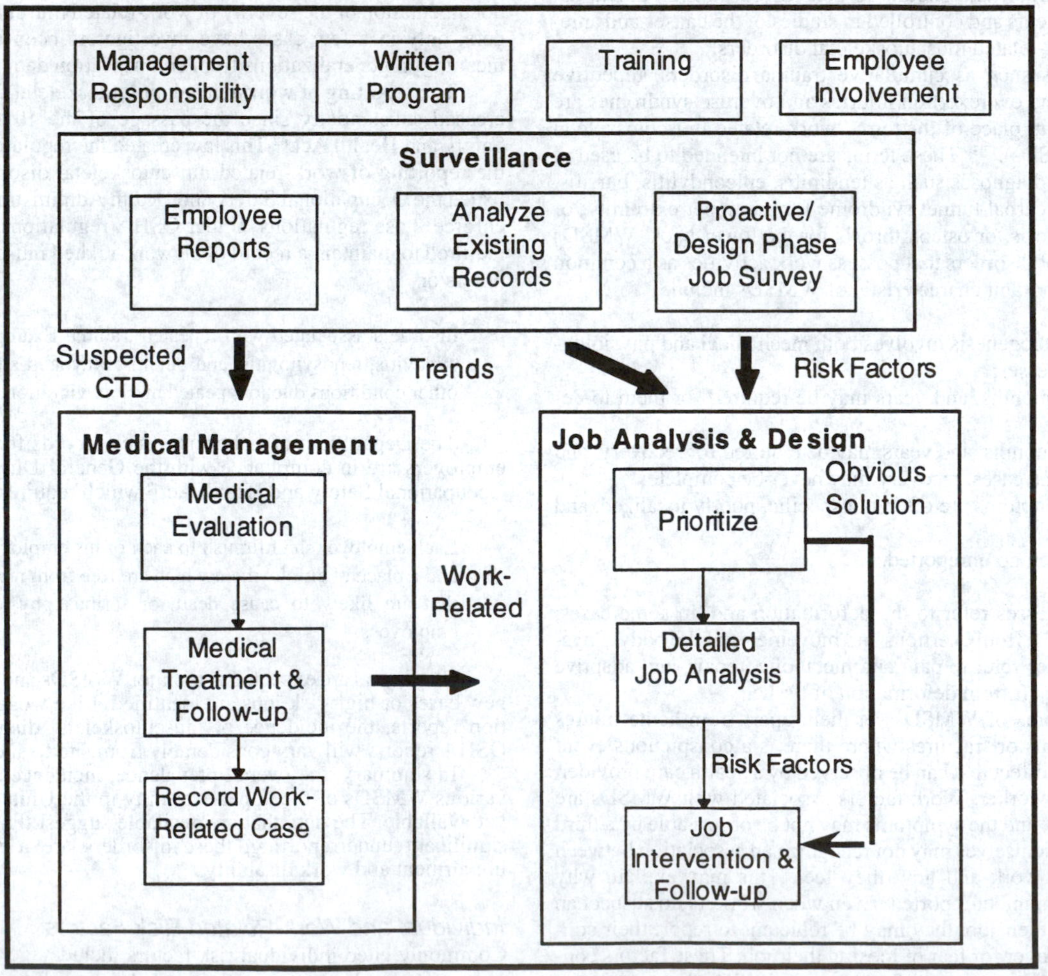

Figure 31-6. A control program for WMSDs.[45]

respective trade organizations and workers compensation carriers for guidance on implementation of a control program.

Surveillance

Surveillance entails (*a*) to the extent possible, identifying and evaluating all musculoskeletal disorders for possible work relatedness; (*b*) periodically reviewing available medical records for musculoskeletal disorders; and (*c*) proactive surveys of the workplace for risk factors at the time of program implementation or following a substantive change in work equipment or procedures. While analysis of available injury and illness data is recommended, it is often difficult to identify areas or processes with statistically elevated risks because of the small numbers of workers.[46,47] For example, to have an 80 percent chance of finding a difference between one population with a 10 percent prevalence rate and a second population with a 20 percent prevalence rate with a with 5 percent chance of a type I error would require 196 persons in each group.[48] In addition, at least several months are generally required for the effects of a given job, method, or tool change to stabilize. Unfortunately, most work populations are not stable enough to rigorously evaluate all possible factors. There is turnover in the workforce, due to work and nonwork causes, changes in production schedules, plant shutdowns, etc. For this reason it is recommended that all cases be identified and investigated.

Surveillance may also be supplemented with worker surveys and medical examinations. Surveys provide information about overall discomfort or morbidity patterns; however, most survey instruments do not yet have sufficient sensitivity or specificity to be used for case screening or medical diagnosis.[49,50]

Analysis of Jobs

The number of jobs at a given work site may vary from only a few to several thousand, and there may not be sufficient resources to examine them all in detail. The level of detail required for analyzing jobs depends on the purpose of the analysis. In some cases, it will be better to obtain a little information about a lot of jobs rather than a lot of information about a few jobs. A walk-through inspection of the production facility may be sufficient to confirm that the production process has not changed since a previous study or to find out about the types of equipment, materials, and methods used. In some cases these walk-through inspections may be supplemented with critiques of representative jobs.[50] If high levels of exposure to risk factors are found, it may be desirable to perform more-detailed analyses to quantify those stresses, understand their causes, and design interventions.[44,46]

Job analysis is divided into four steps: 1) documentation of the job, 2) analysis of stresses, 3) design of interventions, and 4) evaluation of intervention effectiveness. Documentation is the collection of the information necessary to identify and quantify risk factors WMSDs. Documentation is based on traditional industrial engineering work methods analysis and entails collection of data for a systematic evaluation of the job.[51,52] The following items are determined during job documentation:

- *Objective:* why the job is performed.
- *Standards:* production quantity and quality expectations.
- *Staffing:* the number of workers performing the job.
- *Method:* the steps required to perform each task.
- *Workstation layout:* blueprints or a sketch of the workplace with dimensions that can be used to determine reach distances.
- *Materials:* parts and substances used in the production process.
- *Tools:* devices used to accomplish the work.
- *Environment:* conditions at and near the workstation.

Analysis of Work Factors

The ergonomic assessment of work factors entails characterization of stresses that may contribute to WMSDs. Stresses can be identified, ranked, and rated from observations by the analyst.[53,54] Jobs may be analyzed from direct workplace observations and measurements or from video tapes. An advantage of video tapes is that they may be played repeatedly and/or slowed down. A disadvantage is that it may be hard to see the entire job in a video tape. Worker ratings also may be used to quantify physical stresses; however, care should be exercised to not ask workers leading questions.[55] Observations and ratings may be supplemented with measurements of physical parameters of the work such as the cycle time, weights of tools, and locations of work objects. They may also be supplemented with physiological and biomechanical measurements such as muscle activity and joint position.[46,56–58] The best method of assessing work stresses depends on the purpose of the analysis and available resources.

Repeated and Sustained Exertions. The number of exertions per hour or shift can be estimated from the work standard and methods analysis. Assessments of repeated exertions should take into consideration the frequency and speed of exertions as well as the recovery time between exertions. Ratings may be tailored to specific operations such as keyboard work, grinding, welding, assembly, etc. In some cases, the rating can be supplemented with measurements of cycle time, number of exertions per unit time, or instrumental measurements of muscle activity and/or joint motions. Ratings and measurements may be averaged over tasks and breaks.

Forceful Exertions. Forces can be identified by inspecting the work methods for steps that involve resisting gravity, surface finishing operations (e.g., grinding, polishing, or trimming), or tool reaction forces (using a manual or powered tool to tighten a screw or nut). Forces generally vary from the beginning to the end of a work cycle. Consider for example a job in which a worker gets parts one at a time and installs them onto a passing unit on an assembly line. The hand force required to reach for the part is negligible, the force required to transfer the part is 20 percent of maximum muscle strength, and the force required to install the part is 60 percent of maximum strength. The average force across all tasks is 10 percent of maximum strength. Using a 10-point scale for rating force, this job would be given average and peak ratings of 1 and 6, respectively. As pointed out above, most people cannot sustain an average force exertion greater than 10 to 20 percent of maximum strength without excessive fatigue. Force can also be assessed using electromyography and direct measurements. Jonsson has proposed a method in which the normalized EMG measurements (0 to 100 percent of maximum) are presented as a cumulative frequency histogram, called an amplitude probability distribution.[56,57] Armstrong et al.[59] used force gauges under keyboards to measure forces exerted during typing.

Assessments of force requirements should take the following factors into consideration:

- the magnitude of weight, resistance, and reaction forces
- the effects of friction
- balance (well-balanced tools require lower exertions than poorly balanced tools)
- posture (pinch grips require higher exertions than power grips)
- pace
- gloves

Jobs that require workers to get, hold, or use heavy objects will require more force than jobs that require workers to get, hold, or use light objects in the same way. Ratings should be adjusted upward if objects or glove surfaces are slippery, or if objects are poorly balanced or supported with the ends of the fingers. Ratings also should be increased for rapid movements or if stiff or bulky gloves are used.

Posture Stresses. Stressful postures can be identified by inspecting work elements for steps that involve repeated or sustained maximum reaches; elevation of the elbows, reaching behind the torso, full elbow flexion, full forearm rotation, ulnar/radial wrist deviation, wrist flexion, full wrist extension, or a pinch grip. Posture analysis may be performed by directly observing the job or from videotapes that are played back in slow motion. The analysis should examine each joint, e.g., neck, shoulder, elbow, wrist, and hand. Also, it often is possible to predict posture on the basis of the workstation design and tool specifications.[44] Posture stress ratings should be increased as deviation from neutral positions, duration, and frequency increase. Posture, like force, varies from the beginning to the end of the work cycle. Consequently, the minimum, maximum, and average values should be considered in the analysis. Postures can also be assessed with computers using goniometers attached to the joint of interest.[58]

Localized Mechanical Stresses. Localized contact stresses can be calculated as the force acting on the body, divided by the area of contact. Consequently, the average contact stress will be lower if the weight of the arm is distributed over a padded surface than if it is rested on the sharp edge of a work surface. Stresses may not be uniformly distributed due to the irregular shapes of the workstation and tools, as well as the bones. Stresses can be identified by inspecting work methods for steps that involve contact of the body with external objects. Average and peak stresses should be considered in the analysis.

Low Temperature. Exposure to low temperature affects how workers hold and use tools, peripheral circulation, and neurological symptoms of existing nerve disorders. Adverse effects may occur when the skin temperature falls below 20°C. Exposure to low temperatures can be identified by inspecting work methods for steps that result in exposure to cold air, tools, and/or materials. Rankings may be based on temperature, but should be adjusted for thermal conductivity and protective equipment. Ratings also should be adjusted for clothing, as finger skin temperature is affected by the body's core temperature.

Vibration Exposure. Vibration refers to the cyclical displacement of an object and has properties of frequency and amplitude. Available evidence suggests that vibration exerts a direct action on soft tissue and that it affects the way workers hold and use work objects.[16,60] Vibration is often reported as a velocity or an acceleration. Acceleration is often reported because accelerometers are widely used to measure vibration.[60] Instrumental measurements are beyond the scope of this discussion, but vibration exposure can be identified by inspecting work methods for steps that involve the use of stationary or hand-held power tools, impact tools, or controls connected to vibrating equipment. In the absence of proper instrumentation, ratings may be based on the duration and amplitude of contact with vibrating objects. For example, a grinding or buffing job would probably be rated higher in terms of vibration stress than an assembly job that requires periodic use of a powered wrench.

Organizational Factors. Assessment of ergonomic stresses may be supplemented by worker interviews. Interviews should be carefully designed to avoid suggesting to workers how they should feel. Also it is important that all workers be asked the same question. One way of doing this is through the use of surveys in which workers rate discomfort or perceived exertion. An example of a survey in which a visual analog scale was used to assess the weights used in an automobile trim shop is shown in Figure 31-7.[55] These data show a significant increase in ratings towards "too heavy" as the tool mass increases above 2 kg. It cannot be said that workers will not develop WMSDs if they use tools less than 2 kg, but in the absence of better data, worker ratings may be used as a design or selection benchmark. Designing lifting tasks to match acceptable levels of perceived exertion has been reported to reduce the risk of overexertion disorders of the back.[61] While this has not been shown for upper limb disorders, it is a tenable hypothesis.

Intervention and Evaluation of Control Methods

Work elements ranked high in terms of ergonomic stresses should be redesigned to minimize those stresses. Possible strategies may focus on the redesign or modification of methods, tools, workstations, and production processes. Worker training may help workers to select and use tools properly or to properly adjust their workstations, but in many cases ergonomic stresses result from the work requirements and cannot be reduced through training.

As has been previously stated, there are not yet specification standards for acceptable levels of ergonomic stress. Therefore, it is necessary to evaluate interventions to ascertain their effectiveness. Evaluation may be accomplished through reanalysis of the job, measures of localized discomfort or exertion, and ongoing surveillance of health data. These procedures have been described above.

▶ OCCUPATIONAL LOW BACK PAIN

Low back pain is a nonspecific condition that refers to complaints of acute or chronic pain and discomfort in or near the lumbosacral spine that can be caused by inflammatory, degenerative, neoplastic, gynecologic, traumatic, metabolic, and other types of disorders.[62] A large number of disease conditions have been associated with low back pain, including sciatica, lumbago, spondylosis, osteoarthrosis, and degenerative disc disease.[63] However, most episodes of work-related back pain cannot be associated with a specific lesion. Therefore, in most epidemiologic studies of occupational low back pain, the specific cause is not identified. Typically, all categories are grouped together as an idiopathic condition with similar reported symptoms.[64]

Because the causes of back pain are so poorly understood, it is difficult to specify a treatment plan. In most episodes, people with

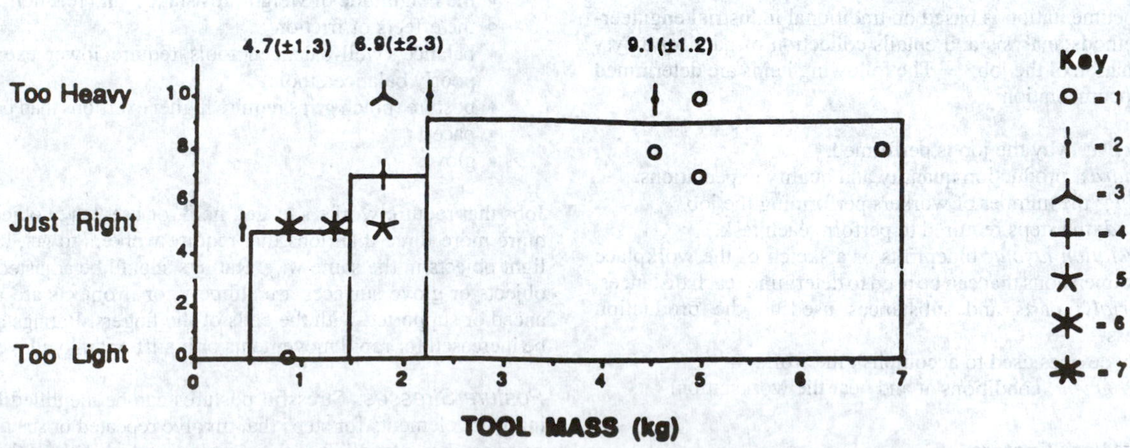

Figure 31-7. Ratings of 33 tools by 22 workers show that tools in excess of 2 kg were considered "too heavy" in an automobile trim shop. (From Armstrong TJ, Punnett L, Ketner P: Subjective worker assessments of hand tools used in automobile assembly. Am Ind Hyg Assoc J 50:639–645, 1989.)

back pain are able to continue working and cope with the problem without seeking medical treatment. Among disabling cases, most resolve themselves within a 2-week period using only conservative treatment (bed rest and pain medication). Isometric abdominal exercises have also been shown to be effective as part of a conservative management strategy. Surgery should not be considered during the first 3 months unless indicated by a specific diagnosis.[65]

Low back pain is one of the most common and costliest health problems in industrialized societies. In Scandinavia, approximately 80 percent of adults experience at least one episode of back pain during their working years (ages 18 to 65).[66] A recent study of workers in an American aircraft manufacturing company showed a lifetime incidence rate of 60 percent for males and 55 percent for females.[67] Because many episodes of low back pain are disabling, it is the most costly occupational health problem in the United States. It is estimated that 2 to 5 percent of U.S. workers file injury claims for back pain each year.[68–70] Direct medical costs for low back pain in the United States during 1990 were estimated at more than $24 billion. When Workers' Compensation indemnity payments and other indirect costs are added to medical expenditures, the total cost of occupational low back pain in the United States is estimated to exceed $50 billion per year.[69]

Occupational risk factors associated with the development of back pain include:

1. *Forceful exertions during manual materials handling*, such as lifting, pushing, and/or pulling of heavy loads;[71–75]
2. *Awkward trunk postures*, such as flexion, lateral bending, axial twisting, and/or prolonged sitting;[75–78]
3. *Whole body vibration*, usually transmitted through a vibrating seat or platform;[79,80]
4. *Repetitive or prolonged exposure* to any of the above risk factors;[64,75,81]
5. *Work-related psychological or psychosocial stress*;[82]
6. *Slips and falls*.[74]

Note: For the first five risk factors listed above, workers are typically exposed on a continuing or ongoing basis, and it may be difficult to associate a back complaint with a specific incident or accident. Back pain complaints associated with slips and falls are different in the sense that the complaint can almost always be associated with a specific event.

Truck drivers experience elevated rates of back pain when compared to other occupational groups.[81] Many truck drivers load and unload their own rigs; this activity often requires heavy lifting combined with awkward posture (e.g., trunk flexion when bending down to grasp an object on the floor of the trailer). Truck drivers also spend a considerable portion of their workday in a sustained seated posture and may be exposed to high levels of whole body vibration if the vehicle and seat suspension systems do not adequately isolate the driver from roadway bumps and shocks. Finally, slips and falls are common in the truck-driving population due to the need to regularly ingress and egress tractors, working and walking outdoors on slippery surfaces in inclement weather, and maneuvering hand trucks on ramps and other irregular surfaces, sometimes with impeded vision (due to the size of packages that can partially block the visual field).

Other high-risk occupations include: nurses and nurses aides, garbage collectors, warehouse workers, and mechanics.[83] All of these occupations require heavy lifting and associated materials handling tasks.

Lifting and Back Pain

Because of the hazards associated with manual lifting, the National Institute for Occupational Safety and Health (NIOSH) developed guidelines for evaluating lifting tasks in 1981.[72] These guidelines were updated in 1993 in a monograph titled *Applications Manual for the Revised NIOSH Lifting Equation*.[84] This document discusses risk factors associated with lifting and describes procedures for analyzing and designing manual tasks to keep biomechanical, physiological, and psychophysical loads within acceptable limits.

To use the NIOSH lifting guidelines, it is necessary to measure the following eight task variables:

1. *Load weight (L):* measured in kilograms.
2. *Horizontal location (H):* the distance from the midpoint of a line connecting the ankles to a point on the floor directly below the load center as shown in Figure 31-8. This distance is measured in centimeters at the origin and destination of the lift.
3. *Vertical location (V):* the location of the hands at the origin of the lift, measured vertically from the floor or working surface in centimeters (Fig. 31-8).
4. *Vertical travel distance (D):* the vertical displacement of the object (origin to destination) over the course of the lift, measured in centimeters.
5. *Asymmetry angle (A):* angular displacement of the load from the front of the body (the midsagittal plane) at the origin and destination of the lift, measured in degrees as shown in Figure 31-9.
6. *Lifting frequency (F):* the average number of lifts per minute.
7. *Duration of lifting activities*: measured in hours.
8. *Coupling classification (C):* Quality of the hand-to-object coupling (i.e., gripping surface), classified as good, fair, or poor.

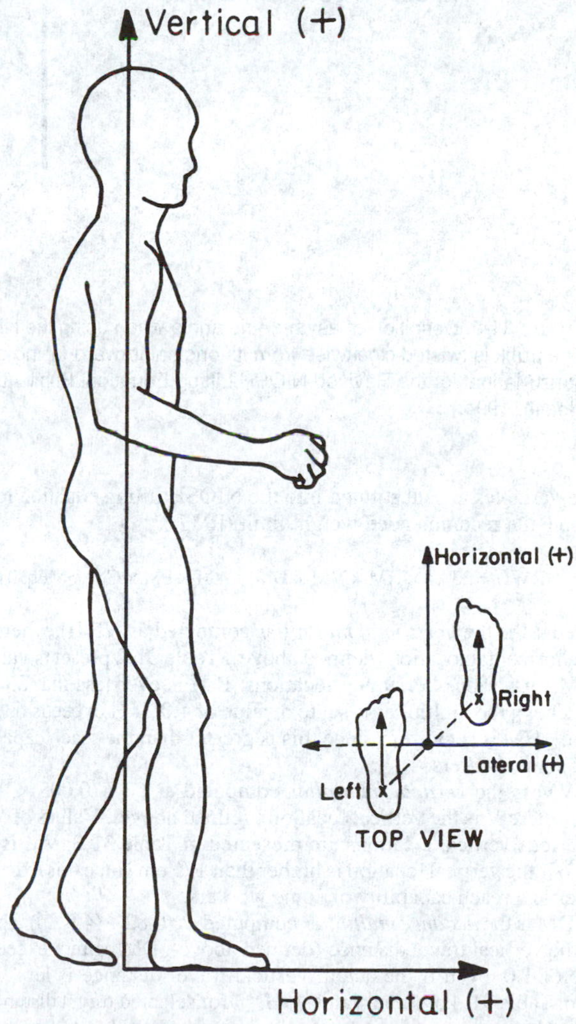

Figure 31-8. Definition of horizontal and vertical locations of the hands when using the NIOSH lifting equation. (Adapted from Waters TR, Putz-Anderson V, Garg A: Applications Manual for the Revised NIOSH Lifting Equation. Publication No. 94-110. Cincinnati: National Institute for Occupational Safety and Health, 1994.)

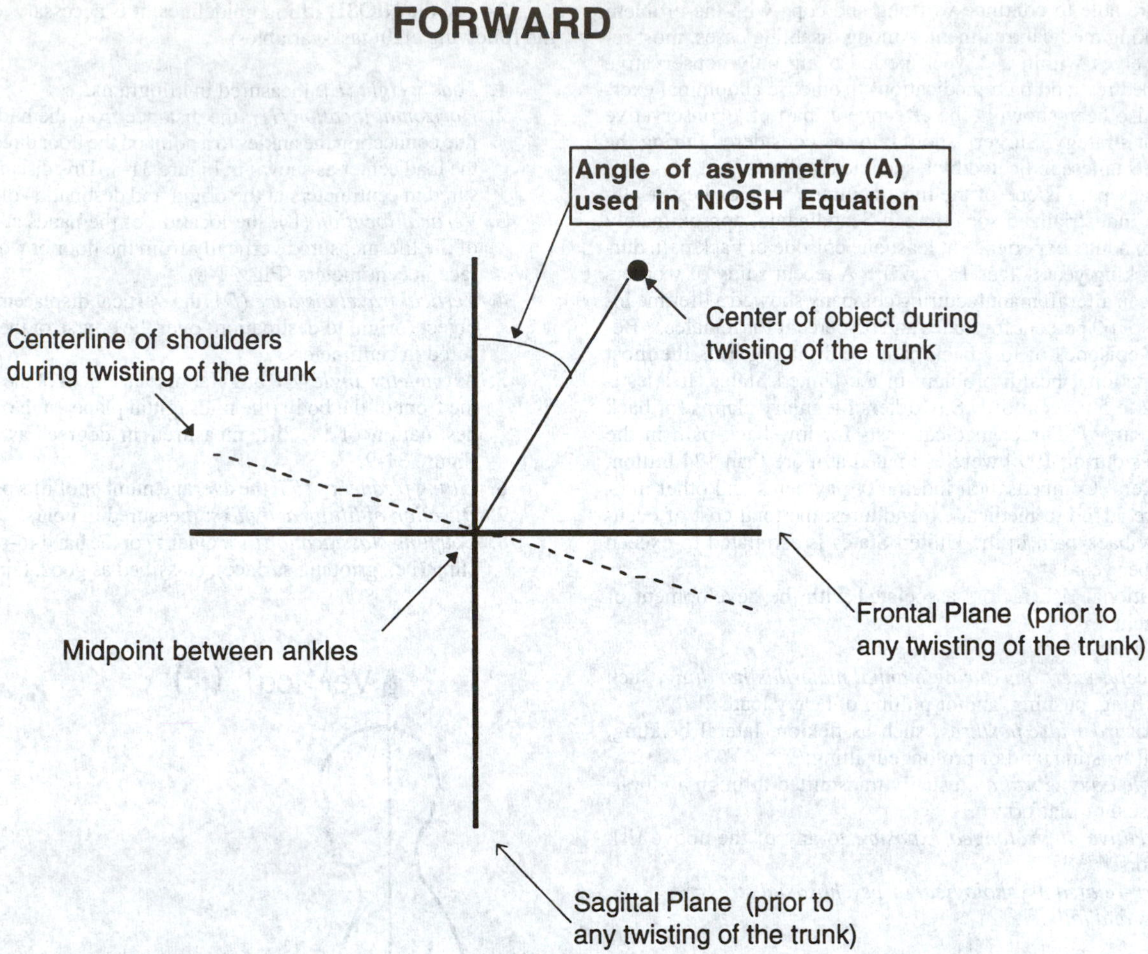

Figure 31-9. Definition of asymmetric angle when using the NIOSH lifting equation. View is looking down on the worker from above. The trunk is twisted clockwise from its original forward-facing orientation. (Adapted from Waters TR, Putz-Anderson V, Garg A: Applications Manual for the Revised NIOSH Lifting Equation. Publication No. 94-110. Cincinnati: National Institute for Occupational Safety and Health, 1994.)

These variables are substituted into the NIOSH lifting equation to compute the recommended weight limit (RWL):

$$RWL = 23\text{ kg} \times HM \times VM \times DM \times AM \times FM \times CM \qquad \text{(Eq. 31-1)}$$

where HM is the *horizontal multiplier* computed as (25/H), where H is the horizontal location (defined above). Table 31-2 presents values of HM for various horizontal locations. If H is ever less that 25 cm (10 inches), the multiplier is set to a value of 1.0. If H exceeds 63 cm (25 in.), HM is set to zero since this is greater than the reach capability of some workers.

VM is the *vertical multiplier* computed as $(1 - (0.003 \times |V - 75|))$, where V is the vertical location (defined above). Values of VM for various vertical locations are presented in Table 31-3. VM is set to zero if the vertical location is higher than 175 cm since this exceeds the vertical reach capability of some workers.

DM is the *distance multiplier* computed as $(0.82 + (4.5/D))$ where D is the vertical travel distance (defined above). DM cannot exceed a value of 1.0, even if the actual vertical travel distance is less than 25 cm. Table 31-4 presents values of DM for selected travel distances.

AM is the *asymmetric multiplier* computed as $(1 - 0.0032 \times A)$, where A is the angle of asymmetry (defined above). Values of AM for selected asymmetry angles are presented in Table 31-5.

FM is the *frequency multiplier* from Table 31-6. The purpose of the frequency multiplier is to adjust for fatigue that results from frequent and/or prolonged lifting. Note that it is necessary to consider both the *frequency* and *duration* of lifting activities to use Table 31-6. It is also necessary to consider the vertical location since low lifts involve lowering and raising the weight of the trunk and the head. This requires additional energy and may contribute to fatigue. (Note: NIOSH has not yet determined multipliers for jobs where the duration of lifting activities exceeds 8 hours.)

CM is the *coupling multiplier*. A "good" coupling (CM = 1.0) exists if the object is equipped with handles or hand-hole cutouts of sufficient size and clearance to accommodate a large hand. For loose objects without handles, a "good" coupling exists if the shape of the object allows the fingers to be comfortably wrapped around the object. A "fair" coupling (CM = 0.95) exists if the object has no handles or hand-holes, but the size, shape, and rigidity are such that the worker can comfortably clamp the fingers under the object (such as when lifting a corrugated case from the floor). "Poor" coupling (CM = 0.90) exists whenever the object is difficult to grasp (e.g., slippery surfaces, sharp edges, nonrigid shape, etc.). Large objects that require a hand separation distance of more than 40 cm are considered to have a poor coupling.

Once all the multipliers have been determined, use Equation 31-1 to compute the recommended weight limit for the lifting task. To estimate the relative level of stress associated with a lifting task, NIOSH defines the lifting index (LI) as the ratio of the load weight to the computed recommended weight limit:

$$LI = L / RWL \qquad \text{(Eq. 31-2)}$$

TABLE 31-2. VALUES OF THE HORIZONTAL MULTIPLIER (HM) FOR VARIOUS HORIZONTAL DISTANCES (H)

Horizontal Distance (H) (inches)	Horizontal Multiplier (HM)	Horizontal Distance (H) (cm)	Horizontal Multiplier (HM)
<10	1.00	<25	1.00
11	0.91	28	0.89
12	0.83	30	0.83
13	0.77	32	0.78
14	0.71	34	0.74
15	0.67	36	0.69
16	0.63	38	0.66
17	0.59	40	0.63
18	0.56	42	0.60
19	0.53	44	0.57
20	0.50	46	0.54
21	0.48	48	0.52
22	0.45	50	0.50
23	0.43	52	0.48
24	0.42	54	0.46
25	0.40	56	0.45
>25	0.00	58	0.43
		60	0.42
		63	0.40
		>63	0.00

Adapted from Waters TR, Putz-Anderson V, Garg A: Applications Manual for the Revised NIOSH Lifting Equation. Publication No. 94-110. Cincinnati: National Institute for Occupational Safety and Health, 1994.

The lifting index can be used to compare the relative hazard of two or more jobs or to prioritize lifting jobs for ergonomic interventions. NIOSH has taken the position that jobs with LI values greater than 1.0 pose an increased risk of lifting-related back pain for some fraction of the workforce. Furthermore, NIOSH believes that jobs should be designed to achieve a LI of 1.0 or less. For additional information on using the NIOSH lifting equation, including numerous detailed examples, refer to the *Applications Manual for the Revised NIOSH Lifting Equation.*[84]

The most effective way for reducing injuries and disorders associated with manual lifting is to implement engineering controls (i.e., changes in equipment, workstation layout, work methods, etc.) that reduce exposure to one or more of the risk factors discussed above. Possible approaches are briefly outlined below:

1. Reduce the weight of lifted items. For example, is it possible to put fewer parts in a tote pan or to resize bags containing bulk materials such as powdered chemicals?
2. If the weight of the load cannot be reduced, use a mechanical assist (e.g., hoist or articulating arm) to reduce the forces exerted by workers.
3. Eliminate low reaches by delivering objects to the worker at knee height or above. Provide an adjustable-height lift table to allow the worker to pick up objects without excessive trunk flexion.
4. Reduce horizontal reach distances by eliminating or relocating barriers that prevent a worker from getting as close to the object as is safely possible prior to starting the lift. Forward reaches should require no trunk flexion.
5. Reduce carrying distances by changing the workstation layout or by installing mechanized equipment (e.g., conveyors). Eliminate twisting by changing the layout or changing the task sequence.

If engineering controls do not reduce the lifting index to less than 1.0, administrative controls should be considered. A rotation scheme that allows workers to alternate between jobs with heavy lifting requirements and jobs with insignificant lifting requirements reduces cumulative exposure to lifting stresses. Although NIOSH does not endorse the use of worker selection tests, a limited number of studies have indicated that strength testing and/or aerobic capacity testing may be used to identify workers who can perform work activities where the lifting index exceeds 1.0 without significantly increasing their risk of work-related injury.[85,86] Employee selection testing, however, is a nontrivial process that requires extensive analysis of job demands and validation of all screening criteria.

Another type of administrative control sometimes suggested as a method for preventing back injuries that result from manual lifting is the industrial lifting support, commonly called a "back belt." Scientific scrutiny of the effectiveness of back belts has been limited. However, based on a review of relevant literature, NIOSH concluded that there is insufficient evidence to support the claim that back belts prevent injuries to healthy workers, and that back belts should not be considered personal protective equipment.[87] One recent study of airline baggage handlers found that worker compliance in wearing back belts is poor, with 58 percent of subjects discontinuing use after 8 months. Furthermore, workers who discontinued wearing belts had higher low back injury experience than a control group who never wore belts.[88]

Awkward Posture and Back Pain

Awkward trunk posture during work activities can be caused by poor workstation layout. The neutral position of the trunk occurs when it is in a vertical upright position with no axial twisting. Trunk flexion (forward bending in the sagittal plane) can usually be attributed to one of two causes: (*a*) reaching down to grasp an object that is lower than the level of the hands when standing with the arms hanging in

TABLE 31-3. VALUES OF THE VERTICAL MULTIPLIER (VM) FOR VARIOUS HORIZONTAL LOCATIONS (V)

Various Horizontal Locations (V) (inches)	Vertical Multiplier (VM)	Various Horizontal Locations (V) (cm.)	Vertical Multiplier (VM)
0	0.78	0	0.78
5	0.81	10	0.81
10	0.85	20	0.84
15	0.89	30	0.87
20	0.93	40	0.90
25	0.96	50	0.93
30	1.00	60	0.96
35	0.96	70	0.99
40	0.93	80	0.99
45	0.89	90	0.96
50	0.85	100	0.93
55	0.81	110	0.90
60	0.78	120	0.87
65	0.74	130	0.84
70	0.70	140	0.81
>70	0.00	150	0.78
		160	0.75
		170	0.72
		175	0.70
		>175	0.00

Adapted from Waters TR, Putz-Anderson V, Garg A: Applications Manual for the Revised NIOSH Lifting Equation. Publication No. 94-110. Cincinnati: National Institute for Occupational Safety and Health, 1994.

TABLE 31-4. VALUES OF THE DISTANCE MULTIPLIER (DM) FOR VARIOUS TRAVEL DISTANCES (D)

Travel Distances (D) (inches)	*Distance Multiplier (DM)*	*Travel Distances (D) (cm.)*	*Distance Multiplier (DM)*
<10	1.00	0	0.78
15	0.94	40	0.93
20	0.91	55	0.90
25	0.89	70	0.88
30	0.88	85	0.87
35	0.87	100	0.87
40	0.87	115	0.86
45	0.86	130	0.85
50	0.86	145	0.85
55	0.85	160	0.85
60	0.85	175	0.85
65	0.85	>175	0.00
70	0.85		
>70	0.00		

Adapted from Waters TR, Putz-Anderson V, Garg A: Applications Manual for the Revised NIOSH Lifting Equation. Publication No. 94-110. Cincinnati: National Institute for Occupational Safety and Health, 1994.

a relaxed vertical position, or (*b*) reaching forward to grasp an object that is too far in front of the body. Lateral bending (in the frontal plane) and axial twisting are usually associated with reaching for objects that are located either to the side or behind a worker's body. Laboratory and field studies have shown that these nonneutral postures are associated with local muscle fatigue and excessive rates of back pain.[23,72,77,78,89,90]

Because working posture is a function of an individual's anthropometry, a workstation layout that is good for one person may not be appropriate for workers who are considerably larger or smaller. For this reason, adjustability should be incorporated into the workstation wherever possible.

TABLE 31-5. VALUES OF THE ASYMMETRIC MULTIPLIER (AM) FOR VARIOUS ANGLES (A)

Angle (A) (degrees)	*Asymmetric Multiplier (AM)*
0	1.00
15	0.95
30	0.90
45	0.86
60	0.81
75	0.76
90	0.71
105	0.66
120	0.62
135	0.57
>135	0.00

Adapted from Waters TR, Putz-Anderson V, Garg A: Applications Manual for the Revised NIOSH Lifting Equation. Publication No. 94-110. Cincinnati: National Institute for Occupational Safety and Health, 1994.

Seated Work and Back Pain

Due to the rapid growth of service and information industries and technological advances in manufacturing methods, an increasing number of workers are spending a major fraction of their workday in a seated posture.[91] Sitting provides many ergonomic benefits, such as a reduction in the amount of body weight borne by the tissues of the feet and lower extremities, a reduction in whole-body energy expenditure due to decreased muscle activity, and stabilization of the body for tasks that require precise manual dexterity. The primary disadvantage of sitting is increased stress on the spine.[8]

TABLE 31-6. VALUES OF THE FREQUENCY MULTIPLIER (FM) FOR VARIOUS LIFTING FREQUENCIES (F)

	Work Duration					
Frequency (F)	*≤ 8 hours*		*≤ 2 hours*		*≤ 1 hour*	
lifts/min	*V < 30*	*V ≥ 30*	*V < 30*	*V ≥ 30*	*V < 30*	*V ≥ 30*
≤0.2	0.85	0.85	0.95	0.95	1.00	1.00
1	0.81	0.81	0.92	0.92	0.97	0.97
2	0.75	0.75	0.88	0.88	0.94	0.94
3	0.65	0.65	0.84	0.84	0.91	0.91
4	0.55	0.55	0.79	0.79	0.88	0.88
5	0.45	0.45	0.72	0.72	0.84	0.84
6	0.35	0.35	0.60	0.60	0.80	0.80
7	0.27	0.27	0.50	0.50	0.75	0.75
8	0.22	0.22	0.42	0.42	0.70	0.70
9	0.18	0.18	0.35	0.35	0.60	0.60
10	0.00	0.15	0.30	0.30	0.52	0.52
11	0.00	0.13	0.26	0.26	0.45	0.45
12	0.00	0.00	0.00	0.23	0.41	0.41
13	0.00	0.00	0.00	0.21	0.37	0.37
14	0.00	0.00	0.00	0.00	0.00	0.34
15	0.00	0.00	0.00	0.00	0.00	0.31
16	0.00	0.00	0.00	0.00	0.00	0.28
	0.00	0.00	0.00	0.00	0.00	0.00

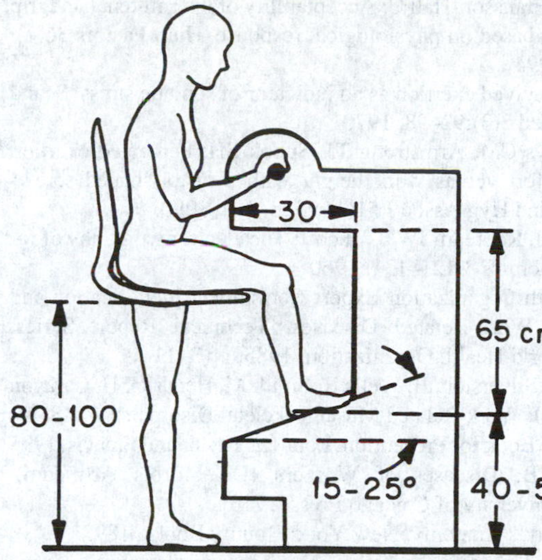

Figure 31-10. Example of a workbench and seat configuration that permits a worker to alternate between standing and sitting. (From Grandjean E.: Fitting the Task to the Man—A Textbook of Occupational Ergonomics. 4th ed. London: Taylor & Francis, 1988.)

Clinical and epidemiological studies have shown that prolonged sitting is associated with increased rates of lower back pain.[76,92] A possible explanation is that when a person moves from a standing to a sitting posture, the pelvis rotates backward, flattening the normal lordotic curve of the lower spine.[93,94] This flattening has the following effects: compression on the anterior portion of the disc, tension on the exterior portion of the disc, increased intradiscal pressure, tension on the apophyseal joint ligaments, and tension on the erector spinae muscles.[95,96] These stresses affect the supply of nutrients to the disc and surrounding tissue and may be related to the development of back disorders.

Spinal stresses associated with sitting are affected by the design of the chair. An important design consideration is the angle between the backrest and the seat pan. As this angle is increased, pelvic rotation and lumbar flattening is reduced.[94] This can be accomplished by tilting the seatpan slightly below the horizontal or by rotating the backrest in a rearward direction from the vertical. Jobs that require the worker to lean forward while sitting (e.g., sewing, many bench assembly tasks, microscope work, etc.) should have forward-slanting seat pans. A recent field study of full-time sewing machine operators found that comfort was enhanced and fatigue reduced by tilting the seat pan to slant forward at an angle 15° below the horizontal.[97] Furthermore, laboratory experiments have demonstrated that intradiscal pressures can be reduced up to 50 percent by increasing the included angle between the seat pan and backrest from 90 to 110°. Adding a lumbar support to the backrest also reduces intradiscal pressure.[98]

The height and shape of the seatpan are also important considerations in chair design. If the seat is too high, the worker's feet dangle, causing pressure on the underside of the thigh. This can interfere with circulation and cause swelling in the feet and lower legs. If the seat is too low, the thighs do not make good contact with the seat pan and an excessive amount of body weight will be borne by the ischial tuberosities and surrounding tissue. This may cause considerable discomfort, particularly if sitting on an unpadded seat or if sitting for a prolonged period. To accommodate the range of body sizes found in the working population, it is suggested that seat height be adjustable between 38 to 53 cm, measured from the floor to the front of the seatpan.[98] This adjustment should be easy to perform and not require any special tools. Ease of adjustment is particularly important if the chair is used by more than one person (e.g., where the same workstation is used by both day-shift and night-shift workers).

Where feasible, the seat and the associated work area should be designed to avoid prolonged static postures.[99] This concept is shown in Figure 31-10. At this workstation, the seat and work bench are designed to allow the user to alternate between standing and sitting postures at will. (Note: The dimensions in this figure show the ranges of adjustability required to accommodate the various body sizes found in the population.) Another method for preventing prolonged sitting is to modify the job description to include occasional tasks that must be performed away from the primary workstation. This allows the worker to periodically stand up and walk during the shift.

When selecting or designing a work seat, it is important to match the characteristics of the chair to the requirements of the job. For example, workers who must periodically reach behind or to the side of the body typically prefer seat pans that swivel while workers who perform precision assembly tasks prefer seat pans that are stable.[100]

▶ MANAGEMENT ISSUES

As discussed above, stresses that result in musculoskeletal disorders of the upper limb and low back can frequently be controlled through redesign of equipment, tools, and/or work methods. While these interventions may reduce the incidence and severity of WMSDs, it is unrealistic to prevent all disorders. They are multifactorial in nature and their causation is not yet understood well enough to achieve zero risk. In addition, there will continue to be some cases due to individual factors. It is necessary to provide for people who experience these impairments so that they do not become long-term disability cases. The details of such a program are beyond the scope of this chapter. It suffices to say that the worker, supervisor, engineer, and health care provider must work together as a team to determine what the worker can do and to find or modify jobs to accommodate any limitations.[101,102]

Control of WMSDs involves health professionals, supervisors, engineers, and workers. Thus an ergonomics program is best managed by a team of persons from each of these areas.[103,104] The team should meet regularly to review health data (new and old cases), set goals, recommend allocation of resources to control ergonomic stresses, and review the progress of ergonomic interventions.

▶ SUMMARY

Many worker health and safety problems can be attributed to failure to anticipate the capacity and behavior of the entire work population. Fatigue, accidents, and back and upper limb disorders are all too common examples of these problems. Ergonomics is the application of epidemiology, anthropometry, biomechanics, physiology, psychology, and engineering to the evaluation and design of work for preventive injury and illness while maximizing productivity. Ergonomics is not yet an exact science; therefore, all interventions should include appropriate evaluations to ascertain their effectiveness.

▶ REFERENCES

1. Kantowitz BH, Sorkin RD: Human Factors: Understanding People—System Relationships. New York: John Wiley & Sons, 1983
2. Adams JA: Human Factors Engineering. New York: Macmillan, 1989
3. Bailey RW: Human Performance Engineering. 3rd ed. Upper Saddle Hill, NJ: Prentice-Hall, 1996
4. VanCott HP, Kincade RG (eds): Human Engineering Guide to Equipment Design. Washington, DC: US Government Printing Office, 1972
5. Pheasant S: Bodyspace—Anthropometry, Ergonomics, and Design. London: Taylor and Francis, 1986
6. Kroemer KHE, Kroemer HB, Kroemer-Elbert KE: Ergonomics: How to Design for Ease and Efficiency. Englewood Cliffs, NJ: Prentice-Hall, 1994

7. Rodahl K: The Physiology of Work. London: Taylor and Francis, 1989
8. Chaffin DB, Andersson GBJ: Occupational Biomechanics. 2nd ed. New York, John Wiley & Sons, 1991
9. Keyserling WM: Occupational safety prevention of accidents and overt trauma. In Levy BS, Wegman DH (eds): Occupational Health—Recognizing and Preventing Work-Related Disease. 3rd ed. Boston: Little, Brown, 1995, pp 145–159
10. National Aeronautics and Space Administration: Anthropometric Source Book. Anthropometry for Designers. Ref. Pub. 1024. Washington, DC: National Aeronautics and Space Administration 1978, vol 1
11. Hagberg M: Local shoulder muscular strain—symptoms and disorders. J Human Ergol (Tokyo) 11:99–108, 1982
12. Roebuck JA, Kroemer KHE, Thomson WG: Engineering Anthropometry Methods. New York: John Wiley & Sons, 1975
13. Drillis R, Contini R: Body Segment Parameters. Department of Health, Education and Welfare, Office of Vocational Rehabilitation, Report No. 1166-03. New York: New York University School of Engineering and Science, 1966
14. Basmajian JV, De Luca CJ: Muscles Alive, Their Functions Revealed by Electromyography. 5th ed. Baltimore: Williams & Wilkins; 1985
15. Lieber RL, Friden J: Skeletal muscle metabolism, fatigue and injury. In Gordon SL, Blair SJ, Fine LJ (eds): Repetitive Motion Disorders of the Upper Extremity. Rosemont, IL: American Academy of Orthopaedic Surgeons, 1995, pp 287–300
16. Friden J, Lieber RL: Biomechanical injury to skeletal muscle from repetitive loading eccentric contractions and vibration. In Gordon SL, Blair SJ, Fine LJ (eds): Repetitive Motion Disorders of the Upper Extremity. Rosemont, IL: American Academy of Orthopaedic Surgeons, 1995, pp 301–312
17. Armstrong TJ, Buckle P, Fine LJ, Hagberg M, Jonsson B, Kilbom A, Kuorinka IAA, Silverstein BA, Sjogaard G, Viikari-Juntura ERA: A conceptual model for work-related neck and upper-limb musculoskeletal disorders. Scand J Work Environ Health 19(2): 73–84, 1993
18. Johansson H, Sojka P: Pathophysiological mechanism involved in genesis and spread of muscular tension in occupational muscle pain and in chronic musculoskeletal pain syndromes—a hypothesis. Med Hypotheses 35:196–203, 1991
19. Rohmert W: Problems in determining rest allowances. Part 1: Use of modern methods to evaluate stress and strain in static muscular work. Appl Ergonomics 4(2):91–95, 1973
20. Carlson BR: Level of maximum isometric strength and relative load—isometric endurance. Ergonomics 12(3):429–435, 1969
21. Armstrong TJ: Circulatory and Local Muscle Responses to Static Manual Work. Ann Arbor, MI: University of Michigan; 1976
22. Lind AR, McNicol GW: Local and central circulatory responses to sustained contractions and the effect of free or restricted arterial inflow on post-exercise hyperaemia. J Physiol 192:575–593, 1967
23. Chaffin DB: Localized muscle fatigue—definition and measurement. J Occup Med 15(4):346–354, 1973
24. Corlett EN, Bishop RP: The ergonomics of spot welders. Appl Ergonomics 9:23–31, 1978
25. Saldana N, Herrin GD, Armstrong TJ, Franzblau A: A computerized method for assessment of musculoskeletal discomfort in the workforce: a tool for surveillance. Ergonomics 37(6):1097–1112, 1994
26. Harms-Ringdahl K: On assessment of shoulder exercise and load-elicited pain in the cervical spine: biomechanical analysis of load-EMG-methodological studies of pain provoked by extreme position. Scand J Rehabil Med Suppl 14:4–34, 1986
27. Sjogaard G, Kiens B, Jorgensen K, Saltin B: Intramuscular pressure, EMG and blood flow during low-level prolonged static contraction in man. Acta Physiol Scand 128:475–484, 1986
28. Bjorkesten M, Jonsson B: Endurance limit of force in long-term intermittent static contractions. Scand J Work Environ Health 3:23–27, 1977
29. Bystrom S, Fransson-Hall C: Acceptability of intermittent handgrip contractions based on physiological response. Hum Factors 36(1): 158–171, 1994
30. Borg G: Perceived exertion as an indicator of somatic stress. Scand J Rehabil Med 2(3):92–98, 1970
31. Ulin S, Ways CM, Armstrong TJ, Snook SH: Perceived exertion and discomfort versus work height with a pistol-shaped screwdriver. Am Ind Hyg Assoc J 51(11):588–594, 1990
32. Lippold OCJ, Redfearn JWT, Vuco J: The electromyography of fatigue. Ergonomics 3:121–131, 1960
33. World Health Organization Expert Committee: Identification and Control of Work-Related Diseases. Technical Report Series. Geneva: World Health Organization, 1985, pp 3–11
34. Hagberg M, Silverstein B, Wells R, Smith M, Hendrick H, Carayon P, Perusse M: Work Related Musculoskeletal Disorders (WMSDs): A Reference Book for Prevention. London: Taylor and Francis, 1995
35. Ramazzini B: Diseases of Workers (De Morbis Artificum). Chicago: University of Chicago Press, 1713
36. Gray H: Gray's Anatomy. New York: Bounty Books, 1893
37. de Quervain: Ueber eine form von chronischer tendovaginitis. Correspondenz-Blatt f Aertzte 25:389–394, 1895
38. Zollinger F: A few remarks on the question of tubercular tendovaginitis and bursitis after an accident. Archiv fur Orthopadische und Unfall-Chirurgie 24:456–467, 1927
39. Conn HR: Tenosynovitis. Ohio State Med J 27:713–716, 1931
40. Fine LJ, Silverstein BA, Armstrong TJ, Anderson C: The detection of cumulative trauma disorders of the upper extremities in the workplace. J Occup Med 28(8):674–678, 1986
41. Franklin GM, Haug J, Heyer N, Checkoway H, Peck N: Occupational carpal tunnel syndrome in Washington State, 1984–1988. Am J Public Health 81(6):741–746, 1991
42. Occupational Safety and Health Administration: Occupational Safety and Health Act of 1970. Washington, DC: US Department Labor, 1970
43. Occupational Safety and Health Administration: Recordkeeping Guidelines for Occupational Injuries and Illnesses. Washington, DC: US Department of Labor, 1986
44. Armstrong TJ, Radwin RG, Hansen DJ, Kennedy KW: Repetitive trauma disorders: job evaluation and design. Hum Factors 28(3):325–336, 1986
45. American National Standards Insitute. Z-365 Control of Work-Related Cumulative Trauma Disorders. Part 1: Upper Extremities. Itaska, IL: National Safety Council, 1996
46. Armstrong TJ, Foulke JA, Joseph BS, Goldstein SA: Investigation of cumulative trauma disorders in a poultry processing plant. Am Ind Hyg Assoc J 43(2):103–116, 1982
47. Armstrong TJ: Control of upper-limb cumulative trauma disorders. Appl Occup Environ Hyg 11(4):275–281, 1996
48. Hennekens CH, Buring JE, Mayrent SL (eds): Epidemiology in Medicine. Boston: Little, Brown, 1987
49. Katz JN, Larson MG, Fossel AH, Liang MH: Validation of a surveillance case definition of carpal tunnel syndrome. Am J Public Health 81(2):189–193, 1991
50. Katz JN, Larson MG, Sabra A, Krarup C, Stirrat CR, Sethi R, Eaton HM, Fossel AH, Liang MH: The carpal tunnel syndrome: diagnostic utility of the history and physical examination findings. Ann Intern Med 112:321–327, 1990
51. Barnes RM: Motion and Time Study—Design and Measurement of Work. 7th ed. New York: John Wiley & Sons, 1978
52. Niebel BW: Motion and Time Study. Homewood, IL: Irwin, 1988
53. Armstrong TJ, Latko WA: Physical stressors: their characterization, assessment, and relationship with physical work requirements. In: Repetitive Motion Disorders of the Upper Extremity. Rosemont, IL: American Academy of Orthopedic Surgeons, 1995, pp 87–98
54. Latko WA, Armstrong TJ, Foulke JA, Herrin GD, Rabourn RA, Ulin SS: Development and evaluation of an observational method for assessing repetition in hand tasks. Am Ind Hyg Assoc J, 58:278–285, 1997

55. Armstrong TJ, Punnett L, Ketner P: Subjective worker assessments of hand tools used in automobile assembly. Am Ind Hyg Assoc J 50:639–645, 1989
56. Jonsson B: The static load component in muscle work. Eur J Appl Physiol 57:305–310, 1988
57. Jonsson B: Quantitative electromyographic evaluation of muscular load during work. Scand J Rehabil Med Suppl 6:69–74, 1978
58. Marras WS, Schoenmarklin RW: Wrist motions in industry. Ergonomics 36(4):341–351, 1993
59. Armstrong TJ, Foulke JA, Martin BJ, Gerson J, Rempel DM: Investigation of applied forces in alphanumeric keyboard work. Am Ind Hyg Assoc J 55(1):30–35, 1994
60. Pelmear PL, Taylor W, Wasserman DE: Hand-Arm Vibration: A Comprehensive Guide for Occupational Health Professionals. New York: Van Nostrand Reinhold, 1992
61. Snook SH, Campanelli RA, Hart JW: A study of three preventive approaches to low back injury. J Occup Med 20:478–481, 1978
62. Snook SH: The cost of back pain in industry. Spine 2:1–5, 1987
63. Burdorf A: Assessment of Postural Load on the Back in Occupational Epidemiology. Alblasserdam, The Netherlands: Thesis Rotterdam, 1992
64. Kelsey JL, Hochberg MC: Epidemiology of musculoskeletal disorders. Ann Rev Public Health 9:379–401, 1988
65. Waddell G: A new clinical model for the treatment of low back pain. Spine 12:632–644, 1987
66. Berquist-Ullman M, Larsson U: Acute low back pain in industry. Acta Orthop Scand Suppl 170, 1977
67. Battie MC, Bigos SJ, Fisher LD, Spengler DM, Hansson TH, Nachemson AL: The role of spinal flexibility in back pain complaints within industry—a prospective study. Spine 15:768–73, 1990
68. Spengler DM, Bigos SJ, Martin NA, Zeh J, Fisher L, Nachemson A: Back injuries in industry: a retrospective study. I. Overview and cost analysis. Spine 11:241–256, 1986
69. Frymoyer JW, Cats-Baril WL: An overview of the incidences and costs of low back pain. Orthop Clin North Am 22:263–271, 1991
70. Battie MC: Minimizing the impact of back pain: workplace strategies. Semin Spine Surg 4:20–28, 1992
71. Snook SH: Approaches to the control of back pain in industry: job design, job placement and education/training. Spine 2:45–59, 1987
72. National Institute for Occupational Safety and Health: Work Practices Guide for Manual Lifting. Publication No. 81-122. Cincinnati: National Institute for Occupational Safety and Health, 1981
73. Bigos SJ, Spengler DM, Martin NA, Zeh J, Fisher L, Nachemson A, Wang, MH: Back injuries in industry—a retrospective study: Part II—injury factors. Spine 11:246–251, 1986
74. National Council on Compensation Insurance. Workers' Compensation Back Pain Claim Study. New York: National Council on Compensation Insurance, 1992
75. Waters TR, Putz-Anderson V, Garg A, Fine LJ: Revised NIOSH equation for the design and evaluation of manual lifting tasks. Ergonomics 36:749–776, 1993
76. Magora A: Investigation of the relation between low back pain and occupation. Ind Med Surg 41:5–9, 1972
77. Punnett L, Fine LJ, Keyserling WM, Herrin GD, Chaffin DB: Back disorders and non-neutral trunk postures of automobile assembly workers. Scand J Work Environ Health 17:337–46, 1991
78. Burdorf A, Govaert G, Elders L: Postural load and back pain of workers in the manufacturing of pre-fabricated concrete elements. Ergonomics 34:909–918, 1991
79. Frymoyer JW: Back pain and sciatica. N Engl J Med 318:291–300, 1988
80. Boshuizen HC, Bongers PM, Hulshof CTJ: Self-reported back pain in tractor drivers exposed to whole-body vibration. Int Arch Occup Environ Health 62:109–115, 1990
81. Kelsey JL, Hardy RJ: Driving motor vehicles as a risk factor for acute herniated lumbar intervertebral disc. Am J Epidemiol 102:63–73, 1988
82. Bigos S, Spengler DM, Martin NA, Zeh J, Fisher L, Nachemson A: Back injuries in industry: a retrospective study. III. Employee-related factors. Spine 11:252–256, 1986
83. Klein BP, Jensen RC, Sanderson LM: Assessment of workers' compensation claims for back sprains/strains. J Occup Med 26:443–448, 1984
84. Waters TR, Putz-Anderson V, Garg A: Applications Manual for the Revised NIOSH Lifting Equation. Publication No. 94-110. Cincinnati: National Institute for Occupational Safety and Health, 1994
85. Keyserling WM, Herrin GD, Chaffin DB: Isometric strength testing as a means of controlling medical incidents on strenuous jobs. J Occup Med 22:332–336, 1980
86. Ayoub MM, Mital A: Manual Materials Handling. London: Taylor and Francis, 1989
87. National Institute for Occupational Safety and Health: Workplace Use of Back Belts: Review and Recommendations. NIOSH Publication No. 94-122. Cincinnati: National Institute for Occupational Safety and Health, 1994
88. Riddell CR, Congleton JJ, Huchingson RD, Montgomery JF: An evaluation of a weight lifting belt and back injury training class for airline baggage handlers. Appl Ergonomics 23:319–329, 1992
89. Andersson GBJ, Ortengren R, Herberts F: Quantitative electromyographic studies of back muscle activity related to posture and loading. Orthop Clin North Am 8:85–96, 1977
90. Snook SH, Ciriello VM: The design of manual handling tasks: revised tables of maximum acceptable weights and forces. Ergonomics 34:1197–1213, 1991
91. Bendix T: Low back pain and seating. In Luder R, Noro K (eds): Hard Facts about Soft Machines. London: Taylor and Francis, 1994
92. Andersson GBJ: Epidemiologic aspects of low back pain in industry. Spine 6:53–60, 1981
93. Keegan JJ: Alterations of the lumbar curve related to posture and sitting. J Bone Joint Surg 35A:589–603, 1953
94. Andersson GBJ, Ortengren R, Nachemson A, Elfstrom S: The Influence of backrest inclination and lumbar support on lumbar lordosis. Spine 4:52–58, 1979
95. Adams MA, Hutton WC, Scott JRR: The resistance to flexion of the lumbar intervertebral joint. Spine 5:245–253, 1980
96. Holm S, Nachemson A: Variation in nutrition of the canine intervertebral disc induced by motion. Spine 8:866–874, 1983
97. Yu C, Keyserling WM: Evaluation of a new work seat for industrial sewing operations: results of three field studies. Appl Ergonomics 20:17–25, 1989
98. Andersson GBJ, Ortengren R, Nachemson A, Elfstrom G: Lumbar disc pressure and myoelectric back muscle activity during sitting. Studies on an experimental chair. Scand J Rehab Med 3:104–114, 1974
99. Grandjean E: Fitting the Task to the Man—A Textbook of Occupational Ergonomics. 4th ed. London: Taylor and Francis, 1988
100. Yu C, Keyserling WM, Chaffin DB: Development of a workseat for industrial sewing operations: results of a laboratory study. Ergonomics 31:1765–1786, 1988
101. Bruening LA, Beaulieu D: The return to work phase for the patient with cumulative trauma. In Hunter JM, Schneider LH, Mackin EJ, Callahan AD (eds): Rehabilitation of the Hand, Surgery and Therapy. Philadelphia: CV Mosby, 1990, pp 1192–1196
102. Berlin S: On-site evaluation of the industrial worker. In Hunter JM, Schneider LH, Mackin EJ, Callahan AD (eds): Rehabilitation of the Hand, Surgery and Therapy. Philadelphia: CV Mosby, 1990, pp 1214–1217
103. Putz-Anderson V: Cumulative Trauma Disorders, A Manual for Musculoskeletal Diseases of the Upper Limbs. New York: Taylor and Francis, 1988
104. Joseph B: Analysis of a program for control of cumulative trauma disorders in the auto industry. In: Ergonomic Interventions to Prevent Musculoskeletal Injuries in Industry. Chelsea: Lewis Publishers, 1987, pp 133–150

Industrial Hygiene

Robert F. Herrick

▸ BACKGROUND

Within the scope of public health practice, industrial hygiene is the health profession devoted to the recognition, evaluation, and control of hazards in the working environment. These include chemical hazards, physical hazards, biological hazards, and ergonomic factors that cause or contribute to injury, disease, impaired function, or discomfort. Throughout the world, the profession that addresses these hazards is known as occupational hygiene; however, the United States has not yet adopted this newer, more accurate term. In this chapter, the term industrial hygiene is used as the equivalent of occupational hygiene.

Industrial hygiene principles have evolved over many years with accelerated development since the Industrial Revolution. Industrial hygiene is a young profession, which traces its name to Hygeia, the goddess of health and prevention, daughter of Aesculapius, god of medicine in Greek mythology. The modern history of industrial hygiene starts with the organization of manufacturing processes into industrial sectors. This history was chronicled by Theodore Hatch, who summarized the "Major Accomplishments in Occupational Health in the Past Fifty Years" on the 50th anniversary of the Division of Occupational Health of the U.S. Public Health Service in 1964. Hatch noted that, prior to World War I (about 1914), the United States was a rural, agricultural society, where the industrial processes were few and conducted by manual labor. The only plastic available was celluloid, petroleum refining dumped most of the product to waste, and Henry Ford had just introduced the radical concept of a $5 daily wage. This was the industrial world that Alice Hamilton discovered when she began to trace the health problems she found among immigrant families back to the husbands' workplaces.

In the 50 years that Hatch reviewed, industrial hygiene had emerged as one of the core disciplines in public health. In 1964, he attributed the progress that had been made in improving workplace conditions to the application of the principle of "epidemiologic assessment of occupational health hazards." Progress in the identification of these hazards resulted from ". . . the joining of skills from the health sciences and medicine on the one hand, and from the physical sciences and engineering on the other, with the two groups cemented together by biostatistics and epidemiology."[1]

This approach taken by the pioneers in industrial hygiene resulted in remarkable progress. Not only did they identify important questions, they had the vision to develop interdisciplinary approaches to solve them. This vision places industrial hygiene in the larger field of public health. The industrial hygienist's work in the recognition, evaluation, and control of hazardous exposures in the work environment is a practice of primary prevention, and the identity of industrial hygienists as public health practitioners is clear. Prevention is the key to a safe and healthful workplace, and industrial hygiene is a practice of primary prevention.

The steps that are involved in the prevention of occupational and environmental diseases are hazard recognition, hazard evaluation, and hazard control/intervention.

Hazard Recognition

The human health hazard resulting from an occupational exposure is determined by both the toxicity of an agent or factor and the extent or magnitude of human exposure. Successful industrial hygiene practice has been defined to include a step that is in some ways preliminary to hazard recognition: the anticipation of hazardous exposures and conditions, before they actually occur. Toxicological testing in animals produces information that is an important component of hazard anticipation and early recognition. In combination with human health data that may be generated through environmental/occupational medicine and surveillance programs, or through epidemiological studies, this information provides the basis for a strategy of hazard anticipation and recognition. For established workplace conditions, surveillance of both exposure and disease provides clues and hypotheses for further evaluation.

Hazard Evaluation

Hazard evaluation is a type of risk assessment, developed from the information gained in the hazard recognition and identification process and the characteristics of the (exposed) population at risk. The series of steps in reaching a conclusion about the degree of hazard associated with a particular exposure or work condition is known as hazard evaluation. Hazard evaluations are essential to determine the need for control measures to minimize exposures and to identify clues to the etiology of an adverse health condition observed in a worker or group of workers.

Hazard Control/Intervention

Primary prevention involves identification and evaluation of environmental hazards that are factors or cofactors in disease production, followed by application of methods to reduce or eliminate human exposures. This is the classical public health approach. Principles and methods for controlling occupational hazards include a range of techniques from substitution or elimination of hazardous materials and processes, to engineering and administrative exposure controls, to exposure reduction using personal protective equipment at the level of individual workers.

▸ RECOGNITION OF OCCUPATIONAL AND ENVIRONMENTAL HAZARDS

Principles of Hazard Recognition

Hazard recognition involves a systematic review of a worker's occupational environment to identify exposures and potential exposures.

This review should include information on the materials used and produced, the characteristics of the workplace including the equipment used, and the nature of each worker's interaction with the sources of workplace hazards. Specific information is obtained on the raw materials used in a process, materials produced or stored, and the by-products formed during the production process. Sources of this information are described in the following section. Hazard recognition also includes gathering information on the types of equipment used in the workplace, the cycle of operation and/or frequency of exposure, and the operational methods and work practices used. Information such as this is available from industrial hygiene reference sources.[2] A workplace review for the purpose of hazard recognition also includes identification of health and safety controls in place, including use of personal protective equipment.

The Occupational Safety and Health Administration (OSHA) Hazard Communication Standard provides a valuable information resource for hazard identification and evaluation. This standard requires employers to: *(a)* develop a written hazard communication program, *(b)* maintain a list of all hazardous chemicals in the workplace, *(c)* make available to workers Material Safety Data Sheets (MSDSs) for each hazardous chemical, *(d)* place labels on containers as to the chemical identity and precautions in handling, and *(e)* provide workers with education and training in the handling of hazardous chemicals.

Classification of Hazards

For purposes of hazard control and disease prevention, contaminants are classified largely on the basis of their physical and chemical characteristics, as these characteristics determine the route of exposure. Workers may be exposed to contaminants by inhalation, by absorption through the skin, by ingestion, or by injection, as in the case of accidental puncture wounds. Inhalation and skin absorption are the primary routes of exposure for most materials in the occupational environment. In cases where poor hygiene practices such as consumption of food and beverages in contaminated work areas are allowed, ingestion may an important source of exposure.

Environmental agents can be classified as either physical hazards or health hazards.

Physical Hazards. In its hazard communication standard, OSHA classifies materials such explosives, flammable or combustible liquids, oxidizers, compressed gases, organic peroxides, pyrophoric materials, unstable (reactive) chemicals or water-reactive chemicals as physical hazards. Other exposures in the workplace such as excessive noise, ionizing and nonionizing radiation, and temperature extremes are other examples of physical hazards.

There is a rapidly growing recognition that ergonomic factors are important causes of injury in the workplace. Repetitive motions, conducted in awkward positions, result in a variety of chronic trauma disorders, including carpal tunnel syndrome.

Health Hazards. Chemical and biological materials capable of producing adverse acute or chronic health effects are defined as health hazards. Exposures to chemical mists, vapors, gases, or airborne particles (dusts and fumes) occur through inhalation, ingestion, or by absorption through the skin. OSHA classifies hazardous chemicals as carcinogens, toxic or highly toxic agents, reproductive toxins, irritants, corrosives, sensitizers, hepatoxins, nephrotoxins, agents that act on the hematopoietic system, and agents that damage the lungs, skin, eyes, or mucous membranes. Biological hazards include exposures to infectious or immunologically active agents such as molds, fungi, and bacteria.

Types of Airborne Contaminants

Aerosols. Liquid droplets or solid particles in a size range that allows them to remain dispersed in air for a prolonged period of time are known as aerosols. Aerosols are also known as airborne particulate matter. The hazard associated with airborne particulate matter is determined by three factors: (*a*) the biological activity of the material, (*b*) concentration of the airborne material, and (*c*) airborne particle size. Particle size is an important determinant of hazard, because it strongly influences the site of deposition within the respiratory system. Many occupational diseases, including silicosis and asbestosis, are associated with material deposited in specific regions of the respiratory tract. Criteria[3] have been developed to define critical size-fractions most closely associated with various health effects and are defined as follows:

- *Inhalable fraction:* This is the fraction of airborne particulate matter that can present a hazard when deposited any place within the respiratory tract. Most particles of diameter less than 100 μm are considered inhalable.
- *Thoracic fraction:* Those particles that are hazardous when deposited anywhere within the lung airways and the gas-exchange region. Particles in this size range are generally less than 25 μm in diameter.
- *Respirable fraction:* Those particles that are a hazard when deposited in the gas-exchange region of the lungs. These particles are less than 10 μm in diameter.

Gases and Vapors. In general, materials are considered gases if they are predominantly in the gaseous state at temperatures and pressures normally found in ambient or occupational environments. Vapors are the gaseous form of substances normally present in the solid or liquid state at room temperature and pressure. Liquids undergo phase transformation to the vapor state by the process of evaporation and mix with the surrounding atmosphere. In the workplace environment, organic solvents volatilize to form vapors at normal temperatures and pressures. In many industrial applications, solvents are heated, which results in increased vaporization and elevated airborne solvent concentrations.

Measures of Airborne Concentration

A number of terms and units are used to describe airborne concentrations and exposures to contaminants. The form of the contaminant and the sampling and analytical method used to measure the airborne concentration dictate the choice of terms that are used. The following terms are used to describe airborne concentrations and exposure:

- ppm (ppb): Parts of vapor or gases per million (or billion) parts of contaminated air by volume at room temperature and pressure.
- mppcf: Millions of particles of a particulate per cubic foot of air.
- mg/m^3 ($\mu g/m^3$): Milligrams (or micrograms) of a substance per cubic meter of air.
- vapor %: Parts of vapor or gas per 100 parts of contaminated air by volume at room temperature and pressure.
- fibers/cc: A measure of the numbers of fibers longer than 5 μm in length per cubic centimeter of air. This measure is used for asbestos and other fibers.

Sources of Hazard Information

Toxicological Reviews. There are many sources of information on hazardous properties of materials found in the workplace environment. These reviews and evaluations are prepared by private organizations as well as government agencies in the United States and internationally. The U.S. National Institute for Occupational Safety and Health (NIOSH) prepares several sets of criteria and recommendations for limiting exposure to occupational hazards. These are not legally enforceable themselves, but NIOSH recommendations are transmitted to OSHA, where they can be used in promulgating legal standards. The Agency for Toxic Substances and Disease Registries (ATSDR) of the U.S. Department of Health and Human Services develops toxicological profiles for compounds commonly found at hazardous waste sites. The National Institute of Environmental Health

Sciences (NIEHS) of the U.S. Department of Health and Human Services prepares an Annual Report on Carcinogens, which reviews and evaluates information on evidence of carcinogenicity. The report provides a listing of chemicals classified on the basis of the strength of the evidence of carcinogenic risk. The American Conference of Governmental Industrial Hygienists (ACGIH) prepares a listing of Threshold Limit Values (TLVs) and Biological Exposure Indices (BEIs), which are updated annually. Several international organizations review scientific information for purposes of evaluating risks resulting from human exposure to chemicals. The International Agency for Research on Cancer (IARC) prepares critical reviews of information on evidence of carcinogenicity for chemicals. The International Programme on Chemical Safety (IPCS) is a joint venture of the United Nations Environment Program, the International Labor Organization, and the World Health Organization. This program develops Environmental Health Criteria Documents, which are summaries and evaluations of the information on toxic effects of specific chemicals and groups of chemicals.

A number of information sources are now available on CD-ROM, the Internet, and the World Wide Web. For example, the OSHA Standards, Letters of Interpretation, Environmental Protection Agency (EPA) Standards, and Hazardous Substances Databanks from the National Library of Medicine, Medline, Toxline, etc. can all be accessed directly from a personal computer. The Internet is currently one of the industrial hygienist's greatest information and communication assets, and in the future it will be central to industrial hygiene practice. For users of the Internet, Blotzer's *Internet User's Guide for Safety and Health Professionals*[4] is an excellent introduction to the Internet and its uses. It also includes 79 pages of site listings for safety and health professionals. Methods for opening an Internet account, logging onto an Internet server, finding sites, etc. are all described. The following list is a sample of some of the readily available information on the World Wide Web:

- MSDSs: hundreds of thousands of material safety data sheets
- Toxicological profiles of thousands of chemicals available from EPA, ATSDR
- Literature searches from the National Library of Medicine, Medline, Toxline, Chemline, Hazardous Substances Database
- Exposure information from NIOSHTIC, National Cancer Institute Surveillance Exposure and Epidemiology Reports (SEER) Data
- OSHA Compliance Reports, Injury and Illness Rates by Industry, etc.
- Training courses, e.g., ATSDR training for lead and radon; notices for upcoming courses, conferences, etc.
- News groups comprised of groups of Internet users with similar interests, e.g., ergonomics, MSDSs, chemical safety
- Complete Federal Regulations and Guidelines (EPA, OSHA, DOT, NIOSH, CDC)
- Governmental and nongovernmental organizations throughout the world, including national institutes, World Health Organization, and universities

Resource Hotlines. A number of emergency response services are in operation, some of which are primarily intended to provide information on environmental aspects of chemical hazards. These services are good sources of information on the toxicity and risk of exposure to a wide range of chemicals, regardless of whether exposure takes place in an environmental or an occupational setting. NIOSH operates a toll-free technical service to provide information on workplace hazards. The service is staffed by technical information specialists who can provide information on NIOSH activities, recommendations and services, or any aspect of occupational safety and health. The number is not a hotline for medical emergencies, but is a source of information and referrals on occupational hazards. The NIOSH toll-free number is 800-35-NIOSH (800-356-4674).

CHEMTREC is a 24-hour hotline to the Chemical Transportation Emergency Center operated by the Chemical Manufacturers Association (800-424-9300). CHEMTREC assists in the identification of unknown chemicals and provides advice on proper emergency response methods and procedures. It does not provide emergency treatment information other than basic first aid, however. CHEMTREC also facilitates contact with chemical manufacturers when further information is required.

The National Pesticides Telecommunications Network Hotline is operated through Oregon State University (800-858-7378). The hotline provides information on pesticide-related health effects on approximately 600 active ingredients contained in over 50,000 products manufactured in the United States since 1947. It is also a source of information on pesticide product formulations, basic safety practices, health and environmental effects, and cleanup and disposal procedures.

Several hotline and information lines are available for response to information requests on toxic materials and environmental issues. The Toxic Substances Control Act (TSCA) Assistance Information Service (TAIS) provides information and publications about toxic substances, including asbestos (202-554-1404). The EPA also operates an Emergency Response Notification System (ERNS), which is a source of information on oil discharges, and releases of hazardous substances (202-260-2342). In addition, each of the 10 USEPA Regional Offices has a hotline telephone number.

▶ EVALUATION OF HAZARDS

The series of steps followed to assess the hazard associated with a particular exposure or work condition is known as hazard evaluation. Hazard evaluations are essential to determine the need for control measures to minimize exposures. They are also conducted in search of clues to the etiology of an adverse health condition observed in a worker or group of workers. Hazard evaluation is founded upon the information gained in the hazard recognition and identification process just described and requires knowledge and information on:

1. Workplace activities and processes, and potential exposures to contaminants.
2. Properties of contaminants and potential routes of human exposure.
3. The actual magnitude and frequency of worker exposures to a contaminant. In the absence of quantitative exposure information, estimates of the potential for human exposure are often useful for hazard evaluation.
4. Potential adverse health effects resulting from an exposure and the approximate level of exposure at which adverse effects occur.

While the techniques for evaluation are tailored to each type of hazard, the principles of evaluation can be generalized. Exposure is evaluated in its role as an underlying cause of disease, so in these investigations, exposure may be regarded the measure of contact with the potential causal agent(s).

Measurements of Environmental Contaminants

Over the range of types of exposures (gases and vapors, aerosols, and biological and physical agents), there are two general classes of measurement techniques. One class is termed the extractive methods, in which the contaminants of interest are removed from the environment for laboratory analysis. With these methods, a sampling device is used to collect the contaminants, usually from air in the vicinity of the worker's breathing zone. This sort of measurement of exposure is termed a personal sample, as it attempts to characterize the composition of the environment at the point the worker contacts it by inhalation. Because of the importance of inhalation exposures, most measurement methods assess airborne contaminants. However, methods to measure contamination of surfaces, as well as the exposure of the skin, are available. These methods are described later in this section.

A large number of sampling and analytical methods are available for measurement of personal exposures. Both NIOSH and OSHA develop and publish methods, and these are considered to be standard for workplace exposure measurements.[5,6]

Direct measurements of contaminants in the atmosphere comprise the second general class of techniques. These approaches are described as monitoring methods, and they have been developed from instrumental methods first used in the laboratory. Examples of these monitoring methods are devices that perform automated chemical analysis or make measurements based upon chromatographic or spectrophotometric approaches. These monitoring methods can measure continuously and report results immediately, which allows the examination of the pattern of exposure as it changes over time. This can be a substantial improvement over the information provided by extractive sampling methods, which accumulate material over the time of sampling and give a result that is time integrated over that period.

Dermal and Surface Contamination

As methods for hazard evaluation have progressed, it has become apparent that inhalation is only one of the significant routes of exposure. Contamination on the skin, as well as on surfaces, may be sources of dermal exposure in the workplace. One approach to measuring this exposure is the placement of cloth patches on the outside of workers' clothing, or by providing workers with thin cotton inspectors' gloves, which are worn while they perform tasks where dermal exposure is of interest. A similar method has been used in which the patches are placed under the workers' clothing to measure the quantity of a contaminant that penetrates the protective clothing. Analysis of the patches or glove material then provides an estimate of the exposure. This approach has also been used to evaluate the performance of protective gloves by wearing the cotton glove under the protective glove. Another techniques used to estimate dermal exposure of the hands is to rinse the hands, or both the inside surface of the protective gloves and the hands, after a worker has performed the task of interest. The volume of rinse solution is collected and analyzed for the contaminant.

The measurement of surface contamination in a working environment can provide another, less direct indication of dermal exposure. Techniques for wipe sampling have been developed to measure surface contamination. These methods have been widely used in industries where exposure may result from resuspension of settled aerosols. For example, surface sampling for lead has been extensively done in industries such as foundries and lead smelters. In cases where the exposure of interest is nonvolatile, such as most metals, and organic chemicals such as polychlorinated biphenyls (PCBs), surface contamination is a useful measure of the likelihood of exposure from skin absorption or ingestion resulting from eating or smoking with contaminated hands. There is a standardized surface wiping method specified by OSHA that describes techniques for collecting samples from contaminated surfaces.[6]

Measurements in Biological Media

Comprehensive hazard evaluation includes the assessment of exposure by several routes. In addition to pulmonary absorption, materials may be cleared from the respiratory tract and swallowed, resulting in uptake from the gastrointestinal tract. Many industrial materials can also be absorbed directly through the skin. Measurement of contaminants in biological media reflects the contributions from these multiple routes of exposure, as well as the variability in absorption, distribution, and metabolism among exposed individuals. Progress in biological monitoring has been driven by the uncertainties in the relationship between measurement of contamination in the workplace environment, such as those made with conventional industrial hygiene air sampling methods, and the actual quantity of a toxic material that may be present in the body.

The measurement made in biological media may be for a particular chemical itself or its metabolites. Another type of measurement used to evaluate workplace exposure is reversible biological change, which is characteristically induced by chemical exposure. These measurements can be made in blood, urine, exhaled breath, or other media. Biological monitoring methods are usually used to complement measurements of inhalation exposures, as they provide information on the total exposure from all sources (nonoccupational and workplace) and by all routes (i.e., skin and gastrointestinal absorption). The medium that is selected for sampling can be chosen to suit a particular purpose, as materials such as organic solvents may be eliminated by several pathways. There are reference values for measurements made in biological media. The ACGIH has prepared these values, known as BEIs, with documentation for their measurement and interpretation of results, for approximately 40 chemicals.[3]

Interpreting Exposure Measurement Information

Exposure measurements are usually compared with a legal or recommended exposure limit. There are several sources of exposure limits, as discussed earlier. While the exposure limit values vary between sources, virtually all these limits are specific to the airborne concentration of a single chemical, and the vast majority set a level that is not to be exceeded as a time-integrated average over an 8- to 10-hour work shift. While this data lends itself to determining compliance with a limit, measurements of levels below a limit should not be considered conclusive for purposes of hazard evaluation. None of the exposure limit values, including the OSHA Permissible Exposure Limits, which are legally enforceable, are intended to be used as fine lines to distinguish between safe and dangerous working conditions. When interpreting the results of exposure measurements, an environment should not be considered to be free from risk when exposure levels are below the limit value. In the case of individual workers in the environment, reported symptoms should not be considered nonwork related only because measured exposure levels are below a limit. The extent of individual variability in response to workplace exposure is not well known, and a conservative approach to the interpretation of exposure is appropriate. The ACGIH has thoroughly described the factors that must be considered in interpreting exposure information, including simultaneous exposure to mixtures of toxic agents, variability in the composition and levels of exposure over time, exposure by multiple routes, and unusual working conditions.[3]

Mixed Exposures

Most exposures in the working environment are comprised of mixtures of potentially hazardous materials. In general, very little is known about the combined effects of exposure to multiple agents. The combined effects of some materials that act upon the same organ system are recognized in the ACGIH Threshold Limit Values for Mixtures. A common example is an atmosphere containing a mixture of solvents. While each solvent may have neurotoxic effects, it may be that no single chemical exceeds its recommended exposure limit. The hazard should be evaluated in consideration of the additive effect of the exposure. The TLVs provide guidelines for assessing the effect of exposure when the components of a mixture have similar toxicological properties.

Exposure Variability

The variability in exposure can be broken down into components. The characteristics of a contaminant in the environment are described by its composition and intensity. The composition, i.e., the chemical makeup, and the distribution of particle sizes changes through time. The intensity of exposure, expressed as its concentration (such as parts of benzene vapor per million parts of air, or number of asbestos fibers per cubic centimeter of air) may also change through time, resulting in a highly variable exposure over a workday. Exposure variability is also introduced by the characteristics of the individuals in the exposure environment. Even for jobs at fixed workstations, where workers perform similar tasks, there can be substantial exposure differences between individuals because of personal work practices.

When interpreting exposure information for hazard evaluation, these sources of exposure variability must be considered. For example, consider two workplaces where benzene exposure is of concern. In one workplace, there is a steady concentration of 1 ppm, so the exposure of a worker spending a full shift in this area would be measured as 1 ppm as an 8-hour time-weighted average exposure. A worker in the second workplace could be in an environment in which the level of exposure to benzene varies widely from periods of no detectable exposure to very high but short-term peaks of exposure. For example, if this second worker experienced a single, high, peak exposure level of 48 ppm of the solvent, for only 10 minutes a day, then spent the remainder of the shift in an unexposed area, this worker's 8-hour time-weighted average exposure would also be 1 ppm. Classifying these two workers as equally exposed could result in an erroneous conclusion in hazard evaluation. When exposure varies widely over time, the time course of exposure must be considered in order to develop an appropriate hazard control strategy. Industrial hygiene sampling methods can be used to measure the high, short-term exposure and identify the work activities that cause it, as well as to measure exposure integrated over the time of sampling.

Exposure by Multiple Routes

While inhalation is an important route of exposure for many occupational hazards, skin exposure may also be a significant route of entry for industrial chemicals. Most exposure guidelines and limits include notations indicating cases in which skin contact may be a significant route of exposure. In the case of the ACGIH-TLVs, this notation appears for approximately 10 percent of the chemicals listed. Unlike measurements of airborne contaminants, the interpretation of information obtained by measuring dermal contact is complicated by the absence of guidelines or reference values. Measurement of skin contact does not necessarily provide a direct indication of the quantity of a chemical that may be absorbed, as the relationship between the material found on the skin and the absorbed amount depends on several factors. The physical and chemical properties of the material, the anatomical area of contact, the duration of contact, and the individual characteristics of the exposed individual can all influence the relationship between the amount of material on the skin and the amount that may be dermally absorbed. The importance of dermal exposure should not be underestimated, however, as in some occupational settings, materials such as pesticides have been shown to enter the body primarily by dermal absorption. In these cases, measurements in biological media can be very helpful in hazard evaluation, as they can integrate the contribution of exposures from a number of routes.

Unusual Working Conditions

Any interpretation of exposure information should recognize that there is uncertainty associated with both the measurement of exposure, as well as the limit value to which it is compared. Information on exposure should be interpreted in view of the overall conditions in the working environment. For example, exposure measurements are generally made with the expectation that the individuals are in the working environment for the "normal" 8-hour day, and 40-hour work week. Many jobs operate on a schedule that varies from this. The potential effect of extended duration on occupational exposure is rarely recognized in exposure limits, however. Of the over 600 materials for which there are OSHA permissible exposure limits (PELs), only the lead standard specifies that the maximum daily allowable exposure level be adjusted down in proportion to the time by which the length of the daily exposure exceeds 8 hours. For purposes of hazard evaluation and decisions about the need for exposure controls, however, duration of exposure should be considered for any exposure situation.

▸ CONTROL OF HAZARDS

Principles and Limitations of Controls

Recalling the public health basis of industrial hygiene practice, exposure control is a means of primary prevention. The elimination or reduction of hazards to the extent feasible is the primary means of prevention for occupational disease and injury. The strategy for effective hazard control is an ordered hierarchy. The three elements of this effectiveness hierarchy of control solutions in order of are:

1. First, prevent or contain hazardous workplace emissions at their source;
2. Next, remove the emissions from the pathway between the source and the worker;
3. Last, control the exposure of the worker with barriers between the worker and the hazardous work environment.[7]

This strategy mandates the use of environmental controls as the primary means of exposure prevention. These controls may take several forms and are frequently used in combinations as part of an overall prevention strategy. Specific control methods include substitution of materials with less hazardous substances, modification of the working environment to contain the source of the hazard, isolation of the worker from the hazardous environment, removal of the hazardous substance by ventilation, modification of work practices to reduce exposure, and use of personal protective equipment to reduce exposure. It should be noted that the use of protective equipment, including respirators, is intentionally mentioned last. Personal protective equipment should be considered the least preferable means of hazard control, implemented only when other means of control are not feasible or effective.

Material Substitution

The practice of reducing risk in the workplace by the removal of a toxic material and its replacement with a less toxic substitute is well established. Elimination or reduction of extremely toxic materials, such as asbestos as an insulating material, or benzene in solvents, adhesives, and gasoline, illustrates the principle of substitution. These examples also illustrate the risk of replacing one hazard with another. As more information is discovered about their toxicity, some of the materials used to replace asbestos as an insulating material, such as artificial mineral fibers and fibrous glass, are suspected of having effects similar to asbestos. The replacement of benzene with another chemical, such as hexane, with similar solvent properties may reduce the risk of exposure to a carcinogen, but increase the hazard of exposure to a neurotoxin. Substitution is an important method of primary prevention of workplace exposures, but it should be practiced with a recognition of the effect the replacement material may have on the work environment. The result of substitution should not be the replacement of one hazard with another.

Process Modification

The application of engineering control technology to modify the design of industrial processes is a very effective method of intervention to reduce exposures. Spray painting is an example of a process in which technology has changed, substantially reducing solvent exposures by using airless atomization systems instead of compressed air spray guns. Many common industrial processes, such as material handling procedures, can be redesigned to minimize the release of contaminants. Exposure control should be included as a central design element at the design stage of a new industrial process or in the modification of existing operations. The anticipation and control of potential hazards at the design stage is more efficient than redesign of existing systems.

Isolation

By considering exposure to be the result of personal contact with a source of contamination, we can easily see the effectiveness of isolation to interrupt the pathway between the source of a hazard and the worker. This approach can be implemented in two ways: by enclosure to isolate a source from the working environment or by isolating the workers from a contaminated environment. Both approaches may be part of a comprehensive exposure control strategy; however, containment of the source is generally preferable. The glove box used in handling infectious materials is a common example of containment for hazard control. This approach is particularly well suited to control individual point sources of contaminants, or physical hazards such as noise. By preventing the release of a hazardous agent into the work environment, exposure is controlled at the source.

Isolation of the workers from the contaminated environment may be preferable, and more feasible, in cases where contaminants are released from multiple sources dispersed through the work environment. While this approach does not prevent the release of the hazard into the environment, it is possible to protect workers through isolation. The use of clean air–supplied control rooms in chemical production facilities is an example of isolation of workers from general environmental contamination.

Ventilation

Ventilation is a very common method of workplace hazard control. There are two general types of ventilation: dilution ventilation (also known as general or comfort ventilation) and local exhaust ventilation. There is some amount of dilution ventilation in any indoor space, even if it is only the natural infiltration of outside air. Most workplace require additional ventilation, known as local exhaust, to capture contaminants at or near their source and remove them from the work environment. Although they are frequently used together, the two types of ventilation are very different in design and performance.

Dilution Ventilation. Dilution (also known as general) ventilation is the replacement of contaminated air with fresh air. In its most simple form, general ventilation is provided by the natural entry of outdoor air through windows, doors, and other openings. Most indoor workplaces require some means of providing mechanical air movement to supplement the natural airflow. Mechanical roof ventilators or wall fans are common in buildings used as workplaces. The human occupants of office buildings may be the primary source of indoor pollution in cases where there are no industrial processes. General building air provided by a heating, ventilation, and air conditioning (HVAC) system may be the only means of controlling the carbon dioxide, water vapor, particulate material, and biological aerosols that are the result of human occupancy. Ventilation guidelines for general dilution are provided by the American Society of Heating, Refrigerating and Air-Conditioning Engineers (ASHRAE) to specify minimum ventilation rates and indoor air quality that provide an acceptable work environment; however, these guidelines are based more on perceptions of comfort by building occupants than on prevention of adverse health effects.

Dilution ventilation is generally not sufficient to provide effective control in workplaces where there are sources of contamination in addition to human occupancy. This is clearly the case where major industrial process are conducted, but it can also be true where the contaminant sources are limited to office equipment such as photocopy machines. The volume of air needed to dilute contaminants to acceptable levels is usually large, requiring large and expensive air handling systems to move the air, as well as to heat and cool it. These systems may reduce the amount of contaminant present in the work environment, but they do not control its release. Local exhaust systems, described in the following section, are generally preferable for a variety of reasons.

Local Exhaust Ventilation. Local exhaust systems differ fundamentally from dilution systems. Rather than allowing contaminants to escape, then reducing their concentration by dilution with clean air, local exhaust ventilation systems capture air contaminants at the source and prevent their dispersion in the environment. By interrupting the pathway between the source of the contaminant and the worker, these local systems control emissions and prevent exposures. These systems typically include a hood, which may partially enclose the source and facilitate the entry of contaminated air entry into the exhaust system. The force to move air into the system is provided by a fan, connected to the hood with duct work. Many systems also include an air cleaning device, such as a filter, to remove contaminants before the air is released to the environment. The design and testing of local exhaust systems is a specialized aspect of industrial hygiene, and the ACGIH's manual[8] and text by Burgess[2] should be consulted as sources of further information.

Personal Protective Equipment

Personal protective devices are at the lowest level of the hierarchy of exposure control methods. These devices are intended to provide a barrier between workers and contaminated environments. They include equipment to protect the eyes (safety glasses, goggles, and face shields); the skin (gloves, aprons, and full body suits made of impervious materials); and the respiratory tract (a wide variety of respiratory protective devices). The selection and use of these devices is largely driven by the particular application, and there is a large number of choices available to protect against chemical, physical, and biological hazards.[9]

The specification and use of respiratory protective devices is more complex than is the case for other personal protective equipment. This is due to the legal requirements, as well as the importance of matching the choice of respiratory protection with both the hazard and the individual respirator user. OSHA has a specific regulation for respirator use (Code of Federal Regulations, 29 CFR 1910.134). In addition, some OSHA standards for specific air contaminants such as asbestos and lead include requirements for respiratory protection programs.

Respiratory protective devices may be classified into two general types. Respirators that operate by removing contaminants from air by filtration, adsorption, or chemical reaction are known as air-purifying respirators. Respirators that supply air from a source other than the surrounding environment (such as from a cylinder of compressed air) are known as atmosphere-supplying respirators. Both types of respirators are tested and certified for use by NIOSH.

NIOSH has developed a full respirator decision logic, which is a recommended procedure to guide to the selection and use of respiratory protection. The correct choice of a respirator requires consideration of the particular contaminants that may be present and the concentrations at which they will be found in the working environment. The ability of an individual worker to wear the respirator in a manner that will provide adequate protection must also be determined as part of a respirator selection and use program. Individual workers vary widely in the degree of protection that a respirator will provide in actual use in the working environment, and the decision logic includes requirements for comprehensive respiratory protection programs with respirator fit testing to ensure that each respirator performs effectively for the individual user.[10]

Education and Training

Worker education and training are essential components of effective programs of primary prevention and exposure control. Any of the control strategies just described function best when workers understand the physical and chemical hazards associated with their work, as well as methods for controlling these hazards. In the OSHA substance-specific regulations (for asbestos, lead, arsenic, cotton dust, etc.), worker education and training are required, although these regulations often lack detailed training specifications. Training requirements also are contained in several OSHA process-specific standards such as the respiratory protection standard, the blood-borne pathogens standard, and the standard concerning process safety management for highly hazardous materials. In addition, the OSHA Hazard Communication Standard, which was promulgated in 1985, establishes generic training requirements for hazardous substances. The OSHA Hazard Communication Standard requires chemical manufacturers and importers to provide hazard information to users of their products. Information must be provided in the form of MSDSs and product labels. The standard requires that employees be provided with information and training on hazardous chemicals in the workplace. Training must include information concerning requirements of the OSHA standard, identification of hazardous materials in the work area, information on the company's written hazard communication standard, methods for detecting presence or release of hazardous chemicals in the work area, specific hazards of chemicals in the workplace, measures to protect workers from exposure to hazardous chemicals, and details concerning the employer's hazard-labeling system for chemicals in the workplace. Although the sort of training required by the hazard communication standard is not legally required for all occupational hazards, it contains the elements of a model program that can be adapted to a variety of workplace situations where hazard control is needed.

▶ REFERENCES

1. Hatch T: Major accomplishments in occupational health in the past fifty years. Ind Hyg J 25:108–113, 1964
2. Burgess WA: Recognition of Health Hazards in Industry. 2nd ed. New York: John Wiley & Sons, 1995
3. American Conference of Governmental Industrial Hygienists (ACGIH): Threshold Limit Value for Chemical Substances and Physical Agents in the Workroom Environment with Intended Changes for 1996. Cincinnati: American Conference of Governmental Industrial Hygienists, 1996
4. Blotzer M: Internet User's Guide for Safety and Health Professionals. Schenectady, NY: Genium Publishing, 1996
5. National Institute for Occupational Safety and Health: NIOSH Manual of Analytical Methods. 4th ed. Cincinnati: National Institute for Occupational Safety and Health, 1994
6. US Department of Labor, Occupational Safety and Health Administration: OSHA Technical Manual. 4th ed. Washington, DC: Government Printing Office, 1996
7. Burgess WA: Philosophy of management of engineering controls. In Cralley LJ, Cralley LV, Harris RJ (eds): Patty's Industrial Hygiene and Toxicology. 3rd ed. New York: John Wiley & Sons, 1994
8. American Conference of Governmental Industrial Hygienists (ACGIH): Industrial Ventilation, A Manual of Recommended Practice. 22nd ed. Cincinnati: American Conference of Governmental Industrial Hygienists, 1995
9. Schwope AD, Costas PP, Jackson JO, Weitzman DJ: Guidelines for Selection of Chemical Protective Clothing. 3rd ed. Cincinnati: American Conference of Governmental Industrial Hygienists, 1987
10. National Institute for Occupational Safety and Health: NIOSH Recommendation for Occupational Health Standards, 1988. MMWR Suppl S-7 37:1–29, 1988

General References

Burgess WA, Ellenbecker MJ, Treitman RD: Ventilation for Control of the Work Environment. New York: John Wiley & Sons, 1989

Di Nardi, S.R. (ed) The Occupational Environment—Its evaluation and control. Fairfax, VA: American Industrial Hygiene Association, 1997

US Department of Labor, Occupational Safety and Health Administration: 29 CFR Part 1910, Air Contaminants, Final Rule. Fed Reg 54(12): 2651–2652, January 19, 1989

33

Surveillance, Monitoring, and Screening in Occupational Health

Larry J. Fein

▶ TYPES AND PURPOSES OF WORKPLACE HEALTH EXAMINATIONS

Health examinations are performed in workplaces for several distinctly different purposes. For example, the most common purpose of the preplacement medical examination, which occurs after an offer of employment has been made but before an individual is placed on a specific job, is to determine if the individual has significant physical or mental impairment that would preclude the individual from performing specific essential duties related to a particular job. While this is one of the principal functions of the preplacement examination, the examination itself may be comprehensive, except in Minnesota due to a state law.[1]

One of the most common purposes of workplace health examinations and one that is most relevant to improving the health of the workforce is to identify toxic health effects at an earlier stage than they would be detected without the examination.[2] This type of screening program is often initiated with a baseline examination and then followed with periodic follow-up examinations. The goal of this type of program is secondary prevention. It may benefit not only the individuals who may have diseases or toxic effects that are detected before they would have sought medical care, but may indirectly benefit other similarly exposed workers since the detection of work-related health effects should trigger an investigation of the workplace. Additionally, if excessive exposures are found, it should lead to efforts to reduce hazardous exposures or change unsafe working conditions. If large groups are tested, the test data can be analyzed to identify group trends. This can lead to the detection of more subtle changes than the evaluation of data solely on a case-by-case basis. This type of screening examination should be voluntary and is intended to benefit the individual worker who is screened. Therefore, the screening tests used in these periodic examinations should be evaluated to ensure that the tests are effective for screening objectives.

A common adjunct to medical monitoring or screening is biological monitoring, which is the measurement of workplace agents or their metabolites in biological specimens, usually blood or urine, for the purpose of monitoring the level of exposure and adsorption. This approach to exposure assessment is particularly useful when adsorption is possible by dermal exposure. Biological monitoring should not be used to replace careful assessment of exposure conditions by other effective methods such as environmental air measurements.

▶ ETHICAL ISSUES IN HEALTH EXAMINATIONS IN THE WORKPLACE

One of the important differences between medical examinations in the occupational setting and those in other settings is that the relationship between the health care provider and the examinee is not, from a legal point of view, the traditional physician-patient relationship. In the traditional physician-patient relationship, the health care provider serves only the interests of the patient and the health care provider's only loyalty is to the patient.[1] When the employer hires or contracts for the occupational health care provider, the provider may have difficulty resolving conflicts of interest between the employer and the employee-patient. This conflict is one of the most important ethical concerns of occupational health.[1] Ethical codes have been developed by both the American College of Occupational and Environmental Medicine (ACOEM) and the International Commission on Occupational Health (ICOH).[3,4] Rothstein has proposed a Bill of Rights of Examinees.[1] ICOH codes explicitly deal with many of the issues related to screening and surveillance activities, and the ACOEM has a position on medical surveillance in the workplace.[5] All of these codes recognize the need to maintain the confidential nature of most medical screening information. This concept is reinforced by the Americans with Disabilities Act (ADA). All medical information must be collected and sorted in separate medical files.[1] Under ADA, management may be informed of workers' restrictions that limit their ability to perform the job duties.[1] In addition to ADA, other federal and state laws or regulations such as the Occupational Safety and Health Act, Department of Transportation examinations for interstate truck drivers, or state laws on human immunodeficiency virus (HIV) or drug testing deal with the issue of medical confidentiality. While the Occupational Safety and Health Administration (OSHA) mandates various preplacement and periodic medical examinations that employers must offer employees, the employees have the right to refuse to participate in these OSHA-mandated examinations unless this is part of the specific employee-employer contract.[6]

One of the best methods to address the ethical issues in workplace examinations and to ensure a high level of voluntary participation in a workplace screening program is to carefully educate workers about the program. Rothstein has suggested a number of issues that should be addressed in any education effort [1] (Table 33-1).

Maintaining the confidentiality of medical data is not only important from the legal and ethical perspective but is critical in facilitating the employee's participation in the program.

TABLE 33-1. CRITICAL INFORMATION ON MEDICAL TESTING PROGRAMS IN THE WORKPLACE[1]

Describe the purpose and nature of the examination.

Explain who is employing the health care provider.

Describe efforts to protect the confidentiality of the collected data.

Describe who will be provided with the results of the examination and how the information will be used, including what actions will be taken to further evaluate possible hazardous workplace exposures.

Describe how the worker will be notified of individual and group test results.

Describe how the worker may have access to his or her health records.

Describe how medical follow-up may be obtained if the test results are positive.

Adapted from Rothstein MA: Legal and ethical aspects of medical screening. Occup Med 11(1):31–39, 1996 and Rempel D: Medical surveillance in the workplace: overview. Occup Med 5(3):435–438, 1990.

▶ SELECTING THE COMPONENTS OF PERIODIC EXAMINATIONS

OSHA standards require periodic examinations for approximately 30 agents. Several common occupational exposures, such as asbestos, benzene, cotton dust, ethylene oxide, formaldehyde, lead, and noise, are covered by these specific OSHA standards. Generally, these examinations are required if a worker is exposed above a specific level of exposure, which is often one-half of the 8-hour permissible exposure limit (PEL).[7] For example, OSHA requires baseline and annual audiometry testing in employees exposed to noise at an average of 85 dBA or above for a typical 40-hour work week. The National Institute of Occupational Safety and Health (NIOSH) recommends periodic testing on a larger list of agents. Table 33-2 illustrates the medical surveillance features of the OSHA Lead Standard 1910.1025.[7]

The first step in deciding whether to institute a program of periodic medical screening is to thoroughly evaluate the occupational exposures of the working population that may be surveyed. In addition to looking to see if there are medical surveillance activities recommended by OSHA or NIOSH, a decision to institute a program can be based on three criteria: the level of exposure; the identification of the most likely types of adverse outcomes; and the availability of a suitable screening test. While there is often substantial scientific uncertainty about the shape of the exposure-effect relationship between many occupational exposures and adverse health outcomes, information about the level of exposure may indicate the probability of identifying a work-related effect is extremely unlikely. In this situation, one may infrequently survey exposed workers to confirm the absence of work-related adverse health effects. In developing a new examination program, one should determine what the adverse health effects are that are most likely to occur with exposure. This is usually based on a review of the animal and human data and the identification of the most sensitive organ system to the specific exposure. The most common adverse health effects are often nonspecific symptoms such as headaches or upper respiratory tract irritation or changes in the respiratory tract that are detectable with simple pulmonary function testing. The components of a medical screening program have been proposed (Table 33-3).[6,7]

The next logical step after the identification of the health effects that should be detected by a screening program is to identify the tests to be included in the program and the frequency of testing of individuals. Most questionnaires and medical tests that are commonly included in occupational screening programs have not been extensively evaluated for their ability to detect those with and those without adverse health effects. An efficient medical screening program should detect most individuals with subclinical adverse health effects (high sensitivity) while not mislabeling any truly healthy individuals (high specificity). When employees are found to have adverse work-related health effects, actions should be undertaken to identify workplace exposures that are hazardous and identify steps to be undertaken to reduce the excessive exposures. These efforts to evaluate exposure should be extended beyond the individual with abnormal test results to other workers with similar exposures. The test must be free of any significant risk for the screened subjects, since the main use of the test is to identify subclinical disease or diseases before an employee would normally seek health care. The test must also be acceptable to the screened population. While medical screening and surveillance are important activities, the most important approach to preventing occupational diseases and injuries is to reduce or eliminate exposure to hazardous agents and unsafe situations in the workplace.

▶ SURVEILLANCE

Definition

The previous discussion is focused on the role of screening and of periodic examinations in occupational health. One of the potential roles of these examinations is to supplement other occupational surveillance. Occupational surveillance is the ongoing and systematic collection, analysis, and interpretation of data related to either occupational exposures (hazard surveillance) or adverse health outcomes (injuries, disorders, or diseases).[8,9] Hazard surveillance should be an important part of occupational surveillance activities. The identification of occupational exposures (hazard surveillance or exposure assessment) before work-related diseases or injuries have developed or occur should trigger further evaluation of the workplace. If high or unsafe levels of exposure are found, then these exposures can be reduced by implementation of either administrative or engineering control activities. The primary goals of surveillance are different from the goals of screening programs. The classic purpose of screening is to identify

TABLE 33-2. OSHA'S MEDICAL SURVEILLANCE PROGRAM FOR LEAD

Initial evaluation: Examination with attention to the teeth, gums, hematologic, gastrointestinal, renal, cardiovascular, and neurological systems; blood pressure; blood sample for blood lead; hemoglobin and hematocrit, red cell indices and peripheral smear morphology, zinc protoporphyrin (ZPP), blood urea nitrogen (BUN), serum creatinine; routine urinalysis (U/A)

Periodic evaluation: Biological monitoring of blood lead and ZPP every 6 months or every 2 months if last blood lead at or above 40 μg/100 g of whole blood; monthly during medical removal; examinations usually for any employee with blood lead at or above 40 μg/100 g during the preceding 12 months

Physician's written statement: To include recommended special protective measures or limitations to be placed upon employee

Special requirements: Allows for multiple physician review of mechanism; provides medical removal protection

TABLE 33-3. COMPONENTS OF A MEDICAL SURVEILLANCE PROGRAM

Exposure assessment and identification of most likely adverse health effects
Selection of medical tests based on evaluation of test characteristics
Identification of employees to be tested and testing frequency
Training of testing staff
Analysis and interpretation of individual and group test results
Actions based on test results
- Verification of test results
- Notification of employees and the employer while protecting confidentiality
- Additional tests or treatment and steps to reduce an individual's exposure
- Exposure evaluation and reeducation of hazardous exposures

Maintenance of records
Evaluation for adequate quality control and revise based on the program performance

patients who have asymptomatic disease in order to initiate therapy early in the natural course of the disease.

Goals

The goals of health or injury surveillance are ideally related to prevention activities. The first goal of surveillance is the identification of new or previously unrecognized problems. Identification will occur with the association of an injury or disease with a specific work process or occupation.[10] This generally happens through two types of surveillance data: either the identification of cases without definite information about the size of the population (the cases are drawn from the sentinel health event); or from a surveillance source of cases that include some information both on the number of cases and the size of the population at risk. An example of the first type of surveillance is a recent report of cases of hypersensitivity pneumonitis with exposure to metalworking fluids.[11] An example of the second type of surveillance is the elevated rate of workers' compensation claims for carpal tunnel syndrome in certain industries in the state of Washington.[12] These two examples illustrate that surveillance activities often involve data such as workers' compensation claims that are collected for other purposes and may be conducted at the level of individual worksite or at a state or national level.

The second goal of surveillance is to determine the magnitude of the problem either at the national, state, or local level. This is one of the most important goals of surveillance from the perspective of prevention. Surveillance data can be used to determine where to focus prevention efforts.

At the national level, surveillance data can be used to identify which industries are at high risk. One of the few sources of national data is collected by the Bureau of Labor Statistics (BLS) in the Department of Labor, which surveys a representative sample of private sector employers with more than 11 employees each year.[15] The number of occupational illnesses and injuries is collected from each surveyed employer. This system was recently revised to improve the classification of occupational diseases and to collect more information about the etiology of diseases and injuries.[16]

Data in Table 33-4 illustrates a characteristic of some occupational surveillance systems. Using industry type, occupation, or job title as a surrogate for the intensity or frequency of exposure has important limitations. Sometimes the industry or job title is an adequate title for exposure; however, more frequently there is substantial variation in the intensity or frequency of exposure within an industry or a common job title. For example, meat packing plants have many highly repetitive jobs that are associated with work-related musculoskeletal injuries of the upper limb; in this case, industry type is an adequate surrogate.[13] Some of the differences between the low- and high-risk industries are possibly the result of a lower ratio of high-risk jobs to low-risk jobs in the lower-risk industries. Despite the limitations of this surveillance system, industries or occupations identified as high risk should be further evaluated.

The magnitude of the occupational injury or disease problem can be estimated at the national, state, or facility (local) level. Local surveillance systems are typically based on one or more of the following data sources: (*a*) OSHA 200 log, an important source of data for the BLS surveillance system; (*b*) in-plant medical records or logs; or (*c*) workers' compensation records. Analyses of surveillance data for the purpose of determining the magnitude of a problem sometimes also suggest a possible cause for the problem. Generally, further research or evaluation is then necessary to thoroughly explore the surveillance-generated hypothesis. Since resources for evaluating exposures and implementing possible prevention strategies are commonly limited, surveillance data identifying the magnitude of the problem should be used to allocate resources for further investigation and preventive activities.

The third goal of surveillance systems is to track trends in the number of workers exposed to occupational hazards, or the number of workers with injuries, disorders, and diseases over time. One of the major uses of this trend data is to qualitatively evaluate the effectiveness of prevention activities. However, an important limitation of surveillance data is that changes in the rate of disorders may be due to changing levels of exposure or changes in the reporting of disorders independent of their level of occurrence. Despite the limitations of

TABLE 33-4. INDUSTRIES WITH HIGH AND LOW RATES OF DISORDERS ASSOCIATED WITH REPEATED TRAUMA, 1990

Industry	*Standard Industrial Classification*[a]	*Incidence Rate*[b]
Meat packing plants	2011	1336
Poultry slaughtering	2015	696
Manufacturing refrigerators	3632	473
Grocery stores	5411-9	2
Manufacturing electronic components	3671-9	2

From Bureau of Labor Statistics. US Department of Labor, November 1991.
[a]Based on a classification system for dividing the economy into different industries, this system is described in *Standard Industrial Classification Manual* (1987). Technical Committee on Industrial Classification, Chairperson: Paul Bugg.
[b]Number of cases per 10,000 full-time workers (40 hours per week for 50 weeks per year).

surveillance data systems, the opportunity they provide for evaluation of preventive efforts is often unique because, while feasible, large-scale research evaluations of intervention programs are difficult and costly to undertake. Surveillance evaluations may involve occupational exposures (hazard) and health outcome data.

Hazard Surveillance

The most effective workplace surveillance system will have a health and a hazard or exposure component. While hazard surveillance may be less common than health surveillance, it is vital. Hazard surveillance provides the opportunity to identify and intervene on hazardous exposures before an injury or disorder develops. When hazardous exposures involve only small groups (less than 25) of workers, most serious work-related health problems will be infrequent. The determination that a disease is work related will often be difficult based on health surveillance alone. In contrast with hazard surveillance data, hazards may be readily identified regardless of the number of exposed workers. The ability of a hazard surveillance system to identify hazardous exposures is less dependent on the number of exposed workers but rather depends on the overall accuracy of methods used to identify the nature and the intensity of the exposures. As with health surveillance information, hazard surveillance information will frequently need validation with more precise data. Hazard surveillance information can be collected by worker interview, walk-through inspections, or environmental sampling. As a result of hazard surveillance and other health surveillance information, jobs can be prioritized for more sophisticated or intensive evaluation to identify hazardous exposures. The purpose of the more sophisticated evaluation is to precisely assess the nature of the exposures and to evaluate possible methods to reduce exposures.[15] Sometimes hazardous exposures identified by the hazard surveillance activities will be so clearly hazardous and ways to reduce the level of exposure will be so obvious that the more sophisticated evaluation will be unnecessary.

With regard to precision in estimating the level of exposure, hazard surveillance activities occupy one end of a spectrum, with sophisticated job analyses at the other end of the spectrum. Hazard surveillance assessments should be completed quickly with modest accuracy by trained nonprofessionals, while sophisticated job analyses will require considerably more time to be completed but will be more accurate in the identification of risk factors. Either approach can be used to assess changes in the level of job exposures after a job has been changed for any reason.

Characteristics of Successful Health Surveillance

One of the features of an effective surveillance program is the use of a standard coding system for recording health outcomes. Standardized coding leads to more homogeneous disease categories. Surveillance systems generally have to be as cost effective as possible to be widely used. The principal advantage of using existing data sources such as workers' compensation records is low cost. Supplementing an existing surveillance system with an additional component such as symptom questionnaires should be considered when observations of the workplace suggest that there are potentially hazardous common exposures, but the existing surveillance data suggests that there are no problems.[13,14] The absence of problems will commonly occur for two reasons: the exposures are not high enough to cause any health complaints and underreporting. Underreporting of problems is likely to be more common where there are obstacles or discentives to the reporting of a possible disorder to supervisors or health professionals. For example, if an organization gives awards to departments without lost time injuries or work-related disorders, either supervisors or coworkers may discourage reporting. In the second situation, more active collection of surveillance data is indicated when there is simply no existing health surveillance information to determine if a problem exists but substantial exposures are common. For example, in many sectors of the economy, OSHA logs are not required.

One of the most common types of actively sought information is the presence of symptoms by use of a questionnaire. Symptom questionnaires may be administered by a number of methods.[13,14] The analysis of questionnaire data requires some training. Generally, the case definition must be defined prior to analysis. The purpose of these definitions is to improve the uniformity or consistency of the data collected, thereby improving the quality of the surveillance data. The goal is to ensure that cases have a common set of characteristics. Symptom questionnaires are generally not used to establish a clinical diagnosis supplemented by other more definitive health examinations.

The analysis of health surveillance data is conceptually similar to the analysis of epidemiological research data.[13] In the analysis of surveillance and epidemiological data, issues of misclassification and random or systematic errors in assessing either exposures or health outcomes should be considered. Errors due to misclassification are likely to be more common in surveillance data compared to epidemiological research data. When the goal of the analysis is to determine if a specific group of workers or jobs is associated with an elevated risk, use of an internal comparison reference group from the same organization rather than some external comparison is useful since the identification of cases within an organization and their reporting are likely to be similar. While random and systematic errors in surveillance data limit the conclusions that can be drawn, these limitations are less important since the goals of the surveillance analyses are less rigorous than in epidemiological research, where the goal is to test a specific hypothesis. Changes in requirements for case reporting may occur over time in surveillance systems, making longitudinal analyses difficult. Surveillance analyses should be interpreted less quantitatively and more qualitatively. Frequently in the analysis of surveillance data, the variation in risk between jobs, departments, or industries is so large that real differences in risk can be characterized by simple statistical analyses and are unlikely to be explained principally by errors in the classification of disease, confounding factors, or random errors. Nevertheless, surveillance data should always be interpreted cautiously, given its limitations. The goal of the analysis of surveillance data is to trigger further investigation if a problem is detected, not to definitively establish its presence or absence.

▸ CONCLUSIONS

One of the most common purposes of workplace health examinations and one that is most relevant to improving the health of the workforce is to identify toxic health effects at an earlier stage than they would be detected without the examination. This type of screening program is often initiated with a baseline examination and then followed with periodic follow-up examinations. The goal of this type of program is secondary prevention.

Health examinations are also performed in workplaces for other purposes. For example, the most common purpose of the preplacement medical examination, which occurs after an offer of employment has been made but before an individual is placed on a specific job, is to determine if the individual has significant physical or mental impairment that would preclude the individual from performing specific essential duties related to a particular job. Most questionnaires and medical tests that are commonly included in occupational screening programs have not been extensively evaluated for their ability to detect those with and without adverse health effects. When employees are found to have adverse work-related health effects, actions should be undertaken to identify workplace exposures that are hazardous, and steps should be undertaken to reduce the excessive exposures.

These efforts to evaluate exposure should be extended beyond the individual with abnormal test results to other workers with similar exposures. The test must be free of any significant risk for the screened subjects since the main use of the test is to identify subclinical disease or diseases before an employee would normally seek health care. The test must also be acceptable to the screened population. The issue of who has access to the medical information collected in a workplace surveillance or screening program is a major ethical concern. Ethical codes have been developed by both the American College of Occupational and Environmental Medicine and the International Commission on Occupational Health.[3,4] Rothstein has proposed a Bill of Rights of Examinees.[1]

The most common surveillance systems used to evaluate occupational health and injury problems are based on the OSHA 200 log data, occupational health service (in-plant medical records), periodic medical examinations, or workers' compensation records. These common surveillance systems have been used to achieve many surveillance goals.

There are three principal surveillance goals. The first goal of surveillance is the identification of new or previously unrecognized problems. The second goal is to determine the magnitude of the occupational health injury or exposure problem either at the national, state, or local level. The third goal is to track trends in the number of workers exposed to occupational hazards, or the number of workers with injuries, and diseases over time. The evaluation of preventive activities is often feasible using surveillance data. While surveillance data needs to be interpreted cautiously given its inherent limitations, surveillance data often correctly identifies hazardous working conditions and can be used successfully to monitor their elimination.

▶ REFERENCES

1. Rothstein MA: Legal and ethical aspects of medical screening. Occup Med 11(1):31–39, 1996
2. Matte TD, Fine LJ, Meinhardt TJ, Baker EL: Guidelines for medical screening in the workplace. Occup Med 5(3):439–456, 1990
3. American College of Occupational and Environmental Medicine: Code of Ethical Conduct, ACOEM, Arlington Heights 1993
4. International Commission on Occupational Health: International Code of Ethics for Occupational Health Professionals, Singapore 1992
5. American College of Occupational and Environmental Medicine: ACOEM Position on Medical Surveillance in the Workplace. American College of Occupational and Environmental Medicine 1989 Report ACOEM, Arlington Heights
6. Rempel D: Medical surveillance in the workplace: overview. Occup Med 5(3):435–438, 1990
7. Jones DL: Occupational health services and OSHA compliance. Occup Med 11(1):57–68, 1996
8. Baker LB, Honeker PA, Fine LJ: Surveillance in occupational illness and injury: concepts and content. Am J Public Health 79(Suppl): 9–11, 1989
9. Thun M, Tanaka S, Smith AB, Halperin WH, et al: Morbidity from repetitive knee trauma in carpet and floor layers. Br J Ind Med 44: 611–620, 1987
10. Halperin W: Occupational health surveillance. Health Environ Dig 8:3–5, 1993
11. Bernstein DI, Lummus ZL, Santilli G, Siskosky J, Bernstein IL: Machine operator's lung: a hypersensitivity pneumonitis disorder associated with exposure to metalworking fluid aerosols. Chest 108:636–641, 1995
12. Franklin GM, Haug J, Heyer N, Checkoway H, Peck N: Occupational carpal tunnel syndrome in Washington state, 1984–1988. Am J Public Health 81(6):741–746, 1991
13. Fine LJ: Surveillance systems. In Nordin M, Andersson G, Pope M (eds): Work-related Musculoskeletal Disorders. St. Louis: Mosby-Year Book, in press
14. American National Standards Institute: ANSI Z-365: Control of Cumulative Trauma Disorders. Draft. Chicago 1994
15. Occupational Safety and Health Administration: Record Keeping Guidelines for Occupational Injuries and Illnesses. O.M.B. No. 1220-0029. Washington, DC: US Department of Labor, Bureau of Labor Statistics, 1986
16. Bureau of Labor Statistics, US Department of Labor: Annual Report. 1993. Washington, DC: Government Printing Office, 1993

34

Occupational Health Problems of Special Working Groups

Workers with Disabilities

Nancy R. Mudrick • Robert J. Weber • Margaret A. Turk

Framework for Defining Disability

The term disability is defined in various ways. In some contexts it is defined in terms of health conditions; in other contexts it is defined in terms of functional limitations; and in still other settings it is defined in terms of activity and role limitations. These varying definitions of disability have in some cases been codified into law, into standardized data collection instruments, and into the practice framework of professionals and organizations that serve people with disabilities. One consequence of the different ways in which disability is defined is that, before the characteristics and needs of people with disabilities can be discussed, the parameters of the disability definition being used must be addressed. Whatever the specific components of the definition, there does appear to be some consensus that a person with a disability is someone who experiences a permanent physical or mental impairment or a chronic health or mental health condition. The health condition or impairment may be one that is visible or it may be invisible. Onset may occur at any age or it may be present at birth. Finally, the severity of disability may vary, even among people with the same condition or impairment, such that some individuals may find it difficult to participate in many life activities, while others experience the effects of disability in a single area.

Among the many definitions of disability used by professionals, government programs, service agencies, and individuals with disabilities, there are three that are most dominant. The first definition involves the extent of limitation in the Activities of Daily Living (ADL) and Instrumental Activities of Daily Living (IADL). The second definition is embodied in the International Code of Impairments, Disabilities, and Handicaps (ICIDH) of the World Health Organization. The third construct for defining disability is based upon a model developed by Saad Nagi that defines disability in terms of the interaction of environment, functional limitation, and impairment.[1,2] As a result of the Disability Rights Movement of the 1970s and 1980s and the passage of the 1990 Americans with Disabilities Act, there appears to be growing consensus in the United States for the use of this third paradigm.

ADL and IADL

The ADL scale measures disability in terms of limitations in the Activities of Daily Living. This scale was developed by Katz and coworkers in the 1950s and has been used extensively by researchers studying the elderly.[3] The ADL scale asks about the need for assistance in the activities of eating, bathing, dressing, transfer, and toileting. A related measure, developed by Lawton and Brody in 1969, is the IADL scale—Instrumental Activities of Daily Living.[3] The items in this scale ask about the need for assistance in such activities as everyday household chores, managing finances, shopping, and getting around outside one's home. More recently, these scales have been used to define levels of disability among adults in general.[4,5] Both the ADL and IADL approach measuring disability by examining tasks or activities that are limited or prevented by an impairment or health condition. The items do not directly address work, although people with ADL and IADL limitations report low rates (approximately 25 percent) of employment.[5]

ICIDH

In 1980 the World Health Organization issued its first edition of a classification of impairments and disabilities, called the International Classification of Impairments, Disabilities, and Handicaps.[6] The intent was to offer a framework comparable to that of the *International Statistical Classification of Diseases, Injuries, and Causes of Death* (ICD) that would be a tool for describing the consequences of disease (as well as injury and other disorders). This disability code, referred to as the ICIDH, uses a framework consisting of four main categories: disease, impairment, disability, and handicap. Disease is not really defined in the ICIDH, but is implicitly based upon the definitions contained in the ICD. *Impairment* is defined as any loss or abnormality of psychological, physiological, or anatomical structure or function, and *disability* is any restriction or lack of ability to perform an activity in a manner or within the range considered normal for a human being. The final category, *handicap*, refers to a disadvantage resulting from an impairment or a disability that limits or prevents the fulfillment of a normal role.[6] While the ICIDH is similar to the Nagi model because it separates the medical condition from its functional and social consequences, it has not been as well accepted. Part of the reason is the lack of conceptual clarity of the different classifications and categories.[7] An additional reason is the objection by many people with disabilities and by disability researchers in the United States to the term, handicap. The Institute of Medicine report explains this by noting that to many people handicap has a negative connotation because it implies "an absolute limitation that does not require for its actualization any interaction with external social circumstances."[2] A revision of the ICIDH has been undertaken and is nearly complete. Representatives of the U.S. Public Health Service have played an active role in the revision process. It is likely that handicap and its related concepts will not be present in the new version. In its place will be a term that identifies the social and environmental barriers that mediate between an impairment and its disabling impact. To date, however, disability research in the United States has generally proceeded without use of the ICIDH framework, especially research focused on disability and work.

Functional Limitation Model

Saad Nagi's work has served as the basis for a model with three components: impairment, functional limitation, and disability.[1] Impairment is defined as the chronic or permanent anatomical or physiological problem (i.e., health conditions) that results from injury or illness. Examples of impairment include paralysis, deafness, or heart damage. Functional limitations are the restrictions or functional inabilities that result from an impairment. Examples of functional limitations include the inability to climb stairs or lift objects weighing more than 20 pounds. Finally, disability is defined as the consequence of functional limitation in terms of the activities of normal or expected roles. Although people have many different roles in their lives, it is the work role—and the ability to maintain the work role—that has been most often used to assess whether impairments and functional limitations are disabling. Thus, someone whose employment is affected by functional limitations is disabled. More recent elaboration of the model has enhanced the consideration of the impact of environment on role performance and quality of life.[2] One implication of this model is that the determination of disability rests very much on the particular activities required by different roles—as well on the presence or absence of environmental barriers that support or impede role (work) performance. In this framework, it is possible for two people with the same impairments and functional limitations to be rated differently in terms of disability.

Work Disability

The most common definition of disability used in the research literature on employment and disability is that of *work disability*. Work disability is present when an individual reports that a mental or physical condition limits the kind or amount of work or prevents work. It is understood from the context that work refers to paid work. This construction of the work disability definition comes out of the functional limitation model and has been used to identify people with disabilities in national surveys since 1966.[8] It is also implicit in the definition of disability used by the Social Security Administration to determine eligibility for income support on the basis of disability. As a result of its wide usage, many of the national statistics on the prevalence of disability in the United States are in fact reporting the status and characteristics of persons with work disability.

While the work disability construct has been useful because it focuses on role performance, not medical condition, as a means of identifying disability, it is increasingly inadequate as the demand for information about the labor market experience of people with disabilities increases. This is because disability is recorded only if employment is limited or prevented by a chronic condition or impairment. In other words, if an assistive device or an employer accommodation result in the ability to work without limits in the kind or amount of work, then no disability may be deemed to be present. From one point of view, this may be an appropriate outcome—the presence of a disability is not noteworthy because it is not a relevant fact about the skills and value of the worker. From another point of view, it prevents a full estimation of the number of working Americans with chronic health or other conditions that constitute disabilities. A second problem with the work disability construct is that it may not sufficiently distinguish work from occupation. That is, asked whether they are limited in the kind or amount of work they can do, do respondents answer with reference to their usual occupation or kind of work, or do they view this as asking about limitations to any kind of work, even work they would not consider doing if there were no disability? The work disability construct may be very vulnerable to the attitudes, aspirations, life experiences, and opportunities of the respondents.

Demographic Characteristics

Using a work disability construct, the 1994 National Health Interview estimates that 11.8 percent of persons age 18 to 69 are limited in the kind or amount of work or unable to work due to an impairment or health problem. An additional 3.8 percent of persons in this age range report that they are not limited in work activities, but are limited in other activities. The distribution of work disability does vary within this broad age group by race, income, education, and age. Table 34-1, which reports these distributions, shows that equal proportions of men and women report that an impairment or health problem limits or prevents work. Because more women than men report a limitation in other activities, a slightly greater proportion of women overall report some limitation. Larger differences can be observed by race. Ten percent of blacks report being unable to work due to an impairment or health problem, in contrast to 6.3 percent of whites. Overall, 14.8 percent of blacks age 18 to 69 report work disability compared to 11.5 percent of whites. Among persons of Hispanic origin (who may be any race), 10.1 percent report having a work disability. From Table 34-1 it is clear that the prevalence of work disability increases with age and decreases with increasing years of education. The prevalence of work disability rises sharply after age 45; among those age 65 to 69, nearly 30 percent report work disability, in contrast to the 8.3 percent of persons age 25 to 44 that report work disability. Work disability prevalence also varies enormously between those with and without college degrees. Approximately 2 percent of those with a college degree or postgraduate education report that they are unable to work because of an impairment or health problem, while 22 percent of those with only an elementary school education and 12.7 percent of those with some high school report that an impairment or health condition makes them unable to work. Finally, there is a greater prevalence of work disability among those with income below the poverty line. Nearly 23 percent of those with income below the poverty line report being work disabled, compared with 9.9 percent of those with household income at or above the poverty line.

These differences in the prevalence of work disability by demographic characteristics illustrate that work disability is very much associated with other social, economic, and environmental factors. Age is a factor not only because health may decline with age, but because older persons have had more years in which to experience an impairment or health problem. While those with higher levels of education may work in occupations that pose fewer risks to health, it is also the case that the occupations associated with higher levels of education are less physical so that many impairments may have no or only a modest impact on the ability to continue working. Thus, much of the racial difference in the prevalence of disability is the result of racial differences in level of education and occupation. When these factors are held constant, the differences in the prevalence of disability by race decrease. The association between poverty status and work disability is influenced by the fact that disability affects earnings and income; nonetheless, low income persons, for a variety of social and economic reasons associated with low income, are also more likely to experience impairments and health problems that have a disabling impact.

Table 34-2 displays the most prevalent conditions that cause work limitation in people age 18 to 69. Musculoskeletal conditions, especially involving the back, are the most common causes of work disability. Heart disease and arthritis and related joint disorders are also prevalent causes of work disability. What is noteworthy about the conditions listed in Table 34-2 is that most of them are conditions with onset in midlife or later. Some of the conditions are the consequence of disease, while others are the result of injury on or off the job. For many of the conditions, there may have been a period of acute illness; however, it is not the case that all people with disabilities are sick. Many of the conditions on Table 34-2 are also "invisible" impairments (e.g., heart disease, asthma, mental disorders, diabetes, and cancer). Finally, it is possible for people to experience more than one disabling condition. An additional risk faced by people with a disability is the onset of a secondary condition that is a consequence or related to the primary condition.[7]

TABLE 34-1. DISTRIBUTION OF WORK DISABILITY BY SEX, RACE, EDUCATION, AGE, AND POVERTY STATUS

	Work Disability Status					
	Total (%)	*Not Limited[a] (%)*	*Unable to Work (%)*	*Limited in Kind/Amount of Work (%)*	*Limited in Other Activities (%)*
All persons 18–69 yrs.	100.0	84.4	6.8	5.0	3.8
Male	100.0	85.0	6.7	5.1	3.3
Female	100.0	83.9	6.9	4.9	4.3
White	100.0	84.5	6.3	5.2	4.0
Black	100.0	82.0	10.3	4.5	3.2
Other race	100.0	88.2	5.8	3.5	2.5
Hispanic origin (any race)	100.0	86.9	7.0	3.1	3.0
1–8 yrs. education	100.0	66.3	22.2	7.1	4.4
9–11 yrs. education	100.0	77.6	12.7	5.6	4.0
12 yrs. (h.s. graduate)	100.0	84.4	6.6	5.4	3.6
1–3 yrs. college	100.0	87.1	4.3	4.8	3.8
4 yrs. (college graduate)	100.0	90.3	2.3	3.6	3.8
5+ yrs. (postgraduate)	100.0	89.6	2.0	4.1	4.3
Age 18–24	100.0	93.3	1.9	2.7	2.0
Age 25–44	100.0	88.5	4.2	4.1	3.2
Age 45–64	100.0	77.3	10.9	6.7	5.1
Age 65–69	100.0	63.2	20.0	9.8	7.1
At or above poverty	100.0	84.8	5.1	4.8	3.8
Below poverty	100.0	73.1	16.8	6.0	4.1
Unknown	100.0	78.6	11.9	5.6	3.9

Source: 1994 National Health Interview, author's calculation.
[a] The "Not Limited" category includes unknowns.

Employment and Disability

The employment rates of people with disabilities are much lower than the employment rates of people without disabilities. This difference is partly the result of differences in labor force participation and partly the result of employment discrimination. Table 34-3 shows that the differences in the labor force participation rates of people with and without disabilities are larger than the differences between men and women in their labor force participation rates. Among white males age 18 to 70, 90 percent with no disability are in the labor force compared with 48 percent of those with a disability. The differences for black males are even larger; approximately 85 percent of black males with no disability are in the labor force compared to 28 percent of black men with a disability. Among women, the patterns are much the same. While the labor force participation rates of women without disabilities are lower than those of men (72 percent for both

TABLE 34-2. MOST PREVALENT CONDITIONS CAUSING WORK LIMITATION, 1992

Main Cause of Limitation	*Number of People (1,000's)*	*% of People with Work Limitation*
All conditions	19,023	100.0
Orthopedic impairments, deformities, and disorders of the spine or back	2,181	11.5
Heart disease	2,071	10.9
Arthritis and allied disorders	1,818	9.6
Orthopedic impairments, deformities, and disorders of other extremities	1,775	9.3
Intervertebral disc disorders	1,479	7.8
Asthma and other respiratory diseases	1,072	5.6
Diseases of the nervous system	1,029	5.4
Mental disorders, excluding learning disability and mental retardation	925	4.9
Speech, hearing, and visual impairments (including disorders of the eye)	743	3.8
Diabetes	624	3.3
Cancer	529	2.8

From LaPlante M, Carlson D: Disability in the United States: Prevalence and Causes, 1992. Disability Statistics Report (7). Washington, DC: US Department of Education, National Institute on Disability and Rehabilitation Research, Table 7a, 1996, pp 120–123.

TABLE 34-3. PERCENTAGE OF PEOPLE IN THE LABOR FORCE WITH AND WITHOUT DISABILITIES BY RACE, HISPANIC ORIGIN, AND GENDER, 1994

	White		Black		Other		Hispanic Origin (Any Race)	
Gender and Disability Status	*% Worked in Past 2 Weeks*	*% in Labor Force*	*% Worked in Past 2 Weeks*	*% in Labor Force*	*% Worked in Past 2 Weeks*	*% in Labor Force*	*% Worked in Past 2 Weeks*	*% in Labor Force*
Males, age 18–70								
With no work disability	85.9	90.0	79.0	84.7	77.8	83.5	82.6	89.0
With a work disability	40.1	48.1	21.7	28.2	34.1	44.4	29.5	40.1
Females, age 18–70								
With no work disability	67.6	72.0	66.0	72.4	60.2	64.7	55.8	61.2
With a work disability	31.9	38.0	20.7	26.7	28.6	35.2	23.2	31.9

From Asch A, Mudrick NR: Disability. In: Encyclopedia of Social Work. 19th ed. June 1997 Update. Washington, DC: National Association of Social Workers, Data from the 1994 Health Interview Survey, 1997.

white and black women), the percent of women with disabilities who are in the labor force is also much lower (38 percent for white women and 27 percent for black women with disabilities). A national survey of people with disabilities conducted by Louis Harris and Associates found that, in addition to the 31 percent of respondents who were working, 23 percent of the respondents reported that they preferred to work and were able to work, but were not employed.[9]

People with disabilities also experience higher rates of unemployment than do people without disabilities.[10] Approximately 35 percent of people with disabilities work part-time compared to the 17.3 percent of people without disabilities who work part-time.[11] Among those who are employed, however, the percentage who are able to work regularly and full-time does not vary with the number of years since the onset of disability.[12]

Economists have also measured a small wage difference between people with and those without disabilities that can be attributed to wage discrimination.[13] Baldwin and Johnson find larger discriminatory wage differentials among men whose impairments are subject to greater prejudice compared to those with impairments associated with less prejudice.[13] Most of the impairments classified in the less prejudiced group are invisible impairments, such as back or spine problems and heart trouble, while those in the more prejudiced group tend to be visible impairments, such as paralysis, and missing legs, feet, arms, hands, or fingers. Also included in the group subject to more prejudice are persons with mental illness, alcohol or drug problems, and cancer. Although some wage discrimination has been measured, Johnson and Baldwin conclude that employment discrimination is the more significant problem for workers with disabilities. In other words, workers with disabilities face greater discrimination in hiring and maintaining employment than in the wages offered them.[13]

When people with disabilities are asked what they believe are the most significant barriers to employment (Table 34-4), they name factors that include the limitations imposed by their impairments, the absence of transportation and accommodations, labor market discrimination, and the concern that employment might cause them to lose their disability and health benefits.[9] Among those who are employed, nearly one-half feel that their jobs do not use the full extent of their talents or abilities.[9] Thirty percent of people with disabilities also report that they have encountered job discrimination, mostly in the form of being refused a job due to disability.

A 1995 survey of corporate employers found that 64 percent reported having hired someone with a disability; this percentage is 2 percent higher than that reported in a similar survey in 1986.[14] Those employers who do have employees with disabilities report satisfaction with the job performance of those employees; 76 percent rate it "pretty good" or "excellent." The reasons most often given for *not* hiring people with disabilities were absence of openings or of qualified applicants. The corporate managers surveyed seldom mentioned concerns about benefit costs, safety, or accommodations as an important reason for not hiring someone with a disability.[14] Twenty-five percent of the managers also said they were "very likely" and 50 percent said they were "likely" to make greater efforts to employ people with disabilities in the next 3 years.

Policies for Workers with Disabilities

Policies for workers with disabilities can be placed in one of three categories: (*a*) policies to protect employment by prohibiting employment discrimination, (*b*) policies to enable employment through rehabilitation and training, and (*c*) policies to replace income for workers no longer able to work. While these policies are implemented at the federal, state, community, and firm level, only the federal policies in these areas will be described below.

TABLE 34-4. REASONS OF WORKING-AGE ADULTS WITH DISABILITIES FOR NOT WORKING OR NOT WORKING FULL-TIME

Problem	*% Reporting*
Disability or health problem severely limits what he or she can do	81
Needs medical treatment of the disability or health problem	58
Employers won't recognize capability to do full-time job	40
Believe that no full-time work is available in his or her line of work or can't find it	35
Doesn't have the skills, education, or training needed to get a full-time job	32
Would risk losing benefits or insurance payments	31
Can't get affordable, convenient, or accessible transportation to and from work, or housing near to work	24
Needs a personal assistant to help get to work and do the job	24
Needs special equipment or devices to work, talk to or hear other workers, or get around	16
Would lose income, health care benefits, or other benefits currently received from private insurance or the government if worked full-time	57

From Louis Harris & Associates: *N.O.D./Harris Survey of Americans with Disabilities.* Commissioned by the National Council on Disability. New York: Louis Harris and Associates, 1994, pp 16–17.

Civil Rights

People with disabilities are protected from discrimination in employment under Title I of the 1990 Americans with Disabilities Act (ADA) and Sections 503 and 504 of the 1973 Rehabilitation Act. While the provisions in the Rehabilitation Act were the first to offer a measure of protection against employment discrimination, the coverage was restricted to people employed in the public sector or by federal contractors and grantees. Much broader coverage is now available under the Americans with Disabilities Act, which applies to employers of 15 or more employees. While the definition of disability in the ADA is modeled after the Rehabilitation Act, the enforcement structure relies on the Equal Employment Opportunity Commission (EEOC) and the methodology developed to enforce the 1964 Civil Rights Act.

The ADA defines those persons protected from disability-based employment discrimination as (*a*) people with a mental or physical impairment that substantially limits a major life activity, (*b*) persons with a record of such impairment, and (*c*) those who are perceived to have such an impairment. Title I protects a "qualified person with a disability," who is someone who can perform, with or without "reasonable accommodation," the "essential functions" of the job. An employer who can show that a requested accommodation would cause the firm undue hardship will not be required to hire the individual and make the accommodation. Undue hardship is judged in terms of the expense of the accommodation in relation to the size of the firm, the extent of change required, and the potential hazard posed to other people. The ADA does not consider someone who is currently using illegal drugs a qualified person with a disability. It also allows an employer to hold someone who is alcoholic to the same performance standard as all other employees, without regard to whether deficits in performance can be attributed to alcohol addiction. These provisions of the ADA require that employers articulate the essential functions of their jobs, take action to ensure that the job application process does not improperly screen out people with disabilities, and have a means through which they can respond to requests for reasonable accommodation.

Between July 1992, when the ADA went into effect, and September 1995, there were 54,690 complaints of discrimination filed with the EEOC under Title I. Of the complaints filed, 51 percent were about discharge, 27 percent involved failure to provide reasonable accommodation, 11 percent included a charge of harassment, with smaller percentages charging discriminatory actions related to benefits, promotion, discipline, or wages; 10 percent were complaints of failure to hire. It is not clear what proportion of the complaints of failure to reasonably accommodate involve newly hired employees versus existing employees with new disabilities. However, the distribution of complaints indicates that the majority of complainants are persons who have been in jobs, rather than persons seeking jobs. This pattern of complaints is probably related to the fact that a large proportion of people with disabilities experience the onset of disability in midlife.[9] Many people are working at the onset of disability. For employers this means that some of the people who already work for them will become people with disabilities, so that compliance with the ADA includes the employer's response to these employees. The pattern of ADA complaints so far suggests that many employees believe that actions their employers have taken toward them are discriminatory and based upon the presence of a disability.

Rehabilitation and Training

A second area of policy for workers with disabilities involves the service system that makes available rehabilitation, job training, and supports for independent living. Rehabilitation services were first authorized under federal and state law to enable veterans with disabilities to obtain and maintain employment. The system of services has been expanded to include all persons with disabilities. While some rehabilitation services are financed by private insurance, either under an individual's health insurance or through Worker's Compensation, many rehabilitation services are financed by public funds at the state and federal level.

The Rehabilitation Act, most recently reauthorized in 1992, is the main vehicle for specifying federal policy and expenditures for rehabilitation services. Various titles under this act support programs that provide job counseling, retraining, and the provision of prosthetic and assistive devices. Many of these rehabilitation services are delivered through a network of state agencies. Supported employment, a service model in which a person with a severe disability works in a private sector job with a job coach who eases the transition to independent employment, is also part of the Rehabilitation Act. Finally, the Rehabilitation Act provides funds to support centers for independent living, community-based self-help agencies that engage in advocacy and other types of support to enable both independent living and self support among people with disabilities.

Initially, the state-federal vocational rehabilitation service system focused its efforts on those with the least severe impairments and those deemed most likely to be able to obtain and maintain employment. This meant that there were few efforts to assist people with more severe disabilities to prepare for employment, even if they desired it. Language in the Rehabilitation Act as reauthorized in 1992 makes it clear that rehabilitation efforts must also be aimed at people with severe levels of impairment.

Finally, while there is no explicit policy to this effect, services for persons with psychiatric disabilities have tended to be funded and provided separately from those aimed at persons with physical impairments. Most states have state offices of mental health and mental retardation that oversee policies, funding, and service agencies for persons with mental or emotional impairments. With a mixture of state and federal funding, services are provided on an in-patient and out-patient basis, although the number of persons in residential institutions is greatly reduced compared to that in the 1950s.

Income Support

For workers whose disabilities prevent continued employment, the main source of replacement income is Social Security Disability Insurance (DI). Coverage for Disability Insurance is earned at the same time that workers earn coverage for the social security retirement benefit. A part of the social security payroll tax (FICA) paid by employers and employees is directed to the Disability Insurance Trust Fund. A worker with a disability will be eligible to collect DI if he or she has worked and contributed to Social Security for 20 of the past 40 quarters (essentially 5 of the past 10 years) and has a condition that meets the medical criteria that prevents "substantial gainful activity." The disability does not need to be the result of a work injury or work-related. However, there is a 5-month waiting period before the start of benefits. Because Disability Insurance defines disability as the inability to engage in substantial gainful activity (measured as earnings in excess of $500 per month), DI essentially requires complete labor force withdrawal to establish eligibility. The size of the benefit is determined by prior earnings using a formula that is a variant of the one used to calculate monthly Social Security retirement benefits. After two years as a DI beneficiary, health insurance coverage under Medicare is available.

There is a requirement in the Disability Insurance program that beneficiaries be assessed for their ability to work and offered rehabilitation if it is deemed appropriate. Refusal to participate in recommended rehabilitation can cause a loss of benefit eligibility. Despite these requirements, less than 1 percent of DI beneficiaries leave the DI rolls each year for employment.[15] The difficulty of establishing eligibility, the work disincentive embodied in the definition of disability used by the program, the severity of the disabilities of most DI beneficiaries, and the lack of vigorous enforcement of the rehabilitation assessment and service provision are all considered factors contributing to the low rate of program termination.[15,16]

Workers with disabilities may also receive income support through Worker's Compensation if their impairments are work-related. Worker's Compensation programs are state laws that require employers to carry insurance to compensate workers for injuries or illness obtained on the job. In some states, employers purchase Worker's Compensation insurance from private insurance carriers or self-insure. In other states, employers must purchase the insurance through a state-run insurance fund. The intent of Worker's Compensation is to replace lost earning capacity. People with a permanent impairment may receive a lump sum or a monthly payment in perpetuity; otherwise workers are paid a portion of their wage for the period they are out of work recovering from the work injury or illness. Worker's Compensation also pays the medical expenses associated with the treatment of the work-related condition.

A small proportion of workers with disabilities may also receive income support from the Supplemental Security Income Program (SSI). SSI is an income-tested public assistance program that provides support to low-income persons with disabilities. Because it is income and asset tested, only workers with low DI benefits are probably also eligible for SSI. Many SSI recipients are persons with little or no work history, or whose work attachment is insufficient to meet the DI coverage criteria. The SSI program is a federal income support program, administered by the Social Security Administration and financed out of general revenues. Some states supplement the federal SSI benefit. SSI recipients are also immediately eligible for health care coverage under the public assistance Medicaid program.

Role of Clinicians

Clinicians play an integral role in the diagnostic, rehabilitation, and return-to-work plan of workers with disabilities. Rehabilitation is a dynamic process, which is most effective when provided through a comprehensive transdisciplinary team approach. Rehabilitation deals not only with physical restoration, but recognizes the importance of psychosocial health and support. The disability evaluation process requires medical evaluation in preparation for hiring, the development and direction of a rehabilitation and return-to-work plan, and the determination of impairment or disability. Of significant importance is recognition that a worker with a disability is not ill or in poor health, but rather can participate in ongoing health maintenance and prevention of further disabilities and secondary conditions.

Acute and Chronic Medical Care

Acute medical management of worker injuries offers the clinician a range of challenges with distinct differences from those posed by chronic management. However, the attitudes, knowledge, and skills required of the practitioner in each area have broad overlap. The process of decision-making and support of worker needs should vary principally in respect to the weight assigned to input elements in each circumstance. The most obvious feature of acute management is the possibility of the abrupt onset of a catastrophic problem that forces an emergency course of treatment. In that circumstance the physician provides triage, diagnosis, and treatment, directing care until stability is restored. This process should ideally lead to the transition into rehabilitation where worker involvement and empowerment become key elements.

The physician's role in the acute management of problems with a less dramatic presentation, such as back injury or repetitive use disorders, is established through the dynamic interaction among worker, physician, employer, and the compensation system. Nonetheless, the worker has the free choice of a clinician in essentially all cases. Thus, the clinician should be attuned to address the worker's interests as he or she individually, or through referral and transfer, moves through the responsibility for triage, diagnosis, treatment, and rehabilitation. Where the worker has knowledge of medical issues, he or she can influence the clinician's role even more significantly. A knowledge of similar worksite problems and workers' experiences increases the likelihood that the worker will use the health care system more effectively, a de facto self-selection of the physician role by the worker. There is no readily available information demonstrating workers' satisfaction with their clinicians' services.

Acute and chronic management of occupational problems share the need for specific knowledge of signs, symptoms, etiology, treatment, rehabilitation, and prognosis of problems encountered in the workplace. While acute management may favor a greater proficiency in some diagnostic and intervention procedure skills, it is in the realm of attitude that clinicians most differ in the spectrum of acute to chronic care. Ideally these differences are masked from the patient since they reflect the gratification that the physician feels as a result of his or her own efforts and outcomes. They derive from the personality structure of the physician and they are reflected also in average personality profile differences observed among specialties. Thus acute care providers tend toward extroversion and gratification in task-related activity, while chronic care/rehabilitation specialists tend toward an introspective and nurturing profile. This corresponds well with the practical aspects of service emphasis in the acute-chronic care spectrum. In the chronic phase, maintenance, adjustment, support and accommodation, and prevention of secondary conditions are more prominent than direct intervention. Worker values, rather than medical pathways, determine the proper course. The physician serves to facilitate and to advise, not to effect change, to intervene only when new factors emerge. This role shift is sometimes a challenge to each party of the relationship.

Rehabilitation

Rehabilitation is an ongoing process that is most effective when it is provided through a comprehensive transdisciplinary team, is introduced as a part of acute medical management, and is continued until there has been a successful return to the workforce. Rehabilitation programs are termed comprehensive when they function in an integrated manner to address the full spectrum of medical, functional, and psychosocial needs of the client throughout the time of need. The transdisciplinary (interdisciplinary) aspect refers to a program organization that fosters the reinforcement, enhancement, and extension of both global and discipline-initiated goals across traditional disciplinary boundaries for services. Core members of comprehensive teams include a rehabilitation physician and nurse, physical, occupational and vocational specialists, psychologist, and social worker. The team develops rehabilitation goals through formal team conferences that meet regularly to update goals, discover and address evolving issues, and devise means to leverage the team via transdisciplinary synergy. Individual service goals to effect the global team goals are developed and shared. The team approach offers benefits through the initiative and knowledge resulting from wide participation and from the efficiency of extending patient learning, reinforcement of skills, endurance, and confidence, building throughout the full day through the close integration of the nursing unit with all services in the total plan.

The rehabilitation process can be separated into two broad conceptual categories. The first is comprised of those cases in which the anticipated rehabilitation outcome is the ability to resume life and work roles with little or no accommodation. The second involves cases for which significant accommodation and perhaps residual disability is likely. In each instance rehabilitation proceeds through three general phases: establishment of goals, worker-focused programming, and transition to the workforce.

Rehabilitation goal setting requires the translation of the medical prognosis into a function-based worker profile, the identification of resources, and the integration of worker options and preferences into practical outcome targets. Defining goals also separates expectations into the broad programmatic categories, and it promotes a rationalization and consistency when selecting among options related to service intensity, intervention risks, and accommodations. Goal setting requires an understanding of both the personal and material resources available for rehabilitation.

The worker-focused phase is the process usually identified as medical rehabilitation—the transdisciplinary delivery of medical, physical, psychosocial, and vocational services to maximize the physical and psychological function of the worker in the context of the established goals. Here specific skill acquisition, adjustment, and the determination of specific vocational targets and accommodation requirements are emphasized.

The transition phase is relatively straightforward where function is well restored. Work site assessment is helpful in ensuring that worker preparation is appropriate or where return to work can be facilitated by minor or temporary accommodations or a phased return. Transition is often a longer process where major accommodation is required. Frequently a gradual shift occurs from a medically directed team management of the program to a vocationally directed one. Here skill assessment and training for the worker, resource acquisition, job site analysis, and negotiation for job site accommodation and its funding take center stage.

Psychological Care

Psychological variables have an effect on the rehabilitation process and outcome and can modify the expression of disability or determine the impact on function. In particular, cognitive impairment and functional limitation as a result of brain injury or mental retardation can determine initiation of or return to work capability. Issues of role or performance change can be difficult for the worker with the disability, the family or other support system, and the employer.

Psychological evaluation of cognitive functioning involves standard intelligence and achievement tests, and batteries or individualized approaches for neuropsychological testing. The evaluation provides information regarding cognitive performance of executive functions, relative strengths and weaknesses, possible direction for cognitive-related services, and useful strategies for cognitive compensation.

A worker with a disability may require psychological support during the acute medical and rehabilitation process. A psychological assessment is a combination of standardized testing and interview information that determines attributes (e.g., personality, intellectual, and cognitive factors) that may influence the rehabilitation process and outcome and identify the presence or magnitude of certain other psychological factors (e.g., depression, anxiety, anger, disinhibition, denial) that may have an impact on return to work. Following a medical event, such psychological forces begin to play an increasingly important role in overall level of disability. Coincident and independent sources of distress from family, employer, or vocational settings can be incorporated into the sense of impairment. The impact of the patient's altered social behavior on families can be substantial. Psychological intervention can be direct counseling, skill building in coping and adjustment strategies, and training in social skills. Families and other support systems should be a part of this process to better understand the psychological status of the patient, reinforce appropriate behaviors or coping strategies, and maintain personal psychological health to continue what may be a prolonged course of impairment and disability.

Assessing the Ability to Work and Accommodations to Enable Work

Determination of work capability requires evaluation of the worker as well as the workplace. The physician becomes involved with issues of work disability in the context of medical evaluations of workers in preparation for hire, for the development and direction of a return-to-work plan, or for the determination of impairment or disability. A workplace assessment involves job description and on-site evaluation.

In the recent past, a number of employers have engaged in selection screening to identify a healthier work force with the use of medical criteria in the selection and maintenance of a work force. This involves worker fitness evaluations (e.g., current health, ability to perform job functions, required modifications) and risk evaluations (e.g., prediction of increased risk for illness or injury based on health history, work history, or behavioral patterns). In most instances, few data exist to support such determinations.[17,18]

The disability evaluation process may require a clinician to assume one or more of three different roles that are potentially in conflict. The physician may act as an advocate and counselor to the patient, a source of information for the agencies that determine benefits, and adjudicator and certifier of impairment or disability.[19] As advocate and counselor, the physician can advise the patient of disease- or injury-specific issues related to initiation of or return to work. In this role the physician can outline the process of rehabilitation and discuss possible accommodations. The physician may also provide information about the advantages and potential pitfalls of the various compensation and rehabilitation programs and make referrals to appropriate services.

For those patients who have applied for benefits, the physician will likely be asked to provide medical records and documentation of impairment. During the phases of reporting on initial, interim, and maximal medical improvement (MMI, the achievement of maximal benefit from intervention with stabilization of impairment), the physician is asked to complete return-to-work status reports, including a date of MMI.

Evaluation of the patient's impairment places the physician in the role of certifier. Impairments can be expressed in terms of functional loss of a unit or to a whole person. The impairment rating system most commonly employed for musculoskeletal impairments is the AMA (American Medical Association) Guides.[20] The AMA Guides have recently been updated (1993) and are anatomically based (description and quantifiable physical examination measurements) and diagnosis related (history plus objective diagnostic findings). However, there are concerns related to validity and reliability,[21,22] inference of functional limitation from anatomically based impairment scales or findings,[20] and the issue of pain as it relates to impairment.[23] In cases involving a dispute between claimant and insurer concerning MMI determination or impairment rating, a physician examiner unfamiliar with the case can review the case records, examine the patient, and render a second opinion, referred to as an Independent Medical Examination (IME).

A number of standardized assessment tools are available to assist the physician in determining physical performance expectations for a disabled worker. A Functional Capacity Evaluation (FCE) is a comprehensive assessment of an individual's strength, flexibility, endurance, and job-specific functional abilities. This is perhaps the most valid predictor of appropriate restrictions to activities throughout the rehabilitation course and at the MMI. When no specific job is available, a more generic Functional Capacity Assessment (FCA) can provide more global information to assist in job placement. A Job Description is a formal listing of the essential job functions and provides the basis of specific performance requirements. A Job Site Evaluation (JSE) determines optimal ergonomic design and validates performance requirements of the job. A JSE in conjunction with a FCE may be useful in determining work restrictions, need for accommodation, and employer/employee willingness to comply.

There is a wide range of possible workplace modifications. Many modifications made for the worker with disabilities also may benefit other workers or even customers. Architectural barriers can be modified with ramps, railings, more easily opened doors, modified bathroom fixtures, and space to accommodate wheelchair turning radius, to name a few. Work site adjustments, such as ergonomic seating, placement of equipment for ease of use or reach, telephone headsets, use of switches, or lift assist devices, can allow improved productivity. Print adjustment (larger size, Braille, raised lettering) and improved lighting will assist persons with vision impairment, and also an aging population. Amplification systems, telephone devices for the deaf (TTD), and the use of vibration or lighting to alert individuals to surrounding activities are among the accommodations helpful to hearing-impaired workers. Schedules to assist with cognitive and physical performance (e.g., focused tasks, routine breaks, routine schedule) and to allow for needed health activities (e.g., intermittent catheterization for healthy urinary management, allowance for position change) must also be considered. The Job Accommodation Network (JAN), a federally financed consultation service, provides specific advice and information about various methods of accommodation. Independent Living Centers, regional ADA information centers, and many of the organizations that focus on a specific condition (e.g., National Spinal Cord Injury Association) also provide advice regarding workplace accommodation.[24]

Prevention and Wellness

With disability ranking among the nation's largest public health problems, application of the prevention model is appropriate. Primary prevention of unintentional injuries, occupationally related injuries or exposures, and other medically or health-related etiologies of disabilities are a part of the national agenda. However, primary prevention of other health issues or secondary conditions of persons with disabilities should be acknowledged. This requires use of traditional public health prevention strategies and the clinician's index of suspicion regarding possible secondary conditions. Secondary prevention is aimed at early recognition of disability or disability-producing activities, with reduction of risk factors for work disabilities and improvement in the quality of life. Disability-related legislation reflects efforts to reduce environmental and social risk factors for worker disability. Appropriate modifications of the workplace for a worker with a disability who has initiated or completed a return to work also is a secondary prevention strategy. Tertiary prevention is centered on the rehabilitation aspects of a return-to-work plan.

Despite the medical complications and implications of disabling conditions, workers with disabilities are not ill or in poor health. There has been a paradigm shift from illness and disease to health and wellness. It is important to recognize health promotion for the worker with a disability, in spite of the disabling condition.

Conclusion

The increasing prevalence of chronic health conditions and impairments with age implies that a substantial proportion of labor force participants are people with disabilities. These workers with disabilities make an important contribution to the support of their families and to the economy as whole. While the focus of care and services for workers with disabilities has in the past often worked to push these individuals out of the labor force, changes in the rehabilitative service system are now more oriented toward facilitating continued employment. These changes are reinforced by the legal requirements of the ADA that prohibit discrimination and require workplace accommodation and by the increasingly wide acceptance of the functional/environmental model and the minority group framework to define disability and disability policy. Challenges remain to more fully include workers with disabilities in the workforce. Among these are increasing insurance coverage for accommodations and assistive devices that are crucial to the maintenance of function, but are not "medical" in nature, and reducing the inaccessibility and inadequacy of transportation systems so that workers with disabilities can reach the workplace. There also is a continuing need to educate employers, coworkers, and other professionals about the positive qualities of the lives and abilities of people with disabilities.

Minority Workers and Communities

Howard Frumkin • E. Darryl Walker

Environmental and occupational hazards do not affect all communities equally. Members of ethnic and racial minorities, whether as working people or as community residents, sustain disproportionate risk from chemical, physical, and biological hazards. This chapter reviews the nature of these disproportionate risks, focusing primarily on the workplace, but considering general environmental exposures as well. It presents evidence for increased exposure, increased susceptibility, and increased resulting illness and injury among members of minority groups.

The U.S. population is becoming more diverse, with minority groups accounting for a growing proportion of the overall population. The Census Bureau projects that, by the year 2000, the U.S. population will reach approximately 275 million, of whom 71.6 percent will be white, 12.8 percent black, 0.9 percent Native American/Eskimo/Aleut, 4.4 percent Asian and Pacific Islander, and 11.3 percent Hispanic (of any race).[1]

Members of minority groups live and work in patterns that distinguish them from the general population and from each other. Minority workers, on average, have less education, lower income levels, inferior housing, worse health status, and less access to services such as health care, compared with white workers. For example, according to 1990 Census Bureau data on the civilian labor force, the proportion of workers who had not completed high school was 14.0 percent for whites, 26.2 percent for blacks, and 44.5 percent for Hispanics. Similarly, the proportion of workers who had completed college was 23.6 percent for whites, 13.1 percent for blacks, and 9.3 percent for Hispanics. The per capita income was $15,265 among whites, $9,017 among blacks, and $8,424 among Hispanics. These and similar data signal persistent disparities in economic opportunities, residential patterns, and other important determinants of health.

Mechanisms of Increased Risk among Minority Workers

Members of minority groups may be at increased risk from occupational and environmental exposures through one or more of several mechanisms. First, they may be disproportionately exposed to hazards. Second, they may be more susceptible to the effects of these exposures. Third, they may receive inferior health care once injured or made ill following an exposure. In discussing these risks, the primary focus will be on blacks, since more data are available than for Hispanics, Native Americans, Asian Americans, and other minority groups.

Increased Exposure to Occupational Hazards

There is ample evidence that members of minority groups have been, and continue to be, concentrated in jobs with lower pay, lower status, and, all too often, higher risk. This is exemplified by one of the watershed occupational health disasters in U.S. history, the construction of the Hawk's Nest Tunnel near Gauley Bridge, West Virginia in 1930–1931. This tunnel was drilled through a mountain rich in silica to transport river water to a power plant. Several hundred tunnel workers lost their lives, some from injuries, but most from acute silicosis. Although the local population was over 80 percent white, the workers hired for the most hazardous jobs—inside the tunnel—were 75 percent black. Accordingly, of over 700 deaths from 1930 to 1935 attributed to work on the tunnel construction, 76 percent occurred among black workers. As the nearby *Fayette Journal* noted in February 1931, "This is a great deal of comments [sic] about town regarding the unusually large number of deaths among the coloured labourers at tunnel works of the New Kanawha Power Company."[2]

In numerous industry-specific studies, similar patterns of disproportionate exposure have continued to be documented. In the chromate industry in the 1940s, 41 percent of the black workers, as compared with 16 percent of the white workers, were assigned to the "dry end" of the process, where exposures to chromate dust were highest.[3] In the steel industry, one of the most hazardous jobs is in the coke plant, due to exposure to carcinogenic polycyclic aromatic hydrocarbons. Among coke plant workers in the 1950s, 89 percent of blacks and 32 percent of whites worked directly at the coke ovens. Among these coke oven workers, 21 percent of blacks and only 8 percent of whites were assigned to the most heavily exposed "full topside" jobs. As a result, 74 percent of full topside workers were black,[4] and black workers were over five times more likely than white workers to be in one of the highest exposure categories.[5] In the textile industry in the 1970s, black workers were concentrated in the dustiest areas of the plants, with a substantially higher risk of byssinosis than their white coworkers.[6] In the rubber industry, black workers were concentrated in the compounding and mixing job categories, where exposures to various carcinogens were highest.[7]

Agricultural work deserves special mention because it is overwhelmingly a minority occupation. Seasonal farm workers are 71 percent Hispanic, and migrant workers are 95 percent Hispanic.[8] Farm work is one of the most dangerous occupations; it employs less than 3 percent of the U.S. workforce, but accounts for 13 percent of workplace fatalities. It is estimated that pesticide toxicity causes 313,000 cases of illness and 1,000 deaths annually among farm workers.[9]

Studies using national databases yield similar conclusions. In a 1974 report based on the 1967 Survey of Economic Opportunity, each of several hundred occupations was categorized in terms of its associated hazardous exposures. Black male workers had a 25 percent greater probability of exposure to at least one hazard than did white male workers, and black female workers had a 93 percent greater probability of exposure to at least one hazard than did their white counterparts.[10] In a 1984 study based on the 1977 Quality of Employment Survey, 47 percent of black workers reported "significant" or "great" exposure to at least one workplace hazard, compared to 37 percent of whites. Blacks reported significantly greater exposure to several specific hazards, including high temperature, dirty conditions, noise, and infectious disease risk. In a risk index based on the workers' compensation experience of various industries, black workers were at 39 percent greater risk than were white workers. (Parallel calculations based on alternative data sources, the 1974 Panel Study of Income Dynamics and the 1977 Current Population Survey, estimated this increased risk to be 52 and 37 percent, respectively.) The effect of race persisted after controlling for education, experience, and other determinants of job selection.[11]

Recent experience can be summarized by comparing the injury/illness rates of the blackest and whitest occupations. Table 34-5 compares all occupations that are more than 25 percent black with those that are less than or equal to 1 percent black, using 1994 data from the Bureau of Labor Statistics and Current Population Survey. With few exceptions, the blackest occupations are more hazardous than the whitest occupations; the weighted average injury/illness rate is approximately three times higher in the blackest occupations.

Another employment-related health hazard, ironically, is the absence of employment. Black unemployment has for some time been approximately twice as high as white unemployment. In 1994, 11 percent of blacks and 5 percent of whites were unemployed.[12] In turn, unemployment is a well-established risk factor for morbidity and mortality.[13] The causal chain operates in both directions. While some of this association occurs because ill people are more likely to become unemployed—the inverse of the "healthy worker effect," well known to occupational epidemiologists—unemployment and its consequences play an important role in contributing to poor health.

Increased Exposure to Environmental Hazards

The association of minority status with hazardous exposures extends beyond the workplace to the general environment as well. Members of minority groups live near more environmental hazards, such as polluting factories and hazardous waste sites, than do whites.[14,15] A considerable body of work in recent years, much of it in the form of correlational studies, small area case studies, and ecological studies using Geographic Information Systems or similar techniques, has demonstrated this pattern.[16–20] This evidence has stimulated further research, government action, and an active community-based "environmental justice" movement.[21]

Minorities sustain disproportionate exposure to air pollution, independent of income and urbanization.[17] For example, as shown in Figure 34-1, blacks and Hispanics are more likely than whites to live in air pollution nonattainment areas.

Hazardous waste exposure demonstrates a similar pattern. Early work by the United Church of Christ showed that race predicted the presence of a hazardous waste facility better than any other community variable.[16] Communities with one hazardous waste facility averaged 24 percent minority population, and communities with two or more hazardous waste facilities averaged 38 percent minority population, compared to a 12 percent minority population in communities without such a facility. In a case study of Houston, six of eight municipal incinerators and all five municipal landfills were located in black neighborhoods.[21a] In a case study of Baton Rouge, the 10 largest white Zip codes contained five hazardous waste sites, while the 10 largest black Zip codes contained 15 hazardous waste sites. Total waste generated was estimated to be 663 times greater in the black neighborhoods than in the white neighborhoods.[22]

Water pollution exposure also varies by race and ethnicity, although fewer data are available than for other media. Exposures to both microbial and chemical contaminants appear to be higher for minority groups. This is well documented in specific situations, such as in migrant worker camps (whose residents are primarily Hispanic), on Indian reservations, and in rural poor counties, whose residents are disproportionately black and Native American.[23]

Lead paint poses the major environmental source of lead exposure to children, now that lead has been removed from gasoline. Black children face substantially greater exposure to lead paint than white children, through living in older, more poorly maintained housing stock.[24–26] Over 50 percent of black children in poverty enter the first grade with blood lead levels above 10 μg/dL, the level at which neurotoxicity has been demonstrated.[27]

Even dietary exposures vary by racial and ethnic background. A well-established example is fish consumption. Since compounds such as dioxins, dibenzofurans, and organometals bioconcentrate in fish, excessive fish consumption may be hazardous. In a study of Michigan anglers, the average daily fish consumption was 17.9 g among whites, 20.3 g among blacks, 19.8 g among "other minorities" (including Hispanics), and 24.3 among Native Americans.[28] While whites tended to fish for recreation, nonwhites fished both for recreation and for food. Among Mohawk Indians in New York State, Mohawk women ate significantly more polychlorinated biphenyl (PCB)-contaminated fish than white women, although the Mohawk women successfully limited their fish consumption during pregnancy thanks to local fish advisories.[29] This pathway is especially worrisome among indigenous and/or poor populations, for whom subsistence fishing may represent a principal source of food.[30]

Exposures to hazards in the ambient environment may be aggravated by problems related to substandard housing, such as absence of air conditioning and appropriate ventilation, and microbiological exposures. Overall, there is a consistent trend that extends from the workplace to the general environment. Members of minority groups are disproportionately exposed to hazards through working in the most dangerous jobs and living in the least wholesome environments.

Increased Susceptibility to Occupational and Environmental Hazards

Independent of increased exposure to occupational and environmental hazards, members of minority groups may be especially susceptible to the effects of hazardous exposures. This could occur through

TABLE 34-5. INJURY/ILLNESS RATES IN THE BLACKEST AND WHITEST OCCUPATIONS, 1994

Occupation	U.S. Census Occupation Code	Percent Black Workers	Injury/Illness Rate (/100 full-time workers/year)
■ **OCCUPATIONS WITH >25% BLACK WORK FORCE**			
Longshore equipment operators	845	54.7	50.00
Winding and twisting machine operators	738	40.4	23.28
Baggage porters and bellhops	464	36.3	57.06
Welfare service aides	465	29.6	40.00
Nursing aides, orderlies, and attendants	447	29.3	74.94
Miscellaneous textile machine operators	749	28.5	40.53
Garbage collectors	875	28.1	100.00
Housekeepers	449	27.9	47.80
Barbers	457	27.6	2.69
Knitting, looping, taping, weaving machine	739	26.5	24.67
Supervisors, computer equipment operators	304	26.2	5.42
Health aides, except nursing	446	25.6	55.05
Bus drivers	808	25.6	36.85
Weighted average			**59.31**
■ **OCCUPATIONS WITH <1% BLACK WORK FORCE**			
Stenographers	314	1.0	20.60
Hand engraving and printing occupations	793	0.9	20.07
Veterinarians	86	0.9	9.95
Aerospace engineers	44	0.9	6.19
Supervisors, painters and paperhangers	556	0.9	3.83
Urban planners	173	0.9	1.80
Physicists and astronomers	69	0.9	0.78
Geologists and geodesists	75	0.9	0.51
Shoe machine operators	745	0.8	29.84
Supervisors, forestry and logging	494	0.8	2.71
Precious stones and metal work	647	0.8	2.54
Hand molders and shapers	675	0.7	111.50
Mechanical controls and valve repair	539	0.7	34.78
Drilling and boring machine operators	708	0.7	25.37
Glaziers	589	0.6	356.40
Miscellaneous woodworking	733	0.6	152.25
Agricultural and food scientists	77	0.3	4.83
Supervisors, extractive workers	613	0.2	31.95
Dental hygienists	204	0.2	12.53
Hoist and winch operators	848	0.1	396.75
Locksmiths and safe repairers	536	0.1	24.08
Weighted average			**20.22**

From Bureau of Labor Statistics, Survey of Occupational Injuries and Illnesses, 1994, and Current Population Survey, 1994 Annual Averages.

one or more of several mechanisms: increased baseline risk of certain diseases to which occupational and environmental exposures further contribute; increased probability of other exposures that may combine with workplace or environmental exposures to harm health; increased genetic susceptibility; and increased general susceptibility to disease through stress, poverty, and decreased social supports.

Increased Baseline Risk of Certain Diseases. Many common illnesses are multifactorial in etiology. While occupational and environmental exposures may contribute to illness, so may a range of genetic, social, environmental, and lifestyle factors. If members of minority groups carry an increased baseline risk for some of these illnesses, then workplace and environmental exposures could pose special hazards for these groups. Several examples are discussed below.

Lung cancer is a leading cause of cancer incidence and mortality for both men and women in the United States in the 1990s. Lung cancer incidence is approximately 50 percent higher in black men than in white men, although black women and white women have comparable incidence rates. Lung cancer mortality is 61 percent higher in black men than in white men, and 13 percent higher in black women than in white women.[31] Other minority groups generally have lower lung cancer incidence and mortality than whites. The black excess is not fully explained by differences in smoking; although the prevalence of smoking is higher among black men than among white men, blacks initiate smoking at a later age and smoke fewer cigarettes compared to whites.[32,33] Possible explanations include dietary differences,[34] genetic and/or metabolic differences,[35,36] and differences in environmental and occupational exposures to lung carcinogens. Based on this increased risk, blacks may be especially susceptible to the effects of further exposures to lung carcinogens in the workplace or general environment.

Asthma is steadily increasing in all U.S. subpopulations, and now affects approximately 13 million Americans.[37] Asthma prevalence and mortality are higher in blacks than in whites; the cumulative prevalence is 122 per 1,000 in blacks and 104 per 1,000 in whites, and asthma mortality is approximately three times higher in blacks than in whites.[37,38] Similarly, asthma prevalence is more than three times higher among Puerto Rican children than among non-Hispanic children.[8] Asthma prevalence and mortality are especially high, and rising, in inner cities, where minority populations are concentrated.[39] The reasons for the increase in asthma are not fully understood; they may include changes in diagnostic practice, health care

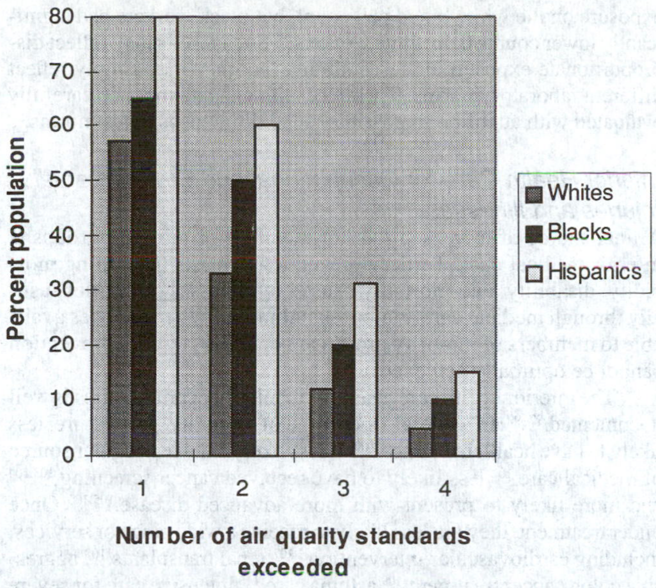

Figure 34-1. Proportion of U.S. population living in air pollution nonattainment areas by race. (Adapted from Wernette DR, Nieves LA: Breathing polluted air: minorities are disproportionately exposed. EPA Journal 18:16–17, 1992.)

access, medication use, environmental exposures and/or immune status. Whatever the reasons, the racial disparity may imply that minority populations are especially susceptible to the effects of any of the hundreds of environmental agents known to cause or aggravate asthma.[40] Moreover, minority workers are concentrated in several occupations, such as health aides and textile workers, with frequent exposure to asthma-causing agents and with elevated asthma mortality.[41] Similarly, since those with asthma are especially susceptible to the effects of certain air pollutants, especially ozone and acid aerosols,[42] and since blacks are disproportionately likely to be asthmatic, excessive exposure to air pollutants may have a disproportionate impact on blacks.

Hypertension continues to cause excess morbidity and mortality among U.S. blacks. Hypertension is between 33 and 50 percent more prevalent in blacks than in whites, and severe hypertension occurs three to seven times more commonly in blacks than in whites.[43,44] Hypertension has important end-organ effects, contributing to the occurrence of renal failure, congestive heart failure, myocardial infarction, and stroke, all conditions that occur at higher rates among blacks.[45–49] The nature of this increased risk is complex and multifactorial. There is evidence of racial differences in salt sensitivity, neurogenic response, and other physiological factors, as well as in diet and social stressors.[43,50,51] Again, whatever the reasons for the increased risk among blacks, they may place blacks at yet further risk when exposed to workplace and environmental factors that contribute to hypertension.

Two such factors are relevant. The first is social factors such as workplace stress and powerlessness, prominent features of the employment experience for minorities. Numerous studies demonstrate that episodes of discrimination on the job and elsewhere contribute to hypertension among blacks.[52–56] Job insecurity and job loss, which are disproportionately common among blacks, also contribute to hypertension.[52,57] Second, a variety of chemical and physical factors may contribute to hypertension directly, or to the end-organ damage caused by hypertension. For example, lead and noise contribute to hypertension. Chronic exposure to neurotoxins such as lead and organic solvents can cause encephalopathy, affecting many of the same functions as multi-infarct dementia. Nephrotoxins such as metals and hydrocarbons may impair kidney function, compounding the effects of hypertension. These exposures, both social and physicochemical, may therefore pose special risks for blacks.

Diabetes disproportionately affects major minority populations in the United States. The prevalence of diagnosed non-insulin-dependent diabetes mellitus (NIDDM) in adults is currently 1.4 times higher in blacks than in whites; by the age of 65 one in six blacks carries the diagnosis. The prevalence of NIDDM is two to three times higher among Mexican Americans than among non-Hispanic whites. Similar findings of increased prevalence have been published for Native American populations, while limited information is available for Asian/Pacific Islanders.[58] Racial and ethnic differences in diabetes mainly reflect genetic and dietary factors, although one or more environmental exposures such as arsenic may play a role.[59,60] As for hypertension, workplace exposures may pose a special risk for persons diagnosed with diabetes, because of a pattern of common end-organ effects. Peripheral neuropathy may be caused by metals, pesticides, and organic solvents. Kidney damage may result from exposure to metals and hydrocarbons. Retinopathy may result from carbon disulfide exposure. Therefore, worker populations with a high prevalence of diabetes, including several minority groups, may face special risk from these occupational exposures.

Infectious diseases have emerged as important occupational disease concerns and exert a disproportionate impact on minorities in varied ways. Tuberculosis increased from the 1980s through the mid-1990s, when the incidence finally began to decrease.[61] Minorities have been disproportionately afflicted.[62] In 1992, tuberculosis incidence was elevated 4-fold among Native Americans, 5-fold among Hispanics, 8-fold among blacks, and 11-fold among Asian Americans, compared with whites; 71 percent of new cases occurred among minorities.[63] In fact, some evidence suggests that blacks may be especially susceptible to *Mycobacterium* infection.[64] Since tuberculosis is well recognized as an occupational hazard among health care workers and certain other occupations,[65–67] black workers in these professions may carry an especially elevated risk of infection. Another infectious disease that bears mention is pneumococcal pneumonia. This is not usually considered an occupational disease. However, pneumonia may increase a person's susceptibility to the effects of air pollutant exposure, such as further respiratory illness and mortality following exposure to particulates.[68] Pneumococcal pneumonia is vaccine preventable, but blacks are much less likely than whites to have been vaccinated.[38] Therefore, blacks may again bear disproportionate risk following such exposures, in this case because of relative lack of a preventive intervention.

Increased Probability of Other Exposures That May Combine with Workplace or Environmental Exposures to Harm Health. Members of minority groups may be excessively exposed to risk factors that aggravate the effects of workplace or environmental exposures. Examples include behavioral factors such as alcohol consumption and exposures in the home environment.

Patterns of alcohol use vary across ethnic and racial groups, as do the health consequences of alcohol abuse. While blacks and whites have generally similar drinking patterns,[69] a recent study using large probability samples showed that 17 percent of Hispanic men, 10 percent of black men, and 7 percent of white men were heavy drinkers.[70] The high prevalence of alcohol abuse among Native Americans has long been recognized.[71,72] Alcohol-related mortality is higher among Native Americans and Hispanics than among whites, and the recent decrease among whites has not been seen in these minority groups.[73] Alcohol abuse may aggravate the effects of workplace and environmental hazards in two ways. First, alcohol intoxication increases the risk of injuries. Second, chronic alcohol exposure may combine with the effects of workplace toxins to cause end-organ damage such as liver dysfunction.

Housing patterns also vary across racial and ethnic groups, with members of minority groups bearing an increased risk of living in substandard housing.[74] As noted above, such housing poses an increased risk of exposure to lead dust. Substandard housing has also been implicated in the etiology of asthma, through exposure to cockroach, dust mite, and other antigens, cooking fuels, and secondary tobacco smoke, compounded by inadequate ventilation.[75] Again, such home exposures could aggravate the effects of workplace and environmental exposures to respiratory hazards.

Increased Genetic Susceptibility. It has long been recognized that several single-gene disorders vary in frequency among different racial and ethnic groups. Among blacks, disorders that are relatively prevalent include glucose-6-phosphate dehydrogenase (G6PD) deficiency, hemoglobinopathies (HbS and HbC), and α- and β-thalassemias.[76] Moreover, differences in the ability to metabolize certain drugs, related to polymorphisms of one or more gene loci, have been associated with racial and ethnic backgrounds. One example is debrisoquin hydroxylase (also known as CYP2D6), a cytochrome P-450 enzyme that catalyzes the oxidation of more than 30 drugs. Compared to whites, blacks and Asians have fewer abnormalities of this enzyme.[77] Mephenytoin metabolism is also controlled by an enzyme for which polymorphisms have been demonstrated, with a much higher frequency in Asians than in whites.[78] Increasingly, with growing success at mapping the human genome, individual genes have been identified that are more common in specific racial or ethnic groups and are associated with specific diseases. Cancer risk is a special area of interest with respect to genetic polymorphisms. Some oncogenes have been reported to vary by race. For example, mutations of the CYP1A1 gene, which is involved with the metabolism of polycyclic aromatic hydrocarbons, are thought to increase the risk of lung cancer among smokers; this abnormality is more common among blacks than among whites.[79,80]

While genetic differences in disease susceptibility are increasingly recognized, their significance in occupational and environmental health remains limited. In the first place, few genetic factors have been clearly demonstrated to increase the risk of specific occupational diseases. Workers with G6PD deficiency are susceptible to hemolytic crises following exposure to oxidants such as naphthalene and trinitrotoluene,[81] but this event is unusual. Perhaps more importantly, job applicants have been excluded from certain jobs because of purported genetic risks, a practice that has been clearly recognized as racial or ethnic discrimination.[82–87] Hence, although genetic bases for susceptibility are being increasingly recognized, an emphasis on primary prevention—decreasing exposures to levels that are safe for all persons—remains the preferred approach.

Increased General Susceptibility to Disease Through Stress, Poverty, and Absent Social Supports. An extensive literature documents the consistent relationship between poverty and poor health. In addition to poverty, members of minority groups are likely to encounter other forms of stress, such as discrimination, uncertainties of income, employment, and housing, and absent social supports. These experiences, of course, vary in nature and intensity among individuals and groups.

Stress has been relatively well studied in this regard. The role of stress, specifically including racial discrimination, is now well established in the etiology of hypertension among blacks.[52,54,56,88,89] Stress is also thought to act more generally, increasing susceptibility to a number of diseases through general effects on immune and other functions.[90–92] Although the medical effects of poverty and stress are not completely understood, it is reasonable to hypothesize that in the aggregate minority groups have heightened susceptibility to adverse health effects, including the effects of workplace and environmental exposures.

Artifacts of Clinical Testing. Finally, minority groups may differ from whites in their clinical test norms, creating the appearance of racial differences in particular health outcomes following exposures. The best recognized example is pulmonary function testing; for a given height, age, and gender, blacks have lower lung volumes compared to whites.[93,94] Another example is the white blood cell count, which is lower among blacks than among whites.[95] Hence, a study of laboratory workers in a petrochemical plant showed no effect of exposure on the white blood cell count, but black workers had significantly lower counts than white workers.[96] Such results may reflect disproportionate exposure or susceptibility, but they may simply reflect different laboratory norms. Therefore, clinical data must be carefully evaluated with attention to possible racial differences in test norms.

Inferior Health Care for Occupational and Environmental Injuries and Illnesses

A final source of increased risk for members of minority groups is inferior medical care. Tertiary prevention consists of limiting morbidity, disability, and mortality caused by illnesses or injuries, usually through medical care and/or rehabilitation. When services available to members of minority groups are deficient, tertiary prevention cannot be optimally achieved.

The inferior health care available to minority communities is well documented.[97–99] In general, members of minority groups are less likely to have health insurance,[100,101] less likely to have a regular source of medical care,[102] less likely to have received cancer screening,[103,104] and more likely to present with more advanced disease.[105,106] Once under treatment, they are less likely to receive a wide range of services, including cardiovascular interventions,[107] renal transplants,[108] aggressive colon cancer treatment,[109] asthma care,[110] intensive care for severe pneumonia,[111] appropriate human immunodeficiency virus (HIV) treatment,[112] and others.[113] When the need arises, minority patients are less likely to gain access to long-term care.[114] These inequities are reflected in a recurring pattern of black-white mortality differences that exceed black-white incidence differences for most major diseases.[115] Members of minority groups receive less medical care, and die earlier and more often of their diseases, than do whites.[116]

While it is likely that this pattern extends to occupational and environmental injuries and illnesses, specific data to document it are not available. There is evidence that nonwhite workers are less likely than white workers to participate in voluntary worksite health promotion programs.[117] There is also evidence that black workers are less likely than white workers to receive workers' compensation benefits, despite higher occupational injury rates.[118] However, the extent to which these findings imply less access to medical care, and worse long-term outcomes, is unclear. Further research is needed to define the disparities in care of occupational and environmental injuries and illnesses and their impact on the health of minorities.

Occupational Mortality, Morbidity, and Disability among Minority Groups

Given the various factors that may place minority workers at increased risk of injury, illness, and death following occupational and environmental exposures, to what extent do data document such outcomes? Many studies of working populations have excluded black and other minority workers on the grounds that they were not numerous enough to permit statistically robust study. In fact, the risk estimates published for minority workers are often unstable, reflecting the smaller numbers of workers available for analysis. This fact reflects a double burden for minority workers: historical exclusions from many occupations, followed by exclusion from research on the health impact of these occupations. However, a considerable body of research from a range of industries is now available, documenting increased morbidity and mortality among minority workers. Environmental data, on the other hand, are almost unavailable, with the exception of information on asthma rates among minority children.

Mortality

Acute mortality is perhaps the most readily measured outcome. According to surveillance data from the National Institute of Occupational Safety and Health (NIOSH) National Traumatic Occupational Fatality system, the occupational fatality rate for blacks during the decade of the 1980s was 6.5 per 100,000 workers per year, compared with 5.8 for whites and 4.9 for workers of other races. In one category, occupational homicides, the rates were 1.6 per 100,000 for workers of other races, 1.4 for blacks, and 0.6 for whites.[119] By the end of the decade, the disparity had narrowed somewhat, with the black workplace death rate at 5.4 per 100,000 per year, compared to 4.8 for whites and 3.9 for other races.[120] Interestingly, localized studies have sometimes found different results. For example, a study of workplace fatalities in New Mexico from 1980 through 1991 found the annual rate to be 8.8 per 100,000 for white workers, 7.3 for Hispanics, and 6.4 for Native Americans.[121]

Mortality from occupational diseases by race is reported in relatively few epidemiologic studies, as has been carefully pointed out with respect to cancer.[122,123] Moreover, racial differences are often difficult to interpret, since exposure data for the different races are rarely available. Published results tend to be variable, and serve mostly to identify areas for future research. For example, a study of occupation and leukemia mortality showed that the black odds ratios exceeded the white ones in several job categories, including technicians and related support workers, mechanics and repairers, and inspectors, testers, samplers and weighers, but this pattern was not evident in many other occupations.[124]

NIOSH has provided data on occupational respiratory disease mortality, showing striking but variable racial differences, as seen in Figure 34-2.[125] Black men have lower mortality rates than white men for asbestosis and coal workers' pneumoconosis. In contrast, black men die of silicosis at twice the rate of white men and of byssinosis at six times the rate of white men (although based on small numbers). These disparities may reflect differences in diagnostic practice or in exposure, but there is some evidence that differences in susceptibility play little role. Although sarcoidosis rates are approximately 10 times higher in blacks and Hispanics than in whites,[38] epidemiologic data do not suggest that minority workers are at increased risk of berylliosis.[126] Similarly, in one study of asbestos workers, blacks sustained heavier asbestos exposure than whites, but had lower mortality from asbestosis.[127]

Morbidity

Morbidity data by race come from industry-specific studies and from larger surveillance efforts. In the Public Health Service study of the chromate industry mentioned above, respiratory cancer was 80-fold elevated among black workers, compared to a 29-fold elevation in the entire workforce. A hallmark lesion of chromate toxicity, perforation of the nasal septum, was found in 76.6 percent of black workers, and in 49.3 percent of white workers.[3] In the steel industry, an approximately 2-fold increase was seen in lung cancer mortality among coke plant workers; it was entirely accounted for by deaths among black workers.[4] In the rubber industry, not only were blacks concentrated in the more heavily exposed compounding and mixing jobs, but blacks in those jobs had higher relative risks of lung cancer than did their white counterparts.[7]

In a 1989 study that used California employers' reports of occupational injuries and illnesses, black male workers were found to have a 17 percent higher risk of workplace injuries and illnesses than white male workers, while for Hispanic male workers the risk was 33 percent higher. Among female workers, blacks had a 31 percent increased risk compared with whites, and Hispanics had a 19 percent increased risk.[128] In contrast, a 1990 study of postal workers revealed that blacks and whites had nearly identical rates of work-related injuries, although whites tended to have higher workers' compensation rates; Asians tended to have lower rates for both outcomes.[129]

A 1993 report from the New Jersey Department of Health compared the occupational health experience of white, black, and Hispanic workers in that state. Minorities composed only 14 percent of the New Jersey population in 1980 and 19 percent in 1990, but they accounted for 28 percent of reported cases of lead toxicity, 20 percent of reported cases of mercury toxicity, and 23 percent of reported cases of occupational asthma during the 1980s. Among New Jersey adults hospitalized for chemical poisoning between 1983 and 1990, in most cases following workplace exposures, the white rate was 6.1 per 100,000 population, the black rate was 13.1, and the Hispanic rate was 11.8.[130]

In summary, available evidence on racial differences in occupational injuries, illnesses, and fatalities is scanty, but consistently suggest that rates for blacks and other minorities are higher than those for whites. Further surveillance and research on the mechanisms of excess minority rates will be required to clarify this issue.

Disability

Recent scholarship has characterized the complex relationship among race and disability status.[131] Much detail has emerged from studies of the University of Michigan's 1992 Health and Retirement Study (HRS).[118,132,133] Data from the HRS not only confirm that minorities are in worse health than whites, but demonstrate substantial differences in disability status as well. Minorities are more likely than whites to identify themselves as unable to work. The differences increase with age and remain after controlling for education, marital status, and health status. Figure 34-3 shows that members of minorities have greater disability than do whites, as measured by several indicators. The extent to which this reflects diseases of occupational or environmental origin is unknown. However, it is clear that disease in general has a greater impact on the employment of minorities than on that of whites, a pattern that is likely to extend to occupational and environmental diseases.

Discussion and Conclusions

Epidemiologic study of occupational illnesses and injuries has often excluded minority groups, creating a serious dearth of data.[122,123,134] This is ironic, since job discrimination by race and ethnicity is such a long-standing, well established fixture of the American workplace. However, an increasing body of evidence suggests that members of minority groups are disproportionately exposed to hazards both at work and in the general environment, and that they suffer a disproportionate burden of morbidity and mortality as a result.

It is essential that preventive interventions be designed and delivered with the needs of minority workers in mind. First, interventions must focus on the most hazardous occupations, often those with a prominent representation of minority workers. Second, training and

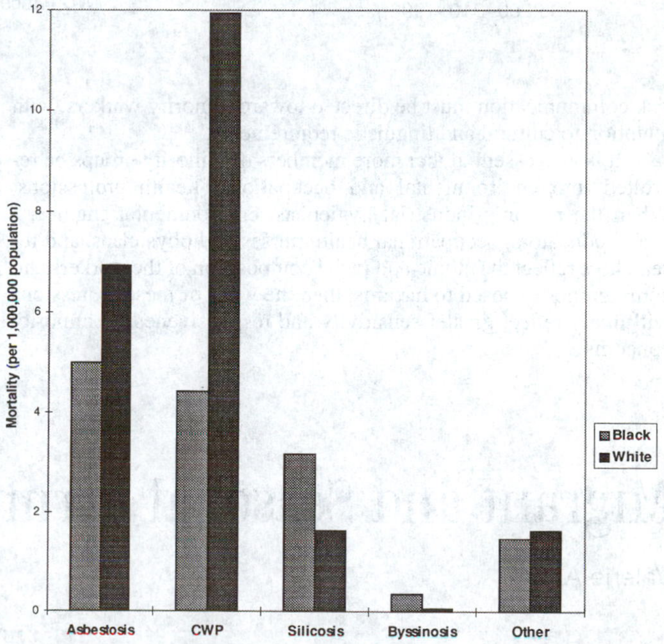

Figure 34-2. Pneumoconiosis mortality by race, U.S. males, 1992. CWP, coal workers' pneumoconiosis; Other, unspecified/other pneumoconioses. (Adapted from National Institute for Occupational Safety and Health: Work-Related Lung Disease Surveillance Report, 1996. DHHS (NIOSH) Publication No. 96-134. Cincinnati: NIOSH, 1996.)

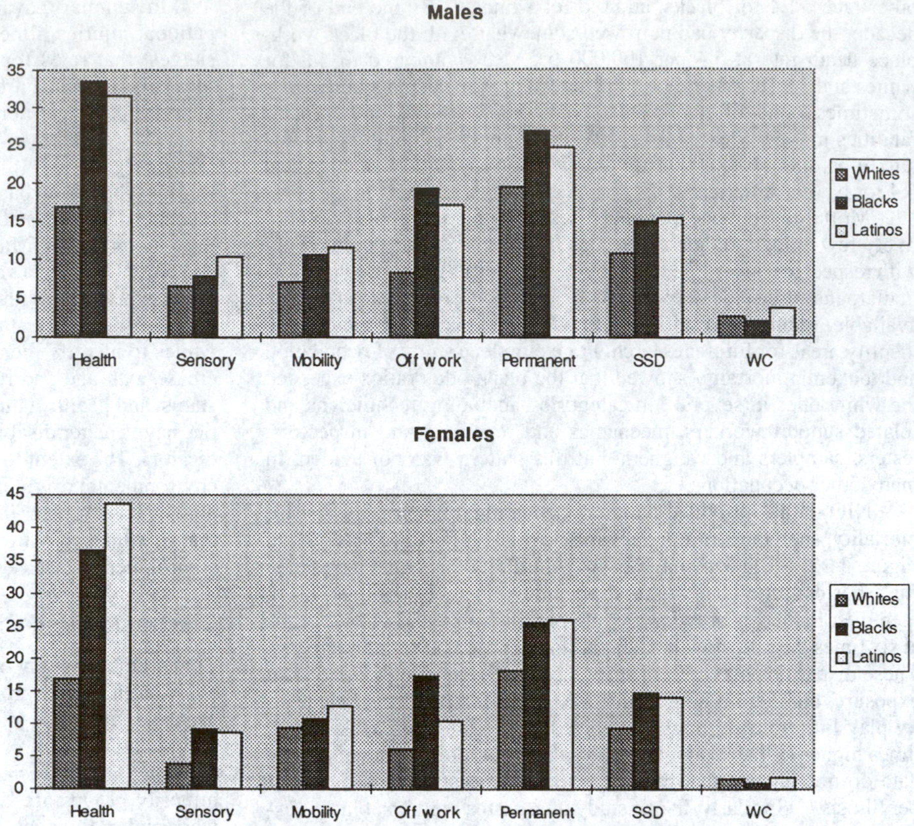

Figure 34-3. Proportion of workers age 50 to 64 with specified measures of disability, by race/ethnicity, 1991. (From Santiago AM, Muschkin CG: Disentangling the effects of disability status and gender on the labor supply of Anglo, black and Latino older workers. Gerontologist 36:299–310, 1996.)

risk communication must be directed toward minority workers, with attention to cultural and linguistic requirements.[135,136]

It is also essential that more members of minority groups be recruited into environmental and occupational health professions. When the nation's industrial hygienists, environmental engineers, health educators, occupational health nurses and physicians, and researchers reflect the ethnic and racial composition of the workers and communities exposed to hazards, then the work of these professions will likely reflect greater sensitivity and responsiveness to minority concerns.

Finally, this chapter has highlighted numerous gaps in knowledge and a consequent need for much further research. What are the morbidity and mortality profiles of various minority groups with respect to hazardous exposures? Do excess injuries and illnesses result from excess exposure, heightened susceptibility, or other factors? How can excess injuries and illnesses be prevented? In public health, the mandates of prevention rarely intersect more strikingly with the mandates of social justice than here. It is essential that we understand, and end, the disproportionate burden of illness and injury caused by hazardous exposures to minority populations.

Migrant and Seasonal Farmworkers

Valerie A. Wilk

Harsh social, economic, and political conditions combine to make migrant and seasonal farmworkers—predominantly people of color—arguably the most at-risk of American workers. These same factors render the traditional analyses of occupational health status inadequate to the task of describing the impact of hazardous working conditions on the health of farmworkers. Discriminatory partial or total exclusions of migrant and seasonal farmworkers from labor and health and safety protections mean that their illnesses and injuries are undercounted in government databases such as workers' compensation data or Occupational Safety and Health Administration (OSHA) 200 logs. In the case of pesticide poisoning, there is no national reporting system to document the extent of the problem or to monitor trends in response to statutory or regulatory changes.

Over the last decade, agriculture has ranked consistently among the three most hazardous U.S. industries. In 1994, agricultural workers ranked second in the rate of work-related fatalities and third in the rate of disabling injuries. Although agriculture accounts for less than 3 percent of the total workforce, it accounted for 18 percent of workplace fatalities that year. In 1994 the death rate in agriculture was 26 per 100,000 workers, 6.5 times greater than the national rate across all industries (4 per 100,000), and a 7 percent increase over 1993. In comparison, the worker mortality rate in mining was 27 per 100,000 workers and 15 per 100,000 in construction. The disabling injury rate in 1994 for farmworkers was 41 per 1,000, behind the 48 per 1,000 for construction workers and 43 per 1,000 for transportation and public utilities workers, respectively, and almost 1.5 times the rate of 29 per 1,000 for all industries combined.[1] In addition to safety hazards, poor sanitation, infectious agents, pesticides, and excessive heat jeopardize the health of farmworkers. Economic necessity for migrant families dictates that children often must work and play in the fields alongside their parents, exposed to an array of potentially life-threatening health and safety hazards such as farm machinery and toxic chemicals.[2–4]

Farmworkers are the lowest paid workers in the country, averaging $6,500 per year.[5] They rarely have health insurance, and the federally funded system of 119 migrant health centers in 34 states reaches less than 17 percent of all farmworkers and their dependents.[6] Migrant farmworkers are forced to live in overcrowded, unhealthy, dilapidated housing or face homelessness as they travel to harvest the crops.[7] The very workers who are closest to our food supply are the ones who most often go hungry.[8]

Federal and state laws that protect most workers from dangerous or oppressive working conditions totally or partially exclude farmworkers. The National Labor Relations Act, which provides legal protection for the unionization and collective bargaining activities of most workers, does not cover farmworkers. Consequently, a mere 2.3 percent of U.S. agricultural wage and salary workers enjoy union representation, compared with 10.9 percent of private nonagricultural workers and 38.7 percent of government employees.[9] Unions secure improved conditions for workers both legislatively and contractually, and farmworkers' harsh working conditions and meager wages and benefits attest to the low rate of unionization.[10]

The workers' compensation laws in more than half of the states exclude from coverage either all or most farmworkers, who then cannot receive payments for lost wages and related medical expenses when they suffer work-related disabilities. The federal Occupational Safety and Health Act, which regulates workplace exposures to hazardous conditions, excludes farms with fewer than 11 employees from its oversight. Consequently, the majority of farmworkers do not enjoy OSHA protection. Moreover, farmworkers are the only workers whose occupational exposure to toxic substances is not regulated by OSHA. This means that, rather than the guaranteed training about the specific pesticides used in their workplace and other protections under the Hazard Communication Act,[11] farmworkers must receive only generic pesticide safety training required under the Environmental Protection Agency's Worker Protection Standard.[12] Additionally, the child labor proscriptions of the federal Fair Labor Standards Act allow even very young children to perform hazardous farmwork such as driving a tractor. Farmworkers do not enjoy the full protection of the act's minimum wage and overtime provisions, nor do they have full rights under the federal Social Security Act, and they are often the victims of employer nonreporting and fraud.[13–15]

Demographic Profile

The U.S. farm labor system is characterized both nationally and regionally by an oversupply of workers. Thus, migrant and seasonal farmworkers face both unemployment and underemployment. Agricultural labor demand is structured into short-term work opportunities, with over half of farm jobs lasting fewer than 13 weeks (one quarter). The extensive use of temporary jobs is largely due to deliberate labor management decisions. Politically, the industry supports expanding the supply of temporary foreign guest workers, which replaces domestic workers with a compliant workforce subject to deportation at the employer's will.[15] The chronic oversupply of farmworkers has led to a pattern of replacement of one group by another. Farmworkers cannot achieve and maintain improved pay and working conditions while employers and intermediaries can recruit newly arrived immigrants willing to work for less. Workers without legal work authorization (about 10 percent of the overall farm work force and nearly one-fourth of migrants) are the most vulnerable to employment abuses and the lowest wages.[5]

By virtue of their mobility, geographic and linguistic isolation, seasonal employment, and, for a segment of the labor force, their undocumented status, migrant and seasonal farmworkers defy accurate census and demographic description. Enumeration difficulties are compounded by definitional differences among government agencies, e.g., whether nonmigratory seasonal workers, undocumented foreign workers, and accompanying dependents are included in counts. Generally, seasonal farmworkers are distinguished from migrants in that the former live and harvest crops in their own communities, whereas the latter travel various distances to find employment. Because many workers shift back and forth between seasonal and migrant status, depending on political, economic, weather, and other conditions, this distinction becomes artificial. The inability to count accurately the farmworker population is significant because underestimations translate into reduced funding for desperately needed health, education, legal, and other service programs targeted to these groups.

There is no universally accepted estimate of U.S. farmworkers. The U.S. Department of Labor uses the Commission on Agricultural Workers' estimate of 2.5 million farmworkers as a benchmark for conducting the quarterly National Agricultural Workers (NAWS) survey.[16] The federal Migrant Health Program estimate of more than 4 million includes workers' dependents.[17] Hired farmworkers are predominantly people of color: Latinos, African Americans, West Indians, Haitians, Southeast Asians, and Native Americans. The work force is relatively young (median age 31, with 17 percent younger than 21), predominantly male (73 percent), and largely Mexican born (55 percent). The median number of years of experience in U.S. farmwork is 8 years, and the median education level is eighth grade. Farmworkers earn an average of $6,500 per year, the lowest income level for any sector of the U.S. labor force. Workers who are hired and paid directly by the grower average $6,900 annually, while those who are recruited, supervised, and paid by farm labor contractors, intermediaries for the growers, average a meager $4,700. Only a minority of workers receive fringe benefits such as health insurance, sick leave, or vacation pay.[5] The two-thirds of migrants who are paid by the hour average $4.47 per hour. When paid by the piece, which rewards productivity, migrant farmworkers average $6.94 per hour.[18] Any injury or illness that interferes with productivity, such as back strain, carpal tunnel syndrome, or "mild" pesticide poisoning, acts directly to depress wages. The 52 percent poverty rate among farmworker households is over four times higher than the national household poverty rate of 12 percent, yet the overwhelming majority of these households (71 percent) receive no form of public assistance.[19] More than three-fourths of undocumented workers live in poverty.[5]

The United States can be divided into three agricultural regions according to seasonal patterns of labor demand: the North, the South, and California. While the North and South have summer and winter seasonal peaks, respectively, California has high labor demand—mostly during the warmer months—for about half the year. The vast majority (70 percent) of migrants originates from international sending areas, such as the Caribbean, Mexico, and Central and South America. A significant minority of migrants (23 percent) is based in California and the South; some of these workers migrate to other regions during the year. All three U.S. regions are highly dependent on international, particularly Mexican-based, migrants.[18]

U.S. Agricultural Production

Increasing consolidation and mechanization, along with intensive chemical usage, have characterized U.S. agricultural production over the last 50 years. While the average fruit, vegetable, and horticultural specialty (FVH) farm is small in comparison with other farms in the United States, intensive production means that profits are more likely to be higher. Corporations control a higher percentage of the land in the FVH sector and account for most of the value of agricultural products sold. The FVH sector is the most labor-intensive, with labor accounting for over 25 percent of total farm expenses, compared to 11.5 percent for all of agriculture.[18] Over 50 percent of hired farmworkers on farms employing more than 10 workers are located in California and Florida, two states with a predominance of high-value, labor-intensive crops. In California, there are approximately 18 farmworkers for every farmer, and over 80 percent of farm work is performed by hired labor.[20] FVH farmworkers—male and female alike—work in a variety of settings, including orchards, vineyards, vegetable farms, nurseries, greenhouses, mushroom sheds, and packinghouses. Workers perform a variety of tasks such as picking, cutting, hoeing, thinning, pruning, weeding, sorting, grading, wrapping, packing, potting and tending ornamental plants, laying and moving irrigation pipes, operating farm machinery, and mixing and applying pesticides.

U.S. agriculture uses 75 percent of the 1.1 billion pounds of "conventional" pesticide products (herbicides, insecticides, and fungicides) sold annually in the United States.[21] Pesticides are chemicals or biological agents used to destroy or control unwanted plants, insects, fungi, rodents, bacteria, and other pests. Some persist in the environment over long periods of time and accumulate in human, animal, and plant tissue. Pesticide formulators combine one or more active ingredients—compounds targeted to control a specific pest—with a number of inert ingredients designed to make the pesticide more effective or usable. Although inert ingredients have no intended pesticidal effect, they are not necessarily biologically, chemically, or toxicologically inactive. Xylenes, for example, can cause eye irritation, impaired short-term memory, hearing loss, infertility, and leukemia. Nonyl phenol is an endocrine disrupter that enhances proliferation of breast cancer cells. There are more than 2,000 chemicals or other substances used as inerts, more than three-fourths of which have "unknown toxicity." These toxic substances often compose the majority of a pesticide product. Yet most inerts are protected as business trade secrets and do not appear on the pesticide label. Evidence also suggests adverse health effects due to the synergistic interaction among inert and active ingredients.[22,23] The pattern of pesticide use has evolved significantly over the past 30 years. The environmentally persistent organochlorine pesticides, popular in the 1950s, were replaced by the less persistent but more acutely toxic organophosphate and carbamate compounds as well as by the pyrethroids and other compounds (see Chapter 26).

General Health Status

Serious deficiencies in sanitation, housing, education, nutrition, and access to health care operating synergistically with hazardous occupational exposures, notably to pesticides and communicable diseases, create a bleak health status picture for the farmworker population.[7,8,10,13,15,20,24–28]

A study of farmworker medical encounters in migrant health centers in Texas, Indiana, and Michigan concluded that migrant farmworkers have different and more complex health problems from those of the general population. Migrant farmworkers suffered more frequently from infectious diseases than the general population and had more clinic visits for diabetes, medical supervision of infants and children, otitis media, pregnancy, hypertension, and contact dermatitis and eczema. Almost half (44 percent) of all farmworkers who visited migrant health clinics had more than one illness. The patterns of significant comorbidity indicate the potential for substantial disability in this population.[29]

The distinction between the living and working conditions of migrants is blurred. When migrating, many workers live in housing units supplied by the employer and often located adjacent to the fields where they work. The quality of housing provided is variable, ranging from relatively comfortable dwellings to crowded barracks with communal sleeping areas and bathrooms to converted chicken coops lacking indoor plumbing, electricity, ventilation, regular garbage removal, and a fresh water supply. Workers also ride to and from the fields in crowded vans and buses. These conditions foster the transmission of infectious diseases like tuberculosis and parasites.[30–32] Workers housed in units adjacent to pesticide-sprayed fields are subject to pesticide drift or even to direct spray. With affordable housing scarce, migrants are even forced to live out in the open, sleeping in cardboard boxes or on plastic sheets in fields, orchards, and groves. For these workers, the occupational hazards described below are ever present.

Farmworkers face a variety of barriers to receiving medical care including: lack of money, health insurance, or transportation from remote labor camps; unfamiliarity with free or sliding scale services in communities where they migrate; unavailability of services during evening or weekend hours when workers have free time and can seek care without losing pay or their job altogether; long waiting times to get an appointment; cultural and linguistic differences between workers and health care providers that impede communication and trust; and fear of detection and deportation of undocumented workers and their families. When migrant families finally do use the health care system, they often must leave the area before they can receive all the necessary follow-up care, e.g., in the case of pregnant patients or those with chronic conditions like diabetes or active tuberculosis. The Migrant Clinicians Network, a national organization of clinicians serving farmworkers at federally funded community and migrant health centers, uses various ways to improve continuity of care for migrant farmworkers including providing patients with a portable medical record and participating in a U.S.-Mexico health data transfer system of patient tracking and education for cases of tuberculosis, leprosy (Hansen's disease), hepatitis, and sexually transmitted diseases.[33]

Farmworker Women's Health

Farmworker women total more than one-quarter of the hired agricultural work force.[18] In recent years, farmworker women have formally organized around issues of family, community, and personal health and are collaborating with researchers, clinicians, and advocates on a range of issues and projects, including prevention of domestic violence,[34] acquired immunodeficiency syndrome (AIDS),[35] and mental health problems such as depression and substance abuse;[36] the promotion of maternal-child health;[36] prevention of pesticide poisonings; and the development of public policy to protect farmworkers.[37]

AIDS is now growing more rapidly in rural than urban areas, and the fastest increase in new cases is among women and children of color. Human immunodeficiency virus (HIV) infection has been increasing dramatically among Hispanic and African American women in the United States, two groups to which the majority of farmworker women belong. Studies show that the rate of HIV infection among migrant and seasonal farmworkers may be as much as 10 times the national rate.[38]

Results of a pilot study of adult migrant farmworker women (most of whom were Hispanic and married), showed farmworker women to be at high risk for domestic violence. More than one-third (35 percent) of the women reported being hurt by their partner within the last year. One-fifth reported forced sexual activity during the last year, and 63 percent reported that their partners used drugs or alcohol.[39] Farmworker women also experience violence in the workplace, from sexual harassment by supervisors and coworkers to physical assault and rape.[37]

The reproductive health effects of pesticides, including during pregnancy, are discussed below. Pregnant workers are at increased risk for heat stress, falls, and pesticide poisonings, and recurrent urinary tract infections can compromise the fetus.[27]

Work-Related Health Problems

Agricultural health and safety was given a boost in 1990 when the U.S. Congress granted monies to the National Institute for Occupational Safety and Health (NIOSH) for a national agricultural program. Part of this initiative included establishment of six NIOSH regional centers (in California, Colorado, Iowa, Wisconsin, Kentucky, and New York) for agricultural research, education, and disease and injury prevention. More recently, NIOSH centers have been added in Texas and Washington state. Information about the work of all centers is accessible through the Internet.[40] During the first 5 years of funding, these centers predominantly focused on studying the health and safety of farm owner/operators and their families. In 1995 NIOSH convened an ad hoc advisory committee of migrant health clinicians, farmworkers, researchers, and policymakers to identify priorities for farmworker surveillance and research. The group ranked ergonomic/musculoskeletal conditions, pesticides, and traumatic injuries as the three most important subjects for both surveillance and research.[41]

Pesticide-Related Illnesses

The primary route of farmworker exposure to most pesticides is through dermal absorption. Inhalation and ingestion are secondary avenues of exposure. Fieldworkers who cultivate and harvest crops are exposed to pesticide residues on foliage, on the crops themselves, and in the dusty soil and decaying organic material that collects in the fields. Aerial and ground pesticide application exposes workers through direct spray and through drift of pesticides sprayed on adjacent fields.

Deficiencies in sanitation in the fields and in nearby labor camps exacerbate pesticide exposures. Pesticide residues contaminate irrigation water that may be used for drinking, cooking, and bathing. The increasing use of chemigation, putting pesticides in the irrigation water, underscores this problem. The lack of adequate toilet and handwashing facilities in the fields means that workers may eat and smoke with pesticide-contaminated hands, use pesticide-contaminated leaves or twigs as a substitute for toilet paper, and contaminate the genital area after elimination because they are unable to wash their hands. Even when children do not accompany their parents to the fields, they can be exposed to pesticide residues via contact with contaminated work clothes.

The Federal Insecticide, Fungicide, and Rodenticide Act (FIFRA) authorizes the Environmental Protection Agency (EPA) to regulate the manufacture, distribution, and use of pesticides. Key provisions of the act include product registration and labeling. As of 1991 EPA had registered approximately 25,000 pesticide products formulated from some 750 active and 2,000 inert ingredients. Most pesticides have not been fully tested and evaluated, however, in accordance with current testing requirements aimed at determining a pesticide's potential for causing cancer, reproductive disorders, birth defects, and other chronic health problems. By 1995 the EPA had completed only 30 percent of its reregistration eligibility decisions.[42]

EPA also regulates farmworkers' exposure to pesticides. More than a decade after acknowledging that existing pesticide regulations were inadequate to protect farmworkers, EPA issued the Worker Protection Standard (WPS) in 1992 and phased in the regulations by 1995. The WPS expands protections beyond fieldworkers doing hand labor to include pesticide mixers, loaders, and applicators; and nursery, greenhouse, and forestry workers. The regulations require employers to: (*a*) train farmworkers about general pesticide safety and first aid; (*b*) provide transportation to a medical facility in case of a poisoning; (*c*) make decontamination water available for use during pesticide emergencies; (*d*) post warning signs in treated areas for the most acutely toxic chemicals; and (*e*) give workers information on pesticide applications and re-entry times.[15] Even before full implementation of these regulations could occur, however, EPA bowed to agribusiness pressure and issued a series of weakening amendments to the WPS.[43]

A key component of the WPS is prevention of exposure through generic restricted entry intervals (REIs) or quarantines of treated areas based on a pesticide's toxicity. The 1995 WPS amendments eroded these protections by allowing extended early entry for various workers and shorter REIs. REIs do not protect workers from the carcinogenic and other chronic effects of pesticide exposure. In addition, a number of studies and case reports demonstrate their inadequacy in preventing acute effects.[44,45] In one case, an outbreak of dermatitis cases among orange pickers was linked to their exposure to a pesticide whose formulation had been modified by the addition of a new inert ingredient intended to prevent leaf burns. The inert ingredient also extended the degradation period of the active ingredient, a known potential skin and eye irritant. Regulators did not adjust the re-entry or preharvest intervals accordingly, and as a result, 114 of 198 exposed workers suffered dermatitis of varying severity. A smaller number suffered eye irritation, with some requiring medical treatment.[46]

Other traditional measures to prevent toxic exposures, such as protective clothing and frequent washing of exposed skin, are unrealistic and ineffective. Growers often fail to supply protective clothing, and workers are loathe to wear the hot, cumbersome gear. The lack of wash water in the fields prevents timely removal of residues.

Adequate data on the extent and magnitude of pesticide-related and other occupational morbidity and mortality among farmworkers are unavailable for a number of reasons. Factors that contribute to underreporting include: the failure and/or inability of farmworkers to get health care; the lack of mandatory workers' compensation coverage for all farmworkers in all agricultural workplaces regardless of size; the lack of adequate training of health care professionals in occupational medicine that allows for the recognition and diagnosis of these illnesses (e.g., pesticide poisoning may be mistaken for gastroenteritis, the flu, or heat stress); health care providers' unfamiliarity with state reporting requirements or processes or an unwillingness on their part to report incidents; difficulties in the verification of incidents and determination of causes because of delays in reporting and the lack of information about the circumstances of injuries or illnesses; and the lack of a national surveillance system to track pesticide or other work-related illnesses.[47] The agricultural industry has lobbied effectively at the national and state levels to limit mandatory pesticide record-keeping and reporting requirements.

There are no reliable data on the extent of farmworker pesticide poisonings. Annual estimates range from 20,000 to over 300,000.[15,28] Few states have mandatory physician reporting of pesticide-related illness; California's system is the most comprehensive, though not without significant problems.[23]

Acute health effects of mild pesticide exposure include increased salivation, tearing, blurred vision, diarrhea, slowed heart rate, weakness, headaches, and listlessness. Severe exposure may cause difficulty in breathing, respiratory failure, paralysis, convulsions, coma, and death. Like nerve gas, the organophosphate and carbamate pesticides attack the nervous system by inhibiting the action of the enzyme cholinesterase. Organophosphates are the most toxic and have been responsible for the great majority of systemic poisonings and deaths in agricultural workers.[23,44,45,48]

Little is known about the magnitude of pesticide-related chronic health effects, and additional research is needed. A number of pesticides can cause allergic dermatitis, a chronic debilitating skin condition that can lead to permanent disability, since even minute exposure to the pesticide can be intolerable.[23] Many commonly used pesticides are known or suspected animal carcinogens. Studies have shown pesticide-exposed farmworkers to be at increased risk for non-Hodgkin's lymphoma, multiple myeloma, leukemia, and cancer of the stomach, prostate, testis, brain, and liver.[49] Studies and case reports have associated pesticides with birth defects, sterility, spontaneous abortion, and menstrual dysfunction.[48,50] More recently, evidence of the estrogenic effects of pesticides and their potential for disrupting the endocrine system has appeared.[51] Pesticides, particularly organophosphates, have been associated with neurological and behavioral abnormalities, including ataxia, tremors, vertigo, drowsiness, anxiety, confusion, defective memory, toxic psychosis, convulsions, coma, and Parkinson's disease.[23,44,48]

Effects of Inadequate Sanitation

The basic public health principle that poor sanitation increases the prevalence of disease has been well understood and universally accepted for over 100 years. Nevertheless, U.S. migrant and seasonal farmworkers have lived and worked under conditions analogous to those faced by third world populations.

After farmworker advocates waged a 15-year battle to win their constituents the same basic sanitation protection afforded to all other workers in this country, OSHA issued a federal field sanitation standard in 1987. The standard requires agricultural employers who hire 11 or more workers to provide them with free drinking water, toilets, and wash water in the fields. OSHA estimates that 36 percent of U.S. field hand laborers are covered by the standard.[52]

The lack of adequate sanitation facilities contributes to farmworkers' increased risk of communicable diseases, heat stress, urinary tract infections (UTIs), and pesticide-related illnesses. Working in hot environments, farmworkers who minimize their fluid intake in an effort to limit the need to urinate risk dehydration and heat stress.[53] Evidence indicates that migrant workers' relative risk of developing a heat-related illness is over four times that of the general working population.[54] Farmworkers, especially women, who try to retain their urine, risk developing urinary tract infections. The rate of UTIs among migrant workers is estimated at 3.5 times that of the general population.[54] The lack of sanitation facilities increases the risk of communicable diseases such as dysentery, hepatitis, typhoid fever, and parasitic infections. Estimates place the rate of parasitic infection among migrants at 20 times that of the general population and the rate of bacterial gastrointestinal infection 11 times greater.[54] A chart audit for fecal-related symptoms conducted in a Utah clinic serving both migrant farmworkers and an urban poor population found that the migrants, who lacked field sanitation facilities, displayed a clinic use rate for diarrhea that was 20 times higher than that of the urban poor. Similar findings applied to other enteric disease symptoms.[55] The impact of sanitary deficiencies on pesticide-related illness has already been discussed.

Dermatitis

Dermatitis is increased in agriculture and may contribute significantly to workplace morbidity, although it is rarely a cause of death.[56] Farmworkers face nearly four times the risk of developing skin disease as workers in other industries.[54] Occupational skin disease accounts for 30 percent of all occupational illnesses nationwide but approximately 70 percent of occupational illnesses in agriculture in California.[57] Pesticides and allergenic plants and crops are the primary culprits. Their effects are exacerbated by constant exposure to the sun, sweat, chapped or abraded skin, and the lack of appropriate protective gear and adequate handwashing facilities. Patch testing generally is necessary to determine whether a rash is chemical- or plant-related. Most pesticide-related skin problems are primary irritant, or contact, dermatitis. Pesticides also can be sensitizers, causing allergic dermatitis. Some workers can be permanently disabled because they cannot tolerate exposure even to minute amounts of pesticides. Sunlight can aggravate the dermatitis, adding to the disability, even leading to convulsions and comas.[23]

Musculoskeletal Problems

Farmworkers face many of the hazards traditionally associated with musculoskeletal problems, including forceful exertions such as lifting, carrying, and hoisting heavy loads overhead; fast-paced, repetitive work; and awkward positions such as stooping, bending, twisting, and leaning over. Redesign of tools or work processes, changes in crop production, regulatory actions, and worker and employer education are some methods to address these problems. For example, the short-handled hoe, el cortito, requires the worker to labor in a doubled-over position and is linked with development of back strain and other ailments. The ban on its use in California was associated with a 34 percent decrease in the rate of sprain and strain injuries among relevant California farmworkers.[57] No national ban on its use has been issued. In 1995 OSHA held a series of stakeholder meetings with employer and worker representatives before publishing a proposed ergonomic standard to cover all industries. Intense employer opposition forced OSHA to halt the rulemaking process.

Injuries

Farmworkers suffer a wide variety of injuries, including acute pesticide poisonings, fractures in falls from ladders, strains from heavy lifting, eye injuries from chemicals and debris ejected by machinery, cuts and lacerations from knives and machetes, and a host of crush, contusion, fracture, and amputation injuries associated with heavy equipment use.[58] Piece work, heat stress, the effects of mild pesticide exposure, long hours, and awkward work positions contribute to the risk of injury. Farmworkers are also at high risk for work-related transportation deaths and injuries because they are often transported by farm labor contractors from central locations to the fields in substandard buses, vans, or pick-up trucks.[24] In 1990, 41 percent of Florida farmworker deaths were transportation-related.[59] Often large distances separate the fields from the nearest health care facility and frustrate the receipt of prompt and appropriate treatment. Lack of health insurance and exclusion from coverage under the state's workers' compensation system contributed to delayed or no care for 65 percent of injured North Carolina migrant farmworkers, including those with more serious injuries. Employers covered medical expenses for only 38 percent of injured workers, and only 20 percent were compensated for lost work.[60] Washington state workers' compensation data showed that farmwork accounted for half of the total number of severe or disabling injuries among claims filed by children under 14 and those age 14 or 15. Researchers noted that these findings indicated underreporting because only those injuries or illnesses that resulted in the filing of a claim were counted.[61]

Recommendations

The secondary legal status of this country's migrant and seasonal farmworkers lies at the heart of their political, social, and economic plight. Changes in labor, health and safety, and social welfare legislation are necessary to combat discrimination and environmental racism and to provide farmworkers and their families with equal legal protections, including the right to organize and bargain collectively.

The existence of laws protecting farmworkers is no guarantee of a safe and healthy workplace. Lack of voluntary employer compliance, poor government enforcement of laws and regulations, and employer intimidation or retaliation against farmworkers who assert their rights mean that even workers well educated about occupational hazards are limited in their ability to protect themselves on the job. The oversupply of labor in agriculture gives workers little economic choice when acting as individuals. Farmworker unions have secured decent wages, benefits, and workplace protections through collective bargaining agreements.[23]

Funding for research on farmworker occupational hazards and their effects must broaden and continue, and a national surveillance system to monitor work-related illnesses and injuries is needed. Feasibility studies funded by the National Cancer Institute are looking at methodological issues such as ways to track farmworkers for long-term prospective studies and to accurately assess lifetime work and pesticide exposure histories. Such efforts should be encouraged.

Farmworkers need to receive culturally and linguistically appropriate worker education materials and training that explain on-the-job hazards and appropriate preventive measures. Workers and their health care providers must have access to complete information about pesticides used in the workplace. A national mandatory pesticide illness reporting system is needed to document the what, where, when, how, and why of the problem.

Clinicians practicing in areas where migrant and seasonal farmworkers live and work cannot serve their patients effectively without a clear picture of their living and working conditions and an understanding of the relationship between these conditions and their patients' health and well-being. Clinicians need training in the importance and methods of taking a thorough occupational and environmental history and in recognition, diagnosis, and treatment of pesticide- and other work-related illnesses and injuries.

Policies and programs that reduce the agricultural industry's dependence on chemicals should be a priority, including promoting known nonchemical alternatives and finding new methods of farming that rely on nontoxic alternatives.

The impact of agricultural hazards is not restricted to farmworkers. The pesticide- and sanitation-related hazards that compromise the health of exposed farmworkers also contaminate produce and ground water and jeopardize the health of consumers and surrounding communities. The growing environmental justice movement is joining farmworkers and their communities with other communities of color and with farmworkers advocates, health care providers, researchers, environmental activists, and concerned consumers to demand safe, fair, and healthy policies and practices in agriculture in the United States and abroad.[62,63]

Women Workers

Karen Messing

About 70 percent of American women are in the paid labor force.[1] Although, overall, women's employment has a positive effect on their health[2] and employed women live longer than unemployed women and housewives,[3,4] risk factors present in some jobs may adversely affect women's health. Action to improve women's occupational health has been slowed by a notion that women's jobs are safe and that any health problems identified among women workers can be attributed to unfitness for the job, hormonal factors, or unnecessary complaining. However, the rise in the number of women in the labor force has sensitized public health practitioners, workers, and scientists to the necessity to include women's concerns in their occupational health activities.

Although it is too soon to speak of convergence of research directions, certain occupational groups have excited the interest of researchers: factory workers in repetitive tasks, hospital workers, and solvent-exposed workers. Particular industries (clothing manufacturing, food-processing) have received attention because health problems have been identified and/or because they employ a large number of women (health care). Methodological questions are emerging: how to analyze data by gender; how to take into account the different life patterns of women and men; and how to identify health problems that arise in women's traditional work and for which strategies may not have been developed. Related social issues arise and must also be dealt with: how to ensure that recognition of health hazards in women's work does not lead to denial of employment opportunities for women; whether men and women should be distributed in a more random way across employment categories or if each gender is more "suited" to a specific type of work.

Despite considerable progress in integrating women into the labor force, women are still found in specific jobs where employment conditions are relatively unfavorable. This sexual division of labor affects women's health in six ways: (*a*) women's jobs have specific characteristics (repetition, monotony, static effort, multiple simultaneous responsibilities), which may lead over time to deleterious effects on physical and mental health; (*b*) spaces, equipment, and schedules designed in relation to the average male body and lifestyle may cause problems for women; (*c*) segregation may cause health risks for women and men by causing task fragmentation and thus increasing repetition and monotony; (*d*) sex-based job assignment may appear to protect the health of both sexes and thus distract from more effective occupational health promotion practices; (*e*) discrimination against women is stressful in and of itself and may affect mental health; and (*f*) part-time workers are excluded from many health-promoting benefits such as adequate sick leave and maternity leave.

Data Collection and Analysis

Before discussing the risks involved in women's work, it is important to present some obstacles to understanding those risks. Although many women such as Alice Hamilton, Harriet Hardy, and Jeanne Stellman have been important pioneers in occupational health, scientists have usually studied traditional men's jobs in mining and manufacturing. The concepts developed were appropriate for men in those jobs, but have in some cases delayed our understanding of problems of women. Women and their work have been excluded from consideration by scientists in occupational health, data collection and analysis have been gender-insensitive, and health outcomes analyzed have not included effects from women's jobs. Filling in the gaps is an important priority for research and intervention in women's health.

Exclusion of Women and Their Work

In the past, women were excluded from studies of occupational health. Greenberg and Dement[5] found a large excess of studies of occupational disease involving only males. A well-documented example is the field of occupational cancer. Zahm et al found that, of 1,233 cancer studies published from 1971 to 1990 in the eight major occupational health journals, only 14 percent presented analyses of data on white women and only 10 percent on nonwhite women.[6] Part of the reason for exclusion is the choice of jobs for study: miners, refinery workers, and foundry workers are almost always men.

These exclusions create a circular situation where there is evidence of health problems only among men, leading to a reluctance to study women because of an impression that not many women get occupational disease. One consequence is that workers are studied as if they were all men. For example, Greenberg and Dement describe the numerous biological differences between women and men that can affect their responses to toxic chemicals. These have not usually been taken into account in standard-setting and exposure assessment.

Problems in Data Collection and Analysis

Problems in data collection can preclude women from being studied. For example, a study of the effects of agricultural exposures was forced to eliminate women since only the husband of a farm family was identified as a farmer in most provincial records.[7] Also, many death certificates have not contained information on women's professions, in part because once a woman has retired she may be considered to be a housewife. Thus, a priority for research in women's (and men's) occupational health is establishment of appropriate databases.

Research instruments and standards that have been derived with all-male populations have sometimes been used without further validation on female populations. An example is the well-known Karasek questionnaire on job demands,[8] or strength testing done with instruments validated on male populations. Some occupational prestige scales and social class scales use the husband's job to ascribe a score to the wife.[9] This causes problems when data on health are adjusted for social class, since some social class influences on health may be mediated through common family-revenue dependent factors such as nutrition, and others may be specific to the individual situation such as education-related health-protective behavior.

When analyzing data, there has sometimes been confusion between male- and female-specific health problems and effects of the sexual division of labor. For example, women have more musculoskeletal problems than men: is this because of their biological "nature" or their different jobs? In fact, women and men are not distributed at random over the labor force, but are segregated into specific industrial sectors and into female-majority jobs within these sectors. The list of the top 20 jobs of women and men is very different, and women are more concentrated into a few professions. About one-third of women are secretaries and clerks. Women are overrepresented in clerical and service jobs and underrepresented in manufacturing and resource generation.[10] There is also vertical segregation in the job market. It is much more common for men to be in positions of higher prestige and authority, as witnessed by the fact that American women who worked full-time during 1994 earned 76 percent of the salary of the average man.[11] (The most recent trend is toward widening rather than narrowing the salary gap between women and men in the United States and Canada.) Women are 3 times as likely as men to work part-time and 3 times as likely to be temporary workers.[12] Also, women are more apt to work in small workplaces employing less than 20 workers.[13]

What jobs do women do? There are five office work professions (secretary, bookkeeper, information clerk, etc.), five personal service professions (cleaner, waiter, hairdresser, etc.), and five caring professions (teacher, nurse, social worker, etc.) among the list of women's top 20 jobs.[10] But a nonnegligible proportion of women are in factories, with job titles too diversified to appear in the list of the top 20. They are not uniformly distributed, but can be found in specific factories and parts of factories. In the clothing industry, women are sewing machine operators making women's clothes, while men's coats are usually sewn by men. Cutters are almost always men while pressers are sometimes women. In the auto industry, women sew seat covers and men install engines. The division in jobs with a manual component usually follows a pattern. On assembly lines, men are found at the beginning and the end, women in the middle where they are pushed by the job behind and pulled by the job ahead.[14]

Even more surprising than the extent of male-female job segregation is that of task segregation. Male cleaners mop and female cleaners dust.[15] Women and men with the same job titles can have very different exposures, a fact which has implications for epidemiological research. For example, male and female gardeners may have different exposures to pesticides because women do more planting and weeding and men do more pruning.[16]

The fact that women and men are treated differently in the workplace makes it inappropriate to consider that women and men with the same job title have the same working conditions. In health research, using job title as a proxy for exposure may introduce inaccuracy and bias according to the gender of the worker. Hsairi et al[17] used expert estimates derived from job titles to classify workers in 13,568 jobs as exposed or not exposed to dust. Workers' reports of their own exposure and self-reports of symptoms of dust exposure (difficulty breathing, asthma, etc.) were correlated with experts' ratings. Self-reports of symptoms were better correlated with self-reports of exposure than with experts' estimates of exposure. Expert estimates were significantly closer to men's self-reports than to women's. The authors interpret these results as implying a "better perception" of exposure by the men, but it is also possible that experts' estimates of exposure according to job title are based on experience with male job-holders.

Women are shorter on average than men and are proportioned differently.[18] Tools and equipment are not always available in the right dimensions for women. Therefore, even the same tasks do not necessarily interact the same ways with men's and women's bodies, and women may develop ways to do specific tasks that are different from those of the average man. Lortie[19] showed that, on average, female hospital orderlies lifted patients differently from men; they found ways to change lifting tasks into pushing and pulling tasks, in accordance with differential distribution of muscle strength. However, in a rigid, repetitive sorting task, where there was little control over task parameters and where certain dimensions of the workstation caused problems for shorter workers, women had more work accidents than did men.[20]

These results would support caution in using job title to estimate exposure for both genders if the job exposure matrix has not previously been validated separately by gender. In addition, it may be unwise to adjust relationships between job title and disease incidence for gender, thus treating gender as a confounder when it may be a proxy for specific exposures.

Underestimation of Women's Problems

Compensated work accidents and injuries are the usual indicators of occupational health problems. Men have from three to 10 times more compensated industrial accidents and illnesses per worker than women.[21–24] Some of this difference is a result of the difference in jobs—when comparisons are made within the same industry, sometimes women have more accidents than men, sometimes fewer. Women average more industrial disease than men,[25] and their problems may be underestimated since many industrial diseases go unrecognized. It is easy to recognize that a leg broken in the workplace is an occupational problem but an allergy or inflammation that develops more slowly is not readily associated with the job.[26] (Québec's Institut de Recherche en Santé et en Sécurité du Travail has compared official work accident and illness statistics with results from the Québec Health Survey and found several professions where they believe that employment-related problems may be underestimated in official statistics.)[27] Women's illness and injury rates may also be artificially lowered by a technical factor. Because women tend to work fewer hours than men at paid jobs, accident rates of women appear lower when, as is usual, the rates are calculated per worker rather than per hour worked. Of 14 studies comparing women and men, only two gave information on person-hours worked.[28]

Since occupational accidents are relatively infrequent in the types of jobs usually held by women, Bourbonnais and colleagues have suggested that certified sick leaves might be a useful indicator of occupational health problems for both sexes. They found that sick leaves of nurses were related to various indicators of work load and to shift work.[29]

Gender Insensitivity and Oversensitivity

Descriptors representing the place of people in society (gender, race, class) pose a special problem for epidemiological research. They may include higher probabilities of some biological characteristics (hormonal status, blood groups, nutritional status), but they also represent probabilities of different occupational exposures. If researchers simply adjust ("control") their analyses for gender, or if they include gender as a variable along with other exposure variables, the effects of gender-specific exposures may disappear from sight. For example, all the studies of carpal tunnel syndrome cited in a major review article[30] adjusted for gender, even though it has been shown that gender is not related to carpal tunnel syndrome if anthropometric measurements related to wrist anatomy and physiology are taken into account.[31] Adjusting or treating gender as an independent variable would be appropriate only if gender were an independent determinant of poor health reports, for example, if women were weaker or complained more than men, or if the health effects had an important independent contribution from sex hormones or other biological differences.

An example is scientific studies on the effects of indoor air pollution. We searched the CISILO database of the International Labor Office in Geneva and found that 13 epidemiological studies related working conditions to symptoms thought to be related to indoor air quality.[32–44] Women by and large suffered 2 to 4 times more symptoms than did men, a fact that was mentioned in almost all of the articles. However, only three articles discussed this difference in symptoms,[35,40,44] and only Stenberg and Wall took into account the gendered division of labor in such a way as to allow us to understand why women had more symptoms: Women in offices probably do more photocopying than men, with consequent increased exposure to ozone, toners, and electrostatic effects; they share offices more often, resulting in more exposure to secondhand smoke and less ventilation per person. Lack of attention to differential exposure leaves the reader with the impression that being female is a cause of the symptoms, perhaps because of weakness or psychological problems.

Gender Implications of Pathology-Based Approaches

Occupational health researchers trained in medicine have often limited their interest to pathologies rather than to indicators, signs, or symptoms of deterioration in physical or mental states, reasoning that the presence of pathology guarantees that the problem examined is worthy of serious consideration. However, a requirement for diagnosed pathology may be premature when studying women's occupational health. Since the aggressors present in women's traditional work have been understudied, and the effects of even well-known conditions on women workers are often unknown, identification of occupational disease in women's work is embryonic. For example, women who handle money report unusual-looking and painful red streaks on their hands. A literature search revealed one article on nickel allergy among cashiers,[45] but no other reference to skin disease among those handling money. It may be years before sufficient research enables us to decide whether to define it as an industrial disease.

The requirement for pathology has two further consequences. First, it forces the researcher to consider events that are rare among populations still at work. This requirement for populations of considerable size is a particular obstacle to identifying women's occupational health problems because women work in very small workplaces.[13] Second and more important, the risks found in women's jobs are often undramatic and diffuse. In fact, obvious danger is a reason for excluding women from particular jobs. Thus, epidemiological studies that seek to link isolated, identifiable risk factors such as chemical exposures to well-defined pathologies are not well-adapted to discovering other types of problems. For example, restaurant workers are found among widely varying stressful conditions, carrying trays of various weights, with diverse scheduling problems and time pressures. Designing a study that isolates these factors is difficult.

Women's Occupational Health Problems

Women's most common health problems are musculoskeletal problems, skin problems, and hypertension.[46] Women are also more likely than men to be hospitalized for mental disorders.[46] Some of these differences can be attributed to specific jobs. One approach has been to examine health problems reported by women according to the sector of the economy where they work. Although employment sector is a poor indicator of job content, this type of gross analysis does suggest a need to study women's jobs. Musculoskeletal problems emerge as a specific risk associated with sales, restaurant, and cleaning work. Psychological distress is found among those in sales, restaurant work, and teaching. Allergies and skin conditions are common in white collar work, especially teaching, and also in personal services such as hairdressing. Heart disease is found among cleaners, personal service workers, saleswomen, and managers.[27]

Musculoskeletal Disorders

The major research area in women's occupational health is probably musculoskeletal problems,[47] the majority of cases of compensated occupational diseases.[26] Although women live longer than men, women and men in many countries can expect to live a similar number of years *in good health*.[3] Put differently, women spend about twice as long as men being disabled. One cause of disability is muscle and joint problems, more often found among women.[46] Women are twice as likely as men to have chronic backache.[48]

Women's working conditions, particularly repetitive work, prolonged standing, and carrying heavy loads may be at the source of some of these musculoskeletal problems. In many jobs assigned to women (as well as some assigned to men), the work cycle[a] is under 10 seconds long, and the same movements are repeated many thousands of times in a day.[49] These movements can individually make trivial demands on the human body, but the enormous degree of repetition makes tiny details of the setup assume primary importance. A chair the wrong height or a counter the wrong width may cause constant oversolicitation of the same tendons or joints, yet the observer sees no problem. This explains why sewing machine operation, classed as light work, is associated with a very high probability of disability.[50]

Many women's jobs require static effort, exerted when muscles are contracted for long periods. This type of effort creates musculoskeletal and circulatory problems due to interference with circulation. Cleaning jobs (dusting high surfaces, bending over toilets) often require this type of posture. Many women's jobs in factories or services in North America (sales, hairdressing, cashiering) require standing for long periods of time, resulting in back and other musculoskeletal problems.[51] These workers usually work sitting down in other countries, namely, in Europe and Latin America.

Although carrying heavy loads is not usually thought to be a characteristic of women's jobs, women working in day care centers, hospitals, and nursing homes are often required to move patients or children. Nursing assistants are particularly at risk for back injuries.[52,53] Guo and colleagues found that, particularly for women workers, professions where back pain had been most studied did not correspond to those reporting most back pain.[54] Cleaners, waitresses, and supermarket clerks were among the neglected groups.

Health Effects of Stress

Any discussion with women (and often men) workers tends to identify "stress" as an important occupational health problem. We can ask whether women "really" have more such problems, but it is undeniable that women consult more health practitioners and take more medication for mental problems than men.[46] Women service workers were particularly likely to experience stress. Secretaries have also been identified by the National Institute for Occupational Safety and Health (NIOSH) as a group particularly prone to stress.[55]

Yassi and coworkers[56] have pointed out that there is sometimes confusion between the notions of "unreal" problems and "mental" problems. In a study of telephone operators, they suggest that a collective stress reaction may be an appropriate response to some working conditions. However, these types of mental health problems are often dismissed as being due to innate characteristics of women rather than to organizational problems in the workplace. For example, a

[a] *The work cycle is the interval between repetitions of a single operation. For a university professor it would be the time between beginnings of successive introductory lectures to the same course (months), for an otorhinolaryngologist it could be the time between beginnings of successive tonsillectomies (hours or days), for a sewing machine operator it is the time between successive pant legs (6 to 10 seconds), for a data entry operator it is the time between characters entered, as little as 0.2 seconds.*

recent study of workplace determinants of depression scored women as depressed at a score of 23 and men at 17 on the same test.[57] Thus, that women had more symptoms of depression was "normalized" and could not be related to working conditions.

Refusing to examine the possibility that women workers' mental health symptoms are linked to jobs rather than to gender has several consequences. First, there may be discrimination in compensation for stress.[55] In American law, women's claims for compensation for physical problems (e.g., heart disease) caused by stress have been refused 4 times as often as men's.[55] Second, there may be reluctance to investigate women's symptoms seriously. For example, women's symptoms of organic solvent exposure have been wrongly attributed to "hysteria."[58] Similar uncertainty surrounds discussions of problems in women's traditional work such as indoor air quality and musculoskeletal disorders.[59]

The work of Karasek and others has related several workplace variables (degree of job control, level of demand) to effects on the cardiovascular system.[60,61] Hall found that jobs assigned to women are characterized by a low level of decision latitude and more likely to be stressful.[8] Unfortunately, most scientists who have studied heart disease by occupation have restricted their samples to men.[b,62] Although coronary artery disease is the most common cause of death among women,[63] and as many women as men report hypertension, heart disease is still thought of as a man's problem and many studies have not been gender-sensitive.[64] Several professions that are commonly held by women are among the 10 professions with the highest diastolic blood pressure: laundry and dry cleaning operatives, food service workers, private child care workers, and telephone operators.[65] Women working on shifts,[66] women with clerical or sales jobs,[67] and women reporting that their work is both hectic and monotonous have a higher incidence of coronary heart disease.[68]

The double workday is another source of stress. Married men with children under 5 years work 18.2 hours per week at domestic tasks and child care compared to 32.2 hours per week for married women with children under 5 and 23.8 for single mothers of children under 5.[69] Walters and colleagues found that female registered nurses (with or without children) reported 24 hours a week spent on homemaking tasks (including car repairs and outdoor tasks) compared to 16 hours for male nurses.[70] Women also assume a major role in eldercare, responsible for 70 to 80 percent of such care. Half of women now between 35 and 64 will have to care for an older relative at some time.[71]

Occupational Cancers

As pointed out in the section on methodologies, women have been excluded from studies on occupational cancer, either to keep samples uniform or because data on their professional exposures is lacking. Recently, women have been increasingly included in studies, and risks are becoming apparent, for example, among cleaners, hairdressers, and health care workers.[72] Exposures to industrial chemicals such as solvents and metals are associated with breast cancer.[73]

In addition, several studies have identified teachers as a group particularly likely to contract breast cancer. This has been explained as a result of delayed childbirth among this occupational group.[74] This points up the necessity to examine the whole issue of delayed childbirth and its effects both on certain cancers and on fertility as an occupational health issue. It may be that childbirth is delayed in some occupations due to an incompatibility between professional and family responsibilities. This is yet another example of how women's social situation is indissociable from their likelihood to suffer from occupational disease.

[b] *A 1991 article by Robert A. Karasek, the pioneering researcher into stress and heart disease, mentions (p. 179) that all the group's studies relating blood pressure to job strain had been done on men, although they intended to expand these studies.*

Reproductive Problems Specific to Women

Menstrual symptoms are among the most commonly diagnosed disorders of women. During the mid-eighties, several researchers suggested that menstrual symptoms might be useful for the study of occupational effects on reproductive health, as well as indicative of health problems that should be addressed.[75,76] Parameters of the menstrual cycle that can be studied in relation to occupation include regularity and length of cycle, length and volume of flow, and symptoms of pain and discomfort associated with the periods. The latter symptoms are common and can be studied in normal populations. Some evidence has now accumulated, both on parameters of the cycle which vary with exposure[77,78] and on variations among working populations.[79,80]

Disorders of the menstrual cycle have been explored in relation to occupational exposures to synthetic hormones,[81,82] organic solvents,[83] carbon disulfide,[84] chemical exposures of hairdressers,[85] and night work,[86] although confounding factors were not examined in these studies. Amenorrhea has been associated with strenuous jobs such as athlete[87] or ballet dancer,[88] but not with styrene exposure.[89] No occupational variables have been considered in relation to cycle length, although exercise has been associated with long cycles among college students.[90] Cycle anomalies were related to working conditions in poultry slaughterhouses; irregular cycles were associated with schedule variability and exposure to cold temperatures at work.[91]

Dysmenorrhea or painful menstruation occurs with increased prostaglandin production. Release by the endometrium during menstruation gives rise to increased abnormal uterine activity that produces ischemia and cramping pelvic pain. There may be other associated symptoms such as leg- or backache or gastrointestinal upset. Menstrual pain can begin before or just after the onset of the menstrual flow.[92,93] Premenstrual syndrome (PMS) is a less well-defined diagnostic category that refers to a group of symptoms thought to occur during the days preceding the onset of menses. Since its diagnosis requires making an association with an event (menstruation) that has not yet occurred, reports of prevalence are not consistent.[94]

Prevalence estimates of perimenstrual symptoms vary greatly between studies, according to age, parity, contraceptive methods, and other demographic characteristics. Severe dysmenorrhea was not associated with work in the reinforced plastics industry[95] or exposure to mercury in Italian lamp factories,[96] or to exposure to toluene,[97] but was associated with shift work and irregular shifts in Japanese hospitals.[98] Dysmenorrhea was found to be associated with several parameters expressing cold exposure and physical work load in poultry slaughterhouses in western France[99] and in Quebec, where increased exposure to cold was associated with increased prevalence of dysmenorrhea and sick leave.[75] It was found at a high level among hairdressers, who are exposed to chemicals and work standing for prolonged periods.[85,100,101] Studies of the prevalence and etiology of back pain, a common occupational health problem among hospital workers, may be confused if perimenstrual back pain is not taken into account.[102]

Pregnancy alters the shape of the body and thus the interaction with the work site.[103–105] A study of precautionary leave or reassignment of pregnant workers exposed to dangerous working conditions showed that ergonomic considerations were the most common reason for giving such leave, with chemical and physical exposures following.[106] In jurisdictions where no such program exists, women may risk health damage due to exposures during pregnancy. For example, it has been found that, during pregnancy, certain working conditions (noise, lifting weights) are associated with higher blood pressure.[107] However, most research on pregnancy has been limited to fetal effects, and little information exists on the effects of conditions during pregnancy on the woman herself.

Information is also lacking on the relation between working conditions and age at menopause or menopausal symptoms.[108] Age at menopause can be an indicator of exposure to environmental pollution, as shown by its relationship to smoking and a possible relationship to carbon disulfide exposure.[109]

Health Hazards of Child Labor

Philip J. Landrigan • Susan H. Pollack • Renate Belville • James Godbold

Child labor is defined in the United States as the paid employment of children younger than 18 years of age.[1] According to data from the U.S. Department of Labor, more than 4 million American children were legally employed in 1988, a substantial increase from a decade earlier.[2] Illegal child labor is also widespread, and at least 1 million children are employed under unlawful and often exploitative conditions. Despite the common belief that the problem of illegal child labor was remedied long ago, the practice has in fact persisted in the United States and appears to be on the rise.[2,3]

Child labor is also a major problem internationally.[4–7] According to the International Labour Office (ILO), at least 200 million children under age 14 are employed worldwide. In some countries, children constitute 15 to 25 percent of the total workforce. Children are employed as rug weavers in the Middle East, as underground tin miners in South America, and as metal workers, fireworks makers, textile weavers, and glass blowers.

Child labor is associated in virtually all countries, industrialized and developing, with poverty, high unemployment, inadequate educational opportunities, and failure to enforce relevant laws and standards. Particularly severe abuses have been documented in so-called free enterprise zones, special industrial areas that have been established in many countries, such as along the Mexico-United States border, where relaxation has been permitted in the enforcement of labor and environmental laws.[4]

Resurgence of Child Labor in the United States

A series of economic and social factors similar to those that produced the major increases in child labor at the beginning of the Industrial Revolution has produced the current resurgence of child labor:[8,9]

- *Increased poverty:* More American children live in poverty today than 20 years ago, and the number below the poverty line increased especially rapidly during the 1980s. For the 20 percent of American children who live in poverty, financial need constitutes a compelling reason to seek employment.
- *Unstable world conditions*, particularly war and poverty in Central America, the Caribbean, and Southeast Asia, have led increasing numbers of immigrants, both legal and undocumented, to enter the United States. These immigrants, particularly children without parents, are highly vulnerable to exploitation in the workplace. Their vulnerability is compounded by their lack of access to health care.
- *Relaxation since 1981 in enforcement of federal child labor law,* including relaxation of provisions limiting maximum permissible hours of work and prohibiting use of dangerous machinery.

Illegal employment of children occurs in all industrial sectors, and often under sweatshop conditions.[10] A sweatshop is defined as an establishment that routinely and repeatedly violates wage, hour, and child labor laws as well as the laws protecting occupational safety and health.

Health and safety conditions in sweatshops are often very dangerous. Fire hazards may be created by blocked exit doors, accumulations of combustible materials, and inadequate lighting and ventilation; electrocution hazards result from overloaded electrical connections, work stations located close to exposed wire, and bare fuse boxes.

Children's Vulnerability to Toxins in the Workplace

Children are uniquely vulnerable to toxins encountered in the workplace.[11] This heightened susceptibility stems from several sources:

- Children have greater exposures to toxins than do adults. Pound for pound of body weight, children drink more water, eat more food, and breathe more air. In consequence, children have substantially heavier exposures pound for pound than adults to any toxins that are present in water, food, or air.
- Children's metabolic pathways are immature compared with those of adults. Children are less able than adults to detoxify and excrete most toxic chemicals and thus are more vulnerable to them.
- Children are undergoing rapid growth and development, and their delicate developmental processes are easily disrupted. Many organ systems in young children—the nervous system in particular—undergo very rapid growth and development in childhood. If cells in the developing brain are destroyed by chemicals encountered in the workplace such as lead, mercury, pesticides, or solvents, or if vital connections between nerve cells fail to form, there is high risk that the resulting neurobehavioral dysfunction will be permanent and irreversible.
- Because children have more future years of life than do most adults, they have more time to develop any chronic diseases that may be triggered by early environmental exposures.

Risks of Child Labor

The hazards of child labor fall into two categories: (*a*) risks of injury, illness, and death; and (*b*) threats to future education and full development.

Health Risks

Work is a major, but insufficiently recognized, contributor to the continuing epidemic of childhood injury in the United States.[12–16] The number of American adolescents killed each year in work-related injuries (110) is comparable to the number killed in falls (103), in fires (126), on bicycles (129), by poisoning (191), and by unintentional firearms injuries (266).[17]

Data from state reporting systems confirm that the health hazards associated with child labor are severe. In New York State each year, more than 1,000 children and adolescents receive workers compensation awards for on-the-job injury, more than 400 are permanently disabled, and 4 to 6 are killed.[9] In Connecticut, a study of work-related injury claims found an injury rate of 150 per 10,000 working 16 and 17 year olds.[18] Similarly, an assessment of state-based workers' compensation claims in nine states by investigators from NIOSH found work-related injury rates of 12.6 per 100 full-time male adolescent workers and of 6.6 per 100 full-time female adolescent workers.[14]

Further evidence of the contribution of occupational injury to the continuing epidemic of adolescent injury in the United States is provided by a recent review of adolescent visits to emergency rooms in Massachusetts for treatment of trauma.[19] This study found that 24 percent of those injuries in adolescents that had occurred in an identified location occurred at work. Occupational injuries resulted in a longer average length of hospital stay than other injuries. By contrast, the proportion of adolescent injuries treated in a Massachusetts emergency room that was related to sports trauma was 17 percent.[17]

Illegal employment is particularly dangerous for children, as is illustrated by the following calculation:[20]

- At least 70 percent of work-related injuries are concentrated in the approximately 1 million children (20 percent of the workforce) who are employed illegally.
- The remaining 30 percent of injuries occur in the 4 million children (80 percent of the total workforce) who are employed under legal conditions.
- The risk of injury is therefore almost 10 times greater among children employed under illegal conditions than among those working in compliance with the law.

Toxic Hazards and Chronic Illness

Little information is available on the incidence or severity of work-related illness caused in children by toxic occupational exposures. Children are, however, known to experience a variety of toxic exposures at work. These include formaldehyde and dyes in the garment industry, solvents in paint shops, pesticides in agriculture plant nursery work and lawn care, asbestos in building demolition, and benzene in pumping unleaded gasoline. It appears likely that some still undefined fraction of adolescent asthma might be related to occupational exposures to dusts or formaldehyde, that some cases of neurotoxicity and developmental impairment may be caused by occupational exposure to solvents or pesticides, or that some cases of leukemia and lymphoma in children and adolescents may be the consequence of occupational exposure to benzene.

Health Risks of Agricultural Child Labor

Agriculture is the least regulated and consequently the most dangerous sector of industry for American children. Rural children are employed extensively in agriculture, both on family farms and in commercial farming operations. The hazards to health associated with agricultural work include lacerations, amputations, and crush injuries from farm machinery; blunt trauma from large animals; motor vehicle accidents involving farm vehicles on public roads; suffocation in grain elevators and silos; and exposures to pesticides, fertilizers, and solvents. Small physical size and inexperience may superimpose additional risk for young workers.

Although the numbers of children working in agriculture are not as large so those employed in other sectors, the potential hazards (especially those involving machinery and large animals), coupled with the historical lack of regulation of agriculture, combine to create an important problem, particularly in rural states. Agriculture has come to surpass mining as the most dangerous occupation, accounting in 1981 for 61 fatalities per 100,000 workers.[37] Perhaps for this reason, much of the scanty literature available on work-related injury and illness in children focuses on agriculture.[21–24]

Risks to Education and Development

Interference with school performance is another serious consequence of child labor. Working children risk having too little time for their school homework and being overtired on school days. Teachers in areas where employment of children is common or industrial homework is escalating have reported declines in the academic performance of previously successful students. These children are described as falling asleep at their desks, and they are unable to learn. Even if they maintain their academic standing, working children are able to participate less than their peers in after-school activities and sports. Child labor also interferes with play, which is important for children's normal development; relaxation and freedom from fatigue are necessary for children to grow and learn.[25]

Finally, perhaps the most important long-term developmental consequence of excessive child labor is that, by interfering with learning, it keeps children from receiving and valuing a good education and thus from moving into well paid, upwardly mobile jobs. These children are at high risk of being trapped in a lifetime of low skills and low wages. They will be less productive and less creative than they could have been if they had not had to work excessively.[26]

Workers in the Global Economy

Howard Frumkin

The increasing integration and globalization of the world economy has been widely noted and debated.[1,2] In the occupational safety and health field, these global trends refocus attention on a long-recognized fact: workers in developing nations face more dangerous conditions, and enjoy fewer protections, than workers in wealthier nations. This chapter reviews the challenges to job safety and health in developing nations in the context of an increasingly global economy and identifies opportunities for advances in this arena of public health.

The term "developing countries" is used to include the poorer nations of the world. These include most of the nations of Latin America and the Caribbean, Africa, Asia, and Oceania, often grouped under the term "third world" or, more recently, "the South." Also included are the transitional economies of the former Soviet block in central and eastern Europe. Some countries, such as the "Asian tigers" (Singapore, South Korea, Taiwan, and Hong Kong), Mexico, and Brazil were "developing" a generation ago and have since made rapid strides toward industrialization, but many of the trends discussed here continue to apply to these countries as well. The common features are relatively low economic indicators such as gross domestic product and per capita income (see Table 34-6), relatively low per capita consumption of energy and goods, and relatively undeveloped infrastructures. Many developing countries also have limited traditions of democracy and labor rights.

In a textbook used primarily by public health students and professionals in developed countries, why include a chapter on workers in developing countries? These workers compose a huge at-risk population that merits special attention, for several reasons:

- *The hazard profile is different.* At one level, this grows out of unique features of geography and natural endowment: the tropical climate, the presence of primary commodities such as tin and copper, and the production of crops such as coffee and bananas. Characteristically, agriculture and primary extractive industries figure prominently in the overall profile of economic activity. Perhaps most significantly, industry in developing countries has fewer financial and technical resources, so hazardous exposures tend to be more common and intense.
- *Resources to control and prevent job hazards are scarce.* Moreover, choices are stark; the need to create and preserve jobs may eclipse the need to improve working conditions,

even more than in developed nations. Therefore, the occupational safety and health advocate has many fewer tools available than in developed nations, and implementing changes may be extremely difficult.

- *The occupational health problems of developed countries are closely linked with those of developing countries.* This creates a special obligation among occupational health professionals in developed countries to assist in addressing the occupational health problems of developing countries.

The Political Economy of Occupational Health in a Global Economy

Economic integration has increased rapidly in recent years, due to advances in electronic telecommunication and communication, liberalization of banking and trade laws, and changes in investment practices. This process has manifested itself in several ways that have a direct impact on occupational health: the growth of multinational companies, the development of free trade zones, and the promulgation of multilateral free trade agreements.

Multinational Companies

Multinational companies have increased in size, wealth, and international reach over recent decades.[3,4] The 200 largest corporations now account for more than a quarter of the world's economic activity, with combined sales that exceed the combined gross domestic product of all countries except the "big nine" (the United States, Japan, Germany, France, Italy, the United Kingdom, Brazil, Canada, and China). The trend toward consolidation of economic activity is continuing; in 1982, the top 200 firms accounted for 24.2 percent of global GDP, and by 1996 this figure had increased to 28.3 percent. The world's top 100 economies—49 nations and 51 multinational companies—are shown in Table 34-7.

Multinational companies have the resources and expertise to implement workplace safety and health practices in their facilities, and in many developing nations they offer the best working conditions available. In some cases, company policy and/or law requires that plants in developing nations observe the same standards of worker protection that apply in the home country. And the economic development heralded by industrialization raises the standard of living, at least for some people. However, as multinational companies locate facilities in countries with lower costs of production, they may take advantage of lax local practice and expose employees to levels of hazards that would be unacceptable in Europe or North America. Moreover, small domestic plants spring up in developing nations to supply the multinational facilities. While these provide employment and strengthen the economic base, small plants may present considerable workplace safety and health risks.

Free Trade Zones

Free trade zones, also known as foreign trade zones, free zones, and export processing zones, are areas established by national governments to encourage international trade. Since their origin in the early 1970s, about 200 free trade zones have been established, now employing approximately 4 million people. About half the world's free trade zones are in China. Free trade zones offer several benefits to manufacturing and trading firms, including tax relief, low or absent customs duties, few if any export controls, land and infrastructure subsidies, a plentiful and tightly controlled labor supply, low wages, and lax social, environmental, and labor regulations. In some free trade zones, national collective bargaining laws are formally suspended. Free trade zones employ a small proportion of the world's workforce. However, they exemplify how occupational safety and health practice may be subordinated to the pressures of development in poor countries.

The U.S.-Mexico border functions as a 2,000-mile-long free trade zone, in which occupational safety and health has received considerable attention.[5–8] The Mexican government established its Border Industrialization Program in 1965 to encourage foreign (usually U.S.) companies to site assembly plants south of the border. The assembly plants, known as *maquiladoras*, grew slowly at first. In the 1980s Mexico joined the General Agreement on Tariffs and Trade (GATT) and liberalized its trade restrictions, and the peso was repeatedly devalued, lowering the cost of Mexican labor. By the mid-1990s, there were over 2,200 maquiladoras, employing approximately 500,000 workers. The maquiladoras produce a wide variety of products, including electrical and electronic equipment, automobile parts, toys, clothing, and others.[9] Labor-intensive assembly processes pose physical hazards such as repetitive motion, awkward work positions, and noise, with risks of musculoskeletal disorders and hearing loss. In cleaning metal parts, fabricating electronic components, and operations such as painting and gluing, exposures to solvents, acids, metals, and other chemicals are common,[10] potentially causing neurotoxicity, dermatitis, cancer, renal and hepatic toxicity, and reproductive dysfunction (important in a workforce that consists predominantly of young women). Work practices such as inadequate breaks increase potential hazards. While epidemiologic surveillance data are unavailable, surveys of maquiladora facilities have suggested that hazards are common.[7] As in free trade zones elsewhere, other features of the U.S.-Mexico border aggravate the effects of occupational exposures. Many of the workers are migrants from elsewhere in Mexico, who arrive without financial resources, education, job skills, or experience. Housing and health services are inadequate, general environmental health risks such as water contamination are prevalent,[10,11] and there is little job security due to the constant influx of new arrivals in search of work. Hence, while stress levels are high among maquiladora employees, they are also high among other workers in the same locations,[6] suggesting that general features of the free trade zone social environment affect workers both in and out of the foreign facilities. This combination of forces has made progress in occupational safety and health extremely difficult to achieve.

TABLE 34-6. AVERAGE HOURLY WAGES IN THE TEXTILE INDUSTRY, 1996

Country	*Hourly wage ($US)*
Germany	18.43
Japan	16.29
Italy	14.32
Canada	9.88
United States	9.56
United Kingdom	9.37
Taiwan	5.10
Brazil	1.92
Malaysia	1.64
Peru	1.39
El Salvador	1.38
Honduras	1.31
Mexico	1.08
Tunisia	0.98
Egypt	0.63
Philippines	0.62
Haiti	0.49
India	0.36
Indonesia	0.34
Bangladesh	0.31
Kenya	0.30
China	0.28
Pakistan	0.26

From Greenhouse S: Voluntary rules on apparel labor proving elusive. New York Times, February 1, 1997, pp 1, 8.

TABLE 34-7. THE WORLD'S TOP 100 ECONOMIES, 1995 (IN MILLIONS OF DOLLARS)[a]

1. United States	6,648,013	51. Daimler-Benz	72,253
2. Japan	4,590,971	52. IBM	71,940
3. Germany	2,045,991	53. Malaysia	70,626
4. France	1,330,381	54. Matsushita Electric	70,454
5. Italy	1,024,634	55. General Electric	70,028
6. United Kingdom	1,017,306	56. Singapore	68,949
7. Brazil	554,587	57. Tomen	67,809
8. Canada	542,954	58. Colombia	67,266
9. China	522,172	59. Mobil	64,767
10. Spain	482,841	60. Philippines	64,162
11. Mexico	377,115	61. Iran	63,716
12. Russian Federation	376,555	62. Nissan Motor	62,618
13. Korea, Republic of	376,505	63. Volkswagen Group	61,487
14. Australia	331,990	64. Siemens Group	60,673
15. Netherlands	329,768	65. Venezuela	58,257
16. India	293,606	66. British Petroleum	56,992
17. Argentina	281,922	67. Bank of Tokyo-Mitsubishi	55,243
18. Switzerland	260,352	68. Chrysler	53,195
19. Belgium	227,550	69. Philip Morris	53,139
20. Austria	196,546	70. Toshiba	53,089
21. Sweden	196,441	71. Ireland	52,060
22. Mitsubishi	184,510	72. Pakistan	52,011
23. Mitsuiand Co.	181,661	73. Chile	51,957
24. Indonesia	174,640	74. Nichimen	50,882
25. Itochu	169,300	75. New Zealand	50,777
26. General Motors	168,829	76. Tokyo Electric Power	50,343
27. Sumitomo	167,662	77. Peru	50,077
28. Marubeni	161,184	78. Kanematsu	49,878
29. Denmark	146,076	79. Unilever	49,638
30. Thailand	143,209	80. Nestlé	47,767
31. Ford Motor	137,137	81. Sony	47,619
32. Hong Kong	131,881	82. Fiat Group	46,467
33. Turkey	131,014	83. VEBA Group	46,278
34. South Africa	121,888	84. NEC	45,593
35. Saudi Arabia	117,236	85. Honda Motor	44,090
36. Toyota Motor	111,139	86. UAP-Union es Assurances	43,929
37. Royal Dutch/Shell	109,853	87. Allianz Worldwide	43,486
38. Norway	109,568	88. Egypt	42,923
39. Exxon	107,893	89. Algeria	41,941
40. Nissho Iwai	97,963	90. Elf Aquitane Group	41,729
41. Finland	97,961	91. Hungary	41,374
42. Wal-Mart	93,627	92. Philips Group	40,146
43. Poland	92,580	93. Fujitsu	39,007
44. Ukraine	91,307	94. Indust. Bank of Japan	38,694
45. Portugal	87,257	95. Deutsche Bank Group	38,418
46. Hitachi	84,233	96. Renault Group	36,876
47. Nippon Tel and Tel	82,002	97. Mitsubishi Motors	36,674
48. AT&T	79,609	98. du Pont de Nemours	36,508
49. Israel	77,777	99. Mitsubishi Electric	36,408
50. Greece	77,721	100. Hoechst Group	36,407

From Anderson S, Cavanagh J: Corporate empires. Multinat Monitor 17(12):26–27, 1996.
[a] Company sales data are for 1995; country GDP data are for 1994.

Free Trade Agreements

Multilateral free trade agreements have developed throughout the world during the second half of the twentieth century. These agreements aim to facilitate international trade by lowering and in some cases removing trade barriers. Increasingly, free trade agreements define the rules of international commerce. To the extent that these agreements incorporate related social issues such as working conditions, they may help advance occupational safety and health. On the other hand, trade agreements that ignore labor standards may have a negative impact. Several major free trade agreements serve as important examples.

The *General Agreement on Tariffs and Trade* (GATT) arose in the years after World War II as a global attempt to regulate trade and limit trade barriers. It has evolved over the last 50 years through a series of eight renegotiation "rounds." The Uruguay Round (1986 to 1993) created a successor organization to GATT, the World Trade Organization (WTO), which broadened its scope from trade in goods to include trade in services and intellectual property as well. GATT and the WTO have been generally silent on issues of worker safety and health, restricting their domain to problems that bear directly on trade. Article XX(b) of GATT authorized nations to enact legislation that is "necessary to protect human, animal or plant life or health," but this clause was never used to support trade challenges based on worker health issues. During the Tokyo Round of negotiations, which began in 1978, Sweden proposed adding a social clause to GATT, which would have acknowledged "the freedom of association, trade union rights, [and] adequate health and safety precautions, social standards and social welfare schemes." However, objections from the United States and certain developing nations blocked the adoption of this clause.[12]

Under WTO, the inclusion of labor standards has continued to be highly controversial. Developed nations, including the United States, have pressed for some consideration of international labor standards. However, India and other developing nations have strongly resisted. They argue that such "social clauses" would amount to a thinly disguised trade restriction, depriving developing nations of their competitive advantage.[13,14] They have insisted that labor standards, including occupational health, be separated from the trade process and handled in such forums as the International Labour Office (ILO). Therefore, the WTO has to date played no role in advancing occupational safety and health.

The process of *European economic integration*, in contrast, has extended well beyond trade issues to incorporate a wide range of social considerations, including occupational safety and health.[12,15–19] The European Economic Community (EC), or Common Market, was established by the Treaty of Rome in 1957. This treaty began to lift trade barriers among member nations and established the EC's organizational structure. There are a civil service and bureaucracy (the Commission of the European Communities), policy-making bodies (the Council of Ministers and the European Parliament), and a judiciary (the Court of Justice). The process of economic integration in Europe has addressed occupational safety and health in three ways: broad declarations of policy, organizational structures, and specific activities.

A clear statement of policy can be found in the Single European Act (SEA) of 1987, which moved to establish a European Free Trade Area. Article 118a of the act holds that member countries

> shall pay particular attention to encouraging improvements, especially in the working environments, as regards the health and safety of workers, and shall set as their objective the harmonization of conditions in this area, while maintaining the improvements made.

This policy was reinforced in 1989 with the adoption of the Social Charter, which includes a clause emphasizing

> the need for training, information, consultation, and balanced participation of workers as regards the risks incurred and the steps taken to eliminate or reduce them.

Also in 1989, the Council promulgated the Framework Directive, the first major policy initiative under the SEA. This directive provided a detailed definition of the EC (now the European Union, or EU) approach to worker safety and health, which member countries must transpose into national law. Public and private employers in member countries are assigned a general "duty to ensure the safety and health of workers in every aspect related to work," and specific duties to:

- Evaluate workplace risks,
- Integrate preventive measures into all aspects of production,
- Inform workers and their representatives of risks and preventive measures taken,
- Consult workers and their representatives in all health and safety matters,
- Provide worker health and safety training,
- Designate workers with specific health and safety responsibilities,
- Provide appropriate health surveillance,
- Protect sensitive risk groups, and
- Maintain injury and illness records.

The Framework Directive adopts a broad view of what workplace factors are relevant to occupational health, including design issues, monotonous work, and piecework. It calls for active worker participation in safety and health programs, including rights to advance consultation with employers on safety and health initiatives, paid time off to perform safety and health functions, meetings with government inspectors, and refusal to work in case of "serious, imminent and unavoidable danger" (subject to national laws).

An organizational structure has also been established to support occupational safety and health initiatives in the EU. Within the Commission is a Directorate General responsible for Employment, Industrial Relations, and Social Affairs. This body, known as DG V, includes a Health and Safety Directorate. An Advisory Committee on Safety, Hygiene and Health Protection at Work (ACSH), established in 1974 to advise the Commission, includes representatives of labor, management, and the governments from each member country and is supported by staff from the DG V Health and Safety Directorate. The ACSH reviews legislative proposals relevant to occupational health, initiates activities on specific hazards, and coordinates joint efforts. The European Foundation for the Improvement of Living and Working Conditions, based in Dublin, and the European Agency for Health and Safety at Work, based in Bilbao, conduct research and provide information and technical assistance.

Finally, specific activities have given form to Europe's involvement in occupational safety and health. In 1978 the Commission introduced the first Action Program on Safety and Health. It focused on hazardous substances, prevention of machinery hazards, monitoring and inspections, and the improvement of attitudes toward safety and health. Since then, successive action programs have been directed at other occupational health concerns, such as ergonomics, occupational health statistics, assistance for small enterprises, and training. These have promoted occupational health solutions throughout the member nations, providing training, technical advice, and written materials. For example, in 1982 the Commission convened an informal group of senior labor inspectors to encourage personnel and information exchanges among the 12 nations, comparison of member countries' practices, and improved practice. Binding policies have also been promulgated. A series of so-called daughter directives issued pursuant to the Framework Directive address the use of personal protective equipment, manual handling of loads, work with video display terminals, and other issues. Such initiatives exemplify how the integration of national economies can have positive effects on the practice of occupational health and safety.

Several problems persist in the European approach to occupational safety and health—reconciling national sovereignty with coordinated progress, monitoring compliance with community directives, reconciling differences between more and less progressive countries, and sharing scarce technical expertise and resources. However, Europe provides the world's most advanced example of linking occupational safety and health with free trade. The process of economic integration has included serious discussion of social issues, and explicit principles have been enunciated that include worker safety and health. There are several agencies with responsibility for workplace safety and health, and a range of activities has promoted job safety and health. It is expected that this process will have an impact beyond EU member nations, since occupational safety and health principles will be part of commercial agreements between the EU and the countries of central and eastern Europe.

The *North American Free Trade Agreement* (NAFTA), ratified by Mexico, Canada, and the United States in 1993 for implementation over the next decade, was designed to abolish most trade restrictions among the three countries. NAFTA is intermediate between the WTO and the EU in terms of its inclusion of labor issues.[9] The process that led to NAFTA differed from the European experience in several ways. NAFTA had a shorter history and was negotiated rapidly. There was no tradition of incorporating social issues into the process. Labor unions and their allies, especially in the United States and Canada, vigorously opposed NAFTA and campaigned more to block the treaty altogether than for specific labor-friendly provisions.

Moreover, all three governments were reluctant to relinquish any sovereignty over their respective labor laws. When NAFTA was ratified, there was a labor side agreement that codified some procedures, but it is relatively narrow, in contrast to a broader, more muscular environmental side agreement.[20]

NAFTA's statement of principles is substantially weaker with respect to occupational health than the corresponding European statements. The labor side agreement, in an annex, defines "guiding principles that the Parties are committed to promote, subject to each Party's domestic law, but do not establish common minimum standards." These principles include prevention of occupational injuries and illnesses, compensation in cases of occupational injuries and illnesses, protection of migrant workers and children, and more traditional labor rights such as freedom of association, the rights to organize, bargain collectively, and strike, and prohibition of forced labor. The emphasis is on information exchange and promoting each country's compliance with its own labor laws.

Consistent with this more limited set of aims, the organizational structure erected by NAFTA is relatively circumscribed. There is a Commission for Labor Cooperation, based in Dallas, with ministerial level representation from each participating government and a small staff. There are liaison offices in each country. The Commission's charge is to adjudicate trade disputes that arise from alleged violations by a member nation of its own labor laws, related to occupational safety and health, child labor, or minimum wages.

Given these limitations, NAFTA has done little to advance occupational safety and health in North America. The focus in NAFTA is on dispute resolution rather than on joint research, training, standard-setting, technology development, and related initiatives. The dispute resolution process, in the view of labor advocates, is cumbersome, time-consuming, and relatively toothless. More importantly, the labor side agreement expresses no shared commitment to upgrading or harmonizing occupational health laws or practices. Its scope is narrow, and although there has been little experience to date, it is likely that the broad European approach to occupational health, extending to such concerns as shiftwork and stress, will not be replicated.

Export of Hazards and the Race to the Bottom

Scholars, public health practitioners, and labor advocates have for some years recognized that increasing international trade may threaten worker health and safety. In the 1980s, considerable attention was devoted to the "export of hazard."[21–25] Concern grew out of observations of double standards;[26] industries from developed nations would relocate plants in developing nations due to lower labor costs, more lax regulatory environments, and in some cases, proximity to raw materials and/or markets.[27] In doing so they would fail to follow the same standards of workplace safety and health that were required in their countries of origin, exposing workers in developing nations to relatively greater risks. Case studies of products such as asbestos,[28–30] pesticides,[31–33] and hazardous wastes[34,35] and high-profile disasters such as the Bhopal explosion[36–39] and the observations of professionals from developed nations who visited and worked with colleagues in developing nations[40–45] all fed concern that workers in developing nations faced serious risks from rapid industrialization.

Ironically, the same process was also recognized as a threat to worker health and safety in industrial nations. North American labor unions forcefully argued this point during the NAFTA debates in the early 1990s.[46–51] Local and national governments, they maintained, would hesitate to enforce regulations for fear of driving plants from their jurisdictions to lower-wage areas and losing needed jobs. Workers, perceiving the same dilemma, would refrain from pressing for safer workplaces. And firms in developed nations, increasingly facing international competitors and seeking the lowest possible costs, would play one location against another. Standards of practice would descend in developed nations toward those of developing nations, exactly as predicted by the factor price equalization theorem that is central to the economics of free trade. This "race to the bottom" would threaten the health and safety of workers in both developed and developing nations.

The extent to which such risks will intensify or abate remains to be seen. Moreover, changing patterns of workplace risks and preventive policies are shaped by other forces than changes in global trading patterns. For example, concurrent changes in macroeconomic policy among many North American and European nations have also had an impact. However, workers in developing nations remain a high-risk population, facing a range of workplace hazards at levels not seen for decades in the industrialized countries and in patterns that seem to be accelerating with the growth of global trade.

Special Problems of Occupational Health and Safety in Developing Countries

Occupational safety and health faces a range of challenges in developing countries. These can be divided into several categories: working conditions, the social organization of work, the workforce, and human resources. These challenges are shown in Table 34-8.

Working conditions in developing nations may present special hazards to workers. The tropical climate that often prevails poses risks of heat exhaustion and heat stroke, especially in hot facilities such as textile plants. The workweek is often well in excess of 40 hours, so exposures to chemical and physical hazards, even if regulated to an intensity considered safe in industrialized nations, may exceed anticipated levels because of duration. Much of the production machinery used in developing nations is imported, sometimes after it is deemed obsolete for use in developed nations. As such the machinery may be old and dangerous, and modifications, replacement parts, and technical backup difficult or unavailable. Moreover, alternatives such as safer machinery may be unavailable or prohibitively expensive on local markets.

The *social organization of work* may also contribute to workplace hazards. In many developing nations, the predominant employment setting is the small firm.[52] These firms have even less access to safe technologies than their larger counterparts and tend to be riskier.[53] In fact, large portions of the workforce in developing countries may work in the informal sector, which consists of smaller, often family-based production units, remote from registration and other government controls and from occupational safety and health services.

TABLE 34-8. CHALLENGES FOR OCCUPATIONAL HEALTH IN DEVELOPING COUNTRIES

Challenges related to working conditions
- Tropical climate
- Long workweeks and workshifts
- Most machinery imported; modifications, replacement parts, and technical backup difficult or unavailable
- Technical alternatives, such as safer machinery, may be unavailable on local markets

Challenges related to the social organization of work
- Preponderance of small firms
- Prominent role of the informal sector
- Absence of an independent labor movement and a tradition of labor rights

Challenges related to the workforce
- Low literacy rates
- Low nutritional levels
- Biological features of the local workforce that increase susceptibility, e.g., small stature (ergonomic risk), genetic factors (chemical exposure risk)

Human resource challenges
- Lack of industrial hygiene expertise
- Lack of epidemiology and occupational medical/nursing expertise

TABLE 34-9. OCCUPATIONAL INJURY RATES IN COLOMBIA AND THE UNITED STATES, SELECTED INDUSTRIES, 1989 (CASES/1,000 FULL-TIME WORKERS)

Industry	*Standard Industrial Classification (SIC) Code*	*Colombian Incidence*	*U.S. incidence*
Coal mining	12	522	110
Construction	15–17	140	142
Beverage manufacturing	208	325	174
Wood and cork product manufacturing	24	134	179
Rubber product manufacturing	30	133	152
Mineral product manufacturing	329	135	128
Primary metal industries	33	262	176
Metallic products manufacturing	34	154	175
Machinery manufacturing	35	203	115

From Nieto-Zapata O: Occupational health in a province of Colombia. In: Reich MR, Okubo T (eds): Protecting Workers' Health in the Third World: National and International Strategies. New York: Auburn House, 1992, pp 67–86; Bureau of Labor Statistics, US Department of Labor: Occupational Injuries and Illnesses in the United States by Industry, 1989. Bulletin 2379. Washington, DC: Bureau of Labor Statistics, 1991.

Moreover, many developing countries lack a significant independent labor movement and a tradition of labor rights, without which one of the major forces for occupational safety and health is absent.

Developing nations also face important occupational safety and health challenges related to the *workforce*. Low literacy rates are an obstacle to effective worker training and risk communication. Workers may be especially susceptible to the effects of workplace hazards due to relative nutritional deficiencies. In Islamic countries, workers who fast during Ramadan may be at increased risk of dehydration while working at hot jobs. Biological features of the workforce may increase susceptibility to various hazards. For example, Asian workers on average have a smaller stature than the European and North American workers for whom much industrial machinery was designed, which may lead to ergonomic risks.[53] African workers have a high prevalence of glucose-6-phosphate dehydrogenase deficiency, which increases susceptibility to certain oxidizing chemicals, and Asian workers have a high prevalence of hepatitis B antigenemia, which may increase susceptibility to hepatotoxins. Endemic parasitic disease in some settings reduces work capacity and immunocompetence and increases susceptibility to a range of diseases.[54] Many of these workforce features can be addressed through modification of jobs.

Finally, developing nations face severe *shortages of trained personnel* essential to occupational safety and health practice. Adequately trained industrial hygienists and safety professionals, who would be able to recognize, assess, and control hazards in the workplace, are scarce. Epidemiologists with skills in surveillance, who would be able to monitor disease and injury trends and identify problem areas, are also scarce. Finally, health care providers such as occupational physicians and nurses are scarce, preventing adequate diagnosis and treatment of work-related illnesses and injuries.

Occupational Injuries and Illnesses in Developing Countries

Rates of occupational injuries and illnesses in developing nations are extremely difficult to quantify. As noted above, much of the economically active population is in the informal sector, where few if any statistics are collected. Among workers in the formal sector, occupational injuries and illnesses may be unrecognized and/or unrecorded. Even when data are recorded, the definitions of occupational injuries vary so much among countries that valid comparison is impossible. For example, some countries define a work-related injury as one that requires medical care, while others have a higher threshold, requiring 4 or more days of lost worktime. Some countries include "commuting" injuries that occur while going to or from work, while others do not. Therefore, while comparative statistics are published annually in the *ILO Yearbook of Labour Statistics*, the occupational injury data that appear are difficult to interpret.

The ILO estimates that there are 125 million workplace injuries daily throughout the world, with 220,000 of them fatal.[55] Country-specific studies give a sense of the magnitude of the problem. For example, a careful study of occupational injuries in the Colombian province of Antioquia, for 1989, showed industry-specific incidences that were in some cases comparable to U.S. rates, but in other cases substantially higher (Table 34-9).

Pesticides remain a serious problem for workers in developing nations, due to the prominence of agriculture in many economies and the absence of adequate controls, training, and safety equipment. Worldwide, according to conservative estimates, an estimated 1 million cases of acute pesticide poisoning occur annually, resulting in 20,000 deaths.[56] However, regional estimates project much higher numbers, as shown on Table 34-10. A study of Costa Rica's pesticide poisoning experience during the 1980s[57] found an annual incidence of symptomatic pesticide poisoning among agricultural workers of 4.5 cases per 1,000 workers per year, with young people and females at especially high risk. A case study of a 1987 outbreak of 548 cases of pesticide poisoning in Nicaragua[58] implicated several contributing factors, which are likely present in many developing countries. These included unsafe working conditions such as manual application of pesticides and the use of backpack sprayers, the introduction of a hazardous powdered formulation of carbofuran, that is highly restricted in the developed world,[33] and agricultural subsidies that encouraged the use of hazardous pesticides. Interestingly, pesticides

TABLE 34-10. ESTIMATED NUMBER OF ACUTE PESTICIDE POISONING CASES IN SELECTED AFRICAN COUNTRIES, 1989

Country	*Population (in millions)*	*% Labor Force in Agriculture*	*Number of Cases*
Sudan	24	80	384,000
Tanzania	23	85	368,000
Kenya	22	80	350,000
Uganda	17	80	272,000
Mozambique	15	70	240,000
Cameroon	11	80	175,000
Zimbabwe	10	80	160,000
Ivory Coast	10	80	160,000
Malawi	8	85	128,000
Senegal	7	80	112,000
Mauritius	2	75	3,200

From Choudhry AW: Health hazard of pesticide use in Africa. In: Lehtinen S et al (eds): Proceedings of the East Africa Regional Symposium on Chemical Accidents and Occupational Health. Helsinki: Institute of Occupational Health, 1989, pp 70–74.[56]

have become a favored means of suicide in many developing nations, presumably because of their ready availability.

As noted above, primary extractive industries are prominent in many developing countries, and these are associated with a considerable burden of workplace injuries and illnesses. For example, Cullen and Baloyi studied several groups of miners in Zimbabwe.[42] Among those with more than 15 years' experience, the prevalence of pneumoconiosis (defined as an ILO radiographic category of 1/0 or greater) was 28 percent for coal miners, 13 percent for nickel miners, 10 percent for copper miners, and 18 percent for gold miners. The risks of mining, milling, and related activities are compounded by inadequate engineering controls, protective equipment, and medical surveillance and by the high prevalence of concurrent diseases such as tuberculosis.

The entire range of occupational injuries and illnesses seen in manufacturing, transport, and other sectors in developed nations occurs in developing nations. As noted above, exposures that are readily recognized, and usually effectively controlled, in developed nations, continue at high levels in developing nations. Matte et al in 1989 provided an instructive example with a study of the Jamaican lead battery industry.[59] They surveyed three manufacturers and 10 battery repair shops and found consistently inadequate engineering, personal protective, and behavioral controls on lead exposure. Of 79 workers who were surveyed, 76 had blood lead levels above 40 μg/dL, 28 of these above 60 μg/dL. With prolonged exposure at these levels, toxicity is not only likely, it is nearly inevitable. Contributing factors in this study included the small size of the shops surveyed and deficiencies of engineering controls, respiratory protection, work practices, medical surveillance, and workplace inspection—all factors that are common in other industries in developing nations.

The risks of industrial work in developing nations are not limited to the injuries, lung diseases, and obvious poisonings of the smokestack era. The intensive use of chemicals has introduced risks of occupational cancer,[60–62] lung disease,[63] and other illnesses. Rapid production demands in labor-intensive assembly operations have introduced ergonomic hazards. In Thailand, Chavalitsakulchai and Shahnavaz surveyed 1,000 women in the garment, fertilizer, pharmaceutical, textile, and cigarette industries, and found that approximately 50 percent complained of musculoskeletal symptoms thought to be related to ergonomic problems at work.[64] Frequently reported exposures included heavy manual handling; prolonged sitting and standing; awkward work postures; poor machine design and operation, including the use of unsuitable imported machinery and highly repetitive and monotonous movements; poor work organization; and unsatisfactory working environments. In such "postindustrial" tasks as data entry, workers in developing nations are demonstrating some of the same musculoskeletal complaints seen in developed nations.[65] Even needlestick injuries among health care workers, a major concern in developed nations, are a hazard for health care workers in poor countries.[66,67] The high prevalence of human immunodeficiency virus (HIV) infection in parts of the developing world, patients with high viral loads due to the absence of medications, and the unavailability of protective equipment such as needleless injection systems increase this risk above that seen in developed nations. Finally, occupational stress affects large numbers of workers in developing nations, related both to job pressure (job insecurity and job tension) and in some cases to the physical and social displacement that accompanies urbanization and industrialization.[68]

This summary, while not comprehensive or systematic, suggests that workers in developing nations face a wide range of hazards and suffer high rates of injury and illness as a result. There continues to be a serious need for better surveillance data, especially among workers in small firms, to document the nature and extent of risks and the most important targets for intervention.

Approaches to Improving Occupational Safety and Health in Developing Countries

While the integrating global economy poses challenges to occupational safety and health, there are also important opportunities. Some of these are policy initiatives, to which occupational safety and health professionals can contribute as advisors and advocates. Others fall within the traditional domain of public health practice, such as training and research.

Policy Initiatives

Policy initiatives include those that are official and legally binding, such as workplace standards promulgated by governments, and those that are voluntary. Official standards may be developed in the context of trade agreements, but as noted above, with the exception of the European Union, this linkage is rare and controversial. More typically, standards are promulgated by national government agencies with jurisdiction over labor affairs.

Two sources of standards are available to the governments of developing nations for this purpose. First, many adopt specific exposure standards used in industrialized nations, especially those of the United States, Germany, Japan, Russia, and the Nordic countries. Of note, such standards are only as effective as their enforcement mechanisms, and enforcement often lags well behind promulgation. Second, developing nations may model their policies on relevant Conventions of the International Labour Office. The ILO Conventions, when ratified by member nations, are legally binding. A number of ILO Conventions are directly relevant to occupational safety and health, as shown in Table 34-11. However, many of these have not been ratified even by leading industrial countries, as shown in Table 34-12, and the ILO has no enforcement power, so the impact of the Conventions is limited.

Voluntary standards for occupational safety and health are also available. A principal example is the International Organization on Standardization (ISO), which has promulgated internationally recognized standards on quality management (ISO 9000) and environmental management (ISO 14000). The ISO considered promulgating a standard for occupational health and safety management systems in the mid-1990s, but this proposal was set aside in late 1996 due to strong opposition from various constituencies.[69] Businesses objected to the prospect of standardization in this arena. In the United States, OSHA raised concerns about the adequacy of U.S. input into the international standard-setting process and the possibility that third-party certification through ISO would exempt companies from OSHA inspection. Representatives of the other leading ISO nations—France, Germany, Japan, and the United Kingdom—also witheld support for the standard. At the same time, the American Federation of Labor and Congress of Industrial Organizations (AFL-CIO) raised questions about the representation of workers in the ISO process. It appears unlikely that this route to voluntary international standardization will yield occupational safety and health standards.

Other voluntary standards or codes of practice have been promulgated by international agencies. For example, the Organization on Economic Co-operation and Development has published *Guiding Principles for Chemical Accident Prevention, Preparedness and Response*, the United Nations Environment Programme (UNEP) has promulgated a *Code of Ethics on the International Trade in Chemicals*, the ILO has promulgated a *Code of Practice on Safety in the Use of Chemicals at Work*, and the International Programme on Chemical Safety (IPCS, a joint program of the ILO, UNEP, and the World Health Organization (WHO)) has published *Health and Safety Guides* for nearly 100 chemicals and *International Chemical Safety Cards*, including handling recommendations, for over 700 chemicals. The recommendations in these documents are readily available to authorities and practitioners in developing nations and are often based on a careful review of evidence available at the time they are prepared. They may be of special use to multinational firms that wish to establish a standard of practice in each of their operating locations. However, the resources to implement them may be out of reach, especially to smaller firms and governments in developing nations.

Some voluntary standards have been issued by industry groups. For example, the International Chamber of Commerce developed the 16-point "Business Charter for Sustainable Development," which was endorsed during its 1991 Rotterdam conference.[70] The Chemical Manufacturers Association introduced its Responsible Care Program in 1988 to improve the industry's safety and environmental performance (Chemical Manufacturers Association, 2501 M Street, NW, Washington, DC 20037). While these initiatives pertain mainly

TABLE 34-11. MAJOR ILO CONVENTIONS RELEVANT TO OCCUPATIONAL SAFETY AND HEALTH

Number	Year	Convention
12	1921	Workmen's Compensation (agriculture)
13	1921	White Lead (painting)
16	1921	Medical Examination of Young Persons (sea)
17	1925	Workmen's Compensation (accidents)
18	1925	Workmen's Compensation (occupational diseases)
19	1925	Quality of Treatment (accidents' compensation)
32	1932	Protection against Accidents (dockers)
42	1934	Workmen's Compensation (occupational diseases)
62	1937	Safety Provisions (building)
77	1946	Medical Examination of Young Persons (industry)
78	1946	Medical Examination of Young Persons (nonindustrial occupations)
113	1959	Medical Examination (fishers)
119	1963	Guarding of Machinery
120	1964	Hygiene (commerce and offices)
121	1964	Employment Injury Benefits
124	1965	Medical Examination of Young Persons (underground work)
134	1970	Prevention of Accidents (seafarers)
136	1971	Benzene
139	1974	Occupational Cancer
148	1977	Working Environment (air pollution, noise, and vibration)
152	1979	Occupational Safety and Health (dock work)
155	1981	Occupational Safety and Health
161	1985	Occupational Health Services
162	1986	Asbestos
164	1987	Health Protection and Medical Care (seafarers)
167	1988	Safety and Health in Construction
170	1990	Chemicals
174	1993	Prevention of Major Industrial Accidents
176	1995	Safety and Health in Mines

to environmental practice rather than to worker safety and health, there is considerable overlap between the two, especially in the chemical industry, and worker safety and health is explicitly mentioned as a priority. The principles are widely available and may be used by occupational health practitioners in developing nations as useful benchmarks.

Voluntary standards and codes have also been issued by nongovernmental organizations. Although these do not have offical status, they may be effective in the context of public education, consumer campaigns, stockholder campaigns, and similar efforts. The Valdez principles, promulgated by a group of environmental organizations in 1989, aims to promote environmentally sustainable operation by companies. One of these principles, "risk reduction," includes a commitment to minimizing workplace hazards by "employing safe technologies and operating procedures and by being constantly prepared for emergencies" (Social Investment Forum, Coalition for Environmentally Responsible Economies (CERES), 711 Atlantic Avenue, Boston, MA 02111). Advocates promote the implementation of Valdez principles by working through stockholders and by encouraging socially responsible investment. Other nongovernmental organizations have issued standards that include safe working conditions and have organized consumer campaigns to promote compliance with these standards through market pressure. Particular attention has been directed at the apparel, carpet, and toy industries. Examples include standards issued by the Clean Clothes Campaign in the Netherlands (van Ostadestraat 233b, 1073 TN Amsterdam; htpp://www.clearclothes.org), the Fairtrade Mark Campaign in the United Kingdom (Fairtrade Foundation, 7th Floor Regent House, 89 Kingsway, London WC2B 6RH; http://www.fairtrade.org/fairtrade), and Co-op America (Co-op America, 1612 K Street NW, Suite 600, Washington, DC 20006; http://www.coopamerica.org).

A final kind of policy relates to investment patterns. Investment in industrial development can be linked to the implementation of sound occupational safety and health policies by lending institutions such as the World Bank and by private lenders. Such linkages are now familiar in the environmental arena, where major projects are contingent on environmental impact statements and proper provisions for environmental safeguards. Lenders can be urged to adapt this approach to protecting worker health as well.

Initiatives by Public Health Professionals

Within the realm of public health work, professionals can promote occupational safety and health in developing nations in several ways. These include training, technical assistance, collaborative research, and advocacy.

Training is an essential activity for occupational health professionals, given the shortages of expertise in industrial hygiene, safety engineering, occupational medicine, occupational health nursing, and related fields noted above. Approaches to training include formal academic study in institutions in industrialized nations, short courses, and distance learning through newsletters and electronic means. One notable example is the extensive training efforts of the Finnish Institute of Occupational Health, through its ILO/FINNIDA African Safety and Health Project and its ILO/FINNIDA Asian-Pacific Regional Programme on Occupational Safety and Health. Regional newsletters published by the Institute are distributed to 6,000 readers in Africa and 4,000 readers in the Asia-Pacific region, covering such topics as information retrieval, small-scale enterprises, and specific

TABLE 34-12. RATIFICATION OF RECENT ILO CONVENTIONS BY CERTAIN MEMBER NATIONS

	Convention Number[a]									
Country	***148***	***152***	***155***	***161***	***162***	***164***	***167***	***170***	***174***	***176***
Algeria										
Argentina										
Australia										
Austria										
Azerbaijan	×									
Belgium	×									
Bolivia					×					
Bosnia and Herzegovina	×		×	×	×					
Brazil	×	×	×	×	×					
Cameroon					×					
Canada					×					
Chile					×					
China								×		
Colombia							×	×		
Congo		×								
Costa Rica	×									
Croatia	×		×	×	×					
Cuba	×	×	×							
Cyprus		×	×		×					
Czech Republic	×		×	×		×	×			
Denmark	×	×	×				×			
Ecuador	×	×			×					
Egypt	×	×								
Ethiopia			×							
Finland	×	×	×	×	×	×				
France	×	×								
Germany	×	×		×		×	×			
Ghana	×									
Greece										
Guatemala				×	×		×			
Guinea	×	×								
Hong Kong										
Hungary	×		×	×		×	×			
Iceland			×							
India										
Indonesia										
Iran										
Iraq	×	×					×			
Ireland			×							
Israel										
Italy	×									
Japan										
Korea										
Kyrgyzstan	×									
Latvia	×		×							
Malaysia										
Malta	P									
Mexico		×	×	×		×	×	×		
Netherlands			×							
New Zealand										
Niger	×									
Nigeria			×							
Norway	×	×	×		×		×	×		
Pakistan										
Peru		×								
Philippines										
Poland										
Portugal	×		×							
Russian Federation	×									
San Marino	×			×						
Saudi Arabia										
Singapore										

TABLE 34-12. RATIFICATION OF RECENT ILO CONVENTIONS BY CERTAIN MEMBER NATIONS (Continued)

	Convention Number[a]									
Country	***148***	***152***	***155***	***161***	***162***	***164***	***167***	***170***	***174***	***176***
Slovakia	×		×	×		×	×			
Slovenia	×		×	×	×					
South Africa										
Spain	P	×	×		×	×				
Sweden	×	×	×	×	×	×	×	×	×	
Switzerland					×					
Tajikstan	×									
Tanzania	×	×								
Thailand										
Turkey										
Uganda					×					
Ukraine										
United Kingdom										
United States										
Uruguay	×		×	×	×					
Venezuela			×							
Vietnam			×							
Yugoslavia	×		×	×	×					
Zambia	×									
Zimbabwe										
Total Ratified	37	18	26	15	20	8	11	5	1	0

From International Labour Office
Abbreviations and symbols: ×, ratification; P, partial ratification.
[a] See Table 34-11 for titles of conventions.

industries. In the United States, the Fogarty International Center of the National Institutes of Health introduced an international training program in environmental and occupational health in 1995. This program brings trainees from developing nations to U.S. institutions for intensive study. Through large-scale efforts such as these, and through more limited training initiatives, needed expertise in occupational safety and health can be transferred to developing countries.

Technical assistance is another important area of effort for public health professionals. Joint investigations of outbreaks, consultancies on occupational safety and health problems, and direct technology transfer can all advance the protection of workers in developing countries. In particular, two practical areas of occupational health and safety activity bear mention. One pertains to *health services delivery*. With a shortage of trained occupational safety and health personnel in developing nations, it is essential to deliver services through existing primary care facilities.[71] The design of such delivery systems, the training of primary care personnel, and implementation of appropriate record-keeping and the linkage of medical care with preventive services at the plant level are all worthwhile efforts. A second area is in implementing preventive measures. The overall strategy of occupational hazard prevention is addressed in Chapter 35. In developing nations, it is essential to emphasize low-cost measures to prevent risk, drawing on the extensive experience of workers and public health practitioners.[72] Designing interventions, installing them, and monitoring their success are also essential.

Collaborative research is a third important activity for occupational safety and health professionals. Would-be researchers in developing nations face daunting challenges: university salaries below subsistence levels, requiring outside employment; lack of infrastructure needs such as libraries, computers, and basic laboratory equipment; lack of domestic sources of research funding; lack of research mentors and collaborators; and the need to address diverse content areas rather than build in-depth specialization. Despite these challenges, there remain important research needs in developing nations.[73–75] One goal of such research, as anywhere in the world, is the *discovery* of unknown exposure-response associations and disease mechanisms. Just as important, however, is the traditional public health research function of *documentation*. Many workplace hazards are well understood, and their effects easily predicted. However, it may require in-country data demonstrating that a hazard is taking a toll on local workers and communities to stimulate government to take action to control the hazard.

Finally, occupational safety and health professionals in developing nations, with the strong support of colleagues in developed nations, need to engage in *advocacy*. In countries where expertise is rare, professionals rarely have the luxury of remaining only practitioners, or researchers, or teachers. Steps must be taken to identify and correct workplace hazards, and working people must be cared for when injured or ill. Relevant data must be assembled, through primary or secondary research. Students must be taught to perform these functions. However, for lasting changes to be made, practical experience, data, and moral conviction must be laid before "those who need to know," including government officials, company officials, and worker representatives, and systematic approaches to protecting worker health must be put in place. Only through such advocacy can the health and safety of a vast and vulnerable population, workers in the developing world, be effectively protected.

▶ REFERENCES

Workers with Disabilities

1. Nagi SZ: Disability and Rehabilitation: Legal, Clinical, and Self-Concepts and Measurement. Columbus, OH: Ohio State University Press, 1969
2. Pope AM, Tarlov AR: Disability in America: Toward a National Agenda for Prevention. Institute of Medicine, Committee on a National Agenda for the Prevention of Disabilities, Division of Health Promotion and Disease Prevention. Washington, DC: National Academy Press, 1991, p 77
3. Katz S: Assessing self-maintenance: Activities of daily living, mobility, and instrumental activities of daily living. J Am Geriatrics Society, 1983; 31(12):721–727

4. LaPlante M, Miller K: People with disabilities in basic life activities in the U.S. In Disability Statistics Abstract. No. 3, April, Disability Statistics Program, University of California, San Francisco. Washington, DC: US Department of Education, National Institute on Disability and Rehabilitation Research, 1992
5. McNeil J: Americans with Disabilities: 1991–92. US Bureau of the Census, Current Population Reports, P70-33. Washington, DC: Government Printing Office, 1993
6. World Health Organization: International Classification of Impairments, Disabilities, and Handicaps. Geneva: World Health Organization, 1980
7. Haber LD: Issues in the definition of disability and the use of disability survey data. In Levine DB, Zitter M, Ingram L (eds): Disability Statistics: An Assessment. Report of a Workshop. National Research Council. Washington, DC: National Academy Press, 1990, Appendix B, 35–51
8. A version of this work disability question appears in the 1966 Survey of the Disabled, the 1972 Survey of Health and Work Characteristics, the 1978 Survey of Disability and Work, the various editions of the Survey of Income and Program Participation, the various waves of the Panel Study of Income Dynamics, the Current Population Survey, and the 1980 and 1990 US Census
9. Louis Harris & Associates: N.O.D./Harris Survey of Americans with Disabilities. Commissioned by the National Council on Disability. New York: Louis Harris & Associates, 1994
10. LaPlante M, Miller S, Miller K: People with work disability in the U.S. In Disability Statistics Abstract. No. 4, May, Disability Statistics Program, University of California, San Francisco. Washington, DC: US Department of Education, National Institute on Disability and Rehabilitation Research, 1992
11. Yelin EH, Katz PP: Labor force trends of persons with and without disabilities. Monthly Labor Review 117(10):36–42, 1994
12. Mudrick NR, Trupin L, LaPlante MP: Patterns of Employment Among People with Work Disabilities. Presented to the American Public Health Association, San Diego, CA, November 1, 1995
13. Johnson WG, Baldwin M: The Americans with Disabilities Act: will it make a difference? Policy Studies Journal 21(4):775–788, 1994
14. Louis Harris & Associates: The N.O.D./Harris Survey on Employment of People with Disabilities. Commissioned by the National Council on Disability. New York: Louis Harris & Associates, 1995
15. U.S. General Accounting Office: Social Security: Disability Rolls Keep Growing, While Explanations Remain Elusive. GAO/HEHS-94-34. Washington, DC: US General Accounting Office, 1994
16. Bound J: The health and earnings of rejected disability insurance applicants. American Economic Review 79(3):482–503, 1989
17. Rothstein MA: Medical Screening and the Employee Health Cost Crisis. Washington, DC: Bureau of National Affairs, 1989
18. Derr PG: Ethical considerations in fitness and risk evaluations. In Himmelstein JS, Pransky GS (eds): Worker Fitness and Risk Evaluations. Occup Med, April–June, 1988
19. Carey TS, Hadler NM: The role of the primary physician in disability determination for Social Security Insurance and workers' compensation. Ann Intern Med 104:706–710, 1986
20. Rondinelli RD: Practical aspects of impairment rating and disability determination. In Braddom RL (ed): Physical Medicine & Rehabilitation. Philadelphia: WB Saunders, 1996
21. Lankhorst GJ, Van de Stadt RJ, Van der Korst JK: The natural history of idiopathic low back pain. Scand J Rehabil Med 17:1–4, 1985
22. Matheson LN: Symptom magnification syndrome structured interview: rationale and procedure. J Occup Rehabil 1:43–56, 1991
23. Osterweis M, Kleinman A, Mechanic D (eds): Pain and Disability: Clinical, Behavioral, and Public Policy Perspectives. Washington, DC: National Academy Press, 1987
24. Veres JG, Sims RR (eds): Human Resource Management and the Americans with Disabilities Act. Westport, CT: Quorum Books, 1995. [Many different resources are listed in the appendix of this book.]

Minority Workers and Communities

1. US Census Bureau: Current Population Reports, Series P25-1104, Population Projections of the United States, by Age, Sex, Race, and Hispanic Origin: 1993 to 2050. Washington, DC: Government Printing Office, 1996
2. Cherniak M: The Hawk's Nest Incident: America's Worst Industrial Disaster. New Haven, CT: Yale University Press, 1986
3. Gafafer WM: Health of Workers in Chromate Producing Industry: A Study. Public Health Service Publication No. 192. Washington, DC: US Public Health Service, 1950
4. Lloyd JW: Long-term mortality study of steelworkers. V. Respiratory cancer in coke plant workers. J Occup Med 13:53–68, 1971
5. Mazumdar S, Redmond C, Sellecito W, Sussman N: An epidemiological study of exposures to coal tar pitch volatiles among coke oven workers. APCA J 25:382–389, 1975
6. Martin C, Higgins J: Byssinosis and other respiratory ailments: a survey of 6,631 cotton textile employees. J Occup Med 18:455–462, 1976
7. McMichael AJ, Spirtas R, Gamble JF, Tousey PM: Mortality among rubber workers: relationship to specific jobs. J Occup Med 18:178–185, 1976
8. Metzger R, Delgado JL, Herrell R: Environmental health and Hispanic children. Environ Health Perspect 103(Suppl 6):25–32, 1995
9. Perfecto I, Velásquez B: Farm workers: among the least protected. EPA Journal 18:13–14, 1992
10. Lucas R: The distribution of job characteristics. Rev Econ Stats 56:530–540, 1974
11. Robinson JC: Racial inequality and the probability of occupation-related injury or illness. Milbank Mem Fund Q 62:567–590, 1984
12. US Census Bureau. Current Population Reports, Series P20-480. The Black Population in the United States, March 1994 and 1993. Washington, DC: Government Printing Office, 1996
13. Sorlie PD, Rogot E: Mortality by employment status in the National Longitudinal Mortality Study. Am J Epidemiol 132:983–992, 1990
14. U.S. Environmental Protection Agency: Environmental Equity: Reducing Risk for All Communities. EPA230-R-92-008. Washington: US Environmental Protection Agency, 1992
15. Soliman MR, Derosa CT, Mielke HW, Bota K: Hazardous wastes, hazardous materials and environmental health inequity. Toxicol Ind Health 9:901–912, 1993
16. United Church of Christ, Commission for Racial Justice: Toxic Waste and Race in the United States: A National Report on the Racial and Socioeconomic Characteristics of Communities with Hazardous Waste Sites. New York: United Church of Christ, 1987
17. Mohai P, Bryant B: Environmental racism: reviewing the evidence. In Bryant B, Mohai P (eds): Race and the Incidence of Environmental Hazards. Boulder, CO: Westview Press, 1992, pp 163–176
18. Sexton K, Gong H, Bailar JC, et al: Air pollution health risks: do class and race matter? Toxicol Ind Health 9:843–878, 1993
19. Bullard RD: Dumping in Dixie: Race, Class, and Environmental Quality. Boulder, CO: Westview Press, 1990
20. Bullard RD (ed): Unequal Protection: Environmental Justice and Communities of Color. San Francisco: Sierra Club Books, 1996
21. Bullard RD, Wright BH: Environmental justice for all: community perspectives on health and research needs. Toxicol Indust Health 9:821–841, 1993
21a. Bullard RD: Unplanned environs: the price of unplanned growth in boomtown Houston. California Sociologist 7:85–101, 1984
22. White HL: Hazardous waste incineration and minority communities. In Bryant B, Mohai P (eds): Race and the Incidence of Environmental Hazards. Boulder, CO: Westview Press, 1992, pp 126–139
23. Calderon RL, Johnson CC Jr, Craun GF, et al: Health risks from contaminated water: do class and race matter? Toxicol Ind Health 9:879–900, 1993

24. Lanphear BP, Weitzman M, Eberly S: Racial differences in Urban children's environmental exposures to lead. Am J Public Health 86:1460–1463, 1996
25. Sargent JD, Brown MJ, Freeman JL, et al: Childhood lead poisoning in Massachusetts communities: its association with sociodemographic and housing characteristics. Am J Public Health 85:528–534, 1995
26. Agency for Toxic Substances and Disease Registry: The Nature and Extent of Lead Poisoning in Children in the United States: A Report to Congress. Atlanta: Agency for Toxic Substances and Disease Registry, 1988
27. Needleman HL: Childhood lead poisoning, a disease for the history texts. Am J Public Health 81:685–687, 1991
28. West PC, Fly JM, Larkin F, Marans RW: Minority anglers and toxic fish consumption: evidence from a statewide survey of Michigan. In Bryant B, Mohai P (eds): Race and the Incidence of Environmental Hazards. Boulder, CO: Westview Press, 1992, pp 100–113
29. Fitzgerald EF, Hwang SA, Brix KA, et al: Fish PCB concentrations and consumption patterns among Mohawk women at Akwesasne. J Expo Anal Environ Epidemiol 5:1–19, 1995
30. Kinloch D, Kuhnlein H, Muir DC: Inuit foods and diet: a preliminary assessment of benefits and risks. Sci Total Environ 122:247–278, 1992
31. Kosary CL, Ries LAG, Miller BA, et al (eds): SEER Cancer Statistics Review, 1973–1992: Tables and Graphs. NIH Publication No. 96-2789. Bethesda, MD: National Cancer Institute, 1995
32. Baquet CR, Gibbs T: Cancer and black Americans. In Braithwaite RL, Taylor SE (eds): Health Issues in the Black Community. San Francisco: Jossey-Bass, 1992, pp 106–120
33. Wynder EL, Muscat JE: The changing epidemiology of smoking and lung cancer histology. Environ Health Perspect 103(Suppl 8):143–148, 1995
34. Block G, Rosenberger WF, Patterson BH: Calories, fat and cholesterol: intake patterns in the US population by race, sex and age. Am J Public Health 78:1150–1155, 1988
35. Wagenknecht LE, Cutter GR, Haley NJ, et al: Racial differences in cotinine levels among smokers in the Coronary Artery Risk Development in (Young) Adults Study. Am J Public Health 80:1053–1056, 1990
36. Harris RE, Zang EA, Anderson JI, Wynder EL: Race and sex differences in lung cancer risk associated with cigarette smoking. Int J Epidemiol 22:592–599, 1993
37. Centers for Disease Control and Prevention, Division of Environmental Hazards and Health Effects, Air Pollution and Respiratory Health Branch: Asthma—United States, 1982–92. MMWR Morb Mortal Weekly Rep 43:952–955, 1995
38. National Heart, Lung and Blood Institute Working Group: Respiratory diseases disproportionately affecting minorities. Chest 108: 1380–1392, 1995
39. Wing JS: Asthma in the inner city—a growing health concern in the United States. J Asthma 30:427–430, 1993
40. Chan-Yeung M, Malo JL: Occupational asthma. N Engl J Med 333:107–112, 1995
41. Schenker MB, Gold EB, Lopez RL, Beaumont JJ: Asthma mortality in California, 1960–89: demographic patterns and occupational associations. Am Rev Respir Dis 147:1454–1460, 1993
42. Koren H: Associations between criteria air pollutants and asthma. Environ Health Perspect 103(Suppl 6):235–242, 1995
43. Saunders E: Hypertension in minorities: blacks. Am J Hypertens 8:115S–119S, 1995
44. Lackland DT, Keil JE: Epidemiology of hypertension in African Americans. Semin Nephrol 16:63–70, 1996
45. Gaines K, Burke G: Ethnic differences in stroke: black-white differences in the United States population. SECORDS Investigators. Southeastern Consortium on Racial Differences in Stroke. Neuroepidemiology 14:209–239, 1995
46. Livingston IL: Renal disease and black Americans: selected issues. Soc Sci Med 37:613–621, 1993
47. Alexander M, Grumbach K, Selby J, et al: Hospitalization for congestive heart failure. Explaining racial differences. JAMA 274: 1037–1042, 1995
48. Centers for Disease Control and Prevention, Division of Chronic Disease Control and Community Intervention, National Center for Chronic Disease Prevention and Health Promotion: Mortality from congestive heart failure—United States, 1980–1990. MMWR 43: 77–81, 1994
49. Gillum RF: Trends in acute myocardial infarction and coronary heart disease death in the United States. J Am Coll Cardiol 23:1273–1277, 1994
50. Calhoun DA, Oparil S: Racial differences in the pathogenesis of hypertension. Am J Med Sci 310(Suppl 1):S86–S90, 1995
51. Weir MR, Hanes DS: Hypertension in African Americans: a paradigm of metabolic disarray. Semin Nephrol 16:102–109, 1996
52. James SA, LaCroix AZ, Kleinbaum DG, Strogatz DS: John Henryism and blood pressure differences among black men, II: the role of occupational stressors. J Behav Med 7:259–275, 1984
53. Krieger N: Racial and gender discrimination: risk factors for high blood pressure? Soc Sci Med 30:1273–1281, 1990
54. James SA: John Henryism and the health of African-Americans. Cult Med Psychiatry 18:163–182, 1994
55. Light KC, Brownley KA, Turner R, et al: Job status and high-effort coping influence work blood pressure in women and blacks. Hypertension 25:554–559, 1995
56. Krieger N, Sidney S: Racial discrimination and blood pressure: the CARDIA study of young black and white adults. Am J Public Health 8:1370–1378, 1996
57. Kasl S, Cobb S: Blood pressure changes in men undergoing job loss: a preliminary report. Psychosom Med 76:184–188, 1970
58. National Diabetes Data Group: Diabetes in America. 2nd ed., NIH Publication No. 95-1468. Bethesda, MD: National Institute of Diabetes and Digestive and Kidney Diseases, 1995, pp 613, 631, 664
59. Lai M-S, Hsueh Y-M, Chen C-J, et al: Ingested inorganic arsenic and prevelance of diabetes mellitus. Am J Epidemiol 139:484–492, 1994
60. Rahman M, Wingren G, Axelson O: Diabetes mellitus among Swedish art glass workers—an effect of arsenic exposure? Scand J Work Environ Health 22:146–149, 1996
61. Centers for Disease Control and Prevention: Tuberculosis morbidity—United States, 1995. MMWR Morb Mortal Weekly Rep 45:365–370, 1996
62. Snider DE Jr, Salinas L, Kelly GD: Tuberculosis: an increasing problem among minorities in the United States. Public Health Rep 104:646–653, 1989
63. Cantwell MF, Snider DE Jr, Cauthen GM, Onorato IM: Epidemiology of tuberculosis in the United States, 1985 through 1992. JAMA 272:535–539, 1994
64. Stead WW, Senner JW, Reddick WT, Lofgren JP: Racial differences in susceptibility to infection by *Mycobacterium tuberculosis*. N Engl J Med 322:422–427, 1990
65. McKenna MT, Hutton M, Cauthen G, Onorato IM: The association between occupation and tuberculosis. A population-based survey. Am J Respir Crit Care Med 154:587–593, 1996
66. Jereb JA, Klevens RM, Privett TD, et al: Tuberculosis in health care workers at a hospital with an outbreak of multidrug-resistant *Mycobacterium tuberculosis*. Arch Intern Med 155:854–859, 1995
67. Bowden KM, McDiarmid MA: Occupationally acquired tuberculosis: what's known. J Occup Med 36:320–325, 1994
68. American Thoracic Society, Environmental and Occupational Health Assembly: Health effects of outdoor air pollution. Part 1. Am Rev Respir Crit Care Med 153:3–50, 1996

69. Herd D: Subgroup differences in drinking patterns among black and white men: results from a national survey. J Stud Alcohol 51:221–232, 1990
70. Caetano R, Kaskutas LA: Changes in drinking patterns among whites, blacks and Hispanics, 1984–1992. J Stud Alcohol 56:558–565, 1995
71. Lamarine RJ: Alcohol abuse among Native Americans. J Community Health 13:143–155, 1988
72. Centers for Disease Control. Alcohol-related hospitalizations—Indian Health Service and tribal hospitals, United States, May 1992. MMWR Morb Mortal Weekly Rep 41:757–760, 1992
73. Gilliland FD, Becker TM, Samet JM, Key CR: Trends in alcohol-related mortality among New Mexico's American Indians, Hispanics, and non-Hispanic whites. Alcohol Clin Exp Res 19:1572–1577, 1995
74. Rosenbaum E: Race and ethnicity in housing: turnover in New York City, 1978–87. Demography 29:467–486, 1992
75. Malveaux FJ, Fletcher-Vincent SA: Environmental risk factors of childhood asthma in urban centers. Environ Health Perspect 103 (Suppl 6):59–62, 1995
76. Polednak AP: Racial and Ethnic Differences in Disease. New York: Oxford University Press, 1989
77. Evans WE, Relling MV, Rahman A, et al: Genetic basis for a lower prevalence of deficient CYP2D6 oxidative drug metabolism phenotypes in black Americans. J Clin Invest 91:2150–2154, 1993
78. Nakamura K, Goto F, Ray WA, et al: Interethnic differences in genetic polymorphism of debrisoquin and mephenytoin hydroxylation between Japanese and Caucasian populations. Clin Pharmacol Ther 38:402–408, 1985
79. Crofts F, Cosma GN, Currie D, et al: A novel CYP1A1 gene polymorphism in African-Americans. Carcinogenesis 14:1729–1731, 1993
80. Shields PG, Caporaso NE, Falk RT, et al: Lung cancer, race, and a CYP1A1 genetic polymorphism. Cancer Epidemiol Biomarkers Prev 2:481–485, 1993
81. Calabrese EJ, Moore G, Brown R: Effects of environmental oxidant stressors on individuals with a G-6-PD deficiency with particular reference to an animal model. Environ Health Persp 29:49–55, 1979
82. Severo R: Genetic tests by industry raise questions on rights of workers. New York Times 3 February, 1980
83. Severo R: Screening of blacks by Du Pont sharpens debate on gene tests. New York Times 4 February, 1980
84. Severo R: Air Force rejects cadets with sickle trait. New York Times 4 February, 1980
85. Severo R: Dispute arises over Dow studies on genetic damage in workers. New York Times 5 February, 1980
86. Hoiberg A, Ernst J, Uddin DE: Sickle cell trait and glucose-6-phosphate dehydrogenase deficiency. Effects on health and military performance in black Navy enlistees. Arch Intern Med 141:1485–1488, 1981
87. Murray RF: Tests of so-called genetic susceptibility. J Occup Med 28:1103–1107, 1986
88. Dressler WW: Lifestyle, stress, and blood pressure in a southern black community. Psychosom Med 52:182–198, 1990
89. Williams DR: Black-white differences in blood pressure: the role of social factors. Ethn Dis 2:126–141, 1992
90. Chrousos GP, Gold PW: The concepts of stress and stress system disorders. Overview of physical and behavioral homeostasis. JAMA 267:1244–1252, 1992
91. McEwen BS, Stellar E: Stress and the individual. Mechanisms leading to disease. Arch Intern Med 153:2093–2101, 1993
92. Sheridan JF, Dobbs C, Brown D, Zwilling B: Psychoneuroimmunology: stress effects on pathogenesis and immunity during infection. Clin Microbiol Rev 7:200–212, 1994
93. Hankinson JL, Kinsley KB, Wagner GR: Comparison of spirometric reference values for Caucasian and African American blue-collar workers. J Occup Environ Med 38:137–143, 1996
94. Glindmeyer HW, Lefante JJ, McColloster C, et al: Blue-collar normative spirometric values for Caucasian and African-American men and women aged 18 to 65. Am J Respir Crit Care Med 151:412–422, 1995
95. Bao W, Dalferes ER Jr, Srinivasan SR, et al: Normative distribution of complete blood count from early childhood through adolescence: the Bogalusa Heart Study. Prev Med 22:825–837, 1993
96. Christian CL, Werley B, Smith A, et al: Comparison of employees' white blood cell counts in a petrochemical plant by worksite and race. J Natl Med Assoc 86:620–623, 1994
97. Council on Ethical and Judicial Affairs, American Medical Association: Black-white disparities in health care. JAMA 263:2344–2346, 1990
98. Council on Scientific Affairs, American Medical Association. Hispanic health in the United States. JAMA;265:248–252, 1991
99. Braithwaite RL, Taylor SE (eds): Health Issues in the Black Community. San Francisco: Jossey-Bass, 1992
100. Short PF, Cornelius LJ, Goldstone DE: Health insurance of minorities in the Unites States. J Health Care Poor Underserved 1:9–23, 1990
101. Seccombe K, Clarke LL, Coward RT: Discrepancies in employer-sponsored health insurance among Hispanics, blacks and whites: the effects of sociodemographic and employment factors. Inquiry 31:221–229, 1994
102. Himmelstein DU, Woolhandler S: Care denied: US residents who are unable to obtain needed medical services. Am J Public Health 85:341–344, 1995
103. Demark-Wahnefried W, Strigo T, Catoe K, et al: Knowledge, beliefs, and prior screening behavior among blacks and whites reporting for prostate cancer screening. Urology 46:346–351, 1995
104. Mickey RM, Durski J, Worden JK, Danigelis NL: Breast cancer screening and associated factors for low-income African-American women. Prev Med 24:467–476, 1995
105. Hunter CP, Redmond CK, Chen VW, et al: Breast cancer: factors associated with stage at diagnosis in black and white women. Black/White Cancer Survival Study Group. J Natl Cancer Inst 85:1129–1137, 1993
106. Zaloznik AJ: Breast cancer stage at diagnosis: Caucasians versus Afro-Americans. Breast Cancer Res Treat 34:195–198, 1995
107. Ford ES, Cooper RS: Racial/ethnic differences in health care utilization of cardiovascular procedures: a review of the evidence. Health Serv Res 30:237–252, 1995
108. Soucie JM, Neylan JF, McClellan W: Race and sex differences in the identification of candidates for renal transplantation. Am J Kidney Dis 19:414–419, 1992
109. Ball JK, Elixhauser A: Treatment differences between blacks and whites with colorectal cancer. Med Care 34:970–984, 1996
110. Halfon N, Newacheck PW: Childhood asthma and poverty: differential impacts and utilization of health services. Pediatrics 91:56–61, 1993
111. Yergan J, Flood AB, LoGerfo JP, Diehr P: Relationship between patient race and the intensity of hospital services. Med Care 25:592–603, 1987
112. Moore RD, Stanton D, Gopalan R, Chaisson RE: Racial differences in the use of drug therapy for HIV disease in an urban community. N Engl J Med 330:763–768, 1994
113. Escarce JJ, Epstein KR, Colby DC, Schwartz JS: Racial differences in the elderly's use of medical procedures and diagnostic tests. Am J Public Health 83:948–954, 1993
114. Falcone D, Broyles R: Access to long-term care: race as a barrier. J Health Polit Policy Law 19:583–595, 1994
115. Clayton LA, Byrd WM: The African-American cancer crisis, Part I: the problem. J Health Care Poor Underserved 4:83–101, 1993
116. Sorlie P, Rogot E, Anderson R, et al: Black-white mortality differences by family income. Lancet 340(8815):346–350, 1992

117. Stange KC, Strogatz D, Schoenbach VJ, et al: Demographic and health characteristics of participants and nonparticipants in a work site health-promotion program. J Occup Med 33:474–478, 1991
118. Santiago AM, Muschkin CG: Disentangling the effects of disability status and gender on the labor supply of Anglo, black and Latino older workers. Gerontologist 36:299–310, 1996
119. National Institute for Occupational Safety and Health: Fatal Injuries to Workers in the United States, 1980–89: A Decade of Surveillance. DHHS (NIOSH) Publication No. 93-108S. Cincinnati: National Institute for Occupational Safety and Health, 1993
120. Stout NA, Jenkins L, Pizatella TJ: Occupational injury mortality rates in the United States: changes from 1980 to 1989. Am J Public Health 86:73–77, 1996
121. Fullerton L, Olson L, Crandall C, et al: Occupational injury mortality in New Mexico. Ann Emerg Med 26:447–454, 1995
122. Kipen H, Wartenberg D, Scully PF, et al: Are non-whites at greater risk for occupational cancer? Am J Ind Med 19:67–74, 1991
123. Zahm SH, Pottern LM, Lewis DR, Ward MH, White DW: Inclusion of women and minorities in occupational cancer epidemiologic research. J Occup Med 36:842–847, 1994
124. Loomis DP, Savitz DA: Occupation and leukemia mortality among men in 16 states: 1985–1987. Am J Ind Med 19:509–521, 1991
125. National Institute for Occupational Safety and Health: Work-Related Lung Disease Surveillance Report, 1996. DHHS (NIOSH) Publication No. 96-134. Cincinnati: National Institute for Occupational Safety and Health, 1996
126. Kreiss K, Mroz MM, Zhen B, et al: Epidemiology of beryllium sensitization and disease in nuclear workers. Am Rev Respir Dis 148:985–991, 1993
127. Dement JM, Brown DP, Okun A: Follow-up study of chrysotile asbestos textile workers: cohort mortality and case-control analyses. Am J Ind Med 26:431–447, 1994
128. Robinson JC: Trends in racial inequality and exposure to work-related hazards, 1968–86. Am Assoc Occup Health Nurses J 37:56–63, 1989
129. Zwerling C, Ryan J, Orav EJ: The efficacy of preemployment drug screening for marijuana and cocaine in predicting employment outcome. JAMA 264:2639–2643, 1990
130. Burnett CA, Lalich NR: Measuring work-related health disparities for minority populations. In: Toward the Year 2000: Refining the Measures. Proceedings of the 1993 Public Health Conference on Records and Statistics, July 19–21, 1993. DHHS Publication PHS 94-1214. Hyattsville, MD: National Center for Health Statistics, 1994
131. Kirkpatrick P: Triple jeopardy: disability, race and poverty in America. Poverty and Race 3:1–8, 1994
132. Bound J, Schoenbaum M, Waidmann T: Race differences in labor force attachment and disability status. Gerontologist 36:311–321, 1996
133. Wray LA: The role of ethnicity in the disability and work experience of preretirement-age Americans. Gerontologist 36:287–298, 1996
134. Swanson GM, Lin CS, Burns PB: Diversity in the association between occupation and lung cancer among black and white men. Cancer Epidemiol Biomarkers Prev 2:313–320, 1993
135. Dula A, Kurtz S, Samper ML: Occupational and environmental reproductive hazards education and resources for communities of color. Environ Health Perspect 101(Suppl 2):181–189, 1993
136. Smith EA: Cultural and linguistic factors in worker notification to blue collar and no-collar African-Americans. Am J Ind Med 23:37–42, 1993

General References

Anonymous: Hispanic environmental health: ambient and indoor air pollution. National Coalition of Hispanic Health and Human Services Organizations (COSSMHO). Otolaryngol Head Neck Surg 114:256–264, 1996

Bryant B, Mohai P: Race and Incidence of Environmental Hazards. Boulder, Co: Westview Press, 1992

Friedman-Jimenez G: Occupational disease among minority workers: a common and preventable public health problem. Am Assoc Occup Health Nurses J 37:64–70, 1989

Montgomery LE, Carter-Pokras O: Health status by social class and/or minority status: implications for environmental equity research. Toxicol Ind Health 9:729–773, 1993

Robinson JC: Exposure to occupational hazards among Hispanics, blacks, and non-Hispanic whites in California. Am J Public Health 79:629–630, 1989

Walker B Jr, Goodwin NJ, Warren RC: Environmental health and African Americans: challenges and opportunities. J Natl Med Assoc 87:123–129, 1995

Migrant and Seasonal Farmworkers

1. National Safety Council: Accidents Facts. Itasca, IL: National Safety Council, 1995
2. Schenker MB, Lopez R, Wintemute G: Farm-related fatalities among Children in California, 1980 to 1989. Am J Public Health 85(1):89–91, 1995
3. Wilk VA: Health hazards to children in agriculture. Am J Ind Med 24:283–290, 1993
4. Lee BC, Gunderson PD (eds): Childhood Agricultural Injury Prevention: Issues and Interventions from Multiple Perspectives. Marshfield, WI: National Farm Medicine Center, 1992
5. US Department of Labor: U.S. Farmworkers in the Post-IRCA Period. Research Report No. 4. Washington, DC: U.S. Government Printing Office, 1993
6. Egan J, Deputy Director of the federal Migrant Health Program, U.S. Department of Health and Human Services: Personal communication, 1996
7. National Advisory Council on Migrant Health: Under the Weather: Farmworker Health. Austin, TX: National Farmworker Health Center, 1993
8. California Rural Legal Assistance Foundation: Hunger in the Heartland. Sacramento, CA: California Rural Legal Assistance Foundation, 1991
9. US Department of Commerce, Bureau of the Census: Statistical Abstract of the United States, 1995. Washington, DC: Government Printing Office, 1995
10. Friedman-Jiménez G, Ortiz JS: Occupational Health. In Molina CW, Aguirre-Molina M (eds): Latino Health in the US: A Growing Challenge. Washington, DC: American Public Health Association, 1994, pp 341–389
11. US Department of Labor, Occupational Safety and Health Administration: Hazard communication; final rule. 29 CFR Parts 1910, 1915, 1917, 1918, 1926, and 1928. Federal Register 52(163):31852–31886, 1987
12. US Environmental Protection Agency: Worker protection standard, hazard information, hand labor tasks on cut flowers and ferns exception; final rule, and proposed rules. 40 CFR Parts 156 and 170. Federal Register 57(163):38102–38176, 1992
13. US General Accounting Office: Hired Farmworkers: Health and Well-Being at Risk. GAO/HRD-92-46. Washington, DC: General Accounting Office, 1992
14. Martin P, Taylor JE: Merchants of Labor: Farm Labor Contractors and Immigration Reform. Washington, DC: Urban Institute, 1995
15. Commission on Security and Cooperation in Europe: Migrant Farmworkers in the United States. Washington, DC: Government Printing Office, 1993
16. Commission on Agricultural Workers: Report of the Commission on Agricultural Workers. Washington, DC: Government Printing Office, 1993

17. Migrant Health Program: An Atlas of State Profiles Which Estimate Number of Migrant and Seasonal Farmworkers and Members of Their Families. Rockville, MD: US Department of Health and Human Services, 1990
18. US Department of Labor: Migrant Farmworkers: Pursuing Security in an Unstable Labor Market. Research Report No. 5. Washington, DC: US Department of Labor, 1994
19. US Department of Labor: The National Agricultural Workers Survey (NAWS): Recent Findings Relevant to Policy Development and Program Planning and Evaluation. Washington, DC: US Department of Labor, 1995
20. Schenker MB: Preventive Medicine and Health Promotion Are Overdue in the Agricultural Workplace. Wellness Lecture Series. Woodland Hills, CA: The California Wellness Foundation, 1995, pp 97–124
21. US Environmental Protection Agency: EPA's Pesticide Programs. Washington, DC: US Environmental Protection Agency, 1991
22. Grier N, Curtis J: Pesticides yield a toxic harvest. Forum for Applied Research and Public Policy 11(1):62–67, 1996
23. Moses M: Farmworkers and Pesticides. In Bullard RD (ed): Confronting Environmental Racism: Voices from the Grassroots. Boston: South End Press, 1993
24. Wilk VA: Farmworker Health and Safety: An Annotated Bibliography 1988–1995. Washington, DC: Farmworker Justice Fund, 1995
25. Meister JS: The Health of Migrant Farm Workers. Occup Med 6(3):503–518, 1991
26. Mobed K, Gold EB, Schenker MB: Occupational health problems among migrant and seasonal farm workers. West J Med 157(3):367–373, 1992
27. Wilk VA: The Occupational Health of Migrant and Seasonal Farmworkers in the United States. Washington, DC: Farmworker Justice Fund, 1986
28. Coye MJ: The health effects of agricultural production: I. The health of agricultural workers. J Public Health Policy 6(3):349–370, 1985
29. Dever GEA: Migrant Health Status: Profile of a Population with Complex Health Problems. Austin, TX: Migrant Clinicians Network, 1991
30. Ciesielski SD, Esposito DH, Protiva J, et al: The incidence of tuberculosis among North Carolina migrant farmworkers, 1991. Am J Public Health 84(11):1836–1838, 1994
31. Ciesielski SD, Seed JR, Esposito DH, Hunter N: The epidemiology of tuberculosis among North Carolina migrant farm workers [published erratum appears in JAMA 266(1):66, 1991]. JAMA 265(13): 1715–1719, 1991
32. Ciesielski SD, Seed JR, Ortiz JC, Metts J: Intestinal parasites among North Carolina migrant farmworkers. Am J Public Health 82(9): 1258–1262, 1992
33. Migrant Clinicians Network: The Guanajuato-Pennsylvania Health Data Exchange Pilot Project. MCN Clinical Supplement May/June 1995. Austin, TX: Migrant Clinicians Network, 1995
34. The Migrant Clinicians Network, Austin, TX, will publish a bilingual (Spanish/English) curriculum on domestic violence for farmworker women trainers in conjunction with the California Farmworker Women's Leadership Project (Líderes Campesinas en California) in 1998. The training manual will also include modules for health care workers dealing with battered women.
35. Marentes A, Treviño-Sauceda M, Wilk VA, Lago M, Parham D: The Farmworker Women's Special Initiative on AIDS. Bethesda, MD: US Department of Health and Human Services, Health Resources and Services Administration, 1995
36. Haines CS, Wilk VA, Harlan C, Wiggins N, Ramirez M, Thompson V: Preventive strategies for health risks in rural women. In: McDuffie HH, Dosman JA, Semchuk K, Olenchock SA, Senthilselvan A (eds): Supplement to Agricultural Health and Safety: Workplace, Environment, Sustainability. Saskatoon, Canada: Center for Agricultural Medicine, University of Saskatchewan, 1994
37. Wilk VA: Farmworker Women Speak Out: Priorities and Policy Recommendations to Improve the Lives of Farmworker Families. Washington, DC: Farmworker Justice Fund, 1994
38. National Commission to Prevent Infant Mortality: HIV/AIDS: A Growing Crisis among Migrant and Seasonal Farmworker Families. Washington, DC: National Commission to Prevent Infant Mortality, 1993 (Available from the National Farmworker Health Center, Austin, TX.)
39. Rodriguez R: Evaluation of the MCN Domestic Violence Assessment Form and Pilot Prevalence Study. MCN Clinical Supplement May/June 1995. Austin, TX: Migrant Clinicians Network, 1995
40. The Universal Resource Locator address for the NIOSH Agricultural Safety and Health Centers' home page and national newsletter is: http://agcenter.ucdavis.edu/agcenter/niosh/niosh.html
41. Dr. Lorraine Cameron, NIOSH, Illness Effects Section, Division of Surveillance, Cincinnati, OH: Personal communication, 1995
42. US Environmental Protection Agency: Office of Pesticide Programs Annual Report for 1995. EPA 730-R-95-002. Washington, DC: US Environmental Protection Agency, 1995
43. US Environmental Protection Agency: Pesticide programs; worker protection standards; final rules and proposed rules. 40 CFR Parts 156 and 170. Federal Register 60(85):21944–21968, 1995
44. US Congress, Office of Technology Assessment: Case studies: exposure to lead, pesticides in agriculture, and organic solvents in the workplace. In: Neurotoxicity: Identifying and Controlling Poisons of the Nervous System. OTA-BA-436. Washington, DC: US Government Printing Office, 1990
45. Centers for Disease Control and Prevention: Occupational pesticide poisoning in apple orchards—Washington, 1993. MMWR 42(51–52): 993–995, 1994
46. Saunders LD, Ames RG, Knaak JB, et al: Outbreak of Omite-CR-induced dermatitis among orange pickers in Tulare County, California. J Occup Med 29(5):409–413, 1987
47. US General Accounting Office: Pesticides on Farms: Limited Capability Exists to Monitor Occupational Illnesses and Injuries. GAO/PEMD-94-6. Washington, DC: General Accounting Office, 1993
48. Moses M: Pesticide-related health problems and farmworkers. Am Assoc Occup Health Nurses J 37(3):115–130, 1989
49. Zahm SH, Blair B: Cancer among migrant and seasonal farmworkers: an epidemiologic review and research agenda. Am J Ind Med 24:753–766, 1993
50. Centers for Disease Control and Prevention, Agency for Toxic Substances and Disease Registry: ATSDR Case Studies in Environmental Medicine #29 Reproductive and Developmental Hazards. Atlanta, GA: Centers for Disease Control and Prevention, 1993
51. Stevens WK: Pesticides may leave legacy of hormonal chaos. New York Times August 23, 1994, pp C1, C6
52. US Department of Labor, Occupational Safety and Health Administration: Field sanitation; final rule. 29 CFR 1928. Federal Register 52(84):16050–16096, 1987
53. US Environmental Protection Agency: A Guide to Heat Stress in Agriculture. EPA-750-b-92-001. Washington, DC: U.S. Environmental Protection Agency, 1993
54. Ortiz JS: Composite summary and analysis of hearing held by the Department of Labor, Occupational Health and Safety Administration on field sanitation for migrant farm workers. Docket No. H-308, October 21, 1985
55. Arbab DM, Weidner BL: Infectious diseases and field water supply and sanitation among migrant farm workers. Am J Public Health 76(6):694–695, 1986
56. Gamsky TE, McCurdy SA, Wiggins P, Samuels SJ, Berman B, Schenker MB: Epidemiology of dermatitis among California farm workers. J Occup Med 34(3):304–310, 1992
57. University of California Agricultural Health and Safety Center at Davis: Case Studies in Agricultural Medicine. Skin Disease in Agriculture (A Self-Instructional Case Study). vol 1. Davis: University of California, 1995

58. Demers P, Rosenstock L: Occupational Injuries and Illnesses among Washington State agricultural workers. Am J Public Health 81(12): 1656–1658, 1991
59. Becker WJ: An Analysis of Agricultural Accidents in Florida—1990. Agricultural Engineering Department, Special Series Report SS-AGE-25. Gainesville, FL: University of Florida, 1991
60. Ciesielski S, Hall P, Sweeney M: Occupational injuries among North Carolina migrant farmworkers. Am J Public Health 81(7):926–927, 1991
61. Heyer NJ, Franklin G, Rivara FP, et al: Occupational injuries among minors doing farm work in Washington State: 1986 to 1989. Am J Public Health 82(4):557–560, 1992
62. Moses M, Johnson ES, Anger WK, Burse VW, Horstman SW, Jackson RJ, et al: Environmental equity and pesticide exposure. Toxicol Ind Health 9(5):913–959, 1993
63. Lee C (ed): Proceedings. The First National People of Color Environmental Leadership Summit—October 24–27, 1991. New York: United Church of Christ Commission for Racial Justice, 1992

Women Workers

1. Ayers L, Cusack M, Crosby F: Combining work and home. Occup Med 8(4):821–831, 1993
2. Doyal L: What Makes Women Sick: Gender and the Political Economy of Health. Waged Work and Well-being. London: Macmillan, 1995, Chapter 6
3. Silman AJ: Why do women live longer and is it worth it? Br Med J 293:1211–1312, 1987
4. Waldron I: Effects of labor force participation on sex differences in mortality and morbidity. In Frankenhaeuser M, Lundberg U, Chesney M (eds): Women, Work and Health. New York: Plenum Press, 1991, pp 17–35
5. Greenberg GN, Dement JM: Exposure assessment and gender differences. J Occup Med 36(8):907–912, 1994
6. Zahm SH, Pottern LM, Lewis DR, Ward MH, White DW: Inclusion of women and minorities in occupational cancer epidemiological research. J Occup Med 36(8):842–847, 1994
7. Semenciew R, Morrison H, Riedel D, Wilkins K, Ritter L, Mao Y: Multiple myeloma mortality and agricultural practices in the prairie provinces of Canada. J Occup Med 35:557–561, 1993
8. Hall EM: Gender, work control and stress: a theoretical discussion and an empirical test. Int J Health Serv 19:725–745, 1989
9. Blishen BR, Carroll WK, Moore C: The 1981 socioeconomic index for occupations in Canada. Canadian Review of Sociology & Anthropology 24:465–488, 1987
10. Stellman J: Where women work and the hazards they may face on the job. J Occup Med 36(8):814–825, 1994
11. US Bureau of Labor Statistics: Employment and Earnings Report for 1994. Washington, DC: US Bureau of Labor Statistics, 1995
12. Armstrong P, Armstrong H: The Double Ghetto: Canadian Women and their Segregated Work, 3rd ed, Toronto: McClelland and Stewart, 1993, pp. 50–54.
13. White J: Sisters and Solidarity. Toronto: Thompson Educational Publishing, 1993, p 168
14. Dumais L, Messing K, Seifert AM, Courville J, Vézina N: Make me a cake as fast as you can: determinants of inertia and change in the sexual division of labour of an industrial bakery. Work, Employment and Society 7:363–382, 1993
15. Messing K, Chatigny C, Courville J: "Light" and "heavy" work: An analysis of housekeeping in a hospital. Applied Ergonomics, in press
16. Messing K, Dumais L, Courville J, Seifert AM, Boucher M: Evaluation of exposure data from men and women with the same job title. J Occup Med 36(8):913–917, 1994
17. Hsairi M, Kauffmann F, Chavance M, Brochard P: Personal factors related to the perception of occupational exposure: an application of a job exposure matrix. Int Epidemiol Assoc J 21:972–980, 1992
18. Pheasant S: Bodyspace. London: Taylor and Francis, 1986, p 111
19. Lortie M: Analyse comparative des accidents déclarés par des préposés hommes et femmes d'un hôpital gériatrique. Journal of Occupational Accidents 9:59–81, 1987
20. Courville J, Vézina N, Messing K: Analyse des facteurs ergonomiques pouvant entraîner l'exclusion des femmes du tri des colis postaux. Le Travail Humain 55:119–134, 1992
21. Pines A, Lemesch C, Grafstein O: Regression analysis of time trends in occupational accidents (Israel, 1970–1980). Safety Science 15:77–95, 1992
22. Robinson JC: Trends in racial inequality and exposure to work-related hazards, 1968–1986. Am Assoc Occup Health Nurses J 37: 56–63, 1989
23. Wagener DK, Winn DW: Injuries in working populations: black-white differences. Am J Public Health 81:1408–1414, 1991
24. Laurin G: Féminisation de la Main d'Oeuvre: Impact sur la santé et la Sécurité du Travail. Montréal: Commission de la Santé et de la Sécurité Travail du Québec, 1991
25. Messing K, Boutin S: La reconnaissance des conditions difficiles dans les emplois des femmes et les instances gouvernementales en santé et en sécurité du travail. Industrial Relations, 52:261–291, 1997
26. Kraut A: Estmates of the extent of morbidity and mortality due to occupational diseases in Canada. Am J Ind Med 25:267–278, 1994
27. Gervais M: Bilan de Santé des Travailleurs Québécois. Montréal: Institut de Recherche en Santé et en Sécurité du Travail du Quebec, 1993
28. Messing K, Courville J, Boucher M, Dumais L, Seifert AM: Can safety risks of blue-collar jobs be compared by gender? Safety Science 18:95–112, 1994
29. Bourbonnais R, Vinet A, Vézina M, Gingras S: Certified sick leave as a non-specific morbidity indicator: a case-referent study among nurses. Br J Ind Med 49:673–678, 1992
30. Hagberg M, Morgenstern H, Kelsh M: Impact of occupations and job tasks on the prevalence of carpal tunnel syndrome. Scand J Work Environ Health 18:337–345, 1992
31. Stetson DS, Albers JW, Silverstein BA, Wolfe RA: Effects of age, sex, and anthropometric factors on nerve conduction measures. Muscle Nerve 15:1095–1104, 1992
32. Skov P, Valbjorn O, Pederson BV: The Danish Indoor Climate Study Group: influence of personal characteristics, job-related factors and psychosocial factors on the sick building syndrome. Scand J Work Environ Health 15:286–295, 1989
33. Skov P, Valbjorn O, Pedersen BV: The Danish Indoor Climate Study Group: influence of indoor climate on the sick building syndrome in an office environment. Scand J Work Environ Health 16: 363–371, 1990
34. Norback D, Michel I, Widstrom J: Indoor air quality and personal factors related to the sick building syndrome. Scand J Work Environ Health 16:121–128, 1990
35. Hodgson MJ, Frohliger J, Permar E, Tidwell C, Traven ND, Olenchock SA, Karpf M: Symptoms and microenvironmental measures in nonproblem buildings. J Occup Med 4:527–533, 1991
36. Harrison J, Pickering CAC, Faragher EB, Austwick PKC, Little SA, Lawton L: An investigation of the relationship between microbial and particulate indoor air pollution and the sick building syndrome. Respir Med 86:225–235, 1992
37. Norback D, Torgen M, Edling C: Volatile organic compounds, respirable dust, and personal factors to prevalence and incidence of sick building syndrome in primary schools. Br J Ind Med 47:733–741, 1990
38. Kelland P: Sick building syndrome, working environments and hospital staff. Indoor Environ 1:335–340, 1992

39. Mendell MJ, Smith AH: Consistent pattern of elevated symptoms in air conditioned office buildings: a reanalysis of epidemiologic studies. Am J Public Health 80:1193–1199, 1990
40. Menzies R, Tamblyn R, Farant J-P, Hanley J, Nunes F, Tamblyn R: The effect of varying levels of outdoor-air supply on the symptoms of the sick building syndrome. N Engl J Med 328:821–827, 1993
41. Franck C, Bach E, Skov P: Prevalence of objective eye manifestations in people working in office buildings with different prevalences of the sick building syndrome compared with the general population. Int Arch Occup Environ Health 65:65–69, 1993
42. Stenberg B, Eriksson N, Mild KHL, Höög Js, Sandström M, Sundell J, Wall S: Facial skin symptoms in visual display terminal workers. A case-referent study of personal, psychosocial, building- and VDT-related risk indicators. Int J Epidemiol 24(4):796–803, 1995
43. Nelson N, Kaufman JD, Burt J, Karr C: Health symptoms and the work environment in four nonproblem United States office buildings. Scand J Work Environ Health 21:51–59, 1995
44. Stenberg B, Wall S: Why do women report "sick building symptoms" more often than men? Soc Sci Med 40(4):491–502, 1995
45. Gilboa R, Al-Tawil NG, Marcusson JA: Metal allergy in cashiers. Acta Derm Venereol 68(4):317–324, 1988
46. Statistics Canada: Women in Canada: A Statistical Report. Cat. No. 89-503E. Ottawa: Statistics Canada, 1995, pp 37–53
47. Hagberg M, Silverstein B, Wells R, Smith MJ, Hendrick HW, Carayon P, Pérusse M: Work-Related Musculoskeletal Disorders: A Reference Book for Prevention. London: Taylor and Francis, 1995
48. Jutras S, Guyon L, Renaud M, Dandurand F, Bouchard P: Comment les Québécois se tirent-ils d'affaire? Sciences sociales et santé 7(4):69–93, 1989
49. Vézina N, Tierney D, Messing K: When is light work heavy? Components of the physical workload of sewing machine operators which may lead to health problems. Applied Ergonomics 23:268–276, 1992
50. Brisson C, Vézina M, Vinet A: Health problems of women employed in jobs involving psychological and ergonomic stressors: The case of garment workers in Québec. Women Health 18(3):49–66, 1992
51. Vézina N, Chatigny C, Messing K: A manual materials handling job: symptoms and working conditions among supermarket cashiers. Chronic Diseases in Canada 15(1):17–22, 1994
52. Stubbs DA, Buckle PW, Hudson MP, et al: Back pain in the nursing profession. Ergonomics 26:755–765, 1983
53. Videman T, Nurminen T, Tola S, et al: Low-back pain in nurses and some loading factors of work. Spine 9:400–404, 1984
54. Guo H-R, Tanaka S, Cameron LL, Seligman PJ, Behrens VJ, Ger J, Wild DK, Putz-Anderson V: Back pain among workers in the United States: national estimates and workers at high risk. Am J Ind Med 28:591–602, 1995
55. Lippel K: Le Stress au Travail. Cowansville, Québec: Les éditions Yvon Blais, 1993, pp 167, 228
56. Yassi A, Weeks JL, Samson K, Raber MB: Epidemic of "shocks" in telephone operators: lessons for the medical community. Can Med Assoc J 140:816–820, 1989
57. Goldberg P, David S, Landre M-F, Fuhrer R, Dassa S, Goldberg M: An epidemiological study of depressive symptomatology and working conditions of prison staff. Proceedings of the 24th International Congress on Occupational Health, 1993, p 110
58. Bowler R, Mergler D, Rauch SS, Bowler RP: Stability of psychological impairment: 2-year follow-up of former microelectronics workers' affective and personality disturbance. Women Health 18(3): 27–48, 1992
59. Lucire Y: Neurosis in the workplace. Med J Aust 145:323–327, 1986
60. Karasek R, Baker D, Marker F, Ahlbom A, Theorell T: Job decision latitude, job demands, and cardiovascular disease: a prospective study of Swedish men. Am J Public Health 71:694–705, 1982
61. Johnson JV, Hall EM: Job strain, workplace social support and cardiovascular disease. Am J Public Health 78:1336–1342, 1988
62. Pickering TG, James GD, Schnall PL, Schlussel YR, Pieper CF, Gerin W, Karasek RA: Occupational stress and blood pressure: studies in working men and women. In Frankenhaeuser M, Lundbergh U, Chesney M (eds) Women, Work and Health: Stress and Opportunities. New York: Plenum Press, 1991, pp 171–186
63. Steingart RM et al: Sex differences in the management of corarary artery disease. N Engl J Med 325:226–230, 1991
64. Doyal L: What Makes Women Sick: Gender and the Political Economy of Health. London: MacMillan Press, 1995, p 17
65. Leigh JP: A ranking of occupations based on the blood pressures of incumbents in the National Health and Nutrition Examination Survey I. J Occup Med 33:853–861, 1991
66. Kwachi I, Colditz GA, Stampfer MJ, Willett WC, Manson JE, Seizer FE, Hennekens CH: Prospective study of shift work and risk of coronary heart disease in women. Circulation 92(11):3178–3182, 1995
67. Haynes S: The effect of job demands, job control and new technologies on the health of employed women. In Frankenhaeuser M, Lundbergh U, Chesney M: 1991. Women, Work and Health: Stress and Opportunities. New York: Plenum Press, 1991, pp 157–169
68. Thorell T: Psychosocial cardiovascular risks—on the double loads in women. Psychother Psychosom 55:81–89, 1991
69. Statistics Canada: Women in the Labour Force. No. 75-507E. Ottawa: Statistics Canada, 1994, Table 6.8
70. Walters V, Beardwood B, Eyles J, French S: Paid and unpaid work roles of male and female nurses. In Messing K, Neis B, Dumais L (eds): Invisible: Issues in Women's Occupational Health and Safety. Charlottetown: gnyergy books, 1995, pp 125–149
71. Guberman N, Maheu P, Maillé C: Travail et soins aux proches dépendants. Montréal: Éditions Remue-mémage, 1994, pp 27–29
72. Pottern LM, Zahm SH, et al: Occupational cancer among women: a conference overview. J Occup Med 36(8):809–813, 1994
73. Cantor KP, Stewart PA, Brinton LA, Dosemeci M: Occupational exposures and female breast cancer mortality in the United States. J Occup Environ Med 37(3):336–348, 1995
74. Rubin CH, Burnett CA, Halperin WE, Seligman PJ: Occupation as a risk identifier for breast cancer. Am J Public Health 83:1311–1315, 1993
75. Mergler D, Vézina N: Dysmenorrhea and cold exposure. J Reprod Med 30:106–111, 1985
76. Harlow SD: Function and dysfunction: a historical critique of the literature on menstruation and work. Health Care Women Int 7:39–50, 1986
77. Messing K, Saurel-Cubizolles M-J, Bourgine M, et al: Menstrual cycle characteristics and working conditions in poultry slaughterhouse and canneries. Scand J Work Environ Health 18:302–309, 1992
78. Harlow SD, Matoski GM: The association between weight, physical activity and stress and variation in the length of the menstrual cycle. Am J Epidemiol 133:38–49, 1991
79. Treloar AE, Boynton RE, Behn BG, Brown BW: Variation in the human menstrual cycle through reproductive life. Int J Fertil 12: 7–125, 1967
80. Shortridge LA: Assessment of menstrual variability in working populations. Rep Toxicol 2:171–176, 1988
81. Mills JL, Jefferys JL, Stolley PD: Effects of occupational exposure to estrogen and progesteogens and how to detect them. J Occup Med 26:269–272, 1984
82. Harrington JM, Stein GF, Rivera RO, Morales AV: The occupational hazards of formulating oral contraceptives. Int Arch Environ Health 1:12–15, 1978
83. Panova Z: Menstrual and reproductive problems and gynaecological morbidity in women occupationally exposed to petrol. Leptosi Na Hiegienno-Epidemiologicinata Sluzba 20:53–56, 1976

84. Zhou SY, Liang YX, Chen ZQ, Wang YL: Effects of occupational exposure to low-level carbon disulfide (CS_2) on menstruation and pregnancy. Ind Health 26:203–214, 1988
85. Blatter BM, Zielhuis GA: Menstrual disorders due to chemical exposure among hairdressers. Occup Medicine 43:105–106, 1993
86. Uehata T, Sasakawan N: The fatigue and maternity disturbances of night workwomen. J Hum Ergol 11:465–474, 1982
87. Toriola AL, Mathur DN: Menstrual dysfunction in Nigerian athletes. Br J Obstet Gynaecol 93:979–985, 1986
88. Frisch RE, Wyshak G, Vincent L: Delayed menarche and amenorrhea in ballet dancers. N Engl J Med 303:17–19, 1980
89. Lemasters G, Hagen A, Samuels SJ: Reproductive outcomes in women exposed to solvents in 36 reinforced plastics companies. I. Menstrual dysfunction. J Occup Med 27:490–494, 1985
90. Harlow SD, Matoski GM: The association between weight, physical activity and stress and variation in the length of the menstrual cycle. Am J Epidemiol 133:38–49, 1991
91. Messing K, Saurel-Cubizolles M-J, Bourgine M, et al: Menstrual cycle characteristics and working conditions in poultry slaughterhouses and canneries. Scand J Work Environ Health 18:302–309, 1992
92. Dawood Y: Dysmenorrhea. Clin Obstet Gynecol 33:168–178, 1990
93. Ylirkorkala O, Dawood Y: New concepts in dysmenorrhea. Am J Obstet Gynecol 130:833–842, 1978
94. Gurevitch M: Rethinking the label: who benefits from the PMS construct? Women Health 23(2):67–98, 1995
95. Lemasters G, Hagen A, Samuels SJ: Reproductive outcomes in women exposed to solvents in 36 reinforced plastics companies. I. Menstrual dysfunction. J Occup Med 27:490–494, 1985
96. Di Rosis F, Anastatasio SP, Selvaggi L, et al: Female reproductive health in mercury lamp factories: effects of exposure to inorganic mercury vapour and stress factors. Br J Ind Med 42:488–494, 1985
97. Ng TP, Foo SC, Yoong T: Menstrual function in workers exposed to toluene. Br J Ind Med 49:799–803, 1992
98. Uehata T, Saskawa N: The fatigue and maternity disturbances of night workwomen. J Hum Ergol 11(Suppl):465–474, 1982
99. Messing K, Saurel-Cubizolles MJ, Kaminski M, Bourgine M: Factors associated with dysmenorrhea among workers in French poultry slaughterhouses and canneries. J Occup Med 35:493–500, 1993
100. Zita JN: The pre-menstrual syndrome: "Dis-easing" the female cycle. In Tuana N (ed): Feminism and Science. Bloomington, IN: Indiana University Press, 1989, pp 188–210
101. Mortola JF, Girton L, Beck L, Yen SC: Diagnosis of premenstrual syndrome by a simple, prospective and reliable instrument: the calendar of premenstrual experiences. Obstet Gynecol 76:302–306, 1990
102. Tissot F, Messing K: Perimenstrual symptoms and working conditions among hospital workers in Québec. Am J Ind Med 27:511–522, 1995
103. Paul JM: Pregnancy and the Standing Working Posture: An Ergonomic Approach. Amsterdam: University of Amsterdam, 1993
104. Paul JA, van Dijk FJH, Frings-Dresen MHW: Work load and musculoskeletal complaints during pregnancy. Scand J Work Environ Health 20:153–159, 1994
105. Paul JA, Frings-Dresen MHW: Standing working posture compared in pregnant and non-pregnant conditions. Ergonomics 37(9):1563–1575, 1994
106. Malenfant R: Le droit au retrait préventif de la travailleuse enceinte ou qui allaite: à la recherche d'un consensus. Sociologie et Sociétés 25(1):61–75, 1993
107. Saurel-Cubizolles MJ, Kaminski M, Du Mazaubrun C, Bréart G: Les conditions de travail professionnel des femmes et l'hypertension artérielle en cours de grossesse. Rev Epidemiol Sante Publique 39:37–43, 1991
108. Sarrel PM: Women, work and menopause. In Frankenhaeuser M, Lundberg U, Chesney M: Women, Work and Health. New York: Plenum Press, 1991, pp 225–237
109. Stanosz S, Kuligowski D, Pieleszek A: Concentration of dihydroepiandrosterone, dihydroepiandrosterone sulphate and testosterone during premature menopause in women chronically exposed to carbon disulphide. Med Pr 46(4):340, 1995

Health Hazards of Child Labor

1. Pollack SH, Landrigan PJ, Mallino DL: Child labor in 1990: prevalence and health hazards. Annu Rev Public Health 11:359–375, 1990
2. Corbin T: Current Trends in Youth Employment. New York State Department of Labor, Division of Research Statistics, 1988
3. Corbin T: Child Labor Law Survey of Teenagers. Working Paper No. 5. Albany: New York State Department of Labor, Division of Research Statistics, 1988
4. Albright J, Kunstel M, McKay R: Stolen Childhood: A Global Report on the Exploitation of Children. Atlanta: Cox Newspaper Enterprises, 1987
5. Anti-Slavery Society: Child Labour Series. Birmingham, United Kingdom: Third World Publ, 1978–1981
6. Waldron HA: Danger: children at work. Br J Ind Med 45:73–74, 1988
7. World Health Organization Study Group: Children at Work: Special Health Risks. Technical Report Series 756. Geneva: World Health Organization, 1987
8. Newman JF, Beyer D, Young AM, Rosenbaum J, Hirsch F, Fajans A, Lopez YC: Child Labor Laws and Youth Employment: A compendium, an analysis, and a design for change. National Child Labor Committee, New York, 1986
9. Belville R, Pollack SH, Godbold JH, Landrigan PJ: Occupational injuries among working adolescents in New York State. JAMA 269:2754–2759, 1993
10. US General Accounting Office: Sweatshops and Child Labor Violations: A Growing Problem in the United States. Washington, DC: Government Printing Office, 1989
11. Landrigan PJ, Carlson JE: Environmental policy and children's health. The Future of Children 5:34–52, 1995
12. Waller AE, Baker SP, Szocka A: Childhood injury deaths: national analysis and geographical variations. Am J Public Health 79:310–315, 1989
13. Centers for Disease Control: Years of Potential Life Lost Before Age 65—United States, 1987. MMWR 38:27–29, 1989
14. Schober SE, Handke JL, Halperin WE, Mill MB, Thun MJ: Work-related injuries in minors. Am J Ind Med 14:585–595, 1988
15. Baker SP: Childhood injuries: the community approach to prevention. J Public Health Policy 2:235–246, 1981
16. Gratz RR: Accidental injury in childhood: a literature review on pediatric trauma. J Trauma 19:551–555, 1979
17. Children's Safety Network. A data book of child and adolescent injury. Washington, DC: National Center for Education in Maternal and Child Health, 1991
18. Banco L, Lapidus G, Braddock M: Work-related injury among Connecticut minors. Pediatrics 89:957–960, 1992
19. Anderka M, Gallagher SS, Azzara CA: Adolescent Work-related Injuries. Presented at Annual Meeting of American Public Health Association, Washington, DC, 1985
20. Landrigan PJ, Belville R: The dangers of illegal child labor [Editorial]. Am J Dis Child 147:1029–1030, 1993
21. Cogbill TH, Busch HM, Stiers GR: Farm accidents in children. Pediatrics 76:562–566, 1988
22. Broste SK, Hansen DA, Strand RL, Steuland DT: Hearing loss among high school farm students. Am J Public Hlth 69:619–622, 1989
23. Karlson T, Noren J: Farm tractor fatalities: the failure of voluntary safety standards. Am J Public Health 69:146–149, 1979

24. Rivara FP: Fatal and nonfatal farm injuries to children and adolescents in the United States. Pediatrics 76:567–573, 1985
25. Cohen S: Social and Personality Development in Childhood. New York: Macmillan, 1976, pp 163–186
26. National Safe Workplace Institute: Sacrificing America's Youth—The Problem of Child Labor and the Response of Government. Chicago: National Safe Workplace Institute, 1992

Workers in the Global Economy

1. Mander J, Goldsmith E (eds): The Case against the Global Economy. San Francisco: Sierra Club Books, 1996
2. Greider W: One World, Ready or Not: The Manic Logic of Global Capitalism. New York: Simon & Schuster, 1997
3. Barnett RJ, Cavanagh J: Global Dreams: Imperial Corporations and the New World Order. New York: Simon & Schuster, 1994
4. Anderson S, Cavanagh J: Corporate empires. Multinational Monitor 17(12):26–27, 1996
5. Hovell M, Sipan C, Hofstetter R, et al: Occupational health risks for Mexican women: the case of the maquiladora along the Mexican-United States border. Int J Health Serv 18:617–627, 1988
6. Guendelman S, Jasis M: The health consequences of maquiladora work: women on the U.S.-Mexico border. Am J Public Health 83: 37–44, 1993
7. US General Accounting Office: U.S.-Mexico Trade: The Work Environment at Eight U.S.-Owned Maquiladora Auto Parts Plants. GAO/GGD-94-22. Washington, DC: General Accounting Office, 1993
8. Moure-Eraso R, Wilcox M, Punnett L, Copeland L, Levenstein C: Back to the future: sweatshop conditions on the Mexico-U.S. border. I. Community health impact of maquiladora industrial activity. Am J Ind Med 25:311–324, 1994
9. Frumkin H, Hernandez Avila M, Espinosa Torres F: The maquiladoras: a case study of free trade zones. Int J Occup Med Environ Health 1(2):21–34, 1995
10. Sánchez RA: Condiciones de vida de los trabajadores de la maquiladora en Tijuana y Nogales. Frontera Norte 2:153–181, 1990
11. Warner DC: Health issues at the U.S.-Mexican border. JAMA 265: 242–247, 1991
12. Frumkin H: Free trade agreements. In: ILO Encyclopaedia of Occupational Health and Safety. 4th ed. Geneva: International Labour Office, 1997, in press
13. Khor M: Why the WTO should not deal with labour standards. Unpublished mimeo, 1994. Third World Network Features. Third World Network, 87 Cantonment Road, Penang 10250, Malaysia. e-mail: twn@igc.org, telephone (604)373511, fax (604)364505
14. Raghavan C: Barking up the wrong tree: trade and social clause links. http://www.southside.org.sg/souths/twn/title/tree-ch.htm. 1996
15. Hunter WJ: EEC legislation in safety and health at work. Ann Occup Hyg 36:337–347, 1992
16. Hecker S: Occupational health and safety policy in the European Community: a case study of economic integration and social policy. Part I—Early initiatives through the Single European Act. New Directions, Summer 59–69, 1993
17. Hecker S: Occupational health and safety policy in the European Community: a case study of economic integration and social policy. Part 2—The framework directive: whither harmonization? New Directions, Fall 57–67, 1993
18. Raworth P: Regional harmonization of occupational health rules: the European example. Am J Law Med 21:7–44, 1995
19. Jackson CL: Social policy harmonization and worker rights in the European Union: a model for North America? NC J Int Law Commercial Regul 21:1–63, 1995
20. Bradsher K: Side agreements to trade accord vary in ambition. New York Times, September 19, 1993, p 1
21. Ives JH: The Export of Hazard: Transnational Corporations and Environmental Control Issues. Boston: Routledge & Kegan Paul, 1985
22. International Labor Rights Education and Research Fund: Trade's Hidden Costs: Worker Rights in a Changing World Economy. Washington, DC: ILRERF, 1988
23. Gaventa JP: From the Mountains to the Maquiladoras: A Case Study of Capital Flight and Its Impact on Workers. New Market, TN: Highlander Center, n.d.
24. Jeyaratnam J: The transfer of hazardous industries. J Soc Occup Med 40:123–126, 1990
25. Hecker S, Hallock M: Labor in a Global Economy. Eugene: University of Oregon Books, 1991
26. Castleman BI: The "double standard" in industrial hazards. Public Health Rev 9:169–184, 1980
27. van Liemt G: Industry on the Move: Causes and Consequences of International Relocation in the Manufacturing Industry. Geneva: International Labour Office, 1992
28. Castleman BI, Vera Vera MJ: Impending proliferation of asbestos. Int J Health Serv 10:389–403, 1980
29. Castleman BI: More on the international asbestos business. Int J Health Serv 11:339–340, 1981
30. Levy BS, Seplow A: Asbestos-related hazards in developing countries. Environ Res 59:167–174, 1992
31. Weir D, Schapiro M: Circle of Poison: Pesticides and People in a Hungry World. San Francisco: Institute for Food and Development Policy, 1981
32. Bull D: A Growing Problem: Pesticides and the Third World Poor. Oxford: Oxfam, 1982
33. Uram C: International regulation of the sale and use of pesticides. Northwestern J Int Law Business 10:460, 1990
34. Third World Network: Toxic Terror: Dumping of Hazardous Wastes in the Third World. Penang: Third World Network, 1988
35. Hilz C: The International Toxic Waste Trade. New York: Van Nostrand Reinhold, 1992
36. Aydelotte C: Bhopal tragedy focuses on changes in chemical industry. Occup Health Saf 54:33–35, 50, 59, 1985
37. Weiss B, Clarkson TW: Toxic chemical disasters and the implications of Bhopal for technology transfer. Milbank Q 64:216–240, 1986
38. Bhopal Working Group: The public health implications of the Bhopal disaster. Report to the Program Development Board, American Public Health Association. Bhopal Working Group. Am J Public Health 77:230–236, 1987
39. Murti CR: Industrialization and emerging environmental health issues: lessons from the Bhopal disaster. Toxicol Ind Health 7:153–164, 1991
40. Christiani DC: Occupational health in the People's Republic of China. Am J Public Health 74:58–64, 1984
41. Elgstrand K: Occupational safety and health in developing countries. Am J Ind Med 8:91–93, 1985
42. Cullen MR, Baloyi RS: Prevalence of pneumonoconiosis among coal and heavy metal miners in Zimbabwe. Am J Ind Med 17:677–682, 1990
43. Frumkin H, Levy BS, Levenstein C: Occupational and environmental health in eastern Europe: challenges and opportunities. Am J Ind Med 20:265–270, 1991
44. Frumkin H, de Camará V: Occupational health in Brazil. Am J Public Health 81:1619–1624, 1991
45. La Botz D: Manufacturing poverty: the maquiladorization of Mexico. Int J Health Serv 24:403–408, 1994
46. Glass, Molders, Pottery, Plastic and Allied Workers International Union, AFL-CIO: Warning: Working in Mexico May Be Dangerous to Your Health. Occupational Health and Safety and the North American Free Trade Agreement. GMPPAWIU, 608 East Baltimore Pike, Media, PA 19063. n.d. (probably 1992)

47. Kochan L: The Maquiladoras and Toxics: The Hidden Costs of Production South of the Border. Publication No. 186-P0690-5. Washington, DC: American Federation of Labor and Congress of Industrial Organizations, no date (probably 1990)
48. Witt M: An injury to one is un agravio a todos: The need for a Mexico-U.S. health and safety movement. New Solutions, Winter 28–31, 1991
49. McGaughey W: A US-Mexico-Canada Free Trade Agreement: Do We Just Say No? Minneapolis: Thistlerose Publications, 1992
50. Moody K, McGinn M: Unions and Free Trade: Solidarity vs. Competition. Detroit: Labor Notes, 1992
51. Cavanagh J, Gershman J, Baker K, Helmke G (eds): Trading Freedom: How Free Trade Affects Our Lives, Work and Environment. San Francisco: Institute for Food and Development Policy, 1992
52. Koh D, Jeyaratnam J: Occupational health services for small scale industries. In: Jeyaratnam J, Chia KS (eds): Occupational Health in National Development. Singapore: World Scientific, 1994, pp 59–73
53. Kogi K: Improving Conditions in Small Enterprises in Developing Asia. Geneva: International Labour Office, 1985
54. van Ee JH, Polderman AM: Physiological performance and work capacity of tin mine labourers infested with schistosomiasis in Zaire. Trop Geogr Med 36:259–266, 1984
55. Taqi A: International safety and health standards: Yesterday, today and tomorrow. Speech to the National Safety Council, October 29, 1996
56. Jeyaratnam J: Acute pesticide poisoning. In: Jeyaratnam J, Chia KS (eds): Occupational Health in National Development. Singapore: World Scientific, 1994, pp 14–26
57. Wesseling C, Castillo L, Elinder CG: Pesticide poisonings in Costa Rica. Scand J Work Environ Health 19:227–235, 1993
58. McConnell R, Hruska AJ: An epidemic of pesticide poisoning in Nicaragua: implications for prevention in developing countries. Am J Public Health 83:1559–1562, 1993
59. Matte TD, Figueroa JP, Burr G, et al: Lead exposure among lead-acid battery workers in Jamaica. Am J Ind Med 16:167–177, 1989
60. Vineis P, Cantor K, Gonzales C, et al: Occupational cancer in developed and developing countries [Review]. Int J Cancer 62:655–660, 1995
61. Pearce N, Matos E: Occupational cancer in developing countries. Introduction. IARC Sci Pub 129:1–3, 1994
62. Pearce N, Matos E: Strategies for the prevention of occupational cancer in developing countries. IARC Sci Pub 129:173–183, 1994
63. Schenker M: Occupational lung diseases in the industrializing and industrialized world due to modern industries and modern pollutants. Tuber Lung Dis 73:27–32, 1992
64. Chavalitsakulchai P, Shahnavaz H: Musculoskeletal disorders of female workers and ergonomics problems in five different industries of a developing country. J Hum Ergol (Tokyo) 22:29–43, 1993
65. Ferraz MB, Frumkin H, Helfenstein M, Gianeschini C, Atra E: Upper extremity musculoskeletal disorders in keyboard operators in Brazil: a cross-sectional study. Int J Occup Med Environ Health 1:239–244, 1995
66. Munjal YP: HIV infection and health care worker. J Indian Med Assoc 92:31–32, 1994
67. Adegboye AA, Moss GB, Soyinka F, Kreiss JK: The epidemiology of needlestick and sharp instrument accidents in a Nigerian hospital. Infect Control Hosp Epidemiol 15:27–31, 1994
68. Shankar J, Famuyiwa OO: Stress among factory workers in a developing country. J Psychosom Res 35:163–171, 1991
69. Dusharme D, Karolyi A: News Digest articles in *Quality Digest*: An ISO standard for occupational health and safety? (August 1996); OSHA and labor: "No" to ISO health and safety standard (September 1996); Support for international health and safety? (October 1996); Conference attendees say "no" to OH&S standard (November 1996)
70. Ember L: Environment protection: Global companies set new endeavor. Chem Engin News 69:4, 1991
71. Jeyaratnam J, Ling SL: Occupational health services and primary health care. In: Jeyaratnam J, Chia KS (eds): Occupational Health in National Development. Singapore: World Scientific, 1994, pp 334–349
72. Kogi K, Phoon WO, Thurman JE: Low-Cost Wasys of Improving Working Conditions: 100 Examples from Asia. Geneva: International Labour Office, 1988
73. Schilling RSF, Andersson N: Occupational epidemiology in developing countries. J Occup Health Saf Austral N Z 2:468–478, 1986
74. Christiani DC, Durvasula R, Myers J: Occupational health in developing countries: review of research needs. Am J Ind Med 17:393–401, 1990
75. Levy BS, Kjellstrom T, Forget G, et al: Ongoing research in occupational health and environmental epidemiology in developing countries. Arch Environ Health 47:231–235, 1992

General References

Castleman BI, Navarro V: International mobility of hazardous products, industries, and wastes. Annu Rev Public Health 8:1–19, 1987

Grinspun R, Cameron MA (eds): The Political Economy of North American Free Trade. New York: St. Martin's Press, 1993

Grunwald J, Flamm K: The Global Factory: Foreign Assembly in International Trade.Washington, DC: Brookings Institution, 1985

Jeyaratnam J (ed): Occupational Health in Developing Countries. Oxford: Oxford University Press, 1992

Jeyaratnam J: Occupational health issues in developing countries. Environ Res 60:207–212, 1993

Jeyaratnam J, Chia KS (eds): Occupational Health in National Development. Singapore: World Scientific, 1994

LeQuesne C: Reforming World Trade: The Social and Environmental Priorities. Oxford: Oxfam Publications, 1996

Ong C-N, Jeyaratnam J, Koh D: Factors influencing the assessment and control of occupational hazards in developing countries. Environ Res 60:112–123, 1993

Organisation for Economic Co-operation and Development: Trade, Employment and Labour Standards. Paris: OECD, 1996

Phoon WO, Ong CN (eds): Occupational Health in Developing Countries in Asia. Tokyo: South-East Asia Medical Information Center (SEAMIC), 1985

Reich MR, Okubo T: Protecting Workers' Health in the Third World: National and International Strategies. New York: Auburn House, 1992

35

Occupational Safety and Health Standards

Eula Bingham

Until 1970 there was almost total reliance on state and local governments and the forces of the market to improve working conditions related to occupational injuries, death, and disease. For more than 50 years state governments had attempted to inspect workplaces and to advise employers about hazards. Few of these programs, however, had adequate enforcement authority to compel abatement of dangerous conditions. In some states, no attempt was made by government to change workplace conditions, either by enforcement or by persuasion. Variations in state legislation resulted in comprehensive, strong regulation in some states (New York and Illinois) and nonexistent regulation in others (e.g., Mississippi). The doctrine of states' rights and a tradition of state regulatory activity in the area of labor standards protected this status quo.

Another traditional approach was to trust market and private sector mechanisms to provide worker protection. Workers' compensation insurance carriers made some attempt to improve workplace safety for economic reasons. Many carriers provided consultative service to their clients and charged lower rates to large companies that were successful in reducing injuries. Then, as well as now, insurance companies' consultative resources are limited and are not available to all who may need them; while it may be possible to provide economic incentives to large firms by basing their premium rates on accident experience, it is not possible to provide this same incentive to small firms, which have few employees to record a statistically significant accident experience. More importantly these economic incentives are inadequate where health problems are concerned because occupational diseases are not often diagnosed as workplace related. Occupational diseases often have complex origins; many years may elapse between exposure and the appearance of symptoms, making physicians and compensation boards reluctant to attribute the symptoms to time spent with specific employers or to the exposure to particular working conditions.

A third approach evolved to cope with occupational safety and health problems; industry-based organizations filled the vacuum by producing guidelines for safe work practices for various types of industrial equipment and processes and for "acceptable" exposure limits to certain harmful substances. These "consensus standards" were adopted by the Occupational Safety and Health Administration (OSHA) in 1972 as federal standards.

Thus a long series of private, voluntary efforts and a slowly evolving pattern of government initiatives (e.g., the Walsh-Healey Act (1936), which authorized sanctions against federal contractors who violated standards) tested a variety of approaches to improving safety and health. These experiences served as the basis for broad federal legislation. As legislators had a record of approaches that had not worked, it became clear that voluntary-compliance approaches and consensus guidelines would have to be backed by a technically experienced federal enforcement staff and that inadequate state safety and health efforts would have to be reshaped to meet national standards of effectiveness. The economic realities of the marketplace had overwhelmed voluntary efforts, and the weak incentives of workers' compensation programs and of the states appeared unable to act effectively because of a need to compete among themselves for industry and jobs.

The Occupational Safety and Health Act was signed into law in 1970. It featured a strong standards-setting authority vested in the Secretary of Labor. The standards-setting process was open to labor, industry, and public inputs at all stages.

The word "standard" connotes uniformity, consensus, and regulatory power. OSHA standards are an attempt, through the federal government's regulatory powers, to set a minimum level of protection for workers against specified hazards and to achieve that level through enforcement, education, and persuasion.

Sections 6 and 3(8) of the Occupational Safety and Health Act govern the standards-setting process. They contain three major schemes under which standards can be promulgated: (*a*) a short-lived authority for adoption of existing consensus standards, (*b*) development and promulgation of new or amended standards, and (*c*) promulgation of temporary emergency standards.

▸ CONSENSUS STANDARDS

At the time the Occupational Safety and Health Act was passed, a large body of consensus standards was already in existence, developed as guidelines by such groups as the American National Standards Institute (ANSI), the National Fire Prevention Association (NFPA), and the American Conference of Governmental Industrial Hygienists (ACGIH). The standards represented industry's agreement on certain reasonable exposures, work practices, and equipment specifications. To establish as rapidly as possible a body of occupational safety and health rules already familiar to employers, Congress required adoption of these standards, but recognized that many were seriously out of date. The legislative history of the act emphasized that the standards would need to be constantly improved and replaced and that new standards were especially needed in the occupational health area.

Many of the consensus standards contained provisions that were irrelevant to safety and health (e.g., several pages of specifications for the wood to be used in ladders). The standards were adopted wholesale, however, without significant deletions, in the interest of speed. Competing priorities made it impossible to evaluate and amend the body of standards within the 2-year deadline allowed by Congress.

Thus, OSHA began with initial standards derived from previous industry use, which had these key weaknesses. They were unduly complex and obsolete. One standard, for example, prohibited the use of ice in drinking water, a rule that dated from a time when ice was cut from contaminated rivers. Certain standards were only tangentially related to the safety or health of workers, e.g., the requirement for coat hooks in toilet stalls.

The consensus standards were guidelines and not designed for enforcement and the adjudicatory process. Provisions that should have been advisory became inflexible law. Threshold limit values reflected industry consensus as to acceptable practice and were not necessarily designed for the greatest protection to workers and often lacked documentation.

By 1978 OSHA removed the most inappropriate of these rules from the books. At that time, 1110 standards provisions were proposed for deletion; after participation by labor and the business community, 927 were finally eliminated. Further improvements have included an updated fire protection standard (1978).

▶ PERMANENT STANDARDS

Section 6(b) of the act outlines the 9-step process for setting permanent safety or health standards:

1. *Decision to initiate standards development project:* The Secretary of Labor may begin the process on the basis of recommendations from the National Institute of Occupational Safety and Health or other governmental agencies, petitions of private parties, research findings from any source, accident and injury data, congressional input, or court decisions.
2. *Drafting the proposal:* Including economic and environmental impact statements to fulfill the requirements of the National Environmental Policy Act of 1969. Economic studies determine whether regulatory analysis will be required.
3. *Advisory committee:* An advisory committee may at the discretion of the Department of Labor be formed to provide help. The statute requires its composition and includes representatives of labor and industry, the safety and health professions, and recognized experts from government or the academic world.
4. *Revision and review:* By technical experts and attorneys. Where appropriate, review by other agencies also occurs.
5. Federal Register *publication of proposal:* The public is invited to comment.
6. *Informal hearings:* May be held to allow further public comment.
7. *Staff analysis of records:* Major issues requiring policy decisions are defined and presented to the assistant secretary. Alternate approaches, if appropriate, are presented.
8. *Final standard:* The staff develops a proposed final standard based on the record of rule making and submits the proposal for internal reviews.
9. *Final publication:* The completed final standard is published in its entirety in the *Federal Register*. A petition for review of the standard may be filed in a federal circuit court of appeals.

This process is only an outline. The length of time between steps may stretch for months or years. At times, proposals are abandoned after first hearings or public comment, and the decision to proceed with a rule making is reevaluated. If appropriate, an entirely new proposal is developed.

▶ TEMPORARY EMERGENCY STANDARDS

The Occupational Safety and Health Act requires that the Secretary of Labor "shall provide . . . for an emergency temporary standard to take immediate effect upon publication in the *Federal Register* if employees are exposed to grave danger from exposure to substances or agents determined to be toxic or physically harmful or from new hazards." These standards are promulgated without the extensive public participation characteristic of permanent standards. The act requires that they be replaced with a permanent standard within 6 months. Emergency temporary standards may be used as a "proposed standard" in the permanent standards proceedings. This provision of the act has been chilled because of unfavorable court decision and is currently rarely used.

▶ CONTENTS OF OSHA STANDARDS

OSHA standards are written to control risks even if exposure continues throughout a person's working life. The effectiveness of the technology available for controlling exposures and the characteristics of the hazard in the particular workplace determine how compliance with the standard will be achieved.

The standards are variable in several areas. The *technical content* necessarily differs according to the hazard being regulated, although it is possible to group related problems in a single standard. A *specification approach* or a *performance approach* may be employed, or the two approaches may be combined.

Specification standards tell precisely what protection an employer must provide. This approach has been used most often in developing safety standards. The advantage of specification standards is that they tell the employer exactly what must be provided to "be in compliance." The disadvantage of the specification standards is that they tend to be inflexible and may restrict an employer's efforts to provide equivalent protection using alternative—and sometimes more satisfactory—methods. In certain instances, employers may be granted a variance by OSHA.

The trend in OSHA regulation is toward performance standards that set exposures but leave the means of compliance largely to the decision of the employer. This greater degree of flexibility allows the employer to consider alternative methods and equipment and choose those most suited to the particular technology. Performance standards, however, do not give the employer carte blanche to substitute less effective means of protection (such as personal protective equipment) for engineering controls of dangerous emissions or other hazards.

Health standards are generally addressed by way of the performance, rather than the specification, approach. While many large corporations prefer performance standards in both the safety and health areas, it is advantageous, at least for small employers, to have an acceptable "specific" method of compliance included in the appendix of a performance standard.

▶ THRESHOLD LIMIT VALUES, PERMISSIBLE EXPOSURE LIMITS, AND ACTION LEVELS

Older occupational health standards (still used in developing countries) were based on *threshold limit values* (TLVs) developed by the ACGIH. In this system, maximum exposures were usually set based on the level of a contaminant known to produce acute effects, allowing some margin for safety and considering what was readily achievable by employers. Unfortunately, such limits do not protect against long-term chronic or subclinical effects on the body, such as changes in blood chemistry, liver function, or the reaction time of the central nervous system. In addition, these values were derived mainly for healthy, young adult, white males, not for the diverse makeup of working populations. In addition these TLVs were not designed to address the problem of irreversible health problems such as cancer.

Permissible exposure limits (PELs) are used in OSHA health standards. The lead standard, for example, contains a PEL of 50 μg of lead per cubic meter of air, averaged over an 8-hour period. PELs are based on consideration of the health effects of hazardous substances.

▶ MEDICAL REMOVAL PROTECTION

Medical removal protection (MRP) is a protective, preventive health mechanism complementing the medical surveillance portion of some OSHA standards. The lead standard, for example, calls for temporary removal for medical purposes of any worker having an elevated blood lead level. During the period of removal, the employer must maintain the worker's earnings, seniority, and other employment rights and benefits as though the worker had not been removed.

Medical removal protection is essential; without it, the major cost of health hazards falls directly on the worker and the worker's family in the event of illness, death, or lost wages. Without a requirement for the protection of workers' wages and job rights, removal could easily take the form of transfer to a lower-paying job, temporary layoff, or termination. A worker who participates in the medical surveillance program might risk losing his or her livelihood. The alternative has sometimes been to resist participation and thereby lose the protection that surveillance offers.

An interesting leveraging effect of MRP is its role as an economic incentive for employers to comply with the OSHA standards. For example, employers who do not comply with the lead standard will have a greater number of removals and thus will have higher labor costs over a long period, while employers who invest in the control technology will experience savings from lowered removal costs.

▶ COMPLIANCE

To comply with the PELs, employers first conduct an industrial hygiene survey, including environmental sampling. This process identifies contaminants, their sources, and the severity of exposure. The employer then devises methods to reduce exposure to permissible levels. Methods commonly employed by industrial hygienists to control exposures fall into three basic categories: engineering controls, work practice controls (including administrative controls), and personal protective equipment.

Engineering controls employ mechanical means or process redesign to reduce exposure. The contaminant may be eliminated, contained, diverted, diluted, or collected at the source. Examples of this type of control include process isolation or enclosure, such as is used in uranium fuel processing. Employee isolation or machine and process enclosure are also used to protect workers from excessive fumes or noise. Closed material-handling systems, product substitution, and exhaust ventilation are also commonly employed.

Work practice controls rely on employees to perform certain activities in a carefully specified manner so that exposures are reduced or eliminated. For example, employers may instruct workers to keep lids on containers, to clean up spills immediately, or to observe specific, required hygiene practices. Such work practices are often required to complement engineering controls. This is particularly true in cases where engineering controls cannot provide complete compliance with the standard. Noise hazards are often controlled by a combination of engineering steps and work practices limiting the amount of time workers are exposed to excessive noise levels.

Personal protective equipment controls exposure by isolating the employee from the emission source. Respirators are a common type of personal protective equipment, used when protection from an inhaled contaminant is required. Personal protective equipment is used to supplement engineering controls and work practices. Often overlooked is the great importance of personal hygiene, which includes the use of protective clothing to provide barriers to both the worker and the worker's family, the provision for shower facilities, and the cleaning of protective clothing so that contaminants are not transferred to others.

Engineering control is the best method for effective and reliable control of worker exposure to many substances. It acts at the source of the emission and eliminates or reduces employee exposure without reliance on self-protective action by the employee. Work practices also act on the source of the emission, but rely on employee behavior, which requires supervision, motivation, and education for effectiveness. While personal protective equipment provides a cheaper alternative to engineering controls, it does so at the expense of safety and reliability. The equipment does not eliminate the source of the exposure, often fails to provide the degree of protection required (or fails to provide it with certainty in all cases), and may create additional hazards by interfering with vision, hearing, and mobility. Feasibility is a mandated requirement by the statute.

Individual differences in employees also affect the acceptability of personal protective equipment. For example, some employees develop infections from some ear-protection devices and respirator face pieces, and some who have impaired breathing cannot safely or comfortably use respirators. Additionally, personal protective equipment is made in standard sizes and facial configurations that may not properly fit female workers and unusually large or small workers.

OSHA should progress from a reactive, priority-setting system to one with an information-based approach. Highest priority must be given to hazards that cause irreversible adverse health effects. Court decisions have required the agency to establish a "reasonably necessary" approach, i.e., determine the number of workers affected and the number protected by the new regulation. This has been translated into a risk assessment requirement. For example, OSHA's cancer policy could be modified to increase the speed with which the particular carcinogens are regulated, with priorities shaped according to the population of the workers exposed, current exposure levels, and the potency of a substance. Consideration should be given to the ways in which these substances are used in actual operations and to the likelihood of substantial accidental exposures.

These same criteria can be applied to other health hazards. In the safety standards area, a parallel process must occur, which should include guidance in the establishment of standards for reducing deaths due to inappropriately designed lock-out procedures, for reducing musculoskeletal injuries, and for controlling the development of stress-related diseases associated with newer technologies. Development of so-called generic standards, e.g., hazard identification, reaches many workers in providing protection. These types of standards are difficult to promulgate because of the divergent industrial sectors and numerous employers coming under the regulation.

Critics of occupational safety and health standards encourage the use of theoretical economic models based on cost-benefit analysis. Common sense indicates that the numbers of workers exposed, the severity of hazards, and the technological feasibility must be considered in setting standards. These factors should be explicit in OSHA's priority-setting processes. Precise costs and benefits, however, cannot be measured.

The costs of standards compliance can be estimated with some precision. New equipment, engineering modifications, and work practices have readily measurable costs. Industry, however, sometimes overestimates these costs by several magnitudes in their testimony against standards: actual costs for vinyl chloride standards compliance turned out to be but a fraction of those indicated in public testimony. More recently, even with the thoroughly worked and reworked estimates of the costs to comply with the cotton dust standard, it appears that costs were overestimated by the government and industry both. OSHA has never had the authority to require facilities to open their financial books in preparing economic feasibility impact studies so must be content with voluntarily divulged economic data.

The benefits of regulation, however, are more difficult to calculate. One cannot count all accidents that were avoided as one can number the accidents and injuries that actually occurred. One cannot precisely identify the health benefits that will accrue in 10, 20, or 30 years from current reduced exposures to toxic substances or carcinogens.

The data for prediction do not exist, and causality mechanisms in occupational disease are too complex to be defined with the same certainty as the costs of a new ventilating system.

The largest problem with cost-benefit analysis, however, is not lack of information—it is the impossibility of weighing lives spared against the dollar costs for prevention. Workers are coming to realize that hazardous-pay differentials are in fact based on a dangerously false assumption that lives can be valued and, in effect, "prorated" on a cash basis. Public debate over regulatory costs can begin to clarify this issue and to uncover the hidden social costs of failure to regulate out of deference to faulty labor market mechanisms. These hidden social costs include not only loss of life and health of workers, but also increased incidence of illness and death among families of workers exposed to some substances such as lead and asbestos, and disruption of family and community life due to death and disability of workers and to local environmental effects of industrial contaminants.

▶ GLOBAL STANDARDS

Particularly important for NIOSH and OSHA is participation in international occupational health and safety forums to achieve full awareness of available research and enforcement experience, including those of the Commission of the European Communities, the International Labor Organization, the World Health Organization, and many foreign national governments. It is critical that the United States shares information internationally and encourages other nations to adopt effective health and safety standards. Without comparable standards in other countries, U.S. industries can choose to export hazardous processes such as asbestos milling or pesticide formulation. This is doubly unacceptable because it not only exposes foreign workers to hazardous conditions but would tend to export jobs along with the hazards. Indeed the failure to participate in the global efforts for health and safety standards could lead U.S. workers backward if U.S. occupational safety and health standards are considered to be a barrier to free trade under trade agreements, e.g., the North American Free Trade Agreement (NAFTA).

▶ CONCLUSION

Standards alone will not guarantee healthful, safe working conditions. Enforcement inspections to determine whether compliance exists is essential. Training and education of workers and employers is also necessary. Government cannot provide direct, constant enforcement of employee protection; this effort must be assisted by employer and employee participation.

Workers' rights to a safe and healthful workplace are facilitated in part by the existence of employer standards, by federal and state enforcement activities, but most of all by the workers' own knowledge and vigilance. The Occupational Safety and Health Act recognizes this fact. It reinforces the workers' rights, with guarantees against reprisals by employers, when workers file and obtain abatement of health and safety hazards. Whether improvements come from voluntary employer action, from direct enforcement, or from labor-management negotiations, health and safety standards are essential to define the necessary levels of protection and the acceptable means of attaining them.

36

Ensuring Food Safety

Douglas L. Marshall • James S. Dickson

The objective of food processing and preparation is to provide safe, wholesome, and nutritious food to the consumer. The responsibilities for accomplishing this objective lie with every step in the food chain, beginning with food production and continuing through processing, storage, distribution, retail sale, and consumption. Producing safe food is a continuum, where each party has certain obligations to meet and certain reasonable expectations of the other parties involved in the process. No single group is solely responsible for producing safe food, and no single group is without obligations in ensuring the safety of food.

Food producers have a reasonable expectation that the food he or she produces will be processed in such a manner that further contamination is minimized. Food producers are an integral part of the food production system, but are not solely responsible for food safety. It is not practical to deliver fresh unprocessed food that is completely free of microorganisms, whether the food in question is apples or livestock. The environment in which the food is produced precludes the possibility that uncontaminated food can be grown or produced. However, appropriate methods can be used to reduce, to the extent possible, this level of background contamination. Alternately, producers have an obligation to use these same reasonable practices to prevent hazards from entering the food chain. As an example, when dairy cattle are treated with antibiotics for mastitis, producers have an obligation to withhold milk from those animals from the normal production lot. Milk from these animals must be withheld for the specified withdrawal time, so that antibiotic residues will not occur in milk delivered to dairies. In contrast, production of salmonellae-free poultry in the United States has been an elusive goal for poultry producers. While it is not a reasonable expectation for producers to deliver salmonellae-free birds to poultry processors, it is reasonable to expect producers to use good management practices to minimize the incidence of *Salmonella* within a flock.

Food processors have reasonable expectations that raw materials delivered to the processing facility are of reasonable quality and not contaminated with violative levels of any drugs or pesticides. In addition, processors have a reasonable expectation that processed food will be properly handled through the distribution and retail chain, and that it will be properly prepared by the consumer. The latter is particularly important, as processors have responsibility for products because they are labeled with the processor's name, even though the food is no longer under processor control once it leaves the processing facility. Processor obligations are to process raw foods in a manner that minimizes growth of existing microorganisms as well as minimizes additional contamination during processing. These obligations extend from general facility maintenance to the use of the best available methods and technologies to process a given food.

Clearly, consumers have an important role in the microbiological safety of foods. However, it is not reasonable to expect every consumer to have a college degree in microbiology. Consumers have a reasonable expectation that foods they purchase have been produced and processed under hygienic conditions. They also have a reasonable expectation that foods have not been held under insanitary conditions, or that foods have not been adulterated by the addition of any biological, chemical, or physical hazards. In addition, consumers have an expectation that foods will be appropriately labeled, so that the consumer has information available on both composition and nutritional aspects of products. These expectations are enforced by regulations that govern production, processing, distribution, and retailing of foods in the United States. The vast majority of foods meets or exceeds these expectations, and the average consumer has relatively little to be concerned with regarding the food they consume.

Some consumers have advocated additional expectations, which may or may not be reasonable. For example, some would argue that raw foods should be free of infectious microorganisms. Initially, this would appear to be reasonable; however, in many cases, technologies or processes do not exist in a legal or cost-effective form to ensure that raw foods are not contaminated with infectious agents. Two recent examples are the outbreaks of *Cyclospora* epidemiologically linked to imported raspberries and *Escherichia coli* O157:H7 in raw ground beef. With the exception of irradiation, technologies do not exist to ensure that either of these foods would be absolutely free of infectious agents while still retaining desirable characteristics associated with raw food. Therefore, in some cases, the expectation that raw foods should be free of infectious agents may not be reasonable.

Consumers have several obligations regarding food safety. As part of the food production to consumption chain, consumers have similar obligations to food processors. Namely, not holding foods under insanitary conditions prior to consumption and not adulterating foods with the addition of biological, chemical, or physical agents. Improper food handling can increase food-borne illness risks by allowing infectious bacteria to increase in numbers or by allowing for cross-contamination between raw and cooked foods. In addition, consumers have an obligation to use reasonable care preparing foods for consumption, as do personnel in food service operations. As an example, consumers should cook poultry until it is "done" (internal temperature at or above 155°F) to eliminate any concerns with salmonellae.

Consumer education on the basics of food safety in the home should be a priority. Every consumer should understand that food is not sterile, and that the way food is handled in the kitchen may affect the health of individuals consuming it. Although our long-term goal is to reduce or eliminate food-borne disease hazards, in the near term we need to remind consumers of what some of the potential risks are and how consumers can avoid them. In the end, it is the consumers who decides what they will or will not eat.

▶ COMMON FOODBORNE DISEASE HAZARDS

Contrary to popular consumer perception about the risk of chemicals in foods, major hazards associated with foodborne illness are clearly of biological origin.[1] The Centers for Disease Control and Prevention (CDC) has published recent summaries of foodborne diseases by etiology for the years 1983 through 1992 (Table 36-1).[2–4] CDC groups foodborne disease agents in four categories: bacterial, parasitic, viral, and chemical. Greater than 95 percent of all reported outbreaks of foodborne illnesses are caused by microorganisms or their toxins. Fully 97 percent of reported cases are likewise linked to a microbial source. Only around 3 percent of the outbreaks and less than 1 percent of cases can be truly linked to chemical (heavy metals, monosodium glutamate, and other chemicals) contamination of foods. Furthermore, 97 percent of reported deaths are due to microbial sources.

Bacterial agents are by far the leading cause of illness, with total numbers estimated as high as 6.5 to 33 million cases per year and deaths as high as 9,000 annually in the United States.[5] Costs are estimated to be $3 to 8 billion annually in medical expenses and lost productivity.[5,6] The high incidence of bacterial foodborne disease is paralleled in other developed countries.[7] Predominant bacterial agents are *Salmonella* spp., *Shigella* spp., and *Clostridium perfringens*. Foodborne bacterial hazards are classified based on their ability to cause infections or intoxications. Foodborne infections are usually the predominant type of foodborne illness reported. Foodborne outbreaks most often occur with foods prepared at food service establishments and at home (Table 36-2).[2–4] Improper holding temperatures and poor personal hygiene were the leading factors contributing to reported outbreaks (Table 36-3).

Bacterial hazards are further classified based upon the severity of risk.[8] Severe hazards are those capable of causing widespread epidemics. Moderate hazards can be those that have potential for extensive spread, with possible severe illness, complication, or sequelae in susceptible populations. Mild hazards can also cause outbreaks but have limited ability to spread. Those involved with food production, processing, and service should pay careful attention to controlling these biological hazards by: (*a*) destroying or minimizing the hazard, (*b*) preventing contamination of food with the hazard, or (*c*) inhibiting growth or preventing toxin production by the hazard. Control steps are described in later sections of this chapter.

TABLE 36-1. REPORTED FOODBORNE DISEASES IN THE UNITED STATES, 1983 TO 1992

	Outbreaks		Cases		Deaths	
Etiologic Agent	***No.***	***%***	***No.***	***%***	***No.***	***per 10,000 Cases***
■ ***BACTERIAL***						
Brucella	2	0.1	38	0.04	1	0.11
Campylobacter	55	2.9	1,459	1.6	3	0.33
Clostridium botulinum	134	7.0	273	0.3	21	2.31
Clostridium perfringens	64	3.4	6,544	7.2	3	0.33
Escherichia coli	18	0.9	884	1.0	4	0.44
Salmonella	891	47.0	52,422	57.6	77	8.46
Shigella	69	3.6	14,759	16.2	2	0.22
Staphylococcus aureus	97	5.1	4,859	5.3	0	<0.1
Streptococcus, Group A	9	0.5	113	1.2	0	<0.1
Streptococcus, other	2	0.1	85	0.09	3	0.33
Bacillus cereus	37	1.9	651	0.7	0	<0.1
Camplybacter/Salmonella	1	0.05	3	0.003	0	<0.1
Listeria monocytogenes	1	0.05	2	0.002	1	0.11
Vibrio cholerae	5	0.26	36	0.04	1	0.11
Vibrio parahaemolyticus	7	0.36	32	0.03	0	<0.1
Vibrio vulnificus	1	0.05	2	0.002	1	0.11
Total bacterial	1,393	73.0	83,185	91.3	117	12.86
■ ***PARASITIC***						
Trichinella spiralis	43	2.3	357	0.4	1	0.11
Giardia lamblia	10	0.5	225	0.2	0	<0.1
Total parasitic	53	2.8	582	0.6	1	0.11
■ ***VIRAL***						
Hepatitis A	72	3.8	3,176	3.5	7	0.77
Norwalk/Norwalk-like	12	0.6	1,456	1.6	0	<0.1
Other	2	0.1	558	0.6	0	<0.1
Total viral	86	4.5	5,190	5.7	7	0.77
■ ***CHEMICAL***						
Ciguatoxin	129	6.8	473	0.5	0	<0.1
Heavy metals	16	0.8	202	0.2	0	<0.1
Mushrooms	19	1.0	67	0.07	2	0.22
Scombrotoxin	159	8.4	820	0.9	1	0.11
Monosodium glutamate	2	0.1	7	0.008	0	<0.1
Shellfish	2	0.1	3	0.003	0	<0.1
Paralytic shellfish poisoning	5	0.3	65	0.08	2	0.22
Other chemical	43	2.3	499	0.5	2	0.22
Total chemical	375	19.8	2,136	2.3	7	0.77
Grand total	1,907		91,093		132	114.5

TABLE 36-2. PLACE WHERE OUTBREAK FOODS WERE EATEN, 1983 TO 1992

	Number	Percentage
Home	997	20.7
Deli, café, restaurant	2,030	42.1
School	217	4.5
Picnic	82	1.7
Church	110	2.3
Other	1,153	23.9
Unknown	174	3.6

When investigating foodborne disease outbreaks, the most important factor is time.[9] Prompt reporting of an outbreak is essential to identifying implicated foods and stopping potentially widespread epidemics. Initial work in the investigation should be inspection of the premises where the outbreak occurred. Look for obvious sources, including sanitation and worker hygiene. Food preparation, storage, and serving should be carefully monitored. Interview those involved in the outbreak. Obtain case histories of victims and healthy individuals. Discuss health history and work habits of food handlers. Collect appropriate specimens for laboratory analysis, including stool samples, vomitus, and swabs of rectum, nose, and skin. Attempt to collect suspect foods, including leftovers or garbage if necessary. Specific tests for pathogens or toxins will depend on potential etiological agents and food type. Analysis of data should include case histories, illness specifics (incubation time, symptoms, and duration), laboratory results, and attack rates. All foodborne disease outbreaks should be reported to local and state health officers and to the CDC.

Bacterial Infections

Predominant bacterial infections transmitted via foods are salmonellosis, campylobacteriosis, yersiniosis, vibriosis, and shigellosis.[10,11] Most are Gram-negative rod-shaped organisms that are inhabitants of the intestinal tract of animals. That foods of animal origin are primary causes of foodborne gastroenteritis is thus not surprising (Table 36-4).[2–4] Indeed, federal and most state regulatory agencies consider foods of animal origin (meat, poultry, eggs, fish, shellfish, milk, and dairy products) potentially hazardous foods. One look at epidemiological data confirms this suspicion.

Salmonellosis

Salmonella resides primarily in the intestinal tract of animals (humans, birds, wild animals, farm animals, and insects).[12] Many people are permanent, often asymptomatic carriers. Salmonellosis varies with species and strain, susceptibility of host, and total number of cells ingested. Several dozen species and serotypes cause food-borne outbreaks. Incubation time is 12 to 36 hours, but may be longer or shorter. Symptoms include nausea, vomiting, abdominal pain, and diarrhea, which may be preceded by headache, fever, and chills. Weakness and prostration may occur. Duration is 1 to 4 days with a low mortality rate. The condition needed for an outbreak is the ingestion of live cells present in the food. For high-fat foods such as chocolate, 50 cells may be a sufficient infectious dose due to enrobement of cells by fat, allowing survival in high-acid gastric fluid during intestinal transit. Foods primarily involved in outbreaks include meat, poultry, fish, eggs, and milk products. *Salmonella enteritidis* is present in raw uncooked eggs even with sound shells.[13] Most often the bacterium is transferred from a raw food to a processed food via cross-contamination. Control of *Salmonella* in foods can be accomplished in several ways. Contamination is avoided by using only healthy food handlers and adequately cleaned and sanitized food contact surfaces, utensils, and equipment. Heat treatment of foods by cooking or pasteurization is sufficient to kill *Salmonella*. Refrigeration temperature at or below 5°C is sufficient, as the minimum temperature for growth is 7 to 10°C. The prevalence of salmonellosis as a foodborne disease has prompted regulatory agencies to adopt a zero tolerance for the genus in ready-to-eat foods. Presence of the bacterium in these foods (luncheon meats, dairy products, pastries, etc.) renders them unwholesome and unfit for consumption. These foods must then be destroyed or reprocessed to eliminate the pathogen.

Shigellosis

Four species are associated with food-borne transmission of dysentery, *Shigella dysenteriae, Shigella flexneri, Shigella boydii*, and *Shigella sonnei*.[10] The disease is characterized with an incubation period of 1 to 7 days (usually less than 4 days). Symptoms include mild diarrhea to very severe with blood, mucus, and pus. Fever, chills, and vomiting also occur. Duration is long, typically 4 days to 2 weeks. *Shigella* spp. have a very low infectious dose of around 10 cells. Foods most often associated with shigellosis are any that are contaminated with fecal material, with salads frequently implicated. Control is best focused on worker hygiene and avoidance of human waste.

Vibriosis

Most vibrios are obligate halophiles that are found in coastal waters and estuaries.[14] Consequently most foodborne outbreaks are associated with consumption of raw or undercooked shellfish (oysters, crabs, shrimp) and fish (sushi or sashimi).[15] *Vibrio parahaemolyticus* causes most vibriosis outbreaks in developed countries and is primarily foodborne. *Vibrio cholerae* is primarily waterborne, but has been associated with foods of aquatic origin.[16] Because *V. cholerae* is halotolerant, it can survive and grow in nonsalt foods. Hence, the bacterium has been spread through foods of terrestrial origin in addition to nonsaline fresh water. *Vibrio vulnificus* is capable of causing very serious infections leading to septicemia and a high mortality rate (30 to 40 percent).[17] Consumption of raw oysters harvested from warm waters (U.S. Gulf Coast) among high-risk individuals (chronic alcoholics, severely immunocompromised individuals) are factors involved with fatalities. Several other *Vibrio* species may be pathogenic.[18] Incubation period for vibriosis is 2 to 48 hours, usually 12 hours. Symptoms include abdominal pain, watery diarrhea, usually nausea and vomiting, mild fever, chills, headache, and prostration. Duration is usually 2 to 5 days. Cholera typically expresses profuse rice water stools as a characterizing symptom. Prevention of vibriosis includes cooking shellfish and fish, harvesting shellfish from approved waters, preventing cross-contamination, and chilling foods to less than 10°C.[19]

Escherichia coli

There are four pathogenic types of *E. coli* associated with food-borne illness.[10,11] The infectious dose for most strains is high (10^6 to 10^8), although for enterohemorrhagic strains it may be much lower. Enteropathogenic (EPEC) strains are serious problems in developing countries but rare in the United States. These strains are a leading cause of diarrhea in neonates in hospitals. Enteroinvasive (EIEC) strains have an incubation period of 8 to 24 hours, with 11 hours most often seen. Symptoms are similar to those of *Shigella* infection, with

TABLE 36-3. CONTRIBUTING FACTORS LEADING TO FOODBORNE OUTBREAKS, 1983 TO 1992

	Number	Percentage
Improper holding temperature	1640	37.3
Inadequate cooking	666	15.2
Contaminated equipment	515	11.7
Food from unsafe source	311	7.1
Poor personal hygiene	863	19.6
Other	401	9.1

TABLE 36-4. TRANSMISSION VEHICLES OF FOODBORNE OUTBREAKS 1983 TO 1992

	Number	Percentage
Beef	114	2.4
Ham	35	0.7
Pork	41	0.9
Sausage	9	0.2
Chicken	71	1.5
Turkey	52	1.0
Other meats and stews	65	1.3
Shellfish	79	1.6
Other fish	335	6.8
Milk	35	0.7
Cheese	16	0.3
Eggs	32	0.7
Ice cream	25	0.5
Other dairy	9	0.2
Baked foods	52	1.1
Fruits and vegetables	123	2.6
Potato salad	30	0.6
Poultry, fish, or egg salad	41	0.9
Other salad	109	2.3
Chinese food	32	0.7
Fried rice	4	0.1
Mexican food	68	1.4
Carbonated drink	13	0.3
Nondairy beverage	27	0.5
Multiple foods	675	14.0
Mushrooms	22	0.5
Unknown	2,707	56.2

bloody diarrhea lasting for several days. Enterotoxigenic (ETEC) strains are a notable cause of traveler's diarrhea. Onset for illness by these strains is 8 to 44 hours, 26 hours normal. Symptoms are similar to cholera, with watery diarrhea, rice water stools, shock, and maybe vomiting lasting a short 24 to 30 hours. Enterohemorrhagic or verotoxigenic strains are the most serious *E. coli* found in foods, especially in the United States. *E. coli* O157:H7 is the predominant serotype among these *Shigella*-like toxin-producing bacteria that cause three syndromes.[20,21] Hemorrhagic colitis (red, bloody stools) is the first symptom usually seen. Hemolytic uremic syndrome (HUS), which is the leading cause of renal failure in children, is characterized by blood clots in kidneys, leading to death or coma in children and the elderly. Rarely, individuals may acquire thrombotic thrombocytopenic purpura (TTP), which is similar to HUS but causes brain damage and has a very high mortality rate. Verotoxic strains have an incubation period of 3 to 4 days. Symptoms include bloody diarrhea, severe abdominal pain, and no fever. Duration ranges from 2 to 9 days. Vehicles of transmission include untreated water, cheese, salads, and raw vegetables. For O157:H7, ground beef, raw milk, and raw apple juice or cider are common vehicles. Prevention of *E. coli* outbreaks includes treatment of water supplies and proper cooking of food. Complete cooking of hamburgers is necessary for destruction of verotoxigenic strains.

Yersiniosis

Most *Yersinia enterocolitica* strains are avirulent; however, pathogenic strains are often isolated from porcine or bovine foods.[22] The disease is predominately serious to the very young or the elderly and is more common in Europe and Canada than in the United States. The incubation period for the disease is 24 to 36 hours with symptoms including severe abdominal pain similar to acute appendicitis, fever, headache, diarrhea, malaise, nausea, vomiting, and chills. It is not uncommon for children involved in outbreaks to experience unnecessary appendectomies. Duration is 1 to 3 days. The majority of foods involved in yersiniosis outbreaks are pork and other meats. Milk, seafood, poultry, and water may also serve as vehicles. Control is achieved by adequate pasteurization and cooking and avoiding cross-contamination. Refrigeration is not adequate because the bacterium is psychrotrophic.

Campylobacteriosis

Three species are linked to foodborne diseases, *Campylobacter jejuni*, *Campylobacter coli*, and *Campylobacter laridis*. Indeed, the incidence of *C. jejuni* infection is thought to rival salmonellosis.[23,24] *Campylobacter* is microaerophilic and is thus sensitive to normal atmospheric oxygen concentrations (21 percent O_2) and very low oxygen concentrations (less than 3 percent). Growth is favored by 5 percent O_2. Disease characteristics are an incubation period of 1 to 10 days, 3 to 5 days normal. Symptoms include fever, abdominal pain, vomiting, bloody diarrhea, and headache, which last for 1 day to several weeks. Relapses are common. The infectious dose is low, 10 to 500 cells. Foods linked to outbreaks include raw milk, animal foods, raw meat, and fresh mushrooms. Control is achieved by adequate cooking, pasteurization, and cooling and by avoiding cross-contamination. The suspected number of cases is much larger than most realize. With improved isolation methods, *Campylobacter* is now isolated at a frequency rivaling that of *Salmonella*.

Listeriosis

Listeria monocytogenes emerged as a cause of food-borne disease in 1981.[1,25] Susceptible humans include pregnant women and their fetuses, newborn infants, the elderly, and immunocompromised individuals, due to cancer, chemotherapy, and the acquired immunodeficiency syndrome (AIDS). The disease has a high 30 percent mortality rate. The incubation period is variable, ranging from 1 day to a few weeks. In healthy individuals, symptoms are mild fever, chills, headache, and diarrhea. In serious cases, septicemia, meningitis, encephalitis, and abortion may occur. The duration is variable. The infectious dose is unknown, but for susceptible individuals it may be as low as 100 to 1000 cells. Foods associated with listeriosis are milk, soft cheeses, meats, and vegetables. Like *Y. enterocolitica*, the bacterium is psychrotrophic and will grow at refrigeration temperatures, though slowly. Control is best done by avoiding cross-contamination and adequately cooking food.

Other Bacterial Foodborne Infections

Many other bacteria have been linked to foodborne diseases including *Plesiomonas shigelloides* (raw seafood), *Aeromonas hydrophila* (raw seafood), *Arizona hinshawii* (poultry), *Streptococcus pyogenes* (milk, eggs), and perhaps *Enterococcus faecalis*.[26] Their contribution to foodborne illness appears to be minimal but they may contribute to opportunistic infections.

Nonbacterial Foodborne Infections

Numerous infectious viruses and parasitic worms are capable of causing foodborne illness.[10] All are easily controlled by proper heat treatment of foods. Difficulty with laboratory confirmation of viral agents as causes of foodborne illness leads to probable underreporting.[27,28]

Infectious Hepatitis

Hepatitis A virus is a fairly common infectious agent having an incubation period of 10 to 50 days, mean 25 days. Symptoms include loss of appetite, fever, malaise, nausea, anorexia, and abdominal distress. Approximately 50 percent of cases develop jaundice that may lead to serious liver damage. The duration is several weeks to months. The infectious dose is quite low, less than 100 particles. The long incubation period and duration of the disease means that affected individuals will shed virus for a prolonged period. Foods handled by an infected worker or those that come in contact with human feces are likely vehicles (raw shellfish, salads, sandwiches, and fruits). Filter-feeding mollusks concentrate virus particles from polluted waters. Control is achieved by cooking food, stressing personal hygiene, and by avoiding shellfish harvested from polluted waters.

Enteroviruses

Coxsackie, ECHO, and Norwalk viruses, and rotavirus, astrovirus, *Calicivirus, Parvovirus*, and adenovirus are being implicated with increasing frequency as agents of foodborne disease.[27,28] Other viruses most certainly are involved but our ability to isolate them from infected consumers and foods is limited. The incubation period is typical for infectious organisms, 27 to 60 hours. Symptoms are usually mild and self-limiting and include fever, headache, abdominal pain, vomiting, and diarrhea. Duration is from 1 to 3 days. The infectious dose for these agents is thought to be very low, 1 to 10 particles. Foods associated with transmission of viral agents are raw shellfish, vegetables, fruits, and salads. Control is primarily achieved by cooking and personal hygiene.

Parasites

Nematodes (roundworms) linked to foodborne illness in humans include *Trichinella spiralis, Ascaris lumbricoides, Trichuris trichiura, Enterobius vermicularis, Anisakis* spp., and *Pseudoterranova* spp. *T. spiralis* can invade skeletal muscle and cause damage to vital organs, leading to fatalities.[8,10]

The incubation period of trichinosis is 2 to 28 days, usually 9 days. Symptoms include nausea, vomiting, diarrhea, muscle pains, and fever. Several days duration is common. Foods linked to the disease are raw or undercooked pork and wild game meat (beaver, bear, and boar). Control in pork is accomplished by: (*a*) cooking to 58.3°C (137°F), (*b*) frozen storage at –15°C (5°F) for more than 20 days, or (*c*) following U.S. Department of Agriculture recommendations for salting, drying, and smoking sausages or other cured pork products. *Anisakis* spp. is found in fish and is a potential problem of consumers of raw fish. The incubation period is several days with irritation of throat and digestive tract as primary symptoms. Control of the nematode is by thoroughly cooking fish or by freezing fish prior to presenting for raw consumption. *A. lumbricoides* is commonly transmitted by use of improperly treated water or sewage fertilizer on crops.[29]

Cestoda (tapeworms) are common in developing countries. Examples include *Taenia saginata* (raw beef), *Taenia solium* (raw pork), and *Diphyllobothrium latum* (raw fish). The incubation period is 10 days to several weeks with usually mild symptoms including abdominal cramps, flatulence, and diarrhea. Control methods are limited to cooking and freezing. Salting has been suggested as an additional control technique.

Protozoa cause a large number of food-borne outbreaks each year. *Entamoeba histolytica, Toxoplasma gondii, Cryptosporidium*, and *Giardia lamblia* cause dysentery-like illness that can be fatal.[30,31] The incubation period is a few days to weeks, leading to diarrhea. Duration can be several weeks, with chronic infections lasting months to years. Those foods that contacted feces or contaminated water are common vehicles. Control is best achieved by proper personal hygiene and water and sewage treatment.

Foodborne Intoxications

Food-borne microbial intoxications are caused by a toxin in the food or production of a toxin in the intestinal tract.[10,11] Normally the organism grows in the food prior to consumption. There are several differences between foodborne infections and intoxications. Intoxicating organisms normally grow in the food prior to consumption, which is not always true for infectious organisms. Organisms causing intoxications may be dead or nonviable in the food when consumed; only the toxin need be present. Organisms causing infections must be alive and viable when food is consumed. Infection-causing organisms invade host tissues and symptoms usually include headache and fever. Toxins usually do not cause fever and toxins act by widely different mechanisms.

Staphylococcus aureus *Enterotoxin*

Certain strains of *S. aureus* produce a heat-stable enterotoxin that is resistant to denaturation during thermal processing (cooking, canning, pasteurization).[32,33] The bacterium is salt (10 to 20 percent NaCl) and nitrite tolerant, which enables survival in cured meat products (luncheon meats, hams, sausages, etc.).[34] Conditions that favor optimum growth favor toxin production, i.e., high protein and starch foods. *S. aureus* competes poorly with other microorganisms, so if competitors are removed by cooking and *S. aureus* is introduced, noncompetitive proliferation is possible. The toxin affects the vagus nerve in the stomach, causing uncontrolled vomiting shortly after consumption (2 to 4 hours). Other symptoms include nausea, retching, severe abdominal cramps, and diarrhea, which clear in 12 to 48 hours. Sources of the bacterium are usually from nasal passages, skin, and wound infections of food handlers. Hence, suspect foods are those rich in nutrients, high in salt, and those that are handled, with ham, salami, cream-filled pastries, and cooked poultry common vehicles. Control is accomplished by preventing contamination, personal hygiene, and no hand-food contact. Refrigeration below 5°C (40°F) prevents multiplication, and heating foods to greater than 60°C (140°F) will not destroy the toxin but will kill the bacterium. Prolific growth of the bacterium is possible in the 5 to 40°C range. Problems with the bacterium occur most frequently with foods prepared at home or at food service establishments, where gross temperature abuse has occurred.

Bacillus cereus *Enterotoxin*

This spore-forming bacterium produces a cell-associated endotoxin that is released when cells lyse upon entering the digestive tract.[10,11] There are two distinct types of disease syndromes seen with this bacterium. The diarrheal syndrome occurs 8 to 16 hours after consumption. Symptoms include abdominal pain, watery diarrhea, with vomiting and nausea rarely seen. Duration is short, 12 to 24 hours. Foods linked to transmission of this syndrome are pudding, sauces, custards, soups, meat loaf, and gravy. The second, emetic, syndrome is similar to *S. aureus* intoxication. The incubation period is very short, 1 to 5 hours. Symptoms commonly are nausea and vomiting, with no diarrhea. Duration again is short, less than 1 day. This syndrome is commonly linked to consumption of fried rice in Oriental restaurants. Other foods include mashed potatoes and pasta. The infectious dose for both is thought to be at least 500,000. Because the bacterium forms spores, prevention of outbreaks is by proper temperature control. Hot foods should be held at greater than 65°C, leftovers should be reheated to greater than 72°C, and chilled foods should be quickly cooled to less than 10°C.

Clostridium perfringens *Enterotoxin*

C. perfringens, also known as *Clostridium welchii* in European literature, is a moderate thermophile showing optimal growth at 43 to 47°C, with a maximum of 55°C.[10,11] Viable cells must be consumed, which then pass through the stomach into the intestine. The abrupt change in pH from stomach to intestine causes sporulation to occur, which releases the toxin. Furthermore, the bacterium can grow in the intestine, leading to a toxicoinfection. The illness is characterized by an incubation period of 8 to 24 hours. Symptoms are abdominal pain, diarrhea, and gas. A cardinal symptom is explosive diarrhea. Fever, nausea, and vomiting are rare. Duration is short, 12 to 24 hours. Infectious dose is high, 500,000, meaning the bacterium must multiply in the food to cause disease. Foods often associated with outbreaks are cooked meats and poultry that have been poorly cooked, gravy (anaerobic environment at bottom of pot), stew, and sauces. Outbreaks frequently occur in food service establishments where large quantities of food are made and poorly cooled. Control is best achieved by rapidly cooling cooked food to less than 7°C, holding hot foods at greater than 60°C, and reheating leftovers to greater than 75°C.

Botulism

This rare disease is caused by consumption of neurotoxins produced by *Clostridium botulinum*.[10,11] This spore-forming bacterium grows anaerobically and sometimes produces gas that can swell improperly processed canned foods. The bacterium produces several types of neurotoxins that are differentiated serologically. The toxins are heat-labile exotoxins. Two main groups (proteolytic and nonproteolytic) are found in nature. Nonproteolytic strains can be psychrotrophic and grow at refrigeration temperatures without the food showing obvious signs of spoilage (no swollen cans or suspect odor).[35] The incubation period is 12 to 36 hours, but may be shorter or longer. Early symptoms, which may be absent, include nausea, vomiting, and occasionally diarrhea. Other symptoms are dizziness; fatigue; headache; constipation; blurred vision; double vision; difficulty in swallowing, breathing, and speaking; dry mouth and throat; and swollen tongue. Later, paralysis of skeletal muscles followed by paralysis of the heart and respiratory system can lead to death due to respiratory failure. Duration is 3 to 6 days for fatal cases, several months for nonfatal cases. Treatment of suspect cases is by immediate administration of antisera, which can be useful if given early. Respiratory assistance is usually required.

Foods frequently linked to botulism are home-canned foods, primarily low-acid vegetables, preserved meats, and fish (more common in Europe), cooked onions, and leftover baked potatoes. The bacterium generally will not grow at a pH of less than 4.6 or at a water activity below 0.85. Thus, high-acid foods, such as tomatoes and some fruits, generally are safer than low-acid foods, such as corn, green beans, peas, etc. Control is by applying a minimum botulinum cook (D_{12}) to all thermally processed foods held in hermetically sealed containers. Each particle of food must reach 120°C (250°F) and be held at that temperature for 3 minutes to reach a D_{12} process. (See High-Temperature Preservation discussed below.) Consumers should reject swollen or putrid cans of food. Properly cured ham, bacon, and luncheon meats should not support growth and toxin production by the bacterium.

A related illness caused by *C. botulinum* is infant botulism. The bacterium can colonize and grow in the intestinal tract of some newborn infants who have not developed a desirable competing microflora. The toxin is then slowly released in the intestines, leading to weakness, lack of sucking, and limpness. Evidence suggests that infant botulism may be associated with sudden infant death syndrome. Consumption of honey by young infants has been linked to this type of disease.

Chemical Intoxications

Chemical hazards are minimally important as etiological agents of food-borne disease (Table 36-1). It should be noted that a number of chemicals, whether naturally occurring or intentionally added, have tolerance limits in foods. These limits are published in the Code of Federal Regulations, Title 21. Informal limits are available through Food and Drug Administration Compliance Policy Guidelines (Center for Food Safety and Applied Nutrition, Washington, D.C.). Prohibited substances (CFR 21, Part 189) are not allowed in human foods either because they have been shown to be a public health risk or because they have not been shown by sound scientific data to be safe.[36] Safe food additives are oftentimes referred to as generally recognized as safe (GRAS) substances.

Although usually considered minor contributors to human illness, toxic chemicals in foods may be significant contributors to morbidity and mortality of consumers.[10] A number of toxic chemicals found in foods are of microbial origin. Mycotoxins are secondary metabolites produced by fungi.[37,38] The aflatoxins were the first fungal metabolite in foods regulated by the U.S. government.[39] Grains and nut products are common carriers of these and other mold toxins. Other fungal toxins not associated with microscopic molds include toxic alkaloids associated with certain mushrooms. In this case direct consumption of wild mushrooms that are frequently confused with edible domesticated species can lead to acute toxicity.[40] There are no current food processing or sanitation methods that can render these mushrooms acceptable as human food.

A number of seafood toxins are naturally associated with shellfish.[41,42] Again, the ultimate cause of these intoxications is traced to the presence of microorganisms. Under favorable environmental conditions, populations of planktonic algae (dinoflagellates) are high (algal bloom) in shellfish-growing waters.[43] The algae are removed from the water column during filter feeding of molluscan shellfish (oysters, clams, mussels, cockles, and scallops). The shellfish then concentrate the algae and associated toxins in their edible flesh. Four primary shellfish intoxications have been identified: amnesic shellfish poisoning (ASP), diarrhetic shellfish poisoning (DSP), neurotoxic shellfish poisoning (NSP), and paralytic shellfish poisoning (PSP). ASP has been linked to mussels; DSP, with mussels, oysters, and scallops; NSP, with oysters and clams; and PSP, with all mentioned shellfish.[8,44] Control of shellfish toxins is best accomplished by monitoring harvest waters for the toxic algae. Postharvest control is not presently possible; however, depuration or relaying may be of some use.

Some marine fish harvested from temperate or tropical climates may contain toxic chemicals. Scombroid fish (anchovy, herring, marlin, sardine, tuna, bonito, mahi mahi, tuna, mackerel, bluefish, and amberjack) under time/temperature abuse during storage can support growth of bacteria that produce histidine decarboxylase.[45] This enzyme releases free histamine from the fish tissues. High histamine levels leads to an allergic response among susceptible consumers. Prompt and continued refrigeration of these fish after harvesting will limit microbial growth and enzyme activity. Fish most often associated with histamine scombrotoxicity are mahi mahi, tuna, mackerel, bluefish, and amberjack. Another form of naturally occurring chemical food poisoning found in tropical and subtropical fish is ciguatera. Like shellfish toxicity, ciguatera results when fish bioconcentrate dinoflagellate toxins though the food chain. Thus, large predatory fish at the top of the food chain can accumulate enough toxin to give a paralysis-type response among consumers. Fish associated with ciguatera poisoning are grouper, barracuda, snapper, jack, mackerel, and triggerfish. Again, monitoring of harvest waters is the essential control step to avoid human illness.

Most human-made chemicals associated with food-borne disease find their way into foods by nonintentional means.[10] Accidental or inadvertent contamination with heavy metals, detergents, or sanitizers can occur.[46] Although infrequently reported to CDC, most chemical intoxications are likely to be short in duration with mild symptoms. CDC does not attempt to link exposure to these chemicals with chronic diseases. There are measurable levels of pesticides, herbicides, fungicides, fertilizers, and veterinary drugs and antibiotics in most foods.[47] In the vast majority of instances where these residues are found, levels are well below tolerance. No instances of foodborne illness have been attributed to these agents when properly used.[48] Heavy metal poisonings have occurred primarily due to leaching of lead, copper, tin, zinc, or cadmium from containers or utensils in contact with acidic foods.[49]

Physical Hazards

Consumers frequently report physical defects with foods, of which presence of foreign objects predominate.[8] Glass is the leading object that consumers report and is evidence of manufacturing or distribution error. Most physical hazards are not particularly dangerous to the consumer, but their obvious presence in a food is disconcerting. Most injuries are cuts, choking, and broken teeth. Control of physical hazards in foods is often difficult, especially when these hazards are a normal constituent of the food, such as bones and shells. Good manufacturing practices and employee awareness are the best measures to prevent physical hazards. Metal detectors and x-ray machines may be installed where appropriate.

▸ ADMINISTRATIVE REGULATION

Several regulatory groups, from local and state agencies to international agencies, are involved in the regulation of food safety and quality standards. Since there is tremendous variation within and between local and state agencies, this discussion is confined to the national and international agencies that regulate food. At the national level, two federal agencies regulate the vast majority of food produced and consumed in the United States, namely, the U.S. Department of Agriculture (USDA) and the Food and Drug Administration (FDA).

U.S. Department of Agriculture

The USDA has responsibility for certification, grading, and inspection of all agricultural products. All federally inspected meat and meat products, including animals, facilities, and procedures, are covered under a series of meat inspection laws that began in 1906 and have been modified on several different occasions, culminating in the latest revisions in 1996.[50] These laws cover only meat that is in interstate commerce, leaving the legal jurisdiction of intrastate meats to individual states. Key elements in meat inspection are examination of live animals for obvious signs of clinical illness and examination of gross pathology of carcasses and viscera for evidence of transmissible diseases. The newest regulations also require the implementation of a hazard analysis critical control point (HACCP) system and microbiological testing of carcasses after chilling. Eggs and egg products are also covered by USDA inspection under the Egg Products Inspection Act of 1970. This act mandates inspection of egg products at all phases of production and processing. All USDA inspection is continuous; that is, products cannot be processed without an inspector or inspectors present to verify the operation.

Food and Drug Administration

The FDA has responsibility for ensuring that foods are wholesome, safe, and have been stored under sanitary conditions, as outlined by the Food, Drug and Cosmetic Act of 1938. This act has been amended to include food additives, packaging, and labeling. The last two issues relate not only to product safety and wholesomeness, but also to nutritional labeling and economic fraud. The FDA is also empowered to act if pesticide residues exceed tolerances set by the Environmental Protection Agency. Unlike USDA inspection, FDA inspection is discontinuous, with food processing plants being required to maintain their own quality control records while inspectors themselves make random visits to facilities.

Milk Sanitation

Perhaps one of the greatest public health success stories of the twentieth century has been the pasteurization of milk. The U.S. Public Health Service drafted a model milk ordinance in 1924, which has been adopted by most local and state regulatory authorities and has become known as the PMO (Pasteurized Grade A Milk Ordinance). This ordinance covers all phases of milk production, including but not limited to animal health, design and construction of milk processing facilities, equipment, and most importantly, the pasteurization process itself. The PMO sets quality standards for both raw and processed milk, in the form of cooling requirements and bacteriological populations. The PMO also standardizes the pasteurization requirements for fluid milk, which ensures that bacteria of public health significance will not survive in the finished product. From a historical perspective, it is interesting to note that neither the public nor the industry initially embraced pasteurization, but that constant pressure from public health officials finally succeeded in making this important advance in public health almost universal.

International Administration

The Codex Alimentarius Commission, created by the Food and Agriculture Organization and the World Health Organization, has the daunting task of implementing food standards on an international scale. These standards apply to both general and specific food categories and also set limits for pesticide residues in foods. Acceptance of these standards is voluntary and at the discretion of individual governments, but acceptance of the standards requires that the country apply them equally to both domestically produced and imported products. The importance of international standards is growing daily as international trade in food expands. Many countries find that they are both importing and exporting foods, and a common set of standards is critical in establishing trade without the presence of nontariff trade barriers.

▸ SANITATION

Sanitation is the fundamental program for all food processing operations, irrespective of whether they are converting raw products into processed food or preparing food for final consumption. Sanitation affects all attributes of processed foods, from organoleptic properties of the food to the safety and quality of the food itself. From a food processor's perspective, an effective sanitation program is essential to producing quality foods with reasonable shelf lives. Without an effective program, even the best operational management and technology will ultimately fail to deliver the quality product that consumers demand.

Sanitation programs are all-encompassing, focusing not only on the details of soil types and chemicals, but on the broader environmental issues of equipment and processing plant design. Many foodborne microorganisms, both spoilage organisms and bacteria of public health significance, can be transferred from the plant environment to the food itself.[51] Perhaps one of the most serious of these microorganisms came to national and international attention in the mid-1980s, when *Listeria monocytogenes* was found in processed dairy products. *Listeria* was considered to be a relatively minor veterinary pathogen until that time, and not even considered a potential foodborne agent. However, subsequent research demonstrated that *L. monocytogenes* was a serious human health concern and, more importantly, was found to be widely distributed in nature. In many food processing plants, *Listeria* was found to be in the general plant environment, and subsequently efforts have been made to improve plant sanitation, through facility and equipment design as well as focusing more attention on basic cleaning and sanitation.

Sanitary Plant Design

Some of the basic considerations of food plant design include the physical separation of raw and processed products, adequate storage areas for nonfood items (such as packaging materials), and a plant layout that minimizes employee traffic between raw and processed areas. While these considerations are easily addressed in newly constructed facilities, they may present challenges in older facilities that have been renovated or expanded. Exposed surfaces, such as floors, walls, and ceilings, in the processing area should be constructed of material that allows for thorough cleaning. Although these surfaces are not direct food contact surfaces, they contribute to overall environmental contamination in the processing area. These surfaces are particularly important in areas where food is open to the environment, and the potential for contamination is greater when temperature differences in the environment result in condensation.[52] As an example, a large open cooking kettle will generate some steam that may condense on surfaces above the kettle. This condensate may, without proper design and sanitation, drip back down into the product, carrying any dirt and dust from overhead surfaces back into the food. Other obvious considerations are basic facility maintenance as well as insect and rodent control programs, as all of these factors may contribute to contamination of food.

Sanitary Equipment Design

Many of the same considerations for sanitary plant design also apply to the design of food processing equipment. Irrespective of its function, processing equipment must protect food from external contamination and from conditions that will allow existing bacteria to grow. The issue of condensate as a form of external contamination has already been raised. Opportunities for existing bacteria to reproduce may be found in the so-called dead spaces within some equipment. These areas can allow food to accumulate over time under conditions that allow bacteria to grow. These areas then become a constant inoculation source for additional product as it moves through the equipment, increasing the bacteriological population within the food. Other considerations of food equipment design include avoiding construction techniques that may allow the product to become trapped within small areas of the equipment, creating the same situation that occurs in the larger dead spaces within the equipment. As an example, lap seams that are tack welded provide ample space for the product to become trapped. Not only does this create a location for bacteria to grow and contaminate the food product, it also creates a point on the equipment that is difficult, if not impossible, to clean.

Cleaning and Sanitizing

Cleaning and sanitizing processes can be generically divided into five separate steps that apply to any sanitation task. The first step is removal of residual food, waste materials, and debris. This is frequently referred to as a "dry" cleanup. The dry cleanup is followed by a rinse with warm (48 to 55°C) water, to remove material that is only loosely attached to surfaces and to hydrate material that is more firmly attached to surfaces. Actual cleaning follows the warm water rinse, which usually involves the application of cleaning chemicals and some form of scrubbing force, either with mechanical brushes or with high-pressure hoses. The nature of the residual food material will determine the type of cleaning compound applied. After this, surfaces are rinsed and inspected for visual cleanliness. At this point, the cleaning process is repeated on any areas that require further attention. Carbohydrates and lipids can generally be removed with warm to hot water and sufficient mechanical scrubbing. Proteins require the use of alkaline cleaners, while mineral deposits can be removed with acid cleaners. Commercially available cleaning compounds generally contain materials to clean the specific type of food residue of concern, as well as surfactants and, as necessary, sequesterants that allow cleaners to function more effectively in hard water.

When surfaces are visually clean, a sanitizer is applied to reduce or eliminate remaining bacteriological contamination. Inadequately cleaned equipment cannot be sanitized, as the residual food material will protect bacteria from the sanitizer. One of the most common sanitizing agents, widely used in small- and medium-sized processing facilities, is hot water. Most regulatory agencies require that, when hot water is used as the sole method of sanitization, the temperature must be at or above 85°C. While heat sanitization in effective, it is not as economical as chemical sanitizers because of the energy costs required to maintain the appropriate temperature. Chlorine-containing sanitizers are economical and effective against a wide range of bacterial species and are widely used in the food industry. Typically, the concentrations of chlorine applied to equipment and surfaces are in the 150- to 200-ppm range. Chlorine sanitizers are corrosive and can, if improperly handled, release chlorine gas into the environment.

Iodine-containing sanitizers are less corrosive than chlorine sanitizers, but are also somewhat less effective. These sanitizers must be used at slightly acidic pH values to allow for the release of free iodine. The amber color of iodine sanitizers can give an approximate indication of concentration, but can also leave residual stains on treated surfaces. Quaternary ammonium compounds (QACs) are noncorrosive and demonstrate effective bactericidal action against a wide range of microorganisms. These sanitizers are generally more costly and not as effective as chlorine compounds, but they are stable and provide residual antimicrobial activity on sanitized surfaces. Food processing plants will frequently alternate between chlorine and QAC sanitizers to prevent development of resistant bacterial populations or will use chlorine sanitizers on regular production days and then apply QACs during periods when the facility is not operating (for example, over a weekend).

Personnel

A final element in food plant sanitation programs are the personnel who perform the sanitation operations as well as the employees who work in the processing area. Sanitation personnel should be adequately trained to understand the importance of their function in the overall processing operation in addition to the training necessary to properly use the chemicals and equipment necessary for them to perform their duties. Personnel who are actually involved in processing operations should also understand the necessity for proper cleaning and sanitation and not simply rely on the sanitation crew to take care of all issues. In addition, all employees must be aware of basic issues of personal hygiene, especially when they are in direct contact with food or food processing equipment. Some key elements, such as handwashing and wearing clean clothing and gloves, should be reemphasized on a periodic basis. This information has been outlined by the U.S. Food and Drug Administration in the Good Manufacturing Practices section of the Code of Federal Regulations.[53]

▶ HAZARD ANALYSIS CRITICAL CONTROL POINT SYSTEM

The basic concept of HACCP was developed in the early 1960s as a joint effort to produce food for the space program. The U.S. Air Force Space Laboratory Project Group, the U.S. Army Natick Laboratories, and the National Aeronautics and Space Administration contributed to the development of the process, as did the Pillsbury Company, which had a major role in developing and producing the actual food products. Since that time, the HACCP system has evolved and been refined, but still focuses on the original goal of producing food that is safe for consumption.[8]

Since development, HACCP principles have been used in many different ways. However, recent interest in the system has been driven by changes in the regulatory agencies, specifically the USDA Food Safety and Inspection Service (FSIS) and the U.S. Food and Drug Administration. The USDA-FSIS recently revised the regulations that govern meat inspection to move all federally inspected meat plants to a HACCP-based system of production and inspection.[50] The FDA has also changed the regulations for fish and seafood, again moving this to a HACCP-based system for production.[54] It is likely, given current trends by federal agencies, that most commercially produced foods will be produced under HACCP systems within the next 10 years.

The goal of a HACCP system is to produce foods that are free of biological, chemical, and physical hazards.[55] HACCP is a preventative system, designed to prevent problems before they occur, rather than trying to fix problems after they occur. Biological hazards fall into two distinct categories, those that can potentially cause infection and those that can potentially cause intoxications. Infectious agents require the presence of viable organisms in the food and may not, depending on the organisms and the circumstances, require that the organism actually reproduce in the food. As an example, *E. coli* O157:H7 has an extremely low infectious dose for humans (possibly less than 100 viable cells), and as such, the mere presence of the bacterium in foods is a cause for concern. In contrast, organisms involved in intoxications usually require higher numbers of the organism in the food to produce sufficient amounts of toxin to cause clinical illness in humans. However, some of the toxins involved in foodborne diseases are heat stable, so that absence of viable organisms in the food is not necessarily an indication of the relative safety of the food. *S. aureus* is a good example, where it typically requires greater than 1,000,000 to 10,000,000 cells per gram of food to produce sufficient toxin to cause illness in humans.[56] However, because the toxin itself is extremely heat stable, cooking the food will eliminate the bacterium but not the toxin, and the food can still potentially cause an outbreak of foodborne illness.

Chemical hazards include chemicals that are specifically prohibited in foods, such as cleaning agents, as well as food additives that are allowed in foods but only at regulated concentrations. Foods containing prohibited chemicals or food additives in levels higher than allowed are considered adulterated. Adulterated foods are not allowed for human consumption and are subject to regulatory action by the appropriate agency (USDA or FDA). Chemical hazards can be minimized by ensuring that raw materials (foods and packaging materials) are acquired from reliable sources that provide written assurances that the products do not contain illegal chemical contaminants or additives. During processing, adequate process controls should be in place to minimize the possibility that an approved additive will be used at levels not exceeding maximum legal limits for both the additive and the food product. Other process controls and Good Manufacturing Practices (GMPs) should also ensure that industrial chemicals, such as cleaners or lubricants, will not contaminate food during production or storage.[53]

Physical hazards are extraneous material or foreign objects that are not normally found in foods. For example, wood, glass, or metal fragments are extraneous materials that are not normally found in foods. Physical hazards typically affect only a single individual or a very small group of individuals, but because they are easily recognized by the consumer, are a source of many complaints. Physical hazards can originate from food processing equipment, packaging materials, the environment, and employees. Physical contaminants can be minimized by complying with good manufacturing practices and by employee training. While some physical hazards can be detected during food processing (e.g., metal by the use of metal detectors), many nonferrous materials are virtually impossible to detect by any means, and so control often resides with employees.

Development of a HACCP plan begins with the formation of a HACCP team.[57] Individuals on this team should represent diverse sections within a given operation, from purchasing to sanitation. The team is then responsible for development of the plan. Initial tasks that the team must accomplish are to identify the food, method of distribution, the consumer, and intended use of the food. Having done this, the HACCP team should construct a flow diagram of the process and verify that this diagram is accurate.

The development of a HACCP plan is based on seven principles or steps in logical order (Table 36-5).[8] With the flow diagram as a reference point, the first principle or step is to conduct a hazard analysis of the process. The HACCP team identifies all biological, chemical, and physical hazards that may occur at each step during the process. Once the list is completed, it is reviewed to determine the relative risk of each potential hazard, which helps identify significant hazards. Risk is the interaction of likelihood of occurrence with severity of occurrence. As an extreme example, a sudden structural failure in the building could potentially contaminate any exposed food with foreign material. However, likelihood of the occurrence of such an event is small. In contrast, if exposed food is held directly below surfaces that are frequently covered with condensate, then the likelihood of condensate dripping on exposed food is considerably higher. An important point in the determination of significant hazards is a written explanation by the HACCP team regarding how the determination of "significant" was made. This documentation can provide a valuable reference in the future, when processing methods change or when new equipment is added to the production line.

TABLE 36-5. SEVEN HACCP PRINCIPLES

Hazard analysis
Identify Critical Control Points (CCP)
Establish critical limits for each CCP
Monitor CCP
Establish corrective action
Record keeping
Verification

The second step in the development of a HACCP plan is the identification of critical control points (CCPs) within the system. A CCP is a point, step, or procedure where control can be applied and a food safety hazard can be prevented, eliminated, or reduced to acceptable levels.[55] An example of a CCP is the terminal heat process applied to canned foods after cans have been filled and sealed. This process, when properly conducted according to FDA guidelines, effectively eliminates a potential food safety hazard, *Clostridium botulinum*. Once CCPs have been identified, the third step in the development of a HACCP plan is to establish critical limits for each CCP. These limits are not necessarily the ideal processing parameters, but the minimum acceptable levels required to maintain the safety of the product. Again, in the example of a canned food, the critical limit is the minimum time and temperature relationship to ensure that each can has met the appropriate standards required by FDA.

The fourth step, following in logical order, is to establish appropriate monitoring requirements for each critical control point. The intent of monitoring is to ensure that critical limits are being met at each critical control point. Monitoring may be on a continuous or discontinuous basis. Presence of a physical hazard, such as metal, can be monitored continuously by passing all of the food produced through a metal detector. Alternately, presence of foreign material can be monitored on a continuous basis by visual inspection. Discontinuous inspection may involve taking analytical measurements, such as temperature or pH, at designated intervals during the production day. Some analytical measurements can be made on a continuous basis by the use of data recording equipment, but it is essential that continuous measures be checked periodically by production personnel.

The fifth step in the development of a HACCP plan is to establish appropriate corrective actions for occasions when critical limits are not met. Corrective actions must address the necessary steps to correct the process that is out of control (such as increasing the temperature on an oven) as well as addressing disposition of the product that was made while the process was out of control. A literal interpretation of the HACCP system and a CCP is that when a CCP fails to meet the critical limits, then the food product is potentially unsafe for human consumption. As a result, food produced while the CCP was not under control cannot be put into the normal distribution chain without corrective actions being taken to that product. Typically this means that the product must be either reworked or destroyed, depending on the nature of the process and the volume of product that was produced while the CCP was out of control. This argues for frequent monitoring, so that the actual volume of product produced during each monitoring interval is relatively small.

The sixth step in the development of a HACCP plan is the establishment of effective record-keeping procedures. In many respects, a HACCP plan is an elaborate record-keeping program. Records should document what was monitored, when it was monitored and by whom, and what was done in the event of a deviation. Reliable records are essential from both a business and regulatory perspective. From the business perspective, HACCP records allow a processor to develop an accurate longitudinal record of production practices and deviations. Reviewing HACCP records may provide insight on a variety of issues, from an individual raw material supplier whose product frequently results in production deviations, to an indication of an equipment or environmental problem within a processing plant. From a regulatory perspective, records allow inspectors to determine if a food processor has been fulfilling commitments made in the HACCP plan. If a processor has designated a particular step in the process as a CCP, then the processor should have records to indicate that the CCP has been monitored on a frequent basis and should also indicate corrective actions taken in the event of a deviation.

The final step in the development of a HACCP plan is verification. Verification can take many forms. Microbiological tests of finished products can be performed to evaluate the effectiveness of a HACCP plan. Alternately, external auditors can be used to evaluate all parts of the HACCP plan to ensure that the stated goals and objectives are being met. A HACCP plan must also be periodically reviewed and updated to reflect changes in production methods and use of different equipment. Another critical aspect of verification is education of new employees on the HACCP plan itself. As HACCP is phased in to many food processing environments, many employees who are unfamiliar with the concepts and goals of HACCP will have to be educated on the necessity of following the plan. In one sense, USDA-FSIS regulations have guaranteed that meat processors will follow HACCP plans, as the penalty for not following the HACCP plan can be as severe as the loss of inspection at an establishment. However, HACCP is an excellent system for monitoring and improving production of food products, and many food processors will discover that HACCP plans offer many benefits, well above and beyond the legal requirements of the regulatory agencies.

▶ FOOD PRESERVATION

Normal microflora of foods are characterized by food type and growing/handling practices. Foods of plant origin have flora on outer surfaces. Animals too have flora on surfaces, but also have intestinal flora and secretion flora. Outside sources, such as soil, dust, water, humans, and equipment, can be significant sources of disease-causing microbes. Use of diseased animals for foods is dangerous because they often carry human pathogens. It should be noted that the inner tissues of plants and animals are generally sterile; however, cabbage inner leaves have lactobacilli and animal intestinal tracts have numerous microbes. Pathogens found on fruits and vegetables are from soil origin (*Clostridium, Bacillus*) or from contaminated water, fertilizer, or food handlers. Some grain and nut products are naturally contaminated in the field with mycotoxin-producing molds. Soil is also a source of contamination of foods from animal origin. Animal feces can harbor coliforms, *C. perfringens*, enterococci, and enteric pathogens. Milk from infected udders (mastitis) can carry disease causing *Streptococcus pyogenes* and *S. aureus*. Nonmastitic udders can shed *Brucella, Rickettsia*, and viruses.

Outside sources of contamination that are not normally associated with food can be important in terms of food safety. Soil and dust contain very large numbers and a large variety of microbes. Many microorganisms responsible for food spoilage come from these sources. Contamination is by direct contact with soil, water, or by airborne dust particles. Air can carry microorganisms from other sources such as sneezing, coughing, dust, and aerosols. Pathogens, mold spores, yeasts, and spoilage bacteria can be then disseminated. Organic debris from plants or animals is an excellent source. Microorganisms can grow on walls, floors, and other surfaces and act as a source of contamination during food processing and preparation. Airborne particles can be removed by filtration or by electrostatic precipitation.

Treated sewage may be used for fertilizer, although due to large amounts of toxic compounds such as heavy metals it is not used often for this purpose.[29] Sewage can be an excellent source of pathogens including all enteric Gram-negative bacteria, enterococci, *Clostridium*, viruses, and parasites. Sewage that contaminates lakes, streams, and estuaries has been linked to many seafood outbreaks. In addition, water used for food must be safe for drinking and must be treated and free of pathogens. Furthermore, water must not contain toxic wastes. Water in food processing is typically used for washing, cooling, chilling, heating, ice, or as an ingredient. Stored water (reservoirs) and underground water (wells) are usually self-purifying.

Numbers and types of microorganisms found in foods depends on: (*a*) the general environment from which the food was obtained, (*b*) quality of raw food, (*c*) sanitary conditions under which the food was processed or handled, and (*d*) adequacy of packaging, handling, and storage of foods. General methods of food preservation are shown in Table 36-6. The Hurdle Concept uses multiple methods (multibarrier approach) to food preservation and is the most common. Examples include pasteurized milk (heat, refrigeration, and packaging) or canned beans (heat, anaerobiosis, and packaging).

Principles of Food Preservation

Principles of food preservation rely on preventing or delaying microbial decomposition.[58,59] This can be accomplished by using asepsis or removal. Preventing growth or activity of microbes with low temperatures, drying, anaerobic conditions, or preservatives can also be done. Killing or injuring microbes with heat, irradiation, or some preservatives is certainly effective. A second principle is to prevent or delay self-decomposition, which is done by destruction or inactivation of enzymes (blanching) or by preventing or delaying autooxidation (antioxidants). The last principle is to prevent physical damage caused by insects, animals, and mechanical forces, which prevents entry of microorganisms into food. Physical barriers (packaging) are the primary means of protection. To control microorganisms in foods, many methods of food preservation depend not on the destruction or removal of microbes but rather on delaying the initiation of growth or hindering growth once it has begun.

TABLE 36-6. METHODS OF FOOD PRESERVATION

Methods	Description
Asepsis	Keeping microorganisms out of foods, "aseptic packaging"
Removal	Limited applications, difficult to do, filtration
Anaerobiosis	Sealed, evacuated container
High temperatures	Sterilization, canning, pasteurization
Low temperatures	Refrigeration, freezing
Dehydration	Drying or tying-up water by solutes and hydrophilic colloids, lower water activity (a_w)
Chemical preservatives	Natural, developed, or added (propionic acid, nisin, spices), acids (lower pH)
Irradiation	γ-Rays (ionizing) or UV (nonionizing)
Mechanical destruction	Grinding, high pressures, etc.—not very useful, nor widely used
Combinations	Most frequently employed, multiple hurdle concept

For food preservation to succeed, one must be able to manipulate the microbial growth curve. Many steps can be done to lengthen the lag phase or positive acceleration phase of a population. These steps include: (*a*) prevent introduction of microbes by reducing contamination (fewer numbers gives a longer lag phase); (*b*) avoid addition of actively growing organisms that may be found on unclean containers, equipment, and utensils; and (*c*) create unfavorable environmental conditions for growth. The last step is the most important in food preservation and can be done by low water activity, extremes of temperature, irradiation, low pH, adverse redox potential, and by adding inhibitors and preservatives (Table 36-6). Some of these steps may only damage or injure microorganisms; hence, the need for multiple barriers becomes essential.[60] For each of these steps to be effective, other factors should be considered. For example, the number of organisms present determines kill rate. Smaller numbers give faster kill rates. Vegetative cells are most resistant to lethal treatments when in late lag or stationary phase and least resistant when in log phase of growth.

Asepsis/Removal

Keeping microorganisms out of food is often difficult during food production. Processing and postprocessing are much easier places to apply asepsis. Protective covering of foods such as skin, shells, and hides are often removed during processing, thereby exposing previously sterile foods to contaminating microbes. Raw agricultural commodities normally carry a natural bioburden upon entering the processing plant. Packaging is the most widely used form of asepsis and includes wraps, packages, cans, etc.

Removal of microorganisms from foods is not very effective. Washing of fruits and vegetables can remove some surface microorganisms. However, if wash water becomes dirty, it can add microbes to the food. Trimming is an effective way to remove spoiled or damaged parts. Filtration is good for clear liquids (juices, beer, soft drinks, wine, and water) but is of little value for solid foods. Centrifugation, such as used in sedimentation/clarification steps, is not useful for removal of bacteria or viruses.

Modified Atmosphere Conditions

Altering the atmosphere surrounding a food can be a useful way to control microbes. Examples include packaging with vacuum, CO_2, N_2, or combinations of inert gases with or without oxygen. Some CO_2 accumulation is possible during fermentations or vegetable respiration. It is important to note that vacuum packaging can lead to favorable environments for proliferation of anaerobic pathogens such as *Clostridium botulinum.*

High-Temperature Preservation

Use of high-temperature processing is based on destroying microbes, but it may also injure certain thermoduric microbes. Not all microorganisms are killed, i.e., spore formers usually survive.[61] Other barriers are combined with a thermal process to achieve adequate safety and product shelf life. Commercial sterilization used in the canning process usually destroys all viable microbes that can spoil the product. Thermophilic spores may survive but will not grow under normal storage conditions.

Several factors affect heat resistance of microorganisms in foods.[59] Species variability and the ability to form spores plus condition of the microbial population can affect heat resistance. Environmental factors such as food variability and presence of other preservative measures employed also dictate thermal resistance. For example, heat resistance increases with decreasing water activity. Hence, moist air heating is better than dry heating. High-fat foods tend to increase resistance of cells. The larger the initial number of microorganisms present means a higher heat resistance. Older (stationary phase) cells are more resistant to heat than are younger cells. Resistance increases as growth temperature increases. A microbe with a high optimum temperature for growth will generally have a high heat resistance. Addition of other inhibitors, such as nitrite, will decrease resistance. Likewise high-acid foods (pH less than 4.6) will not generally support growth of pathogens. There is a time-temperature relationship that is a very important factor governing heat resistance of a microbial population. As temperature increases, the time needed for a given kill decreases. The relationship is dependent on type and size of food container. Larger containers require longer process times. Metal conducts heat better than glass, which can lower process times.

Microorganisms are killed by heat at a rate nearly proportional to the numbers present. This is a log order of death, which means that under a constant temperature the same percentage of a population will die at a given time interval regardless of the population size (Fig. 36-1). For example, 90 percent die in 30 seconds, 90 percent of remaining in the next 30 seconds, and so on. Thus, as the initial number of organisms increases, then the time required for the reduction of all organisms at a given temperature also increases. Food microbiologists express this time-temperature relationship by calculating a number of constants. D value is the time required to reduce a population by one log cycle at a given temperature. Thermal death time (TDT) is the time needed to kill a given number of organisms at a given temperature. Thermal death point (TDP) is the temperature needed to kill a given number of organisms at a set time (usually 10 minutes; D_{10}).

In food canning, the time-temperature profile must be calculated for each size of container, for each food type, and for each retort used. When done correctly, these time-temperature conditions provide a large margin of safety since one rarely knows the numbers and types of microbes in a given container, but one must assume that *C. botulinum* is present. To ensure safety, inoculated pack studies are done using *Clostridium sporogenes* PA 3679, which is six times more heat resistant than *C. botulinum*. A known number of PA 3679 are added

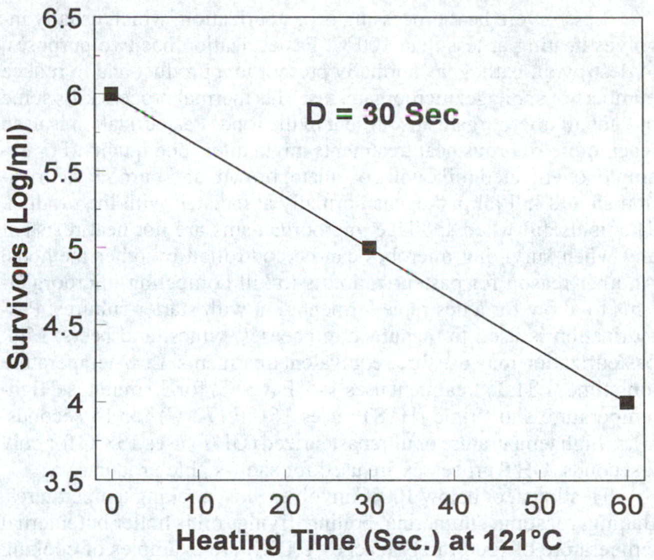

Figure 36-1. Typical heat inactivation curve for a bacterial population.

to cans fitted with thermocouples. Cans are then processed to 120°C (250°F) and held for various time periods. Survivors are enumerated to construct a thermal death curve for that particular food and a D value calculated. For canned foods a 12D margin of safety is used. Thus, heat at a given temperature is applied for a time equal to D times 12 log cycle reductions of PA 3679. Therefore, if a can had 10^9 spores only 1 in 1000 cans would have a viable spore. Thus, the probability of survival for *C. botulinum* would be 1 in 10^{12} if a can is heated at 250°F for 3 minutes. A minimum botulinum cook is one where every particle of food in a container reaches 250°F and remains at that temperature for at least 3 minutes.

Several factors affect heat transfer and penetration into food packages. Food type (liquids, solids, size, and shape) determine mixing effects during heating. Conduction occurs with solid foods (pumpkin) and results in slow heat transfer because there is no mixing of contents. Convection gives liquids (juice) faster heat transfer due to mixing by currents or mechanical agitation. Combination of conduction and convection is observed with particles in liquid (peas), though heating is primarily by convection and depends on viscosity of liquid component. Container size, shape, and composition are important. Tall thin cans transfer heat faster than short round cans. Large cans take longer than small cans. Metal (tin, steel, and aluminum) containers transfer heat faster than glass, resulting in shorter process times. Plastics can have rapid heat transfer due to thinness. Retort pouches, which are laminates of foil and plastic, have rapid heat transfer; however, pinhole problems can occur. Preheating foods prior to filling containers and preheating retort will shorten process time. Rotation or agitation of cans during processing increases convection, giving faster heating.

Canning is the preservation of foods in hermetically sealed containers, usually by heat treatments. The typical sequence in canning is as follows. Freshly harvested good-quality foods are washed to remove soils. Next, a blanch or mild heat treatment is applied to set color of fruits and vegetables, inactivate enzymes, purge dissolved gases, and kill some microorganisms. Clean containers are then filled to leave some head space. Hot packing is filling with preheated food to give faster processing, although cold packing can be done. Containers are sealed under vacuum then placed into a retort. The retort is sealed and heated with pressurized steam. After heating, cans should be rapidly cooled to avoid overcooking and to prevent growth of thermophiles. Cooling is done by submerging cans in a sanitized water bath, which can cause problems if pinhole leaks are present, allowing water to enter containers.

Less severe heat processing is pasteurization, which usually involves heating at less than 100°C. Pasteurization has two purposes, to destroy all pathogens normally present in a product and to reduce numbers of spoilage microorganisms. This thermal process kills some but not all microorganisms present in the food. Pasteurization is used when more rigorous heat treatments might alter food quality. For example, overheated milk will coagulate, brown, and burn. Pasteurization should kill all pathogens normally associated with the product. This is useful when spoilage microorganisms are not heat resistant and when surviving microbes can be controlled by other methods. Another reason for pasteurization is to kill competing microorganisms to allow for a desirable fermentation with starter cultures. Pasteurization is used to manufacture cheeses, wines, and beers. Milk pasteurization may use three equivalent treatments. Low-temperature long time (LTLT) treatment uses 145°F (63°C) for 30 minutes. High-temperature short time (HTST) uses 161°F (72°C) for 15 seconds. Ultra high temperature or ultrapasteurized (UHT) uses 138°C for only 2 seconds. UHT processes are used for shelf-stable products.

Heating at or below 100°C involves most cooking temperatures. Baking, roasting, simmering, boiling, frying (oil is hotter but internal temperature of food rarely reaches 100°C) are examples of cooking methods. All pathogens are usually killed except spore formers. Microwaving does not exceed 100°C and can result in uneven heating. Microwave cooking should allow an equilibration time after removal from the oven for more even heating.[60,61]

Low-Temperature Preservation

Low temperatures retard chemical reactions, and refrigeration slows microbial growth rates. Freezing prevents growth of most microorganisms by lowering water activity. Several psychrotrophic pathogens *(Listeria monocytogenes, Yersinia enterocolitica*, and nonproteolytic *Clostridium botulinum)* are able to multiply at refrigeration temperatures.[62] Among factors influencing chill storage, temperature of the compartment is critical.[63] Temperature of food products should be held as low as possible. Relative humidity should be high enough to prevent dehydration but not too high to favor growth of microorganisms. Air velocity in coolers helps to remove odors, control humidity, and maintain uniform temperatures. Atmosphere surrounding food during chill storage can affect microbial growth. Modified atmosphere packaging can help ensure safe chill-stored foods. Some plant foods respire, resulting in removal of O_2 and release of CO_2. Ultraviolet irradiation can be used to kill microorganisms on surfaces and in the air during chill storage of foods.

For chill storage to be effective in controlling microorganisms, the rate of cooling should be done rapidly. Temperature should be maintained as low as possible for refrigerated foods (less than 40°F). Thawing of frozen foods presents special problems because drip loss provides ample nutrients for microorganisms. In addition, thawing should be done as rapidly as possible and the food used as quickly as possible to avoid opportunity for microbial growth. Often, thawing is done at room temperature over many hours, which can lead to exposure of surfaces to ambient temperatures for extended periods. Another problem is incomplete thawing of large food items (turkeys). By cooking a large item that is not completely thawed, the internal temperature may not reach lethal levels to kill even the most heat-sensitive enteric pathogen. In fact, a spike in the number of salmonellosis and camplyobacteriosis outbreaks occurs every Thanksgiving and Christmas holidays because of consumption of undercooked turkey and stuffing.

Drying

Foods can be preserved by removing or binding water. Any treatment that lowers water activity can reduce or eliminate growth of microorganisms. Some examples include sun drying, heating, freeze drying, and addition of humectants. Humectants act not by removing water but rather by binding water to make it unavailable to act as a solvent. Humectants in common use are salt, sugars, and sugar alcohols (sorbitol). Intermediate moisture foods are those that have 20 to 40 percent moisture and a water activity (a_w) of 0.75 to 0.85. Examples include soft candies, jams, jellies, honey, pepperoni, and country ham. These foods often require antifungal agents for complete stability.

Preservatives

Food preservatives can be extrinsic (intentionally added), intrinsic (normal constituent of food), or developed (produced during fermentation).[58,59] Factors affecting preservative effectiveness include: (*a*) concentration of inhibitor; (*b*) kind, number, and age of microorganisms (older cells more resistant); (*c*) temperature; (*d*) time of exposure (if long enough some microbes can adapt and overcome inhibition); and (*e*) chemical and physical characteristics of food (water activity, pH, solutes, etc.). Preservatives that are cidal are able to kill microorganisms when large concentrations of the substances are used. Static activity results when sublethal concentrations inhibit microbial growth.

Some examples of inorganic preservatives are NaCl, nitrate and nitrite, and sulfites and SO_2. NaCl lowers water activity and causes plasmolysis by withdrawing water from cells. Nitrites and nitrates are curing agents for meats (hams, bacons, sausages, etc.) to inhibit *C. botulinum* under vacuum packaging conditions. Sulfur dioxide (SO_2), sulfites (SO_3), bisulfite (HSO_3), and metabisulfites (S_2O_5) form sulfurous acid in aqueous solutions, which is the antimicrobial agent. Sulfites are widely used in the wine industry to sanitize equipment and reduce competing microorganisms. Wine yeasts are resistant to sulfites. Sulfites are also used in dried fruits and some fruit juices. Sulfites have been used to prevent enzymatic and nonezymatic browning in some fruits and vegetables (cut potatoes).

Nitrites can react with secondary and tertiary amines to form potentially carcinogenic nitrosamines during cooking; however, current formulations greatly reduce this risk. Nitrates in high concentrations can result in red blood cell functional impairment; however, at approved usage levels they are safe.[64,65] Sulfiting agents likewise can cause adverse respiratory effects to susceptible consumers, particularly asthmatics.[66,67] Therefore, use of these two classes of agents is strictly regulated.

A number of organic acids and their salts are used as preservatives. These include lactic acid and lactates, propionic acid and propionates, citric acid, acetic acid, sorbic acid and sorbates, benzoic acid and benzoates, and methyl and propyl parabens (benzoic acid derivatives). Benzoates are most effective when undissociated; therefore, they require low pH values for activity (2.5 to 4.0). The sodium salt of benzoate is used to permit ease of solubility in foods. When esterified (parabens), benzoates are active at higher pH values. Benzoates are primarily used in high-acid foods (jams, jellies, juices, soft drinks, ketchup, salad dressings, and margarine). They are active against yeast and molds, but minimally so against bacteria. They can be used at levels up to 0.1 percent.

Sorbic acid and sorbate salts (potassium is most effective) are effective at pH values less than 6.5 but at a higher pH than benzoates. Sorbates are used in cheeses, baked or nonyeast goods, beverages, jellies, jams, salad dressings, dried fruits, pickles, and margarine. They inhibit yeasts and molds, but few bacteria except *C. botulinum*. They prevent yeast growth during vegetable fermentations and can be used at levels up to 0.3 percent.

Propionic acid and propionate salts (calcium is most common) are active against molds at pH values less than 6. They have limited activity against yeasts and bacteria. They are widely used in baked products and cheeses. Propionic acid is found naturally in Swiss cheese at levels up to 1 percent. Propionates can be added to foods at levels up to 0.3 percent.

Acetic acid is found in vinegar at levels up to 4 to 5 percent. It is used in mayonnaise, pickles, and ketchup, primarily as a flavoring agent. Acetic acid is most active against bacteria, but has some yeast and mold activity, though less active than sorbates or propionates. Lactic acid, citric acid, and their salts can be added as preservatives, to lower pH, and as flavorants. They are also developed during fermentation. These organic acids are most effective against bacteria.

Some antibiotics may be found in foods. Although medical compounds are not allowed in human food, trace amounts used for animal therapy may occasionally be found. Bacteriocins, which are antimicrobial peptides produced by microorganisms, can be found in foods. An example of an approved bacteriocin is nisin, which is allowed in process cheese food as an additive. Some naturally occurring enzymes (lysozyme and lactoferrin) can be used as preservatives in limited applications where denaturation is not an issue. Some spices, herbs, and essential oils have antimicrobial activity, but such high levels are needed that the food becomes unpalatable. Ethanol has excellent preservative ability but is underutilized because of social stigma. Wood smoke, whether natural or added in liquid form, contains several phenolic antimicrobial compounds in addition to formaldehyde. Wood smoke is most active against vegetative bacteria and some fungi. Bacterial endospores are resistant. Activity is correlated with phenolic content. Carbon dioxide gas can dissolve in food tissues to lower pH and inhibit microbes. Developed preservatives produced during fermentation include organic acids (primarily lactic, acetic, and propionic), ethanol, and bacteriocins. All added preservatives must meet government standards for direct addition to foods. All preservatives added to foods are GRAS, generally recognized as safe.

Irradiation

Foods can be processed or preserved with a number of types of radiation. Nonionizing radiations used include ultraviolet, microwave, and infrared. These function by exciting molecules. Ionizing radiations include γ-rays, x-rays, β-rays, protons, neutrons, and α-particles. Neutrons make food radioactive, while β-rays (low-energy electrons), protons, and α-particles have little penetrating ability and are of little practical use in foods. Ionizing γ-rays, x-rays, and high-energy electrons produce ions by breaking molecules and can be lethal to microorganisms.

Ultraviolet (260 nm) lamps are used to disinfect water, meat surfaces, utensils, air, walls, ceilings, and floors. UV can control film yeasts in brines during vegetable fermentations. UV effectiveness is dose dependent. Longer exposure time increases effectiveness. UV intensity depends on lamp power, distance to object, and amount of interfering material in its path. For example, humidity greater than 60 percent reduces intensity. UV will not penetrate opaque materials and is good only for surface decontamination. Infrared heats products, but has little penetrating power. Microwaves cause rapid oscillation of dipole molecules (water) and result in the production of heat. Microwaves have excellent penetrating power. However, there are problems with the time-temperature relationship because microwaves cause foods to reach hot temperatures too quickly. Also, microwave-treated foods rarely exceed 100°C. Thus, instances of microbial survival in these foods has been reported.[60,61]

X-rays have excellent penetrating ability but are quite expensive. They are not widely used in the food industry. γ-Rays from radioactive sources (Cs^{135} and Co^{150}) have good penetration and are widely used to pasteurize and sterilize foods. Electron beam generators also are gaining appeal as ionizing sources of radiation to process foods. Food irradiation is much more widespread in countries other than the United States. There is much untapped potential to use ionizing radiations to reduce or eliminate microbial pathogens in foods.[68,69] This technology remains underexploited due to consumer wariness about the safety of the technology.[70–72]

Fermentation

A number of foods use beneficial microorganisms in the course of their processing.[59] Bread, cheeses, pickles, sauerkraut, some sausages, and alcoholic beverages are made by the conversion of sugar to organic acids, ethanol, or carbon dioxide. These three byproducts not only serve as desirable flavors but also provide a significant antimicrobial barrier to pathogens. There have been instances where poorly fermented foods have been linked to food-borne illness. Furthermore, cheese made from unpasteurized milk has a distinctly higher risk of carrying pathogens than cheese made from pasteurized milk. Proper acid development and avoidance of cross-contamination are essential control steps in manufacturing fermented foods. Alcoholic beverages have not been linked to food-borne disease other than excess consumption leading to ethanol toxicity.

▶ REFERENCES

1. Smith JL, Fratamico PM: Factors involved in the emergence and persistence of food-borne diseases. J Food Prot 58:696–716, 1995
2. Centers for Disease Control: Foodborne disease outbreaks, 5-year summary, 1983–1987. MMWR 39:SS-1, 1990
3. Centers for Disease Control and Prevention: Summary of notifiable diseases, United States, 1995. MMWR 44(53):4–9, 74–77, 1995
4. Centers for Disease Control and Prevention: Foodborne disease outbreaks, 5-year summary, 1988–1992. MMWR 45:SS-5, 1996
5. Council for Agriculture Science and Technology: Foodborne Pathogens: Risks and Consequences. Ames, IA: Council for Agriculture Science and Technology, 1994
6. Archer DL, Kvenberg JE: Incidence and cost of foodborne diarrheal disease in the United States. J Food Prot 48:887–894, 1985
7. Todd ECD: Foodborne disease in Canada—a 10 year summary from 1975–1984. J Food Prot 55:123–132, 1992
8. Pierson MD, Corlett DA: HACCP; Principles and Applications. New York: Chapman & Hall, 1992
9. Bryan FL: Risks of practices, procedures and processes that lead to outbreaks of foodborne diseases. J Food Prot 51:663–673, 1988
10. Cliver DO: Foodborne Diseases. San Diego, CA: Academic Press, 1990
11. Doyle MP: Foodborne bacterial pathogens. New York: Marcel Dekker, 1989
12. Tauxe RV: *Salmonella*: A postmodern pathogen. J Food Prot 54: 563–568, 1991
13. Humphrey JJ, Baskerville A, Mawer S, Rowe B, Hopper S: *Salmonella enteritidis* phage type 4 from the contents of intact eggs: a study involving naturally infected hens. Epidemiol Infect 103:415–423, 1989
14. Hackney CR, Dicharry A: Seafood-borne bacterial pathogens of marine origin. Food Technol 42(3):104–109, 1988
15. Holmberg SD: Cholera related illnesses caused by *Vibrio* species and *Aeromonas*. In Gorbach SL, Bartlett, JG, Blacklow NR (eds): Infectious Disease. Philadelphia: WB Saunders, 1992, pp 605–611
16. Popovic T, Olsvik O, Blake PA, Wachsmuth K: Cholera in the Americas: foodborne aspects. J Food Prot 56:811–821, 1993
17. Tacket CO, Brenner F, Blake PA: Clinical features and an epidemiological study of *Vibrio vulnificus* infections. J Infect Dis 149:558–561, 1984
18. Blake PA, Weaver RE, Hollis DG: Diseases of humans (other than cholera) caused by vibrios. Annu Rev Microbiol 34:341–367, 1980
19. Recommendations by the National Advisory Committee on Microbiological Criteria for Foods: microbiological criteria for raw molluscan shellfish. J Food Prot 55:463–480, 1992
20. Tarr PI: *Escherichia coli* O157:H7: overview of clinical and epidemiological issues. J Food Prot 57:632–637, 1994
21. Padhye NV, Doyle MP: *Escherichia coli* O157:H7: epidemiology, pathogenesis, and methods for detection in food. J Food Prot 55:555–565, 1992
22. Lee WH: An assessment of *Yersinia enterocolitica* and its presence in foods. J Food Prot 40:486–489, 1977
23. Blaser MJ, Berkowitz ID, LaForce FM, Cravens J, Reller LB, Wang W-LL: *Campylobacter* enteritis: clinical and epidemiological features. Ann Intern Med 91:179–185, 1979
24. The National Advisory Committee on Microbiological Criteria for Foods: *Campylobacter jejuni/coli*. J Food Prot 57:1101–1121, 1994

25. Farber JM, Peterkin PI: *Listeria monocytogenes*, a food-borne pathogen. Microbiol Rev 55:476–511, 1991
26. Buchanan RL, Palumbo SA: *Aeromonas hydrophila* and *Aeromonas sobria* as potential food poisoning species: a review. J Food Safety 7:15–29, 1985
27. Cliver DO: Viral foodborne disease agents of concern. J Food Prot 57:176–178, 1994
28. Cliver DO: Epidemiology of viral foodborne diseases. J Food Prot 57:263–266, 1994
29. Jelinek CF, Braude GL: Management of sludge use on land. J Food Prot 41:476–480, 1978
30. Smith JL: *Cryptosporidium* and *Giardia* as agents of foodborne disease. J Food Prot 56:451–461, 1993
31. Smith JL: Documented outbreaks of toxoplasmosis: Transmission of *Toxoplasma gondii* to humans. J Food Prot 56:630–639, 1993
32. Minor TE, Marth EH: *Staphylococcus aureus* and staphylococcal food intoxications. A review. III. Staphylococci in dairy foods. J Milk Food Technol 35:77–82, 1972
33. Minor TE, Marth EH: Staphylococci and Their Significance in Foods. New York: Elsevier, 1976
34. Centers for Disease Control: Staphylococcal food poisoning associated with Genoa and hard salami—United States. MMWR 28:179–180, 1979
35. Centers for Disease Control: International outbreak of Type E botulism associated with ungutted, salted whitefish. MMWR 36:812–813, 1987
36. Biehl ML, Buck WB: Chemical contaminants: their metabolism and their residues. J Food Prot 50:1058–1073, 1989
37. Bullerman LB, Buchanan RL: Mycotoxins other than aflatoxins—their relationships to food safety. Introduction. J Food Prot 44:701, 707, 1981
38. Harrison MA: Presence and stability of patulin in apple products: a review. J Food Safety 9:147–153, 1989
39. Labuza TP: Regulation of mycotoxins in foods. J Food Prot 46: 260–265, 1983
40. Gecan JS, Cichowicz SM: Toxic mushroom contamination of wild mushrooms in commercial distribution. J Food Prot 56:730–734, 1993
41. Ahmed FA: National Academy of Sciences: Seafood Safety. Washington, DC: National Academy Press, 1991
42. Taylor S: Marine toxins of microbial origin. Food Technol 42(3): 94–98, 1988
43. Graneli E, Sundstrom B, Edler L, Anderson DM: Toxic marine phytoplankton. New York: Elsevier, 1990
44. Todd ECD: Domoic acid and amnesic shellfish poisoning—a review. J Food Prot 56:69–83, 1993
45. Taylor SL: Histamine food poisoning: toxicology and clinical aspects. Crit Rev Toxicol 17:91–128, 1986
46. Reilly C: Metal Contamination of Food. London: Applied Science Publishers, 1980
47. Petersen B, Chaisson C: Pesticides and residues in food. Food Technol 42(7):59–64, 1988
48. Centers for Disease Control: Aldicarb food poisoning from contaminated melons—California. MMWR 35:254–258, 1986
49. Harris RW, Elsea WR: Ceramic glaze as a source of lead poisoning. JAMA 202:544–546, 1967
50. US Department of Agriculture, Food Safety and Inspection Service: Pathogen reduction; hazard analysis and critical control point (HACCP) systems; action: Final rule with request for comments. 9 CFR Parts 304, 308, 310, 320, 327, 381, 416, and 417. Federal Register 61(144):38805, 1996
51. Food and Drug Administration/Milk Industry Foundation/International Ice Cream Association: Recommended guidelines for controlling environmental contamination in dairy plants. Dairy Food Environ Sanitation 8:52–56, 1988
52. Gabis D, Faust RE: Controlling microbial growth in food processing environments. Food Technol 42(12):81–83, 1988
53. Food and Drug Administration: Current good manufacturing practice in manufacturing, processing, packing, or holding human food. Part 110, Title 21, Code of Federal Regulations, 1995
54. Food and Drug Administration: Procedures for the safe and sanitary processing and importing of fish and fishery products; final rule. 21 CFR Parts 123 and 1240. Federal Register 60(242):65096, 1995
55. Stevenson KE, Bernard DT: HACCP: Establishing Hazard Analysis Critical Control Point Programs. Washington, D.C.: The Food Processors Institute, 1995
56. Noleto AL, Bergdoll MS: Production of enterotoxin by a *Staphylococcus aureus* strain that produces three identifiable enterotoxins. J Food Prot 45:1096–1097, 1982
57. American Meat Institute Foundation: HACCP: The Hazard Analysis Critical Control Point System in the Meat and Poultry Industry. Washington, DC: American Meat Institute Foundation, 1994
58. Potter NN, Hotchkiss JH: Food Science. 5th ed. New York: Chapman & Hall, 1995
59. Jay JM: Modern Food Microbiology. 5th ed. New York: Chapman & Hall, 1996
60. Sawyer CA, Naidu YM, Thompson S: Cook/chill foodservice systems: microbiological quality and endpoint temperature of beef loaf, peas and potatoes after reheating by conduction, convection and microwave radiation. J Food Prot 46:1036–1043, 1983
61. Fruin JT, Guthertz LS: Survival of bacteria in food cooked by microwave oven, conventional oven, and slow cookers. J Food Prot 45:695–698, 1982
62. Lechowich RV: Microbiological challenges of refrigerated foods. Food Technol 42(12):84–89, 1988
63. Scott VN: Interaction of factors to control microbial spoilage of refrigerated foods. J Food Prot 52:431–435, 1989
64. Nitrite Safety Council: A survey of nitrosamines in sausages and dry-cured meat products. Food Technol 34:45–53, 1980
65. Hotchkiss JH, Cassens RG: Nitrate, nitrite, and nitroso compounds in foods. Food Technol 41(4):127–134, 1987
66. Stevenson DD, Simon RA: Sensitivity to ingested metabisulfites in asthmatic subjects. J Allergy Clin Immunol 68:26, 1981
67. Schwartz HJ: Sensitivity to ingested metabisulfite: variations in clinical presentation. J Allergy Clin Immunol 71:487–489, 1983
68. Ingram M, Roberts TA: Ionizing irradiation. In Microbial Ecology of Foods. vol 1. New York: Academic Press, 1980, pp 46–47
69. Radomyski T, Murano EA, Olson DG, Murano PS: Elimination of pathogens of significance in food by low-dose irradiation: a review. J Food Prot 57:73–86, 1994
70. World Health Organization: Wholesomeness of Irradiated Food. World Health Organization Technical Report Series, No. 659. Geneva: World Health Organization, 1981
71. Institute of Food Technologists: Radiation preservation of foods. Food Technol 37:55–60, 1983
72. Skala JH, McGown EL, Waring PP: Wholesomeness of irradiated foods. J Food Prot 50:150–160, 1987

37

Water Quality Management

John B. Conway[a]

Water is a necessity for human survival. Wholesome and abundant, it supports and enriches life. Unwholesome or scarce, it is a threat to health and to life itself. This chapter concerns the adequacy and quality of water in the service of people.

The amount of water in the world is fixed, some 3.59×10^{20} gallons in all. Only about 0.2 percent of this is fresh water, readily available for use. Fresh waters run to the sea and become saline, but evaporation of water from the seas and precipitation on land, the hydrologic cycle, restores these fresh waters continuously so that the quantity of fresh water is relatively fixed.

Water resources were sufficient for all purposes in early settlements, yet there were still instances where communities disappeared because of declining water supplies. The current water crisis has arisen from population growth and urbanization, which puts pressure on the fixed sources of fresh water available locally. These pressures have created problems in maintaining the quantity and quality of the water supply. An increasing investment will be necessary to provide a safe water supply and to maintain its quality. This chapter discusses the provision of a safe and adequate water supply and the sanitary removal of wastewaters from communities.

▶ USES OF WATER

The uses of water include (*a*) drinking and culinary purposes; (*b*) personal cleanliness, including bathing and laundering; (*c*) household cleanliness; (*d*) heating and air conditioning; (*e*) urban irrigation; (*f*) street cleaning; (*g*) recreational purposes, including swimming pools and the watering of playing fields; (*h*) amenity purposes, such as public fountains and ornamental ponds; (*i*) power production from hydropower and steam power; (*j*) commercial and industrial purposes, including industrial process waters and cooling; (*k*) fire protection; (*l*) agricultural purposes, including irrigation; and (*m*) carrying away wastes from all manner of establishments.

The quantities required for each use vary substantially. In a typical American community, the average per capita consumption is between 50 and 100 gallons per day (Tables 37-1 and 37-2). In summer, the demand may increase by 50 percent, mainly because of increased urban irrigation. It has been suggested that this per capita water usage can be substantially reduced and this is illustrated in Table 37-3. In Asia and Africa, per capita consumption may be only 13 gallons per day.

[a] *This chapter is an edited version of the chapter previously prepared by Daniel A. Okun.*

▶ WATER SYSTEMS

To serve these uses, communities require sources of water, transmission pumps and mains, treatment plants, and distribution systems for delivering water to each user. Transmission systems and treatment plants should be designed for the maximum day, which occurs generally in summer and is about 150 percent of the average demand. The distribution system should meet the peak demand during the day, which may be 150 to 300 percent of the maximum day demand, being larger for smaller communities where the peak is determined by requirements for fire protection. Also necessary is a sewerage system for collecting the wastewaters from each user in the community and treatment facilities for rendering the wastewaters suitable for disposal or reuse. Some 80 percent of the population of the United States in more than 60,000 communities is served by water supply and sewerage systems. The remaining population, not always in rural areas, is served by individual wells and on-site disposal systems, generally septic tanks and tile fields for percolation of the septic tank effluents.

▶ PROPERTIES OF WATER

Water is a unique substance. "Pure" water is a clear, colorless, tasteless, and odorless fluid. It is a strong solvent, and in nature it washes gases from the atmosphere, dissolves minerals and humic substances from the soil through which it flows, and carries substantial quantities of silt. Many of the uses to which water is put further affect its quality. Accordingly, water is seldom useful without some kind of treatment. In addition, microorganisms find their way into waters and, depending on circumstances, may prosper or die. Some of these microorganisms are beneficial or at least not harmful. Others may be pathogenic. Many scourges of mankind have been waterborne, and the potential for spread of enteric disease is always present.

At normal atmospheric pressure, water freezes at 0°C and boils at 100°C. Because it has its greatest density at 4°C, ice floats on the surface, keeping bodies of water from freezing solid, an important phenomenon that keeps aquatic creatures alive and permits lakes and reservoirs to serve as sources of water even at subfreezing temperatures. The specific heat of water is high, resulting in the ameliorating effects of large water bodies on climate and temperature. The surface tension of water is also high, resulting in the concentration of many contaminants on its surface in monomolecular layers.

Water is an important constituent of living matter, constituting about 70 percent of the weight of the human body. It is a medium for transferring nutrients and waste materials as well as maintaining thermostability through heat transfer and evaporation. The water intake of an adult varies from 1 to 3 quarts per day, about half of which is lost through the skin and lungs and the other half in feces and urine.

TABLE 37-1. WATER USE IN U.S. COMMUNITIES

Use	%
Residential	40
Commercial	15
Industrial	25
Public	5
Unaccounted for	15
Total	100

It is this latter half that needs to be managed properly if adequate sanitation is to be maintained and the spread of disease avoided. Water management involves protecting water supplies for people from damage by people.

▶ SOURCES OF WATER

Water may be abstracted for use from any one of a number of points in its movement through the hydrological cycle shown in Figure 37-1. The specific source to be developed for any community depends on the quantity and quality of the source and its case of development. The selection of the most suitable source can come from any of the various options available. The most common sources of water are listed below.[1]

Rainwater

Rainwater is the source of all fresh water. It may be collected directly from roofs and other prepared catchments and stored in cisterns. Because catchment areas for the direct capture of rainwater are necessarily limited in size, such supplies are useful only for individual households or small communities. Households in the Southwest are examples of the former, and paved catchments in Gibraltar are examples of the latter. The quality of rainwater is generally good, being free of minerals, but it may be contaminated by gases and particles it washes out of the atmosphere and by the accumulation of dust and other debris on the catchments. For example, gaseous sulfur and nitrogen oxides are emitted from power plants that use fossil fuels. These gases react with atmospheric water, forming dilute solutions of sulfuric and nitric acids. The precipitation of these acids ("acid rain") has begun to have serious impacts on surface water quality and on the biota that depend upon water.

TABLE 37-2. ALLOCATION OF INTERIOR RESIDENTIAL WATER USE

Use	%
Drinking and cooking	5
Bathing	30
Toilet flushing	40
Laundering	15
Dishwashing	5
Miscellaneous	5
Total	100

Surface Water

The earliest sources of water for large communities were rivers and lakes, which readily afforded the quantity needed. The large drainage areas required for such run-of-river or lake supplies inevitably sub-

TABLE 37-3. COMPARISON OF AVERAGE DAILY, PERSONAL WATER USE EMPLOYING WATER CONSERVATION PRACTICES OR FIXTURES VERSUS NORMAL WATER USE[a]

Activity	*Frequency*	*Circumstances*	*Water Used*	*Total*
Toilet	4 flushes/day	Ultra-low flush toilet	1.6 gal./flush	6 gal.[b]
		Conventional toilet	3.5–7 gal./flush	14–28 gal.
Shower	Once/day for 5 min	Low-flow showerhead	2.5 gal./min.	12 gal.[b]
		Conventional head	3–8 gal./min.	15–40 gal.
Bath	Once/day	Tub ¼ to ⅓ full	9–12 gal.	9–12 gal.
		Full tub	36 gal.	36 gal.
Shaving	Once/day	1 full basin	1 gal.	1 gal.[b]
		Open tap	5–10 gal.	5–10 gal.
Brushing teeth	Twice/day	Brush and rinse	¼–½ gal.	½–1 gal.[b]
		Open tap	2–5 gal.	4–10 gal.
Washing hands	Twice/day	1 full basin	1 gal.	2 gal.[b]
		Open tap	2 gal.	4 gal.[b]
Cooking[c]	Washing produce	1 full kitchen basin	1–2 gal.	1–2 gal.[b]
		Open tap	5–10 gal.	5–10 gal.
Automatic dishwasher	Once/day full load	Short cycle	8–13 gal.	8–13 gal.
		Standard cycle	10–15 gal.	10–15 gal.
Manual dishwashing	Once/day	Full basin/wash and rinse	5 gal.	5 gal.[b]
		Open tap	30 gal.	30 gal.
Laundry[d]	⅓ load/day	Portion of full load	35–50 gal./Full load	10–15 gal.[b]
Lawn, trees, and shrubs	Watering requirements vary with plant species, type of turf, season, region, and soil type. Consult your local nursery or county horticulture agent.			
Car washing	Twice/mo.	5 full, 2-gal. buckets	20 gal./mo.	⅓ gal.
		Hose with shut-off nozzle	100 gal./mo.	⅗ gal.

[a] Numbers are based on approximate, average household use. Water use will vary with individual habits and lifestyles, differing water pressure, and the age and model of appliances.

[b] Total = about 40 gallons, plus 10 gallons for outdoor use = 50 gallons per day.

[c] Real cooking figure will be higher to include boiling water, rinsing utensils, and other uses.

[d] Laundry figure is based on two full loads per person, per week.

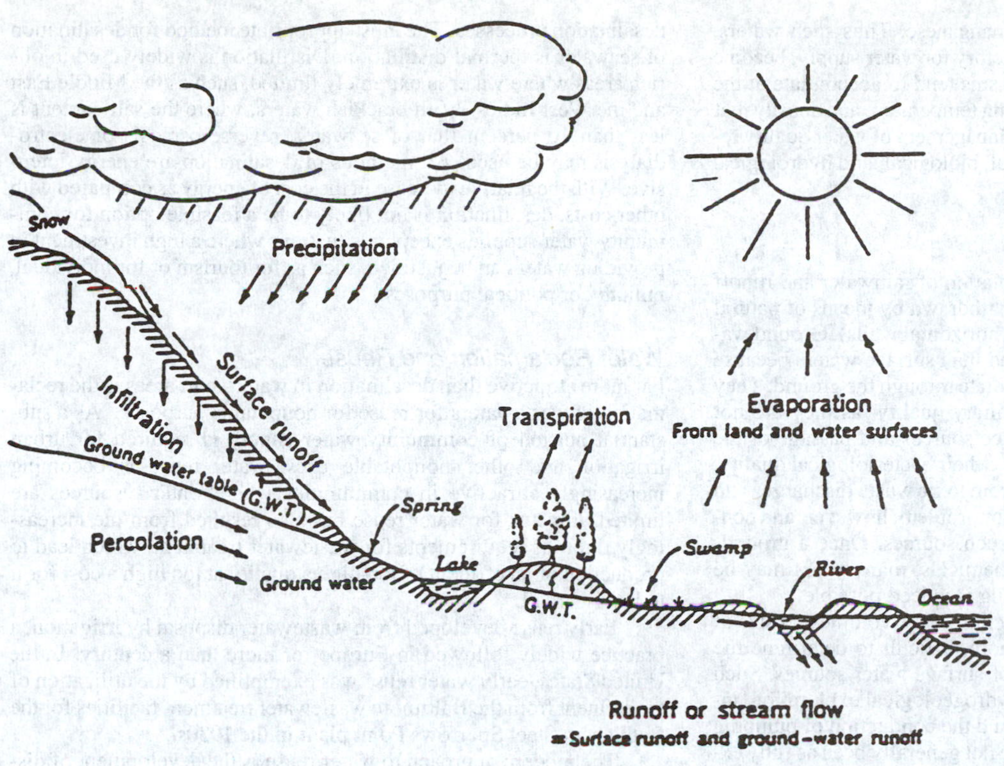

Figure 37-1. The water cycle. (From Fair GM, Geyer J, Okun DA: Elements of Water Supply and Wastewater Disposal. New York: John Wiley & Sons, 1971.)

ject them to activities, such as urban and industrial development, that results in quality degradation. Water supplies for Philadelphia, Cincinnati, and New Orleans are typical of run-of-river supplies. Such supplies have historically been the source of waterborne epidemics (e.g., in the nineteenth century) and still pose disease hazards in situations where treatment is inadequate, as in the developing countries of Asia, Africa, and Latin America. The development of filtration and disinfection of water by chlorination at about the turn of the century rendered such waters free of pathogenic organisms and suitable for community supplies. Since the onset of the chemical revolution beginning in the mid-twentieth century, waters obtained from large watersheds, such as those of the Ohio and Mississippi rivers, inevitably contain numerous synthetic organic chemicals used in cities, industry, and on farms, some of which have been identified as being carcinogenic, mutagenic, teratogenic, or otherwise toxic. These chemicals are not easily removed in wastewater or water treatment or in the environment during passage downstream, so that use of such sources is once again brought into question. It was the identification of many synthetic organic chemicals in the lower Mississippi River that provided the impetus for the passage of the Safe Drinking Water Act (PL 93-523) in 1974. The groundwork for this act has been laid by the Community Water Supply Survey conducted by the Public Health Service (PHS) in 1969,[2] which indicated that many public water supplies, particularly those serving small communities, were not providing adequate service and were not in a position to meet the requirements of the 1962 PHS Drinking Water Standards.

A safer option is the use of smaller watersheds, which do not have naturally sustained flows during all periods of the year, but by the storage of wet-weather flows in impounding reservoirs, can provide substantial quantities of water for use during dry periods. Such small watersheds are generally found in upland areas and are often free of the major urban and industrial development that results in the chemical pollution that is now a growing concern.

Boston, New York, and San Francisco are examples of cities that have developed upstream sources. The quality of these upstream sources has often been so high that up to now the only treatment required is disinfection. Pressure for development of such heretofore protected watersheds is now threatening to degrade them, and special efforts will be required in the future to identify such protected watersheds and preserve them. The watershed area serving New York City is currently undergoing extensive evaluation, and increased protection measures may have to be implemented.

Natural and human-made lakes may improve or degrade waters drawn from their watersheds. Storage in a lake provides opportunities for coagulation and sedimentation of colloidal and suspended solids that are tributary to the lake. Some measure of disinfection is accomplished by exposure to sunlight, provided there is time for biochemical stabilization of organic matter and for die-away of microorganisms. Furthermore, storage in a lake or reservoir attenuates high levels of contaminants that may result from rainstorms or accidents on the watershed, such as spills from tankers.

On the other hand, storage in lakes or reservoirs may degrade water quality through eutrophication, biomagnification, and thermal stratification. Eutrophication, or overnourishing, of a water body occurs naturally as a result of the influent of nutrient materials, particularly phosphorus and nitrogen, which support the growth of algae. In a standing body of water with adequate sunlight, these nutrients tend to accumulate in the algae. As the algae settle, the lake tends slowly to fill, a process that naturally might take a considerable length of time. Development on a watershed, particularly urbanization and agriculture, adds significantly to sediment and nutrient input to the lake; the former reduces the capacity of lakes, and the latter accelerates the process of eutrophication to the point where many of the uses of the lake are adversely affected. The increasing concentrations of algae are difficult to remove in water treatment, and they often impart unpleasant taste and odors to the water. Another impact of storage is the bioaccumulation of small concentrations of chemicals and other contaminants that are taken up by aquatic life in the lake. These may affect the quality of fish taken from the lake and may also increase the levels of these contaminants beyond what they would be in a slowing river.

Lake quality is further affected by thermal stratification. During the summer, the warmer, lighter water accumulates in the upper layers of the lake. The density difference is sufficient to interfere with mixing, thereby preventing the lower layers of the lake from obtaining atmospheric oxygen. Organic matter reduces the dissolved oxygen in the lower levels of the lake, often resulting in anaerobic conditions, with the accumulation of hydrogen sulfide and carbon dioxide, and because of the increasing acidity under such circumstances, increasing solution of such metals as iron and manganese. Thus such waters, which may otherwise have been satisfactory for water supply, become exceedingly troublesome. Microorganisms tend to accumulate at the thermocline, the zone of rapidly changing temperature and density that separates the upper and lower layers. Management of water quality requires an understanding of the chemical, biological, and hydrological phenomena that occur in such waters.

Ground Water

Ground waters are recharged by percolation of rainwater and runoff through the ground. Ground water is withdrawn by means of natural springs, wells, or infiltration galleries (horizontal wells). Ground waters tend to be more highly mineralized than surface waters because of the solution of minerals as they percolate through the ground. They are, however, generally of higher sanitary quality, as they are not nearly so subject to pollution as surface sources and passage of the water through the soil serves to improve their bacteriological quality. Ground-water pollution, particularly from toxic waste discharges and leaching of landfills, has become a major problem, however, and considerable care is required to protect such sources. Once a ground-water aquifer is contaminated with chemicals, many years may be required for it to be cleansed, if cleaning is indeed possible.

Yields of ground waters are a function of the volume and size of soil interstices. In general, it is far more difficult to determine the yields of ground-water sources than of surface water sources. Such determinations depend on extensive hydrogeological exploration, including the construction of test wells and the conduction of pumping tests. Accordingly, ground waters have not generally been as fully exploited as they might be and have been used primarily for smaller communities. On the other hand, some ground-water supplies have been overpumped, or "mined," where withdrawals have exceeded recharge. This has resulted in a steady lowering of the elevation of the water surface underground, the *water table*, diminishing the amount that can be withdrawn and increasing the cost of pumping. Such excessive withdrawals have also had a bearing on the ground above, threatening structures and increasing the potential for flooding.

The use of ground waters in association with surface waters is only now beginning to be explored. Underground reservoirs have major advantages over surface water reservoirs: they do not lose water through evaporation; their quality is not so likely to be deleteriously affected by natural or urban and industrial pollution; and they do not require the expropriation of large areas of land. Also, they may be located nearer to the points of use than are surface impoundments. In a combined use, water would be drawn from surface sources during wet periods while ground-water reservoirs are recharged. During dry periods, withdrawal would be from underground. Planning for such combined use requires engineering and hydrological study.

A special category of underground source is the artesian aquifer, a confined aquifer under pressure. Such an aquifer is recharged at a higher elevation some distance away. When it is tapped by a well, the water in the well rises above the confining layer and may often be free flowing. Flowing springs originate from artesian aquifers because they are under pressure. Artesian aquifers are less likely to be contaminated than unconfined aquifers.

Wells are constructed in a variety of ways and configurations, depending on the nature of the aquifer from which the water is to be withdrawn. Special precautions are required, however, to ensure that wells are protected from surface water runoff by being encased properly, with the casing extending above ground surface.

After construction, wells must be disinfected before being tested for water quality. Sampling of water from a well is, however, pointless if the *sanitary survey* indicates that the well is not protected from contamination by surface runoff. A sample taken during a dry period may show good quality, but the water will inevitably be contaminated by surface runoff if the well is not adequately protected.

Ocean and Brackish Waters

These are unsuitable for water supply but, in conditions of dire necessity, fresh water can be obtained from them by one of several desalination processes. The most appropriate method for desalination of seawater is thermal distillation. Distillation is widely used in oil-rich areas where water is extremely limited, such as the Middle East and the West Indies. With brackish waters, where the salt content is less than 10 percent that of seawater, reverse osmosis or electrodialysis may be used. All methods of desalination are energy intensive. With the relative increase in the cost of energy as compared with other costs, desalination is not likely to be a feasible option for community water supplies except in situations where a high investment in providing water can be justified, such as for tourism or for individual, military, or political purposes.

Water Reclamation and Reuse

Far more attractive than desalination in water-short areas is the reclamation of wastewaters for reuse for nonpotable purposes.[3] As a substantial portion of community water supply is required for urban irrigation and other nonpotable uses, water reuse is becoming increasingly attractive in communities where water resources are limited. Impetus for water reuse has also resulted from the increasingly rigorous requirements for wastewater treatment, which lead to production of an effluent of too high a quality at too high a cost for it to be discarded.

Early reuse developed from wastewater disposal by irrigation, a practice widely followed in Europe for more than a century. In the United States, early water reuse was exemplified by the utilization of the effluent from the Baltimore wastewater treatment facilities for the Bethlehem Steel Sparrows Point plant in the 1930s.

The modern approach to water reuse is the development of distribution systems for nonpotable waters for a variety of purposes, including urban irrigation, residential, and industrial use. Such dual distribution systems were pioneered in Colorado Springs, Colorado; Pomona and Irvine, California; and St. Petersburg, Florida. In these instances, the nonpotable distribution systems carry secondary wastewater effluent additionally treated by coagulation, filtration, and disinfection, processes used for treatment of potable waters drawn from polluted sources. Inadvertent ingestion of water from such a nonpotable system would not be a source of waterborne disease. The main difference between the potable and nonpotable waters would be that the nonpotable waters, having as their source the wastewaters of a community, would not be free of the chemicals that are inevitably present in such wastewaters and that are not removed in wastewater or water supply treatment, but that are hazardous if ingested over a long period of time.

In 1958 the United Nations Economic and Social Council stated, "No higher quality water, unless there is a surplus of it, should be used for a purpose that can tolerate a lower grade."[4] This policy is beginning to be adopted in water-short areas of the United States. In Florida, for example, where consumptive use permits are required for all abstractions of water, the policy is that a permit will not be issued if a lower-quality water can be used and is available. Nonpotable reuse is becoming so widely adopted that the American Water Works Association has published a *Manual on Dual Distribution Systems*,[5] and some 14 states have adopted regulations for water reclamation and reuse.

In San Diego, California, at least one builder will provide a collection system for gray water from showers, bath tubs, and washing machines that can then be used to flush toilets, water the lawn, etc. The cost of this additional plumbing is less than $2,000.

Selection of Sources

A community and its engineers facing the need to provide a community's water supply must recognize that each situation is unique. Topography, climate, the availability of untapped water resources, population density, land use, and myriad other characteristics help differentiate one situation from another; none is precisely like that of any other community. The guiding principle in the selection of the source is provided in the National Interim Primary Drinking Water Regulations promulgated by the U.S. Environmental Protection Agency (EPA) in 1976:

> Production of water that poses no threat to the consumer's health depends on continuous protection. Because of human frailties associated with protection, priority should be given to the selection of the *purest source*. Polluted sources should not be used unless other sources are economically unavailable, and then only when personnel, equipment, and operating procedures can be depended on to purify and otherwise continuously protect the drinking water supply.[6] (Emphasis added.)

Earlier drinking water standards established by the U.S. Public Health Service expressed similar sentiments. Because the primary concern with water quality had been transmission of waterborne infectious disease, and because conventional filtration and disinfection with chlorine had ensured protection against such disease, many cities throughout the United States opted for run-of-river supplies that were conveniently available, even though they did not constitute the "purest" source. The relatively new threat to health arising from the "chemical revolution," with the creation of many new long-lasting synthetic organic chemicals, has given new meaning to the concern for selecting the purest source, particularly because methods of monitoring for many of these chemicals are not yet available. Given options in the selection of sources, prudence dictates a search for the purest source. This might mean development of ground waters or upstream sources free of urban and industrial pollution. Where these are not adequate in quantity to provide all the water required in a community, consideration must be given for potable purposes; and polluted sources or reclaimed wastewaters, for nonpotable purposes.

Protection of Sources

Where high-quality sources of water supply are available, whether surface or underground, they are subject to despoliation from development on the watershed or recharge areas. Only in rare instances is the land on the watershed or recharge area under the control of the water purveyor; these areas are generally the responsibility of the local authorities that have planning jurisdiction. Even where the water purveyor owns the land or the local authority that has dominion over the land is served by the water supply, the pressure of development can lead to degradation of the water supply.

In a landmark case, water companies in Connecticut sought to sell off portions of their wholly owned protected watersheds for development. After considerable study, legislation was enacted that forbade the sale of watershed lands for development. In response to a suit against the State of Connecticut by the water companies, the U.S. District Court upheld the State:

> . . . the obvious purpose of the legislation is the protection of the health and welfare of the State's inhabitants . . . watershed properties are critical to water purity . . . the State is ensuring the ability of the water companies to provide pure water to its customers.[7]

More generally, local authorities have planning jurisdiction over watershed lands and recharge areas, and they must work closely with the water purveyor in developing land use strategies that would protect the integrity of the water supplies. Such strategies would include regulations specifying maximum densities, limits for impervious areas, setbacks from the banks of streams and reservoirs, permissible activities, etc.[8,9] The promulgation and enforcement of such regulations require great courage and leadership on the part of elected and appointed officials because they sharply curtail the opportunities for financial profit from development.

While the greatest attention is generally given to the numerical limits for specific contaminants, far more attention needs to be given to the "sanitary survey," which can ensure a high quality of water and its adequate handling and distribution to the user. The regulations state:

> Knowledge of physical defects or of the existence of other health hazards in the water supply system is evidence of a deficiency in protection of the water supply. Even though water quality analysis have indicated that the quality requirements have been met, the deficiencies must be corrected before the supply can be considered safe.[6]

Obvious deficiencies include pollution of the source, inadequate treatment, cross-connections with sources of contamination, inadequate capacity resulting in low pressure, and inadequate operation of the facilities, including inadequate disinfection and failure to provide standby facilities in the event of power or other equipment failure.

In contention is whether or not the discharge of a pollutant upstream of the water intake is a deficiency. While many laws exist directed to the prevention of the discharge of toxic substances into the environment in general and water bodies in particular, implementation of these laws is uncertain at best. Little assurance can be given that a water supply drawn from a source that drains large urban and industrial areas will, in fact, be free of potentially harmful chemicals. The best course is to avoid discharging wastes above water supply intakes and to avoid installing intakes below waste discharges.

▶ POTABLE WATER QUALITY

In the United States, protection of the public health was initially a responsibility of the states, with federal initiatives only where interstate activities were concerned. The U.S. Public Health Service Drinking Water Standards were first adopted in 1914 to protect the health of the traveling public. These standards were often adopted by individual states and came to be applicable to water supplies generally. Initially, because of their limited application, primary emphasis was on physical and bacterial parameters, the first to ensure esthetic quality and the second to prevent the transmission of waterborne disease. These standards were updated periodically. In 1962, the standards were extensively revised to include chemicals and radioactivity for the first time. The only chemicals for which limits were established were heavy metals. Recognition of the problem of synthetic organic chemicals surfaced with the establishment of an upper limit for carbon chloroform extract (CCE). This served as a comprehensive, gross surrogate for synthetic organic chemicals, although it could not distinguish between those chemicals that are innocuous and those harmful to health. These standards required systems that have adequate capacity to meet peak demands without development of low pressures or other health hazards, that the quality be assessed at the free-flowing outlet of the consumer, and that the facilities be under the responsible charge of personnel whose qualifications are acceptable to the regulatory agency.

It was not until passage of the Safe Drinking Water Act (SDWA) in 1974 that public water supply systems in the United States came under the federal aegis. Under this law, the National Interim Primary Drinking Water Regulations were established and maximum contaminant levels (MCLs) were set. They are summarized in Table 37-4.[6] Contaminants not directly related to safety but only to esthetic quality are called secondary maximum contaminant levels (SMCLs) and are summarized in Table 37-5. For the first time, six synthetic organic chemicals, all well-known biocides, were included. However, no measure of total synthetic organic chemical concentration was called for. The 70,000 chemicals now in commercial production and the thousand or so introduced each year, many of which reach water sources, were ignored.

The SDWA mandated that the National Academy of Sciences (National Research Council) conduct studies on the health effects associated with contaminants found in drinking water. A series of nine reports has been published under the title *Drinking Water and Health*.[10] The first, published in 1977, is a 939-page compendium of health effects associated with microbiological, radioactive, particulate, inorganic, and organic chemical contaminants found in drinking water, including risk assessments for cancer resulting from exposure to chemical contaminants in drinking water. The others, published through 1989, add information on chlorination and disinfection byproducts in water, toxicology, epidemiological risks, risk assessments

TABLE 37-4. NATIONAL INTERIM PRIMARY DRINKING WATER REGULATIONS (MAXIMUM CONTAMINANT LEVELS)

Contaminant	MCL
■ **INORGANIC CHEMICALS**	
Arsenic	0.05 (mg/L)
Barium	1
Cadmium	0.010
Chromium	0.05
Fluoride	1.4–2.4
Lead	0.05
Mercury	0.002
Nitrate (as N)	10
Selenium	0.01
Silver	0.05
□ **ORGANIC CHEMICALS**	
Chlorinated hydrocarbons	
Endrin	0.0002
Lindane	0.004
Methoxychlor	0.1
Toxaphene	0.005
Chlorophenoxys	
2,4-D	0.1
2,4,5-T, Silvex	0.01
■ **TRIHALOMETHANES**	0.100
■ **TURBIDITY**	1 unit
■ **MICROBIOLOGIC CONTAMINANTS**	1 coliform bacterium/100 mL as the arithmetical mean of all samples/month
■ **RADIOACTIVITY**	
Combined radium 226 and radium 228	5 pCi/L
Gross α particle activity (including radium 226 but excluding radon and uranium)	15 pCi/L
Average annual concentration of β particle and photon radioactivity not to produce annual dose	not to produce annual dose equivalent greater than 4 mrem per year
Tritium	20,000 pCi/L
Strontium 90	8 pCi/L

on additional chemicals, pharmacokinetics, and suggested no-adverse-response levels (SNARLs) for acute and chronic exposures to chemicals in drinking water.

In 1981, an MCL was added for trihalomethanes (THMs), including chloroform, formed by the reaction of chlorine used for disinfection with water containing organics. An interesting aspect of the THM standard was that it was not to apply to communities of less than 10,000 population because the technology involved in meeting and monitoring for the standard was believed to be beyond the resources of such small communities, which make up more than 95 percent of community water supplies in the United States.

Troubled by the slow pace of establishment of new MCLs, the Congress enacted amendments to the Safe Drinking Water Act in 1986, which represented a quantum increase in requirements for the regulation of the quality of drinking water. The principal revision was that new contaminants are to be added to the regulations in a timely fashion, with a total of 83 by 1989 and at least 25 new contaminants every 3 years thereafter. In addition, MCL goals (MCLGs) are to be established for each contaminant at a level at which no known adverse effects on health would occur and that allows an adequate margin of safety. For known carcinogens, MCLGs are set at zero. The MCL is to be as close to the MCLG as is feasible. The promulgation of these MCLs and MCLGs is behind schedule.

Only the contaminants listed in Table 37-6, all volatile organic chemicals, had been added by 1989. Other contaminants have been proposed for regulation, including a priority list that may be considered for inclusion in the regulations in the future. A major problem for water purveyors and local regulatory authorities is that the new regulations are published piecemeal, as they are approved, in the *Federal Register* and no single publication that codifies all the regulations is available 14 years after the Interim Regulations[6] were published.

Other regulations mandated by the 1986 Amendments to the SDWA include:

- The establishment of the best available technology (BAT) to meet the MCLs and MCLGs promulgated;
- Prohibition of the use of lead materials in water supply systems or in plumbing used to convey drinking water, with a requirement for public notice where lead is present and/or where the water is sufficiently corrosive to cause leaching of lead;
- Regulations for the protection of ground-water sources;
- Regulations specifying criteria under which filtration will be required for surface water sources, including quality of the source, vulnerability of the watershed to pollution, and protection offered by watershed management practices.

Among the criteria established to avoid filtration are the following:

- Fecal coliform ≤ 20/100 mL or total coliform ≤ 100/100 mL 90 percent of the time;
- Turbidity ≤ 5 nephelometric + urbidity unit (NTU) immediately before disinfection;
- Maintenance of a watershed control program that minimizes the potential for contamination by *Giardia lamblia* and viruses;
- Performance of an annual sanitary survey;
- Contiguous monitoring of disinfectant residual and maintenance of no less than 0.2 mg/L in the distribution system.

Altogether, regulations for the assurance of safe water are expected to be in continuous flux for the foreseeable future.

▶ CHEMICAL CONTAMINANTS

Maximum contaminant levels in drinking waters have been set for eight metals, nitrates, and fluorides and six organic chemicals plus trihalomethanes (THMs), as shown in Table 37-4. In arriving at MCLs,

TABLE 37-5. INTERIM NATIONAL SECONDARY DRINKING WATER REGULATIONS (SECONDARY MAXIMUM CONTAMINANT LEVELS)

Contaminant	SMCL
Chloride	250 mg/L
Color	15 color units
Copper	1 mg/L
Corrosivity	Noncorrosive
Foaming agents	0.5 mg/L
Hydrogen sulfide	0.5 mg/L
Iron	0.3 mg/L
Manganese	0.05 mg/L
Odor	3 threshold odor number
pH	6.5–8.5
Sulfate	250 mg/L
TDS	500 mg/L
Zinc	5 mg/L

TABLE 37-6. VOLATILE ORGANIC CHEMICAL ADDITIONS TO PRIMARY DRINKING WATER REGULATIONS IN TABLE 37-4

Contaminants	*MCL (mg/L)*	*MCLG (mg/L)*
Benzene	0.005	0
Carbon Tetrachloride	0.005	0
p-Dichlorobenzene	0.075	0.075
1,2-Dichloroethane	0.005	0
1,1-Dichloroethylene	0.007	0.007
1,1,1-Trichloroethane	0.20	0.20
Trichloroethane	0.005	0
Vinyl chloride	0.002	0

the total environmental exposure of humans to the specific toxin is considered. An attempt is made to set lifetime limits at the lowest practical level to minimize the amount of toxicant carried by water, particularly when other sources such as food or air are known to represent the major exposure. The toxicological basis for each of the limits is provided in the appendix of the Drinking Water Regulations and in the *Federal Register* from time to time as new contaminants are proposed for regulation.[6] Limits are not given for every toxicant or undesirable contaminant that might be in the public water supply, as scientific data are not available for many of the chemicals of concern. Also, the analytic burden for assessing the presence and concentration of all the chemicals of concern would be inordinately great. As it is, the determination of these chemicals requires experienced analysis and sophisticated instrumentation. Most larger water supply laboratories are equipped with atomic absorption spectrophotometers for determination of the metals. The gas chromatograph-mass spectrometers required for determination of the synthetic organics are many times more costly, however; and fewer laboratories are equipped for these determinations. Utilities with the more protected sources will have fewer monitoring problems.

Heavy Metals

Among the classes of contaminants, the MCLs for the heavy metals appear to rest on the firmest basis; however, the data on the health effects of many individual metals are not adequate, and the significance of combinations of contaminants has not been addressed. The MCLs for several metals, such as chromium and arsenic, are being re-evaluated, and even so ubiquitous a metal as aluminum, which is used as a coagulant in water treatment, is being examined for possible neurological significance.

Of all the heavy metals, lead is of greatest concern. The heaviest concentrations of lead in water supplies result from the use of lead service piping. Water remaining in lead pipes overnight, particularly soft waters, dissolve considerable lead. Lead is no longer authorized for piping, and existing lead-containing services should be gradually replaced. Meanwhile, customers with lead service pipes should allow the first flush of water each day to be wasted. Lead also originates from developments on watersheds, its load being a function of the length of streets in the area. The evidence is strong that even very low concentrations of lead are neurologically damaging to children, so that a reduction in the MCL for lead is expected in the next regulations. Also, an MCL and an MCLG of 1.3 mg/L for copper is being proposed.

Synthetic Organic Chemicals

Some 1,000 specific synthetic organic chemicals (SOCs), at nanogram to microgram per liter concentrations, have been identified in drinking water supplies in the United States. These compounds result from industrial and municipal discharges, urban road runoff, and reaction of chlorine in water treatment with natural organics.

The problem of the synthetic organic chemicals that originate from industrial and municipal discharges and urban runoff is far less tractable because of their vast number, their highly variable concentrations, and the uncertainty as to their presence.

Most of the organic chemicals identified in drinking water have not yet been examined for their health effects, and the National Research Council indicates that only about 10 percent of the organic chemicals in water have been identified. Where effects have been established, these are generally based on animal studies on individual contaminants, and there is uncertainty as to the actual risk posed to humans who ingest very low concentrations of combinations of contaminants over an extended period of time. Such epidemiological studies as have been made are far from definitive. The National Research Council studies[10] offer ample evidence of the uncertainties involved in establishing acceptable levels of trace contaminants. What can be stated with certainty is that the situation with regard to acceptable levels of synthetic organic chemicals in drinking water is constantly changing and will undergo continuous reassessment.

Accordingly, the most prudent approach lies in selecting sources of water that are free of urban and industrial pollution. Although this does not guarantee that they would not be subject to airborne contaminants and runoff from the land, these contaminants may be more readily identified and managed.

Chlorine Reaction Products. The problem of chlorine reaction products, and other disinfectant reaction products as well, is also troublesome. The MCL for THMs, 0.100 mg/L, had been established as an expedient, rather than on the same health-risk basis as for other contaminants, one additional death per 1 million population over 70 years' exposure. This MCL is expected to be lowered to 0.025 or 0.050 mg/L, which will still allow it at higher risk than other contaminants. Another chlorine reaction product, 3-chloro-4-(dichloromethyl)-5-hydroxy-2(5H)-furanone (labeled MX), has been found in drinking waters drawn from surface waters. Although present only at nanogram levels, its high mutagenicity (more than 1 millionfold greater than the THMs) makes MX potentially a far more serious reaction product than THMs, accounting for an estimated 15 to 60 percent of the total mutagenicity of chlorinated waters. One problem with MX is that it is nonvolatile and therefore is not easily measured.

The epidemiological significance of chlorine reaction products was established in a case-control study by the National Cancer Institute.[11] Through examination of some 8,000 persons, including 2,805 with bladder cancer, a significantly higher cancer risk was found for people who drank chlorinated surface tap water for at least 40 years than for people who drank unchlorinated ground water. Those who drank the most chlorinated water had twice the risk as the lowest tap water users. Among nonsmokers, the relative risk for more than 60 years' exposure was 3.1 as compared with nonsmokers using unchlorinated water. From these data, it was inferred that 12 percent of bladder cancer in the study population was caused by the chlorinated surface water.

Nitrates

A temporary blood disorder, methemoglobinemia, has occurred in infants after ingestion of well waters containing nitrates in concentrations greater than 10 mg/L of nitrogen. Some 2,000 cases of this disease have been reported in North America and Europe, with a 7 to 8 percent mortality rate. The disease results from the conversion in the gastrointestinal tract of innocuous nitrates to nitrites, which then convert hemoglobin to methemoglobin (which cannot transport oxygen), resulting in suffocation. Nitrites in water do not themselves pose a problem because they are unstable and are not present in sufficient concentrations to be troublesome. The disease has not been associated with ingestion of high-nitrate surface waters, although the reasons for this have not yet been established. Since only infants are at risk and then only for a few months, a convenient solution where the public water supply cannot easily conform with the standards is to provide bottled water for infants during this brief period of risk.

Consumers of water supply systems that contain excessive nitrates or, for that matter, exceed any of the maximum contaminant levels established in the primary drinking water regulations, must be informed by the purveyor through the media and by direct notification.

Fluorides

Fluoride is a normal constituent of all diets and is an essential nutrient. When the concentration is optimum, no ill effects result and the caries rate in children is 60 to 65 percent below the rates in communities with little or no fluorides in their water supplies. Excessive fluorides in drinking water supplies produce unsightly dental fluorosis, which increases with increasing fluoride concentration. The optimal fluoride level in drinking water differs from place to place, varying with amounts of fluoride in food and with climatic conditions, because the amount of water and therefore the amount of fluoride ingested by children is influenced by temperature. In the interim primary regulations, the optimum fluoride content varied from 0.7 to 1.2 mg/L with MCLs of 1.4 to 2.4 mg/L, with the higher values at temperatures below 12°C and the lower values at temperatures above 26.3°C. Currently the MCL for fluorides is 4 mg/L.

Some water supplies in the United States, particularly in the Southwest, contain fluorides naturally at or near the optimum level and have achieved the benefits of fluorides without intervention. Many communities throughout the country with water supplies containing less than the optimum level of fluorides have provided fluoride supplementation, although the decision to adopt fluoridation has not been without controversy. Communities with excessively high fluoride levels tend to reduce the concentrations by partial defluoridation, by changing the water source, or by adding a low-fluoride water to attain the optimum. The health effects of fluoridation have been studied intensively, and no side effects have been associated with optimum levels of fluoride in water. Although there is no scientific basis for considering added fluorides any different from naturally occurring fluorides, the issue continues to be examined.

Asbestos

While it has long been recognized that workers exposed to asbestos through inhalation may have marked increases in rates of lung cancer and pleural and peritoneal mesothelioma, and regulations to limit inhalation exposures to asbestos have been promulgated, asbestos is not mentioned in the Drinking Water Regulations.[6] Volume 1 of *Drinking Water and Health* suggests, however, that the possibility of long-delayed effects of the ingestion of asbestos through drinking water cannot be ignored, and volume 5, published 6 years later, concludes that an excess of gastrointestinal (GI) tract cancers is associated with occupational exposure to asbestos.[10] Although animal asbestos-ingestion studies have not produced convincing evidence of GI tumors, epidemiological studies did lead to the conclusion that ingestion of asbestos in drinking water increases the risk of cancer. Assuming a daily consumption of 2 L of water, a concentration of 110,000 fibers, as measured by transmission electronic microscopy (TEM), per liter may lead to one additional GI tract cancer per 100,000 persons exposed over a 70-year lifetime.

The possibility of the presence of asbestos should be considered in the evaluation and selection of water sources and treatment. More than 20 percent of 365 cities surveyed in the United States had water containing more than 1 million TEM fibers per liter and more than 10 percent had more than 10 million fibers per liter. Much of this asbestos originates on watersheds and can be removed by filtration. Some, however, is attributed to the use of asbestos-cement pipes, but its significance is yet to be established.

Radionuclides

Radioactivity in public water supplies may be naturally occurring or human-made. Radium 226, among the more important of the naturally occurring radionuclides, is found in ground water as a result of geological conditions. Human-made radioactivity, on the other hand, finds its way into surface waters as a result of fallout from weapons testing and releases from nuclear power plants and users of radioactive materials.[12]

The establishment of limits for radioactivity suffers from the same uncertainties as those inherent in establishment of limits for synthetic organic chemicals, i.e., the assumptions that there is no threshold below which any dose is considered to be harmless and that health effects are proportional to the dose. Attempts are made, in establishing limits, to weigh the cost of achieving certain levels, both in uses of radioactivity forgone and in water supply decisions, as against the expected risks and benefits in reduced radiation exposures to the population.[13]

Some hint of the order of magnitude of the allowable concentrations can be ascertained by comparing the maximum contaminant levels permitted in the standards with dose levels established by the Federal Radiation Council.[4] The annual dose of human-made radionuclides, β and photon emitters, via the drinking water route is limited to 4 mrem/year by the EPA as compared with 170 mrem specified by the Federal Radiation Council from all sources except radiation received for medical purposes and that due to natural background. An exposure of 4 mrem/year corresponds to a lifetime cancer risk increase of 0.025 percent in exposed groups.

In the case of natural radioactivity, primarily radium 226 and radium 228, the allowance for drinking water amounts to half the recommended daily intake via all routes.

The maximum contaminant level for gross α particle activity, 15 picocouries (pCi)/L, is based on the conservative assumption that, if the radium concentration is 5 pCi/L, which is its limit, and the balance of the α particle activity is due to the most radiotoxic α particle–emitting chain, the total dose to bone would be equivalent to less than 6 pCi/L of radium 226.

Because its control is less tractable, the natural radium contamination in drinking water is often of more concern than human-made radioactivity, particularly because it affects the small water supplies that draw from ground waters. Some concentrations as large as 50 pC/L have been reported, and some 500 community water supply systems deliver water that exceeds the standard. If other sources of water cannot be found, the radium can be removed by ion exchange, although this increases the concentration of sodium and may be of concern to that portion of the population requiring low-sodium diets.

Radon, a daughter product of radium, is a naturally occurring radionuclide in ground water. Surveys indicate that about 70 percent of ground water supplies have detectable radon, but only about 10 percent exceed 1000 pCi/L and, of these, fewer than 1 percent occur in communities of more than 500 people.[14] An MCL for radon is being considered, possibly between 500 and 1,000 pCi/L. Aeration is an effective and simple method for removing radon from community water supplies. Granular activated carbon (GAC) filters may be used for absorption of radon for private supplies serving individual households, but the buildup of radioactivity on the GAC may present problems. Accordingly, while radon is not likely to pose a problem for larger community supplies, it may be a problem for individual or very small supplies.

Secondary Maximum Contaminant Levels

There are no direct health consequences from exceeding the levels shown in Table 37-5. Effects are primarily of esthetic or economic concern. Waters high in hydrogen sulfide, iron, manganese, color, or odor may, even if satisfactory from a health standpoint, encourage a user to seek another less offensive source, which may not be safe. Corrosive action resulting from low pH and low alkalinity may have significant economic consequences as well as discoloring the water and imparting stains to clothing and fixtures.

Hardness in water is due primarily to the carbonate and sulfate salts of calcium and magnesium. More soap is required for bathing and laundering with hard water than with soft water. While no limit is specified for hardness or the constituents associated with hardness, many water supplies have incorporated softening to reduce the economic burden on customers who would otherwise be required to use excessive amounts of soap. With the development of synthetic detergents, which contain softening agents, hardness poses much less of a problem and softening may not be economically justified. Furthermore, epidemiological studies have suggested that there is an inverse relationship between the hardness of water and the cardiovascular disease mortality rate. While these studies are not conclusive, and there is not yet a basis for adding hardness to water supplies or for selecting a source based on higher hardness, there does appear to be less justification today for softening public water supplies. Individual large consumers, such as laundries, may find softening of their own supplies advisable.

Sulfates in drinking water are cathartic. The laxative dose for Epsom salt ($MgSO_4 \cdot 7H_2O$) is about 2 g. This dose would be obtained by ingesting 2 liters of water containing 390 mg/L of sulfate. This laxative effect of waters high in sulfates is more pronounced in occasional users, as those who ingest such waters continuously apparently become acclimated. A safeguard is that waters containing sulfate salts in concentrations that may have laxative properties also impart a slight taste that is noticeable to the occasional user if not to the chronic user. Hence there is considered to be no serious health consequence from the presence of high levels of sulfates in water.

Sodium is ingested as sodium chloride, table salt, in fairly liberal quantities, ranging from 4 to 24 g/day and averaging 10 g/day for American males. This represents a sodium intake of 1,600 to 9,600 mg/day. Intakes at these levels are considered to have no adverse effect on normal persons. Consequently, the sodium ion concentration in water supplies is of little consequence to the normal person. A sodium survey of 2,100 public water supplies in 1963 indicated that 95 percent of the samples contained a sodium ion concentration under 250 mg/L, with almost 50 percent under 20 mg/L. At a 2-L intake per day, the 250 mg/L concentration would represent only a small portion of the total salt intake. Sodium levels are important, however, in the control of several disease conditions, including congestive heart failure and hypertension, which affect some 25 million Americans. A restricted sodium intake is recommended for these people. Water supplies with high concentrations of sodium might well furnish their entire daily allowance, permitting no salt ingestion with food. Although there is now no limit on sodium, water purveyors who furnish waters high in sodium should advise physicians in their service areas of the concentrations they can expect.

Softening of water, particularly by ion exchange, adds significant concentrations of sodium, which would be of consequence to that portion of the population on low-sodium diets. The use of home softeners, which are all based on ion exchange, adds substantial concentrations of sodium to water delivered in the home, concentrations of which consumers may not be aware. This constitutes another argument for a policy requiring water quality problems to be addressed centrally rather than in individual homes, where the costs for treatment are substantially higher and where the impacts on quality are uncertain.

Analytic Methods of Analysis

Methods of analysis for water quality, published in *Standard Methods for the Examination of Water and Wastewater*[15] by the American Public Health Association and other organizations, are updated every 5 years. These are being improved continually, with better methods replacing older technologies and with new methods for contaminants that are only recently being considered for regulation. These newer methods appear in the journals, but those being introduced before publication in *Standard Methods* are published in the *Federal Register*.

▶ MICROBIOLOGICAL QUALITY

Five categories of pathogens are found in water: bacteria, viruses, protozoa, worms, and fungi. The principal bacterial waterborne diseases are typhoid, cholera, and shigellosis (bacillary dysentery), all of which attacked populations in the industrialized countries of the world in the mid-nineteenth century and are still major causes of morbidity and mortality in Asia, Africa, and Latin America.

The coliform determination that has been used as a measure of fecal contamination since the early twentieth century is valuable, not because the coliform organisms are pathogenic but because they are always present in the normal intestinal tract of humans and other warm-blooded animals and are found in great numbers in fecal wastes. Thus, while their presence may not signify that a water is a health hazard, their absence provides reasonable evidence of bacteriologically safe water.

Some bacteria included in the total coliform group have wide distribution in the environment but are not evident in all fecal discharges. Other coliforms may be found in fecal discharges but usually in smaller numbers than *Escherichia coli*, the predominant coliform in humans and other warm-blooded animals. Various coliforms have different survival times in the environment, and an assessment of the presence of these different species may indicate the nature of the water contamination. In waters recently contaminated by fecal discharges, however, the fecal coliform organisms are present in large numbers and the fecal coliform count is a useful test to affirm the presence of fecal pollution.

Nevertheless, the presence of any type of coliform organism in treated water suggests either inadequate treatment or contamination of the treated water. Coliform bacteria, whether fecal or nonfecal, should not be present in significant numbers in any potable water supply.

Unfortunately, coliform determinations are somewhat tedious and time consuming, despite recent simplifications of the methods and modifications that produce results within 24 hours. By the time the results of the bacterial analyses are in hand, the water sampled will already have been ingested. For quality-control purposes, the frequent determination of turbidity levels and disinfectant residuals, which can be on-line in real time, are now used for quality control in addition to periodic coliform determinations. The product of the disinfectant residual concentration (C) and the time of contact (T), or CT in milligrams per liter-minutes, to achieve a specified degree of inactivation of a target pathogen in water at a given pH and temperature, is becoming the basis for disinfection regulations in the United States. For example, in the current regulations for drinking water derived from surface sources, the target organism for disinfectant CT values is the protozoan cyst *Giardia lamblia*. Table 37-7 indicates CT values for selected temperatures, pH values, and disinfectants based on *G. lamblia*, the most resistant. The additional 2-log inactivation required by the regulations is expected to be achieved by filtration before disinfection. For drinking water derived from surface sources, filtration is recommended before disinfection to reduce turbidity to better remove pathogens and also to reduce disinfection requirements.

Turbidity interferes with the effectiveness of disinfection, and many pathogens and indicator organisms in water are associated with the particulate matter composing turbidity. For this reason, a turbidity standard is included in the primary drinking water regulations. The standard has been modified from the 5 units in the 1962 standards and the 1 unit in the 1976 regulations by relating the turbidity limit of drinking water produced from surface sources to the options for filtration. Filtered water supplies must achieve a turbidity of less than 1 unit, although turbidity up to 5 units is allowed in exceptional cases for unfiltered or slow sand-filtered waters. The requirement in the 1989 regulations for filtration (and associated pretreatment, such as coagulation and flocculation) as well as disinfection of drinking water produced from surface sources is intended to adequately control contamination by *G. lamblia* as well as by enteric viruses, bacteria, and turbidity.

Viruses of human origin have been identified as causative agents of waterborne disease. The viruses of concern include the enteroviruses (hepatitis A virus, polioviruses, Coxsackieviruses, and echoviruses), rotaviruses, reoviruses, adenoviruses, and the Norwalk-type gastroenteritis viruses ("small, round viruses" or SRVs). In all, more than 100 different human enteric viruses are recognized, and new ones continue to be discovered. Numerous outbreaks of hepatitis A and Norwalk gastroenteritis, a few outbreaks of rotavirus gastroenteritis, and possibly some of poliomyelitis have been identified as waterborne, some from waters that were thought to be treated to satisfactory standards, although this is not yet well established.

However, there is no MCL standard for viruses in the regulations because virology techniques have not yet been perfected to the point where they can be used for the routine monitoring of water quality re-

TABLE 37-7. CT[a] VALUES FOR 1-LOG INACTIVATION OF *GIARDIA LAMBLIA*[b]

		Temperature (°C)			
	pH	***0.5***	***5***	***10***	***15***
Free chlorine[c]	6	49	35	26	19
	7	70	50	37	28
	8	101	72	54	36
	9	146	146	78	59
Ozone		0.97	0.63	0.48	0.32
Chlorine dioxide		2.1	8.4	7.4	6.3
Chloramines, preformed		1,270	730	620	500

From Environmental Protection Agency: Part II 40 CFR Parts 141 and 142. Federal Register June 29, 1989.
[a] C, concentration of disinfectant (mg/L); *T*, contact time (minutes).
[b] Prefiltration removes about 2 logs of *G. lambia.*
[c] Based on free chlorine of 2 mg/L; varies somewhat with other concentrations.

quired for regulation. As viruses in substantial numbers are expected to be present where polluted sources are used or where wastewater reclamation is practiced, technology-based standards designed to control viruses continue to be the basis for regulations until a reliable viral indicator system is developed or the procedures for enteric virus examination become simple, reliable, and rapid.

In untreated wastewaters and fecal material some 50,000 to 100,000 coliform organisms can be expected per virus unit, although this ratio can be substantially different during virus disease outbreaks. Viruses survive longer in natural waters and are more resistant to treatment processes than coliforms are.

The role of waterborne viruses in the spread of disease is yet to be adequately quantified. There is a hypothesis that polluted waters that are inadequately treated, but that meet present drinking water standards, may in fact contain low levels of human viruses that might cause subclinical infections and illness in susceptible persons. This, in turn, might result in spread of the virus by person-to-person contact. Epidemiological studies of waterborne viral disease, other than during epidemics, are difficult to mount, and it may be many years before the relationship between viral contamination of water and health can be established.

Protozoan infections, particularly amebic dysentery, are estimated to affect up to 10 percent of the U.S. population. Because of the small number of cysts excreted and their ready removal in nature and in treatment, relatively massive pollution is required for the initiation of waterborne outbreaks of amebic dysentery.

Giardiasis, caused by a flagellated protozoa, *G. lamblia*, has emerged as one of the most important waterborne infectious diseases in the United States, with over 100 outbreaks causing over 25,000 cases, more than for any other waterborne disease of known etiology. Most outbreaks have been attributed to the ingestion of surface waters without adequate treatment. Because of their ability to survive for long periods in natural waters, waterborne *G. lamblia* may be a problem where *Giardia* is endemic in wild animal populations. Apparently, meeting coliform standards without effective coagulation and filtration in addition to chlorination does not ensure the destruction of *Giardia* cysts. This has become another reason for recommending filtration of all surface waters.

Another protozoan now recognized as being responsible for waterborne disease is *Cryptosporidium*, a coccidian protozoan that is fecally excreted and present in polluted water as a highly resistant, relatively small (3 to 6 pm diameter) oocyst. The natural history of this agent is similar to that of *G. lamblia*. A recent outbreak in Milwaukee, Wisconsin, indicates that conventional treatment may be inadequate to prevent waterborne outbreaks by this agent if the source water is heavily contaminated. This outbreak, which affected over 400,000 persons, serves to emphasize the importance of protecting source waters from excessive fecal contamination by animal as well as human sources.[16]

Worm infections generally result from unsanitary disposal of fecal material and, as they are not a function of the distribution of water, are not generally addressed through water treatment. Worm infections are caused by pollution of the soil on which people, particularly children, walk barefoot (hookworm) or by irrigation or fertilization with wastewaters or fecal material of vegetable crops that are eaten raw. The most important of the worm infections is schistosomiasis. While water supply has been shown to reduce schistosomiasis by making available proper bathing and laundering facilities, which reduce exposure to polluted waters, in general the control of schistosomiasis requires the sanitary disposal of human wastes and the control of the snail hosts. While schistosomiasis does not occur in the United States, the snail hosts and larvae of schistosomes that cause swimmer's itch do occur in some parts of the country, where they are transported from one body of water to another by infected waterfowl.

Bacteriological Examination of Drinking Waters

Determination of coliform organisms in drinking water is routinely required by the purveyor, the regulatory agency, or both. Because the number of coliform organisms in drinking water is small and the organisms are not necessarily randomly distributed, the 1989 coliform MCL is based on the frequency of positive 100-mL samples collected over time. No more than 5.0 percent of the samples collected per month can be positive for coliform, and if fewer than 40 samples are collected monthly, no more than 1 can be positive for coliform. The number of samples required each month is based on the size of the populations served by the water supply, with larger service populations requiring larger numbers of samples. A coliform-positive sample requires the collection of repeat samples for coliform analysis within 24 hours of obtaining positive results. Furthermore, cultures from coliform-positive samples must be further analyzed for fecal coliforms or *E. coli*, that, if positive, are considered to represent a serious violation requiring notification of the state agency and further investigative and corrective actions.

Four alternative tests can be used for coliform analysis of water, but the total sample size must be 100 mL in all cases. The basis of all tests is to detect aerobic or facultative anaerobic, Gram-negative rod-shaped, non-spore–forming bacteria that ferment lactose with the production of acid and gas within 24 to 48 hours of incubation at 35°C. The multiple-tube fermentation technique is done by adding 10-mL portions of the sample to 10 separate tubes of lactose-containing medium (or 20-mL portions to five separate tubes of medium). Positive (growth plus gas production) tubes after 48 hours of incubation at 35°C are transferred to confirmatory medium, and, if any are positive, the sample is confirmed positive for coliforms. The membrane filter test (MFT) is done by filtering a 100-mL sample through a membrane filter that retains the bacteria. The membrane is placed on the surface of coliform medium in a petri dish and incubated for 24 hours at 35°C. If coliforms are present, they will produce characteristic-appearing colonies on the surface of the membrane that can be readily counted with the unaided eye or under a low-power microscope. The presence-absence (P-A) coliform test is done by using a single 100-mL sample. Growth with the production of acid or acid plus gas is presumptively positive, and these cultures are transferred as in the MFT test for confirmation. Another coliform test that can be performed with multiple tubes or a single P-A container uses a nonlactose–containing medium in which coliforms are detected because they grow by 24 hours at 35°C on a minimal medium containing the substrate ortho-nitrophenyl-galactoside (ONPG). Growth causes hydrolysis of this substrate and acid production, which is detected by a dye in the medium that changes color when acidified.

Microbiology of Recreational Waters

Until 1986 the bacteriological quality of bathing waters recommended by the EPA was based on a fecal coliform level not exceeding a log mean of 200/100 mL over a 30-day period.[17] This criterion, which was used by some 95 percent of the states and territories of the United States, was first proposed in 1968 and was based on only the sketchiest of epidemiological data. Furthermore, it provides regulatory officials with a "go–no go" number of doubtful validity.

From 1972 to 1982 the EPA engaged in a long-term recreational water quality research program that examined the relationship between water quality and swimming-associated acute infectious disease, first in marine bathing areas[18] and then in fresh-water bathing areas.[19,20] In both types of water, a linear relationship was found between *E. coli* and enterococci density and swimming-associated gastrointestinal symptoms rates, such as shown in Figure 37-2. Fecal coliforms did not exhibit such a relationship.

Measurable health effects were associated with enterococcus or *E. coli* densities in seawater as low as 10/100 mL via a route in which 10 to 50 mL of water is ingested. At equivalent indicator densities, the health effects were approximately one-third as great as in fresh water.

The best use of these relationships is in the selection of acceptable risks, followed by estimates of relevant bacterial densities and their translation into effluent guidelines for degree of wastewater treatment and location of outfalls. Much more information is needed, however, particularly with regard to die-away of both indicators and pathogens and identification of the pathogens responsible for gastrointestinal illness.

EPA produced guidelines in 1986 recommending that the states adopt the enterococcus criterion for marine waters and either the enterococcus or *E. coli* criterion for fresh waters. While the states were left to select appropriate bacterial densities, the EPA recommended a geometric mean of about 35/100 mL for both waters, corresponding to a geometric mean of 200/mL fecal coliform.[21]

Water Standards As Applied in Developing Countries

High infant mortality rates in developing countries, often more than 10-fold greater than in industrialized countries, are attributed in good part to inadequate water supply and sanitation. That some 1.5 billion people are estimated to lack reasonable access to safe water led the United Nations, on November 10, 1980, to inaugurate the International Drinking Water Supply and Sanitation Decade (1981 to 1990). An excellent reference, *Water and Human Health*, on the relationship between water and disease in developing countries was prepared by McJunkin.[22]

Considerable controversy has arisen concerning the standards to be applied to community water supplies in developing countries. It has been argued that the availability of water for household use and personal cleanliness may be more important than the quality of that water. The cost of ensuring quality such as is required in the United States and other industrialized countries may be so great as to militate against the installation of any water supply facilities at all. Thus, there is pressure to relax drinking water standards in developing countries. On the other hand, bacterial standards must necessarily be a function of the incidence of bacterial disease. The success of water-sanitation programs in the United States in the twentieth century has resulted in the virtual disappearance of waterborne typhoid and cholera. Consequently, U.S. bacterial standards could be relaxed considerably without much likelihood of any increase in waterborne disease. On the other hand, in countries where typhoid and cholera are endemic and periodically epidemic, if water is not to be a vehicle for the spread of the diseases, the bacterial standards may have to be somewhat more stringent. Health status, water use habits, and economic circumstances should all help determine the standards that are most appropriate.[23]

Chemical standards may be of less importance in the developing countries because these chemicals are not likely to be present in large numbers or concentration and chronic disease resulting from long-term exposure to low concentrations of SOCs is not likely to be a problem in the face of high rates of enteric disease.

The World Health Organization (WHO) had adopted separate drinking water standards for Europe and the developing countries of Asia, Africa, and Latin America. Recognizing that these standards were used primarily as guides to countries for establishing their own standards, WHO has published *Guidelines for Drinking Water Quality*.[24] It considers all health effects issues but also the practical application of the guidelines to developing countries. The guidelines comprise three volumes: volume 1 includes recommended values for all contaminants, including SOCs, together with guidelines for their application and attainment; volume 2 provides the health effects criteria on which volume 1 is based; and volume 3, "Drinking Water Quality Surveillance for Small Community Supplies" contains guidelines for developing countries, emphasizing microbiological rather than chemical problems.

However, the introduction of oral rehydration therapy (ORT), a relatively new and simple ministration that averts many child deaths from diarrhea, has diverted attention from water supply and sanitation (WS&S). The principal attractiveness of ORT is its apparent low cost per diarrheal death averted as compared with WS&S. However, WS&S provides many more benefits that are essential to sustaining the lives saved by ORT and vital to maintaining and enhancing the lives of both children and adults.[25] WS&S *prevents* diarrhea, and many other diseases as well, releases women from the heavy and time-consuming burden of carrying water from distant possibly contaminated sources, and improves the quality of life in the community.

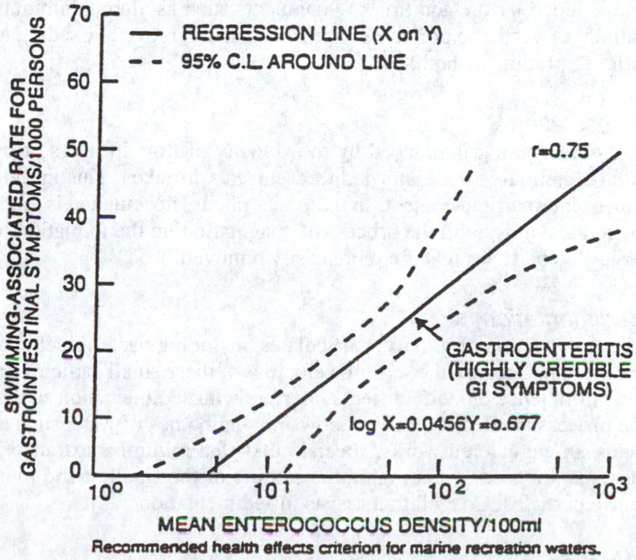

Figure 37-2. Recommended health effects criteria for marine recreation waters. (From Cabelli VJ: Health Effects Criteria for Marine Recreational Waters. EPA-600/1-80-031. Washington, DC: Environmental Protection Agency, August 1983.)

WS&S is a long-term investment in preventive health, while ORT is a response to an immediate life-threatening situation. The costs are not high, and, without WS&S and hygiene education, ORT programs are not likely to improve child health status.

▶ TREATMENT OF WATER AND WASTEWATER

The treatment of waters to make them suitable for subsequent use requires physical, chemical, and biological processes.[1] These processes may take place in nature. When natural processes cannot be ensured of a desired quality, these processes need to be engineered in water treatment plans.[26–28]

Engineering processes are increasingly necessary, in part because the contamination that impairs the quality of water is increasingly human-made and resistant to nature's purification process and in part because of growth of population and its activity in the face of fixed natural resources. The processing steps used for purifying water for drinking are described below, while those used for treating wastewater are described under Bacterial Examination of Drinking Waters.

Distillation

Evaporation and condensation maintain the hydrologic cycle. Engineered distillation is used for desalination and for other applications where special water quality may be needed. Distillation produces the purest water of any of the processes listed, with only volatile organics persisting.

Gas Exchange

Oxygen is added to waters, and dissolved gases such as carbon dioxide and hydrogen sulfide are removed. This helps in reducing taste and odors and may also assist in the oxidation of iron and manganese, making them more easily removable. Aeration is an important natural process, helping to restore water quality in polluted rivers and other bodies of water. It is also used in water purification and wastewater treatment.

Coagulation

Colloidal and suspended particles are brought together to form large *flocs* that settle more easily. This occurs in nature in lakes and other bodies of water, but it is an important process in water purification and is aided by the addition of coagulants such as alum (aluminum sulfate) or synthetic polymers. The floc is then removed by sedimentation, filtration, or both.

Flocculation

In nature, mixing is induced by the velocity of flow in rivers or by wind-, thermal-, or density-induced currents in lakes. This mixing causes interparticle contact. In treatment plants, flocculation is engineered and aids, with the process of coagulation, in the formation of large-floc particles that are more easily removed.

Sedimentation

Under the action of gravity, particulates, including bacteria, settle to the bottom. Because the settling velocities of these small particles are low, turbulence or swift currents interfere with sedimentation so that the process is effective only in slow-moving bodies of water such as lakes. In engineered works, special tanks that minimize extraneous currents are used, encouraging the settling of the smallest and most dense particles. Coagulation assists in sedimentation.

Filtration

Water passes through granular media, and fine particulates are removed by the adhesion to the grains and by sedimentation in the pore spaces. Removal of particles by filtration is not accomplished by straining, as the particles removed are generally much smaller than the spaces between the grains of the medium. In some instances, biological growth on the filter helps with the removal of particles and assists with biochemical degradation of the adsorbed organic matter. Natural filtration occurs as water percolates through the soil.

Adsorption

While some adsorption takes place in filtration, often special media designed to adsorb contaminants may be used. Activated carbon, both in granular form as filters and in powdered form as an additive to water, is used to adsorb taste and odors and a wide variety of organic chemicals.

Ion Exchange

Resins, both natural and synthetic, are used to remove specific ions. The most common are zeolites used for removing calcium and magnesium, two hardness-producing ions, and replacing them with sodium.

Disinfection

A wide variety of disinfection procedures is available for the destruction of microorganisms that may cause disease. Sterilization is not intended or necessary. The most common disinfection procedure is chlorination.

Other processes are available for specific purposes, such as treatment to help prevent corrosion and processes for the handling of the solids (sludge) that accumulate in treatment. The handling and disposal of sludge is a difficult problem, particularly at wastewater treatment plants where the sludge is often noxious and can constitute a health hazard. Other processes may be required for the removal of specific substances such as ammonia, phosphorus, radioactivity, or specific contaminants. In general, one or more of the unit processes mentioned will be used.

Where the aim is a potable water, the selection of the treatment process is dependent on the quality of the water source. For example, ground waters may require only aeration and disinfection, while heavily polluted surface waters may require all the processes. Community wastewaters, except for the presence of industrial wastewater discharges, tend to be much the same, and the treatment processes are selected to provide an effluent that protects the receiving water and the subsequent uses to which the water may be put. If the effluent is to be discharged into an ocean, fewer processes are likely to be required than if the effluent is intended for discharge into a small, fragile stream or for reuse for nonpotable purposes.

▶ ENGINEERED WATER PURIFICATION

The conventional sequence of processes for the purification of surface water for potable purposes includes flocculation and coagulation, sedimentation, filtration, and disinfection. This treatment removes color, turbidity, microorganisms, colloidal particles, and some dissolved substances. Some of these processes may be omitted where the waters are drawn from a protected source and are free of color and turbidity. On the other hand, the conventional treatment is not directed to dissolved synthetic organic chemicals and is only moderately effective in the removal of heavy metals and radioactivity. If these constitute a problem, additional processes, such as adsorption on granular activated carbon, may be required. The following sections describe, and Figure 37-3 illustrates, the principal unit processes required in most water purification plants.

Coagulation

The processes described here include chemical addition, rapid mixing, and flocculation. The purpose is to remove finely divided suspended material, colloidal material, microorganisms, and to some extent dissolved substances, particularly those of larger molecular size, by bringing them together into flocs sufficiently large to be removed by sedimentation, filtration, or both. The raw water may be highly colored and free to turbidity or turbid and free to color. The particles responsible for the color and turbidity are not discernible to the naked eye. After coagulation, however, the individual floc particles are easily observed, being on the order of 1 to 2 mm in diameter.

The principal coagulants are alum, aluminum sulfate ($Al_2(SO^4)^3$ $14H_2O$) available in solid or liquid form, and ferric salts such as ferric sulfate. These aluminum and iron salts, on solution, form trivalent aluminum and ferric ions. These ions react with alkalinity, which may be naturally present or, if not, may be provided through the addition of lime or soda ash.

$$Al_2(SO_4)_3 + 6HCO_3 = 3SO_4 + 2A1(OH)_3 + 6CO_2$$

The addition of these coagulants reduces the pH of the water. Since optimum coagulation is a function of pH, coagulation may require pH adjustment.

While the aluminum hydroxide is essentially insoluble and forms a loosely bound gelatinous structure, which might appear to be the basis for the floc formation, the process is one in which the trivalent ions interact with the materials in the water to reduce the forces of repulsion among them, allowing them to come together in larger and larger aggregates, which then grow by accretion. As natural colloids are largely negatively charged, the positive ions are effective in neutralizing and allowing their coagulation.

Where large amounts of coagulants are required, the pH is reduced, tending to make the water somewhat more corrosive. The use of natural or synthetic polymers can reduce coagulant requirements 10-fold. The proper amount of coagulant and polymer and the optimum pH are determined by jar tests or by pilot plant studies prior to the design of the facility. Jar tests are then run routinely as a guide to the adjustment of chemical dosages with changing temperature and quality of the raw water.

Chemical feeding equipment selection is based on the needed chemical, the required precision of feeding, and the variety of dosages necessitated by changing quality, which is generally gradual, or the changing flow, which may be sudden and frequent.

After the chemicals are added to the water, it is customary to provide rapid mixing equipment to be certain that the chemicals are distributed uniformly in the water. Turbine or propeller mixers are commonly used, although if the water is to be pumped, the chemical may be added on the suction side of the pump, using the pump as the mixer. Hydraulic mixing may be used. Pipes themselves can be used if there are sufficient bends to ensure the necessary turbulence, or stators may be inserted in a pipe. The time required for rapid mixing is only seconds.

The coagulation process is aided by flocculation produced in special tanks, where mechanical paddles or diffused air stirs in water gently, promoting the conjunction of suspended particles. The resulting large flocs then settle easily. Where sufficient head is available, the flocculation can take place in baffled tanks. This method is suited to developing countries, where the use of imported mechanical equipment is to be minimized. Generally, the more flexible power-driven mechanical devices are used in industrialized countries. The parameter of concern in the design of such tanks is the velocity gradient, the velocity variation across an element of water. In practice, the velocities in flocculation tanks vary from about 1 m/s at the entrance to the tanks, decreasing to about 0.2 m/s near the outlet, with a retention time of 30 minutes. Specific requirements vary with different raw waters and variations in temperature, so that the flocculator is designed to accommodate the worst situation, which generally occurs in winter.

Sedimentation

The effluent from the flocculation tanks with large but variable-sized flocs is led into sedimentation tanks, where the flocs are encouraged to settle. The detention time, again depending on the water to be treated, varies from about 2 to 6 hours. The required capacity is divided into two or more units to permit one unit to be out of service without requiring shutdown of the plant. Commonly, these tanks are rectangular in plan and about 4 to 5 m deep. Where the rate of accumulation of floc at the bottom of the tanks is expected to be too great to be easily removed manually, mechanical sludge collectors may be installed. Where the sludge can be stored at the bottom of the tank for several months without creating problems in treatment, and removed manually, mechanical sludge collectors can be dispensed with, saving the cost of equipment and maintenance.

Another useful configuration, particularly where space is at a premium, is the upward flow or sludge blanket clarifier, in which the water after flocculation moves up through a floc blanket, which is suspended in the tank by the upward velocity. The impurities are removed in the blanket, and the effluent is clear. These upward flow units were initially developed for softening, but their economics have encouraged their use in conventional treatment as well. A compact arrangement for the upflow unit in combination with the flocculator is in concentric tanks, the flocculator in the center and sedimentation on the outside. Unless first-class supervision of operation can be ensured, however, the conventional horizontal-flow sedimentation tank is preferred because it is far less subject to upset.

An improvement in the efficiency of these sedimentation tanks can be obtained by increasing the area on which the floc can settle. Initially, this was done by installing intermediate bottoms in horizontal-flow tanks. A more effective approach is the installation of a series of sloping plates or tubes installed in the top of the sedimentation tank through which the floc-bearing waters must flow before reaching the effluent weirs. The flocs settle on the plates or in the tubes and then fall to the bottom of the tank. Such settlers can be installed in existing tanks to improve their performance.

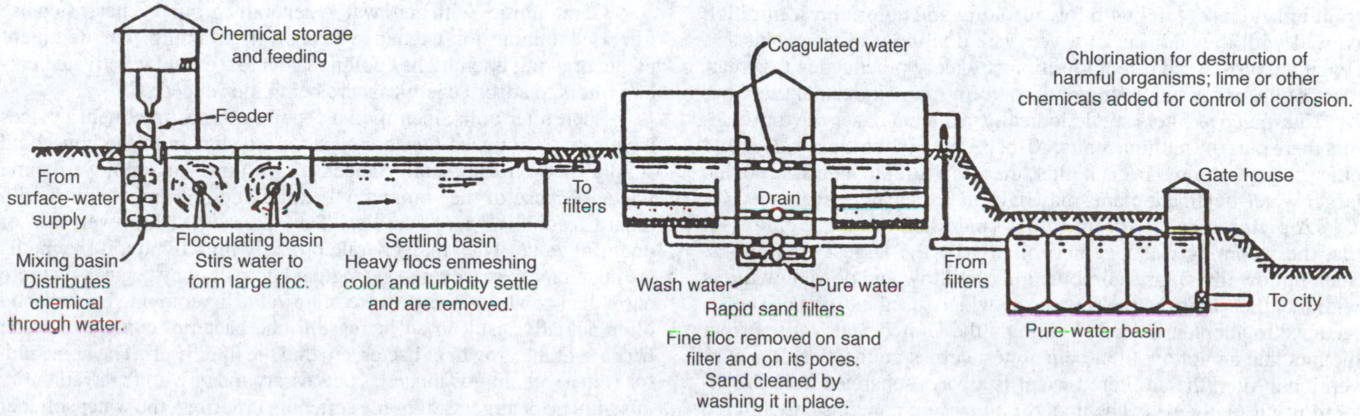

Figure 37-3. Typical water treatment plant profile. (From Fair GM, Geyer J, Okun DA: Elements of Water Supply and Wastewater Disposal. New York: John Wiley & Sons, 1971.)

Management of Sludge

The material that falls to the bottom of the tank, sludge, is now identified as a *residual* to encourage its recovery as a by-product of the treatment process. At one time this sludge was returned to the river whence the raw water was drawn, but today it is considered a pollutant and must be reclaimed or disposed of properly. Discharge to the sewerage system, if a sewer is available, for final handling and disposal at the wastewater treatment plant is an expeditious solution. Otherwise, transport by truck to a landfill or other acceptable place for disposal may be required. In such instances, dewatering of the sludge is appropriate to reduce the cost of transportation. For this purpose, sand drying beds, vacuum filtration, filter presses, or centrifuges, all processes similar to those used for handling sludges in wastewater-treatment plants, may be used. Where alum and/or lime is used in the water-treatment process, their recovery may be economical.

Filtration

Floc particles that escape the sedimentation tank are removed in filters. The conventional filter is about 1 m in depth and is made up of sand grains varying in size from 0.5 to 1.0 mm. The granular material rests on a bed of graded gravel or on a specially designed underdrain system made of porous plates or false bottoms of various types with small orifices to ensure uniform backwashing. As water passes down through the filter beds, the floc settles in the interstices or is adsorbed onto the surface of the sand grains. When the amount of floc accumulated in the filter is sufficiently great to impede the flow of water by increasing the head loss to 2 to 3 m, the filter is backwashed, using filtered water sometimes accompanied by air. A filter run may last 48 hours, and the filter washing takes about 10 minutes. Three to 5 percent of the filtered water is required for backwashing, and the dirtied backwash water can be retained and returned to the plant influent. The cleansing of the filter is accomplished by expanding the sand bed with water introduced into the bottom of the filter. On completion of the wash, the sand settles back into place with the finest particles at the top and the coarsest at the bottom. This configuration of particles limits the effectiveness of the filter, as the top layer tends to remove most of the floc particles and the remainder of the depth of the filter goes unused. One approach now widely accepted to help alleviate this situation is the use of dual media or even multimedia filters, where granular materials of different specific gravity are used. Most common is the dual media filter, where coarser anthracite grains with a specific gravity of about 1.5 rest on top of a silica sand with a specific gravity of 2.65. In backwashing such a filter, the larger grains of the lighter anthracite always remain on the top of the filter, permitting the full depth of the bed to be more effectively used.

The rate of application to the filters range from 4 to 10 m/h, depending on the quality of the water. The engineer selects the sizes and loadings of the pretreatment and filter units to minimize the overall cost. Where the raw waters are of high quality and coagulation and sedimentation are not required, as is the case when water is drawn from upland reservoirs with low turbidity and color, direct filtration is used with the addition of a very small amount of coagulant and coagulant aids. Such direct filtration is widely practiced in the treatment of water for swimming pools and for many industrial uses.

Inasmuch as filters are periodically taken out of service for washing, there must be multiple units. Also, because of the many valves and other fittings required in each filter, there is a limit to their size, so that larger water-treatment plants may have many separate filter units.

A preferred mode for operating sand filters would be upflow so that the incoming water is met initially by the largest sand grains. Such upflow filters, or a combination of upflow and downflow filters with the filter drains in the center, are widely used in Europe. The reluctance to adopt such upflow units in the United States arises from the fact that an upflow filter constitutes a cross-connection. In a conventional filter, the unfiltered water is always separated from the filtered water by the bed. The underdrain system contains only filtered water, which is used for backwashing. The dirtied wash water on top of the filters after washing should not mix with the filtered water. Any wash water that remains on top of the filter is refiltered, so there is never an occasion when the underdrains receiving the filtered water can be contaminated by unfiltered or wash water. On the other hand, the purified effluent from upflow filters occupies the same space above the filters as is occupied by the wash water during washing, and contamination of the filtered water is quite possible. In many European plants, where filters are used primarily to remove iron and manganese from ground waters and there is no bacterial contamination, such cross-connections are of little consequence. Also, in the reclamation of wastewaters where the production of potable water is not intended, upflow filters may be used.

The earliest filters, introduced in the middle of the nineteenth century for use without pretreatment by coagulation and sedimentation, were slow sand filters. The rate of application to the slow sand filter is approximately 0.15 m/h, requiring an area about 50 times greater than conventional filters. The slow sand filter operates by the creation on its top layer of a film of material removed from the water, including microorganisms, called a *schmutzdecke*. It is this living filter that removes color, turbidity, and bacteria. The top layer is easily clogged, however, and the top 3 to 5 cm of sand is removed periodically for washing. Immediately after removal of the schmutzdecke, the performance of the filter may be somewhat poorer, but it is quickly restored. Several cleanings take place before the washed sand is restored to the filter. Slow sand filters have much to commend them in small communities and in developing countries, because they require a minimum of mechanical equipment and much less skilled supervision than conventional rapid sand filters. In fact, slow sand filters are used exclusively in treating the water from the rivers Thames and Lee for the city of London. Many cities in Europe that draw from polluted sources use slow sand filters. To permit somewhat greater loads on slow sand filters, it is customary to precede the slow sand filtration with pretreatment by rapid sand filters or microstrainers, drums made of finely woven steel mesh that remove algae and other large particles, permitting the slow sand filters to operate for longer periods between cleanings. Chemical coagulants are not used.

Diatomaceous earth filters are used for industrial water supplies and many specialized applications. The water to be filtered is mixed with diatomaceous earth and forced through a porous septum in a pressure shell, forming a filtering layer several millimeters thick on the surface of the septum. When the filter is clogged, the flow is reversed, the diatomaceous earth is dislodged and washed away, and a new cycle of operation is initiated. Filters of considerable capacity can be provided in a small space, so such units are particularly suitable for mobile installations, swimming pools, and many industrial water supplies. However, they are not well suited for handling coagulated waters because they clog quickly. More important, the small thickness of diatomaceous earth does not provide the security against breakthroughs of unfiltered water that is provided by the meter depth of sand in conventional filters. Hence, they have not been widely adopted in municipal practice.

Communities with hard water, generally ground water, often use filters containing ion-exchange resins for softening. For treatment plants drawing upon highly polluted sources, granular activated carbon filters to adsorb chemicals are being introduced.

Such filter units, identified as "point-of-use" treatment devices have been introduced for home use for attachment to the household supply or even to a single faucet. These units have enjoyed some vogue because of the commercial exploitation of uncertainties with regard to public water supplies. They are costly, however, and of doubtful value. They may operate properly initially, but if the media are not replaced or recharged at regular intervals, they begin to do more harm than good. These filters are of no value in removing bacteria and often actually result in an increase in the bacterial content of water because of the growth of bacteria within the filter itself. The home unit for water softening is much less necessary today with the availability of synthetic detergents. If home softening is desired, the water softener is best attached to the household hot water tank and the washing machines, rather than softening the entire supply.

Home remedies are uncertain and costly, and they can be afforded by only the relatively well-to-do segment of the population. The growing use of household filters and bottled water, a sign that the public has lost faith in the quality of the water supply, should stimulate corrective action by water purveyors and regulatory agencies.

Disinfection

Disinfection with chlorine has been the single most important process for ensuring the bacteriological safety of potable water supplies. Waterborne epidemics have virtually disappeared in the industrialized countries of the world. Such waterborne outbreaks as have occurred have generally been traced to failures in chlorination.

To be used in water treatment, water disinfectants must possess the following properties:

1. They must destroy bacteria, viruses, and amebic cysts in water within a reasonable time despite all variations in water temperature, composition, and concentration of contaminants.
2. They must not be toxic to humans and domestic animals, unpalatable, or otherwise objectionable.
3. They must be reasonable in cost and safe and easy to store, transport, handle, and apply.
4. Their residual concentration in the treated water must be easily, and preferably automatically, determinable.
5. They must be sufficiently persistent so that the disappearance of the residual would be a warning of recontamination.

As it is not feasible to continuously monitor bacteriological or virological quality of water and to have the results before the water is distributed to the consumer, the ability to detect a residual concentration of a known bactericidal disinfectant (C) after exposure for a certain time (T) at a certain pH and temperature is the key quality-control test. Table 37-7 shows CT values for various conditions and disinfectants.

The use of chlorine or one of its derivatives meets these requirements most economically; however, other methods of disinfection are sought for two reasons: (*a*) chlorine added to some waters imparts an undesirable taste and odor, particularly where phenol is present; and (*b*) the reaction of chlorine with organic matter, even where these organics are not themselves of health significance, has resulted in the formation of a wide range of reaction products. One group of these, trihalomethanes, including chloroform, has been shown to cause cancer in animals. The problems created by the use of chlorine have been exacerbated because chlorine is a useful oxidant that can remove taste and odors economically and which, when added at the beginning of a treatment process, facilitates subsequent treatment by reducing the concentration of microorganisms that can cause difficulty in sedimentation tanks and filters. Because of the wide use of prechlorination, particularly with waters drawn from polluted sources such as the Mississippi and Ohio rivers, many water supplies do not meet the trihalomethane standard of 100 pg/L. This problem is rapidly addressed by the use of better sources of water or by adequate treatment before the disinfecting dose of chlorine is added. Humic organics, phenols, and other precursors of the trihalomethanes should be removed before the addition of chlorine. This requires abandoning the process of prechlorination. While the removal of natural organics through coagulation, sedimentation, and filtration can be readily accomplished, the removal of synthetic organic chemicals in polluted waters is more difficult.

The adoption of substitutes for chlorine must be initiated with great care. Other disinfectants may themselves produce compounds of which far less is known than of the trihalomethanes. Also, some of the other methods of disinfection, such as chloramination, do not provide the same level of microbiological safety as chlorine. Nevertheless, knowledge of all methods of disinfection might help reveal a combination that provides the required safety while minimizing the undesirable side effects. For example, the use of another method for disinfection, such as those described below with chlorine added primarily to ensure bacterial safety by providing the water with a measurable chlorine residual, may be suitable.

A wide range of other methods of disinfection, including the use of strong oxidants, is available. Boiling water will disinfect it, but this is suitable only as an emergency measure for individual consumers. It is not a reasonable community approach.

While sunlight is a natural disinfectant, irradiation by ultraviolet light is an engineered process that can be tailored to the need. A mercury vapor arc lamp emitting invisable light of 25 to 37 Å applied to a water free of light-absorbing substances, particularly suspended matter that will protect microorganisms against the light, is a useful method of disinfection. There is no way of continuously monitoring the effectiveness of the process, however, and therefore it has not yet found application in municipal potable water supply practice in the United States, although it is used in the Soviet Union.

Silver ions are bactericidal at concentrations as low as 15 μg/L, but the action is quite slow. Larger concentrations that speed up the process are unacceptable because of possible side effects from the silver. Furthermore, silver ions are neither viricidal nor cysticidal in appropriate concentrations, and silver is expensive. Nevertheless, silver-coated sand may be appropriate for specialized installations. Copper ions are strongly algicidal, and copper sulfate is often used for algae control in lakes and reservoirs. However, copper is not bactericidal.

Pathogenic bacteria do not survive in highly acid or alkaline waters, below 3 or above 11 pH. Where the treatment process brings the water to these pH levels, as might be the case through the use of lime, some disinfection benefits accrue. Otherwise, the use of acids or alkalis as disinfectants is not feasible.

Oxidizing Chemicals

Oxidizing chemicals include the halogens (chlorine, bromine, iodine), ozone, and other oxidants, such as potassium permanganate and hydrogen peroxide. Potassium permanganate has found wide use as a replacement for chlorine for taste and odor control, but it is not as effective as a disinfectant. Ozone is useful for destroying odors and color and is also an effective disinfectant, but it suffers from the fact that it leaves no residual suitable for monitoring. Among the halogens, gaseous chlorine and a wide variety of chlorine compounds are economically most useful. Bromine and iodine have been employed on a limited scale for the disinfection of swimming pool waters as well as in tablets for disinfecting small quantities of drinking water in the field.

Ozone

Ozone is produced on site by the corona discharge of high-voltage electricity into dry air or oxygen. Ozone is corrosive and toxic, and strong concentrations in the atmosphere, from its photochemical genesis in conjunction with hydrocarbon vapors from automobile exhaust, are responsible for oxidant smogs that are eye, throat, and lung irritants. In the vicinity of a plant using ozone, its effect can often be seen on vegetation. Nevertheless, ozone is used effectively and efficiently as an oxidant, a deodorant, a decolorant, and a disinfectant in both drinking water and wastewaters. Because the production of ozone is expensive and energy-intensive, and because ozone residuals disappear rapidly from water and are not available for quality control, ozone is used for special applications and not as a general replacement for chlorine. The combination of ozone for pretreatment while providing some disinfection, to be followed by chlorination, has become a popular sequence in Europe and is beginning to be used in the United States to reduce the level of THMs in finished water. Intensive research into the characteristics, biocidal efficiency, and reaction products of ozone is being undertaken, although it is not expected that it will replace chlorine entirely because it leaves no residual.

Chlorine

Chlorinated lime (CaClOl) was the first chlorine disinfectant used for public water supplies. It is a hygroscopic white powder that rapidly absorbs both moisture and carbon dioxide from the air with the loss of chlorine. Because it is unstable, it was rapidly replaced by hypochlorites. This was shortly followed by elemental chlorine (Cl_2), produced by the electrolysis of brine, in liquid form for storage and transmission in steel cylinders. Liquid chlorine is still by far the most common form of chlorine to be used for water supply and wastewater disinfection. Calcium hypochlorite ($Ca(OCl)_2$) is stable and is used for small installations. It is easily stored in solid form in small containers, and 1 to 3 percent solutions can be made up as needed. Sodium hypochlorite (NaOCl) is also used for small installations and increasingly for large installations where the transportation of liquid chlorine is considered too hazardous because of the danger of leakage. Chlorine is heavier than air and is extremely toxic, so that all handling and dosing of liquid and gaseous chlorine must be done with care. Chlorine dioxide (ClO_2) is used in special instances, particularly where tastes and odors may be a problem. It is produced directly in water by the reaction of elemental chlorine with sodium chlorite ($NaClO_2$).

The on-site generation of hypochlorite by electrolysis of brine may be appropriate for communities in isolated locations where power is available but the delivery of chlorine may be difficult.

When chlorine or its derivatives are added to water in the absence of ammonia or organic nitrogen, hypochlorous acid (HOCl), hypochlorite ion (OCl^-), or both are formed, with the distribution between the two depending on pH. These are referred to in practice as free available chlorine. When ammonia or organic nitrogen is present, monochloramine (NH_2Cl_2), dichloramine ($NHCl_2$), and nitrogen trichloride (NCl_3) may be formed, the distribution among the species again being a function of pH. Generally, the first two of these prevail and are referred to as chloramines of combined available chlorine. Because the disinfecting power of each of these varies widely, the chemistry of chlorination must be fully understood so that the chlorine may be used effectively and disinfection assured.

Although the purpose of adding chlorine is to destroy microorganisms, most of the substances in water that react with the chlorine are inert organic materials, both natural and human-made, as well as other reducing substances. To the extent that the organic matter and other chemicals that cause chlorine demand can be removed from water by treatment before the addition of chlorine, both the required addition of chlorine and the formation of chlorinated organic compounds will be reduced.

When chlorine is added to water, it is hydrolized immediately and completely, according to the following reaction:

$$Cl_2 + H_2O \rightarrow HOCl + H^+ + Cl^-$$

Hypochlorous acid ionizes in part into H^+ and OCl^-. At pH below 5, the chlorine exists almost entirely as HOCl; and above pH 10, as OCl^-. Between these two pHs, the percent of chlorine added as HOCl at 20°C is

$$\frac{100}{1 + 2.5 \times 10^{pH}/10^8}.$$

At pH 7, 80 percent of the chlorine is in the form of HOCl. The distribution is important because HOCl has a much higher killing power than OCl^-. Figure 37-4 indicates that at pH 10 some 50-fold greater chlorine residuals are required for a 99 percent kill of *E. coli* in 30 minutes at 2 to 5°C, as compared with requirements at pH 7.

When ammonia or its salts are present in chlorinated water, chloramines are formed. Monochloramine is formed in the pH range of 6 to 8, while dichloramine predominates at lower pH values. The chloramines appear as part of the residual chlorine, but as they are considerably less effective disinfecting agents than hypochlorous acid, it is important to differentiate them in analysis. To ensure adequate disinfection, a free residual must be formed: this requires the addition of more than enough chlorine to react with all the ammonia and organic compounds present. The great advantage of obtaining free available chlorine is that most tastes and odors that can be oxidized by chlorine are destroyed, and rigorous disinfection, even to the inactivation of viruses, can be ensured as long as the proper combination of chlorine residual concentration, pH, time of contact, and temperature are observed.

While hypochlorites can be added with solution feeders much as any other chemical solutions are added in water treatment, special equipment is required for adding elemental chlorine. Chlorine is transported in liquid form in steel cylinders, but chlorine gas also exists within the cylinder, and it is the gas that is drawn off for solution in a water stream, feeding into the water to be treated. For large rates of use, particularly in wastewater treatments where the amounts of chlorine used are substantially greater than in water supply disinfection, the chlorine may be withdrawn from the steel tank as a liquid and vaporized in special evaporation equipment. The solubility of chlorine gas in water is about 7300 mg/L at 20°C at 1 atm. Below 9.5°C, chlorine combines with water to form chlorine hydrate, chlorine ice, which may obstruct feeding equipment. Therefore, it is important that chlorine feeding equipment and the water that may come in contact with the gas be kept above this temperature.

Because chlorine is highly toxic, it must be handled with great care and under adequate safeguards. Its odor threshold is about 3.5 ppm by volume. Concentrations of 30 ppm or more induce coughing, and exposures for 30 minutes to concentrations of 40 to 60 ppm are dangerous, with 1,000 ppm being rapidly fatal. Because chlorine gas is heavier than air, it concentrates in tunnels and lower levels of buildings at the water treatment plants. Therefore, special facilities are provided for handling chlorine, with separate entrances to feeding and weighing rooms, adequate automatic ventilation, and safety equipment, including appropriate gas masks stored nearby.

Inasmuch as chlorine is the most important safeguard for microbiological safety, no breakdown in chlorine feeding can be tolerated. Thus, units must be adequate in size and be duplicated so that failure of any single unit would not interfere with continuous chlorination. An ample number of filled cylinders must be available, with at least two cylinders on-line at all times so that an empty cylinder can be replaced without interfering with chlorination. Most chlorinators operate under vacuum to prevent leakage of chlorine gas. The vacuum is created by the feed water being pumped under pressure through a venturi throat in the feeder. The pressure of water required for this feed water line must be substantially greater than the water pressure in the line being fed. Accordingly, separate pumps are re-

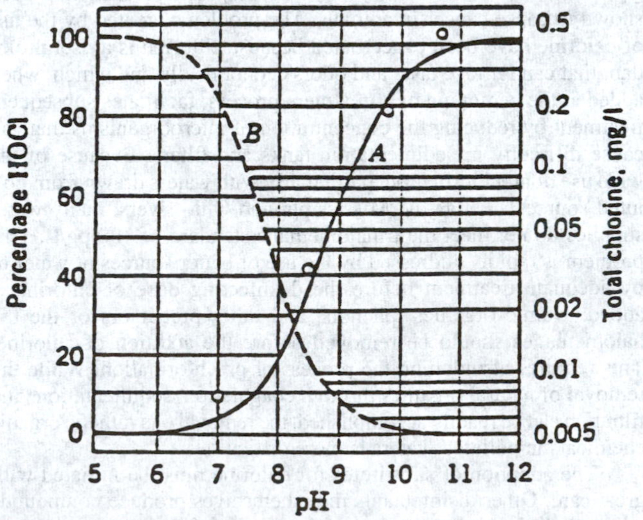

Figure 37-4. Observed concentration of free available chlorine required for 99 percent kill of *E. coli* in 30 min at 2 to 5°C (*curve A* and *right-hand scale*) and percentage of HOCl in the total chlorine (*curve B* and *left-hand scale*). (From Fair GM, Geyer J, Okun DA: Elements of Water Supply and Wastewater Disposal. New York: John Wiley & Sons, 1971.)

quired. Failure of these pumps because of a power failure would mean the cessation of chlorination. Therefore, suitable alarms with provision for standby power can help ensure continuous operation.

Portable chlorinators that operate off the pressure in the cylinders may be used for emergency chlorination of water mains, wells, tanks, and reservoirs in the field.

After the chlorine is added, sufficient contact time, which depends on the particular water but is generally approximately 30 minutes, must be provided. The product of the concentration, C, and time of contact, T, the CT, is the operating parameter (Table 37-7). In water treatment plants, this can be done in a clear well at the plant. In wastewater treatment plants, on the other hand, special chlorine contact chambers are constructed. It may be that sufficient treated water transmission mains exist to provide adequate contact time before the first customer is reached even at highest flows. This would make a contact chamber unnecessary; however, it is then necessary to be able to sample for chlorine residual at a point at least 30-minutes flow distant from the point of addition.

Chlorination is now routinely automated to permit automatic variation of dosage to account for variations in flow and chlorine demand and to maintain a constant chlorine residual. The chlorine dosages and residuals are recorded, and it is common to maintain an alarm to give warning of any departure from the required chlorine residual.

Corrosion Inhibition

The treated water may be more corrosive because of the addition of coagulants and chlorine, both of which reduce pH. Also, many natural waters are quite soft and corrosive. To avoid corrosion of pipelines, hot water heaters, and plumbing fittings, it is general practice to reduce the corrosivity of the water. This is done either by adding sufficient alkalinity and raising the pH to render the water noncorrosive or by adding a hexametaphosphate sequestering agent, which tends to form a light coating in the pipes and mitigates the effect of any corrosion that might occur. Corrosion control is also important to minimize lead concentrations in water where lead is present in household water plumbing.

Adsorption

Depending on the source of water, a treatment plant may use one or more of the processes described. None of these processes, however, are directed against the SOCs present in waters that drain urban and industrial areas, although some removal of these organics can be expected when powdered activated carbon is used for taste and odor control. The organics in water were initially characterized by passing the water sample through activated carbon filters on which the organics are adsorbed and then dissolving these organics with chloroform. The 1962 U.S. Public Health Service Drinking Water Standards had a limit of 0.2 mg/L for this carbon chloroform extract. It was recognized that many of the organics adsorbed on the filter were of no health concern and that many organics that might be of health concern were not adsorbed at all. The use of GAC filters for treating water drawn from polluted sources is now being introduced in an attempt to remove some, if not all, of these refractory organic chemicals. Pilot plants have been built but there is little experience with the long-term full-scale use of these GAC filters. They have limited capacity, require recharging, and may release contaminants into the finished water. In time, the larger cities that draw from polluted sources, such as the lower Delaware, Hudson, Ohio, and Mississippi rivers, are likely to incorporate GAC filters into their treatment. This represents a small proportion of the total water supplies in the country. Smaller supplies that draw from polluted sources will be constrained in their adoption of GAC filters because of their inadequate operating and monitoring capabilities. One beneficial effect of requiring such additional treatment may be that water purveyors now drawing on polluted sources will examine other options. For example, Vicksburg, Mississippi, which had been drawing its water supply from the Mississippi River prior to passage of the SDWA, switched to ground water. This possibility does exist for other cities and may be more attractive than trying to monitor for and remove the myriad SOCs present in these rivers. Also, the cost of installation and operation of GAC filters, together with the cost of monitoring, may make higher-quality sources a more attractive option.

▸ WATER DISTRIBUTION

A water supply system, including the treatment plant, is designed to meet the average demand on the maximum day. Use, however, varies from hour to hour and may reach a peak during a fire. Accordingly, the distribution system, which includes the high lift pumps that deliver the treated water to the system, the transmission mains for the treated water, the piping in the streets that serves the individual houses, hydrants on the system for firefighting, and service reservoirs, must be based on peak demand requirements. Each customer is served by a connection to the main in the street generally through a meter. To ensure continuity of service, pumps are selected so that, if any single pump is down for repairs, the remaining pumps can handle the requirements. Also, it is customary to provide standby power, generally through diesel engines. Distribution system piping, most commonly cement-lined ductile cast-iron pipe, is 6 inches and larger in diameter. This minimum size is required for fire protection. The pipe network is designed with sufficient interconnections so that, if any pipe breaks, the service, including water for fire protection, can be provided via other routes. The system is designed to maintain a minimum pressure of 20 psi (about 280 kg/cm^2) during peak flows to permit service to be maintained at least to the second floor of homes without creating a backdraft that might pollute the supply. Higher buildings need to be served by their own pumping stations. Elevated service reservoirs are used to help maintain these pressures by storing water for peak hours, firefighting, or an emergency.

The introduction of dual water supply systems, potable and nonpotable, requires that the two systems be kept physically separate and easily distinguishable. This is accomplished by using different materials and colors for the pipe and hydrants and different-shaped valve boxes.[5]

The operation and maintenance of the distribution system so that it may perform in an emergency is an obligation of the water supply authority. It is to the credit of the water industry in the United States that power failures occur with considerably greater frequency than failure of water services.

▸ WASTEWATER COLLECTION AND DISPOSAL

In common with other living organisms, humans discharge to the environment waste substances that, in turn, re-energize the endless cycle of nature. With urbanization and industrialization, waste products have increased in volume and in kind, and their impact on the environment has intensified.

Human wastes are discussed under two headings: so-called night soil and wastewaters. Each exerts its influence on specific environmental resources; night soil, principally on the soil; water-carried wastes, principally on water; but both, in some degree on the atmosphere and in some places or in some ways on soil and water together. Some of the effects on the environment have, in turn, reacted on our health and general well-being.

Night Soil

The expression *night soil* is used to describe human body wastes, excreta, or excrement, or the combination of feces and urine voided by humans. The terms itself derives from the practice of carting away accumulations of human ordure at night. Night soil is one of several components of urban refuse in parts of the developing world. In industrialized countries, except in parts of Japan, night soil no longer exists as such, because excreta are flushed away by water into sewerage systems.

The disposal of night soil is a problem of economy, convenience, general cleanliness, and personal hygiene. The danger of exposure to infectious diseases is proportional to the concentration of the causative agents, which tends to be high in countries that do not yet have sewerage systems. The unsightliness of excrement does not injure the public health and neither do the odors disseminated by decomposing urine and feces. Yet they are offensive to the senses and interfere with the enjoyment of an otherwise attractive environment. From this standpoint alone, their elimination is important.

Night soil is the source of a wide variety of GI infections. Its safe disposal has important public health implications, and it is understandable why this has become a concern of official health agencies even though needed operations are commonly left to other departments of local government.

Composition and Quantities. The two components of night soil—feces and urine—vary much in amount (but only slightly in composition) with the diet and age distribution of the general population and the consumption of water and other liquids. Fecal matter contains food residues, the remains of bile and intestinal secretions, cellular substances from the alimentary tract, and bacterial cells in large numbers. The per capita amount of fecal matter excreted daily is estimated at about 90 g for well-fed people, ranging up to an average of 150 g for adult males. It becomes lower, more or less in proportion to body weight, in populations that are not so fully nourished.

On the basis of wet solids, fecal matter contains about 1 percent nitrogen, much the same relative amount of phosphoric acid, and approximately one-fourth that weight of potash. The number of coliform organisms alone is well in excess of 100×10^9, and there is a wide variety of other bacteria in fecal discharges. Bacterial cells, indeed, make up about one-fourth of the weight of feces.

The infective danger of human feces is illustrated by the isolation of more than 100×10^9 *Salmonella typhosa* from some carriers of typhoid fever bacilli, in the millions of cysts of *Entamoeba histolytica* from carriers of amebic dysentery, and of similar numbers of virus units of poliomyelitis in the stools of those infected with this virus. Viral hepatitis A is the most important, if the least understood, of the viral diseases transmitted from the feces of infected persons. The eggs of intestinal parasites vary in number with the degree of infection, but the per capita figures do not come anywhere near the magnitude of bacterial pathogens. Of particular importance in certain tropical parts of the world is the discharge in feces of the eggs of the blood fluke that causes schistosomiasis.

The principal components of urine are water, urea, and mineral ash. The weight of urine excreted is about 1000 g per capita daily, up to 1500 g in adult males. Compared with fecal matter, however, urine is richer in fertilizing elements; daily per capita production of nitrogen is almost 10 times as great; of phosphoric acid, perhaps two times; and of potash, about eight times. It follows that urine constitutes the most agriculturally valuable part of human excreta. At the same time, urine is normally sterile, in fact, destroys bacteria in fecal matter with which it is left in contact for any length of time. It is quite salty because of a daily per capita excretion of 5 to 9 g of chlorides.

As chemical fertilizers have become economical in industrial parts of the world, the use of human excreta as fertilizer has been abandoned with mounting zeal and in clear opposition to established folkways. It is doubtful that education in hygiene and esthetics could have done as much in so short a time. With increasing cost of chemical fertilizers, primarily because of the high energy costs involved in their manufacture, interest in using human wastes for fertilizer is being revived.

The circulation of enteric pathogens in the environment is a function of many things, including the prevalence of the causative agents through cases and carriers, the rate of survival of the excreted organisms in different environments and climates, the nature of the infection, and the minimum infective dose with due consideration of immunological factors. Operating in favor of control are low incidence, rapid die-off, warm climates (except for the production of insects that may serve as vectors of disease), and protection of possible vehicles of infection, such as drinking water, natural ice, shellfish, bathing waters, and the soil, including foods raised upon it.

Collection and Disposal. In some parts of the world—or regionally in some countries—night soil is disposed of on site; in others it is collected and emptied into a sewerage system or dumped into an open water course or treated by itself or jointly with wastewater. On-site disposal is often primitive. A clump of bushes or trees satisfies the urge for privacy for defecation, and excreta are scattered over the ground in disregard of religious injunctions such as the Mosaic law of burial (Deuteronomy 23:12,13).

Most common in on-site disposal is the pit privy, which provides privacy but may neglect sanitation. Four common types of privy are shown in Figure 37-5.

Privies that are not properly built or well maintained may constitute as much of a hazard as their absence. The vault and pail privies require regular and frequent emptying, which has worked satisfactorily when well-managed in villages and the unsewered outskirts of sewered communities. Poorly operated, these systems can be a nuisance and a threat to health.

Because it is successful in operation and low in cost, the earth pit privy has found wide use in rural areas. The pit is usually shallow enough to lie above groundwater, yet deep enough to be shunned by flies because of its darkness and large enough to hold its accumulation for a year or two. A concrete slab floor includes either a riser with self-closing seat or an opening and foot rests, and a screened vent that prevents moisture from condensing on the underside of seat and lid.

The danger of contaminating ground-water supplies must be clearly recognized for deep pit privies. No arbitrary rules can be laid down for the minimum safe distance of any privy from a well. Everything depends on the height and direction of ground-water flow and the nature of the soil. In sand, a distance of 50 feet or more should intervene for safety. No safe distance can be prescribed where the privy

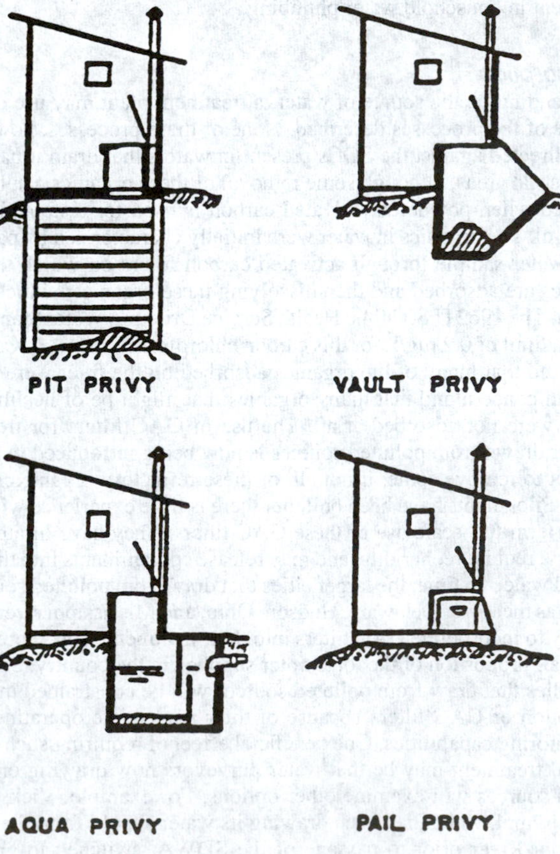

Figure 37-5. Types of privies.

is in a limestone or similar aquifer from which drinking water is drawn. Pollution of ground water can be prevented by using watertight concrete vaults, which must be cleaned out at suitable intervals.

For vacation or other homes in isolated areas, electric toilets that incinerate the fecal material are available. For aircraft, pleasure boats, and similar situations, recirculating chemical toilets are used, with provision made for their emptying into sewerage systems or treatment facilities.

The sanitary privy can be the instrument for materially reducing the incidence of intestinal diseases, particularly in developing countries. It cannot, however, be considered a satisfactory method of excreta disposal in densely populated villages or congested urban slums.

Water Pollution

Household wastes from kitchen, bathroom, and laundry are conveniently flushed away by water as domestic wastewater, and manufacturing wastes are discarded as industrial wastewaters. The system of underground pipes and appurtenances into which wastewaters are poured is called the sewerage system.

Cities built sewers initially to protect their street and lowlying areas from inundation by flooding rainstorms—not to carry away human body wastes. The sewers were storm-water drains, not sanitary sewers. The *cloaca maxima*, which drained the Roman Forum to the Tiber, is such a sewer and continues in service to this day. Water carriage of wastes of human activity did not come into purposeful use until the nineteenth century. Then, under the impact of the Industrial Revolution, the explosive growth of urban communities placed so sudden and heavy a burden on existing waste storage and vehicular transport for its removal that storm-water drains were pressed into service for domestic wastes, creating a combined sewerage system. When summers grew hot and waste loads great, the streams into which the sewers emptied began "to seethe and ferment under a burning sun," because the oxygenating capacity of their waters had been surpassed. One remedy was the construction of intercepting sewers along the banks of larger bodies of water. These conduits were made big enough to transport the dry weather flow and deliver it beyond the town to points of possible disposal without nuisance. Storm waters had to be spilled, together with their share of municipal wastes, into the otherwise protected waters. This weakness of the combined system of sewerage is as yet unresolved in the older cities of the United States. Separate systems of sewerage did not come in significant use until the beginning of the twentieth century, when the treatment of wastewater was introduced. The reasons for this are patent: protection of water courses within the community against pollution and treatment of all the wastewaters unaffected by rainwater.

Understandably, the need for reducing the burden of waste matters imposed upon the waters in streams was established first in densely settled industrial communities. Depending on the capacity of the waters to receive the wastes and stabilize them without nuisance, removal progressed from the separation of gross, generally settleable pollutional constituents (primary treatment) to the separation of fine or dissolved, generally nonsettleable, pollutional components by biological treatment (secondary treatment) and ultimately to the removal of the small concentration of specific classes of residual pollutants (tertiary treatment).

The disposal of water-carried domestic and industrial wastes involves collection through plumbing systems of the wastes in houses and other buildings, followed either by on-site disposal of these wastes or their delivery to the public sewer; collections of the wastes emptied into public sewers; treatment of the communal and industrial wastewaters; and their ultimate disposal onto or into receiving waters.

Modern wastewater treatment in the United States began in the 1920s and for a half-century was devoted to protecting the best uses of the waters into which the wastewaters were discharged. The classes of uses were as follows:

A. Drinking water and protection of shellfish beds
B. Bathing waters
C. Aquatic life
D. Industrial and agricultural water supply
E. Navigation and disposal of wastewaters without nuisance

Standards were established for each of these classes, and the treatment required was then established to maintain these standards. For example, class A and B waters for drinking and bathing have rigorous bacterial standards, which are not applicable to waters for other purposes. Treatment facilities discharging to class A and B waters were required to provide bacterial removal. Dissolved oxygen levels did not need to be so high in waters used for industry and agriculture as in waters for aquatic life. Accordingly, the treatment to remove biochemical oxygen demand needed to be greater when discharges were to class C waters, intended for protecting aquatic life, than when they were to class D waters.

These standards were the responsibility of the individual states. Some states were more rigorous in their implementation of standards than others. Accordingly, some streams were allowed to become highly polluted and unfit for any use. The environmental movement originating in the 1960s addressed this problem, leading to passage of Public Law 92-500, the Federal Water Pollution Control Act Amendments of 1972, which, with its 1977 amendments, is called the Clean Water Act. Among the goals of this act were that water quality in the nation's waters provide for the protection and propagation of fish, shellfish, and wildlife and provide for recreation in and on the waters, all to be achieved by 1983. This eliminated classification D and E. Another national goal stated in the act was that the discharge of pollutants into navigable water be eliminated by 1983, a goal that was recognized by professionals as being unattainable and that has since come to be recognized by all as unfeasible. The environmental movement focused far more on the quality of the aquatic environment (i.e., fishable and swimmable) than on public health, and little in Public Law 92-500 was directed to preservation of receiving waters for potable water supplies. In the United States, the greatest threat to the public health from pollution of water sources is from the nondegradable SOCs. Not even tertiary treatment of wastewaters addresses these chemicals; nor are waters routinely monitored for them. In some instances, fish have been found to contain dangerously high levels of chemicals discharged from industries upstream, and proscriptions against the eating of these fish have been established by health authorities. Similar concern has not yet been expressed by public agencies about drinking waters drawn from streams in which these contaminated fish swim. With the growing concern about the relationship between drinking water and health, however, more attention is now being devoted to this problem. Meanwhile, the arbitrary separation, both in legislation and administration, of water pollution control and drinking water protection militates against a comprehensive attack on this issue.

One important provision of the Clean Water Act is the requirement for National Pollution Discharge Elimination System (NPDES) permits for all sewered, so-called point-source, discharges. The permits list the conditions that have to be met by the discharges, and together they afford a useful tool for wastewater management. The problems of nonpoint-source wastewaters, such as urban and agricultural runoff, however, remain less tractable, although a permit system is being considered for urban runoff, initially targeted at communities of 100,000 population or more.

Drainage of Buildings. The plumbing system of dwellings and other buildings is the terminus of water supply and the beginning of wastewater disposal. As shown in Figure 37-6, the central components of house drainage systems are a vertical stack and a connecting, nearly horizontal house drain leading to the house sewer that leads to the street sewer or to an on-site method of disposal. For tightness, all piping, with the exception of the house sewer, is metallic or rigid plastic.

Each fixture drains into the system through a trap in which a sealing depth of water prevents air within the piping from seeping into the building. Usually malodorous, this air may at times contain toxic and flammable contaminants. Fixture traps also keep out vermin. Accordingly, the seal of traps are intended to remain intact. To prevent their being siphoned by aspiration or blown by back-pressure because of water rushing through them or past them in pipes or stacks, the traps are vented.

Important hygienically is the proper relating of water supply to drainage in the manifold fixtures within dwellings, hotels, hospitals, mercantile establishments, and industrial buildings. For full safety, water inlets must discharge well above the high-water mark of the fixture to keep its waters from being sucked or forced back into the water system by backflow. If an adequate air gap cannot be provided, special backflow preventers must be installed in the supply pipe. Although water supply systems are normally under higher pressure than drainage systems, pressures are reduced drastically at times of high draft, e.g., during fires or when pipes break. The pressure in the water system may then drop below atmospheric pressure and the resulting negative (in relation to barometric) pressure differential may pull dangerous pollutants into the system.

Drainage of Towns. Sewerage systems, whether separate or combined, are in a sense vascular systems of underground conduits that collect the spent water of the community for treatment and disposal.[29] Sewers begin in the high-lying parts of the town and point progressively downhill. They increase in size as they take in more and more wastewaters from larger and larger tributary areas. In the United States, street sewers are at least 8 inches in diameter and house sewers at least 6 inches. Sanitary and combined sewers are laid deep enough to drain the lowest fixtures in the properties they serve. However, when basements are very deep, as in tall buildings, their wastewaters are lifted into the street sewer by pumps or ejectors. Sewers are generally of vitrified tile or concrete, with joints of premolded rubber or plastic to maintain watertightness.

The slopes on which sewers are laid are set more or less by existing street grades. If the town is flat, sewers must still be laid on minimum grade, becoming quite deep, and pumping stations must lift the wastewater back to minimum depth, making for a costly system. Alternative systems, using vacuum or pressure sewers to avoid the need for laying sewers to grade, have application in special situations.

For inspection and cleaning, sewer access holes are generally built into the system at changes in grade and direction and also at intermediate points in long, straight runs.

Rainwater enters combined or storm sewers through street inlets with catch basins necessary for combined sewerage systems. The outlets of catch basins to their sewers are trapped to contain the air in the sewer and to keep sand and gravel out of it. Street inlets in separate storm systems are left untrapped.

Quantity and Composition of Wastewater. During dry weather, the volume of wastewater[1] is about 70 percent of water used. The flow fluctuates by the day, the week, and the seasons. Maximum rates are as much as 200 percent greater than the daily average. Some industrial uses introduce still greater differences. In wet weather and for some time after, ground water adds to flow, depending upon the tightness of the sewers and the wetness of the ground.

Intercepting sewers for combined systems are designed to carry as much water as can be economically and technologically justified. Where rains are steady and gentle (in England, for example), interceptors are designed for up to six times the dry weather flow, because spills are then rare. Where most storms are intense and of short duration, as they are in the United States, the frequency and volume of stormwater overflow is not altered much by oversizing the interceptors to carry more than the peak dry weather flow.

Wastewater shares the fundamental quality of the water supply but is debased by the waste load imposed upon it, by influx of ground water, and in combined sewers by varying quantities of rainwater and

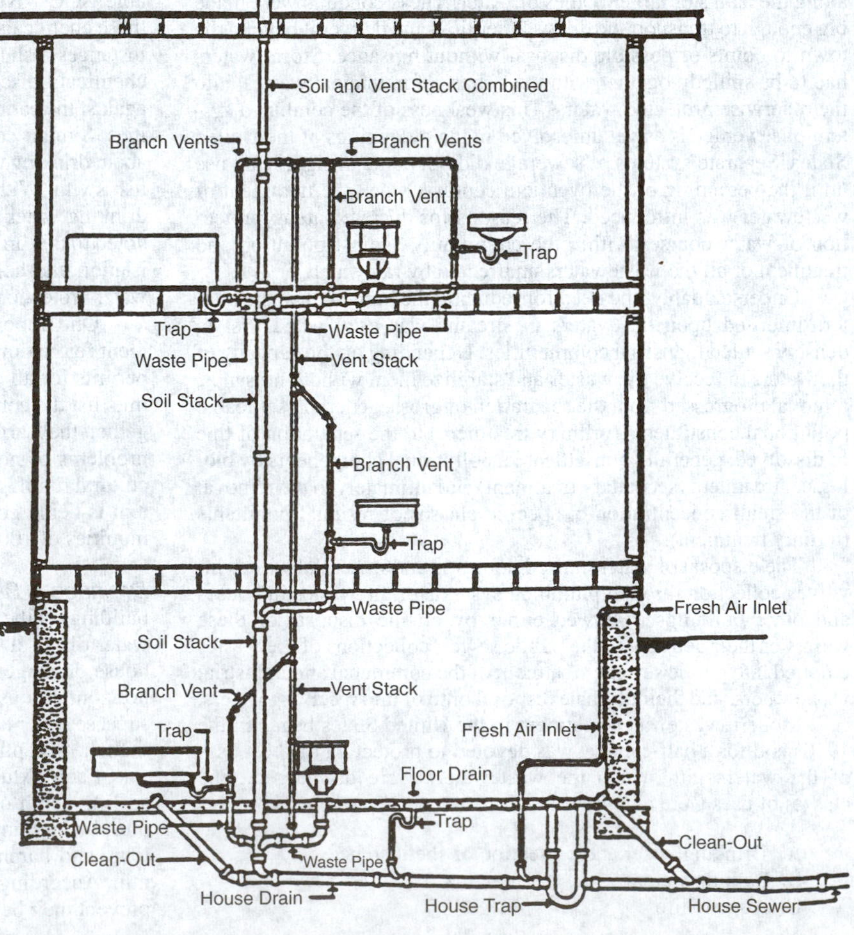

Figure 37-6. House plumbing system.

street wash. The longer it flows or stands, the more its constituents disintegrate; fecal matter and paper become unrecognizable as such; bacteria and other saprophytes multiply enormously; and the respiration of living organisms and incidental biochemical changes reduce the oxygen originally dissolved in the water, so that fresh sewerage becomes first stale and then anaerobic or septic. Wastewater is obnoxious to the senses when it purifies; it is dangerous to health when it contains pathogenic microorganisms.

In general, wastewater is analyzed for the purpose of ascertaining or predicting its effects on bodies of water into which it is to be discharged and for evaluating the performance of treatment processes. The test for biochemical oxygen demand (BOD) is worthy of special mention. This test measures the oxygen requirements of bacteria and other organisms as they feed upon and bring about the decomposition of organic matter. These requirements are important because they decree whether the receiving body of water remains aerobic (oxygen present) or anaerobic (oxygen exhausted). Hence, the BOD test is a measure of the putrescible load placed on treatment works and on bodies of water into which treatment plants empty.

In the United States, the per capita contribution of 5-day 20°C BOD to domestic wastewater averages 54 g, of which 42 g is in suspension, 19 g is settleable from suspension, and 12 g is dissolved. This compares with a per capita contribution of 250 g of solids, of which 90 g are suspended, 54 g are settleable, and 160 g are dissolved. Industrial wastes may add to these amounts appreciably. Their relative strength is conveniently expressed in terms of the number of people who would exert an equivalent BOD load. Especially high BODs are added to municipal wastewater by breweries, canneries, distilleries, packinghouses, milk plants, tanneries, and textile mills.

Industrial Wastewaters

Because BOD characterizes only organic wastes typical of human discharges, where industrial wastes are present, the chemical oxygen demand (COD) or the total organic carbon (TOC) determination may be useful. Where industrial organics or heavy metals are suspected, these too must be monitored in wastewater streams and treatment plant effluents, particularly where wastes are discharged into waters to be used for drinking or that provide the environment for edible fish.

Many industrial wastewaters interfere with treatment processes by imposing heavy loads on the plants or by impairing biological treatment because of toxic components in the wastewaters. Accordingly, industries may be required to pretreat their wastes before being permitted to discharge them to a municipal sewerage system. In addition, they are often required to reimburse the municipality for handling these wastewaters, generally in accordance with their volume and strength.

Many industrial wastewaters are discharged directly into receiving waters, thereby requiring NPDES permits under the Clean Water Act. These wastewaters contain myriads of contaminants of all types. Two approaches have been taken together to address this problem. The first is based on technology, the requirement for the use of the best available technology economically achievable, with guidelines established by EPA for each of the 21 industrial categories. The second is based on monitoring polluting chemical compounds; initially 65 compounds and classes of compounds were identified, which could include thousands of individual pollutants. This was refined to a list of 129 so-called "priority pollutants." Establishing standards for these, as well as monitoring procedures, is a formidable and expensive task, so it can be expected that they will need to be addressed on a selective basis. For example, the establishment of an MCL for a particular compound in drinking water would strongly suggest consideration of including it among those to be regulated in effluents that discharge to waters that are drawn upon for potable supplies.

Wastewater Treatment

With few exceptions, water purification and wastewater treatment processes are alike in concept and in kind.[1] They differ only in the amounts of pollutants they must remove and in the degree of purification they must accomplish.

The key operations in wastewater treatment plants are directed to the separation of the imposed load from the carrying water. The unloaded solids constitute sewerage sludge or, in the current vernacular, residuals. The desired phase separation or mass transfer of removable solids is set in motion in a number of different ways that include physical, chemical, and biological unit operations. Moreover, since wastewater is rich in nutrients, it is understandable that air or oxygen must be introduced into some treatment processes if the wastes are to be kept fresh and odorless. This, too, is a form of mass transfer—in this case as aeration or gas transfer, accompanied coincidentally by a sweeping out of gases and odors of decomposition. By contrast, anaerobic conditions may favor the degradation of putrescible matter in the dewatering and stabilization of sewage sludge.

The common unit operations and their useful combinations are as follows:

Preliminary Treatment. Screens or comminutors are often placed at the influent of treatment plants to remove or macerate rags and other large objects that may interfere with subsequent treatment units. Similarly, grit chambers remove heavy sand and grit that may be troublesome in the plant, if not in a receiving stream.

Sedimentation. The workhorse of wastewater treatment plants is the settling tank. In it, settleable solids are removed by sedimentation. These are similar to sedimentation tanks in water treatment except that, because the settled sludge can become quickly putrescible, mechanical sludge-removal equipment is always provided.

Primary sedimentation tanks hold the sewage for 1 to 2 hours. During this time, 50 to 70 percent of the influent suspended solids, including 30 to 50 percent of the influent BOD, are deposited on the tank bottom. The sludge is bulky because it contains about 95 percent water and is putrescible because its solids are volatile (organic) to the extent of about 72 percent on a dry basis.

Intermediate and secondary or final sedimentation tanks remove the flocs or sludges formed in biologically treated wastewaters. When wastewater treatment was first introduced, a recognized goal was the introduction of at least primary treatment in all the industrialized countries. In the United States, Public Law 92-500 mandates a minimum of secondary treatment (i.e., biological treatment), although the need for more than primary treatment for discharges to the ocean or to large rivers is questioned. In general, primary sedimentation is a precursor to biological treatment.

Chemical Coagulation and Flocculation. This is similar to water treatment, although the amount of aluminum and iron salts required may range as high as 100 mg/L. Reductions as high as 80 to 90 percent in suspended solids and 70 to 80 percent in BOD are obtained. The sludges from chemical treatment are generally more troublesome than primary treatment sludges.

Biological Treatment. Biological treatment units are designed to encourage a high rate of growth and activity of scavenging microorganisms. The physical result is 2-fold: (*a*) conversion of finely divided, colloidal, and dissolved organic matter into settleable cell substance by biosynthesis; and (*b*) reduction of the energy level of much of the remaining organic matter by bioanalysis, degradation, or oxidation. The wastes must not be toxic to bacteria and other microorganisms. As already mentioned, secondary or biological treatment is the minimum treatment to be provided by U.S. communities, with but few exceptions. This treatment removes about 85 percent of the BOD, resulting in an effluent BOD of about 30 mg/L.

Two unique biological treatment operations have continued in wide service over the years: trickling filtration and activated-sludge aeration. Diagrams for treatment works that include, respectively, high-rate trickling filters and activated-sludge units are shown in Figure 37-7. A third treatment approach finding favor today is the rotating biological contactor, which provides for the establishment of biological growths on a fixed medium while not requiring the large areas necessary for trickling filters.

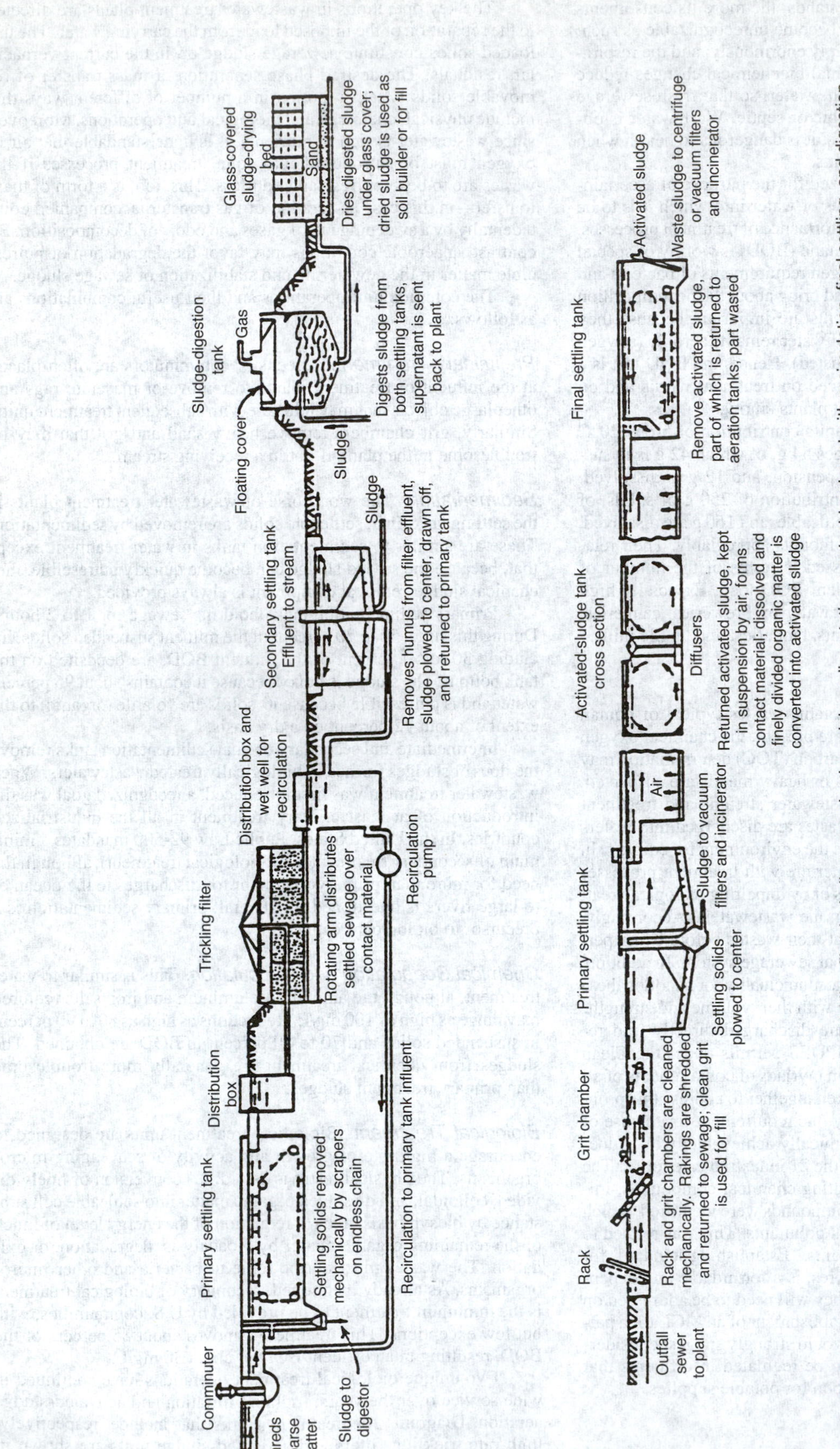

Figure 37-7. Typical wastewater treatment plants. **A**, Trickling filter including comminution, plain sedimentation, contact treatment with recirculation, final settling, and digestion and drying of sludge. **B**, Activated-sludge plant, including coarse screening, grit removal, plain sedimentation, contact treatment, and final settling. Sludge is partly dewatered by centrifugation or on vacuum filters and then incinerated. (From Fair GM, Geyer J, Okun DA: Elements of Water Supply and Wastewater Disposal. New York: John Wiley & Sons, 1971.)

Trickling Filters. Structurally, trickling filters are beds of stone or plastic media 1 to 4 m deep. The beds have extensive surfaces to which microorganisms adhere as zoogleal slimes or biomasses that are supplied (*a*) with nutrients by the wastes trickling over them from top to bottom and (*b*) with oxygen by air sweeping up or down of its own accord through the filter bed.

The wastewaters are distributed over the circular filters from arms rotating over the bed, propelled—in much the same way as an ordinary lawn sprinkler—by their own jets issuing horizontally from rows of nozzles.

The filter effluent is collected by a system of underdrains large enough to carry the flows from the bed and to transmit enough air to the zoogleal slimes to keep the operation aerobic. The biomass that builds up in the filter is kept in balance by sloughing into the filter effluent for capture in the secondary settling tank. The effluent of modern filters is normally recycled for dilution of influent and greater efficiency. For strong wastes or high loadings, two or more units may be placed in series.

Trickling filters can produce effluents containing, after sedimentation, less than 20 mg of BOD and suspended solids per liter. Their performance is not greatly affected by transient shocks of strong or toxic wastes, implying that the filter slimes have a large reserve capacity that is not easily destroyed. Because of this, trickling filters are sometimes introduced as "shock absorbers" in advance of activated sludge units, which are less rugged in their response to taxing changes in the applied wastewater. Sludge produced is about 0.05 to 0.1 percent of the flow treated. Ordinarily, this sludge contains 92 to 95 percent water and 60 to 70 percent organic matter on a dry basis. Because of the great area occupied by such plants, they are not used in large cities.

Activated Sludge Units. Structurally, activated sludge units are tanks 10 to 15 feet deep in which the wastewater is mixed and aerated together with previously formed biomasses or flocs that are returned to the tank influent. The flocs play the part of the trickling-filter slimes. Aerobic conditions are maintained by the injection of compressed air or oxygen or by absorption of oxygen from the atmosphere at the air-water interface, which is continuously renewed by mechanical stirring or air diffusion. The flocculant solids, the activated sludge, are then removed in final settling tanks.

The biomass that builds up in the aeration unit is maintained by returning a useful amount of sludge to the process from the final settling tank. Therefore, recycling is built into the activated sludge process. Transfer of organic matter to the zooglean flocs by adsorption and its stabilization and oxidation take several hours. Sludge return of approximately 25 percent by volume of incoming sewage produces about 2500 mg of suspended solids per liter of the mixed liquor.

Because it is watery, the activated sludge wasted from the process is large in bulk. Because it consists principally of living cells, it is highly putrescible. About 0.5 percent of the flow is wasted as sludge.

Modern activated-sludge plants are flexible, making it possible to vary returned sludge and air in quantities and ways that meet changing needs and experience. Three variants of the conventional process serve as examples. In *modified aeration*, the period of aeration is shortened, and the concentration of suspended solids in the mixed liquor is reduced. Less air is required, but the degree of treatment is reduced. In *step aeration* or *step loading*, the returned sludge is added to a fraction of the inflowing sewage, the remainder being introduced at equal distances along the path of the mixed liquor. The returning sludge renews its activity without being overwhelmed. In *complete mixing*, the influent is introduced transverse to the flow. This avoids "shock loading" of the sludge even more effectively than step loading. Sludge may be kept in circulation within the aeration unit until it is no longer degradable, a practice favored in small plants or when the organic substances in the wastes being treated are completely soluble. Milk-processing wastes are of this kind.

Stabilization Ponds. A system of stabilization ponds is like a river wound up in one spot. The ponds are constructed in porous or tight soil as rude basins about 1 m deep. They expose large surfaces to air and light. Putrescible wastewaters are held in them for several weeks. During this time, settleable solids sink to the bottom, and organic matter decomposes. Under favorable climatic conditions, carbon dioxide, nitrogen, phosphorus, and other nutrients are released to the water during decomposition and stimulate profuse algal growths. During daylight hours, oxygen is produced by photosynthesis and helps keep the ponds aerobic. At night, carbon dioxide is lost to the atmosphere. Seepage and evaporation are not great.

Except in winter at high latitudes, when they are covered with ice, properly dimensioned ponds remain aerobic, and both BOD and coliforms are reduced to acceptable levels. Climatic and operational factors enter into the performance of stabilization ponds so greatly that allowable loadings cannot be set with certitude. Depending on circumstances, winter loadings may be no more than 20; summer loadings, as high as 400 persons per 1,000 m^2. The green alga *Chlorella* is a common bloom. Its small spherical cells are not easily separated from the effluent, but the incentive remains to convert waste nutrients into useful algal proteins that can be harvested safely and economically as animal feeds.

Because of their large area, stabilization ponds are introduced where waste volumes are not too large and land is not too costly. The ponds themselves are simple to construct and are particularly suitable in developing countries.

Tertiary Treatment. In many instances, secondary treatment is insufficient to maintain water quality in receiving streams and lakes, and tertiary treatment is required. When tertiary treatment involves physical-chemical treatment, it is characterized as advanced waste treatment (AWT). Often the tertiary treatment is required to remove additional BOD, which can be accomplished by adding a second stage of biological treatment or by carrying the process to nitrification, which oxidizes the oxygen-demanding ammonia, relieving oxygen pressures on receiving streams. Other tertiary treatment processes are for the removal of phosphorus and/or nitrogen. Phosphorus is generally removed chemically, while nitrogen can be removed biologically or by ammonia stripping, a gas-exchange process. It should not be necessary to remove both phosphorus and nitrogen. These are nutrients that stimulate eutrophication, or fertilization, in lakes and other still or slow-moving bodies of water. Generally, one or the other of these nutrients is limiting, and its removal may control eutrophication.

Unfortunately, these nutrients originate also in nonpoint sources, such as from runoff from fertilized urban and agricultural lands, which are more difficult to control. Removal of phosphorus and nitrogen from wastewaters may then not be sufficient to effect any improvement in receiving waters.

Where wastewater reclamation is intended, filtration may be introduced for polishing the effluent, increasing its clarity, and reducing the chlorine demand for disinfection. In some special instances, the filter may be activated carbon to reduce the color and the concentration of synthetic organics.

As the efficiency of removal of pollutants is increased, the cost of removing each additional unit of pollution increases exponentially. After secondary treatment achieves 85 percent removal, an additional 10 percent removal may cost much more than removal of the first 40 percent. Going from 97 to 99 percent removal may cost as much as the entire effort of going from 0 to 97 percent. Moreover, the operation and energy costs are exceedingly high. Accordingly, authorities should demonstrate ample justification in public benefits, including public health, before selecting treatment levels.

Disinfection of Wastewaters

Chlorine is the principal disinfectant, with contact times of at least 15 minutes at maximum flow rates, and residuals of 0.2 to 1.0 mg/L. For 99.9 percent reduction of coliform organisms, chlorine dosages range from 5 to 25 mg/L.

Chlorination is called for only where effluents are to be discharged into waters used for drinking, bathing, or shellfish growing. Chlorination of effluents may create three problems: (*a*) chloramines are formed, which may be toxic to aquatic life; (*b*) in reaction with organics, chlorinated hydrocarbons of potential health significance may be formed; and (*c*) beneficial microorganisms, as well as pathogens, are destroyed, thereby reducing the ability of the receiving water to biochemically stabilize the organic matter remaining. In contrast with the United States, where EPA had initially mandated chlorination for every effluent, no effluents are chlorinated in Great Britain, even where they discharge into waters to be used for drinking. Disinfection of effluents needs to be evaluated carefully in each instance.

An alternative to chlorination of effluents is the use of ultraviolet light, which eliminates the impact on aquatic life and the possibility of the creation of chlorinated hydrocarbons. To be successful, however, UV light requires an effluent of consistently low turbidity, implying the need for tertiary filtration.

Sludge Management

Sludge is the settled solids removed from the flow during its passage through primary sedimentation tanks with or without the benefit of coagulating chemicals, or after biological treatment. Sludge accumulates most of the living organisms that find their way into wastewaters. Sludge teems with predators such as the ciliated protozoa that feed upon bacteria and thereby accelerate the die-away of bacterial pathogens. Sludge drying deprives the organisms of moisture needed for survival.

Fresh primary-tank solids are the most dangerous, solids from biological treatment units less so, solids that have been subjected to biological decomposition still less, and air-dried solids the least. Heat-dried solids are microbiologically safe. The period of survival of enteric viruses in sludge is still unknown; for enteric bacteria, such as the typhoid bacillus, it is reported as about 1 week. Viable cysts of *E. histolytica* have been isolated from sludge held for 10 days at 30°C, and viable hookworm eggs after 41 days. For sludge held 6 months, a 10 percent survival of *Ascaris* eggs was noted; but when pulverized sludge was heated to 103°C for 3 minutes, all eggs were destroyed.

Treatment. Generally speaking, sludge is of little value and is disposed of in the cheapest possible way. In normal circumstances, however, it is neither feasible nor economical to get rid of the large volumes of sludge generated without dewatering it, destroying its organic (putrescible) constituents, or both. Why it pays to reduce the water content of sludge is exemplified by the fact that reducing the moisture content of sludge from 98 percent (2 percent solids) to 96 percent (4 percent solids) doubles the proportion of solid matter and, in consequence, halves the volume of sludge to be handled. Dewatering and destruction of organic matter are indeed the primary objectives of sludge treatment. The wide range of options for the handling of sludges is illustrated in Figure 37-8.

Sludge Digestion. Sludge is an abundant source of food for saprophytic bacteria and other organisms. Different groups of living things use different types of nutrients originally contained in the sludge or produced in the course of decomposition. As the nutritive elements are used up, the sludge becomes stable and, in its final state of degradation, inoffensive to sight and smell. The sludge is then well digested. The end products of digestion are gases, liquids, and residues of mineral and conservative organic substances. Losses by gasification and liquefaction, destruction of water-binding colloids, and physical compaction of solids reduce the bulk of the sludge and prepare it for dewatering.

Organic solids digest under both aerobic and anaerobic conditions. They do so in swamps and river deposits. In the preparation of sludge for land disposal, however, it is simpler and more economical to digest the solids anerobically. The principal gas released during aerobic decomposition is carbon dioxide; during anaerobic digestion it is combustible methane (65 to 80 percent by volume). The potential heat energy of the methane is a prime factor in the economy of anaerobic sludge digestion. The gas may be burned under a boiler or in a gas engine. The power released as heat and mechanical energy is put to use for the heating of buildings and digestion units, air compression, pumping, and minor laboratory purposes. On a per capita basis, the normal daily volume of gas generated is about 0.03 m^3 from primary settling tanks and nearly the same amount again from biological treatment units. Ground garbage and some organic industrial wastes increase the gas yield appreciably. The fuel value of the gas is about 24,000 kJ (BTUs)/m^3, more than that of most synthetic illuminating gases.

Anaerobic sludge digestion units are heated, covered, insulated tanks in which the sludge is stored until it is dense, essentially odorless, and readily dewatered. The temperature of the sludge mass is kept at an optimal operating value—normally about 35°C. In modern, high-rate installations, digestion is promoted by stirring as well as by heating. Digestion tank capacity requirements range from 0.07 m^3 per capita for sludge from primary treatment up to twice that for all the sludge from an activated sludge plant.

Where sludge treatment is by mechanical dewatering and heat-drying or incineration, sludge digestion is not necessary; where it is practiced, capacities may be much less than indicated above because digestion need not be complete. The destruction of organic matter at high temperatures and pressures by wet combustion is finding some application.

Sludge Drying. For small works, the cheapest and therefore the most common method of dewatering sludge is drying it in the open air. To this purpose, digested sludge is run or pumped onto beds of

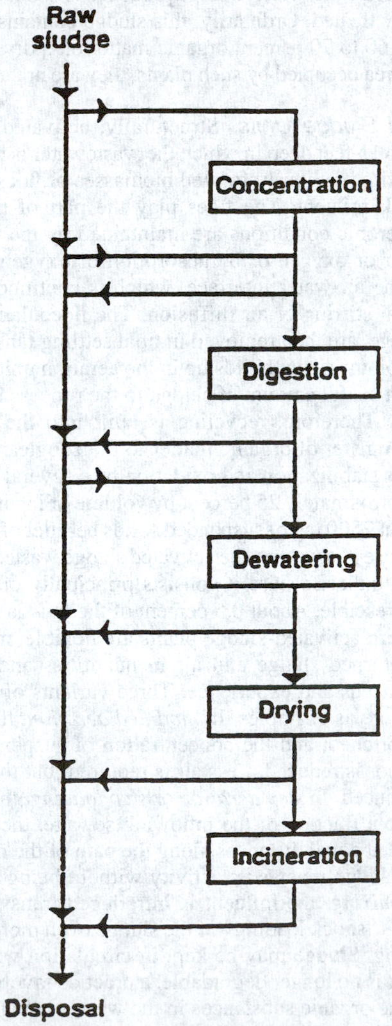

Figure 37-8. Flow diagram for the handling of wastewater treatment plant sludges, with arrows indicating possible flow paths. (From Okun DA, Ponghis G: Community Wastewater Collection and Disposal. Geneva: World Health Organization, 1975.)

sand and gravel or other suitable porous material. Part of the sludge moisture evaporates at its surface, and part seeps through the supporting bed into underdrains. Drying times vary with climate and character of sludge. The required area is about 0.1 m^2 per capita for well-digested primary sludge and twice that amount for biological sludges. When sludge has lost enough moisture to become a spadable cake, it is removed from the drying beds for final disposal.

In works of moderate and large size, it pays to dewater sludge mechanically.

Sludge Disposal. Some seacoast towns pump wet sludge to sea; others load partially dewatered sludge onto vessels or scows and carry it out to dumping grounds at sea. This practice is being re-evaluated.

Dewatered sludge is a suitable material for disposal in a properly designed landfill by itself or in combination with municipal refuse. Wet sludge can provide useful moisture, humus, and nutrients for composting operations. The use of sludge as a fertilizer may be warranted as a measure of nitrogen and phosphorus conservation and soil building. To this purpose, some municipalities are able to dispose of wet sludge, or sludge cake, to farmers. Tank trucks with fixed nozzles that plow and discharge the liquid sludge into the soil have become popular. In general, only commercially dry (heat-dried to less than 10 percent moisture) activated sludge has been found sufficiently marketable in the United States—for use on lawns and golf greens—to meet the expense of dewatering and heating.

Because of the low cost and the convenience of chemical fertilizers, however, the production of heat-dried sludge for sale is seldom economically rewarding. This may change, though, as rising energy costs increase the costs of chemical fertilizers. In the few instances where heat-dried activated sludge is marketed, as from Milwaukee, the capital investment in the facilities has already been paid off and further capital investment is not warranted. Where suitable sites for sludge disposal are not economically available, the sludge must be incinerated, leaving only the ash for disposal. In some communities, incineration of sludge with municipal refuse has been found feasible.

The ultimate disposal of wastewater sludges, particularly when they may contain pathogens, heavy metals, and synthetic organic chemicals, has raised many questions. All of the methods of disposal, whether by discharge to sea, application to agricultural land, burying in landfills, composting, or incineration have come under attack. The EPA has been wrestling with this problem since passage of the 1977 Clean Water Act Amendments. The regulations involve contaminant limits for heavy metals and organics in the sludges, in milligrams per kilogram, and loading rates, in kilograms per hectare, for various land applications, as well as technology, monitoring, and reporting requirements. Ultimate disposal will likely be by land application and landfills for communities that have such land available to them, and for larger cities, incineration. With land applications, a major concern is the potential for impact in water supplies.

Wastewater Disposal

Outfall sewers are used to discharge the treated wastewater into the receiving body of water. If outfalls are to be effective, they must be designed and situated to disperse the effluent quickly and thoroughly throughout the receiving water. In streams, this is not difficult; in lakes, tidal estuaries, and the ocean it is not simple. Outfall locations must be chosen with an eye to waterworks intakes, shellfish layings, bathing beaches, and recreational areas. This calls for the study of water movements of all kinds: normal currents, wind-induced and tidal movements, and eddy diffusion created by differences in the density of the sewerage and the receiving water. Density is a function of water temperature and the concentration of dissolved solids, or salinity.

Wastewaters are generally warmer and lighter than the water into which they are discharged. Emptied into a receiving body of water near its surface—especially the brackish waters of tidal estuaries—the wastewater rides on top of the diluting water, does not mix appreciably, and tends to form a slick, noticeable for many miles. Nevertheless, the temperature-density equilibria are so delicate that every situation and season must be handled individually. Under some conditions, for example, subsurface discharge of wastewaters into a deep fresh-water lake may build up a large mass of undispersed wastes around the outfall. Otherwise, subsurface and submarine outfalls are widely used. The lighter liquid rises like a smoke plume through the receiving body of water, and there is good dispersion. This is stepped up further by discharging the wastes through a number of outlets (diffuser), spaced so as to not interfere with one another.

The purification accomplished in streams can be improved by engineering works that either supply water for dilution during periods of low flow, lengthen the time of downstream passage of the receiving water, or introduce air into the flowing water, either directly by injection or indirectly by agitation. In low-water regulation, water is released from upland reservoirs in the same or neighboring catchment areas, or water is pumped back or recycled from the more voluminous flows of lower river reaches or other water courses. Times of travel and self-purification are normally lengthened by impoundages within the polluted stretches of the stream. The reservoirs are not made so deep that they stratify and undergo eutrophication. Compressed air has been introduced with some success into critical reaches of polluted streams from stationary compressors and piping or from floating, occasionally self-propelled, barges.

A somewhat unusual example of controlled dilution of wastewaters is the construction of fish ponds in which effluent is mixed with clean river water to create an ecosystem favorable for the cultivation of fish and the raising of ducks. Large crops of organisms that serve as food for fish and ducks are raised in the aquatic meadows of these ponds. Both impoundages and fish ponds are variations on stabilization ponds that receive raw or treated wastes without the benefit of diluting waters.

On-Site Disposal of Domestic Wastewaters. Where running water has been introduced into kitchens, bathrooms, laundries, and outbuildings of farms and fringe-area houses but there is no public sewerage, the wastewaters must be disposed of on site. Usually, this is done through septic tanks or cesspools, which involve simple settling and subsurface leaching. For success, the amount of sewage cannot be large in relation to the leaching area, and the soil must be porous. Where the volume of wastewater is high or the soil is tight, more sophisticated and costly treatment methods patterned after municipal processes must be introduced. Of special concern is the contamination, both chemical and biological, of nearby wells. Septic tanks derive their name from the septic or anaerobic condition created by the decomposition of the settling solids or accumulating sewage sludges. All septic tanks must be emptied of accumulated sludge periodically. Septage is generally disposed of in community wastewater treatment plants.

The ability of soil to absorb settled sewage is explored by digging test holes, filling them with water, and clocking the time required for the water to drop a given distance in the stratum in which leaching is to take place. In some states, soil profiles are used to determine the ability of the soil to absorb settled sewage.

Septic tanks and tile fields may be suitable for truly rural areas, but they have been adopted by builders for housing developments, where they inevitably cause trouble, generally because the tile fields become clogged and the septic tanks overflow, creating a local health hazard. Even where soil conditions are suitable, septic tanks and tile fields should not be used unless at least about 4000 m^2 (1 acre) is available per dwelling unit.

Housing developments constructed in periurban areas not accessible to municipal sewerage systems have led to the proliferation of package plants for wastewater treatment. These plants do conform to most modern practices, often providing tertiary treatment, and they may be obliged, by their NPDES permits, to meet exacting effluent standards. However, their operation and maintenance becomes the responsibility of the home owners, who have little capacity to manage such facilities. Even where private utility companies are employed to operate these plants, their performance record is abysmal. The quality of personnel and the cost of monitoring for small plants are little different than for large plants. The diseconomies that accompany such small facilities militate against collecting sufficient funds for proper management of package plants. It is preferable that densities of development be low enough to permit septic tanks or, where greater densities are desired, the development must be obligated to arrange for sewerage service from a nearby large municipality. Package plants are particularly to be avoided on water supply watersheds.

Where dense housing is developed without sewers, retrofitting an area with sewers is exceedingly expensive. This is a serious problem facing the urban areas of Asia, Africa, and Latin America, which were provided with water supplies but no adequate means of wastewater disposal. Alternatives to costly sewerage are being sought, and many on-site methods of disposal have been found satisfactory for rural communities, but to date no suitable alternative to sewerage has been developed for urban areas.

Wastewater Reclamation

Wastewaters are a water resource, and their reclamation for reuse serves both to conserve limited quantities of fresh water and to reduce the load of pollution on receiving bodies of water. The following purposes have been served by wastewater reclamation.[3]

1. Irrigation, both agricultural and urban
2. Industrial use, both process and cooling
3. Recreation, through establishment of lakes and ponds
4. Nonpotable residential and commercial use, including toilet flushing

Reclamation for potable purposes is not recommended, as sound drinking water practice requires that priority should be given to the purest source. Treatment and monitoring technology are not adequate to ensure safety where wastewaters are to be used directly for potable purposes.

Reclamation for irrigation and land disposal of wastewaters are different. Irrigation is the beneficial use of wastewaters for growing crops or lawns. Land disposal is a method of wastewater disposal where harvesting of crops is incidental. Many of the constraints and benefits are the same.

Land disposal may be useful in smaller communities where ample land is available and the soil conditions are appropriate. Where the nutrients in wastewaters would be troublesome if discharged to a body of water, on land they constitute an important plus, particularly as chemical fertilizers become more costly. Land disposal provides a method for removing the nutrients in the soil, to be picked up by harvested crops.

Each situation is unique, permitting certain rates of application and requiring specific treatment. Because the wastewaters are produced year-round, but cannot be applied to the land during periods of heavy rainfall or freezing, seasonal storage is required. Soil scientists can make useful contributions to resolution of these problems.

Where wastewaters are to be reused, the treatment needs to be tailored to the specific reuse, with more intensive treatment and more stringent standards as the uses become of greater public health concern. The California Department of Health has prepared *Wastewater Reclamation Criteria*, which guides the regulation of many hundreds of reclamation projects in the state. The highest degree of treatment is for nonpotable distribution systems, which include urban irrigation, toilet flushing, industry, etc., as well as spray irrigation of food crops and nonrestricted recreational impoundments (i.e., those that permit body contact). On the basis of the Pomona Study, an appropriate quality would appear to be produced by secondary wastewater treatment followed by coagulation, direct filtration, and disinfection with chlorine.

Essential to such reclamation are reliability of operation of the treatment facilities and continuous monitoring of effluent quality with a capacity to automatically reject effluent that does not meet the bacterial, turbidity, and chlorine residual standards.[30]

▶ ORGANIZATION FOR WATER QUALITY MANAGEMENT

Human ecology is distinguished from the ecology of other biological systems by our ability to reason, inquire, and invent. As a result, we have developed the means for adjusting the environment to ourselves. This is a never-ending task, as development continues to interfere with the environment, often creating new hazards to health. We must continue efforts to protect ourselves against disease processes that have environmental causes. Among other things, this requires the collaboration of persons with many different skills.

Engineers have long been members of public agencies that have as one of their responsibilities the initiation, approval, and control of public works related in one way or another to human health and well-being. In England, the start was made through the promotion of the "sanitary idea," which found expression in the sanitation of growing industrial towns. In the United States, it was begun at the state level for the protection of the purity of inland waters and continued at the federal level for the safety of interstate travelers and the protection of interstate waters. At the international level, water sanitation has been promoted by international treaty; examples are the control of oil pollution of international waters in the seas and oceans of the world and the maintenance of acceptable standards of water quality in international bodies of fresh water such as the Rhine, the Rio Grande, and the chain of lakes and rivers along the boundary between the United States and Canada.

At another level, municipal, county, or regional authorities are generally responsible for the provision and operation of water supply and wastewater treatment facilities. Regulation through monitoring of water quality, review of plans for treatment works, and data from their operations is the responsibility of state agencies. At one time, this responsibility almost always rested with the state health agency, but gradually separate pollution control agencies were established. At the federal level, the EPA administers the national water supply and water pollution control programs.

Because the waters of the earth know no political boundaries—although they often become international and interstate borders by political choice—some countries have found it expedient to establish national water authorities.

As revealed by the PHS Community Water Supply Survey,[2] one of the problems with the quality of water service arises from the excessive fragmentation of the water supply industry. More than half the water supply systems in the United States serve fewer than 1,000 people. The same is true for sewerage and wastewater disposal. Such small systems cannot afford the quality of design and operation of complex facilities that large communities can, and yet the needs are much the same. Moreover, smaller communities are in competition with each other for limited water resources, and they lose the advantages of the economies and efficiencies of scale.

One clear solution is the regionalization of water management, which has been approached in a revolutionary way by England and Wales with the creation of 10 regional water authorities based on hydrological boundaries.[31] Each authority owns, operates, and finances all the facilities for water supply, wastewater collection and disposal, and water-based recreation. The success of this approach is revealed by the fact that more than 99 percent of the population is served by public water supplies and by the way in which England met the 1975–1976 drought, the most severe in a millennium. While the integrated approach to water management was abandoned in 1989 by privatization of the water supply, sewerage, and wastewater disposal functions of the authorities, this regional approach can be studied with profit, and elements of it adopted, by all who are responsible for water quality management. Whatever form of organization is adopted, its ultimate task is to manage water resources in the service of people while protecting their health and the quality of the environment.

▸ REFERENCES

1. Fair GM, Geyer J, Okun DA: Elements of Water Supply and Wastewater Disposal. New York: John Wiley & Sons, 1971
2. US Public Health Service: Commmunity Water Supply Survey, 1969. Summarized in McCabe L, et al: Study of community water supply systems. J Am Water Works Assoc 62:670, 1970
3. Camp, Dresser & McKee, Inc: Guidelines for Water Reuse. 600/8-80-036. Washington, DC: Environmental Protection Agency, 1980
4. United Nations Economic and Social Council: Water for Industrial Use. Report No. E-3058 ST/ECA/50. New York: United Nations Economic and Social Council, 1958
5. American Water Works Association: Manual on Dual Distribution Systems, No. M 24. Denver: American Water Works Association, 1983
6. Environmental Protection Agency: National Interim Primary Drinking Water Regulations. Washington, DC: Environmental Protection Agency, 1976
7. US District Court, District of Connecticut: Bridgeport Hydraulic Co. et al. vs. The Council on Water Company Lands of the State of Connecticut et al., Civil No. B-75-212, December 1977
8. University of North Carolina: Protecting Drinking Water Supplies Through Watershed Management: A Guidebook for Devising Local Programs. Chapel Hill, NC: Center for Urban and Regional Studies, 1982
9. Burby RJ, Okun DA: Land use planning and health. Annu Rev Public Health 4:47–67, 1983
10. National Research Council: Drinking Water and Health. Washington, DC: National Academy Press, vol 1, 1977; vols 2 and 3, 1980; vol 4, 1982; vol 5, 1983; vol 6, 1986; vols 7 and 8, 1987; vol 9, 1989
11. Cantor KP, Hoover R, et al: Bladder cancer, drinking water source, and tap water consumption: a case-control study. J Natl Cancer Inst 19(6):1269–1279, 1987
12. Cothern CR: Radioactivity in Drinking Water. EPA 570/9-81-002. Washington, DC: Environmental Protection Agency, 1981
13. National Academy of Sciences–National Research Council: The Effects on Populations of Exposure to Low Levels of Ionizing Radiation. Washington, DC: Government Printing Office, 1972
14. Longtin JP: Radon, Radium and Uranium Occurrence in Drinking Water from Groundwater Sources. Proceedings of National Conference of American Water Works Association, June 1987. Denver: American Water Works Association, 1987
15. Standard Methods for the Examination of Water and Wastewater: American Water Works Association, American Public Health Association, 19th ed. Washington, DC: American Water Works Association, 1995
16. Bryan RT, Pinner RW, Berkelman RL: Emerging infectious diseases in the United States. Improved surveillance, a requisite for prevention. Ann NY Acad Sci 740:346–361, 1994
17. Craun GF: Surface water supplies and health. J Am Water Works Assoc 80:40, 1988
18. Cabelli VJ: Health Effects Criteria for Marine Recreational Waters. EPA-600/1-80-031. Washington, DC: Environmental Protection Agency, August 1983
19. Colbourne JS: Thames Water Authority's experience with *Cryptosporidium*. Proceedings of 1989 Water Technology Conference, American Water Works Association, Denver 1990
20. Dufour AP: Health Effects Criteria for Fresh Recreational Waters. EPA-600/1-84-004. Washington, DC: Environmental Protection Agency, August 1984
21. Environmental Protection Agency: Part II 40 CFR, Parts 141 and 142, Federal Register, June 29, 1989
22. McJunkin FE: Water and Human Health. Washington, DC: US Agency for International Development, July 1982
23. Thomas HA Jr: The animal farm. J Am Water Works Assoc 56:1087, 1964
24. World Health Organization: Guidelines for Drinking Water Quality. 3 vols. Geneva: World Health Organization, 1984
25. Okun DA: The value of water supply and sanitation development: an assessment. Am J Public Health 78:1463, 1988
26. American Water Works Association: Water Quality and Treatment. New York: McGraw-Hill, 1971
27. American Society of Civil Engineers, American Water Works Association, Conference of State Sanitary Engineers: Water Treatment Plant Design. Denver: American Water Works Association, 1989
28. Water Pollution Control Federation and American Society of Civil Engineers: Wastewater Treatment Plant Design. New York: American Society of Civil Engineers, 1977
29. Water Pollution Control Federation and American Society of Civil Engineers: Design and Construction of Sanitary and Storm Sewers. Alexandria, VA: Water Pollution Control Federation, 1969
30. California Department of Health Services: Wastewater Reclamation Criteria. California Administrative Code, Title 22, Division 4, 1978
31. Okun DA: Regionalization of Water Management: A Revolution in England and Wales. Essex, England: Applied Science Publishers, 1977

38

Solid and Radioactive Waste Disposal

William A. Suk

Waste has pervaded our environment for centuries and will continue to contaminate our surroundings in the foreseeable future. Although waste is a by-product of lifestyle, not all the problems that waste creates has been dealt with effectively. The challenge is to better understand these contaminants, and to determine under which conditions and at which levels they pose a threat to human health and the environment.

▸ HAZARDOUS WASTES

Definitions of Waste

Wastes may be classified by their physical, chemical, and biological characteristics. An important classification criterion is their consistency. Solid wastes are waste materials having less than approximately 70 percent water. This class includes municipal solid wastes such as household garbage, industrial wastes, mining wastes, and oil-field wastes. Liquid wastes are usually wastewaters, including municipal and industrial wastewaters, that contain less than 1 percent suspended solids. Such wastes may contain high concentrations (greater than 1 percent) of dissolved species, such as salts and metals. Solid waste, as defined under the Resource, Conservation, and Recovery Act (RCRA) is any solid, semisolid, liquid, or contained gaseous materials discarded from industrial, commercial, mining, or agricultural operations and from community activities. Solid waste includes garbage, construction debris, commercial refuse, sludge from water supply or waste treatment plants, material from air pollution control facilities, and other discarded materials. Solid waste does not include solid or dissolved materials in irrigation return flows or industrial discharges. Sludge is a class of wastes intermediate to solid and liquid wastes. Sludges usually contain between 3 and 25 percent solids, while the rest of the material is water-dissolved species. These materials, which have a slurrylike consistency, include municipal sludges, which are produced during secondary treatment of wastewaters, and sediments found in storage tanks and lagoons.

Federal regulations classify wastes into three different categories, based on hazard criteria: (*a*) nonhazardous, (*b*) hazardous, and (*c*) special. Nonhazardous wastes are those that pose no immediate threat to human health and/or the environment, for example, municipal wastes such as household garbage and many high-volume industrial wastes. Hazardous wastes are of two types: (*a*) those that have characteristic hazardous properties, i.e., ignitability, corrosivity, or reactivity, and (*b*) those that contain leachable toxic constituents. Other hazardous wastes include liquid wastes, which are identified with a particular industry or industrial activity. The third category from industry is classified generically as special wastes by origin, and are regulated with waste-specific guidelines. Examples include mine spoils, oil-field wastes, spent oils, and radioactive wastes. In the United States, all hazardous wastes are regulated under Subtitle C of RCRA.

Hazardous waste has been defined as a myriad of substances that causes toxicity to living organisms. For all practical purposes, toxic waste and hazardous waste are interchangeable. As indicated, hazardous waste is defined as solid waste that is acutely toxic or possesses one or more of the following criteria: ignitability, corrosivity, reactivity, or toxicity.[1] Traditionally, when discussing radioactive or medical waste, the term "mixed waste" is used (see section on Radioactive and Mixed Wastes). Toxic substances occur naturally in soil, water, and air; however, thousands of toxic substances are anthropogenic. The anthropogenic substances are of particular concern because of the quantities that are produced, their dissemination and persistence, and because, historically, their release into the environment has not been well controlled. Furthermore, most anthropogenic compounds are organic and are readily absorbed by living organisms.

Hazardous Wastes

Hazardous waste is a subset of solid wastes that poses substantial or potential threats to public health or the environment. It is specifically listed as a hazardous waste by exhibiting one or more of the characteristics of hazardous waste (i.e., ignitability, corrosivity, reactivity, and/or toxicity), is generated by the treatment of hazardous waste, or is contained in a hazardous waste. Some environmental laws list specific materials as hazardous waste. For example, hazardous waste can exist in the form of a solid, liquid, or sludge and can include materials such as polychlorinated biphenyls (PCBs), chemicals, explosives, gasoline, diesel fuel, organic solvents, asbestos, acid, metals, and pesticides. Environmental laws also list materials that must be treated and managed as hazardous.

The true amount of hazardous wastes generated is not known, although the approximate amount is 400 million tons a year. The Organization for Economic Cooperation and Development (OECD) estimates that, on average, a consignment of hazardous wastes crosses the frontier of an OECD nation every 5 minutes of every day all year. More than 2 million tons of those wastes are estimated to cross national frontiers of OECD European countries annually on the way to disposal sites. Other movements, which are illegal, are motivated by the possibility of important gains in transferring the problem to places where controls or standards are less strict. Another motive may be that vast territory and scant resources in countries that import products make any attempt at serious surveillance impossible. Some countries also prefer to manage their hazardous waste problem by transporting it at lower cost to other countries.

The quantity of generated wastes of all kinds is still increasing, and the rapid pace of industrialization worldwide will necessitate careful attention. In response to growing recognition of health and environmental risks associated with hazardous wastes, governments have brought into force a series of national laws to control the generation, handling, storage, treatment, transport, disposal, and recovery of these wastes. To mitigate such potential threats, urgent measures should be taken to avoid or reduce generation of hazardous wastes, optimize environmentally sound recovery of wastes, reduce to a minimum or eliminate transboundary movements of hazardous wastes, manage wastes in an environmentally sound and efficient way, and dispose of wastes as close as possible to the place where they are generated.

In exceptional cases, exporting hazardous wastes to a country capable of eliminating them properly may be safer for human health and the environment if adequate storage or treatment is not possible in the generating country or until appropriate technology and adequate infrastructure are available. Increased international cooperation is necessary to help developing countries manage and treat the wastes they generate in an environmentally sound way. There have been a number of conferences and workshops to assess and evaluate hazardous waste exposures and to provide a framework for future research and collaborative efforts to address these problems.[2,3]

Thousands of new chemicals are being developed and introduced annually into commerce. Only a small fraction of these substances have been tested for toxicity. Hundreds of millions of tons of hazardous waste are generated annually and the quantities are increasing.[4] A small fraction of toxic waste in the environment is from household use; the greatest production comes from industry, particularly the chemical and petroleum industries.[5] Another leading generator, the agricultural chemical manufacturing industry, produces chemicals, such as pesticides, that by their very nature are toxic not only to their targets, but also to other life forms. The magnitude of problems created by toxic substances is immense and ubiquitous, while the impact is, to a great extent, unknown.

Transportation of Hazardous Wastes

Toxic substances and other contaminants know no borders and, as such, the issues surrounding them have gained a presence in international forums. In 1972, 70 governments met in Sweden for the United Nations Conference on the Human Environment. This conference brought environmental issues to an international level. Since that time more than 170 international environmental treaties have been signed,[6] demonstrating the global commitment to the issue. In 1976 the United Nations Environment Program's International Register of Potentially Toxic Chemicals was established. This Register collects information on hazardous waste and distributes it to anyone who requests it. The Basil Convention, 1989, established the Control of Transboundary Movement of Hazardous Wastes and Their Dispersal. With more than 100 signatories on this treaty, the movement of wastes is now managed throughout much of the world. A pivotal conference sponsored by the United Nations held in Rio de Janeiro, Brazil, in 1992, United Nations Conference on Environment and Development (Rio Earth Summit), focused on the issues of biodiversity and sustainable development.[7] This report included a chapter on both toxic waste and hazardous waste, thus demonstrating the priority of the effective control and management of such releases into the environment. Protection of the environment in conjunction with economic development are closely related in any proposals that support future global welfare.

Policies Managing the Fate of Toxic Substances

In the 1960s the United States Congress began its journey in establishing environmentally oriented laws. In 1966, the Division of Environmental Health Science was established in the Department of Health, Education and Welfare to study the health effects of environmental agents. In 1969, it was elevated to Institute status (National Institute of Environmental Health Sciences (NIEHS)), thus emphasizing the importance of environmental implications on human health. In the same year the United States Congress passed the National Environmental Policy Act, requiring federal agencies to assess the impact of their actions on the environment. A year later the U.S. Environmental Protection Agency (EPA) was established. EPA is responsible for working with state and local governments to control and prevent pollution in areas of solid and hazardous waste, pesticides, water, air, drinking water, and toxic and radioactive substances. Since that time numerous other acts, including the Toxic Substance Control Act (1976) (TSCA), have been passed with the goal of maintaining a healthy environment. TSCA requires that producers of toxic substances be held accountable for the release of these substances into the environment. In 1976 the Resource, Conservation, and Recovery Act (RCRA) gave EPA authority to control hazardous waste from "cradle-to-grave." This control includes the minimization, generation, transportation, treatment, storage, and disposal of hazardous waste. RCRA also set forth a framework for the management of nonhazardous solid wastes. RCRA focuses only on active and future facilities and does not address abandoned or historical sites. The National Toxicology Program was established in 1978 as an interagency organization to provide toxicological information on potentially hazardous chemicals to regulatory and research agencies and to the public.

The Comprehensive, Emergency Response, and Compensation and Liability Act (CERCLA (also known as Superfund)) was passed in 1980, to address immediate and long-term threats to the public health and the environment from abandoned or active sites contaminated with hazardous or radioactive materials. Under the Superfund program, EPA has the authority to clean up the nation's worst hazardous waste sites, using money from a trust fund supported primarily from a tax on chemical feedstocks used by manufacturers. Companies or individuals responsible for the wastes are identified by EPA, if possible, and made to pay for the cleanups. The Superfund Amendments and Reauthorization Act (SARA) of 1986 reauthorized CERCLA to continue cleanup activities around the country. Several site-specific amendments, definitions, clarifications, and technical requirements were added to the legislation, including additional enforcement authorities. Also under the SARA, the Superfund Hazardous Substances Basic Research Program (Superfund Basic Research Program) was established. The Superfund Basic Research Program is a multidisciplinary program administered by the NIEHS. This Program is committed to advancing the state-of-the-science, reducing the amount and toxicity of hazardous substances and, ultimately, preventing adverse human health effects.

Assessing Potential Adverse Health Effects of Hazardous Waste

Studies of the adverse health effects of hazardous waste must contend with many challenges. Exposure is usually ill defined and often misclassified, historical data may not be available or are otherwise problematic, and mixed chemical exposures are likely and may not always be uniform across a population. The exposed population is often small or incompletely determined. Resources for study may also be limited. The endpoints to be studied may be uncertain, leading to consideration of multiple endpoints.

The many types of hazardous wastes and the variety of their origination make this a difficult field to study. In addition to designated chemical dumps, other sites include illegal chemical dumps, mining waste sites, pesticide-contaminated sites, municipal dumps, leaking underground waste storage tanks, dumps in federal facilities, radioactive release sites, underground injection wells, municipal gas facilities, and wood-preserving plants. Furthermore, hazardous wastes sites may contain many environmental contaminants: PCBs, pesticides, trichlorethylene and other volatile organic chemicals (VOCs), dioxanes, herbicides, metals (e.g., lead), and simple and complex mixtures of chemicals.

Despite these complications, several studies have indicated that serious health effects from hazardous wastes can occur. Various routes of exposure may be relevant, including inhalation, dermal contact, and ingestion. Health outcomes that should be considered as endpoints include asthma and respiratory hypersensitivity, lung dysfunction and growth, degenerative neurologic diseases, neurobehavioral and developmental problems, birth defects, reproductive health problems in males and females, immunologic and endocrine diseases such as diabetes, and cancer including leukemia. The availability of toxicologic studies on a chemical or complex mixtures may be valuable in determining health outcomes to be considered as endpoints. Some studies provide useful information to communities, public health officials, and researchers about specific exposures in local areas and general health problems potentially associated with exposures from hazardous wastes.

Exposure assessment is an important element of the studies on hazardous wastes. It involves techniques to measure or estimate the contaminant; to learn its source, the environmental media of exposure (e.g., air, water, soil), routes of transport through each medium, whether chemical and physical transformation of chemicals has occurred, paths of entry into the body, the degree and frequency of contact with chemicals, and their spatial and temporal concentration patterns; and to measure the contaminant or its transformation products in body fluids or excreta. Records of ambient pollutant concentrations can sometimes provide a surrogate for exposure, but direct measures of past human exposure have not usually been recorded and must be estimated with models. In addition, the biologically relevant dose absorbed by subjects should be determined wherever possible and related to individual susceptibility.

Biologic markers may assist in several ways and are increasingly being evaluated for their use in such studies. Such markers may prove valuable in assessing individual susceptibility and biologically relevant exposure as well as serving as predictors of outcome. Examples include changes in liver enzymes, DNA and protein adducts, changes in neurobehavioral patterns, and changes in sperm motility. When coupled with epidemiologic studies, i.e., molecular epidemiology, biologic markers may be critical to the assessment and evaluation of exposure, susceptibility, internal dose, and effect.

Metals and Organics in Soil and Water

All medias, particularly soil and water, have small amounts of essential trace metals needed for plant growth, but they may also contain variable amounts of potentially toxic heavy metals. Metals of particular concern include Zn, Cu, Cd, Ni, Pb, Hg, Mo, and As. The amount of metal contaminants in a particular media depends on the amount of industrial inputs.

The soil environment also influences the toxicity of metals. Soils with high pH have lower plant-available metal concentrations than do low-pH soils because the water solubility of most metals increases as pH decreases. Thus, one management strategy to reduce metal mobility and toxicity in plants is to lime soils to a neutral or alkaline pH. The organic matter content of soils also affects metal availability. In general, soils with high organic matter content (greater than 5 percent) exhibit relatively low metal uptake by plants, as metals are sorbed and complexed by the polymer-like organic carbon structure of organic matter. Once metals are introduced into soil, their bioavailability and mobility can be manipulated by changing the valence state of the metal or by altering the soil factors that influence their solubilities. While short-term effects of metal additions to soil can be beneficial, the long-term fate of these metals is more difficult to predict because metal pollutants do not biodegrade and therefore continue to accumulate in the soil environment.

Toxic organic compounds that originate from household wastes or industrial wastewaters can be found in all medias. All municipal sludges contain trace amounts of the most common organic chemicals, such as pesticides, polyaromatic hydrocarbons (PAHs), plasticizers, volatile organics, and solvents. Depending on the magnitude of the inputs, many of these organics are degraded in the wastewater-treatment processes. However, the more refractory and insoluble compounds, such as chlorinated pesticides, as well as complex mixtures, can pass through wastewater treatment plants without degrading.

New regulations for disposal of wastes on land require periodic monitoring not only of metals but also organic pollutants (Table 38-1). The degradation, bioavailability, and mobility of these chemicals are largely dependent on soil type and soil organic-matter content. Other general soil physical and chemical conditions, such as particle size distribution, pH, oxygen levels, and soil moisture, also affect their degradation. Therefore, the long-term effects of these chemicals are hard to predict, particularly since many can accumulate in the soil environment.

As substances move through the environment, they are subject to chemical, physical, and biological interactions. Some toxic substances are naturally degraded by the environment; when nature's thresholds are reached, however, the ability to degrade the substance is erased. The environmental fate of the toxicant then changes. Not only does the contaminant persist in the environmental milieu in which it was being degraded, but it is subject to moving into other milieus. For example, a contaminant may be completely degraded by microbes (or fungi) in soil; when the soil's threshold is met, however, the contaminant overwhelms or kills the microbes. At that point the remaining contaminant may then begin to leach into ground water.

TABLE 38-1. MAJOR GROUPS OF ORGANIC CHEMICALS

Pollutants by Group	*Origins and Comments*
Aldrin/dieldrin, heptachlor, DDT/DDE/DDD lindane, toxaphene, malathion, hexachloro-2,4-dichlorophenoxyacetic acid (2,4-D), hexachlorobutadiene	Pesticides and herbicides. Some are found in household chemicals. Many chlorinated pesticides have been banned from use.
Benzo[*a*]pyrene, benzo[*a*]anthracene, phenanthrene	Motor oils and diesel fuel. These occur naturally as by-products of fuel combustion.
Polychlorinated biphenyls (PCBs)	Electrical and chemical manufacturing. PCBs are banned.
Dioxins, furans	By-products from the synthesis of phenol-based pesticides, such as 2,4-D
Phenol	Household products and disinfectants
Pentachlorophenol	Wood preservative. Pentachlorophenol is very persistent in the environment.
Benzene, methylene chloride, methyethyl ketone tetrachloroethylene, trichloroethylene, hexachlorobutadiene	Some household products such as paints. These chlorinated solvents are very volatile.
Vinyl chloride, bis(2-ethyhexyl)phthalate, tricresyl phosphate, dimethylnitrosamine, benzidine, 3-3′-dichlorobenzidine	Plastics and plasticizers

Source: Title 40, Code of Federal Regulations. Part 257

Need for Multidisciplinary Research

Research focused on hazardous wastes is driven by the need to protect human health; however, a positive outcome can be attained only if the full life cycle of the contaminant is understood. It is evident that hazardous substances are capable of moving through the environment from one stratum to another, interacting with microbes, plants, animals, and humans. Each step of the process must be elucidated and related to the steps before and after. Thus many scientific disciplines must be integrated. In doing so the procedures of characterizing and evaluating risks of hazardous wastes can be scrutinized and revised as directed by new research findings.

From a public health perspective, disease prevention and reduction of risk and exposure is fundamentally affected by the bioavailability and transformation of hazardous wastes in various medias. Therefore, it is important to support the development of environmental technologies that allow for the treatment of environmental contaminants so that potential human health effects are ameliorated, or indeed prevented.[8] Basic and applied research needs to be funded on the premise that these research developments will one day be used to decrease or prevent the risk to human health associated with hazardous wastes. It is important to recognize that the cleanup of contaminated soils, sediments, and groundwater is not only for improvement of the environment, but it is also a means by which human exposure and human health risks can be reduced. To this end, promoting and strengthening basic and applied research in environmental technologies integrated within a framework of health-related research and development is essential.

▸ RADIOACTIVE AND MIXED WASTES

Approximately 800 thousand cubic feet of low-level radioactive waste was disposed in 1993, a 45 percent decrease from the preceding year. Industry efforts to minimize waste generation and to reduce the volume of waste by compaction and incineration have contributed to the decrease. The Nuclear Regulatory Commission (NRC) has developed a classification system for low-level waste (LLW) based on its potential hazards and has specified disposal and waste form requirements for each of the three general classes of waste—A, B, and C. Class A waste contains lower concentrations of radioactive material than Class C waste. The volume and radioactivity of waste vary from year to year based on the types and quantities of waste shipped each year.

The disposal of high-level radioactive waste requires a determination of acceptable health and environmental impacts over thousands of years. Current plans call for the ultimate disposal of the waste in solid form in a licensed deep, stable geologic structure.

There are basically two types of by-product materials. The first type is produced by a nuclear reactor. More precisely, this is any radioactive material or made radioactive by exposure incident to the process of producing or using special nuclear material. The second type is produced by the uranium and thorium mining process as well as the tailings or wastes produced by the extraction or concentration of uranium or thorium from ore processed primarily for its source material content, including discrete surface wastes resulting from uranium solution extraction processes.

The radioactive waste material that results from the reprocessing of spent nuclear fuel, including liquid waste produced directly from reprocessing and any solid waste derived from the liquid that contains a combination of transuranic and fission product nuclides in quantities that require permanent isolation, is referred to as high-level waste (HLW). HLW is also a mixed waste because it has highly corrosive components or has organics or heavy metals that are regulated under RCRA. HLW may include other highly radioactive material that NRC, consistent with existing law, determines by rule requires permanent isolation.

Definitions of Radioactive Wastes

Radioactive waste is solid, liquid, or gaseous waste that contains radionuclides. The Department of Energy (DOE) manages four categories of radioactive waste: high-level waste, transuranic waste, low-level waste, and uranium mill tailings.

HLW is highly radioactive material from the reprocessing of spent nuclear fuel. HLW includes spent nuclear fuel, liquid waste, and solid waste derived from the liquid. HLW contains elements that decay slowly and remain radioactive for hundreds or thousands of years. HLW must be handled by remote-control from behind protective shielding to protect workers.

Transuranic (TRU) waste contains human-made elements heavier than uranium that emit α radiation. TRU waste is produced during reactor fuel assembly, weapons fabrication, and chemical processing operations. It decays slowly and requires long-term isolation. TRU waste can include protective clothing, equipment, and tools.

Uranium mill tailings are by-products of uranium mining and milling operations. Tailings are radioactive rock and soil containing small amounts of radium and other radioactive materials. When radium decays, it emits radon, a colorless, odorless radioactive gas. Released into the atmosphere, radon gas disperses harmlessly, but the gas is harmful if a person is exposed to high concentrations for long periods of time under conditions of limited air circulation.

LLW is any radioactive waste not classified as high-level waste, transuranic waste, or uranium mill tailings. LLW often contains small amounts of radioactivity dispersed in large amounts of material. It is generated by uranium enrichment processes, reactor operations, isotope production, medical procedures, and research and development activities. LLW is usually made up of rags, papers, filters, tools, equipment, discarded protective clothing, dirt, and construction rubble contaminated with radionuclides.

Mixed waste is defined as radioactive waste contaminated with hazardous waste regulated by the RCRA. A large portion of the Department of Energy's mixed waste is mixed low-level waste found in soils. No mixed waste can be disposed of without complying with RCRA's requirements for hazardous waste and meeting RCRA's Land Disposal Restrictions, which require waste to be treated before disposal in appropriate landfills. Meeting regulatory requirements and resolving mixed waste questions related to different regulations is one of DOE's most significant waste management challenges.

▸ REFERENCES

1. Anderson FR, Mandelker DR, Tarlock AD: Environmental Protection: Law and Policy. Boston: Little, Brown, 1984, 558
2. Carpenter DO, Suk WA, Blaha K, Cikrt M: Hazardous wastes in eastern and central europe. Environ Health Perspect. 104 (Suppl 3): 244–248, 1996
3. Carter DE, Pena C, Varady R, Suk WA: Environmental health and hazardous waste issues related to the U.S.-Mexico border. Environ Health Perspect, 104(Suppl 6):590–594, 1996
4. Rummel-Bulska I: The Basil Convention: a global approach for the management of hazardous wastes. In Andrews JS, Frumkin H, Johnson BL, Mehlman MA, Xintaras C, Bucsela JA (eds): Hazardous Waste and Public Health: International Congress on the Health Effects of Hazardous Waste. Princeton, New Jersey: Princeton Publishing Company, 1993, pp 139–145
5. Darnay AJ (ed): Statistical Record of the Environment. Washington, DC: Gale Environmental Library, 1991
6. Brown LR, Denniston D, Flavin C, French H, Kane H, Lenssen N, Renner, M, Roodman D, Ryan M, Sachs A, Starke L, Weber P, Young J: State of the World. New York: W.W. Norton, 1995, p 172
7. Report of the United Nations Conference on Environment and Development, Rio de Janeiro, Brazil, June 3–14, 1992 New York: United Nations, 1992, Chapter 19
8. Young L, Suk WA (eds): Biodegradation: its role in reducing toxicity and exposure to environmental contaminants. Environ Health Perspect 103(Suppl 5):, 1995

39

Aerospace Medicine

Roy L. DeHart

▸ DEFINITION

Aerospace medicine is "that specialty of medical practice within preventive medicine that focuses on the health of a population group defined by the operating aircrews and passengers of air and space vehicles, together with the support personnel who are required to operate them."[1] The practice of aerospace medicine tends to reverse the usual order of traditional or curative medicine. Normally the physician is treating abnormal physiology (illness) in a normal (terrestrial) environment. The physician concerned with the care of the aviator or astronaut most frequently deals with a normal (perhaps supernormal) individual in an abnormal (aeronautical) environment.

Since its earliest beginnings, flight has required people to adapt to or to protect themselves from multiple environmental stressors. Progress in flight has required continuing improvement in adaptation or in the devices used for protection. Such progress has always been marked by the sacrifices made by those who push the envelope of aeronautical and astronautical activity. On December 17, 1903, on a windswept beach in Kitty Hawk, North Carolina, the Wright brothers succeeded in accomplishing sustained powered flight for 12 seconds over a distance of 40 m. In less than 15 years, thousands of these powered flying machines swarmed over the battlefields of the "Great War." During this rapid expansion of military aviation, the seed of aviation medicine sprouted, took root, and grew. Aviation medicine developed with the expansion of aviation. The department of space medicine was officially established at the United States Air Force School of Aerospace Medicine under the directorship of Dr. Hubertus Strughold on February 9, 1949.[2]

The first human operated flight in space, circumnavigating the globe, was performed by Soviet cosmonaut Yuri Gagarin on April 12, 1961. In February 1962 American astronauts joined the Soviets with the successful orbital flight of John Glenn.

Biomedical oversight for the United States' space program is headquartered at the National Aeronautics and Space Administration's facility at the Johnson Space Center, Houston, Texas. Following successful lunar flights and space laboratory missions, the United States entered into a nearly routine operation with the space transportation system or "shuttle." The loss of *Challenger* in 1986, however, is a reminder of the operational hazards of space flight. Medical planning is well under way toward the continuing human habitation of an orbiting space station.

The Specialty of Aerospace Medicine

Shortly after World War II the Aero Medical Association initiated activities for the establishment of a training program for medical specialists in the field of aviation medicine. In 1953 the American Board of Preventive Medicine (ABPM) approved the decision to authorize certification in aviation medicine. The first group of physicians was certified in the specialty that same year. As of 1996, 1,142 physicians have been certified in the specialty.

With the advent of space flight, both the association and the specialty changed names to appropriately reflect their activities in both the aeronautical and astronautical environments. The name of the specialty was officially changed by the ABPM to aerospace medicine.

Recently the ABPM initiated the development of a Certificate of Added Competency in Undersea Medicine. This is of interest to aerospace medicine as it is related to the hyperbaric environment, an environment used to treat dysbarism or aviator's bends.

▸ TRAINING AND EDUCATION

Few physicians have the opportunity to gain experience in aerospace medicine until their postgraduate years. Typically, physicians are introduced to the specialty via one of two routes. Those practitioners with an interest in aviation may turn to the Federal Aviation Administration (FAA) for orientation and training as an aviation medical examiner (AME) to support general aviation. Each year the FAA conducts postgraduate educational courses for new physicians who are becoming AMEs and refresher training for established AMEs. The second route is via the military, as the three services conduct their own training programs for flight surgeons. These courses are basically introductory and focus on the clinical preventive medical aspects of evaluation and care of the aviator. Historically, most physicians who have entered the field of aerospace medicine have done so via the military route.

Residency Programs

Aerospace medicine is one of the smallest specialty training programs in the United States, both with regard to training sites and number of residents. Its program is similar in structure to other training programs in preventive medicine. Two programs are under the Department of Defense (DoD) sponsorship. The Air Force program is headquartered at the United States Air Force School of Aerospace Medicine, San Antonio, Texas, and the Navy program is managed at the Naval Aerospace Medical Institute, Pensacola, Florida. The only civilian program is housed at Wright State University, College of Medicine, Dayton, Ohio. A new program is to be introduced at the University of Texas College of Medicine, Galveston. Fewer than 50 residents are in training at any one time, with 25 to 30 candidates sitting for the specialty board examination annually.

▸ THE AEROSPACE ENVIRONMENT

The characteristic that distinguishes aerospace medicine from other medical fields is the complex environment in which flight takes place.

Stressors that impinge on humans in this unique environment, either singularly or in combination, include hypoxia, reduced atmospheric pressure, thermal extremes, brief and sustained acceleration fields, ionizing radiation, and null gravity fields. For men and women to perform successfully in this potentially hazardous environment, the principles of preventive medicine apply in the selection, health maintenance, and engineering protection of aircrew.

The Biosphere

The chemical and physical properties of the atmosphere vary with the attained altitude. Although the properties are frequently described in terms of altitude, it must be appreciated that the atmosphere is dynamic in that specific characteristics are altered by season, the earth's rotation, and latitudes. For practical purposes the components and their relative percentage of the atmosphere remain relatively constant up to an altitude of approximately 90 km. The major constituents of the atmosphere are nitrogen (78 percent) and oxygen (21 percent). The remaining 1 percent of the atmosphere consists of argon, carbon dioxide, helium, krypton, xenon, hydrogen, and methane. The actual percentages of these constituents vary with the water content of the atmosphere, which is altitude-dependent. As one ascends, the air becomes dryer.

Regardless of the altitude within the aeronautical frame of reference, the percentage of oxygen available to an individual at sea level is basically the same as that found at 90 km. The difference is that the partial pressure of oxygen is much reduced at altitude. Consequently the physiological availability of oxygen is likewise reduced.

One constituent of the atmosphere has received considerable attention in recent years because of concern for potential adverse health effects should it be reduced. Ozone is produced in the upper atmosphere by the photodissociation of molecular oxygen. Ozone attains maximum density at an altitude of approximately 22 km but is present in measurable concentrations from 10 to 35 km. Reduction in the ozone concentration would increase the level of ultraviolet radiation reaching the earth's surface (See Chapter 41).

At sea level the column of air creates an atmospheric pressure of 760 mm Hg, 760 torr, or 1013.2 millibars. As one ascends in altitude, there is less of a column of air and thus less air pressure; however, this relationship is not linear: the density of the air decreases exponentially. Consequently, at a height of 5.5 km the air density is one-half that found at sea level, and at 11 km the density is one-quarter. In practice the actual heights are somewhat greater because of the effects of temperature.

Oxygen Systems

Hypoxia, which may have any one of several causes, has devastating effects on normal physiological function. In aviation, one is faced with the potential for hypoxia resulting from a deficiency in alveolar oxygen exchange. This oxygen deficiency is due to a reduction in the oxygen partial pressure in inspired air, which occurs at altitude because of reduced oxygen in the ambient air. The alveolar partial pressure of oxygen is the most critical factor in this problem. In aviation, two factors must be considered in understanding hypoxia at altitude.

Not only may the partial pressure of oxygen be low, for example, the available oxygen is reduced by half in the ambient air at 6 km, but the ambient pressure may be insufficient to permit gas exchange at the alveoli. Considering that water vapor at normal body temperature is 47 mm Hg and the residual alveolar carbon dioxide pressure is 40 mm Hg, then for any air exchange to occur in the lung, the ambient pressure must exceed 87 mm Hg. Even if the aviator is breathing 100 percent oxygen, if the ambient pressure of that oxygen is no higher than 87 mm Hg, it would be impossible to overcome the gas pressures already present at the alveoli and thus provide oxygen.

Hypoxia is particularly dangerous because its signs and symptoms produce little discomfort and no pain. Between 2,000 and 3,000 m the subtle symptoms may produce deficiencies in night vision and some drowsiness. Unfortunately, intellectual impairment can be an early manifestation of hypoxia, thus compromising the ability of an individual to behave rationally. Thinking is slow and calculations are difficult. Both memory and judgment are faulty, and reaction time is delayed. This condition can be rapidly treated by administering oxygen at altitudes between 3,000 and 10,000 m and adding positive pressure oxygen up to 14,000 m or by enclosing the individual in a pressurized system with available oxygen at altitudes out to space.

To avoid discomfort and potential hazard in flying at altitude, the most logical solution is to carry your terrestrial environment with you. Although it is not the usual case, the same principle applies for many aircraft systems, particularly passenger-carrying aircraft. The body of the aircraft becomes a pressure vessel in which the air pressure and oxygen availability are similar to that at sea level. For a number of practical reasons, such as passenger comfort, avoiding clinical hypoxia for most passengers, and the additional cost of maintaining a sea level environment, the actual cabin altitude for most commercial aircraft is set at approximately 2500 m. Although passengers will note some pressure changes in the ears or sinuses, the change is gradual and rarely causes pain or discomfort. In most cases the passenger is not even aware of these pressure changes. The altitude is set so that most passengers are able to fly without experiencing any hypoxic symptoms. Occasionally, passengers with a compromised pulmonary or cardiovascular system may require supplemental oxygen, since their reserve is inadequate to compensate for the relatively small changes in oxygen partial pressure.

In the absence of a pressurized cabin the aviator may be forced to adapt by wearing a self-contained pressure system. Although the public is most familiar with "space suits" from television reporting, similar suits have been used for nearly a half century by military aviators flying high-altitude missions.

Provided the ambient pressure is adequate, supplemental oxygen systems permit high altitude flying and provide a safety factor for passengers on commercial airliners. Most systems employ an oxygen storage system of either pressurized gas or liquid oxygen. The source of oxygen is then connected through a regulator or metering device to an oxygen mask worn by the user. Another less commonly used oxygen storage system uses solid chemicals that, when activated, release oxygen. Two devices have been developed recently to provide onboard oxygen generation systems. The fuel-cell concept has been developed for space flight and is basically an electrolysis system freeing oxygen from water. A second system uses the reversible absorption properties of fluomine for oxygen. In this technology, pressurized air is forced over a fluomine bed, and the pressure is then reduced, allowing the absorbed oxygen to be released. Other techniques have included the molecular sieve device, which is used to filter oxygen from air; a similar technology employs a permeable membrane that passes oxygen preferentially to other constituents of the atmosphere.

Biodynamics

The first powered flight aviation death occurred in the United States when an army lieutenant sustained fatal injuries while flying with Orville Wright. Since that initial accident, there has been an ever-increasing sophistication in the science of aircraft accident prevention and aircrew and passenger protection.

Acceleration occurs whenever the velocity of an object changes. This change may occur either in direction or in magnitude. For convenience, transitory acceleration in aerospace applications is expressed in terms of "g" and is defined as the magnitude of acceleration when the velocity change approximates 9.8 m/s^2. Transitory acceleration is of such a short duration that the body does not reach a steady-state status. Protection from transitory acceleration has generally centered around two technologies: the development of restraint devices, such as lap belts and shoulder harnesses, and the design of crew space to reduce the possibility of contact.

Accident protection technology has been employed in the design of the airframe to absorb energy and improvements in the seat structure to reduce mechanical failure.

Primarily in military aviation, escape systems have been designed that often impart a new acceleration field. Ejection seats and capsules are designed to carry the occupant free of the aircraft envelope even on the ground at zero speed or in adverse conditions during uncontrolled descent. These new components of acceleration are specifically designed to remain within human tolerance.

During World War I, fighter pilots began reporting visual changes when they engaged in a pull-out or during aerial combat. Research work using a human centrifuge demonstrated, in 1935, the effects of blackout during sustained acceleration. Sustained acceleration is achieved when the body has sufficient time to reach equilibrium with the effects of the acceleration. In this context, g has been used to reflect a ratio of weight. Consequently, a pilot flying a maneuver in an aircraft in which he or she sustains 4 g would likewise experience an increase in body weight from 175 to 700 pounds. In such an acceleration, a flight helmet with equipment weighing 10 pounds becomes a mass of 40 pounds. As any mass exposed to such a field will experience a proportionate increase in weight, this has dynamic effects on the body's hydrostatic column and thus on cardiovascular function. For example, the hydrostatic column from the heart to the eye in a normal terrestrial environment is 30 cm; when exposed to a plus 6 g acceleration environment, it becomes 180 cm. In this example the body's blood pressure would be unable to overcome the hydrostatic pressure, and blood flow to the level of the eyes would cease.

Because of the hydrostatic pressure of the eyeball, a pilot will experience blackout wherein vision is lost but consciousness is maintained. When tested on a centrifuge using a standard protocol, the typical aviator, relaxed and without any protective devices, experienced blackout between 4 and 5.5 g. The same aviator, when allowed to strain to increase blood pressure, was able to increase his tolerance 0.5 g to 1.5 additional g. Two critical factors impact the degree of tolerance: the rate of onset of the acceleration and its duration.

Further protection is available using mechanical devices such as an anti-g suit. The suit is basically a lower torso device with bladders to press on the abdomen, thighs, and calves. These bladders inflate when a sensor is stimulated by acceleration. Such devices increase the g tolerance by 2 g. Research performed over two decades ago demonstrated that an anti-g suit properly worn during performance of a straining maneuver can increase g tolerance from approximately 4 g to about 9 g. Another mechanism used to enhance acceleration tolerance for pilots has included body positioning to orient the long axis of the body more perpendicular to the acceleration vector. Positive pressure breathing is also shown to be helpful in increasing tolerance, as it increases intrathoracic pressure.

The biomechanical force environments in aerospace systems can be enormous, with generation of severe noise and vibration. Human exposure to these forces may affect performance and contribute to adverse health outcomes. Prevention is the key to proper management of these stressors.

Vibration is a series of oscillations of velocity that involve displacement and acceleration. The frequency of these vibrations is described in terms of the numbers of complete cycles of motion taking place in 1 second. Amplitude of vibration is defined as the maximum displacement about a position of rest. The vibration field may be generated by mechanical devices, such as engines, or from aerodynamically induced mechanisms. Mechanical transmission of vibration to the body usually occurs in the frequency range below 100 Hz. Each major body segment and internal organ system has its own frequency to which it is most susceptible. For example, the thoracoabdominal viscera are most susceptible to vibration in the 2- to 12-Hz range. Excessive vibration and noise can have adverse effects on motor performance, vision, and communications.

Spatial Disorientation

The complex neurosensory system that we terrestrials use to maintain our orientation in the three-dimensional plane of our normal existence is inadequate for the three-dimensional dynamic environment of aerospace.

The vision sensory system is by far the most important modality for providing us input to maintain spatial orientation. Visual information processing, however, is acted on by the vestibular system and, to some degree, by proprioception and motion.

Vestibular function in maintaining spatial orientation is not as clearly defined or evident as vision. Once we are deprived of visual cues, the vestibular system becomes a major source of orientation cues in our normal environment. The visual-vestibular interface is important in fine-tuning our spatial orientation activities. However, an individual with a nonfunctional vestibular system is able to perform well as long as visual cues are adequate.

In the environment of flight, the aviator is exposed to far more complex motion inputs than the physiological system is designed to process. Not infrequently, visual cues may be in conflict with apparent motion and velocity cues processed by the vestibular system. These conflicting cues may lead to severe spatial disorientation or induce episodes of motion sickness. In flight the visual system may be subjected to various illusions, which may cause the pilot to assume a position in free space that is inaccurate. At night or in inclement weather the pilot may not have any external visual cues.

Vestibular illusions are often severe and may produce a fatal outcome. These illusions are generally produced by velocity changes that generate input from the semicircular ducts and otolith organs.

Disorientation accidents in military aircraft account for approximately 18 percent of fatal mishaps. Measures that may be employed to prevent these accidents include modifying flight procedures to reduce the opportunity for disorientation; improving the ease of interpretation of information presented by flight instruments; increasing proficiency in instrument flying, which will permit the pilot to overcome false sensory input; and educating the pilot regarding his or her own physiological frailty and the need for dependence on and acceptance of flight instrument information.

Space

The transition from the terrestrial to the space environment is not a well-demarcated line but rather a continuum that varies with altitude depending upon the parameter discussed. Human operated flight and near-earth orbit at altitudes in excess of 240 km require a self-contained vehicle sealed from the near vacuum of space. At this altitude the air density is so low that there is no practical method for compressing the gases to supply both pressure and oxygen to the craft's inhabitants. Although the sun's radiation may heat the vehicle, occupants must be protected from the extreme cold of the ambient environment. While in orbital flight, the astronaut experiences a nearly gravity-free, or weightless, environment. This occurs when the gravitational force vector is counterbalanced by the centrifugal force imparted to the vehicle as it travels tangential to the earth's surface. Long-term exposure to this near-null gravity environment has important biomedical ramifications that as yet are not fully defined.

The earth's atmosphere serves as an insulator to shield us from many of the potential dangers of space radiation. Once a person is in space, this protection is no longer available, and ionizing radiation must be a concern. Three types of radiation present hazards: primary cosmic radiations, geomagnetically trapped radiation (also known as the Van Allen belts), and radiation produced by solar flares. The environment of space is similar in many ways to the aeronautical environment; however, the duration of exposure is much more prolonged in space, and null-gravity is unique.

▶ OPERATIONAL AEROSPACE MEDICINE

The physician practicing aerospace medicine as a clinical specialty must be an astute clinician in the office setting and also a practitioner able to grasp the nuance of the environment of flight.

The stressors impinging on aircrew vary with the type of flight vehicle, whether a single-seat private plane or a multicrew space habitat. Consequently the physician serving as an AME or flight surgeon (FS) must be cognizant of the aircrew's flight environment. For ease of discussion these operational flight environments are defined as civil aviation, military aviation, and space operations.

Civil Aviation

This category of flight operations includes commercial aviation and private or recreational flying. Airlines represent an international industry with aircraft worldwide transporting nearly 12,000 million passengers over 1,300 billion air miles per year. With the deregulation of the airline industry in the United States, air taxi and air commuter operations have grown to fill the vacuum left when airlines pulled out of small airport terminals. Most large corporations in the United States either own or lease aircraft for business purposes. Other commercial activities include air ambulance service, flight training, aerial application, air cargo, and the new growth industry of commercial parcel delivery.

In the United States there are approximately 639,000 active pilots, 170,000 general aviation aircraft, 18,700 air carrier aircraft, and 18,000 airports.

The magnitude of preventive medicine intervention by the aerospace physician takes on added meaning when one realizes that all U.S. licensed aviators are required to have an initial medical examination prior to issuance of their license and periodic assessments as long as they continue to fly. To examine these aviators, the FAA has designated 5,300 physicians as AMEs. These physicians have undergone special training conducted under the auspices of the FAA; they may have had experience as military flight surgeons and frequently are private pilots themselves. The examination is performed to a rigorous protocol, and detailed physical standards have been promulgated.

The periodicity and sophistication of the examination is dictated in part by the class of the license exercised by the aviator. The airline captain must meet a more stringent standard, more frequently, than is required of the private pilot. In all cases the medical examination is reviewed by medical personnel at the FAA's Civil Aeromedical Institute (CAMI). Approximately 17,000 medical examinations are received each business day by the office. This represents one of the largest longitudinal medical databases in the country; unfortunately, resources to use the tools of epidemiology for fully studying this wealth of data have not been available.

Another employment category required to meet flight medical standards is air traffic controller. These 12,000 federal employees stationed throughout the United States must meet, as a minimum, the physical standards required of private pilots, and just as with pilots, these examinations are repeated periodically.

CAMI also has responsibility for conducting research to address issues of health and safety for flight deck and cabin crew as well as for the private aviator and passengers. Toward this goal the institute has conducted research and recommended standards on emergency aircraft lighting, egress systems, restraint systems, breathing equipment, emergency breathing devices, and flotation systems.

Military Aviation

The Air Force has by far the widest range of aeronautical activities. Low and slow describes some Air Force missions, while others are truly into the fringes of space. Current fighter aircraft are capable of readily exceeding the physiological tolerance of the pilot with rapid onset, high g. The response of fighter aircraft is so fast that controls are now electronic rather than hydraulic or mechanical. Large transport aircraft are capable of nearly endless flight with air-to-air refueling. With rest facilities and multiple crew, the aircraft can simply keep on flying; the only restriction is the crew rest requirements of its human operators. For over two decades, it had been predicted that aeronautical design would take aircraft performance beyond the performance of the pilot. That time has arrived, as aeronautical engineers are now forced to curtail performance characteristics because the human operator can fail.

Army aviation medicine has for some years concentrated on unique facets of rotary wing operations and pilot adaptability. In past years, helicopter crashes that were survivable in terms of impact force frequently ended in fire and death of the occupants. With intense research and redesign, this hazard has been significantly reduced. The military necessity of helicopter operations in adverse weather conditions and at night have created human factor challenges that have only in part been successfully addressed by technology.

The unique challenge for naval aviation medicine is related to aircraft carrier operations. The flight surgeon is responsible not only for health maintenance of the flight crews but also for maintaining health surveillance for the 5,000 people on board the carrier. The word "independent" has been used to describe a prominent characteristic of this medical service. The flight surgeon is the public health officer for this isolated community and oversees all aspects of hygiene, epidemiological surveillance, health maintenance, and medical disaster preparedness aboard ship.

The Navy has celebrated the fiftieth anniversary of the Thousand Aviator Program,[3] one of the first large cohort, longitudinal health surveillance programs undertaken in the United States. More than 1,000 aviators and aviation cadets were examined using psychological and physiological assessment procedures. This ongoing study has reviewed cardiovascular status, overall morbidity and mortality rates, and the effects of the aviation experience on the overall health of the individual.

Space Operations

The United States piloted space program has enjoyed successes; unfortunately, it has also experienced several disasters that continue to remind one that space operations are neither routine nor free from potential catastrophic failures. The Soviet Union likewise has experienced success and disaster in space.

As experience has accumulated with human-days in space and monitoring of increasing numbers of astronauts in the space environment, medical concerns have focused on the physiological effects of null gravity. Based on our current experience for short duration flights, the biomedical challenges include space adaptation syndrome (space motion sickness), cardiovascular deconditioning, loss of red cell mass, and bone mineral loss. For shuttle operations the first two concerns are primary. Space adaptation syndrome has been experienced by up to one-third of the shuttle crew. This syndrome occurs in the early segments of orbital flight and may adversely affect early mission performance.

Fluid shift and deconditioning effects occur even during the relatively short duration of the shuttle orbital missions. Performance during orbit does not appear to be compromised, but with the increasing g upon reentry, performance decrements are possible.

As preparations proceed for a continuous habitat in space, the remaining biomedical challenges will become important. Russia has successfully maintained cosmonauts in orbit for over a year.

The space station operation introduces additional challenges for maintaining astronauts on long duration missions. The environmental control systems must be able to maintain potable water and uncontaminated air reliably for long periods. Microbe overgrowth must be prevented. Food and sanitation issues need to be addressed with resupply providing only one solution. Health maintenance surveillance and emergency medical treatment will require attention. Crew work-rest cycles and psychological considerations remain challenges, as do biologically efficient extravehicular activities.

▸ PERSONNEL, PASSENGERS, AND PATIENTS

In general the people most involved in the aerospace industry are flight crews, cabin personnel, and ground staff; passengers, who represent the chief revenue source for commercial aviation and patients, who may be transported either by an airline or air ambulance service.

Personnel

American flag carrier airlines are responsible for the direct employment of approximately 500,000 workers, including 60,000 flight deck and 85,000 cabin crew members.[3] The remaining employees make up the maintenance teams, counter servicing and baggage personnel, and those engaged in administration and management. The preventive health surveillance and medical monitoring of these individuals are provided via a variety of health service mechanisms. A number of the larger airlines maintain modern, sophisticated medical departments providing both occupational and aviation medicine services to the workforce. Other airlines have elected to keep only a minimal medical presence in-house and to contract for or otherwise provide services to employees. Smaller airlines have found it successful to hire the periodic services of an aeromedical consultant and to contract out health services. Less common is contracting all health services without the benefit of corporate medical oversight.

Airlines providing comprehensive aviation medical services will provide many, if not all, of the services detailed in Table 39-1.

Many of the activities for either flight crew or ground personnel are clinical preventive medicine services. The sophistication of the preemployment examination depends on the job description of the future employee. In part, because of the enormous training investment in pilots, airlines try to select pilots who are free of active disease, who have few precursors to chronic illness, and who do not exhibit high-risk lifestyle behavior.

Prior to the promulgation of the regulation dealing with urine drug screening by the Department of Transportation, many airlines had already initiated such a policy. Recognizing their obligation to public safety, airline companies began by the mid-1980s to implement a drug-free work policy. From the perspective of public health and preventive medicine, two components of this policy are essential—education and treatment. Broad-based educational programs were initiated for all employees, including flight personnel, maintenance crews, and management. Individuals who recognized their own drug dependency were encouraged to step forward and receive treatment and support. Management then worked with employee representatives to establish guidelines and rules for implementing a drug abuse protection program. Most airlines established a drug screening component to their preemployment processing. Drug testing for cause was also implemented; however, fewer airlines established a no-notice urine drug screening program. These programs continue to evolve, and both legislation and litigation will clearly modify the process.

Approximately two decades ago, airlines in association with the Airline Pilots Association and with cooperation from the FAA, initiated a model alcoholic rehabilitation program. With few exceptions it had been the FAA policy to revoke the medical certificate of airline pilots who had alcoholism. Such a practice was devastating, requiring counseling, support, and treatment for those whose licenses were revoked. Once identified as an alcoholic, the pilot, even when seeking help, lost his or her livelihood. The new program encouraged self-identification since treatment was now available and because, if it was successful, the pilot would be able to return to the cockpit. The rehabilitation program involved supervisors, peers, medical personnel, FAA supervision, and, perhaps most importantly, close affiliation with Alcoholics Anonymous. Hundreds of pilots have successfully completed the recovery programs and have returned to the cockpit. This program provides an excellent model for industry in general and clearly recognizes the importance of continuing support to the recovering alcoholic.

TABLE 39-1. AIRLINE AVIATION MEDICAL SERVICES

Preemployment medical examination	Employee assistance program
	Acute care
Drug abuse testing	Emergency response service
Psychological profile or personality inventory	Periodic medical assessment
	Job-related illness or injury monitoring
Physiological training	
Wellness or health maintenance program	Return to work assessment
	Aircraft accident team

Although many pilots earn their livelihood in commercial aviation, most aviators in the United States are private pilots who fly for recreation or business. Whether the aircraft is a wide-bodied, multi-engine, commercial passenger airliner, a high-performance jet fighter, or a single-engine private aircraft, the aviation environment and its potential adverse effects on human physiology remain. Although the level to which stress is imposed on the aviator is determined in large measure by the flight profile of the aircraft, all aviators are exposed to some adverse environmental factors associated with flight. Prevention or amelioration of adverse effects resulting from the flight environment continues to be a key component of the practice of aerospace medicine. Flight personnel whose health and well-being may be compromised by illness or by self-imposed stress compromise their performance as aviators and thus have a potential adverse effect on flight safety.

Illness and Disease. Aviation is among those few avocations or vocations where the incapacitation of the operator could have dire effects. Once airborne, the aircraft is dependent on the pilot to safely complete the flight. Although there are many assists to the aviator both in the aircraft and on the ground, the number of aircraft capable of fully automated flight is small. Consequently, public safety dictates that the potential for pilot incapacitation be minimized.

There are many physical afflictions an aviator may have without undue risk to flight safety. However, certain medical conditions are currently considered incompatible with safe flight. The clinical skills of the aerospace medicine specialist are most tested in diagnosing occult disease and determining the risk such a condition may impose on flight safety and the aviation activities of the aviator.

Unexplained loss of consciousness or epilepsy are examples of conditions that may create an unacceptable risk to the pilot and to the public. Diabetes mellitus requiring medication and exertional angina are other examples where the risk to public safety may take precedence over the individual pilot's desire to continue flying. *Clinical Aviation Medicine* addresses most common afflictions and their aeromedical implications.[4]

Therapeutic Medications. Physicians write nearly 2 billion prescriptions for therapeutic medications each year in the United States. An even greater number of over-the-counter medications are purchased annually. With this degree of drug ingestion among the U.S. population, it is most probable that medication is being taken by a substantial percentage of aviators. Both therapeutic effects and adverse side effects may create situations that adversely affect flight performance. Common side effects of medications include drowsiness and loss of concentration. A pilot on a long, uneventful flight must be vigilant to fight boredom and inattention. He or she may also be experiencing mild hypoxia. If one adds to this scenario the side effects of medication, the results could be tragic. Most studies have shown that adverse effects of medications are enhanced by the flight environment. Recognizing that pilots may be unaware of some of the common adverse effects of medication, Mohler published a guide written in layman's terms specifically addressing this issue for pilots.[5]

The DoD, because it supervises the health care of its pilots, simply removes the aviator from flight duty until completion of the therapeutic regimen. For long-term or chronic disease requiring therapy, such as mild hypertension, limited prescription medications are available, provided a prior trial has demonstrated that the pilot experiences no adverse side effects. In the civilian sector, such control of health care is essentially nonexistent. This is true even for commercial airlines that may attempt to monitor the health status of their pilots. Consequently both the physician providing treatment and the pilot taking medication must be educated to the potential dangers of adverse side effects in flight.

Nontherapeutic Drugs. Two commonly used nontherapeutic drugs are cigarettes and alcohol. Although the incidence of alcohol-related aircraft accidents has fallen in response to an extensive educational effort on the part of the FAA, alcohol continues to be associated with approximately 13 percent of accidents. Alcohol and altitude are synergistic, both in the effects upon the central nervous system and with respect to slowing metabolic clearance rates. Ground-based simulation and actual in-flight performance have demonstrated that blood alcohol levels as low as 0.04 percent (40 mg/dL) adversely compromise flight performance.

Habitual cigarette smokers commonly have blood carbon monoxide levels in excess of 5 percent. This represents a reduction in the blood oxygen level equal to that of a nonsmoker at an altitude of 2200 m. Consequently the aviator who smokes is placing his or her body physiologically at a higher altitude than indicated and thus compromises altitude tolerance.

Work-Rest Cycles. Numerous factors in the aerospace environment enhance the onset of fatigue. One of the more significant of these factors is the erratic schedule many aviators maintain while flying. Weather remains the greatest cause for flight schedule disruption in private, business, or commercial aviation. Although larger, more expensive aircraft are now equipped with electronic measures to reduce the impact of weather on flight schedules, problems remain. There are regulatory controls, work rules, and common sense methods in place to reduce inadvertent or intentional fatigue factors. Although a pilot may fly only the prescribed number of hours over a particular time period, there is no assurance that there will be either the opportunity or ability to obtain adequate rest in the interval.

The excitement of a new place, insomnia in a strange bed, circadian rhythm asynchrony, and work-related anxiety may contribute to restless sleep and inadequate rest. Then a new workday begins, which may, in fact, be in the middle of the pilot's biological night. Such circumstances are not infrequent and do lead to both acute and chronic fatigue for aircrew members.

For the private pilot, time schedules are frequently self-imposed, which initially may have been realistic but become severely disrupted with the passage of a storm front. Frequently, the individual attempts to reach the next destination, ignoring the length of time without rest and the manifestations of fatigue. Fatigue is rarely cited as the primary cause of an aircraft accident; however, it often appears as a contributing factor.

Aging. For a number of years, the FAA has had in place the Age 60 Rule. This rule directs that air transport pilots flying for commercial airlines may not serve as pilots beyond age 60 years. This is not a medical regulation but one promulgated through operations. There is no such age limitation for other categories of flying. All others, regardless of age, may continue aviation activities as pilots as long as a current medical certificate is maintained and other evaluation requirements of the license are met.

The Age 60 Rule had its origin some years ago before sophisticated medical diagnostic techniques were available and predated the advanced simulators, which are now able to measure subtle performance decrements. It was recognized that the risk for sudden incapacitation in flight increased with age, particularly cerebral vascular accidents and heart attacks. The wisdom at the time said such a rule was necessary to reduce the potential for such events by controlling the population at risk. Although the rule is currently being sustained in the courts, considerable epidemiological evidence is being put forward in an attempt to overturn what some have described as age discrimination.

Passengers

Commercial airlines have both an obligation and a commitment to provide safe, reliable, and comfortable service to their passengers. In general this is the experience of millions of passengers flying each year. Table 39-2 provides comparative accident data for road, rail, and air travel. Travel by domestic airlines remains one of the safest forms of transportation.

Safety. Many of the safety features in modern commercial aircraft go unrecognized by the passengers. The number of emergency exits are specified to ensure rapid evacuation in case of an emergency. Both airline seats and seat belts are designed to sustain considerable impact force in order to protect and restrain the passenger. Other than the preflight demonstration, few passengers have seen the emergency oxygen masks, which are available at every seat location in aircraft flying at substantial altitudes. Emergency lighting has been designed to provide illumination in case of power failure and floor level track lighting leading to the emergency evacuation routes. The most important safety features is not equipment but the cabin attendant. Although most passengers look to these individuals to make the flight more comfortable by providing service and assistance, the cabin attendant's primary purpose is to provide safety instructions and to help passengers in case of emergencies.[6]

Circadian Asynchronization ["Jet Lag"]. Transmeridian flights commonly are disruptive to the passenger's awake-sleep cycle. There is considerable individual variability to disruption of the normal body rhythm. Time shifts of 3 to 4 hours often will alter the body's homeostasis. The recovery time is dependent not only on the number of time zones crossed but also on the direction of flight. Body cycle disruptions occurring after crossing 6 or more time zones appear to be relatively persistent when one is flying east, lasting upward of 11 days; symptoms from flying west persist for no more than 1 or 2 days. Measures recommended to reduce the impact of this circadian asynchronization include adjusting daily activities several days before the flight, changing meals to the new time, eating light meals, avoiding alcohol, and using hypnotics during and following the flight, as well as allowing specific rest periods on arrival at the destination. More recent work suggests bright light and melatonin may help in resetting the "body clock."

Patients

There are few absolute contraindications to transporting patients by air. Patients who suffer from dysbarism, acute myocardial infarction, pneumothorax, or air embolism can be moved with relative safety, provided appropriate precautions are taken and preparations made. Assuming that maximum effort has been made to stabilize the patient, the question should be asked, "Are the benefits of air transportation real, and do they justify the clinical risks and financial costs?" The DoD has the greatest experience with transporting seriously ill and injured patients. The military aeromedical evacuation system employing the McDonnell-Douglas C-9A represents the nation's main resource for fixed-wing medical transport.

Commercial air ambulance services are available in all large communities in the United States. To date, there are no federally mandated air ambulance standards, and consequently the quality of service varies over a wide spectrum. Recognizing the potential problem, the industry itself has developed standards to enhance the service to the patient through improved training of personnel and placement of specialized equipment aboard the aircraft. Most visible is the medical center helicopter used to transfer critically ill and injured patients and neonates to tertiary medical facilities.

TABLE 39-2. COMPARATIVE ACCIDENT DATA FOR ROAD, RAIL, AND AIRLINE TRAVEL 1975–1993

Passenger Fatalities Per 100 Million Passenger-Miles				
Year	*Automobiles and Taxis*	*Buses*	*Passenger Trains*	*Domestic Scheduled Aircraft*
1975	1.40	0.15	0.08	0.08
1980	1.32	0.15	0.04	0.01
1985	0.96	0.04	0.03	0.07
1990	0.99	0.02	0.02	0.003
1993	0.82	0.01	0.42	0.01

From the National Safety Council: Accident Facts. Washington, DC: US Government Printing Office, 1996.

Medical conditions requiring particular insight into the physiology and environment of flight are air embolism and pressure change–induced decompression sickness, or dysbarism. In the transfer of such patients, it is imperative that pressure changes routinely experienced in flight be avoided. Some aircraft, such as the Hercules C-130, can be overpressurized to maintain the cabin below sea level pressure provided flight is at a relatively low altitude.

Airline companies are frequently called upon to make special provisions for the transfer of ill or injured patients in the normal cabin environment of an airliner. Provided such a transfer does not represent a hazard to other passengers, stretchers are available that extend over three airline seats. The patient must be accompanied by at least one attendant. The expense is significant because of the block of seats required by the stretcher apparatus.

Prevention is the hallmark of aeromedical support to personnel, passengers, and patients: prevention of disease and risk behaviors that might compromise the longitudinal health of air-crew personnel; prevention of injury or death to passengers through safety design of aircraft and safe airline operations; and prevention of further complications to the air-transported patient through planning, training, and equipping aeromedical transportation systems.

▸ COMMUNITY AND INTERNATIONAL HEALTH

Aerospace flight operations have the potential for disrupting the environment and serving as a mechanism for the introduction of disease. Within the United States, regulations have helped reduce the impact of flight operations on the environment. The potential for disease transmission has been reduced with the implementation of international sanitary regulations and other control mechanisms.

Disease Transmission

The spread of epidemics by movement of populations has been well-documented throughout history. In days past, an infected individual traveling by land or sea usually became symptomatic, and thus the disease was apparent before the person reached his or her destination. With today's high-speed jet traffic it is not only possible but likely that an individual infected with a communicable disease could be asymptomatic yet incubating the disease at the time of arrival at the destination. Today it is possible to fly to nearly any destination on the globe with 24 hours. Roberts[7] implicates the aircraft in the spread of cholera, penicillin-resistant gonorrhea, influenza, rubella, and Lassa fever. Shilts, in *And The Band Played On*, describes how a flight attendant, with his ability to move rapidly from city to city, may have served as a vector of the human immunodeficiency virus.[8]

Recognizing the potential importance of the aircraft as a mechanism to spread disease and vectors, the first sanitary convention for aerial navigation convened in 1933. The convention's focus was curtailment of the spread of yellow fever, including limiting the distribution of the mosquito vector *Aedes aegypti*. This convention eventually became the World Health Organization (WHO) Committee on Hygiene and Sanitation in Aviation. International airlines are required to comply with the International Health Regulations published by WHO, which primarily address the following:

1. Promulgation of the application of epidemiological principles
2. Enhancement of sanitation at international airports
3. Reduction or elimination of factors contributing to the spread of disease
4. Elimination of disease vector transportation
5. Enhancement of epidemiological techniques to halt the introduction or establishment of a foreign disease

Vector Control

Disinfection procedures vary from airline to airline. The principal objective of these procedures is to kill mosquitoes and other insect vectors of disease. At one time it was common when one was flying to or from tropical areas to have cabin attendants pass through the aircraft with activated aerosol cans spraying insecticide. Another procedure, which was less obvious, was to disseminate an insecticide vapor from several fixed stations in the aircraft. Current regulations permit residual treatment of the aircraft with permethrin. A common practice was the "blocks-away" disinsection technique, in which insecticide would be introduced into the passenger cabin immediately after the aircraft was closed and was taxiing to take off. An alternative method was to use aerosol insecticide prior to arrival at the destination airport. In any case, to be effective, it is necessary that insecticides be used before unloading passengers, cargo, and luggage. It is becoming more common for live animal cargo to be transported by air. The issues of disease and vectors must be addressed with such cargo.

Large pieces of expensive equipment are also being transported by air. When the equipment has been used in the field, it is extremely difficult to ensure that all fomite contamination has been removed prior to air transportation to another country. Washing and steam cleaning of the exterior of such equipment has become regular practice. The use of some form of pesticide is commonly required before the equipment is allowed to be unloaded after it has crossed international borders.

Airline Community Health

A commercial airliner, whether traveling domestic or international routes, provides a partially closed, self-contained environment. Air is brought on board, filtered, condensed, warmed, and if necessary, neutralized for irritants such as ozone and oxides of nitrogen. Potable water must be available as well as beverages safe for human consumption. The catering service must provide food items, which frequently include both preprepared meals and other items requiring some degree of preparation. Provisions must be made for the generation of solid and hazardous waste. Toilet facilities must be provided that require retention tanks to hold sewage until servicing can be provided on the ground. Arrangements for the collection of trash and sewage and its proper disposal on arrival must be made. These details may prove relatively simple in the domestic environment but may become extremely complex with international flights. In some international situations, all food products must be incinerated at the destination airport to ensure no introduction of a plant or animal disease.

▸ THE ENVIRONMENT

Noise

One of the more noticeable features of aerospace operations is noise. The Department of Transportation estimates that approximately 3 percent of the U.S. population, 9 million persons, have been exposed to a potentially hazardous level of aircraft noise. The Environmental Protection Agency (EPA) is authorized under the Noise Pollution and Abatement Act (1970) and the Noise Control Act (1972) to institute noise control abatement procedures around airports. The FAA has also been assigned responsibilities to reduce environmental noise. Regulatory requirements set goals and timelines for airport operators to submit and comply with noise compatibility programs.

Since the implementation of these laws, efforts have been undertaken by airframe manufacturers to control aircraft noise at its source. Numerous design changes have been made in engines primarily to reduce noise. Airports may require specific landing and departure patterns including engine power adjustments to comply with abatement controls. Some airports have found it necessary to curtail nighttime operations to satisfy objections by the community surrounding the airport. All levels of government have taken an active role in ensuring the compatibility of land use around airfields, both with regard to safety and noise control.

The "Greenhouse Effect" and Ozone Depletion

Aerospace operations contribute approximately 1 percent to the nation's total emissions of hydrocarbons, oxides of nitrogen, and carbon monoxide. In certain areas such as Atlanta and Chicago where aircraft operations are intense, emission levels have increased to approximately 3 percent of the average level. Under the Clean Air Act, airlines have markedly reduced the practice of inflight fuel dumping. Economics have also dictated a change in this policy. The principal environmental problem of the fuel is its contribution to photochemical pollution. The formation of the condensation trail, or con-trail, results from the emissions of the aircraft's engines condensing and freezing in the cold ambient temperature of altitude. It has been suggested that heavy jet traffic may cause weather changes in areas surrounding major airport hubs.

Ozone depletion is receiving an appropriate international response. In the 1970s there was much concern that oxides of nitrogen would serve as catalysts for ozone depletion at the high altitudes of the supersonic transport (SST) flights. It was estimated that an SST fleet of 100 aircraft would decrease the ozone layer by 10 percent. This concern played an important role in the decision by this country to withdraw from the SST commercial competition. With additional research and a better understanding of the high-altitude atmospheric chemical relationship, the fears of ozone depletion from this source were shown to be exaggerated.

▸ THE FUTURE

As we approach the twenty-first century, all projections point to more people flying higher and faster. The technology of aerospace systems will continue to improve, and the degree of automation of both air and space craft will continue to increase. Large numbers of men and women will be required to maintain and operate the expanding fleet of aerospace vehicles. New exotic materials will be introduced by the aerospace industry, requiring special medical surveillance programs to ensure the safety and health of those working with these new substances.

The challenges to public health and the environment will continue. With the continued expansion of international commerce via rapid air and space transport, the potential for transporting disease, vectors, and fomites will continue. Increasing air traffic in finite, three-dimensional space will result in some compromise to environmental factors. Airports will continue to expand, challenging community aesthetics and introducing social and environmental concerns.

With all of the opportunities and challenges of the future, aerospace medicine will continue to have an important niche in the ecology of health services.

▸ REFERENCES

1. Directory of Graduate Medical Education Programs. Chicago: American Medical Association, 1995
2. Peyton G: Fifty years of Aerospace Medicine. Washington, DC: US Government Printing Office, 1967
3. Lampl R (ed): The Aviation and Aerospace Almanac. Washington, DC: TAB Books, 1995
4. Rayman RB: Clinical Aviation Medicine. 2nd ed. Philadelphia: Lea & Febiger, 1989
5. Mohler SR: Medication and Flying: A Pilot's Guide. Boston: Boston Publishing, 1982
6. Rayman RB: Aircrew Health Care Maintenance. In DeHart RL (ed): Fundamentals of Aerospace Medicine. 2nd ed. Baltimore: Williams & Wilkins, 1996
7. Roberts MA: Role of the Aircraft in Transmission of Disease. In DeHart RL (ed). Fundamentals of Aerospace Medicine. 2nd ed. Baltimore: Williams & Wilkins, 1996
8. Shilts R: And the Band Played On. New York: St. Martin's Press, 1987

General References

DeHart R (ed). Fundamentals of Aerospace Medicine. 2nd ed. Baltimore: Williams & Wilkins, 1996

Ernsting J, King PF (eds). Aviation Medicine. 2nd ed. London: Butterworth, 1988

Hawkins FH: Human Factors in Flight. London: Grover Technical Press, 1987

Nocogassian AE, Huntoon CL, Pool SL (eds): Space Physiology and Medicine. 3rd ed. Philadelphia: Lea & Febiger, 1994

40

Housing and Health

John M. Last

All humans need shelter: protection against the elements, somewhere to store food and prepare meals, and a secure place to raise offspring. The effects of housing conditions on health have been known since antiquity. Deplorable living conditions in urban slums became a political issue in the nineteenth century when vivid descriptions by journalists, novelists, and social reformers aroused public opinion. Osler's *Principles and Practice of Medicine* (1892) and Rosenau's *Preventive Medicine and Hygiene* (1913) noted the association between overcrowding and common serious diseases such as tuberculosis and rheumatic fever.

▸ OVERVIEW OF HOUSING CONDITIONS IN THE WORLD

Housing conditions have greatly improved in the affluent industrial nations throughout the second half of the twentieth century, but more than two-thirds of the households in the world are in developing countries, the great majority of them in rural areas; the most prevalent indoor environment in the world is the same now as throughout history—huts in rural communities.[1] But this is changing. Urbanization is rapidly transforming the distribution of populations in the developing world, where the proportion living in urban areas rose from less than 25 percent to over 33 percent between 1970 and 1985; by the beginning of the new millennium, the proportion living in urban areas in the world will exceed 50 percent,[2] and in the world as a whole the urban population will compose 65 percent or more by 2025. Many cities will be very large (see Table 41-8).

Many of these new urban dwellers have terrible living conditions. In the last 30 years there has been a great increase in the numbers of people living in periurban slums in developing countries. They often lack sanitation, clean water supplies, access to health care, and other basic services such as elementary education. The proportion of people in such circumstances ranges between 20 to more than 80 percent in most cities throughout Africa, Latin America, and South, Southeast, and Southwest Asia. The plight of children is especially deplorable; infant mortality rates exceed 100 in many places.[3] Children are often abandoned by parents who cannot provide for them and must fend for themselves from ages as young as 5 or 6 years; many turn to crime and child prostitution to survive.

These shantytowns and periurban slums endanger the health and security of many millions in Latin America, Africa, and many parts of Asia. They are ideal breeding places for disease and social unrest. Accurate numbers are impossible to obtain because the missing services include enumeration by census-takers and because situations change so rapidly, but in Mexico City, Lima, Santiago, Rio de Janeiro, São Paulo, and Bogota, well over half the total population live in the periurban slums. In the mid-1990s, there were as many as 40 million periurban slum-dwellers in these six cities alone. Others are even worse off; worldwide, an estimated 100 million people are entirely homeless, living on the streets without possessions, often from infancy onward. Although this is a problem mainly in developing countries, homeless people have increased in numbers in the most affluent industrial nations in the last decade, often forced out of their homes by hard economic times. Public health departments in large cities such as New York and London have been obliged to spend increasing proportions of their budgets on emergency shelter for growing numbers of homeless destitute families.

Increasing numbers, an estimated 22 million in 1995, live in refugee communities[4] in Africa and the Middle and Far East where housing conditions are equally deplorable, sometimes worse than in periurban slums. Refugee communities may have health services, but these are seldom adequate; supplies and continuity of services are often precarious; the safety and security of the inhabitants is often threatened by hostilities, and their long-term prospects for a better life are poor.

Industrially developed nations are experiencing other challenging new health problems related to housing conditions. Rising land values and the need to provide cheap housing for expanding populations have led to proliferation of high-rise, high-density apartment housing. Publicly supported housing projects economize by restricting living space and providing few amenities. This kind of dwelling creates new sets of problems: emotional tensions attributable to living too close to the neighbors, inadequate play areas for children, poor services, and defective elevators and communal washing machines. Only a small minority of people, predominantly the educated professional classes (such as many readers of this book), enjoy comfortable, aesthetically pleasing, healthy living conditions.

▸ INDOOR ENVIRONMENT

Indoor climate and indoor air pollution, biological exposure factors, and various physical hazards encountered inside the home are encompassed by the term *indoor environment*.

The indoor climate may be the same as that out of doors, or it may be modified by heating, cooling, or adjustment of humidity levels, and often in sealed modern buildings, by all of these.

Physical Hazards

Physical hazards in the indoor environment include toxic gases, respirable suspended particulates, asbestos fibers, ionizing radiation, notably radon and "daughters," nonionizing radiation, and tobacco smoke.

Indoor air may be contaminated with dusts, fumes, pollen, and microorganisms. The principal indoor air pollutants in industrially developed nations are summarized in Table 40-1. Many of these pollutants are harmful to health. Some occur mainly in sealed office buildings, and others, such as tobacco smoke, in private dwellings.

In developing countries, indoor air pollution with products of biomass fuel combustion is a pervasive problem (Table 40-2). The

TABLE 40-1. SOURCES AND POSSIBLE CONCENTRATIONS OF INDOOR POLLUTANTS

Pollutant	*Sources*[a]	*Range of Concentrations*
Respirable particles	Tobacco smoke, stoves, aerosol sprays	0.05–0.7 mg/m^3
Carbon monoxide	Combustion equipment, stoves, gas heaters	1–115 mg/m^3
Nitrogen dioxide	Gas cookers, cigarettes	0.05–1.0 mg/m^3
Sulfur dioxide	Coal combustion	0.02–1.0 mg/m^3
Carbon dioxide	Combustion, respiration	600–9,000 mg/m^3
Formaldehyde	Particle board, carpet adhesives, insulation	0.06–2.0 mg/m^3
Other organic vapors (benzene, toluene, etc.)	Solvents, adhesives, resin products, aerosol sprays	0.01–0.1 mg/m^3
Ozone	Electric arcing, UV light sources	0.02–0.4 mg/m^3
Radon and "daughters"	Building materials	10–3,000 Bq/m^3
Asbestos	Insulation, fireproofing	1 + fiber/cm^3
Mineral fibers	Appliances	100–10,000/m^3

[a]Tobacco smoke, benzene, radon and daughters, asbestos, and possibly formaldehyde are carcinogens: most others on this list are respiratory or conjunctival irritants. Carbon dioxide is an asphyxiant; carbon monoxide is a lethal poison.

fumes from cooking fires include high concentrations of respiratory irritants that cause chronic obstructive pulmonary disease (COPD) and that sometimes contain carcinogens too. Premature death from COPD is common among women who from their childhood have spent many hours every day close to primitive cooking stoves, inhaling large quantities of toxic fumes.[5]

The toxic gases specified in Table 40-1 come from many sources. Formaldehyde is emitted as an off-gas from particle board, carpet adhesives, and urea-formaldehyde foam insulation; it is a respiratory and conjunctival irritant and sometimes causes asthma. It is not emitted in sufficient concentrations to constitute a significant cancer risk. Although rats exposed to formaldehyde do demonstrate increased incidence of nasopharyngeal cancer, there is only weak evidence of elevated cancer incidence or mortality rates even among persons occupationally exposed to far higher concentrations than occur in domestic settings. Nonetheless, urea-formaldehyde foam insulation has been banned in many jurisdictions on the basis of the evidence for carcinogenicity in rats. Gases and vapors from volatile solvents, such as cleaning fluids, have diverse origins. There is a wide range of other pollutants, such as many organic substances, oxides of nitrogen, sulfur, carbon, ozone, benzene, and terpenes.[6] All such toxic substances can be troublesome, especially in sealed air-conditioned buildings and most of all when the air is recirculated to conserve energy used to heat or cool the building. In combination with fluorescent lighting, these gases and suspended particulate matter can produce an irritating photochemical smog that may cause chronic conjunctivitis and nasal congestion.

Imperfect ventilation can become a serious hazard if it leads to accumulation or recirculation of highly toxic gas such as carbon monoxide; this is especially likely when coal or coke is used as cooking or heating fuel in cold weather, and vents to the outside are closed to conserve heat.

Asbestos was used for many years as a fire retardant and insulating substance in both domestic and commercial buildings. Its dangers to health have led to restriction or banning of its use and to expensive renovations aimed at removing it (see Chapter 19). Fibrous glass insulation may present hazards similar to those of asbestos but less severe.

Ionizing radiation, in particular radon and "daughters," can be a health hazard, especially if houses are sealed and air recirculated, in which case there is greater opportunity for higher concentrations to accumulate. Sources of radon include trace amounts of radioactive material incorporated in cement used to construct basements. Radon can also be emitted from soil or rocks in the environment where the houses are built.

Extremely low frequency electromagnetic radiation (ELF) has attracted much attention since the observation of cancer incidence at higher rates than expected among children living close to high-voltage power lines.[7] No convincing relationship has been demonstrated between childhood cancer and exposure to ELF from domestic appliances, with the possible exception of electric blankets.[8] Microwave ovens and television screens are safe. The nature of the relationship, if any, between ELF and cancer remains controversial, however.

TABLE 40-2. INDOOR AIR POLLUTION FROM BIOMASS FUEL COMBUSTION IN DEVELOPING COUNTRIES

	GPM (mg/m^3)	*BaP (mg/m^3)*	*CO (mg/m^3)*	*NO_2 (μg/m^3)*	*Other*
Nigeria, Lagos	—	—	1,076	15,168	SO_2, 38 ppm Benzene, 66 ppm
Papua New Guinea	0.84	—	35.5	—	HCHO, 1.2 ppm
Kenya Highlands	4.0	145	—	—	BaH, 224 μg/m^3 Phenols, 1.0 μg/m^3 Acetic acid, 4.6 μg/m^3
India, Ahmedabad					
Cattle dung	16.0	8,250	—	144	SO_2, 242 μg/m^3
Dung and wood	21.1	9,320	—	326	SO_2, 269 μg/m^3
India, Gujarat	2.7–10	2,220–6,070			
Monsoon	56.6	19,300			

BaP = benz-a-pyrene; SPM = suspended particulate matter.

Data from de Koning HW, Smith KR, Last JM: Biomass fuel combustion and health. Bull WHO 63:11–26, 1985 and World Health Organization: *Air Quality Guidelines.* Regional Reports series 23. Copenhagen: World Health Organization, 1987.

Tobacco smoke is often the greatest health hazard attributable to physical factors in the indoor environment. Infants and children are significantly more prone to respiratory infections, and nonsmoking spouses are more prone to chronic respiratory illnesses and to tobacco-related respiratory cancer when living in the same house as a habitual cigarette smoker. Cigarette smoking is a hazard in another way as well: about 20 to 25 percent of deaths in domestic fires are a result of smoking.

Biological Hazards

Biological hazards in the indoor environment include many varieties of pathogenic microorganisms. *Mycobacterium tuberculosis* survives for long periods in dark and dusty corners. *Legionella* lives in air conditioners, water-cooled air conditioning systems, stagnant water pipes, and shower stalls, for example. Mites that live on mattresses, cushions, and infrequently swept floors cause asthma, as may many organic dusts and pollens. Many other infections, especially those spread by the fecal-oral route, occur most often when homes are dirty, verminous, or rat infested. Food storage and cooking facilities should be kept scrupulously clean at all times because many varieties of disease-carrying vermin are attracted by filth and because food scraps can be an excellent culture medium for many pathogens that cause food poisoning or other diseases.

Socioeconomic Conditions

Socioeconomic conditions are related to the quality of housing in many ways, some already alluded to. Crowding always is greater among the poor than among the rich; this increases risks of transmitting communicable diseases and often imposes additional emotional stress that probably contributes to domestic violence. Street accidents involving children are more common in poor than in wealthy neighborhoods because the children often have no other place than the street to play. Poor people generally live in poorly equipped and maintained homes, adding to the risk of domestic accidents ranging from falls down poorly lit stairwells to electrocution. Lead poisoning is a particular hazard for children in dilapidated houses where they are likely to ingest dried-out flakes of lead-based paint. Emissions from factory smelter stacks contribute to environmental lead and other toxic metal contamination and are more often present in poor than in well-to-do neighborhoods because the former are more often located in or close to heavily industrialized areas.

▸ HOUSING CONDITIONS AND MENTAL HEALTH

Many descriptive studies by social epidemiologists and psychiatrists have demonstrated a consistent association between mental disorders and urban living conditions.[9] There is also a close relationship between mental health and social class.[10] Those who cannot cope with the competitive pressures of industrial and commercial civilization because they suffer from such disorders as schizophrenia, alcoholism, or mental retardation and have inadequate family and social support systems drift downward to the lowest depths of the slums or become homeless street people. There are estimated to be between 500,000 and 2 million homeless mentally ill persons in the United States.[11] Schizophrenia and alcoholism have maximum prevalence in slums and "skid row" districts, and depression, manifested by attempted and accomplished suicide, is clustered in neighborhoods where a high proportion of the people live in single-room rented apartments.[12] Adolescent delinquency, vandalism, and underachievement at school have high prevalence in dormitory suburbs occupied mainly by low-paid workers, where recreational facilities for young people are often inadequate and schools are often of inferior quality. Bad housing does not cause these problems; they are usually symptoms of more complex social pathology. A different set of factors contribute to the syndrome called "suburban neurosis," which occurs among women who remain housebound for much of the time while their husbands are at work and their children are at school;[13] this condition has been alleviated by television, which by bringing faces and voices into the house relieves loneliness. It has also been alleviated by changing work patterns, with increasing proportions of married women joining the workforce.

▸ HOUSING STANDARDS

Public health workers are directly concerned about the quality of housing because of the many ways it can affect health. Local health officials have special powers to intervene when health is threatened by inadequate housing conditions. A handbook frequently revised by the Centers for Disease Control and Prevention and the American Public Health Association, *Housing and Health; APHA-CDC Recommended Minimum Housing Standards,*[14] sets out specific details on basic equipment and facilities, fire safety, lighting, ventilation, thermal requirements, sanitation, space requirements (occupancy standards), and the special requirements for rooming houses. This valuable reference spells out general guidelines that can be used by local authorities as the basis for regulations, but there are no universal legally enforcible standards until local jurisdictions introduce them. *Health Principles of Housing,*[15] a WHO manual, gives guidance on a wide range of behavioral factors that can influence health in relation to housing conditions, for example, by providing guidelines on ways to reduce psychological and social stresses by ensuring privacy and comfort and on the housing needs of populations at special risk such as pregnant women, the handicapped, and the elderly infirm. Both booklets should be part of the library of every local health officer.

▸ STATISTICAL INDICATORS OF HOUSING CONDITIONS

Health planning requires every kind of information pertinent to community health, including statistics on housing conditions. Useful information is routinely collected at the decennial census on density of occupancy (persons per bedroom), cooking and refrigerating facilities, and sanitary conditions. Perusal of tables showing these and other housing statistics enables health planners to identify neighborhoods at high risk of diseases associated with crowding and poor sanitation.

Census tables also enable health planners to identify less obtrusive health hazards, such as proportions of elderly persons living alone, whether in small apartments or multiple-room dwellings that perhaps were once the family home before all the others in the family moved away or died, leaving an elderly person as sole resident. Once such neighborhoods are identified, public health nurses and other community health workers can more easily locate the individuals at risk, who may need but have not yet asked for help.

In addition to census tables, there are other useful sources of information on neighborhoods with a high incidence of social pathology. Fire departments record false alarms and fires deliberately lit; police departments record details of vandalism and calls to settle domestic disturbances; and schools record absenteeism and truancy. All can be analyzed by area, thus pinpointing high-risk neighborhoods; this method has been used as part of a program aimed at improving the chances of getting a good start in life for children from disadvantaged homes. There is a high correlation between these indicators of social pathology in a neighborhood, such as a high-rise, high-density apartment complex for low-income families, and the incidence of emotional disturbances and similar behavioral upsets among young and teenaged children.[16]

▸ HEALTHY COMMUNITIES AND HEALTHY CITIES

As part of the initiative for "Health for all by the year 2000" that followed resolutions passed at the World Health Assembly in 1977,[17] health planners in many nations, notably in the European region of the World Health Organization (WHO), began active planning for health promotion (to be distinguished from disease prevention). Health promotion (see Chapter 1) requires action by many individuals and groups not usually identified with care of the sick or prevention of disease. The definition of health promotion, "the process of enabling people to increase control over and improve their health," implies that people may often have to take action aimed at improving their living conditions. The Healthy Cities movement is a coordinated program involving community health workers, local elected officials in urban affairs, and a wide variety of community groups who collectively seek to upgrade living conditions. Initially, some of the participating cities were relatively healthy places to live (e.g., Toronto, Canada) while others, (e.g., Liverpool, England) were not. The Healthy Cities initiative emphasizes activities that could be expected to enhance good health, such as provision of improved recreational facilities, services for children and their mothers (including basic education for the mothers as well as the children), and aggressive action to eradicate urban wasteland, industrial pollution, toxic dump sites, and other forms of urban blight.[18] From modest beginnings the Healthy Cities movement has spread all over the world and in some places has extended beyond cities to embrace rural communities.[19] Since the environment in which people live, grow, work, and play so manifestly influences their health and happiness, the Healthy Cities initiative is potentially among the most valuable means at our disposal to make this environment healthful.

► SPECIAL HOUSING NEEDS

Elderly and disabled people require accommodation that has been adapted to enable easier access (ramps, handrails, wide doors to permit passage of wheelchairs), to facilitate storage and preparation of food (low-placed cupboards and stoves with front-fitted switches, which are inadvisable in homes where there are small children), and with special equipment for bathing and toileting (strong handrails, wheelchair access). Special accommodation of this type is often segregated, which tends to set the occupants apart in an urban ghetto for the elderly and disabled. Integrated special housing is preferable, as examples in Denmark, Sweden, and the United Kingdom have demonstrated; in this setting, elderly, infirm, and younger disabled persons live among nondisabled people, a situation that many of them prefer and that helps to accustom nondisabled people to making allowances for their disabled fellow-citizens.

► CONCLUSION

This is a brief summary of a complex and diverse field. The essential requirements of the domestic environment have been stressed, along with some of the obvious adverse effects of unsatisfactory housing.

The home should provide more than mere shelter and a safe place to raise children. It should be the setting in which the family lives and grows together, where bonds of affection and mutual trust are formed and strengthened, where socialization into the prevailing culture and intellectual stimulation are occurring, and where privacy is available when it is wanted and needed. Doxiadis[20] coined the term *ekistics*, meaning the science of human settlements, to encompass the many interactive factors that make living space compatible with good physical, mental, emotional, and social health and well-being. The arrangement of dwelling units, their relationship to the natural and to the human-made environment, and their interior structure and function all play a part in creating a housing environment conducive to good health. Many less easily described and unmeasurable factors, such as the innumerable ways that people can interact, also contribute to the ambience of the living space. These intangible factors would receive more attention in a better world than this if we were really intent on applying all possible means to the end of promoting and preserving the public's health.

► REFERENCES

1. de Koning HW, Smith KR, Last JM: Biomass fuel combustion and health. Bull WHO 63:11–26, 1985
2. Tabibzadeh I, Rossi-Espagnet A, Maxwell R: Spotlight on the cities; improving urban health in the developing world. Geneva: World Health Organization, 1989
3. World Resources; A Guide to the Global Environment: The Urban Environment 1996–97. (A UNEP/UNDP/World Bank/WRI Monograph. New York: Oxford University Press, 1991
4. UNHCR: State of the World's Refugees, 1996. Geneva: UNHCR, 1996
5. Last JM: Biomass fuels. In Environmental Determinants of Health Associated with the Production, Distribution and Use of Energy, Geneva: World Health Organization, 1991
6. Indoor air quality: organic pollutants. WHO Regional Office for Europe, Euro Reports and Studies No. 111, 1987
7. Wertheimer N, Leeper E: Electrical wiring configurations and childhood cancer. Am J Epidemiol 109:273–284, 1979
8. Savitz D, John EM, Kleckner RC: Magnetic field exposure from electric appliances and childhood cancer. Am J Epidemiol 131:763–773, 1990
9. Srole L, Langner TS, Michael ST, et al: Mental Health in the Metropolis: the Mid-town Manhattan Study. New York: McGraw-Hill, 1962
10. Dohrenwend BP, Dohrenwend BS: Social status and psychological disorder: a causal inquiry. New York: John Wiley & Sons, 1969
11. American Psychiatric Association Report on the Homeless Mentally Ill. Washington, DC: The Association, 1984
12. Hare EH: Mental Illness and social conditions in Bristol. J Ment Sci 102:349–357, 1956
13. Hare EH, Shaw GK: Mental health on a new housing estate. Oxford: Oxford University Press, 1965
14. Wood EW: Housing and Health: APHA-CDC Recommended Minimum Housing Standards, Washington, DC: APHA, 1995
15. Health Principles of Housing. Geneva: World Health Organization, 1989
16. Offord DR, Barrette PA, Last JM: A comparison of school performance, emotional adjustment and skill development of poor and middle-class children. Can J Public Health 76:157–163, 1985
17. Resolution 30.43. World Health Assembly. Geneva: World Health Organization, 1977
18. Ashton J (ed): Healthy Cities. Milton Keynes, Philadelphia: Open Universities Press, 1992
19. Lacombe R: Villes et villages en sante: l'experience Quebecoise. Can J Public Health 80:3–5, 1989
20. Doxiadis CA: Action for Human Settlements. New York: Norton, 1977

41

Human Health in a Changing World

John M. Last

Throughout its 4 billion year life the earth's atmospheric composition and climate have changed many times. Sometimes air and ocean currents that determine climate and weather have been altered by tectonic plate movements. The impact of large meteors or massive volcanic activity that blocks sunlight by filling the air with dust and gases such as sulfur dioxide have occasionally produced sudden climate changes leading to great extinctions.[1] Variation in solar radiation, oscillation of the earth's axis, or passing clouds of interstellar dust may induce ice ages and periods of interglacial warming.[2] Minor seasonal fluctuations are associated with many intervening variables that make weather forecasting the most inexact of all sciences.

Recently a consensus has developed among scientists in the relevant disciplines that human activity is adversely affecting the earth's climate;[3] and there is compelling evidence that human activity is changing the biosphere in other ways besides climate. The changes represent a new scale of human impact on the world unlike anything in recorded history. Collectively the changes endanger human health and future prospects for many other living creatures. Global warming and stratospheric ozone depletion have attracted the most attention, but the changes go beyond these two processes. The term *global change* covers several interconnected phenomena:[4] global warming ("climate change"); stratospheric ozone attenuation; resource depletion; species extinction and reduced biodiversity; serious and widespread environmental pollution; desertification; and macro and micro ecosystem changes, including some that have led to emergence or re-emergence of dangerous pathogens (Table 41-1). These phenomena are mostly associated with industrial processes or are due to the increased pressure of people on fragile ecosystems.[5] All are interconnected and some are synergistic—some processes reinforce others.

Underlying them all is a population explosion. In little more than the length of an average lifetime, the population has quadrupled, from about 1.6 billion in 1900 to an estimated 6.4 billion by the year 2000.[6] It is not clear whether our numbers have already reached or even exceeded the earth's carrying capacity; but responsible opinion inclines to the view that we have reached the limits for comfortable human existence. The earth might sustain for a while many millions more than the present number, but life for all but a very small minority would be of greatly diminished quality, and long-term sustainability would be at best a precarious possibility.[7]

Some evidence on the causes and consequences of global change was published by the Intergovernmental Panel on Climate Change (IPCC) in 1990[8,9] and in subsequent supplementary reports and other documents. The situation is described and discussed in greater detail in the Second Assessment Report of IPCC, *Climate Change 1995, Impacts, Adaptations and Mitigation of Climate Change; Scientific-Technical Analysis*.[10] Much of the information in this chapter is taken from that Report, and from *Climate Change and Human Health*,[11] also published in 1996. There have been many other reports: by national governments,[a,12] scientific articles,[13,13a] and documents produced by nongovernmental agencies such as the Union of Concerned Scientists,[14] Friends of the Earth, the Worldwatch Institute,[15] and the Sierra Club.

In the late 1980s when concerns about global warming and other aspects of global change began to attract widespread public interest, some contrary views and rebuttals were published,[16,17] sometimes but not always sponsored by organizations that opposed actions aimed at mitigating global change. As the empirical evidence mounted, these contrary views have become more muted.

Every component of global change merits discussion; I also mention some of the complex interconnections among them in this brief account. Readers are urged to consult the sources I cite. The health, social, economic, and other impacts of global change have been the topic of many important reports.[18,19,19a] There are some obvious actions we should take to enhance readiness to deal with public health aspects of global change and implications for public policy generally.

▸ GLOBAL WARMING

Svante Arrhenius recognized in 1896 that the earth's mantle of atmosphere acts like a greenhouse, allowing passage of short-wavelength solar radiation into the biosphere, trapping longer wavelength infrared radiation. Without the greenhouse effect, the earth's surface temperature would swing from over 50°C in strong sunlight to –40°C at dawn. The concentration of greenhouse gases in the troposphere has risen rapidly since the beginning of the industrial era because several of these gases, notably carbon dioxide, are products of fossil fuel combustion and other human activities (Table 41-2). Industrial activity and the combustion of petroleum fuels in automobiles have increased exponentially since the 1950s, accelerated by industrial and commercial development in India, China, South Korea, Taiwan, Indonesia, Thailand, Brazil, Mexico, and other countries. Currently about 6 billion metric tons of CO_2, the principal greenhouse gas, are added to the troposphere annually, increasing amounts every year (Fig. 41-1). This is despite the promises made by most national leaders at the UN Conference on Environment and Development[20] (UNCED) in Rio de Janeiro in 1992, to stabilize carbon emissions at or below 1990 levels. Moreover, tropical rain forests, perhaps the most important carbon sink, are being rapidly depleted often by slash-burning and this adds even more carbon gases to the greenhouse. Phytoplankton, another important carbon sink, are damaged

[a] *Government-sponsored scientific committees in the United Kingdom, the Netherlands, Canada, Sweden, and Australia have produced multiple reports since approximately 1985. In the United States, the National Academy of Sciences has produced several reports.*

TABLE 41-1. HEALTH-RELATED FEATURES OF GLOBAL CHANGE

Feature	*Quality of Evidence*	*Impact*
Global warming	Fair to good: based on models and empirical observation	Entire world
Ozone depletion	Good: based on observations	Entire world
Resource depletion	Fair to good	Hits developing countries hardest
Environmental pollution	Good, but health impacts not always firmly linked to pollutants	Mainly regional, e.g., eastern Europe, former Soviet Union, industrializing nations
Demographic changes	Good, but many details based on estimates	Developing countries, especially Africa
Emerging, re-emerging pathogens	Good	Varies; HIV and some others are global, some are regional
Other factors: rise of transnational corporations; advances in technology and communication; political volatility; religious fundamentalism; regional conflicts	Fair to good	Mainly regional, but some is global in scope

by increased ultraviolet radiation (UVR) flux due to depletion of stratospheric ozone, an example of reinforcement of one form of global change by another. When they signed the 1995 Framework Convention on Climate Change, most national leaders reiterated their earlier promises, and the 1995 IPCC Reports add a sense of urgency to the need for action.

In 1995, the atmospheric concentration of carbon dioxide reached a higher level than at any time in the last 140,000 years, and the average ambient atmospheric temperature was the highest since record-keeping began[21] (Fig. 41-2). It is estimated by global climate models using a variety of methods that the average global ambient temperature will rise by about 0.5°C in the first half of the twenty-first century and may rise 2°C by 2100.[2] These are conservative estimates. Moreover, these are *average* temperatures; the increase, and seasonal and diurnal swing, are expected to be greater, as much as 6–8°C, in temperate zones, and perhaps even more near the poles. If arctic permafrost thaws as a result, a great deal of methane will be released, adding to the existing burden of atmospheric greenhouse gases and accelerating the warming process.

Global warming has direct and indirect and predominantly adverse effects on health (Fig. 41-3). Although heat-wave deaths are dramatic and obvious, in terms of overall health impact, the largest factor is vector-borne disease. Increased average ambient temperatures extend the range, distribution, and abundance of insect vectors such as mosquitoes, allow the pathogens they carry to breed more rapidly, and may enhance their virulence. Malaria, for instance, is expected to become prevalent in temperate zones and at altitudes in tropical and subtropical regions from which it is now absent, notably large highland cities and periurban slums in East Africa (Nairobi, Harare, Soweto, etc.), where an additional 20–30 million people will be at risk; there will be many millions more at risk of malaria annually in Indonesia and other populous South and Southeast Asian nations. Other tropical and subtropical vector-borne diseases also will increase in incidence, prevalence, and perhaps mortality (Table 41-3). In North America, several arbovirus diseases (e.g. viral encephalitis and hemorrhagic dengue fever) will occur more frequently.

The indirect effects of global warming include a sea-level rise of up to 50 cm by the year 2050, due to melting of polar and alpine ice-caps and thermal expansion of the seawater mass. This will disrupt many coastal ecosystems, jeopardize coastal and perhaps some ocean fisheries, salinate river estuaries that are an important source of drinking water, and displace scores of millions of people from low-lying coastal regions in many parts of the world, including the Netherlands, Bangladesh, much of South China, parts of Japan, and small island states (Vanu Atu, the Maldives, etc.) that face inundation and obliteration. Up to 10–15 million people along the eastern seaboard of the

TABLE 41-2. KEY GREENHOUSE GASES INFLUENCED BY HUMAN ACTIVITY

	CO_2	*CH_4*	*CFC-11*	*CFC-12*	*N_2O*
Preindustrial atmospheric concentration	280 ppmv	0.8 ppmv	0	0	288 ppbv
Current atmospheric concentration (1990)[a]	353 ppmv	1.72 ppmv	280 pptv	484 pptv	310 ppbv
Current rate of annual atmospheric accumulation[b]	1.8 ppmv (0.5%)	0.015 ppmv (0.9%)	9.5 pptv (4%)	17 pptv (4%)	0.8 ppbv (0.25%)
Atmospheric lifetime (years)[c]	(50–200)	10	65	130	150

From World Meteorological Organization: *Climate Change, the IPCC Scientific Assessment.* Cambridge, United Kingdom: Cambridge University Press, 1990.

NOTES: Ozone has not been included in the table because of lack of precise data. Abbreviations: ppmv, parts per million by volume; ppbv, parts per billion by volume; pptv, parts per trillion by volume.

[a] The 1990 concentrations have been estimated on the basis of an extrapolation of measurements reported for earlier years, assuming that the recent trends remained approximately constant.

[b] Net annual emissions of CO_2 from the biosphere not affected by human activity, such as volcanic emissions, are assumed to be small. Estimates of human-induced emissions from the biosphere are controversial.

[c] For each gas in the table, except CO_2, the "lifetime" is defined as the ratio of the atmospheric concentration to the total rate of removal. This time scale also characterizes the rate of adjustment of the atmospheric concentrations if the emission rates are changed abruptly. CO_2 is a special case because it is merely circulated among various reservoirs (atmosphere, ocean, biota). The "lifetime" of CO_2 given in the table is a rough indication of the time it would take for the CO_2 concentration to adjust to changes in the emissions.

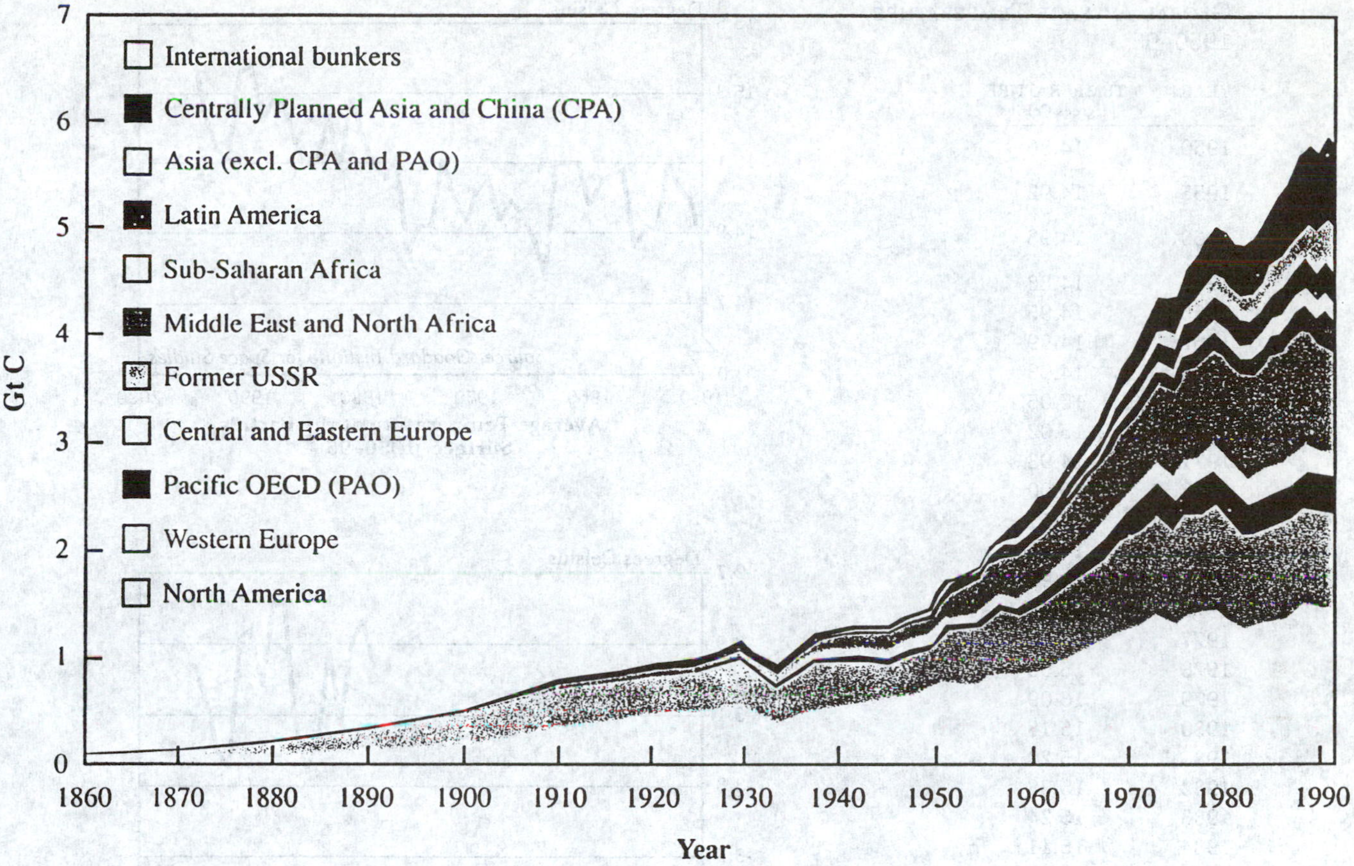

Figure 41-1. Global energy-related CO_2 emissions by major world region in Gigatonnes (Gt) C/yr. (Source: Reference 10.)

United States may be affected. Many of those displaced will become "environmental refugees" in third-world megacities or drift into urban squalor in the rich industrial nations.

Another effect of global climate change with implications for human health is anomalous weather—notably, more frequent and severe weather emergencies such as catastrophic floods, hurricanes and tornadoes, and heat waves. Atmospheric physicists and climatologists believe that some unusual weather events in the 1986–1995 decade may be attributable to global climate change. These anomalous weather events have already extracted a heavy financial toll from the insurance industry and from national disaster funds in the United States and elsewhere (Table 41-4).

The impact of global warming on food security could be very serious; here the interconnection of global warming with resource depletion and desertification is important. Global warming will jeopardize the viability of crops in some of the world's most important grain-growing regions because it will alter rainfall patterns and soil moisture levels and hasten desertification of marginal grazing and agricultural land, as it has already done in much of the West African Sahel, parts of northeast Brazil, and elsewhere in Africa (Ethiopia, Sudan, Angola, Zimbabwe, etc.). An increase in surface-level ultraviolet radiation flux, discussed below, will make matters worse if it impairs plant reproduction or growth. Predictions are difficult when so many variables are involved, but the models developed by agronomists suggest that, while some grain crops might benefit from warmer climate and higher levels of atmospheric CO_2, the overall impact is likely to be a decline in world grain crop production[22] (Table 41-5).

Desertification is made worse by unsound and inappropriate agricultural methods. The "green revolution" that dramatically increased agricultural output in the 40 years following the end of World War II is over: many forms of agricultural output have remained stationary or have declined in the past 5 to 10 years, raising troubling questions about the earth's carrying capacity.

Global warming is probably the principal cause of the retreat of alpine glaciers that has been observed since the late nineteenth century. This could reduce the ice-melt component of many river systems, which contribute by irrigation and/or seasonal flooding to productivity of food-producing regions. The deficit is compensated in part at least by increased rainfall, but in the long term, river flow could decline. Shortages of fresh water for irrigation and drinking may be the most critical limiting factor on further population growth in many parts of the world.

▶ STRATOSPHERIC OZONE ATTENUATION

In 1974 Molina and Rowland, two atmospheric physicists, predicted that chlorofluorocarbons (CFCs) a widely used class of chemicals, would permeate the upper atmosphere where they would break down under the influence of solar radiation to produce chlorine monoxide.[23,23a] Chlorine monoxide destroys ozone; each molecule of chlorine monoxide is capable of destroying over 10,000 ozone molecules. Rowland and Molina were awarded the Nobel Prize for Physics in 1995 in recognition of their work. Other atmospheric contaminants that destroy stratospheric ozone include other halocarbons and perhaps oxides of nitrogen, e.g., in exhaust emissions of high-flying supersonic jet aircraft. Volcanic eruptions sometimes release chlorine compounds into the atmosphere, so natural as well as human-induced processes can contribute to stratospheric ozone attenuation.

Rowland and Molina's predictions soon began to come true. In 1985, Farman and coworkers observed extensive attenuation (a "hole") in the stratospheric ozone layer over Antarctica during the

Global Average Temperature, 1950–95

Year	Temperature (degrees Celsius)
1950	14.86
1955	14.92
1960	14.98
1965	14.88
1966	14.95
1967	14.99
1968	14.93
1969	15.05
1970	15.02
1971	14.93
1972	15.00
1973	15.11
1974	14.92
1975	14.92
1976	14.84
1977	15.11
1978	15.06
1979	15.09
1980	15.18
1981	15.29
1982	15.08
1983	15.24
1984	15.11
1985	15.09
1986	15.16
1987	15.27
1988	15.28
1989	15.22
1990	15.38
1991	15.36
1992	15.11
1993	15.14
1994	15.23
1995 (prel)	15.39

Sources: Goddard Institute for Space Studies, New York, January 19, 1996.

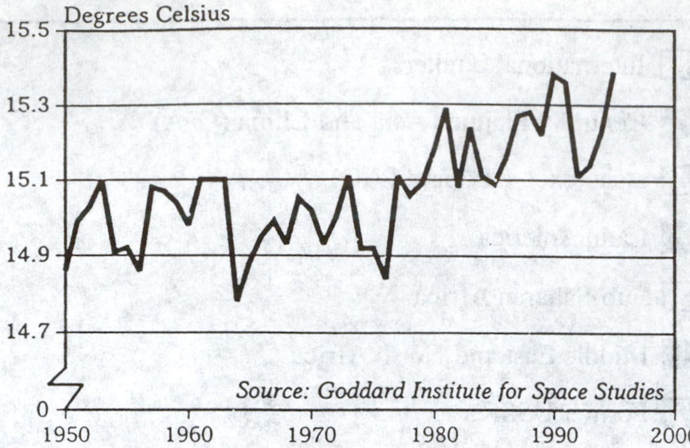

Average Temperature at the Earth's Surface, 1950–95

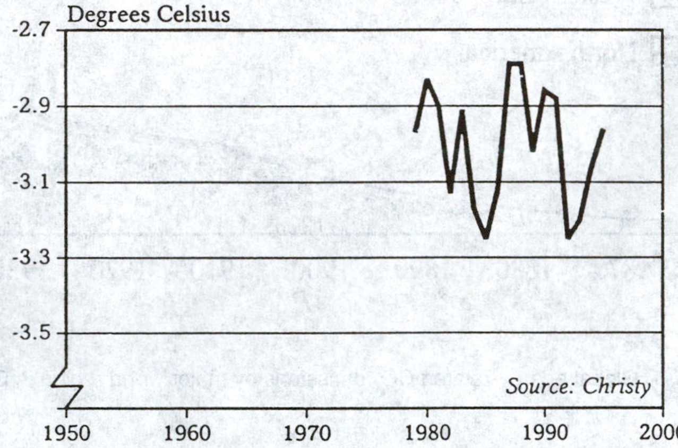

Average Temperature of the Lower Atmosphere Based on Satellite Measurements, 1979–95

Figure 41-2. Global average temperature trends. (From Intergovernmental Panel on Climate Change: Climate Change 1995; Impacts, Adaptations and Mitigation; Summary for Policymakers. Geneva: WMO, World Health Organization, United Nations Environment Programme, 1996.)

Southern Hemisphere spring.[24] This has recurred annually; since 1990, seasonal ozone depletion has been observed in the Northern Hemisphere too, greatest over parts of Siberia and northeastern North America. Stratospheric ozone depletion was correlated by Kerr and colleagues at the Canadian Climate Centre in 1993 with increased surface level UVR flux.[25] Ozone depletion so far is about 3 to 4 percent of total stratospheric ozone and increasing annually.

The stratospheric ozone layer protects the biosphere from exposure to lethal levels of ultraviolet radiation. The gravity of this progressive loss of stratospheric ozone was recognized almost immediately and led many industrial nations to adopt the Montreal Protocol, calling for a moratorium on manufacture and use of CFCs.[26] CFCs were widely used as solvents in manufacture of microprocessors for computers, foaming agents in polystyrene packing, propellants in spray cans, and as Freon gas in air conditioners and refrigerators; their supposed chemical inertness made them a popular choice. But because they are inert they have, on average, an atmospheric half-life of about 100 years, so stratospheric ozone depletion will continue to be a serious problem well into the twenty-second century. Stratospheric ozone must not be confused with toxic surface-level air pollution with ozone that contaminates fumes from some industrial processes or as a result of the action of sunlight on automobile exhaust fumes ("photochemical smog").

Stratospheric ozone depletion permits greater amounts of harmful UVR to enter the biosphere, where it has adverse effects on many biological systems and on human health (Table 41-6). The principal effects of increased UVR are disruption of the reproductive capacity and vitality of small and single-celled organisms, notably phytoplankton at the base of marine food chains, pollen, amphibians' eggs, many insects, and the sensitive growing ends of green leaf plants. Increased UVR also has direct adverse effects on human health: it in-

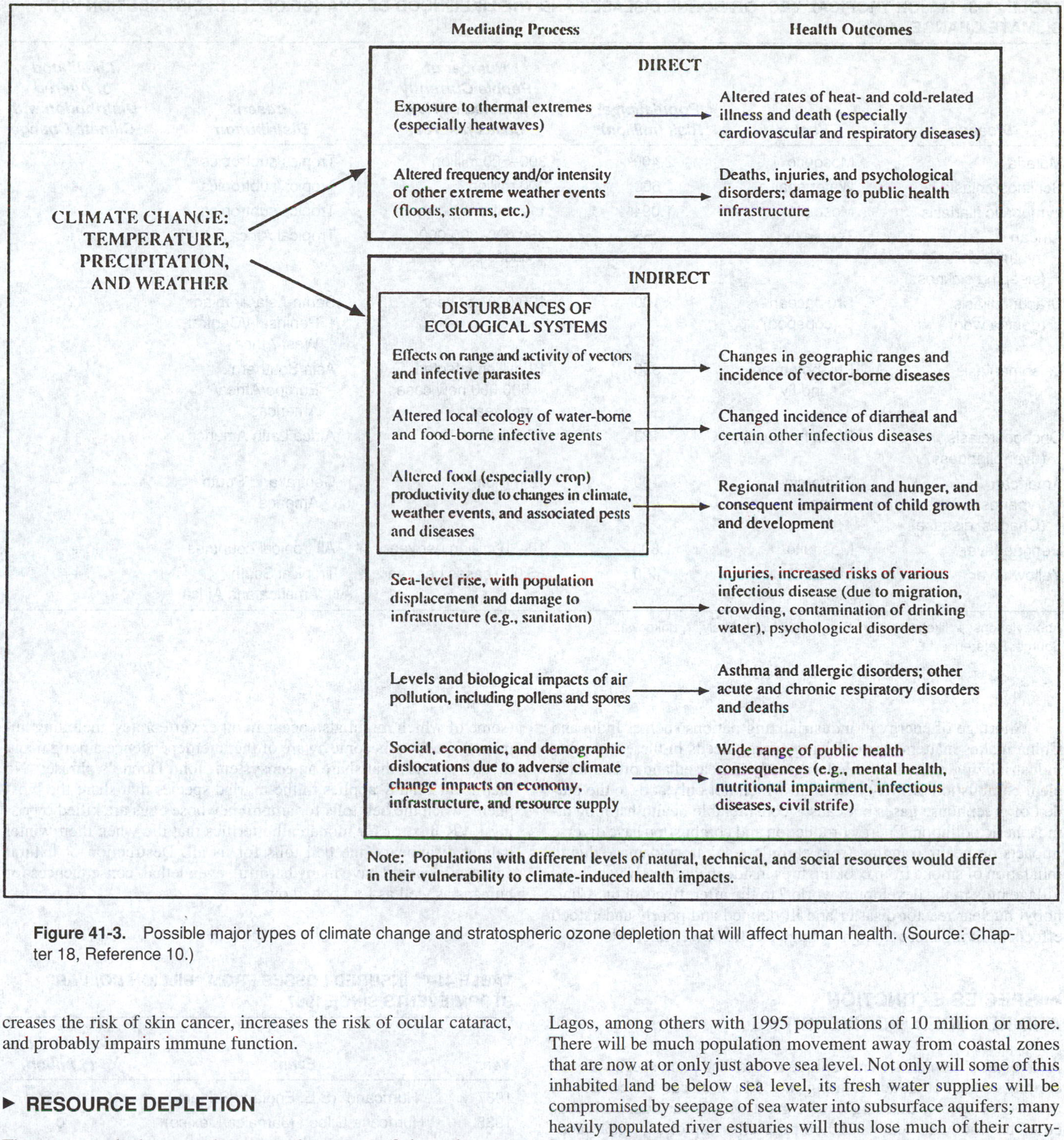

Figure 41-3. Possible major types of climate change and stratospheric ozone depletion that will affect human health. (Source: Chapter 18, Reference 10.)

creases the risk of skin cancer, increases the risk of ocular cataract, and probably impairs immune function.

▸ RESOURCE DEPLETION

The more people there are, the greater the stress on finite and scarce resources. Two resources are essential for survival—fresh water for drinking and irrigation, and food. Water shortages in some parts of the world are associated with conflicts, and in the next 50 years as the shortages spread to other countries and regions, these conflicts probably will be exacerbated (Table 41-7). Threats to water security are a primary cause of some of the most intractable conflicts in the world.[27] The IPCC *Summary for Policymakers* suggests that water shortages will be an important limiting factor on growth and development in some regions, notably much of the Middle East, Southern Africa, parts of Brazil, and the Southwest of the United States.[28] Sea-level rise due to global warming and salination of river estuaries and water tables close to seacoasts will threaten some of the largest human settlements on earth: Tokyo, Shanghai, Calcutta, Bombay, Jakarta, and Lagos, among others with 1995 populations of 10 million or more. There will be much population movement away from coastal zones that are now at or only just above sea level. Not only will some of this inhabited land be below sea level, its fresh water supplies will be compromised by seepage of sea water into subsurface aquifers; many heavily populated river estuaries will thus lose much of their carrying capacity. Desertification of grazing lands and marginal cultivated agricultural land would further threaten food security.

Another critical limiting factor is shortage of ocean and coastal fish stocks. This was seen in the early 1990s in dramatic form in the collapse of many of the world's ocean fisheries, mainly due to almost criminally irresponsible overfishing; but it was aggravated by changes in marine ecosystems accompanying disappearance of coastal wetlands, disruption of river outflows by massive dams (e.g., the Aswan High Dam), pollution with chemicals, oil spills, etc. Other factors were changes in ocean temperature and flow of currents such as El Niño, which affect marine ecology. Fish provide about 20 to 25 percent of human protein needs, considerably more in coastal-dwelling populations in South and Southeast Asia. It is not clear where replacement protein will come from.[29]

TABLE 41-3. MAJOR TROPICAL VECTOR-BORNE DISEASES AND THE LIKELIHOOD OF CHANGE OF THEIR DISTRIBUTION WITH CLIMATE CHANGE

Disease	Vector	Population at Risk (million)[a]	Number of People Currently Infected or New Cases per Year	Present Distribution	Likelihood of Altered Distribution with Climate Change
Malaria	Mosquito	2,400[b]	300–500 million	Tropics/subtropics	+++
Schistosomiasis	Water snail	600	200 million	Tropics/subtropics	++
Lymphatic filariasis	Mosquito	1,094[c]	117 million	Tropics/subtropics	+
African trypanosomiasis (sleeping sickness)	Tsetse fly	55[d]	250,000–300,000 cases per year	Tropical Africa	+
Dracunculiasis (guinea worm)	Crustacean (copepod)	100[e]	100,000 per year	South Asia/Arabian Peninsula/Central-West Africa	?
Leishmaniasis	Phlebotomine sand fly	350	12 million infected, 500,000 new cases per year[f]	Asia/Southern Europe/Africa/Americas	+
Onchocerciasis (river blindness)	Black fly	123	17.5 million	Africa/Latin America	++
American trypanosomiasis (Chagas' disease)	Triatomine bug	100[g]	18 million	Central and South America	+
Dengue fever	Mosquito	1,800	10–30 million per year	All tropical countries	++
Yellow fever	Mosquito	450	<5,000 cases per year	Tropical South America and Africa	++

Abbreviations: +, likely; ++, very likely; +++, highly likely; ?, unknown.
Source: Reference 11

Shortage of energy in industrializing nations such as India and China makes matters worse. Rising energy needs in these and other industrializing nations have led to greatly increased and often inefficient combustion of low-grade coal, which not only adds to the burden of greenhouse gases but causes considerable health-harming atmospheric pollution. Energy production and combustion have diverse impacts on health, ranging from chronic respiratory damage due to inhalation of smoke from cooking fires inside inadequately ventilated village huts in the developing world[30] to the aftereffects of the Chernobyl nuclear reactor disaster and ill-defined and poorly understood effects of living close to high-voltage electic power lines.[31,31a]

▸ SPECIES EXTINCTION AND REDUCED BIODIVERSITY

As a result of human activity, unique animal and plant species are becoming extinct at an accelerating rate. Much discussion centers on the loss of species that might have great benefit for humans if they could be studied in detail and their properties exploited, e.g., as anticancer agents. This view of species extinction is anthropocentric, a narrow view that considers only the possible direct benefits of biodiversity for humans. Subtle features of biodiversity matter more, especially the loss of genetic diversity.[32] It may be very hazardous to proceed on our present course of increasing reliance on monocultures of high-yielding grain crops. Entire yields could be wiped out by an epidemic plant disease to which that strain is vulnerable; if a genetically diverse grain crop is struck by plant disease, some strains at least are likely to survive. We have long understood that widespread pesticide use on insects that damage crops killed large numbers of useful arthropod species such as bees and led to death or reproductive failure of many species of birds.[33] Fat-soluble dioxins and PCBs that concentrate as they move through food chains have adverse effects on reproductive outcomes, e.g., by causing lethal deformities (some of which might also occur in other vertebrates, including humans). We have become aware of the interdependence among many diverse species that share an ecosystem. John Donne's phrase, "No man is an island" applies to the myriad species that share the biosphere; when the bell tolls for amphibia whose eggs are killed by rising UVR flux, or for monarch butterflies that die when their winter habitat disappears, the bell tolls for us all. Destruction of natural ecosystems could have many harmful, even lethal, consequences for humans as well as for spotted owls.

TABLE 41-4. INSURED LOSSES FROM "BILLION DOLLAR" STORM EVENTS SINCE 1987

Year	Event	Insured Loss ($ billion)
1987	"Hurricane" (S.E. England/Brittany)	2.5
1988	Hurricane Gilbert (Jamaica/Mexico)	0.8
1989	Hurricane Hugo (Puerto Rico/ South Carolina)	5.8
1990	European storms (4 total)	10.4
1991	Typhoon Mireille (Japan)	4.8
1992	Hurricane Andrew (Florida)	16.5
1993	"Storm of the Century" (Eastern United States)	1.7
1994	Winter storms in Germany	2.0

From Munich Reinsurance Company: Windstorm—New Loss Dimensions of a Natural Hazard. Munich: Munich Reinsurance Company, 1990; Leggett J: Climate change. Presentation to the 26th Annual Meeting of the Reinsurance Association of America. April 29, 1994, Laguna Niguel, CA, Greenpeace International.

TABLE 41-5. SELECTED CROP STUDY RESULTS FOR 2 × CO_2-EQUIVALENT EQUILIBRIUM GCM SCENARIOS[a]

Region	*Crop*	*Yield Impact (%)*	*Comments*
Latin America	Maize	–61 to increase	Data are from Argentina, Brazil, Chile, and Mexico; range is across GCM scenarios, with and without CO_2 effect.
	Wheat	–50 to –5	Data are from Argentina, Uruguay, and Brazil; range is across GCM scenarios, with and without CO_2 effect.
	Soybean	–10 to +40	Data are from Brazil; range is across Global Climate Model (GCM) scenarios, with CO_2 effect.
Former Soviet Union	Wheat Grain	–19 to +41 –14 to +13	Range is across GCM scenarios and region, with CO_2 effect.
Europe	Maize	–30 to increase	Data are from France, Spain, and northern Europe; with adaptation and CO_2 effect; assumes longer season, irrigation efficiency loss, and northward shift.
	Wheat	Increase or decrease	Data are from France, United Kingdom, and northern Europe; with adaptation and CO_2 effect; assumes longer season, northward shift, increased pest damage, and lower risk of crop failure.
	Vegetables	Increase	Data are from United Kingdom and northern Europe; assumes pest damage increased and lower risk of crop failure.
North America	Maize Wheat	–55 to +62 –100 to +234	Data are from United States and Canada; range is across GCM scenarios and sites, with/without adaptation and with/without CO_2 effect.
	Soybean	–96 to +58	Data are from United States; less severe or increase with CO_2 and adaptation.
Africa	Maize	–65 to +6	Data are from Egypt, Kenya, South Africa, and Zimbabwe; range is over studies and climate scenarios, with CO_2 effect.
	Millet	–79 to –63	Data are from Senegal; carrying capacity fell 11–38%.
	Biomass	Decrease	Data are from South Africa; agrozone shifts.
South Asia	Rice Maize Wheat	–22 to +28 –65 to –10 –61 to +67	Data are from Bangladesh, India, Philippines, Thailand, Indonesia, Malaysia, and Myanmar; range is over GCM scenarios, with CO_2 effect; some studies also consider adaptation.
China	Rice	–78 to +28	Includes rainfed and irrigated rice; range is across sites and GCM scenarios; genetic variation provides scope for adaptation.
Other Asia and Pacific Rim	Rice	–45 to +30	Data are from Japan and South Korea; range is across GCM scenarios; generally positive in north Japan, and negative in south.
	Pasture	–1 to +35	Data are from Australia and New Zealand; regional variation.
	Wheat	–41 to +65	Data are from Australia and Japan; wide variation, depending on cultivar.

[a] For most regions, studies have focused on one or two principal grains. These studies strongly demonstrate the variability in estimated yield impacts among countries, scenarios, methods of analysis, and crops, making it difficult to generalize results across areas or for different climate scenarios. (See Chapter 13 Reference 10.)

▸ DESERTIFICATION

Conversion of marginal agricultural land into desert is a widespread problem. Land that was suitable for light grazing was inappropriately used in attempts to grow crops. Thin soil on mountain slopes that held native vegetation capable of resisting erosion in annual spring snowmelt was cleared and cultivated, leading to rapid erosion—the soil slid down steep mountain slopes leaving only bare rock on which nothing grows. Trees and shrubs have been stripped from arid zone savannah and from many mountain slopes to provide fuelwood, with the same result.[34] Sometimes the climate has changed, as in parts of formerly tropical rain forest in Central and South America that have been cleared as grazing land for beef cattle or in attempts to grow wheat or rice. The hydrologic cycle from tropical rain forest to rivers and lakes to clouds that precipitate as heavy rain is disrupted when trees are cut. Within a decade or less, rainfall is reduced, and soil moisture levels decline precipitously.[35] The Sahara Desert was at least partly covered with rain forest as recently as 2000 years ago; once the trees were cut, conversion to desert proceeded rapidly and has shown no signs of recovery. Similar processes are at work in other parts of the world; the consequence is declining potential to produce food. Formerly bountiful land that desertifies might take from a few hundred to a few hundred-thousand years to become fertile again.

▸ ENVIRONMENTAL POLLUTION

Environmental pollution can be localized, regional, or global; all forms adversely affect human health and the integrity of the environment. Those that fall into the category of "global change" include major environmental disasters and catastrophes: the Chernobyl nuclear accident in the former Soviet Union;[36] massive oil spills in maritime accidents involving supertankers (*Torrey Canyon*, *Exxon Valdez*, etc.); and insidious permeation of the entire biosphere by stable toxic chemicals that enter and are transmitted from one species to another through marine and terrestrial food chains.

The collapse of the former Soviet Union and its satellites has revealed gross environmental destruction that could take many centuries to be healed. This regional pollution has had adverse effects on health, such as occurrence of high levels of birth defects and severe respiratory damage.[37]

Some forms of chemical pollution are global in scope: PCBs, dioxins, and DDT, fat-soluble chemicals that travel through food chains, have permeated the entire world. Heavy metals, e.g., lead and mercury, occur in trace amounts in emissions from coal-burning power generators and ore smelting plants (which may emit other toxic chemicals such as arsenic). These contaminants occur in trace amounts, but the total burden worldwide, falling on land and into the

TABLE 41-6. BIOLOGIC AND HUMAN HEALTH EFFECTS OF UV RADIATION

■ ***BIOLOGIC EFFECTS***
DNA damage
Ecologically important
Impaired photosynthesis
Impaired plant growth
Impaired motility of phytoplankton
Agriculturally important
Impaired reproductive capacity
Damage to nitrogen-fixing soil bacteria
Impaired plant and animal health
■ ***HUMAN HEALTH EFFECTS***
Immunosuppression
Enhanced susceptibility to infection (epidemics)
Cancer proneness
Dermatological
Sunburn
Loss of elasticity (premature aging)
Photosensitivity
Neoplasia
Melanocytic (malignant melanoma)
Squamous and basal cell cancer
? Cancer of the lip
Ocular
Cataract
? Pterygium

sea, amounts to millions of metric tons annually. These toxic chemicals all concentrate in food chains.

Lead and mercury concentration in cormorants' feathers has been assayed in museum specimens prepared by taxidermists before the Industrial Revolution and compared to present-day levels; modern levels are up to 1,000 to 10,000 times greater than before the Industrial Revolution.[38] Pregnant women who eat much fish risk causing mercury poisoning of their fetus.

▶ DEMOGRAPHIC CHANGE

Underlying all the above features of global change are several aspects of population dynamics. The most obvious is population growth, which since approximately the 1950s has accelerated in an unprecedented surge almost all over the world.[39] After many millennia of stable world population in the hunter-gatherer era of human existence, the development of agriculture about 10,000 years ago led to the first spurt in population growth and subsequently to slow but generally steady arithmetical increase in numbers of humans. Roughly coinciding with the Industrial Revolution and European colonization of the Americas and Oceania, the pattern of growth became approximately exponential about 200 years ago, leading to the sharp increase that has occurred in the last 100 years, which was followed by a hypergeometric population explosion that coincided with and was probably in part caused by the "green revolution" and greatly increased agricultural productivity in the two to three decades after World War II. The reasons for the increase are complex and controversial. The efficacy of public health measures (environmental sanitation, vaccination, etc.) played a part, but ecological and behavioral causes, such as optimism about the future and earlier age at marriage, probably were more important. In the nineteenth and early twentieth centuries agricultural development provided more food, and the population expanded to approach the available supply of food. Not all causes of the population explosion are well understood.[40,40a]

As well as the surging increase in numbers, unprecedented movements of people have occurred since the late nineteenth century. Long-term migration has been very large, e.g., an estimated 30 to 40 million people from Europe into the Americas and Australasia in the period from 1850 to 1910, and perhaps larger undocumented migrations within Asia, e.g., of ethnic Chinese into many parts of Southeast Asia, over a longer period dating from some time in the last millennium.[41,41a,41b] Seemingly perpetual wars and widespread political unrest have contributed to migrations, but the main factor has been economic: many who migrate have perceived that their opportunities for work and a good life would be better elsewhere than where they were born and raised.

Rapid urban and industrial growth is an important parallel sociodemographic phenomenon. The proportion of people living in cities will exceed 50 percent of total global population by the year 2000.[b,42] In rich industrial nations, urban land shortage, real estate values, new building techniques, and personal preferences have led to enormous growth of high-rise apartment dwelling. In developing nations, megacity shantytown slums with populations of 10 million or more have proliferated; these lack sanitary and other essential services and create an ideal breeding ground for disease and social unrest. This aspect of global change has far-reaching effects on health.

The movement of large numbers of people from rural to urban regions is attributable to industrialization, mechanization of agriculture, attraction of rural subsistence farmers and landless peasants to prospects for more lucrative work in cities, and in many parts of the world, flight from oppression by powerful rich landowners, banditry, or overt armed conflict.

We can regard these massive people movements as a biological process, a form of tropism that has attracted people toward places where they can grow and develop, and away from places where growth and development were inhibited. This perspective comes close to considering humans as a parasitic infestation of the biosphere,[43] a harsh judgment, but one for which there is some empirical support.

Another form of movement with important health implications is short-term international air travel. International Air Transport Authority (IATA) statistics show present annual air travel between countries and continents to be 600 to 700 million persons; they travel on business or pleasure or for seasonal employment.[44] Rapid air travel allows people who may be incubating communicable diseases to travel to destinations where large numbers of people may be susceptible to the pathogens introduced in this way.

▶ EMERGING AND RE-EMERGING INFECTIONS

Another way in which the world has changed is in the emergence and re-emergence of lethal infectious pathogens.[45,45a,45b,45e] The human immunodeficiency virus (HIV) pandemic is the most obvious; it is linked to a resurgence of two old plagues, tuberculosis and syphilis, which find fertile soil in immunocompromised hosts and often now are due to resistant strains of pathogens. These three diseases are endemic in megacity slums in the developing world and in the counterpart of these slums in rich industrial nations, among the homeless, disenfranchised, urban underclass. Other emerging infections are due to organisms such as Ebola virus, hantavirus, *Borrelia burgdorferi* (Lyme disease), *Legionella pneumophila* (Legionnaire's disease), etc. Others are due to expansion of old diseases, such as hemorrhagic dengue fever, into regions from which such diseases had been eliminated generations ago, only to return now because of the combination of climate change and the introduction of hardy vector species such as *Aedes albopictus*.

▶ OTHER RELEVANT CHANGES

Complex economic, social, industrial, and political factors accompany the above processes and contribute to the difficulty of finding

[b] *United Nations Statistical Office, World Bank, and United Nations Demographic Yearbooks give details.*

TABLE 41-7. PER CAPITA WATER AVAILABILITY (M^3/YEAR, PER CAPITA) IN 2050[a]

Country	*1990*	*No Climate Change—2050*	*GFDL 2050*	*UKMO 2050*	*MPI 2050*
Cyprus	1,280	770	470	180	1,100
El Salvador	3,670	1,570	210	1,710	1,250
Haiti	1,700	650	840	280	820
Japan	4,430	4,260	4,720	4,800	4,480
Kenya	640	170	210	250	210
Madagascar	3,330	710	610	480	730
Mexico	4,270	2,100	1,740	1,980	2,010
Peru	1,860	880	830	690	1,020
Poland	1,470	1,200	1,160	1,150	1,140
Saudi Arabia	310	80	60	30	140
South Africa	1,320	540	500	150	330
Spain	2,850	2,680	970	1,370	1,660

[a] Assumptions about population growth are from the IPCC IS92a scenario based on the World Bank (1991) projections; the climate data are from the IPCC WGII TSU climate scenarios (based on transient model runs of Geophysics Fluid Dynamics Laboratory (GFDL), Max-Planck Institute (MPI) and UK Meteorological Office (UKMO)). The results show that in all developing countries with high rate of population growth, future "per capita" water availability will decrease independently of the assumed climate scenario.

solutions that work. Global economies have supplanted national and regional ones. Transnational corporations, owing allegiance to no nation and seemingly driven by the desire for a profitable balance sheet in the next quarterly report, move capital and production from places where obsolete plant and equipment, tough labor and environmental laws, and political systems may impede them, to countries without these restraining influences, thus maximizing short-term profits.[46]

TABLE 41–8. GLOBAL URBAN POPULATION GROWTH

	Population (millions)	*Growth Rate 1990–1995 (%)*
Tokyo, Japan	26.8	1.41
São Paulo, Brazil	16.4	2.01
New York, United States	18.3	0.34
Mexico City, Mexico	15.6	0.73
Bombay, India	15.1	4.22
Shanghai, China	15.1	2.29
Los Angeles, United States	12.4	1.60
Beijing, China	12.4	2.57
Calcutta, India	11.7	1.67
Seoul, Republic of Korea	11.6	1.95
Jakarta, Indonesia	11.5	4.35
Buenos Aires, Argentina	11.0	0.68
Tianjin, China	10.7	2.88
Osaka, Japan	10.6	0.23
Lagos, Nigeria	10.3	5.68
Rio de Janeiro, Brazil	9.9	0.77
Delhi, India	9.9	3.80
Karachi, Pakistan	9.9	4.27
Cairo, Egypt	9.7	2.24
Paris, France	9.5	0.29
Manila, Philippines	9.3	3.05
Moscow, Russia	9.2	0.40
Dhaka, Bangladesh	7.8	5.74
Istanbul, Turkey	7.8	3.67
Lima, Peru	7.5	2.81

From: United Nations Population Division, 1996

Political revolts against local and regional taxation have undermined the effectiveness and efficiency of public health and other essential infrastructures in some rich industrial nations, most of all in the United States. For many years there have been no new investments, little maintenance, no salary increases (sometimes reductions of pay and benefits), and serious staff reductions in many public health services.

Television "sound-bites" and fragmentary news reporting deprive people of information that is necessary to enable them to make intelligent decisions about such matters as public health services and environmental sustainability. Many people regard elected officials with contempt, which deters them from voting—a dangerous trend that has the potential for the political agenda to be captured by determined single-issue interests. All too frequently, those who are elected lack the political courage to make the tough decisions—such as raising taxes on fossil fuels—that the state of the world demands if the climatic trends are to be halted and ultimately reversed before irreversible harm is done.

▶ PUBLIC HEALTH RESPONSES

Perhaps never before have public health workers and their services faced such challenges as they do now. Actions of several kinds are required (Table 41-9). Some obvious and simple measures can be initiated at once, e.g. protection of fair-skinned infants and children against excessive sun exposure. We need to establish or strengthen our surveillance of insect vectors and the pathogens they can carry. Needed research strategies are also summarized in Table 41-9.

Effective responses are hampered by many factors. The decay of infrastructures and erosion of morale, as dedicated staff are laid off and salaries frozen or cut, have inhibited meaningful efforts to prepare for any but immediate emergencies. Yet some obvious preparations to cope would cost little. Disaster planning must be maintained at a high level of preparedness; nothing is more certain than that there will be increasingly frequent, and probably more severe, weather emergencies. Large cities and towns on flood plains or in places where there can be tidal surges are increasingly vulnerable. Insurance companies have recognized this by reluctance to insure against some natural disasters. Some public health agencies and local government departments have disaster plans, but many do not.

There are many simple actions that public health services can carry out to mitigate the adverse effects of global change on human

TABLE 41-9. PUBLIC HEALTH RESPONSE TO GLOBAL CHANGE

Monitoring
Migrant, refugee movements
Food production, distribution
Acute sunburn
Heat-related illness
Epidemiologic surveillance
Water quality
Vectors, pathogens
Infectious diseases
Fecal-oral
Respiratory
Vector-borne
Cancer
Malignant melanoma
Nonmelanoma skin cancer
Other cancer
Cataract
Surveys
Sun-seeking, sun-avoiding
Attitudes to sustainability
Epidemiologic studies
Case-control, cohort studies to assess UV risk
RCTs[a] of sunscreen ointments
RCTs of UV-filtering sunglasses
Public health action
Advisory messages about sun exposure
Standard-setting for protective clothing, etc.
Health education directed at behavior change
Health care of migrant groups
Disaster preparedness
Public health policy
National food and nutrition policies
Research priorities

[a]RCT—Randomized Controlled Trials

health. For instance, weather reports now often mention the level of UVR flux and offer advice about sun avoidance.

▶ GROUNDS FOR OPTIMISM

Faced with the array of problems outlined above, it would be easy to admit defeat. But there are grounds for optimism about our situation. Humans are robust, a very hardy species: we have demonstrated considerable ability to adapt to a wide range of harsh environments. We are resourceful, intelligent, and often at our best in a crisis. We are now, perhaps, entering the greatest crisis we have ever faced. Its insidious onset has lulled us into complacency, if we think at all about the nature of the global changes that endanger us. There is also an element of denial, akin to the reluctance of a cancer patient to accept the seriousness of the condition, or of the risk-taking adolescent to whom death or permanent disability due to dangerous behavior is unimaginable.

Epidemiology and other public health sciences can do much to induce greater recognition of the need for changes in values and behavior. Precedents in the history of public health since the second half of the nineteenth century[47] are encouraging. The necessary sequence for control of any public health problem is: awareness that the problem exists, understanding what causes it, capability to control it, a sense of values that the problem matters, and political will. All but the last of these exist now. We have the basic science evidence that enables us to predict what will happen. Empirical evidence to support the predictions is rapidly mounting and soon will comprise an incontrovertable body of knowledge and understanding that even the most obtuse self-interested group will be unable to deny or rebut. Increasing numbers of important interest groups, such as the insurance industry and leaders in some resource-based industries, are recognizing the need for action. Increasing numbers of thoughtful people are aware of the need to conserve resources rather than squandering them wantonly as we did in the 1950s and 1960s with "disposable" products. A few more dramatic disasters due to the collapse or major disruption of established weather systems would help to galvanize public opinion and lead to pressure for change that even the most complacent political leaders would be unable to ignore.

Environmental protection laws and regulations have remained substantially intact. This suggests that the change of values required as a necessary prerequisite for action to mitigate global change is already begining. It will undoubtedly help if the health impacts of global change are given greater attention in the media. Public health workers and epidemiologists can contribute by emphasizing the health effects of global change, and actions needed to minimize their impact.

▶ ENVIRONMENTAL ETHICS AND THE PRECAUTIONARY PRINCIPLE

The change of values that I believe is already under way is leading to recognition of the need to observe a code of conduct for the environment, an ethic of environmental sustainability. Environmental movements are gathering strength in many countries and "Green" parties are seen increasingly as "respectable" and in the mainstream of politics. They are beginning to influence the political agenda despite pressure from powerful industrial and commercial interest groups that have long been able to achieve their ends by control of political decisions. The pressure often comes first from grass-root levels, perhaps because of a proposal to establish a toxic waste dump or a polluting industry; but its origins may matter less than its increasingly successful efforts to influence the outcome.

Another hopeful sign is recognition of the Precautionary Principle: when there is doubt about the possible environmental harm that may arise from an industrial or commercial development, a nuclear power station, an oil refinery, an open-cast coal mine, or other environmentally damaging activities, people and communities who will be most affected are increasingly often given the benefit of the doubt, because of the Precautionary Principle. A few years ago this almost never happened. Now it is commonplace.

▶ MITIGATION OPTIONS

The 1995 IPCC Report discusses several mitigation options (Table 41-10): energy-efficient industrial processes and means of transportation; reduction of human settlement emissions; sound agricultural conservation and rehabilitation policies; forest management policies and strategies, etc. The Framework Convention on Climate Change that was adopted by most national leaders early in 1996, spells out ways in which industries that contribute heavily to greenhouse gas accumulation can and must change. These changes are not without cost, although experience has often demonstrated that conserving energy, like all other conservation measures, is cost-effective. An obvious change that would benefit all who share the earth is introduction of deterrent taxes that would discourage use of private cars for all but truly essential purposes. Political leaders everywhere are reluctant to enact this unpopular measure and are equally reluctant to spend large capital sums on new or upgraded public transport systems in an era when reducing taxes is what got many of them elected in the first place. This is unlikely to change until a climatic emergency or other environmental crisis forces large numbers to come to their senses and realize that the time for action rather than rhetoric has arrived. Public health workers should be preparing to take the initiative in the event of climatic emergencies or environmental crises and should have cogent arguments ready to state the case for action toward environmental sustainability.

Our situation resembles that depicted by the clock on the cover of the *Bulletin of the Atomic Scientists*, with hands pointing to a few

TABLE 41-10. MITIGATION OPTIONS

Energy supply
- Reduce greenhouse emissions
  - Convert efficiently
  - Suppress emissions
  - Decarbonize fuels
  - Switch to nuclear fuel
  - Switch to renewable sources of energy

Industry
- Technical abatement options
  - Fuel substitution (low carbon, electric, renewable, hydrogen fuel, energy-efficient fuel, etc.)
- Policy options
  - Fostering technology transfer
  - Energy audits
  - Technical innovations
  - Recycling, etc.

Transportation
- Reducing emissions
  - Energy-intensive innovations
  - Alternative fuels
- Transport policy shifts

Human settlements
- Residential buildings
  - Space conditioning (heating, cooling)
  - Water heating, lighting, cooking, appliances
  - Potential for residential energy savings
- Commercial buildings
  - Space conditioning
  - Lighting, heating, office equipment, etc.
  - Potential for energy savings
- Community-level
  - Reducing heat islands
  - Methane emissions from waste dumps
- Policy options for buildings, heat islands, etc.

Agricultural and forestry options
- Abatement of CO_2, methane, etc.
- Conservation, reforestation, etc.

minutes before midnight. The analogy is a calendar from which all but a few days near the end of the year have been torn. The imperative need for action is urgent.

▶ REFERENCES

1. Tudge C: The Time before History. New York: Scribner, 1996
2. Eddy JA: Climate and the role of the sun. In Rotberg RI, Rabb TK (eds): Climate and History. Princeton, NJ: Princeton University Press, 1981, pp 145–167
3. Houghton JT, Filho LGM, Callander BA, Kattenburg A, Maskell K (eds): Climate Change 1995—The Science of Climate Change. Volume 1 of the Report of the Intergovernmental Panel on Climate Change. Cambridge: Cambridge University Press, 1996
4. Canadian Global Change Program. Ottawa: Royal Society of Canada, 1992
5. McMichael AJ: Planetary Overload: Global Environmental Change and the Health of the Human Species. Cambridge: Cambridge University Press, 1993
6. Annual Population Statistics and Projections. New York: UN Statistical Office, 1995
7. Cohen JE: How Many People Can the Earth Support? New York: Norton, 1995
8. Intergovernmental Panel on Climate Change: Scientific Assessment of Climate Change. A Report by Working Group I. Geneva: World Health Organization and United Nations Environmental Programme, 1990
9. Intergovernmental Panel on Climate Change: Impact Assessment; A Report to IPCC from Working Group II. Canberra: Australian Government Printing Office, 1990
10. Watson RT, Zinyowera MC, Moss RH, Dokken DJ (eds): Climate Change 1995—Impacts, Adaptations and Mitigation of Climate Change: Scientific-Technical Analysis. Cambridge: Cambridge University Press, 1996 (Contributions of Working Group II to the Second Assessment Report of the Intergovernmental Panel on Climate Change)
11. McMichael AJ, Haines A, Sloof R, Kovats S (eds): Climate Change and Human Health. Geneva: World Health Organization/WMO/ United Nations Environmental Programme, 1996
12. Deleted in proof
13. Haines A, Fuchs C: Potential impacts on health of atmospheric change. J Public Health Med 13:69–80, 1991

13a. Last JM: Global change; ozone depletion, greenhouse warming and public health. Annu Rev Public Health 14:115–136, 1993

14. Union of Concerned Scientists: World Scientists' Warning Briefing Book. Cambridge, MA: Union of Concerned Scientists, 1993
15. Worldwatch Institute: State of the World, Annual Reports since 1985. Washington DC: Worldwatch Institute
16. Brookes WT: The global warming panic. Forbes 144(14):96–102, 1989
17. Lindzen RS: Some remarks on global warming. Environ Sci Technol 24:424–426, 1990
18. Our Planet, Our Health. Report of the WHO Commission on Health and Environment. Geneva: World Health Organization, 1992 (with Annexe volumes on Food and Agriculture, Energy, Urbanization, and Industry)
19. Silver CS, DeFries RS (eds): One Earth, One Future. Washington DC: National Academy Press, 1990

19a. Yoda S (ed): Trilemma; Three Major Problems Threatening the World Survival. Report of the Committee for Research on Global Problems. Tokyo: Central Research Institute of Electric Power Industry, 1995

20. United Nations Conference on Environment and Development (the Rio Summit). New York: United Nations, 1992 ("Agenda 21")
21. Patz JA, Epstein PR, Burke TA, Balbus JM: Global climate change and emerging infectious diseases. JAMA 275:217–223, 1996
22. Parry ML, Rosenzweig C: Health and climate change; food supply and risk of hunger. Lancet 342:1345–1347, 1993
23. Molina MJ, Rowland FS: Stratospheric sink for chloro-fluoromethanes; chlorine atom-catalyzed destruction of ozone. Nature 249:810–814, 1974

23a. Rowland FS, Molina MJ: Estimated future atmospheric concentrations of CCl_3F (fluorocarbon-11) for various hypothetical tropospheric removal rates. J Phys Chem 80:2049–2056, 1976

24. Farman JC, Gardiner BG, Shanklin JD: Large losses of total ozone in Antarctica reveal seasonal ClO_x/NO_x interaction. Nature 315:207–210, 1985
25. Kerr JB, McElroy CT: Evidence for large upward trends of ultraviolet-B radiation linked to ozone depletion. Science 262:523–524, 1993
26. United Nations Environmental Programme (UNEP): Montreal Protocol on Substances That Deplete the Ozone Layer. Montreal, September 16, 1987
27. Homer-Dixon TF, Percival V: Environmental Scarcity and Violent Conflict; Briefing Book. Washington, DC and Toronto: American Association for the Advancement of Science and University of Toronto, 1996
28. Intergovernmental Panel on Climate Change: Climate Change 1995; Impacts, Adapatations and Mitigation; Summary for Policymakers. Geneva: World Meterological Organization, World Health Organization, United Nations Environmental Programme, 1995
29. Food and Agriculture Organization: State of the World's Fisheries (Annual Report). Rome: Food and Agriculture Organization, 1995
30. de Koning HW, Smith KR, Last JM: Biomass fuel combustion and health. Bull WHO 63:11–26, 1985

31. WHO Commission on Health and Environment: Report of the Panel on Energy. Geneva: World Health Organization, 1992
31a. Nakicenovic N et al: Energy primer. In: Climate Change 1995; Impacts, Adaptations and Mitigation; Summary for Policymakers. Geneva: WMO, World Health Organization, United Nations Environmental Programme, 1995, pp 75–92
32. Wilson EO: The Diversity of Life. Cambridge, MA: Harvard University Press, 1992
33. Carson R: Silent Spring. Boston: Houghton Mifflin, 1962
34. Aggarwal AR: Cold hearths and barren slopes. London: Zed Books, 1986
35. Almandares J, Anderson PK, Epstein PR: Critical regions; a profile of Honduras. Lancet 342:1400–1402, 1993
36. Anderson TW: Health problems in Ukraine related to the Chernobyl accident. Washington DC: World Bank, Natural Resources Management Division, 1992
37. Herzman C: Environment and Health in Central and Eastern Europe; a Report for the Environmental Action Programme for Central and Eastern Europe. Washington, DC: World Bank, 1995
38. Nriagu JD: A history of global metal pollution. Science 272:223–226, 1996
39. Cohen JE: How Many People Can the Earth Support? New York: Norton, 1995, p 25–31
40. McKeown T, Brown RG: The modern rise of population. Pop Stud 9:119–137, 1995
40a. Cohen JE: How Many People Can the Earth Support? New York: Norton, 1995, pp 25–106
41. UN Demographic Yearbooks and historical demographic records
42. Deleted in proof
43. Hern WM: Why are there so many of us? Description and diagnosis of a planetary ecopathological process. Pop Environ 12(1):9–37, 1990
44. International Air Transport Authority: Annual Air Movements Statistics. Montreal: International Air Transport Authority, 1995
45. Lederberg J: Infection emergent. JAMA 275:243–244, 1996
45a. Roizman B (ed): Infectious Diseases in an Age of Change; The Impact of Human Ecology and Behavior on Disease Transmission. Washington, DC: National Academy Press, 1995
45b. Garrett L: The Coming Plague; Newly Emerging Diseases in a World Out of Balance. New York: Farrar Straus Giroux, 1995
45c. Horton R: The infected metropolis. Lancet 347:134–135, 1996
46. Kennedy P: Preparing for the 21st Century. New York: Random House, 1993
47. Last J: New pathways in an age of ethical and ecological concern. Int J Epidemiol 23:1:1–4, 1994

IV

Behavioral Factors Affecting Health

Edited by Jonathan E. Fielding

42

Social Determinants of Disease

S. Leonard Syme • Jennifer L. Balfour

The prevention of disease is a major goal of public health programs. In developing and implementing prevention programs, environmental factors are increasingly recognized as important components. In part, this recognition is based on the fact that many diseases of concern involve large numbers of people and that it is simply more cost-effective to prevent such diseases at an environmental level than at a one-to-one, individual level. Interest in environmental factors also has developed because of the difficulty in getting individuals to change their behaviors; in many cases, it is more efficient to change the environment than to encourage individuals, one at a time, to change their behavior. Yet a third reason for the increasing interest in environmental factors is that the distribution of many diseases remains relatively constant over time even though individuals come and go from the population; this constancy of rate suggests that there is something about the environment that elicits a characteristic rate of disease in different population groups.

This chapter is concerned with the influence of social factors in the environment on health. This limited focus is not meant to suggest that the social environment stands alone in its relationship to health and disease. The term "environment" is a very general one describing many different conditions and influences under which any person or thing lives or develops. This term has been used to describe many phenomena including the air we breathe, the water we drink, the geographic regions and buildings in which we live, the groups to which we belong, and the climatic conditions that we experience.[1,2] While one can distinguish between the human-made environment, the natural environment, and the social and cultural environment, none of these aspects exists independently of the others: the environment is the result of the continuing interaction between natural and human-made spatial forms, social processes, and the relationships between individuals and groups. In spite of these interconnections, it nevertheless often is useful to examine closely specific components of the whole.

In this chapter, we first discuss the overall rationale for an environmental approach to disease prevention before focusing in more detail on the social environment. In discussing the social environment, we review research findings showing a link between social factors and the incidence and severity of disease and then consider some of the implications of these findings for disease prevention.

▶ RATIONALE FOR AN ENVIRONMENTAL APPROACH TO DISEASE PREVENTION

Magnitude of the Disease Problem

The first reason for the consideration of environmental factors in efforts to prevent disease is based on the sheer magnitude of many of the diseases with which we are concerned (including coronary heart disease, cancer of various sites, arthritis, mental illness, diabetes, and stroke). Consider, for example, the case of coronary heart disease, a disease of substantial prevalence in all of the developed nations of the world. In the United States, over 8 million people now have one or another form of this disease.[3] If a permanent cure were available for this disease that was 100 percent effective (with no relapses), the treatment of these 8 million patients would require 28 percent of available physician time during that year.

While the cost of this program in terms of physician time is relatively high, it might be acceptable, except that enormous numbers of *new* people would continue to develop heart disease for the first time since the treatment program did nothing to deal with people "at risk" to becoming ill. If these at-risk people were included, this expanded program would require 91 percent of available physician time. Even the higher cost of this activity might be considered acceptable since it could achieve a permanent and completely effective cure for a major disease. However, it must be noted that, while this program virtually exhausts all available physician resources, it does not solve the problem because it has not dealt with those forces in society that brought about the problem in the first place: about 1 percent of healthy people over the age of 30 in the United States (over 1 million people) are expected to become at risk for the first time each year because they start smoking, become overweight, or develop elevated levels of a risk factor.

While a one-to-one approach to diseases of great prevalence clearly is of value to patients, families, and friends, it does little to alter the distribution of disease in the population because new people develop disease even as sick people are cured. Thus, an individual approach exhausts substantial medical care resources but does little to address those environmental factors that have initiated the problem. In this circumstance, an environmental approach to prevention clearly is more efficient.

The Patterning of Disease Rates

The continual swell of new at-risk people in the population leads to the second reason for considering environmental factors in disease prevention research and programs: groups often have a characteristic pattern of disease over time even though individuals come and go from these groups. This pattern indicates that there may be something about the group that either promotes or discourages disease among individuals in those groups.

One example of patterning of disease rates occurs with immigration into the United States. Breast cancer rates are far higher in the United States than in many Asian countries. In 1980, the breast cancer incidence rate for white women living in the United States was two to four times higher than for women living in China, Japan, and the Philippines.[4] Yet when women from Asia immigrate to the United States, their breast cancer rates rise compared to those in their country of origin. In the first generation of immigrants, the elevation of rates is only modest, but by the second and third generation, the rates of breast cancer in the migrant families have risen until they are equal to that of the entire population of U.S. women.[5,6] A similar pattern occurs for many other diseases. It seems reasonable to suppose that something about the environment of the United States causes people who settle here to slowly (or sometimes not so slowly) adopt the endemic rates of disease in the United States.

This example of patterned consistency of disease rates across geography and social and cultural groups emphasizes the potential importance of environmental factors in the study of disease etiology. A considerable amount of research has been done to identify environmental factors so that interventions might be developed to prevent or control disease. However, the reasons for differences in disease rates between groups are not well understood.

Success of Environmental Approach with Infectious Disease

That environmental factors might be involved in the etiology and prevention of a broad range of diseases has been forcefully suggested both by McKeown[7] and by McKinlay and McKinlay.[8] These scholars have concluded that the dramatic decline since 1900 in overall mortality in both Britain and the United States cannot be explained by the introduction and use of medical interventions. Indeed, many medical measures against disease (both chemotherapeutic and prophylactic) were introduced several decades after a marked decline in mortality from those diseases already had taken place. McKinlay and McKinlay cite five diseases that in their view did benefit from medical intervention: influenza, pneumonia, diphtheria, whooping cough, and poliomyelitis. They note, however, that, even if all of the decline in these diseases were attributable to medical measures, at best they account for only 3.5 percent of the total decline in mortality. In assessing these statistics, McKeown has argued that most of the decline in mortality since the second half of the nineteenth century was primarily due to improvements in hygiene and to rising standards of living, especially improved nutrition. With changes in living standards and discovery that many common diseases arise from infectious agents, disease could be prevented by altering the environmental conditions in which the infectious agents flourished and spread.

With the decline of infectious disease, however, noninfectious diseases such as heart disease, cancer, and diabetes have become a major source of morbidity and mortality. These diseases, perhaps because they are not infectious or contagious, are often thought of as being caused by individual behavior. The primary etiologic research and intervention strategies have been to pinpoint which individual lifestyle choices are associated with disease. The environment that allows these lifestyle choices to develop (in much the same way as infectious agents breed) has remained comparatively unexamined.

Difficulties in Changing Behavior

A fourth reason for the consideration of environmental factors in disease prevention is that the prevention of so many diseases requires that people change their behavior. To prevent disease, we increasingly ask people to begin to do things that they have not done previously, to stop doing things they have been doing for years, and to do more of some things and less of others. This behavioral approach to disease prevention contrasts with programs that attempt to do something "to" people. While some diseases and conditions can be prevented best by injection, surgery, or other nonbehavioral manipulations, most chronic diseases cannot. Chronic diseases and conditions such as cancer, diseases of the cardiovascular system, cirrhosis, and chronic respiratory diseases to a greater or lesser degree are associated with particular behaviors and hopefully can be prevented or treated by behavior change.[9,10]

Of course, it is one thing to identify a risk behavior and another thing to ensure that people will actually change that behavior. It is of little value to identify a hazardous behavior if people will not change it. While there certainly are examples of successful programs to change behavior, the evidence suggests that behavior change is a very difficult and complex challenge.[11] While many different factors need to be considered in helping people change their behavior, one factor rarely considered is that of the environment. It is difficult to expect that people will change their behavior easily when many forces in the social, cultural, and physical environment conspire against such change.[12–14] If successful behavior modification programs are to be developed to prevent diseases, more attention will need to be given not only to the behavior and risk profiles of individuals, but also to the environmental context within which people live.

Even if all these people with risk factors were totally successful in changing behaviors to lower risk, the impact of this on the distribution of disease in the community would be limited. This minimal success can be illustrated by referring once again to the case of coronary heart disease. Several collaborative long-term community studies in the United States involving several thousand middle-aged people have shown that high serum cholesterol, high blood pressure, and cigarette smoking are important risk factors for the development of coronary heart disease.[15] After adjusting for age, men with all three of these risk factors have over six times the chance of developing a first major coronary attack than men with none of the risk factors; the relative risks for people having one or two of these risk factors compared to men with none are 2.4 and 4.5, respectively.[16]

However, as Marmot and Winkelstein have shown,[17] only 14 percent of people with all three of these risk factors actually developed coronary heart disease during 10 years of observation in these community studies; 86 percent did not have a coronary event. Of people with one or two risk factors, only 5 and 9 percent, respectively, had an event in the 10-year period of study. Thus, even though these three risk factors clearly are associated with an increased relative risk of disease, few people with the risk factors actually develop disease. Looked at another way, of all the people who developed coronary heart disease in these community studies over the 10-year follow-up period, only 17 percent had all three risk factors, and only 58 percent had two or more risk factors. Therefore, many people develop coronary heart disease for reasons not entirely explainable by these three risk factors. While this observation should not lead to a de-emphasis on the importance of the three established risk factors, it does suggest that other factors also may be involved in the etiologic process.

The emphasis on the importance of environmental factors in the etiology and control of diseases has a long history.[18] In the case of infectious disease, focus on the environment has led to a disease classification system based on mode of transmission; diseases are categorized as airborne, waterborne, food-borne, and vector-borne. This classification system is based directly on the environmental conditions that allow the disease to spread and in turn allows prevention programs to be formulated at the environmental level.

In spite of this long concern with the environment among researchers studying infectious diseases, most work on the prevention, treatment, and control of noninfectious diseases has focused, in one way or another, on the individual. As a consequence, we have very little specific and precise information about how the environment affects the incidence, severity, and persistence of noninfectious diseases and even less information about how they can be prevented by environmental interventions. Since chronic diseases are common and have consistent patterns in population groups, and since lifestyle risk factors associated with chronic disease are widespread and difficult to change, seeking understanding of disease etiology and disease prevention at the level of the environment seems a wise strategy.

▶ SOCIAL FACTORS AND THE INCIDENCE OF DISEASE

The first modern argument for the inclusion of social factors in environmental studies of disease etiology was that offered by Emile Durkheim in his classic research on suicide. Durkheim's book, *Le Suicide*, was published in France in 1897, but was not translated into English until 1951.[19] This work is among the very first examples of the systematic and organized use of the statistical method to further the sociocultural investigation of disease. In this research, Durkheim noted that, while suicide is one of the most individualistic acts imaginable, it can be understood only in terms of the social setting within which it takes place. At the time Durkheim wrote, it was known that suicide varied among different groups and among different time periods. Suicide rates were higher for Protestants than for Catholics, higher for the unmarried than for the married, higher for soldiers than for civilians, higher for noncommissioned officers than for enlisted men, higher in times of peace than in times of war and revolution, and higher in times of both prosperity and recession than in times of economic stability.

Durkheim acknowledged that there were many different individual reasons for committing suicide (e.g., economic problems, sickness, personal failure); he pointed out, however, that suicide rates differ among social groups and that such differences persist over time and cultural setting, even though individuals may come and go and even though individual problems may vary within the groups. To explain this difference in group rates, Durkheim argued, one must refer to social factors. He reasoned that, if different groups have different suicide rates, there must be something about the social organization of the groups that encourages or deters individuals from suicide. Durkheim's research led him to conclude that the major factor affecting suicide rates was the degree of social integration of groups. He suggested that the extent to which the individual was integrated into group life determined whether he or she would be motivated to commit suicide. As will be seen, this emphasis on the importance of social ties is a theme that also emerges from current research. Aside from Durkheim's substantive contribution regarding suicide, however, is the important epidemiological observation that systematic, patterned differences in disease rates between groups must be explainable in group terms. This idea continues to be the major rationale for research on social factors in disease etiology.

During the last 40 years, research evidence has accumulated regarding the role of many social factors in disease etiology. While most of this work has been done in reference to coronary heart disease, other diseases also have been studied. From this work, several themes can be identified that are supported by a relatively large body of consistent empirical evidence. As the research has developed, ideas have changed and transformed. Below, each general topic begins with a discussion of the evidence accumulated through early research and moves to discussing research areas now being pursued.

Socioeconomic Status

One of the most persistent disease patterns observed in public health research is that people in the lowest socioeconomic groups have the highest rates of morbidity and mortality. In a comprehensive review of 30 studies on this topic, Antonovsky noted the consistency of this finding dating from the twelfth century.[20] Further, this differential has been observed throughout the world, regardless of whether the dominant diseases of death and disability were attributed to infectious or noninfectious causes and regardless of the specific methods used to assess socioeconomic status.[21,22]

In a massive nationwide survey of mortality in the United States, Kitagawa and Hauser[23] found that mortality rates varied dramatically among socioeconomic groups for both men and women, whether socioeconomic status was studied in relation to education, income, or occupation: the lower the socioeconomic level, the higher the death rate. In addition, Kitagawa and Hauser found that those in lower socioeconomic groups had higher death rates for every cause of death except, among women, cancer of the breast and motor vehicle accidents. Higher rates of morbidity also have been observed among those in lower socioeconomic groups. These higher morbidity rates include virtually every disease, as well as mental illnesses and conditions such as schizophrenia, depression, unhappiness, worry, anxiety, and hopelessness.[21–24] In spite of the fact that socioeconomic status is such a well-recognized and important risk factor for disease, we know little of the reasons for its importance. There are at least two explanations for this. One is that socioeconomic status is so powerful a risk factor that we almost always statistically control for its influence in research in order to study other factors of interest. If we did not do this, the effect of socioeconomic status would overwhelm everything else under study. In consequence, rarely has socioeconomic status been studied as a phenomenon in its own right. The second explanation is more subtle: we tend to study risk factors that we think we can do something about and socioeconomic status does not seem readily amenable to intervention. However, it is inappropriate to conclude that we cannot intervene on socioeconomic status without first knowing its essential elements. If the important element in socioeconomic status is income, interventions may indeed be difficult. On the other hand, if the important element is education or a way of looking at the world, there may be things we *can* do to intervene. In any case, without an understanding of the components involved in socioeconomic status, it seems unwise to decide ahead of time that interventions are impossible. As a result of the past 40 years of research, some of the essential elements of socioeconomic status are now being uncovered.

The research done by Marmot and his colleagues[25] on British civil servants provided an opportunity to study socioeconomic status in detail. As shown in Figure 42-1, these investigators have demonstrated that British civil servants in the highest grade (administrators) have the lowest rate of coronary heart disease while those in the lowest grade (mainly unskilled manual workers) have rates four times as high. After account had been taken of such coronary heart disease risk factors as serum cholesterol, cigarette smoking, blood pressure, physical activity, glucose intolerance, and social support, the differences in rate between those at the top and bottom of the graded hierarchy was reduced to three times. However, about 60 percent of the difference in coronary heart disease rates among civil service grades remained unexplained after this adjustment. More interesting is the fact that workers in professional and executive jobs (grade 2) and in clerical jobs (grade 3) have coronary heart disease rates 2 and 3.2 times as high as administrators. This finding poses a challenge. While it is reasonably simple to propose possible explanations for why those at the bottom have higher rates than those at the top, these explanations do not account for why those *close* to the top have higher rates of disease than those *at* the top. Factors such as inadequate medical care, unemployment, low income, race, poor nutrition, poor housing, and poor education may account for higher rates of disease among those in class 5 but they do not explain why professionals and executives in the British civil service have rates twice as high as administrators.

This gradient of disease is not unique to British civil servants. It has been observed in a wide variety of populations in many different countries, and it is not confined to a single disease entity or age group.[24–26] The gradient has been observed for many body systems including the digestive, genitourinary, respiratory, circulatory, nervous, blood, and endocrine systems. It has been observed also for most malignancies, congenital anomalies, infectious and parasitic diseases, accidents, poisoning and violence, perinatal mortality, diabetes, and musculoskeletal impairments. In addition, the gradient has been observed for early stages of and progression to carotid atherosclerosis.[27]

Recent research has explored the shape of the gradient, the consistency of the gradient across life span, and the potency of the gradient at different life stages. Blacklund and colleagues[28] explored the nature of the gradient in a different population and using a different measure of socioeconomic status (SES). Using data from the National Longitudinal Mortality Study, they report that income is strongly and inversely related to risk of mortality. However, unlike the study done by Marmot, Backlund et al did not find a linear relationship; as income rose above $25,000 (in 1980 dollars) the relationship between income and mortality remained only for men ages 45 to 64 years. Earlier studies, such as the British Civil Service Study, may not have discovered this curvilinear relationship because they studied men of working age.

The strength of the association between socioeconomic status and poor health is not consistent across the life span, and it decreases in those older than 65 years.[28,29] One explanation for this is selective mortality; those lower on the social scale are more likely to die at an earlier age, leaving only those survivors who are hardy. Another explanation is that traditional measures of socioeconomic status, in-

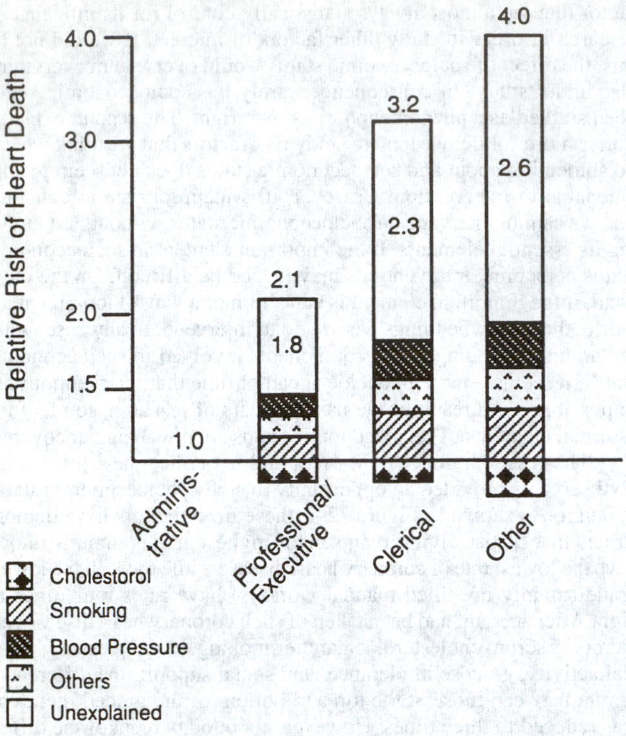

Figure 42-1. Relative risk of coronary heart disease death by civil service rank—male civil service workers, London, England. *Number at top of column,* unadjusted relative risk; *number in column,* adjusted relative risk. (Adapted from Marmot MG, Rose G, Shipley M, Hamilton PJS: Employment grade and coronary heart disease in British civil servants. J Epidemiol Community Health 3:244–249, 1978.)

come and education, are less sensitive in the elderly, who rely primarily on fixed incomes after retirement. Accumulated wealth such as property and investment wealth may be a more appropriate measure of socioeconomic status in older age groups.

Recent evidence also suggests that socioeconomic status may have its most lasting and potent effect during childhood and that many sequelae are a result of this early exposure. The rationale for this view is that many of the risk factors we study in adults have their origins in childhood and may "track" into adult years. Children with high blood pressure tend more often to be hypertensive as adults.[30,31] Obese children tend more often to become obese adults.[32] The same pattern exists for serum cholesterol, height, and respiratory function.[33,34] Furthermore, during childhood and adolescence, these same risk factors are inversely graded by socioeconomic status.[35]

Kaplan and Salonen have shown that childhood socioeconomic status is a more powerful predictor of heart disease in adult men than is adult socioeconomic status,[36] and Gliksman and colleagues[37] have found that low socioeconomic status during childhood is associated with cardiovascular disease in adult women. Using data from the Kuopio Ischemic Heart Disease Risk Factor Study, Lynch and colleagues[38] have shown that a large number of health behaviors and psychosocial orientations are graded, in adulthood, according to socioeconomic status in childhood, adolescence, and adulthood. Barker[39] has suggested an even narrower time span of importance: that many chronic diseases, and particularly heart disease, have their origins in utero. This hypothesis suggests that if in utero environment is related to the socioeconomic status of the mother, the most important impact of socioeconomic status on health could occur during gestation. In spite of the fact that early years of life offer great potential for targeted intervention, little research has been done on the origins of disease in infancy and childhood; the implications of this are discussed later in this chapter.

Other research on socioeconomic status seeks to examine factors that underlay the socioeconomic status gradient. This research has been approached in two ways. One approach tries to explain the gradient by more detailed study of disease risk factors. Many studies have confirmed the results reported by Marmot that adjustment for disease risk factors fails to attenuate the socioeconomic status-health gradient.[40–42] However, a number of new risk factors with potential to explain the association between socioeconomic status and poorer health have been identified since Marmot's original and pioneering work.[43–45] A recent study using data from the Kuopio Ischemic Heart Disease Risk Factor Study retested the proposition that the associations between socioeconomic status and all-cause and cardiovascular mortality were independent of all known risk factors.[46] After adjustment for a very wide range of risk factors, the gradient for all-cause and cardiovascular mortality was much reduced and found to be not significant statistically. Risk factors included in this detailed analysis were: age; 13 biological risk factors (plasma fibrinogen, serum high density lipoproteins, serum apolipoprotein B, blood leukocyte count, serum copper, mercury deposits in hair, serum ferritin, blood hemoglobin, serum triglycerides, systolic blood pressure, body mass index, height, and cardiorespiratory fitness); three behavioral risk factors (cigarette smoking, alcohol consumption, and conditioning physical activity); three psychological risk factors (depression, hopelessness, and cynical hostility); and three social risk factors (participation in organizations, quality of social support, and marital status). This study offers strong evidence that the association between socioeconomic status and all-cause and cardiovascular mortality may be explained by adjustment for known risk factors.

In this view, socioeconomic status is not a mystical force. It operates by changing our biology, behavior, psychological responses, and social situations. Although adjustment for a full range of biological, behavioral, psychological, and social variables offers evidence of the routes through which socioeconomic status may affect mortality, there nevertheless remains a major explanatory problem: adjusting for other major risk factors does not address the fact that each of these risk factors is graded by socioeconomic status.[47] These risk factors are likely to be part of the pathway between socioeconomic status and disease.

Further, behavior changes are adopted at a greater rate by more socially advantaged groups, and, even with overall behavioral improvements, the relative disadvantage in health risks between high and low social class groups is maintained.[48,49] If social class acts as a force that shapes the adoption of healthy behaviors and that changes the physiologic risk markers for disease, psychological responses, and coping strategies, then it is possible that all of these factors are part of a chain of causation linking social status to disease.[50–52] To formulate a more effective explanation for the effect of socioeconomic status on health, we need to move toward an explanation of the link between socioeconomic status and health; therefore, we need to address the clustering patterns of risk factors as well as of diseases.

The second approach to study of the socioeconomic gradient is based, not on efforts to explain the gradient, but rather on efforts to discover the reasons for patterning of both risk factors and disease. The concept of "control of destiny" has been suggested as a possible hypothesis for this phenomenon. It could be postulated, for example, that the lower down one is in the socioeconomic status hierarchy, the less control one has over the factors that affect life and living circumstance. This hypothesis is very general, and it does not specify whether control involves money, power, information, prestige, experience, or something else. Over the years, many social scientists have studied different concepts related to the idea of control of destiny and it may be of value to look for common denominators in that work. The list of such concepts includes mastery, self-efficacy, locus of control, learned helplessness, controllability, predictability, desire for control, sense of control, powerlessness, hardiness, competence, and so on. If these ideas, or something like them, are supported by research evidence, an avenue for intervention might become available that is more precise and understandable than simply to suggest that we change "socioeconomic status."[53]

Research on job stress supports the usefulness of this approach. For many years, researchers have tried unsuccessfully to demonstrate the existence of a relationship between "job stress" and disease. It was only after Karasek,[54] Theorell,[55] and their associates added the idea of job latitude and discretion to that of job stress that such a link was shown: occupational stressors have consequences for health primarily when workers do not have sufficient latitude and discretion for coping with these stressors. When workers have little control over work pace and methods, higher rates of catacholamines are seen as well as higher rates of mental strain, coronary heart disease, and other health problems. The implications for prevention are clear when one is able to focus on such concepts as worker discretion, latitude, and involvement instead of on concepts such as socioeconomic status. In doing so, the focus is placed on the work environment and the characteristics of the jobs rather than the individual in that job.

An example of the efficacy of control of destiny in a more general setting than a workplace is offered by the *California Wellness Guide*. This Guide was specially designed to help people find solutions to life problems. In straightforward language, it attempts to share with people ways to "work the system" and offers advice on where to get help and how best to present oneself for such help. The Guide was distributed to 100,000 mothers in the California Women, Infants and Children program. Compared to a control group, mothers who received the Guide displayed significantly greater wellness-related knowledge, improved wellness-related attitudes, and healthful behavior changes.[56] If socioeconomic status produces an environment that, throughout the life span, limits the ability of people to control their destiny or to adopt the skills needed to do so, using the type of approach employed by the *California Wellness Guide* explicitly addresses the gradient between socioeconomic status and health.

Control of destiny may be encouraged primarily through individual changes, but there is an environmental component. First, the genesis for the content of the Guide began and ended in the community rather than with professionals. This means that the definition of the problem is recognizable and vital to those who use the Guide rather than imposed from outside. Second, the content of the Guide addressed a wide range of issues relating to both health and life problems, over a wide variety of age and social groups, rather than being targeted toward one disease or behavior. Thus, the Guide was designed for multiple problems and suggests that strategies employed solving one problem may be useful to solve future problems. Third, an environmental change was effected because a community service telephone listing was developed and standardized in all telephone books throughout the state of California for use in the Guide. The consequence of this has been the creation of a statewide referral and resource network.

Even though there are environmental components in studies of job latitude and in projects such as the *California Wellness Guide*, socioeconomic status has been primarily conceptualized as an individual trait. It is typically measured as a factor associated with one person: his or her income, education, or occupational status. This view of socioeconomic status ignores patterns of exposure, opportunities, and resources that occur by social class level. Socioeconomic status defines where one stands vis-à-vis the group, and, since people cluster together by class in geographic and social groups, socioeconomic status also is an environmental concept. Socioeconomic status defines what is available to the group, as well as to an individual within the group.

Quality of the Socioenvironment

Socioeconomic status has the effect of grouping individuals and of nesting them within geographic, social, and occupational environments. Obviously, not all environments are equal. They are more or less desirable places to live or work for a variety of reasons: more or fewer public and private resources; better or poorer housing and infrastructure; different organization into patterns used for work, residence, play, waste, and nature; higher or lower levels of social capital;[56a] and more or less evenly distributed wealth. These environmental differences are patterned by socioeconomic status. Yet, as noted above, socioeconomic status is often treated as if it was a quality of individuals. Poverty, richness, and social status are qualities of environments as well as of people.

Evidence that area socioeconomic status has an independent relationship with mortality, over and above individual socioeconomic status, has emerged in the last decade. Haan and colleagues showed that residents in a federally designated poverty area experienced elevated age-, race-, and sex-adjusted mortality over a follow-up period compared to that of residents of a nonpoverty area.[57] In this study, the heightened risk of death persisted after adjustment for a wide range of demographic, behavioral, social, psychological, and health characteristics. Haan and colleagues concluded that some qualities of the social environment contributed to the association between low socioeconomic status and excess mortality, independent of individual factors. Recently, other analyses have supported these results on a nationwide scale.[58]

Further support for this observation comes from England, where Blaxter[59] investigated a wide variety of health outcomes in manual and nonmanual workers living in different types of areas. Blaxter concludes that type of living area does affect health, but that the association is complex; "good" and industrial residential areas have larger social class differences in health than do rural neighborhoods. The interaction between social class of area of residence and individual social class characteristics was also reported by Yen and Kaplan,[60] and Shouls and colleagues.[61] Both studies found that poverty area of residence, together with individual characteristics, affect illness and adoption of risk behaviors.

Another approach to the study of area quality, one that focuses on economic patterns, involves attention to equality of income distribution, a concept that has no equivalent measure at the individual level. In recent years, evidence has accumulated to suggest that, within populations of developed countries, it is the relative socioeconomic position as well as the absolute level of income that is associated with health.[61] Wilkinson has shown that, in a sample of industrialized countries, life expectancy increases as the distribution of income in the country becomes more egalitarian. Data from the Luxembourg Income Study revealed a correlation of 0.86 between life expectancy and the proportion of the total net income received by the least well-off 70 percent of the population. In addition, when changes in income distribution and life expectancy were compared over time, increases in equality of income distribution were associated with greater increases in life expectancy.

Two other recent studies have explored the association between income distribution and mortality and morbidity within the United States.[62,63] Although these studies used different measures of income distribution, they report similar results: as the equality of the income distribution increases, the age-adjusted rates of all-cause mortality decreases (Fig. 42-2). Kennedy and colleagues report similar relationships between state income equality and mortality from heart disease, malignant neoplasms, cerebrovascular disease, and homicide. Kaplan and colleagues report strong, significant correlations between greater income equality and lower rates of all-cause and age-specific mortality, other health indicators (including rates of low-birth weight, violent crimes, disability, per capita expenditures on protection, sedentary behavior, and current smoking), other social indicators (proportions of unemployed, prisoners, those receiving Aid to Families with Dependent Children, and those without health insurance), and educational indicators. The results reported in these two studies were not changed by adjusting for the wealth of the state as measured either by proportion of the population in poverty or by the state median income. Kaplan and colleagues also reported that equality of income in states in 1980 was associated with more favorable mortality rates in those states in 1990.

Results from these studies are striking and consistent, but more work needs to be done to understand the role of macroeconomic income distribution and the health of the population. Governments, through policies on taxation, income transfers, and benefits, alter the distribution of income; if these policies affect the health of populations,

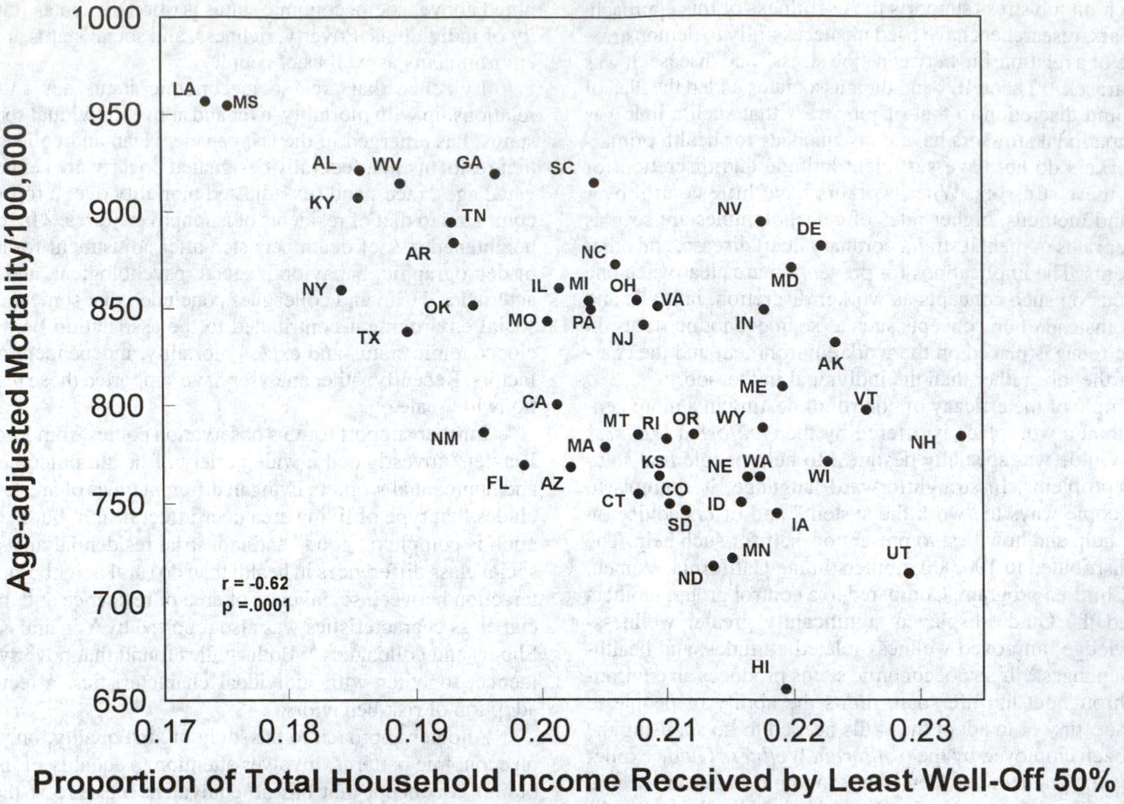

Figure 42-2. Equality of income distribution and age-adjusted all-cause mortality in the United States, 1990. (From Kaplan GA, Pamuk ER, Lynch JW, Cohen RD, Balfour JL: Inequality in income and mortality in the United States: analysis of mortality and potential pathways. Br Med J 312:999–1003, 1996.)

the magnitude of such effects needs to be known so that health outcome may be considered when economic policy is made. This is all the more important because of the reported increase in inequality of income distribution in the United States during the last decade.[64]

The results of these early studies suggest that we need to explore the attributes of neighborhoods and areas that might affect health. Very little work has been done to examine differences in the areas themselves rather than in the composition of the population living there. One study examined the services and resources available in poverty areas of San Francisco and found that life was more difficult, more expensive, and took more time because of differences in housing, services, infrastructure, transportation, and economic policies.[65] An ongoing study in Glasgow, Scotland, by Macintyre and colleagues is classifying four areas according to a wide variety of characteristics in order to study them over time for health outcomes.[66,67] The rationale behind this study is to develop interventions at the community level so that individuals will find it easier to adopt healthful behaviors. This, of course, is in direct contrast to our usual approach of focusing on individuals in the hope that this will lead to healthier communities.

While it is unfortunate that socioeconomic status remains so poorly understood, the increased attention to the gradient between socioeconomic status and disease and risk factors; the effect of lifestage; and consideration of socioeconomic status at an environmental level may help us develop more effective public health interventions.

Race and Ethnicity

Another pervasive and persistent patterned regularity in the study of health and disease is seen between race and ethnic groups. For example, young and middle-aged black Americans have disproportionately high morbidity and mortality rates.[68] McCord and Freeman[69] have estimated that black men living in Harlem in 1980 had less chance of surviving to the age of 65 than men in Bangladesh, and recent data from a nationwide study by Geronimus[70] show that this situation was even worse in 1990. Those data indicate that about half of the higher mortality rate in blacks is due to poverty but that the other half is not explained by this factor. Other possible explanations include lifestyle factors, use of medical care, and biologic differences. Exploration of the relative importance of these factors is complicated by the fact that "race" is such an imprecise term. Biologically, race is an indicator of the distribution of gene frequencies accross populations, but, as Susser et al[26] point out, this distribution of genes is deeply conflated with geographic, social class, and cultural distinctions. Many physical anthropologists prefer to dispense with the term altogether because it is so vague.

Neverthless, race clearly has social meaning. People react differently to people of different races and this has health consequences. In an innovative and pioneering study, Kreiger and Sidney[71] studied the consequences of racial discrimination on blood pressure in 5,115 young adults in four cities: Birmingham, Chicago, Minneapolis, and Oakland. Eighty percent of black men and women reported experiences of racial discrimination and these were associated with elevations of blood pressure.

Race influences behavior: it influences how people interact with one another, where people live, what jobs they have, and how much education they have. It has impact on life choices and opportunities. Racial categories are associated with differences in life expectency, diasability, cirrhosis, infant mortality, birth weight, arthritis, diabetes, hypertension, anemia, and virtually every cause of death among adults. These are important and complex issues that deserve a high priority in our research agenda. As in the case of socioeconomic status, epidemiologists tend to control for race in reporting research results because, if they did not, it would overwhelm all other findings. Recent research on race, especially that focusing on black-white differences, is providing important new findings.[72–74] It is clear that this issue deserves serious and continued attention directed to a wider range of race and ethnic groups.

Social Support and Social Connection

Historically, one of the earliest areas of interest in the social patterning of disease has been the beneficial effect of marital status on health. While this research area yielded interesting results, it also has branched out to new research areas of social support and social connection.

It has been known for many years that people who are not married—whether single, separated, widowed, or divorced—have higher mortality rates than married people.[72–74] These differences in rate cannot be explained by an increase in any one cause or death. Ortmeyer,[73] using national data, has reported that divorced and single white men and women have higher mortality rates compared to those who are married. Adjustment for risk factors such as serum cholesterol, systolic and diastolic blood pressure, and obesity did not diminish the mortality differences observed for marital status in a sample of 6,672 adults with and without coronary heart disease from the U.S. Health Examination Survey.[75]

Not only is having a spouse beneficial to health, but loss of spouse to death is particularly detrimental. Some research suggests that this burden of excess mortality operates only during the first 6 months,[76,77] while other research suggests that the impact of widowhood extends many years after the death of the partner.[78] While considerable attention was given to this issue, and especially to the effect of different types of work on women in various marital circumstances and to the way in which these relationships are affected by variations in socioeconomic status, the effect of marital status on health remains largely unexplained.

Common to marital status research is the theme of social support and social connection. In an influential article written in 1976, Cassel[79] pointed out that lack of social connection, such as disruption of marriage or moving to a new social setting, was associated with a wide range of disease outcomes. According to Cassel's hypothesis, the essential element in these situations was lack of social connection or support. In the absence of social connections a person becomes generally susceptible to illness, the specific type of disease being determined by that person's particular risk situation.

One of the first studies on social support was done in 1972 by Nuckolls et al[80] on complications of pregnancy and delivery among 107 women with a similar demographic background. Women reported on life changes both before and during pregnancy as well as on the presence or absence of social supports. Women with frequent life changes before and/or during pregnancy had no more complications than those with few life changes. However, among women who experienced frequent life changes and who *also* reported poor social support, 90 percent had one or more complications of pregnancy. While this study was done in a small population, it nevertheless generated interesting findings that also were consistent with the observations made by Durkheim in 1897 regarding the importance of supportive interpersonal relations for health and well-being.

The concept of social support subsequently was studied in a much larger community sample in Alameda County, California.[81] In that study, an increased mortality rate was observed among persons previously identified as having fewer friends and social relationships. This study was conducted among a random sample of 6,928 adults whose mortality experience was monitored for 9 years following the baseline interview. Social ties were assessed in terms of marital status, contact with friends and relatives, church membership, and organizational affiliations. Persons with more social ties had lower mortality rates than those with fewer ties, and this relationship existed in all age groups and for both sexes. While the relative risk associated with social networks was slightly reduced after account had been taken of relative weight, cigarette smoking, alcohol consumption, physical activity, health practices, and health status at baseline, those with weak networks still had mortality rates 2 to 3 times higher than those with strong ties (Fig. 42-3).

Since the Alameda County study, several other studies have been done to test the social support hypothesis. The results from this research are generally, but not completely, supportive of the findings from California. In Tecumseh, Michigan, House and his colleagues[82] studied 2,754 men and women who had originally been interviewed and medically examined in 1967–1969. The mortality experience of this group was followed until 1978–1979. Using a measure of social networks similar but not identical to that used in Alameda County, these investigators found basically the same relationship between networks and mortality as in Alameda County for men, but not for women (again, after adjusting for such factors as age, smoking, alcohol consumption, education, employment status, occupation, height/weight, and several measures of health status as determined at the baseline examination).

In Evans County, Georgia, Schoenbach et al[83] attempted to replicate the Alameda County results in a study of 2,059 men and women followed from 1967–1969 to 1980. Using a measure of social networks generally comparable to that used in Alameda County and in Tecumseh, these investigators found that two network measures were only modestly related to this outcome. In all comparisons, however, the influence of networks on mortality was weaker than that observed in Alameda County.

In their study of 7,639 Japanese American men living in Hawaii, Reed and his colleagues[84] found an inverse relationship between coronary heart disease and social support in a prevalence design, but failed to confirm that observation in a study of incidence. In a follow-up on these men from 1965–1968 through 1978, no significant association was observed between social networks and various measures of coronary heart disease. On the other hand, results from a study in Durham County, North Carolina,[85] among 331 men and women over 65 years of age showed a strong relationship between social networks and mortality during a 30-month follow-up period (after account had been taken of age, race, sex, economic resources, physical health, activities of daily living, stressful life events, smoking, and several psychological traits).

In a recent study of social support and social networks in eastern Finland, Kaplan and his colleagues[86] found a strong association between networks and mortality from all causes of death. This study involved a survey of a representative sample of 13,301 men and women followed for 5 years. After adjustments for age, serum cholesterol, blood pressure, smoking, obesity, education, residence, health status, and family history, the most isolated men had an all-cause death rate twice as high as those most socially connected. The odds ratios for death from cardiovascular and ischemic heart disease were 1.6 and 1.7, respectively. In striking contrast to these findings for men, no increase in mortality rate associated with social connections was seen for women.

As is evident from this brief account, several large studies have shown that weak social ties are associated with an increased risk of disease, but results from Michigan, Georgia, and Finland are only partially consistent with this conclusion, and those from Hawaii are not at all supportive.

Several reviews[87–89] have critically assessed this literature and have concluded that something of importance is going on but that the precise elements of this "something" are not yet clear. One possible explanation for the inconsistent pattern of findings may be that a few simple questions about relationships (e.g., about marriage, clubs, and number of friends) may be enough to separate those with ties from those without ties in a large, urban area like Alameda County, but they are not precise enough in smaller, more rural communities,[82] particularly for women. Thus, it may be that more sensitive, detailed, and culturally appropriate questions about relationships may be necessary in small towns like Tecumseh, Michigan, in rural areas like Evans County, Georgia, and North Karelia, Finland, and in close-knit groups such as Japanese American men in Hawaii. It is hoped that the research now under way on this issue will provide clarity on this interesting point.

Another important dimension in research on social support is the effort to define it more precisely. Research has focused on such

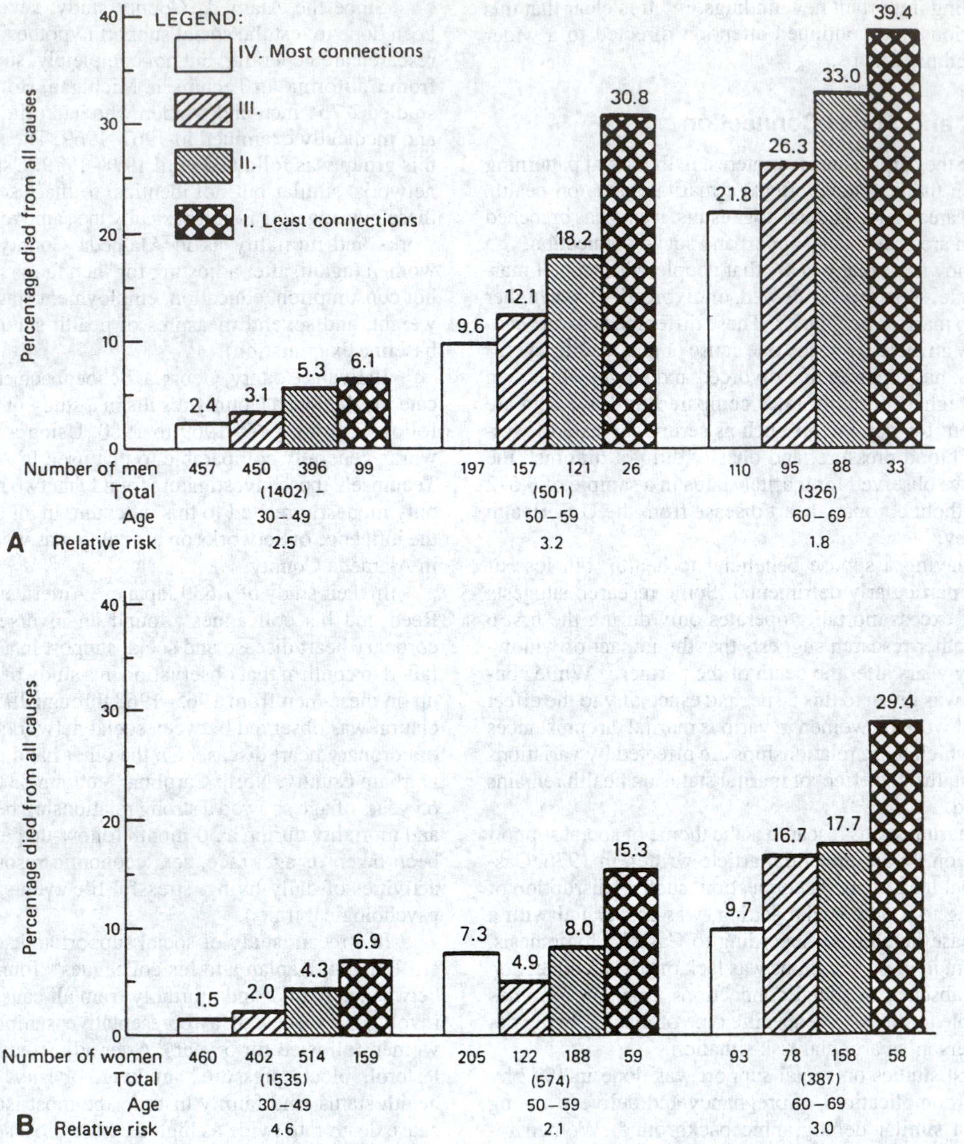

Figure 42-3. Social ties and 9-year mortality in Alameda County, California. **A,** Men. **B,** Women. (From Berkman L, Syrne SL: Social networks, host resistance, and mortality: a nine year follow-up study of Alameda County residents. Am J Epidemiol 109:186–204, 1979.)

aspects as number of friends, number of close friends, frequency of seeing people, satisfaction with the quantity and quality of relationships, and so on. In one approach to the study of this issue, Seeman and Syme[90] compared the relative importance of several different social support and network components in a study of men and women undergoing coronary angiography. In assessing the predictive power of these various components, the most powerful was the instrumental dimension. Compared to other definitions of social support, less coronary atherosclerosis was seen among people who could count on specific people to help them when they needed specific kinds of help (for example, to borrow money, help with household repairs, advice on problems). Further work will be necessary to better define the importance of various dimensions of social networks and social support for health and well-being.

Environmental Stress and Psychoneuroimmunology

The idea that chronic stress may have an effect on the health of the body was first suggested in modern times by Hans Selye.[91] Building on the long research tradition that stemmed from this observation, McEwan and Stellar[92] recently proposed that a combination of environmental factors and genetic predispositions lead to susceptibility to stress and perhaps to disease. The proposed model argues that stress results in measurable, cumulative damage that leads to increased mortality and morbidity.[93] One research area that investigates this model is psychoneuroimmunology.

The field of psychoneuroimmunology[94] examines the interactions among the central nervous system, the endocrine system, and immune function. As a result of work in this field, “immune response is being re-examined in the context of an integrated system and no longer as a body system which operates independently in a vacuum.”[95] Thus, psychoneuroimmunology examines, explicitly, a pathway by which the environment might “get under the skin”: psychological response to stressors in the environment impacts the central nervous system, and the central nervous system, in turn, modulates immune response.

Evidence is accumulating that many social conditions are associated with changes in immune function. Marital interruption, whether from death or divorce, is associated with downregulation of the immune system.[96–99] Immune function is also impaired in the presence of other short-term and chronic stressors. The most extensively studied commonplace stressor is examination periods of graduate students. When immune response during examination periods is compared with immune response measured at an earlier time, changes in immune response include decline in activity of and decrease in number of natural killer cells,[100,101] depression of the ability of cellular immune response to maintain control over latent herpes viruses,[102] and changes in T-lymphocyte numbers and ratios and mitogen responsiveness.[103] Immunologic changes have also been observed during acute psychological stressors that are laboratory-induced.[95] Presence of at least one type of chronic stressor, caring for a family member with Alzheimer's disease, is associated with generally poorer immune function.[104] Evidence suggests that this immune deficit persists during and beyond the cessation of the stressor.[105]

Quality of social relationships also have a role on immune function. Reported loneliness has direct affects on immune response, and those who are above average on a scale of loneliness show lower natural killer cell activity, depressed ability to control latent viral infection, and poorer T-cell proliferative response.[95] In addition, certain patterns of marital discord are associated with changes in endocrine function of wives,[106] and research suggests that immune function of women and men may be affected as well.[98,99] Some evidence suggests that social support also moderates the association between chronic stressors and immune response. The depressed immune response seen in Alzheimer's caregivers is reduced in those caregivers and former caregivers who report more positive emotional and tangible support.[107] Easterling and colleagues also suggest that the lower levels of social support that continue after cessation of caregiving may be responsible for the continuing depression of immune response.

An impressive body of research supports the influence of the social environment and behavior on immune response. However, it is still unclear whether the observed immune changes actually lead to morbidity and mortality. Only a few prospective studies have shown psychosocial stressors leading to health changes in the presence of immunologic alterations.[95]

In epidemiology we have a history of research areas that had the implicit or explicit goal of investigating levels of stress and their effect on health. One area of early research was concerned with the impact of various types of mobility on the occurrence of disease. Many studies found an increased rate of disease among mobile persons but others failed to do so. The way in which social mobility affected the incidence of disease was never clear, in part due to the fact that social mobility was never a clear concept. The common link between studies seemed to be that the participants were experiencing change in some large environmental setting: geographic, social, occupational, or cultural change.

Closely related to research on mobility was work attempting to establish a link between stressful life events and disease. In 1967, Holmes and Rahe[108] developed a Social Readjustment Rating Scale to record such life events as change in residence, injury, job changes, death of loved ones, and birth of children. Again, the common theme around the life events is change, and like mobility research, results from life events research were mixed.[109] The retrospective nature of most life events studies added further problems to the field. However, prospective studies investigating the increase in incidence of relatively minor diseases did show similar results.[110–112]

It is clear that the relationship between social mobility, life events, and disease is difficult to understand. One of the reasons for the inconsistency of the results may stem from the inaccuracy of the measurement of life events and mobility as a proxy for stressors and stress responses. The impact of mobility and life events are most likely mediated by personality, perception, previous experiences, social context, and coping styles, and these data are unavailable in most of the studies. Another reason for inconsistency and difficulties of this research stems from the embryonic measurement of risk: both life events and mobility attempt to measure many types of stressors simultaneously. These global measurements may obscure relationships that exist in specific situations, such as bereavement.

Epidemiologic attempts to study the effect of environmental stressors on health have met with mixed results. Psychoneuroimmunology, by approaching the association from a specific point within the disease pathway, is having better success. It is hoped that this success will lead to new research areas or techniques in studying the association between stress and health at the population level.

Psychological Traits and Mental Health

Of all the research that has been done on the ways people cope with stressful life events, most early attention was focused on "Type A" behavior. This behavior pattern was said to be exhibited by individuals engaged in a relatively chronic and excessive struggle to obtain an unlimited number of things from the environment in the shortest period of time and/or against the opposing efforts of other persons or things.[113]

For almost 30 years, Friedman, Rosenman, Jenkins, Brand, and others published a series of papers showing an increased rate of coronary heart disease among men characterized by this behavior pattern. The most compelling evidence from this group was based on the study of 3,524 men in the Western Collaborative Group Study (WCGS),[114] a prospective investigation with an 8½-year follow-up. Men judged on interview to have behavior pattern A had twice as much coronary heart disease as men with behavior pattern B. The apparent relative risk of about two persisted after adjustment for major coronary risk factors.

Following these initial studies, several long-term follow-up investigations have been completed on the WCGS cohort. Two of the studies showed that Type A behavior was not associated with elevated coronary heart disease mortality.[115,116] A third study of this cohort found that Type A men, ages 61 to 81, reported better health than Type B men after 22 years of follow-up.[117]

Negative evidence regarding Type A behavior comes from the Multiple Risk Factor Intervention Trial (MRFIT)[118] and the Aspirin Myocardial Infarction Study (AMIS).[119] Data from MRFIT showed that Type A behavior, assessed in ways closely similar to the method used in the WCGS, was unrelated to the incidence of coronary heart disease among 3,110 men at high risk to develop the disease. Similarly, data from AMIS showed that Type A men who survived a first myocardial infarction were at no greater risk of a second infarction than Type B men who also had survived a first infarction. It is not yet clear how seriously to regard these negative reports since, in both cases, only men at very high risk to develop disease were studied. On the other hand, both studies were carefully done in large populations and, in both cases, the identification of Type A behavior demonstrated not even modest predictive power.

One of the ways to evaluate the importance of a suspected risk factor is to see if the incidence of disease is reduced after the risk factor is removed. A major intervention project to alter Type A behavior yielded interesting results. In this study,[120] 862 postmyocardial infarction patients received general cardiologic counseling, but an experimental group consisting of 592 patients also received counseling to reduce Type A behavior. After 3 years of follow-up, patients in the experimental group experienced half the amount of coronary heart disease than that experienced by those in the control group (7.2 percent incidence versus 13 percent incidence, respectively).

Mixed findings from research on Type A behavior has led to a new generation of research focused on particular components of the behavior patterns rather than on the global phenomenon. Most component research has been directed toward "hostility." Assessing hostility from the Type A structured interview, positive relationships with coronary heart disease have been observed in prospective[121] and angiography studies.[122,123] Using the Cook-Medley Hostility Inventory, positive findings between hostility and coronary heart disease have been found in a number of prospective studies.[124–126] A recent meta-analysis and literature review confirmed this conclusion.[127,128]

It has been proposed that three aspects of hostility—cognitive, affective, and behavioral—should be considered in order to examine whether each shares the same association with poor health. In a recent study investigating the association between separate components of hostility and progression of atherosclerosis, cynical distrust and anger-control predicted significant change after adjusting for established risk factors.[129]

Evidence from behavior pattern research has led to the study of other forms of psychological response, including antagonism and resentment,[130] time urgency,[131] anger,[132–134] need for control,[135] self-involvement,[136] self-esteem,[137] hardiness,[138] and cynicism. Another new area of psychological response is hopelessness. A growing body of evidence supports the belief that giving up hope has adverse health consequences.[139] In a 12-year cohort study of 2,800 healthy men and women participating in the National Health Examination Follow-up survey, hopelessness predicted fatal and nonfatal ischemic heart disease.[140] These results were supported by evidence from a 6-year cohort of Finnish men, where a high level of hopelessness was associated with incident myocardial infarction and cancer, all-cause mortality, and cardiovascular mortality.[141] Controlling for traditional risk factors had little impact on the association. Using the same cohort of Eastern Finnish men, Everson and colleagues examined levels of hopelessness and 4-year progression of atherosclerosis.[142] A high level of hopelessness exacerbated atherosclerotic progression, but primarily in men who had increased arterial wall thickening at baseline.

Many of the psychological responses investigated in current research are maladaptive responses to high allostatic load from the environment. Individuals, interacting with their environment, develop psychological, behavioral, and physiological responses that have a generic and cumulative effect on health. The complexities involved in this research are formidable and it will be of interest to observe continuing developments in this important field.

▸ ENVIRONMENTAL INTERVENTIONS

This chapter has been concerned primarily with the prevention of disease. It has been argued that, while disease prevention can and should be encouraged as we work with both healthy and sick individuals, more attention now must be given to an environmental approach to prevention. Environmental approaches have a long history in public health and have been of great importance in the control of infectious diseases. They have been much less prominent with reference to noninfectious diseases. There are many reasons for this, but one important factor may be our reluctance to encourage environmental interventions for fear they may preempt individual freedom and choice by limiting options and by allowing the few to dictate to the many. In fact, environmental interventions can be seen in precisely the opposite way—as increasing freedom of choice and options. For example, teenagers can hardly be considered free agents when the tobacco industry provides enormous pressure on them to smoke. By providing structural alternatives, teenagers would have more options for making choices than are now possible. Similarly, when a food market has a wide selection of unhealthful foods prominently and attractively displayed at cheap prices (while healthy foods are more expensive and hidden on the bottom shelf), the consumer hardly has a full range of options equally available. The environmental pressures now in place often favor unhealthful interests; introduction of healthful environmental changes can be seen as redressing the balance by providing people with greater freedom of choice among a broader range of alternatives.

In the past two decades, intervention studies that included environmental changes have been conducted. Several large-scale heart disease intervention programs, such as the Stanford Five-City Coronary Heart Disease Project,[143] the Minnesota Health Program,[144] and a community-based program in North Karelia, Finland,[145] have had mixed results. No reduction in heart disease mortality and very few changes in health behaviors were reported by the Stanford and Minnesota studies, but the North Karelia project reported significant changes in both coronary heart disease mortality rates and in risk behaviors. Similarly, a nationwide Community Intervention Trials for Smoking Cessation (COMMIT) project[146] showed no difference in smoking prevalence or quit rates for heavy smokers between treatment and intervention communities.

The disappointing results from many community intervention trials makes it imperative that we examine those studies that do work. What was different about the North Karelia project? One substantial difference between the North Karelia intervention study and those in the United States was that the instigation, planning, and design for the intervention was initiated by a citizen activist group. Community involvement may be a vital component of successful community intervention.

The involvement of community members in public health planning, implementation, and evaluation is not new. For at least 15 years it has been a central feature of the so-called "new public health," which addresses a broad range of health-related issues and involves communities in defining problems and their solutions.[147–150] When those most directly concerned with an issue are involved in defining interventions that *they* consider most likely to solve that problem, they have a stake in the process.[56] Although evaluations of projects in which community participation is a central feature are still infrequent, results are beginning to demonstrate the power of community participation to create more effective programs.[151–154]

▸ TOWARD A MORE APPROPRIATE SOCIAL EPIDEMIOLOGY

While several social factors have been identified in this chapter as increasing risk to disease, some of the evidence presented is conflicting and contradictory. One possible explanation for this inconsistency is that investigators have used different research designs in different populations, that they have defined concepts differently and that they have used crude, imprecise, and noncomparable assessment tools. These are problems typical of many research fields, and they tend to be resolved in time as research experience accumulates. Nevertheless, in view of these design and measurement problems, it is especially interesting to note that research on social factors has yielded as consistent a pattern of findings as it has.

There are at least three other possible explanations for this uneven pattern of research findings. One is that we have been using an inappropriate disease classification system yielding findings that are misleading and incomplete. The second possible explanation is that we have for the most part been studying disease in adults when, as noted earlier, a more useful strategy would instead have been to study the early years of life. And the third is that we have been studying disease in individuals and ignoring the contribution group factors may make toward understanding distribution and etiology of disease in populations.

The Use of an Appropriate Disease Classification Scheme

The possibility that social epidemiology may be using an inappropriate disease classification scheme was powerfully suggested by John Cassel.[79] In that paper, Cassel noted that a wide variety of disease outcomes was associated with similar circumstances. For example, he cited the remarkably similar set of risk factors that characterize people who develop tuberculosis and schizophrenia, become alcoholics, and are victims of multiple accidents or commit suicide. Cassel also noted that this phenomenon had generally escaped comment. To explain this, he suggested that investigators usually are "concerned with only one clinical entity, so that features common to multiple disease manifestations have tended to be overlooked."

When researchers focus on one or another clinical entity, they are, consciously or unconsciously, adopting a clinical classification scheme that may be useful in clinical settings but that may not be as useful in studies of disease etiology. The clinician uses a classification scheme that has proven useful in the treatment of diseases and in making prognostic estimates for such diseases. However, when epidemiologists observe that several different clinical entities have one risk factor in common, it is not unreasonable to consider a new disease classification that unifies these disparate clinical entities based on the features they have in common.

This is not a new idea. Infectious disease epidemiologists have for many years grouped together different clinical entities based on their similarities in modes of transmission. Thus, as noted earlier, different clinical conditions have been grouped together according to whether they are waterborne, airborne, vector-borne, or food-borne. These environmental classifications may not be of direct value in the treatment of sick people, but they certainly are of value in identifying those aspects of the environment to which interventions can be directed. A comparable set of environmental categories for noninfectious diseases does not exist. The reasons for this are not clear, but it may be that diseases such as coronary heart disease, cancer, and arthritis often are viewed as being diseases "of the individual" and not diseases influenced by environmental factors. As we have seen, the fact that so many diseases exhibit patterned consistencies in populations suggests that there may indeed by environmental factors associated with the occurrence of these diseases.

An illustration of this environmental perspective is provided by a research project currently under way among bus drivers in San Francisco.[155] Several previous studies have noted that bus drivers have a higher prevalence of hypertension as well as diseases of the gastrointestinal tract and of the musculoskeletal system, compared with workers in other occupations. These results have been obtained from studies of different transit systems, under different conditions, and in several countries.[156–161] Based on these findings, it has been suggested that certain aspects of the occupation of bus drivers may create an increased risk of disease for workers in that occupation.

From a clinical viewpoint, it is of value to identify drivers with disease in order to treat them. It would also be of value to teach drivers about better posture, more healthful eating habits, and about alternative ways of dealing with job stress. However, from an environmental perspective, it would perhaps be more useful to identify those aspects of the job itself that might be changed to prevent diseases by identifying characteristics of the job that are associated with increased disease risk.

In this study of drivers, the exposure of drivers to noise, vibration, and carbon monoxide fumes is being monitored but particular attention is being paid to the social environment of the driver.[162] For example, in preliminary studies of drivers, the "tyranny of the schedule" has been forcefully brought to attention. Drivers must keep to a specific schedule, but, in almost every instance, this schedule is arranged without realistic reference to actual road conditions and, in fact, cannot be met. If this and other characteristics of the job of bus driving can be identified that are associated with disease, it may be possible to introduce interventions, not merely among bus drivers, but directly on those environmental factors associated with the job. For example, it may be that, by changing the way in which schedules are arranged, the bus company will be able to earn more money than it loses because of lower rates of absenteeism, sickness, accidents, and in particular, turnover of employees. In the case of bus drivers, a clinical focus either on hypertension, gastrointestinal diseases, or musculoskeletal disorders clearly is useful. However, from an environmental and preventive perspective, it might be more useful to group together these different diseases and conditions associated with a common work exposure so that they can be studied as related phenomena. If this is not done, the circumstances they share in common will not likely be appreciated.

In spite of the usefulness of looking at groups of diseases in this way, almost all research on noninfectious disease is directed more or less exclusively toward one or another clinical entity. While this is understandable (not only because of the enormous influence of the clinical tradition but also because funding for research is so firmly focused on well-established and recognized clinical entities), it has serious consequences. One consequence is that the power of our research is compromised: if a risk factor is associated with several diseases and if we study it only with reference to one disease, its more general importance is not likely to be appreciated and, in fact, may be missed entirely.[163]

The concept of social support provides an illustration of this problem. As noted earlier, the absence of social support is moderately related to an increased risk of coronary heart disease, complications of pregnancy and delivery, suicide, and several other diseases and conditions. It also is associated with an increased rate of all-cause mortality. If we could study all of the disease consequences associated with inadequate social support, we might develop a much clearer understanding of its importance for disease etiology. Indeed, by studying social support in relation to only one or another disease, we may be missing what is most important about the concept.

Let us pursue this example one step further. The fact that those with weak social supports have higher rates of many different diseases and conditions is not immediately plausible biologically. Two models come to mind to account for this observation. One model is that the concept of social support includes many diverse elements and that each of these elements separately influences the likelihood of different diseases. This often is the explanation offered to account for the higher rate of so many diseases associated with cigarette smoking. The second model is that social support affects bodily defenses so that with weak supports people are more vulnerable to a wide range of disease agents.[164–172] In this case, the presence of specific viruses, bacteria, or air pollutants would not result in disease unless the person was vulnerable to them. For this reason, the presence of weak social support would predict whether or not people got sick, but not what disease they got. This latter model is attractive because it would account for the fact that several psychosocial factors are related to many different diseases (involving many organ systems) as well as that most well-recognized disease-specific risk factors are only modestly predictive of those diseases.

The use of the concept of social support in this way is of course merely illustrative. As noted above, a new area of research referred to as psychoneuroimmunology is now emerging showing the link between a wide range of psychosocial factors and immunologic function. This field is growing rapidly and promises to expand our understanding in this important field. One of the central debates in this work is whether one should study the relationship between a psychosocial variable such as anger or hardiness and a specific disease or whether it is more appropriate to study a generalized bodily response.[173,174] The results of this debate will eventually provide information useful not only for studies of disease etiology but for intervention programs as well.

The Study of Appropriate Age Groups

As noted earlier, it is disappointing that, after almost 40 years of epidemiologic research on noninfectious diseases, we are not further along in our understanding of their risk factors. We have only an imperfect knowledge of psychosocial risk factors, but our knowledge of other risk factors is limited as well. In addition, even when we have identified risk factors, we have had substantial difficulty in getting people to change behavior to lower that risk. Part of the explanation for this state of affairs is that we are dealing with complex issues that are difficult to define and measure. Part of the difficulty also is that our most powerful research method, the experiment, is difficult to use in human populations. Both of these explanations are reasonable. But one of our problems may also be that we typically study adults when we ought to be studying infants and children.

One of the most intriguing findings in this area involves a follow-up study of children involved in an early education program. This study reported a 22-year follow-up of low income children, 3 and 4 years of age, from Ypsilanti, Michigan.[175] These children had been randomly assigned either to a program offering special education prior to enrollment in regular school or no program. As shown in Table 42-1, children who had 1 or 2 years of early education were more likely than those in the control group to complete high school and be employed and were less likely to have been arrested, been on public assistance, and, for girls, to have had a teenage pregnancy. Since these children were assigned at random to the program, these reported differences are probably attributable to the program itself and not to such other factors as motivated parents or differences in baseline intellectual level. It is interesting that 1 or 2 years of exposure to an early education program would, at age 19, make such a difference in living circumstance.

TABLE 42-1. EFFECTS OF PRESCHOOL THROUGH AGE 19—PERRY PRESCHOOL STUDY[a]

Outcome	No. Responding	Preschool Group	No Preschool	p
Employed	121	59%	32%	0.032
High school graduation	121	67%	49%	0.034
College or vocational training or both	121	38%	21%	0.029
Ever detained/arrested	121	31%	51%	0.022
Females: Teen pregnancies per 100	49	64	117	0.084

[a] Adapted from Berrueta-Clement JR, Schweinhart LJ, Barrett WS, Epstein AS, Weikart DP: Changed Lives: The Effects of the Perry Preschool Program on Youths through Age 19. Ypsilanti, MI: High/Scope Press, 1984.

It is hardly original to suggest that experiences in early life are important for later life. In spite of the fact that this relationship is well-known, it is difficult to find solid research evidence demonstrating this phenomenon. Many pediatricians and child development experts feel that early experiences are important but base their view on personal experience and on intuition. It is not surprising that they have so little data to rely on because it is difficult to do follow-up research covering 40 or 50 years. Nevertheless, if one could review the data already available in many long-term data sets, it might be possible to document more precisely how much tracking really occurs and with what strength. If certain physical or psychological traits track, are we doomed as adults? What other factors modify the impact of early experiences?[176] One interesting study of high-risk children in Kauai, Hawaii,[177] for example, suggests that subsequent life events can buffer or ameliorate earlier experiences and that childhood "high-risk" status can in fact be modified.

If it could be established more clearly that certain risk factors are initiated early in life, it might be more appropriate to initiate interventions at that time instead of many years later. While this might make intuitive sense, it is difficult to shift the financial and organizational resources necessary to do this without a sound body of research evidence to support it. In any case, given our difficulty in making sense of risk factors in the adult years and of developing effective intervention programs, it may be useful now to at least explore this issue as a practical and reasonable alternative.

Examination of Group-Level Risk

In a recent methodological discussion paper, Susser argues that studies that try to account for individual processes while ignoring the effects of pairings, families, peer groups, schools, communities, cultures, and laws will fail: "With these contexts unmeasured, neither patterns of mortality and morbidity, nor epidemic spread, nor sexual transmission can be explained."[178] Attention has also been directed toward the possibility of a reverse ecologic fallacy. If it is possible to have error when inferring from group associations to individuals within those groups, then when models contain only individual variables, we have potential error in assuming there is no group association. If characteristics of the social or structural group environment help shape health outcomes, and if we fail to measure them, we are, at the very least, overestimating the strength of the individual factors. This overestimation might lead to many failed interventions that attempt to change risk by changing each person.

Why and how are risk factors clustered in certain socioeconomic groups? Kaplan argues that "[p]rogress will require considerably more data collection on the daily experiences of individuals, on material and symbolic demands which challenge them, on the personal and community resources to meet these challenges, and on the macroeconomic forces which impact both the individual and the community.[50]

Conclusion

A more appropriate social epidemiology would take advantage of current discrepancies and inconsistencies in the research evidence by developing better research methods and instruments, by thinking about more appropriate disease classification systems, by exploring more precisely the ways in which psychosocial factors affect immune function, by considering more systematically the possibility that what happens early in life may hold an important key to understanding what happens later in life, and by moving beyond models that do not consider disease pathways beyond those of an individual.

The importance of social factors in the etiology of many diseases is becoming increasingly clear. The evidence for some factors is weak and for others it is still unclear. Nevertheless, it is impressive that an increasingly large body of consistent findings is being generated in spite of these major methodologic problems. We may not be ready now to use the data emerging from this research in public health programs, but it is clear that we will need to use them soon. The reason for this is that most serious diseases today are importantly influenced by the social environment. For these reasons, interventions in the social environment clearly are necessary, and continued research on social factors therefore must become an important priority in both public health planning and program development.

▶ REFERENCES

1. Lindheim R, Syme SL: Environments, people and health. Annu Rev Public Health 4:335–459, 1983
2. Taylor SE, Repetti RL, Seeman T: Health psychology: what is an unhealthy environment and how does it get under the skin? Annu Rev Psychol 48:411– 447, 1997
3. US Department of Health and Human Services: Vital and Health Statisics: Current Estimates form the National Health Interview Survey, 1993
4. Parkin DM, Muir CS, Whelan SL et al (eds): Cancer Incidence in Five Continents. vol 4. IARC Publ No 120. Lyon, France: International Agency for Research on Cancer, 1992
5. Ziegler RG, Hoover RN, Pike MC, Hildesheim A, Nomura AMY, et al: Migration patterns and breast cancer risk in Asian-American women. J Natl Cancer Inst 85:1819–1827, 1993
6. Thomas DB, Karagas MR: Cancer in first and second generation Americans. Cancer Res 47:5771–5776, 1987
7. McKeown T: The Role of Medicine: Dream, Mirage or Nemesis. London: Nuffield Provincial Hospitals Trust, 1976
8. McKinlay JB, McKinlay SM: The questionable contribution of medical measures to the decline of mortality in the United States in the twentieth century. Health and Society, Summer, 405–428, 1977
9. Hamburg D: In Elliot GR, Parron DL (eds): Health and Behavior: Frontiers of Research in the Biobehavioral Sciences. Washington, DC: National Academy Press, 1982
10. Lalonde M: A New Perspective on the Health of Canadians: A Working Document. Ottawa: Information Canada, 1974
11. Syme SL: Strategies for health promotion. Prev Med 15:492–507, 1986
12. Leventhal H, Cleary PD: The smoking problem: a review of the research and theory in behavioral risk modification. Psychol Bull 88:370–405, 1980

13. Dekker E: Youth culture and influences on the smoking behavior of young people. In: Smoking and Health. Proceedings of the Third World Conference. Washington, DC: Public Health Service, 1975, pp 381–392
14. Syme SL, Alcalay R: Control of cigarette smoking from a social perspective. Annu Rev Public Health 3:179–199, 1982
15. Pooling Project Research Group: Relationship of blood pressure, serum cholesterol, smoking habit, relative weight and ECG abnormalities to incidence of major coronary events: final report of the Pooling Project. J Chron Dis 31:201–306, 1978
16. Inter-Society Commission for Heart Disease Resources: Primary prevention of the atherosclerotic diseases. Circulation 42:A55–A95, 1970
17. Marmot M, Winkelstein W Jr: Epidemiologic observations on intervention trials for prevention of coronary heart disease. Am J Epidemiol 101:177–181, 1975
18. Rosen G: From Medical Policy to Social Medicine: Essays on the History of Health Care. New York: Science History Publications, 1974
19. Durkheim E: Suicide: A Study in Sociology. Simpson G (ed and trans). Glencoe, IL: Free Press, 1951
20. Antonovsky A: Social class, life expectancy and overall mortality. Milbank Mem Fund Q 45:31–73, 1967
21. Syme SL, Berkman LF: Social class, susceptibility and sickness. Am J Epidemiol 104:1–8, 1976
22. Feinstein JS: The relationship between socioeconomic status and health: a review of the literature. Milbank 71:279–322, 1993
23. Kitagawa EM, Hauser PM: Differential Mortality in the United States. Cambridge, MA: Harvard University Press, 1973
24. Haan MN, Kaplan GA, Syme SL: Socioeconomic status and health: old observations and new thoughts. In Bunker JP, Gomby DF, Kehrer BH (eds): Pathways to Health: The Role of Social Factors. Palo Alto, CA: H.J. Kaiser Family Foundation, 1989
25. Marmot MG, Rose G, Shipley M, Hamilton PJS: Employment grade and coronary heart disease in British civil servants. J Epidemiol Community Health 3:244–249, 1978
26. Susser MW, Watson W, Hopper K: Sociology in Medicine. New York: Oxford University Press, 1985
27. Lynch J, Kaplan GA, Salonen R, Cohen RD, Salonen JT: Socioeconomic status and carotid atherosclerosis. Circulation 92:1786–1792, 1995
28. Blacklund E, Sorlie PD, Johnson NJ: The shape of the relationship between income and mortality in the United States: evidence from the national Longitudinal Mortality Study. Ann Epidemiol 6:1–9, 1996
29. House JS, Lepkowski JM, Kinney AM, Mero RP, Kessler RC, Herzog AR: The social stratification of aging and health. J Health Soc Behav 35:213–234, 1994
30. Kuller LH, Crook M, Almes MJ: Dormont High School (Pittsburgh, PA) blood pressure study. Hypertension 2 (Suppl 1): 109–116, 1980
31. Rosner B, Hennekens CH, Kass EH, Miall WE: Age-specific correlation analysis of longitudinal blood pressure data. Am J Epidemiol 106:306–313, 1977
32. Clarke WR, Woolson RF, Lauer RM: Changes in ponderosity and blood pressure in childhood: The Muscatine Study. Am J Epidemiol 124:195–206, 1986
33. Venters MH: Family life and cardiovascular risk: implications for the prevention of chronic disease. Soc Sci Med 22:1067–1074, 1986
34. Samet JM, Tager IB, Speizer FE: The relationship between respiratory illness in childhood and chronic air-flow obstruction in adulthood. Am Rev Respir Dis 127:508–523, 1983
35. Lowry R, Kann L, Collins JL, Kolbe LJ: The effect of socioeconomic status on chronic disease risk behaviors among U.S. adolescents. JAMA 276:792–797, 1996
36. Kaplan GA, Salonen JT: Socioeconomic conditions in childhood are associated with ischaemic heart disease during middle age. Br Med J 301:1121–1123, 1990
37. Gliksman MD, Kawachi I, Hunter D, Colditz GA, Manson JE, Stampfer MJ, Speizer FE, Willett WC, Hennekens CH: Childhood socioeconomic status and risk of cardiovascular disease in middle aged US women: a prospective study. J Epidemiol Community Health 49:10–15, 1995
38. Lynch JL, Kaplan GA, Salonen JT: Why do poor people behave poorly? Variation in adult health behaviors and psychosocial characteristics by stages of the socio-economic lifecourse. Soc Sci Med, in press
39. Barker DJ: Intra-uterine programming of the adult cardiovascular system. Current Opinion in Nephrology and Hypertension 6(1): 106–110, 1997
40. Pocock SJ, Shaper AG, Cook DG, et al: Social class differences in ischemic heart disease in British men. Lancet 2:197–201, 1987
41. Davey-Smith G, Shipley MJ, Rose G: Magnitude and causes of socioeconomic differentials in mortality: further evidence from the Whitehall study. J Epidemiol Community Health 44:265–70, 1990
42. Lundberg O: Causal explanation for class inequality in health—an empirical analysis. Soc Sci Med 32:385–393, 1991
43. Markowe HLJ, Marmot MG, Shipley MJ, et al: Fibrinogen: a possible link between social class and coronary heart disease. Br Med J 291:1312–1314, 1985
44. Marmot MG, Theorell T: Social class and cardiovascular disease: the contribution of work. Int J Health Serv 18:659–689, 1988
45. Williams DR: Socioeconomic differentials in health: a review and redirection. Soc Psychol Q 53:81–99, 1990
46. Lynch JL, Kaplan GA, Cohen RD, Tuomilehto J, Salonen JT: Do known risk factors explain the relationship between socioeconomic status, risk of all-cause mortality, cardiovascular mortality and acute myocardial infarction? Am J Epidemiol, in press
47. Mackenbach JP: Socio-economic health differences in the Netherlands: a review of recent empirical findings. Soc Sci Med 34:213–226, 1992
48. Bennett S: Cardiovascular risk factors in Australia: trends in socioeconomic inequalities. J Epidemiol Community Health 49:363–372, 1995
49. Winkelby M: The future of community-based cardiovascular disease prevention studies. Am J Public Health 84:1369–1372, 1994
50. Kaplan GA: People and places: contrasting perspectives on the association between social class and health. Int J Health Serv 26: 507–519, 1996
51. Krieger N: Epidemiology and the web of causation: has anyone seen the spider? Soc Sci Med 39:887–903, 1994
52. Lynch JL: Social position and health [Editorial]. Ann Epidemiol 6:21–23, 1996
53. Syme SL: Control and health: a personal perspective. In Steptoe A, Appels A (eds): Stress, Personal Control and Health. New York: John Wiley, 1989
54. Karasek R, Baker D, Marxer F, Ahlbom A, Theorell T: Job decision latitude, job demands, and cardiovascular disease: a prospective study of Swedish men. Am J Public Health 71:694–705, 1981
55. Theorell T, Alfreddson L, Knox S, Persk A, Svensson J, Waller D: On the interplay between socioeconomic factors, personality and work environment in the pathogenesis of cardiovascular disease. Scand J Work Environ Health 10:373–380, 1984
56. Neuhauser L, Schwab M, Obarski S, Syme SL, Bieber M: Community participation in health promotion: Evaluation of a statewide wellness guide. Health Promotion International, in press, 1998
57. Haan M, Kaplan GA, Camacho T: Poverty and health: prospective evidence from the Alameda County Study. Am J Epidemiol 125:989–998, 1987
58. Anderson RT, Sorlie P, Backlund E, Johnson N, Kaplan GA. Mortality effects of community socioeconomic status. Epidemiology 8(1):42–47, 1997
59. Blaxter M: Health and Lifestyles. London: Routledge, 1990
60. Yen I, Kaplan GA: Poverty area residence and prospective change in risk behavior: evidence for the Alameda County Study. Presented at the Society for Epidemiologic Research Meeting, Boston, June 1996

61. Shouls S, Congdon P, Curtis S: Modelling inequality in reported long term illness in the UK: combining individual and area characteristics. J Epidemiol Community Health 50:366–376, 1996
61a. Wilkinson RG: Income distribution and life expectency. Br Med J 304:165–168, 1992
62. Kennedy BP, Kawachi I, Prothow-Stith D. Income distribution and mortality: cross sectional ecological study of the Robin Hood index in the United States. BMJ 312(7037):1004–1007, 1996
63. Kaplan GA, Pamuk ER, Lynch JW, Cohen RD, Balfour JL: Inequality in income and mortality in the United States: analysis of mortality and potential pathways. Br Med J 312:999–1003, 1996
64. Wolff EN: Top heavy: a study of the increasing inequality of wealth in America. New York: Twentieth Century Fund, 1995
65. Troutt DD: The thin red line: how the poor still pay more. San Francisco: West Coast Regional Office of Consumers Union, 1994
66. Macintyre S, MacIver S, Sooman A: Area, class and health: should we be focusing on places or people? J Soc Pol 22:213–234, 1993
67. Sooman A, Macintyre S, Anderson A: Scotland's health—A more difficult challence for some? The price and availability of healthy foods in socially contrasting localities in the West of Scotland. Health Bull 51:276–284, 1993
68. Lillie-Blanton M, Parsons PE, Gayle H, Dievler A: Racial differences in health: not just Black and White, but shades of gray. Annu Rev Public Health 17:411–448, 1996
69. McCord C, Freeman HP: Excess mortality in Harlem. N Engl J Med 322:173–177, 1990
70. Geronimus AT: The weathering hypothesis and the health of African-American women and infants: evidence and speculations. Ethn Dis 2:207–221, 1992
71. Kreiger N, Sidney S: Racial discrimination and blood pressure: the CARDIA study of young black and white adults. Am J Public Health 86:1370–1378, 1996
72. Carter H, Glick PC: Marriage and Divorce: A Social and Economic Study. Cambridge, MA: Harvard University Press, 1970
73. Ortmeyer CF: Variations in mortality, morbidity, and health care by marital status. In Erhardt LL, Berlin VE (eds): Mortality and Morbidity in the United States. Cambridge, MA: Harvard University Press, 1974, pp 159–188
74. Thiel HG, Parker D, Bruce T: Stress factors and the risk of myocardial infarction. Psychol Res 17:43–57, 1973
75. Weiss NS: Marital status and risk factors for coronary heart disease: the United States Health Examination Survey of Adults. Br J Prev Soc Med 27:41–43, 1973
76. Jacobs S, Ostfeld A: An epidemiological review of the mortality of bereavement. Psychosom Med 39:344–357, 1977
77. Martikainen P, Valkonen T: Mortality after the death of a spouse: rates and causes of death in a large Finnish cohort. Am J Public Health 86:1087–1093, 1996
78. Helsing K, Szklo M, Comstock G: Factors associated with mortality after widowhood. Am J Public Health 71:802–809, 1981
79. Cassel J: The contribution of the social environment to host resistance. Am J Epidemiol 104:107–123, 1976
80. Nuckolls KB, Cassel J, Kaplan BH: Psychosocial assets, life crises, and the prognosis of pregnancy. Am J Epidemiol 95:431–441, 1972
81. Berkman LF, Syme SL: Social networks, host resistance, and mortality: a nine year follow-up study of Alameda County residents. Am J Epidemiol 109:186–204, 1979
82. House JS, Robbins C, Metzner HL: The association of social relationships and activities with mortality: prospective evidence from the Tecumseh Health study. Am J Epidemiol 116:123–140, 1982
83. Schoenbach VJ, Kaplan BH, Fredman L, Kleinbaum DG: Social ties and mortality in Evans County, Georgia. Am J Epidemiol 123:577–591, 1986
84. Reed D, McGee D, Yano K, Feibleib M: Social networks and coronary heart disease among Japanese men in Hawaii. Am J Epidemiol 117:384–396, 1983
85. Blazer D: Social support and mortality in an elderly community population. Am J Epidemiol 115:684–694, 1982
86. Kaplan GA, Salonen JT, Cohen RD, Brand RJ, Syme SL, Puska P: Social connections and mortality from all causes and cardiovascular disease: prospective evidence from Eastern Finland. Am J Epidemiol 128:370–380, 1988
87. Broadhead WE, Kaplan BH, James SA, Wagner EH, Schoenbach VJ, Grimson R, Heyden S, Tibblin G, Gehlbach SH: The epidemiologic evidence for a relationship between social support and health. Am J Epidemiol 117:521–537, 1983
88. Cohen S, Syme SL (eds): Social Support and Health. New York: Academic Press, 1985
89. House JS, Landis KR, Umberson D: Social relationships and health. Science 241:540–545, 1988
90. Seeman TE, Syme SL: Social networks and coronary artery disease: a comparison of the structure and function of social relations as predictors of disease. Psychosom Dis 49:341–354, 1987
91. Selye H: The Stress of Life. New York: McGraw-Hill, 1956
92. McEwan BS, Stellar E: Stress and the individual: mechanisms leading to disease. Arch Intern Med 153:2093–2101, 1993
93. Seeman TE, Bruce ML, McAvay G: Social network characteristics and onset of ADL disability: MacArthur studies of successful aging. J Gerontol B Psychol Sci Soc Sci 51:S191–S200, 1996
94. Ader R, Felten DL, Cohen N (eds): Psychoneuroimmunology. 2nd ed. New York: Academic Press, 1991
95. Kiecolt-Glaser JK, Glaser R: Stress and immune function in humans. In Ader R, Felten DL, Cohen N (eds): Psychoneuroimmunology. 2nd ed. New York: Academic Press, 1991, pp 849–867
96. Irwin M, Daniels M, Smith TL, Bloom E, Weiner H: Impaired natural killer cell activity during bereavement. Brain Behav Immun 1:98–104, 1987
97. Schliefer SJ, Keller SE, Camerino M, Thornton JC, Stein M: Suppression of lymphocyte stimulation following bereavement. JAMA 250:374–377, 1983
98. Kiecolt-Glaser JK, Fisher L, Ogrocki P, Stout JC, Speicher CE, Glaser R: Marital quality, marital disruption and immune function. Psychosom Med 49:13–34, 1987
99. Kiecolt-Glaser JK, Kennedy S, Malkoff S, Fisher L, Speicher CE, Glaser R: Marital discord and immunity in males. Psychosom Med 50:213–229, 1988
100. Kiecolt-Glaser JK, Garner W, Speicher CE, Penn G, Glaser R: Psychosocial modifiers of immunocompetence in medical students. Psychosom Med 46:7–14, 1984
101. Glaser R, Rice J, Speicher CE, Stout JC, Kiecolt-Glaser JK: Stress depresses interferon production by leukocytes concomitant with a decrease in natural killer cell activity. Behav Neurosci 100:675–678, 1986
102. Glaser R, Kiecolt-Glaser JK, Speicher CE, Holliday JE: Stress, loneliness, and changes in herpesvirus latency. J Behav Med 8:249–260, 1985
103. Kiecolt-Glaser JK, Glaser R, Strain E, Stout J, Tarr K, et al: Modulation of cellular immunity in medical students. J Behav Med 9:5–21, 1986
104. Kiecolt-Glaser JK, Glaser R: Caregiving, mental health, and immune function. In Light E, Lebowitz B (eds): Alzheimer's Disease Treatment and Family Stress: Directions for Research. Washington, DC: National Institute of Mental Health, 1989
105. Easterling BA, Kiecolt-Glaser JK, Bodnar JC, Glaser R: Chronic stress, social support, and persistent alterations in the natural killer cell response to cytokines in older adults. Health Psychol 13: 291–298, 1994
106. Kiecolt-Glaser JK, Newton T, Cacioppo JT, MacCallum RC, Glaser R, Malarkey WB: Marital conflict and endocrine function: are men really more physiologically affected than women? J Consult Clin Psychol 64:324–332, 1996
107. Easterling BA, Kiecolt-Glaser JK, Glaser R: Psychosocial modulation of cytokine-induced natural killer cell activity in older adults. Psychosom Med 58:264–272, 1996

108. Holmes TH, Rahe RH: The Social Readjustment Rating Scale. J Psychosom Res 11:213–218, 1967
109. Dohrenwend BS, Dohrenwend BP: Stressful Life Events: Their Nature and Effects. New York: Wiley-Interscience, 1974
110. Parens H, McConville BJ, Kaplan SM: Prediction of frequency of illness from the response to separation: a preliminary study and replication attempt. Psychosom Med 28:162–176, 1966
111. Thurlow HJ: Illness in relation to life situation and sick-role tendency. J Psychosom Res 15:73–88, 1971
112. Spilken AZ, Jacobs MA: Prediction of illness behavior from measures of life changes. J Psychosom Res 14:410– 406, 1970
113. Dembroski TM (ed): Proceedings of the Forum on Coronary-Prone Behavior. DHEW Publication No. NIH 78-1451. Washington, DC: Government Printing Office, 1977
114. Rosenman RH, Brand RJ, Jenkins CD, Friedman M, Straus R, Wurm M: Coronary heart disease in the Western Collaborative Group Study: final follow-up experience of 8½ years. JAMA 233: 872–877, 1975
115. Ragland DR, Brand RJ: Coronary heart disease mortality in the Western Collaborative Group Study: follow-up experience of 22 years. Am J Epidemiol 127:462–475, 1988
116. Ragland DR, Brand RJ: Type A behavior and mortality from coronary heart disease. N Engl J Med 318:65–69, 1988
117. Shoham-Yakubovich I, Ragland DR, Brand RJ, Syme SL: Type A behavior pattern and health status after 22 years of follow-up in the Western Collaborative Group Study. Am J Epidemiol 128:579–588, 1988
118. Shekelle RB, Hulley SB, Neaton JD, Billings JH, Borhani NO, Gerace TA, Jacobs DR, Lasser NL, Mittlemark MB, Stamler J: The MRFIT behavior pattern study II: Type A behavior and incidence of coronary heart disease. Am J Epidemiol 122:559–570, 1985
119. Aspirin Myocardial Infarction Study Research Group. A randomized, controlled trial of aspirin in persons recovered from myocardial infarction. JAMA 243:661–668, 1980
120. Friedman M, Thoresen CE, Gill JJ, Powell LH, Ulmer D, Thompson L, Price VA, Rabin DD, Breall WS, Dixon T, Levy R, Bourg E: Alteration of Type A behavior and reduction in cardiac recurrences in post myocardial infarction patients. Am Heart J 108:237–248, 1984
121. Matthews KA, Glass DC, Rosenman RH: Competitive drive, pattern A, and coronary heart disease: a further analysis of some data from the Western Collaborative Group Study. J Chronic Dis 30: 489–498, 1977
122. MacDougall JM, Dembroski TM, Dimsdale JE: Components of Type A, hostility and anger: Further relationships to angiographic findings. J Health Psychol 4:137–152, 1985
123. Dembroski TM, Mac Dougall JM, Williams RD: Components of Type A, hostility and anger: relationship to angiographic findings. Psychosom Med 47:219–233, 1985
124. Shekelle RB, Gale M, Ostfeld AM: Hostility, risk of coronary heart disease and mortality. Psychosom Med 45:109–114, 1983
125. Barefoot JC, Dahlstrom WG, Williams RB: Hostility, CHD incidence and total mortality: a 25 year follow-up study of 255 physicians. Psychosom Med 45:59–63, 1983
126. Dembroski TM, Costa PT: Assessment of coronary-prone behavior: a current overview: Ann Behav Med 10:60–63, 1988
127. Matthews KA: Coronary heart disease and type A behaviors: update on and alternative to the Booth-Kewlwy and Freidman quantitative review. Psychol Bull 104:373–380, 1988
128. Goldstein MG, Niaura R: Psychological factors affecting physical condition: cardiovascular disease literature review. Psychosomatics 33:134–155, 1992
129. Julkenen J, Salonen R, Kaplan GA, Chesney MA, Salonen JT: Hostility and progression of carotid atherosclerosis. Psychosom Med 56:519–525, 1994
130. Hecker MH, Chesney MA, Black GW: Coronary-prone behavior in the Western Group Collaborative Study. Psychosom Med 50: 153–164, 1988
131. Kanner AD, Coyne JC, Schaefer C, et al: Comparison of two modes of stress management: daily hassles and uplifts vs. major life events. J Behav Med 4:1–38, 1981
132. Kahn HA, Medalie JH, Newfeld HN, et al: The incidence of hypertension and associated factors: the Israeli Ischemic Heart Disease Study. Am Heart J 84:171–182, 1972
133. Haynes SG, Feinleib M, Kannel WB: The relationship of psychosocial factors to coronary heart disease in the Framingham study: eight-year incidence of coronary heart disease. Am J Epidemiol 111:37–58, 1980
134. Kawachi I, Sparrow D, Spiro A, Vokonas P, Weiss ST: A prospective study of anger and coronary heart disease: the normative aging study. Circulation 94:2090–2095, 1996
135. Glass DC: Behavior Patterns, Stress and Coronary Disease. Hillsdale, NJ: Lawrence Erlbaum, 1977
136. Scherwitz L, Berton K, Leventhal H: Type A behavior, self-involvement, and cardiovascular response. Psychosom Med 40: 593–609, 1978
137. Matthews KA: Psychological perspectives on the Type A behavior pattern. Psychol Bull 91:293–323, 1982
138. Kobasa SC, Maddi SR, Kahn S: Hardiness and health: a prospective study. J Pers Soc Psychol 42:168–177, 1982
139. Scheier MF, Carver CS: Optimism, coping and health: assessment and implications of generalized outcome expectencies. Health Psychol 4:219–247, 1985
140. Anda R, Williamson D, Jones D, Macera C, Eaker E, Glassman A, Marks A: Depressed affect, hopelessness, and the risk of ischemic heart disease in a cohort of U.S. adults. Epidemiology 4:285–294, 1993
141. Everson SA, Goldberg DE, Kaplan GA, Cohen RD, Pukkala E, Tuomilehto J, Salonen JT: Hopelessness and risk of mortality and incidence of myocardial infarction and cancer. Psychosom Med 58:113–131, 1996
142. Everson SA, Kaplan GA, Goldberg DE, Salonen R, Salonen JT: Hopelessness and 4-year progression of carotid athersclerosis: the Kuopio Ischemic Heart Disease Risk Factor Study. Atherosclerosis, Thrombosis, and Vascular Biology, 17(8):1490–1495, 1997
143. Farquhar JW, Fortmann SP, Flora JA, Taylor CB, Haskell WL, et al: Effects of community-wide education on cardiovascular disease risk factors. JAMA 264:359–365, 1990
144. Luepker RV, Murray DM, Jacobs DR, Mittelmark MB, Bracht N, et al.: Community education for cardiovascular disease prevention: risk factor changes in the Minnesota Heart Health Program. Am J Public Health 84:1383–1393, 1994
145. Puska P, Nissinen A, Tuomilehto J, Salonen JT, Koskela K, et al: The community-based strategy to prevent coronary heart disease: conclusions from the ten years of the North Karelia Project. Annu Rev Public Health 6:147–193, 1985
146. Community Intervention Trial for Smoking Cessation (COMMIT): II. Changes in adult cigarette smoking prevalence. Am J Public Health 85:193–200, 1995
147. McBeath WM: Health for all: a public health vision. Am J Public Health 81:1560–1565, 1990
148. Tonon MA: Concepts in community participation: a case of sanitary change in a Guatamalan village. Int J Health Ed 23S:1–16, 1980
149. Whyte WF: Participatory approaches to agricultural research and development: a state-of-the-art paper. Ithaca, NY: Center for International Studies, Cornell University, 1981
150. Martin PA: Community Participation in Primary Health Care. Washington DC: American Public Health Association, 1983
151. Minkler M: Building supportive ties and sense of community among the inner-city elderly: the Tenderloin Senior Outreach project. Health Ed Q 12:303–314, 1985

152. Eng E, Briscoe J, Cunningham A: Participation effect from water projects on EPI. Soc Sci Med 30:1349–1358, 1990
153. Green L, Kreuter M: Health Promotion Planning: An Educational and Environmental Approach. Mountain View, CA: Mayfield, 1991
154. Kegeles SM, Hays RB, Coates TJ: The empowerment project: a community-level prevention intervention for young gay men. Am J Public Health 86:1129–1135, 1996
155. Ragland DR, Winkelby MA, Schwalbe J, Holman BL, Morse L, Syme SL, Fisher JM: Prevalence of hypertension in bus drivers. Int J Epidemiol 16:208–214, 1987
156. Morris JN, Kagen A, Pattison DC, Gardner MJ, Raffle PAB: Incidence and prediction of ischaemic heart disease in London busmen. Lancet 2:553, 1966
157. Netterstrom B, Laursen P: Incidence and prevalence of ischaemic heart disease among urban bus drivers in Copenhagen. Institute of Social Medicine, University of Copenhagen, Denmark. Scand J Soc Med 2:75–79, 1981
158. Berlinguer G: Maladies and Industrial Health of Public Transportation Workers. Italian Institute of Social Medicine, 1962
159. Pikus VG, Taranikkova VA: Hypertension disease in drivers of passenger motor transport. Ter Arkh 47:135, 1975
160. Garke C: Health and Health Risks Among City Bus Drivers in West Berlin. Institute for Social Medicine and Epidemiology of the Ministry of Health, 1980
161. Winkelby MA, Ragland DR, Fisher JM, Syme SL: Excess risk of sickness and disease in bus drivers: a review and synthesis of epidemiologic studies. Int J Epidemiol 17:124–134, 1988
162. Winkelby MA, Ragland DR, Syme SL: Self-reported stressors and hypertension: evidence of an inverse association. Am J Epidemiol 127:124–134, 1988
163. Syme SL: Rethinking disease: where do go from here? Ann Epidemiol 6:463–468, 1996
164. Bartrop RW, Lockhurst E, Lazarus L, Kiloh HG, Penny R: Depressed lymphocyte function after bereavement. Lancet 1:834–836, 1977
165. Jackson GG, Dowling HF, Anderson TO, Riff L, Saporta J, Turek M: Susceptibility and immunity to common upper respiratory viral infection—the common cold. Ann Intern Med 53:719–738, 1960
166. Jemmott JB III, Borysenko JZ, Borysenko M, McClelland DC, Chapman R, Meyer D, Benson H: Academic stress, power motivation, and decrease in salivary secretory immunoglobulin and secretion rate. Lancet 1:1400–1402, 1983
167. Kiecolt-Glaser JK, Garner W, Speisher C, Penn GM, Holliday J, Glaser R: Psychosocial modifiers of immuno-competence in medical students. Psychosom Med 46:7–14, 1984
168. Schleifer SJ, Keller SE, Camerino M, Thornton JC, Stein M: Suppression of lymphocyte stimulation following bereavement. JAMA 250:374–377, 1984
169. Totman RG, Kiff J: Life stress and susceptibility to colds. In Oborne DJ, Gruneberg MM, Eiser JR (eds): Research in Psychology and Medicine. vol 1. New York: Academic Press, 1979, pp 141–149
170. Sklar LS, Anisman H: Stress and coping factors influence tumor growth. Science 205:513–515, 1979
171. Visitainer MA, Volpicelli JR, Seligman MEP: Tumor rejection in rats after inescapable shock. Science 216:437– 439, 1982
172. Laudenslager ML, Ryan SM, Drugan RC, Hyson RL, Maier SF: Coping and immunosuppression: inescapable but not escapable shock suppresses lymphocyte proliferation. Science 221:568–571, 1983
173. Syme SL: Control and health: an epidemiologic perspective. In Schaie KW, Rodin J, Schooler C (eds): Self-Directedness: Cause and Effects throughout the Life Course. Hillsdale, NJ: Erlbaum, in press
174. Cohen S: Control and the epidemiology of physical health: where do we go from here? In Schaie KW, Rodin J, Schooler C (eds): Self-Directedness: Cause and Effects throughout the Life Course. Hillsdale, NJ: Erlbaum, in press
175. Berrueta-Clement JR, Schweinhart LJ, Barrett WS, Epstein AS, Weikart DP: Changed Lives: The Effects of the Perry Preschool Program on Youths through Age 19. Ypsilanti, MI: High/Scope Press, 1984
176. Richmond JB, Beardslee WR: Resiliency: research and practical implications for pediatricians. Dev Behav Pediatr 9:157–163, 1988
177. Werner E: High-risk children in young adulthood: a longitudinal study from birth to 32 years. Am J Orthopsychiatry 59:72–81, 1989
178. Susser M: The logic in ecological: I. The logic of analysis. Am J Public Health 84:825–829, 1994

43

Health Behavior

Kristi J. Ferguson

While estimates of the relative contribution of lifestyle factors to health problems vary, it is clear that many of the major public health problems of our time have a significant individual decision-making/behavior component. With one exception, the 22 areas covered by the Healthy People 2000 Objectives all include components pertaining to individual behavior.[1] In addition, according to the *Clinician's Handbook of Preventive Services*, "Many of the most serious disorders encountered in clinical practice can be prevented or postponed by immunizations, chemoprophylaxis, and healthier lifestyles, or detected early with screening and treated effectively."[2] For example, Healthy People 2000 states elimination of measles as a goal (Objective 20.1). Aggressive campaigns to increase compliance with immunization against childhood diseases have required proof of immunization to enter school, yet measles has experienced a resurgence from its all-time low of 1,500 cases in 1983 to 16,000 cases in 1989. The prevalence of diseases such as pneumococcal pneumonia and hepatitis B[3] could be substantially reduced with broader utilization of available vaccines.

Almost 12 million cases of sexually transmitted diseases occur annually in the United States[1] and most could be prevented by condom use. Transmission of viral and bacterial diseases in day-care settings could potentially be reduced by frequent hand-washing, and transmission of food-borne diseases could be prevented by safer handling of foods. Health risks associated with pesticides could be reduced by safer handling of pesticides, and harm-causing noise pollution could be reduced through use of personal protective equipment.

The morbidity and mortality associated with chronic diseases such as cancer, heart disease, hypertension, and diabetes mellitus could be significantly reduced through lifestyle modification. For example, the proportion of fat in the average American diet is well above recommended levels and most Americans do not engage in regular physical activity.[1] Deaths due to motor vehicle accidents could be reduced by proper use of seat belts, observing speed limits, and avoiding drinking and driving. Finally, unintentional injuries could be reduced by properly installing fire alarms and regularly changing the batteries.

In summary, modifiable health-related behavior contributes substantially to excess morbidity and mortality. Although developing interventions to change behavior is no simple matter, the potential benefits are great.

▶ ENVIRONMENTAL AND SOCIAL CONTEXT

While individual behavioral factors contribute significantly to most major health problems, the behavior takes place in an environmental and societal context. Some have argued that focusing exclusively on the individual ignores societal and group factors that significantly influence health and in essence blame the victim.[4–6] Others have suggested that researchers and those developing programs use a multilevel approach to include both individual and societal factors.[7] In the case of smoking, for example, legislation can influence norms regarding smoking, employers can support treatment or change worksite policies, and insurance companies can provide reimbursement for treatment.[8]

Healthy People 2000 suggests that reduction of morbidity and mortality is a shared responsibility of the individual, family, community, health professionals, media, and government.[1] The degree to which this responsibility is shared depends to some extent on the nature of the change, the privacy rights of the individual, and the likelihood of success when various components have major responsibility for reducing morbidity and mortality.

Planning models such as PRECEDE, which addresses predisposing, enabling, and reinforcing variables, explicitly include factors in the community that reinforce individual behavior and/or enable it.[9] For example, having healthy alternatives available for school lunches will not guarantee that students will select those choices, but it increases the likelihood that students will eat healthy foods. Alternatively, providing hepatitis B vaccinations at the worksite and covering the cost for health care workers can favorably influence vaccination rates.

In addition, the degree to which health professionals or policymakers are willing to intrude in an individual's life varies. On the one hand, some health professionals or government officials believe that society's responsibility is only to educate people and that the ultimate decision-making belongs to the individual. On the other hand, there are those who mandate legislative or policy changes as the most effective and efficient strategy, as, for example, requiring air bags in new automobiles and thereby removing responsibility from the individual. When legal steps are taken, however, there should be very strong evidence that they are the most effective means to achieve the desired outcome.

Health care professionals who favor individual approaches believe it is not society's role to wrest decision-making and responsibility from the individual. "Empowerment" is a popular term in health education and it implies that the primary outcome should be to empower individuals to make decisions that they perceive are in their best interest, rather than to get them to do what the health care provider dictates. The self-regulation approach, in which individuals learn to observe their own behavior, make judgments about whether a particular action has been effective (e.g., whether they are satisfied with the level of disease control), and then make adjustments, has shown encouraging results in reducing morbidity associated with asthma.[10]

The degree to which society is willing to take steps to control an individual's behavior depends on a number of considerations.[11] Public health approaches to such problems as sexually transmitted disease and tuberculosis have argued that the individual's rights can be abrogated when that individual can harm others directly. It is less clear whether society has the right to declare harm or assign economic responsibility when such effects are indirect, as in the case of careless behavior such as not wearing a motorcycle helmet. Enforcement of the resource issue is problematic for a number of reasons. First, denying treatment would be harsh if the individual could not afford to pay. Second, the idea of seeking financial reimbursement or exacting penalties raises questions of science and evidence, namely, whether a certain proportion of the responsibility can clearly be shown to rest with the individual versus what was purely due to chance. Third, this approach raises the potential that intervening variables may be as much to blame as the individual's own behavior. Finally, putting health care providers in the role of enforcer of this approach removes them from the role of healer.

In addition to philosophical or ethical considerations, deciding which alternatives give the best result in terms of effectiveness and efficiency is important. Some would argue that societal or community-level change is the only effective way to implement lasting change. Others would suggest that even societal changes should be accompanied by interventions addressed to individuals. An example of a multifaceted approach would be smoking reduction, which has included efforts to reduce youth access to tobacco, increase taxes, provide school-based education programs about the hazards of smoking, develop practitioner-based interventions to help individuals stop smoking, and promote public, media-based education about the hazards of smoking.

A multifaceted approach has also been used to reduce alcohol-related traffic deaths. Advocacy organizations have lobbied for stricter laws about drunk driving, policymakers have adopted changes in the legal drinking age, educational approaches have been directed toward school-age children, and health care providers have encouraged insurance carriers to increase resources for substance abuse treatment.

Models of Health Behavior

Health Belief Model

A number of models have been developed to explain health-related behavior from the individual perspective. The Health Belief Model, for example, was originally developed from value expectancy theory to explain the likelihood that an individual would obtain an immunization.[12] The initial model included four major variables: perceived susceptibility, or the individual's perception about his or her own likelihood of contracting a condition; perceived severity, or the seriousness the individual would assign to such a condition were it to happen; perceived benefits of the proposed action, or the individual's perception about the likelihood that a given action would succeed in reducing or eliminating harm; and perceived barriers, or factors that would interfere with the individual's taking the desired action.

A review of studies of the Health Belief Model showed that perceived susceptibility and perceived barriers were most strongly associated with preventive health behavior, while perceived severity, perceived benefits, and perceived barriers were most strongly associated with sick role behavior or behavior related to treatment for a known condition such as taking medication for hypertension.[13] The Health Belief Model has been quite successful in predicting a variety of behaviors in cross-sectional studies. Efforts to modify an individual's health beliefs in order to modify behavior have not been as common, however.

Theory of Reasoned Action

Another model that has been used to study health behavior is Fishbein and Ajzen's Theory of Reasoned Action.[14] As originally formulated, the Theory of Reasoned Action examined an individual's attitudes toward a particular behavior (perceived advantages and disadvantages) and subjective norms about the behavior (the individual's perceptions about whether significant individuals would approve or disapprove of the behavior) to explain intention to behave in a particular way. Intention is a strong predictor of how the individual will ultimately behave. Ajzen later added the idea of the individual's ability to exercise volitional control over the behavior. This control includes both internal factors (e.g., possessing the skill to monitor blood glucose and administer insulin injections) or external factors (e.g., having resources to buy healthy foods).

A review of 58 studies of Planned Behavior Theory concluded that the model had substantial predictive power across a range of behaviors (addictive behaviors, clinical screening, driving, eating, exercising, human immunodeficiency virus (HIV)/acquired immunodeficiency syndrome (AIDS), and oral hygiene).[15] The study also concluded that the addition of perceived control significantly benefited the model. One drawback, however, was that there were measurement issues related to what was meant by perceived control, i.e., in some instances it meant how effective the individual perceived himself or herself to be in executing the desired behavior while in others it pertained more to external barriers to success.

Transtheoretical Model (Stages of Change Model)

A third model that has been used fairly extensively in health behavior research is the Transtheoretical Model by DiClemente and colleagues (originally called the Stages of Change Model).[16] The Transtheoretical Model was developed because existing models were believed to be too static, i.e., they did not adequately represent individual shifts from one stage of readiness to another. This model was originally developed from a large cross-sectional study of smokers who had attempted to stop smoking on their own. The Precontemplation Stage represented individuals who were not planning to quit smoking in the next 6 months. The Contemplation Stage included those who were planning to quit within the next 6 months. The Action Stage was for those who had started to quit smoking but had not yet completed the process. The Maintenance Stage included those who had quit smoking but had maintained it for less than 1 year. The Preparation Stage was added later for those who were planning to quit smoking within the next month and had begun the process but had not yet stopped completely.

In the Transtheoretical Model, individuals move from one stage to the other based on their assessment of the advantages (pros) and disadvantages (cons) of a particular action, termed "decision balance." In an application of the Transtheoretical Model to prevention of HIV infection, pros accounted for more of the variance in movement across stages while cons remained constant.[17]

In a study of 12 behaviors, Prochaska and others noted that the relative strengths of pros and cons differ for different behaviors and at different stages.[18] For example, the cons were higher than the pros in the Precontemplation Stage for all behaviors except smoking, while the pros were higher than the cons for the Action and Maintenance Stages except for cocaine and smoking.

Relapse Prevention Model

The Relapse Prevention Model of Marlatt and Gordon has guided recent research into addictive behaviors.[19,20] Their approach includes perceived self-efficacy as a significant mediator for relapse prevention. Those who successfully avoid relapse have identified situations in which relapse has occurred for them in the past and have developed a plan for dealing with potential relapse situations in the future.[21] How individuals attribute responsibility for lapses (called the "abstinence violation effect") determines whether they interpret a lapse as temporary or as the first step in a permanent relapse.

While relapse prevention research began in dealing with addictive behavior, extending it to health behaviors such as weight control and exercise programs has proven fruitful. For example, individuals who successfully lost weight and maintained the weight loss viewed deviations from their dietary goals as temporary slips that could be made up for, rather than as evidence of a personal failure.[22] In the case of exercise, increasing awareness of obstacles to exercise and developing appropriate strategies for addressing them show small but consistent benefits.[23]

Social Learning Theory

Social Learning Theory is widely cited and used in research about health behavior.[24] Two particularly important concepts in the field of health behavior research came out of this theory. One concept is social modeling. In social modeling interventions, someone demonstrates (either live or through videotape) an example of the desired behavior. Observers then attempt to apply or practice the technique and are reinforced for appropriate responses. Many educational campaigns, both school-based and media-based, use this approach. Small group exercises in which students practice dealing with situations they are likely to face, for example, refusing an offer of a cigarette, are developed from social learning theory.

Another important concept in Social Learning Theory is that of self-efficacy. According to Bandura, "An efficacy expectation is the conviction that one can successfully execute the behavior required to produce the outcomes."[24] Outcome expectations, on the other hand, refer to the individual's belief that undertaking a particular behavior will lead to a desired outcome. For example, self-efficacy related to exercise would indicate that the individual believes himself or herself to be capable of initiating and maintaining an exercise program, while outcome expectations would indicate the expectation that engaging in an exercise program would lead to better health.

Although self-efficacy and self-esteem may be related, self-efficacy is distinct from self-esteem in that it describes self-perception in relation to a specific behavior or objective rather than a general view of one's self-worth. A review of studies relating self-efficacy to behavior change suggests that an individual's self-efficacy can be modified and that doing so has potential benefit in implementing and maintaining behavior change.[25]

A recent review compared four models of health behavior: the Health Belief Model, the Theory of Reasoned Action, Protection Motivation Theory, and Subjective Expected Utility Theory.[26] The review concluded that all of the models had four basic concepts: severity of the result given no action, probability or likelihood of that result happening to a given individual, the expected effect (benefits), and the cost. Self-efficacy was considered separately in some models and as another barrier to action in others. Weinstein argues that the one problem with research in health behavior is that mathematical models are not adequately specified.[26] Other factors of interest may be the familiarity or novelty of the behavior, whether one is initiating or stopping a behavior, whether the consequences are imminent versus delayed, and whether other variables intervene between intentions and actions.

Decision-making Theory

The literature on decision-making has relevance for those interested in studying health behavior. A classic book by Janis and Mann pulled together existing literature to develop a conflict model of decision-making that consisted of five stages.[27] In Stage 1, appraising the challenge, the individual decides whether the risks are serious if he or she does not change. In Stage 2, surveying alternatives, the individual decides whether an alternative is acceptable and whether all alternatives have been considered. In Stage 3, weighing alternatives, the individual decides which alternative is best and whether certain essential requirements of a particular decision have been met. In Stage 4, deliberating about commitment, the individual decides whether to act and whether to let others know. In Stage 5, adhering despite negative feedback, the individual decides whether the benefits outweigh the risks.

One review of decision-making theory related to health suggests that the ideal decision-maker would gather all available information about the situation, calculate the costs and benefits of every feasible option, and then decide on the optimal choice.[28] In contrast to the ideal, however, people reach judgments based on simplifying heuristic rules and search until they find an acceptable solution, not necessarily the best solution. One decision-making concept related to health behavior is the notion of categorical safety and danger. Humans tend to categorize an entity as either "dangerous" or "safe" without recognizing that low and high levels of exposure can have different or even opposite effects. For example, some people still fear that even the most trivial contact with anyone having AIDS is dangerous.

Another decision-making concept that has relevance for health behavior is the idea of "zero risk." People often discriminate more sharply than is appropriate between interventions that eliminate a risk and interventions that merely reduce it. While lessening the odds is the realistic aim in most cases, it has far less appeal than the illusion of perfect safety, e.g., the risk of getting AIDS from a blood transfusion today is very low, but it is not zero. Helping individuals understand very small probabilities requires listing concrete events that have similar likelihoods; for example, one in 20,000 corresponds to the chance that a person will live more than 100 years and one in 200,000 to the chance that an airline flight will be highjacked.

Measurement Issues

Measuring Health-Related Behavior

Definition of the target behavior is an important first step in planning an educational program geared to changing people's health-related behavior. While program planners may not have the resources to collect the depth and breadth of information normally collected in intervention studies, doing assessments regarding the prevalence of target behaviors, attitudes, and the level of readiness to change can significantly influence the development of programs.

In the Theory of Reasoned Action, defining the behavior involves four elements: action, target, time, and context.[14] Epidemiologic data can help determine behaviors most likely to have public health consequences. So in a public health intervention program to reduce risk behavior related to sexually transmitted diseases, for example, examples of the target behavior might be as follows: "To use (action) a condom (target) during the next sexual intercourse (time) with a new partner who takes contraceptive pills (context)." Another example might be: "To reduce the amount of saturated fat in the diet from 30 g/day to 20 g/day within 6 weeks." A third example: "To increase exercise from 20 minutes three times a week to 30 minutes 3 times per week in the first month by adding mall walking when the weather is not conducive to outdoor activity."

Other dimensions to consider in defining health behavior include whether it is an acquisition behavior change (e.g., condom use) or a termination behavior (e.g., smoking cessation), whether it is addictive or nonaddictive, how often it occurs (many times/day to yearly or even once), whether it is legal or illegal, public or private, socially acceptable or not socially acceptable.[29] All of these dimensions have implications for the type and level of intervention.

Measuring Attitudes

The next step is assessment of attitudes that might be expected to influence the behavior. These might include perception of risk, decisional balance, and perceptions about the tradeoffs involved in changing behavior. Different theories use different terminology for these concepts. In the Health Belief Model, they are called perceived benefits and perceived barriers. In the Theory of Reasoned Action, they are called the advantages and disadvantages; and in the Transtheoretical Model, pros and cons. But they all share the same general rationale, i.e., that individuals weigh the positive and negative aspects involved in making a behavior change and behave in ways that will maximize the potential benefit while minimizing the potential harm.

In listing the advantages and disadvantages of the desired behavior (pros and cons), one can also list influential individuals who might approve or disapprove of the recommended action.[3] This can be especially helpful when planning public education campaigns in which one wants credible sources of information to deliver the health information. Another dimension to consider is the potential affective benefits of *unhealthy* behaviors. For example, some unhealthy behaviors have mood enhancing characteristics (they help the individual unwind or relax) while others have mood-diminishing characteristics (they reduce anxiety or reduce shyness) which may make them more resistant to change.

In a study that looked at general contraceptive use and condoms, researchers selected five pros and five cons for each behavior and asked respondents to rate importance on a five-point scale.[30] They also assessed self-efficacy in specific situations; for example, they asked respondents to rate their own confidence in handling certain circumstances such as when a partner might get angry at the suggestion of using a condom. That same study examined pros and cons of condom use. Examples of specific items for pros for condoms would be: "I would be safer from disease." "It is easily available." "It protects my partner as well as myself." Examples of cons would be: "It would be too much trouble." "My partner would be angry." "My partner would think that I do not trust him."[17]

Positive or negative wording about gains and losses can significantly influence individual perceptions and therefore decisions. Psychological research has shown that people are often sensitive to the presentation of problems and that they fail to realize the extent to which their preferences can be altered by an inconsequential change in formulation.[28] For example, one could say that of 100 patients undergoing surgery for lung cancer, 90 live through the postoperative period, and 34 are alive at the end of 5 years. Alternatively, 10 die during the postoperative period and 66 die by the end of 5 years. A recent study showed that the difference between 10 percent mortality and 0 percent mortality was more impressive to patients considering lung surgery than the difference between 90 percent survival and 100 percent survival.[28]

In discussing "decisional balance," Janis and Mann categorize pros and cons according to whether they are gains or losses for self, gains or losses for significant others, self-approval or self-disapproval, and approval or disapproval of others.[27] Others have simply listed pros and cons without distinguishing those related to self versus others. Questions related to decisional balance can be answered in terms of their importance for making a decision to change a specified problem behavior (rated on a five-point Likert scale ranging from 1, not important, to 5, extremely important). A study of exercise behavior assessed potential obstacles to exercise by the following questions: "What is the probability it will rain this weekend?" and "If it rains this weekend, what are the chances that I will participate in the planned cycling tour with my friends?"[31]

Examples of attitudes toward breast self-examination might include: "If I have breast cancer, I can find it with breast self-examination." "I'll get early, effective treatment, and I'll be cured, extending healthy productive life." "I will do breast self-examination regularly" (intention).[32] Examples of a pro of contraceptive use: "I would be safer from pregnancy."

Measuring Readiness to Change

Measuring an individual's readiness to change can allow educational and behavioral interventions to be specifically targeted. As Prochaska notes, "The vast majority of our behavior change programs are designed for the small minority of the people who are ready to take action on their health behavior problems."[33] Using a seven-point scale ranging from "extremely sure I will" to "extremely sure I won't" can help determine an individual's readiness, as can asking for a time frame regarding when a behavior change is planned.

In one study of contraception, for example, those in the Precontemplation Stage had neutral or negative intent to start using contraception regularly.[30] Those in the Contemplation Stage intended to start using contraception within 6 months, while those in the Preparation Stage planned to use contraceptives all of the time and reported some use. Individuals in the Action Stage used contraceptives every time or all of the time for less than 6 months, and individuals in the Maintenance Stage had used contraceptives for 6 months or more.

Intervention Strategies

Several important decisions need to be made when developing interventions to change health behavior. Whether one targets an individual, policies, laws, or some combination is a first step. In targeting individuals, whether one addresses knowledge, attitudes, skills, or all three is also important. Deciding on the content of the educational message is key, as is determining the method of delivering the program.

Decision to Target Individual or Policies

Abby King, in a discussion of physical activity, compares individual and community approaches and suggests ways to broaden individually targeted interventions to involve the community.[34] For example, she describes a worksite program to increase use of stairs. Encouraging building design that makes stairs more convenient to use than elevators is another way to enhance physical activity.

While some interventions focus more on the individual than others, it is helpful whenever feasible to measure both community and individual variables in order to assess the relative contributions of each to the outcome. Von Korff and colleagues discuss dental caries as being a problem of individual factors (genetic or behavioral), social factors (dietary or hygiene practices), and environment (fluoridated water supply).[7]

Smoking is another behavior that has required intervention on multiple fronts to reduce its prevalence. Reducing youth access, regulating smoking in public areas, eliminating advertising from television, educating the public about the hazards of smoking and the benefits of quitting, teaching school-age children to resist pressure to smoke, offering cessation counseling, and developing effective nicotine replacement therapy when indicated have all played a role in reducing morbidity and mortality related to smoking.

Decision to Target Knowledge, Attitudes, or Skills

A common mistake in public health education is to assume that simply arming people with more information will solve the problem. While lack of information can be a contributing factor, favorable attitudes and skills may also be required. Another mistake is the tendency to give information in very large doses, which is not very effective since the information is often not absorbed or retained.

Effective education should be relevant for a given individual, the message should be personalized, the individual should receive feedback about performance, progress should be reinforced, and written materials should be provided.[35] Readiness to change is an important attitude to consider in designing interventions. Different strategies are more appropriate for different stages of change. For example, effort directed toward individuals in the Precontemplation Stage should be geared toward persuading individuals regarding the benefits of changing their behavior relative to the risk of not doing so. Efforts for individuals in the Action Stage should be directed toward implementing a plan for changing the behavior. Motivation can be enhanced by getting the individual to articulate potential benefits of change rather than imposing one's own ideas.

Deciding on the Message Itself

Health education campaigns may attempt to increase an individual's willingness to change by raising the level of concern about potential consequences. While this can be effective in terms of moving individuals toward a greater state of readiness to change, it can have a deleterious effect if the individual simply avoids thinking about the behavior or if the anxiety level becomes too uncomfortable.[36] Therefore construction of the content and presentation of a health-related message is extremely important. Another consideration is whether to present counterarguments to the main message in order to rebut them. In many instances, anticipating the counterarguments and providing alternate evidence can prepare individuals to resist pressure from those with opposing viewpoints, a process termed "inoculation."[37] A final concept to consider in the design of educational messages concerns the order in which information is presented, called "primacy/ recency." People tend to remember best the part of the message that they hear first or last.[37]

Deciding on the Method of Delivery

Most health education messages are delivered through individuals who are believed to be authoritative about a particular health issue.[37]

In some cases, that individual is a health care provider. In others, it may be a volunteer or someone who is paid to deliver an educational message. Several questions should be considered in deciding the most appropriate source of information. For example, is the individual credible, that is, does he or she have the expertise necessary to make the statements that are proposed? Second, is the source trustworthy, or does he or she have anything to gain from presenting information in a certain way (e.g., are there potential financial benefits to recommending a particular course of treatment?). Finally, to what degree will those viewing or hearing the message believe that the information source is like them and therefore understands how they would weigh the pros and cons of a recommended action?

Conclusion

While policy changes can produce significant and lasting change in morbidity and mortality related to disease, many public health interventions still require individual changes in behavior for them to succeed. Focusing exclusively on individual factors, on the other hand, ignores societal and group factors that significantly influence health. The degree to which responsibility for health problems and their solutions is shared by the individual and society depends to some extent on the nature of the recommendation, the privacy rights of the individual, and the likelihood of success associated with different approaches to assigning responsibility to the individual or society.

Several models have been developed to explain individual health behavior and to suggest ways to change it. Each model has its strengths and the decision about which model or models to apply in a particular situation depends on the nature of the problem being studied or changed, on the focus of the individual or organization doing the study or intervention, and on the stated purpose of organizations involved in funding the study or the intervention. As yet there is no theory that works perfectly in every context.

Those interested in developing educational interventions should develop assessment tools to determine the prevalence of attitudes and behaviors that are the targets for the intervention, to assess the impact of the intervention, and to aid in planning subsequent programs. When this information is not collected, programs can waste time teaching information that participants already know or trying to develop materials that do not correspond to the level of readiness in the target population.

A final step in developing educational interventions is to set reasonable expectations about what can be accomplished. While those who deliver health services would not expect a brief exposure to a single medication to resolve a health condition, those involved in health education should not expect a very brief exposure to a single educational approach to change behavior that has been established over a lifetime.

▸ REFERENCES

1. US Department of Health and Human Services: Healthy People 2000: National Health Promotion and Disease Prevention Objectives. Washington, DC: Government Printing Office, 1991
2. US Department of Health and Human Services: Clinician's Handbook of Preventive Services. Washington, DC: Government Printing Office, 1994
3. Doebbeling BN, Ferguson KJ, Kohout FJ: Predictors of Hepatitis B vaccine acceptance in health care workers. Med Care 34(1):58–72, 1996
4. Ryan W: Blaming the Victim. New York: Random House, 1976
5. Kirscht JP: Some issues for health behavior and health education. In Glanz K, Lewis FM, Rimer BK (eds): Health Behavior and Health Education. San Francisco: Jossey-Bass, 1990
6. Becker MH: The tyranny of health promotion. Public Health Rev 14(1):15–23, 1986
7. Von Korff M, Koepsell T, Curry S, Diehr P: Multi-level analysis in epidemiologic research on health behaviors and outcomes. Am J Epidemiol 135(10):1077–1082, 1992
8. Smoking Cessation Clinical Practice Guideline Panel and Staff: The Agency for Health Care Policy and Research smoking cessation clinical practice guideline. JAMA 275(16):1270–1280, 1996
9. Green L, Kreuter MW, Deeds SG, Partridge KD: Health Education Planning: A Diagnostic Approach. Mountain View, CA: Mayfield, 1980
10. Clark NM, Starr-Schneidkraut NJ: Management of asthma by patients and families. Am J Respir Crit Care Med 149:S54–S66, 1994
11. Morreim EH: Lifestyles of the risky and infamous: from managed care to managed lives. Hastings Cent Rep 25(6):5–12, 1995
12. Rosenstock IM: The health belief model: explaining health behavior through expectancies. In Glanz K, Lewis FM, Rimer BK (eds): Health Behavior and Health Education. San Francisco: Jossey-Bass, 1990, pp 39–62
13. Janz NK, Becker MN: The health belief model: a decade later. Health Educ Q 11(1):1–47, 1984
14. Fishbein M, Ajzen I: Belief, attitude, intention and behavior. New York: Addison-Wesley, 1975
15. Godin G, Kok G: The theory of planned behavior: a review of its applications to health-related behaviors. Am J Health Promotion 11(2):87–98, 1996
16. DiClemente CC, Fairhurst SK, Velasquez MM, Prochaska JO, Velicer WF, Rossi JS: The process of smoking cessation: an analysis of precontemplation, contemplation, and preparation stages of change. J Consult Clin Psychol 59(2):295–304, 1991
17. Prochaska JO, Redding CA, Harlow LL, Rossi JS, Velicer WF: The transtheoretical model of change and HIV prevention: a review. Health Educ Q 21(4):471–486, 1994
18. Prochaska JO, Velicer WF, Rossi JS, Goldstein MG, Marcus BH, Rakowski W, Fiore C, Harlow LL, Redding CA, Rosenbloom D, Rossi SR: Stages of change and decisional balance for 12 problem behaviors. Health Psychol 13(1):39–46, 1994
19. Marlatt GA: Relapse prevention: theoretical rationale and overview of the model. In Marlatt GA, Gordon JR (eds): Relapse Prevention. New York: The Guilford Press, 1985
20. Marlatt GA: Situational determinants of relapse and skill-training interventions. In Marlatt GA, Gordon JR (eds): Relapse Prevention. New York: The Guilford Press, 1985
21. Marlatt GA: Lifestyle modification. In Marlatt GA, Gordon JR (eds): Relapse Prevention. New York: The Guilford Press, 1985
22. Ferguson KJ, Brink PJ, Wood M, Koop P: Characteristics of successful dieters as measured by guided interview responses and restraint scale scores. J Am Diet Assoc 92(9):1119–1121, 1992
23. Belisle M, Roskies E, Levesque JM: Improving adherence to physical activity. Health Psychol 6(2):159–172, 1987
24. Bandura A: Social Learning Theory. Englewood Cliffs, NJ: Prentice-Hall, 1977
25. Strecher VJ, DeVellis BM, Becker MH, Rosenstock IM: The role of self-efficacy in achieving health behavior change. Health Educ Q 13(1):73–92, 1986
26. Weinstein ND: Testing four competing theories of health-protective behavior. Health Psychol 12(4):324–333, 1993
27. Janis IL, Mann L: Decision Making: A Psychological Analysis of Conflict, Choice, and Commitment. New York: The Free Press, 1977
28. Redelmeier DA, Rozin P, Kahneman D: Understanding patients' decisions: cognitive and emotional perspectives. JAMA 270(1):72–76, 1993
29. Prochaska JO: Strong and weak principles for progressing from precontemplation to action on the basis of twelve problem behaviors. Health Psychol 13(1):47–51, 1994
30. Galavotti C, Cabral RJ, Lansky A, Grimley DM, Riley GE, Prochaska JO: Validation of measures of condom and other contraceptive use among women at high risk for HIV infection and unintended pregnancy. Health Psychol 14:570–578, 1995

31. Godin G: Theories of reasoned action and planned behavior: usefulness for exercise promotion. Med Sci Sports Exerc 26(11):1391–1394, 1994
32. Miller SM, Hurley K, Shoda Y: Applying cognitive-social theory to health-protective behavior: breast self-examination in cancer screening. Psychol Bull 119(1):70–94, 1996
33. Prochaska JO: Assessing how people change. Cancer 67(3):805–807, 1991
34. King AC: Community and public health approaches to the promotion of physical activity. Med Sci Sports Exerc 26(11):1405–1412, 1994
35. Simons-Morton DG, Mullen PD, Mains DA, Tabak ER, Green LW: Characteristics of controlled studies of patient education and counseling for preventive health behaviors. Patient Education and Counseling 19:175–204, 1992
36. Basler H-D: Patient education with reference to the process of behavioral change. Patient Education and Counseling 26:93–98, 1995
37. Wilde GJS: Effects of mass media communications on health and safety habits: an overview of issues and evidence. Addiction 88: 983–996, 1993

44

Tobacco: Health Effects and Control

Jonathan E. Fielding • Corinne G. Husten • Michael P. Eriksen

Tobacco drieth the brain, dimmeth the sight, vitiateth the smell, hurteth the stomach, destroyeth the concoction, disturbeth the humours and spirits, corrupteth the breath, induceth a trembling of the limbs, exsiccateth the windpipe, lungs, and liver, annoyeth the milt, scorcheth the heart, and causeth the blood to be adjusted.

——Tobias Venner (*Via recta ad vitam Longam*, 1638)

This very night I am going to *leave off tobacco*!
Surely there must be some other world in which this unconquerable purpose shall be realized.

——Charles Lamb, 1815

The custom of smoking dried tobacco leaves spread from America to the rest of the world after European colonization began in the sixteenth century. Given the deleterious effects of tobacco on cardiovascular, respiratory, and other body systems, coupled with its addictive properties and widespread use, it is perhaps the most dangerous of all psychoactive drugs. Its effects are soothing and tranquilizing, and under appropriate circumstances there is also a stimulant action. Physiological and psychological dependence occur, and there are severe withdrawal symptoms and a craving for tobacco that make this among the most refractory of all addictions.

People smoke for several reasons. Some smoke for enjoyment or social reinforcement, and some to alleviate stress. Many young people perceive smoking as an attribute of maturity or sexual desirability. Nicotine is the psychoactive compound in tobacco. Pharmacological factors interact with stimuli in the social environment (social reinforcers) so that after many thousands of repetitions of inhaling tobacco fumes, confirmed smokers are inseparable from their cigarettes. Tolerance, the need for increasing amounts to achieve the same physiological response, develops to some but not all effects of nicotine. Heavy smokers who abruptly cease smoking experience a withdrawal syndrome of irritability, aggressiveness, hostility, depression, and difficulty in concentrating. These symptoms may last several days or even weeks and are accompanied by electroencephalographic changes. Many smokers who have such symptoms relapse if they try to quit.

▸ TOLL OF SMOKING

Excess Mortality

Cigarette smoking has been identified as the single most significant cause of preventable morbidity and premature death.[1] One of two continuing smokers will die of a smoking-related disease.[2,3] The estimated annual excess mortality from cigarette smoking in the United States is nearly 440,000 (more than the total number of American lives lost in all wars during the twentieth century).[4] If current patterns of smoking persist, an estimated 5 million U.S. persons age 1 to 17 years in 1995 will die prematurely from smoking-related diseases.[5] Because of its importance as a cause of morbidity and mortality in the United States, the prevalence of cigarette smoking is now one of the conditions designated as reportable by states to the Centers for Disease Control and Prevention (CDC). This marks the first time a behavior, rather than a disease or illness, has been considered nationally reportable.[6]

Coronary heart disease (CHD), cancer, and various respiratory diseases account for the majority of excess mortality related to cigarette smoking.[7] Of the 489,000 deaths from ischemic heart disease in 1990, an estimated 99,000 (20 percent) were attributable to smoking. Furthermore, 148,000 (29 percent) of the 505,000 cancer deaths in 1990 were attributable to smoking. Lung cancer caused 146,000 deaths in 1990 (29 percent of all cancers), and 83 percent of these deaths were attributed to smoking.[7,8] Other cancers caused by smoking are those of the oral cavity, esophagus, and larynx; smoking is a contributing cause of cancers of the pancreas, bladder, kidney, and cervix.[9,10] Chronic obstructive pulmonary diseases (COPD), such as chronic bronchitis and emphysema, account annually for another 64,000 smoking-related deaths.[7] Smokers average a 16-fold increased risk of acquiring lung cancer, a 12-fold increased risk of acquiring COPD, and a 2-fold increased risk of having a myocardial infarction (MI) in comparison with nonsmoker.[2,11]

It has been estimated that an average of 7 minutes of life is lost for each cigarette smoked—about the time taken to smoke it. This estimate is based on an average reduction in life expectancy for cigarette smokers of 6.6 years.[12] For a 25-year-old man smoking one pack per day (20 cigarettes), the reduction averages 4.6 years; for a man of the same age smoking 2 packs per day (40 cigarettes), 8.3 years of expected life are lost. The reduction in life expectancy is also affected by the age of smoking initiation. A person who begins smoking at the age of 15 years has an average of 8 years of reduced longevity, and one starting after 25 years of age faces an average 4-year reduction.[11] Historical gender differences in smoking prevalence are responsible for at least part of the gender difference in life expectancy in the United States.

Economic Costs

The annual economic toll of smoking can be divided into direct and indirect costs. The total direct health care cost associated with smoking in 1993 was an estimated $50 billion.[13] The total indirect cost attributable to smoking because of lost productivity and earnings as a result of excess morbidity, disability, and premature death is estimated at $47.2 billion annually.[14] These figures translate into an annual per capita social cost of approximately $391 directly attributable to smoking.[15] In addition, pregnant smokers account for a sizable economic burden on the medical care system: medical costs associated with smoking during pregnancy were estimated to be $1.4 billion in 1995.[15a]

Part of the cost of smoking is due to cigarette-caused fires, although this cost was not included in the calculations cited above. Smoking is the leading cause of deaths due to fire.[16] In the United States, fires caused by smoking claim more than 1,000 lives and injure another 3,400 people annually.[17] Data from the National Fire Data Center show that 7 percent of fires in residential structures result from smoking,[16] causing about $320 million in property losses each year.[17] Overall, smoking accounts for about $400 million annually in direct property damage.[17] Smoking materials were the cause of 5 percent of fires on national forest lands in 1979 through 1988, with an average yearly loss of 11,570 acres.[18]

▸ CARDIOVASCULAR DISEASE

Coronary Heart Disease

CHD is related to several risk factors, one of which is tobacco use. Of the various disease manifestations associated with tobacco use, CHD is the leading cause of excess death and disability in the United States. In 1990 more than 40 percent of the 2,148,463 deaths in the United States were due to diseases of the cardiovascular system.[19] Of cardiovascular deaths, 489,000 were due to ischemic heart disease.[19] On the basis of data from a very large U.S. study, smoking was estimated to cause 46 and 37 percent, respectively, of ischemic heart disease deaths of men and women less than 65 years of age, with 20 and 12 percent being the corresponding percentages for men and women 65 years of age and older.[7,19]

In early investigations, cigarette smoking, along with several other characteristics, was observed to be strongly associated with CHD. On the basis of this observation, cohort studies were set up to determine the nature and degree of CHD risk attributable to smoking. These studies each revealed a higher incidence of MI and death from CHD in cigarette smokers than in nonsmokers. The 1990 Surgeon General's Report provides a summary of studies (to 1988) that estimates both the risk of CHD from smoking and the decrease in risk with smoking cessation. This report concluded that, on the basis of both cohort and case-control studies, "cigarette smoking is firmly established as an important cause of coronary heart disease, arteriosclerotic peripheral vascular disease, and stroke. Eliminating smoking presents an opportunity for bringing about a major reduction in the occurrence of CHD, the leading cause of death in the United States."[20] These studies demonstrated similar findings, whether in the United States, Canada, the United Kingdom, Scandinavia, or Japan.[9] In a more recent American Cancer Society prospective study (Cancer Prevention Study II) (ACS CPS-II) with 1.2 million participants, smokers had CHD mortality approximately 85 percent greater than nonsmokers did.[2] Similarly, the 40-year follow-up of the British Physicians' Study reported a doubling of risk for heavy smokers.[3] In the U.S. Veterans Study, a study of 293,958 male war veterans, the risk of death from CHD and cardiovascular disease increased directly with usual daily cigarette consumption (Fig. 44-1).[21] Even among past smokers, risk of death due to CHD and cardiovascular disease was associated with previous usual daily cigarette consumption.[9]

Smokers have a higher death rate from CHD at all ages, and the increase in mortality with age is more rapid among smokers, probably

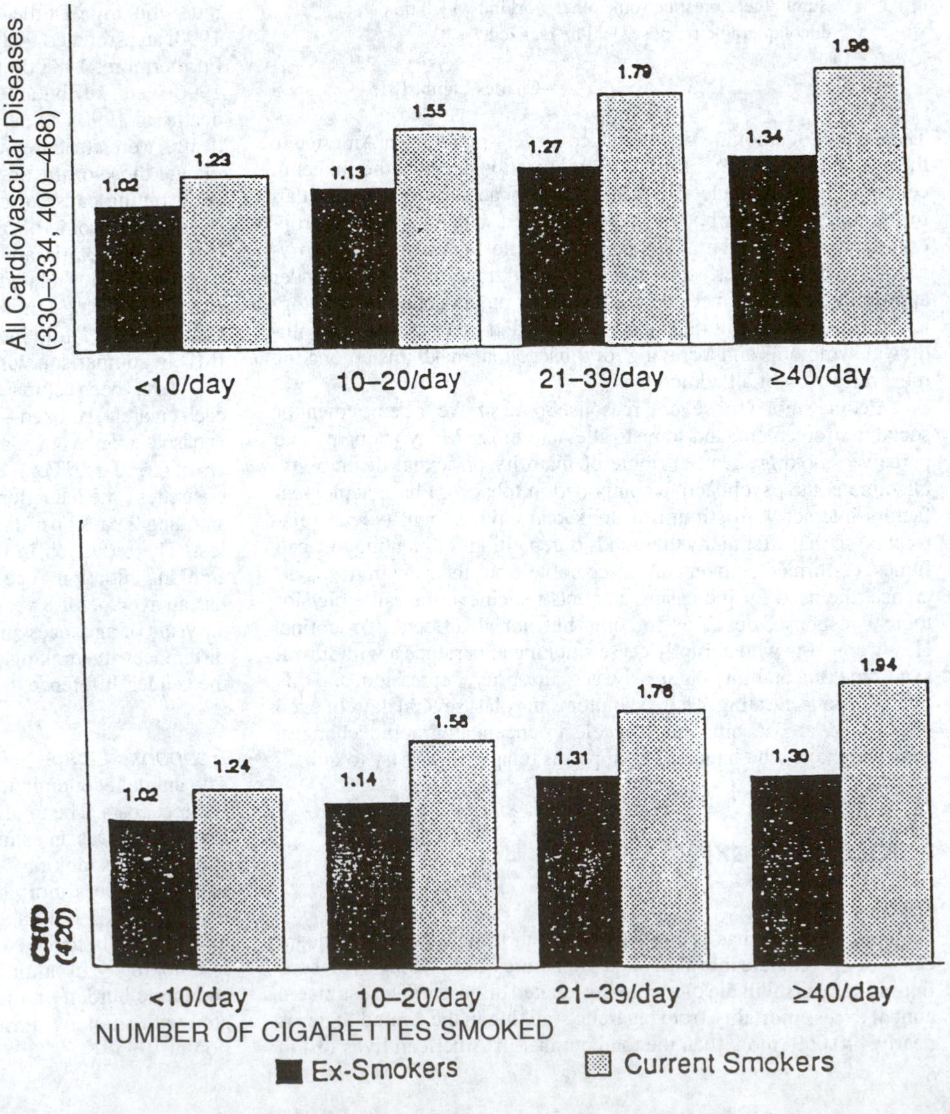

Figure 44-1. Mortality ratios for all cardiovascular diseases and coronary heart disease, by daily cigarette consumption, U.S. Veterans Study, 1954 to 1969. *Ex-smokers* designation includes only former cigarette smokers who stopped smoking for reasons other than physician's orders. (From Centers for Disease Control, Office on Smoking and Health: The Health Benefits of Smoking Cessation: A Report of the Surgeon General. DHHS Publication No. (CDC) 90-8416. Washington, DC: Centers for Disease Control, 1990.)

because of cumulative physiological damage from smoking. However, since the incidence of CHD increases sharply with age for both smokers and nonsmokers, the relative risk peaks for men age 40 to 44 years and for women age 45 to 49 years. The percentage of CHD deaths attributable to smoking is 84 percent for men age 40 to 44 years and 26 percent for men age 75 to 79 years. Among women, the smoking attributable percentage for CHD deaths is 85 percent for women age 45 to 49 years and 23 percent for women age 80 years and older.[22]

Although most investigations of smoking-related risk of CHD have used male subjects, multiple prospective studies indicate that women who smoke are also at increased risk for CHD.[2,23–27] Data from the ACS CPS-II indicated relative risks of CHD of 3.0 among female smokers age 35 to 64 years and 1.6 among female smokers age 65 years and older.[9] The Nurses Health Study, which examined a cohort of 121,000 women, indicated a relative risk among current smokers of 4.13 for fatal CHD, 3.88 for nonfatal MI, and 3.93 for CHD overall. The risk increased with number of cigarettes smoked per day: the adjusted relative risk was 2.53 for women smoking 1 to 14 cigarettes per day (cpd), 4.79 for women smoking 15 to 24 cpd, and 5.49 for women smoking 25 cpd or more.[25] Thus, women smokers who adopt smoking patterns similar to those of men have a similar increased risk of death from CHD in comparison with nonsmokers.[28]

Results from cohort studies clearly demonstrate that the risk of death from CHD is increased by early smoking initiation, number of cigarettes smoked per day, and depth of smoke inhalation. For example, data from the Nurses Health Study show that, although the risk of CHD is increased for all smokers regardless of age of smoking initiation, the risk is higher for women who started smoking before age 15 (Table 44-1). After adjustment for potential confounders, including number of cigarettes smoked daily, the relative risk for those starting to smoke before age 15 was 9.2. Among former smokers, women who started smoking before age 15 years were also at highest risk for CHD, but this finding was based on a small number of cases.[25]

Smoking in combination with other CHD risk factors appears to have a synergistic effect on CHD mortality.[29] For example, in the Pooling project, the 10-year incidence of first major coronary event was 54 per 1,000 for smokers, 92 to 103 per 1,000 for smokers with one other risk factor (hypertension or hypercholesterolemia), and 189 per 1,000 for persons with all three risk factors.[30] Diabetes also confers an increased risk of CHD that is further increased if the person smokes.[31,32]

In studies of women using high-dose oral contraceptives, increased cardiovascular risk was reported among women who smoke;[33–35] it is unclear if this risk occurs with the newer low-dose pills.

Data from cohort studies show that pipe and cigar smokers generally have a substantially lower risk of a major coronary event and subsequent CHD than do cigarette smokers. The risk of CHD-related death for pipe and cigar smokers is in the range of 1.02 to 1.40 compared with that for nonsmokers, with deeper smoke inhalation increasing the risk.[28] A Swedish study reported that pipe smokers and cigarette smokers had similar risk of death from ischemic heart disease; this finding was attributed to there being a similar proportion of smoke inhalers among the pipe smokers and cigarette smokers.[36] The Copenhagen City Heart Study found no difference in risk for first MI among pipe, cigar/cheroot, or cigarette smokers.[37] Pipe and cigar smokers who are former cigarette smokers tend to inhale the smoke and to have much higher venous blood carboxyhemoglobin levels than do those who have never smoked cigarettes, and they are likely to be at higher risk for CHD.[38]

The positive effect of smoking cessation on both primary and secondary prevention of CHD has been extensively studied and validated. The 1990 Surgeon General's Report evaluated this research and concluded that, compared with continued smoking, cessation substantially reduces the risk of CHD among men and women of all ages. The excess risk of CHD is reduced by about half after 1 year of abstinence and then declines gradually. After 15 years of abstinence, the risk of CHD is similar to the risk in those who have never smoked. Among persons with diagnosed CHD, smoking cessation markedly reduces the risk of recurrent MI and cardiovascular death. In many studies, this reduction has been 50 percent or more.[20,39,40]

Peripheral Arterial Occlusive Disease

The most powerful risk factor predisposing persons to atherosclerotic peripheral arterial occlusive disease is cigarette smoking.[20,34,41] Cigarette smoking has been shown to be directly related to lower extremity atherosclerotic disease of both large and small arteries.[42] Smoking prevalence is high among victims of aortoiliac (98 percent) and femoropopliteal (91 percent) disease.[43,44] One epidemiological study found that, in smokers consuming fewer than one pack of cigarettes per day, the relative risk of acquiring peripheral arterial occlusive disease was 11.53 compared with that in nonsmokers, and the relative

TABLE 44-1. AGE AT STARTING SMOKING AMONG CURRENT AND FORMER SMOKERS AND AGE-ADJUSTED AND MULTIVARIATE RELATIVE RISKS (RRS) OF TOTAL CHD COMPARED WITH NEVER SMOKERS [a]

		Age at Starting Smoking[b]				
Event	***Never Smoker***	***<15***	***15–17***	***18–21***	***22–25***	***≥26***
■ ***TOTAL CHD (CURRENT SMOKERS)***						
No.	215	21	66	336	73	40
RR[c]	1.00	7.17	3.21	4.17	3.91	3.19
		(4.88–10.53)	(2.47–4.17)	(3.55–4.89)	(3.06–5.00)	(2.32–4.40)
RR[d]	1.00	9.25	3.41	4.53	4.30	3.17
		(5.27–16.23)	(2.38–4.89)	(3.59–5.71)	(3.03–6.12)	(2.10–4.78)
■ ***TOTAL CHD (FORMER SMOKERS)***						
No.	215	4	25	140	28	12
RR[c]	1.00	1.72	1.35	1.57	1.44	1.34
		(0.65–4.58)	(0.89–2.03)	(1.27–1.94)	(0.97–2.13)	(0.75–2.39)
RR[e]	1.00	7.55	1.42	1.66	1.83	1.67
		(2.54–22.45)	(0.84–2.40)	(1.28–2.16)	(1.12–2.98)	(0.83–3.36)

[a] Numbers in parentheses are 95 percent confidence intervals.
[b] Age at starting smoking was missing for five current smokers and five former smokers.
[c] Age-adjusted RR.
[d] Adjusted for age in 5-year intervals, follow-up period (1976 to 1978, 1978 to 1980 . . . 1986 to 1988), history of hypertension, diabetes, high cholesterol levels, body mass index, past use of oral contraceptives, postmenopausal estrogen therapy, and number of cigarettes smoked daily.
[e] Adjusted for above coronary heart disease risk factors plus time since quitting smoking.
From Kawachi I, Colditz GA, Stampfer MJ, et al: Smoking cessation and time course of decreased risks of coronary heart disease in middle-aged women. Arch Intern Med 154:169–75, 1994.

risk in those who smoked more than one pack per day was 15.56 compared with the risk in nonsmokers. Severe intermittent claudication is more frequent among nondiabetic smokers who consume 15 cpd or more than among nonsmokers and lighter smokers.[45] Limited studies of smokeless tobacco use have not demonstrated a high incidence of peripheral vascular disease in users. An elevated risk of peripheral vascular disease is also not evident in cigar or pipe smokers.[28]

Studies show a lower risk of peripheral arterial occlusive disease among former smokers than among current smokers. A recent cohort study found that current smoking was associated with a 50 percent increase in the progression of atherosclerosis over 3 years compared with never smokers, and past smoking was associated with a 25 percent increase compared with never smokers.[46] There is also a consistent reduction in complications of peripheral vascular disease among patients who quit smoking: those who stop smoking have improved performance and overall survival.[20] Smoking cessation can also significantly reduce the risk of peripheral arterial occlusive disease for persons with diabetes.[44] However, progression of atherosclerosis was not associated with current or past smoking after adjustment for number of pack-years of smoking, suggesting that some adverse effects may be cumulative and irreversible.[46]

An autopsy study of atherosclerotic plaque in smokers found that the complexity and extent of plaque in the abdominal aorta increased with the number of cigarettes smoked.[47] This study provides a rationale for the findings of several cohort studies that smokers have a higher abdominal aortic aneurysm mortality rate than do nonsmokers.[28] Several studies have also shown an increased risk of aortic aneurysm among pipe and cigar smokers,[9,48] and an autopsy study indicated that men who smoked cigars, pipes, or both had more complex patterns of atherosclerotic plaques than did men who had never smoked cigars or pipes regularly.[47] Five cohort studies that analyzed risk of death due to aortic aneurysm for current and former smokers compared with never smokers found that, among men, excess risk among former smokers is two to three times higher than that among never smokers and that excess risk is about 50 percent lower among former smokers than among current smokers. Patterns are similar for women.[20]

Cerebrovascular Disease

Both ischemic and hemorrhagic cerebrovascular diseases are major causes of death in the United States. Although stroke deaths have declined substantially during the past two decades, ischemic and hemorrhagic strokes accounted for approximately 144,000 (7 percent) of deaths in the United States in 1990.[19] Each year there are more than 400,000 new events.[20] The risk of stroke increases with age.

Smoking has been well demonstrated as a causal factor in stroke.[9,49] A meta-analysis of 32 studies found that the risk of cerebral infarction was 1.9, the risk for cerebral hemorrhage was 0.7, and the risk of subarachnoid hemorrhage was 2.9 among current smokers compared with never smokers; a positive dose-response relationship between number of cigarettes smoked and relative risk for stroke was also noted.[50]

Female smokers who use high-dose oral contraceptives are reported to be at increased risk of stroke.[51] However, the low-dose oral contraceptives used today may have different risk than that observed for the early high-dose formulations.[20,34]

Compared with continued smoking, smoking cessation reduces the risk of both ischemic stroke and subarachnoid hemorrhage. After smoking cessation, the risk of stroke returns to the level of never smokers. In some studies this return has occurred within 5 years, but in other studies this level was not reached until up to 15 years of abstinence.[20]

Mechanisms of Cardiovascular Disease Development Related to Smoking

The mechanisms by which smoking contributes to the development and clinical manifestation of cardiovascular disease are not completely understood. The development of CHD includes at least five interrelated processes: atherosclerosis, thrombosis, coronary artery spasm, cardiac arrhythmia, and reduced oxygen-carrying capacity of the blood. The exact components of cigarette smoke that cause these changes are not known. Smoking is associated with atherosclerosis: data from animal studies suggest that nicotine causes endothelial damage, and data from humans indicate that smoking increases the number of damaged endothelial cells. Smoking also appears to stimulate smooth muscle cell proliferation by increasing the adherence of platelets to arterial endothelium. Smoking decreases high-density lipoprotein cholesterol, which has been shown to be protective for ischemic heart disease. Smoking may also increase thrombus formation: fibrinogen levels have been shown to be elevated in smokers, and other clotting abnormalities that tend to promote thrombus formation have been observed in smokers. Cigarette smoking also has a vasoconstrictor effect on coronary arteries. Coronary artery spasm can cause acute myocardial ischemia and may promote thrombus formation. Arrhythmias can precipitate heart attacks and can increase the case fatality rate of MI; smoking has been shown to lower the threshold for ventricular fibrillation. Cigarette smoking increases myocardial oxygen demand by increasing peripheral resistance, blood pressure, and heart rate. In addition, the capacity of the blood to deliver oxygen is reduced by increased carboxyhemoglobin, greater viscosity, and higher coronary vascular resistance. Reduced oxygen-carrying capacity may contribute to infarction in the presence of significant atherosclerotic narrowing of the vessels.[20]

The strong association between smoking and peripheral vascular disease is likely to be mediated through the mechanisms that promote atherosclerosis as described above. The peripheral vasoconstrictive effects of smoking probably also play an important role.[20]

The association of smoking with ischemic stroke is likely to occur through the mechanisms that promote atherosclerosis and thrombus formation.[52] Cigarette smoking appears to increase the risk of stroke by decreasing cerebral blood flow.[53] In smokers with other risk factors for stroke, cerebral blood flow is reduced in an additive manner compared with that in nonsmokers with similar risk factors.[54] The mechanism for the strong relationship between smoking and subarachnoid hemorrhage is currently unknown.[20]

▸ CANCER

Lung Cancer

In the United States, carcinoma of the lung is the leading cancer cause of death for both men and women.[55] Lung cancer mortality rates, as measured by ACS CPS-I from 1959 to 1965 and ACS CPS-II from 1982 to 1988 increased over time, from 26 to 155 per 100,000 women and from 187 to 341 per 100,000 men over this period.[2] The number of lung cancer deaths in the United States has also risen sharply, from 18,300 in 1950 to 61,800 in 1969, and an estimated 160,100 in 1998.[56] In 1990, lung cancer accounted for 28 percent of cancer deaths and 7 percent of all deaths in the United States.[19] Eighty-three percent of lung cancer deaths were directly attributable to smoking.[5,19]

Ninety percent of malignant lung tumors belong to four major cell types: squamous cell, oat cell, large cell, and adenocarcinoma, which are commonly designated bronchogenic carcinoma. Smoking induces all four major histologic types of lung cancer. Smoking is most strongly associated with squamous cell and oat cell carcinomas, but dose-response relationships for adenocarcinomas and other types of lung cancer have been reported.[57] It has been suggested that the increasing incidence of adenocarcinoma may be related to the switch to low-tar, filtered cigarettes.[58,59] Lung cancer has a propensity to metastasize early and widely. Once the patient is symptomatic and the cancer is unresectable, the patient has a 5-year survival rate of 13 percent; the 5-year survival rate is 15 percent with regional disease at diagnosis and 2 percent with distant disease at diagnosis.[60] The survival rate from lung cancer has increased only slightly in the past 20 years.[61]

The rise in lung cancer rates in male smokers preceded that of female smokers. In 1959–1961, the male/female ratio of death rates

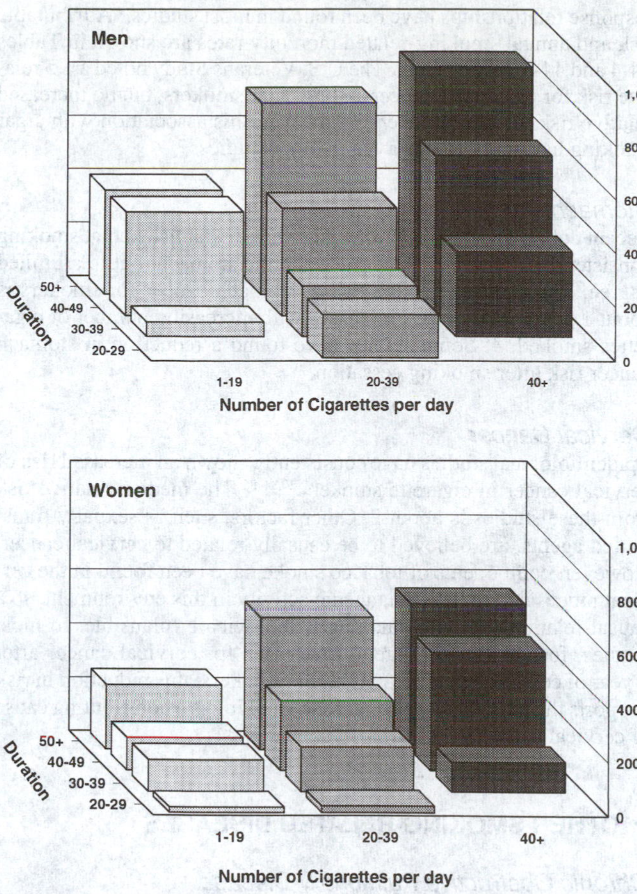

Figure 44-2. Death rates from lung cancer among persons age 60 to 69, by amount and duration (in years) of cigarette smoking: Duration progresses over time. ACS Cancer Prevention Study II. (From Thun MJ, Myers DG, Day-Lally C, et al: Age and exposure-response relationships between cigarette smoking and premature death in Cancer Prevention Study II. In Burns DM, Garfinkel L, Samet J (eds): Changes in Cigarette–Related Disease Risks and Their Implication for Prevention and Control. Smoking and Tobacco Control Monograph No. 8. Rockville, MD: National Cancer Institute, 1997 NIH Publication No. 97-4213.)

from lung cancer was 6.7:1. Whereas the incidence rate in men appears to have peaked in 1984, the rate for women has continued to increase by 2 percent per year. By 1989–1991, the male-female ratio had declined to 2.4:1.[60] Current lung cancer rates for women approximate those for men of three decades ago. Lung cancer has replaced breast cancer as the leading cause of cancer death among both white and black American women.[55] An estimated 93,100 men and 67,000 women will die of lung cancer in 1998.[56]

Although the 1964 Surgeon General's Report was the first official U.S. statement on the relationship of smoking and lung cancer, the question of an association was first raised much earlier, in the late 1920s. Case control, cohort, and animal studies performed in the 1950s showed a clear association between smoking and lung cancer.[62–64] The study most influential in drawing medical attention to this relationship was the preliminary results from a 1956 cohort study of 40,000 British physicians 36 years of age and older. This study demonstrated that the age-adjusted death rate for lung cancer increased from 7 per 100,000 for nonsmokers to 166 per 100,000 for heavy smokers.[65]

Other cohort studies in various parts of the world further demonstrated the consistency, specificity, strength, coherence, and temporal nature of the association between smoking and lung cancer. The 1990 Surgeon General's Report provides an outline of the lung cancer mortality ratios for current, former, and never smokers from prospective studies. Although the mortality ratios vary among studies, smoker mortality rates for lung cancer ranged from 4 to 27 times those of nonsmokers.[20] The relative risk has increased over time, doubling for men and quadrupling for women from ACS CPS-I from 1959–1965 to ACS CPS-II from 1982–1988.[2] Strength of association was further demonstrated by the dose-response relationship clearly illustrated in the ACS CPS-II (Fig. 44-2).[22] The figure demonstrates the gradient of increasing risk of death from lung cancer as the number of cigarettes smoked per day increases. Increased consumption of cigarettes per day, whether filtered or nonfiltered, results in an increased relative risk for both male and female smokers.[66–67]

Data from ACS CPS-II also confirm a direct relationship between number of years of smoking and lung cancer mortality (Fig. 44-2). Lung cancer incidence appears to increase with the square of the amount smoked daily, but with the duration of smoking raised to a power of four or five.[68] Smoking mechanics also affect lung cancer mortality: the degree of inhalation varies directly with smoking-associated mortality.[9] However, even smokers who report slight inhalation or none have a relative risk of cancer as much as 8-fold that for nonsmokers.[69] Both case-control and cohort studies have demonstrated some reduction in lung cancer risk in smokers who switched from nonfiltered to filtered cigarettes.[9,70] For those who have always smoked filtered cigarettes, the risk of lung cancer is still high, but may be 10 to 30 percent lower than that for lifelong smokers of nonfiltered cigarettes (Table 44-2).[71]

For persons who stop smoking cigarettes, the decrease in lung cancer mortality is related to smoking history (e.g., dose, duration, type of cigarette, and depth of inhalation) as well as the number of years since cessation. Risk reduction is gradual, and after 10 years the risk is about 30 to 50 percent the risk for continuing smokers.[20]

Several case-control and cohort studies have reported an increased risk of lung cancer among those who smoke pipes, cigars, or both.[72–75] In general, the risk of lung cancer is much less for pipe and

TABLE 44-2. ADJUSTED ODDS RATIOS AND 95 PERCENT CONFIDENCE INTERVALS FOR MEN IN THE AMERICAN HEALTH FOUNDATION CASE-CONTROL STUDY, BY LEVEL OF FILTER SMOKING

	Tumor Type			
	Kreyberg I		Kreyberg II	
Pattern of Smoking	*Odds Ratio*	*95% Confidence Interval*	*Odds Ratio*	*95% Confidence Interval*
Nonfilter only	1.00	—	1.00	—
Switchers (1–9 years)	0.83	0.59–1.17	0.96	0.61–1.51
Switchers (10+ years)	0.66	0.49–0.90	0.79	0.53–1.18
Filter only	0.69	0.37–1.27	0.87	0.43–1.54

Source: Wynder and Kabat, 1988

From Samet JM. The changing cigarette and disease risk: Current status of the evidence. In: The FTC Cigarette Test Method for Determining Tar, Nicotine, and Carbon Monoxide Yields of U.S. Cigarettes: Report of the NCI Expert Committee. Smoking and Tobacco Control Monograph No. 7. NIH Publication No. 96-4028. Bethesda, MD: National Cancer Institute, 1996.

cigar smokers than for cigarette smokers, but greater than for nonsmokers. An estimated 825 Americans died in 1991 from lung cancer as a result of pipe smoking.[76] Among pipe and cigar smokers, lung cancer death rates also exhibit dose-response relationships to smoking.[20] Chemical analysis of the smoke from pipes, cigars, and cigarettes shows that carcinogens are found at comparable levels in the smoke of all these tobacco products; the lower risk of lung cancer among pipe and cigar smokers compared with cigarette smokers is due to the lesser amount of tobacco smoked and the lower degree of inhalation.[20] In Denmark and Sweden, where the style of smoking pipes and cigars involves deeper inhalation than is generally practiced in the United States, the rate of lung cancer for pipe and cigar smokers approaches that for cigarette smokers.[36,67]

Although research during the past 25 years has led to a greatly expanded knowledge of the major factors contributing to the toxicity and carcinogenicity of cigarette smoke, the mechanisms responsible for lung tumor initiation from tobacco smoke constituents are complex and not yet completely understood. Tobacco smoke contains numerous carcinogens that have both cancer-initiating and cancer-promoting activity. The bronchial epithelia of smokers show progressive abnormal changes; the frequency and intensity of epithelial changes increase with the amount smoked. The number of cells with atypical nuclei decreases with number of years since smoking cessation. There have also been reports describing an association between smoking and the presence of DNA adducts.[20] For example, a carcinogen in cigarette smoke (benzo[*a*]pyrene) forms adducts at specific codons on the p53 gene; these adducts are at the same locations as mutations associated with lung cancer.[77]

Oral, Laryngeal, and Esophageal Cancer

Large numbers of cohort and case-control studies from many countries support the conclusion that smoking is a cause of oral, laryngeal, and esophageal cancer. For these cancers, the mortality ratios for smokers—regardless of whether they smoke cigarettes, pipes, or cigars—are similar.[9] The estimated numbers of deaths attributable to smoking for these cancers, other cancers, and other diseases are shown in Table 44-3; Table 44-4 displays the attributable risks. For both men and women, most cases of these three cancers are attributable to smoking, with strong dose-response relationships at each of these sites.[9] Smokeless tobacco use is also a cause of oral cancer.[78]

Alcohol appears to play a synergistic role with smoking for each of these cancers.[56,60] In one study of oral cancer risk, for nonsmokers who consumed 7 ounces or more of alcohol per week, the relative risk of death from oral cancer was 2.5 compared with that for nondrinkers. Those who consumed the same amount of alcohol and smoked one-half pack of cigarettes or less per day had approximately double the risk, but the relative risk rose to 24 if the smoker consumed one pack or more per day.[79]

Smoking cessation halves the risk of oral and esophageal cancer within 5 years of quitting; the risk is reduced further with longer abstinence. The risk of laryngeal cancer is reduced after 3 to 4 years of abstinence, but it remains higher than that for never smokers.[20]

Bladder and Renal Cancer

As seen in Tables 44-3 and 44-4, about 45 percent of bladder cancer cases in men and 30 percent in women are attributable to smoking, accounting for more than 4,000 deaths per year. Relative risks for bladder cancer are 2 to 3, and have a clear dose-response relationship. Smoking cessation reduces the risk of bladder cancer by half after only a few years.[20,80,81]

Corresponding risks attributable to smoking and corresponding numbers of annual deaths are shown in Tables 44-3 and 44-4 for renal cancer. Relative risks from a variety of studies have ranged from 1 to 5, and most studies have demonstrated a clear dose-response relationship.[9]

Pancreatic Cancer

In both men and women, smoking increases the risk of pancreatic cancer. Relative risks range from 2 to 3 in most studies, and dose-response relationships have been found in most studies.[9] Attributable risk and annual smoking-related mortality rates are shown in Tables 44-4 and 44-3, respectively. The U.S. Veterans Study noted a 1.5 relative risk for pancreatic cancer among cigar smokers, but no increased relative risk for pipe smokers;[10] however, this association with cigar smoking has not been observed in other studies.[82]

Stomach Cancer

Recent cohort and case-control studies have established that smoking consistently increases risk of cancer of the stomach, but to a limited degree. The average relative risk of stomach cancer for smokers is about 1.5; the relative risk increases with increasing number of cigarettes smoked.[9,83] Some studies have found a reduction in stomach cancer risk after smoking cessation.[20]

Cervical Cancer

Epidemiological studies have consistently shown an increased risk of cervical cancer in cigarette smokers.[20,84–86] The median relative risk from these studies is about 2. Other factors, such as sexually transmitted agents, are believed to be causally related to cervical cancer. However, components of tobacco smoke have been found in the cervical mucus and to have mutagenic activity in this environment, so a causal relationship with smoking is biologically plausible. In most studies, former smokers are at lower risk for cervical cancer after 1 year of cessation than are continuing smokers; this reduction in risk supports the hypothesis that cigarette smoking is a contributing cause of cervical cancer.[20]

▸ OTHER SMOKING-RELATED DISEASES

Chronic Obstructive Pulmonary Disease

An estimated 87,000 Americans died of COPD in 1990; 79 percent of these deaths were attributable to smoking.[5,19] The death rates from COPD increased with age, and in 1990, they were 1.9 times higher in men than in women and 1.2 times higher in whites than in African Americans.[19] Mortality from COPD has paralleled lung cancer mortality, increasing progressively over the past 25 years.[9] A recent decline in COPD mortality at younger ages is consistent with lower smoking prevalence among younger cohorts of Americans.[9] The 1990 Surgeon General's Report summarized the studies of smoking and COPD to 1989: data from case-control and cohort studies consistently demonstrate a higher COPD mortality among cigarette smokers than among nonsmokers, with the mortality ratio as high as 32 for persons smoking 25 cpd or more.[20] Updates of the British Physicians' Study[3] and the ACS CPS-II[2] have since been published. In the update of the British Physicians' Study, the risk of COPD among smokers was found to be almost as strong as the risk of lung cancer. Dose-response relationships have been consistently observed, with the risk of death from COPD influenced not only by the number of cigarettes smoked per day but also by the depth of smoke inhalation and by the age at smoking initiation.[67,87,88]

Abnormal lung function (especially expiratory airflow) occurs as early as 2 years after smoking initiation.[89–91] Smokers exhibit a more rapid decline in forced expiratory volume at 1 second (FEV_1) with age than do nonsmokers,[92] and the aggregate loss correlates well with cumulative pack-years of consumption of cigarettes.[93,94] Decline in lung function begins with inflammation in the small airways, although inflammation in the lung parenchyma is also a major factor in the development of COPD. Symptoms of such inflammation are not always a reliable indicator of smokers who will subsequently have symptomatic COPD. However, those smokers with a fast annual decline in FEV appear to constitute a high-risk group for COPD development.[92,95]

Studies have identified the likely mechanisms by which cigarette smoking induces COPD. The current model suggests that after a long latency period, COPD develops because of a more rapid

TABLE 44-3. RELATIVE RISKS (RR) FOR DEATH ATTRIBUTED TO SMOKING AND SMOKING-ATTRIBUTABLE MORTALITY (SAM) FOR CURRENT AND FORMER SMOKERS, BY DISEASE CATEGORY AND SEX, UNITED STATES, 1990[a]

	Men			Women			
	RR			RR			
Disease Category (ICD-9 code)[b]	Current Smokers	Former Smokers	SAM	Current Smokers	Former Smokers	SAM	Total SAM
■ ***ADULT DISEASES (PERSONS AGE ≥35 YRS)***							
Neoplasms							
Lip, oral cavity, pharynx (140–149)	27.5	8.8	5,033	5.6	2.9	1,442	6,475
Esophagus (150)	7.6	5.8	5,668	10.3	3.2	1,616	7,284
Pancreas (157)	2.1	1.1	2,667	2.3	1.8	3,447	6,114
Larynx (161)	10.5	5.2	2,379	17.8	11.9	611	2,990
Trachea, lung, bronchus (162)	22.4	9.4	81,179	11.9	4.7	35,741	116,920
Cervix uteri (180)	NA[c]	NA	NA	2.1	1.9	1,294	1,294
Urinary bladder (188)	2.9	1.9	3,046	2.6	1.9	980	4,026
Kidney, other urinary (189)	3.0	2.0	2,866	1.4	1.2	353	3,219
Cardiovascular diseases							
Hypertension (401–404)	1.9	1.3	3,299	1.7	1.2	2,151	5,450
Ischemic heart disease (410–414)							
Persons age 35–64 yrs	2.8	1.8	26,431	3.0	1.4	7,701	34,132
Persons age ≥65 yrs	1.6	1.3	38,918	1.6	1.3	25,871	64,789
Other heart diseases (390–398, 415–417, 420–429)	1.9	1.3	23,295	1.7	1.2	12,019	35,314
Cerebrovascular diseases (430–438)							
Persons age 35–64 yrs	3.7	1.4	4,557	4.8	1.4	4,114	8,671
Persons age ≥65 yrs	1.9	1.3	10,421	1.5	1.0	4,189	14,610
Atherosclerosis (440)	4.1	2.3	3,737	3.0	1.3	2,675	6,412
Aortic aneurysm (441)	4.1	2.3	5,913	3.0	1.3	1,382	7,295
Other arterial disease (442–448)	4.1	2.3	2,032	3.0	1.3	1,115	3,147
Respiratory diseases							
Pneumonia and influenza (480–487)	2.0	1.6	11,292	2.2	1.4	7,881	19,173
Bronchitis, emphysema (491–492)	9.7	8.8	9,324	10.5	7.0	5,541	14,865
Chronic airway obstruction (496)	9.7	8.8	30,385	10.5	7.0	18,597	48,982
Other respiratory diseases (010–012, 493)	2.0	1.6	787	2.2	1.4	668	1,455
■ ***PEDIATRIC DISEASES (PERSONS AGE <1 YR)***							
Short gestation, low–birth weight (765)	1.8		285	1.8		222	507
Respiratory distress syndrome (769)	1.8		219	1.8		141	360
Other respiratory conditions of newborn (770)	1.8		214	1.8		160	374
Sudden infant death syndrome (798)	1.5		288	1.5		182	470
■ ***BURN DEATHS***[d]			863			499	1,362
■ ***ENVIRONMENTAL TOBACCO SMOKE DEATHS***[e]			1,055			1,945	3,000
Total			276,153			142,537	418,690

From Centers for Disease Control and Prevention: Cigarette smoking-attributable mortality and years of potential life lost—United States, 1990. MMWR 42(33):645–649, 1993.

[a] Relative risk means relative to never smokers.

[b] *International Classification of Diseases.* 9th revision.

[c] Not applicable.

[d] Source: National Fire Protection Association, 1993.

[e] Deaths among nonsmokers from lung cancer attributable to environmental tobacco smoke (Environmental Protection Agency, 1992).

decline in lung function during adulthood or because of a reduction in maximal lung growth in childhood and adolescence. The age at which smoking has the greatest influence on COPD pathogenesis is currently unknown. Studies have also confirmed that atopy and increased airway responsiveness are associated with a more rapid decrease in pulmonary function, and cigarette smoking is a cause of exaggerated airway responsiveness. Finally, the protease-antiprotease hypothesis suggests that an imbalance between proteolytic and nonproteolytic enzymes in the lung can result in the destruction of lung tissue and emphysema. Cigarette use may enhance protease enzyme action (through neutrophil and macrophage elastase) and decrease antiprotease activity through smoke-induced oxidents.[92,97–100]

Smokers have more respiratory symptoms than do nonsmokers. The principle chronic respiratory symptoms are chronic cough, phlegm, wheezing, and dyspnea. Smoking contributes to these symptoms by decreasing tracheal mucous velocity, increasing mucous secretion, causing chronic airway inflammation, increasing epithelial permeability, and damaging parenchymal cells.[20]

Cigar smokers and pipe smokers who inhale are reported to have a higher rate of decline of FEV_1 than cigarette smokers.[101] Cigar smokers and pipe smokers are also reported to have a higher preva-

TABLE 44-4. ATTRIBUTABLE RISKS FOR SELECTED CAUSES OF DEATH IN CIGARETTE SMOKERS, UNITED STATES, 1990

Disease Category (ICD-9 Code)[a]	Smoking Attributable Risk Men	Women	Total
■ NEOPLASMS			
Lip, oral cavity, pharynx (140–149)	0.89	0.52	0.77
Esophagus (150)	0.78	0.64	0.75
Pancreas (157)	0.22	0.27	0.24
Larynx (151)	0.80	0.83	0.81
Trachea, lung, bronchus (162)	0.89	0.71	0.83
Cervix uteri (180)	NA[b]	0.28	0.28
Urinary bladder (188)	0.44	0.29	0.39
Kidney, other urinary (189)	0.46	0.09	0.31
■ CARDIOVASCULAR DISEASES			
Ischemic heart disease (410–414)			
Persons age 35–64 yrs	0.46	0.37	0.43
Persons age ≥65 yrs	0.20	0.12	0.16
Cerebrovascular diseases (430–438)			
Persons age 35–64 yrs	0.49	0.51	0.50
Persons age ≥65 yrs	0.22	0.05	0.12
Atherosclerosis (440)	0.54	0.24	0.36
Aortic aneurysm (441)	0.55	0.25	0.44
■ RESPIRATORY DISEASES			
Pneumonia and influenza (480–487)	0.31	0.18	0.24
Bronchitis, emphysema (491–492)	0.84	0.72	0.79
Chronic airway obstruction (496)	0.85	0.72	0.79

From CDC: Cigarette smoking-attributable mortality and years of potential life lost—United States, 1990. MMWR. 42(33):645–649, 1993; US Department of Health and Human Services: Vital Statistics Data Tapes, 1990.

[a] International Classification of Diseases. 9th revision.

[b] NA, not applicable.

lence of chronic cough and phlegm than never smokers.[102] Several large cohort studies have found that pipe smokers and cigar smokers have an approximately 2-fold increase in COPD mortality compared with nonsmokers, but the case fatality rate for these groups of smokers is lower than that for cigarette smokers.[92] However, a large prospective study in Scandinavia found that the lower mortality risk compared with the risk with cigarette smoking was markedly diminished after adjustment for smoke inhalation.[67] In 1991, an estimated 145 persons in the United States died from COPD as a result of pipe smoking.[76]

After smoking cessation the rate of reduction of COPD excess risk is determined by prior smoking patterns (duration and daily consumption) and number of years since cessation. Smoking cessation reduces respiratory symptoms and respiratory infections. Smokers who quit have better pulmonary function than continuing smokers.[94] For persons without overt COPD, smoking improves pulmonary function about 5 percent within a few months of quitting. Cigarette smoking accelerates the age-related decline in lung function; with abstinence, the rate of decline returns to that of never smokers. With sustained abstinence, the COPD mortality rate is lower than that for continuing smokers.[20] For example, in the U.S. Veterans Study, the mortality ratio for current smokers was about 12; this ratio was reduced to 10 among ex-smokers 10 years after cessation. After more than 20 years of abstinence, the mortality rate was twice that of nonsmokers.[21] Persons with destructive lung changes can often stabilize after cessation but do not regain lost lung function.[92]

Gastrointestinal Disease

Cigarette smoking is epidemiologically associated with symptomatic gastroesophageal reflux disease. Compared with nonsmokers, smokers have reduced lower esophageal sphincter pressure and reduced salivary function, which contributes to a longer acid clearance time.[103]

Smokers of both genders have a high prevalence of peptic ulcer disease, with a clear dose-response relationship.[104] The ACS CPS-I found that the relative risk of mortality for peptic ulcer among men was 3.1 for current smokers and 1.5 for former smokers compared with lifetime nonsmokers.[9] Duodenal ulcers heal more slowly among smokers than among nonsmokers, even with therapy. Both gastric and duodenal ulcers are also more likely to recur among smokers. Smoking cessation is associated with fewer duodenal ulcers, improved short-term healing of gastric ulcers, and reduced recurrence of gastric ulcers.[20]

Diseases of the Mouth

Epidemiological studies from several countries have shown that cigarette smokers have more periodontal disease than do nonsmokers, suggesting a possible causal role for cigarette smoking in the development of periodontal disease.[11,105–109] An analysis of 2,948 persons who participated in the first National Health and Nutrition Examination survey (NHANES I) found that smoking has an independent, direct association with periodontal disease.[107] A strong association has been noted between both the duration of smoking and cumulative consumption and the level of periodontal disease.[110,111]

Leukoplakia or gum recession occurs in 40 to 60 percent of smokeless tobacco users[112] and can occur even among young people.[113,114] Gum recession commonly occurs in the area of the mouth adjacent to where the smokeless tobacco is held. Among adult users of smokeless tobacco or snuff, the risk of oral disease has been well documented, and changes in the hard and soft tissues of the mouth, discoloration of teeth, and decreased ability to taste and smell have been reported.[115–117] One study of smokeless tobacco users in a high school population reported that 49 percent of these teenage users (averaging 1.7 years of smokeless tobacco use) had soft tissue lesions, periodontal inflammation, or both, or erosion of dental hard tissues.[118]

In Utero Effects of Maternal Smoking

The effects on the fetus of maternal smoking have been extensively studied.[20,40] It is well documented that infants born to women who smoke during pregnancy weigh an average of 200 g less than those born to nonsmokers.[20,119] The incidence of low–birth weight (less than 2,500 g) in infants born to mothers who smoke is twice that in infants born to nonsmokers.[20,120] The relationship between maternal smoking and low–birth weight is dose dependent and independent of other factors known to influence birth weight, including race, parity, maternal body weight and height, socioeconomic status, gender of child, and gestational age.[40] An estimated 17 to 26 percent of low–birth weight births could be prevented by eliminating smoking during pregnancy.[20] Women who stop smoking before becoming pregnant have infants of the same birth weight as never smokers do. In addition, pregnant smokers who quit in the first 3 to 4 months of pregnancy and remain abstinent through the rest of the pregnancy have normal birth weight infants. Pregnant women who stop smoking before the 30th week of gestation have infants with higher birth weight than do continuing smokers.[20]

Preterm delivery is associated with maternal smoking (relative risk of 1.5). An estimated 7 to 10 percent of preterm deliveries could be prevented by eliminating smoking during pregnancy. However, smoking affects birth weight primarily by retarding fetal growth. The risk for a small-for-gestation-age infant is 3.5 to 4 times higher among women who smoke during pregnancy than among nonsmoking women.[20] In 1985, the Centers for Disease Control defined the fetal tobacco syndrome as follows: (*a*) the mother smoked 5 cpd or more a day throughout the pregnancy; (*b*) the mother had no evidence of hypertension during pregnancy, specifically no pre-eclampsia and documentation of normal blood pressure at least once after the first trimester; (*c*) the newborn infant had symmetrical growth retardation at term, 37 weeks, defined as birth weight less than 2,500 g and a ponderal index (weight in grams divided by length) greater than 2.32; and (*d*) there is no obvious cause of intrauterine growth retardation, such as congenital malformation or infection.[9] Several mechanisms are thought to cause the reduction in fetal growth, including impaired maternal weight gain and increased cyanide exposure (leading to impaired vitamin B_{12} metabolism). The primary mechanism, however, is thought be intrauterine hypoxia, which is caused by increased carboxyhemoglobin production from carbon monoxide exposure and vasoconstriction of the umbilical arteries.[20] Although fetal growth is diminished among maternal smokers, placenta-to-birth weight ratios are larger in comparison with those of maternal nonsmokers,[121] probably because of the larger placental surface necessary to provide adequate fetal oxygenation in smokers.

Maternal smoking is associated with higher fetal, neonatal, and infant mortality, independent of sociodemographic factors for such mortality.[20] Some data support an association between smoking and increased risk of spontaneous abortion.[9,122,123] Smoking during pregnancy also increases the risk of placenta previa and abruptio placentae.[20] One large study showed adjusted infant mortality rates of 15.1 per 1,000 for white nonsmokers and 23.3 per 1,000 for white women who smoked more than one pack per day. Comparable infant mortality rates for black women were 26.0 and 39.9 per 1,000, respectively.[124] A strong risk factor for sudden infant death syndrome (SIDS) is maternal smoking during pregnancy. Studies have consistently shown a 2- to 4-fold increased risk of SIDS among infants whose mothers smoked during pregnancy compared with infants of nonsmoking mothers, even after other risk factors were controlled for. Most hypotheses about possible mechanisms center around the effects of maternal smoking on fetal oxygenation and fetal development.[125–127] One animal study reported that fetal exposure to nicotine leads to reduced tolerance of hypoxic episodes and increased mortality.[128]

The few studies that have examined the long-term consequences of maternal smoking in offspring suggest a slight increase in the incidence of mental retardation, cerebral palsy, epilepsy, hyperactivity, shortened attention span, lower test scores, and electroencephalographic abnormalities.[129–132] However, these studies are limited by small numbers and infrequency of events of interest, making any conclusion premature.

Health Effects on Young People

Although many of the adverse health effects from tobacco occur later in life, smoking also has health implications for young people. High school seniors who are regular cigarette smokers are more likely to report shortness of breath when not exercising, cough, productive cough, or wheezing and gasping, even after statistical adjustment for sex, other drug use, and parental education.[134] Cigarette smoking during adolescence also appears to reduce the rate of lung growth and the level of lung function that can be achieved. Young smokers are more likely to be less physically fit than nonsmokers. Smoking by children is also associated with an increased risk for early atheromatous lesions and increased cardiovascular risk factors. Smokeless tobacco use by children is associated with halitosis, periodontal degeneration, and soft tissue lesions.[113] Cigarette smoking is also associated with other high-risk behaviors among young people, including other drug use, fighting, and high-risk sexual behavior.[113]

Most young people who smoke regularly are already addicted to nicotine. For example, at least one symptom of nicotine withdrawal was reported by 92 percent of daily cigarette smokers and 93 percent of daily smokeless tobacco users age 12 to 22 years who had previously tried to quit.[135] In another study using different measures of nicotine dependence, 91 percent of daily cigarette users (smoked daily for 2 consecutive weeks or more in the past year), 48 percent of daily alcohol users, 60 percent of daily marijuana users, and 79 percent of daily cocaine users reported one or more indicators of dependence on that drug.[136]

▸ HEALTH RISKS OF ENVIRONMENTAL TOBACCO SMOKE

Constituents of Environmental Tobacco Smoke

Evidence for adverse health effects from environmental tobacco smoke (ETS), which is sometimes called secondhand smoke or passive smoke, is strong. ETS is a diluted mixture of "mainstream" smoke exhaled by smokers and "sidestream" smoke from the burning end of a cigarette or other tobacco product. However, it is chemically similar to the smoke inhaled by smokers and contains a complex mix of over 4,000 chemicals, including a number of cancer-causing chemicals and toxic substances such as nicotine, carbon monoxide, and nitrogen.[137] Sidestream smoke is the major component of ETS, providing nearly all of the vapor-phase constituents and more than half the particulate matter. Sidestream and mainstream smoke are different in their temperature of combustion of the tobacco, pH, and degree of dilution in air, which occurs in conjunction with a decline in temperature. All of the five known human carcinogens, nine probable human carcinogens, and three animal carcinogens are emitted at higher levels in sidestream smoke than in mainstream smoke. In addition, many toxic compounds, such as ammonia and carbon monoxide, are emitted at higher levels in sidestream smoke.[137]

Considerable work has been done to develop sensitive and specific markers of exposure to passive smoking. Vapor-phase nicotine and respirable suspended particulate matter have been identified as markers for the presence and concentration of ETS in the environment, and cotinine (a metabolite of nicotine), and to a lesser degree nicotine itself, are widely used biomarkers of ETS exposure and uptake.[137] The dose-response correlation between urinary cotinine levels and self-reported exposure to tobacco smoke is strong.[137–139] Biomarker data show that levels of ETS constituents encountered indoors by nonsmokers are large enough to be absorbed and result in measurable doses in exposed persons.[137] For example, a study of a large nationally representative sample of persons age 4 years and older indicated that 88 percent of nontobacco users had detectable levels of serum cotinine, although only 37 percent of adults and 43 percent of children were aware they were exposed to ETS in the home or at work.[140]

Environmental Tobacco Smoke and Children's Health

One-third to one-half of adult current cigarette smokers have children living in the home, and 70 percent allow smoking in some or all areas of the home.[141] Urinary cotinine concentrations in infants and young children correlate with the number of smokers reported in the home[137,142–144] and the number of cigarettes smoked by the mother during the prior 24 hours.[145] Studies in the early 1970s suggested an association between ETS exposure in the home and respiratory conditions among children. More than 100 epidemiological studies on the health effects of ETS exposure among children have been published; more than 50 have been added since the 1986 Surgeon General's Report[146] and 1986 National Academy of Science's National Research Council (NRC) review,[147] both of which concluded that ETS is a major contributor to impaired respiratory health among children, especially young children. After extensive review of the literature, the U.S. Environmental Protection Agency (EPA) concluded that ETS is causally associated with an increased risk of lower respiratory infections (e.g., bronchitis and pneumonia) in children and that an estimated 150,000 to 300,000 cases each year among infants and young children up to 18 months of age are attributable to ETS exposure. The EPA also concluded that ETS exposure is causally associated with increased prevalence of fluid in the middle ear, symptoms of upper respiratory tract irritation, and a small but significant reduction in lung function in children. In addition, ETS is causally associated with additional episodes and increased severity of asthma in children—an estimated 200,000 to 1,000,000 asthmatic children have their condition exacerbated by exposure to ETS—and is a risk factor for new cases of asthma among children who have not previously been symptomatic.[137]

Children exposed to ETS have an average 1.87 more days of restricted activity, 1.06 more days in bed, and 1.45 more days absent from school than do children not exposed to ETS. Nationwide, children have 18 million days of restricted activity, 10 millions days of bed confinement, and 7 million days of school absence attributable to daily ETS exposure.[148]

Environmental Tobacco Smoke and Sudden Infant Death Syndrome

Several studies have shown an association between infant exposure to ETS and SIDS independent of the effect of maternal smoking during pregnancy. This relationship has been found for maternal smoking, paternal smoking, and smoking by others in the household. A dose-response relationship was noted with increasing numbers of cigarettes, increasing number of smokers, and increasing duration of exposure to ETS.[125–127] In 1997, the California Environmental Protection Agency reported that there was sufficient evidence to conclude that there was a causal association between ETS and SIDS.[149]

Environmental Tobacco Smoke and Adults

Among healthy adults, the most common complaints after exposure to ETS are irritant effects. The main irritant effects of ETS occur in the eye conjunctiva and in the mucous membranes of the nose, throat, and lower respiratory tract. The primary eye symptoms include reddening, itching, and tearing; the primary respiratory tract symptoms are itching, cough, and sore throat.[146] Exposure to ETS both precipitates and aggravates allergic attacks in some individuals with respiratory allergies and exacerbates other symptoms associated with allergies such as eye irritation, nasal symptoms, headaches, cough, wheezing, sore throat, and hoarseness.[146,149a]

Environmental Tobacco Smoke and Lung Cancer

In 1985 three major bodies were independently convened to consider the evidence for health impacts of passive smoking. These three bodies, the U.S. Public Health Service, the NRC, and the Interagency Task Force on Environmental Cancer, Heart, and Lung Disease, reached a consensus that a substantial number of lung cancer deaths among nonsmokers can be attributed to involuntary smoking.[146,147,150]

At least three prospective studies and 15 case-control studies were reviewed in detail in the 1986 Surgeon General's Report[146] and the 1986 NRC review.[147] Most of the studies reported a positive association between ETS and lung cancer, which was statistically significant in six of the studies. Because of the consistency of the results and supporting evidence, both reports concluded that ETS is causally associated with lung cancer in nonsmokers. The EPA reviewed the scientific evidence on ETS and lung cancer in a report published in 1993. Thirty epidemiological studies (four prospective and 26 case-control) conducted in eight countries and using a variety of study designs were reviewed; these studies comprised 3,000 lung cancer cases. Twenty-four of the 30 studies reported a higher risk of lung cancer among never smokers exposed to ETS than among never smokers not exposed to ETS, the higher risk was statistically significant in nine of the studies. The 17 studies that reported levels of spousal smoking showed an increased risk among nonsmoking spouses most heavily exposed to ETS, and the increase was statistically significant in nine of the studies despite small sample sizes. Of the 14 studies with dose-response information, 10 demonstrated a statistically significant dose-response relationship. On the basis of the weight of this evidence, the EPA concluded that exposure to ETS causes lung cancer in nonsmokers and estimated that 3,000 deaths occur among U.S. nonsmokers each year as a result of exposure to ETS. The EPA report also classified ETS as a "Group A" (known human) carcinogen, a classification that includes asbestos and benzene.[137] Since the release of the EPA report, several other U.S. studies have been published. Two found no overall increased risk of lung cancer from ever being exposed to ETS, although one of these studies showed an increased risk for persons most intensely exposed to ETS.[151,152] Another study found an increased risk among those ever exposed to ETS, which was not statistically significant, and a significant increased risk among the more intensely exposed.[153] The largest U.S. case-control study to date found a statistically significant increase of lung cancer among women ever exposed to ETS and a dose-response relationship.[154] In the ACS CPS-II, a nonsignificant increased risk of lung cancer of about 20 percent was found for nonsmoking women married to smokers.[155]

Environmental Tobacco Smoke and Other Diseases

The effect of ETS smoking on chronic respiratory symptoms or disease in adult nonsmokers is difficult to measure. The EPA concluded that ETS exposure may result in increased frequency of respiratory symptoms in adults and estimated that respiratory symptoms are 30 to 60 percent higher in nonsmokers exposed to ETS than in nonsmokers not exposed to ETS.[137]

Both the 1986 Surgeon General's Report and the 1986 NRC report reviewed the evidence available on ETS and respiratory disease in adults. The Surgeon General's Report concluded that healthy adults exposed to ETS may have small changes in pulmonary function tests, probably because of the irritants in ETS, but are not likely to have significant reductions in pulmonary function as a result of exposure to ETS as an adult.[146] The NRC concluded that it was difficult to determine how a single factor such as ETS affects lung function, but reported that ETS may add to the burden of environmental insults that can cause chronic lung disease.[147] The EPA report also reviewed six additional studies of ETS and adult lung function and respiratory symptoms and concluded that ETS exposure may result in small decreases (2.5 percent) in lung function among adult nonsmokers.[137] Whether these reductions translate into overt health problems in otherwise healthy individuals or even in those with preexisting respiratory problems remains unknown.

Epidemiological evidence of an association between ETS and cardiovascular disease among nonsmokers has been increasing: at least 15 studies have examined the association between heart disease and exposure to ETS in nonsmokers.[156–162] Almost all of these studies have reported an increased risk of heart disease among these persons. Many of the studies controlled for other cardiovascular risk factors and several demonstrated a positive dose-response relationship between ETS exposure and cardiovascular disease. A 1994 meta-analytic review of 12 of these studies concluded that there was a 23 percent higher CHD mortality among never smokers exposed to ETS than in never smokers not exposed to ETS.[163] The most recent and the largest study, which used data from the ACS CPS-II, controlled for other cardiovascular risk factors and found about a 20 percent higher CHD mortality among never smokers exposed to ETS; however, a consistent dose-response trend was not found.[162] A recent cohort study found that ETS exposure increased the progression of atherosclerosis by 20 percent compared to those not exposed to ETS.[46] In 1997, the California Environmental Protection Agency reported that there was sufficient evidence to conclude that there was a causal association between ETS and cardiovascular disease.[149]

Various experimental and clinical studies suggest possible mechanisms for the effects of ETS on cardiovascular disease. ETS appears to cause increased platelet aggregation, increased thrombosis, decreased oxygen supply, and increased oxygen demand—all effects consistent with the mechanisms found for active smoking. Many of the effects are believed to be caused by nicotine and carbon monoxide in ETS, but other agents may also be important.[164]

► TRENDS IN TOBACCO USE

Prevalence of Cigarette Consumption among Adults and Teenagers

Annual per capita consumption of cigarettes reached a peak of 4,345 in 1963, a year before the first Surgeon General's Report was published, and, except for an increase from 1971 through 1973, steadily declined (Fig. 44-3). Per capita cigarette consumption was 2399 in 1997. Overall numbers of cigarettes sold in the United States declined from 640 billion in 1981 to 475 billion in 1997.[166]

From 1964 to the late 1980s, smoking prevalence in the United States decreased an average of 0.5 percent per year; since the early

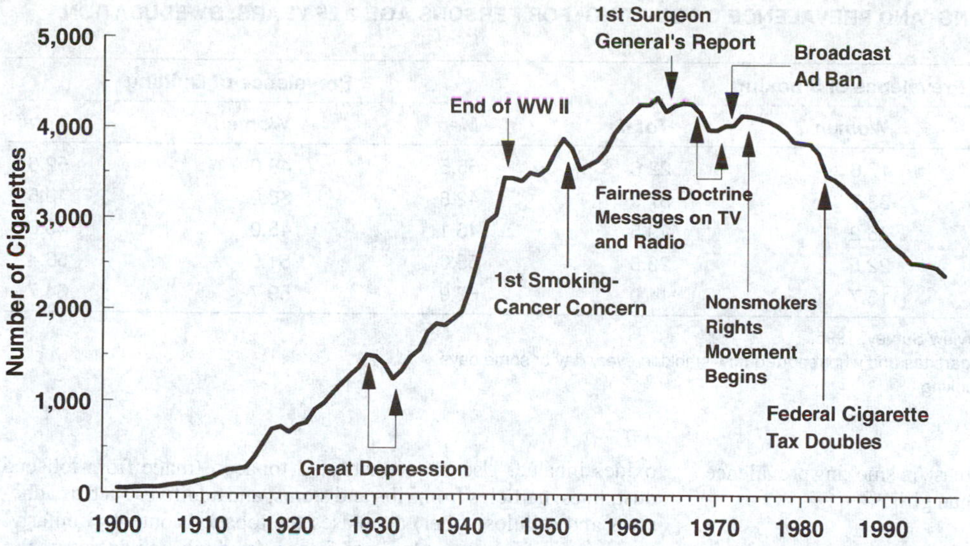

Figure 44-3. Adult per capita cigarette consumption and major smoking and health events, United States, 1900 to 1997 (1997 estimate is preliminary). (From Centers for Disease Control, Office of Smoking and Health: Reducing the Health Consequences of Smoking: 25 Years of Progress. A Report of the Surgeon General. DHHS Publication No. (CDC) 89-8411. Rockville, MD: Centers for Disease Control, Office of Smoking and Health, 1989 and U.S. Dept. of Agriculture. Tobacco Situation and Outlook Report: USDA Pub No TBS-239. Washington, DC: US Dept of Agriculture, Economic Research Source Commercial Agriculture Division, 1997).

1990s, the prevalence has remained essentially unchanged.[167,168] In the 1995 National Health Interview Survey (NHIS), 24.7 percent of adults (persons 18 years of age and older) were reported to be current smokers. The recent slowing of the reduction in smoking prevalence is of concern, as are the differences by age, gender, race, education, and socioeconomic status. This analysis examined prevalence and cessation rates.

Smoking prevalence was higher for men (27.0) than for women (22.6 percent). Smoking prevalence was highest in the 25- to 44-year age group (28.6 percent), followed by those 45 to 64 years of age (25.5 percent) and 18 to 24 years of age (24.8 percent). Americans age 65 years and older continued to smoke at a lower rate (13.0 percent).[168]

Among both women and men, the trend in smoking prevalence has been downward, both for white and black populations. In 1965, smoking prevalence was higher for men (52 percent) than for women (34 percent). From 1965 to 1983, the decline in smoking prevalence was greater for men (16.8 percentage points) than for women (4.4 percentage points); however, from 1983 to 1995, the decline in smoking prevalence was comparable for women and men (7 to 8 percentage points).[167–169] In 1995, the prevalence of quitting among those who ever smoked continued to be higher for men (50 percent) than for women (46 percent).[170] This has sometimes been interpreted to mean that women are less likely to quit smoking than men. Because men are more likely than women to switch to or continue to use other tobacco products when they stop smoking cigarettes, the gender difference is less for quitting any tobacco use. In addition, from 1965 to 1994, the prevalence of quitting among ever smokers increased 27 percentage points for women but 23 percentage points for men. The patterns in the prevalence of quitting among ever smokers is consistent with the historical patterns of smoking among women and men: men began quitting in greater numbers in the 1950s, but this pattern did not occur for women until the 1960s. Thus, the comparable trend with the higher absolute value for men reflects that early quitters were predominantly male.[169] Other data show that women are as likely as men to quit for a day and to remain abstinent.[171,172]

In 1978, the first year data were available from the NHIS for whites, blacks, and Hispanics, smoking prevalence was lower among Hispanics (32 percent) than among whites (34 percent) or blacks (37 percent).[167] In 1995, smoking prevalence was 17 percent among Asians and Pacific Islanders, 18 percent among Hispanics, 26 percent among whites, 26 percent among blacks, and 36 percent among American Indians and Alaska Natives.[168] The prevalence of quitting among ever smokers in 1995 was 50 percent for whites, 36 percent for blacks, and 47 percent for Hispanics.[170] Unlike the gender differences, which are explained by historical patterns in smoking behavior, the lower prevalence of quitting among blacks reflects differences in quitting behavior: blacks are more likely than whites to try to quit smoking and are less likely to succeed, even after adjustment for demographic differences.[171,173] This difference remains even after adjustment for other tobacco use.[20]

Formal educational attainment exhibits a striking association with smoking prevalence and cessation rates. However, this relationship is not linear. The "less than high school graduate" category consists of two groups with distinct smoking patterns: persons with 0 to 8 years of education and persons with 9 to 11 years of education. Smoking prevalence and cessation for persons in the former group are similar to persons having 12 years of education, whereas persons in the latter group are the most likely to be current, ever, and heavy smokers, and the least likely to have quit smoking. After 11 years of education, the likelihood of smoking decreases with each successive year of education. These results persist after adjustment for age, sex, ethnicity, poverty status, employment status, marital status, geographic region, and year of survey.[173] In 1995, smoking prevalence was highest for persons with 9 to 11 years of education (38 percent) and lowest for persons with 16 years of education or more (14 percent) (Table 44-5).[168] Similarly, the prevalence of quitting among ever smokers was lowest among persons with 9 to 11 years of education (41 percent) and highest among persons with 16 years of education or more (65 percent).[170]

Persons who are unemployed; blue-collar workers; persons who are widowed, separated, or divorced; and those below the poverty level are more likely to have ever smoked or to be current smokers and to be heavy smokers (15 cpd or more).[168,174,175]

In 1997, 47 percent of 8th graders, 60 percent of 10th graders, and 65 percent of 12th graders had tried cigarette smoking.[176] The prevalence of current smoking (defined as smoking within the past 30 days) among high school seniors decreased from 39 percent in 1976 to 29 percent in 1981. The prevalence was then relatively stable until 1992. However, current smoking prevalence then increased to 36 percent by 1997 (Fig. 44-4). Between 1991 and 1997, the prevalence of smoking increased from 21 to 30 percent among 10th graders and from 14 to 19 percent among 8th graders. Similar patterns were seen for daily smoking: the prevalence among high school seniors decreased from 29 percent in 1976 to 17 percent in 1992, but then increased to 25 percent by 1997. Daily smoking increased from 1991 to 1997 among 8th and 10th graders as well. Among high school seniors, smoking prevalence was higher for girls than for boys until the late 1980s; since 1990, current and daily smoking prevalences have been comparable for girls and boys.[176] A larger decline in current smoking prevalence occurred among black high school seniors from 1977 (36.7 percent) to 1992 (8.7 percent).[167] However, smoking prevalence among black high school students increased from 1992 to

TABLE 44-5. PREVALENCE OF SMOKING[a] AND PREVALENCE OF QUITTING[b] FOR PERSONS AGE ≥ 25 YEARS, BY EDUCATION, UNITED STATES, 1995

	Prevalence of Smoking			Prevalence of Quitting		
Education (yr)	*Men*	*Women*	*Total*	*Men*	*Women*	*Total*
≤8	28.4	17.8	22.6	55.5	48.0	52.6
9–11	41.9	33.7	37.5	42.8	38.0	40.5
12	33.7	26.2	29.5	46.1	45.0	45.6
13–15	25.0	22.5	23.6	55.6	51.0	53.4
≥16	14.3	13.7	14.0	67.9	59.7	64.7

From CDC, MMWR, 1997; National Health Interview Survey, 1995.
[a] Persons who reported having smoked ≥100 cigarettes and who reported now smoking every day or some days.
[b] Percentage of ever smokers who have quit smoking.

1996, from 8.7 to 14.3 percent.[176] The increase in smoking prevalence was greater for African American boys than girls.[177]

The Changing Cigarette

Tar is a complex mixture of compounds, including a number of identifiable carcinogens and cocarcinogens; nicotine is generally accepted as the principal constituent responsible for a smoker's pharmacological response.[9,11,178] In the early 1950s, when smoking was first associated with lung cancer, a majority of Americans smoked unfiltered (plain) high-tar cigarettes, with a sales-weighted average tar and nicotine content per cigarette of 38 mg and 2.7 mg, respectively, in 1954. By 1993, the sales-weighted average tar and nicotine content per cigarette had dropped to 12 mg and 0.95 mg, respectively. The reductions have resulted through the use of efficient filters, highly porous cigarette paper, and changing the composition of the tobacco blend. However, the measurements are based on yields from cigarettes as measured by the U.S. Federal Trade Commission (FTC) smoking machine under standardized laboratory conditions, which do not reflect the actual smoking patterns of persons who smoke filtered cigarettes.[179]

A major reason for the decline in sales-weighted tar and nicotine levels is the widespread acceptance of filtered cigarettes. Their use increased from 0.56 percent in 1955 to more than 97 percent since 1993. Filters are generally composed of cellulose acetate, although some also have charcoal. Filters reduce the amount of tar inhaled and selectively reduce some of the volatile components of cigarette smoke. Since 1968, filters increasingly have contained perforations (which may or may not be visible) which allow air to dilute the smoke.[180]

Other measures used to reduce the tar and nicotine content yields on the standard smoke assays include the use of porous cigarette paper, which reduces the tar, carbon monoxide, and nitrogen oxides inhaled. Use of reconstituted tobacco (made from tobacco dust, fines, particles from ribs and stems, and additives such as adhesives and cellulose fiber) decreases the tobacco content. Similarly, the use of puffed, expanded, and freeze-dried tobacco decreases the amount of tobacco needed to fill a cigarette. Increasing the length of the cigarette allows more air to enter the paper and for more of the volatile components to diffuse out of the cigarette; increasing the filter length decreases the amount of tobacco in the cigarette, and decreasing the cigarette circumference reduces the amount of tobacco available for burning. Finally, using a more coarsely cut tobacco means the tobacco burns less efficiently.[179,181]

The progression from unfiltered high-tar, to filtered high-tar, to filtered middle-tar, and to filtered low-tar cigarettes has also been observed in most industrialized countries, although at a slower pace and 5 to 10 years after the introduction of these changes in the United States.[179] Since their introduction to the U.S. cigarette market in the late 1960s and early 1970s, the so-called low-tar and low-nicotine cigarettes, have had rapid increases in market share. The market share of cigarettes yielding 15 mg of tar or less increased from 2 percent in 1967 to 73 percent by 1995. In addition, since their introduction in the late 1970s, the cigarette brands with less than 10 mg of tar, have captured 27 percent of the U.S. market.[182] Similar patterns of consumption of low-tar cigarettes also occurred in Canada during this period.[183] The significant growth of the low-tar cigarette market in the past two decades is attributable to increased public awareness that cigarette smoking, particularly exposure to tar and nicotine, is detrimental to health.

Because of the widespread acceptance of cigarettes lower in tar and nicotine content, several studies were conducted to ascertain the health consequences associated with reductions in cigarette tar and

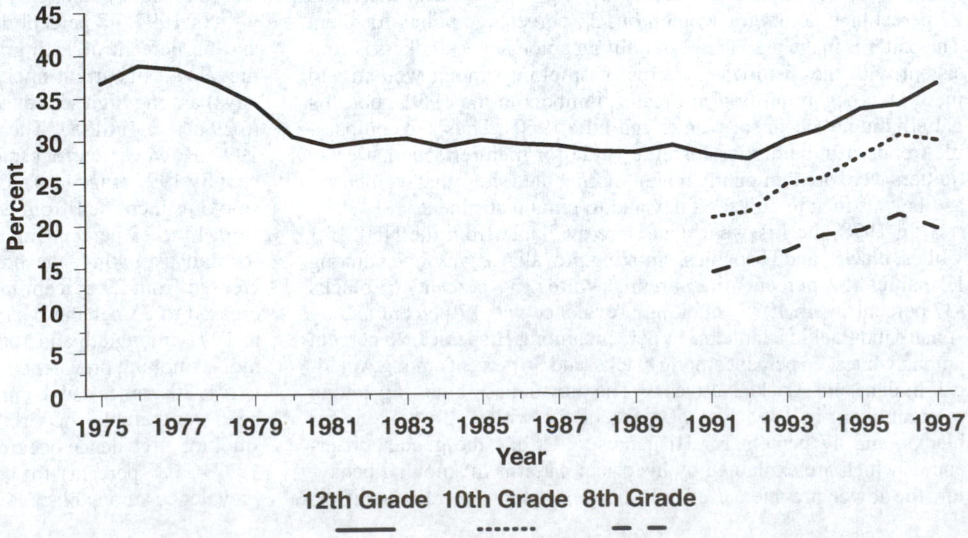

Figure 44-4. Trends in cigarette smoking anytime in the past 30 days (i.e., smoking one or more cigarettes during the previous 30 days) by grade in school, United States, 1975 to 1997. (From Anonymous: Cigarette smoking rates may have peaked among younger teens. Ann Arbor, MI: The University of Michigan, News and Information Services, 1997.)

nicotine yields. One study followed more than 1 million people for 12 years and reported that those persons who smoked medium-tar brands (at that time defined as cigarettes having 17.6 to 25.8 mg of tar per cigarette) had a 9 percent lower overall mortality rate and those smoking low-tar cigarettes (defined then as cigarettes having less than 17.6 mg of tar per cigarette) had a 16 percent lower overall mortality rate than did smokers of high-tar cigarettes (defined as cigarettes having 25.8 to 35.7 mg of tar per cigarette).[184]

Results from the same study indicated that smokers of low-tar brands had a 26 percent reduction in lung cancer mortality rates compared with smokers of high-tar brands. Despite these reductions, lung cancer mortality and overall mortality among smokers of low-tar cigarettes were much greater than those of nonsmokers.[184] Adenocarcinoma has replaced squamous cell as the leading cause of lung cancer death in the United States. A recent analysis suggests that this increase in incidence parallels changes in smoking behavior and cigarette design. It has been hypothesized that the smoke from high-tar, unfiltered cigarettes was too irritating to be inhaled deeply and was deposited in the central bronchi where squamous cell carcinomas occur. Smoke from milder filtered cigarettes could be inhaled more deeply, allowing for the development of the more peripheral adenocarcinomas.[58,59]

With respect to heart disease, a large cohort study reported a significant reduction (14 percent) in CHD mortality among low-tar cigarette smokers, but evidence from the Framingham Study suggests that smokers of low-tar, low-nicotine cigarettes and of filtered cigarettes do not have a lower CHD incidence than smokers of high-tar, unfiltered brands.[184–186] This latter finding has been corroborated in later case-control studies, one of which reported the relative risk for nonfatal MI among young men (30 to 54 years of age) smoking low-tar cigarettes to be 2.8 compared with the relative risk for nonsmokers.[187]

Evidence is unavailable on the relative risks of developing COPD from the smoking of low-tar, low-nicotine cigarettes. An autopsy series study indicated that autopsies on smokers performed from 1970 to 1977 found fewer airway changes at comparable smoking levels than those performed from 1955 to 1960, suggesting that lower tar cigarettes had less effect on the lungs than did higher tar cigarettes. However, the existing evidence does not support a relationship between tar yield and lung function: in two studies (one cohort and one cross-sectional), there was no association between tar level and FEV_1.[70] It appears from a number of studies, however, that the prevalence of cough and phlegm may be halved among smokers of very-low-tar cigarettes compared with that of smokers of high-tar cigarettes.[70,92]

Although there appear to be some differences in human nicotine exposure between high-yield cigarettes and low-yield cigarettes, these differences are small and do not correspond to the magnitude of difference in the yields as measured by the FTC smoking machine. Similarly, studies have generally found no relationship between carbon monoxide levels in the human body and FTC machine yields. In addition, studies suggest that the published tar-to-nicotine ratio based on the FTC machine test does not correspond to the actual tar-to-nicotine ratios absorbed by smokers. Thus, the published tar-to-nicotine ratios cannot be used to estimate the tar exposure for smokers. In general, the FTC method underestimates human exposure to the chemicals in cigarette smoke.[188] The FTC machine takes 2-second, 35-mL puffs every 60 seconds until the cigarette is smoked to 3 mm of the filter overwrap, whereas humans, on average, take puffs of greater than 35 mL over 1.8 seconds and take a puff every 34 seconds. The FTC method underestimates by a greater degree the amount of smoke drawn from low-yield cigarettes than from high-yield cigarettes.[189] In addition, since the FTC machine smokes to within 3 mm of the overwrap, lengthening the overwrap can decrease the apparent yield, even though the remaining tobacco can be smoked. A common but apt suggestion is that smoking machine parameters and methods used by the U.S. Federal Trade Commission to determine cigarette yields be updated to approximate more closely the patterns of human smoking behavior. The FTC is proposing changes in the laboratory method of determining the smoke yield of tar, nicotine, and carbon monoxide. As of January 1998, the FTC was soliciting public comment on these proposed changes.[190]

It is reported that changes in smoking methods are related to smokers' self-regulation of their blood nicotine level[191] and that higher yields of nicotine can be obtained by alternating the frequency and depth of inhalation,[192] increasing the number of cigarettes smoked, or mechanically compressing filter tips and blocking air channels with the lips or fingers.[9,180,189,193,194] One study of participants who spontaneously switched cigarette brands to ones with a lower reported yield compared the smokers' cotinine levels before and after the switch. Although the nicotine yield was reduced from 1.09 to 0.68 mg, the serum cotinine levels were unchanged.[195] Another study found that even persons smoking ultra-low–yield cigarettes could be exposed to high levels of nicotine and carbon monoxide.[196] Therefore, smokers need to be informed that they may not be deriving any health benefit from low-tar products and strongly advised to quit smoking completely.

Cigars and Pipes

In the United States, total consumption of cigars decreased yearly from 8,108 million cigars in 1970 to 2,138 million cigars in 1993, then increased 68 percent to 3,589 million cigars in 1997; the level in 1997 was comparable to that in 1983.[197] This recent increase corresponds with an aggressive marketing campaign that glamorizes cigar use.

A 1996 national survey found that 27% of adolescents (aged 14 to 19 years) had smoked a cigar in the past year. Similarly, a 1996 Massachusetts study found that 5 percent of 6th graders, 14 percent of 7th and 8th graders, and 28 percent of high school students had smoked a cigar in the past year.[197a]

Cigar smoke contains the same toxic and carcinogenic constituents as cigarette smoke, and it is associated with significant health risks, including lung cancer and COPD.[28,36,37,67] Although the 1983 Surgeon General's Report on the health consequences of smoking on cardiovascular disease concluded that smokers who have used only cigars do not have a greater risk of CHD than do nonsmokers, a large recent study suggests an association between cigar smoking and CHD, particularly if the user inhales the smoke.[37] Because cigars are addictive, their use by young people may lead to the chronic use of tobacco products, with potential switching to other products such as cigarettes.

From 1965 to 1991, the prevalence of pipe smoking decreased from 14 to 2 percent among men. Pipe smoking has never been common among women. In 1991, men age 45 years and older were the primary pipe smokers. Most men who smoke pipes often previously used another form of tobacco, particularly cigarettes.[76] Pipe smoking is also associated with significant health risks, including lung cancer and COPD.[28,36,37,67] The 1983 Surgeon General's Report concluded that smokers who have used only pipes are not at greater risk for CHD than nonsmokers, but some recent studies suggest an association between pipe smoking and CHD, particularly if the smoke inhalation patterns mimic that for cigarettes.[36,37]

Smokeless Tobacco

Smokeless, "spit," or oral tobacco (chewing tobacco or snuff) contains tobacco leaves plus sweeteners, flavorings, and scents. Chewing tobacco may be in the form of strands, cakes, or shreds and is either chewed or placed in the mouth. Snuff, which is marketed in a small round can, or tin, is supplied dry or moist, and is held ("dipped") between the gingiva and the lip or cheek. Whereas the smoking of tobacco has declined, the overall prevalence of smokeless tobacco use among U.S. adults has changed little during the past 20 years. The NHIS found that the prevalence of smokeless tobacco use was 5 percent in 1970 and 6 percent in 1991 for men and 2 percent in 1970 and less than 1 percent in 1991 for women.[167] The prevalence tends to be lower in the Northeast and higher in the South.[198] Although the overall prevalence of smokeless tobacco use has remained low for the past two decades, the demographics of smokeless tobacco use have changed dramatically. The behavior was formerly found predominantly among older people, particularly older black men and women and older white men; since the late 1980s, smokeless tobacco use, particularly snuff use, has been seen primarily among young white males.[167] In 1995, the prevalence of smokeless tobacco use among high school boys overall was 20 percent: it was 25 percent among whites, 4 percent among African Americans, and 6 percent among Hispanics.[177]

Long-term smokeless tobacco use increases the risk of periodontal disease and oral leukoplakia.[199,200] There is also strong evidence that smokeless tobacco use causes cancer in humans. The association is strongest for cancers of the oral cavity, particularly among snuff users. One cohort study reported that smokeless tobacco users are also at increased risk of dying from cardiovascular disease.[201] Smokeless tobacco is addictive, its use may predispose those who try it to become smokers of tobacco. Starting in 1986, smokeless tobacco products and advertisements were required by federal law to carry warning labels about the health hazards of their use.

Other Tobacco Products

Tobacco companies have introduced novel, nontherapeutic nicotine-delivery devices. For example, the Favor Smokeless Cigarette, a nicotine inhaler, was introduced in 1985. The U.S. Food and Drug Administration (FDA) determined that this device delivered a drug, and the inhaler was withdrawn from the market. In 1987, the Pinkerton Tobacco Company introduced Masterpiece Tobacs, a chewing gum containing shreds of tobacco. Although the FDA determined that chewing gum is a food product, tobacco had not been approved as a food additive and the product was withdrawn from the market. In 1987, the R.J. Reynolds Tobacco Company introduced Premier, a device that the company claimed heated tobacco rather than burned it. Adverse publicity and consumer complaints about the taste and difficulty lighting the product caused the company to withdraw the product before the FDA could determine whether the product was a drug delivery device.[181] In 1996, the company test marketed Eclipse, which was promoted as a low-smoke cigarette and which, like Premier, the company claims heats tobacco. As of early 1997, the FDA had not determined the regulatory status of Eclipse.[202,203]

► TOBACCO INTERVENTIONS

Treatment for Tobacco Use/Nicotine Dependence

Reduced prevalence of smoking suggests, and many national surveys confirm, that millions of smokers (nearly half of ever smokers) have quit smoking. In addition, 68 percent of current smokers want to stop smoking completely, and 46 percent of current daily smokers stopped smoking for at least 1 day in the preceding 12 months.[168] Of those who have achieved long-term abstinence, the vast majority have stopped without the help of any formal programs, materials, or clinical interventions.[204] The stimuli for cessation differ substantially among individual smokers. Among stimuli reported by ex-smokers as contributing to their cessation and abstinence are health problems, such as emphysema or an MI; strong family pressures, both from spouses and children; peer pressure from friends and coworkers; cost of cigarettes, especially for lower-income individuals; fear of potential adverse effects on personal health or on the health of children; the likelihood of their children starting to smoke; and concern for cleanliness and social acceptance.[9,205–207]

In 1996, the Agency for Health Care Policy and Research (AHCPR) published clinical guidelines on tobacco-use cessation that were based on the systematic review of the scientific literature from 1976 through 1994. Meta-analyses of randomized controlled trials that contained at least 5 months of follow-up served as the basis for most of the recommendations. The guidelines provide recommendations for primary care providers, cessation specialists, and health care systems.[208]

For primary care providers, the guideline recommendations emphasize the importance of (*a*) systematically identifying all tobacco users (so that every patient at every clinic visit has his or her tobacco use documented), (*b*) strongly advising (in a personalized manner) all tobacco users to quit, and (*c*) determining the patient's willingness to quit. The primary care intervention is designed to be brief. Patients not willing to quit should receive a motivational intervention to promote later quit attempts. For patients willing to make a quit attempt, the provider should help the patient set a quit date, prepare the patient for quitting, encourage nicotine replacement therapy, provide self-help materials, and provide key advice on dealing with problem situations. The health care provider should refer the patient to more intensive treatments if appropriate (e.g., the patient has relapsed repeatedly) or if the patient prefers more intensive treatment. All patients attempting to quit should have scheduled follow-up contacts in person or by telephone. These AHCPR recommendations assume that office systems will be implemented to institutionalize tobacco use cessation assessment and intervention.

Cessation specialists are those who view tobacco use cessation as a critical professional role. Cessation specialists often provide intensive treatment programs, train nonspecialists, and develop and evaluate cessation programs. Some AHCPR recommendations are of particular use to cessation specialists. (*a*) Patient assessment should determine whether a tobacco user is motivated to quit with the help of an intensive cessation program. (*b*) Because there is a strong dose-response relationship between counseling intensity and cessation success, there should be at least four sessions, each lasting 20 to 30 minutes, occurring over at least 2 weeks (and preferably more than 8 weeks). (*c*) Multiple types of clinicians should be used. (*d*) Individual counseling, group counseling, or both may be used (use of adjuvant self-help materials is optional), and follow-up should be provided. (*e*) Counseling should include problem-solving and skills training and provide within-treatment social support. (*f*) Except in special circumstances, every smoker should be offered nicotine replacement. (*g*) Intensive intervention programs may be used with all tobacco users willing to enter such programs. Although specialists have an important role to play in tobacco use cessation efforts, the effect of intensive cessation programs is limited because few smokers participate in these programs.[204]

Administrators, insurers, and purchasers of health care delivery can also promote the treatment for tobacco use/nicotine dependence. Administrators can help ensure that institutional changes to promote cessation interventions are systematically and universally implemented. Insurers should consider making effective treatments a covered benefit. Purchasers should consider making tobacco use assessment, counseling, and treatment a contractual obligation. The AHCPR guidelines recommend that (*a*) a tobacco use identification system be implemented in every clinic; (*b*) education, resources, and feedback to promote intervention be provided to clinicians; (*c*) staff be dedicated to provide effective cessation treatment, and the delivery of this treatment be assessed in performance evaluations; (*d*) hospital policies support the provision of cessation services; (*e*) effective smoking cessation treatment (both pharmacology and counseling) be included as paid services in health insurance packages; and (*f*) clinicians be reimbursed for providing effective cessation treatments, and these interventions be among the defined duties of salaried clinicians.

The AHCPR guidelines are consistent with other published recommendations, including those from the National Cancer Institute[209] and the American Medical Association.[210] Similarly, in 1996, the U.S. Preventive Services Task Force recommended that regular tobacco cessation counseling be provided for all persons who use tobacco products; nicotine replacement therapy be prescribed as an adjunct for selected patients; pregnant women and parents be counseled on the potentially harmful effects of ETS on the health of the fetus and children; and antitobacco messages be used during the health promotion counseling of children, adolescents, and young adults.[211]

The AHCPR also evaluated the cost-effectiveness of implementing the guidelines. Their conclusions were similar to previous studies:[211a,212] tobacco treatment is extremely cost-effective, and less costly than other preventive interventions, such as screening mammography, screening for hypertension, and treatment for hypercholesterolemia. Although all types of recommended treatment were cost-effective, those involving more intensive counseling and nicotine replacement therapy were the most cost-effective.[213] Other data suggest that there are cost savings from the treatment of tobacco use, even in the first year, as a result of the rapid decline in risk of acute myocardial infarction and stroke.[214]

Treatment for Tobacco Use in a Managed Care Setting

Quality assurance measures allow comparisons between managed care plans. For example, a majority of plans have adopted at least some of these measures in the Health Plan Employer Data Information Set (HEDIS) and are reporting statistics according to HEDIS specifications.[215] A measure of a plan's smoking cessation activities was first included in December 1996, when HEDIS 3.0 was released. Under this survey measure, managed care plans report the proportion of smokers or recent quitters (within the past year) who had been seen in the plan during the previous year and who had received advice to quit smoking.[216] In 1996, the plan average for smokers reporting receipt of advice to quit in the previous year was 61%; however, advice rates were as low as 30% for some plans.[217]

One managed care plan found that tobacco treatment interventions not only improve quality of care, but also decrease use of medical services: after 1 year of cessation, an ex-smoker's medical costs drop progressively and can reach levels comparable to that of a never smoker's.[218] This plan also found that systematically implementing tobacco treatment interventions accelerated the reduction in smoking prevalence among plan members compared with the general population.[218a] In addition, provision of preventive services in a health plan is associated with increased patient satisfaction with the plan.[218b]

Community Intervention Programs

Community trials for cardiovascular disease prevention, which have tried to decrease cigarette smoking as one of several risk factors, have provided mixed results. In areas where risk factor levels are stable and high and where there is no social movement to produce secular changes in the risk factors (such as Finland's North Karelia project,[219] South Africa's Coronary Risk Factor Study,[220] and the Stanford Three Communities Study[221]), community interventions have produced favorable results. However, in the Stanford Five Cities Project,[222] the Multiple Risk Factor Intervention Trial,[223] the Minnesota Heart Health Program,[224] and the Pawtucket Heart Health Program,[225] the results were mixed or not statistically significant. In these studies, unanticipated secular changes in the control group or inappropriate or inadequate interventions may have produced these results. It is also possible that effects may not be observable except in the very long term.

The Community Intervention Trial for Smoking Cessation (COMMIT) was a community-level intervention designed specifically to increase smoking cessation rates. This multichannel, 4-year intervention consisted of proactive efforts to reach smokers through existing social institutions. COMMIT focused on heavy smokers, although it was assumed that any multichannel communitywide strategy would reach light to moderate smokers as well. The quit rate changed significantly among light to moderate smokers but not among heavy smokers in the intervention communities. No significant differences in smoking prevalence in the intervention or control communities among heavy smokers or overall were observed.[226]

Currently, there are several demonstration projects in the states (the District of Columbia is treated as a state for this discussion) for community tobacco control activities. ASSIST (the American Stop Smoking Intervention Study for Cancer Prevention), which is funded by the National Cancer Institute (NCI) and conducted in collaboration with the ACS, funds 17 state health departments to form community-based tobacco coalitions. These coalitions are responsible for developing and implementing comprehensive state plans for tobacco use prevention and control. The CDC funds 33 state health departments in the non-ASSIST states through its IMPACT (Initiatives to Mobilize for the Prevention and Control of Tobacco Use) program. California has its own statewide initiative funded by tobacco taxes. As a result of these initiatives, all states now have a tobacco control coordinator, a state plan for tobacco prevention and control, and community-based tobacco coalitions.[227] In addition, as of Jan 1998 the Robert Wood Johnson Foundation funds 31 state agencies and organizations to develop programs to reduce tobacco use, particularly among children and youth, and other states besides California have developed statewide initiatives funded by tobacco taxes.

In 1994, Mississippi became the first state to sue the tobacco industry for medical expenses incurred under Medicaid for the treatment of tobacco-related illnesses; by January 1998, 39 other states had also sued. In June, 1997, the tobacco industry proposed, in conjunction with some of the state Attorneys General, a national settlement in exchange for industry immunity against class-action lawsuits or punitive damages for past activities. As of January 1998, the industry had settled with three states (for amounts ranging from $3.4 billion in Mississippi to $15.3 billion in Texas), and Congress was considering several proposals for national legislation on tobacco.

Government and Private Sector Measures

Nonsmokers are increasingly able to breathe smoke-free air in indoor environments. The U.S. Congress and federal agencies have taken action to reduce exposure to ETS. In 1988, the U.S. Department of Health and Human Services instituted a smoke-free policy, and in 1994, the U.S. Department of Defense prohibited smoking in its facilities worldwide. In addition, the Pro-Children Act of 1994 banned smoking in indoor facilities that regularly or routinely are used to provide services to children (e.g., school, library, day care, health care, and early childhood development settings). Also, the Occupational Safety and Health Administration has proposed standards that restrict exposure to ETS in workplaces.[228] In August, 1997, the President issued an Executive Order making all Federal facilities of the executive branch smokefree; thus, smoking is banned in all interior space owned, rented, or leased by the executive branch unless there are separately-ventilated smoking areas.[229]

As of June 30, 1997, 48 states had some restriction on smoking indoors. Three (Alabama, Kentucky, North Carolina) had no legislation and 2 (KY, NC) also had legislation that pre-empted localities from enacting laws to restrict smoking in public places. Forty-one states had laws restricting smoking in state government worksites; however, only nine either completely banned smoking or required designated smoking areas with separate ventilation. Only 21 states had laws restricting smoking in private worksites, and only California required either no smoking or separate ventilation for smoking areas. Of the 21 states that restricted smoking in private worksites, seven mandated designated smoking areas only in worksites with a minimum number of employees. Thirty-one states had laws regulating smoking in restaurants, but only three either banned smoking or required separately ventilated smoking areas. In addition, many state laws exempt small restaurants from smoking regulations. California became a leader in assuring a smoke-free environment for its citizens when all workplaces, including restaurants and bars, became smoke-free on January 1, 1998.[230] More than half of states had laws restricting smoking in child day care centers, but only 12 prohibited smoking at all times or required separately ventilated areas. In addition 43 states restricted smoking in hospitals, 42 on selected forms of public transportation, 30 in grocery stores, and 23 in enclosed arenas.[170,228]

Some states use regulations rather than legislation to offer the public additional protection from exposure to ETS. For example, regulations adopted in Maryland prohibit smoking or limit it to separately ventilated areas in many worksites. Many local governments have also enacted laws to reduce the public's exposure to ETS.[228] In 1995, New York City strengthened the Clean Indoor Air Act by restricting smoking in public places, including restaurants with more than 35 seats.[231]

As of September 1992, 543 cities and counties nationwide had restrictive smoking laws.[228] However, the tobacco industry has successfully promoted pre-emptive state laws that prevent local jurisdictions from enacting restrictions more stringent than the state law. As of June 30, 1997, 18 of the state laws on smoke-free indoor air contained pre-emptive language.[170,228] In addition to reducing the number and degree of protection of local regulations, pre-emption prevents the education of the public that occurs as a result of the public debate and community organization around the issue.[231a]

Effective in 1994, the Joint Commission on the Accreditation of Healthcare Organizations required hospitals to be smoke free.[232] Nonsmoking rental cars, sections of hotels and motels reserved for nonsmokers, and nonsmoking airlines provide a constant reinforcement that many people wish to reduce their exposure to smoke at every possible opportunity.[233] In 1990, smoking was banned on all U.S. domestic flights of less than 6 hours' duration. Some airlines are now offering smoke-free international flights. Delta Airlines made all of its flights smoke free as of January 1, 1995,[234] and other airlines have banned smoking on their trans-Atlantic flights.[235]

Insurance companies are increasingly recognizing the overall impact of smoking on premature death and illness. For example, the Task Force on Smoker/Nonsmoker Mortality of the Society of Actuaries of America used the collective experience of five life insurance companies in developing a set of smoker-nonsmoker mortality ratios for men, varying by age. Smoker-nonsmoker ratios were determined to be 1.50 at the age of 25 years, increasing to a peak of 2.5 at the age of 45 years and decreasing thereafter with increasing age. Results of this and other studies have prompted almost all major life insurance underwriters (more than 200 companies) to offer premium discounts ranging from 10 to 30 percent for policyholders who have never smoked or have stopped for at least 12 months.[236] However, as of 1985, only about 15 percent of companies offering health and disability insurance provided nonsmoker discounts.[237] The trend in nonsmokers' discounts is slowly extending to fire, home owner, and automobile insurance policies; Farmers Insurance Group reports offering a 10 to 25 percent discount to drivers who have never smoked or have not smoked for at least 2 years.[233]

Since the Surgeon General's first report on smoking and health in 1964, public and private health agencies have engaged in a broad variety of activities designed to reduce the prevalence of smoking. Although the impact of any single such effort is difficult to establish, growing evidence suggests a collective demonstrable effect, particularly on the prevalence of smoking. In the absence of the antismoking campaign, an estimated additional 42 million more Americans would have smoked in 1992. As a result of these campaign-induced decisions not to smoke, an estimated 1.6 million Americans postponed death between 1964 and 1992, gaining an average of 21 years of additional life expectancy, and an estimated additional 4.1 million deaths will be avoided or postponed between 1993 and 2015.[238] Such analyses must be interpreted cautiously, however, because they rely heavily on assumptions of what would have occurred in the absence of antismoking campaigns.

One mechanism available to influence the consumption of tobacco is the taxation of cigarettes and other tobacco products. In the year ending June 30, 1996, the federal cigarette tax was 24 cents per pack. However, federal and state taxes as a percentage of retail price declined from 51.4 percent in 1965 to 30.5 percent in 1996.[239] By the end of 1997, state excise taxes ranged from 2.5 cents per pack in Virginia to 100.0 cents in Alaska, with an average state tax of 38.1 cents per pack.[170,228] In addition, 46 states imposed general sales taxes on cigarettes as of 1996. In 1994, the federal tax on smokeless tobacco was only 2.7 cents per can of snuff and 2.3 cents per package;[240] in addition, in 1996 40 states taxed smokeless tobacco.[239]

A California initiative petition to increase cigarette taxes by 25 cents per pack passed in 1988 and 20 percent of the increase was dedicated to tobacco control activities. In 1992, Massachusetts increased its excise tax on cigarettes by 25 cents and dedicated the increase to tobacco control and health education.[241] Arizona in 1994 and Oregon in 1996 also increased tobacco taxes with a proportion of the money dedicated to tobacco prevention and control activities.[180] Even a small percentage of funds dedicated to tobacco control results in a large infusion of money into state tobacco control activities. These funds have resulted in innovative media campaigns and other activities. The combination of a tax increase and a comprehensive tobacco control program reduced the prevalence of smoking in California by 2.7 percent and in Massachusetts by 2.2 percent over 3 years (1993 to 1996); in the 41 other states that measured smoking prevalence during these years, the reduction was 0.8 percent.[241]

Taxation increases price, which in turn reduces consumption. A large body of literature has developed regarding the demand-based price elasticity of cigarettes. In 1993, an NCI consensus panel reviewed the existing studies on the price elasticity of cigarettes and concluded that the price elasticity in most studies was between –0.3 and –0.5 (i.e., that for every 10 percent increase in price, cigarette consumption will decrease 3 to 5 percent). An estimated two-thirds of the decreased consumption is due to people choosing not to smoke (both increased smoking cessation and decreased smoking initiation).[242] Tobacco taxes in the United States are lower than in nearly all industrialized nations: the tax comprises 30 percent of the price of cigarettes in the United States, but more than 60 percent in other industrialized countries (Fig. 44-5).[243,244]

Advertising and Promotion

In 1970, the tobacco industry spent $360 million on advertising and promotion, two-thirds of which was for television and radio advertising. In the United States, broadcast media advertising was banned as of January 1, 1971. In 1975, the tobacco industry spent $490 million on advertising and promotion, two-thirds in newspapers, magazines, and outdoor ads. In 1995, the industry spent $4.9 billion in advertising and promotion, with 79 percent being used for promotions, speciality items, and coupons.[182]

Tobacco companies have maintained in the past that none of their advertising and promotions are intended to appeal to teenagers or preteen children. However, on March 20, 1997, one tobacco company (Liggett Group, Inc.), as part of a settlement of state lawsuits, acknowledged that the tobacco industry markets to youth under 18 years of age.[245] Similarly, documents released in January 1998 show that in 1975, R.J. Reynolds Tobacco wanted to increase the market share of Camel filter cigarettes among young people 14–24 years of age "who represent tomorrow's cigarette business."[246]

The nature of the activities promoted (often popular musical events and sporting events) as well as the effort in advertisements has to associate smoking with maturity, glamour, and self-confidence has a strong appeal with youth. In a 1993 national study, 86 percent of adolescents who bought their own cigarettes bought Malboro, Camel, or Newport, the three most heavily advertised brands; only 35 percent of adult smokers bought those brands.[247] One study found that the cartoon camel was as familiar to 6-year-old children as Mickey Mouse's silhouette.[248] Since the Joe Camel cartoon character was introduced in 1988, Camel's share of the adolescent cigarette market increased from 2 percent in 1978–1980, to 8 percent in 1989, to more than 13 percent in 1993.[113,247] The Joe Camel campaign was one of the tobacco industry's most heavily criticized advertising campaigns, and there was increased pressure to drop the campaign after the Federal Trade Commission (FTC) filed suit against the company in May of 1997, alleging that the Joe Camel symbol enticed children to smoke. In July of 1997, R.J. Reynolds announced that they were discontinuing the Joe Camel in the United States, although they still planned to use the cartoon character for overseas advertising.[249] In addition, the

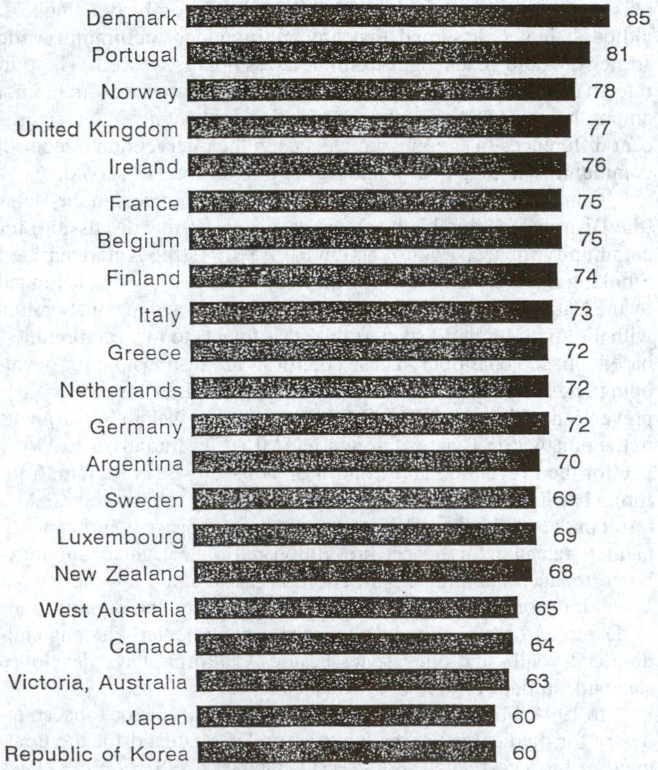

Figure 44-5. Percentage of the price of 20 cigarettes that is tax, selected countries, 1995. (From Non-smokers' Rights Association, Ottawa, Canada.)

promotions of televised sporting and entertainment events heavily expose youth to tobacco advertising.

Several studies have looked at the effect of tobacco advertising on smoking, particularly among young people. One study examined the relationship between the intensity of brand-level cigarette advertising and the effect on brand market shares for adults and adolescents. The model allowed for both current and historical effects of advertising and for the effects of brand advertising relative to total advertising. The study concluded that brand choices among adolescents are related to brand advertising and that the relationship between brand choices and brand advertising is stronger among adolescents than among adults.[250] Another study modeled adolescent susceptibility to smoking and assessed the relative influence of receptivity to advertising, family members smoking, and peer smoking. This study found that tobacco marketing may be a stronger influence in encouraging adolescent smoking initiation than is exposure to peers or family members who smoke or sociodemographic variables.[251] Other studies have found a correlation between cigarette advertising campaigns and increased smoking initiation among young people.[252–254]

Tobacco company marketing efforts have also targeted women and minorities. In 1990, after the Secretary of the Department of Health and Human Services, Dr. Louis Sullivan, denounced R.J. Reynolds for "slick and sinister advertising" and for "promoting a culture of cancer," the company abruptly decided to cancel the launch of Uptown, their new cigarette aimed at blacks.[255] Only a month later, the same company was preparing to introduce a new cigarette aimed at young, poorly educated, blue-collar women.[256] This cigarette, called Dakota, was also withdrawn after public outcry. These examples suggest that new tobacco product introductions aimed at young and minority populations are likely to be aggressively attacked as exploitative.

Some other countries have very broad advertising restrictions. For example, Canada passed legislation in 1988 to ban all tobacco advertising in newspapers and magazines published in Canada as well as all point-of-sale tobacco advertising and promotion. In Europe, a number of countries have enacted similar restrictions on the use of graphics in tobacco advertising. In the United States, the federal Public Health Cigarette Smoking Act of 1969 pre-empted most state advertising restrictions.[257] As of June 1997, only nine states had laws restricting the advertising of tobacco products. These laws included restricting advertising on lottery tickets or video games, prohibiting advertising within certain distances of schools, and requiring warning labels on billboards advertising smokeless tobacco products. In August of 1996, the FDA issued a rule that all tobacco advertising must be in black-and-white text only except when it appears in adult publications or in locations inaccessible to young people. In addition, billboards were banned within 1,000 feet of schools and playgrounds; events, teams, and entries could be sponsored only in the corporate name, not a brand name; brand name nontobacco items, such as t-shirts, were banned; gifts and items provided in exchange for proof of purchase were banned; and use of nontobacco names on tobacco items was banned.[258] The FDA rule was being challenged in federal court as of early 1998.

Evidence for the effectiveness of advertising bans comes primarily from international data.[259] One study used multiple regression analysis to evaluate the effectiveness of advertising restrictions, price, and income on tobacco consumption in 22 countries from 1960 to 1986. Above threshold levels, both advertising restrictions and higher prices were effective in decreasing tobacco consumption.[260] However, an analysis of the 1971 U.S. broadcast media ban did not show an effect.[261] This apparent lack of effect may be due in part to these bans being frequently circumvented, such as during the promotions of televised sporting and entertainment events. For example, during a Marlboro Grand Prix telecast, the Marlboro logo was seen or mentioned nearly 6,000 times and was visible for 46 of the 94-minute broadcast.[262] In addition, after the broadcast ban went into effect in the United States, tobacco advertising merely shifted to other media—newspapers, magazines, outdoor, transit, point of sale, and a variety of promotions—at much higher expenditure levels.[182] If the broadcast ban resulted in the industry being more efficient and targeted in its marketing, this could also account for the broadcast media ban's lack of effectiveness.

Evidence for the effectiveness of counteradvertising comes from both national and international data. An econometric analysis of the U.S. Fairness Doctrine (which required one antismoking message for every three to five tobacco advertising messages) concluded that counteradvertising substantially deterred smoking.[263] Another study of the Fairness Doctrine concluded that the number of people who successfully quit smoking tripled during the period that the doctrine was in effect.[264] An evaluation of an Australia paid media campaign against smoking found that there was a marked decrease in smoking prevalence attributable to the campaign.[265] An evaluation of a Greek media campaign showed that the annual increase in tobacco consumption was reduced to nearly zero as a result of the campaign. When the campaign stopped, consumption again rose at the precampaign rate.[266]

Tobacco Use Prevention

The 1994 Surgeon General's Report on preventing tobacco use among young people concluded that (*a*) most Americans strongly favor policies that discourage tobacco use among young people; (*b*) comprehensive school-based prevention programs work when they occur in conjunction with supportive community activities; (*c*) smoking cessation programs have low success rates, and it is difficult to attract and keep adolescents in such programs; (*d*) illegal sales of tobacco to minors are common; and (*e*) increases in the real price of cigarettes reduce cigarette smoking among young people.[113]

Evidence that knowledge of adverse and long-term health effects did not translate into reduced smoking among youth led to focusing on susceptibility of youth to peer pressure in the development of health behaviors.[267] Since the mid-1960s, increasing attention has been given to developing valid theoretical models of smoking initiation and related prevention programs. There are thought to be five stages to smoking initiation among children and adolescents: (*a*) preparatory stage where attitudes and beliefs about the utility of smoking develop and smoking may be viewed as having positive benefits even though no smoking has yet occurred; (*b*) trying stage, which includes the first two or three times an adolescent tries to smoke (usually in a situation involving peers); (*c*) experimentation, or repeated but irregular smoking, where smoking is usually in response to a particular situation; (*d*) regular use, that is, at least weekly smoking across a variety of situations; and (*e*) nicotine dependence, which is a physiological need for nicotine.[113] Baseline susceptibility (the lack of a firm decision not to smoke) was a strong predictor of experimentation, even after adjustment for other risk factors.[268] Current recommendations on quality school-based smoking prevention programs emphasize helping children understand and effectively cope with social influences associated with smoking, on highlighting the immediate negative social consequences (including correcting student perceptions that smoking is common in their peer group), and on inoculating youth against the effects of continued pressure.[9,269–271] Theoretical underpinnings to these curricula include social, psychological, and behavioral theories.[113,272,273]

Most current prevention programs focus on students in grades 6 to 8, the time of greatest increase in smoking experimentation.[274] A review of a large number of prevention curricula showed that common features of programs with some effects include a focus on students in junior high and middle grades, multiple sessions, material to correct misimpressions of the social significance and prevalence among peers, emphasis on short-term reasons not to smoke, education on a variety of social factors influencing smoking, practicing of resistance skills, involvement of peers as leaders or role models, and public commitment (not to smoke) procedures.[113,274,275] Those curricula that focus on life skills also generally include education to enhance decision-making, social competence, and self-esteem.[276]

A number of these social influence-based curricula, when applied in the context of well-designed research studies, have been shown to delay smoking experimentation and progression to regular smoking, although the effect size differs widely among programs.[275,277,278] The effects of these programs have not been sustained without additional educational interventions or supportive community programs. Thus, although school-based skills training are important for preventing smoking, more sustained and comprehensive interventions may be necessary for long-term success.[113] Awaited are longitudinal studies to assess whether the delay in smoking translates into lower prevalence throughout young adult life. If smoking is a gateway behavior to other drug use, evaluating the effect of decreased or delayed smoking initiation on reducing the age-specific incidence of other drug use merits attention.

Community-based programs, including media-based prevention efforts, appear to be necessary complements to school-based programs.[113,279] Data on the effectiveness of media interventions alone on youth smoking behavior are limited. One study reported that mass media intervention can prevent cigarette smoking when it is carefully targeted at high-risk youths and shares educational objectives with existing school health programs.[280] Similarly, an evaluation of a California media campaign concluded that the campaign was successful in stopping the rise in teen smoking in the state; however, this campaign occurred in the context of other interventions, including school prevention programs.[281] In contrast, a Minnesota media campaign, which occurred without a strong school-prevention component, did not have any effect on adolescent smoking behavior.[282]

An additional mechanism to prevent tobacco use among youth is to increase the price of tobacco products. In 1993, an NCI consensus panel concluded that an increase in cigarette excise taxes may be the most effective single intervention to reduce tobacco use by youth, since youth consumption appears to be influenced by prices at least as much as adult consumption does. For example, one study concluded that youth consumption may be three times more sensitive to price increases than is adult consumption.[242] Another analysis of the cigarette excise tax concluded that an increase in the federal cigarette excise tax would encourage an additional 3.5 million Americans to forego smoking, including more than 800,000 teenagers and almost 2 million young adults age 20 to 35 years.[283] Anything resulting in an increase in real price can be expected to have similar effects.

Another approach to discouraging smoking among youth is the establishment of strong no-smoking policies in schools. Such policies not only directly discourage smoking by youth but increase the likelihood that their teachers, who are role models, will not be seen smoking. However, in 1995, only 28.5 percent of school districts provided tobacco-free environments in middle, junior, or senior high schools.[284]

Commercial tobacco outlets are the most common source of cigarettes and smokeless tobacco for minors.[285] Since 1986, numerous published studies involving purchase attempts by minors confirm that, despite state and local laws banning such sales, minors can easily buy tobacco from over-the-counter outlets and vending machines.[113,285] However, active enforcement of tobacco laws increases retailer compliance[113,227] and may also reduce smoking prevalence among minors.[286,287] Unfortunately, in recent years, as states have developed minors' access laws, some have developed weak laws that include pre-emptive language preventing stronger local legislation. As of June 30, 1997, 20 states had such pre-emptive language in their minors' access legislation.[170,228]

In 1992, Congress responded to the problem of minors' access to tobacco by enacting the Synar amendment. This federal statute, and its implementing regulations issued in 1996, require every state to have a law prohibiting tobacco sales to minors under age 18, enforce the law, conduct annual statewide inspections of tobacco outlets to assess the rate of illegal tobacco sales to minors, and develop a strategy and time frame to reduce the statewide illegal sales rate to 20 percent or less.[288,289] In August of 1996, the FDA issued regulations that prohibit the sale of tobacco to persons less than 18 years of age, require retailers to obtain photo identification to verify the age of all persons under 27 years of age, ban vending machines and self-service displays except in facilities where only adults are allowed, ban sales of single cigarettes and packages with fewer than 20 cigarettes, and ban free samples.[258] As of early 1998, the FDA rule was being challenged in federal court by the tobacco industry.

Smoking and the Workplace

Employee smoking is very costly to employers. Smokers increase absenteeism, health insurance and life insurance costs and claims, worker's compensation payments and occupational health awards, accidents and fires (and related insurance costs), property damage (and related insurance costs), cleaning and maintenance costs, and illness and discomfort among nonsmokers exposed to ETS.[290–293] The Control Data Corporation reported that when employee data were trichotomized into risk categories based on smoking behavior, the excess claims cost for the high-risk group over the low-risk group was 118 percent.[290] One frequently cited estimate of the excess costs of employing a smoker is $1,300 per year (1991 dollars).[292,293] A male smoker incurs approximately $11,000 in additional health costs over his lifetime than a male who has never smoked; for a female smoker, the excess medical expenditures are approximately $13,000.[238] The total economic cost of smoking for the United States, including direct medical costs and loss of productivity, is about $100 billion per year.[13,14,238] The direct medical costs associated with smoking were $50 billion in 1993, or 7.1 percent of direct medical expenditures for the United States.[13]

Although the percentage of employees who smoke has decreased, certain subpopulations, including blue-collar and service workers, continue to smoke at higher levels than average. For 1987 to 1990, roofers (58 percent) and crane and tower operators (58 percent) had the highest prevalences of cigarette smoking, and physicians (5 percent) and clergy (6 percent) had the lowest prevalences of cigarette smoking.[175]

In the 1992 National Survey of Worksite Health Promotion Activities, 40 percent of private firms with 50 employees or more reported offering some type of smoking cessation assistance. Smoking cessation assistance was offered by 32 percent of work sites with 50 to 99 and 79 percent of work sites with 750 employees or more.[294]

Employers can support employees who want to quit tobacco use by offering (or offering referral to) a variety of cessation assistance options, including self-help programs, formal cessation programs, counseling from a health care provider, and pharmacological aids. Work-site smoking-cessation assistance may be provided on-site or off-site, may be run by outside or in-house personnel, and may be an isolated activity or integrated into a comprehensive employee health promotion program. Company incentives to support employee cessation efforts may include full or partial payment of any costs, including pharmacological agents, time released from work to get cessation assistance, and lower employee contributions to health benefit costs for nonsmokers.[293] Literature reviews suggest that cessation assistance programs can help participating employees achieve long-term abstinence, but design and methodological limitations of many studies preclude a judgment on an expected cessation rate for most work-site programs. Approaches that appear to enhance program success include strong management support, good employer-employee relations, and employee choice of type of cessation program. Incentives, competition, and public feedback on progress appear to have less influence on program results.[295,296] One comprehensive work-site health promotion program that included smoking cessation, Live for Life (LFL), reported a verified decline among the entire work-site population of 22.6 percent for 2 years; at comparison work sites, the reduction in health-profile-only groups was 17.4 percent. In the LFL companies, 32 percent of smokers at high-risk for cardiovascular disease quit versus 12.9 percent in the health-profile-only companies.[291]

Workplace smoking policies, originally implemented primarily for safety reasons, have been adopted increasingly because of health concerns about the effects of ETS.[293,297,298] In 1992, 97 percent of nonsmokers and 79 percent of current smokers agreed that ETS exposure is a health hazard for healthy adults.[299] The percentage of Americans who support some type of restriction on smoking in the workplace increased from 81 percent in 1983 to 94 percent in 1992.[293] The 1992 National Survey of Worksite Health Promotion Activities, a survey of work sites with 50 or more employees, found that 59 percent of private employers had either smoke-free policies or permitted smoking only in separately ventilated smoking areas. A smaller 1994 survey of businesses with up to 25,000 employees found that 54 percent had smoke-free policies and only 7 percent had no smoking policy at all.[293] A survey of 100,00 workers conducted in 1992 to 1993 found that although 82 percent of workers reported that their workplace had an official policy that addressed smoking, 54 percent were not covered by a smokefree workplace policy.

Among young workers (aged 15–19), only 32 percent reported that their workplace had a smoke-free policy. In addition, nearly 79 percent of food service workers reported that they were covered by no policy or by a policy that permitted smoking in the workplace.[300]

▸ TOBACCO ECONOMICS

In 1996 consumers in the United States spent more than $50 billion on tobacco products, equal to 0.9 percent of personal disposable income.[301] The industry directly accounted for about 353,000 jobs in 1993 (tobacco farming, auctioning and warehousing, manufacturing, wholesaling, and retail or vending).[302] In 1996, U.S. tobacco farmers produced an estimated 1.6 billion pounds of tobacco leaf with a value of $3 billion,[303] and U.S. cigarette manufacturers produced an estimated 754 billion packs of cigarettes, 32 percent of which was exported.[165] In monetary value, domestic tobacco exports (cigarettes, other manufactured tobacco products, and unmanufactured tobacco) account for 0.7 percent of the total export earnings of the United States.[244] Cigarette production in the United States is highly concentrated; five major cigarette manufacturers produce nearly all the cigarettes in this country.[304]

In large part because of a price support control program first introduced in the 1930s, in the United States both the number of tobacco producers and the quantity of tobacco produced are regulated through a complex system of quotas. The tobacco price support program leads to a higher price of tobacco for tobacco farmers. In 1995 the estimated gross income per acre for tobacco was $3,479.40, compared with $218.54 for corn and $321.98 for soybeans.[305] In 1996, the federal government spent approximately $97 million administering the tobacco price support program and providing crop insurance, disaster payments to farmers, and other services for tobacco producers.[301]

▸ INTERNATIONAL PERSPECTIVE ON TOBACCO

Tobacco use is a major preventable cause of death worldwide. The World Health Organization (WHO) estimates that there are about 1.1 billion smokers in the world, about one-third of the global population age 15 years and older. Most of these smokers are in developing countries (800 million), and are men (700 million). Smoking prevalence for men (based upon the most recent survey data available for each country) ranges from 60 percent in the Western Pacific to 29 percent in Africa; for women, smoking prevalence is highest in Europe (26 percent) and the Americas (22 percent) and lowest in Africa, the eastern Mediterranean, and Southeast Asia (all 4 percent).[244] From 1970–1972 to 1990–1992, per capita cigarette consumption decreased in the Americas (an average annual decrease of 1.5 percent), remained unchanged in Europe, increased in Africa (average annual increase of 1.2 percent), the eastern Mediterranean (1.4 percent), Southeast Asia (1.8 percent), and the Western Pacific (3 percent). In most European and Western Pacific countries, smoking prevalence is at U.S. levels or slightly higher (Table 44-6).[244] China is a good example of the size and scope of the tobacco problem because it is the largest producer and consumer of cigarettes in the world. An estimated 300 million Chinese smoke (61 percent of men and 9 percent of women), the same number as in all the developed countries combined. By 2025, an estimated 2 million Chinese men will die annually

TABLE 44-6. ESTIMATED SMOKING PREVALENCE AMONG MEN AND WOMEN AGE 15 YEARS AND OVER, BY SELECTED COUNTRIES, LATEST AVAILABLE YEAR (TOP 10 AND BOTTOM 10 RANKS)

Rank in Order of Male Prevalence				Rank in Order of Female Prevalence			
Rank No.	*Country*	*Men*	*Women*	*Rank No.*	*Country*	*Women*	*Men*
1	Republic of Korea (1989)	68.2	6.7	1	Denmark (1993)	37.0	37.0
2	Latvia (1993)	67.0	12.0	2	Norway (1994)	35.5	36.4
3	Russian Federation (1993)	67.0	30.0	3	Czech Republic (1994)	31.0	43.0
4	Dominican Republic (1990)	66.3	13.6	4	Fiji (1988)	30.6	59.3
5	Tonga (1991)	65.0	14.0	5	Israel (1989)	30.0	45.0
6	Turkey (1988)	63.0	24.0	5	Russian Federation (1993)	30.0	67.0
7	China (1984)[a]	61.0	7.0	7	Canada (1991)	29.0	31.0
8	Bangladesh (1990)	60.0	15.0	7	Netherlands (1994)	29.0	36.0
9	Fiji (1988)	59.3	30.6	7	Poland (1993)	29.0	51.0
10	Japan (1994)	59.0	14.8	10	Greece (1994)	28.0	46.0
				10	Iceland Papua New (1994)	28.0	31.0
				10	Ireland (1993)	28.0	29.0
				10	Guinea (1990)	28.0	46.0
78	United States of America (1991)	28.1	23.5	78	Bahamas (1989)	3.8	19.3
79	Pakistan (1980)	27.4	4.4	79	Mauritius (1992)	3.7	47.2
80	Finland (1994)	27.0	19.0	80	India (1980s)	3.0	40.0
81	Turkmenistan (1992)	26.6	0.5	81	Singapore (1995)	2.7	31.9
82	Nigeria (1990)	24.4	6.7	82	Egypt (1986)	1.0	39.8
83	Paraguay (1990)	24.1	5.5	82	Lesotho (1989)	1.0	38.3
84	Bahrain (1991)	24.0	6.0	82	Uzbekistan (1989)	1.0	40.0
84	New Zealand (1992)	24.0	22.0	85	Sri Lanka (1988)	0.8	54.8
86	Sweden (1994)	22.0	24.0	86	Turkmenistan (1992)	0.5	26.6
87	Bahamas (1989)	19.3	3.8	87	Saudi Arabia (1990)	N/A	52.7

From World Health Organization, 1996; data comes from surveys that were conducted in individual countries meeting the following criteria: a methodologically sound nationally representative survey or a survey of a large segment of the national population.

[a] More recent data collected in 1991 on the smoking habits of men and women in the context of a prospective study of the health effects of smoking in China suggests that there has been little change in smoking prevalence since 1984.

from smoking.[306] Before the middle of this century, very few developing countries either produced tobacco or had significant consumption of manufactured cigarettes. In the late 1950s, cigarette manufacturers, sensing a shrinking domestic market because of the growing controversy surrounding smoking and lung cancer, sought to establish new markets in the developing countries. These countries, with more than half of the world's population, who may be unaware of the health problems associated with tobacco use, represented a huge, potentially untapped resource for tobacco cultivation, cigarette manufacture, and cigarette marketing. Currently, all 15 countries that devote more than 1 percent of their total import expenses to purchasing tobacco are either developing countries or countries of Central and Eastern Europe. In these 15 countries, expenditures on tobacco imports are a significant cost to economic development.[244]

Currently, more than 100 countries are involved in the growth, development, and processing of tobacco and its related products, athough 25 countries account for 90 percent of the global tobacco production.[244] Export earnings from tobacco exceed 1 percent of total export earnings in 14 countries, all but one being a developing country or a former Soviet country of Central or Eastern Europe. Two countries are particularly dependent on tobacco exports as a major source of export earnings: in 1993, 64 and 23 percent of export earning came from tobacco exports for Malawi's and Zimbabwe, respectively.[244]

Many tobacco-producing countries are poor and lack the resources to grow or import sufficient quantities of food for their populations; yet they divert agricultural land that could be used for growing staple crops, such as sorghum and maize, to tobacco cultivation. One explanation for this growth of a deadly industry is that the governments have been eager to emulate the practices of their more successful and wealthy neighbors in the industrialized world. In addition, they may perceive tobacco production as (*a*) a relatively simple mechanism for raising substantial revenue from taxation of tobacco products, (*b*) an easy way to generate foreign exchange necessary to buy commodities from abroad and to improve their balance of trade, and (*c*) a significant source of rural employment and wage production.[307]

The short-run economic advantages of tobacco growth and consumption come at a high real cost. Most obvious are the direct, well-documented health problems associated with tobacco use. Moreover, other indirect effects of tobacco production include destruction of agricultural lands and forests and improper use of insecticides by rural farmers.

According to United Nations sources, the deforestation problem in many developing countries may soon become a "poor man's energy crisis."[308] This problem is traceable in large part to the need for wood to fuel fires that flue-cure many varieties of tobacco at high temperatures for about a week. Tobacco farmers in developing countries, most of whom are dependent on wood as their sole source of energy, use approximately 2 hectares of trees for each ton of tobacco cured, equivalent to two trees for every 300 cigarettes, or 15 packs of cigarettes, produced.[309] A direct result of deforestation is soil erosion, which in hilly rural areas may lead to silt-filled rivers and dams during the rainy season and denuded croplands during growing seasons. In addition, because tobacco grows well in sandy soils and many developing countries are located in semi-arid lands bordering deserts, tobacco is often grown on agricultural fringe land bordering deserts. As trees in nearby forests are cut down to provide fuel for the curing process, desertification is accelerated and farmers are forced to move into other, less arid regions, where cultivation of tobacco displaces staple food crops, leading to lost food production.[308]

Further, the lack of adequate education among rural area tobacco farmers regarding proper use of modern insecticides often leads to indiscriminate dispersal of the products in lakes and rivers. The resultant pollution endangers water sources of rural villagers and surrounding wildlife. Failure to use gloves and protective garments designed to limit exposure to toxic chemicals in insecticides also places rural tobacco farmers at an increased long-term risk of occupationally related diseases such as skin, lung, and bladder cancer.[309]

The major health consequences associated with smoking (e.g., cancer, heart disease, and COPD), which are well established in developed countries, are becoming increasingly prevalent in the developing world. In 1995, an estimated 1.4 million men in developed countries and 1.6 million men in developing countries (with more than half of these occurring in China) died from smoking-related diseases. Tobacco use also caused an estimated 475,000 deaths among women in developed countries, and an estimated 250,000 deaths among women in developing countries (including 20,000 to 30,000 deaths from smokeless tobacco) in 1995. WHO estimates that smoking caused 3.8 million deaths globally in 1995 (7 percent of all deaths). Tobacco will cause an estimated 2 to 3 million deaths yearly in developing countries by the year 2000, and the number of deaths caused by smoking will increase dramatically in developing countries after the year 2000. Unless a large number of current smokers in developing countries quit, it is estimated that smoking will be causing 10 million deaths per year worldwide by the 2020s or early 2030s, of which 7 million will be in developing countries.[244]

There are disturbing parallels between the advertising and promotion techniques used to sell cigarette smoking in the United States and other developed countries in the late 1910s and throughout the 1920s and the current efforts to promote smoking as a pleasurable status symbol in developing countries. There is also a tragic difference. In the 1920s, neither producer, consumer, nor government knew of the direct adverse health effects of tobacco use. Today, the scientific evidence is incontrovertible, and yet the developed countries, through their silence, trade, and foreign policies, implicitly encourage the growth of the tobacco industry in these countries.

In 1986, the World Health Assembly unanimously adopted a resolution for member states to consider a comprehensive national tobacco control strategy containing nine elements:

1. Measures to ensure that nonsmokers receive effective protection, to which they are entitled, from involuntary exposure to tobacco smoke in enclosed public places, restaurants, transport, and places of work and entertainment.
2. Measures to promote abstention from the use of tobacco to protect children and young people from becoming addicted.
3. Measures to ensure that a good example is set in all health-related premises and by all health personnel.
4. Measures leading to the progressive elimination of those socio-economic, behavioral, and other incentives that maintain and promote the use of tobacco.
5. Prominent health warnings, which might include the statement that tobacco is addictive, on cigarette packets and containers of all types of tobacco products.
6. The establishment of programs of education and public information on tobacco and health issues, including smoking cessation programs, with active involvement of the health professions and the media.
7. Monitoring of trends in smoking and other forms of tobacco use, tobacco-related diseases, and the effectiveness of national smoking-control action.
8. The promotion of viable economic alternatives to tobacco production, trade, and taxation.
9. The establishment of a national focal point to stimulate, support, and coordinate all the above activities.[244]

In 1990, the World Health Assembly passed another resolution urging all member states to:

1. Implement multisectoral comprehensive tobacco control strategies that contain at least the nine elements outlined above and
2. Consider including in their tobacco control strategies plans for legislation or other effective government measures providing for effective protection from ETS in indoor workplaces, enclosed public places, and public transport, with special attention to risk groups such as pregnant women and children; progressive financial measures to discourage the use of tobacco; and progressive restrictions and concerted actions to eventually eliminate all direct and indirect advertising, promotion, and sponsorship concerning tobacco.[244]

In 1996, the World Health Assembly passed a third resolution requesting the Director-General to initiate the development of an International Framework Convention for Tobacco Control. The convention involves:

1. A preparatory process to define the degree to which the convention can become a legally binding instrument acceptable to Member States, and how the Convention can best support national and international efforts in tobacco control; and
2. A strategy to encourage Member States to progress towards the adoption of comprehensive tobacco control policies, as well as address aspects of tobacco control that transcend national boundaries.[310]

In the early 1990s, about 25 countries had laws prohibiting the sale of cigarettes to minors. However, few countries had effective enforcement of these laws. Many jurisdictions also had laws that ban or restrict smoking in public places, workplaces, and transit vehicles. By 1990, 27 countries had passed laws to ban all or most tobacco advertising; however, the number subsequently decreased to 18 countries. In addition, these bans are frequently circumvented. For example, after a 1976 law in France banned tobacco advertising, the ads were replaced by advertisements for matches and lighters with the tobacco names and logos until a law banning both direct and indirect advertising was passed. In the early 1990s, about 80 countries required health warnings to appear on tobacco product packages. However, in most countries, the warnings were small and ineffective. By the mid-1990s, a number of countries had adopted more stringent warnings, including more direct statements of risk, multiple messages, and large and rotating messages. Such warnings are required in Australia, Canada, Iceland, Norway, Singapore, South Africa, and Thailand. Internationally, taxes on cigarettes are generally 60 to 80 percent of the retail price. A number of countries use part of the revenue generated to operate their comprehensive tobacco control programs.[244]

Many countries have had difficulty implementing comprehensive tobacco control measures. However, good examples of successful implementation exist. Finland, Iceland, Norway, Portugal, and Singapore have comprehensive tobacco control policies that have developed since the 1970s. Australia, France, New Zealand, Sweden, and Thailand have more recently implemented comprehensive tobacco control programs. Generally, countries with comprehensive tobacco control policies have tobacco consumption rates that have been low and stable or that are declining.[244] One study used multiple regression analysis to evaluate the effectiveness of advertising restrictions, price, and income on tobacco consumption in 22 countries from 1960 to 1986.[260] Above threshold levels, both advertising restrictions and higher prices were effective in decreasing tobacco consumption. In addition, the most comprehensive tobacco control programs that included high prices, comprehensive bans on advertising, and stringent health warnings had the greatest effect on decreasing tobacco consumption. It was estimated that banning tobacco advertising, requiring strong and varied health warnings on packages, and implementing a 36 percent increase in real price would decrease tobacco consumption by 13.5 percent.

In 1992, the World Bank developed a formal five-part tobacco policy. (*a*) World Bank activities in the health sector discourage the use of tobacco products. (*b*) The World Bank does not lend directly for, invest in, or guarantee investments or loans for tobacco production, processing, or marketing. For those countries where tobacco constitutes more than 10 percent of the exports, the World Bank is more flexible, but works toward helping these countries diversify away from tobacco. (*c*) The World Bank does not lend indirectly for tobacco production activities to the extent practical. (*d*) Unmanufactured and manufactured tobacco, tobacco-processing machinery and equipment, and related services are not included among imports financed under World Bank loans. (*e*) Tobacco and tobacco-related producer or consumer imports may be exempt from borrowers' agreements with the World Bank that try to liberalize trade and reduce tariff levels.[311]

However, powerful economic forces will continue to militate against a strong tobacco control policy in developing countries. Only a concerted effort by international organizations (i.e., the WHO, the International Monetary Fund, the Food and Agriculture Organization, UNICEF, and NGOs) is likely to be effective in helping developing countries assign a high priority to tobacco prevention and reduction.

▶ CHALLENGES IN TOBACCO PREVENTION AND CONTROL

Lessons from the considerable progress achieved in tobacco prevention and control during the past 25 years can serve to confront remaining challenges successfully. Despite considerable progress, smoking remains the largest cause of preventable death in the United States and most of the industrialized world, and it is rapidly becoming a major cause of death in developing countries as well.

The growth of knowledge about adverse health effects of tobacco has been substantial. Public education campaigns have helped to translate scientific knowledge into improved public awareness of some smoking-caused problems, such as lung cancer, COPD, and cardiovascular disease, but awareness of other smoking-caused cancers and reproductive effects is still limited. ETS is increasingly appreciated as a health problem, and smokers in the United States are becoming more sensitive to the concerns of the nonsmokers with whom they interact. In 1992, 97 percent of nonsmokers and 79 percent of current smokers agreed that exposure to ETS is harmful to healthy adults.[299]

Public information efforts in support of tobacco prevention and control have also benefited from the insatiable public desire for health information, which is reflected in television health programming, routine coverage of health issues as part of broadcast news, and expanded health coverage and columns in newspapers and general interest magazines.

Smokers are concerned that their addiction is likely to adversely affect their health. In the United States, nearly half of all persons who have ever smoked have quit,[168] and most continuing smokers have tried to quit. Market responses to consumer concerns have included the filter cigarette, substantial reductions in average tar and nicotine content, and new delivery systems. However, if these innovations are perceived as "safer," smokers who are concerned about health issues may switch to these products and may continue to smoke rather than quit tobacco use entirely. In addition, smokers may derive little or none of the purported health benefit from the newer products due to compensation (e.g., increased number of cigarettes smoked, increased depth of inhalation, smoking more of the cigarette, vent blocking, etc.). Ultimately, tobacco users must realize that there is no safe way to use tobacco and that they need to quit.

Tobacco companies spend large amounts of money to advertise and promote cigarettes ($823 million and $4,072 million, respectively, in 1995).[182] Although the effects of these activities on overall cigarette consumption are difficult to assess, they are likely to make smoking more attractive to youth, to make continuing smokers less motivated to attempt cessation, and perhaps to increase recidivism by providing omnipresent clues that smoking is fun and relaxing and contributes to conviviality. The inverse correlation between the percentage of health articles discussing smoking and cigarette advertising revenues as a percentage of total advertising revenue[312–315] suggests that the presence of cigarette advertising affects editorial decisions.

Limited experience with cigarette counteradvertising in broadcast media in the late 1960s strongly suggests that counteradvertising can depress consumption, even in the presence of severalfold greater brand-specific procigarette advertising.[263] More recent data from the United States and other countries suggest that counteradvertising through the mass media can significantly reduce per capita consumption of cigarettes and smoking prevalence.[265,266] Some data also suggest that broad bans on tobacco advertising are also effective in reducing tobacco consumption.[244]

From 1970 to 1995, the percentage of cigarette advertising and expenditures allocated to promotion increased from 15 to 83 percent.[182] Many of the promotional dollars sponsor sports events that are associated with being healthy, being fit, and being outdoors. The subliminal message is that smoking contributes to health and fitness. Other tobacco company promotional money goes to blockbuster exhibitions at leading art museums, promoting the association of smoking with culture, sophistication, and artistic achievement. This support may buy silence, if not active opposition to smoking control proposals. For example, in 1994, the arts organizations in New York, which had been recipients of tobacco philanthropy, spoke out against an ordinance to ban smoking in public places.[316,317]

Of all targets of opportunity, continuing the process of changing social norms offers the greatest promise. Nonsmoking is an accepted norm in many socially defined groups in the United States. Rapid growth of community, state, and federal legislation and administrative actions limiting or banning smoking in places of public assembly, coupled with growing and increasingly stringent public and private employer restrictions on workplace smoking, should further limit smoking opportunities and increase the perceived benefits of quitting to the individual. Public health agencies and preventive medicine practitioners can help accelerate social pressure not to smoke by supporting enactment of strict clean indoor air legislation, and particularly enforcement, which is often lax.

Economic incentives can significantly affect cigarette consumption. Lower-income Americans, overrepresented among current smokers, may be especially sensitive to price increases in tobacco products. Although the addiction to nicotine may blunt the price elasticity of demand compared with other consumer products, data from the United States and other countries demonstrate that consumption decreases with escalating real prices. The enactment of an increase in cigarette taxes in California and Massachusetts, with all or part of the revenues being used for tobacco control and education, has led to an accelerated decrease in cigarette consumption.[241] These initiatives also provide an excellent opportunity to better understand the price elasticity among different sociodemographic groups. Other states have initiated or are considering similar actions.

As the 68 percent of current smokers who want to quit smoking[168] attempt cessation, both public and private health organizations should be prepared to assist them. Referral to programs screened for their effectiveness should be encouraged. Physicians and other health care professionals should invariably assess for tobacco use and advise tobacco users to quit. Cessation assistance, including nicotine replacement therapy and follow-up, should be provided. Health professionals should provide positive reinforcement of the individual's ability to quit.

Psychosocial prevention programs have demonstrated the ability to delay age-specific smoking initiation for students in grades 6 to 10. These curricula deserve broad dissemination and modification to target the highest-risk groups, including students from the lower socioeconomic backgrounds and those most likely to drop out of school. However, the impact of these curricula is likely to be limited unless they are reinforced through additional educational interventions and supportive community programs. These supportive community programs could include mass media efforts that make smoking appear unattractive, socially unpopular, and sexually unappealing. Communication should also stress that tobacco is a very addictive drug. Tobacco use is associated with increased risk of other drug use,[113] another potentially powerful message for parents and youth.

Similar issues are rapidly becoming important in developing countries. Exportation of tobacco and the role that American-based tobacco companies play in promoting use of their tobacco products in third world countries, almost all having a real increase in per capita cigarette consumption, deserve to be viewed as exportation of a serious health threat to the citizens of countries we claim to want to help.

With the declines in overall U.S. consumption and adult smoking prevalence slowing in the 1990s and the concurrent increase in adolescent smoking, strategies to prevent tobacco-use initiation and promote cessation among users need to be intensified. These efforts will involve the widespread use of known effective strategies, reducing barriers to the use of these proven interventions, and the development of innovative strategies, particularly regarding tobacco use among youth.

▸ REFERENCES

1. McGinnis JM, Foege WH: Actual causes of death in the United States. JAMA 270(18):2207–2212, 1993
2. Thun MJ, Day-Lally CA, Calle EE, Flanders WD, Heath CW: Excess mortality among cigarette smokers: changes in a 20-year interval. Am J Public Health 85(9):1223–1230, 1995
3. Doll R, Peto R, Wheatley K, et al: Mortality in relation to smoking: 40 years' observations on male British doctors. Br Med J 309:901–922, 1994
4. Centers for Disease Control and Prevention: Smoking-attributable mortality and years of potential life lost—United States, 1984. MMWR 46(20):444–451, 1997
5. Centers for Disease Control and Prevention: Projected smoking-related deaths among youth—United States. MMWR 45(44):971–974, 1996
6. Centers for Disease Control and Prevention: Addition of prevalence of cigarette smoking as a Nationally Notifiable Condition—June 1996. MMWR 45(25):537, 1996
7. Centers for Disease Control and Prevention: Cigarette smoking-attributable mortality and years of potential life lost—United States, 1990. MMWR 42(33):645–649, 1993
8. National Center for Health Statistics: Final Mortality Statistics Data Tape. Rockville, MD: Centers for Disease Control and Prevention, National Center for Health Statistics, 1990.
9. Centers for Disease Control, Office of Smoking and Health: Reducing the Health Consequences of Smoking: 25 Years of Progress. A Report of the Surgeon General. DHHS Publication No. (CDC) 89-8411. Rockville, MD: Public Health Service, 1989
10. Public Health Service, Office of Smoking and Health: The Health Consequences of Smoking: Cancer. A Report of the Surgeon General. DHHS Publication No. (PHS) 82-50179. Washington, DC: Public Health Service, 1982
11. Public Health Service, Office on Smoking and Health: Smoking and Health: A Report of the Surgeon General. DHEW Publication No. (PHS) 7950066. Washington, DC: Public Health Service, 1979
12. Lew EA, Garfinkel L: Differences in mortality and longevity by sex, smoking habits, and health status. J Soc Actuaries 39:107–130, 1987
13. Centers for Disease Control and Prevention: Medical-care expenditures attributable to cigarette smoking—United States, 1993. MMWR 43(26):469– 472, 1994
14. Herdman R, Hewitt M, Lashober M: Smoking-Related Deaths and Financial Costs: Office of Technology Assessment Estimates for 1990—OTA Testimony Before the Senate Special Committee on Aging. Washington, DC: US Congress, Office of Technology Assessment Testimony, 1993
15. Statistical Abstract of the United States, 1996. 116th ed. Washington, DC: US Bureau of the Census, 1996

15a. Centers for Disease Control and Prevention. Medical-care expenditures attributable to cigarette smoking during pregnancy—United States, 1995. MMWR 46(44):1048–1050, 1997.

16. Fire in the United States, 1983—1990. Emmitsburg, MD: United National Fire Data Center, 1993
17. Stewart LJ: The US Smoking-Material Fire Problem through 1993: The Role of Lighted Tobacco Products in Fire. Quincy, MA: National Fire Protection Association, 1996
18. US Forest Service: Fire and Aviation Management. Unpublished data, 1990
19. National Center for Health Statistics: Advance Report of Final Mortality Statistics, 1990. Monthly Vital Statistic Report 41(7, Suppl). Rockville, MD: Centers for Disease Control and Prevention, 1993
20. Centers for Disease Control, Office on Smoking and Health: The Health Benefits of Smoking Cessation: A Report of the Surgeon General. DHHS Publication No. (CDC) 90-8416. Washington, DC: Public Health Service, 1990

21. Rogot E, Murray JL: Smoking and causes of death among U.S. veterans: 16 years of observation. Public Health Rep 95(3):213–222, 1980
22. Thun MJ, Myers DG, Day-Lally C, et al: Age and the exposure-response relationships between cigarette smoking and premature death in Cancer Prevention Study II. In: Burns DM, Garfinkel L, Samet JM (eds): Changes in Cigarette-Related Disease Risks and Their Implication for Prevention and Control. Smoking and Tobacco Control Monograph No. 8. Rockville, MD: National Cancer Institute, 1997 NIH Pub No 97-4213
23. Hammond EC, Garfinkel L: Coronary heart disease, stroke, and aortic aneurysm. Arch Environ Health 19:167–182, 1969
24. Doll R, Gray R, Hafner B, Peto R: Mortality in relation to smoking: 22 years' observations on female British doctors. Br Med J 280: 967–971, 1980
25. Kawachi I, Colditz GA, Stampfer MJ, et al: Smoking cessation and time course of decreased risks of coronary heart disease in middle-aged women. Arch Intern Med 154:169–175, 1994
26. Cederlof R, Friberg L, Hrubec Z, Lorch U: The Relationship of Smoking and Some Social Covariables to Mortality and Cancer Morbidity: A 10-Year Follow-Up in a Probability Sample of 55,000 Swedish Subjects age 18–69. Stockholm: Karolinska Institute, Department of Environmental Hygiene, 1975
27. Freund KM, Belanger AJ, D'Agostino RB, Kannel WB: The health risks of smoking. The Framingham study: 34 years of follow-up. Ann Epidemiol 3:417–424, 1993
28. Public Health Service, Office on Smoking and Health: The Health Consequences of Smoking: Cardiovascular Disease. A Report of the Surgeon General. DHHS Publication No. (PHS) 84-50204. Washington DC: Public Health Service, 1983
29. Miettinen TA, Gulling H: Mortality and cholesterol metabolism in familial hypercholesterolemia: long-term follow-up of 96 patients. Arteriosclerosis 8:163–167, 1988
30. Pooling Project Research Group: Relationship of blood pressure, serum cholesterol, smoking habit, relative weight, and-ECG abnormalities to incidence of major coronary events: final report of the Pooling Project. J Chronic Dis 31:201–306, 1978
31. Suarez L, Barrett-Connor E: Interaction between cigarette smoking and diabetes mellitus in the prediction of death attributed to cardiovascular disease. Am J Epidemiol 120:670–675, 1984
32. Stamler J, Vaccaro O, Neaton JD, et al: Diabetes, other risk factors, and 12-yr cardiovascular mortality for men screened in the Multiple Risk Factor Intervention Trial. Diabetes Care 16(2):434–443, 1993
33. Mishell DR: Use of oral contraceptives in women of older reproductive age. Am J Obstet Gynecol 158:1652–1657, 1988
34. McBride PE: The health consequences of smoking. Med Clin North Am 76(2):333–353, 1992
35. Rosenberg L, Kaufman DW, Helmrich SP, et al: Myocardial infarction and cigarette smoking in women younger than 50 years of age. JAMA 253(20):2965–2969, 1985
36. Carstensen JM, Pershagen G, Eklund G: Mortality in relation to cigarette and pipe smoking: 16 years' observations of 25000 Swedish men. J Epidemiol Community Health 41:166–172, 1987
37. Nyboe J, Jensen G, Appleyard M, Schnohr P: Smoking and the risk of first myocardial infarction. Am Heart J 122(2):438–447, 1991
38. Castieden CM, Cole PV: Inhalation of tobacco smoke by pipe and cigar smokers. Lancet 2(819):21–23, 1973
39. Centers for Disease Control, Office of Smoking and Health: Smoking and Health: A National Status Report, 2nd ed. A Report to Congress. DHHS Publication No. (CDC) 87-8396 (revised 02/90). Washington, D.C.: Public Health Service, 1987
40. US Department of Health and Human Services, Office on Smoking and Health: The Health Consequences of Smoking for Women. A Report of the Surgeon General. Washington, DC: Public Health Service, 1980
41. Stokes J, Kannel WB, Wolf PA, et al: The relative importance of selected risk factors for various manifestations of cardiovascular disease among men and women from 35 to 64 years old: 30 years of follow-up in the Framingham Study. Circulation 75(5):V-65–73, 1987
42. Criqui MH, Fronek A, Klauber MR, et al: Peripheral arterial disease in large vessels is epidemiologically distinct from small vessel disease [Abstract]. CVD Epidemiology Newsletter 37:67, 1985
43. Tomatis LA, Fierens EE, Verbrugge GP: Evaluation of surgical risk in peripheral vascular disease by coronary arteriography. Surgery 71:429–435, 1972
44. Levy LA: Smoking and peripheral vascular disease. Clin Podiatr Med Surg 9(1):165–171, 1992
45. Weinroth LA, Hertzstein J: Relation of tobacco smoking to arteriosclerosis obliterans in diabetes mellitus. JAMA 131:205–209, 1946
46. Howard G, Wagenknecht LE, Burke GL, et al: Cigarette smoking and progression of atherosclerosis. JAMA 279(2):119–124, 1998
47. Auerbach O, Garfinkel L: Atherosclerosis and aneurysm of aorta in relation to smoking habits and age. Chest 78(6):805–809, 1980
48. Strachan DP: Predictors of death from aortic aneurysm among middle-aged men: the Whitehall study. Br J Surg 78:401–404, 1991
49. Wolf PA, D'Agostino RB, Kannel WB, et al: Cigarette smoking as a risk factor for stroke: the Framingham Study. JAMA 259:1025–1029, 1988
50. Shinton R, Beevers G: Meta-analysis of relation between cigarette smoking and stroke. Br Med J 298(6676):789–794, 1989
51. Bronner LL, Kanter DS, Manson JE: Primary prevention of stroke. N Engl J Med 333(21):1392–1400, 1995
52. Cruickshank JM, Neil-Dwyer G, Dorrance DE, et al: Acute effects of smoking on blood pressure and cerebral blood flow. J Hum Hypertens 3:443–449, 1989
53. Yamashita K, Kobayashi S, Yamaguchi S, et al: Effect of smoking on regional cerebral blood flow in the normal aged volunteers. Gerontology 34(4):199–204, 1988
54. Rogers RL, Meyer JS, Shaw TG, et al: Cigarette smoking decreases cerebral blood flow suggesting increased risk for stroke. JAMA 250:2794–2800, 1983
55. Centers for Disease Control and Prevention: Mortality trends for selected smoking-related cancers and breast cancer—United States, 1950–1990. MMWR 42:857, 863–866, 1993
56. Cancer Facts and Figures—1998. Atlanta: American Cancer Society, 1998
57. Blot WJ, Fraumeni JF: Cancers of the lung and pleura. In: Schottenfeld D, Fraumeni JF (eds): Cancer Epidemiology and Prevention. 2nd ed. New York: Oxford University Press, 1996
58. Levi F, Franceschi S, La Vecchia C, et al: Lung carcinoma trends by histologic type in Vaud and Neuchatel, Switzerland, 1974–1994. Cancer 79(5):906–914, 1997
59. Thun MJ, Lally CA, Flannery JT, Calle EE, Flanders WD, Heath CW: Cigarette smoking and changes in the histopathology of lung cancer. J Natl Cancer Inst 89(21):1580–1586, 1997
60. Cancer Facts and Figures—1995. Atlanta: American Cancer Society, 1995
61. Ries LA, Miller BA, Hankey BF, et al (eds): Seer Cancer Statistics Review, 1973–1991: Tables and Graphs. NIH Publication No. 94-2789. Bethesda, MD: National Cancer Institute, 1994
62. Ochsner A: Corner of history. My first recognition of the relationship of smoking and lung cancer. Prev Med 2:611–614, 1973
63. Wynder EL, Graham EA: Tobacco smoking as a possible etiologic factor in bronchiogenic carcinoma: a study of six hundred and eighty-four proved cases. JAMA 143:329–336, 1950
64. US Department of Health, Education, and Welfare: Smoking and Health: Report of the Advisory Committee to the Surgeon General of the Public Health Service. PHS Publication No. 1103. Washington D.C.: Public Health Service, 1964

65. Doll R, Hill AB: Lung cancer and other causes of death in relation to smoking: a second report on the mortality of British doctors. Br Med J 2:1071–1081, 1956
66. Wynder EL, Stellman SD: Impact of long-term filter cigarette usage on lung and larynx cancer risk: a case-control study. J Natl Cancer Inst 62:471–477, 1979
67. Lange P, Nyboe J, Appleyard M, et al: Relationship of the type of tobacco and inhalation pattern to pulmonary and total mortality. Eur Respir J 5:1111–1117, 1992
68. Doll R, Peto R: Cigarette smoking and bronchial carcinoma: dose and time relationships among regular smokers and lifelong non-smokers. J Epidemiol Community Health 32:303–313, 1978
69. Hammond EC: Smoking in relation to the death rates of one million men and women. In Haenszel W (ed): Epidemiological Approaches to the Study of Cancer and Other Chronic Diseases. National Cancer Institute Monograph No. 19. Washington, DC: Public Health Service, 1966
70. Samet JM: The changing cigarette and disease risk: current status of the evidence. In: The FTC Cigarette Test Method for Determining Tar, Nicotine, and Carbon Monoxide Yields of US Cigarettes: Report of the NCI Expert Committee. Smoking and Tobacco Control Monograph No. 7. NIH Publication No. 96-4028. Bethesda, MD: Public Health Service, 1996
71. Wynder EL, Kabat GC: The effect of low-yield cigarette smoking on lung cancer risk. Cancer 62(6):1223–1230, 1988
72. Lubin JH, Richter BS, Blot WJ: Lung cancer risk with cigar and pipe use. J Natl Cancer Inst 73:377–381, 1984
73. Higgins IT, Mahan CM, Wynder EL: Lung cancer among cigar and pipe smokers. Prev Med 17:116–128, 1988
74. Chow WH, Schuman LM, McLaughlin JK, et al: A cohort study of tobacco use, diet, occupation, and lung cancer mortality. Cancer Causes Control 3:247–254, 1992
75. Doll R, Peto R: Mortality in relation to smoking: 20 years' observations on male British doctors. Br Med J 2:1525–1536, 1976
76. Nelson DE, Davis RM, Chrismon JH, Giovino GA: Pipe smoking in the United States, 1965–1991: prevalence and attributable mortality. Prev Med 25:91–99, 1996
77. Denissenko MF, Pao A, Moon-shong T, Pfeifer GP: Preferential formation of benzo[a]pyrene adducts at lung cancer mutational hotspots in P53. Science 274(18):430–432, 1996
78. Winn DM, Blot WJ, Shy CM, et al: Snuff dipping and oral cancer among women in the southern United States. N Engl J Med 304(13): 745–749, 1981
79. Wynder EL, Mushinski MH, Spivak JC: Tobacco and alcohol consumption in relation to the development of multiple primary cancers. Cancer 40:1872–1878, 1977
80. McLaughlin JK, Mandel JS, Blot WJ, et al: A population-based case-control study of renal cell carcinoma. J Natl Cancer Inst 72: 275–284, 1984
81. Zahm SH, Hartge P, Hoover R: The National Bladder Cancer Study: employment in the chemical industry. J Natl Cancer Inst 79:217–222, 1987
82. Farrow DC, Davis S: Risk of pancreatic cancer in relation to medical history and the use of tobacco, alcohol and coffee. Int J Cancer 45:816–820, 1990
83. Gajalakshmi CK, Shanta V: Lifestyle and risk of stomach cancer: a hospital-based case-control study. Int J Epidemiol 25(6):1146–1153, 1996
84. Winkelstein W Jr, Shillitoe EJ, Brand R, Johnson KK: Further comments on cancer of the uterine cervix, smoking, and herpes virus infection. Am J Epidemiol 119:1–8, 1984
85. Baron JA, Byers T, Greenberg ER, et al: Cigarette smoking in women with cancers of the breast and reproductive organs. J Natl Cancer Inst 77:677–680, 1986
86. Brinton LA, Schairer C, Haenszel W, et al: Cigarette smoking and invasive cervical cancer. JAMA 255:3265–3269, 1986
87. Dean G, Lee PN, Todd GF, Wicker AJ: Report on a second retrospective mortality study in North-east England. Part 1. Factors related to mortality from lung cancer, bronchitis, heart disease and stroke in Cleveland County, with a particular emphasis on the relative risks associated with smoking filter and plain cigarettes. Research Paper No. 14. London: Tobacco Research Council, 1977
88. Hirayama T: Smoking and cancer in Japan: a prospective study on cancer epidemiology based on census population in Japan: results of 13 years follow-up. In Tominaga S, Aoki K (eds): The ULCC Smoking Control Workshop. Japan: The University of Nagoya Press, 1981, pp 2–8
89. Beck GJ, Doyle CA, Schachter EN: Smoking and lung function. Am Rev Respir Dis 123:149–155, 1981
90. Niewoehner DE, Kleinerman J, Rice B: Pathologic changes in the peripheral airways of young cigarette smokers. N Engl J Med 291: 755–758, 1974
91. Walter S, Jeyaseelan L: Impact of cigarette smoking on pulmonary function in non-allergic subjects. Natl Med J India 5(5):211–213, 1992
92. US Department of Health and Human Services, Office on Smoking and Health: The Health Consequences of Smoking: Chronic Obstructive Lung Disease. A Report of the Surgeon General. DHHS Publication No. (PHS) 84-50205. Washington, DC: Public Health Service, 1984
93. Dockery DW, Spaizer FE, Ferris BG Jr, et al: Cumulative and reversible effects of lifetime smoking on simple tests of lung function in adults. Am Rev Respir Dis 137:286–292, 1988
94. Higgins MW, Enright PL, Kronmal RA, et al: Smoking and lung function in elderly men and women: the Cardiovascular Health Study. JAMA 269(21):2741–2748, 1993
95. Buist AS, Burrows B, Eriksson S, et al: The natural history of air flow obstruction in PiZ emphysema. Am Rev Respir Dis 127:435–445, 1983
96. Sherman CB: The health consequences of cigarette smoking. Med Clin North Am 76(2):355–375, 1992
97. Janoff A, Raju L, Dearing R: Levels of elastase activity in bronchoalveolar lavage fluids of healthy smokers and nonsmokers. Am Rev Respir Dis 127:540–544, 1983
98. Gadek JE, Fells GA, Zimmerman RL, et al: The anti-elastases of the human alveolar structures: implications for the protease-antiprotease theory of emphysema. J Clin Invest 68:889–898, 1981
99. Lonkey SA, McCurren J: Neutrophil enzymes in the lung: regulation of neutrophil elastase. Am Rev Respir Dis 127:59, 1983
100. Janoff A, Carp H, Laurent P, Raju L: The role of oxidative processes in emphysema. Am Rev Respir Dis 127:531–538, 1983
101. Lange P, Groth S, Nyboe J, et al: Decline of the lung function related to the type of tobacco smoked and inhalation. Thorax 45(1): 22–26, 1990
102. Brown CA, Woodward M, Tunstall-Pedoe H: Prevalence of chronic cough and phlegm among male cigar and pipe smokers: results of the Scottish Heart Health Study. Thorax 48;1163–1167, 1993
103. Kahrilas PH: Cigarette smoking and gastroesophageal reflux disease. Dig Dis 10:61–71, 1992
104. Kato I, Nomura AMY, Stemmermann GN, Chyou PH: A prospective study of gastric and duodenal ulcer and its relation to smoking, alcohol, and diet. Am J Epidemiol 135(5):521–530, 1992
105. Bastiaan RJ, Waite IM: Effects of tobacco smoking on plaque development and gingivitis. J Periodontol 49:48, 1978.
106. Sheiham A: Periodontal disease and oral cleanliness in tobacco smokers. J Periodontol 42:259–263, 1971
107. Mandel I: Smoke signals: an alert for oral disease. J Am Dental Assoc 125:872–878, 1994
108. Akef J, Weine FS, Weissman DP: The role of smoking in the progression of periodontal disease: a literature review. Compend Contin Educ Dent 13:526–531, 1992

109. Haber J, Kent RL: Cigarette smoking in a periodontal practice. J Periodontol 63(2):100–106, 1992
110. Ismail AI, Burt BA, Eklund SA: Epidemiologic patterns of smoker and periodontal disease in the United States. J Am Dent Assoc 106:617–621, 1983
111. Fox CH: New considerations in the prevalence of periodontal disease. Current Opinion in Dentistry 2:5–11, 1992
112. National Cancer Institute: Tobacco Effects in the Mouth: A National Cancer Institute and National Institute of Dental Research Guide for Health Professionals. NIH Publication No. 93-3330. Bethesda, MD: National Institutes of Health, National Cancer Institute, 1993
113. Centers for Disease Control and Prevention, Office on Smoking and Health: Preventing Tobacco Use among Young People: A Report of the Surgeon General. Atlanta: Centers for Disease Control and Prevention, 1994
114. Greene JC, Ernster VL, Grady DG, et al: Oral mucosal lesions: clinical findings in relation to smokeless tobacco use among US baseball players. In: Smokeless Tobacco or Health: An International Perspective. Smoking and Tobacco Control Monograph No. 2. Bethesda, MD: National Cancer Institute, 1992
115. Christen AG, Swanson BZ, Glover ED, Henderson AH: Smokeless tobacco: the folklore and social history of snuffing, sneezing, dipping, and chewing. J Am Dent Assoc 105:821–829, 1982
116. Christen AG, Armstrong WR, McDaniel RK: Intraoral leukoplakia, abrasion, periodontal breakdown, and tooth loss in a snuff dipper. J Am Dent Assoc 98:584–586, 1979
117. NIH Consensus Development Panel: National Institutes of Health consensus statement: health implications of smokeless tobacco use. Biomed Pharmacother 42:93–98, 1988
118. Greer RO, Poulson TS: Oral tissue alterations associated with the use of smokeless tobacco by teenagers. Oral Surg Oral Med Oral Pathol 56:275–284, 1983
119. Comstock GW, Shah FK, Meyer MB, Abbey H: Low birth weight and neonatal mortality rate related to maternal smoking on socioeconomic status. Am J Obstet Gynecol 111(1):53–59, 1971
120. Meyer MB, Jonas BS, Tonascia JA: Perinatal events associated with maternal smoking during pregnancy. Am J Epidemiol 103:464–476, 1976
121. Wingerd J, Christianson R, Lovitt WV, Schoden EJ: Placental ratio in white and black women: relation to smoking and anemia. Am J Obstet Gynecol 124:671–675, 1976
122. Stein Z, Kline J, Levin B, Susser M, Warburton D: Epidemiologic studies of environmental exposures in human reproduction. In Berg GG, Maillie HD (eds): Measurement of Risks. New York: Plenum Press, 1981, pp 163–183
123. DiFranza JR, Lew RA: Effect of maternal cigarette smoking on pregnancy complications and sudden infant death syndrome. J Fam Pract 40(4):385–394, 1995
124. Kleinman JC, Pierre MB Jr, Madans JH, Land JH, Schramm WF: The effects of maternal smoking on fetal and infant mortality. Am J Epidemiol 127:274–282, 1988
125. Klonoff-Cohen HS, Edelstein SL, Lefkowitz ES, et al: The effect of passive smoking and tobacco exposure through breast milk on sudden infant death syndrome. JAMA 273(10):795–798, 1995
126. Schoendorf KC, Kiely JL: Relationship of sudden infant death syndrome to maternal smoking during and after pregnancy. Pediatrics 90(6):905–908, 1992
127. Blair PS, Fleming PJ, Bensley D, et al: Smoking and the sudden infant death syndrome: results from 1993–5 case-control study for confidential inquiry into stillbirths and deaths in infancy. Br Med J 313:195–198, 1996
128. Slotkin TA, Lappi SE, McCook EC, et al: Loss of neonatal hypoxia tolerance after prenatal nicotine exposure: implications for sudden infant death syndrome. Brain Res Bull 38(1):69–75, 1995
129. Rantakallio P, Koiranen M: Neurological handicaps among children whose mothers smoked during pregnancy. Prev Med 16:597–606, 1987
130. Naeye RL, Peters EC: Mental development of children whose mothers smoked during pregnancy. Obstet Gynecol 64:601–607, 1984
131. Dunn HG, McBurney AK, Ingram S, Hunter CM: Maternal cigarette smoking during pregnancy and the child's subsequent development. II. Neurological and intellectual maturation to the age of 6½ years. Can J Public Health 68:43–50, 1977
132. Drews CD, Murphy CC, Yeargin-Allsopp M, Decoufle P: The relationship between idiopathic mental retardation and maternal smoking during pregnancy. Pediatrics 97(4):547–553, 1996
133. Weitzman M, Gortmaker S, Sobol A: Maternal smoking and behavior problems of children. Pediatrics 90(3):342–349, 1992
134. Arday DR, Giovino GA, Schulman J, et al: Cigarette smoking and self-reported health problems among US high school seniors, 1982–89. Am J Health Promotion 10(2):111–116, 1995
135. Centers for Disease Control and Prevention: Reasons for tobacco use and symptoms of nicotine withdrawal among adolescent and young adult tobacco users—United States, 1993. MMWR 43(41): 45–50, 1994
136. Centers for Disease Control and Prevention: Symptoms of substance dependence associated with use of cigarettes, alcohol, and illicit drugs—United States, 1991–1992. MMWR 44(44):830–831, 837–839, 1995
137. Respiratory Health Effects of Passive Smoking: Lung Cancer and Other Disorders. The Report of the U.S. Environmental Protection Agency. NIH Publication No. 98-3605. Bethesda, MD: National Institutes of Health and US Environmental Protection Agency, Office of Research and Development, Office of Air and Radiation, 1993
138. Wald NJ, Boreham J, Bailey A, et al: Urinary cotinine as marker of breathing other people's tobacco smoke. Lancet 1:230–231, 1984
139. Foliart D, Benowitz NL, Becker CE: Passive absorption of nicotine in airline flight attendants. N Engl J Med 308:1105, 1983
140. Pirkle JL, Flegal KM, Bernert JT, et al: Exposure of the US populations to environmental tobacco smoke. JAMA 275(16):1233–1240, 1996
141. State-specific prevalence of cigarette-smoking among adults, and children's and adolescents' exposure to environmental tobacco smoke—United States, 1996. MMWR 46(44):1038–1043, 1997
142. Coultas DB, Howard CA, Peake GT, Skipper BJ, Samet JM: Salivary cotinine levels and involuntary tobacco smoke exposure in children and adults in New Mexico. Am Rev Respir Dis 136:305–309, 1987
143. Jarvis MJ, Russell MAH, Feyerabend C, et al: Passive exposure to tobacco smoke: saliva cotinine concentrations in a representative population sample of non-smoking schoolchildren. Br Med J 291: 927–929, 1985
144. Hoffmann D, Haley NJ, Adams JD, Brunnemann KD: Tobacco sidestream smoke: uptake by nonsmokers. Prev Med 13:608–617, 1984
145. Greenberg RA, Haley NJ, Etzel RA, Loda FA: Measuring the exposure of infants to tobacco smoke: nicotine and cotinine in urine and saliva. N Engl J Med 310:1075–1078, 1984
146. Centers for Disease Control, Office on Smoking and Health: The Health Consequences of Involuntary Smoking: A Report of the Surgeon General. DHHS Publication No. (CDC) 87-8398. Rockville, MD: Public Health Service, 1986
147. National Research Council, Committee on Passive Smoking: Environmental Tobacco Smoke. Measuring Exposures and Assessing Health Effects. Washington, DC: National Academy Press, 1986
148. Mannino DM, Siegel M, Husten C, et al: Environmental tobacco smoke exposure and health effects in children: results from the 1991 National Health Interview Survey. Tobacco Control 5:13–18, 1996

149. California Environment Protection Agency: Health effect of exposure to environmental tobacco smoke. Sacramento CA: California Environmental Protection Agency, Office of Environmental Health Hazard Assessment, 1997
149a. Speer F: Tobacco and the nonsmoker: a study of subjective symptoms. Arch Environ Health 16:443–446, 1968
150. Environmental Protection Agency: Environmental Cancer and Heart and Lung Disease: Annual Report to Congress (8th). Rockville, MD: Environmental Protection Agency, Task Force on Environmental Cancer and Heart and Lung Disease, 1985
151. Brownson RC, Alavanja MC, Hock ET, Loy TS: Passive smoking and lung cancer in nonsmoking women. Am J Public Health 82(11): 1525–1530, 1992
152. Kabat GC, Stellman SD, Wynder EL: Relation between exposure to environmental tobacco smoke and lung cancer in lifetime nonsmokers. Am J Epidemiol 142(2):141–148, 1995
153. Stockwell HG, Goldman AL, Lyman GH, et al: Environmental tobacco smoke and lung cancer risk in nonsmoking women. J Natl Cancer Inst 84(18):1417–1422, 1992
154. Fonthan ETH, Correa P, Reynolds P, et al: Environmental tobacco smoke and lung cancer in nonsmoking women: a multicenter study. JAMA 271(22):1752–1759, 1994
155. Cardenas VM, Thun MJ, Austin H, et al: Environmental tobacco smoke and lung cancer mortality in the American Cancer Society's Cancer Prevention Study II. Cancer Causes Control 8:57–64, 1997
156. Gillis CR, Hole DJ, Hawthorne VM, Boyle P: The effect of environmental tobacco smoke in two urban communities in the west of Scotland. Eur J Respir Dis 133(Suppl):121–126, 1984
157. Svendsen K, Kulier LH, Martin MI, Ockene JK: Effects of passive smoking in the Multiple Risk Factor Intervention Trial. Am J Epidemiol 126:783–795, 1987
158. Hirayama T: Passive smoking: a new target of epidemiology. Tokai J Exp Clin Med 10:287–293, 1985
159. Garland C, Barett-Connor E, Suarez L, Criqui MH, Wingard DL: Effects of passive smoking on ischemic heart disease mortality of nonsmokers: a prospective study. Am J Epidemiol 121:645–650, 1985
160. Helsing KJ, Sandler DP, Comstock GW, Chee E: Heart disease mortality in nonsmokers living with smokers. Am J Epidemiol 127: 915–922, 1988
161. Steenland K: Passive smoking and the risk of heart disease. JAMA 267(1):94–99, 1992
162. Steenland K, Thun M, Lally C, Heath C: Environmental tobacco smoke and coronary heart disease in the American Cancer Society CPS-II cohort. Circulation 94(4):622–628, 1996
163. Wells AJ: Passive smoking as a cause of heart disease. J Am Coll Cardiol 24:546–554, 1994
164. Glantz SA, Parmeley WW: Passive smoking and heart disease: mechanisms and risk. JAMA 273:1047–1053, 1995
165. US Department of Agriculture: Tobacco Situation and Outlook Report. USDA Publication No. TBS-236. Washington DC: US Department of Agriculture, Economic Research Service, Commercial Agriculture Division, 1996
166. US Department of Agriculture: Tobacco Situation and Outlook Report. USDA Publication No. TBS-239. Washington DC: US Department of Agriculture, Economic Research Service, Commercial Agriculture Division, 1997
167. Giovino GA, Schooley MW, Zhu BP, et al: Surveillance for selected tobacco-use behaviors—United States, 1990–1994. MMWR 43 (SS-3):1–43, 1994
168. Centers for Disease Control and Prevention: Cigarette smoking among adults—United States, 1995. MMWR 46(51):1217–1220, 1997
169. Husten CG, Chrismon JH, Reddi MN: Trends and effects of cigarette smoking among girls and women in the United States, 1965–1993. J Am Med Women's Assoc 51:11–18, 1996
170. Centers for Disease Control and Prevention, Office on Smoking and Health: Unpublished data
171. Centers for Disease Control and Prevention: Smoking cessation during previous year among adults—United States, 1990 and 1991. MMWR 42: 504–507, 1993
172. Jarvis MJ: Gender differences in smoking cessation: real or myth? Tobacco Control 3:324–328, 1994
173. Zhu BP, Giovino GA, Mowery PD, Eriksen MP: The relationship between cigarette smoking and education revisited: implications for categorizing persons' educational status. Am J Public Health 86(11): 1582–1589, 1996
174. Novotny TE, Warner KE, Kendrick JS, Remington PL: Smoking by blacks and whites: socioeconomic and demographic differences. Am J Public Health 78:1187–1189, 1989
175. Nelson DE, Emont SL, Brackbill RM, et al: Cigarette smoking prevalence by occupation in the United States: a comparison between 1978 to 1980 and 1987 to 1990. J Occup Med 36(5):516–525, 1994
176. Anonymous: Cigarette smoking rates may have peaked among younger teens. Ann Arbor MI: The University of Michigan, News and Information Services, 1997
177. Kann L, Warren CW, Harris WA, et al: Youth risk behavior surveillance—United States, 1995. MMWR 45(SS-4):1–84, 1996
178. Centers for Disease Control, Office on Smoking and Health: The Health Consequences of Smoking: Nicotine Addiction. A Report of the Surgeon General. Washington, DC: Centers for Disease Control, Office on Smoking and Health, 1988
179. Hoffmann D, Djordjevic MV, Brunnemann KD: Changes in cigarette design and composition over time and how they influence the yields of smoke constituents. In: The FTC Cigarette Test Method for Determining Tar, Nicotine, and Carbon Monoxide Yields of U.S. Cigarettes: Report of the NCI Expert Committee. Smoking and Tobacco Control Monograph No. 7. NIH Publication No. 96-4028. Bethesda, MD: National Institutes of Health, 1996
180. Centers for Disease Control and Prevention: Filter ventilation levels in selected US cigarettes, 1997. MMWR 46(44):1043–1047, 1997
181. Slade J: Nicotine delivery devices. In Orleans CT, Slade J (eds): Nicotine Addiction: Principles and Management. New York: Oxford University Press, 1993
182. Federal Trade Commission Report to Congress for 1995: Pursuant to the Federal Cigarette Labeling and Advertising Act. Washington, DC: Federal Trade Commission, 1997
183. Rickert WS, Robinson JC: Yields of selected toxic agents in the smoke of Canadian cigarettes, 1969 and 1978: A decade of change? Prev Med 10:353–363, 1981
184. Hammond EC, Garfinkel L, Seidman H, Lew EA: "Tar" and nicotine content of cigarette smoke in relation to death rates. Environ Res 12:263–274, 1976
185. Lee PM, Garfinkel L: Mortality and type of cigarette smoked. J Epidemiol Community Health 35:16–22, 1981
186. Castelli WP, Dawber TR, Feinlab M, et al: The filter cigarette and coronary heart disease: the Framingham Study. Lancet 2:109–113, 1981
187. Kaufman DW, Helmrich SP, Rosenberg L, et al: Nicotine and carbon monoxide content of cigarette smoke and the risk of myocardial infarction in young men. N Engl J Med 308:407–413, 1983
188. Benowitz NL: Biomarkers of cigarette smoking. In: The FTC Cigarette Test Method for Determining Tar, Nicotine, and Carbon Monoxide Yields of U.S. Cigarettes: Report of the NCI Expert Committee. Smoking and Tobacco Control Monograph No. 7. NIH Publication No. 96-4028. Bethesda, MD: National Institutes of Health, 1996
189. Zacny JP, Stitzer ML: Human smoking patterns. In: The FTC Cigarette Test Method for Determining Tar, Nicotine, and Carbon Monoxide Yields of U.S. Cigarettes: Report of the NCI Expert Committee. Smoking and Tobacco Control Monograph No. 7. NIH Publication No. 96-4028. Bethesda, MD: National Institutes of Health, 1996

190. Federal Register. Federal Trade Commission. Cigarette Testing; Request for Public Comment; Notice, 62 Fed. Reg. 48157, 1997
191. Herning RI, Jones RT, Benowitz NC, Mines AH: How a cigarette is smoked determines blood nicotine levels. Clin Pharmacol Ther 33:84–90, 1983
192. Sutton SR, Russell MAH, Iyer R, et al: Relationship between cigarette yields, puffing patterns and smoke intake: evidence for tar compensation. Br Med J 285:600–603, 1982
193. Kozlowski LT, Frecker RC, Khouw V, Pope MA: The misuse of "less hazardous" cigarettes and detection: hole-blocking of ventilated filters. Am J Public Health 70:1202–1203, 1980
194. Kozlowski LT, Pillitteri J: Compensation for nicotine by smokers of lower yield cigarettes. In: The FTC Cigarette Test Method for Determining Tar, Nicotine, and Carbon Monoxide Yields of U.S. Cigarettes: Report of the NCI Expert Committee. Smoking and Tobacco Control Monograph No. 7. NIH Publication No. 96-4028. Bethesda, MD: National Institutes of Health, 1996
195. Lynch CJ, Benowitz NL: Spontaneous cigarette brand switching: consequences for nicotine and carbon monoxide exposure. Am J Public Health 78:1191–1194, 1978
196. Kozlowski LT, Heatherton TF, Frecker RC, et al: Self-selected blocking of vents on low-yield cigarettes. Pharmacol Biochem Behav 33:815–819, 1989
197. US Department of Agriculture: Tobacco Situation and Outlook Report. USDA Publication No. TBS-240. Washington, DC: US Department of Agriculture, Economic Research Service, 1998
197a. Centers for Disease Control and Prevention: Cigar smoking among teenagers—United States, Massachusetts, and New York, 1996. MMWR 46(20):433–440, 1997
198. Substance Abuse and Mental Health Services Administration: National Household Survey on Drug Abuse: Population Estimates 1994. DHHS Publication No. (SMA) 95-3063. Rockville, MD: Public Health Service, 1995
199. Public Health Service, Office on Smoking and Health: The Health Consequences of Using Smokeless Tobacco: A Report of the Advisory Committee to the Surgeon General. NIH Publication No. 86-2874. Bethesda, MD: Public Health Service, 1986
200. National Institutes of Health: Smokeless Tobacco or Health: An International Perspective. Smoking and Tobacco Control Monograph 2. NIH Publication No. 92-3461. Bethesda, MD: National Institutes of Health, 1992
201. Bolinder G, Alfredsson L, Englund A, de Faire U: Smokeless tobacco use and increased cardiovascular mortality among Swedish construction workers. Am J Public Health 84:399–404, 1994
202. Schwartz J: New cigarette clears the smoke, but the heat is still on. Wall Street Journal, May 28, 1996
203. Hwang S, Noah T: RJR is planning final market test for new cigarette. Wall Street Journal, April 8, 1996
204. Fiore M, Novotny TE, Pierce JP, et al: Methods used to quit smoking in the United States: do cessation programs help? JAMA 263(20): 2760–2765, 1990
205. Public Health Service: Healthy People: The Surgeon General's Report on Health Promotion and Disease Prevention. Rockville, MD: Public Health Service, 1979
206. Schwartz JL: Myths and realities of smoking cessation. NY State J Med 83:1355–1357, 1983
207. Halpern MT, Warner KE: Motivations of smoking cessation: a comparison of successful quitters and failures. J Subst Abuse 5(3): 247–256, 1993
208. Public Health Service: Smoking Cessation: Clinical Practice Guideline. AHCPR Publication No. 96-0692. Rockville, MD: Agency of Health Care Policy and Research and Centers for Disease Control and Prevention, 1996
209. Glynn TJ, Manley MW: How To Help Your Patients Stop Smoking: A National Cancer Institute Manual for Physicians. NIH Publication No. 90-3064. Bethesda, MD: National Institutes of Health, National Cancer Institute, 1990
210. American Medical Association: How To Help Patients Stop Smoking: Guidelines for Diagnosis and Treatment of Nicotine Dependence. Chicago, IL: American Medical Association, 1994
211. U.S. Preventive Services Task Force: Guide to Clinical Preventive Services. 2nd ed. Baltimore, MD: Williams & Wilkins, 1996
211a. Tsevat J: Impact and cost-effectiveness of smoking interventions. Am J Med 93(suppl a):43s–47s, 1992
212. Cummings SR, Rubin SM, Oster G: The cost-effectiveness of counseling smokers to quit. JAMA 261(1):75–79, 1989
213. Cromwell J, Bartosch WJ, Fiore MC, Hasselblad V, Baker T: Cost-effectiveness of the clinical practice recommendations in the AHCPR guideline for smoking cessation. JAMA 278(21):1759–1766, 1997
214. Lightwood JM, Glantz SA: Short-term economic and health benefits of smoking cessation. Myocardial infarction and stroke. Circulation 96(4):1089–1096, 1997
215. Sennett C: An introduction to HEDIS—The Health Plan Employer Data and Information Set. J Clin Outcomes Management 3(2):59–61, 1996
216. Committee on Performance: HEDIS 3.0. Washington, DC: National Committee for Quality Assurance, 1996
217. National Center for Quality Assurance: Quality Compass™. Washington DC: National Center for Quality Assurance, 1997
218. Wagner EH, Curry SJ, Grothaus L, Saunders KW, McBride CM: The impact of smoking and quitting on health care use. Arch Intern Med 155(16):1789–1795, 1995
218a. McAfee T, Wilson J, Dacey S, Sofian N, Curry S, Wagener B. Awakening the sleeping giant: mainstreaming efforts to decrease tobacco use in an HMO. HMO Pract 9(3):138–143, 1995
218b. Schauffler HH, Rodriguez T: Availability and utilization of health promotion programs and satisfaction with health plan. Med Care 32(12):1182–1196, 1994
219. Puska P, Salonen J, Nissinen A, et al: Change in risk factors for coronary heart disease during 10 years of a community intervention programme (North Karelia project). Br Med J 287(17):1840–1844, 1983
220. Rossouw JE, Jooste PL, Chalton DO, et al: Community-based intervention: the Coronary Risk Factor Study (CORIS). Int J Epidemiol 22(3):428–438, 1993
221. Farquhar JW, Wood PD, Breitrose H, et al: Community education for cardiovascular health. Lancet 1(8023):1192–1195, 1977
222. Farquhar JW, Fortmann AP, Flora JA, et al: Effects of community-wide education on cardiovascular disease risk factors: the Stanford Five-City Project. JAMA 264(3):359–365, 1990
223. Multiple Risk Factor Intervention Trial Research Group. Multiple Risk Factor Intervention Trial: risk factor changes and mortality results. JAMA 248(12):1465–1477, 1982
224. Lando HA, Pechacek TF, Pirie PL, et al: Changes in adult cigarette smoking in the Minnesota Heart Health Program. Am J Public Health 85(2):201–208, 1995
225. Carleton RA, Lasater TM, Assaf AR, et al: The Pawtucket Heart Health Program: community changes in cardiovascular risk factors and projected disease risk. Am J Public Health 85(6):777–785, 1995
226. The COMMIT Research Group: Community Intervention Trial for Smoking Cessation (COMMIT): I. Cohort results from a four-year community intervention. Am J Public Health 85(2):183–192, 1995
227. Lynch BS, Bonnie RJ (eds): Growing Up Tobacco Free: Preventing Nicotine Addition in Children and Youths. Washington, DC: National Academy Press, 1994
228. Shelton DM, Alciati MH, Chang MM: State laws on tobacco control—United States, 1995. MMWR 44(SS-6):1–28, 1995
229. Executive Order #13058: Protecting federal employees and the public from exposure to tobacco smoke in the Federal workplace, August 9, 1997
230. California Chapter 989 Labor Code, Section 6404.5, September 27, 1996

231. Tobacco Law—Clean Indoor Air Act. New York State—PH Law 1399 N-X, New York City—AC 17-501-514. City law revised: Tobacco Law—Smoke-free Air Act, New York City Local law No. 5 of 1995, April 10, 1995
231a. Conlisk E, Siegel M, Lengerich E, et al: The status of local smoking regulations in North Carolina following a state preemption bill. JAMA 273(10):805–807, 1995
232. Joint Commission on Accreditation of Healthcare Organizations: Smoking standards of the Joint Commission on Accreditation of Healthcare Organizations. Joint Commission Perspectives Nov/Dec: 12–14, 1991
233. "Non-smoking, please": a money-saving proposition [News Features]. NY State J Med 83:1361–1363, 1983
234. Anonymous: Delta Air Lines is the first smokefree US airline worldwide. Wall Street Journal Nov 15, 1994, p A15
235. Jones D: Airlines join forces to ban trans-Atlantic smoking. USA Today Jan 25, 1995, p B1
236. Warner KE, Murt HA: Economic incentives for health. Annu Rev Public Health 5:107–133, 1984
237. National Association of Insurance Commissioners: Life and Health Actuarial (Ex5) Task Force results of field test of the Smoker/Nonsmoker Experience Exhibit. NAIC-Proceedings 1987 2:687–705, 1987
238. Office for Disease Prevention and Health Promotion, Centers for Disease Control and Prevention: For a Healthy Nation: Returns on Investment in Public Health. Washington, DC: Office for Disease Prevention and Health Promotion and Centers for Disease Control and Prevention, 1994
239. The tax burden on tobacco, 1996. Tob Inst 31:1–254, 1997
240. Public Health Service: Healthy People 2000: Midcourse Review and 1995 Revisions. Washington, DC: Public Health Service, 1996
241. Centers for Disease Control and Prevention: Cigarette smoking before and after an excise tax increase and an antismoking campaign—Massachusetts, 1990–1996. MMWR 45(44):966–970, 1996
242. National Cancer Institute: The impact of cigarette excise taxes on smoking among children and adults: summary report of a National Cancer Institute Expert Panel. Washington, DC: National Cancer Institute, 1993
243. Sweanor D, Warner KE: The role of federal state excise taxes. In: Tobacco Use: An American Crisis. Washington DC: American Medical Association, 1993
244. Tobacco or Health Programme: Tobacco or Health: First Global Status Report. Geneva: World Health Organization, 1996
245. Attorneys General Settlement Agreement. In Glob@Link; Resources on Tobacco Control—North American [online database] (cited 20 March 1997)
246. Meier B: Files of R.J. Reynolds Tobacco show effort on youths. The New York Times, Jan 15, 1998
247. Centers for Disease Control and Prevention: Changes in the cigarette brand preferences of adolescent smokers—United States, 1989–1993. MMWR 43(32):577–581, 1994
248. Fischer PM, Schwartz MP, Richards JW, et al: Brand logo recognition by children aged 3 to 6 years. JAMA 266(22):3145–3148, 1991
249. Ono Y, Ingersoll B: RJR retires Joe Camel, adds sexy smokers. Wall Street Journal, July 11, 1997, p. B1.
250. Pollay RW, Siddarth S, Siegel M, et al: The last straw? Cigarette advertising and realized market shares among youth and adults, 1979–1993. J Marketing 60:1–16, 1996
251. Evans N, Farkas A, Gilpin E, et al: Influence of tobacco marketing and exposure to smokers on adolescent susceptibility to smoking. J Natl Cancer Inst 87(20):1538–1545, 1995
252. Pierce JP, Gilpin EA: A historical analysis of tobacco marketing and the uptake of smoking by youth in the United States: 1890–1977. Health Psychol 14(6):500–508, 1995
253. Pierce JP, Gilpin E, Burns DM, et al: Does tobacco advertising target young people to start smoking? Evidence from California. JAMA 266(22):3154–3158, 1991
254. Pierce JP, Lee L, Gilpin EA: Smoking initiation by adolescent girls, 1944 through 1988: an association with targeted advertising. JAMA 271(8):608–611, 1994
255. Ramirez A: Reynolds, after protests, cancels cigarette aimed at black smokers. New York Times, Jan 20, 1990
256. Freedman AM, McCarthy MJ: New smoke from RJR under fire. Wall Street Journal, Feb 20, 1990
257. The Public Health Cigarette Smoking Act of 1969. Public Law 91-222
258. US Food and Drug Administration: Regulations restricting the sale and distribution of cigarettes and smokeless tobacco products to protect children and adolescents—final rule. Federal Register 61: 41, 314–375, 1996
259. Smee C, Parsonage M, Anderson R, Duckworth S: Effect of Tobacco Advertising on Tobacco Consumption. A Discussion Document Reviewing the Evidence. London: Department of Health, Economics and Operational Research Division, 1992
260. Laugesen M, Meads C: Tobacco advertising restrictions, price, income and tobacco consumption in OECD countries, 1960–1986. Br J Addict 86:1343–1354, 1991
261. Warner KE: Selling health: a media campaign against tobacco. J Public Health Policy 7:434–439, 1986
262. Blum A: The Marlboro Grand Prix—Circumvention of the television ban on tobacco advertising. N Engl J Med 324:913–917, 1991
263. Hamilton JL: The demand for cigarettes: advertising, the health scare, and the cigarette advertising ban. Rev Econ Stat 54:401–411, 1972
264. Horn D: Who Is Quitting—and Why. Progress in Smoking Cessation. Proceedings of the International Conference on Smoking Cessation. New York: American Cancer Society, 1978
265. Pierce JP, Macaskill P, Hill DJ: Long-term effectiveness of mass media anti-smoking campaigns in Australia. Am J Public Health 80:565–569, 1990
266. Doxiadis SA, Trihopoulos DV, Phylactou HD: Impact of a nationwide anti-smoking campaign. Lancet 2(8457):712–713, 1985
267. Flay BR, D'Avernas JR, Best JA, Kersell MW, Ryan KB: Cigarette smoking: why young people do it and ways of preventing it. In McGrath P, Firestone P (eds): Pediatric and Adolescent Behavioral Medicine. vol. 10. New York: Springer, 1983
268. Pierce JP, Choi WS, Gilpin EA, et al: Validation of susceptibility as a predictor of which adolescents take up smoking in the United States. Health Psychol 15(5):355–361, 1996
269. McAlister AL, Percy C, MacCoby N: Adolescent smoking: onset and prevention. Pediatrics 63:650–658, 1979
270. Centers for Disease Control and Prevention: Guidelines for school health programs to prevent tobacco use and addiction. MMWR 43(RR-2):1–18, 1994
271. National Institutes of Health: School Programs to Prevent Smoking: The National Cancer Institute Guide to Strategies that Succeed. NIH Publication No. 90-500. Bethesda, MD: National Institutes of Health, 1990
272. Flay BR, Ditecco D, Schlegal RP: Mass media in health promotion. Health Educ Q 7:127–143, 1980
273. Bandura A: Social Learning Theory. Englewood Cliffs, NJ: Prentice-Hall, 1977
274. Flay BR: Psychosocial approaches to smoking prevention: a review of findings. Health Psychol 4:449–488, 1985
275. Flay BR: What we know about the social influences approach to smoking prevention: Review and recommendations. In Bell CS, Battjes R (eds): Prevention Research: Deterring Drug Abuse Among Children and Adolescents. NIDA Research Monograph 63. DHHS Publication No. (ADM) 85-1334. Washington, DC: Alcohol, Drug Abuse and Mental Health Administration, National Institute on Drug Abuse, 1985
276. Botvin GJ, Wills TA: Personal and social skills training: Cognitive behavior approaches to substance abuse prevention. In Bell CS, Battjes R (eds): Prevention Research: Deterring Drug Abuse Among Children and Adolescents. NIDA Research Monograph 63.

DHHS Publication No. (ADM) 85-1134. Washington, DC: Alcohol, Drug Abuse, and Mental Health Administration, National Institute on Drug Abuse, 1985
277. Best JA, Thomson SJ, Santi SM, Smith EA, Brown KS: Preventing cigarette-smoking among schoolchildren. Annu Rev Public Health 9:161–201, 1988
278. Biglan A, Ary DV: Methodological issues in research on smoking prevention. In Bell CS, Battjes R (eds): Prevention Research: Deterring Drug Abuse Among Children and Adolescents. NIDA Research Monograph 63. DHHS Publication No. (ADM) 85-1134. Washington, DC: Alcohol, Drug Abuse, and Mental Health Administration, National Institute on Drug Abuse, 1985
279. Flay BR: Mass media linkages with school-based programs for drug abuse prevention. J School Health 56:402–406, 1986
280. Flynn BS, Worden JK, Secker-Walker RH, et al: Prevention of cigarette smoking through mass media intervention and school programs. Am J Public Health 82:827–834, 1992
281. Pierce JP, Evans N, Farkas AJ, et al: Tobacco Use in California. An Evaluation of the Tobacco Control Program, 1989–1993. La Jolla, CA: University of California, San Diego, 1994
282. Murray DM, Prokhorov AV, Hart KC: Effects of a statewide antismoking campaign on mass media messages and smoking beliefs. Prev Med 23:54–60, 1994
283. Warner KE: Smoking and health implications of a change in the federal cigarette excise tax. JAMA 225:1028–1032, 1986
284. Centers for Disease Control and Prevention: Healthy People 2000 Review 1995–96. DHHS Publication No. (PHS) 96-1256. Hyattsville, MD: National Center for Health Statistics, 1996
285. Centers for Disease Control and Prevention: Tobacco use and usual source of cigarettes among high school students—United States, 1995. MMWR 45(20):413–418, 1996
286. Jason JA, Ji PY, Anes MD, Birkhead SH: Active enforcement of cigarette control laws in the prevention of cigarette sales to minors. JAMA 266(22):3159–3161, 1991
287. DiFranza JR, Carlson RP, Caisse RE: Reducing youth access to tobacco. Tobacco Control 1(1):58, 1992
288. Substance Abuse and Mental Health Services Administration: Final regulations to implement section 1926 of the Public Health Service Act, regarding the sale and distribution of tobacco products to individuals under the age of 18. Federal Register 13:1492–1500, 1996
289. US Department of Health and Human Services: Synar Regulation Guidance Series: Sampling, Inspection, and Change Strategies. Rockville MD: Substance Abuse and Mental Health Services Administration, 1996
290. Brink SD: Health Risks and Behavior: The Impact on Medical Costs. Milwaukee: Milliman & Robertson, 1987
291. Shipley RH, Orleans CT, Wilbur CS, et al: Effect of the Johnson & Johnson Live for Life Program on employee smoking. Prev Med 17:25–34, 1988
292. Kristein MM: How much can business expect to profit from smoking cessation? Prev Med 12:358–381, 1983
293. Centers for Disease Control and Prevention: Making your workplace smokefree: a decision maker's guide. Atlanta: Centers for Disease Control and Prevention, 1996
294. US Department of Health and Human Services: 1992 National Survey of Worksite Health Promotion Activities. Washington, DC: Public Health Service, 1993
295. Hallett R: Smoking intervention in the workplace: review and recommendations. Prev Med 15:213–231, 1986
296. Klesges RC, Glasgow RE: Smoking modification in the worksite. In Cataldo MF, Coates TJ (eds): Health and Industry: A Behavioral Medicine Perspective. New York: John Wiley & Sons, 1986
297. Schilling RS, Letai AD, Hui SL, et al: Lung function, respiratory disease, and smoking in families. Am J Epidemiol 106:274–283, 1977
298. Walsh DC, McDougall V: Current policies regarding smoking in the workplace. Am J Indust Med 13:181–190, 1988
299. The Gallup Organization: Survey of the public's attitudes toward smoking. Princeton, NJ: The Gallup Organization, 1992
300. Gerlach KK, Shopland DR, Hartman AM, Gibson JT, Pechacek TF: Workplace smoking policies in the United States: results from a national survey of more than 100,000 workers. Tobacco Control 6:199–206, 1997
301. US Department of Agriculture: Tobacco Situation and Outlook Report. USDA Publication No. TBS-239. Washington, DC: Department of Agriculture, Economic Research Service, 1997
302. Warner K: The employment implications of declining tobacco product sales for the regional economies of the United States. JAMA 275(16):1241–1246, 1996
303. U.S. Department of Agriculture: Unpublished data, 1996
304. US Federal Trade Commission: Competition and the financial impact of the proposed tobacco industry settlement. Washington DC: Bureau of Economics, Competition, and Consumer Protection, Federal Trade Commission, September 1997
305. U.S. Department of Agriculture: Unpublished data, 1995
306. Yu JJ, Mattson ME, Boyd GM, et al: A comparison of smoking patterns in the People's Republic of China with the United States: an impending health catastrophe in the Middle Kingdom. JAMA 264: 1575–1579, 1990
307. Muller M: Preventing tomorrow's epidemic: the control of smoking and tobacco production in developing countries. NY State J Med 83:1304–1309, 1983
308. Whelan EM: A smoking gun: how the tobacco industry gets away with murder. Philadelphia: George F. Stickley, 1984, pp 166–176
309. Madeley J: The environmental impact of tobacco production in developing countries. NY State J Med 83:1310–1311, 1983
310. Forty-ninth World Health Assembly: International framework convention for tobacco control, May 25, 1996. WHA49.17.
311. Barnum H: The economic burden of the global trade in tobacco. Tobacco Control 3:358–361, 1994
312. Dale KC: ACSH survey: which magazines report the hazards of smoking? ACSH News and Views 3:1,8–10, 1982
313. White L, Whelan EM: How well do American magazines cover the health hazards of smoking? The 1986 survey. ACSH News and Views 7:1,7–11, 1986
314. Warner KE, Goldenhar LM, McLaughlin CG: Cigarette advertising and magazine coverage of the hazards of smoking: a statistical analysis. N Engl J Med 326(5):305–309, 1992
315. Warner KE, Goldenhar LM: The cigarette advertising ban and magazine coverage of smoking and health. J Public Health Policy. Spring: 32–42, 1989
316. Qunidlen A: Quid pro quo. New York Times, Oct 8, 1994
317. Hicks JP: In council, bill gains to restrict smoking. New York Times, Dec 8, 1994, p B2

45

Alcohol-Related Health Problems

Brian L. Cook • J. Alberto Abreu

The abuse of alcohol is more common than any other form of drug abuse throughout the world. The consequences of alcohol use are pervasive in society. From a public health prospective, alcohol use presents a unique dilemma, referred to as the "prevention paradox."[1] This paradox stems from the observation that health and economic consequences resulting from alcohol use are far greater due to hazardous drinking than drinking patterns that constitute a formal diagnosis of alcohol dependence.[2] This paradox is further complicated by findings that suggest that low to moderate levels of alcohol use may play a role in reducing mortality for certain disorders, such as cardiovascular disease.[3] To better understand this paradox and the risk of alcohol use, it is helpful to stratify alcohol use and risk along a continuum. This continuum stretches from abstinence to alcohol dependence.

Categories of Alcohol Use along the Drinking Continuum

"Safe" (Low-Risk) Drinking

Based on the concept of a continuum of risk, some organizations have proposed guidelines for safe (low-risk) drinking, some of which include both the characteristics and circumstances of the drinker as well as levels of consumption. American guidelines for safe drinking generally recommend no more than two drinks per day for men and one drink per day for nonpregnant women.[4–6] Slightly higher limits are proposed by U.K. authorities.[7]

One example of safe drinking guidelines that also include characteristics of the drinker as well as levels of consumption is contained in the report of the Australian National Health and Medical Research Council (NHMRC),[8] "Is there a safe level of daily consumption of alcohol for men and women? Recommendations regarding responsible drinking behavior," in which it is recommended that:

> responsible drinking be considered as the consumption of the least amount of alcohol that will meet an individual's personal and social needs and in any case:
>
> (a) that men should not exceed 4 units or 40 grams of absolute alcohol per day on a regular basis, or 28 units per week; that 4–6 units per day or 28–42 units per week be considered as hazardous and that greater than 6 units per day or 42 units per week be regarded as harmful;
>
> (b) that women should not exceed 2 units or 20 grams of absolute alcohol per day on a regular basis, or 14 units per week; that 2–4 units per day or 14–28 units per week be considered as hazardous and that greater than 4 units per day or 28 units per week be regarded as harmful because of the biological differences between men and women;
>
> (c) that abstinence be promoted as highly desirable during pregnancy;
>
> (d) that persons who intend to drive, operate machinery or undertake activities in hazardous or potentially hazardous situations should not drink;
>
> (e) that in any given situation it is difficult to say that there is an absolute safe level of consumption and thus in situations of any doubt people should not drink.

In this report, a unit or standard drink was equivalent to 8 to 10 g of alcohol compared with Canada and the United States, where one unit or standard drink contains approximately 13.6 g of alcohol.

In essence, no level of alcohol consumption will always be safe for all individuals under all conditions. Rather, increasing levels of consumption hold a progressively increasing risk of causing either acute or chronic damage. Moreover, the level at which risk occurs and its significance are influenced by a combination of personal and environmental factors that render the individual more or less vulnerable to damage from alcohol.

Hazardous Drinking

The term "hazardous drinking" has been used to describe levels of alcohol consumption that expose the drinker to a high risk of physical complications.[9] Under certain circumstances, relatively low levels of consumption on isolated occasions may result in damage to the individual drinker. There is evidence as well that levels of consumption far below those found in people diagnosed as alcohol dependent are linked with increased risks of adverse health consequences.[10,11] A special case involves the survival and normal development of the fetus of the drinking pregnant woman.[12] In this instance, some authorities would assert that there is no safe level of consumption, or that it may be impossible to define such a level.[13] As information grows on how alcohol is hazardous to health, we find ourselves less secure in defining what is safe.[14,15] Rather, alcohol use involves a continuum of risk, defined by host and environmental factors as well as by the levels of alcohol consumption.

▸ ALCOHOL ABUSE AND ALCOHOL DEPENDENCY DEFINITIONS

The definitions of alcohol abuse and dependency have evolved over time, and differ somewhat between various organizations, e.g., the World Health Organization (WHO) as compared with the American Psychiatric Association (APA). The WHO has recently published its 10th edition of the *International Classification of Diseases* (ICD-10),[16] while The APA recently published its 4th edition of the *Diagnostic and Statistical Manual of Mental Disorders* (DSM-IV).[17] The definitions differ primarily in the number and definition of symptoms required before a diagnosis of alcohol abuse or dependency are met. The ICD-10 and DSM-IV were compared in a study by

Caetano.[18] The 1-year prevalence rate of alcohol dependence was higher (5.5 versus 3.9 percent) when ICD-10 criteria were applied as compared to the DSM-IV criteria. Predictors of meeting ICD-10 versus DSM-IV criteria were slightly different in the study, thus highlighting differences in these two criteria sets, which should be considered in epidemiological research. The DSM-IV definition is most widely used in alcohol use disorder research in the United States at this time.

The DSM-IV defines alcohol abuse as a maladaptive pattern of alcohol use leading to clinically significant impairment or distress, as manifested by one or more of the following, occurring within a 12-month period: (*a*) recurrent alcohol use resulting in failure to fulfill major role obligations at work, school, or home; (*b*) recurrent alcohol use in situations in which it is physically dangerous; (*c*) recurrent alcohol-related legal problems; (*d*) continued alcohol use despite having a persistent or recurrent social or interpersonal problem caused or exacerbated by the effects of alcohol.

The DSM-IV defines alcohol dependence as a maladaptive pattern of alcohol use, leading to clinically significant impairment or distress, as manifested by three (or more) of the following occurring at any time in the same 12-month period: (*a*) tolerance; (*b*) withdrawal; (*c*) alcohol use in greater quantity or for a longer period than intended; (*d*) persistent desire or unsuccessful efforts to cut down or control alcohol use; (*e*) a great deal of time spent acquiring, using, or recovering from alcohol's effects; (*f*) important social, occupational, or recreational activities given up or reduced because of alcohol use; (*g*) alcohol use continued despite knowledge of having a persistent or recurrent physical or psychological problem that is likely to have been caused by or exacerbated by alcohol use.

In the DSM-IV classification, once an individual meets dependency criteria, the diagnosis of alcohol abuse should no longer be used for that individual. Course specifiers should be used to describe the individual after no criteria for dependence have been met for at least 1 month. The course specifiers include early full remission, early partial remission, sustained full remission, sustained partial remission, on agonist therapy, or in a controlled environment.

Several observations are important regarding the DSM-IV classification system. The DSM-IV classification emphasizes the central role that alcohol comes to play in the life of a dependent individual, not simply the physiological changes associated with heavy alcohol use. Thus, an individual can be classified as alcohol dependent without classic signs or symptoms of physical tolerance and resultant withdrawal upon abrupt discontinuation of alcohol. Also, complete abstinence is not required before the remission course specifiers can be used. If none of the seven dependence criteria symptoms are met during a period of a month or longer, a form of remission is reached that is defined as either partial or full. If continued drinking does not result in full return of three or more dependence criteria symptoms, but does cause at least one dependence symptom, the remission is considered partial. If the full dependence criteria are not met for 12 months or more, the remission category is considered sustained. The utility and predictive validity of these categories remain to be established.

▶ EPIDEMIOLOGY OF ALCOHOL ABUSE AND DEPENDENCY

Alcohol is regularly consumed by roughly half of the adult United States population. A detailed account of alcohol consumption, along with DSM-IV prevalence rates of alcohol abuse and dependence, were reported by Grant in 1994.[19] This study used data gathered during a nationally representative survey of alcohol use and alcohol-related problems sponsored by the National Institute on Alcohol Abuse and Alcoholism (NIAAA), which was conducted in 1988. In this survey, the majority of Americans were classified as current drinkers (51.4 percent). Over 27 percent of the sample reported drinking more than three times/week, and the mean number of drinks used per drinking occasion was 2.9. The 1-year prevalence rate of alcohol abuse and dependency in this survey was about 9 percent. A similar study was conducted in 1992 during the National Longitudinal Alcohol Epidemiologic Survey (NLAES), again sponsored by the NIAAA.[20] In the 1992 survey, the 1-year prevalence rate of alcohol abuse and dependence in the United States was 7.41 percent. Prevalence was greater for nonblacks (7.68 percent) than among blacks (5.28 percent). Males overall outnumbered females by nearly 3-fold, 11.0 versus 4.0 percent. Prevalence rates were highest in the under 45-year-old age categories. Interestingly, in the youngest age category of 18- to-29-year-olds, the male-to-female ratio was only 2:1 in nonblack respondents.

Large population-based studies have demonstrated that the lifetime prevalence of alcohol use disorders (abuse and dependence) are even more common. The Epidemiologic Catchment Area (ECA) study demonstrated that, among community dwelling, nontreatment seeking individuals, the lifetime prevalence of alcohol dependency was 13.7 percent.[21] Results from the National Comorbidity Survey (NCS) by Kessler et al demonstrated a lifetime prevalence of alcohol abuse plus dependency of 14.6 percent in females and a prevalence of 23.5 percent in males.[22]

Given these 1-year and lifetime prevalence rates, a conservative estimate of the number of individuals directly affected by alcohol use disorders is at least 20 to 30 million in the United States at any given time. Additionally, it should be remembered that the number of individuals affected by those with alcohol use disorders through marriage and family, the work site, and the highways is far greater than the number of individuals with alcohol use disorder.

Surveys done in health care settings present a startling example of alcohol-related costs. In a primary care outpatient setting, problem drinking rates of 8 to 20 percent are seen, and between 20 and 40 percent of patients admitted to general medical hospitals have a history of alcohol use disorders.[23] This extent of medical morbidity obviously translates into significant mortality. United States data from the Centers for Disease Control National Center for Health Statistics provide estimates of 105,095 deaths in the United States related to alcohol use (4.9 percent of deaths from all causes in 1987).[24] This estimate is considered an underestimate, as many deaths which are associated with alcohol use are not coded as such on death certificates. A review of studies across multiple nations examining alcohol-related mortality demonstrated that alcoholics lose on average more than 20 years of potential life.[25]

The price tag for alcohol-related disorders far exceeds $100 billion annually in the United States.[26] Economic costs to industry alone in the United States have been estimated at $136 billion for 1990.[27] Such costs include absenteeism, sick leave, decreased worker efficiency, and employee replacement costs through workers quitting, being fired, or dying prematurely.

These summary statistics can be further broken down into risk indicators that are more useful for preventive health purposes, e.g., to focus screening and prevention efforts. Alcohol use disorders are more common in males than in females, with the ratio of affected males to females being approximately 2–3:1. While rates of females affected with alcohol use disorders are lower, health-related consequences of alcohol use in females who do not meet diagnostic criteria for alcoholism are more severe than in males. Review of health-related consequences of alcoholism in females later in this chapter will include medical risks associated with alcohol use in nonalcohol-dependent drinkers.

Age is another factor that can be used to point to risk. Alcohol use disorders typically are most common in those under 45 years of age. Health-related morbidity is different across the age span, with more unnatural deaths (e.g., accidents, suicides, homicides) observed in younger age groups and more chronic disorders seen in the older age groups. Screening tools and definitions of alcohol use disorders in the elderly are less satisfactory than in middle age, and thus rates of alcohol use disorders in the elderly may be underestimated.

Alcohol use disorders are seen across all socioeconomic groups. Alcohol use disorders cluster weakly in lower socioeconomic groups, but this may simply be secondary to alcohol's effect upon poor school and job performance. Persons of Asian descent have lower rates of alcohol-related disorders, presumed related to their tendency toward decreased alcohol-metabolizing enzymes leading to a flush reaction, tachycardia, and headache. Differences between blacks and nonblacks are significant, generally with nonblack rates being lower in both males and females. Drinking is most prevalent in urban America, and geographically in the Northeast.

The comorbidity of alcohol use disorders and other psychiatric disorders is very common. The ECA study found that about half of individuals with alcohol use disorders had a concomitant psychiatric disorder.[21] The most commonly observed psychiatric comorbidities include antisocial personality disorder, mood disorders, and anxiety disorders.

▶ GENERAL MECHANISMS OF ALCOHOL-RELATED DYSFUNCTION AND DAMAGE

A general schema of the mechanisms involved in alcohol-related tissue injury is provided in Figure 45-1. Tissue in this context refers to either a single type of cell or a single organ. Besides having direct toxic effects on target tissue, alcohol also may act indirectly through a variety of mechanisms. Other alcohol-associated behaviors involving tobacco, risky sexual behavior, illicit drugs, and other drugs and chemicals as well as nonalcohol-related disease processes may contribute as cofactors to the development, course, and outcome of alcohol-induced primary damage. In addition, alcohol may act as a factor influencing the development, course, and outcome of coincidental diseases.

Much of the tissue damage that occurs in association with alcohol use has been attributed, at least in part, to direct toxic effects; for example, alcoholic hepatitis, cardiomyopathy, and neuronal degeneration. New findings, however, suggest that excitotoxicity mediated through alterations in glutamate neurotransmission may be responsible for many of the central nervous system (CNS) degenerative processes associated with alcoholism (e.g., Wernike-Korsakoff syndrome, cerebellar degeneration, dementia associated with alcoholism).[28] The effects on the CNS are also of great importance in the development of various alcohol-related problems associated with acute intoxication and withdrawal from alcohol, as well as alcohol dependence.[28,29] Acute effects are particularly important in circumstances under which drinkers may injure themselves or others.[30]

Alcohol also may act indirectly through the production of metabolic disturbances, endocrine changes,[31] immune system changes,[32] aggravation of obstructive sleep apnea,[33] and displacement of dietary nutrients or impairment of their absorption or use,[34] as well as through the effects of diseases caused by alcohol.

Obstructive sleep apnea, a complication of alcohol use that occurs as a result of acute intoxication, is potentially important as a direct cause of morbidity and mortality.[33] It may contribute also to the course and outcome of other alcohol- as well as nonalcohol-related diseases. This disturbance and its precipitation and aggravation by alcohol have been recognized only recently.[35–37]

When an alcohol-related health problem does occur, its course and outcome may be influenced by whether or not the affected individual continues to be exposed to alcohol and alcohol-related hazards. Furthermore, course and outcome may be influenced by whether or not he or she seeks, has access to, receives, and adheres to effective treatment, not only for the complications of alcohol use but also for the drinking behavior itself.

A summary of the etiological significance of alcohol and associated variables that contribute to the excess mortality of heavy drinkers is provided in Table 45-1.

▶ MORBIDITY AND MORTALITY

The important health problems related to alcohol use were reviewed by the Institute of Medicine.[38] The major health problems associated with alcohol use named in this report included alcohol withdrawal syndrome, psychosis, hepatitis, cirrhosis, pancreatitis, thiamine

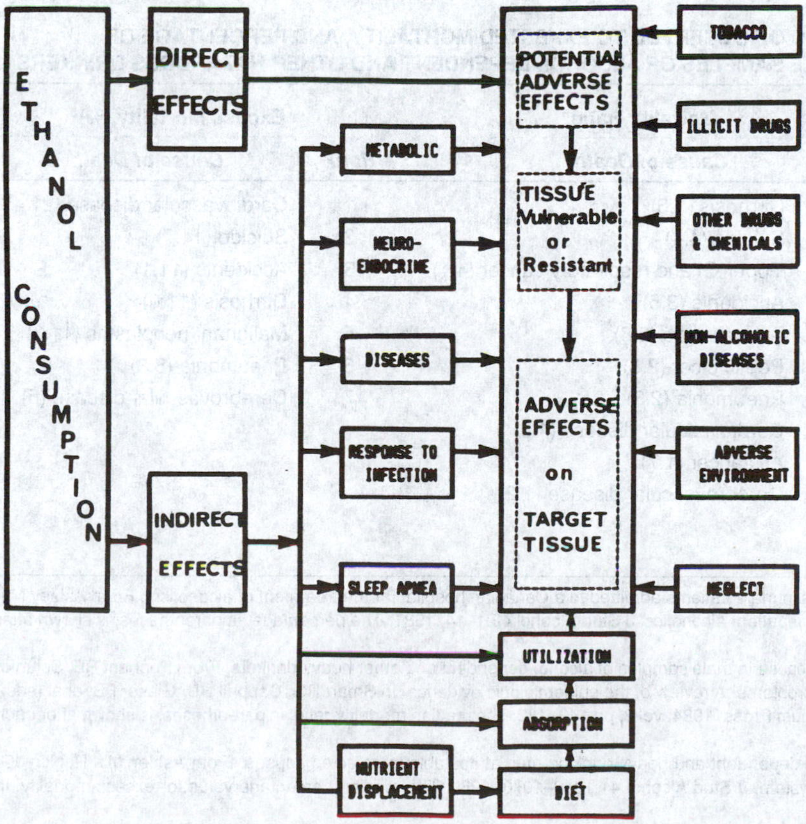

Figure 45-1. Schematic representation of the general mechanisms involved in the development of alcohol-related tissue injury.

TABLE 45-1. ETIOLOGICAL SIGNIFICANCE OF ALCOHOL AND ASSOCIATED VARIABLES IN THE EXCESS MORTALITY OF CHRONIC HEAVY DRINKERS

Cause of Death	*Effects of Alcohol*	*Heavy Tobacco Smoking*	*Emotional Problems*	*Poor Food Habits*	*Other Personal Neglect*	*Increased Environmental Hazards*
Tuberculosis		X		X	X	X
Carcinoma						
Mouth	XX	XX				
Larynx	XX	XX				
Pharynx	XX	XX				
Esophagus	XX	XX				
Liver	X					XX
Lung	X	XX				
Alcoholic cardiomyopathy	XX					
Other cardiovascular disease	XX	XX		X	X	
Pneumonia	XX	XX			XX	XX
Peptic ulcers	XX	X		X	X	
Liver cirrhosis						
Alcoholic	XX			X		
Nonalcoholic	X					XX
Suicide	XX		XX			
Accidents	XX	XX	X		X	X

Modified from Popham RE, Schmidt W, Israelstam S: Heavy alcohol consumption and physical health problems. A review of the epidemiologic evidence. In Smart RG, Cappell HD, Glaser FB, et al (eds): Research Advances in Alcohol and Drug Problems. New York: Plenum Press, 1984, vol 8, pp 149–182.

X, probably indicated; XX, clearly indicated. Where a space is left blank, either the factor is probably of no significance or its role, if any, is unknown.

deficiency, neuropathy, dementia, and cardiomyopathy. Alcohol use also plays a key role in injury and accidents, suicide, and homicide. Also important is a range of adverse pregnancy outcomes and fetal abnormalities caused by the embryotoxic and teratogenic effects of alcohol.

The most common medical problems in alcohol-dependent and heavy drinking men, in terms of decreasing lifetime incidence, are trauma, acute alcoholic liver disease, peptic ulceration, chronic obstructive lung disease, pneumonia, hypertension, gastritis, epileptiform disorders, acute brain syndromes, peripheral neuritis, ischemic heart disease, and cirrhosis (Table 45-2).[39] This pattern of lifetime morbidity contrasts greatly with the ranking in terms of excess mortality, namely, cardiovascular disease, suicide, accidents, cirrhosis, malignant neoplasms, pneumonia, and cerebrovascular disease.[40]

TABLE 45-2. RANKING OF LIFETIME INCIDENCE, RATIO OF OBSERVED TO EXPECTED MORTALITY, AND PERCENTAGE OF EXCESS MORTALITY FOR SELECTED CAUSES IN MALE SAMPLES OF ALCOHOL-DEPENDENT AND OTHER HAZARDOUS DRINKERS

Lifetime Incidence (%)[a]		Mortality Ratio[b]		Excess Mortality (%)[c]	
Rank	*Disease*	*Rank*	*Cause of Death*	*Rank*	*Cause of Death*
1	Trauma (81.9)[a]	1	Cirrhosis (7.6)[b]	1	Cardiovascular disease (21.4)[c]
2	Acute alcoholic liver disease (49.9)	2	Suicide (4.4)	2	Suicide (14.7)
3	Peptic ulcer (22.8)	3	Upper GI and respiratory cancer (4.1)	3	Accidents (11.1)
4	Obstructive lung disease (19.0)	4	Accidents (3.5)	4	Cirrhosis (11.0)
5	Pneumonia (16.8)	5	Tuberculosis (2.8)	5	Malignant neoplasms (11.8)
6	Hypertension (12.4)	6	Peptic ulcer (2.8)	6	Pneumonia (8.8)
7	Gastritis (11.5)	7	Pneumonia (2.3)	7	Cerebrovascular disease (5)
8	Epileptic disorders (10.9)	8	Cardiovascular disease (1.8)		
9	Acute brain syndromes (7.7)	9	All cancer (1.7)		
10	Peripheral neuritis (7.1)	10	Cerebrovascular disease (1.2)		
11	Ischemic heart disease (8.1)				
12	Cirrhosis (6.4)				

[a] Based on lifetime incidence of certain diseases and complications in male patients admitted to a Canadian hospital for the treatment of alcoholism. From Ashley MJ, Olin JS, le Riche WH, et al: The physical disease characteristics of inpatient alcoholics. J Stud Alcohol 42:1–14, 1981. The percentage, in parentheses, is shown after each disease or complication.

[b] Based on analyses of ratios of observed to expected mortality by cause in male samples of alcohol-dependent and other heavy drinkers. From Popham RE, Schmidt W, Israelstam S: Heavy alcohol consumption and physical health problems. A review of the epidemiologic evidence. In Smart RG, Cappell HD, Glaser FB, et al (eds): Research Advances in Alcohol and Drug Problems. New York: Plenum Press, 1984, vol 8, pp 149–182. The median mortality ratio, in parentheses, is shown after each cause of death.

[c] Based on analyses of percentages of excess mortality in alcohol-dependent and heavy drinking men attributable to selected causes. From Ashley MJ, Rankin JG: Hazardous alcohol consumption and diseases of the circulatory system. J Stud Alcohol 41:1040–1070, 1980. The median percentage value for excess mortality, in parentheses, is shown after each cause of death.

These differences in patterns of morbidity and mortality are related to the lethality of the conditions, the risk of this population dying from these disorders compared with the community-at-large,[41] and the frequency of the conditions in the general adult population. The three most common causes of excess mortality, i.e., cardiovascular disease, suicide, and accidents, occur as acute problems, associated with sudden and usually unexpected death, whereas cirrhosis of the liver is the main chronic physical health problem in terms of incapacity and excess mortality.

Alcohol use in females exposes them to all of the risks reviewed for men. Several consequences of drinking are more common in females, often with less quantity of alcohol use than in males. In females, accidents and suicidal mortality predominate in adolescence and young adulthood as health consequences of drinking. In middle age, breast cancer and osteoporosis become issues of concern. The risk of breast cancer due to alcohol use is not clear, but several studies have raised concerns in this regard.[42–44] Drinking appears to be more detrimental to women than men with respect to liver disease. Higher cirrhosis rates among female alcoholics as compared to male alcoholics, with females having lower consumption rates, has been observed in a variety of studies.[45–47] Alcohol is also the most widely used substance associated with domestic violence. Females are most commonly the battered party, and both their use of alcohol and their partner's use of alcohol appears to increase risk. The risk of human immunodeficiency virus/acquired immunodeficiency syndrome (HIV/AIDS) and alcohol use presents similar concerns in females as well as males. Use of alcohol may influence risk of acquiring HIV infection both through direct effects on the immune system, as well as increased likelihood of unsafe sexual behavior during periods of intoxication.

▶ ESTIMATING THE PUBLIC HEALTH IMPORTANCE OF ALCOHOL-RELATED PROBLEMS

In alcohol-consuming nations, the public health importance of alcohol-related health problems usually is considered by each country to be significant.[48] There are differences, however, from country to country, concerning the impact of alcohol-related health problems on the total burden of ill health and with regard to what are perceived to be the major alcohol-related health problems.

The impact of alcohol-related health problems is felt, both directly and indirectly, by many different groups. This includes those with alcohol-related health problems, their families, other individuals or groups who may suffer injury or loss due to the use of alcohol by others, those who provide services for the prevention and treatment of alcohol-related problems, and the community-at-large. Many of the effects are tangible but immeasurable, such as the pain and suffering experienced by the alcohol-damaged individual and his or her family. However, other manifestations of alcohol-related problems are suitable for empirical study, for example, the incidence and prevalence of alcohol-related heath problems, the costs of health and social services attributable to these problems, the number of people who are disabled or die from alcohol-related problems, and the economic costs of illness, disability, and death.

It may be possible to make reasonably good estimates for specific aspects of mortality and morbidity, e.g., the burden of alcoholic psychoses in specialized institutions. Unfortunately, such directly related consequences are only a small part of the total problem. This is illustrated in a report on alcohol-related deaths in Canada in 1980 (Table 45-3). Of the almost 18,000 such deaths (10.5 percent of all deaths), the vast majority (88 percent) were classified as indirectly related, i.e., they were due to accidents, cancers, and circulatory and respiratory diseases in which alcohol was a contributing factor.[49] This problem is further exemplified by U.S. studies in which only about 3 percent of recorded deaths were officially attributable to alcohol, 1.9 percent were attributable to an alcohol-related condition, and the remaining 1.2 percent had an alcohol-related condition listed along with the specified cause of death.[50] These figures are small when compare with estimates that alcohol dependence is responsible for 1 in 10 deaths in the United States,[51] and when follow-up studies demonstrate high alcohol-related mortality.[52]

Despite such shortcomings in available statistics, there is no doubt about the serious toll of morbidity and mortality that alcohol use exacts from alcohol-consuming societies, such as the United States and Canada. These countries rank as moderate consuming nations, and one can assume that the toll is higher in heavier consuming nations. Selected indicators of the public health impact of alcohol use in Canada (Table 45-3)[49,53] illustrate this clearly.

In the period of these studies, 1979 to 1980, of Canadians 15 years and over, at least 12 percent were regularly consuming enough alcohol to be at increased risk of health consequences, 5 percent of current drinkers were alcohol-dependent, and almost 10 percent experienced at least one alcohol-related problem. More than 1 in 10 deaths were alcohol-related. In an earlier study of premature deaths

TABLE 45-3. SELECTED INDICATORS OF THE PUBLIC HEALTH IMPACT OF ALCOHOL USE IN CANADA

Indicator	Year	Selected Findings		
Population 15 years and over drinking 14+ drinks per week[53]	1978–1979	Overall 12%	Males 19.4%	
			Females 4.8%	
		Age group 20–24	Males 31.0%	
			Females 8.1%	
Alcohol-dependent persons[49]	1980	600,000 persons; 1 in 19 (5.3% of) current drinkers		
Current drinkers 15 years and older with alcohol-associated problem[49]	1978–1979	Tension or disagreement with family or friends		6.1%
		Problems with health		2.3%
		Difficulty with driving		1.5%
		Injury to self or other		1.3%
		Trouble with the law		1.3%
		Trouble with school or work		1.2%
Current drinkers 15 years and over with at least one alcohol-associated problem[49]	1978–1979	Overall 9.7%	Males 12.4%	
			Females 6.1%	
Alcohol-related deaths[49]	1980	17,974 (10.5%) of all deaths		
		Directly related deaths: 2,110[a]		
		Indirectly related deaths: 15,864[b]		

[a] Deaths due to alcohol-related cirrhosis, alcohol dependency syndrome, the nondependent abuse of alcohol, alcoholic psychoses, and accidental poisoning by alcohol.
[b] Deaths due to motor vehicle accidents, falls, fires, drownings, homicides, suicides (5,554 in 1980), as well as circulatory and respiratory diseases and certain types of cancer (e.g., oral, esophageal, and laryngeal) totaling 10,310 in 1980.

and potential years of life lost in Canada in 1974, it was concluded that no other risk factor was responsible for more premature mortality than either smoking or hazardous drinking.[54] The adverse health consequences of drinking remain a major health problem, despite evidence since this period of study and in association with a plateauing and modest fall in alcohol consumption that there has been a significant decline in various indicators of alcohol-related health problems in Canada.[55,56] Furthermore, tobacco and alcohol continue to rate first and second as risk factors responsible for premature mortality.

A different approach to quantifying the effects of alcohol-related health problems is to express them in monetary terms. Such an approach is useful because it provides an estimate of the relative distribution of the costs, for example, across organ systems or various health and social services, as well as a measure of total costs. Thus, these figures can be used to compare the costs of alcohol-related problems with other health problems as a basis for focusing the attention of the community or making policy decisions regarding the funding of prevention, treatment, and research.

An example of an economic approach to measuring the magnitude of alcohol-related problems is contained in Table 45-4, which provides an estimate of the costs of alcohol-related problems in the United States in 1983.[57,58] First, notice that the total cost is large, $116.875 billion. Of this amount, 89.0 percent was attributable to core costs, including losses in productivity associated with disability and death (76.2 percent) and costs incurred in the treatment and care of people with alcohol-related health problems (12.8 percent). Total alcohol-related health costs ranked a close second to heart and vascular disease, as the prime health cause of economic loss and were well ahead of cancer and respiratory disease. In this analysis, other related costs covered nonhealth alcohol-related costs attributable to motor vehicle crashes and fires, highway safety and the fire protection, and the criminal justice and social welfare systems. The costs of alcohol-related problems were equal to 3.54 percent of the gross national product, and the direct costs for health services were equal to 4.22 percent of the total costs of health services. Although these figures are large, very likely they are underestimates of the true economic costs of alcohol-related problems.

▶ PREVENTION STRATEGIES

The public health approach to disease prevention was first classified in 1957 as proposed by the Commission on Chronic Illness.[59] Primary, secondary, and tertiary prevention techniques were defined. In this model, primary prevention is geared toward efforts to decrease new cases of a disorder (incident cases), secondary prevention is designed to lower the rate of established cases (prevalent cases), and tertiary prevention seeks to decrease the amount of disability associated with existing disorder or illness. Gordon[60,61] later proposed an alternative classification system that incorporated the concept of the risks and benefits in the evaluation of prevention efforts. His categories of prevention strategies consisted of universal measures, selective measures, and indicated measures. Universal prevention measures are measures of low cost and low risk for which benefits outweigh costs when they are applied to everyone in an eligible population. Selective measures are desirable only for a select population at above-average risk of development of a disorder. Indicated preventive measures are applied to individuals who, upon screening examination, demonstrate high risk of development of a disorder.

The Institute of Medicine (IOM) noted that both of these classification systems were designed and worked best for traditional medical disorders,[62] but that their application to mental disorders was not straightforward. An alternative system, proposed by the IOM, is referred to as the Mental Health Intervention Spectrum for Mental Illness. This system incorporates the whole spectrum of interventions for mental disorders, from prevention, through treatment, to maintenance. Table 45-5 outlines this spectrum. The term prevention is reserved for those interventions that occur before the initial onset of the disorder, and it incorporates many of Gordon's concepts such as universal, selective, and indicated measures.

TABLE 45-4. ESTIMATED COSTS OF ALCOHOL-RELATED PROBLEMS IN THE UNITED STATES IN 1983

		$Billion	%
■ ***CORE COSTS***			
Direct	Treatment	13.457	
	Health support services	1.549	
	Subtotal	15.006	12.8
Indirect	Mortality	18.151	
	Reduced productivity	65.582	
	Lost employment	5.323	
	Subtotal	89.056	76.2
Total core costs		104.062	89.0
■ ***OTHER RELATED COSTS***			
Direct	Motor vehicle crashes	2.697	
	Crime	2.631	
	Social welfare administration	0.049	
	Other	3.673	
	Subtotal	9.050	7.8
Indirect	Victims of crime	0.194	
	Incarceration	2.979	
	Motor vehicle crashes	0.590	
	Subtotal	3.763	3.2
Total other related costs		12.813	11.0
■ ***TOTAL COSTS***		116.875	100.0

Adapted from US Department of Health and Human Services: Sixth Special Report to the US Congress on Alcohol and Health from the Secretary of Health and Human Services. DHHS Publication No. (ADM) 871519. Rockville, MD: US Government Printing Office, 1987 and US Bureau of the Census: Statistical Abstract of the United States, 106th ed. Washington, DC: US Bureau of the Census, 1985.
Gross national product (GNP) in 1983: $3305.0 billion; costs of alcohol-related problems: 3.54% of GNP.
Total costs of health services in 1983: $355.4 billion; cost of direct services for alcohol-related problems: 4.22% of total costs of health services.

TABLE 45-5. MENTAL HEALTH INTERVENTION FOR MENTAL DISORDERS[62]

1. Prevention
   - Universal
   - Selective
   - Indicated
2. Treatment
   - Case identification
   - Standard treatment for known disorders
3. Maintenance
   - Compliance with long-term treatment
   - After-care

Universal Prevention Efforts

A significant amount of evidence suggests that early use of alcohol along with underachievement, school problems, and aggressive behavior predict future problem drinking. While some of this risk may be due to genetic vulnerability to alcohol use disorders (covered under Selective Intervention Efforts below), clearly genetic-environmental interactions are likely. Broader community context factors external to the individual are also strong predictors of alcohol use and problems. Community use patterns, availability of alcohol (including legal drinking age, cost, and enforcement), and peer group behavior affect the use and abuse of alcohol.

Universal prevention efforts have been tried in various forms. Community-based programs for the prevention of alcohol abuse and alcohol-related problems were recently reviewed by Aguirre-Molina and Gorman.[63] This review summarized studies concerned with changing the behavior of individuals rather than environmental changes such as altering availability. Data analysis for many such studies is ongoing and hence their final overall impact is unknown.

Community-based studies designed to change behavior of individuals are difficult to design, implement, and complete. A more direct universal prevention strategy involves limiting availability, increasing enforcement of laws pertaining to alcohol use, legislating stricter laws and community standards, and increasing the cost of alcoholic beverages through taxation.

A substantial body of evidence now supports the view that increases in overall or per capita consumption are associated with higher rates of heavy drinking and, consequently, with increased frequencies of alcohol-related health problems.[64–68] Studies of relationships between per capita alcohol consumption and alcohol-related morbidity and mortality have focused on cirrhosis, where a strong positive correlation has been established.[69] Per capita consumption also has been correlated positively with total mortality in men,[70] international variations in deaths from diabetes mellitus,[71] deaths from alcohol-related disease,[72] alcoholism death rates,[73] and hospital admission for alcohol dependence, alcoholic psychosis, liver cirrhosis, pancreatitis,[74] Wernicke's encephalopathy, and Korsakoff's psychosis.[75]

Recognition of the relationships among per capita alcohol consumption, rates of heavy use, and the incidence of alcohol-related health problems has focused attention on universal prevention strategies aimed at the drinking population, generally with the principal objective of reducing per capita alcohol consumption. Critical reviews suggest that measures addressing the economic and physical accessibility of alcohol are among the most effective in this regard.[76]

Economic Accessibility

Price Controls. Numerous studies, reviews, and reports have examined the use of price control via taxation in reducing alcohol consumption and alcohol-related problems. The accumulated evidence indicates that price control could be effective and, in some instances, powerful, both in relation to other measures and in combination with them.[9,57,77–80] According to Cook[81,82] and Cook and Tauchen,[83] doubling the federal tax on liquor in the United States would reduce the cirrhosis mortality rate by at least 20 percent. An effect on automobile fatalities also was postulated.[81] Holder and Blose[84] used a system dynamics model to study the effect of four prevention strategies: raising the retail price of all alcoholic beverages by 25 percent once, indexing the price of alcoholic beverages to the consumer price index (CPI) each year, raising the minimum drinking age to 21 years, and reducing high-risk alcohol consumption through state-of-the-art public education on alcohol-related family disruptions and alcohol-related work problems, against a background of business as usual in three counties of the United States. Although both outcome measures were modestly sensitive to one-time changes in price, the largest effect was obtained by instituting a community education effort concurrently with indexing the prices of alcoholic beverages to the CPI. From an analysis of the price of beer and spirits, other economic and sociodemographic factors, and various regulatory control variables, Ornstein[85] concluded that price was the most important policy tool available to regulators in the United States. A similar conclusion arose from a study of the effects of various regulatory measures on the consumption of distilled spirits in the United States over a 25-year period.[86] Levy and Sheflin,[87] using methods intended to overcome the problem of beverage substitution when price control is not directed at all beverages, estimated that the price elasticity for total alcohol consumption, although less than 1 (implying that demand is inelastic), was large enough for price policies to be effective in reducing alcohol consumption. Others,[88–93] however, have been more guarded in their support for price manipulation as a control measure, pointing out the methodological limitations in econometric analyses, the modest or conflicting implications of some findings, and the possible role of countervailing forces.

In a study of individual drinkers, Kendell and colleagues[94,95] found that overall consumption and associated adverse effects fell 18 and 16 percent, respectively, among 463 "regular drinkers" in the Lothian region of Scotland when prices were increased via the excise duty. Heavy and dependent drinkers reduced their consumption at least as much as light and moderate drinkers, with fewer adverse effects as a result. Clinical data also show that alcohol-dependent persons reduce their alcohol consumption as a function of beverage costs.[96,97] Further, in an experimental study of price reductions during afternoon happy hours, Babor and associates[98] found that such reductions significantly increased alcohol consumption by both casual and heavy drinkers. With the reinstatement of standard prices, drinking in both groups returned to previous levels. These findings and others[78,82,83,99] seriously challenge the previously held view that a reduction in overall consumption does not affect consumption by the heaviest drinkers. Further, liver cirrhosis mortality rates, which are considered the most accurate indicator of the prevalence of heavy drinking, respond directly and rather quickly to major restrictions on availability, including economic ones, that produce declines in per capita consumption.[9,64,82] Indeed, the recent leveling off and decrease in cirrhosis mortality rates in Canada[49] and the United States[100] may be, in part, the result of current economic conditions affecting the price of alcohol relative to personal disposable income[77] and, consequently, the consumption of all drinkers, including heavy drinkers.

Price elasticities of alcoholic beverages vary among themselves, across time, and among countries.[9] In the United States, as in Canada and the United Kingdom, beer tends to be relatively price inelastic.[64,101,102] However, this general inelasticity does not hold in certain age groups. Grossman and colleagues[102–106] estimated the effects on young people of increases in alcoholic beverage prices with regard to alcohol use and motor vehicle mortality. They showed that for beer, the alcoholic beverage of preference in the young, the price elasticity was considerably higher than that usually reported: a 10-cent increase in the price of a package of six 12-ounce cans resulted in an 11 percent decrease in the number of youths drinking beer and a 15 percent decrease in the number of youthful heavy beer drinkers (three to five drinks per day).[103] Further, they predicted that a national policy simultaneously taxing the alcohol in beer and distilled spirits at the same rates and offsetting the erosion in the real beer tax since 1951 would reduce the number of youths 16 to 21 years old who drink beer frequently (four to seven times a week, about 11 percent of youths) and fairly frequently (one to three times a week, about 28 percent of all youths) by 32 and 24 percent, respectively.[112,113] Additional analyses showed dramatic effects of excise tax policies on motor vehicle accidents in youths.[104–106] In a multivariate analysis, it was estimated that a policy that fixed the federal beer tax in real terms since 1951 would have reduced the number of motor vehicle fatalities in youths ages 18 to 20 in the period 1975 to 1981 by 15 percent, and a policy that taxed the alcohol in beer at the same rate as the alcohol in liquor would have lowered fatalities by 21 percent. A combination of the two policies would have caused a 54 percent decline in the number of youths killed. In contrast, the enactment of a uniform drinking age of 21 years in all states would have reduced such fatalities by 8 percent, with considerable additional costs in enforcement. Since the principal objective of price control in the public health context is universal prevention, a differentially higher price sensitivity among young drinkers for beer is an especially important finding.

Price control via taxation has been recommended repeatedly as a strategy for stabilizing or reducing per capita consumption and, thereby, preventing alcohol-related health problems.[80,107–109] In the United States, recent public opinion polls indicate clear majority support for excise tax increases on alcohol for public health purposes.[80] However, federal excise taxes on distilled spirits, wine, and beer remained constant in nominal terms (current dollar value) between November 1, 1951, and the end of fiscal year 1985.[104] In 1985, the federal excise tax on distilled spirits was raised slightly (as a deficit reduction measure), but federal tax rates on beer and wine were not changed. Thus, the real price of alcoholic beverages has actually declined in recent years, such that between 1960 and 1980 the real price of liquor declined 48 percent, beer 27 percent, and wine 20 percent.[81] A similar situation has been documented in Ontario, Canada, where a taxation policy that would maintain a reasonably constant relationship between the price of alcohol and the consumer price index has been a key element in a long-proposed, but unimplemented, prevention strategy.[107]

Physical Availability

The relationship between the physical availability of alcohol and alcohol consumption and related problems is multifaceted and complex. It is difficult to show the effect of small changes and to untangle the effects of changes in physical availability that take place simultaneously with others, either nonspecific changes (e.g., in the general economy) or specific changes (e.g., in the economic and legal accessibility of alcohol). It is not surprising, therefore, that the evidence concerning the effectiveness of limitations on physical accessibility is mixed.[9,48,64,110–115] Taken together, there is considerable evidence that controls on physical availability can reduce alcohol-related problems and that the consumption of both heavy and moderate drinkers can be reduced.

Prohibition is successful in reducing consumption and attendant health risks.[9,48,64,113] Such a situation prevails in some countries today.[113] With the institution of Prohibition in the United States earlier in this century, cirrhosis mortality rates fell dramatically and remained well below their former levels during the earlier years and to a considerable extent even in the later years, indicative of greatly decreased consumption.[64] On repeal of Prohibition and the subsequent increase in the availability of alcohol, consumption rose, and cirrhosis mortality rates gradually increased toward previous levels. Similar trends have been observed in the face of other severe limitations on availability, for example, in Paris during the two World Wars[9,67] and during some strikes and periods of rationing.[48,110,112,113] Under such conditions, the consumption of both heavy and moderate drinkers is reduced.[110–113]

Similarly, sudden, marked relaxation in the availability of alcohol is associated with increases in overall consumption, heavy drinking, and alcohol-related problems. The Finnish experience, which included a very marked increase in overall consumption in connection with liberalizing legislation that led to an extensive and rapid increase in outlets in previously dry areas, has been detailed[116] and summarized[113] elsewhere.

A number of additional factors play a role in physical accessibility to alcohol. These factors include the times of sale permitted, the types, characteristics, and location of outlets, and the distribution system of alcoholic beverages. Different positive and negative consequences may be seen across even subtle changes. For example, while restricting the number of outlets may lead to decreased consumption, a rise in automobile crashes associated with alcohol use can be seen due to driving after acquiring the beverage of choice, as location of purchase is related to where it is consumed.[117] The rapidity with which community changes are made are also of importance upon the outcome of the change.[48,110,113] As previously discussed, if multiple outlets for alcohol sale are added in formerly dry areas, there is a subsequent marked increase in overall consumption.[110,116] These examples all point to the need for careful consideration and monitoring of changes made in the physical availability of alcohol in society.

Legal Accessibility

Age limitations represent a legal barrier to alcohol. Most countries have age restrictions on its purchase or consumption or both.[48] Although the data are neither unflawed nor entirely consistent, there is much evidence that the lower the drinking age, the higher the consumption of alcohol[48,104,118–121] and the incidence of alcohol-related problems, particularly among teenagers.[48,111,113,118,119,122,123] Lowered blood alcohol content (BAC) limits for legal driving are currently being proposed in many states in the United States. The effect of such measures on automobile crashes and automobile fatalities will be an important outcome measure. The tradeoff of increased costs, potential social stigma, and consequent increased rates of alcohol use disorder diagnoses for individuals caught with the lowered alcohol blood levels has not been factored into decisions to lower the legal driving limits, but obviously some price will be paid.

Selective Intervention Efforts

Selective intervention efforts are those efforts geared toward individuals at greater than average risk of development of alcohol use disorders. The strongest predictor of who will develop alcohol dependency comes from the genetic literature. Family studies of alcoholics have clearly demonstrated that alcohol dependency is familial.[124] First-degree offspring of an alcohol-dependent parent are 3- to 4-fold more likely to develop alcohol dependence that those without such a parent. Family studies are not useful in separating environmental factors from genetic factors important to the development of alcohol dependency. Studies of twins[125,126] and adoptees[127,128] have produced evidence for such genetic factors, although at this time no alcohol dependency gene has been found. While a gene for alcohol dependency awaits discovery, the results of the adoptee studies have demonstrated that heterogeneity in alcohol dependency exists, i.e., there exists at least two types of alcohol dependence. The two types of alcoholism have been referred to as milieu-limited alcoholism, which requires the presence of environmental factors for alcoholism to develop (type I alcoholism), and male-limited alcoholism (type II alcoholism), which does not.[129] These forms of alcohol dependency differ in terms of age of onset and associated symptoms. Type II alcoholism has an early age of onset and often serious legal manifestations such as driving while intoxicated and fighting. Furthermore, there is evidence of various biological markers that potentially may prove valuable for targeting high-risk populations for intervention trials that have been discovered through various family and genetic studies of alcoholism.[130]

If a strong family history of alcohol dependence is discovered, it is important to educate unaffected individuals in the pedigree of their enhanced risk. This educational component should be added to the other interventions described below.

Indicated Intervention Efforts

Indicated intervention efforts are targeted toward high-risk individuals who are identified through screening to have hazardous drinking or early symptoms of alcohol dependence that have gone undetected. Screening methods are also important to uncover undiagnosed individuals with alcohol dependence, but who are able to mask such symptoms from others.

Screening for Alcohol Dependence

Assessing patients for alcohol use disorders in a busy primary care setting is difficult. The importance of screening for alcoholism in primary care settings is essential to public health efforts to reduce the burden of alcohol-related problems. To ascertain a full history of alcohol use and to assess whether an individual meets DSM-IV criteria for alcohol abuse or dependency are generally considered too time consuming by many clinicians, and some doubt exists among clinicians of the validity of self-report regarding use of alcohol. Because of these constraints, a variety of screening tools have been proposed. The most commonly used tools are screening questionnaires and laboratory values. The most common screening questionnaires include the Michigan Alcoholism Screening Test (MAST),[131] the abbreviated Brief-MAST,[132] and the CAGE instrument.[133] Several newer instruments include the Alcohol Use Disorders Identification Test (AUDIT)[134] and the TWEAK instrument.[135] Laboratory screening tests include blood alcohol levels, liver enzymes elevations, erythrocyte mean corpuscular volume, lipid profiles, and carbohydrate-deficient transferrin.

Screening Questionnaires. A number of review articles are available that describe the use of alcohol use screening questionnaires. The U.S. Preventive Services Task Force recently published a Guide to Clinical Preventive Services, 2nd edition,[136] which provides a detailed review of the sensitivity and specificity for the MAST (84 to 100 percent and 87 to 95 percent, respectively), Brief-MAST (66 to 78 percent and 80 percent, respectively), CAGE (74 to 89 percent and 79 to 95 percent, respectively for alcohol abuse and dependence; but only 49 to 73 percent sensitivity for heavy alcohol use), and the AUDIT (96 and 96 percent, respectively, in an inner city clinic; but only 61 and 90 percent in a rural setting). These sensitivity and specificity figures are for middle-age adults. Adolescents and the elderly may not be as adequately screened by these instruments. Other limitations of these screening instruments include the MAST being rather lengthy for routine use (25 questions) and the CAGE being most sensitive for alcohol abuse or dependency and not heavy drinking. Both the CAGE and MAST fail to distinguish current from lifetime problems due to alcohol. The AUDIT is very sensitive and specific for "harmful and hazardous drinking," but uses a 1-year time frame for screening and hence is less sensitive for past drinking problems.

Allen et al[137] offer guidelines for selection of screening tests in primary care. Based upon their review of the literature, use of the AUDIT, CAGE, or MAST were recommended. Because of time constraints in primary care, the AUDIT or CAGE were first-choice recommendations, and the TWEAK was recommended for pregnant women. For adolescents, the Adolescent Drinking Index (ADI)[138] was suggested as a good choice.

In the elderly, two studies[139,140] point to deficiencies in the CAGE as a screening tool and suggest the need for development of more sensitive and specific tools in this population. Adams et al[140] suggests asking about quantity and frequency of alcohol use in addition to the CAGE to increase the detection of elderly hazardous drinking.

Laboratory Screening Tools. Alcohol induces a number of laboratory abnormalities. Unfortunately, to date laboratory tests for screening have not been as sensitive nor as specific for alcohol use disorders when compared to the screening questionnaires reviewed above.

Liver enzymes, including γ-glutamyltransferase (GGT), aspartate aminotransferase (AST), alanine aminotransferase (ALT), and alkaline phosphatase have all been used as screening tests. The GGT is the most useful of the liver tests. It demonstrates a sensitivity of 50 to 90 percent for ingestion of 40 to 60 g of alcohol daily (three to four standard drinks).[141] The GGT rises most rapidly in response to heavy alcohol use, and with abstinence it returns to normal most rapidly. Other liver enzyme tests such as the AST, ALT, and alkaline phosphatase are less specific and sensitive than the GGT. Some have suggested use of the AST:ALT ratio of 1.5–2:1 as being an indicator of liver damage being more likely due to alcohol than other causes. While the AST and ALT are not adequately sensitive or specific to be recommended as screening laboratory tests, they have some utility as supportive tests. The GGT may be most useful as a marker for return to heavy drinking after a period of abstinence in which the GGT has returned to normal. If the GGT rises by 20 percent, a high likelihood for return to drinking can be assumed.

Increase in mean corpuscular volume (MCV) is less sensitive to alcohol use than elevation in the GGT, but it is quite specific to heavy alcohol intake (up to 90 percent).[142] Utility of the MCV is much like that of the AST and ALT, i.e., helpful as supporting evidence, but not as a screening tool.

The BAC is useful and can even support a diagnosis of alcohol dependence as outlined by the National Council on Alcoholism (NCA).[143] A BAC of 100 mg/100 mL is considered a legally intoxicated level in most states and is conclusive evidence for a driving-while-intoxicated charge. Individuals nontolerant to alcohol will generally appear intoxicated at such levels. A BAC of 150 mg/100 mL without gross evidence of intoxication suggests significant tolerance to alcohol and fulfills criteria for alcohol dependence according to the NCA. A BAC of 100 mg/100 mL during a routine physical examination is highly suggestive of alcohol use problems according to the NCA. Thus, screening of BAC in patients who may appear intoxicated or smell of alcohol during a clinic visit can be very useful. A breath analysis of BAC is also a useful tool and can be used to screen for individuals too impaired to drive home from emergency rooms or clinic visits if intoxication is suspected and serum BAC cannot be readily performed or if patients refuse blood drawing.

Carbohydrate-deficient transferrin (CDT), a protein associated with iron transport, appears to effectively distinguish alcoholics consuming large amounts of alcohol from light social drinkers or abstinent individuals. Allen et al[144] reviewed the available data from over 40 studies that used this laboratory marker. While excellent sensitivity and specificity could be demonstrated in the overwhelming majority of the studies, technical problems and expense may keep this tool from widespread use. This laboratory marker at present is still under investigation and cannot be recommended for screening purposes.

Presently, none of the laboratory markers reviewed offer advantages in sensitivity or specificity over the screening questionnaires reviewed. However, in a general medical setting, liver enzymes and MCV are often ordered as part of the medical workup for individuals presenting for care. The laboratory studies in combination with screening questionnaires can be useful in discussions with patients regarding the health consequences of their alcohol use.

▸ TREATMENT INTERVENTIONS

While prevention strategies are the focus of the chapter, unless primary care clinicians become aware of their potential impact on reducing hazardous and problem drinking, it is doubtful that prevention strategies will be emphasized. Similarly, physicians are unlikely to inquire about alcohol use if they feel they lack the skills to intervene or if they feel interventions are unsuccessful. In a survey of Australian medical trainees in internal medicine, psychiatry, and general practice, there was a high level of agreement that alcohol use history should be obtained from all patients and that problem drinking should be managed, but views on treatment were less positive.[145] There was considerable uncertainty regarding treatment modalities most readily available to the primary care physician, i.e., brief advice and cognitive-behavioral therapies. In this study, the trainees were most certain that Alcoholics Anonymous (AA) techniques for treatment were well supported in the literature.

While AA has been a well-supported and beneficial treatment for alcohol-dependent individuals since its beginnings in 1935, its fellowship is most appropriate for individuals who are alcohol dependent and less likely to be an acceptable treatment modality for patients who are nondependent, but who are displaying hazardous drinking styles. This distinction is imperative, as the hazardous drinking population far exceeds the dependent population of drinkers and, as previously noted, contributes greatly to the societal burdens of alcohol use problems. The hazardous, but nondependent, population of drinkers is also more likely to respond to brief interventions for alcohol problems. Another reason the primary care physician should be familiar with brief intervention techniques involves the lack of many alcohol-dependent individuals to follow through on recommendations to seek more formal treatment on referral. In a study of 1,200 emergency room patients diagnosed as alcohol dependent and advised to seek treatment, only 5 percent did so.[146] A similar finding was noted in a study of U.S. veterans screened for at-risk drinking. Of those who were identified as having at-risk drinking, only 5 percent followed advice to return for a single consultation session regarding their drinking.[147] These studies point to the need for the primary care physician to be skilled in office-based techniques to help patients modify and reduce or stop their alcohol use.

Effective Intervention

Recent evidence strongly suggests that brief interventions in the early stages of heavy drinking are both feasible and effective.[147,148] Edwards and colleagues,[149] in a controlled clinical trial of intensive inpatient-outpatient treatment versus brief advice for alcoholism, found the latter to be more effective in nondependent alcohol abusers after 2 years of follow-up,[150] whereas physically dependent patients achieved better results with more intensive treatment. In a randomized controlled trial of general practitioner intervention in patients with excessive alcohol consumption, Wallace and associates[151] showed that advice on reducing alcohol consumption was effective. If the results of their study were applied to the United Kingdom, intervention by general practitioners in the first year could reduce to moderate levels the alcohol consumption of some 250,000 men and 67,500 women who currently drink to excess. Other studies have shown the effectiveness of brief intervention in socially stable, healthy, problem drinkers who do not have a high degree of alcohol dependence and whose histories of problem drinking are short.[152–156] A careful assessment of alcohol dependence in detected heavy drinkers underpins the determination of the appropriateness of brief intervention.[157]

The degree of alcohol dependence also is crucial in determining whether the treatment goal should be moderation (i.e., controlled drinking) or abstinence.[148,157,158] Moderation appears to be a realistic alternative in problem drinkers who are not heavily alcohol dependent, as is often the case in the early-stage heavy drinkers.[148,153,157,159–161] It may be a more acceptable treatment goal, particularly in environments where alcohol use is especially diffuse[191] and among young drinkers, who may perceive the costs of abstinence to outweigh the risks from continued drinking.[157,162]

A five-step early intervention and treatment strategy for use in clinical practice settings has been developed,[157] along with self-help manuals[148] and procedures for teaching moderate drinking and abstinence.[163] Evaluations of brief interventions conducted as part of a general health screening project,[164] among problem drinkers in a general hospital,[165,166] in community referral centers for referred problem drinkers,[159,167] and in a family practice setting[168] are promising. This approach may be applicable beyond the clinical setting, for example, in the workplace, with considerable potential for public health impact.[152,159] A review of 32 controlled studies of brief interventions demonstrate effectiveness of such techniques across 14 nations.[147]

Skinner[169] has discussed the reasons why early detection and effective intervention strategies deserve major emphasis. To summarize: most heavy drinkers do not seek treatment for their alcohol problems, socially stable persons at early stages of problem drinking have a better prognosis, health professionals in primary care settings are in an excellent position to identify problem drinkers, and brief intervention by health professionals can be effective in reducing heavy alcohol use. Skinner cited reasons why early detection and effective intervention are not occurring, namely, widespread pessimism among health professionals about being able to intervene effectively, confusion regarding responsibility for confronting alcohol problems, uncertainly about the target population, lack of appreciation of what are appropriate interventions, and deficiencies in the practical skills and techniques to carry them out. He suggested that simple strategies be adopted that included recommendations that training materials and opportunities be readily available and incorporated into core education programs and that strenuous efforts be made to convince key people in the health professions to give early detection and effective intervention a high priority.

▶ SUMMARY

Alcohol use problems are not restricted to those with alcohol abuse or dependency. Recognition of hazardous drinking as being linked to many health-related and societal burdens of alcohol is a first step toward a rational public health policy. Primary care providers are asked to screen for and be able to treat many different disorders. Alcohol use problems have for too long been viewed as either untreatable or needing specialty management. Evidence exists that office screening tools, combined with relatively brief interventions, can be powerful methods to help assist a large population at risk. While the alcohol screening must compete with many disorders for primary care providers' attention, it is hoped that the data presented in this chapter will raise the priority of alcohol use disorder in the minds of those caregivers.

▶ REFERENCES

1. Kreitman N: Alcohol consumption and the prevention paradox. Br J Addict 81:353–363, 1986
2. Davidson DM: Cardiovascular effects of alcohol. West J Med 151:430–439, 1989
3. National Institute on Alcohol Abuse and Alcoholism: Moderate drinking. Alcohol Alert No. 16. Bethesda, MD: US Department of Health and Human Services, 1992
4. US Department of Health and Human Services: The surgeon general's report on nutrition and health. Publication no. PHS-88-50210. Washington, DC: Government Printing Office, 1988
5. US Department of Agriculture and US Department of Health and Human Services: Dietary guidelines for Americans. Washington, DC: US Department of Agriculture, 1992
6. Dietary Guidelines Advisory Committee: Report of the dietary guidelines advisory committee on the Americans, 1995, to the Secretary of Health and Human Services and the Secretary of Agriculture. Washington DC: US Department of Agriculture, 1995
7. Secretary of State for Health: The Health of the Nation: A Strategy for Health in England. London: Her Majesty's Stationery Office, 1992
8. Pols RG, Hawks DV: Is there a safe level of daily consumption of alcohol for men and women? Recommendations responsible drinking behavior. Technical Report for the National Health and Medical Research Council, Health Care Committee. Canberra: Australian Government Publishing Service, 1987
9. Bruun K, Edwards G, Lumio M, et al: Alcohol Control Policies: Public Health Perspective. The Finnish Foundation for Alcohol Studies. vol 25. Helsinki: Finnish Foundation for Alcohol Studies, 1975
10. Kreitman N: Alcohol consumption and the prevention paradox. Br J Addict 81:353–363, 1986
11. Péquignot G, Tuyns A: Rations d'alcool consommées "declarées" et risques pathologiques. In INSEAM. Paris: INSEAM, 1975, pp. 1–15

12. Streissguth AP, Clarren SK, Jones KL: Natural history of the fetal alcohol syndrome. Lancet 2:85–92, 1985
13. Little RE, Streissguth AP: Effects of alcohol on the fetus: impact and prevention. Can Med Assoc J 125:159–164, 1981
14. Lieber CS: Medical disorders of alcoholism. N Engl J Med 333(16): 1058–1065, 1995
15. Popham RE, Schmidt W: The biomedical definition of safe alcohol consumption: a crucial issue for the researcher and the drinker. Br J Addict 73:233–235, 1978
16. World Health Organization (WHO): The ICD-10 Classification of Mental and Behavioural Disorders. Geneva: World Health Organization, 1992
17. American Psychiatric Association: DSM-IV: Diagnostic and Statistical Manual of Mental Disorders. Washington, DC: American Psychiatric Association, 1994
18. Caetano R, Tam TW: Prevalence and correlates of DSM-IV and ICD-10 alcohol dependence: 1990 US national alcohol survey. Alcohol Alcohol 30:177–186, 1995
19. Grant BF: Alcohol consumption, alcohol abuse and alcohol dependence. The United States as an example. Addiction 89:1357–1365, 1994
20. Grant BF, Harford TC, Dawson DA, et al: Prevalence of DSM-IV alcohol abuse and dependency: United States 1992. Alcohol Health Res World 18(3):243–248, 1994
21. Helzer J: Psychiatric diagnoses and substance abuse in the general population: the ECA data. NIDA Res Monog 81:405–415, 1988
22. Kessler RC, McGonagle KA, Shanyang Z, et al: Lifetime and 12-month prevalence of DSM-III-R psychiatric disorders in the United States: results from the national comorbidity survey. Arch Gen Psychiatry 51:8–19, 1994
23. Allen JP, Maisto SA, Connors GJ: Self-report screening tests for alcohol problems in primary care. Arch Intern Med 155(16):1726–1730, 1995
24. Centers for Disease Control and Prevention: Alcohol-related mortality and years of potential life lost—United States, 1987. MMWR 39(11):173–178, 1990
25. Poldrugo F, Chick JD, Moore N, et al: Mortality studies in the long-term evaluation of treatment of alcoholics. Alcohol Alcohol Suppl 2:151–155, 1993
26. Angell M, Kassirer JP: Alcohol and other drugs-toward a more rational and consistent policy. N Engl J Med 331:537–539, 1994
27. Burke TR: The economic impact of alcohol abuse and alcoholism. Public Health Rep 103:564–568, 1988
28. Tsai G, Gastfriend DR, Coyle JT: The glutamatergic basis of human alcoholism. Am J Psychiatry 152(3):332–340, 1995
29. Gross MM: Psychobiological contributions to the alcohol dependence syndrome: a selective review of recent research. In Edwards G, Gross MM, Keller M, et al (eds): Alcohol Related Disabilities. Geneva: World Health Organization, 1977, pp 107–131
30. Borkenstein RF, Crowther RF, Shumate RP, et al: The Role of the Drinking Driver in Traffic Accidents. Bloomington, IN: Department of Police Administration, Indiana University, 1964
31. Lieber CS: Medical disorders of alcoholism. Pathogenesis and treatment. In Smith LH Jr (ed): Major Problems in Internal Medicine. vol 22. Philadelphia: WB Saunders, 1982
32. Kronfol Z, Nair M, Hill E, et al: Immune function in alcoholism: a controlled study. Alcohol Clin Exp Res 17:279–283, 1993
33. Remmers JE: Obstructive sleep apnea. A common disorder exacerbated by alcohol. Am Rev Respir Dis 130:153–155, 1984
34. Rankin JG: Alcohol—A specific toxin or nutrient displacer. In Hawkens WW (ed): Drug-Nutrient Interrelationships: Nutrition & Pharmacology—An Interphase of Disciplines, Miles Symposium III. Hamilton, Ontario: McMaster University, 1974, pp 71–87
35. Issa FQ, Sullivan CE: Alcohol, snoring and sleep apnea. J Neurol Neurosurg Psychiatry 45:353–359, 1983
36. Bonora M, Shields GI, Knuth SL, et al: Selective depression by ethanol of upper airway respiratory activity in cats. Am Rev Respir Dis 130:156–161, 1984
37. Krol RC, Knuth SL, Bartlett D Jr: Selective reduction of genioglossal muscle activity by alcohol in normal human subjects. Am Rev Respir Dis 129:247–250, 1984
38. Institute of Medicine: Causes and Consequences of Alcohol Problems: An Agenda for Research. Washington, DC: National Academy Press, 1987
39. Ashley MJ, Olin JS, le Riche WH, et al: The physical disease characteristics of inpatient alcoholics. J Stud Alcohol 42:1–14, 1981
40. Ashley MJ, Rankin JG: Hazardous alcohol consumption and diseases of the circulatory system. J Stud Alcohol 41:1040–1070, 1980
41. Popham RE, Schmidt W, Israelstam S: Heavy alcohol consumption and physical health problems. A review of the epidemiologic evidence. In Smart RG, Cappell HD, Glaser FB, et al (eds): Research Advances in Alcohol and Drug Problems. vol 8. New York: Plenum Press, 1984, pp 149–182
42. Harvey EB, Schairer C, Brinton LA, et al: Alcohol consumption and breast cancer. J Natl Cancer Inst 78:657–661, 1987
43. LaVecchia C, Decarli A, Franceschi S, et al: Alcohol consumption and the risk of breast cancer in women. J Natl Cancer Inst 75:61–65, 1985
44. Rosenberg L, Shapiro S, Slone D, et al: Breast cancer and alcoholic-beverage consumption. Lancet 1:267–270, 1982
45. Pequignot G, Chabert C, Eydoux H, et al: Increased risk of liver cirrhosis with intake of alcohol. Rev Alcohol 20:191–202, 1974
46. Wilkinson P, Santamaria JN, Rankin JG: Epidemiology of alcoholic cirrhosis. Australas Ann Med 18:222–226, 1969
47. Loft S, Olesen KL, Dossing M: Increased susceptibility to liver disease in relation to alcohol consumption in women. Scand J Gastroenterol 22:1251–1256, 1987
48. Moser J: Prevention of Alcohol-related Problems: An International Review of Preventive Measures, Policies, and Programmes. Published on behalf of the World Health Organization. Toronto: Alcoholism and Drug Addiction Research Foundation, 1980
49. Health and Welfare Canada: Alcohol in Canada. A National Perspective, 2nd ed. Ottawa: Health and Welfare Canada, 1984
50. Van Natta P, Malin H, Bertolucci D, et al: The influence of alcohol abuse as a hidden contributor to mortality. Alcohol 2:535–539, 1985
51. US Department of Health and Human Services: Fifth Special Report to the US Congress on Alcohol and Health from the Secretary of Health and Human Services. DHHS Publication No. (ADM) 841291. Washington DC: US Government Printing Office, 1983
52. Finney JW, Moos RH: The long-term course of treated alcoholism: I. Mortality, relapse, and remission rates and comparisons with community controls. J Stud Alcohol 52(1):44–54, 1991
53. Ableson J, Paddon P, Strohmenger C: Perspectives on Health. Ottawa: Statistics Canada, 1983
54. Ouellet BL, Romeder J-M, Lance J-M: Premature mortality attributable to smoking and hazardous drinking in Canada. Am J Epidemiol 109:451–463, 1979
55. Smart RG, Mann RE: Large decreases in alcohol-related problems following a slight reduction in alcohol consumption in Ontario 1975–83. Br J Addict 82:285–291, 1987
56. Mann RE, Smart RG, Anglin L: Reductions in liver cirrhosis mortality in Canada: demographic differences and possible explanations. Alcohol Clin Exp Res 12:1–8, 1988
57. US Department of Health and Human Services: Sixth Special Report to the US Congress on Alcohol and Health from the Secretary of Health and Human Services. DHHS Publication No. (ADM) 871519. Rockville, MD: US Government Printing Office, 1987
58. US Bureau of the Census: Statistical Abstract of the United States, 106th ed. Washington, DC: US Bureau of the Census, 1985
59. Commission on Chronic Illness: Chronic Illness in the United States. Cambridge, MA: Harvard University Press, 1957, vol. 1

60. Gordon R: An operational classification of disease prevention. Public Health Rep 98:107–109, 1983
61. Gordon R: An operational classification of disease prevention. In Steinberg JA, Silverman MM (eds): Preventing Mental Disorders. Rockville MD: US Department of Health and Human Services, 1987, pp 20–26
62. Institute of Medicine: Reducing Risks For Mental Disorders. Washington DC: National Academy Press, 1994
63. Aguirre-Molina M, Gorman DM: Community-based approaches for the prevention of alcohol, tobacco, and other drug use. Annu Rev Public Health 17:337–358, 1996
64. Popham RE, Schmidt W, de Lint J: The effects of legal restraint on drinking. In Kissin B, Begleiter H (eds): The Biology of Alcoholism. vol 4. Social Aspects of Alcoholism. New York: Plenum Press, 1976, pp 579–625
65. Terris M: Epidemiology of cirrhosis of the liver. Am J Public Health 57:2076–2088, 1967
66. Mäkelä K: Concentration of alcohol consumption. Scand Studies Ciminol 3:77–88, 1971
67. Schmidt W: Cirrhosis and alcohol consumption: an epidemiologic perspective. In Edwards G, Grant M (eds): Alcoholism: New Knowledge New Responses. London: Croom Helm, 1977, pp 15–47
68. Schmidt W, Popham RE: An approach to the control of alcohol consumption. In Rutledge B, Fulton EK (eds): International Collaboration: Problems and Opportunities. Toronto: Addiction Research Foundation of Ontario, 1977, pp 155–164
69. Schmidt W: The epidemiology of cirrhosis of the liver: a statistical analysis of mortality data with special reference to Canada. In Fisher MM, Rankin JG (eds): Alcohol and the Liver. New York: Plenum Press, 1976, pp 1–26
70. Ledermann S: Alcool, Alcoolisme, Alcoolization: Mortalité, Morbitité, Accidents du Travail Institut National d'Etudes Démographiques, Travaux et Documents, Cahier. No 41. Paris: Presses Universitaires de France, 1964
71. Keilman PA: Alcohol consumption and diabetes mellitus mortality in different countries. Am J Public Health 73:1316–1317, 1983
72. La Vecchia C, Decarli A, Mezzanotte G, et al: Mortality from alcohol-related disease in Italy. J Epidemiol Community Health 40:257–261, 1986
73. Imaizumi Y: Alcoholism mortality rate in Japan. Alcohol Alcohol 21:159–162, 1986
74. Poikolainen K: Increasing alcohol consumption correlated with hospital admission rates. Br J Addict 78:305–309, 1983
75. Truswell AS, Apeagyei F: Incidence of Wernicke's encephalopathy and Korsakoff's psychosis in Sydney. Presented at Alcohol, Nutrition and the Nervous System, Coppleston Postgraduate Medical Institute, University of Sydney, March 18, 1981
76. Ashley MJ, Rankin JG: A public health approach to the prevention of alcohol-related health problems. Annu Rev Public Health 9:233–271, 1988
77. Mäkelä K, Room R, Single E, et al: Alcohol, Society, and the State I: A Comparative Study of Alcohol Control. Toronto: Addiction Research Foundation, 1981
78. Popham RE, Schmidt W, de Lint J: The prevention of alcoholism: epidemiological studies of the effects of government control measures. Br J Addict 70:125–44, 1975
79. Rush B, Steinberg M, Brook R: The relationship among alcohol availability, alcohol consumption and alcohol-related damage in the Province of Ontario and the State of Michigan 1955–1982. Adv Alcohol Subst Abuse 5:33–44, 1986
80. Wagenaar AC, Farrell S: Alcohol beverage control policies: their role in preventing alcohol-impaired driving. In Surgeon General's Workshop on Drunk Driving. Background Papers, Washington DC, December 14–16, 1988. Rockville, MD: Office of the Surgeon General, 1989
81. Cook PJ: The effect of liquor taxes on drinking, cirrhosis and auto accidents. In Moore MH, Gerstein DR (eds): Alcohol and Public Policy: Beyond the Shadow of Prohibition. Washington, DC: National Academy, 1981
82. Cook PJ: Alcohol taxes as a public health measure. Br J Addict 77:245–250, 1982
83. Cook PJ, Tauchen G: The effect of liquor taxes on heavy drinking. Bell J Econ 13:379–390, 1982
84. Holder HD, Blose JO: Reduction of community alcohol problems: computer simulation experiments in three counties. J Stud Alcohol 48:124–135, 1987
85. Ornstein SI: A survey of findings on the economic and regulatory determinants of the demand for alcoholic beverages. Subst Alcohol Actions Misuse 5:39–44, 1984
86. Hoadley JF, Fuchs BC, Holder HD: The effect of alcohol beverage restrictions on consumption: a 25-year longitudinal analysis. Am J Drug Alcohol Abuse 10:375–401, 1984
87. Levy D, Sheflin N: New evidence on controlling alcohol use through price. J Stud Alcohol 44:929–937, 1983
88. Davies P: The relationship between taxation, price and alcohol consumption in the countries of Europe. In Grant M, Plant M, Williams A (eds): Economics and Alcohol: Consumption and Controls. London: Croom Helm, 1983
89. Maynard A: Modeling alcohol consumption and abuse: the powers and pitfalls of economic techniques. In Grant M, Plant M, Williams A (eds): Economics and Alcohol: Consumption and Controls. London: Croom Helm, 1983
90. Walsh BM: The economics of alcohol taxation. In Grant M, Plant M, Williams A (eds): Economics and Alcohol: Consumption and Controls. Croom Helm, 1983
91. McGuinness T: The demand for beer, spirits and wine in the UK, 1956–79. In Grant M, Plant M, Williams A (eds): Economics and Alcohol: Consumption and Control. London: Croom Helm, 1983
92. Heien D, Pompelli G: Stress, ethnic and distribution factors in a dichotomous response model of alcohol abuse. J Stud Alcohol 48:450–455, 1987
93. Walsh BM: Do excise taxes save lives? The Irish experience with alcohol taxation. Accid Anal Prev 19:433–448, 1987
94. Kendell RE, de Roumanie M, Ritson EB: Effect of economic changes on Scottish drinking habits, 1978–82. Br J Addict 78:365–379, 1983
95. Kendell RE, de Roumanie M, Ritson EB: Influence of an increase in excise duty on alcohol consumption and its adverse effects. Br Med J 287:809–811, 1983
96. Bigelow G, Liebson I: Cost factors controlling alcohol drinking. Psychol Record 22:305–314, 1972
97. Mello NK: Behavioural studies of alcoholism. In Kissin B, Begleiter H, (eds): The Biology of Alcoholism. vol 3. Physiology and Behaviour. New York: Plenum, 1972
98. Babor TF, Mendelson, JH, Greenberg I, et al: Experimental analysis of the "happy hour." Effects of purchase price on alcohol consumption. Psychopharmacology 58:35–41, 1978
99. Moore MH, Gerstein DR: Alcohol and Public Policy: Beyond the Shadow of Prohibition. Washington, DC: National Academy Press, 1981, p 116
100. Grant BF, Zobeck TS, Chan Ng M-J: Liver cirrhosis mortality in the United States, 1971–1985. Surveillance Report No. 8. Alcohol Epidemiologic Data System, Division of Biometry and Epidemiology, National Institute on Alcohol Abuse and Alcoholism. Washington, DC: Alcohol, Drug Abuse, and Mental Health Administration, 1988
101. Duffy M: The influence of prices, consumer incomes and advertising upon the demand for alcoholic drink in the United Kingdom. Br J Alcohol Alcohol 16:200–208, 1981
102. Ornstein SI: Control of alcohol consumption through price increases. J Stud Alcohol 41:807–818, 1980

103. Grossman M, Coate D, Arluck GM: Price sensitivity of alcoholic beverages in the United States. In Holder HD (ed): Control Issues in Alcohol Abuse Prevention: Strategies for Communities. Greenwich, CT: JAI Press, 1987
104. Coate D, Grossman M: Change in alcoholic beverage prices and legal drinking ages: effects on youth alcohol use and motor vehicle mortality. Alcohol Health Res World 12:22–25, 59, 1987
105. Saffer H, Grossman M: Beer taxes, the legal drinking age, and youth motor vehicle fatalities. J Legal Stud 16:351–374, 1987
106. Saffer H, Grossman M: Drinking age laws and highway mortality rates: Cause and effect. Econ Inquiry 25:403–418, 1987
107. Schmidt W, Popham RE: Alcohol Problems and Their Prevention. A Public Health Perspective. Toronto: Addiction Research Foundation, 1980
108. Mosher JF, Beauchamp DE: Justifying alcohol taxes to public officials. J Public Health Policy 4:422–439, 1983
109. Vernberg WB: Alcohol Tax Reform. Proposed Position Paper, American Public Health Association. The Nation's Health August 1986
110. Addiction Research Foundation: Alcohol, Public Education and Social Policy. Report of the Task Force on Public Education and Social Policy. Toronto: Addiction Research Foundation, 1981
111. Single E: International perspectives on alcohol as a public health issue. J Public Health Policy 5:238–256, 1984
112. Room R: Alcohol control and public health. Annu Rev Public Health 5:293–317, 1984
113. Farrell S: Review of National Policy Measures to Prevent Alcohol-related Problems. Geneva: World Health Organization, 1985
114. Smith DI: Effectiveness of restrictions on availability as a means of reducing the use and abuse of alcohol. Aust Alcohol Drug Rev 2:84–90, 1983
115. MacDonald S, Whitehead P: Availability of outlets and consumption of alcoholic beverages. J Drug Issues 13:477–486, 1983
116. Mäkelä K, Osterberg E, Sulkunen P: Drink in Finland: increasing alcohol availability in a monopoly state. In Single E, Morgan P, de Lint J (eds): Alcohol, Society and the State. 2. The Social History of Control Policy in Seven Countries. Toronto: Addiction Research Foundation, 1981
117. Ryan BE, Segars L: Mini-marts and maxi-problems. The relationship between purchase and consumption levels. Alcohol Health Res World 12:26–29, 1987
118. Smart RG, Goodstadt MS: Effects of reducing the legal alcohol purchasing age on drinking and drinking problems. A review of empirical studies. J Stud Alcohol 38:1313–1323, 1977
119. Vingilis ER, DeGenova K: Youth and the forbidden fruit: Experiences with changes in the legal drinking age in North America. J Criminal Justice 12:161–172, 1984
120. Williams TP, Lillis RP: Changes in alcohol consumption by 18-year-olds following an increase in New York State's purchase age to 19. J Stud Alcohol 47:290–296, 1986
121. Engs RC, Hanson DJ: Age-specific alcohol prohibition and college students drinking problems. Psychol Rep 59:979–984, 1986
122. Smith DI, Burvill PW: Effect on juvenile crime of lowering the drinking age in three Australian states. Br J Addict 82:181–188, 1986
123. Cook PJ, Tauchen G: The effect of minimum drinking age legislation on youthful auto fatalities, 1970–1977. J Legal Stud 13: 169–190, 1984
124. Cotton NS: The familial incidence of alcoholism. J Stud Alcohol 40:89–116, 1979
125. Hrubec Z and Omenn GS: Evidence of genetic predisposition to alcohol cirrhosis and psychosis: twin concordances for alcoholism and its biological end points by zygosity among male veterans. Alcohol Clin Exp Res 5:207–212, 1981
126. Schuckit MA: Twin studies on substance abuse: an overview. In Gedda L, Parisi P, Nance W, (eds): Twin Research 3: Epidemiological and Clinical Studies. New York: Alan R Liss, 1981, pp 61–70
127. Goodwin DW: Alcoholism and genetics. Arch Gen Psychiatry 42:171–174, 1985
128. Bohman M, Sigvardsson S, Cloninger R: Maternal inheritance of alcohol abuse: cross-fostering analysis of adopted women. Arch Gen Psychiatry 38:965–969, 1981
129. Cloninger CR, Sigvardsson S, Gilligan SB, et al: Genetic heterogeneity and the classification of alcoholism. In Gordis E, Tabakoff B, and Linnoila M (eds): Alcohol Research from Bench to Bedside. New York: Haworth Press, 1989, pp 3–16
130. Tabakoff B, Hoffman P, Lee J, et al: Differences in platelet enzyme activity between alcoholics and nonalcoholics. N Engl J Med 318:134–139, 1988
131. Selzer ML: Michigan Alcoholism Screening Test: the quest for a new diagnostic instrument. Am J Psychiatry 127:89–94, 1971
132. Pokorny AD, Miller BA, Kaplan HB: The brief MAST: a shortened version of the Michigan Alcoholism Screening Test. Am J Psychiatry 129:342–345, 1972
133. Mayfield D, McLeod G, Hall P: The CAGE questionnaire: validation of a new alcoholism screening instrument. Am J Psychiatry 131:1121–1123, 1974
134. Babor TF, Grant M: From clinical research to secondary prevention: international collaboration in the development of the Alcohol Use Disorders Identification Test (AUDIT). Alcohol Health Res World 13:371–374, 1989
135. Russell M, Martier SS, Sokol RJ, et al: Screening for pregnancy risk-drinking. Alcohol Clin Exp Res 18:1156–1161, 1994
136. US Preventive Services Task Force: Guide to Clinical Preventive Services, 2nd ed. Baltimore: Williams & Wilkins, 1996
137. Allen JP, Maisto SA, Connors GJ: Self-report screening tests for alcohol problems in primary care. Arch Intern Med 155(16): 1726–1730, 1995
138. Harrell AV, Wirtz PW: Screening for adolescent problem drinking: validation of a multidimensional instrument for case identification. Psychol Assess 1:61–63, 1989
139. Fink A, Hays RD, Moore AA, et al: Alcohol-related problems in older persons. Determinants, consequences, and screening. Arch Intern Med 156(11):1150–1156, 1996
140. Adams WL, Barry KL, Fleming MF: Screening for problem drinking in older primary care patients. JAMA 276(24):1964–1967, 1996
141. Magruder-Habib K, Durand AM, Frey KA: Alcohol abuse and alcoholism in primary health care settings. J Fam Pract 32:406, 1991
142. Skinner HA, Holt S, Schuller R, et al: Identification of alcohol abuse using laboratory tests and a history of trauma. Ann Intern Med 101:847–851, 1984
143. Criteria Committee, National Council on Alcoholism: Criteria for the diagnosis and alcoholism. Am J Psychiatry 129:127–135, 1972
144. Allen JP, Litten RZ, Anton RF, et al: Carbohydrate-deficient transferrin as a measure of immoderate drinking: remaining issues. Alcohol Clin Exp Res 18(4):799–808, 1994
145. Saunders JB: Management and treatment efficacy of drug and alcohol problems: what do doctors believe? Addiction 90(10): 1357–1366, 1995
146. Chafetz ME, Blane HT, Abram HS, et al: Establishing treatment relations with alcoholics. J Nerv Ment Dis 134:385–409, 1062
147. Bien TH, Miller WR, Tonigan JS: Brief interventions for alcohol problems: a review. Addiction 88(3):315–335, 1993
148. Babor TF, Ritson EB, Hodgson RJ: Alcohol-related problems in the primary health care setting: a review of early intervention strategies. Br J Addict 81:23–46, 1986
149. Edwards G, Orford J, Egert S, et al: Alcoholism: a controlled trial of "treatment" and "advice." J Stud Alcohol 38:1004–1031, 1977
150. Orford J, Oppenheimer E, Edwards G: Abstinence or control: the outcome for excessive drinkers two years after consultation. Behav Res Ther 14:397–416, 1976

151. Wallace P, Cutler S, Haines A: Randomized controlled trial of general practitioner intervention in patients with excessive alcohol consumption. Br Med J 297:663–668, 1988
152. Sanchez-Craig M, Leigh G, Spivek K, et al: Superior outcome of females over males after brief treatment for the reduction of heavy drinking. Br J Addict 84:395–404, 1989
153. Sanchez-Craig M, Annis HM, Bornet AR, et al: Random assignment to abstinence and controlled drinking: evaluation of a cognitive-behavioural program for problem drinkers. J Consult Clin Psychol 52:390–403, 1984
154. Skutle A, Berg G: Training in controlled drinking for early-stage problem drinkers. Br J Addict 82:493–501, 1987
155. Zweben A, Pearlman S, Li S: A comparison of brief advice and conjoint therapy in the treatment of alcohol abuse: the results of the marital systems study. Br J Addict 83:899–916, 1988
156. Sannibale C: Differential effect of a set of brief interventions on the functioning of a group of "early-stage" problem drinkers. Aust Drug Alcohol Rev 7:147–155, 1988
157. Skinner HA, Holt S: Early intervention for alcohol problems. J R Coll Gen Pract 33:787–791, 1983
158. Stockwell T: Can severely dependent drinkers learn controlled drinking? Summing up the debate. Br J Addict 83:149–152, 1988
159. Babor TF, Treffardier M, Weill J, et al: Early detection and secondary prevention of alcoholism in France. J Stud Alcohol 44: 600–616, 1983
160. Alden LE: Behavioural self-management controlled-drinking strategies in a context of secondary prevention. J Consult Clin Psychol 56:280–286, 1988
161. Taylor JR, Heizer JE, Robins LN: Moderate drinking in ex-alcoholics: recent studies. J Stud Alcohol 47:115–121, 1986
162. Rush BR, Ogborne AC: Acceptibility of nonabstinence treatment goals among alcoholism treatment programs. J Stud Alcohol 47:1 46–150, 1986
163. Sanchez-Craig M: A Therapist's Manual for Secondary Prevention of Alcohol Problems. Procedures for Teaching Moderate Drinking and Abstinence. Toronto: Addiction Research Foundation, 1984
164. Kristenson H, Hood B: The impact of alcohol on health in the general population: a review with particular reference to experience in Malmo. Br J Addict 79:139–145, 1984
165. Chick J, Lloyd G, Crombie E: Counselling problem drinkers in medical wards: a controlled study. Br Med J 290:965–967, 1985
166. Elvy GA, Wells JE, Baird KA: Attempted referral as intervention for problem drinking in the general hospital. Br J Addict 83:83–89, 1988
167. Chick J: Secondary prevention of alcoholism and the Centres D'Hygiene Alimentaire. Br J Addict 79:221–225, 1984
168. Mcintosh M, Sanchez-Craig M: Moderate drinking: an alternative treatment goal for early-stage problem drinking. Can Med Assoc J 131:873–876, 1984
169. Skinner HA: Early detection of alcohol and drug problems—why? Aust Drug Alcohol Rev 6:293–301, 1987

46

Prevention of Drug Abuse

C. Roberts Schuster • M. Marlyne Kilbey

In Western society we would like to believe that the only factor limiting an individual's ability to enjoy a healthy life is that set by one's genes. However, abuse of psychoactive drugs is a major threat to the realization of that birthright.

▸ HEALTH AND COST IMPACT

The cost of drug abuse may be measured in adverse health effects that are reflected in expenditures for treatment of drug abuse and associated disorders as well as premature mortality and morbidity of persons abusing drugs. Besides these direct costs of drug abuse, there are also related costs that arise from lost productivity, crime, apprehension and incarceration, and rehabilitative social welfare programs. Adolescence is the only segment of our population that has not experienced improved health over the past 30 years.[1] In large part, this results from the disproportionate representation of adolescents among the drug-abusing segment of our population. Homicides, suicide, and accidents account for over 77 percent of adolescent deaths, and drug abuse is implicated in over half of these deaths.[1]

In 1988, the economic impact of drug abuse was $58.3 billion including $2.9 billion for direct treatment of drug abusers.[2] Another dimension of the cost of drug abuse comes from the link between intravenous (IV) drug use and seropositivity for the human immunodeficiency virus (HIV). As of December 1995 the Centers for Disease Control and Prevention estimated that there were 184,359 cases of acquired immunodeficiency syndrome (AIDS) directly or indirectly associated with IV drug use.[3] The cost of treating an AIDS patient from onset of AIDS to death was estimated to be $69,000.[4] Thus, the cost of treating these patients is approximately $14 million. This estimate does not include the cost of treating these patients from the point of seroconversion to onset of AIDS, estimated to be $50,000/patient,[4] or the cost of treatment with retroviral medications, which may double the lifetime cost of treating AIDS patients.[5]

Much of the economic cost of drug abuse comes from crime (cost of losses to nondrug-abusing citizens and lost productivity of persons incarcerated, for example). Rice and her colleagues[2] estimate these costs at a staggering 78 percent of the total economic burden for drug abuse whereas crime-associated costs represent less than 18 percent of the costs of alcohol abuse and less than 4 percent of the costs of mental disorders. Clearly, preventing drug abuse would result in significant health improvement and economic savings in addition to improving the quality of life for those living in neighborhoods threatened by drug-related crime.

▸ DEFINITIONS

The term "psychoactive drug" refers to the various classes of exogenous substances that affect the central nervous system, inducing responses that generally are recognized subjectively as calming, energizing, or pleasurable. Legal restrictions on the production and distribution of psychoactive substances vary from being nonexistent (e.g., caffeine) to being highly restrictive (e.g., morphine), and both possession and use of psychoactive substances can be legal (e.g., nicotine) or illegal (e.g., cocaine). Control of the availability of psychoactive substances is a fundamental approach to substance abuse prevention.[6]

One way the availability of psychoactive substances is controlled in the United States is through regulation under Title II of the Comprehensive Drug Abuse Prevention and Control Act of 1970, generally referred to as the Controlled Substances Act (CSA).[7] The act establishes five schedules of decreasing control from schedule I through V. It regulates possession and distribution of drugs and establishes penalties for individuals who violate the regulations. Schedule assignment is made based on the drug's potential for abuse as well as any current or historical pattern of abuse. Current medical use and safety, as well as the psychological and physiological dependence-producing properties of the drug are considered. Table 46-1 lists five major types of drugs based on their pharmacological actions and shows their scheduling under the CSA, trade names of common drugs in the class, important medical uses, and certain physical and psychological dependence characteristics.

For controlled substances, drug abuse may be defined as any use in a nonprescribed manner, and for noncontrolled substances, drug abuse may be thought of as continued use in the face of recurrent, adverse consequences. For example, any use whatsoever of lysergic acid diethylamide (LSD) constitutes abuse, whereas for tobacco and alcohol, only use by minors or excessive use of alcohol by adults may be termed abuse. Clearly, the definition of drug abuse is dependent on culture and historical period.[8,9] Drug dependence is defined as "a state of psychic or physical dependence, or both, on a drug, arising in a person following administration of that drug on a periodic or continuous basis."[10] Psychoactive substance abuse disorders involving excessive and compulsive use of drugs that results in tolerance and withdrawal are conceptualized as mental disorders.[11]

▸ PHARMACOLOGY OF DRUGS OF ABUSE

An understanding of the pharmacological properties of drugs is essential in the design of prevention efforts. Three processes are important in the development of drug dependence: (*a*) physical dependence, conceptualized as "an adaptive state that manifests itself by intense physical disturbances when the administration of a drug is suspended,"[10] (*b*) psychological dependence, conceptualized as a condition in which there is "a feeling of satisfaction and a psychic drive that requires periodic or continuous administration of the drug to produce pleasure or to avoid discomfort,"[10] and (*c*) tolerance,

TABLE 46-1. CONTROLLED SUBSTANCES—USES AND EFFECTS

Drugs/ CSA Schedules	Trade or Other Names	Medical Uses	Dependence: Physical	Dependence: Psychological	Tolerance	Duration (Hours)	Usual Methods of Administration	Possible Effects	Effects of Overdose	Withdrawal Symptoms
■ ***NARCOTICS***										
Morphine II	MS-Contin, Roxanol Oramorph-SR	Analgesic	High	High	Yes	3–6	Oral, smoked, injected	Euphoria, drowsiness, respiratory depression, constricted pupils, nausea	Slow and shallow breathing, clammy skin, convulsions, coma, possible death	Water eyes, runny nose, yawning, loss of appetite, irritability, tremors, panic, cramps, nausea, chills and sweating
Codeine II III V	Tylenol w/Codeine, Empirin w/Codeine Robitussan A-C, Fiorinal w/Codeine, APAP w/Codeine	Analgesic, antitussive	Moderate	Moderate	Yes	3–6	Oral, injected Oral			
Heroin I	Diacetylmorphine Horse, Smack	None in U.S.	High	High	Yes	3–6	Injected, sniffed smoked			
Hydromorphone II	Dilaudid	Analgesic	High	High	Yes	3–6	Oral, injected			
Methadone I, II and LAAM	Dolophine, Levo-Alpha-Acetyl-methadol, Levo-methadyl Acetate, Methodose	Analgesic, treatment of dependence	High	High	Yes	12–72	Oral, injected			
Other narcotics II, III, IV, V	Percodan, Percocet, Tylox, Darvon, Talwinᵇ, Opium, Buprenorphine, Meperdine (Pethidine), Demerol, Roxicet, Roxicodone	Analgesic, antidiarrheal	High–low	High–low	Yes	Variable	Oral, injected			
■ ***DEPRESSANTS***										
Chloral Hydrate IV	Noctec, Somnos, Felsules	Hypnotic	Moderate	Moderate	Yes	5–8	Oral	Slurred speech, disorientation, drunken behavior without odor of alcohol	Shallow respiration, clamerry skin, dialated pupils, weak and rapid pulse, coma, possible death	Anxiety, insomnia, tremors, delirium, convulsions, possible death
Barbiturates II, III, IV	Amytal, Fiorinal, Nembutal, Seconal, Tuinal, Phenobarbital, Pentobarbital	Anesthetic, anticonvulsant, sedative, hypnotic, veterinary euthanasia agent	High-moderate	High-moderate	Yes	1–16	Oral, injected			
Benzodiazepines IV	Ativan, Dalmane, Diazepam, Librium, Xanax, Serax, Valium, Tranxexe, Veratran, Versed, Halcion, Paxipam, Restoril	Antianxiety, anticonvulsant, sedative, hypnotic	Low	Low	Yes	4–8	Oral, injected			
Glutethimide II	Doriden	Sedative, hypnotic	High	Moderate	Yes	4–8	Oral			
Other depressants I, II, III IV	Equanil, Miltown, Noludar, Placidyl, Valmid, Methaqualone	Antianxiety, sedative, hypnotic	Moderate	Moderate	Yes	4–8	Oral			

■ ***STIMULANTS***										
Cocaine[a]-II	Coke, Flake, Snow, Crack	Local anesthetic	Possible	High	Yes	1–2	Sniffed, smoked, injected	Increased alertness, excitation, euphoria, increased pulse rate and blood pressure, insomnia, loss of appetite	Agitation, increase in body temperature, hallucinations, convulsions, possible death	Apathy, long periods of sleep, irritability, depression, disorientation
Amphetamines Methamphetamine II	Biphetamine, Desoxyn, Dexedrine, Obetrol, Ice	Attention deficit disorders, narcolepsy, weight control	Possible	High	Yes	2–4	Oral, injected, smoked			
Methylphenidate II	Ritalin	Attention deficit disorders, narcolepsy	Possible	High	Yes	2–4	Oral, injected			
Other stimulants I, II, III, IV	Adipex, Didrex, Ionamin, Melfiat, Plegine, Captagon, Sanorex, Tenuate, Tepanil, Prelu-2, Preludin	Weight control	Possible	High	Yes	2–4	Oral, injected			
■ ***HALLUCINOGENS***										
LSD I	Acid, Microdot	None	None	Unknown	Yes	8–12	Oral	Illusions and hallucinations, altered perception of time and distance	Longer, more intense "trip" episodes, psychosis possible death	Unknown
Mascaline and Peyote I	Mescal, Butions, Cactus	None	None	Unknown	Yes	8–12	Oral			
Amphetamine variants I	2, 5-DMA, STP, MDA, MDMA, Ecstasy, DOM, DOB	None	Unknown	Unknown	Yes	Variable	Oral, injected			
Phencyclidine and analogs I, II	PCE, PCPy, TCP, PCP, Hog, Loveboat, Angel Dust	None	Unknown	High	Yes	Days	Smoked, oral			
Other hallucinogens I	Bufotenine, Ibogaine, DMT, DET, Psilocybin, Psilocyn	None	None	Unknown	Possible	Variable	Smoked, oral, injected, sniffed			
■ ***CANNABIS***										
Marijuana I	Pot, Acapulco Gold, Grass, Reefer, Sinsemilla, Thai Sticks	None	Unknown	Moderate	Yes	2–4	Smoked, oral	Euphoria, relaxed inhibitions, increased appetite, disorientation	Fatigue, paranoia, possible psychosis	Occasional reports of insomnia, hyperactivity, and decreased appetite
Tetrahydrocannabinol I, II	THC, Marinol	Antinauseant	Unknown	Moderate	Yes	2–4	Smoked, oral			
Hashish and Hashish oil, I	Hash, Hash oil	None	Unknown	Moderate	Yes	2–4	Smoked, oral			
■ ***ANABOLIC STEROIDS***										
Testosterone (Cypionate, Enanthate) III	Depo-testosterone, Delatestryl	Hypogonadism	Unknown	Unknown	Unknown	14–28 days	Injected	Virilization, acne, testicular atrophy, gynecomastia, aggressive behavior, edema	Unknown	Possible depression
Nandrolone (Decanote, Phenpropionate) III	Nortestosterone, Durabolin, Deca-Durabolin, Deca	Anemia, breast cancer	Unknown	Unknown	Unknown	14–21 days	Injected			
Oxymetholone III	Anadrol-50	Anemia	Unknown	Unknown	Unknown	24 hours	Oral			

[a] Designated a narcotic under the CSA.
[b] Not designated a narcotic under the CSA.

conceptualized as the need for increasingly higher doses of a drug to recapture the original effect of a drug.[12] All three of these processes reflect the pharmacological characteristics of a drug, individual characteristics of the person using it, and environmental characteristics particular to the setting(s) in which the drug is used. Psychopharmacological research is designed to gain a better understanding of the processes themselves, the ways in which they interact, and their contribution to drug dependence. It should be noted, however, that drug abuse may exist in the absence of tolerance or dependence. A person engaging in initial use of an illicit drug or repeatedly driving an auto under the influence of alcohol could be an example of this.

On initial use of a psychoactive drug, an individual is exposed to the reinforcing or pleasurable characteristics of the drug. The reinforcing-reward characteristic is an important factor in the initiation and maintenance of drug abuse. The more reinforcing the drug is, the more likely it is to be abused. This characteristic, termed the abuse liability of a drug, can be assessed in animal self-administration models. Work over the past 20 years has shown a strong correlation between the drugs that animals will self-administer and those that humans abuse.[13,14] With knowledge of its abuse liability, a drug can be scheduled under the CSA in a manner to minimize its availability. Availability of a drug is seen as one of the principal determinants of the number of people who will try a drug and possibly go on to use it in a regular or compulsive fashion.[15,16] However, evaluation of abuse liability, although diagnostic of potential abuse, is not foolproof. For example, hallucinogens, such as mescaline, are not self-administered by animals,[17] but they are abused by humans. Nevertheless, knowledge of the general pharmacology and abuse liability of substances and the control of their distribution and use are useful steps in curtailing the amount of drug abuse that occurs. Both basic research that establishes a drug's characteristics and governmental regulation that assigns a drug to a schedule are essential aspects of drug abuse prevention.

Narcotics

Narcotics include drugs ranging from heroin, which has no accepted medical use in the United States, to such drugs as morphine and codeine, which are used commonly for their analgesic or antitussive properties. This class of drugs is widely abused. The degree of abuse depends on many factors, including the relative potency of the available formulations of the drug and economic and social factors.

Drugs listed under narcotics in Table 46-1 have opium-like or morphine-like properties. These properties are shared with naturally occurring neuroactive peptides, for example, enkephalins and endorphins, which are active at certain brain sites[18] and coexist with norepinephrine, serotonin, and other transmitters.[19] Narcotic drugs appear to be active in brain systems that mediate positive mood where they mimic neuropeptides that may have evolved to guarantee that such essential acts as eating and sexual intercourse are repeated, thus increasing the probability of survival of the individual and the species.

Opium, the prototypical opioid, is extracted from the poppy plant and has been known to humanity since ancient times. Its medical analgesic uses were well established by the mid-sixteenth century, and opium smoking for purely subjective effects was an established practice in Asia by the eighteenth century.[20] Morphine, an alkaloid of opium, was isolated in 1806, and its structure has been known since 1925. Synthetic derivatives are made by simple modifications of morphine's structure or that of thebaine, another opium alkaloid. The effects of opioids are diverse, depending on many factors, and include altered endocrine and autonomic nervous system functions, changes in mood and pain perception, decreased gastrointestinal motility, drowsiness, nausea, respiratory depression, and vomiting.

Several types of brain receptors for opioid drugs have been identified, with morphine like drugs appearing to prefer one subtype, the μ receptor. The site and mechanism of action of opioids and their relation to abuse and dependence are a focus of much current work by neuropharmacologists and other neuroscientists.[20,21] Recently an endogenous molecule, orphanin, has been identified that blocks the effects of morphine and other opiates.[22] A further appreciation of its properties may be a key to understanding physical dependence and withdrawal.

One of the key characteristics of repeated administrations of narcotics is development of tolerance, dependence, and withdrawal. It should be emphasized that these phenomena reflect changes in pharmacokinetics and pharmacodynamics of the drug that result from an interaction of its pharmacological characteristics and the individual's biology, behavior, and environment. This principle is made clear in experiments in which the lethality of heroin has been shown to increase radically when rodents in a novel setting are given a heroin dose that they had tolerated previously in a familiar setting.[23] Furthermore, tolerance to the many effects of a narcotic does not develop uniformly. For example, differentially greater tolerance to the euphoric effects of heroin in comparison to its respiratory depressive characteristics may underlie at least some of the deaths associated with heroin overdoses.

Depressants

These include the drugs listed in Table 46-1 and alcohol, which is covered in Chapter 45. In general, the drugs shown under this heading share sedative and hypnotic properties and are used medically to produce drowsiness, sleep, and muscle relaxation and to prevent convulsions. In addition, barbiturates have anesthetic properties. The effects of these drugs are dose dependent, progressing from relaxation to sedation through hypnosis to stupor. In the 1950s, benzodiazepines were developed with high anxiolytic and low central nervous system depressant properties. This permitted relief of anxiety symptoms without impairment of cognitive, attention, or motor functions. Depressants have complex effects, and their pharmacological properties have been reviewed recently.[24] Depressants' relative degree of safety, tolerance, and dependence vary from the benzodiazepines, assigned to schedule IV, to those barbiturates, which are associated with toxicity and high abuse liability, assigned to schedule II. Tolerance for and dependence on the various drugs of this class generalize within the class and across classes to some opiates and alcohol. This is termed cross-tolerance and cross-dependence. Since, in our society, alcohol often is not recognized as a depressant drug, its use with sedative-hypnotic drugs results in stupor and death more frequently than might be the case were alcohol's depressant characteristics more fully appreciated.[25]

Stimulants

Stimulant drugs generally are classified as excitatory in recognition of their main effect on the central nervous system. At low doses, stimulants are associated with feelings of increased alertness, euphoria, vigor, motor activity, and appetite suppression. At high doses, they cause convulsions. Changes in thought have been characterized on a continuum from hyper-vigilance through suspicion to paranoia. Amphetamine and cocaine-induced psychoses are described in chronic abusers.[26–28] Paranoid ideation generally is reported in persons with histories of chronic stimulant abuse, but transient psychotic symptoms have been reported with initial use of high doses,[29] and instances of psychoses associated with use of medically prescribed doses have been reported.[30] With repeated use, tolerance to some drug effects occurs, for example, euphoria and appetite suppression, whereas for other effects, for example, increased motor activity, stereotypy, and possibly paranoia, sensitization, an increased response to the drug, occurs.[31] Cocaine has various toxic effects especially upon the cardiovascular system,[32] and, when cocaine and alcohol are taken together, cocaethylene is produced, which is even more lethal than cocaine.[33] Thorough discussions[34] are available of the general pharmacology of amphetamine and other sympathomimetic amines, including the various receptor systems at which they act. A comprehensive review of cocaine's behavioral pharmacology relevant to issues of abuse[35] is available also.

Hallucinogens

Hallucinogens, unlike many abused drugs, have no accepted medical use. These drugs share an ability to distort perception and induce delusions, hallucinations, illusions, and profound alterations of mood.

Mescaline and psilocin-containing plants have been used ceremonially for centuries, and LSD was synthesized by Hoffman in 1925. Under certain conditions, drugs from a variety of classes, in addition to those listed as hallucinogens in Table 46-1, show hallucinogenic properties. Because of similarities between experiences of persons ingesting hallucinogens and those of mentally ill persons and persons reporting profound religious experiences, these drugs also are called psychotomimetics or psychedelics.

Hallucinogens can be classified as indolealkylamines, phenylethylamines, or phenylisopropylamines, based on their structure and pharmacology. Their effects reflect activity at receptors of the serotonergic, cholinergic, and possibly other systems. Tolerance occurs with repeated use of all hallucinogens. As is true for other psychoactive substances, differential tolerance to their various effects can be demonstrated. For example, tolerance to the subjective effects of hallucinogens is greater than that seen for cardiovascular effects. Considerable cross-tolerance exists among drugs in this category. Symptoms of physical dependence after abrupt withdrawal of phencyclidine have been described,[36] but similar reports for LSD do not exist. Jaffe[12] has discussed the pharmacology of hallucinogens in relation to their abuse.

Cannabis

Cannabis is obtained from the flowering top of the hemp plant. More than 60 cannabinoids have been isolated from the hemp plant, and 1-delta-9-tetrahydrocannabinol (Δ-9-THC) has been identified as the constituent responsible for most of the characteristic effects of this category of drugs.[37] Cannabis affects cognition, memory, mood, motor coordination, self-perception, and sense of time and, under some conditions, produces feelings of relaxation and well-being. Tolerance is clearly seen after high doses and/or sustained use. Differential tolerance occurs to the various effects as well as cross-tolerance to some hallucinogens.[38] Withdrawal symptoms characterized by irritability, restlessness, nervousness, decreased appetite, weight loss, and insomnia as well as delusions, paranoid ideation, and hallucinations have been reported.[12] Cannabis affects the cardiovascular system by increasing heart rate and differentially altering standing and supine blood pressure. Disruption of performance[39] and withdrawal symptoms[40] have been noted after discontinued use of Δ-9-THC. A fuller discussion of the pharmacology of cannabis relative to its abuse is provided by Jaffe.[12]

▶ EPIDEMIOLOGY

An understanding of the extent, nature, and duration of use and abuse of psychoactive drugs is a necessary prerequisite for developing effective and efficient drug abuse prevention and treatment programs. Three valuable sources of data are the National Household Survey on Drug Use, the Monitoring the Future Study, and the National Comorbidity Survey. The first survey is sponsored by the Substance Abuse and Mental Health Services Administration (SAMHSA); the second by the National Institute on Drug Abuse (NIDA); and the final one by NIDA, the National Institute of Mental Health, and the W.T. Grant Foundation.

National Household Survey

The National Household Survey is based on responses to a structured interview of a stratified, multistage area probability sample of people 12 years of age or older who are living in households.[41–43] Neighborhoods were chosen to overrepresent black and Hispanic residents to permit statistical analysis by ethnicity. The survey covers use of marijuana, cocaine, inhalants, hallucinogens, heroin, nonmedical use of four classes of psychotherapeutic drugs (stimulants, sedatives, tranquilizers, and analgesics) and anabolic steroids, cigarettes and smokeless tobacco, and alcohol. Separate answer sheets are provided for sections with questions that respondents may hesitate to answer orally. Additional information gathered includes sex, race or ethnicity, region of residence and density of population, educational attainment, employment status, perceptions of drug use and problems associated with use. Use is reported for the past month, past year, and the respondent's lifetime. The 1994 survey interviewed 17,809 persons, of whom 48.6 percent were white, 22.5 percent black, and 26.4 percent Hispanic. As shown in Table 46-2, approximately 37.6 percent of the population had used some illicit drug over their lifetime, and approximately 6 percent had used an illicit drug in the past month. Marijuana was the single most commonly used illicit drug, with 34.1 percent reporting lifetime use and 4.7 percent reporting current use.

Reports of lifetime use differed by age. The lifetime use of marijuana and hashish was highest in 1994 for those age 26 to 34 (52.7 percent) in comparison to those age 18 to 25 (41.9 percent), over 35 (25.4 percent), and 12 to 17 (13.6 percent). Marijuana use peaked between 1979 and 1982 for all age groups, but the 1990s have seen a steady increase in marijuana use. Of special interest was the statistically significant increase in the percentage of youth (age 12 to 17) reporting lifetime, past year, and past month use of marijuana in 1993 and 1994. Twice as many males as females reported marijuana use in the past month (6.7 versus 3.1 percent), although at younger ages the difference was not as great (6.8 versus 5.2 percent at ages 12 to 17). When all ages are considered, blacks reported more current marijuana use than whites or Hispanics (13.1 versus 9.1 versus 7.4 percent), although among 18 to 25 year olds, a higher percent of whites report marijuana use than other groups (13.3 versus 12 percent for blacks and 7.7 percent for Hispanics; see Table 3.3 in Reference 42).

Marijuana use in the past month was greatest in the unemployed (10.8 percent) compared to those employed full-time (5.5 percent) or part-time (5.4 percent). For people 18 or older, marijuana use was also lowest in college graduates (4.0 versus 5.5 percent in those having some college education, 4.6 percent in high school graduates, and 6.4 percent in those who did not graduate from high school).

Cocaine use was less frequent than marijuana use, but 9.7 percent of those surveyed reported having used it at least once, 1.9 percent used it in the past year, and 0.6 percent used it in the past month.

TABLE 46-2. PERCENTAGE OF USERS OF ILLICIT DRUGS AND TOBACCO IN THE U.S. CIVILIAN, NONINSTITUTIONALIZED POPULATION AGE 12 AND OLDER IN THEIR LIFETIME, PAST YEAR, AND THE PAST MONTH

	Time Period		
Drug	**Lifetime (%)**	**Past Year (%)**	**Past Month (%)**
Any illicit drug use	37.6	12.4	5.8
Marijuana/hashish	34.1	9.2	4.7
Cocaine	9.7	1.9	0.6
Crack	1.8	0.4	0.2
Inhalants	5.1	1.3	0.7
Hallucinogens	8.1	1.4	0.3
Phencyclidine (PCP)	4.3	0.2	0.1
Heroin	1.1	0.2	0.1
Nonmedical use of any psychotheraputic	10.1	3.4	0.8
Stimulants	5.5	0.7	0.1
Sedatives	3.5	0.8	0.8
Tranquilizers	4.1	1.2	0.2
Analgesics	5.0	1.9	0.6
Cigarettes	71.2	28.1	23.4
Smokeless tobacco	15.0	4.7	3.0

From Substance Abuse and Mental Health Services Administration: National Household Survey on Drug Abuse: Main Findings 1994. DHHS Publication No. (SMA) 96-3085. Washington, DC: Government Printing Office, 1996.

Lifetime crack use was 1.8 percent with 0.4 percent past year use and 0.2 percent past month use. Male use of cocaine and crack in the past year was over twice that of females (2.4 versus 1.1 percent and 0.9 and 0.4 percent for cocaine and crack, respectively). Use of both cocaine (2.9 percent) and crack (1.6 percent) in the past year was higher for blacks than for Hispanics (2.4 percent, cocaine; 0.7 percent, crack) or whites (1.5 percent, cocaine; 0.5 percent, crack). Use of both was highest among those who did not graduate from high school and the unemployed (see Tables 4.2 and 4.8 in Reference 42). The higher rate of crack use by blacks reflects social conditions, as when the data were examined by neighborhoods; holding constant characteristics such as drug availability, use rates of blacks and whites did not differ.[44] It is the disproportionately larger percent of blacks living in such neighborhoods that account for their higher prevalence of crack use.

The National Household Survey also inquires about some of the consequences of drug use, and a large proportion of drug users report concerns about their drug use (see Tables 9.1 and 9.2 in Reference 42). Of those who used marijuana, monthly or more frequently over the past year, 48.5 percent reported wanting to cut down their use, and 18.1 percent reported that their marijuana use caused problems at home or at work. Among those who used cocaine monthly or more frequently over the past year, 56.5 percent reported a desire to cut down, and 47.5 percent reported home or work problems caused by cocaine use. These data suggest that a significant percentage of frequent users of illicit drugs is concerned about their drug use; yet only 5.6 percent of respondent who frequently used marijuana and 22.5 percent of those who frequently used cocaine reported that they received treatment for drug abuse in the past year. Motivational factors may account for the failure to enter treatment in some cases, but clearly economic and political factors also contribute to the unavailability of drug abuse treatment for many of those who need and desire it.

Although the percentage of the sample reporting use of some drugs may appear small, the total numbers of persons involved is not trivial. For example, the 0.9 percent of men and 0.3 percent of women age 12 and above who reported using cocaine on 12 or more days in 1994 represents over 1.25 million people.[43] Overall, the National Household Survey data show that use is greatest for licit drugs, while nonmedical use of psychotherapeutic drugs is much lower, and use of illicit drugs is lower still. Based on these data it is possible to assert that current scheduling and prescribing practices successfully limit the availability of psychotherapeutic drugs and that criminal penalties for production, distribution, and use of illicit drugs result in even less availability and use. Moreover, review of the trends for use by comparing these data over a two-decade period shows that use and abuse of all drugs is down from historic high levels. However, there is a disturbing trend in the most recent years of significant increases in marijuana use in 12 to 17 year olds.

Monitoring the Future

The Monitoring the Future Study annually surveys approximately 17,000 seniors, 15,000 tenth graders, and 18,500 eight graders in 125 to 140 public and private schools. Students complete the pencil and paper survey, and a representative sample of eight graders and seniors are followed in ensuing years. A review of the 1975 to 1994 data outlines the study design and procedures and presents a summary of key findings.[45] The survey covers use of 18 types of drugs at four periods: lifetime, annual, past month, and daily (see Table 1 in Reference 45). As might be expected from the younger mean age of the respondents, a higher proportion of the sample report lifetime illicit drug use (45.6 percent of seniors and 57.5 percent of young adults) compared to the National Household Survey.

As in the National Household Survey, marijuana was the most frequently used illicit drug. The percentage of seniors reporting marijuana use (39 percent for lifetime and 19 percent for past month) was exceeded only by the percentage reporting cigarette use (62 percent for lifetime and 31 percent for past month). Compared to other groups, women and all college-bound seniors have lower rates of illicit drug use, and black seniors have lower rates of use of both illicit and licit drugs (see Tables 6 and 10 in Reference 45).

Lifetime prevalence of drug use by senior students has declined over the past 10 years. The year in which use peaked varied from 1979 for marijuana to 1985 for cocaine and 1986 for inhalants. While the proportion of students who use illicit drugs remains below historic peak levels, increased use has been seen since 1992 for many illicit drugs, including marijuana, stimulants, inhalants, sedatives, barbiturates, hallucinogens, and cigarettes. In 1978 10.7 percent of high school seniors reported daily use of marijuana; by 1991 this had dropped to 2.0 percent, but by 1994 it had risen to 3.6 percent. Similarly, the proportion of students who report cocaine and crack use increased in 1993 and 1994.

Continuation, defined as the percentage of lifetime users of a specific drug who continue its use in the year surveyed, varies by drug class. Less than half of the lifetime users of inhalants and heroin continues use. Higher rates of continuation (52 to 60 percent) are seen among users of PCP, stimulants, sedatives, and steroids. Even higher rates of continuation are seen among marijuana (80.4 percent) and cigarette users (85.1 percent). While continuation rates have been relatively stable for many drugs, the present high rate of continuation for marijuana represents an increased from the continuation rate of 72.3 percent reported in 1987. Continuation rates for more experienced users (10 or more times in their lifetime) are much higher than for the total group of users. For example, in 1994, the continuation rate for marijuana was 95.0 percent for the more experienced group compared to 80.4 percent for all users. For cocaine, continuation rates were 77.1 percent for the more experienced group compared to 57.6 percent for the all users (see Tables 16 and 17, Reference 45).

Johnston and colleagues[45] theorize that decline in drug use follows an increased perception of adverse effects and peer disapproval of use. As supporting evidence, they report that the percentage of students who perceive smoking marijuana regularly as being a "great risk" had increased from less than 40 percent in 1978 to over 70 percent in 1987, and that the percentage who disapprove of regular smoking of marijuana increased from 67.5 to 89.2 percent over the same period. During this same period, the percentage of students reporting marijuana use fell from 59.2 to 50.2 percent. They report that perceived risk began to drop in 1992, and that in 1993 and 1994 sharp increases in use were seen (see Figures 21a and 21b and Table 11 in Reference 45).

The 30-day prevalence of marijuana use reported by Johnston and associates[45] for young adults (14.1 percent) is similar to the National Household Survey finding that 12.1 percent of the 18- to 25-year group used marijuana in the past 30 days. This indicates that self-report data are reliable over these surveys. The question of validity of self-reports is, of course, crucial to an understanding of these survey data. An excellent overview of this issue is presented by Rouse and colleagues.[46] It is worth noting that the increases and decreases that have been reported by seniors in marijuana use since 1977 have taken place in the context of an almost universal perception of the availability of marijuana (85 to 90 percent of seniors annually report marijuana to be "fairly easy" or "very easy" to get). Johnston and his colleagues[45] argue that supply reduction has little influence on student use of illicit drugs in the face of positive drug beliefs and a pro-drug social milieu. Thus, they see perceived danger from use and perceived peer disapproval of use as major determinants of abstinence.

It should be noted that large variations exist in drug use patterns within specific subgroups and from one local community to another. It is desirable to supplement national surveys with local surveys. Good discussions and examples of this point and other methodological considerations are available.[47–49] Beauvais and Oetting[48] emphasize that surveys of local drug use patterns must be completed for effective prevention programs to be tailored to the local community's needs.

Finally, review of the trends for use by comparing these data obtained from high school students over an extended period shows that use and abuse of drugs is down from historic high levels. However, there is a disturbing trend for increased use of many drugs in the most

TABLE 46-3. THIRTY-DAY PREVALENCE OF USE (PERCENTAGES) OF 18 TYPES OF DRUGS BY SUBGROUPS, CLASS OF 1994

	Marijuana	*Inhalants*[a]	*Hallucinogens*	*LSD*	*Cocaine*[b]	*Crack*[b]	*Other Cocaine*[b]	*Heroin*	*Other Opiates*	*Stimulants*[c] *(Adjusted)*	*Barbiturates*	*Tranquilizers*	*Cigarettes*
All seniors	19.0	2.7	3.1	2.6	1.5	0.8	1.3	0.3	1.5	4.0	1.7	1.4	31.2
Sex													
Male	23.0	3.6	4.3	3.6	1.9	1.1	1.5	0.4	1.8	4.1	2.0	1.7	32.9
Female	15.1	1.9	1.7	1.6	1.1	0.5	1.0	0.2	1.2	3.8	1.4	1.1	29.2
College plans													
None or <4 yr	21.6	3.0	3.7	3.5	2.4	1.5	2.2	0.5	2.0	5.8	2.4	1.6	40.9
Complete 4 yr	17.7	2.6	2.7	2.2	1.1	0.5	0.9	0.2	1.3	3.5	1.5	1.3	28.0
Region													
Northeast	22.7	3.9	4.4	3.2	1.3	0.7	1.2	0.4	1.2	3.4	2.0	1.4	33.2
North Central	19.3	3.6	3.7	3.3	1.7	0.9	1.8	0.4	2.0	5.2	1.5	1.3	36.2
South	17.3	2.1	2.2	2.1	1.3	0.7	1.0	0.3	1.5	3.6	1.9	1.7	30.7
West	18.6	1.7	2.7	2.1	1.6	1.1	1.0	0.1	1.1	4.0	1.3	1.0	24.0
Population density													
Large SMSA	21.6	2.8	3.3	2.7	1.3	0.6	0.9	0.1	1.7	3.4	1.7	1.6	29.3
Other SMSA	19.7	2.8	3.7	3.1	1.6	1.0	1.4	0.4	1.5	3.9	1.8	1.4	30.7
Non-SMSA	15.7	2.6	1.7	1.4	1.3	0.7	1.2	0.2	1.3	4.9	1.5	1.3	33.8

Abbreviation: SMSA, Standard metropolitan area.
[a] Unjustified for known underreporting of certain drugs.
[b] Cocaine data based on five questionnaire forms; crack data based on two questionnaire forms; and other cocaine data based on one questionnaire form.
[c] Based on the data from the revised question, which attempts to exclude the inappropriate reporting of nonprescription stimulants.

recent years. This finding coupled with the National Household Survey finding of increased use of marijuana by 12 to 17 year olds emphasize the need for continued and improved prevention programs.

National Comorbidity Survey (NCS)

The NCS has provided estimates of the proportion of people who have a drug abuse or drug dependency disorder and co-occurring mental disorders. Kessler and his associates[50] adapted the Composite International Diagnostic Interview, based on DSM-III-R criteria,[11] to identify the prevalence of drug abuse, drug dependency, and co-occurring mental disorder in a stratified, multistage area probability sample of persons between 15 and 54 years of age living in households. Prevalence for both substance dependence and mental disorders was ascertained for both lifetime and within the past 12 months (current). While the NCS included alcohol and tobacco use, this discussion is limited to findings related to use of illicit drugs (i.e., illegal drugs, inhalants, and nonmedical use of psychotropic medications). Lifetime and 12-month prevalence rates for illicit drug dependency disorder were 7.5 and 1.8 percent, respectively. Among users, the current dependence rate was 3.5 percent, and among the lifetime dependent it was 23.8 percent. Males were more likely than females to report both lifetime and current use and dependence. Other demographic correlates associated with significantly higher rates of dependence included age under 45, race (white), being a homemaker or unemployed, high school education or less, low income, and living in a metropolitan or urban area or in the western United States. Religious affiliation of all types was associated with less risk for dependence.[51]

Lifetime history of use was highest for cannabis (46.3 percent), followed by cocaine (16.2 percent), stimulants (15.3 percent), anxiolytics, sedatives, and hypnotics (12.7 percent), hallucinogens (10.6 percent), inhalants (6.8 percent) and heroin (1.5 percent). Dependence rate among users for these drugs was highest for heroin (23.1 percent), followed by cocaine (16.7 percent), stimulants (11.2 percent), anxiolytics (9.2 percent), cannabis (9.1 percent), psychedelics (4.9 percent), and inhalants (3.7 percent). By comparison, tobacco use was reported by 75.6 percent of the population, and its use was associated with the highest rate of dependence (31.9 percent).[52]

The epidemiology of co-occurring addictive and mental disorders has been addressed specifically in the NCS sample.[50] Over half (52.8 percent) of the NCS respondents with current drug dependence had at least one of the affective or anxiety disorders surveyed (see Table 2 in Reference 50). Respondents with a history of co-occurring addictive and mental disorders were asked to recall retrospectively which began first. Nine of 10 drug-dependent persons with co-occurring conduct disorder or adult antisocial behavior disorder reported that symptoms of these disorders preceded drug use. Likewise, eight of 10 drug-dependent persons with co-occurring anxiety disorder reported that its symptoms preceded drug use.

Less than half the current drug-dependent persons received treatment (46.8 percent), and treatment rates were even lower for those meeting the criteria for drug abuse but not dependence (12.7 percent). For those with drug abuse, having a co-occurring mental disorder did not improve the likelihood of receiving treatment. However, current drug-dependent persons were more likely to receive treatment if they had a co-occurring mental disorder (63.1 versus 25 percent), and they were most likely to receive treatment in a specialized mental health setting rather than a substance abuse setting.[50]

In summary, the epidemiological data establish that drug abuse and drug dependence in varying degrees of severity affects much of the general population. It is clear, for example, that substance disorders are the most prevalent form of mental disorder. Nevertheless, they have historically received less attention and resources for prevention and treatment than other mental disorders. Trend analyses show that, although drug use has declined from the historic high levels seen in the 1970s (marijuana) and 1980s (cocaine), rates of use generally have risen over the past 5 years. The data also reveal differential rates and patterns of use and dependence, suggesting that not all persons are equally at risk for drug use or, given use, drug dependence. Information on correlates of drug use suggest that variables associated with drug use include age, sex, race, employment, education, and perception of adverse effects of drugs.[42–45] Dependence rates among users indicate that those drugs that activate the brain's rewarding mechanism and that are administered by routes that produce immediate effects are most likely to be associated with dependence (i.e., smoking tobacco, IV injection of heroin, smoking crack cocaine). Nevertheless, even for these drugs the majority of users do not proceed to dependence. Correlates of dependence on illicit drugs include initiation of drug use before age 17, daily smoking, and neuroticism.[52,53] Finally, the NCS data strongly suggest that persons with a history of an affective, anxiety, conduct disorder, or adult antisocial behavior are at increased risk for substance abuse disorders and that likewise people with substance abuse disorders are at increased risk for other mental disorders.[52] Respondents in these surveys generally report that symptoms of mental disorders precede initial illicit drug use. However, one cannot presume that if these symptoms were treated illicit substances would not be used. The "self-medication" hypothesis is appealing, but it needs to be tested through further research to clarify the ways in which psychiatric and substance use comorbidities develop. It should be clear, however, that once either has developed, treatment is needed. As noted, at present, the majority of drug-dependent persons with co-occurring psychiatric disorders are not treated, and only one in 10 substance abuser receives treatment.

▸ ETIOLOGY

An understanding of the causal factors that lead to the initiation and maintenance of drug abuse is fundamental to the development of prevention and treatment strategies. Substance use, abuse, and dependence are considered to result from complex interactions of biological, sociological, and psychological factors. A detailed discussion of the current major conceptualizations of drug abuse and the investigations they generate is beyond the scope of this chapter. However, since discussion of prevention activities is facilitated by an understanding of their relation to etiologic models of drug abuse, a brief discussion is warranted.

Behavioral Genetics Studies

Behavioral genetics provides the framework for one line of etiologic investigations. These studies use two experimental designs to look at the relationships among genetic factors, environmental factors, and an outcome behavior. The twin design compares identical twins and fraternal twins for similarity on a behavioral end point. The adopted-away design compares twins adopted away at birth or shortly thereafter with those raised by their natural parents for similarity on a behavioral end point when adoptive or natural parents do or do not have the behavioral end point (e.g., alcoholism). Heritability, a statistical description of the portion of the variability in the behavior that can be ascribed to genetic factors, can be determined by both approaches. These designs can clarify the contribution of genetic and environmental factors to behavioral outcomes that have been shown to be familial, that is, their occurrence differs across families historically.[54] Intelligence, personality, temperament, psychopathology, and alcoholism—and, to a lesser extent, other forms of substance abuse—have been shown to be influenced by genetic factors using these experimental designs. However, it would appear that few complex behaviors are under the control of a single gene. A recent review of behavioral genetic work concluded that "genetic effects on behavior are polygenic and probabilistic, not single gene and deterministic" and that "genetic influence on individual differences in behavioral development is usually significant and often substantial," but "nongenetic factors are responsible for more than half of the variance for most complex behaviors."[55] Environmental factors, i.e., nongenetic factors, may themselves lead to substance use, abuse, and dependency, or they may affect the manifestation of a genetic predisposition for these outcomes.

Behavioral Genetics of Substance Abuse

Most of the information we have about genetic contributions to substance abuse has come from studies of alcoholism. In this work, other forms of drug abuse generally were not considered. Cadoret and colleagues[56] reviewed twin studies that indicated a greater concordance for alcoholism in monozygotic twins than in dizygotic twins. However, the 40 to 50 percent discordance in alcoholism seen in monozygotic twins suggests a strong influence of environmental factors in the development of alcoholism. Adopted-away studies of alcoholism have clearly established that sons of alcoholic mothers or fathers are at risk for increased rates of alcoholism (23 versus 10 percent in the general population).[57] For daughters, a biological mother with alcoholism significantly increased the rate of alcoholism (10.3 percent). Rates (3.5 percent) for women with an alcoholic biological father were not significantly higher that those (2.8 percent) found in women whose biological parents were not alcoholic.[58] Cloninger and coworkers have been leaders in this field and note "an important general principle in genetic epidemiology is that disorders as prevalent as alcoholism have complex patterns of development involving the interaction of many genetic and environmental influences."[59] Genetic predisposition toward alcoholism is moderated by two types of factors, those that increase and those that decrease risk.[60–63] The identification of these factors and the ways in which they interact with any inherited factors is important to our understanding of alcoholism, and similar information about drug abuse would be very useful.

Little research has been done on the behavioral genetics of use of illicit drugs. Genetic and environmental factors in initiation of drug use and the transition to drug abuse have been examined in two "adopted-away" studies,[64] and an additional twin study has studied illicit drug abuse.[65] In the "adopted-away" studies, alcohol abuse and drug abuse/dependence co-occurred at a high rate, as 78 percent of those meeting criteria for drug abuse/dependence also met criteria for alcohol abuse compared to 8.7 percent of those with no history of illicit drug use. Interviews with the adoptive parents provided information about possible etiologic factors related to childhood and adolescent behaviors, and information about the biological parents' use of alcohol provided information about possible genetic factors. Information about use of illicit drugs by the biological parents was not available. An antisocial adoptive sibling, "bad friends," childhood and adolescent aggression, and alcohol problems in the biological parents predicted drug use. The aggression and parental factors also predicted drug abuse/dependence. While this work did not separate alcohol abuse and dependence, other work has shown that genetic influences are stronger for dependence than abuse.[65] In the recent study of illicit drug abuse in twins, a higher concordance of illicit drug abuse was found in monozygotic than in dizygotic twins, but the differences were not statistically significant.[65] Clearly, much work remains to be done if we are to understand the role of genetic factors in illicit substance abuse.

Familial Transmission Studies

Familial transmission of illicit drug abuse has received somewhat more attention than genetic transmission. Studies of the occurrence of drug abuse within families allow one to determine if there is a higher probability for drug abuse across successive generations in some family lines than in others. Although this design does not allow separation of environmental and biological factors, positive findings can be further explored through twin or adopted-away studies. Four studies have looked at opioid dependence and alcoholism in relatives of opioid-dependent probands.[66–69] Maddux and Desmond[69] reviewed the earlier studies and concluded that they support the clustering of opioid dependence, but not alcoholism, within families of addict probands. In this regard, the aggregate data support earlier work,[68] suggesting that alcoholism tended to cluster in families of alcoholics and opioid abuse in families of opioid abusers, thus raising the possibility that vulnerability to abuse of a specific drug is transmitted genetically. Additional support for the hypothesis of a genetic vulnerability to abuse of a specific drug put forth by Hill and colleagues[68] has been reported more recently.[70] Substance use and psychiatric disorders were studied in the siblings of opiate users. This group had high rates of illicit substance use (varying between 23 percent for solvents to 65 percent for marijuana), and over 90 percent of those who used were abusers. In logistic regression analyses of variables correlated with substance abuse, paternal illicit drug abuse contributed significantly to illicit drug abuse and parental alcohol abuse contributed significantly to alcohol abuse in this group.

Maddux and Desmond[69] also looked at opioid dependence and alcoholism in the parents and siblings of 235 opioid-dependent persons whose use of alcohol also was evaluated. These opioid abusers had a 56 percent lifetime prevalence of alcoholism, which is elevated over the 14 percent lifetime prevalence for males estimated by the NCS.[52] The alcoholism rate for fathers of these opioid abusers (33.2 percent) also exceeded the NCS projections, whereas those for their mothers (4.3 percent), brothers (9.9 percent), and sisters (1.3 percent) did not. Siblings' rate of opioid dependence (16.6 percent for brothers and 2.2 percent for sisters) was greater than the NCS estimated lifetime prevalence of 0.4 percent in the general population, whereas parental rate of opioid dependence (0.4 percent for fathers and zero for mothers) was not. The authors conclude that their study demonstrates familial clustering for opioid abuse but argue that this is not equivalent to familial transmission of susceptibility to abuse of a specific drug. In Maddux and Desmond's opinion, if familial transmission is operating, it consists of a generalized predisposition to either alcoholism or opioid dependence, with the principal substance of abuse being influenced by availability and peer influences.

Codependency and Comorbidity

Two factors that complicate consideration of the etiology of drug abuse are the presence of polydrug abuse (codependency) and the co-occurrence of drug abuse and a psychological disorder (comorbidity) including other substance use disorders. In a review of 75 studies that evaluated the co-occurrence of alcoholism, drug abuse, or antisocial personality, these three conditions were found to be highly associated.[71] Of the 44 studies that examined the relationship between alcoholism and drug abuse, 80 percent described positive associations. Positive associations also were reported for 76 percent of the studies examining antisocial personality and drug abuse relationships and for 79 percent of the studies investigating antisocial personality and alcoholism relationships. Another study found increased alcoholism in opiate addicts—35 versus approximately 15 percent in the local community in which the study was carried out—and 54 percent of the addicts were diagnosed as having a major depressive disorder, whereas 27 percent were found to have an antisocial personality disorder.[72] A general population study has provided evidence of codependency in that regular smoking for a month or more, as well as nicotine dependence, was found to be associated with higher rates of illicit substance abuse/dependence.[53] The NCS has also provided evidence of comorbidity in that conduct disorder and adult antisocial behavior disorder co-occurred at high rates with substance abuse and dependence.[50]

Little is known about the natural history of codependency and comorbidity in drug abusers. The NCS has not addressed the specific question of co-occurrence of multiple substance abuse disorders, but rather focuses on the co-occurrence of substance use and mental disorders which are found to be common.[50] The only prospective report detailing the natural history of drug abuse from adolescence through midlife did not evaluate psychiatric status.[73] If prevention efforts are to be based on an understanding of the etiology of drug abuse, psychiatric epidemiology and natural history studies are needed to clarify how codependency and comorbidities develop and their individual and shared risk factors. These issues are of such importance that both the National Research Council and the Institute of Medicine have recently conducted studies focusing on methodological issues and potential directions such work might take.[49,74]

Risk Factor Studies. Over the past 15 years, a number of risk factors, in addition to those discussed previously, have been identified as facilitating the initiation or augmentation of drug abuse in adolescents and young adults and the development of dependence. The following risk factors have been identified relatively consistently.

- Parents' drug use[75–77]
- Parents' educational level[78]
- Parental monitoring[79,80]
- Family strife[77,81]
- Peer drug use[82,83]
- Early drug use[52,77,84]
- Sensation seeking[85,86]
- Deviance[77,87,88]
- Poor school grades[89,90]
- Low self-esteem[77,91]
- Depression[77,92]
- Aggression[93,94]
- Age[73,95]
- Low socioeconomic status[96]

Older age of initiation of drug use, employment, and marriage are factors that are associated with decreased drug use in young adults.[93,97,98]

To understand the progression of drug use from its initiation to the point where a drug abuse or drug dependency disorder develops, many factors have been evaluated to determine if their presence can be causally linked to continued drug use, drug abuse/drug dependency disorders, other psychological disorders, or criminal behavior. Kandel and coworkers outlined developmental periods of risk for drug abuse, progression patterns, and predictors of progression.[95,99,100] Data derived from a longitudinal sample of New York high school students, who were first interviewed in the 10th or 11th year of school and again 9 years later, indicated that 90 percent of use began by age 18 for alcohol, by age 19 for cigarettes, and by age 20 for marijuana. Most use of other illicit drugs, except cocaine, was initiated before age 21. The pattern of drug abuse involvement for most of the sample consisted of progression from alcohol or cigarettes to marijuana and, subsequently, to other illicit drugs or to prescription drugs. Peers' use of marijuana was identified as an important factor for marijuana initiation. Current use of marijuana or prescription psychoactive drugs was strongly related to initiation of use of other illicit drugs. Initiation of prescription psychoactive drug use was related to multiple factors, including current or former use of illicit drugs, depression symptoms, maternal use of psychoactive drugs, and dropping out of school. Persistence of illicit drug use in young adulthood was related to the same factors that predict initiation in adolescence: peer use, delinquency, and unconventionality.[101] Important age effects in the initiation, escalation, persistence, and cessation of drug abuse and dependence have been identified.[95,98–100] Age effects must be considered in conjunction with the period and cohort trends in drug use,[102] since the modal pattern of drug abuse across age may be subject to cultural influence. In addition, the modal pattern of drug abuse combines many subpopulations with differential risks of drug abuse. Identification of the factors that separate these subgroups is critical if prevention programs are to be targeted to the needs of the specific groups.

The importance of environmental variables as risk factors has been shown in work prospectively evaluating the role of parental monitoring in children's initiation and continued use of drugs.[79,80] In a sample of elementary school children, the incidence of drug sampling, primarily initial use of alcohol and tobacco, was four times higher in the children with the least parental monitoring compared to those with the most, and this association remained significant even when other risk factors of peer use and antisocial behavior were considered. While level of parental monitoring does not influence licit drug use in older youth (older than 11) it is associated with less initiation of illicit drugs (marijuana and cocaine) and inhalants.[79]

Other work has found a highly significant linear relation between number of risk factors and extent of drug use in a high school population.[77,103] In a group of 994 adolescents, 8 percent used marijuana daily. Of these, 56 percent had 7 or more risk factors and only 1 percent had zero risk factors.

Oetting and coworkers[82,104,105] have proposed that the peer cluster, which they define as the small intimate group who shares beliefs and values, mediates the influence of other psychosocial variables on drug abuse. Furthermore, peer cluster effects are robust across various ethnic groups, whereas the importance of other variables, notably the mediating influence of anger and self-esteem, appears to vary from culture to culture in the direction and strength of their influence on drug abuse.[106]

The various studies of the etiology of drug abuse clearly indicate that primary prevention efforts should be targeted for certain populations distinguished on the basis of demographic or personal characteristics or both, especially those identified in the epidemiological studies reviewed earlier. In addition, since the probability of drug abuse may be related linearly to the number of risk factors present, intensity and content of prevention programs should be improved by tailoring them to both the extent and type of risk factors found in the population to whom the program is being delivered.

▸ PREVENTION

Research on primary prevention of drug abuse may be said to have begun in the mid-1970s with school-based programs to prevent smoking. In the ensuing two decades, research has expanded to include programs, delivered in a variety of settings, aimed at preventing illicit drug use. Bukoski[107] has provided a summary of the various models of drug abuse prevention, including public health, communicable disease, and risk factor models. In Bukoski's view, research findings support the use of a combination of prevention strategies based on the level of the individual's psychosocial development and the extent of his or her drug use. In this model, termed comprehensive prevention, various prevention strategies are focused at four levels: individual, family, peer group, and community. As they have developed over the past two and a half decades, prevention strategies have been based on theories related to: risk-factors, developmental factors, social influence, and community-specific factors. Prevention strategies have been applied to the general or a targeted population. An extensive review of primary drug abuse prevention activity is beyond the scope of this chapter. Readers who are interested in a detailed historical account of prevention research in the United States may wish to consult our chapter in the 13th edition of this book.[108] To provide a brief overview of primary prevention, we discuss several meta-analyses of outcome effects for prevention programs,[109–112] a recent evaluation sponsored by the National Research Council[49] of what is known about primary prevention, and an Institute of Medicine study of opportunities in drug abuse research.[74]

Meta-analysis of Prevention Studies

Meta-analysis allows the evaluations of programs to be merged and their overall effect sizes computed. An effect size is a ratio computed by dividing the difference between the mean of a group who received an intervention and a group who did not by the pooled standardized deviation. Thus, it contrasts mean differences between the two groups with a measure of the variation that exists within the groups when they are combined. Several meta-analyses of drug prevention programs have been carried out, and they provide the strongest available scientific evidence about the success or failure of drug prevention programs. The earliest of these studies[109] demonstrated the utility of using peers to influence, teach, counsel, and facilitate the delivery of primary prevention programs to groups of young people. Outcome measures were compared for 143 programs employing five major program modalities: (*a*) knowledge only, (*b*) affective only (designed to enhance self-esteem or general competency), (*c*) peer programs incorporating refusal skills or social skills and life skills, (*d*) knowledge plus affective, (*e*) alternative programs dealing with activities or competence. The outcome measures included knowledge, attitudes and values about drugs, decision-making, assertiveness, and refusing drugs. Changes in knowledge and attitudes about drugs were observed in several types of programs without concomitant changes in drug use. However, compared to other modalities, peer programs had significantly more influence on use of alcohol, tobacco, and illicit drugs. Tobler[109] pointed out that use of peers facilitates positive outcomes in programs designed for the average student, but that programs using alternative strategies delivered with high intensity proved to be useful with special populations, including minority ethnic groups, adolescents with poor school performance, and those who already were using drugs.

Bangert-Drowns[110] criticized Tobler on methodological grounds and applied a more stringent criterion to identify programs for inclusion in a meta-analysis of the effectiveness of school-based primary prevention programs. As a result, only data from 33 school-based prevention programs were used to evaluate the effect of prevention education on three outcome criteria: drug knowledge, drug attitudes, and drug behavior. While significant changes were found for knowledge and attitudes, no significant effects of prevention programs on drug behavior were found. In response to this criticism, Tobler conducted an analysis including only 91 programs of the original set and focused solely on drug use outcome data. Her conclusions were similar to those of the original study—that is, only peer programs provided significant effects on drug use behavior (Tobler, 1989, cited in Reference 49, pp. 79–83).

Recently Tobler and Stratton[111] examined school-based drug prevention to determine the effect sizes attributable to various characteristics of the programs. As in her earlier analysis, interactive programs that emphasize exchange of information between peers in comparison to nonparticipatory programs utilizing didactic instruction were more effective. Both noninteractive and interactive programs were effective in increasing knowledge about drug use, but the interactive programs had a much larger effect than noninteractive programs in facilitating antidrug use attitudes and decreased use. Significant findings for the interactive programs were observed for all adolescents, including minority populations, and were equal for tobacco, alcohol, marijuana, and illicit drugs. Program size was an important consideration, as larger programs had less success in preventing drug use regardless of type. For example, when high-quality experimental programs were examined by size, large programs were less effective in countermanding prodrug social influences and building comprehensive life skills. Other research[113] has suggested that program quality measures suffer when large-scale prevention programs are instituted, and this may explain the effect of program size observed by Tobler and Stratton. The authors argue that the data show that noninteractive programs should be replaced by interactive programs, as this would increase the effectiveness of school-based programs by 8.5 percent.[111] To place the success rate of the interactive programs (9.5 percent) versus the noninteractive programs (1 percent) in perspective, the authors note that a recent study of aspirin's effect on heart attacks was terminated so that aspirin could be offered to the control group when a success rate of 3.5 percent was found.

Unfortunately the most commonly implemented school-based drug prevention program relies heavily on expert instruction. Project DARE[112] has been adopted by approximately 59 percent of the local school districts nationwide. A meta-analysis of the effects of these programs[112] compared their outcomes to those of both interactive and noninteractive programs because, while DARE relies on lectures by police personnel, it does include group discussion and role playing, i.e., some peer interactive elements. Because there are few longer-term studies of DARE's effectiveness, only outcome measures obtained immediately after the course (generally 17 weeks in length) were included. Drug knowledge and attitudes, social skills, and use of tobacco, alcohol, and marijuana were examined pre- and post-intervention. The DARE intervention was superior to the noninteractive programs for all measures except drug use. Compared to the interactive programs, DARE effects were far less, ranging from being only one-third as effective in preventing drug use and fostering antidrug attitudes to being approximately one-fourth as effective in developing social skills. For drug knowledge, DARE was almost as effective as the interactive programs (mean effect size of 0.42 versus 0.53). Besides shortcomings in terms of its mode of instruction, the DARE curriculum does not use the "bogus pipeline" technique (discussed below) to validate drug use self-report, which raises questions about its validity. While the maximum impact of any widely implemented school-based prevention program has not been determined, it would appear worthwhile to replace "expert" instruction in the DARE curriculum with peer-delivered information.

In general, the analyses cited above indicate that program content, process, and size all influence the outcome of prevention efforts. The value of an interactive process and the problems of wholesale implementation have been discussed. We now turn our attention to a brief review of research on the content of prevention programs, especially social influences and comprehensive life skills programs whose effectiveness has been demonstrated,[111] and the comprehensive programs that constitute the leading edge of current research efforts.

Social Inoculation

Much of the program content for current drug abuse prevention programs comes from research, begun in the mid-1970s, on ways to enable young people to resist peer and media forces that promote use of cigarettes and alcohol. Although use of these drugs is legal for adults, it should be remembered that their purchase is illegal for youngsters, and thus, use of cigarettes and alcohol can be considered abuse in a young population. Early research on resistance skills training was conducted by Evans and coworkers[114–116] and showed that the rate of smoking initiation (8.6 and 10 percent) in nonsmokers who had participated in either of two forms of a prevention program was approximately half that of a control group (18.3 percent).

Flay[117] reviewed four generations of work on social inoculation-peer resistance techniques in which the content of the material presented is closely linked to substance use behavioral end points. The Evans work was described as "first generation." Fourth-generation studies are large-scale field trials with numerous classrooms assigned to each intervention. In these studies, participation in the prevention program was clearly related to noninitiation of smoking that did not erode over a 2-year period.[118–120] When children who had never smoked before the intervention (early in 6th grade) were surveyed at the end of 8th grade, 60 percent of the children who had taken part in the prevention program had not initiated smoking compared to 47 percent of the children in the control program. Furthermore, children who were at high risk for smoking, as defined by having parents, siblings, and friends who smoked, appeared to benefit most from the intervention. High-risk children, who had not smoked before the intervention, were retested at the end of 8th grade. Sixty-seven percent of the high-risk children who were in the prevention program still had not initiated smoking, whereas only 22 percent of the high-risk control group remained nonsmokers.

Besides pointing out specific research design and analysis issues, the work on drug abuse resistance skills training suggests that prevention can be enhanced by the development of objective, noninvasive measures of use. This point was demonstrated clearly by Evans and associates,[116] who found that presentation of a short film demonstrating that nicotine could be detected in saliva improved the accuracy of smoking self-reports. This procedure of convincing people that an objective measure of truthfulness of self-reports is available to the researcher is known as the "bogus pipeline" procedure, and it has become a standard feature of much smoking research. The improved validity and reliability associated with it strongly suggest that the development of relatively innocuous methods of testing for the presence of illicit drugs would strengthen drug abuse prevention research by allowing the bogus pipeline procedure to be used to enhance the validity of self-reports of drug use.

In their review of social influence approaches to prevention of drug use, the Committee on Drug Abuse Prevention Research pointed to several methodological shortcomings that weaken the findings of these studies.[49] These include that, in the main, studies of social inoculation prevention programs have more participant attrition than is experienced in longitudinal epidemiologic studies. In addition, social influence studies often reported differentially higher drug use in those who drop out of the studies (and school), and this attrition is not appropriately considered in evaluating the effects of the intervention on drug use. The studies also suffer from a lack of statistical power and failure to describe the extent to which the control group is exposed to drug prevention content from sources not under the control of the researchers (see Reference 49, pp. 109–110 for discussion of these issues).

Comprehensive Life Skills

Review of nine recent studies using the same basic social learning-persuasive communication theoretical framework as that reviewed by Flay[117] but concentrating on transmitting more general skills indicates that this model is an effective way of preventing drug abuse.[121] Although the nine studies shared some intervention strategies, others were unique to specific programs. Thus, the programs could be designated by their unique intervention elements, such as social assertiveness skills training,[122] cognitive-behavioral skills training,[123] decision skills training,[124] and life training skills.[125] All nine studies showed positive outcomes on one or more measures of smoking, and three reported significant effects on alcohol or marijuana use. The magnitude of the effects was "relatively large" demonstrating "that generic skills approaches to substance abuse prevention can produce about a 50 percent reduction in the incidence of substance use behavior."[121] One of these programs, the Life Skills Training curriculum is administered over 15 sessions in two forms to 7th grade students and followed up with 10 booster sessions given in 8th grade and 10 in 9th grade. The program has been evaluated for effectiveness 1, 2, and 6 years after the initial sessions. Booster sessions followed the collection of self-reports of drug use and breath samples that were used to measure expired carbon monoxide; a measure of smoking that is used to improve validity of self report. Significant reductions in smoking and marijuana use were reported for both intervention groups compared to the control group at years 1 and 6. At year 6 the prevention effect for marijuana smoking was not found.[126,127] The significantly lower polydrug use involving weekly use of tobacco and marijuana or tobacco, marijuana, and alcohol in the intervention groups provided evidence that the program was effective in preventing escalation of drug use.[127]

Comprehensive Model of Prevention

Prevention research has adopted a goal of developing theoretically based, multimodal interventions that can be disseminated on a communitywide basis without the loss of impact and at a reasonable cost. One program that promises to meet these criteria has been developed by Pentz and associates.[128] This program includes mass media programming, school-based training of drug use resistance skills, parent involvement and education, community organization, and health policy components. The research project consists of a quasi-experimental design introduced sequentially to the entire adolescent population of 15 Kansas City metropolitan area communities and replicated with a randomized experimental design in Indianapolis. In the first 2 years of the study, 22,500 children, enrolled in the 6th or 7th grade in 42 Kansas City area schools, were surveyed. Base rates of drug use were essentially equal between prevention and control classrooms. At the 1-year follow-up, prevalence rates of cigarette, marijuana, and alcohol use were significantly lower for children enrolled in schools with prevention programs (17 versus 24 percent for cigarette, 7 versus 10 percent for marijuana and 11 versus 16 percent for alcohol for the prevention and control groups, respectively). At the 2-year follow-up, 12 percent of students receiving the intervention versus 19 percent of those not receiving it reported smoking in the prior week.[129] Five-year follow-up data from the Kansas City site indicated that 24 percent of the students who received the intervention reported smoking cigarettes versus 32 percent of the control students. Alcohol was used in the preceding month by 36 percent of the students who had received the intervention and 50 percent of those who had not. Marijuana use in the past month was reported by 14 percent of the intervention students and 20 percent of the control students. In a subset of students tracked over time, 1.6 percent of the intervention students and 3.7 percent of the control students reported past month use of cocaine. In the eyes of the Committee on Drug Abuse Prevention Research, "... results from the Midwestern Prevention Project in Kansas City indicate solid, statistically significant effects on all three gateway drugs: cigarettes, alcohol, and marijuana. These effects seem to have persisted for up to 5 years following the intervention. These are the most unequivocal results produced by any social influence (or any other kind of) prevention program to date. (reference 49, pg. 101)." Future development of this model should provide guidelines to communities for providing cost-efficient effective prevention measures to school-age children, who compose one of the largest populations at risk for drug abuse.

The measure of drug use that has been most affected by school- and community-based prevention programs appears to be the onset of tobacco, marijuana, and alcohol use. The majority of students who have received prevention interventions have been white, middle-class students. However, there is some evidence that programs may be generalized to other youth. The Life Skills Training program has been implemented with black urban youth who at the 3-month follow-up had a 56 percent reduction in smoking prevalence.[130] It has also been provided to a predominately Hispanic school population in the New York City area where preliminary evidence indicated that it was effective.[131]

Future work must further address the generalizability of prevention programs to various subpopulations. Likewise, future work will need to design early intervention programs for children with specific risks for drug abuse and employ long-term follow-up measures to determine the effect of the interventions on substance abuse. For example, Kellam and coworkers have initiated a prevention program with shy-aggressive early elementary age children who are at risk for drug abuse as teenagers.[132] This work and similarly designed studies will determine whether delaying the onset of smoking influences the onset of use of other drugs and whether or not nonuse of these substances during preteen and teenage years protects high-risk persons from abuse of drugs at later stages of life.

Once drug use is begun, frequency of use is an important variable in predicting whether or not it will be continued. Kandel and associates studied persons, identified at age 15 or 16 as having used illicit drugs at least 10 times, for their drug use at ages 24 or 25. Continuance rates of 80 percent for marijuana and 75 percent for other illicit drugs were found for men, and for women these rates were 71 percent for marijuana and 59 percent for other illicit drugs.[93] Thus, these data indicate that a large number of persons, particularly males, who use an illicit drug 10 or more times are likely to continue drug use. The household survey data indicate that people who use drugs are concerned about it. Taken together, these studies indicate a need for research on the transition from light to heavier drug use and the development of intervention programs targeted at people who are already abusing drugs but in whom the drug use pattern has not become so severe as to warrant a diagnosis of drug abuse/drug dependence disorder. Furthermore, the data suggest that intervention programs sensitive to the circumstances of males in low socioeconomic groups, which includes many racial and ethnic minorities, are especially needed given the picture of continuation, and perhaps escalation, of drug use in this group.

Finally, much work remains to be done on the questions of codependency among the various forms of drug abuse and comorbidity with other mental disorders to determine the degree to which prevention of drug abuse must be conceptualized as an activity independent of other preventive mental health activities.

▶ TREATMENT OF DRUG ABUSE

The major goal of treatment is to eliminate or reduce drug use and its associated morbidity among drug abusers and drug-dependent persons and to prevent their relapse to drug use after treatment. Psychoactive substance use disorders[11] are characterized by maladaptive behavioral changes associated with more or less regular use of the substance or irregular use in amounts that impair functioning. Classification of psychoactive substance abuse disorders has undergone continual revision and refinement over the past 30 years and reflects the growth of empirical knowledge about the behavioral pharmacology of abused drugs and clinical experience with populations who abuse them. Psychoactive substance use disorders have been defined for 10 categories of drugs: alcohol, amphetamine, cannabis, cocaine, hallucinogen, inhalant, nicotine, opioid, phencyclidine, and sedative, hypnotic, or anxiolytic drugs. In general, two subcategories exist for each disorder: abuse and dependence. In addition, polydrug dependence and abuse of other unspecified psychoactive substances is recognized. It is estimated that approximately 3.6 million Americans have psychoactive substance use disorders, other than alcohol abuse/dependence, severe enough to warrant treatment.[133]

Most of the 72 million persons who indicated use of illicit drugs in the 1994 NIDA Household Survey do not use amounts of drugs or suffer consequences of use that characterize drug abuse or meet the diagnostic criteria for psychoactive substance use disorders. Most of these people do not require assistance to cease using illicit drugs beyond the kind of information and social sanctions that are widely available. Another sizable group of persons whose use of illicit drugs becomes a problem finds the help they need to change their behavior in self-help groups, such as the 12-step programs or through personal resources, such as family, friends, and church. A small portion of the people who initiate use of an illicit psychoactive substance, who nonetheless compose a large number of people, go on to use drugs in ways that are troublesome to them and their families and find that they are unable to initiate or maintain the behavior changes necessary to become drug free without the aid of a treatment program. The proportion of people who escalate from substance use to dependence varies with the class of drug used[52] as well as with other environmental and organismic (e.g., genetic) variables.[134]

Over the past 30 years, treatment programs designed to provide services to drug abusers have been established by federal, state, and local governments. Public treatment programs can be categorized by the primary treatment modality offered: methadone-maintenance; outpatient drug-free programs; therapeutic communities and chemical dependency programs that are provided generally in three settings, outpatient, residential, and hospital inpatient. Private, nonprofit, or for-profit facilities also are available, which usually are residential, inpatient programs that treat clients who pay for the service directly or through health insurance. The National Drug and Alcoholism Treatment Unit Survey (NDATUS) conducted by SAMHSA is a voluntary survey of various aspects of treatment provided by private and public treatment facilities. This survey reported that almost 1 million people were in treatment for a substance use disorder in the year 1993.[135] Of these, approximately 20 percent were in treatment for illicit drug use, and an additional 30 percent were in treatment for illicit drug abuse/dependence in combination with an alcohol problem. The remaining 50 percent were in treatment for alcohol dependence only. Thus, of the 3.6 million people who are estimated to be in need of treatment for an illicit substance use disorder only approximately 0.5 million were enrolled in 1993. There are a variety of reasons why so few people in need are receiving treatment for illicit drug abuse/dependence including lack of motivation compounded by waiting lists for vacancies in overcrowded underfunded public treatment programs. Regardless of the reasons, it is safe to say that many people who need treatment for drug abuse are not receiving it.

Treatment Evaluation

Two large-scale treatment evaluation programs have been carried out from the early 1970s to the present. They have unequivocally established that drug abuse treatment is successful in reducing illicit drug use and in improving the functioning of clients.

Drug Abuse Reporting Program (DARP)

This was the first nationally based evaluation of the effectiveness of drug abuse treatment. The study obtained data from clients entering detoxification, methadone maintenance, residential, or drug-free treatment between 1969 and 1973 and at periods thereafter for up to 12 years. DARP included 44,000 clients from 52 programs, and the findings were reported in detail.[136–138] Hubbard and colleagues[139] concluded that these studies provided convincing evidence of drug abuse treatment effectiveness in reducing drug use and criminal activity associated with drug use. The length of time spent in treatment was the variable most predictive of success in treatment, and the modalities of treatment did not have different success rates. The DARP study clearly identified the chronic nature of drug abuse, since approximately 80 percent of the clients who were included in the 12-year follow-up study had re-entered treatment in the interval following the conclusion of their initial treatment.

Treatment Outcome Prospective Study (TOPS)

TOPS evaluated treatment received between 1979 and 1981.[139] The study used a longitudinal, prospective cohort research design. Approximately 10,000 clients who entered 37 urban treatment programs representing three modalities of treatment—methadone maintenance, residential, and outpatient drug-free—were interviewed at intake, at 3-month intervals during treatment, and at 3 months and 1, 2, 3, and 5 years posttreatment. Not all former patients were selected at each follow-up period, but between 70 and 80 percent of the large number of clients designated were interviewed at each data collection point. TOPS patients may be considered as representative of the national treatment population.[140,141] Patient characteristics differed across the three treatment modalities in terms of previous treatment history for drug abuse, alcohol abuse, or mental illness, as well as in terms of referral to treatment through the criminal justice system. The length of time clients spent in treatment varied by type of program, with methadone clients averaging 38.4 weeks; residential clients, 21.3 weeks, and outpatient drug free clients, 14.6 weeks. Dropout rates for clients in the first month were 41.2 percent for outpatient drug-free, 32.1 percent for residential, and 19.1 percent for methadone programs. However, half the clients who stayed in outpatient drug-free and methadone programs 3 months or more completed treatment, as did 38 percent of those who remained in residential programs for this length of time. Clients in all programs were predominantly young, poorly educated men.

The most important predictor of success in treatment was length of time in the program, with 6 to 12 months of treatment being necessary to produce positive outcomes on drug use variables. One-year abstinence rates and improvement rates for clients in all three types of programs were similar for heroin, cocaine, and nonmedical use of psychoactive drugs. Between 40 and 50 percent of all clients remained abstinent at 1 year, and 70 to 80 percent improved at 1 year in comparison to their pretreatment pattern of use. Marijuana use proved resistant to treatment, however. Between 55 and 65 percent of those clients who remained in treatment for 3 or more months used marijuana regularly in the year before entering treatment. At 1, 2, 3, and 5 years posttreatment, between 30 and 45 percent of these clients continued its regular use. Marijuana use was particularly persistent in young male clients. Heavy drinking in the year before entering treatment was characteristic of approximately one-fourth of the methadone clients and one-third of the clients in residential and outpatient drug-free programs. Three to 5 years later, heavy drinking had decreased by 6 to 8 percent.

Duration of treatment also predicted success on several other outcome measures. Clients who stayed in outpatient drug-free treatment for at least 6 months or in residential treatment for at least 1 year were approximately twice as likely to be employed full-time in the year after treatment as were those whose stays were shorter. Methadone clients who completed treatment or remained in long-term treatment were 50 percent more likely to be employed full-time than methadone clients who dropped out of treatment. Suicidal indicators in clients treated for more than 3 months decreased by one-third to one-half in the 3- to 5-year posttreatment period compared with the year before entering treatment.

A more recent study[142] has confirmed the importance of time in treatment for positive outcomes but in addition found large differences between programs in the percentage of methadone clients who became abstinent from cocaine and heroin use while in treatment. In the six programs studied, the percentage of clients who continued drug use while in treatment varied by a factor of 11 for heroin and of 8 for cocaine. The authors related continued use to program deficiencies, low methadone maintenance dosage, and length of time in program.

In the year before entering treatment, 33.3 percent of the methadone and outpatient drug-free clients and 60 percent of the residential clients in the TOPS study had committed one or more predatory crimes, that is, aggravated assault, robbery, burglary, theft, auto theft, forgery or embezzlement, and sale of stolen property. At 3- to 5-years posttreatment, less than 10 percent of the residential treatment clients was engaged in any predatory crime. Rates of predatory crime involvement also were decreased by approximately 18 percent for clients of the methadone programs and by 20 percent for residential program clients. Length of time in treatment was associated with significantly decreased predatory crime for clients in all three types of programs. Economic analyses indicate that the costs of treatment are offset by the savings to society from the decreased amount of crime committed by these clients during and after treatment.[143]

Re-entry to treatment was very characteristic of the clients included in TOPS. Within a year of concluding the course of treatment that had brought them into contact with TOPS, almost one-third had returned to treatment, with the average interval for returning being 3 months. Methadone program clients were more likely than clients of other programs to re-enter treatment. This pattern, of course, emphasizes the chronic nature of drug abuse problems seen in persons dependent on licit[144] as well as illicit drugs.

In summary, the TOPS data conclusively show that, for those who stay in treatment for reasonable lengths of time, the process leads to decreased drug use for most drugs, decreased predatory crime and suicidal intention, and improvement on a number of other variables associated with productive lives and that these benefits last for a significant period of time after treatment is concluded. On the other hand, it is obvious that not all clients who enter treatment programs become abstinent during that particular course of treatment and that a large number of people who terminate a course of treatment return for additional treatment.

Treatment Research

The information from the two large studies on the usefulness of treatment points to several problems that are the focus of much basic research on treatment processes. One major question concerns the nature of relapse—Why does a person who becomes free of drugs revert to their use? What constitutes psychological dependence and how is this related to relapse? Are there ways to maximize the probability that a person will remain free of drug use? Much of the work in this field examines the contributions of learned factors in drug dependence.

Several investigators have concentrated on the role of environmental cues in relapse to drug use,[145,146] showing that when confronted with cues associated with drug use, abstinent abusers exhibit conditioned craving and withdrawal. These responses can be reduced by exposing the addict repeatedly to conditioned stimuli in the absence of drug, that is, in an extinction procedure.[147,148] Childress and coworkers[149] have designed treatments for methadone outpatients, detoxifying methadone inpatients, abstinent opioid users, and abstinent cocaine users. Stimuli associated with an individual's specific craving and withdrawal responses are identified and extinguished, better enabling the client to encounter these stimuli in the environment without discomfort or the desire to use drugs. This approach promises to decrease relapse in clients. For example, these investigators presented data on treatment of craving in clients being treated for cocaine abuse. Cue exposure in combination with psychotherapy proved better than other treatments in retaining the clients in treatment and decreasing the likelihood that their urine samples would be found to contain cocaine.

To improve treatment, laboratory and clinical studies have been conducted to investigate the role of pharmacological and behavioral variables controlling drug-seeking and drug-taking behavior (see chapter 2 of Reference 74 for further review of this issue). Many successful studies have investigated the role of contingency management procedures for reinforcing drug abstinence. In one study,[150] for example, methadone clients were permitted to take home their medication provided their urine tests did not show evidence of abuse of drugs. Under these conditions, illicit drug use was decreased. More recently, contingency management treatment programs using vouchers exchangeable for goods and services, which were contingent upon cocaine-free urines, have been shown to be highly effective in assisting cocaine-dependent clients to initiate and maintain cocaine abstinence.[151,152]

Medication Development

Another line of ongoing research aimed at improving treatment of drug abusers focuses on developing medications that may be useful in attenuating the reinforcing effects of drugs, in alleviating the craving for drugs once the person becomes drug free, or in lessening the adverse effects of drug withdrawal. Methadone has been available for treatment of opiate-dependent persons since the 1960s, and, as discussed above, methadone treatment is successful in reducing drug use and improving other areas of functioning. Since 1984, naltrexone, an opiate antagonist that blocks the euphoric effects of heroin, has been available for treatment. Its use has been limited, however, and additional research is needed to evaluate the circumstances under which it will be useful.[153] In 1993 1-α-acetylmethadol (LAAM) received approval by the Food and Drug Administration (FDA) for the treatment of opiate dependence. It has been found to be as effective as methadone and, because of its long-acting active metabolite, it needs only to be administered three times weekly. Guidelines for its use were published in 1995 by the SAMHSA.[154] Buprenorphine, a methadone-type drug with less potential for toxicity and dependence-producing properties will soon be approved by the FDA for the treatment of opiate dependence.[155,156] In addition, medications are needed that will block cocaine's euphoric properties as well as reduce cocaine craving. Initial work indicated that desipramine treatment assists clients to abstain from cocaine use better than does lithium or a placebo.[157] Unfortunately this has not been confirmed by subsequent studies,[158] and there are currently no accepted medications for the treatment of cocaine abuse/dependence. The National Institute on Drug Abuse has established medication development as a research priority, and it is hoped that this action will lead to the development of medications that will enable clinicians to treat those drug abusers who are not helped by current methods.

Aftercare

In the same way that increasing life skills decreases the initiation of drug use (see Prevention), the acquisition of life skills helps former drug abusers to prevent relapse to drug use once treatment is completed. One current research program employs four modules—recovery training, self-help meetings, weekend and holiday recreational and social activities, and a network of senior ex-addicts—to specifically address factors that are related to relapse. The program is provided in an outpatient group setting for a 26-week period after discharge from a primary treatment program. The significant reduction in relapse to illicit opiates and increase in the percentage of persons holding jobs reported for the clients in this program[159] emphasize the high priority that should be given to aftercare in planning treatment programs.

▸ CONCLUSION

Recent research on the epidemiology and etiology of drug abuse, as well as its prevention and treatment, has been presented. Epidemiological studies have provided information on the extent and pattern of drug abuse in the United States, and within the general population the use of illicit drugs is clearly down from historic high levels of the 1970s and 1980s. In the past few years there has been, however, a small but consistent rise in illicit drug use as revealed by the epidemiologic data review earlier. Although the rates of drug use are still relatively low when compared to peak years in the 1970s and 1980s, this recent upward trend is still a matter of concern. The decreases in the prevalence rates of illicit drug abuse seen from the period of 1985 through the early nineties are thought to reflect the improved methods for delivering primary prevention programs that have evolved over the past 20 years. For example, meta-analysis of school-based prevention intervention programs indicates clearly that drug use is decreased when students are actively involved in program activities. The recent upward trend makes it clear that there is a need to continue these programs and the research that leads to their improvement so that we can prevent a continued increase in the prevalence of illicit drug use. Along with interactive school-based primary prevention programs, there is a need to develop effective programs that can be delivered in other settings, e.g., college-based or work-group based.

There are additional concerns that drug abuse is a problem that has become endemic in certain portions of our general population, notably the educationally, economically, and socially disadvantaged. Besides these demographic risk factors, numerous other risk factors have been identified that suggest the need to tailor prevention, intervention, and treatment programs to specific groups in the future.

In contrast to the opinion held by many people that treatment for drug abuse is futile, outcome studies demonstrate that treatment of drug abuse is useful in reducing abuse of drugs, drug-related antisocial behavior, and other adverse consequences of drug use. However, the high proportion of persons who drop out of treatment demonstrates the need for improved methods of treatment, including pharmacological methods of treating cocaine abuse and improving treatment of opiate abusers. Finally, the high relapse rate for drug abuse suggests the need for the design and delivery of intensive aftercare programs for persons who successfully complete drug abuse treatment.

▸ REFERENCES

1. Blum R: Contemporary threats to adolescent health in the United States. JAMA 257:3390–3395, 1987
2. Rice DP, Kelman S, Miller LS: Estimates of economic costs of alcohol and drug abuse and mental illness, 1985 and 1988. Public Health Rep 106:280–292, 1991
3. Centers for Disease Control and Prevention: AIDS associated with injecting-drug use—United States, 1995. MMWR 45:392–398, 1996
4. Hellinger FJ: The lifetime cost of treating a person with HIV. JAMA 270:474–478, 1993
5. Moore RD, Hidalgo J, Bareta JC, Chaisson RE: Zidoverdine therapy and health resource utilization in AIDS. J Acquir Immune Defic Syndr 7:349–354, 1994
6. Ashley MJ, Rankin JC: A public health approach to the prevention of alcohol-related health problems. Annu Rev Public Health 9:233–271, 1988
7. Gibson C (ed): Drugs of Abuse. US Department of Justice, Drug Enforcement Administration. Washington, DC: Government Printing Office, 1996
8. Falk JL, Feingold DA: Environmental and cultural factors in the behavioral action of drugs. In Meltzer HY (ed): Psychopharmacology: The Third Generation of Progress. New York: Raven Press, 1987, pp 1503–1510
9. Brecher EM: Licit and Illicit Drugs: The Consumers Union Report on Narcotics, Stimulants, Depressants, Inhalants, Hallucinogens and Marijuana—Including Caffeine, Nicotine and Alcohol. Boston: Little, Brown, 1972
10. Eddy NB, Halbach H, Isbell H, Seevers MH: Drug dependence: its significance and characteristics. Bull World Health Organ 32: 721–733, 1965
11. American Psychiatric Association: Diagnostic and Statistical Manual of Mental Disorders. 4th ed. Washington, DC: American Psychiatric Association, 1994
12. Jaffe JH: Drug addiction and drug use. In Gilman AG, Goodman S, Rall TW, Murad F (eds): The Pharmacological Basis of Therapeutics. New York: Macmillan, 1985, pp 532–581
13. Johanson CE, Balster RL: A summary of the results of a drug self-administration study using substitution procedures in rhesus monkeys. Bull Narc 30:43–54, 1978
14. Johanson CE, Schuster CR: Animal models of drug-self administration. In Mello NK (ed): Advances in Substance Abuse: Behavioral and Biological Research, vol 11. Greenwich, CT: JAI Press, 1981, pp 219–297
15. Cohen S: Coca paste and freebase: new fashions in cocaine use. Drug Abuse Alcohol News 9, 1980
16. Robins LN: The interaction of setting and predisposition in explaining novel behavior: drug initiations before, in, and after Vietnam. In Kandel DB (ed): Longitudinal Research on Drug Use. Washington, DC: Hemisphere, 1978, pp 179–196
17. Deneau G, Yanagita T, Seevers MH: Self-administration of psychoactive substances by the monkey: a measure of psychological dependence. Psychopharmacologia 16:30–48, 1969
18. Hughes J, Smith TW, Kosterlitz HW, et al: Identification of two related pentapeptides from the brain with potent opiate agonist activity. Nature 258:577, 1975
19. Cooper IR, Bloom FE, Roth RH: The Biochemical Basis of Neuropharmacology. New York: Oxford University Press, 1986
20. Reisine T, Pasternak, G. Opioid analgesics and antagonists. In Hardman JG, Gilman AG, Limbird, L (eds): Goodman & Gilman's The Pharmacological Basis of Therapeutics. 9th ed. New York: McGraw-Hill, 1996, pp 521–555
21. Koob GF, Bloom FE: Cellular and molecular mechanisms of drug dependence. Science 242:715–723, 1988
22. Mogil JS, Grisel JE, Reinscheid RK, Civelli O, et al: Orphanin FQ is a functional anti-opioid peptide. Neuroscience 75:333–337, 1996
23. Siegel S, MacRae J: Environmental specificity of tolerance. Trends Neurosci 7:140–142, 1984
24. Hobbs WR, Rall TW, Verdoorn TA: Hypnotics and sedatives; ethanol. In Hardman JG, Gilman AG, Limbird, L (eds): Goodman & Gilman's The Pharmacological Basis of Therapeutics. 9th ed. New York: McGraw-Hill, 1996, pp 361–396
25. Sellers EM, Busto U: Benzodiazepines and ethanol: assessment of the effects and consequences of psychotropic drug interactions. J Clin Psychopharmacol 2:249–262, 1982
26. Ellinwood EH Jr: Amphetamine psychosis. 1. Description of the individuals and process. J Nerv Ment Dis 144:273–283, 1967

27. Gawin FH, Ellinwood EH: Cocaine and other stimulants: actions, abuse and treatment. N Engl J Med 318:1173–1182, 1988
28. Manschreck TC, Allen DF, Neville M: Freebase psychosis: cases from a Bahamian epidemic of cocaine abuse. Comp Psychiatry 28:555–564, 1987
29. Jeri FR, Sanchez CC, del Pozo T, et al: Further experience with the syndromes produced by coca paste smoking. Bull Narc 30:1–11, 1978
30. Lesko LM, Fischman MW, Javaid JI, Davis JM: Iatrogenous cocaine psychosis. N Engl J Med 307:1153, 1982
31. Kilbey MM, Ellinwood EH Jr: Reverse tolerance to stimulant-induced behavior. Life Sci 20:1063–1076, 1977
32. Benowitz NL: How toxic is cocaine? Ciba Found Symp 166: 125–148, 1992
33. Hearn WL, Rose S, Wagner J, et al: Cocaethylene is more potent than cocaine in mediating lethality. Pharmacol Biochem Behav 3:531–533, 1991
34. Weiner N: Norepinephrine, epinephrine, and the sympathomimetic amines. In Gilman AG, Goodman LS, Rall TW, Murad F (eds): The Pharmacological Basis of Therapeutics. New York: Macmillan, 1985, pp 145–180
35. Johanson CE, Schuster CR: Cocaine. In Bloom FE, Kupfer DJ (eds): Psychopharmacology: The Fourth Generation of Progress. New York: Raven Press, 1995, pp 1685–1697
36. Balster RL, Wessinger WD: Central nervous system depressant effects of phencyclidine. In Kamenka JM, Domino EF, Geneste P (eds): Phencyclidine and Related Arylcyclohexylamines: Present and Future Applications. Ann Arbor, MI: NPP Books, 1983, pp 291–309
37. Mechoulam R: Marihuana chemistry. Science 168:1159–1166, 1970
38. Harris LS, Dewey WL, Razdan RK: Cannabis: its chemistry, pharmacology, and toxicology. In Martin WR (ed): Drug Addiction 11: Amphetamine, Psychotogen, and Marihuana Dependence. vol. 45. Handbuch der Experimentellen Pharmakologie. Berlin: Springer-Verlag, 1977, pp 371–429
39. Beardsley PM, Balster RL, Harris LS: Dependence on tetrahydrocannabinol in rhesus monkeys. J Pharmacol Exp Ther 239:311–319, 1986
40. Jones RT: Cannabis tolerance and dependence. In Fehr KO, Kalant H (eds): Cannabis and Health Hazards. Toronto: Addiction Research Foundation, 1983, pp 617–689
41. Substance Abuse and Mental Health Services Administration: The Development and Implementation of a New Data Collection Instrument for the 1994 National Household Survey on Drug Abuse. DHHS Publication No (SMA) 96-3084. Washington, DC: Government Printing Office, 1996
42. Substance Abuse and Mental Health Services Administration: National Household Survey on Drug Abuse: Main Findings 1994. DHHS Publication No. (SMA) 96-3085. Washington, DC: Government Printing Office, 1996
43. Substance Abuse and Mental Health Services Administration: National Household Survey on Drug Abuse: Population Estimates, 1994. DHHS Publication No. (SMA) 95-3063. Washington, DC: Government Printing Office, 1995
44. Chilcoat H, Schutz C: Racial/ethnic and age differences in crack use within neighborhoods. Addiction Research 3:103–111, 1995
45. Johnston LD, O'Malley PM, Bachman JG: National Survey Results on Drug Use from The Monitoring the Future Study, 1975–1994. NIH Publication No 95-4026. Washington, DC: Government Printing Office, 1995
46. Rouse BA, Kozel NJ, Richards LG (eds): Self-Report Methods of Estimating Drug Use: Meeting Current Challenges to Validity. NIDA Research Monograph No 57, (ADM) 85-1402. Washington, DC: Government Printing Office, 1985
47. Murray DM, Perry CL, O'Connell C, Schmid L: Seventh-grade cigarette, alcohol, and marijuana use: distribution in a north central U.S. metropolitan population. Int J Addict 22:357–376, 1987
48. Beauvais F, Oetting ER: Adolescent drug use: findings of national and local surveys. J Consult Clin Psychol 58(4):385–394, 1990
49. Gerstein DR, Green LW (eds): Preventing Drug Abuse: What Do We Know? Washington DC: National Academy Press, 1993
50. Kessler RC, Nelson CB, McGonagle KA, et al: The epidemiology of co-occurring addictive and mental disorders: Implications for prevention and service utilization. Am J Orthopsychiatry 66:17–31, 1996
51. Warner LA, Kessler RC, Hughes M, et al: Prevalence and correlates of drug use and dependence in the United States. Arch Gen Psychiatry 52:219–229, 1995
52. Anthony JC, Warner LA, Kessler RC: Comparative epidemiology of dependence on tobacco, alcohol, controlled substances, and inhalants: basic findings from the National Comorbidity Survey. Experimental & Clinical Psychopharmacology 2:244–268, 1994
53. Breslau N, Kilbey MM: Nicotine dependence, major depression and anxiety in young adults. Arch Gen Psychiatry 48:1069–1074, 1991
54. Cotton NS: The familial incidence of alcoholism: a review. J Stud Alcoholism 40:89–116, 1979
55. Plomin R: Environment and genes: determinants of behavior. Am Psychol 44:105–111, 1989
56. Cadoret RJ, Cain CA, Grove WM: Development of alcoholism in adoptees raised apart from alcoholic biologic relatives. Arch Gen Psychiatry 37:561–563, 1980
57. Bohman M, Cloninger R, Sigvardsson S, von Knorring AL: The genetics of alcoholismis and related disorders. J Psychiatr Res 21:447–452, 1987
58. Bohman M, Sigvardsson S, Cloninger CR: Maternal inheritance of alcohol abuse: cross fostering analysis of adopted women. Arch Gen Psychiatry 38:965–969, 1981
59. Cloninger CR, Sigvardsson S, von Knorring AL, Bohman M: The Swedish studies of the adopted children of alcoholics: a reply to Littrell. J Stud Alcohol 49:500–509, 1988
60. Cloninger CR, Bohman M, Sigvardsson S: Inheritance of alcohol abuse: cross-fostering analysis of adopted men. Arch Gen Psychiatry 38:861–868, 1981
61. Cloninger CR, Bohman M, Sigvardsson S, von Knorring AL: Psychopathology in adopted-out children of alcoholics. The Stockholm adoption study. Recent Dev Alcohol 3:37–51, 1985
62. Wolin S, Bennett L, Noonan D: Family rituals and the recurrence of alcoholism over generations. Am J Psychiatry 136:589–593, 1979
63. Wolin S, Bennett L, Noonan D, Teitelbaum M: Disrupted family rituals: a factor in the intergenerational transmission of alcoholism. J Stud Alcohol 41:199–214, 1980
64. Cadoret RJ: Genetic and environmental factors in initiation of drug use and transition to abuse. In M Glantz, R Pickens (eds): Vulnerability to Drug Abuse. Washington DC: American Psychological Association, 1992, pp 99–113
65. Pickens R, Svikis D, McGue M, et al: Heterogeneity in the inheritance of alcoholism: a study of male and female twins. Arch Gen Psychiatry 48:19–28, 1991
66. Ellinwood EH, Smith WG, Vaillant GE: Narcotic addict males and females: a comparison. Int J Addict 1:33–55, 1966
67. O'Donnell JA: Narcotic Addicts in Kentucky. National Institute on Drug Abuse. DHHS Publication No 1881. Washington, DC: Government Printing Office, 1969
68. Hill SY, Cloninger CR, Ayre FR: Independent familial transmission of alcoholism and opiate abuse. Alcohol Clin Exp Res 1:335–342, 1977
69. Maddux JF, Desmond DF: Family and environment in the choice of opioid dependence or alcoholism. Am J Alcohol Abuse 15:117–134, 1989
70. Marikangas KR, Rounsaville BJ, Prusoff BA: Familial factors in vulnerability to substance abuse. In Glantz M, Pickens R (eds) Vulnerability to Drug Abuse. Washington DC: American Psychological Association, 1992, pp 75–97

71. Grande TP, Wolf AW, Schubert DSP, et al: Associations among alcoholism, drug abuse and antisocial personality: a review of the literature. Psychol Rep 55:455–474, 1984
72. Kosten TR, Rounsaville BJ, Kleber HD: Parental alcoholism in opioid addicts. J Nerv Ment Dis 173:461–469, 1985
73. Chen K, Kandel DB: The natural history of drug use from adolescence to the mid-thirties in a general population sample. Am J Public Health 85:41–47, 1995
74. Committee on Opportunities in Drug Abuse Research: Pathways of Addition: Opportunities in Drug Abuse Research. Washington DC: National Academy Press, 1996
75. Kandel DB: Adolescent marijuana use: role of parents and peers. Science 181:1067–1070, 1973
76. Newcomb MD, Huba GJ, Bentler PM: Mother's influence on the drug use of their children: confirmatory tests of direct modeling and mediational theories. Dev Psychol 19:714–726, 1983
77. Newcomb MD, Maddahian E, Bentler PM: Risk factors for drug use among adolescents: concurrent and longitudinal analyses. Am J Public Health 76:525–531, 1986
78. Robinston TN, Killen JD, Taylor CB, et al: Perspectives on adolescent substance use: a defined population study. JAMA 258:2072–2076, 1987
79. Chilcoat H, Anthony J: Impact of parent monitoring on initiation of drug use through late childhood. J Am Acad Child Adolesc Psychiatry 35:91–100, 1996
80. Chilcoat H, Dishion T, Anthony J: Parent monitoring and the incidence of drug sampling in urban elementary school children. Am J Epidemiol 141:25–31, 1995
81. Pandina RJ, Schuele J: Psychosocial correlates of adolescent alcohol and drug use. J Stud Alcohol 44:950–973, 1983
82. Oetting ER, Beauvais F: Peer cluster theory: drugs and the adolescent. J Couns Dev 65:17–22, 1986
83. Hawkins JD, Catalano RF, Miller JY: Risk and protective factors for alcohol and other drug problems in adolescence and early adulthood: implications for substance abuse prevention. Psychol Bull 112:64–105, 1992
84. Tennant FS, Detels R, Clark V: Some childhood antecedents of drug and alcohol abuse. Am J Epidemiol 102:377–384, 1975
85. Huba GJ, Newcomb MD, Bentler PM: Comparison of canonical correlation and interbattery factor analysis on sensation seeking and drug use domains. Appl Psychol Meas 5:291–306, 1981
86. Segal B, Huba GJ, Singer JL: Prediction of college drug use from personality and inner experience. Int J Addict 15:849–867, 1980
87. Jessor R, Jessor SL: Problem Behavior and Psychosocial Development. New York: Academic Press, 1977
88. Jessor R, Jessor SL: Theory testing in longitudinal research on marijuana use. In Kandel DB (ed): Longitudinal Research on Drug Use: Empirical Findings and Methodological Issues. Washington, DC: Hemisphere, 1978, pp 41–71
89. Gossett JT, Lewis JM, Phillips VA: Psychological characteristics of adolescent drug users and abstainers: some implications for prevention education. Bull Menninger Clin 36:425–435, 1972
90. Mills CJ, Noyes HL: Patterns and correlates of initial and subsequent drug use among adolescents. J Consult Clin Psychol 52:231–243, 1984
91. Kaplan HB: Increase in self-rejection as an antecedent of deviant responses. J Youth Adolesc 4:438–458, 1975
92. Aneshensel CS, Huba GJ: Depression, alcohol use, and smoking over one year: a four-wave longitudinal causal model. J Abnorm Psychol 92:134–150, 1983
93. Kandel DB, Simcha-Fagan O, Davies M: Risk factors for delinquency and illicit drug use from adolescence to young adulthood. J Drug Issues 16:67–90, 1986
94. Kellam SG, Brown CH, Rubin BR, Ensminger ME: Paths leading to teenage psychiatric symptoms and substance use: developmental epidemiological studies in Woodlawn. In Guze SB, Earls FJ, Barrett JE (eds): Childhood Psychopathology and Development. New York: Raven Press, 1983, pp 17–51
95. Kandel DB, Logan JA: Patterns of drug use from adolescence to young adulthood: I Periods of risk for initiation, continued use, and discontinuation. Am J Public Health 74:660–666, 1984
96. Auslander G: Social networks and the functional health status of the poor. J Community Health 13:197–209, 1988
97. Bachman JG, O'Malley PM, Johnston LD: Drug use among young adults: the impacts of role status and social environments. J Pers Soc Psychol 47:629–645, 1984
98. Breslau N, Peterson EL: Smoking cessation in young adults: age at initiation of cigarette smoking and other suspected influences. Am J Public Health 86:324–220, 1996
99. Yamaguchi K, Kandel DB: Patterns of drug use from adolescence to young adulthood: II Sequence of progression. Am J Public Health 74:668–672, 1984
100. Yamaguchi K, Kandel DB: Patterns of drug use from adolescence to young adulthood: III Predictors progression. Am J Public Health 74:673–681, 1984
101. Kandel DB, Raveis VH: Cessation of illicit drug use in young adulthood. Arch Gen Psychiatry 46:109–116, 1989
102. O'Malley PM, Bachman JG, Johnston LD: Period, age and cohort effects on substance use among American youth. Am J Public Health 74:682–688, 1984
103. Bry BH, McKeon P, Pandina RJ: Extent of drug use as a function of number of risk factors. J Abnorm Psychol 91:173–279, 1982
104. Oetting ER, Beauvais F: Peer cluster theory, socialization characteristics and adolescent drug use: a path analysis. J Couns Psychol 34:205–213, 1987
105. Swaim RC, Oetting ER, Edwards RW, Beauvais F: Links from emotional distress to adolescent drug use: a path model. J Consult Clin Psychol 57:227–231, 1989
106. Oetting ER, Swaim RC, Edwards RW, Beauvais F: Indian and Anglo adolescent alcohol use and emotional distress: path models. Am J Alcohol Drug Abuse 15:153–172, 1989
107. Bukoski WJ: A definition of drug abuse prevention research. In Donohew L, Sipher HE, Bukoski WJ (eds): Persuasive Communication and Drug Abuse Prevention. Hillsdale, NJ: Lawrence Erlbaum Associates, 1991, pp 3–19
108. Schuster CR, Kilbey MM: Prevention of drug abuse. In Last JM, Wallace RB (eds): Maxcy-Rosenau-Last Public Health & Preventive Medicine. 13th ed. Norwalk, CT: Appleton & Lange, pp 769–786, 1992
109. Tobler NS: Meta-analysis of 143 adolescent drug prevention programs: quantitative outcome results of program participants compared to a control or comparison group. J Drug Issues 16:537–567, 1986
110. Bangert-Drowns RL: The effects of school-based substance abuse education—a meta-analysis. J Drug Educ 18:243–264, 1988
111. Tobler NS, Stratton H: Effectiveness of school-based drug prevention programs: a meta-analysis of the research. J Prim Prev, 18, 71–128, 1997
112. Ennett ST, Tobler NS, Ringwalt CL, Flewelling RL: How effective is drug abuse resistance education? A meta-analysis of project DARE outcome evaluations. Am J Public Health 84:1394–1401, 1994
113. Botvin G, Baker E, Filazolla A, Botvin E: A cognitive behavioral approach to substance abuse prevention: one year follow up. Addict Behav 15:47–73, 1990
114. Evans RI: How can health lifestyles in adolescents be modified? Some implications from a smoking prevention program. In Routh DK (ed): Handbook of Pediatric Psychology. New York: Guilford Press, 1988, pp 321–331
115. Evans RI, Dratt LM, Raines BE, Rosenberg SS: Social influences on smoking initiation: importance of distinguishing descriptive versus mediating process variables. J Appl Soc Psychol 18:925–943, 1988

116. Evans RI, Handon WB, Mittelmark MB: Increasing the validity of self-reports of smoking behavior in children. J Appl Psychol 62:521–523, 1977
117. Flay BR: What we know about the social influences approach to smoking prevention: review and recommendations. In Bell CS, Battjes R (ed): Prevention Research: Deterring Drug Abuse Among Children and Adolescents. DHHS Publication No. (ADM) 86-1334. Washington, DC: Government Printing Office, 1986, pp 67–111
118. Best JA, Flay BR, Towson SMJ, et al: Smoking prevention and the concept of risk. J Appl Soc Psychol 14:257–273, 1984
119. Flay BR, d'Avernas JR, Best JA, et al: Cigarette smoking: why young people do it and ways of preventing it. In McGrath P, Firestone P (eds): Pediatric and Adolescent Behavioral Medicine. New York: Springer, 1983, pp 132–183
120. Botvin GI, Wills TA: Personal and social skills training: cognitive-behavioral approaches to substance abuse prevention. In Bell CS, Battjes R (eds): Prevention Research: Deterring Drug Abuse Among Children and Adolescents. DHHS Publication No. (ADM)86-1334. Washington, DC: Government Printing Office, 1986, pp 8–49
121. Best JA, Thompson SJ, Santi SM, et al: Preventing cigarette smoking among school children. Annu Rev Public Health 9:161–201, 1988
122. Pentz MA: Prevention of adolescent substance abuse through social skills. In Glynn TJ, Leukefeld CG, Ludford JP (eds): Preventing Adolescent Drug Abuse: Intervention Strategies. DHHS Publication No. (ADM)83-1280, 1983, pp 195–232
123. Schinke SP, Gilchrist LD: Primary prevention of tobacco smoking. J School Health 53:416–419, 1983
124. Wills TA: Stress, coping, and tobacco and alcohol use in early adolescence. In Shiffmans S, Wills TA (eds): Coping and Substance Use. Orlando, FL: Academic Press, 1985, pp 67–94
125. Botvin GJ, Eng A, Williams CL: Preventing the onset of cigarette smoking through life skills training. Prev Med 9:135–143, 1980
126. Botvin GJ, Baker E, Dusenbury L, Tortu S, Botvin EM: Preventing adolescent drug abuse through a multi-modal cognitive-behavioral approach: results of a 3 year study. J Consult Clin Psychol 58:437–446, 1990
127. Botvin GJ, Baker E, Dusenbury L, Botvin EM, Diaz T: Long-term follow-up results of a randomized drug abuse prevention trail in a white middle-class population. JAMA 273:1106–1112, 1995
128. Pentz MA, Dwyer JH, MacKinnon DP, et al: A multicommunity trial for primary prevention of adolescent drug use: effects on drug use prevalence. JAMA 261:3259–3266, 1989
129. Dwyer JH, MacKinnon DP, Pentz MA, Flay BR, Hansen WB, Wang EYI, Johnson CA: Estimating intervention effects on longitudinally observed health behaviors: the Midwestern Prevention Project. Am J Epidemiol 120:781–795, 1989
130. Botvin GJ, Batson HW, Witts-Vitale S, Bess V, Baker E, Dusenbury L: A psychosocial approach to smoking prevention for urban black youth. Public Health Rep 104:573–582, 1989
131. Botvin G, Dusenbury L, James-Ortiz S, Kerner J: A skills training approach to smoking prevention among Hispanic youth. J Behav Med 12:279–296, 1989
132. Kellam SG, Anthony JC, Brown CH, et al: Prevention research on early risk behaviors: a cross-cultural study. In Schmidt MH, Remschmidt H (eds): Needs and Prospects of Child and Adolescent Psychiatry. Gottingen, Germany: Verlag-Hans Huber, 1989
133. Office of National Drug Control Policy: National Drug Control Strategy, 1996. Washington, DC: Office of National Drug Control Policy, 1996
134. Chilcoat H, Johanson C-E: Vulnerability to cocaine abuse. In Higgins ST, Katz JL (eds): Cocaine Abuse Research: Pharmacology, Behavior, and Clinical Applications. San Diego: Academic Press, in press
135. Substance Abuse and Mental Health Services Administration: The Role of Current Status of Patient Placement Criteria in the Treatment of Substance Use Disorders. Treatment Improvement Series (TIP) 13. DHHS Publication No. (SMA) 95-3021. Washington, DC: Government Printing Office, 1995
136. Sells SB (ed): Effectiveness of Drug Abuse Treatment. Cambridge, MA: Ballinger, 1974, vols 1 and 2
137. Sells SB, Simpson DD (eds): Effectiveness of Drug Abuse Treatment. vols 3–5. Cambridge, MA: Ballinger, 1976
138. Simpson DD, Joe GW, Lehman WEK, Sells SB: Addiction careers: etiology, treatment, and 12-year follow-up outcomes. J Drug Issues 16:107–121, 1986
139. Hubbard RL, Marsden ME, Rachal JV, et al: Drug Abuse Treatment: A National Study of Effectiveness. Chapel Hill, NC: University of North Carolina Press, 1989
140. Hubbard RL, Bray RM, Cavanaugh ER, et al: Drug Abuse Treatment Client Characteristics and Pretreatment Behavior in 1979–1981 TOPS Admission Cohorts. DHHS Publication No. (ADM)861453. Washington, DC: Government Printing Office, 1986
141. Allison M, Hubbard RL, Rachal JV: Treatment Process in Methadone, Residential and Outpatient Drug Free Programs. DHHS Publication No. (ADM)85-1411. Washington, DC: Government Printing Office, 1985
142. Ball JC, Ross A, Jaffe JH: Cocaine and heroin use by methadone maintenance patients. In LS Harris (ed): Problems of Drug Dependence, 1989. DHHS Publication No. (ADM)90-1663. Washington, DC: Government Printing Office, 1990, p 328
143. Harwood HJ, Napolitano DM, Kristiansen PL, Collins JJ: Economic Costs to Society of Alcohol and Drug Abuse and Mental Illness: 1980. Report 2734/00-01FR. Rockville, MD: Alcohol, Drug Abuse and Mental Health Administration, Office of Program Planning and Coordination, 1984
144. Cohen S, Lichtenstein E, Prochaska JO, et al: Debunking myths about self-quitting. Am Psychol 44:1355–1365, 1989
145. Siegel S: Drug anticipation and the treatment of dependence. In Ray BA (ed): Learning Factors in Substance Abuse. DHHS Publication No. (ADM)88-1576. Washington, DC: Government Printing Office, 1988, pp 1–24
146. O'Brien CP, Childress AR, McLellan AT, et al: Types of conditioning found in drug-dependent humans. In Ray BA (ed): Learning Factors in Substance Abuse. DHHS Publication No. (ADM)88-1576). Washington, DC: Government Printing Office, 1988, pp 44–61
147. Childress AR, McLellan AT, Ehrman R, O'Brien CP: Classically conditioned responses in opioid and cocaine dependence: a role in relapse? In Ray BA (ed): Learning Factors in Substance Abuse. DHHS Publication No. (ADM)88-1576. Washington, DC: Government Printing Office, 1988, pp 25–43
148. Childress AR, McLellan AT, O'Brien CP: Nature and incidence of conditioned responses in a methadone population: a comparison of laboratory, clinic and naturalistic setting. In Harris L (ed): Problems of Drug Dependence, 1985: Proceedings of the 47th Annual Scientific Meeting, The Committee on Problems of Drug Dependence, Inc. DHHS Publication No. (ADM)86-1448. Washington, DC: Government Printing Office, 1986, pp 366–372
149. Childress AR, Hole AV, Ehrman R, Robbins SJ, et al: Cue reactivity and cue reactivity interventions in drug dependence. NIDA Res Monogr 127:73–95, 1995
150. Higgins ST, Stitzer ML, Bigelow GE, Liebson IA: Contingent methadone delivery: effects on illicit opiate use. Drug Alcohol Depend 17:311–322, 1986
151. Higgins ST, Budney AJ, Bickel WK, Foerg FE, et al: Incentives improve outcome in outpatient behavioral treatment of cocaine dependence. Arch Gen Psychiatry 51:568–576, 1994
152. Silverman K, Higgins ST, Brooner RK, Montoys ID, et al: Sustained cocaine abstinence in methadone maintenance patients through voucher-based reinforcement therapy. Arch Gen Psychiatry 53:409–415, 1996

153. Kleber HD, Topazian M, Gaspari J, et al: Clonidine and naltrexone in outpatient treatment of heroin withdrawal. Am J Drug Alcohol Abuse 13:1–17, 1987
154. Substance Abuse and Mental Health Services Administration: LAAM and the Treatment of Opiate Addiction. Treatment Improvement Protocol (TIP) Series 22. Rockville, MD: Substance Abuse and Mental Health Services Administration, 1995
155. Bickel WK, Stitzer ML, Bigelow GE, et al: A clinical trial of buprenorphine: comparison with methadone in detoxification of heroin addicts. Clin Pharmacol Ther 43:72–78, 1988
156. Bickel WK, Stitzer ML, Bigelow GE, et al: Buprenorphine: dose related blockage of opioid challenge effects in opioid dependent humans. J Pharmacol Exp Ther 247:47–53, 1988
157. Gawin FH, Kleber HD, Byck R, et al: Desipramine facilitation of initial cocaine abstinence. Arch Gen Psychiatry 6:117–121, 1989
158. Mendelson JH, Mello NK: Management of cocaine abuse and dependence. N Engl J Med 334:965–972, 1996
159. McAuliffe WE, Ch'ien JMN: Recovery training and self-help: a relapse-prevention program for treated opiate addicts. J Subst Abuse Treat 3:9–20, 1986

47

Community Intervention Programs

John E. Ferguson

Morbidity and mortality resulting from communicable diseases have greatly declined during the later half of the twentieth century. Correspondingly there has been greater professional and public interest in lowering morbidity and mortality attributable to noncommunicable diseases, such as cancers and cardiovascular diseases, as well as to the harmful effects of alcohol and drug abuse, and to accidents, suicide, and violence. Analysis of health in terms of four dimensions—environment, health care organization, human biology, and lifestyle[1]—has attributed as much as half of all premature deaths in the United States to lifestyles.[2] During the past twenty-five years, community-based intervention programs have become fashionable for addressing these kinds of problems, usually by promoting lifestyle changes.[3–13]

These interventions are generally characterized by attempts to achieve multiple changes in the policies, practices, and behaviors of diverse social, economic, and political sectors of a community, usually lead by community members and institutions, for a particular health or social outcome.

A general definition of community intervention as a procedure in public health is the process of reducing preventable sickness, disability and death through a combination of behavior-oriented prevention activities (e.g., health education, behavioral modifications) and situation-oriented prevention activities (e.g., health promotion at schools and at work sites). In order for community intervention to demonstrate its efficacy for public health more convincingly, practitioners need to define as precisely as possible what contribution each behavioral component and situational component is intended to make, to examine how these components are more efficient in combination, to measure how far these objectives have been met, and to suggest how to improve on these results in the future.

There are several advantages for describing a health-related project as community based. First, the "community" is inherently persuasive to others and refers both to the existing state of affairs as well as to a longed-for alternative.[14] Second, the notion of "community" is usually and intuitively understood, even if it has proven extremely difficult to define operationally.[15,16] Third, the popularity of an intuitive approach to community activism has grown over the last twenty-five years. "This movement was, and is, based on the belief that the urgent need was for action with and by communities, not debate about them, for engagement with them, not analysis of them."[14] In short, proposing an ostensibly new mode of intervention encompassing the community had the potential for garnering interest and support. Early advocates for community-based approaches often were convinced of their value and were likewise often convinced that the programs will benefit others."[17] However, this confidence needed to be tempered with evidence from the education, health, or social science literature concerning the efficacy of such measures.

There does seem to be implicit consensus on two points. First, many discussions of community and community-based intervention tend to be normatively prescriptive, emphasizing its contribution to human well-being.[14] Second, there is an expectation that these settings or systems are more likely to be relatively placid so that change is somewhat predictable, rather than to be so turbulent that change is unpredictable.[18] "An inherent assumption is that . . . [these] systems are long-lasting, functionally interdependent, and relatively stable."[19] Otherwise, community-based intervention would be impracticable.

Published descriptions of community-based interventions indicate that they regularly take place in a population that occupies a common geographical area and shares some concerns, needs, and problems, as well as economic, political, and sociocultural characteristics. They also report that a community generally has constituent units, that is, its population participates in various formal and informal organizations within that area, and that the community itself may be a constituent unit for another level of organization, such as the nation-state.

There is sometimes a lack of specificity about the target for an intervention mode. For example, a definition for community might be as simplistic as "a group of people with some things in common (and) who are aware of those commonalities."[17] Sometimes the discussion refers to a specific human population within conventional geographical and political boundaries. At other times the population may share a common condition, set of interests, or problem. The community may be characterized by accentuating the homogeneity within the population and strong ties creating identity among constituents, but occasionally the emphasis is on heterogeneity and weak social ties, providing little integration.[20]

▸ VANTAGE POINTS FOR COMMUNITY INTERVENTIONS

There are two contrasting points from which participants view community-based intervention, that from within and that from outside the community. Members of the target community have relatively specific concerns about whether this mode of intervention is feasible within their community and how they can implement it effectively there. On the other hand, those outside the community have relatively general concerns about whether this mode of intervention is universally feasible and how they can implement it effectively anywhere. These perspectives are not necessarily incompatible.[21] Both have a stake in the success of a project and tend to view community intervention primarily as a means to an end. As one commentator observed, "What community approaches . . . need is more articulated research that tests which *kinds* of community approaches have which *kinds* of effects."[22,p159] There are differences in emphasis among adherents of community-based intervention. Some have an orientation toward social change, others to the process of intervention, and still others to the targets for intervention. As a result, there are often different strategies for designing an intervention.

With regard to the orientation toward social change, some advocates see power relationships as structured pluralistically with multiple spheres for decision making and suggest that programs often founder when addressing these problems becomes adversarial. Their preferred community organization techniques correspond to Rothman's[23] models "A" [locality development] and "B" [social planning]. The theoretical models shaping a program are primarily behavioral. Others see power relationships as structured pyramidally with a few top decision makers and suggest that addressing these problems often will become adversarial. Their preferred community organization techniques correspond to Rothman's model "C" [social action]. The theoretical models shaping a program are primarily political.

With regard to the process for intervention, some advocates argue that the appropriate process for addressing these problems is a bottom up or "grassroots" intervention, which begins with ordinary citizens. In its unadulterated form, funding for such an intervention would not be contingent upon addressing expert-determined health or social issues, implementing a predetermined protocol, and progressing along bureaucratically set timelines. If experts are involved, they contribute technical assistance and serve as catalysts, expediters, or facilitators. Others argue that the appropriate process is a top down or "professional" intervention, which begins with specialists and decision-making officials, continues with formation of a partnership between organizers and those being organized, and progresses to a transfer of responsibilities to those who have been successfully organized.[12] Experts serve several roles, which may involve "doing with" the community but most of which involve "doing for" or "doing to" the community.[24]

With regard to the target for intervention, some proponents argue that the social system and its underlying risk conditions, such as poverty, powerlessness, and unemployment, should be the target for interventions to reduce morbidity and mortality. Others argue the target should be the individual and his or her particular risk factors, such as alcohol intake, sexual habits, fat consumption, and tobacco use.[25] The public health perspective, which focuses on the interaction between agent, environment, and host, usually an individual, offers a potential bridge to close the gap between risk condition and risk factor proponents and some have advocated community-based intervention as being appropriate for both types of programs.[26]

In addition to the enthusiasm of advocates championing community-based approaches, official endorsement for the fundamental principle of community involvement in disease prevention and health promotion has been one of the driving forces behind community-based intervention. The Alma Alta Declaration[33] and the Ottawa Charter for Health Promotion[34] mandate "community participation." Subsequently, not only the World Health Organization (WHO) but also the national governments of Australia, Canada, the United Kingdom, and the United States have endorsed community-based approaches as important vehicles for local self-determination and self-reliance.[35]

These various international and national proclamations probably have had the most impact on those people and organizations engaged in health education and human services. Those recommendations serve "as a constant reminder to them that 'community' is formally on the agenda, the term has officially sanctioned currency, as well as being one to which, in turn, their own activities may contribute. Indeed, the term may be part of their job descriptions and occupational titles."[14]

The ideals of "empowerment" or "enabling" ordinary citizens are obviously attractive to "grassroots" activists. Similarly, the ideal of "decentralization" is potentially attractive to opponents of unlimited government. However, governmental and other funding agencies have been more receptive to proposals that focus on risk factors and individual lifestyle than on social change. They have been much less receptive to "grassroots" than to "expert" designs. Program planners have tended to go "where the money is," either through choice or necessity.[36]

Several circumstances in recent decades have contributed to official and personal affirmations of decentralization, empowerment, and enabling as ideals. In addition to the community activism movement, there have been various other, occasionally overlapping social movements, such as the civil rights, self-care, and women's movements, which demanded a transfer of authority and resources from the powerful to the powerless.[37] There has been dwindling public satisfaction with conventional medical approaches to health, while public fascination with nutrition, physical exercise, and "alternative" approaches to health, such as holistic practices encompassing mental, social, and spiritual qualities of life has grown. Perhaps most significantly, there has been an increase in the number of professional personnel having a health education or human services orientation.[29]

▶ GENERAL CONSIDERATIONS FOR COMMUNITY INTERVENTION

Beginning with the landmark North Karelia Study in Finland, where community-based approaches to coronary heart disease prevention were undertaken, encouraging reports emerged from other community-based interventions, but they often showed relatively modest results. Some commentators raised questions on technical issues as well as on the feasibility of applying a similar type of protocol in other communities.[27,28] Nevertheless, the proponents for this mode of intervention succeeded in generating excitement, innovation, and the exploration of alternative approaches.[24] However, given the mixed results of early *clinical trials* in reducing coronary heart disease, a few early skeptics had urged caution in intemperately shifting health care resources to seemingly inexpensive but unproven mass interventions with whole populations, including community-based interventions. They insisted on the importance of maintaining financial support for basic biomedical research and proven, if seemingly expensive, specific interventions with individuals identified as being at high risk.[29]

How to allocate resources efficiently to individual and mass interventions is extremely difficult to decide. Investments in promoting the health of the majority divert resources from investments to improve the quality of life for the minority of high-risk individuals. Moreover, there is what Rose terms the prevention paradox: "A preventive measure that brings large benefits to the community affords little to each participating individual."[30,p3] Thus community-based intervention has to produce sufficient if small improvements to many persons in order to bring discernible and important benefits to the community. Community-based intervention must produce a sufficiently large, statistically significant absolute difference between the target and reference populations. Such results would reduce questions about the efficacy of community-based intervention.[31]

Perhaps the major difficulty in evaluating the efficacy of community-based interventions is that effects of spontaneous social change in a population are highly unpredictable. Particularly challenging is the possibility of large, favorable population changes occurring at the same time as an intervention. For example, the impact initially attributed to community-based intervention, such as the 5.6% decrease in serum cholesterol for the intervention area of North Karelia in contrast to a 1.6% decrease in a comparison area of Finland, is less impressive when the difference narrows over time as a result of larger secular trends.[32]

Another challenge to community-based intervention is the pragmatic consideration of persuading people and organizations to participate, especially in large-scale campaigns or programs. A campaign or program addressing an issue or a problem targeted by experts, especially one originating "outside" the community, may not only have difficulty mobilizing ordinary citizens at its beginning but also with sustaining this mobilization. "[W]ith evangelical zeal, health educators have, on occasion, become manipulative and forced decisions and programs on an unprepared public. . . . As leaders in the profession recognized the image that was developing, they began to stress the concepts of community organization. This emphasis, which started in the 1960s, . . . has resulted in . . . an improved image.[17]

Consequently, "institutionalization" (incorporation into a system), "ownership," and "participation" have become cardinal precepts for community mobilization: "[L]arge-scale behavioral change requires the people heavily affected by a problem . . . be involved in defining the problem, planning and instituting steps to resolve the problem, and establishing structures to ensure that the desired change is maintained . . . *Ownership* means that local people must have a sense of responsibility [for a program], so they will continue to support [it] after the initial organizing effort."[19]

Sometimes public health agencies and programs have legal sanctions available to punish noncompliance, but they seldom have the authority or sufficient financial resources to offer more than small incentives or rewards for compliance. For example, children in the United States usually must be vaccinated for certain communicable diseases in order to attend public schools, and health care providers may receive a subsidy to provide these vaccinations to the poor for little or no out-of-pocket cost. Consequently, public health agencies and programs mainly rely on health education as a means to obtain voluntary compliance from the public.[37] When large-scale health education is the means for a disease prevention program or a health promotion campaign, a community-based intervention is a practical approach for boosting participation.

Cost-cutting in health programs may be one factor contributing to the interest in community-based intervention. One possible impetus for community-based intervention is the possibility that such approaches would be more cost effective than other techniques. Several circumstances in recent decades have contributed to this expectation. Mass telecommunications technologies have made large-scale, low-cost per capita disease prevention and health promotion programs possible. There is the prospect that future public investments in medical care and public health will produce diminishing returns. Political concerns worldwide about cost containment and inflation have led to reductions in governmental expenditures not only on high-priced, high-technology medical care but also on social programs. The recognized link between chronic disease occurrence and personal behavior has stimulated a search for inexpensive ways to alter lifestyle.[37]

Community-based intervention would be impressively cost effective if it could produce greater cumulative effects than previous techniques for a lower cost. However, it would still be more cost effective if it could either produce cumulative effects equivalent to previous techniques for a lower cost or greater cumulative effects at the same cost. The belief that such approaches would be more cost effective than previous techniques is based on several fundamental assumptions. One premise is that community-based intervention would not produce any significant negative side effects. Although drugs and medical procedures have documented side effects, there is scant information about what kinds of side effects community-based intervention might have. Perhaps because most discussions of community have been normatively prescriptive, it seems to be taken for granted that this mode of intervention will not cause short- or long-term harm for either the population as a whole, or its constituents, but this remains to be proven.

Another premise is that community-based intervention has an economy of scale because of its potential per unit discounting and synergy. If intervention cost per unit (families, organizations, persons, subcommunities) in time, effort, and resources is neither constant nor will increase as the number of units reached goes up, then cost per unit goes down as more units are reached. When the intervention design targets multiple risk factors or conditions at minimal additional cost per unit, "bundling" or "piggybacking" is obviously less costly than separate interventions. If a multiple component or multifaceted design proves to be synergistic, so that its total result is greater than the sum of results for its separate components, then the intervention is extremely cost effective. Social marketing and social learning theory imply synergy is possible because exposure to multiple media, messages, and reinforcers can be more effective than exposure to a single source. Research in social marketing and social learning has emphasized the potency of incorporating several complementary components into intervention design. Paradoxically, although a community-based intervention may eventually achieve such an economy of scale, initially there may be an enormous diseconomy of scale: "The complexities grow exponentially with each additional [participant]. . . . In short, a truly orchestrated large-scale program—as distinct from numerous replications of a small-scale program—requires additional planning and coordination for each unique unit added, multiplied by (not merely added to) the number of variations in prior units added."[38,p797]

There is also the simple operational assumption that the etiologic fraction or population attributable risk is helpful as a guideline for choosing a population intervention over an alternative approach. Population attributable risk is an estimate of the proportion of the disease rate in a population attributable to a risk factor.[39] Its magnitude varies according to the prevalence of the risk factor in a population and the relative risk associated with that factor. The population attributable risk has a small value when both prevalence and relative risk are very low. Therefore, unless an alternative approach is disproportionately expensive, there would not be a clear cut advantage for community-based intervention. When the prevalence of a risk factor (e.g., smoking) is not small, the larger the relative risk, the more the potential population impact of reducing the risk factor warrants a community-based intervention.[10] However, even when the relative risk is small, the larger the prevalence of a risk factor (e.g., sedentary lifestyle), the more the potential population impact of reducing the risk factor warrants a community-based intervention. "A large number of people exposed to a small risk may generate more—many more cases than a small number exposed to a high risk."[30]

Finally, because behavior is grounded in social structures and cultural contexts, interventions focusing on changing individual behavior by increasing awareness, knowledge, and motivation should presumably be supplemented with social and environmental supports to enhance their effectiveness. Health education research has extensively documented that individuals often revert to previous behavior when their surroundings do not reinforce the new behavior. One theoretical approach to community-based intervention is primarily behavioral, that is, based on the adoption-diffusion model,[40] the belief-intention model,[41] the communication-persuasion model,[42] the social learning model,[43] or the social marketing model,[44] and social factors have an auxiliary role, as tools or reinforcers for individual level change.[25]

Another theoretical approach incorporates social factors as having a more complementary role. For example, the "new 'community' approach argues that permanent, large-scale behavior change is best achieved by changing the standards of acceptable behavior in the community; that is, by changing community norms about health-related behavior."[19,p45] There is relative consensus within the community about norms, and behavior conforms to norms.

▶ EXAMPLES OF COMMUNITY-BASED INTERVENTION PROJECTS

The first community-based projects attempting to reduce the morbidity and mortality of chronic diseases were the Stanford Three-Community Study in California[6] and the North Karelia Project in Finland.[8] Reports from these projects generated interest in community-based intervention, especially for applications of research that was already compatible with or seemed adaptable to this innovative approach. Beginning in the late 1970s, four other major projects received funding: the Stanford Five-City Project (1978),[6,45,46] the Pawtucket Heart Health Project (1980),[7,47,48] the Minnesota Heart Health Program (1980),[8,49] and the Community Intervention Trial for Smoking Cessation [COMMIT] (1986).[50–52]

All six of these community intervention projects were based in relatively different community contexts.[10] They varied in where the human populations were located geographically as well as in the size and sociodemographic composition; the economic, political, and sociocultural characteristics; the formal and informal organizations; and the concerns, needs, and problems of those populations.

Most of these projects planned their intervention using a hybrid model incorporating two or more theoretical orientations toward changing lifestyles (an adoption-diffusion model, a belief-intention model, a communication-persuasion model, a social learning model, or a social marketing model). Each developed its own approach to community organizing.

North Karelia, Finland

North Karelia was one of the regions sampled in the Seven Countries Study begun in the late 1950s. This study confirmed that its population had one of the highest, if not *the* highest, rates of ischemic heart disease mortality in the world. The North Karelia Project commenced in 1971 after a parliamentary petition by elected officials from the region. The population at that time was approximately 180,000. Relative to other areas of Finland, it was mainly rural, with low socioeconomic status (SES) and high unemployment. The study was designed to compare North Karelia to a neighboring and demographically similar reference region, Kuopio, that did not receive the intervention program. The theoretical model incorporated an adoption-diffusion model, a belief-intention model, and a social learning model. The community organizing approach targeted mass media, political leaders, and a variety of formal and informal organizations (business associations, health care and social service organizations, labor unions, sports groups, and voluntary associations).

Stanford Three-Community Study

The Stanford Three-Community Study started in 1972 in the northern California towns of Tracy, Gilroy, and Watsonville. The population of each town at that time was around 12,000 to 15,000. The English-speaking populations were predominately middle class, while the Spanish-speaking populations tended to be lower SES. The later population composed nine to twenty-six percent of the population, and a separate Spanish-language campaign was implemented with this group. The study was designed to compare three conditions: no intervention (Tracy), a mass media health education program (Gilroy), and a high-intensity program (Watsonville) that added face-to-face communication to the mass media program for people identified through screening as being in the highest quartile of cardiovascular risk. The social learning model was the primary theoretical input and the community organizing approach targeted the home, worksite, and various community settings.

Stanford Five-City Project

The later Stanford Five-City Project was initiated in 1978 in the northern California cities of Modesto, Monterey, Salinas, San Luis Obispo, and Santa Maria. The total population at that time was composed of approximately 330,000 people. The study was designed to compare two conditions in demographically similar cities: no intervention (Modesto, San Luis Obispo, Santa Maria) with the comprehensive intervention (Monterey, Salinas). The theoretical model added an adoption-diffusion model, a belief-intention model, a communication-persuasion model, and a social marketing model to the social learning model employed in the earlier project. The social marketing model guided the educational messages developed using the other models. The community organizing approach was similar to the earlier project with the addition of institutionalization.

Pawtucket Heart Health Project

The Pawtucket Heart Health Project began in 1980 in Pawtucket, Rhode Island. The total population at that time comprised approximately 71,000 people. The study was designed to compare Pawtucket with a demographically similar reference city. The intervention component started in 1982 following baseline data collection and planning. The theoretical model included the adoption-diffusion model, the belief-intention model, the communication-persuasion model, the social learning model, and the social marketing model. The community organizing approach tried to incorporate three patterns or styles [Rothman], making extensive use of volunteers and working with churches.

Minnesota Heart Health Program

The Minnesota Heart Health Program was initiated in 1980 in the central upper Midwest. The project has three pairs of demographically similar communities in Minnesota, North Dakota, and South Dakota. One set of intervention and comparison communities consists of small towns with populations of 25,000 to 40,000, another consists of larger, free-standing cities with populations of 75,000 to 80,000, and the third set consists of metropolitan areas with populations of 80,000 to 115,000. A five-year intervention phase was followed by a two-year transition period, in which resources and responsibilities were transferred to local organizations. Its theoretical model also included the adoption-diffusion model, the belief-intention model, the communication-persuasion model, the social learning model, and the social marketing model. The community organizing approach tried to involve local leaders as well as local organizations to create interest in continuing project activities after funding ended.

The Community Intervention Trial for Smoking Cessation (COMMIT)

The Community Intervention Trial for Smoking Cessation [COMMIT] commenced in 1988 in one Canadian and ten American regions. COMMIT was unique in that it randomly assigned communities to be targeted for intervention. Also, it included a sufficient number of matched community pairs (eleven) to provide good statistical power for detecting intervention effects on smoking cessation rates, using community as the unit of analysis. The study's purpose was to test "the systematic application of previously tested risk factor reduction programs with randomized trials using large, well-defined population samples drawn from entire workforces, neighborhoods, health care plans or communities."[50] COMMIT was a Phase IV trial in a programmatic approach to prevention. The ultimate level, Phase V, involved disseminating the risk reduction program broadly enough to have an impact on national disease rates. COMMIT broadly defined community to include portions of well-defined metropolitan areas and geographically linked multiple smaller cities as well as individual cities. A prospective research center proposed a potential pair of communities that were matched with each other in smoking prevalence, population size and other sociodemographic characteristics, and capacity to implement the protocol. The smallest set of intervention and comparison communities had populations of 58,000 and 54,000, while the largest set had populations of 167,000 and 163,000. This unevenness resulted from the distribution of research centers.

The theoretical model for COMMIT also included the adoption-diffusion model, the belief-intention model, the communication-persuasion model, the social learning model, and the social marketing model. It "incorporated virtually all key features of past community trials."[45] In addition, it combined components from previously tested risk factor reduction programs into a mandated activities protocol and systematically applied the protocol. The community organizing approach also involved the implementation of a community mobilization protocol, requiring an initial planning group and development of an administrative community board and various specific task forces to guide the application of the activities protocol.

▶ PROJECT OUTCOMES

These community-based projects have successfully demonstrated that this approach is not feckless. First, not only is it possible to set up relatively simple activities within smaller populations, but it is also possible to implement a variety of relatively complex protocols within larger populations. Community-based projects have confirmed that previously tested risk factor reduction programs can be applied systematically in a community milieu, delivering an intervention to populations through multiple activities involving not only such accepted auspices as educational and health care settings but also other settings including neighborhoods, workplaces, and other kinds of community settings. Second, these projects have shown that interventions originally set in motion by specialists and decision-making officials cannot only mobilize community members but also can sustain this mobilization for several years. The initial collaboration between organizers and those being organized may progress eventually to a transfer of responsibilities to those who have been organized successfully. Third, these projects have confirmed that intervention ingredients reached a large number of people within the targeted population. These individuals, families, neighborhoods, and organizations have been exposed to or received intervention messages as well as participated in activities and events designed to change behavior and reinforce behavior change as well as to change social norms.

Although these community-based projects were partially successful, counter to intuitions that this approach would ultimately be more cost effective than alternative smaller scale approaches, none has even partially validated this belief convincingly. Even from the beginning of community-based intervention in North Karelia, reports from community-based projects showed relatively modest results concerning the reduction of morbidity and mortality. However, progress reports from ongoing projects were encouraging enough for its proponents to hope that eventually there would be sufficiently large outcomes to demonstrate the strength for this mode of intervention.

By 1995, the publication of results from COMMIT, the Heart Health Programs in Minnesota and Pawtucket, and the Stanford Five-City Project brought an end to the optimism.[46–53] At best their results were mixed.[24] At worst their results were disappointing.[22,54] An analysis of the program effectiveness in eight community-based programs targeting alcohol abuse and alcohol-related problems similarly found an inability to impact upon community level processes.[55] In addition, there was generally a failure to generate much community involvement in the design and implementation of program activities. From its inception community-based intervention had been touted as cost effective, but so far the size of effects have usually been meager in relation to effort expended. Often, no beneficial change or only modest gains could be attributed to the intervention program. Even when there were modest improvements, they were not necessarily sustained over time. In summary, results to date from community-based projects have neither justified the optimistic predictions nor the underlying assumptions. In the case of COMMIT, the trial results left little doubt that the particular protocols for activities and community mobilization did not work as well as predicted.

COMMIT served as an example, at least in the investigative setting, of the potential costs of community-based programs. Project costs were high because there were several mandated internal organizational bodies [5] to be coordinated in addition to the large number of mandated activities [58] to be implemented throughout the target communities. Each intervention community received an average of $220,000 per year for 4 years, including staff salaries necessary for coordination and facilitation.[52] In the eleven communities after four years, a total of more than 3,000 smokers (in the target age interval of 25 to 64 years) were induced to quit beyond the naturally occurring secular trend.[52] Each of these smokers represented an average input of more than $3,000.

However, possibly even these results have not been so disappointing as to warrant abandoning this mode of intervention entirely. Greater effects might have been observable in a few more years, having been deferred through a period of latency. Whether these particular protocols could have produced greater results under other conditions at some other time is unknown. It is intriguing to speculate how much the secular trends affecting cessation diminished the impact. In commenting on COMMIT, Susser observed "[w]here the starting levels [in risk factors] are high and stable and as yet untouched by a vigorous social movement, . . . then intervention has been seen to produce effects."[54] It is also tantalizing to speculate whether the impact would have been heightened by having a variety of nicotine replacement products not only available over the counter but also heavily advertised and placed in high-traffic displays.

In commenting on COMMIT, Fisher suggested a different strategy: testing a defined approach to community organization, not a defined intervention. "The distinction rests not on whether key components are well-defined but on what components are considered key."[22,p159] Such an "approach might focus definition not on specifying intervention and governance but on defining the *process* by which an intervention is developed or defining the range of *choices* communities make. [A protocol] could standardize the authority of local groups to (1) rank program objectives . . . , (2) choose among intervention characteristics (program materials, program settings, or staging sites), (3) identify the range of groups which might be invited into program planning, (4) strike alliance with other groups pursuing other health or social objectives . . . , or (5) choose among channels of influence. . . . "[22,p159]

▸ CONCLUSIONS

Various completed and evaluated community-based projects have demonstrated that this approach is not futile. It is undeniable that "we have much to learn about how to change group behavior to accomplish [desired] effects. Future trials will need to draw on a deeper understanding, now lacking, of methods for bringing about social change."[54,158] An observation about living systems provides a clue for why community-based intervention has so far remained impractical. The complex relationships between system constituents evolve nonlinearly, that is, recursively or in loops with feedback. An intervention package may introduce a change, that is, a perturbation or disturbance into a system or subsystem. Nonlinearity permits huge variations in the consequences of a given perturbation or disturbance. In comparison to linear relationships, sometimes the effects of a perturbation may be disproportionately large or disproportionately small. Within the present context, massive changes in some interdependencies may leave the organization of the system undisturbed, only to be followed by a tiny change that triggers the change in the organization of the systems through a bandwagon process or domino effect.

Perhaps the simplest explanation for why community-based intervention has so far remained impractical is the short-term stability of living systems [homeostasis]. One of the most basic observations about systems is that they can maintain regularity despite irregularity in the systems' environments. Systems are self-regulatory, converting any difference into actions that will keep the differences small. If a community has the properties of a system, especially one with constituent subsystems, intervention activities may produce only slight disturbances temporarily or introduce change in some subsystems but not others. For example, in the Stanford Five-City Project there was evidence of differential response among community subgroups. In the case of the Minnesota Heart Health Program, the investigators concluded that changing the risk levels of individuals exposed to particular interventions was less difficult than changing the risk levels of the community. In the case of COMMIT, the less educated subgroup of light-to-moderate smokers seemed more responsive to the intervention than college-educated smokers.

A straightforward explanation for why community-based intervention has not been more practical may be the extreme difficulty of predicting secular trends and the extraordinary complexity of not only human behavior but also the social environment. As a result, initial diseconomies of scale may have been underestimated, along with how long it might take to "turn a profit" by surpassing a break-even point for results relative to the resources invested.

Program planners have faced limited opportunities for funding and by necessity have designed programs to these specifications. They undoubtedly had considerable knowledge about the particular area of health behavior that they were attempting to change and expertise in specific techniques (such as smoking cessation in the case of COMMIT). They were also undoubtedly familiar with prior and concurrent community-based projects in public health. Good research guarantees scientifically relevant results, and the community intervention projects described here were worth conducting and evaluating. Perhaps a quotation from Helen Hayes cited at the start of a review of health education campaign is appropriate: "It's what you learn after you know it all that really counts."[56] Further research is necessary to demonstrate the value of community intervention for prevention more convincingly.

▶ REFERENCES

1. Lalonde M: A New Perspective on the Health of Canadians. Ottawa: Information Canada, 1974
2. The Leading Causes of Death in the United States. Atlanta: Centers for Disease Control,
3. Blackburn H: Research and demonstration projects in community cardiovascular disease prevention. J Public Health Policy 4: 398–421, 1983
4. Elder JP, Schmid TL, Dower P, Hedund S: Community heart health programs: Components, rationale and strategies for effective intervention. J Public Health Policy 4:463–479, 1983
5. Carlaw R, Mittelmark M, Bracht N, Luepker R: Organization for a community cardiovascular health program. Health Educ Q 11:242–252, 1984
6. Maccoby N, Farquhar J, Wood P: Reducing the risk of cardiovascular disease: Effects of a community-based campaign on knowledge and behavior. J Community Health 3:100–114, 1977
7. Lefbvre R, Lasater T, McKinlay S, Carleton R: Theory and the delivery of health programming in the community: The Pawtucket Heart Health Program. Preventive Medicine 16:80–95, 1987
8. McAllister A, Puska P, Salonen J: Theory and action for health promotion: Illustrations from the North Karelia Project. Am J Public Health 72:43–50, 1982
9. Pentz MA, Dwyer JH, MacKinnon DP, Flay BR, Hansen WB, Wang EY, Johnson CA: A multicommunity trial for primary prevention of adolescent drug abuse. JAMA 261:3259–3266, 1989
10. Shea S, Basch CE: A review of five major community-based cardiovascular disease prevention programs: Part 1. Rationale, design and theoretical framework. Am J Health Promotion 4:203–213, 1990
11. Tarlov A, Kehrer B, Hall D, Samuels S, Brown G, Felix M, Ross J: Foundation work: The health promotion program of the Henry Kaiser Family Foundation. Am J Health Promotion 2:74–80, 1987
12. Thompson B, Wallack L, Lichtenstein E, Pechacek T: Principles of community organization and partnership for smoking cessation in the Community Intervention Trial for Smoking Cessation [COMMIT]. Int Q Health Education 11:187–204, 1990–1991
13. Vincent M, Clearie A, Schluchter M: Reducing adolescent pregnancy through school and community-based education. JAMA 257:3382–3386, 1987
14. Jewkes R, Murcott A: Meanings of community. Soc Sci Med 43: 555–563, 1996
15. Hillery GA: Definitions of community: Areas of agreement. Rural Sociology 20:111–123, 1955
16. Bell C, Newby H: Community Studies. London: George Allen and Unwin, 1971
17. Breckon DJ, Harvey JR, Lancaster RB: Community Health Education: Settings, Roles and Skills for the 21st Century. 3rd ed. Gaithersburg, MD: Aspen, 1994
18. Emery FE: Toward a social ecology: Contextual appreciation of the future in the present. New York: Plenum Press, 1973
19. Thompson B, Kinne S: Social change theory: Applications to community health. In Bracht N (ed): Health Promotion at the Community Level. Newbury Park: Sage, 1990
20. Granovetter M: The strength of weak ties. Am J Sociology 78:1361–1380, 1973
21. Dunbar RL, Ahlstorm D: Seeking the institutional balance of power: Avoiding the power of a balanced view. Acad Manag Rev 20:171–192, 1995
22. Fisher EB: Editorial: The results of the COMMIT trial. Am J Public Health 85:159–160, 1995
23. Rothman J: Three models of community organization practice. Social Work Practice. 1968. New York: Columbia University Press, 1968
24. Altman D: Sustaining interventions in community systems: On the relationship between researchers and communities. Health Psychology 14:526–536, 1995
25. Shiell, Hawe P: Health promotion, community development and the tyranny of the individual. Health Economics 5:241–247, 1996
26. Green LW, Kreuter MW: Health Promotion Planning: An Educational and Environmental Approach. Toronto: Mayfield Publishing, 1991
27. Kasl SV: Cardiovascular risk reduction in a community setting: Some comments. J Consulting Clinical Psych 48:143–149, 1980
28. Leventhal H, Cleary PD, Safer MA, Gutman M: Cardiovascular risk modification by community-based programs for life-style change: Comments on the Stanford Study. J Consulting Clinical Psych 48:150–158, 1980
29. Oliver MF: Prevention of coronary heart disease—propaganda, promises, problems, and prospects. Circulation 73:1–9, 1986
30. Rose G: The Strategy of Preventive Medicine. Oxford: Oxford University Press, 1992
31. Mattson ME, Cummings KM, Lynn WR, Giffen C, Corle D, Pechacek T: Evaluation plan for the Community Intervention Trial for Smoking Cessation [COMMIT]. Int Q Health Education 11:271–290, 1990–1991
32. Puska P, Nissinen A, Toumilehto J: The community-based strategy to prevent coronary heart disease: Conclusions from the first ten years of the North Karelia project. Annu Rev Public Health 6:147–159, 1985
33. World Health Organization: Alma Alta 1978: Primary Health Care. Geneva: WHO, 1978
34. World Health Organization: The Ottawa charter for health promotion. Health Promotion 1:iii–v, 1986
35. Guldan GS: Obstacles to health promotion. Soc Sci Medicine 43: 689– 695, 1996
36. Pearce N: Traditional epidemiology, modern epidemiology, and public health. Am J Public Health 86:678–683, 1996
37. Green LW, Raeburn J: Community wide change: Theory and practice. In Bracht N (ed): Health Promotion at the Community Level. Newbury Park: Sage, 1990
38. Green LW: Prevention and health education. In Last JM, Wallace RB (eds): Maxcy-Rosenau-Last Public Health and Preventive Medicine. (13th ed) Norwalk, CT: Appleton and Lange, 1992
39. Rothenberg RB, Hahn RA: Measures of attribution. In Haddix AC, Teutsch SM, Shaffer PA, Duñet DO (eds): Prevention Effectiveness: A Guide to Decision Analysis and Economic Evaluation. New York: Oxford University Press, 1996
40. Rogers E: Diffusion of Innovations. (3rd ed). New York: Free Press, 1982
41. Ajzen I, Fishbein M: Understanding Attitudes and Predicting Social Behavior. Englewood Cliffs, NJ: Prentice Hall, 1980
42. Flay B, diTecco D, Schlege R: Mass media in health promotion: An analysis using an extended information processing model. Health Educ Q 7:127–147, 1980
43. Bandura A: Social Foundations of Thought and Action. Englewood Cliffs, NJ: Prentice Hall, 1986
44. Kotler P (ed): Marketing for Nonprofit Organizations. (2nd ed). Englewood Cliffs, NJ: Prentice Hall, 1975
45. Lynn WR, Thompson B, Pechacek TF: Community intervention trial for smoking cessation: Development of the intervention. In Community Based Intervention for Smokers: The COMMIT Field Experi-

ence [Smoking and Tobacco Control Monograph 6]. Washington, DC: NCI Smoking and Tobacco Control Monograph Series, 1995

46. Winkleby MA, Flora JA, Kraemer HC: A community-based cardiovascular disease prevention project: Predictors of change. Am J Public Health 84:767–772, 1994
47. Winkleby MA: The future of community-based cardiovascular disease intervention studies. Am J Public Health 84:1369–1372, 1994
48. Mittelmark MB, Hunt MK, Heath GW, Schmidt TL: Realistic outcomes: Lessons from community-based research and demonstration programs for the prevention of cardiovascular disease. J Public Health Policy 4:437–462, 1993
49. Carleton RA, Lasater TM, Assaf AR, Feldman HA, McKinaly S: The Pawtucket Heart Health Program: Community changes in cardiovascular risk factors and projected disease risk. Am J Public Health 85:777–785, 1995
50. Luepker RV, Murray DM, Jacobs DR, Mittelmark MB, Bracht N, Carlaw R, Crow R, Elmer P, Finnegan J, Folsom AR, Grimm R, Hannan PJ, Jeffrey R, Lando H, McGovern P, Mullis R, Perry CL, Pechacek T, Pirie P, Sprafka JM, Weisbrod R, Blackburn H: Community education for cardiovascular disease prevention: Risk factor changes in the Minnesota Heart Health Program. Am J Public Health 84:1383–1393, 1994
51. Lichtenstein E, Wallack L, Pechacek T: Introduction to the Community Intervention Trial for Smoking Cessation [COMMIT]. Int Q Health Education 11:173–186, 1990–1991
52. COMMIT Research Group Community intervention trial for smoking cessation: I. Cohort results from a four-year community intervention. Am J Public Health 85:183–192, 1995
53. COMMIT Research Group Community intervention trial for smoking cessation: II. Changes in adult cigarette smoking prevalence. Am J Public Health 85:193–200, 1995
54. Susser M: Editorial: The tribulations of trials—intervention in communities. Am J Public Health 85:156–168, 1995
55. Gorman DM, Speer PW: Preventing alcohol abuse and alcohol-related problems through community interventions: A review of evaluation studies. Psych and Health 11:95–131, 1996
56. Backer TE, Rogers EM, Sopory: Designing Health Education Campaigns: What Works. Newbury Park: Sage, 1992
57. Rangan VK, Sohel K, Sandberg: Do better at doing good. Harvard Business Rev May–June:42–54, 1996

48

Prevention and Health Education in Clinical, School, and Community Settings

Lawrence W. Green

Advances in biomedical and behavioral sciences have complicated the messages and methods of health education. No longer is the task simply one of informing and admonishing people about discrete actions they could take to protect themselves against single organisms or vectors of infectious diseases. Supplanting the germ theory with multicausal explanations of chronic and degenerative diseases meant replacing proscriptions with probabilities and single actions with lifelong behavioral development and lifestyle change. Demographic and living conditions, at least in western countries, shifted the emphasis of health education from survival and security to performance and productivity, from physical prowess to physical fitness, from mental hygiene to mental efficiency, from healthy people to healthful environments and policies.

These shifts occurred in the objectives of health education within the context of health promotion for the population at large. Still, large segments of the population have yet to achieve the full benefit of the first epidemiological revolution. Poor people continue to suffer premature death and preventable morbidity from infectious diseases, nutritional imbalances, unsafe work and residential environments, limited access to health care, and inadequate knowledge and organization in their communities. Public health and preventive medicine carry a frontline responsibility to reach these underserved segments of the population with a more basic health education in the context of organizational, economic, and environmental supports for behavior and conditions of living conducive to health.

New perspectives on the meaning of health and on the demand for behavioral and environmental interventions have called traditional health education into question as being too narrow in concept and too soft in method. I review how recent advances in the science and art of health education have been applied in practical ways within medical and other settings for prevention and public health. Even where the goals are too ambitious for health education alone, as with health promotion for complex lifestyle changes, health education remains an indispensable and primary component of organizational, economic, and environmental interventions designed to channel, support, or restrain behavior.

▶ DEFINITIONS

The terms health education, patient education, self-care education, school health education, and health promotion are distinguished from each other as follows.

Health education is any combination of learning experiences designed to predispose, enable, and reinforce voluntary adaptations of individual or collective behavior conducive to health.[1]

Patient education is initiated by medical care personnel to strengthen the motivation and ability of patients to adhere to prescribed medical or self-care regimens, including preparation for hospitalization, surgery, and rehabilitation.[2]

Self-care education is designed to predispose, enable, and reinforce individuals (not necessarily patients) or groups in diagnosing, managing, and monitoring their own health care needs. It differs from health education only in the sense that it refers more specifically to the judgments and actions for which people traditionally have depended on professionals.[3]

School health education is initiated and directed by personnel in preschool, school, or college to develop the motivation and skills required by students to cope with challenges to health and to build the foundation of knowledge required to comprehend the further health learning scheduled for their future. This definition is intended to narrow the range of behavioral and health objectives for which schools are accountable and to emphasize outcomes to which schools will be most responsive.[4]

Similar definitions can be framed for other setting-specific, disease-specific, or behavior-specific enterprises, such as occupational health education, nutrition education, physical education, cancer education, diabetes education, or dental health education. Each may be seen as a subset of health education or of school health education, depending on the setting, function, or target population.

Health promotion is any combination of educational, organizational, economic, and environmental supports for behavior and conditions of living conducive to health. Health promotion thus goes beyond health education when the behavior in question is beyond the control of the individual or group at risk. Health promotion is a component of public health and preventive medicine. The U.S. national strategy in disease prevention and health promotion, for example, includes three components: health promotion directed at behavioral causes of health, health protection directed at environmental causes, and preventive health services directed at the organization of medical resources and services.[5] Health education is a subset or strategy within each of these but is the primary and dominant strategy in health promotion (Fig. 48-1).

Most health education activities are embedded in other programs, and many are not identified as health education. Indeed, persons responsible for programs or studies sometimes attempt to distinguish

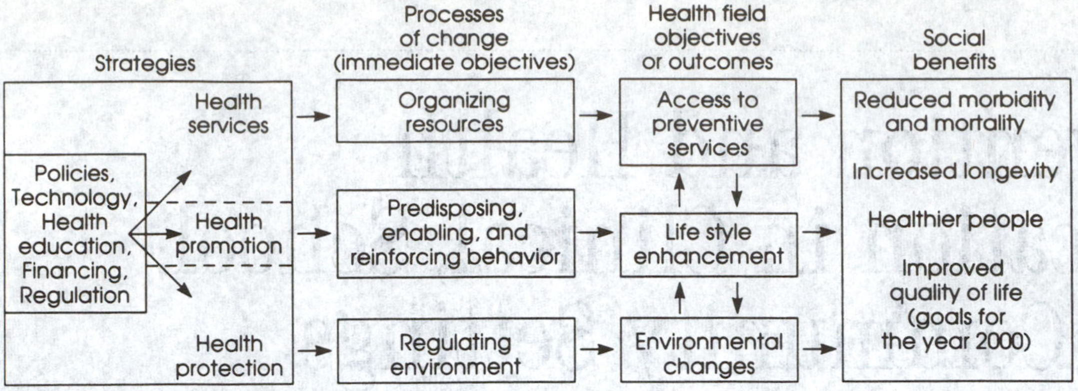

Figure 48-1. Functional relationships of health education strategies to immediate and long-term goals of health services, health promotion, and health protection.

their efforts as more innovative, modern, technological, behavioristic, client-centered, or scientific than they perceive health education to be. Alternative labeling occurs even when the methods employed clearly derive their approaches from education, educational psychology, educational technology, or health education itself.[6] Variations on self-care education, for example, have been referred to variously as "cognitive assessment and intervention procedures for relapse prevention,"[7] "self-monitoring . . . to provide feedback . . . in helping individuals assume more responsibility for their own care,"[8] and "helping people maximize their abilities to self-regulate [to] promote maintenance of behavior changes despite fluctuations in the physical and social environment."[9]

The varied labels used for health education programs and activities reveal the scope and diversity of educational applications in areas concerned with health.

Motivation

The term "motivation" refers to that which drives behaviors from within the individual, not to something done to the person to influence behavior. Interventions can appeal to or reward people's motives, not motivate them.[10] This term has been used incorrectly in some programs to refer to the activities generally included in health education and to incentive schemes used in "social marketing" to appeal more directly to economic and other nonhealth motives for behavioral change.[11]

Behavior Modification

Like motivation, the term "behavior modification" has expanded from its original applications by behaviorist psychologists to refer to a wider range of educational and political strategies for which the priority objectives are changes in behavior.[12] Most of the cognitive and training components of behavior modification, including self-monitoring, are essentially educational.

Health Counseling

This term and its variants (e.g., genetic counseling, diet counseling, patient counseling) represent an approach to voluntary change in health behavior. Most counseling methods of education have theoretical and philosophical roots in ego psychology, which is at extreme variance with behaviorism. Counseling is outside the scope of health education when it is more psychotherapeutic than informational in its method and content. Studies of doctor-patient interaction suggest a variety of purposes and tasks served by the reciprocal exchange of a counseling session besides educational purposes.[13]

Communications

The impact of communications on behaviors are studied in every sphere of human endeavor. Their applications in relation to health behaviors are usually within the scope of health education programming, except when they are used to advertise or promote products or causes that are inconsistent with the health needs of consumers.[14]

These examples of alternative labels used for health education activities illustrate what various programs may have in common and how they differ. Figure 48-2 provides an incomplete representation of these methods and techniques in relation to health education, suggesting aspects or applications of each that do not qualify as educational. The defining characteristic of health education is the voluntary participation of individuals in determining their own health practices. This is not merely a philosophical tenet. The durability of cognitive and behavioral changes is proportional to the degree of active rather than passive participation of the learner.[15]

Government and voluntary agencies adhere to this usage of health education to avoid public resistance or reaction to programs that might be perceived as propaganda or as being manipulative, coercive, politically or commercially directed, threatening, or paternalistic.[16]

Other forms of health education that define its scope are community organization, community development, policy advocacy, in-service training, consultation, group work, computer-assisted instruction (CAI), other teaching machines and audio-visual methods, bibliotherapy, patient teaching, health fairs, exhibits, libraries, conferences, and social marketing.

Planning for disease prevention and health promotion in several countries has applied these methods in community, medical, occupational, and school settings. Health promotion is seen as the broader enterprise of creating a supportive environment for behaviors conducive to health. Health promotion must necessarily include health education but may require more structural, financial, technological, and even coercive interventions (e.g., regulatory or tax penalty laws) to influence behavior when it is deemed that such behavior threatens the health of others—as with reckless driving, irresponsible alcohol or drug use, marketing of harmful food products to young children, or smoking in crowded public places.[17]

Health education applies to that range of behavior that is voluntary, self-directed, and relatively self-controlled. To the extent that the health outcomes to which health education may be addressed are not entirely controlled by behavior, health education may require the additional supports of medical services and resources and environmental controls over toxic and infectious agents, as suggested by Figure 48-1. Even where organizational, economic, or environmental supports for behavior or health outcomes are paramount, health education helps to gain the cooperation of political and administrative decision makers, directors and staffs of agencies dispensing services or resources, and the voting public.

Health education occurs through the mass media and in various settings: worksites (occupational health and safety, employee health promotion), medical (patient education, health education in primary care settings and hospitals), community agencies (voluntary health organizations, health fairs, health promotion events), and schools.

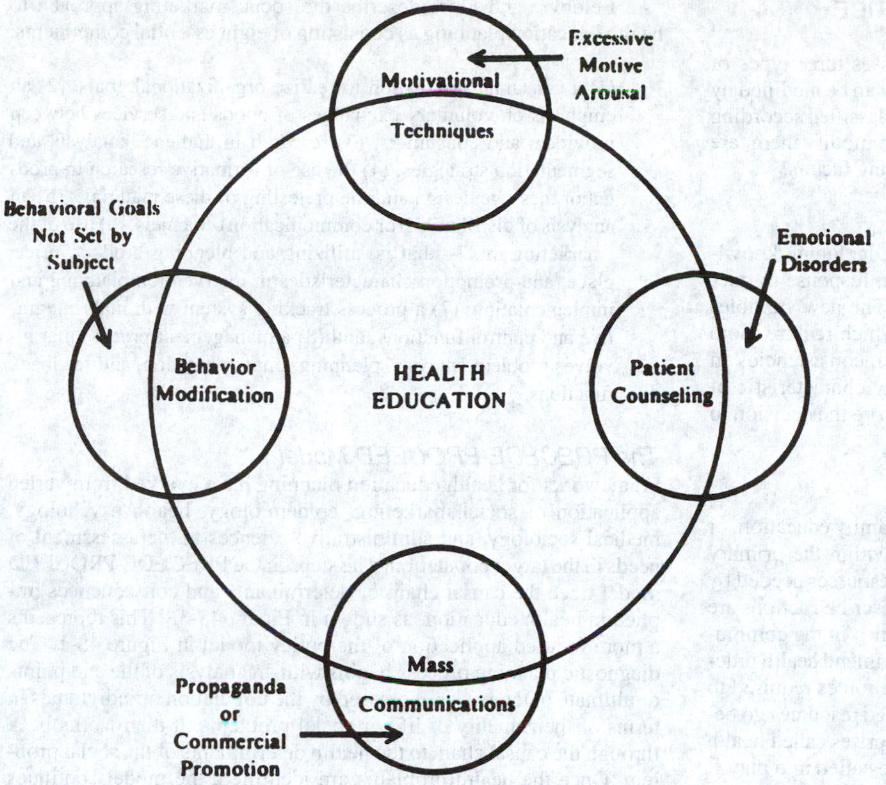

Figure 48-2. Examples of overlapping technologies for changing health-related behavior, showing the aspects of the technologies that fall outside the definition of health education.

Patient education represents health education centered in medical care settings, but not necessarily limited to clinics or hospitals, to the patients themselves, or to diagnosed health problems. It may include education to prevent the onset of symptoms, and it may be directed at family members.[18]

Because classrooms are the primary locus of school health education and because children or adolescents are the major target groups, the methods of school health education are largely pedagogical, and concentration is on the health and behavioral problems of children and youth. The other distinguishing characteristic of school health education is its limited focus on educational outcomes.

> It is taken as a task of school health education . . . that children at each age or grade should be helped to master those health maintenance skills necessary to cope with potential threats to their health in the coming age or grade, and those additional foundation skills necessary to benefit from the instructions next year in relation to the potential health problems of the year after that.[19]

▸ THE CHANGING CIRCUMSTANCES OF HEALTH EDUCATION

In the earliest practice of health education, the health outcomes of primary concern were injuries and infectious diseases. The behavior required of children, youth, and adults was largely assumed to be in the sphere of personal safety or hygienic practices. Such practices were equated with good manners and moral development. By associating personal hygiene with socially acceptable behavior, a causal link was implied between personal responsibility for social good and the communicable nature of diseases spread by contact, or between behaving recklessly and endangering public safety.[20]

As the infectious diseases gave way to chronic, degenerative, developmental, and violent causes of death and disability, contagion no longer served as the underlying rationale for health education. Proper health behavior no longer can be prescribed entirely on the basis of the common good or family welfare. Unhealthful behavior must be prescribed in relation to increasingly personal, distant, and improbable or seemingly inevitable morbid events in the future. In contrast with the past, current generations are told that virtually every substance they consume and every pleasure they seek has some chance of harming them. In short, probabilities have replaced precept, data have replaced dictum, decision-making skills have replaced definitions of proper health conduct. The behavioral sciences have influenced understanding of the forces affecting behavior so that health educators today are expected to design their programs with traditional attention to knowledge, attitudes, and skills but also with methods and materials that take into account the circumstances that enable behavior to occur and that provide for rewards that will reinforce the desired behavior.[21] Attention to circumstances is understood to be especially important in health promotion, where the behaviors of increasing concern are heavily embedded in lifestyle and social learning. Weight loss, for example, will not yield to simplistic lesson plans that drill patients on food groups,[22] nor will smoking be prevented simply by increasing the percentage of students who know it may cause cancer.[23]

These changes in the problems and patterns of health education have broadened the assumptions concerning cause-and-effect relationships between intervention and potential health benefits. Some educators and evaluators continue to emphasize content in health education and content mastery in testing, although the content itself has changed. Most health educators, however, have come to grips with the value-laden and socially charged issues of lifestyle changes, acquired immunodeficiency syndrome (AIDS), teenage pregnancy, drug abuse, and smoking by placing greater emphasis on factors beyond factual knowledge. Bending too far from factual knowledge and understanding, however, has resulted in some programs achieving expedient change at the expense of durable change.[24] People will make token changes in response to token rewards or social influence, but unless they also understand and believe in the personally relevant reasons for maintaining the change, they will return to their former behavior as soon as the token rewards are withdrawn or the socially influential person is out of sight.[25]

▶ NEW SCOPE OF THEORY AND PRACTICE

Contemporary practice of health education addresses three types of factors that may influence health behaviors and that can be modified by educational intervention. The three sets of factors, classified according to the types of interventions or methods required to modify them, are predisposing factors, enabling factors, and reinforcing factors.

Predisposing Factors

These include the traditional targets of education, including knowledge, attitudes, and beliefs, which often change in response to one-way didactic and mass communication methods. The new variables in this category include values and perceptions, which require more interactive communication to clarify and adjust inconsistencies in values and misperceptions of reality. The defining characteristic of predisposing factors is their motivational force before the decision to take a given health action.[26]

Enabling Factors

These call for some community health education, family education, or staff education and organizational development within the primary care setting, worksite, or school to assure that the resources needed by patients, employees, or students to carry out the prescribed actions are accessible. The accessibility of resources or facilities in the community or the institution must concern those who recommend health practices that are blocked by circumstances. When the forces required to change these circumstances or to mobilize the needed resources go beyond education, strategies within the broader enterprises called health promotion, health services, or health protection are called into play.[27]

Reinforcing Factors

These have become more prevalent in health education where the assumed causes of the behavior are largely social, such as peer influence. These factors may include token rewards (e.g., certificate of achievement) or tangible rewards (e.g., money) for successful trials or test performances, but more significant reinforcing factors are those associated with social learning.[28] One of the most fruitful lines of theory and research in recent health education efforts directed at the problems of smoking, drug abuse, and adolescent sexuality has been with concepts of *inoculation* against peer pressure: children are reinforced for demonstrating skills in declining or resisting the offer of a cigarette or pressure to engage in sexual activity, against their better judgment.

The most effective health education programs combine learning experiences directed at all three sets of factors influencing behavior, based on an educational diagnosis of the predominant variables in each category. A behavior that is highly motivated and reinforced will be frustrated if it is not also enabled. A motivated and enabled behavior that meets with social punishment or ridicule rather than reinforcement will not persist. Any review of contemporary research can be organized around the three sets of factors influencing health behavior.

Planning and Evaluation Models for Health Education

Social Marketing

Divorced from its public health or medical context, health education planning can be seen as a social marketing research task.[29] As defined by Kotler, social marketing is "The analysis, planning, implementation and control of carefully formulated programs designed to bring about voluntary exchanges of values with target markets for the purpose of achieving organizational objectives."[30] Insert "health" in this definition and it would define health education as an organizational strategy to engage the public in helping achieve the organization's objective. Manoff took the social marketing concepts and methods closer to health education by subtitling his book on the subject, New Imperative for Public Health.[31] His applications and examples of social marketing methods are taken from nutrition education, family planning, and other health education campaigns in developing countries.

Lefebvre and Flora describe the social marketing approach to health education planning as consisting of eight essential components:

> (1) a consumer orientation to realize organizational goals, (2) an emphasis on voluntary exchanges of goods and services between providers and consumers, (3) research in audience analysis and segmentation strategies, (4) the use of formative research in product or message design and the pretesting of these materials, (5) an analysis of distribution (or communication) channels, (6) use of the "marketing mix"—that is, utilizing and blending product, price, place, and promotion characteristics in intervention planning and implementation, (7) a process tracking system with both integrative and control functions, and (8) a management process that involves problem analysis, planning, implementation, and feedback functions.[32]

The PRECEDE-PROCEED Model

Frameworks for health education planning have evolved from varied application of social marketing, epidemiology, health psychology, medical sociology, and administrative sciences in the assessment of needs in the target population. The steps in the PRECEDE-PROCEED model trace the causal chain of determinants and consequences implied in health education, as shown in Figure 48-3.[33] This represents a more focused application of the policy model in Figure 48-1. The diagnostic planning process begins with an analysis of the end points or ultimate outcomes as expressed by the population or individuals in terms of their quality of life or social problems. It then works back through the causal chain to the health determinants of the social problem. Once the health problems are identified, the model continues with an analysis of the behavioral determinants of each health problem. As with each preceding step, critical selection of the behaviors that are most important and potentially changeable must eliminate from further analysis those factors that fail to meet both criteria, or else the process becomes too cumbersome.

The next step is to identify the factors determining the behaviors previously identified. Finally, the administrative diagnosis identifies the educational resources and interventions that can be deployed to initiate the process of predisposing, enabling, and reinforcing behavior conducive to health.

The PRECEDE-PROCEED framework helped in the formulation of targeted and focused health education programs where earlier programs had been diffuse and inefficiently scattered over too many objects and processes of change. The acronym PRECEDE stands for *predisposing, reinforcing, and enabling constructs in educational diagnosis and evaluation*. It was intended to emphasize the repeated etiological search for what precedes the problem at hand.

Critics of the original PRECEDE framework pointed out that it left environmental determinants of health dangling in a residual category, implying that the responsibility for health should fall entirely on the people whose behavior was errant, regardless of their environmental circumstances. The framework also left the political, regulatory, and organizational context for implementation of programs to the imagination of the user. These concerns became increasingly important during the 1980s as the new policies in health promotion provided opportunities for health education to be teamed with more regulatory and organizational interventions, such as smoking ordinances and company arrangements for release time or facilities for employee participation in health programs. Such policies, regulations, and organizational arrangements supplement the educational interventions directed at enabling factors and environmental barriers to change.

With the health promotion movement, PRECEDE evolved an additional set of appendages and steps in the planning and evaluation process referred to as PROCEED. This acronym refers to *policy, regulatory, and organizational constructs in educational and environmental development*. PROCEED, as seen in Figure 48-4, continues where PRECEDE leaves off, but with implementation rather than planning as the focus.

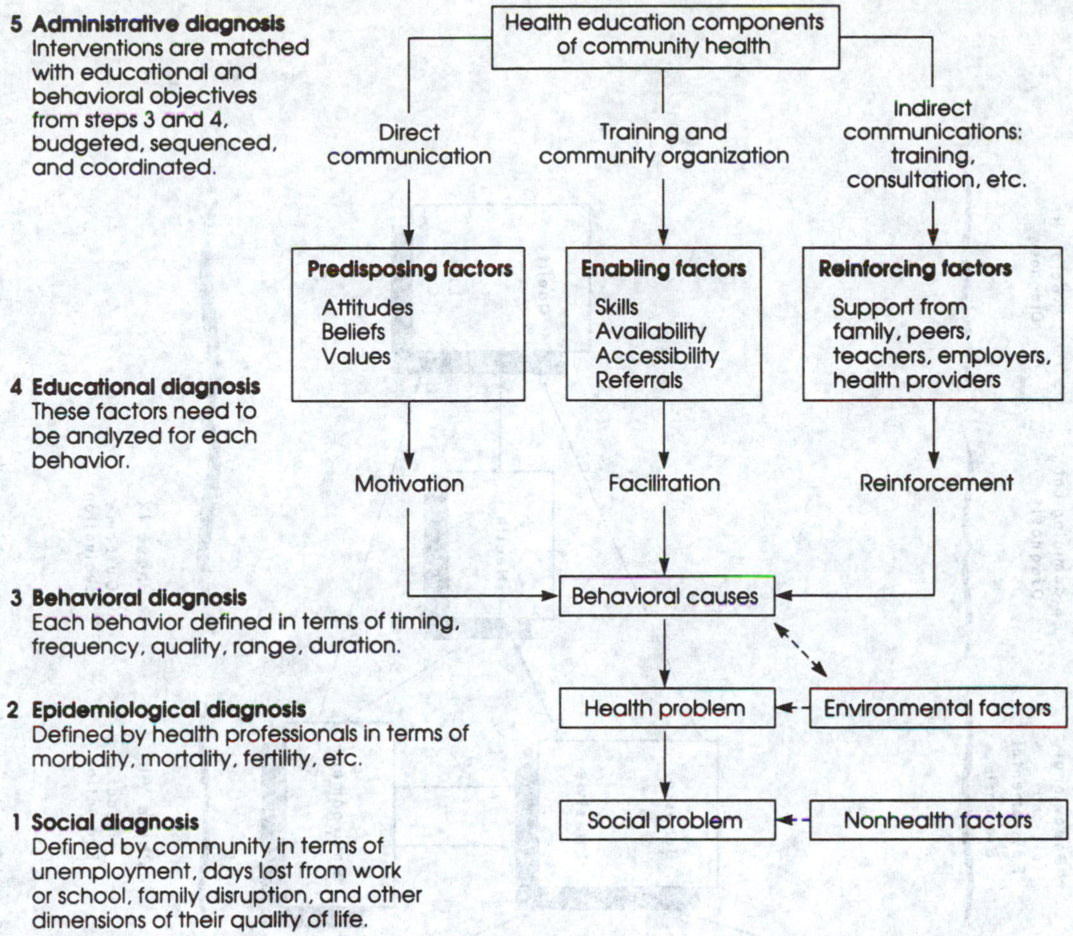

Figure 48-3. The five steps preceding the development of a specific plan of health education, related to the determinants of each level of outcome in a hierarchy of objectives for health programs, referred to as the PRECEDE framework.

Social Learning Model

Of the three sets of factors—predisposing, enabling, and reinforcing—those that reinforce (reward or punish) health behavior are likely to be the most influential in relation to the development of complex behavior that must be maintained. Reinforcing factors determine whether a behavior that is motivated and enabled will occur or persist once it has been contemplated or tried. Depending on the social models demonstrating the behavior and the quality of feedback received in response to the behavior, the pattern of behavior will be more or less likely to develop and persist. Social learning theory has elaborated the reinforcing factors important to health education by showing how they can occur before the behavior has been enacted. These include efficacy expectations (Can I do it?) and outcome expectations (What benefit will it bring me?).[34] The theory also emphasizes vicarious learning and self-reinforcement as ways in which individuals can learn without necessarily receiving direct, external rewards.[35]

The most important sources of reinforcement are beyond the control of clinical personnel. These sources include the family, mass media, and peer influences, in that order of dominance for children. Peer influences, however, increase with age and eventually surpass the family in social influence on adolescents and young adults.[36] With advancing age, organizational, economic, and environmental factors play an increasing role in enabling and reinforcing health behavior.

Even where family influence, mass media, and peer pressure are beyond the direct control of the primary care setting and the school, these institutional centers can still prepare children and adults to recognize and to be able to resist mass media and peer pressures to adopt unhealthful practices. This approach has yielded impressive results in the delay of onset of smoking, alcohol, and drug use in children and adolescents.[37]

In summary, the evidence strongly supports the employment of methods in health education that help people resist social pressures for unhealthful behavior, especially those of family and the mass media. The appropriate level of parental involvement, however, is in dispute. It appears to be most effective to involve parents while the children are young, but some authorities emphasize the need for children to learn independent, adult-free decision making about health matters at younger ages.[38]

▸ SELF-CARE EDUCATION IN MEDICAL SETTINGS

Immediate and compelling opportunities for health education to influence behavioral risk factors exist with patients in medical care settings. The evidence for effective interventions is stronger from randomized trials in this arena than from others. Especially well documented through meta-analyses are studies in preoperative counseling to improve postoperative outcomes[39] and in patient education to reduce drug errors[40] and quit smoking.[41]

Patients can play a major role in the maintenance and management of their own health and disease. The increasing prevalence of chronic and degenerative disease, the increasing costs of medical care, and the increasing importance of patient behavior as a determinant of health outcomes all have forced growing attention on self-care education as an inescapable component of secondary prevention.[42]

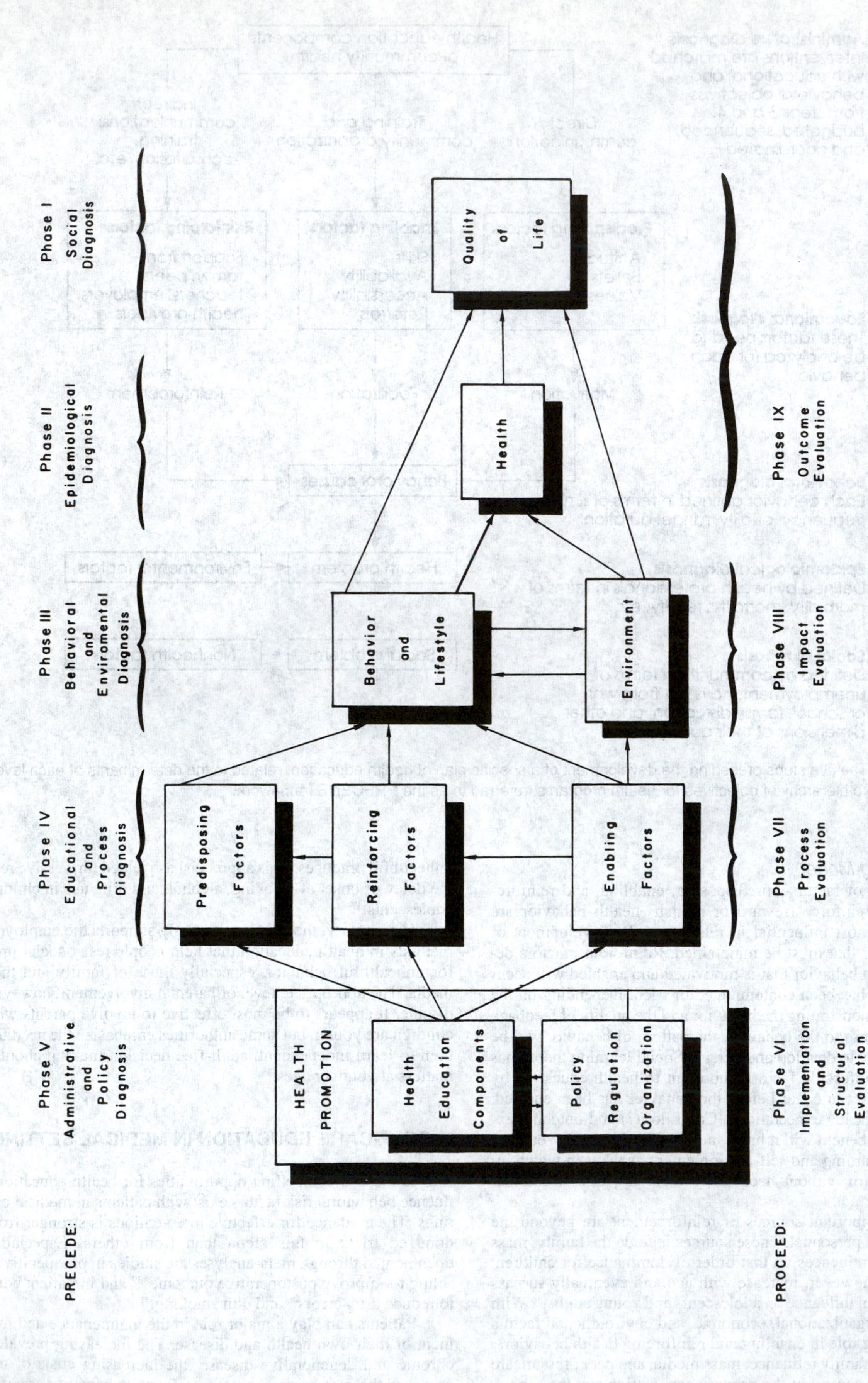

Figure 48-4. Phases of PRECEDE and PROCEED models for health education and health promotion.

The questions center not on whether to allow self-care but on how to organize and support it. How can the physician, for example, organize a medical practice that turns responsibility over to patients for a larger role in their own care without abrogating the physician's function? How can a medical practice devote sufficient resources to self-care education to be effective without stretching its resources so thin that medical procedures are compromised? How can the transfer to patients of responsibility for their own care provide for the necessary monitoring and surveillance of responsible medical care and secondary prevention?

The Role of the Clinical Setting

Conceding that self-care education is necessary still leaves open to debate whether health care workers in clinical settings should assume responsibility for it. Some have argued that self-care education belongs outside the medical sector, that nonmedical agencies can provide it at lower cost, with fewer conflicts of interest, and at less sacrifice to frank medical services. This argument is most credible with regard to the concerns of primary prevention or health promotion where the temptation to medicalize lifestyle issues draws the health care worker into some complex social, economic, and ethical arenas. How far should the physician or nurse go, for example, in pressing patients to stop smoking or to change eating habits that are highly interwoven with family, occupational, or ethnic ties? Should physicians extend the scope of their practice to intervene effectively on alcohol consumption, stress management, and physical fitness?

Some clinicians hedge the stridency of their advice to patients and some patients avoid a physician who advocates changes in health-related behavior without considering other dimensions of their life circumstances.[43]

These issues apply also to nonmedical settings, but the costs relative to the risks and benefits can be lowered by educating people in groups, thus reducing overhead costs and unit costs of educational personnel, media, and facilities. Locating these educational functions outside the clinical practice of medicine also conserves the expensive time of the physician for more strictly medical problems, including the supervision of self-care in secondary prevention. Just as the hospital is not an ideal setting for the efficient and cost-effective provision of primary medical care, the primary care setting is less than ideal for the continuing supervision and education of most people (not to say patients) in their struggle with habits of daily living related to primary prevention.[44]

Clinical settings, nevertheless, provide ideal venues in which to offer habituated patients a number of positive reinforcements. These can include initial encouragement, a medical rationale to help them perceive the benefits of behavioral change, the credibility of medical expertise and familiarity with their history, suggestions for strategies of behavioral change that fit their medical and economic circumstances, an authoritative referral for outside help, and periodic support of their progress with the habit on subsequent medical encounters. Physicians also can stimulate social support for their patients by asking family members to come in with the patients for health education or, better still, by treating the family as a unit. Physicians can in this way use their position in the community to coordinate lifestyle modification with agencies better equipped than they are to offer some types of health education and social support economically and effectively.[45]

Secondary prevention, on the other hand, requires early and effective response to signs or symptoms. Self-care education then does represent a larger opportunity for an effective and economical role for the clinical setting. The research on this aspect of patient education indicates that it holds the potential for large savings in unnecessary medical care costs, emergency room visits, hospitalization, absenteeism, disability days, and premature deaths and for improved quality of life for patients with chronic conditions.[46] It also may have the side benefits of reducing malpractice suits and broken appointments and of increasing patient satisfaction.[47] These and other benefits are achieved by enhancing patient understanding and participation in the development of the treatment or maintenance regimen and enhancing adherence to the prescribed regimen.[48]

The possible tradeoffs of increased self-care education in primary care include the time and opportunity costs of the physician and other personnel that might have been devoted to more lucrative medical activities, the production or purchase costs of educational materials, the increased independence of patients, who make less frequent office visits, and the potential risks of mismanagement in less competent patients. The control of these costs and potential risks are discussed in the following paragraphs.

Implementation of Patient Education

Medical care personnel resist implementing self-care education in primary care in part because they fear that it will become a bottomless pit of counseling on an array of psychological and social problems. The best way to overcome this barrier is to classify the major problems and needs of patients into categories that are broad enough to allow an initial triage of patients into a few educational categories for each disease or self-care task. This will help to control the array. To control the sense of a bottomless pit, a stepped approach to each triage group is needed. These two strategies, applied in sequence, can limit the costs and can maximize the benefits of self-care education in primary care and in hospitals.

One approach to triage is to identify which source of support for the prescribed behavior is lacking. This educational diagnosis sorts patients into one of three groups where (*a*) personal motivation is lacking, (*b*) there is motivation, but a self-care skill or other resource is lacking, or (*c*) personal motivation and skill are both present, but there is little or no support for patients at home, school, or work. As seen in Figure 48-5, this classification yields a hierarchy of three categories of patients for whom qualitatively different educational objectives and methods can be drawn from the growing accumulation of health education literature organized around predisposing, enabling, and reinforcing factors.[49]

The first category of patients can be educated through direct communication to alter the predisposing beliefs, attitudes, and perceptions. Counseling the patients on three health beliefs in particular can be expected to provide the best motivational foundation to predispose them to take a more active role in self-care: (1) the belief that they are susceptible to the consequences of not following the prescribed regimen of self-care, (2) the belief that the consequences might be severe, and (3) the belief that the benefits of the recommended self-care methods outweigh the costs and inconvenience.[50]

Patients in the second group face the enabling factors of skill or resources as their primary barrier to self-care practice. These patients are motivated, but they will be frustrated if they are expected to carry out complicated or expensive self-care procedures without specific forms of help. The essential ingredients in the health care worker's initial responsibility to these patients are basic instruction and training to build the necessary skills, coupled with an appropriate payment plan or a referral to a specific community source of resources or support.[51]

The third group of patients has predisposing and enabling factors already in place, but their continuing practice of the recommended behavior is threatened by one or more social or environmental factors in the home or workplace. These factors will punish the patients for self-care, making the immediate social costs and inconvenience of the behavior outweigh the more distant medical rewards. The best educational antidote for patients in this group is to invite family members, with the permission of the patients, to discuss ways in which they can support the patients in following the self-care regimen. An alternative (for this group and others) is to form patient groups that meet periodically with or without invited partners to exchange self-care experiences and to provide mutual support and reinforcement. This, of course, is more economical and also provides the third category of patients a substitute form of social reinforcement for self-care when the home or work environment cannot be altered.

Medical and nursing care can be most helpful in referring patients to community organizations and resources, such as self-help groups, weight-control programs, voluntary agencies, and health education centers. These resources can provide the additional education, training, facilities, and social support necessary to predispose,

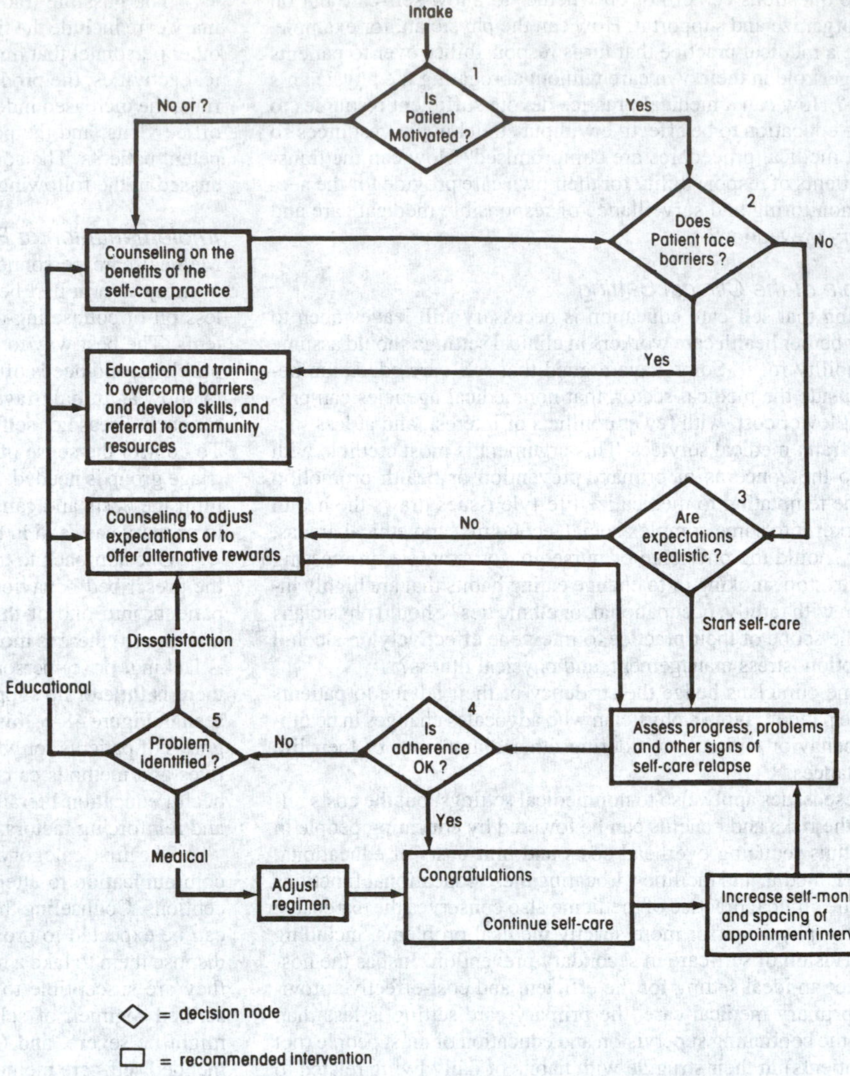

Figure 48-5. Algorithm for the triage and stepped approach to self-care education for patients in clinical settings.

enable, or reinforce the self-care practice. Return appointments to see patients after the referral can provide a responsible means of ensuring that the needed help is being received in a form consistent with the medical indications for the recommended self-care. A follow-up appointment provides the patient with an additional incentive to pursue the referral and to act on the recommended self-care practices. It also identifies the strengths and weaknesses of community organizations in providing medically sound self-care education and support. The physician then can participate more effectively as a professional member of the community in correcting deficiencies in health education resources, services, and facilities.

Monitoring Patient Education

Return appointment enable the physician to verify the diagnosis, to evaluate progress of the treatment, and to correct any deficiencies in the treatment. The same principle applies in self-care, but it needs to be put in an operational form that takes into account the greater complexity and duration of the usual self-care regimen in secondary prevention (e.g., hypertension medications, weight control, sodium intake). A stepped-care approach is recommended for the systematic transfer of responsibility to patients and for the responsible monitoring of self-care practices.

A stepped-care approach can proceed from the triage method outlined in the previous section, moving the patients in group 1 to group 2 and from group 2 to group 3. Once patients are receiving the necessary environmental and social support for the recommended self-care practice, the next step can be to wean them from dependency on health professional supervision of the self-care practice. This can be accomplished with a minimum of risk only if patients learn to observe the same primary signals that physicians and other health professionals use in detecting an irregularity in the results of self-care (e.g., blood pressure readings in hypertensive patients, blood sugar readings in diabetic patients).

The means and the ends in self-care are as much self-monitoring as they are self-treatment. For example, educating hypertensive patients to take their own blood pressure readings at home or at work makes it possible to transfer not only the perfunctory aspects of following a rigid self-treatment regimen but also the evaluative function of monitoring and recording changes in the resulting blood pressure. The self-monitoring function can become a major source of reinforcement of proper self-treatment, so that two forms of self-care behavior are strengthened and become mutually reinforcing in a continuous feedback loop. This can make patients less dependent on the physician for evaluation. It also makes them less dependent on family and friends for social reinforcement of self-care behavior.

The ultimate step in a stepped-care program of self-care education establishes a truly collaborative relationship between the health care professional and the patient for treatment and monitoring. The health care professional assesses the quality of patient self-care and reduces the frequency of office visits according to the validation of patient self-assessments. Office visits may be more frequent if patients have multiple risk factors or medical, social, and economic complications. Some fail-safe signals should be included in the protocol for patient self-monitoring to ensure that patients call in response to some symptoms. Periodic mailing of self-monitoring records and a tickler file in the office can assure patients that they are not forgotten by the physician, but reinforce their independence and interdependence rather than their dependence.

The procedure for initiating stepped care would assign most patients to group 2 ideally for skill training unless they obviously are unmotivated or already are skilled in self-treatment. Those who show little interest or motivation for self-treatment would be assigned to group 1 for education on the three health beliefs. Those who have the necessary skills and resources to carry out the regimen can be advanced to group 3.

The health care professional can make reasonable assessments and assignments, even without standardized instruments for educational triage, by asking patients such questions as: What do you know about your illness? Do you have any specific fears or concerns about it? How serious do you think it is? What are your goals for the treatment of your condition? What are your feelings about the prescribed therapeutic regimen? Can you describe how you will go about your self-treatment? Do you expect to have any problems with family, friends, or employers in carrying out these procedures?

The additional education needed for self-monitoring can be built into the same three phases of predisposing, enabling, and reinforcing education as suggested in Figure 48-5.

In summary, two conditions ensure that the benefits of self-care education in clinical settings will outweigh the costs. One is that the behavior in question is related to a diagnosed medical condition rather than to a general health habit embedded in the lifestyle of patients. The second is that the predisposing and enabling barriers for patients are not so great as to render them ineffective in trying to carry out the recommended self-care practices.

Even in primary prevention, the health care workers in clinical settings can encourage patients, present data on the expected benefits of behavioral change, explore the costs of attempting to change behavior, offer strategies for minimizing these costs, refer patients to community resources and programs, and follow-up with reinforcement for any progress the patients have made at the time of subsequent office visits.

▶ HEALTH EDUCATION IN SCHOOL SETTINGS

The object of much attention in health education and preventive health services, evaluations of school programs appear to have produced some disappointment with the outcomes. The disappointments stem largely from expectations that these programs and services should have given us more spectacular gains in health outcomes (i.e., morbidity and mortality reductions). In contrast to expectations, the 15- to 24-year age group, representing the immediate fruits of school health programs and services, was the only age group in the United States to experience an increased death rate in recent decades.[52] In addition, substance abuse and sexually transmitted diseases have increased, and injuries from automobile crashes and violence remain highest in the secondary school ages.

Health care services as we know them today cannot be expected to have prevented these problems, any more than school health education alone could have prevented them. A renewed partnership of health services with community social and educational agencies and private organizations would emphasize a different set of outcomes than those of primary importance to the health services. These mutually beneficial outcomes would be more in line with educational models than with those of medicine and public health.[53] They would also gain greater hospitality in the education sector.

Public Health Models of Health Education Applied to Schools

Most health programs have had only marginal utility in schools because their end points (health outcomes) do not address the primary function of schools, namely, education. School health services and curricula have been supported or hosted by the educational establishment only to the extent that the health outcomes (or health problems prevented) were believed to have enhanced the educational mission of the schools.[54]

Within public health, health education has required more complex and difficult-to-test models because of the necessary linkages of cognitive, environmental, and behavioral variables, each of which is variously and sometimes tenuously related to the others and to health outcomes. A generic health education model is one that contains, by definition, a combination of interventions designed to predispose, enable, and reinforce voluntary adaptations of behavior conducive to health.

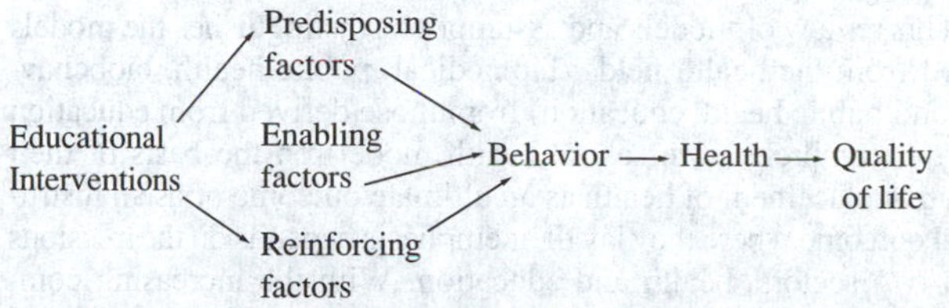

(A)

School Health Education Models

After decades of little or no evaluation, an impressive record of school health education impact on health behavior began to accumulate in the 1980s. The most thoroughly documented is with improvements in knowledge, attitudes, and skills assumed to be important in the subsequent development of health behavior. In this hierarchy and sequencing of effects, an implicit model is imposed on, rather than inherent in, school health education.

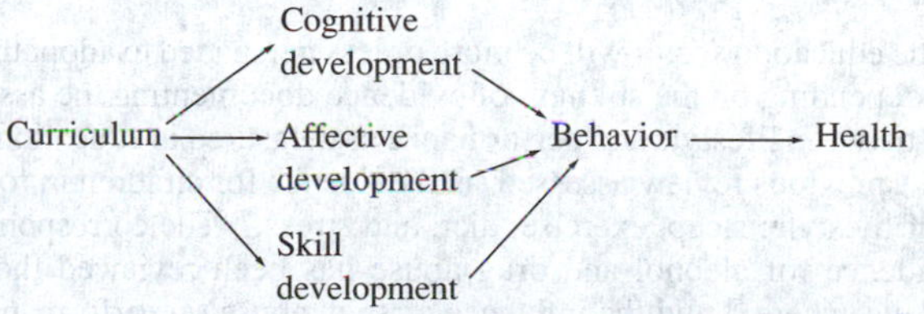

(B)

This model, derivative of the public health education model (A), places ultimate importance on health outcomes and the behaviors necessary to achieve them. The problem is that schools are neither medical institutions nor public health agencies and have never adopted the same mission and goals. School health educators have worked valiantly to live up to the expectations of their public health education colleagues, but they have been fighting an uphill battle within the education sector in recent years with the back-to-basics movement. The schools simply cannot be held accountable for solutions to all the ills of society. The line is now being drawn more severely but also more creatively between the primary educational mission of the schools and the functions that other agencies would like them to serve through school-linked integrated human services.[56]

The Comprehensive School Health Program Model

Recognition that the classroom alone cannot be expected to accomplish behavioral and health outcomes led to a return to a basic model of school health programs, one that was not derivative of public health education but rather of education in general. This model combines health teaching with school and community health services and environment to produce a level of health necessary to ensure that students can perform effectively in school and achieve academically. The two significant departures of this model from the preceding models are (*a*) the combination of education with school and community services and environmental interventions to promote health and (*b*) the emphasis on health as a means to educational ends.

The comprehensive school health program model would approximate the following:

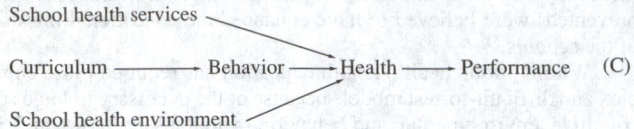

School health services ↘
Curriculum ⟶ Behavior ⟶ Health ⟶ Performance (C)
School health environment ↗

The education sector is not obliged to justify its attention to performance and achievement in terms of its contribution to health, just as senior citizen centers are not obliged to justify their recreational programs in terms of their contribution to health. Yet both contribute to health and, therefore, could be construed as health services or health programs.

This review of models and assumptions distinguishes the models derived from the health fields (biomedical, public health, biobehavioral, and public health education) from those derived from education (e.g., the comprehensive school health model) on the basis of their respective placement of health as an ultimate outcome or as an instrumental outcome where they lay their emphasis depends on the missions of the two sectors, health and education. With the increasing complexity of etiologies and causal pathways for specific diseases and health problems, the health establishment seems ready to entertain more complex and time-lapsed models of intervention as related to health outcomes. The growing interest in disease prevention and health promotion attests to this. At the same time, the schools and their constituencies are demanding greater time on task and improved achievement scores of their students. The convergence of these trends suggests a new rationale for health education in schools in which behavioral and performance variables are targeted for the short-term outcomes.

Intervention ⟶ Lifestyle ⟶ Performance ⟶ Achievement (D)

The education sector will be more or less persuaded to adopt this model depending on the strength of evidence documenting the association between lifestyle and performance as measured in educational terms. A previous review assessed such evidence for children in four areas of lifestyle: sleep, exercise, diet, and stress.[57] The corresponding evidence for alcohol and drug abuse has been reviewed thoroughly elsewhere,[58] and the influence of such abuse on performance in school is hardly in doubt.

To sustain the interest and possible support of the health establishment, this model needs to be extended to show its potential contribution to health outcomes. The main argument affirming the relevance of this model to health is the pervasive and inescapable correlation between educational attainment and health.[59] The connection of educational attainment to health is explained most logically in behavioral terms, although genetic and economic factors undeniably enter into both the educational attainment and the health behavior of children and their parents. The empirical evidence supporting the causal link between educational attainment and health behavior is consistent but tenuous, in that it is not experimental. Similarly, the link between health behaviors and long-term health outcomes is widely documented and accepted but nearly impossible to establish experimentally.

With these caveats in mind, the following model would seem to place health education (curriculum) most appropriately within the context of schools.

School health services ↘
Health Curriculum ⟶ Lifestyle ⟶ Performance ⟶ Achievement ⟶ Health (E)
School environment ↗

This highly simplified model leaves out a variety of exogenous influences. These include aspects of the curriculum on performance, factors other than performance on achievement, and factors outside the school, including coordinated community health services and community health promotion efforts, on all the outcomes. The purpose of this model is simply to specify the essential elements linking school health education and related interventions with health outcomes in a causal chain that recognizes and gives primacy to the educational outcomes, which are the main, if not the sole, concern of the schools.

▶ HEALTH PROMOTION IN THE COMMUNITY

Comprehensive school health as modeled in (C) approximates at the school level what has come to be associated with health promotion at the community and national level in two ways. First, the combination of health education with organizational and environmental services and resources in support of health behavior, in both the school health model and in the health promotion model, relieves some of the unrealistic expectation of health education alone to accomplish behavioral and health outcomes. Second, the recognition that health is not necessarily an end in itself but may serve other values and social goals or quality-of-life concerns is in keeping with the positive concepts of health as "physical, mental, and social well-being" inherent in the earliest approaches to health education in the World Health Organization (WHO)[60] and in the more recent formulations of policy in health promotion.[61]

This instrumental function of health is reflected in the resolution of the World Health Assembly of 1977: "The main social target of Governments and WHO in the coming decades should be the attainment by all the citizens of the world, by the year 2000, of a level of health that will permit them to lead a socially and economically productive life." Where the WHO, the U.S. Surgeon General, and private industries initiating worksite health promotion programs speak of productivity, the schools speak of performance and academic achievement. Where the school health models speaks of combining education with school health services and interventions in the school environment, national policy combines health promotion with health services and health protection, as reflected in Figure 48-1.

The health promotion movement also has forced health professionals to recognize more immediate benefits to be appreciated from lifestyle modification than most of them would normally count as health outcomes. Some would not be counted because they are too subjective, such as "feeling good," and "feeling more energetic." Others would not be counted because they are considered to have more to do with cosmetics, economics, or social norms than with objectively defined health. These include such outcomes of "healthier" lifestyle as weight control, agility, endurance, concentration, efficiency of movement, muscle tone, and independence in activities of daily living.[62]

These and related intangibles make up a large part of the quality-of-life or social concerns that were considered consequences of health in the public health education model (A). They were given prominence there because public health education begins "where the people are" as a practical matter similar to that of social marketing. Educational research, especially on adult populations,[63] has demonstrated also that the commitment of people to the goals of a program increases the probability of their participation, cooperation, or behavioral response to a program.[64] Recognizing that the priority concerns of a population are seldom expressed in terms of health, public health education typically has worked to show people how health can contribute to their quality-of-life or social interests.

▶ LARGE-SCALE CAMPAIGNS AND COMMUNITY PROGRAMS

Large-scale campaigns and programs in communities are, of course, bigger than their counterparts at the clinical, school, or worksite levels. But is there a qualitative difference in community or multicommunity programs from their component interventions in medical and other institutional settings, or do they merely represent the sum of these parts? Besides coordination of the pieces, what makes community programs run? Other than the additive effects of small-scale programs, what makes large-scale programs more or less effective?

At the heart of a public health approach to health education and health promotion, these questions defy simplistic answers that would merely distinguish community approaches from institutionally based programs in terms of magnitude, scope, or volume. There is something more than critical mass that holds such community or multi-community programs together over time. They are more than medical models writ large, more than pedagogic methods transferred to the media, more than a step up the bureaucratic ladder from town to county or from province to nation.

Community or large-scale programs, even within large institutions, require a shift in perspective and employment of a distinct set of analytical and programmatic tools from those used with patients, clients, or customers. The differences reflect a blend of the distinctions between clinical and epidemiological methods of analysis, between strictly psychological and social-psychological theories, between counseling and mass media methods of communication, and between intraorganizational and interorganizational levels of intervention and management.

Three Generalizations and Propositions

Implications to be drawn from the experience and data on large-scale campaigns and community health education programs are as follows:

1. Large-scale health education and health promotion efforts require, above all, more planning and coordination than small-scale programs. More participants in the planning and execution means more meetings and telephone calls to achieve consensus, more letters and documents to convey concepts and procedures to more varied actors. The complexities grow exponentially with each additional organization or community added to the roster of participants, at least up to a point where added organizations or communities can be matched or clustered according to their similarities. Typically, such a point is not reached until many dissimilar organizations or communities have been accumulated. In short, a truly orchestrated large-scale program—as distinct from numerous replications of a small-scale program—requires additional planning and coordination for each unique unit added, multiplied by (not merely added to) the number of variations in prior units added.
2. As the number of units (organizations, communities) reaches a point where newcomers are more and more likely to be similar to some previous comers, large-scale programs begin to realize an economy of scale, which means that for each newcomer, the job of planning and coordination gets easier because it is more and more likely to be (or seem to be) repetitious. The cost in time, effort, and resources per unit of production or service goes down as the number of organizations and people reached goes up. Some programs never reach their threshold level because their initial planning, production of materials, or coordination failed in the early stages to satisfy early participants, establish a reputation, and ensure the diffusion of the program.
3. Diffusion of a new program depends both on satisfying the early adopters and on timing and placing interventions strategically according to stages in the natural history of the diffusion process. The natural history of the diffusion process as applied to organizations follows a logistic curve similar to the diffusion of innovations or ideas in populations.[65] Theories associated with the curve can describe and explain three important features of the diffusion process: (*a*) It helps us understand the characteristics and distribution of individuals or organizations according to their relative time of adoption as identified by their place in the diffusion curve. (*b*) A second understanding we gain concerns the lag time between awareness and adoption and how this lag time differs between early adopters and late adopters. (*c*) The third implication of diffusion theory is an understanding of the forces pushing the diffusion process forward and the forces holding it back, at each stage of time.

Using the Classification and Distribution of Adopters in Planning and Evaluation

Figure 48-6*A* shows the normal distribution of adoption over time, with the curve divided into standard deviations from the theoretical midpoint of the program or diffusion process. This curve has a vertical axis of numbers of new people or organizations adopting an idea or program at a given point in time. It is, therefore, an incidence curve, in epidemiological terms. The same phenomena and numbers can be expressed as a prevalence curve showing, as in Figure 48-6*B*, the cumulative number who have adopted up to a point in time. Here the same people who were adopting within one of the standard deviation categories of the incidence curve can be located and labeled on a segment of the cumulative S-shaped prevalence curve in Figure 48-6*B*.

Few, if any, government-sponsored programs could honestly claim to have entered at time zero on the adoption curve to which they sought to contribute. Usually they enter at a later stage. It is no criticism of government to say that in economies with free enterprise and extensive communication and marketing networks, the innovators and early adopters, and often the early majority, have been skimmed, like cream off milk, by commercial interests by the time government is called on to take action. Indeed, the relative deprivation of those who could not avail themselves of privately sponsored programs or services is often the impetus for government initiative in health. The previous adoption by the affluent and the middle majority causes an innovation related to health to be perceived more and more as a benefit, first negotiated in collective bargaining, then demanded as a right. Whether in the interest of equity or in the interest of health as a right, government agencies undertake large-scale programs in public health when previously acceptable circumstances have been redefined in the public's perception as unacceptable. As Sir Geoffrey Vickers said, "The history of public health might well be written as a record of successive redefinings of the unacceptable." Health education has a large role in affecting the public's perception of acceptable and unacceptable circumstances.

Entering late on the diffusion curve has several implications for public health campaigns. Some of these distinguish such government programs from large-scale commercial marketing efforts. Much has been said in the professional literature in recent years about the need to apply marketing principles and strategies in public health. The implicit criticism that public health has failed where commercial marketing has succeeded oversimplifies the task public health faces. It equates a percentage point commercial gain in the early-adopter phase with a percentage point health behavior gain in the late-adopter phase.

A first implication of the point of intervention on the diffusion curve has to do with the classification and distribution of people or organizations according to their order of adoption. Innovators and early adopters typically are more affluent and keyed in to national media. They are cosmopolitans who know the most about health and can afford the most in private purchase of health care products and services and least need some of the health products and services they buy. They are the upscale market of Madison Avenue in New York or of Bay Street in Toronto or of the Zona Rosa of Mexico City. They are the social models for the majority. Mass media alone can suffice in reaching them.

Those who will adopt with the early and late majorities attend less to national media and more to local media, and they respond less to media in general than to interpersonal influence. This is why most large-scale programs have put so much emphasis on involving the local media and organizational channels of communication rather than depending on network broadcasts or national publications. This middle majority is the primary target group of those public health programs addressing problems for which everybody is at some risk, such as food sanitation, fitness, stress, nutrition, and injury-control programs. All these relate to socially and culturally conditioned behaviors embedded in a complex web of lifestyle. This fact, in addition to the characteristics of people in this phase of the diffusion process, makes organizational and institutional channels essential to the health promotion and social modeling strategies required to support changes in their behavior. Media alone no longer suffice.

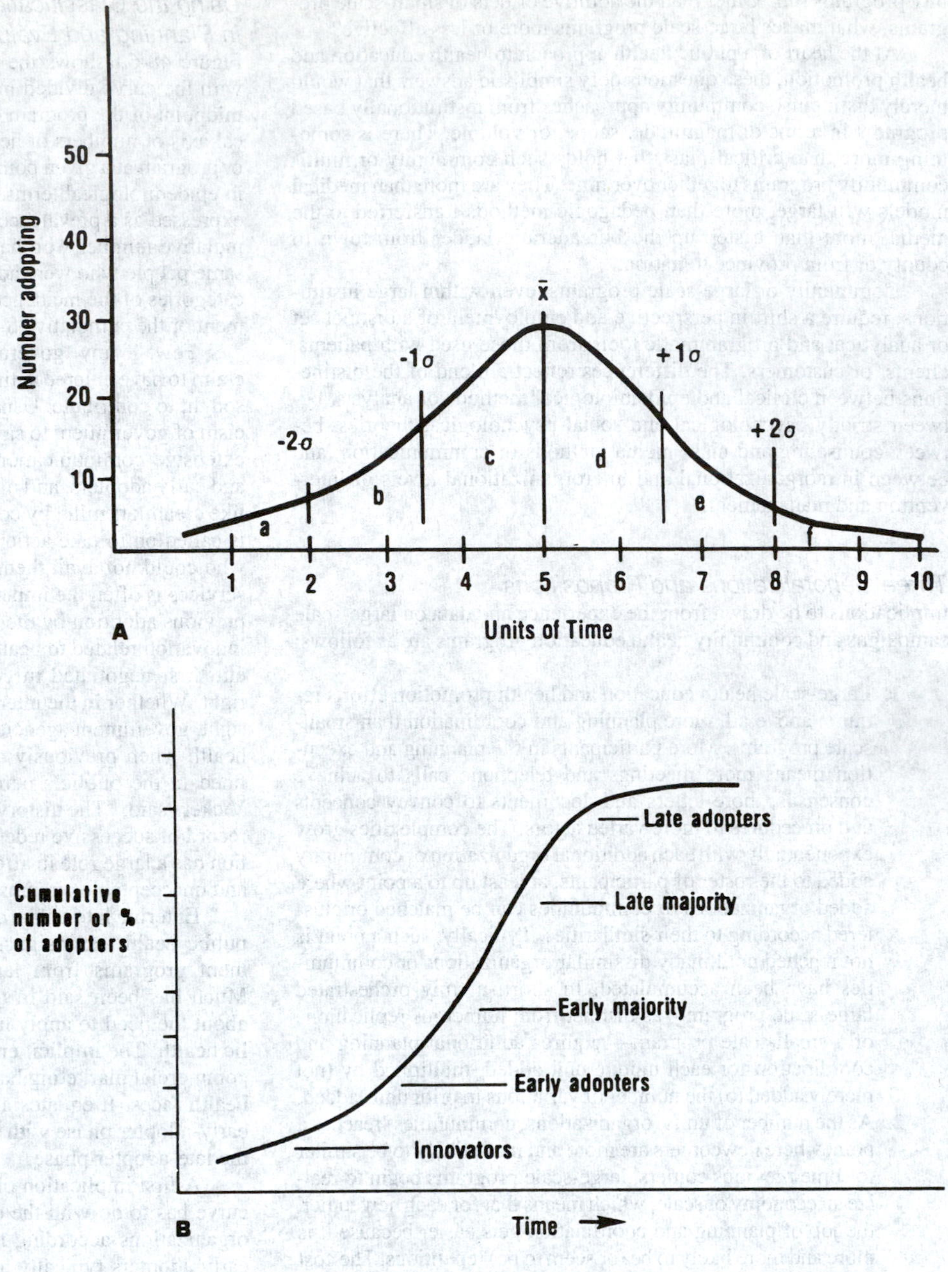

Figure 48-6. A, The incidence of adoption over time. **B**, The prevalence of adoption over time.

Finally, the late adopters and hard-to-reach are even more likely to be the primary targets of public health campaigns, especially in preventive health services, such as hypertension, immunization, maternal and child health, family planning, and occupational health and safety. The people and organizations in these late-adopter categories typically are disadvantaged in economic or status terms and are more isolated or alienated socially. They tend to be suspicious of organizations, including government agencies, purporting to help them. Their use of media is more exclusively for entertainment, and their membership in organizations or coalitions is sporadic and limited in comparison with the earlier adopters. Reaching these people and organizations requires more expensive and labor-intensive forms of community organization, communication, and outreach. The payoff in health outcomes often is greater because of their high risk, but the cost per unit of service effectively delivered is necessarily higher.

Evaluating the Gap between Exposure and Adoption

The second implication of the point at which health education programs enter the diffusion curve is the delay between intervention and results. For commercial marketing directed at innovators, early adopters, and the early majority, the lapses between awareness and interest, between interest and trial, and between trial and adoption or rejection are brief. As illustrated in Figure 48-7, the time elapsed in the decision and adoption stages represented by gaps *e*, *f*, and *g* at the early stages tends, on the average, to be shorter than the corresponding gaps *a*, *b*, and *c* for later adopters. Following these theoretical curves up the scale to the latest group to become aware of the innovation or program, the horizontal lines one might draw to connect the awareness curve with the adoption curve might be infinitely long on the time scale. It falls to public health education to overcome or offset this natural history of diffusion and adoption at this end of the curve.

Accomplishing a percentage point increment in adoption at the public health end of the diffusion curve requires a great deal more effort and expense, as well as time, than an equal increment in the commercial marketing segments of the curve. This can be seen at a theoretical level just by contrasting the slope of the curve at the early-adopter stage, where the rate of adoption is increasing, with the

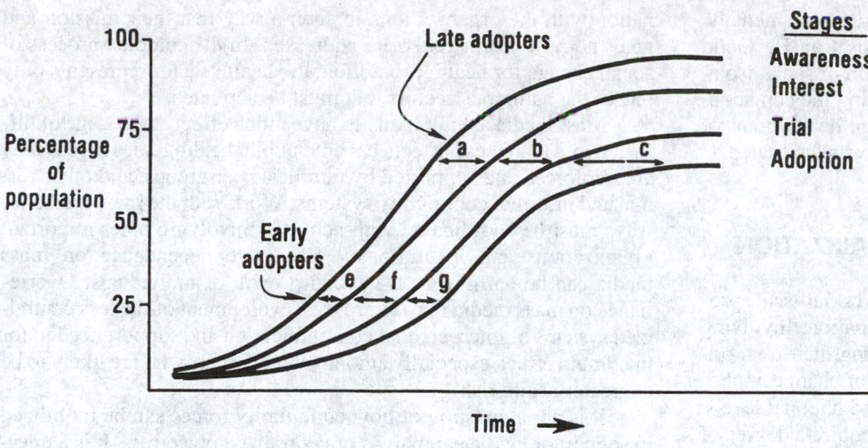

Figure 48-7. Differential time gaps between the stages of adoption for early adopters and late adopters. *(From Green L, McAlister A: Macro-intervention to support health behavior: some theoretical perspectives and practical reflections. Health Educ Q 11(3):323–339, 1984.)*

slope at the late-adopter segments, where the rate of adoption is declining. This disparity in the boost of natural diffusion rates at the two ends of the time scale for a product, program, or service makes the simple comparisons of percentage points gained by commercial marketing and by public health campaigns manifestly unequal.

Using or Resisting the Forces Operating on the Diffusion Curve

Figure 48-8 illustrates how a variety of forces stimulate or retard the rate of growth of adopters in a population. These forces need to be taken into account in large-scale programs as advantages to be exploited or barriers to be overcome. Most of these may be seen as inevitable natural forces, but even those that cannot be changed might be hastened or delayed in their impact. The nature of the services offered or the design of the program might be modified strategically to accommodate the forces impinging on the diffusion process at various points in time.

Communication channels and health education messages need to be adapted to the forces operating variously at successive stages of large-scale programs. Recognizing that many of the forces pushing or inhibiting the diffusion and adoption process are not strictly cognitive or motivational, health promotion programs seek to mobilize organizational, economic, and environmental supports for the behavior advocated.

Examples of these strategies complementing the communications in the large-scale programs in the United States are the health styles, high blood pressure, and alcohol campaigns of recent years. Particular attention has been given to mobilization of community organizations and the channeling of communications through worksites

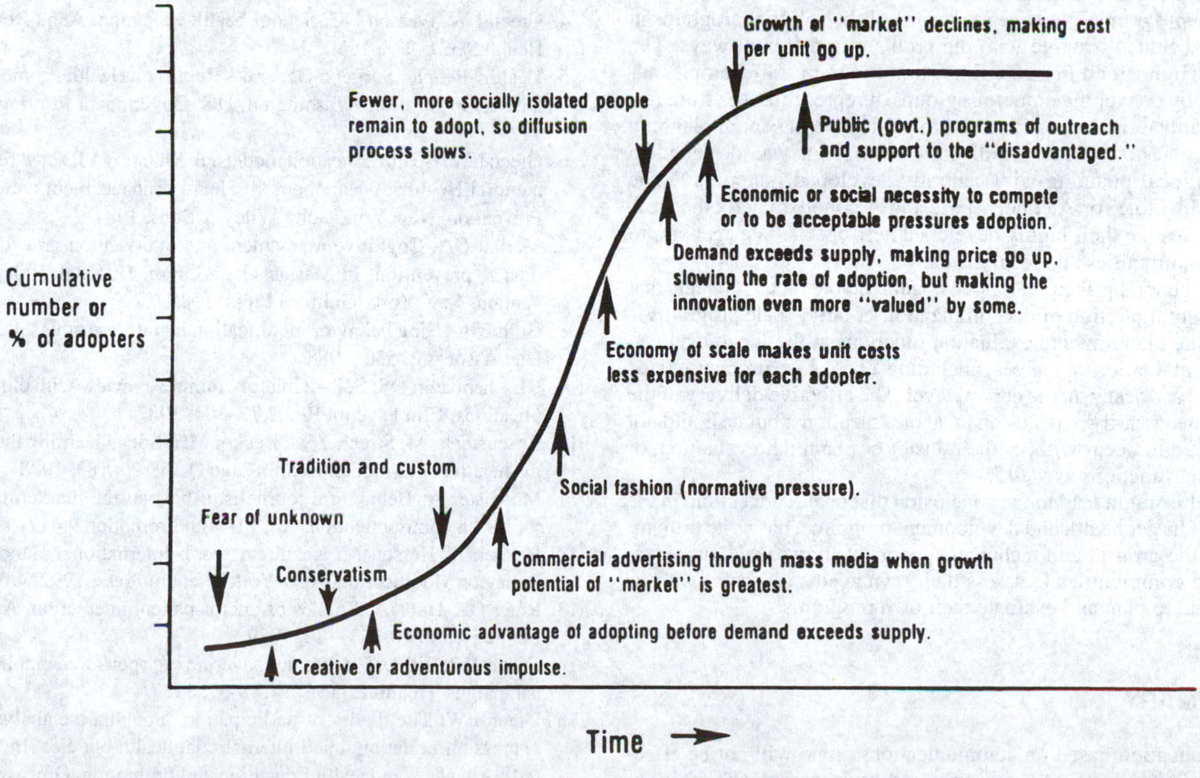

Figure 48-8. Examples of forces pushing the diffusion and adoption process up and those holding the process back at slower phases. *(From Green L, McAlister A: Macro-intervention to support health behavior: some theoretical perspectives and practical reflections. Health Educ Q 11(3):323–339, 1984.)*

and other settings where interpersonal influence could complement the formal communications of the media. The "Friends Can Be Good Medicine" campaign in California made the reduction of social isolation both a means and an end in itself. By encouraging the contact of people with their social support networks, the mental health goals of the program were served, and the diffusion process was facilitated.[66]

▶ CENTRALIZATION VERSUS DECENTRALIZATION

One thing that does not differ between large-scale and small-scale programs is the importance of the principle of participation. Involving people actively in identifying their own needs, setting their own priorities and goals, and planning their own programs of change applies equally at the individual, classroom, community, and national levels. The paradox for large-scale programs is that they require a degree of centralization of authority and responsibility almost by definition. Does this mean that large-scale programs should be avoided in favor of localized planning, implementation, and evaluation in all cases?

This policy question has stalemated implementation of the World Health Organization's primary health care approach in many countries where centralized planning is deeply ingrained in their systems. It also has limited the degree to which the community-based cardiovascular risk-reduction programs, such as those funded centrally by the National Institutes of Health (NIH) and managed regionally by the Stanford University and University of Minnesota research teams, have been able to achieve truly community-based initiatives.

Decentralization has occurred most commonly in the implementation of large-scale programs, not in their planning or evaluation. This has given the concept of community participation a bad reputation in some circles as a form of exploitation, cooptation, or cheap labor for central agencies.

Communities and organizations asked to implement programs planned elsewhere and evaluated on someone else's terms might cooperate, but usually with a limited commitment to the goals and methods of the programs. We have seen some of the national programs in the United States struggle with the problem in different ways. The National High Blood Pressure Education Program, for example, addressed it by convening numerous groups of representatives from far-flung organizations or communities to participate in central planning processes.[67] The federal Health Styles campaign was designed to stimulate local planning with centrally developed materials.[68] The National Institute for Alcohol Abuse and Alcoholism and other federal agencies tap their highly developed network of state agencies to engage communities and local media.[69]

As a general principle, if not a documentable fact, it appears that the ideal configuration of decentralization of large-scale programs is to place the planning and evaluation functions at the local level and the implementation resources, including expensive productions of media and advocacy, at the central level. The effective delivery of the program necessarily depends on local organizations, but it should not be expected to occur without the transfer of planning, evaluation, or monitoring functions as well.[70]

All this might lead to the conclusion that health education, in the context of larger health and development programs, has as its primary function the arousal and technical support of individuals, organizations, and communities to assess their own needs, set their own priorities, and to plan and evaluate their own programs.

▶ SUMMARY

Health education based on communications alone will not be effective unless organizational, economic, and environmental changes enable, and interpersonal communications reinforce, the behavioral change objectives. Systematic plans for organizations and communities to support behavioral objectives need to be developed in coordination with the organizations in such a way that their mission and goals not just health goals, are addressed. In the complex process of social change for health promotion, the health sector represents only one of the numerous sectors that must be activated.

Mass media are not likely to have much effect at the stage of diffusion in which these effects become public health issues unless they are reinforced and supported by families, peer groups, and other formal and informal community systems. Work with the mass media always must be coordinated with activities involving other important organizations and institutions.[71] Excessive dependence on mass media can be harmful to the social growth of individuals. Overreliance on mass media may retard the development of the less centralized systems of interpersonal communication and support needed for maximum effect, especially among later adopters who are likely to be at greater health risk.

It is not a question of how community forces can be mobilized in support of media campaigns or centralized objectives. It is a question of how the mass media can be used and supported by central agencies most appropriately and effectively in pursuit of *community* objectives. Large-scale programs still need to be seen as community-based programs. National and state objectives and resources still need to be adapted and tailored to communities. Communities, in turn, must adapt their resources and objectives down to institutional, organizational, neighborhood, family, and individual needs.

▶ REFERENCES

1. Green LW, Ottoson JM: Community and Population Health. 8th ed. New York: McGraw-Hill, 1998
2. Green LW, Kreuter MW: Health Promotion Planning: An Educational and Environmental Approach. 3rd ed. Mountain View, CA: Mayfield Publishing, 1998
3. Lewis FM: The concept of control: a typology and health-related variables. In Ward W (ed): Advances in Health Education and Promotion. Greenwich, CT: JAI Press, 1987, vol 2
4. Green LW, Iverson DC: School health education. Annu Rev Public Health 3:321–338, 1982
5. Healthy People: Surgeon General's Report on Health Promotion and Disease Prevention. Washington, DC: Government Printing Office, 1979
6. Green LW: Health education models. In Matarazzo JD et al (eds): Behavioral Health: A Handbook of Health Enhancement and Disease Prevention. New York: John Wiley & Sons, 1984
7. Marlatt GA: Cognitive assessment and intervention procedures for relapse prevention. In Marlatt GA, Gordon JR (eds): Relapse Prevention. New York: Guilford Press, 1985
8. Holli BB: Using behavior modification in nutrition counseling. J Am Diet Assoc 88:1530, 1988
9. Kirschenbaum DS: Self-regulatory failure: a review with clinical implications. Clin Psychol Rev 7:77–104, 1987
10. Rosenstock IM, Strecher VJ, Becker MH: Social learning theory and the health belief model. Health Educ Q 15:175–183, 1988
11. McAlister A: Behavioral journalism: beyond the marketing model for health communication. Am J Health Promotion 9:417–420, 1995
12. Bellack A, Hersen M, Kazdin A (eds): International Handbook of Behavior Modification, New York: Plenum Press, 1992, vol 2
13. Roter DL, Hall JA: Studies of doctor-patient interaction. Annu Rev Public Health 10:163–180, 1989
14. Faden RR: Ethical issues in government sponsored public health campaigns. Health Educ Q 14:27–37, 1987
15. Green LW: The theory of participation: a qualitative analysis of its expression in national and international health policies. In Ward W (ed): Advances in Health Education and Promotion. Greenwich, CT: JAI Press, 1986, vol 1
16. Green LW: Program Planning and Evaluation Guide for Lung Associations. New York: American Lung Association, 1987

17. Green LW, Richard L, Potvin L: Ecological foundations of health promotion. Am J Health Promotion 10:270–281, 1996
18. Mullen PD: Health promotion and patient education benefits for employees. Annu Rev Public Health 9:305–332, 1988
19. Green LW, Heit P, Iverson D, Kolbe LJ, Kreuter MW: The school health curriculum project: its theory, practice and measurement experience. Health Educ Q 7:14–34, 1980
20. Wikler D: Who should be blamed for being sick? Health Educ Q 14:11–25, 1987
21. Stokols D: Establishing and maintaining healthy environments: toward a social ecology of health promotion. Am Psychol 47:6–22, 1992
22. Foreyt JP, Goodrick GK: Impact of behavior therapy on weight loss. Am J Health Promotion 8:466–468, 1994
23. Flay BR: Social psychological approaches to smoking prevention: review and recommendations. In Ward W (ed): Advances in Health Education and Promotion. Greenwich, CT: JAI Press, 1987, vol 2
24. Green LW, Wilson AW, Lovato C: What changes can health promotion achieve and how long will these changes last? Prev Med 15:508–521, 1986
25. Green LW: The trade-offs between the expediency of health promotion and the durability of health education. In Maes S, et al (eds): Topics in Health Psychology. New York: John Wiley & Sons, 1988
26. Becker MH, Rosenstock IM: Comparing social learning theory and the Health Belief Model. In Ward W (ed): Advances in Health Education and Promotion. Greenwich, CT: JAI Press, 1987, vol 2
27. Schwartz R, Goodman R, Steckler A: Policy advocacy interventions for health promotion and education: advancing the state of practice. Health Educ Q 22:421–426, 1995
28. Best JA, et al: Preventing cigarette smoking among school children. Annu Rev Public Health 9:161–201, 1988
29. De Pietro R: A marketing research approach to health education planning. In Ward W (ed): Advances in Health Education and Promotion, Greenwich, CT: JAI Press, 1987, vol 2
30. Kotler P: Marketing for Nonprofit Organizations. 2nd ed. Englewood Cliffs, NJ: Prentice-Hall, 1982
31. Manoff RK: Social Marketing: New Imperative for Public Health. New York: Praeger, 1985
32. Lefebvre RC, Flora JA: Social marketing and public health intervention. Health Educ Q 15:299–315, 1988
33. Green LW, Kreuter MW: Health Promotion Planning: An Educational and Environmental Approach. Mountain View, CA: Mayfield Publishing, 1991
34. Rosenstock IM, Strecher V, Becker M: Social learning theory and the Health Belief Model. Health Educ Q 15:175–183, 1988
35. Clark NM: Social learning theory in current health education practice. In Ward W (ed): Advances in Health Education and Promotion. Greenwich, CT: JAI Press, 1987, vol 2
36. Lau RR, Quadrel MJ, Hartman KA: Development and change of young adult's preventive health beliefs and behavior: influence from parents and peers. J Health Soc Behav 31:240–259, 1990
37. Worden JK, Flynn BS, Carpenter JH: Using mass media to prevent cigarette smoking among adolescent girls. Health Educ Q 23:453–468, 1996
38. Cohen RY, Felix MRJ, Brownell KD: The role of parents and older peers in school-based cardiovascular prevention programs: implications for program development. Health Educ Q 16:245–253, 1989
39. Devine EC, Cook TD: A meta-analytic analysis of effects of psychoeducational interventions on length of postsurgical hospital stay. Nurs Res 32:267–274, 1983
40. Mullen PD, Green LW, Persinger G: Clinical trails of patient education for chronic conditions: a comparative meta-analysis of intervention types. Prev Med 14:753–781, 1985
41. Kottke TE, Battista RN, DeFriese G, et al: Attributes of successful smoking cessation interventions in medical practice. JAMA 259: 2883–2889, 1988
42. Vickery DM, Kalmer H, Lowry D, et al: Effect of self-care education program on medical visits. JAMA 250:2952–2956, 1983
43. Mann KV, Putnam RW: Barriers to prevention: physician perceptions of ideal versus actual practices in reducing cardiovascular risk. Can Fam Physician 36:665–670, 1990
44. Green LW: Modifying lifestyle to improve health. In Kelton WD, Osterweis M (eds): Promoting Community Health: The Role of Academic Health Centers. Washington, DC: Association of Academic Health Centers, 1993, pp 54–69
45. Green LW, Cargo M, Ottoson JM: The role of physicians in supporting lifestyle changes. Med Exerc Nutr Health 3:119–130, 1994
46. Kernaghan SG, Giloth BE: Tracking the Impact of Health Promotion on Organizations: A Key to Program Survival. Chicago: American Hospital Association, 1988
47. Green LW: Toward cost-benefit evaluations of health education: Some concepts, methods and examples. Health Educ Mongr 2(suppl): 34–64, 1974
48. Green LW: Refocusing health care systems to address both individual care and population health. Clin Invest Med 17:133–141, 1994
49. Green LW: What physicians can do to increase participation and maintenance of patients in self-care. West J Med 147:346–349, 1987
50. Harrison JA, Mullen PD, Green LW: A meta-analysis of studies of the Health Belief Model. Health Educ Res 7:107–116, 1992
51. Mullen PD, Green LW: Educating and counseling for prevention: from theory and research to principles. In Goldbloom RB, Lawrence RS (eds): Preventing Disease: Beyond the Rhetoric. New York: Springer-Verlag, 1990, pp 474–479
52. Fingerhut LA, Kleinman JC: Mortality among children and youth. Am J Public Health 79:899–901, 1989
53. Kolbe LJ: Indicators for planning and monitoring school health programs. In Kar SB (ed): Health Promotion Indicators and Actions. New York: Springer, 1989
54. MacDonald M, Green LW: Health education. In Lewy A (ed): International Encyclopedia of Education. London: Pergamon Press, 1994
55. Rundall TG, Bruvold WH: A meta-analysis of school-based smoking and alcohol use prevention programs. Health Educ Q 15:317–334, 1988
56. Wagner MM, Gomby DS: Evaluating a statewide school-linked services initiative: California's Healthy Start. New Directions for Evaluation 69:51–67, Spring 1996
57. Kolbe LJ, Green LW, Foreyt J, et al: Appropriate functions of health education in schools. In Krasnagor N, Arasteh J, Cataldo M (eds): Child Health Behavior. New York: John Wiley & Sons, 1985
58. Gerstein D, Green LW (eds): Preventing Drug Abuse: What Do We Know. Washington, DC: National Academy Press, 1993
59. Green LW, Simons-Morton D, Potvin L: Education and life-style determinants of health and disease. In Holland WW, Detels R, Knox G (eds): Oxford Textbook of Public Health. 3rd ed. London: Oxford University Press, 1996
60. World Health Organization: Expert Committee on Health Education of the Public. WHO Technical Report Series No. 89. Geneva: World Health Organization, 1954
61. Pederson A, O'Neill M, Rootman I (eds): Health Promotion in Canada: Provincial, National and International Perspectives. Toronto: WB Saunders Canada, 1994
62. Green LW: The health promotion research agenda revisited. Am J Health Promotion 6:411–413, 1992
63. Nyswander D: Education for health: some principles and their application. Calif Health 14:65–70, 1956
64. Ottoson JM: Reclaiming the concept of application: from social to technological process and back again. Adult Educ Q 46:17–30, 1995
65. Green LW, Johnson JL: Dissemination and utilization of health promotion and disease prevention knowledge: theory, research and experience. Can J Public Health 87(Suppl 1):511–517, 1996

66. Hersey JC, Kilbanoff LS, Lam DJ, Taylor RL: Promoting social support: the impact of California's Friends Can Be Good Medicine campaign. Health Educ Q 11:293–311, 1984
67. Rocella EJ, Ward GW: The national high blood pressure education program: a description of its utility as a generic program model. Health Educ Q 11:225–242, 1984
68. Davis M, Iverson D: An overview and analysis of the HealthStyles campaign. Health Educ Q 11:253–272, 1984
69. Dejong W, Atkin CK: A review of national television PSA campaigns for preventing alcohol-impaired driving, 1987–1992. J Public Health Policy 16:59–80, 1995
70. Frankish CJ, Green LW: Organizational and community change as the social scientific basis for disease prevention and health promotion policy. Adv Med Soc 4:209–233, 1994
71. Chapman S, Lupton D: The Fight for Public Health: Principles and Practice of Media Advocacy. London: BMJ Publishing Group, 1994

V

Noncommunicable and Chronic Disabling Conditions

Elizabeth Barret-Connor

49

Screening for Early and Asymptomatic Conditions

Robert B. Wallace

One major activity in the prevention armamentarium is screening. The purpose of screening is either to detect individuals with risk factors that predispose to disease development, in which case, specific preventive interventions would be invoked, or to identify persons with early or asymptomatic (latent) disease that can be effectively treated, leading to a better health outcome. In general, screening is applied to a population of individuals with an overall low probability of the risk factor or disease prevalence relative to individuals with symptoms of the condition.

There are several criteria that aid in selecting and applying an appropriate screening test.[1] (*a*) The disease should be common enough to warrant a search for its risk factors or latent stages because screening for excessively rare diseases may result in unacceptable cost-benefit ratios. (*b*) The morbidity or mortality (i.e., burden of suffering) of the untreated target condition must be substantial. (*c*) An effective preventive intervention or therapy must exist and should not encumber a more beneficial outcome when applied to the presymptomatic rather than to the symptomatic stage. (*d*) The screening test should be acceptable to the population and suitable for routine application. Many other criteria for an effective screening test could be added, such as maintenance of test accuracy over time and freedom from screening-related adverse effects.

Even with concerted application of these screening criteria, major pitfalls may cause an erroneous assessment of a screening program's value. An example is *lead time bias*, the interval between presymptomatic disease detection by a screening test and symptom onset.[2] If the natural history of a disease is variable or not thoroughly understood during the presymptomatic and symptomatic stages, a screening test may identify a presymptomatic condition earlier and increase the interval to overt morbidity but not change the ultimate outcome. *Length bias* occurs when there is a correlation between the duration of disease latency and the natural history of the symptomatic phase.[2] If the mild form of a disease has a longer latency and is hence more easily found on screening than are more severe forms of disease, the screening test may appear falsely beneficial. These pitfalls can be fully resolved only through controlled trials of a screening procedure with long-term follow-up, as in the 18-year follow-up of the Health Insurance Plan clinical trial of mammography for detecting breast cancer.[3]

Selection and interpretation of screening tests require a combination of subjective and objective criteria. Objective criteria include operating characteristics, predictive value, and cost-effectiveness of the tests, which are tempered by subjective evaluations of individual and public acceptability and financing.

The operating characteristics of a test are its sensitivity and specificity. These characteristics apply to laboratory test data as well as other information collected from the medical history and physical examination. *Sensitivity* is the proportional detection of individuals with the disease of interest in the tested population, expressed as follows:

$$\text{Sensitivity (\%)} = \frac{\text{True positives}}{\text{True positive + False Negatives}} \times 100$$

True positives are individuals with the disease and whose test result is positive. False negatives are individual whose test result is negative despite having the disease. *Specificity* is the proportional detection of individuals without the disease of interest, expressed as follows:

$$\text{Specificity (\%)} = \frac{\text{True negatives}}{\text{True negatives + False positive}} \times 100$$

True negatives are individuals without the disease and whose test result is negative. False positives are those who have a positive test result but do not have the disease. Sensitivity is limited by the proportion of cases missed by the test (false negatives) and specificity is limited by the proportion of noncases found to be positive (false positives). Ideally, a test would have a 100 percent sensitivity and specificity, but few if any tests have achieved this. Unfortunately, sensitivity and specificity are often inversely related. This relationship has been expressed as the receiver operating characteristic (ROC)[4] of a numerically continuous test result. The ROC allows optimal specification of test sensitivity and specificity. The sensitivity, or true-positive ratio, is displayed along the ordinate, and the specificity, or false-positive ratio, is exhibited on the abscissa. As the sensitivity increases, so does the false-positive ratio in most instances. When a ROC has been established for a test, any one of several sensitivity and specificity combinations may be evaluated for suitability in test application and contrasted with potential alternate tests. Alternative summary indices of ROCs have been proposed.[5]

Sensitivity and specificity values from the literature are most applicable to populations and test conditions similar to those under which the values were established. It is possible that test properties may differ according to mode of administration (e.g., telephone versus mail questionnaire) or by any demographic feature of the target population, and thus, further generalization or extrapolation of these values can be misleading. For example, it has been suggested that the increasingly common use of hormone replacement therapy among postmenopausal women may decrease the sensitivity and specificity of mammographic screening.[6]

Whereas the operating characteristics of a test are of major help in selecting a screening test, the predictive value of a test is a major aid in interpretation of a result. The *predictive value* of a *positive test* is the proportion of all individuals with positive tests who have the disease and is expressed as follows:

$$\text{Positive predictive value (\%)} = \frac{\text{True positives}}{\text{True positives + False positives}} \times 100$$

The predictive value of a negative test is the proportion of all individuals with negative tests who are nondiseased. This is expressed as follows:

$$\text{Negative predictive value (\%)} = \frac{\text{True negatives}}{\text{True negatives + False negatives}} \times 100$$

Predictive values are dependent on both the operating characteristics and the prevalence of the disease in the target population. For any given set of operating characteristics, the positive predictive value is directly related to prevalence, and the negative predictive value is inversely related to prevalence. Therefore, in screening situations where the prevalence is relatively low, the operating characteristics must be very high to avoid low positive predictive values. In most screening situations for serious fatal conditions, such as cancer, the test or test sequence offering the highest sensitivity ordinarily will be preferred. This has the effect of finding as many cases as possible but may correspondingly increase the number of false positives. The effect of sensitivity, specificity, and prevalence on predictive values has been clearly demonstrated.[7]

Cost-effectiveness is especially important in screening programs because of the number of asymptomatic individuals who must be evaluated for the relatively small number of diseased cases. Formal cost-effectiveness analysis[8–10] should be undertaken before program initiation. The program's value must include an assessment of all costs and a realistic appraisal of effectiveness. Positive predictive values are usually well below 50 percent for most initial screening situations, so that secondary diagnostic evaluation is nearly always required to eliminate false positives, adding substantially to program cost.

Exhaustive reviews of the efficacy of clinically applicable screening programs have been undertaken by the Canadian Task Force on the Periodic Health Examination,[11] and the United States Preventive Services Task Force[12] have been undertaken including recommendations weighted in part by consideration of cost-effectiveness. Many other sets of useful recommendations exist,[13–15] in addition to those related to specific clinical subspecialties. On the other hand, public screening, or mass screening, may have inherent advantages from the standpoint of efficiency. The tests and procedures selected for use are often highly standardized and can be administered more inexpensively than they can in clinical or more specialized settings, and generally they can be applied without the need for direct physician supervision. To enjoy the efficiency of mass screening, such programs must be carefully organized and managed. Recipients of both normal and abnormal test results must be considered. Those with abnormal test results must have a properly organized follow-up evaluation protocol, and those with normal results should be informed of the predictive value of a normal test to avoid false reassurance. Even with the inherent efficiency of mass screening, most such programs must still be focused on populations with sufficient disease or risk factor prevalence to maximize program efficiency.

Another application of screening programs is in the clinical context where patients have active clinical problems. Examples include screening on the first evaluative ambulatory clinic visit or at hospital admission. Comprehensive clinical screening with routine physical examinations or laboratory tests, or both, remains controversial, largely because there is very little if any evidence in the scientific literature concerning the efficacy or effectiveness of standard screening tests in the face of existing clinical illness. For example, is mammography effective in persons with active insulin-dependent diabetes, or cholesterol screening in the face of an active carcinoma? These are questions yet to be addressed in research. In the past, so-called "multiphasic" screening programs had been proposed for persons being admitted to the hospital. It now appears that these procedures have limited utility and high cost primarily because of numerous false-positive tests and irrelevant findings and should be discarded in favor of diagnostic and therapeutic activities directed at the immediate clinical problems.[16–18] However, inpatient hospital services have been used as opportunities for categorical screening programs such as undiagnosed human immunodeficiency virus infection,[19] alcoholism,[20] or nutritional problems among the elderly.[21] Multiphasic biochemical screening is still being proposed as a useful inpatient tool.[22]

▶ REFERENCES

1. Wilson JMG, Jungner G: Principles and practice of screening for disease. Public Health Pap 34, 1968
2. Pelikan S, Moskowitz M: Effects of lead time, length bias, and false negative assurance on screening for breast cancer. Cancer 71: 1998–2005, 1993
3. Chu KC, Smart CR, Tarone RE: Analysis of breast cancer mortality and stage distribution by age for the Health Insurance Plan clinical trial. J Natl Cancer Inst 80:1125–1132, 1988
4. Swets JA: Measuring the accuracy of diagnostic systems. Science 240:1285–1293, 1988
5. Lee W-C, Hsiao CK. Alternative summary indices for the receiver operating characteristic curve. Epidemiology 7:605–611, 1996
6. Laya MB, Larson EB, Taplin SH, White E: Effect of estrogen replacement therapy on the sensitivity and specificity of screening mammography. J Natl Cancer Inst 88:643–649, 1996
7. Galen RS, Gambino SR: Beyond Normality: The Predictive Value and Efficiency of Medical Diagnosis. New York: John Wiley, 1975
8. Schmid GP: Understanding the essentials of economic evaluation. J Acquir Immune Defic Syndr Hum Retrovirol 10(Suppl 4):S6–S13, 1995
9. Johannesson M: The relationship between cost-effectiveness analysis and cost-benefit analysis. Soc Sci Med 41:483–489, 1995
10. Gold MR, Siegel JE, Russell LB, Weinstein MC (eds): Cost Effectiveness in Health and Medicine. New York: Oxford University Press, 1996
11. Canadian Task Force on the Periodic Health Examination: Canadian guide to clinical preventive health care. Ottawa: Canada Communication Group, 1994
12. US Preventive Services Task Force: Guide to Clinical Preventive Services. 2nd ed. Baltimore: Williams & Wilkins, 1996
13. Eddy DM (ed): Common Screening Tests. Philadelphia: American College of Physicians, 1991
14. American Medical Association: AMA guidelines for adolescent preventive services (GAPS): recommendations and rationale. Chicago: American Medical Association, 1994
15. American Academy of Family Physicians: Age charts for periodic health examination. Reprint no. 510. Kansas City, MO: American Academy of Family Physicians, 1994
16. Whitehead TP, Wotton IDP: Biochemical profiles for hospital patients. Lancet 2:1439, 1974
17. Korvin CC, Pearce RH, Stanley J: Admissions screening: clinical benefits. Ann Intern Med 83:197, 1975
18. Burbridge TC, Edwards F, Edwards RG, Atkinson M: Evaluation of benefits of screening tests done immediately on admission to hospital. Clin Chem 22:968, 1976
19. Trepka MJ, Davidson AJ, Douglas JM Jr: Extent of undiagnosed HIV infection in hospitalized patients: assessment by linkage of seroprevalence and surveillance methods. Am J Prev Med 12:195–202, 1996
20. Bothelho RJ, Richmond R: Secondary prevention of excessive alcohol use: assessing the prospects for implementation. Fam Pract 13:182–193, 1996
21. Cotton E, Zinober B, Jessop J: A nutritional tool for older patients. Professional Nurse 11:609–612, 1966
22. Ferguson RP, Kohler FR, Chavez J, et al: Discovering asymptomatic abnormalities on a Baltimore internal medicine service. M Med J 45:543–546, 1996

50

Cancer

Diana C. Farrow • David B. Thomas

Neoplasms are diseases characterized by abnormal proliferation of cells. If the proliferating cells do not invade surrounding tissues, the resultant tumor is benign; if they do, it is malignant. Some benign neoplasms may be fatal, including histologically benign brain tumors that grow and displace normal brain tissue in the confined space of the skull, and hepatocellular adenomas that rupture and cause bleeding into the peritoneal cavity. Some benign tumors such as intestinal polyps are considered premalignant lesions and confer a high risk of progression to malignancy. The term cancer usually implies a malignant tumor (malignancy), but refers also to brain tumors and some other benign neoplasms.

▸ DESCRIPTIVE EPIDEMIOLOGY

Classification

Cancers are classified according to their organ or tissue of origin (site or topography code) and histological features (morphology code). A number of classification schemes have been developed, the most recent and widely used of which appears in Chapter 2 of the *International Classification of Diseases,* 9th revision (ICD-9), which is largely a topography code[1] and the *International Classification of Diseases for Oncology* (ICD-O), which contains an expanded version of the topography code in ICD-9 as well as a detailed morphology code.[2]

Sources of Incidence and Mortality Rates

Mortality rates are calculated from death certificate records and population census data. Mortality rates from various countries have been compiled periodically.[3] Cancer mortality rates for the United States are published by the U.S. National Cancer Institute (NCI).[4–6]

Population-based tumor registries, which have been established in many countries, provide information on incidence rates. These have been compiled in "Cancer in Five Continents," which is jointly published periodically by the International Agency for Research on Cancer (IARC) and the International Association of Cancer Registries (IACR).[7] The best source of cancer incidence rates for the United States is the Surveillance, Epidemiology, and End Results (SEER) program of the NCI, which supports a network of 10 population-based cancer registries throughout the country. Results from this program are published annually and more detailed monographs are published periodically.[4–6] Both incidence and mortality statistics for the United States are summarized for the lay public and published annually by the American Cancer Society.[8]

A North American Association of Central Cancer Registries (NAACCR) was established in 1987, and beginning in 1991 the Centers for Disease Control and Prevention (CDC) made funds available to individual states for cancer registration. The NAACCR and CDC programs have encouraged the establishment of a cancer registry in each state and promulgated uniform guidelines and standards for registry operations; cancer incidence rates for most states and all provinces of Canada from 1988 to 1992 have been published.[9] The cost of collecting high-quality data on a sufficiently large proportion of all cases in a defined population is considerable, and cancer registration efforts may not warrant sufficiently high priority for continued funding in regions with limited resources, especially if they are not well utilized for research or cancer control purposes.

Magnitude of the Cancer Problem

In the aggregate, cancer is second only to heart disease as a cause of death in the United States and accounts for about 23 percent of all deaths.[10] Approximately 206 deaths from cancer occur per 100,000 people per year, compared with about 287 per 100,000 from heart disease, 58 per 100,000 from stroke, and 34 per 100,000 from accidents.[10] Based on U.S. mortality and incidence rates for 1990 to 1992, the lifetime probabilities of developing cancer have been estimated to be 47.1 percent in men and 38.4 percent in women; the lifetime probabilities of dying of cancer are estimated at 23.7 percent in men and 20.5 percent in women.[4] The National Cancer Institute estimates the direct medical costs of cancer to be $40 billion annually, or about 10 percent of the total health care costs in the United States.[11]

Relative Importance of Specific Neoplasms

Age-adjusted incidence, mortality, and 5-year survival rates in men and women in the United States are shown in Table 50-1.[4] The most common cancers in men are those of the prostate, lung, colon and bladder, and non-Hodgkin's lymphoma; the cancers causing the most deaths per capita are those of the lung, prostate, colon and rectum, and pancreas. In women, breast cancer is by far the most common neoplasm, followed by cancers of the lung, colon, corpus uteri, and ovary. However, because of the more favorable survival of women with breast than lung cancer, mortality rates of lung cancer exceed those for breast cancer in the United States. The other cancers that are among the most important causes of death in American women are those of the colon, ovary, and pancreas.

Another way to judge the importance of a malignancy is by the number of years of life lost due to its occurrence in a population. This measure reflects the incidence of the cancer, the fatality rate in those who develop it, and the age at which the cancer tends to occur. This measure gives more weight to childhood cancers than overall mortality rates, and because of its economic implications can be of value in setting priorities for research and prevention. In order of estimated years of life lost, the 10 most important cancers in the United States are lung, breast, colon and rectum, pancreas, leukemia, non-Hodgkin's lymphoma, prostate, brain, ovary, and stomach.[4]

TABLE 50-1. AVERAGE ANNUAL AGE-ADJUSTED (1970 STANDARD) INCIDENCE AND MORTALITY RATES (1988 TO 1992) AND 5-YEAR RELATIVE SURVIVAL RATES (1986 TO 1991 CASES) BY PRIMARY SITE AND SEX, ALL RACES, ALL SEER AREAS COMBINED (EXCEPT PUERTO RICO AND NEW JERSEY)

	Rates (per 100,000)				5-Year Relative Survival (%)	
	Incidence		Mortality			
Site	Male	Female	Male	Female	Male	Female
Buccal cavity and pharynx	16.2	6.2	4.6	1.7	48.4	60.2
Digestive system	96.7	61.8	52.3	31.3	42.0	45.0
Colon and rectum	58.2	40.0	23.1	15.6	61.6	60.4
Colon	40.2	29.7	—	—	62.7	60.8
Rectum and rectosigmoid	17.9	10.2	—	—	59.3	59.4
Pancreas	10.4	8.0	10.0	7.2	3.2	4.0
Stomach	11.4	4.9	6.8	3.1	17.2	24.9
Esophagus	6.5	1.8	6.0	1.5	10.1	9.7
Respiratory system	92.2	44.0	77.6	32.2	17.5	17.7
Lung and bronchus	81.7	41.5	74.4	31.4	12.1	15.4
Larynx	7.9	1.7	2.5	0.5	66.9	61.3
Bones and joints	1.0	0.8	0.5	0.3	57.9	68.2
Soft tissues (including heart)	2.6	1.8	1.3	1.1	62.3	66.7
Skin (excluding basal and squamous cell carcinoma)	21.2	10.9	4.4	1.9	53.1	89.9
Melanomas of skin	13.8	9.9	3.1	1.5	83.4	90.1
Breast	0.9	109.6	0.2	27.1	83.9	83.2
Female genital system	—	48.0	—	14.9	—	67.6
Cervix uteri (invasive only)	—	8.6	—	3.0	—	68.3
Corpus uteri	—	20.9	—	1.8	—	83.9
Ovary	—	15.1	—	7.8	—	44.1
Male genital system	146.9	—	26.5	—	86.3	—
Prostate gland	141.4	—	26.0	—	85.8	—
Testis	4.5	—	0.3	—	94.9	—
Urinary system	43.1	14.1	10.8	4.1	75.7	66.0
Urinary bladder	29.7	7.6	5.6	1.7	83.3	73.6
Kidney and renal pelvis	12.3	6.1	5.0	2.3	58.3	57.2
Eye and orbit	0.8	0.6	0.1	0.1	75.6	75.7
Brain and nervous system	7.5	5.2	5.1	3.5	28.1	29.9
Endocrine system	3.3	7.1	0.7	0.6	85.6	93.4
Thyroid	2.6	6.6	0.3	0.4	92.4	96.0
Lymphomas	21.5	14.3	8.6	5.5	52.9	60.7
Non-Hodgkin's	18.3	11.8	7.8	5.1	47.1	55.3
Hodgkin's	3.2	2.5	0.7	0.4	77.2	83.4
Multiple myeloma	5.6	3.7	3.7	2.5	29.3	26.4
Leukemias	13.4	7.8	8.4	4.9	41.0	38.7
All sites	485.0	345.0	219.6	141.5	52.3	60.1

Data from National Cancer Institute: Cancer Mortality in the United States: 1950–1977. National Cancer Institute Monograph 59, NIH Publication No. 82-2435. Bethesda, MD: National Cancer Institute, 1982.

The incidence rates of all cancers vary among the various regions of the world, and the cancers of most importance in developing countries are different from those in developed countries such as the United States. In order by numbers of cases, the 10 most common cancers in developing countries are those of the cervix uteri, stomach, mouth and pharynx, esophagus, breast, lung, liver, colon and rectum, the lymphomas, and the prostate.[12]

Age

Cancers most probably arise from undifferentiated stem cells that are capable of mitotic division and differentiation. In adults, most cancers are carcinomas that arise from basal epithelial cells of ectodermal or endodermal origin. In children, most cancers are of mesodermal origin and consist largely of leukemias and lymphomas that arise from hematopoietic and lymphoid stem cells and sarcomas that probably develop from undifferentiated cells of embryonal origin.

Incidence rates for the most common childhood cancers in the United States are shown in Table 50-2.[4] The morality rates for even the most frequent cancers in children are many times lower than the rates of comparable tumors for all ages (Table 50-1), which largely reflect rates in adults.

With some notable exceptions (e.g., cancers of the female breast and uterine cervix), there is an exponential increase in incidence rates with age for most adult malignancies. The median age at which cancer was diagnosed from 1988 to 1992 was 68.0 for males and 67.0 for females, and most cancers develop in the sixth, seventh, and eighth decades of life.[4]

Sex

Most major cancers occur more frequently in men than in women, exceptions being carcinomas of the thyroid, gallbladder, and extrahepatic

TABLE 50-2. ANNUAL INCIDENCE OF SELECTED CANCERS IN CHILDREN UNDER AGE 15, 1988 TO 1992

	Ages 0–14	
Site	*Male*	*Female*
All sites	15.0	12.9
Bone and joint	0.6	0.8
Brain and other nervous	3.6	3.0
Hodgkin's disease	0.7	0.5
Kidney and renal pelvis	0.8	0.8
Leukemias	4.6	3.8
Acute lymphocytic	3.7	2.9
Non-Hodgkin's lymphomas	1.2	0.4
Soft tissue	0.8	0.8

Data from SEER program of the National Cancer Institute. Rates are per 100,000 and are age-adjusted (by 5-year age groups) to the 1970 U.S. Standard population.

bile ducts. Smoking-related cancers, described in detail subsequently, occur more frequently in men, at least in part because of their earlier and greater exposure to tobacco smoke. Some other cancers, such as carcinomas of the bladder and mesotheliomas, are more frequent in men, at least in part because of their greater occupational exposure to various chemical carcinogens and asbestos, respectively. Other cancers that occur more frequently in men include the lymphomas and leukemias, malignant melanomas, sarcomas of the bone, and carcinomas of the nasopharynx, stomach, kidney, pancreas, colon, rectum, parotid gland, and liver. The reasons for the excess of these cancers in males is unknown. Women could be either constitutionally less susceptible to these neoplasms or less exposed to whatever (largely unknown) environmental factors contribute to their development.

Race and Geography

Within individual races, incidence and mortality rates of all cancers vary considerably from one geographic region to another; migrants from one country to another, or their descendants, tend to eventually develop most cancers at rates more similar to those in their country of adoption than to those in their country of origin.[13] These observations imply that environmental factors play a large role in the etiology of most cancers. The frequency of occurrence of many cancers also varies among racial groups residing in the same country. This variation may be due to either genetic differences among the races or to factors related to their distinct cultural patterns, social behavior, or economic status.

Some cancers appear to be related to a "Western" lifestyle. Cancers that tend to occur at lower rates in developing countries and migrants from these countries than in lifelong residents of such areas as North America and Western Europe include cancers of the colon and rectum, which may be related to diets rich in animal products; cancers of the prostate, ovary, corpus uteri, and breast, which have to some extent also been related to high consumption of meats and fats, as well as to endocrinological and reproductive factors; Hodgkin's disease, which has been hypothesized to be due to a common infectious agent, probably the Epstein-Barr virus that, like polio viruses, may cause clinically overt disease with a frequency directly related to age at initial infection; and non-Hodgkin's lymphomas and neoplasms of the brain and testis, the causes of which are largely unknown. Other cancers occur more frequently in developing countries and in migrants from these countries. For example, compared to white populations of the United States and Western Europe, migrants from Asian countries have higher rates of stomach cancer, possibly related to intake of preserved foods and infection with *Helicobacter pylori*; liver cancers, which may, in part, be caused by the production of aflatoxins in contaminated foods and by hepatitis B and C viruses; cancers of the nasopharynx, caused in part by the Epstein-Barr virus (EBV); and cancer of the uterine cervix, which is caused by some types of human papillomaviruses.

Cancers that are strongly related to smoking occur with a frequency commensurate with the smoking habits in the population. Thus, cancers of the lung, larynx, bladder, kidney, and pancreas have tended to occur more frequently in developed than developing countries, but rates of these neoplasms are increasing in developing countries where more widespread cigarette smoking has accompanied economic changes.

In the United States, the patterns of cancer occurrence in recent immigrants reflect the cancer patterns in their countries of origin and become less distinct as these groups become more acculturated with the passage of time. The overall incidence and mortality rates and the ratio of mortality to incidence in various social and ethnic groups in the United States are shown in Table 50-3.[14] Variations in overall cancer incidence reflect the mix of cancers in the different groups. Variations in mortality are due to variations in both incidence and survival. The differences in the ratio of mortality to incidence rates provide a rough indicator of differences in overall survival from cancer. These are a reflection of both the types of cancer that predominate in the different groups and the level of utilization of screening and treatment services by their members. Less advantaged groups have the highest ratios of mortality to incidence, clearly indicating that improvement of services could have an impact on the cancer burden in these populations.

Time Trends

Figure 50-1, *A* and *B*, shows trends in mortality rates for various cancers in the United States from 1930 to 1992, for men and women.[8] The striking increase in rates of lung cancer is largely due to cigarette smoking. The reason for the marked decline in rates of stomach cancer is unknown but may be related to changes in dietary habits, with consumption of less preserved and more fresh and frozen foods. Mortality rates of uterine cancer largely reflect deaths due to cancer of the cervix, because invasive neoplasms arising from that site have a considerably poorer prognosis than endometrial cancers. The decline in mortality from uterine cancer is probably due to a real drop in incidence resulting from the use of cytological screening, as well as to a decrease in the number of women with a uterus due to an increase in rates of hysterectomies for nonneoplastic conditions. The decline in liver cancer rates is, at least in part, due to improvements over time in diagnosis, with fewer individuals with cancers of other sites that have metastasized to the liver erroneously diagnosed as having primary liver cancer. Breast and prostate cancer incidence, but not mortality, have increased dramatically in recent years, probably as a result of mammography and prostate-specific antigen (PSA) screening, respectively. There has been either no change or only gradual and sometimes erratic changes over time in the mortality rates of such major cancers as those of the pancreas, breast, and prostate, and the leukemias. This indicates that the major environmental determinants of these cancers are likely to be temporally stable factors that are well ingrained into the social and cultural environment. The unremarkable changes in mortality over time also indicate that there has been little or no improvement in survival from many of the major cancers in the past several decades, although the small decline in breast cancer mortality rates in recent years may be an indication of the impact of mammographic screening.

Temporal trends in mortality from cancer in children are much more encouraging. From 1973 to 1992, mortality rates in children under age 15 declined 51.8 percent for leukemia, 65.6 percent for non-Hodgkin's lymphoma, 69.4 percent for Hodgkin's disease, 47.2 percent for sarcomas of the bone, 53.7 percent for kidney cancer (largely Wilms' tumor), and 43.4 percent for all cancer sites combined.[4] There has been little change in the incidence of these neoplasms in children, and these reductions in mortality are a result of prolonged survival due to improved therapy.

TABLE 50-3. AGE-ADJUSTED INCIDENCE AND MORTALITY RATES OF ALL CANCERS COMBINED IN RACIAL AND ETHNIC GROUPS IN THE UNITED STATES, 1988 TO 1992[a]

	Men			Women		
	Rates per 100,000		Mortality Ratio of to Incidence	Rates per 100,000		Mortality Ratio of to Incidence
Race/Ethnic Group	Incidence	Mortality		Incidence	Mortality	
Alaska Native	372	225	0.60	348	179	0.51
American Indian[b]	196	123	0.63	180	99	0.55
African American	560	319	0.57	326	168	0.52
Chinese	282	139	0.49	213	86	0.40
Filipino	274	105	0.38	224	63	0.28
Hawaiian	340	239	0.70	321	168	0.52
Japanese	322	133	0.41	241	88	0.37
Korean	266	NA[c]	—	180	NA[c]	—
Vietnamese	326	NA[c]	—	273	NA[c]	—
White	469	213	0.45	346	40	0.40
Hispanic (total)	319	129	0.40	243	85	0.35
White Hispanic	336	134	0.40	256	89	0.35
White non-Hispanic	481	217	0.45	354	143	0.40

[a] Age-adjusted to 1987 U.S. Standard Incidence rates from SEER areas, mortality rates for United States.
[b] New Mexico.
[c] Rates not calculated when based on less than 25 cases.

Goals for the Year 2000

In 1984, the NCI set a goal to halve the cancer mortality rate by the year 2000.[15] This goal was a theoretical possibility because if the incidence rate of each cancer in the United States were reduced to equal the lowest rate in the world observed for the same cancer, then the overall cancer burden in the country would be reduced by about 80 percent.

The four major areas in which improvements in cancer mortality were projected are smoking cessation, dietary fat and fiber modification, breast and cervical cancer screening, and treatment (Table 50-4). Despite some improvements in each of the four areas, the goals for 2000 will not be met.

Although the goal of a 50 percent reduction in cancer mortality has been criticized as overly ambitious and unrealistic, it continues to be of use for establishing priorities for funding activities of basic and

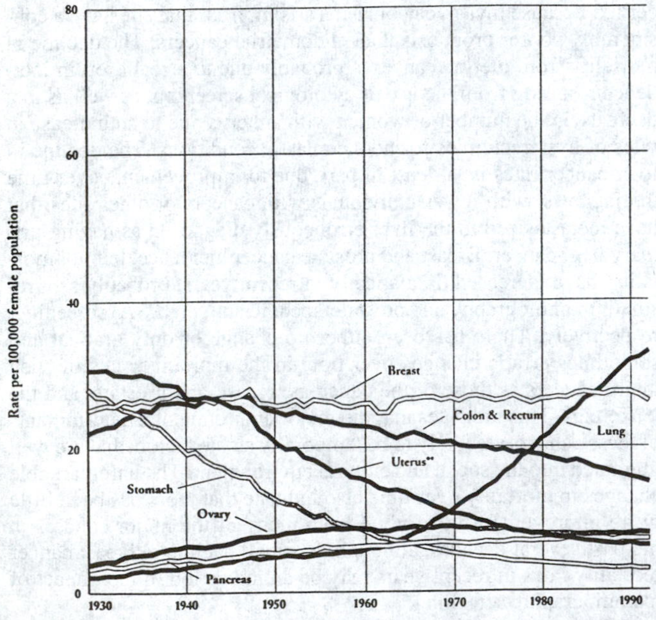

A

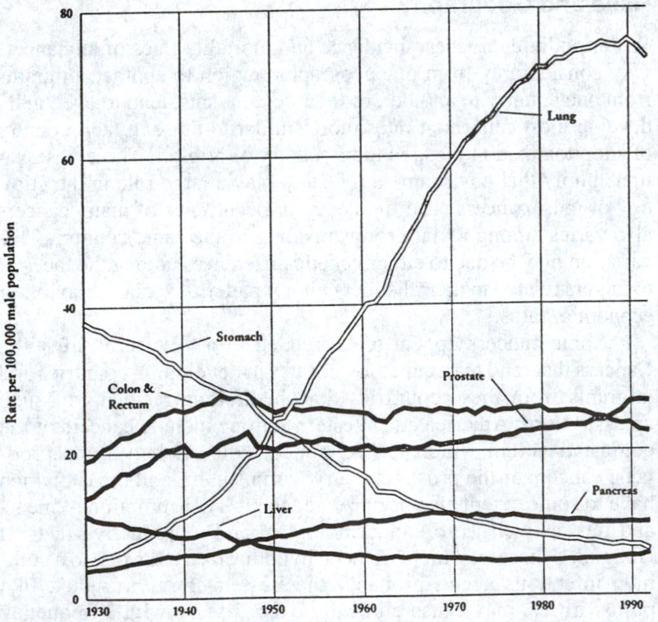

B

Figure 50-1. A, Age-adjusted cancer death rates, females by site, United States, 1930–1992. **B**, Age-adjusted cancer death rates, males by site, United States, 1930–1992. Rates are per 100,000 and are age-adjusted to the 1970 standard population. Uterine cancer death rates are for cervix and corpus combined. *Note:* Due to changes in ICD coding, numerator information has changed over time. Rates for cancer of the liver are particularly affected by these coding changes. Denominator information for the years 1930–1967 and 1991–1992 is based on intercensal population estimates, while denominator information for the years 1968–1990 is based on postcensal recalculation of estimates. Sources: Vital Statistics of the United States, 1995. (From American Cancer Society: Cancer Facts and Figures—1996. New York: American Cancer Society, 1996.)

TABLE 50-4. NATIONAL CANCER INSTITUTE'S GOALS FOR IMPROVED CANCER MORTALITY BY THE YEAR 2000

Factor	*Goal*	*Reduction in Mortality if Goal Met (%)*
Smoking	Reduce prevalence to 16% by 1990	15
	by 2000	8
Diet	Reduce fat to 30% of calories and increase fiber to 20–30 g/day	8
Screening	Mammograms in 80% of 50–70 year olds	
	Pap smears in 90% of 20–39 year olds; 80% of 40–70 year olds	3
Treatment	Increase use of state-of-the-art therapy	10–26

clinical scientists, epidemiologists, health planners and administrators, and community cancer control specialists.

▶ ETIOLOGY AND PRIMARY PREVENTION

Criteria for Causality

Primary cancer prevention is prevention of the initial development of a neoplasm or its precursor. This can be accomplished only if one or more causes of the neoplasm are known, and it is achieved by reducing or preventing exposure to the causative agent. An agent is considered a cause if reducing or removing a population's exposure to it would result in a decrease in the amount of disease occurring in that population.

To determine whether an agent is a cause of a particular disease in humans, information from all relevant studies must be assessed critically. In making such an assessment, evidence for causality is strengthened if the criteria listed in Chapter 2 are met. Additional criteria include evidence that risk is reduced following a reduction in exposure and that the disease associated with the substance has unusual features (such as a specific histological type).

Attempts to determine whether an agent is carcinogenic in humans must often be made without information on all of these criteria; yet assessment of whatever evidence is available must frequently be made. Investigators must examine existing evidence to identify additional questions that should be addressed by further studies, physicians must assess available evidence to be able to give their patients adequate advice, and public officials must assess the evidence to determine needs for laws and regulations to limit exposure. Each must weigh the evidence for a causal relationship and consider the consequences of falsely implicating a substance as being carcinogenic when it is not and of failing to identify as carcinogenic a substance that is. All must also be willing to alter their opinions as results of additional investigations become available. Errors of judgment can be minimized by a clear understanding of basic epidemiologic principles and by careful examination of available evidence using the above-referenced criteria for assessing causality.

General Etiological Considerations

At the level of the cell, cancer is a genetic disease. The development of a cancer appears to involve a multistep accumulation of genetic damage, leading eventually to the development of an abnormal clone of cells with a selective advantage over normal cells, and finally to an incipient tumor that acquires the ability to invade surrounding tissue.[16] Molecular genetic technology has led to the identification of at least 100 genes that play a role in carcinogenesis.

For each organ site, a tumor is the end result of multiple genetic aberrations that may be caused by multiple agents, and the same endpoint may be reached via different pathways. As a result, multiple risk factors are observed for all cancers, and only a small proportion of individuals who are exposed to most known carcinogens develop cancer. For example, a factor may increase cancer risk if it contributes directly to DNA damage, alters the ability of the cell to recognize or repair damage, inhibits apoptosis, encourages cell proliferation, enhances vascularization of the incipient tumor, or otherwise confers a selective advantage to that clone of cells. Similarly, agents that inhibit tumor development might act by reducing epithelial absorption of carcinogens, inhibiting the enzymatic activation of procarcinogens, enhancing the metabolic destruction of carcinogenic agents, promoting DNA repair, or causing cell differentiation or apoptosis and thereby reducing the number of stem and intermediate cells susceptible to the effects of carcinogens.

Most of the genes in which mutations appear to play a mechanistic role in carcinogenesis are categorized as either oncogenes or tumor suppressor genes, or are involved directly in DNA repair. Most identified oncogenes are mutated forms of genes (proto-oncogenes) that code for proteins involved in signal transduction, the regulation of gene expression, or growth-regulating mechanisms such as growth factors or growth factor receptors; overexpression of these genes results in enhanced cell proliferation. Most known tumor suppressor genes function as negative regulators of cell proliferation. The tumor suppressor gene p53, for example, is mutated in a majority of epithelial tumors.

Other contributors to the carcinogenic process probably include genes affecting angiogenesis, metastasis, and other components of the process such as the ability to evade or disable the immune response.

The latent period between exposure to some agent and the development of a neoplasm is dependent in part on the mechanism by which the agent operates. For example, mesothelioma follows exposure to asbestos only decades after exposure; the same is true of breast cancers following radiation to the chest, suggesting that these agents act early in the carcinogenic process. On the other hand, endometrial cancers can occur within 2 years of exposure to exogenous estrogens, suggesting a late-stage effect of these hormones. Reticulum cell sarcomas have developed within just months of exposure to immunosuppressive drugs in persons with renal transplants. A single exposure may act at one or more points in the progression to neoplasia, and its mechanism of action may vary across cancer sites. For example, epidemiologic evidence suggests that tobacco acts early in the carcinogenesis of esophageal and gastric adenocarcinoma, late in pancreatic tumors, and at both early and late stages in lung tumors.

It must be emphasized, however, that a risk factor can represent a cause in the public health sense, as defined previously, whether or not its precise mode of action is known. For example, we have only incomplete knowledge of the exact mechanisms by which tobacco smoke increases a smoker's risk of lung cancer. For the purpose of primary prevention, however, the mechanisms of action are unimportant. Cessation of smoking will prevent lung cancer, and that is what we need to know to take preventive action.

Some of the known causes of various cancers are described below. The best source of additional information is this chapter's Reference 17.

Tobacco

Smoking and associated cancer risks are also discussed in Chapter 44. Use of tobacco is responsible for about 30 percent of all cancer deaths, which is more than all other known causes of cancer combined. For cancers at nine sites, Table 50-5 shows the estimated relative risk in cigarette smokers compared to relative risk in nonsmokers, the estimated proportion of cases that would be prevented in the absence of exposure (the population-attributable risk percent), and the annual number of deaths in the United States attributable to tobacco.[18,19] Population-attributable risks such as these are dependent

TABLE 50-5. ASSOCIATION OF CIGARETTE SMOKING WITH CANCERS AT SELECTED SITES

Cancer Site	Relative Risk	Smoking Attributable Risk %	1994 Deaths Due to Smoking
Lung	10.0	85.1	130,163
Larynx	8.0	80.9	3,074
Oral cavity	4.0	79.0	6,259
Esophagus	3.0	75.4	7,845
Bladder	2.0	40.1	4,252
Pancreas	2.0	28.5	7,386
Stomach	1.8	35.7	5,000
Kidney	1.5	32.9	3,722

on the proportion of people in the population who use tobacco, the relative risk of the particular cancer in users of tobacco, and the presence of other causes of the cancers of interest in the population. Estimates of population-attributable risks thus vary among populations, and the values for the United States are different from values for other parts of the world.

In addition to the cancer sites shown in Table 50-5, for which the associations with tobacco are well established, a growing body of evidence implicates cigarette smoking as a contributor to the risk of colon and rectum cancers.[20] Case-control studies have also shown a possible association between smoking and cancer of the uterine cervix, although this may be a spurious observation due to incomplete control for the confounding effects of sexual behavior.

Relative risk estimates in Table 50-5 are for individuals who have ever smoked; relative risks for heavy smokers of long duration are higher. Many of these estimates are based on studies of individuals who smoked cigarettes that were popular decades ago. Relative risks in comparable smokers of the newer filter and low-tar products are lower but still appreciable. Furthermore, the number of puffs per cigarette and the number of cigarettes smoked per hour are inversely proportional to the amount of nicotine in the tobacco. Low levels of nicotine therefore result in an increased exposure to carcinogens in tobacco smoke. There is no safe cigarette.

Risks of a variety of neoplasms are also increased in users of other forms of tobacco. Compared to nonsmokers, risk in pipe and cigar smokers is approximately doubled for lung cancer, increased 4-fold for cancer of the larynx, and doubled or tripled for neoplasms of the esophagus, oral cavity, and pharynx. Pipe smoking approximately triples one's risk of lip cancer, and chewing tobacco or using snuff results in a 4-fold increase in the risk of oral cancer.[21]

Sidestream smoke contains some carcinogens in higher concentration than mainstream smoke, and nonsmokers exposed to tobacco smoke by living with a smoker are at an estimated 30 to 50 percent increased risk of lung cancer.[19,22–24] Passive smoking may account for much of the lung cancer not due to smoking or industrial exposures.

Alcohol

The risk of several human neoplasms is clearly associated with alcohol consumption.[25] Risk of hepatocellular carcinomas is increased in heavy drinkers, but the extent to which this is due to the unusually high prevalence of hepatitis B and C in alcoholics is unknown. These tumors tend to develop in alcoholics with macronodular cirrhosis, probably as a result of the rapid regeneration of liver cells in such individuals. If alcohol is a cause of liver cancer, it is an uncommon complication of its use, because these tumors are rare in countries such as the United States where exposure to alcohol is common.

With the exception of the liver, cancer risk is definitely increased only in those tissues that come in direct contact with undigested alcohol. Risk is thus increased for squamous cell carcinomas of the mouth (buccal cavity and pharynx), esophagus, and supraglottic larynx, but not, for example, of the lung or bladder. Esophageal, oral, and laryngeal squamous cell cancers are all also related to smoking, and most studies show the effect of smoking on the risk of these tumors to be greater in drinkers than in nondrinkers. Alcohol thus appears to potentiate the carcinogenic effect of tobacco smoke. It is not known whether alcohol use increases risk of these neoplasms in the absence of tobacco smoke or other carcinogens. The effect of alcohol on these neoplasms may also be greater in individuals with marginal nutritional status than in better nourished individuals. In the United States, alcohol and tobacco account for about 80 percent of these cancers.

Adenocarcinomas of the lower esophagus, gastroesophageal junction, and gastric cardia have also been consistently associated with alcohol use, but the relationship is not as strong as for the squamous cell carcinomas of the upper aerodigestive tract. Risks of cancer of the distal stomach, pancreas, colon, and rectum have not been consistently related to alcohol use, but observed associations between beer and rectal cancers and between heavy drinking and pancreatic cancer warrant further study. An association between alcohol intake and breast cancer has been observed in multiple investigations, even after controlling for known risk factors for breast cancer; additional studies of this relationship should be conducted.

Approximately 4 percent of all male cancer deaths and 2 percent of all female cancer deaths in the United States can be attributed to alcohol use. Most alcohol-related neoplasms develop as a result of smoking as well as drinking, and cessation of smoking would have nearly the same impact on the occurrence of these neoplasms as cessation of drinking.

Industrial Exposures

In 1972, the International Agency for Research on Cancer in Lyon, France, initiated a series of monographs on the evaluation of carcinogenic risks to humans. As of 1996, 65 multidisciplinary committees of experts have reviewed the published literature on approximately 900 suspect chemicals, industrial processes, drugs, and infectious agents and classified them as to their likely carcinogenicity in animals and humans.[26–49] Of the over 800 chemical and industrial processes evaluated, the available evidence was considered sufficient to clarify 22 specific exposures and 13 industrial processes with multiple exposures as carcinogenic to humans (Group 1). These, and the neoplasms most strongly and consistently associated with them, are shown in Table 50-6. Over 50 other chemicals and industrial processes were judged to be probably carcinogenic to humans (Group 2A), and over 100 others were considered possibly carcinogenic to humans (Group 2B). The remaining chemicals and industrial processes were considered not classifiable as to their carcinogenicity to humans (Group 3).

There has been considerable controversy in recent years as to the proportion of cancers that are attributable to known occupational exposures. Although estimates of over one-third have been published, those in the range of 2 to 5 percent are more generally accepted for the United States.[50]

Environmental Pollution

The evidence that the agents shown in Table 50-6 are carcinogenic in humans comes from studies of relatively high exposure in the workplace. Exposures outside the workplace to most of these agents are sufficiently rare or at such low levels as to be of little importance. Exposures outside the industrial setting to point sources of arsenic, chromium, and nickel from industrial pollutants and to vinyl chloride and asbestos indoors are, however, causes for concern.

Numerous efforts have been made to assess the impact of ambient air pollution on lung cancer risk.[51] Although rates of lung cancer are higher in urban than in rural areas, smoking is also more prevalent in urban areas. Case-control and cohort studies, in which attempts were made to control for the confounding effects of smoking, have

TABLE 50-6. OCCUPATIONAL CAUSES OF CANCER

Specific Exposures	Site or Tumor Type
SPECIFIC EXPOSURES	
4-Aminobiphenyl	Bladder
Arsenic and arsenic compounds	Lung, skin
Asbestos	Lung, mesothelioma
Benzene	Leukemia
Benzidine	Bladder
Beryllium and beryllium compounds	Lung
Bis(chloromethyl)ether and chloromethyl methyl ether	Lung
Cadmium and cadmium compounds	Lung
Chromium compounds	Lung, sinonasal
Coal tar pitches	Skin, lung, bladder
Coal tars	Skin
Erionite	Mesothelioma
Ethylene oxide	Leukemia, lymphoma
Mineral oils, untreated and mildly treated	Skin
Mustard gas (sulphur mustard)	Lung, larynx
2-Naphthylamine	Bladder
Nickel and nickel compounds	Sinonasal, lung
Shale oils	Skin
Soots	Skin, lung
Talc containing asbestiform fibers	Lung
Vinyl chloride	Liver, lung, brain, leukemia, lymphoma
Wood dust	Sinonasal
INDUSTRIAL PROCESS	
Aluminum production	Lung, bladder, lymphosarcomas and reticulosarcomas
Manufacture of auramine	Bladder
Boot and shoe manufacture and repair	Nose, bladder
Coal gasification	Lung, bladder, skin
Coke production	Lung, bladder, skin
Furniture and cabinetmaking	Nose
Hematite mining, underground, with exposure to radon	Lung
Occupational exposure to strong—inorganic—acid mists containing sulfuric acid	Lung, larynx, nasal sinus
Iron and steel founding	Lung
Isopropyl alcohol manufacture, strong acid process	Nasal sinus
Manufacture of magenta	Bladder
Painters	Lung, larynx, esophagus, stomach, bladder, leukemia, lymphoma
Rubber industry	Bladder, leukemia, lymphoma

yielded inconsistent estimates of relative risk of lung cancer in relation to residence in an urban setting, distance from a point source of pollution, or levels of specific pollutants in the ambient air; these studies have generally not controlled for the potential confounding effect of passive smoking. On balance, however, most studies have shown a small increase in risk of lung cancer in relation to polluted ambient air. This exposure has been estimated by various investigators to account for 0.2 to 4 percent of all lung cancers in the United States. The lower figure is more likely correct, especially today, because there have been improvements in air quality since the time of the studies on which these estimates were made.

Drugs

Two classes of drugs are strongly and consistently associated with excess risks of subsequent cancer development. They include certain cancer chemotherapeutic drugs, particularly alkylating agents such as melphalan and chlorambucil, which can cause acute nonlymphocytic leukemia, and immunosuppressive drugs given to organ transplant recipients and to treat autoimmune diseases. The risk of non-Hodgkin's lymphoma is increased approximately 50-fold following aggressive immunosuppressive therapy in transplant patients. Risks of other cancers including skin cancers, sarcomas, and malignant melanoma are increased to a lesser degree.

Other drugs have been implicated as causes of cancer, often followed by withdrawal of the drug from the market and attempts to replace it with safer agents. Examples include chlornaphazaine, used to treat polycythemia vera and Hodgkin's disease, but found to cause bladder cancer; and topical nitrogen mustard, used to treat mycosis fungoides and psoriasis, but a cause of squamous cell carcinomas of the skin. Other drugs that are likely causes of skin cancer include arsenic compounds (Fowler's solution) used systemically and topically, coal tar ointments, and methoxysporalens used with ultraviolet light to treat psoriasis. The analgesic phenacetin has been strongly implicated as a cause of carcinomas of the renal pelvis and bladder. Studies are currently being conducted to assess whether the use of thiazide diuretics increases subsequent risk of kidney cancer and whether calcium channel blockers are contributors to cancer risk.[52]

Studies of medication use and cancer are complicated by the fact that the underlying condition for which a medication is prescribed may be an independent contributor to cancer risk. It may be difficult to distinguish the effect of the medication from the effect of the condition itself.

Recent evidence suggests that certain medications may also decrease the risk of cancer. Foremost among these drugs are aspirin and other nonsteroidal anti-inflammatory drugs (NSAIDs), which appear to decrease the risk of cancers of the colon and rectum and possibly other sites.[53]

Overall, drugs account for less than 1 percent of cancer in the United States. Furthermore, most of the known leukemogenic and carcinogenic drugs are used to treat conditions sufficiently life threatening to warrant accepting the associated risk of subsequent neoplasia. The identification of drugs that cause cancer is, nonetheless, of obvious importance to the practicing oncologist; and the problem of drug-induced neoplasia will probably become greater in the future as more patients survive for longer periods of time and as more potentially carcinogenic and leukemogenic drugs come into use. The practicing physician should be aware of the known risks of subsequent neoplasia in patients receiving various chemotherapeutic agents and should support formal epidemiological efforts to monitor new and existing drugs for their potential long-term carcinogenic effects.

Ionizing Radiation

Ionizing radiation can cause a variety of human neoplasms.[54] Most of the evidence for this comes from studies that followed individuals exposed to moderate or high doses from nuclear explosions, medical treatments, and occupational sources. Exposures have been both external and internal and have included x-rays, γ-rays, neutrons, α-particles, and β-particles.

Studies of individuals who have received total body radiation from external sources have shown that some organs are more susceptible to the carcinogenic effects of radiation than others. In the atomic bomb survivors in Japan, there were large increases in rates of carcinomas of the anatomically exposed thyroid and mammary glands and of leukemias arising from the highly susceptible cells of the bone marrow; lesser increases in rates of lymphomas and carcinomas of the stomach, esophagus, and bladder were observed; and risks of cancer at other sites were either not altered or the increases were too small to measure with certainty. Risk of leukemia was also increased in early radiologists who took few precautions to reduce their general exposure to radiation and probably also in individuals exposed *in utero* to x-rays from pelvimetry.

External sources of radiation directed at specific sites have resulted in a variety of neoplasms. Breast cancer was induced in women treated with x-rays for a variety of benign breast conditions and in women who received multiple fluoroscopies of the chest in conjunction with pneumothorax treatment of tuberculosis. Individuals treated with x-rays for ankylosing spondylitis have had increased rates of leukemia and lung cancer and, like the atomic bomb survivors, lesser increases in rates of lymphomas and cancers of the stomach and esophagus. An increased risk of lung cancer has been observed in women who received radiation following mastectomy for breast cancer. Children treated with x-rays for tinea capitis and enlarged thymus have developed leukemia and neoplasms of the salivary and thyroid glands. Those treated for an enlarged thymus have also had an increased risk of leukemia, and those with tinea capitis developed more brain tumors than expected.

Internal exposures to radiation have likewise resulted in increased risks of cancer at specific sites. Inhalation of radioactive dusts contributed to the increased rates of lung cancer in the atomic bomb survivors, and inhalation of radon and its decay products resulted in elevated rates of lung cancer in miners of uranium, iron, and fluorspar. Radium inadvertently swallowed by radium-dial watch painters and administered for treatment of ankylosing spondylitis was concentrated in osseous tissues and caused high rates of bone cancers. Individuals exposed to iodine-131 (I-131) in fallout from a hydrogen bomb test and in emissions from the nuclear power plant accident at Chernobyl subsequently had increased rates of thyroid cancer. The radiopaque contrast material thorotrast that was used to x-ray the liver has resulted in hepatic cancers, as well as leukemias and lung carcinomas. Women receiving cervical radium implants and other forms of pelvic radiation for a variety of gynecological conditions have had increased rates of cancers of the colon, rectum, and possibly small bowel, as well as leukemia.

The results of most studies show a linear increase in risk of neoplasms with the amount of radiation received over a wide range of observed doses, with a possible decrease in the slope of the dose-response curve at very high levels of exposure (perhaps due to cell killing). These observations are based primarily on studies of individuals who received from tens to hundreds of rads. Doses commonly received today are orders of magnitude lower, and it is uncertain whether the dose-response curve should be linearly extrapolated to these low levels to provide an estimate of the associated risk. There may be a threshold level below which radiation does not induce neoplasms, perhaps because mechanisms of DNA repair are adequate. If so, linear extrapolation would yield estimates of risk to low levels of radiation that are too high. Conversely, chronic exposure to low levels of radiation might be more carcinogenic, rad for rad, than acute exposure at a higher dose. If so, linear extrapolations would underestimate the risk of low doses. Since there is little evidence for the latter possibility, most authorities believe that it is reasonable, as well as prudent, to assume a linear, nonthreshold dose-response relationship.

Approximately half of all ionizing radiation received by individuals in the United States comes from natural background sources, which deliver about 80 mrem of ionizing radiation per year to a person living at sea level, and about twice this amount in individuals living at high altitudes, or where concentrations of radium in the ground are unusually high. Radium decays to a radioactive gas, radon-222, which can seep into houses and accumulate under conditions of poor ventilation. Radon-222 is likely the cause of lung cancer in uranium miners, but it is uncertain whether the lower doses found in some homes contribute appreciably to the lung cancer burden.[55] Approximately 43 percent of all ionizing radiation is received from medical sources; largely from diagnostic x-rays. These result in an annual exposure of about 92 mrem per year for the average U.S. citizen. Most other exposures have been from mining and processing radioactive ores (2 to 3 percent), fallout from nuclear weapons (2 to 4 percent), and such consumer products as television sets and smoke detectors (1 to 4 percent).

The average person living at sea level in the United States thus receives about 180 mrem of ionizing radiation per year. This is roughly equivalent to that received during an upper or lower gastrointestinal (GI) series, whereas only about 10 mrem are received from a chest x-ray.

Based on a linear, nonthreshold dose-response model, it has been estimated that approximately 1 percent of all cancer in the United States may be attributable to radiation from other than background sources. Because most of the preventable radiation-induced neoplasms result from medical exposures, the responsibility for preventing them rests primarily with members of the medical profession. Political efforts to reduce the likelihood of environmental contamination from nuclear power plants and nuclear weapons would also obviously reduce the risk of radiation-induced neoplasms.

Nonionizing Radiation

Sunlight is definitely a cause of squamous and basal cell carcinomas of the skin, as evidenced by the observations that these tumors tend to occur on exposed parts of the body, risk increases with the amount of sun exposure, and incidence rates are greater in light- than dark-skinned individuals.

The relationship of malignant melanomas of the skin to sunlight is more complicated.[56] Incidence rates are highest in low altitudes with sunny climates, and in individuals with little natural skin pigmentation. Unlike other skin cancers, rates are not increased in individuals who regularly work outside, and although there is some tendency for these tumors to occur on exposed parts of the body, many do not. The results of some studies suggest that episodic exposures to the sun and sunburns increase risk, and an investigation of migrants to Australia provided evidence that exposure at an early age may be of particular importance.[56] In the white U.S. population, incidence rates of melanomas of the skin approximately doubled between 1973 and 1992, which is due in part to destruction of the ozone layer in the upper atmosphere and to changes in diagnostic criteria and enhanced awareness of the importance of early evaluation of melanotic lesions. This rise in incidence now appears to be slowing.[57]

Because nonmelanotic skin cancers are common and largely attributable to sun exposure, sunlight accounts for approximately 10 percent of all neoplasms. It accounts for only about 2 percent of cancer deaths, however, both because these neoplasms are infrequently fatal and because the more fatal melanomas are related less strongly to sun exposure. All individuals, but particularly those with light skin who burn easily, should be encouraged to avoid excessive direct exposure to intense sunlight and to use sunshades and sunscreens.

Recent studies have focused public attention on the possible association between exposure to electric and magnetic fields (EMF), particularly from electric power lines and appliances, and risk of cancer. This association is observed most consistently in studies of childhood leukemia, but the findings remain inconclusive. Study of this issue is made particularly difficult by our inability to identify and accurately measure the relevant exposure. A number of reviews of the subject have been published.[58,59]

Exogenous Sex Hormones

Diethylstilbestrol (DES) was used in the 1940s and 1950s to treat between one-half and 5 million women in the United States for threatened abortion. Approximately 80 percent of the female offspring who were exposed to DES while in utero have been found to have glandular epithelium resembling that of the endometrium, and presumably of Müllerian origin, in the vagina or cervix. This is referred to as adenosis. A small portion of women with this condition have developed clear cell adenocarcinomas of the vagina or (less frequently) the cervix when in their teens or twenties.[60] Fortunately, the risk of carcinoma is small, about one case per 100,000 exposed women by the age of 34 years. This represents a small proportion of total cancers, but a high proportion of neoplasms in this age group, including virtually all vaginal cancers. Women exposed in utero to DES with vaginal or cervical adenosis should be followed carefully for the development of clear cell carcinoma. Boys exposed in utero to DES are at increased risk of cryptorchidism, which is a risk factor for testicular cancer; several studies have implicated prenatal DES exposure as a rare cause of testicular cancer. These neoplasms represent the first documented instances of transplacental carcinogenesis in humans. This experience, along with that of leukemia in children following *in utero* exposure to radiation from pelvimetry, emphasizes the vulnerability of the growing fetus and the importance of minimizing in utero exposures to any suspected mutagens or carcinogens.

In some countries, DES is used as a "morning after" pill to prevent pregnancy. It has also been used to treat menopausal symptoms. Care must be exercised not to give DES inadvertently for these or other purposes to women who may be pregnant.

In considering the effects of exogenous female sex hormones on the risk of neoplasms in the women who take them, it is useful to categorize these substances according to their net estrogenic or progestogenic pharmacological effect. At one end of the spectrum are the pure progestational agents, such as depot-medroxyprogesterone acetate (DMPA), which is used as a long-acting injectable contraceptive in many countries and to treat malignant and benign proliferative disorders of the endometrium. Other progestational contraceptives include the so-called mini-pills; the injectable contraceptive, norethindrone; and subcutaneous implants, such as Norplant. At the other end of the spectrum are the pure estrogen preparations. The most common of these are the conjugated "natural" estrogens (e.g., Premarin), used largely to treat or prevent symptoms and conditions associated with the menopause, and the nonsteroidal synthetic estrogen, DES, mentioned previously. Between these two ends of the estrogen-progestin spectrum are the previously used sequential oral contraceptives, which contained only an estrogen in pills taken for 2 weeks of a cycle and which had a net estrogenic effect; and the commonly used combined oral contraceptives with an estrogen and a progestin in each pill, and therefore a net pharmacological effect more progestational than the sequential pills. Most epidemiologic studies of cancer and combined oral contraceptives that have been conducted to date assessed the influence on cancer risks of products that were marketed in the 1970s and 1980s. More recently introduced products differ from these older formulations in dosage and in the types of estrogens and progestins that they contain. Although the findings from studies conducted through the mid-1990s may not be applicable to these newer contraceptive agents, it would seem prudent to assume that they do until results of additional epidemiologic investigations provide evidence to the contrary.

Risk of endometrial cancer is increased in women who have received estrogens for menopausal conditions and other reasons and in women who took sequential oral contraceptives.[61,62] Tamoxifen, which is used as adjuvant therapy for breast cancer, has an estrogenic effect on the uterus and has also been shown to increase the risk of endometrial cancer.[63] On the other hand, risk is decreased in users of combined oral contraceptives[64] and in users of DMPA[65] because of their net progestational effect on the endometrium. To reduce the risk of endometrial cancer in users of estrogens, a progestin is often given, either continuously with the estrogen or cyclically for a specified number of days each month, and this has been shown to markedly reduce the risk of endometrial cancer, although a small residual increase in risk may remain.

Studies of breast cancer in women given both high and more modest doses of DES for threatened abortion have yielded equivocal and inconsistent results.[66] Studies of breast cancer in relation to estrogens given at menopause have also yielded inconsistent results, but most show no increase in risk in women who have used these products for less than 5 years. A small increase in risk with years of use beyond 5 years has been observed in most studies (30 to 80 percent increase after 10 years of use), with a decline in risks to that of nonusers from 2 to 5 years after cessation of use.[67] A recent collaborative reanalysis of 51 studies[67a] on this issue found that during or shortly after use, there was a relative risk of 1.023 for each year of use for those with 1–4 years of use, and 1.028 for those with more than five years of use. Limited evidence to date suggests that the addition of a progestin to the regimen does not alter its effect (if any) on breast cancer risk. Tamoxifen, which has antiestrogenic properties in the breast, has been shown to reduce the risk of breast cancer in the contralateral breast of a woman who receives this substance as adjuvant therapy for primary breast cancer.

The effect of combined oral contraceptives on risk of breast cancer was addressed in a 1995 meta-analysis of most of the existing epidemiologic data on this subject.[68] Risk of having breast cancer diagnosed was found to be increased by about 25 percent in current users and to decline to that of nonusers by about 10 years after cessation of use. The relative risk in women who ever used oral contraceptives was estimated to be 1.07. Tumors tended to be more localized in users than in nonusers, suggesting enhanced surveillance in recent and current users as an explanation for the increased risk. Even if the findings do represent a causal phenomenon, use of oral contraceptives would result in few additional cases of breast cancer, because most current and recent users of oral contraceptives are young women with a low background rate of this disease. A combined analysis of two studies of DMPA and breast cancer similarly found an increase in risk in recent and current users of this progestational agent, but no increase in risk after 5 years since last use, and an overall relative risk of 1.1 in women who had ever used this agent.[69] The small possible increase in risk of breast cancer in users of steroid contraceptives must be weighed against the many benefits of these products.

Use of estrogens for menopausal indications has not consistently been shown to alter risk of ovarian cancer. Oral contraceptives clearly reduce the risk of epithelial ovarian cancer.[70] Risk in women who have ever used combined oral contraceptives is about 60 percent that of nonusers, and the risk decreases with duration of use. A single study showed no effect of DMPA on risk of ovarian cancer.

Studies of cervical cancer and menopausal estrogens have not been conducted. Most studies of oral contraceptives and invasive cervical cancer have shown risk of both squamous cell and adenomatous histologic types to increase with duration of oral contraceptive use, even after taking into account the possible confounding effects of sexual activity and infection with oncogenic types of human papilloma viruses (HPV). Oral contraceptives provide hormonal conditions favorable to the persistence of HPV infection[48] or transformation of infected cells.

Combined oral contraceptives have clearly been shown to cause benign hepatic cell adenomas and focal nodular hyperplasia. These are highly vascular tumors that can rupture, bleed into the peritoneal cavity, and cause death. Fortunately, they are a rare complication of oral contraceptive use, occurring at a rate of less than 3 per 100,000 women-years in women under 30 years of age. Case-control studies conducted in developed countries have shown that primary hepatocellular carcinomas are also rare complications of oral contraceptive use.[71] Some of these studies, plus investigations conducted largely in developing countries, provided evidence that this adverse effect is not mediated by enhancing the influence of other factors such as hepatitis B or C on risk.

Both case-control and cohort studies have failed to confirm earlier reports that risk of malignant melanoma is increased by use of oral contraceptives.[64] Isolated reports of associations between oral contraceptives and pituitary adenomas, choriocarcinomas, gallbladder carcinomas, and thyroid tumors have also appeared, but these observations have not been convincingly confirmed by epidemiological investigations.[64]

The proportion of cancers caused by exogenous hormones is unknown. Rates of endometrial cancer have declined since the mid-1970s, following a reduction in the use of unopposed estrogens that resulted from the discovery that estrogens caused carcinomas of the endometrium. Few estrogen-related breast cancers will occur with these changes in estrogen usage unless the addition of progestins to replacement therapy regimens unexpectedly is shown to adversely affect risk of breast cancer. The small increases in risks of some cancers must be considered in the larger context of the putative benefits of estrogen replacement therapy, particularly the reduction in risks of *cardiovascular diseases* and osteoporosis. In developed countries, the protective effects of oral contraceptives against benign breast diseases and cancers of the ovary and endometrium outweigh the increased risks of liver tumors and cancers of the breast and cervix. In developing countries where cervical cancer rates are high, the risks of oral contraceptive use are still far outweighed by the benefits of an effective means of contraception. DMPA, on balance, probably has a net beneficial effect on risk of neoplasia and appears to be at least as safe in this respect as combined oral contraceptives. The newer oral contraceptives have been subject to epidemiologic evaluation, but the long term effects with respect to cancer are uncertain. Until evidence from such studies becomes available, it is reasonable to assume that the effect of these products on risks of various cancers will be no greater than those observed for combined oral contraceptive and DMPA, respectively.

Infectious Agents

Both DNA and RNA viruses have been shown to cause a variety of neoplasms in animals. The DNA viruses that have been most strongly linked to cancers in humans include the EBV, hepatitis B and C (HBV and HCV), and the HPV.

EBV has been strongly related to African Burkitt's lymphoma and nasopharyngeal carcinomas.[72] Almost 100 percent of persons with these diseases have antibodies against EBV, compared with much lower percentages in unaffected persons, and antibody titers are higher in these cases. A cohort study clearly showed EBV infection to precede the development of African Burkitt's lymphomas. In addition, the EBV genome has been demonstrated in tumor cells from most African Burkitt's lymphomas and virtually all nasopharyngeal carcinomas. Only a small proportion of individuals infected with EBV develop either of these neoplasms, however, and the worldwide distributions of the two malignancies are different. Therefore, other factors must also be operative in conjunction with EBV for these tumors to develop. Chronic malaria and the resultant immunosuppression or antigenic stimulation may play a role in African Burkitt's lymphoma. Cofactors for nasopharyngeal carcinoma are unknown but may include human leukocyte antigen (HLA) type, other nasopharyngeal diseases, chemical exposures (e.g., the smoke from tobacco or cooking fires), and dietary factors such as salted fish. EBV is not a necessary factor for Burkitt's lymphoma, because only 15 to 25 percent of the cases outside Africa have evidence of prior EBV infection.

EBV probably also contributes to the development of Hodgkin's disease.[72] It is known to cause infectious mononucleosis, and persons with a history of this disease have a 2- to 3-fold increase in risk of Hodgkin's disease. Compared to controls, cases of Hodgkin's disease more frequently have antibodies against EBV and higher antibody titers. However, EBV DNA or gene products can be demonstrated in only half of cases, and only 30 to 40 percent of cases have anti-EBV antibodies, suggesting either the existence of causal pathways not including EBV or loss of EBV infection after tumor development.

Although rare in the United States, hepatocellular carcinoma is the most common cancer in some places, including parts of Africa and China. There is strong evidence that hepatitis B and C viruses are causes of this disease, and an IARC working group has judged that both of these viruses are carcinogenic to humans.[43] The disease appears to develop in individuals who become chronic carriers of one of these viruses. Determinants of the chronic carrier states are not fully understood. In high-risk areas, transmission of HBV to the child from the mother at or soon after birth, before immune competence is fully developed, appears to result in the child becoming a carrier. In adults, factors causing immunosuppression may play a role. It is uncertain whether these viruses directly cause hepatomas or whether they cause chronic hepatitis and liver cirrhosis, which lead to repeated periods of cell death and regeneration, which in turn increase risk, perhaps in the presence of other carcinogens such as aflatoxins.

In 1995, an IARC working group[48] concluded that HPV types 16 and 18 are carcinogenic to humans (Group 1), that types 31 and 33 are probably carcinogenic to humans (Groups 2A), and that several other types (including 35, 39, 45, 51, 52, 56, and 58) are possibly carcinogenic to humans. The strongest evidence implicates type 16 as a cause of carcinomas of the uterine cervix, anus, vulva (poorly keratinized type), and penis, and type 18 as a cause of cervical cancer (especially adenocarcinomas). But other types also very likely are causes of a small proportion of these neoplasms. These viruses are transmitted primarily through sexual contact, perhaps with enhanced efficiency in the presence of epithelial abrasions. Most infections are cleared, but in individuals in whom infection persists for a prolonged period of time, intraepithelial lesions develop, some of which eventually progress to invasive carcinomas. The factors responsible for viral persistence and lesion progression are not well defined, but may include hormonal factors (parity and steroid contraceptives), nutritional factors (e.g., folate, vitamin C, carotenoids), immunodeficiency (human immunodeficiency virus (HIV) infection, immunosuppression for renal transplantation), and possibly chemical factors (e.g., cigarette smoking) and other infectious agents (e.g., *Chlamydia trachomatis*, human T-cell leukemia virus-type 1 (HTLV-1)). HPV DNA can be demonstrated in over 90 percent of invasive cervical carcinomas, and in high proportions of the other anogential neoplasms, suggesting that most of these neoplasms are caused, at least in part, by one or more types of HPV. Women who belong to identifiable groups at increased risk for the acquisition of sexually transmitted diseases should receive high priority for cervical cancer screening.

Individuals with acquired immunodeficiency syndrome (AIDS), caused by infection by HIV, an RNA virus, are at greatly increased risk of Kaposi's sarcoma and of non-Hodgkin's lymphomas.[73] (See also Chapter 8.) Many of the latter are extranodal, often involving the brain. Rates of intraepithelial cervical and anal squamous cell carcinomas are also increased in AIDS patients, but increased rates of invasive cancer at these sites have not been observed. Testicular seminomas also occur more frequently in AIDS patients, and there are unconfirmed reports of increased risks of testicular teratocarcinoma, malignant melanoma, leiomyosarcoma, non–small cell lung cancer, multiple myeloma, hepatocellular carcinoma, and Hodgkin's disease.

HTLV-1 has been strongly implicated as a cause of T-cell leukemias and lymphomas, particularly in some areas of Japan, the South Pacific, the Caribbean, and Africa that are endemic for this virus, but this agent probably is of little current importance in the United States.

There are no proven methods of preventing any neoplasms of viral etiology, but prospects for prevention by means of vaccines against some of the oncogenic viruses are promising. An inactivated HBV vaccine was shown to prevent the development of the chronic hepatitis B surface antigen carrier state in infants born to mothers who were carriers, and efforts are under way to develop vaccines against HCV, EBV, HTLV-1, HIV, and specific types of HPV. Barrier methods of contraception may reduce rates of transmission of sexually transmitted agents and could theoretically help prevent HPV- and HIV-related cancers. Some studies have documented reduced risks of cervical cancer in monogamous women whose promiscuous husbands used condoms when visiting prostitutes.[74]

Four infectious agents other than viruses have been strongly implicated as causes of human cancers. In 1994, an IARC working group[45] judged that *Shistosoma haematobium* was a definite cause of bladder cancer (Group 1), that the liver flukes *Opisthorchis viverrini* and *Clonorchis sinensis* were definitely (Group 1) and probably (Group 2) causes of cholangiocarcinomas of the liver, respectively, and that the bacteria *Helicobacter pylori* was a carcinogen for the stomach (Group 1). Only the relationship of *H. pylori* to gastric cancer is of potential importance in developed countries. This pathogen has been associated with both intestinal and diffuse histologic types, and most strongly with tumors developing outside the cardia.[75]

The proportion of cancers due to infectious agents has not been reliably estimated. Given the enhanced proportion of specific cancers caused by known infectious agents, we estimate that about 3.5 percent of all cancers are due to an oncogenic virus. It is likely that an additional 0.9 percent of cancers are attributable to *H. pylori* infection, for a total of 54,900, or 4.4 percent of all cancers in the United

States (3.5 and 5.2 percent of all cancers in men and women, respectively). Of the estimated 547,000 deaths due to cancer in the United States in 1995, 3.9 percent were similarly estimated to be due to viral agents, and 1.3 percent to *H. pylori*, for a total of 5.2 percent of all cancer deaths due to cancers with a known infectious etiology.

Nutrition and Physical Activity

Reasons for the large international differences in the incidence of most cancers are unknown. Studies of rates in migrants have clearly shown that they are largely due to variation in environmental factors, not in genetic predisposition or susceptibility to carcinogens. Correlational studies have been conducted to identify factors that vary across countries in accordance with variations in the rates of various cancers. These studies have shown a variety of dietary components to be related to a number of different neoplasms. To investigate these associations further, many case-control studies and several large cohort studies have been conducted,[76] a variety of laboratory investigations have been performed to elucidate possible mechanisms for observed epidemiological findings, and randomized trials of dietary supplements or modifications have been conducted or are under way.

Epidemiological studies of diet and cancer are difficult for a variety of reasons. One common problem in all epidemiological approaches is that many individual dietary constituents are highly correlated. For example, diets that are poor in animal protein are also likely to be poor in animal fat and high in carbohydrates and fiber. Under such circumstances, it is difficult to determine which of the interrelated dietary constituents (if any) is responsible for observed variations in risk. Another difficulty is that diet many years prior to the development of a neoplasm may be of the greatest etiological relevance. Such information is difficult (although not impossible) to obtain in case-control studies. Cohort studies can theoretically overcome this problem, but must include large numbers of subjects and must be continued for decades, and hence require large commitments of time and money. Despite these methodological problems, results of recent research strongly suggest that dietary factors contribute to the etiology of a variety of neoplasms. Some of the more likely mechanisms are briefly summarized in the following paragraphs.

Food items may be contaminated by preformed carcinogens. Aflatoxins produced by fungi that can grow in grains and other crops in warm, moist climates have been linked to liver cancers in some parts of the world. In China, mutagens have been detected in fermented pancakes and vegetable gruels, and these have been related to both esophageal cancer in humans and neoplasms of the gullet in chickens; and nasopharyngeal carcinomas have been related to consumption of salted fish and fermented food during infancy.

Carcinogens may be formed in the body by bacteria. Nitrites may be ingested in small amounts with preserved meats and fish or formed in larger quantities from dietary nitrates, either spontaneously before being eaten or in the presence of bacteria in the body; and carcinogenic *N*-nitroso compounds may then be produced from ingested amines and nitrites by bacteria in the stomach of people with chronic gastritis, in the bladder of individuals with urinary tract infection, or in the normal colon and mouth to produce cancers of the stomach, bladder, colon, and esophagus, respectively.

Smoked and cured foods, charcoal-broiled meats, and some fruits and vegetables from contaminated areas may contain carcinogenic polycyclic aromatic hydrocarbons.

A high-fat diet may increase bile production and produce an environment in the large bowel conducive to the growth of bacteria capable of forming carcinogens, and perhaps steroid hormones, from bile salts. Production of such substances provides one plausible explanation for the observed associations between a high-fat diet and cancers of the colon, breast, and prostate.

Overnutrition, leading to obesity, has been associated with endometrial and postmenopausal breast cancers. A possible mechanism is tumor promotion by excess endogenous estrogens. In postmenopausal women, estrogens are derived from androgens produced by the adrenal gland. This reaction takes place in adipose tissue and is enhanced in obese women. Also, early menarche is a risk factor for breast cancer, late menopause is a risk factor for both breast and endometrial cancers, and both of these factors have been directly or indirectly related to overnutrition.

Although the epidemiologic evidence is not completely consistent, regular exercise appears to reduce the risk of breast cancer, perhaps because of the effects of physical activity on body weight. There is also evidence that exercise exerts an independent effect on the risk of colon cancer, possibly by decreasing stool transit time and therefore the duration of exposure to carcinogens in the gut.

Dietary constituents may also protect against cancer. Diets high in fresh fruits and raw vegetables have been associated with decreased risks of carcinomas of virtually all sites within the gastrointestinal and respiratory systems, the uterine cervix, and (less consistently) other tissues. Foods rich in retinol (preformed vitamin A) have also been associated with reduced risks of some epithelial cancers. Levels of many of the potentially protective micronutrients are highly correlated in human diets, making it difficult to determine which micronutrients are most strongly associated with reduced risks, and the specific substances in fruits and vegetables responsible for the apparent protective effects have therefore not been conclusively identified. It is likely that different micronutrients or combinations of micronutrients operate at different sites, and a variety of protective mechanisms have been suggested. For example: the reduced risks of stomach and esophageal carcinomas may be due to inhibition by vitamin C of *N*-nitroso compound formation; vegetables of the *Brassicaceae* family have been hypothesized to induce activity of mixed-function oxidases, which may detoxify ingested carcinogens responsible for colon cancer development; and vitamins C, E, and β-carotene quench free radicals that cause oxidative damage to DNA.

Dietary fiber may increase the bulk of the bowel contents, dilute intraluminal carcinogens, and enhance transit time through the gut. These mechanisms would reduce contact of the colonic mucosa with carcinogens and explain the inverse association between dietary fiber and the risk of colon cancer.

Certain plant foods also contain phytoestrogens. These weak estrogens may reduce the risk of hormonally mediated cancers by binding competitively to estrogen receptors and thereby exerting antiestrogenic effects.

Although the evidence that a diet high in fruits and vegetables decreases cancer risk has been used as one rationale for marketing vitamin supplements, there is no evidence that such products are protective against any neoplasm, and some evidence that they may even be harmful. For example, a number of studies have linked high fruit and vegetable intake, as well as high serum β-carotene levels, with a reduced risk of lung cancer, but recent clinical trials of β-carotene supplementation in individuals at high risk of lung cancer found *increased* lung cancer rates among supplemented patients.[77] These findings serve as a reminder that our current understanding of the constituents of fruits and vegetables, and their mechanisms of action, is incomplete. Nonetheless, the bulk of current knowledge suggests the elements of a prudent diet: compared to the average Western diet, it would be lower in meats and animal fats and higher in fresh fruits, vegetables, and fiber. Citrus fruits with high levels of vitamin C, vegetables of the *Brassicaceae* family, and vegetables rich in β-carotene might be of particular importance. Smoked, charred, or cured meats would be avoided or used in moderation, as would alcoholic beverages. Caloric intake would be optimized to avoid obesity. This diet would do no harm, probably reduce the risk of cancers, and be compatible with diets advocated to reduce risks of cardiovascular and cerebrovascular diseases. There is little evidence that supplementation of a prudent diet with vitamins would have a beneficial effect on cancer risk.

Reproductive Factors

Nulliparous women are at increased risk of cancers of the ovary, endometrium, and breast. Risk of ovarian and endometrial cancers decreases with increasing number of pregnancies, whereas pregnancies beyond the first have a lesser protective effect against breast cancer. Risk of breast cancer increases strongly with age at first full-term birth, but risks of ovarian and endometrial cancer probably do not. Earlier age at menarche and late age at menopause are associated with an increased risk of cancers of the breast and possibly endometrium, but not the ovary. Lactation, which suppresses ovarian function, has not consistently been shown to alter risk of breast cancer. Ovulation suppression by lactation is maximal soon after delivery, and short-term lactation probably has a small protective effect against ovarian cancer, although prolonged lactation does not seem to confer an additional benefit. Risk of endometrial cancer may be inversely related to duration of lactation, but the effect is short term so that there is little or no protection in the postmenopausal years, when most endometrial cancers occur. Induced abortion may enhance risk of breast cancer, but studies to date have yielded inconsistent findings.

Mechanisms for these associations are not fully understood, but they undoubtedly involve endogenous pituitary and ovarian hormones. The development of epithelial ovarian tumors is probably promoted by gonadotropin stimulation and reduced by suppression of gonadotropins during pregnancy and lactation. Nulliparous women may, on average, be less fertile than parous women and have more anovulatory menstrual cycles, and hence more constant production of estrogens without cyclic progesterone each month; this relative excess of estrogens could promote endometrial tumor development. Several mechanisms for the relationship of breast cancer to age at birth of first child have been proposed, but none appears adequate. Studies of the endocrinological events associated with childbearing and other endocrinological studies in women at varying risks of cancers of endocrine target organs have been conducted, and others are in progress, to attempt to explain more fully the mechanisms by which factors related to childbearing alter risk.

An increase in risk of cervical cancer with parity has been fairly consistently observed, even after taking into account possible confounding by HPV infection. The mechanism for this association is not understood, but pregnancies, like oral contraceptives, may provide hormonal conditions conducive to persistence of HPV infection or transformation of infected cervical tissue to precancerous or cancerous lesions.

The observed association with breast cancer of maternal age at birth of first child at least theoretically suggests a means of primary prevention. Women who have their first child before age 20 have approximately one-third the risk of women whose first child is born when they are over 35. Although many other factors must obviously be considered when a woman decides to have a child, women should be informed of the strong protective effect of an early first birth so that this issue can be considered when decisions to have children are made.

Genetic Factors

Early investigations of the role of genetic factors in cancer etiology focused on determining the extent to which cancers clustered in families. Such studies pointed out that the risk of many cancers, including cancers of the breast, ovary, colon, lung, brain, and prostate, was increased severalfold in individuals with a history of the disease in a first-degree relative.[78] Segregation analysis suggested that for many of these cancer sites one or more rare autosomal genes was associated with increased cancer susceptibility.

Recent work has identified inherited cancer susceptibility genes for cancers of the breast (BRCA1 and 2), colon (APC, HNPCC), and for other sites. Inherited mutations in a cancer susceptibility gene predispose the affected individual to develop cancer at an early age. Familial retinoblastoma, the prototype of such a condition, arises because an individual inherits a germline mutation in one allele of the Rb gene, which is then followed by a somatic mutation in the other allele.[79] Somatic mutations at both alleles of the gene are required to cause sporadic cases of retinoblastoma.

Inherited BRCA1 mutations affect risk of breast and ovarian cancer; the gene has received intense public attention because breast cancer is a common disease and because the penetrance of the gene is very high, i.e., a large proportion of individuals with the gene mutation will develop cancer. Commercially available screening tests to identify affected women have been developed. Nonetheless, the prevalence of mutations among women with breast cancer and in the general population is low, and BRCA1 mutations are unlikely to account for more than a small percent of all breast or ovarian cancers.

Although only a small proportion of cancers appears to be caused by inherited mutations at single loci, it is increasingly clear that genetic factors play an important role in many, or even all, tumors. Some individuals exposed to known carcinogens develop cancer and others with apparently identical exposure do not. This variability is probably due in part to inherited polymorphisms in genes that code for enzymes that affect the body's ability to metabolize or detoxify carcinogens or potential carcinogens. Polymorphisms have been identified in a number of such genes, including those that code for the glutathione *S*-transferases (GST), cytochrome P-450 enzymes (CYP), and *N*-acetyltransferases (NAT). Some of the presumed high-risk genotypes are highly prevalent and may contribute substantially to the overall cancer risk within populations. For example, 40 to 50 percent of Caucasians have the glutathione *S*-transferase M1 (GSTM1) null genotype, which appears to confer a severalfold increased risk of lung and bladder cancer and possibly other tumors.

Summary of Known Causes and Preventive Measures

Table 50-7 summarizes estimates of the proportion of new cancer cases and cancer deaths in the United States that are most likely due to various confirmed causes. The actual percentages shown are obviously rough approximations only, but they serve to indicate where preventive efforts should be directed to achieve the greatest reduction in incident cases and deaths. Efforts to reduce all forms of tobacco use should receive the highest priority. Elimination of all tobacco products would, in time, prevent twice as many cancer deaths as the elimination of all other known causes of cancer combined.

A second important point demonstrated in Table 50-7 is that almost half of the cancers in men and almost two-thirds of those in women are not explained by any of the known causes. Because the rate-limiting factors are known from migrant studies to be environmental, the unknown causes are most likely factors to which people are subjected as a result of their style of living. These may include other infectious or chemical agents and factors related to diet and reproduction.

Table 50-7 does not include factors that are protective against cancers. The proportion of cancers attributed to exposure to exogenous hormones is not shown because the protective effects of oral contraceptives and other exogenous sources of hormones on cancers of the endometrium and ovary probably outweigh the adverse effect on cancer risk. Also, although dietary factors clearly influence rates of many cancers, no quantitative estimate of the effect on cancer risks of

TABLE 50-7. PERCENTAGE OF U.S. CANCER CASES AND DEATHS MOST PROBABLY ATTRIBUTABLE TO VARIOUS ACCEPTED CAUSES OF CANCER

Cause	New Cases Male	New Cases Female	Total Cancer Deaths
Tobacco	30	20	30
Alcohol and tobacco	4	2	3
Occupation	5	2	4
Drugs	<1	<1	<1
Ionizing radiation	1	1	1
Sunlight	10	10	2
Infectious agents	3	5	5
Total percentage	<54	<41	46

specific dietary patterns or constituents are shown because many of the observed associations appear to be protective rather than causal.

Prospects seem bright for ultimately preventing many cancers. There is already much that can be done. The following is a summary of actions that can be taken:

1. Urge all users of tobacco to stop using this substance in any form, and encourage all nonusers not to start (especially the young).
2. Advise use of alcohol in moderation, if at all, especially by smokers.
3. Support efforts to reduce exposures to known carcinogens in the workplace.
4. Support efforts to identify and reduce exposures outside the workplace to known carcinogens such as arsenic, chromium, nickel, vinyl chloride, and asbestos.
5. Avoid unnecessary use of drugs that are known or suspected to be carcinogenic.
6. Use diagnostic x-rays prudently.
7. Urge individuals to avoid excess exposure to sunlight, especially if they are light skinned and easily sunburned, and to use sunscreen.
8. When estrogens are prescribed, use the lowest dose necessary to achieve the therapeutic objective and include a progestin in the regimen. Avoid giving estrogens to pregnant women.
9. Caution women that nonmonogamous sexual behavior (of both themselves and their partners) enhances their risk of cervical and other anogenital cancers. Suggest use of barrier contraceptives to reduce risk of infection.
10. Caution men that homosexual behavior is associated with anal cancer and AIDS, which can lead to Kaposi's sarcoma and other malignancies. Suggest use of condoms.
11. Avoid exposure to blood or blood products in settings outside the medical care system.
12. Suggest a diet lower in fats and meats and higher in fresh fruits, vegetables, and fiber than the average American diet. Avoid blackened, charred, or smoked foods.
13. Urge obese individuals to lose weight and others not to become overweight. Encourage regular exercise.
14. Apprise women of the protective effect against breast cancer of an early first full-term pregnancy.

▶ SCREENING AND SECONDARY PREVENTION

Secondary prevention is the prevention of progression of a disease to a fatal outcome by means of early detection followed by definitive treatment. Screening is one component of early detection, which in turn is one aspect of secondary prevention. Secondary prevention against a cancer can be achieved only if there is a stage of that cancer that is amenable to cure, and if there is a means of detecting the cancer at that stage.

Planning a Screening Program

A number of factors must be considered before initiating a screening program:[80,81]

1. *The sensitivity and specificity of the tests or procedures used for screening:* The number of diseased people that will be missed (false negatives) increases as the sensitivity of the test decreases, and the number of well people that will erroneously be considered possibly diseased (false positives) increases as the specificity of the test decreases.
2. *The target population:* Individuals at highest risk for the disease should be identified, and special efforts should be made to screen such persons.
3. *The prevalence of the disease in the target population:* For any test of given sensitivity and specificity, numbers of false-positive and false-negative tests are functions of the prevalence of the disease in the target population. More false-negative tests occur if the disease is common, and more false-positives if the disease is rare. The latter is of particular importance in screening for cancer.
4. *The predictive value of a positive test:* This is the proportion of individuals with a positive test who actually have the disease. This proportion declines only slightly as test sensitivity decreases but declines markedly as test specificity declines. In addition, the predictive value of a positive test declines as the prevalence of the disease diminishes. For example, if we have a test of high sensitivity (e.g., 95 percent) and high specificity (e.g., 98 percent), and if the prevalence of the cancer in the target population is 1 per 1,000, then only 4.6 percent of the individuals with a positive test will actually be found to have the disease on further evaluation. The rest will have a false-positive test.
5. *The consequences of false-positive tests:* A false-positive test is a false alarm. The consequences of this for the individual, the medical care system, and the screening program must be considered. How much inconvenience or psychological trauma will the individual erroneously screened have to bear? Are there sufficient facilities and personnel to provide the necessary diagnostic tests to determine who actually has the disease? What are the costs of these services and who will pay them? Is morbidity associated with further testing (such as biopsies of the breast) acceptable? Do physicians want to have referred to them large numbers of healthy people for diagnostic evaluation? Will possible adverse reactions to the screening program by those falsely screened positive or their physicians have a negative impact on the screening program itself?
6. *Consequences of a false-negative test:* A false-negative test gives the person screened a false sense of security, and the neoplasm may then progress to a noncurable stage and kill the patient. This could have medical-legal implications, particularly if a more sensitive test could have been used. One missed case can result in unfavorable publicity that can have an adverse impact on the screening program.
7. *Applicability of the test:* Can the test be administered to the people in the target population? Are special equipment or special resources needed (e.g., electrical power, water, a mobile van, transportation for the potential screenees)? Can the test be administered rapidly?
8. *Acceptability of the test:* Having made the test available to people in the target population, will the people agree to be screened? What kind of publicity should be given? Are there esthetic or cultural barriers? Is the cost to those being screened acceptably low?
9. *Adverse consequences of the test:* Is there a possibility that the test will do harm? This issue had originally been a great concern in using mammography to screen for breast cancer. The breast is a radiosensitive organ, high doses of ionizing radiation are known to cause breast cancer, and early mammographic techniques resulted in considerable levels of exposure. This controversy had an adverse impact on breast cancer screening programs, with many women fearing mammography. Similar problems should be anticipated with any future radiographic screening techniques.
10. *The evaluability of the program:* Public and private resources are all too often spent on service programs that are never evaluated, and program evaluators are all too often called upon to assist in program evaluation after a project is fully under way or even completed. The time to begin program evaluation is when the program is being planned.

Evaluation of Methods of Secondary Prevention

The aim of secondary prevention is the prevention of fatal outcome. This implies that a method of secondary prevention of a disease should reduce mortality from that disease, and reduction in mortality should be the measure used to evaluate the method. This is not always done. Two other forms of evaluation have commonly been used, both of which can give misleading results.

One of these is the comparison of cases detected at screening with cases detected by other means, with respect to their stage at diagnosis. It is not surprising that those detected at screening tend to be at a less advanced stage. This does not indicate whether the early detection altered the course of the disease, however. This method of evaluation is based on the assumptions that early lesions have the same natural history as symptomatic lesions and that treatment of early lesions alters the course of the disease. Neither assumption is necessarily correct. For example, not all carcinomas *in situ* of the uterine cervix progress to invasive disease, and individuals with early lung cancer detected at screening with chest x-rays do not have a more favorable prognosis than persons with lung cancer diagnosed later after development of symptoms.

The other misleading method of evaluating secondary prevention is by comparing survival rates, or time to death, in cases detected at screening and cases detected by other means. There are two problems with this method. One is that the time from diagnosis to death may be longer for individuals who have been screened, not because their death is postponed but only because their disease is diagnosed earlier. This is referred to as lead-time bias. The other problem is known as length-bias sampling and results from the fact that neoplasms grow at varying rates: at any point in time (when screening is performed), there will exist more tumors that are progressing slowly than rapidly. Therefore, compared to tumors in symptomatic cases, a higher proportion of tumors detected at screening will be slow growing, so that survival from time of detection will tend to be longer in screened than symptomatic patients, even if early detection does not result in a prolongation of time to death.

Because of the problems of lead-time and length-bias sampling, there is no way of knowing from a comparison of survival rates or survival times whether a secondary prevention program results in a prolonging of life. This can be done only by comparing risks of dying (or risks of advanced disease as a surrogate for mortality) in screened and unscreened individuals.

Individuals who volunteer to be screened may differ from those who do not with respect to factors related to risk of death, and these factors must be taken into consideration when comparing mortality rates in screened and unscreened persons. This can be done in two ways: It is preferable to conduct a randomized trial of the secondary prevention method to be evaluated. The other method is to control statistically for differences between the screened and unscreened during data analysis.

A classic example of a randomized trial of a procedure for secondary prevention is the study of mammography conducted among members of the Health Insurance Plan (HIP) in New York.[82] In 1963, approximately 62,000 women between the ages of 40 and 64 were randomly allocated to one of two groups. Approximately half were offered a series of four annual screenings by mammography and breast palpation (the experimental group). The other half served as a control group and received their usual medical care. Not all women in the experimental group agreed to participate. To eliminate a possible bias due to the remainder being volunteers, the mortality rate due to breast cancer in the entire experimental group was compared to the breast cancer mortality rate in the control group. Inclusion of those not screened in the experimental group gave a conservative estimate of the impact of the program on breast cancer mortality, which represented a combined evaluation of the efficacy and the acceptability of the screening procedures. After 5 years of follow-up, in women in their fifties there was over a 50 percent reduction in mortality from breast cancer; breast cancer mortality was reduced by one-third in women older than 50. Although there was no beneficial effect on breast cancer mortality in women under 50 after 5 years, follow-up for 18 years showed a small reduction in mortality from breast cancer in these women as well. This observation demonstrates the importance of long-term follow-up in studies of secondary prevention.

Once a screening technique is widely believed to be useful, regardless of whether or not it has been rigorously tested, a randomized trial becomes ethically questionable and operationally impossible. Other less satisfactory methods of evaluation must then be used. This is exemplified by the Pap smear for early detection of cervical cancer. When this technique was first introduced, it was greeted with such enthusiasm that suggestions for a randomized trial were not taken. The need to evaluate this procedure subsequently became evident, but by then it was too late for a randomized trial. As a result, a large number of less satisfactory epidemiological studies have been conducted to attempt to measure the effectiveness of the Pap smear.[83] Correlational studies have shown that mortality rates from cervical cancer in many populations have declined following the introduction of screening programs, that the magnitude of the decline is correlated with the amount of screening, and that the decline within some of the populations was greatest in those racial and age groups that received the most screening. Case-control studies of women with invasive cervical cancer have shown that, compared with normal control subjects, fewer of the cases had prior Pap smears; and a cohort study showed, after controlling for socioeconomic differences between women who enrolled in a screening program and women who did not, that there was a decline in cervical cancer mortality rates in the screened women compared to an increase in rates in those not screened. None of these methods to evaluate the Pap smear are as satisfactory as a randomized trial would have been, although in the aggregate they do provide strong evidence that the procedure reduces mortality.

Current Status of Secondary Prevention of Selected Cancers

Mammographic screening in women over age 50 years has clearly been shown in multiple randomized trials to reduce subsequent mortality from breast cancer by 30 to 40 percent,[84] and annual mammograms beginning at age 50 are generally recommended. Eight randomized trials of mammography in women 40 to 49 years of age at entry into the trial have yielded inconsistent results, with none showing a statistically significant reduction in breast cancer mortality after 5 to 18 years of follow-up. A meta-analysis of data from these trials yielded an estimated 16 percent reduction in risk of dying from breast cancer, which was of borderline statistical significance.[85] Mammography is less efficacious in women under age 50 than in older women: Breast tissue of women under age 50 is radiographically more dense than that of older women, and early neoplasms are more difficult to visualize on mammographic films. Also, relatively fewer malignancies and more benign lesions occur in younger women, resulting in more false-positive screenings. The small benefit that may be derived by screening women in their forties or younger must be weighed against the costs and the consequences of more frequent false-positive screenings. There is currently no consensus among experts regarding mammographic screening in women under age 50.

Physical examination of the breast by a medical practitioner has been shown to result in the detection of some malignancies missed by mammography and may therefore be of value as a screening modality in conjunction with mammographic screening. Tumors detected by physical examination or by women practicing breast self-examination have been shown in some studies to be less advanced at diagnosis than symptomatic cancers, but the efficacy of these procedures as primary screening modalities in reducing mortality from breast cancer has not been demonstrated. Randomized trials of both breast self-examination and physical examination of the breast are currently being conducted in areas of the world where mammographic screening is not available.

Cancer of the cervix has also been shown beyond a reasonable doubt to be amenable to secondary prevention. Results of a critical review of cytologic screening for cervical cancer were published in

1986.[86,87] By combining data from 10 screening programs in eight countries, it was shown that two negative cytologic smears were more effective than one in reducing mortality from cervical cancer (presumably because of a reduction in false-negative diagnoses) and that the protective effect did not decline until 3 years after a second negative smear. Based on these findings, it is generally believed that screening for cervical cancer every 3 years is sufficient after a woman has had two normal smears. Some women, however, do develop invasive disease soon after an apparently normal smear, and studies are needed to determine what proportion of such events are a result of prior false-negative smears and how many (if any) represent a rapidly progressing form of the disease.

Fecal occult blood testing (FOBT) and sigmoidoscopy are both used to screen for colorectal cancer. Recent randomized trials suggest that use of FOBT leads to a reduction in colon cancer mortality.[88,89] Recently published screening guidelines for colorectal cancer recommend annual FOBT or sigmoidoscopy for individuals age 50 and older, but suggested that evidence is insufficient to determine which test is more effective or whether the use of both tests together would produce additional reductions in mortality.[90] However, the level of reduction conferred by FOBT is small, and a large proportion of positive tests are false positives, resulting in many unnecessary clinical follow-up evaluations. The cost-benefit ratio of this procedure is therefore low, as is its acceptability, given the aversion that some people have to fecal testing.

Prostate specific antigen (PSA) has been widely incorporated into medical practice as a screening test for prostate cancer and has resulted in a recent apparent increase in prostate cancer incidence rates. However, use of the test has not been accompanied by a reduction in prostate cancer mortality. Although PSA testing may prevent deaths by identifying tumors at a treatable stage, there is concern that the test may also identify tumors that would have remained clinically irrelevant during the remainder of a patient's lifetime and thereby may lead men to undergo invasive and potentially unnecessary treatment. The American Cancer Society recommends annual PSA screening in conjunction with digital rectal examination in men ages 50 and over, but the recently published screening guidelines from the U.S. Preventive Health Services Task Force recommend against routine screening by PSA.[90] This disagreement will not be resolved without substantial further research.

A variety of other techniques has been developed for the early detection of cancer. Some have not been rigorously evaluated, and some that have do not show great promise. For example, three trials with sputum cytology and x-rays have demonstrated that lung cancer screening is not effective. Studies in industrial settings of urinary cytology for bladder cancer have not yielded encouraging results, and although NCI guidelines recommend oral examination by medical practitioners to screen for oral cancer, the effectiveness of the technique is questionable because of the poor compliance of those individuals at highest risk of the disease.[91]

Barium swallow and x-ray have been used in Japan to detect early stomach cancer. Survival has been found to be better in those detected at screening than in other cases, and mortality rates from stomach cancer decreased in those screened but not in the general population. The disease is sufficiently rare in the United States that large-scale screening is not recommended.

α-Fetoprotein (AFP) blood levels have been used to screen for primary hepatocellular carcinoma in individuals serologically positive for hepatitis B surface antigen (HB_sAg) in areas where hepatitis B is endemic and liver cancer highly prevalent. A study from China showed improved survival in asymptomatic persons with small tumors detected by this method, but studies to determine whether it reduces mortality from liver cancer have not been completed.

Despite considerable interest in the development of ovarian cancer screening using transvaginal ultrasonography or the circulating tumor marker CA-125, neither method is clearly associated with reduced mortality from this disease.[92]

Improved cancer screening must be a part of any long-term strategy to reduce cancer mortality. These efforts must include both the evaluation of new screening methods and research into the most effective ways to implement the techniques that are of demonstrated benefit.

▶ REFERENCES

1. ICD-9-CM: The International Classification of Diseases, 9th revision, Clinical Modification. Salt Lake City: Med-Index, 1991
2. World Health Organization: International Classification of Diseases for Oncology. 2nd ed. Geneva: World Health Organization, 1990
3. Coleman MP, Esteve J, Damiecki P, Arslan A, Renard H: Trends in cancer incidence and mortality. IARC Scientific Publ. No. 121. Lyon: International Agency for Research on Cancer, 1993
4. Kosary CL, Ries LAG, Miller BA, Hankey BF, Harras A, Edwards BK (eds): SEER Cancer Statistics Review, 1973–1992: Tables and Graphs. NIH Publication No. 96-2789. Bethesda, MD: National Cancer Institute, 1995
5. National Cancer Institute: Cancer Statistics Review 1973–1986. NIH Publication No. 89-2789. Bethesda, MD: National Cancer Institute, 1989
6. National Cancer Institute: Cancer Mortality in the United States: 1950–1977. National Cancer Institute Monograph 59, NIH Publication No. 82-2435. Bethesda, MD: National Cancer Institute, 1982
7. Parkin DM, Muir CS, Whelan SL, Gao YT, Ferlay J, Powell J (eds): Cancer in Five Continents. IARC Scientific Publication No. 120. Lyon: International Agency for Research on Cancer, 1992, vol 6
8. American Cancer Society: Cancer Facts and Figures—1996. New York: American Cancer Society, 1996
9. Howe HL, Lehnherr M, Derrick L, eds. Cancer Incidence in North America, 1988–1992. Sacramento, CA: North American Association of Central Cancer Registries, April 1996
10. National Center for Health Statistics: Annual summary of births, marriages, divorces, and deaths: United States, 1993. Mon Vital Stat Rep 42(13), 1994
11. Bailes JS: The economics of cancer care. Cancer 76:1886–1887, 1995
12. Parkin DM, Pisani P, Ferlay J: Estimates of the worldwide incidence of eighteen major cancers in 1985. Int J Cancer 54:594–606, 1993
13. Thomas DB, Karagas MR: Migrant studies. In Schottenfeld D, Fraumeni JF Jr (eds): Cancer Epidemiology and Prevention. Philadelphia: W.B. Saunders, 1996
14. National Cancer Institute: Racial/Ethnic Patterns of Cancer in the United States 1988–1992. NIH Publication No. 96-4104. Bethesda, MD: National Cancer Institute, 1996
15. Greenwald P, Sondik EJ: Cancer Control Objectives for the Nation: 1985–2000. NIH Publication No. 86-2880. Washington, DC: Government Printing Office, 1986
16. Nowell PC: The clonal evolution of tumor cell populations. Science 194:23–28, 1976
17. Schottenfeld D, Fraumeni JF Jr (eds): Cancer Epidemiology and Prevention. Philadelphia: WB Saunders, 1996
18. Office on Smoking and Health, US Department of Health and Human Services: The Health Consequences of Smoking: Cancer. A Report of the Surgeon General. Washington, DC: Government Printing Office, 1982
19. Shopland DR, Eyre HJ, Pechacek TF: Smoking-attributable cancer mortality in 1991: is lung cancer now the leading cause of death among smokers in the United States? J Natl Cancer Inst 82:1142–1148, 1991
20. Heineman EF, Zahm SH, McLaughlin JK, Vaught JB: Increased risk of colorectal cancer among smokers: results of a 26-year follow-up of U.S. veterans and a review. Int J Cancer 59:728–738, 1995
21. National Cancer Institute: The Health Consequences of using Smokeless Tobacco. A Report of the Advisory Committee to the Surgeon General. NIH Publication No. 86-2874. Bethesda, MD: National Cancer Institute, 1986

22. U.S. Department of Health and Human Services: The health consequences of involuntary smoking. A Report of the Surgeon General, 1986. DHHS Publ. No. (PHS) 87-8398. Washington, DC: Government Printing Office, 1987
23. National Research Council: Environmental Tobacco Smoke: Measuring Exposure and Assessing Health Effects. Washington, DC: National Academy Press, 1986
24. U.S. Environmental Protection Agency: Respiratory health effects of passive smoking: Lung cancer and other disorders. The Report of the Smoking and Tobacco Control Monograph No. 4. NIH Publication No. 93-3605. Bethesda, MD: U.S. Environmental Protection Agency, 1993
25. Thomas DB: Alcohol as a cause of cancer. Environ Health Perspect 103(Suppl 8):153–160, 1995
26. Overall evaluations of carcinogenicity: an updating of IARC Monographs Volumes 1 to 42. IARC Monogr Eval Carcinog Risks Hum Suppl 7, 1987
27. Manmade minerals, fibers and radon. IARC Monogr Eval Carcinog Risks Hum 43, 1988
28. Alcohol drinking. IARC Monogr Eval Carcinog Risks Hum 44, 1988
29. Occupational exposures in petroleum. IARC Monogr Eval Carcinog Risks Hum 45, 1989
30. Diesel and gasoline engine exhaust and some nitroarenes. IARC Monogr Eval Carcinog Risks Hum 46, 1989
31. Some organic solvents, resin monomers, related compounds, pigments, and occupational exposures in paint manufacture and painting. IARC Monogr Eval Carcinog Risks Hum 47, 1989
32. Some flame retardants and textile chemicals, and exposures in the textile manufacturing industry. IARC Monogr Eval Carcinog Risks Hum 48, 1990
33. Chromium, nickel, and welding. IARC Monogr Eval Carcinog Risks Hum 49, 1990
34. Pharmaceutical drugs. IARC Monogr Eval Carcinog Risks Hum 50, 1990
35. Coffee, tea, mate, methylxanthines and methyl glyoxal. IARC Monogr Eval Carcinog Risks Hum 51, 1991
36. Chlorinated drinking water; chlorination by-products; some other hydrogenated compounds, cobalt and cobalt compounds. IARC Monogr Eval Carcinog Risks Hum 52, 1991
37. Occupational exposures in insecticide application, and some pesticides. IARC Monogr Eval Carcinog Risks Hum 53, 1991
38. Occupational exposures to mists and vapours from strong inorganic acids and other industrial chemicals. IARC Monogr Eval Carcinog Risks Hum 54, 1992
39. Solar and UV radiation. IARC Monogr Eval Carcinog Risks Hum 55, 1992
40. Some naturally occurring substances. IARC Monogr Eval Carcinog Risks Hum 56, 1993
41. Occupational exposures of hairdressers and barbers and personal use of hair colorants; some hair dyes, cosmetic colourants, industrial dyestuffs and aromatic amines. IARC Monogr Eval Carcinog Risks Hum 57, 1993
42. Beryllium, cadmium, mercury and exposures in the glass manufacturing industry. IARC Monogr Eval Carcinog Risks Hum 58, 1993
43. Hepatitis viruses. IARC Monogr Eval Carcinog Risks Hum 59, 1994
44. Some industrial chemicals. IARC Monogr Eval Carcinog Risks Hum 60, 1994
45. Schistosomes, liver flukes and *Helicobacter pylori*. IARC Monogr Eval Carcinog Risks Hum 61, 1994
46. Wood dust and formaldehyde. IARC Monogr Eval Carcinog Risks Hum 62, 1995
47. Dry cleaning, some chlorinated solvents, and other chemicals. IARC Monogr Eval Carcinog Risks Hum 63, 1995
48. Human papillomaviruses. IARC Monogr Eval Carcinog Risks Hum 64, 1995
49. Printing processes and printing inks, carbon black and some nitro compounds. IARC Monogr Eval Carcinog Risks Hum 65, 1996
50. Higginson J: Proportion of cancers due to occupation. Prev Med 9:180–188, 1980
51. Shy CM: Air pollution. In Schottenfeld D, Fraumeni JF Jr (eds): Cancer Epidemiology and Prevention. Philadelphia: WB Saunders, 1996, pp 406–417
52. Pahor M, Guralnik JM, Ferrucci L, Corti M-C, Salive ME, Cerhan JR, Wallace RB, Havlik RJ: Calcium-channel blockade and incidence of cancer in aged populations. Lancet 348:493–497, 1996
53. Baron JA, Adami H-O: A broad anticancer effect of aspirin? Epidemiology 5:133–135, 1994
54. Boice JD, Land CE, Preston DL: Ionizing radiation. In Schottenfeld D, Fraumeni JF Jr (eds): Cancer Epidemiology and Prevention. Philadelphia: WB Saunders, 1996, pp 319–354
55. Lubin JH, Boice JD: Lung cancer risk from residential radon: meta-analysis of eight epidemiologic studies. J Natl Cancer Inst 89(1):49–57, 1997
56. Gallagher RP, Elwood JM: Recent progress in the epidemiology of malignant melanoma. In Gallagher RP, Elwood JM (eds): Epidemiological Aspects of Cutaneous Malignant Melanoma. Boston: Kluwer Academic Publishers, 1994, pp 3–12
57. Roush GC, McKay L, Holford TR: A reversal in the long-term increase in deaths attributable to malignant melanoma. Cancer 69: 1714–1720, 1992
58. Heath CW: Electromagnetic field exposure and cancer: a review of the epidemiologic evidence. CA Cancer J Clin 65:29–44, 1996
59. Washburn EP, Orza MJ, Berlin JA, Nicholson WJ, Todd AC, Frumkin H, Chalmers TC: Residential proximity to electric transmission and distribution equipment and risk of childhood leukemia, childhood lymphoma, and childhood nervous system tumors: systematic review, evaluation, and meta-analysis. Cancer Causes Control 5:299–309, 1994
60. Herbst AL, Ulfelder H, Poskanzer DC: Adenocarcinoma of the vagina: association of maternal stilbestrol therapy with tumor appearance in young women. N Engl J Med 284:878–881, 1971
61. Weiss NS: Epidemiology of endometrial cancer. In Lilienfeld AM (ed): Reviews in Cancer Epidemiology. New York: Elsevier, 1983, vol 2
62. Grady D, Ernster VL: Endometrial Cancer. In Schottenfeld D, Fraumeni JF Jr (eds): Cancer Epidemiology and Prevention. Philadelphia: WB Saunders, 1996, pp 1058–1089
63. Curtis RE, Boice JD Jr, Shriner DA, Hankey BF, Fraumeni JF: Second Cancers After Adjuvant Tamoxifen Therapy for Breast Cancer. J Natl Cancer Inst 88:832–834, 1996
64. Prentice RL, Thomas DB: On the epidemiology of oral contraceptives and disease. Adv Cancer Res 49:285–401, 1987
65. The WHO Collaborative Study of Neoplasia and Steroid Contraceptives: Depot-medroxyprogesterone acetate (DMPA) and the risk of endometrial cancer. Int J Cancer 49:186–1901, 1991
66. Colton T, Greenberg ER, Noller K, Resseguie L, Van Bennekom C, Heeren T, Zhang Y: Breast cancer in mothers prescribed diethylstilbestrol in pregnancy: further follow-up. JAMA 296(16):2096–2100, 1993
67. Ewertz M: Hormone therapy in the menopause and breast cancer risk—a review. Maturitas 23:241–246, 1996
67a. Beral V, et al.: Breast cancer and hormone replacement therapy-collaborative reanalysis of data from 51 epidemiological studies of 52,705 women with breast cancer and 108,411 women without breast cancer. Lancet 350:1047–1059, 1997
68. Collaborative Group on Hormonal Factors in Breast Cancer: Breast cancer and hormonal contraceptives: collaborative reanalysis of individual data on 53,297 women with breast cancer and 100,239 women without breast cancer from 54 epidemiological studies. Lancet 347:1713–1727, 1996
69. Skegg DCG, Noonan EA, Paul C, Spears GFS, Meirik O, Thomas DB: Depot medroxyprogesterone acetate and breast cancer: a pooled analysis of the World Health Organization and New Zealand studies. JAMA 273:799–804, 1995

70. Weiss NS, Cook LS, Farrow DC, Rosenblatt KA: Ovarian cancer. In Schottenfeld D, Fraumeni JF Jr (eds): Cancer Epidemiology and Prevention. Philadelphia: WB Saunders, 1996, pp 1040–1057
71. Thomas DB: Exogenous steroid hormones and hepatocellular carcinoma. In Tablr E, Di Biceglie AM, Purcell RH (eds): Etiology, Pathology, and Treatment of Hepatocellular Carcinoma in North America. Advances in Applied Biotechnology Series, vol 13. Houston: Gulf Publishing Company, 1990, pp 77–89
72. Mueller NE, Evans AS, London WT: Viruses. In Schottenfeld D, Fraumeni JF Jr (eds): Cancer Epidemiology and Prevention. Philadelphia: WB Saunders, 1996, pp 502–531
73. Schulz TF, Boshoff CH, Weiss RA: HIV infection and neoplasia. Lancet 348:587–591, 1996
74. Thomas DB, Ray RM, Pardthaisong T, Chutivongse, S, Koetsawang S, Silpisornkosol S, Virutamasen P, Christopherson WM, Melnick JL, Meirik O, Farley TMM, Riotton G: Prostitution, condom use, and invasive squamous cell cervical cancer in Thailand. Am J Epidemiol 143:779–786, 1996
75. Muñoz N: Is *Helicobacter pylori* a cause of gastric cancer? An appraisal of seroepidemiological evidence. Cancer Epidemiol Biomarkers Prev 3:445–453, 1994
76. Hunter DJ, Spiegelman D, Adami H-O, et al: Cohort studies of fat intake and the risk of breast cancer—a pooled analysis. N Engl J Med 334:356–361, 1996
77. Omenn GS, Goodman GE, Thornquist MD, Balmes J, Cullen MR, Glass A, Keogh JP, Meyskens FL, Valanis B, Williams JH, Barnhart S, Hammar S: Effects of a combination of beta carotene and vitamin A on lung cancer and cardiovascular disease. N Engl J Med 334:1150–1155, 1996
78. Muller H, Weber W (eds): Familial Cancer. Basel: Karger, 1985
79. Knudson AG: Mutation and cancer: statistical study of retinoblastoma. Proc Natl Acad Sci 68:820–823, 1971
80. Lilienfeld AM: Some limitations and problems of screening for cancer. Cancer 33(Suppl):1720–1724, 1974
81. Cole P, Morrison AS: Basic issues in population screening for cancer. J Natl Cancer Inst 64:1263–1272, 1980
82. Shapiro S: Statistical evidence for mass screening for breast cancer and some remaining issues. Cancer Detect Prev 1:347–363, 1976
83. Shingleton HM, Patrick RL, Johnston WW, Smith RA: The current status of the Papanicolaou smear. CA Cancer J Clin 45:305–320, 1995
84. Hurley SF, Kaldor JM: The benefits and risks of mammographic screening for breast cancer. Epidemiol Rev 14:101–130, 1992
85. Smart CR, Hendrick RE, Rutledge JH, Smith RA: Benefit of mammography screening in women ages 40 to 49 years. Cancer 75:1619–1626, 1995
86. Hakama M, Miller AB, Day NE: Screening for Cancer of the Uterine Cervix. IARC Scientific Publication No. 76. Lyon: International Agency for Research on Cancer, 1986
87. IARC Working Group on Evaluation of Cervical Cancer Screening Programmes: Screening for squamous cervical cancer: duration of low risk after negative results of cervical cytology and its implication for screening policies. Br Med J 293:659–664, 1986
88. Kronborg O, Fenger C, Olsen J, Jorgensen OD, Sondergaard O: Randomised study of screening for colorectal cancer with faecal-occult-blood test. Lancet 348:1467–1471, 1996
89. Hardcastle JD, Chamberlain JO, Robinson MHE, Moss SM, Amar SS, Balfour TW, James PD, Mangham CM: Randomised controlled trial of faecal-occult-blood screening for colorectal cancer. Lancet 348:1472–1477, 1996
90. US Preventive Services Task Force: Guide to Clinical Preventive Services: Report of the U.S. Preventive Services Task Force. 2nd ed. Baltimore: Williams & Wilkins, 1996
91. Prorock PC, Chamberlain J, Day NE, et al: UICC workshop on the evaluation of screening programmes for cancer. Int J Cancer 34:1–4, 1984
92. NIH Consensus Development Panel on Ovarian Cancer: NIH consensus conference: ovarian cancer. Screening, treatment, and follow-up. JAMA 273:491–497, 1995

51

Heart Disease

Russell V. Luepker

Cardiovascular diseases (CVDs) are public health concerns around the world, particularly coronary or ischemic heart disease (CHD), hypertensive heart disease, and rheumatic heart disease. CHD remains the leading cause of adult death in industrial societies, although its incidence differs widely and the mortality ascribed to it is changing dramatically (Figs. 51-1 and 51-2). While deaths from CHD are rising in many populations, they are falling in others. The decline of age-adjusted U.S. deaths ascribed to CHD continues for men and women, white and nonwhite (Fig. 51-3). The exact causes of the decline are not established, but much is now known about U.S. trends in out-of-hospital deaths, in-hospital case fatality, and longer-term survival after acute myocardial infarction.[1] Parallel to the CHD mortality trends are improvements in medical diagnosis and treatment, in population levels of risk factors, and in lifestyle.[2] Nevertheless, the critical explanatory data, including incidence trends from representative populations, are few. This deficiency, along with the difficulty of measuring change in diagnostic custom and in severity of CHD, or of its precursor, atherosclerosis, leaves considerable uncertainty about the causes of the mortality trends. Systematic surveillance is now in place in many countries to improve the future detection, prediction, and explanation of trends in CVD rates.[1–4]

Deaths ascribed to hypertensive heart disease have diminished over recent decades in many industrialized countries.[5] In West Africa, Latin America, and the Orient, however, the high prevalence still found in hospitals and clinics indicates the continued worldwide importance of hypertension.

Rheumatic fever and rheumatic valvular heart disease remain public health concerns in many developing countries and are still seen among disadvantaged peoples in affluent nations. On the other hand, syphilitic heart disease, a worldwide scourge until the 1940s, is now rare. Cardiomyopathies, often of unknown or infectious origin, constitute a common cause of heart disease in many regions, particularly Africa and Latin America. Finally, congenital heart disease continues to contribute to the heart disease burden among youth and adults of all countries.

The worldwide potential for primary prevention of most CVD is established by several salient facts: (*a*) the large population differences in CVD incidence and death rates; CVD is rare in many countries and common in others; (*b*) dynamic national trends in CVD deaths, both upward and downward; (*c*) rapid changes in CVD risk among migrant populations; (*d*) the identification of modifiable risk characteristics for CVD among and within populations; and (*e*) the generally positive results of preventive trials. There is much evidence that the risk of whole populations, as opposed to individual risk, is predominantly determined by mass sociocultural characteristics, which are in turn subject to change and to public policy.

▸ CORONARY HEART DISEASE

CHD remains the leading cause of adult deaths in many industrial societies. Much about its causes and prevention has been learned from diverse research methods, including clinicopathological observations, laboratory-experimental studies, population studies, and clinical trials. The evidence of causation from all these disciplines is largely congruent. As a result, several ubiquitous cultural characteristics described below are now established as powerful influences on population risk of CHD. These influences and risk factors appear to be safely modifiable for individuals and for entire populations.[6–9]

The sum of evidence suggests that there is widespread human susceptibility to atherosclerosis and, consequently, that CHD is maximally exhibited when the environment is unfavorable. These ubiquitous susceptibilities, exposures, and behaviors lead eventually to the mass precursors of CHD found among so many people in high-incidence societies. The rationale and the potential for preventive practice, as well as for public policy in prevention, are based on several well-established relationships: between risk factor levels and CHD, between health behaviors and risk factor levels, and between culture and mass health behaviors.

Epidemiology

We summarize here what we consider to be the salient observations about CHD:

- Population comparisons show large differences in CHD incidence and mortality rates (Fig. 51-1) and in the extent of its underlying vascular disease, atherosclerosis.
- Population differences in the mean levels and distributions of CHD risk characteristics (particular blood lipoprotein levels) are strongly correlated ecologically with population differences in CHD rates.
- Within populations, several risk characteristics (blood cholesterol and blood pressure levels and smoking habits) are strongly and continuously related to future individual risk of a CHD event.
- Population differences in average levels of CHD risk characteristics are already apparent in youth. Individual values of children tend to "track" into adult years.
- CHD risk characteristics and incidence in migrants rapidly approach levels of the adopted culture.
- Trends in CHD mortality rates, both upward and downward, occur over relatively short periods of 5 to 10 years. These trends tend to be associated with changes in medical care and case-fatality rates as well as with trends in incidence and in population distributions of risk characteristics.

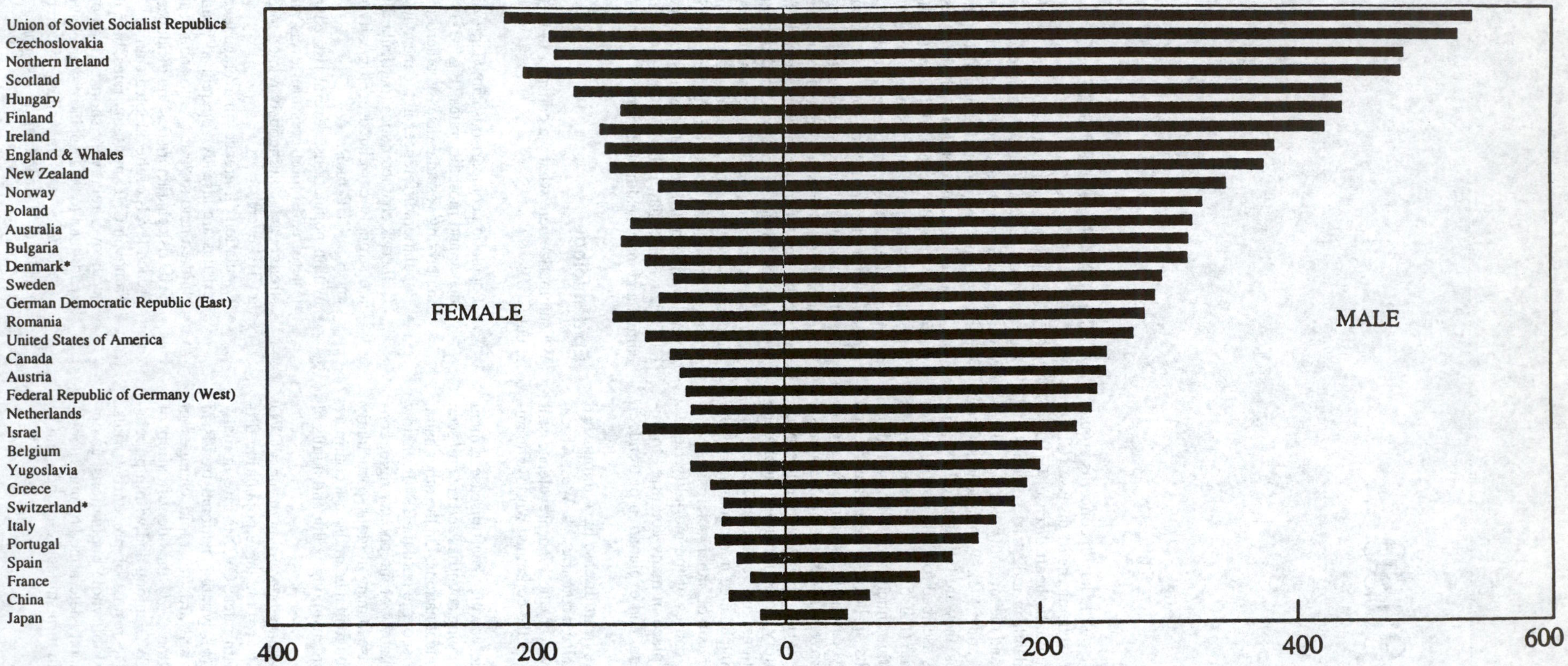

Figure 51-1. Death rates for CHD, age 35 to 74, by country and sex, 1990. (*Source:* National Heart, Lung, and Blood Institute. Morbidity and Mortality Chartbook on Cardiovascular, Lung, and Blood Diseases. Bethesda, Maryland, 1994; NIH Publication.)

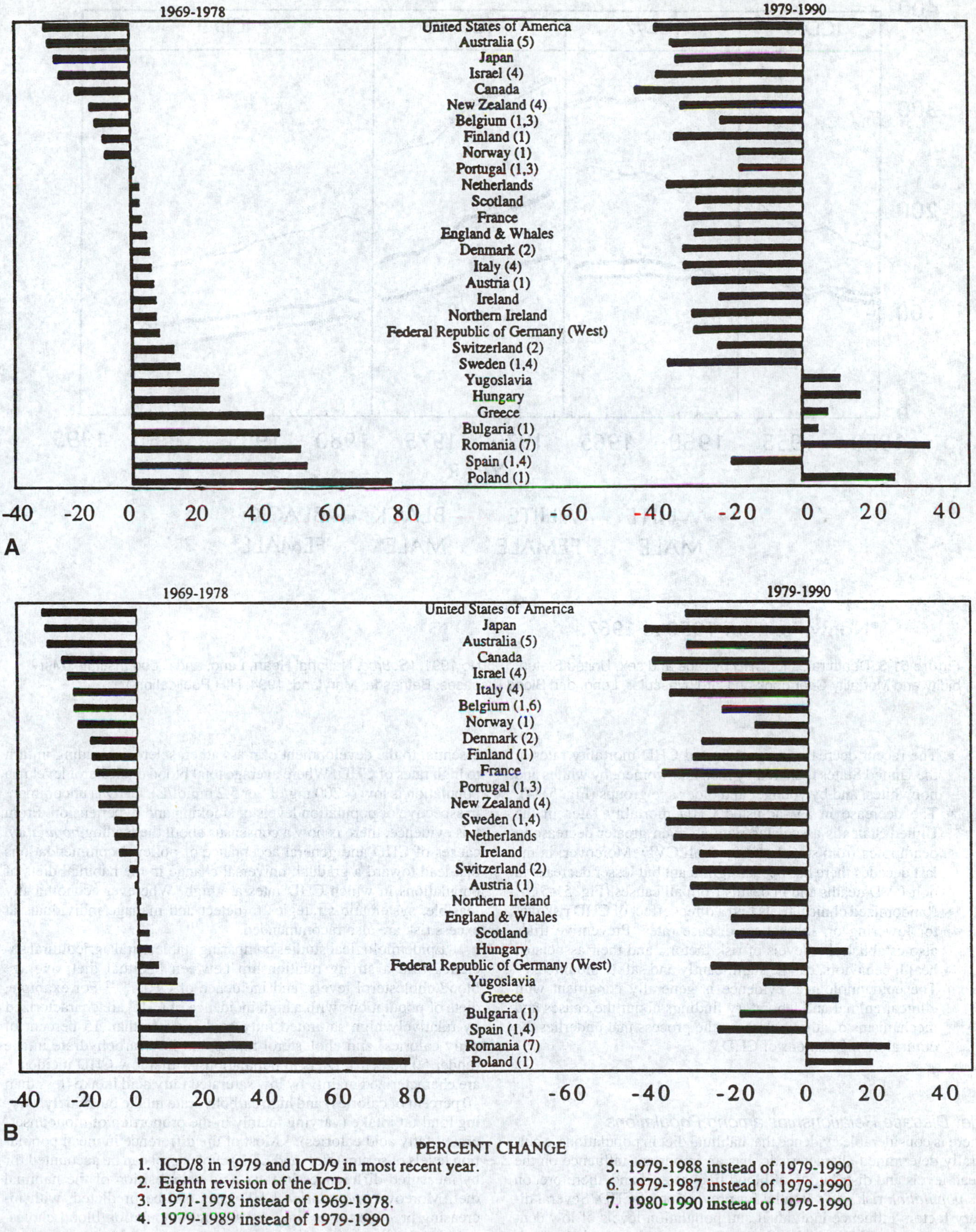

Figure 51-2. A. Percent change in death rates for CHD in men age 35 to 74 by country, 1979 to 1990. **B**. Percent change in death rates for CHD in women age 35 to 74 by country, 1979 to 1990. (*Source:* National Heart, Lung, and Blood Institute. Morbidity and Mortality Chartbook on Cardiovascular, Lung, and Blood Diseases. Bethesda, Maryland, 1994; NIH Publication.)

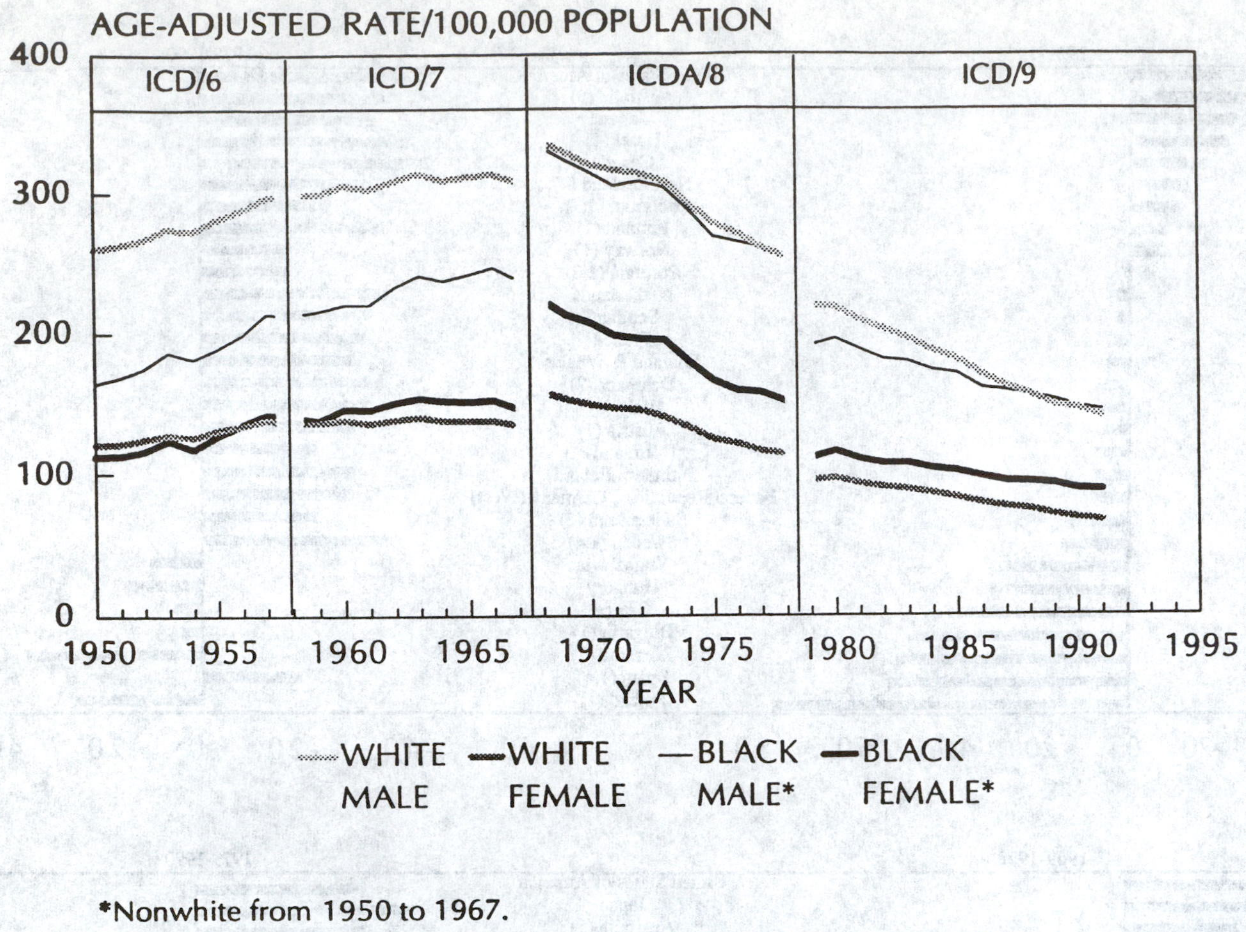

Figure 51-3. Death rates for CHD by race and sex, United States, 1950 to 1991. (*Source*: National Heart, Lung, and Blood Institute. Morbidity and Mortality Chartbook on Cardiovascular, Lung, and Blood Diseases. Bethesda, Maryland, 1994; NIH Publication.)

- The recent decrease in age-adjusted CHD mortality rates in the United States is shared by men and women, by whites and nonwhites, and by younger and older age groups (Fig. 51-4).
- The decrease in age-adjusted CHD mortality rates in the United States is associated with an even greater decrease in death rates from stroke and from all CVD. Moreover, in the last decades there has been a significant but lesser decrease in non-CVD deaths and in deaths from all causes (Fig. 51-5).
- Randomized clinical trials find a direct effect of CHD risk factor lowering on subsequent disease rates. Preventive trials also establish that levels of risk factors, and their associated health behaviors, can be significantly and safely modified.
- The epidemiological evidence is generally congruent with clinical animal and laboratory findings about the causes and mechanisms of atherosclerosis, the process that underlies the clinical manifestations of CHD.

Diet

Diet-Disease Relationships among Populations

There is considerable evidence that habitual diet in populations, a culturally determined characteristic, has an important influence on the mean levels and distribution of blood lipoproteins and, therefore, on the *population* risk and potential for prevention of CHD. Several dietary factors influence individual and population levels of low density lipoproteins (LDL) in the blood, a leading pathogenetic factor in atherosclerosis. These include particular fatty acids and dietary cholesterol, the complex carbohydrates of starches, vegetables, fruits and their fibers, alcohol, and caloric excess. Many investigators consider that the cholesterol-raising properties of some habitual diets are essential to the development of mass atherosclerosis, leading in turn to high rates of CHD. Where average total blood cholesterol level in a population is low (<200 mg/dL, or 5.2 mmol/L), CHD is uncommon, irrespective of population levels of smoking and hypertension. From this evidence, there is now a consensus about the leading *population* causes of CHD and general acceptance of policy recommendations that lead toward a gradual, universal change in the habitual diets of populations in which CHD rates are high. Wherever economically feasible, systematic strategies to detect and manage individuals at excess risk are also recommended.

Epidemiological studies comparing stable, rural agricultural societies find a strong relationship between habitual diet, average blood cholesterol levels, and incidence of CHD.[10–12] For example, diets of populations with a high incidence of CHD are characterized by relatively high saturated fatty acid (greater than 15 percent of daily calories) and cholesterol intake and low carbohydrate intake (under 50 percent). Diets in populations with a low CHD incidence are characterized mainly by low saturated fatty acid intake (less than 10 percent of calories) and high carbohydrate intake but widely varying total fat intake (varying mainly in the proportion of monounsaturated fatty acid calories).[11] Most of the difference in mean population levels of serum total (and LDL) cholesterol can be accounted for by measured differences in fatty acid composition of the habitual diet. Moreover, *population* CHD rates can be predicted, with increasing precision over time, by average population blood cholesterol levels.[13]

Cross-cultural comparisons of diet versus postmortem findings of atherosclerosis reveal a strong correlation between habitual dietary fat intake of a population and the frequency and extent of advanced atherosclerotic lesions.[14]

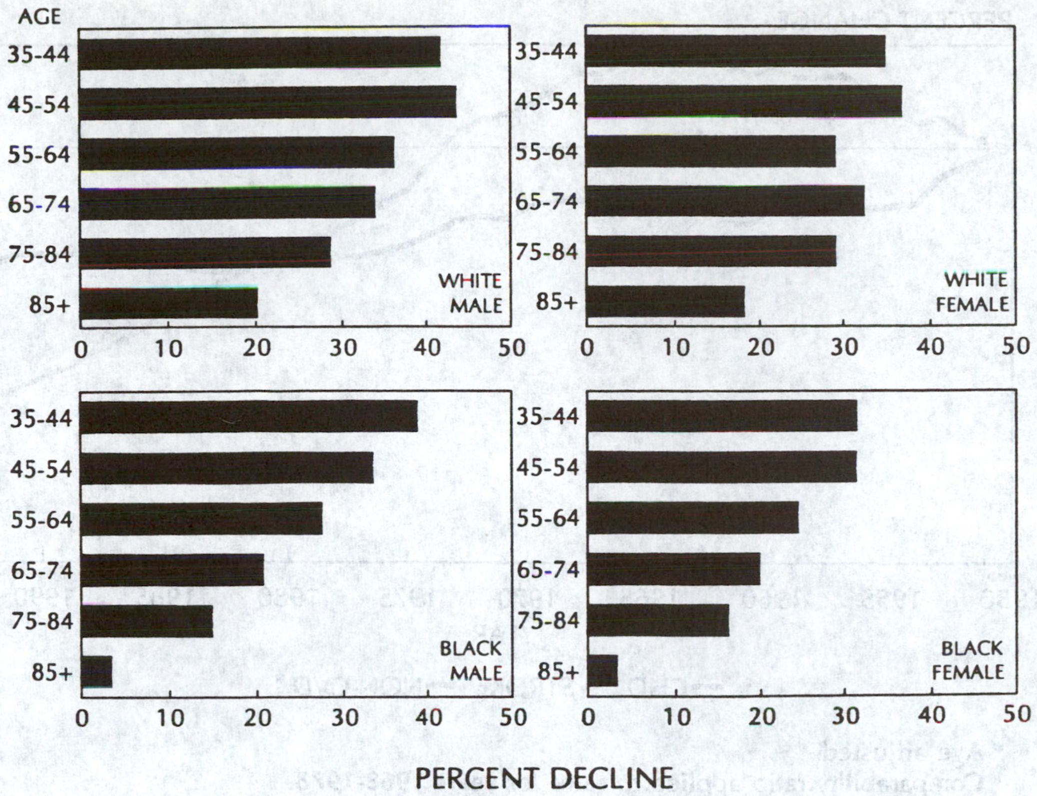

Figure 51-4. Percent decline in death rates for CHD by age, race, and sex, United States, 1981 to 1991. (*Source:* National Heart, Lung, and Blood Institute. Morbidity and Mortality Chartbook on Cardiovascular, Lung, and Blood Diseases. Bethesda, Maryland, 1994; NIH Publication.)

Studies of migrant populations indicate the predominance of sociocultural influences, including diet, in trends of risk and CHD among migrants. For example, Japanese who migrate to California become taller, heavier, more obese, and more sedentary; their diet changes dramatically; they eat more meat and dairy products, saturated fatty acids and cholesterol, and consume less complex carbohydrate and less alcohol than their counterparts in the Nagasaki-Hiroshima area.[15] They develop higher risk profiles and disease rates within a generation. With few exceptions, migrant Hawaiian Japanese have risk factor values intermediate between mainland and California Japanese, and the CHD rate in migrants generally parallels their mean values for risk factor levels.

The rapid evolving national trends in CHD deaths are another indication of the predominance of culture in the population causes and prevention of CHD, as disease occurrence changes more rapidly than any genetic characteristics. Nevertheless, systematic explanatory studies of trends in CHD mortality are very recent, and current attempts to estimate the relative contribution of cultural versus medical care contributions are quite tentative.[1–3,16,17] In a number of countries on an upward slope of CHD mortality, smoking and calorie and fat consumption are increasing and physical activity is decreasing, while cardiological practice is probably becoming less effective.[18] In many other industrial countries, including the United States, decreasing CHD mortality rates parallel improved cardiac care and significant reductions in average risk characteristics.[1,2,16,19] Standardized measurements of risk and disease trends are not generally available for comparisons among countries, but the public health implications of these simultaneous trends in behaviors, risk, disease rates, and medical care are immense.

Another feature of diet, the relative excess of calorie intake over expenditure, influences health through the metabolic maladaptations of hyperlipidemia, hyperinsulinism, and hypertension.[20] This caloric imbalance occurs in sedentary cultures and results in mass obesity. With or without mass obesity, however, high salt intake and low potassium intake in populations appear to encourage the wide exhibition of hypertensive phenotypes. Other cations (e.g., magnesium, calcium) may also be significant dietary influences on population levels of blood pressure, while alcohol intake is clearly involved (see below).

Anthropological Aspects of Diet

Anthropology and paleontology provide insights into the probable effects of rapid cultural change, including modern diets, from the lifestyle to which humans adapted during earlier periods of evolution. Until 500 or so generations ago, all humans were hunter-gatherers. The habitual eating pattern likely involved alternating scarce and abundant calories and a great variety of foods. It surely included lean wild game and usually a predominance of plant over animal calories, a relatively low sodium and high potassium intake, and of course there was universal breast-feeding of infants. Observations of the eating patterns among extant hunter-gatherer tribes confirm the varied nature and the adequacy (or near adequacy) of such an eating pattern for growth and development, as well as for the potential of longevity and the absence of mass phenomena such as atherosclerosis and hypertension.[21–23] Although modern humans can scarcely return to such subsistence economies, the anthropological observations suggest that current metabolic maladaptations derived from affluent eating and exercise patterns imposed rapidly on a very different evolutionary legacy result in the mass precursors of cardiovascular diseases found in modern society.[22]

Diet-Disease Relationships within Populations

Despite the generally strong population (ecological) correlations between diet, blood lipid levels, and CHD rates, these correlations are often absent for individuals within high-risk industrial societies.[24] This apparent paradox does not negate the causal importance of diet in mass hypercholesterolemia and atherosclerosis. Consider, for example, the

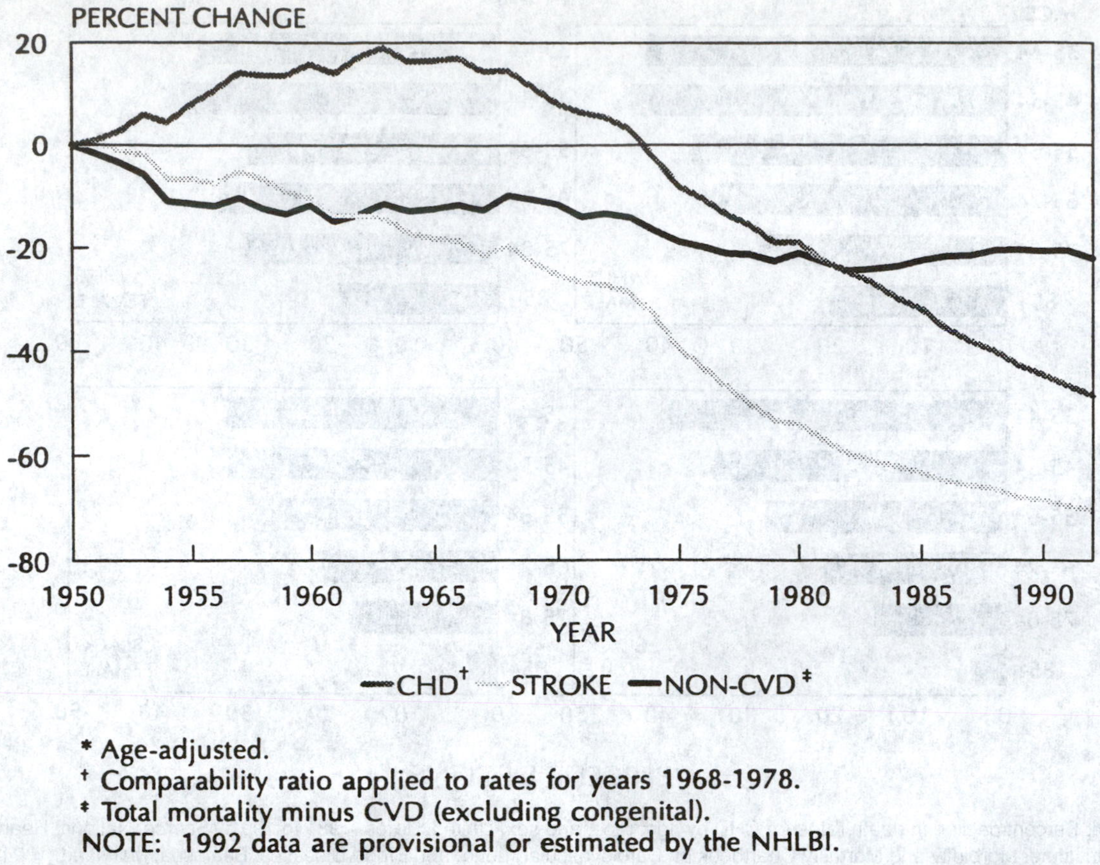

Figure 51-5. Percent change in death rates (age-adjusted) since 1950, United States, 1950 to 1992. (*Source:* National Heart, Lung, and Blood Institute. Morbidity and Mortality Chartbook on Cardiovascular, Lung, and Blood Diseases. Bethesda, Maryland, 1994; NIH Publication.)

simple additive model of Table 51-1, which suggests the powerful influence, in the individual, of inherent lipid regulation. Different individual lipoprotein genotypes may develop widely different adult risk phenotypes and different serum cholesterol levels, while consuming the same U.S.-type diet. Other individuals may have similar blood cholesterol levels while subsisting on very different diets. In contrast, the population model of Table 51-2 makes the assumption that the multiple genes that influence lipid metabolism are randomly and similarly distributed throughout large heterogeneous populations. Under this condition, population means and distributions of blood lipids are seen to be influenced predominantly by the cholesterol-raising or lowering properties of the habitual diet of the population.[25,26] The range and degree of this dietary influence are estimated from short-term controlled diet experiments.[27–29]

TABLE 51-1. A MODEL OF INDIVIDUAL DIET–SERUM CHOLESTEROL (TC) RELATIONS WITH INDIVIDUAL EXAMPLES

Genotypic TC Value (mg/dL)	Mean Diet–TC Effect (mg/dL)				
	0	*+25*	*+50*	*+75*	*+100*
75	75	100	125	150	175
150	150	175	200	225	250
300	300	325	350	375	400

Derived from Blackburn H: The concept of risk. In Pearson TA, Criqui MH, Luepker RV, Oberman A, Winston M (eds): Primer in Preventive Cardiology. Dallas: American Heart Association, 1994, pp 25–41; and Keys A, Grande F, Anderson JT: Bias and misrepresentation revisited—"perspective" on saturated fat. Am J Clin Nutr 27:188–212, 1974.

It is assumed that an intrinsic lipid regulatory base exists for each individual and is expressed in the first year of life. On this genotype is superimposed the effect of habitual diet, which is either neutral or cholesterol-raising according to properties determined in controlled Minnesota diet experiments, resulting, in this simple additive model, in the adult phenotypes values.

TABLE 51-2. A MODEL OF POPULATION DIET–SERUM CHOLESTEROL (TC) RELATION WITH POPULATION EXAMPLES

	Mean Diet–TC Effect (mg/dL)				
	Japan 0	*Greece +25*	*Italy +50*	*United States +75*	*Finland +100*
Population mean TC	75	100	125	150	175
Lower limit (2.5%)	150	175	200	225	250
Upper limit (97.5%)	300	325	350	375	400

Derived from Keys A, Grande F, Anderson JT: Bias and misrepresentation revisited—"perspective" on saturated fat. Am J Clin Nutr 27:188–212, 1974; and Keys A (ed): Coronary heart disease in seven countries. Circulation 41–42 (Suppl I), 1970.

In this oversimplified model, it is assumed that uncommon single gene effects and widespread polygenic determinants of blood cholesterol levels are randomly and usually distributed among large hetergeneous populations, such that a mean population TC value of 150 mg/dL would prevail (SD ± 37.5 mg/dL) in the presence of a habitual average diet having neutral properties in respect to cholesterol. On this mean and population distribution of intrinsic responsiveness is superimposed the average habitual diet effect for a population, which is either neutral or cholesterol-raising according to the country's measured diet composition and properties.

Recently, several well-conducted cohort studies have provided evidence of diet-CHD relationships within societies in which CHD risk is high.[30–33] With particular care to reduce variability and increase validity of individual dietary intake assessments, all of these studies were able to demonstrate small but significant and often independent prediction of CHD risk based on entry nutrient intake or other dietary characteristics. In our view, this evidence is less persuasive than the powerful synergism of diet, blood lipid levels, and CHD risk so firmly established over 30 years, but it is clearly confirmatory.

With this logic, habitual diet has come to be considered the *necessary* factor in mass hypercholesterolemia and, thus, in the mass atherosclerosis that leads to high rates of CHD. The population data are, however, equally compatible with another idea, that *all three* of the major risk factors (i.e., elevated population averages of blood cholesterol, blood pressure, and smoking) are essential for a high population burden of CHD.

Congruence of Evidence about Diet

The relationship of habitual diet to population levels of blood lipids and blood pressure, and to CHD and CVD rates, is largely congruent with clinical and experimental observations. First, experimental modification of diet has a predictable effect on group blood lipid levels. When calories and weight are held constant in controlled diet experiments and diet composition is varied, the largest dietary contributions to serum total and LDL cholesterol level are (*a*) the proportion of calories consumed as saturated fatty acids, (*b*) dietary cholesterol, both of which raise cholesterol levels, and (*c*) polyunsaturated fatty acids, which have a cholesterol lowering effect. The role of monounsaturates is debated, with some suggesting a neutral effect while others a cholesterol-lowering effect.[27–29,34] Although this is debated, these clinical experiments confirm the broader relation found between long-term habitual diet and population mean levels of blood lipids.[10,11]

Animal experiments are not treated here but are relevant to the human diet-CHD relationship in that lesions resembling the human plaque are produced by dietary manipulations of blood lipoprotein levels; the fatty components of these animal plaques are reversible with dietary manipulations to lower blood lipoprotein levels.[35,36]

Preventive Trials

Plasma cholesterol-lowering preventive trials, which tend to complete the overall evidence for causation, indicate the feasibility and safety of changing risk factors and demonstrate the actual lag times between such change and its effect on CHD rates.[37] The synthesis of results of *all* these trials and their implications for the public health are central because carrying out the "definitive diet-heart trial" is not considered feasible. Therefore, experimental "proof" of the role of diet in the primary prevention of CHD is not likely to be established.

Lipid-lowering trials demonstrate that substantial lowering of blood lipid levels is feasible, that the progress of arterial lesions is arrested, and that CHD morbidity and mortality are reduced, all in proportion to the cholesterol lowering achieved and its duration. These trials, carried out mainly in middle-aged men with moderately elevated blood lipids, have usually involved cholesterol-lowering medication plus diet. However, because they specifically tested the cholesterol-lowering hypothesis and because their effects are congruent with the observational evidence cited here in support of that hypothesis, these experimental findings have been extrapolated by many authorities to the potential for prevention in the broader population, including women, younger age groups, and those with lower lipid and risk levels.[7] Many consider, also, that the results of randomized clinical trials, because of their congruence with the other evidence, may be extrapolated to the larger public health, including the potential for CHD prevention by long-term change in eating patterns of the population as a whole, and, finally, to the prevention of elevated risk in the first place. Because the intervention trials have concentrated on one or two risk factors only, in a disease that has multiple causal influences, because they have been carried out in middle-aged subjects with respect to a disease that develops over decades, and because they have been performed only in the fraction of the adult population at highest risk, it is estimated that cholesterol lowering across the *entire* population *will* have a greater influence than that found in clinical trials, where it nevertheless appears relatively safe and effective within a very few years.

Dietary Protein

International vital statistics on deaths correlated with national food-consumption data indicate that, as with fat consumption, strong ecologic correlations exist between animal protein intake and death rates from CHD, but there is little evidence that this association is causal. Anitschkow[38] found originally that it was dietary lipid rather than protein that resulted in hyperlipidemia and atherosclerosis in his experimental rabbits. Controlled metabolic ward studies in men under isocaloric conditions, with fat intake held constant while protein intake was varied between 5 and 20 percent of daily calories, found no change in blood cholesterol level (Laboratory of Physiological Hygiene, University of Minnesota, unpublished data).

Neither clinical, experimental, nor epidemiological evidence is now sufficient to attribute a *specific* effect of dietary protein on either blood lipid levels or CHD risk. The overall importance of the consumption of meats from domesticated animals and of fatty milk products is therefore thought to rest mainly in their saturated fatty acid content rather than their protein content, at least with respect to CHD risk.

Dietary Carbohydrate

There is generally a positive ecologic association between population intake of refined sugars and CHD mortality and a negative relationship between complex carbohydrates and CHD mortality. Although these diet components are seriously confounded with other dietary factors that are strongly associated with carbohydrate intake, the effect of certain fibers, including the pectins in fruit, bran fiber, and the guar gum of numerous vegetables and legumes, on blood sugar and on blood lipid regulation has recently attracted greater interest. This is particularly so now that the fatty acid effects are well delineated; yet they fail to explain all of the observed population differences in blood lipid or all the lipid changes seen during experiments involving different nutrient composition.

More important, however, is that plausible mechanisms of atherogenesis are not established for sugars. The broader issue of plant foods (fruits, vegetables, pulses, legumes, and seeds), their complex carbohydrates, protein, other nutrients, and fibers is nevertheless of great public health interest because their consumption may affect the risk of cancers as well as of CVD.

Our summary view is that the different amounts of sugars consumed in "natural diets" around the world do not account for the important differences found in population levels of blood lipids and their associated CHD risk. High carbohydrate intake is confounded with low fat intake (since protein intake is relatively comparable), and both are associated with low rates of CHD. More study is needed on the matter of fibers.

Alcohol

Positive correlations between alcohol consumption and blood pressure levels found for individuals in population studies appear to be dose-related and independent of body weight and smoking habits.[39,40] Evidence is also consistent with respect to the positive relationship of alcohol consumption to blood high density lipoprotein (HDL) cholesterol level and of change in alcohol consumption to change in HDL cholesterol level. Substitution of alcohol for carbohydrates in a mixed U.S. diet results in a rise in HDL, mainly the HDL_3 subfraction, one that may not be strongly related to CHD risk.[41]

Experimentally, myocardial metabolism and ventricular function are affected by relatively small doses of alcohol. In addition, neurohormonal links are established between alcohol-stimulated catecholamine excretion and myocardial oxygen requirements. These effects could act as contributory factors to the clinical manifestations of ischemia.

The epidemiological evidence from longitudinal studies about the relation of alcohol to CHD risk is, however, conflicting.[42–44]

Inverse relationships of alcohol intake and CHD are found in some studies, whereas a U-shaped, linear, or no relationship is found in others. Positive relationships, when found, are usually independent of tobacco, obesity, and blood pressure levels.[44]

Reasons for these inconsistent findings in the alcohol–coronary disease relationship may involve the poor (self-report) measurement for alcohol intake as well as misclassification of the cause of death among heavy drinkers who are known to die of sudden, unexplained causes. Moreover, there are many possible confounding factors, including blood pressure levels, cigarette smoking, and diet.

Preventive practice with respect to alcohol is, therefore, based on its social and public health consequences rather than on any possible direct effect, favorable or otherwise, on cardiovascular disease risk. A major concern about regular alcohol use is, however, its enhancement of overeating, underactivity, and smoking, along with its intrinsic caloric density. Given these several relationships, public health recommendations for alcohol are not indicated in *any* quantity, as a "protective measure" for heart diseases.

Salt Intake

Salting of food, primarily for preservation, began with civilization and trade. Now salting is based mainly on acquired taste and is likely a "new" phenomenon in an evolutionary sense. Moreover, the mammalian kidney probably evolved in salt-poor regions where the predominantly plant and wild game diet was likely very low in sodium and rich in potassium. Thus survival of humans and other mammals in salt-poor environments may have rested on an evolutionarily acquired and exquisite sodium-retaining mechanism of the kidney. The physiological need for salt under ordinary circumstances is approximately only 1 to 2 g of sodium chloride per day. It is hypothesized that this mechanism is now overwhelmed by the concentrated salt presented to modern humans in preserved meats and pickled foods, in many processed foods, and in the strong culturally acquired taste for salt.[22,45]

Clinical, experimental, and epidemiological links between salt intake and hypertension are increasingly well forged[45,46] (see Chapter 52). Marked sodium depletion dramatically reduces blood pressure in persons with severe hypertension. Sodium restriction enables high blood pressure to be controlled with lower doses of antihypertensive drugs. In many patients, salt restriction may result in adequate control of mild to moderate hypertension without drugs. Weight reduction and salt restriction appear to be independently important in lowering high blood pressure. In summary, a culture with high salt consumption appears to encourage maximal exhibition of an inherent human susceptibility to hypertension. Because potassium tends to reduce the blood pressure–raising effects of sodium, the sodium-potassium ratio of habitual diets also may be important in the public health.[47]

Surveys consistently find strong relationships between average population blood pressure and salt intake.[46,48,49] High blood pressure is usually prevalent in high-salting cultures, irrespective of the prevalence of obesity. In contrast, hypertension is usually absent in low-salting cultures, despite frequent obesity. Moreover, rapid acculturation to greater salt intake among South Pacific islanders who migrate to industrialized countries is associated with an increased frequency of hypertension and elevated mean blood pressure.[50] Even within high-salting cultures, when special efforts are made to reduce the measurement error for blood pressure and to characterize individual sodium intake with maximum precision, significant individual salt–blood pressure correlations are usually found.[50,51]

Despite all this evidence, neither preventive practice nor public health policy on reduction of salting is well advanced. This may be due in part to professional skepticism, based perhaps on the relatively weak individual correlations of salt intake and blood pressure. Admittedly, modification of salt intake by traditional dietary counseling has not been very successful. However, when interventions are attempted in a supportive and systematic way, change in salting behavior is readily achievable.[52] In the United States, wider education has significantly and widely influenced food processing and marketing of products with lower salt content, and a great deal of voluntary public health action has been taken by food companies.

Current U.S. national dietary goals recommend no more than 4.5 to 6.0 g of salt daily.[37] For individuals, this is achievable by not salting foods at the table, by adding no salt in cooking, and by avoidance of salt-rich foods, particularly canned, processed, and pickled foods. Despite the absence of a strong policy, preventive practice and public health approaches to reduced salt consumption are increasing. Significant public health effects of such population changes might be expected in high-salting societies, in light of recent trends in blood pressure and stroke observed in Japanese populations.[53]

Soft Water and Minerals

The effects of other minerals, cations, and trace elements on cardiovascular function and disease are the subject of active research because of their important role in many basic metabolic reactions, because of the need to define their daily requirements for good nutrition, and because of the wide variation of their concentration in foods and water sources. Significant associations are found between water softness and rates of hypertension and CHD mortality. Plausible mechanisms are not established, however, and the epidemiological associations are inconsistent and confounded.[54–56] Leaching of minerals from the soil, composition of water supplies, and the tissue effects of minerals and trace elements are all areas of current research. Interest is centered on the intake of calcium, iron, magnesium, manganese, lead, cadmium, the zinc-copper ratio, and selenium.

Blood Lipoproteins

Clinical, experimental, and epidemiological evidence of the relationship between certain blood lipoproteins, atherosclerosis, and incidence of CHD is strong, consistent, and congruent. Because much knowledge is available, we present here only a summary of what we regard as the salient facts in this relationship, along with a few key references. The subject was recently reviewed in detail.[57]

- Mean levels and distributions of total serum cholesterol and other blood lipids vary widely among populations.[10,11,57]
- Associations are consistently strong between mean population levels of total serum cholesterol and measured CHD incidence.[10,11]
- Associations are generally weak and variable between mean population levels of fasting serum triglycerides and coronary disease rates.[57–59]
- Total serum cholesterol levels at birth have similar means and ranges in many cultures.[60]
- Average levels and distributions of total serum cholesterol differ widely for populations of school-age children.[60] They tend to parallel the differences found in adult population distributions of blood lipid levels, that is, means and distributions are found to be elevated in youth when they are elevated in adult populations.[60]
- Means and distributions of total serum cholesterol of migrants rapidly approach those of the adopted country, whether higher or lower than the country of origin.[15]
- Blood lipids measured in cohorts of healthy adults followed over time show consistently positive relationships, usually with a continuously rising individual risk of CHD according to the entry levels of total serum cholesterol (and LDL), at least until late middle age.[7,61,62]

- Computation of the population risk attributable to blood cholesterol levels indicates that the majority of excess CHD cases occurs in the central segment of the population distribution, that is, 220 to 310 mg/dL, whereas only 10 percent derive from values above 310.[6,25]
- In healthy cohorts, a strong inverse relationship between individual HDL cholesterol level and its ratio to total cholesterol is found with subsequent CHD risk. It is relatively stronger at older ages and within populations that have a relatively high CHD risk overall.[34,59,63]
- Large-scale experiments indicate the feasibility and apparent safety of blood cholesterol lowering from moderate changes made in dietary composition, with and without weight loss.[9,34,64]
- Clinical trials of lipid lowering alone in middle-age, high-risk populations indicates a reduction of CHD risk according to the degree and duration of exposure to the lowered cholesterol level.[8,9,65–67] Further, clear evidence has emerged that a class of lipid-lowering agents, the "statins" can reduce the risk of further CHD morbidity and mortality when coronary disease is already clinically apparent.[67a,67b]
- There has probably been a significant drop, of approximately 10 to 15 percent, in the U.S. mean total serum cholesterol level in the last 20 years, which is partly explained by changes in composition of the habitual diet during this period.[68]
- The downward trends observed in CHD mortality in the United States cannot be attributed directly to the lowered population levels of risk factors. The findings are compatible with causation, however, because the decline in out-of-hospital CHD mortality, a crude reflection of incidence, is occurring, and falling incidence is observed in some studies.[2]

The effect of improved coronary care on CHD mortality trends is documented by the decrease in hospital case-fatality from myocardial infarction and by improved long-term survival.[1,2,69,70]

Consensus from these facts has resulted in a vigorous population strategy of reduction in blood lipid level in the United States. Major recommendations are now in place for a change in eating pattern among North Americans.[34,71] Moreover, the U.S. National Cholesterol Education Program has apparently increased both public and professional awareness and has improved the medical practice of lowering blood cholesterol.[72–75]

Overweight and Obesity

Whatever the physiological or cosmetic disadvantages of obesity and overweight, their relationship to CVD risk and mortality remains interesting, difficult to dissect, and basically unsettled. From a clinical perspective, extreme obesity is associated with manifest physical limitations and a propensity for many disabilities and illnesses. Beyond this, however, associations with cardiovascular diseases are not consistent throughout most of the distribution of relative weight or skin-fold measurements.[76]

Overweight and weight gain tend to raise risk factor levels, and correction of the many metabolic disorders that accompany obesity is prompt and substantial when weight loss is achieved, with or without an increase in physical activity. When weight loss is carried out primarily through increased physical activity, appetite is generally "self-regulated" and body fat is lost, lean body mass is better maintained, insulin activity is lowered, glucose tolerance is improved, LDL and very low density lipoprotein (VLDL) levels are lowered, HDL level is raised, and cardiovascular efficiency is enhanced. As we shall review here, however, the status of obesity and weight gain and loss as risk factors for CVD is complex and uncertain.

Obesity is arbitrarily considered to be present when the fat content of the body is greater than 25 percent of body mass in men and 30 percent in women. Overweight is equally arbitrarily chosen as greater than 130 percent relative weight, according to life insurance build and mortality tables, or on a body mass index (wt/ht^2) greater than 26. "Ideal weight" criteria are often based on standards associated with the lowest mortality risk in life insurance experience. The prevalence of overweight (and obesity) in U.S. adults is variously estimated at from 20 to 50 percent, depending on the measurement used and the definition chosen, as well as by age, sex, and race classification.

A most salient fact about overweight in the United States is that average weight and relative body weight are increasing, according to national health surveys. Mean body mass index (wt/ht^2) in men (20 to 74 years of age) rose from 25.1 kg/m^2 in 1960 to 1962 to 26.3 kg/m^2 in 1988 to 1991. In women, similar changes have occurred, with mean body mass index in 1960 to 1962 being 24.4 kg^2, rising to 26.1 kg/m^2 in the later survey.[77] The prevalence of extreme overweight is increasing at a greater rate than is average weight.[77] Finally, relative obesity increases with age, even in a setting of stable body weight, because, as people grow older, muscle is replaced with fat.

The causes of *mass obesity* in populations are only partly understood. Widespread abundance, availability, and low cost of calorie-dense foods, along with many environmental cues to appetite, encourage overeating in relation to physiologic need. These environmental "facilitators" act on an apparently widespread genetic susceptibility to obesity. This, in turn, may be an evolutionary legacy from hunter-gatherer lifestyles. Moreover, there are other factors that enhance excess calorie intake relative to need. For example, dietary fat is more efficiently stored as adipose tissue than is carbohydrate under conditions of excess calorie intake.[34] Refined sugars have less satiety value than the complex carbohydrates of fruits and vegetables. And alcohol is cheap and available in many societies.

Nevertheless, a major "cause" of mass obesity in Western populations appears to be the increase of relative sedentariness. Americans are, on average, heavier now than they were earlier in this century when, in fact, they consumed significantly more calories per day.[34] The stable, rural, laboring populations that consume (and expend) more energy are, in turn, the leaner populations.[10] Unfortunately, however, sedentariness in populations is largely confounded with calorie density and other differences in eating patterns.

CHD and Obesity among Populations

Comparisons among and within populations in the Seven Countries Study illustrate the complexity of the relationship of overweight and obesity to CHD and to death from all causes.[10,11] Among populations, CHD incidence is not correlated with any measure of obesity or overweight. The population distributions of skin-fold obesity are, however, strikingly different. They almost fail to overlap, for example, between the highest skin-fold values found among Serbian farmers and the lowest values among sedentary U.S. rail clerks.[10] Obesity is, therefore, a mass phenomenon and is apparently strongly determined by (*a*) the average energy expenditure of the population and (*b*) the composition (caloric density) of the diet.

CHD and Obesity within Populations

Within populations the picture is highly variable. In East Finns, with high CHD rates, incident CHD cases are evenly distributed across the entry distribution of skin-fold fatness and overweight. In another population with a high CHD incidence—U.S. railroad workers—the relationship between skin-fold obesity and CHD death is weakly positive, in contrast to an insignificant and opposite relationship for relative body weight. In another population with a high CHD incidence, consisting of rural Dutch men, there is a strongly positive linear relationship between CHD incidence and overweight and obesity throughout the wide range of values found there. Among men from the southern Mediterranean regions of Italy, Greece, and Yugoslavia, there is a U-shaped relationship between overweight or obesity and CHD risk, as well as with deaths from all causes. There the thinnest individuals as well as the heaviest and fattest have the higher disease rates; lowest disease risk is found for those with intermediate weight values.[10,11]

Multivariate analysis in the Seven Countries Study, used to adjust for the many confounding variables related alike to body mass and to CHD, shows no consistent relationship of 10-year CHD incidence with either relative weight or fatness.[11] In most of these populations there is a tendency for CHD incidence to be slightly higher in the upper than in the lower half of the fatness distributions, but this tendency disappears when other variables are simultaneously considered. Similarly, except for men at the extremes of the distribution, within generally high-incidence and overweight U.S. populations, there is little relationship between obesity or overweight and risk of CHD or death in men.

Within populations, several other longitudinal studies, including the Framingham Heart Study,[78] the Evans County Study,[79] and the Manitoba Study,[80] suggest that an independent contribution of relative weight to risk in a society with high CHD incidence may be reflected only in very long-term CHD risk. In Framingham, in addition, weight gain since youth is a risk predictor for CHD.[78] Finally, in the Evans County Study, initial overweight and weight gain over time are also strongly related to the 7-year incidence of new hypertension.[79]

The ability to distinguish CVD risk according to the body distribution of obesity, usually measured as the ratio of waist to hip circumference (WHR), is relatively new.[81] WHR is positively related to risk of CHD, premature death, non-insulin–dependent diabetes mellitus, and cancers in women, as well as to established CVD risk factor levels. The finding that several diseases correlate better with fat distribution than with general measures of overweight or obesity has raised major new hypotheses about possible separate metabolic entities and about the pathogenesis, risk, and treatment of obesity.[82,83]

Results of autopsy studies are inconclusive. The International Atherosclerosis Project concluded that the degree and severity of atherosclerosis were not consistently associated with overweight and obesity.[84]

Finally, a major gap exists in our knowledge of the effect of weight reduction on disease risk in a relatively overweight society at high risk from combined CHD risk factors. This hugely confounded question, as well as the effects of weight cycling, remains to be clarified.[85]

In summary, obesity and overweight are centrally involved with the many metabolic maladaptations related to diabetes mellitus, hypertension, blood lipids, and probably atherogenesis. These maladaptations are particularly amenable to correction by weight loss, with or without increased physical activity. The epidemiological evidence indicates, however, that relative body weight and obesity have a different disease-related significance in different populations and cultures. This may be due in part to different composition of the diets by which individuals and populations become obese, as well as to coexisting elevated distributions of other CVD risk characteristics. In most societies with high CHD incidence in which the issue has been systematically studied, the relationship between overweight, obesity, and CHD risk is seen mainly at the extremes of relative weight and over the longer term. Inconsistent disease associations and the obvious and dramatic declines in CVD deaths in the United States over the last 20 years, despite the clearly increased average U.S. body mass, indicate the primary importance for population CVD risk of factors other than overweight and obesity.

Physical Inactivity

Two primal human activities are the obtaining and consuming of food. Only since the advent of agriculture, and more recently of urbanization and industrialization, has the sustained subsistence activity of humans changed dramatically. In affluent industrial societies with automated occupations, motorized transport, and sedentary leisure, reduced energy expenditure is one of the more profound changes in human behavior. Aside from its likely importance as a fundamental departure from evolutionary adaptations and its apparently determining effect on mass obesity, the evidence specifically linking physical activity to chronic and CVD disease risk is difficult to obtain and interpret. It defies effective analysis because, in Western society, there are simply no "unselected" active and inactive groups to compare. Moreover, a definitive, long-term controlled experiment on habitual activity with respect to CVD risk is not considered feasible.[86] We attempt here a brief synthesis of the evidence relating habitual activity to CHD risk.

The caliber of the coronary arteries at autopsy is larger in very active people, but limitations of design, method, feasibility, and cost have prevented a satisfactory study of the effect of exercise training on changes in coronary angiograms or functional measures of ischemia.

Clinical trials of cardiac rehabilitation after myocardial infarction, including the effects of exercise training, have been difficult. Nevertheless, Oldridge and colleagues[87] carried out a meta-analysis on the "better-designed" studies, noting first that many of the trials demonstrated an effect of exercise on levels of risk factors and exercise tolerance. They used rigorous criteria for inclusion of 10 trials in their statistical summary, which estimated a 24 percent reduction in deaths from all causes in patients undergoing cardiac rehabilitation and a 25 percent reduction in CVD mortality. Both estimates were statistically significant and clinically important. The incidence of nonfatal myocardial infarction, however, was 15 percent higher (not statistically significant) in all the treatment groups combined and 32 percent higher ($P = 0.058$) in the groups in which cardiac rehabilitation was begun early (i.e., within 8 weeks after infarction). Thus, cardiac rehabilitation with exercise apparently had no overall effect on risk of nonfatal infarction and, when initiated early, may even have increased the incidence of nonfatal infarction. A prudent approach, therefore, would be to avoid the premature institution (within 8 weeks) of vigorous exercise as a component of rehabilitation.[88]

In addition to fatal and morbid outcomes, there is a growing consensus on the benefits of physical activity among patients with clinically significant cardiovascular diseases including myocardial infarction, angina pectoris, peripheral vascular disease, and congestive heart failure. Symptom reduction, improved exercise tolerance and functional capacity, and improvement in psychological well-being and quality of life are among the benefits.[89]

The major source of information about the primary prevention of CHD is indirect, from observational studies. These usually involve attempts to identify the confounding effects of lifestyle characteristics *other* than physical activity.[88] A recent synthesis by Powell and colleagues[90] concluded that the majority of observational studies meeting their criteria found a significant and graded relationship between physical inactivity and the risk of first CHD event and that studies with a stronger design were more likely to show an effect. These authors calculated a median risk ratio of 1.9, that is, a 90 percent excess risk of CHD among physically inactive persons.

We analyzed the subset of 16 studies from the review of Powell et al that measured individual levels of physical activity, and we added recent studies from the Multiple Risk Factor Intervention Trial (MRFIT) and U.S. railroad workers.[88,91,92] All 18 studies showed that habitual physical activity was inversely related to death from CHD or death from all causes. The more recent studies adjusted for confounding risks and this adjustment usually diminished, but did not abolish, the risk associated with physical inactivity. Several studies found that the relation was largely "explained" by the level of physical fitness, in that the gradient of risk with the level of physical activity largely disappeared when measures of fitness were controlled. In a cohort study, fitness measured by a maximal exercise treadmill test predicted all-cause mortality for men and women, independently of other risk characteristics.[93]

The duration, frequency, and intensity of physical activity that may be "protective" against CHD remain, nevertheless, at issue. Recent studies suggest that an energy expenditure of 150 to 300 kcal daily, in activity of moderate intensity such as walking and working around the house, is associated with lower risk, as is a moderate amount of vigorous physical activity.[89,91,92,94] Anthropologic observations suggest that healthy farmers and herdsmen the world over rarely work at a pace that leads to shortness of breath or exhaustion. Systematic observations in the Seven Countries Study indicate that even a substantial amount of regular, vigorous physical activity does not necessarily protect an individual or a population from CVD risk, particularly if other risk factors such as mass hypercholesterolemia are prevalent. In that study, farmers and loggers in eastern Finland were found to be the most physically active of men, and yet they had the highest rates of CHD; there was little less risk among the more physically active within that population.[10,11]

The interpretation of these many observations is that habitual, current physical activity very likely protects against coronary death.[89] A basic uncertainty that remains is whether the apparent benefit is due to physical activity itself or to genetic factors. People tend to exercise if they are able to and if they feel good when they exercise. Fitness, a component strongly determined by constitution, may be a major contributor to an apparently protective effect of physical activity. It is possible that fitness determines both who will be active and who will be protected from CHD.

At least two other pieces of evidence suggest that constitution is *not* the major operant. Any protective effect of having once been a college athlete, and thus presumably genetically superior, disappears with time after graduation, whereas current physical activity is associated with lower risk.[95] Moreover, it seems that genetic factors are likely to be less important to participation in moderate exercise than to participation in vigorous exercise, but both carry a lower risk of CHD.

Finally, safety should be the foremost consideration both in prescribing exercise for individuals and in making recommendations for the public health. Several studies have found an excess risk of primary cardiac arrest during and shortly after strenuous exercise in all subjects, regardless of their level of habitual physical inactivity, despite a much lower overall risk of sudden coronary death in habitually active subjects.[96,97] They concluded that the reduced risk of sudden death due to regular physical activity was greater than the excess risk of sudden death during vigorous activity. This view, important for the public health, would be small comfort, however, to the families of those stricken while running. The evidence suggests that brisk walking or other moderately vigorous activity is the more reasonable exercise prescription, at least for sedentary and middle-aged people who have not maintained their fitness from youth.[89]

Diabetes, Hyperglycemia, Hyperinsulinism

Since the insulin era began, enabling persons with diabetes to survive, a strong relationship between diabetes and atherosclerosis risk has emerged. In addition, there are important mechanistic interrelations between insulin-glucose regulation, lipoprotein and uric acid metabolism, obesity and hypertension, on the one hand, and atherosclerosis on the other.

The association of clinical diabetes mellitus with CHD and atherosclerotic manifestations is documented clinically, pathologically, and epidemiologically.[98,99] It is thought that hyperinsulinemia, hypoglycemic episodes, or both in treated diabetics, coupled (formerly) with the common prescription of a high-fat, low-carbohydrate low-fiber diet, increases vascular complications. Cross-cultural comparisons suggest that the risk of atherosclerosis and CVD in diabetic patients is indeed related to factors other than the glucose-insulin disorder itself. For example, apparently low rates of atherosclerosis exist in diabetic eastern Jews, Chinese, and Southwest American Indians.[98,99] The Pima Indians of Arizona are thought to be an example of the theoretical "thrifty genotype," that is, a population only recently (in evolutionary terms) exposed to calorie abundance, that frequently (±50 percent of adults) develops an obese, diabetic phenotype but nevertheless manifests little CVD.[100]

In longitudinal studies among cohorts, clinical diabetes mellitus is associated with excess CHD risk and severity of CHD, and many studies confirm the excess of fatal myocardial infarction in women with diabetes.[101] The excess risk among diabetics is not always differentiated by the degree of hyperglycemia or the degree of control. Much of the excess CHD risk in diabetics is, in fact, accounted for by associated risk variables.[98,99] More severe atherosclerosis, diabetic cardiomyopathy, and a hypercoagulable state are also thought to contribute to the excess risk of diabetes.[99] Finally, in most autopsy studies, coronary artery disease and the frequency and severity of myocardial infarction are greater in diabetics than in control subjects.[98,99]

Diabetic treatment by the control of blood glucose levels is the mainstay of therapy. However, the role of glucose control in the reduction of cardiovascular and other complications has been controversial. The University Group Diabetes Program (UGDP) reported an increased rate of myocardial infarction with the use of first-generation sulfonyl ureas despite effective blood glucose control.[102] These effects are not seen with later agents.[103] The Diabetes Control and Complications Trial (DCCT) studied "tight" glucose control in insulin-dependent diabetics. Findings included significant reduction in retinopathy, microalbuminuria, and clinical neuropathy. Elevated LDL cholesterol levels were also reduced with tight control.[104] Cardiovascular and peripheral vascular disease was also reduced, but did not reach significance.

In healthy persons glucose intolerance alone is weakly and inconsistently associated with CVD risk.[99,105] However, high insulin activity was found to be a significant independent predictor of coronary events in cohorts studied in Australia, France, and Finland,[99] and it has also been proposed as a cause of excess atherosclerosis in Asian migrants.[106]

In summary, the relationship between diabetes, atherosclerosis, and coronary disease is well established among persons with clinical diabetes living under the conditions of affluent Western culture. Data from other cultures suggest, however, that other factors, such as physical activity, body weight, blood pressure, blood lipid levels, dietary composition, and smoking habits, greatly affect the risk of CHD among diabetics. This, plus evidence that the metabolic disorders of middle-age persons with diabetes can be significantly improved through exercise and modified by diet and weight loss, provide a sound rationale for preventive practice. More study of these complex issues is needed to develop an effective preventive approach to noninsulin-dependent diabetes mellitus itself.

Elevated Blood Pressure: Hypertension

The epidemiology, control, and prevention of hypertension and its complications are discussed in detail in Chapter 52 and therefore are only summarized here.

It is estimated that hypertension contributes to more than one-half of adult deaths in the United States. It is a strong and independent risk factor for CHD and stroke, and there are plausible mechanisms for its effects on atherosclerosis and vascular disease. Patients with CHD have higher average blood pressure than control subjects. Experimental atherosclerosis induced in animals is directly related to pressure levels within the arterial system. In cohort studies, elevated blood pressure is positively, continuously, and independently related to CHD risk, according to increasing level of systolic or diastolic blood pressured. The relationship of elevated blood pressure to risk of cerebrovascular hemorrhage and congestive heart failure is even stronger than the relationship to risk of CHD and thrombotic stroke.

Population comparisons suggest, however, that hypertension accounts for relatively little of the great variation in CHD incidence found *among* populations, despite the fact that it is significantly related to individual CHD risk *within* populations. For example, there is a remarkable difference in CHD rates between Mediterranean populations and northern Europeans, in which average blood pressures are little different.[10,11]

The preventive potential for hypertension control is illustrated by drug trials that have demonstrated a significant decrease in rate of stroke and heart failure. Most recently the Systolic Hypertension in the Elderly Project (SHEP) demonstrated the importance of systolic blood pressure control in this group.[107] Results of other trials suggest that CHD risk is lowered by control of hypertension, but most have had insufficient power to study this question.[108]

Blood pressure control has greatly improved in the United States in the last 15 to 20 years, according to surveys showing a substantial decrease in the proportion of hypertensive persons unidentified or not under control.[109,110] These trends have occurred in parallel with downward trends for both CHD and stroke mortality, although a direct relationship cannot be established. In fact, the mortality rate from stroke was diminishing long before safe and effective antihypertensive therapy was widely used. Moreover, stroke death rates in the United States fell during the 1950s and 1960s, when CHD death rates were rising sharply.[1]

Estimated changes in death rates for CHD and stroke, based on models of hypertension control, suggest a large potential for the prevention of CVD. Primary prevention of hypertension would likely have even more impressive effects on the public health.

Present challenges to preventive practice lie mainly in more effective control of elevated blood pressure in the elderly and in finding the ideal combination of drug and hygienic management for correction of mild or borderline levels of high blood pressure. The larger public health challenge lies in improvement of populationwide correlates of hypertension, such as physical inactivity, overweight, and high salt and alcohol intake. Such primary preventive and public health approaches promise to minimize the exhibition of high blood pressure, since human populations are apparently widely susceptible.

Tobacco Smoking

The broader relationship of tobacco to disease and health is detailed in Chapter 44. Much of the clinical evidence of a direct relationship between cigarette smoking and coronary disease was, until recently, anecdotal. Experimentally, ischemic pain, angiographic coronary spasm, and electrocardiographic findings are now demonstrated during smoking in patients with compromised coronary circulation.[111]

For individuals living within societies with a high CHD incidence, smoking is consistently found to be a strong and independent risk factor for myocardial infarction and sudden death.[93–95] The risk is continuous from persons who have never smoked, to ex-smokers, to those who smoke even in small amounts and is also related to duration of the habit.[112,113] Interactions with other risk factors are also important, as indicated by the weak association of smoking with CHD risk in low-risk societies.[10,11] For example, the observed incidence of CHD in populations that do not have a base of relative mass hypercholesterolemia is much lower than the risk predicted with multiple regression equations derived from U.S. or northern Europe data.[112] The Japanese, for example, with a heavy prevalence of smoking and substantial amounts of hypertension, but without hypercholesterolemia, show much less coronary heart disease than would be predicted.[10,11]

As is the case with serum cholesterol level, most of the CHD cases attributable to smoking derive from the central part of the distribution, that is, light and moderate smokers; the prevalence of heavy smokers is low. A 17 percent population-attributable risk fraction for smoking and CHD deaths in the United States was estimated (conservatively) in the Carter Report.[114] Smoking is particularly significant in CHD risk among women.[115]

Smoking cessation is associated with lower CHD rates according to years of cessation.[116] While those who have never smoked have the best disease experience, long-term quitters approximate their rates, and even temporary quitters have a better risk experience than persistent smokers.[117] Improvement in the prognosis of survivors of myocardial infarction who quit smoking also tends to confirm the harmful cardiovascular effects of cigarettes and supports the potential for CHD prevention by reduction of tobacco use.[113,118]

Synthesis of this evidence, therefore, suggests that cigarette smoking is neither a primary nor a necessary factor in determining *population* rates of CHD. It is, rather, a strong and independent risk factor for CHD and vascular disease among individuals living in high-incidence populations where there is a significant background of coronary and peripheral atherosclerosis.

Mechanisms presumed to be important in CHD include the physicochemical effects of tobacco, that is, increased heart rate and myocardial contractility and greater myocardial oxygen demand due to raised catecholamine levels, decreased oxygen-carrying capacity of the blood, elevated fibrinogen levels, and platelet-aggregating effects. Other possible mechanisms include elevated fasting blood glucose levels and white blood cell counts and lower HDL levels, all found among smokers.[111]

A public health policy to foster so-called safer cigarettes, at least with respect to lowering CVD risk, is not supported by the evidence of persistent high exposure to gas-phase toxins in "low-yield" cigarette users.[111] Moreover, the promotion and adoption of Western-type cigarettes and smoking patterns in developing countries augurs ill for the future CVD risk in those populations. In contrast, smoking prevalence has decreased substantially in the United States, where large numbers of educated adults in particular have stopped smoking. This is attributed to increased community awareness of the health need to stop smoking, to social pressure and legislation for "clean air" and "smoke-free" environments, and to a greater access to the support and skills needed for quitting. The downward U.S. trend in smoking is not as evident, however, among lower socioeconomic groups and heavy smokers.[119]

Under "ideal" supportive circumstances, such as that given high-risk participants in the MRFIT, smoking cessation success rates approximate 40 percent in the first year, with maintenance of this rate for up to 4 years among volunteer participants. Thus a long-standing medical pessimism about helping patients stop smoking might be replaced by optimism for cessation programs that are systematically applied. Moreover, communitywide educational and legislative efforts are increasingly effective.[120,121] The results of all these efforts and the population trends downward in smoking frequency provide a rational basis for more public programs and for a more focused national policy to reduce cigarette smoking and tobacco production. It is equally possible that the currently declining rate of cigarette smoking will level off, unless educational programs and wider social support for nonsmoking behavior reach the lower socioeconomic classes, heavy smokers, women, and youth.

Hemostatic Factors

For decades, arguments have existed about the relative predominance of the role of blood lipids versus thrombosis in the pathogenesis of atherosclerosis and CHD. A more unified theory now joins the effects of diet and blood lipids, physical activity and smoking, and diabetes and insulin levels to atherosclerosis and to thrombosis. The interaction between chronic arterial wall disease and the blood properties leading to coagulation continues to be a major subject for research as it becomes clear that a critical fixed obstructive lesion is not necessary for myocardial infarction. The components of the coagulation system found so far to be of major interest are fibrin, which forms when cell walls are damaged and which contributes to fibrin platelet masses, and platelet aggregation.[122–125]

Of the several hemostatic variables measured with respect to subsequent CHD risk, fibrinogen has received the most attention. Several investigators conclude that an elevated fibrinogen level is likely to be causally associated with CHD but that its elevation overall may be due primarily to smoking.[122]

Anticoagulant trials appear to reduce short-term mortality in the hospital phase of acute myocardial infarction,[125] but long-term results are inconclusive. The reduction of reinfarction appears to be more likely than the reduction in deaths.

As for primary prevention of CHD events with low-level anticoagulation, such as with small doses of aspirin, this appears now to be established for nonfatal myocardial infarction.[126]

Hyperuricemia

A weak but consistent association between hyperuricemia, obesity, hypertension, hyperlipidemia, and coronary disease has been noted in clinical and epidemiological studies. Most evidence suggests that there is no significant independent association of serum uric acid level with coronary events after adequately accounting for confounding variables. A public health issues has emerged, however, in the combined effects on serum uric acid, glucose levels, and blood lipids of thiazide diuretics used widely in the control of hypertension. These drugs elevate LDL and HDL levels as well as uric acid and glucose levels.[127] Preventive practice among people with hypertension now requires, therefore, careful tailoring of antihypertensive therapy with lower dosages of diuretics or other medications, when hyperuricemia, hyperlipidemia, or glucose intolerance accompany hypertension.

Physical Environment

The weather, particularly the influx of cold fronts and rapid falls in barometric pressure, has been correlated with new hospital admissions for coronary events and sudden death.[128] Reasonable preventive practice includes advice to avoid exposure, in particular the combination of isometric work and cold, and to use light face masks to maintain a favorable personal air temperature and humidity.

Similarly, atmospheric inversions and air pollution are related to hospitalization and death rates from pulmonary and cardiovascular diseases, particularly in the elderly. Because most circumstances of the physical environment are so confounded by other risks in atherosclerosis, useful studies and preventive strategies are difficult to devise.

Behavior Pattern, Personality, and Stress

Emotional states of anger and aggression, fear and anxiety, and hyperactivity and depression are associated with overt metabolic and physiological reactions, symptoms, and signs. Pervasive popular and professional impressions are that they influence all the major diseases of modern life. Causal connections between stress and behavior and coronary events and sudden death remain, however, unestablished. Laboratory study is limited by poor definition and measurement of "stress" and the components of stress reactions. Personality type, habitual behavior, and reactions to external stress have not been tied together effectively into a theoretical model susceptible of testing or amenable to preventive practice. Nevertheless, major psychosocial issues are being investigated actively, including type A behavior, hostility, and social support. Because of a long and considerable controversy in this area, and because of a wealth of new information about it, we consider these relationships here in some detail.

Type A Behavior

Type A behavior was accepted by many to be a strong psychosocial risk factor for CHD until the early 1980s. The major studies first establishing the relationship were the Western Collaborative Group Study and the Framingham Study.[129,130]

The Western Collaborative Group Study was a prospective study of more than 3,000 men in whom the type A behavior pattern was assessed by its originators, using their structured interview method. The relative risk of CHD (both fatal and nonfatal incident events) among type A men was about 2.[129] The Framingham Study used a paper-and-pencil instrument to assess type A behavior in men and women, again with both fatal and nonfatal events as endpoints. The relative risk of CHD among type A persons was greater than 2 for incident events in both sexes.[130]

The relationship between type A behavior and CHD was also examined in many coronary angiographic studies in which behavior pattern was assessed before angiography. A summary of 14 such studies found about an equal balance of positive and absent associations.[131]

Several studies in the early 1980s failed to demonstrate the expected relationship to CHD.[132–135] These differed from the earlier, population-based studies on several counts: they used high risk subgroups; for the most part, they used the Jenkins Activity Survey, another paper-and-pencil instrument; and they generally examined "harder" endpoints (CHD death or definite myocardial infarction). The MRFIT study, however, used the structured interview in a subset of participants and also found no significant relationship to risk. The Honolulu Heart Study used the Jenkins Activity Survey and found no relationship between type A behavior and incidence of disease but did find a relationship to prevalence of angina pectoris.[136]

At least one study among high-risk populations found a positive relationship between behavior pattern and CHD; the Recurrent Coronary Prevention Project reported that intervention in the behavior pattern reduced the risk of recurrent CHD.[137] These results have not been replicated.

Two publications based on follow-up of the original Western Collaborative Group data have also raised questions as to whether type A behavior is, in fact, a risk factor for CHD.[138,139] At present, we consider that clear evidence for a type A/B relationship to CHD risk is not established.

Hostility

Several studies have broken down type A behavior into components and attempted to examine their relationships to CHD. Both Matthews et al[140] and Hecker et al[141] identified hostility as a "coronary-prone" component within the Western Collaborative Group population. "Hostility" was assessed by independent raters evaluating audiotapes of baseline structured interviews.

Another approach uses the "Cook-Medley" hostility subscore of the Minnesota Multiphasic Personality Index (MMPI), a well-constructed and standardized instrument that is part of the MMPI, with data available on many populations. Six prospective studies using the Cook-Medley instrument have now been published; three have found associations of hostility with CHD and three have not.[142–147] On the other hand, hostility has been found related to CHD in several coronary angiographic studies.[148–150]

In summary, there is evidence relating hostility to CHD in men; little investigation has been carried out in women. The reasons are unclear for the discrepant results among the six methodologically similar prospective studies. Thus further investigations of hostility and CVD risk appear warranted.

Social Support

Several prospective population-based studies have established social support or "social connectedness" as a factor associated with *reduced* risk of death. Two large studies—one from Finland[151] and one from Sweden[152]—examined CVD disease risk. The pattern of results suggests a relationship between social support and mortality, at least in men. Whether this is a causal relationship or is attributable to a confounding variable such as baseline health or to personality characteristics such as hostility is unclear, and this line of investigation might well be continued.

Attempts have been made to change psychosocial characteristics experimentally and to measure CHD risk factors and disease changes. In our view, however, the problems of measurement, the relative absence of plausible linking mechanisms, and the limited techniques for modifying behavioral characteristics are all at a stage where a public health strategy is not feasible. Nevertheless, attempts at modifying individual behavior in preventive practice appear to be appropriate and safe.

Gender and Estrogens

The excess risk of CHD and atherosclerosis in white men is documented throughout affluent Western society. The sex differential is much less prominent, however, in nonwhite populations and in areas where the overall incidence is relatively low.[153] The particular susceptibility of men is only partly explained by their higher risk factor configurations between the ages of 25 and 60. On the other hand, the relative protection from CHD among premenopausal women is assumed to be related to hormones, although the effect of early oophorectomy, menopause, or estrogen replacement therapy on known risk factor distributions in women fails to completely explain these differences. In countries with a high incidence of CHD, where there is relative mass hyperlipidemia much more of the plasma cholesterol is carried in the HDL fraction in women. Recent experimental evidence concerning mechanisms of LDL and HDL function, related to cell receptors and lipid transport in and out of the arterial wall, confirm this particular biological difference as a likely cause for some of the sex difference in CHD risk.

In contrast, women have a proportionately greater risk of angina pectoris than of myocardial infarction or sudden death. While they have less severe atherosclerosis in the coronary arteries, the sex difference is not as apparent in cerebral, aortic, and peripheral vessels. The male-female ratio of coronary disease prevalence and incidence is almost absent among persons with clinical diabetes.[101] Survival of women after myocardial infarction is poorer in-hospital, although this is balanced by greater out-of-hospital death for men.

Finally, trends in CHD deaths in the United States indicate that the age-specific decline in mortality is proportionately greater in women than in men.[1] Similarly, the rise in CHD death rates among women in eastern Europe, where CVD deaths overall are increasing rapidly, is proportionately greater in women and in young women.[154]

The excess risk of thromboembolism, stroke, and myocardial infarction in women taking oral contraceptives (OCs), and the interaction of OCs with age and smoking, are well established. Young women taking OCs have systematically higher serum lipid levels, higher blood pressure, and impaired glucose tolerance compared with control subjects.[155]

Numerous epidemiologic studies have evaluated the use of postmenopausal estrogen in the primary prevention of cardiovascular disease.[156] Meta-analysis suggests a relative risk of 0.50 to 0.65 for coronary artery disease in estrogen users.[157] The mechanism for this apparent benefit may be the positive shifts in lipids (increased HDL cholesterol and lower LDL cholesterol) or other factors associated with use.[158] Recent randomized clinical trials support this view.[159]

In summary, the sex differential for atherosclerosis and cardiovascular disease events and their time trends is not completely explained on the basis of known effects of hormones on the level of risk factors. More study is needed. The widespread therapeutic use of hormones may turn out to have profound public health importance.

Hereditary Factors

Much current work is opening up the understanding of host-environmental relationships. The relative contribution of genes to disease risk of populations can be exaggerated, however, by studies of gene effects when limited to homogeneous, high-risk cultures where exposure is great and universal. Most of the lack of understanding, and much of the difficulty in identification of susceptible persons, lies in the unavailability of specific genetic markers for CVD and the incapacity of family studies to discriminate intrinsic components without such markers. Recent findings of the gene loci for apolipoprotein regulation hold great promise of an improved understanding of individual differences in blood lipoproteins and their response to diet. There is, for example, evidence of the genetic inheritance of LDL subclasses HDL, apo-B and apo-E.[160] A substantial proportion of the variation in apo-B levels (43 percent) may be explained by a major locus.[161] A major gene controlling LDL subclasses may account for much of the familial aggregation of blood lipids and CHD risk.[162]

Most intrinsic blood lipoprotein regulation, however, is clearly polygenic and strongly interactive with the environment, especially with composition of the habitual diet. Controlled experiments in metabolically normal people suggest that there is a normal distribution of individual blood lipid responses to a known dietary change.[163]

The rare major gene effects that cause extreme manifestations of the hyperlipidemias are increasingly well characterized, but they account for only a small fraction of the mass phenomenon of hypercholesterolemia found in affluent cultures. Thus most atherosclerotic complications and most of the excess CHD events in the general population cannot be attributed to major gene effects. Nevertheless, gene-culture interactions remain important to preventive practice for better detection and individualized therapy of patients who have elevated blood lipid values.

A potentially important aspect of genetically determined diet responses now under investigation is the response of individual lipoprotein fractions to specific dietary factors, mainly fatty acids and cholesterol. A wider issue, however, is the relative magnitude of the contribution of intrinsic regulation to the large population differences found for average blood lipid values and their distributions. For the time being, this contribution remains speculative.

Genetic control of CVD risk factors *other* than blood lipids is even less well known.[164] For example, not yet identified are genetic traits that might affect individual sensitivity to salt intake, to the atherogenic effect of cigarette smoking, or to the regulation of blood insulin and glucose levels, arterial wall enzymes, or personality type.

The public health view that a favorable environment assures minimal expression of phenotypic risk provides the rationale for a population approach to prevention. This rationale has not been effectively challenged, but neither has it been universally accepted.

Combined Risk Factors

Clinical, laboratory, and epidemiological studies of CVD risk factors have been oriented mainly toward determining individual causal roles for each factor. Cardiovascular diseases are clearly related, however, in both individuals and communities, to *multiple* factors operating together over time. Multiple-factor risk is firmly established and actually is quantified for both CHD and stroke. Based mainly on Framingham and Pooling Project analysis, a consistent, independent, and at least additive contribution is found for each of the major risk factors: cigarette smoking, arterial blood pressure, and total serum cholesterol level.[61] The risk ratio between highest and lowest categories for *combined* risk within populations is approximately 8- to 10-fold, in contrast to the risk ratio for single risk factors, which is approximately 2- to 4-fold.

Prediction regressions derived from follow-up experience in European men, with the use of four major risk factors at baseline, when applied to men in the United States, show the multiple-risk concept to be "universal." That is, the regressions define a continuum of CHD risk among individual U.S. men in a society that has quite different CHD rates overall.[165] The slope of the relationship (regression) between the combined risk factors and disease, however, is much steeper in the United States than in the European population. At any given level of multiple risk, U.S. rates are twice those in Europe. This cultural difference in the "force" of risk factors indicates that a sizable influence on population differences in CHD risk remains unknown. Nevertheless, since these few risk factors operate universally and explain a substantial part of individual and population risk differences, public health action on that part of the difference now explained is both promising and indicated.

Still another interpretation of the evidence of combined risk of CHD is that the synergism between risk characteristics leads to a major potential for preventive effects in the population by achieving relatively small shifts in the means and distributions of the multiple risk factors. This does not exclude the possibility of a population threshold for risk factors, below which population risk is remote. That is indicated by the relative scarcity of mass atherosclerosis and CHD in societies in which average serum total cholesterol levels are less than 200 mg/dL. Nor does it exclude the concept of *necessary* versus *contributory* causes. In the absence of the presumed necessary factor (i.e., mass hypercholesterolemia), population risk is negligible. It may be that the departures from perfect prediction, found with the use of multiple regression analysis, are due in part to their failure to include the duration of exposure to, or the directionality of, a particular risk level.

▸ ACUTE RHEUMATIC FEVER AND RHEUMATIC HEART DISEASE

Rheumatic fever and rheumatic heart disease are important public health problems in parts of the world where poverty, overcrowding, malnutrition, and inadequate medical care are commonplace.[166,167] Even in industrialized societies, a relatively high prevalence of rheumatic fever persists in pockets of poverty, and outbreaks have been reported recently in affluent areas.[168–170] Despite that rheumatic fever is demonstrably preventable and rheumatic heart disease has declined dramatically in most industrialized nations, this condition remains a major public health problem internationally.

For more than 40 years it has been known that group A streptococcus infection underlies initial and recurrent attacks of rheumatic fever (see Chapter 9). The immunologic mechanisms and circumstances by which infection with this organism produces rheumatic fever and rheumatic heart disease and acute and chronic glomerulonephritis are well understood.[171] In some surveys, as many as 3 percent of patients, rheumatic fever develops after known streptococcal infections.[172] As many as 50 percent of those who have once had rheumatic fever will, if untreated, experience attacks after a subsequent streptococcal infection. This suggests that host factors significantly determine susceptibility. Age is also an obvious factor, for example, infants do not develop rheumatic fever even though they are susceptible to streptococcal infection and glomerulonephritis. Such differences in susceptibility are clearly developmental, such as the variation with age, but others may have a genetic basis. The tendency of rheumatic fever to cluster in families, however, may be explained by shared environment as well as genes.

During the 1960s, the incidence of acute rheumatic fever per 100,000 urban children 2 to 14 years of age in the United States ranged from 23 to 28 for whites and 27 to 55 for blacks. The incidence was still higher in Puerto Ricans. Currently it is closer to 2 per 100,000 with most cases among the underprivileged.

In other parts of the world, the lowest rates of rheumatic fever have been observed in Scandinavia, with 1.3 cases per 100,000. In underdeveloped nations, the rates are much higher. Prevalence among school-age children in South America ranges from 1 to 10 percent.[176]

Mortality from rheumatic fever and rheumatic heart disease has fallen significantly in the United States in this century. It was 14.8 per 100,000 in 1950, 7.3 in 1970, and 2.7 in 1986, a decline of 82 percent.

The diagnosis of acute rheumatic fever is made principally from clinical findings with the revised Jones criteria (see Chapter 9).[173] These may be insufficiently sensitive, however, to detect mild cases, particularly in Western countries where clinical patterns have changed so that arthritis is often the only presenting manifestation; chorea, subcutaneous nodules, and erythema marginatum are now rarely seen. Diagnosis may be complicated by the lack of a preceding sore throat or an apparent infection.[174]

Rapid antigen tests for the "diagnosis" of group A streptococcal throat infections are highly specific but less sensitive. A positive test indicates the need for treatment, but a negative test indicates the need for a throat culture.[175] Antibody tests can confirm a recent group A streptococcal infection (e.g., antistreptolysin O).

Current recommendations for the primary prevention of acute rheumatic fever and rheumatic heart disease are as follows: throat cultures should be made for all patients with tonsillopharyngitis, and those with a positive culture for group A streptococci should be treated when the diagnosis is made.[176] Treatment effectively prevents rheumatic fever, even when started several days after the onset of the acute illness. The recommended treatment schedule of the American Heart Association is seen in Table 51-3. In the United States, mass throat cultures in schools have been advocated because many children with streptococcal infections have no symptoms or seek no care when symptoms are present. Such programs may be of particular value in economically depressed areas, where inaccessibility of medical care and lack of health awareness in the population are barriers to the detection and treatment of streptococcal infections.

It has long been known that initial attacks of rheumatic fever can be prevented by adequately treating the preceding streptococcal infection. More recently, a study of the incidence of hospitalized cases of rheumatic fever among black children in Baltimore indicates that incidence decreased 60 percent in areas with comprehensive care clinics but remained unchanged in other areas.[172] The decline was limited to cases of rheumatic fever that followed symptomatic pharyngitis.

A program of mass throat cultures of children in the schools of Wyoming resulted in a decrease in positive culture rates for β-streptococci, from 10 percent positive at the beginning of each school year to below 5 percent at the end of the year, along with an apparent decrease in incidence of acute rheumatic fever.[177] The cost was about $1 per pupil per year.

All acute streptococcal infections should be treated. Recurrent rheumatic fever can usually be prevented, and progressive valvular damage avoided, by the eradication of streptococcal infection. For long-term chemoprophylaxis, sulfadiazine given orally in a dose 1,000 mg daily (500 mg for small children) has proved effective, as has oral penicillin V, 250 mg twice daily, or benzathine penicillin, 1.2 million units intramuscularly every 4 weeks. Erythromycin given orally 250 mg twice a day may be used in penicillin-sensitive individuals. The major problem with long-term chemoprophylaxis is non-

TABLE 51-3. PRIMARY PREVENTION OF RHEUMATIC FEVER (TREATMENT OF STREPTOCOCCAL TONSILLOPHARYNGITIS)

Agent	*Dose*	*Mode*	*Duration*
Benzathine penicillin G	600,00 units for patients <60 lb 1,200,000 units for patients >60 lb *or*	Intramuscular	Once
Penicillin V (phenoxymethyl penicillin)	250 mg 2–3 times daily	Oral	10 days
■ ***FOR INDIVIDUALS ALLERGIC TO PENICILLIN***			
Erythromycin estolate	20–40 mg/kg per day 2–4 times daily (maximum 1 g per day) *or*	Oral	10 days
Erythromycin ethylsuccinate	40 mg/kg per day 2–4 times daily (maximum 1 g per day)		

The following agents are acceptable but are usually not recommended: amoxicillin, dicloxacillin, oral cephalosporins, and clindamycin. The following are not acceptable: sulfonamides, trimethoprim, tetracyclines, and chloramphenicol.

*Adapted from Pediatrics 1995;96:758–764.

compliance. Prophylaxis for patients who have had rheumatic carditis and valvular disease should be lifelong. In patients with a history of rheumatic fever without rheumatic carditis, prophylaxis should continue until the patient is in the early twenties and for at least 5 years after the last attack.[175]

► CONGENITAL HEART DISEASE

Malformations of the cardiovascular system are among the more frequently occurring congenital defects. They result from developmental errors caused by inherent defects in the genetic material of the embryo, environmental factors, or both.[178–183]

Family studies suggest that the offspring of parents with congenital heart disease have malformation rates ranging from 1.4 to 16.1 percent.[184] Identical twins are both affected 25 to 30 percent of the time. While these and other findings of familial aggregation suggest polygenic factors, common environment may also play a role.[183] Chromosomal aberrations or gender mutations account for less than 10 percent of all congenital cardiovascular anomalies. In addition, noncardiac disorders produce cardiovascular defects; these include Marfan's syndrome, Friedreich's ataxia, glycogen storage disease, and Down's and Turner's syndromes.

Maternal viral infections during pregnancy are estimated to cause up to 10 percent of all congenital cardiac malformations. Rubella in the first 2 months of pregnancy is associated with congenital malformations in about 80 percent of live births and is thought to account for 2 to 4 percent of all congenital heart disease. Patent ductus arteriosus and pulmonic stenosis are the most common defects. Subclinical Coxsackievirus infections may be related to congenital heart disease. Acute hypoxia, residence at high altitudes, high carboxyhemoglobin levels, and uterine vascular changes from cigarette smoking are other potential causes.[182] Maternal x-ray exposure results in an increased incidence of Down's syndrome and possibly other congenital defects.[181] Maternal metabolic defects, such as diabetes mellitus and phenylketonuria, are associated with increased incidence of congenital heart defects.

Animal investigations, which have not been substantiated in humans, indicate that dietary deficiencies in the mother may result in congenital malformations. Obstetric problems are associated with congenital heart disease, including association of advanced maternal age with Down's syndrome and a history of vaginal bleeding (threatened abortion) during the first 11 weeks of gestation with prematurity. The teratogenic potential of drugs, such as thalidomide and folic acid antagonists, is well documented. In addition, dextroamphetamines, anticonvulsants, lithium chloride, alcohol, and progesterone/estrogen are highly suspected teratogens acting in the first trimester of pregnancy, as are certain pesticides and herbicides (see Chapter 26).[185]

Data on the true incidence of congenital heart disease are limited. The chief sources of information are birth certificate and hospital birth data.[179,180] Birth certificate data usually underestimate the true rate.

A U.S. multicenter collaborative study in 1970 yielded the following incidence rates for congenital heart disease: 8.1 per 1,000 total births, 7.6 per 1,000 live births, and 16.5 per 1,000 twin births.[186] Most are correctable by modern medical and surgical methods, including cardiac transplantation; it is estimated that only one child per 1,000 cannot be helped by such approaches.[187]

Although the overall incidence of congenital heart disease has apparently remained stable, the distribution of types of defects may be shifting. This includes unexplained increases in ventricular septal defects and patent ductus arteriosus. A decline in the number of infants born with rubella-caused defects may be explained by vaccination programs.[186]

Primary prevention of congenital heart disease includes the following established measures:[179]

1. Genetic counseling of potential parents and families with congenital heart disease
2. Rubella immunization programs
   a. Identification of susceptible women of childbearing age by serologic examination
   b. Immunization of susceptible women
   c. Avoidance of pregnancy for 2 months after rubella vaccination
3. Avoidance of exposure to viral diseases during pregnancy
4. Administration of all usual vaccines to all children to eliminate reservoirs of infection
5. Avoidance of radiation during pregnancy
6. Avoidance of exposure to gas fumes, air pollution, cigarettes, alcohol, pesticides, herbicides, and high altitude during the first trimester of pregnancy
7. Avoidance of drugs of any kind during the first trimester of pregnancy, especially drugs of known or suspected teratogenic potential.

► CARDIOMYOPATHIES AND MYOCARDITIS

Cardiomyopathies are a broad group of cardiac diseases that involve the heart muscle. Although less common in industrialized nations, they account for 30 percent or more of heart disease deaths in some developing countries.[188] They are of diverse etiology and are usually classified by the functional results of their effects on the myocardium: dilated or congestive, hypertrophic and restrictive. Recent recommendations suggest that the term *cardiomyopathy* be reserved for disease of unknown origin involving heart muscle.[188] However, the common use of the term still associates it with specific causal syndromes when these are known.

Some cardiomyopathies are diagnosed in their acute phase, where inflammation of the myocardium is common (myocarditis). While myocarditis is particularly difficult to categorize, diagnosis has been facilitated by the widespread use of endomyocardial biopsy.[189] These techniques have suggested that an inflammatory reaction is more common than was previously suspected. Identified causes include infectious, metabolic, toxic, allergic, and genetic factors.[190] Myocarditis and cardiomyopathy may be mild and undetected but also can be rapidly fatal through progressive heart failure.

In industrialized nations, cardiomyopathies appear to be increasing in prevalence, although it is unclear whether there is an actual increase or an increase in professional awareness and improved diagnostic techniques.[191] The latter include use of the echocardiogram, Doppler flow studies, and catheter-based endomyocardial biopsy. A study of death certificates in the United States in 1982 found 10,345 deaths assigned to cardiomyopathy.[191] The majority of these (87 percent) were coded to "other primary cardiomyopathy," with cause unspecified. Surveillance of Olmsted County, Minnesota, found an incidence of idiopathic dilated cardiomyopathy of 6 per 100,000 person years. Overall prevalence was 35.3 per 100,000 population.[192] In these and other studies, cases of cardiomyopathy are distributed evenly across ages and sexes.[193]

Alcohol abuse is an important cause of cardiomyopathy, accounting for approximately 8 percent of all cases in the United States.[191,194] Alcohol causes myocardial damage by several mechanisms.[195,196] These include (*a*) a direct toxic effect, (*b*) effects of thiamine deficiencies, and (*c*) effects of additives such as cobalt in alcoholic beverages. Abstinence from alcohol may halt or reverse the cardiomyopathy.[197]

Another major cause of cardiomyopathy in industrialized countries is viral infection, particularly Coxsackie B virus, echovirus, influenza, and polio,[198] often beginning as a viral myocarditis. Subclinical viral disease is thought to be more common than was previously suspected, with many patients recovering without sequelae. More severe forms, however, result in dilated cardiomyopathy and death due to congestive heart failure or arrhythmias. Recent research has suggested an autoimmune component and indicated that immunosuppressive therapy may be helpful in modifying the disease.[199] However, early clinical trials have shown little beneficial effect for corticosteroids.[200]

Hypertrophic cardiomyopathy is less common as a cause of death.[201] Largely undetected until the advent of echocardiographic techniques, it is becoming increasingly clear that this condition rarely causes difficulty for patients and is usually well managed with pharmacologic therapy.[201]

In South and Central America, trypanosomiasis (Chagas' disease) is endemic; an estimated 20 million people are afflicted.[202] Extensive chronic myocarditis with heart failure may be observed years after the initial infection with the trypanosome. An acute infectious phase, characterized by fulminant and fatal myocarditis, occurs mainly in children. In most cases, however, an average of 20 years passes before Chagas' cardiomyopathy becomes clinically apparent. An autoimmune process may play some role in the disease.[203] Diagnosis is made by means of serologic study or a xenodiagnostic test. Although antiparasitic agents, such as nitroimidazole derivatives, can alter the acute infestation, there is little evidence that they are effective for the cardiomyopathy.[188]

Schistosomiasis is a major public health problem in the Nile and Yangtze basins where the parasitic infection is endemic, involving 85 percent of the population in certain areas. Chronic pulmonary embolization leads to pulmonary hypertension and right heart failure, but direct involvement of the myocardium is rare. New antiparasitic agents can limit the infection, but the main preventive strategy is a public health approach to controlling the vectors.

▶ SYPHILITIC HEART DISEASE

Although the prevalence and patterns of syphilis worldwide have been altered significantly in the antibiotic era, it remains an important public health problem in many nations. Recent reports indicate a rise in reported cases of primary and secondary syphilis in the United States, and surveys in developing nations indicate continued high incidence and prevalence rates.[204] An increase in reported cases and a general decline in medical alertness to this condition encourage a continuing reservoir for late complications. Life-threatening tertiary syphilis is found in approximately 25 to 30 percent of untreated cases.[205] Approximately 10 percent of those are cardiovascular syphilis, manifest predominantly as uncomplicated syphilitic aortitis, aortic aneurysm, aortic valvulitis with regurgitation, and coronary ostial stenosis.[206] Although a course of antibiotic therapy is indicated when cardiovascular syphilis is diagnosed, there is little evidence that it alters the course of the cardiovascular disease.

Because syphilis remains preventable, detectable, and treatable in the early stages, public health approaches should lead to eradication of the late effects of syphilis, including those in the cardiovascular system.[207]

▶ PREVENTIVE STRATEGIES

A population approach to CVD prevention has been formally outlined by the World Health Organization.[6] It embraces both the systematic practice of screening and education for high risk, where national priorities can afford such practices, and broad public health policy and programs in health promotion for communities.

Strategies for preventive practice are now widely available. Community-based strategies, programs, and materials are becoming available. National programs are under way in blood pressure control, diet and blood lipids, and smoking. Finally, health-promotion resource centers are now established for training in the design and dissemination of preventive programs. The student and the health worker are referred to these sources: Division of Nutrition, Chronic Disease Prevention and Health Promotion at the Centers for Disease Control and Prevention, Atlanta, GA; and the Henry J. Kaiser Family Foundation, Menlo Park, CA, and the Office of Prevention, Education and Control, National Heart Lung and Blood Institute, Bethesda, MD.

▶ REFERENCES

1. Higgens M, Luepker R (eds): Report of a conference on trends and determinants of coronary heart disease mortality: international comparisons. Int J Epidemiol 18(Suppl 1), 1989
2. McGovern PG, Pankow JS, Shahar E, et al: Recent trends in acute coronary heart disease: mortality, morbidity, medical care, and risk factors. N Engl J Med 334:884–890, 1996
3. World Health Organization MONICA Project Principal Investigators: The WHO MONICA Project: a major international collaboration. J Clin Epidemiol 41:105–114, 1988
4. Tunstall-Pedoe H, Kuulasmaa K, Amouyel P, Arveiler D, Rajakangas AM, Pajak A: Myocardial infarction and coronary deaths in the World Health Organization MONICA Project: registration procedures, event rates, and case-fatality rates in 38 populations from 21 countries in four continents. Circulation 90:583–612, 1994
5. World Health Organization: World Health Statistics Annual. Geneva: World Health Organization, 1986, 1987, 1988
6. World Health Organization: Prevention of Coronary Heart Disease: Report of a WHO Expert Committee. WHO Technical Report Series, No. 678. Geneva: World Health Organization, 1982
7. Inter-Society Commission for Heart Disease Resources: Optimal resources for primary prevention of atherosclerotic diseases. Circulation 70:153A–205A, 1984
8. The Lipid Research Clinic Program: The lipid research clinic's coronary primary prevention trial results. 11. The relationship of reduction in incidence of coronary heart disease to cholesterol lowering. JAMA 251:365–374, 1984
9. The Multiple Risk Factor Intervention Trial Research Group: Mortality after 16 years for participants randomized to the Multiple Risk Factor Intervention Trial. Circulation 94:946–951, 1996
10. Keys A (ed): Coronary heart disease in seven countries. Circulation 41–42 (Suppl I), 1970
11. Keys A: Seven Countries: Death and Coronary Heart Disease in Ten Years. Cambridge, MA: Harvard University Press, 1979
12. Gordon T, Garcia-Palmieri MR, Kagan A, Kannel WB, Schiffman J: Differences in coronary heart disease mortality in Framingham, Honolulu and Puerto Rico. J Chronic Dis 27:329–344, 1974
13. Rose G: Incubation period of coronary heart disease. Br Med J 284:1600–1601, 1982
14. McGill HC Jr (ed): Geographic Pathology of Atherosclerosis. Baltimore: Williams & Wilkins, 1968
15. Marmot MG, Syme SL, Kagan A, et al: Epidemiologic studies of coronary heart disease and stroke in Japanese men living in Japan, Hawaii and California: prevalence of coronary and hypertensive heart disease and associated risk factors. Am J Epidemiol 102:514–525, 1975
16. Blackburn H: Trends and determinants of CHD mortality: changes in risk factors and their effects. Int J Epidemiol 18 (Suppl 1): S210–S215, 1989
17. Stern MP: The recent decline in ischemic heart disease mortality. Ann Intern Med 91:630–640, 1979
18. Cooper R: Rising death rates in the Soviet Union: the impact of coronary heart disease. N Engl J Med 304:1259–1265, 1981
19. Luepker RV: Epidemiology of atherosclerotic disease in population groups. In Pearson TA, Criqui MH, Luepker RV, Oberman A, Winston M (eds): Primer in Preventive Cardiology. Dallas: American Heart Association, 1994 pp 1–10
20. Elmer PJ: Obesity and cardiovascular disease: practical approaches for weight loss in clinical practice. In Pearson TA, Criqui MH, Luepker RV, Oberman A, Winston M (eds): Primer in Preventive Cardiology. Dallas: American Heart Association, 1994, pp 189–204
21. Truswell AS: Diet and nutrition of hunter-gatherers. In Elliott K, Whelan J (eds): Health and Disease in Tribal Societies. Ciba Found Symp 49 213–222, 1977

22. Blackburn H, Prineas RJ: Diet and hypertension: anthropology, epidemiology, and public health implications. Prog Biochem Pharmacol 19:31–79, 1983
23. Eaton SB, Konner M: Paleolithic nutrition: a consideration of its nature and current implications. N Engl J Med 312:283–289, 1985
24. Jacobs DR, Anderson J, Blackburn H: Diet and serum cholesterol: do zero correlations negate the relationships? Am J Epidemiol 10:77–88, 1979
25. Blackburn H: The concept of risk. In Pearson TA, Criqui MH, Luepker RV, Oberman A, Winston M (eds): Primer in Preventive Cardiology. Dallas: American Heart Association, 1994, pp 25–41
26. Blackburn H, Jacobs DR: Sources of the diet-heart controversy: confusion over population versus individual correlations. Circulation 70:775–780, 1984
27. Keys A, Grande F, Anderson JT: Bias and misrepresentation revisited—"perspective" on saturated fat. Am J Clin Nutr 27:188–212, 1974
28. Hegsted DM, McGandy RB, Myers ML, Stare FJ: Quantitative effects of dietary fat on serum cholesterol in man. Am J Clin Nutr 17:281–295, 1965
29. Connor WE, Stone DB, Hodges RE: The interrelated effects of dietary cholesterol and fat upon human serum lipid levels. J Clin Invest 43:1691–1696, 1964
30. Shekelle RB, Shryock AM, Paul O, et al: Diet, serum cholesterol, and death from coronary heart disease: the Western Electric Study. N Engl J Med 304:65–70, 1981
31. Kromhout D, de Lezenne Coulander C: Diet, prevalence and 10-year mortality from coronary heart disease in 871 middle-aged men: the Zutphen study. Am J Epidemiol 119:733–741, 1984
32. McGee DL, Reed DM, Yano K, Kagan A, Tillotson J: Ten-year incidence of coronary heart disease in the Honolulu Heart Program: relationship to nutrient intake. Am J Epidemiol 119:667–676, 1984
33. Kushi LH, Lew RA, Stare FJ, et al: Diet and 20-year mortality from coronary heart disease: the Ireland-Boston Diet-Heart Study. N Engl J Med 312:811–818, 1985
34. Mattson FH, Grundy SM: Comparison of effects of dietary saturated, monounsaturated, and polyunsaturated fatty acids on plasma lipids and lipoproteins in man. J Lipid Res 26:194–202, 1985
35. St. Clair RW: Atherosclerosis regression in animal models: current concepts of cellular and biochemical mechanisms. Prog Cardiovasc Dis 26:109–132, 1983
36. Clarkson TB, Bond MG, Bullock BC, McLaughlin KJ, Sawyer JK: A study of atherosclerosis regression in Macaca mulatta: V. Changes in abdominal aorta and carotid and coronary arteries from animals with atherosclerosis induced for 38 months and then regressed for 24 or 48 months at plasma cholesterol concentrations of 300 or 200 mg/dl. Exp Mol Pathol 41:96–118, 1984
37. The Lipid Research Clinic Program: The Lipid Research Clinic's coronary primary prevention trial results. 1. Reduction in incidence of coronary heart disease. JAMA 251:351–364, 1984
38. Anitschkow N: Experimental atherosclerosis in animals. In Cowdry EV (ed): Arteriosclerosis. New York: Macmillan, 1983, p 271
39. Wallace RB, Lynch CF, Pomrehn PR, Criqui MH, Heiss G: Alcohol and hypertension: epidemiologic and experimental considerations. Circulation 64:41–47, 1981
40. Dyer AR, Stamler J, Paul O, et al: Alcohol, cardiovascular risk factors and mortality: the Chicago experience. Circulation 64:20–27, 1981
41. Haskell WL, Comargo C, Williams PT, et al: The effect of cessation and resumption of moderate alcohol intake on serum high density lipoprotein subfractions. N Engl J Med 310:805–810, 1984
42. Kagan A, Yano K, Rhoads G, McGee D: Alcohol and cardiovascular disease: the Hawaiian experience. Circulation 64:27–31, 1981
43. Klatsky AL, Friedman GD, Siegelaub AB: Alcohol use and cardiovascular disease: the Kaiser-Permanente experience. Circulation 64:32–41, 1981
44. Kaelber CT, Barboriak J (eds): Symposium on alcohol and cardiovascular diseases. Circulation 64(Suppl 3), 1981
45. Kare MR, Fregly MJ, Bernard RA (eds): Biological and Behavioral Aspects of Salt Intake. New York: Academic Press, 1980
46. Freis ED: Salt, volume and the prevention of hypertension. Circulation 53:589–595, 1976
47. Meneely GR, Battarbee HD: High sodium–low potassium environment and hypertension. Am J Cardiol 38:768–785, 1976
48. Gleibermann L: Blood pressure and dietary salt in human populations. Ecol Food Nutr 2:143–156, 1973
49. INTERSALT Cooperative Research Group: INTERSALT: an international study of electrolyte excretion and blood pressure: results for 24 hour urinary sodium and potassium excretion. Br Med J 297:319–328, 1988
50. Joseph JG, Prior IAM, Salmond CE, Stanley D: Elevation of systolic and diastolic blood pressure associated with migration: the Tokelau Island Migrant Study. J Chronic Dis 36(7):507–516, 1983
51. Kesteloot H, Vuylsteks M, Costenoble A: Relationship between blood pressure and sodium and potassium intake in a Belgian male population group. In Kesteloot K, Joossens J (eds): Epidemiology of Arterial Blood Pressure. The Hague: Nijhoff, 1980, pp 345–351
52. Grimm RH Jr, Kofron PM, Neaton JD, et al: Effect of potassium supplementation combined with dietary sodium reduction on blood pressure in men taking antihypertensive medication. J Hypertens 6:S591–S593, 1988
53. Shimamoto T, Komachi Y, Inada H, et al: Trends for coronary heart disease and stroke and their risk factors in Japan. Circulation 79:503–515, 1989
54. Sharrett AR, Feinleib M: Water constituents and trace elements in relation to cardiovascular diseases. Prev Med 4:20–36, 1975
55. Liao Y, Cooper RS, McGee DL: Iron status and coronary heart disease: negative findings from the NHANES I Epidemiologic Follow-up Study. Am J Epidemiol 139:704–712, 1994
56. Sempos CT, Looker AC, Gillum RF, Makuc DM: Body iron stores and the risk of coronary heart disease. N Engl J Med 330: 1119–1124, 1994
57. Wallace RB, Anderson RA: Blood lipids, lipid-related measures, and the risk of atherosclerotic cardiovascular disease. Epidemiol Rev 9:95–119, 1987
58. Hulley SB, Rosenman RH, Banol RD, Brand RJ: Epidemiology as a guide to clinical decisions: the associations between triglycerides and coronary heart disease. N Engl J Med 302:1383–1389, 1980
59. NIH Consensus Development Panel: Triglyceride, high density lipoprotein, and coronary heart disease. JAMA 269:505–510, 1993
60. Conference on Blood Lipids in Children: Optimal levels for early prevention of coronary artery disease. Prev Med 12:725–905, 1983
61. The Pooling Project Research Group. Relationship of blood pressure, serum cholesterol, smoking habits, relative weight and ECG abnormalities to incidence of major coronary events: final report of the Pooling Project. J Chronic Dis 31:201–306, 1978
62. Stamler J, Wentworth D, Neaton JD: Is the relationship between serum cholesterol and risk of premature death from coronary heart disease continuous and graded? Findings in 356,222 primary screenees of the Multiple Risk Factor Intervention Trial (MRFIT). JAMA 256:2823–2828, 1986
63. Gordon T, Castelli W, Hjortland MC, Kannel WB, Dawber TR: High density lipoprotein as a protective factor against coronary heart disease. Am J Med 62:707–714, 1977
64. National Diet-Heart Study Research Group: The National Diet-Heart Study: final report. Circulation 37:1–428, 1968
65. Frick MH, Elo O, Haapa K, et al: Helsinki Heart Study: primary prevention trial with gemfibrozil in middle-aged men with dyslipidemia. N Engl J Med 317:1237–1245, 1987

66. Shepherd J, Cobbe SM, Ford I, et al, for the West of Scotland Coronary Prevention Study Group: Prevention of coronary heart disease with provastatin in men with hypercholesterolemia. N Engl J Med 333:1301–1307, 1995
67. Scandinavian Simvastatin Survival Study Group: Randomized trial of cholesterol lowering in 4444 patients with coronary heart disease: the Scandinavian Simvastatin Survival Study (4S). Lancet 344:1383–1389, 1994
67a. Kiekshus H, Pedersen TR: Reducing the risk of coronary events: evidence from the Scandinavian Simvastatin Survival Study. American Journal of Cardiology 76:64C–68C, 1995
67b. Pfeffer MA, Sacks FM, Move LA, et al: Cholesterol and recurrent events: a secondary prevention trial for normolipidemic patients. CARE Investigators. American Journal of Cardiology. 76:98C–106C, 1995
68. Johnson CL, Rifkind BM, Sempos CT, et al: Declining serum total cholesterol levels among US adults. JAMA 269:3002–3008, 1993
69. Gomez-Marin O, Folsom AR, Kottke TE, et al: Improved long-term survival of patients hospitalized with acute myocardial infarction, 1970–1980: the Minnesota Heart Survey. N Engl J Med 316:1353–1359, 1987
70. Gillum RF, Folsom AR, Blackburn H: Decline in coronary heart disease mortality. Am J Med 76:1055–1065, 1984
71. US Department of Health and Human Services, Public Health Service: The Surgeon General's Report on Nutrition and Health. DHHS (PHS) Publication No. 88-50210. Washington DC: Government Printing Office, 1988
72. The Expert Panel: Report of the National Cholesterol Education Program Expert Panel on Detection, Evaluation, and Treatment of High Blood Cholesterol in Adults. Arch Intern Med 148:36–69, 1988
73. National Cholesterol Education Program: Second Report of the Expert Panel on Detection, Evaluation, and Treatment of High Blood Cholesterol in Adults (Adult Treatment Panel II). Circulation 89:1329–1445, 1994
74. National Cholesterol Education Program: Report of the Expert Panel on Population Strategies for Blood Cholesterol Reduction. Arch Intern Med 151:1071–1084, 1991
75. National Cholesterol Education Program: Report of the Expert Panel on Blood Cholesterol Levels in Children and Adolescents. Pediatrics 89:525–584, 1992
76. Barrett-Connor EL: Obesity, atherosclerosis and coronary heart disease. Ann Intern Med 103:1010–1019, 1985
77. Kuczmarski RJ, Flegal KM, Campbell SM, Johnson CL: Increasing prevalence of overweight among US adults: the National Health and Nutrition Examination Surveys, 1960 to 1991. JAMA 272:205–211, 1994
78. Hubert HB, Feinlieb M, McNamara PM, Castelli WP: Obesity as an independent risk factor for cardiovascular disease: a 26-year followup of participants in the Framingham Heart Study. Circulation 67:968–977, 1983
79. Tyroler HA, Heyden S, Hames CG: Weight and hypertension: Evans County studies of blacks and whites. In Paul O (ed): Epidemiology and Control of Hypertension. New York: Grune & Stratton, 1975
80. Rabkin SW, Mathewson FAC, Hsu PH: Relation of body weight to the development of ischemic heart disease in a cohort of young North American men after a 26-year observation period: the Manitoba study. Am J Cardiol 39:452–458, 1977
81. Larsson B, Svardsudd K, Welin L, Wilhelmsen L, Bjorntorp P, Tibblin G: Abdominal adipose tissue distribution, obesity, and risk of cardiovascular disease and death: 13-year follow-up of participants in the study of men born in 1913. Br Med J 288:1401–1404, 1984
82. Donahue RP, Abbott RD, Bloom E, Reed DM, Yano K: Central obesity and coronary heart disease in men. Lancet 1:821–824, 1987
83. Bjorntorp P: The associations between obesity, adipose tissue distribution and disease. Acta Med Scand 723:121–134, 1988
84. Montenegro MR, Solberg LA: Obesity, body weight, body length, and atherosclerosis. Lab Invest 18:594–603, 1968
85. Lissner L, Bengtsson C, Lapidus L, Larsson B, Bengtsson B, Brownell K: Body weight variability and mortality in the Goteborg prospective studies of men and women. In Bjorntorp P, Rossner S (eds): Proceedings of the European Congress of Obesity. London: John Libbey, 1989, pp 55–60
86. Taylor HL, Buskirk ER, Remington RD: Exercise in controlled trials of the prevention of coronary heart disease. Fed Proc 32: 1623–1627, 1973
87. Oldridge NB, Guyatt GH, Fischer ME, Rimm AA: Cardiac rehabilitation after myocardial infarction: combined experience of randomized clinical trials. JAMA 260:945–950, 1988
88. Blackburn H. Jacobs DR: Physical activity and the risk of coronary heart disease [Editorial]. N Engl J Med 319:1217–1219, 1988
89. NIH Consensus Development Panel on Physical Activity and Cardiovascular Health: Physical activity and cardiovascular health. JAMA 276:241–246, 1996
90. Powell KE, Thompson PD, Caspersen CJ, Kendrick JS: Physical activity and the incidence of coronary heart disease. Annu Rev Public Health 8:253–287, 1987
91. Leon AS, Connett J, Jacobs DR Jr, Rauramaa R: Leisure-time physical activity levels and risk of coronary heart disease and death: the Multiple Risk Factor Intervention Trial. JAMA 258:2388–2395, 1987
92. Slattery ML, Jacobs DR Jr, Nichaman MZ: Leisure time physical activity and coronary heart disease death: the U.S. Railroad Study. Circulation 79:304–311, 1989
93. Blair SN, Kohl HW, Paffenbarger RS Jr, Clark DG, Cooper KH, Gibbons LW: Physical fitness and all-cause mortality: a prospective study of healthy men and women. JAMA 262:2395–2401, 1989
94. Paffenbarger RS Jr, Wing AL, Hyde RT: Physical activity as an index of heart attack risk in college alumni. Am J Epidemiol 108:161–175, 1978
95. Paffenbarger RS Jr, Hyde RT, Wing AL, Steinmetz CH: A natural history of athleticism and cardiovascular health. JAMA 252:491–495, 1984
96. Siscovick DS, Weiss NS, Fletcher RH, Lasky T: The incidence of primary cardiac arrest during vigorous exercise. N Engl J Med 311:874–877, 1984
97. Mittleman MA, Maclure M, Tofler GH, et al: Triggering of acute myocardial infarction by heavy physical exertion: protection against triggering of regular exertion. N Engl J Med 329:1677–1683, 1993
98. West KM: Epidemiology of Diabetes and Its Vascular Lesions. New York: Elsevier,1978, pp 375–402
99. Pyorala K, Laakso M, Uusitupa M: Diabetes and atherosclerosis: an epidemiologic view. Diabetes Metab Rev 3:463–524, 1987
100. Knowler WC, Bennett PH, Hammon RF, Miller M: Diabetes incidence and prevalence in Pima Indians: a 19-fold greater incidence than in Rochester, MN. Am J Epidemiol 108:497–505, 1978
101. Barrett-Connor E, Wingard DL: Sex differential in ischemic heart disease mortality in diabetics: a prospective population-based study. Am J Epidemiol 118:489–496, 1983
102. University Group Diabetes Program: A study of the effects of hypoglycemic agents on vascular complications in patients with adult onset diabetes. V. Evaluation of phenoformin therapy. Diabetes 24:65–184, 1975
103. United Kingdom Prospective Diabetes Study Group: United Kingdom prospective diabetes study (UKPDS) 13: relative efficacy of randomly allocated diet, sulphonylurea, insulin, or metformin in patients with newly diagnosed non-insulin dependent diabetes followed for three years. Br Med J 310:83–88, 1995
104. The Diabetes Control and Complications Trial Research Group: The effect of intensive treatment of diabetes on the development

and progression of long-term complications in insulin-dependent diabetes mellitus. N Engl J Med 329:977–986, 1993
105. Stamler R, Stamler J, Lindberg HA, et al: Asymptomatic hyperglycemia and coronary heart disease in middle-aged men in two employed populations in Chicago. J Chronic Dis 32:805–815, 1979
106. Hughes LO: Insulin, Indian origin and ischemic heart disease [Editorial]. Int J Cardiol 26:1–4, 1990
107. SHEP Cooperative Research Group: Prevention of stroke by antihypertensive drug treatment in older persons with isolated systolic hypertension. JAMA 265:3255–3264, 1991
108. Hypertension Detection and Follow-Up Group: The effect of treatment on mortality in "mild" hypertension. N Engl J Med 307: 976–980, 1982
109. Folsom AR, Luepker RV, Gillum RF, et al: Improvement in hypertension detection and control: the Minnesota Heart Survey experience. JAMA 250:916–921, 1983
110. Joint National Committee on Detection, Evaluation, and Treatment of High Blood Pressure: The Fifth Report of the Joint National Committee on Detection, Evaluation, and Treatment of High Blood Cholesterol (JNC V). Arch Intern Med 153:154–183, 1993
111. McGill HC Jr: Potential mechanisms for the augmentation of atherosclerosis and atherosclerotic disease by cigarette smoking. Prev Med 8:390–403, 1979
112. Kannel WB, McGee DL, Castelli WP: Latest perspectives on cigarette smoking and cardiovascular disease: the Framingham Study. J Cardiovasc Rehab 4:267–277, 1984
113. Wilhelmsen L: Coronary heart disease: epidemiology of smoking and intervention studies of smoking. Am Heart J 115:242–249, 1988
114. Amler RW, Dull HB (eds): Closing the Gap: The Burden of Unnecessary Illness. New York: Oxford University Press, 1987
115. Willett WC, Green A, Stampfer MJ, et al: Relative and absolute excess risks of coronary heart disease among women who smoke cigarettes. N Engl J Med 317:1303–1309, 1987
116. Doll R, Hill AB: Mortality in relation to smoking: ten years' observations of British doctors. Br Med J 1:1399–1410, 1964
117. Freidman GD, Petitti DB, Bawol RD, Siegelaub AB: Mortality in cigarette smokers and quitters: effect of base-line differences. N Engl J Med 304:1407–1410, 1981
118. Aberg A, Bergstrand J, Johansson S, et al: Cessation of smoking after myocardial infarction: effects on mortality after ten years. Br Heart J 49:416–422, 1983
119. Luepker RV, Rosamond WD, Murphy R, et al: Socioeconomic status and coronary heart disease risk factor trends: the Minnesota Heart Survey. Circulation 88:2172–2179, 1993
120. Luepker RV, Murray DM, Jacobs DR Jr, et al: Community education for cardiovascular disease prevention: risk factor changes in the Minnesota Heart Health Program. Am J Prev Med 84:1383–1393, 1994
121. Public Health Service, Office on Smoking and Health: Report of the Surgeon General. Reducing the Health Consequences of Smoking: Twenty-Five Years of Progress. Rockville, MD: US Department of Health and Human Services, 1989
122. Meade TW: Clotting factors and ischemic heart disease. In Meade TW (ed): The Epidemiological Evidence from Anti-coagulants in Myocardial Infarction: A Reappraisal. New York: John Wiley & Sons, 1984
123. Ernst E, Resch KL: Fibrinogen as a cardiovascular risk factor: a meta-analysis and review of the literature. Ann Intern Med 118:956–963, 1993
124. Meade TW, Brozovich M, Chakrabarti RR, et al: Hemostatic function and ischemic heart disease: principal results of the Northwick Park Heart Study. Lancet 2:533–537, 1986
125. Chalmers TC, Matta RJ, Smith H. Kunzler AM: Evidence favoring the use of anti-coagulants in the hospital phase of acute myocardial infarction. N Engl J Med 297:1091–1096, 1977
126. Steering Committee of the Physicians' Health Study Research Group HMS: Preliminary report: findings from the aspirin component of the ongoing Physicians' Health Study. N Engl J Med 318:262–264, 1988
127. Grimm RH Jr, Leon AS, Hunninghake DB, et al: Effects of thiazide diuretics on plasma lipids and lipoproteins in mildly hypertensive patients. Ann Intern Med 94:7–11, 1981
128. Beard CM, Fuster V, Elveback LR: Daily and seasonal variation in sudden cardiac death, Rochester, Minnesota, 1950–1975. Mayo Clin Proc 57:704–706, 1982
129. Rosenman RH, Brand RJ, Jenkins CD, et al: Coronary heart disease in the Western Collaborative Group Study: final follow-up experience of 8½ years. JAMA 233:872–877, 1975
130. Haynes SG, Feinleib M, Kannel WB: The relationship of psychosocial factors to coronary heart disease in the Framingham Study. III. Eight-year incidence of coronary heart disease. Am J Epidemiol 111:37–58, 1980
131. Matthews KA, Haynes SG: Type A behavior pattern and coronary disease risk. Am J Epidemiol 123:923–960, 1986
132. Dimsdale JE, Gilbert J, Hutter AM, et al: Predicting cardiac morbidity based on risk factors and coronary angiographic findings. Am J Cardiol 47:73–76, 1981
133. Case RB, Heller SS, Case NB, et al: Type A behavior and survival after acute myocardial infarction. N Engl J Med 312:737–741, 1985
134. Shekelle RB, Gale M, Norusis M: Type A score (Jenkins Activity Survey) and risk of recurrent coronary heart disease in the Aspirin Myocardial Infarction Study. Am J Cardiol 56:221–225, 1985
135. Shekelle RB, Hulley SB, Neaton JD, et al: The MRFIT behavior pattern study. II. Type A behavior and incidence of coronary heart disease. Am J Epidemiol 122:559–570, 1985
136. Cohen JB, Reed D: Type A behavior and coronary heart disease among Japanese men in Hawaii. J Behav Med 8:343–352, 1985
137. Friedmann M, Thorensen CE, Gill JJ, et al: Alteration of type A behavior and reduction in cardiac recurrences in post-myocardial infarction patients. Am Heart J 108:237–248, 1984
138. Ragland DR, Brand RJ: Type A behavior and mortality from coronary heart disease. N Engl J Med 318:65–69, 1988
139. Ragland DR, Brand RJ: Coronary heart disease mortality in the Western Collaborative Group Study: follow-up experience of 22 years. Am J Epidemiol 127:462–475, 1988
140. Matthews KA, Glass DC, Rosenman RH, et al: Competitive drive, pattern A, and coronary heart disease: a further analysis of some data from the Western Collaborative Group Study. J Chronic Dis 30:489–498, 1977
141. Hecker MHL, Chesney MA, Black GW, Frautsch N: Coronary prone behaviors in the Western Collaborative Group Study. Psychosom Med 50:153–164, 1988
142. Barefoot JC, Dahlstrom WG, Williams RB: Hostility, CHD incidence, and total mortality: a 25-year follow-up study of 255 physicians. Psychosom Med 45:59–63, 1983
143. Shekelle RB, Gale M, Ostfeld AM, Paul O: Hostility, risk of coronary heart disease, and mortality. Psychosom Med 45:109–114, 1983
144. Barefoot JC, Dodge KA, Peterson BL, Dahlstrom WG, Williams RB: The Cook-Medley hostility scale: item content and ability to predict survival. Psychosom Med 51(1):46–57, 1989
145. McCranie EW, Watkins LO, Brandsma JM, Sisson BD: Hostility, coronary heart disease (CHD) incidence, and total mortality: lack of an association in a 25-year follow-up study of 478 physicians. J Behav Med 9:119–125, 1986
146. Leon GR, Finn SE, Murray D, Bailey JM: Inability to predict cardiovascular disease from hostility scores of MMPI items related to type A behavior. J Consult Clin Psychol 56:597–600, 1988
147. Hearn MD, Murray DM, Luepker RV: Hostility, coronary heart disease, and total mortality: a 33-year follow-up study of university students. J Behav Med 12:105–121, 1988
148. Dembroski TM, MacDougall JM, Williams RB, Haney TL, Blumenthal JA: Components of type A, hostility, and anger-in:

relationship to angiographic findings. Psychosom Med 47:219–233, 1985
149. MacDougall JM, Dembroski TM, Dimsdale JE, Hackett TP: Components of type A, hostility, and anger-in: further relationship to angiographic findings. Health Psychol 4:137–152, 1985
150. Williams RB, Haney TL, Lee KL, Kong Y, Blumenthal JA, Whalen RE: Type A behavior, hostility, and coronary atherosclerosis. Psychosom Med 42:539–549, 1980
151. Kaplan GA, Salonen JT, Cohen RD, Brand RJ, Syme SL, Puska P: Social connections and mortality from all causes and from cardiovascular disease: prospective evidence from Eastern Finland. Am J Epidemiol 128:370–380, 1988
152. Orth-Gomer K, Johnson JV: Social network interaction and mortality: a six year follow-up study of a random sample of the Swedish population. J Chronic Dis 40:949–957, 1987
153. McGill HC Jr, Stern MP: Sex and atherosclerosis. In Paoletti R, Gotto AM Jr (eds): Atherosclerosis Reviews. New York: Raven Press, 1979, vol 4, pp 157–242
154. Demirovic J: Recent trends in coronary heart disease mortality among women in Yugoslavia. CVD Epidemiology Newsletter 44:96–97, 1988
155. Wahl P, Walden C, Knopp R, et al: Effect of estrogen/progestin potency on lipid/lipoprotein metabolism. N Engl J Med 308:862–867, 1983
156. Grady D, Rubin SM, Petitti DB, et al: Hormone therapy to prevent disease and prolong life in postmenopausal women. Ann Intern Med 117:1016–1037, 1992
157. Stampfer MJ, Colditz GA: Estrogen replacement therapy and coronary heart disease: a quantitative assessment of the epidemiologic evidence. Prev Med 20:47–63, 1991
158. Gilligan DM, Quyyumi AA, Cannon RO III: Effects of physiological levels of estrogen on coronary vasomotor function in postmenopausal women. Circulation 89:2545–2551, 1994
159. The Writing Group for the PEPI Trial: Effects of estrogen or estrogen/progestin regimens on heart disease risk factors in postmenopausal women: the Postmenopausal Estrogen/Progestin Interventions (PEPI) Trial. JAMA 273:199–208, 1995
160. Austin MA, King MC, Bawol RD, Hulley SB, Friedman GD: Risk factors for coronary heart disease in adult female twins: genetic heritability and shared environmental influences. Am J Epidemiol 125:308–318, 1987
161. Hasstedt SJ, Wu L, Williams RR: Major locus inheritance of apolipoprotein B in Utah pedigrees. Genet Epidemiol 4:67–76, 1987
162. Austin MA, King MC, Vranizan KM, Newman B, Krauss RM: Inheritance of low-density lipoprotein subclass patterns: results of complex segregation analysis. Am J Hum Genet 43:838–846, 1988
163. Jacobs DR, Anderson JT, Hannan P, Keys A, Blackburn H: Variability in individual serum cholesterol response to change in diet. Arteriosclerosis 3:349–356, 1983
164. Hunt SC, Hasstedt SJ, Kuida H, Stults BM, Hopkins PN, Williams RR: Genetic heritability and common environmental components of resting and stressed blood pressures, lipids, and body mass index in Utah pedigrees and twins. Am J Epidemiol 129:625–638, 1989
165. Keys A, Aravanis C, Blackburn H, et al: Probability of middle-aged men developing coronary heart disease in five years. Circulation 45:815–828, 1972
166. Strasser T: Rheumatic fever and rheumatic heart disease in the 1970s. Public Health Rev 5:207–234, 1976
167. World Health Organization: Intensified program: action to prevent rheumatic fever/rheumatic heart disease. WHO Document WHO/CVD/84.3. Geneva: World Health Organization, 1984
168. Veasy LG, Tani LY, Hill HR: Persistence of acute rheumatic fever in the intermountain area of the United States. J Pediatr 124:9–16, 1994
169. Hoffman JIE: Congenital heart disease. Pediatr Clin North Am 37:25–43, 1990
170. Zangwill KM, Wald ER, Londino AV: Acute rheumatic fever in western Pennsylvania: a persistent problem into the 1990s. J Pediatr 118:561–563, 1991
171. Wannamaker LW, Matsen JM (eds): Streptococci and Streptococcal Diseases: Recognition, Understanding, and Management. New York: Academic Press, 1972
172. Gordis L, Lilienfeld A, Rodriguez R: Studies in the epidemiology and preventability of rheumatic fever. II. Socio-economic factors and the incidence of acute attacks. J Chronic Dis 21:655–666, 1969
173. Dajani AS, Ayoub EM, Bierman FZ, et al: Guidelines for the diagnosis of rheumatic fever: Jones criteria, updated 1992. JAMA 268:2069–2073, 1992
174. Wannamaker LW: The chain that links the heart to the throat. Circulation 48:9–18, 1973
175. Dajani AS, Bisno AL, Chung KJ, et al: Prevention of rheumatic fever: a statement for health professionals by the Committee on Rheumatic Fever, Endocarditis, and Kawasaki Disease of the Council on Cardiovascular Disease in the Young, the American Heart Association. Circulation 78:1082–1086, 1988
176. Pan American Health Organization: Fourth Meeting of the Working Group on Prevention of Rheumatic Fever. Quito, Ecuador, 1970
177. Phibbs B, Taylor J, Zimmerman RA: A community-wide streptococcal control project: the Natrona County Primary Prevention Program. JAMA 214:2018–2024, 1970
178. Elliot RS, Edwards JE: Pathology of congenital heart disease. In Hurst JW ed: The Heart. New York: McGraw-Hill, 1978
179. Congenital Heart Disease Study Group: Primary prevention of congenital heart disease. In Wright IS, Fredrickson DT (eds): Cardiovascular Diseases, Guidelines for Prevention and Care. Reports of the Inter-Society Commission for Heart Disease Resources. Washington, DC: Government Printing Office, 1972, p 116
180. Higgins ITT: The epidemiology of congenital heart disease. J Chronic Dis 18:699, 1965
181. Nora JJ: Etiologic factors in congenital heart diseases. Pediatr Clin North Am 18:1059–1074, 1971
182. Fredrich J, Alberman ED, Goldsteen H: Possible teratogenic effect of cigarette smoking. Nature 231:529, 1971
183. Rose V, Gold RJM, Lindsay G, et al: A possible increase in the incidence of congenital heart defects among the offspring of affected parents. J Am Coll Cardiol 6:376–382, 1985
184. Ferencz C: Offspring of fathers with cardiovascular malformations. Am Heart J 111:1212–1213, 1986
185. Zierler S: Maternal drugs and congenital heart disease. Obstet Gynecol 65:155–165, 1985
186. NHLBI Working Group on Heart Disease Epidemiology: Report. NIH Report 79-1667. Washington, DC: Government Printing Office, 1979
187. Bailey NA, Lay P. New horizons: infant cardiac transplantation. Heart Lung 18:172–178, 1989
188. World Health Organization: Cardiomyopathies: Report of a WHO Expert Committee. WHO Technical Report Series, No. 697. Geneva: World Health Organization, 1984
189. Fowles RE: Progress of research in cardiomyopathy and myocarditis in the USA. International Symposium on Cardiomyopathy and Myocarditis. Heart Vessels Suppl 1: 5–7, 1985
190. Olsen EGJ: What is myocarditis? International Symposium on Cardiomyopathy and Myocarditis. Heart Vessels Suppl 1:1–3, 1985
191. Shabeter R: Cardiomyopathy: how far have we come in 25 years? How far yet to go? J Am Coll Cardiol 1:252–263, 1983
192. Gillum RF: Idiopathic cardiomyopathy in the United States, 1970–1982. Am Heart J 111:752–755, 1986
193. Codd MB, Sugrue DD, Gersh BJ, Melton J III: Epidemiology of idiopathic dilated and hypertrophic cardiomyopathy: a population-based study in Olmsted County, MN, 1975–1984. Circulation 80:564–572, 1989

194. Okada R. Wakafuji S: Myocarditis in autopsy. International Symposium on Cardiomyopathy and Myocarditis. Heart Vessels Suppl 1:23–29, 1985
195. Rubin E: Alcoholic myopathy in heart and skeletal muscle. N Engl J Med 301:28–33, 1979
196. Alexander CS: Cobalt-beer cardiomyopathy: a clinical and pathological study of twenty-eight cases. Am J Med 53:395–417, 1972
197. Regan TJ, Haider B, Ahmed SS, et al: Whisky and the heart. Cardiovasc Med 2:165, 1977
198. Levine HD: Virus myocarditis: a critique of the literature from clinical, electrocardiographic and pathologic standpoints. Am J Med Sci 277:132–143, 1979
199. McAllister HA Jr: Myocarditis: some current perspectives and future directions. Tex Heart Inst J 14:331–334, 1987
200. Parrillo JE, Cunnion RE, Epstein SE, et al: A prospective, randomized, controlled trial of prednisone for dilated cardiomyopathy. N Engl J Med 321:1061–1068, 1989
201. Wigle ED: Hypertrophic cardiomyopathy 1988. AHA-Mod Concepts Cardiovasc Dis 57:1–6, 1988
202. Hagar JM, Rahimtoola SH: Chagas' heart disease. Curr Probl Cardiol 20:825–924, 1995
203. World Health Organization: Report of the WHO Consultation on Cardiomyopathies: Approaches to Prevention and Early Detection. WHO Document, WHO/CVD/85.6. Geneva: World Health Organization, 1985
204. Centers for Disease Control: Summary of Notifiable Diseases—United States. MMWR 36:54–58, 1988
205. Clark EG, Danbolt N: The Oslo study of the natural course of untreated syphilis: an epidemiologic investigation based on a re-study of the Boeck-Bruusgaard material. Med Clin North Am 48:613, 1964
206. Musher DM: Syphilis. Infect Dis Clin North Am 1:83–95, 1987
207. Jackman JD Jr, Radolf JD: Cardiovascular syphilis. Am J Med 87:425–433, 1989

52

Hypertension

Darwin R. Labarthe

Hypertension, or high blood pressure, is a chronic condition of concern in much of the world due to the role of hypertension in the causation of coronary heart disease, stroke, and other vascular complications with a combined mortality that in some countries exceeds 50 percent of the total deaths. The added morbidity and the personal and societal burdens of treatment contribute further to an immense cost in compromised duration and quality of life, as well as economic cost. Treatment is effective, however, and the detection and long-term management of those at risk present substantial opportunities. In addition, prevention of high blood pressure itself poses a major challenge for public health and preventive medicine worldwide.

For these reasons the World Health Organization has convened expert committees whose reports provide a broad perspective on the prevention of hypertension[1] and in particular on the importance of both research and preventive programs concerning blood pressure in childhood and youth.[2,3]

▸ DEFINITION

Definitions of hypertension have varied with evolving concepts of its natural history, and accepted indications for its treatment have changed. Because risks of morbidity and mortality are graded continuously in relation to blood pressure levels, any demarcation to classify individuals along the continuum as "normal" or "hypertensive" is arbitrary, and persons with hypertension should no longer be viewed as a discrete subgroup.

In a committee report from the U.S. National High Blood Pressure Education Program, which appeared in 1985,[4] it was proposed that both risk and evidence of treatment response should be incorporated in a definition most appropriate for community diagnosis and for decision-making about intervention; that the lowest risk in the population, rather than the average risk, should be taken as the reference or target value; and that multistage rather than single-occasion screening should be incorporated (see discussion of Screening below). Both systolic and diastolic pressure should be included because, although they are highly correlated, each contributes to risk.

Especially within the United States the recommendations of the Joint National Committee on Detection, Evaluation, and Treatment of High Blood Pressure (also of the High Blood Pressure Education Program) are widely recognized. Their most recent (1993) classification of blood pressure for adults is presented in Table 52-1.[5]

▸ MEASUREMENT

Definitions in terms of blood pressure values are strictly meaningful only when the measurement of blood pressure is reliable. The importance of this fact increases as refinement of the objectives of screening requires increasing stratification of populations or groups of patients into multiple discrete classes. Accuracy of classification of the individual on any single occasion of blood pressure measurement depends upon control of potential influences of the circumstances, the equipment and procedures used, and characteristics of the observer. For many years, recommended procedures for blood pressure measurement have been published by the American Heart Association.[6] Training materials for standardization of observers in community blood pressure control programs and for multicenter research programs have also been developed.[7] It is hoped that conformity with such recommendations will eventually become the standard of clinical and public health practice.

A contemporary view of hypertension is not restricted to the upper extreme of the population distribution of blood pressure, where treatment has been shown effective in reducing risks, but encompasses the whole distribution as it varies by age and other attributes within and among populations. Of concern is not only adulthood, where established hypertension is common, but also childhood and youth, where absolute values are lower but are expected to progress to higher values with increasing age in most populations. Accordingly, the natural history and effects of intervention on blood pressure are addressed here, both in adulthood and in childhood and youth.

▸ NATURAL HISTORY IN ADULTS

Prevalence

The prevalence of hypertension in populations is assessed by cross-sectional surveys, with typical results as depicted in Figure 52-1.[8] The frequency distribution of diastolic blood pressure among adults at the first stage of screening for a very large population-based trial (the Hypertension Detection and Follow-up Program (HDFP)) demonstrates a modal value at 80 to 84 mm Hg and the typical skewing toward higher values. The prevalence of "hypertension," if this were based on a single occasion and diastolic pressure alone, would depend on the blood pressure criterion selected, as shown. From the highest values down to 90 mm Hg, the prevalence roughly doubles for each reduction of 5 mm Hg in the criterion value. Obviously, estimates of prevalence depend importantly on the definition used. However defined, prevalence varies among groups by age, sex, and ethnicity. For example, twice as many blacks as whites in the United States exceed each of the criterion values indicated in the figure.

Although variation in blood pressure levels with age follows generally similar patterns by race or ethnicity in the United States, blacks most consistently exhibit the highest values (Fig. 52-2).[9]

Screening

When surveys are conducted for the purpose of identifying individuals for possible intervention, as in the example above from the HDFP,

TABLE 52-1. CLASSIFICATION OF BLOOD PRESSURE FOR ADULTS AGE 18 YEARS AND OLDER[a]

Category	Systolic (mm Hg)	Diastolic (mm Hg)
Normal[b]	<130	<85
High normal	130–139	85–89
Hypertension[c]		
Stage 1 (mild)	140–159	90–99
Stage 2 (moderate)	160–179	100–109
Stage 3 (severe)	180–209	110–119
Stage 4 (very severe)	≥210	≥120

From National High Blood Pressure Education Program: The Fifth Report of the Joint National Committee on Detection, Evaluation, and Treatment of High Blood Pressure. NIH Publication No. 93-1088. Bethesda, MD: National Institutes of Health, National Heart, Lung, and Blood Institute, 1993.

[a] Not taking antihypertensive drugs and not acutely ill. When systolic and diastolic pressures fall into different categories, the higher category should be selected to classify the individual's blood pressure status. For instance, 160/92 mm Hg should be classified as stage 2, and 180/120 mm Hg should be classified as stage 4. Isolated systolic hypertension (ISH) is defined as systolic blood pressure (SBP) ≥ 140 mm Hg and diastolic blood pressure (DBP) < 90 mm Hg and staged appropriately (e.g., 170/85 mm Hg is defined as stage 2 ISH).

[b] Optimal blood pressure with respect to cardiovascular risk is SBP < 120 mm Hg and DBP < 80 mm Hg. However, unusually low readings should be evaluated for clinical significance.

[c] Based on the average of two or more readings taken at each of two or more visits following an initial screening.

Note: In addition to classifying stages of hypertension based on average blood pressure levels, the clinician should specify presence or absence of target-organ disease and additional risk factors. For example, a patient with diabetes and a blood pressure of 142/94 mm Hg plus left ventricular hypertrophy should be classified as "stage 1 hypertension with target-organ disease (left ventricular hypertrophy) and with another major risk factor (diabetes)." This specificity is important for risk classification and management.

more than one occasion of measurement is required. This is because individual variability of blood pressure results in identification of some persons with only transient elevations when a single occasion is observed.

How many persons in the United States have hypertension? There are large differences in estimates, reflecting differences in approaches to screening and the criteria for classification. The estimate of 43.2 million American adults age 20 to 74 years as of the early 1990s was limited to the civilian, noninstitutionalized population. Addition of these other population groups would of course increase the total number.[9]

Incidence

Incidence of hypertension is more difficult to estimate than prevalence. This is because changes in blood pressure levels over time must be determined in a fixed cohort, taking both inaccuracy of measurement and intraindividual variability into account. The possibility that treatment may be initiated by those who have been found hypertensive between study examinations must also be addressed. Such an investigation has been reported from the HDFP, cited above, in which persons not definitely hypertensive at initial screening were classified as to the presence or absence of diastolic pressures of 95 mm Hg or greater after two-stage rescreening 3 years later (Table 52-2).[10]

The overall incidence rate of 3 percent per year included rates of about 2 percent per year for white men and women and rates more than twice as great for blacks, especially black men. The incidence rates were closely related to initial blood pressure values, as would be expected, and for those with values from 80 to 94 mm Hg at initial screening the incidence was 5 percent per year. This result emphasizes the potential importance, for prevention of hypertension, of the early recognition of those at intermediate risk.

Incidence of hypertension was previously investigated among whites and blacks in Evans County, Georgia, and was found to relate strongly to both overweight at the baseline examination and to weight gain of 10 pounds or more in the 7-year interval of analysis.[11] The greater incidence in blacks than in whites, in each class of baseline weight and weight gain, predicted the results observed in the HDFP.

Secular Trends

The distribution of blood pressure values in successive national surveys in the United States from 1960–1962 to 1988–1991 has shifted downward, as illustrated for selected age groups in Figure 52-3.[12] Not only the ninetieth percentile values but also the median values decreased. This indicates a general shift in the whole distribution and not only an effect of treatment of high blood pressure, which would specifically affect the upper extreme values.

Risks

The importance of blood pressure as a public health problem results from its contribution to the risks of morbidity and mortality. Early recognition of this fact stimulated research by the Society of Actuaries, beginning early in the twentieth century, on the relation of blood pressure to mortality among life insurance policyholders. Such studies

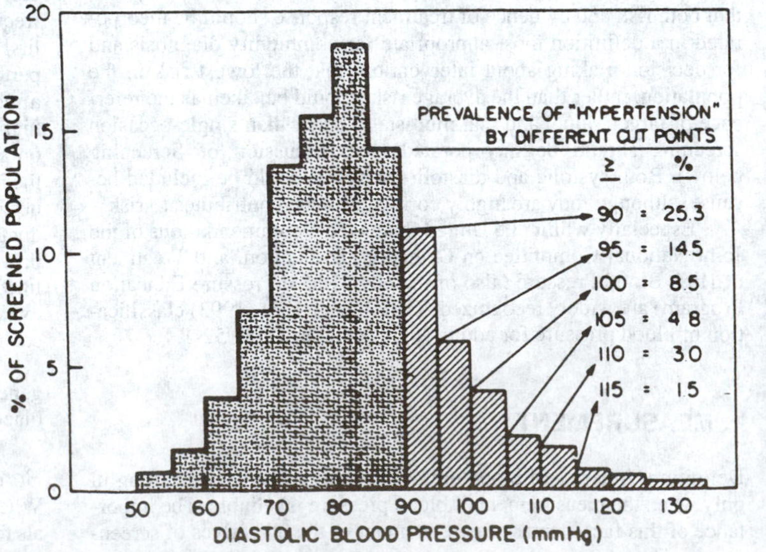

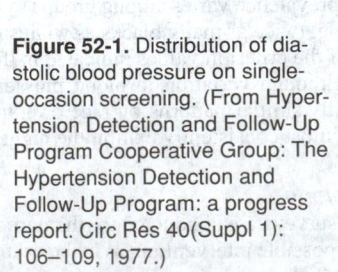

Figure 52-1. Distribution of diastolic blood pressure on single-occasion screening. (From Hypertension Detection and Follow-Up Program Cooperative Group: The Hypertension Detection and Follow-Up Program: a progress report. Circ Res 40(Suppl 1): 106–109, 1977.)

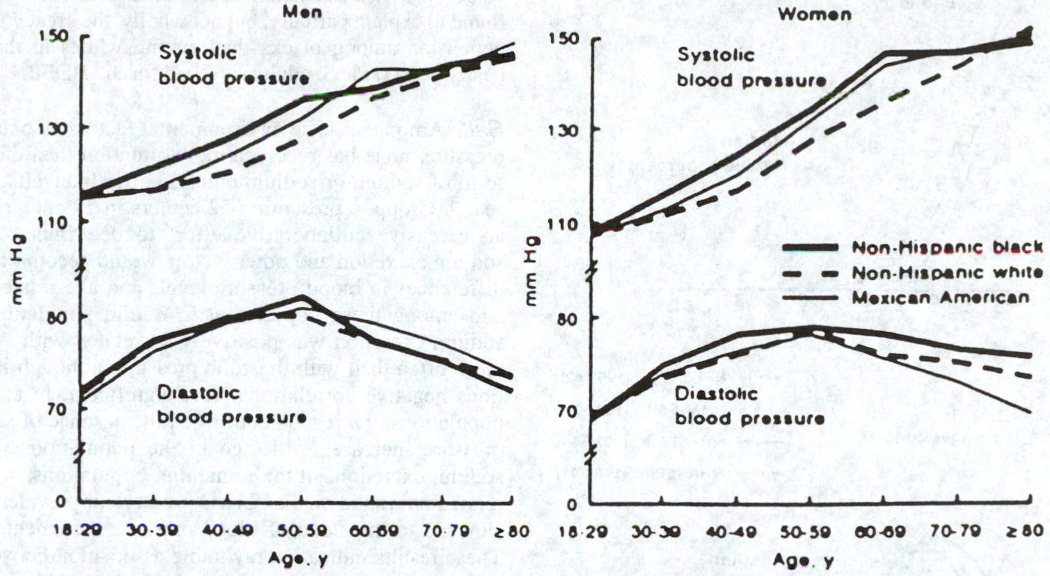

Figure 52-2. Mean systolic and diastolic blood pressure by age and race/ethnicity for men and women. U.S. population 18 years of age and older. (From Burt VL, Whelton P, Rocella EJ, et al: Prevalence of hypertension in the US adult population. Results from the Third National Health and Nutrition Examination Survey, 1988–1991. Hypertension 25:305–313, 1995.)

have demonstrated independent contributions to risk for both systolic and diastolic pressure (Fig. 52-4).[13]

In addition, data from five long-term cohort studies of cardiovascular diseases in American adults were pooled to estimate the risk of several specific fatal or nonfatal cardiovascular events in relation to prior blood pressure levels (Fig. 52-5).[14] These data demonstrate strong gradients of risk associated with increasing blood pressure values. The same data were further analyzed by the Working Group on Risk and High Blood Pressure, whose report indicated risks for several cardiovascular endpoints which were 1.5 to 2 times as great among persons with baseline diastolic pressures from 80 to 89 mm Hg as for those with lower values.[4]

Determinants

Age, Race, Sex and Education. The relation of blood pressure levels to age, alluded to above, is common to most, though not all, adult populations for which cross-sectional survey data are available. These observations were summarized 25 years ago by Epstein and Eckoff, who schematically represented patterns of mean systolic blood pressure by age in many populations around the world (Fig. 52-6).[15]

Commonly, the upward slope of mean systolic pressure was a few millimeters of mercury per decade. This increase in the population mean by age was rarely absent. However, the existence of exceptions has been interpreted to indicate that hypertension in adults reflects not aging itself but more specific environmental influences. Sex

TABLE 52-2. THREE-YEAR INCIDENCE OF HYPERTENSION

	A Incidence	B % of A on Treatment	C Incidence of Treated Case (A × B)	D Remaining Cases (A – C)	E Confirmation Rate	F Percent New Confirmed Cases (D × E)	G Two-stage Incidence of Hypertension (C + F)
■ ***RACE AND SEX***							
Black men	28.6	39.6	11.3	17.3	53.4	9.2	20.5 6.8/yr
Black women	23.3	49.5	11.5	11.8	41.8	4.9	16.4 5.5/yr
White men	8.2	53.0	4.4	3.8	47.6	1.8	6.2 2.1/yr
White women	9.6	73.1	7.0	2.6	29.8	0.8	7.8 2.6/yr
■ ***BASELINE DBP (MM HG)***							
<80	5.0	65.1	3.3	1.7	29.7	0.5	3.8 1.3/yr
80–94	16.8	78.8	13.2	3.6	46.3	1.7	14.9 5.0/yr
Labiles	41.8	51.2	21.4	20.4	46.2	9.4	30.8 10.3/yr
Total	11.8	57.4	6.8	5.0	43.6	2.2	9.0 3.0/yr

From Apostolides AY, Cutter G, Daugherty SA, et al: Three-year incidence of hypertension in 13 U.S. communities. Prev Med 11:487–499, 1982.

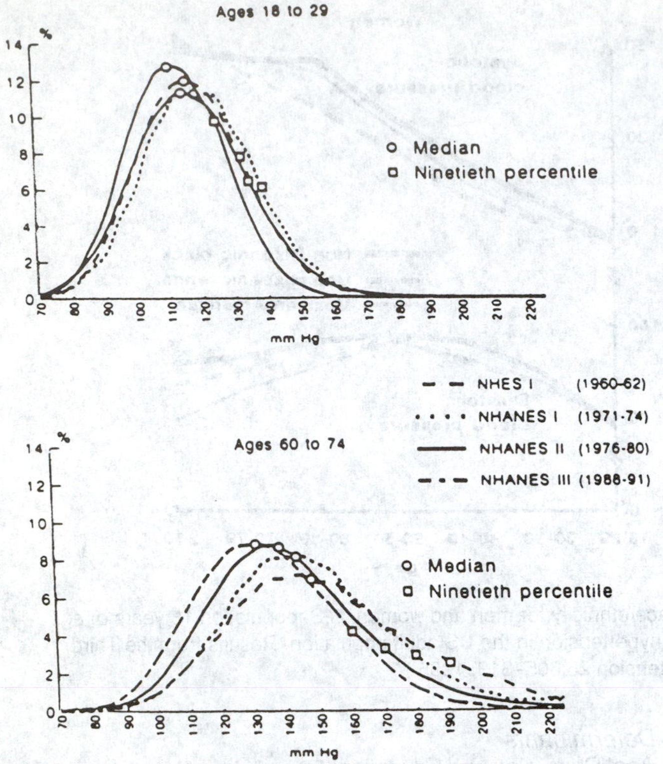

Figure 52-3. Smoothed weighted frequency distribution, median, and 90th percentile of systolic pressure for populations 18 to 29 years and 60 to 74 years of age in the United States, 1960 to 1991. (From Centers for Disease Control and Prevention, National Center for Health Statistics.)

differences in the distribution of systolic blood pressure are also age-related; values for women are lower in early adulthood and higher in later adulthood than for men. Differences among sex-race groups in incidence of hypertension have already been noted.[10] Socioeconomic status has generally been found to relate inversely to blood pressure values in adults. Education, as a marker of socioeconomic status, was found to explain partially, but not wholly, the greater frequency of hypertension among blacks than among whites in the population of nearly 160,000 U.S. adults screened for the HDFP.[16]

Salt. Among specific environmental factors associated with blood pressure, none has received more attention than dietary salt in the form of sodium or sodium chloride. The Intersalt Cooperative Research Group, representing 52 centers in 29 countries, reported on an extensive collaborative effort to determine whether urinary sodium excretion and other factors would account for the expected differences in blood pressure levels and age-related slopes within and among these populations.[17] Within populations, the urinary sodium excretion was positively correlated with systolic pressure more often than with diastolic pressure, although in some populations negative correlations were significant. In analyses between populations, the results confirmed the absence of significant blood pressure increases with age in the populations with the lowest sodium excretion. In the remaining populations, sodium excretion related not to the median blood pressure or prevalence of hypertension but to the slope of blood pressure increments by age group. These results indicate a favorable association between low salt intake and change in blood pressure with age. The urinary sodium-potassium ratio was similarly related to the blood pressure indices in these populations. The confrontation between commercial and health interests over recommendations concerning salt intake has been dramatic.[18]

Other Dietary Factors. Detailed and extensively documented reviews of dietary factors in relation to health have been presented in the United States by both the National Research Council and the Surgeon General.[19,20] In relation to blood pressure, in addition to sodium and potassium, attention is given to calcium, chloride, lead, magnesium, trace elements, carbohydrates, fiber, fat (especially polyunsaturates and the ratio of polyunsaturated to saturated fats), protein, caffeine, and overall caloric balance. Recommendations in the Surgeon General's report include improvements in food labeling, food services, food processing by manufacturers, and advice to populations at special risk of hypertension.[20] Both reports address research priorities, as many questions remain concerning the role of these specific aspects of diet and their possible implications for tailoring of dietary

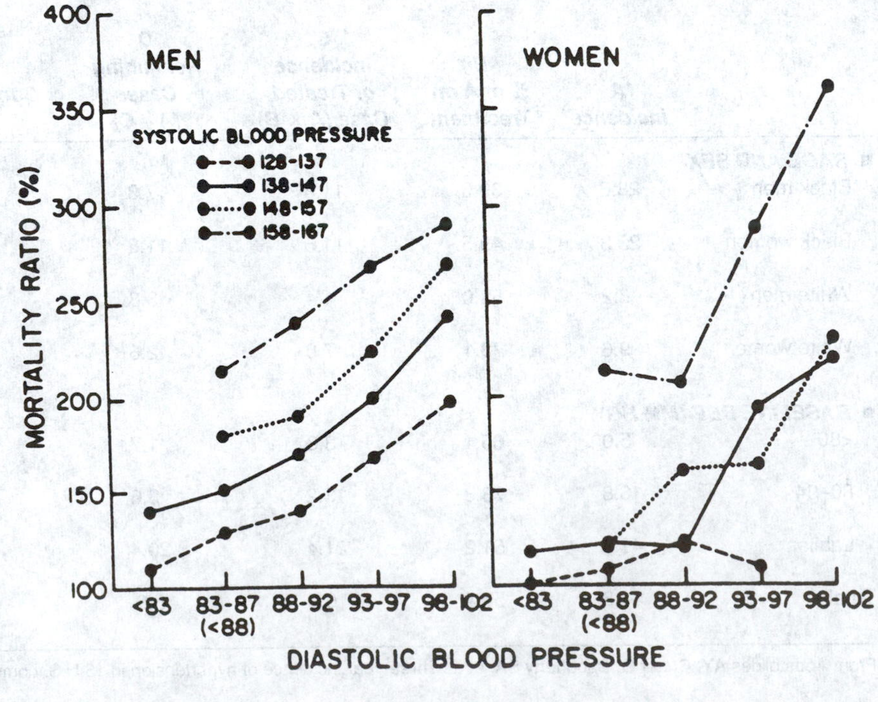

Figure 52-4. Mortality risks related to systolic and diastolic blood pressure. (From Labarthe DR: The cardiovascular complications of hypertension; natural history. In Onesti G, Klimt C (eds): Hypertension—Determinants, Complications, and Intervention. New York: Grune & Stratton, 1977.)

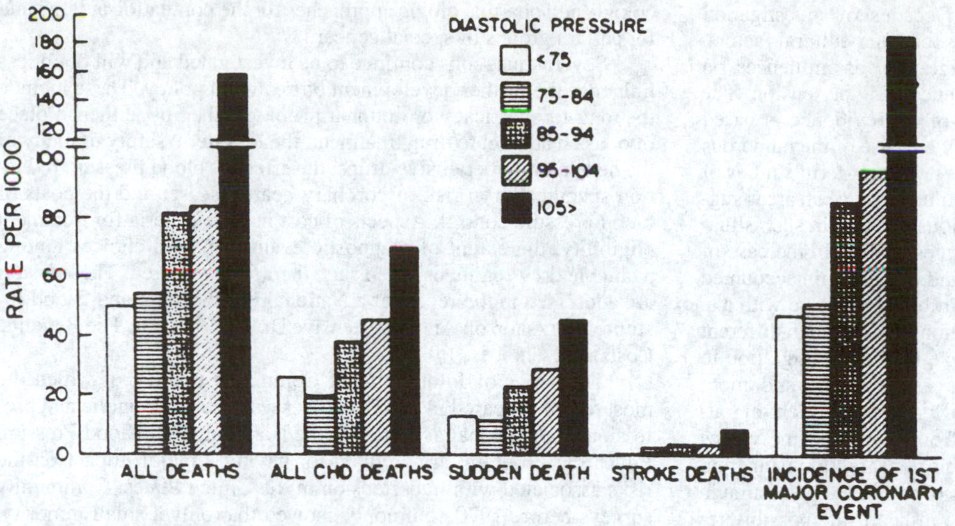

Figure 52-5. Cardiovascular risks related to diastolic blood pressure. (From The Pooling Project Research Group: Relationship of blood pressure, serum cholesterol, smoking habit, relative weight and ECG abnormalities to incidence of major coronary events: final report of the Pooling Project. J Chronic Dis 31:201–306, 1978.)

recommendations to the actual food sources available to particular populations.

Weight, Weight Gain, and Obesity. The relation of weight and weight gain to incidence of hypertension was discussed above and is consistent with other observations in both cross-sectional and longitudinal studies.[11] In the Intersalt Cooperative Research Group study just described, body mass index (weight in kilograms per square of height in meters) was strongly correlated with blood pressure within and across populations.[17]

Alcohol. Alcohol intake has also been found to be strongly related to blood pressure levels and is addressed in the reports cited above.[17,19–20] The nature of the relation between alcohol and blood pressure has been examined carefully by Criqui.[21] He demonstrated both a pressor or blood pressure-raising effect of alcohol consumption (possibly due to the alcohol-withdrawal state at the time of measurement rather than a direct effect) and the widely recognized observation that cardiovascular mortality was least not for nondrinkers but for those who reported consuming about two drinks per day. It appears that alcohol, by raising blood pressure, does contribute to cardiovascular mortality and reduces the possible beneficial action of moderate alcohol intake, which may operate through a different pathway involving lipid metabolism. For this and other reasons, it would be a dubious public health policy to encourage the use of alcohol for the purpose of reducing cardiovascular disease risk.

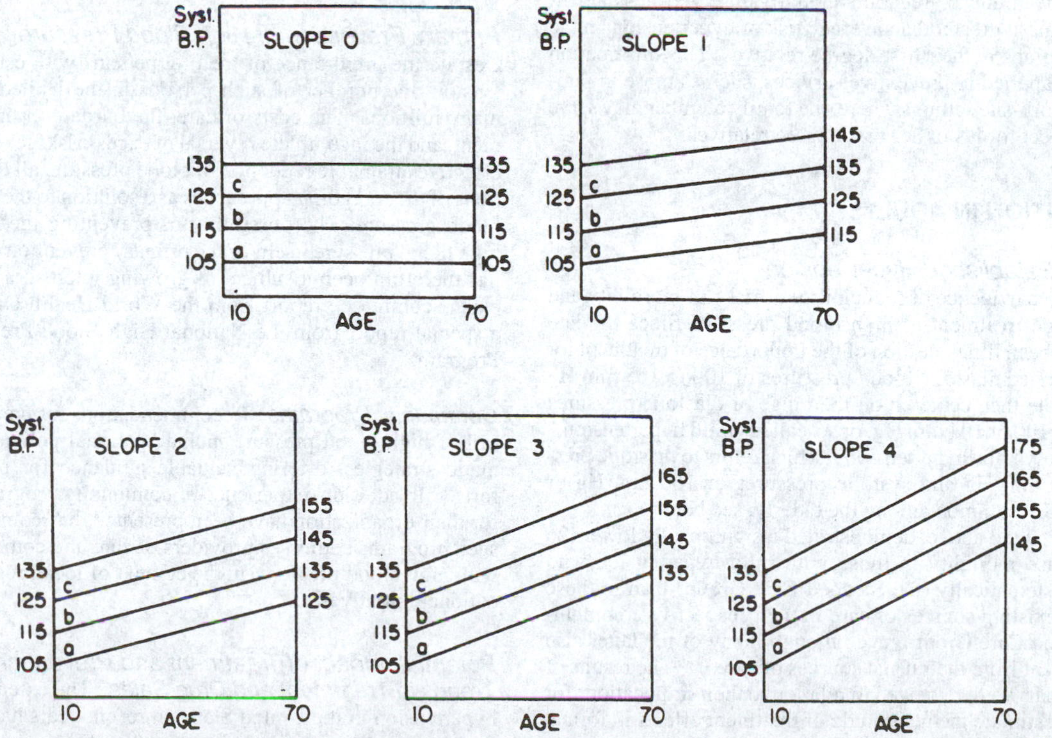

Figure 52-6. Patterns of blood pressure by age in adults. (From Epstein FH, Eckoff RD: The epidemiology of high blood pressure—geographic distributions and etiologic factors. In Stamler J, Stamler R, Pullman T (eds): The Epidemiology of Hypertension. New York: Grune & Stratton, 1967.)

Psychosocial and Cultural Factors. Decades of investigation have contributed abundant data on psychosocial and cultural factors, including stress, culture change, and migration, as influences on blood pressure distributions or the prevalence of hypertension. The population comparisons on which much of this evidence is based have often been difficult to interpret clearly because of the numerous uncontrolled factors in such comparisons. Two long-term studies of groups migrating from remote rural environments to urban areas suggest that the blood pressure changes previously found in such situations may be strongly determined by changes in diet. In the case of Tokelau Islanders migrating to New Zealand, weight gain accounted for most of the observed excess increase in blood pressure with age in migrating versus nonmigrating men, although for women different patterns were observed.[22] In the Luo people in Kenya, migration to Nairobi was accompanied by an abrupt increase in systolic and (more gradually) in diastolic pressure, and the differences between migrating and nonmigrating men and women from their baseline values were explained largely by weight gain. This appeared to result from fluid retention caused by an increased ratio of sodium to potassium in the diet. In addition, however, an increase in heart rate possibly reflecting psychological factors was also observed on the first postmigration examination after only about 1 month in Nairobi.[23]

Genetics and Family History. The nature of the genetic contribution to blood pressure levels in individuals has long been debated, most notably by Pickering[24] and by Platt[25] some 30 years ago. Pickering's argument for polygenic inheritance of blood pressure determinants, with multiple environmental influences, has prevailed. Within families, resemblance of blood pressure levels among first-degree relatives (parents, siblings, and offspring) is commonly observed and is consistent with genetic contributions; the influence of common environmental factors within such closely related individuals cannot be entirely separated from genetic aspects, however.[26,27] Evidence from studies of blood pressure resemblance in monozygotic versus dizygotic twins provides the clearest quantitation of genetic influence.[28] The specific mechanisms by which the genetic makeup contributes to blood pressure levels have yet to be established. Nonetheless, the familial aggregation regularly observed aids in identifying individuals at greater than average risk of hypertension on the basis of observations in their first-degree relatives. This information can be usefully applied in preventive services, such as those in family practice or work-site settings where one family member may serve as an index subject for his or her first-degree relatives.

▸ INTERVENTION IN ADULTS

Treatment of Established Hypertension

There is extensive evidence of reducibility of risks of morbidity and mortality through treatment of high blood pressure. Since the late 1960s there has been little question of the importance of treatment for those with sustained diastolic blood pressures of 100 to 105 mm Hg or greater. Debate then centered on the range of diastolic pressures between 90 and 100 or 104 mm Hg, or so-called "mild hypertension," and on "isolated systolic hypertension," which refers to diastolic pressures below 90 mm Hg and systolic pressures of 160 mm Hg or greater (especially common among the elderly, see below).

The HDFP, cited above, demonstrated a significantly lower (26 percent) all-cause mortality in those with mild hypertension who were treated systematically (the Stepped Care Group) than in those referred to the existing sources of care in their respective communities (the Referred Care Group), even though many of the latter also received treatment from their usual sources of care.[29,30] The results of this and other trials were reviewed in relation to their implications for policy[31] and to estimate the magnitude of treatment effects in formal meta-analyses (e.g., Cutler et al, and others[32–34]). These results are also reflected in the current recommendations of the Joint National Committee on Detection, Evaluation, and Treatment of High Blood Pressure, which address in detail treatment through both nonpharmacologic and pharmacologic approaches for the population at large and for certain groups of special concern.[5]

Several questions continue to be investigated and will doubtless influence the further development of treatment policy. These include the long-term efficacy of nonpharmacologic therapy, either in place of or as an adjunct to drug treatment; the long-term safety of many of the newer antihypertensive drugs; the effect of blood pressure reduction specifically on risk of coronary heart disease; and the costs of blood pressure control. Aspects of cost include criteria for treatment eligibility, the extent of diagnostic evaluation, and choices among available drug regimens when such therapy is required. These issues are addressed in the report of a National Heart, Lung, and Blood Institute Workshop on Antihypertensive Drug Treatment: The Benefits, Costs, and Choices.[35]

The series of Joint National Committee reports, of which the most recent appeared in 1993, together with the other public and professional educational activities of the National High Blood Pressure Education Program, are credited for having a major impact on the risks associated with hypertension in the United States. Community surveys before 1970 commonly showed that only a small minority, about one-eighth, of those with hypertension were detected, under treatment, and controlled, and a major public health strategy of the 1970s and 1980s was the conduct of community screening programs for case detection and for monitoring of progress in blood pressure control. The Joint National Committee now de-emphasizes programs for case detection and suggests instead community services to ensure follow-up of the cases already known and currently being detected so as to maintain their long-term medical management.[5]

The particular problem of blacks in the United States, and of course other population groups in many other settings, may still require special detection efforts, however, and local programs should be designed with such considerations in view. Evidence from diverse studies, such as the HDFP based on sampling of whole communities to estimate the impact of blood pressure control and the North Karelia Project in East Finland, demonstrates that integrated efforts to reduce the population risks attributable to hypertension can be highly effective.[29–30,36]

Primary Prevention of High Blood Pressure

Despite the importance of treating persons with established hypertension, the number of such persons in the United States alone is many millions. The costs of care, the burden on those under treatment, and the incomplete reversal of excess risks, even with the most effective attainable reduction of blood pressure, all constitute limitations of the foregoing approaches as a solution to the problem of high blood pressure. The possibility of preventing the development of high blood pressure itself, or the primary prevention of hypertension, has therefore been a subject of growing interest, as reflected in an expert committee report from the World Health Organization[1] and a special report from the National High Blood Pressure Education Program.[37]

Community Programs. Recommendations for prevention and control of high blood pressure include national policies and programmatic strategies, offering valuable guidance for public health efforts.[1,3] In addition, experience of community programs and a model for their organization have been presented.[38] A composite model for such programs addresses providers of care and community members with high blood pressure, in the context of local, regional, state, and national initiatives.

Potential Impact of Treatment and Prevention

Trends in Treatment and Drug Sales. The extent of treatment of hypertension in the United States in recent years has been estimated from surveys of use of ambulatory care and from prescription data for antihypertensive medications. The National Ambulatory Care Survey of the National Center for Health Statistics indicated from 408 to 441 visits per 1,000 persons 45 to 64 years of age for survey periods from

1975–1976 to 1985 or more than twice the number of visits for either ischemic heart disease or diabetes.[39] Drug-use data suggested an increase in the number of prescriptions for antihypertensive medications, from approximately 128 million in 1973 to 209 million in 1985.[40] Even with allowance for population increase in the most affected age groups, greater intensity of medication is suggested by these data. This fact reinforces concern about the problem of high blood pressure control from the viewpoint of health care costs.

Mortality Trends in the United States. The decline in mortality from cardiovascular diseases and stroke in the United States over recent decades has been attributed in part to the improved rates of detection and control of hypertension. The pattern of decreasing mortality for cerebrovascular disease from 1950 to 1985 suggests a steeper downward slope beginning in the early 1970s, when drug therapy for hypertension became increasingly common.[41] However, because stroke mortality has declined in the United States since early in the twentieth century, factors other than treatment of hypertension have been important. Data from observational studies and from clinical and community trials all predict a beneficial impact of blood pressure reduction on these trends, but quantitation of its specific contribution to mortality trends remains uncertain.

Older Persons

The special problem of hypertension in older persons has been noted above. As characterized by the Joint National Committee report, a large proportion of persons over age 65 in the United States have both systolic and diastolic blood pressure elevations that warrant treatment.[5] A study of isolated systolic hypertension, the Systolic Hypertension in the Elderly Program (SHEP), demonstrated clear benefit of antihypertensive drug therapy in persons age 60 years and above, with minimal adverse effects.[42] Total stroke incidence was reduced by 36 percent and all-cause mortality by 13 percent. This study offset much of the prior concern that lowering blood pressure in the elderly would result in adverse events due to reduced coronary and cerebral blood flow. Because the elderly constitute a large and expanding segment of the United States population, the recommendations emerging from this and related studies will potentially have a great impact on the extent of treatment for hypertension in this country.[43]

Blacks

For blacks in the United States, as addressed earlier, the incidence and prevalence of hypertension are greater than for whites, and morbidity and mortality are correspondingly high. Although the importance of the problem of hypertension is proportionately even greater for blacks than for whites, rates of detection and effective treatment have been lower, especially for black men. Effective response to treatment can be expected in blacks, although some classes of drugs are said to be less effective in blacks than in whites. The need for improved public health programs to reach this target population is evident. Whether other racial and ethnic groups similarly require special consideration in the design of programs has not been established but is suggested for Mexican Americans.[9]

▶ NATURAL HISTORY IN CHILDREN

Concepts of hypertension and of blood pressure distributions have different meanings in childhood, or more broadly, the period from birth through adolescence, from those that apply in adulthood. Although levels of blood pressure that reflect hypertension are sometimes observed, usually due to a demonstrable pathologic condition, the primary focus of public health attention is the relative level of blood pressure and the question of its implications for the risk of essential hypertension in adulthood. The potential for early influences to determine the later development of blood pressure levels is the reason for growing interest in blood pressure in youth from the perspective of preventive medicine and public health.[1–3]

Prevalence

The distribution of blood pressure in childhood has been studied extensively. The published reports on children from around the world have been reviewed to permit comparison of the situations of childhood and adulthood in their patterns of blood pressure levels by age.[44] The results indicated that in nearly all populations the age-specific mean systolic blood pressure values by sex were within 5 percent of the pooled values shown in Figure 52-7. Values for boys and for girls were the same until ages corresponding to the onset of puberty, after which those for boys were consistently higher; by the late teen years the values for boys showed no further increase, while those for girls actually decreased. Similar patterns were observed for fourth-phase diastolic pressure, but much less increase by age was found for fifth-phase values, and no decrease in the later teen years was found for girls. Unlike the situation in adulthood, then, childhood populations were quite similar in their overall patterns of blood pressure increase by age, at least within the school-age period.

On the basis of such survey results, it is possible to construct curves of selected percentile values of systolic and diastolic pressure for use as reference values in assessment of individual children in screening or practice settings. For this purpose, a Task Force on Blood Pressure Control in Children has, for the United States, presented reference values and detailed recommendations for detection and management of relatively high blood pressure values in children.[45] In principle, those children whose values are above the 90th or 95th percentile on repeated occasions of measurement are considered to have "hypertension" and to require special long-term manage-

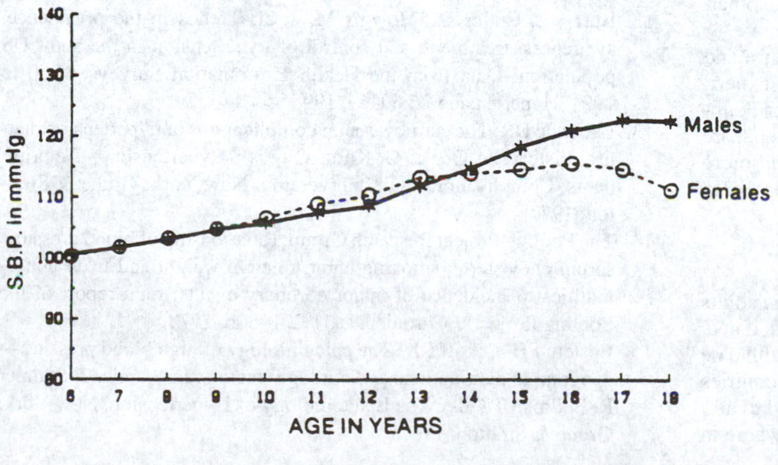

Figure 52-7. Patterns of blood pressure by age in children. (From Brotons C, Singh P, Nishio T, Labarthe DR: Blood pressure by age in childhood and adolescence: a review of 129 studies worldwide. Int J Epidemiol 18:824–829, 1989.)

ment. Those in the range from the 90th to the 95th percentile who are also above the 90th percentile for height are considered to have normal blood pressure. This qualification is based on the strong relation of blood pressure to measures of growth and maturation during this period of life; hence more mature children exhibit higher levels of blood pressure.

Incidence

Just as percentile rank replaces prevalence in considering blood pressure in childhood, the concept of "tracking" replaces incidence. Tracking is often defined as persistence in relative blood pressure rank with increasing age. While for some purposes tracking is of interest at all levels of the blood pressure distribution, special attention is usually given to the persistence of relatively high blood pressure values, which may be predictive of hypertension in adulthood or may require intervention at current ages. A number of studies of tracking and an example of the longitudinal development of blood pressure in several successive cohorts of children are given by Szklo[46] and by Hofman et al,[47] respectively.

Determinants

As noted above, prominent determinants of blood pressure levels in childhood include influences of growth and maturation. The close resemblance of patterns of blood pressure with age in diverse populations of children may reflect predominance of these largely intrinsic and universal influences in childhood and adolescence. Other factors, such as genetic differences, energy balance, and specific dietary components, are also found to contribute as in adulthood. Very early effects of diet and of general health conditions, even in fetal life, have been demonstrated or suggested by recent studies.[48,49] Further research on the natural history of blood pressure development in the perinatal period and infancy, as well as in later childhood and adolescence, may be very fruitful.

► INTERVENTIONS FOR CHILDREN

Approaches to interventions of blood pressure control in childhood are outlined in the Joint National Committee report[5] and the report of the Task Force on Blood Pressure Control in Children.[45] Pharmacologic therapy should be used rarely in this age group. Suggested interventions are primarily related to energy balance—toward weight reduction, or control of weight gain, and reduction in sodium intake.

The concept that even the early development of the major risk factors for cardiovascular diseases, including blood pressure, could be averted was expressed by Strasser with the term "primordial prevention."[50] The target of primordial prevention includes the conditions that foster development of the risk factors, such as energy imbalance leading to excess weight gain, attributable to eating and activity patterns that may accompany economic and social development. One implication of this view is that interventions for whole populations may modify these conditions and thereby slow, arrest, or reverse the otherwise expected undesirable shift in distributions of the risk factors.

Several studies of interventions to modify blood pressure and other risk factors in children have been reported, such as the experience of the Know Your Body Program of the American Health Foundation.[51] The results to date have offered some encouragement but are modest and inconsistent. Longer-term evaluation, earlier and more intensive intervention, or a combination of these may be necessary to observe the expected benefits.

Potential Impact of Prevention and Treatment

It is clear from a discussion of the problem of blood pressure in adults in the United States that the impact of effective prevention and, if necessary, early treatment on adult morbidity, mortality, and health care needs could be great. The United States and many other countries have experienced epidemics of cardiovascular disease related to atherosclerosis and hypertension in the twentieth century; elsewhere in the world, especially in developing countries, epidemic atherosclerosis, emerging or anticipated, and hypertension are already a serious problems.[52,53] The concept that improved living conditions—through better-controlled development, with attendant optimization of habits related to health—could allow many populations to avert this epidemic of cardiovascular diseases poses an international public health challenge of large proportions. It remains to be seen whether knowledge of natural history and approaches to intervention, both in adults and in children, can be joined with the necessary social and political forces to realize this goal.

► REFERENCES

1. World Health Organization: Primary prevention of essential hypertension. WHO Technical Report Series, No. 686. Geneva: World Health Organization, 1983
2. World Health Organization: Blood pressure studies in children. WHO Technical Report Series, No. 715. Geneva: World Health Organization, 1985
3. World Health Organization: Prevention in childhood and youth of adult cardiovascular diseases. WHO Technical Report Series, No. 792. Geneva: World Health Organization, 1990
4. Working Group on Risk and High Blood Pressure: An epidemiological approach to describing risk associated with blood pressure levels. Hypertension 7:641–651, 1985
5. National High Blood Pressure Education Program: The Fifth Report of the Joint National Committee on Detection, Evaluation, and Treatment of High Blood Pressure. NIH Publication No. 93-1088. Bethesda, MD: National Institutes of Health, National Heart, Lung, and Blood Institute, 1993
6. Frohlich ED, Grim C, Labarthe, DR, et al: Report of a special task force appointed by the Steering Committee, American Heart Association: recommendations for human blood pressure determinations by sphygmomanometers. Hypertension 11:209A–222A, 1988
7. Curb JD, Labarthe DR, Cooper SP, et al: Training and certification of blood pressure observers. Hypertension 5:610–614, 1983
8. Hypertension Detection and Follow-Up Program Cooperative Group: The Hypertension Detection and Follow-Up Program: a progress report. Circ Res 40(Suppl 1):106–109, 1977
9. Burt VL, Whelton P, Rocella EJ, et al: Prevalence of hypertension in the US adult population. Results from the Third National Health and Nutrition Examination Survey, 1988–1991. Hypertension 25:305–313, 1995
10. Apostolides AY, Cutter G, Daugherty SA, et al: Three-year incidence of hypertension in 13 U.S. communities. Prev Med 11:487– 499, 1982
11. Tyroler H, Heyden S, Hames C: Weight and hypertension: Evans County studies of blacks and whites. In Paul O (ed): Epidemiology and Control of Hypertension. New York: Stratton Intercontinental Medical Book Association, 1975
12. Burt VL, Cutler JA, Higgins M, et al: Trends in the prevalence, awareness, treatment, and control of hypertension in the adult US population. Data from the Health Examination Surveys, 1960 to 1991. Hypertension 26:60–69, 1995
13. Labarthe DR: The cardiovascular complications of hypertension: natural history. In Onesti G, Klimt C (eds): Hypertension—Determinants, Complications, and Intervention. New York: Grune & Stratton, 1977
14. The Pooling Project Research Group: Relationship of blood pressure, serum cholesterol, smoking habit, relative weight and ECG abnormalities to incidence of major coronary events: final report of the Pooling Project. J Chronic Dis 31:201–306, 1978
15. Epstein FH, Eckoff RD: The epidemiology of high blood pressure—geographic distributions and etiologic factors. In Stamler J, Stamler R, Pullman T (eds): The Epidemiology of Hypertension. New York: Grune & Stratton, 1967

16. Hypertension Detection and Follow-Up Program Cooperative Group: Race, education and prevalence of hypertension. Am J Epidemiol 106:351–361, 1977
17. Intersalt Cooperative Research Group: Intersalt: an international study of electrolyte excretion and blood pressure: results for 24 hour urinary sodium and potassium excretion. Br Med J 297:319–328, 1988
18. Godlee F: The food industry fights for salt. Br Med J 312:1239–1240, 1996
19. Committee on Diet and Health, Food and Nutrition Board, Commission on Life Sciences, National Research Council: Diet and Health: Implications for Reducing Chronic Disease Risk. Washington DC: National Academy Press, 1989
20. US Department of Health and Human Services, Public Health Service: The Surgeon General's Report on Nutrition and Health, 1988. DHHS (PHS) Publication No. 88-50210. Washington, DC: Government Printing Office, 1988
21. Criqui MH: Alcohol and hypertension: new insights from population studies. Eur Heart J 8(Suppl B):19–26, 1987
22. Salmond CE, Prior IAM, Wessen AF: Blood pressure patterns and migration: a 14-year cohort study of adult Tokelauans. Am J Epidemiol 130:37–52, 1989
23. Poulter N, Khaw KT, Mugambi M, et al: Longitudinal study of migrants from a "low blood pressure population." Abstract presented at the Second International Conference on Preventive Cardiology, Washington, DC, June 22, 1989
24. Pickering G: The inheritance of arterial pressure. In Stamler J, Stamler R, Pullman T (eds): The Epidemiology of Hypertension. New York: Grune & Stratton, 1967
25. Platt R: The influence of heredity. In Stamler J, Stamler R, Pullman T (eds): The Epidemiology of Hypertension. New York: Grune & Stratton, 1967
26. Tyroler HA: The Detroit Project studies of blood pressure: a prologue and review of related studies and epidemiologic issues. J Chronic Dis 30:659–670, 1977
27. Schull WJ, Harburg E, Schork MA, et al: Heredity, stress and blood pressure, a family set method. III. Family aggregation of hypertension. J Chronic Dis 30:659–670, 1977
28. Biron P, Mongeau JG, Bertrand D: Familial aggregation of blood pressure in 558 adopted children. Can Med Assoc J 115:773–774, 1976
29. Hypertension Detection and Follow-Up Program Cooperative Group: Five year findings of the Hypertension Detection and Fol-low-Up Program. I. Reduction in mortality of persons with high blood pressure including mild hypertension. JAMA 242:2562– 2571, 1979
30. Hypertension Detection and Follow-Up Program Cooperative Group: Five year findings of the Hypertension Detection and Follow-Up Program. II. Mortality by race-sex and age. JAMA 242: 2572–2577, 1979
31. Labarthe DR: Mild hypertension: the question of treatment. Annu Rev Public Health 7:193–215, 1986
32. Cutler JA, MacMahon SW, Furberg CD: Controlled clinical trials of drug treatment for hypertension: a review. Hypertension 13(Suppl I):I-36–I-44, 1989
33. MacMahon S, Peto R, Cutler J, et al: Blood pressure, stroke, and coronary heart disease. Part 1, prolonged differences in blood pressure: prospective observational studies corrected for the regression dilution bias. Lancet 335:765–774, 1990
34. Collins R, Peto R, MacMahon S, et al: Blood pressure, stroke, and coronary heart disease. Part 2, short-term reductions in blood pressure: overview of randomised drug trials in their epidemiological context. Lancet 335:827–838, 1990
35. Cutler JA, Horan MJ, Roccella EJ, Zusman RM (eds): The National Heart, Lung, and Blood Institute Workshop of Antihypertensive Drug Treatment: the benefits, costs, and choices. Hypertension 13 (Suppl I), 1989
36. Nissinen A, Tuomilehto J, Korhonen HJ, et al: Ten-year results of hypertension care in the community: follow-up of the North Karelia Hypertension Control Program. Am J Epidemiol 127:488–499, 1988
37. National High Blood Pressure Education Program: Working Group Report on Primary Prevention of Hypertension. Arch Int Med 153:186–208, 1993
38. McClellan W, Wilber JA: A decade's experience with hypertension control programs in the United States: the empirical basis for a model of community control programs. In Rosenfeld JB, Silverberg DS, Viskiper R (eds): Hypertension Control in the Community. London: John Libbey, 1985
39. Kovar MG, Collins JG, Delozier J, et al: Trends in the availability and use of medical care for coronary heart disease and related diseases. In Higgins MH, Luepker RV (eds): Trends in Coronary Heart Disease Mortality: The Influence of Medical Care. New York: Oxford University Press, 1988
40. Gross TP, Wise RP, Knapp DE: Antihypertensive drug use: trends in the United States from 1973 to 1985. Hypertension 13(Suppl I): I-113–I-118, 1989
41. Higgins MH, Luepker RV: Preface. In Higgins MH, Luepker RV (eds): Trends in Coronary Heart Disease Mortality: The Influence of Medical Care. New York: Oxford University Press, 1988
42. SHEP Cooperative Research Group: Prevention of stroke by antihypertensive drug treatment in older persons with isolated systolic hypertension. Final results of the Systolic Hypertension in the Elderly Program (SHEP). JAMA 265:3255–3264, 1991
43. Smith WMcF: Epidemiology of hypertension in older patients. Am J Med 85(Suppl 3B):2–6, 1988
44. Brotons C, Singh P, Nishio T, Labarthe DR: Blood pressure by age in childhood and adolescence: a review of 129 studies worldwide. Int J Epidemiol 18:824–829, 1989
45. Task Force on Blood Pressure Control in Children: Report of the Second Task Force on Blood Pressure Control in Children—1987. Pediatrics 79:1–25, 1987
46. Szklo M: Epidemiologic patterns of blood pressure in children. Epidemiol Rev 1:143–169, 1979
47. Hofman A, Valkenburg HA, Maas J, Groustra FN: The natural history of blood pressure in childhood. Int J Epidemiol 14:91–96, 1985
48. Hofman A, Hazebroek A, Valkenburg A: A randomized trial of sodium intake and blood pressure in newborn infants. JAMA 250:370–373, 1983
49. Barker DJP, Osmond C, Golding J et al: Growth in utero, blood pressure in childhood and adult life, and mortality from cardiovascular disease. Br Med J 298:564–567, 1989
50. Strasser T: Reflections on cardiovascular diseases. Interdisc Sci Rev 3:225–230, 1978
51. Walter HJ, Hofman A, Vaughan RD, Wynder EL: Modification of risk factors for coronary heart disease: five-year results of a school-based intervention trial. N Engl J Med 318:1093–1100, 1988
52. Dodu SRA: Emergence of cardiovascular diseases in developing countries. Cardiology 75:56–64, 1988
53. The WHO MONICA Project: Geographical variation in the major risk factors of coronary heart disease in men and women aged 35–64 years. World Health Stat Q 41:115–140, 1988

53

Renal and Urinary Tract Disease

Rebecca L. Hegeman

Rates and patterns of renal and urinary tract diseases differ among populations and are constantly changing. With development and industrialization, diseases related to infections, crowding, and poor nutrition recede, and those associated with affluence, aging, "overnutrition," medical interventions, drugs, addictions, and other exposures become prominent. Complex relationships between many renal and urinary tract diseases and socioeconomic, racial, cultural, and behavioral factors are becoming more apparent. The diseases of westernized societies are the main focus of this chapter with emphasis on those that cause the most morbidity. Challah and Wing[1] provide a more comprehensive international perspective.

Rates of most renal diseases and of end-stage renal disease (ESRD) in westernized societies rise with age, and increased longevity enhances the expression of both. More males than females are affected by many renal diseases, and more males enter ESRD treatment programs. Some groups recently absorbed into westernized societies, such as U.S. blacks, North American Indians, Hispanics and Mexican Americans, urban South African blacks, Australian aborigines, Pacific Islanders, and New Zealand Maoris, have especially high rates of renal disease, in part from conditions such as hypertension and diabetes that were rare in their forebears. ESRD treatment programs themselves have produced a whole new set of clinical, economic, and sociological perspectives and concerns.

Renal and urinary tract diseases are frequently asymptomatic, and diagnosis is frequently dependent on laboratory and radiologic studies. Clinical renal disease may be manifested by blood, protein, or white blood cells in the urine, sometimes with hypertension. Heavy protein excretion, decreased levels of serum albumin, hyperlipidemia, and edema characterize the "nephrotic syndrome." Excretory renal function can be normal or impaired and can remain stable or progress to renal failure. Renal impairment generates, and is exacerbated by, hypertension. ESRD defines a situation of chronic irreversible renal failure in which prolonged survival is not possible without dialysis or renal transplantation.

Specific diseases are diagnosed by history and clinical findings; biochemical, serological, imaging, and urodynamic studies; and sometimes by biopsy of the kidneys, bladder, or prostate. Kidney biopsy specimens are examined by light, immunofluorescent, and electron microscopy to aid in diagnosis and prognosis. The serum creatinine level provides an approximate measure of renal insufficiency, although it varies with muscle mass and diet, underestimates renal insufficiency in the elderly, is relatively insensitive to loss of the first 50 percent of renal function, and is less sensitive to progressive loss of function in severe renal failure. Glomerular filtration rate, precisely measured by iothalamate and inulin clearances, can be estimated from the reciprocal of the serum creatinine or by creatinine clearance. In some persons, changes in these parameters or in the logarithm of the serum creatinine follow a fairly consistent course, so that rates or renal functional deterioration can be expressed quantitatively.[2]

Although specific interventions for many diseases are not yet available, progressive renal damage may be modulated by a few standard maneuvers, thereby avoiding or postponing the development of ESRD. Control of coexisting or secondary hypertension, moderate dietary protein restriction, and in diabetics, strict control of blood glucose levels and angiotensin converting enzyme inhibitors are of proven value.[3–5] Other strategies recommended include control of hyperlipidemia, control of obesity, reduction of left ventricular hypertrophy, cessation of tobacco use, and improved nutritional status including a low-sodium diet.[6]

▸ SPECIFIC RENAL DISEASES

Diabetic Renal Disease

Diabetic nephropathy is the leading cause of ESRD in the United States, accounting for approximately one-third of all patients on dialysis.[7] Of the estimated 13 million diabetic individuals in the United States, 5 to 10 percent have insulin-dependent diabetes mellitus (IDDM) and 90 to 95 percent have noninsulin-dependent diabetes mellitus (NIDDM). The cumulative risk of developing nephropathy in IDDM is approximately 30 to 40 percent, peaking after approximately 18 to 20 years. The cumulative risk in NIDDM is less well defined, but because most patients with diabetes have NIDDM, the majority of patients in dialysis units have NIDDM.[8] The incidence of ESRD caused by diabetic nephropathy is increased in certain racial and ethnic groups including Hispanics, African Americans, and American Indians. Most of the increase in these groups seems to be caused by NIDDM. Familial clustering of diabetic nephropathy has also been noted and may be due to genetic inheritance, shared environment, or both.[9,10]

The pathogenesis of diabetic nephropathy is not yet fully understood. Early on, the glomerular and tubular basement membranes thicken, and there is accumulation of extracellular matrix in the glomerular mesangium. Over time the glomerular capillary lumina are obliterated and the glomerular filtration rate eventually declines. Functionally, there is an initial increase in the glomerular filtration rate with glomerular hypertension, followed by the development of proteinuria and systemic hypertension with an eventual decline in renal function. Hyperglycemia is the central factor, which is presumably initiating the above events. Current studies are focusing on the role of advanced glycosylation end-products (AGEs), the polyol pathway, transforming growth factor-β, and endothelins (as well as several others) in the accumulation of the extracellular matrix and other histochemical abnormalities that eventually lead to the decline of renal function in diabetics.[11]

The most important clinical marker of diabetic nephropathy is microalbuminuria, or "dipstick-negative" urinary albumin excretion. This corresponds to a urinary albumin excretion rate of 30 to 300 mg/day or 20 to 200 μg/min.[12] Unfortunately, it is a late marker for diabetic nephropathy in that irreversible kidney damage may have already occurred by the time it is detected. It is also a risk factor for increased overall mortality. Identification of diabetics with microalbuminuria is important because patients with microalbuminuria progress to develop overt diabetic nephropathy (excretion of more than 300 mg protein per 24 hours) and eventually ESRD.[8]

Several major clinical trials have recently been completed that provide guidance for therapy in diabetics to prevent diabetic nephropathy and the complications associated with it. Treatment of overt diabetic nephropathy with an angiotensin-converting enzyme (ACE) inhibitor in patients with IDDM has been shown to delay (but not totally halt) the rate of deterioration of renal function. This effect is independent of the effect of ACE inhibition on the treatment of blood pressure.[13]

The recently completed Diabetes Control and Complications Trial (DCCT) has demonstrated the beneficial effects of intensive insulin therapy on the development of diabetic nephropathy. In the DCCT, the mean adjusted risk of microalbuminuria (more than 28 μg/min) was reduced by 34 percent in the group of patients on intensive insulin therapy with no baseline retinopathy. Unfortunately, intensive insulin therapy did not show a significant benefit in preventing the development of overt diabetic nephropathy in patients who already had microalbuminuria.[14]

Hypertension is more common in diabetics with microalbuminuria, especially in patients with NIDDM, and is both a predictor and a consequence of nephropathy in NIDDM. Hypertension has been shown to increase the rate at which diabetic nephropathy progresses, and antihypertensive therapy has been shown to slow its course.[15]

Although the incidence of diabetic nephropathy among patients who have had IDDM for 25 years or more is falling, the increasing population of elderly patients with NIDDM marks diabetic nephropathy as a continued major cause of morbidity and mortality.[16] For this reason, annual screening for microalbuminuria is recommended for all diabetics older than 12 years. If microalbuminuria is present and persists, ACE inhibitor therapy is appropriate in both normotensive and hypertensive patients. Serum potassium and creatinine will need to be monitored, and females of child-bearing age will need to be cautioned about becoming pregnant due to the known adverse effects of ACE inhibition on the fetus. Glycemic control should be monitored on a regular basis as well as blood pressure control. In addition, microalbuminuria is frequently associated with elevated levels of cholesterol and triglycerides, so dietary restriction of cholesterol and weight reduction should be emphasized. Cigarette smoking has also been associated with the development and progression of microalbuminuria and should be discouraged.[8]

While significant advances have been made in the approach to patients with diabetic nephropathy, we await the results of ongoing basic science research studies and clinical trials that will increase the knowledge and improve the management of diabetic nephropathy, eliminating, it is hoped, or at least significantly reducing the requirement for renal replacement therapy with its attendant comorbidity in this population.

Hypertensive Renal Disease

Hypertension can both produce and complicate renal disease, and its contribution to renal insufficiency is probably underestimated. Hypertensive renal disease was the most common diagnosis for African Americans receiving ESRD treatment in the United States from 1989 to 1993 and the second leading diagnosis for whites, constituting 39.9 and 30.3 percent of new ESRD cases, respectively.[7]

Primary hypertensive renal disease can be of two kinds. The more common, sometimes called "nephrosclerosis," is a form of chronic renal insufficiency associated with long-standing blood pressure elevation. The second, a form of accelerated renal failure associated with malignant hypertension, is now rare where treatment of hypertension is widespread.

Race and ethnic group are powerful risk factors for hypertensive nephropathy, through mechanisms that are not yet clear. Rates of treated hypertensive ESRD in U.S. blacks are more than seven times those of whites (higher in some regional studies), although essential hypertension is only about twice as common,[8] and hypertensive ESRD in Texas Mexican Americans is 2.6 times more frequent than in non-Hispanic whites, although their rates of hypertension are not higher.[17] ESRD attributed to hypertension is rare in Native American groups studied to date, but blood pressure elevations in the last few decades might contribute to their high rates of renal failure from type 2 diabetes and glomerulonephritis.[18–20] Additional risk factors for nephropathy in hypertensive persons include the height of the systolic and diastolic blood pressures, the presence of diabetes, male sex, increasing age, and high normal serum creatinine levels.[21–23]

Although widespread treatment of hypertension has reduced other hypertensive morbidities, its effects on hypertensive renal disease are not yet clear. Two regional studies in the United States show that renal damage can progress in some treated hypertensive persons despite "adequate" blood pressure control,[22,24] and the community-based Hypertension Detection and Follow-up Program (HDFP) confirms this phenomenon.[23] However, most seasoned practitioners feel that blood pressure control is mitigating much hypertensive renal disease, and the HDFP suggests the superiority of aggressive control over a more relaxed treatment approach. A fall in the incidence of treated hypertensive ESRD is not yet apparent from nationwide U.S. data, but data from Jefferson County, Alabama, show that the age of onset of hypertensive ESRD in blacks has been delayed by nearly a decade over the last 15 years and that older females rather than younger males now dominate the hypertensive ESRD treatment group.[25]

The definition of "adequate" blood pressure control in this context might be critical; "safe" blood pressure limits for populations at high risk of renal disease and for those with already established renal impairment might be lower than the accepted "normal" range for the Caucasian population. Retrospective and prospective analyses of large cohorts of hypertensive subjects and comparisons of therapeutic regimens will help clarify some of these issues.

Glomerulonephritis

Glomerulonephritis (GN) encompasses several syndromes with a variety of pathological changes in the renal glomerulus. Injury to the glomeruli is manifest by variable degrees of hematuria and/or proteinuria, red blood cell casts, hypertension, edema, oliguria/anuria, and renal insufficiency. This injury is categorized by morphological or clinical features, precipitating events, or associated conditions. Susceptibility is enhanced by infections, malnutrition, and poor living conditions, and rates fall as these conditions improve.[1] Most forms of GN are probably immunologically mediated, and genetic predispositions to some are suggested by family clusters and by associations with certain human leukocyte antigen (HLA) types. Associations with specific infections are well established, especially in the developing world, but few precursors or etiologic factors are recognized in the common forms of GN that persist in westernized countries.

GN is the most common cause of renal failure and renal death in the developing world. It is the leading cause of treated ESRD in western Europe and Australia/New Zealand and has only recently fallen to third place in the United States, as diabetic and hypertensive nephropathies have increased.[7] Pathological diagnosis relies on renal biopsy, which has risks and is expensive. Little is known about the distribution or natural history of mild GN or the extent to which subclinical GN might be eroding renal function in the broader community.

This discussion addresses the major histological categories of idiopathic GN, idiopathic IgA nephropathy, and poststreptococcal GN (PSGN).

Chronic Idiopathic GN

The major morphological categories of idiopathic GN are minimal change disease (MCD), focal segmental glomerular sclerosis (FSGS), mesangial proliferative GN, membranous GN (MGN), and membranoproliferative GN (MPGN). There are probably interfaces among these categories. Each can afflict subjects of all ages, but the distributions are dependent on age. MCD is the most common lesion in children, whereas adults have a broader distribution of all these forms of GN. Idiopathic GN may be associated with infections such as hepatitis B or C or malignancies. MCD has the best prognosis, with remission usual before adulthood; MGN often remits but leads to renal failure after 10 to 15 years in perhaps 50 percent of subjects, whereas FSGS and MPGN have fewer remissions and a more relentless course. A reduction in proteinuria usually occurs with corticosteroid treatment of MCD, but response to steroids and cytotoxic drugs is less predictable in other disease.[26–30]

Risk factors for progression of idiopathic MGN, and probably other forms of GN, include elevated serum creatinine, hypertension, male gender, age more than 50, renal biopsy evidence of glomerular sclerosis and/or interstitial fibrosis, and the persistence of heavy proteinuria. Progression is rare if protein excretion remains mild or falls toward normal, whether spontaneously or with treatment. With progressive proteinuria, it is highly probable that patients will progress to ESRD.

IgA Nephropathy

IgA nephropathy is considered to be the most common form of glomerular disease in the world. It is more common in the western Pacific rim where prevalences approaching 50 percent of all glomerular diseases have been reported,[31] while in Europe and the United States, lower prevalence rates (2 to 30 percent) have been reported. Local variability in health screening practices and indications for kidney biopsy will influence these statistics. Males predominate by at least 2:1, and, unlike with other glomerular diseases, the prevalence is low in African Americans. There have been reports of familial clustering.

The pathogenesis of IgA nephropathy remains unknown, but it is associated with abnormal deposition of IgA in the glomerular mesangium. The clinical presentation may be quite variable and includes several syndromes. Most patients present with microscopic or macroscopic hematuria. In 30 to 40 percent of patients there may be proteinuria usually associated with microscopic hematuria, and in less than 10 percent of patients there is acute renal insufficiency, edema, and hypertension on presentation. Skin lesions (Henoch-Schönlein purpura) develop more often in children, and these patients may have skin, joint, and intestinal involvement. Glomerular IgA deposition is associated with several disorders including hepatic cirrhosis, gluten enteropathy, human immunodeficiency virus (HIV) infection, Wegener's granulomatosis, systemic lupus erythematosus, minimal change disease, and membranous nephropathy.

IgA nephropathy usually has an indolent course with about 30 percent of patients reaching ESRD after 20 years. Patients who present with hypertension, heavy proteinuria, or an elevated creatinine are at higher risk for progression to ESRD. There is currently no satisfactory treatment available. Efforts should be directed at controlling hypertension and hyperlipidemia if present. Angiotensin-converting enzyme inhibitors[32] and/or fish oil[33] may offer benefits related to control of intraglomerular pressure, particularly in patients with proteinuria. A National Institutes of Health (NIH)-sponsored trial is currently being conducted evaluating prednisone and fish oil in children and young adults with IgA nephropathy.[34] Allograft survival in patients who receive a kidney transplant is good.

Poststreptococcal Glomerulonephritis

The epidemiology and pathogenesis of PSGN are well defined.[35] It is characterized by the onset of hematuria, proteinuria, hypertension, and sometimes oliguria and renal insufficiency 7 to 15 days after a streptococcal upper respiratory infection and 21 to 40 days after a streptococcal skin infection. Most common in children, it can occur at all ages. Epidemic disease occurs in crowded and unhygienic living conditions and is common in tropical countries and third world populations, especially in association with anemia, malnutrition, and intestinal parasites. It may occur in seasonal patterns and sometimes in cycles separated by several years. Epidemic disease is now uncommon in most westernized countries, although sporadic cases continue.[36] Asymptomatic disease is more common than clinical disease in most studies. Males predominate among patients with clinical but not subclinical disease. Only certain strains of streptococci have nephritogenic potential; nontypeable group A streptococci may also have that potential. It has been estimated that an average of 15 percent of infections with nephritogenic strains result in PSGN, with fully 90 percent of cases being subclinical, but the proportion varies with site of infection, the epidemic (if any), and the strain. Recurrence is uncommon.

PSGN is due to glomerular immune complex deposition, although the constituent streptococcal antigens are still being identified. A genetic predisposition is evidenced by attack rates in siblings of index cases of up to 37.8 percent after throat infections and 4.5 percent after skin infections. A streptococcal origin of acute GN is suggested if cultures or antigen tests have been positive for streptococci, or serum levels of antistreptolysin O (ASO) antibodies are elevated after throat infections (60 to 80 percent of cases), or if antihyaluronidase and anti-deoxyribonuclease antibodies are elevated after skin infections. A transient depression of serum complement helps differentiate PSGN from some other forms of GN. Renal biopsy is rarely indicated.

Prevention of PSGN involves improved nutrition, hygiene, and living conditions. Antibiotic treatment of streptococcal infections does not prevent PSGN, although it can confound the diagnosis by reducing ASO antibody production. Treatment does, however, reduce spread of streptococci to contacts and lessen their risk of getting PSGN. Prophylactic treatment for subjects at risk is recommended during epidemics and for siblings or families of patients with PSGN.

Urine abnormalities may persist for months after the acute attack. However, with follow-up limited to 10 to 15 years, studies of broad populations rather than of subjects initially hospitalized show complete recovery for most children, with rapidly progressive acute disease in less than 0.1 percent and chronic renal failure in less than 1 percent. Adults have about twice the rate of long-term urine abnormalities as do children, and chronic renal failure is more common, although still exceptional. Superimposed hypertension, renal changes with aging, and the hyperperfusion phenomenon might contribute to such a course.

Autosomal Dominant Polycystic Kidney Disease

Autosomal dominant polycystic kidney disease (ADPKD) is one of the most common inherited diseases and is characterized by fluid-filled cysts in the kidney, which can compress surrounding tissue and cause renal insufficiency. It occurs in every 1 of 400 to 1,000 live births, and an estimated 500,000 people have the disease in the United States.[37] Most families with ADPKD have an abnormality on chromosome 16 (PKD1 gene locus), but two other genes have been found that produce clinically similar ADPKD.[38] The abnormal gene on chromosome 16 has almost complete penetrance; however, the disease is often clinically silent and undiagnosed.

Abnormalities in the regulation of cell growth, epithelial fluid secretion, and extracellular matrix metabolism contribute to the clinical problems associated with ADPKD. Renal manifestations of ADPKD include hematuria, urinary tract infections, flank pain, nephrolithiasis, hypertension, and the most serious, renal failure. Approximately 45 percent of patients will have end-stage renal disease by 60 years of age. Although there is no treatment for ADPKD, control of hypertension and treatment of urinary tract infections are important to optimize renal function.

Extrarenal manifestations include hepatic cysts, cardiac valve abnormalities, colonic diverticula, hernias, and intracranial saccular aneurysms. Rupture of the intracranial aneurysms is associated with high morbidity and mortality, and screening is recommended for high-risk patients, such as those with a positive family history of intracerebral bleed, warning symptoms, a previous rupture, or a high-risk occupation where loss of consciousness would place the patient or others at risk.

The diagnosis of ADPKD has traditionally been done by ultrasound or CT evaluation of the kidneys. The sensitivity of these tests is not very high when used in patients under 20 to 25 years of age. Gene-linkage studies may be done in high-risk patients with no radiographically defined cysts; however, these studies will not detect non-PKD1 ADPKD, and they do not predict the clinical course. Genetic counseling is very important for patients with this disorder.[39]

Analgesic Nephropathy

Analgesic nephropathy (AAN) is a slowly progressive renal disease caused by the long-term ingestion of analgesics, classically a combination of agents including aspirin, acetaminophen, caffeine, and/or codeine. While the prevalence of AAN has decreased secondary to the removal of phenacetin from the market, the disease has not been completely eliminated and was named as the cause of renal failure in 0.8 percent of the incident ESRD cases from 1989 to 1993 in the United States.[7] The prevalence of AAN has been studied more extensively in Australia and Europe, where it appears to be more prevalent and is reported to be the cause of renal failure in up to 30 percent of the ESRD population.[40]

The pathogenesis of AAN is not well understood. Examination of the kidneys reveals chronic interstitial inflammation and papillary necrosis. In more advanced cases, cortical scarring occurs, most pronounced over the necrotic papillae, and gross examination of the kidneys reveal them to be small and nodular. Involvement of the medulla and papillae is felt to be secondary to increased concentration of the drugs in these areas with the generation of oxygen radicals and reduction of medullary bloodflow due to inhibition of prostaglandins.

AAN is more common in women. Individuals who have chronic pain for which analgesics may be consumed regularly and those with a history of peptic ulcer disease or gastric complaints are more likely to have a history of analgesic consumption. The patients may not be taking the medications at the time of presentation, but it is estimated that at least 1 to 2 kg of an offending agent need to have been ingested at some time to cause significant renal disease. The urinalysis may be normal or show pyuria, bacteriuria, and proteinuria, which is usually mild. Reduced ability to concentrate urine and renal tubular acidosis may occur, and there may be evidence for papillary necrosis when the kidneys are imaged as well as the reduced size and nodularity previously noted.

In addition to being the sole cause of ESRD in some cases, analgesic use contributes to more minor degrees of renal dysfunction in many other cases, and it is very probable that it contributes to the decline in renal function in patients with other underlying causes of renal insufficiency.

The nephrotoxicity of nonsteroidal anti-inflammatory agents (NSAIDs) is a more recently recognized phenomenon and is characterized by one of several presentations: acute renal failure secondary to renal vasoconstriction, interstitial nephritis with or without nephrotic syndrome and minimal change disease, hyperkalemia, sodium and water retention, and papillary necrosis. People with underlying volume depletion and/or those with chronic renal insufficiency have a higher risk of developing problems. Most of these conditions are reversible.

AAN is preventable, and renal disease has been shown to decrease with decreased availability of agents such as phenacetin. The National Kidney Foundation recently published a position paper regarding analgesic use. It has been recommended that over-the-counter combination analgesics be eliminated and all prescription combination analgesics have a warning on them regarding the risk of renal damage.[41] Aspirin as a single agent does not appear to impair renal function when used in therapeutic doses, especially the small doses recommended for prevention of cardiovascular events. There is an increased risk of larger doses leading to reversible deterioration of renal function in patients with underlying renal disease, and renal function should be monitored. For patients without liver disease, acetaminophen remains the nonnarcotic analgesic of choice, particularly for patients with underlying renal disease. Habitual consumption should be discouraged, as a case-control study done in Maryland, Virginia, West Virginia, and Washington, D.C., suggests that there may be an increased risk of renal insufficiency in patients who have taken large amounts over a lifetime.[42] Prolonged regular use of NSAIDs should be discouraged, and renal function should be monitored if regular use is necessary. NSAIDs should be avoided altogether in pregnancy. Use of NSAIDs in combination with other analgesics needs to be prospectively evaluated and should be avoided at this time.

Acute Renal Failure

Acute renal failure (ARF) is characterized by a relatively acute deterioration in renal function. Because defining the exact rate and nature of the deterioration is difficult to do, ARF is not well defined and therefore it is difficult to compare rates and outcomes.

Most cases of community-acquired ARF have a single, treatable cause of renal failure that is either prerenal (secondary to vomiting, poor intake, diarrhea, glycosuria, gastrointestinal bleeding, and diuretics) or postrenal (secondary to prostate enlargement from hyperplasia or carcinoma).[43] It is not very common and the prognosis is usually good.

Greater than 60 percent of patients with hospital-acquired ARF have had more than one renal insult. Hospital-acquired ARF develops in between 2 and 5 percent of patients in a general medical-surgical environment and is frequently caused by decreased renal perfusion usually secondary to volume contraction, poor cardiac output, and sepsis. In one study postoperative patients accounted for 18 percent of all ARF, and contrast media and aminoglycosides combined accounted for another 19 percent. Prognosis appears to correlate with the severity of renal insufficiency and degree of oliguria/anuria.[44]

The frequency of ARF in intensive care units ranges from 6 to 23 percent. Nearly all of these patients have had multiple renal insults, and it is frequently seen in the context of multiorgan failure. Survival is significantly reduced in these patients (10 to 30 percent), especially in the presence of multiorgan failure.

ARF caused by blood loss and crush injuries is common during war and natural disasters. ARF secondary to general trauma has declined from 11.3 percent of all ARF cases in 1960 to 1969 to 2.8 percent in 1980 to 1988.[45] Pregnancy-related ARF has declined in the United States from 10 to 20 percent of all ARF in the 1960s to being rare since 1980. Abortion contributed to much of the ARF in the past, and now preeclampsia/eclampsia and uterine hemorrhage cause the majority of pregnancy-related ARF. ARF is being seen more commonly now in patients with AIDS, malignancy, and sepsis. The use of NSAIDs and angiotensin-converting enzyme inhibitors may also contribute to the development of ARF in patients with underlying renal hypoperfusion. ARF rates secondary to contrast and antibiotics appears to be stable.

Despite increasing awareness of the etiology of ARF and advancing technology, the mortality of ARF has not decreased significantly over the last several decades. Several explanations have been offered to explain this including the increasing age of patients with ARF, the presence of multiple medical problems and/or organ failure in patients with ARF, and lack of efficacy of new renal replacement techniques. While the exact reason for the above is not clear, it is clear that many episodes of ARF can be avoided by limiting the use of diagnostic and therapeutic nephrotoxic agents, particularly in susceptible patients such as those with volume depletion, poor cardiac function, and sepsis.

Renal Disease and Illicit Drugs

Renal disease related to drug abuse is being recognized more frequently as a cause of renal disease and has great social and economic impact; in a survey reported in 1983 more than 10 percent of ESRD dialysis populations between 18 and 45 years in some large U.S. metropolitan areas had this diagnosis.[46] Several syndromes are recognized.

Focal segmental glomerulosclerosis (FSGS) occurs in intravenous heron addicts, with heavy proteinuria and progression to renal failure in a few months to years. There is no effective treatment. An immunologic mechanism is postulated, mediated through a response to heroin itself, to adulterants, or to infectious agents. FSGS associated with drug abuse occurs in all ethnic groups, but rates are especially high in young black males, leading to the hypothesis that parental drug abuse unmasks a genetic predisposition to FSGS in blacks. In a study from Buffalo, New York, rates of FSGS were 29 times higher in black addicts than in other blacks, and ESRD rates were 18 times higher.[46]

Renal deposition of amyloid, associated with chronic inflammation and infection, occurs in skin poppers.[47] Proteinuria and sometimes renal failure are diagnosed at an average age of 41 years, 10 years older than FSGS patients. In a New York City autopsy series, 5 percent of addicts and 26 percent of addicts with suppurative skin infections had unsuspected renal amyloidosis.[48]

Other renal diseases related to drug abuse include immune-complex GN associated with infectious endocarditis or hepatitis B antigenemia, membranoproliferative GN and cryoglobulinemia associated with hepatitis C, necrotizing vasculitis related most strongly to amphetamine abuse, tubular dysfunction and occasionally acute renal failure in solvent sniffers, acute renal failure due to muscle breakdown, and the renal syndromes of human immunodeficiency virus infection.

Treatment of addicts with ESRD is often complicated by noncompliance, communicable diseases such as hepatitis B, hepatitis C, and acquired immunodeficiency syndrome (AIDS), and, with continued drug abuse, infection and clotting of vascular access and recurrence of disease in kidney transplants. Because of the interfaces of drug addiction with crime, some of these subjects are incarcerated. Such problems accentuate dilemmas about responsibility for personal health and allocation of limited resources.

Renal Disease and the Human Immunodeficiency Virus

The understanding of renal disease associated with HIV infection continues to evolve. Renal disease may occur at all stages of HIV illness including the asymptomatic stage, but many complications are associated with acute illness. Patients may develop fluid and electrolyte disorders, acid-base disturbances, and/or acute renal failure secondary to volume depletion, infections, drugs, and/or abnormal adrenal steroid synthesis and secretion. There is also a pathologically unique nephropathy associated with HIV called HIV nephropathy. Patients with this disorder usually have nephrotic range proteinuria accompanied by renal insufficiency, which progresses fairly rapidly to ESRD (within 3 to 6 months).[49] On examination there is frequently no significant peripheral edema or hypertension, and the kidneys are normal to increased in size despite being highly echogenic. This may be contrasted to heroin-associated nephropathy in which hypertension is frequently present, the kidneys are small, and progression to ESRD is a slower process. Although it is not always possible to distinguish HIV-associated disease from other forms of glomerulosclerosis, the following pathological findings are felt to be very suggestive of HIV nephropathy and include focal to global glomerulosclerosis, collapse of the glomerular tuft, severe tubulointerstitial fibrosis with some inflammation, microcyst formation, tubular degeneration, and characteristic tubuloreticular inclusions.[49]

While HIV nephropathy was initially noted to be more prevalent in young, black males who were IV drug users, it is now known that it can occur in most risk groups. It has even been reported in children of HIV-infected mothers, where vertical transmission accounts for infection. Development of HIV nephropathy does appear to be more likely in blacks and males.

Patients who are HIV positive and develop acute renal failure due to acute tubular necrosis (ATN) tend to be younger than the non-HIV–positive patient with ATN, and frequently the ATN is associated with sepsis. Treatment consists of conservative, supportive care, and hemodialysis may be used until kidney function returns. Much of the ATN associated with HIV disease is preventable if patients receive adequate volume support prior to use of nephrotoxic agents or during episodes of hypovolemia and if attention is paid to medication/antibiotic dosing.[50]

There is no proven effective treatment of HIV nephropathy. Preliminary reports suggest that antiviral therapy with azidothymidine (AZT) may slow the progression of HIV nephropathy. Symptom-free HIV-positive subjects with chronic renal failure can do quite well on dialysis, but chronic dialysis of subjects with clinical AIDS is complicated by concomitant illness, cachexia, infectious hazards, and prolonged hospitalizations, and survival is usually short.

Hemolytic Uremic Syndrome (HUS)

HUS is one of several clinical syndromes that affects the vasculature of the kidney, producing a thrombotic microangiopathy. It is discussed here in relationship to a bacteria, *Escherichia coli* O157:H7, which has emerged as a major cause of diarrhea, particularly bloody diarrhea, in North America. Several studies[51] have now shown that this *E. coli* is responsible for most cases of HUS in children, which is a major cause of acute renal failure. While it has been isolated in many parts of the world, its prevalence is unknown. Infections are more common in warmer months, and transmission may occur via undercooked beef, fecally contaminated water, and person-to-person. Infection has also been associated with unpasteurized commercial apple juice.[52]

Patients typically present with abdominal cramping, diarrhea (nonbloody or bloody), nausea, and vomiting. HUS has been reported to occur in about 6 percent of patients with infection and is diagnosed from 2 to 14 days after the onset of the diarrhea. It is more likely to affect young children and the elderly. It is characterized by microangiopathic hemolytic anemia, thrombocytopenia, and renal failure. Central nervous system manifestations may be present. The renal pathologic lesions include edematous intimal expansion of arteries, fibrinoid necrosis of arterioles, and edematous subendothelial expansion in glomerular capillaries.[53]

There is no specific therapy that has proven to be effective for HUS secondary to *E. coli* infection. Treatment involves supportive therapy with red blood cell transfusions, control of hypertension, and dialysis if necessary. The prognosis for typical childhood HUS is usually good. Neurological involvement, prolonged oliguria, elevated white blood cell count, age under 2 years, and atypical presentations have been associated with a poorer prognosis. The mortality rate is 3 to 5 percent, and about 5 percent of patients who survive have severe sequelae, including ESRD.

To prevent *E. coli* infection, patients should be counseled about the risk of eating undercooked ground beef. A thorough history should be taken in suspected cases, and cases should be reported early to prevent spread. Hand washing is essential in institutions such as day care centers and nursing homes, and children with a known infection should be kept at home.

▸ URINARY TRACT DISEASES

Urinary Tract Infections

Urinary tract infections (UTIs) are one of the most common types of infection encountered in clinical medicine. They account for more than 7 million physician visits and necessitate or complicate over 1 million hospital admissions annually in the United States.[54] They are most frequent in young, sexually active women, and it is estimated that one in five women will have a UTI in her lifetime. UTIs are also common in preschool girls, in postmenopausal women, and in elderly men and women, especially those who are institutionalized and those with indwelling urinary catheters. UTIs in older men are often associated with urinary retention, urethral strictures, calculi, and debilitating illness. Boys and men with normal urinary tracts are not often affected, but men can acquire bacterial UTIs through heterosexual or homosexual intercourse, and recurrent UTI is the hallmark of chronic prostatitis.[55]

Most infections are localized to the bladder and urethra, but some involve the kidneys and renal pelves (pyelonephritis) or the prostate. UTIs rarely lead to renal damage or failure unless they are associated with diabetes, pregnancy, reflux, obstruction, or neurogenic bladder. Diabetic persons with UTIs risk papillary necrosis and sepsis; abortion and other complications can result from UTIs in pregnancy; and morbidity and mortality of UTIs increase greatly in the elderly and in those with complicating conditions, such as spinal cord injury.

Most UTIs in young women are new events, uncomplicated, and caused by *E. coli* and other bowel organisms that enter the bladder through the short female urethra. Subjects with recurrent UTIs have increased density of bacterial receptors on epithelial cell surfaces in the vagina and bladder. Women with blood groups A and AB who are nonsecretors of blood group substance are at greater risk. Intercourse, diaphragm use, and failure to void after intercourse all increase risk. Women who have closely spaced recurrent infections with the same organisms or who have pyelonephritis should be evaluated for urinary tract abnormality, as should men with persistent infection.

In the presence of symptoms, white cells and bacteria in a clean-void midstream specimen of urine usually indicate a UTI. The usual bacterial count considered diagnostic on urine culture is more than 100,000/mL, but many patients have lower counts, including half of those with cystitis and most patients with urethral syndromes. Enterobacteriaceae colony counts as low as 100/mL have a sensitivity and a specificity for UTI of 94 and 85 percent. An easy and relatively inexpensive dip slide urine culture technique can be performed by subjects with recurrent UTIs, and self-treatment under medical guidance can be initiated. Many uncomplicated UTIs are treated on the basis of symptoms and pyuria alone.

Screening for bacteriuria in symptom-free persons is not cost-effective and may lead to inappropriate treatment, drug reactions, and selection of resistant organisms. Treatment of asymptomatic bacteriuria is not generally recommended, except in pregnant women, diabetics, and children with vesicoureteral reflux. Symptomatic infections are treated by antimicrobials, and infections associated with sexual intercourse can usually be prevented by single-dose prophylactic therapy. Repeated or prolonged antibiotic treatment can select antibiotic-resistant organisms. Some broad-spectrum antimicrobial agents may not pose this threat and are sometimes used for prophylaxis in subjects with chronic infections.

UTIs are the leading form of nosocomial infection and are especially common in nursing homes. Spread can be reduced by separation of catheterized patients from others who are debilitated or catheterized, and by washing the hands after patient contact. For subjects who require temporary catheterization, risks of infection can be reduced by aseptic insertion, curtailed duration of catheterization, and meticulous care of the patient and the drainage system. However, infection remains very common in persons with chronic indwelling catheters. The bacterial flora in the urine of catheterized subjects is in flux, colonization is often asymptomatic, and repeated courses of treatment are not advised.

Interstitial cystitis is a syndrome of unknown etiology and pathogenesis with symptoms similar to UTIs. It is characterized by nocturia, urgency, and suprapubic pressure and pain with filling of the bladder. It is more common in women and may be the cause of multiple outpatient physician visits. Therapy is frequently not completely effective, and it can occasionally lead to a significant decrease in quality of life.

Urinary Stone Disease

Urinary stone disease has been recognized since antiquity and continues to be a major cause of morbidity. The incidence is increasing not only in the United States, but in Sweden and Japan, and is felt to be related to increased dietary animal protein intake. It is estimated that 500,000 Americans suffer from stone episodes each year and up to 12 million Americans will develop stones in their lifetime.[56] In 1986, more than $2 billion was spent on the treatment of kidney stones.[57] Men are affected about four times as often as women, and the initial stone usually presents in the third to fifth decade. Urinary stone disease is relatively uncommon in underdeveloped countries, where bladder stones predominate.

Most kidney stones (82 percent) contain calcium, primarily in the form of calcium oxalate (60 percent of all stones). The remaining stones contain uric acid, struvite, cystine, and/or small amounts of other compounds. The content of the stone may give clues to the underlying physiological problem, especially in the case of stones without calcium. Disorders associated with stone disease include primary hyperparathyroidism, renal tubular acidosis, enteric hyperoxaluria, sarcoidosis, cystinuria, and urinary tract infection or obstruction. Risk factors associated with calcium stone formation include low urinary volume, hypercalciuria, hyperoxaluria, hypocitraturia, and hyperuricosuria.

Most patients present with flank pain radiating into the groin which is abrupt in onset and frequently severe. Gross or microscopic hematuria, dysuria, frequency, nausea, and vomiting can be present. Occasionally, patients will have an ileus. Most kidney stones pass spontaneously, and the patient can be supported with analgesics. Urological intervention may be required, including extracorporeal shock-wave lithotripsy (ESWL) and percutaneous nephrolithotomy. These two procedures have reduced the costs, morbidity, and hospitalization rates compared with surgery.

The primary objective of therapy is to prevent the formation of recurrent stones. Conservative management includes adequate fluid intake (2 L or more/day) and dietary sodium restriction. Oxalate restriction, reduction of animal protein intake, thiazide diuretics, and other agents may also be recommended, depending on the patient's underlying medical condition and the cause of stone formation. Studies looking at dietary modification of calcium intake have produced conflicting results,[57] but calcium restriction is frequently recommended.

Prostate Cancer

Prostate cancer, a disease of aging men, is becoming an increasingly important public health problem in the United States. It is the most commonly diagnosed cancer in men in the United States and is the second leading cause of male cancer deaths.[58] The incidence, prevalence, and mortality rates from prostate cancer increase with age, particularly after age 50 years. One estimate predicted that a 50-year-old American man has an approximately 40 percent chance of developing microscopic prostate cancer during his lifetime, a 10 percent chance of being diagnosed with the disease, and a 2 to 3 percent chance of dying of prostate cancer.[59] Age-adjusted incidence rates and mortality rates vary from country to country. In 1988, the age-adjusted death rates per 100,000 population were 15.6 for men in the United States and 3.5 for men in Japan.[60]

While the presence of histologic cancer appears to be related to age, both genetic and environmental risk factors appear to increase the development of clinical prostate cancer. Asian men have a lower incidence of and mortality due to clinical prostate cancer, while Scandinavian men have a higher incidence. Men tend to take on the risk of their host country, but race is also a factor. African American men have a higher incidence than do black men in Africa or Asia and a higher incidence than white men. African American men are also diagnosed with later-stage disease, and their survival rates are shorter. In general, socioeconomic status is not felt to explain the incidence differences between African Americans and whites. There is an increased risk of prostate cancer for men with a family history, and cadmium exposure is felt to weakly increase the risk. While both prostate cancer and benign prostatic hypertrophy (BPH) appear to be androgen dependent, it has been difficult to determine whether or not BPH is a risk factor for prostate cancer because both are common in men as they age. Associations with venereal disease, sexual activity, and smoking have been proposed but not proven. Studies have been conflicting, but it appears that vasectomy may increase the risk of prostate cancer. It has been suggested that this is mediated through the increased levels of testosterone seen in men after vasectomy. A high intake of dietary fat also seems to be a risk factor, and it has been suggested that this is mediated through endogenous hormones. Recent reports suggest that a gene on the long arm of chromosome 1 may be the first major gene identified which predisposes men to prostate cancer.[61]

Patients typically present with symptoms of urinary tract obstruction (urgency, nocturia, frequency, and hesitancy) from an enlarged prostate gland causing bladder-neck obstruction. These symptoms are essentially the same as those seen with BPH. Other less common signs and symptoms include back pain from vertebral metastases and new onset of impotence. A few patients may have symptoms related to urinary retention caused by bladder-neck obstruction, bilateral hydronephrosis from periaortic lymph node enlargement, or spinal cord compression from epidural extension. Rarely, patients may present with an enlarged supraclavicular node or elevation of liver tests.

Many of the small, well-differentiated carcinomas remain confined to the prostate and are detected only at autopsy (latent or autopsy cancers). The majority never become active, but how to predict which tumors will become so has not been determined. Management of prostate cancer may include watchful waiting, hormonal therapy, prostatectomy, and radiation therapy, depending on the stage of the cancer. Treatment considerations should include age, life expectancy, comorbid conditions, side effects, and costs. Urinary incontinence, impotence, and radiation morbidity compose the treatment-related adverse effects. Multiple clinical trials are currently under way that should help identify the best therapy for the various stages of prostate cancer.

Measuring serum prostate-specific antigen (PSA), a glycoprotein produced almost exclusively by prostatic epithelial cells, has been used with increasing frequency as a screening tool in the detection of prostate cancer in conjunction with digital rectal examinations and transrectal ultrasonography. While PSA is elevated in men with prostate cancer and has been shown to correlate with tumor burden in men with established cancer, it is not specific for prostate cancer. Concerns have been raised about its use as a screening tool, leading to increased detection of insignificant cancers with an increase in expense but not reduction in mortality. A recent prospective study looking at the pathological features of prostate cancer detected via PSA concluded that most of the cancers detected via PSA screening were clinically important.[62] Randomized, prospective trials are currently being conducted to attempt to identify the most appropriate use of the various screening techniques, including the PSA.

Prostatic Hyperplasia

Benign prostatic hypertrophy is extremely common in older men. It has been reported that BPH can be found in 88 percent of autopsies in men 80 or more years of age and that nearly 50 percent of men 50 or more years of age have symptoms compatible with BPH.[63] Three men in 10 may ultimately require surgery.[64]

The cause of BPH is not known. Necessary conditions are the presence of androgens and aging. No associations with sociocultural factors, sexual behavior, use of tobacco or alcohol, or other diseases have been consistently demonstrated, and there is no firm evidence that BPH is a precursor of prostate cancer.

In BPH subjects, a period of rapid prostate enlargement occurs, usually after the age of 50, followed by stabilization. Clinical symptoms result from variable compression of the bladder outlet, with difficulties in urinating, and the potential for infection, complete obstruction, and bleeding. The determinants of clinical symptoms are poorly understood, but they might correlate better with horizontal cross-sectional features of the prostate around the bladder neck and urethra than with total prostate weight.[65] The natural history of symptoms can vary greatly. Many subjects have mild symptoms for years, with no change, and many do not require surgical intervention. Evaluation consists of rectal examination, blood chemistry studies, urinalysis and culture, measurement of residual urine volume after voiding, cystourethroscopy, urodynamic evaluation, and imaging or contrast studies of the kidneys and ureters.

Many patients can be observed while monitoring for progression. α-Adrenergic blocking agents and androgen suppressants are currently being studied for patients with mild to moderate symptoms. For more severe symptoms, prostatectomy is the standard of care. Indications for surgery vary, need better definition, and should be weighed against the comorbidities, complications, outcomes, and costs. Firm indications are acute urinary retention, hydronephrosis, recurrent urinary infections, severe hematuria, severe outflow obstruction, and urgency incontinence. Persistence of symptoms and impotence can result from surgery in a significant minority of subjects. Newer procedures are being developed including the use of prostatic stents, balloon dilation of the prostate, laser prostatectomy, and microwave hyperthermia.[66]

▸ END-STAGE RENAL DISEASE

ESRD can be caused by many renal diseases and by some urinary tract diseases when they are complicated by chronic obstruction or infection. In the United States, diabetic nephropathy accounted for 37.2 percent of treated incident ESRD from 1989 to 1993, followed by hypertensive nephropathy (30.3 percent), glomerulonephritis (12.3 percent), cystic kidney disease (3.0 percent), interstitial nephritis (3.0 percent), collagen vascular diseases (2.2 percent), and obstructive nephropathy (2.0 percent).[7]

At the end of 1993, approximately 220,000 ESRD patients were being treated in the United States and its territories. Both the incidence rate and the prevalence rate of ESRD increase with age until 65 to 74 years, at which point the rate declines. The average age of incident ESRD patients was 60 years for the period from 1991 to 1993, while the average age of prevalent ESRD patients was 54.4 years. Definite gender and racial differences exist. While blacks constitute 12.5 percent of the general population in the United States, they constitute 29.1 percent of the ESRD population, a rate 4-fold higher than that of whites. The ESRD incidence and prevalence rates for Asian/Pacific Islanders and Native Americans are between those of whites and blacks. ESRD is also slightly more common in men than in women, with 54 percent of the incident and prevalent ESRD population comprised of men.

The first patient with chronic renal disease was dialyzed in 1960 by Belding Scribner. During the 1960s the development of vascular access, chronic peritoneal dialysis catheters, and improved immunosuppressive therapies allowed patients to choose between some form of hemodialysis, peritoneal dialysis, or renal transplantation. With the enactment of the Social Security Amendments of 1972 (effective in July 1973), treatment became available for all patients with ESRD. Currently, patients choose one of the above therapeutic modalities based on a combination of medical and social factors. Transplantation is regulated by national and local policies, physician and patient preference, and availability of donor organs.

Relatively recent advances in the treatment of ESRD patients include high flux, bicarbonate hemodialysis using biocompatible membranes, automation of peritoneal dialysis, use of vitamin D derivatives for treatment of renal osteodystrophy, and genetically engineered erythropoietin for treatment of anemia, reducing the need for blood transfusions. Continued advancements in the development of immunosuppressive agents have improved the 1-year first-time cadaveric transplant survival from 70 percent in 1984 to 83 percent in 1993.

Despite improvements in dialysis technology, mortality remains high. For example, at age 44 the expected remaining lifetime of a white male with ESRD on dialysis is 6.3 years compared with 35.4 years for a white male from the general population. Survival for patients receiving a transplant cannot be directly compared to that for dialysis patients due to selection factors; however, in the example above, survival extends to 9.6 years when including all patients with ESRD including those who received a renal transplant. Gross mortality rates of dialysis patients in the United States have been the highest in any surveyed country and were continuing to rise until recently. Age, primary diagnosis, acceptance of patients with multiple comorbid conditions, transplantation rates, dose of dialysis delivered, patient compliance, nutrition, and predialysis therapy all may contribute to this phenomenon.

The total Medicare payment per patient-year (average for all ESRD patients of all ages) is estimated to be $36,700 for the years 1991 to 1993. Transplantation costs are less than those for dialysis patients, $17,600 per year versus 43,700 per year. This does not include the cost of organ procurement for transplantation patients. Annual costs for all ESRD patients rise with age, primarily due to the decline in transplantation rate for elderly patients. Diabetic patients with ESRD are more costly to treat than nondiabetics.[7]

Current efforts are being directed at determining the reasons for the significant mortality rates in United States dialysis patients.[67] In addition, the Health Care Financing Agency is sponsoring a national study to determine whether more effective ESRD care can be provided using a capitated system.

▶ THE FUTURE

Progress has been made in several areas of renal and urinary tract diseases as evidenced by the decrease in death rate from hypertensive renal disease, renal infections, and renal congenital abnormalities. However, Eberhardt et al found that death rates from diabetes with renal involvement increased 102 percent from 1979 to 1990, and death rates associated with other selected renal conditions also increased. Mortality associated with nephritis or ESRD and renal cancer also increased, but to a lesser extent. During the same period, changes in hospital discharge rates and doctor's office visit rates mirrored changes in mortality rates, except for hypertensive renal disease, for which hospital discharge rates increased 70 percent and doctor's office visit rates increased 190 percent.[68]

While progress has been made, the number of patients reaching ESRD continues to increase. The total estimated direct medical payments for ESRD by public and private sources was $11.13 billion during 1994 with the estimated total federal spending being $8.31 billion, or 75 percent of the total estimated cost.[7] It is clear that the current challenge in westernized societies, many of which have made a large commitment to life support for subjects with irreversible renal failure, is to better understand the factors that contribute to ESRD. The public health perspectives of many of these diseases remain poorly defined and the distributions and natural histories of many remain obscure. While progress has been made in identifying specific prevention and treatment strategies, many diseases continue to lack specific strategies, and the prevalence of ESRD will continue to increase.

Epidemiological and health services research in renal and urinary tract diseases is expanding rapidly. In the United States, the National Institutes of Diabetes, Digestive and Kidney Diseases have collated existing data on rates, morbidities, mortalities, resource utilization, and costs. They are supporting studies on diabetic renal disease, hypertension, progressive glomerular sclerosis, progression of renal failure, urinary tract obstruction, prostatic hyperplasia, prostatic cancer screening, and urinary incontinence. They have also established research initiatives in interstitial cystitis, HIV-associated renal disease, the genetic basis of polycystic kidney disease, and renal disease and hypertension in minorities. The National Health and Nutrition Examination Survey–1988 to 1994 will yield estimates of rates of kidney stones, UTIs, interstitial cystitis, prostate disease, bladder dysfunction, microalbuminuria, and elevated serum creatinine levels. The newly established United States Renal Data System promises valuable longitudinal data.

The results of these initiatives should invigorate the practice of nephrology, guide judicious apportionment of limited resources, support formulation of rational health policy, and improve the overall outcomes for patients with renal and urinary tract disease.

▶ REFERENCES

1. Challah S, Wing AJ: The epidemiology of genitourinary disease. In Holland WW, Detels R, Knox G (eds): The Oxford Textbook of Public Health. Oxford, England: Oxford University Press, 1985, chap. 11, vol. 4
2. Levey AS, Perrone RD, Madias NE: Serum creatinine and renal function. Annu Rev Med 39:465–490, 1988
3. Pedrini MT, Levey AS, et al: The effect of dietary protein restriction on the progression of diabetic and nondiabetic renal diseases: a meta-analysis. Ann Intern Med 124:627–632, 1996
4. Klahr S, Levey AS, et al: The effects of dietary protein restriction and blood pressure control on the progression of chronic renal disease. N Engl J Med 330(13):877–884, 1994
5. The Diabetes Control and Complications (DCCT) Research Group: Effect of intensive therapy on the development and progression of diabetic nephropathy in the Diabetes Control and Complications Trial. Kidney Int 47:1703–1720, 1995
6. Striker G: Report on a workshop to develop management recommendations for the prevention of progression in chronic renal disease. J Am Soc Nephrol 5(7):1537–1540, 1995
7. Excerpts from United States Renal Data System 1996 Annual Data Report. Am J Kidney Dis 28(3(S2)):1996
8. Bennett PH, Haffner S, et al: Screening and management of microalbuminuria in patients with diabetes mellitus: Recommendations to the Scientific Advisory Board of the National Kidney Foundation from an ad hoc committee on the Council on Diabetes Mellitus of the National Kidney Foundation. Am J Kidney Dis 25(1):107–112, 1995
9. Borch-Johnsen K, Norgaard K, et al: Is diabetic nephropathy an inherited complication? Kidney Int 41:719–722, 1992
10. Selby JV, FitzSimmons SC, et al: The natural history and epidemiology of diabetic nephropathy. JAMA 263(14):1954–1960, 1990
11. Mogyorosi A, Ziyadeh FN: Update on pathogenesis, markers and management of diabetic nephropathy. Curr Opin Nephrol Hypertens 5:243–253, 1996
12. Messent JWC, Elliott TG, Hill RD, et al: Prognostic significance of microalbuminuria in insulin-dependent diabetes millitus: a twenty-three year follow-up study. Kidney Int 41:836–839, 1992
13. Lewis EJ, Hunsicker LG, et al: The effect of angiotensin-converting-enzyme inhibition on diabetic nephropathy. N Engl J Med 329:1456–1462, 1993
14. The Diabetes Control and Complications Trial Research Group: The effect of intensive treatment of diabetes on the development and progression of long-term complications in insulin-dependent diabetes mellitus. N Engl J Med 329(14):977–986, 1993
15. Clark CM Jr, Lee DA: Prevention and treatment of the complications of diabetes mellitus. N Engl J Med 332(18):1210–1217, 1995
16. Bojestig M, Arnqvist HJ, et al: Declining incidence of nephropathy in insulin-dependent diabetes mellitus. N Engl J Med 330:15–18, 1994
17. Pugh JA, Stern MP, et al: Excess incidence of treatment of end-stage renal disease in Mexican Americans. Am J Epidemiol 27:135–144, 1988
18. Megill DM, Hoy WE, Soodruff SD: Rates and causes of end stage renal disease in Navajo Indians, 1971–1985. West J Med 149:178–182, 1988

19. Hoy WE, Megill DM: Mesangial proliferative glomerulonephritis in Southwestern Native Americans. Transplant Proc 21:3909–3912, 1989
20. Sievers ML: Historical overview of hypertension among American Indians and Alaskan Natives. Ariz Med 43:607–610, 1977
21. McClellan W, Tuttle E, Issa A: Racial differences in the incidence of hypertensive end stage renal disease are not entirely explained by differences in the prevalence of hypertension. Am J Kidney Dis 12:285–290,1988
22. Tierney WM, McDonald CJ, Luft FC: Renal disease in hypertensive adults: effect of race and type 2 diabetes mellitus. Am J Kidney Dis 13:485–493, 1989
23. Schulman NB, Ford CE, Hall WD, et al: Prognostic value of serum creatinine and effect of treatment of hypertension on renal function: results from the Hypertension Detection and Follow-up Program. Hypertension 13(suppl):180–193, 1989
24. Rostand SG, Brown G, Kirk KA, et al: Renal insufficiency in treated essential hypertension. N Engl J Med 320:684–688, 1989
25. Qualheim RE, Rostand SG, Kirk KA, et al: Changing patterns of end-stage renal disease due to hypertension. Kidney Int 37:244, 1990
26. Schwartz MM, Korbet SM: Primary focal segmental glomerulosclerosis: pathology, histological variants, and pathogenesis. Am J Kidney Dis 22(6):874–883, 1993
27. Schwartz MM, Korbet SM, Lewis EJ: Primary focal segmental glomerulosclerosis: clinical course and response to therapy. Am J Kidney Dis 23(6):773–783, 1994
28. Austin HA, et al: Membranous nephropathy. Ann Intern Med 116(8): 672–682, 1992
29. Glassock RJ: The therapy of idiopathic membranous glomerulonephritis. Semin Nephrol 11(2):138–147, 1991
30. Imperiale TF, Goldfarb S, Berns JS: Are cytotoxic agents beneficial in idiopathic membranous nephropathy? A meta-analysis of the controlled trials. J Am Soc Nephrol 5:1553–1558, 1995
31. Galla JH: IgA nephropathy. Kidney Int 47:377–387, 1995
32. Cattran DC, Greenwood C, Ritchie S: Long-term benefits of angiotensin-converting enzyme inhibitor therapy in patients with severe immunoglobulin A nephropathy: a comparison to patients receiving treatment with other antihypertensive agents and to patients receiving no therapy. Am J Kidney Dis 23(2):247–254, 1994
33. Donadio JV, Bergstralh EJ, et al: A controlled trial of fish oil in IgA nephropathy. N Engl J Med 331:1194–1199, 1994
34. Hogg RJ: A randomized, placebo-controlled, multicenter trial evaluating alternate-day prednisone and fish oil supplements in young patients with immunoglobulin A nephropathy. Am J Kidney Dis 26(5): 792–796, 1995
35. Rodriguez-Iturbe B: Acute poststreptococcal glomerulonephritis. In Schrier RW, Gottschalk CW (eds): Diseases of the Kidney. 4th ed. Boston: Little, Brown, 1986, chap 63
36. Cameron JS: The long term outcome of glomerular diseases. In Schrier RW, Gottschalk CW (eds): Diseases of the Kidney. 4th ed. Boston: Little, Brown, 1986, chap 69
37. Gabow PA: Autosomal dominant polycystic kidney disease. N Engl J Med 329(5):322–342, 1993
38. Grantham JJ: The etiology, pathogenesis, and treatment of autosomal dominant polycystic kidney disease: recent advances. Am J Kidney Dis 28(6):788–803, 1996
39. Lieske JC, Toback FG: Autosomal dominant polycystic kidney disease. J Am Soc Nephrol 3:1442–1450, 1993
40. Eknoyan G: Current status of chronic analgesic and nonsteroidal anti-inflammatory nephropathy. Curr Opin Nephrol Hypertens 3:182–188, 1994
41. Henrich WL, Agodoa LE, Barrett B, et al: Analgesics and the kidney: summary and recommendations to the Scientific Advisory Board of the National Kidney Foundation from an ad hoc committee of the National Kidney Foundation. Am J Kidney Dis 27(1):162–165, 1996
42. Perneger TV, Whelton PK, Klag MJ: Risk of kidney failure associated with the use of acetaminophen, aspirin, and nonsteroidal anti-inflammatory drugs. N Engl J Med 331(25):1675–1679, 1994
43. Kaufman J, Dhakal M, et al: Community-acquired acute renal failure. Am J Kidney Dis 17:191–198, 1991
44. Elasy TA, Anderson RJ: Changing demography of acute renal failure. Semin Dialysis 9(6):438–443, 1996
45. Turney JH, Marshall DH: The evolution of acute renal failure, 1956–1988. Q J Med 74:83–104, 1990
46. Cunningham EE, Zielezny MA, Venuto RC: Heroin associated nephropathy, a nationwide problem. JAMA 250:2935–2936, 1983
47. Neugarten J, Gallo GR, et al: Amyloidosis in subcutaneous heroin abusers ("skin poppers' amyloidosis"). Am J Med 81:635–640, 1986
48. Menchel S, Cohen D, Gross E, et al: AA protein-related renal amyloidosis in drug addicts. Am J Pathol 112:195–199, 1983
49. Humphreys MH: Human immunodeficiency virus-associated glomerulosclerosis. Kidney Int 48:311–320, 1995
50. Rao TKS, Friedman EA: Outcome of severe acute renal failure in patients with acquired immunodeficiency syndrome. Am J Kidney Dis 25(3):390–398, 1995
51. Boyce TG, Swerdlow DL, Griffin PM: *Escherichia coli* O157:H7 and the hemolytic-uremic syndrome. N Engl J Med 333(6):364–368, 1995
52. Morbidity and Mortality Weekly Report: Outbreak of *Escherichia coli* O157:H7 infections associated with drinking unpasteurized commercial apple juice. JAMA 276(23):1865, 1996
53. Remuzzi G, Ruggenenti P: The hemolytic uremic syndrome. Kidney Int 47:2–19, 1995
54. Stamm WE, Hooton TM: Management of urinary tract infections in adults. N Engl J Med 329(18):1328–1334, 1993
55. Neu HC: Urinary tract infections. Am J Med 92(4A):63S–70S, 1992
56. Pak CYC: Etiology and treatment of urolithiasis. Am J Kidney Dis 18(6):624–637, 1991
57. Curhan GC, Willett WC, Rimm EB, Stampfer MJ: A prospective study of dietary calcium and other nutrients and the risk of symptomatic kidney stones. N Engl J Med 328(12):833–838, 1992
58. Pienta KJ, Esper PS: Risk factors for prostate cancer. Ann Intern Med 118:793–803, 1993
59. Garnick MB: Prostate cancer: screening, diagnosis, and management. Ann Intern Med 118:804–818, 1993
60. Boring CC, Squires TS, Tong T: Cancer statistics, 1992. CA 42: 19–39, 1992
61. Health agencies update: gene for prostate cancer. JAMA 276(23): 1864, 1996
62. Humphrey PA et al: Prospective characterization of pathological features of prostatic carcinomas detected via serum prostate specific antigen based screening. J Urol 155(3):816–820, 1996
63. Napalkov P, Maisonneuve P, Boyle P: Worldwide patterns of prevalence and mortality from benign prostatic hyperplasia. Urology 46(3 Suppl A):41–46, 1995
64. Boyle P: New insights into the epidemiology and natural history of benign prostatic hyperplasia. Prog Clin Biol Res 386:3–18, 1994
65. Watanabe H: Natural history of benign prostatic hypertrophy. Ultrasound Med Biol 12:567–571, 1986
66. Hollander JB, Diokno AC: Prostatism: benign prostatic hyperplasia. Urol Clin North Am 23(1):75–86, 1996
67. Morbidity and mortality of renal dialysis: An NIH consensus conference statement. Ann Intern Med 121:62–70, 1994
68. Eberhardt MS, Wagener DK, et al: Trends in renal disease morbidity and mortality in the United States, 1979 to 1990. Am J Kidney Dis 26(2):308–320, 1995

54

Diabetes

Trevor J. Orchard • Ronald E. LaPorte • Janice S. Dorman

Diabetes is an important chronic disease both in terms of the number of persons affected and the considerable associated morbidity and early mortality. In this review we focus on the epidemiology and public health implications of diabetes.

Diabetes is a chronic disease in which there is a deficiency in the action of the hormone insulin. This may result from a quantitative deficiency of insulin, an abnormal insulin, resistance to its action, or a combination of deficits. Two major forms of the disease are recognized: insulin-dependent diabetes mellitus (IDDM), which composes about 10 percent of all cases, and non-insulin–dependent diabetes mellitus (NIDDM), which accounts for about 90 percent of the cases. The criteria for the definition of diabetes are shown in Table 54-1 and are those of the National Diabetes Data Group (NDDG).[1] Diabetes may occasionally occur as a result of other diseases: endocrine diseases, such as acromegaly and Cushing's syndrome, or metabolic disorders, such as hemochromatosis. Diabetes can also be drug induced, for example, by steroids and possibly by the thiazide diuretics and oral contraceptives. Finally, diabetes may occur secondary to disease processes directly affecting the pancreas, such as cancer or chronic pancreatitis, which destroy the insulin-producing β cells in the pancreatic islets (of Langerhans). However, these are relatively rare causes of diabetes.

In addition to these primary and secondary types of diabetes, two further classifications of abnormalities of glucose tolerance are of note, namely, gestational diabetes and impaired glucose tolerance (IGT). Gestational diabetes occurs during pregnancy but typically remits shortly after delivery. IGT is a condition with high blood sugars after glucose challenge that are not elevated enough to be classified as diabetic but nonetheless may carry some increased risk of large vessel (e.g., coronary heart) disease.[1,2] Both gestational diabetes[3] and IGT[4] carry an increased risk for the subsequent development of NIDDM.

▸ DIAGNOSIS

The diagnosis of IDDM, also known as type I diabetes or juvenile onset diabetes, is fairly straightforward. IDDM often, though by no means always, has its onset in childhood. Classically the child will have symptoms of excessive thirst (polydipsia), excessive urination (polyuria), and weight loss. In a child with a high blood sugar these symptoms almost invariably point to IDDM. This type of diabetes is called insulin dependent because patients lose virtually all capacity to produce insulin. Without treatment they develop severe metabolic disturbances, including ketoacidosis and dehydration, which can lead to death. As death from ketoacidosis is largely preventable, the continuing though small number of deaths from this cause represents a challenge to our preventive health services.[5,6] In an international study, wide variations in mortality from acute diabetes complications were noted, with high rates in Japan and low rates in Finland. This variation was thought to reflect disease incidence (low in Japan and high in Finland) and resulting availability of skilled health care.[7]

NIDDM, also known as type II, usually presents in adulthood. In the past the terms *maturity-onset* and *mild diabetes* have been used. These terms are somewhat misleading, since NIDDM may present in youth, albeit rarely, and the complications may be far from mild. Patients with NIDDM, however, produce some insulin, although its secretion is often delayed, and there is usually some resistance to its action in the peripheral tissues. This resistance is often associated with elevated concentrations of insulin, particularly in newly recognized cases. However, concentrations are now recognized to be low in many NIDDM subjects, especially after accounting for obesity and using more specific assays.[8] In 1993, 7.8 million persons, or approximately 3 percent of the population, in the United States were estimated to have been diagnosed with diabetes according to the National Health Interview Survey.[9] This prevalence is strongly related to age and increases from 1.3 percent for 18 to 44 year olds to 6.2 percent for 45 to 64 year olds and 10.2 for 65 to 74 year olds. It is also estimated that almost as many cases of NIDDM are undiagnosed as are clinically recognized. This is made clear by data from the National Health and Examination Survey[10] where the overall prevalence of diabetes in the adult U.S. population (20 to 74 years old) is estimated to be about 6.7 percent (Table 54-2). This includes a small proportion (0.23 percent) who have IDDM, 3.4 percent who are recognized to have NIDDM, and a further 3.2 percent of the population with undiagnosed type II diabetes. A further 11.2 percent of the population probably suffer from impaired glucose tolerance according to World Health Organization (WHO) criteria. Thus, combining all three groups, diagnosed diabetes, undiagnosed diabetes, and IGT, over 28 percent of 45 to 74 year olds are affected.[11]

In NIDDM, often the diagnosis is not made on the basis of classic diabetic symptoms but rather on the presentation of one of the complications of diabetes. Such complications can be macrovascular (accelerated atherosclerosis with coronary artery, peripheral vascular, or cerebrovascular manifestations), microvascular (with disease of the small vessels in the kidneys or the eyes), or neuropathic (which may take the form of a variety of neurological syndromes). In addition, the disease may also be recognized as a result of routine screening for elevated blood sugar or by the presence of sugar in the urine. Some cases, however, may be diagnosed because of classic diabetic symptoms.

Over the years both the diagnostic criteria and dose of glucose in the oral glucose tolerance test (OGTT) have varied. The effect of these different criteria on the prevalence of diabetes has been studied by many investigators.[12] Compared to many earlier criteria, the current NDDG criteria (Table 54-1) represent a relatively strict set of limits requiring a higher degree of hyperglycemia before a diagnosis of diabetes is made.[13]

TABLE 54-1. CRITERIA FOR THE CLASSIFICATION OF DIABETES

Classification	*Adults*	*Children*
Diabetes[a]	A. Symptoms with unequivocal hyperglycemia *or* B.[b] Fasting glucose ≥ 140 mg/dL (venous plasma) or ≥ 120 mg/dL (venous or capillary whole blood) *or* C.[b] Fasting glucose < B, but at 2 h plus an intervening value,[d] glucose ≥ 200 mg/dL (venous plasma or capillary whole blood) *or* ≥ 180 mg/dL (venous whole blood)	A. Symptoms with random plasma glucose ≥ 200 mg/dL *or* B.[b] Fasting glucose ≥ 140 mg/dL (venous plasma) *or* ≥ 120 mg/dL (venous/capillary whole blood) *and* 2 h plus an intervening value[e] ≥ 200 mg/dL (venous plasma/capillary whole blood) *or* ≥ 180 mg/dL (venous whole blood)
Impaired glucose tolerance[c]	1. Fasting glucose < 140 mg/dL (venous plasma) *or* < 120 mg/dL (venous capillary whole blood) *and* 2. ½ h, 1 h, or 1½ h glucose[d] ≥ 200 mg/dL (venous plasma or capillary whole blood) *or* ≥ 180 mg/dL (venous whole blood) *and* 3. 2 h glucose[d] between 140 and 200 mg/dL (venous plasma or capillary whole blood) *or* between 120 and 180 mg/dL (venous whole blood)	1. Fasting glucose < 140 mg/dL (venous plasma) *or* < 120 mg/dL (venous or capillary whole blood) *and* 2. 2 h glucose[e] > 140 mg/dL (venous plasma) *or* > 120 mg/dL (venous or capillary whole blood)
Gestational diabetes	*Two or more of the following values after a 100-g oral glucose load:* Fasting ≥ 105 mg/dL (venous plasma) 1 h ≥ 190 mg/dL (venous plasma) 2 h ≥ 165 mg/dL (venous plasma) 3 h ≥ 145 mg/dL (venous plasma)	 90 mg/dL (venous or capillary whole blood) 170 mg/dL (venous or capillary whole blood) 145 mg/dL (venous or capillary whole blood) 125 mg/dL (venous or capillary whole blood)
Normal glucose values (nonpregnant individuals)	Fasting < 115 mg/dL (venous plasma) < 110 mg/dL (venous or capillary whole blood) ½ h,[d] 1 h,[d] 1½ h[d] < 200 mg/dL (venous plasma/capillary whole blood) < 180 mg/dL (venous whole blood) 2 h[d] < 140 mg/dL (venous plasma/capillary whole blood) < 120 mg/dL (venous whole blood)	Fasting < 130 mg/dL (venous plasma) or < 115 mg/dL (venous or capillary whole blood) 2 h[e] < 140 mg/dL (venous plasma/capillary whole blood) *or* < 120 mg/dL (venous whole blood)

From National Diabetes Data Group: Criteria for the classification of diabetes. Diabetes 28:1039–1054, 1979.

[a] Diabetes is subclassified as:

IDDM (type I): insulin is needed to preserve life.

NIDDM (type II): further classed as (1) nonobese NIDDM and (2) obese NIDDM.

Gestational: Diabetes or impaired glucose tolerance is first recognized during pregnancy. Usually remits postpartum.

Other: Diabetes that develops secondary to or in association with other conditions, e.g., pancreatic disease; hormonal, drug, or chemical induced; insulin receptor abnormalities; and genetic syndromes.

[b] Criteria need to be present on at least two occasions.

[c] For epidemiological purposes, an adult may be assigned to this classification if criteria 1 and 3 are met and other blood samples are not available.

[d] Following 75 g of oral glucose.

[e] Following glucose 1.5 g/kg body weight; maximum 75 g.

The reasons for choosing the current criteria are 2-fold. First, studies in several high-risk populations, especially among the Pima Indians,[14] have shown that the distribution of blood sugars in these populations may be bimodal rather than the unimodal pattern found in a typical U.S. white population and that the second upper distribution is characterized by plasma glucose concentrations approximately equal to the NDDG suggested limits. Second, the specific complications of diabetes, for example, retinopathy, also appeared to occur primarily among individuals who had blood sugars that exceeded these limits.

Thus in reviewing studies done in previous years, it is important to remember that the criteria of diabetes were often less stringent and that the relationship between diabetes and subsequent risk of disease may have been quite different from that based on the current definitions. Also, because of these changes in the criteria for the diagnosis of NIDDM, estimates of the prevalence and temporal trends of NIDDM are difficult if not impossible to evaluate. Furthermore, the different criteria for NIDDM used by different research groups and countries make geographical comparisons difficult. As major efforts are made to identify the specific genetic abnormalities in diabetes and to define the disease on the basis of genotypic rather than phenotypic expression, such as hyperglycemia and insulin levels, there may soon be yet another way of classifying diabetes. Furthermore, the development of glycosylated hemoglobin (GHb),[15] which provides an integrated measure of hyperglycemia over the prior 2 to 3 months, represents another dimension that may add to the ability to define diabetes. For example, some patients may show a "diabetic" response to an oral glucose challenge but experience little hyperglycemia in their normal life, where such glucose loads are rare. Such patients may therefore have "diabetes" but may have normal GHb and conceivably a lower risk of developing complications. Because of these developments, and

TABLE 54-2. PERCENT OF POPULATION (STANDARD ERROR) OF PREVIOUSLY DIAGNOSED AND OF UNDIAGNOSED DIABETES IN THE U.S. POPULATION AGE 20 TO 74 YEARS (NHANES II) FROM 1978 TO 1980

	Age				
	20–74	*20–44*	*45–54*	*55–64*	*65–74*
■ ***MEDICAL HISTORY OF DIABETES***[a]					
All races					
Both sexes	3.4 (.14)	1.1 (.11)	4.3 (.53)	6.6 (.66)	9.3 (.45)
Male	2.9 (.25)	.6 (.12)	4.3 (.82)	5.6 (.64)	9.7 (.71)
Female	3.8 (.24)	1.5 (.22)	4.3 (.67)	7.4 (1.10)	8.9 (.56)
White					
Both sexes	3.2 (.16)	1.0 (.12)	4.2 (.55)	6.0 (.58)	8.9 (.49)
Male	2.8 (.27)	.5 (.15)	4.5 (.92)	5.3 (.66)	9.1 (.78)
Female	3.6 (.23)	1.4 (.22)	3.9 (.60)	6.6 (.91)	8.8 (.64)
Black					
Both sexes	5.2 (.49)	2.2 (.58)	5.7 (1.46)	13.1 (2.65)	13.6 (1.35)
Male	4.5 (.60)	1.8 (.63)	3.6 (1.48)	9.2 (2.55)	17.2 (2.87)
Female	5.9 (.99)	2.6 (1.00)	7.5 (2.33)	16.3 (4.03)	10.8 (1.51)
■ ***UNDIAGNOSED DIABETES (NDDG CRITERIA)***[b]					
All races					
Both sexes	3.2 (.35)	0.9 (.31)	4.2 (.81)	6.2 (1.03)	8.4 (.85)
Male	2.8 (.41)	0.8 (.39)	3.6 (1.28)	4.0 (1.03)	9.5 (1.42)
Female	3.6 (.42)	1.0 (.38)	4.7 (1.14)	8.1 (1.68)	7.6 (.89)
White					
Both sexes	3.0 (.38)	0.7 (.31)	4.0 (.90)	5.9 (1.24)	8.0 (.85)
Male	2.5 (.36)	0.5 (.27)	3.2 (1.25)	3.8 (1.00)	9.0 (1.38)
Female	3.4 (.52)	0.8 (.40)	4.6 (1.25)	7.9 (2.08)	7.3 (.95)
Black					
Both sexes	4.4 (.91)	0.9 (.68)	7.2 (3.05)	7.7 (3.75)	12.3 (3.94)
Male	4.0 (1.72)	1.0 (.98)	7.5 (6.40)	5.2 (3.94)	12.2 (7.23)
Female	4.6 (1.35)	0.9 (.91)	7.0 (3.70)	9.1 (5.92)	12.3 (4.50)

From Harris MI, Hadden WC, Knowler WC, Bennett PH: Prevalence of diabetes and impaired glucose tolerance and plasma glucose levels in the U.S. population aged 20–74 yr. Diabetes 36(4):523–534, 1987.

[a] Based on a self-report that the persons had been told by a doctor that they had diabetes, plus current or past use of diabetic therapy.

[b] Based on the results of a 75-g oral glucose tolerance test conducted in the morning after an overnight 10- to 16-hour fast in persons with no medical history of diabetes.

the recognition that few doctors use the OGTT to diagnose diabetes, except in association with pregnancy,[5] both the WHO and the American Diabetes Association are actively (at the time of writing) re-examining the diagnostic and classification criteria for diabetes with an increased focus on fasting blood sugar levels and GHb, both of which appear in Pima Indians to predict NIDDM complications as well as the 2 hour OGTT.[16,16a]

Heterogeneity in Primary Diabetes

Although two different primary types of diabetes have been described, the classification of diabetes into these two groups is not simple. For example, there may be varying types of insulin-dependent diabetes according to the human leukocyte antigen (HLA) types with which they are associated, particularly HLA-DR3 and HLA-DR4, which are common in IDDM.[17,18] It is also possible that some cases of childhood diabetes are in fact better classified as being "maturity-onset diabetes of youth (MODY)" or "Mason"-type diabetes, the latter named after the family in England first described with this variety.[19] MODY or Mason are types of diabetes characterized by a familial abnormality of glucose tolerance inherited in an autosomal dominant pattern who often have a low frequency of complications and ketoacidosis. Children in such families, however, are often treated with insulin, although they are not strictly insulin dependent. Thus there are probably further subcategories beyond the insulin- and non-insulin–dependent types, which themselves may not be totally distinct entities. For example, data from Pittsburgh[20] and from the Joslin Clinic[21] show an increased risk for the development of IDDM in families where a relative has NIDDM, suggesting that these two types of diabetes may not be totally independent of each other. Although some of this increased risk may be explained by ascertainment bias,[20] this does not seem to be the entire explanation. The possibility of an "incomplete" IDDM process of autoimmune cell destruction, which may give rise to a clinically intermediary type of diabetes, therefore exists.[5,22] This possibility has gained further strength with reports of anti-GAD antibodies (a marker of IDDM) being present in the sera of some clinically non-insulin–dependent diabetic subjects.[23]

Insulin-Dependent Diabetes Mellitus

One of the most important observations related to insulin-dependent diabetes is the marked geographic variability of the disease. Figure 54-1 presents the incidence of IDDM for the various registries around the world. The annual risk for developing IDDM varies from over 35/100,000 in Finland to 0.5/100,000 in Korea and China. Overall there is approximately a 50-fold difference between countries for developing IDDM (Fig. 54-1).[24,25]

In the United States the risk for developing IDDM is about 15/100,000/year[26,27] during childhood. About 12,000 children per year develop IDDM in the United States. The estimated prevalence of IDDM is about 1.6/1,000 school-age children.[27,28]

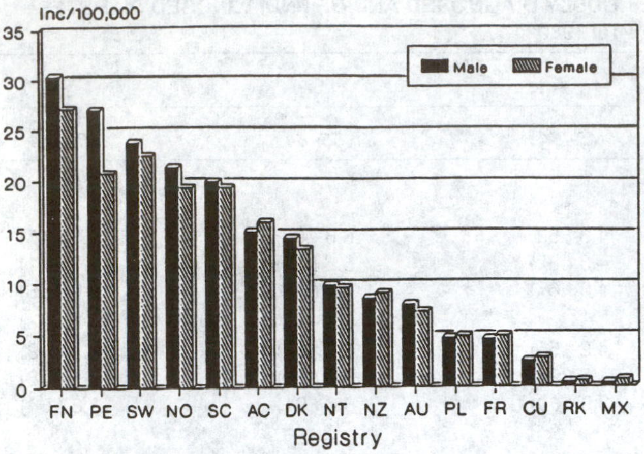

Figure 54-1. Age-standardized incidence rates of IDDM under age 15 years (per 100,000). *FN,* Finland; *PE,* Prince Edward Island, Canada; *SW,* Sweden; *NO,* Norway; *SC,* Scotland; *AC,* Allegheny County, Pennsylvania, United States; *DK,* Denmark; *NT,* The Netherlands; *NZ,* New Zealand; *AU,* Austria; *PL,* Poland; *FR,* France; *CU,* Cuba; *RK,* Republic of Korea; *MX,* Mexico. (From Reivers M, LaPorte RE, King HOM, Tuomilehto J: Trends in the prevalence and incidence of diabetes: insulin-dependent diabetes mellitus in childhood. World Health Stat Q 41:179–190, 1988.)

In addition to the marked geographic differences in incidence, IDDM has a distinctive demographic pattern. There is little difference in the overall incidence rates for males and females.[26] Whites have about 1.5 times the incidence rate of blacks. The incidence increases with age, peaking at adolescence, followed by a marked decline. This adolescent peak is likely to be related to puberty or to a growth spurt–associated phenomenon, since in females this peak occurs earlier than in males in a way similar to the onset of puberty. The incidence patterns by age are virtually identical across countries except for a very unusual pattern in Finland[29] where, other than age 0, the incidence is about the same thoughout childhood and very high. The environmental agent may be a super antigen. Most HLA diseases have distinctive epidemiologic patterns. A super antigen is the product of viral or bacterial agents, which can stimulate whole families of T cells (e.g., 30 percent) in contrast with a usual agent that may stimulate 1/10,000 T cells.[30] Recently, several HLA-associated disorders, including lupus,[31] toxic shock syndrome,[32] and Kawasaki disease,[33] in addition to IDDM[34] appear to have the features of a super antigen–mediated disease, which may explain their epidemiologic characteristics.

In the United States there was no evidence for a changing incidence with IDDM from 1965 to 1985.[35] However, in Allegheny County, Pennsylvania, there was an extensively rapid increase in incidence from 1985 to 1989, especially in young males.[36] The increase was most evident in nonwhites from 1990 to 1994, such that the rate in nonwhites was higher than for whites.[37]

Several European countries have also experienced an increase.[38] There is also a seasonal pattern of the onset of IDDM, with a consistent decline in the number of cases presenting during the summer months.[26] The pattern of seasonality has been identified in essentially all registry studies and is similar in high-risk as well as in low-risk countries.[35] The seasonality pattern has primarily been attributed to a viral cause of the disease or to an acute stress precipitating the clinical disease.[39] Recently it has been argued that the geographic patterns, seasonality, changes of incidence over time, and the migrant studies all strongly imply major environmental determinants of the disease.[40] It has been estimated that at least 70 percent and perhaps up to 95 percent of IDDM can be attributed to an environmental cause.

One of the most intriguing aspects of IDDM is the strong associations with the HLA region of chromosome 6. During the 1980s, most studies evaluating serological HLA markers have confirmed that IDDM susceptibility is highly related to specific alleles at the HLA-DR locus. Approximately 95 percent of all IDDM patients are HLA-DR3, HLA-DR4, or both.[41] Children with these antigens, particularly the DR3-DR4 heterozygotes, have a greater risk of developing IDDM than individuals without the high-risk alleles have.

With the current advances in molecular biology, the associations between IDDM and the HLA region are now being studied at the DNA level. Early restriction fragment length polymorphism (RFLP) studies show a strong association between some HLA-DQ β-fragment patterns and IDDM.[42] The molecular HLA studies have begun to focus on the DQ locus in search of possible "diabetogenic" genes. It has been demonstrated that an amino acid other than aspartate in position 57 of the HLA-DQ β chain (non-Asp-57; ND), coded for by the DQB1 gene is highly associated with IDDM susceptibility, whereas an aspartic acid in this position (Asp-57) appears to protect against the development of the disease.[43,44] These relationships are particularly striking among individuals who also carry DQA1 alleles (which code for the DQ α chain) that contain DNA sequencer for arginine in position 52 (non-Arg-52; R).[45,46] The HLA-DQ and DR loci are tightly linked with linkage disequilibrium between the DQA1*R and DQB1*ND alleles, and both DR3/DR4. Thus, the molecular associations observed for DQ appear to reflect, in part, the well-documented relationships with DR.

The risk within families also appears to be associated with the presence of HLA susceptibility genes. The differential risk of developing IDDM for the sibling of a proband depends on the number of HLA haplotypes the individual shares.[41] In normal populations, siblings have a 25 percent likelihood of sharing both haplotypes, a 50 percent likelihood of sharing only one, and a 25 percent probability of not sharing any haplotypes. Evaluation of DQ allele sharing in multiple-case families has revealed that 87.5 percent of affected sibling pairs shared both DQ alleles with the proband, 4.2 percent shared one, and 8.3 percent shared zero.[41] Among the nonaffected siblings in these families, the distribution was 27.3, 45.4, and 27.3 percent, respectively, for sharing two, one, and zero alleles with the proband. The strong associations between IDDM and the HLA-DQ alleles, as well as the increase in risk for siblings who are HLA-identical with the index case, suggest that molecular genetic screening of siblings of an IDDM patient could provide useful information about risks among the siblings. High-risk children could then be monitored for early signs of glucose intolerance and autoimmunity.[47] Those with HLA susceptibility alleles and islet-cell antibodies are most likely to subsequently develop IDDM.[48] However, sometimes these antibodies disappear prior to disease onset.[49]

Screening the general population to identify genetically at-risk individuals is not advised. The frequency of diabetes is low even among those who are genetically susceptible. Among caucasians, for example, the overall annual incidence of IDDM among whites is approximately 15 to 20/100,000. However, in the general population those who are homozygous for DQA1*R and DQB1*ND alleles have less than 5 percent chance of developing diabetes.[49] Thus the risk of developing IDDM, even in those who are genetically susceptible, is low and it would seem unlikely that a screening program, especially since there is no preventive approach, would be advantageous.

With recent advances in molecular genetics, several investigators have undertaken several genomewide screens of multiple IDDM case families.[50] These studies have revealed that at least six additional loci are involved in IDDM susceptibility. However, with the exception of the insulin gene region on chromosome 11p15, little is known about the nature of these additional genes, or their interaction, in contributing to IDDM risk. Although future research will obviously focus on the confirmation and characterization of these genes, it is also known that immunological markers are good predictors of IDDM, particularly in susceptible individuals.

The treatment of new cases of IDDM with immunosuppressive agents such as cyclosporin or oral insulin is being evaluated to try to arrest the development of disease. This approach, however, is strictly experimental at present.[51]

Non-Insulin–Dependent Diabetes Mellitus

NIDDM is difficult to define. The rates among and within countries vary dramatically, partially depending on the specific classification criteria used for NIDDM.

Estimates of the prevalence of NIDDM between populations vary from a low of less than 2/10,000 to a high of 4,000/10,000 in the Pima Indians.[52] NIDDM occurs in all races, but the prevalence tends to be high among American Indians, Micronesians, Polynesians, U.S. black women, and Mexican Americans.[53] The prevalence of diabetes (known and unknown) in the United States is intermediary, about 6 percent for whites and about 10 percent for blacks (Table 54-2).[10]

Certain key factors that account for these marked geographic and ethnic differences in diabetes have been suggested. One of the critical risk factors appears to be change in socioeconomic status.[53] In communities where there has been rapid economic development, such as in Korea[54] and among the Pima Indians,[52] there appears to be a marked and rapid increase in the incidence and prevalence of NIDDM.[52–54] Two factors have been suggested to account for this rapid rise in NIDDM. When the food sources in a population become more plentiful, a rapid rise in body weights of individuals and a decline in physical activity may occur, with a corresponding increase in the rates of NIDDM. A pattern of increasing mean weight of the population and increasing prevalence of NIDDM has been noted.[55] Similarly within a population there is a strong correlation between degree of obesity and risk of NIDDM.[52,56,57] Interestingly, within a country such as the United States, one generally finds an inverse relationship between obesity and socioeconomic class,[58] as well as higher rates of NIDDM in lower socioeconomic groups.[59] Many studies have determined that obesity is independently associated with the risk of NIDDM. Approximately 80 percent of non-insulin–dependent diabetics are obese. Controversy is related to the specific type of calories responsible for this excess. There is relatively little evidence that increased sugar, per se, in the diet is a risk factor for diabetes. There are also questions about the effects of high fiber and its role in the diet and the risk of developing diabetes. Some studies suggest that there is relatively little difference in the blood sugar response to simple sugar compared with starch among both normal individuals and those with diabetes,[60] while the hypothesis that a high-fiber diet protects against diabetes also remains unsubstantiated.[61] Nonetheless, the value of increasing fiber in the diet to reduce the blood glucose response to food among diabetics is well established.[62] Accumulating evidence suggests that dietary fat may be the dietary component most likely to play a role in the pathogenesis of NIDDM.[63] At present, low caloric intake and weight reduction (including fat restriction) are suggested for prevention of NIDDM.

A number of recent studies have clearly demonstrated that the distribution of body fat, independent of obesity, is a further predictor of subsequent diabetes.[64,65] An increased central deposition of fat (i.e., "android" as opposed to "gynoid"), often measured as an increased waist-hip girth ratio, or waist circumference, appears to predict not only diabetes but also cardiovascular disease (see below). Central adiposity, which is an indirect measure of visceral adiposity, may be associated with a different metabolic state linked to insulin resistance.[66]

The second primary risk factor for NIDDM associated with the increase in socioeconomic status is physical activity. As socioeconomic status increases, the overall level of physical activity generally declines, especially that related to work. Thus, at the same time that caloric intake is increasing, physical activity is decreasing, and there is an increased prevalence of obesity within the population. Data from the South Pacific suggest that physical activity itself may be an independent risk factor for NIDDM, separate from obesity,[67] while a recent prospective study in the United States also suggests that reduced physical activity predicts NIDDM.[68] The recognition of other risk factors (such as inactivity) is important since not all obese individuals develop NIDDM. In some populations there is little increase in the prevalence of diabetes despite a substantial increase in the degree of obesity.[53]

Genetic factors play an extremely important role in the development of NIDDM. In a large study of twins, Pyke and colleagues found that the concordance rates for NIDDM among monozygotic twins was over 90 percent compared with 50 percent for IDDM.[69] Twin studies, however, do not provide the complete story. In recent years there have been numerous studies of the relationship of genetic markers to the development of NIDDM as well as of IDDM. Although HLA genes are related primarily to the risk of developing IDDM, they may also play a role in NIDDM.[70] Several candidate genes have been found to contribute to NIDDM susceptibility, including mutations in the insulin gene,[71] the glucokinase gene,[72] and mitochondrial gene.[73] However, it is unlikely that any of these alterations explain the genetic susceptibility to NIDDM on a population basis. Thus family and pedigree studies are still needed to determine the contribution of these genetic markers to the development of NIDDM.

The prevention of NIDDM may be possible in the future. Further analyses of the insulin gene structure and its relationship to both insulin secretion and insulin structure may provide a technique for identifying high-risk individuals, at least within specific families. A consensus is growing that development of NIDDM is a two-stage process, with the first stage being resistance to insulin's action (probably exacerbated by obesity and physical inactivity) and the second stage being failure of the pancreas to increase insulin secretion enough to compensate. This theory receives support from a number of reports including one from the Pima Indians, which showed differing predictive values of fasting and post challenge insulin values for developing NIDDM consistent with a hyperinsulinemic phase followed by eventual insulinopenia.[74]

Weight loss is strongly recommended to improve glucose tolerance among NIDDM patients[75] and will substantially improve glucose tolerance among nondiabetic individuals.[76] Similarly, increased physical activity leads to improved insulin sensitivity and glucose tolerance.[77] As obesity and inactivity are major risk factors for NIDDM, they have been adopted as the basis of a lifestyle intervention arm in a new U.S. government–sponsored trial to determine whether NIDDM can be prevented. This trial, called the Diabetes Prevention Program (DPP), will also include in addition to a placebo group, two drug arms, namely metformin and troglitazone in a massive undertaking involving 4,000 subjects with impaired glucose tolerance. DPP is not scheduled to be completed until 2002.[78]

Persons with impaired glucose tolerance, the entry qualification for DPP, have both an increased risk of subsequent diabetes and appear to be at increased risk for cardiovascular disease compared with individuals with normal glucose tolerance, according to the large Whitehall[2] and Paris[79] studies. However, despite an increasing body of evidence linking this subgroup with hyperinsulinemia, another Cardiovascular Disease (CVD) risk factor (see below), there is no evidence to date that intervention to correct impaired glucose tolerance is beneficial. A secondary objective of DPP is, therefore, to determine if the interventions will help to reduce cardiovascular risk.

▶ MORBIDITY AND COMPLICATIONS OF DIABETES

Prior to the introduction of insulin in 1922 by Banting and Best, life expectancy of patients with IDDM was about 1 to 2 years. After the development and widespread use of insulin, there was a dramatic increase in life expectancy for patients with IDDM. Suddenly those with insulin-dependent diabetes could lead relatively normal lives. However, 20 to 30 years later the long-term sequelae of IDDM began to become evident.

Both IDDM and NIDDM patients are at risk for these long-term complications. These come mainly from disorders of the circulation, either macrovascular, including accelerated atherosclerosis resulting in stroke, heart, and peripheral vascular disease, or microvascular disorders of the kidney and retina, as well as neuropathy. The complications appear to be similar for both IDDM and NIDDM, although the prevalence may be somewhat higher in IDDM, especially of renal disease. The relationships with age and duration also vary between the two types of diabetes, partly because of the younger age of onset of IDDM (which leads to complications at a younger age) and the difficulty of determining the onset of NIDDM (which means complications are often present at the onset of known disease). However, careful analysis controlling for these time-dependent variables suggests that the incidence of the microvascular complications is remarkably similar by true duration.[80] The following discussion will mainly focus on IDDM, since these data are more complete.

In an international study, Diabetes Epidemiology Research International (DERI), mortality in young cohorts of IDDM cases from four different countries (the United States, Israel, Japan, and Finland) was investigated. The study showed tremendous variation in diabetes-related mortality. In addition to the high mortality from acute complications, the Japanese cohort also has a high mortality from renal disease (276/100,000/year) compared with Finland (16/100,000/year, $P < 0.05$).[81] The importance of renal disease is highlighted by data from the Steno Memorial Hospital in Copenhagen, which suggests that renal disease (as identified by proteinuria) is the chief risk factor for coronary disease in IDDM.[82]

Mortality rates in diabetes, especially IDDM, appear to be falling.[82,83] Data from Pittsburgh suggest that cohorts who were diagnosed in the 1960s and 1970s have a lower mortality than those diagnosed in the 1950s.[83] Much of the decline in mortality has been the result of a reduction in deaths at onset, but there also has been an improvement in long-term life expectancy among insulin-dependent diabetics.[82] In Japan, where the disease is rare, mortality rates are also falling rapidly as medical care for IDDM improves and expands (Fig. 54-2).[84]

Diabetic Retinopathy

After 20 years of IDDM, virtually 100 percent of patients show some evidence of damage to the retina, called background retinopathy. Similar prevalence rates are seen in NIDDM for patients treated with insulin, although rates are lower (around 55 percent) for those not on insulin.[85] In addition, as many as 70 percent of IDDM[86] and 30 percent of NIDDM[85] on insulin may develop proliferative changes in the eyes that may lead to blindness.

Diabetes is the leading cause of blindness in the 20- to 74-year age group in the United States. Each year approximately 6,000 diabetics become legally blind (corrected visual acuity less than 20/200 in the better eye). The prevalence of blindness due to diabetes is estimated at 40,000 individuals. Diabetes is associated with a 6-fold greater risk of blindness compared with that in the general population.[87]

The Diabetic Retinopathy Study has demonstrated that individuals with severe diabetic retinopathy can be treated successfully and their vision preserved with laser photocoagulation therapy.[88] Retinopathy was the primary outcome of a major U.S. study called Diabetes Control and Complications Trial (DCCT).[89] This landmark study clearly demonstrated the value of intensive therapy (with normal blood sugars as a goal) for IDDM subjects in preventing or delaying the microvascular complications. Progression of retinopathy was reduced by 54 percent in the intensive therapy group compared with conventional therapy over a mean follow-up period of 6.5 years.[89]

Because diabetic retinopathy can be detected before it threatens vision, blindness due to diabetic retinopathy can be prevented in many cases. It is thus important that patients and physicians be educated about the need for frequent eye examinations and that adequate clinical treatment for diabetic retinopathy be available in the community.

Diabetic Renal Disease

Diabetic renal disease is a major cause of morbidity and mortality among those with diabetes.[5,81,87,90,91] Diabetes is currently the leading cause of treatment for end-stage renal disease,[87] accounting for 25 percent of the 4,000 new end-stage renal disease patients each year. About 8,000 such diabetic patients are currently receiving treatment. Diabetes increases the risk of renal failure 17- to 20-fold, while approximately 40 percent of patients with IDDM[82,91] eventually develop significant clinical proteinuria and renal disease. Studies from Pittsburgh[86] suggest that approximately 70 percent of IDDM subjects will have some degree of renal damage (i.e., including those with microalbuminuria—a more modest degree of abnormal urinary albumin excretion that is predictive of more advanced disease).

Prevalence rates are somewhat lower in NIDDM overall, partly because the later age of onset means that many patients may have died from heart disease before there has been sufficient duration to develop renal disease. The relative risk of mortality from renal disease for persons with diabetes compared with the general population is highest for those in the 15- to 44-year age group, consistent with a higher prevalence and severity in IDDM.[90] Despite recent advances in the diagnosis and treatment of renal failure in diabetes, the problem has not been resolved. The presence of microalbuminuria appears to predict the subsequent development of diabetic nephropathy and end-stage renal failure.[92] Of particular note is the value of angiotensin-converting enzyme (ACE) inhibitors in reducing the risk of renal failure and/or progression of nephropathy in IDDM subjects with proteinuria,[93] and more recently in slowing the progression from microalbuminuria to overt proteinuria/nephropathy.[94] This effect of ACE inhibitors appears to be independent of any blood pressure–lowering effect. Hypertension, which may be primary or secondary to the renal disease, also accelerates the development of renal failure. Lipid disturbances may also predict the development of microalbuminuria.[95] The major predictor, however, of the development of early diabetic renal disease is poor glycemic control,[96] and the value of an intensive therapy regimen was also clearly demonstrated in the DCCT.[89] Several further reports, largely based on IDDM patients, have suggested that drug treatment of hypertension (or even mildly elevated blood pressure) and protein restriction, as well as intensified glucose control, may reduce albumin excretion in the early stages.[92]

Neuropathy

Another major complication of diabetes is neuropathy. Clinically significant neurological disability usually does not occur until at least 5 years after the diagnosis of diabetes. The major consequences of diabetic neuropathy are pain, weakness, and loss of sensation. Parallel disorders of the autonomic nervous system may lead to problems of sexual function and urinary and gastrointestinal abnormalities. Research has focused on the metabolic causes of the nerve damage and the specific biochemical lesions that lead to neurological changes.[97] One recent epidemiological study has demonstrated both a high prevalence of distal symmetrical neuropathy in IDDM, 70 percent after 30 years,[86] and a strong relationship with cardiovascular risk factors, for example, lipid disturbances, cigarette smoking, and especially

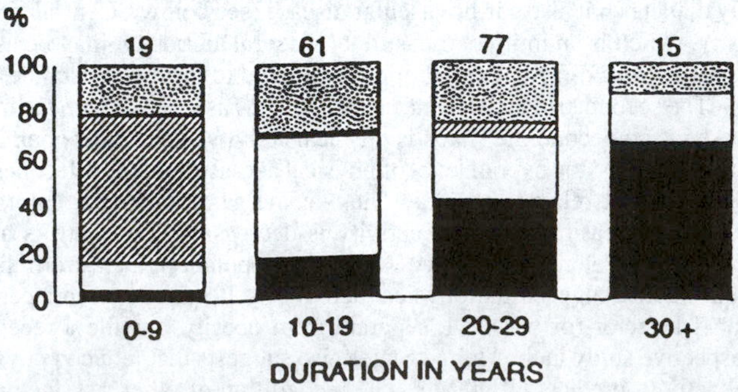

Figure 54-2. EDC Study: causes of death by duration in years. ■, cardiovascular; □, renal; ▨, other diabetes-related; ▩, non-diabetes-related causes. (From Orchard TJ: From diagnosis and classification to complication and therapy: DCCT Part II? The Kelly West Lecture. Diabetes Care 17(4):326–338, 1994.)

hypertension.[98] A major problem in diabetic neuropathy is how to measure it. Multiple techniques are currently advocated.[99,100]

It has long been recognized that strict control of blood sugar may improve neural function, for example, peripheral nerve conduction.[101] The recent DCCT results also confirm the value of lower blood sugar levels in preventing/delaying clinical neuropathy.[89] The above findings concerning blood pressure and lipids suggest that studies to evaluate the benefits of controlling these factors may also be worthwhile. Another area that has been investigated recently is the role of a new group of drugs called aldose reductase inhibitors. Although the results have been variable, most trials to date have involved late-stage neuropathy.[102] A greater benefit might be seen if these metabolically active drugs were used earlier.

Macrovascular Disease and Atherosclerosis

Atherosclerosis, a multifactorial process, is still not clearly understood. Many of the putative risk factors, or elements in the process, are altered to varying degrees in the diverse manifestations of glucose intolerance discussed earlier. The most convincing epidemiological evidence for increased cardiovascular disease in diabetes comes from large-scale prospective studies, many of which were primarily designed to study cardiovascular disease in the general population. The reader is referred to recent reviews for details.[103,104] Briefly, studies like Framingham[105] have demonstrated that the diabetic individual (uniquely defined in Framingham as "glucose intolerant") has a greatly enhanced risk and that cardiovascular disease is the leading cause of death in those with diabetes.[106,107] Diabetes leads to a greater than normal risk for all manifestations of atherosclerosis, including coronary, cerebrovascular, and peripheral vascular disease.[104,105] The latter is so common in diabetes that half of all lower extremity amputations in the United States occur in persons with diabetes.[59] In the general population, women have a lower risk of coronary heart disease (CHD) than men do, but this advantage is lost in women with diabetes, who have rates approaching those of men.[103,104,108,109] However, data from a mortality follow-up of individuals from a nationwide study[110] suggests that males with diabetes do have a greater risk of death from CHD than do women with diabetes, although this finding is based on a reported history of diabetes that may be biased.[111] A recent meta-analysis suggests that a reduction in the gender differential for CHD in diabetes is true for CHD mortality but not for morbidity.[112] The survival of diabetic patients, especially women, after a cardiac event also appears to be less than that seen in the general population.[113,114]

Although, when it occurs, atherosclerosis is often more extensive in diabetic[115,116] than in nondiabetic subjects, not all studies are in agreement.[117,118] Divergent opinions also are apparent in terms of the role of blood sugar in the nondiabetic range. Some studies have shown the group with IGT to have a greater than normal risk of CVD.[2,79] Other studies have failed to show a relationship between blood glucose levels in the nondiabetic range and CVD.[119] Of further interest is that the IGT stage is often characterized by hyperinsulinemia and insulin resistance. In the Paris study, in multivariate analyses, insulin concentration rather than diabetic IGT status was the stronger predictor of CHD.[120] A further factor linked with hyperinsulinemia is central adiposity, which was discussed earlier as a risk factor for the development of diabetes.[64,65] Central adiposity is also a risk factor for CVD independent of obesity,[121] a finding most clearly shown in women. Consequently, a male type of fat deposition (especially in women) may be associated with hyperinsulinemia[122] and thus may provide a marker for a metabolic derangement predisposing to both diabetes and CVD generally and the relatively poorer cardiovascular prognosis of diabetic women.

Unlike the other diabetes complications, duration of diabetes is not strongly related to CVD in NIDDM in most studies,[80,107,123] although in Pima Indians,[124] in Finland,[125] and in IDDM, a relationship with duration is seen.[126] This lack of a duration effect has led to the suggestion that diabetes per se is not a risk factor for heart disease but rather that a deranged metabolic state, which predisposes to heart disease, also leads to diabetes in some cases.[127] This hypothesis, proposed by Jarrett, is also consistent with the findings of disturbed lipoprotein concentrations in offspring of NIDDM patients with mild glucose intolerance[128] and the predictive power of CVD risk factors, notably lipoproteins, for the development of diabetes. Whether insulin resistance might explain this joint predisposition to diabetes and CVD remains controversial.[129–131]

As lipoproteins are altered in diabetes, it is tempting to hypothesize that these changes account for the increased CVD risk seen in diabetes. Many studies[105,106,108] have shown that serum cholesterol levels relate to CVD risk in those with diabetes in a way similar to that seen in the general population. However, total and LDL cholesterol levels are not greatly elevated in many diabetics, so the role of cholesterol in explaining the *increased* risk in diabetes is limited.[132] Data from the Multiple Risk Factor Intervention Study,[133] which screened over 360,000 men for CVD risk factors and subsequently followed them for mortality, suggests that diabetic men had rates three times higher than nondiabetics all along the cholesterol curve. The MRFIT data is exclusively NIDDM. In IDDM, as indicated earlier, it appears that the major determinant of CVD risk is proteinuria[82] although recent data suggest that hypertension, HDL cholesterol, waist-hip ratio, physical activity, and depressive symptoms may also be important.[134]

As cholesterol concentration has a limited role to play, other lipid measures may be of greater importance in diabetes. Reports suggest that triglyceride level is an independent risk factor for CVD in diabetes.[126,135] Furthermore, alterations in HDL concentration and lipoprotein composition occur in diabetes, which may further increase cardiovascular risk.[136] Insulin itself, beyond its effect on the lipids, can have direct effects on the arterial wall that promote atherogenicity.[137–139] Hyperinsulinemia has also been related to blood pressure elevation.[140–143] The importance of insulin is also shown by its demonstration as an independent risk factor for CVD in some,[144–147] but not all,[148–150] prospective studies of men in the general population.

Many studies have demonstrated altered hemostatic factors, including platelets and fibrinogen, which may provide yet another mechanism for the enhanced CVD risk in diabetes.[151,152] Thus it is abundantly clear that those with diabetes have severe handicaps to face in terms of cardiovascular risk beyond the lipoprotein disturbances.

Diabetes and Pregnancy

Although the data concerning the prevalence of diabetic pregnancy are limited, it has been estimated that 10,000 babies are born each year to women with overt diabetes.[153] Another 90,000 babies are born to women who develop gestational diabetes, a disorder discussed earlier.[154] The sequelae of diabetes mellitus in the pregnant woman include both increased maternal and fetal morbidity and fetal wastage.[155] However, there has been substantial improvement in the treatment of the pregnant diabetic patient, with maternal morbidity and perinatal survival approaching normal. Nevertheless, an excess of birth defects still exists. Studies have generally shown that the rate of major malformations is three times higher in the offspring of a diabetic compared with those of a nondiabetic mother, and fetal malformations are six times more common.[156] In the Collaborative Perinatal Project (CPP), 18 percent of the infants of white diabetic mothers had major malformations compared with 8 percent of the infants of white nondiabetics mothers.[156] The major malformations most commonly associated with diabetes usually occur around 7 to 8 weeks of gestation.[157]

Currently the major question is whether improved metabolic control of diabetes, especially early control, will reduce or prevent the development of congenital malformations in the fetus. It is important to recognize that these malformations occur so early in fetal development that most of the women will not have sought obstetrical care at the time of highest risk.[157] Thus, if the current studies demonstrate that good metabolic control reduces the frequency of malformations (circumstantial evidence suggests this may be true),[158,159] it will be necessary to develop preventive programs that identify the IDDM women prior to pregnancy and ensure metabolic control early in the pregnancy.

In recent years the relationship between metabolic control during pregnancy and adverse pregnancy outcome has become even more muddled. Data from Cincinnati indicate that women who subsequently go on to have malformed infants have higher HbA_{1c} levels during the first trimester than do those who do not subsequently have malformed infants.[158] In contrast, the data from the Diabetes and Early Pregnancy Study[159,160] reveal no increased risk for spontaneous abortion among women who have IDDM compared with that for nondiabetic women.[159] Women who have diabetes are at markedly increased risk for severe malformations.[160] However, there is no evidence that glycemic control early in the pregnancy is related to the increased incidence of malformations. Thus the contribution of metabolic control early in pregnancy to the incidence of severe malformations is still unclear.[161]

Patients with gestational diabetes who enter pregnancy without clinically detectable vascular disease and who acquire no new complications during pregnancy, such as pyelonephritis and pregnancy-induced hypertension, achieve pregnancy outcomes no different from those of the nondiabetic patient.[156] The effect of pregnancy on the complication status of IDDM women appears to be small despite previous concerns. A recent study showed that, despite a suggestion that neuropathy and possible retinopathy may be accelerated in the short term, the long-term effect of parity was negative.[162]

► THE FUTURE PREVENTION OF COMPLICATIONS

While the DCCT has put beyond question the value of intensive therapy to lower blood sugar levels in terms of the so-called triopathy of IDDM complications (retinopathy, nephropathy, and neuropathy), questions remain as to the applicability of these results to NIDDM patients and to the latter macrovascular complications where the glycemic relationship is less clear.[163] Unfortunately, though suggestive, the DCCT data were insufficient to address the macrovascular question.[89] A recent epidemiological study failed to find that GHb levels had a predictive role for CHD[134] in IDDM, while both a previous controversial NIDDM trial[164] and a recent pilot study for intensive therapy with insulin in NIDDM subjects[165] failed to show that vigorous lowering of blood sugar per se would prevent CHD. As intensive therapy with insulin also increases the risk of severe hypoglycemia[89] and is difficult to translate into general practice, it would seem prudent to also focus on other CVD risk factors to prevent these complications in NIDDM.

Fortunately, a recent study using simvastatin to lower cholesterol levels provides clear evidence of benefit for the secondary prevention of recurrent CHD and total mortality in NIDDM subjects.[166] More such studies, particularly in the primary prevention area, are now needed.

► REFERENCES

1. National Diabetes Data Group: Classification and diagnosis of diabetes mellitus and other categories of glucose intolerance. Diabetes 128:57, 1979
2. Fuller JH, Shipley MJ, Rose G, Jarrett RJ, Keen H: Coronary-heart-disease risk and impaired glucose tolerance: the Whitehall study. Lancet 1:1373–1376, 1980
3. O'Sullivan J: Quarter century study of glucose intolerance: incidence of diabetes mellitus by USPHS, NIH, and WHO criteria. In Eschwege E (ed): Advances in Diabetes Epidemiology. Amsterdam: Elsevier Biomedical Press, 1982, pp 123–131
4. Jarrett RJ, Keen H, McCartney P: Worsening of diabetes with impaired glucose tolerance: ten-year experience in the Bedford and Whitehall Studies. In Eschevege E (ed): Advances in Diabetes Epidemiology. Amsterdam: Elsevier Biomedical Press, 1982, pp 95–102
5. Orchard TJ: From diagnosis and classification to complication and therapy: DCCT part II? The 1993 Kelly West Lecture. Diabetes Care 17:326–338, 1994
6. Holman RC, Herron CA, Sinnock P: Epidemiologic characteristics of mortality from diabetes with acidosis or coma, United States, 1970–78. Am J Public Health 73:1169–1173, 1983
7. Diabetes Epidemiology Research International Mortality Study Group, LaPorte RE: Major cross-country differences in risk of dying for people with IDDM. Diabetes Care 14:49–54, 1991
8. Temple RC, Luzio SD, Schneider AE, et al: Insulin deficiency in non-insulin-dependent diabetes. Lancet 1:293–295, 1989
9. Kenny SJ, Aubert RE, Geiss LS: Prevalence and Incidence of Non-Insulin-Dependent Diabetes. In Harris ML, Cowie CC, Stern MP, Boyko EJ, Reiber GE, Bennett PH (eds): Diabetes in America. Washington, DC: National Institute of Diabetes and Digestive and Kidney Diseases, 1995, pp 47–67
10. Harris MI, Hadden WC, Knowler WC, Bennett PH: Prevalence of diabetes and impaired glucose tolerance and plasma glucose levels in U.S. population aged 20–74 yr. Diabetes 36:523–534, 1987
11. Fletcher J, Mijovic C, Odugbesan O, Jenkins D, Bradwell AR, Barnett AH: Trans-racial studies implicate HLA-DQ as a component of genetic susceptibility to type 1 (insulin-dependent) diabetes. Diabetologia 31:864–870, 1988
12. Sasaki A: Assessment of the new criteria for diabetes mellitus according to 10-year relative survival rates. Diabetologia 20:195–198, 1981
13. Ito C, Mito K, Hara H: Review of criteria for diagnosis of diabetes mellitus based on results of follow-up study. Diabetes 32:343–351, 1983
14. Pettitt DJ, Lisse JR, Knowler WC, Bennett PH: Development of retinopathy and proteinuria in relation to plasma-glucose concentrations in Pima Indians. Lancet 2:1050–1052, 1980
15. Duncan BB, Heiss G: Nonenzymatic glycosylation of proteins—a new tool for assessment of cumulative hyperglycemia in epidemiologic studies, past and future. Am J Epidemiol 120:169–189, 1984
16. McCance DR, Hanson RL, Charles M-A, et al: Comparison of tests for glycated haemoglobin and fasting and two hour plasma glucose concentrations as diagnostic methods for diabetes. Br Med J 308: 1323–1328, 1994

16a. Anonymous. American Diabetes Association: clinical practice recommendations 1997. Diabetes Care 20 Suppl 1:S1–S70, 1997

17. Sverjgaard A, Platz P, Ryder L: HLA and disease—1982: a survey. Immunol Rev 70:193, 1983
18. Rotter JI, Rimoin DL: The genetics of the glucose intolerance disorders. Am J Med 70:116, 1981
19. Tattersall R, Pyke D, Nerup J: Genetic patterns in diabetes mellitus. Hum Pathol 11:273–283, 1980
20. Wagener D, Kuller L, Orchard T, LaPorte R, Rabin B, Drash A: Pittsburgh diabetes mellitus study II. Secondary attack rates in families with insulin-dependent diabetes mellitus. Am J Epidemiol 115:868–878, 1982
21. Gottlieb MS: Diabetes in offspring and siblings of juvenile- and maturity-onset-type diabetics. J Chronic Dis 33:331–339, 1980
22. Anonymous: Insulin-dependent? [Editorial]. Lancet 2:809–810, 1985
23. Tuomi T, Groop LC, Zimmet PZ, Rowley MJ, Knowles W, Mackay IR: Antibodies to glutamic acid decarboxylase reveal latent autoimmune diabetes mellitus in adults with a non-insulin-dependent onset of disease. Diabetes 42:359–362, 1993
24. Diabetes Epidemiology Research International Group: Geographic patterns of childhood insulin-dependent diabetes mellitus. Diabetes 37:1113–1119, 1988
25. Rewers M, LaPorte RE, King HOM, Tuomilehto J: Trends in the prevalence and incidence of diabetes: insulin-dependent diabetes mellitus in childhood. World Health Stat 41:179–190, 1988
26. LaPorte RE, Cruickshanks KJ: Incidence and risk factors for insulin-dependent diabetes. In Harris MI, Cowie CC, Stern MP, Boyko EJ, Reiber GE, Bennett PH (eds): National Diabetes Data Group: Diabetes in America, Data Compiled 1984. Washington, DC: US Department of Health and Human Services, 1985, pp 1–12

27. LaPorte RE, Matsushima M, Chang Y-F: Prevalence and incidence of insulin-dependent diabetes. In Harris MI, Cowie CC, Stern MP, Boyko EJ, Reiber GE, Bennett PH (eds): Diabetes in America. Washington, DC: National Institute of Diabetes and Digestive and Kidney Diseases, 1995, pp 37–46
28. LaPorte RE, Tajima N: Prevalence of insulin-dependent diabetes. In Harris MI, Cowie CC, Stern MP, Boyko EJ, Reiber GE, Bennett PH (eds): National Diabetes Data Group: Diabetes in America, Data Compiled 1984. Washington, DC: US Department of Health and Human Services, 1985, pp 1–8
29. Toumilehto J, Virtala E, Karvonen M, et al: Increase in incidence of insulin-dependent diabetes mellitus among children in Finland. Int J Epidemiol 25:984–992, 1995
30. Marrack P, Kappler J: The streptococcal endotoxins and their relatives. Science 248:705–711, 1990
31. Portairova JP, Kotzin BL: Lupus-like autoimmunity graft versus host disease. Concepts Immunopathol 6:119–140, 1988
32. Choi Y, Lafferty JA, Clements JR: Selective expansion of T-cell expressing VB2 in toxic shock syndrome. J Exp Med 172:981–984, 1990
33. Leung DYM: Immunologic aspects of Kawasaki disease. J Rheumatol 17:15–18, 1990
34. Conrad B, Weldmann E, Trucco G, et al: Evidence for a superantigen involvement insulin-dependent diabetes mellitus aetiology. Nature 371:351–355, 1994
35. Tajima N, LaPorte RE, Hibi I, Kitagawa T, Fujita H, Drash AL: A comparison of the epidemiology of youth-onset insulin-dependent diabetes mellitus between Japan and the United States (Allegheny County, Pennsylvania). Diabetes Care 8:17–23, 1985
36. Dokheel TM, for the Pittsburgh Diabetes Epidemiology Group: An Epidemic of Childhood diabetes in the United States? [Abstract]. Diabetes Care 16:1606–1611, 1993
37. Libman IM. Was there an epidemic of diabetes in non-whites in Allegheny County? Abstract #308, Proceedings of IDEG Symposium. Finland, 1997
38. Diabetes Epidemiology Research International Group: Secular trends in incidence of childhood IDDM in 10 countries. Diabetes 39:858–864, 1990
39. Fishbein HA, LaPorte RE, Orchard TJ: The Pittsburgh insulin dependent diabetes mellitus (IDDM) registry: seasonal incidence of IDDM by the host characteristics. Diabetologia 23:83–85, 1982
40. Diabetes Epidemiology Research International Group: Preventing insulin dependent mellitus: the environmental challenge. Br Med J 295:479–481, 1987
41. Cavender DE, Wagener DK, Rabin BS, et al: The Pittsburgh insulin-dependent diabetes mellitus (IDDM) study. HLA antigens and haplotypes as risk factors for the development of IDDM in IDDM patients and their siblings. J Chronic Dis 37:555–568, 1984
42. Schreuder G, Tilanus M, Bontrop R, et al: HLA-DQ polymorphism associated with resistance to type I diabetes detected with monoclonal antibodies, isoelectric point differences and restriction fragment length polymorphism. J Exp Med 164:938, 1986
43. Todd JA, Bell JI, McDevitt HO: HLA-DQ-beta gene contributes to susceptibility and resistance to insulin-dependent diabetes mellitus. Nature 329:559, 1987
44. Morel PA, Dorman JS, Todd JA, McDevitt HO, Trucco M: Aspartic acid at position 57 of the HLA-DQ β chain protects against type I diabetes: a family study. Proc Natl Acad Sci USA 85:8111–8115, 1988
45. Khalil I, Deschamps I, Lepage V: Dose effect of *cis-* and *trans-* encoded HLA-DQaB heterodimers in IDDM susceptibility. Diabetes 41:378–384, 1992
46. Gutierrez-Lopez MD, Bertera S, Chantres MT, et al: Susceptibility to Type I (insulin-dependent) diabetes mellitus in Spanish patients correlates quantitatively with expression of HLA-DQalpha Arg 52 and HLA-DQbeta non-Asp 57 alleles [Abstract]. Diabetologia 35:583–588, 1992
47. Trucco G, Fritsch R, Giorda R, Trucco M: Rapid detection of IDDM susceptibility with HLA-DQ β-alleles as markers. Diabetes 38: 1617–1622, 1989
48. Srikanta S, Ganda OP, Eisenbarth GS, Soeldner JS: Islet-cell antibodies and beta-cell function in monozygotic triplets and twins initially discordant for type I diabetes mellitus. N Engl J Med 308: 322–325, 1983
49. Spencer KM, Dean BM, Tarn A, Lister J, Bottazzo GF: Fluctuating islet-cell autoimmunity in unaffected relatives of patients with insulin-dependent diabetes. Lancet 1:764–766, 1984
50. Owerbach D, Gabbay KH: The search for IDDM susceptibility genes: the next generation. Diabetes 45:544–551, 1996
51. Lipton RB, LaPorte RE, Becker DJ, et al: Cyclosporine therapy for the prevention and cure of insulin-dependent diabetes: an epidemiologic perspective of benefits and risks. Diabetes Care 13:776–784, 1990
52. Bennett PH, Rushforth NB, Miller M, LeCompte PM: Epidemiologic studies of diabetes in the Pima Indians. Recent Prog Horm Res 333–376, 1976
53. Zimmet P: Epidemiology of diabetes and its macrovascular manifestations in Pacific populations: the medical effects of social progress. Diabetes Care 2:85–90, 1979
54. Min HK, Yoo HJ, Lee HK, Kim EJ: Changing patterns of the prevalence of diabetes mellitus in Korea. In Minuira A, Baba S, Goyo Y, Kobberling J (eds): Clinico-genetic Genesis of Diabetes Mellitus. Amsterdam: Excerpta Medica, 1982
55. Medalie JH: Risk factors other than hyperglycemia in diabetic macrovascular disease. Diabetes Care 2:77–84, 1979
56. Van Itallie TB: Obesity: adverse effects on health and longevity. Am J Clin Nutr 32:2723–2733, 1979
57. Keen H: The incomplete story of obesity and diabetes. In Howard A (ed): Recent Advances in Obesity Research: 1. Proceedings of the 1st International Congress on Obesity. London: Newman Publishing, 1975
58. Rimm IJ, Rimm AA: Association between socioeconomic status and obesity in 59,556 women. Prev Med 3:543–572, 1974
59. Palumbo PJ, Melton JL III: Peripheral vascular disease and diabetes. In Harris MI, Cowie CC, Stern MP, Boyko EJ, Reiber GE, Bennett PH (eds): Diabetes in America. Washington, DC: National Institute of Diabetes and Digestive and Kidney Diseases, 1995, pp 401–408
60. Slama G, Haardt MJ, Jean-Joseph P, Costagliola D: Sucrose taken during mixed meal has no additional hyperglycemic action over isocaloric amounts of starch in well-controlled diabetics. Lancet 2: 122–124, 1984
61. Trowell HC: Diabetes mellitus and dietary fiber of starchy foods. Am J Clin Nutr 31:53–57, 1978
62. American Diabetes Association: Nutritional recommendations and principles for individuals with diabetes mellitus: 1986. Diabetes Care 10:126–132, 1987
63. Marshall JA, Hoag S, Shetterly S, Hamman RF: Dietary fat predicts conversion from impaired glucose tolerance to NIDDM. The San Luis Valley Diabetes Study. Diabetes Care 17:50–56, 1994
64. Ohlson LO, Larsson B, Svardsudd K: The influence of body fat distribution on the incidence of diabetes mellitus: 13.5 years of follow-up of the participants in the study of men born in 1913. Diabetes 34:1055–1058, 1985
65. Haffner SM, Stern MP, Hazuda HP, Rosenthal M, Knapp JA, Malina RM: Role of obesity and fat distribution in non-insulin-dependent diabetes mellitus in Mexican Americans and non-Hispanic whites. Diabetes Care 9:153–161, 1986
66. Williams B: Insulin resistance: the shape of things to come. Lancet 344:521–524, 1994
67. Taylor RJ, Bennett PH, LeGonidec G, et al: The prevalence of diabetes mellitus in a traditional-living Polynesian population: the Wallis Island Survey. Diabetes Care 6:334–340, 1983

68. Manson JE, Nathan DM, Krolewski AS, Stampfer MJ, Willett WC, Hennekens CH: A prospective study of exercise and incidence of diabetes among US male physicians. JAMA 268:63–67, 1992
69. Barnett AH, Eff C, Leslie RDG, Pyke DA: Diabetes in identical twins: a study of 200 pairs. Diabetologia 20:87–93, 1981
70. Tuomilehto-Wolf E, Tuomilehto J, Cepaitis Z, Lounamaa R, DIME Study Group: New susceptibility haplotype for Type I diabetes [Abstract]. Lancet 2:299–302, 1989
71. Bell GI, Karem JH, Rutter WJ: Polymorphic cDNA region adjacent to the 5′ end of the human insulin gene. Proc Natl Acad Sci USA 78:5759–5763, 1981
72. Vionnet N, Stoffel M, Takeda J, et al: Nonsense mutation in the glucokinase gene causes early-onset non-insulin-dependent diabetes mellitus. Nature 356:721–722, 1992
73. Reardon W, Ross RJM, Sweeney MG, et al: Diabetes mellitus associated with a pathogenic point mutation in mitochondrial DNA. Lancet 340:1376–1379, 1992
74. Saad MF, Knowler WC, Pettitt DJ, Nelson RG, Mott DM, Bennett PH: The natural history of impaired glucose tolerance in the Pima Indians. N Engl J Med 319:1500–1506, 1988
75. American Diabetes Association: The physician's guide to type II diabetes (NIDDM). New York: KPR International Media Corp, 1984
76. Olefsky J, Reaven GM, Farquhar JW: Effects of weight reduction on obesity: studies of lipid and carbohydrate metabolism in normal and hyperlipoproteinemic subjects. J Clin Invest 53:64–76, 1974
77. Zinman B, Zuniga-Guajardo S, Kelly D: Comparison of the acute and long-term effects of exercise on glucose control in type I diabetes. Diabetes Care 7:515–519, 1984
78. Diabetes Prevention Program Research Group: Diabetes Prevention Program (DPP) Protocol. Springfield, VA: National Technical Information Service, 1996
79. Eschwege E, Ducimetiere P, Papoz L, Claude JR, Richard JL: Blood glucose and coronary heart disease. Lancet 1980, pp 472–473
80. Knuiman MW, Welborn TA, McCann VJ, Stanton KG, Constable IJ: Prevalence of diabetic complications in relation to risk factors. Diabetes 35:1332–1339, 1986
81. Diabetes Epidemiology Research International Mortality Study Group, Orchard TJ: International evaluation of cause-specific mortality and IDDM. Diabetes Care 14:55–60, 1991
82. Borch-Johnsen K, Kreiner S: Proteinuria: value as predictor of cardiovascular mortality in insulin dependent diabetes mellitus. Br Med J 294:1651–1654, 1987
83. Portuese E, Orchard TJ: Mortality in Insulin-Dependent Diabetes. In Harris MI, Cowie CC, Stern MP, Boyko EJ, Reiber GE, Bennett PH (eds): Diabetes in America. Washington, DC: National Institute of Diabetes and Digestive and Kidney Diseases, 1995, pp 221–232
84. Nishimura R, Matsushima M, Tajima N, et al: A major improvement in the prognosis of individuals with IDDM in the past 30 years in Japan. Diabetes Care 19:758–760, 1996
85. Klein R, Davis MD, Moss SE, Klein BEK, DeMets DL: The Wisconsin epidemiologic study of diabetic retinopathy: a comparison of retinopathy in younger and older onset diabetic persons. In Vranic M, Hollenberg CH, Steiner G (eds): Comparisons of Type I and Type II Diabetes Advances in Experimental Medicine and Biology. New York: Plenum Press, 1985, pp 321–335
86. Orchard TJ, Dorman JS, Maser RE, et al: The prevalence of complications in insulin dependent diabetes mellitus by sex and duration: Pittsburgh Epidemiology of Diabetes Complications Study—II. Diabetes 39:1116–1124, 1990
87. National Diabetes Advisory Board: Progress and Promise in Diabetes Research. Report of the Second National Diabetes Research Conference. NIH Publication No. 84-661. Bethesda, MD: National Institutes of Health, 1984
88. Diabetic Retinopathy Study Group: Photocoagulation treatment of proliferative diabetic retinopathy. Clinical Application of Diabetic Retinopathy Study (DRS) Findings, DRS Report No. 8. Ophthalmology 88:583, 1981
89. The Diabetes Control and Complications Trial Research Group: The effect of intensive treatment of diabetes on the development and progression of long-term complications in insulin-dependent diabetes mellitus. N Engl J Med 329:977–986, 1993
90. Geiss LS, Herman WH, Teutsch SM: Diabetes and renal mortality in the United States. Am J Public Health 75:1325–1326, 1985
91. Knowles HC: Magnitude of the renal failure problem in diabetic patients. Kidney Int 6:52–57, 1974
92. Viberti G: Etiology and prognostic significance of albuminuria in diabetes. Diabetes Care 11:840–845, 1988
93. Lewis EJ, Hunsicker LG, Bain RP, Rohde RD: The effect of angiotensin-converting-enzyme inhibition on diabetic nephropathy. N Engl J Med 329:1456–1462, 1993
94. The Microalbuminuria Captopril Study Group: Captopril reduces the risk of nephropathy in IDDM patients with microalbuminuria. Diabetologia 39:587–593, 1996
95. Coonrod BA, Ellis D, Becker DJ, et al: Predictors of microalbuminuria in individuals with IDDM: Pittsburgh Epidemiology of Diabetes Complications Study. Diabetes Care 16:1376–1383, 1993
96. Lloyd CE, Becker DJ, Ellis D, Orchard TJ: Incidence of complications in insulin-dependent diabetes mellitus: a survival analysis. Am J Epidemiol 143:431–441, 1996
97. Winegrad AI, Morrison AD, Greene DA: Late complication of diabetes. In DeGrott LJ, Cahill GF, Martini L (eds): Endocrinology. New York: Grune & Stratton, 1979
98. Forrest KY, Maser RE, Pambianco G, Portuese EI, Orchard TJ: Hypertension as a risk factor for diabetic neuropathy: a prospective study. Diabetes 1997, in press
99. American Diabetes Association, American Academy of Neurology: Report and recommendations of the San Antonio conference on diabetic neuropathy. Diabetes Care 11:592–597, 1988
100. Maser RE, Neilson VK, Bass EB, et al. Measuring diabetic neuropathy: an assessment and comparison of a clinical examination and quantitative sensory testing. Diabetes Care 12:270–275, 1989
101. Ward JD, Fisher DJ, Barnes CG, Jessop JD: Improvement in nerve conduction following treatment of newly diagnosed diabetics. Lancet 1:428, 1971
102. Boel E, Selmer J, Flodgaard HJ, Jensen T: Diabetic late complications: will aldose reductase inhibitors or inhibitors of advanced glycosylation endproduct formation hold promise? J Diabetes Complications 9:104–129, 1995
103. Wingard DL, Barrett-Connor E: Heart disease and diabetes. In Harris M, Cowie C (eds): Diabetes in America. Washington, DC: Government Printing Office, 1995
104. Donahue RP, Orchard TJ: Diabetes mellitus and macrovascular complications. Diabetes Care 15:1141–1155, 1992
105. Kannel WB, McGee DL: Diabetes and glucose tolerance as risk factors for cardiovascular disease: The Framingham Study. Diabetes Care 2:120–126, 1979
106. Barrett-Connor E, Wingard DL: Sex differential in ischemic heart disease mortality in diabetics: a prospective population-based study. Am J Epidemiol 118:489–496, 1983
107. Panzram G: Mortality and survival in type 2 (non-insulin-dependent) diabetes mellitus. Diabetologia 30:123–131, 1987
108. Jarrett RJ, McCartney P, Keen H: The Bedford Survey: ten year mortality rates in newly diagnosed diabetics, borderline diabetics and normoglycaemic controls and risk indices for coronary heart disease in borderline diabetics. Diabetologia 22:79–84, 1982
109. Barrett-Connor EL, Cohn BA, Wingard DL, Edelstein SL: Why is diabetes mellitus a stronger risk factor for fatal ischemic heart disease in women than in men? JAMA 265:627–631, 1991
110. Kleinman JC, Donahue RP, Harris MI, Finucane FF, Madans JH, Brock DB: Mortality among diabetics in a national sample. Am J Epidemiol 128:389–401, 1988

111. West KM: Epidemiology of Diabetes in Its Vascular Lesions. Amsterdam: Elsevier Science, 1978, pp 231–248
112. Orchard TJ: The impact of gender and general risk factors on the occurrence of atherosclerotic vascular disease in NIDDM. Ann Med 28:323–333, 1996
113. Abbott RD, Donahue RP, Kannel WB, Wilson PWF: The impact of diabetes on survival following myocardial infarction in men vs. women. JAMA 260:3456–3460, 1988
114. Donahue RP, Goldberg RJ, Chen Z, Gore JM, Alpert JS: The influence of sex and diabetes mellitus on survival following acute myocardial infarction: a community-wide perspective. J Clin Epidemiol 46:245–252, 1993
115. Waller BF, Palumbo PJ, Lie JT: The heart in diabetes mellitus as viewed from a morphologic perspective. In Scott C (ed): Clinical Cardiology and Diabetes. Mount Kisco, NY: Futura Publishing, 1981, pp 83–125
116. Dortimer AC, Shenoy PN, Shiroff RA: Diffuse coronary artery disease in diabetic patients. Circulation 57:133–336, 1978
117. Barrett-Connor E, Orchard TJ: Diabetes and heart disease. In National Diabetes Data Group: Diabetes in America. Washington, DC: National Diabetes Data Group, 1985, pp 1–41
118. Waller BF, Palumbo PJ, Lie JT, Roberts WC: Status of the coronary arteries at necropsy in diabetes mellitus with onset after age 30 years. Am J Med 69:498–506, 1980
119. The International Collaborative Group: Joint discussion. J Chronic Dis 32:829–837, 1979
120. Eschwege E, Richard JL, Thibult N: Coronary heart disease mortality in relation with diabetes, blood glucose, and plasma insulin levels: the Paris Prospective Study, ten years later. Horm Metab Res Suppl 15:41–46, 1985
121. Lapidus L, Bengtsson C, Larsson B: Distribution of adipose tissue and risk of cardiovascular disease and death: a 12 year follow-up of participants in the population study of women in Gothenburg, Sweden. Br Med J 289:1257–1261, 1984
122. Peiris AN, Mueller RA, Struve MF: Splanchnic insulin metabolism in obesity: influence of body fat distribution. J Clin Invest 78:1648–1658, 1986
123. Jarrett RJ, Shipley MJ: Type 2 (non-insulin-dependent) diabetes mellitus and cardiovascular disease—putative association via common antecedents; further evidence from the Whitehall Study. Diabetologia 31:737–740, 1988
124. Nelson RG, Sievers ML, Knowler WC, et al: Low incidence of fatal coronary heart disease in Pima Indians despite high prevalence of non-insulin-dependent diabetes. Circulation 81:987–995, 1990
125. Kuusisto J, Mykkänen L, Pyörälä K, Laakso M: NIDDM and its metabolic control predict coronary heart disease in elderly subjects. Diabetes 43:960–967, 1994
126. Janka HU: Five-year incidence of major macrovascular complications in diabetes mellitus. Horm Metab Res Suppl 15:15–19, 1985
127. Jarrett RJ: Type 2 (non-insulin-dependent) diabetes mellitus and coronary heart disease—chicken, egg or neither? Diabetologia 26: 99–102, 1984
128. Ganda OP, Soeldner JS, Gleason RE: Alterations in plasma lipids in the presence of mild glucose intolerance in the offspring of two type II diabetic patients. Diabetes Care 8:254–260, 1985
129. Jarrett RJ: Is insulin atherogenic? Diabetologia 31:71–75, 1988
130. Orchard TJ: Is insulin atherogenic? Diabetologia 31:404–405, 1988
131. Wingard DL, Barrett-Connor EL, Ferrara A: Is insulin really a heart disease risk factor? Diabetes Care 18:1299–1304, 1995
132. Orchard TJ: Dyslipoproteinemia and diabetes. Endocrinol Metab Clin North Am 19:361–380, 1990
133. Stamler J, Vaccaro O, Neaton JD, Wentworth D: Diabetes, other risk factors, and 12-yr cardiovascular mortality for men screened in the Multiple Risk Factor Intervention Trial. Diabetes Care 16:434–444, 1993
134. Lloyd CE, Kuller LH, Becker DJ, Ellis D, Wing RR, Orchard TJ: Coronary artery disease in IDDM: gender differences in risk factors, but not risk. Arterioscler Thromb Vasc Biol 16:720–726, 1996
135. West KM, Ahuja MMS, Bennett PH, et al: The role of circulating glucose and triglyceride concentrations and their interactions with other "risk factors" as determinants of arterial disease in nine diabetic population samples from the WHO multinational study. Diabetes Care 6:361–369, 1983
136. Howard BV: Lipoprotein metabolism in diabetes mellitus. J Lipid Res 28:613–628, 1987
137. Stout RW, Bierman EL, Ross R: Effect of insulin on the proliferation of cultured primate arterial smooth muscle cells. Circ Res 36: 361–327, 1975
138. Stout RW: The effect of insulin and glucose on sterol synthesis in cultured rat arterial smooth muscle cells. Atherosclerosis 27:271–278, 1977
139. Porta M, LaSelva M, Molinatti P, Molinatti GM: Endothelial cell function in diabetic microangiopathy. Diabetologia 30:601–609, 1987
140. Christlieb AR, Krolewski AS, Warran JH: Insulin and diastolic hypertension. Circulation 70:61, 1984
141. Donahue RP, Orchard TJ, Becker DJ, Kuller LH, Drash AL: Sex differences in the coronary heart disease risk profile. A possible role for insulin. The Beaver County Study. Am J Epidemiol 125:650–657, 1987
142. Modan M, Halkin H, Almog S, et al: Hyperinsulinemia: a link between hypertension obesity and glucose intolerance. J Clin Invest 75:809–817, 1985
143. Ferrannini E, Buzzigoli G, Bonadonna R, et al: Insulin resistance in essential hypertension. N Engl J Med 317:350–357, 1987
144. Ducimetiere P, Eschwege E, Papoz L, Richard JL, Claude JR, Rosselin G: Relationship of plasma insulin levels to the incidence of myocardial infarction and coronary heart disease mortality in a middle-aged population. Diabetologia 19:205–210, 1980
145. Pyörälä K: Relationship of glucose tolerance and plasma insulin to the incidence of coronary heart disease: results from two population studies in Finland. Diabetes Care 2:131–141, 1979
146. Welborn TA, Wearne K: Coronary heart disease incidence and cardiovascular mortality in Busselton with reference to glucose and insulin concentrations. Diabetes Care 2:154–159, 1979
147. Despres J, Lamarche B, Mauriege P, et al: Hyperinsulinemia as an independent risk factor for ischemic heart disease [Abstract]. N Engl J Med 334:952–957, 1996
148. Ferrara A, Barrett-Connor EL, Edelstein SL: Hyperinsulinemia does not increase the risk of fatal cardiovascular disease in elderly men or women without diabetes: the Rancho Bernardo study, 1984–1991. Am J Epidemiol 140:857–869, 1994
149. Orchard TJ, Eichner JE, Kuller LH, Becker DJ, McCallum LA, Grandits GA: Insulin as a predictor of coronary heart disease: interaction with Apo E phenotype. A report from MRFIT. Ann Epidemiol 4:40–45, 1994
150. Welin L, Eriksson H, Larsson B, Ohlson L-O, Svärdsudd K, Tibblin G: Hyperinsulinaemia is not a major coronary risk factor in elderly men. Diabetologia 35:766–770, 1992
151. Colwell JA, Winocour PD, Halushka PV: Do platelets have anything to do with diabetic microvascular disease? Diabetes 32:14–19, 1983
152. Jensen T, Stender S, Deckert T: Abnormalities in plasmas concentrations of lipoproteins and fibrinogen in type 1 (insulin-dependent) diabetic patients with increased urinary albumin excretion. Diabetologia 31:142–145, 1988
153. North AF, Mazumdar S, Logiuilo VM: Birth weight, gestational age and perinatal deaths in 5,471 infants of diabetic mothers. J Pediatr 90:444–447, 1977
154. Freinnkel N: Gestational diabetes 1979: philosophical and practical aspects of a major public health problem. Diabetes Care 3:399–401, 1980

155. Wheeler FC, Gollmar CW, Deeb LC: Diabetes and pregnancy in South Carolina: prevalence, perinatal mortality and neonatal morbidity in 1978. Diabetes Care 5:561–565, 1982
156. Chung LS, Myrianthopoulos NC: Factors affecting risk of congenital malformations. 11. Effect of maternal diabetes. Birth Defects 11:10, 1975
157. Mills JL, Baker L, Goldman AS: Malformations in infants of diabetic mothers occur before the gestational week. Diabetes 28:292–293, 1979
158. Miodovnik M, Mimouni F, St. John Dignan P, et al: Major malformations in infants of IDDM women: vasculopathy and early first-trimester poor glycemic control. Diabetes Care 11:713–718, 1988
159. Mills JL, Simpson JL, Driscoll SG, Jovanovic-Peterson L, Van Allen M: Incidence of spontaneous abortion among normal women and insulin-dependent diabetic women whose pregnancies were identified within 21 days of conception. N Engl J Med 319:1617–1623, 1988
160. Mills JL, Knopp RH, Simpson JL, Jovanovic-Peterson L, Metzger BE, Holmes LB: Lack of relation of increased malformation rates in infants of diabetic mothers to glycemic control during organogenesis. N Engl J Med 318:671–676, 1988
161. Mills JL: Summary and Comment—Can prepregnancy care of diabetic women reduce the risk of abnormal babies? [Abstract]. Diabetes Spectrum 4:218, 1991
162. Hemachandra A, Ellis D, Lloyd CE, Orchard TJ: The influence of pregnancy on IDDM complications. Diabetes Care 18:950–954, 1995
163. Steinberg D, Parthasarathy S, Carew TE, Khoo JC, Witztum JL: Beyond cholesterol: modifications of low-density lipoprotein that increase its atherogenicity. N Engl J Med 320:915–924, 1989
164. Seltzer HS: A summary of criticisms of the findings and conclusions of the University Group Diabetes Program (UGDP). Diabetes 21: 976–979, 1972
165. Abraira C, Johnson N, Colwell J, VA CSDM Group: VA cooperative study on glycemic control and complications in type II diabetes (VA CSDM): results of the completed feasibility trial. Diabetes 43:59A, 1994
166. Scandinavian Simvastatin Survival Group: Randomised trial of cholesterol lowering in 4444 patients with coronary heart disease: the Scandinavian Simvastatin Survival Study (4S). Lancet 344: 1383– 1389, 1994
167. The Expert Committee on the Diagnosis and Classification of Diabetes Mellitus: Report of the Expert Committee on the Diagnosis and Classification of Diabetes Mellitus. Diabetes Care 20(7): 1183–1197, 1997

55

Respiratory Disease Prevention

David B. Coultas • Jonathan M. Samet

Diseases of the respiratory system are an important public health problem in all countries. The respiratory system, which includes the lungs and the upper airway that joins the trachea to the larynx, is exposed to a wide range of potentially injurious agents (Table 55-1). On average, an adult inhales about 5 L of air per minute; with exercise, the amount may increase 20-fold or more. With 10,000 to 20,000 L of air inhaled daily, agents present even in low concentrations may be toxic. The respiratory system is equipped with a remarkably effective system of defense mechanisms against inhaled particles and gases. Disease may result, however, if an acute exposure overwhelms the defenses (e.g., toxic gas inhalation), if an agent is particularly toxic even at low concentrations (e.g., toluene diisocyanate), if exposure is sustained (e.g., cigarette smoking), or if the exposed person is particularly susceptible (e.g., asthmatics).

In the United States in 1990, more than 190,000 deaths were due to nonmalignant respiratory diseases (Table 55-2).[1] Chronic lung diseases were the fourth leading cause of death in 1990.[2] Respiratory tract infections continue to cause substantial morbidity and mortality. For example, in the United States in 1994, an estimated 80.5 acute respiratory tract conditions were experienced per 100 persons,[3] and acute respiratory tract infections and influenza directly caused over 79,000 deaths in 1990.[1] Worldwide, 4 to 6 million children are estimated to die annually of acute respiratory infections.[4] Environmental and occupational respiratory exposures also cause an enormous burden of potentially preventable disease. In the United States, for example, over 400,000 total deaths were attributed to cigarette smoking in 1990.[5] In many countries, environmental and occupational agents that cause disease have become subject to regulation to ensure that workplaces are healthful and that neither outdoor nor indoor air causes adverse effects. Such regulations are not in place throughout the world, however, and where they do exist, enforcement and compliance are variable.

▸ INTERNATIONAL DISTRIBUTIONS

The occurrence of respiratory system diseases varies widely around the world (Table 55-3).[6,7] Among children under 5 years of age, about 33 percent of all deaths, or 4.1 million deaths in 1990, were due to acute respiratory tract infections;[8] over 95 percent of these deaths are among children from developing countries. The markedly higher childhood mortality from acute respiratory tract infections in developing countries as compared with those in developed countries probably reflects poorer nutrition and immunization practices and more frequent low birth weight, crowding, and indoor and outdoor air pollution.[4]

Chronic diseases of the respiratory system and respiratory tract cancer are major causes of morbidity and mortality among adults. On average, the proportion of deaths due to bronchitis, emphysema, and asthma is about 40 percent worldwide, but this figure varies widely, from about 7 percent in Thailand to 60 percent in Australia.[9] Internationally, the rates of occurrence of respiratory tract cancer and of nonmalignant chronic diseases of the respiratory system can be directly related to patterns of cigarette smoking.[10] However, inconsistencies in the association between mortality from chronic obstructive pulmonary disease (COPD) and cigarette smoking have been found.[11] These inconsistencies may be partly explained by differences among countries in reporting of COPD mortality and smoking prevalence. Indoor air pollution from domestic wood burning for cooking has been associated with an increased risk of chronic bronchitis and chronic airflow obstruction.[12]

▸ PEDIATRIC RESPIRATORY DISEASES

Respiratory Distress Syndrome

Respiratory distress syndrome (RDS) in the newborn results primarily from surfactant deficiency associated with lung immaturity.[13] Because of surfactant deficiency, the lung does not effectively exchange oxygen and carbon dioxide after birth, and positive pressure ventilation is frequently required to maintain life. Bronchopulmonary dysplasia, characterized by persistent pulmonary dysfunction and oxygen dependence beyond the age of 1 month, occurs as a frequent sequela of RDS.[14]

Between 60 and 70 thousand cases of RDS are reported annually in the United States and about 5,000 children per year die from RDS, accounting for 20 percent of all neonatal deaths.[15] Of infants who survive RDS, estimates of the proportion in whom bronchopulmonary dysplasia develops vary from 10 to 45 percent.[14,16]

Several risk factors have been established for RDS, including prematurity, male sex, white race, cesarean section, and perinatal asphyxia.[13] The incidence of RDS is inversely related to gestational age and birth weight, both measures of fetal prematurity. Among infants less than 28 weeks gestation, the incidence of RDS is approximately 80 percent, declining to about 60 percent after 29 weeks gestation, and is less than 1 percent at 39 weeks gestation.[13]

Prevention of premature birth represents the most effective method for reducing the morbidity and mortality associated with RDS.[17] However, because prematurity is frequently a result of poor socioeconomic conditions, and therefore not directly amenable to medical intervention, prematurity and RDS will remain public health problems until underlying causes can be remedied.

Prenatal identification of fetuses at high risk for RDS can be accomplished by analysis of amniotic fluid phospholipids.[13] As the fetus matures, amniotic fluid lecithin concentration increases while sphingomyelin concentration remains constant. Ratios of lecithin to sphingomyelin (L/S) of 2:1 or greater are associated with low risk for RDS. The probability of RDS is 40 percent with a L/S ratio less than 1.5, 33 percent with a ratio of 1.5–2, and 10 percent with a ratio of 2 or greater.[13] However, the L/S ratio may not predict lung maturity in diabetic mothers.[13]

TABLE 55-1. MECHANISMS OF LUNG INJURY AND EXAMPLES OF INJURIOUS AGENTS AND ASSOCIATED DISEASES

	Example	
Mechanism of Injury	***Agent***	***Disease***
Infection	Respiratory syncytial virus	Bronchiolitis
	Streptococcus pneumonia	Pneumonia
Carcinogenesis	Cigarette smoke	Lung cancer
	Asbestos	Mesothelioma
Immunologic	Thermophilic actinomycetes	Hypersensitive pneumonitis
Inflammation	Cigarette smoke	COPD
	Oxides of nitrogen	Silo-fillers' lung
Fibrogenesis	Asbestos	Asbestosis
	Coal dust	Coal workers' pneumoconiosis
Other	Plicatic acid	Western red cedar workers' asthma
	Cotton dust	Byssinosis

Medical interventions including antenatal corticosteroids[18] and surfactant replacement[19] provide partial solutions for the prevention of RDS and its complications. The administration of corticosteroids to the mother has been shown to decrease the frequency of RDS by approximately 50 percent.[18] Antenatal corticosteroids also decrease the severity and improve survival of neonates who develop RDS.[18] Surfactant replacement with either natural extracts or synthetic forms has proven effective for decreasing complications associated with RDS with an overall 40 percent reduction in mortality.[19] However, controversy remains about whether to use prophylactic therapy in neonates at high risk of developing RDS compared to treatment of premature infants with established RDS.[19]

▶ CYSTIC FIBROSIS

In the United States, cystic fibrosis is the most common lethal genetic disease in whites of Northern European descent, estimated to occur in about 1 in 3,500 live births in 1990.[20] The disease occurs less frequently in other racial and ethnic groups in the United States with estimates of 1 in 14,000 black births; 1 in 11,500 Hispanic births; 1 in 10,500 American Indian and Alaska Native births; and 1 in 25,500 Asian births.[20] Cystic fibrosis is transmitted as an autosomal recessive trait, and the heterozygote frequency in persons of Northern European descent is about 1 in 25.[21]

More than 400 mutations of the cystic fibrosis transmembrane conductance regulator (CFTR) gene on chromosome 7 have been characterized since the gene was identified in 1989, and one mutation (delta F508) accounts for about 70 percent of all cases.[22] The CFTR gene mutations result in an inability of epithelial cells to secrete chloride ions and the production of an abnormally thick mucus. This defect affects the lungs, intestines, and exocrine glands and may result in diverse clinical manifestations, but patients invariably develop chronic obstructive pulmonary disease from repeated infections that destroy lung tissue.[22] Pulmonary involvement has been reported in over 90 percent of all patients with cystic fibrosis and accounts for the majority of hospital admissions and deaths.[23]

The prognosis for patients with cystic fibrosis has improved markedly over the last 30 years.[20] Based on data from the National Cystic Fibrosis Patient Registry, the median survival in the United States has increased from 14 years in 1969 to 28 years in 1990.[20] In 1990, male patients had longer median survival compared with females, 30 and 25 years, respectively. The improving prognosis of cystic fibrosis probably reflects the beneficial effects of early recognition, nutritional support, and antibiotic therapy.[23]

Because cystic fibrosis is a fatal genetic disease, prenatal diagnosis with early termination of affected pregnancies offers one method for control. However, acceptance of this method for prevention of cystic fibrosis has varied widely among couples, ranging from 20 to 65 percent.[24] The most accurate method for prenatal diagnosis is identification of CFTR mutations from chorionic villous biopsy at 10 weeks gestation.[24] This method of prenatal diagnosis can be offered only to the pregnant woman who has previously had a child with cystic fibrosis. Since 80 percent of children with the disease are born into families without a history of cystic fibrosis,[24] using this method of prenatal screening will have little impact on the incidence of the disease.

Screening of the general population for carriers of CFTR gene mutations with genetic counseling to guide reproductive decisions offers another method to prevent cystic fibrosis.[24,25] However, because all mutations cannot be detected and the number of trained genetic counselors is limited, populationwide screening remains controversial. Further, little is known about the cultural and economic impacts of screening. A number of projects to examine the appropriateness of population screening are in progress worldwide.

The early diagnosis of cystic fibrosis in newborn children by screening of dried blood spots for trypsin levels may lessen morbidity; however, the benefits of early detection are debatable.[24] Results from several studies suggest that screened infants have shorter hospital

TABLE 55-2. NUMBER OF DEATHS FROM RESPIRATORY DISEASES IN THE UNITED STATES IN 1990

Disease (ICD-9)[a]	***Number***
■ ***DISEASES OF NEWBORNS***	
Respiratory distress syndrome (769)	2,858
Other respiratory conditions of newborns (770)	3,048
■ ***NONMALIGNANT RESPIRATORY DISEASES***	
Pneumonia and influenza (480–487)	79,513
Chronic bronchitis (491)	2,985
Emphysema (492)	15,706
Asthma (493)	4,819
Chronic airway obstruction, NEC (496)	61,599
Pneumoconioses and other lung diseases due to external agents (500–508)	9,108
Interstitial lung disease (515–516)	6,367
Pulmonary embolism (415.1)	9,472
Total disease of respiratory system (460–519)	192,533
■ ***MALIGNANT RESPIRATORY DISEASES***	
Larynx (161)	3,710
Trachea, bronchus, lung (162)	141,285

From National Center for Health Statistics: Mortality, Part A. In: Vital Statistics of the United States, 1990. DHHS Publication No. PHS 95-1101. Washington, DC: Government Printing Office, 1994, vol. 2.

[a] International Classification of Diseases, 9th revision.

TABLE 55-3. MORTALITY RATES (PER 100,000) IN SELECTED COUNTRIES FOR VARIOUS RESPIRATORY DISEASES AGE-STANDARDIZED TO WORLD POPULATIONS

		Malignant Neoplasms of Trachea, Bronchus, and Lung (162)[a]		*Diseases of the Respiratory System (460–466, 470–478, 480–519)*[a]		*Chronic and Unspecified Bronchitis, Emphysema, and Asthma (490–493)*[a]	
African Region		**1987**	**1994**	**1987**	**1994**	**1987**	**1994**
Mauritius	Total	10.2[b]	8.9[c]	90.1	75.1	39.9	27.0
	Male	17.8	15.6	116.4	108.8	55.2	38.7
	Female	4.0	4.4	68.1	52.4	29.2	19.9
Americas Region							
Guatemala	Total	1.5[d]	—	164.4	—	10.0	—
	Male	0.9	—	177.8	—	11.3	—
	Female	2.0	—	152.1	—	9.0	—
United States	Total	36.3[d]	39.2[e]	37.2	41.2	5.5	6.0
	Male	56.9	57.2	54.1	55.4	7.9	7.6
	Female	20.4	25.4	26.0	32.2	3.9	5.0
European Region							
Portugal	Total	13.0[b]	15.9[c]	40.7	39.8	11.0	6.5
	Male	24.3	29.8	58.8	59.4	16.8	10.3
	Female	4.1	4.8	27.9	26.4	7.1	4.1
England and Wales	Total	38.6[f]	—	56.7	—	15.2	—
	Male	64.9	—	83.5	—	25.5	—
	Female	19.3	—	41.0	—	9.1	—
Eastern Mediterranean							
Kuwait	Total	14.4[b]	—	40.9	—	7.4	—
	Male	20.6	—	45.3	—	9.9	—
	Female	7.2	—	37.3	—	4.7	—
Western Pacific							
Australia	Total	27.8[f]	25.6[g]	39.8	34.3	11.0	7.7
	Male	48.0	40.9	62.0	49.7	16.4	10.4
	Female	11.5	12.8	25.5	23.9	7.5	5.7
Japan	Total	16.1[f]	17.8[c]	38.1	43.4	7.3	6.2
	Male	27.6	30.9	56.6	67.1	11.5	10.2
	Female	7.7	8.2	26.0	28.1	4.5	3.6
Singapore	Total	34.0[b]	31.8[g]	107.5	91.4	9.2	8.1
	Male	49.9	49.9	157.4	123.5	11.9	10.8
	Female	19.7	16.0	75.1	65.2	7.4	6.1

From World Health Organization: World Health Statistics Annual, 1987.
Geneva: World Health Organization, 1987
Geneva: World Health Organization, 1995a.
[a] International Classification of Diseases, 9th revision.
[b] Age-standardized to 1986 world population.
[c] Age-standardized to 1993 world population.
[d] Age-standardized to 1984 world population.
[e] Age-standardized to 1991 world population.
[f] Age-standardized to 1985 world population.
[g] Age-standardized to 1992 world population.

stays, but few other differences have been found. Although clinical benefits of early detection are limited, the psychological health of families may benefit from early detection.[24] The sweat chloride test is the gold standard for diagnosis of cystic fibrosis, but this test is not suited for mass screening.[24]

As noted previously, the improving survival among persons with cystic fibrosis has been attributed to better medical care. However, the relative contributions of the various components of care to the improvement cannot be readily established. The details of management of cystic fibrosis are beyond the scope of this review and have been discussed extensively elsewhere.[22,23]

Respiratory Tract Infection

In the twentieth century, respiratory tract infections are the main cause of morbidity and mortality among children living in developing countries and, although a much less frequent cause of death, the predominant source of morbidity among children living in developed countries.[4] Respiratory viruses are responsible for most childhood respiratory tract infections, although bacteria, *Mycoplasma*, and *Chlamydia* cause some infections at particular ages. Respiratory tract infections in childhood may plausibly have long-term sequelae, including loss of lung function after severe episodes of lower respiratory tract infection, the development of asthma, the development of bronchiectasis, and an increased risk of developing COPD in adulthood.[26,27]

In developed countries the predominant clinical syndromes associated with childhood respiratory tract infection include colds (infections of the upper respiratory tract), epiglottitis (infection of the epiglottis), croup or laryngeotracheobronchitis (infection of the larynx and large airways), bronchiolitis (infection of the small airways), and pneumonia (infection of the lung tissues). Rhinoviruses are most closely associated with colds, parainfluenza viruses with croup, respiratory syncytial virus with bronchiolitis, and various viruses, including respiratory syncytial virus and the parainfluenza viruses, with pneumonia.[28,29] Bacteria cause epiglottitis. Epiglottitis, croup, bronchiolitis, and pneumonia may be severe and cause death through respiratory failure. In less developed countries, measles and whooping cough may be important causes of severe respiratory tract infection.[30]

Childhood respiratory tract infections are extremely common. Surveillance data for general population samples worldwide show that children experience five to nine respiratory illnesses during the first year of life;[4] by the teenage years children still have about two or three respiratory illnesses annually.[31] Mortality from childhood respiratory tract infections is low in the United States and other more developed countries, about 0.1 deaths annually per 1,000 children from birth through the age of 5 years.[32] However, mortality rates for this same age group are more than 100 times greater in some developing countries.

Many risk factors for respiratory tract infection have been identified. In developing countries, overcrowded dwellings, poor nutrition, low birth weight, and possibly intense smoke pollution underlie the high rates.[4] Studies in developed countries have shown that males have higher rates of infection, as do younger siblings of school-age children who introduce infections into households. Children from homes of lower socioeconomic status also tend to have more respiratory infections. Maternal cigarette smoking has also been causally linked to increased occurrence of respiratory tract infections during the first years of life.[33] Attendance at day care centers also increases the occurrence of respiratory tract infections among preschool children.[4] Some studies indicate that breast-feeding decreases risk and that use of a gas-fueled stove increases risk, but the evidence of these associations is conflicting.[34–36]

Present understanding of risk factors for respiratory tract infection in childhood indicates several approaches for primary prevention. In developing countries, improved living conditions, better nutrition, and reduction of smoke pollution indoors should reduce the burden of morbidity and mortality associated with respiratory tract infections. In developed countries, mothers should be encouraged to stop smoking or to avoid smoking in the presence of their children. We lack approaches for controlling the emerging problem of excess respiratory tract infections associated with day care. Vaccines are now available for *Haemophilus influenzae*, the bacteria that causes epiglottitis. However, effective vaccines have not yet been developed for the common respiratory viruses.

Asthma

Numerous investigations of the occurrence of asthma in children have been conducted worldwide.[37] In the United States, data from nationwide samples and survey populations indicate that asthma is a common disease in children, with an overall prevalence nationwide of about 5 percent in 1992, an increase from about 3 percent in 1982.[38] Data from Tucson, Arizona,[39] and Rochester, Minnesota,[40] show a sharp decline in the incidence of asthma from early childhood to adolescence (Fig. 55-1). The prevalence may vary widely between racial and ethnic groups[41] and is higher in blacks compared with whites.[38] Rates are particularly high in children living in inner cities. Worldwide, data from cross-sectional surveys indicate a wide range for the prevalence of childhood asthma.[37,42] Gregg[42] summarized the findings of surveys of children and adolescents and noted that the prevalence varied from near 0 to 75 percent. Methodological differences among the surveys may partially explain this range, but variation in the distributions of risk factors may also be important.[43] Prevalence estimates from developed countries are similar to those for the United States.[42] Generally, asthma is less common in developing countries.[37]

The natural history of wheezing illnesses and childhood asthma have been described in longitudinal studies; most of the studies have been conducted retrospectively in developed countries on patients from office practices or hospital clinics. In a longitudinal study of 826 newborns, Martinez et al[44] found that about 30 percent of children develop a wheezing illness during the first 3 years of life, and of these children about 60 percent are symptom-free at age 6. Few prospective population-based studies of children with asthma have been carried out.[45–47] These studies have shown that between 30 and 70 percent of asthmatic children become symptom-free or show improvement by adolescence or early adulthood.

Many endogenous and exogenous risk factors have been identified for asthma (Table 55-4). Studies of familial aggregation of asthma and twins show a strong familial influence on the prevalence of asthma,[48] but these studies do not separate genetic from common environmental effects. Descriptive studies of childhood asthma have consistently shown an increased prevalence in males,[45,49] which may be explained by differences in airway geometry.[50] Atopy, defined by positive skin tests to common aeroallergens, predicts increased risk of asthma if present in the parents or child.[51] Exposure to the common aeroallergen house dust mite during infancy is associated with a marked excess risk of asthma by age 11 years.[52] More severe episodes of lower respiratory tract infection are associated with subsequent asthma and increased airway reactivity.[53] Involuntary exposure to tobacco smoke, particularly maternal smoking, is independently associated with asthma.[54–56] Involuntary exposure to tobacco smoke has also been shown to exacerbate asthma.[33] Ambient air pollution may exacerbate asthma,[57,58] but it has not been established as a causal risk factor for childhood asthma.

Although risk factors for childhood asthma have been identified, few investigations of the primary prevention of asthma have been conducted, and most preventive strategies have been directed at secondary prevention with pharmacologic and other interventions

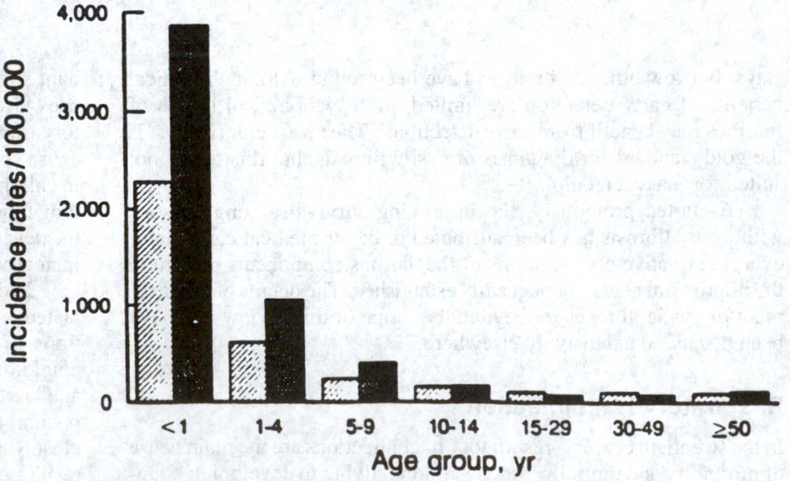

Figure 55-1. Annual incidence rates per 100,000 person-years by sex and age for definite and probable asthma cases among Rochester residents, 1964 through 1983. Hatched bars = females; shaded bars = males. (From Yunginger et al. 1992.[40])

TABLE 55-4. RISK FACTORS FOR CHILDHOOD ASTHMA

Familial and genetic factors
Male gender
Atopy
Environmental factors
Respiratory tract infection
Ambient air pollution
Environmental tobacco smoke
Bronchial hyperreactivity

to lessen morbidity. In a randomized trial of 120 infants, Arshad et al[59] found that measures to limit allergen exposures of the infants during the first 12 months of life were effective in lowering the occurrence of asthma at 12 months of age. The use of bronchodilators, corticosteroids, and disodium cromoglycate greatly reduces morbidity from asthma. Speight et al[60] found that school absenteeism, an important measure of morbidity, fell 10-fold after effective treatment among 31 asthmatic children who had been having more than 12 attacks per year.

Many nonpharmacological interventions have been examined, including environmental control, prevention of sensitization in infancy and childhood, immunizations, allergen immunotherapy, physical training, chest physiotherapy, and education.[61–63] In the United States, a national strategy for asthma education has been developed to prevent morbidity and mortality from asthma.[64]

Death from childhood asthma, although infrequent, is well documented and potentially preventable. Childhood mortality rates from asthma vary from country to country and by age, sex, and race in the United States. In the United States, annual age-adjusted mortality rates for asthma among persons 5 to 34 years of age increased 42 percent during the period 1982 through 1991, from 3.4 per million to 4.9 per million, respectively.[38] During this period the mortality rates were approximately five times higher for blacks compared with whites.

Findings from retrospective studies suggest that clinical severity of asthma predicts risk of death.[65] Factors that are suspected to affect mortality include failure on the part of patients and physicians to recognize severity, behavioral patterns, underuse of inhaled or oral corticosteroids, overuse and overdependence on nebulizers, and additive toxicity from combined use of theophylline and β-agonists. For individual children, however, the predictive value of these factors is limited.

▸ ADULT RESPIRATORY TRACT DISEASES

Asthma

Worldwide, the occurrence of asthma is lower in adults than in children.[37] Incidence is highest in children less than 5 years of age, declines during adolescence, and then remains constant through adulthood (Fig. 55-1).[39,40] In a population-based sample of U.S. residents[66] including 14,404 adults 25 to 74 years of age, the overall prevalence of active asthma was estimated at 2.6 percent. The cumulative incidence of new-onset asthma was 2.1/1,000/year. In contrast to children, among adults female gender was associated with a 40 percent increase in incidence. However, the higher incidence in women may partly be explained by physician bias in labeling obstructive lung disease in women as asthma rather than COPD.[39]

Although the occurrence of asthma is lower in adults than in children, in the United States the economic impact of asthma is greatest among persons 18 years of age and older.[67] In 1985, the overall costs for asthma in the United States were estimated at $4.5 billion with approximately 66 percent of the costs associated with persons 18 years of age and older. Emergency room use, hospitalizations, and death accounted for 43 percent of the total economic impact of asthma, suggesting that asthma costs could be reduced by interventions targetting these three areas.

While death from asthma is uncommon, the majority of asthma deaths occur in adults,[68] and during the past 10 to 15 years asthma mortality rates among adults have increased worldwide.[69,70] Among asthmatics fewer than 5 percent die from asthma.[68,71] Population-based investigations have provided conflicting results on survival among adults with asthma that may be partly explained by methodologic differences.[68,71] Impaired lung function is associated with increased mortality.[71]

Overall, strategies for asthma management and prevention in adults differ little from those in children and incorporate pharmacological and other interventions. For adults, occupational asthma is of special concern, with approximately 250 causative agents identified.[72] Among adult asthmatics, about 15 percent of cases are attributed to occupational exposures.[72] Early recognition of the relationship between an occupational exposure and asthma is important, since prompt removal from exposure correlates best with full resolution of asthma.[72] Certain occupations may be associated with an increased risk of death from asthma.[73]

Chronic Obstructive Pulmonary Disease

COPD is a clinically applied term for persistent and generally symptomatic obstruction to airflow within the lungs. The lungs of most persons with COPD display a mixture of emphysema, enlargement and destruction of the air spaces, and inflammation and narrowing of the smaller airways, although in some persons emphysema or airway abnormalities may predominate.[74] Emphysema reduces the driving pressure for airflow, and the airway abnormalities increase the resistance to airflow.

A small number of cases of COPD, distinguished by severe emphysema, occur in smokers and nonsmokers with deficiency of α-antitrypsin, a substance that defends against injury by proteolytic enzymes;[74] however, most cases result from cigarette smoking.[74] Occupational agents can also contribute to the development of COPD.[75] Other postulated risk factors for COPD include childhood respiratory tract infection[26,27] and hyperresponsiveness of the airways of the lung.[76,77]

The natural history of COPD generally follows a slow but progressive course that offers a lengthy time window for intervention. The results of epidemiological studies suggest that impaired lung growth from smoking during childhood and adolescence[78] and sustained loss of ventilatory function beyond that expected from aging alone causes clinically evident COPD (Fig. 55-2).[74] The rate of decline in smokers tends to increase with the amount smoked, and smoking cessation results in a slower rate of decline compared with that in smokers unable to quit.[79] Among smokers with mild airflow obstruction, moderate to marked airways hyperreactivity is more common in women (48 percent) compared with men (25 percent)[80] and is associated with accelerated decline in lung function.[77] However, only a minority of smokers develop COPD.

Clinicians make the diagnosis of COPD in patients with sufficient chronic airflow obstruction to result in shortness of breath and limitation of exercise capacity. In epidemiological studies COPD is considered to be present if lung function tests demonstrate a specified degree of impairment or if a physician's diagnosis is reported. Although prevalence can be readily assessed with the use of these criteria, incidence cannot be described over short periods because of the slow evolution of impairment in persons developing COPD.

Epidemiological data from throughout the world show that COPD is common among adults, with prevalence estimates ranging from about 1 to 15 percent.[2,74,81] The prevalence is greater among men than among women and increases with the extent of smoking.

Mortality rates for COPD, although subject to well-described limitations,[82] provide another measure of occurrence. Unfortunately, procedures and codes for classifying COPD as the underlying cause of death have not been consistent across this century. Consequently, mortality trends must be interpreted cautiously. Moreover, attribution of a death to COPD ordinarily requires contact with a clinician and diagnosis of the disease. In spite of the limitations of death certificates in investigating COPD, mortality data for the United States document a dramatic increase in deaths from COPD. In 1950, 3,157 deaths were attributed to categories related to COPD; by 1990 the number of deaths from COPD was 80,290. Worldwide, mortality rates among countries are highly variable, and from 1979 through 1988 most countries had a decline or no change in mortality rates among men, but a rise in mortality rates for women.[11]

The 1984 Report of the Surgeon General concluded that 80 to 90 percent of COPD in the United States is attributable to cigarette smoking.[74] Similarly high attributable risks for smoking would be anticipated for other developed countries. The slow evolution of COPD provides an opportunity to identify and to target for intervention the smokers in whom the disease is developing. With sustained smoking, lung function in smokers, declining at a more rapid rate (Fig. 55-2), tends to drop below normal levels. Lung function testing of chronic smokers can identify individuals whose function has dropped below the range of normal values but not yet reached the degree of impairment associated with frank COPD.[83] These at-risk persons could then be targeted for intensive smoking cessation interventions.[79]

Acute Respiratory Distress Syndrome

The clinical syndrome of acute respiratory distress syndrome (ARDS) was originally described in the late 1960s; it represents a diffuse response of the lung to a wide variety of causative factors including sepsis, trauma, aspiration and other inhalational injuries, pancreatitis, multiple transfusions, and drug overdose.[84] The clinical picture comprises pulmonary edema that does not have a cardiac basis and respiratory failure. Of the few studies describing the incidence of ARDS in the general population, most estimates have ranged from about 2 cases per 100,000 per year to 8 cases per 100,000 per year.[85] Overall, about 25 percent of patients with any one of the risk factors will develop ARDS, ranging from 13 percent among patients with drug overdose to 43 percent among patients with sepsis.[84] Mortality from ARDS is high, about 60 percent of patients do not survive,[84] but is highly variable ranging from 33 percent among patients with near-drowning to 70 percent among patients with sepsis and multiple transfusions. The ninth revision of the *International Classification of Diseases* includes a code (518.5) for "pulmonary insufficiency following trauma and surgery" including ARDS. However, this code would not capture all cases of ARDS.

In summary, acute respiratory distress syndrome occurs as a consequence of severe lung injury by diverse and distinct agents and often represents the most proximal cause of death. Preventive strategies must be directed toward the causative factors (e.g., motor vehicle accidents and drug abuse).

Pulmonary Thromboembolism

Each year in the United States more than 600,000 persons suffer from pulmonary thromboembolism, and 50,000 to 100,000 premature deaths are estimated to result from pulmonary thromboembolism, comprising about 5 to 10 percent of all deaths in U.S. hospitals.[86] Despite the public health impact of the problem, it is often undiagnosed and, if untreated, has a mortality rate of about 30 percent.[87] A high index of suspicion is necessary for making the diagnosis of pulmonary thromboembolism.

Identification of risk factors for pulmonary thromboembolism (Table 55-5)[86] is the key for making a correct diagnosis. Over 90 percent of patients treated for thromboembolism have one or more risk factors (Table 55-5), and among patients with clinically significant pulmonary embolism more than 90 percent result from deep venous thrombosis in the lower extremities.

Because of the high frequency of pulmonary thromboembolism and the difficulties of diagnosis, prevention has been a major area of investigation. Numerous methods have been assessed for preventing venous thromboembolism in hospital patients.[86] Most information has come from surgical patients, for whom administration of subcu-

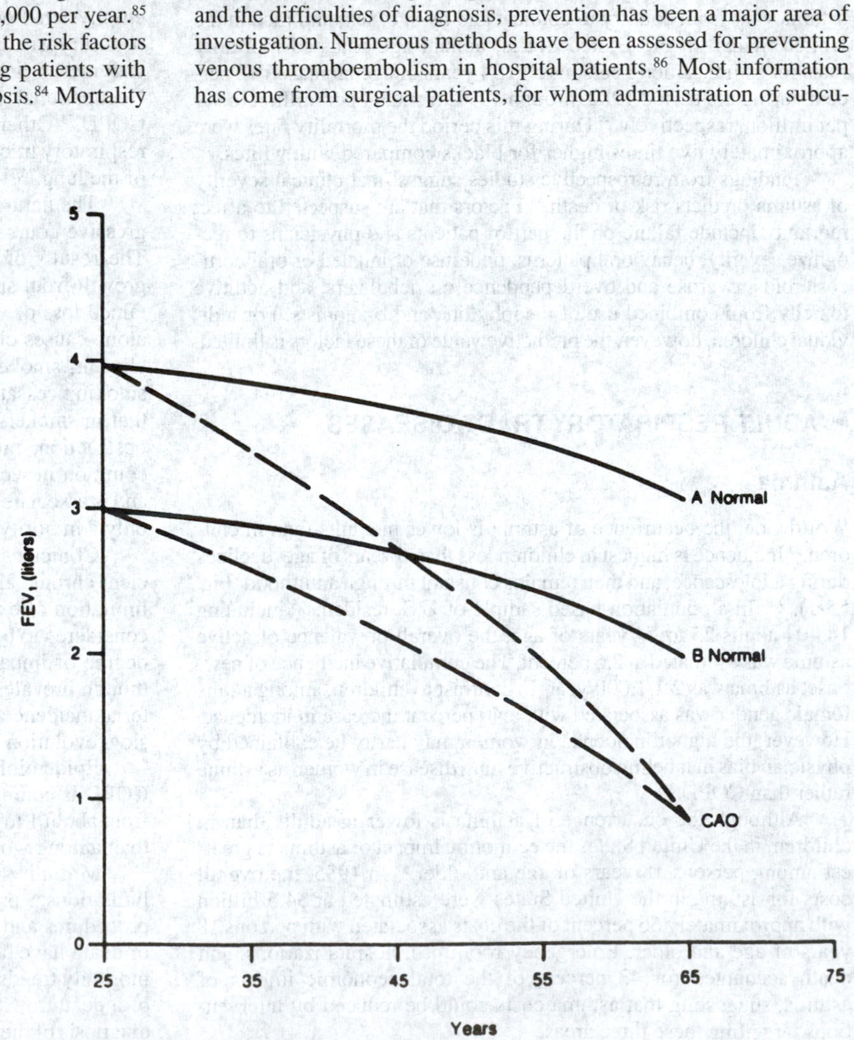

Figure 55-2. Decline of FEV_1 at normal rate (*solid line*) and at an accelerated rate (*dashed line*). **A**, Person who has attained a "normal" maximal FEV_1 during lung growth and development; **B**, Person whose maximal FEV_1 has been reduced by childhood respiratory infection. CAO = chronic airflow obstruction (From US Department of Health and Human Services: The Health Consequences of Smoking. Chronic Obstructive Pulmonary Disease. DHHS Publication No. (PHS) 84-50205, Rockville, MD: Office on Smoking and Health, 1984.)

TABLE 55-5. RISK FACTORS FOR VENOUS THROMBOEMBOLISM

Age 40 years or more	Stroke
Obesity	Malignant disease
History of venous thromboembolism	Trauma
Heart disease	Major surgery
Myocardial infarction	Pelvic and lower extremity surgery
Congestive heart failure	Pregnancy or puerperium
Atrial arrhythmia	Exogenous estrogen
Mural thrombosis	Immobility

Adapted from Anderson FA Jr, Wheeler HB: Venous thromboembolism. Risk factors and prophylaxis [Review]. Clin Chest Med 16(2):235–251, 1995.

taneous heparin has proved efficacious. Although less information is available on the use of subcutaneous heparin in nonsurgical patients, there is evidence of efficacy in patients with other medical conditions, including acute myocardial infarction, congestive heart failure, and acute paraplegia, quadriplegia, and stroke. Other methods that may be useful for the prevention of venous thromboembolism include intermittent pneumatic compression and aspirin.

Interstitial Lung Diseases

The interstitial lung diseases are a heterogeneous group of disorders comprising more than 130 entities that damage the pulmonary interstitium (Table 55-6).[88] However, in the general population only six major diagnostic categories of these diseases are usually seen, including occupational and environmental, drug and radiation induced, pulmonary hemorrhage syndromes, connective tissue diseases, idiopathic pulmonary fibrosis, and sarcoidosis.[89] Idiopathic pulmonary fibrosis composes the single-largest category, accounting for 51 percent of all incident cases. Interstitial lung diseases of known cause (e.g., asbestosis, coal workers' pneumoconiosis, silicosis, hypersensitivity pneumonitis, drug induced) compose only about 15 percent of incident cases in the general population.

In the United States, interstitial lung diseases are commonly encountered by pulmonary physicians. A 1972 Respiratory Diseases Task Force report from the National Institutes of Health[90] estimated that interstitial lung diseases accounted for about 15 percent of a pulmonary physician's practice. In a population-based investigation of the occurrence of interstitial lung diseases the overall prevalence was higher in men compared with that in women, 81 per 100,000 and 67 per 100,000, respectively.[89] The overall incidence was 32 per 100,000/year among men and 26 per 100,000/year among women.[89]

Both endogenous and environmental factors have been proposed as determinants of interstitial lung diseases of unknown causes.[91] With regard to endogenous factors, inherited interstitial lung disease, association with human lymphocyte antigen (HLA) types, and airway and lung dimensions suggest that genetic factors may influence the development of some interstitial lung diseases because of altered lung clearance, lung defenses, or lung immunoregulation.

Inhalation of environmental agents and exposure to drugs account for most interstitial lung diseases of known cause, and a growing number of recent investigations have found associations between environmental exposures and idiopathic pulmonary fibrosis.[92–96] Examples of environmental factors that have been associated with idiopathic pulmonary fibrosis include cigarette smoking, working with livestock, wood dust, and metal dust. Infectious agents, viruses,[94] and *Mycoplasma*[97] have been implicated as causes of pulmonary fibrosis, indistinguishable from idiopathic pulmonary fibrosis, but the importance of these agents as causes of interstitial lung disease in the general population is not known. Exposure to environmental agents may also alter risk of development of interstitial lung diseases of known or unknown cause; cigarette smoking decreases the risk of hypersensitivity pneumonitis[98] and increases the risk of histiocytosis X.[99]

Because most interstitial lung diseases are of unknown cause, little can be offered for prevention now. However, growing evidence suggests that exposure to environmental agents is associated with idiopathic pulmonary fibrosis, the most common interstitial lung disease. As evidence accumulates to fulfill the criteria for causation for specific exposures and determinants of individual susceptibility are identified, specific recommendations for prevention will be possible.

Sleep Apnea

The sleep apnea syndrome is characterized by excessive daytime sleepiness, snoring, and many episodes of cessation of breathing during sleep. In the majority of cases, the syndrome results from recurrent collapse of the pharynx with blockage of the passage of air.[100] Because of recurrent apneas, significant lack of oxygen may develop and cause fragmented sleep and secondary complications. The excessive daytime sleepiness may result in a number of psychosocial problems and substantially increases the risk of automoble accidents.[101] If untreated, moderate to severe sleep apnea syndrome results in excess mortality.[100]

Based on a number of surveys that have been conducted worldwide, the prevalence of the sleep apnea syndrome in the general population is estimated to be less than 5 percent.[100] The prevalence is higher among men, habitual snorers, and obese persons and increases with age. Because of the high prevalence of the syndrome in the general population and the potential morbidity and mortality, the sleep apnea syndrome presents a major public health problem,[101] but its long-term consequences remain uncharacterized.

Little information is available on the prevention of morbidity and mortality from the sleep apnea syndrome, and the long-term benefits of treatment remain to be established.[102] For moderate to severe sleep apnea, continuous positive airway pressure through a nasal mask is the main treatment modality. Because obesity is often associated with the syndrome, weight reduction is frequently recommended but offers limited improvement unless body weight is substantially reduced.[103] Alcohol avoidance is recommended because it can cause sleep apnea in persons who simply snore and can worsen the severity of apnea among patients with the sleep apnea syndrome.[101]

▸ CONCLUSIONS

Respiratory diseases are common causes of morbidity and mortality worldwide, and many of these diseases can be prevented. Because the occurrence of the various respiratory diseases may vary widely in dif-

TABLE 55-6. INTERSTITIAL LUNG DISEASES

▪ *KNOWN CAUSES*	▪ *UNKNOWN CAUSES*
Inorganic dusts	Idiopathic pulmonary fibrosis
Organic dusts	Collagen-vascular disorders
Gases, fumes, vapors, aerosols	Sarcoidosis
Drugs	Histiocytosis X
Poisons	Goodpasture's syndrome
Radiation	Idiopathic pulmonary hemosiderosis
Infectious agents	Wegener's granulomatosis
Chronic pulmonary edema	Vasculitides
Chromic uremia	Inherited disorders
	Lymphocytic infiltrative disorders
	Others

Adapted from Crystal RG, Gadek JE, Ferrans VJ, Fulmer JD, Line BR, Hunninghake GW: Interstitial lung disease: current concepts of pathogenesis, staging and therapy [Review]. Am J Med 70(3):542–568, 1981.

ferent geographic locations, epidemiologic data are important for development of prevention strategies. Of particular public health concern is tobacco smoking, a major cause of avoidable respiratory disease from the prenatal period through adulthood.

▶ REFERENCES

1. National Center for Health Statistics: Mortality, Part A. In: Vital Statistics of the United States, 1990. DHHS Publication No. PHS 95-1101. Washington, DC: Government Printing Office, 1994, vol 2
2. Goldring JM, James DS, Anderson HA: Chronic Lung Diseases. In Brownson RC, Remington PL, Davis JR (eds): Chronic Disease Epidemiology and Control. Washington, DC: American Public Health Association, 1993
3. National Center for Health Statistics: Current Estimates from the National Health Interview Survey. Vital and Health Statistics Series 10. Washington, DC: Government Printing Office, 1995
4. Graham NMH: The epidemiology of acute respiratory infections in children and adults: a global perspective [Review]. Epidemiol Rev 12:149–178, 1990
5. Nelson DE, Kirkendall RS, Lawton RL, et al: Surveillance for smoking-attributable mortality and years of potential life lost, by state—United States, 1990. MMWR 43(SS-1):1–8, 1994
6. World Health Organization: World Health Statistics Annual 1987. Geneva: World Health Organization 1987
7. World Health Organization: World Health Statistics Annual 1994. Geneva: World Health Organization 1995a
8. World Health Organization: The World Health Report 1995. Bridging the Gaps. Geneva: World Health Organization, 1995b
9. Bouvier MH, Guidevaux M: Mortality from disorders of the respiratory system throughout the world between 1950 and 1972. World Health Stat Q 32(3):174–197, 1979
10. Stanley K, Stjernsward J: Lung cancer—a worldwide health problem [Review]. Chest 96(Suppl 1):1S–5S, 1989
11. Brown CA, Crombie IK, Tunstall-Pedoe H: Failure of cigarette smoking to explain international differences in mortality from chronic obstructive pulmonary disease. J Epidemiol Community Health 48:134–139, 1994
12. Perez-Padilla R, Regalado J, Vedal S, et al: Exposure to biomass smoke and chronic airway disease in Mexican women: a case-control study. Am J Respir Crit Care Med 154:701–706, 1996
13. Verma RP: Respiratory distress syndrome of the newborn infant [Review]. Obstet Gynecol Surv 50(7):542–555, 1995
14. Bancalari E, Gerhardt T: Bronchopulmonary dysplasia [Review]. Pediatr Clin North Am 33(1):1–23, 1986
15. Wegman ME: Annual summary of vital statistics—1989. Pediatrics 86(6):835–847, 1990
16. Horbar JD, Soll RF, Sutherland JM, et al: A multicenter randomized, placebo-controlled trial of surfactant therapy for respiratory distress syndrome. N Engl J Med 320(15):959–965, 1989
17. Stahlman MT: Medical complications in premature infants: is treatment enough? [Editorial]. N Engl J Med 320(23):1551–1553, 1989
18. Gardner MO, Goldenberg RL: Use of antenatal corticosteroids for fetal maturation [Review]. Curr Opin Obstet Gynecol 8:106–109, 1996
19. Soll RF: Appropriate surfactant usage in 1996 [Review]. Eur J Pediatr 155(Suppl 2):S8–S13, 1996
20. FitzSimmons SC: The changing epidemiology of cystic fibrosis [Review]. Pediatrics 122(1):1–9, 1993
21. Collins FS: Cystic fibrosis: molecular biology and therapeutic implications [Review]. Science 256:774–779, 1992
22. Davis PB, Drumm M, Konstan MW: Cystic fibrosis [Review]. Am J Respir Crit Care Med 154:1229–1256, 1996
23. Ramsey BW: Management of pulmonary disease in patients with cystic fibrosis [Review]. N Engl J Med 335(2):179–188, 1996
24. Ryley HC, Goodchild MC, Dodge JA: Screening for cystic fibrosis [Review]. Br Med Bull 48(4):805–822, 1992
25. U.S. Congress Office of Technology Assessment: Cystic Fibrosis and DNA Tests: Implications of Carrier Screening. OTA-BA-532. Washington, DC: Government Printing Office, 1992
26. Samet JM, Tager IB, Speizer FE: The relationship between respiratory illness in childhood and chronic air-flow obstruction in adulthood [Review]. Am Rev Respir Dis 127(4):508–523, 1983
27. Barker DJ, Godfrey KM, Fall C, Osmond C, Winter PD, Shaheen SO: Relation of birth weight and childhood respiratory infection to adult lung function and death from chronic obstructive airways disease. Br Med J 303(6804):671–675, 1991
28. Wright AL, Taussig LM, Ray CG, Harrison HR, Holberg CJ: The Tucson children's respiratory study. II. Lower respiratory tract illness in the first year of life. Am J Epidemiol 129(6):1232–1246, 1989
29. Glezen P, Denny FW: Epidemiology of acute lower respiratory disease in children. N Engl J Med 288(10):498–505, 1973
30. Chretien J, Holland W, Macklem P, Murray J, Woolcock A: Acute respiratory infections in children. A global public-health problem. N Engl J Med 310(15):982–984, 1984
31. Monto AS, Ullman BM: Acute respiratory illness in an American community. The Tecumseh study. JAMA 227(2):164–169, 1974
32. Smith KR: Biofuels, air pollution, and health: a global review. New York: Plenum Press, 1987
33. US Environmental Protection Agency: Respiratory Health Effects of Passive Smoking: Lung Cancer and Other Disorders. EPA/600/6-90/006F. Washington, DC: Government Printing Office, 1992
34. Bauchner H, Leventhal JM, Shapiro ED: Studies of breast-feeding and infections. How good is the evidence? [Review]. JAMA 256(7):887–892, 1986
35. Samet JM, Marbury MC, Spengler JD: Health effects and sources of indoor air pollution. Part I [Review]. Am Rev Respir Dis 136(6):1486–1508, 1987
36. Samet JM, Lambert WE, Skipper BJ, et al: Nitrogen dioxide and respiratory illnesses in infants. Am Rev Respir Dis 148:1258–1265, 1993
37. Cookson JB: Prevalence rates of asthma in developing countries and their comparison with those in Europe and North America. Chest 91 (Suppl 6):97S–103S, 1987
38. Centers for Disease Control and Prevention: Asthma—United States, 1982–1992. MMWR 43:952–955, 1995
39. Dodge R, Cline MG, Burrows B: Comparisons of asthma, emphysema, and chronic bronchitis diagnoses in a general population sample. Am Rev Respir Dis 133(6):981–986, 1986
40. Yunginger JW, Reed CE, O'Connell EJ, Melton J, O'Fallon WM, Silverstein MD: A community-based study of the epidemiology of asthma. Am Rev Respir Dis 146:888–894, 1992
41. Coultas DB, Gong H Jr, Grad R, et al: Respiratory diseases in minorities of the United States [published erratum appears in Am J Respir Crit Care Med 1994 Jul; 150(1):290] [Review]. Am J Respir Crit Care Med 149(3 Pt 2):S93–S131, 1994
42. Gregg I: Epidemiological aspects. In Clark TJH, Godfrey S (eds): Asthma. London: Chapman & Hall, 1983, p 242
43. Weiss KB, Gergen PJ, Wagener DK: Breathing better or wheezing worse? The changing epidemiology of asthma morbidity and mortality [Review]. Annu Rev Public Health 14:491–513, 1993
44. Martinez FD, Wright AL, Taussig LM, et al: Asthma and wheezing in the first six years of life. N Engl J Med 332:133–138, 1995
45. Schachter EN, Doyle CA, Beck GJ: A prospective study of asthma in a rural community. Chest 85(5):623–630, 1984
46. McNicol KN, Williams HB: Spectrum of asthma in children. I. Clinical and physiological components. Br Med J 4:7–11, 1973
47. Godden DJ, Ross S, Abdalla M, et al: Outcome of wheeze in childhood. Symptoms and pulmonary function 25 years later. Am J Respir Crit Care Med 149(1):106–112, 1994

48. Sandford A, Weir T, Pare P: The genetics of asthma. Am J Respir Crit Care Med 153:1749–1765, 1996
49. Horwood LJ, Fergusson DM, Shannon FT: Social and familial factors in the development of early childhood asthma. Pediatrics 75(5):859–868, 1985
50. Taussig LM: Maximal expiratory flows at functional residual capacity: a test of lung function for young children. Am Rev Respir Dis 116(6):1031–1038, 1977
51. Weiss ST, Tager IB, Munoz A, Speizer FE: The relationship of respiratory infections in early childhood to the occurrence of increased levels of bronchial responsiveness and atopy. Am Rev Respir Dis 131(4):573–578, 1985
52. Sporik R, Holgate ST, Platts-Mills TA, Cogswell JJ: Exposure to house-dust mite allergen (Der p I) and the development of asthma in childhood. A prospective study. N Engl J Med 323(8):502–507, 1990
53. McConnochie KM, Roghmann KJ: Bronchiolitis as a possible cause of wheezing in childhood: new evidence. Pediatrics 74(1):1–10, 1984
54. Martinez FD, Cline M, Burrows B: Increased incidence of asthma in children of smoking mothers. Pediatrics 89(1):21–26, 1992
55. Infante-Rivard C: Childhood asthma and indoor environmental risk factors. Am J Epidemiol 137(8):834–844, 1993
56. Stoddard JJ, Miller T: Impact of parental smoking on the prevalence of wheezing respiratory illness in children. Am J Epidemiol 141(2):96–102, 1995
57. American Thoracic Society: Health effects of outdoor air pollution. Part 1 [Review]. Am J Respir Crit Care Med 153:3–50, 1996
58. American Thoracic Society: Health Effects of Outdoor Air Pollution. Part 2 [Review] Am J Respir Crit Care Med 153:477–498, 1996
59. Arshad SH, Matthews S, Gant C, Hide DW: Effect of allergen avoidance on development of allergic disorders in infancy. Lancet 339(8808):1493–1497, 1992
60. Speight AN, Lee DA, Hey EN: Underdiagnosis and undertreatment of asthma in childhood. Br Med J 286(6373):1253–1256, 1983
61. Abramson MJ, Puy RM, Weiner JM: Is allergen immunotherapy effective in asthma? A meta-analysis of randomized controlled trials. Am J Respir Crit Care Med 151:969–974, 1995
62. Blessing-Moore J: Does asthma education change behavior? To know is not to do. Chest 109:9–11, 1996
63. Welch MJ, Ostrom NK, Meltzer EO, Orgel HA: Nonpharmacologic approaches to the management of asthma. In Tinkelman DG, Naspitz CK (eds): Childhood Asthma. Pathophysiology and Treatment. 2nd ed. New York: Marcel Dekker, 1993
64. National Asthma Education Program: Guidelines for the Diagnosis and Management of Asthma. Publication No. 91-3042. Bethesda, MD: National Heart, Lung, and Blood Institute, 1991
65. Strunk RC: Death due to asthma. New insights into sudden unexpected deaths, but the focus remains on prevention [Editorial]. Am Rev Respir Dis 148:550–552, 1993
66. McWhorter WP, Polis MA, Kaslow RA: Occurrence, predictors, and consequences of adult asthma in NHANESI and follow-up survey. Am Rev Respir Dis 139(3):721–724, 1989
67. Weiss KB, Gergen PJ, Hodgson TA: An economic evaluation of asthma in the United States. N Engl J Med 326:862–866, 1992
68. Silverstein MD, Reed CE, O'Connell EJ, Melton LJ, O'Fallon WM, Yunginger JW: Long-term survival of a cohort of community residents with asthma. N Engl J Med 331(23):1537–1541, 1994
69. Nakamura Y, Labarthe DR: Secular trends in mortality from asthma in Japan, 1979–1988: comparison with the United States. Int J Epidemiol 23(1):143–147, 1994
70. Lang DM, Polansky M: Patterns of asthma mortality in Philadelphia from 1969 to 1991. N Engl J Med 331(23):1542–1546, 1994
71. Lange P, Ulrik CS, Vestbo J: Mortality in adults with self-reported asthma. Copenhagen City Heart Study Group. Lancet 347(9011): 1285–1289, 1996
72. Chan-Yeung M, Malo J-L: Occupational asthma. N Engl J Med 333(2):107–112, 1995
73. Schenker MB, Gold EB, Lopez RL, Beaumont JJ: Asthma mortality in California, 1960–1989. Demographic patterns and occupational associations. Am Rev Respir Dis 147:1454–1460, 1993
74. US Department of Health and Human Services: The Health Consequences of Smoking. Chronic Obstructive Pulmonary Disease. DHHS Publication No. (PHS)84-50205. Rockville, MD: Office on Smoking and Health, 1984
75. Becklake MR: Occupational pollution [Review]. Chest 96(Suppl 3): 372S–378S, 1989
76. O'Connor GT, Sparrow D, Weiss ST: The role of allergy and nonspecific airway hyperresponsiveness in the pathogenesis of chronic obstructive pulmonary disease [Review]. Am Rev Respir Dis 140(1):225–252, 1989
77. Tashkin DP, Altose MD, Connett JE, Kanner RE, Lee WW, Wise RA: Methacholine reactivity predicts changes in lung function over time in smokers with early chronic obstructive pulmonary disease. The Lung Health Study Research Group. Am J Respir Crit Care Med 153:1802–1811, 1996
78. Gold DR, Wang X, Wypij D, Speizer FD, Ware JH, Dockery DW: Effects of cigarette smoking on lung function in adolescent boys and girls. N Engl J Med 335:931–937, 1996
79. Anthonisen NR, Connett JE, Kiley JP, et al: Effects of smoking intervention and the use of an inhaled anticholinergic bronchodilator on the rate of decline of FEV_1. The Lung Health Study. JAMA 272(19):1497–1505, 1994
80. Kanner RE, Connett JE, Altose MD, et al: Gender difference in airway hyperresponsiveness in smokers with mild COPD. The Lung Health Study. Am J Respir Crit Care Med 150(4):956–961, 1994
81. Higgins MW, Thomas T: Incidence, prevalence, and mortality: intra- and intercountry differences. In Hensley MJ, Saunders NA (eds): Clinical Epidemiology of Chronic Obstructive Pulmonary Disease. New York: Marcel Dekker, 1989
82. Feinleib M, Rosenberg HM, Collins JG, Delozier JE, Pokras R, Chevarley FM: Trends in COPD morbidity and mortality in the United States. Am Rev Respir Dis 140:S9–S18, 1989
83. Fletcher C, Peto R: The natural history of chronic airflow obstruction. Br Med J 1(6077):1645–1648, 1977
84. Hudson LD, Milberg JA, Anardi D, Maunder RJ: Clinical risks for development of the acute respiratory distress syndrome. Am J Respir Crit Care Med 151:293–301, 1995
85. Thomsen GE, Morris AH: Incidence of the adult respiratory distress syndrome in the state of Utah. Am J Respir Crit Care Med 152: 965–971, 1995
86. Anderson FA Jr, Wheeler HB: Venous thromboembolism. Risk factors and prophylaxis [Review]. Clin Chest Med 16(2):235–251, 1995
87. Dalen JE, Paraskos JA, Ockene IS, Alpert JS, Hirsh J: Venous thromboembolism. Scope of the problem. Chest 89(Suppl 5):370S–373S, 1986
88. Crystal RG, Gadek JE, Ferrans VJ, Fulmer JD, Line BR, Hunninghake GW: Interstitial lung disease: current concepts of pathogenesis, staging and therapy [Review]. Am J Med 70(3):542–568, 1981
89. Coultas DB, Zumwalt RE, Black WC, Sobonya RE: The epidemiology of interstitial lung diseases. Am J Respir Crit Care Med 150(4):967–972, 1994
90. National Institute of Health, Respiratory Diseases Task Force: Report of Problems, Research, Approaches and Needs. DHEW Publication No. (NIH) 76-432. Bethesda, MD: National Institutes of Health, 1972
91. Coultas DB: Epidemiology of idiopathic pulmonary fibrosis. Semin Respir Med 14(3):181–196, 1993
92. Scott J, Johnston I, Britton J: What causes cryptogenic fibrosing alveolitis? A case-control study of environmental exposure to dust. Br Med J 301:1015–1017, 1990

93. Iwai K, Mori T, Yamada N, Yamaguchi M, Hosoda Y: Idiopathic pulmonary fibrosis. Epidemiologic approaches to occupational exposure. Am J Respir Crit Care Med 150:670–675, 1994
94. Egan JJ, Stewart JP, Hasleton PS, Arrand JR, Carroll KB, Woodcock AA: Epstein-Barr virus replication within pulmonary epithelial cells in cryptogenic fibrosing alveolitis. Thorax 50:1234–1239, 1995
95. Hubbard R, Lewis S, Richards K, Johnston I, Britton J: Occupational exposure to metal or wood dust and aetiology of cryptogenic fibrosing alveolitis. Lancet 347:284–289, 1996
96. Baumgartner KB, Samet JM, Stidley CA, et al: Cigarette smoking: a risk factor for idiopathic pulmonary fibrosis. Am J Respir Crit Care Med 155:242–248, 1997
97. Tablau OC, Reyes MP: Chronic interstitial pulmonary fibrosis following *Mycoplasma pneumoniae* pneumonia. Am J Med 79(2): 268–270, 1985
98. Morgan DC, Smyth JT, Lister RW, et al: Chest symptoms in farming communities with special reference to farmer's lung. Br J Ind Med 32(3):228–234, 1975
99. Hance A, Basset F, Soler P, et al: The role of cigarette smoking in the pathogenesis of pulmonary histiocytosis X. Am Rev Respir Dis 131:A369, 1985
100. Bresnitz EA, Goldberg R, Kosinski RM: Epidemiology of obstructive sleep apnea [Review]. Epidemiol Rev 16(2):210–227, 1994
101. Phillipson EA: Sleep apena—a major public health problem [Editorial]. N Engl J Med 328:1271–1273, 1993
102. Gonzalez-Rothi RJ, Block AJ: Mortality and sleep apnea. The trouble with looking backward [Editorial]. Chest 94(4):678–679, 1988
103. Kales A, Vela-Bueno A, Kales JD: Sleep disorders: sleep apnea and narcolepsy [Review]. Ann Intern Med 106(3):434–443, 1987

56

Gastrointestinal Tract Disorders

Cedric F. Garland • Frank C. Garland • Edward D. Gorham

This chapter presents recent advances in the epidemiology and possible prevention of five diseases of the gastrointestinal tract: duodenal ulcer, gastric ulcer, chronic gastritis, ulcerative colitis, and Crohn's disease.

The epidemiology of duodenal and peptic ulcers has been changing markedly. Rates of the two types of ulcers have declined considerably in men, but only slightly in women, producing nearly equal hospitalization,[1] mortality,[2] and prevalence[3] rates in the two sexes.

Research on *Helicobacter pylori*, a common bacterium that colonizes the stomach,[4,5] has increased understanding of the etiology and pathogenesis of duodenal and peptic ulcers. The organism has a prevalence rate of 10 to 20 percent in adults in the United States, 10 to 35 percent in most other developed countries, and is almost universal in third world populations.[6–8]

The most common serious chronic disorders of the lower gastrointestinal system are ulcerative colitis and Crohn's disease. Incidence rates of ulcerative colitis were stable during the last three decades of the twentieth century, while rates of Crohn's disease steadily rose from the late 1930s until the 1980s, then stabilized in the United States at rates similar to those of ulcerative colitis.[9,10] Dietary factors[11–13] and viral agents possibly transmitted during childhood[14,15] have been investigated as risk factors for ulcerative colitis and Crohn's disease.

▸ GASTRIC AND DUODENAL ULCER

Detailed reviews are available of the epidemiology of gastric and duodenal ulcer.[16,17] Investigation of the role of *H. pylori* has stirred more interest in the field than any other development related to the etiology of gastric and duodenal ulcer.[18–24]

Peptic ulcer (ICD9 Codes 531–532) accounted for 6,088 deaths in the United States in 1994 (including 1,757 from gastric ulcer, 1,993 from duodenal ulcer, and 2,338 from unspecified peptic ulcer),[2] and for 82,525 hospitalizations (34,528 for gastric ulcer and 47,997 for duodenal and unspecified peptic ulcer in 1990).[1] The self-reported annual period prevalence of peptic ulcer in the United States (both sites combined) was approximately 2 percent in 1988 and was approximately equal in men and women.[3]

Duodenal ulcers are associated with being in the top two thirds of the population in maximal acid secretion[25] and with high serum levels of pepsinogen I, an indirect marker of pepsinogen I level in the stomach.[26,27] A possible role of pancreatic bicarbonate deficiency, with reduced buffering of gastric acid reaching the duodenum through the pylorus, has been suggested.[28] By contrast, gastric ulcers usually are associated with low gastric acidity.[29] Both environmental and genetic factors contribute to the incidence of ulcers.

Trends

From 1960 to 1994, duodenal and gastric ulcer mortality rates declined from about 2.0 per 100,000 population for each to about 0.7 for each per 100,000 in the United States,[2] with a similar decline in the United Kingdom.[30] The death rate for duodenal ulcer in 1994 in the United States was 1.2 times higher for men than for women, but that for gastric ulcer was 1.2 times higher for women.[2] Sex ratios of mortality rates are currently close to 1.0 in England[30] and Germany.[31] This represents an important trend, since death rates from both types of ulcer were once much higher for men in these three countries. In the United States, the historical preponderance of self-reported peptic ulcer in men ended with the convergence of rates for men and women at the end of the 1970s (Fig. 56-1). Hospitalization rates for duodenal ulcer with hemorrhage or perforation remained stable for the past three decades, while hospitalization rates for uncomplicated duodenal ulcers declined markedly during the same interval (Fig. 56-2).

Hospitalization rates for gastric ulcers with hemorrhage more than doubled between 1980 and 1987, then declined slightly (Fig. 56-3). Hospitalization rates for gastric ulcer with perforation remained stable, while rates for uncomplicated gastric ulcer declined.

The use of effective H_2-receptor antagonists[32,33] after 1975 apparently contributed to the subsequent decline in hospitalizations[34] and surgery[35] for duodenal ulcer, and possibly to a decline in the hospitalization rate for uncomplicated gastric ulcer, but did not appear to influence hospitalization rates for ulcers with hemorrhage or perforation. Use of antacids also may have contributed.[36] The rise in hospitalization rates for gastric ulcer with hemorrhage (Fig. 56-3) requires further investigation.

Risk Factors

Apart from *H. pylori* infection, known risk factors for both types of peptic ulcer (duodenal and gastric) include cigarette smoking, use of nonsteroidal anti-inflammatory drugs by persons 55 years and older, and family history of ulcer at the same site. Risk factors specific to duodenal ulcer include, in addition to gastric hyperacidity,[25] blood group O,[37] and blood group nonsecretor status,[37] while those specific to gastric ulcer include aspirin use[38] and diet high in salt.[39] Aspirin use is associated with risk of bleeding duodenal ulcer,[38] but not with overall risk of duodenal ulcer.[40] The effect of aspirin on incidence of and severity of gastrointestinal bleeding is dose-dependent.[41] Known cofactors and risk factors are summarized in Table 56-1.

H. pylori, a strong correlate and probable cause of most chronic gastritis, mainly acts as a cofactor in peptic ulcer. *H. pylori* is a ubiquitous bacterium that eludes hydrolysis by colonizing the zone between the mucous layer and the gastric mucosal surface, an area of nearly neutral pH.[21] The prevalence of the helically shaped, curved,

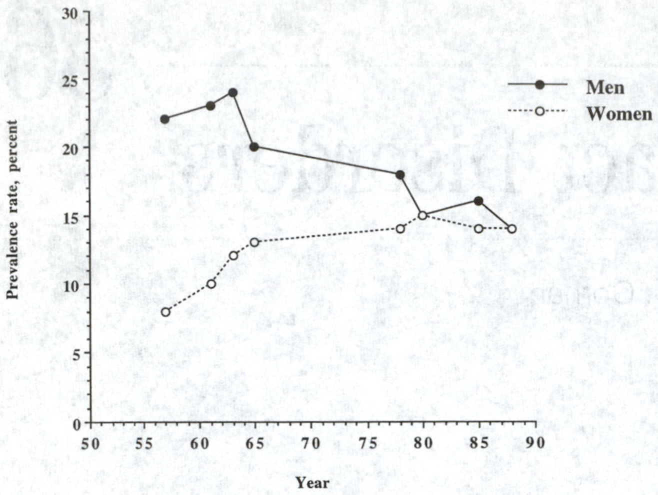

Figure 56-1. Self-reported annual period prevalence rate of peptic ulcer (gastric and duodenal combined), by sex, United States, 1957–1988. (Source: U.S. National Center for Health Statistics, Health Interview Surveys, 1974–1988.)

often multiflagellated Gram-negative microaerophilic organism is 10 to 50 percent in the normal-appearing gastric mucosa of asymptomatic people in developed countries. Prevalence of colonization in the general population varies by region; it is generally lowest in the United States and Europe (10 to 50 percent) and nearly universal in the third world.[19] Prevalence rates in the United States are lowest in whites, intermediate in Hispanics, and highest in blacks and in the lowest socioeconomic strata.[19]

Cigarette Smoking

Peptic ulcers are about twice as prevalent in smokers as in nonsmokers,[52,74–76] a finding that is paralleled by ulcer mortality rates despite competing risks from other adverse effects of smoking.[77] There is a dose-response relation between number of cigarettes smoked, duration of smoking, and inhalation habits and risk of peptic ulcer.[48] Nicotine and tar levels are less important than number of cigarettes smoked.[78]

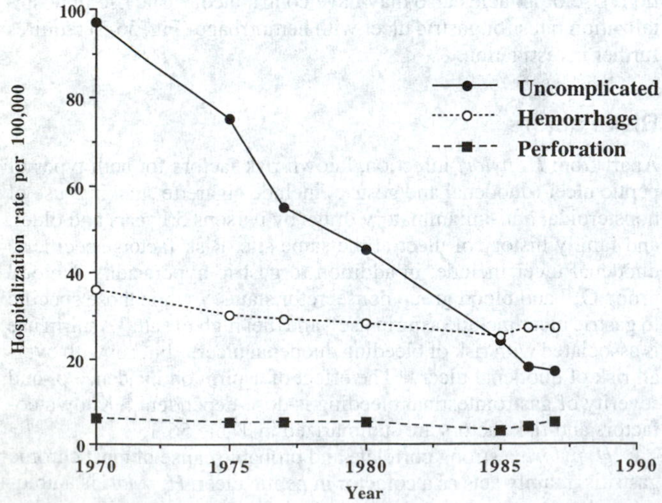

Figure 56-2. Annual duodenal ulcer hospitalization rate per 100,000 population, United States, 1970–1987. (Source: U.S. National Center for Health Statistics, 1970–1987.)

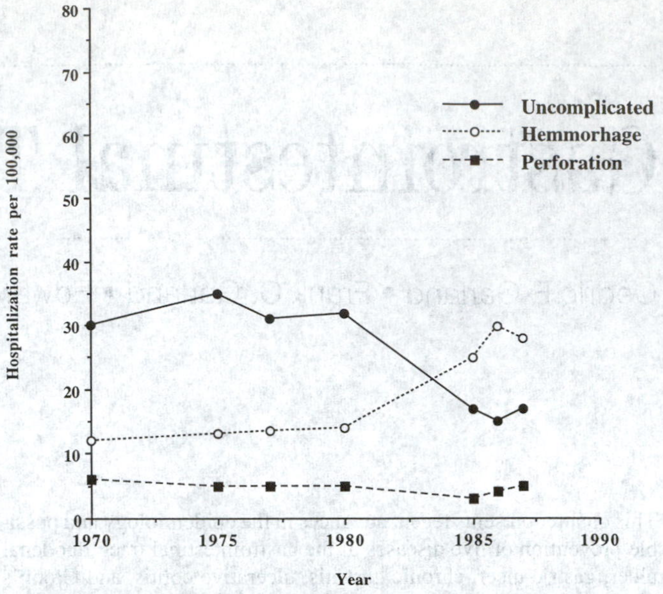

Figure 56-3. Annual gastric ulcer hospitalization rate per 100,000 population, United States, 1970–1987 (Source: U.S. National Center for Health Statistics, 1970–1987.)

Effects of treatment with H_2-receptor antagonists and antacids are diminished,[48,79,80] and duodenal or gastric ulcers heal more slowly and recur at higher rates in smokers.[51,81,82] However, the recurrence rate of duodenal ulcer after eradication of *H. pylori* infection is low regardless of smoking status.[53] Smoking increases gastric acid output in a dose-related manner[83–85] and reduces pancreatic bicarbonate output.[28] Smoking also diminishes perfusion of the gastric mucosa.[85,86] Pyloric sphincter tone is reduced in smokers, which may allow reflux of bile acids into the stomach, and possibly allow increased transport of gastric acid from the stomach to the duodenum.[87]

Nonsteroidal Anti-inflammatory Drugs

Aspirin. Aspirin use is associated with development of gastric, but apparently not duodenal, ulcer.[41,88,89] Heavy users of aspirin (4 or more days per week for 12 weeks) had three times the risk of gastric ulcer as nonusers, but no excess of duodenal ulcer.[88] Heavy and chronic use of aspirin injures the gastric mucosa.[90–92] Although aspirin use is not associated with an increase in risk of duodenal ulcer in general,[40] it is associated with an increase in risk of bleeding duodenal ulcer.[38] While aspirin plays an etiological role in gastric ulcers, its role in duodenal ulcers appears to be mainly one of increasing liability of bleeding from the ulcer crater, probably due to the effect of acetylsalicylic acid on platelet aggregation.[94]

Other Nonsteroidal Anti-inflammatory Drugs. Other nonsteroidal anti-inflammatory drugs (NSAIDs), which are widely used in treating headache, rheumatoid arthritis, and various inflammatory disorders, also increase risk of gastric ulcer.[56,57,95,96] Non-aspirin, nonsteroidal anti-inflammatory drugs had been taken nearly three times as often by patients with bleeding ulcers as by population control subjects.[56] The association was present for both gastric and duodenal ulcer in both sexes.

Coffee

Epidemiological evidence does not support the role of coffee in the etiology of peptic ulcer[52] although physiological studies show that both regular and decaffeinated coffee stimulates excessive gastric acid secretion, increases esophageal reflux, and exacerbates dyspepsia.[97] Early epidemiological studies implicating coffee failed to con-

TABLE 56-1. SUMMARY OF ESTABLISHED AND POSSIBLE RISK FACTORS FOR DUODENAL AND GASTRIC ULCER

	Ulcer Type	
Risk Factor or Cofactor	***Duodenal***[a]	***Gastric***[b]
Helicobacter pylori infection	Cofactor with prevalence ratio of approximately 3 for duodenal ulcer.[42] A cross-sectional association has previously been established.[43] Eradication of infection usually heals ulcers except those due to NSAIDs.[44,45] Recurrence rate after eradication is ≤1% annually.[44]	Cofactor with prevalence ratios from 1.0,[42] 1.6,[46] to 3.0[47] for gastric ulcer, the latter for previously undetected ulcer in infected but apparently healthy volunteers compared to uninfected healthy volunteers. A cross-sectional association has been established.[43] Eradication of infection usually heals ulcer except those due to NSAIDs.[44,45] Recurrence rate after eradication is ≤10% annually.[44]
Cigarette smoking	Increased risk (RR = 2)[48–50] with dose-response; increased recurrence (RR = 3);[51] retarded healing.[52] Smoking does not contribute to duodenal ulcer relapse after *H. pylori* eradication.[53]	Increased risk (RR = 2);[48,49] dose-response; increased recurrence (RR = 3) and retarded healing.[52] Smoking is not associated with *H. pylori* infection.[54]
Aspirin	No established association[40] for duodenal ulcer, but RR = 3–9 for bleeding duodenal ulcer.[38]	Increased risk (RR = 2–6),[43] for nonbleeding gastric ulcer and similar increased risk for bleeding gastric ulcer.[38] *H. pylori* is not a cofactor.[55] There is a dose-response relation for bleeding.[41]
Other nonsteroidal anti-inflammatory drugs	Increased risk at ages 55+ yr (RR = 2–6).[56,57] *H. pylori* is not a cofactor when NSAID use is the etiological factor.[43,55]	Increased risk, mainly at ages 55+ yr (RR = 2–6).[48,56,57] *H. pylori* is not a cofactor.[43,55]
Familial aggregation	Increased risk if first-degree relative has duodenal ulcer (RR = 3).[50,58,59]	Increased risk if first-degree relative has gastric ulcer (RR = 3).[50,58,59] Number of siblings is not related to risk of *H. pylori* infection.[60]
Blood group O	Relative risk = 1.3[37]	No established association
Blood group nonsecretor	Relative risk = 1.5[37]	No established association
Serum hyperpepsinogenemia I	Increased in cases.[27] Elevation is an autosomal dominant trait.[61]	No established association
Familial aggregation	Increased risk in first-degree relatives of duodenal ulcer patients (RR = 3).[27,58]	Increased risk in first-degree relatives of gastric ulcer patients (RR = 3).[27,58]
Gastric acidity	Associated with elevated gastric acidity (lower pH), RR = 7 in the 2 highest tertiles of maximal acid output (MAO) compared with the lowest tertile.[25]	Associated with low gastric acidity (higher pH)[25]
Alcohol use	No independent association has been established.[43,48,52]	No independent association has been established.[48,52] Alcohol use is unrelated to prevalence of *H. pylori* infection.[54,60]
Coffee	Equivocal[48,62]	Equivocal[48,62]
Diet	No established association at present[63]	Association with high-salt diet[39,64]
Emotional stress	No independent association has been established, except for stressful occupation.[16,65]	No independent association has been established, except for stressful occupation.[16,65]
Occupation	Slight excess of peptic ulcer in foremen and executives,[66] air traffic controllers[67,68] and shift workers.[69]	Slight excess of peptic ulcer in foremen and executives,[66] air traffic controllers,[67,68] and shift workers.[69]
Prostaglandin E_2 deficiency	Case reports and laboratory results are suggestive of an adverse effect of deficiency in patients taking NSAIDs.[70–72]	Case reports, laboratory results, and pharmacological data are supportive of an adverse effect of deficiency in patients taking NSAIDs[70–72]

Abbreviations: NSAIDs, nonsteroidal anti-inflammatory drugs; RR, relative risk.
[a] ICD9 Code 532.
[b] ICD9 Code 531.

trol for cigarette smoking, which is strongly associated with coffee intake and risk of ulcer.[98] A study of current coffee consumption among more than 35,000 members of a health maintenance organization found no relationship between coffee intake and risk of peptic ulcer.[48]

Alcohol

Although patients with alcoholic cirrhosis of the liver are at excess risk of peptic ulcer,[99] moderate alcohol ingestion is not associated with increased risk of peptic ulcer.[48,62] Concentrated ethanol lowers mucosal resistance to gastric acid, but moderate alcohol intake suppresses gastric acid production.[63]

Diet and Eating Habits

Although there is no evidence suggesting that a bland diet decreases ulcer incidence, prevents recurrence, or promotes healing,[52] improvement of symptoms in ulcer patients on a bland diet has been historically recognized.[100,101] Surveys in India, Bangladesh, and South Africa describe elevated incidence rates of duodenal ulcer in population groups with high intake of rice[102] or yams,[103] and low incidence in groups with high intake of wheat or corn.

Stress and Occupation

It has not been established that psychological factors are causally related to duodenal or gastric ulcer, despite belief that they are important.[65] Problems with the study of psychological factors as the cause of ulcer include difficulties in achieving consensus on definition and measurement of psychological stress and in measuring differences in the responses of individuals to stressful situations.[65]

One approach to studying the role of stress in the development of ulcer has been to study occupations considered to be stressful. Air traffic controllers were shown to have moderately elevated rates of peptic ulcer.[67,68] Foremen and executives also had a higher than expected prevalence of ulcers.[66] These studies did not control for cigarette smoking, which is associated with self-reported subjective occupational stress.[104,105] There are marked individual differences in the tendency to increase or decrease cigarette smoking in response to varying levels of stress.[104]

A case-control study of 132 patients with prepyloric and duodenal ulcers and an equal number of population control subjects reported no relation between factors such as personal worries or a psychologically demanding occupation and these ulcers.[106] However, smoking, low income, and low educational level were more common in cases than in control subjects. Manual labor as compared with office labor carried a relative risk of 1.6 for gastric ulcer and of 2.0 for duodenal ulcer in German workers,[107] but this finding was not adjusted for cigarette smoking. Shift workers were reported to have approximately twice the prevalence rates of gastric and duodenal ulcer as other workers,[95] although this finding was not adjusted for cigarette smoking or education.

Feldman and associates reported that peptic ulcer was not associated with the number of life events occurring in the previous year.[108] Cross-sectionally, ulcer patients had more negative personality traits such as depression and anxiety and a diminished coping ability. Walker and associates developed a theoretical model linking psychosocial and behavioral risk factors in a multifactorial concept of the cause of ulcer.[109] They suggested that stress as a factor in ulcer is not as much related to the number of life events as the way that individuals react to the events. It has been suggested that urbanization is a factor in risk of ulcers,[110] but no clear role for urbanization was found in a controlled study of patients with duodenal ulcer who moved from small towns in South Africa to a large urban area.[111]

Genetics

Duodenal or gastric ulcers tend to aggregate in families, but both do not aggregate in the same families.[50,58,59] Each type of ulcer also is associated with genetic markers not shared by the other type.[112,113] A simple pattern of inheritance does not exist for either type of ulcer, although hyperpepsinogenemia I is a Mendelian dominant trait present in 30 to 40 percent of people with duodenal ulcer.[26,27] The preponderance of evidence suggests that, while the etiology of ulcers is largely environmental, genetic predisposition plays some contributory role.

First-degree relatives of patients with gastric ulcer have a 3-fold excess risk for gastric ulcer but no increased risk for duodenal ulcer.[58] Similarly, first-degree relatives of patients with duodenal ulcer have a 3-fold excess risk for duodenal, but not gastric, ulcer.[58]

Further evidence for a genetic basis of familial aggregation comes from twin studies. The concordance for ulcer among monozygotic twin pairs is greater than for dizygotic twins.[114] Overall, studies of genetic studies and environmental risk factors suggest that duodenal and gastric ulcers are different diseases, with some risk factors specific to each and some relevant to both.[115,116]

H. pylori Eradication

H. pylori colonization of the stomach can be detected with a urease breath test.[117] The organism is generally eradicated with a 14-day course of bismuth subsalicylate (525 mg q.i.d.), metronidazole (250 to 500 mg, t.i.d. or q.i.d), and tetracycline (500 mg q.i.d.).[118] Clarithromycin can be substituted for metronidazole for individuals who previously have taken metronidazole or if metronidazole specifically is contraindicated.[117] Therapy also generally includes an H_2-antagonist started at the same time and continued for 4 to 6 weeks.[118] Eradication of *H. pylori* usually heals peptic ulcers, but does not heal ulcers associated with use of aspirin or other NSAIDs.

Ulcers and Cancer

Individuals with a history of gastric ulcer have twice the incidence rate of stomach cancer as those without such a history, while duodenal ulcer is associated with a 50 percent reduction in risk of gastric malignancy.[73] The favorable association with duodenal ulcer is reversed in patients who have had gastrectomy for ulcer.[119–122]

Prevention

The principal means of preventing both gastric and duodenal ulcers are avoidance of cigarette smoking and of chronic use of nonsteroidal anti-inflammatory drugs. Eradication of *H. pylori* infection in the general population in the United States would not be justified at present as a means of preventing gastric or duodenal ulcer.[123] However eradication of *H. pylori* in the elderly might be cost-effective, since widespread *H. pylori* colonization of the stomach has been reported in institutional settings,[124] ulcer treatment is more difficult, and fatal complications of ulcer are more common in older adults. Death rates for gastric and duodenal ulcer in men 75 to 84 years old are 30 times higher than in middle-aged men, although some of the age difference may be due to a birth cohort effect.[16]

Results of the urease breath test for *H. pylori* colonization agree adequately with histology and culture of the organism from endoscopic biopsies.[42] A serological test also is available for detection for *H. pylori* antibody; in one study of blood donors in Italy, 94 percent of individuals who were positive for serum antibodies had histologic evidence of infection at endoscopy; 20 percent of the seropositive individuals had an ulcer (20 duodenal, 5 gastric) and 2 had gastric cancer.[125] The yield from serological testing in the United States has been lower.[123]

▸ CHRONIC GASTRITIS

Risk factors for chronic gastritis are shown in Table 56-2. The disorder involves a range of inflammatory changes in the gastric mucosa. Two common sites of gastritis have been identified, fundal (type A) and antral (type B), but most population-based studies have not been specific for site. *H. pylori* is believed to be the principal pathogenic agent of the antral and probably the fundal forms. The organism is present in 90 percent or more of patients with chronic gastritis.[126]

Patients with chronic gastritis have *H. pylori* present in the gastric mucosa from 5 to 100 times times more frequently than healthy control subjects, depending on the population studied.[19,20,22,23]

The Sydney System of classification has been developed to describe and grade the microscopic features of gastritis, i.e., chronic or acute inflammation, degree of atrophy of mucosal glands, degree of intestinal metaplasia of the gastric mucosa, and presence or absence of *H. pylori* in endoscopic biopsy specimens.[126]

Similarities of DNA sequence between isolates from family members strongly support the idea that *H. pylori* infections commonly are acquired in households during childhood and persist throughout life if not eradicated.[130] In the United States, *H. pylori* gastritis is most common in cohorts born in the early decades of the twentieth century.[126]

Mass endoscopic screening for chronic or atrophic gastritis has not been done in the United States, but has been performed in Japan in an effort to prevent gastric cancer. A possible role of screening for chronic gastritis should be evaluated for high-risk populations in the United States, such as older immigrants from areas where chronic and

TABLE 56-2. SUMMARY OF ESTABLISHED AND POSSIBLE RISK FACTORS OR CO-FACTORS FOR CHRONIC GASTRITIS[a]

Risk Factor or Cofactor	Comment
H. pylori infection	Agent associated with most chronic gastritis worldwide. Estimated prevalence of *H. pylori* infection in individuals with gastritis is 90% or higher, compared with 10 to 20% of the general population in the United States and 10 to 35% in most other developed countries.[54,126,127]
Age	Chronic gastritis can be present at any age, but usually is first detected during adulthood. The atrophic form is generally limited to adults 55 years and older.[54,126,127]
Geographic region	Chronic gastritis is common in residents of, or migrants from, Japan, China, Southeast Asia, India, Mexico, Central and South America, and the third world.[7]
Alcohol	Persistent excessive intake of alcohol is associated with chronic gastritis.[63,99]
Diet	A diet high in salt is positively associated.[39,64]
Familial aggregation	The pattern of familial aggregation indicates a mainly environmental rather than genetic etiology. Risk of chronic gastritis is not related to gastritis in parents, but is related to gastritis in the spouse and siblings.[128]

Abbreviation: RR, relative risk.
[a] ICD9 Code 535.0–535.5.

atrophic gastritis is relatively common and risk of malignancy is high (Table 56-2).

Prevention

Most cases of chronic gastritis, particularly the antral form, can be prevented or cured by pharmacological eradication of *H. pylori* infection. Eradication should be considered in older adults from ethnic groups or countries of origin where *H. pylori* infection is common and for those living in institutions where the infection is widespread. Severity of chronic gastritis associated with heavy use of nonsteroidal anti-inflammatory drugs can be reduced by contemporaneous administration of synthetic prostaglandins such as misoprostol.

Ultimately, immunization may provide the only feasible approach to large-scale eradication of *H. pylori* infection and its complications.[131–133] High rates of protection against *H. pylori* have been achieved in mice, using antigens ranging from whole cells to purified recombinant proteins.[131]

▸ ULCERATIVE COLITIS AND CROHN'S DISEASE

Ulcerative colitis (ICD9 Code 556) and Crohn's disease (ICD9 Code 555) were responsible for 5,556 deaths from ulcerative colitis and 404 from Crohn's disease in the United States in 1994.[2] There were 34,528 hospitalizations for ulcerative colitis and 47,997 for Crohn's disease in the United States in 1990, the latest year for which data were available from the National Center for Health Statistics.[1]

▸ ULCERATIVE COLITIS

Comprehensive reviews of the epidemiology of ulcerative colitis are available.[134–141] First distinguished in the nineteenth century from colitis caused by bacteria and parasites, ulcerative colitis is characterized by a gradual onset of chronic diarrhea, colicky abdominal pain, weight loss, and blood or mucus in the stool.[134] Ulcerative colitis affects the rectum, often encompassing the sigmoid and descending colon, and occasionally the entire colon. Microscopically, there is inflammation with neutrophilic infiltration of the surface mucosal cells, crypt epithelium, and submucosa.[142] Most observational studies have been based on relatively few cases. Many of the findings regarding this disease should be considered as indicative of general trends or patterns, rather than as findings that have reached a particular criterion of statistical significance. Also, unless otherwise specified, the incidence rates given are unadjusted for age. Ulcerative colitis is a disease of public health importance since it is difficult to treat successfully, it occurs in young, otherwise healthy people, it raises the risk of colorectal malignancy,[145] and it is responsible for a considerable number of deaths annually.[2]

Incidence

The highest reported annual incidence rate of ulcerative colitis was in Northeastern England, 15 per 100,000 population[146] (Table 56-3). Elsewhere, incidence rates were high in Norway,[147,148] Minnesota,[149] Scotland,[151] the Faroes,[152] Iceland,[153] and Denmark.[154] Intermediate rates were reported in central and southern Europe.[159,160] Low rates were reported in the mid-to-southern United States,[9,10] Italy,[168] and Kuwait.[170] Kuwait had the lowest reported annual incidence rate, 1 per 100,000 population.[170]

With some exceptions, the incidence rate of ulcerative colitis appears to vary directly with latitude. The highest reported rates generally occur in areas distant from the equator (Fig. 56-4). Latitude accounts for nearly 40 percent of the geographic variation in incidence rates. The main exception was Japan which is between 31 and 45°N. The geographic distribution of ulcerative colitis parallels that of colorectal cancer.[171]

The latitude gradient in incidence of ulcerative colitis has not always been a feature of this disease. For example, rates in Norway have climbed steeply since the 1960s.[180] The trend is especially evident in western Norway; northeastern Scotland, including the Orkney and Shetland Islands;[151] and in the Faroes, where the incidence rate rose from 2 per 100,000 population during 1964 to 1968 to 13 during 1979 to 1983 ($P < 0.01$).[152]

Incidence Rates in Jews

Incidence rates in the Jewish population groups vary widely (Table 56-4). The incidence rate in the Jewish population in Baltimore was the highest ever reported in Jews,[163] about four times the incidence in the non-Jewish population.[171] Low incidence rates in Jews in Israel are consistent with the latitude gradient characteristic of ulcerative colitis. High rates previously reported in Jews in Cape Town, South Africa[173] may partly be due to incidence in Jews who migrated from Germany and other European countries at high latitudes.

Trends in Incidence Rates

International secular trends in incidence of ulcerative colitis have been reviewed in detail.[10] The only published longitudinal incidence data from the early half of the twentieth century are from Rochester, Minnesota,[176] where the age-adjusted incidence rate for ulcerative colitis doubled between 1935 and 1964, and from Czechoslovakia, where the incidence of ulcerative colitis increased between 1935 and 1963.[177]

The principal data on trends in incidence rates of ulcerative colitis in the United States are from the Baltimore, Maryland, metropolitan area.[10] Annual age-adjusted incidence rates of ulcerative colitis in whites, estimated from first hospitalizations, were stable at 5.0/100,000 during 1960 to 1963 and 5.1/100,000 during 1973, but dropped to 2.3/100,000 during 1977 to 1979.[10] The first hospitalization rates in all three periods were obtained using the same diagnostic criteria and research protocols. A review of cases from earlier periods showed that the decline in incidence rates was not due to the classification of a higher proportion of chronic colitis cases as

TABLE 56-3. ANNUAL CRUDE INCIDENCE RATES OF ULCERATIVE COLITIS PER 100,000 POPULATION, SELECTED AREAS, 1960 TO 1994[a]

Authors, Reference	*Location*	*Period*	*Rate*
Devlin et al.[146]	Northeastern England	1971–77	15
Haug et al.[147]	Norway	1984–85	15
Moum et al.[148]	Southwestern Norway	1990–93	14
Stonnington et al.[149]	Minnesota, United States	1960–79	14
Stewenius et al.[150]	Malmo, Sweden	1982	13
Sinclair et al.[151]	Scotland	1967–76	11
Berner and Kiaer[152]	Faroes	1983	11
Bjørnsson and Thorgeirsson[153]	Iceland	1980	7
Binder et al.[154]	Denmark	1962–78	7
Srivastava et al.[155]	Cardiff, Wales	1978–87	6
Hiatt and Kaufman[156]	Northern California, United States[b]	1971–82	6
Eason et al.[157]	New Zealand[a]	1969–78	5
Brandes et al.[158]	West Germany	1962–75	5
Tragnone et al.[159]	Bologna, Italy	1988–89	5
Tsianos et al.[160]	Northwest Greece	1991	5
Nordenvall et al.[161]	Sweden	1975–79	4
Shivananda et al.[162]	Holland	1979–83	4
Monk et al.[163]	Maryland, United States[b]	1960–63	4
Garland et al.[9]	United States, 15 areas[b]	1973	4
Latour et al.[164]	Liege, Belgium	1993–94	4
Gower-Rousseau et al.[165]	Northern France	1988–90	3
Dirks et al.[166]	Western Ruhr, Germany	1980–84	3
Mate-Jimenez et al.[167]	Central Spain		
	Urban	1981–88	3
	Rural	1981–88	3
Calkins et al.[10]	Maryland, United States[b]	1977–79	2
LaFranchi et al.[168]	Italy	1972–73	2
Morita et al.[169]	Japan	1991	2
Al-Nakib et al.[170]	Kuwait	1984	1

[a] ICD9 Code 556.
[b] Whites.

Crohn's colitis during 1977 to 1979. Some of the apparent decline could reflect more frequent management of mild cases outside hospitals, but there are no data to support this possibility. Trends were similar in men and women.

Age-adjusted annual incidence rates in nonwhite men in Baltimore dropped from 1.0/100,000 population in 1960 to 1963 to 0.7 in 1973 and then rose slightly to 1.3 in 1977 to 1979. The incidence rate in nonwhite women rose from 1.7 in 1960 to 1963 to 4.1 in 1973, then dropped slightly to 2.9 in 1977 to 1979.

Only limited long-term data on incidence rates are available elsewhere. Hiatt and Kaufman[156] reported no changes in first hospitalization rates for ulcerative colitis and Crohn's disease in a large northern California group practice during the period from 1971 to 1982. Hospitalization rates in Japan remained stable from 1954 to 1974 at their characteristically low levels.[178]

Migrant Studies

Incidence of ulcerative colitis is related to migration. For example, the incidence of ulcerative colitis was twice as high in Jews who migrated to Israel from Europe and the United States as in Jews born in Israel; the difference was most pronounced from ages 15 through 29 years, where the incidence rate in migrant Jews was three times that of resident Jews.[179]

Studies performed to date cannot rule out the possibility that the observed differences might be due, at least in part, to genetic differences. In the United States, Jews of central European ancestry were more likely to develop ulcerative colitis (and Crohn's disease) than those of Russian or Polish ancestry.[179] However, genetic factors would not explain an observed convergence of incidence rates at older ages in migrants at young ages to Israel with those of the native-born.

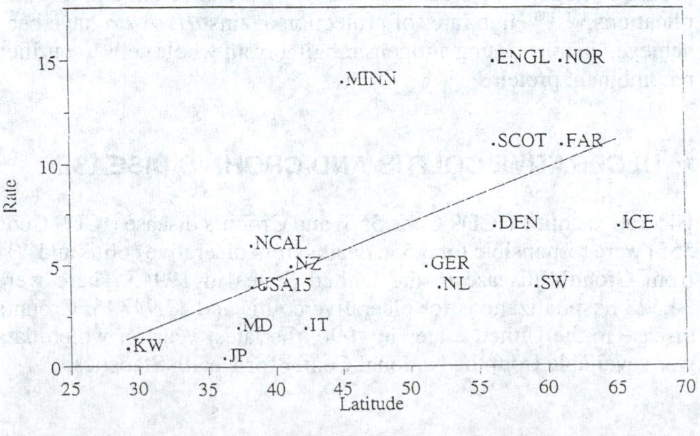

Figure 56-4. Annual incidence rates of ulcerative colitis per 100,000 population, by latitude. *DEN*, Denmark; *ENGL*, England; *FAR*, Faroes; *GER*, Germany; *ICE*, Iceland; *IT*, Italy; *JP*, Japan; *KW*, Kuwait; *MD*, Maryland; *NCAL*, Northern California; *NL*, Netherlands; *NOR*, Norway; *NZ*, New Zealand; *MINN*, Minnesota (Olmstead County); *SCOT*, Scotland; *SW*, Sweden; *USA15*, United States (15 areas).

TABLE 56-4. ANNUAL INCIDENCE RATES OF ULCERATIVE COLITIS PER 100,000 JEWISH POPULATION, SELECTED AREAS, 1960 TO 1984

Authors, Reference	Location	Period	Rate
Wright et al.[173]	Cape Town, South Africa	1980–1984	17
Monk et al.[163]	Maryland, United States	1960–1963	13
Jacobsohn and Levine[174]	Jerusalem, Israel	1973–1980	6
Odes et al.[175]	Beer Sheva, Israel	1980–1984	6

Risk Factors

Age

Incidence of ulcerative colitis generally peaks at ages 25 through 35 years and again at ages 70 and older. Most studies of ulcerative colitis have reported bimodal age incidence, although some studies have reported a unimodal pattern.[134]

The most prominent bimodal pattern of incidence has been reported from the United States, with incidence peaks at approximately ages 25 and 75 years in men, and at 35 years and again in later life in women.[9] Another U.S. study reported prominent peaks at about age 25 and 65 years in men and 35 and 70 years and older in women.[10]

Seasonality

Self-reported relapses of ulcerative colitis have a distinct seasonality, with the greatest occurrence in fall and winter.[181]

Smoking

Since Heatley et al.[182] and Harries et al.[183] noticed that there were few patients with ulcerative colitis who were current smokers of cigarettes, a number of case-control studies have verified these observations.[184] The inverse association is strong. One study reported an odds ratio of 0.16 (95 percent confidence interval, 0.09 to 0.29) for current smokers at time of diagnosis compared with those who never smoked.[185] An analysis of 12 case-control studies reported a Mantel-Haenszel odds ratio of 0.25 ($P < 0.01$) in current smokers compared with nonsmokers.[186] The effect was also strong for smoking at the time of first diagnosis, with an odds ratio of 0.3 for nonsmokers compared to ever-smokers (95 percent confidence interval, 0.1 to 0.7).

In several studies it was noted that former smokers were at higher risk for ulcerative colitis than those who had never smoked or those who smoked currently.[187–189] A study based on patients in a large group practice, reported an odds ratio of 2.0 (95 percent confidence interval, 1.1 to 3.7) for former smokers compared with those who never smoked.[190] Another case-control study reported an odds ratio of 2.7 (95 percent confidence interval, 1.5 to 4.9) for former smokers compared with nonsmokers.[189] A meta-analysis of 12 case-control studies reported a combined odds ratio of 1.33 for former smokers compared with those who never smoked ($P < 0.01$).[186] However, some studies showed former smokers to be at similar or only slightly higher risk than those who never smoked.[185,191]

The association between not smoking and ulcerative colitis is strong and highly reproducible, suggesting that there may be an agent in tobacco smoke that reduces the incidence and severity of the disease.[184] The agent has not yet been identified. Inhaling cigarette smoke depletes arachidonic acid,[192] so less of this substrate is available for synthesis of inflammatory mediators that may play a causal role.

Person-to-Person Transmission

Presently there is no evidence of person-to-person horizontal or vertical transmission of ulcerative colitis. Although there are rare reports of spouse pairs concordant for the disease[193] no such pairs have been reported from large population-based observational studies of inflammatory bowel disease, which have included thousands of married couples.[134,180] The occurrence of ulcerative colitis (or Crohn's disease) in spouses of patients appears to be no more common than would be expected on the basis of chance.[193,194] Mother-child case pairs are no more common than other pairs of equal consanguinity,[195] suggesting that vertical transmission is uncommon or nonexistent.

There is no evidence of time or space clustering of either ulcerative colitis or Crohn's disease[196,197] although a lymphocytotoxic antibody was reported to occur at higher levels in household contacts of patients than in relatives of equal consanguinity living outside the household.[198] There is no known relationship between any particular species of *Mycobacterium* and ulcerative colitis.[199]

A major international case control study of ulcerative colitis and Crohn's disease in patients who had onset of the disease before age 20 years showed that there had been no increased contact with animals or with other persons who had ulcerative colitis or Crohn's disease. In addition, no correlation was shown with birth order, number of siblings, or a history of having been breast-fed.[200]

Genetics

Genetic factors in ulcerative colitis have been reviewed previously.[134,194,195] From a genetic viewpoint, ulcerative colitis and Crohn's disease sometimes behave as a single disease.[195] The incidence of ulcerative colitis or Crohn's disease in close family members of patients (parents, siblings, or children) with inflammatory bowel disease has been reported as two to three times the expected rate. This estimate may be high, however, because some studies have accepted unvalidated reports of inflammatory bowel disease in relatives.[196] Incidence of inflammatory bowel disease appears to decrease with decreasing consanguinity to the patient.[194] Sixteen identical twin pairs in which at least one twin had ulcerative colitis were identified among 25,000 same-sex pairs in the Swedish twin registry, based on a central national diagnosis registry. Only one of the twin pairs was concordant for the disease.[201] Twenty pairs of same-sex fraternal twins in which at least one twin had ulcerative colitis were identified, but there were no pairs in which both twins had the disease. Discordance between twins was not accounted for by differences in smoking habits.

Despite the tendency for inflammatory bowel disease to occur in families, 60 to 90 percent of patients have no first-degree relative with the disease[202] and pedigree studies have failed to detect any known Mendelian pattern.[195] Rapid variations in incidence of ulcerative colitis[10,135,147] suggest that, although it is likely that a genetic predisposition to the disease exists, environmental factors must largely control incidence.

Religions Other Than Jewish

An excess of ulcerative colitis prevalence is present in Mormons in the United Kingdom, compared to non-Mormons in the United Kingdom.[203] Incidence in Mormons may be associated with rules prohibiting smoking or with dietary practices. In Utah only 10 percent of Mormon men and 5 percent of Mormon women smoke, compared with 35 and 38 percent, respectively, of non-Mormons in Utah.[204]

Psychological Factors

The influence of psychological factors on ulcerative colitis has been reviewed.[140] Case-control studies have reported no correlation between the number of stressful life events and incidence of the disease, either in children[200] or in adults.[205] There are no personality traits that reliably differentiate people with ulcerative colitis from the unaffected population or those with Crohn's disease.[140]

Oral Contraceptives

The risk of ulcerative colitis is about twice as high in users of oral contraceptives as in control subjects, but the small number of cases reported and lack of statistical significance limits a definite conclusion.[188,206,207] Ulcerative colitis has been reported to improve on discontinuation of oral contraceptives.[208] Interestingly, there was a

3.5-fold increase in age-adjusted incidence of ulcerative colitis in black women in Baltimore during the decade following introduction of oral contraceptives in the early 1960s, while no increase occurred in black men during the same time interval.

Diet

Dietary studies of ulcerative colitis and Crohn's disease have been reviewed.[134] Specific adverse dietary factors have not been identified, and most dietary studies have been negative. There is little evidence to date that dietary deficiency of insoluble fiber is a factor in ulcerative colitis (or in Crohn's disease). Japan, where polished rice is consumed in preference to that containing bran, has a low incidence rate of ulcerative colitis.[169] Intake of saturated fat also may not explain the geographic pattern, since New Zealand Maoris, in whom ulcerative colitis is rare,[209] are believed to consume a large proportion of calories as saturated fat. Intake of coffee is unrelated to risk of ulcerative colitis.[210]

Complications

Patients with longer than a 10-year duration of extensive disease are at high risk for colorectal cancer.[145] Patients with ulcerative colitis should have colonoscopy every 1 or 2 years, with biopsies every 10 cm, including samples from normal-appearing mucosa. Colectomy may become necessary if malignancy or multifocal or persistent high-grade dysplasia is detected.[145]

Prevention

There is no known way to prevent ulcerative colitis. Attentive medical care can relieve many symptoms, minimize complications, and allow detection of colorectal cancer while it is still localized. Avoidance of oral contraceptives might reduce the incidence of ulcerative colitis or a syndrome that mimics it. Future studies should consider whether restriction of intake of dietary arachidonic acid and its precursors such as linoleic acid, which occurs primarily in vegetable oils, might reduce incidence rates by reducing levels of the substrate required for synthesis of inflammatory mediators. Alternatively, increased dietary intake of nutrients that inhibit synthesis of prostaglandins may be of preventive value. These nutrients include eicosapentaenoic and docosahexaenoic fatty acids, which are present in most fatty marine fish and fish oil. The latitude gradient of incidence rates and the seasonality of hospitalization rates suggest that vitamin D deficiency may play some role as a cofactor in ulcerative colitis. Addressing vitamin D deficiency on a populationwide basis with a modest nutritional dose of vitamin D (400 IU/day in children, 800 to 1000 IU/day in adults) as one aspect of prophylaxis has no known adverse effects, would have other benefits, and should receive further evaluation. Despite the association with smoking, advising it in an effort to prevent or treat ulcerative colitis would be unwise, because the absolute risk of lung cancer and heart disease are much higher in smokers than nonsmokers.

▶ CROHN'S DISEASE

Incidence rates of Crohn's disease have been reviewed previously.[134,135] There is considerable geographic variation in incidence rates (Table 56-5). The highest incidence rate of Crohn's disease is in Spokane, Washington.[211] Trends in incidence rates of Crohn's disease have been reviewed in detail previously, and a clear rise in incidence is evident in most studies.[134] Notably, the age-adjusted incidence rate doubled in Olmsted County, Minnesota, between 1945 and 1975.[214]

In Baltimore, the incidence of Crohn's disease in white men rose from 2.6/100,000 population during 1960 to 1963 to 3.9 in 1973 but then declined slightly to 3.4 during 1977 to 1979; in white women, incidence rose from 1.3/100,000 population during 1960 to 1963 to 3.6 in 1973, remaining at approximately that level during 1977 to 1979.[10] Crohn's disease, like ulcerative colitis, has a bimodal age distribution in most populations.[10,134] Despite a persistent search for contributing factors, no risk factors other than family history,[195] a positive association with smoking,[218] and Jewish religion[219] have been clearly identified. The positive association of smoking with Crohn's disease contrasts with the inverse association of smoking with ulcerative colitis. This suggests that there may be an ischemic component to Crohn's disease associated with smoking, but the issue remains unresolved.

Measles and Crohn's Disease

Wakefield et al. recently proposed that Crohn's disease is a chronic granulomatous vasculitis due to persistent infection by measles virus in the vascular endothelium.[14] Measles immunization also has been reported as a risk factor for both Crohn's disease and ulcerative colitis,

TABLE 56-5. ANNUAL CRUDE INCIDENCE RATES OF CROHN'S DISEASE PER 100,000 POPULATION, SELECTED AREAS, WHITES (UNLESS OTHERWISE NOTED), 1964 TO 1994[a]

Authors, Reference	Location	Period	Rate
Nunes and Ahlquist[211]	Spokane, Washington, United States	1981	9
Lee and Costello[212]	Blackpool, England	1968–80	7
Latour et al.[164]	Liege, Belgium	1993–94	6
Gower-Rousseau et al.[165]	Northern France	1988–90	5
Munkholm et al.[213]	Copenhagen County, Denmark	1979–87	4
Garland et al.[9]	United States, 15 areas	1973	4
Dirks et al.[166]	West Germany	1980–84	4
Gollop et al.[214]	Minnesota, United States	1943–82	4
Calkins et al.[10]	Baltimore, United States, white	1977–79	4
Calkins et al.[10]	Baltimore, United States, nonwhite	1977–79	3
Shapira and Tamir[215]	Israel, Jews	1980–90	3
	Israel, Arabs	1980–90	0
Tragnone et al.[159]	Bologna, Italy	1988–89	3
Berner and Kiaer[152]	Faroes	1964–83	2
Krawiec et al.[216]	Beer-Sheva, Israel	1976–80	2
Morita et al.[169]	Japan	1991	0.5
Tsianos et al.[160]	Northwest Greece	1991	0.3
Kimura et al.[217]	Japan	1980–81	0.2

[a] ICD9 Code 555.

with odds ratios in the range of 3.0 to 5.0.[220,221] There was a higher incidence of Crohn's disease in people born during measles epidemics in Sweden, where epidemics occurred at approximately 2-year intervals from 1945 to 1954.[15] Other evidence includes detection of persistent measles virus in intestinal tissue of patients with Crohn's disease according to immunochemistry for measles nucleocapsid protein, *in situ* hybdridization for measles genomic RNA, and electron microscopy.[14]

Prevention

There is no known means of prevention of Crohn's disease, except possibly for avoidance of cigarette smoking and oral contraceptives. Increased dietary intake of long-chain fatty acids in marine fish and fish oil inhibits synthesis of leukotrienes and some prostanoids and may be of preventive value. In a 1-year randomized trial, patients who took fish oil (550 mg/day) had 28 percent relapse rate compared with 69 percent in those who took a placebo ($P < 0.001$).[222]

Measles immunization with attenuated live virus does not protect against Crohn's disease and has been reported to adversely affect risk.[220,221] Eradication of measles would be difficult on anything other than a worldwide basis.

A case-control study in Germany observed lower serum 25-hydroxyvitamin D in patients with inflammatory bowel disease than that in control subjects, with a mean serum concentration of 23 ng/mL in patients and 45 ng/mL in normal control subjects ($P < 0.05$).[13] Patients with Crohn's disease in Finland had significantly lower serum 25-hydroxyvitamin D levels than did healthy control subjects ($P < 0.001$).[223] Neither study proves an etiologic role of vitamin D deficiency, since differences in absorption may have contributed nevertheless, combined with the latitude gradient of the disease, these studies suggest that vitamin D deficiency should be evaluated as a possible cofactor in Crohn's disease.

► REFERENCES

1. Centers for Disease Control and Prevention, National Center for Health Statistics: Hospital discharge survey data. CDC WONDER. World Wide Web address http://www.cdc.gov
2. Centers for Disease Control and Prevention, National Center for Health Statistics. Mortality data. CDC WONDER. World Wide Web address http://www.cdc.gov
3. National Center for Health Statistics: Current estimates from the National Health Interview Survey, 1988. Vital and Health Statistics Series 10. DHHS Publication No. (PHS) 89-1501. Washington, DC: Government Printing Office, 1989
4. Marshall BJ, Warren JR: Unidentified curved bacilli in the stomach of patients with gastritis and peptic ulceration. Lancet 1:1311–1314, 1984
5. Marshall BJ: *Helicobacter pylori*. Am J Gastroenterol 89(Suppl 8): S116–128, 1994
6. Communicable disease report. CDR review. London: PHLS Communicable Disease Surveillance Centre, 1992
7. Genta RM, Gurer IE, Graham DY: Geographical pathology of *Helicobacter pylori* infection: is there more than one gastritis? Ann Med 27:595–599, 1995
8. Lin JT, Wang JT, Wang TH, Wu MS, Lee TK, Chen CJ: *Helicobacter pylori* infection in a randomly selected population, healthy volunteers, and patients with gastric ulcer and gastric adenocarcinoma. A seroprevalence study in Taiwan. Scand J Gastroenterol 28:1067–1072, 1993
9. Garland C, Lilienfeld AM, Mendeloff AL, Markowitz JA, Terrell KB, Garland FC: Incidence rates of ulcerative colitis and Crohn's disease in fifteen areas of the United States. Gastroenterology 81:1115–1124, 1981
10. Calkins BM, Lilienfeld AM, Garland CF, Mendeloff AL: Trends in incidence rates of ulcerative colitis and Crohn's disease. Dig Dis Sci 29:913–920, 1984
11. Levine J: Exogenous factors in Crohn's disease. J Clin Gastroenterol 14:216–226, 1992
12. Epidemiology Group of the Research Committee on Inflammatory Bowel Disease in Japan: Dietary factors in inflammatory bowel disease in Japan. J Gastroenterol 30(Suppl 8):9–12, 1995
13. Vogelsang H, Klamert M, Resch H, Ferenci P: Dietary vitamin D intake in patients with Crohn's disease. Wien Klin Wochenschr 107: 578–581, 1995
14. Wakefield AJ, Pittilo RM, Sim R, Cosby SL, Stephenson JR, Dhillon AP, Pounder RE: Evidence of persistent measles infection in Crohn's disease. J Med Virol 39:345–353, 1993
15. Ekbom A, Wakefield AJ, Zack M, Adami HO: Perinatal measles infection and subsequent Crohn's disease. Lancet 344:508–510, 1994
16. Sonnenberg A: Temporal trends and geographic variations of peptic ulcer disease. Aliment Pharmacol Ther 9(Suppl 2):3–12, 1995
17. Kurata JH: Epidemiology of peptic ulcer disease. In: Swabb EA, Szabo S (eds): Ulcer Disease: Investigation and Basis for Therapy. New York: Marcel Dekker, 1991, pp 31–53
18. Marshall BJ, McGechie DB, Francis GJ, Utley PJ: Pyloric campylobacter serology. Lancet 2:281, 1984
19. Tytgat GNJ, Rauws EAJ, de Koster E: *Campylobacter pylori*: diagnosis and treatment. J Clin Gastroenterol 11(Suppl 1):S49–S53, 1989
20. Yardley JH, Paull G: *Campylobacter pylori*: a newly recognized infectious agent in the gastrointestinal tract. Am J Surg Pathol 12 (Suppl 1):89–99, 1988
21. Blaser MJ: Gastric *Campylobacter*-like organisms, gastritis, and peptic ulcer disease. Gastroenterology 93:371–383, 1987
22. Slomiany BL, Bilski J, Sarosiek J, et al: *Campylobacter pyloridis* degrades mucin and undermines gastric mucosal integrity. Biochem Biophys Res Commun 144:307–314, 1987
23. Goodwin CS, Armstrong JA, Marshall BJ: *Campylobacter pyloridis*, gastritis, and peptic ulceration. J Clin Pathol 39:353–365, 1986
24. Marshall BJ, Armstrong JA, Mc Gechie DB, Glancy RJ: Attempt to fulfill Koch's postulates for pyloric *Campylobacter*. Med J Aust 142:436–439, 1985
25. Leoci C, Ierardi E, Chiloiro M, Piccioli E, Di Matteo G, Misciagna G, Giorgio I: Incidence and risk factors for duodenal ulcer. A retrospective cohort study. J Clin Gastroenterol 20:104–109, 1995
26. Rotter JI, Jones JQ, Samloff IM, et al: Duodenal-ulcer disease associated with elevated serum pepsinogen 1. An inherited autosomal dominant disorder. N Engl J Med 300:63–66, 1979
27. Taylor IL, Calan J, Rotter JI, et al: Family studies of hyper pepsinogenomic I duodenal ulcer. Ann Intern Med 95:421–425, 1981
28. Kikendall JW, Evaul J, Johnson LF: Effect of cigarette smoking on gastrointestinal physiology and non-neoplastic digestive disease. J Clin Gastroenterol 6:65–78, 1984
29. Kuipers EJ, Thijs JC, Festen HP: The prevalence of *Helicobacter pylori* in peptic ulcer disease. Aliment Pharmacol Ther 9(Suppl 2): 59–69, 1995
30. Coggon D, Lambert P, Langman MJS: Twenty years of hospital admissions for peptic ulcer in England and Wales. Lancet 1:1302, 1984
31. Sonnenberg A, Fritsch A: Changing mortality of peptic ulcer disease in Germany. Gastroenterology 84:1553–1557, 1983
32. Wyllie JH, Clark CG, Alexander-Williams J, et al: Effect of cimetidine on surgery for duodenal ulcer. Lancet 2:1307–1308, 1981
33. Grossman MI, Kurata JH, Rotter JI, et al: Peptic ulcer: new therapies, new diseases. Ann Intern Med 95:609–627, 1981
34. O'Connor PC, Griffiths K, Shanks RG: Trends in peptic ulcer related diseases from 1972 to 1980: hospital activity analysis data and general practice cimetidine prescribing levels. Eur J Clin Pharmacol 24:435–440, 1983
35. Fineberg HV, Pearlman L: Surgical treatment of peptic ulcer in the United States. Lancet 1:1305, 1981
36. Peterson WL, et al: Healing of duodenal ulcer with an antacid regimen. N Engl J Med 297:341–345, 1977
37. Langman MJS: Blood groups and alimentary disorders. Clin Gastroenterol 2:497–506, 1973
38. Coggin D, Langman MJS, Spiegelhalter D: Aspirin, acetominophen, and hematemesis and melena. Gut 23:340–344, 1982

39. Sonnenberg A: Dietary salt and gastric ulcer. Gut 27:1138–1142, 1986
40. Turnberg LA, Rees WD: Aspirin, ulcer and intestinal bleeding: what do the data show? Gastroenterology 83:726–727, 1982
41. Ranke C, Creutzig A, Luska G, Wagner HH, Galanski M, Bode-Boger S, Frolich J, Avenarius HJ, Hecker H, Alexander K: Dose-dependent side effects of acetylsalicylic acid therapy. Results of a prospective randomized clinical study in patients with peripheral arterial occlusive disease. Med Klin 88:571–567, 1993
42. Prasad S, Mathan M, Chandy G, Rajan DP, Venkateswaran S, Ramakrishna BS, Mathan VI: Prevalence of *Helicobacter pylori* in southern Indian controls and patients with gastroduodenal disease. J Gastroenterol Hepatol 9:501–506, 1994
43. Schubert TT, Bologna SD, Nensey Y, Schubert AB, Mascha EJ, Ma CK: Ulcer risk factors: interactions between *Helicobacter pylori* infection, nonsteroidal use, and age. Am J Med 94:413–418, 1993
44. Rauws EJ, Tytgat GN: *Helicobacter pylori* in duodenal and gastric ulcer disease. Baillieres Clin Gastroenterol 9:529–547, 1995
45. National Institutes of Health (NIH) Consensus Development Conference on *H. pylori*, Bethesda MD: 1994
46. The San Marino Study: *Helicobacter pylori* infection in a European country: relations with gastrointestinal diseases. Gut 36:838–844, 1995
47. Anand BS, Raed AK, Malaty HM, Genta RM, Klein PD, Evans DJ Jr, Graham DY: Low point prevalence of peptic ulcer in normal individuals with *Helicobacter pylori* infection. J Gastroenterol 91(6): 1112–1115, 1996
48. Friedman GS, Siegelaub AB, Seltzer CC: Cigarettes, alcohol, coffee, and peptic ulcer. N Engl J Med 290:469, 1974
49. Menzel M, Hogel J, Allmendinger G, Schmid E: Relative risks of age, gender, nationality, smoking, and *Helicobacter pylori* infection in duodenal and gastric ulcer and interactions. Z Gastroenterol 33:193–197, 1995
50. Leoci C, Ierardi E, Chiloiro M, Piccioli E, Di Matteo G, Misciagna G, Giorgio I: Incidence and risk factors of duodenal ulcer. A retrospective cohort study. J Clin Gastroenterol 20:104–109, 1995
51. Sontag S, Graham DY, Belsito A, et al: Cimetidine, cigarette smoking, and recurrence of duodenal ulcer. N Engl J Med 311:689–693, 1984
52. Isenberg JL: Peptic ulcer: epidemiology, nutritional aspects, drugs, smoking, alcohol, and diet. J Fam Pract 18:141–151, 1984
53. Borody TJ, George LL, Brandl S, Andrews P, Jankiewicz E, Ostapowicz N: Smoking does not contribute to duodenal ulcer relapse after *Helicobacter pylori* eradication. Am J Gastroenterol 87:1390–1393, 1992
54. Battaglia G, Di Mario F, Pasini M, Donisi PM, Dotto P, Benvenuti ME, Stracca-Pansa V, Pasquino M: *Helicobacter pylori* infection, cigarette smoking and alcohol consumption. A histological and clinical study on 286 subjects. Ital J Gastroenterol 25(8):419–424, 1993
55. Laine L, Marin-Sorensen M, Weinstein WM: Nonsteroidal antiinflammatory drug-associated gastric ulcers do not require *Helicobacter pylori* for their development. Am J Gastroenterol 87: 1398–1402, 1992
56. Somerville K, Faulkner G, Langman MJS: Non-steroidal anti-inflammatory drugs and bleeding peptic ulcer. Lancet 1:462–464, 1986
57. Taylor RT, Huskinson EC, Whitehouse GH, et al: Gastric ulceration occurring during indomethacin therapy. Br Med J 4:734–737, 1968
58. Doll R, Kellock TD: The separate inheritance of gastric and duodenal ulcers. Ann Eugen 16:231, 1951
59. Rotter JI, Rimoin DL: Peptic ulcer disease—a heterogenous group of disorders? Gastroenterology 73:604, 1977
60. Tsugane S, Tei Y, Takahashi T, Watanabe S, Sugano K: Salty food intake and risk of *Helicobacter pylori* infection. Jpn J Cancer Res 85:474–478, 1994
61. Samloff IM, Stemmermann GN, Heilbrun L, Nomura A: Elevated serum pepsinogen I and II levels differ as risk factors for duodenal and gastric ulcer. Gastroenterology 90:570–575, 1986
62. Paffenbarger RS, Wing AL, Hyde RT: Chronic disease in former college students. XIII. Early percursors of peptic ulcer. Am J Epidemiol 100:307–315, 1974
63. Sleisenger MD, Fordtran JS: Gastrointestinal disease; pathophysiology, diagnosis, treatment. 3rd ed. Philadelphia: WB Saunders, 1983, p 655
64. Stemmermann G, Haenszel W, Locke F: Epidemiological pathology of gastric ulcer and gastric carcinoma among Japanese in Hawaii. J Natl Cancer Inst 58:13–19, 1977
65. Sturdevant RAL: Epidemiology of peptic ulcer: report of a conference. Am J Epidemiol 104:9–14, 1976
66. Dunn JP, Cobb S: Frequency of peptic ulcer among executives, craftsmen, and foremen. J Occup Med 4:343–348, 1962
67. Cobb S, Rose RM: Hypertension, peptic ulcer and diabetes in air traffic controllers. JAMA 224:489–492, 1973
68. Grayson RR: Peptic ulcer in air traffic controllers. IMJ 142:111–152, 1972
69. Segawa K, Nakazawa S, Tsukamoto Y, et al: Peptic ulcer is prevalent among shift workers. Dig Dis Sci 32:449–453, 1987
70. Hinsdale JG, Engel JJ, Wilson DE: Prostaglandin E in peptic ulcer disease. Prostaglandins 6:495, 1974
71. Wright JP, Young GO, Klaff LJ, et al: Gastric mucosal prostaglandin E levels in patients with gastric ulcer disease and carcinoma. Gastroenterology 82:263–267, 1982
72. Sharon P, Cohen F, Zifroni A, et al: Prostanoid synthesis by cultured gastric and duodenal mucosa: possible role in the pathogenesis of duodenal ulcer. Scand J Gastroenterol 18:1045–1049, 1983
73. Hansson LE, Nyren O, Hsing AW, Bergstrom R, Josefsson S, Chow WH, Fraumeni JF Jr, Adami HO: The risk of stomach cancer in patients with gastric or duodenal ulcer disease. N Engl J Med 335: 242–249, 1996
74. Harrison AR, Elashoff JD, Grossman ML: Peptic ulcer disease. In: Smoking and Health: A Report by the Surgeon General. DHEW Publication No. (PHS) 79-50066, Washington, DC: U.S. Government Printing Office, 1979
75. Stemmermann GN, Marcus EB, Buist AS, MacLean CJ: Relative impact of smoking and reduced pulmonary function on peptic ulcer risk. Gastroenterology 96:1419–1424, 1989
76. Elashoff JD, Grossman MI: Trends in hospital admissions and death rates for peptic ulcer in the United States from 1970–78. Gastroenterology 78:280–285, 1980
77. Hammond EG: Smoking in relation to death rates of 1 million men and women. Monogr Natl Cancer Inst 13:127, 1966
78. Petitti DB, Friedman GD, Kahn W: Peptic ulcer disease and the tar and nicotine yield of currently smoked cigarettes. J Chron Dis 35:503–507, 1982
79. Korman MG, Shaw G, Hansky J, et al: Influence of smoking on healing rate of duodenal ulcer in response to cimetidine or high dose antacid. Gastroenterology 239:39–42, 1981
80. Hasan M, Sircus W: The factors determining success or failure of cimetidine treatment of peptic ulcer. J Clin Gastroenterol 3:225–229, 1981
81. Ippoliti A, Elashoff J, Valenzuela J: Recurrent ulcer after successful treatment with cimetidine or antacid. Gastroenterology 85:875–880, 1983
82. Sonnenberg A, Muller-Lissner S, Vogel E, et al: Predictors of duodenal ulcer healing and relapse. Gastroenterology 81:1061–1067, 1981
83. Murthy SNS, Dinoso UP, Clearfield HR, et al: Simultaneous measurement of basal pancreatic gastric acid secretion, plasma gastrin and secretin during smoking. Gastroenterology 73:758–761, 1977
84. Navis BH, Marks IN, Bank S, Sloan AW: The relation between gastric acid secretion and body habitus, blood groups, smoking, and the

subsequent development of dyspepsia and duodenal ulcer. Gut 14: 107–112, 1973
85. Sonnenberg A, Husmer N: Effect of nicotine on gastric musosal blood flow and acid secretion. Gut 23:532–535, 1982
86. Naitove A, Constantian MB, Arkins T: Gastric hemodynamic effects of smoking and nicotine. Gastroenterology 58:1058, 1970
87. Valenzuela JE, Defilippi C, Csendes A: Manometric studies on the human pyloric sphincter. Effect of cigarette smoking, metoclopramide and atropine. Gastroenterology 70:481–483, 1976
88. Levy M: Aspirin use in patients with major upper gastrointestinal bleeding and peptic-ulcer disease. N Engl J Med 290:1158–1162, 1981
89. Piper DW: The treatment of chronic peptic ulcer. Front Gastrointest Res 6:109, 1980
90. Lanza FL, Royer GL, Nelson RS: Endoscopic evaluation of the effects of aspirin, buffered aspirin, and enteric-coated aspirin on gastric and duodenal mucosa. N Engl J Med 303:136–137, 1980
91. Douthwaite HA, Lintott GAM: Gastroscopic observation of the effect of aspirin and certain other substances on the stomach. Lancet 2:1222–1225, 1938
92. Silvoso GR, Ivey KS, Butt JH: Incidence of gastric lesions in patients with rheumatic disease on chronic aspirin therapy. Ann Intern Med 91:517–520, 1979
93. Hennekens C, Buring J: Aspirin in primary prevention of cardiovascular disease. Cardiol Clin 12:443–450, 1994
94. Shorrock CJ, Langman MJ: Nonsteroidal anti-inflammatory drug-induced gastric damage: epidemiology. Digest Dis 13(Suppl 1):3–8, 1995
95. McIntosh JH, Fung CS, Berry G, Piper DW: Smoking, nonsteroidal anti-inflammatory drugs, and acetaminophen in gastric ulcer. Am J Epidemiol 128:761–770, 1988
96. Soll AH, Kurata J, McGuigan JE: Ulcers, nonsteroidal anti-inflammatory drugs, and related matters. Gastroenterology 96:561–568, 1989
97. Cohen S, Booth GH: Gastric acid secretion and lower esophageal sphincter pressure in response to coffee and caffeine. N Engl J Med 1975 293:897
98. Kurata JH, Elashoff JD, Grossman ML: Inadequacy of the literature on the relationship between drugs, ulcers, and gastrointestinal bleeding. Gastroenterology 82:373–382, 1982
99. Cooke AR: Ethanol and gastric function. Gastroenterology 62:501, 1972
100. Welsh J: Diet therapy and peptic ulcer disease. Gastroenterology 72:740, 1977
101. Spiro HM: Is milk all that bad for the ulcer patient? J Clin Gastroenterol 3:219, 1981
102. Tovey FI: Progress report: peptic ulcer in India and Bangladesh. Gut 20:329–347, 1979
103. Tovey FI, Tunstall M: Progress report: duodenal ulcer in black populations in Africa south of the Sahara. Gut 16:564–576, 1975
104. Conway TL, Ward HW, Vickers RR, Rahe RH: Occupational stress and variation in cigarette, coffee, and alcohol consumption. J Health Soc Behav 22:155–165, 1981
105. Cummings S: Stress, cigarettes, and ulcers. Gastroenterology 85: 1232, 1983
106. Adami HO, Bergstrom R, Nyren O, et al: Is duodenal ulcer really a psychosomatic disease? Scand J Gastroenterol 22:889–896, 1987
107. Sonnenberg A, Haas J: Joint effects of occupation and nationality on the prevalence of peptic ulcer in German workers. Br J Ind Med 43:490–493, 1986
108. Feldman M, Walker P, Green JL, Weingarden K: Life events, stress and psychosocial factors in men with peptic ulcer disease: a multidimensional case-control study. Gastroenterology 91:1370–1379, 1986
109. Walker P, Luther J, Samloff MI, Feldman M: Life events and stress and psychosocial factors in men with peptic ulcer disease. II. Relationships with serum pepsinogen concentrations and behavioral risk factors. Gastroenterology 94:323–330, 1988
110. Susser M, Stein Z: Civilization and peptic ulcer. Lancet 1:115–118, 1962
111. Segal I, Unterhalter B, Rosenbush H: Further observations on social factors associated with duodenal ulcer in Soweto. Soc Sci Med 23:417– 422, 1986
112. Ellis A, Woodrow JC: HLA and duodenal ulcer. Gut 20:760, 1979
113. Rotter JL, Rimoin DL, Gursky JM, et al: HLA-B5 associated with duodenal ulcer. Gastroenterology 73:438, 1977
114. Almy TP, Mendeloff AI, Rice D: Prevalence and significance of digestive diseases. Gastroenterology 68:1351–1371, 1975
115. Ivey KJ: Drugs, gastritis, and peptic ulcer. J Clin Gastroenterol 3(Suppl 2):29–34, 1981
116. Rotter JI: The genetics of gastritis and peptic ulcer. J Clin Gastroenterol 3(Suppl 2):35–43, 1981
117. Walsh JH, Peterson WL: The treatment of *Helicobacter pylori* infection in the management of peptic ulcer disease. N Engl J Med 333:984–991, 1995
118. Drug Information Service, University of California, San Diego Medical Center: *Helicobacter pylori* standard eradication protocol, 1997
119. Saegesser F, James D: Cancer of the gastric stump after partial gastrectomy (Billroth II principle) for ulcer. Cancer 29:1150–1159, 1972
120. Nicholls JC: Carcinoma of the stomach following partial gastrectomy for benign gastroduodenal lesions. Br J Surg 61:244–249, 1974
121. Tersmette AC, Goodman SN, Offerhaus GJ, et al: Multivariate analysis of the risk of stomach cancer after ulcer surgery in an Amsterdam cohort of postgastrectomy patients. Am J Epidemiol 134: 14–21, 1991
122. Greene FL: Neoplastic changes in the stomach after gastrectomy. Surg Gynecol Obstet 171:477–480, 1990
123. Sonnenberg A: Cost-benefit analysis of testing for *Helicobacter pylori* in dyspeptic subjects. Am J Gastroenterol 91:1773–1777, 1996
124. Quiros A, Quiros E, Gonzalez I, Bernal MC, Piedrola G, Maroto MC: *Helicobacter pylori* seroepidemiology in risk groups. Eur J Epidemiol 10:299–301, 1994
125. Vaira D, Miglioli M, Mule P, Holton J, Menegatti M, Vergura M, Biasco G, Conte R, Logan RP, Barbara L: Prevalence of peptic ulcer in *Helicobacter pylori* positive blood donors. Gut 35:309–312, 1994
126. Sipponen P: *Helicobacter pylori*: a cohort phenomenon. Am J Surg Pathol 19(Suppl 1):S30–36, 1995
127. Banatvala N, Feldman R: The epidemiology of *Helicobacter pylori*: missing pieces in a jigsaw. Commun Dis Rep CDR Rev 3(4):R56–59, March 26, 1993
128. Zhao L, Blot WJ, Liu WD, Chang YS, Zhang JS, Hu YR, You WC, Xu GW, Fraumeni JF Jr: Familial predisposition to precancerous gastric lesions in a high-risk area of China. Cancer Epidemiol Biomarkers Prev 3:461–464, 1994
129. Hirai M, Azuma T, Ito S, Kato T, Kohli Y, Fujiki N: High prevalence of neutralizing activity to *Helicobacter pylori* cytotoxin in serum of gastric-carcinoma patients. Int J Cancer 56:56–60, 1994
130. Haubrich T, Boeing H, Gores W, Hengels KJ, Scheuermann W, Wahrendorf: Prevalence of *Helicobacter pylori* and gastritis in southern Germany: results of a representative cross-sectional study. Z Gastroenterol 31:432–436, 1993
131. Lee A, Buck F: Vaccination and mucosal responses to *Helicobacter pylori* infection. Aliment Pharmacol Ther 10(Suppl 1):129–138, 1996
132. Sellman S, Blanchard TG, Nedrud JG, Czinn SJ: Vaccine strategies for prevention of *Helicobacter pylori* infection. Eur J Gastroenterol Hepatol 7(Suppl 1):S1–6, 1995
133. Fennerty MB: Polio and small pox: diseases of historical interest because of vaccines. Will this also apply to *Helicobacter pylori*? Am J Gastroenterol 91:170–171, 1996

134. Calkins B, Mendeloff AI: Epidemiology of inflammatory bowel disease. Epidemiol Rev 8:60–91, 1986
135. Mayberry JF: Recent epidemiology of ulcerative colitis and Crohn's disease. Int J Colorectal Dis 4:59–66, 1989
136. Binder V: Epidemiology, course and socio-economic influence of inflammatory bowel disease. Schweiz Med Wochenschr 118:738–742, 1988
137. Sonnenberg A: Geographic variation in the incidence of and mortality from inflammatory bowel disease. Dis Colon Rectum 29: 854–861, 1986
138. Mendeloff AI, Calkins B, Lilienfeld AM, Garland CF, Monk M: Inflammatory bowel disease in Baltimore, 1960–79: hospital incidence rates, bimodality, and smoking factors. Front Gastrointest Res 11:88–93, 1986
139. Hellers G: Ulcerative colitis: epidemiology. Top Gastroenterol 12: 129–139, 1985
140. Zuckerman MJ, Briones DF: Inflammatory bowel disease: overview and psychosomatics. Tex Med 85:32–36, 1989
141. Koutroubakis I, Manousos ON, Meuwissen SG, Pena AS: Environmental risk factors in inflammatory bowel disease. Hepatogastroenterology 43:381–393, 1996
142. Myren J, Bouchier AD, Watkinson G, et al: The Organization Mondiale de Gastroenterologie (OMGE) multinational inflammatory bowel disease survey 1976–1982. Scand J Gastroenterol 19(Suppl 95):1–27, 1984
143. Brostrom O: Ulcerative colitis in Stockholm County—a study of epidemiology, prognosis, mortality, and cancer risk with social reference to a surveillance program. Acta Chir Scand Suppl 534, 1986
144. Rotegard J, Ahsgren L, Janunger K-G: Ulcerative colitis: mortality and surgery in an unselected population. Acta Chir Scand 154:216–220, 1988
145. Isbell G, Levin B: Ulcerative colitis and colon cancer. Gastroenterol Clin North Am 17:773–791, 1988
146. Devlin HB, Datta D, Dellipiani AW: The incidence and prevalence of inflammatory bowel disease in North Tees Health District. World J Surg 4:183–193, 1980
147. Haug K, Schrumpf E, Barstad S, Fluge G, Halvorsen JF, and the Study Group of Inflammatory Bowel Disease in Western Norway: Epidemiology of ulcerative colitis in Western Norway. Scand J Gastroenterol 23:517–522, 1988
148. Moum B, Vatn MH, Ekbom A, Aadland E, Fausa O, Lygren I, Sauar J, Schulz T, Stray N: Incidence of ulcerative colitis and indeterminate colitis in four counties of southeastern Norway, 1990–93. A prospective population-based study. Scand J Gastroenterol 31:362–366, 1996
149. Stonnington CM, Phillips SF, Melton LJ, Zinsmeister AR: Chronic ulcerative colitis: incidence and prevalence in a community (Rochester MN). Gut 28:402–409, 1987
150. Stewenius J, Adnerhill I, Ekelund G, Floren CH, Fork FT, Janzon L, Lindstrom C, Mars I, Nyman M, Rosengren JE: Ulcerative colitis and indeterminate colitis in the city of Malmo, Sweden. A 25-year incidence study. Scand J Gastroenterol 30:38–43, 1995
151. Sinclair TS, Brunt PW, Mowat NA: Nonspecific proctocolitis in Northeastern Scotland: a community study. Gastroenterology 85: 1– 11, 1983
152. Berner J, Kiaer T: Ulcerative colitis and Crohn's disease on the Faroe islands 1964–83: a retrospective epidemiological survey. Scand J Gastroenterol 21:188–192, 1986
153. Bjørnsson S, Thorgeirsson T: Colitis ulcerosa i Island (Iceland): epidemiologisk undersokning 1950–1979. Nord Med 98:298–301, 1983
154. Binder JH, Cocco A, Crossley RJ, et al: Cimetidine in the treatment of duodenal ulcer. A multicenter double blind study. Gastroenterology 74:380–388, 1978
155. Srivastava ED, Mayberry JF, Morris TJ, Smith PM, Williams GT, Roberts GM, Newcombe RG, Rhodes J: Incidence of ulcerative colitis in Cardiff over 20 years: 1968–87. Gut 33:256–258, 1992
156. Hiatt RA, Kaufman L: Epidemiology of inflammatory bowel disease in a defined northern California population. West J Med 149: 541–546, 1988
157. Eason RJ, Lee SP, Tasman-Jones C: Inflammatory bowel disease in Auckland, New Zealand. Aust N Z J Med 12:125–131, 1982
158. Brandes JW, Lorenz-Meyer H: Epidemiologische Aspekte zur Enterocolitis regionalis Crohn und Colitis ulcerosa in Marburg Lohn (FRG) Zwischen 1962 und 1975. Z Gastroenterol 21:69–78, 1983
159. Tragnone A, Hanau C, Bazzocchi G, Lanfranchi GA: Epidemiological characteristics of inflammatory bowel disease in Bologna, Italy—incidence and risk factors. Digestion 54:183–188, 1993
160. Tsianos EV, Masalas CN, Merkouropoulos M, Dalekos GN, Logan RF: Incidence of inflammatory bowel disease in north west Greece: rarity of Crohn's disease in an area where ulcerative colitis is common. Gut 35:369–372, 1994
161. Nordenvall B, Brostrom O, Berglund M, et al: Incidence of ulcerative colitis in Stockholm county, 1955–1979. Scand J Gastroenterol 20:783–790, 1985
162. Shivananda S, Pena AS, Mayberry F, et al: Epidemiology of proctocolitis in the Region of Leiden, the Netherlands: a population study from 1979 to 1983. Scand J Gastroenterol 22:993–1002, 1987
163. Monk M, Mendeloff AL, Siegel CL, et al: An epidemiological study of ulcerative colitis and regional enteritis among adults in Baltimore. 1. Hospital incidence and prevalence. Gastroenterology 53:198–210, 1967
164. Latour P, Belaiche J, Louis E, et al: Incidence of inflammatory bowel disease in the province of Liege (Belgium). Acta Gastroenterol Belg 59:3–6, 1996
165. Gower-Rousseau C, Salomez JL, Dupas JL, Marti R, Nuttens MC, Votte A, Lemahieu M, Lemaire B, Colombel JF, Cortot A: Incidence of inflammatory bowel disease in northern France (1988–1990). Gut 35:1433–1438, 1994
166. Dirks E, Forster S, Goebell H: Incidence and prevalence of chronic inflammatory bowel disease in a prospective study from an industrial area in West Germany. Dig Dis Sci 31(Suppl 83):323, 1986
167. Mate-Jimenez J, Munoz S, Vicent D, Pajares JM: Incidence and prevalence of ulcerative colitis and Crohn's disease in urban and rural areas of Spain from 1981 to 1988. J Clin Gastroenterol 18:27–31, 1994
168. LaFranchi GA, Michelini A, Brignola C, Campieri M, Cortini C, Marzio L: Uno studio epidemiologico sulle malatie inflammatorie intestinale nella provincia di Bologna. Clin Med 57:235–245, 1976
169. Morita N, Toki S, Hirohashi T, Minoda T, Ogawa K, Kono S, Tamakoshi A, Ohno Y, Sawada T, Muto T: Incidence and prevalence of inflammatory bowel disease in Japan: nationwide epidemiological survey during the year 1991. J Gastroenterol 30(Suppl 8):1–4, 1995
170. Al-Nakib B, Radhakrishnan S, Jacob GS, Al-Liddawi H, Al Ruwaih A: Inflammatory bowel disease in Kuwait. Am J Gastroenterol 79:191–194, 1984
171. Garland CF, Garland FC: Do sunlight and vitamin D reduce the risk of colon cancer. Int J Epidemiol 9:227–231, 1980
172. Mendeloff AI, Monk M, Siegel CI, Lilienfeld AM: Some epidemiological features of ulcerative colitis and regional enteritis. Gastroenterology 51:748–752, 1966
173. Wright JP, Froggatt J, O'Keefe EA, et al: The epidemiology of inflammatory bowel disease in Cape Town 1980–1984. S Afr Med J 70:10–15, 1986
174. Jacobsohn WZ, Levine Y: Incidence and prevalence of ulcerative colitis in the Jewish population of Jerusalem. Isr J Med Sci 22:559–563, 1986
175. Odes HS, Fraser D, Krawiec J: Incidence of idiopathic ulcerative colitis in Jewish population subgroups in the Beer Sheva region of Israel. Am J Gastroenterol 82:854–858, 1987
176. Sedlack RE, Nobrega FR, Kurland LT, et al: Inflammatory colon disease in Rochester, Minnesota, 1935–1964. Gastroenterology 62:935–941, 1972

177. Nedbal J, Maratka Z: Ulcerative proctocolitis in Czechoslovakia. Am J Proctol 19:106–114, 1968
178. Ishikawa M, Watanabe H, Yamagishi G, et al: Crohn's disease, nonspecific ulcers of the small intestine, and idiopathic proctocolitis in a Japanese university hospital from 1954 to 1974. Tohoku J Exp Med 118:97–109, 1976
179. Roth MP, Petersen GM, McElree C, et al: Geographic origins of Jewish patients with inflammatory bowel disease. Gastroenterology 7:900–904, 1989
180. Myren J, Gjone E, Hertzberg JN, et al: Epidemiology of ulcerative colitis and regional enterocolitis (Crohn's disease) in Norway. Scand J Gastroenterol 6:511–514, 1971
181. Myszor M, Calam J: Seasonality of ulcerative colitis [Letter]. Lancet 2:522–523, 1984
182. Heatley RV, Thomas P, Prokipchuk EJ, Gauldie J, Sieniewicz DJ, Bienstock J: Pulmonary function abnormalities in patients with inflammatory bowel disease. Q J Med 203:241–250, 1982
183. Harries AD, Baird A, Rhodes J: Non-smoking: a feature of ulcerative colitis. Br Med J 284:706, 1982
184. Calkins B: A meta-analysis of the role of smoking in inflammatory bowel disease. Digest Dis Sci 34:1841–1854, 1989
185. Tobin MV, Logan RFA, Langman MJS, McConnell RB, Gilmore IT: Smoking and inflammatory bowel disease [Abstract]. Gut 26:A1155, 1985
186. Cope GF, Heatley RV, Kelleher J, Lee PN: Cigarette smoking and inflammatory bowel disease: a review. Hum Toxicol 6:189–193, 1987
187. Logan RFA, Edmond M, Somerville KW, Langman MJS: Smoking and ulcerative colitis. Br Med J 288:751–753, 1984
188. Vessey M, Jewell D, Smith A, Yeates D, McPherson K: Chronic inflammatory bowel disease, cigarette smoking, and use of oral contraceptives: findings of a large cohort study of women of child bearing age. Br Med J 292:1101–1103, 1986
189. Franceschi S, Panza E, La Vecchia C, Parazzini F, DeCarli A, Porro GB: Nonspecific inflammatory bowel disease and smoking. Am J Epidemiol 125:445–452, 1987
190. Boyko EJ, Koepsell TD, Perera DR, Inui TS: Risk of ulcerative colitis among former and current cigarette smokers. N Engl J Med 316:707–710, 1987
191. Benoni C, Nilsson A: Smoking habits in patients with inflammatory bowel disease. Scand J Gastroenterol 22:1130–1136, 1987
192. Borgeat P, Samuelsson B: Metabolism of arachidonic acid in polymorphonuclear leukocytes. J Biol Chem 254:7865–7869, 1979
193. Craxi A, Olive L, Distefano G: Ulcerative colitis in a married couple. Ital J Gastroenterol 11:184–186, 1979
194. Farmer RG, Michever WM, Mortimer EA: Studies of family history among patients with inflammatory bowel disease. Clin Gastroenterol 9:271–278, 1980
195. McConnell RB: Inflammatory bowel disease: newer views of genetic influences. In Berk JE (ed): Developments in Digestive Diseases. Philadelphia: Lea & Febiger, 1980, vol 3, pp 129–137
196. Miller DS, Keighley A, Smith PG, et al: Crohn's disease in Nottingham: a search for time and space clustering. Gut 16:454–457, 1975
197. Miller DS, Keighley A, Smith PG, et al: A case-control method for seeking evidence of contagion in Crohn's disease. Gastroenterology 71:385–387, 1976
198. Korsmeyer SJ, Williams RC, Wilson ID, et al: Lymphocytotoxic antibody in inflammatory bowel disease. N Engl J Med 293:1117–1120, 1975
199. Graham DY, Markesich DC, Yoshimura HH: Mycobacteria and inflammatory bowel disease. Gastroenterology 92:436–442, 1987
200. Gilat T, Hacohen D, Lilos P, Langman MJS: Childhood factors in ulcerative colitis and Crohn's disease: an international cooperative study. Scand J Gastroenterol 22:1009–1024, 1987
201. Tysk C, Lindberg E, Jarnerot G, Floderus-Myrhed B: Ulcerative colitis and Crohn's disease in an unselected population of monozygotic and dizygotic twins: a study of heritability and the influence of smoking. Gut 29:990–996, 1988
202. Singer HC, Anderson JGO, Fischer H, et al: Familial aspects of inflammatory bowel disease. Gastroenterology 61:423–430, 1971
203. Penny WJ, Penny E, Mayberry JF, Rhodes J: Prevalence of inflammatory bowel disease amongst Mormons in Britain and Ireland. Soc Sci Med 21:287–290, 1985
204. West DW, Lyon JL, Gardner JW: Cancer risk factors: an analysis of Utah Mormons and non-Mormons. J Natl Cancer Inst 65:1083–1095, 1980
205. Helzer JE, Stillings WA, Chammas S, et al: A controlled study of the association between ulcerative colitis and psychiatric diagnoses. Dig Dis Sci 27:513–518, 1982
206. Calkins B, Mendeloff AL, Garland C: Inflammatory bowel disease in oral contraceptive users. Gastroenterology 91:523–524, 1986
207. Logan RFA, Kay CR, Scott L: The pill, smoking, and inflammatory bowel disease—results from the Royal College of General Practitioners (RCGP) oral contraception study. Gut 27:A127, 1986
208. Bernardino ME, Lawson TL: Discrete colonic ulcers associated with oral contraceptives. Dig Dis Sci 21:503–506, 1976
209. Wigley RD, MacLaurin BP: A study of ulcerative colitis in New Zealand showing a low incidence in Maoris. Br Med J 3:228–231, 1962
210. Boyko EJ, Perera DR, Koepsell TD, et al: Coffee and alcohol use and the risk of ulcerative colitis. Am J Gastroenterol 84:530–534, 1989
211. Nunes GC, Ahlquist RE: Increasing incidence of Crohn's disease. Am J Surg 145:578–581, 1983
212. Lee FL, Costello FT: Crohn's disease in Blackpool—incidence and prevalence, 1968–80. Gut 26:274–278, 1985
213. Munkholm P, Langholz E, Nielsen OH, Kreiner S, Binder V: Increased incidence of Crohn disease in the county of Copenhagen. Ugeskr Laeger 155:3199–3202, 1993
214. Gollop JH, Phillips SF, Melton CJ, et al: Epidemiologic aspects of Crohn's disease: a population-based study in Olmsted County, Minnesota, 1943–1982. Gut 29:49–56, 1988
215. Shapira M, Tamir A: Crohn's disease in the Kinneret sub-district, Israel, 1960–1990. Incidence and prevalence in different ethnic subgroups. Eur J Epidemiol 10:231–233, 1994
216. Krawiec J, Odes HS, Lasry Y, et al: Aspects of the epidemiology of Crohn's disease in the Jewish population in Beer Sheva, Israel. Isr J Med Sci 20:16–21, 1984
217. Kimura A, Sasagawa T: Incidence of Crohn's disease in Japan. In Shiratori T, Nakano H (eds): Japan Medical Research Foundation Publication 22: Inflammatory Bowel Disease. Tokyo: University of Tokyo Press, 1984, pp 191–200
218. Calkins B, Lilienfeld A, Mendeloff A, Garland C: Smoking factors in ulcerative colitis and Crohn's disease [Letter]. Am J Epidemiol 120:498, 1984
219. Acheson ED: The distribution of ulcerative colitis and regional enteritis in United States veterans with particular reference to the Jewish religion. Gut I:91–93, 1960
220. Thompson NP, Montgomery SM, Pounder RE, Wakefield AJ: Is measles vaccination a risk factor for inflammatory bowel disease? Lancet 1995;345:1071–1074
221. Thompson NP, Montgomery SM, Begg N, Pounder RE, Wakefield AJ: Measles vaccination: a risk factor for inflammatory bowel disease? Gastroenterology 108:A928, 1995
222. Belluzzi A, Brignola C, Campieri M, Pera A, Boschi S, Miglioli M: Effect of enteric-coated fish-oil preparation on relapses in Crohn's disease. N Engl J Med 334:1557–1560, 1996
223. Silvennoinen J: Relationships between vitamin D, parathyroid hormone, and bone mineral density in inflammatory bowel disease. J Int Med 239:131–137, 1996

57

Musculoskeletal Disorders

Jennifer L. Kelsey

Musculoskeletal disorders are common, affect all age groups, and are associated with a great deal of disability, impairment, and handicap. About 12 million people in the United States have their activity limited by musculoskeletal disorders, a figure greater than for any other disease category (Fig. 57-1).[1] Musculoskeletal impairments affect about 12 percent of the population, with the spine most commonly involved, followed by the lower extremity or hip and the upper extremity or shoulder (Table 57-1).[2] Each year about 14 percent of the population in the United States experience a musculoskeletal injury, including fractures, dislocations, sprains, and strains, severe enough that medical care is sought or activity is restricted for at least one-half a day.[2] The estimated total economic cost to the United States of musculoskeletal conditions was estimated to be over $126 billion in 1988,[2] second only to diseases of the circulatory system. Indirect costs from lost earnings and services represent a particularly high proportion of this cost, since many people are affected during their most productive years.

▸ DISORDERS PRIMARILY OF ADULTS

Low Back and Neck Pain

From 60 to 80 percent of the population experience low back pain at some time during their lives.[3] Most episodes of low back pain are not seriously incapacitating. Among people seeking care from family physicians for low back pain, almost 50 percent improve in a week, and close to 90 percent are better within a month, regardless of treatment.[4] The small proportion of cases that become chronic account for a high proportion of the cost; one study found that 25 percent of the cases accounted for 90 percent of the costs.[5]

The specific lesion responsible for low back pain usually is not known.[6] It is likely that the different conditions composing the category "low back pain" (e.g., sprains and strains, disc herniations, spondylosis and spondylolisthesis, facet abnormalities) have in part different etiologies. However, until these specific conditions are identified and differentiated in epidemiologic investigations, the category "low back pain" as a whole must generally be considered.

Low back pain is more common in people who do heavy manual work than in those whose work is sedentary. Jobs that involve heavy lifting (e.g., of objects weighing 25 pounds or more) are associated with an increase in risk for back pain, but there is little evidence of increased risk in most people when objects lighter than this are lifted. Factors that appear to increase the risk for both herniated disc and low back pain also include frequent lifting of heavy objects while bending and twisting the body, holding heavy objects away from the body while lifting, and failing to bend the knees while lifting.[3,6–9] Several studies have found an association between cigarette smoking and low back pain and between smoking and herniated disc, probably because of the pressure exerted by frequent coughing or the decreased diffusion of nutrients into the intervertebral disc, both of which are associated with smoking.[3,6,9] Prolonged sitting in one position is also thought to increase the risk, but evidence is conflicting.[3,6] Finally, motor vehicle driving and exposure to other forms of whole body vibration are detrimental to the spine.[3,6,9–11] Some evidence suggests that tallness is a risk factor for low back pain, that heavy body weight has little or no effect, and that a narrow spinal canal increases the risk, at least for lumbar disc herniation.[12] Although psychological factors are often said to play a role in the etiology of back pain, there is little firm evidence to support or refute this belief. However, one cohort study[12] did find a 2-fold increase in risk of subsequent disc herniation among people experiencing psychologically stressful symptoms.

The percentage of the population having neck pain has been found to be 40 to 80 percent, which is somewhat lower than those having low back pain. However, the number of neck pain cases appears to be increasing. This increase is thought to be attributable to the lower percentage of the workforce participating in heavy manual work and the greater number of people sitting for long periods in front of video display terminals. Neck pain is also related to a variety of different lesions. Little is known of risk factors. Prolonged exposure to awkward postures appears to be associated with mild neck pain, and some evidence indicates that heavy lifting, cigarette smoking, frequent aquatic diving from a board, motor vehicle driving, and exposure to other sources of whole body vibration increase the risk for prolapsed cervical intervertebral disc.[13]

One useful approach to the prevention of low back pain is modification of factors in the workplace.[3,5] First, there can be selection of workers for jobs involving heavy manual work. Although low back x-rays and medical examinations have not proved useful as routine screening tests for selection of workers, selection on the basis of strength testing for specific jobs appears to reduce the likelihood of back injury. Training workers to bend the knees while lifting does not seem to have reduced the number of back injuries, partly because of poor compliance. Other lifting methods that workers may find more acceptable are keeping objects close to the body and lifting slowly, smoothly, and without twisting. Redesigning jobs to minimize bending and twisting motions and to reduce the amount of weight lifted can decrease the number of back injuries and also may allow an injured worker to return to work sooner.

Other methods of primary prevention are improved physical fitness, cessation of smoking, moving around from time to time in situations requiring prolonged exposure to one position, vibration dampening, and use of motor vehicles with good seat positioning and lumbar support.

As mentioned above, most back pain resolves without any specific therapy. Predictors of disability from low back pain include long duration of the pain, a history of past disability and hospitalizations, low educational level, psychosocial factors, heavy physical demands on the job, dissatisfaction with the job, whether insurance payments are being received, the perception of fault, and whether a lawyer has

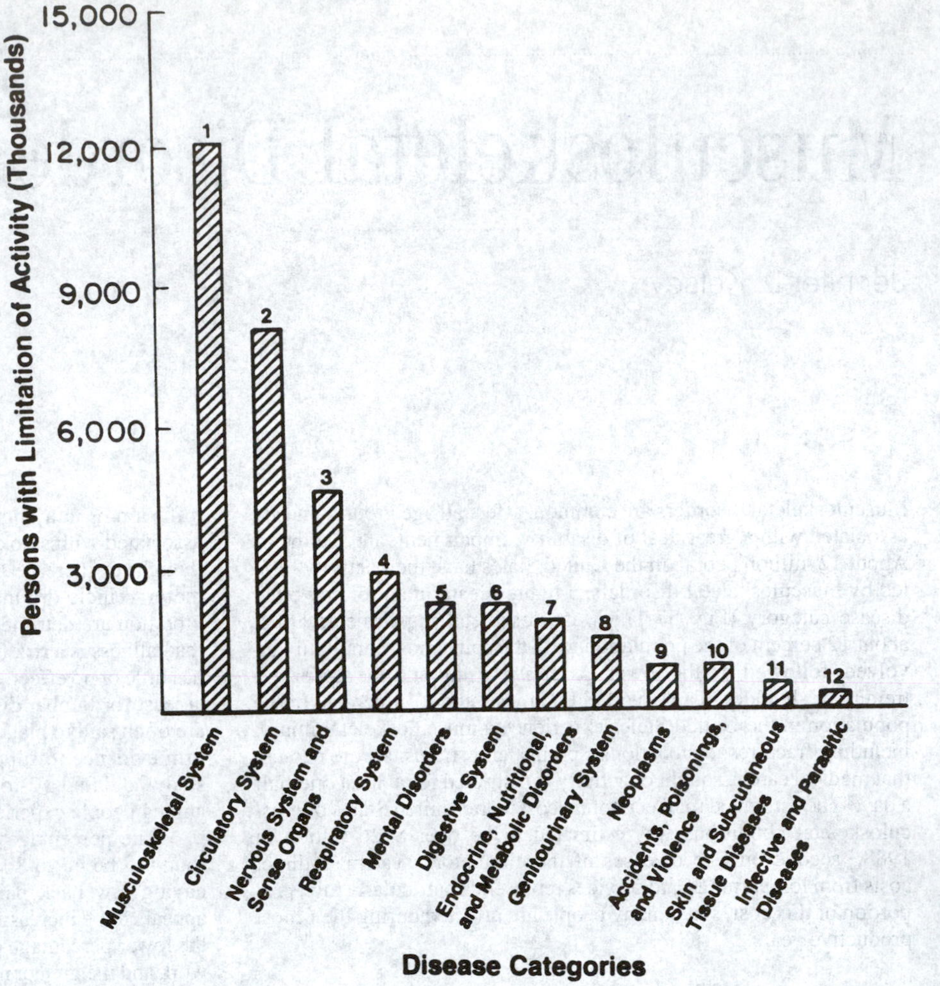

Figure 57-1. Estimated number of persons in the United States in 1984 with limitation of activity attributable to specific disease categories. (From Holbrook TL, Grazier K, Kelsey JL, Stauffer RN: The Frequency, Occurrence, Impact, and Cost of Musculoskeletal Conditions in the United States. Chicago: American Academy of Orthopaedic Surgeons, 1985.)

been retained.[3,10,14,15] Because surgical treatment is often unsatisfactory, conservative approaches such as physical therapy and back schools frequently are used for tertiary prevention. The primary aims of back schools are to decrease pain and illness behavior while increasing function through self-involvement and self-reliance.[16,17] Although schools have different emphases, most (*a*) teach patients enough about spinal mechanics so that they can use their backs effectively and avoid pain and damage, (*b*) try to effect attitude changes through psychological approaches, and (*c*) offer exercise and physical fitness programs. There have been no definitive evaluations of the efficacy of back schools, but available evidence suggests that they are effective for patients with back pain of recent onset but not for those whose pain is chronic.[18] Also important in tertiary prevention for many people with acute low back pain is a continuation of normal activities to the extent tolerated[19] and a prompt return to work, most commonly after a short period of rest.[15,20] On first returning to work after having had an episode of low back pain, the worker should avoid lifting heavy objects, bending, twisting, sitting in a low chair, and remaining in the same position for long periods of time. Individuals should also be advised to stand close to their work and use a lumbar support and armrests while sitting.

Osteoporosis

The reduction of bone mass in osteoporosis causes the bones to be susceptible to fracture. Fractures of the hip, vertebrae, and distal radius are particularly common. Although osteoporosis may occur secondarily to such conditions as hormonal defects, connective tissue disorders, or certain drug therapies, most cases are idiopathic. Heredity is an important determinant of bone mass when it is at its peak in early adulthood, but the role of genetics on rates of bone loss with aging or after menopause is less clear.[21]

American blacks have higher bone mass than non-Hispanic whites, Hispanic whites, and Asian Americans.[22] After about age 40 to 50, bone mass is lost in both men and women of all racial and ethnic groups, but a particularly rapid decrease occurs in women in the years following menopause. It has been estimated that a white woman of age 50 has a 17 percent chance of fracturing a hip, a 16 percent chance of fracturing a distal forearm, and a 16 percent chance of having a clinically diagnosed vertebral fracture during the remainder of her lifetime.[23] Hip fracture incidence rates are higher in non-Hispanic

TABLE 57-1. PREVALENCE OF MUSCULOSKELETAL IMPAIRMENTS IN THE UNITED STATES IN 1988

Type of Impairment	*Estimated No. of Affected Individuals*	*% of Population*
All musculoskeletal impairments	29,866,000	12.4
Back or spine	15,431,000	6.4
Lower extremity or hip	11,126,000	4.6
Upper extremity or shoulder	3,309,000	1.4

Modified from Praemer A, Furner S, Rice DP: Musculoskeletal Conditions in the United States. Park Ridge, IL: American Academy of Orthopaedic Surgeons, 1992.

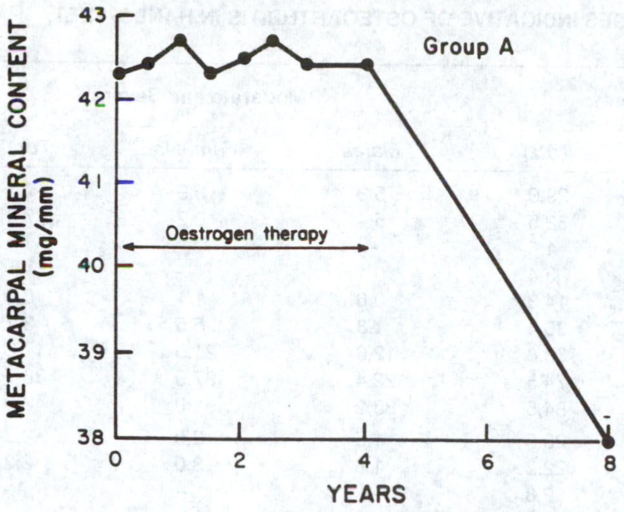

Figure 57-2. Effects of estrogen on bone mineral content of metacarpal and of withdrawal of estrogen after 4 years of active treatment. (From Lindsay R, Hart DM, MacLean A, Clark AC, Kraszewski A, Garwood J: Bone response to termination of estrogen treatment. Lancet 1:1325–1327, 1978.)

white women than in Hispanic white and Asian women, with black women having the lowest rates.

The relatively rapid rate of bone loss in middle-aged and older women has been related to a decrease in estrogen production. Women who have had an oophorectomy have earlier loss of bone mass than other women. Figure 57-2 shows that estrogen-replacement therapy protects against bone loss for as long as it is being administered. However, loss of bone mass continues when estrogen use ceases.[24] Replacement estrogen also protects against osteoporotic fractures, but available data suggest that recent use is needed for this protection.[25] On the average, the lower the endogenous estrogen concentration around the time of menopause, the higher the rate of bone loss.[25] Thin women are at higher risk than obese women, partly because of their lower estrogen production, their lower concentration of circulating estrogens, and the decreased mechanical stress on their bones. Also, fat padding around the hip gives some protection during a fall. Long hip-axis length (distance from the greater trochanter to the inner pelvic rim) is associated with an increased risk for hip fracture independent of bone mass.[26]

Some studies have shown an association between low levels of dietary calcium and osteoporosis, and calcium supplementation in the adult years appears to afford some protection against loss of cortical bone.[27,28] Some evidence suggests that the amount of dietary calcium consumed during childhood and the teen years and during old age may be especially important.[27,29] Adequate vitamin D intake also may be protective, but available data are contradictory. It is known that prolonged immobilization may result in osteoporosis, while the effect of moderate physical activity among healthy adults is uncertain, and probably is at most only slightly protective.[30] Again, adequate physical exercise during childhood and adolescence may be critical. Cigarette smoking increases the risk for osteoporosis, probably through a lowering of estrogen levels.[31] Heavy alcohol consumption also may increase the risk for osteoporosis and related fractures, but data are inconsistent.[31] Use of thiazide diuretics is associated with increased bone mass and decreased risk of hip fracture.[25]

Primary prevention includes measures that will promote adequate bone mass at an early age, such as a diet adequate in calcium, sufficient physical activity, and not smoking. Once the osteoporotic process has begun, administration of estrogens (with or without progestin) will limit further loss of bone mass, but the other benefits and risks of hormone replacement therapy need to be considered as well. New bisphosphonate agents are also useful in decreasing loss of bone mass.[32] However, these agents have to be taken in a rather strict manner to avoid unpleasant gastrointestinal side effects, and are generally used in people who have already lost a substantial amount of bone. Although the effect of supplemental calcium is not nearly as strong as that of estrogen, it is believed to have no long-term detrimental effects among persons with no specific contraindications (e.g., kidney stones). Moderate physical activity, such as brisk walking, is often recommended for older people to reduce bone loss, but there is little firm evidence to support this recommendation.

In recent years, screening women in the perimenopausal and immediate postmenopausal period for high fracture risk by measuring their bone mass, most commonly by dual energy x-ray absorptiometry or single photon absorptiometry, has been undertaken with increasing frequency. However, many questions remain about the appropriateness of screening, such as who should be screened, whether multiple measurements over time are needed, what other information on risk should be obtained along with the measure of bone mass, and what therapy should be recommended for those with various degrees of low bone mass.[33] Ultrasonography, which is usually applied to the heel bone, and which may provide information about the architecture and elasticity of bone as well as about bone mineral density, has been found to predict hip fracture.[34] Since ultrasound is less expensive, faster, and radiation-free compared with other methods commonly used to measure bone density, it may be increasingly used as a screening tool over the next several years.

Reducing the likelihood of falls among those with osteoporosis may be an important way to prevent fractures. Possible preventive measures include balance and gait training, muscle strengthening exercises, training in transfer skills, correction of visual and hearing problems, avoidance of long-acting sedative or centrally acting medications, and home safety improvements.[35,36] A randomized trial in a nursing home population has shown that wearing protective hip pads substantially reduces the risk for hip fracture,[37] although compliance may be a problem.

Arthritis

Osteoarthritis

Osteoarthritis, also known as degenerative joint disease, is characterized by degeneration of articular cartilage with proliferation and remodeling of subchondral bone. The usual clinical manifestations include pain and stiffness, accompanied by loss of function.[38] The diagnosis of osteoarthritis in most population surveys has been made using radiographic criteria as defined in the Atlas of Standard Radiographs of Arthritis.[39] These criteria are based on typical radiographic changes, including osteophytes, bony spurs, joint space narrowing, subchondral cysts, and bony remodeling. A new scale has been developed for grading osteoarthritis of the hands; this scale has been tested for reliability and validity in a sample of participants in the Baltimore Longitudinal Study on Aging.[40,41] Recently, high-frequency ultrasound has been found to provide highly accurate and reproducible measurement of the thickness and subsurface characteristics of articular cartilage.[42]

Osteoarthritis may be classified as either primary/idiopathic or secondary.[43] Subsets of the idiopathic condition include localized involvement of single joint groups as well as the syndrome of generalized osteoarthritis. Generalized osteoarthritis is characterized by involvement of three or more joint groups and typically affects perimenopausal and postmenopausal women.[44] Secondary osteoarthritis develops after the occurrence of an identifiable traumatic, congenital, developmental, or systemic disorder that has previously involved the joints.[45]

Approximately 30 percent of adults between the ages of 18 to 79 years have radiographic evidence of some degree of osteoarthritis in their hands (Table 57-2); 24 percent of the affected cases are classified as moderate or severe (grade III or IV).[46,47] About 4 percent of adults age 25 to 74 have osteoarthritis of the knee, and 1 percent of adult males have osteoarthritis of the hip.[46,48] Many people with

TABLE 57-2. PERCENT PREVALENCE PER 100 OF RADIOLOGIC CHANGES INDICATIVE OF OSTEOARTHRITIS IN HANDS, FEET, KNEES, AND HIPS, BY AGE AND SEX

		Mild, Moderate, and Severe			Moderate and Severe		
Part of Body	***Ages (yr)***	***Males***	***Females***	***Total***	***Males***	***Females***	***Total***
Hands[a]	18–79	29.4	30.4	29.9	5.3	9.9	7.1
	25–74	32.0	33.0	32.5	5.4	0.2	7.9
	18–24	2.8	0.4	1.6	—	—	—
	25–34	4.8	2.1	3.4	0.1	—	—
	35–44	17.5	11.3	14.3	0.6	1.1	0.9
	45–54	39.0	34.0	36.4	1.8	5.5	3.7
	55–64	56.6	68.8	63.0	12.6	21.5	17.3
	65–74	71.0	77.1	74.5	22.4	37.0	30.7
	75–79	78.7	88.4	84.5	33.2	51.0	43.9
Feet[a]	18–79	19.8	21.3	20.6	1.5	2.9	2.2
	25–74	21.1	23.2	22.2	1.6	3.0	2.3
	18–24	4.5	1.2	2.8	—	—	—
	25–34	9.7	4.4	7.0	—	—	—
	35–44	17.3	11.2	14.1	0.4	0.4	0.4
	45–54	22.8	25.0	23.9	1.5	1.9	1.7
	55–64	29.0	44.1	36.9	3.4	6.9	5.2
	65–74	40.3	47.1	44.2	5.8	9.1	7.7
	75–79	48.6	53.1	51.3	4.8	14.6	10.7
Knees[b]	25–74	2.6	4.9	3.8	0.5	1.3	0.9
	25–34	—	0.1	0.0	—	0.0	0.0
	35–44	1.7	1.5	1.6	0.1	0.5	0.3
	45–54	2.3	3.6	3.0	0.2	0.5	0.4
	55–64	4.1	7.3	5.7	1.0	0.9	0.9
	65–74	8.3	18.0	13.8	2.0	6.6	4.6
Hips[b]	25–74	1.3	—	—	0.5	—	—
	25–34	0.4	—	—	0.2	—	—
	35–44	0.1	—	—	—	—	—
	45–54	0.7	—	—	0.1	—	—
	50–54	—	0.8	—	—	0.1	—
	55–64	2.6	2.8	2.7	0.7	1.6	1.2
	65–74	4.6	2.7	3.5	2.3	1.2	1.7
	55–74	3.5	2.8	3.1	1.4	1.4	1.4

[a] Data from the National Health Examination Survey, 1960–1962.
[b] Data from the National Health and Nutrition Examination Survey, 1971–1975.
From Lawrence RC, Hochberg MC, Kelsey JL, et al: Estimates of the prevalence of selected arthritic and musculoskeletal diseases in the United States. J Rheumatol 16:427–441, 1989, with permission.

radiographic evidence of osteoarthritis have no symptoms or disability. For example, in the First National Health and Nutrition Examination Survey (NHANES-I), only about half of the people with severe osteoarthritis of the hip or knee reported significant pain on most days for at least 1 month.[48] Studies in persons with osteoarthritis of the knee have identified the following factors as predictive of knee pain: severity of radiographic changes, presence of morning stiffness, crepitus on passive range of motion, and a feeling of low spirits.[49]

Prevalence rates of osteoarthritis and the proportion of cases that are moderate or severe increase with age.[46–48,50,51] Age-specific prevalence rates are higher in men below the age of 45 and in women above the age of 55. Women have a greater number of joints involved[51] and more frequent reports of morning stiffness, joint swelling, and nocturnal pain.[52] The more common occurrence of Heberden's nodes in women is believed to be related to a single autosomal gene that is dominant in women and recessive in men.[53] Studies using techniques of recombinant DNA analysis have demonstrated linkage of a polymorphism of the type II collagen gene (Col2A1) with generalized osteoarthritis in two families.[54] Other genetic abnormalities in cartilage matrix may also exist.[55] No striking racial, ethnic, regional, or urban-rural differences in disease prevalence have been noted in the United States. Asian populations, including Indians and Hong Kong Chinese, have been reported to have a lower prevalence of osteoarthritis of the hip than whites.[56]

It is generally accepted that osteoarthritis develops when the articular cartilage and subchondral bone are normal but excessive mechanical stress on the joint causes tissue damage, or when the mechanical stress is not unusual but the cartilage or subchondral bone is abnormal. The loss of cartilage matrix in osteoarthritis is thought to involve enzymes such as lysosomal proteases and metalloproteinases that are synthesized by the chondrocyte.[55]

Several studies have suggested that repetitive joint trauma associated with occupational activity may predispose to osteoarthritis.[57–59] For instance, high prevalence rates are found in the elbows and knees of miners,[60] in the fingers of cotton pickers,[61] in the hips of farmers,[62] and in the fingers, elbows, and knees of dock workers.[63] Jobs requiring a great deal of knee bending, squatting, kneeling, stair climbing, heavy lifting, and mechanical loading increase the risk for osteoarthritis of the knee.[59,64] One study showed that a history of unilateral knee injury was strongly associated with ipsilateral but not contralateral osteoarthritis of the knee in both sexes.[65] Recreational low-impact physical activity, including running, does not appear to be associated with osteoarthritis of the knees in most people,[66] but elite athletes[67] and recreational runners who already have abnormal or injured joints[68] are at increased risk for osteoarthritis.

Obesity is another factor that is known to increase the risk for osteoarthritis of several joints.[58,69–72] Other nonoccupational risk factors for osteoarthritis of the knee include knee injury, meniscectomy, and the presence of Heberden's nodes.[73] Osteoarthritis of the hip is more weakly associated with obesity, hip injury, and Heberden's nodes, but is rather strongly associated with developmental disorders that may affect the shape of the hip joint, including congenital dislocation of the hip and slipped capital femoral epiphysis.[64] Several studies, although not all, have noted an inverse association between osteoarthritis and osteoporosis.[58]

Osteoarthritis of the knee is associated with excess mortality and decreased survival in persons age 55 and older.[49] The likely explanations for this observation include the association of obesity with both osteoarthritis and mortality and possibly with adverse effects of treatment with nonsteroidal anti-inflammatory drugs (NSAIDs). One study noted excess proportionate mortality from gastrointestinal diseases in subjects with osteoarthritis,[74] while another demonstrated an increased incidence of gastroduodenal ulcers in subjects with osteoarthritis and knee pain.[49] Finally, osteoarthritis of the knee, especially with concomitant pain, is predictive of increased risk of long-term disability characterized by activity and mobility limitation.[49]

Regarding primary prevention, several potentially modifiable risk factors have been identified, including obesity and repetitive joint usage and trauma. Weight loss can lower risk for the development of osteoarthritis and probably also slow disease progression.[75] Reduction of the number of injuries and reduction of exposure to repetitive mechanical stress on the joints in the workplace should be beneficial. Early treatment of conditions such as congenital dislocation of the hip, slipped epiphysis, and various other developmental and acquired bone and joint disorders may prevent the development of or at least limit the extent of secondary osteoarthritis.

Screening tests for osteoarthritis are not available at present. Rather, secondary prevention strategies are primarily aimed at controlling the early symptoms of pain and stiffness. A variety of non-pharmacologic measures are now recommended in the treatment of early osteoarthritis.[55,76] Patients should be instructed in how to rest or unload affected joints, to protect affected joints through changes in their immediate environment and through learning appropriate methods of lifting and bending, and to maintain and improve muscle strength and flexibility. Isometric exercises and provision of social support may be helpful in reducing pain and improving mobility. If medication is to be used, acetaminophen is generally the first choice rather than nonsteroidal anti-inflammatory drugs (NSAIDs) because of the lower frequency of side effects, particularly of the gastrointestinal system. If NSAIDs are used, they should be started in low doses. Ibuprofen is often recommended because it can be given in low doses for short durations, has been associated with lower occurrence of gastrointestinal side effects, and is inexpensive. An agent that has shown promise in animals is tetracyclines, which may slow the rate of cartilage breakdown in osteoarthritis.[77] Also, of apparent benefit in dogs and cats are nutritional supplements containing glucosamines, which stimulate the synthesis of synovial fluid and cartilage matrix, chondroitin sulfate, which inhibits degradative enzymes, and manganese, which is needed for the biosynthesis of proteoglycans.[78]

Rheumatoid Arthritis

Rheumatoid arthritis is a chronic inflammatory joint disease, generally thought to be of autoimmune etiology, characterized by proliferative synovitis that results in destruction of articular cartilage and bony erosion; this gives rise to typical articular deformities. The usual clinical symptoms include stiffness, pain, and swelling of multiple joints, most commonly the small joints of the hands and wrists. The arthritis usually develops over time in a symmetric fashion. It also may be associated with a variety of extra-articular manifestations and has many characteristics of a systemic disease.[79] Although rheumatoid arthritis often results in considerable pain, activity limitation, and disability, recent studies suggest that in many cases the course of the disease is more benign than previously thought.[80]

Prevalence surveys of rheumatoid arthritis have relied primarily on two sets of criteria for case definition: the 1958 American Rheumatism Association (ARA) criteria[81] and the New York criteria.[82] With the 1958 ARA criteria, cases are divided into probable, definite, and classic rheumatoid arthritis. Two independent studies have noted that the majority of persons classified as having probable rheumatoid arthritis in population surveys do not have clinical rheumatoid arthritis but rather have other arthritides, most often generalized osteoarthritis.[83,84] Therefore, the following discussion will emphasize definite rheumatoid arthritis, as defined by 1958 ARA criteria, with the term "definite" including classic rheumatoid arthritis as well. It should be noted that the 1958 ARA criteria have been replaced by the 1987 revised criteria (Table 57-3); the major differences are (*a*) the deletion of the categories of possible and probable rheumatoid arthritis, (*b*) the combination of definite and classical rheumatoid arthritis into a single category, and (*c*) the deletion of the list of exclusion diagnoses.[85]

Based on the U.S. Health Examination Survey of 1960–1962, the prevalence of definite rheumatoid arthritis is almost 1 percent among persons age 18 years and older (Table 57-4).[86] A similar prevalence estimate of 0.8 percent was found from physical examinations done by physicians in NHANES-1 conducted from 1971 through 1975.[87]

Incidence rates of rheumatoid arthritis in the United States have been estimated over the 25-year interval from 1950 through 1974 from the Rochester (MN) Epidemiology Program Project.[88] The average annual incidence rates for persons age 15 and older were 40 per 100,000 for men, and 83 per 100,000 for women. Declining incidence rates among women, but not men, were noted between the periods 1960 through 1964 and 1970 through 1974 in Rochester;[88] this finding was consistent with a protective effect of oral contraceptives first reported by the Royal College of General Practitioners Oral Contraceptive Study.[89] However, not all studies have found a decrease in incidence rates over time among women, and it is possible that the inclusion of possible and probable cases in some studies is responsible for the apparent decline.[90]

Prevalence and incidence rates of rheumatoid arthritis increase with age in both sexes, at least through age 65 years and are between two and three times greater in women than in men. No striking differences in morbidity rates have been noted between American blacks and whites. However, several Native American tribes have particularly high prevalence rates of rheumatoid arthritis; these include the Yakima of central Washington State[91] and the Mille-Lac Band of Chippewa in Minnesota.[92] Asians, including Japanese and Chinese, appear to have lower prevalence rates than whites.[93,94]

Genetic factors have an important role in rheumatoid arthritis. The disease exhibits familial aggregation and a higher concordance rate in monozygotic than in dizygotic twins.[95] Studies have demon-

TABLE 57-3. THE 1987 AMERICAN RHEUMATISM ASSOCIATION REVISED CRITERIA FOR THE CLASSIFICATION OF RHEUMATOID ARTHRITIS[a]

Item	*Definition*
1	Morning stiffness, lasting at least 1 hour
2	Arthritis involving at least three joint groups simultaneously
3	Arthritis involving at least one area in the hands or wrists
4	Simultaneous involvement of the same joint area on both sides of the body
5	Presence of subcutaneous nodules
6	Presence of serum rheumatoid factor
7	Presence of typical radiographic features (juxta-articular osteopenia and/or erosions) on hand and wrist films

Modified from Arnett FC, Edworthy SM, Bloch DA, et al: American Rheumatism Association 1987 revised criteria for the classification of rheumatoid arthritis. Arthritis Rheum 31:315–324, 1988.

[a] Positive classification requires at least four of the seven criteria.

TABLE 57-4. PERCENT PREVALENCE OF DEFINITE RHEUMATOID ARTHRITIS IN THE UNITED STATES: U.S. HEALTH EXAMINATION SURVEY [1960–1962]

Age (yr)	*Males*	*Females*
18–24	—	—
25–34	—	—
35–44	—	0.9
45–54	0.2	1.1
55–64	1.9	2.9
≥65	1.8	4.9
Total	0.7	1.6

From National Center for Health Statistics: Rheumatoid arthritis in adults, 1960–1962. Vital Health Stat 11:17, 1966.

strated a strong association between the class II major histocompatibility antigen HLA-DR4 and rheumatoid arthritis; in whites, the relative risk for this association exceeds 4.0.[96,97] This association crosses ethnic and racial bounds, with just a few exceptions, including the Yakima Indians of Washington State, Asian Indians, Greeks, and Israeli Jews. In whites who lack HLA-DR4 and in these other ethnic and racial groups, there is an association between rheumatoid arthritis and HLA-DR1. HLA-DR10 and HLA-DR14 may also be associated with rheumatoid arthritis.[98] Recent work has identified a shared common epitope in the third hypervariable region of these alleles;[98,99] in almost all cases, rheumatoid arthritis is associated with the sequence stretch QKRAA or QRRAA.[98] This shared epitope may be involved in interactions between the antigen(s) that causes rheumatoid arthritis and other immunocompetent cells, especially T lymphocytes. This epitope is a strong marker for more severe disease.

Current evidence suggests that HLA is not so much associated with the onset of the disease as with its severity and progression.[100,101] It is likely that what is currently called rheumatoid arthritis is actually several diseases with somewhat similar clinical phenotypes, but with different or only partially overlapping genetic and environmental risk factors. The largest proportion of cases is associated with HLA-DR4 and other DRB1 alleles positive for the shared epitope.[101] About 8 to 10 percent of cases have an autoimmune condition in which type II collagen is the autoantigen and in which HLA-DR3 and HLA-DR7 are involved. Another relatively small group of cases may be associated only with HLA-DR1 and not with HLA-DR4. Non-HLA genes may also be involved, and candidate genes such as transporter in antigen processing (TAP) genes are currently being explored.[98,101]

The role of infectious agents as etiological factors in rheumatoid arthritis has been extensively explored, but no specific agent has been implicated.[102]

Finally, considerable attention has been directed toward the relation of oral contraceptive use and rheumatoid arthritis, and the possible mechanism of hormonal modulation of the immune response.[103] In a meta-analysis of 11 published analytical epidemiological studies, Spector and Hochberg[104] confirmed a protective effect of oral contraceptive use on the development of rheumatoid arthritis, with a pooled relative risk of 0.70. These authors concluded, however, that it was more likely that oral contraceptives, and possibly noncontraceptive hormone replacement therapy, modified the course of rheumatoid arthritis by preventing the progression of mild to severe disease, rather than preventing the development of disease itself.

Rheumatoid arthritis is associated with excess mortality and decreased survival; the standardized mortality ratio approximates 170, and there is reduced relative survival compared to age- and sex-matched general population control subjects.[105,106] Causes of death that are more frequent in rheumatoid arthritis patients include respiratory and infectious diseases, gastrointestinal disorders, and complications of rheumatoid arthritis. It is likely that some of the excess mortality is related to complications of therapy for the disease. Persistent synovitis, the presence of rheumatoid factor, extra-articular involvement, functional losses, low levels of education, and the "RA epitope" have been associated with increased mortality or excess disability.[90,107,108]

Methods of primary prevention or screening for rheumatoid arthritis are not currently available. First-line medical therapy consists of salicylates or NSAIDs.[108–110] These drugs are anti-inflammatory, analgesic, and antipyretic, and lead to a quick improvement in pain and swelling. However, there is no evidence that they affect the underlying disease process. It is now recommended that second-line therapies, which may modify the course of the disease, be initiated early in the course of the disease in patients with persistent synovitis.[108] Such therapies include antimalarials, sulfasalazine, methotrexate, intramuscular gold, penicillamine, azathioprine, and cyclosporin A. These drugs may be used alone or in combination. Oral corticosteroids probably have a role in management of the rheumatoid arthritis patient as an adjunct to remittive therapy.[111]

Physical therapy is another secondary prevention strategy, the goals of which are relief of pain, prevention of deformity, and maintenance of function. Modalities employed by the therapist include rest, splinting, heat and cold, and instruction in an exercise program, including energy-conservation and joint-protection techniques and range of motion and muscle-strengthening exercises.[112] The physical therapy program needs to be individualized for specific diseases and for individual patients with each disorder. In addition, patient education and social support mechanisms are important. Education may include behavioral instruction, provision of information about the disease, relaxation training, biofeedback, problem-solving strategies, energy conservation behaviors, stress reduction and coping strategies, and social support.[113] When used in conjunction with NSAIDs, patient education has a beneficial effect on pain relief, improvement in functional ability, and reduction in the number of tender joints.[113]

Foot Disorders in Older Adults

About three-fourths of fully active older adults complain of painful feet.[114–116] Among institutionalized adults, foot problems are one-fifth as common, indicating an important etiological role for stress on the feet from ordinary physical activity. Over half of noninstitutionalized older adults have corns and calluses, one-fourth have bunions, one-third have painful toenails, and one-fourth have cold feet, often as a result of circulatory disorders. A variety of static and functional deformities of the feet, such as hallux valgus, digiti flexus, and trophic changes, are related to degenerative disease; their prevalence rates increase with age. Foot strain from walking and standing is also common. The majority of painful conditions of the foot seen by orthopedists originate in soft tissues such as muscles, ligaments, tendons, nerves, and blood vessels. Articular and skeletal disorders of the feet may result from congenital abnormalities, infections, neoplasms, or trauma,[117] as well as from osteoarthritis, rheumatoid arthritis, and, less commonly, gout.

Prevention at all levels includes wearing proper shoes, wearing socks or stockings, bathing the feet frequently, avoidance of obesity, protection against infection and trauma to the feet, and proper care of toenails.[115,118] Once foot problems occur, soft, well-padded shoes should be worn to relieve pressure in sore areas. Pads, moleskin, lamb's wool, and hammer-toe pads applied to localized areas of soreness may be helpful. In most instances, these simple methods can reduce much of the discomfort associated with foot problems.[115] In some cases, rest, application of heat and cold, specific exercises, and use of special corrective shoes may be needed.[117] Almost half of the people with foot disorders are not receiving care for the problem.[116]

Paraplegia and Quadriplegia

The most common cause of paraplegia and quadriplegia in Western countries is vertebral fractures and dislocation from trauma. Complete transection of the spinal cord results in paralysis of all muscles supplied by motor neurons below the level of the lesion and in the loss of skin sensation in all areas supplied by sensory neurons below the lesion. Because neurons in the central nervous system do not regenerate, both motor and sensory paralysis is permanent.

The effect on the patient, family, and friends is immediate and enormous. Most affected individuals were previously independent and must learn to cope with partial or complete paralysis, loss of sensation in major parts of the body, and loss of voluntary control over body functions, frequently including bowel and bladder dysfunction, and loss of sexual function. The patient's work, marriage, family, and social relationships are likely to be substantially altered.[119]

In the United States about 238,000 people have traumatic spinal cord injuries, with 11,000 new cases occurring each year.[120] Spinal cord injuries occur most frequently in persons age 15 to 20 years and are more common in males than in females and in blacks than in whites.[121] Motor vehicle accidents, especially those involving motorcycles, are by far the leading cause of these injuries. Other major causes are falls from heights, acts of violence (gunshot wounds and stabbings), and sports and recreational activities such as diving in shallow water, injuries sustained during gymnastics, and hard contact sports.[121,122] One study[123] found that among those whose spinal cord injury occurred as a result of being in a motor vehicle, 70 percent were involved in a vehicle rollover, and 39 percent were ejected from the vehicle. Only 25 percent reported using seat belts. In another study,[122] drugs and alcohol had been used before the injury in at least 25 percent of cases. Nontraumatic causes include infections, vascular diseases, congenital abnormalities, tumors, intervertebral disc lesions, and neuromuscular diseases.[124]

The most important primary prevention measures are those that reduce the likelihood of motor vehicle accidents and lessen the risk of injury if accidents do occur. These include not driving after drinking alcoholic beverages, reducing speed limits, using seat belts and headrests, and the wearing of helmets by motorcyclists. Prevention of falls in the elderly and safety measures in occupational and recreational settings are also important. For instance, in high school and collegiate football, rules banning "spearing" or initial contact with the top of the helmet when making a tackle have markedly reduced the frequency of permanent cervical quadriplegia resulting from participation in that sport. Changes in neck conditioning, playing techniques, and equipment might reduce the frequency of such injuries in other sports as well.[125,126]

The number of survivors with paraplegia and quadriplegia has greatly increased because of medical and surgical advances. Since most of those injured are in their late teens and early adult years, enormous costs and very long-term severe disability ensue. In addition to psychological problems, the greatest difficulties are in self-care, locomotion, obtaining employment, and medical complications. The main object of tertiary prevention is to return the affected person to maximum physical and social functioning. Both physical and psychological adjustments are needed. Accordingly, in addition to specialists in orthopedic and neurological surgery, other specialists that should be involved in therapy of these patients include occupational and physical therapists, psychiatrists, orthotics specialists, urologists, and vocational counselors. Long leg braces, crutches, and gait training may help highly motivated paraplegics with low-level lesions return to walking and may even enable them to become self-supporting. Because many paraplegics drive cars, wheelchair accessibility of public buildings is becoming increasingly important.[127] Sexual counseling also may be helpful for many.

▶ DISORDERS PRIMARILY OF CHILDREN

Scoliosis

Scoliosis, or abnormal lateral curvature of the spine associated with rotation of the vertebrae, is the most common cause of spinal deformity in North American children.[128] Of the various forms of scoliosis, the most common and serious is adolescent idiopathic scoliosis. About 2 to 3 percent of children develop curves of 10° or more before growth ceases, and about 2 to 3 per 1,000 children develop curves of 30° or more.[129,130] Persons left with significant curvature frequently develop spinal osteoarthritis in adulthood; lung and heart complications may occur. Also, further curve progression sometimes takes place in adults.

Scoliosis is most frequently diagnosed around the ages of 11 to 14 years in girls and 14 to 16 years in boys. The ratio of female to male cases seen at surgery is as high as 5 to 1, but mild curves of less than 15° are found with almost equal frequency in both sexes. Although surgical series have indicated that scoliotic curves are most common at the thoracic level, screening programs identifying children who do not necessarily seek medical care have found that the peak frequency is at the thoracolumbar level.[131]

The risk for scoliosis in first-degree relatives of cases is about three to four times higher than in other children.[132] Little is known of other risk factors for development of the disease. Some evidence suggests that children who are skeletally more mature at the onset but not at the end of puberty are most likely to be affected and that individuals with scoliosis tend to be taller and leaner than others of their age at the beginning but not at the end of adolescence.[133,134] Once girls have reached menarche, their risk for developing scoliosis is reduced.[134] Impaired visual and vestibular functioning, defects in proprioceptive postural control, asymmetric muscle activity, unequal leg length, high concentrations of calcium in paraspinal muscles, and collagen disorders may be etiologically involved, but evidence is not conclusive.[135,136] Children with scoliosis appear to have mothers of older age than do other children of the same age.[132]

Some risk factors for progression of existing curves have been identified: double curves as opposed to single curves, thoracic curves as opposed to curves at lower levels, curves of greater magnitude, female sex, absence of a sacral tilt, limb length inequality, early chronological age, and skeletal immaturity.[137,138]

Because so little is known of the etiology of adolescent idiopathic scoliosis, primary prevention is not feasible. However, detection of early disease by screening is being undertaken in many places and screening for scoliosis is required by law in some states. It is assumed that with early detection affected children can be treated by conservative means and thereby avoid surgery. The traditional screening test for scoliosis has been the forward-bend test. In this test, the child's back is examined while he or she bends forward from the waist. The rotation that accompanies the lateral curvature in scoliosis results in posterior prominence of the ribs on the concave side of the curvature, so that a "rib hump" is often apparent on forward bending. In a more recently developed screening method, Moiré topography, a photograph of the back is used to measure the degree of topographic asymmetry. The forward-bend test has good specificity but fairly low sensitivity. Moiré topography has sensitivity of greater than 95 percent, but it picks up many minor curves.[139] The inclinometer (scoliometer), which measures trunk asymmetry as an indicator of trunk rotation, has been reported to have high sensitivity and fairly good specificity, but it has not been used much. Most school screening programs use the forward-bend test.

In the United States, school screening programs are identifying large numbers of children with possible spinal curvatures. Positive screening tests are followed up with x-ray examination for more definitive diagnosis. Curves of over 5° are monitored by further x-ray examination every few months. Should a curve progress to 20–25°, treatment is generally indicated to prevent further progression and may consist of exercises, braces, external or internal muscle stimulators, or, in severe cases, surgery.

Many questions have arisen about the desirability of widespread screening for scoliosis.[140,141] First, it is uncertain that school screening programs have brought about a reduction in the prevalence of severe deformities and thereby the number of operations needed. In particular, the efficacy of conservative treatment in preventing progression is uncertain. Also, many children screened as positive are not subsequently seen for definitive diagnosis. On the other hand, many false positives occur, resulting in referral for far too many x-ray examinations, and a great deal of medical expense and anxiety. In addition, most cases identified through screening do not progress, and not enough is known about factors that predict which curves will progress. The optimal ages for screening and whether males should be screened at all have not been determined. Criteria for referral for diagnosis and treatment should be reconsidered, and better training and evaluation of the nurses who do the screening may be needed.[130,140] Because of these uncertainties about the effectiveness of screening for scoliosis, the U.S. Preventive Services Task Force was unable to recommend for or against routine screening of adolescents for scoliosis.[142]

Slipped Capital Femoral Epiphysis

Slipped epiphysis of the head of the femur, in which epiphysis of the head of the femur is displaced backward and downward off the diaphysis, is primarily a disease of adolescents. It is closely related to the adolescent growth spurt and does not occur once the epiphysis is fused to the shaft of the femur. In the northeastern United States about 1 in 800 males and 1 in 2,000 females will be diagnosed as having a slipped epiphysis before they reach 25 years of age.[143]

The median age at diagnosis is 13 years for males and 11 years for females, the earlier age in females corresponding to their earlier onset of puberty. Males are affected more frequently than females; however, the magnitude of the excess varies from one geographical area to another and appears to have decreased over time. Blacks are affected more frequently than whites. In most studies in Northern latitudes, symptoms begin more frequently in spring and summer than in fall and winter.[144–146]

A large proportion of children with slipped epiphysis are markedly overweight;[147,148] about half are at or above the 95th percentile for their age Fig. 57-3.[147] Children with slipped epiphysis tend to have undergone slower-than-average skeletal maturation and to be tall for their age at the time of diagnosis.[149] At maturity, however, their heights are almost normal for their chronological age.[145] Familial aggregation of cases has been reported,[150] but it is not clear whether this aggregation is primarily attributable to inherited characteristics or to common environmental factors.

Many of these risk factors are related either to a weakening of the epiphyseal plate, such as occurs during periods of rapid growth, or to increased shearing stress on the plate. Animal experiments indicate that a deficit of sex hormones relative to growth hormone brings about the widening of the epiphyseal plate and a reduction in the shearing force necessary to displace the epiphysis.[151] Estrogens protect against slipped epiphysis, whereas androgens are protective only in large doses after prolonged exposure. Children with the unusual combination of being overweight and undergoing slow maturation would appear to be at high risk, and these children should be carefully watched for slipped epiphysis.

The only known means of primary prevention is prevention of obesity in adolescents. No screening tests for slipped epiphysis exist,

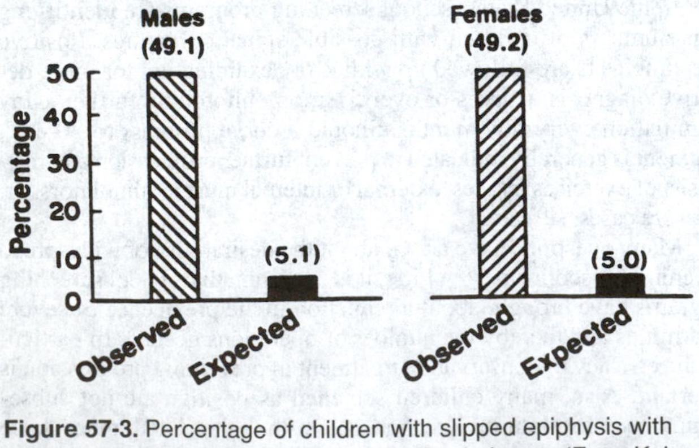

Figure 57-3. Percentage of children with slipped epiphysis with weights at or above the 95th percentile for their age. (From Kelsey JL, Acheson RM, Keggi KJ: The body builds of patients with slipped capital femoral epiphysis. Am J Dis Child 124:276–281, 1972.)

but the diagnosis should be suspected in adolescents who have a limp and hip or knee discomfort, especially if there is restriction of internal rotation of the hip. X-ray examination should be performed immediately to confirm the diagnosis. Since the condition is bilateral in 20 to 25 percent of cases, the contralateral hip of children with slipped epiphysis on one side should be carefully monitored, especially those whose first slipped epiphysis occurred at an early age.[148,152] Slight degrees of slippage that are treated early by hip pinning have a favorable prognosis, whereas cases diagnosed late and that involve severe displacement generally are associated with early onset of osteoarthritis of the hip and permanent disability despite treatment.

Fractures in Children

Each year almost 1 in 20 to 25 children fracture or dislocate a bone in some part of the body.[153,154] Sites fractured with high frequency in children relative to other age groups include the lower forearm, clavicle, tibia, fibula, and elbow (including supracondylar fractures and fractures of the capitulum of the humerus). A fall on an outstretched hand is a frequent cause of fractures of the clavicle, radius, ulna, and supracondylar region of the humerus; blows to the forearm frequently cause fractures of the radius and ulna; falls on the elbow may result in fractures of the capitulum of the humerus; and angulating or rotational forces are the main cause of fractures of the tibia and fibula. Motorcycle accidents, sports injuries, and accidents related to bicycles also are frequent causes of fractures of the tibia and fibula. In general, primary prevention of fractures in children depends on reducing the number of automobile and bicycle accidents, falls, child-battering injuries, sports and recreational injuries, and other childhood traumas.[155–157]

Fractures usually heal rapidly in children; the younger the age, the more rapid the healing. However, if the growth plate is involved in the fracture, growth in that bone may be adversely affected, particularly if a crushing injury has occurred. Other complications are rare but may include infection, delayed union, nonunion, avascular necrosis, and malunion. Prevention of these complications involves thorough cleansing and removal of all dead and contaminated tissue from an open (compound) fracture and competent initial treatment of the fracture.[158]

Congenital Dislocation of the Hip

In congenital dislocation of the hip, the head of the femur is displaced completely or partially out of the acetabulum. Partial displacement is sometimes referred to as congenital subluxation of the hip. In about 80 percent of cases the diagnosis is made shortly after birth, and in the remaining cases the diagnosis is made later, especially when the child starts to walk. Although it is possible that some of these late-diagnosed cases may represent dislocations that were missed around the time of birth, there is good evidence that some dislocations actually do develop after birth.[159]

The prevalence of congenital dislocation of the hip varies considerably from one geographic area to another. Rates ranging from 1 per 1,000 to 10 per 1,000 births have been reported in most North American and Western European populations and in Israel, Australia, and New Zealand. Higher rates of from 10 per 1,000 to 100 per 1,000 have been observed in the Navajo, Apache, and Cree-Ojibwa of North America, in the Lapps, and in the populations of Hungary, northern Italy, Brittany, and the Faroe Islands. Congenital dislocation of the hip is rare among blacks in South Africa, the West Indies, and Uganda, as well as among Chinese living in Hong Kong.[135] Although the frequency of congenital dislocation of the hip has been reported to be rising in certain areas, much of the apparent rise may be attributable to more extensive screening after birth and to increased awareness by physicians.[160]

In North America, girls are affected more frequently than boys in the ratio of about 6 to 1. Rates are also higher in whites than in blacks. In most areas, a greater than expected number of cases is encountered in children born in late fall and winter than in summer.[161]

Familial aggregation of cases occurs; both hereditary and environmental factors contribute to the familial excess.[162,163] Maternal relatives of cases have a higher risk than paternal relatives.[164] On average, infants with congenital dislocation of the hip have had longer gestation periods than other infants and are considerably more likely to have been born by breech delivery than other infants.[161,163,165]

The reasons for these epidemiologic characteristics are not known with certainty. Position in utero may be involved, since breech position in utero elongates the ligament of the hip joint capsule by persistent upward pressure of the greater trochanter.[166] Ligamentous and capsular laxity are also probably predisposing factors.[167] No feasible methods of primary prevention are known.

In regard to secondary prevention, examination of newborn infants for congenital dislocation of the hip is now accepted as a routine procedure. Without prompt treatment the affected leg may be shorter, the child may limp, surgery may be required, and osteoarthritis of the hip is likely to occur in young adulthood. Two screening tests have generally been used: the Ortolani and the Barlow. The Ortolani test involves placing the hip in flexion and gently adducting and then abducting the hip. The test is considered positive if a palpable jerk and audible clunk are heard as the head of the femur returns to the acetabulum. Some practitioners also consider an audible click to constitute a positive test. In the Barlow test, gentle downward pressure is exerted over the lesser trochanter with the hip in flexion and adduction; the unstable hip shifts from the acetabulum, and a sensation similar to the Ortolani sign is produced. When the leg is allowed to abduct, the hip is reduced.

About half of the hips noted to be unstable at birth become stable spontaneously within 3 weeks;[168] thus, these tests are often repeated at that time. Infants showing positive results on these tests are treated with braces, splints, or harnesses for 2 to 4 months. X-ray examination of the hip is of limited value in the newborn, but is an important diagnostic tool in children past the age of 3 months. Routine checks on hips of these infants should be done until they are walking well. If the disease is diagnosed after the neonatal period, surgery is generally required, and the prognosis is poorer.[169]

Despite the routine use in many locales of screening tests for congenital dislocation of the hip, many questions have arisen regarding the effectiveness of the screening by the Ortolani and Barlow tests.[170,171] First, it appears that incidence rates of congenital dislocation of the hip requiring prolonged treatment are no lower now than they were before screening became widespread. Both the sensitivity and specificity of the screening tests are poor. In one study[170] only one-third of genuine cases were detected, and the ratio of false positives to true positives was 10 to 1. Thus, for every one infant who benefits from splinting as a result of a positive test, 10 infants undergo unnecessary splinting. Furthermore, there is no consensus on indications for treatment, the timing of treatment, and the type of splint to be used. The question has arisen as to whether the screening procedures may themselves induce hip dislocation. Although these screening tests require experienced examiners for proper performance and interpretation, inexperienced examiners often are used, thus increasing both false-positive and false-negative rates. Better knowledge of which hips will spontaneously stabilize would allow better decisions about the cases that should receive immediate treatment. Disagreement exists about the significance of a soft audible or palpable click without evidence of abnormal movement between the femoral head and acetabulum.[172] Some physicians feel that such infants should be followed closely and given x-ray examination, while others feel that the likelihood of these infants actually developing congenital dislocation of the hip is too low to warrant the expense, exposure to x-rays, and anxiety. More data are needed to resolve these issues.

In recent years, ultrasound, which provides a defined image of the bony and cartilaginous neonatal hip, has become widely available for screening for congenital dislocation of the hip. Although it was initially believed that it might alleviate some of the problems with the Barlow and Ortolani tests,[173,174] its use as a routine screening test in all infants has not been found to be cost-effective. Even its use as a screening test in high-risk infants is controversial. Among its limitations as a screening test are its high cost, the low prevalence of congenital dislocation of the hip, the large proportion of hips testing positive on screening that develop normally, and the tendency of some cases to occur after the neonatal period.[175–177] In addition, while adequate interobserver agreement in reading ultrasound scans may be obtained with proper training, producing the scans is subject to even more variability. Thorough training and more attention to detail are needed to improve this situation.[178]

▶ CONCLUSION

The extent to which musculoskeletal disorders may be prevented varies considerably from one disorder to another. Some methods of primary prevention are possible for back disorders, osteoporosis, osteoarthritis, foot disorders, paraplegia and quadriplegia, slipped epiphysis, and fractures. However, these preventive measures frequently involve changes in individual behavior that are difficult to achieve. Screening tests for scoliosis, congenital dislocation of the hip, and osteoporosis are available. Although the tests for scoliosis and congenital dislocation of the hip are widely used at present, many questions regarding their efficacy remain unresolved.

Secondary and tertiary prevention are the levels more frequently used for the major musculoskeletal disorders of adults. However, with the exception of reconstructive joint surgery, secondary and tertiary prevention for such common problems as back pain and the arthritic disorders often has met with only limited success. Because of the chronicity of most of the common musculoskeletal conditions and the frequent reliance on only partially successful secondary and tertiary prevention measures, it is not surprising that musculoskeletal disorders have such a major effect on the quality of life and are associated with such high individual and societal costs. Improving the quality of life of affected individuals and further development and evaluation of screening tests will remain important in the management of musculoskeletal disorders, but it is also hoped that more emphasis will be placed on identification of feasible ways of preventing these disorders from occurring in the first place. Since the elderly are most frequently affected by musculoskeletal disorders and since the numbers of elderly will be increasing greatly over the next several decades, development of better methods of prevention at all levels is an urgent public health concern.

▶ REFERENCES

1. Holbrook TL, Grazier K, Kelsey JL, Stauffer RN: The Frequency of Occurrence, Impact, and Cost of Musculoskeletal Conditions in the United States. Chicago: American Academy of Orthopaedic Surgeons, 1985
2. Praemer A, Furner S, Rice DP: Musculoskeletal Conditions in the United States. Park Ridge, Il: American Academy of Orthopaedic Surgeons, 1992
3. Kelsey JL, Golden AL, Mundt DJ: Low back pain/prolapsed lumbar intervertebral disk. Epidemiology of Rheumatic Diseases 16:699–716, 1990
4. Dixon A St J: Progress and problems in back pain research. Rheumatol Rehabil 12:165–174, 1973
5. Snook SH: Low back pain in industry. In White AA III, Gordon SL (eds): Symposium on Idiopathic Low Back Pain. St. Louis: CV Mosby, 1982
6. Riihimäki H: Low-back pain, its origin and risk indicators. Scand J Work Environ Health 17:81–90, 1991
7. Andersson GB: Epidemiologic aspects of low-back pain in industry. Spine 6:53–60, 1981
8. Kelsey JL, Githens PB, White AA III, et al: An epidemiologic study of lifting and twisting on the job and risk for acute prolapsed lumbar intervertebral disc. J Orthop Res 2:61–66, 1984

9. Lüra JP, Shannon HS, Chambers LW, Haines TA: Long-term back problems and physical work exposures in the 1990 Ontario Health Survey. Am J Public Health 86:382–387, 1996
10. Frymoyer JW: Back pain and sciatica. N Engl J Med 318:291–300, 1986
11. Kelsey JL, Githens PB, O'Connor T, et al: Acute prolapsed lumbar intervertebral disc: an epidemiologic study with special reference to driving automobiles and cigarette smoking. Spine 9:608–613, 1984
12. Heliovaara M: Epidemiology of Sciatica and Herniated Lumbar Intervertebral Disc. Helsinki: Publications of the Social Insurance Institution, Finland, 1988
13. Kelsey JL, Githens PB, Walter SD, et al: An epidemiologic study of acute prolapsed cervical intervertebral disc. J Bone Joint Surg 66A:907–914, 1984
14. Deyo RA, Diehl AK: Psychosocial predictors of disability in patients with low back pain. J Rheumatol 15:1557–1564, 1988
15. Cats-Baril WL, Frymoyer JW: Identifying patients at risk of becoming disabled because of low-back pain. The Vermont Rehabilitation Engineering Center predictive model. Spine 16:605–607, 1991
16. Fish JR, DiMonte P, Courington SM: Back schools: past, present, and future. Clin Orthop 179:18–23, 1983
17. Hall H, Iceton JA: Back school: an overview with specific reference to the Canadian back education units. Clin Orthop 179:10–17, 1983
18. Lankhurst GJ, Van de Stadt RJ, Vogelaar TW, Van de Korst JK, Prevo AJH: The effect of the Swedish back school on chronic idiopathic low back pain. Scand J Rehabil Med 15:141–145, 1983
19. Malmivaara A, Häkkinen U, Aro T, et al: The treatment of acute low back pain—bed rest, exercises, or ordinary activity? N Engl J Med 332:351–355, 1995
20. Nachemson A: Work for all: those with back pain as well. Clin Orthop 179:77–85, 1983
21. Sambrook PN, Kelly PJ, White CP, Morrison NA, Eisman JA: Genetic determinants of bone mass. In Marcus R, Feldman D, Kelsey J (eds): Osteoporosis. San Diego: Academic Press, 1996
22. Villa ML, Nelson L: Race, ethnicity and osteoporosis. In Marcus R, Feldman D, Kelsey J (eds): Osteoporosis. San Diego: Academic Press, 1996
23. Melton LJ III, Chrischilles EA, Cooper C, Lanc AW, Riggs BL: How many women have osteoporosis? J Bone Miner Res 7:1005–1010, 1992
24. Lindsay R, Hart DM, MacLean A, Clark AC, Kraszewski A, Garwood J: Bone response to termination of estrogen treatment. Lancet 1:1325–1327, 1978
25. Cauley JA, Salamone LM, Lucas FL: Postmenopausal endogenous and exogenous hormones, degree of obesity, thiazide diuretics, and risk of osteoporosis. In Marcus R, Feldman D, Kelsey J (eds): Osteoporosis. San Diego: Academic Press, 1996
26. Faulkner KG, Cummings SR, Black D, Palermo L, Glüer CC, Genant HK: Simple measurement of femoral geometry predicts hip fracture: the study of osteoporotic fractures. J Bone Miner Res 8:1211–1217, 1993
27. Heaney RP: Nutrition and risk for osteoporosis. In Marcus R, Feldman D, Kelsey J (eds): Osteoporosis. San Diego: Academic Press, 1996
28. Cumming RG: Calcium intake and bone mass: a quantitative review of the evidence. Calcif Tissue Int 47:194–201, 1990
29. Chapuy MC, Arlot ME, Duboeuf F, et al: Vitamin D_3 and calcium to prevent hip fractures in elderly women. N Engl J Med 327:1637–1642, 1992
30. Snow CM, Shaw JM, Matkin CC: Physical activity and risk for osteoporosis. In Marcus R, Feldman D, Kelsey J (eds): Osteoporosis. San Diego: Academic Press, 1996
31. Seeman E: The effects of tobacco and alcohol use on bone. In Marcus R, Feldman D, Kelsey J (eds): Osteoporosis. San Diego: Academic Press, 1996
32. Kelsey JL, Marcus R: Intervention trials concerned with disease prevention in women. In Casper RC (ed): Women's Health: Hormones, Emotions and Behavior. Cambridge, England: Cambridge University Press, in press
33. Slemenda CW, Johnston CC, Hui SL: Assessing fracture risk. In Marcus R, Feldman D, Kelsey J (eds): Osteoporosis. San Diego: Academic Press, 1996
34. Hans D, Dargent-Molina P, Schott AM, et al: Ultrasonographic heel measurements to predict hip fracture in elderly women: the EPIDOS prospective study. Lancet 348:511–514, 1996
35. Tinetti ME, Baker DI, McAvay G, et al: A multifactorial intervention to reduce the risk of falling among elderly people living in the community. N Engl J Med 331:821–827, 1994
36. Grisso JA, Capezuti E, Schwartz A: Falls as risk factors for fractures. In Marcus R, Feldman D, Kelsey J (eds): Osteoporosis. San Diego: Academic Press, 1996
37. Lauritzen JB, Petersen MM, Lund B: Effect of external hip protectors on hip fractures. Lancet 341:11–13, 1993
38. Hochberg MC: Osteoarthritis. Postgrad Adv Rheumatol 3:1–12, 1988
39. Council for International Organizations of Medical Sciences: Atlas of Standard Radiographs of Arthritis. In: The Epidemiology of Chronic Rheumatism. Oxford: Blackwell, 1963, vol 2
40. Kallman DA, Wigley FM, Scott WW Jr, Hochberg MC, Tobin JD: New grading scales for radiographic hand osteoarthritis: reliability for determining prevalence and progression. Arthritis Rheum 32:1584–1591, 1989
41. Kallman DA, Wigley FM, Scott WW Jr, Hochberg MC, Tobin JD: The longitudinal course of hand osteoarthritis in a male population. Arthritis Rheum 33:1323–1332, 1990
42. Myers SL, Dines K, Brandt DA, Brandt KD, Albrecht ME: Experimental assessment by high frequency ultrasound of articular cartilage thickness and osteoarthritic changes. J Rheumatol 22:109–116, 1995
43. Altman RD, Asch E, Bloch DA, et al: Development of criteria for the classification and reporting of osteoarthritis: classification of osteoarthritis of the knee. Arthritis Rheum 29:1039–1049, 1986
44. Kellgren JH, Moore R: Generalized osteoarthritis and Heberden's nodes. Br Med J 1:181–187, 1952
45. Schumacher HR: Secondary osteoarthritis. In Moskowitz RW, Howell DS, Goldberg WM, Mankin HJ (eds): Osteoarthritis: Diagnosis and Management. Philadelphia: WB Saunders, 1984
46. Lawrence RC, Hochberg MC, Kelsey JL, et al: Estimates of the prevalence of selected arthritic and musculoskeletal diseases in the United States. J Rheumatol 16:427–441, 1989
47. National Center for Health Statistics: Osteoarthrosis in adults by selected demographic characteristics: United States, 1960–1962. Vital Health Stat 2:20, 1966
48. National Center for Health Statistics: Basic data on arthritis: knee, hip and sacroiliac joints in adults aged 25–74 Years: United States, 1971–1975. Vital Health Stat 11:213, 1979
49. Hochberg MC, Lawrence RC, Everett DF, Cornoni-Huntley J: Epidemiologic associations of pain in osteoarthritis of the knee. Semin Arthritis Rheum 18(Suppl 2):4–9, 1989
50. Butler WJ, Hawthorne VM, Mikkelsen WM, et al: Prevalence of radiographically defined osteoarthritis in the finger and wrist joints of adult residents of Tecumseh, Michigan, 1962–65. J Clin Epidemiol 41:467–473, 1988
51. Lawrence JS, Bremner JM, Bier F: Osteoarthrosis, prevalence in the population and relationship between symptoms and x-ray changes. Ann Rheum Dis 25:1–24, 1966
52. Acheson RM, Chan Y-K, Clemett AR: New Haven Survey of Joint Diseases. XII. Distribution and symptoms of osteoarthrosis in the hands with reference to handedness. Ann Rheum Dis 29:275–286, 1970
53. Stecher RM: Heberden's nodes: a clinical description of osteoarthritis of the finger joints. Ann Rheum Dis 14:1–10, 1955

54. Palotie A, Vaisanen P, Ott J, et al: Predisposition to familial osteoarthrosis linked to Type II collagen gene. Lancet 1:924–927, 1989
55. Brandt KD: Nonsurgical management of osteoarthritis, with an emphasis on nonpharmacologic measures. Arch Fam Med 4:1057–1064, 1995
56. Scott JC, Hochberg MC: Epidemiologic insights into the pathogenesis of hip osteoarthritis. In Hadler NM (ed): Clinical Concepts in Regional Musculoskeletal Illness. Orlando, FL: Grune & Stratton, 1987
57. Felson DT: Epidemiology of hip and knee osteoarthritis. Epidemiol Rev 10:1–28, 1988
58. Peacock DJ, Cooper C: Epidemiology of the rheumatic diseases. Curr Opin Rheumatol 7:82–86, 1995
59. Cooper C, McAlindon T, Cockburn T, Egger P, Dieppe P: Occupational activity in osteoarthritis of the knee. Ann Rheum Dis 53:90–93, 1994
60. Lawrence JS: Rheumatism in coalminers. Part 3. Occupational factors. Br J Ind Med 12:249–261, 1955
61. Lawrence JS: Rheumatism in cotton operatives. Br J Ind Med 18:270–276, 1961
62. Croft P, Coggon D, Cruddas M, Cooper C: Osteoarthritis of the hip: an occupational disease in farmers. Br Med J 304:1269–1272, 1992
63. Partridge REH, Duthie JJR: Rheumatism in dockers and civil servants: a comparison of heavy manual and sedentary workers. Ann Rheum Dis 27:559–568, 1968
64. Cooper C: Occupational activity and the risk of osteoarthritis. J Rheumatol 22(Suppl 43):10–12, 1995
65. Davis MA, Ettinger WH, Neuhaus JM, Cho SA, Hauch WW: The association of knee injury and obesity with unilateral and bilateral osteoarthritis of the knee. Am J Epidemiol 130:279–288, 1989
66. Panush RS, Schmidt C, Caldwell JR, et al: Is running associated with degenerative joint disease? JAMA 255:1152–1155, 1986
67. Kujala UN, Kaprio J, Sarna S: Osteoarthritis of weight bearing joints of lower limbs in former elite male athletes. Br Med J 308:231–234, 1994
68. Lane NE: Exercise: a cause of osteoarthritis. J Rheumatol 22(Suppl 43):3–6, 1995
69. Hartz AJ, Fischer ME, Bril G, et al: The association of obesity with joint pain and osteoarthritis in the HANES data. J Chronic Dis 39:311–319, 1986
70. Davis MA, Ettinger WH, Neuhaus JM, Hauck WW: Sex differences in osteoarthritis of the knee: the role of obesity. Am J Epidemiol 127:1029–1030, 1988
71. Carmen WJ, Sowers M, Hawthorne VM, Weissfeld LA: Obesity is a risk factor of osteoarthritis of the hand and wrist: a prospective study. Am J Epidemiol 139:119–129, 1994
72. Davis MA, Ettinger WH, Neuhaus JM: The role of metabolic factors and blood pressure in the association of obesity with osteoarthritis of the knee. J Rheumatol 15:1827–1832, 1988
73. Cooper C, McAlindon T, Snow S, et al: Mechanical and constitutional risk factors for symptomatic knee osteoarthritis: differences between tibiofemoral and patellofemoral disease. J Rheumatol 21: 307–313, 1994
74. Monson RR, Hall AP: Mortality among arthritics. J Chronic Dis 28:459–467, 1976
75. Felson DT, Ahange Y, Anthony JM, Naimark A, Anderson JJ: Weight loss reduces the risk for symptomatic knee osteoarthritis in women. Ann Intern Med 116:535–539, 1992
76. Griffin MR, Brandt KD, Liang MH, Pincus T, Ray WA: Practical management of osteoarthritis. Arch Fam Med 4:1049–1055, 1995
77. Brandt KD, Schumacher HR: Osteoarthritis and crystal deposition diseases. Curr Opin Rheumatol 8:235–237, 1996
78. Nutramax Laboratories, Inc., Veterinary Science Division: Cosequin
79. Firestein GS: Etiology and pathogenesis of rheumatoid arthritis. In Kelley WN, Harris ED Jr, Ruddy S, Sledge CB (eds): Textbook of Rheumatology. Philadelphia: WB Saunders, 1997
80. Gabriel SE: Update on the epidemiology of the rheumatic diseases. Curr Opin Rheumatol 8:96–100, 1996
81. Ropes MW, Bennett GA, Cobb S, Jacox R, Jessar RA: Revision of diagnostic criteria for rheumatoid arthritis. Bull Rheum Dis 9:175–176, 1958
82. Bennett PH, Burch TA: New York symposium on population studies in the rheumatic disease: new diagnostic criteria. Bull Rheum Dis 17:453–458, 1967
83. Lawrence JS: Rheumatism in Populations. London: Heinemann Medical Books, 1977
84. O'Sullivan JB, Cathcart ES: The prevalence of rheumatoid arthritis: follow-up examination of the effect of criteria on rates in Sudbury, Massachusetts. Ann Intern Med 76:572–577, 1972
85. Arnett FC, Edworthy SM, Bloch DA, et al: American Rheumatism Association 1987 revised criteria for the classification of rheumatoid arthritis. Arthritis Rheum 31:315–324, 1988
86. National Center for Health Statistics: Rheumatoid arthritis in adults, 1960–1962. Vital Health Stat, 11:17, 1966
87. Cunningham LS, Kelsey JL: Epidemiology of musculoskeletal impairments and associated disability. Am J Public Health 74:574–579, 1984
88. Linos A, Worthington JW, O'Fallon WM, Kurland LT: The epidemiology of rheumatoid arthritis in Rochester, Minnesota: a study of incidence, prevalence and mortality. Am J Epidemiol 111:87–98, 1980
89. Wingrave S, Kay CR: Reduction in incidence of rheumatoid arthritis associated with oral contraceptives. Lancet 1:569–571, 1978
90. Alarcón GS: Epidemiology of rheumatoid arthritis. Rheum Dis Clin North Am 21:589–604, 1995
91. Beasley RP, Wilkens RF, Bennett PH: High prevalence of rheumatoid arthritis in Yakima Indians. Arthritis Rheum 16:743–747, 1973
92. Harvey J, Lotze M, Arnett FC, et al: Rheumatoid arthritis in a Chippewa band: II. Field study with clinical, serologic and HLA-D correlations. J Rheumatol 10:28–32, 1983
93. Kato H, Duff IF, Russell WJ, et al: Rheumatoid arthritis and gout in Hiroshima and Nagasaki, Japan: a prevalence and incidence study. J Chronic Dis 23:659–679, 1971
94. Beasley RP, Bennett PH, Lin CC: Low prevalence of rheumatoid arthritis in Chinese: prevalence survey in a rural community. J Rheumatol 10(Suppl 10):11–15, 1983
95. del Junco DJ, Luthra HS, Annegers JF, Worthington JW, Kurland LT: The familial aggregation of rheumatoid arthritis and its relationship to the HLA-DR4 association. Am J Epidemiol 119: 813–829, 1984
96. Goldstein R, Arnett FC: The genetics of rheumatic disease in man. Rheum Dis Clin North Am 13:487–510, 1987
97. Grennan DM, Sanders PA: Rheumatoid arthritis. Baillieres Clin Rheumatol 2:585–601, 1988
98. Weyand CM, Goronzy JJ: Inherited and noninherited risk factors in rheumatoid arthritis. Curr Opin Rheumatol 7:206–213, 1995
99. Gregersen PK, Silver J, Winchester RJ: The shared epitope hypothesis: an approach to understanding the molecular genetics of the susceptibility to rheumatoid arthritis. Arthritis Rheum 30:1205–1213, 1987
100. Weyand CM, Hicok KC, Conn DL, Goronzy JJ: The influence of HLA-DRB1 genes on disease severity in rheumatoid arthritis. Ann Intern Med 117:801–806, 1992
101. Ollier WER, MacGregor A: Genetic epidemiology of rheumatoid disease. Br Med Bull 51:267–285, 1995
102. Albani S, Carson DA: Etiology and pathogenesis of rheumatoid arthritis. In Koopman WJ (ed): Arthritis and Allied Conditions. A Textbook of Rheumatology. Baltimore: Williams & Wilkins, 1997
103. Silman AJ, Vandenbroucke J (eds): Female sex hormones and rheumatoid arthritis. Br J Rheumatol 28(Suppl):1–73, 1989
104. Spector TD, Hochberg MC: The protective effect of oral contraceptives on the development of rheumatoid arthritis: an overview of

analytic epidemiologic studies with a meta-analysis. J Clin Epidemiol 43:1221–1230, 1990
105. Kelsey JL, Hochberg MC: Epidemiology of chronic musculoskeletal disorders. Annu Rev Public Health 9:379–401, 1988
106. Kirwan JR, Silman AJ: Epidemiologic, sociological, and environmental aspects of rheumatoid arthritis and osteoarthritis. Baillieres Clin Rheumatol 1:467–489, 1987
107. Pincus T, Callahan LF: Formal education as a marker for increased mortality and morbidity in rheumatoid arthritis. J Chronic Dis 38:973–984, 1985
108. Weinblatt ME: Treatment of rheumatoid arthritis. In Koopman WJ (ed): Arthitis and Allied Conditions. A Textbook of Rheumatology. Baltimore: Williams & Wilkins, 1997
109. Hochberg MC: NSAIDs: mechanisms and pathways of action. Hosp Pract 24:185–198, 1989
110. Hochberg MC: NSAIDs: Patterns of usage and side effects. Hosp Pract 24:167–174, 1989
111. Weiss MM: Corticosteroids in rheumatoid arthritis. Semin Arthritis Rheum 19:9–21, 1989
112. Navarro AH: The role of the physical therapist. In Riggs GK, Gall EP (eds): Rheumatic Diseases: Rehabilitation and Management. Boston: Butterworth, 1984
113. Superio-Cabuslay E, Ward MM, Lorig KR: Patient education interventions in osteoarthritis and rheumatoid arthritis: a meta-analytic comparison with nonsteroidal antiinflammatory drug treatment. Arthritis Care Res 9:292–301, 1996
114. Evanski PM: The geriatric foot. In Jahss MH (ed): Disorders of the Foot. Philadelphia: WB Saunders, 1982
115. Caillet R: Foot and Ankle Pain. Philadelphia: FA Davis, 1983
116. Elton PJ, Sanderson SP: A chiropodial survey of elderly persons over 65 years in the community. Public Health 100:219–222, 1986
117. Helfand AE: At the foot of South Mountain. A 5-year longitudinal study of foot problems and screening in an elderly population. J Am Podiatr Assoc 63:512–521, 1973
118. Edelstein JE: Foot care for the aging. Phys Ther 68:1882–1886, 1988
119. Smart CN, Sanders CR: The Costs of Motor Vehicle Related Spinal Cord Injuries. Washington, DC: Insurance Institute for Highway Safety, 1976
120. Ergas Z: Spinal cord injury in the United States: a statistical update. Cent Nerv Syst Trauma 2:19–32, 1985
121. Stover SL, Fine PR. The epidemiology and economics of spinal cord injury. Paraplegia 25:225–228, 1987
122. Woodruff BA, Baron RC: A description of nonfatal spinal cord injury using a hospital-based registry. Am J Prev Med 10:10–14, 1994
123. Thurman DJ, Burnett CL, Beaudoin DE, Jeppson L, Sniezek JE: Risk factors and mechanisms of occurrence in motor vehicle-related spinal cord injuries: Utah. Accid Anal Prev 27:411–415, 1995
124. Brashear HR Jr, Raney RB Sr: Handbook of Orthopaedic Surgery. St. Louis: CV Mosby, 1986
125. Torg JS, Vesgo JJ, Sennett B, Das M: The National Football Head and Neck Injury Registry: 14-year report on cervical quadriplegia, 1971 through 1984. JAMA 254:3439–3443, 1985
126. Cantu RC: Head and spine injuries in youth sports. Clin Sports Med 14:517–532, 1995
127. Sutton RA, Bentley M, Castree B, Mattinson R, Pattinson J, Smith R: Review of the social situation of paraplegic and tetraplegic patients rehabilitated in the Hexham Regional Spinal Injury Unit in the north of England over the past four years. Paraplegia 20:71–79, 1982
128. Winter RB: Spinal problems in pediatric orthopaedics. In Morrissey RT (ed): Lovell and Winter's Pediatric Orthopaedics. Philadelphia: JB Lippincott, 1990, vol 2
129. Shands AR, Eisberg HB: The incidence of scoliosis in the state of Delaware. J Bone Joint Surg 37A:1243–1249, 1955
130. Morais T, Bernier M, Turcotte F: Age- and sex-specific prevalence of scoliosis and the value of school screening programs. Am J Public Health 75:1377–1380, 1985
131. Brooks HL, Azen SD, Gerberg E, Brooks R, Chan L: Scoliosis: a prospective epidemiological study. J Bone Joint Surg 57A:968–972, 1975
132. Wynne-Davies R: Familial (idiopathic) scoliosis. A family survey. J Bone Joint Surg 50B:24–30, 1968
133. Willner S: A Study of height, weight, and menarche in girls with idiopathic structural scoliosis. Acta Orthop Scand 46:71–83, 1975
134. Hazebroek-Kampschreur AAJM, Hofman A, Van Dijk AP, Van Linge B: Determinants of trunk abnormalities in adolescence. Int J Epidemiol 23:1242–1247, 1994
135. Kelsey JL: Epidemiology of Musculoskeletal Disorders. New York: Oxford University Press, 1982
136. Keessen W, Crowe A, Hearn M: Proprioceptive accuracy in idiopathic scoliosis. Spine 17:149–155, 1992
137. Dickson RA, Stamper P, Sharp A-M, Harker P: School screening for scoliosis: cohort study of clinical course. Br Med J 2:265–267, 1980
138. Lonstein JR: Natural history and school screening for scoliosis. Orthop Clin North Am 19:227–237, 1988
139. Laulund T, Sojbjerg JO, Horlyck E: Moiré topography in school screening for structural scoliosis. Acta Orthop Scand 53:765–768, 1982
140. Williams JI. Criteria for screening: are the effects predictable? Spine 13:1178–1186, 1988
141. US Preventive Services Task Force: Screening for adolescent idiopathic scoliosis [Review article]. JAMA 269:2667–2672, 1993
142. US Preventive Services Task Force: Screening for adolescent idiopathic scoliosis [Policy statement]. JAMA 269:2664–2666, 1993
143. Kelsey JL: Incidence and distribution of slipped capital femoral epiphysis in Connecticut. J Chronic Dis 23:567–587, 1971
144. Kelsey JL: Epidemiology of slipped capital femoral epiphysis: a review of the literature. Pediatrics 51:1042–1050, 1973
145. Hansson LI, Hagglund G, Ordeberg G: Slipped capital femoral epiphysis in southern Sweden, 1910–1982. Acta Orthop Scand 226: 1–67, 1987
146. Loder RT: A worldwide study on the seasonal variation of slipped capital femoral epiphysis. Clin Orthop 322:28–36, 1996
147. Kelsey JL, Acheson RM, Keggi KJ: The body builds of patients with slipped capital femoral epiphysis. Am J Dis Child 124:276–281, 1972
148. Loder RT: The demographics of slipped capital femoral epiphysis. An international multicenter study. Clin Orthop 332:8–27, 1996
149. Sorenson KH: Slipped upper femoral epiphysis. Acta Orthop Scand 39:499–517, 1968
150. Rennie AM: Familial slipped upper femoral epiphysis. J Bone Joint Surg 49B:535–539, 1967
151. Morscher E: Strength and morphology of growth cartilage under hormonal influence of puberty. Reconstr Surg Traumatol 10:3–104, 1968
152. Hurley JM, Betz RR, Loder RT, Davidson RS, Alburger PD, Steel HH: Slipped capital femoral epiphysis. The prevalence of late contralateral slip. J Bone Joint Surg 78A:226–230, 1996
153. National Center for Health Statistics: Current estimates from the National Health Interview Survey, United States, 1987. Vital Health Stat 10:166, 1988
154. Rivara FD, Calonge N, Thompson RS: Population-based study of unintentional injury incidence and impact during childhood. Am J Public Health 79:990–994, 1989
155. Buhr AJ, Cooke AM: Fracture patterns. Lancet 1:531–536, 1959
156. Garraway WM, Stauffer RN, Kurland LT, O'Fallon WM: Limb fractures in a defined population: frequency and distribution. Mayo Clin Proc 54:701–707, 1979
157. Rockwood CA Jr, Wilkins KE, Beaty RE (eds): Fractures in Children. Philadelphia: Lippincott-Raven, 1996
158. Adams JC: Outline of Fractures. Edinburgh: Churchill-Livingstone, 1987
159. Bjerkedal T: Congenital dislocation of the hip in Norway: a clinical-epidemiological study. J Oslo City Hosp 26:79–90, 1976

160. Leck I: Rising rates of congenital dislocation of the hip. Lancet 1:372, 1976
161. Robinson GW: Birth characteristics of children with congenital dislocation of the hip. Am J Epidemiol 87:275–284, 1968
162. Record RC, Edwards JH: Environmental influences related to the aetiology of congenital dislocation of the hip. Br J Prev Soc Med 12:8–22, 1958
163. Gunther A, Smith SJ, Maynard PV, Beaver MW, Chilvers CED: A case-control study of congenital hip dislocation. Public Health 107: 9–18, 1993
164. Kramer AA, Berg K, Nance WE: Familial aggregation of congenital dislocation of the hip in a Norwegian population. J Clin Epidemiol 41:91–96, 1988
165. Cyvin KB: Congenital dislocation of the hip joint. Acta Paediatr Scand 263:1–67, 1977
166. Jones DH: The early diagnosis of congenital dislocation of the hip joint. Br J Clin Pract 19:443–449, 1965
167. Carter CO, Wilkinson J: Persistent joint laxity and congenital dislocation of the hip. J Bone Joint Surg 46B:40–45, 1964
168. Katz JF, Challenor YB: Childhood orthopedic syndromes. In Downey JA, Low NL (eds): The Child with Disabling Illness. Philadelphia: WB Saunders, 1974
169. Cunningham KT, Beningfield SA, Moulton A, Maddock CR: A clicking hip in a newborn baby should never be ignored. Lancet 1:668–670, 1984
170. Knox EG, Armstrong EH, Lancashire RJ: Effectiveness of screening for congenital dislocation of the hip. J Epidemiol Community Health 41:283–289, 1987
171. Leck I: An epidemiological assessment of neonatal screening for dislocation of the hip. J R Coll Physicians Lond 20:56–62, 1986
172. Fulton MJ, Barer ML: Screening for congenital dislocation of the hip: an economic appraisal. Can Med Assoc J 130:1149–1156, 1984
173. MacFarlane A: Screening for congenital dislocation of the hip. Br Med J 294:1047, 1987
174. Berman L, Klenerman L: Ultrasound screening for hip abnormalities. Preliminary findings in 1001 neonates. Br Med J 293:719–722, 1986
175. Geitung JT, Rosendahl K, Sudmann E: Cost-effectiveness of ultrasonographic screening for congenital hip dysplasia in newborns. Skeletal Radiol 25:251–254, 1996
176. Hernandez RJ, Cornell RG, Hensinger RN: Ultrasound diagnosis of neonatal congenital dislocation of the hip. A decision analysis assessment. J Bone Joint Surg Br 76:539–543, 1994
177. Rosendahl K, Markestad T, Lie RT: Ultrasound screening for developmental dysplasia of the hip in the neonate: the effect on treatment rate and prevalence of late cases. Pediatrics 94:47–52, 1994
178. Rosendahl K, Aslaksen A, Lie RT, Markestad T: Reliability of ultrasound in the early diagnosis of developmental dysplasia of the hip. Pediatr Radiol 25:219–224, 1995.

58

Neurological Disorders

James C. Torner • Robert B. Wallace

Neurological disorders include many diseases and conditions of acute and chronic development. The etiology of these disorders can be infectious, toxic, genetic, traumatic, ischemic, and related to other chronic pathophysiology. The occurrence may be at birth, which may confer a lifelong disability, or may occur in middle or late life, which may result in progressive disability and death. Neurological disorders may have an insidious onset or have symptoms that are nonspecific with classification difficult. Early stages of some disorders are characterized by a variable presentation or by subtle signs and symptoms that are difficult to detect or that go unrecognized. Individuals often ignore symptoms until function is impaired. Some disorders in children may be developmental and may go undetected until the children reach the age at which deficits could be assessed. Hence, recognition, diagnosis, and progression of neurological symptoms may affect the true magnitude and onset of neurological disorders.

Diagnosis of neurological disorders requires not only recognition of symptoms but confirmation with a neurological examination. The neurological examination may be specific to symptoms and to onset. Diagnostic tests have changed with advances in imaging and electrophysiological testing. The use of computerized tomographic scanning, magnetic resonance imaging, cerebral blood flow measurement, and positron emission tomography have increased the certainty of diagnosis. Additional cognitive tests developed by neuropsychologists have aided in the diagnosis of cognitive decline. Hence the evaluation of incidence and prevalence over time is difficult due to changing diagnostic criteria and the likelihood of changing classification and inclusion of milder or early onset disease.

Mortality, Incidence, and Prevalence of Neurological Disorders

Mortality rates of neurological disorders are low with the exception of cerebrovascular conditions. Cerebrovascular disease remains as a major cause of death with a rate of nearly 60 per 100,000 persons (Fig. 58-1). Rates of death of progressive neurological disorders such as Parkinson's disease and Alzheimer's disease increase as the population becomes older. Poor survival following the occurrence of malignant brain neoplasms accounts for 4.6 deaths per 100,000 population.[1] Table 58-1 includes mortality data of neurological conditions for the United States for 1990.

Few population-based registries of neurological disorders exist. The Rochester Epidemiologic Project has focused research on neurological conditions with data of cases observed in Olmstead County, Minnesota, from 1945 to the late 1980s.[2,3] The consistency of documentation and the evaluation of diagnostic change can be elucidated in this unique registry of medical records. Rates of infrequent neurological conditions may require analysis over decades to accumulate enough cases. However, a limitation is the size and diversity of the population. Also the demographic composition of Olmstead County limits generalizability to minorities and urban populations. The following sections in this chapter include data and rates from this unique resource.

Using discharge diagnoses as measure of the magnitude of neurological disorders on the health care system from the National Hospital Discharge Survey of 1990 shows that discharge rate for epileptic seizures, migraine, multiple sclerosis, and malignant brain neoplasm were highest when the first-listed diagnosis was used.[4] (Fig. 58-2) However, for all admissions epilepsy, Parkinson's disease, Alzheimer's disease, migraine, and toxic neuropathies were the highest (Table 58-2). These reflect the prevalence and progressive nature of these disorders associated with other medical conditions and repeat follow-up and treatment of these conditions.

The National Ambulatory Medical Care Survey of 1991–1992 examined the 7,253,000 visits to neurologists that were reported by respondents.[5] The rate of visits was 2.9 per 100 persons per year. Only 6 percent of the visits were referred and 15.5 percent were new patients. Most of the visits (81 percent) were due to symptoms, with 43 percent of those from nervous system problems and 23 percent from musculoskeletal complaints. The main reasons for the visit were headaches (18 percent), seizures (9 percent), and sensory disturbances (5.5 percent). Only 36 percent of the visits resulted in a diagnosis of nervous system disorders, 21 percent were symptoms and signs, 15 percent were musculoskeletal conditions, 8 percent were mental disorders, and 7 percent were injuries or poisonings. The National Ambulatory Care Survey of 1993 showed visits to neurologists increasing to 8,393,000 (1.2 percent of total visits), but there were 22,556,000 (3.1 percent) total visits of symptoms from the nervous system and 77,737,000 (10.8 percent) visits with a principal diagnosis of nervous system or sense organ disorders. Headache accounted for 10,736,000 visits (1.5 percent).[6]

The 1990–1992 National Health Interview Survey asked respondents about conditions causing the highest percentage of limitation of activity.[7] Neurological disorders reported were migraine headache (40.2/1,000 persons), other headache (40.2/1,000), cerebrovascular disease (12.1/1,000), mental retardation (6.3/1,000), epilepsy (5.0/1,000), impairment of sensation (4.6/1,000), and multiple sclerosis (0.7/1,000).

The magnitude of neurological disorders is wide ranging in incidence, prevalence, and mortality as well as across ages and etiologies. The remainder of the chapter describes several neurological disorders that are a public health problem and with some the etiology is yet to be identified.

Cerebral Palsy

Cerebral palsy (CP) is a group of nonprogressive motor impairment syndromes that arise during brain development and is recognized early in life as the child develops.[8] CP is classified based on the

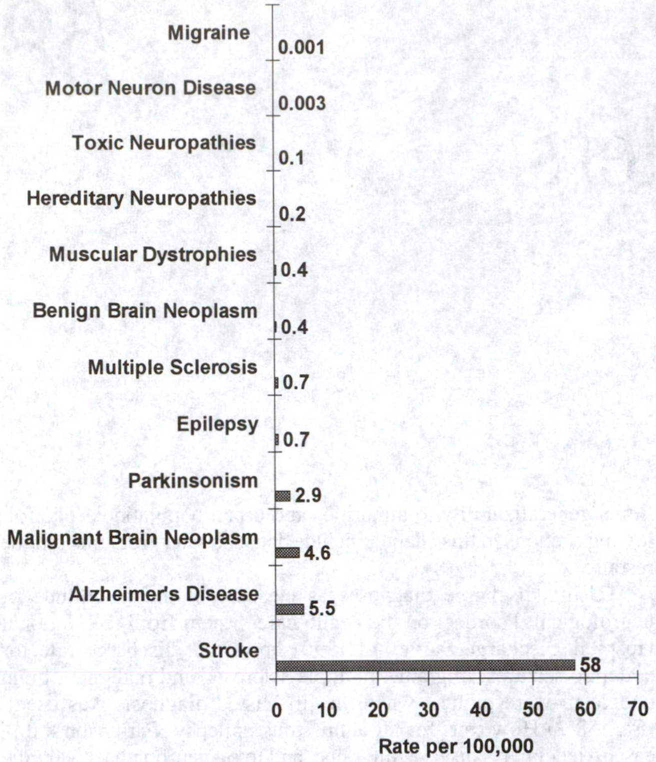

Figure 58-1. United States death rates for 1990 of selected neurological diseases. (From National Center for Health Statistics: Mortality, Part A. In: Vital Statistics of the United States, 1990. Bethesda, MD: US Department of Health and Human Services, 1990, vol 2.)

extremities involved and the neurological dysfunction (spastic, athetotic, hypotonic, dystonic, or combined). The most common form is spastic CP, which is present in about 80 percent of prevalent cases. The presence of other neurological disabilities, such as mental retardation, seizure disorders, and sensory problems, are more common in persons with CP. The Metropolitan Atlanta Developmental Disabilities Surveillance Program in 1991 found that 48 percent of 599 CP children in their study had vision impairment, 8 percent had hearing impairment, and 17 percent had mental retardation.[9]

Cerebral palsy occurs between 1.5 and 2.5 of every 1,000 live births. However, this rate depends on definition and inclusion based on impairment.[8] Because CP is developmental, it may present in a variety of forms and severities and may disappear with growth. Case ascertainment may require surveillance using multiple sources. The Disabilities Education Act allows surveillance through special education programs in school systems. In Atlanta over 90 percent of children with developmental disabilities could be identified through education sources.[9] Prevalence then may be a better measure than incidence. CP has been identified by early school age in 1.4 to 5.1 per 1,000 children. In Atlanta the prevalence rate was 2.4 per 1,000 in age 3 to 10 years, and the rate was lowest in the younger ages (2.0/1,000) for both disabling and nondisabling CP. There are slightly more males and blacks among affected persons in Atlanta. However, ethnicity is not consistently related to CP.

Data from several studies have demonstrated an increase in CP births due to an increase in low–birth weight infants, but there is some controversy on the impact on total CP incidence.[9–12]

Innate genetic factors may play a role in CP occurrence. Several studies have reported positive familial history and genetic risk in CP children. Twins are at higher risk but they share a common pregnancy and birthing process.[13] Other risk factors include maternal factors prior to pregnancy such as long menstrual cycles and a history of spontaneous abortions and stillbirths. Low socioeconomic status increases the risk of CP. During pregnancy, factors that may increase risk include hyperthyroidism, thyroid hormone drugs, and exogenous estrogen. An association with occurrence of other congenital malformations has also been observed.[9,10,14] Low–birth weight and immaturity at birth are among the most consistent risk factors for CP. Several factors may contribute to early delivery or low–birth weight. These include intrauterine infection and congenital malformations. Intracranial hemorrhage in premature infants is associated with CP. The increase in survival of infants with very low–birth weight has increased the causal distribution of CP. A study by Pharoah et al showed that low–birth weight infants account for nearly 50 percent of cases of CP.[10] Physical injury during the perinatal and postnatal period such as intrauterine exposure to heavy metals, neonatal hyperbilirubinemia, and exposure to benzyl alcohol may be related to CP occurrence.[15] Severe asphyxia at birth may account for about 10 percent of all CP.[16–18] Difficult birth is associated with increased risk of CP only among children who have neurological symptoms in the neonatal period. Postnatal causes of CP include neonatal encephalopathy, trauma, or occlusion of a cerebral artery or vein. These may account for 12 to 21 percent of cases.

Most of the risk factors for CP are before birth in the prenatal period. The decreased use of isoimmunization for Rh factors has been associated with a decrease of CP of the athetoid type. Improvements in obstetric and neonatal care and an increasing frequency of obstetric interventions have not been associated with a decrease in incidence of CP.[8,19,20] Recent studies have shown a possible protective effect of administration of magnesium sulfate preceding delivery for protection against cerebral hemorrhage and development of CP.[21] The paucity of information about causal factors for the majority of CP that is not attributable to birth events limits severely the development of strategies for prevention.

Human Immunodeficiency Virus Infection

Since 1981 when the human immunodeficiency virus (HIV) type 1 and the acquired immunodeficiency syndrome (AIDS) first appeared in the United States, the epidemic has increased to nearly a half million people.[22] Almost half have died from this devastating infection. HIV has manifestations in neurological disorders also. Neurological manifestations include HIV dementia, myelopathies, neuromuscular disorders, and CNS infections of cryptococcal meningitis, toxoplasmosis, progressive multifocal leukoencephalopathy, cytomegalovirus, *Myocabacterium tuberculosis*, neurosyphilis, and primary CNS lymphoma. Meningitis, neuropathy, and myopathy can occur before the AIDS-related complex is present. Dementia, myelopathies, and opportunistic infections are present as the disease progresses as AIDS.[23–25]

Estimates of incidence and prevalence of the neurological manifestation of HIV are problematic. Many of the studies are retrospective based on autopsy or clinical populations.[23] The estimates vary widely depending on the population and the definition used. Most often the diagnosis is based on clinical findings without verification. Some estimates are based on HIV-AIDS cohorts, but generalizability between locations and severity of illness is problematic.

HIV dementia is characterized by cognitive and memory impairment. It is associated with the onset of AIDS and it is estimated that approximately 3 percent of AIDS patients present with dementia as their first symptom. Its prevalence varies by type of study from 7 to 66 percent.[26–28] An estimate derived from Centers of Disease Control and Prevention (CDC) data is that 2.8 percent of AIDS cases have dementia.[26] The Multicenter AIDS Cohort Study found a 3.3 percent figure. They also found that after AIDS has developed there was a 7 percent incidence per year of dementia.[27] Factors associated with HIV dementia include lower CD4+ cell counts, anemia, low–body mass index, older age, and other systemic AIDS symptoms.[27] The proportion of AIDS cases with dementia has not changed, but there is some indication of improvement with zidovudine treatment.[29,30]

Inflammatory demyelinating polyneuropathies may occur either in acute or chronic form. The estimates are that from 0.5 to 3.0 percent of patients have these conditions.[23,31] Other neuropathies may occur.

TABLE 58-1. NUMBER OF DEATHS AND DEATH RATE OF NEUROLOGICAL DISORDERS IN U.S. POPULATION, 1990

ICD-9	Description	Number	Rate per 100,000
042	HIV	24,289	9.8
043.10	HIV causing diseases of CNS	90	0.036
191	Malignant neoplasm of brain	11,355	4.6
225	Benign neoplasm of brain to other parts of nervous system	896	0.4
225.2	Cerebral meninges	711	0.3
320	Bacterial meningitis	564	0.2
322	Meningitis of unspecified cause	453	0.2
323	Encephalitis, myelitis, and encephalomyelitis	272	0.2
331.0	Alzheimer's disease	13,744	5.5
331.4	Obstructive hydrocephalus	596	0.2
332	Parkinson's disease	7,254	2.9
333	Other extrapyramidal disease and abnormal movement disorders	654	0.3
340	Multiple sclerosis	1,647	0.7
342	Hemiplegia	157	0.1
343	Infantile cerebral palsy	773	0.3
344	Other paralytic syndromes	658	0.3
345	Epilepsy	1,627	0.7
346	Migraine	3	0.001
348.1	Anoxic brain damage	1,933	0.8
348.3	Encephalopathy, unspecified	480	0.2
349	Other and unspecified disorders of the nervous system	331	0.1
351	Facial nerve disorders	4	0.002
354	Mononeuritis of upper limb and mononeuritis multiplex	7	0.003
355	Mononeuritis of lower limb	46	0.02
356	Hereditary and idiopathic peripheral neuropathy	450	0.2
357	Inflammatory and toxic neuropathy	220	0.1
358	Myoneural disorders	407	0.2
359	Muscular dystrophies and other myopathies	918	0.4
430	Subarachnoid hemorrhage	6,815	2.7
431	Intracerebral hemorrhage	17,852	7.2
432	Other and unspecified intracranial hemorrhage	2,723	1.1
433	Occlusion and stenosis of precerebral arteries	1,256	0.5
434	Occlusion of cerebral arteries	18,912	7.6
435	Transient cerebral ischemia	336	0.1
436	Acute but ill-defined cerebrovascular disease	80,745	32.5
437	Other and ill-defined cerebrovascular disease	9,325	3.7
438	Late effects of cerebrovascular disease	6,124	2.5
721	Spondylosis and allied disorders	81	0.03
722	Intervertebral disc disorders	34	0.014
723	Other disorders of cervical region	11	0.004
724	Other and unspecified disorders of back	31	0.13
742	Other and congenital anomalies of nervous system	1,150	0.5
756	Other congenital musculoskeletal anomalies	633	0.3

Sensory neuropathy occurs in the later stages of HIV infection.[32] Toxic neuropathy associated with antiretroviral agents also occurs.[33,34] The manifestation of these disorders is severe pain and impaired walking ability. It is estimated from a clinical population that 13 percent of the patients may be affected. There appears to be an increasing prevalence of the neuropathies associated with HIV.

Opportunistic infections are a hallmark of AIDS progression. Infections can affect the central nervous system. Cryptoccocal meningitis is present in about 10 percent of AIDS cases and is associated with a drop in CD4+ count below 200 cells/mm^3.[35,36] A common cause of mass lesion abscesses is toxoplasmosis. The prevalence varies with location. CNS infection is a result of latent reactivation and may be inhibited by prophylactic treatment of pneumonia. CMV infection can lead to retinitis and encephalitis in patients with HIV.[37–39] CMV retinitis is common in patients with CMV infection, causing visual loss or blindness in 15 to 28 percent of AIDS patients. Encephalitis presents with confusion, disorientation, and memory loss and may occur in approximately 2 percent of AIDS patients. Primary CNS lymphoma is rare but has been increasing due to immunosuppression frequency.[40] Up to 3 percent of AIDS patients

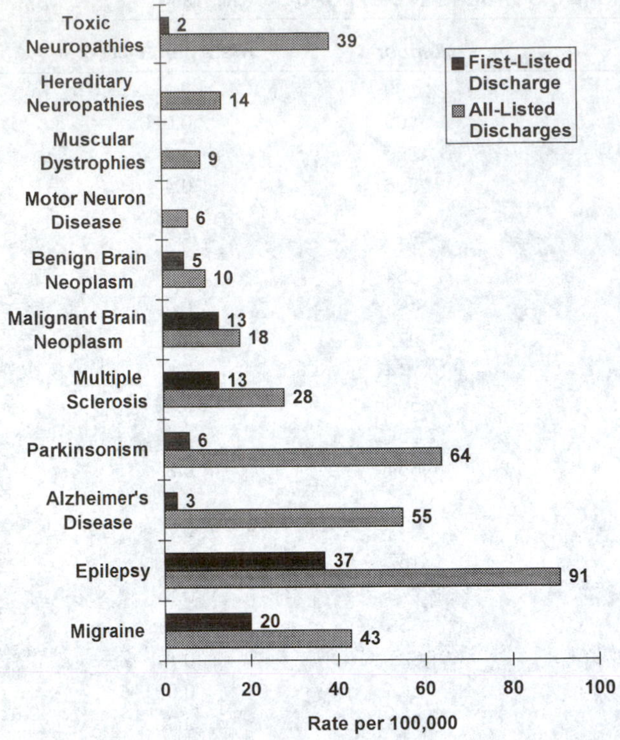

Figure 58-2. United States discharge rates from the National Hospital Discharge Survey of 1990 for selected neurological diseases. (From Graves EJ: Detailed Diagnoses and Procedures, National Hospital Discharge Survey, 1990. Data from the National Health Survey, Series 13, No. 113. Hyattsville, MD: National Center for Health Statistics, 1992.)

develop CNS lymphoma. Many of these patients are diagnosed at autopsy. Prior AIDS-related illness and low CD4+ count are linked to lymphoma occurrence.[41]

The public health burden of HIV and AIDS remains a challenge. With increasing survival the prevalence of HIV or AIDS neurologic conditions will increase.

Seizure Disorders

Seizures are an alteration in consciousness associated with an above-normal discharge of neurons of the brain. Seizures can be classified based on etiology as acute symptomatic (provoked) seizures and unprovoked seizures. Unprovoked, recurrent seizures are considered epilepsy. Seizures are classified by onset as simple or complex partial seizures or generalized major motor, absence, or myoclonic seizures. EEGs are used to verify the diagnosis and to determine the electrical activity pattern.[42–44]

Epilepsy occurs mostly in the young and the old. The overall incidence in the Rochester, Minnesota, population studies for 50 years was 44 per 100,000 persons.[45] All convulsive disorders had an incidence of 130 per 100,000 persons. The incidence of partial seizures cases was observed to be 25/100,000 and generalized onset to be 19/100,000. Generalized seizures are highest during the first year of life, decrease throughout childhood, and increase again in the elderly. Partial seizures have a relative constant rate up to age 65 and then increase sharply. For generalized seizures with onset in early life, females are at higher risk, and for later life seizures, males are at higher risk. For partial seizures, the rates are similar until age 65 at which age men are at higher risk. There has been a slight decrease in incidence of epilepsy over time but an increase in the elderly. The prevalence of epilepsy varies widely among populations from 27 to 40 per 1,000. In Rochester, the prevalence in 1980 was 6.8 per 1,000. Sixty percent are partial seizures and 75 percent are of unknown etiology. The prevalence in several studies is higher in blacks in the 20 to 66 year age range.[46]

A number of factors have been associated with epilepsy and are related to development of definable brain lesions. These include severe head injury, stroke, CNS infection, brain tumors, and CNS degenerative diseases.[47,48] Factors that are clearly casually related are associated at birth with brain development, such as mental retardation and cerebral palsy. Febrile seizures are related to increased seizure risk. These may occur in 2.3 to 4.7 percent of children. Other factors that have shown a relationship but without a direct causal pathway are drug abuse, e.g., heroin, and medical conditions such as asthma, hypertension, and depression. Suggested but unproven risk factors include prenatal or perinatal adverse events and immunizations. Positive family history has also been associated with development of epilepsy.

Seizure control can be obtained in a majority of patients. Recurrence rates show that 25 percent will suffer a recurrence in the 2 years following first seizure, but this rate varies by the presence of risk factors.

Headaches

Headache is the most common neurological disorder. Based on a telephone interview in a population-based study, 90 percent of men and 95 percent of women reported a headache in the last year. From 65 to 71 percent of women and 48 to 50 percent of men report one headache per month. Headache is one of the most common symptoms prompting people to seek medical care.[49,50] It is estimated that 5.5 million days of activity restriction can be attributed to headache each year by adults in the United States.[51,52]

Headaches may be primary or secondary to another disorder such as brain tumor, stroke, or vasculitis. Primary headaches can be classified into tension-type, migraine, and cluster. Diagnosis is based on clinical presentation. Classification criteria were established by the International Headache Society.[53,54] Distinguishing aspects of migraine include unilateral onset with associated anorexia and sometimes nausea and vomiting. The presence of a warning (aura) has also been described as a prodromal change in mood and is used as part of the diagnosis.

The incidence of migraine depends on gender, age, and type. The lifetime prevalence of migraine has been estimated to be 8 percent with women having a prevalence of 25 percent. A 1-year prevalence is 6 percent for men and 15 percent for women. In general, women have more migraine than men do, particularly with aura and occurring most frequently in young adult life. The incidence of migraine from the Rochester, Minnesota, population was 294 per 100,000 for women and 137 per 100,000 for men using data from 1979 to 1981. Between age 5 and puberty the incidence probably approximates 10 percent per year.[55] The incidence increases in females with the onset of menses. The peak age for women is between 20 and 24 years of age. The incidence returns to the male level about the age of 40. In both women and men, the incidence appears to decrease, beginning in the early forties. Prevalence of migraine headache may vary in populations and may be increasing. This may be due to varying definitions. Using the International Headache Society criteria, the prevalence of migraine in four population-based studies was from 13 to 15 percent in women and 4 to 6 percent in men.[56] Data from Rochester, Minnesota, showed an increase from 25.8/1,000 to 41/1,000 from 1981 to 1989 in both sexes combined.

While migraine was thought to occur more often in high socioeconomic groups, data from the American Migraine Society shows the opposite. Data also from the National Health Interview Survey showed also the low socioeconomic and middle socioeconomic groups may have similar rates. Rates of clinically diagnosed migraine may be higher due to higher rates of physician diagnosis in the high socioeconomic population.[52,57]

Migraine may have a familial component, but this may be over estimated due to biases in ascertainment.[49] The strongest evidence of a genetic association is from the higher concordance in monozygotic

TABLE 58-2. NATIONAL HOSPITAL DISCHARGE SURVEY, 1990

ICD-9	*Description*	*First Diagnosis (in thousands)*	*All Diagnosis (in thousands)*
042	HIV	19	93
191	Malignant neoplasm of brain	30	44
198.0	Secondary malignant neoplasm of other specified sites:		
198.3	Brain and spinal cord	32	78
225	Benign neoplasm of brain to other parts of nervous system	13	25
225.2	Benign neoplasm of cerebral meninges	8	17
320	Bacterial meningitis	11	16
322	Meningitis of unspecified cause	7	14
323	Encephalitis, myelitis, and encephalomyelitis	5	10
331.0	Alzheimer's disease	7	138
331.4	Obstructive hydrocephalus	6	30
332	Parkinson's disease	14	159
333	Other extrapyramidal disease and abnormal movement disorders	10	40
340	Multiple sclerosis	32	71
342	Hemiplegia	20	340
343	Infantile cerebral palsy	<5	44
344	Other paralytic syndromes	14	147
345	Epilepsy	92	228
346	Migraine	50	107
348.1	Anoxic brain damage	6	39
348.3	Encephalopathy, unspecified	10	44
349	Other and unspecified disorders of the nervous system	15	52
351	Facial nerve disorders	6	23
353	Nerve root and plexus disorders	10	16
354	Mononeuritis of upper limb and mononeuritis multiplex	31	59
354.0	Carpal tunnel syndrome	20	40
354.2	Lesion of ulnar nerve	7	10
355	Mononeuritis of lower limb	11	35
356	Hereditary and idiopathic peripheral neuropathy	<5	34
357	Inflammatory and toxic neuropathy	6	98
358	Myoneural disorders	<5	15
359	Muscular dystrophies and other myopathies	<5	22
430	Subarachnoid hemorrhage	20	25
431	Intracerebral hemorrhage	59	71
432	Other and unspecified intracranial hemorrhage	15	23
433	Occlusion and stenosis of precerebral arteries	86	210
434	Occlusion of cerebral arteries	240	316
435	Transient cerebral ischemia	165	245
436	Acute but ill-defined cerebrovascular disease	163	229
437	Other and ill-defined cerebrovascular disease	45	174
438	Late effects of cerebrovascular disease	18	354
721	Spondylosis and allied disorders	61	218
722	Intervertebral disc disorders	425	552
723	Other disorders of cervical region	31	61
724	Other and unspecified disorders of back	163	349
742	Other and congenital anomalies of nervous system	7	31
756	Other congenital musculoskeletal anomalies	11	39
800	Fracture of vault of skull	13	17
801	Fracture of base of skull	21	30
803	Other and unqualified skull fractures	6	8
805	Fracture of vertebral column without spinal cord injury	72	117
806	Fracture of vertebral column with spinal cord injury	7	10
847	Sprains and strains of joints and adjacent muscles	40	96
850	Concussion	83	122

(continued)

TABLE 58-2. (CON'TINUED)

ICD-9	Description	First Diagnosis (in thousands)	All Diagnosis (in thousands)
851	Cerebral laceration and contusion	12	19
852	Subarachnoid, subdural, and extradural hemorrhage, following injury	20	28
853	Other and unspecified intracranial hemorrhage following injury	5	8
854	Intracranial injury of other and unspecified nature	64	87
320–326	Inflammatory diseases	30*	45
330–337	Hereditary and degenerative diseases	59*	509
340–349	Other disorders	250*	1119
350–359	Disorders of peripheral nervous system	64*	300

* Grouped categories

than in dizygotic twins. If genetic factors contribute to a person's propensity to migraine, then other factors, usually exogenous, are likely to play an important role in determining the occurrence and frequency. Risk factors for headache onset in women are related to menstrual flow or the use of oral contraceptives. Other factors include ingestion of some foods (those with tyramine, including chocolate and aged cheeses) or alcoholic beverages (red wines, particularly). Psychosocial characteristics appear to be associated with headache occurrence. These include characteristics of perfectionism, inflexibility, and hypochondriasis, as well as propensity to anxiety and depression. Stress and psychosocial events may be important. The consequences of migraine are not viewed as life threatening, but migraine may be associated with hypertension, atherosclerotic heart disease, and stroke.[58]

In contrast to migraine are cluster headaches, which occur in groups most often in the spring and fall. These occur more in men than in women. Onset is also in midlife but later than migraine. The incidence is 15.6/100,000 for men and 4.0/100,000 for women.[59] Smoking may be associated with cluster headaches but personality characteristics may play a role. Cluster headache occurrence appears to be related to peptic ulcer occurrence as well as cancer-related deaths.

The cost of headaches is enormous. The restricted activity and disability, the use of medications, and the number of physician visits for diagnosis and treatment is large. The annual productivity lost for migraine alone is estimated at $1 billion per year.[60]

Multiple Sclerosis

Multiple sclerosis (MS) is one of the demyelinating diseases and is characterized by white matter lesions.[61] Classification of MS is dependent on clinical criteria that feature multiple lesions in the CNS separated in multiple locations and symptomatic attacks. Clinical presentation occurs in midlife and is highly variable. Symptoms include sensory, visual, and motor dysfunction. The disease is generally progressive and is characterized by clinical remissions and exacerbations.

Onset of multiple sclerosis occurs between ages 15 and 65 years. The median ages at onset for cases identified in Rochester, Minnesota, were 34 years for men and 32 years for women.[62] Incidence was 7.7 per 100,000 for women and 3.4 per 100,000 for men. Multiple sclerosis shows a north-south geographical distribution. Another disease, which had a differential geographic pattern, was poliomyelitis. However, with MS the Northern Hemisphere has distinct high-risk zones. Prevalence increases as latitude increases. This has been observed in the United States and Europe. High-risk areas have prevalence rates of multiple sclerosis of greater than 50 per 100,000; low-risk areas have less than 5 per 100,000.

Studies among migrants suggest that persons who move from an area of high prevalence to one of low prevalence take on the risk level of their new environment. The country (latitude) and the age of migration appear to an important determinant in MS risk.[63,64] Migration before the early adolescence (before age of 15) shifts the risk to the new country. With migration after 15 years, the individual has the risk of the former country. Kurtzke in studies of the Faroe Islands felt that a minimum exposure time of 2 years was necessary to confer susceptibility.[65–67]

After 50 years of studying MS the cause is still unknown. The hypothesis is that gene and environmental factors are necessary for MS occurrence. Ethnic background may play a role since the highest rates are in areas populated by those with a northern European/Scandinavian background. Clusters and epidemics of multiple sclerosis have been reported. Clusters have been reported in Canada, Norway, and Florida. Epidemics have occurred in the Faroe Islands and in Iceland.[65–67] No cases of MS were apparent before 1945. Since then cases have been reported with peaks in 1945, 1955, and 1965.

Infectious agents have been studied extensively, but no single agent has yet been identified. Measles virus and canine distemper virus have received the most attention. Case-control studies have demonstrated a relationship of dog ownership. Infection may also be related to immunologic change to increase susceptibility. Ecological studies have shown associations with low temperature, plants, soil, industrialization, meat consumption, type of meats, and dairy foods. Other factors also that have been investigated with conflicting results include trauma and exposure to trace elements and heavy metals, such as zinc and lead. A possible role for genetic factors in the etiology of multiple sclerosis has also been investigated. Caucasians of European descent are at highest risk. There has been familial aggregation of MS reported in several studies.[68] Familial aggregation may be due to shared environment or genetic susceptibility. Twin studies have generally found a greater concordance for multiple sclerosis among monozygotic twins than among dizygotic twins. The risk to family members is low, with 4 percent for siblings and 2 to 4 percent for children, depending on gender. Since northern Europeans have a higher frequency of HLA-DR2, haplotype studies of human lymphocyte antigens (HLA) in MS have been inconclusive possibly due to methodological errors.[69] Further candidate genes still are being evaluated.

The incidence of MS may be increasing as reported in Rochester, Minnesota.[62] Changes in diagnostic studies may lead to improved ascertainment but few longitudinal, population-based databases exist.

Survival is longer for women than for men. Approximately 75 percent of MS persons will survive 25 years or more. The rate of progression and disability is variable. Many patients even with progression remain ambulatory for many years. There is currently no definitive therapy for multiple sclerosis that affects the ultimate course of the disease, but steroid or ACTH therapy is used for acute exacerbations. β-Interferon and azathioprine may be helpful in preventing relapses, but data on rate of progression are inconclusive.

Myasthenia Gravis

Myasthenia gravis, a disorder at the neuromuscular junction, is a neurological disease with progressive muscle weakness with worsening at activity. The clinical presentation is varied with involvement of ocular muscles in the majority of cases. Diagnosis is based on clinical symptoms, electromyography, and measurement of circulating acetylcholine receptor (AChR) activity.[70,71]

Mortality rates and incidence rates increase with age and are consistently higher for males. Mortality rates are higher in whites in the United States, but prevalence rates in Virginia were higher in blacks.[72] Case ascertainment and misdiagnosis may explain these differences. Incidence rates of myasthenia gravis are between 2 and 6 per million. There has been an increase in incidence if all studies are considered, but no trend has been observed in Norway.[73] Improved diagnosis and case finding may explain this discrepancy and the increase. Prevalence also shows an increase to nearly 60 per million population. Prolonged survival may account as well as increasing incidence for this change.[74]

Risk factors may include autoimmune disease, genetic predisposition due to a positive familial association, and viral etiology.[75] No conclusive studies have demonstrated a cause. Further case-control studies are needed. Early identification and treatment by anticholinesterase drug therapy or thymectomy may improve the course but further studies are needed.

Stroke

Cerebrovascular disease, or stroke, is a major cause of death and disability. Stroke is the third leading cause of death and ranks eleventh in disabling conditions that restrict activity. The major types of stroke are cerebral thrombosis, cerebral embolism, intracerebral hemorrhage, and subarachnoid hemorrhage. Thromboembolic, ischemic stroke accounts for nearly 80 percent of all strokes. Hemorrhagic stroke has a different epidemiology and prognosis than ischemic stroke. Distinguishing among subtypes requires neurologic examination and use of neuroimaging of computerized tomography and magnetic resonance imaging.

Mortality from stroke varies by country, with the highest rates reported for Japan and the lowest rates for Switzerland and Canada.[76] Change has occurred in stroke occurrence in most countries with the exception of eastern Europe. There are also marked differences in stroke mortality between whites and blacks in the United States.[77] Overall death rates are approximately twice as high in blacks as in whites.

As has been observed for diseases of the heart, there has been a striking decline in mortality rates for stroke in the past several decades. Reductions in mortality rates have been observed for both sexes and all race groups. The decline has been attributed primarily to a decreasing incidence of stroke due to efforts to control hypertension and, to a lesser extent, to a reduction in case fatality.[78,79]

Data from the Rochester Epidemiology Project have shown that the incidence rates of stroke in 1985 to 1989 are lower than in the 1950s and 1960s but stabilized over the last two decades.[79] The incidence rate for 1985 to 1989 was 145 per 100,000. A higher incidence was observed for men than women (174 versus 122) but overall more women than men had stroke. Stroke subtype specific incidence rates were 120 per 100,000 for cerebral infarction, 15.5 per 100,000 for intracerebral hemorrhage, and 7.5 per 100,000 for subarachnoid hemorrhage.

The primary prevention of stroke is through control of hypertension. Hypertension is the major risk factor for ischemic stroke and intracerebral hemorrhage. Studies have shown a consistent reduction in stroke occurrence with blood pressure control and most recently for the elderly.[80–82] Other risk factors for ischemic stroke include diabetes mellitus, transient ischemic attacks, and cardiac disease.[83] In contrast diabetes mellitus and cholesterol level are not associated with increased risk of hemorrhagic stroke. Migraine headaches may be associated with stroke. A case-control study indicated that women under the age of 45 had 4.3-fold increased risk with migraine.[84] In the Physicians Health Study the relative risk for migraine and ischemic stroke in all participants was 2.0.[85] Cigarette smoking has been associated in some studies with risk of both ischemic and hemorrhagic stroke.[85] It may be the leading risk factor for cerebral aneurysms and subarchnoid hemorrhage. Data from the Nurses Health Study suggest that smoking cessation can reduce the risk of stroke.[87] The role of alcohol consumption in increasing risk of stroke is less certain and may vary by type of stroke.[88] One study in women found that moderate consumption of alcohol was associated with a lower risk of ischemic strokes but with an increased risk of subarachnoid hemorrhage.[89,90] The role of binge drinking and stroke has also been demonstrated. Drugs of abuse, particularly stimulants and diet pills, have been associated with stroke occurrence.

Secondary prevention of stroke through antiplatelet therapy (aspirin and ticlopidine) in patients with transient ischemic attacks and minor strokes has been shown to be effective in prevention of recurrent events and severe strokes.[91,92] Treatment of patients with nonvalvular atrial fibrillation with aspirin or warfarin has been shown also to prevent ischemic stroke occurrence.[93] In patients who have major stenosis or occlusion of the carotid arteries also there is benefit from surgical carotid endarterectomy in prevention of future stroke events.[94–96] For tertiary prevention the use of thrombolytic therapy has been shown to be effective in decreasing the disability from stroke if administered within 3 hours of onset.[97,98] Several clinical trials of neuroprotective agents are under way.

Parkinson's Disease

Parkinson's disease is a progressive neurological disorder with bradykinesia, resting tremor, rigidity, and postural reflex. The disorder is due to progressive loss of pigmented neurons associated with loss of dopamine. The onset is insidious, progression tends to be gradual, and the course of the disease is usually prolonged. Diagnosis is based on clinical criteria, which has changed over time due to changes in clinical practice. Misdiagnosis with depression and multiple system involvement leads to variable case determination. Parkinson's disease may occur with dementia in 10 to 25 percent of cases.[99]

Incidence rates for Parkinson's disease are varied and reported to range from 4 to 20 per 100,000. In Rochester, Minnesota, the incidence was 20.5 per 100,000, and in a study in northern Manhattan the rate was 13 per 100,000.[100,101] The incidence rates increase with age with the highest rates in 70- to 79-year-olds. Prevalence of Parkinson's disease has varied widely with the range from 31.4 to 347 per 100,000.[102] Differences in case ascertainment using clinical, drug usage, and survey data may account for this variation. There has been little change in the age-adjusted incidence in Parkinson's disease over time, but with increasing age and survival the number of affected individuals is likely to increase.

Parkinsonism may be a direct result from exposure to toxins (e.g., carbon monoxide or manganese), drugs (e.g., phenothiazides), traumatic or vascular lesions of the brain, or tumors. Arteriosclerosis, when present, is most likely a concurrent disease rather than a subtype of parkinsonism. Postencephalitic parkinsonism is well recognized but accounts for a relatively small and decreasing proportion of all prevalent cases. However, the majority of cases are of unknown cause. The cause of most cases of Parkinson's disease remains obscure. Age is a known risk factor because the occurrence is dependent upon loss of neurons, which indicates a chronic onset. Whether or not men or women are at greater risk is difficult to establish. Population studies have suggested that men are at higher risk, but the prevalence may be higher in women due to their longer survival.

The debate of genetic predisposition versus environmental exposure is unresolved. Several studies of familial aggregation suggest that a positive family history of Parkinson's disease is present from 16 to 41 percent of idiopathic cases. However, twin studies do not show a relationship with clinical Parkinson's disease or f-dopa uptake analysis.[103]

Environmental exposures are suggested by variation in the geographic distribution of the disease and by associations from analytical studies.[104] Parkinson's disease is more common in Europe and North America.[102] In population studies the rates are higher for whites and Hispanics than for blacks. However, a door-to-door survey in Copiah County, Mississippi, found no difference in rates.[105] Ethnic differences in the clinical manifestations of Parkinson's disease or in diagnosis rates may explain some of this situation.

Etiological studies using a variety of case ascertainment methods have suggested that rural residence, farming, well water drinking, and herbicide/pesticide exposure are related to Parkinson's disease.[104] Infectious agents have been evaluated, particularly focusing on the epidemic of 1918. However, no agents or relationship has been found. Coronavirus titers have been found to be elevated in Parkinson's patients who may indicate an animal exposure. Other factors that have been suggested but unproven include head trauma and emotional stress.[105,106] Recent studies suggest that diet may be important. Animal fat and protein intake may increase risk. Antioxidants have demonstrated inconsistent results as a protective factor.[107,108] Numerous studies have reported a lower risk of Parkinson's disease among cigarette smokers. Various explanations for this observation have been proposed, but whether the inverse association between cigarette smoking and risk of Parkinson's disease has biological significance or behavioral relationship remains controversial.[102,109] The observation that drug abusers exposed to the meperidine derivative MPTP sometimes have a syndrome clinically indistinguishable from advanced Parkinson's disease, as well as subsequent studies using animal models of MPTP toxicity, supports the hypothesis that environmental exposures may be important in causing Parkinson's disease.[110,111]

Parkinson's disease remains an increasing problem with the advancing age of the population. The disease leads to progressive disability. Agents have demonstrated efficacy in limiting the symptoms and disability. The etiology still has yet to be determined.

Dementias

Dementia is a relatively heterogeneous clinical syndrome characterized by a decline in memory and other cognitive functions such as reasoning, judgment, calculation, abstraction, and language. In addition to the decline in cognitive abilities, there are clear decrements in everyday functioning such as activities of daily living and social activities. The diagnosis of dementia requires that there be no coexisting disturbances of consciousness[112] or any other acute conditions or situations that preclude clinical or psychological evaluation of cognitive performance. There is no universal agreement on the criteria for the dementia syndrome, but several useful published criteria exist in the *International Classification of Diseases* and elsewhere.[112–114] The dementia syndrome has many known causes, including a variety of concurrent nonneurologic diseases, medications, and toxic environmental exposures;[115] some dementia patients with defined environmental or anatomic causes have syndromes that are at least partially reversible. However, it is generally felt that over half of clinical dementia cases are due to Alzheimer's disease (AD), with the next most common being related to cerebrovascular disease and Parkinson's disease.[115] Human immunodeficiency virus is neurotropic,[116] and an AIDS-related dementia syndrome has been identified as the most common neurologic complication of this disease. However, AIDS is associated with increased risk of other important central nervous system conditions, some of which may have dementia-like clinical features, and the differential diagnostic possibilities must be kept in mind.[117]

The epidemiology of the dementias and AD suggests that they are an important and growing public health problem, particularly among older persons. While community surveys of the prevalence and incidence of dementia and AD can be methodologically challenging, it appears that the prevalence of dementia in persons 85 years and older and residing in the community may be as high as 40 to 50 percent.[118,119] Accurate geographically based prevalence and incidence surveys of dementia surveys are sometimes hampered by several factors, including frequent supervening of substantial clinical illness, the refusal or inability of demented patients to participate in surveys, and the increased likelihood that dementia patients will be institutionalized. Nonetheless, the general magnitude of the problem is understood. Less well-studied but of clear importance is the epidemiology of cognitive decline and impairment before achieving the "case" stage.[120] Attention to environmental and host factors associated with cognitive change could lead to enhanced quality of life and improved function.

Because it is the most common form of dementia, AD has received substantial attention in terms of etiology, pathogenesis, and prevention. As dementia in general, AD increases in incidence with increasing age among older persons.[121,122] In addition, several putative risk factors for AD have been identified, such as prior head trauma and aluminum exposure, but few have received consensual agreement as to being true causes, and no known risk factors could yet form a specific prevention strategy.[123] Recent interest in the possible preventive effects of exogenous estrogen use[124] and the discovery of genetic factors in both familial and nonfamilial AD[125] are examples of how progress in prevention is possible. However, in general, there seems to be little evidence at this time for suggesting routine universal screening of ostensibly normal persons for the possibility of dementia or AD,[126] as proven, effective interventions are not yet available.

Conclusion

The incidence of neurological conditions has remained constant for most disorders while the prevalence appears to be increasing due to aging of the population and longer survival. This has profound impact on the magnitude of disability and impairment in the population. As yet, there are many neurological conditions for which early detection and prevention are not justified or possible.

▶ REFERENCES

1. National Center for Health Statistics: Mortality, Part A. In: Vital Statistics of the United States, 1990. Bethesda, MD: US Department of Health and Human Services, 1990, vol 2
2. Kurland LT, Brian DD: Contributions to Neurology from Records Linkage in Olmsted County, Minnesota. In Schoenberg BS (ed): Advances in Neurology. New York: Raven Press, 1978, vol 19
3. Melton LJ: History of the Rochester Epidemiology Project. Mayo Clin Proc 71:266–274, 1996
4. Graves EJ: Detailed Diagnoses and Procedures, National Hospital Discharge Survey, 1990. Data from the National Health Survey, Series 13, No. 113. Hyattsville, MD: National Center for Health Statistics, 1992
5. Schappert SM: Office visits to neurologists: United States, 1991–1992. Advance Data from Vital and Health Statistics, No. 267. Hyattsville, MD: National Center for Health Statistics, 1995
6. Wodwell DA, Schappert SM: National Ambulatory Medical Care Survey: 1993 summary. Advance Data from Vital and Health Statistics, No. 270. Hyattsville, MD: National Center for Health Statistics, 1995
7. Collins JG: Prevalence of selected chronic conditions, United States, 1990–92. Advance Data from Vital and Health Statistics, No. 194. Hyattsville, MD: National Center for Health Statistics, 1997
8. Kubak KCK, Leviton A: Cerebral palsy. N Engl J Med 330:188–195, 1994
9. Boyle CA, Yeargin-Allsopp M, Doernberg NS, et al: Prevalence of selected developmental disabilities in children 3–10 years of age: the Metropolitan Atlanta Developmental Disabilities Surveillance Program, 1991. MMWR 45(SS-2); 1–14, 1996
10. Pharoah POD, Cooke T, Rosenblood I, Cooke RWI: Trends in the birth prevalence of cerebral palsy. Arch Dis Child 62:379–389, 1987
11. Pharoah PO, Platt MJ, Cooke T: The changing epidemiology of cerebral palsy. Arch Dis Child 75(3):F169–F173, 1996
12. Meberg A, Broch H: A changing pattern of cerebral palsy. Declining trend for incidence of cerebral palsy in the 20-year period 1970–1989. J Perinat Med 23(5):395–402, 1995
13. Nelson KB, Ellenberg JH: Childhood neurological disorders in twins. Paediatric and Perinatal Epidemiology 9:135–145; 1995

14. Grether JK, Cummins SK, Nelson KB: The California Cerebral Palsy Project. Paediatr Perinat Epidemiol 6:339–351, 1992
15. Benda GI, Hiller JL, Reynolds JW: Benzyl alcohol toxicity: impact on neurologic handicaps among surviving very low birth weight infants. Pediatrics 77:507–512, 1986
16. Nelson KB, Ellenberg JH: Antecedents of cerebral palsy: multivariate analysis of risk. N Engl J Med 315:81–86, 1986
17. Blair E, Stanley FJ: Intrapartum asphyxia: a rare cause of cerebral palsy. J Pediatr 122:575–579, 1988
18. Nelson KB, Ellenberg JH: Antecedents of cerebral palsy: univariate analysis of risks. Am J Dis Child 139:1031–1038, 1985
19. Stanley JK, Watson L: The cerebral palsies in Western Australia: trends, 1968 to 1981. Am J Obstet Gynecol 158:89–93, 1988
20. Emond A, Golding J, Peckham C: Cerebral palsy in two national cohort studies. Arch Dis Child 64:848–852, 1989
21. Nelson KB, Grether JK: Can magnesium sulfate reduce the risk of cerebral palsy in very low birth weight infants? Pediatrics 95:263–269, 1995
22. Centers for Disease Control and Prevention: US HIV and AIDS reported through December 1994. HIV/AIDS Surveillance Report 6:1–9, 1994
23. Dal Pan GJ, McArthur JC: Neuroepidemiology of HIV Infection. Neurol Clin 14:359–381, 1996
24. Johnson RT, McArthur JC, Narayan O: The neurobiology of human immunodeficiency virus infection. FASEB J 2:2970–2981, 1988
25. McArthur JC: Neurologic manifestations of AIDS. Medicine (Baltimore) 66:407–437, 1987
26. Janssen RS, Nwanyanwu, Selik RM, et al: Epidemiology of human immunodeficiency virus encephalopathy in the United States. Neurology 42:1742–1746, 1992
27. McArthur JC, Hoover DR, Bacellar H, et al: Dementia in AIDS patients: incidence and risk factors. Neurology 43:2245–2253, 1993
28. Navia BA, Jordon BD, Price RW: The AIDS dementia complex. I. Clinical features. Ann Neurol 19:517–524, 1986
29. Arendt G, Hefter, Buescher L, et al: Improvement of motor performance of HIV-positive patients under AZT therapy. Neurology 42:891–895, 1992
30. Pizzo PA, Eddy J, Falloon J, et al: Effect on continuous intravenous infusion of zidovudine (AZT) in children with symptomatic HIV infection. N Engl J Med 319:889–896, 1988
31. Fuller GN, Jacobs JM, Guilloff RJ: Nature and incidence of peripheral nerve syndromes in HIV infection. J Neurol Neurosurg Psychiatry 56:372–381, 1993
32. Cornbalth DR, McArthur JC: Predominantly sensory neuropathy in patients with AIDS and AIDS-related complex. Neurology 38:794–796, 1988
33. Blum A, Dal Pan G, Raines C, et al: ddC-related toxic neuropathy: risk factors and natural history Neurology 4(Suppl 2):A190, 1993
34. Lambert JS, Seidlin M, Reichman RC, et al: 2′,3′-dideoxyinosine (dI) in patients with the acquired immunodeficiency syndrome or AIDS-related complex: a phase I trial. N Engl J Med 322:1333–1340, 1990
35. Chuck SL, Sande MA: Infections from cryptococcus neoformans in acquired immunodeficiency syndrome. N Engl J Med 321:794–799, 1989
36. Larsen RA, Leal MA, Chan LS: Fluconazole compared with amphotericin B plus flucytosine for cryptococcal meningitis in AIDS: a randomized trial. Ann Intern Med 113:183–197, 1990
37. Jabs DA, Green WR, Fox R, et al: Ocular manifestations of acquired immunodeficiency syndrome. Ophthalmology 96:1092–1099, 1989
38. Degans J, Portegies P: Neurological complications of infection with human immunodeficiency virus type 1: a review of literature and 241 cases. Clin Neurol Neurosurg 91:199–219, 1989
39. Guiloff RJ, Fuller GN, Roberts A, et al: Nature, incidence and prognosis of neurological involvement in the acquired immunodeficiency syndrome in central London. Postgrad Med J 64:919–925, 1988
40. Eby NL, Grufferman S, Flannelly CM, et al: Increasing incidence of primary brain lymphoma in the U.S. Cancer 62:2461–2465, 1988
41. Rosenbloom ML, Levy RM, Bredesen DE, et al: Primary central nervous system lymphomas in patients with AIDS. Ann Neurol 23:S13–S16, 1988
42. Commission on Classification and Terminology of the International League Against Epilepsy: A revised proposal for the classification of epilepsy and epileptic syndromes. Epilepsia 30:268–278, 1989
43. Commission on Epidemiology and Prognosis, International League Against Epilepsy: Guidelines for epidemiologic studies on epilepsy. Epilepsia 34:592–596, 1993
44. Commission on Classification and Terminology of the International League Against Epilepsy: A proposal for revised clinical and electroencephalographic classification of epileptic seizures. Epilepsia 22:489–501, 1981
45. Hauser WA, Annegers JF, Rocca WA: Descriptive epidemiology of epilepsy: contributions of population-based studies from Rochester, Minnesota. Mayo Clin Proc 71:576–586, 1996
46. Haerer AF, Anderson DW, Schoenberg BS: Prevalence and clinical features of epilepsy in a biracial United States population. Epilepsia 27:66–75, 1986
47. Hauser WA: Epidemiology of epilepsy. In Gorelick PB, Alter M (eds): Handbook of Neuroepidemiology. New York: Marcel Dekker, 1994, pp 315–356
48. Annegers JF, Rocca WA, Hauser WA: Causes of epilepsy: contributions of the Rochester Epidemiology Project. Mayo Clin Proc 71:570–575, 1996
49. Silberstein SD, Lipton RB: Headache epidemiology. Emphasis on migraine. Neurol Clin 14:421–434, 1996
50. Leviton A: Epidemiology of headache. Adv Neurol 19:341–353, 1978
51. National Center for Health Statistics: Advance data. Vital and Health Statistics, No. 53. Hyattsville, MD: National Center for Health Statistics, 1979
52. Stang PE, Osterhaus JT: Impact of migraine in the United States: data from the National Health Interview Survey. Headache 33: 29–35, 1993
53. International Headache Society: Classification and diagnostic criteria for headache disorders, cranial neuralgias, and facial pain. Cephalalgia 8:1, 1988
54. Olesen J, Lipton RB: Migraine classification and diagnosis: International Headache Society criteria. Neurology 44(Suppl 4):S6–S10, 1994
55. Stang PE, Yanagihara T, Swanson JW, et al: Incidence of migraine headache: a population-based study in Olmsted County, Minnesota. Neurology 42:1657–1662, 1992
56. Stewart WF, Shechter A, Rasmussen BK: Migraine prevalence. A review of population-based studies. Neurology 44(Suppl 4): S17–S23, 1994
57. Lipton RB, Stewart WF: Migraine in the United States: a review of use. Neurology 43(Suppl 3): 6–10, 1993
58. Couch JR, Hassanein RS: Headache as a risk factor in atherosclerosis-related diseases. Headache 29:49–54, 1989
59. Swanson JW, Yanagihara T, Stang PE, et al: Incidence of cluster headaches: a population-based study in Olmsted County, Minnesota. Neurology 44:433–437, 1994
60. Osterhaus JT, Gutterrnan DL, Plachetka JR: Healthcare resources and lost labor costs of migraine headaches in the U.S. Pharmacoeconomics 2:67, 1992
61. McFarlin DE, McFarland HF: Multiple sclerosis. Parts I and 2. N Engl J Med 307:1183–1188, 1246–1251, 1982
62. Wynn DR, Rodriguez M, O'Fallon WM, Kurland LT: A reappraisal of the epidemiology of multiple sclerosis in Olmsted County, Minnesota. Neurology 40:780–786, 1990
63. Alter M, Leibowitz U, Speer J: Risk of multiple sclerosis related to age of immigration to Israel. Arch Neurol 15:234–237, 1966

64. Dean G: Annual incidence, prevalence and mortality of multiple sclerosis in white South African-born and in white immigrants to South Africa. Br Med J 2:724–730, 1967
65. Kurtzke JF, Hyllested K: Multiple sclerosis in the Faroe Islands I. Clinical and epidemiological features. Ann Neurol 5:6–21, 1979
66. Kurtzke JF, Hyllested K: Multiple sclerosis in the Faroe Islands II. Clinical update, transmission, and the nature of MS. Neurology 36:307–328, 1985
67. Kurtzke JF, Hyllested K: Multiple sclerosis in the Faroe Islands III. An alternative assessment of the three epidemics. Acta Neurol Scand 76:317–339, 1987
68. Weinshenker BG: Epidemiology of multiple sclerosis. Neurol Clin 14:291–308, 1996
69. Poser CM: The epidemiology of multiple sclerosis: a general overview. Ann Neurol 36(S2):S180–S193, 1994
70. Osserman KE, Kaplan LI. Rapid diagnostic test for myasthenia gravis: increased muscle strength without fasciculations, after intravenous administration of edrophonium (Tensilon) chloride. JAMA 150:265, 1958
71. Lindstrom JM, Seybold ME, Lennon VA, Whittingham S, Duane DO: Antibody to acetylcholine receptor in myasthenia gravis prevalence, clinical correlates, and diagnostic value. Neurology 26:1054–1059, 1976
72. Phillips LH, Torner JC, Anderson MS: The epidemiology of myasthenia gravis in Central and Western Virginia. Neurology 42:1088–1093, 1992
73. Storm-Mathisen A: Epidemiology of myasthenia gravis in Norway. Acta Neurol Scand 70:274–84, 1984
74. Phillips LH, Torner JC: Epidemiologic evidence for a changing natural history of myasthenia gravis. Neurology 47:1233–1238, 1996
75. Treves TA, Rocca WA, Meneghini F: Epidemiology of myasthenia gravis. In Anderson DW (ed): Neuroepidemiology: A Tribute to Bruce Schoenberg. Boca Raton, FL: CRC Press, 1991, pp 297–309
76. Bonita R, Beaglehole R: Stroke mortality: In JP Whisnant (ed): Stroke: Populations, Cohorts, and Clinical Trials, Oxford: Butterworth-Heinemann, 1993, pp 59–79
77. American Heart Association: Heart and Stroke Facts. 1995 Statistical Supplement. Dallas: American Heart Association, 1995, pp 11–12
78. Broderick JP, Phillips SJ, Whisnant JP, et al: Incidence rates of stroke in the eighties: the decline in stroke. Stroke 20:577–582, 1989
79. Brown RD, Whisnant JP, Sicks JD, et al: Stroke incidence, prevalence, and survival: secular trends in Rochester, Minnesota, through 1989. Stroke 27:373–380, 1996
80. Collins R, Peto R, MacMahon S, et al: Blood pressure, stroke, and coronary heart disease. Part 2, Short-term reductions in blood pressure: overview of randomized drug trials in their epidemiological context. Lancet 335:827–838, 1990
81. SHEP Cooperative Research Group: Prevention of stroke by antihypertensive drug treatment in older persons with isolated hypertension: final results of the Systolic Hypertension in Elderly Program (SHEP). JAMA 265:3255–3264, 1991
82. Meissner 1, Whisnant JP, Garraway WM: Hypertension management and stroke recurrence in a community (Rochester, Minnesota, 1950–79). Stroke 19:459–463, 1988
83. Dyken ML: Stroke risk factors. In Norris JW, Hachinski VC (eds): Prevention of Stroke. New York: Springer-Verlag, 1991, pp 83–102
84. Tzourio C, Iglesias S, Hubert JB, et al: Migraine and risk of ischaemic stroke: a case-control study. Br Med J 307:289–292, 1993
85. Buring JE, Hebert P, Romero J, et al: Migraine and subsequent risk of stroke in the Physicians' Health Study. Arch Neurol 52:129–134, 1995
86. Shinton R, Beevers G: Meta-analysis of relation between cigarette smoking and stroke. Br Med J 25:298:784–794, 1989
87. Kawachi I, Colditz GA, Stampfer MJ, et al: Smoking cessation and decreased risk of stroke in women. JAMA 269:232–236, 1993
88. Stampfer MJ, Colditz GA, Willet WC, Spaizer FE, Hennekens CH: A prospective study of moderate alcohol consumption and the risk of coronary disease and stroke in women. N Engl J Med 319: 267–273, 1988
89. Longstreth WT Jr, Koepsell TD, Yerby MS, et al: Cigarette smoking, alcohol use, and subarachnoid hemorrhage. Stroke 23:1242–1249, 1992
90. Torner JC: Epidemiology of subarachnoid hemorrhage. Semin Neurol 4:354–369, 1984
91. Antiplatelet Trialists' Collaboration: Collaborative overview of randomized trials of antiplatelet treatment. Part I: Prevention of death, myocardial infarction, and stroke. By prolonged antiplatelet therapy in various categories of patients. BMJ 304:81–106, 1994
92. Hass WK, Easton JD, Adams HP Jr, et al for the Ticlopidine Aspirin Stroke Study Group: A randomized trial comparing ticlopidine hydrochloride with aspirin for the prevention of stroke in high-risk patients. N Engl J Med 321:501–507, 1989
93. Stroke Prevention in Atrial Fibrillation Investigators: Stroke Prevention in Atrial Fibrillation Study—final results. Circulation 84:527–539, 1991
94. North American Symptomatic Carotid Endarterectomy Trial Collaborators: Beneficial effect of carotid endarterectomy in symptomatic patients with high-grade stenosis. N Engl J Med 325:445–453, 1991
95. Executive Committee for the Asymptomatic Carotid Atherosclerosis Study: Endarterectomy for asymptomatic carotid artery stenosis. JAMA 273:1421–1428, 1995
96. Moore WS, Barnett HJ, Beebe HG, et al: Guidelines for carotid endarterectomy. A multidisciplinary consensus statement from the ad hoc committee, American Heart Association. Stroke 26:188–201, 1995
97. The National Institute of Neurological Disorders and Stroke rt-PA Stroke Study Group: Tissue plasminogen activator for acute ischemic stroke. N Engl J Med 333:1581–1587, 1995
98. Adams HP, Brott TG, Furlan AJ, et al: Guidelines for thrombolytic therapy for acute stroke: a supplement to the guidelines for the management of patients with acute ischemic stroke. Circulation 94:1167–1174, 1996
99. Aarsland D, Tandberg E, Larsen JP, Cummings JL: Frequency of dementia in Parkinson's disease. Arch Neurol 53:538–542, 1996
100. Mayeux R, Marder K, Cote L, et al: The frequency of idiopathic Parkinson's disease by age, ethinic group and sex in northern Manhattan, 1988–1993. Am J Epidemiol 142:820–827, 1995
101. Rajput AH, Offord KP, Beard CM, et al: A case-control study of smoking habits, dementia, and other illnesses in idiopathic Parkinson's disease. Neurology 37:226–232, 1987
102. Tanner CM, Goldman SM: Epidemiology of Parkinson's disease. Neurol Clin 14:317–335, 1996
103. Tanner CM, Chen B, Wang WZ, Peng ML, Liu ZL, Liang XL, Kao LC, Gilley DW, Schoenberg BS: Environmental factors in the etiology of Parkinson's disease. Can J Neurol Sci 14:419–423, 1987
104. Bharucha NE, Stokes L, Schoenberg BS, et al: A case-control study of twin pairs discordant for Parkinson's disease: a search for environmental risk factors. Neurology 36:284–288, 1986
105. Piccini P, Burn D, Sawle G et al: Dopaminergic function in relatives of Parkinson's disease patients: a clinical and PET study. Neurology 45(Suppl 4):A203, 1995
106. Goetz CG, Stebbins GT: Effects of head trauma from motor vehicle accidents on Parkinson's disease. Ann Neurol 29:191–193, 1991
107. Logroscino G, Marder K, Cote L, et al: Dietary lipids and antioxidants in Parkinson's disease: a population-based, case-control study. Neurology 39:89–94, 1996

108. Fahn S, Cohen G: The oxidant stress hypothesis in Parkinson's disease: evidence supporting it. Ann Neurol 32:804–812, 1992
109. Mayeux R, Tang MX, Marder K, et al: Smoking and Parkinson's disease. Mov Disord 9:207–212, 1994
110. Le Witt PA: Clinical trials of neuroprotection in Parkinson's disease: long-term selegiline and alpha-tocopherol treatment. J Neural Transm Suppl 43:171–181, 1994
111. Kopin IJ, Markey SP: MPTP toxicity: implications for research in Parkinson's disease. Annu Rev Neurosci 11:81–96, 1988
112. McKhann G, Drachman D, Folstein M, Katzman R, Price D, Stadlan EM: Clinical diagnosis of Alzheimer's disease: report of the NINCDS-ADRDA Work Group. Neurology 34:939–944, 1984
113. National Institutes of Health Consensus Development Conference: Differential diagnoses of dementing diseases. JAMA 258:3411–3419, 1987
114. American Psychiatric Association: Diagnostic and Statistical Manual of Mental Disorders. 4th ed. Washington, DC: American Psychiatric Association, 1994
115. Larson EB, Kukull WA, Katzman RA: Cognitive impairment: dementia and Alzheimer's disease. Annu Rev Public Health 13:431–449, 1992
116. Oster S, Christoffersen P, Gundersen HJ, Nielsen JO, Pedersen C, Pakkenberg B: Six billion neurons lost in AIDS. A stereologic study of the neocortex. APMIS 103:525–529, 1995
117. Simpson DM, Tagliati M: Neurologic manifestations of HIV infection. Ann Intern Med 121:769–785, 1994
118. Jorm AF, Korten AE, Henderson AS: The prevalence of dementia, a quantitative integration of the literature. Acta Psychiatr Scand 76:456–479, 1987
119. Bachman DL, Wolf PA Linn R, et al: Prevalence of dementia and probable senile dementia of the Alzheimer type in the Framingham study. Neurology 42:115–119, 1992
120. Colsher P, Wallace RB: Epidemiologic in studies of cognitive function in the elderly: methodology and non-dementing acquired dysfunction. Epidemiol Rev 13:1–27, 1991
121. Evans DA, Funkenstein HH, Alberts, M, et al: Prevalence of Alzheimer's disease in community population of older persons. JAMA 262:2551–2556, 1989
122. Evans DA: Estimated prevalence of Alzheimer's disease in the United States. Milbank Q 68:267–279, 1990
123. Larson EB, Kukull WA: Prevention of Alzheimer's disease—a perspective based on successes in the prevention of other chronic diseases. Alzheimer Dis Assoc Disord 10(Suppl):9–12, 1996
124. Tang MX, Jacobs D, Stern Y, et al: Effect of oestrogen during menopause on risk and age at onset of Alzheimer's disease. Lancet 348:429–432, 1996
125. Rao VS, Cupples LA, Vanduijn CM, et al: Evidence for major gene inheritance of Alzheimer disease in families with and without apolipoprotein E Epsilon-4. Am J Hum Genet 59:664–675, 1996
126. U.S. Preventive Services Task Force: Guide to Clinical Preventive Services. 2nd ed. Baltimore: Williams & Wilkins, 1996

59

Disabling Visual Disorders

Dawn M. Oh • Kean T. Oh

Although the prevalence of blindness worldwide is not precisely known, conservative estimates from 1990 World Health Organization (WHO) data report at least 38 million blind people in the world. This figure is based on the standard international definition of blindness: a visual acuity of less than 3/60 or corresponding visual field loss in the better eye with best possible correction. This high frequency of blindness also corresponds to loss in disability-adjusted life years. The causes of blindness and visual loss, most preventable through primary intervention or secondary therapy, include a small core of major diseases including: cataract, glaucoma, diabetic retinopathy, macular degeneration, trachoma, onchocerciasis, and xerophthalmia (Fig. 59-1). However the fraction of the blindness burden for each disease differs from region to region.

The total disease burden of blindness also varies geographically (Fig. 59-2) with the largest impact occurring in regions least able to afford the loss in human resources or address economic costs of treatment; e.g., of the 13.5 million unoperated cases of cataract in the world, greater than 95 percent are found in developing countries. Age is the primary risk factor associated with most blinding disorders, regardless of etiology (Fig. 59-3). The vast majority (88.8 percent) of the blindness in people over 60 is also found in the developing countries of the world, even though the overall populations of these countries are younger. This age-related distribution has been further deepened by an aging world population.

Other visual disorders, while not major causes of blindness worldwide, represent significant medical cost, and, without treatment, significant loss of daily life functions, as in the case of uncorrected refractive error. Another area of public health interest among the less-blinding disorders is international emphasis on screening children for amblyopia, treatable only in childhood. Furthermore, minor visual complications may characterize populations at increased risk for developing blinding visual diseases; e.g., myopics are at increased risk for retinal detachments and glaucoma.

Major recent research has provided new insights into causes, risk factors, and treatments of most visual disorders. This research reinforces the need for multidisciplinary, and often development-oriented, consideration and intervention in the area of visual health. The need for sufficient and appropriate data to make such policy decisions has generated new methodologies for measurement, such as WHO programs that use a standardized method of low-cost, small-scale field surveys to provide more reliable blindness data than were previously available. These new research approaches are even more crucial as more diseases are found to have multifactoral causes, and the traditional areas of public health interest, such as health behavior patterns (smoking and cataracts or age-related macular degeneration (AMD)), nutrition (vitamin A and xerophthalmia, antioxidants and AMD), and education (trachoma and public health education), are drawn into the circle of causation for blinding disorders.

This chapter reviews the major causes of blindness in the world, defines additional visual disorders, and finally, reviews historically relevant examples of the interaction of technology and public health intervention.

Cataract

Unoperated cataract is the main cause (estimated 16 million cases) of visual loss globally.[1] Primarily a disease of aging, cataract describes the opacification of the lens of the eye. This gradually blinding process is associated in its most common form ("senile cataracts") with an increase in the weight and thickness of the lens and a decrease in accommodation as new layers of cortical fibers are laid down, hardening the lens nucleus. While not subject to primary prevention in most cases, effective surgery for the removal of the lens and its replacement have been developed and refined. The most desirable treatment is now phacoemulsification of the lens. The international lack of access to trained ophthalmologists and issues of surgical cost, however, leave the statistics of blindness from cataract high, despite this effective treatment.

Outside of the primary risk factor of age, some environmental, physical, and nutritional risks have also been associated with earlier onset or progression of cataracts. These include: exposure to UV-B light, diabetes, high blood pressure, corticosteroid therapy, smoking, protein energy malnutrition, and dehydration.[2] These last two risk factors may indicate an antioxidant relationship with cataracts and suggest that studies in antioxidants may implicate dietary protective factors. Cataracts secondary to high-grade myopia or glaucoma surgery have also been reported in the literature.

Current international focus is on the development of low-cost intraocular lenses, sutures, and other equipment used in cataract surgery, as well as the training of human resources for surgery in many of the world's least developed countries, which carry high disease burdens. Regular ophthalmologic examinations are also encouraged for proper identification of cataracts and eventual surgery.

Glaucoma

With an estimated disease burden of 67 million cases expected worldwide by the year 2000, primary glaucoma is currently responsible for at least 5.2 million blind people (15 percent of the total world blindness burden).[3] The total numbers affected by glaucoma are evenly split between primary angle closure glaucoma (PACG) and primary open angle glaucoma (POAG). The overwhelming majority of cases of PACG are in Asia and Asian-descent populations, while POAG is distributed evenly throughout the world. The rate of occult glaucoma is roughly equal to that of detected disease even in developed nations, making it a further public health challenge.

Like cataract and AMD, glaucoma is predominantly a disease of aging, with prevalence rates increasing dramatically over the age of 65, with especial public health implications as populations age. There has been considerable change in the understanding of POAG in recent

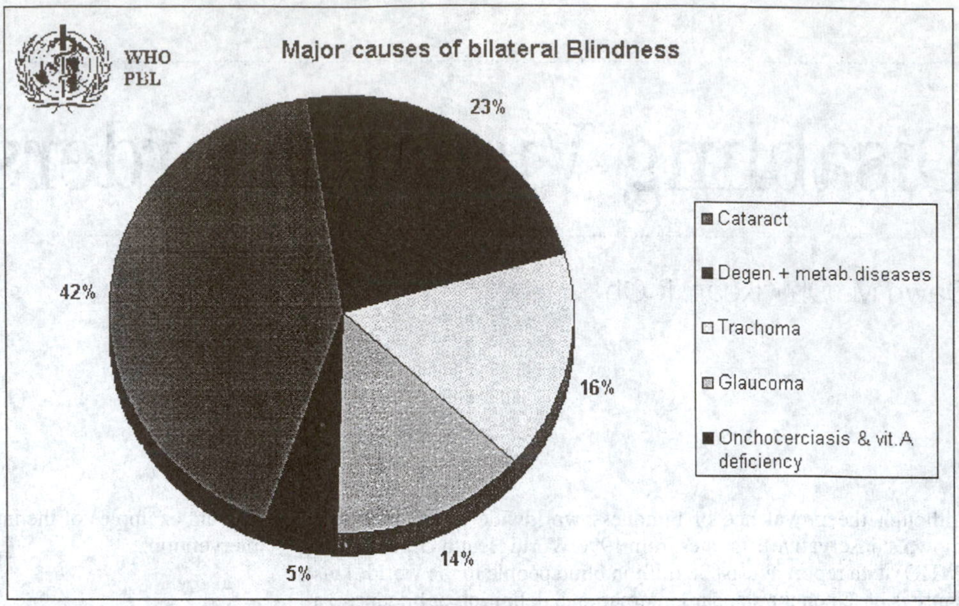

Figure 59-1. Causes of blindness. (From Thylefors B et al: Global data on blindness. Bull World Health Organ 73(1):115–121, 1995.)

years.[4] Previously elevated intraocular pressure (IOP) was considered the cause and part of the definitive diagnosis of the disease, but it is now known that elevated IOP (ocular hypertension) may be associated with as little as 10 percent of POAG. The characteristic visual field loss that describes glaucoma has remained constant, however, for over a century, with progressive damage of optic nerve fibers causing a loss of vision from peripheral to central vision in a spiraling pattern. This damage is related to changes in vascular perfusion of the optic nerve head and is worsened by elevated IOP. Progression of the disease can be prevented in many cases by trabeculectomy or topical drug treatments, which lower IOP. However, often patients do not present for treatment until substantial permanent visual loss has already occurred. Clearly glaucoma is a prime target for early intervention measures; unfortunately, making an early diagnosis is problematic, especially when characteristic field loss, often not noticeable until 80 percent or more of the optic nerve is permanently damaged, is now considered the definitive diagnostic tool. Other measurements of optic nerve head signs, such as cup-to-disc ratios, cup asymmetry, and splinter hemorrhages, although useful supplemental information, lack both sensitivity and specificity.

While epidemiologic studies of POAG are limited by their differing disease definitions, small sample sizes, and questionable sampling methods, they suggest a number of risk factors for the development of POAG, with or without elevated IOP (sometimes called "normal or low-tension glaucoma"). Age is the most constant risk factor, with the incidence over 60 years being 7 times that of the under 40 age group. Race is another factor, with the risk for blacks shown to be 4 times greater than that for whites in both the United States and United Kingdom, and with most glaucoma in blacks occurring at a younger age. Family history of glaucoma is also a risk factor, with approximately 13 to 26 percent of cases having a genetic component. Other putative risk factors include diabetes (via increased IOP); myopia; hypertension; inconsistent associations with modifiable risk factors including smoking and an atherosclerotic diet; and protective effects from vitamin B_{12}, ω-3 fatty acid, magnesium, and exercise. Glaucoma is a serious public health challenge, as efforts center on

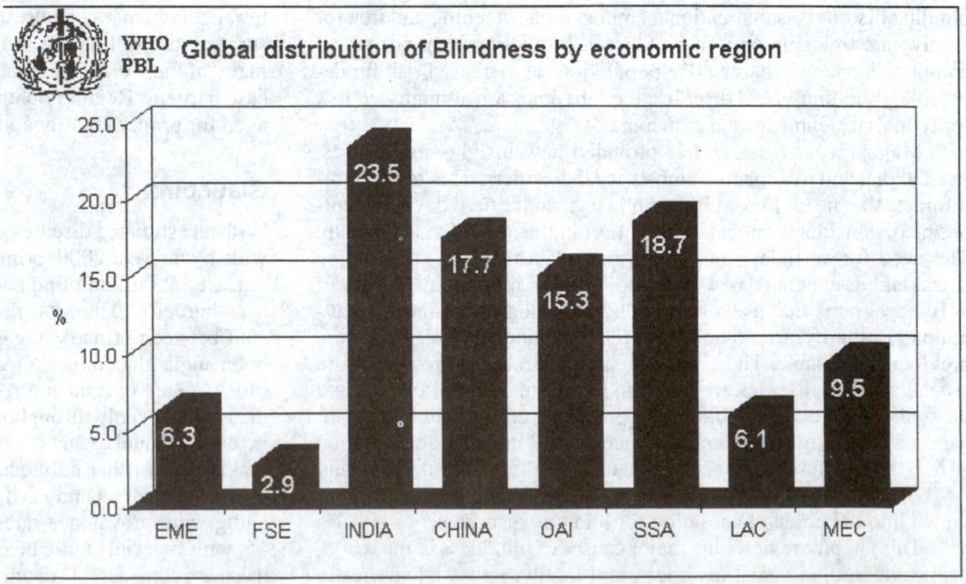

Figure 59-2. Geography of blindness. (From Thylefors B et al: Global data on blindness. Bull World Health Organ 73(1):115–121, 1995.)

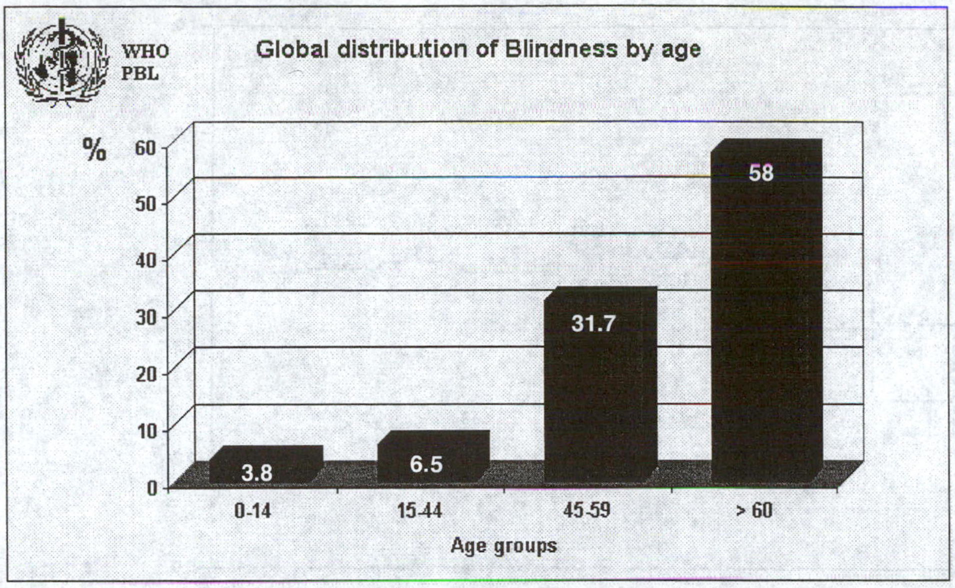

Figure 59-3. Age and blindness. (From Thylefors B et al: Global data on blindness. Bull World Health Organ 73(1):115–121, 1995.)

identifying causes that may help prevent the disease as well as developing more useful screening techniques, especially for international field work.

Macular Degenerations and Dystrophies

A wide spectrum of macular disease contributes significantly to blindness in the United States and worldwide, encompassing known hereditary dystrophies and acquired disorders such as presumed ocular histoplasmosis syndrome. For other degenerations, such as age-related macular degeneration, the etiology, although probably multifactorial, remains enigmatic. Without accurate understanding of the disease process, primary intervention may be misguided and ineffective.

Recent progress in molecular genetics has allowed many hereditary macular dystrophies to be mapped, and in some instances, the specific gene causing the disease has been defined. While little may be offered from a curative standpoint to patients with hereditary dystrophies such as Best's disease or X-linked retinoschisis, primary intervention may take the form of genetic counseling for involved families.

Age-Related Macular Degeneration

AMD is the leading cause of blindness for people older than 65 years in the United States and Europe. AMD is best defined as diffuse morphologic changes at the level of the retinal pigment epithelium (RPE), shown to be associated with a reduction in visual acuity.[5] AMD is divided morphologically into *dry* or *atrophic, nonexudative* AMD and *wet* or *exudative* AMD. Although no incidence rates are available for AMD, studies in the U.S. population have reported prevalences ranging from 6.4 to 16 percent in the elderly and rates of nearly 20 percent in the oldest old.[5,6] It is believed that the number of AMD cases in the United States will be 7.5 million by the year 2030, up from 2.7 million in 1973.[6]

Despite this high prevalence, the pathophysiology of macular degeneration is poorly understood. Proposed mechanisms have included oxidant stress and atherosclerosis[7,8] with reported risk factors including age,[2] sex, family history, iris color,[4] cardiovascular disease,[3] body mass index,[9] smoking,[10] light exposure, and nutritional deficiency in antioxidants and zinc. Primary prevention once included wearing UV blocking sunglasses, but recent studies have not shown any correlation between light exposure and AMD prevalence.[11,12] Earlier recommendations for the use of supplemental antioxidants and zinc are also equivocal. Current studies show only weak protective effects of zinc and no correlation between dietary carotenoids or tocopherols and AMD.[13] Thus, recommendations now include increasing dietary forms of antioxidants (e.g., green leafy vegetables) but not the use of supplements.[14] Mounting evidence suggests that dietary and environmental risk factors associated with atherosclerosis and high body mass index, such as smoking and dietary fat, also carry increased risk for AMD. Thus, dietary modification and smoking cessation may be a strategy for primary prevention of AMD.

The only means of treatment of AMD at this time is photocoagulation of choroidal neovascular membranes, which occur in exudative AMD and are the primary cause for decreased vision in these patients. The Macular Photocoagulation Study (MPS), a multicenter trial examining photocoagulation treatment efficacy,[15–17] has shown that the 10 percent of patients with wet AMD who are seen in time for macular photocoagulation treatment according to its protocols[18] have a better visual prognosis than those with untreated AMD. Nevertheless, the overall visual prognosis for both treated and nontreated patients is not promising. (Fig. 59-4) Treated eyes remain at high risk for persistence or recurrence of choroidal neovascularization, mostly in the direction of central vision. Unfortunately, no proven form of treatment is currently available for individuals with the dry, atrophic form of AMD, who represent over 90 percent of all AMD cases.

Presumed Ocular Histoplasmosis Syndrome (POHS)

POHS is defined by a characteristic clinical appearance of atrophic chorioretinal scars in the periphery of the fundus ("histo spots"), peripapillary atrophy, and macular choroidal neovascularization (CNV). This disorder is characterized in the United States by a characteristic geographic distribution: the Ohio and Mississippi River valleys. Patients are younger than individuals with AMD (median age of 30 to 40 years) and have a high prevalence of histoplasmin skin sensitivity. Annual incidence rates for POHS-associated macular CNV have been predicted between 2.0 to 12.0 percent in endemic areas. Patients with characteristic histo spots within the macula are at high risk for the eventual development of CNV, which in turn is the cause of vision loss in POHS. Patients with histo spots warrant screening for early detection of CNV. The MPS also examined the treatment of choroidal neovascularization in POHS, demonstrating that patients treated with photocoagulation had better long-term visual prognosis than patients without treatment. Furthermore, because CNV develops in younger people with healthier overall retinal pigment epithelium, subfoveal surgery for removal of CNV has been shown to be an effective means of treatment, though this mode of therapy is still undergoing debate and development. Ideally, primary prevention would involve control of exposure to *Histoplasma capsulatum*, but the ubiquity of this organism in the endemic region precludes effective exposure control

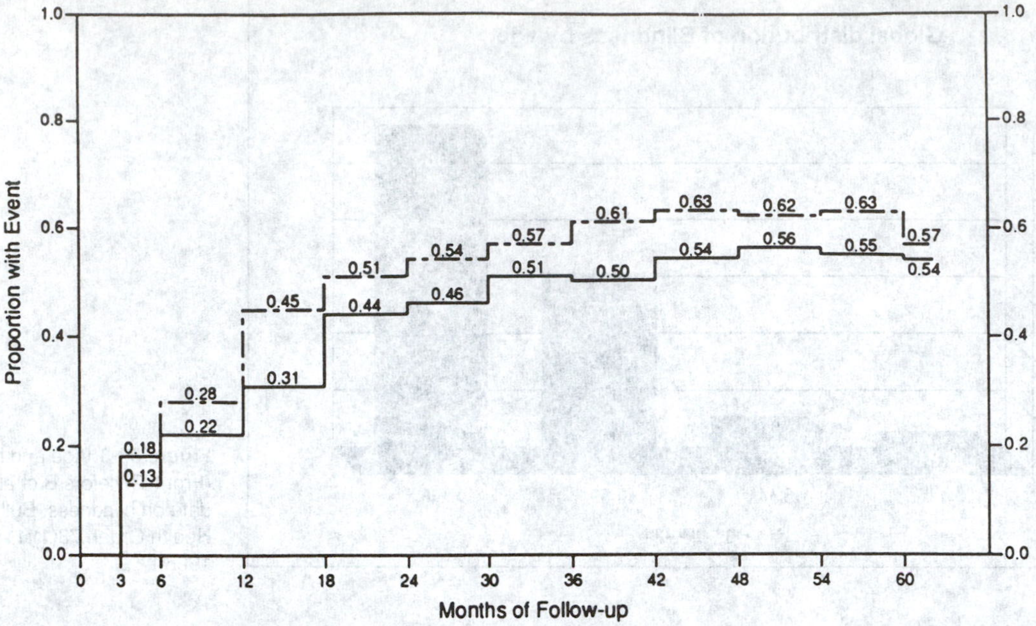

Figure 59-4. Mean change in lines of visual acuity from baseline at each specified time. *Broken line* indicates no-treatment group; *solid line*, treatment group. All eyes had juxtafoveal CMV secondary to age-related macular degeneration at time zero. (From Macular Photocoagulation Study Group: Krypton laser photocoagulation for neovascular lesions of age-related macular degeneration. Results of a randomized clinical trial. Arch Ophthalmol 108:816–824, 1990. Copyright 1990, American Medical Association.)

measures. Thus, major preventive issues involve screening and following patients known to have this condition for the development of choroidal neovascularization.

Retinal Vascular Disease

Diabetic retinopathy is the leading cause of blindness in the United States among individuals 20 to 74 years old, accounting for 12 percent of all new cases of blindness each year. This retinal vascular disease causes visual morbidity through the proliferation of neovascular fronds and the development of macular edema. There are roughly 700,000 Americans with proliferative retinopathy and more than 500,000 with macular edema.[19]

Primary prevention of diabetic retinopathy is based on good diabetic and hypertensive control. The Diabetes Control and Complication Trial (DCCT) demonstrated a 60 percent reduction in the risk of retinopathy with intensive control (versus standard treatment) of insulin-dependent diabetes mellitus (IDDM). After 3.5 years, the risk of progression was more than five times lower with intensive control.[20] Although the intensive treatment of hyperglycemia is impractical from a compliance standpoint in average patients, the results of the DCCT indicate that careful control of blood sugars in all diabetics will retard the onset of diabetic retinopathy. Screening for the presence of diabetic retinopathy is a very important first step to secondary management, and guidelines have been established for both IDDM and non-insulin–dependent diabetes mellitus (NIDDM) patients. Treatment of diabetic retinopathy has been guided by a series of well-designed multicenter trials. Initial studies demonstrated that panretinal photocoagulation reduced the risk of severe visual loss by greater than 50 percent over no treatment.[21] Later multicenter trials established firm definitions and guidelines for the treatment of clinically significant diabetic macular edema. Focal photocoagulation reduced visual loss from diabetic macular edema by about 50 percent as well.[22]

The second most common retinal vascular disease involves *retinal vein occlusion.* Risk factors for retinal vein occlusion include hypertension, cardiovascular disease, diabetes mellitus, increasing age, and glaucoma.[23] Branch retinal vein occlusion (BRVO) causes decreased vision primarily by cystoid macular edema, neovascularization, and ischemia. Focal photocoagulation for macular edema resulted in 65 percent gains in visual acuity among treated patients. Scatter laser photocoagulation was found to lower the risk of vitreous hemorrhage following the development of neovascularization.[24,25] Central retinal vein occlusion, however, did not demonstrate any visual improvement in macular edema following focal photocoagulation, though panretinal photocoagulation was an effective means of treatment for iris and angle neovascularization following an ischemic CRVO.

Retinal vascular disease is a common cause of visual morbidity in the U.S. and worldwide. Because risk factors involve systemic disease, prevention of major retinal vascular disease involves control of these systemic diseases. Large multicenter trials have studied and established the management of these diseases following their development.

Trachoma

Responsible for 15 percent of world blindness, trachoma, unlike the above visual disorders, is an infectious disease, concentrated in poor and rural areas of the world.[26] *Chlamydia trachomatis*, the causative microorganism, and eye-seeking flies, the vector of transmission, are endemic in Central America, Brazil, Africa, the Eastern Mediterranean, and several Asian nations. *C. trachomatis* causes an inflammation in the eye, resulting in the formation of follicles in the conjunctiva which scar the eyelid until it turns inwards with the lashes rubbing the eye, gradually leading to blindness. This process can be halted at the primary level by the improvement of living standards and hygiene in endemic areas, as proper face-washing with clean water is protective. This control may be supplemented by the new availability of the long-acting azithromycin as an effective but extremely expensive treatment and by surgery on underturned lids to prevent progression to blindness. Limited success after 50 years of global public health efforts to eradicate trachoma has emphasized that, without improvement in the sanitation, water, population densities, economies, and attention to literacy and cultural appropriateness in public education programs, no secondary interventions will be successful in completely controlling the disease.

Onchocerciasis

In endemic regions of Africa, the Arabian peninsula, and the Americas, onchocerciasis, or "river blindness," is the second leading infectious cause of blindness. Of the 18 million people currently infected, approximately 99 percent are in Africa, with blindness occurring in 270,000 persons. While the dermatologic effects of onchocerciasis are more common among the infected (6 million people), the blindness is nevertheless an important issue in visual health. The disease, caused by the parasite *Onchocerca volvulus*, is spread through the black fly population in endemic areas, and the intensity of infection is the best indicator of risk for developing blindness. Unfortunately, onchocerciasis is a public health example where development projects have assisted in the proliferation of the disease by increasing vector breeding sites (near fast-flowing rivers or streams). Current international efforts at eradication are focused on both controlling the vector and the use of a recently developed suppressive drug, ivermectin, which is being distributed with WHO efforts. Based on past experience with problems of access, understanding of the disease, and cultural appropriateness of development projects, these efforts are now targeted at developing local initiatives and community-based prevention plans.

Xerophthalmia

The leading cause of blindness in children worldwide is now blinding malnutrition, also known as xerophthalmia, with 70 percent of the 500,000 new cases annually of childhood blindness resulting from vitamin A deficiency. An additional 14 million children currently show signs of clinical xerophthalmia, from eye dryness to ulceration. In this case, the micronutrient deficiency leads to irreversible blindness in the young. Current recommendations include exclusive breastfeeding for the first 4 to 6 months of life and complementing diets with food items high in vitamin A. Preventive interventions include programs to distribute high doses of vitamin A to infants and children in areas with high rates of micronutrient deficiency. In the case of xerophthalmia, the nutritional deficiency leading to blindness also represents an increased risk for other childhood illnesses and mortality.

AIDS and the Eye

AIDS is an increasing world health problem, and more than 200,000 individuals are affected by it in the United States. Because of its overall increasing prevalence, it has also become a significant cause of visual morbidity. Between 40 and 70 percent of all AIDS patients exhibit ocular disease, and postmortem examinations have found evidence of ocular disease in greater than 95 percent of cases.[27,28] AIDS may involve the eye directly by causing a microangiopathy, characterized by the presence of cotton wool spots, or by opportunistic infection, or neoplastic and neuro-ophthalmologic manifestations. Anterior segment manifestations include common diseases, such as molluscum contagiosum, as well as rare diseases, such as microsporadal keratitis and Kaposi's sarcoma. The most common posterior segment opportunistic infection is cytomegalovirus (CMV) retinitis. It affects between 5 and 40 percent of AIDS patients. CMV rarely causes retinal disease unless the CD4 count falls below 50 cells/mm^3. Initially, CMV retinitis may be asymptomatic or present with trivial symptoms. Hence, screening this population is important to identify patients requiring initiation of therapy. Current antivirals for CMV have been shown in the studies for ocular complications of AIDS (SOCA) to prolong the life of AIDS patients. As AIDS patients survive longer with treatment, the incidence of CMV-associated retinal detachments has subsequently risen. Currently, the incidence of CMV retinitis–associated retinal detachment is 24 percent at 1 year. Hence patients diagnosed with AIDS require regular ophthalmologic screening to allow early initiation of therapy for CMV retinitis. Following diagnosis and therapy, the patient should be co-managed by an ophthalmologist for monitoring the disease course and to watch for retinal detachment.

Retinopathy of Prematurity

Retinopathy of prematurity (ROP) is a multifactorial disorder of premature infants that affects 1,300 children each year.[29,30] Between 85 and 90 percent of low–birth weight children exposed to oxygen will demonstrate some evidence of ROP, though relatively few infants suffer severe visual impairment.[1,2,31] It is estimated that only 6 percent of infants reach a stage of ROP requiring treatment.[32] Time of oxygen exposure and to a lesser degree oxygen concentration, low–birth weight, and short gestation are key risk factors for the development of ROP. Exposure to high concentrations of oxygen interferes with the process of retinal vascularization in premature infants. Consequently, neovascularization, vitreous hemorrhage, and tractional retinal detachment by fibrovascular proliferation results in visual morbidity.[33,34] It was previously felt that careful management of arterial oxygen could prevent the onset of ROP, but increased ability of neonatologists to keep smaller, more premature infants alive has resulted in a resurgence of ROP in spite of careful oxygen control. It is now evident that ROP is driven by multiple factors in addition to oxygen exposure.

Because of the high incidence of ROP in low–birth weight infants, careful screening is an important step in the management of this disease. Current recommendations call for infants below 1,500 g birth weight to be carefully screened at specific intervals. Cryotherapy for patients who reach a well-described threshold stage has reduced the risk for retinal detachment in these infants by 50 percent.[4] For patients who develop subtotal retinal detachments, scleral buckling surgery has a high rate of success. Without this surgery, 85 percent of patients will progress slowly. Once total retinal detachments develop, they are often complicated and require extensive surgical intervention.[4]

Thus, advances in neonatology have resulted in an increased incidence of ROP in spite of careful oxygen management. Primary prevention of ROP must address means of reducing premature and low–birth weight infants. Studies have examined vitamin E as a prevention strategy for ROP, but this supplementation has been shown to only possibly reduce the severity of disease. Once ROP is identified, however, management guidelines allow prevention of visual morbidity in the majority of infants.

Other Visual Problems

Although we have considered the most common blinding disorders, the most common ocular complaint is loss of sight due to refractive error. In the case of myopics, this means that distant objects are focused anterior to the retina because of a longer eye and cannot be seen clearly. In contrast, hyperopics have a shorter eye where focus falls behind the retina, making closer objects difficult to view. Finally, presbyopia is a loss of accommodative functioning, where the eye cannot adjust to bring near objects into focus; this accommodative loss is primarily associated with aging. The majority of cases of refractive error can be corrected through glasses; however, severe myopics are also at increased risk (regardless of refractive correction) for retinal detachments and glaucoma, both potentially blinding.

Another common visual disorder that has been subject to extensive public health intervention at the screening level is amblyopia. Amblyopia describes the preferential use of one eye. This imbalance in use occurs from different refractive errors or muscle balance in each eye during the first 6 years of life. The most effective treatment remains early patching of the dominant eye, with cases being identified as early as possible. To reach these cases, vision-screening is recommended worldwide at the preschool and elementary levels.

Visual disorders span a large range of effects, from the inconvenience of refractive error, to infectious diseases, to blinding degenerative disorders. In each case, however, appropriate identification and intervention remains the international challenge of the public health community.

▶ REFERENCES

1. Thylefors B, Negrel AD, Pararajasegaram R, Dadzie KY: Global data on blindness. Bull World Health Organ 73(1):115–121, 1995
2. Krumpaszky HG, Klaus V: Epidemiology of the causes of blindness. Opthalmologica 210:1–84, 1996
3. Quigley H: Number of people with glaucoma worldwide. Br J Ophthalmol 80:389–393, 1996
4. Tielsch JM: The epidemiology and control of open angle glaucoma: a population-based perspective. Annu Rev Public Health 17:121–136, 1996
5. Sarks SH, Sarks JP: Age related macular degeneration: atrophic form. In Ryan SJ (ed): Retina. 2nd ed. St. Louis: CV Mosby, 1994, pp 1071–1102
6. Hyman LG, Lilienfeld AM, Ferris FL, Fine SL: Senile macular degeneration: a case control study. Am J Epidemiol 118:213–227, 1983
7. Katz ML, Parker KR, Handelman GJ, Bramel TL, Dratz EA: Effects of antioxidant nutrient deficiency on the retina and retinal pigment epithelium of albino rats: a light and electron microscopy study. Exp Eye Res 34:339–369, 1982
8. Gass JDM: Pathogeness of disciform detachment of the neuroepithelium. I: General concepts and classification. Am J Ophthalmol 63: 573–585, 1967
9. Hirvela H, Luukinen H, Laara E, Laatikainen L: Risk factors for age related maculopathy in a population 70 years of age or older. Ophthalmology 103:871–877, 1996
10. Schwartz D: The Beaver Dam Eye Study: the relation of age related maculopathy to smoking. Surv Ophthalmol 39:84–85, 1994
11. Cruikshanks KJ, Klein R, Klein BEK: Sunlight and age related macular degeneration: the Beaver Dam Eye Study. Arch Ophthalmol 111:514–518, 1993
12. The Eye Disease Case-Control Study Group: Risk factors for neovascular age-related macular degeneration. Arch Ophthalmol 110: 1701–1708, 1992
13. Mares-Perlman JA, Brady WE, Klein BE, et al: Serum antioxidants and age related macular degeneration in a population based case control study. Arch Ophthalmol 113:1518–1523, 1995
14. Seddon JM, Ajani UA, Sperduto RD, et al: Dietary carotenoids, vitamins A, C, and E and advanced age-related macular degeneration. Eye Disease Case-Control Study Group. JAMA 272:1413–1420, 1994
15. Macular Photocoagulation Study Group: Argon laser photocoagulation for neovascular maculopathy after five years. Results from randomized clinical trials. Arch Ophthalmol 109:1109–1114, 1991
16. Macular Photocoagulation Study Group: Laser photocoagulation of subfoveal neovascular lesions of age-related macular degeneration. Updated findings from two clinical trials. Arch Ophthalmol 111:1200–1209, 1993
17. Macular Photocoagulation Study Group: Laser photocoagulation of subfoveal recurrent neovascular lesions in age related macular degeneration. Results of a randomized clinical trial. Arch Ophthalmol 109:1242–1257, 1991
18. Berkow JW: Subretinal neovascularization in senile macular degeneration. Am J Ophthalmol 97:143–147, 1984
19. Patz A, Smith RE: The ETDRS and Diabetes 2000 [Editorial]. Ophthalmology 98:739–740, 1991
20. Diabetes Control and Complications Trial: The Effects of Intensive Diabetes Treatment on the Progression of Diabetic Retinopathy in Insulin Dependent Diabetes Mellitus. Arch Ophthalmol 113:36, 1995
21. Diabetic Retinopathy Study Research Group: Photocoagulation treatment of proliferative diabetic retinopathy: clinical application of Diabetic Retinopathy Study (DRS) findings. DRS Report 8. Ophthalmology 88:583–600, 1981
22. Early Treatment Diabetic Retinopathy Study Research Group: Photocoagulation for retinal macular edema. ETDRS Report No. 4. Int Ophthalmol Clin 27:265–272, 1987
23. Gutman FA: Evaluation of a patient with central retinal vein occlusion. Ophthalmology 90:481–483, 1983
24. Branch Retinal Vein Occlusion Study Group: Argon laser photocoagulation for macular edema in branch retinal vein occlusion. Am J Ophthalmol 98:271–282, 1984
25. Branch Retinal Vein Occlusion Study Group: Argon laser scatter photocoagulation for prevention of neovascularization and vitreous hemorrhage in branch retinal vein occlusion. Arch Ophthalmol 104:34–41, 1986
26. World Health Organization: WHO Press Release (WHO/45) 17 Jun 1996
27. Jabs DA, Green WR, Fox R, et al: Ocular manifestations of acquired immune deficiency syndrome. Ophthalmology 96:1092–1099, 1989
28. Pepose JS: Ophthalmic manifestations of HIV infection. Current Topics in AIDS 2:191–206, 1989
29. Patz A, Payne JW: Retinopathy of Prematurity. In Duane TD (ed): Clinical Ophthalmology. Philadelphia: Harper & Row, 1983, vol 3, chap 20, pp 1–19.
30. Patz A: Symposium on retrolental fibroplasia. Summary. Ophthalmology 86:1761–1763, 1979
31. Flynn JT, O'Grady GE, Herrera J, Kushner BJ, Cantolino S, Milam W: Retrolental fibroplasia: I. Clinical Observations. Arch Ophthalmol 95:217–223, 1977
32. Cryotherapy for Retinopathy of Prematurity Cooperative Group: Multicenter trial of cryotherapy for retinopathy of prematurity: preliminary results. Arch Ophthalmol 106:471–479, 1988
33. Palmer EA: Retinopathy of Prematurity. Focal Points: Clinical Modules for Ophthalmologists. San Francisco: American Academy of Ophthalmology, 1993, vol 11, module 3
34. James S, Lanman JT: History of oxygen therapy and retrolental fibroplasia. Prepared by the American Academy of Pediatrics Committee on Fetus and Newborn, with collaboration of special consultants. Pediatrics 57:591–642, 1976

60

Psychiatric Disorders

Evelyn J. Bromet

Psychiatric disorders occur in every socioeconomic, racial, and cultural group in the world. In the United States, the estimated current prevalence of mental disorders is 10 to 15 percent in children[1,2] and 15 percent in adults.[3] The rate of dementia increases from 1.4 percent in persons aged 65 to 69 to more than 20 percent in people over 80 years old.[4] In the last 50 years, a great deal has been learned about the distribution of psychiatric disorders in the population; biological, social, and psychological factors associated with their occurrence and prognosis; and effective treatments.

Psychiatric disorders account for a large proportion of all chronic health problems. Moreover, an individual's mental state greatly influences general health status and ability to access needed health care services. Four issues underscore the importance of mental health issues for public health: (*a*) quality of life is largely determined by a person's mental state; (*b*) a large proportion of people who need medical care have psychiatric or brain disorders; (*c*) many physical disorders have an important mental component; and (*d*) as the risk of premature death recedes, the risk of chronic impairment rises. Given the significance of mental health problems, the search for causes is urgent. If environmental factors play a large role, prevention can be a potent force.

The methods used for psychiatric public health work are fundamentally no different from public health methods used for other disorders. However, some specific features distinguish mental health from other aspects of public health. Mental disorders are not usually listed as a direct cause of death on death certificates and are not often detectable on autopsy. Thus, mortality statistics shed little light on the burden of mental disorder in the population. On the other hand, two features of mental disorders make morbidity data more accessible for statistical summaries of community diagnosis than is so for other nonfatal conditions.

First, the care of the seriously mentally ill has long been a government responsibility. Except for tuberculosis and acute communicable diseases, no other branch of medicine has such a long history of official state responsibility. Consequently, substantial data have accumulated on the hospitalization of mentally disordered individuals. The National Institute of Mental Health (NIMH) developed a national system for recording hospitalizations for mental illness and analyzing national statistics for mental illness.[5] These hospitalization rates are one measure of the statistics of public mental health.

A second unique feature of psychiatric epidemiology is that personal interviews must be used to obtain direct access to mental life. Questions about such experiences as depression, headaches, phobias, and hallucinations are best directed at the subjects of a population survey (although interview data can be compromised if the question has not been understood or if the respondent's memory or accuracy is flawed).

The classification of mental disorders has a long history. Current concepts are rooted in the diagnostic characterizations of Kraepelin and Bleuler.[6] In the United States, the current state of classification is recorded in the American Psychiatric Association's *Diagnostic and Statistical Manual of Mental Disorders*, now in its 4th edition (DSM-IV).[7] This document reflects a consensus about the types of mental disorders present throughout the life cycle and the constellation of features encompassed in each type. In making a diagnosis, a clinician depends mainly on the results of a comprehensive mental examination, which focuses on the patient's (*a*) intellectual ability; (*b*) current state of consciousness, confusion, or contact; (*c*) mood or affect; (*d*) lack of connectedness of thought patterns, hallucinations, delusions, or distortion of thoughts and ideas; (*e*) personality (e.g., passivity, aggression, helplessness, rebelliousness); (*f*) behavior patterns; and (*g*) the complaint bringing the patient into treatment. In epidemiologic research, these domains are systematically evaluated using structured or semistructured diagnostic instruments.

Epidemiologic research aimed at establishing the incidence and prevalence of mental disorders in the United States has evolved during the twentieth century.[8] Three generations were identified: (*a*) the period before World War II, in which the median prevalence rate was 3.6 percent based on information from key informants and agency records; (*b*) World War II to the 1970s, in which the median rate was 20 percent, based on direct interviews with representative samples using psychological and psychosomatic symptom inventories to determine degree of "impairment"; and (*c*) 1970s to the present, in which lifetime rates of close to 30 percent in the Epidemiologic Catchment Area studies[9] and almost 50 percent in the National Comorbidity Study[10] were reported based on structured diagnostic interviews and formal diagnostic criteria.

This chapter focuses on findings from recent diagnostic studies, although important earlier results and classic studies are described. For a more detailed historical account of the epidemiology of mental disorders, see recent reviews.[8,11] Before presenting an overview of psychiatric epidemiology, however, it is important to describe the key developments in psychiatry that led to current diagnostic techniques for ascertaining cases of mental disorder. In the early 1960s, hospital admission rates for schizophrenia and depression differed widely between the United States and England.[12] This observation foreshadowed the first international study of diagnosis (the U.S.-U.K. project), in which systematic interviewing techniques and comparable diagnostic criteria were applied, and similar diagnostic distributions were obtained.[13] The World Health Organization's (WHO) program of research on schizophrenia also demonstrated the importance of uniform, structured assessment of patients within and outside the formal treatment network.[14,15] In the United States the need to define homogeneous patient populations for clinical drug trials and multicenter collaborative research also propelled the development of structured assessment procedures.[16] As part of the Collaborative Program on the Psychobiology of Depression, the Schedule for Affective Disorders and Schizophrenia[17] (SADS), a semistructured diagnostic interview schedule, was designed for use by experienced clinicians, along with the Research Diagnostic Criteria[18] (RDC), a set of operational criteria for diagnosis. The Structured Clinical Interview for Diagnosis

(SCID) was subsequently created for clinically experienced raters to match DSM-III-R and now DSM-IV criteria.[19]

Studies using clinician-administered interview schedules are costly. Although two-stage designs have been used, they often result in inadequate response rates. Hence, in the late 1970s, NIMH developed the Diagnostic Interview Schedule[20] (DIS), a fully structured instrument that could be administered by nonclinical raters, or lay interviewers. The DIS has been administered in several community surveys in the United States and has been translated into many languages for use in other countries. The largest U.S. study administering the DIS is the Epidemiologic Catchment Area (ECA) study of nearly 20,000 individuals from catchment areas in New Haven, St. Louis, Baltimore, Los Angeles, and Piedmont, North Carolina.[21] A subsequent instrument, the Composite International Diagnostic Interview (CIDI), was developed by the World Health Organization to permit diagnoses to be formulated according to multiple diagnostic systems. The CIDI was modified at the University of Michigan and administered to more than 8,000 respondents in the National Comorbidity Survey.[10] Structured diagnostic interview schedules have also been developed for children.[22]

This chapter is organized around Morris' framework on the "uses" of epidemiology[23] and provides an overview of public health psychiatry, summarizing information on the epidemiology, treatment, and prevention of mental disorders.

▶ COMMUNITY DIAGNOSIS

General Prevalence Studies

The prevalence and incidence rates of specific psychiatric disorders have been estimated from national probability samples and from studies conducted in specific communities. While national studies provide information on overall rates and demographic and geographic correlates, studies of specific communities, or catchment areas within communities, provide prevalence data useful for planning and evaluating mental health services.

The first U.S. prevalence study of mental illness (insanity, as it was then called) was conducted in Massachusetts in 1854 by Edward Jarvis,[24] who undertook a census of the "insane" by gathering information from general practitioners, other key informants such as clergymen, and records of mental hospitals and other official agencies. He identified 2,632 "lunatics" and 1,087 "idiots" needing "the care and protection of their friends or of the public for their support, restoration or custody." This method of using key informants to identify cases of mental illness was the method of choice for psychiatric epidemiology until after World War II.

After the war, a number of studies were conducted in specific communities using symptom-based inventories to determine rates of psychological impairment. For example, the Midtown Manhattan study[25] included a large, representative sample of adults assessed with a detailed symptom inventory. The symptom data were then reviewed by psychiatrists who rated the level of impairment of each respondent. As noted above, the rate of severe impairment was more than 20 percent. The first U.S. national morbidity study was conducted in the 1950s by investigators at the University of Michigan.[26] When asked: "Have you ever felt that you were going to have a nervous breakdown?" approximately 20 percent of the sample (N = 2,460) responded affirmatively. Since 1964, national studies have also been conducted on drinking patterns and alcohol-related problems, with about 12 percent of respondents being classified as "heavy drinkers."[27]

The first large-scale study using modern assessment techniques to determine specific psychiatric diagnoses (as opposed to impairment) was the ECA study of catchment areas in five U.S. communities.[28] Face-to-face assessments using the DIS were conducted at baseline and at 1-year follow-up, along with 6-month follow-up telephone information on interim patterns of medical and psychiatric service use. The 1-year incidence rates[29] and 1-month,[3] 6-month,[30] and lifetime[31] prevalence rates of selected disorders are provided in Table 60-1. Table 60-2 gives a summary of the DSM-III criteria for each disorder. The most prevalent DIS/DSM-III disorders across the five sites were substance abuse, phobias, and major depression. The least common were schizophrenia, mania, and somatization. There were several important findings, in addition to estimates of the incidence and prevalence of mental disorders. They included: only a minority of respondents with a diagnosable mental disorder received care, particularly from mental health providers; almost one-third of those with a mental disorder had a comorbid substance use disorder; and the rate of depression, as well as several other conditions, was inversely related to age.

The ECA findings on the prevalence of schizophrenia merits separate comment. The differential diagnosis of schizophrenia versus another psychotic condition is sometimes difficult even for experienced psychiatrists to make. Thus the reliability of this diagnosis in the ECA turned out to be particularly poor. In the Baltimore site, only

TABLE 60-1. AVERAGE RATES OF PSYCHIATRIC DISORDER IN THE EPIDEMIOLOGIC CATCHMENT AREA STUDY (N = 18,571), CONDUCTED IN SELECTED CATCHMENT AREAS OF NEW HAVEN, CT; DURHAM, NC; ST. LOUIS, MO; BALTIMORE, MD; AND LOS ANGELES, CA

Disorder	*Lifetime Prevalence*	*6-mo Prevalence*	*1-mo Prevalence*	*1-yr Incidence*
Alcohol abuse/dependence	13.3	4.7	2.8	1.8
Phobia	12.5	7.7	6.2	4.0
Drug abuse/dependence	5.9	2.0	1.3	1.1
Major depressive episode	5.8	3.0	2.2	1.6
Obsessive-compulsive	2.5	1.5	1.3	0.7
Antisocial personality	2.5	0.8	0.5	—
Panic	1.6	0.8	0.5	0.6
Cognitive impairment	1.3	1.3	1.3	1.2
Schizophrenia	1.3	0.8	0.6	—
Mania	0.8	0.5	0.4	—
Somatization	0.1	0.1	0.1	—

Prevalence rates adapted from Regier DA, Boyd JH, Burke JD, et al: One-month prevalence of mental disorders in the United States based on five epidemiologic catchment area sites. Arch Gen Psychiatry 45:977–986, 1988; and incidence rates are from Eaton WW Jr, Kramer M, Anthony JC, Dryman A, Shapiro S, Locke BZ: The incidence of specific DIS/DSM-III mental disorders: data from the NIMH Epidemiologic Catchment Area Program. Acta Psychiatr Scand 79:163–178, 1989.
Incidence rates do not include data from the New Haven site. Rates of cognitive impairment reflect current impairment at the time of interview only. Clinical data are based on the Diagnostic Interview Schedule and DSM-III. Rates are expressed as percentages.

TABLE 60-2. A SYNOPSIS OF DSM-III CRITERIA

Alcohol or drug abuse	A.	Pattern of pathological use (e.g., unable to cut down; binges; blackouts; use despite serious physical disorder)
	B.	Impairment in social or occupational functioning due to alcohol or drug use
	C.	Duration at least 1 month
Alcohol or drug dependence	A.	Pattern of pathological use or impairment of social or occupational functioning
	B.	Tolerance or withdrawal
Phobia	A.	Persistent irrational fear causing avoidance of certain situations
	B.	Significant distress; recognition that fear is irrational
Major depression	A.	Depressed mood, vegetative symptoms, fatigue, impaired concentration, or suicidal ideation
	B.	Duration at least 2 weeks
Obsessive-compulsive disorder	A.	Persistent ideas, images, or impulses invade consciousness, or stereotyped behaviors are repeated compulsively
	B.	Obsessions or compulsions cause distress or interfere with functioning
Antisocial personality	A.	Childhood history of delinquency, school or family problems, or illegal behavior
	B.	Adult inability to function responsibly or within the law
Panic disorder	A.	3+ discrete periods within a 3-week period of fear, accompanied by palpitations, dizziness, feeling faint, and the like
Cognitive impairment	A.	Severe impairment in cognitive abilities such as orientation, attention, recall, and language
Schizophrenia	A.	Delusions, hallucinations, or thought disorder accompanied by deterioration in functioning
	B.	Duration at least 6 months
Mania	A.	Elevated, expansive mood characterized by restlessness, thought racing, grandiosity, reduced need for sleep, and involvement in reckless activities
	B.	Duration at least 1 week
Somatization	A.	History of complaints of multiple physical symptoms not explainable by a physician
	B.	Onset before age 30

20 percent of individuals diagnosed with schizophrenia in the community interview were confirmed as having this diagnosis by an independent psychiatric assessment.[32] Thus readers interested in ascertaining the prevalence of schizophrenia should rely on other sources of information. For example Link and Dohrenwend[33] suggested that, since most schizophrenic patients use formal psychiatric services, treatment data are a useful source of information. The best source of treatment data is the case registry. Crude annual incidence rates from registries around the world range from 0.11/1000 in Salford, United Kingdom, to 0.70/1000 in Maryland.[32]

The ECA focused on DSM-III disorders in selected catchment areas in five sites. In contrast, 10 years later, Kessler and colleagues undertook the first national probability sample study of the distribution of DSM-III-R disorders.[10] In this study, known as the National Comorbidity Survey (NCS), a modified version of the CIDI was administered to 8,098 individuals age 15 to 54 from the 48 contiguous states. The response rate was 82.6 percent, and special efforts were made to study the impact of nonresponse and to recruit initial nonrespondents. Several diagnostic conditions were studied, along with their patterns of comorbidity. Because psychotic disorders were shown in the ECA to have poor reliability and validity when assessed by nonclinicians, NCS respondents endorsing psychotic symptoms were reinterviewed by telephone by a clinician with the SCID. Table 60-3 presents the 1-year prevalence rates of a number of NCS disorders. Because of differences in recruitment and assessment methods, especially attention given to memory priming, the NCS rates are higher than those of the ECA. Overall, almost 50 percent met criteria for a psychiatric disorder in their lifetime, and about one-quarter in the past 12 months. The most prevalent conditions were depression, anxiety, and substance use disorders. While 21 percent of the sample experienced a single disorder, 14 percent met criteria for three or more disorders. Moreover, among respondents meeting criteria for a DSM-III-R disorder, most had more than one condition.

Comparative Studies

Research comparing the rates of mental illness across geographic areas dates back to the pioneering work of Faris and Dunham,[34] who showed that hospitalization rates for schizophrenia in Illinois state institutions decreased progressively with distance away from the center of Chicago. Forty-six percent of the cases were from the inner city area, compared with 13 percent from the outermost districts. Faris and Dunham hypothesized that the inner city environment elicited mental illness, rejecting the alternative explanation that social selection or drift was responsible for these higher rates (see below). Since then, studies conducted in other urban areas have consistently shown the same pattern.

Urban-rural differences in rates of treated mental illness also have been studied extensively. Dohrenwend and Dohrenwend's classic review[35] concluded that neuroses and personality disorder were more prevalent in urban areas, schizophrenia rates were similar, and other psychoses were relatively more frequent in rural areas. While some subsequent evidence supported these conclusions in both adults[36–39] and children,[40,41] these patterns have not been reported consistently. For example, Eaton[42] found that the hospital admission rate for schizophrenia was three times higher in an urban area than in a nearby rural area of Maryland. Most importantly, no significant urban-rural differences were found in the NCS.[10] Urban-rural differences have also been evaluated in relation to dementia. Three Scandinavian studies reported significantly lower rates in rural versus urban areas.[43]

TABLE 60-3. TWELVE-MONTH PREVALENCE RATES OF DSM-III-R PSYCHIATRIC DISORDERS FOR MALES AND FEMALES IN THE NATIONAL COMORBIDITY STUDY (N = 8,098), CONDUCTED BETWEEN SEPTEMBER 1990 AND FEBRUARY 1992 WITH A NATIONAL PROBABILITY SAMPLE DRAWN FROM THE 48 CONTINUOUS STATES

DSM-III-R Disorder	*Males (%)*	*Females (%)*	*Total (%)*
Affective disorders			
Major depressive episode	7.7	12.9	10.3
Manic episode	1.4	1.3	1.3
Dysthymia	2.1	3.0	2.5
Any affective disorder	8.5	14.1	11.3
Anxiety disorders			
Panic disorder	1.3	3.2	2.3
Agoraphobia without panic disorder	1.7	3.8	2.8
Social phobia	6.6	9.1	7.9
Simple phobia	4.4	13.2	8.8
Generalized anxiety disorder	2.0	4.3	3.1
Any anxiety disorder	11.8	22.6	17.2
Substance use disorders			
Alcohol abuse without dependence	3.4	1.6	2.5
Alcohol dependence	10.7	3.7	7.2
Drug abuse without dependence	1.3	0.3	0.8
Drug dependence	3.8	1.9	2.8
Any substance abuse/dependence	16.1	6.6	11.3
Nonaffective psychosis	0.5	0.6	0.5
Any disorder	27.7	31.2	29.5

Data are from Kessler RC, McGonagle KA, Zhao S, et al: Lifetime and 12-month prevalence of DSM-III-R psychiatric disorders in the United States. Arch Gen Psychiatry 51:8–19, 1994.
Among the respondents with a disorder in the prior 12-months, the proportions having 1, 2, and 3+ disorders were 17.4, 23.1, and 58.9 percent, respectively.

International variations in rates of mental disorders and substance use disorders have also been the focus of recent research. Weissman et al.[44] reported that the rates of lifetime depression in a selection of studies using similar methodologies ranged from 1.5 percent in Taiwan to 19 percent in Beirut, Lebanon. Regardless of the actual rates, the two most common symptoms in each site were insomnia and loss of energy. The rates of alcoholism were also compared across studies with similar methodologies from 10 regions around the world.[45] The rates ranged from 5 percent in Taiwan to 22 percent in Korea. As with depression, the symptom pictures were similar across the studies, with the mean age of onset in the early twenties, the mean number of symptoms about four, and males having significantly higher rates than females.

▶ INDIVIDUAL RISKS AND CHANCES

Several individual risk factors are associated with the occurrence of psychiatric disorders, including gender, age, social class, marital status, ethnicity, physical health, family history of mental disorder, and for schizophrenia, season of birth.

Gender

Gender differences in rates of substance abuse, anxiety disorders, and depression have been confirmed in community samples, primary care patients, and treatment samples in psychiatric and substance abuse clinics. The male-female ratios are approximately 6:1 for alcoholism, 1:2 for depression, and 1:2 to 1:3 for phobias. Table 60-3 shows the rates of these disorders for males and females in the NCS. Many social and biological factors have been hypothesized to underlie these differences. These include gender differences in recurrence risk,[46] drinking habits, expressing emotion, social roles, role performance, and role-related strains, as well as professional biases in diagnosis.[47] In contrast, there is no overall gender difference in the prevalence of dementia or schizophrenia. However, in schizophrenia, the age at first hospitalization is earlier in males (late teen to early twenties) than in females (late twenties).[32]

Psychopathology is twice as common in prepubertal boys than in girls, but this 2:1 sex ratio reverses itself during adolescence. A new field of developmental psychiatric epidemiology has emerged, and research is being designed to help explain why the sex ratio changes with puberty.[48]

Age

The ECA and NCS both noted that affective and anxiety disorders were higher in those 18 to 35 years of age than in the older populations.[10,31] This pattern occurred for lifetime as well as more recent episodes. Although the peak period of heavy drinking is the early twenties,[49] the rate of alcoholism peaks in the early forties. Finally, dementia is rare in people under age 60. However, after age 60, the rate essentially doubles every 5 years.[43]

Social Class

Numerous studies have been undertaken of the relationship between social class and mental illness. As noted above, the ecological studies, starting with that of Faris and Dunham, emphasized the importance of social class in relation to schizophrenia and argued that something in the physical or social environment of poor neighborhoods caused the higher than expected numbers of patients from those areas. Other nonecological studies also suggested an environmental explanation. For example, Hollingshead and Redlich found that among psychiatric patients higher rates of schizophrenia occurred in the lower social classes.[50] Most of these patients had lived in poor areas of the city all of their lives. Moreover, 90 percent of their families of origin were in the same social class, suggesting to the authors that downward social mobility could not explain the findings. More recent studies, however, indicate that social selection rather than social causation is the more plausible explanation. For example, in one study, the occupational attainment of schizophrenic patients was lower than that of their fathers and lower than that predicted from their school careers.[51] Currently in schizophrenia research, the recent genetics findings have tipped the balance in favor of the social selection rather than the social causation hypothesis.

Lower social class status is also associated with higher rates of depressive symptoms, alcohol abuse or dependence, drug abuse or dependence, and antisocial personality disorder.[10,52] In addition, lower social class status is a risk factor for many psychiatric disorders of both childhood[53] and old age.[54]

Ethnicity

The NCS[10] reported no ethnic differences in rates of anxiety disorders. However, whites had higher rates of affective disorders, substance use disorders, and lifetime comorbidity than did African Americans. Costello and colleagues also reported no difference in rates in children in a general population sample, with the exception of a higher rate of enuresis in African American than white children.[53]

Research on suicide has consistently shown that whites have significantly higher rates than nonwhites, particularly white males. Later in this chapter we discuss the recent increase in suicide rate in young white males. Here it is important to note that the age-adjusted suicide rates for Native Americans and Chinese Americans are higher than those for whites. In fact, the rate for Native American youth is 2.3 times greater than that of their same-age peers.[55]

Research on psychosis has shown that some ethnic groups have higher than expected rates of schizophrenia, including the indigenous populations of specific regions of Croatia[56,57] and western Ireland.[58] In early studies of psychiatric patients in the United States, African American patients were disproportionately diagnosed with schizophrenia and were hospitalized at a younger age and for longer periods of time than whites. However, these findings are generally attributed to clinical bias. In the NCS, the odds ratios for ethnicity (white, black, Hispanic, other) were not significant when clinician-derived diagnoses of nonaffective psychosis were analyzed.[59]

Marital Status

Being single is associated with several psychiatric disorders, although whether it is a cause or a consequence is unknown. In schizophrenia, being single at the time of first hospitalization is associated with a poorer prognosis. However, in this case the findings on marital status may be a reflection of both gender and age. That is, the single patients tend to be predominantly male and young.

The association of marital status with nonpsychotic disorders is also complex. Individuals who are recently separated or divorced have higher rates of depression and alcoholism than those who are currently married. It is unclear from these cross-sectional findings whether these disorders are a result or a cause (or both) of marital problems and marital dissolution. Community studies have also found that, while married men are less depressed than unmarried men, married women are more symptomatic than unmarried women.[25] This suggests that being married may be a protective factor for men but not for women.

Physical Health Status

Several sources of evidence point to a link between physical and mental health. First, psychiatrically ill individuals have a higher than expected mortality rate than the nonpsychiatrically ill. In one study, the adjusted death rate of psychiatric patients was elevated 2- to 3-fold.[60] Another study reported that 6 percent of patients reporting to a psychiatric emergency service died within 2 years of the visit, whereas the expected rate was 1.6 percent.[61] In a community sample age 55 and older, the odds of dying over a 15-month period was four times higher for people with affective disorder than for persons who did not have affective disorder.[62]

A second source of evidence is the finding of elevated rates of psychiatric disorders in hospital patients. It has long been known that infectious diseases can produce serious mental disorders. In addition, high rates of major depression and depressive symptoms have been found in patients with such chronic conditions as multiple sclerosis, cancer, diabetes mellitus, cardiovascular disease, thyroid disease, and chronic pain.[63] One study reported that 61 percent of severely ill hospital patients were depressed compared with 21 percent of less ill patients.[64] Whether depression is a consequence of disease or of its concomitant disability is difficult to determine. Regardless, depression is also predictive of a shortened life expectancy.

Third, outpatient primary care patients have high rates of psychiatric symptoms.[63] In the ECA, 22 percent of respondents who had recently used a medical care facility met criteria for a DSM-III disorder compared with 17 percent of nonusers.[65] Affective disorders were the most common diagnoses in women, and alcohol abuse or dependence was the most common diagnosis in men. A review of British studies of psychiatric morbidity in general practice patients concluded that 20 to 25 percent suffered from a psychiatric disturbance primarily affective in nature.[66] Recently, a WHO-sponsored international study of more than 5,000 patients in 15 primary care centers reported that 24 percent of the patients were diagnosed with a psychiatric or substance use disorder.[67] Despite the high prevalence of psychiatric disorders, especially depression, medical patients are often undiagnosed or are misdiagnosed, in part because both physicians and patients focus on somatic symptoms and possible physical diagnoses.

Familial Aggregation

Considerable research on familial aggregation of psychopathology has been conducted. In schizophrenia, monozygotic twins have a concordance rate for schizophrenia between 33 and 78 percent compared with 8 to 28 percent for dizygotic twins. The risk for developing schizophrenia, given the presence of an affected first-degree relative, is approximately 10 percent (compared with an overall prevalence of less than 1 percent).[68] Weissman[69] reviewed findings from family studies of depression and reported a 2- to 3-fold increase in major depression in adult first-degree relatives of patients with depression. Weissman's study of the offspring of depressed parents also found a 3-fold increase in risk for psychiatric disorder (24 percent with any psychiatric disorder compared with 8 percent among control subjects).[70] The preponderance of evidence regarding alcoholism deriving from family, twin, and adoption studies also points to a genetic vulnerability for developing this disease.[71]

Season of Birth

Seasonal variation has been a well-documented phenomenon in stillbirths, neonatal deaths, and congenital rubella, although it has been suggested that the impact of seasonal variation has diminished over time.[72] In England, Scandinavia, and the United States, patients with schizophrenia are disproportionately likely to have been born during the winter or spring months. Possible explanations for this phenomenon include nutritional factors during pregnancy, environmental factors such as lead exposure, genetic factors, and exposure to infectious or viral agents.[73]

▶ CAUSES

New understandings of the origins and course of mental disorder emerge when clinical research, laboratory studies, sociological inquiries, and epidemiology interact. A dramatic illustration occurred early in the twentieth century, when pellagra psychosis accounted for almost 10 percent of the admissions to mental hospitals. In South Carolina during the early 1920s, Goldberger et al[74] showed that pellagra was associated with a nutritional deficiency, although the specific items missing from the diet could not be identified. As a result of dietary changes, pellagra psychosis became rare in the United States, although it remains endemic in parts of Africa and India.

The causal role of both social and physical environmental agents are discussed in this section. Although technically a causal factor must predate the onset of a disorder—that is, its presence increases the risk for developing a disorder—the insidious onset of many psychiatric disorders often makes it difficult to separate risks from consequences. Thus it is more parsimonious at times to describe the findings about environmental factors as correlates rather than as causes of mental disorder.

Social Environment

The aspect of the social environment that has been linked to a variety of mental disorders is stress, defined here as a set of disruptive environmental presses or stimuli. Two types of studies demonstrate that higher levels of stress are associated with increased rates of psychiatric disorder and subclinical psychiatric symptoms: studies of communitywide traumas and studies of personal adversities and persistent strains.

Communitywide Traumas

Communitywide stressors expose large numbers of people to uncontrollable events and provide an opportunity to understand both short-term and long-term psychological sequelae. Such a situation arose following the Three Mile Island (TMI) nuclear plant accident of March 1979. Like many disasters, TMI was not an acute, time-limited event but entailed a sequence of interrelated stressful occurrences that unfolded over a long period of time, including the initial crisis, intermittent radiation leaks, and difficulties surrounding the clean-up operations. It differed from other disasters, however, in that there were no deaths or property damage. In a longitudinal study of mothers of preschool children living within 10 miles of the plant, the rate of major depression and generalized anxiety during the year after the accident was double that of an unexposed comparison group.[75] Two to 3 years later, the comparison site underwent widespread unemployment, and the mental health impact of it turned out to be remarkably similar to the stress-effects of the TMI accident.[76] Over the next 10 years, the women near Three Mile Island continued to report higher than expected affective symptomatology.[77]

The psychiatric sequelae of such natural disasters as floods, tornadoes, and earthquakes have also been investigated. Recent studies have focused not only on affective and anxiety conditions but also on the emergence of posttraumatic stress disorder (PTSD). This disorder is defined as a response to an unusual stressor in which an individual re-experiences the traumatic event through recurrent thoughts or dreams, experiences psychic numbing, and has symptoms such as sleep disturbance, survivor guilt, difficulty concentrating, hyperarousal, avoidance of activities associated with the event, and an intensification of symptoms if re-exposed to a similar event. Such studies generally find an acute effect of these stressors, particularly during the first year after their occurrence.[78] The only consistent risk factors for adverse mental health outcomes are gender, prior history of psychiatric disturbance, and greater involvement in the disaster in terms of loss of life or property.[78,79]

Studies of combat show that such trauma can engender short-term and long-term adverse mental health consequences even in healthy individuals. One of the first such observations occurred during the two world wars, when soldiers prescreened for adequate mental health often suffered from combat stress reaction when faced with extremely adverse circumstances or to deprivation. Since the Vietnam War, there has been considerable interest in establishing the prevalence of PTSD among combat veterans. A national study of Vietnam veterans conducted in the late 1980s reported a point prevalence rate of 15.2 percent and a lifetime rate of 31 percent.[80] These high rates led the Department of Veterans Affairs to increase research and treatment programs for this vulnerable group.

Personal Adversities and Strains

Studies employing life event checklists to assess stress typically find that such events play a minor and transient role in eliciting psychiatric symptoms in general populations samples. However, in vulnerable populations, these events may be more important. In schizophrenia, life events may trigger psychotic episodes, particularly in patients with inadequate social network support.[81] Adverse life events may play a causal role in the occurrence of some forms of depression in vulnerable populations.[82] Brown and Harris found that working class women may be at particular risk, especially when they lack a confiding relationship with their husbands, are not employed outside the home, have three or more children under the age of 6 years, and endured the loss of their own parents in childhood.[83]

Two specific events that have been studied in depth are unemployment[84] and bereavement.[85] Both were shown to produce short-term deleterious effects in more than 50 percent of exposed individuals. Several factors have been evaluated as potential moderators or mediators, including social support, good physical health, and pre-existing financial security.

The mental health effects of chronic strain at work and at home have also been studied. With regard to the work environment, employees in jobs characterized by high levels of demand, little autonomy over decision-making, conflicting requirements, and task-related ambiguity have been found to experience higher levels of psychological symptoms and alcohol abuse than employees experiencing less occupational strain.[86] The combination of high demands and low decision latitude is particularly stressful.[87,88]

Earlier in the chapter, we described the high rate of depression and alcoholism in recently separated and divorced individuals. Clinicians have long been aware of the links between depression and marital conflict. Empirical evidence from research on depressed patients and on general populations has confirmed this association, although the causal direction is difficult to disentangle. A stressful family environment is also a well-documented risk factor for behavioral problems in children. Children reared in families with high levels of conflict, abuse, or neglect are at risk for a range of health problems, including depression, sleep disorders, developmental delay, generalized anxiety, school behavior problems, phobias, and antisocial behavior.[89]

Physical Environment

Three aspects of the physical environment are described in this section: toxic exposures in the work environment, lead exposure among children, and homelessness.

Occupational Exposures

Exposure to lead, mercury, carbon monoxide, carbon disulfide, and the like may cause serious central nervous system (CNS) disturbances. In *Alice in Worderland*, Lewis Carroll immortalized the well-known hallucinations, delusions, and mania produced by high-level mercury exposure in the character the Mad Hatter. Since the nineteenth century, dramatic case reports have described cognitive and neurasthenic symptoms and even suicide in workers exposed to a variety of solvents.

An issue of ongoing public health concern is the potential health effect of low-level exposure to neurotoxic agents. Lead and solvents are two neurotoxic exposures that have been investigated extensively. Early studies of low-level lead exposure often reported cognitive and psychological sequelae, but the studies were based on volunteer samples, poorly matched controls, and nonblind raters. In recent epidemiological research, in contrast, no significant effects on neuropsychological or psychiatric impairment were reported.[90] The findings for low-level solvent exposure are more complex. Several Scandinavian studies of male workers chronically exposed at threshold or subthreshold levels reported significantly more CNS symptoms (headaches, fatigue, depression, dizziness, memory disturbances), nonspecific somatic complaints (nausea, abdominal pain, skin problems, and aches and pains), and impaired performance on cognitive tasks compared with that found of unexposed controls.[91–94] Because these studies contain some serious methodological flaws,[95] further confirmation from epidemiologic research is needed. In one recent study of *female* workers,[96] low-level solvent exposure was significantly associated with increased depressive symptomatology, CNS disturbance, and an array of nonspecific somatic complaints. However, women have rarely been studied, and more research is needed to understand the impact of solvent exposure in this group.

It has been hypothesized that the combination of low-level exposure and high occupational stress might be especially deleterious, although empirical findings have so far been mixed.[97–99] In this regard, it is interesting to note that mass psychogenic illness has been found to occur in several female workforces in which both high stress and low-level solvent exposures were present.[100]

Lead Exposure in Children

Environmental exposure to lead was shown to have a significant effect on the cognitive performance of children. Needleman et al conducted a classic epidemiologic study using tooth samples from elementary school children. They showed that, after controlling for 39 factors, including social class and parental IQ, increased exposure was significantly related to lower intelligence test scores.[101] In an 11-year follow-up study of these children, higher dentin lead levels continued to be predictive of both school performance and whether the child dropped out of school.[102] Although this study was the object of considerable controversy, the central findings were confirmed in reanalyses of the data set as well as in subsequent research.

Homelessness

Rates of mental illness among homeless adults and children are alarmingly high. In one study, more than one-quarter of homeless individuals were found to have a major chronic mental illness such as schizophrenia or substance abuse.[103] Compared with socioeconomically matched control subjects, homeless children have more overt health problems and more psychiatric risk factors such as abuse, neglect, and elevated blood lead levels.[104] In some cities, deinstitutionalization of the mentally ill from state mental hospitals contributed significantly to the problem of homelessness. The risk of homelessness among discharged state hospital patients was as high as 28 percent in New York City.[105] It is beyond the scope of this review to detail the numerous studies showing a significant correlation between homelessness and mental illness. For a scholarly review of this research, see Reference 106.

▶ HISTORICAL TRENDS

Historical trends have been difficult to study because of temporal changes in diagnostic criteria and service provision. However, temporal changes in rates of psychosis, depression, and adolescent suicide have received considerable attention.

Psychosis

A major debate centers on whether schizophrenia increased as a function of industrialization. A pioneering analysis by Goldhamer and Marshall[107] focused on mental hospital admission rates for psychosis from 1840 to 1940. They concluded that, although a progressive increase in hospital admissions occurred among the elderly, the rates of psychosis (primarily schizophrenia) among young and middle-age groups changed very little. Eaton, however, extended the time period to 1970 and concluded that the prevalence of psychosis had increased.[108] To date, the debate is unresolved and is perhaps unresolvable, although two recent pieces of evidence support the original tenet of no change. First, an examination of Australian mental hospital admissions over a 130-year period found that, when historical changes in diagnosis were taken into account, admission rates were relatively stable.[109] Second, the extensive WHO program of research found similar rates of psychosis in industrialized and nonindustrialized countries.[15]

While it may be impossible to settle the argument definitively, if the rates are shown to change as a function of industrialization, research will be needed to explain the change. Häfner[110] delineated several potential explanatory factors, including environmental exposures, changes in infant mortality and longevity, lifestyle changes associated with industrialization, and/or artifactual variables such as changes in who enters the treatment system or availability of services.

Depression

Evidence has also accumulated regarding an increase in depression since World War II. In Lundby, Sweden, a longitudinal study was initiated in 1947[111] in which direct interviews by psychiatrists, information from key informants, and medical records were used to determine psychiatric diagnoses of the entire population. Based on follow-up interviews by psychiatrists in 1957 and 1972 with 97 percent of the original cohort, a significant increase in the incidence of nonpsychotic depression was detected.

Although the Lundby study is the only direct source of evidence regarding an increase in depression, other important, albeit indirect, evidence also suggests that depression has increased. Hospital admission rates for affective disorder have risen since World War II. In epidemiologic studies, the rate of lifetime depression is inversely related to age. That is, older respondents have lower rates of lifetime depression than do younger respondents.[112] This increased rate in birth cohorts born after World War II was observed in the United States and in several other countries. As with psychosis, firm conclusions about changes in depression are difficult to draw because of artifacts such as differential mortality, changes in diagnostic criteria, reporting biases, and changing attitudes about depression in society. Nevertheless, the NIMH became so concerned about the prevalence of depression that it instituted the Depression/Awareness, Recognition, and Treatment Program (D/ART). The D/ART program is aimed at mental health professionals, general medical practitioners, and the general population, and its ultimate aim is to reduce the level of morbidity associated with depression and to prevent its occurrence through early detection.[113] The final source of evidence for an increase in depression is the rise in suicide rate discussed below.

Suicide in Adolescents and Young Adults

Between 1955 and 1980 the rate of suicide tripled in people 15 to 24 years of age, increasing from 2.6/100,000 population to 8.5/100,000 population, making suicide the second leading cause of death in this age group.[114] The group at highest risk is white males. (Other risk factors are prior suicide attempts, substance abuse, mental illness, and familial depression.) One study found that adolescent suicide victims with detectable blood alcohol concentrations were more likely to use firearms, a method likely to result in a completed suicide.[115] Thus it appears likely that the increasing substance abuse in young people is contributing to the observed increase in completed suicides.

▶ COMPLETING THE CLINICAL PICTURE

Since most individuals with psychiatric disorders are not in mental health treatment, community studies can markedly alter our understanding of the clinical signs and prognosis of some disorders. Recent studies applying formal diagnostic criteria to untreated populations have helped complete the clinical picture by pointing out that the syndromes of depression and alcoholism, for example, may be different in treated and untreated groups. A study of white collar employees found that 25 percent met DSM-III-R criteria for depression, and 10 percent met criteria for alcoholism.[116] Nevertheless, these individuals continued to function on their jobs, albeit with some difficulty in concentration and with occasional missed deadlines. Most of the alcohol-related episodes occurred years before, and the vast majority of these "cases" became normal drinkers with no serious legal, social, occupational, or clinical consequences. These findings suggest that community respondents meeting diagnostic criteria for depression and alcoholism may not have the significant social and occupational impairment usually noted in clinical samples, despite experiencing the same intensity of symptoms experienced by patient populations during their episodes.

When a condition does come to clinical attention, representative samples of first-episode patients can be studied longitudinally to learn more about the natural course of the condition. In fact, such follow-up studies have provided more optimistic predictions about the long-term prognosis of many disorders.[117] The poor prognosis noted for conditions such as alcoholism and schizophrenia is in part because of the clinician's illusion, which derives from treating chronic cases who stay in the service system.

Another important issue is comorbidity. Psychiatric patients in treatment often meet criteria for more than one psychiatric disorder, sometimes labeled primary and secondary disorders. For example, patients with primary alcoholism often develop secondary depression during the course of the alcoholism. Schizophrenic patients discharged after their first lifetime admission often develop depression during the subsequent year. Patients with major depression often suffer from an accompanying anxiety disorder such as phobia or panic disorder. However, people often enter treatment precisely because they have more than one disorder (Berkson's fallacy). Epidemiologic studies were needed to complete the clinical picture regarding comorbidity. In this case, recent epidemiological findings confirmed that multiple psychiatric disorders co-occur in the general population as well.[10] Examples of highly comorbid conditions include alcoholism with drug abuse, alcoholism with antisocial personality, obsessive-compulsive personality with panic disorder, and depression with somatization.[118] A similar pattern of comorbidity is also found in children.

▸ IDENTIFYING NEW SYNDROMES

By systematizing clinical observations, epidemiologists can potentially identify new syndromes. Until recently, depression was viewed as an adult disorder that rarely occurred during childhood. Several factors converged to stimulate the need to define depressive disorders of childhood as a separate entity: the increasing rate of adolescent suicide and suicide attempts, the increased frequency with which childhood depressions were being noted in pediatric and psychiatric settings, and the high rates of depression reported in studies of the offspring of clinically depressed parents. Recent findings suggest that the rate of depression using DSM-III-R criteria is approximately 2 percent in preadolescent children and 5 to 10 percent in adolescents.[119]

Epidemiological studies of occupational exposures identified syndromes associated with specific toxic chemicals such as lead, cyanide, carbon monoxide, carbon disulfide, and mercury.[120] For example, the constellation of symptoms resulting from carbon monoxide exposure (occurring in blast furnace workers, firefighters, fork-lift truck operators, and others) includes disturbances in concentration and memory, impulsivity, and lack of insight into one's behavior. As noted, the phrase "mad as a hatter" stemmed from observations of specific types of tremors among workers in the hatting industry who were exposed to high levels of mercuric nitrate in Europe during the nineteenth century.

▸ EVALUATING MENTAL HEALTH SERVICES

Studies of the provision of mental health services help to explain why some patients are in the visible (treated) tip of the iceberg, while many others are undiagnosed, untreated, and unknown to treatment agencies. Evaluation of mental health services involves assessing not only ongoing treatment efforts but also preventive interventions aimed at reducing levels of morbidity in high-risk populations. This section considers three issues: a brief historical overview of American psychiatric service delivery, a discussion of factors associated with entry into treatment, and efforts to prevent mental disorders.

Historical Overview of American Psychiatric Care

In 1841, when Dorothea Lynde Dix began her crusade on behalf of the mentally ill, there were only 18 hospitals in the United States devoted exclusively to the care of the mentally ill. The vast majority of psychiatrically ill individuals were in jails and poorhouses, kept at home, boarded out, or auctioned off to the highest bidder. Echoing Horace Mann's 1828 plea that the mentally ill be declared "wards of the state," Dix convinced the Massachusetts legislature that local communities had shown themselves incapable of caring for the mentally ill. Like other reformers, she did not hesitate to reinforce her arguments with the economic lure that decent treatment in state hospitals small and geographically isolated from the stresses of daily life would cure psychiatrically disturbed individuals quickly, making them productive members of society instead of drains on the public purse. In 1843, the legislators voted to make all of the indigent mentally ill wards of the Commonwealth of Massachusetts and to enlarge Worcester State Hospital, a mental hospital established as a result of Horace Mann's efforts a decade before.

The Dix-Mann doctrine that the mentally ill should be wards of the state reached its most explicit expression with the passage of the New York State Care Act of 1890. This legislation provided for removal of the mentally ill from local poorhouses and jails to state hospitals, where they were to be supported and treated at state expense. The law further required each state hospital to admit all cases of mental illness from its district, regardless of prognosis. Following its initiation in New York, other states adopted the Dix-Mann principle of complete state care for the seriously mentally ill. A major consequence of this action was the isolation of mental patients and of psychiatry from the mainstream of medicine.

Although some state hospitals in the United States were established explicitly as custodial institutions, most attempted to apply moral treatment, and some closely approached that ideal. Even the best-managed hospitals, however, did not long continue to function as the small, rural, therapeutic retreats that Dix and Mann had envisioned. New asylums were built as older ones overflowed, and the demand for accommodation always seemed to exceed capacity. As chronic cases accumulated and new admissions rose, overcrowding led to deterioration in the standards of care. At the turn of the century, the "cult of curability" yielded to the notion, "once insane, always insane"; moral treatment precepts were forgotten, and patients' behavior was controlled with physical restraints and seclusion.

The National Association for Mental Hygiene was founded in 1909, with the aim of improving the care and treatment of patients in mental hospitals. After World War I, the mental hygiene movement turned its attention to prevention by early detection and treatment of mental disorders, a strategy exemplified by its active support for the development of child guidance clinics and parental education. The rapid growth of child guidance clinics and other outpatient psychiatric services marked the beginning of organized community-based psychiatry in the United States, which had begun in the late nineteenth century in Europe. By the mid-1930s, nearly all state mental hospitals had at least one outpatient clinic.

In 1946, Congress passed the National Mental Health Act (Public Law 79-487), thereby creating the National Institute of Mental Health. For the first time, the federal government took responsibility for research, training of personnel, and assisting the states in prevention, diagnosis, and treatment of serious psychiatric disorders.

Having grown at a steady rate for over a century, the resident patient population reached an all-time high of 560,000 in 1955. The slow decline of resident mental patients that began in 1956 has been credited to three factors: the introduction of neuroleptic drugs, which accelerated management and sometimes even recovery and enabled some patients to be treated at home; the introduction of the therapeutic community, or community-oriented treatment within the hospital, which reduced the demoralization of custodial care; and the geographic decentralization of large state mental hospitals, which led to closer relationships between state hospitals and local communities. Around 1960, a systematic policy of releasing patients was initiated, based on successful reforms in England, where a reduction of the patient census had preceded the use of neuroleptic drugs. Criteria for both admission and release were liberalized. That is, less severe symptoms were needed for admission, and more symptoms were allowed at the time of release. Length of stay was shortened for acute admissions, and the resident patient census dropped. However, the actual number of admissions increased, in part transforming the custodial hospitals into short-term intensive therapy centers. The introduction of this "revolving door" policy highlighted the need for expanded community treatment. Mental hospital censuses decreased from 560,000 in 1955 to 214,065 in 1981.[121]

In 1955, Congress enacted the Mental Health Study Act (Public Law 84-182) to evaluate the "human and economic problems of mental illness." This act led to the establishment of the Joint Commission on Mental Illness and Health. The Commission's final report, Action for Mental Health, recommended funding basic and applied research, training, and expanded services to the mentally ill. The Commission recommended establishing (*a*) outpatient mental health facilities in communities to provide immediate care for acutely disturbed patients, (*b*) one clinic per 50,000 population, (*c*) inpatient psychiatric units in every general hospital with 100 or more beds, (*d*) maximum occupancy in state mental hospitals of 1,000 beds, and (*e*) expanded mental health education to reduce the stigma associated with mental illness. In 1963, President Kennedy delivered a message to Congress on mental illness and mental retardation in which he proposed a national federally funded program for setting up comprehensive community mental health centers and for improving care in state hospitals. This set the stage for the passage of the Community Mental Health Centers Act of October 1963. The newly mandated community mental health centers had to provide five essential services: inpatient care, outpatient care, emergency services, partial hospitalization, and consultation and education. Over time, five additional services were to be added: diagnostic services, rehabilitation services, precare and aftercare services, training, and research and evaluation. The centers were to serve geographically defined catchment areas of 75,000 to 200,000 people. By 1980, 717 community mental health centers had been funded across the country (2,000 had been envisaged), with the federal government investing more than 1.5 billion dollars.

In 1977, President Carter signed an executive order establishing the President's Commission on Mental Health to review and make new recommendations on the mental health needs of the nation. Among its 100 recommendations were the following: improving linkages between community support networks and mental health facilities; expanding services to children, minorities, the elderly, and the chronically mentally ill; the continued phasing down of large state mental hospitals; and the development of a case management system by the states. In 1980, President Carter signed the resulting Mental Health Systems Act (Public Law 96-398) into law. However, the subsequent Omnibus Budget and Reconciliation Act of 1981 (Public Law 97-35) rescinded continued federal management and turned responsibility for provision of community mental health services to the states through the block grant. At present, in New York and other states, treatment of the chronically mentally ill, both young and old, is the primary focus of community mental health centers.

In the mid-1990s, the direct cost associated with care for mental disorders is more than $50 billion[121] and was estimated to constitute 10 percent of all health care costs in the United States.[122] Overall, considering indirect costs associated with absence from work, unemployment, social services, related accidents, and crime, the estimated cost associated with all mental illness is more than $200 billion.[121] Treatment studies are under way in mental health and in primary care settings to identify methods to improve patients' outcomes and reduce this cost.

Preventive Interventions

Preventive medicine divides prevention activities into primary, secondary, and tertiary categories. These divisions also are useful in identifying psychiatric problems that can be prevented totally (and thus eliminated) from those for which early detection and treatment may avert or minimize the progression of the disease. The priority assigned to each type of prevention will change as our knowledge of etiology becomes more certain.

Primary prevention can be carried out when the etiology of the disease is understood and the environmental cause is eliminated. Two disorders have essentially been eradicated through primary prevention efforts: pellagra psychoses and brain damage from measles and rubella.

In the workplace, as noted earlier, high-level exposure to heavy metals such as lead and mercury resulted in psychiatric disorders. Standards such as the U.S. Occupational Safety and Health Administration's Lead Standard have reduced exposure to levels at which neuropathy or encephalopathy rarely occur. Similarly, concerns regarding childhood lead poisoning resulted in the passage of laws to reduce lead in paints, a primary source of exposure. It is important to point out, however, that, in many countries in South America, Africa, Asia, and Eastern Europe, environmental exposure is poorly regulated. High levels of contaminants produce exposures comparable to those described in nineteenth century Europe and the United States.

In addition to environmental factors, other primary prevention efforts have focused on asymptomatic individuals in high-risk groups. For example, as a consequence of the recent increase in suicide rates in adolescents and young adults, there has been a growth in school-based programs aimed at preventing teenage suicide.[123] The goals of these programs are to heighten awareness of the problem, to promote the identification of students at risk, and to provide information about mental health resources. Shaffer et al[123] studied 1,000 13- to 18-year-old students from six high schools who were exposed to one of three programs. Although the three programs used significantly different techniques, the authors felt that they were not differentially effective, concluding that the true value of the programs was their screening function, in which 3 percent of the students reported that they were suicidal and in need of professional help.

Early detection is the cornerstone of secondary prevention. The most famous example in psychiatry has been the elimination of general paresis (syphilitic psychoses) through antibiotic therapy. Secondary prevention programs have been implemented in the early phases of a variety of high-risk situations. These programs were aimed at reducing psychological difficulties in recently separated couples; substance abuse and delinquency in young adolescents with a history of poor academic performance and disruptive behaviors; and depression in Mexican American women, in low-income mothers, and in adults undergoing major life changes.[124] Recently, Kessler advocated developing interventions for secondary disorders, given the high rate of comorbidity in the population.[125]

A report by the U.S. Preventive Services Task Force identified several psychiatric disorders in which screening for early detection has been considered, namely, dementia, depression, suicide, abnormal bereavement, and alcohol and drug abuse.[126] The Task Force did not recommend screening for these conditions in asymptomatic populations because of the uncertain sensitivity and specificity of available screening tools.

The workplace also has become a focal point for secondary intervention programs. Many companies established Employee Assistance Programs and the like to assist troubled employees. The goal of these programs is to detect mental health problems at an early stage and offer an intervention that might avert a full-blown psychiatric episode. Similarly, health programs aimed at reducing physical symptoms (e.g., smoking, obesity, high blood pressure) also are proliferating in occupational settings. In light of the significant relationship between physical and mental health, it has been suggested that these programs will also have an indirect impact on the psychological well-being of employees.

Clinical trials focused on psychotherapeutic medications or other forms of therapy are examples of tertiary prevention efforts focused on minimizing disability and handicap in patients with a history of mental illness. For example, the NIMH D/ART program described above[113] is based on the premise that depressive disorders are treatable in 80 to 90 percent of cases. The program is aimed at educating psychiatrists, general practitioners, and the lay public about the symptoms and treatments for affective disorders. A review of the vast psychiatric treatment literature is beyond the scope of this chapter; however, clinical drug trials currently are being conducted for an array of medications presumed to alleviate symptoms associated with schizophrenia, depression, obsessive-compulsive disorder, panic disorder, and other mental illnesses.

▶ CONCLUSION

Considerable progress has occurred in research on the epidemiology of mental disorders. In the last few years, new textbooks[127,128] as well as a special issue of *Epidemiologic Reviews*[129] were published. Although most of the achievements have occurred at the level of descriptive epidemiology, analytic findings on variables associated with onset and course have also begun to appear. Recent advances in molecular genetics, brain imaging techniques, statistical methods, and measurement of disorder and risk factors are having a major impact on the scope and focus of current research. Ultimately, the goal of psychiatric epidemiology is to advance our understanding of mechanisms that are modifiable and lend themselves to preventive interventions.

▶ REFERENCES

1. Institute of Medicine: Research on Children and Adolescents with Mental, Behavioral, and Developmental Disorders: Mobilizing a National Initiative. Washington, DC: National Academy Press, 1989
2. Verhulst FC, Koot HM: Child Psychiatric Epidemiology. Newbury Park CA: Sage Publications, 1992
3. Regier DA, Boyd JH, Burke JD, et al: One-month prevalence of mental disorders in the United States based on five epidemiologic catchment area sites. Arch Gen Psychiatry 45:977–986, 1988
4. Henderson AS: Alzheimer's disease in its epidemiological context. Acta Neurol Scand Suppl 149:1–3, 1993
5. National Institute of Mental Health, Division of Biometry and Applied Sciences: Mental Health Stat Notes, various years
6. Kendall RE: The Role of Diagnosis in Psychiatry. Oxford: Blackwell Scientific Publications, 1975
7. American Psychiatric Association: Diagnostic and Statistical Manual of Mental Disorders. 4th ed. Washington, DC: American Psychiatric Association, 1994
8. Dohrenwend BP, Dohrenwend BS: Perspectives on the past and future of psychiatric epidemiology: The 1981 Rema Lapouse Lecture. Am J Public Health 72(11):1271–1279, 1982
9. Regier D, Burke J: Psychiatric disorders in the community: the Epidemiologic Catchment Area study. In Hales R, Frances A (eds): American Psychiatric Association Annual Review. Washington, DC: American Psychiatric Press, 1987, vol 6, ch 27
10. Kessler RC, McGonagle KA, Zhao S, et al: Lifetime and 12-month prevalence of DSM-III-R psychiatric disorders in the United States. Arch Gen Psychiatry 51:8–19, 1994
11. Grob GN: The origins of American psychiatric epidemiology. Am J Public Health 75(3):229–236, 1985
12. Kramer M: Some problems for international research suggested by observations on differences in first admission rates to the mental hospitals of England and Wales and of the United States. In: Proceedings of the Third World Congress of Psychiatry. Montreal: University of Toronto Press, 1961, vol 3, pp 153–160
13. Cooper JE, Kendell RE, Gurland BJ, Sharpe L, Copeland JRM: Psychiatric Diagnosis in New York and London: A Comparative Study of Mental Hospital Admissions. Maudsley Monographs, No. 20. London: Oxford University Press, 1972
14. World Health Organization: Schizophrenia: A Multinational Study. Geneva: World Health Organization, 1975
15. Sartorius N, Jablensky A, Korten A, et al: Early manifestations and first-contact incidence of schizophrenia in different cultures: a preliminary report on the initial evaluation phase of the WHO Collaborative Study on Determinants of Outcome of Severe Mental Disorders. Psychol Med 16:909–928, 1986
16. Feighner JP, Robins E, Guze SB, et al: Diagnostic criteria for use in diagnostic research. Arch Gen Psychiatry 26:57–63, 1972
17. Endicott J, Spitzer R: A diagnostic interview: the Schedule for Affective Disorders and Schizophrenia. Arch Gen Pyschiatry 35:837–844, 1978
18. Spitzer R, Endicott J, Robins E: Research diagnostic criteria: rationale and reliability. Arch Gen Psychiatry 35:773–782, 1978
19. Spitzer R, Williams B, Gibbon M, First M: The Structured Clinical Interview for DSM-III-R (SCID): I. History, rationale, and description. Arch Gen Psychiatry 49:624–629, 1992
20. Robins LN, Helzer JE, Croughan J, Ratcliff KS: National Institute of Mental Health Diagnostic Interview Schedule. Arch Gen Psychiatry 34:129–133, 1977
21. Eaton WW, Kessler LG (eds): Epidemiologic Field Methods in Psychiatry: The NIMH Epidemiologic Catchment Area Program. Orlando, FL: Academic Press, 1985
22. Jensen P, Roper M, Fisher P, et al: Test-retest reliability of the Diagnostic Interview Schedule for Children (DISC 2.1). Arch Gen Psychiatry 52:61–71, 1995
23. Morris JN: Uses of Epidemiology, 2nd ed. London: Livingstone, 1964
24. Jarvis E: Insanity and Idiocy in Massachusetts: Report of the Commission on Lunacy, 1855. Cambridge, MA: Harvard University Press, 1971
25. Srole L, Langner TS, Michael ST, Kirkpatrick P, Opler MK, Rennie TAC: Mental Health in the Metropolis: The Midtown Manhattan Study. New York: Harper & Row, 1962
26. Gurin G, Veroff J, Feld J: Americans View Their Mental Health. New York: Basic Books, 1960
27. Cahalan D: Understanding America's Drinking Problem: How to Combat the Hazards of Alcohol. San Francisco: Jossey-Bass, 1987
28. Eaton WW Jr, Regier DA, Locke BZ, Taube CA: The Epidemiologic Catchment Area Program of the National Institute of Mental Health. Public Health Rep 96(4):319–325, 1981
29. Eaton WW Jr, Kramer M, Anthony JC, Dryman A, Shapiro S, Locke BZ: The incidence of specific DIS/DSM-III mental disorders: data from the NIMH Epidemiologic Catchment Area Program. Acta Psychiatr Scand 79:163–178, 1989
30. Myers JK, Weissman MM, Tischler GL, et al: Six-month prevalence of psychiatric disorders in three communities. Arch Gen Psychiatry 41:959–967, 1984
31. Robins LN, Heizer JE, Weissman MM, et al: Lifetime prevalence of specific psychiatric disorders in three sites. Arch Gen Psychiatry 41:949–958, 1984
32. Eaton WW Jr, Day R. Kramer M: The use of epidemiology for risk factor research in schizophrenia: an overview and methodologic critique. In Tsuang MT, Simpson JC (eds): Nosology, Epidemiology and Genetics of Schizophrenia. New York: Elsevier, 1988, ch 9
33. Link B, Dohrenwend BP: Formulation of hypotheses about the ratio of untreated to treated cases in the true prevalence studies of functional psychiatric disorders in adults in the United States. In Dohrenwend BP, Dohrenwend BS, Gould MS, et al (eds): Mental Illness in the United States: Epidemiological Estimates. New York: Praeger, 1980
34. Faris R, Dunham H: Mental Disorders in Urban Areas: An Ecological Study of Schizophrenia and Other Psychoses. New York: Hafner, 1939
35. Dohrenwend BP, Dohrenwend BS: Psychiatric disorders in urban settings. In Arieti S (ed): American Handbook of Psychiatry, vol 2:

Child and Adolescent Psychiatry, Sociocultural and Community Psychiatry. New York: Basic Books, 1974
36. Mueller DP: The current status of urban-rural differences in psychiatric disorder: an emerging trend for depression. J Nerv Ment Dis 169(1):18–27, 1981
37. Brown GW, Davidson S, Harris T, Maclean U, Pollock S, Prudo R: Psychiatric disorder in London and North Uist. Soc Sci Med 11:367–377, 1977
38. Blazer W, Oeorge LK, Landerman R, et al: Psychiatric disorders: a rural/urban comparison. Arch Gen Psychiatry 42:651–656, 1985
39. Blazer DG, Crowell BA, George LK, Landerman R: Urban-rural differences in depressive disorders: does age make a difference? In Barrett J, Rose RM (eds): Mental Disorders in the Community: Progress and Challenge. New York: The Guilford Press, 1986, ch 3
40. Rutter M, Yule B, Quinton D, Rowlands O, Yule W, Berger M: Attainment and adjustment in two geographical areas: III. Some factors accounting for area differences. Br J Psychiatry 125:520–533, 1974
41. Offord D, Boyle M, Szatmari P, et al: Six-month prevalence of disorder and rates of service utilization. Arch Gen Psychiatry 44: 832–836, 1987
42. Eaton WW Jr: Residence, social class and schizophrenia. J Health Soc Behav 15:289–299, 1974
43. Jorm AF, Korten A, Henderson AS: The prevalence of dementia: a quantitative integration of the literature. Acta Psychiatr Scand 76:465–479, 1987
44. Weissman MM, Bland R, Canino G, et al: Cross-national epidemiology of major depression and bipolar disorder. JAMA 276:293–299, 1996
45. Helzer JE, Canino GJ (eds): Alcoholism in North America, Europe, and Asia. New York: Oxford University Press, 1992
46. Kessler RC, McGonagle KA, Nelson CB et al: Sex and depression in the National Comorbidity Survey. II: Cohort effects. J Affect Disord 30:15–26, 1994
47. Bebbington P: The origins of sex differences in depression: bridging the gap. Int Rev Psychiatry 8:295–332, 1996
48. Rutter M: Epidemiological approaches to developmental psychopathology. Arch Gen Psychiatry 45:486–495, 1988
49. Cahalan D, Cisin IH: American drinking practices: summary of findings from a national probability sample. 1. Extent of drinking by population subgroups. In Ward DA (ed): Alcoholism, Introduction to Theory and Treatment. Dubuque, IA: Kendall Hunt, 1980, ch 8
50. Hollingshead AB, Redlich FC: Social Class and Mental Illness: A Community Study. New York: John Wiley & Sons, 1958
51. Goldberg E, Morrison S: Schizophrenia and social class. Br J Psychiatry 109:785–802, 1963
52. Schwab JJ, Schwab ME: Sociocultural Roots of Mental Illness: An Epidemiologic Survey. New York: Plenum, 1978
53. Costello EJ, Angold A, Burns BJ, et al: The Great Smoky Mountains study of youth: goals, design, methods, and the prevalence of DSM-III-R disorders. Arch Gen Psychiatry 53:1129–1136, 1996
54. Berkman LF, Berkman CS, Kasl S, Freeman DH, Leo L, Ostfeld AM, Cornoni-Huntley J, Brody JA: Depressive symptoms in relation to physical health and functioning in the elderly. Am J Epidemiol 124:372–387, 1986
55. May P: Suicide and self-destruction among American Indian youths. Am Indian Alsk Native Ment Health Res 1:52–69, 1987
56. Kulcar Z, Crocetti GM, Lemkau PV, Kesic B: Selected aspects of the epidemiology of psychoses in Croatia, Yugoslavia: 11. Pilot studies of communities. Am J Epidemiol 94:118–125, 1971
57. Crocetti GM, Lemkau PV, Kulcar Z: Selected aspects of the epidemiology of psychoses in Croatia, Yugoslavia: III. The cluster sample and the results of the pilot survey. Am J Epidemiol 94:126–134, 1971
58. Walsh D, O'Hare A, Blake B, Holpenny J, O'Brien P: The treated prevalence of mental illness in the Republic of Ireland. The three county case register study. Psychol Med 10:465–470, 1980
59. Kendler KS, Gallagher TJ, Abelson JM, Kessler RC: Lifetime prevalence, demographic risk factors, and diagnostic validity of nonaffective psychosis as assessed in a US community sample. Arch Gen Psychiatry 53:1022–1030, 1996
60. Babigian HM, Odoroff CL: The mortality experience of a population with psychiatric illness. Am J Psychiatry 126:470–480, 1969
61. Munoz RA, Marten S, Gentry KA, et al: Mortality following a psychiatric emergency room visit: an 18-month follow-up study. Am J Psychiatry 128:220–224, 1971
62. Bruce ML, Leaf PJ: Psychiatric disorders and 15-month mortality in a community sample of older adults. Am J Public Health 79:727–730, 1989
63. Katon W: The epidemiology of depression in medical care. Int J Psychiatry Med 17:93–112, 1987
64. Moffic H. Paykel E: Depression in medical inpatients. Br J Psychiatry 126:346–353, 1975
65. Kessler LG, Burns BJ, Shapiro S, Tischler GL, George LK, Hough RL, Bodison D, Miller RH: Psychiatric diagnoses of medical service users: evidence from the Epidemiologic Catchment Area Program. Am J Public Health 77:18–24, 1987
66. Blacker CVR, Clare AW: Depressive disorder in primary care. Br J Psychiatry 150:737–751, 1987
67. Üstün TB, Sartorius N: Mental Illness in General Health Care: An International Study. New York: John Wiley & Sons, 1995
68. Kendler KS: The genetics of schizophrenia: an overview. In Tsuang MT, Simpson JC (eds): Nosology, Epidemiology and Genetics of Schizophrenia. New York: Elsevier, 1988, ch 18
69. Weissman MM: Advances in psychiatric epidemiology: rates and risks for major depression. Am J Public Health 77:445–451, 1987
70. Weissman MM, Prusoff BA, Gammon GD, et al: Psychopathology in the children (ages 6–18) of depressed and normal parents. J Am Acad Child Psychiatry 23(1):78–84, 1984
71. Merikangas KR: The genetic epidemiology of alcoholism. Psychol Med 20:11–22, 1990
72. Hare E: Aspects of the epidemiology of schizophrenia. Br J Psychiatry 149:554–561, 1986
73. Bromet EJ, Dew MA, Eaton W: Epidemiology of psychosis with special reference to schizophrenia. In Tsuang M, Tohen M, Zahner G (eds): Textbook in Psychiatric Epidemiology. New York: John Wiley, 1995, ch 14
74. Goldberger J, Waring CH, Tanner WF: Pellagra prevention by diet in institution inmates. Public Health Rep 38:2361–2368, 1925
75. Bromet EJ, Parkinson D, Schulberg HC, Dunn L, Gondek PC: Mental health of residents near the TMI reactor: a comparative study of selected groups. J Prev Psychiatry 1:225–275, 1982
76. Dew MA, Bromet EJ, Schulberg HC: A comparative analysis of two community stressors' long-term mental health effects. Am J Community Psychol 15:167–184, 1987
77. Dew MA, Bromet EJ: Predictors of temporal patterns of psychiatric distress 10 years following the nuclear accident at Three Mile Island. Soc Psychiatry Psychiatr Epidemiol 28:49–55, 1993
78. Bromet E, Dew MA: Review of psychiatric epidemiologic research on disasters. Epidemiol Rev 17:113–119, 1995
79. Solomon S: Research issues in assessing disaster's effects. In Gist R. Lubin B (eds): Psychosocial Aspects of Disaster. New York: John Wiley & Sons, 1989, ch 12
80. Kulka RA, Schlenger WE, Fairbank JA, et al: Trauma and the Vietnam War generation: report of findings from the National Vietnam Veterans Readjustment Study. New York: Brunner/Mazel, 1990
81. Zubin J, Steinhauer R, Day R, van Kammen D: Schizophrenia at the crossroads: a blueprint for the 80s. Compr Psychiatry 26:217–240, 1985
82. Paykel E: Contribution of life events to causation of psychiatric illness. Psychol Med 8:245–253, 1978
83. Brown G, Harris T: Social Origins of Depression: A Study of Psychiatric-Disorder in Women. New York: The Free Press, 1978

84. Kates N, Greiff BS, Hagen DQ: The Psychosocial Impact of Job Loss. Washington, DC: American Psychiatric Press, 1990
85. Jacobs S, Hansen F, Berkman L, et al: Depressions of bereavement. Compr Psychiatry 30:218–224, 1989
86. Kasl S: Epidemiological contributions to the study of work stress. In Cooper C, Payne R (eds): Stress at Work. New York: John Wiley & Sons, 1978, ch 1
87. Karasek R: Job demands, job decision latitude, and mental strain: implications for job redesign. Administrative Science Quarterly 24:285–306, 1979
88. Phelan J, Schwartz JE, Bromet EJ, et al: Work stress, family stress and depression in professional and managerial employees. Psychol Med 21:999–1012, 1991
89. Garfinkel B, Carlson G, Weller E (eds): Psychiatric Disorders in Children and Adolescents. Philadelphia: WB Saunders, 1990
90. Parkinson D, Ryan C, Bromet EJ, Connell M: A psychiatric epidemiologic study of occupational lead exposure. Am J Epidemiol 123:261–269, 1986
91. Elofsson S, Gamberale F, Hindmarsh T, et al: Exposure to organic solvents. Scand J Work Environ Health 6:239–273, 1980
92. Husman K: Symptoms of car painters with long-term exposure to a mixture of organic solvents. Scand J Work Environ Health 6:19–32, 1980
93. Larsen F, Leira H: Organic brain syndrome and long-term exposure to toluene: a clinical, psychiatric study of vocationally active printing workers. J Occup Med 30:875–878, 1988
94. Orbaek P, Risberg J, Rosen I, et al: Effects of long-term exposure to solvents in the paint industry. Scand J Work Environ Health 11(Suppl 2):1–28, 1985
95. Errebo-Knudsen E, Olsen F: Organic solvents and presenile dementia (the painter's syndrome): a critical review of the Danish literature. Sci Total Environ 48:45–67, 1986
96. Parkinson DK, Bromet EJ, Cohen S, et al: Health effects of long-term solvent exposure among women in blue collar occupations. Am J Ind Med 17:661–675, 1990
97. House J, McMichael A, Wells J, et al: Occupational stress and health among factory workers. J Health Soc Behav 20:139–116, 1979
98. Bromet EJ, Ryan CM, Parkinson DK: Psychosocial correlates of occupational lead exposure. In Lebovits AH, Baum A, Singer JE (eds): Advances in Environmental Psychology, vol 6: Exposure to Hazardous Substances: Psychological Parameters. Hillsdale, NJ: Lawrence Erlbaum Associates, 1986, ch 2
99. Bromet EJ, Dew MA, Parkinson DK, et al: Effects of occupational stress on the physical and psychological health of women in a microelectronics plant. Soc Sci Med 34:1377–1383, 1992
100. Colligan M, Murphy L: Mass psychogenic illness in organizations: an overview. J Occup Psychol 52:77–90, 1979
101. Needleman HL, Gunnoe C, Leviton A, Reed R, Peresie H, Maher C, Barrett P: Deficits in psychologic and classroom performance of children with elevated dentine lead levels. N Engl J Med 300(13):689–695, 1979
102. Needleman HL, Schell A, Bellinger D, Leviton A, Allred EN: The long-term effects of exposure to low doses of lead in childhood: An 11-year follow-up report. N Engl J Med 322(2):83–88, 1990
103. Koegel P, Burnam A, Farr RK: The prevalence of specific psychiatric disorders among homeless individuals in the inner city of Los Angeles. Arch Gen Psychiatry 45:1085–1092, 1988
104. Alperstein G, Rappaport C, Flanigan JM: Health problems of homeless children in New York City. Am J Public Health 78:1232–1233, 1988
105. Susser E, Lin S, Conover S, Struening E: Childhood antecedents of homelessness in psychiatric patients. Am J Psychiatry 148:1026–1030, 1991
106. Fisher PJ, Breakey WR: The epidemiology of alcohol, drug, and mental disorders among homeless persons. Am Psychol 46:1115–1128, 1991
107. Goldhamer H, Marshall A: Psychosis and Civilization. Glencoe, IL: Free Press, 1955
108. Eaton WW Jr: The Sociology of Mental Disorders. New York: Praeger, 1980
109. Krupinski J, Alexander L: Patterns of psychiatric morbidity in Victoria, Australia in relation to changes in diagnostic criteria 1848–1978. Soc Psychiatry 18:61–67, 1983
110. Häfner H: Are mental disorders increasing over time? Psychopathology 18:66–81, 1985
111. Hagnell O, Lanke J, Rorsman B, Ojesjo L: Are we entering an age of melancholy? Depressive illnesses in a prospective epidemiological study over 25 years: the Lundby Study, Sweden. Psychol Med 12:279–289, 1982
112. Klerman GL, Weissman MM: Increasing rates of depression. JAMA 261:2229–2235, 1989
113. Regier D, Hirschfeld R, Goodwin F, Burke J, Lazar J, Judd L: The NIMH Depression Awareness, Recognition, and Treatment Program: structure, aims, and scientific basis. Am J Psychiatry 145: 1351–1357, 1988
114. Rosenberg ML, Smith JC, Davidson LE, Conn JM: The emergence of youth suicide: an epidemiologic analysis and public health perspective. Am Rev Public Health 8:417–440, 1987
115. Brent DA, Perper JA, Allman CJ: Alcohol, firearms, and suicide among youth: temporal trends in Allegheny County, Pennsylvania, 1960 to 1983. JAMA 257:3369–3372, 1987
116. Bromet EJ, Parkinson D, Curtis EC, et al: Epidemiology of depression and alcohol abuse/dependence in a managerial and professional workforce. J Occup Med 32:989–995, 1990
117. Cohen P, Cohen J: The clinician's illusion. Arch Gen Psychiatry 41:1178–1182, 1984
118. Robins LN, Regier DA (eds): Psychiatric Disorders in America. New York: Free Press, 1991
119. Weller E, Weller R: Depressive disorders in children and adolescents. In Garfinkel B, Carlson G, Weller E (eds): Psychiatric Disorders in Children and Adolescents. Philadelphia: WB Saunders, 1990, ch 1
120. Collier HE: The mental manifestations of some industrial illnesses. Occup Psychol 113:89–97, 1939
121. Burke JD Jr: Mental health services research. In Tsuang M, Tohen M, Zahner G (eds): Textbook in Psychiatric Epidemiology. New York: John Wiley, 1995, ch 8
122. National Advisory Mental Health Council: Health care reform for Americans with severe mental illnesses. Am J Psychiatry 150:1447–1465, 1993
123. Shaffer D, Garland A, Gould M, Fisher P, Trautman P: Preventing teenage suicide: a critical review. J Am Acad Child Adolesc Psychiatry 27:675–687, 1988
124. Price RH, Smith SS: A Guide to Evaluating Prevention Programs in Mental Health. Washington, DC: Government Printing Office, 1984
125. Kessler RC: Epidemiology of psychiatric comorbidity. In Tsuang M, Tohen M, Zahner G (eds): Textbook in Psychiatric Epidemiology. New York: John Wiley, 1995, ch 7
126. U.S. Preventive Services Task Force: Guide to Clinical Preventive Services: An Assessment of the Effectiveness of 169 Interventions. Baltimore: Williams & Wilkins, 1989
127. Tsuang M, Tohen M, Zahner G (eds): Textbook in Psychiatric Epidemiology. New York: John Wiley, 1995
128. Henderson AS: An Introduction to Social Psychiatry. New York: Oxford University Press, 1988
129. Anthony JC, Eaton WW, Henderson AS (eds): Looking to the future in psychiatric epidemiology. Epidemiol Rev 17:240–242, 1995

61

Mental Retardation

Maureen S. Durkin • Nicole Schupf • Zena A. Stein • Mervyn W. Susser

Mental retardation is a condition with enormous public health implications for at least four reasons. One is its relative frequency; with prevalence rates of 2 percent or greater in most populations, mental retardation is among the most common disabilities occurring in childhood.[1–3] Another is its early onset and frequent life-long duration. A third is its socioeconomic impacts, which include adverse impacts on productivity and quality of life of affected individuals and caregivers as well as increased expenditures for medical care and residential services. A fourth reason is that prevention, whether primary, secondary, or tertiary, is attainable via public health interventions for nearly all forms of mental retardation. Examples of primary prevention include prenatal screening, genetic counseling, dietary supplementation of iodine and folate, and immunization programs. Early identification followed by therapeutic interventions for conditions such as phenylketonuria (PKU) and lead toxicity are examples of secondary prevention of mental retardation. Examples of tertiary prevention include early cognitive stimulation, special education, and habilitation to enhance functioning.

One of the new challenges mental retardation poses to public health is that certain prevention strategies, highly effective in one respect, have had the paradoxical side effect of increasing the occurrence of mental retardation in the population in terms of either incidence (new cases) or prevalence (by means of improved survival). Examples of this paradox include mental retardation associated with inborn errors of metabolism, Down syndrome, and premature birth. These and other specific topics in mental retardation are discussed below, following an overview of definitions and prevalence.

▸ DEFINITION AND CLASSIFICATION

Mental retardation implies significant deficits, with onset early in life, in intelligence (as measured by standardized intelligence tests) and in adaptive behavior (e.g., communication, self-care, social interaction, school and/or work).[4] The deficits are recognized in the performance of social roles and age-appropriate tasks. The infant and preschool child may fail to achieve developmental milestones of sitting, responding to familiar faces, walking, talking, and sphincter control at expected ages. The schoolchild falls short of social expectations for classroom behavior and for reading, writing, and arithmetic. The adult may have difficulty in the performance of work roles within and outside the home, in communication skills, or in the understanding of money, transport, and locality.

Functional limitations in mental retardation can potentially be identified at three levels: *impairment* (altered brain structure and/or function), *disability* (deficits in intellectual function and adaptive behavior), and *handicap* (limitations in social roles and opportunities experienced by persons with disabilities due environmental conditions).[5,6] One-to-one correlations between currently understood causes, identifiable impairments, and levels of disability and handicap appear to be the exception rather than the rule. For example, in people with mental retardation, identifiable neuropathological lesions often correlate weakly or not at all with specific causes and/or clinical/functional attributes.[7,8]

The dominant approach to defining and classifying mental retardation is by severity of disability rather than by cause. The *International Classification of Diseases* (ICD-9, ICD-10)[9,10] as well as the *Diagnostic and Statistical Manual* (DSM-IV)[11] and former versions of the American Association on Mental Retardation classification[4] distinguish four grades of severity defined in terms of IQ (Table 61-1). The most recent version of the American Association on Mental Retardation's classification system has moved away from distinguishing grades of intellectual deficit and toward defining severity in terms of the level of support required for optimal functioning (e.g., intermittent, limited, extensive, and pervasive levels of support).[12]

Classification based on etiology is increasingly used, as advances in cytogenetics, molecular genetics, and brain imaging improve our ability to determine specific causes. Etiologic classifications have clear advantages for epidemiologic research and for primary prevention. They may also be preferable to functional classifications for assessing specific needs for appropriate medical care, rehabilitation, and other services.[13] However, even with recent advances in knowledge and diagnostic capabilities, most cases of mental retardation cannot be attributed with certainty to a specific cause. Table 61-2 provides an outline of the categories of known causes of mental retardation.

▸ INCIDENCE AND PREVALENCE

Studies of the true incidence of mental retardation are not possible because only a minority of cases survive long enough to be identified and because the onset and recognition of disability are often insidious during the course of a child's development.[14,15] The descriptive epidemiology of mental retardation is based largely on prevalence (the number of existing cases in a population at a given time) rather than incidence (the number of newly occurring cases during a given time period).

In describing the prevalence of mental retardation, it is useful to combine moderate, severe, and profound grades of intellectual disability into a single category of *severe* mental retardation (IQ below 50 or 55) and distinguish this from *mild* mental retardation (IQ between 50 or 55 and 70 or 75). Table 61-3 contrasts the major epidemiologic characteristics of these two classes. In developed countries the prevalence of severe mental retardation in childhood is consistently found to range from 3 to 5 per 1,000 (Table 61-4) and more than 50 percent of cases are attributed to genetic causes. Mild mental retardation in developed countries varies widely in prevalence, is generally more frequent than severe forms, is strongly associated with low socioeconomic status, and is rarely associated

TABLE 61-1. CLASSIFICATION OF MENTAL RETARDATION BY GRADE OF SEVERITY OF INTELLECTUAL DEFICIT

Severity	ICD-9[a] Code	ICD-10[b] Code	Approximate IQ Range[c]
Mild	317.00	F70.9	50–55 to 70–75
Moderate	318.00	F71.9	30–35 to 50–55
Severe	318.10	F72.9	20–25 to 35–40
Profound	318.20	F73.9	<20–25
Unspecified	319.00	F79.9	

[a] World Health Organization: International Classification of Diseases. 9th ed. Geneva: World Health Organization, 1980.
[b] World Health Organization: International Classification of Diseases. 10th ed. Geneva: World Health Organization, 1992.
[c] Precise IQ cut-points may vary to allow for differences between tests. Guidelines of the American Association on Mental Deficiency[4] and the *Diagnostic and Statistical Manual* (DSM-IV) of the American Psychiatric Association[11] recommend the use of these or similar cut-points as well as clinical judgment and assessment of adaptive skills in the diagnosis and classification of severity of mental retardation.

with known causes or with other neurologic disorders. A male excess is observed in both severe and mild mental retardation, due in part to the contribution of X-linked forms of mental retardation (discussed below). The few estimates available from less developed countries point to elevated prevalence rates of severe mental retardation (Table 61-4). This may be due to the higher frequency in those settings of nutritional, traumatic, and infectious causes of brain damage.[16]

Low socioeconomic status is the strongest and most consistent predictor of mild mental retardation but has little or no association with the prevalence of severe mental retardation (Table 61-3).[17,18] This pattern points to the role of poverty and social disadvantage in the etiology of mild mental retardation. Preschool programs providing social and intellectual stimulation may boost IQ and reduce the risk of mild mental retardation in vulnerable groups.[19–22]

Several cross-sectional studies of age-specific prevalence rates conducted in different decades and populations are consistent in showing, for both severe and mild mental retardation, increasing prevalence rates with age during childhood followed by declining rates with advancing age throughout adulthood.[1] Severe mental retardation is much more likely than mild to be diagnosed during infancy. The increasing prevalence with age during childhood could be due to increases with age in the use of specialty services and in the probability of being included in agency records[1] as well as the likelihood of exposure to postnatal causes (infections, trauma). For severe mental retardation, excess mortality is responsible for the decline in prevalence with age after childhood. For mild mental retardation, the decline may be due in part to mortality, but a more important factor is that societies do not universally require of adults the cognitive skills they require of school children. A degree of recovery is also probable. Thus, many persons categorized as mildly retarded in school become indistinguishable from the general population during adulthood.

► SELECTED CAUSES

Chromosomal Anomalies

Chromosomal anomalies, including structural and numerical anomalies, are a major cause of severe mental retardation. Structural changes result from breakage and rearrangement of chromosome parts and can be induced by a variety of exposures, including ionizing radiation and certain viral infections and toxic substances. Numerical anomalies arise through nondisjunction during meiosis or mitosis or through lagging of chromosomes at anaphase of cell division. Among several types of abnormalities of chromosome number that occur, trisomies play the largest role in the etiology of mental retardation. Chromosomal anomalies as a whole contribute more to fetal loss than to live births and mental retardation. About 40 percent of miscarriages, 6 percent of stillbirths, and less than 1 percent of live births are chromosomally aberrant.[23] After 8 weeks gestational age, the proportion of chromosomal aberrations lost by miscarriage exceeds 90 percent for all but trisomy 21 (Down syndrome), XXX, XXY (Klinefelter's syndrome), and XYY.[23] Chromosomal anomalies, primarily Down syndrome, cause more than 30 percent of prevalent cases of severe mental retardation in developed countries.[24–26]

Down Syndrome

Down syndrome is the most common genetic cause of mental retardation and the leading known cause of severe mental retardation in developed countries.[27] All cases of Down syndrome result from partial or complete duplication of chromosome 21 in the genome.[28] The most common form (95 percent of cases at birth) is standard trisomy, involving duplication of chromosome 21. In over 90 percent of these cases, the extra chromosome is of maternal origin, due to nondisjunction during meiosis.[29–31] Translocation of chromosome 21 material to another chromosome (usually 13 or 18) and mosaicism (trans-

TABLE 61-2. MAJOR CATEGORIES OF KNOWN CAUSES OF MENTAL RETARDATION WITH SPECIFIC EXAMPLES OF EACH

Causal Category	Specific Examples
Chromosomal	Down syndrome
	Cri-du-chat
Single gene	Phenylketonuria (PKU)
	Fragile X syndrome
Hormonal	Hypothyroidism
Specific nutritional	Iodine
Deficiency/dietary factor (prenatal)	Folate
	Maternal PKU
Infection	
Prenatal	Rubella
	Toxoplasmosis
Perinatal	Syphilis
	Human immunodeficiency virus
Postnatal	Measles encephalitis
Toxic exposure	
Prenatal	Ionizing radiation
	Fetal alcohol syndrome
	Lead
Postnatal	Lead
Traumatic brain injury, anoxia	
Perinatal	Prolonged, obstructed labor
	Premature birth
Postnatal	Motor vehicle collision
	Fall
	Near drowning

TABLE 61-3. EPIDEMIOLOGIC CHARACTERISTICS OF SEVERE AND MILD MENTAL RETARDATION

	Severe	***Mild***
Prevalence range in childhood (/1000):		
Populations with advanced medical care	2.5–5.0	2.5–40.0
Less developed countries	5.0–25.0	(Estimates not available)
Life expectancy	Considerably shorter than general population	Somewhat shorter than general population
% with other neurodevelopmental or sensory disorders	About 85%	About one-third
% with other psychiatric disorders	Higher frequency than general population	Higher frequency than general population
% with known genetic cause	About 50%	Small percentage
% with unknown cause	Minority	Majority
Usual age at recognition	Infancy or preschool years	School age
Duration	Lifelong	May be restricted to school age
Male-Female ratio	Male excess (1.1 to 1.4:1)	Male excess (1.1 to 1.8:1)
Major demographic risk factors	Maternal age is a strong predictor of trisomies, which cause about 30% of severe mental retardation	Low socioeconomic status
Association with social class	Prevalence is relatively even across the social classes	Occurs predominantly in children of low social class

Sources: Alberman E: Main causes of major mental handicap: prevalence and epidemiology. Ciba Found Symp 59:3–16, 1978; Eyman RK, Grossman HJ, Chaney et al: The life expectancy of profoundly handicapped persons with mental retardation. N Engl J Med 323:584–589, 1990; Kaveggia EG, Durkin MV, Pendleton E, et al: Genetic studies on 1,224 patients with severe mental retardation. In: Proceedings of the Third Congress of the International Association for the Scientific Study of Mental Deficiency. Warsaw: Polish Medical Publishers, 1975, pp 82–93; Kiely M: The prevalence of mental retardation. Epidemiol Rev 9:194–218, 1987; Murphy CC, Yeargin-Allsopp M, Decoufle P, Drews CD: The administrative prevalence of mental retardation in 10-year-old children in metropolitan Atlanta, 1985 through 1987. Am J Public Health 85(3):319–323, 1995.

mission of a cryptic trisomy 21 cell line from an unaffected parent) are rare causes of Down syndrome.[32,33]

The most striking epidemiologic characteristic of Down syndrome is the marked increase in risk with increasing maternal age, from 1 per 1,550 live births at ages 20 to 24 to 1 per 700 live births at ages 30 to 34 to 1 per 50 live births at ages 41 to 45.[34] Increased availability of effective birth control in the 1960s was followed by reductions in the number and proportion of births to older women and corresponding reductions in the prevalence of Down syndrome at birth.[33] Also contributing to reductions in the frequency of Down syndrome births, but to a lesser extent, is the availability of prenatal diagnosis followed by selective abortion. A comparative study of 19 populations found this to be responsible for an average 6 percent reduction in the number of infants with Down syndrome.[35] However, the era of decreased prevalence at birth has also been an era of increased longevity of persons with Down syndrome. The net effect of these two trends has been a rise in the prevalence of Down syndrome in adolescents and adults. It has been estimated that even with improved screening and assuming increased use of selective abortion to prevent Down syndrome births, prevalence rates will be higher in the twenty-first century than ever before.[27]

Despite the strong association between Down syndrome risk and maternal age, most Down syndrome births are to women under 35 because these women contribute the great majority of births. Thus, the current practice in some countries of restricting prenatal screening for Down syndrome to women 35 and over (using amniocentesis or chorionic villus sampling) will detect and potentially prevent no more than 15 to 20 percent of affected births.[36,37] The discovery of safer and more practical methods of screening for this anomaly during the first trimester of pregnancy is, therefore, an important public health goal. The method of "triple analyte" screening (based on α-fetoprotein, human chorionic gonadotropin, and unconjugated estriol levels in maternal serum) used in conjunction with maternal age and ultrasound estimation of gestational age may have a sensitivity of up to 70 percent for Down syndrome.[38,39] Analysis of amniotic fluid when a pregnancy has screened positive for Down syndrome may also detect a comparable number of fetuses with other chromosomal abnormalities, including other autosomal trisomies, sex chromosome abnormalities, and structural rearrangements.[40]

About one-third of children with Down syndrome have congenital heart defects and 2 to 5 percent have duodenal obstruction. Other conditions that occur with increased frequency in Down syndrome are childhood leukemia, recurrent infections, hypothyroidism, and seizure disorders. Mental retardation is virtually always present and the majority of children function in the moderate to profound range of intellectual disability. Adults with Down syndrome show a variety of age-related changes in physical and functional capacities suggestive of premature or accelerated aging,[41] including changes in skin tone, hypogonadism, increased frequency of cataracts, increased frequency of vision and hearing loss, hypothyroidism, seizures, degenerative vascular disease, and early and severe Alzheimer's disease.[42–46] The increased life span of individuals with Down syndrome and accompanying age-associated morbidity have important consequences for medical care and community services as well as sustained support from family members who are facing new concerns about the need for prolonged care of offspring with Down syndrome.

X-Linked Mental Retardation

Sex-linked disorders arise from differences in the expression of genes on the sex chromosomes between males and females. Only in males

TABLE 61-4. SEVERE MENTAL RETARDATION IN CHILDHOOD: SELECTED ESTIMATES OF PREVALENCE

Location	Reference	Data Source	Age	Prevalence[a]
Aberdeen, Scotland	Birch et al, 1970[b]	Follow-up of births	8–10	3.70
Isle of Wight, England	Rutter et al, 1970[c]	Population screening, evaluations	5–14	3.40
Quebec, Canada	McDonald, 1973[d]	Agency records	10	3.84
Netherlands	Stein et al, 1976[e]	Birth cohort, military records	19	3.73
United Kingdom	Peckham and Pearson, 1976[f]	Birth cohort, examinations, interviews	7	2.40
			11	3.30
			16	3.40
Uppsala County, Sweden	Gustavson et al, 1977[g]	Registry, agency, vital records	11–16	2.88
Salford, England	Fryers and Mackay, 1979[h]	Agency records	5–15	4.50
Karnataka, India	Narayanan, 1981[i]	Household survey, evaluations	5–9	12.40
Karachi, Pakistan	Hasan and Hasan, 1981[j]	Household survey, evaluations	11–15	24.30
Kuruma City, Japan	Shiotsuki et al, 1984[k]		7–12	4.90
Beijing, China	Zuo et al, 1986[l]	Household survey, evaluations	0–14	2.94
New Brunswick,	McQueen et al, 1987[m]	Agency records	7–10	4.61
Nova Scotia, Canada				2.82
North West Spain	Diaz-Fernandez, 1988[n]	Registry	5–9	2.71
			10–14	4.08
May Pen, Jamaica	Thorburn et al, 1992[o]	Household survey, evaluations	2–9	17.00
Bangladesh	Zaman et al, 1992[p]	Household survey, evaluations	2–9	5.28
Atlanta, Georgia, United States	Murphy et al, 1995[q]	School and other record review	10	3.60
Karachi, Pakistan	Durkin et al, 1998[r]	Household survey, evaluations	2–9	19.00

[a] Prevalence per 1000.
[b] Birch HG, Richardson SA, Baird D, et al: Mental Subnormality in the Community: A Clinical and Epidemiologic Study, Baltimore: Williams & Wilkins, 1970.
[c] Rutter M, Tizard J, Whitmore K (eds): Education, Health and Behaviour. London: Longman, 1970.
[d] McDonald AD: Severely retarded children in Quebec: prevalence, causes and care. Am J Mental Defic Res 78:205–215, 1973.
[e] Stein ZA, Susser MW, Saenger G, Marolla F: Mental retardation in a national population of young men in The Netherlands: 1. Prevalence of severe mental retardation. Am J Epidemiol 103:477–489, 1976.
[f] Peckham C, Pearson R: The prevalence and nature of ascertained handicap in the National Child Development Study (1958 cohort). Public Health 90:111–121, 1976.
[g] Gustavson KH, Hagberg B, Hagberg G, Sars K: Severe mental retardation in a Swedish county. I. Epidemiology, gestational age, birth weight and associated CNS handicaps in children born 1959–1970. Acta Paediatr Scand 66:373–379, 1977.
[h] Fryers T, MacKay RI: The epidemiology of severe mental handicap. Early Hum Dev 3:277–294, 1979.
[i] Narayanan HS: A study of the prevalence of mental retardation in southern India. Int J Ment Health 10:28–36, 1981.
[j] Hasan Z, Hasan A: Report on a population survey of mental retardation in Pakistan. Int J Ment Health 10:23–27, 1981.
[k] Shiotsuki Y, Matsuishi T, Toshimura K, et al: The prevalence of mental retardation in Kurume City. Brain Dev 6:487–490, 1984.
[l] Zuo QH, Zhang ZX, Li Z, et al: An epidemiological study on mental retardation among children in Chang-Qiao area of Beijing. Chin Med J 99(1):9–14, 1986.
[m] McQueen PC, Spence MW, Garner JB, Pereira LH, Winsor EJT: Prevalence of major mental retardation and associated disabilities in the Canadian maritime provinces. Am J Ment Defic 91(5):460–466, 1987.
[n] Diaz-Fernandez F: Descriptive epidemiology of registered mentally retarded persons in Galicia (Northwest Spain). Am J Ment Retard 92(4):385–392, 1988.
[o] Thorburn M, Desai P, Paul TJ, Malcolm L, Durkin M, Davidson L: Identification of childhood disability in Jamaica: the ten question screen. Int J Rehabil Res 15: 115–127, 1992.
[p] Zaman SS, Khan NZ, Durkin MS, Islam S: Childhood Disabilities in Bangladesh. Dhaka: Protibondhi Foundation, 1992.
[q] Murphy CC, Yeargin-Allsopp M, Decoufle P, Drews CD: The administrative prevalence of mental retardation in 10-year-old children in metropolitan Atlanta, 1985 through 1987. Am J Public Health 85(3):319–323, 1995.
[r] Durkin MS, Hasan ZM, Hasan Z: Prevalence and correlates of mental retardation among children in Karachi, Pakistan. Am J Epidemiol 147(3):1–8, 1998.

are the genes located on the X chromosome fully expressed. In females, random inactivation in each cell of either the maternal or paternal X chromosome occurs early in embryonic development. Thus, if a female is heterozygous for an X-linked mutant gene, on the average approximately half her cells have the normal and half the abnormal allele as the functional member. This averaging of the effects of the two X chromosomes protects females from certain disorders transmitted on the X chromosome, such as hemophilia. Genes on the X chromosome are associated with a number of neurologic and cognitive disorders, including Lesch-Nyhan syndrome, Duchenne muscular dystrophy, X-linked hydrocephalus, Menkes' syndrome (kinky hair disease), and fragile X syndrome. Of these, fragile X syndrome is the most common form of inherited mental retardation.

Fragile X Syndrome

A fragile site on the X chromosome, fra(X), was first identified in males from families with X-linked mental retardation. In cytogenetic studies, Lubs[47] described a constriction on the long arm of the X chromosome. Sutherland[48] showed that the fragile X site could be routinely observed as a gap or break in the X chromosome when culture media deficient in folate or thymidine were used, and the site has been localized to Xq27.3. The proportion of cells showing the fragile X site in cytogenetic studies is quite variable and may be characteristic of each individual. About 80 percent of male carriers of the mutation and about 30 percent of female carriers show some degree of mental retardation.[49,50]

In 1991, the isolation of the fra(X) locus (FRAXA) located at the beginning of the FMR-1 gene permitted direct diagnosis at the DNA level.[51–53] Understanding of the inheritance of this condition has changed accordingly and affords a unique opportunity to examine the influence of a genetic factor on development. An unusual pattern of inheritance emerged from segregation analysis of families affected with FRAXA, which followed the intergenerational passage of the gene.[49,54] About 20 percent of males who carry the genotype are clinically unaffected and do not express the fragile site on cytogenetic testing. Mothers of these nonpenetrant males are rarely affected. These nonpenetrant normal transmitting males (NTMs) transmit the mutation to daughters who, although unaffected themselves, will have affected children. Thus, grandsons of NTMs are often mentally retarded and granddaughters may show some cognitive impairment.[49,54]

That the risk of mental retardation of individuals depends upon generation position within the family is known as the Sherman paradox: mothers and daughters of nonpenetrant males, both obligate carriers of the gene and phenotypically similar, have differing risks in their offspring. Brothers of NTMs are at low risk (approximately 9 percent) while grandsons and great grandsons are at high risk (approximately 40 to 50 percent).

The molecular basis of the Sherman paradox has now been elucidated. At the molecular level the FRAXA site contains an exon of the FMR-1 gene responsible for the fragile X mental retardation. This exon includes a repetitive CGG sequence that demonstrates length variation in normal and in fra(X) individuals, and a cytidine phosphate guanosine (CpG) island that shows preferential methylation in fra(X) cases.[55,56] The length of the CGG repeat in genomic DNA is correlated with risk for the fragile X syndrome.[52] Normal individuals have a CGG repeat of 90 to 150 base pairs (bp). NTMs and carrier females have a "premutation," which is seen as length variation of the CGG repeat in the range of 150 to 500 bp. Affected individuals, however, show dramatic amplification of the CGG repeat (from 500 to 3,000 bp) and hypermethylation of the adjacent "CpG island" region, which is associated with lack of expression of FMR-1 mRNA.[51,55,57,58] It appears that methylation is critical for expression of the phenotype.

Expansion of the premutation to the full mutation occurs only in female meiotic transmission;[51,59,60] risk for expansion to the full mutation in oogenesis increases with the number of repeats.[61] Hence daughters of NTMs inherit only the premutation and are not affected,[51,59] yet they may transmit an expanded allele to their offspring, increasing the risk of fra(X). As amplification of the gene increases, it becomes more unstable, leading to mitotic instability as well as meiotic instability.[51,57,61] In addition, several cases have been found with atypical mutations at the FRAXA site, two involving a deletion and one a point mutation in the FMR-1 gene.[62,63] Other fragile sites (FRAXD, FRAXE, FRAXF) are found close to the FRAXA site. FRAXE is associated with learning disabilities, but is caused by a different expanding trinucleotide repeat.[64]

While the correlation between the full mutation and the occurrence of mental retardation has been established, differences in cognitive ability have not been found in females or males with premutations of varying repeat sizes.[65] A high proportion of females with the full mutation, though not necessarily mentally retarded, exhibit selective cognitive deficits, but only if the mutation was inherited maternally.[66] Additional population-based studies are needed to determine the prevalence of structural rearrangements of the fragile X gene in the population and their relationship to cognitive performance, especially in females who may be nonretarded carriers of the gene.

Prevalence of the Fragile X Syndrome. Prevalence studies in defined populations have employed cytogenetic testing for fragile X among individuals with mental retardation. As Sherman[67] points out, cytogenetic testing may be sufficient for ascertainment in affected males, because most will have overt mental retardation of varying degrees. Females, however, will have milder mental retardation and be less likely to express the FRAXA site. Thus, current estimates of the prevalence of the fragile X syndrome in the population are undoubtedly too low, especially for females. The prevalence of fragile X syndrome has been estimated to be one in 1,000 among males and one in 2,000 to 2,500 among females. One in 700 females are thought to be carriers.[68–71]

The full spectrum of X-linked mental retardation may involve many distinct pathogenic mechanisms. Recent work has suggested that approximately 95 different X-linked learning disorders may exist,[72] although most are rare and have been observed only in studies of single families. Because many X-linked learning disorders are not associated with additional phenotypic features (i.e., are nonsyndromic) and can only be identified by genetic mapping, the full extent and diversity of X-linked mental retardation will be determined only with genetic screening of all affected individuals.

Autosomal Genetic Causes

Autosomally inherited disorders are rare but important causes of mental retardation. Autosomal dominant disorders causing cognitive disability in childhood include tuberous sclerosis and neurofibromatosis. The most common mode of transmission is through autosomal recessives. A number of metabolic disorders transmitted in this fashion, including phenylketonuria, are marked by progressive mental retardation with systemic manifestations.

Phenylketonuria

This rare defect of amino acid metabolism occurs in 1 in 15,000 Caucasian live births, with somewhat lower rates in other races. Deficient metabolism of phenylalanine causes accumulation, which, untreated, leads to hyperphenylalaninemia, damages the developing brain, and results in severe mental retardation in most cases. Neonatal screening permits early treatment by a special diet that diminishes phenylalanine levels. The diet must be continued through puberty to achieve the maximum protective effect. In countries with routine neonatal screening programs and effective follow-up of affected children, the condition is now rarely seen.

A new problem resulting from the success of neonatal screening programs for PKU is the rising prevalence of maternal PKU in women successfully treated in childhood.[73] Themselves of normal or near normal intelligence, at childbearing age they still have high blood levels of phenylalanine. Their surviving offspring are at increased risk of mental retardation, microcephaly, congenital heart disease, and low–birth weight.[74–76] Severe mental retardation is typically observed in children of mothers with classic PKU (defined as blood phenylalanine level of more than 1,200 μmol/L). Less severe cognitive deficit may affect children of mothers with atypical PKU (elevations of blood phenylalanine between 594 to 1,194 μmol/L),[76] while maternal mild hyperphenylalaninemia (blood phenylalanine less than 400 μmol/L) does not appear to have serious consequences for the fetus.[77] Dietary restrictions during pregnancy to reduce maternal blood phenylalanine levels and prevent phenylalanine metabolite accumulation can improve the outcome in offspring if started prior to conception and maintained throughout pregnancy. Routine umbilical cord blood screening, while it cannot prevent cases, can detect women with hyperphenylalaninemia and thus prevent recurrence in future pregnancies. From a public health perspective, the problem is to identify and locate the population of women at risk prior to their first pregnancies. The experience of the New England Maternal PKU Project suggests that the majority of women with classic PKU can be found, but a much lower proportion of those with atypical hyperphenylalaninemia are likely to be identified in time to permit primary prevention in their first-born children.[78]

Nutritional Causes

Iodine Deficiency

Cretinism is a form of mental retardation resulting from hypothyroidism and typically is complicated by hearing loss, motor impairment, and abnormal growth and physical development. Sporadic congenital hypothyroidism occurs in about one in 3,500 births. Newborn screening programs currently in operation throughout the developed world permit early detection and treatment of this condition, which, in turn, prevent the damage to the brain that results in sporadic cretinism.

A far more common cause of cretinism in some populations occurs prenatally due to maternal hypothyroidism associated with dietary deficiency of iodine. Iodine deficiency, defined for adults as an average daily iodine intake of less than 100 μg, is endemic in large populations throughout the world, particularly in mountainous areas and interior regions where iodine has been leached from the soil.[79]

Recent estimates suggest that nearly 1 billion people worldwide are at risk for iodine deficiency disorders.[80] In addition to endemic cretinism, which affects an estimated 3.2 million people and is a leading cause of mental retardation worldwide, the spectrum of iodine disorders includes spontaneous abortion, stillbirth, infant mortality, goiter, and impaired cognitive functioning (apart from that associated with frank cretinism).[81]

Prevention of iodine deficiency and endemic cretinism is achieved in many developed countries by means of fortification of dietary salt at a level of one part of iodide per 10,000 to 50,000 parts salt. In nonindustrialized communities, where the distribution of iodinized salt often proves infeasible, prevention of endemic cretinism can be achieved by annual administration to women of childbearing age of high doses of iodine in an oil solution taken either orally or by intramuscular injection.[82] Effective prevention of prenatally acquired cretinism requires that maternal iodine deficiency and hypothyroidism be corrected very early in pregnancy or preferably before conception. Considerable international pressure is now being exerted against the problem of iodine lack. Ongoing efforts in this regard will be needed to bring about full prevention of this important cause of mental retardation.

Folate Deficiency

Spina bifida is one of the commonest and most disabling birth defects worldwide. Prevalence at birth varies geographically and over time with peaks among the poorest classes and during times of famine and economic strife. Among children born with spina bifida in the developed world, approximately 75 percent survive past infancy. Hydrocephalus is a regular accompaniment, usually treated with an intracranial shunt to preserve brain tissue and prevent mental retardation. A wide range of intellectual function is found among survivors; fewer than half have severe intellectual disability and many have normal levels of intelligence. Physical accompaniments, including limitations in mobility and in sphincter control, create major nursing problems. The pathogenesis of spina bifida, as in neural tube defects for which survival is rare (anencephalus, encephalocele, iniencephaly), apparently involves failure of the embryonic neural tube to fuse completely, a process that should be completed by the 20th post conceptional day.

It is now clear that preconceptional and periconceptional folate consumption of the mother influences the incidence, an observation with enormous potential for primary prevention.[83] It remains likely that there still is a genetic influence, such that genetically predisposed mothers or offspring are sensitive to relatively mild deficiency, while a much bigger component of the population are sensitive to severe deficiency. The knowledge we have today suggests that at least half of present-day births with spina bifida in the United States could be prevented if mothers were to take 4 mg of folate preconception and periconception. Prevention currently hinges around how and no longer about whether to deliver the necessary supplement. An unavoidable problem is that the folate should be taken at a time that the woman will not usually know she is pregnant (as is probably also true for iodine supplement). One strategy, similar to that used to prevent iodine deficiency, is to supply the whole population, for example in the bread flour. Folates are present in the normal diet, in leafy vegetables, but whether dietary advice alone would result in consumption of sufficient amounts by those who need it is doubtful. Not all neural tube defects will disappear given preventive policies based on current knowledge, even though we can be confident that the incidence will decrease by at least half. Future research should clarify residual causes.

Prenatal screening for neural tube defects is now done routinely and with increasing accuracy in settings with advanced levels of prenatal care. Effective prenatal diagnosis involves screening maternal serum at 16 weeks gestation for elevated levels of α-fetoprotein (AFP) and following positive screening results with ultrasound anomaly scans and/or amniocentesis to detect elevated AFP levels in amniotic fluid.[84] Several difficulties persist with the procedure, apart from the hazards associated with amniocentesis. Even in the most experienced laboratories, the procedure is not entirely specific: other conditions raise AFP levels, and sometimes even with very high levels the fetus is apparently normal. Testing of AFP is also not entirely sensitive; affected fetuses, especially those with closed spina bifida but occasionally other types too, may not be detected. When a positive diagnosis is made, prevention involves induced abortion. This course may be less acceptable than in Down's syndrome because the risk of a false-positive result (and the consequent termination of a normal pregnancy) is much higher (up to 3 percent or more depending on cutoff levels and gestational age).[84]

Premature Birth

Infants born prematurely and at very low–birth weight (less than 1,501 g) are surviving with increased frequency due to advances in perinatology and neonatal medicine. Survivors of very low–birth weight carry a high risk of mental retardation as well as cerebral palsy (especially spastic diplegia), epilepsy, and vision and hearing impairments. Increases in the prevalence of cerebral palsy have been observed in several developed countries since the 1970s and been attributed to concomitant improvements in the survival of very preterm infants.[85] The impact of this trend on the prevalence of mental retardation per se is not clear, though follow-up studies of very low–birth weight infants are consistent in showing an inverse association between gestational age at birth and the risk of cognitive disability in childhood.[86] Although prematurity is an important risk factor for mental retardation, up to 75 percent of survivors of even very preterm birth (e.g., less than 33 weeks gestation) exhibit a normal course of development and functioning in childhood.[86,87]

Recent studies have identified two specific factors associated with premature birth to be strongly predictive of which infants will have poor developmental outcomes: white matter lesions observable neonatally on cranial ultrasound scans[88–91] and transient hypothyroxinemia of prematurity.[92] Further study is needed to determine the specific mechanisms by which these factors come to be associated with neurodevelopmental disability as well as the potential for interventions to prevent their occurrence. Recent studies have also identified a possible neuroprotective role of magnesium sulfate used in the treatment of preeclampsia and preterm labor.[93,94] Here too, further research, possibly including randomized trials, is needed to confirm the possibility that prenatal administration of magnesium sulfate can prevent mental retardation and other neurodevelopmental disorders in infants born prematurely.

Infections

At least 20 different infectious agents can cause brain damage and mental deficiency in children. Congenital syphilis, the first congenital disorder to be linked to an infectious cause, is now a rare and preventable cause of mental retardation. Rubella, like syphilis, is a fetal infection. It affects the fetus only if the mother contracts the disease between the 8th and 13th weeks of pregnancy. It has been virtually eliminated as a cause of mental retardation in vaccinated populations. Brain damage from other intrauterine infections (toxoplasmosis, cytomegalovirus, varicella) may follow either prenatal or perinatal transmission. When exposure occurs during the first or second trimester of pregnancy, several impairments are recognizable at birth and may include microcephaly, hydrocephaly, growth retardation, cataracts, seizures, rashes, jaundice, and hepatosplenomegaly.[95] Exposure late in pregnancy or during delivery may result in inapparent infection at birth and onset of developmental delay during infancy or childhood. Inapparent toxoplasmosis infection at birth, for example, is reported to result in neurodevelopmental disabilities in 80 to 90 percent of cases by age 20 years.[96–98]

Postnatally acquired meningitis and encephalitis associated with a variety of infectious agents also leave a proportion of children with permanent cognitive disability, particularly in less developed countries where access to vaccination and treatment is more limited and often delayed. Adverse reactions to the pertussis vaccine causes encephalitis and residual mental retardation in children, but the risk is likely to be lower than the risk of death from pertussis infection in unvaccinated populations.[99,100]

Estimates of the risk of vertical transmission of the human immunodeficiency virus (HIV) from infected mothers to offspring range from 15 to 25 percent in European and North American populations and from 30 to 40 percent in African populations. The effects of HIV infection on the neurodevelopment of the child are devastating.[101] It is now recognized that HIV infection of the central nervous system, independent of coexisting infections, causes CNS impairment, acquired microcephaly, and cognitive and movement disabilities in virtually all cases of pediatric acquired immunodeficiency syndrome (AIDS). HIV infection has become a leading, if fatal, cause of mental retardation in high-risk populations. Prevention efforts must focus on curtailing maternal infection as well as maternal-infant transmission.

Environmental Toxins

Lead

Lead absorbed from a variety of sources has long been known to cause the serious and often fatal condition of *lead encephalopathy* in children. Survivors were regularly severely mentally retarded and could be found in populations and institutions housing retarded persons. In recent decades, neuropsychologic impairments of various kinds have been recognized even in children with moderately raised lead levels, well below levels that cause acute lead encephalopathy. Current evidence suggests a dose-response relation of lead exposure in early childhood to mental performance and perhaps also to hyperactivity. The United States government now considers levels higher than 10 μg/dL to be potentially neurotoxic and estimates that more than 17 percent of young children have levels in this range.[102]

In many populations, socioeconomic status and iron deficiency are confounded with and may interact with lead poisoning in its effect on IQ. In the United States the effects are more marked on urban children living in poverty. Prevention is not simple but is certainly feasible and, in the long run, is likely to be cost-effective when balanced against reduced health costs and improved school performance and quality of work.[103] What is required is control of industrial processes, removal of lead from gasoline and paint, maintaining low lead levels in soil, monitoring residences (many houses still have the remains of lead paint, within and without), screening young children, and possibly, environmental lead abatement. For those with raised lead levels, removal from the source of exposure and possibly chelation treatment to increase the level excretion are indicated. The cost-effectiveness of mandatory screening as well as therapeutic and environmental interventions on neuropsychological outcomes of children with mild and moderate blood lead levels are controversial and require further study.[102,104]

Alcohol

Heavy alcohol abuse during pregnancy is associated with *fetal alcohol syndrome* in offspring. This syndrome includes mild to moderate cognitive disability, low–birth weight, microcephaly, stunting, flattened nasolabial facies, and narrow palpebral tissues. Incidence and prevalence of fetal alcohol syndrome vary with the frequency of alcohol abuse in pregnancy. A minimum rate of 1 per 6,000 live births was determined retrospectively among 55,000 consecutive United States maternity cases in which a history of alcohol intake was not specifically sought. A frequency at birth of 1 per 600 was observed in Gothenburg, Sweden,[105] a population in which nearly 10 percent of the cases of mild mental retardation in school children was attributed to this cause.[106] Prevention is easier to prescribe than to execute. In view of evidence that alcohol consumption during pregnancy is associated with a variety of adverse fetal outcomes other than mental retardation, abstinence or restricted drinking during pregnancy has become a worthwhile public health objective.

Trauma

Traumatic brain injury is an important preventable cause of intellectual deficiency.[107] The annual incidence of head injury (with loss of consciousness) in the United States is about 2.3 per 1,000 in children under 15 years and increases to 60 per 1,000 among 15- to 19-year-old boys.[108] The major causes are motor vehicle collisions, falls, and assaults. Throughout childhood, boys have a 2-fold risk of severe head injury relative to girls. It has been estimated that 5 to 10 percent of all cases are fatal and that another 5 to 10 percent result in a wide range of neuropsychologic sequelae.[109] Permanent declines in IQ and adaptive function are observed in a proportion of cases but population-based studies of the frequency, predictors, and prevention of these outcomes have not yet been done.

▸ PREVENTION

Clearly, mental retardation has many causes. Preventive strategies must focus on each in turn. Sometimes, as with prenatal screening, there are exemplary preventive programs, which can be applied wherever the administrative and economic structure can support them. Programs involving prenatal diagnosis followed by selective abortion or gene therapies call for a high level of organization; for some, they will also involve a conflict of values. Programs that require intensification of the educational input for many children over a prolonged period call for a major allocation of funds and human resources.

Twelve recommendations for prevention have been compiled by the Joint Commission of the International Association for the Scientific Study of Mental Deficiency and the International League of Parents of Retarded Children and accepted by the World Health Organization:

1. Genetic counseling, prenatal diagnosis, early identification, and proper treatment are important in preventing mental retardation of genetic origin.
2. Prevention of infections and parasitic diseases contributes significantly to the prevention of mental retardation.
3. Monitoring the environment to protect against pollutants and other chemical and physical hazards is an important part of prevention programs.
4. Safe environments for young children and the prompt treatment of injuries should reduce accidental causes of mental retardation.
5. The nutrition of mothers and children is of importance, especially in developing countries.
6. Good obstetrics and good care of the newborn reduce the incidence of mental and physical handicap. Good care includes adequate treatment of maternal illness, such as diabetes or toxemia; prompt recognition of obstetrical abnormalities; adequate monitoring of the fetus; immediate resuscitation of the infant; prediction, prevention, and treatment of biochemical disorders, such as respiratory distress syndrome, hypoglycemia, anoxia, and all causes of cerebral damage.
7. Social and educational stimulation is essential for proper mental growth and development. It is an important element in prevention of mental retardation, especially for mild mental retardation. Suitable interventions are needed for children whose families do not provide this stimulation.
8. In more severely retarded persons, proper stimulation, modern principles of rehabilitation, and good remedial service can also reduce disability and prevent the development of secondary handicaps.
9. Improvements of living standards and the general health of the population constitutes an important element of nonspecific prevention of mental retardation. Preventive programs for mental retardation should form an integral part of all general health planning and programs.
10. The patterns of preventive programs and the speed with which they are implemented will vary according to resources, but high priority should be given to the problem in all countries.
11. International cooperation on many levels is necessary to speed up the development of effective preventive measures.

12. Research into the causes of mental retardation should be encouraged and facilitated. The effectiveness of preventive measures should be tested and monitored continuously. Special attention should be given to evaluative research in the biomedical and psychosocial spheres.

► CARE: COMMUNITY SERVICES FOR MENTAL RETARDATION

Many mentally retarded persons achieve considerable self-reliance with maturity and training, so that the deficit even when severe is seen as relative rather than absolute. The early years are often those for which the family of birth provides basic care and support, while for the later years the community does this increasingly. A family with a mentally retarded child experiences major impacts. There is shock and pain, when the diagnosis is imparted, and a time of emotional turbulence and readjustment to a new kind of parental role often follows. The turbulence is often compounded by concern about effects on other family members, especially siblings; painful embarrassment before friends, neighbors, and strangers; and economic strain. The strain is not limited to the early years. A mentally retarded person may remain emotionally and physically dependent on parents long after the departure of other children. With improved medical care and increasing longevity of persons with severe mental retardation, dependence may continue into a phase when parents lack the physical, psychological, and economic resources to provide adequate care.

For some families, residential placement of the child at an early age is the most suitable arrangement. For many others, the family home is preferred. Whichever course is followed, cooperative arrangements between a family and appropriate community services work best. Types of services needed change over the life course of the individual. In adulthood, there is often a continued need for sheltered living, work, and recreational services. Families play an important role in planning transitions in services, recognizing that the rights of retarded people, who may be limited in arguing their own case, need special protection. Increasingly, persons with mental retardation themselves are being consulted.

► CONCLUSION

Today, the field of mental retardation involves public health in some of the most critical issues facing society. The selected issues touched on here are intended to serve as an introduction to the potential role of public health. Societal forces will shape future public health views and actions, as they have in the past. Scientific and technologic advances bring new opportunities for prevention and change in the balance between incidence and prevalence. In these emerging circumstances, the choices societies make among the forms of prevention and care can have profound effects.

► REFERENCES

1. Kiely M: The prevalence of mental retardation. Epidemiol Rev 9: 194–218, 1987
2. Power C: A review of child health in the 1958 birth cohort: National Child Development Study. Paediatr Perinat Epidemiol 6:81–110, 1992
3. Chen J, Simeonsson RJ: Prevention of childhood disability in the People's Republic of China. Child Care Health Dev 19(2):71–88, 1993
4. Grossman HJ (ed): Classification in Mental Retardation. Washington, DC: American Association on Mental Deficiency, 1983
5. Susser MW, Watson W: Sociology in Medicine. Oxford, England: Oxford University Press, 1971
6. World Health Organization: International Classification of Impairments, Disabilities and Handicaps. Geneva: World Health Organization, 1980
7. Epstein CJ: The Consequences of Chromosome Imbalance. Cambridge, England: Cambridge University Press, 1986
8. Shaw CM: Correlates of mental retardation and structural changes of the brain. Development 9:1–8, 1987
9. World Health Organization: International Classification of Diseases. 9th ed. Geneva: World Health Organization, 1980
10. World Health Organization: International Classification of Diseases. 10th ed. Geneva: World Health Organization, 1992
11. American Psychiatric Association: Diagnostic and Statistical Manual of Mental Disorders, Fourth Edition (DSM-IV). Washington, DC: American Psychiatric Association, 1994
12. Luckasson R, Coulter DL, Polloway EA, et al: Mental Retardation: Definition, Classification, and Systems of Supports. 9th ed. Washington, DC: American Association on Mental Retardation, 1992
13. Burack JA, Hodapp RM, Zigler E: Issues in the classification of mental retardation: differentiating among organic etiologies. J Child Psychol Psychiatry 29(6):765–779, 1988
14. Hook EB: Incidence and prevalence as measures of the frequency of birth defects. Am J Epidemiol 116:743–747, 1982
15. Stein ZA, Susser MW: The epidemiology of mental retardation. In Butler NR, Connor BD (eds): Stress and Disability in Childhood. Bristol, England: Wright, 1984, pp 21–46
16. Stein ZA, Durkin MS, Belmont L: Serious mental retardation in developing countries: an epidemiologic approach. In Wisniewski H, Snider D (eds): Mental Retardation and Developmental Disabilities: Research, Education and Technology Transfer. Annals of the New York Academy of Sciences. New York: New York Academy of Sciences, 1986, vol 477, pp 8–21
17. Stein ZA, Susser MW, Saenger G: Mental retardation in a national population of young men in the Netherlands: 2. prevalence of mild mental retardation. Am J Epidemiol 104:159–169, 1976
18. Stein ZA, Susser MW, Saenger G, Marolla F: Mental retardation in a national population of young men in the Netherlands: 1. prevalence of severe mental retardation. American Journal of Epidemiology, 103:477–489, 1976
19. Stein ZA, Susser MW: The mutability of intelligence and the epidemiology of mild mental retardation. Reviews in Education Research 40:29–67, 1970
20. Garber H, Heber R: The Milwaukee Project: early intervention as a technique to prevent mental retardation. The University of Connecticut Technical Papers. Storrs, CT: University of Connecticut, 1973
21. McKay H, Sinisterra L, McKay A, et al: Improving cognitive ability in chronically deprived children. Science 200:270–278, 1978
22. Ramey CT, Bryant DM, Wasik BH, Sparling JJ, Fendt KH, LaVange LM: The Infant Health and Development Program for low birth weight, premature infants: program elements, family participation and child intelligence. Pediatrics 89:454–466, 1992
23. Kline J, Stein Z, Susser M: Conception to Birth: Epidemiology of Prenatal Development. New York: Oxford University Press, 1989
24. Gustavson KH, Hagberg B, Hagberg G, Sars K: Severe mental retardation in a Swedish county. I. Epidemiology, gestational age, birth weight and associated CNS handicaps in children born 1959–1970. Acta Paediatr Scand 66:373–379, 1977
25. Gustavson KH, Hagberg B, Hagberg G, Sars K: Severe mental retardation in a Swedish county: etiological and pathogenic aspects of children born 1959–1970. Neuropadiatrie 8:293–304, 1977
26. Hagberg B: Severe mental retardation in Swedish children born 1959–1970: Epidemiological panorama and causative factors. In: Major Mental Handicap: Methods and Costs of Prevention. Ciba Found Symp 59:29–51, 1978
27. Nicholson A, Alberman E: Prediction of the number of Down's syndrome infants to be born in England and Wales up to the year 2000 and their likely survival rates. J Intellect Disabil Res 36:505–517, 1992
28. Holtzman DM, Epstein CJ: The molecular genetics of Down syndrome. Molec Genet Med 2:105–120, 1992

29. Hassold T, Chiu D, Yamane JA: Parental origin of autosomal trisomies. Ann Hum Genet 48:129–144, 1984
30. Stewart GD, Hassold TJ, Berg A, Watkins P, Tanzi R, Kurnit DM: Trisomy 21 (Down syndrome): studying nondisjunction and meiotic recombination by using cytogenetic and molecular polymorphisms that span chromosome 21. Am J Hum Genet 42:227–236, 1988
31. Sherman SL, Takaesu N, Freeman SB, et al: 1991 Trisomy 21: association between reduced recombination and nondisjunction. Am J Hum Genet 49:608–620, 1991
32. Hook EB: Epidemiology of Down syndrome. In Pueschel SM, Rynders JE (eds): Down Syndrome: Advances in Biomedicine and the Behavioral Sciences. Cambridge, MA: Ware Press, 1982, pp 11–88
33. Staples AJ, Sutherland G, Haan EA, Clisby S: Epidemiology of Down syndrome in South Australia, 1960–89. Am J Hum Genet 49:1014–1024, 1991
34. Cuckle HS, Wald NJ, Thompson SG: Estimating a woman's risk of having a pregnancy associated with Down's syndrome using her age and serum alpha-fetoprotein level. Br J Obstet Gynaecol 94:387–402, 1987
35. Kallen B, Knudsen LB: Effect of maternal age distribution and prenatal diagnosis on the population rates of Down syndrome—a comparative study of nineteen populations. Hereditas 110:55–60, 1989
36. Adams MM, Erickson JD, Layde PM, Oakley GP: Down's syndrome: recent trends in the United States. JAMA 246(7):758–760, 1991
37. Steele J, Stratford B: The United Kingdom population with Down syndrome: present and future projections. Am J Ment Retard 99:664–682, 1995
38. Phillips OP, Elias S, Shulman LP, et al: Maternal serum screening for fetal Down syndrome in women less than 35 years of age using alpha-fetoprotein, hCG, and unconjugated estriol: a prospective 2-year study. Obset Gynecol 80(31):353–358, 1992
39. Wald NJ, Kennard A: Prenatal biochemical screening for Down's syndrome and neural tube defects. Curr Opin Obstet Gynecol 4(2): 302–307, 1992
40. Benn PA, Horne D, Birganti S, Greenstein RM: Prenatal diagnosis of chromosome abnormalities in a population of patients identified by triple-marker testing as screen positive for Down syndrome. Am J Obstet Gynecol 173:496–501, 1995
41. Martin GM: Genetic syndromes in man with potential relevance to pathobiology of aging. Birth Defects Original Articles Series 14: 5–39, 1978
42. Sare Z, Ruvalcaba RH, Kelly VC: Prevalence of thyroid disorder in Down syndrome. Clin Genet 14:154–158, 1978
43. Oliver C, Holland AJ: Down syndrome and Alzheimer's disease: a review. Psychol Med 16:307–322, 1986
44. Wisniewski KE, Wisniewski HM Wen GY: Occurrence of Alzheimer neuropathology and dementia in Down syndrome. Ann Neurol 17: 278–282, 1985
45. Schupf N, Silverman WP, Sterling RC, Zigman WB: Down syndrome, terminal illness and risk for dementia of the Alzheimer type. Brain Dysfunction 2:181–188, 1989
46. Zigman WB, Schupf N, Lubin RA, Silverman WP: Premature regression of adults with Down syndrome. Am J Ment Defic 92: 161–168, 1987
47. Lubs HA: A marker-X chromosome. Am J Hum Genet 21:231–244, 1969
48. Sutherland GR: Fragile sites on human chromosomes. Demonstration of their dependence on the type of tissue culture medium. Science 197:265–266, 1977
49. Sherman SL, Morton NE, Jacobs PA, Turner G: The fragile X syndrome. A cytogenetic and genetic analysis. Ann Hum Genet 48: 21–37, 1984
50. Chudley AE, Knoll J, Gerrard JW, Shepel L, McGahey E, Anderson J: Fragile (X) X-linked mental retardation. I Retardation between age and intelligence and the frequency of expression of fragile (X) (q28). Am J Med Genet 14:699–712, 1983
51. Oberle I, Rousseau F, Heitz D, et al: Instability of a 550-base pair DNA segment and abnormal methylation in fragile X syndrome. Science 252:1097–1102, 1991
52. Kremer EJ, Pritchard M, Lynch M, et al: Mapping of DNA instability at the fragile X to a trinucleotide repeat sequence p(CCG)n. Science 252:1711–1714, 1991
53. Verkerk AJMH, Pieretti M, Sutcliffe JS, et al: Identification of a gene (FMR-1) containing a CGG repeat coincident with a breakpoint cluster region exhibiting length variation in fragile X syndrome. Cell 65:905–914, 1991
54. Sherman SL, Jacobs P, Morton NE, Froster-Iskenius J, Howard-Peebles PN, Nielson KB, Partington MW, Sutherland GR, Turner G, Watson M: Further segregation analysis of the fragile-X syndrome with special reference to transmitting males. Human Genetics 69:289–299, 1985
55. Bell MV, Hirst MC, Nakahori Y, et al: Physical mapping across the fragile X: hypermethylation and clinical expression of the fragile X syndrome. Cell 64:861–866, 1991
56. Vincent A, Heitz D, Petit C, Krietz C, Oberle I, Mandel JL: Abnormal pattern detected in fragile X patients by pulsed field gel electrophoresis. Nature 349:624–626, 1991
57. Pieretti M, Zhang F, Fu YH, Warren ST, Oostra BA, Caskey ST, Nelson DL: Absence of expression of the FMR-1 gene in fragile X syndrome. Cell 66:817–822, 1991
58. Sutcliffe JS, Nelson DL, Zhang F, Pieretti M, Caskey CT, Saxe D, Warren ST: DNA methylation represses FMR-1 transcription in fragile X syndrome. Hum Mol Genet 1(6):397–400, 1992
59. Yu S, Pritchard M, Kremer E, et al: Fragile X genotype characterized by an unstable region of DNA. Science 252:1179–1181, 1991
60. Smits A, Smeets D, Dreesen J, Hamel B, de Haan A, van Oost B: Parental origin of the Fra(X) gene is a major determinant of the cytogenetic expression and the CGG repeat length in female carriers. Am J Med Genet 43:261–267, 1992
61. Fu YH, Kuhl DPA, Pizzuti A, et al: Variation of the CGG repeat at the fragile X site results in genetic stability: resolution of the Sherman Paradox. Cell 67:1047–1058, 1991
62. Gedeon AK, Baker E, Robinson H, et al: Fragile X syndrome without CCG amplification has an FMR1 deletion. Nat Genet 1:341–344, 1992
63. Wohrle D, Kotzot D, Hirst MC, et al: A microdeletion of less than 250 kb, including the proximal part of the FMR-1 gene and the fragile site, in a male with the clinical phenotype of fragile X syndrome. Am J Hum Genet 51:299–306, 1992
64. Feldman EJ: The recognition and investigation of X-linked learning disability syndromes. J Intellect Disabil Res 40:400–411, 1996
65. Rousseau F: The fragile X syndrome: implications of molecular genetics for the clinical syndrome. Eur J Clin Invest 24:1–10, 1994
66. Hinton VJ, Halperin JM, Dobkin CS, Ding XH, Brown WT, Miezejeski CM: Cognitive and molecular aspects of fragile X. J Clin Exp Neuropsychol 17:518–528, 1995
67. Sherman S: Epidemiology. In Hagerman RJ, Silverman AC (eds): Fragile X syndrome diagnosis, treatment and research. Baltimore: Johns Hopkins University Press, 1991, pp 69–97
68. Gustavson KH, Blomquist HK, Holmgren G: Prevalence of the fragile-X syndrome in mentally retarded boys in a Swedish county. Am J Med Genet 23:581–587, 1986
69. Kahkonen, M, Alitalo T, Airaksinen E, Matilainen R, Launiala K, Autio S, Leisti J: Prevalence of the fragile X syndrome in four birth cohorts of children of school age. Hum Genet 77:85–87, 1987
70. Turner G, Robinson H, Laing S, Purvis-Smith S: Preventive screening for the fragile X syndrome. N Engl J Med 315:607–609, 1986
71. Webb TP, Bundy S, Thake A, Todd J: The frequency of the fragile X chromosome among school children in Coventry. J Med Genet 23:396–399, 1986

72. Schwartz CE: X-linked mental retardation: in pursuit of a gene map. Invited Editorial. Am J Hum Genet 52:1025–1031, 1993
73. Levy HL, Waisbren SE: Effects of untreated maternal phenylketonuria and hyperphenylalaninemia on the fetus. N Engl J Med 309(21):1269–1274, 1983
74. Lenke RR, Levy HL: Maternal phenylketonuria and hyperphenylalanemia: an international survey of the outcome of treated and untreated pregnancies. N Engl J Med 303:1202, 1980
75. Rohr FJ, Doherty LB, Waisbren SE, Bailey IV, Ampola MG, Benacerraf B, Levy HL: New England Maternal PKU Project: prospective study of untreated and treated pregnancies and their outcomes. J Pediatr 10(3):391–398, 1987
76. Waisbren SE, Levy HL: Effects of untreated maternal hyperphenylalaninemia on the fetus: further study of families identified by routine cord blood screening. J Pediatr 116(6):926–929, 1990
77. Levy HL, Waisbren SE, Lobbregt D, Allred E, Shuler A, Trefz FK, Schweiter SM, Walter JH, Barwell BE, Berlin CM, Leviton A: Maternal mild hyperphenylaninaemia: an international survey of offspring outcome. Lancet 344:1589–1594, 1994
78. Waisbren SE, Doherty LB, Bailey IV, Rohr FJ, Levy HL: The New England Maternal PKU Project: identification of at-risk women. Am J Public Health 78(7):789–791, 1988
79. Delange F: The disorders induced by iodine deficiency. Thyroid 4:107–128, 1994
80. Delange F, Dunn JT, Glinoer D: Iodine Deficiency in Europe: A Continuing Concern. New York: Plenum Press, 1993
81. Hetzel BS: Iodine deficiency disorders (IDD) and their eradication. Lancet 2:1126–1128, 1983
82. Hetzel BS: The Story of Iodine Deficiency: An International Challenge in Nutrition. Oxford: Oxford University Press, 1989
83. Milunsky A, Jick H, Jick SS, Bruell CL, Maclaughlin DS, Rothman KJ, Willett W: Multivitamin/folic acid supplementation in early pregnancy reduced the prevalence of neural tube defects. JAMA 262:2847–2852, 1989
84. Cuckle HS, Thornton JG: 1995 Antenatal diagnosis and management of neural tube defects. In Levene MI, Lilford RJ (eds): Fetal and Neonatal Neurology and Neurosurgery. Edinburgh: Churchill Livingstone, 1995, pp 295–309
85. Bhushan VG, Paneth N, Kiely JL: Impact of improved survival of very low birth weight infants on recent secular trends in the prevalence of cerebral palsy. Pediatrics 91:1094–1100, 1993
86. Escobar GJ, Littenberg B, Petitti DB: Outcome among surviving very low birthweight infants: a meta analysis. Arch Dis Child 66: 204–211, 1991
87. Paneth N, Rudelli R, Kazam E, Monte W: Brain Damage in the Preterm Infant. Clinics in Developmental Medicine No. 131, London: Mac Keith Press, 1994
88. DeVries LS, Eken P, Groenendaal F, vanHaastert IC, Meiners LC: Correlation between degree of periventricular leukomalacia diagnosed using cranial ultrasound and MRI later in infancy with cerebral palsy. Neuropediatrics 24:263–268, 1993
89. Paneth N, Rudelli R, Kazam E, Monte W: Brain Damage in the Preterm Infant. In: Clinics in Developmental Medicine No. 131. London: Mac Keith Press, 1994
90. Pinto-Martin JA, Riolo S, Cnaan A, Holzman C, Susser M, Paneth N: Cranial ultrasound prediction of disabling and nondisabling cerebral palsy at age two in a low birth weight population. Pediatrics 95:249–254, 1995
91. Whitaker AH, Feldman JF, VanRossem R, Schonfeld IS, Pinto-Martin JA, Torre C, Blumenthal SR, Paneth NS: Neonatal cranial ultrasound abnormalities in low birth weight infants: relation to cognitive outcomes at age six. Pediatrics 98:719–729, 1996
92. Reuss ML, Paneth N, Pinto-Martin JA, Lorenz JM, Susser M: The relation of transient hypothyroxinemia in preterm infants to neurologic development at two years of age. N Engl J Med 334:821–827, 1996
93. Nelson KB, Grether JK: Can magnesium sulfate reduce the risk of cerebral palsy in very low birth weight infants? Pediatrics 95: 263–269, 1995
94. Schendel DE, Berg CJ, Yeargin-Allsopp M, Boyle CA, Decoufle P: Prental magnesium sulfate exposure and the risk for cerebral palsy or mental retardation among very low birth weight children aged 3 to 5 years. JAMA 276:1805–1810, 1996
95. Ramer JC, Miller G: Overview of mental retardation. In Miller G, Ramer JC (eds): Static Encephalopathies of Infancy and Childhood. New York: Raven Press, 1992, pp 1–10
96. Koppe J, Loewer-Sieger D, de Roever-Bonnet H: Results of 20 year follow-up of congenital toxoplasmosis. Lancet 1:254–256, 1986
97. Wilson C, Remington J: Development of adverse sequelae in children born with subclinical congenital *Toxoplasmosis* infection. Pediatrics 66:767–774, 1980
98. Koskiniemi M, Lappalainen M, Hedman K: *Toxoplasmosis* needs evaluation: an overview and proposals. Am J Dis Child 143:724–728, 1989
99. Hinman AR, Koplan JP: Pertussis and pertusis vaccine: reanalysis of benefits, risks and costs. JAMA 251:3109–3113, 1984
100. Cody CL, Baraff LJ, Cherry JD, et al: Nature and rates of adverse reactions associated with DPT and DT immunizations in infants and children. Pediatrics 68(5):650–660, 1981
101. Belman AL: AIDS and pediatric neurology. Neurol Clin 8(3):571–602, 1992
102. Weitzman M, Aschengrau A, Bellinger D, Jones R, Hamlin JS, Beiser A: Lead-contaminated soil abatement and urban children's blood lead levels. JAMA 269(13):1647–1654, 1993
103. Needleman HL: Childhood lead poisoning: a disease for the history texts. Am J Public Health 81(6):685–687, 1991
104. Ruff HA, Bijur PE, Markowitz M, Yeou-Cheng M, Rosen JF: Declining blood levels and cognitive changes in moderately lead-poisoned children. JAMA 269(13):1641–1646, 1993
105. Hagberg B: Pre- and perinatal environmental origin in mild mental retardation. Ups J Med Sci Suppl 44:178–182, 1987
106. Hagberg B, Hagberg G, Lewerth A, Lindberg U: Mild mental retardation in Swedish school children: prevalence. Acta Paediatr Scand 70:441–444, 1981
107. Chadwick O, Rutter M, Brown G, Shaffer D, Traub M: A prospective study of children with head injuries: II. cognitive sequelae. Psychol Med 11:49–61, 1981
108. Annegers JF, Grabow JD, Kurland LT, Laws ER: The incidence, causes, and secular trends of head trauma in Olmsted County, Minnesota, 1935–1974. Neurology 30:912–919, 1980
109. Frankowski RF, Annegers JF, Whitman S: Epidemiologic and descriptive studies part 1: the descriptive epidemiology of head trauma in the United States. In Becker DP, Povlishock JT (eds): Central Nervous System Trauma Status Report. Bethesda, MD: National Institute of Neurological Diseases and Stroke, 1985, pp 33–43

► GENERAL REFERENCES

Birch HG, Richardson SA, Baird D, et al: Mental Subnormality in the Community: A Clinical and Epidemiologic Study. Baltimore: Williams & Wilkins, 1970

Casiro OG, Moddemann DM, Stanwick RS, Cheang MS: The natural history and predictive value of early language delays in very low birth weight infants. Early Hum Dev 26(1):45–50, 1991

Lehrke RG: X-linked mental retardation and verbal disability. Birth Defects 10:1–100, 1974

Lewis EO: Report on an investigation into the incidence of mental deficiency in six areas, 1925–1927. In: Report of the Mental Deficiency Committee, Being a Joint Committee on the Board of Education and Board of Control. London: H. M. Stationery Office, 1929, part 4

Whitaker A, Johnson J, Sebris S, et al: Neonatal cranial ultrasound abnormalities: association with developmental delay at age one in low birth weight infants. J Dev Behav Pediatr 11(5):253–260, 1990

Zaman SS, Khan NZ, Durkin MS, Islam S: Childhood Disabilities in Bangladesh. Dhaka: Protibondhi Foundation, 1992

62

Prevention of Disability in Older Persons

William H. Barker

Increased risk of disease, disability, and death are well-known accompaniments of old age. While disease incidence and death are the conventional indices of a society's health status and targets of health care interventions, functional disability is perhaps the most consequential index when dealing with health in old age. This chapter defines the character and magnitude of disability in old age, reviews preventive and restorative approaches to specific and general causes of disability among the elderly, and examines the role of health care organization in facilitating the delivery of such services.

▶ DIMENSIONS OF THE PROBLEM

Concept and Measurement of Disability

Conceptually, disability has been classified by the World Health Organization as part of a continuum of measures of disease impact that include:[1]

- *Impairment:* the loss or abnormality of psychological, physiological, or anatomical integrity at the level of specific organ systems.
- *Disability:* the inability to perform an activity within the range considered normal for a human being, hence a functional limitation experienced at the level of the person as a whole.
- *Handicap:* a disadvantage resulting from an impairment or disability that, if not addressed, limits an individual's ability to fulfill certain desired social roles.

Collectively this continuum of stages of dysfunction has been referred to as the "disablement model." Figure 62-1 depicts the conditions that characterize dysfunction at each of the three stages of the model and the types of functional assessment and medical, restorative, and social intervention appropriate to maintaining and improving function and limiting disability at each stage.

A wide variety of systems have been developed for measuring functional ability/disability.[2] The best-known of these are the Activities of Daily Living (ADL) and the Instrumental Activities of Daily Living (IADL) indices. The ADL index, first introduced by Katz and colleagues, classifies limitations in six fundamental sociobiological functions of daily living: bathing, dressing, toileting, transferring from bed or chair, continence, and feeding.[3] Lawton and Brody broadened the scope with the IADL concept, which incorporates measures of more complex adaptive or self-maintaining functions such as housekeeping, money management, and grocery shopping.[4] In addition to screening and care planning for individual patients, these measurement systems have been very useful for describing the disability status of the elderly population, estimating community and institutional service needs, and evaluating outcomes of interventions designed to limit disability.

The emerging concept of "preclinical disability" focuses on identifying stages in the natural history of functional loss that precede the onset of overt ADL or IADL dependencies. This phenomenon has been measured in terms of adaptive modifications in the performance of common tasks such as doing heavy housework, getting out of bed, and walking up or down stairs.[5]

Magnitude of Aging and Disability

The aging of populations is occurring in all parts of the world, most profoundly in developed areas, as illustrated in estimates compiled by the United Nations (Fig. 62-3). Furthermore, in the United States and other countries, the greatest proportionate growth is occurring among those over age 80.

The magnitude and distribution of disabled elderly Americans living both in the community and in nursing homes in the last quarter of the twentieth century has been estimated from a variety of statistical sources. In the early 1980s, approximately 6.3 million, or 22 percent, of older persons were partially or completely disabled, 1.3 million of whom were residents of nursing homes, while more than three times as many (4.9 million) lived in the community (Table 62-1). Among community-dwelling disabled elderly, the most common ADL dependencies include bathing and transferring, while dependence on assistance with eating is least common. Shopping and meal preparation are the most common IADL dependencies. All domains of ADL and IADL limitation increase dramatically with age, from "young old" (65 to 74) to "old old" (85 and older), and are generally more prevalent in women than in men (Table 62-2).

There is a strong association between ADL limitation and the presence of chronic medical conditions, both of which increase dramatically with age in men and women.[6] With few exceptions such as stroke and hip fracture, it has been difficult to establish direct cause-and-effect relationships between specific morbidities (diseases) or combinations of morbidities and the onset of disability. Nonetheless, it is reasonable to presume that a substantial amount of disability is attributable to physical and physiologic impairments resulting from specific chronic diseases.[7,8] In turn, the prevention of such impairments and consequent disability would be largely dependent on the success with which major chronic diseases are prevented or controlled using techniques reviewed in other chapters in this volume. A substantial amount of disability in old age may also be explained and potentially

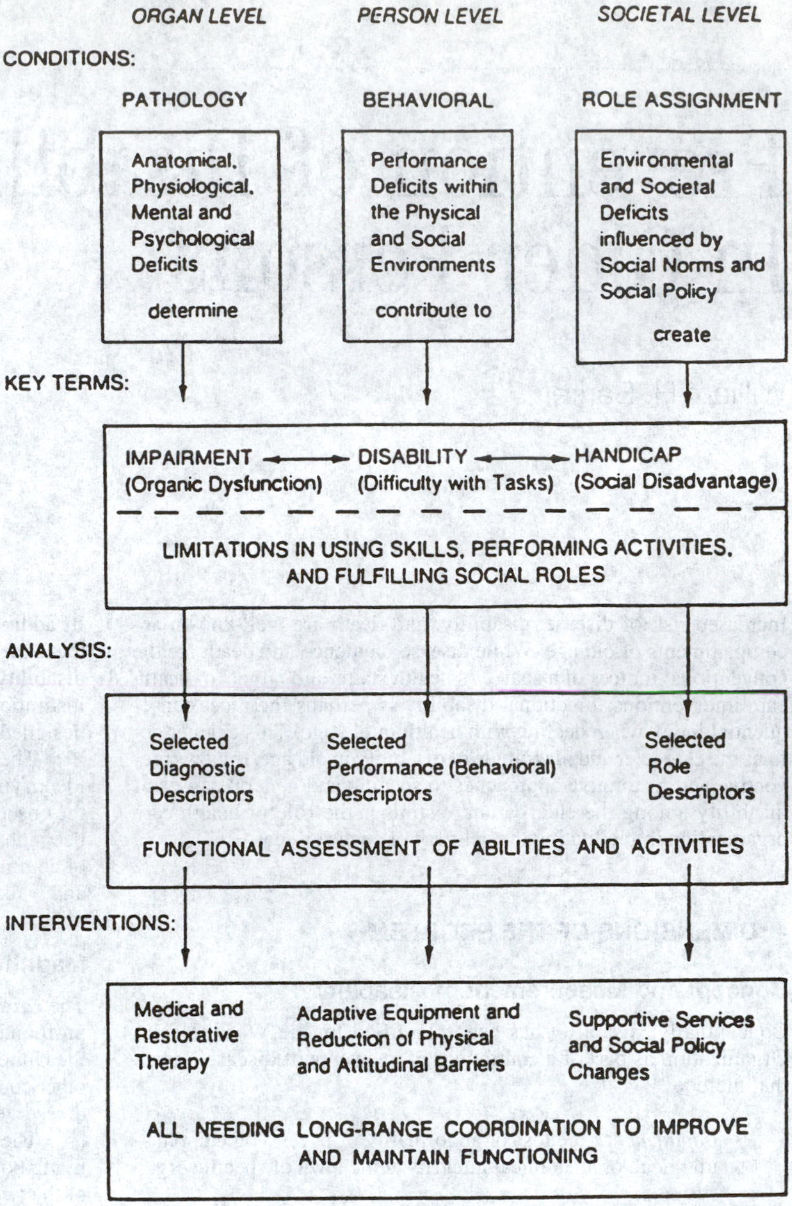

Figure 62-1. The functional approach to medical care and the disablement model. (From Granger CV. Gresham GE: Functional Assessment in Rehabilitation Medicine. Baltimore: Williams & Wilkins, 1984, p 20.)

prevented by attention to changes in physical, psychological, and social support factors that are related to the functional integrity of older persons. Comprehensive strategies of health promotion, multidisciplinary assessment and rehabilitation, and environmental adaptation constitute the armamentarium of preventive approaches to such factors.

A further dimension of the social impact of disability in old age is the strong relationship between functional impairment and use of acute and subacute health services and long-term care. Based on the 1984 U.S. Household Health Interview Survey, dividing respondents over age 65 into those with severe impairment (major limitation in two or more ADLs), moderate impairment (some difficulty performing one or more ADLs), and no significant impairment, average number of physician contacts per year were 9.9, 7.7, and 4.2, respectively, and annual hospital admission rates were 90, 55, and 23 per 100, respectively.[9]

Future Trends

Of great interest and consequence to the future provision of health and social services is the increased life expectancy among older persons that has occurred in many industrialized societies in the final quarter of the twentieth century.[10,11] This phenomenon, along with general decline in birth rates throughout the century, will result in an ever-increasing proportion of persons over age 65, with the largest proportionate increases involving those over age 80, among whom functional disability is most prevalent.

These demographic developments have given rise to a number of forecasts with respect to the burden of disability to be anticipated. At one extreme is Fries's "compression of morbidity" thesis that, with reference to Figure 62-3, argues that age of onset of chronic disease among the elderly is being postponed or prevented as a result of a variety of risk-reducing and health-promoting measures.[12] Under these circumstances, prevalence rates of disability associated with chronic disease would be expected to diminish, relative to current rates. At the other extreme is the "failure of success" thesis promulgated by Gruenberg[13] and others that argues that prolongation of life expectancy among the elderly is largely the result of advances in medical technology, which, with reference to Figure 62-3, results in increase in the average duration of certain chronic disabling diseases. This phenomenon would result in expanded future need for chronic care services. Others have suggested that the increased life expectancy reflects a combination of both of these phenomena, resulting in delayed

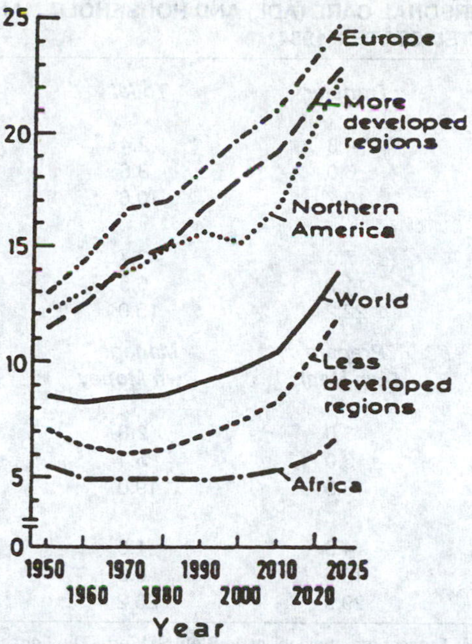

Figure 62-2. Percentage of population 60 years and over in different regions of the world. UN data and predictions 1950 to 2025. (From Davies AM: Epidemiology and the Challenge of Aging. In Brody JA, Maddox GL (eds): Epidemiology and Aging. New York: Springer, 1988.)

age of onset of chronic disease and disability but not substantially reducing the overall health service burden.[14]

Various longitudinal population studies to empirically assess trends in the burden of disability among older persons are in progress in the United States,[15] Sweden,[16] and elsewhere. Common to such studies is a quest to identify and quantify determinants of disability-free aging, variably referred to as "active life expectancy"[17] or "successful aging."[18]

The National Long Term Care Survey (NLTCS), a 12-year longitudinal study involving sequential cohorts of older Americans, has documented a decline of one to two percentage points in the prevalence of chronic disability in this population between 1982 and 1989. This translates into an estimated 540,000 fewer older persons with chronic disabilities than would have been expected in 1989. The NLTCS has documented concurrent significant declines in prevalence of 10 of 16 potentially disabling chronic medical conditions, including arthritis, hypertension, and cancer.[19] Further decline in prevalence of disability has been reported through 1994.[20]

▸ HEALTH PROMOTION AND PREVENTION

In considering approaches to prevention of disability in the aging population, and in the aging individual, it is useful to bear in mind several phenomenon that are involved. These include on the one hand the contributions to disability attributable, respectively, to biologic changes of aging, pathologic disease process, and disuse or deconditioning. On the other hand are the roles of health promotion and therapeutic, rehabilitative, and environmental intervention in preventing or reversing disability.

Impairments and Losses

Old age is associated with increased occurrence of a wide array of physiologic, physical, mental, and social impairments or losses, which may contribute independently or collectively to disabilities. These include elevated blood pressure; decreased immune response; reduced visual, auditory, and olfactory acuity; loss of muscle and bone mass; fragility of the skin; slowing of mental response; decreased cognitive ability; loss of spouses and companions; reduced income; and loss of social roles and autonomy.

Some of these changes and their consequences are intrinsic to the biology of aging. Examples include age-related decline in the individual's maximum oxygen consumption (Vo_2max), a fundamental index of capacity for physical activity; decrease in muscle mass (sarcopenia); modifications of lens protein leading to cataract formation and loss of vision; decrease in bone density with resultant osteoporosis and heightened risk of fracture; stiffening of arterial

TABLE 62-1. NUMBER AND DISTRIBUTION OF DISABLED ELDERLY, BY PLACE OF RESIDENCE, 1985

Category	Total Number of Elderly (millions)	Nursing Home		Community		Total		Disabled Elderly as a Percentage of Number of Elderly in Each Category		
		Number (millions)	%	Number (millions)	%	Number (millions)	%	Nursing Home	Community	All Disabled
Age (yr)										
65–74	16.9	0.2	15.4	2.1	41.9	2.3	36.5	1.3	12.3	13.6
75–84	9.1	0.5	38.5	2.0	40.9	2.5	40.0	5.6	22.1	27.7
85 and over	2.7	0.6	46.2	1.0	19.7	1.6	25.0	22.1	36.1	58.2
Sex										
Male	11.4	0.3	23.1	1.7	35.3	2.1	33.2	2.9	15.2	18.2
Female	17.2	1.0	76.9	3.3	66.2	4.3	68.0	5.7	19.1	24.8
Race										
White	25.9	1.2	92.3	4.2	84.0	5.4	85.9	4.7	16.1	20.8
Black	2.3	0.1	7.7	0.6	13.0	0.7	11.6	3.5	27.6	31.2
Number of ADL dependencies										
Fewer than three	—	0.4	28.5	3.3	67.0	3.7	58.9	1.3	11.6	12.9
Three or more	—	0.9	71.5	1.6	33.2	2.6	41.3	3.3	5.7	9.0
Total	28.6	1.3	100.0	4.9	100.0	6.3	100.0	4.6	17.3	21.9

From Rivlin AM, Wiener JM: Caring for the Disabled Elderly. Who Will Pay? Washington, DC: The Brookings Institution, 1988, p 6.

TABLE 62-2. PERCENTAGE OF PERSONS WHO HAVE DIFFICULTY WITH PERSONAL CARE (ADL) AND HOUSEHOLD MANAGEMENT (IADL) TASKS BECAUSE OF CHRONIC CONDITIONS, BY AGE AND SEX, UNITED STATES, 1984[a]

■ *PERSONAL CARE (ADL)*	*Bathe*	*Dress*	*Transfer*	*Toilet*	*Eat*
Men					
65–74	5.7	4.4	4.8	2.4	1.5
75–84	9.2	7.3	6.0	3.6	2.5
85+	23.1	14.1	12.7	10.0	4.3
Women					
65–74	6.9	4.2	7.0	2.7	0.9
75–84	14.2	7.7	11.2	6.5	2.4
85+	30.1	17.7	22.2	15.9	4.4
■ *HOUSEHOLD MANAGEMENT (IADL)*	*Shop*	*Light Housework*	*Prepare Own Meals*	*Manage Own Money*	*Use Telephone*
Men					
65–74	4.6	3.5	3.0	2.8	3.5
75–84	9.6	6.2	6.0	5.4	7.9
85+	26.8	15.2	18.5	19.0	18.4
Women					
65–74	7.8	5.0	4.8	1.8	2.0
75–84	18.4	10.5	10.5	6.8	4.8
85+	41.6	27.4	29.5	26.2	17.1

Data from Supplement on Aging, National Health Interview Survey, 1984. From Verbrugge LM: The iceberg of disability. In Stahl SM (ed): The Legacy of Longevity. Newbury Park, CA: Sage, 1990.

[a] For activities of daily living (ADL), "by yourself and without using special equipment." For instrumental (ADL), "by yourself." People who said they don't do an activity are in the denominator but not the numerator and are thus effectively considered nondisabled in these rates.

walls, causing increased systolic blood pressure and risk of disabling cerebrovascular accident.

A growing body of evidence indicates that many physiologic, physical, and mental changes as well as virtually all social changes associated with old age are not intrinsic to the aging process but are in significant part due to potentially modifiable extrinsic or self-induced factors that contribute to disability and dependence.

Disuse/Deconditioning

The first level of preventable extrinsic factors in functional decline is discontinuation of usual activity referred to as "disuse" or "deconditioning."[21] This may occur insidiously as older persons with–draw from usual activities either voluntarily in response to a sense of "growing old" or involuntarily as a consequence of intercurrent acute illness, retirement from work, etc. The best-studied model of global disuse/deconditioning, and one to which older persons are particularly prone on their own volition or their physician's or family's bidding, is extended bed rest. Going to bed for a prolonged period of time may lead to a litany of physiologic adaptations and potentially disabling consequences, as listed in Table 62-3. Of particular concern because of their potential contribution to limitation of mobility and risk of falls and fractures are physiologic and structural changes in muscle, bone, and joint tissues. Rate of decrease in muscle strength may be as high as 5 percent per day in the bedfast individual, with leg muscles tending to lose strength faster than arm muscles. Disuse osteoporosis results from both cessation of bone synthesis and increased resorption and tends to predominantly affect weight-bearing bones. Immobility and loss of weight-bearing forces on joints contribute to changes in both periarticular and articular tissue structure, which may lead to joint contractures.[22]

Also contributing directly or indirectly to bed rest–induced disability are atelectasis and other pulmonary changes that predispose to pneumonia, slowing of peristalsis with resulting constipation, bladder-emptying difficulties leading to urinary incontinence, sustained pressure on fragile skin predisposing to pressure sores, and sensory deprivation leading to an array of negative affective and cognitive effects.

Clearly an essential principle is to avoid taking to bed in old age, except as necessitated by medical problems. Instances of the latter should be minimized, with emphasis on progressive mobilization of bed-bound patients, first from bed to chair, then to ambulation with or without assistance. This should include purposeful activity such as ambulating to the toilet or to meals and dressing in normal clothing and footwear as opposed to institutional bed clothing. These principles, well known to progressive geriatric medicine services (see below), will prevent or reverse much of the potentially disabling deconditioning associated with prolonged bed rest.

Exercise

Regular physical exercise is perhaps the single most important health promotional activity for preventing many of the dysfunctional consequences of aging. Numerous studies have demonstrated that older persons, like their younger counterparts, can significantly increase physical fitness, as reflected in Vo_2max, by engaging in regular aero-

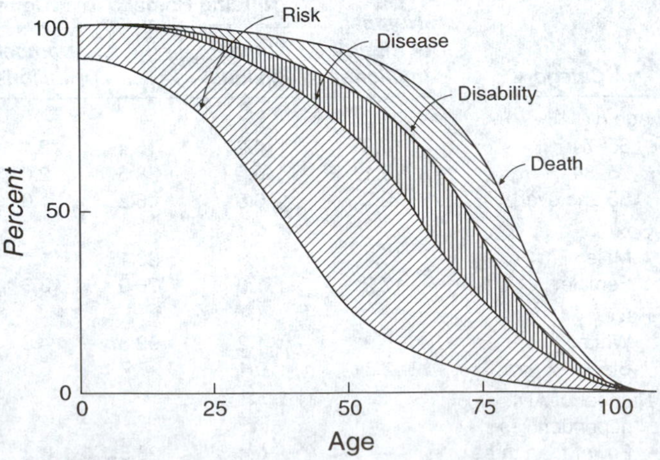

Figure 62-3. Conceptual relationship between age and percentage of the population remaining free of the respective stages in the natural history of chronic disabling disease.

TABLE 62-3. COMPLICATIONS OF BEDREST

Cardiovascular	Decreased cardiac output, contributing to decreased aerobic capacity
	Orthostatic intolerance
	Venous thrombophlebitis
Respiratory	Atelectasis
	Relative hypoxemia
	Pneumonia
Musculoskeletal	Muscle atrophy and loss of strength
	Decreased muscle oxidative capacity, contributing to decreased aerobic capacity
	Bone loss (osteoporosis)
Gastrointestinal	Constipation
Genitourinary	Incontinence
	Renal calculi
Skin	Pressure sores
Functional	Impaired ambulation
Psychological	Sensory deprivation

From Harper CM, Lyles YM: Physiology and complications of bed rest. J Am Geriatr Soc 36: 1047–1054, 1988.

bic exercise. Furthermore, there is clear experimental evidence involving older subjects that progressive resistance training can both retard and reverse losses of muscle mass and strength as well as bone density.[23,24] Several controlled trials have demonstrated improvements in gait speed, stair climbing, rising from a chair, and other significant physical tasks following participation in exercise programs conducted among frail nursing home residents.[25,26]

The application of such experimental observations to preventing disability is captured in the concept of "threshold levels" as follows:

> Strength, aerobic power and other indices of physical ability change on continuous scales whereas functional and quality of life changes are quantal. Thus a very small strength gain may be accompanied by a considerable functional improvement if it takes the patient from being just unable to transfer independently to being just able to do so. This also applies in reverse: A gradual loss of strength may not be apparent until the patient is suddenly unable to perform a crucial function.[27]

Added to the experimental and conceptual case favoring exercise in old age is the finding from longitudinal observations of community-dwelling elderly persons of a clear association between the lack of regular exercising and subsequent decline in ability to perform certain simple physical tasks.[28]

In spite of the demonstrated benefits of regular physical activity, the majority of older Americans live essentially sedentary lives, which has prompted the Public Health Service to set a national goal of reducing to less than 25 percent the proportion of persons over age 65 who engage in no leisure-time physical activity.[29] The Surgeon General's recommendations issued in 1996 call for 30 minutes of moderate activity a day, which may consist of walking, gardening, cycling, swimming, or other activities and which must be sustained for benefits to accrue.

▶ EARLY INTERVENTIONS AND REHABILITATION

Despite the best efforts of primary and secondary prevention and health promotion, the majority of older persons will develop one or more potentially disabling medical conditions. Under these circumstances the goals of health care, where possible, will be early medical or surgical intervention and rehabilitation or continuing supportive care to limit disability and provide for highest level of independence of individuals and their caregivers. Components of such tertiary prevention include both specific interventions for individual disabling conditions and comprehensive geriatric medicine services.

▶ SELECTED DISABLING CONDITIONS

Falls and Fractures

Falls occur among approximately 20 to 30 percent of community-dwelling elderly persons per year and an even greater percent of nursing home residents, with attendant risks of fracture, soft tissue injury, and psychological compromise to independence. Risk of falling increases with the number and type of chronic disabling conditions present and medications being taken. Visual and proprioceptive abnormalities, musculoskeletal and neurological diseases, depression, dementia, and hypotension-inducing conditions (biologic and iatrogenic) are particularly important. A fall risk index has been successfully used to guide preventive interventions.[30] A variety of exercise and balance training programs have also been found to reduce incidence of falling.[31]

To avoid certain secondary consequences of falls such as hypothermia or pressure sores from prolonged immobility, recurrent fallers should be provided with portable alarm systems as well as instructions for effectively maneuvering to right themselves following a fall. Wearing an external protective device over the hip has been shown to reduce frequency of fracture among fall-prone frail elderly persons.[32]

More than a million fractures occur in older persons in the United States each year, the three most common sites being vertebrae, proximal hip, and distal forearm (Colles' fracture). The principle contributing factor is osteoporosis or loss of bone mass, a progressive natural process that begins in the fourth or fifth decade of life and renders aging individuals increasingly susceptible to fracture associated with relatively minor trauma. Osteoporosis is accentuated in women following menopause, and age-specific risks of osteoporotic fractures are markedly higher among older women versus men (Fig. 62-4). Osteoporosis is significantly retarded by postmenopausal estrogen replacement therapy, by oral bisphosphonates, and probably by regular exercise and supplemental calcium intake throughout adulthood.[33]

Hip fractures are associated with more deaths, disability, and medical costs than all other osteoporotic fractures combined. Over 250,000 occur annually in the United States, at estimated direct medical and long-term care costs of $8 to 10 billion,[34] and there is evidence that the age-specific incidence of hip fracture may be increasing in some industrialized societies.[35] Between 10 and 20 percent of patients who have fractured their hips die within 6 months, and a substantial percentage of survivors are destined for long-term nursing home

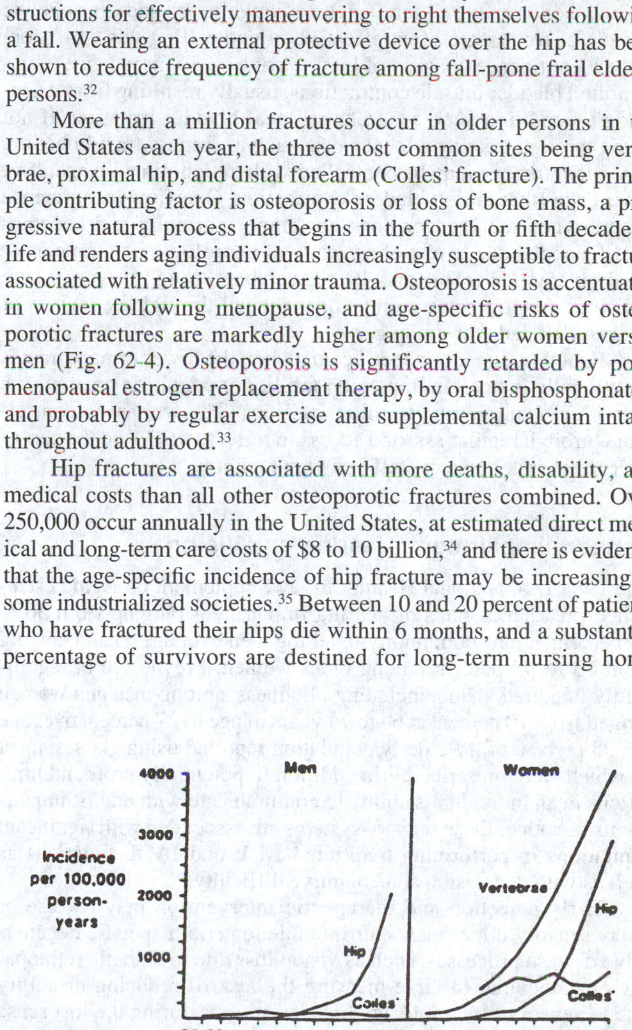

Figure 62-4. Incidence rates for the three common osteoporotic fractures (Colles', hip, and vertebral) in men and women, plotted as a function of age at the time of the fracture. (From Riggs BL, Melton LJ: Involutional osteoporosis. N Engl J Med 314:1676–1686, 1985.)

placement. There is, however, considerable potential for reducing mortality and institutional placement and restoring mobility, with or without assistive devices, if patients receive timely surgical, medical, and particularly rehabilitative care (see below under "Geriatric Strategies").

Incontinence

Urinary incontinence is defined as "the involuntary loss of urine so severe to have social and/or hygienic consequences." A symptom with multiple causes, rather than a discrete disease process, incontinence affects 15 to 30 percent of community-dwelling elderly and at least half of all nursing home residents. In addition to its immense psychosocial burden on afflicted individuals and their caretakers, the costs of managing urinary incontinence in the United States are estimated at over $10 billion dollars annually. This disabling condition of old age can in many instances be cured or effectively controlled through appropriate medical and nursing assessment and intervention.[36]

There are several subtypes of incontinence, each representing a distinctive pathophysiological mechanism. Stress incontinence, a particularly common form in women, results from dysfunction at the bladder outlet, allowing urine leakage during times of increase in intra-abdominal pressure, such as coughing or sneezing. Pelvic muscle exercises are often effective in controlling this condition. Urge incontinence consists of loss of urine as a consequence of uninhibited bladder muscle contractions, usually resulting from a neurologic condition such as stroke or local bladder irritation. If not cured through treating a local cause such as urinary tract infection, urge incontinence may be controlled with anticholinergic agents or other drugs that inhibit bladder contraction. Overflow incontinence occurs when the bladder does not empty normally and becomes overdistended due to one of a variety of neurologic impairments or local obstructions. This may be correctable through surgery where indicated (e.g., prostatectomy) or managed through a program of intermittent catheter drainage.

Functional incontinence occurs when the lower urinary tract is functionally intact, but impaired mobility or cognition prevents the individual from getting to toilet facilities. This variant is controllable through regular assisted access to toilet facilities on the part of the caretaker at home or staff in a nursing home.

Sensory Impairment: Hearing and Vision

The 1984 U.S. National Health Survey Supplement on Aging established prevalence rates of hearing impairment ranging from 30 to 60 percent among community-dwelling men over age 65 and ranging from 13 to 45 percent among older women. Prevalence of significantly impaired vision, including blindness, among men and women ranged from 10 percent at 64 to 74 years of age to 27 percent over age 85; 95 percent of the elderly population reported using glasses, most of which were prescribed.[37] In addition to potentially profound limitations in an individual's ability to communicate with others, impairments in both of these sensory systems are associated with significant limitations in performing traditional ADL and IADL functions as well as with depression and cognitive difficulty.

Early detection and therapeutic intervention may reverse or delay sensory impairments attributable to certain specific degenerative disease processes, such as visual loss due to diabetic retinopathy or glaucoma. In large measure the task of reducing disability due to sensory loss in old age focuses upon restoring the lost sense as in surgical treatment of senile cataract or prosthetic treatment in presbycusis. Cataract surgery with lens implantation has been shown to improve physical function as well as vision.[38] Hearing aides, voice amplifying devices, and lip reading represent the mainstays of hearing rehabilitation, which, if used effectively, can reverse physical and particularly psychosocial disability associated with hearing loss.

Depression and Dementia

Mental and psychological disability among the elderly are major societal concerns, particularly in long-term care institutions where the majority of residents have mental or behavioral problems that require continuing staff attention. Depression and dementia constitute the most prominent forms of affective and cognitive disorders encountered in old age. Both conditions may result from multiple causes and, while generally not preventable, the impact of depression and dementia on affected individuals or their caregivers may be alleviated through judicious intervention.

Major depression as defined by the *Diagnostic and Statistical Manual of Mental Disorders*, 3rd edition, revised (DSM-III-R), is found in fewer than 5 percent of older persons in the community, while distressing depressive symptoms associated with physical illness and adjustment to life changes occur in 10 to 20 percent.[39] A variety of antidepressant drugs as well as electroconvulsive therapy are effective in treating depression of old age, though these carry risks of serious side effects.[40]

Broadly defined by the DSM-III-R as "a loss of intellectual abilities sufficient to interfere with social or occupational functioning," dementia is a disabling mental condition, well known to aging societies, which increases dramatically in prevalence from 2 to 3 percent at age 65 to 30 percent or above at age 85 (Fig. 62-5). The most common pathologic subtypes of dementia are Alzheimer's disease and multi-infarct dementia. A small percent of cases of potentially reversible dementia occur secondary to treatable causes including hypothyroidism, subdural hematoma, drug toxicity, and others.

An increasing number of licensed and experimental drugs show promise of alleviating if not reversing the symptoms of dementia and a number of epidemiologic studies suggest that postmenopausal estrogen replacement therapy and nonsteroidal anti-inflammatory drugs (NSAIDs) may protect against development of Alzheimer's disease.[41]

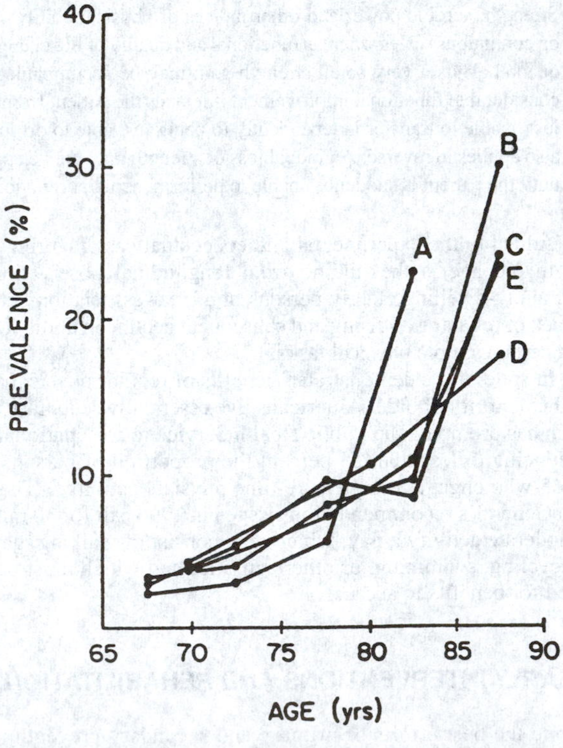

Figure 62-5. Age-specific prevalence rates for moderate or severe dementia in five studies: England (1970), United States (1978), Denmark (1963), Finland (1985), and New Zealand (1983). (From Mortimer JA, Hutton JT: Epidemiology and etiology of Alzheimer's disease. In Hutton JT, Kenny AD (eds): Senile Dementia of the Alzheimer Type. New York: Alan R. Liss, 1985.)

A variety of intervention strategies have been developed with the twin goals of maintaining independence and dignity for dementia patients and providing social and psychological support for their caregivers.[42] These invariably involve a multidisciplinary approach. Patient care includes continuing attention to basic medical and nursing needs, with particular emphasis on adequate nutrition, assistance with toileting and grooming, and prevention or early treatment of minor infections and skin breakdown. Regularly scheduled occupational and recreational therapy help to maintain patient morale. Support for caregivers in the community includes counseling and education about the natural course and management of dementia, particularly the characteristic and highly stressful memory loss and aberrant behavior; assistance with obtaining legal, financial and safety advice; and provision of temporary relief through day care or short-term residential respite care. To ensure appropriate and effective care for patients with advanced disease, often accompanied by wandering and abusive behavior, special care dementia units have been widely and successfully introduced in nursing homes in the United States and elsewhere.[43]

In addition to the burden suffered directly by patients and their caregivers, Alzheimer's and related disorders pose an immense monetary cost, estimated in the early 1990s at approximately $67 billion annually in the United States. The largest portion of this goes to long-term care.[44]

Stroke and Parkinson's Disease

Stroke and Parkinson's disease represent two of the most common disabling neurologic conditions of old age, both of which are candidates for early preventive or rehabilitative intervention.

Stroke, or cerebrovascular disease, comprises a heterogeneous group of pathological entities all of which carry a high risk of residual disability. While age-specific stroke mortality rates have declined dramatically and levels of disability among survivors of incident stroke have improved in the past two decades,[45] stroke remains the third leading cause of death and the most common disabling condition of old age with a prevalence of some 500 to 600 per 100,000 in the United States. Among acute stroke survivors 30 to 40 percent become dependent in self care, with most functional recovery occurring 3 to 6 months poststroke; over 50 percent experience significant depression and social isolation, and 20 to 30 percent are institutionalized for continuing care.[46] A number of randomized trials have found that hospital-based special stroke units, which combine acute medical-nursing expertise and multidisciplinary rehabilitation, yield decreased mortality and in some instances decreased long-term disability and institutional placement when compared with stroke management on general medical units.[47] Among a number of recent trials of thrombolytic therapy in acute ischemic stroke, significantly lower rates of poststroke disability have been observed in patients treated within 3 hours of onset of stroke. Some trials, however, have observed excess mortality and/or complications among treated cases compared with controls; hence use of this potential disability-reducing treatment is recommended with caution and within strict guidelines.[48]

Parkinson's disease (PD) is a degenerative condition resulting largely from deficiency of the neurotransmitter substance dopamine in the midbrain and causing generalized movement and postural abnormalities. Disabling manifestations include tremulous hands, shuffling gait with tendency to fall, plus some dulling of the intellect. Increasingly common with aging, the prevalence is estimated at 500 to 1,000 per 100,000 over age 60, with more than half of prevalent cases being over 70 years of age. Some Parkinsonism among older persons is drug-induced by neuroleptic agents and may resolve when the offending drug is discontinued. Conventional treatment to ameliorate manifest disability in PD consists of one of a variety of dopamine replacement regimens plus physical therapy.[49] Initial studies that reported delayed development of disability when treating PD patients early with the antioxidant deprenyl have unfortunately not borne up over time.[50]

Implants of fetal adrenal gland tissue as well as pallidotomy represent evolving surgical interventions with potential for reversing the pathophysiologic effects of PD.

Congestive Heart Failure and Chronic Obstructive Pulmonary Disease

Congestive heart failure (CHF) and chronic obstructive pulmonary disease (COPD) constitute the two most common disabling chronic cardiopulmonary conditions of old age. From a public health perspective, the impact of both conditions on society at large in the United States and elsewhere is manifest by increasing mortality and morbidity rates for both conditions among older persons since the 1980s. From a clinical perspective, impact of these conditions on patient functional status and quality of life has been shown to be partially controllable through use of selected medical and rehabilitative interventions.

CHF is the most common reason for hospitalization among persons over age 65 in the United States, with rates rising steeply between the seventh and ninth decades of life. Increasing incidence and prevalence of CHF is attributed to increased numbers of surviving patients with ischemic heart disease who are at high risk of developing CHF.[51] While CHF was formerly a condition with very poor prognosis, a number of randomized clinical trials in the past decade have shown significant improvement in survival and in functional capacity among patients treated with angiotensin-converting enzyme inhibitors.[52] Additionally, physician–nurse practitioner coordinated care has been shown to reduce hospitalizations and improve quality of life among community-dwelling older patients with chronic CHF.[53]

COPD, the end stage of prolonged insult to the bronchi, bronchioles, and lung parenchyma from tobacco smoke and other atmospheric pollutants, is the fifth commonest cause of death in the United States, with prevalence rates and death rates rising among persons over 70 years of age in recent decades.[54] Loss of capacity for physical activity and psychological distress due to oxygen deprivation are the main functional impacts of COPD on the individual. A variety of inpatient, outpatient, and home-based respiratory rehabilitation programs have been developed to assist in long-term management of patients with COPD. A meta-analysis of 14 randomized trials of rehabilitation programs offered to patients with activity limitation attributable to COPD found clinically significant improvement in health-related quality of life measures and functional capacity when compared with conventional care.[55] While physical exercise is considered the central pillar of these programs, it is likely that attention to nutrition and psychosocial status and other programtic activities also contribute to the positive results.

Transitions: Retirement, Bereavement, Relocation

Certain discrete transitions in social status place older persons at increased risk of onset or worsening of disabling physical and mental health problems. Most prominent among these transitions are retirement, loss of spouse, and residential relocation. These events are commonly associated with loss of autonomy and control over one's life, as well as loss of the social and psychological support that contributes to physical and mental well-being.

The major impacts of retirement on well-being relate to reduction in income and attendant increase in various mental health problems. Loss of spouse and the accompanying experience of loneliness and bereavement are associated with increased likelihood of a variety of nonspecific mental and physical symptoms as well as excess mortality. The excess mortality is more common in men than in women and peaks during the first 6 months of bereavement. Residential relocation, particularly placement in a nursing home, represents an unusually stressful event, depriving the old person of a familiar social and physical environment as well as much of his or her sense of autonomy. The nursing home experience is commonly aggravated further by the excessive use of physical and chemical restraints, which diminish or distort mental performance and increase the risk of iatrogenic illness or injury. Such untoward effects as well as increased risk of death tend to be concentrated in the early months following residential relocation.[18]

Reduction in the ill health risks and increased mortality associated with social transitions may be achieved through various supportive and autonomy-enhancing interventions. Providing material assistance, medical attention as needed, and companionship are fundamental supportive approaches. Teaching, encouraging, and enabling are important autonomy-enhancing approaches, in contrast to excessive cautioning and "doing for," which may induce a sense of helplessness. A number of observations in nursing homes have demonstrated improvement in mental health and other health status indices among residents maintained free of unnecessary restraints and encouraged to exercise initiative in choice of daily activities.

At the level of primary prevention directed to social transitions of aging, a society's or community's existing policies and practices may be altered with respect to both retirement and nursing home placement.[56] Normative, if not legally mandated, retirement age can and has been increased in some settings. Rehabilitative and community-based services can and have been successfully implemented as alternatives to custodial placement in nursing homes. Such continuing care alternatives have been most fully developed in societies with comprehensive health care systems.[57]

▸ HEALTH CARE DELIVERY

The Geriatric Medicine Movement

The breadth of threats to health and independent functioning in old age and the attendant potentials for preventive interventions, as reviewed above, constitute a major challenge to develop suitable prevention-oriented health care delivery systems. In recognition of this challenge, the World Health Organization convened an expert panel in 1974 on "Planning and Organization of Geriatric Services." This body recommended that countries develop integrated health services for older persons, including "elements of medical and social prevention, multidisciplinary assessment, home and institutional curative treatment, rehabilitation, long-term care and supportive social welfare."[58] This spectrum of services, with dedicated professionals and resources, constitutes the essence of the modern geriatric medicine movement, which was pioneered in Great Britain and has now developed in many other parts of the world.[59] The principal focus of this field of medicine, captured in the motto, "adding life to years," is the provision of timely interventions to treat and prevent unnecessary disease, disability, and dependency at all stages. Translating this concept into practical terms, comprehensive health services for older persons include an array of community, hospital, and institutional continuing care elements and academic commitments such as developed in Great Britain and summarized in Table 62-4.

Geriatric Strategies

Comprehensive geriatric assessment (CGA) represents the core clinical activity of geriatric medicine. Practiced in inpatient and outpatient settings on the part of geriatricians, nurses, social workers, rehabilitation therapists, and others working in collaboration, geriatric assessment identifies the vulnerable elderly patient's medical, psychosocial, and functional capabilities and problems and leads to appropriate preventive, curative, rehabilitative, and long-term care.[60] In a meta-analysis of 28 controlled trials of geriatric assessment programs, the odds of surviving and living in the community, as well as showing improvement in physical or mental status at 6- to-12-month follow-up, are generally more favorable for patients managed by CGA programs. Programs that include control over implementing medical recommendations and provide extended ambulatory follow-up are more likely to be successful.[61]

The need for progressive geriatric care is particularly evident in the acute hospital sector, where older patients not only constitute the largest constituency of admissions, but are at particularly high risk of experiencing decline in physical and mental function. Such strategies have been incorporated into hospitals in various ways in Great Britain, the United States, and elsewhere, as shown in Figure 62-6. The simplest approach (*C* in the figure) involves referral for consultation by a multidisciplinary geriatrics team. The modality labeled *T* in the figure consists of a special hospital-based or affiliated unit to which patients are transferred for geriatric rehabilitation following acute care on a medical or surgical service. The third modality (*A* in the figure), involves designating part of an inpatient medical service as an acute geriatric admitting unit.[57]

Among the documented successes of hospital-based geriatric programs, three prototypic experiences are particularly illustrative. The first of these, based at the Sepulveda Veterans Administration Medical Center in Los Angeles, comprised a 15-bed geriatric unit operated by a full-time medical, nursing, and social work team, with part-time participation by rehabilitation therapists and others. In a randomized trial, older hospitalized patients who were transferred to the geriatric unit, when compared with control subjects who were managed on a general medical unit, were found to experience significantly lower mortality (24 versus 49 percent), a reduced likelihood of nursing home admission (27 versus 47 percent), fewer overall acute hospital and nursing home days over a 1-year follow-up, significantly greater improvement in functional status and morale, and lower average cost of care.[62]

The second experience involved a collaborative geriatric orthopedic rehabilitation unit (GORU) developed in Sterling, Scotland,

TABLE 62-4. SOME SPECIFIC ELEMENTS OF COMPREHENSIVE HEALTH SERVICES FOR THE ELDERLY IN GREAT BRITAIN

■ ***COMMUNITY***

Enrollment in primary care practice
- General practitioner
- Attached community nurses
- Home visiting by general practitioners

Social service liaisons
- Home help
- Meals on wheels
- Domiciliary occupational therapy

■ ***GENERAL HOSPITAL***

Acute geriatric services
- Defined catchment population
- Geriatric medicine specialists, house officers
- Multidisciplinary teams
- Rehabilitation emphasis
- Home visiting
- Day hospital
- Respite admissions

Liaison consultation with other hospital services
- Medicine
- Orthopedics
- Psychiatry

■ ***INSTITUTIONAL CONTINUING CARE***
- Medical surveillance, avoid frequent transfer to hospital
- Multidisciplinary rehabilitation, maintenance of function
- Social and recreational activities

■ ***EDUCATION***
- Academic departments of geriatric medicine
- Required curriculum in medical schools
- Formal postgraduate specialty training

From Barker WH. Adding Life to Years: Organized Geriatrics Services in Great Britain and Implications for the United States. Baltimore: Johns Hopkins University Press, 1987, p 170.

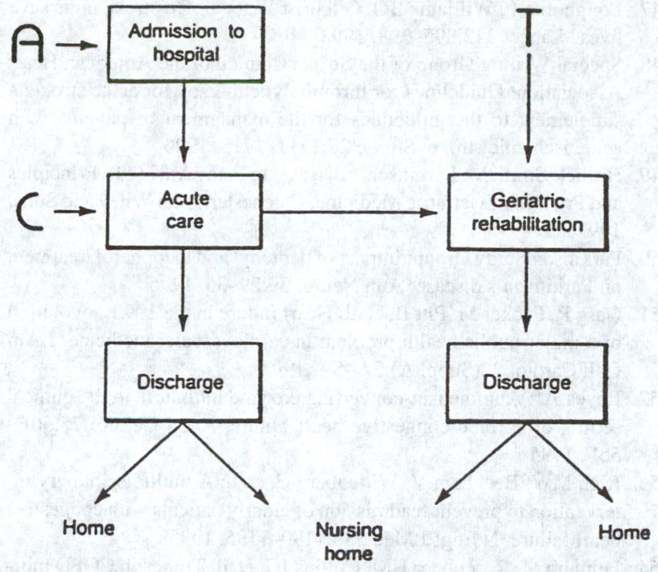

Figure 62-6. Potential intervention by special geriatrics services in the course of acute hospital admission in the United States. *A*, admit to acute geriatrics service; *C*, geriatric consultation on acute medical and surgical services; *T*, postacute transfer to special geriatric rehabilitation unit. (From Barker WH: Adding Life to Years: Organized Geriatrics Services in Great Britain and Implications for the United States. Baltimore: Johns Hopkins University Press, 1987, p 131.)

in which elderly female patients with hip fracture were transferred postoperatively to the care of a multidisciplinary service headed by a geriatrician. In a randomized trial comparing patients managed by the GORU with those managed by the orthopedic service, median length of acute and postacute hospital stay was shorter (24 versus 41 days), fewer patients were discharged to long-term institutional care (10 versus 32 percent), and more patients attained high levels of independence in activities of daily living at time of discharge (76 versus 46 percent).[63]

The third experience is the Acute Care for the Elderly (ACE) unit developed at the Case Western Reserve Medical Center in Cleveland, Ohio. Designed to avoid the cascade of "hazards of hospitalization" for older patients,[64] the ACE unit incorporates a set of explicit geriatric care principles into routine acute care, beginning at the time of admission to the hospital. These include patient-centered care protocols to maintain or restore continence, mobility, skin integrity, mental health, etc., and daily rounds by a multidisciplinary team led by medical and nursing directors. A randomized trial showed significantly better functional status at discharge and lower rate of posthospital nursing home placement for the ACE unit patients, with comparable lengths of stay and hospital bills for these patients and control patients admitted to acute general medicine units.[65]

Comprehensive Health Services

Successful provision of geriatric assessment, rehabilitation, and continuing care with a preventive orientation is most likely to occur in a comprehensive health care program in which the various elements listed in Table 62-4 are linked together under one system of financing. Such systems have developed in Great Britain, Scandinavian countries, and a number of other societies with national health programs.[57] In the United States, fragmentation among health care providers and payors and an excessive reliance on costly institutional services (acute hospitals and nursing homes) has left many gaps in the provision of services that could prevent or alleviate disability and dependency in old age. This problem was recognized and addressed in a number of national health policy proposals developed during the 1980s and early 1990s, but no comprehensive national system has evolved. A number of demonstration projects, including the PACE/On Lok Program for All-Inclusive Care of the Elderly, the Social Health Maintenance Organization (SHMO), and a number of public/private integrated care systems sponsored by members of the National Chronic Care Consortium, as well as the Veterans Administration health services, have developed model comprehensive programs for older persons in the United States.[66] At such time that a national health program should evolve in the coming century, policymakers will be well provided with these model experiences to draw upon in ensuring progressive comprehensive services for society's oldest and most vulnerable members.

▶ REFERENCES

1. International Classification of Impairments, Disabilities and Handicaps (ICIDH): Geneva: World Health Organization, 1980
2. Andresen EM, Rothenberg BM, Zimmer JG: Assessing Health Status among Older Adults, New York: Springer, 1997
3. Katz S, Ford AB, Moskowitz RW, et al: Studies of illness in the aged. The index of ADL. JAMA 185:914–919, 1963
4. Lawton MP, Brody EM: Assessment of older people: self-maintaining and instrumental activities of daily living. Gerontologist 9:179–186, 1969
5. Fried LP, Herdman SJ, Kuhn KE, et al: Preclinical disability: hypotheses about the bottom of the iceberg. J Aging Health 3:285–300, 1991
6. Guralnik JM, LaCroix AZ, Everett DF, et al: Aging in the eighties: the prevelance of comorbidity and its association with disability. Advancedata 170:1–8, 1989
7. Boult C, Kane RL, Louis TA, et al: Chronic conditions that lead to functional limitation in the elderly. J Gerontol 49:M28–M36, 1994
8. Ettinger WH, Fried LP, Harris T, et al: Self-reported causes of physical disability in older people: the Cardiovascular Health Study. J Am Geriatr Soc 42:1035–1044, 1994
9. Rowland D, Lyons B: Disability and disease: medical care use by the impaired elderly. Gerontologist 29:237A, 1989
10. Cohen RA, VanNostrand J: Trends in health of older Americans: United States, 1994. National Center for Health Statistics. Vital Health Stat 3 (30), 1995. Chapter 3. Trends in Mortality
11. Heikkinen E: Health implications of population aging in Europe. World Health Stat Q 40:22–40, 1987
12. Fries JF: Aging, natural death, and the compression of morbidity. N Engl J Med 303:130–135, 1980
13. Gruenberg EM: The failures of success. Milbank Mem Fund Q 55: 3–24, 1977
14. Manton KG: Changing concepts of morbidity and mortality in the elderly population. Milbank Mem Fund Q 60:183–244, 1982
15. Manton KG: A longitudinal study of functional change and mortality in the United States. J Gerontol 43:153–161, 1988
16. Svanborg A: Cohort differences in the Gothenberg studies of Swedish 70-year-olds. In Brody JA, Maddox GL (eds): Epidemiology and Aging. New York: Springer, 1988
17. Katz S, Branch LG, Branson MH, et al: Active life expectancy. N Engl J Med 309:1218–1224, 1983
18. Rowe JW, Kahn RL: Human aging: usual and successful. Science 237:143–149, 1987
19. Manton KG, Sallard E, Corder LS: Changes in morbidity and disability in the U.S. elderly population: evidence from the 1982, 1984, and 1989 national long term care surveys. J Gerontol 50B:S194–S204, 1995
20. Manton KG, Corder L, Stallard E: Chronic disability trends in elderly United States populations: 1982–1994. Proc Nat Acad Sci 94: 2593–2598, 1997
21. Bortz WM: Disuse and aging. JAMA 248:1203–1208, 1982

22. Harper CM, Lyles YM: Physiology and complications of bed rest. J Am Geriatr Soc 36:1047–1054, 1988
23. Fiatarone MA, Evans WJ: The etiology and reversibility of muscle dysfunction in the aged. J Gerontol 47:77–83, 1993
24. Evans WJ: Effects of exercise on body composition and functional capacity of the elderly. J Gerontol 50A:147–150, 1995
25. McMurdo ME, Rennie L: A controlled trial of exercise by residents of old people's homes. Age Ageing 22:11–15, 1993
26. Fiatarone MA, O'Neill EF, Ryan ND, et al: Exercise training and nutritional supplementation for physical frailty in very elderly people. N Engl J Med 330:1769–1775, 1994
27. Young A: Exercise and physiology in geriatric practice. Acta Med Scan Suppl 711:227–232, 1986
28. Mor V, Murphy J, Masterson-Allen S, et al: Risk of functional decline among well elderly. J Clin Epidemiol 42:895–904, 1989
29. Centers for Disease Control and Prevention: State-specific changes in physical inactivity among persons ≥ 65 years. United States 1987–1992. MMWR 44:663–673, 1995
30. Tinetti ME, Baker DI, McAvay G, et al: A multifactorial intervention to reduce the risk of falling among elderly people living in the community. N Engl J Med 331:821–827, 1994
31. Province MA, Hadley EC, Hornbrook MC, et al: The effects of exercise on falls in the elderly. A preplanned meta-analysis of the FICSIT trials. JAMA 273:1341–1347, 1995
32. Lauritzen JB, Peterson MM, Lund B: Effect of external protectors on hip fractures. Lancet 341:11–13, 1993
33. Raisz LG: The osteoporosis revolution. Ann Intern Med 126: 458–462, 1997
34. Herthoff KA, Lohr KN (eds): Hip Fracture: Setting Priorities for Effectiveness Research. Washington, DC: National Academy Press, 1990
35. Melton JL, O'Fallon WM, Riggs L: Secular trends in the incidence of hip fractures. Calcif Tissue Int 41:57–64, 1987
36. Resnick NM, Ouslander JG: Urinary incontinence: Where do we stand and where do we go from here? J Am Geriatr Soc 38:263–264, 1990
37. Havlik RJ: Ageing in the eighties, impaired senses for sound and light in persons age 65 years and over. Advancedata 125:1–8, 1986
38. Applegate WB, Miller ST, Elam JT, et al: Impact of cataract surgery with lens implantation on vision and physical function in elderly patients. JAMA 257:1064–1066, 1987
39. Blazer D: Depression in the elderly. N Engl J Med 320:164–166, 1989
40. Katz I, Alexopoulos GS (eds): Consensus Update Conference: diagnosis and treatment of late-life depression. Am J Geriatr Psychiatry 4(Suppl 1):S1–S95, 1996
41. Marx J: Searching for drugs that combat Alzheimer's. Science 273: 50–53, 1996
42. Mace NL, Rabins PV: The 36-Hour Day. Baltimore: Johns Hopkins University Press, 1991
43. Maslow K: Current knowledge about special care units: findings of a study by the U.S. Office of Technology Assessment. Alzheimer Dis Assoc Disord 8(Suppl 1):S14–S40, 1994
44. Ernst RL, Hay JW: The U.S. economic costs of Alzheimer's disease revisted. Am J Public Health 84:1261–1264, 1994
45. Barker WH, Mullooly JP: Stroke in a defined elderly population, 1967–1985. A less lethal and disabling but no less common disease. Stroke, in press
46. Dombovy ML: Rehabilitation and the course of recovery after stroke. In Whisnant JP (ed): Stroke: Populations, Cohorts, and Clinical Trials. Oxford: Butterworth Heinemann, 1993, pp 218–237
47. Longhorne P, Williams BO, Gilchrist W, et al: Do stroke units save lives? Lancet 342:395–398, 1993
48. Special Writing Group of the Stroke Council of the American Heart Association: Guidelines for thrombolytic therapy for acute stroke: a supplement to the guidelines for the managment of patients with acute ischemic stroke. Stroke 27:1711–1718, 1996
49. Hildick-Smith M: Parkinson's disease. In Pathy MSJ (ed): Principles and Practice of Geriatric Medicine. Chichester: John Wiley and Sons, 1997
50. Parkinson Study Group: Impact of deprenyl and tocopherol treatment on Parkinson's disease. Ann Neurol 39:29–36, 1996
51. Garg R, Packer M, Pitt B, et al: Heart failure in the 1990s: evolution of a major public health problem in cardiovascular medicine. J Am Coll Cardiol 22(Suppl A):3A–5A, 1993
52. Reyes AJ: Angiotensin-converting enzyme inhibitors in the clinical setting of chronic congestive heart failure. Am J Cardiol 75:50F–55F, 1995
53. Rich MW, Beckham V, Wittenberg C, et al: A multidisciplinary intervention to prevent readmission of elderly patients with congestive heart failure. N Engl J Med 333:1190–1195, 1995
54. Feinleib M, Rosenberg HM, Collins JG, et al: Trends in COPD mortality and morbidity in the United States. Am Rev Respir Dis 140:S9–S18, 1989
55. Lacasse Y, Wong E, Guyatt GH, et al: Meta-analysis of respiratory rehabilitation in chronic obstructive pulmonary disease. Lancet 348: 1115–1119, 1996
56. Townsend P: The structured dependency of the elderly: A creation of social policy in the twentieth century. Ageing Soc 1:5–28, 1981
57. Barker WH: Adding Life to Years: Organized Geriatrics Services in Great Britain and Implications for the United States. Chapters 9–11. Baltimore: Johns Hopkins University Press, 1987
58. World Health Organization: Planning and Organization of Geriatric Services. World Health Organizational Technical Report Series No. 548. Geneva: World Health Organization, 1974
59. Barker WH: Geriatrics internationally. In Fox R, Horan M, Puxity J (eds): Medicine in the Elderly: A Problem Solving Approach. London: Edward Arnold, 1990
60. NIA Conference on Assessment. J Am Geriatr Soc 31:636–765, 1983
61. Stuck AE, Siu AL, Wieland D, et al: Comprehensive geriatric assessment a meta-analysis of controlled trials. Lancet 342:1032–1036, 1993
62. Rubenstein LZ, Josephson KR, Wieland GD, et al: Effectiveness of a geriatric evaluation unit: a randomized clinical trial. N Engl J Med 311:1664–1670, 1984
63. Kennie DC, Reid J, Richardson IR, Kiamari AA, Kelt C: Effectiveness of geriatric rehabilitative care after fracture of the proximal femur in elderly women: a randomized clinical trial. Br Med J 297:1083–1086, 1988
64. Creditor MC: Hazards of hospitalization of the elderly. Ann Int Med 118:219–223, 1993
65. Landefield SC, Palmer RM, Kresevic DM, et al: A randomized trial of care in a hospital medical unit especially designed to improve the functional outcomes of acutely ill older patients. N Engl J Med 332:1338–1344, 1995
66. Evashwick CJ: The Continuum of Long-Term Care. Albany: Delmar Publishers, 1996, Chapters 3 and 14.
67. Barker WH: "Geriatrics in North America." Chapter 108 in Brocklehurst J, Tallis R, Fillet H (editors) Geriatric Medicine and Gerontology, 5th edition. London: Churchill and Livingstone International, 1998

63

Genetics and the Public Health

Patricia A. Baird • Charles R. Scriver

Social policies, public health, and medicine, in that general descending order of importance, improved human well-being and longevity in the twentieth century, yet disease continues, in the form of sick populations and sick individuals,[1] and unhealthy longevity is a macroeconomic problem.[2] Naturally, there has been a response—one composed of social policies, public health, and medicine. In Canada, a major milestone in this response was the government document *A Perspective on the Health of Canadians*,[3] which outlined the Health Field Concept. Reasonable, thoughtful, and provocative, this document espoused a four-pronged attack on disease, and it welded ideas on lifestyle, environment, health care organization, and human biology into an approach to address disease more effectively. Considerable attention has been paid to the first three but rather less has been heard about the fourth component, namely, the biological basis of disease. This chapter addresses that particular theme. Our topic is genetic determinants of disease. We believe them to be important because they explain both incidence and causes; they also explain some examples of clustering of disease in geographic regions.

Health is a state of homeostasis, and it is maintained in the face of a changing and shifting environment. The central tendencies of metrical traits (mean values) are the quantitative measures of homeostasis (e.g., level of blood glucose, cholesterol, phosphorus, osmolarity, blood pressure, and so on).[4] The polypeptide mediators of homeostasis (enzymes, transporters, channels, receptors, etc.) that are essential to this process of homeostasis are encoded by genes, descended to homo sapiens through the evolutionary process. Individuals retain health if experience does not overwhelm homeostasis or mutation does not undermine it.

In the conventional medical model, disease manifestations (symptoms and signs) are the product of a process (pathogenesis) that has an origin (cause). The manifestations of disease dominate the practice of medicine. Consideration of cause, incidence, and distribution of cases constitutes the public health focus. In medicine the emphasis is on the case; in public health it is on the population. But when adverse infectious and nutritional experiences (the major agents of genetic selection in human evolution) are well controlled, the causes of persistent disease may be of that form that undermines homeostasis rather than of the type that overwhelms it; that is, they may be intrinsic, or genetic, causes. If so the "heritability" of disease in the population has increased; further, it implies that the biological basis of disease is important and that the health care system must accommodate genetic causes of disease.

Rather than thinking of the determinants of disease as outside ourselves, our genetic individuality should be seen as a potential ingredient in the origin of health. Because each individual has a different risk for disease, progress will be optimized if this fact is recognized, taken into account, and applied. Socioeconomic and environmental factors are important determinants of health, but, given a particular environmental factor, *who* gets sick may be determined by genotype. If environmental causes of disease are examined without taking genetic predisposition into account, we not only are getting an incomplete picture but also may be missing the chance to identify, and target with preventive programs, the most "vulnerable" groups.

In this chapter we start with the premise that genetic causes of disease have implications for public health because they either explain cases or identify persons predisposed to disease under disadvantageous circumstances. Since most diseases have two histories, one biological and the other cultural, it is likely that genes have entered different populations because of those populations' different histories. This means that in some populations the genes may have reached such a frequency that they may now exhibit "clustering" of related disease. When diseases have significant genetic determinants, there is an opportunity for prevention through counseling. To explain cases and thus understand why a particular person has a particular genetic disease at a certain time, we summarize the rules of inheritance. If diseases associated with inheritance of biological determinants reach particular high frequencies in a population, it is through one or several historical mechanisms: genetic drift (founder effect), selective advantage, high mutation rate, reproductive compensation, or several genes associated with a common, shared phenotype. These mechanisms are examined in this chapter because they are relevant to public health. They are helpful in our understanding of the impact and relevance of particular population screening programs to current and future disease incidence.

A completed human gene map (both genetic and physical) is an important resource in medicine and for public health; we therefore describe its relevance. Finally, medical screening is a conventional activity in public health; genetic screening is a new form of it. The rationales, principles, and practices of genetic screening are therefore examined as well. Because innovations on the horizon (e.g., DNA tests) will change the way health care professionals view sick individuals and sick populations, we discuss the implications for public health and for society in general of the new genetic technology.

▸ GENES IN POPULATIONS

Inheritance and Distribution

Since the beginning of Western medicine, it has been recognized that physical traits and some diseases are inherited. A conceptual basis for the mechanism of inheritance was provided by Mendel,[5] and this concept of a unit of inheritance—the gene—has been richly borne out by a great deal of animal and plant experimental data as well as by empirical human data. The advent of recombinant DNA approaches has borne out the use of this concept even further.

As a species we have a long evolutionary history, and natural selection has ensured that most genes we possess are useful and advantageous. However, deleterious genes certainly exist and cause major problems for their possessors. What determines the frequency of such genes? Will modern medical care for people with deleterious genes (relaxed selection) mean that as a species we will accumulate an increasing genetic load of such mutant genes? The question of what determines the frequency of mutant genes is therefore an important one.

It has been estimated[6–8] that a human being has between 50,000 and 100,000 structural genes. In general, except for those on the sex chromosomes in males, humans have two copies of every gene, and therefore each specific function in an individual is usually coded for by two genes—one from the mother, one from the father. If both copies in a gene pair code for fully functional gene products, the individual will have normal function. If both copies code for defective products that normally are essential for life, the individual will have a lethal disease. If one member of the pair is normal and the other defective, the person's fate will depend on whether the normal gene has sufficient product to allow healthy function. Alternative forms of a given gene are called *alleles* of that gene. An individual who has identical alleles in a gene pair is said to be homozygous. If the alleles in a pair are different—that is, they code for different (although similar in structure) products—that individual is said to be heterozygous.

In thinking about the frequency of genes in a population, that population can be considered as a pool of genes, a pool from which any individual draws two alleles for each gene pair. Consider a population with random mating where a given gene may exist in the form of allele A or of allele a. The chance that a person will draw any one of three possible combinations (AA, Aa, aa) depends on the frequency of A compared with a in the gene pool.

If p is the frequency of A, and q is the frequency of a, then

$$p + q = 1$$

and

$$p = 1 - q$$

and the relative proportion of the three possible combinations will be

$$p^2(AA) + 2pq(Aa) + q^2(aa)$$

This formula for the distribution of genes in a population[9,10] is known as the Hardy-Weinberg equilibrium, since this relationship holds only as long as there is no mitigating influence (e.g., *AA*s have twice the number of children). In the absence of any factor disturbing the equilibrium, the proportions of the genotypes will remain the same from generation to generation. Thus, if one knows how often a disease due to two defective alleles (a recessive disorder) occurs, it is possible to calculate the frequency of heterozygotes (or carriers) in the population. For example, if a given recessive disorder (aa) appears in 1 in 10,000 liveborn individuals, the frequency of carriers (Aa) in that population will be approximately 1 in 50.

It is clear from this illustration that there are far more copies of the gene in carriers than occur in affected individuals. There is a shortcut in the calculation for diseases of this kind, which have a low frequency, where P is very close to 1: the carrier frequency will be twice the square root of the disease frequency. For example, in cystic fibrosis, which occurs about 1 in 2,000 births in white populations, approximately 1 in 22 individuals will carry the gene.

Changing Gene Frequencies

What may disrupt this equilibrium and change the frequency of genotypes (and resulting phenotypes) in a population? A rise in the frequency of a particular phenotype (due to changing gene frequencies) may be caused by one or more of the following five factors, which disturb the Hardy-Weinberg equilibrium.

1. Nonrandom Mating

If mating is random, the only thing determining the probability of a genotype's occurring is the relative frequency of the genes in the population pool. This condition may not be met if there is preferential mating due to traits wholly or partly genetically determined. Assortative mating (like with like) exists for several human traits.

2. Selection

A mutant allele that is harmful to the individual will be less likely to be passed on to the next generation, since its possessor is less likely to have children. In other words, it will be selected against and become less frequent. If the allele is *dominant* (i.e., just one copy of it is harmful), selection may be quite rapid, particularly if it means that all individuals with the gene are unable to reproduce; then no copies will be passed on to the next generation. In this situation, if the disorder occurs in the next generation, it does so by new mutation. Thus the proportion of cases of a dominant genetic disorder that are inherited depends on the effects of the gene on the likelihood of reproduction by its possessor. Selection against *recessive* alleles is much less effective, since most copies of the gene exist in carriers who are normal and able to pass the mutant gene on. Even if selection is complete against reproduction in the homozygote, it would take 10 generations (about 300 years) to reduce a gene frequency of 0.10 to 0.05. The less frequent the allele, the slower the decline in frequency. From a health policy point of view, it is important to note that going in the opposite direction—that is, removing selection—acts just as slowly. Successful therapy for phenylketonuria, for example, would take many generations to raise the frequency of the gene to any appreciable extent.

If an X-linked allele affects the male so that he does not reproduce, only the genes in female carriers are passed on to the next generation. Females carry about two-thirds of all such mutations. About one-third of all cases of a disease are due to new mutation, with two-thirds inherited. If affected males are able to have children, then a greater proportion of cases in the next generation are inherited. Treatment of males with hemophilia, for example, would be expected to cause some increase in the frequency of this condition in the absence of any other measure (such as prenatal diagnosis).

3. Mutation

A mutation is a change in the genetic material (DNA). The term can be used in a broad sense to encompass any change, including chromosomal deletions or rearrangements. However, it is usually used to mean a change in the DNA sequence of a gene so that the gene product is different (a point mutation), and that is how it is used here.

Mutations are the raw material of evolution and, in a changing environment, give a species the ability to adapt. However, most mutations cannot be expected to be beneficial, since they occur in an exquisitely coordinated system of genetic information that has taken eons to develop. A random change is not likely to be helpful. Many new dominant mutations are lethal either in utero or very early in life, so that the cases actually observed in human populations represent only a proportion of those that occur.

It is difficult to estimate with any accuracy[11] the current mutation rate in humans. It is probably quite different for different gene loci. An "average" spontaneous mutation rate in humans would be about 1 in 100,000 per locus per gamete per generation. Since mutation is usually a stochastic event, the longer the time elapsed, the greater the likelihood that a mutation will have occurred. Thus it could be predicted that parents who are older at conception would have an increased risk for a child with a dominant mutation, and this in fact is borne out by data. There is increased paternal age in fathers of children with dominant disorders (e.g., achondroplasia) that have never before occurred in the family.[12,13]

4. Heterozygote Advantage

It is possible that a gene that is harmful in the homozygous state may be advantageous in the carrier. This is the case with the genes for thalassemia and sickle-cell anemia, which in carriers may protect against malaria.[14] The gene for Tay-Sachs disease is frequent in Ashkenazi Jews, and it has been suggested that under ghetto conditions[15] it confers an advantage in the carrier. The occurrence of such genes in populations has importance in terms of health planning and in evaluating whether screening programs are appropriate for particular groups within the larger population.

5. Genetic Drift and Founder Effect

When people migrate to new regions, they may develop "new" diseases or express "old" disease at higher frequencies. This phenomenon reflects either new experiences or "old" genes expressed at altered frequencies in the settlers.[16] How many susceptible persons there are in the newly resident population after migration of the "founder" depends on the number of incoming mutant genes borne by the founders and on factors that favor their spread through the population (rates of natural increase, degree of consanguinity, and mode of inheritance). Accordingly, demographic history and structure of genetic variation may explain clustering of cases.

Methods of Measuring Mutation Rates

In theory, simply counting all individuals in a population of births who have a disease known to be due to a dominant gene, at the same time by family history evaluating how many are not inherited, should give the mutation rate for that locus. In practice, even with excellent population-based disease registries, this is extremely difficult to carry out in a large population. In addition to the logistical difficulties of collecting complete information on a large number of individuals, it is complicated by such factors as nonpaternity, mild cases that are missed, patients who die before ascertainment, and similar conditions that may be wrongly categorized. Indirect approaches to estimating the mutation rate for recessive disorders use the fact that the frequency of the recessive disease can be counted and that the reproductive "fitness" (the proportion of mutant to normal alleles passed on) can be measured in affected individuals. These are related as follows:

$$\text{Mutation} = (1 - \text{Fitness}) \times \text{Disease frequency}$$

These methods have yielded a range of estimates and may differ according to gene locus and sex.[17] In any case, determining frequencies in humans is difficult.[18]

▶ INCIDENCE AND PREVALENCE OF GENETIC DISEASE

Measuring the frequency of genetically determined diseases in a population is also difficult. Onset may occur at any time in the life cycle, and there is a gradation from diseases due to genes that do not permit normal function in any environment to those in which genetic predisposition is expressed only in certain environments. Statistics are usually available on a population only for aspects such as mortality by categories of cause or hospital admissions for diseases coded to the International Classification of Disease (ICD). This classification does not allow the frequency of genetic disease to be estimated because it is not a classification by etiology. For these reasons, at present it is not possible to quantify accurately the contribution of genetic disease to death and sickness.

However, population-based registries offer a mechanism for counting the occurrence of various disorders that may be exploited to answer this question. Registries provide the basic information on disease incidence and prevalence necessary for planning health and other special programs and facilities such as health professional and other personnel needs. If a registry receives information from multiple sources over individuals' lifetimes (especially if this can be linked into sibship and family groupings), some classification of disease in a population by etiology is possible. Additional coding for classification of cases by etiology is needed. With this approach it is possible to get some estimate of the relative importance of genetics to health.[19,20] Some estimates on the role of genes at different stages of life are provided:

Conception to Birth

Between 50 and 70 percent[21] of pregnancies in healthy women fail to produce liveborn babies. Genetic causes are a major factor in failed pregnancies, especially those during the first trimester. Chromosomal abnormalities are found in half of early spontaneous abortions.[22]

From Infancy to Young Adulthood

At least 5.3 percent of liveborn individuals in a large population of over a million consecutive births were found to have diseases with an important genetic component before age 25 years.[19] If congenital anomalies (some of which have a genetic cause) are also included, then 7.9 percent of the population has been identified by age 25 as having a genetic disorder. A sampling of over 12,000 admissions to a pediatric hospital found that 11.1 percent were "genetic"; 18.5 percent were for congenital malformations, and 2 percent were "probably" genetic.[23] These findings have been confirmed in other studies.[24,25]

The relative contribution of genetic disorders to all causes of disease in our population has likely increased markedly in this century for many conditions. As environmental causes of death and disease have declined, such as for infant mortality,[26] genetic causes assume more prominence. As the nutritional causes of rickets have declined, the proportion due to genetic defects in vitamin D metabolism have increased[27] and the heritability of the conditions has increased. This is but one example of several thousand different genetic diseases,[28] many of which are likely to have also increased in heritability as the environment has changed.

From Middle to Late Adulthood

We have very limited knowledge about the effects of genetic factors on the overall health of people after 25 years of age. The incidence of multifactorial disorders of late onset may be up to 60 percent if such conditions as diabetes, hypertension, myocardial infarction, ulcers, and thyrotoxicosis are included.[29] Including certain cancers makes this figure even higher.

If age-specific mortality rates are examined, a characteristic "U-shaped" mortality curve is obtained, with rates highest at each end of the age spectrum. The causes of death composing the two arms of the curve are not the same.[30] Those in early life are characterized by abnormal development and difficulty in adaption to life after birth. Mendelian disorders are characteristically diseases of prereproductive life,[31] with over 90 percent being apparent by the end of puberty. They reduce the life span and usually cause psychosocial handicaps. Those in the other "limb" of the curve are mainly diseases associated with specific environments, patterns of living, particular occupations, and advancing senescence.

The genetic variability of a cohort decreases as it moves through the life span and selection operates. The most disadaptive genes are the first to be deleted. After puberty the remaining genes contributing to disease are likely to be disadaptive only in certain environmental circumstances. In contrast, the variability of experience with environmental sources of disease determinants must increase throughout life. These reciprocal trends may be reflected in a diminution of heritability of the diseases that affect the cohort as it ages. Aging is associated with a decline in homeostatic competence of the various organ systems. This may set the stage for genes that previously had been harmless to become disadaptive. Genes are expressed differentially in ontogeny, and so new phenotypes will be revealed to selection as different stages of life are entered. This means diseases may have their own separate timetable for onset, and it will not be a general uniform decline in heritability for all diseases throughout life.

Several predictions follow from the assumption that heritability of disease declines with increasing age[30]:

1. Persons with early onset are more likely to have severe disease and to have affected first-degree relatives.
2. Age-specific age at onset should reach a peak and decline, since by some age most of those with the relevant genes will already have the disease.

3. There should be multigenic diseases that do not require a specific environment.
4. Migration, socioeconomic status, and other environmental change may change age of onset and the likelihood of the disease's clustering in families.
5. If one sex is less often affected, early onset, severity, and increased incidence in affected relatives should characterize it.
6. Concordance in monozygotic twins should be greatest when disease onset is early.
7. Patients with late-onset have milder disease that is more responsive to prevention and treatment.

For disease categories with a wide range of age of onset, monogenic forms are more likely to be found among the early-onset cases, multifactorial subtypes should characterize adult and middle age, and in the very old the disease should likely be due to environmental determinants. Single-gene disorders of early onset carry heavier burdens than those of later life and are relatively resistant to treatment.[32] There may be an irreducible minimum of genetic contribution to disease and death that feasible environmental manipulation cannot prevent, and the genetic variation in the population may determine the limits to what can be achieved by any environmental measures. However, with the advent of a greater understanding of genetic pathophysiology, it may become possible to tailor "microenvironments" to fit particular genotypes.

Determining the role of genetics in disease will require better methods of classifying disease and processing health data. Computerized record linkage will be increasingly important, not only to build longitudinal health histories on individuals but to link these into sibships and family groupings. Administrative and other health data sets that already exist can be combined to evaluate if familial clustering occurs. If familial clustering is found, then various methodologies may be used to untangle whether this is due to genetic or shared environmental factors or, more likely, an interaction between the two.

▶ CATEGORIES OF GENETIC DISEASE

Given that genetic disease has a substantial impact on health, it is of interest to examine the various categories of genetic disease that occur in humans, their frequencies, and the strategies currently available to deal with them. Several categories may be used when thinking about genetic disease, although at some level these are artefactual and imposed to organize the reality, which is a continuum.

Chromosomal Disorders

One in 200 liveborn infants has a chromosomal error, making this a common category of disorder. All are potentially detectable by prenatal diagnosis, but since only those subgroups of women identified as being at higher risk (because of age or family history) are screened prenatally, there is the opportunity to avoid only a proportion of such conditions at present. Errors may occur in the number of chromosomes (too many or too few) or in their structure (deletions or duplications of parts of chromosomes). Two texts cover this topic in depth.[33,34] Many of these errors are incompatible with survival to term; for example, almost half of all recognized spontaneous abortions in the first trimester have chromosomal abnormalities.[35] The proportion of stillborn infants with chromosomal errors is about 6 percent.[36,37]

Autosomal Chromosome Disorders

If an extra chromosome occurs for a given pair, this is called trisomy. Trisomy has not been observed in living infants for most chromosomes, although it is compatible with life for the sex chromosomes and chromosomes 13, 15, and 21. The latter, Down's syndrome, is the most frequent trisomy in liveborn humans. It occurs approximately once in 1,000 births, the exact frequency depending on the age composition of reproducing women in the population and whether prenatal diagnostic programs for its detection are in place. It is the most common recognizable cause for mental retardation in Western populations and is thus of relevance to public health and planning. Its occurrence is very strongly related to maternal age;[38] prenatal diagnostic programs are usually offered to detect chromosomal abnormalities in pregnant women over 35 years of age. Even though these programs are shown to be cost-effective in terms of health resources, they can reduce the birth incidence of Down's syndrome only to a limited degree.[39] This is because, even though young women have a much lower risk individually, they contribute a far greater number of births than women over 35, so that most Down's syndrome infants are born to young women. It is important that couples with an increased recurrence risk are made aware of the option of prenatal diagnosis in future pregnancies. It used to be thought that survival to adulthood in Down's syndrome was very poor, but recent data[40,41] show that over 70 percent of afflicted individuals survive to their thirties and about half to their late fifties. This obviously has implications for programs planning to integrate affected individuals into community, educational, vocational, and residential settings.

The other autosomal trisomies (15 and 18) are less frequent (1 in 5,000 to 7,000 and 1 in 8,000 livebirths, respectively) and result in infants with multiple congenital anomalies who often fail to thrive and die relatively young. It is important to make the diagnosis so that the parents may be counseled regarding the etiology, prognosis, and recurrence risk. Deletions (or duplications) may occur in any chromosome and occur anywhere along the chromosome. The size will vary among patients and give rise to a whole array of abnormal conditions. Some correlations of particular chromosomal abnormalities with particular clinical pictures have been made, for instance, deletion of part of the short arm of chromosome 5 with the cri-du-chat syndrome. Such chromosomal abnormalities explain many infants and children who are retarded, fail to thrive, and have birth defects.

Sex Chromosome Disorders

Recognition of sex chromosome disorders is important so that there is opportunity for avoidance of abnormal offspring and so that the affected individual can receive proper management to avoid known complications. Turner's syndrome was described in 1938[42] in girls who were short and sexually immature. It was later[43] discovered that this clinical picture was found in girls missing the second X chromosome in at least some of their cells. This condition occurs once in 5,000 livebirths and does not occur more frequently in the offspring of older mothers; the recurrence risk is negligible. Klinefelter's syndrome occurs in newborn surveys in about 1 in 500 males. This term is used to refer to males who have at least one extra X in at least some of their cells. The classic case has an XXY constitution, but there are other variants. The more Xs present, the more likely are mental retardation and additional physical stigmata. If Klinefelter's syndrome is not detected during childhood, afflicted males may learn that they have the syndrome when they attend an infertility clinic as an adult.

The XYY syndrome probably occurs about 1 in 500 males. This condition was sensationalized in the lay press for a time because of a theory that the extra Y made these males taller, aggressive, and antisocial. A study in the Danish population of army inductees[44] with this condition showed that crimes of violence against another person were not higher, although the total rate of criminal convictions was greater. The intelligence and educational level of XYY individuals was lower than control subjects, and it is possible that they may not commit crimes more often but get caught more often. The triple X female has been given the misnomer "superfemale" by some; however, retardation and infertility are increased in these women, although most are probably never diagnosed. If the diagnosis is made, prenatal diagnosis should be offered, since they are at increased risk for bearing XXY and XXX offspring.

Autosomal Dominant Disorders

This is the first of four categories that fall into the "single gene" or mendelian disorder group. It is important to understand the mechanism of their transmission, so that opportunities for prevention can be incorporated into planning and that the differing impact of preventive programs on the future frequency of these disorders be understood. In total, by 1997, over 5,000 mendelian disorders had been documented, with another 3,000 conditions thought to be in this category. Most of the identified loci (4,917) were on autosomes with less than 300 being X linked.[45] Although individually each is uncommon, there are so many that they have in toto a substantial impact on the health care system.

If an allele is always expressed, whether that person is homozygous or heterozygous at that locus, it is said to be dominantly inherited. If a gene is expressed in the phenotype only when it is homozygous, that trait is said to be recessively inherited. This distinction between dominant and recessive inheritance is an operational one for convenience in many ways. As better techniques are found, more recessive genes in the heterozygote can be detected. Thus, the line between dominance and recessivity is an artificial, albeit useful, concept in practice.

What sorts of disease are inherited in an autosomal dominant fashion? Included in this category are such entities as Huntington's chorea, neurofibromatosis, achondroplasia, tuberous sclerosis, and Marfan syndrome. If the affected person reproduces, the abnormal gene will be passed on average to half his or her children, who will also be affected. If a person does not receive the gene, then that branch of the family is "in the clear" from then on. Dominant disorders can change frequency rapidly in the population with intervention, making genetic diagnosis and counseling crucial.

Several factors make counseling families for dominant disorders very difficult at a practical level, despite the seemingly simple mechanism of transmission—"like tossing a coin." Although many dominantly inherited disorders follow the pattern described, where males and females are equally likely to be affected and to pass it on, and where on average half the offspring are affected, there are also many where additional aspects must be taken into account *before* one can give accurate and informed advice. First, some dominantly inherited disorders are due to new mutations. It is important to establish if a given case is familial or due to a new mutation, since once it has occurred, it will breed true and have a 50 percent chance of being passed on to a child. The important practical consequence is that siblings and other relatives will not be at increased risk.

Variable expressivity must also be considered before counseling is given. Each dominantly inherited disorder has a recognized profile; one disorder may have a very narrow range clinically with little variation in expression, whereas another may typically differ between persons even within a family. If an individual has the gene for a disorder where variable expressivity is not a feature, it is safe to reassure the apparently normal sibling that his or her children will not be at increased risk. However, for dominant disorders where there is great variation in severity, such as osteogenesis imperfecta, this reassurance must be tempered with caution. If a couple asks advice about risk for children when this disorder is segregating in their family, a detailed and sophisticated examination is indicated.

Another recently identified factor is "imprinting," which is imposed on the genetic information during gametogenesis.[46–49] This imprinting persists in a stable fashion throughout DNA replication and cell division in an individual, to be erased in the germ line and then be differentially established once more in the sperm (or egg) genomes of that individual. It has the consequence that expression of a given disease gene can depend on whether it is inherited from the mother or the father. Other factors to consider are reduced penetrance (where some individuals with the gene will show no clinical effect) and variation in age of onset. All genetic disease is not congenital. Many genetic disorders do not become clinically evident until adulthood or midlife. Genetic heterogeneity is a common phenomenon that must be taken into account, not just for dominant disorders but for all categories of genetic disease. A genetic disorder that appears to be the same in different families may in fact be due to different lesions in the same gene or to a different mutation at another locus that affects the same pathway and therefore leads to a similar clinical endpoint. When a case is sporadic and no other individual in the family is affected, the clinical endpoint observed may have been reached by other means than a single gene mechanism, such as an environmental insult in development.

Autosomal Recessive Disorders

Most recessive disorders are individually rare, each with a birth prevalence of 1 in 15,000 to 100,000. However, since there are so many, they have a considerable impact, with 1 in 500 liveborn individuals being identified as having one of these disorders before age 25 years. They often have their onset in early life, and there are population screening programs at birth for several of them, based on biochemical testing. Rapid advances in DNA technology will make it possible to offer population screening programs in a public health context for some of these disorders. Examples include phenylketonuria (which results in retardation and seizures but can be treated by diet), adenosine deaminase deficiency (which results in severe immune deficiency and early death), and cystic fibrosis, which is one of the commonest recessive disorders in white populations (approximately 1 in 22 people carry this gene).

Since genes segregate in families, the rarer the particular recessive allele for a disorder, the more likely that consanguinity is observed in the parents of an affected child case or that the individual will be born into a religious or geographical isolate. An allele for a particular recessive disorder may be so common in some subgroups that an appreciably increased risk of affected offspring occurs. It is therefore desirable to offer carrier or prenatal testing to these groups (e.g., Tay-Sachs disease in Ashkenazi Jews; thalassemia testing for populations of Mediterranean or Asian descent). For disorders with a very high carrier rate in the population (such as hemochromatosis, which has a carrier rate of about 1 in 10 people),[50] cases may appear in succeeding generations, a feature not usually observed for recessive disorders.

Just as with dominant disorders, genetic heterogeneity may occur. For example, a couple, both deaf because of being homozygous for a recessive gene that causes hearing loss, may have normal children if the genetic lesion in one parent is not allelic to that in the other. There is also variability seen in recessive disorders, just as in dominantly inherited disorders. This may be because of molecular heterogeneity—that is, the lesion in the gene is different on the two chromosomes—or because the recessive genes act on different backgrounds of other genes.

In an increasing number of recessive disorders, prenatal detection is now possible. Unfortunately, a particular couple usually does not realize the need for prenatal detection until they have had one affected child; however, they may wish to have the opportunity to avoid having another affected child. In some disorders that cause severe shortness of stature or particular morphological abnormalities, x-ray or ultrasound studies may be diagnostic. In others with a known biochemical defect, enzyme activity or other metabolites can be measured either directly in the amniotic fluid or in cultured fetal cells. In yet others, DNA diagnosis is possible. An enzyme deficiency has already been demonstrated in about a third of the known recessive disorders in humans.[28] Two alternatives that should be mentioned to couples who do not wish to take the 1 in 4 risk of an affected child and for whom prenatal diagnosis is not possible are adoption and gamete donation.

X-linked Recessive Disorders

Some examples of X-linked single-gene disorders are hemophilia and Duchenne's muscular dystrophy. In X-linked recessive disorders, the problem gene is located on the X chromosome. Since females have two Xs, if one is normal, that female will be healthy. Since males only have one X, if this has the X-linked disease gene, the male will be affected. In these families, therefore, females may be healthy, unaffected carriers of the gene, but half of their sons will have the disease. Carrier detection tests for the female relatives of male patients are very important in giving them the option to avoid having affected sons, and prenatal diagnosis is becoming available for an increasing number.

X-linked Dominant Disorders

There are fewer disorders in this category, with some examples being familial (XL) hypophosphatemia with rickets, and Alport's syndrome (hereditary nephropathy and deafness). X-linked dominant disorders occur in females as well as in males, and an affected female transmits the gene to half her daughters and half her sons, whereas an affected male transmits it only to his daughters, all of whom will have the gene. There is no male-to-male transmission.

Mitochondrial Disorders

The mitochondria in human cells have circular chromosomes that contain genes that code for proteins involved in oxidative phosphorylation, providing the cell with energy. Since the mitochondria are cytoplasmic organelles, these are always inherited from the mother. A characteristic of cytoplasmic inheritance is that segregation ratios characteristic of mendelian disorders are not observed, but many offspring in the maternal line are affected. By 1997, 37 mitochondrial loci had been identified.[45] Some clinical entities identified with mitochondrial mutations are Leber's optic atrophy, infantile bilateral striatal neurosis, and Kearns-Sayre syndrome. The situation is complex in that a wide range of abnormality is possible, depending on the numbers of abnormal mitochondria included in the egg and the differential multiplication of these organelles in different tissues.[51] They may explain some errors of development and congenital malformations, as well as later-onset disorders.[52]

Multifactorial Disorders

In this group, interactions between environmental factors and the genes of an individual cause disease in ways only partly understood. Some examples are common congenital malformations such as neural tube defects (spina bifida and anencephaly), congenital dislocated hips, and some adult-onset disorders such as atherosclerosis, hypertension, schizophrenia, and some cancers. It is likely that most chronic diseases of adult onset with a major impact on health care and social systems fall into this group. This is by far the largest category of disease where genetics plays a role; it appears that even by age 25 at least 1 in 20 individuals in the population is affected by multifactorial disorders; over a lifetime probably a much greater number are affected.[19] The situation is not simple, and at the population level a given disease category is likely to consist of individuals who have reached that endpoint by a variety of genetic "routes," some interacting with environmental factors.

It is likely that many individuals with a common disease such as Alzheimer's disease, atherosclerosis, manic depression, or diabetes have a gene that determines whether external influences will result in illness. In the future, the use of DNA markers may give the opportunity to prevent expression of the disease. For example, 1 to 2 percent of the population has a single gene type of hyperlipidemia. These individuals constitute over a quarter of individuals with heart attack at less than 60 years.[37] Such individuals may avoid this by early detection, followed by diet and medication. Since genes underlying predisposition to these "multifactorial" conditions cluster in families, there is an opportunity to identify and pull out of the larger group subsets of individuals (and members of their families) who are identifiable as being at increased risk.

Noninherited "Genetic" Disorders

Individuals who are normal at birth may acquire diseases in which clear genetic abnormalities arise in a particular type of cell. Genes may be damaged or the genome in some cells altered by environmental agents such as radiation, chemicals, or viruses. Examples of such diseases are cancer and acquired immunodeficiency syndrome (AIDS). In the future, it is also possible that many of the changes associated with aging may be found to be acquired genetic changes at the somatic cell level.

▸ THE HUMAN GENE MAP AND GENE SEQUENCING

A detailed knowledge of the structures of genes would open the door to diagnosis and treatment of human genetic disease. A collaborative project—the Human Genome Project[8]—to obtain such knowledge for all human genes, by determining the sequence of the DNA in all 23 different human chromosomes, has been undertaken by human and molecular geneticists worldwide.

Several remarkable technological developments have made it possible to determine the human sequence and to "map" the location of any gene. The first is "molecular cloning," the insertion of a stretch of DNA of interest from one source into another DNA molecule that can reproduce itself independently in special strains of laboratory bacteria. This allows the collection of purified DNA molecules in very large amounts that could not be obtained from their original sources. Another is "DNA sequencing," the ability to determine the order of the bases for any stretch of DNA that has been cloned, and automation of that sequencing.

Several complementary and useful approaches to developing the human gene map include somatic cell hybridization, in situ hybridization, cell sorting, deletion and duplication mapping, linkage development of yeast artificial chromosomes, and sequence scanning.[8] These methods are even more powerful and informative when used in a complementary way.

▸ METHODS USED IN EVALUATING THE ROLE OF GENETICS IN DISEASE

Several levels of questions can be asked about whether genetic determinants contribute to occurrence of a particular disease category or endpoint. Historically, perhaps the first question that has been asked is, "Does a given disease cluster in families?"

Various methods for assessing this question are discussed below. Given that a disease *is* found to show familial clustering, the consequent logical question to ask is whether this is caused by a common environmental exposure or a biologically inherited determinant. The second section will outline several methods that have been used in genetics to elucidate the answer to this. If in fact the disorder is found to be inherited, the next step is to clarify the particular mechanism of inheritance. Several approaches that are used in genetics to evaluate this will be discussed in the third and final section. We have taken an approach similar to that in the very useful detailed review of this topic by King et al.[53]

Evidence for Clustering in Families

Obviously, if a disease is common, it may occur in more than one member of a family simply by chance. Several features, if present, provide evidence that the familial clustering is nonrandom:

1. Healthy individuals who have a family history of the disorder when followed over time develop that condition more often than other comparable individuals without any family history.
2. The relatives of afflicted individuals have a greater frequency of the disorder than comparable control subjects.
3. The relatives of afflicted individuals have a greater frequency of the disorder than is found in the general population.
4. If the trait can be quantitatively measured (e.g., blood pressure), there is a positive correlation between pairs of related individuals.

It is essential that the endpoint or disease being evaluated for familial clustering is as homogeneous as possible. If the disease being evaluated is actually a clinical picture that can be reached in several different ways (some with a genetic determinant, others where an environmental factor is the main determinant), then a very confused picture may result, with some studies finding familial clustering and others not.

There are many common diseases in adults that by the foregoing criteria have been shown to aggregate in families. For example, coronary heart disease shows familial clustering even after all known risk factors have been adjusted for (e.g., smoking, weight, serum lipids, blood pressure, diabetes, behavior pattern). There is also evidence for familial clustering of each of these risk factors.[54] Several birth defects, neurological and behavioral disorders, and cancers also cluster in families by the usual criteria. Identification of this clustering is the first step in untangling the complex web to elucidate the genetic components that determine a disease. Clustering in families may be due not to sharing of genes but to sharing of a common environment or to cultural transmission of disease determinants. Even showing that correlation in the disease frequency is greater the closer the genetic relationship is not sufficient, since shared environmental and cultural factors may also increase as the relationship gets closer.

Methods to Elucidate Cause of Familial Clustering

Usually several methods are used because they are complementary.

Twin Studies

Monozygotic (MZ) twins are genetically identical; they result from the splitting of one fertilized ovum. Dizygotic (DZ) twins are only as genetically alike as any two siblings. This allows comparison of genetically identical and genetically different individuals who are usually raised in a similar environment. It therefore makes possible an estimation of the degree of genetic influence on the disease. It is also possible to look at identical twins reared apart and together to help estimate the effect of environmental factors.

If a disease were completely determined by gene(s), then the concordance rate in MZ twins should be 100 percent and the concordance in DZ twins should be the same as in the other siblings of a proband. Studies in MZ and DZ twins for many common adult disorders show much higher concordance in MZ than in DZ pairs. This is true for schizophrenia, multiple sclerosis, alcoholism, affective disorders, epilepsy, the neuroses, non-insulin–dependent diabetes mellitus, and allergies, clearly demonstrating a genetic contribution. However, the concordance rate in these studies in MZ twins is less than 100 percent, demonstrating that an environmental component is also present. Interestingly, the concordance rate for DZ twins in these studies is often greater than that shown between twin probands and their other siblings, which could reflect a greater similarity in environment of DZ twins compared with other siblings or could reflect some selection bias.

Heritability Studies

Heritability (h^2) in the narrow sense is defined as the contribution of additive genes to the phenotype of interest. It will be the proportion of variance in a population for the trait contributed by additive genes (V_A) compared with the total population variance for the phenotype (V_p).

$$h^2 - \frac{V_A}{V_p}$$

In genetic aspects of human disease this definition of heritability is usually broadened to

$$h^2 - \frac{VG}{V_P}$$

where VG refers to the total genotypic variance including nonadditive interactions, such as dominance or epistasis, between genes. (Epistasis is the synergistic effect of genes at different loci.) Estimates of heritability of a trait relate to the particular conditions under which it is measured. For example, if the environment changes, it is no longer valid. Estimates of heritability have been made for many quantitative human traits. They should be interpreted only as indicators of whether the role of genes is relatively large or small in the population and of the circumstances in which the condition is measured.[55]

Adoption Studies

If individuals are raised by adopting parents, it gives the opportunity to examine given traits or disorders in adopted individuals for resemblance to the biological and the rearing families and thus address the "nature-nurture" issues. This approach has been followed for a number of traits such as blood pressure and for disorders such as schizophrenia[56] and alcoholism.[57]

Path Analysis

Studies of individuals give little information about causal hypotheses but analysis of pairs of relatives are much more informative (e.g., father-son pairs, brother-sister pairs). Path analysis was created by Sewall Wright as an aid in analysis of causation. It is a way of deriving consequences of linear causal assumptions and then testing these assumptions on correlation structures such as pairs of relatives.[58]

Analysis of Familial Common Environmental Exposures

Familial clustering may be due to clustering of culturally transmitted behaviors or family practices that result in particular exposures (e.g., dietary or smoking habits).[59] Kuru, for example, was a disease thought to be genetic but in reality is due to an infection perpetuated by ritual cannibalism. It is likely that diseases such as lung cancer or alcoholism involve cultural inheritance of exposure behavior as well as genetically inherited determinants.

Associations between Genotype and Susceptibility

Humans differ in an identifiable way in their human leukocyte antigen (HLA) system and their ABO blood group systems, thus allowing evaluation of existing genotypes in these systems. Different genotypes within these systems are associated with the occurrence of any one of a variety of diseases. Increasingly, recombinant DNA polymorphisms will be evaluated and correlated with a variety of disease outcomes in the same way. There are now a number of well-documented examples where having a particular identifiable genotype is associated with disease susceptibility (or resistance).

Methods for Determining Mode of Inheritance

Most common diseases that cluster in families do not show simple mendelian inheritance, since they result from an interaction of both genes and environmental factors. A number of methods elucidate the mode of inheritance of the genetic susceptibility.

Multifactorial Model Analysis

The genetic component to determination of a disease with a multifactorial etiology could be equal additive effects of many genes or a few or one gene of large effect. Either model explains why individuals could be put over a threshold in the continuum of liability and thus show disease.

The introduction of methods to detect single genes (HLA typing, DNA polymorphisms, sophisticated statistical pedigree analysis) has in recent years shown that it is likely that one or a very few genes of major effect are involved in the multifactorial pathway.[60] This finding is relevant to diabetes mellitus, rheumatoid arthritis, and some hyperlipidemias. Increasingly there will be opportunities to identify predisposed individuals, and the study of families (particularly those of early onset cases) may give the opportunity to target to clusters of higher-risk individuals. The model where many genes of small effect are relevant (polygenic) may apply to pyloric stenosis.

Segregation Analysis

If a single gene has a major effect on disease susceptibility, it is essential to clarify how it is inherited—autosomal dominant, autosomal recessive, or X-linked. These alternative modes of inheritance give different disease risks for different classes of relatives (e.g., 50 percent of children are affected if dominant, compared with a low risk for the children of an individual with a recessive disorder). By comparing the observed disease incidence in each class with that expected based on alternative genetic models, it is possible to see how well these agree.

Analysis of Maternal Effects

As discussed previously, the DNA of the mitochondria is inherited only from the mother. This means that diseases that appear to affect both males and females but are transmitted only by the mother are candidates for this mechanism of inheritance,[51] and data may be analyzed with this hypothesis in mind.

Linkage Analysis

If segregation analysis shows that inheritance of a single gene may be responsible for disease susceptibility, it is possible to look at whether a wide variety of genetic markers (including DNA polymorphisms) segregate along with the disease susceptibility. Already this approach has indicated that a dominant susceptibility allele may exist in linkage to particular DNA markers in certain families for Alzheimer's disease,[61] manic depression,[62,63] and breast cancer.[64]

Sibling Pair Methods

These are particularly relevant where data on genetic haplotype (usually for the HLA region) is available in siblings. On the hypothesis that there is a disease susceptibility gene close (linked) to the HLA region, this gene should usually be inherited along with a particular haplotype. Thus, siblings who share this HLA haplotype are more likely to have also both inherited the susceptibility allele. This method evaluates coinheritance of HLA haplotype and disease. Siblings who are both affected with the disease would be expected to share the same haplotype more often. With sufficient data on affected sibling pairs, it is possible to evaluate the mode of inheritance of the disease-predisposing allele.[65]

The goal of epidemiology is to understand how diseases are distributed in the population. Most common diseases today are likely due to interaction between the genotype and environmental factors, so that progress will be made by studies that control for one class of these influences while investigating the other.

Genetic methods are increasingly allowing us to identify genetically susceptible individuals. Tools from classic epidemiology can then be profitably used to compare environmental factors in affected and unaffected genetically susceptible individuals. Conversely, the other approach to disentangling the interaction is first to identify those individuals who have the environmental factor present and then compare the unaffected and affected in that group, looking for particular genetic subgroups. The new molecular genetic techniques now allow particular DNA sequences to be evaluated in patients and in control subjects and hold out the hope of more fruitful progress.

▶ SCREENING

Genetic screening may serve several objectives. A program may exist to identify individuals with a particular genotype so they may receive an intervention or treatment. Newborn screening programs are of this category. A program may exist to identify individuals who are at risk of having children affected by a genetic disease. Examples of such programs are Tay-Sachs screening in Ashkenazi Jews and amniocentesis for prenatal karyotyping in women over 35 years of age. A screening program may also exist to gather needed epidemiological information. Useful reviews of this topic are contained in a report of a Workshop on Population Screening[66] and a report of the Office of Technology Assessment.[67]

Newborn Screening Programs

Screening for phenylketonuria, congenital hypothyroidism, and other inborn errors such as galactosemia is widely practiced in the Western world by using a small blood spot obtained by heel stick at a few days of age. Many of these programs are mandated by law, and appropriate resources must be provided to ensure that follow-up study and counseling are available as necessary and also to ensure laboratory quality and accuracy.[68] An abnormal screening test is not diagnostic but is the signal for rapid and appropriate medical and biochemical evaluation as well as parental counseling.

Urine samples taken in the first month of life on filter paper are also used in some screening programs. The compliance rate is high, but the cost effectiveness has been questioned.[69] There is the possibility of adding neuroblastoma testing, which may make it more effective.[70] With the advent of recombinant DNA approaches, a variety of additional screening tests have been suggested, including those for Duchenne's muscular dystrophy, hyperlipidemias, and cystic fibrosis. Some of the ethical and social issues raised by screening programs are discussed later.

Screening in Special Groups

Screening targeted groups is the public health response to the phenomenon of clustering that has a genetic explanation. Testing close relatives of individuals with autosomal recessive disorders may be helpful if such carrier tests are available and accurate. This is especially true for those disorders where the carrier frequency in the population is high. For example, the normal sibling of a patient in the United States with sickle-cell anemia has a two-thirds chance of being a carrier. If two married individuals are found to be carriers of the same recessive gene (e.g., by having an affected child), then they should receive counseling.

Particular genes occur in higher frequency in a number of subgroups. One such gene is that for Tay-Sachs disease in Ashkenazi Jews. Between 1970 and 1980, over 300,000 Jewish adults were voluntarily screened.[71] Screening for carrier detection for cystic fibrosis, now that the gene has been located,[72] is likely to develop rapidly. This disorder is common (1 in 2,000 to 2,500 births) in individuals of northern European extraction. Thalassemia screening is offered to people from southeast Asia and China, since the frequency of this gene is similar to that of the cystic fibrosis gene in northern Europeans. Populations of Mediterranean origin may be screened for β-thalassemia.[73]

▶ PRENATAL DIAGNOSIS

Prenatal diagnostic techniques are used to diagnose genetic disorders and birth defects that result in marked disability or death early in life. Although usually the option that it permits is termination of the affected fetus, in a few disorders diagnosis permits therapy in utero or special management during pregnancy and delivery to minimize further damage to a vulnerable infant. For example, for a fetus with methylmalonic acidemia, the mother will be given vitamin B_{12}; for a galactosemic infant, the mother may receive a low-galactose diet.

There are a number of indications for prenatal diagnosis, and the test that is done prenatally is targeted specifically to the indication for prenatal testing. For example, a mother with a previous child with Tay-Sachs disease will have hexosaminidase A measured in the amniotic fluid sample, whereas a woman who is at risk because of increased age will have chromosome analysis of the fetal cells obtained at sampling. Because some disorders are common and inexpensive to test for once a sample is obtained, they are done on any pregnant woman who is already being subject to sampling. For example, α-fetoprotein in the amniotic fluid sample is usually measured regardless of the indication. Several indications for prenatal screening are discussed below.

Increased Maternal Age

As maternal age increases, so does the risk of Down syndrome,[74] and this is also true for the other trisomies. For this reason many jurisdictions offer prenatal diagnosis to pregnant women 35 years and over. Such testing can decrease the birth incidence of Down syndrome by approximately 25 percent in most North American populations.[75]

Neural Tube Defects

These birth defects, anencephaly and spina bifida, are relatively common, occurring in approximately 1 in 700 births in many North American populations.[76] Once a couple has had an affected child, the recurrence risk in subsequent pregnancies is about 2 percent.[77] Other close relatives may be at increased risk.[78]

Family History of Specific Disorders

A previous child may have had a mendelian disorder, chromosome anomaly, or birth defect. Also, the family history may indicate that the woman may be a carrier for an X-linked disorder. If a test is available (biochemical, cytogenetic, or DNA) or it is possible to evaluate for abnormal morphological findings (e.g., short limbs), then this testing is offered. For example, maternal exposure to a known teratogen (e.g., valproic acid) or a maternal disorder (diabetes mellitus) may justify offering prenatal diagnosis in some cases.

▶ GENETIC SERVICES

Genetic services, both diagnosis and counseling, are offered only to those who have been identified as in need, by their physicians or by themselves. There are two main avenues for service receipt: by having had an individual in the family with a genetic disorder or being identified as "at risk" by a population screening program.

Genetic service programs usually have arisen in association with a university or teaching hospital, fostering a research-service interaction. All provinces and states have at least one center, often many. However, the availability and expertise differs from one region to another. There is a useful directory of such programs published by the March of Dimes Birth Defects Foundation.[79] Many university centers also have associated training programs.[80]

The process of genetic consultation and counseling is complex and time-consuming and has not yet been well integrated into the clinical practice of medicine. Funding mechanisms for provision of this service are not satisfactory in many jurisdictions and differ from place to place, having grown in an "ad hoc" fashion. If the rapidly escalating new insights into human diseases being made in genetics are to be brought to practical use, we will need a cadre of trained individuals to deliver these services in the coming decades. Already it is not possible to offer on a population level many beneficial genetic programs (e.g., DNA diagnosis for a variety of mendelian disorders).[13]

An important principle in genetic medicine is the need for diagnostic accuracy and precision. Genetic heterogeneity is a complicating issue in many disorders. Accuracy of diagnosis may be especially difficult to achieve in the sporadic case, when the possibilities of new dominant mutations or phenocopies exist. Paternity is an issue that must be borne in mind, since in a significant proportion of cases (which will differ with the particular population) the husband cannot be assumed to be the father. This needs sensitive and empathetic handling. If the genetic mechanism leading to the particular condition diagnosed is known, it is possible to quantitate risk precisely for different relatives. If the genetic mechanism is not clear, as is the case for many "multifactorial" conditions (e.g., congenital malformations, mental retardation, schizophrenia), then if a thorough evaluation of the family history, pregnancy history, medical history, and physical findings reveals no specific etiology, empirical risk figures can be given regarding recurrence risk. These should be employed with caution, and communication of their meaning and limitations is not a simple process.

▶ OPPORTUNITY AND DANGER: SOME SOCIAL AND ETHICAL IMPLICATIONS

We have known for a long time that many common diseases are familial, but the genetic aspects have been ill-defined. It is clear that most common diseases are genetically heterogeneous, but susceptibility is due to major genes in many cases. Genotypes relatively unusual in the population may come to make up a large proportion of those with common diseases. Individuals at risk may soon be identified by DNA testing for intervention, and there may be ample time to intervene. For example, the immunological process in diabetes can precede onset of symptoms by many years; carcinogenesis also takes many years. The phenotype of disease, what we observe clinically, is somewhat removed from the primary action of the particular gene. This means that there may be considerable modulation possible. Rather than ignore the internal genetic component of disease causation, we should evaluate the genetic input and then attempt to tailor preventive or therapeutic programs to take it into account. If the new molecular genetic capability is incorporated into health care planning, it could allow public health to enter a new era of prevention. Through this new technology, rather than exposing the whole population to the same preventive medical programs, they could be directed to those individuals at risk, with relevant health messages focused to particular individuals.

The path to planning how the new capabilities in genetic risk identification might best be used in prevention and treatment is not simple. Although it has the potential to better the human condition, it is essential that enthusiasm for this approach be tempered with the realization that it is possible to cause great harm because we have not carefully weighed the pitfalls, ramifications, and dangers of this approach.[81,82] Well-designed research projects should be undertaken before there is any implementation at the population level.[83] These should address aspects such as psychological and family impact, confidentiality, long-term outcome, compliance, safety, cost benefits, and appropriate laboratory quality control procedures. It is also important that genetic risk identification not be offered before the personnel and facilities to provide appropriate counseling and follow-up study are identified and funded.

The new capabilities raise many questions that will require scrutiny, relating, for example, to ownership of the information on genetic makeup.[84] With regard to confidentiality, policies and procedures must be put in place on who should have access to genetic test results so that the values of personal privacy and autonomy are respected. There may be potential situations where the public good may override the value of personal confidentiality, but these must be thoroughly considered before inclusion in policy.

As we become able to identify individuals in whom the disease outcome is less clear because of unpredictable gene-environment interactions, we may need guidelines to evaluate whether such programs should be offered. We might cause harm by identifying individuals as having a genetic vulnerability. Much of illness is perception and attitude, and it is important to avoid harm by causing identified individuals to view themselves as ill. In addition to stringent guidelines regarding data confidentiality, policies to avoid possible discrimination against identified individuals are also needed.

All of us are genetically unique, and all of us have weaknesses and strengths. This realization has the potential to break down the current generally held perception of the distinction between the majority "normal" population and the small minority with "genetic diseases." A better perception—that everyone is vulnerable in his or her own way—would weaken or remove any basis for stigmatization of those with "genetic diseases." However, genetic identification could also be negative if it created a population each of whose members was aware of and continuously concerned about a particular genetic predisposition and the likelihood of becoming ill.

Some specific issues of legal and social consequence raised by DNA testing are discussed below. DNA testing can identify each individual (except for identical twins) uniquely. It can also be used to identify genetic relationships with unprecedented accuracy. These new abilities raise issues in several areas.

Paternity

The paternity tests that were previously available could disprove paternity when a child had a genetic factor that wasn't present either in the mother or in the putative father. It could not usually prove that a particular man was the father. The new DNA testing can achieve levels of probability that establish beyond any reasonable doubt (1 in 100 million) the real father, if the tests are of high quality. This has been accepted as evidence in a number of courts. At the same time it means that quality control of laboratory tests and procedures to safeguard against human error, such as mislabeled samples, are also necessary.

Immigration

In Great Britain, as in some other countries, resident immigrants can ask for resident status for certain relatives. DNA fingerprinting has been used to test if a claimed relationship is true.

Forensic Identification

DNA fingerprinting may be used to identify with great certainty whether a tissue sample found at the scene of a crime belongs to a particular suspect. DNA fingerprinting seems to provide evidence that is acceptable to British courts of law. In the United States, DNA data have been considered as evidence in criminal, rape, and murder trials in most states.[85] DNA testing for forensic purposes will probably increase markedly over the next decade.[86,87]

Workplace Testing

DNA testing can also be used to identify persons at risk in situations where costs may be incurred, for example, by an employer or an insurance carrier. DNA testing could show predisposition to cancer, emphysema, hemolysis, ischemic artery disease, hypertension, and so on with implications for both the employer's cost and the insurance carrier's profits. For many U.S. companies, offering health benefits adds substantially to the costs of production, and this added cost is becoming important in an increasingly competitive global market. Employers may therefore wish to screen potential employees so that their medical and life insurance plan costs will be lower. Appropriate safeguards against discrimination and misuse must be put in place.

Individuals differ in the metabolic machinery they have inherited for dealing with chemicals in the home and work environments. Some individuals have genes that make them less able to handle particular pollutants, so that they are more likely to develop lung disease or other problems after exposure. This could mean that those individuals genetically vulnerable to particular exposures may be refused employment. Another danger is that a strategy of employing only "resistant" individuals may allow industries to relax expensive environmental controls.

Insurance

Laws may be needed to address how the new genetic knowledge should be limited in its application by the insurance industry as well as by employers. Guidelines or legislation may be required for medical and life insurance companies concerning genetic testing before coverage. It is possible that insurance companies could require testing before coverage and then charge higher premiums or refuse coverage to those at higher risk because of their genotype. Because the principle of insurance is to spread risk over many individuals, it seems unjust to disadvantage individuals who through no fault of their own are likely to become ill. This is not as dramatic a problem in Canada, which has a universal health care system, but it could be a very important problem in the United States. If the U.S. insurance industry is not regulated in this regard in some way, it may be necessary for government to set aside funding for health care of such noninsurable individuals.

▶ SUMMARY AND CONCLUSIONS

It is evident that the new DNA technology will affect many areas of our society and will pose often difficult choices. It presents an opportunity and a useful tool if it is used wisely and humanely, but it is also a danger if the implications for social justice of its use are not thought through. Screening programs, in particular, if applied prematurely may cause harm and waste resources. However, if done well and with fully informed communication, they could decrease disease and better the human condition. The new DNA technology opens up questions that have wide-ranging social, ethical, and legal ramifications. Our new abilities with the technology often highlight the difficulty of balancing the individual's and the group's rights.[88,89] These issues require ongoing discussion by scientists, public health practitioners, lawyers, politicians, and the public.[90,91]

▶ REFERENCES

1. Rose G: Sick individuals and sick populations. Int J Epidemiol 14:32–35, 1985
2. Gori GB, Richter BJ: Macroeconomics of disease. Prevention in the United States. Science 200:1124–1130, 1978
3. Canada Department of National Health and Welfare: A New Perspective on the Health of Canadians: A Working Document. Ottawa: Canada Department of National Health and Welfare, 1974
4. Murphy EA, Pyeritz RE: Homeostasis VII. A conspectus. Am J Med Genet 24:745–751, 1986
5. Mendel G: Experiments in plant hybridization. In Peters JA (ed): Classic Papers in Genetics. New York: Prentice-Hall, 1959
6. O'Brien SJ: On estimating functional gene number in eukaryotes. Nature 242:52–54, 1973
7. Bishop JO: The gene numbers game. Cell 2:81–95, 1974
8. Cutter MAG, Drexler E, McCullough LB, McInerney JD, Murray JC, Rossiter B, Zola J: Mapping and sequencing the human genome: science, ethics, and public policy. Chicago: BSCS, Colorado, and the American Medical Association, 1992
9. Hardy GH: Mendelian proportions in a mixed population. Science 28:49–50, 1908
10. Weinberg W: Uber den Nachweis der Venerbungbeim Menschen jahreshefte des Vereins fur Vaterlandische. Naturkunde in Wurttenberg 64:368–382, 1908
11. Neel JV, Satoh C, Goriki K, Asakawa J, Fujita M, Takahashi N, Kageska T, Hazama R: Search for mutations altering protein charge and/or function in children of atomic bomb survivors: final report. Am J Hum Genet 42:663–676, 1988
12. Stoll C, Roth MP, Bigel P: A reexamination of parental age effect on the occurrence of new mutations dysplasias. In Papdatos CJ, Bartsocas CS (eds): Skeletal Dysplasias. New York: Alan R. Liss, 1982, pp 419–426
13. Riccardi VH, Dobson CE II, Chakraborty R, Bontke C: The pathophysiology of neurofibromatosis. IX. Paternal age as a factor in the origin of new mutations. Am J Med Genet 18:169–176, 1984
14. Alison AC: Notes on sickle-cell polymorphism. Ann Hum Genet 19:39, 1954
15. Petersen GM, Rotter JI, Cantor RM, Field LL, Greenwald S, Lim JST, Roy C, Schoenfeld V, Lowden JA, Kaback MM: The Tay-Sachs disease gene in North American Jewish populations: geographic variations and origin. Am J Hum Genet 35:1258–1269, 1983
16. Scriver CR: New experiences: Old genes—lessons from the Mennonites [Editorial]. Clin Invest Med 12:142–143, 1989
17. Francke U, Felsenstein J, Gartler SM, Migeon BR, Dancis J, Seegmiller JE, Bakay F, Nyhan WL: The occurrence of new mutants in the X-linked recessive Lesch-Nyhan disease. Am J Hum Genet 28:123–137, 1976
18. Neel JV: Should editorials be peer-reviewed? Am J Hum Genet 43:981–982, 1988
19. Baird PA, Anderson TW, Newcombe HB, Lowry RB: Genetic disorders in children and young adults. Am J Hum Genet 42:677–693, 1988

20. Baird PA: Measuring birth defects and handicapping disorders in the population: the British Columbia Health Surveillance Registry. Can Med Assoc J 136:109–111, 1987
21. Opitz JM: Study of the malformed fetus and infant. Pediatr Rev 3:57–64, 1981
22. Carr DH: Detection and evaluation of pregnancy wastage. In Wilson JG, Fraser FC (eds): Handbook of Teratology, New York: Plenum Press, 1977, vol. 3, pp 189–213
23. Neal JL, Saginur R, Clow A, Scriver CR: The frequency of genetic disease and congenital malformations among patients in a pediatric hospital. Can Med Assoc J 108:1111–1115, 1973
24. Day N, Holmes LB: The incidence of genetic disease in a university hospital population. Am J Hum Genet 25:237–246, 1973
25. Hall JE, Powers EK, McIlvaine RT, Ean VH: The frequency of familial burden of genetic disease in a pediatric hospital. Am J Med Genet 1:417–436, 1978
26. Kaback MM: Medical genetics. An overview. Pediatr Clin North Am 25:395–409, 1978
27. Scriver CR, Tenenhouse HJ: On the heritability of rickets, a common disease. (Mendel, mammals and phosphate). Johns Hopkins Med J 149:179–187, 1981
28. McKusick VA: Mendelian Inheritance in Man. Catalogues of Autosomal Dominant, Autosomal Recessive, and X-Linked Phenotypes. 8th ed. Baltimore: Johns Hopkins University Press, 1988
29. UNSCEAR Report: Genetic and somatic effects of ionizing radiation. New York: United Nations, 1986
30. Childs B, Scriver CR: Age at onset and causes of disease. Perspect Biol Med 29(3):437–460, 1986
31. Costa T, Scriver CR, Childs B: The effect of mendelian disease on human health: a measurement. Am J Med Genet 21:231–242, 1985
32. Hayes A, Costa T, Scriver CR, Childs B: The impact of mendelian disease in man. Effect of treatment: a measurement. Am J Med Genet 21:243–255, 1985
33. Schinzel A: Catalogue of Unbalanced Chromosome Aberrations in Man. Berlin: Walter de Gruyter, 1984
34. DeGrouchy J, Turleau C: Clinical Atlas of Human Chromosomes, 2nd ed. New York: John Wiley & Sons, 1984
35. Clendenin TM, Benirschke K: Chromosome studies on spontaneous abortions. Lab Invest 12:1281–1291, 1963
36. Hook E: Human teratogenic and mutagenic markers in monitoring about point sources of pollution. Environ Res 25:178–203, 1981
37. Vogel F, Motulsky A: Human Genetics: Problems and Approaches. 2nd ed. Berlin: Springer-Verlag, 1986
38. Trimble BK, Baird PA: Maternal age and Down syndrome. Age-specific incidence rates by single year intervals. Am J Med Genet 2:1–5, 1978
39. Baird PA, Sadovnick AD: Maternal age-specific rates for Down syndrome: changes over time. Am J Med Genet 29:917–927, 1988
40. Baird PA, Sadovnick AD: Life expectancy in Down syndrome. J Pediatr 110:849–854, 1987
41. Baird PA, Sadovnick AD: Life expectancy in Down syndrome adults. Lancet 2:1354–1356, 1988
42. Turner HH: A syndrome of infantilism, congenital webbed neck and arbitus valgus. Endocrinology 25:566, 1938
43. Ford CE, Miller OJ, Polari PE, Almeida JC, de Briggs JH: A sex chromosome anomaly in a case of gonadal dysgenesis (Turner's syndrome). Lancet 1:886, 1959
44. Witkin HA, Sarnoff AM, Schulsinger F, Bakkestrom E, Christiansen KO, Goodenough DR, Hirschhorn K, Lundsteen C, Owen DR, Pilip J, Rubin DB, Stocking M: Criminality in XYY and XXY men. Science 193:547–555, 1976
45. Online Mendelian Inheritance in Man, OMIM™. Bethesda, MD: Center for Medical Genetics, Johns Hopkins University and National Center for Biotechnology Information, National Library of Medicine, 1996. World Wide Web URL: http://www3.ncbi.nlm.gov/omim/
46. Monk M: Genomic imprinting: memories of mother and father. Nature 328:203–204, 1987
47. Reik W: Genomic imprinting and genetic disorders in man. Trends Genet 3:331–336, 1989
48. Hall JG: Genomic imprinting: review and relevance to human diseases. Am J Hum Genet 46:857–873, 1990
49. Nicholls RD: New insights reveal complex mechanisms involved in genomic imprinting. Am J Hum Genet 54:733–740, 1994
50. Bothwell TH, Charlton RW, Motulsky AG: Idiopathic hemochromatosis. In Stanbury JB, Wyngoarden JB, Fredrickson DS, Goldstein JL, Brown MS (eds): The Metabolic Cases of Inherited Disease, 5th ed. New York: McGraw-Hill, 1983, pp 1269–1298
51. Wallace DC: Mitochondrial DNA mutations and neuromuscular disease. Trends Genet 5:9–13, 1989
52. Wallace DC: Mitochondrial DNA variation in human evolution, degenerative disease, and aging. Am J Hum Genet 57:201–223, 1995
53. King MC, Lee GM, Spinner NB, Thomson G, Wrensch MR: Genetic epidemiology. Annu Rev Public Health 5:1–52, 1984
54. Neufeld HN, Goldbourt U: Coronary heart disease: genetic aspects. Circulation 67:643–654, 1983
55. Cavalli-Sforza LL, Bodmer WF: The Genetics of Human Populations. San Francisco: WH Freeman, 1971
56. Kety SS, Rosenthal D, Wedner PH, Schulsinger F: Studies based on a total sample of adopted individuals and their relatives: why they were necessary, what they demonstrated and failed to demonstrate. Schizophr Bull 2:413–428, 1976
57. Goodwin DW: Genetic component of alcoholism. Annu Rev Med 32:93–99, 1981
58. Rao DC, Morton NE, Gottesman II, Lew R: Path analysis of qualitative data on pairs of relatives. Application to schizophrenia. Hum Hered 31:325–333, 1981
59. Cavalli-Sforza LL, Feldman MW, Chen KH, Dornbusch SM: Theory and observation in cultural transmission. Science 218:19–27, 1982
60. Motulsky AG: Approaches to the genetics of common disease. In Rotter JI, Samloff IM, Rimoin DL (eds): The Genetics and Heterogeneity of Common Gastrointestinal Disorders. New York: Academic Press, 1980, pp 3–10
61. St. George-Hyslop PH, Tanzi RE, Polinsky RJ, Haines JL, Nee L, Watkins PC, Myers CH, Feldman RB et al: The genetic defect causing familial Alzheimer's disease maps on chromosome 21. Science 235:885–890, 1987
62. Egeland JA, Gerhard DS, Pauls DL, Sussex JN, Kidd KK, Allen CR, Hustetter AM, Housman DE: Bipolar affective disorders linked to DNA markers on chromosome 11. Nature 325:783–787, 1987
63. Hodgkinson S, Sherrington R, Gurling H, Marchbanks R, Reeders S, Mallet J, McInnis M, Petursson H, Brynjolfsson J: Molecular genetic evidence for heterogeneity in manic depression. Nature 325: 805–806, 1987
64. King MC, Go RC, Lynch HT, Elston RC, Terasaki PI, Petrakis NL, Rodgers GC, Lattanzio D, Baily-Wilson J: Genetic epidemiology of breast cancer and associated cancers in high-risk families. II. Linkage analysis. J Natl Cancer Inst 71:463–467, 1983
65. Thomson G: A review of theoretical aspects of HLA and disease associations. Theor Pop Biol 20:168–201, 1981
66. Scriver CR: Population screening: report of a workshop. Progr Clin Biol Res 163B:89–152, 1985
67. US Congress Office of Technology Assessment: Cystic fibrosis and DNA testing: Implications of carrier screening OTA-BA-532. Washington, DC: Government Printing Office, 1992
68. Scriver CR, Holtzman NA, Howell RR, Mamunes P, Nadler HL: Committee on Genetics: New issues in newborn screening for phenylketonuria and congenital hypothyroidism. Pediatrics 69:104–106, 1982
69. Wilcken B, Smith A, Brown DA: Urine screening for aminocidopathies: is it beneficial? J Pediatr 97:492–497, 1980

70. Lemieux B, Avray-Blais C, Giguere R, Shapcott D, Scriver CR: Newborn urine screening experience with over one million infants in Quebec Network of Genetic Medicine. J Inher Metab Dis 2:45–55, 1988
71. Kaback MM: Heterozygote screening. In Emery AH, Remoin DL (eds): Principles and Practice of Medical Genetics, New York: Churchill Livingstone, 1983, vol. 2, pp 1451–1457
72. Kerem B, Rommens JM, Buchanan JA, Markiewicz D, Cox TA, Chakravarti A, Buchwald M, Tsui LC: Identification of the cystic fibrosis gene: genetic analysis. Science 245:1073–1080, 1989
73. Mitchell JJ, Capua A, Clow C, Scriver CR: Twenty-year outcome analysis of genetic screening programs for Tay-Sachs and β-thalassemia disease carriers in high schools. Am J Hum Genet 59:793–798, 1996
74. Trimble BK, Baird PA: Maternal age and Down syndrome. Age-specific rates by single year intervals. Am J Med Genet 2:1–5, 1978
75. Sadovnick AD, Baird PA: The impact of prenatal chromosomal diagnosis offered to older gravidas in the population incidence of severe mental retardation. Am J Obstet Gynecol 143:486–487, 1982
76. Trimble BK, Baird PA: Congenital anomalies of the central nervous system. Incidence in British Columbia, 1952–72. Teratology 17: 43–49, 1978
77. McBride M: Sib risks of anencephaly and spina bifida in British Columbia. Am J Med Genet 3:377–387, 1979
78. Sadovnick AD, Baird PA: A cost-benefit analysis of prenatal diagnosis for neural tube defects selectively offered to relatives of index cases. Am J Med Genet 12:63–73, 1982
79. Paul NW (ed): International Directory of Genetic Services. 9th ed. New York: March of Dimes Birth Defects Foundation, 1990
80. American Society of Human Genetics: Guide to North American Graduate and Postgraduate Training Programs in Human Genetics. Bethesda, MD: American Society of Human Genetics, 1994
81. Andrews LB, Fullarton JE, Holtzman MA, Motulsky AG (eds): Assessing Genetic Risks: Implications for Health and Social Policy. Washington, DC: National Academy Press, 1994
82. Kitcher P: The Lives to Come: The Genetic Revolution and Human Possibilities. New York: Simon & Schuster, 1996
83. Baird PA: Opportunity and danger: Medical, ethical and social implications of early DNA screening for identification of genetic risk of common adult onset disorders. In Knoppers BM, Laberge CM (eds): Genetic Screening: From Newborns to DNA Typing. New York: Elsevier Science Publishers B. V. (Biomedical Division), 1990, pp 279–288
84. Baird PA: Identifying people's genes: ethical aspects of DNA sampling in populations. Perspect Biol Med 38(2):159–166, 1995
85. Barinaga M: Pitfalls come to light. Science 339:89, 1989
86. Housman DE: DNA on trial—the molecular basis of DNA fingerprinting. N Engl J Med 332(8):534–535, 1995
87. McEwen JE: Forensic DNA data banking by state crime laboratories. Am J Hum Genet 56:1487–1492, 1995
88. Proceed with Care: Final Report of the Royal Commission on New Reproductive Technologies. Ottawa: Canada Communications Group-Publishing, 1993
89. Baird PA: Proceed with Care: new reproductive technologies and the need for boundaries. J Asst Reprod Genet 12(8):491–498, 1995
90. Knoppers BM, Chadwick R: The Human Genome Project: under an international ethical microscope. Science 265:2035–2036, 1994
91. Baird PA: Ethical issues of fertility and reproduction. Annu Rev Med 47:107–116, 1996

64

Nutrition in Public Health and Preventive Medicine

Marion Nestle

The role of nutrition in public health and preventive medicine is self-evident: people must eat to live. Both inadequate and excessive food intake lead to adverse health consequences and contribute to major causes of morbidity and mortality in industrialized as well as developing nations. Because all individuals consume food and, therefore, are interested in diet, nutrition is an unusually accessible entry point into health education and service intervention programs. Because food intake is determined not only by individual choice but also by cultural norms, socioeconomic variables, and agricultural policies, public health approaches to dietary intervention are especially useful and desirable.

This chapter discusses diet and nutrition within the broad context of public health. It describes the health impact of dietary intake both below and above recommended levels of energy and essential nutrients. It reviews current guidelines for patterns of food intake that best meet nutritional requirements, improve nutritional status, and promote health in the population. Finally, it suggests public health strategies to address behavioral and environmental barriers to consumption of healthful diets by individuals and populations.

▸ DIETARY REQUIREMENTS AND ALLOWANCES

People require a continuous supply of external food sources of energy and essential nutrients to maintain life, to grow, and to reproduce.[1,2] By definition, essential nutrients are those that cannot be synthesized in adequate amounts by the body; their dietary or metabolically induced deficiency causes recognizable symptoms that disappear when the nutrients are replaced. The list of nutrients essential or otherwise useful to human physiology is long, complex, and almost certainly incomplete. It includes the more than 40 distinct substances listed in Table 64-1: sources of energy, amino acids, fatty acids, vitamins, minerals, trace elements, fiber, and water. As indicated in the table, other nutrients also may be required under certain conditions.

Malnutrition refers to excessive and unbalanced—as well as deficient—intake of essential nutrients. Fat-soluble vitamins and virtually all of the mineral elements cause disease symptoms when consumed or absorbed in excess. The adverse effects of overconsumption of energy, fat, cholesterol, sodium, sugar, and alcohol are important public health concerns. For each nutrient, a certain range of intake meets physiologic requirements but does not induce harmful symptoms.[3]

Optimal levels of intake of specific nutrients, however, can only be estimated. Individuals vary in nutrient requirements, and research on human nutritional requirements is incomplete. In the United States, estimates of levels of nutrient intake "adequate to meet the known nutritional needs of practically all healthy persons" have been published at approximately 5-year intervals by the National Research Council as Recommended Dietary Allowances (RDAs).[4] The 1989 edition of this report recommended intake levels for protein, 11 vitamins, and seven minerals according to age, body size, gender, and developmental stage. The report also presented estimates of "safe and adequate" intake ranges for seven additional nutrients for which research is too limited to define an RDA. Allowances for energy, however, reflected average needs of individuals of varying heights and weights, ages, and activity levels. These levels were similar to dietary standards for other industrialized countries but typically exceed those for populations of developing nations.[1]

Because RDAs were used to assess dietary adequacy, interpret dietary analyses, establish levels of food assistance, evaluate the nutritional status of individuals and populations, label food products, and develop nutrition counseling guidelines, their limitations required careful attention. In the United States, RDAs were established at levels that exceed the requirements of 97 percent of the population; most individuals can meet nutrient requirements at lower levels of intake. Because RDAs were established at levels that will prevent deficiencies, they did not address issues of overconsumption. This omission led to difficulties in translating RDA standards into universally applicable diet plans, and was the impetus for developing new standards, Dietary Reference Intakes (DRIs), that also encompass nutrient excesses. DRIs have been issued for four minerals and one vitamin.[5]

▸ NUTRITIONAL DEFICIENCIES: CAUSES AND CONSEQUENCES

Inadequate dietary intake is only one cause of nutrient deficiency. Symptoms also result from conditions that interfere with appetite; impair nutrient digestion, absorption, or metabolism; or substantially increase nutrient requirements or losses. Deficiencies may appear clinically as starvation, protein-energy malnutrition, syndromes of deficiency of single nutrients (e.g., pellagra, scurvy, iron-deficiency anemia), or as a wide range of less specific symptoms.[1,2]

The number of people throughout the world who suffer from nutritional deficiencies can only be estimated. Some economists believe that approximately 800 million people are chronically undernourished, a figure representing 20 percent of the developing world's population (range: 12 percent in the Near East to 33 percent in Africa). Such figures, based on a food supply cut point of 2,300 kcal/day, do not include estimates from industrialized nations.[6] Widespread nutritional deficiencies most often occur when income, education, and housing are inadequate and where water supplies are contaminated

TABLE 64-1. DIETARY COMPONENTS GENERALLY CONSIDERED TO BE ESSENTIAL OR BENEFICIAL FOR HUMAN HEALTH

Category	Specific Examples
Energy sources	Carbohydrate, fat, protein, alcohol[a]
Essential amino acids	Isoleucine, leucine, lysine, methionine, phenylalanine, threonine, tryptophan, valine, histidine[b]
Essential fatty acids	Linoleic acid, linolenic acid[c]
Vitamins	
Water-soluble	Ascorbic acid, biotin,[d] cobalamin, folacin, niacin, pantothenic acid, pyridoxine, riboflavin, thiamin
Fat-soluble	Vitamin A,[e] vitamin D,[f] vitamin E, and vitamin K[d]
Minerals	Calcium, chloride, magnesium, phosphate, potassium, sodium
Trace elements	Chromium, cobalt,[g] copper, fluoride, iodine, iron, manganese, molybdenum, selenium, zinc[h]
Fiber[i]	
Water	

NOTE: See References 1 and 2.
[a] Carbohydrates (starches and sugars), proteins, fat, and alcohol contribute about 4, 4, 9, and 7 kcal/g, respectively.
[b] Essential for infants; adult requirement uncertain; arginine, taurine, ornithine, and carnitine may also be required under certain circumstances.
[c] Other fatty acids in the ω-3 series may have essential functions.
[d] Synthesized by intestinal microorganisms; dietary requirement uncertain.
[e] Includes β-carotene.
[f] Mainly synthesized from the action of sunlight on precursors of the vitamin in skin.
[g] Incorporated as part of cobalamin.
[h] Arsenic, boron, nickel, silicon, tin, and vanadium are required by certain animal species, but human requirements are uncertain.
[i] Evidence supports health benefits, but no specific requirement has been determined.

with infectious organisms that induce diarrheal diseases.[7] In such situations, more than one-half of children under the age of 5 years may suffer from some degree of malnutrition.[8] These problems are direct consequences of poverty. Except in the very poorest countries, food production is adequate to meet energy requirements, but the segments of the population most in need are not able to purchase or use foods appropriately.

In industrialized countries, dietary deficiencies are less prevalent. Hunger, as defined by inadequate access to food assistance, has been reported to affect 20 million children and adults in the United States, and numerous surveys have identified nutrient intakes below RDAs among poverty groups.[9] Such findings, however, are accompanied only rarely by clinical signs of nutrient deficiencies. When clinical signs do occur, they are usually associated with the additional nutritional requirements of pregnancy, infancy, early childhood, or aging; the toxic effects of alcohol or drug abuse; or illness, injury, or hospitalization.[1,2]

Regardless of cause, inadequate dietary intake profoundly affects human function. It induces: rapid and severe losses of body weight and electrolytes, decreases in blood pressure and metabolic rate, electrocardiogram abnormalities, losses in muscle strength and stamina, and gastrointestinal and behavioral changes.[1] The result is a generalized lack of vigor, alertness, and vitality that reduces productivity and impairs the ability of people to escape the consequences of poverty. Of special concern is the loss of immune function that accompanies starvation. Malnourished individuals lose cellular immune competence and demonstrate poor resistance to infectious disease. Infections, in turn, increase nutrient losses and requirements, and, in the absence of adequate nutrient intake, induce further malnutrition. This cycle is the principal cause of death among young children in developing countries and is an important cause of morbidity in malnourished children and adults everywhere.[10]

Protein-energy malnutrition is the collective term for the clinical effects of this cycle on young children. Survivors display typical effects of starvation: depression, apathy, irritability, and growth retardation. Protein-energy malnutrition usually is classified into two entities—kwashiorkor and marasmus—on the basis of clinical signs and on the relative intake of protein to energy. Kwashiorkor is characterized by edema and fatty infiltration of the liver and is associated with a relative deficit of protein to energy. Marasmus is manifested as generalized wasting due to overall nutritional deprivation. In practice, such distinctions blur. Undernourished children exhibit symptoms that fall between the two extremes and similar diets contribute to either form.[1,11]

Numerous methods to prevent poverty-associated malnutrition in adults and children by improving household food security have been demonstrated to be effective in developing countries. Among them are programs that redistribute income, subsidize food prices, promote agricultural production, provide food supplements, and educate. Improvements in sanitation and in primary health care are also essential components of programs to reduce nutritional deficiencies.[12]

► DIET AND CHRONIC DISEASE

As nutritional deficiencies decline in prevalence in industrialized as well as developing countries, they are replaced rapidly by chronic conditions of dietary excess and imbalance. In the late 1980s, three comprehensive reports reviewed the entire spectrum of evidence linking diet to chronic diseases and estimated the incidence and prevalence, cost to society, and overall public health impact of these conditions in the United States and Europe.[13–15] In today's rapidly changing sociopolitical environment, populations in developing countries also exhibit rising rates of chronic diseases, but these are superimposed on classic patterns of malnutrition.[16]

In the United States, five of the 10 leading causes of death—coronary heart disease, cancer, stroke, diabetes, and liver cirrhosis—are chronic diseases related in part to diets containing excessive energy, fat, saturated fat, cholesterol, salt, or alcohol, and too little fiber[17] or too sedentary a lifestyle.[18] Diet-related conditions account for about two-thirds of the more than 2 million annual deaths.[19] When data from 32 European countries are considered together, more than half the annual deaths are due to cardiovascular and cerebrovascular diseases, cancers, and digestive diseases related in part to diet.[20] Table 64-2 lists dietary factors associated with the principal chronic diseases. Dietary factors, singly or in combination with physical activity, also affect risks for hypertension, obesity, dental diseases, osteoporosis, and renal and other diseases.[1,2]

Although the proportion of disease prevalence attributable to diet and activity patterns can only be estimated, it is certainly significant. Early estimates suggested that 30 percent of cancer incidence (range: 10 to 70 percent) was due to dietary factors and another 3 percent to alcohol,[21] with similar percentages suggested for coronary heart disease.[22] A more recent and conservative analysis argues that inappropriate patterns of diet, activity, and alcohol use account for 400,000 (or 19 percent) of annual deaths in the United States.[23]

Uncertainties in such estimates are due to difficulties in the design, conduct, and evaluation of research on diet and disease. Nutrition research is complicated by individual variations in dietary requirements, limitations in the ability of investigators to obtain accurate information about the dietary intake of individuals or populations, and by other endlessly debated methodologic issues.[24] Dietary changes over time are especially difficult to estimate.[25] Proof of dietary causality is exceedingly difficult to demonstrate for diseases affected by so many other genetic, environmental, and behavioral risk factors.

TABLE 64-2. DIETARY FACTORS ASSOCIATED DIRECTLY OR INDIRECTLY WITH INCREASED CHRONIC DISEASE RISK[a]

	Dietary Factor				
Leading Cause of Death	***Excess Energy (kcal)***	***Excess Fat***	***Inadequate Fiber***	***Excess Sodium***	***Excess Alcohol***
Coronary heart disease	×	×	×	×	×
Cancer	×	×	×	×	×
Stroke	×	×		×	×
Diabetes	×	×	×		
Atherosclerosis	×	×	×	×	×
Liver cirrhosis					×
Digestive diseases	×	×	×		×

[a] The evidence that supports these associations is reviewed in References 13, 14, 35–39, and 57.

Instead, investigators identify associations between diet and disease from studies of laboratory animals and from biochemical, epidemiologic, and clinical investigations in humans. Because each of these methods has limitations, diet-disease associations are usually inferred from the totality of available evidence and are considered most compelling when data from all sources are consistent, strongly correlated, highly specific, dose-related, and biologically plausible.[26] Despite these difficulties, authorities repeatedly reach the same conclusion: the preponderance of evidence supports the associations listed in Table 64-2.[27] They consider most compelling the evidence for fat (especially saturated fat) and coronary heart disease; the evidence for the other associations also is considered strongly suggestive, if not always entirely convincing.

▶ DIETARY RECOMMENDATIONS

The ideal diet should provide energy and essential nutrients within optimal ranges from foods that are available, affordable, and palatable. Until the mid-1970s, governmental and health agencies in the United States advised the public to select diets from specific groups of foods (e.g., dairy, meat, fruits and vegetables, grains) in order to ensure adequate intake of nutrients most likely to be consumed at below-standard levels.[28] As the role of dietary risk factors for chronic diseases became increasingly apparent, the focus of dietary recommendations shifted to prevention of these highly prevalent conditions.

Dietary Goals and Guidelines

The first American report to reflect this new focus established numerical targets for dietary changes to reduce chronic disease risk: reduce intake of fat (to 30 percent or less of total energy), saturated fat (10 percent), sugar (10 percent), cholesterol (300 mg/day or less), and salt (5 g/day); increase intake of foods containing starch, fiber, and naturally occurring sugars (48 percent); consume alcoholic beverages in moderation; and balance energy intake and expenditure to maintain appropriate body weight. To achieve these targets, the report advised the public to consume more fruits, vegetables, and grains, and to select meat and dairy foods low in fat.[29]

As discussed below, such advice elicited intense controversy, and subsequent federal dietary guidance policy has generally omitted explicit numerical targets when recommending dietary changes for disease prevention. Recently, however, the Public Health Service has revised its nutrition objectives to include 30 percent of energy from fat as a national target.[30] Current policy is expressed in the general Dietary Guidelines for Americans: eat a variety of foods; balance the food you eat with physical activity—maintain or improve your weight; choose a diet with plenty of grain products, vegetables, and fruits; choose a diet low in fat, saturated fat, and cholesterol; choose a diet moderate in sugars; choose a diet moderate in salt and sodium; if you drink alcoholic beverages, do so in moderation.[31] This policy statement includes numerical targets in the text of the guideline for intake of fat (30 percent kcal or less) and cholesterol (300 mg/day or less).

Similar goals for intake of fat, saturated fat, and cholesterol also are embedded in the information about daily portions provided by the food guide pyramid,[32] the U.S. Department of Agriculture's implementation guide to the Dietary Guidelines. As illustrated in Figure 64-1, the pyramid emphasizes the importance of plant foods—grains, vegetables, fruit—in the daily diet, and minimizes intake of meat, dairy foods, and foods high in sugar and fat. The pyramid also elicited controversy when first released, but is now the most widely used nutrition guide in the United States.[33]

Despite the controversy, more specific numerical targets continue to be recommended by agencies concerned with prevention or treatment of coronary heart disease,[34,35] cancer,[36,37] diabetes,[38] and hypertension.[39] Similar guidelines also have been issued by agencies in many other countries throughout the world.[1,27]

The Current Consensus

Since the mid-1950s, when coronary heart disease was first recognized as a major public health problem, dietary guidelines for chronic disease prevention have advised people to eat more fruit, vegetables, and grains, to choose low-fat meat and dairy foods, to balance energy intake with expenditure, and to consume alcohol in moderation, if at all. From the outset, such guidelines encountered opposition from the food industry and certain scientific and medical groups who argued that such advice was economically unwise, unjustified by the evidence, and inappropriate for the general public.[40] Despite such considerations, consensus appeared to have been achieved in the late 1980s.[13–15]

More recently, further research and more pronounced economic concerns have led to a renewal of the debates, particularly about guidelines that suggest restrictions on intake of any type of food or product. One reason for the continued controversy may be the limitations of research studies involving single nutrients such as folic acid, transsaturated fat, or antioxidants. Scientists may disagree about the significance of research studies on single risk factors, but the benefits of adhering to overall recommendations for dietary intake or physical activity patterns are well established.

The international consensus on dietary guidelines for chronic disease prevention firmly establishes the need for public policies to promote their implementation.[41] The recent increase in the prevalence of obesity,[42] for example, focuses attention on the need for public health approaches to improving diet and activity patterns among people of all ages, as does evidence that the food and nutrient supplies of many countries do not promote achievement of national nutrition recommendations.[43]

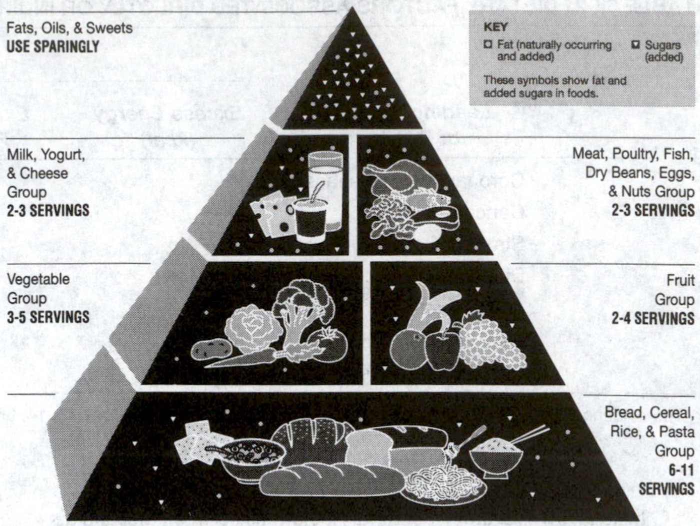

Figure 64-1. This federal implementation guide to the Dietary Guidelines for Americans illustrates the idea that grains, vegetables, and fruits constitute the basis of diets that best promote health and prevent chronic as well as deficiency diseases.[32]

▶ BARRIERS TO IMPLEMENTATION

Although the ultimate decisions targeted by dietary recommendations are personal food choices, people make such choices within the context of the social, economic, and cultural environment in which they live. Adults prefer foods that taste, look, and smell good, are familiar, and provide variety, but these preferences are influenced strongly by family and ethnic background, levels of education and income, age, and gender. Food availability, advertising, and the demand for convenience also influence food choices and create barriers to dietary change.[41]

Food Availability

Food production, distribution, and marketing in the United States have undergone significant changes that affect food availability and, therefore, consumption patterns. Since the mid-1930s, the number of farms in the United States has declined by half but their average size has nearly tripled. This trend has been accompanied by an increase in the proportion and number of foods for home use purchased in supermarkets; from 1980 to 1993, the average number of items in a supermarket rose from about 14,000 items to 25,000.[44] In 1994 alone, manufacturers introduced more than 15,000 new food products, among them more than 1,300 dairy products, 1,600 baked goods, 2,250 beverages, and 2,400 candies, chewing gums, and snacks.[45] In 1995, 3,000 such products were developed to "improve" nutrient content, half for the purpose of reducing fat, whether or not they reduced energy content.[46]

Food Advertising

Advertising enhances the sales of such products to adults and influences the eating habits of children.[47] It promotes consumption of entire categories of foods; stimulates food production, processing, and marketing; and builds brand loyalty.[48] Nearly 80 percent of the more than $500 billion spent in the United States for food in 1994 paid for marketing costs that included labor, packaging, transportation, other business costs, and profit. Advertising costs were estimated at nearly $30 billion,[49] much of it for television commercials for food and beverages purchased outside the home.[50] The influence of food commercials on consumption patterns, particularly of children, is of great concern as the advertisements rarely display foods consistent with dietary guidelines.[51] For example, advertisements for alcoholic beverages have been found to promote drinking among school-age children.[52]

Demand for Convenience

More than half of American women with children under 1 year of age work outside the home, a trend sufficient to explain why convenience is so prominent a motive for food selection and why, among adults age 20 to 29, men consumed nearly 41 percent of energy outside the home, and women 34 percent in 1994.[53] Higher disposable incomes in two-income families and less leisure time also contribute to demands for convenience. Thus, expenditures on commercial foodservice nearly doubled from 1984 to 1994; they more than doubled on foods purchased in fast food outlets, which now account for more than half of all food consumed outside the home. McDonald's alone accounted for nearly $24 billion in sales from nearly 10,000 domestic sites and nearly 5,000 foreign sites in 1994.[54]

Such barriers account at least in part for observations that overall patterns of food consumption in the United States are responding slowly, if at all, to dietary recommendations. Health messages to consume more fruits, vegetables, and grains, for example, must counteract powerful societal barriers.[55]

▶ CONTRADICTIONS BETWEEN KNOWLEDGE OF NUTRITION AND BEHAVIOR

Americans are increasingly well informed about the relationship between diet and health. In 1970, for example, only 8 percent of survey respondents were aware of the link between fat intake and heart disease, but the proportion had increased to 55 percent by 1988.[56] Federal surveys in 1989 to 1991 reported that very high proportions of women respondents were aware of health problems related to fat (79.6 percent), saturated fat (65.1 percent), cholesterol (86.7 percent), salt or sodium (87.8 percent), and being overweight (90.7 percent).[57] In 1994, more than half of respondents to a survey believed that eating fruits and vegetables could reduce cancer risk.[58] Recent surveys also report that consumers say they are making significant dietary changes to improve health, such as eating more fruits and vegetables (94 percent), less fat (63 percent), and less red meat (32 percent), and that nutrition is an important factor in their food selections (76 percent).[59]

Despite these impressive reports of knowledge and positive attitudes, only a small fraction of the population appears to be following dietary recommendations, perhaps because of confusion about dietary messages,[58] or because alterations in dietary preferences may require deviations from accepted patterns of food intake and be perceived as demanding increased skills, costs, or efforts in preparation.[60] For

TABLE 64-3. EXAMPLES OF POPULATION SURVEY ELEMENTS FOR NUTRITIONAL STATUS EVALUATION

Nutritional History	*Medical History and Physical Examination*
■ ***DIETARY INTAKE***	■ ***SIGNS OF UNDERNUTRITION***
Food record	Low weight-for-height
24-hour recall	Recent weight loss
Food frequency	Clinical signs of malnutrition
Diet history	Chronic or acute conditions that increase nutrient requirements or needs
Use of supplements	Medication use
Eating habits	Substance abuse
■ ***RELATED SOCIAL FACTORS***	■ ***CHRONIC DISEASE RISK***
Income	Elevated blood glucose
Educational level	High blood pressure
Ethnicity	High blood cholesterol
Use of food assistance	Overweight
Medications	
Activity levels	
Anthropometric Measurements	***Laboratory Tests***
Height	Hemoglobin, hematocrit
Weight	Iron and iron-binding
Skinfolds	Serum vitamin and mineral levels
Head circumference	Serum albumin
Elbow breadth	Blood glucose
Waist circumference	Blood cholesterol
Bioelectrical impedance	Lipoproteins

example, the major sources of saturated fat in the United States diet in 1994 were meat (26 percent) dairy foods (24 percent), and fats and oils (41 percent).[61] Advice to consume no more than 10 percent of total energy as saturated fat requires consumers to eat less red meat, to select low-fat dairy foods, and to replace energy contributed by fats and oils with that from fruits, vegetables, and grains.

Food supply data (an indirect measure of dietary intake) do indicate a slight decrease in the use of red meat since the 1970s, along with substantial replacement of whole with low-fat and skim milk, and significant increases in use of fruits and vegetables. The availability of saturated fat in the U.S. food supply, however, has remained at a relatively constant level, largely because of increased use of poultry, cheese, and shortenings. The availability of total fat has risen steadily throughout this century; virtually all of this increase can be accounted for by greater use of vegetable fats in salad dressings and table spreads.[62] Similar data have been used to compare trends in food availability in countries throughout the world.[63]

Trends in actual dietary intake are more difficult to evaluate due to methodologic differences among the various surveys. To the extent that determination is possible, levels of intake of total and saturated fat did not appear to change significantly between the early 1970s and 1990s, but the data suggest a weak trend toward reduced intake, at least of total fat.[25,64]

Such observations reflect the environment of food intake in the United States. Consumers are increasingly well informed about nutrition and health and will, on occasion, choose diets based on this information. People who do adhere to dietary guidelines tend to be older, better educated, and of higher income.[57] On a daily basis, however, convenience in eating takes precedence over nutritional quality, meals are increasingly consumed from restaurant, fast food, and take-out establishments, and the food industry actively produces, markets, and advertises alcohol and foods high in calories, fat, cholesterol, sugar, and salt. Public health planning and evaluation strategies to improve dietary patterns are especially valuable in this type of environment.

► ASSESSMENT OF NUTRITIONAL STATUS

As with any other public health campaign, the first step in development of a dietary intervention is to identify the nutritional problems and, therefore, the needs of the population at risk.[65] As noted earlier, malnutrition includes not only deficiency conditions resulting from overall or specific inadequacies in food or nutrient intake, but also from conditions of excessive or unbalanced consumption. Evaluation of either form of malnutrition is complicated by the many genetic, medical, behavioral, and environmental factors that influence development of diet-related conditions, by the multiplicity of signs and symptoms of malnutrition, by the lack of suitable biochemical or clinical markers for many of these signs and symptoms,[1,2] and by lack of precision in available assessment methods.[66] Assessment is also complicated by the variety of personal, cultural, and socioeconomic factors that influence dietary intake.

Assessment Methods: Individuals and Populations

To date, no single, independent measurement of dietary, biochemical, or clinical status has been found adequate to confirm the nutritional status of individuals or populations. Instead, nutritional risk is defined by a combination of methods: nutritional history, medical history and physical examination, anthropometric measurements, and laboratory tests.[67] Table 64-3 lists examples of elements of these methods used in population surveys. In practice, surveys rarely use the full range of nutritional assessment methods; many of them are too imprecise, inconvenient, or expensive for frequent use. Most assessments are based on professional judgment of the severity of selected nutritional risk factors.

Short of duplicate meal analysis (and even this method has limitations), techniques to determine the usual dietary intake of individuals are imprecise; standard methods produce approximations that cannot be interpreted too literally. These include a record of foods consumed during a specified time period (food record), retrospective recall of foods consumed within a recent time period (24-hour recall or longer), and measures of the frequency of consumption of specific index foods (food frequencies). The nutrient content of diets described by these methods is obtained from tables of food composition and compared to standards of nutrient intake such as the RDAs,[4] RDIs,[5] or patterns of food consumption described by dietary goals[29,30] or guidelines.[31]

Each of these methods, used singly or in combination, must balance strengths and weaknesses. All yield useful, if imprecise, information.[67] Demographic and socioeconomic data are especially useful as indirect indicators of nutritional risk in community surveys where detailed diet histories, physical examinations, and laboratory tests would be impractical.

The simplest and most useful indication of undernutrition in individuals or populations is low weight for height. Other clinical signs listed in Table 64-3 are useful for assessment of the nutritional status of hospital patients.[1] Evaluation of chronic disease risk is accomplished through measurements of blood glucose, blood pressure, blood cholesterol, and body weight. The high prevalence of these risk factors is the basis of large-scale campaigns to reduce them among the general population.[35,39] The fact that no simple screen is as yet available for evaluation of diet-related cancer risk is one reason for promotion of healthier diets as a prevention strategy.[36,37]

National Nutrition Monitoring

The prevalence of diet-related risk factors and conditions in the United States is determined through a series of national surveys mandated by legislation in 1990 and known collectively as the National Nutrition Monitoring and Related Research Program. This program plans and coordinates the monitoring activities of 22 federal agencies and includes about 40 distinct surveys that measure health and nutritional status, food and nutrient consumption, food composition, dietary knowledge and attitudes, foods available for purchase, and sociodemographic and economic indicators related to dietary intake.[68] Some historical concerns about the limited ability of the program to provide data on trends in dietary intake patterns, hunger prevalence, and dietary patterns of minority groups[69] have been addressed in recent monitoring surveys.[57] The most comprehensive of these surveys is the National Health and Nutrition Examination Survey (NHANES), which collects data from dietary interviews, physical examinations, and biochemical and hematological tests conducted on a large probability sample of the U.S. population. NHANES surveys were conducted in 1971–1974 (NHANES I), 1976–1980 (NHANES II), and 1988–1991 (NHANES III, Phase I). NHANES III is continuous and oversamples minority groups and older Americans. It has already produced important information about the increasing prevalence of obesity in the United States[42] and will eventually provide information about even more data elements than those listed in Table 64-3.

Community Nutrition Assessment

Methods for assessment of the nutritional needs of communities vary only slightly from conventional means of community health assessment. Table 64-4 lists the principal data elements used to evaluate the level of nutritional risk in communities. These elements include geographical, demographic, socioeconomic, and health descriptors. They also include descriptors of food and nutrition resources in the community, utilization rates for such resources, and indicators of food availability, intake, and nutritional status obtained from nutrition monitoring surveys.

In developing countries with high rates of clinically apparent conditions of undernutrition, investigators have selected elements from this list to develop rapid, convenient, and relatively inexpensive screening instruments to evaluate nutritional risk under field conditions.[70] These methods, which range from a graded series of bracelets to measure arm circumference to comprehensive surveys, have been used successfully to identify children and adults at high nutritional risk who can be targeted for intervention.[71]

Since the early 1980s, more than 250 communities in the United States have correlated data on poverty levels, nonparticipation of eligible persons in food assistance programs, and the rapid expansion of private-sector soup kitchens and food pantries to document the need for expansion of federal food assistance programs.[9] Also in the United States, encouragement of local screening campaigns for high blood cholesterol is a key implementation strategy of the National Cholesterol Education Program.[35]

▸ POLICY RECOMMENDATIONS AND IMPLEMENTATION STRATEGIES

The quantity, strength, and consistency of evidence that relates dietary factors to chronic diseases, and the substantial impact of these conditions on health, are reasons enough to promote policies to improve the availability of healthful diets. Such policies should address environmental as well as behavioral barriers to dietary change and should be directed not only to the general public and to individuals at risk of chronic disease, but also to health professionals, health care service providers, the food-service industry, food manufacturers, the government, and research investigators.

The General Public

Education of individuals has been demonstrated to improve nutrition knowledge, attitude, and behavior and to help reduce chronic disease risk factors.[60] The most effective counseling interventions involve subjects in the design, conduct, and evaluation of their own dietary plans, employ multiple educational strategies, and use a team approach.[72,73] In the United States, broad public health campaigns to reduce chronic disease risk factors have proven effective;[35,39] the National 5-A-Day Campaign to increase public consumption of fruits and vegetables has great potential to improve dietary patterns.[74] These separate drives to reduce distinct chronic disease risk factors could well be joined into a single, universal campaign that encourages the public to follow overall diet and activity recommendations.

High-Risk Groups

Pregnant women, infants, young children, and the elderly are most vulnerable to nutritional deficiencies, especially when they are poor. Members of racial and ethnic minority groups bear a disproportionate burden not only of undernutrition but also of chronic disease—largely as a consequence of poverty, inadequate access to health care, and educational disadvantage. The contribution of diet to chronic disease risk in these groups is difficult to evaluate. Available data do not permit identification of consistent associations between dietary

TABLE 64-4. DATA ELEMENTS FOR COMMUNITY NUTRITION ASSESSMENT

■ ***COMMUNITY DESCRIPTORS***
Geographical boundaries, area
Population within boundaries, density
Community agencies and services
Community health care programs and services
Hospitals and clinics
Educational institutions

■ ***POPULATION DESCRIPTORS***
Age, gender, racial, and ethnic distribution
Income level
Educational level
Employment level
Length of time in location
Primary language
Health status indicators
- Infant mortality
- Low–birth weight
- Life expectancy
- Leading causes of death
- Chronic disease rates

■ ***NUTRITIONAL STATUS INDICATORS***
See Table 64-3

■ ***FOOD AND NUTRITION RESOURCES***
Federal food assistance programs
- Utilization rates
- Nonparticipation rates for eligible persons

Community food assistance programs
- Soup kitchens
- Food pantries
- Food banks

Food markets
- Supermarkets
- Grocery stores
- Farmers' markets

Food service institutions
Nutrition education and training programs
Food and nutrition advocacy groups
Food assistance outreach programs
Weight-control programs
Worksite wellness programs

patterns and disease risk in minority populations; they also find few consistent differences in dietary intake patterns between minority and majority populations.[75]

Community-based, media-oriented public education ("social marketing") campaigns that transmit culturally sensitive messages designed to address the needs and attitudes of specific target groups have been applied successfully to promote breast-feeding and other dietary improvements in developing countries.[76] In the United States, preliminary use of these techniques has shown promise in improving the nutritional status of low-income homemakers, increasing the prevalence of breast-feeding, and improving health and function among the elderly and minority groups.[77] Whether such methods achieve long-term educational goals is uncertain, however.[78] In the interim, education methods that empower community members to determine their own dietary needs and interventions appear most likely to be effective.

Health Professionals

Despite decades of public, professional, and governmental demands for expanded and improved nutrition training of physicians and other health professionals, progress has been slow.[79] The necessary curriculum is well established: basic principles of nutrition, the role of diet in disease prevention, methods for assessment of nutritional status, therapeutic diets, behavioral aspects of dietary counseling, and the role of nutritionists in health care.[13,80] One optimistic view of current trends toward managed health care is that they will promote greater interest in disease prevention as a cost-containment strategy and, therefore, in the nutrition training of health care personnel.

Health Care Providers

The focus on reduction of health care costs emphasizes the need for greater attention to preventive services.[81] Thus, it seems logical that nutrition services should be routinely integrated into health care delivery programs. Such services should include dietary counseling and prescription, referral to community nutrition and food assistance programs, and monitoring of patient progress; they also should address barriers to access and to the effective organization and delivery of nutritional care.[72,73]

The Food Service Industry

The trend toward eating meals away from home illustrates the need to shift the targets of dietary recommendations from homemakers to food providers—restaurants, schools, worksites, hospitals, nursing homes, child care centers, and other institutions. With this shift, the nutritional quality of professional food service takes on increasing importance. Meals served in restaurants increasingly should and do reflect health concerns.[82] In food-service institutions less driven by market considerations, implementation of dietary recommendations may well require federal intervention or other incentives, especially since improvements are likely to require substantial education and training of kitchen personnel.

Food Manufacturers

The interest of consumers in health is one factor that motivates development of new food products,[46] but the food industry needs stronger encouragement to increase the production and marketability of foods that contribute to overall patterns of healthful dietary intake, to convey appropriate messages about the sizes of food portions, and to exercise greater responsibility in use of health claims. To date, mandatory food labeling and public education campaigns have stimulated consumption of low-fat products, but have been less successful in promoting more complex dietary messages that may conflict with economic concerns.

The Government

Food Labels

The Nutrition Labeling and Education Act (NLEA) of 1990 became fully effective in 1994; it requires nutrition information on the labels of nearly all packaged foods and instructs the FDA to set and enforce standards for serving sizes, product descriptors ("light," "reduced"), and health claims on product labels.[83] International authorities also have proposed such rules.[84] U.S. food labels now include information about key nutrients in chronic disease prevention—energy, fat, saturated fat, cholesterol, and added salt and sugar, and are used frequently by consumers to select packaged foods, particularly those low in fat. The effectiveness of the NLEA has led to opposition by food industry and dietary supplement groups that have worked through Congress to weaken federal labeling authority in general, and restrictions on health claims in particular.[85]

Food Assistance Programs

All individuals should have access to a sufficient and appropriate diet. For many years, industrialized and developing countries have supported policies and programs that have improved the availability of food to their populations.[86] In the United States, despite federal expenditures of nearly $40 billion annually for U.S. Department of Agriculture (USDA) programs alone, demands for food assistance continue to increase.[87] Recent welfare legislation has weakened federal authority over food assistance programs by delegating funding to the states. The effect of this change on families in poverty has yet to be determined, but the new rules on funding restrictions and work requirements seem unlikely to improve the "safety net" that had been in place since the 1940s.[88]

Nutrition Monitoring

National health surveillance systems should collect systematic data on food availability, dietary intake, and the nutritional status of the general population and of targeted high-risk groups in order to establish a rational foundation for development of public policies in education, services, and research. In the United States, the 1990 legislation has led to improvements in the coordination and focus of federal food and nutrition monitoring activities and has stimulated significant research and publication.[57,68] Many other countries are developing similar initiatives, especially to address rising worldwide rates of chronic diseases.[89]

Research Investigators

Various organizations and agencies have proposed research agendas to address needs for more information about food,[90] food safety,[91] dietetics,[92] and nutrition education.[60] Of particular public health relevance is the pressing need to identify effective methods for encouraging people to make appropriate changes in diet and exercise behavior. More adequate funding and institutional support is needed for applied research in epidemiology, behavioral science, prevention, and dietary intervention.[93] Such data would establish a more rigorous basis for policies and programs to improve the nutritional health of the population.

▸ REFERENCES

1. Shils ME, Olson JA, Shike M (eds): Modern Nutrition in Health and Disease. 8th ed. Philadelphia: Lea & Febiger, 1994, (vols 1 and 2)
2. Ziegler EE, Filer LJ (eds): Present Knowledge in Nutrition. 7th ed. Washington, DC: ILSI Press, 1996
3. Mertz W: The essential trace elements. Science 213:1332–1338, 1981
4. National Research Council, Food and Nutrition Board: Recommended Dietary Allowances. 10th ed. Washington, DC: National Academy of Sciences Press, 1989

5. Institute of Medicine, Food and Nutrition Board: Dietary Reference Intakes for Calcium, Phosphorus, Magnesium, Vitamin D, and Fluoride. Washington, DC: National Academy Press, 1997
6. Missiaen M, Shapouri S: Food shortages in developing countries continuing. FoodReview Jan–Apr:24–31, 1995
7. Institute of Medicine: Nutrition Issues in Developing Countries. Part I: Diarrheal Diseases. Washington, DC: National Academy Press, 1992, pp 5–69
8. Bellamy C: The State of the World's Children. New York: UNICEF (Oxford University Press), 1998
9. Nestle M, Guttmacher S: Hunger in the United States: rationale, methods, and policy implications of state hunger surveys. J Nutr Educ 24:18s–22s, 1992
10. Karp RJ (ed): Malnourished Children in the United States: Caught in the Cycle of Poverty. New York: Springer, 1993
11. Scrimshaw NS, Schurch B (eds): Protein-Energy Interactions. Proceedings of an I/D/E/C/G/ Workshop, October 21–25, 1992, Lausanne: Nestle Foundation, 1992
12. Maxwell S, Frankenberger TR: Household Food Security: Concepts, Indicators, Measurements: A Technical Review. New York and Rome: United Nations Children's Fund and International Fund for Agricultural Development, 1992
13. Department of Health and Human Services, Public Health Service: The Surgeon General's Report on Nutrition and Health. DHHS (PHS) Publication No. 88-50210. Washington, DC: Government Printing Office, 1988
14. National Research Council: Diet and Health: Implications for Reducing Chronic Disease Risk. Washington, DC: National Academy Press, 1989
15. James WPT: Healthy Nutrition: Preventing Nutrition-Related Diseases in Europe. WHO Regional Publications, European Series, No. 24, Copenhagen: World Health Organization, 1988
16. Popkin BM: The nutrition transition in low-income countries: an emerging crisis. Nutr Rev 52(9):285–298, 1994
17. Frazao E: The American diet: health and economic consequences. Agriculture Information Bulletin No. 711. Washington, DC: US Department of Agriculture, 1995
18. U.S. Department of Health and Human Services: Physical Activity and Health: A Report of the Surgeon General. Atlanta: Centers for Disease Control and Prevention, 1996
19. Singh GK, Kochanek KD, MacDorman MF: Advance report of final mortality statistics, 1994. Centers for Disease Control and Prevention/National Center for Health Statistics Monthly Vital Stat Rep 45(3) suppl, 1996
20. WHO Study Group: Diet, Nutrition, and the Prevention of Chronic Diseases. WHO Technical Report 797. Geneva: World Health Organization, 1990
21. Doll R, Peto R: The causes of cancer: quantitative estimates of avoidable risks of cancer in the United States today. J Natl Cancer Inst 66:1191–1308, 1981
22. Goldman L, Cook EF: The decline in ischemic heart disease mortality rates: an analysis of the comparative effects of medical interventions and changes in lifestyle. Ann Intern Med 101:825–836, 1984
23. McGinnis JM, Foege WH: Actual causes of death in the United States. JAMA 270:2207–2212, 1993
24. Willett WC, Buzzard IM (eds): Dietary assessment methods. Am J Clin Nutr 59 (1 Suppl):143s–306s, 1994
25. Nestle M, Woteki C: Trends in American dietary patterns: research issues and policy implications. In Bronner F (ed): Nutrition and Health—Topics and Controversies. Boca Raton, FL: CRC Press, 1995, pp 1–44
26. Lilienfeld DE, Stolley PD: Foundations of Epidemiology. 3rd ed. New York: Oxford Press, 1994
27. Cannon G: Food and Health: The Experts Agree. London: Consumers' Association, 1992
28. Nestle M, Porter DV: Evolution of federal dietary guidance policy: from food adequacy to chronic disease prevention. Caduceus 6(2): 43–67, 1990
29. Select Committee on Nutrition and Human Needs, United States Senate: Dietary Goals for the United States. 2nd ed. Washington, DC: Government Printing Office, 1977
30. US Department of Health and Human Services: Healthy People 2000: Midcourse Review and 1995 Revisions. Washington, DC: US Public Health Service, 1995
31. US Department of Agriculture and US Department of Health and Human Services: Nutrition and Your Health: Dietary Guidelines for Americans. 4th ed. HG 232. Washington, DC: Government Printing Office, 1995
32. Human Nutrition Information Service: The Food Guide Pyramid. HG 252. Hyattsville, MD: US Department of Agriculture, 1992, rev.1996
33. Nestle M: Dietary advice for the 1990s: the political history of the food guide pyramid. Caduceus 9:136–153, 1993
34. Krauss RM, Deckelbaum RJ, Ernst N, et al: Dietary guidelines for healthy American adults. Circulation 94:1795–1800, 1996
35. National Cholestrol Education Program: Second Report of the Expert Panel on Detection, Evaluation, and Treatment of High Blood Cholesterol in Adults (Adult Treatment Panel II). NIH Publication No. 93-3095. Bethesda, MD: National Institutes of Health, 1993
36. American Cancer Society 1996 Advisory Committee on Diet, Nutrition, and Cancer Prevention: Guidelines on diet, nutrition, and cancer prevention: reducing the risk of cancer with healthy food choices and physical activity. CA Cancer J Clin 46(6):325–341, 1996
37. Potter JD, ed: Food, Nutrition, and the Prevention of Cancer: a Global Perspective. Washington, DC: World Cancer Research Fund/American Institute for Cancer Research, 1997
38. Franz MJ, Horton ES, Bantle JP, et al: Nutrition principles for the management of diabetes and related complications. Diabetes Care 17:126–132, 1994
39. Joint National Committee on Detection, Evaluation, and Treatment of High Blood Pressure: Fifth Report. NIH Publication No. 93-1088. Bethesda, MD: National Institutes of Health, 1994
40. Nestle M: Food lobbies, the food pyramid, and U.S. nutrition policy. Int J Health Serv 23:483–496, 1993
41. Thomas PR (ed): Improving America's Diet and Health: From Recommendations to Action. Washington, DC: National Academy Press, 1991
42. Kuczmarski RJ, Flegal KM, Campbell SM, Johnson CL: Increasing prevalence of overweight among US adults. JAMA 272:205–211, 1994
43. Posner BM, Franz M, Quatromoni P, and the INTERHEALTH Steering Committee: Nutrition and the global risk for chronic diseases: the INTERHEALTH nutrition initiative. Nutr Rev 52:201–207, 1994
44. Kaufman P: Fewer but larger supermarkets. FoodReview 18:26–29, 1995
45. Gallo AE: Food marketing sales, mergers, and new product introductions rose in 1994. FoodReview 18(2):24–25, 1995
46. Frazao E, Allshouse JE: Sales of nutritionally improved foods outpace traditional counterparts. FoodReview 18(3):2–6, 1995
47. Sylvester GP, Achterberg C, Williams J: Children's television and nutrition: friends or foes? Nutr Today 30(1):6–15, 1995
48. Hollingsworth P: Betcha can't watch just one: food advertising trends. Food Technol 50(10):59–62, 1996
49. Elitzak H: Food marketing costs rose less than the farm value in 1995. FoodReview 19(3):6–10, 1996
50. Sun TY, Blaylock JR, Allshouse JE: Dramatic growth in mass media food advertising in the 1980's. FoodReview 16(3):36–40, 1993
51. Kotz K, Story M: Food advertisements during children's Saturday morning television programming: are they consistent with dietary recommendations? J Am Diet Assoc 94:1296–1300, 1994

52. Grube JW, Wallack L: Television beer advertising and drinking knowledge, beliefs, and intentions among schoolchildren. Am J Public Health 84:254–259, 1994
53. Cleveland LE, Goldman JD, Borrud LG: Data tables: results from USDA's 1994 Continuing Survey of Food Intakes by Individuals and 1994 Diet and Health Knowledge Survey. Riverdale, MD: US Department of Agriculture, 1996
54. Price CC: Sales of food away from home expanding. FoodReview 18(2):30–32, 1995
55. Nestle M: Dietary guidance for the 21st century: new approaches. J Nutr Educ 27:272–275, 1995
56. Frazao E: Consumer concerns about nutrition: opportunities for the food sector. Agriculture Information Bulletin No. 705. Washington, DC: US Department of Agriculture, 1994
57. Life Sciences Research Office: Third Report on Nutrition Monitoring in the United States. Washington, DC: Government Printing Office, 1995, vol 1
58. Gallup Organization: How Are Americans Making Food Choices?—1994 Update. Washington, DC: American Dietetic Association and International Food Information Council, 1994
59. Opinion Research Corporation: Trends in the United States: Consumer Attitudes and the Supermarket 1994. Washington, DC: Food Marketing Institute, 1994
60. Contento I, Balch GI, Bronner YL, et al (eds): The effectiveness of nutrition education and implications for nutrition education policy, programs, and research: a review of research. J Nutr Educ 27:276–422, 1995
61. Gerrior SA, Bente L: Nutrient content of the U.S. food supply, 1909–94. Home Economics Research Report No. 53. Washington, DC: US Department of Agriculture, 1997
62. Putnam JJ, Allshouse JE: Food Consumption, Prices, and Expenditures, 1970–94. Statistical Bulletin No. 939. Washington, DC: US Department of Agriculture, 1997
63. Scott L, Shapouri S: World food consumption up, but not everywhere. FoodReview 18(2):48–54, 1995
64. Daily dietary fat and total food-energy intakes—Third National Health and Nutrition Examination Survey, Phase 1, 1988–91. MMWR 43(7):116–117, 123–125, 1994
65. Jelliffe DB: The Assessment of the Nutritional Status of the Community. Geneva: World Health Organization, 1966
66. Lee RD, Nieman DC: Nutritional Assessment. 2nd ed. St. Louis, MO: Mosby, 1996
67. Thompson FE, Byers T: Dietary assessment resource manual. J Nutr 124(11 Suppl):2245s–2317s, 1994
68. Kuczmarski MF, Moshfegh A, Briefel R: Update on nutrition monitoring activities in the United States. J Am Diet Assoc 94:753–760, 1994
69. Nestle M: National nutrition monitoring policy: the continuing need for legislative intervention. J Nutr Educ 22:141–144, 1990
70. Collins S: Using middle upper arm circumference to assess severe adult malnutrition during famine. JAMA 276:391–395, 1996
71. Beghin I, Cap M, Dujardin B: Health and Community: Nutritional Assessment Guide. Geneva: World Health Organization, 1988
72. US Preventive Services Task Force: Guide to Clinical Preventive Services. 2nd ed. Alexandria, VA: International Medical Publishing, 1996
73. Woolf SH, Jonas S, Lawrence RS (eds): Health Promotion and Disease Prevention in Clinical Practice. Baltimore, MD: Williams & Wilkins, 1996
74. Havas S, Heimendinger J, Reynolds K, et al: 5 A Day for better health: a new research initiative. J Am Diet Assoc 94:32–36, 1994
75. Kumanyika S: Diet and chronic disease issues for minority populations. J Nutr Educ 22:89–96, 1990
76. Manoff RK: Social Marketing: New Imperative for Public Health. New York: Praeger, 1985
77. Glanz K, Lewis FM, Rimer BK (eds): Health Behavior and Health Education: Theory, Research, and Practice. 2nd ed. San Francisco: Jossey-Bass, 1996
78. Vanden Heede FA, Pelican S: Reflections on marketing as an inappropriate model for nutrition education. J Nutr Educ 27:141–145, 1995
79. Bruer RA, Chapel T, Schmidt RE: Nutrition education for physicians: a review of the issues. Silver Spring, MD: Macro International, 1992
80. American Dietetic Association: Position of the American Dietetic Association: nutrition—an essential component of medical education. J Am Diet Assoc 94:555–557, 1994
81. Tucker HN, Miguel SG: Cost containment through nutrition intervention. Nutr Rev 54:111–121, 1996
82. Warshaw HS: America eats out: nutrition in the chain and family restaurant industry. J Am Diet Assoc 93:19–20, 1993
83. Mermelstein NH: A guide to the new nutrition labeling proposals. Food Technology 46(1):56–62, 1992
84. Porter DV: Dietary supplements: recent regulations and related activities. Nutr Today 31(3):127–130, 1996
85. Silverglade B: The Nutrition Labeling and Education Act: a public health milestone is now under attack. J Nutr Educ 28:251–253, 1996
86. Scrimshaw NS, Wallerstein MB (eds): Nutrition Policy Implementation: Issues and Experience. New York: Plenum, 1982
87. Oliveira V: Food-assistance spending held steady in 1996. FoodReview 20(1):49–56, 1997
88. Voichek J (ed): Welfare reform and nutrition education. J Nutr Educ 28(2):58–128, 1996
89. Posner BM, Quatromoni PA, Franz M: Nutrition policies and interventions for chronic disease risk reduction in international settings: the INTERHEALTH nutrition initiative. Nutr Rev 52:179–187, 1994
90. Research Committee of the Institute of Food Technologists: America's food research needs: into the 21st century. Food Technology 47(3 Suppl):1s–40s, 1993
91. National Science and Technology Council Committee on Health, Safety, and Food: Meeting the challenge: a research agenda for America's health, safety, and food. Washington, DC: Executive Office of the President, 1996
92. American Dietetic Association: The Research Agenda for Dietetics, Conference Proceedings, May 14 and 15, 1992, Chicago, IL. Chicago: American Dietetic Association, 1993
93. Wynder EL: Invited commentary: studies in mechanism and prevention. Am J Epidemiol 139:457–549, 1994

65

Dental Public Health

R. Gary Rozier

The mouth contains a number of different tissues, some of which are found throughout the body. As a result of infection, trauma, degeneration, or neoplastic changes, these tissues can be affected by up to 265 categories of diseases or conditions.[1] Of greatest importance to oral health are two specialized tissues—the teeth and their supporting (periodontal) structures. The majority of oral health services are directed toward the prevention and control of diseases and conditions affecting these two tissues.

Oral diseases are important considerations in public health, preventive dentistry, and preventive medicine for several reasons. First, they are of almost universal prevalence. Rarely if ever does anyone go unaffected by at least one of these diseases, and most people are affected by several during their lifetimes. Second, most oral diseases do not undergo remission or termination if left untreated, as do many diseases, but accumulate a backlog of unmet needs that can ultimately end in loss of teeth. Third, these diseases usually require technically demanding, expensive, and time-consuming professional treatment. Expenditures for dental care in the United States totaled an estimated $45.8 billion in 1995.[2] For every $4 spent for physician services, about $1 is spent for dental services. However, the relative burden on individuals for costs of dental care are more than for physician services because 48 percent of national dental expenditures are out-of-pocket, compared to only 18 percent for physician services. This large difference is due to the virtual absence of dental care coverage in Medicare, the limited number of services available in Medicaid, particularly for adults, and the limited use of Medicaid services by either children or adults. Less than 4 percent of total national dental expenditures in 1995 were from public sources, compared with 32 percent of those for physician services.

Oral diseases also are important for consideration because they are in large measure preventable. Because of a rich tradition of research and development, dentistry has at its disposal a large and sound science base for use in the prevention and control of most oral conditions, particularly dental caries and periodontal diseases. Evidence available since the mid-1970s clearly indicates that oral health promotion and disease prevention services implemented in industrialized countries beginning in the 1940s have had a dramatic effect on disease levels, particularly in children. Yet current information suggests that further improvements in oral disease prevention are necessary to eliminate the continuing effects of disease on an excessive number of individuals. Available community and individual strategies, if fully implemented and maintained, could reduce oral diseases to insignificant levels in society.

Oral diseases and conditions also merit consideration because of the effect they can have on the physical health of the remainder of the body and because of the manifestation of systemic health in the oral cavity. This bidirectionality of the relationship between the health of the mouth and the rest of the body has been emphasized by findings, for example, that periodontal disease might be a risk factor for cardiovascular disease[3] and that periodontal disease is a sixth complication of diabetes.[4] The mouth is of essential importance in the overall health of the body and can serve as an indicator of general health.

Finally, oral diseases affect the quality of life. A healthy, pain-free mouth is important as an outcome in its own right, but it also can have a significant impact on the quality of life because disease results in dysfunction, discomfort, or disability. In one group of elderly individuals, 30 percent said that their teeth had a bad effect on chewing and biting; 19 percent, on feeling comfortable; 11 percent, on smiling and laughing; and 10 percent, on having confidence.[5] In a given year, dental-related illnesses can account for as much as 6.4 million days of bed disability, 14.3 million days of restricted activity, and 20.9 million lost work days.[6] Surgeon General C. Everett Koop commented several years ago that "Without oral health you are not healthy," a statement that is only now being fully appreciated because of scientific investigations into oral health and its impact on physical conditions and the quality of life.

The purpose of this chapter is to review the magnitude of oral diseases and the strategies available for their prevention and control. Its focus is on dental caries, periodontal diseases, and oral cancers—dental caries and periodontal diseases because of their widespread nature and the effectiveness of available prevention strategies, and oral cancers because of their devastating effects. Other oral health problems such as cleft lip and palate, malocclusion, or problems resulting from trauma to the mouth or face are not considered in this chapter but are nevertheless important considerations in any comprehensive public health program.

▸ DENTAL CARIES

Pathogenesis and Etiology

Dental caries is defined as the destruction of the tooth resulting from a series of complex biochemical events occurring at a localized site on the enamel, dentin, or cementum.[7–9] Minerals actively leave and re-enter the tooth surface, a dynamic process of demineralization and remineralization resulting from microbial metabolism on the tooth surface. Demineralization occurs when the pH is lowered by microorganisms that are organized into plaque, a soft, sticky film that coats the teeth, are exposed to fermentable carbohydrates, particularly sugars. Calcium and phosphates leave the enamel due to the lowered pH. Under favorable circumstances, the surface area is "repaired" by remineralization. This ongoing demineralization-remineralization process is affected by a number of intraoral factors including the type of bacteria present, type of diet, saliva secretion rate, saliva buffering capacity, and fluorides. One theory suggests that this process might even be random, and that the clinical signs resulting from this process are the accumulation of numerous episodes and an imbalance

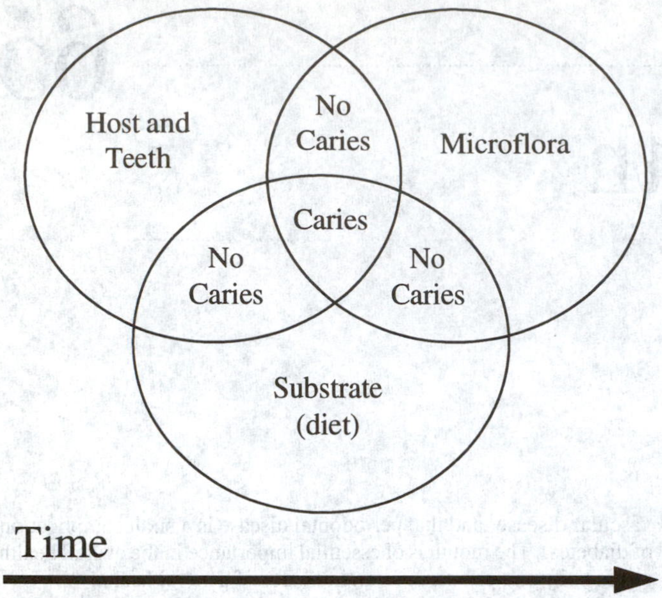

Figure 65-1. Etiologic model for dental caries. (Adapted from Keyes PH: Recent advances in dental caries research. Bacteriology. Bacteriological findings and biological implications. Int Dent J 12: 443–464, 1962; and Newbrun E: Cariology. 3rd ed. Chicago: Quintessence, 1989.)

in the dynamic equilibrium between tooth mineral and surrounding plaque fluid brought on by many factors.[9]

When the demineralization process predominates for long enough, a clinically detectable lesion can develop. In its early stages, the process can be reversed with therapeutic agents such as high concentrations of fluoride applied directly to the lesion. As demineralization progresses, a "cavity" develops and the damage cannot be repaired biochemically, but requires treatment interventions of some sort. At this point, the tooth begins a cycle that often requires repeated repairs with larger and larger fillings, sometimes resulting in tooth loss and a cycle of tooth replacement with prosthetic devices.

Some of the offending microorganisms are more important than others in the pathogenesis of dental caries, supporting a specific plaque hypothesis.[9] *Streptococcus mutans* is generally associated with the initial development of both coronal caries and root caries. *Lactobacillus* is implicated in the disease because of its association with *S. mutans* in lesions and might be important in the further development of the lesion. *Actinomyces* has been considered important in root surface caries; however, most recent studies fail to find an association between this bacteria species and root caries. A particular virulent subspecies of *Actinomyces* might be more important than others, however.

The interrelationships of the multiple factors involved in the etiology of dental caries are depicted in Figure 65-1.[10,11] Only when all three factors, a susceptible surface, caries-specific bacteria, and a cariogenic substrate or diet, are present and interacting for a sufficient length of time does dental caries develop. This model should be kept firmly in mind in the prevention and control of dental caries, since prevention strategies must be directed toward one or more of these factors.

The different surfaces of teeth exhibit different risks for caries attack. The occlusal, or biting, surfaces of the crowns of teeth are at high risk to attack (pit and fissure caries) and are usually affected first because microorganisms become entrapped in the pits and fissures soon after the teeth erupt into the mouth, and the microorganisms cannot be removed easily with usual oral hygiene methods. Smooth crown surfaces are affected soon thereafter (smooth surface caries) and are particularly protected by fluorides. Root surface caries is generally confined to exposed root surfaces and therefore occurs later in life because it is dependent on previous periodontal disease causing a loss of periodontal structures and exposure of tooth cementum.

Early childhood caries is a form of rampant decay affecting the primary teeth in infants and young children.[12,13] Current theory holds that it is a dietary carbohydrate-modified infectious disease.[14] One manifestation of this condition, nursing caries or baby bottle tooth decay, has received considerable attention in recent years. The process results from the use of solutions such as milk sweetened with sugar, sugared water, fruit juices, and carbonated or noncarbonated beverages in the nursing bottle, from the use of a pacifier sweetened with a substance such as honey, or from at-will breast feeding in an infant infected with *S. mutans*. In those affected, exposure to carbohydrates usually is for prolonged periods of time, particularly at night, resulting in an unremitting cariogenic attack caused by the constant supply of fermentable carbohydrates. It is a particularly virulent and difficult form of decay to control, with devastating effects on infants and preschool children. Its clinical appearance is unique because the maxillary incisors, those teeth usually at low risk for decay in very young children, show the greatest carious destruction, while the mandibular incisors show the least. This pattern of decay is due in part to the protection that the tongue affords the mandibular incisors during infant sucking. Nursing caries is further characterized by its very rapid development and the involvement of many primary teeth. Treatment often requires hospitalization, and lack of treatment can lead to serious and painful medical complications. Those affected are at increased risk for caries in permanent teeth later in life.

Epidemiology

Several exciting developments in the epidemiology of dental caries have occurred since the mid-1970s. First, and perhaps most significant, has been a decline in the prevalence of dental caries, affecting large numbers of children and young adults from around the world. The second is an increase in the study of various types of dental caries other than coronal caries, such as nursing caries and root surface caries. Third, with the study of the decline of coronal caries, the distribution of caries within population groups has come under closer scrutiny, resulting in the knowledge that the disease is concentrated in a small percentage of children. With this finding has come increased attention to the study of risk indicators, beginning confirmation of some of these indicators as risk factors through longitudinal epidemiological studies, and consideration of the use of targeting for the delivery of oral health services, for both individuals and populations.

Measurement of Dental Caries for Epidemiological Studies

Dental epidemiologists have developed reliable and valid clinical measures for coronal caries in the primary and permanent dentitions.[15] Dental caries is universally measured by the DMF Tooth (T) or Surface (S) Index.[16] Each of the 32 permanent tooth spaces is scored as to whether it is normal or has been diseased. If ever diseased, the tooth must exhibit one of three conditions. It can (*a*) have an untreated (decayed) cavitated lesion; (2) show evidence of surgical treatment (missing); or (3) show evidence of restorative treatment (filled). The DMF index for an individual is the sum of either teeth or surfaces having these three conditions. The index is appealing because it is nonreversible and determines someone's lifetime experience with caries. The index does become less valid in adults because teeth may be missing for reasons other than dental caries, primarily periodontal diseases and the extraction of remaining sound teeth for placement of dentures. For the primary teeth, the index usually is modified to include only decayed (d) and filled (f) teeth. The df tooth or surface index does not include missing teeth because of the difficulty in distinguishing primary teeth lost as a result of caries from those lost by natural exfoliation.

Compared with coronal caries, there is less consensus on diagnostic criteria and reporting for root caries.[17,18] Nevertheless, indices are available and consensus is beginning to emerge as measurement issues are debated and investigators gain more field experience in their use.[19] Reporting of the condition is generally based on the number of exposed root surfaces decayed or filled, with some consideration of the number of surfaces present in the mouth and at risk to caries.

Trends

The World Health Organization (WHO) Global Oral Health Data Bank, initiated in 1969, has identified three different worldwide trends in dental caries.[20–24] The first clear trend affecting large numbers of countries was identified in 1974 and signaled an increase in caries prevalence in developing countries, particularly in urban centers. Increases were noted in countries such as American Samoa, Ethiopia, Nigeria, Uganda, and Zambia. For the first time ever, children in developing countries, where 80 percent of the world's children live, were found to have a higher prevalence of dental caries than those in industrialized countries.[25] In many third world populations, dental caries can now be considered a ubiquitous disease.[26] Of recent concern are the potential effects of political, social, and economic changes occurring in Central and Eastern Europe.[27] The oral health of populations of the new states that emerged in the 1990s are faced with unemployment, inflation, a decline in family income, privatization of health services, and in some cases, discontinuation of water fluoridation, all of which can adversely affect the oral health of these populations.

The second clear trend emerged from the WHO Data Bank in 1978 and was confirmed by other sources of data at approximately the same time. Industrialized countries, known to have high rates of dental caries, were found to be experiencing a decline. This second group of countries has received a considerable amount of study during the 1980s and 1990s. At the First International Conference on the Declining Prevalence of Dental Caries in June 1982, reports from nine countries (Denmark, England, Ireland, The Netherlands, New Zealand, Norway, Scotland, Sweden, United States) were presented.[28] Based on this conference, our knowledge of these trends has been summarized as follows: (*a*) the number of decayed and missing permanent teeth has declined dramatically; (*b*) caries prevalence in primary teeth has also declined; (*c*) the percentage of caries-free children has increased; (*d*) the percentage reductions in decay have been much greater in anterior and premolar teeth than in molars; (*e*) the percentage reductions in proximal and in buccal and lingual surfaces have been much greater than in occlusal surfaces; (*f*) caries declines have occurred in fluoride-deficient as well as fluoridated areas; and (*g*) significant declines have occurred in time periods as short as 3 to 5 years.[29]

A principal question from the time of the initial discovery of the decline in caries was whether it would continue, flatten out, or even reverse and begin to rise. This question was answered by the Second International Conference on Changing Caries Prevalence held in London. Evidence presented during the conference provided no indication that this downward trend in caries in permanent teeth has subsided, and the large variation in prevalence among countries observed in the 1970s has narrowed. Murray summarized information presented on 12-year-old children from 14 countries.[30] All countries were well below the WHO goal for the year 2000 of a mean DMF value of less than 3 (Table 65-1). At the age of 12 years, mean DMFT scores of 1.0 per person or below seem attainable. By the early part of 1990, England and Wales, Finland, and portions of The Netherlands and Switzerland had achieved very low levels of dental caries. Declines in Spain, Portugal, Western and Eastern Germany, and France are well documented. Of the large, populous Western continental countries, only Italy has no documented decline in caries.

In the United States, the decline in dental caries in schoolchildren, first observed nationwide at the end of the 1970s and estimated at 32 percent, was confirmed by second and third national epidemiological surveys completed in 1987 and 1988–1991, respectively.[31,32] In the 20-year span between the first and latest national surveys a 65 percent reduction in caries experience occurred in permanent teeth, and 35 percent occurred in primary teeth.

With respect to adults, there is limited current information on caries experience. However, available data provide relatively consistent findings, suggesting that at least young adults are experiencing a decline in caries prevalence, with fewer teeth being lost as treatment shifts to maintenance and repair rather than extractions.[33] Older adults, because of high past disease experiences, have not yet attained appreciable reductions in caries experience. The treatment needs of older adults will continue to command considerable attention for years to come.

The third worldwide trend in dental caries that has emerged, but less well documented than the other two, is that in some countries, such as Mexico, the prevalence of dental caries has remained unchanged.

Epidemiology of Coronal Caries in Children

In 1988–1991, 55 percent of U.S. children 5 to 17 years of age had never had a cavity in their permanent teeth, a substantial increase in caries-free children since 1971–1974, when the comparable estimate was 26 percent (Table 65-2). The percentage of children caries-free varies inversely with age, however. By 17 years, 84 percent of children surveyed in 1986–1987 had experienced disease. Overall, the average child had 2.5 DMF surfaces in the most recent survey, and 16 percent of this disease was untreated; 5- to 9-year-olds had an average of 4.1 df surfaces in their primary teeth.[32] Besides the decline in its prevalence to rather low levels, other key features of the epidemiology of dental caries in children are that: (*a*) the relative distribution on different tooth surfaces has changed so that it is now a pit and fissure, or molar, disease; (*b*) the annual increment of coronal caries in permanent teeth of U.S. children has declined and appears to be less than 1.0 DMF surface; (*c*) its rate of progression, once initiated, has slowed, and cavitation occurs later in the natural history of the disease; and (*d*) the distribution in the population has changed so that only a few individuals (20 percent) are moderately-to-severely affected. Today, most children show little evidence of disease, and it can be considered a disease that affects selected teeth within the mouth—the pits and fissures of molars. These features have had an impact on the delivery of community- and clinical-based dental services.

TABLE 65-1. DATA FROM 14 COUNTRIES PROVIDING DMFT VALUES FOR 12-YEAR-OLD CHILDREN

Country	Year	Mean DMF	% Caries Free
England and Wales	1993	1.1	50
Denmark	1991	1.3	49
Finland	1991	1.2	30
Iceland	1991	2.5	23
Norway	1991	2.2	36
Sweden	1991	1.6	43
Belgium	1990	2.7	25
Germany	1993	2.5	
Netherlands			60
Eire			
GHB	1992	1.5	
WHBF	1992	1.6	
WHB non-F	1992	2.1	
Switzerland	1992	1.1	
Canada	1990	1.5	
Australia	1992	1.2	55
China (Beijing)	1993	1.3	50

From Murray JJ: Comments on results reported at the Second International Conference "Changes in Caries Prevalence." Int Dent J 44 (Suppl 1):457–458, 1994.

TABLE 65-2. TRENDS IN DENTAL CARIES IN U.S. SCHOOLCHILDREN

	Primary Dentition[a]			Permanent Dentition[b]		
Year	*Severity (Mean dfs)*	*% Caries Untreated*	*% Children Caries Free*	*Severity (Mean DMFS)*	*% DMFS Occlusal Caries*	*% Caries Untreated[c]*
1971–1974	6.3		26.0	7.1	49.3	29.9
1979–1980	5.3	37	36.6	4.8	54.9	16.8
1986–1987	3.9	28	49.9	3.1	57.7	13.4
1988–1991	4.1	34	54.7	2.5	56.0	16.0

Data from Brunelle JA, Carlos JP: Recent trends in dental caries in U.S. children and the effect of water fluoridation. J Dent Res 69:723–727, 1990; and Kaste LM, Selwitz RH, Oldakowski RJ, Brunelle JA, Winn DM, Brown LJ: Coronal caries in the primary and permanent dentition of children and adolescents 1–17 years of age: United States, 1988–1991. J Dent Res 75:631–641, 1996.

[a] 5- to 9-year-old children.

[b] 5- to 17-year-old children.

[c] Mean number of decayed surfaces (ds or DS) per person divided by mean number of affected surfaces (dfs or DMFS).

Edelstein and Douglass[34] have warned against being overly optimistic about the extent to which dental caries is no longer a significant problem in U.S. children. They suggest the statement claiming that "one-half of U.S. schoolchildren have never experienced tooth decay," which was adopted by both the popular and scientific press after the 1986–1987 national survey, misrepresents the true situation, primarily because it ignores dental disease in the primary dentition, is based on conservative epidemiologic diagnostic criteria and techniques that underreport disease levels, and is an overall average for the 5- to 17-year-old age span, which includes a large number of young children who are at reduced risk of disease simply because all their teeth have yet to erupt. They conclude that dental caries remains the single most common disease of childhood that is not self-limiting or amenable to a course of antibiotics.

Their warning has merit. Data on preschool children are scarce because of the difficulty in accessing representative samples for clinical examination. However, evidence from surveys of Head Start children suggest that caries affects children of low-income families early in their lives, reaches a high prevalence, and in many children, goes untreated. Surveys of young children from several countries suggest that the downward decline has leveled off. The strongest evidence is available from Great Britain and the United States. An 11 percent deterioration in DMFT scores and a 30 percent increase in untreated decay was observed between 1989–1990 and 1993–1994 in Scotland.[35] The National Health and Nutrition Examination Survey III (NHANES III) in the United States suggests that the caries trend has leveled off. Of perhaps greater concern is that 81 percent of this disease goes untreated in 2- to 4-year-olds, a figure that varies little by race.[32]

With the downward trend in industrialized countries, some factors associated with dental caries appear to have changed as well, most notably socioeconomic status (SES) and race. Historically, the relationship between SES and DMF has been in a positive direction. More recent studies have reported a reversal in this relationship, and epidemiologists now generally acknowledged that caries rates are higher among children as well as young and middle-age adults of lower social class.[36] Caries prevalence and treatment also have been strongly associated with race. For example, U.S. blacks traditionally have had a lower prevalence but more untreated disease than whites. With the overall changes in caries prevalence, this relationship, similar to SES, has changed, and blacks now have about the same or more disease than do whites in permanent teeth.[29] The severity level of affected primary tooth surfaces in 2- to 9-year-old Mexican Americans (mean DFS = 6.2) is particularly high compared to non-Hispanic whites (mean DFS = 2.5) and non-Hispanic blacks (mean DFS = 2.7). The net effect of trends in dental caries according to SES and race-ethnicity, which are most likely related, has been a shift in the burden of disease from those most able to get treatment to those least able to do so.

Traditional sex and geographic differences in caries prevalence persist. Caries prevalence in the primary dentition is similar in boys and girls. Most likely due to earlier eruption, DMFS scores in the permanent dentition are higher in females than in males.[29]

To date, epidemiologists have not been able to establish a clear or consistent relationship between oral hygiene levels and dental caries prevalence.[36] Although it may be possible for an individual to prevent caries with meticulous oral hygiene, there is little epidemiological evidence that good oral hygiene actually reduces caries rates. The use of fluoride-containing dentifrices and their positive effects on dental caries make oral hygiene easily justified, as does its effect on gingival health and personal appearance.

The consumption of sugars is probably the most important factor in the etiology of dental caries.[37] National data in the United States have indicated that the frequency of soft drinks and other sugar products between meals are related to increased caries risk, even when controlling for age, race, income, and education.[38] The role of dietary habits such as the amount, kinds, and frequency of sugar exposures in caries increments quickly are becoming less clear, however, because of the low prevalence of caries and the relatively small differences in dietary patterns in children, complicating recommendations related to the emphasis that should be place on this aspect of preventive dentistry.[39]

In a review of physical and environmental factors associated with dental caries, Graves et al.[40] found that some factors, particularly past caries experience in primary and permanent teeth, have relatively strong associations with caries increments. More limited data also show an association between molar occlusal morphology and caries risk—the deeper the pits and fissures, the greater the risk. Weak associations with caries appear to exist for malocclusion and nutritional and genetic differences. Undoubtedly, the most important environment factor associated with caries is past and present exposure to fluoride—systemic, topical, or both—which has consistently shown an inverse relationship to caries prevalence or increment.

There is no question that caries is an infectious and transmissible disease.[41] A considerable body of data has shown a direct correlation between caries prevalence or increment and *Lactobacillus* or *S. mutans* counts. In addition, some data have shown an indirect relationship between age of infection and caries risk—the younger the child at time of infection, the greater the risk. No single salivary component, such as flow rate, sugar clearance, buffering capacity, or enzyme activity has been related to caries, with the exception of extreme reduced salivary flow, consistently related to high caries risk.

Epidemiology of Coronal and Root Caries in Adults

Dental caries is a common problem in U.S. adults; virtually every adult (93.8 percent) in the United States shows evidence of having experienced dental caries.[42] Overall, U.S. adults 18 years of age and older with at least one remaining natural tooth had on average 43.8 DMF coronal surfaces per person in 1988–1991 (Table 65–3). About one-half of these surfaces were missing (the difference between DMFS

TABLE 65-3. CORONAL AND ROOT CARIES EXPERIENCE FOR THE DENTATE UNITED STATES POPULATION AGE 18 AND OVER, 1988–1991

		Coronal Caries			Root Caries		
Age Group	*% Dentate*	*Mean DMFS*	*Mean DFS*	*% Caries Untreated*[a]	*% >0 DFS*	*Mean DFS*	*% Caries Untreated*[a]
18–24	100.0	11.5	9.9	16.2	6.9	0.3	100.0
25–34	99.0	23.6	16.5	12.7	13.6	0.6	83.3
35–44	96.0	39.5	23.3	8.2	20.8	1.0	70.0
45–54	89.3	57.7	29.4	5.4	28.7	1.2	66.7
55–64	79.4	69.5	29.2	5.5	38.2	1.7	58.8
65–74	71.5	73.1	30.8	5.2	47.0	2.2	40.9
75+	56.8	80.9	25.1	6.8	55.9	3.1	48.4
Overall[b]	89.4	43.8	22.2	8.1	25.1	1.2	58.3

[a] Mean number of decayed surfaces (DS) per person divided by mean number of affected surfaces (DFS).
[b] Standardized to sex and age distribution of total NHANES III adult sample.
From Winn DM, Brunelle JA, Selwitz RH, Kaste LM, Oldakowski RJ, Kingman A, Brown LJ: Coronal and root caries in the dentition of adults in the United States, 1988–1991. J Dent Res 75:642–651, 1996.

and DFS). The percentage of past and current coronal caries that was untreated was relatively small at 8.1 percent overall. Differences in caries experience occur by age, sex, and race-ethnicity. The association between DFS and age followed an inverse U–shaped curve; females had higher scores than males. Non-Hispanic whites had about twice the number of DFS (24.3) as non-Hispanic blacks (11.9) or Mexican Americans (14.1); and non-Hispanic blacks (29 percent) and Mexican Americans (25 percent) had much more untreated disease than non-Hispanic whites (6.2 percent).

A wide variation in root surface caries has been reported among different populations, possibly because of differences in the diagnostic and survey methods as well as to the effect of dentists' treatment decisions and inherent differences in the prevalence of the condition. A large proportion of the adult population is affected, perhaps approaching 100 percent if inactive, recurrent, and root surface restorations are considered. Overall, about 25 percent of U.S. adults have one or more carious or filled root surface in 1988–1991 when using standard epidemiologic criteria, which measure lesions at the cavitated level. The estimate varied greatly by age, however, ranging from 6.9 percent at age 18 to 24 years to 55.9 percent at age 75 and older (Table 65-3). The mean number of decayed and filled root surfaces was slightly higher for males (1.4 DFS per person) than for females (1.0); and non-Hispanic blacks (1.6) and Mexican Americans (1.4) had more than non-Hispanic whites (1.1). Other key features of root caries is its low severity (1.2 surfaces per person) and low level of treatment (58.3 percent of affected surfaces untreated), particularly in comparison to coronal caries.

Root caries increments appear to be low, probably averaging about one DF surface every 3 to 4 years.[43] Although low, the problem is much more substantial when the number of teeth at risk is taken into account. When coronal and root caries are both considered, the total caries increment for adults in industrialized countries may now be greater than coronal caries in children. Further, similar to coronal caries, a minority of people have most of the root caries. The growing number of elderly who are retaining more teeth will probably increase the root caries problem in the future.

Beyond age, which is related to increasing risk due to exposure of root surfaces because of periodontal breakdown, there are very few variables consistently found to be strongly associated with prevalence of root caries. Those with the greatest potential of being risk predictors and risk factors are number of teeth, coronal caries, fluoridated water, dental behaviors, medications, and a number of social and function status indicators such as social class and impaired cognitive functions.

Epidemiology of Early Childhood Caries

Lack of a universally accepted definition of early childhood caries and the difficulty of surveying infants and children have made it difficult to estimate its prevalence. Based on a review of 35 studies, Milnes[13] estimated the prevalence of nursing caries to be between 1 and 12 percent in developed countries. He also observed that in some disadvantaged populations, such as Native Americans and preschool children in developing countries, the prevalence could be as high as 70 percent.

Caries in Special Populations

Even with the decline in dental caries, the prevalence remains high in special subgroups of the population. Included among those who need special attention through organized community and individual services are the poor, minorities, the disabled, and the institutionalized. Further, while dental caries has declined overall, some communities have very high caries rates. For example, in one statewide survey representative of all schoolchildren 5 to 17 years of age, the prevalence of dental caries varied by as much as 500 percent from one community to another.[44]

Individual and Community Caries Risk Assessment

Epidemiologic knowledge that dental caries is concentrated in a smaller segment of the population resulted in considerable interest among the research and practice communities in trying to identify those factors that contribute to placing someone, particularly children, at high risk for dental caries.[45–48] A large number of studies designed to develop prediction models and identify risk factors were undertaken. The accuracy of these caries prediction models has varied based on the prevalence of dental caries, the definition of high caries rates, and the number and type of risk factors included in the models.

The state-of-the-science for caries risk assessment was reviewed in the late 1980s at two conferences on risk assessment in dentistry, both of which reached roughly the same conclusions.[45,46] Proceedings indicate that: (*a*) a single, highly accurate diagnostic test for the detection of the degree of risk an individual has for the development of dental caries does not exist; (*b*) it would be naive to expect such a test to emerge, both because of the intrinsic variability among individuals within groups and because of the multifactorial nature of the caries process; and (*c*) the use of multifactorial models combining several factors offers the potential for making relatively good predictions.

Results of studies to date suggest that using available diagnostic methods about 60 and 80 percent of those at risk and not at risk of developing caries, respectively, can be identified accurately when the cutoff for the percentage of the population that is high risk is set at approximately 25 percent. In a comprehensive review, Hausen concluded, somewhat pessimistically, that none of the markers aimed at assessing the risk for coronal caries have predictive power, which reaches a reasonable target of combined sensitivity and specificity of 160 percent.[48] The predictive power of even the strongest markers of high caries risk was modest, and none of the reported measures for assessing caries risk were accurate enough to be relied on mechanically when targeting caries preventive measures.

Even with the realization that the prediction of a multifactorial disease such as dental caries is at best difficult, epidemiologic and risk assessment research during the last decade have had a profound effect on the practice of dentistry and public health. Current practice guidelines for preventive dentistry are encouraging clinicians to base their services on an assessment of an individual's risk so that they will be cost-effective (Table 65-4). Little actual research has been done to develop prediction models for communities, even though the large variation from community to community justifies such an approach. Nevertheless, public health programs are moving toward an assessment of community needs and the specific targeting of appropriate services to whole communities based on these findings.

Prevention and Control of Dental Caries

A large number of well-proven, safe and cost-effective methods are available for use by the public, clinicians, and public health practitioners for the prevention and control of dental caries. Community water fluoridation along with individual use of toothpaste with fluoride provide the background foundation against which other methods build. Guidelines for the use of methods other than water fluoridation have been specified by an expert committee of the American Dental Association. The need for these different methods, which are discussed in the following pages, vary according to the risk of each individual to dental caries (Table 65-5).

Prevention and Control with Fluorides

Comprehensive reviews of the public health benefits and risks of fluoride in drinking water and other sources have been completed by as many as 12 major independent expert panels.[49] Their conclusions are unanimous in support of both the safety and benefits of fluorides. In the United States, recent extensive evaluations by the Public Health Service[50] and the National Research Council[51] confirmed its benefits to the public as well as its safety. Other comprehensive reviews focusing primarily on the dental benefits of fluorides have affirmed their effectiveness as both a public health and individual measure in contributing to the health of the public. The U.S. Preventive Services Task Force[52] and a comparable committee in Canada[53] reviewed methods for preventing the more common oral diseases and make recommendations for interventions to be used by physicians, dentists, and other clinicians. Both judged all major methods for providing fluorides, both systemic and topical, to be well supported by scientific evidence. The goals of fluoride use are to maximize the prevention and control of dental caries, while minimizing the occurrence of enamel fluorosis.

Mechanisms of Action. Fluoride's anticaries properties have been attributed to several characteristics, three of which have received the most support over the years.[54–56] One theory is that fluoride available in plaque and saliva inhibits demineralization of the enamel and en-

TABLE 65-4. CARIES RISK CLASSIFICATION GUIDELINES

	Age Category for Recall Patients[a]	
Risk Category	***Child/Adolescent***	***Adult***
Low	No carious lesions in last year Coalesced or sealed pits and fissures Good oral hygiene Appropriate fluoride use Regular dental visits	No carious lesions in last 3 years Adequately restored surfaces Good oral hygiene Regular dental visits
Moderate	One carious lesion in last year Deep pits and fissures Fair oral hygiene Inadequate fluoride White spots and/or interproximal radiolucencies Irregular dental visits Orthodontic treatment	One carious lesion in last 3 years Exposed roots Fair oral hygiene White spots and/or interproximal radiolucencies Irregular dental visits Orthodontic treatment
High	≥2 carious lesions in last year Past smooth surface caries Elevated *S. mutans* count Deep pits and fissures No/little systemic and topical fluoride exposure Poor oral hygiene Frequent sugar intake Irregular dental visits Inadequate saliva flow Inappropriate bottle-feeding or nursing (infants)	≥2 carious lesions in last 3 years Past root caries; or Large number of exposed roots Elevated *S. mutans* count Deep pits and fissures Poor oral hygiene Frequent sugar intake Inadequate use of topical fluoride Irregular dental visits Inadequate saliva flow

From American Dental Association: Caries diagnosis and risk assessment. A review of preventive strategies and management. J Am Dent Assoc 126(Suppl):1S–24S, 1995.

[a] At initial visit for new patients, if time of last caries experience cannot be determined, a person with no decayed, missing, or filled surfaces (DMFS = 0) would be classified as low risk. A person with past caries experience (DMFS > 0) and/or one active lesion would be classified as moderate risk. A person with past caries experience and/or two active caries or one smooth surface lesion would be classified as high risk.

Parents of young children and expectant parents need additional counseling on inappropriate nursing or bottle-feeding practices, which can lead to the development of baby bottle tooth decay. Parents and caregivers should be advised to introduce children to a cup in an effort to discontinue use of the bottle by the age of 1 year. Also, parents and caregivers should be advised never to place anything other than plain water in a naptime or nighttime bottle. Children should not be allowed to bottle feed at will and should be weaned from the bottle by the age of 1 year.

Many medically compromised individuals are likely to be assessed in the higher risk categories because of their use of certain medications and possible xerostomia.

TABLE 65-5. CARIES PREVENTION MODALITIES BY RISK STATUS AND AGE GROUP: PREVENTIVE OPTIONS FOR RISK CATEGORIES

	Age Category	
Risk Category	***Child/Adolescent***	***Adult***
Low	Educational reinforcement re: good oral hygiene and use of fluoride dentifrice 1-year recall	Educational reinforcement re: good oral hygiene and use of fluoride dentifrice 1-year recall
Moderate	*Pit and Fissure Caries* Sealants *Smooth Surface, Recurrent, and Root Caries* Educational reinforcement Dietary counseling Fluoride mouthrinse[a] Professional topical fluoride Sealants Brush with fluoride dentifrice 6-month recall Fluoride supplements[b]	*Pit and Fissure Caries* Sealants *Smooth Surface, Root, and Recurrent Caries* Educational reinforcement Dietary counseling Fluoride mouthrinse Professional topical fluoride Sealants Brush with fluoride dentifrice 6-month recall
High	*Pit and Fissure Caries* Sealants *Smooth Surface, Recurrent, and Root Caries* Educational reinforcement Brush with fluoride dentifrice Sealants Home fluoride (mouthrinse/1.1% sodium fluoride gel[a]) Professional topical fluoride at each visit 3–6-month recall Dietary counseling Monitoring *S. mutans* count Antimicrobial agents Fluoride supplements[b]	*Pit and Fissure Caries* Sealants *Smooth Surface, Root, and Recurrent Caries* Educational reinforcement Brush with fluoride dentifrice Sealants Home fluoride (mouthrinse/1.1% sodium fluoride gel[a]) Professional topical fluoride at each visit 3–6 month recall Monitoring *S. mutans* count Antimicrobial agents Dietary counseling

From American Dental Association: Caries diagnosis and risk assessment. A review of preventive strategies and management. J Am Dent Assoc 126(Suppl):1S–24S, 1995.
[a] Not for children under 6 years of age.
[b] Age considerations and fluoride content of primary water supply (refer to section on Interventions, Fluoride Supplementation).

hances remineralization, that is, enhances repair, after an acid attack. A second is that fluoride has several antibacterial properties. Its concentration in plaque can be sufficiently high to disrupt bacterial enzyme systems, thus resulting in less acid production and possible prevention of bacterial adhesion to the enamel surface. A third theory holds that, when fluoride is available from systemic sources during tooth development and before teeth erupt into the mouth, it is incorporated into enamel, making its crystalline structure less soluble during acid attack. This traditional theory of how fluoride works has received less support in recent years. Most likely, fluoride works by a combination of these mechanisms, but its topical effects dominate. Thus fluoride works best to prevent dental caries when it is ever-present in the oral cavity at low levels; the source is not as important as its availability.

Fluoridation of Drinking Water. Fluoridation is the process of adding a carefully measured amount of a fluoride compound to drinking water at a level that is optimum for the prevention of dental caries. In the United States and other places with temperate climates, the optimal fluoride levels for community drinking water supplies are between 0.7 and 1.2 parts per million, depending on a community's annual mean maximum daily air temperature. In rural areas without a central community water supply, fluoridation of a school's drinking water is an alternative to community water fluoridation. Because children spend only 5 to 7 hours a day in school, the optimal concentration of fluoride for the school water supply is 4.5 times the optimal level recommended for community water fluoridation for that locale. These programs have many of the benefits of community fluoridation programs, yet have not been utilized extensively, primarily because of the need for personnel with water engineering skills to install and maintain equipment and the need for trained school personnel to monitor the system on a daily basis. In 1992, only slightly more than 100,000 children were attending schools with independent water systems that were fluoridated, and many of these systems have been discontinued since then.

The fluoride story represents one of the true successes in public health. In the United States the story began in 1901 when Dr. Frederick McKay arrived in Colorado Springs, Colorado, to establish his private dental practice. He immediately noticed that many of his patients, particularly those who had lived in the area all their lives, had a permanent stain on their teeth, which he called mottled enamel. A desire to find the cause so that his patients could be helped led to almost three decades of work in which McKay developed two very important hypotheses: that the source of the etiologic agent was most likely the water supply and that those with mottling also appeared to have no increased susceptibility to dental caries, even though the enamel was defective. McKay was joined in his work in 1931 when H. Trendley Dean, a U.S. Public Health Service dentist, was assigned to full-time research on mottled enamel. By 1938, Dean and McKay had documented the prevalence of mottled enamel, which they renamed fluorosis, and provided direct evidence that fluoride in the domestic water was the primary cause.[57] Dean then set about to explore the relationship between fluoride in drinking water and dental caries. His efforts culminated in publication of the famous

TABLE 65-6. POPULATION SERVED BY FLUORIDE-ADJUSTED AND NATURALLY FLUORIDATED WATER, UNITED STATES, 1992

Type of Fluoridation	Population (in millions)	Systems	Communities
Adjusted	134.6	10,567	8,572
Natural	10.0	3,784	1,924
Both	144.6	14,351	10,496

From US Department of Health and Human Services: Fluoridation Census, 1992. Atlanta: Centers for Disease Control and Prevention, Division of Oral Health, 1993, Table II.

"21-cities study," which showed clearly the relationships between increasing fluoride concentration and both decreasing dental caries prevalence and increasing fluorosis.[58] The scientific foundation was laid for the experimental studies on the benefits and safety of adjusting fluoride levels in community water supplies.

Worldwide Status. International statistics on community water fluoridation are difficult to obtain. About 34 countries practice controlled water fluoridation.[59] In some of these countries, such as Australia, Brazil, Canada, Ireland, and New Zealand, large segments of the population are participating.

The latest national data on community water fluoridation for the United States reflect the status of fluoridation as of 1992 (Table 65-6).[60] About 144.6 million people, or 62 percent of the population on public water supplies, consume water with optimal fluoride levels. Of that total, roughly 134.6 million people were on public water systems that were adjusting the fluoride content to optimum levels, while approximately 10 million people consumed water from community systems with adequate natural fluoride levels. To these totals can be added those special populations served by fluoridated systems, including schoolchildren benefiting through fluoridated school water supplies, American Indian and Alaskan Natives on reservations with fluoridated water systems, and residents of American military bases with fluoridated systems. Of the 50 largest cities in the United States, 42 are currently fluoridated.

As the population has increased, a steady increase in the total U.S. population served by fluoridation has occurred over the first 50 years of its implementation. While many states and large cities were quick to implement fluoridation programs in the 1950s and 1960s, the trend thereafter began to level off. In the absence of categorical funding, Congress deferred fluoridation decisions to the states, which in turn largely left the responsibility to enact such measures to local governments and city councils. The net effect has been that the gap between the total population on public water systems and the population on those systems with fluoride has not closed in recent years. Forty-four percent of the U.S. population does not drink fluoridated water, about 88 million of whom are drinking public water that does not have fluoride added to it. Those not benefiting from fluoridation are geographically concentrated in certain states and regions of the country. Located within California are 93 of the 153 largest nonfluoridated cities and 99 of the 253 nonfluoridated water systems serving populations greater than 50,000 in the United States. Twenty-five more of these 253 cities are in the northeast corridor of the United States (New Jersey, New York, Maine, Rhode Island, Delaware, Vermont, New Hampshire, Massachusetts, Pennsylvania, and West Virginia).[61]

To stimulate adoption of fluoridation and help reach the national year 2000 fluoridation objective of having 75 percent of people using public drinking water that is fluoridated, a National Fluoridation Plan To Promote Oral Health has been developed by the U.S. Public Health Service (PHS).[61] This Plan, published in 1996, reaffirms the commitment of federal health agencies to community water fluoridation and describes coordinated policy and research efforts that should be undertaken by various public agencies and the private sector to ensure that all Americans benefit from appropriate exposure to fluorides. Early successes are evident. As part of this effort, a PHS field office was established in California to assist in the promotion of community water fluoridation. In October 1995, the Governor of California signed into law a bill mandating statewide water fluoridation, and the private sector has provided funds to help support this effort.

Benefits of Water Fluoridation. The first city in the world to adjust fluoride in its water supply to optimal levels was Grand Rapids, Michigan, United States, in 1945.[62] Grand Rapids was quickly followed by other U.S. cities: Newburgh, New York, in the same year and by Evanston, Illinois, and in Canada by Branford, Ontario, in 1946. These four cities became part of a pioneering effort to evaluate the benefits of fluoridation. Dental caries rates in all of these cities were compared to matched control cites, Muskegon, Kingston, Oak Park, and Sarnia, respectively, in the early years of the trial. However, Grand Rapids and Evanston lost the comparison city to fluoridation in subsequent years, and a historical control was used. Results at the end of the study period are presented in Table 65-7[63] and demonstrate reductions of 48 to 70 percent in caries experience of adolescents after lifetime exposure.

In an extensive review of the results of 95 studies conducted between 1945 and 1978, Murray and Rugg-Gunn reported the modal percentage caries reduction following controlled water fluoridation to be 40 to 50 percent for primary teeth and 50 to 60 percent for permanent teeth.[64] Newbrun reviewed studies conducted during the 1980s, limiting his review to those with concurrent control groups because of the decline in dental caries.[65] Over 60 comparisons for fluoride-deficient and fluoridated communities, including studies in the United

TABLE 65-7. DMF TEETH AND MISSING TEETH PER CHILD, FIRST FOUR COMMUNITY FLUORIDATION TRIALS

City	Year	DMFT	Difference (%)	MT	Difference (%)
Grand Rapids	1944	9.58		0.84	
Ages 12–14	1959	4.26	−55.5	0.29	−65.5
Evanston	1946	9.03		0.19	
Ages 12–14	1959	4.66	−48.4	0.06	−68.4
Sarnia	1959	7.46		0.75	
Branford Ages 12–14	1959	3.23	−56.7	0.22	−70.7
Kingston	1960	12.46		0.92	
Newburgh Ages 13–14	1960	3.73	−70.1	0.10	−89.1

From Ast DB, Fitzgerald B: Effectiveness of water fluoridation. J Am Dent Assoc 65:581–587, 1962.

States, Australia, Britain, Canada, Ireland, and New Zealand, as well as several age groups, consistently demonstrated the present-day effectiveness of water fluoridation. The range of caries reductions for children and adolescents in fluoridated as compared with fluoride-deficient communities is now approximately 20 to 40 percent. Fluoridation benefits also are evident in studies of middle-age adults and seniors, ranging from 20 to 30 percent and 17 to 35 percent, respectively. Benefits to adults and seniors include reductions in the prevalence of both coronal and root caries.

The evidence pointing to smaller differences in dental caries experience between those individuals now living in fluoridated and nonfluoridated communities compared to the results obtained from studies done from 1945 to 1978 does not mean that the effectiveness of water fluoridation has declined. Rather, this situation is due to two primary factors—the diffusion effects of fluoridated water and the dilution effects of other sources of fluoride, both of which have contributed to a decline in caries in the usual comparison nonfluordiated populations.[66] Many beverages and foods are prepared with fluoridated water and distributed to nonfluoridated areas, providing a diffusion of fluoridation benefits beyond those living in fluoridated areas. With the exception of fluoride supplements, most fluoride products are designed for use by both those drinking and not drinking fluoridated water. These fluoride rinses, gels, and toothpastes are all in common use by professionals or the public and are known to be effective in lowering the prevalence of dental caries, particularly in those populations at high risk for decay such as those drinking fluoride-deficient water. Essentially, the effect of these two trends in fluoride exposures is to eliminate the possibility of a true comparison group in studies of the dental benefits of water fluoridation.

Other evidence on the benefits of fluoridation comes from studies of populations where fluoridation has ceased. Studies in the United States, Germany, and Scotland have shown that, when fluoridation is withdrawn, caries rates increase. In Wick, Scotland, which started water fluoridation in 1969 but stopped it in 1979, the caries prevalence in 5- to 6-year-olds increased by 27 percent between 1979 and 1984, despite a national decline in caries and increased availability of fluoride-containing dentifrices.[67]

Costs and Cost-Effectiveness of Fluoridation. The smaller differences now being found in the prevalence of dental caries between those living in fluoridated compared to fluoride-deficient communities have raised questions about the possible reduced cost-effectiveness of water fluoridation. The increase in environmental fluorides since water fluoridation was first introduced in 1945, particularly from fluoride-containing toothpastes, mouthrinses, foods and drinks, and professional sources, generally provides the basis for this issue, along with the evidence of declining caries. Water fluoridation continues to be a cost-effective strategy for caries prevention, even in those areas where the overall caries level has declined and where the cost of implementing water fluoridation has increased.[68,69]

The annual cost of fluoridation per person is estimated to be from 12 to 21 cents in large communities (more than 200,000), 18 to 75 cents for medium-sized communities (10,000 to 200,000), and 60 cents to $5.41 for small communities (less than 10,000). The larger variability in small communities is due to the high degree of sensitivity to changes in capital investment, labor, number of injection points, and type of fluoride material used. Of all persons receiving optimally fluoridated drinking water, 85 percent are served by water systems for which the annual per capita cost of fluoridation is 12 to 75 cents.[68] The Centers for Disease Control and Prevention (CDC) has estimated that each $1 spent on water fluoridation results in a savings of $80 in dental treatment.[69] Water fluoridation provides cost savings, a rare characteristic of public health promotion and disease prevention strategies.

Safety of Fluoridation. Over the years, fluoridation has been attacked as being part of a variety of conspiracies and the cause of numerous diseases.[49] The most persistent question raised about the safety of fluoridation is its role in various types of cancers. Extensive reviews, expert commissions, and numerous studies have failed to find a link between fluoride and cancer. An animal study directed by the U.S. National Toxicology Program (NTP), a unit of the National Institute of Environmental Health Sciences and charged with developing and evaluating scientific information about potentially toxic and hazardous chemicals, revived the controversy over fluoride's cancer-causing potential in 1990.[70] The results of this 2-year study were evaluated extensively by an expert panel of external reviewers and by the interested community. The panel of reviewers agreed with the final conclusion of the NTP that there was no evidence or that the evidence was too weak to attribute any detrimental health effects to fluoride administration. A subsequent review by the PHS confirmed that there is no indication that fluoride causes cancer in humans.[50] The report recommended that communities continue to add fluoride to water supplies for preventing dental caries when less than optimal levels of this ion are present. Subsequently, the Assistant Secretary of Health and the Surgeon General jointly signed a policy statement in support of water fluoridation. Today, the U.S. Public Health Service and virtually every other national health organization in the United States support the use of fluorides for the prevention of dental caries.[71]

The PHS review of fluorides noted that the prevalence of enamel fluorosis has increased in both fluoridated and nonfluoridated communities over the last several years, signaling an increase in total fluoride intake in infants and young children. Fluorosis is considered an esthetic problem in a small percentage of those who are affected, but has no other health affects. Public and professional use of fluoride products such as toothpastes, mouthrinses, gels, and dietary supplements have increased since water fluoridation began. All of these must be used according to recommended guidelines to prevent excessive fluoride intake.

Public Policy and Fluoridation. The legality of fluoridation in the United States has been thoroughly tested in our court system, and no court of last resort has ever rendered an opinion against fluoridation. The highest courts of more than a dozen states have confirmed the constitutionality of fluoridation. The U.S. Supreme Court has denied review of fluoridation on every occasion—more than 12 times—citing that no substantial federal or constitutional questions were involved.[72]

States vary considerably in their constitutional provisions on how fluoridation laws are enacted. Nine states currently mandate community water fluoridation (California, Connecticut, Georgia, Illinois, Michigan, Minnesota, Nebraska, Ohio, and South Dakota). Some of these states (Delaware, Maine, Nevada, New Hampshire, and Utah) require a public vote before fluoridation can be instituted. In the remaining states, authorization to fluoridate a public water supply can be established by administrative decision, by governing body legislation, or by voter initiative. The most effective means to implementing fluoridation at the community level, in the absence of a state mandate, is to pursue promotion with the local governing body or officials rather than through a referendum. Of those community fluoridation decisions made from 1980 to 1989, 78 percent were successful when only a governing body was involved in the decision-making, while only 37 percent were successful when subjected to voter referenda.[73]

Summary. Today, community fluoridation is viewed as the single most cost-effective, practical, and safe public health measure available to prevent dental caries. Water fluoridation continues to be the cornerstone of community oral disease prevention. It is specifically identified as a critical technology for protecting the public's health in the "population-based core functions."[74] Research conducted over virtually the entire twentieth century has proven fluoridation to be an ideal public health measure. Its characteristics can be summarized as follows: it is the least expensive and most effective way to reduce dental caries; it is eminently safe; it benefits adults as well as children; it provides benefits that last a lifetime when consumption of the water continues; it reduces the cost of children's dental treatment; it is the fairest way for everyone in a community to benefit, regardless of income, education, or the financial ability to seek dental care services;

and it requires no individual effort or direct action by those who will benefit.[62] Yet, considerable work remains to be done in extending the benefits of fluoridation to all communities.

Dietary Fluoride Supplements

Dietary fluoride supplements in the form of fluoride-containing vitamins, drops, or tablets are an alternative way to provide systemic and topical fluorides to those children not benefiting from community or school water fluoridation. Fluoride supplements are available to individuals only by prescription and can be taken at home beginning at 6 months of age. They also can be administered to groups of children in community programs, usually school-based programs. While there are a number of supplement programs run by public health agencies, the majority of supplements are prescribed by physicians or dentists in private-practice settings. Of primary care physicians and dentists, physicians prescribe the majority of supplements.

Over 50 reports on the effectiveness of fluoride tablets or drops have appeared in the literature indicating that their use is effective in preventing dental caries in both the primary and permanent dentitions.[55] Estimates of effectiveness vary considerably because of differences in study design, age at which subjects started taking supplements, and compliance, particularly with home-based administration where cooperation can fall off dramatically. Historically, estimates of effectiveness for home administration range from 40 to 80 percent if supplementation begins before 2 years of age. Combining fluoride and vitamin supplementation does not appear to have any effect on the caries inhibiting effect of supplements. For school-based programs, effectiveness appears to be lower and variable, with an average of approximately 30 percent. School-based programs are highly effective in preventing caries in permanent teeth in high-risk children when administration is tightly controlled and when children are instructed to let the fluoride tablets dissolve slowly in their mouths each school day to ensure as high an intraoral topical fluoride level as possible. The most recent dietary fluoride supplement study is now almost a decade old, so the actual number of cavities prevented in children and the reduction compared to control subjects is probably lower than those provided in existing reviews. In locations where caries rates are low, public health programs have moved away from fluoride supplement programs, primarily based on cost-effectiveness and practical concerns, and some expert panels have suggested that they have limited to no use in public programs.[54,75,76]

Prenatal fluoride supplements are not recommended. Claims have been made to their effectiveness, but only one double-blind study has been done. In this study, 1,400 pregnant women living in communities without fluoridation were allocated to either a prenatal fluoride supplementation group (1 mg F tablet daily during the last 6 months of pregnancy) or one where identical placebo preparations were taken. Postnatally all were provided with the same fluoride-containing supplement for distribution to their infants whose primary teeth were examined for dental caries at 5 years of age. While there was a trend in favor of the prenatal group, a statistically significant difference between groups was not achieved.[77]

Prescribing of fluoride tablets or drops for children, often in association with vitamins, is widespread in the United States. Brunelle and Carlos reported that in 1986–1987, 54.2 percent of U.S. children ages 5 to 17 years living in communities without fluoridation reported use of supplemental fluorides.[31] State and national surveys indicate that 32 to 86 percent of physicians and 21 to 93 percent of dentists prescribe supplements.[78,79] These studies also showed that some practitioners are unaware of the proper dosage guidelines for supplementation, the contraindications for their use, and the actual fluoride concentration in water supplies where they practice. Of note was the finding that 14.8 percent of U.S. children 5 to 17 years of age drinking fluoridated community water also reported use of fluoride supplements.[31] Also of concern are the results of a study by Levy and Carrell in which compliance by health care providers with the recommended fluoride supplement protocol was determined in patients for whom water fluoride analyses were performed prior to prescription of fluoride tablets or drops.[79] Even in patients with assay results available to the prescribing provider, one-third of child patients and one-half of their siblings did not receive the correct supplement dosage based on age and fluoride content of their drinking water. The seriousness of the inappropriate prescription of supplements is illustrated by results of a study by Pendrys et al.[80] They found a 23-fold increase in risk of mild-to-moderate enamel fluorosis associated with the use of fluoride supplements by children living in optimally fluoridated areas.

Supplement Protocol. With the increased availability of fluorides from sources such as diet, toothpaste, and the dilution of concentrated or powdered baby formulas with fluoridated water, adherence to the appropriate protocol in fluoride supplementation is critical to provide maximum protection without risks of fluorosis. Before a fluoride supplement is prescribed, it is essential that adequate fluoride histories be taken. If the fluoride content of the patient's home or school water supply is unknown, for example, if the patient drinks water from a private well or it cannot be determined if the patient is on a public water system, major sources of the patient's drinking water must be obtained and assayed for fluoride content. Natural fluorides occur in many geographic areas, and within any one area its concentration in water can be highly variable. Many state health departments and dental schools provide assay services at a nominal fee. Services also are available from commercial laboratories. Once the fluoride levels in drinking water are determined and a prescription written, the patient must be monitored to encourage compliance and to make adjustments in the dosage should the patient's fluoride exposure change.

Dosage Schedule. At least 18 different dosage schedules for fluoride tablets and drops have been published for different countries around the world. In recent years there has been a tendency to revise schedules and reduce the dosage for young children. These revisions are a direct result of concerns about the contribution that fluoride supplements make to the prevalence of fluorosis. The fluoride supplement dosage for the United States was recently revised by the American Dental Association, the American Academy of Pediatric Dentistry, and the American Academy of Pediatrics (Table 65-8).[47] The major change from the previous 1979 schedule is that the recommended dosage schedule is reduced for children younger than 6 years of age.

Other Sources of Therapeutic Fluorides

A number of fluoride-containing gels, solutions, pastes, foams, and varnishes are available for topical application. These fluorides fall into two categories: those applied by professionals and those that are self-applied at home or in other settings such as elementary schools, generally as part of public health programs. Topical fluoride products designed for professional use generally have high concentrations of fluoride, while those designed for self-application have low concentrations.

TABLE 65-8. DIETARY FLUORIDE SUPPLEMENT DOSAGE SCHEDULE

	Fluoride in Water (ppm)		
Age of Child	*<0.3*	*0.3–0.6*	*>0.6*
Birth to 6 months	None	None	None
6 months to 3 years	0.25 mg/d	None	None
3 to 6 years	0.50 mg/d	0.25 mg/d	None
6 to 16 years	1.00 mg/d	0.50 mg/d	None

From American Dental Association: Caries diagnosis and risk assessment. A review of preventive strategies and management. J. Am Dent Assoc 126 (Suppl):1S–24S, 1995.

Professionally Applied Topical Fluorides. Pioneering efforts testing the effectiveness of solutions containing sodium fluoride (NaF), stannous fluoride, and acidulated phosphate fluoride (APF) in preventing dental caries were conducted by Bibby, Muhler et al, and Brudevold and Chilton, respectively, beginning with Bibby's work in 1943.[81–83] Many controlled clinical trails conducted during the 1940s through the 1970s documented their benefits. Few studies of their effectiveness have been done in the United States in the last few years, particularly with groups of children having low risks for caries similar to today's levels. Several excellent reviews of the effectiveness of these three compounds have been published.[84–87] In general, there are no clear data supporting the superiority of one of these fluoride compounds over another.

The initial use of these fluoride compounds in aqueous solutions has given way since the 1960s to gels, an aqueous solution with an added organic compound to provide increased stickiness and viscosity. Their popularity is based upon their handling characteristics, which make them easy to use in a mouth-tray or in brush-on techniques, and upon patient acceptance. There are currently two types of topical fluoride gel products available for professional use in the United States: APF and NaF compounds with 12,300 ppm (1.23 percent fluoride) and 9,040 ppm F (2 percent fluoride), respectively.

The APF technique has proven to reduce dental caries in permanent teeth of children by about 30 percent in fluoridated and in fluoride-deficient communities even though the absolute reduction in dental caries is less in fluoridated communities. Little information is available on the effect of topical fluoride applications on root caries in adults. Collectively, however, these studies support their value for the prevention of root caries.

With the decrease in dental caries, the application of topical fluorides should not be performed routinely on everyone, but should be based on caries risk assessments of the individual. Generally, individuals drinking fluoridated water do not need topical fluoride application. Children and adults who are caries active should receive topical applications about every 6 months, regardless of their exposure to systemic fluorides. Individuals with rapidly progressing caries brought on by radiation to the head and neck, developmental disabilities, eating disorders, or drastic caries promoting life-style changes might need more frequent applications. Topical fluorides are more effective on newly erupted teeth. A prophylaxis is not required before fluoride application. Fluoride prophylaxis pastes, although widely used in clinical settings, have not been adequately tested in clinical trials to support their efficacy an a means for providing topical fluoride treatments. Currently, they are not recommended for use in school programs in countries with low caries levels.

Fluoride varnishes, first introduced in 1968, are used extensively in Europe. They are viscous, resinous lacquers painted onto teeth. Since the varnish adheres to the enamel surface for prolonged periods (up to 12 hours or more) there is increased retention of fluoride in the mouth resulting in greater fluoride uptake in plaque and enamel compared to solutions or gels. Reviews suggest that the two older products, Duraphat (2.26 percent fluoride) and Fluor Protector (0.7 percent fluoride), are caries inhibitory. Carex (1.8 percent fluoride), a new product, has been tested in Norway and found equivalent to Duraphat. The American Dental Association has not approved their use in the United States, although the U.S. Food and Drug Administration approved in 1994 the marketing of DuraFlor, the name for Duraphat chosen for marketing in the United States. Like other topicals, they should be used for high-risk individuals only, and application frequency should be every 3 to 6 months. They have the advantage over other topicals in that they can be used safely in very young children and in the disabled. For this reason, several public health programs are testing the feasibility of their use in the treatment of early childhood caries.

Self-Applied Topical Fluorides. A number of fluoride gels and rinses are available for use by individuals for self-application, along with fluoride-containing dentifrices. These products are a safe means of providing caries protection to children and adults.

Fluoride rinses were developed during the 1960s as a public health measure to be used primarily in school settings. They were a direct result of the high expense associated with professional applications in school settings and the poor patient acceptance of brush-on fluoride pastes. As a result of extensive study, three fluoride rinse systems, 0.2 percent sodium fluoride (900 ppm F) used once per week, 0.05 percent sodium fluoride (225 ppm F) used daily, and 0.2 percent APF fluoride (225 ppm F) used daily were approved by the U.S. Food and Drug Administration[88] and accepted by the American Dental Association.[89] With favorable results derived from a 17-community national demonstration project funded by the National Institute of Dental Research, as many as 12 million U.S. schoolchildren were participating in supervised weekly fluoride mouthrinse programs (10-mL dose of 0.2 percent NaF) at their height.[90] These school-based rinse programs are popular because they are inexpensive and require little professional supervision or time—5 to 10 minutes once every week. With the declining prevalence of dental caries becoming more pronounced, the cost-effectiveness of these programs is reduced and generally are not recommended for use in low–caries risk communities. These fluoride mouthrinse programs also are not recommended for preschool children, and 5 mL of solution is used for kindergarten children because they often are unable to prevent swallowing of the solution.

Low fluoride concentration (0.05 percent neutral sodium fluoride or 0.1 percent stannous fluoride) and high-frequency (daily) rinses designed for home use are available over-the-counter. Other rinses and gels (some with as much as 5,000 ppm fluoride) are available by prescription for home use. Several trials evaluating fluoride mouthrinse in combination with fluoride dentifrices suggest that for most children fluoride rinses offer little benefit over the use of fluoride dentifrices alone. Thus all of these fluoride products are recommended only for adolescents and adults at moderate or high risk for caries, especially those individuals undergoing head and neck radiation, orthodontic treatment, or taking medications or with diseases that decrease salivary flow.

Fluoride-containing dentifrices are clearly an important component of efforts to prevent and control dental caries. These dentifrices are ideal for caries control because of their ease of use, ability to produce significant reductions in dental caries, and low cost. The decline in dental caries has been attributed in part to their widespread use because the daily use of this product is in keeping with current theories of the role that fluoride plays in the de-remineralization phenomenom.[91] First marketed in the United States in 1955, they gained approval from the Council of Dental Therapeutics of the American Dental Association in 1964. The different brands containing fluoride now represent about 95 percent of sales in countries where dentifrices are sold. The clinical efficacy of the fluoride agents used in most dentifrices (SnF_2, Na_2PO_3F, NaF, amine F) is undisputed, and a review of clinical studies shows them to be at least similar in effectiveness. Use of these dentifrices in a fluoride-deficient community can result in reductions in dental caries of from 15 to 40 percent. Benefits also can be expected from their use in fluoridated communities.[87] While less well documented in clinical trials, they also are thought to be effective in the prevention of root caries in adults. They are recommended for daily use by all patients, regardless of risk category.

Of concern from a public health standpoint is the possibility of fluoride ingestion by young children when using fluoride-containing dentifrices. Since the fluoride concentration in dentifrices is approximately 1,000 ppm, it is possible for a child to consume 1 mg or more of fluoride per day from inadvertent ingestion. Children who have a habit of ingesting their dentifrice and who also reside in an optimally fluoridated community or are receiving dietary fluoride supplements can have a total fluoride consumption capable of producing enamel fluorosis. An estimated 71 percent of mild-to-moderate fluorosis cases in fluoridated communities can be explained by a history of brushing more than once a day with an amount of toothpaste greater than the recommended amount throughout the first 8 years of life.[92] Young children should not be restricted in their use of fluoride toothpastes. Rather, parents should be careful to place a small amount of toothpaste on the child's brush (about a pea-sized amount) and to supervise brushing of children younger than 6 years of age.

Prevention and Control with Pit and Fissure Dental Sealants

Fluoride is most effective in preventing dental caries on smooth tooth surfaces and least effective on those surfaces with pits and fissures. These numerous pits and fissures, primarily on biting surfaces of the teeth, are at high risk for dental caries because they retain food debris and microorganisms that are hard to remove by cleaning. Dental sealants, first introduced in the late 1960s and given full acceptance by the American Dental Association in 1976,[93] are plastic materials that are applied as a thin coating over the pits and fissures of the teeth and are effective in protecting them from caries attack. Most of the dozen products approved by the American Dental Association contain no therapeutic agent but work by providing a physical barrier, thus preventing microorganisms and food particles from collecting within the pits and fissures and initiating the acid conditions necessary for caries to begin. To be most effective, their placement is required in young children who are at risk for decay soon after the teeth erupt, but they can be needed throughout a wide age span because risk for caries can continue unabated in an individual or change from low to high risk as one goes through life. Dental sealants are an ideal conservative procedure because they require no removal of tooth structure. The epidemiology of dental caries provides a strong rationale for sealant use. Presently, biting surfaces represent 56 percent of permanent tooth surfaces affected with dental caries, but if the pits and fissures on the cheek and tongue side of teeth are included, from 80 to 90 percent of surfaces can benefit from sealants.[32] Ripa has argued that the need for sealants might even be greater than before because pit and fissure surfaces of permanent molars are the most susceptible surfaces and teeth, and the slower progression of lesions has extended caries susceptibility beyond the first few years after tooth eruption.[94]

Several comprehensive reviews of sealant retention and the amount of caries prevented by their use are available.[95–98] The most recent of these reviews pooled results from 44 studies and found that 71 percent of caries is avoided by use of autopolymerized sealants.[97] Three studies have followed sealant retention and caries prevention for 10 years or more.[99–101] The longest running of these found that a one-time application of sealants reduced occlusal caries by 52 percent after 15 years.[101] Evidence suggests that sealants can be up to 100 percent effective when fissures are resealed as needed.[100] When combined with other dental caries preventive strategies, sealants have the potential to virtually eliminate dental caries in children. The cost-effectiveness and cost savings of dental sealants have not been evaluated extensively. However, studies by Simonsen[101] and Weintraub et al.[102] provide an indication that sealants might not only be cost-effective, but perhaps can be included in that select group of preventive procedures that provide cost savings if used in high-risk individuals.

Dentists have been slow to adopt sealants despite their proven effectiveness and safety. By the end of the 1980s, fewer than two of every 10 children in the United States had any sealants in their permanent teeth, leaving a great deal of work to be done during the next decade to reach the 50 percent sealant prevalence targeted for 8- and 14-year olds for the year 2000.[103] Reasons given by dentists for not using them include a preference for amalgam restorations, concerns about retention and sealing in caries, patients' difficulties in understanding their value, and the perception that insurance programs do not include sealants among their covered services. All of these concerns are unfounded. Even the sealing of small cavities is now recommended as a conservative treatment that arrests decay and can prevent the need for fillings, a more expensive and invasive dental procedure.[104,105]

A number of initiatives in the early 1990s brought attention to dental sealants and their underutilization as a preventive procedure.[105] The U.S. Surgeon General issued a policy statement in strong support of their use; the federal Maternal and Child Health (MCH) Bureau made sealants one of 28 national MCH objectives that states are charged with addressing through their Title V MCH Block Grant funds; all 50 states had included sealants as a benefit in their Medicaid programs; a national resource center providing a comprehensive school-based sealant program manual, videotapes, and reprints of pertinent articles and recommendations was established (National Maternal and Child Oral Health Resource Center in Arlington, VA); and new guidelines for their use in private practice and in public programs had been published.

As a result of these initiatives, the use of sealants is increasing in dental offices and community settings. Over 90 percent of dentists report using sealants, and more than one-half the states have implemented school-based or school-linked sealant programs. Sealants can play an important role in further gains in caries reductions in the next century. However, public and professional efforts need to continue to promote their use according to guidelines, which will help ensure their cost-effective use in private and community settings.

Dietary Control

Health professionals and the public generally are aware of the potential for frequent consumption of refined carbohydrates to result in caries in both children and adults. Less awareness appears to exist about the cause of nursing caries in toddlers and its control. In a survey of expectant parents attending prenatal classes in the Boston area, 54 percent thought that a bottle of milk at other than regular feeding times would not harm the teeth of the infant, and 84 percent had never heard of nursing caries.[106] An estimated 16.7 percent, or 3.5 million U.S. children age 6 months through 5 years have been put to sleep at bedtime or naptime with a bottle with contents other than water, and thus are at risk for severe early childhood caries. About 8 percent of those age 2 through 5 years still used a bottle with contents other than water. The main strategy for preventing nursing caries is to alert prospective parents and new parents about the condition and its causes and to clinically monitor children so that early signs of the condition can be followed with intensive preventive regimens. High-risk groups, or those in which more than 50 percent of children have inappropriate feeding practices every day, and thus should be targeted for intervention, include: parents with less than a high school education, Hispanics, those with a family income of $7,000 to $14,000, and those who had no dental visit during the year for children 2 through 5 years of age. Intervention programs that can be used in these efforts have been described.[107]

▸ PERIODONTAL DISEASES

Pathogenesis and Etiology

The term *periodontal disease* is used to refer to a collection of diseases of the hard and soft tissues surrounding the teeth. The majority of adults show residual signs of past infection or current signs, ranging from swollen gums that bleed under gentle pressure to deep, bacteria-infested gingival crevices that compromise the attachment of the teeth. Plaque-associated gingivitis is the most common of the periodontal diseases. It is an inflammation of the gingiva (gum tissue) and is characterized clinically by redness, gingival bleeding, edema or enlargement, and gingival sensitivity and tenderness. Periodontitis is an inflammation of the supporting tissues of the teeth, usually a progressively destructive change leading to loss of bone and periodontal ligament. Destructive periodontal diseases can be thought of as a series of episodic infections that affect single or multiple periodontal sites within the oral cavity. Destruction of the underlying supporting tissues can occur rapidly, followed by periods of remission of disease activity. Gingivitis and periodontitis are two separate but related diseases. Gingivitis does not always progress to periodontitis but periodontitis has not yet been reported without a preceding gingivitis. Once periodontitis is initiated, gingivitis is not necessary for the destruction of deeper periodontal structures to continue. Left untreated, periodontal diseases can result in formation of periodontal "pockets," a deepening of the space between the tooth and gums, called the gingival crevice, loosening of the teeth, and their ultimate loss.

The 1989 World Workshop in Clinical Periodontics identified five types of destructive periodontal diseases: adult periodontitis, early-onset periodontitis, periodontitis associated with systemic disease, necrotizing ulcerative periodontitis, and refractory periodontitis.[108] Adult periodontitis is by far the most common of these and is the one dealt with in this chapter. In their early stages, these diseases generally go unnoticed by the public because they are painless and do not interfere with function.

Bacteria organized into plaque, the soft, sticky film that coats the tooth surface within hours of brushing, are the primary causes of gingivitis and the various forms of periodontitis. Classic studies by Loe and his colleagues in the early 1960s demonstrated the cause-and-effect relationship between plaque and gingivitis.[109] Until the early 1960s, the amount of dental plaque rather than its composition was considered to be the most important etiologic factor in disease. Based on knowledge at the time, etiologic models of periodontal disease emphasized an overgrowth of plaque. These models evolved into those that suggest that the amount of plaque is less important than the specific pathogens or groups of pathogens in the plaque. Recent etiologic models emphasize the multifactorial nature of the disease, with the role of host and environmental factors being elevated in importance. Because several studies found that less than 20 percent of disease can be explained by levels of specific microorganisms, periodontal diseases are best thought of now as "specific mixed infections which cause periodontal destruction in the appropriately susceptible host."[110,111]

Of over 300 species of microorganisms that comprise the oral microbiota, about 30 are suspected of being pathogenic of destructive disease. Difficulties in studying the microbiology of periodontal diseases have slowed progress in determining specific periodontal pathogens, but the etiologic evidence is considered strong for three microorganisms—*Actinobacillus actinomycetemcomitans, Porphyromonas gingivalis,* and *Bacteroides forsythus.*[111] The first of these most often is found in early-onset periodontitis, whereas the other two are found more frequently in adult onset periodontitis. Initial to moderate evidence exists for the importance of more than a dozen other microorganisms in the etiology of periodontitis.

Offenbacher[110] has described an eight-step model of periodontal disease pathogenesis, which helps define the critical path for disease expression (Fig. 65-2). This model incorporates the primary role of both virulent microorganisms capable of evading neutrophil clearance and the host response and is based on the biology of infections within the body. It also can account for the possibility of periodontal disease being a risk factor for systemic conditions such as cardiovascular disease and pregnancy complications. The model places more emphasis on the host response to neutrophil-evading organisms than some etiologic models that emphasize the development of an imbalance in an otherwise stable oral flora. Offenbacher's model specifies

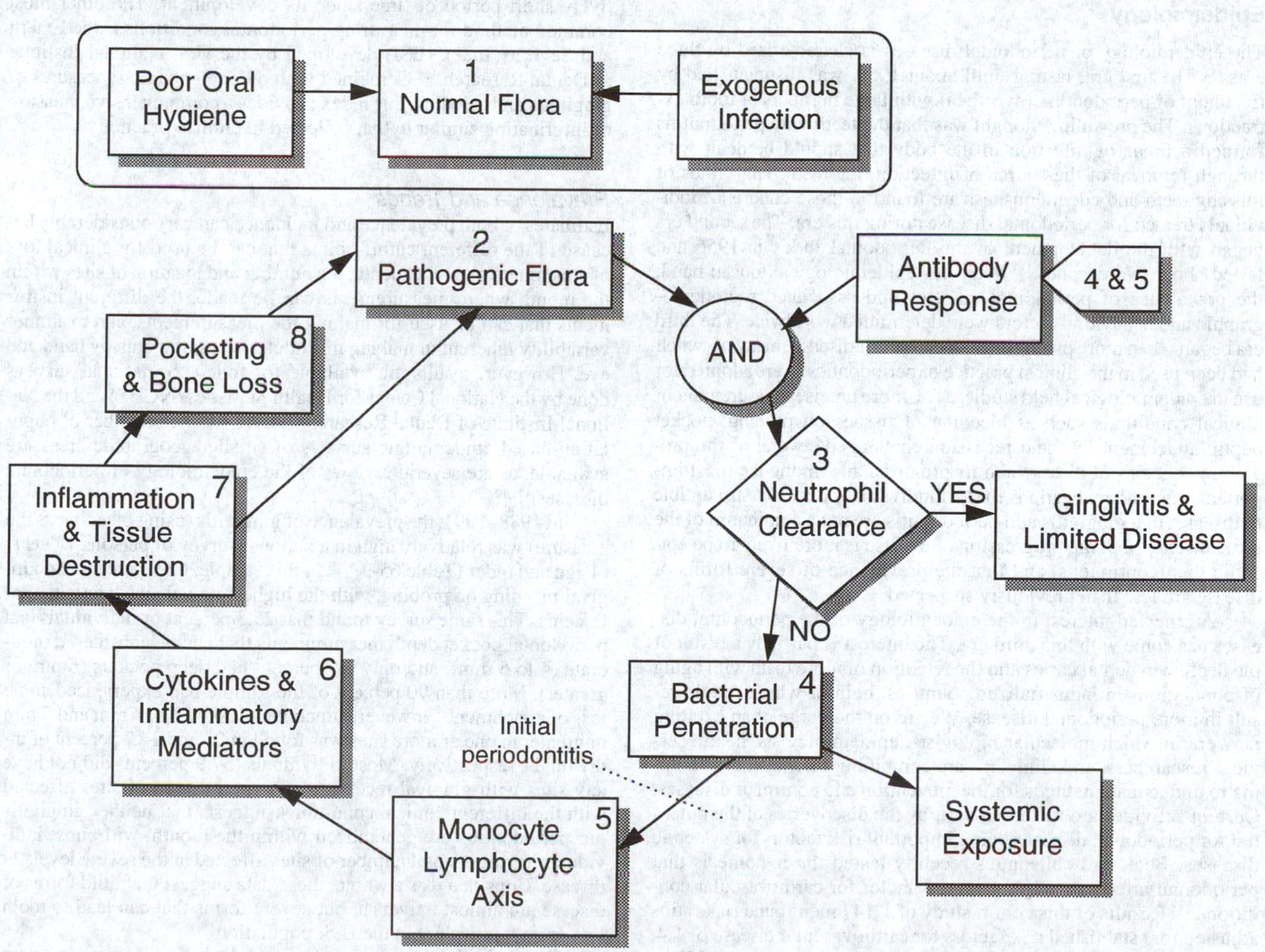

Figure 65-2. Critical pathway model of pathogenesis for periodontal diseases. (From Offenbacher S: Periodontal diseases: pathogenesis. Ann Periodontol 1:821–878, 1996.)

that with normal flora (step 1) the pathogenic cycle will not develop. If microorganisms (step 2) are acquired through either a bacterial overgrowth from poor oral hygiene or an exogenous source and these organisms are capable of evading neutrophil clearance (or the host neutrophil is dysfunctional) (step 3), then the disease can progress beyond gingivitis. The host response (steps 4 and 5) to gingivitis is characteristic of a superficial infection probably because the neutrophil is capable of controlling the infection, but with deeper bacterial penetration of the tissues (step 4) periodontitis is initiated and the body mounts a more aggressive antibody response (step 5), the degree of the response being affected by genetic differences in MO/T-cell response traits. The bacterial lipopolysaccharides (LPS) challenge to the monocytic/lymphocytic axis results in the secretion of catabolic cytokines and inflammatory mediators (step 6). These inflammatory mediators will elicit clinical signs of inflammation, connective tissue destruction, and attachment loss with pocketing and bone loss (steps 7 and 8). Inflammation and pocketing provide both nutrients and an ideal growth environment for continuation of the cycle. Host stress, genetic traits, and risk factors such as diabetes or smoking can affect key nodes in the pathway and result in changes such as impaired neutrophil clearance or enhanced inflammatory response and more clinical inflammation and disease. The model allows for the possibility that periodontal infection also can serve as a reservoir of "periotoxins" such as LPS, prostaglandin E_2 (PGE_2), tumor necrosis factor (TNF), and interluekin-1 (IL-1) that might have systemic effects.

Epidemiology

The epidemiology of periodontal diseases is characterized by three eras.[112] The first era, lasting until about 1950, was distinguished by treatment of periodontitis (pyorrhea) with large numbers of tooth extractions. The prevailing thought was that the teeth with periodontitis formed a focus of infection in the body that should be dealt with through removal of the source of infection, the teeth. High rates of missing teeth and edentulousness are found in those cohorts of individuals treated for periodontal disease during this era. The second era began with the development of the Periodontal Index in 1956 and lasted about two decades.[113] With this epidemiological tool in hand, the prevalence of periodontal diseases and associated sociodemographic and behavioral factors were determined worldwide. The third era began when more precise measurements of disease, many of which had been used in the clinical practice of periodontics, were adopted for use in epidemiological field studies. The more precise measurement of clinical conditions such as bleeding of tissues on probing, pocket depth, attachment loss and recession challenged several of the prevailing concepts of disease and its progression. Among the most important were the realizations that all individuals were not susceptible to disease, that gingivitis and periodontitis are not a continuum of the same disease, that the progression of disease is more likely to be episodic than continuous, and that the prevalence of severe forms of disease are less than previously suspected.

A renewed interest in the epidemiology of the periodontal diseases has come with this third era. The interest is partially a result of the decline in dental caries and the retention of more teeth with aging of populations in industrialized countries, both of which should result in more periodontal disease. We are on the verge of an exciting new era in which molecular biologists, epidemiologists, health services researchers, and clinicians are combining their talents in helping to understand methods for the prevention and control of diseases. Current activities are fueled, in part, by the discoveries of the potential for periodontal diseases being important risk factors for systemic diseases. Beck and colleagues recently tested the hypothesis that periodontal infections might be a risk factor for cardiovascular conditions.[114] Results of this cohort study of 1,147 men found risk ratios adjusted for established risk factors for cardiovascular disease of 1.4, 1.6, and 2.1 for bone loss and total coronary heart disease (CHD), fatal CHD, and stroke, respectively. In a case-control study of pregnancy complications and periodontal diseases, Offenbacher et al found that mothers with preterm low–birth weight babies were 7.9 times more likely to have periodontal disease than those mothers without periodontal disease.[115] Hypothesized relationships between periodontal diseases and many other medical conditions are being developed and tested.

Measurements for Epidemiological Studies

Early indices for periodontal diseases were based on the concept that it was a single disease, with gingivitis and periodontitis representing different stages in its progression.[113,116] Indices were calculated as composite scores, usually as weighted averages of scores given to each of several signs of periodontal disease. The most common clinical signs included in these early efforts were visual signs of gingival inflammation, pocket formation, and tooth mobility as an indication of severe pocket formation. The most widely used of these indices was Russell's PI index.[113] In response to current theories of pathogenesis of periodontal diseases, epidemiologists have taken a disaggregated approach to recording signs of disease rather than a composite one. Clinical signs, usually gingival bleeding, loss of supporting structure as a measure of past disease (recession or loss of attachment), pocket formation, and sometimes calculus as a contributing risk factor, are scored separately and presented as such. The Community Periodontal Index of Treatment Needs (CPITN) developed by the World Health Organization provides an indication of the presence of bleeding, calculus, shallow and deep pockets, as well as treatment needed for the observed conditions.[117] This index has been adopted around the world for use in hundreds of surveys in the relatively short period of time since its development. The other most common method for measuring periodontal conditions is the Extent and Severity Index (ESI) developed by the U.S. National Institute of Dental Research.[118] Combined with other companion measures of gingivitis and calculus, this index provides a comprehensive measure of information similar to that collected in clinical practice.

Prevalence and Trends

Estimates of both prevalence and incidence can vary considerably because of the different cutoff points that can be used for clinical loss of attachment or pocket depth, the number and location of sites within the mouth where measurements can be made, the different instruments that can be used for making the measurements, and examiner variability inherent in making millimeter measurements by hand and eye. However, results are available for four U.S. national surveys done by the National Center for Health Statistics (NCHS) and the National Institute of Dental Research (NIDR).[119,120] A number of population-based epidemiolgic surveys of smaller geographic areas are available, as are several reviews of the epidemiology of periodontal diseases.[121,122]

In 1988–1991, the prevalence of gingivitis (using bleeding as the measure) was relatively high in a national survey of persons 13 years of age and older (Table 65-9).[120] In this sample, 62.9 percent had gingival bleeding on probing, with the highest prevalence being in adolescents. This same survey found that 25.3 percent of individuals had periodontal pocket depth measurements that can be considered moderate (4 to 5 mm), and only 3.9 percent had deep pockets (6 mm or greater). More than 90 percent of the sample had experienced some loss of attachment. However, attachment loss of 3 to 4 mm and 5 mm or greater in one or more sites was found in 25 and 14.7 percent of individuals, respectively. Most individuals (57.9 percent) did not have any sites with gingival recession. The percentage of sites affected with the different clinical conditions suggests that neither gingivitis nor periodontitis are generalized within the mouth, with most individuals having a small number of sites affected at the severe levels of disease. Considered as a whole, these data suggest that mild forms of disease are almost universal, but severe forms that can lead to tooth loss are not prevalent in the U.S. population.

Trends in the prevalence of periodontal diseases are less clear than those occurring for dental caries because of the different methods used in their measurement in national surveys. Using the National

TABLE 65-9. PERIODONTAL CONDITIONS OF UNITED STATES POPULATIONS AGES 13 YEARS AND OLDER, 1988–1991

	% Subjects		% Sites	
Condition	**Severity Categories (in mm)**	**Prevalence**	**Severity Categories (in mm)**	**Prevalence**
Gingivitis		62.9		12.0
Pocket depth	≤3	70.8	≤1	54.9
	4–5	25.3	2–3	41.6
	≥6	3.9	≥4	3.4
Loss of attachment	0	7.5	0	37.5
	1–2	52.8	1	38.7
	3–4	25.0	2–3	18.3
	≥5	14.7	≥4	5.5
Recession	0	57.9	0	89.0
	1–2	27.3	1–2	8.1
	≥3	14.8	≥3	2.9

From Brown LJ, Brunelle JA, Kingman A: Periodontal status in the United States, 1988–1991: prevalence, extent, and demographic variation. J Dent Res 75:672–683, 1996.

Center for Health Statistics (NCHS) examination surveys conducted in 1960–1962 and in 1971–1974, Capilouto and Douglass concluded that the proportions in both sexes and all ages of U.S. adults with no disease increased due primarily to less gingivitis (disease without pockets).[119] Overall there was little change in pockets but a slight trend toward a decrease in the proportions with the more severe disease. They concluded that older adults continue to exhibit more disease and greater levels of disease than the younger age groups. A recent review commissioned by the American Academy of Periodontology likewise concluded that the prevalence of gingivitis had improved by 1985, and periodontitis had not declined much, but that its severity probably had.[121] The recent NHANES III survey results found that 21 percent of people age 35 to 44 years of age had one or more sites with 4 or more mm of attachment loss.[120] This estimate is only slightly better than the 25 percent who had this level of periodontitis in 1985–1986, but seems to be on track for achieving the rather modest national *Healthy People 2000* objective of 15 percent in the year 2000. The improvement in periodontal disease levels are consistent with national trends of improved oral hygiene, improved income and education levels, increased dental care utilization, cessation of smoking habits, increased exposure to fluoride, increased general use of systemic antibiotics, and a decrease in tooth loss.[119]

Data on the prevalence of periodontal conditions based on the CPITN and from the WHO Global Oral Health Data Bank for 35- to 44-year-olds have been presented for 34 countries.[123] Subjects with completely healthy periodontal tissues were virtually nonexistent. Calculus and shallow pocketing, periodontal conditions that require self-care combined with professional oral hygiene instruction and cleaning of teeth, were of notable magnitude in adult populations around the world. Nevertheless, with a few exceptions the percentages of persons with severe disease (deep pockets) were less than 20 percent. Tooth loss because of periodontal diseases did not seem to be a frequently encountered phenomenon in the studied age group. Previously assumed differences between industrialized and developing countries with regard to the prevalence of severe periodontal diseases were not reflected in these survey data. For the majority of populations studied, the progress of periodontal diseases seems to have been slowed. In worldwide studies of older adults from 90 countries, the progress of disease is not reflected in an increase in CPITN scores, but an increase in tooth loss. Like populations with dental caries, there are populations with high levels of severe periodontal disease that have severe consequences, one of which is tooth loss.[124]

Incidence of Periodontal Diseases

When clinical measurements are averaged across the many sites within the mouth, the increment of disease appears low. Goodson put the average loss of attachment at 0.12 mm per year in untreated populations.[125] At this rate, the average person would not loose enough periodontal support over a large number of years to jeopardize tooth retention, a conclusion that obviously is not in keeping with clinical observations. The view that periodontal disease progression is episodic and site specific led epidemiologists to define a case at the person level, with definitions usually based on some combination of number of sites affected by some level of attachment loss. Studies are few in number because of the difficulties in completing these longitudinal studies in representation samples. Also, the definition of disease has varied in these few studies. Thus the estimates of incidence vary considerably. In a community-based sample of an elderly population in five counties in North Carolina, Brown et al found a disease increment over 18 months of 24 percent for blacks and 16 percent for whites using 3 mm or more attachment loss in three or more sites as the definition of a case, a fairly conservative definition of disease.[126] Wennstrom et al provided 12-year increments of periodontal disease in randomly selected patients 18- to 65-years-old selected from 12 community dental clinics in a county in Sweden.[127] Almost all subjects (96 percent) showed at least one site with 2 mm or more of attachment loss during the study period. When the threshold value was set at 3 mm or greater, 72 percent experienced disease.

Factors Associated with Prevalence and Incidence

Numerous descriptive epidemiological studies have identified factors associated with the variation of periodontal diseases, some of which have proven to be true risk factors for the disease. To summarize the sociodemographic indicators, the prevalence of periodontal diseases tends to increase with age, is higher in males than in females, is higher in low socioeconomic groups compared to other groups, and is affected by race. A study of an elderly population found striking differences between whites and blacks, confirming similar findings in state and national surveys.[128] The NHANES III survey found that non-Hispanic whites exhibited better periodontal health than either non-Hispanic blacks or Mexican Americans.[120] Multivariable analyses that controlled for socioeconomic status and other variables generally explain only a small portion of the black-white differences in periodontal status. Other than sociodemographic variables, a large number of possible risk factors have been identified for the periodontal diseases.[129] Even though few population-based, longitudinal studies have been done to confirm putative risk factors, the evidence supports both type I and type II diabetes, smoking, and the three periodontal bacteria discussed previously in this chapter as being causal of periodontal disease.[130] Diabetics are at particularly high risk for periodontal disease if they do not maintain good oral hygiene, have a long history of diabetes, demonstrate complications of diabetes other than periodontal disease, have a history of poorly controlled diabetes, and are either teenagers or pregnant women.[131] The risk of periodontitis appears to be 2.5 to 6.0 times greater in tobacco users compared to that in nonusers.[132] Some evidence suggests that the risk for disease is decreased when smokers stop tobacco use.[133] Less evidence exists for a genetic predisposition, immunosuppression from diseases, stress, and nutrition being risk factors, and definitive studies are needed.[130]

Conclusions

The more precise measurement of periodontal diseases in the 1980s and an increase in the number of population-based surveys provide useful information in defining the epidemiology of periodontal diseases. Although periodontal diseases are still considered widespread, these new measurement techniques have allowed a clearer distinction between the prevalence of disease and its severity. While periodontal disease is very prevalent, the severity is less than once thought. Further, the disease is not as generalized within the mouth as previous measurement methods indicated. Fewer sites are affected and the estimated amount and type of treatment needed requires fewer resources based on these findings. Nevertheless, millions of individuals are affected and efforts need to be directed toward prevention and control of the disease. In the U.S. alone, a large proportion of adult Americans have experienced periodontal disease; more than half have gingivitis, and millions have periodontal pockets that may need treatment.[134] As with dental caries, the current epidemiology of the periodontal diseases suggests that identification of risk factors should be pursued further, but strong evidence supports the role of smoking, diabetes, and some specific microorganisms in its cause.

Prevention and Control

Prevention of plaque-associated periodontal diseases requires consideration of their pathogenesis and risk factors. Gingivitis is highly correlated with plaque, and its prevention and control requires the thorough and frequent removal of bacterial buildup on the teeth. Plaque control can be accomplished through a combination of personal oral hygiene and professional care. Methods for personal oral hygiene include mechanical means, such as toothbrushing and flossing, and the use of chemotherapeutic or pharmacological agents contained in dentifrices or mouthrinses. Professional care includes cleaning and early diagnosis, which is easily accomplished by detection of signs of gingival bleeding during clinical examination. Plaque has a weak correlation with periodontitis, and its role in the initiation of this disease is poorly understood. Only approximately 30 percent of those with gingivitis get periodontitis, so the prevention of periodontitis and its progression requires a consideration of bacterial, host, and environmental risk factors in addition to the amount of plaque buildup or gingival bleeding. New understandings of the pathogenesis and epidemiology of periodontal diseases have provided a strong rationale for risk assessment for periodontal diseases, yet the methods are not as well developed as for dental caries.[135,136] Nevertheless, risks such as cigarette smoking, diabetes mellitus, and certain other systemic conditions should be considered in the prevention and control of moderate to severe periodontitis. The 1996 World Workshop on Periodontics did not recommend testing for specific bacteria or biochemical markers, based on the evidence at the time, even though many show promise.

Unfortunately, there are no public health interventions for the prevention and control of periodontal diseases similar to fluorides for dental caries. No comprehensive community trials directed toward the prevention and control of periodontal diseases have been done in the United States, as has been done for cardiovascular diseases, for example. As an alternative, some efforts have been directed toward dental practitioners to ensure their attention to the periodontal tissues. These efforts have met with some success, but they reach only that segment of the population who are already users of dental services.[137,138]

Mechanical Methods for Personal Plaque Control

Self-care is essential for maintenance of periodontal health. A successful preventive regimen requires the thorough removal of plaque every 24 to 48 hours. The toothbrush alone cannot successfully clean all surfaces of a tooth, particularly between the teeth, and its use must be supplemented with dental floss, interproximal brush, or wood point.[139]

With the confirmation of plaque as the primary etiologic agent in gingivitis, through well-designed clinical trials, efforts were made in public programs to extend plaque control to a number of groups, particularly public schoolchildren. Results of these efforts, based on supervised group brushing combined with some degree of education, proved to be equivocal.[140] While improvements in knowledge, attitudes, and behavior were achieved in these demonstration programs and clinical trials, any improvements in plaque levels and gingivitis were usually short-lived. These self-care, group plaque control strategies cannot be recommended for public health settings in the absence of more comprehensive oral or general health education and access programs.

Chemical and Antibiotic Methods for Plaque Control

For more than 30 years, dental researchers have sought chemical means to control plaque—enzymes to loosen and dissolve the plaque mass so that it can be washed away, topical antibiotic rinses to eliminate certain bacteria in a narrowly focused attack, and antiseptics that work against a broad spectrum of bacteria. Significant reductions in gingival inflammation have been demonstrated for chlorhexidine, triclosan with copolymer or zinc citrate, essential oils, and stannous fluoride. Of these, chlorhexidine has the most evidence for its effectiveness. Peridex, containing 0.12 percent chlorhexidine gluconate as its active ingredient, is a commercial product accepted by the American Dental Association and is approved by the U.S. Food and Drug Administration. It has been used in Scandinavia and other European countries for 20 years and provides short-term reductions in gingivitis averaging 60 percent. Three long-term studies have shown reductions in plaque averaging 55 percent and reductions in gingivitis averaging 45 percent. Peridex is available by prescription only, is not recommended for long-term use, and should be used only under the careful supervision of a dentist. Listerine, a mouthrinse containing a mixture of essential oils and available over the counter, also is effective in the reduction of plaque and gingivitis. Because mouthrinses do not penetrate appreciably into the gingival crevice, their value is limited to the management of plaque above the gingiva and thus to the prevention and control of gingivitis. None of these chemical agents offer a substantial benefit for the treatment of periodontitis. Sodium benzoate prebrushing rinses and rinses containing cetylpyridinium chloride, the active agent in many commercial rinses, have yet to demonstrate any effectiveness in plaque or gingivitis reductions.[136]

Combined Personal and Professional Care

While maintenance of periodontal health depends on daily self-care, professional care also is essential, particularly when disease has caused a deepening of the periodontal crevice. Two recent long-term studies provide evidence of the effectiveness of professional preventive measures supplemented by personal preventive measures in preventing periodontal disease.[141,142] In a 15-year longitudinal study, adults assigned to an experimental group ($n = 375$) were provided with instruction and practice in effective self-performed tooth cleaning with emphasis on interproximal cleaning, dental prophylaxis including scaling, polishing, and application of topical fluoride. Patients were recalled every 2 to 3 months during the first 6 years and once a year, or more frequently, depending on need, during the remainder of the trial. The control group was recalled every 6 months for routine care. After 6 years, the experimental group demonstrated a mean gain of 0.2-mm attachment per subject, while the control group presented a mean loss of attachment of 1.2 mm. At 15 years, clinical attachment levels continued to improve from the gain of 0.2 mm noted at 6 years to 0.3 mm. In the other study, 3,928 subjects located in three geographically isolated villages in the Kingdom of Tonga were followed for 3 years. One village served as the control and received nothing other than annual evaluations. One village received a self-care program that included periodic health education by dental personnel and village counselors. The third village received all the health education plus tooth cleanings twice a year. After 3 years, bacterial plaque, gingival bleeding, calculus, and periodontal pockets of 4 mm or greater were less common in the village where people received the more comprehensive program. The authors concluded that the minimal professional care provided added significantly to the improvement of the periodontal health of the participants.

Early pocket formation requires the removal of bacteria from the gingival crevice through professional intervention. This condition is usually responsive to scaling (removal of bacteria, calculus, and other debris), root planing (smoothing the root to help prevent recolonization of bacteria), and effective plaque control. Professional scaling and root planing with manual instruments decreases gingival inflammation by 40 to 60 percent, decreases probing depth, and facilitates gain in clinical attachment levels. As pockets deepen, scaling and root planing as well as plaque control become less effective, but still are valuable for reducing inflammation and bacteria and increasing the tissue's prognosis for repair and reattachment. Sustained-release antimicrobials are sometimes indicated as an adjunct to scaling and root planing, although the systemic administration of antibiotics do not offer sufficient benefit to overcome risks such as drug sensitivity and emergence of antibiotic-resistant pathogens, except in the most refractory cases of periodontitis.[136]

Summary

An array of mechanical and chemical means are available to prevent and control periodontal diseases. In the average person, gingivitis is easily controlled with conscientious oral hygiene practices and regular visits to the dental office. However, the motivation of the public to perform these measures at the level required to prevent disease is not sufficient to make further major gains in the prevalence of the disease. Etiologic studies to identify and quantify risk, new diagnostic methods to identify those at risk of disease, and studies to better understand the natural history of the disease are all under way.[143] These advances should yield new methods, some of which might allow community-based interventions to be mounted.

▸ ORAL CANCERS

The term *oral cancer* generally includes squamous cell carcinomas of the lip (internal and external), tongue, floor of the mouth, palate, buccal mucosa and vestibule, gingiva, other unspecified parts of the mouth, and the pharynx. However, in some analyses and presentations, all pharyngeal tumors except the oropharynx are excluded in a desire to limit cancers to those that can be detected in a clinical screening such as is done by a dentist in a dental office. This approach is particularly important in studies of detection rates or stage of diagnosis. In other instances, presentations include the larynx so that most head and neck cancers can be included. A number of precancer lesions have clinical importance, but their incidence and prevalence is difficult to determine. The most important lesions are leukoplakia, erythroplakia and lichen planus, which probably affect about 5 percent of the population over 40 years of age in industrialized populations. They have a low rate of transformation, estimated at 4 percent or less in industrialized countries.[144]

Epidemiology

Incidence and Mortality

In the United States, cancers of the lips, tongue, floor of the mouth, palate, gingiva, buccal mucosa, and pharynx account for about 30,000 new cases of cancer and about 8,000 deaths each year. These oral cancers are 2.2 percent of all cancers in the United States. Squamous cell carcinoma represents about 90 percent of those cancers that occur. About 85 percent of all oral cancers occur at four sites—the tongue, oropharynx, lips, and floor of the mouth.[145]

Age-adjusted Surveillance, Epidemiology, and End Results program (SEER) incidence and NCHS mortality rates for the period 1988–1992, and incidence and mortality trends from 1973 to 1992 for oral and pharyngeal cancers, are presented by race and sex in Table 65-10. The annual age-adjusted incidence in 1988–1992 was 10.7 cases per 100,000. The male-female ratio for incidence was 2.6. Black males had the highest incidence at 23.2 per 100,000. The annual mortality rate for the overall population in 1988–1992 was 2.9 per 100,000, being more than twice as high in males and blacks compared to that in females and whites, respectively. A total of 41,000 deaths occurred during the period.

Between 1973 and 1992, the incidence of oral and pharyngeal cancers decreased by 6.4 percent overall. Over one-half of cases, however, are diagnosed at advanced stages, and trends by race are dramatically different. In this same 20-year period, the incidence of oral and pharyngeal cancers increased 20.2 percent in blacks compared to an 8.3 percent decrease in whites. The racial difference is even larger among males, with an increase of 32.6 percent in black men compared to a 12.3 percent decrease in white men. A similar trend according to race is found in mortality. From 1973 to 1992, mortality decreased 21.1 percent in the overall population; however,

TABLE 65-10. AGE-ADJUSTED SEER INCIDENCE AND U.S. MORTALITY RATES FOR ORAL AND PHARYNGEAL CANCERS, 1988 TO 1992, PER 100,000 POPULATION, AND INCIDENCE AND MORTALITY TRENDS FROM 1973 TO 1992 BY SEX AND RACE

	All Races			Whites			Blacks		
	Total	*Males*	*Females*	*Total*	*Males*	*Females*	*Total*	*Males*	*Females*
Age-adjusted SEER incidence rates, 1988 to 1992									
All ages	10.7	16.2	6.2	10.4	15.6	6.1	13.9	23.2	6.6
Age-adjusted U.S. mortality rates, 1988 to 1992									
All ages	2.9	4.6	1.7	2.7	4.1	1.6	5.2	9.2	2.2
Age-adjusted SEER incidence trends, 1973 to 1992									
% change[a]	−6.4	− 9.2	−2.7	−8.3	−12.3	−3.6	20.2	32.6	3.4
EAPC[b]	−0.4[c]	− 0.6[c]	− 0.1	− 0.5[c]	− 0.8[c]	− 0.1	0.9[c]	1.6[c]	− 0.4
Age-adjusted U.S. mortality trends, 1973–1992									
% change[a]	−21.1	−25.1	−13.2	−25.2	−30.4	−14.6	5.3	10.9	− 2.1
EAPC[b]	−1.4[c]	−1.7[c]	− 0.9[c]	−1.7[c]	−2.1[c]	−1.1[c]	0.1	0.3	−0.2

From Swango PA: Cancers of the oral cavity and pharynx in the United States: an epidemiologic overview. J Public Health Dent 56:309–318, 1996.

[a] Percent change is the percent increase or decrease in mortality rates between 1973 and 1992.

[b] EAPC is the estimated annual percent change over the time interval.

[c] EAPC is significantly different from zero ($P < 0.05$).

it increased 10.9 percent among black males compared to a 30.4 percent decline in white males. The male-female ratio in mortality, which was about 6:1 in 1950, is now about 2:1. The most likely explanation for this change in sex ratios is the increase in the use of tobacco among women.

Survival

Most oral cancers, exclusive of those occurring on the lip, are advanced when diagnosed. According to the American Cancer society, oral cancers in 1989 had the fifth lowest survival rate of 13 selected sites.[146] About half of all patients with oral cancer die of their disease within 5 years. This figure is even higher if lip cancers, 87 percent of which are localized when discovered, were excluded. These survival rates did not improve between 1973 and 1984, despite advances in radiation therapy, surgical management, and chemotherapy. Silverman and Gorsky underscored the importance of early diagnosis.[147] More than 79 percent of the oropharyngeal lesions showed regional lymph node metastases at the time of diagnosis. For cancers of the tongue, 73 percent were already advanced. Survival varies by race. In 1974–1976, 5-year survival was significantly shorter among blacks (36.4 percent) than among whites (54.9 percent); in 1986–1991 this difference had widened further, being 32.9 percent for blacks and 54.7 percent for whites.

Risk Factors

Besides race and sex, which have already been mentioned, age is directly associated with oral cancer. The average age at diagnosis is between 60 and 65 years. As the population in industrialized countries ages, the magnitude of the problem may increase. The two main risk factors for oral cancer are tobacco use and alcohol consumption.[148–150] It is more common among persons who either smoke or use smokeless tobacco, and especially among those who also are heavy drinkers of alcohol. During the 1980s, concern developed over the increased use of smokeless tobacco among American youth. User rates as high as 30 to 40 percent were reported among boys in some junior and senior high schools.[151] The health effects of smokeless tobacco have been examined in a report by the U.S. Surgeon General, which concluded that, far from being a safe substitute for smoking cigarettes, smokeless tobacco can cause cancer and a number of noncancerous oral conditions such as gingivitis, periodontitis, and gingival recession and can lead to nicotine addiction and dependence.[152] The excess risk of cancer of the cheek and gum may reach nearly 50-fold among long-term users.[153] Exposure to sunlight is a major risk factor for lip cancer, with fair-skinned, outdoor workers being at the greatest risk. Pipe smoking also is a risk factor for lip cancer.

One of the characteristic epidemiologic features of oral cancer is the wide disparity in rates in different parts of the world. The disease is very common in parts of Central and Southeast Asia, where it constitutes as much as 30 to 50 percent of all diagnosed malignancies. The geographical variation in rates reflects local conditions and habits, which influence the degree of exposure to etiologic factors. A high incidence in India is due to betel-quid chewing; and in Bas-Rhin, France, to high consumption of crudely distilled spirits.

Prevention and Control

A strong rationale for public health programs directed toward oral cancers exists.[154] The main risk factors for oral cancer are known, and changes in behaviors can reduce or eliminate exposures. The majority of oral and pharyngeal precancerous and cancerous lesions are particularly amenable to early detection because the sites of involvement are accessible by clinical examination, a well-accepted noninvasive procedure. It takes several years for an oral cancer to reach its full-blown invasive potential, making it possible to prevent it or interfere with its progression at an early stage. Furthermore, most people are in contact with physicians and dentists. Hence, the disease is amenable to prevention and control through health promotion programs that help reduce exposures to tobacco, alcohol, and sunlight. As many as 13 objectives in the different sections of *Healthy People 2000* are related to the prevention, detection, and control of oral cancers, signaling the need for cooperation among health professionals for their prevention and control.

Even with the importance of the disease, primary and secondary prevention has been lacking in the United States. Only 8.7 percent of adults reported having had an examination for oral cancer by a dentist or hygienist and 2.7 percent by a physician during the 3 years prior to 1992.[155] Less than one of every four adult patients who smoke report receiving smoking cessation counseling from dentists; and just over one-half, from physicians. More surprising than the low screening statistics for professionals are data from Scotland[156] and from England and Wales[157] documenting a pronounced upward trend in the incidence and mortality from oral cancer. A thorough analysis of barriers to addressing the oral cancer problem has documented additional factors that prevent progress toward national goals, including the knowledge, opinions, and practices of both professionals and the public.[154]

Programs that lead to a reduction in the use of tobacco products are important in the prevention and control of oral cancers. The role that tobacco use plays in oral cancers, as well as other cancers, should be emphasized in education programs for the public. Early detection through careful and periodic examinations also is important, and these education programs need to emphasize the importance of early detection for oral cancer. For those patients who use tobacco, at least annual examinations for early detection of premalignant or malignant lesions are recommended.[158]

Health professionals can be effective smoking cessation counselors, play an important role in oral cancer prevention, and potentially affect the smoking status of millions of patients. Dentists and dental hygienists are in a particularly unique and favorable position to modify the smoking behavior of their patients. Each year more than half of the population visits a dental office, and a substantial proportion of these patients will make a series of such visits, often as part of an ongoing relationship of several years' standing. Further, many of these patients will be adolescents, a population group underrepresented in physicians' offices and the age group in which smoking usually begins. For young people some detrimental aesthetic consequences of smoking, discolored teeth and restorations, bad breath, and hairy tongue, can possibly provide more powerful motivation to stop than the fear of remote health consequences such as heart disease or cancer. The dental profession has a historically strong preventive orientation, which increases the potential for adoption of smoking cessation interventions by providers. Dental hygienists devote almost all of their treatment time to preventive procedures, of which a large portion consists of patient education. Dental providers generally have positive attitudes toward providing smoking cessation counseling in their practices, and a clinical trial has shown them to be effective counselors.[159] A number of materials have been developed by the National Cancer Institute for use by dental professionals in helping their patients to stop using tobacco.

To date, public health programs directed toward oral cancer have been few in number and have not undergone rigorous evaluation. Questions remain as to: why there has been only a modest improvement in oral cancer incidence (6.4 percent) over the last 20 years or so compared with impressive improvements in cancers of other sites such as the cervix (38.1 percent); why most cancers are diagnosed in such an advanced stage; what accounts for the differences between blacks and whites in incidence, mortality, stage at diagnosis, and survival; and what is an appropriate screening schedule for oral cancers. In 1996, a number of public and private entities under the leadership of the Centers for Disease Control and Prevention and other federal agencies developed a comprehensive national agenda for the fight against oral cancer in the United States.[160,161] Efforts in implementing parts of this agenda are just beginning. In the same year, the National Institute of Dental Research and the National Cancer Institute cofunded four oral cancer research centers. Both of these initiatives represent expressions of interest in the promotion of public and professional initiatives targeted toward oral cancer prevention and control. The next decade should see progress toward reducing the oral cancer burden in the United States.

▶ CONCLUSIONS

Efforts by the public, health professionals, and researchers have all contributed to improving trends in oral health, most notably, for dental caries in children. Other conditions have remained stable or improved only slightly, while some serious conditions, such as oral cancer, may even be increasing in some segments of society.

Community and individual methods for the primary prevention of dental caries, periodontal diseases, oral cancers, and other conditions are available. These methods, among others, include a wide array of systemic and topical fluorides, dental sealants, regular professional care, plaque control, and avoidance of tobacco and alcohol. The scientific evidence supporting these interventions as safe and effective is in large measure overwhelming. The cost-effectiveness of some of these methods, such as community water fluoridation, are among the best of any preventive strategies available to the public health practitioner.

Much remains to be done in extending the benefits of these preventive services to larger segments of society. *Healthy People 2000: National Health Promotion and Disease Prevention Objectives* provides realistic oral health benchmarks for the end of the century.[162] The midpoint evaluation of the 16 oral health objectives in this document found that seven targets will likely be achieved by the year 2000.[163] However, this evaluation also found that achieving these objectives will not come easily. Successful efforts must be maintained and new initiatives begun in order to extend the benefits of the twentieth century into the next.

▶ REFERENCES

1. World Health Organization: Application of the International Classification of Diseases to Dentistry and Stomatology. Geneva: World Health Organization, 1996
2. Levit KR, Lazenby HC, Braden BR, Cowan CA, McDonnell PA, Lekha S, Stiller JM, Won DK, Donham CS, Long AM, Stewart MW: National health expenditures, 1995. Health Care Financ Rev 18:175–214, 1996
3. DeStefano F, Anda FR, Kahn S, Williamson DF, Russell CM: Dental disease and risk of coronary health disease and mortality. Br Med J 306:688–691, 1993
4. Katz PP, Wirthin MR, Szpunar SM, Selby JV, Sepe SJ, Showstack JA: Epidemiology and prevention of periodontal disease in individuals with diabetes. Diabetes Care 14:375–385, 1991
5. Strauss RP, Hunt RJ: Understanding the value of teeth to older adults: influences on the quality of life. J Am Dent Assoc 124: 105–110, 1993
6. Resine S, Miller J: A longitudinal study of work loss related to dental diseases. Soc Sci Med 21:1309–1314, 1985
7. Emilson CG, Krasse B: Support for and implications of a specific plaque hypothesis. Scand J Dent Res 93:96–104, 1985
8. Fejerskov O, Clarkson BH: Dynamics of caries lesion formation. In Fejerskov O, Ekstrand J, Burt BA (eds): Fluoride in Dentistry. 2nd ed. Copenhagen: Munksgaard, 1996, pp 187–213
9. Fejerskov O: Concepts of dental caries and their consequences for understanding the disease. Community Dent Oral Epidemiol 25:5–12, 1997
10. Keyes PH: Recent advances in dental caries research. Bacteriology. Bacteriological findings and biological implications. Int Dent J 12: 443–464, 1962
11. Newbrun E: Cariology. 3rd ed. Chicago: Quintessence, 1989
12. Ripa LW: Nursing caries: a comprehensive review. Pediatr Dent 10:268–282, 1988
13. Milnes AR: Description and epidemiology of nursing caries. J Public Health Dent 56:38–50, 1996
14. Berkowitz R: Etiology of nursing caries: a microbiologic perspective. J Public Health Dent 56:51–54, 1996
15. World Health Organization: Oral Health Surveys: Basic Methods, 3rd ed. Geneva: World Health Organization, 1987
16. Klein H, Palmer CE, Knutson JW: Studies on dental caries: I. Dental status and dental needs of elementary school children. Public Health Rep 53:751–765, 1938
17. DePaola PF, Soparker PM, Kent RL Jr: Methodological issues relative to the quantification of root surface caries. Gerodontology 8:3–8, 1989
18. Beck J: The epidemiology of root surface caries. J Dent Res 69: 1216–1221, 1990
19. Katz RV: The RCI revisited after 15 years: used, reinvented, modified, debated, and natural logged. J Public Health Dent 56:28–34, 1996
20. Barmes DE, Infirri JS: WHO activities in oral epidemiology. Community Dent Oral Epidemiol 5:22–29, 1977
21. Barmes DE: Epidemiology of dental disease. J Clin Periodontol 4:80–93, 1979
22. Infirri JS, Barmes DE: Epidemiology of oral diseases—differences in national problems. Int Dent J 29:183–190, 1979
23. Heleo LA, Haugejorden O: "The rise and fall" of dental caries: some global aspects of dental caries epidemiology. Community Dent Oral Epidemiol 9:296–299, 1981
24. Barmes DE: Indicators for oral health and their implications for developing countries. Int Dent J 33:60–66, 1982
25. Sheiham A: Changing trends in dental caries. Int J Epidemiol 13:142–147, 1984
26. Manji F, Fejerskov O: Dental caries in developing countries in relation to the appropriate use of fluoride. J Dent Res 69:733–741, 1990
27. Marthaler TM: The prevalence of dental caries in Europe 1990–1995. Caries Res 30:237–255, 1996
28. Glass RL (ed): The first international conference on the declining prevalence of dental caries. J Dent Res 61:1304–1383, 1982
29. Graves RC, Bohannan HM, Disney JA, Stamm JW, Bader JD, Abernathy JR: Recent dental caries and treatment patterns in U.S. children. J Public Health Dent 46:23–29, 1986
30. Murray JJ: Comments on results reported at the Second International Conference "Changes in Caries Prevalence." Int Dent J 44:457–458, 1994
31. Brunelle JA, Carlos JP: Recent trends in dental caries in U.S. children and the effect of water fluoridation. J Dent Res 69:723–727, 1990
32. Kaste LM, Selwitz RH, Oldakowski RJ, Brunelle JA, Winn DM, Brown LJ: Coronal caries in the primary and permanent dentition of children and adolescents 1–17 years of age: United States, 1988–1991. J Dent Res 75:631–641, 1996
33. Brown LJ, Swango PA: Trends in caries experience in US employed adults from 1971–74 to 1985: cross-sectional comparisons. Adv Dent Res 7:52–60, 1993
34. Edelstein BL, Douglass CW: Dispelling the myth that 50 percent of U.S. schoolchildren have never had a cavity. Public Health Rep 110:522–530, 1995
35. Pitts NB, Davies JA: The Scottish Health Board's Dental Epidemiological Programme: initial surveys of 5- and 12-year-olds. Br Dent J 172:408–413, 1992
36. Hunt RJ: Behavioral and sociodemographic risk factors for caries. In Bader JD (ed): Risk Assessment in Dentistry. Chapel Hill: University of North Carolina Dental Ecology, 1990, pp 29–34
37. Newbrun E: Sugar and dental caries: a review of human studies. Science 217:418–423, 1982
38. Ismail AI: Food cariogenicity in Americans aged 9 to 29 years assessed in a national cross-sectional survey, 1971–74. J Dent Res 65:1435–1440, 1986

39. Burt BA, Eklund SA, Morgan KJ, et al: The effects of sugar intake and frequency of ingestion on dental caries increment in a three-year longitudinal study. J Dent Res 67:1422–1429, 1988
40. Graves RG, Disney JA, Stamm JW, Abernathy JR, Bohannan HM: Physical and environmental risk factors in dental caries. In Bader JD (ed): Risk Assessment in Dentistry. Chapel Hill: University of North Carolina Dental Ecology, 1990, pp 37–47
41. Krasse B: Microbiological and salivary risk factors. In Bader JD (ed): Risk Assessment in Dentistry. Chapel Hill: University of North Carolina Dental Ecology, 1990, pp 51–61
42. Winn DM, Brunelle JA, Selwitz RH, Kaste LM, Oldakowski RJ, Kingman A, Brown LJ: Coronal and root caries in the dentition of adults in the United States, 1988–1991. J Dent Res 75:642–651, 1996
43. Clarkson JE: Epidemiology of root caries. Am J Dent 8:329–334, 1995
44. Amstutz R, Rozier RG: Community risk indicators for dental caries in schoolchildren. Community Dent Oral Epidemiol 23:129–137, 1995
45. Bader JD (ed): Risk Assessment in Dentistry. Chapel Hill: University of North Carolina Dental Ecology, 1990
46. Johnson NW (ed): Risk markers for oral diseases. vol 1, Dental caries. Markers of high and low risk groups and individuals. Cambridge, England: Cambridge University Press, 1991
47. American Dental Association: Caries diagnosis and risk assessment. A review of preventive strategies and management. J Am Dent Assoc 126(Suppl):1S–24S, 1995
48. Hausen H: Caries prediction—state of the art. Community Dent Oral Epidemiol 25:87–96, 1997
49. Newbrun E: The fluoridation war: a scientific dispute or a religious argument? J Public Health Dent 56:246–252, 1996
50. US Public Health Service: Report of the ad hoc subcommittee on fluoride of the committee to coordinate environmental health and related programs. Review of fluoride benefits and risks. Washington, DC: US Department of Health and Human Services, 1991
51. National Research Council: Health effects of ingested fluoride. Washington, DC: National Academy Press, 1993
52. Greene JC, Louie R, Wycoff SJ: Preventive dentistry, I: dental caries. JAMA 262:3459–3463, 1989
53. Lewis DW, Ismail AI: Periodic health examination, 1995 update: 2. Prevention of dental caries. Can Med Assoc J 152:836–846, 1995
54. World Health Organization: Fluorides and oral health. Geneva: World Health Organization, 1994
55. Murray JJ, Naylor MN: Fluorides and dental caries. In Murray JJ (ed): Prevention of Oral Disease. 3rd ed. Oxford, England: Oxford University Press, 1996
56. Fejerskov O, Ekstrand J, Burt BA: Fluoride in Dentistry. 2nd ed. Copenhagen: Munksgaard, 1996
57. Dean HT, McKay FS: Production of mottled enamel halted by a change in common water supply. Am J Public Health 29:567–575, 1939
58. Dean HT, Arnold FA Jr, Elvove E: Domestic water and dental caries, V. Additional studies of the relation of fluoride domestic waters to dental caries experience in 4425 white children aged 12–14 years, of 13 cities in 4 states. Public Health Rep 57:1155–1179, 1942
59. Federation Dentaire Internationale: Basic Fact Sheets. London: Federation Dentaire Internationale, 1987
60. US Department of Health and Human Services: Fluoridation Census, 1992. Atlanta: Centers for Disease Control and Prevention, Division of Oral Health, Sept 1993
61. US Public Health Service: Report of the U.S. Public Health Service Oral Health Coordinating Committee. National fluoride plan to promote oral health. Washington, DC: US Department of Health and Human Services, 1996
62. Horowitz HS: Grand Rapids: the public health story. J Public Health Dent 49:62–63, 1989
63. Ast DB, Fitzgerald B: Effectiveness of water fluoridation. J Am Dent Assoc 65:581–587, 1962
64. Murray JJ, Rugg-Gunn AJ: Fluorides and Dental Caries. 2nd ed. Bristol, England; Wright, 1982
65. Newbrun E: Effectiveness of water fluoridation. J Public Health Dent 49:279–289, 1989
66. Ripa LW: A Half-century of community water fluoridation in the United States: review and commentary. J Public Health Dent 53:17–44, 1993
67. Stephen KW, McCall DR, Tallis JI: Caries prevalence in northern Scotland before, and 5 years after, water defluoridation. Br Dent J 163:324–326, 1987
68. Burt BA (ed): Proceedings for the workshop: cost effectiveness of caries prevention in dental public health. J Public Health Dent 49:251–344, 1989
69. Division of Oral Health: Public health focus: fluoridation of community water systems. MMWR Morb Mort Wkly Rep 41:372–381, 1992
70. Marshall E: The fluoride debate: one more time. Science 247:276–277, 1990
71. Statement by James O. Mason, MD, Assistant Secretary for Health, April 26, 1990
72. Block LE: Antifluoridationists persist: the constitutional basis for fluoridation. J Public Health Dent 46:188–198, 1986
73. Easley MW: The status of community water fluoridation in the United States. Public Health Rep 105:348–353, 1990
74. US Public Health Service: Health care reform and public health. A paper on population-based core functions. The Core Functions Project. Washington, DC: US Public Health Service, 1993
75. Clarkson J: A European view of fluoride supplementation: meeting matters. Br Dent J 172:357, 1992
76. Ismail AI: Fluoride supplements: current effectiveness, side effects and recommendations. Community Dent Oral Epidemiol 22:164–172, 1994
77. Leverett DH, Adair SM, Vaughn BW, Proskin HM, Moss ME: Randomized clinical trial of the effect of prenatal fluoride supplements in preventing dental caries. Caries Res 31:174–179, 1997
78. Levy SM: Expansion of the proper use of systemic fluoride supplements. J Am Dent Assoc 112:30–34, 1986
79. Levy SM, Carrell AF: Compliance by health care providers with recommended systemic fluoride supplementation protocol. Clin Prev Dent 9:19–22, 1987
80. Pendrys DG, Katz RV, Morse DE: Risk factors for enamel fluorosis in a fluoridated population. Am J Epidemiol 140:461–471, 1994
81. Bibby BG: A consideration of the effectiveness of various fluoride mixtures. J Am Dent Assoc 34:26, 1947
82. Muhler JC, Radike AW, Nebergall WH, Day HG: A comparison between the anticariogenic effect of dentifrices containing stannous fluoride and sodium fluoride. J Am Dent Assoc 51:556–559, 1955
83. Brudevold F, Chilton NW: Comparative study of a fluoride dentifrice containing soluble phosphate and a calcium-free abrasive. Second year report. J Am Dent Assoc 72:889–894, 1966
84. Ripa LW: An evaluation of the use of professional (operator-applied) topical fluorides. J Dent Res 69:786–796, 1990
85. Johnston DW: Current status of professionally applied topical fluorides. Community Dent Oral Epidemiol 22:159–163, 1994
86. Stookey GK, Beiswanger BB: Topical fluoride therapy. In Harris NO, Christen AG (eds): Primary Preventive Dentistry. 4th ed. Norwalk, CT: Appleton & Lange, 1995, pp 193–233
87. Horowitz HS, Ismail AI: Topical fluorides in caries prevention. In Fejerskov O, Ekstrand J, Burt BA (eds): Fluoride in Dentistry. 2nd ed. Copenhagen: Munksgaard, 1996, pp 311–327
88. Fine SD: Topical fluoride preparations for reducing incidence of dental caries. Notice of status. Fed Reg 39:17245
89. Council on Dental Therapeutics: Council classifies fluoride mouthrinses. J Am Dent Assoc 91:1250–1252, 1975

90. Miller AJ, Brunelle JA: A summary of the NIDR community caries prevention demonstration program. J Am Dent Assoc 107:265–269, 1983
91. Renson CE, Crielaers, PJA, Ibikunle SAJ, Pinto VG, Ross CB, Infirri JS, Takazoe I, Tala H: Changing patterns of oral health and implications for health manpower: Part I. Int Dent J 35:235–251, 1985
92. Pendrys DG: Risk of fluorosis in a fluoridated population. Implications for the dentists and hygienist. J Am Dent Assoc 126:1617–1624, 1995
93. Council on Dental Materials and Devices: pit and fissure sealants. J Am Dent Assoc 93:134, 1976
94. Ripa LW: Has the decline in caries prevalence reduced the need for fissure sealants in the UK? A review. J Paediatr Dent 6:131–140, 1990
95. Rock WP: The effectiveness of fissure sealant resins. J Dent Educ 48(Suppl):27–31, 1984
96. Weintraub JA: The effectiveness of pit and fissure sealants. J Public Health Dent 49:317–330, 1989
97. Llodra JC, Bravo M, Delgado-Rodriguez M, Baca P, Galvey R: Factors influencing the effectiveness of sealants—a meta-analysis. Community Dent Oral Epidemiol 21:261–268, 1993
98. Ripa LW: Sealants revisited: an update of the effectiveness of pit and fissure sealants. Caries Res 27(Suppl 1):77–82, 1993
99. Wendt L-K, Koch G: Fissure sealant in permanent first molars after 10 years. Swed Dent J 12:181–185, 1988
100. Romcke RG, Lewis DW, Maze BD, Vickerson RA: Retention and maintenance of fissure sealants over 10 years. J Can Dent Assoc 56:235–237, 1990
101. Simonsen RJ: Retention and effectiveness of dental sealants after 15 years. J Am Dent Assoc 122:34–42, 1991
102. Weintraub JA, Stearns SC, Burt BA, Beltran E, Eklund S: A retrospective analysis of the cost-effectiveness of dental sealants in a children's health center. Soc Sci Med 36:1483–1493, 1993
103. Selwitz RH, Winn DM, Kingman A, Zion GR: The prevalence of dental sealants in the US population: findings from NHANES III, 1988–91. J Dent Res 75:652–660, 1996
104. Siegal MD, Farquhar CL, Bouchard JM: Dental sealants. Who needs them? Public Health Rep 112:98–106, 1997
105. Proceedings of the Workshop on Guidelines for Sealant Use. J Public Health Dent 55:259–313, 1995
106. Kaste LM, Gift HC: Inappropriate infant bottle feeding. Arch Pediatr Adolesc Med 149:786–791, 1995
107. Shelton PG, Berkowitz RJ, Forrester DJ: Nursing bottle caries. Pediatr 59:777–778, 1977
108. American Academy of Periodontology: Proceedings of the World Workshop in Clinical Periodontics. Chicago: American Academy of Periodontology, 1989
109. Loe H, Theliade E, Jensen SB: Experimental gingivitis in man. J Periodontal 36:177–187, 1965
110. Offenbacher S: Periodontal diseases: pathogenesis. Ann Periodontol 1:821–878, 1996
111. Consensus Report: Periodontal diseases: pathogenesis and microbial factors. Ann Periodontol 1:926–932, 1996
112. Burt BA: The status of epidemiological data on periodontal diseases. In Guggenheim B (ed): Periodontology Today. Basel: Karger, 1988, pp 68–76
113. Russell AL: A system of classification and scoring for prevalence surveys of periodontal disease. J Dent Res 35:350–359, 1956
114. Beck JD, Garcia R, Heiss G, Vokonas PS, Offenbacher S: Periodontal disease and cardiovascular disease. J Periodontol 67:1112–1137, 1996
115. Offenbacher S, Katz VL, Fertik GS, et al: Periodontal infection as a risk factor for preterm low birth weight. J Peirodontol 67:1103–1112, 1996
116. Ramfjord SP: The periodontal disease index. J Periodontal 38 (Suppl):30–38, 1967
117. Cutress TW, Ainamo J, Sardo, Infirri J: The Community Periodontal Index of Treatment Needs (CPITN) procedure for population groups and individuals. Int Dent J 37:222–233, 1987
118. Carlos JP, Wolfe MD, Kingman A: The extent and severity index: a simple method for use in epidemiological studies of periodontal disease. J Clin Periodontal 13:500–505, 1986
119. Capilouto ML, Douglass CW: Trends in the prevalence and severity of periodontal diseases in the US: a public health problem? J Public Health Dent 48:245–251, 1988
120. Brown LJ, Brunelle JA, Kingman A: Periodontal status in the United States, 1988–1991: prevalence, extent, and demographic variation. J Dent Res 75:672–683, 1996
121. American Academy of Periodontology: Position paper. Epidemiology of periodontal diseases. J Periodontol 67:935–945, 1996
122. Papapanou PN: Periodontal diseases: epidemiology. Ann Periodontol 1:1–36, 1996
123. Pilot T, Barnes DE: An update on periodontal conditions in adults, measured by CPITN. Int Dent J 37:169–172, 1987
124. Pilot T, Miyazaki H, Lectercq M-H, Barmes DE: Profiles of periodontal conditions in older age cohorts, measured by CPITN. Int Dent J 42:23–30, 1992
125. Goodson JM: Selection of suitable indicators of periodontitis. In Bader JD (ed): Risk Assessment in Dentistry. Chapel Hill: University of North Carolina Dental Ecology, 1990, pp 69–74
126. Brown LF, Beck JD, Rozier RG: Incidence of attachment loss in community-dwelling older adults. J Periodontol 65:316–323, 1994
127. Wennstrom JL, Serino G, Lindhe J, Eneroth L, Tollskog G: Periodontal conditions of adult regular dental care attendants. A 12-year longitudinal study. J Clin Periodontol 20:714–722, 1993
128. Beck JD, Koch GG, Rozier RG, Tudor GE: Prevalence and risk indicators for periodontal attachment loss in a population of older community-dwelling blacks and whites. J Periodontol 61:521–528, 1990
129. Haffajee AD, Oliver RC: Periodontal diseases working group summary and recommendations. In Bader JD (ed): Risk Assessment in Dentistry. Chapel Hill: University of North Carolina Dental Ecology, 1990, pp 306–308
130. Consensus Report: Periodontal diseases: epidemiology and diagnosis. Ann Periodontol 1:216–222, 1996
131. Katz PP, Wirthin MR Jr, Szpunar SM, Selby JV, Sepe SJ, Showstack JA: Epidemiology and prevention of periodontal disease in individuals with diabetes. Diabetes Care 14:375–385, 1991
132. Bergstrom J, Preber H: Tobacco use as a risk factor. J Periodontol 96:34–39, 1994
133. Haber J, Wattles J, Crowley M, Mandell R, Joshipura K, Kent RL: Evidence for cigarette smoking as a major risk factor for periodontitis. J Periodontol 64:16–23, 1993
134. Brown LJ, Oliver RC, Loe H: Evaluating periodontal status of U.S. employed adults. J Am Dent Assoc 121:226–232, 1990
135. Page RC, Beck JD: Risk assessment for periodontal diseases. Int Dent J 47:61–87, 1997
136. Jeffcoat MK, McGuire M, Newman MG: Evidence-based periodontal treatment. Highlights form the 1996 World Workshop in Periodontics. J Am Dent Assoc 128:713–724, 1997
137. Brown LF, Spencer AJ: Special report—continuing education in periodontology—the Adelaide study. Periodontol 10:12–13, 1989
138. Bader JD, McFall WT Jr, Rozier RG, Sams DH, Ramsey DL: Short-term change in dental providers' diagnostic data recording behavior following an educational intervention. J Contin Educ Health Prof 9:267–276, 1989
139. Federation Dentaire Internationale: The prevention of dental caries and periodontal disease. Int Dent J 34:141–158, 1984
140. Frazier JP: A new look at dental health education in community programs. Dent Hygiene 52:176–186, 1978
141. Axelsson P, Lindhe J, Nystrom B: On the prevention of caries and periodontal disease. Results of a 15-year longitudinal study in adults. J Clin Periodontol 18:182–189, 1991

142. Cutress TW, Powell RN, Kilisimasi S, Tomiki S, Holborow D: A 3-year community-based periodontal disease prevention programme for adults in a developing nation. Int Dent J 41:323–324, 1991
143. Jeffcoat MK: Prevention of periodontal diseases in adults: strategies for the future. Prev Med 23:704–708, 1994
144. Downer MC. Oral cancer. In Pine CM (ed): Community Oral Health. Oxford, England: Wright, 1997, pp 88–94
145. Swango PA: Cancers of the oral cavity and pharynx in the United States: an epidemiologic overview. J Public Health Dent 56:309–318, 1996
146. Silverman S Jr: Oral Cancer. 3rd ed. Atlanta, GA, American Cancer Society, 1989
147. Silverman S, Gorsky M: Epidemiologic and demographic update in oral cancer: California and national data—1973–1985. J Am Dent Assoc 120:495–499, 1990
148. Blot WJ, McLaughlin JK, et al: Smoking and drinking in relation to oral and pharyngeal cancer. Cancer Res 48:3282–3287, 1988
149. Marshall JR, Graham S, Haughey BP, et al: Smoking, alcohol, dentition and diet in the epidemiology of oral cancer. Eur J Cancer B Oral Oncol 28:9–15, 1992
150. Johnson NW, Warnakulasuriya KAAS: Epidemiology and aetiology of oral cancer in the United Kingdom. Community Dent Health 10(Suppl 1):13–29, 1993
151. Office of the Inspector General, Office of Analysis and Inspections: Youth Use of Smokeless Tobacco: More than a Pinch of Trouble. Dallas: US Department of Health and Human Services, 1986
152. National Institutes of Health: The Health Consequences of Using Smokeless Tobacco: A Report of the Advisory Committee to the Surgeon General. Publication No. (NIH) 86-2874. Bethesda, MD: Department of Health and Human Services, 1986
153. Winn DM, Blot WJ, Shy CM, Pickle LW, Toledo A, Fraumeni JR Jr: Snuff dipping and oral cancer among women in the Southern United States. N Engl J Med 304:745–749, 1981
154. Horowitz AM: The need for health promotion in oral cancer prevention and early detection. J Public Health Dent 56:319–330, 1996
155. Martin LM, Bouquot JE, Wingo PA, Heath CW: Cancer prevention in the dental practice: oral cancer screening and tobacco cessation advice. J Public Health Dent 56:336–340, 1996
156. Boyle P, Macfarlane GJ, Scully C: Oral cancer: necessity for prevention strategies. Lancet 342:1129, 1993
157. Hindle I, Nally F: Oral cancer: a comparative study between 1962–67 and 1980–84 in England and Wales. Br Dent J 170:15–19, 1991
158. Green JC, Louie R, Wycoff SJ: Preventive dentistry. II. Periodontal diseases, malocclusion, trauma, and oral cancer. JAMA 263: 421–425, 1990
159. Cohn SJ, Stookey GK, Katz BP, Drook CA, Christen AG: Helping smokers quit: a randomized controlled trial with private practice dentists. J Am Dent Assoc 118:41–45, 1989
160. New strategies to fight oral cancer. JAMA 14:276, 1996
161. Jacob JA: ADA oral cancer prevention efforts honored this month. National conference plots strategies for future work. ADA News 27:1,3, 1996
162. Public Health Service: Healthy People 2000: National Health Promotion and Disease Prevention Objectives. Conference Edition. Washington, DC: US Department of Health and Human Services, 1990
163. Gift HC, Drury TF, Nowjack-Raymer RE, Selwitz RH: The state of the nation's oral health: mid-decade assessment of Healthy People 2000. J Public Health Dent 56:84–91, 1996

VI

Health Care Planning, Organization, and Evaluation

Edited by F. Douglas Scutchfield

66

The American Health Care System: Structure and Function

F. Douglas Scutchfield • Stephen J. Williams

This chapter reviews the organization and operation of the nation's health care system. A systems approach to health care is used to emphasize the interdependencies among the parts of the system and between the system's "hard assets" and the organizational and financial arrangements that allow the system to function. A solid understanding of the system is essential for all participants: provider, consumer, payer, and policymaker.

▶ SYSTEMS APPROACH

A systems approach to health care services creates a topology to guide the review of the components of the system and places each element in context. The system uses resources such as facilities (e.g., hospitals), personnel (e.g., physicians), and technology.[1] These resources are organized by financing mechanisms to produce services for consumers.

The system is dynamic with many feedback loops among the components. This allows for change in the system. The system is interdependent. Modification of one element will impact other elements. It is impossible to change one part of the system without causing reactions in other elements.

The dynamic and interactive nature of the system frequently is forgotten in policymaking. Efforts to improve services to consumers often are based on modifying a single element within the system without recognizing the impact of that modification on other components. Thus each element, and the system as a whole, must be examined and understood.

The system does not operate in isolation from the environment within which it functions. The external environment dramatically influences the function of the health care system. For example, the changing demographic composition of the United States, with an aging population and a growing proportion of minorities, influences the location and types of services that need to be provided. Changes in the economy also dramatically impact health care; for example, job creation increases demand for insurance products and care while recession decreases demand.

The changing nature of disease also provides a dramatic illustration of interaction of health care with the external environment. In the early 1900s the leading causes of death were infectious diseases with acute, frequently self-limited courses. In 1990, by contrast, the major causes of death are the chronic diseases of an aging population. These diseases are more closely linked to lifestyle than to such fundamental environmental concerns as water quality and sewage disposal, as was the case in the early 1900s. Thus today's health policy decision-makers must focus on health behavior and health behavioral change to address contemporary health issues, unlike those of previous generations who needed to focus on such issues as clean water and sewage disposal.

Even since 1950 dramatic changes have occurred in the patterns of disease and illness to which the system must respond.[2] Death rates from cardiovascular and cerebrovascular disease have declined while those from most malignant neoplasms have increased. Overall, reductions in death rates have resulted in greater longevity, which in itself has placed financial and political stress on other aspects of our society, including the Social Security system, Medicare, housing, and education.

The changing nature of the external environment, patterns of illness, and of the system's necessary responses has been outlined by William and Torrens.[1] The problems addressed by the health care system and the nature of the system's changes over the years have been dramatic. There is little doubt that the future will hold even more dramatic and rapid change.

Within the larger system are a multitude of subsystems. Many of these subsystems are informal, put together by the consumer or provider, and some are more formal, put together by insurers and governments. Existing subsystems range from community preventive services to personal care for illness and injury, to mental illness care, to care for aging or debilitated patients. These subsystems vary for each individual. There may be little coordination between providers of each service, and subsystems may be affected by the patient's ability to pay. In general, managed care is increasingly serving as the focal point of the coordination and operation of these systems.

▶ PURPOSE OF HEALTH CARE

The universal goal of the health care system is to ensure adequate access to quality care at a reasonable price. The components of this goal include access, quality, and price. Again, each of these factors cannot be dealt with in isolation. Increasing access may have a negative impact on quality and costs. Decreasing costs often has an adverse impact on access or quality. In the best of all worlds, each component would be maximized with the goal of improving health. However, our nation has a tendency to focus on only one component. A major concern in the 1960s was ensuring access to care; the major concern in the 1990s is containing the cost of that care. We have not been especially successful in achieving our health care goals while at the same time adequately addressing the issues of access, quality, and cost. That is the challenge we faced in the 1990s and will continue to face in the years to come.

► COMPONENTS OF THE SYSTEM

The individual parts of the system are discussed in the next few sections. They are described and then analyzed in their relation to the entire system. The final parts of this chapter address the integration and control of the subsystems, such as control of the flow of dollars spent on care through various insurance programs, that put the pieces together into a "system." Although not every component of the system is addressed in detail, the major parts are covered.

Institutional Care: The Hospital

The hospital is the predominant institutional health care provider. The hospital consumes the largest single share of personal health care resources and in some respects is the most visible and central organization in modern health care. Recently, the growth of ambulatory care, especially within the context of technological advances and cost pressures, is causing the hospital to lose its historical pre-eminence.

The hospital has not always been held in high esteem. The hospital had its origins in the religious orders of medieval times who would provide care for the sick poor. In the United States the earliest hospitals were the almshouses and pest houses, a legacy of the British tradition. They were dark, smelly facilities, unappealing and to be avoided whenever possible. Only people without homes and families were housed in them; anyone of means was cared for in their home by their family.

The first modern U.S. hospital was the Pennsylvania Hospital, founded in Philadelphia in 1751. Slowly throughout the 1800s, other large facilities were built, such as the Massachusetts General Hospital. It was not until the middle 1900s, however, that the modern hospital became a common and central component of the system. The rise of the contemporary hospital resulted from changes in the way medicine was practiced.

The Changing Hospital Environment

The first influence on the growth of the modern hospital was the ability to perform surgical procedures successfully. This was the result of two important scientific advances. The first was the discovery of anesthesia in the 1850s. Before anesthesia, the very best surgeon was the speediest one; complicated procedures could not be performed because of the pain associated with them. The advent of anesthesia ushered in the golden age of surgery in the late 1800s.

The second major advance was the discovery of sepsis. Patients undergoing surgery frequently developed postoperative infections. With the knowledge of sepsis, the danger of postoperative infection was substantially reduced. These two advances allowed surgery to become a major force in the care of patients. One need only consider that over 40 percent of total hospital beds are surgical beds to understand the impact of these discoveries. The more recent advances in outpatient surgical procedures probably represent another turning point in the influence of surgery on the system.

The late 1800s saw the emergence of the biological revolution. The new science of microbiology ushered in a new understanding of disease. The notion of the etiologic agent as the cause of disease required fundamental rethinking of diagnosis and treatment. New technology to assist in the diagnosis and treatment of patients developed rapidly during that period. The discovery of the electrocardiograph and the x-ray illustrate the expanding role of technology.

The early laboratories and machines of this technological revolution were primitive by today's standards and were physically very large. It made sense to provide a central place, the hospital, where all physicians could have access to this new technology. To this day, the hospital continues to serve a major role as the repository of technology for the community, although presently much is being done to move this technology into noninstitutional locations.

A third major development occurred in the nursing profession. Inmates provided what nursing care was available in the early almshouses. In the mid-1800s, during the Crimean War, Florence Nightingale demonstrated the advantages of professional nursing services on mortality. She later developed nurse training programs in Britain, and hospitals in the United States followed suit. The availability of well-trained nursing personnel made hospitals much safer and more pleasant places.

The training of physicians also has changed dramatically, and this has been an important factor in the development of hospitals. Before 1900, medical education in the United States was seriously deficient. Most physicians were trained in proprietary apprenticeships, with many lectures and little exposure to patients.

The development of professional licensure was important in the reformation of American medical education. Licensing was based on an examination and required graduation from an approved school. A second contributing factor was the Flexner Report. The Carnegie Foundation, at the urging of the American Medical Association, hired a nonphysician educator, Abraham Flexner, to visit the nation's medical schools and to provide recommendations for their reform. Flexner reported that the existing medical schools were grossly inadequate. One school, however, stood out. This school, Johns Hopkins University, served as an example for the others. The positive features of this school were: (*a*) students were required to have a college degree before they were admitted; (*b*) the medical curriculum was 4 years in duration, with 2 years dedicated to basic sciences and 2 years to work with full-time clinical instructors; (*c*) the medical school was an integral part of a comprehensive university; and (*d*) faculty of the school were actively engaged in medical research; and (*e*) the university owned and operated its own hospital where clinical instruction of students and medical residents occured.[3]

Another development that was critical to the modern hospital was the increasing number of individuals who had health insurance. Health insurance was relatively unknown until the 1930s. During the 1940s, there was a rapid increase in the proportion of people who were covered. In addition, the advent of public insurance programs during the 1960s, specifically Medicare and Medicaid, provided a guaranteed source of support for the hospital.

Types of Hospitals

Hospitals can be classified by length of stay, ownership, and number of beds (Table 66-1). There are short- and long-term hospitals; the dividing point is an average length of stay of 30 days. Hospitals also are characterized by type of service, the most common being the general hospital. There are also children's, eye, and other specialized hospitals. A third classification of hospitals is by ownership: governmental, not-for-profit, and proprietary (also known as for-profit) or investor-owned.

Governmental hospitals, in turn, are classified as federal, state, and local. Federal hospitals serve groups eligible as the result of some type of legislative entitlement. Indian Health Service hospitals, for example, meet treaty obligations, and Veterans Administration hospitals serve certain eligible veterans.

State facilities generally are either mental or tuberculosis hospitals. Increasingly, these hospitals have been closed, as states attempt to control their budgets and as treatment for mental illness and tuberculosis moves to outpatient settings. In some cases, states share responsibility with local government as a hospital provider of last resort for patients without financial resources.

Local governmental hospitals include city or county hospitals that provide care to those individuals without the resources to pay. They are usually under local political government supervision. They are often large and overburdened, may have inadequate physical plants, and are usually affiliated with a medical school that provides all or a portion of their medical staff. Local government hospitals have gone through troubled times. With the advent of Medicaid it was thought that these hospitals would be abandoned by the urban poor who could then buy care elsewhere. But this did not happen, and the growth in the uninsured population has put severe stresses on these hospitals in an era of declining financial and political support.

Another type of local hospital, popular in the western United States, is the public authority hospital, which is financed in part by a

TABLE 66-1. SHORT-STAY HOSPITALS, BEDS, AND OCCUPANCY RATES, ACCORDING TO TYPE OF OWNERSHIP AND SIZE OF HOSPITAL: UNITED STATES[a]

Type of Ownership and Size of Hospital	*1960*	*1970*	*1980*	*1993*
■ ***HOSPITALS***				
All ownerships	5,768	6,193	6,229	5,579
Federal	361	334	325	290
Nonfederal	5,407	5,859	5,904	5,289
Nonprofit	3,291	3,386	3,339	3,163
Proprietary	856	769	730	717
State-local government	1,260	1,704	1,835	1,409
Size of hospital				
6–99 beds			2,953	2,436
100–199 beds			1,436	1,398
200–299 beds			742	760
300–499 beds			724	653
500 beds or more			374	332
■ ***BEDS***				
All ownerships	73,451	935,724	1,080,164	992,375
Federal	96,394	87,492	88,144	71,868
Nonfederal	639,057	848,232	992,020	920,507
Nonprofit	445,753	591,937	692,929	651,560
Proprietary	37,029	52,739	87,033	98,964
State-local government	156,275	203,556	212,058	169,983
Size of hospital				
6–99 beds			155,259	127,377
100–199 beds			203,023	197,729
200–299 beds			180,047	186,059
300–499 beds			276,201	247,355
500 beds or more			265,634	233,855
■ ***OCCUPANCY RATE***		***PERCENT OF BEDS OCCUPIED***		
All ownerships	75.7	77.9	75.6	65.1
Federal	82.5	77.5	77.8	73.8
Nonfederal	74.7	78.0	75.4	64.4
Nonprofit	76.6	80.1	78.2	66.4
Proprietary	65.4	72.2	65.2	51.1
State-local government	71.6	73.2	70.7	64.6
Size of hospital				
6–99 beds		60.6	49.2	
100–199 beds		71.6	59.4	
200–299 beds		77.3	64.7	
300–499 beds		80.0	68.8	
500 beds or more		81.9	75.0	

From National Center for Health Statistics: Health, United States, 1995. Hyattsville, MD: US Public Health Service, 1996.
[a] Data are based on reporting by a census of hospitals.

hospital assessment district similar to a water or fire district. These hospitals receive tax money and are controlled by an elected board. Many of these facilities, however, serve relatively affluent suburbs.

Not-for-profit hospitals are public corporations exempt from taxation. Any excess revenue over expenses is retained to expand services. Many not-for-profit hospitals are affiliated with religious orders. In several states these facilities are increasingly being called upon to justify their tax exempt status, as in many cases they function much like proprietary hospitals.

Proprietary hospitals have been around for many years. Early in the century prominent physicians would build a hospital for their own use. The number of such facilities has declined over the years. The 1960s saw the development of large "chains" of investor-owned facilities. These hospitals are owned by stockholders, who receive a return on their equity as in other publicly held companies. These entities have seen rapid growth as companies built, bought, or developed management contracts with an increasing number of hospitals. There is considerable controversy regarding the relative efficiency and quality of care of not-for-profit versus for-profit hospitals. However, both types of hospital ownership seem to serve the consumer adequately.

In response to the growth of these corporations and the need to have access to capital and to achieve economies of scale, other multihospital systems have developed. Some are small, some focus on rural hospitals, and many are comprised of not-for-profit hospitals. As occupancy rates have fallen, hospitals have had to become more competitive. They also have diversified, adding new programs and services. Hospitals have developed market niches through specialized programs and have established joint ventures with each other and with physicians to attract dollars, physicians, and patients. But the most striking development of all has been the overall move toward consolidation and affiliation primarily in response to the pressure of the managed care environment.

Structure of the Hospital

There are three competing sources of authority in the hospital: the governing board, administration, and medical staff. The governing board has the ultimate responsibility for the hospital. They set policy, hire and fire the administrator, and appoint members of the medical staff. They also have ultimate responsibility for the quality of care; as a result, many hospitals have added members of the medical staff to the board and most have increased quality assurance activities. In some corporate arrangements, hospital governance may become the responsibility of the parent company. In the United States there usually is not a direct financial relationship between hospitals and physicians, although some physicians need a hospital to practice in and hospitals need physicians to admit patients. The mutual dependence is represented by the governing bylaws of the medical staff, which define the rules and regulations governing physician interaction with the hospital. Election and duties of the medical staff officers and committees and processes for awarding and maintaining privileges are defined by these bylaws.

The growth in the size and complexity of the hospital mandates a well-educated administrator who can provide leadership and professional management. The administrator now is often termed the president or chief executive officer to reflect the new corporate orientation of the contemporary hospital.

Challenges Facing the Hospital

The hospital faces many complex problems;[4] these problems are especially severe for small and rural hospitals. The rising cost of hospital care, consuming the largest proportion of the health-care dollar, has prompted programs to control the use of hospital beds. Some of these mechanisms, such as diagnosis-related groups (DRGs), have substantial impact on hospital decision-making. Employers and insurers negotiate with hospitals for discounted rates for their employees or subscribers. Managed care arrangements may force significant price concessions. Avenues for recovery of funds for nonpaying patients and for subsidized indigent care are declining, especially with less cost shifting. The federally mandated Peer Review Organizations (PRO) review care provided to recipients of Medicare benefits for appropriateness of use.

Another issue is overbedding. After World War II, the Health Facilities and Planning (Hill-Burton) Act was passed. Although successful, this program and subsequent hospital construction has resulted in excess capacity. In addition, out-of-hospital care, technological advances in diagnosis and treatment, and quicker recovery of patients have shortened hospital stays (Table 66-2). Excess capacity contributes to higher costs as the fixed costs of operating an empty bed is borne by the consumer in the filled beds.

A third, and related, issue is the changing nature of hospital use. Patients who previously would have been hospitalized now are being treated on an outpatient basis; those remaining in the hospital are sicker and require more technology and care. These increases in intensity also contribute to nursing stresses and shortages.

TABLE 66-2. DISCHARGES, DAYS OF CARE, AND AVERAGE LENGTH OF STAY IN SHORT-STAY HOSPITALS, ACCORDING TO SELECTED CHARACTERISTICS: UNITED STATES, 1964 AND 1994[a]

	Discharges[b]		Days of Care		Average Length of Stay[c]	
Characteristics	*1964*	*1994*	*1964*	*1994*	*1964*	*1994*
Total	109.1	87.5	970.9	549.4	8.9	6.3
■ ***AGE***						
Under 15 years	67.6	40.7	45.7	237.2	6.0	5.8
5–14 years	94.3	67.7	731.1	423.7	7.8	6.3
15–44 years	100.6	60.6	760.7	326.8	7.6	5.4
45–64 years	146.2	121.9	1,559.3	711.5	10.7	5.8
65 years or over	10.0	268.8	2,292.7	2,086.2	12.1	7.8
65–74 years	181.2	230.1	2,150.4	1,648.7	11.9	7.2
75 years and over	206.7	324.2	2,560.4	2,711.6	12.4	8.4
■ ***SEX***						
Male	103.8	86.6	1,010.2	605.8	9.7	7.0
Female	113.7	89.0	933.4	502.7	8.2	5.6
■ ***RACE***						
White	112.4	85.1	961.4	518.7	8.6	6.1
Black	84.0	111.6	1,062.9	746.5	12.7	6.7
■ ***FAMILY INCOME***						
Less than $14,000	102.4	134.6	1,051.2	969.9	10.3	7.2
$14,000–$24,999	116.4	103.4	1,213.9	747.5	10.4	7.2
$25,00–$34,999	110.7	81.9	939.8	446.4	8.5	5.5
$35,000–$49,999	109.2	76.9	882.6	446.2	8.1	5.8
$50,000 or more	110.7	60.6	918.9	320.4	8.3	5.3
■ ***GEOGRAPHIC REGION***						
Northeast	98.5	82.6	993.8	626.0	10.1	7.6
Midwest	109.2	92.2	944.9	539.0	8.7	5.8
South	117.8	98.2	968.0	577.7	8.2	5.9
West	110.5	70.0	985.9	439.6	8.9	6.3
■ ***LOCATION OF RESIDENCE***						
Within MSA	107.5	82.8	1,015.4	549.0	9.4	6.6
Outside MSA	113.3	104.3	871.9	559.4	7.7	5.4

From National Center for Health Statistics: Health, United States, 1995. Hyattsville, MD: US Public Health Service, 1996.

[a] Data are based on household interviews of a sample of the civilian noninstitutionalized population.

[b] Number per 1,000 population.

[c] Number of days.

Ambulatory Care

Ambulatory care includes a wide range of practitioners, settings, and services for the "walking" or noninstitutionalized patient. Ambulatory care services play a central role as the initial and continuing point of contact with the system for most people. Ambulatory services provide intake for patients, serve as their point of contact for follow-up and ongoing care, and serve a broker function as the center of the referral network for specialized hospital and physician services, an especially visible role in managed care programs.

Types of Care Provided

Public health services, discussed in more detail in the following chapter, include services designed to avoid the occurrence of disease in populations. Although these services do not involve the direct provision of health care, they are critical to the improvement of health; they include protection of the workplace through accident avoidance and safety efforts and protection of the food and water supplies. Clinical preventive services include the direct provision of care to avoid disease. These services include counseling interventions, disease screening, and immunizations and chemoprophylaxis.

Primary care includes the daily routine care that individuals receive from the health care system for diagnosis, counseling, follow-up, and therapy for the most common conditions. More complex care is termed secondary care. Considerable secondary care is provided on an ambulatory basis by specialty physicians in their offices or in specialized centers such as ambulatory surgical centers. Tertiary care includes the most highly complex services, such as open-heart surgery, and is provided in sophisticated medical centers.

Historical Perspective

Historically, most medical care has been provided on an ambulatory care basis. Ambulatory care services traditionally have been provided by individual medical practitioners providing care in their offices and in patients' homes and by public clinics operating primarily for poor and medically indigent patients. The general practitioner who made house calls and offered what treatment was available was typical of the primary care provider before World War II.

Since World War II, fewer physicians have been able to spend the time required traveling to the patient's home, and many can no longer carry with them the specialized resources available in the office. The growth of technology and specialization has led to the rapid expansion of newer settings for providing care, such as group practices and hospital clinics. For the poor, care often has been limited to public or philanthropic clinics or dispensaries. These public care providers eventually evolved into public hospitals and clinics.

Use of Ambulatory Care Services

Quantitative information on the use of ambulatory care resources consists mostly of data on physician utilization. These data reflect greater use of hospital outpatient departments by blacks than by whites, and by lower income than by higher income people. This would suggest that office-based care may be less accessible to the poor and to minorities than to the nonpoor and to whites.

Most of the ambulatory care that people receive is provided in office-based practice settings, as reflected in Table 66-3. Although a significant amount of care is provided in hospital settings, the predominant source of care is the physician's office, including solo, group, and noninstitutional clinic practices.

The two predominant settings or organizational forms of practice are solo and group practice. Solo practice means a single private practitioner. Group practice is the combination of three or more practitioners in a medical or other office-based practice. True group practice involves the sharing of income, expenses, staff, medical records, and other resources. Sometimes physicians share only physical space or staff. This arrangement does not constitute a formal group.

Most ambulatory care services traditionally have been provided by physicians in solo office-based practice. From the provider's perspective, solo practice offers an opportunity to avoid organizational dependence and to be self-employed. Philosophically, solo practice is most closely aligned with the traditional economic orientations that have characterized medicine. Although solo practice still accounts for substantial ambulatory services, group practice and hospital-based services are expanding dramatically. Changing lifestyles, the growth of managed care and other contracting arrangements, the cost of establishing a practice, and other pressures on practitioners also have adversely affected the traditional dominance of solo practice.

National Ambulatory Care Survey

An ongoing national study of all private office-based physicians, the National Ambulatory Medical Care Survey (NAMCS), has been conducted by the federal government.[5] The NAMCS involves a random sample of the nation's office-based nonfederal physicians who are asked to complete a data collection form for each patient treated during a brief time period. The most common care provided is routine care. Follow-up or ongoing care and the prominence of relatively simple primary care problems is striking. Limited examinations, laboratory tests, and blood pressure checks are the most common diagnostic services provided, whereas counseling is the most common therapeutic service provided, exclusive of drugs.

Group Practice

Some of the earliest group practices in the United States were started by industries that needed to provide care to employees in rural sites where medical care was unavailable. The Mayo Clinic in Rochester, Minnesota, was the first successful nonindustrial group practice. The Mayo Clinic, originally organized as a single specialty group practice in 1887 and later broadened into a multispecialty group, represented a reputable model for group practice. In 1931 the Committee on the Costs of Medical Care issued a report suggesting a major role for group practice, especially those associated with hospitals, in providing comprehensive care. Unfortunately the far-sighted recommendations contained in that report were never implemented, in large measure due to the vigorous opposition of organized medicine.

Developments in medical practice, especially increasing specialization and expansion of technology, has also spurred the group practice movement. More complex and expensive facilities, equipment, and personnel were needed, and group practice provided a structure for sharing the costs associated with this increased complexity. Multispecialty groups could provide patients with more of their health care under one roof and thus reduce problems of physical access to care. Group practice was seen by many as facilitating referral arrangements and shared after-hours coverage, providing more flexible working hours, and requiring less financial risk for the physician while also benefiting the patient.

The American Medical Association conducts a periodic survey of physician-oriented medical group practices in the United States. There are currently over 16,000 group practices in the country.[6] Most are relatively small, with an average of slightly under 10 physicians, but the prevalence of larger multispecialty groups is growing. Recent evidence indicates the increasing preference of group practice, especially by younger physicians and in the managed care environment. Furthermore, physicians are increasingly practicing in a more corporate-oriented environment as employees rather than owners.[7]

The increasing integration of the health care system raises interesting questions regarding the affiliations of group practices with other organizations. Increasing numbers of groups are affiliated with a hospital through ownership or affiliation arrangements. There is a growing tendency for the creation of alliances between physicians and hospitals in the form of Physician Hospital Organizations (PHOs) or Medical Service Organizations (MSOs). By development of these alliances, hospital and physician organizations may more effectively compete for contracts with insurance and managed care organizations.

From a community perspective, groups may reduce the geographic dispersion of providers and thus increase difficulties of

TABLE 66-3. PHYSICIANS' CONTACTS, ACCORDING TO PLACE OF CONTACT AND SELECTED PATIENT CHARACTERISTICS: UNITED STATES, 1994[a]

Characteristics	Total	Place of Contact: Doctor's Office	Hospital Outpatient Department	Telephone	Home	Other
		Percent Distribution				
Total	100.0	56.8	13.6	13.2	3.5	12.8
AGE						
Under 15 years	100.0	60.6	13.1	14.3	0.8	11.1
Under 5 years	100.0	59.2	12.7	15.4	0.9	11.8
5–14 years	100.0	62.1	13.5	13.1	0.8	10.5
15–44 years	100.0	55.7	14.1	13.1	1.8	15.2
45–64 years	100.0	55.1	15.0	14.2	3.6	12.2
65 years or over	100.0	53.4	10.1	8.6	18.6	9.3
65–74 years	100.0	55.4	11.9	9.4	12.4	10.9
75 years and over	100.0	51.1	7.9	7.8	25.8	7.4
SEX						
Male	100.0	55.4	15.6	11.7	3.5	13.9
Female	100.0	57.7	12.2	14.3	3.5	12.2
RACE						
White	100.0	58.4	12.5	14.1	3.3	11.8
Black	100.0	47.9	20.3	8.1	4.2	19.4
FAMILY INCOME						
Less than $14,000	100.0	43.9	19.0	11.9	5.7	19.5
$14,000–$24,999	100.0	53.8	16.6	13.0	3.9	12.7
$25,000–$34,999	100.0	61.5	12.1	12.7	2.0	11.6
$35,000–$49,999	100.0	56.9	11.6	16.3	3.9	11.2
$50,000 or more	100.0	63.8	9.4	15.5	1.6	9.8
GEOGRAPHIC REGION						
Northeast	100.0	59.0	13.0	12.8	4.0	11.2
Midwest	100.0	55.8	14.0	15.1	2.2	12.9
South	100.0	58.4	14.0	12.5	4.3	10.8
West	100.0	54.1	13.5	12.8	3.2	16.5

From National Center for Health Statistics: Health, United States, 1995. Hyattsville, MD: US Public Health Service, 1996.
[a] Data are based on household interviews of a sample of the civilian noninstitutionalized population.

physical access to care. In addition groups may reduce competition in the health care marketplace by consolidating what would otherwise be competing providers.

Hospital-based Ambulatory Care

An increasing number of people have sought primary care from hospitals, sometimes as a result of lack of access to other care, taxing the ability of many facilities to respond. The result has been overcrowded facilities; the wrong mix of services, equipment, and personnel to respond to patient needs; and extremely dissatisfied consumers and providers. Many hospitals have now successfully expanded outpatient services and hired full-time providers to staff redesigned hospital ambulatory facilities. A hospital-sponsored or hospital-based group practice can provide comprehensive and accessible care and remove primary care patients from emergency rooms. These groups also increase the use of the hospital inpatient and ancillary services. Hospitals with ambulatory care resources can negotiate contracts for providing a wide range of both inpatient and outpatient services. They are also better able to control the use of services and costs. Increasing competition is forcing many hospitals to enter this business.

Hospitals have long been involved with the construction of medical office buildings and are now moving into new businesses such as joint ventures with physicians and others, development of health plans, and purchases of medical practices. The success or failure of these ventures will not be measurable for some time, but they place the hospital at greater financial risk as hospitals become more dependent on their successful administrative and financial involvement in other ventures.

Freestanding Ambulatory Centers

A further innovation in hospital-based care has been the development of ambulatory surgery centers that provide 1-day surgical care. In the early 1970s, freestanding ambulatory surgery centers were opened independent of hospitals. Many physicians perform surgery in their offices as well; specialties such as oral surgery, plastic surgery, and ophthalmology use office-based facilities extensively. Freestanding emergency centers also have opened in many cities. These emergency centers sometimes provide a wide range of primary care in addition to responding to urgent problems. The future of specialized ambulatory centers, in both hospitals and as freestanding facilities, will include further expansion into other areas of health care, ranging from sports medicine to women's health care.

Governmental and Noninstitutional Programs

Governmental programs have been designed to increase the availability of health care resources. Neighborhood Health Centers, first funded in 1965, are freestanding group practices that predominantly serve the medically indigent in urban areas. The combination of former "free" clinics, neighborhood health centers, public agency clinics, and some hospital clinics and groups now form an informal "safety net" of providers for individuals who lack private insurance or access to other sources of care, or who simply need care. Some of these providers also contract to provide care under local governmental entitlement programs.

The federal government also operates health care facilities. The Veterans Administration includes one of the largest health services system under a unified management structure in the United States. The military services provides health care to millions of people in the armed forces, and the Indian Health Service is charged with ensuring access to medical care to the Native American population.

Many other services help to meet the needs of a community. The list is nearly endless. Home health services are provided by visiting nurse associations, proprietary companies, some hospitals, public health departments, and other agencies. Rural health care has required unique and innovative solutions in many communities, especially in the absence of adequate supplies of physicians and facilities, and remains a challenging test of the ingenuity and resourcefulness of the health services system. Other community health services include school health services; prison health services; vision care; dental care provided by solo, group, and institutionally based practitioners; foot care from podiatrists; and drug-dispensing from pharmacists.

Long-Term Care

Long-term or chronic care represents, along with mental health services, perhaps our greatest challenge for the future in health care. Although other countries have successfully implemented long-term care innovations, the United States has been slow to innovate and to address the underlying problems of those people in need of long-term care.

Long-term care encompasses a wide spectrum of services, termed the continuum of care. Long-term care includes skilled nursing, intermediate, and respite care; certain acute care services such as rehabilitation; ambulatory care, including both traditional services and more targeted care such as adult day care and substance abuse programs; home health care; and outreach, health promotion, and recreational and housing services. Among the problems our nation faces in the area of long-term care are coordinating each component of the continuum and ensuring access to those services that meet the specific needs of each patient. Financing for many components of the system is currently inadequate.

The nursing home is the most costly component of the continuum of care and the one that attracts the most visibility. There are nearly 1.5 million residents of the nation's more than 23,000 nursing homes. Most residents are over age 75, are female, have multiple health problems, and have severe mobility and independence difficulties (Table 66-4). Although many nursing homes are small, there is an increasing trend toward larger homes and toward ownership by multihome not-for-profit and for-profit entities.

Because Medicare generally does not cover care in nursing homes, patients must rely on their own financial resources until these are depleted and then must rely on Medicaid. Financial support for nursing home care generally is inadequate to provide the level of services, activities, physical environment, and staff care responsibility needed for all patients to receive high quality care. Financing of long-term care services remains oriented toward short-term interventions, especially for insurance plans; government, especially at the local level, remains the provider of last resort. Complex legal and social issues related to patient rights, to the obligations of providers, and to the role of society are constantly evolving; many issues have not been adequately addressed.

Other progress is being made in the continuum of long-term care. The hospice provides services to terminally ill patients in a caring and medically supportive environment using a multispecialty approach in institutional and home settings. Home health services have expanded rapidly over the past few years. Various types of retirement and "life care" communities are being developed, although some earlier attempts were not financially successful. The financing, administrative, and coordinating requirements to adequately address these long-term care needs remains far too limited. The availability of increased financial support would likely lead to great success in meeting the needs of the long-term care patient.

TABLE 66-4. NURSING HOME AND PERSONAL CARE HOME RESIDENTS 65 YEARS OF AGE AND OVER AND RATE PER 1,000 POPULATION, ACCORDING TO AGE, SEX, AND RACE: UNITED STATES, 1985[a]

Characteristics	*Residents*	*Residents per 1,000 Population*
■ ***AGE***		
All ages	1,318,300	46.2
65–74 years	212,100	12.5
75–84 years	509,000	57.7
85 years and over	597,300	220.3
■ ***SEX AND AGE***		
Male	334,400	29.0
65–74 years	80,600	10.8
75–84 years	141,300	43.0
85 years and over	112,600	145.7
Female	983,900	57.9
65–74 years	131,500	13.8
75–84 years	367,700	66.4
85 years and over	484,700	250.01
■ ***RACE AND AGE***		
White	1,227,400	47.7
65–74 years	187,800	12.3
75–84 years	473,600	59.1
85 years and over	566,000	228.7
Black	82,000	35.0
65–74 years	22,500	15.4
75–84 years	30,600	45.3
85 years and over	29,000	141.5

From National Center for Health Statistics: Health, United States, 1995. Hyattsville, MD: US Public Health Service, 1996.

[a] Data are based on a sample of nursing homes.

Mental Health Services

Mental health care shares some similar characteristics with long-term care, but it also requires some unique considerations of its own. Financing is inadequate in this arena as well, and many insurers and governmental programs provide only limited reimbursement for these services. Unfortunately the trend is probably toward even further restrictions, with the possible exception of substance abuse treatment.

Mental health services involve a number of somewhat unique issues. Services are generally provided through parallel public and private subsystems, with those individuals having insurance or self-pay capacity receiving care through the private route. These patients are more likely to obtain care from psychiatrists and private mental health hospitals and facilities. Public hospitals and clinics are the providers of last resort and have a higher predominance of psychologists. Mental health professionals, particularly psychiatrists, psychologists, and social workers also compete for certain patient care responsibilities. Increasingly, biomedical progress and clinical interventions, primarily pharmacological, may shift the balance of power further to physicians in mental health.

As with long-term care, our society has yet to accept responsibility for solving the problems involving the mental health of our nation's citizens. Although the technology for clinical intervention is in a relatively young but hopeful stage of development, with considerable long-term progress likely, the financial, political, and administrative challenges continue to beg for attention.

▸ HEALTH CARE PERSONNEL

The health care system is a major employer. There are numerous professions that are involved in health services. Physicians are the most powerful of these professionals, and they have the most important role in making decisions about the use of resources, most notably especially since the evolution of a scientific approach to clinical medicine starting early in the twentieth century.[3]

The Physician

In the early 1960s there was a perception that a shortage of physicians existed. National policy resulted in the growth of medical school classes and the building of new medical schools. Foreign medical school graduates were viewed as an additional source of physician personnel for United States.

In 1963 the Health Professions Educational Assistance Act was passed to provide funds to medical schools based on enrollments and for grants and loans for the construction of new medical education facilities. This legislation marked the first instance of direct federal involvement in medical education. Previous attempts by the federal government had been opposed by both organized medicine and medical schools themselves, based on a concern that the federal government might regulate medical education.

The incentives contained in the Health Professions Assistance Act were effective in increasing the number of medical school graduates. From 1965 to 1980 the number of medical schools and graduates doubled (Table 66-5).

Immigration policy preferentially allowed foreign medical school graduates to enter the country. An influx of physicians from many foreign countries resulted from this policy, with a notable representation from third world countries. Many hospitals used these physicians to fill residency training programs and to staff the hospital. At its peak, foreign medical graduates received nearly half of the annual new licenses issued.

By the mid-1980s these policies may have overcorrected physician supply, and a surplus may now exist. It is projected that there will be more than 700,000 active physicians by the year 2000. In 1980 the Graduate Medical Education National Advisory Committee (GMENAC) suggested that by 1990 there would be an excess of 70,000 physicians.[8] With the pendulum now swinging the other way, medical school class sizes have shrunk, and immigration laws no longer allow preferential treatment for foreign medical graduates.

By 1988 the Council on Graduate Medical Education (COGME) concluded that the nation had more physicians than it needed. More recent COGME reports have reiterated that concern, especially in light of the growth of managed care, and have suggested methods for dealing with the physician excess.[9] Regardless, there remains some controversy regarding the current balance between supply and demand.[10] In spite of the excess, applicants are still drawn to medical school. While there was a modest dip in the number of applicants in the 1980s, there continues to be an increase in the number of individuals who apply to medical school. The number of women choosing careers in medicine has increased.[11] Much less success has been achieved with minority enrollments.

There is also concern about specialty distribution (Table 66-6). There is a perception of a shortage of primary care physicians and an excess of specialists. Managed care, in particular, has emphasized an increasing role for and use of primary care physicians.[12] Efforts to correct specialty imbalances have included federal training grants for residency training in primary care specialties. The COGME identified the shortage of primary care, geriatric, and preventive medicine specialists as a national problem. COGME has also suggested mechanisms for paying for postgraduate medical education to redress the specialty maldistribution and increase the proportion of physicians who provide primary care.

Another issue has been physician geographic distribution. Rural and inner city areas have had difficulty attracting physicians because of income differentials, ambiance, lack of peer interaction, and other factors. The physician is a well-educated professional who wants the amenities of education, cultural opportunities, and an appealing environment for his or her family. There has been speculation that the increase in the number of physicians would result in physicians locating in shortage areas and, to some extent, this has occurred, although deficiencies still exist.

Some states have loan programs for students who agree to practice in medically underserved areas. The Federal National Health Service Corps also was developed to support medical students who agreed to practice in shortage areas. Other programs exposed medical students and residents to rural and urban underserved areas. The Area Health Education Center program, for example, provides experiences in undeserved areas. Unfortunately, most of these programs have had only limited success.

Nursing

The nursing profession is in transition. The development of the professional nurse contributed to the rise of the modern hospital. Florence Nightingale validated the tremendous impact of good nursing on mortality. Dorthea Dix had a similar impact on the nursing profession during the U.S. Civil War. The first nursing training programs associated with hospitals were 3 years in length, and graduates, who received a diploma, were eligible to take state registered nurse (RN) examinations. To assist the registered nurse, another auxiliary profession, the licensed practical nurse, was created. The licensed practical nurse trains for about 1 year in a vocational program. Hospital-trained diploma nurses registered by the state as RNs and 1-year licensed practical or vocational nurses were predominant until the 1950s. During the 1950s and 1960s the nursing profession sought a more professional role. The nursing profession promoted university-educated nurses

TABLE 66-5. ACTIVE PHYSICIANS, ACCORDING TO TYPE OF PHYSICIAN AND NUMBER PER 10,000 POPULATION: UNITED STATES AND OUTLYING U.S. AREAS, SELECTED YEARS 1950, 1960, 1970, 1980, 1990 AND PROJECTIONS FOR THE YEAR 2000

	Number of Physicians			
Year	***All Active Physicians***	***Doctors of Medicine***	***Doctors of Osteopathy***	***Active Physicians per 10,000 Population***
1950	219,900	209,000	10,900	14.1
1960	259,500	247,300	12,200	14.0
1970	326,500	314,200	12,300	15.6
1980	457,500	440,400	17,100	19.7
1990	589,500	561,400	28,100	23.4
2000	724,200	682,400	41,800	26.2

From National Center for Health Statistics: Health, United States, 1995. Hyattsville, MD: US Public Health Service, 1996.

TABLE 66-6. PHYSICIANS, ACCORDING TO ACTIVITY AND PLACE OF MEDICAL EDUCATION: UNITED STATES AND OUTLYING U.S. AREAS, SELECTED YEARS 1975 AND 1994

Activity and Place of Medical Education	*1975*	*1994*
Doctors of medicine	393,742	684,414
Professionally active	340,280	605,468
Place of medical education		
U. S. medical graduates		467,092
International medical graduates		138,376
Activity		
Nonfederal	312,089	583,014
Patient care	287,837	538,437
Office-based practice	213,334	407,044
General and family practice	46,347	58,210
Cardiovascular diseases	5,046	12,917
Dermatology	3,442	6,709
Gastroenterology	1,696	6,707
Internal medicine	28,188	67,897
Pediatrics	12,687	31,474
Pulmonary diseases	1,166	4,631
General surgery	19,710	24,209
Obstetrics and gynecology	15,613	28,211
Ophthalmology	8,795	15,297
Orthopedic surgery	8,148	15,580
Otolaryngology	4,297	6,856
Plastic surgery	1,706	4,313
Urological surgery	5,025	7,779
Anesthesiology	8,970	21,962
Diagnostic radiology	1,978	12,079
Emergency medicine		10,604
Neurology	1,862	7,131
Pathology, anatomical/clinical	4,195	8,715
Psychiatry	12,173	22,551
Radiology	6,970	5,885
Other specialty	15,320	27,327
Hospital-based practice	74,503	131,393
Residents and interns	53,527	86,832
Full-time hospital staff	20,976	44,561
Other professional activity	24,252	44,577
Federal	28,191	22,454
Patient care	24,100	19,101
Office-based practice	2,095	0
Hospital-based practice	22,005	19,101
Residents and interns	4,275	
Full-time hospital staff	17,730	16,658
Other professional activity	4,091	3,353
Inactive	21,449	63,285
Not classified	26,145	14,283
Unknown address	5,868	1,378

From National Center for Health Statistics: Health, United States, 1995. Hyattsville, MD: US Public Health Service, 1996.

who received baccalaureate degrees and could assume overall patient care responsibility. A second group were nurses trained in a 2-year technical program. Both the "professional" nurse and the "technical" nurse were eligible for the registration examination.

Since the 1980s the nursing profession has suggested that only the baccalaureate nurse should be eligible for the RN examination. The number of diploma graduates has decreased, and the number of baccalaureate and associate degree nurses has increased, although these changes have not been without controversy.

Although there are more nurses than any other health professional group, many nurses have left the field because of salary and work condition constraints and other more attractive opportunities. With an increase of hospitalized patients there is an increased demand for more clinical training on the part of nursing personnel. In addition, the continued downsizing of the hospital industry suggests that we may be producing too many nurses, as hospitals are currently the largest employer of nursing personnel. The nursing profession has also indicated its willingness to assume more responsibility for primary care, if primary care physicians are not available to provide needed service.

Dental Personnel

There are approximately 50,000 dentists licensed to practice in the United States. Dentistry has achieved great success in prevention, but also has become a troubled profession. Dentistry is largely a discretionary service and under some economic conditions people have a tendency to postpone using dental services. Dental conditions frequently are not fully covered by insurance, increasing its price sensitivity. Advances in dentistry such as fluoridation of the public water supply and better oral hygiene have decreased the incidence of tooth decay and other oral health problems, thereby decreasing the need for dental practitioners.

Dentists have changed the way they practice by using auxiliary personnel more effectively to increase the volume of services they provide. The use of "four-handed dentistry" also has improved productivity. Like medicine, dentistry benefited from the Health Professions Education Assistance Act, which resulted in an increased number of schools and class sizes. However, the current surplus of dentists has led to the closure of some schools and a downturn in the number of applicants to dental schools.

Auxiliary Personnel

During the 1960s and 1970s, in response to a perceived shortage of physicians, especially in primary care, and geographic maldistribution of physicians, there were suggestions that other nonphysician personnel could meet these needs. These personnel included nurse practitioners and physician assistants. Nurse practitioners are registered nurses who receive 1 or 2 years of additional specialized clinical training leading to a certificate and sometimes a master's degree.

These programs provide the skills to do histories and physical examinations, to follow protocols for diagnosing common illnesses, and to provide limited clinical care, including prescribing certain medications. Increased access to care was intended to result from the decision of these professionals to practice in areas where a physician was unavailable or where a practice could efficiently use such practitioners.[13]

The use of nurse practitioners and physician assistants has been limited by clinical and political struggles over where and under what conditions they can practice. State practice statutes and insurance billing procedures also have hindered their role. The increasing supply of physicians is leading to turf battles and a decreased role for some of these personnel, except for some prepaid settings and in physician practices where they clearly increase the incomes and productivity of the physicians.[14] Finally, the quality of care provided by these individuals and patient satisfaction with them appear to be quite good when supervision is adequate.

▸ FINANCING AND THE COST OF MEDICAL CARE

The United States spends over 13.5 percent of its gross domestic product on health care, or nearly a trillion dollars per year (Table 66-7). The hospital is the largest user of health care dollars (Table 66-8). Although physicians account for under 20 percent of total health care expenditures, they control many other resources. The United States spends a greater percentage of gross domestic product on health care than any other nation, though the international differences have not always been as great as they are now.

TABLE 66-7. TOTAL HEALTH EXPENDITURES AS A PERCENT OF GROSS DOMESTIC PRODUCT AND PER CAPITA HEALTH EXPENDITURES IN DOLLARS: SELECTED COUNTRIES AND YEARS[a]

Country	*1960*	*1970*	*1980*	*1990*	*1993*
Australia	4.9	5.7	7.3	8.2	8.5
Austria	4.4	5.4	7.9	8.4	9.3
Belgium	3.4	4.1	6.6	7.6	8.3
Canada	5.5	7.1	7.4	9.4	10.2
Denmark	3.6	6.1	6.8	6.5	6.7
Finland	3.9	5.7	6.5	8.0	8.8
France	4.2	5.8	7.6	8.9	9.8
Germany	4.8	5.9	8.4	8.3	8.6
Greece	2.9	4.0	4.3	5.3	5.7
Iceland	3.3	5.0	6.2	7.9	8.3
Ireland	3.8	5.3	8.7	6.7	6.7
Italy	3.6	5.2	6.9	8.1	8.5
Japan	3.0	4.6	6.6	6.8	7.3
Luxembourg		3.8	6.3	6.5	6.9
Netherlands	3.8	5.9	7.9	8.0	8.7
New Zealand	4.3	5.2	7.2	7.4	7.7
Norway	3.3	5.0	6.6	7.5	8.2
Portugal		2.8	5.8	6.6	7.3
Spain	1.5	3.7	5.7	6.9	7.3
Sweden	437	7.1	9.4	8.6	7.5
Switzerland	3.3	5.2	7.3	8.4	9.9
Turkey		2.5	3.4	2.9	2.7
United Kingdom	3.9	4.5	5.6	6.01	7.1
United States	5.1	7.1	8.9	12.1	13.6

From National Center for Health Statistics: Health, United States, 1995. Hyattsville, MD: US Public Health Service, 1996.
[a] Data compiled by the Organization for Economic Cooperation and Development.

Questions have been raised as to whether longevity and morbidity differences between nations justify the great differences in national resources allocated to health care. The rapid escalation of health care costs and the increasing percentage of national productive resources required for health care has been a continuing serious concern throughout the twentieth century.

The largest payer of medical care expenses is government (about 40 percent), with private health insurance close behind (about 33 percent). Among governments, the federal government through the Medicare program has borne the greatest financial burden, although state and local resources have also been stressed severely by health care costs.

TABLE 66-8. NATIONAL HEALTH EXPENDITURES, PERCENT DISTRIBUTION, AND AVERAGE ANNUAL PERCENT CHANGE, ACCORDING TO TYPE OF EXPENDITURE: UNITED STATES, SELECTED YEARS 1960, 1970, 1980, 1990, 1994[a] (in billions)

Type of Expenditure	*1960*	*1970*	*1980*	*1990*	*1994*
Total	$26.9	$73.2	$247.2	$697.5	$949.4
% of Distribution					
All expenditures	100.0	100.0	100.0	100.0	100.0
Health services and supplies	93.7	92.7	95.3	96.5	96.8
% of Distribution					
Personal health care	88.0	87.1	87.8	88.1	87.6
Hospital care	34.5	38.2	41.5	36.8	35.7
Physician services	19.7	18.5	18.3	21.0	19.9
Dentist services	7.3	6.4	5.4	4.5	4.4
Nursing home care	3.2	5.8	7.1	7.3	7.6
Other professional services	2.3	1.9	2.6	5.0	5.2
Home health care	0.2	0.3	1.0	1.9	2.8
Drugs and other medical nondurables	15.8	12.0	8.7	8.6	8.3
Vision products and other medical durables	2.4	2.2	1.5	41.5	1.4
Other personal health care	2.6	1.8	1.6	1.6	2.3
Program administration and net cost of health insurance	4.3	3.7	4.8	5.5	6.2
Government public health activities	1.4	1.8	2.7	2.8	3.0
Research and construction	6.3	7.3	4.7	3.5	3.2
Noncommercial research	2.6	2.7	2.2	1.8	1.7
Construction	3.7	4.6	2.5	1.8	1.5

From National Center for Health Statistics: Health, United States, 1995. Hyattsville, MD: US Public Health Service, 1996.
[a] Data are compiled by the Health Care Financing Administration.

A number of factors have contributed to the tremendous increase in the costs of medical care. Medical care is as sensitive as other goods and services to general inflationary pressures. The aging of the population, with elderly people using more health services, has increased costs. The growth in health insurance has also increased the use of the system because people with health insurance are more likely to use services (moral hazard in insurance terminology). Major technological innovations are now available to the consumer, such as growth in the number of intensive care beds and imaging techniques.

Reimbursement to Professionals

Physicians can be reimbursed through three mechanisms: fee-for-service, capitation, and salary. The predominant mode of reimbursement in the United States has been fee-for-service, where a physician renders care and the patient or third party (insurance company) reimburses the physician on a per service basis. This reimbursement frequently is computed based on usual, customary, and reasonable, or prevailing, fees. The physician receives a fee based on the physician's own fee history and/or on what other physicians in the community usually charge for the same service.

Capitation is more common in other countries, though with the growth in managed care there is an increase in the number of U.S. physicians who are paid on a capitated basis. With capitation a primary care physician (or other providers or provider system) receives a per capita payment based on the number of patients in their "panel." This is usually computed on a per member per month (PMPM) basis. In exchange for this prospective payment the physician is obligated to provide all benefits required by the contract between the physician and the insurer. This tends to decrease use of services by the physician, and it provides a powerful incentive to decrease the use of unnecessary or marginal services. It also may lower quality of care if physicians underuse services that might otherwise be in the patient's best interest. The shift of risk to providers, using capitation and other mechanisms, is a central tenet of managed care.

Salary usually is combined with some form of incentive reimbursement tied to productivity. Salary is more common outside the United States. In England, for example, the consulting physician, the hospital-based specialist, is paid on a salary basis. In the United States as staff model Health Maintenance Organizations (HMOs) pay their physicians on a salaried basis.

Recently, physician reimbursement has received careful scrutiny. The usual, customary, and reasonable fees paid by insurance carriers are based on physicians' historical charge data and may overvalue procedural as compared with cognitive services. In addition, some procedures that formerly were complex have become less so, but fees have not been reduced to reflect this change. Fee schedules based on the resources required to provide a specific service now have been developed. These fees consider the time and effort required, complexity of services, and any associated administrative costs. These resource-based relative value scales (RBRVSs) have changed physician reimbursement by the federal government under Medicare and are also being used by other payers as well.

One of the most difficult problems with preventive medicine is that preventive activities, such as screening, counseling, and immunizations, are not always covered benefits. The struggle to ensure that Medicare, for example, covered screening services and paid for influenza immunization was long and difficult, as discussed in a subsequent chapter. In most cases, to receive reimbursement for a medical service, the service has only to demonstrate that it is safe and effective. In the case of preventive procedures, the cost-benefit tradeoff of the intervention has to be demonstrated, holding preventive interventions to a higher standard.

Institutional Reimbursement

Hospitals may be reimbursed based on charges. Patients (or less often insurers) receive an itemized bill representing all services obtained. Note that charges differ from costs. Hospitals cross-subsidize some services. For example, nursing care generally does not pay its way, and pharmacy, laboratory, and radiology often are "profit" generating. Patients are not charged the true costs of "hotel services," but they pay more for ancillary services to subsidize nursing. Costs reflect the institution's true cost of providing each service; charges reflect a somewhat arbitrary price assigned to each service.

Under prospective payment, a facility receives a negotiated payment that is determined before services are rendered. A form of this type of payment is the hospital reimbursement provided by Medicare Part A, using DRGs.

Until the mid-1980s, retrospective cost reimbursement was common. Hospitals would determine their costs for providing care and would then bill insurance carriers and Medicare that proportion of total costs that carrier's subscribers incurred. This method has been criticized because it provides no incentives to contain costs.

Conversely, prospective reimbursement schemes have been praised for the incentives they provide to contain costs. The quality of care, especially as it pertains to access restrictions, underutilization, and early discharge, has been inadequately addressed, however.

Health Insurance

Most individuals have some health insurance (Table 66-10). Health insurance does not easily fit the classic insurance model, which is oriented to infrequent, undesirable, and unwanted events. Insurance companies developed health care policies primarily so that they could offer a full line of products to customers.

The providers of health services themselves initiated the health insurance industry. The depression of the 1930s profoundly affected the hospital industry, as patients were unable to pay their bills. In response, a Texas hospital developed a health insurance plan for schoolteachers, the forerunner of Blue Cross. This concept was adopted by other hospital associations who developed Blue Cross plans in their own states.

Medical societies adopted these hospital industry concepts to develop insurance to provide reimbursement to physicians. Blue Shield was thus developed. Blue Cross and Blue Shield, developed by the hospitals and physicians, were termed provider-sponsored plans. Although originally controlled by the providers, most provider-sponsored plans now have boards that are representative of the subscribers, with a minority representation of providers.

During World War II, prices and wages were frozen. Unions negotiated for fringe benefits rather than for wage increases. Also, during this time the commercial insurance companies entered the health care field as they saw the opportunity to expand their business line.

Utilization of a plan in services or benefits is termed the experience of the group. Experience such as 280 bed days of hospital care per enrollee is used to compute the premium. Adverse selection occurs when a plan attracts enrollees who are unusually high users. Premium rating based on a community experience is termed community rating. Premiums based on the experience of a specific group in the community is termed experience rating.

Financial arrangements between the enrolled, insurer, and providers vary as well. In indemnity plans, consumers (or employers) pay the premium to the plan. Providers bill the consumer who then submits a claim to the plan; there is no contractual relationship between the plan and the provider. The provider may bill the consumer more or less than the plan will pay. The contractual relationships are between the plan and the consumer, and the consumer and the provider.

The exception is when the provider accepts assignment, under which the consumer assigns the right to the claim to the provider. Under assignment, the plan pays the provider directly. The provider may agree to accept the assignment as payment in full for the service. In some instances, the providers may bill the patient for the difference between the charge and what the plan pays (balance billing).

A service plan involves a more complex contractual arrangement. The consumer (or employer) pays the premium to the plan. When the consumer visits the provider, the provider bills the plan; the plan pays the provider. Generally, the provider agrees, in advance, to accept the reimbursement as payment in full for the bill, except for any required copayments or deductibles. These arrangements provide

TABLE 66-9. HEALTH CARE COVERAGE FOR PERSONS UNDER 65 YEARS OF AGE, ACCORDING TO TYPE OF COVERAGE AND SELECTED CHARACTERISTICS: UNITED STATES, 1994[a]

	Percent of population		
Characteristic	**Private Insurance**	**Medicaid**	**Not covered**
Total, age adjusted	70.1	10.2	17.8
Total, crude	70.5	9.4	18.3
■ ***AGE***			
Under 15 years	63.0	19.8	16.1
Under 5 years	57.9	25.8	15.1
5–14 years	65.8	16.7	16.6
15–44 years	69.9	6.7	22.0
45–64 years	80.5	3.6	12.2
■ ***SEX***			
Male	70.6	8.6	18.8
Female	69.7	11.7	16.9
■ ***RACE***			
White	73.6	7.7	16.9
Black	52.0	23.9	21.5
■ ***HISPANIC ORIGIN AND RACE***			
All Hispanic	48.7	17.4	32.9
Mexican American	45.8	16.1	37.2
Puerto Rican	49.1	32.8	17.4
Cuban	63.6	8.4	27.4
Other Hispanic	52.2	14.7	31.5
White, non-Hispanic	77.4	6.2	14.6
Black, non-Hispanic	52.4	23.8	21.1
■ ***FAMILY INCOME***			
Less than $14,000	24.7	38.0	35.0
$14,000–$24,999	54.0	12.3	30.4
$25,000–$34,999	78.4	3.5	15.6
$35,000–$49,999	88.5	1.3	8.7
$50,000 or more	92.7	0.7	5.6
■ ***GEOGRAPHIC REGION***			
Northeast	74.8	10.2	14.7
Midwest	77.3	9.4	12.3
South	65.3	10.2	21.4
West	65.4	11.0	21.2

From National Center for Health Statistics: Health, United States, 1995. Hyattsville, MD: US Public Health Service, 1996.
[a] Data are based on household interviews of a sample of the civilian noninstitutionalized population.

for much greater control over providers, through the terms of the contractual arrangements, especially under managed care.

The Uninsured and Underinsured

Although a large proportion of the population has some health insurance coverage, currently over 30 million people are without any coverage (Table 66-9). This fact, combined with other concerns about health insurance coverage, such as the portability of health insurance from job to job, prompted the Clinton administration to attempt health system reform. For a variety of reasons, as in many previous attempts to provide universal health insurance, the effort was a failure. Many of the uninsured are employed or are dependents of employed individuals, often minimum wage earners. The problems associated with ensuring financial access to care for this population is a continuing national issue, though one that looks as if it will be addressed on an incremental basis rather than through sweeping reform.

A second consideration is the extent of coverage by those who have health insurance. Hospital care is covered more frequently than outpatient physician services, which is covered more frequently than pharmacy benefits. Most plans have coinsurance requirements, a fixed portion of the bill that must be paid by the patient, or deductibles, an initial payment responsibility paid by the patient before coverage begins. Some indemnity plans leave patients responsible for fees charged in excess of allowable reimbursements. Thus, nearly one-third of all medical care costs are still paid out-of-pocket by the consumer.

Managed Care

There has been a rapid growth in the proportion of the U.S. population who receive their medical care through managed care organizations (Table 66-10). To illustrate, the number of individuals who received their care through HMOs grew from 33 million in 1990 to 46.2 million in 1995. A good definition of managed care is Iglehart's, drawn from his 1992 *New England Journal of Medicine* article:

> Managed care is a system that integrates financing and delivery of appropriate medical care by means of the following features: contracts with selected physicians and hospitals that furnish comprehensive services to enrolled members, usually for a predetermined premium; utilization and quality controls that contracting providers agree to accept; financial incentives to use providers and facilities associated with the plan; assumption of some financial risk by doctors, thus fundamentally altering their roles from serving as an agent for the patient's needs against the need for cost control—or moving from "advocacy to allocation."

TABLE 66-10. HEALTH MAINTENANCE ORGANIZATIONS (HMOs) AND ENROLLMENT, ACCORDING TO MODEL TYPE, GEOGRAPHIC REGION, AND FEDERAL PROGRAM: UNITED STATES, SELECTED YEARS 1976, 1990, AND 1995[a]

Plans and Enrollment	1976	1990	1995
		Number	
All plans	174	572	550
Model types[b]			
Individual practice association	41	360	323
Group	122	212	107
Mixed	—	—	120
Geographic region			
Northeast	29	115	99
Midwest	52	160	154
South	23	176	190
West	70	121	107
		Number of Persons in Millions	
Total enrollment	6.0	33.0	46.2
Model type			
Individual practice association	0.4	13.7	17.4
Group	5.6	19.3	12.9
Mixed	—	—	15.9
Federal program			
Medicaid	—	1.2	3.5
Medicare	—	1.8	2.9
		Percent of HMO Increases	
Model type			
Individual practice association	6.6	41.6	37.6
Group	93.4	58.4	27.9
Mixed	—	—	34.5
Federal program			
Medicaid	—	3.5	10.0
Medicare	—	5.4	8.0
		Percent of Population Enrolled in HMOs	
Total enrollment	2.8	13.4	17.7
Geographic region			
Northeast	2.0	14.6	20.9
Midwest	1.5	12.6	14.4
South	0.4	7.1	11.2
West	9.7	23.2	29.0

From National Center for Health Statistics: Health, United States, 1995. Hyattsville, MD: US Public Health Service, 1996.
[a] Data are based on a census of health maintenance organizations.
[b] Eleven HMOs with 35,000 enrollment did not report model type in 1976.

The simplest type of managed care is the preferred provider organization (PPO).[15] A PPO is basically a discounted fee-for-service arrangement, where the provider agrees to accept a lower fee in exchange for access to the insurer's patients. Patients have financial incentives to see only providers who have contracted with the PPO, as they pay the difference in the fee charged by the provider outside the plan and what would be paid to the PPO provider. An exclusive provider organization (EPO) is similar to a PPO, except the insurer will not pay anything to a nonplan provider, leaving the entire payment as a consumer out-of-pocket cost.

The other major type of managed care organization is the HMO. HMOs in turn have several organizational patterns. The first and largest is the independent practice association (IPA). In an IPA the health plan contracts with solo and small group practice to provide care to their subscribers with the provider assuming some risk. Either they are capitated, that is, paid a set amount per member per month for which they are to provide a contracted set of services, or through a withhold, where a portion of their fee is held back and a portion returned to the provider, depending on the success of the plan in containing costs.

A network model is very much like an IPA, but the plan contracts with a few large group practices. In a staff model HMO, the providers are all employees of the health plan. In a group model HMO, the plan contracts with one group practice and that group practice has an exclusive arrangement with one plan. Another type of HMO is the mixed model or point-of-service plan. This allows HMO patients to use out-of-plan physicians, but requires a much larger premium and copay/deductible for that benefit. Out-of-plan care is used by less than 10 percent of eligible patients and, generally, is a mechanism to allow a concerned patient to make the transition from an indemnity plan to an HMO.

In general, compared with fee-for-service plans, HMOs tend to use less hospital resources and more ambulatory resources, have better rates of disease screening activities, and use less expensive alternative diagnostic and therapeutic services. In general, patients in managed care are satisfied with their financial arrangements, but less so with the care provided.[16]

There is a tendency for not-for-profit plans to convert to for-profit status to achieve better access to capital. A larger portion of the population in the west are in HMOs. Increasingly, recipients of public insurance programs, Medicaid, and Medicare are also being covered by managed care organizations as both the federal and state governments attempt to control the spiraling cost of these programs.

Concerns regarding the quality of care provided by managed care organizations continue to surface, as plans can increase their "bottom line" by restricting access and reducing the use of specialty services and by providing a lesser quality of care to enrollees. To address that concern, the National Committee on Quality Assurance (NCQA) was formed to accredit managed care organizations. NCQA is also responsible for the creation of a "report card" that it uses in this process. This report card is called the Health Employers Data and Information Set (HEDIS). HEDIS is important to preventive medicine, as many of the quality-of-care indicators are preventive in nature, such as proportion of enrollees who have had screening Pap smears and mammography.

Governmental Insurance Programs

In addition to private insurance, two major public insurance plans operate in the United States: Title 18 (Medicare) and Title 19 (Medicaid) of the Social Security Act. These programs were enacted in the mid-1960s with the intention of providing financial access to medical care for the nation's poor and elderly. Both programs have been revised many times in response to cost containment pressures, quality and utilization concerns, and various political factors.

Medicare is a federal program with two parts: A and B Medicare eligibility generally includes those people age 65 years and older, the permanently and totally disabled, and people with end-stage renal disease. Part A is mandatory and is financed by a Medicare trust fund comprised of contributions from employers and employees. Part B is voluntary and is financed by a monthly premium for enrollees and general federal funds. Part A was established to resemble Blue Cross, and Part B was established to resemble Blue Shield. Originally, Part A reimbursed hospitals on a service plan basis, based on retrospective costs. In 1986 the method of reimbursement was changed to prospective payment. All diagnoses and conditions were categorized based on resource requirements for the inpatient care in nearly 500 DRGs. Hospitals are paid a prospectively determined fixed dollar amount based on a patient's DRG category. If the hospital can provide the required care for less than the reimbursement, it keeps the difference. If more money is required to care for the patient, the hospital is required to provide that care with no additional reimbursement, except for certain "outliers," or special cases of justified extra care.

Part B of Medicare originally reimbursed physicians based on a percentage of the usual, customary, and prevailing fee, like an indemnity plan. Medicare now reimburses using the RBRVSs instead of usual and customary reimbursement. This system is intended to increase financial rewards for primary care physicians doing cognitive work and decrease rewards for physicians who do procedures, such as surgeons, as well as reflect the actual resources required to treat the patient and not just historical charges.

Because of the program's benefits, deductibles, co-insurance, and premiums, Medicare pays for only approximately 50 percent of the total cost of medical care for the eligible population. There is minimal coverage for nursing home care, a serious concern for this population group.

Medicaid is a joint federal-state program. The states administer and jointly, with the federal government, fund Medicaid programs and agree to provide a minimum set of services to recipients in order to receive the federal funds. These minimum services include inpatient and outpatient care, physician's office care, laboratory, x-ray, family planning services, mental health benefits, and early periodic diagnostic screening and treatment services. The federal government requires that these services be provided to the categorically needy, a determination based on income levels. The proportion of the federal government's financial participation is based on a formula that considers the state's wealth and other factors.

States may expand the scope of benefits beyond the minimum, with the federal government paying its proportion of costs associated with such expanded services as ambulance services, durable medical equipment, and chiropractic care, for example. The states' eligibility levels for Medicaid benefits are subject to certain federal guidelines. States may elect to cover the medically needy as well as the categorically needy. There is limited uniformity between the states in the Medicaid programs, which has led to considerable inequity across the nation.

The categorically needy are people who receive cash payments under the Supplemental Security Income (SSI-welfare payments) program. These people include those who are blind, those who are permanently and totally disabled, the aged, and those who receive aid to families with dependent children. People in these categories who are not poor are ineligible for Medicaid; people who are poor but do not fit one of the categories also are not eligible. The medically indigent can be covered at the election of the state. This category is comprised of individuals who have more income than the official poverty level and fit one of the SSI categories, but whose medical expenses put them below the official poverty level.

The range of benefits and eligibility requirements across the country under the Medicaid program is complex and confusing. Moreover, these programs are frequently so underfunded that providers receive only limited reimbursement. These concerns, and the paperwork involved in claims, is such that many providers do not participate in Medicaid programs at all. Although these programs were intended to provide a "safety net" for the poor, their success has been somewhat limited.

The Medicaid program represents a substantial portion of many states' budgets. In addition, there is concern that the Medicare Trust Fund, which provides for Part A payments, is in difficult financial straits. The advent of the baby boom cohort's eligibility for Medicare has substantial financial implications. One of the efforts to deal with this situation is to move both Medicaid and Medicare patients into managed care to at least make expenditures in these two public programs predictable. It is likely that both will undergo more profound change with time.

▶ THE FUTURE

It is obvious that there are problems with the health care "system." Many of these problems will require action by policymakers. The pendulum swings between the competing issues of ensuring access to quality care and providing such care at a reasonable cost.[17] The major concerns of the 1980s have surrounded the costs of health care. For a brief time in the early 1990s we were concerned about access to health insurance. The continued growth of the cost of medical care has ushered in a period of major growth for managed care organizations and the advent of an increase in for-profit hospitals and managed care corporations.

Changes in reimbursement policy have changed how providers are doing business. Hospitals have closed, multihospital systems have been created, joint ventures by physicians and hospitals is popular, group practice has grown, and managed care has proliferated. There will continue to be new experiments in the delivery of health care, especially to further address issues of the cost of care. But serious access problems continue to exist. The aging of the population also represents a challenge that must be dealt with, especially as regards long-term care and the solvency of Medicare.

National health policy has been developed for many years on a fragmented, incremental basis. The marketplace is moving rapidly toward increased consolidation and market concentration. Various forms of managed care are forming the predominant structure of the system with ongoing evolution in form and function. Technological advances are also increasingly influencing the structure of the system with tremendous growth in ambulatory services. Underlying demographic change, patterns of disease and illness (for example, as illustrated in Table 66-11), social and economic trends, and national politics all heavily affect the system as well.

Efforts at governmental health reform demonstrated our concern, as a nation, with having government intimately involved with decisions about health care. However, it is likely that government will continue to be involved in the decision-making about how health care is organized, delivered, and paid for. Our nation must choose wisely to ensure both high quality care and access for all of our citizens.

TABLE 66-11. PROVISIONAL DEATH RATES FOR SELECTED CAUSES OF DEATH: UNITED STATES, 1994[a]

Cause of Death	*Age-Adjusted Death Rate*	*Rank*
All causes	508.4	
Diseases of heart	140.0	1
Ischemic heart disease	92.4	
Cerebrovascular diseases	26.7	3
Malignant neoplasms	132.1	2
Respiratory system	40.1	
Breast	21.0	
Chronic obstructive pulmonary disease	20.9	4
Pneumonia and influenza	13.1	6
Chronic liver disease and cirrhosis	7.9	10
Diabetes mellitus	12.7	7
Nephritis, nephrotic syndrome and nephrosis	4.4	12
Septicemia	3.9	13
Human immunodeficiency virus infection	15.1	8
Unintentional injuries	29.8	5
Motor vehicle crashes	16.0	
Suicide	11.6	9
Homicide and legal intervention	9.7	11
Firearm injuries	15.4	

From National Center for Health Statistics: Health, United States, 1995. Hyattsville, MD: US Public Health Service, 1996.

[a] Data are based on a 10-percent sample of death certificates from the National Vital Statistics System.

▶ REFERENCES

1. William SJ, Torrens P: Introduction to Health Services. 4th ed. Albany NY: Delmar Publishers, 1993
2. National Center for Health Statistics: Health, United States, 1995. Hyattsville, MD: US Public Health Service, 1996
3. Flexner A: Medical Education in the United States and Canada: A Report to the Carnegie Foundation for the Advancement of Teaching. Bulletin No 4. New York: The Carnegie Foundation, 1910
4. Feldman R et al: Effects of HMOs on the creation of competitive markets for hospital services. J Health Econ 9(2):207–222, 1990
5. Schappert SM: National Ambulatory Medical Care Survey: 1994 Summary. Advance Data No. 273: April 10, 1996. Washington, DC: US Department of Health and Human Services, 1996
6. AMA Medical Groups in the U.S. 1996 edition. Chicago, IL
7. Kletke PR, Emmons DW, Gillis KD: Current trends in physicians' practice arrangements from owners to employees. JAMA 276 (7): August 21, 1996
8. Report of the Graduate Medical Education National Advisory Committee; Summary Report. Washington, DC: US Department of Health and Human Services, 1981
9. Rivo M, Satcher D: Improving access to health care though physician workforce reform: directions for the 21st century. JAMA 270(9): 1074–1078, 1993
10. Hurley RE, Freund DA, Gage BJ: Gatekeeper effects on patterns of physician use. J Fam Pract 32(2):167–174, 1991
11. Kletke PR, Marder WD, Silbeger AB: The growing proportion of female physicians: implications for U.S. physician supply. Am J Public Health 80:300–304, 1990
12. Council on Graduate Medical Education Sixth Report. Managed Health Care: Implications for the Physician Workforce and Medical Educations. Washington, DC: US Department of Health and Human Services, 1995
13. Bledsoe T: Physician assistants and nurse practitioners: needed more than ever. HMO Pract 4(5):155–156, 1990
14. Hooker RS, Freeborn DK: Use of physician assistants in a managed health care system. Public Health Rep 106(1):90–94, 1991
15. Langwell KM: Structure and performance of health maintenance organizations: a review. Health Care Finan Rev 12(1):71–79, 1990
16. Dolinsky AL, Caputo RK: An assessment of employers' experiences with HMOs: factors that make a difference. Health Care Manage Rev 16(1):25–31, 1991
17. Hughes EFX (ed): Perspectives on Quality in American Health Care. Washington, DC: McGraw-Hill, 1988

67

Structure and Function of the Public Health System in the United States

F. Douglas Scutchfield • C. William Keck

John Last defines public health in his dictionary of epidemiology as, "Efforts organized by society to protect, promote and restore the people's health. It is the combination of science, skills and beliefs that is directed to the maintenance and improvement of the health of all the people through collective or social actions."[1] These efforts organized by society are focused on, "creating conditions in which people can be healthy"—the mission of public health as defined by the Institute of Medicine (IOM) in its Report on the Future of Public Health.[2]

Public health is practiced in a variety of settings and agencies and by a variety of professionals. The work of many community-based organizations or major not-for-profit voluntary organizations can certainly be characterized as the practice of public health. Their programs fit Last's definition and are consistent with the mission statement articulated by the IOM. However, when we think of public health activities we most often envision the constellation of activities of governmental public health agencies at the federal, state, and particularly the local level. This is especially true since it is only official public health agencies that have statutory responsibility for the health status of the populations they serve. Legal authority for this responsibility is based on a variety of federal, state, and local ordinances, including the granting of police powers.

▶ THE FEDERAL PUBLIC HEALTH ROLE

The federal government's role in promoting and protecting the health of the public has evolved significantly over time. One of the best current descriptions of the federal role comes from the IOM.

As Defined by the Institute of Medicine

The IOM report defines the responsibility of the federal government toward public health services as:

- Support of knowledge development and dissemination through data gathering, research, and information exchanges;
- Establishment of nationwide health objectives and priorities, and stimulation of debate on interstate and national public health issues;
- Provision of technical assistance to help states and localities determine their own objectives and to carry out action on national and regional objectives;
- Provision of funds to states to strengthen state capacity for services, especially to achieve an adequate minimum capacity, and to achieve national objectives; and
- Assurance of actions and services that are in the public interest of the entire nation such as control of acquired immunodeficiency syndrome (AIDS) and similar communicable diseases, interstate environmental actions, and food and drug inspection.[2]

Organization

The federal government is divided into three branches; the legislative, judicial, and executive. The legislative and judicial branches do play substantial roles in public health, but it is usually the activities of the executive branch that come to mind when considering the federal government's role in improving the public's health. Within the executive branch, it is the Department of Health and Human Services (DHHS) that is the primary site of public health activities. Many of those activities are centered in one of the DHHS's component parts, the U.S. Public Health Service (PHS). There are, nonetheless, significant activities related to public health that occur in other branches of the executive branch. Examples include the Women, Infants and Children Program (WIC) run by the Department of Agriculture (the largest public health program in the country in terms of dollars spent), the many pollution and contamination control programs run by the Environmental Protection Agency (EPA), the workplace safety programs run by the Occupational Safety and Health Administration (OSHA), which is part of the Department of Labor, and the health care and public health services provided to active-duty military personnel by the Department of Defense.

The Department of Health and Human Services

The DHHS is currently going through a major restructuring because of the administration's reinventing government initiative, the removal of the Social Security Administration from DHHS and congressional efforts to diminish the size of the federal government. It is difficult, therefore, to predict the ultimate organizational structure of DHHS. It is likely that current functions will remain fairly intact, however, regardless of the agency's eventual structure.

The PHS had its origins in the Marine Hospital Service in the late 1700s, created to meet the health care needs of Merchant Marine seamen. The Marine Health Service continued relatively unchanged until the turn of the twentieth century, when it was renamed the Public Health Service and took on new responsibilities, most notably providing states with expertise to deal with major infectious disease epidemics.[3]

The PHS eventually became an arm of the DHHS after that cabinet department was formed, originally as the Department of Health, Education and Welfare. The PHS consists of a series of operating agencies that have remained relatively intact through many changes in the federal executive establishment. The current operational arms of the PHS include the National Institutes of Health (NIH), the Centers for Disease Control and Prevention (CDC), the Health Resources and Services Administration (HRSA), the Indian Health Service (IHS), the Food and Drug Administration (FDA), the Agency for Toxic Substances and Disease Registry (ATSDR) (administered by the CDC) and the Substance Abuse and Mental Health Administration (SAMHA). These major agencies are subdivided into centers, institutes, and branches staffed with both commissioned officers of the PHS and civilian employees of the federal government.

▶ THE STATE PUBLIC HEALTH ROLE

The role of the states and territories in public health, as with the role of the federal government, has evolved over time. The IOM has also defined these responsibilities well.

As Defined by the Institute of Medicine

The IOM report describes the duties of the state health department as:

- Assessment of the health needs in the state based on statewide data collection;
- Assurance of an adequate statutory base for health activities in the state;
- Establishment of statewide health objectives, delegating power to locals as appropriate and holding them accountable;
- Assurance of appropriate organized statewide effort to develop and maintain essential personal, educational, and environmental health services; provision of access to necessary services; and solution of problems inimical to health;
- Guarantee of a minimum set of essential health services; and
- Support of local service capacity, especially when disparities in local ability to raise revenue and/or administer programs require subsidies, technical assistance or direct action by the state to achieve adequate service levels.[2]

Organization

To fulfill these functions, the 50 states and five trusts (Guam, District of Columbia, American Samoa, Puerto Rico, and the Virgin Islands) have developed agencies to address them. In many cases these are not departments, so the Association of State and Territorial Health Officers refers to them as state health agencies (SHAs). There is substantial variability in the organizational structures of these agencies. In some cases the SHA is a cabinet-level office reporting directly to the governor, an arrangement encouraged by the IOM. In other circumstances the SHA functions are subsumed as part of a larger administrative organization, which often includes social services functions as well as health. These "umbrella" or "superagencies" carry titles such as Cabinet for Human Resources or Department of Health and Human Services. They are frequently led by political appointees who often have no substantive health expertise. These individuals report to their governors and are cabinet-level officers. In 1990, 19 states had the SHA in a superagency. This number decreased from 22 states in 1980, reversing a 40-year trend toward the establishment of superagencies.[4]

State Health Agency Activities

The activities of SHAs vary considerably. For example, the IOM report recommended that Medicaid, environmental programs and mental health services should be a part of the SHAs function.[2] That, however, is not the norm. In only four states is the SHA responsible for mental health services,[4] and in only five states and three territories is the SHA responsible for Medicaid.[5] In most states Medicaid management is the responsibility of the welfare agency. A case can certainly be made that subsuming the large budgets of Medicaid under the aegis of the SHA would allow the SHA to more closely integrate its public health functions with that of payment for medical care services. In fact, the group receiving the largest amount of public health services is women and children. Women and children also receive the biggest proportion of Medicaid expenditures, thus providing opportunity for synergy between these two governmental functions.

Environmental health was traditionally a part of the SHA's responsibility until the 1960s. At that point, growing concern about environmental degradation led special interest groups and policymakers to give special attention to many environmental issues. The federal government had made the decision to create the Environmental Protection Agency in response to those same concerns, and most states followed the federal lead by creating a state environmental protection agency separate from the SHA with responsibility for many environmental issues. All states were given the opportunity to designate a lead environmental health agency. While some initially designated the SHA as the lead agency, the number so designated fell from 19 in 1978 to only 8 in 1991. Even though most major environmental concerns are dealt with by state environmental protection agencies, most SHAs have retained responsibility for some environmental health issues, such as food service, recreation facility inspections, investigation of chronic disease clusters that might have an environmental etiology, etc.

State Boards of Health

One of the strong recommendations of the IOM regarded state boards of health. They believed that ". . . each state should have a state health council that reports regularly on the health of the state's residents, makes health policy recommendations to the governor and legislature, promulgates regulations, reviews the work of the state health department, and recommends candidates for director of the department."[2] In 1990, 23 states had boards of health that were responsible for making policy, while 17 had boards that were advisory. It is more likely that existing boards of health have a policymaking function in states with a free-standing SHA than in those with a superagency. Only four states had a board that appointed the director of the SHA in 1992.[6] The growing centralization of policymaking in the executive branch and the perception that special interest groups, especially physicians, have "captured" them have led to a decline in the power and influence of state boards of health.

Public Health Directors

In the earlier half of the century, the director of health was a physician, frequently trained in public health, who held the job for a protracted period of time. In fact, many states had statutes that required the director to be a physician. That has changed over the years to the point that in 1992 only 28 states had that requirement, and only 15 required public health training.[6] In many cases there is no statutory blockage to the governor appointing his or her cardiologist or campaign manager to the post. The "politization" of the position in many places has led to substantial turnover and a diminished desire on the part of qualified individuals to take such a position.

▶ THE LOCAL PUBLIC HEALTH ROLE

Local health departments are the governmental entities closest to the populations needing services. The IOM believed that, ". . . no citizen from any community, no matter how small or remote, should be without protection, which is possible only through a local component of the public health delivery system."[2] This is a more modern reaffirmation of the need for "a governmental presence at the local level (AGPALL)."[7]

As Defined by the Institute of Medicine

The IOM defined the functions of official local public health agencies as assessment, policy development, and assurance. By assessment, the IOM meant the responsibility to develop or collect data and information that allows for analysis and understanding of the health status of the communities for which the agencies are responsible. The policy development function requires that public health agencies take the lead in developing policies and making decisions based on the best available scientific knowledge. Finally, the official public health agency has the responsibility to ensure that services necessary to achieve agreed-upon health goals are provided.[2] This can be done by providing the required services directly or by encouraging their delivery by other agencies, groups, or individuals in the community.

The three public health "core functions" described by the IOM have subsequently been expanded and rewritten by public health practitioners to express them in programmatic and service terms that can be more easily understood by both public health professionals and the general public. They have evolved into a list of 10 "Essential Public Health Services":

1. Monitoring the community's health status, to identify and solve community health problems;
2. Diagnosing and investigating health problems and health hazards in the community;
3. Informing, educating, and empowering people about health issues;
4. Mobilizing community partnerships and action to solve health problems;
5. Developing policies and plans that support individual and community health efforts;
6. Enforcing laws and regulations that protect health and ensure safety;
7. Linking people to needed personal health services and ensuring the provision of health care when otherwise unavailable;
8. Ensuring a competent workforce for both personal care and public health services;
9. Evaluating the effectiveness, accessibility, and quality of personal and population-based health services;
10. Doing research to develop new insights and innovative solutions to health problems.[8]

These essential public health functions should be part of every local health department, or at least be present in every community, if that community is to reach the highest health status possible. Almost every health department will be involved in activities that might not fit under one of the 10 functions listed above, of course. Additional services and programs offered will depend on the needs of each community and decisions made locally about where those services can best be located.

Size of Local Health Departments

State health agencies vary considerably from state to state, but there is even more variability in the approximately 3,000 local public health departments in the United States. A periodic survey conducted by the National Association of County and City Health Officials (NACCHO) allows us to characterize the structure and function of local health departments (LHDs).

Generally, LHDs serve small populations. Two-thirds of LHDs serve a jurisdiction containing fewer than 50,000 people. In fact, 44 percent of LHDs serve less than 25,000 people. According to the survey, 56 percent of LHDs are county, 11 percent are multicounty, 13 percent are city/county, 7 percent are city, and 11 percent are town/township jurisdictions. Not surprisingly, the smaller jurisdictions have the fewest employees. Of the LHDs that serve a population less than 50,000, 74 percent have fewer than 10 employees.[9]

▶ ORGANIZATION AND STRUCTURE

The organizational relationships between the SHA and the LHDs also vary considerably. In 11 states the SHA is the LHD or directly operates the LHD. Of these 11, four are very small states (Hawaii, Delaware, Rhode Island, and Vermont). In seven states, control is shared between the county and the state. Sixteen states are totally decentralized with local government operating the LHD, and another 16 states have a mix, where large jurisdictions run their own LHD, but the state directly runs smaller, more rural, LHDs.[9]

The IOM recommended that a single jurisdiction in a community be given the responsibility for providing public health services to decrease duplication and/or prevent confusion about responsibilities. As a corollary, it also recommended that jurisdictions too small to support an effective LHD consider linking with other communities to create district health departments.[2]

The IOM also recommended that boards of health should exist at the local level with responsibilities comparable to those it recommended for state boards.[2] In 1992–1993 approximately 73 percent of LHDs had a board of health, a slight increase from 70 percent in 1989.[9]

Funding

Local health departments accounted for about $8 billion ($32 per capita) of spending annually in the United States in 1993. At the same time, total expenditures for health in this country exceeded $800 billion.[10] It is apparent, therefore, that less than 1 percent of the money spent on health is spent on local public health activities.

As noted previously, many LHDs are small, so it isn't surprising that half of all LHDs spend less than $500,000 annually. Available dollars come from a variety of sources. States provide, on average, 40 percent of the funds spent locally, including federal dollars that are "passed through." Local government contributes about 34 percent of the funding. The rest of the money comes from a mixture of places, including about 6 percent from direct federal funding, 7 percent from Medicaid reimbursement for service, and varying amounts from other fees, grants, and contracts. The actual mix of funding is different from place to place, however, reflecting the wide range of services and responsibilities among LHDs.[9]

Leadership

Leadership at the local level is more stable than it is in SHAs. Over 50 percent of LHD leaders have been in office longer than 5 years. In general, the smaller jurisdictions have the longest tenure, and the largest health departments experience turnover rates comparable to those in SHAs. Approximately 37 percent of LHD directors have doctoral degrees, and only have 17 percent have public health practice degrees (MPH or DrPH).[9]

Services

Despite the recommendation that a group of essential public health services be evident in every LHD, the evidence shows that there is great disparity in services offered. Most LHDs offer clinical preventive services, such as childhood immunizations (96 percent) and well child clinics (79 percent). Most assess the extent to which clinical preventive services are provided in their communities (76 percent), and provide programs to fill gaps in those services (83 percent). Communicable disease control is commonly present. Eighty-two percent of LHDs have an infectious disease surveillance system of some type, 86 percent are responsible for tuberculosis control, and 68 percent do human immunodeficiency virus (HIV) counseling and testing. Only 42 percent have chronic disease surveillance systems.[9]

Almost all public health departments provide some personal health services. In many cases, the health department is the provider of last resort, filling gaps in the private medical care system. Reimbursement for Medicaid-eligible clients often provides the funding base required for the department to maintain its services to the uninsured population. The growing trend in states to mandatory Medicaid managed care arrangements is moving paying clients out of health departments into the private sector without reducing the need for care for the growing numbers of uninsured. This threatens the viability of one of our society's "last resort" systems for the medically disenfranchised and challenges both the private and public sectors to develop collaborative arrangements to ensure continued access to needed personal health services.

Environmental issues are more clearly identified at the local level as the responsibility of the health department, in general, than they are at the state level. Most LHDs enforce state environmental laws (restaurant inspections, trailer park inspections, etc.), regulate private water and sewage systems, and enforce other local environmental ordinances. Confusion does sometimes occur when LHDs receive environmental complaints about problems when jurisdiction for dealing with those problems lies with others. It is then the job of the LHD to coordinate the response and ensure that the state or federal agency with jurisdiction follows through on investigation and resolution of the problem.

▸ FUNDING FOR PUBLIC HEALTH

It has been said that the federal government has the money, state government has the authority, and local government has the responsibility. The federal government is a major source of funding for local public health programs. These dollars are distributed in two major forms: categorical grants and block grants.

Categorical Grants

Categorical grants are created by Congress to address very specific problems in a targeted fashion. These grants are often the creatures of special interests who successfully lobby for funding to address their area(s) of interest. These grants may be "passed through" the SHA or be given directly to a LHD or other local nonprofit organization. These grants are usually competitive, meaning that applications for funding are solicited and judged on merit. A limited number of applicants are subsequently funded. It is easy to ensure accountability for these monies, as the specific objectives to be achieved by the project are well spelled out at the onset.

Block Grants

Block grants, on the other hand, are delivered for expenditure in broad categories with a minimum of oversight by the Federal Government. During the Reagan administration there was an effort to roll funding for all categorical health programs into one large block grant. Vigorous resistance to this approach resulted in a compromise effort that created a series of more "categorical" block grants, such as maternal and child health, primary care, and mental health. The major assumption underlying these grants is that the states and local governments can best determine their own priorities for spending within these broad categories. Dollars generally flow from the federal government to the SHA, which then determines the distribution pattern for these funds. Critics complain of the new layer of state bureaucracy added by this approach and the increased power it provides for the executive and legislative branches of state government.

Accountability for these funds is more difficult than it is for categorical grants. Specific outcome expectations are missing at the federal level, so there is no uniform reporting requirement in most cases. This makes it difficult to assess the impact of the funding, and that reality jeopardizes future levels of resources. Moreover, there is always concern that these funds might be used by SHAs to replace state dollars rather than augment them, thus diminishing the impact of federal funding. The loss of federal discretion over program goals and objectives is a source of concern for federal employees responsible for determining the impact of this spending.

Concern over these accountability issues has led to tighter requirements for reporting in some block grants in the recent past. The newest approach to block grant accountability is the formation of "performance partnerships." The intent of this arrangement is to allow the states to make decisions about how the money is to be spent, but to require that specific health objectives be developed that describe the outcomes anticipated. The requirement for specific objectives and outcome reporting is then transmitted from the state to the local agencies funded to implement the programs.

▸ ASSESSMENT AND MANAGEMENT TOOLS

Public health has benefited from the movement of a number of management tools from the private to the public sector over the past two to three decades. It has increased its capacity in recent years to deal with public health issues by successfully marrying good management mechanisms with new tools to describe and develop solutions for community health problems.

Setting National Objectives for 1990

One of the most important steps taken was to apply management by objectives and total quality management to public health. The notion to use measurable objectives to enhance the productivity of public health efforts at the federal level dates to the publication in 1979 of *Healthy People: The Surgeon General's Report on Health Promotion and Disease Prevention*. This document laid out a series of goals for mortality reductions to be achieved in the United States by 1990 for four age groups:

1. A 35 percent reduction in infant mortality;
2. A 20 percent reduction in mortality for children ages 1 to 14 years;
3. A 20 percent death rate reduction for those between 15 and 24 years of age;
4. A 25 percent reduction in adult mortality for those age 25 to 65 years.

For those above age 65, it called for a reduction in disability days.[11]

The Public Health Service began examining health status determinants and developed information on 15 disease prevention/health promotion areas. With the help of outside experts, in 1979 the first draft of specific objectives for these 15 priority areas was developed. After considerable outside review, *Health Promotion/Disease Prevention: Objectives for the Nation* was published in 1981. It contained 226 objectives with targets for achievement by 1990 that were linked to the 15 priority areas. The objectives were grouped as improvement in health status, reduction of risks to health, increased awareness, improved and expanded preventive health services, and improved surveillance.[12]

This effort was moderately successful. Three of the four mortality-related goals were met or exceeded. Specifically, the infant and adult mortality goals were met, and the childhood mortality target was significantly exceeded. The mortality goal for adolescents was not met. Failure to achieve the goal was directly due to high rates of both unintentional (motor vehicle accidents) and intentional (homicide) fatal injuries in this age group.[13]

Thirty-two percent of the 228 objectives set for 1990 were met. Progress was made toward an additional 30 percent, and ground was either lost or no progress made in another 15 percent. Insufficient data was available to determine the status of the remaining 23 percent of the objectives.[13]

In general, however, the success of this project was remarkable. It established an agenda that the public health community could rally around and served to energize and empower those who were committed to improving community health status.

Setting National Objectives for 2000

Because this project was so well received, the PHS began work in the late 1980s toward the establishment of a new set of objectives for the year 2000. It sought input even more broadly than it had previously and in September 1990 distributed *Healthy People 2000: The National Health Promotion and Disease Prevention Objectives*. This document contains three overarching goals:

- Increase the span of health life;
- Reduce health disparities among Americans;
- Achieve access to preventive services for all Americans.[13]

The 332 objectives contained in *Healthy People 2000* address health promotion, health protection, preventive services, and surveillance and data systems. They are grouped into 22 priority areas (see Table 67-1). Surveillance and data systems was included in this new version of national objectives in order to provide the foundation for tracking all of the objectives in an effort to minimize the problem of not being able to determine progress made on some of them.

The objectives listed in *Healthy People 2000* are of three types:

1. *Health status:* objectives to reduce death, disease, and disability;
2. *Risk reduction:* objectives to reduce the prevalence of risks to health or to increase behaviors known to reduce such risks;
3. *Services and protection:* objectives to increase comprehensiveness, accessibility, and/or quality of preventive services and preventive interventions.[13]

TABLE 67-1. HEALTHY PEOPLE 2000 PRIORITY AREAS

■ ***HEALTH PROMOTION***	
1.	Physical activity and fitness
2.	Nutrition
3.	Tobacco
4.	Alcohol and other drugs
5.	Family planning
6.	Mental health and mental disorders
7.	Violent and abusive behavior
8.	Educational and community-based programs
■ ***HEALTH PROTECTION***	
9.	Unintentional injuries
10.	Occupational safety and health
11.	Environmental health
12.	Food and drug safety
13.	Oral health
■ ***PREVENTIVE SERVICES***	
14.	Maternal and infant health
15.	Heart disease and stroke
16.	Cancer
17.	Diabetes and chronic disabling conditions
18.	HIV infection
19.	Sexually transmitted diseases
20.	Immunization and infectious diseases
21.	Clinical preventive services
■ ***SURVEILLANCE AND DATA SYSTEMS***	
22.	Surveillance and data systems

From: Public Health Service: Healthy People 2000: National Health Promotion and Disease Prevention Objectives. Washington, DC: US Department of Health and Human Services, 1990.

A 1993 review of progress in tracking these objectives based on data from 1992 yielded the following information: Four percent of the objectives were already met, progress was made on 28 percent, ground was lost on 15 percent, 4 percent were showing mixed results, 10 percent had no baseline data, and 28 percent lacked sufficient data to track results.[14] The establishment of measurable national health objectives coupled with regular tracking of progress made toward their accomplishment has proven to be a very effective way to focus the nation's attention on health status. The objectives have brought a variety of governmental agencies together to determine approaches to protecting and improving health. They have also provided an opportunity for contributions to the process by non–public health organizations and agencies, resulting in a prevention agenda that has a wide range of national support.

Setting Local Objectives

Setting national objectives is a very important step in preparing for an ordered process of allocating resources where the impact is likely to be greatest. It is the translation of those national objectives into action at the local level that actually ensures progress toward meeting them.

Assessment Protocol for Excellence in Public Health

Local health departments are at the vanguard of the effort to effect that translation. To assist LHDs with that task, the National Association of County Health Officials spearheaded a collaborative process in league with the CDC, the United States Conference of Local Health Officers, the American Public Health Association, the Association of State and Territorial Health Officials, and the Association of Schools of Public Health to develop the *Assessment Protocol for Excellence in Public Health (APEX/PH).*[15] The APEX/PH program is designed to help LHDs involve their communities in a process to assess community health status, identify and prioritize public health problems, and create a community plan for action. It contains three phases. Phase I is an assessment of internal organizational capacity of the department intended to identify strengths and weaknesses, particularly as they pertain to a department's capacity to take the lead in the broader community assessment effort. Working with an internal staff team, it allows the health department's director to grade the department's authority to operate, its administrative capacity, and its ability to develop policy and do a community assessment.

Phase II, intended to be initiated after the department addresses weaknesses or concerns identified in Phase I, is the actual community assessment portion. This part of APEX/PH is designed to involve the community in determining its public health needs. It depends on the identification and involvement of key community participants in the review of objective and subjective data on community health status, and it is expected that decisions will be made by the community representatives, not the public health professionals. The expected product of Phase II is a community health plan that is data based and includes the concerns of the community.

Phase III is the implementation of the community health plan under the leadership of the LHD. The health officer is expected to combine the results of Phase I and Phase II in a manner that enhances the capacity of the health department to lead the community in directing its resources to most appropriately address the problems identified.

Planned Approach to Community Health

During the 1980s the CDC, encouraged by the evidence that community-based prevention programs were effective in reducing coronary heart disease risk factors, developed a protocol that could be locally applied to develop community-based health promotion programs. The *Planned Approach to Community Health (PATCH)* was designed as a working partnership between the CDC, SHAs, and communities to focus resources and activities on health promotion. There are five phases to the PATCH process:

1. *Mobilizing the community*: establishing a strong core of representative local support and participation in the process;
2. *Collecting and organizing data*: gathering and analyzing local community opinion and health data for the purpose of identifying health priorities;
3. *Choosing health priorities*: setting objectives and standards to denote progress and success;
4. *Intervention*: design and implementation of multiple intervention strategies to meet objectives;
5. *Evaluation*: continued monitoring of problems and intervention strategies to evaluate progress and detect need for change.[16]

PATCH training has been provided by the CDC to 39 states and territories, and there are at least 130 operational programs.

Healthy Cities

The idea of *Healthy Cities* also emerged in the 1980s as a demonstration project of the European office of the World Health Organization. The project creates public, private, and voluntary partnerships that focus collective energies into coordinated, broad-based approaches to the resolution of community health problems. Each project is expected to attain four major goals: ensure organizational capacity, enhance information, establish initiatives, and create networks.[17]

Healthy Communities 2000: Model Standards

One of the most valuable tools available for translating locally identified health problems into measurable objectives is *Healthy Communities 2000: Model Standards*.[18] The third edition of this manual was published in 1991 immediately following the publication of *Healthy People 2000*. It represents a collaborative effort among the American Public Health Association, the Association of State and Territorial Health Officials, the National Association of City and County Health Officials, the Association of Schools of Public Health, and the CDC. The manual is keyed to each of the objectives in *Healthy People 2000*. It helps communities choose the objectives they wish to address and to specify the level of achievement they wish to attain. It has several key features that make it particularly useful:

- It uses a "fill-in-the-blanks" format for objectives with the same wording that is in *Healthy People 2000*, permitting the insertion of local data to match national concerns;
- The chapters and topic areas match those in *Healthy People 2000*;
- Recommended steps to setting community objectives are included;
- Sample indicators are provided for the use of local data to measure objective achievement.[18]

▶ THE FUTURE

The health status of citizens of the United States has improved dramatically over the past several centuries. The bulk of that improvement is due to public health policies and actions.[19] The major causes of disease and death have changed during that period, however, from communicable disease agents to behavioral and environmental factors that cause chronic illnesses or injuries. Approximately 70 percent of the resultant premature mortality currently suffered by the population of the United States is amenable to control using population-based strategies.[11] The future of public health lies in efforts for minimizing the use of tobacco, alcohol, and other harmful substances; increasing physical activity; reducing intentional and unintentional violence; promoting sexual behaviors that protect health; developing healthful environments, including promoting ecological balance; and encouraging other similar activities that promote health and prevent disease and injury.

The Place of Public Health in an Evolving System

The United States is currently enduring a restructuring of its illness care system. Change is evolving based on a series of governmental and private policy decisions aimed at controlling illness care costs by applying market strategies to health care. The central components of this evolution are managed care and the expansion of for-profit hospitals. Little attention is being paid to the more than 40 million Americans without health care insurance or to the public health infrastructure.

If our concern was for the health status of our population, reform of our "system" would be based on what should be done to create the healthiest population possible. Following that concern to its logical end would lead to the realization that improved health status depends on both illness care reform and public health reform. It is the responsibility of public health practitioners to help society understand that both disciplines are important, and that they should be integrated to provide a seamless web of services from health promotion through disease prevention to illness diagnosis and treatment accessible to all Americans. No one should be denied access to illness care, but it is population-based services that have the greatest potential to improve health status.

Strengthening Public Health for the Future

Public health departments face an operational environment that is more fluid than it has perhaps ever been. Rapid advances in technology and understanding of risks to health challenge agencies with minimal funding, training, and technical capacity to incorporate new methods into time-honored, traditional modes of operation. Federal and state comparative inattention to public health needs coupled with the shift of resources and some responsibilities to managed care companies in many, especially urban, localities create crises of role definition and funding.

As often occurs, however, this period of relatively rapid change presents opportunities. The description of the core functions of public health has made basic public health roles and functions more easily understood and appreciated. The ascendency of managed care brings new players to the scene who should be philosophically in tune with population risk reduction. The growing technical capacity to store, transmit, and analyze large bits of information brings new opportunities for interaction among public health professionals and between the public health profession and the community. If public health departments can be flexible and adjust their services and activities to match the needs and opportunities now apparent, they will be in good position to serve well the communities that fund them.

Basic to the successful LHD of the future will be its position as the health intelligence center of its constituency. The LHD must be the source of epidemiologically based thinking and analysis of its community's approach to health problem solving. It must be the facilitator of strong and meaningful community participation in the assessment and prioritization of community health problems and issues. It must be a major participant in public policy decision-making relative to health, and it must deliver, and broker the delivery of, services needed by its constituency to maintain or regain health. And, of course, it must focus on health outcomes as the measure of the impact of interventions.

It will be the rare LHD that has the resources available to it that are needed to carry out its community's full public health agenda. To be successful, LHDs will have to build strong collaborative and cooperative linkages with a variety of other community agencies and institutions. These linkages might take the form of joint programming efforts, service and referral arrangements, contracts for services, conduits for funding, information-sharing agreements, etc. By acting as a broker to bring needed services together to meet identified community needs, the LHD can complete its role in ensuring that the community will have access to the services it needs.

The proliferation of private, organized health care delivery systems puts health departments into the position of deciding whether or not to partner with emerging managed care companies and/or to monitor their activities to ensure that personal health services are available to all who need them in the community. It is far from clear how, or even if, this dual role can be successfully carried out. Circumstances are different community by community, and the many ways these issues will be addressed should be followed closely and evaluated rigorously. At the very least, essential public health services should not be compromised in the meantime.

Also important for success will be the development of stronger linkages between public health agencies and their academic bases, particularly schools and programs of public health. This should be pursued in a manner that the technical capacity of public health workers is improved and the knowledge of community public health problems is advanced. Students and faculty from educational settings teaching public health–related disciplines should be welcomed into LHDs for pragmatic practice experiences and for access to data and systems to carry out research. Likewise, educational institutions should seek out the participation of practitioners in their teaching and research activities. Local health department's should be supportive of their employees who wish to receive further training while employed.

▶ CONCLUSION

Significant systems change is occurring in both the illness care system and the public health system. No one is clearly in charge of either. Consequently, there are remarkable opportunities for entrepreneurial efforts to reshape each. Those efforts are clearly evident in the illness care system. They are also present in the public health system, although not as visibly. If the public health leadership of the United States can move the public health system out of old molds that no longer serve it well, there is every reason to believe that public health can provide a valuable set of services to communities, and be recognized as having done so. Steady, measurable gains in community health status will be the ultimate marker of success.

▶ REFERENCES

1. Last JM: A Dictionary of Epidemiology. 2nd ed. New York: Oxford University Press, 1988
2. Institute of Medicine, Committee for the Study of the Future of Public Health: The Future of Public Health. Washington, DC: National Academy Press, 1988
3. Fee E: History and development of public health. In Scutchfield FD, Keck CW (eds): Principles of Public Health Practice. Albany, NY: Delmar Publishers, 1997, pp 10–30
4. Public Health Practice Office, Division of Public Health Systems: Profile of State and Territorial Public Health Systems: United States, 1990. Atlanta: Centers for Disease Control, 1991
5. Public Health Foundation: Public Health Agencies 1991: An Inventory of Programs and Block Grant Expenditures. Washington, DC: Public Health Foundation, 1991
6. Degnon GK, Morelli V: 1992 Salary Survey. Washington, DC: Association of State and Territorial Health Officials, 1992
7. American Public Health Association: Model Standards: A Guide for Community Preventive Services. 2nd ed. Washington, DC: American Public Health Association, 1985, p 4
8. Baker EL, Melton RJ, Stange PV, et al: Health Reform and the Health of the Public. JAMA. 272:1276–1282, 1994
9. National Association of County and City Health Officials: 1992–1993 National Profile of Local Health Departments. Washington, DC: National Association of County and City Health Officials, 1995
10. Office of Health Promotion and Disease Prevention, Centers for Disease Control and Prevention: For a Healthy Nation: Returns on Investments in Public Health. Washington, DC: Office of Health Promotion and Disease Prevention and the Centers for Disease Control and Prevention, 1995
11. Public Health Service: Healthy People: The Surgeon General's Report on Health Promotion and Disease Prevention. Washington, DC: US Department of Health and Human Services, 1979
12. Public Health Service: Health Promotion/Disease Prevention: Objectives for the Nation. Washington, DC: US Department of Health and Human Services, 1981
13. Public Health Service: Healthy People 2000: National Health Promotion and Disease Prevention Objectives. Washington, DC: US Department of Health and Human Services, 1990
14. Public Health Service: Healthy People 2000 Review, 1992. Hyattsville, MD: US Department of Health and Human Services, 1993
15. National Association of County Health Officials: APEX/PH Assessment Protocol for Excellence in Public Health. Washington, DC: National Association of County Health Officials; 1991
16. US Department of Health and Human Services: Planned Approach to Community Health (PATCH). Washington, DC: US Department of Health and Human Services, November 1993
17. World Health Organization: Promoting Health in the Urban Context, Five Year Planning Framework, A Guide to Assessing Health Cities. Copenhagen: World Health Organization, 1988
18. American Public Health Organization: Healthy Communities 2000: Model Standards. Guidelines for Community Attainment of the Year 2000 National Health Objectives. Washington, DC: American Public Health Association, 1991
19. McKeown T: Medicine in Modern Society—Medical Planning Based on Evaluation of Medical Achievement. London: Allen & Vawin, 1966

68

International Health

John M. Last

It has long been realized that epidemic infectious disease is not stopped by national frontiers. International conferences aimed at standardizing quarantine regulations and procedures have been held at intervals since 1851; these led in 1907 to the establishment of the Office International d'Hygiene Publique (OIHP), which was the precursor of the Health Office of the League of Nations. In 1948 the functions of the Health Office were assumed by the World Health Organization (WHO), which soon was recognized as the most important international health agency.

There are several good reasons why we should be concerned about international health. The most obvious is self-interest: some of the world's health problems endanger us all. Those of us who live in rich industrial nations can easily become complacent or indifferent to the poverty and malnutrition, the preventable disease and premature death of children, and of women in their reproductive years, that occur in many developing nations. Of course similar problems exist in parts of many rich nations. These deplorable conditions influence the health and well-being of us all, wherever we live. They are at the roots of some of the political unrest that threatens the world with new outbreaks of violence. Many infectious diseases can be exported to other nations and can threaten people from affluent nations when they travel to or work in the developing world. Political unrest and warfare in many parts of the third world disrupt public health services, adding to the risk that dangerous epidemics will occur and spread. Other reasons for international health programs include the scientific challenge of unsolved health problems, and the altruistic impulse that leads some people to devote their lives to improving the lot of others less fortunate than themselves. This has been an important motive for medical missionaries; hospitals and clinics run by religious orders provide the only health care available in some communities in developing countries.

Classifications of Nations

The terms "developing" and "developed" country are loosely used in relation to gross national product (GNP). The World Bank classifies nations into low-income economies (including the two most populous nations on earth, India and China) with per capita GNPs of about $350 in 1991 U.S. dollars; lower-middle income nations with per capita GNPs up to $2,500; upper-middle income nations with per capita GNPs up to $3,500; and high-income nations, most of them members of the Organization for Economic Cooperation and Development (OECD), with per capita GNPs on average of $21,500.[1] A further classification is into severely indebted nations and oil-exporting nations, recognition of the dependence of all nations on oil-derived energy (Table 68-1). About 3.1 billion people, well over half the world's population, live in countries in the poorest group. A further 1.4 billion live in the lower-middle income nations and 630 million in the upper-middle income nations. About 820 million people live in the high-income nations, which are rich at least in part because of their ability to exploit resources such as oil, minerals, and food from the poorer nations. Putting it another way, over 80 percent of the world's people live in nations that collectively have less than 20 percent of the world's wealth and productive capacity. An even more striking fact is that the poorest 40 percent of the world's people collectively have less wealth than the world's richest 400 people. Moreover, the gap between rich and poor nations (and people) is getting wider.

Another collective term sometimes used to describe the developing nations is the "third world"; this term originated in French (*tiers monde*) and evokes memories of the time soon after the end of World War II when the world became divided along geopolitical lines into the so-called "free world," the communist and socialist nations that were politically aligned with the USSR, and the rest, the "third world," sometimes also called nonaligned nations. The Brandt Commission[2] gave us another concept, a division of the world into the "North," the industrially developed nations, nearly all in the Northern Hemisphere, and the "South," comprising almost all of Africa, Latin America, and South, Southeast, and Southwest Asia, which are industrially and economically less developed or undeveloped. The United Nations' Childrens Fund (UNICEF) simply ranks the nations in order of their infant and early child mortality rates—which correlate closely with per capita GNP.[3] Clearly all descriptive terms for the nations of the world have limitations.

Economic and social development and health improvement are hard to achieve among the poorest nations. In the mid-1990s, many nations in Africa south of the Sahara and in parts of the former Soviet Union are deteriorating; some are suffering because of inadequate natural resources that have to be shared among too many people, some because of poor planning and misuse of available resources, some because of corruption or political or military turmoil.[4] The prospects for improvement in the short term are not bright for many of the worst-off nations, which often are poor because they lack the natural resources that ultimately produce wealth.

Agencies Involved in International Health[5]

International and national agencies under the control of governments, nongovernmental organizations (NGOs), and private voluntary organizations are all active in international health. The government-sponsored international agencies include several United Nations (UN) organizations, the best known of which is the World Health Organization (WHO). Other UN agencies with well-defined and important health-related roles are UNICEF, the United Nations Development Programme (UNDP), the Food and Agriculture Organization (FAO), the United Nations Fund for Population Activities (UNFPA), the Office of the UN High Commissioner for Refugees (UNHCR), the UN Fund for Drug Abuse Control (UNFDAC), and

TABLE 68-1. POPULATION AND SOCIOECONOMIC INDICATORS, 1991–1993

	Population 1991 (Millions)	*GNP (per capita) 1991 ($U.S.)*	*Life Expectancy 1991*	*% Growth 1991 to 2000*	*% Urban 1991*
Low income economies					
China, India	2,016	350	66	1.5	46
32 others	1,111	350	55	2.4	28
Low-mid income economies	773	1,590	67	1.8	54
Upper-mid income economies	627	3,530	69	1.1	73
Severely indebted economies	486	2,350	67	1.8	68
Fuel exporting economies	262	14,820	66	3.0	52
High income economies	822	21,050	77	0.5	77

From World Bank: World Development Report, 1993; Investing in Health. New York: Oxford University Press, 1993.

the International Bank for Reconstruction and Development, better known as the World Bank. The most important international NGO is probably the International Commission of the Red Cross/Red Crescent (ICRC). Several high-income nations have their own agencies that provide direct financial and logistical support for health-related activities in the developing world. These bilateral agencies include the U.S. Agency for International Development (USAID), the Swedish International Development Authority (SIDA), the Canadian International Development Agency (CIDA), and similar agencies based in Switzerland, Japan, Saudi Arabia, Australia, and a few other nations. Many agencies, both governmental and NGOs, are affiliated with WHO; examples include the U.S. Centers for Disease Control and Prevention, the Public Health Laboratory Service in the United Kingdom, the Canadian Addiction Research Foundation, and some international and national professional health-related associations.

The NGOs and private voluntary organizations provide funds and human and technical resources for international health work of many kinds, mainly supported by voluntary subscriptions and donations. Many churches and missionary groups also play a prominent role; their activities include general and specific programs, such as hospital and community-based therapeutic and preventive services, aid for persons with specific diseases such as leprosy, trachoma, and cataract and aid for destitute children. Several foundations, notably the Rockefeller, Milbank, and Ford Foundations, have a long record of contributions to the advance of medical research and education in developing countries.

WHO is supported by all nations and is concerned with all aspects of human health. Its achievements since 1948 have been impressive. WHO has made at least one contribution of lasting historical importance, the eradication of smallpox;[6] this was accomplished in 1979 after an international collaborative effort that was supervised, coordinated, and directed by WHO. WHO aspires to eradicate poliomyelitis and dracunculosis and to eliminate leprosy and several other diseases by 2000.[7]

Communicable disease control is much emphasized among the activities of WHO; there are programs aimed at controlling all the principal communicable diseases of developing and tropical countries—malaria, schistosomiasis, onchocerciasis, leprosy, leishmaniasis, trypanosomiasis, yaws, tuberculosis, yellow fever, parasitic diseases, sexually transmitted diseases, viral hemorrhagic fevers, zoonoses, and emerging infections including, of course, human immunodeficiency virus (HIV) disease.[8] WHO's Global Programme on acquired immunodeficiency syndrome (AIDS) became a direct UN agency in 1993. There are programs on maternal and child health, nutritional disorders, occupational and environmental health problems, mental disorders, etc. Other programs deal with education and training of health workers, information and technology transfer, and quality control of biological products and pharmaceutical preparations. A section is concerned with epidemiologic surveillance, health status analysis, and trend assessment, health statistics, disease classification systems, etc.[9]

An activity often done in collaboration with ICRC and UNHCR is emergency and disaster relief. Natural or human-made disasters often displace large numbers of people, rendering them homeless and depriving them of means to subsist and survive. In the mid-1990s there are an estimated 20 million refugees and another 50 million displaced persons, i.e., displaced from their normal place of residence but still within the borders of their own country. These include people affected by natural as well as human-made disasters, mostly living in refugee communities in various parts of the world.[10] It is difficult to find any aspect of health affairs that is not dealt with somewhere within the scope of work of WHO.

The work of WHO is conducted at the headquarters in Geneva, in the six regional offices (Fig. 68-1), at country offices, and in the field. All offices have permanent staff, reinforced by temporary advisers, short-term consultants, and technical experts.

The activities of WHO took a new direction after a resolution approved by the World Health Assembly in 1977 and an international conference in Alma-Ata, USSR, in 1978.[11] At this conference, it was agreed that a realistic target to aim for would be the provision of primary health care for all the world's people by 2000. This goal, summarized in the slogan "Health for all by the year 2000," induced much effort and thought about ways to achieve better health for people everywhere. Internationally recognized experts on every aspect of health and disease considered how to achieve "health for all." Strategies and tactics were formulated at national, regional, and international levels, and action began on them. Within the regions of WHO, specific objectives were set, relating to the existing health problems and health resources; the objectives of the mainly rich and developed European region differed from those of the mainly developing African and Southeast Asian regions.

Unfortunately the work of WHO has been severely compromised by defaulting donor nations that collectively owe more than $2 billion to this and other UN agencies.[12] The United States is by far the largest defaulter with outstanding debts of about $1.4 billion in 1996. One reason for failure to pay is perception of excessive waste and bureaucracy that have often been the topic of adverse criticism. The combination of severe budget cuts and widespread criticism contributes to low morale of WHO staff, which of course makes matters worse.[13] Many people believe a change in leadership and radical administrative reorganization are needed, but these are opposed by some member states on grounds of national pride and politics.

► THE STATE OF THE WORLD IN THE MID-1990s

Spectacular improvements in health have occurred since the beginning of the twentieth century; many are attributable to advances of medical science and application of public health measures such as sanitation and clean water. Some formidable obstacles to good health and well-being, however, still persist. Wars and political instability are at the heart of some of the most intractable problems. Some resurgent infections are due to organisms, or their vectors, that are resistant to antibiotics or pesticides. Other problems are due to uncontrolled excesses in exploiting the environment, destroying what was

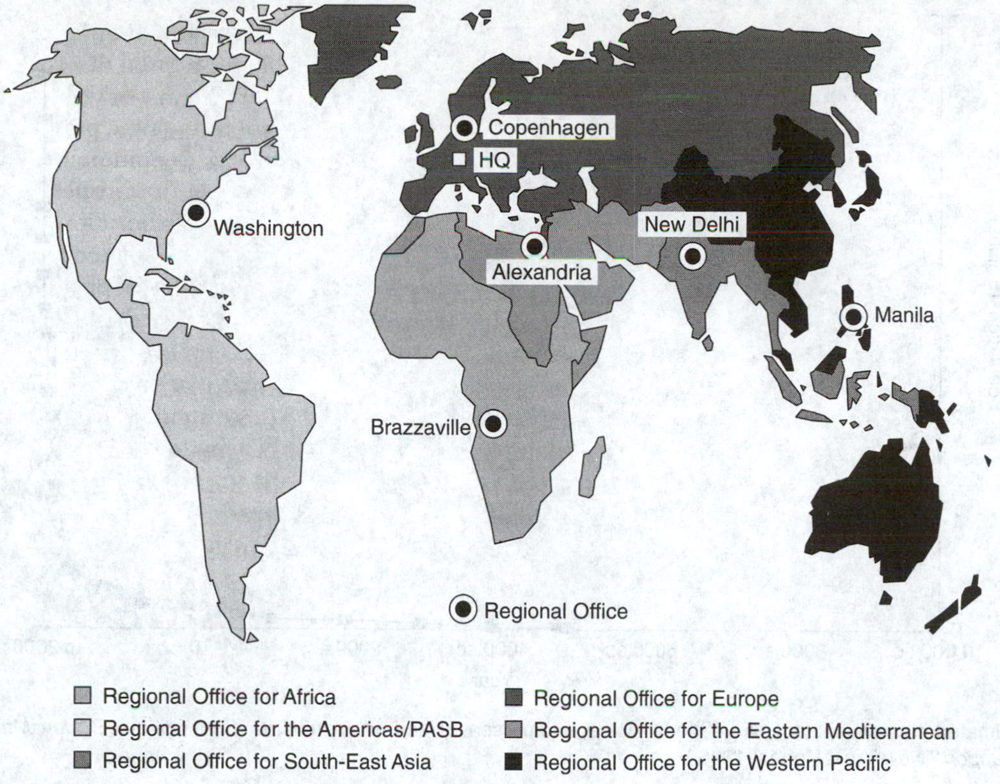

Figure 68-1. WHO regions and the areas they serve as of December 1994. (Used with permission from World Health Report 1995.)

naturally present, and poisoning vegetation, wildlife, even human communities. We cannot consider the health problems of the developing world in isolation from those of the industrial nations. All are interconnected.

Population Growth

Throughout history and probably since long before recorded history, the growth rate of human numbers was linear, except for occasional disruptions such as the fourteenth century epidemics of plague, which killed about a third of the population of Europe. At varying times from the late eighteenth century onward, the rate of growth became exponential, and since about 1950 is has become hyperexponential[14] (Fig. 68-2). These trends have been observed all over the world, beginning in the late eighteenth century in western Europe, the early nineteenth century in eastern Europe, and the early twentieth century in Africa, South and Southeast Asia, and Latin America.[15] Birth rates began to greatly exceed death rates early in the nineteenth century in the United States. The causes of this surge in numbers are debated by demographers. Some believe that improved nutrition, related to favorable climatic conditions and opening up to agriculture of vast areas in the Americas and Australasia, was the primary determinant; others think the reasons are more complex, including reduced risks of infant death from infections, related to ecological changes. The transition to an exponential growth rate preceded most of the modern advances of medical science.[16] It therefore was not due initially to control of infectious disease by antibiotics and immunization programs, although these helped to accelerate the trends, first in the industrial countries, then in much of the developing world. The hyperexponential growth in the second half of the twentieth century may be due to a combination of optimism about the future after World War II (giving rise to the "baby boom"), earlier age at childbearing, and effects of vaccines, antibiotics, and, in developing countries, child-survival strategies such as oral rehydration therapy for infant diarrhea.

This cannot continue indefinitely. Other living creatures fluctuate in numbers according to the supply of needed nutriment and the pressure from predators. Humans are subject to the same biological laws and, like all other living creatures we must strike a balance between reproductive rates and the supply of food and other essentials. The difference between humans and the other life forms whose reproductive performance has been studied is that humans have greater capacity to adapt to a wide range of environmental conditions. This has made it possible for humans to settle all over the planet on a scale unmatched by any other species; but it has also meant that almost no part of the earth's surface has remained untouched (and unspoilt) by human occupation. Humans have transformed the planetary ecology as a result. Human health cannot be sustained at its present level unless environments required for survival are sustainable too.[17] There is a growing consensus that there will be serious adverse ecological effects of the recent population explosion, probably soon. We may have to pay a heavy price for our reproductive success.

Migrations and Rural-Urban Shifts

Several times in human history there have been massive movements of large numbers of people about the earth, great redistributions, probably related to imbalance between numbers and the supply of needed resources of food, fuel, raw materials, or valued commodities. Evidence from archeology and folklore suggests considerable migration from Asia to Southeastern Europe about 2000 B.C.; another migration probably played a role in the fall of the Roman Empire (200 to 600 A.D.) when an invasion of people from Asiatic Russia to Europe took place. The most recent mass migrations began with the initial European colonization of the Americas, gathered momentum toward the end of the nineteenth century with large scale migration from Europe to the Americas and Australasia, and continues until the present, interrupted only by the two world wars. This movement includes not only a massive flow of people from many European

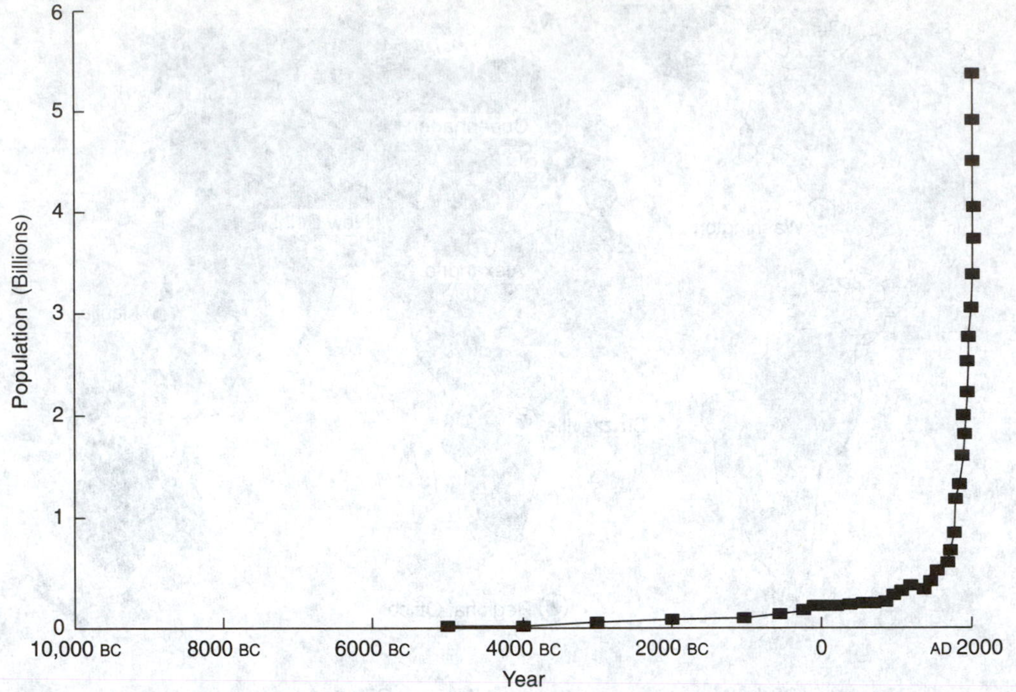

Figure 68-2. Estimated human population from the last ice age to present. (Used with permission from Cohen JE: *How Many People Can the Earth Support?* New York: Norton, 1996.)

nations to other parts of the world, but also at least as much movement, perhaps more, between certain Asian nations, from Asian nations to Europe and the Americas, from Latin America into the United States, and within Africa. Much of the migration is not documented in detail, though the approximate numbers and their origins and destinations are known. This poorly understood feature of modern times has had and continues to have profound effects on the well-being and health of people in many countries. Environmental stress, when too many people attempt to extract a living from a fragile ecosystem, causes many conflicts;[18] the 1995 genocide in Rwanda may have been an extreme example or a sentinel event.

Within many developing and developed nations there has also been a massive redistribution from rural to urban areas. In the early twentieth century, well over half, often over 90 percent of the population, lived in rural areas. By 2000, the proportion of people living in urban areas will exceed the proportion in rural areas.[19] By the mid-1980s about 45 percent of the world population was urbanized. Some of this rural-urban movement has been due to drought or other natural disasters that have led people to flee from the land in search of work in cities. In India and Pakistan, Southeast Asia, much of Latin America, and many African nations, it has been due in part to economic and political disturbances sometimes with warfare or rural banditry. Many millions of dispossessed subsistence farmers and displaced or unwanted rural agricultural laborers have moved to squalid shanty towns on the outskirts of third world cities, swelling the urban populations and overloading already inadequate water supply and sanitary services. Whenever they can, people living under such conditions as these seek to escape by migrating—legally or illegally—to industrially developed nations in Europe or North America.

The growth of cities, especially in the developing nations, is an oppressive problem. The population living in cities of 10 million in 1995 is shown in Table 68-2; even cities in affluent industrial nations do not function well nor are they pleasant places for most people to live when they reach such a size. In developing nations, water and food supplies, sanitary services, fuel, and shelter are often inadequate to cope with such numbers. These megacities are excellent breeding grounds for infectious diseases, drug abuse, and social unrest. Moreover, the rural areas of many of the developing nations in which these cities are located are experiencing equal or greater rates of population growth and cannot relieve the pressure.

Health Problems of Developing Nations

A useful way to arrange and classify the nations of the world, suggested by former UNICEF Director-General James Grant,[3] is according to their prevailing infant mortality rates. Infant mortality rates correlate closely with levels of economic development, literacy, housing conditions, access to pure water supplies, and several other variables dependent upon economic development; the availability of health care is not directly related to infant mortality rates, though it is often related to the level of economic development.

Table 68-3, which arranges selected nations in order of infant mortality, also shows their growth rates, per capita GNP, literacy levels, access to clean water, and the supply of doctors. The World Bank's recognition of the relationship between economic development and health[1] is an important contribution if it leads to greater investment in material and human resources to improve health. The low status of women,[20] leading to female illiteracy and poor understanding of ways to protect their infants' health, must also be dealt with.

Interaction of Infection, Malnutrition, and Population Growth

Many health problems of the developing world arise from the interaction of three forces: infectious diseases, especially of infants and young children, malnutrition, and uncontrolled population growth.

Infectious diseases take a terrible toll. There are about a billion cases each year of some of the common infectious diseases—diarrhea, respiratory infections, malaria, schistosomiasis, tuberculosis, and intestinal parasites. More than a million deaths occur each year from malaria alone in Africa. About 3 million children die each year

TABLE 68-2. BASIC INDICATORS, SELECTED COUNTRIES, IN DESCENDING ORDER OF MORTALITY RATES FOR CHILDREN UNDER FIVE

Country	*Mortality Rate (under 5)* 1960	1994	*Infant Mortality Rate (under 1)* 1960	1994	*Total Population (millions)* 1994	*GNP per capita (U.S. $)* 1993	*Life Expectancy at Birth (years)* 1994
Angola	345	292	208	170	10.7	700	46
Sierra Leone	385	284	219	164	4.4	150	39
Nigeria	204	191	122	114	108.5	300	50
Zaire	286	185	167	120	42.6	220	52
Uganda	218	185	129	111	20.6	180	45
Pakistan	221	137	137	95	136.7	430	61
Ghana	213	131	126	76	16.9	430	56
India	236	119	144	79	918.6	300	60
Nepal	290	118	190	84	21.4	190	53
Bangladesh	247	117	151	91	117.8	220	55
Indonesia	216	111	127	71	194.6	740	62
Kenya	202	90	120	61	27.3	270	56
Brazil	181	61	118	51	159.1	2930	66
Egypt	258	52	169	41	61.6	660	63
Iran, Islamic Republic of	233	51	145	40	65.8	2200	67
Viet Nam	219	46	147	35	72.9	170	65
China	209	43	140	35	1208.8	490	68
Thailand	146	32	101	27	58.2	2110	69
Mexico	148	32	103	27	91.9	3610	71
Russian Federation	n.a.	31	n.a.	28	147.4	2340	68
Sri Lanka	130	19	90	15	18.1	600	72
Hungary	57	14	51	13	10.2	3350	69
Cuba	50	10	39	9	11.0	1170	75
United States	30	10	26	8	260.6	24740	76
Spain	57	9	46	8	39.6	13590	78
France	34	9	29	7	57.8	22490	77
Israel	39	9	32	7	5.5	13920	76
Australia	24	8	20	7	17.9	17500	77
Italy	50	8	44	7	57.2	19840	77
Netherlands	22	8	18	6	15.4	20950	77
Norway	23	8	19	6	4.3	25970	77
Canada	33	8	28	6	29.1	19970	77
United Kingdom	27	7	23	6	58.1	18060	76
Switzerland	27	7	22	6	7.1	35760	78
Germany	40	7	34	6	81.3	23560	76
Denmark	25	7	22	6	5.2	26730	75
Japan	40	6	31	4	124.8	31490	79
Finland	28	5	22	4	5.1	19300	76
Sweden	20	5	16	4	8.7	24740	78

(Source: UNICEF, 1996.)

from diarrhea, 4 million die from respiratory infections, and another 3 million from a combination of malnutrition and vaccine-preventable diseases, especially measles.[21] About 150,000 deaths are due to neonatal tetanus. There are also about half a million maternal deaths each year in the developing world, and many of these, leaving infants motherless, are followed by the death of these infants.

Malnutrition is almost universal in some of the poorest nations, notably those affected by droughts and famine in Africa, where matters have been made worse by civil unrest and warfare. All forms of malnutrition occur—protein-calorie shortage, marasmus, and vitamin deficiency diseases. Malnutrition enhances susceptibility to infection, and infection enhances metabolic demand for protein and calorie intake, so there is a vicious circle in the infection/malnutrition complex that causes many premature deaths in developing countries.

Children continue to die of measles and diarrhea, despite the fact that there are inexpensive ways to prevent and treat these diseases. As part of the "Health for All" strategy, the Expanded Programme on Immunization set targets to be achieved in immunization coverage of infants and children. Considerable progress has been made in many countries, but this must be a continuing effort, for new generations of susceptible infants are added each year. Some countries lag far behind in immunization coverage, and since the collapse and breakup of the former Soviet Union, immunization programs, along with other parts of a previously efficient public health infrastructure, have broken down and diphtheria, for instance, has returned.

Oral rehydration therapy—a simple and inexpensive supplement that replaces fluid and electrolytes lost during bouts of diarrhea—has saved many lives; this technique is easily taught even to illiterate village women. International health agencies have justifiably invested much effort in teaching women about oral rehydration therapy, and the benefits are apparent in many rural communities. The program has the virtue of being easily applied by minimally trained health workers.

The fact that so many children now live where previously children died helps to persuade parents that fewer children have to be conceived to provide the workforce needed to maintain farms or paddy fields. Protecting and preserving the lives of infants and chil-

TABLE 68-3. LARGE URBAN AGGREGATIONS, 1994–1996.

	Population (Millions)	Rate of increase Percent/annum
Populations over 10 million		
Tokyo, Japan	26.8	1.41
São Paulo, Brazil	16.4	2.01
New York, USA	16.3	0.34
Mexico City, Mexico	15.6	0.73
Bombay, India	15.1	4.22
Shanghai, PRC	15.1	2.29
Los Angeles, USA	12.4	1.60
Beijing, PRC	12.4	2.57
Calcutta, India	11.7	1.67
Seoul, Korea	11.6	1.95
Jakarta, Indonesia	11.5	4.35
Buenos Aires, Argentina	11.0	0.68
Tienjin, PRC	10.7	2.88
Osaka, Japan	10.6	0.23
Lagos, Nigeria	10.3	5.68
Populations 7.5 – 10 million		
Rio de Janeiro, Brazil	9.9	0.77
Delhi, India	9.9	3.80
Karachi, Pakistan	9.9	4.27
Cairo, Egypt	9.7	2.24
Paris, France	9.5	0.29
Manila, Philippines	9.3	3.05
Moscow, Russia	9.2	0.40
Dhaka, Bangladesh	7.8	5.74
Istanbul, Turkey	7.8	3.67
Lima, Peru	7.5	2.81

Source: United Nations Population reference bureau

dren is the first step toward dealing with the most urgent problem of all, uncontrolled human reproduction.

The rate of population growth is influenced by complex cultural factors, religious beliefs, and levels of education and literacy, especially female literacy, which depends on the status of women. In some nations there is a long way still to go, however. Once they are able to read, women are better able to understand the basic principles of contraception; they are also better able to understand that disease and premature death are not inevitable facts of life. The education that is needed to change traditional values is another urgent priority. Television can play a valuable role by contributing to the education and value changes needed to improve the status of women.

Special efforts are needed in some nations to improve the status of women. In many rural agrarian societies, women's lives are determined for them by the elders of the family or tribe; most are destined to spend their lives in a combination of childbearing and heavy manual labor, working crops, carrying fuelwood and water long distances, crouching over smoky cooking fires in ill-ventilated village huts, inhaling toxic fumes in greater amount than if they smoked 40 cigarettes a day.[22] In African countries where AIDS has had a heavy toll, many able-bodied men have already died or are dying, leaving women on their own (often infected with HIV) to till the land, harvest the crops, and raise the children.[23] The ultimate legacy of the AIDS epidemic in many developing countries will be a generation of orphans.

High population density favors the spread of communicable diseases, so population pressure not only drains food resources and leads to widespread malnutrition, but also sets the stage for epidemics. The three problems, population pressure, malnutrition, and infection, thus, constantly reinforce one another. Economic development and education of women may best help to break these vicious circles by concentrating on the control of infections, but the control of infections cannot achieve much without opportunities for employment—which requires improved education and higher levels of literacy. The solution is as challenging as the problem is complex.

New Problems

The combination of population pressure, malnutrition, and infection has sapped the vitality of the developing nations for generations. Now there are new problems. Industrial development, often without the restraining laws and regulations of the rich industrial nations, is causing serious environmental damage and occupational diseases. And some of the worst health-harming habits of the industrial nations, notably cigarette smoking and traffic injury, are increasingly common.[24]

Industrial development is needed but unfortunately many multinational corporations seek a supply of cheap labor and avoidance of regulations and laws that protect health and preserve environmental quality. Factories in the developing nations frequently employ children and women for low wages, have no workers' compensation, and few if any occupational health and safety standards. Environmental quality is often damaged by unrestrained discharge of toxic waste products.

The habits and customs we recognize as harmful to health are eagerly embraced by many people in developing nations. Women are persuaded that artificial formula is better than breast-feeding; transnational infant formula manufacturers promote infant formulas, even though it is well known that mothers in rural villages lack the means to purchase, sterilize, or store formula under safe and hygienic conditions.[25] Despite campaigns by UNICEF, public health, and child care agencies, some manufacturers of breast milk substitutes continue to promote infant formula rather than breast milk.

Addiction to cigarette smoking is probably the worst of the unhealthy practices of industrially developed nations to be exported. The tobacco companies are able to promote their deadly product without restraint in most developing nations.[26] Tobacco is securely established as a lucrative cash crop, displacing badly needed subsistence agriculture, and trees are depleted to provide fuel for flue-curing tobacco to make cigarettes.

Another problem is the export to developing countries of pharmaceutical preparations that have been denied a licence in the country where they were manufactured, usually because of doubts about their safety or efficacy.[27] In cities in Latin America and Southeast Asia, these drugs are often sold in open stalls in marketplaces. Apart from the harm they may do, some of these drugs are broad-spectrum antibiotic combinations that help to produce resistant strains of pathogenic microorganisms.

There has always been a heavy toll of accidental death and injury in developing countries, e.g., from burns and scalds that occur when cooking is done over open fires inside village huts. With the influx of automobiles, often on roads never built to carry them and with drivers who have never been properly taught to drive, the toll of traffic injury and premature death is also rising. Industrial accidents also occur with increasing frequency because untrained workers and unsafe machinery are a dangerous combination. For all these reasons, the burden of accidental death and injury is rapidly increasing.

▶ FAILURES OF PLANNING AND ORGANIZATION

The solutions to many health problems in developing nations are elusive, at least in part because of poor planning, inadequate organization, and misplaced values. These human factors contribute to several problems, of which the following are the most obvious, although this is not an all-inclusive list.

Inequitable Access to Health Care

The poor, especially the rural poor, frequently have great difficulty gaining access to any form of health care other than traditional village healers.

Treatment Gets Higher Priority Than Prevention

Of course this is not unique to developing countries. In developing countries, however, expensively equipped modern hospitals to treat complex and difficult medical and surgical cases can do harm because they attract not only an unfair share of the small budget available for health services, but also a disproportionate share of skilled and well-trained health care workers.

Maldistribution among the Health Professions

In many countries, there is serious maldistribution between the branches of health care practice.[28] There may be a surplus of physicians and a shortage of nurses, as well as greater numbers of specialist than generalist physicians.

Inappropriate Investment in High Technology

Political decisions may lead to investment in expensive technical devices such as electron microscopes and diagnostic imaging equipment, which is not only expensive and requires expensively trained technical staff, but is even more expensive to maintain—but there may be no funds for maintenance, or persons qualified to do repairs, so the investment is wasted.

Inappropriate Training Programs

Although international planners sponsored by WHO and other agencies have recommended emphasis on training primary health care workers, many training programs remain set in the pattern of the United States or Western Europe. Graduates of such training programs are attracted to nations where they can practice the kind of medicine or nursing that they have been taught and are reluctant to work in the rural areas of their own countries where there is more need for their services. Yet there is an understandable reluctance to train indigenous health workers to supposedly lower standards than those prevailing in rich nations. This situation requires a value change, recognition that training programs for primary health care workers are not of a lower, but a different, standard.

Lack of Health Information

Sometimes the population and its distribution are not accurately known, let alone their diseases and causes of death. A high priority is to establish and maintain comprehensive health information systems, or if this is not feasible, at least to set up registration areas in which the numbers of persons, diseases, premature deaths, and disabilities can be accurately and continuously ascertained.

Administrative Deficiencies

Sometimes there is no trained cadre of administrators. Some former colonies of European nations were left with no civil service when the colonists departed. Sometimes the administration is corrupt, further aggravating the situation.

Breakdown of Communication

All forms of communication may be faulty—road and rail communication from the center to the periphery, the posts, telephone service, even contact between professionals in different sections of the service.

Wrong Priorities

National budgets may be meager, and often funds are misallocated. There is an imbalance between expenditures on social and health services and on military weapons in many developing countries (as there is in the world as a whole). Since the 1960s, the scale of expenditure on armed services, and imports of sophisticated armaments from the industrial nations to the developing nations, has sharply increased.[29]

Chronic so-called low-intensity warfare is another pervasive problem. On average, more than 400,000 people have died in wars every year since the end of World War II, almost all of them in developing countries. Increasing proportions are noncombatant women and children. In several combat zones, children not yet even in their teens, often kidnapped or captured when their parents have been killed or their villages overrun, have been pressed into military service.[30] Another consequence of these conflicts is the terrible toll in death and maimed limbs due to landmines that continue to kill indiscriminately long after hostilities have ceased and "peace" is restored.

Problem-Solving in the Developing World

Probably because the problems are tangible rather than a reflection of prevailing values, progress toward solutions is sometimes more impressive in developing than in industrial nations. There is much to inspire confidence and hope.

"Health for All" gave a focus to what were previously rather aimless efforts. The Expanded Programme on Immunization and oral rehydration therapy have achieved measurable results already; infant and early child mortality rates have declined sharply since the early 1980s. The tropical disease research program, chasing elusive goals such as vaccines against malaria and schistosomiasis, has achieved more than optimists could have hoped for a few years ago. Less glamorous but as important, the infrastructure of primary care services and health information systems in developing countries is beginning to work. Instrumental in this is collaboration between WHO, other official agencies and NGOs, which have responded to the challenge of meeting specific goals with finite deadlines. A significant achievement has been the shift of emphasis of leadership from the international agencies to local communities, giving control over their own health affairs back to the people who will directly benefit. A central feature of this reorientation of aims and methods has been the development of primary health care—a direct and explicit reaction to the "Health for All" initiatives. A few years ago, many developing countries had virtually no primary health care workers other than traditional healers; now increasingly there are battalions of rural health workers, often modeled on the Chinese barefoot doctor pattern. One of the most valuable forms of development assistance that industrial nations can offer to the third world is to help with these training programs for primary health care workers.

Another priority is to promote the concept of global interdependence, recognizing that actions of groups, communities, and nations in one part of the world affect those who live at a distance, perhaps ultimately reacting on us all wherever we may live. All agree that despoiling the environment and profligate consumption of nonrenewable resources will ultimately harm us and our descendants, especially if this is accompanied by pollution and destruction of other living creatures with which humans are interdependent. But little can be done about this when people must clear tropical rain forests to ensure their immediate need to grow food required for survival, and when elected leaders plan with a time horizon no further off than the next election.

Another priority is to focus attention on major problems, rather than attempting to deal superficially with a great many at once, including perhaps some of little consequence. Programs that protect the health of infants and children have the highest priority in developing countries.

▶ REFERENCES

1. World Bank: World Development Report, 1993; Investing in Health. New York: Oxford University Press, 1993
2. Brandt Commission Reports: Common Crisis: North-South Cooperation for World Recovery. London: Pan Books, 1983
3. Grant J (ed): The State of the World's Children, 1983. New York: UNICEF and Oxford University Press, 1983
4. Kaplan RD: The Ends of the Earth: a Journey at the Dawn of the 21st Century. New York: Random House, 1996
5. Basch PF: Textbook of International Health. New York: Oxford University Press, 1989, pp 326–354
6. Henderson DA: The eradication of smallpox. In Last JM (ed): Maxcy-Rosenau Public Health and Preventive Medicine. 11th ed. New York: Appleton-Century-Crofts, 1980, pp 95–110
7. World Health Organization: World Health Report, 1996. Geneva: World Health Organization, 1996
8. World Health Organization: Ninth General Programme of Work. Geneva: World Health Organization, 1995

9. World Health Organization: World Health Situation Analysis and Trend Assessment. Geneva, World Health Organization, 1995
10. Office of the United Nations High Commission for Refugees: Annual Report, 1995. Geneva: United Nations High Commission for Refugees, 1995
11. World Health Organization, UNICEF: Primary Health Care. Geneva and New York: World Health Organization/UNICEF, 1978
12. Godlee F: The World Health Organization; WHO in crisis. BMJ 309:1424–1428, 1994 [and subsequent articles]
13. Ermakov V: Reform of the World Health Organization. Lancet 347:1536–1537, 1996
14. Cohen JL: How Many People can the Earth Support? New York: Norton, 1996
15. McEvedy C, Jones R: Atlas of World Population History. London: Allen Lane, Penguin Books, 1977
16. McKeown T: The Role of Medicine; Dream, Mirage or Nemesis. Princeton, NJ: Princeton University Press, 1979
17. King M: Health is a sustainable state. Lancet 336:664–667, 1990
18. Homer-Dixon TF: Environmental changes as causes of acute conflict. International Security 16:76–116, 1991
19. United Nations Statistical Office: Population Statistics and Projections. New York: United Nations, 1995
20. United Nations Development Programme: Human Development Report, 1995. New York: Oxford University Press, 1995
21. Bellamy C (ed): State of the World's Children 1996 (UNICEF Annual Report). New York: Oxford University Press, 1996
22. de Koning HW, Smith KR, Last JM: Biomass fuel combustion and health. Bull World Health Organ 63:1:11–26, 1989
23. Gupta GR, Weiss E, Whelan D: HIV/AIDS among women. In Mann J, Taratola D (eds): AIDS in the World. New York: Oxford University Press, 1996, vol 2, pp 215–228
24. World Health Organization: Bridging the Gaps: The World Health Report 1995. Geneva: World Health Organization, 1995
25. World Health Organization: Women, Health and Development. A Report by the Director-General. Publication No. 90. Geneva: World Health Organization, 1985
26. World Health Organization: WHO's Tobacco Control Programme. Geneva: World Health Organization, 1995
27. Silverman M, Lee PR, Lydecker M: Prescriptions for death: the drugging of the third world. Berkeley: University of California Press, 1982
28. Bankowski Z, Fülop T: Health Manpower out of Balance. Report of the XXth CIOMS Conference, Acapulco, 1986. Geneva: CIOMS/World Health Organization, 1986
29. Sivard RL: World Military and Social Expenditures. Washington, DC: World Priorities, 1994
30. Children in War. In Bellamy C (Ed): State of the World's Children 1996. New York: Oxford University Press, 1996, pp 12–41

69

Public Health Law

Edward P. Richards, III • Katharine C. Rathbun

Core public health—food and water sanitation, sewage and refuse disposal, vermin control, and the management of zoonosis and communicable diseases—depends on law as much as on science. From the Roman sewers and public water systems and the Venetian 40-day interregnum for ships entering port, to the recent eradication of smallpox, public health depends on the power of the state. Public health authorities must seize property, close businesses, destroy animals, treat involuntary individuals, or even lock them away. Without the coercive power of the state, public health and modern society would be impossible.

In all societies, public health authority is derived from the basic power of the state to preserve itself: the right of societal self-defense.[1] Public health law must address the societal, as well as the biological dimensions of epidemic disease. The disruption of societal institutions has done as much as direct deaths from contagion to destroy indigenous populations throughout the world and to change the face of European culture.[2] Even when the public health power has been used for actions that were later found to be scientifically worthless, the assertion of authority was valuable because it lessened the political disorder that accompanies public health crises.

This chapter focuses on public health law in the United States. The United States puts more limits on the state's power to protect the public health and safety than most other countries.[3] These limits protect the rights of individuals against restrictions by the state, but at the cost of increased risk to the community from communicable diseases and other public health threats. While other countries may have a different balance point, the tension between individual autonomy and community protection is the heart of public health law everywhere.

Historic Basis of Public Health Law

Given the current emphasis on individual liberties rather than community obligations, the breadth of public health authority allowed under the Constitution is surprising. It becomes more understandable when public health authority is considered in historical perspective. Pestilence was part of everyday colonial life, a constant threat that contributed to a life expectancy of only 25 years.[4] Soon after the Constitution was ratified, an epidemic of yellow fever raged in New York and Philadelphia. The prevalent attitude of that period toward disease was captured in an argument before the Supreme Court:

> For ten years prior, the yellow-fever had raged almost annually in the city, and annual laws were passed to resist it. The wit of man was exhausted, but in vain. Never did the pestilence rage more violently than in the summer of 1798. The State was in despair. The rising hopes of the metropolis began to fade. The opinion was gaining ground, that the cause of this annual disease was indigenous, and that all precautions against its importation were useless. But the leading spirits of that day were unwilling to give up the city without a final desperate effort. The havoc in the summer of 1798 is represented as terrific. The whole country was roused. A cordon sanitaire was thrown around the city. Governor Mifflin of Pennsylvania proclaimed a non-intercourse between New York and Philadelphia.[5]

These extreme actions, including isolating the federal government which was sitting in Philadelphia at the time, were accepted as necessary. It was this personal experience with the reality of epidemic disease that caused the drafters of the United States Constitution to leave the states almost unfettered in their authority to deal with threats to the public health:

> Every state has acknowledged power to pass, and enforce quarantine, health, and inspection laws, to prevent the introduction of disease, pestilence, or unwholesome provisions; such laws interfere with no powers of Congress or treaty stipulations; they relate to internal police, and are subjects of domestic regulation within each state, over which no authority can be exercised by any power under the Constitution, save by requiring the consent of Congress to the imposition of duties on exports and imports, and their payment into the treasury of the United States.[6]

These are called the police powers. The term police does not refer to police departments, which did not exist in their present form until much later. It refers to the older meaning of the word "police"—to keep order. The state's police powers deal with general issues of public health and safety, not the punishment of criminals. Most public health police powers are exercised by health officers, fire marshals, sheriffs, and judges.

Legal Foundation of Public Health Agencies

Constitutional Limits

The primary limitation on governmental action is the United States Constitution. Public health measures potentially violate the prohibitions against unreasonable searches and seizures, taking property without due process of law and compensation, or punishment without trial by jury. In practice, however, the courts seldom hold a public health regulation unconstitutional. There are three reasons for this deference. First, judges and juries do not have the expertise to make technical decisions, so the courts delegate these to an agency or individual with expertise:

> It is not for the courts to determine which scientific view is correct in ruling upon whether the police power has been properly exercised. The judicial function is exhausted with the discovery that the relation between means and ends is not wholly vain and fanciful, an illusory pretense . . .[7]

The second reason for this deference is cost-effectiveness. Legal process costs money and extensive due process requirements thwart government regulation. For example, allowing every disgruntled would-be food handler to have his or her day in court, with a full legal review of the facts and basis of the health department's decisions, would increase the cost of a food handling permit to many thousands of dollars. This cost would have to be borne by either the public or the permitted food handlers. As the cost becomes too high, the agency will end the permitting process or will make it a sham by giving a permit to every applicant with the resources to fight the agency in court. Either solution endangers the public health.

The third, and most important reason for deference is time. Court procedures take time, while disasters and diseases spread quickly. Time is the critical limitation on an individual's right to legal process. A person who has been arrested for a crime is entitled to elaborate and lengthy court proceeding to determine guilt, and is punished only if found guilty. That same person, armed and resisting arrest, may be shot and killed with no legal process, save a later administrative review of the situation to ensure that the shooting was justified.

Hearings cost public health agencies valuable time. The person subject to the order has to be served with a notice of the hearing and given time to hire an attorney to present a defense. It can take several weeks to get both parties before a judge. As courts have recognized in their rejection of requests for bail by persons under disease control orders, you cannot allow the disease carrier to go free while you litigate the restriction:

> To grant release on bail to persons isolated and detained on a quarantine order because they have a contagious disease which makes them dangerous to others, or to the public in general, would render quarantine laws and regulations nugatory and of no avail.[8]

Punishment Versus Prevention

Unlike police departments which function to capture and punish individuals who have already committed crimes, public health agencies function to prevent future harm. The United States Supreme Court has held that it is the intent to punish, rather than the nature of the agency action itself, that triggers criminal law due process protections. This was addressed directly in claims by persons detained prior to trial:

> Not every disability imposed during pretrial detention amounts to "punishment" in the constitutional sense, however. . . . Traditionally, this has meant confinement in a facility which, no matter how modern or how antiquated, results in restricting the movement of a detainee in a manner in which he would not be restricted if he simply were free to walk the streets pending trial. Whether it be called a jail, a prison, or a custodial center, the purpose of the facility is to detain. Loss of freedom of choice and privacy are inherent incidents of confinement in such a facility. And the fact that such detention interferes with the detainee's understandable desire to live as comfortably as possible and with as little restraint as possible during confinement does not convert the conditions or restrictions of detention into "punishment."[9]

Because public health actions are not intended to punish, and because public health officials often must confront new threats, the courts have held that public health powers are broad and flexible to allow for quick action. Constitutional protections against unreasonable searches and seizures and deprivations of liberty or property without due process of law still apply to public health actions, but the standards for determining the reasonability of searches and seizures and what constitutes deprivations of liberty and property are very different for public health officers than they are for police officers.

Since police power actions get less judicial scrutiny than do criminal prosecutions, legislatures sometimes masquerade a punishment as a public health restriction. This would allow the state to avoid giving the target of the law proper due process protections. While the courts generally accept the legislature's determination that a law is intended to protect the public health, they will examine the law and, if the law is found to punish without due process, it will be struck down.

Public health laws will also be invalidated if they are discriminatory or if they improperly interfere with interstate commerce. The courts have rejected special health regulations for Chinese because there was no evidence that Chinese were at any greater risk of contracting or spreading disease.[10] Public health laws can be constitutional even if they have a differential impact on otherwise protected groups if the disease is more prevalent in a specific racial or ethnic group. This is commonly seen in screening programs for genetic diseases, which can affect blacks, Jews, Amish, and other genetically distinct groups at very different rates.

State laws that use public health enforcement to discriminate against out-of-state businesses are unconstitutional. Courts have struck down laws that imposed more stringent sanitary restrictions on out-of-state milk processors. Even if the restrictions are the same for in-state and out-of-state businesses, the courts will strike down the law if it unnecessarily discriminates against the out-of-state business.[11] For example, a requirement that milk must be processed and delivered within 24 hours would put out-of-state dairies out of business. This law would be improper if there was no evidence that the 24-hour rule was necessary to protect the public's health. Conversely, a Texas law that banned the import of Louisiana cattle was constitutional because Texas could show a real risk of anthrax in the Louisiana cattle.[12]

General Authority

Public health agencies operate under general grants of authority that allow them to develop new rules to deal with unexpected circumstances. The public health codes usually state a general authority to take any steps necessary to protect the public's health if there is a danger that was not anticipated by the legislature. In contrast, the criminal justice system can only enforce laws passed by the legislature. These laws must be specific and written to put potential violators on notice of their provisions. They can apply only to future violations. The legislature cannot pass an ex post facto law to punish past behavior. An individual cannot be punished for a new type of behavior until a law has been passed against that behavior.

Enforcement Powers

While the public health laws are intended to prevent future harm rather than to punish past behavior, these laws do have provisions for forcing compliance. Public health officials have four primary enforcement tools:[13]

1. Permits, licenses, and registrations;
2. Administrative orders;
3. Civil penalties; and
4. Injunctions.

Permits

Permits, licenses, and registrations are used to regulate routine activities that may pose a threat if they are carried out improperly. Food establishment permits are the most common public health example. Permits pose the fewest legal issues because they are prospective—the establishment must show that it meets the requirements before the permit is issued. The standards for the permitted activity are established by the legislative body, which usually specifies that the regulation will follow an approved national code and that special situations will be handled by the public health officer. To qualify for a permit, the applicant must agree to be bound by the standards for maintaining the permit. The applicant must agree to allow entry by the health inspectors, without notice or a warrant, to ensure compliance with the applicable standards. The health officer will determine if the applicant meets the standards for a permit and whether a permit should be revoked or denied because the permittee has violated these standards.

Administrative Orders

Administrative orders are orders issued by the public health agency directly to an individual or a business requiring that actions be taken to mitigate a threat to the public health. These can range from an order to clean up garbage in a vacant lot to an order to show up for tuberculosis treatment. There may be a fine for violating an administrative order, but most enforcement by administrative orders depends on the cooperation of the affected individuals or businesses. Administrative orders are most effective when the violator holds a permit that may be suspended for not complying with the order. In other cases, if the violator does not comply with the order, the agency must ask a court to enforce the order.

Public health agencies can use administrative orders to empower private entities to act in situations where they would otherwise be legally unable to act. As an example, the federal regulations on managing tuberculosis in hospitals require that the hospital have a process for quickly identifying and isolating persons with active tuberculosis. Assume a coughing patient is admitted to the hospital with respiratory distress. The history and x-ray are consistent with active pulmonary tuberculosis. The patient is put into respiratory isolation, but refuses to stay in the isolation room, preferring to pass the time drinking coffee in the cafeteria.[14] The hospital has no legal right to isolate the patient against the patient's will. The agency can order that the patient be isolated and direct the hospital to carry out the agency's orders.

Fines and Other Punishments

Persons who violate public health administrative orders or statutes can be fined or jailed, after appropriate legal process. In most public health cases the fines are too small to be a deterrent and the municipal court judges who hear these cases are usually unwilling to jail a person for a public health violation. (As health officers quickly learn, it is hard to get judges to take "dog law" cases seriously.) However, fines and imprisonment are important enforcement tools for state and federal environmental quality laws because the fines can run to millions of dollars and the federal judges have no hesitation in ordering jail sentences.

Injunctions

When a violator ignores administrative orders, when the violator has been incarcerated but the hazard has not been abated, or when the public health agency wants to mitigate a hazard prospectively, the proper remedy is an injunction. Unlike other legal proceedings where the court can only order fines or imprisonment, an injunction allows the court to give specific orders on what must be done or what is prohibited. In addition, the agency can often select the judge that will rule on the injunction. Courts can and do use fines, imprisonment, and other coercive strategies to enforce their injunctions.

Courts may grant an injunction to prevent irreparable harm—harm that cannot be remedied by awarding monetary damages. For example, if a logging company mistakenly enters your land and begins to cut the trees, the court could order them to stop rather than just ensuring that you get the market value of the wood. When a public health agency seeks an injunction, the courts will usually grant it if the agency has substantial evidence (usually based on the expertise of the agency) that the condition threatens the public health and that the injunction will remove this threat.

If there is an immediate threat, the court can order a temporary injunction on the evidence presented by the agency without waiting to hear from the other party. These are called ex parte proceedings. The court will order a hearing as soon as possible to allow the enjoined party to contest the injunction. Such emergency actions are used for threats such as tainted food or water or a hazard such as a fire-weakened structure that threatens to fall on a neighboring building. If the threat does not require emergency action, the opposing party must be given notice and be allowed to be heard in a court hearing before an injunction is granted. After the opposing party has been heard, the court may either dissolve the temporary injunction or enter a permanent injunction. Permanent injunctions are very important in public health enforcement because they are often the only way to deal with recalcitrant violators.

Entry onto Private Property

Public health officials must enter onto private property to do routine inspections and to assess potential health hazards. This can be controversial when public health authority is used to enter and close criminal premises such as crack houses. Following the general distinction between punishment and prevention, the public health agency has broader authority to enter private property than do the police. With certain exceptions for crimes in progress or the hot pursuit of a felon, the police cannot enter private property without a search warrant. The warrant must be approved by a judge who has been shown probable cause to enter the premises. If the police violate this rule, the evidence they find cannot be introduced in court and the criminal will usually go free.

The courts do not require specific warrants for public health inspections, as long as there is no threat of criminal prosecution based on the evidence found during the search. Thus, inspecting a crack house for rats does not require a search warrant. The state cannot prosecute the owner for possession of cocaine found during the search, but if there is a significant rat problem, the crack house can be closed as a nuisance. When a public health agency wants to bring criminal charges, such as prosecution for toxic waste dumping, the agency must meet the same standards for a search warrant as do the police.

Public health agencies do not have an unlimited right to enter private property. Fearing the potential for harassment, the courts have required some showing of public health purpose for a search. This purpose is assumed for permitted or licensed premises because inspections are a condition for the license or permit. If the owner believes the agency is entering the licensed premises for improper reasons, the owner can seek redress from the courts. When the public health agency wants to enter property that is not covered with a license or permit, the showing of public health purpose can be satisfied by having a general plan for the inspections (called an area warrant) that describes which buildings will be searched and why.[15] If evidence of a crime is found during an inspection under an area warrant, it cannot be used in a criminal prosecution of the owner.

Contesting Public Health Actions

The traditional check on public health authority is habeas corpus, the "Great Writ" from the English common law that means "bring me the body." Habeas corpus requires that persons detained by the state be given a chance to answer the charges against themselves at a hearing before a judge, and that the state be required to show cause why the person should not be released. The Constitution and traditional courts allowed public health agencies to act without a hearing, subject only to later habeas corpus review if the person they restricted wanted to contest the restriction. This same standard of post-action review is applied to time-sensitive environmental health actions such as condemning tainted food.

Post-action review is less of a burden on an agency than a pre-action court hearing because it is used only when the target of the action contests it. Most persons restricted by public health orders do not contest the restriction. In the vast majority of cases involving individuals, the person is only temporarily confined for a medical evaluation or to begin treatment or suffers some other minor inconvenience. Businesses are reluctant to challenge an order after the fact because the chance of winning a damage award is too low to justify paying an attorney to bring the action. Holding hearings before enforcing routine or uncontested public health orders diverts limited resources from other public health agency functions and makes it easier for politically powerful interests to escape regulation. Public health agencies should resist providing constitutionally unnecessary legal process.

If a post-action hearing determines that the agency acted improperly, the agency (local, state, or federal) can be required to reverse their action. If that is not possible, then the agency may have to pay monetary damages to compensate for the value of the property destroyed. Agency personnel generally have personal immunity from claims related to the work done in their official capacity. This immunity does not extend to actions that are outside the scope of the agency powers or that otherwise violate state or federal law. For example, an agency employee could not be sued personally for closing a restaurant, even if the restaurant did not deserve closing. The inspector could be sued personally for civil rights violations if he or she intentionally closed only Indian restaurants.

Since the 1960s there has been increasing pressure to pass state laws requiring hearings and court orders before taking public health actions that effect individuals or businesses. In some cases disease control laws have been amended to require court hearings before public health orders are issued against individuals.[16] While some public health officials support such expanded due process requirements, these requirements come at the cost of effective disease control programs. No health departments have enough lawyers on staff to have a court hearing before every enforcement action. Most health departments depend on understaffed city or county legal departments where public health enforcement actions usually have a low priority.

Environmental Health

Enforcement Strategies

Public health began with sanitation, what is now called environmental health. The Bible contains some of the earliest food sanitation laws.[17] The Romans built large-scale aqueducts and sewers to improve the aesthetics of their communities and reduced waterborne illness in the process. Laws to ensure the safety of food and drinking water, the safe disposal of wastewater, and the control of rats and other vermin have been mainstays of public health since earliest times. As the federal and state governments began to pass laws dealing with air and water pollution, health departments added these to their traditional responsibility for sanitation and formed modern environmental programs. In health departments that are charged with enforcing these state and federal regulations, environmental health will be the largest enforcement program.

Food Handling

Food-borne illness still causes many preventable deaths in the United States, and the control of spoilage and vermin means the difference between plenty and famine in much of the world. Food-handling laws are concerned with whether the food is unfit because of spoilage or contamination with filth, whether it has been adulterated, and whether it is what it is purported to be. The Food and Drug Administration (FDA) and the Department of Agriculture regulate what pesticides and herbicides can be used on crops and their allowable residues, the drugs and supplements used to medicate and stimulate animal growth, and the slaughter and packaging of meat. These federal agencies have extensive powers to order the seizure of noncompliant food.

State and local health departments inspect food-handling facilities in their jurisdiction, sharing jurisdiction with the federal agencies for businesses that ship food products in interstate commerce. Most state and local enforcement activities involve restaurants and are done through a permit system. These permits can be suspended or denied for violations without a court hearing. Most jurisdictions provide for some appeal of denials or suspensions of permits, usually to a political body such as a city council. Violators can also challenge the department's actions in court, subject to the usual deference to the department's expertise. In either case it is important that the inspection reports detail the violations in ways that are understandable to laypeople. An agency action is much less likely to be overturned if the inspection discusses easily understood violations such as rat droppings on the food preparation area or spoiled food in the cooler.

Long before current concerns with the effect of pollution on health, society was concerned that the miasma from swamps, tanneries, and other fetid locations would upset the humors and lead to disease. These, and more immediate threats, such as a sinkhole on a traveled road, were classed as nuisances. The common law allows private parties to bring lawsuits to abate a nuisance. Private lawsuits are still used, but the party bringing the suit has to pay the legal costs and will not get the deference due the public health agency. Public health agencies abate nuisances by obtaining injunctions that force the property owners to clean up the nuisance. In some cases where the owner is unable to act, or is unavailable, the agency will abate the nuisance and put a lien on the property. Modern environmental laws evolved from the power to abate nuisances.

While the United States Constitution requires that property not be taken without due process of law, and that owners be paid a fair price for property taken for public purposes, this does not apply to the abatement of nuisances. The key issue in public health enforcement is whether the property is taken for public purposes or whether it is seized as a nuisance or a threat to the public health. The leading constitutional case involved the seizure and destruction of chicken stored in a cold storage plant that had lost its refrigeration. The owners of the plant demanded a hearing to determine whether the chicken was really spoiled and compensation for the chicken that was destroyed. The court ruled that there was no right to a hearing before the destruction of dangerous property and that dangerous property had no value, so the owners were entitled to no compensation.[18]

Public Health Reporting

Disease Registries and Vital Statistics

Disease registries are used for background epidemiological data rather than immediate disease control interventions. Reporting to registries is generally voluntary, but state laws vary and some reports may be mandatory. Since incomplete registry data can mask serious health threats, health care providers should treat registry reporting as if it were required by statute.

Vital statistics are birth and death records that are kept on a statewide basis. All states require physicians or others who officially attend births or deaths to report these events on standard forms. Unlike disease registries, vital statistics reports are mandatory. There has been substantial progress toward standardizing state laws on keeping vital statistics, but there are still differences between states. The registrar of vital statistics at the state health department is the best source of information about the laws of a particular state.

It is important that a birth attendant file the birth certificate promptly. The certificate must be filed before a certified copy can be issued. The child cannot get a social security number without the certified copy of the birth certificate. This is particularly important if the family receives any type of public assistance. Federally funded assistance programs limit the time that children may be carried on the program without their own social security number.

Birth certificates pose two important legal questions: what is the child's name and who is the child's father. State laws on choosing children's surnames vary substantially. Some states allow the mother to choose any surname; others allow any surname except that of a putative but unacknowledged father; some require that the child be given the surname of a legally recognized relative. While the lower courts in two states have found a constitutional right to name your child anything you please, the only federal appeals court to consider this issue held that a state could require that a child be named for a legal parent.[19] The name on the birth certificate does not establish the child's paternity. It may be evidence of paternity if the named father agreed to the use of his name, but it does not affect the state's legal procedures for establishing paternity. Anyone attending births should find out the specific laws for the state.

States may have a specific form for filing a report of stillbirth. Other states require the birth attendant to file both a birth certificate and a death certificate. The gestational age that constitutes a stillbirth differs from state to state but is usually around 20 weeks. In some cases, an induced abortion may require registration. The stillbirth certificate may be the appropriate form even if the child is born alive. Separate birth and death certificates are usually required only if the child is potentially viable and lives for some period. If a fetus of any gestational age shows signs of life such as a heartbeat or respiratory effort, it may be necessary to file separate certificates.

Death certificates are important legally for time and cause of death. The time of death can affect inheritances and is an important fact in criminal cases. The cause of death is important in criminal proceedings. In civil litigation it may determine who will be compensated for an accident or whether the insurance company will pay on a policy. The causes of death listed should match the codes in the *International Classification of Disease*. Unfortunately, the actual cause of the death is often not clear. A death certificate that lists cardiac arrest as the cause of death and respiratory arrest following shock as the contributing causes may be for a patient who died of a gunshot wound, a terminal cancer patient, or a patient with underlying heart disease. The cause of death should indicate what killed the patient, not what the terminal events were.

Reports to Law Enforcement

As injury prevention has become a recognized public health issue, there has been an increase in the conditions that must be reported to law enforcement agencies. Generally, these laws require reporting of assaults, child abuse, elder abuse, family violence, and certain criminal activity. The health care provider's duty is to report suspicious circumstances, not to do the police job of investigating the situation. For example, whenever a health care provider suspects that a child has been abused or neglected, that suspicion must be reported immediately.[20] Trying to investigate may confuse the evidence and make it more difficult for law enforcement to protect the child.[21] Child abuse interventions should be left to experts.[22]

Many states require the reporting of violent or suspicious injuries, including all gunshot wounds, knifings, poisonings, serious motor vehicle injuries, and any other questionable wounds. Even if the state does not require a specific report, reports may be made under the general right to report crimes to the police. If the patient is brought to the hospital in the custody of the police or from the scene of a police investigation, then the health care provider may safely assume that the police have been notified.

Disease Reporting

All states and the federal government require health care providers to report public health-related diseases, injuries, and conditions to a public health authority. Most reports are made to local or state officials,[23] who forward certain information to the Centers for Disease Control and Prevention (CDC) or other federal agencies, but some reports must be made to the CDC directly.[24] Depending on the subject of the required report, these duties extend to physicians, nurses, dentists, veterinarians, laboratories, hospitals, employers, schools, and other institutions. In the case of child abuse, the duty extends to the general public. All states share a common core of about 50 reportable diseases, plus the federal requirements. Most states add several diseases to the core list based on local conditions or politics, including work-related injuries and conditions.

Health agencies will also accept reports of diseases and conditions that are not on the state list if these may pose a threat to the public health or safety. The one exception is human immunodeficiency virus (HIV) infection. Some states still do not recognize HIV infection as a reportable condition and will not accept or investigate voluntary reports of HIV infection.

Health care providers do not need the patient's consent or a medical records release to make reports to the health agency, nor may the patient veto these reports. Patients have no right to be informed that they are the subject of a report to the health department, and the source of all information in the report is kept strictly confidential. It may be a good practice to inform patients about reports on syphilis or other diseases that may trigger a visit from the health agency. However, there are many situations, particularly child abuse, when such a warning can cause injury to others.

As with all legally mandated reports, knowingly reporting false information to the public health agency can be a crime. While some agencies tolerate or even encourage false reports, the reporter can be liable for any injuries caused by the false report, including the spread of infection to third parties or injuries caused by dangerous persons. The reporter may rely on the information provided by the patient if the provider does not know the information is false. However, outside of some sexually transmitted disease clinics, health care providers usually know their patients' correct names and addresses. It is a very rare patient who pays cash for all their medical care and never requires a prescription.

Right to Privacy

These reporting measures raise questions about the individual's right to privacy and the right of personal autonomy. Unlike traditional privileges such as the lawyer-client or priest-penitent privilege, which allow the lawyer or priest to withhold information from the state, there was no common law physician-patient privilege. Since there is no specific right of privacy stated in the Constitution, public health reporting raised no legal issues for the first 150 years. When the Supreme Court found an implied right of privacy in the Bill of Rights,[25] it severely limited that right where public health is at issue:

> Unquestionably, some individuals' concern for their own privacy may lead them to avoid or to postpone needed medical attention. Nevertheless, disclosures of private medical information to doctors, to hospital personnel, to insurance companies, and to public health agencies are often an essential part of modern medical practice even when the disclosure may reflect unfavorably on the character of the patient. Requiring such disclosures to representatives of the State having responsibility for the health of the community, does not automatically amount to an impermissible invasion of privacy.[26]

While many state legislatures and Congress, under pressure from individual rights advocates, have chosen to limit health agency access to epidemiological data,[27] these limitations are not required by the Constitution. If the information is used only for public health activities, and not criminal law prosecutions, anyone can be required to report, even if the information was gained in otherwise privileged communications.

Disease Control

Disease control is the management of communicable disease in the community. Historically, most disease control was done with administrative orders that mandated vaccination and restricted infected individuals to keep them from spreading their disease. With the advent of antimicrobial agents, individuals infected with bacterial diseases could be treated and did not have to be restricted. Mandated treatments are usually beneficial to the patient, as with penicillin therapy for syphilis, or at least harmless, as with erythromycin therapy for pertussis, which makes the patient noninfectious but does not alter the course of the disease. Vaccines pose some, although very low, risks to the individual: the vaccine that prevents thousands of cases of polio does so at the cost of an occasional case of vaccine-related paralytic polio. Legally, treatments and immunizations are mandated even if they benefit only society and pose a risk to the individual. As the United States Supreme Court held in a case brought by a man who did not want to be vaccinated against smallpox because he was afraid of the risks (not insignificant) of the smallpox vaccine:

> We are not prepared to hold that a minority, residing or remaining in any city or town where smallpox is prevalent, and enjoying the general protection afforded by an organized local government, may

> thus defy the will of its constituted authorities, acting in good faith for all, under the legislative sanction of the state. If such be the privilege of a minority, then a like privilege would belong to each individual of the community, and the spectacle would be presented of the welfare and safety of an entire population being subordinated to the notions of a single individual who chooses to remain a part of that population.[28]

Disease control poses the most difficult questions in public health law because it often requires direct assaults on personal autonomy such as involuntary testing, forced treatment, and restrictions on personal behavior. The courts will uphold these actions if they are necessary to protect the public health, as long as the state has not passed laws that limit the authority of the health officer. Unfortunately, the most severe limitation on public health authority for disease control is political. Health officers serve at the whim of political officials who are loath to do anything that has significant political opposition.

Testing, Screening, and Contact Tracing

Involuntary testing and screening are key strategies in assessing populations at risk for communicable disease. Screening systems are necessary to learn the prevalence of a disease in the community, to investigate specific outbreaks, and to identify individuals for treatment or restrictions. While there are strict limits on involuntary testing for drugs and on other tests intended to assist in criminal prosecutions, public health agencies have great latitude to test for diseases.[29] In most cases, testing is done under regulation or an administrative order and is voluntary in that the individual does not contest the testing in court. If the individual does refuse testing, the health officer can seek an injunction or court order to enforce the testing requirement. Unfortunately, involuntary testing has fallen into disfavor, and many states have passed laws limiting its use for HIV.

Contact tracing (partner notification) is the process of finding who an individual was infected by and who the individual may have infected. Contact tracing is very efficient, especially for sexually transmitted diseases, because it tends to identify the persons who are most active in spreading the disease.[30] Contact tracing begins when disease reporting or testing identifies an infected individual.[31] An investigator interviews the patient, family members, physicians, nurses, or anyone else who might know the patient's contacts. As contacts are identified, they are warned that they have been exposed to a communicable disease and are offered testing and treatment, if available.

Contact tracing has been attacked as an invasion of privacy. This would be true if it were carried on by a private individual, but the state has the right to search for individuals who may pose a threat to the public health or who themselves may be in need of treatment or counseling. Contact tracing interviews are always voluntary. Individuals are not coerced to divulge the name of their contacts. In most cases infected individuals cooperate because it will help their contacts get medical care and because most people want to prevent the spread of disease.

In the last 15 years there has been great concern about breaches of confidentiality, particularly for the contacts of persons with sexually transmitted diseases such as HIV. Disease investigators are trained never to identify one individual to another when doing contact tracing. In the United States, there has been no documented evidence of significant breaches of confidentiality by public health agencies. The courts have not found this concern over confidentiality a valid ground for limiting contact tracing. When breaches of confidentially have been investigated, they are usually from the patient's own disclosures, from other individuals whom the patient has told of the condition, or, in a smaller number of cases, disclosures ancillary to routine medical care.[32]

The primary attack on contact tracing and other intrusive disease control measures is that they are not perfect—that contact tracing does not find every contact, that screening will not locate every case, that restrictions on prostitutes will not keep every infected prostitute off the streets. Since these techniques cannot eradicate the diseases, they are not worth the cost to the restricted individuals. The courts, however, defer to the public health agency's determination that these techniques are valuable.[33] The courts generally accept that public health activities can manage diseases, but often cannot eradicate them. Even smallpox eradication, the paradigmatic public health success, was not achieved by immunizing every person on earth. Instead, very intrusive contact tracing was used to find infected individuals, who were then isolated, and all the persons in the surrounding village were vaccinated.[34]

Immunizations and Mandated Treatment

A health officer may issue an administrative order to treat an individual who refuses treatment for a communicable disease. The officer or agency can seek a court order if their jurisdiction does not allow administrative orders for treatment.[35] Most agencies try to avoid using physical force on a person who refuses treatment. Rather, the individual is incarcerated until he or she consents to the treatment. If the individual believes that he or she has a valid reason to not be treated, the incarceration can be reviewed through a habeas corpus proceeding.

The United States Supreme Court has held that it does not impermissibly interfere with religion to require health and safety measures of members of religions that oppose these measures.[36] This specifically includes immunizations.[37] Most states do provide exceptions from immunizations for persons with religious objections, but the courts have upheld state laws that require all children to be vaccinated.[38] Religious exceptions tend to undermine immunization laws because the courts cannot allow them to be restricted to "mainstream" religions, greatly increasing the number of children exempted.[39] Since these unimmunized children are brought together in the churches or in church schools, rather than being randomly distributed in the community, they have no herd immunity and are at much higher risk of catching and spreading the disease.

Special Problems of Pregnant Women and Infants

Pregnant women pose special legal problems because the interests of the mother and the fetus are not always the same. Once the child is born, the state has almost unlimited authority to protect it from abuse and neglect, including taking it away from the mother. Before the child is born the interest in protecting the baby must be balanced against the mother's right of autonomy. This is a public health issue because the fetus can be harmed if the mother is infected with diseases such as syphilis or HIV and they are not treated.

Untreated syphilis kills approximately 50 percent of fetuses in utero and leaves many of the rest with a congenital syndrome that includes malformations and brain damage.[40] If the woman's syphilis is treated early in pregnancy, these complications can be avoided. For many decades states have required health care providers caring for pregnant women to test those women for syphilis as early as possible in the pregnancy.[41] If the woman has syphilis but refuses treatment, the health officer can issue an administrative order for treatment or request a court order. This seldom is necessary because it is almost unheard of to refuse treatment for syphilis.

Like syphilis, HIV infection in the mother can infect her fetus. Approximately 30 percent of infants born to women with HIV are infected in utero or at birth, and go on to die of HIV-related illnesses. With screening for HIV early in pregnancy and treatment of infected women, the rate of transmission to the fetus is less than 10 percent. Unless this screening is mandated by the public health laws, health care providers can screen for HIV only with the patient's permission. This puts babies at unnecessary risk, and, given the propensity of juries to award money to innocent babies who are injured, puts the obstetricians at substantial malpractice risk. Unfortunately, many states prohibit screening for HIV without elaborate informed consents that allow the screening to be refused. Legally, there is no distinction between HIV screening and syphilis screening. States have the power, and the obligation to order both.

Personal Restrictions

Public health practice has always included personal restrictions. From Leviticus and the Koran, to quarantine in fourteenth century Venice[42] to the contemporary federal regulations on tuberculosis control,[43] public health practice depends on the authority to impose restrictions on individuals to prevent them from spreading disease in the community. The common law provided severe punishment, including death, for breaking quarantine. The legal authority (if not the punishment) was preserved in the Constitution. While antibiotics, antitubercular drugs, and immunizations have reduced the need for them, restrictions are still routinely used. As bacteria and viruses become resistant to antimicrobials[44] and new emerging infections appear, it can be expected that personal restrictions and isolation will again be a core strategy in public health.[45]

Personal restrictions pose two legal problems: they violate an individual's right of autonomy, and they can be an invasion of privacy to the extent that they must be publicly known. Typhoid Mary is an example. She was a typhoid carrier who posed a risk only if she was involved in food preparation. Unfortunately, she refused to stop working as a cook. Whenever she was found, usually through the investigation of a typhoid outbreak, she would disappear, change her name, and get a job elsewhere. She infected more than 100 people, killing several, before she was put under permanent house arrest. In a later case, a typhoid carrier challenged a typhoid control law that disclosed the identity of typhoid carriers when necessary to prevent their handling food. The court upheld the law:

> The Sanitary Code which has the force of law . . . requires local health officers to keep the State Department of Health informed of the names, ages and addresses of known or suspected typhoid carriers, to furnish to the State Health Department necessary specimens for laboratory examination in such cases, to inform the carrier and members of his household of the situation and to exercise certain controls over the activities of the carriers, including a prohibition against any handling by the carrier of food which is to be consumed by persons other than members of his own household. . . . Why should the record of compliance by the County Health Officer with these salutary requirements be kept confidential? Hidden in the files of the health offices, it serves no public purpose except a bare statistical one. Made available to those with a legitimate ground for inquiry, it is effective to check the spread of the dread disease. It would be worse than useless to keep secret an order by a public officer that a certain typhoid carrier must not handle foods which are to be served to the public.[46]

As a constitutional matter, public health officers still have broad powers to restrict individuals to protect the public. Unfortunately these powers have been weakened in several states through lobbying by civil liberties organizations and HIV advocacy groups. Fearing screening for HIV and the persecution of HIV carriers, they persuaded states such as Texas to prevent health officers from using isolation and mandatory treatment for any disease without expensive and time-consuming court review. Most troublingly, the legislature did away with deference to the health officer and made the determination of disease control methods a jury question: "The jury shall determine if the person is infected with or is reasonably suspected of being infected with a communicable disease that presents a threat to the public health and has refused or failed to follow the orders of the health authority."[47]

This standard makes it nearly impossible to restrict persons with communicable diseases, and can be directly linked to outbreaks of drug-resistant tuberculosis.[48] Even in states that have not weakened their disease control laws, there is little political support for isolation and other personal restrictions. Many public health agencies are headed by personal health services physicians who have never used restrictions and are reluctant to do so. Their focus is on individual patient care services, not community health and safety. Public health professionals encourage government to strengthen public health agencies and to revise disease control laws to meet the new threats posed by emerging infectious diseases.

▸ REFERENCES

1. Richards EP: The jurisprudence of prevention: society's right of self-defense against dangerous individuals. Hastings Constitutional Law Quarterly 16:329, 1989
2. McNeill WH: Plagues and Peoples. New York: Doubleday, 1976
3. Richards EP, Rathbun, KC: Law and the Physician: A Practical Guide. Boston: Little, Brown, Boston (1993).
4. Shattuck L: Report of the Sanitary Commission of Massachusetts 1850. Cambridge, MA: Harvard University Press, 1948 [Facsimile edition]
5. Smith v Turner, 48 US (7 How) 283, 340–41 (1849)
6. Holmes v Jennison, 39 US (14 Pet) 540, 616 (1840)
7. City of New York v New Saint Mark's Baths, 497 NYS 2d 979, 983 (1986)
8. Varholy v Sweat, 153 Fla 571, 575, 15 So 2d 267, 270 (1943)
9. Bell v Wolfish, 441 US 520 (1979)
10. Yick Wo v Hopkins, 118 US 356 (1886)
11. Baldwin v G. A. F. Seelig, Inc., 294 US 511 (1935)
12. Smith v St. Louis & S.W. Ry. Co., 181 US 248 (1901)
13. Grad, FB: The Public Health Law Manual. 2nd ed. Washington, DC: American Public Health Association, 1990
14. Dooley SW, Villarino ME, Lawrence M, Salinas L, Amil S, Rullan JV, Jarvis WR, Bloch AB, Cauthen GM: Nosocomial transmission of tuberculosis in a hospital unit for HIV-infected patients. JAMA 267:2632, 1992
15. Camara v Municipal Court of City and County of San Francisco, 387 US 523 (1967)
16. Tex Health & Safety Code § 81.151, et seq (1996)
17. Leviticus 11–16
18. North American Cold Storage Co. v Chicago 211 US 306 (1908)
19. Henne v Wright 904 F 2d 1208 (CTA 8 1990)
20. Gaus SM: Reporting child abuse. "Whistle blower protection" and physician responsibility. Mich Med 87(4):191–193, 1988
21. Johnson CF, Showers J: Injury variables in child abuse. Child Abuse Negl 9(2):207–215, 1985
22. Morris JL, Johnson CF, Clasen M: To report or not to report. Physicians' attitudes toward discipline and child abuse. Am J Dis Child 139(2):194–197, 1985
23. Chorba TL, Berkelman RL, Safford SK, Gibbs NP, Hull HF: Mandatory reporting of infectious diseases by clinicians. JAMA 262:3018–3026, 1989
24. Centers for Disease Control and Prevention: Manual of Procedures for the Reporting of Nationally Notifiable Diseases to CDC. Atlanta: Centers for Disease Control and Prevention, 1995
25. Griswold v Connecticut, 381 US 479 (1965)
26. Whalen v Roe, 429 US 589, 602 (1977)
27. Richards EP, Rathbun KC: A review of Private Acts, Social Consequences by Ronald Bayer. Family Law Quarterly 23:137, 1989
28. Jacobson v Massachusetts, 197 US 11 (1905)
29. Ex parte Woodruff, 210 P 2d 191 (Okla Crim App, 1949); Ex parte Fowler, 184 P 2d 814 (Okla Crim App, 1947)
30. Hethcote HW, Yorke JA: Gonorrhea Transmission Dynamics and Control. New York Springer-Verlag, 1984
31. Potterat JJ, Meheus A, Gallwey J: Partner notification: operational considerations. Int J STD AIDS 2:411–415, 1991
32. Association of State and Territorial Health Officers: Guide to Public Health Practice: Principles to Protect HIV-Related Confidentiality and Prevent Discrimination. Washington, DC: Association of State and Territorial Health Officers, 1988
33. Potterat JJ, Spencer NE, Woodhouse DE, Muth JB: Partner notification in the control of human immunodeficiency virus infection. Am J Public Health 79(7):874, 1989
34. Carrell S, Zoler ML, Defiant diseases: hard-won gains erode. Medical World News 31(12):20, 1990

35. Reynolds v McNichols, 488 F 2d 1378 (10th Cir [Colo], Dec 13, 1973)
36. Braunfeld v Brown, 366 US 599, 6 L Ed 2d 563, 81 S Ct 1144 (1961)
37. U.S. v Chadwell, 36 CMR 741 (NBR, Oct 25, 1965)
38. Wright v DeWitt School Dist. No. 1 of Arkansas County, 238 Ark 906, 385 SW 2d 644 (1965)
39. Sherr v Northport-East Northport Union Free School Dist., 672 F Supp 81 (EDNY 1987)
40. Rathbun KC: Congenital syphilis [Review]. Sex Transm Dis 10: 93–99, 1983
41. Rathbun KC: Congenital syphilis: a proposal for improved surveillance, diagnosis, and treatment. Sex Transm Dis 10:102–107, 1983
42. Bolduan C, Bolduan N: Public Health and Hygiene: A Students' Manual. 3rd ed. Philadelphia, WB Saunders, 194.
43. Guidelines for Preventing the Transmission of Mycobacterium Tuberculosis in Health-Care Facilities, 59 FR 54242 (1994)
44. Haley CE, McDonald RC, Rossi L, et al: Tuberculosis epidemic among hospital personnel. Infect Control Hosp Epidemiol 10:204, 1989
45. Woodhouse DE, Muth JB, Potterat JJ, Riffe LD: Restricting personal behaviour: case studies on legal measures to prevent the spread of HIV. Int J STD AIDS 4(2):114–117, 1993
46. Thomas v Morris, 286 NY 266, 269, 36 NE 2d 141, 142 (1941)
47. Tex Health & Safety Code Chapter 81.170 (1989)
48. Centers for Disease Control: Outbreak of multidrug-resistant tuberculosis—Texas, California, and Pennsylvania. Morb Mortal Wkly Rep 39:369–372, 1990

70

Public Health Management Tools

Planning

K. Michael Peddecord

▸ DEFINING PLANNING: THE PROBLEM WITH ALL THOSE WORDS

Planning is the future-oriented, systematic process of determining a direction, setting a goal, and taking actions to reach that goal. Planning is a basic management function essential to the function of all levels of an organization. This chapter provides an overview of planning definitions, issues, and tools and techniques. Major health and medical care policy planning initiatives at the state and local level are described. A brief overview of the history of formal federal health planning initiatives is presented. A second goal of this chapter is that readers develop an appreciation for the ambiguous nature of the planning vocabulary and recognize the need for clarifying discussions related to planning. While planning can be described in the terms of techniques and tools, it is also a very complicated social process that must be mastered by the successful manager and thriving organization. While every manager may realize the need to plan, there are few prescriptions for effective planning. Gaps that exist between public expectations and how an institution, sector of government, or the society actually functions may point to inadequate planning or lack of planning, rather than poor leadership and implementation.

Planning As a Political Process

Planning is as much a social and political as a technical process. A complete discussion of organizational behavior and the politics of planning is beyond the scope of this chapter. However, it is essential to recognize that all participatory planning takes place in the context of an organizational culture and a history of relationships between the planning parties (both organizations and individuals).[1,2] Complications and conflicts often arise over disagreements on the scope of planning, strategies, and specific actions necessary to achieve goals. Combine conflicting economic incentives and egos and the politics of planning takes on a life all its own.

Planning As a Systematic Management Function: Planning, Implementation, Evaluation Model

Planning is core in what professionals, managers, and executives do. Separating planning from other management processes may be useful for convenience and discussion. Without planning and the formulation of explicit goals and objectives, evaluation becomes difficult in larger organizations and communities. Another view of planning is that of a continuous improvement process that involves the iterative gathering of data, translating it into useful information, and using that information to make decisions.[3]

▸ HISTORICAL OVERVIEW OF PLANNING INITIATIVES

Planning for Health: Hill Burton Act, Comprehensive Health Planning Act, and Health System Agencies

Hill Burton Act

The Hill Burton Act is one of several significant federal initiatives that have helped to shape our current medical care and public health system. The act, which began in the late 1940s, was the first federal, state, and local strategy that provided federal matching funds to local public and nonprofit entities in order to increase local hospital and other health service resources. In addition to providing funds for hospital facilities, the Hill Burton Act and amendments stimulated formal facilities planning. For states to participate, they were required to develop a facilities plan, which served as the basis for resource allocation.[4]

Comprehensive Health Planning Act

The Partnership for Health era in the late 1960s included, among many other initiatives, the Comprehensive Health Planning (CHP) Act. This voluntary program provided grants to states and local planning agencies. With the growth of the Medicare program in the early 1970s, emphasis of these voluntary planning programs began to shift from improving the health care access and resource planning to cost control. Some state and local CHP agencies developed programs known as "certificate of need" (CON) to publicly review requests for facilities. To obtain a CON, the hospital that wanted to expand or purchase expensive technology (such as a computed tomography scanner) was required to document the "community's need" for the proposed expenditures. While some program planning efforts were useful, most policy analysts regarded the CHP cost containment efforts as a failure.[3,4]

National Health Planning and Resources Development Act of 1974

A new generation of grant-funded state and local health planning agencies replaced the CHPs. The National Health Planning and Resources Development Act of 1974 was an ambitious federal program requiring states to implement their own planning laws, which included, at a minimum, a state planning agency, a comprehensive statewide facilities plan, and a certificate-of-need law. Local "health system" agencies (HSAs) usually covered multicounty areas, reflecting political rather than actual health care market boundaries. These agencies used a systematic planning process to produce comprehensive 5-year "health systems plans." The HSAs were also charged with producing annual implementation plans whose goal was to improve the health and the functioning of the local health system. Given the incentives, the complexity of the law, lack of funding for implementation, and often an adversarial CON role, most HSAs were disconnected from local public health departments, hospitals, and other personal health care services.[a] To no one's surprise, the agencies never reached goals envisioned by policymakers.[5] Dwindling funds in the late 1970s and the movement toward reliance on the "market" rather than on "systems planning" caused HSAs in most states to fade away. All states still have a state planning agency and a few still maintain certificate of need laws, legacies of almost 50 years of federal planning initiatives.[4]

The 1980s and 1990s: Categorical Planning, Market Forces, and Voluntary Planning As Needed

The decline of federally initiated planning in the 1980s did not lessen the need to plan at local levels. The acquired immunodeficiency syndrome (AIDS) epidemic was the single most important event in the 1980s and 1990s that helped to align the interests and actions of public health, medical care, and community-based agencies. Community planning initiatives to more effectively deal with AIDS were often centered in community-based organizations and sometimes coordinated within health departments. While planning efforts were often fraught with fear, politics, limited resources, and the complications of multiple levels of government, some observers point to the success of efforts in many communities.[6]

Medicaid Managed Care

As states seek to limit the growth of Medicaid expenditures, they have almost uniformly adopted a managed care strategy. While many states have had health maintenance organizations (HMOs) as options for years, numerous states are now requiring all members of major categories of recipients to enroll in some form of managed care. In some states this shift to managed care has resulted in competition between health departments, public hospitals, traditional safety net providers, and private-sector HMOs. The reaction is often planning and collaboration mixed with the threat of chaos and bankruptcy. Such planning often has a sense of urgency and a concern for the health and welfare of large numbers of Medicaid patients and the organizations and people who served them. Such urgent planning is seldom a thoughtful deliberate process of gathering information, setting goals, and agreeing on actions. Rather, it is ad hoc, expedient, and usually lacking good information; however, the relationships formed may survive and continue planning into the future.

Trends: Community Benefit Planning—the Not-for-Profit Institutions Respond

The 1980s and 1990s have also been a period of expanding for-profit enterprises into health care.[7] Some of the debate over the contributions of for-profit and not-for-profit institutions has led some to question the extent to which some not-for-profit community hospitals are earning their tax exempt status. Several states have enacted laws requiring hospitals to document and quantify the community benefit that they provide. While all hospitals have been heavily involved in institutional (survival) planning, California's law (Senate Bill 697) requires nonprofit hospitals to assess the "health needs" of their community and to submit plans to the state to document how they are assisting in meeting the health needs of the community.

▸ INSTITUTIONAL VERSUS COMMUNITY-BASED PLANNING

Scope and Philosophy of Planning

Planning, direction, and control are the basic functions of managers. It is somewhat artificial to separate planning from the day-to-day operations of an organization or the implementation of programs. However, as organizations become larger and work needs to be differentiated, planning may become a specialized task. While every management and supervisory text has chapters devoted to planning, the primary focus of planning texts for health facilities is on broader institutional or "strategic" functions.[8,9] Planning is also an important topic in other specialized books that focus on marketing[10] or quality improvement.[11] Texts on health program planning[12] and community health needs assessment are also available and can provide greater detail on concepts, models, and methods.[12]

System View of Complex Systems: Comprehensive Versus Narrow Planning?

Systems theory can provide useful guidance to think how parts of the whole (subsystems) are connected.[3,13] The concept is that, at some level, everything is connected to everything else. Realistically, however, it is impossible to plan for the "system" as a whole. However, spending time to describe and understand the workings and interactions of the entire system is a useful investment. After planners have a sense of how things work, the problem may then be broken down into smaller parts for planning. The planning of "subsystems" or subtasks then proceeds. Making sure all of the "parts" still work together is no small task. This systems approach is described in detail in the next part, "Public Health Leadership."

Institutional and Community-Based Planning

The two types of planning described here are institutional and community. The most common planning is that based in institutions. Institutions and organizations must plan for their day-to-day operations, programs they operate, and their short-term goals and long-term survival. Institutions operate in communities; therefore, some planning must take place across institution boundaries. Community-based planning may originate in the community, in community-based organizations, or in public agencies. Participants, called stakeholders, may be a large and varied number of organizations and individuals. Such planning is often complex, laden with politics, and frustrating for participants who often have very different values, goals, and expectations of the planning process. Community planning activities may include volunteers, single-issue advocates, interested community members, elected officials, community opinion leaders, professional planners, and medical and social services professionals with narrow professional self-interests. The variety of participants in community planning may serve as a source of frustration to professional managers who are most comfortable in well-defined organizations with clear lines of authority and power.[b] Whether managing, facilitating, or participating in community planning, it may be helpful to consult a textbook that details the literature from community-development models, political science, social psychology, public relations, and voluntary participation.[1] Important aspects that differentiate community from institutional planning is provided in Table 70-1. In the left column of Table 70-1 is a list of selected characteristics (attributes or steps) in a planning process. The columns for institutional and community-based planning point out some of the differ-

[a] *These are generalizations. A few HSAs were part of the local health department. Federal law did not mandate integration with local health departments. Many local health departments did not see HSAs as highly relevant to traditional public health because of their role in hospitals and CON.*

[b] *As described below, the "level" of planning is also divided into categories for discussion. These are usually hierarchical with strategic planning at the top, programmatic planning in the middle, and operational planning at the most basic level.*

TABLE 70-1. INSTITUTIONAL VERSUS COMMUNITY PLANNING

Selected Characteristics, Attributes, or Steps in a Planning Process	*Institutional*	*Community Based*
Main focus or reason for planning	Furthering that organization's goals: profit, survival, improving services to the market that is served	Concerned with the health and welfare of an entire defined population (e.g., cross-institutional planning, safety-net planning)
Who does planning? Which organizations or groups?	All organizations, both public and private, must plan for institutional success and survival.	Health and public welfare agencies, public school districts, community-based organizations with broad mandates
Are strategic issues (issues that relate to the core concerns or values of the business or community) addressed?	Yes, but only within the context of the organization's goals	Yes, but terms such as community of health system may be used
Short time frame (months)	Yes	Community planning may need to be rapid. Some planning goes on for years.
Long time frame (years)	Yes	Yes
Need for political savvy	Essential in large organizations. Many factions must be reconciled.	Essential. Many groups must be satisfied or dealt with. Self-interest of groups may make consensus difficult or impossible.
Information needs and use	Information from inside and outside the organization is needed.	Information may be complex and from many sources. Difficult to find information for some concerns
Examples of management science or planning techniques used	Budgets, operations research, cost analysis models, statistical process control may be useful for program or operational plans.	Group management techniques and nominal group process may be useful.
Assessment of needs	Usually termed "marketing" or "market research" in an institution situation	Often done in a community context: which services are needed and by whom? etc.
Implementation: operational planning and program planning	Most planning done at this level by supervisors, workers	Not an emphasis. Institutions that have resources usually do implementation
Results or outputs of the planning process	Organizations develop action plans, business plans, or program plans to implement programs, finance operations, raise money.	Community-based planning groups may not have an organizational base or resources, but may provide recommendations to policymakers and organizations that provide services.
Emphasis on written documents	May be little emphasis on the written plan per se. More emphasis on policies, procedures, action plans, budgets, or business plans that implement the agreed-upon strategy	Well-detailed plans may be needed to communicate to those who can influence public policy or implement action.

ences that might be expected when focusing on institutional versus community priorities.

Planning Models and Planning Jargon

Jargon is a fact of modern life and planning has adopted an array of often ambiguous sounding terms. The term **strategic planning** derives from military jargon. It implies a planning process of significance, usually done by high-level decision-makers, that will result in setting the organization's overall direction. It is often coupled with "long term or long range" to create an important-sounding "long-range strategic planning," which implies a systematic (information-driven) periodic process that sets the overall business strategy of the organization for the years ahead.[8]

Operational planning, the most common type of planning, is engaged in by managers, supervisors, and every member of an organization in routine, yet essential, day-to-day activities. Besides being most common, it is crucial to providing the services and products in health and human service organizations. When objectives are clearly defined and resources known, operational planning is straightforward. Office automation, computerized scheduling systems, spread sheets, voice mail, and electronic mail all provide tools to better planning and implementation.

Tactical planning, another term having military origins, is "how to," or implementation, planning. Program and project planning are other planning types that deal with implementation. Tactical planning implies a broader scope and somewhat longer time horizon than operational planning. Projects can be as massive as a new hospital or a nationwide immunization campaign or as limited as implementing a re-engineered care process or new computer software system. Numerous management tools and techniques, such as decision support and project planning software, exist to aid in monitoring progress and optimizing project implementation.

▶ METHODS AND TOOLS FOR PLANNING

Planning: Information and the Scientific Method

Information is at the core of all planning, and a variety of collection techniques may be useful. The emphasis in selecting and executing various qualitative and quantitative data-gathering methods are pragmatic. The cost and quality of data needs to be matched to the importance of decisions that are involved. Some market research studies might be rated poor with respect to their "scientific rigor" but may be acceptable for planning decisions. In fact, for some planning information needs, a "scientifically rigorous" study would provide more accurate and precise information than is actually needed for decisions being made. Conversely, poor information from poorly designed or poorly executed studies may have devastating long-term consequences when incorrect decisions are made based on flawed studies and poor information. Again, the effective leader must balance the costs and quality issues related to information. It should be noted that information is "created" when data is organized into a usable form. Good data that is poorly organized may be worse than no data at all.

Gathering and transforming data into information that is useful in making decisions is at the core of any systematic planning process. Information may come from formal and informal sources or systems. For example, a formal system includes vital statistics systems and disease surveillance information systems.[14] Much of the information from programs comes from management information systems. Such systems, automated or manual, are seldom adequate to meet all of an organization's needs for planning information. Strategic planning and marketing texts describe the need for a comprehensive system to gather "market" intelligence; such a system uses both formal and informal data.[8,10] An example of informal information includes information on the current and predicted political and economic realities that exist in a community. Executives and staff may read newspaper reports and attend public meetings to gather this "informal" intelligence. The importance of this informal information should not be underestimated, particularly for strategic and long-range planning. Several strategic planning texts suggest that in "strategic" decision-making the most important information is informal rather than formal.[2,8]

All organizations need to gather formal statistical data and information to answer specific questions and make tactical or strategic decisions. Formal data collection techniques using epidemiological studies are described elsewhere in this text (see Chapters 2 and 33). Planning also relies on less rigorous qualitative research methods. Planning may depend on interviews or surveys of "key informants" to gather information. Nurses, physicians, social workers, and hospital or clinic clerks may be regarded as key informants. In theory, these people are able to synthesize or filter the "raw" data inexpensively and rapidly, thereby provide the planner with information.

Mathematical Modeling and Quality Planning

In recent years, various methods/models for improving the quality of products and services have become popular in health care settings.[11] In many situations, organizations and communities must make decisions for the future with little information. Statistical modeling is among the useful techniques in such situations. Mathematical models are often essential because we may be unable to wait for even preliminary empirical data that could aid our decisions. Relatively simple deterministic models,[10] more complex mathematical models such as simulation Markov models, or decision theory may be useful in planning where it is not possible to pilot-test alternative interventions in a systematic manner.[15] Cost-effectiveness analysis may also be useful in selecting interventions and assisting in making strategic, tactical, or policy decisions.[16] For more on quality planning approaches see the chapter part, "Quality Assurance and Quality Improvement."

Integrated Planning, Budgeting, and Improvement Approaches

Over the years management science, industrial engineering, and organizational development specialists have developed systems designed to integrate and improve various management functions including planning. Management by objectives (MBO) swept businesses in the 1970 with the promise of quantitatively linking the performance of every member of the organization with the organization's goals by using a system of quantifiable objectives.[17] Large organizations developed their own approaches including zero-based budgeting, which President Carter attempted to introduce to the public sector.[18] While many management systems have proved to be short-term fads, other systems and management tools have been successful and worthy of long-term adoption.

▶ GUIDEPOSTS, BENCHMARKS, AND MODELS FOR PLANNING HEALTH AND PREVENTION

Implicit in all of these sections is that we decide for *what* we are planning. Since health is a state of individual and community well-being, it is among the most difficult things to plan. Of the many initiatives designed to improve the health status of individuals, our communities, and our nation, *Healthy People 2000* "provides a vision for achieving improved health for all Americans"[19] and represents the continuation of a cooperative effort lead by the U.S. Public Health Service. *Healthy People 2000* is without doubt the most important set of quantified guideposts (benchmarks) for measuring and improving health. Most states and many local communities have used this framework to establish goals and priorities for local health monitoring and improvement initiatives.[20] Hospital and managed care providers as well as their accreditation organizations also use *Healthy People 2000* guidelines in selecting indicators to monitor performance of personal health care services.[21] Other guidelines, standards, and planning models are also available. While there are currently no accrediting agencies for public health departments, a set of *Model Standards: A Guide for Community Preventive Health Services* is available.[22]

During the last decade, the public health community and its professional organizations have taken the lead to provide assistance to health departments and other segments of the community to plan for the improvement of health. Several resource packages have been developed to provide frameworks, training resources, background material, and even workbooks for community-based health planning initiatives. The Assessment Protocol for Excellence in Public Health (APEX-PH) includes both an internal capacity assessment for health departments as well as a template for community health assessment. A seven-stage planning and resource development model is the framework for this assessment. The Planned Approach for Community Health (PATCH) provides a model that uses a community-based approach and follows a classic planning, implementation, and evaluation strategy.[23] All of these are discussed in more detail in Chapter 67.

▶ IMPROVING PLANNING: BOTH LEADERSHIP AND TECHNICAL SKILLS ARE NEEDED FOR THE FUTURE

Organizations that plan well at both the strategic and programmatic level are likely to be the most successful. Some have suggested that governmental public health departments must be more concerned with "steering" rather than "rowing,"[24] and should be primarily responsible for providing leadership to improve community health rather than providing direct services in the future.[25] In this leadership role, the ability to engage other organizations and individuals in the community and to plan effectively becomes even more essential. At the local level there will be more emphasis on community-based rather that institutional and program planning. Without political and interpersonal skills, in addition to technical planning skills, it will be difficult to establish the credibility of the health department as a leader in community health improvement.

This chapter part presents an overview of health planning history, approaches, current planning guidelines, and models that may be useful at the community level. Other chapter parts on evaluation, policy development, and quality improvement provide additional tools and frameworks for planning. This text includes many epidemiological techniques that are indispensable tools for planning sound programs that are designed to improve community health. Effective planning is essential to improving the health of our communities and the effective operation of programs, small and large. Devoting the necessary time and resources for planning is a challenge that leaders must meet if they are to improve the quality of our services and the health status of our communities.

Public Health Leadership: Current Constraints and a Vision of the Future

John C. Lammers

Since the 1990 Institute of Medicine report, *The Future of Public Health*,[1] a number of efforts around the country have arisen to renew and strengthen the leadership of public health enterprises at the federal, state, and local levels. Several states have established leadership institutes for the development of their executives, and the national-level Public Health Leadership Institute is in its 6th year of providing leadership development training for top state and local managers.[2] Also, recent changes in the health care system, pushing indigent medical care and the state-federal Medicaid programs toward the privately managed sector, have caused both public health leaders and the public to reflect once again upon the question, what is public health? The development of the *Journal of Public Health Management and Practice* reflects the growing awareness that public health work requires management skills of a generic nature as well as practices that may be particular to public health purposes. This section outlines briefly the generic and field-specific areas of public health leadership.

Traditional public health training and practice has emphasized skills, knowledge, and abilities in epidemiology, disease prevention, health education, and population and family health. There is a relatively scant literature on leadership and management in public health.[3,4] In assessing the needs and concerns of public health leaders, four areas of practice lie outside these traditional public health areas. These include the recognition that public health as a field requires (*a*) the advocacy of its leadership, (*b*) collaboration with other public and private sectors, (*c*) development of a vision for its own corps, and (*d*) a strengthened pattern of renewal as an integral part of the nation's health system.

Advocacy activities on the part of public health leaders have until lately been dominated with concerns for medical services to the underserved. More recently, population-based services have received renewed attention. Public health leaders have used the notions of media advocacy (framing key health concerns to sustain their presence in the mass media),[5] and social marketing (viewing health behaviors as products to be sold to consumers).[6]

As population-based services have arisen as a key concern for the public's health, leaders have recognized that progress can be made only in collaboration with other organizations. Systems thinking is one method for identifying the social, institutional, and organizational elements in the networks of concern to public health leaders.[4,7] Collaborative leadership has been successfully argued by several authors.[8] Like systems thinking, collaborative leadership takes into account the requirement that change in the health system necessitates change in organizations and systems to which it is linked. One process for identifying the elements of the broader system, and for working with representatives of that system, is known as team learning, or dialogue.[9]

The benefits of a strong public health system are often taken for granted in U.S. society. Public health leaders have recognized that maintaining and strengthening the public health corps requires the key activity of leadership known as visioning.[10] An organizational vision is a realistic, credible, attractive future for an organization—that its members can strive to attain.[10] Elements of developing an organization's vision include assessing the present state of the organization, identifying constituencies, building scenarios to generate alternative visions, and packaging the vision for practice within and beyond the organization.[10]

Relatedly, developing scenarios for planning has also gained credence in public health work. Scenarios are detailed alternative futures.[11] Developing scenarios involves eight steps: identifying focal issue(s); describing key forces in the environment; identifying driving trends; ranking trends by importance and uncertainty; selecting scenario logics; fleshing out scenario descriptions; developing the implications of the scenarios; and identifying leading indicators and signposts.

Renewal is the leadership activity that concerns both the personal renewal of individual energies of leaders and managers as well as the vitality of whole organizations. The pressures of public health work, given its urgency as well as its political context, have made cynics of many of its managers. Personal considerations of career choice and value development have therefore become important in developing leaders. Senge uses the term "personal mastery" to refer to this activity of personal reflection and development.[7] Gardner is more concerned with the renewal of public enterprises broadly and highlights the necessity of bringing young people into public service.[12]

Each of theses four areas, advocacy, collaboration, vision, and renewal, are receiving increasing attention in public health curricula and executive level training.

Policy Development

Helen H. Schauffler

There are many different avenues for influencing policy development for public health and preventive medicine. In addition to policy decisions made by the U.S. Congress (the legislative branch of the federal government), public policy decisions affecting preventive medicine and public health are also made at the federal level in the executive branch (the Department of Health and Human Services, the Centers for Disease Control and Prevention, the Surgeon General's Office, the Food and Drug Administration, etc.), at the state level in both the executive (governor's office, state health department) and legislative branches, at the city and local levels of governments, and in the private sector in private associations, representing health care organizations and professionals, and among health plans and employers.

Agenda Setting

The process of agenda setting is key to initiating the policy development process.[1,2] The formal policy agenda is defined as those issues to which policymakers will pay attention and take action. Thus, the first step in any policy development process is to get an issue on the formal policy agenda. Two of the most commonly used strategies for getting an issue on the policy agenda include: (*a*) gaining *inside access* to decision-makers in the policy arena, and (*b*) organizing an *outside initiative* through grass-roots mobilization or coalition building to call the issue to the attention of policymakers.[1] These agenda-setting strategies can be used alone or in combination. Recently, both have been used successfully to influence the policy agenda for public health and preventive medicine.

Using Inside Access to Influence Policy-making

During the 103rd Congress, effective inside access was achieved by state and local public health officials who met individually with their elected representatives in Congress to discuss the importance of securing stable and adequate funding for the core functions of public health under a reformed health care system. Public health officials, both as constituents and leaders in their state and communities, bring credibility and lend importance to an issue and can facilitate translation of public health issues in terms that make them locally relevant to individual elected representatives.[3]

Using Outside Initiative Strategies to Influence Policy-making

In 1994, the National Breast Cancer Coalition and other women's groups organized a massive and effective postcard-writing campaign from women at the grassroots level all over the country regarding the importance of covering mammography screening as a health insurance benefit under health care reform in the 103rd Congress. U.S. Senators and Representatives reported receiving hundreds of postcards from their constituents calling their attention to this issue. Legislators care most about how an issue affects their constituents and will pay more attention to an issue if it comes from the grassroots.

The state of Washington provides a model for how states may proceed, in the absence of reforms at the federal level, to put together a coalition of all of the key stakeholders in public health and engage in a productive planning process that produces tangible results. Washington state developed its own Public Health Improvement Plan in 1994, which was submitted to the state legislature and enacted into law in 1995.[4] The plan was developed by the Washington state Department of Health and a Public Health Improvement Plan Steering Committee, representative of a broad coalition of public health and health care organizations in the state. The coalition included representatives of the Department of Health, the state medical association, the association of community clinics, consumers, public health nursing directors, state legislators, schools of public health, labor unions, the state nurses' association, local public health officials, the hospital association, the health care purchasers' association, and the Indian Health Service. The purpose of the plan was to help achieve three goals—stabilization of health care costs, assurance of universal access to health care, and improvement of population health. The plan includes comprehensive recommendations for public health capacity, finance and governance of the public health system, and standards and strategies for addressing key public health problems. It served as the blueprint for state legislation enacted to reform Washington state's public health system.

Difficulties in Getting Public Health and Preventive Medicine on the Policy Agenda

For the last 10 to 15 years, public health and preventive medicine have had difficulty getting attention on either the public or private sector policy agendas, unless there was a perceived crisis that required immediate attention. And even in crisis situations, such as the acquired immunodeficiency syndrome (AIDS) epidemic, the government has been slow to respond.

The relative importance of public health and preventive medicine in health policy development over the last decade is illustrated by estimates that less than 1 percent of total health expenditures in the United States is spent on population-based public health and prevention programs.[5] There are many reasons for this neglect, including the bias toward the medical model in health policy development. One example that illustrates this struggle was the experience in trying to add preventive care as a benefit to the Medicare program.

Incremental Policy Development: Adding Prevention Benefits to the Medicare Program

Perhaps the best example of how policy development for preventive medicine proceeds incrementally are the efforts over the last 30 years to add preventive services benefits to the Medicare program. The amendments to the Social Security Act, which authorized the Medicare program in 1965, include a provision (Section 1862) that prohibits reimbursement for any preventive care. The original Medicare program was based on the Blue Cross and Blue Shield programs operating at that time, where preventive care was not considered medically necessary. Preventive care is also neither unpredictable nor high cost, thus it was not considered to be appropriate for insurance coverage.

Between 1965 and 1980, over 350 bills were introduced into the U.S. Congress proposing to add preventive care benefits under Medicare before one bill finally passed adding the pneumococcal vaccine as a covered benefit.[5] Only incrementally and within the context of huge budget reconciliation bills were additional screening and immunization benefits added to the Medicare program between 1980 and 1992. And the only benefits that were added were those for which research had demonstrated not only their effectiveness, but their relative cost-effectiveness. The pneumococcal vaccine was shown to be cost-saving to the Medicare program, while mammography and Pap smears were added later only when studies from the Office of Technology Assessment showed that they were relatively cost-effective.[6]

Key Factors Influencing Health Insurance Coverage of Preventive Care

The key factors associated with successful policy development for adding prevention benefits in the Medicare program include an incremental approach of adding only one benefit at a time, documented and scientific evidence of the effectiveness and cost-effectiveness of the preventive service, and sponsorship and leadership of key policymakers. Factors associated with failure include lack of active support from beneficiaries and health professionals, projected increases in costs to the medical care system associated with adding the benefit, and competing priorities on the policy agenda.

Predicting the Outcomes and Designing Successful Strategies for Prevention Policy

One of the most useful models for predicting the likely success or failure of proposed policies, and one that is also useful for designing more effective strategies for influencing the policy-making process, is James Q. Wilson's model of concentrated and diffuse cost and benefits (Table 70-2).[7]

To apply Wilson's model to a particular policy, one must identify the intended effects of the policy—who will benefit from the policy and who will bear the costs. In each case, one must also assess if the benefits and costs are concentrated or diffuse. Concentrated costs are those that are imposed on a well-organized, relatively small number of individuals or groups where the cost will be strongly felt. An example of a concentrated cost would be a tax policy requiring hospitals to contribute to a pool to support local public health activities. A diffuse cost, in contrast, is one where the cost burden is widely distributed among a large group of relatively unorganized individuals or groups, where the impact of the cost is relatively small. An example of a diffuse cost would be a small increase in the income tax or in

TABLE 70-2. JAMES Q. WILSON MODEL OF CONCENTRATED AND DIFFUSE COST AND BENEFITS

	Concentrated Benefits	*Diffuse Benefits*
Concentrated costs	(±) Alternating victories. Equally matched opponents. Battles between organized interest groups.	(–) A losing policy. Organized opposition with little organized support. Need to reframe policy effects to get out of this box.
Diffuse costs	(+) A winning policy. Organized support with little organized opposition.	(±) Incremental policy development, without strong, organized support or opposition.

From Wilson JQ: The Politics of Regulation. New York: Basic Books, 1980, pp 357–394.

insurance premiums to pay to support public health activities. Policies that rely on concentrated costs are always more difficult to adopt, as the group targeted to bear the cost is likely to organize strong opposition to the policy and will, more often than not, be successful in defeating it. The only case where this is not true is when the benefits are also concentrated and the group who will benefit is equally well organized and prepared to support the policy proposal. In this case, the victories are likely to be alternating. Policies that have concentrated benefits and diffuse costs are almost always winners, as the proponents are well organized, while those bearing the cost are not. Policies that have both diffuse benefits and costs proceed incrementally without strong or well-organized support or opposition.

To be successful in developing policy for public health and preventive medicine, it is best to frame the policy and its impacts as having diffuse costs and concentrated benefits. Conversely, in trying to defeat a proposed policy, it is best to frame the policy's effects as having concentrated costs. The central challenge for public health is rooted in the fact that most public health programs, by definition, have diffuse benefits, making it very difficult to successfully organize political support for them.

Importance of Problem Definition in Policy Development

Also key to influencing the policy agenda is how a problem is defined.[8] In times of budget constraint, programs that are seen as inexpensive or cost-saving are particularly popular among policymakers.[2] If reforming and/or increased investment in public health and preventive medicine are portrayed as contributing toward lowering health care costs, advocates may be more successful in capturing the attention of policymakers.[9] In contrast, if public health is viewed as contributing toward increasing government expenditures and enlarging the role of government, it will be difficult to get the attention of policymakers in a political environment that seeks to reduce the role and size of government.

The Role of Evidence-Based Guidelines for Preventive Medicine Policy: The U.S. Preventive Services Task Force Report

One of the greatest influences on health insurance policy for preventive medicine was the 1989 release of the U.S. Preventive Services Task Force Report, which established national guidelines for clinical preventive services.[11] The report was prepared for the Department of Health and Human Services, and the Task Force recommendations were based on a rigorous review of the scientific evidence on the efficacy and effectiveness of 169 clinical preventive services. The reasons this report has been so influential are (*a*) the recommendations are grounded in health services research demonstrating the effects of preventive medicine, and (*b*) the report was developed by an independent task force, not associated with any one special interest or professional group. Clinical trials demonstrating the effectiveness and cost-effectiveness of specific preventive care measures are one of the most powerful tools for influencing purchaser and health plan decisions to pay for and cover preventive medicine.

The Task Force report has also had an influence in the development of quality measures to assess the performance of health plans. The National Committee for Quality Assurance (NCQA) defined seven of its nine quality measures in its Health Plan Employer Data and Information Set (HEDIS) 2.0, based on the recommendations for specific screening and immunization services in the U.S. Preventive Services Task Force Report.[12] Employers, as purchasers of health care, have also relied on the U.S. Preventive Services Task Force Report to define standard benefits packages to be offered by health plans and to define performance standards for assessing the performance of health plans and the quality of care delivered to their employees.[8]

The Importance of Population-Based Data and Goals for Public Health Policy: *Healthy People 2000*

Also important to furthering the development of public health policy in the last 10 years has been the development and release of the *Healthy People 2000* goals and objectives for the nation.[10] It not only documents the current health status of the U.S. population, but it establishes population-based goals to improving population health. *Healthy People 2000* has provided the basis for establishing data systems at the national, state, and local levels for collecting and reporting on population data and has served as the benchmark against which to measure the influence of public health programs and health care policies. The goals and objectives were developed between 1987 and 1990 using an extensive consultative and hearings process by the U.S. Public Health Service in partnership with the National Academy of Science and the Institute of Medicine.[13]

The impact of the goals and objectives has been far-reaching. Congress has enacted three laws that incorporate the objectives, and 40 states have issued their own *Healthy People 2000* plans, which have been used to build coalitions to improve public health and to improve data systems to monitor the health status of the population.[10] The goals have also been widely adopted at the local level and by private and voluntary agencies. Even the quality measures for health plans developed by the National Committee for Quality Assurance were based in part on the *Healthy People 2000* objectives to reward health plans for keeping populations healthy.[14]

New Opportunities for Policy Development in an Era of Accountability

Perhaps the greatest opportunities for policy development that promotes public health and preventive medicine is the recent shift toward defining the problems in the health care systems as ones of quality and accountability. As quality and "value" in the health care system are increasingly defined as maintaining and improving the health of the population, monitoring changes in the health status of the population is necessary to ensure quality and accountability, and public health and preventive medicine become important players in the solution. Public health and preventive medicine offer expertise and experience in community-based prevention programs and population-based data collection and can take a leadership role in policy development in these areas.

The clearest example of this shift toward increased accountability is the development of HEDIS measures by NCQA. The majority of the quality measures in HEDIS 2.0, 2.5 and 3.0 address provision of clinical preventive services in accordance with the U.S. Preventive Services Task Force recommendations. Health maintenance organizations (HMOs) all over the country are being evaluated against these measures, and their performance is being published in report cards made available to employers and the general public. In some instances, employers are requiring that HMOs guarantee their performance in meeting quality standards by placing a percentage of their premium at risk.[9] Building requirements for collecting data, meeting performance standards, and adding economic incentives for performance guarantees into the contracts between HMOs and purchasers, including private employers, state Medicaid agencies, and federal Medicare contracts, may be the most effective policy tools currently available for increasing appropriate provision of preventive care to the insured population.

Additional Public Policy Tools for Promoting Prevention and Public Health

There are many additional policy tools that are effective in promoting population health.[15] Taxation of unhealthy products (e.g., cigarettes and alcohol), regulation of individual and industry behaviors that will promote health and prevent disease (e.g., regulating helmet use and industrial environmental pollution), and public health education (e.g., media campaigns promoting good nutrition and physical activity) are all important tools that can contribute toward a more effective health care system that promotes and maintains health.[16] It is essential that policy for prevention and public health be developed at the national, state, local, and institutional levels and that it is developed based on a comprehensive model with policies that seek to influence the medical care system, communities, and governmental policies to promote population health and prevent disease.[16]

Quality Assurance and Quality Improvement

Richard S. Kurz

In this section, two approaches to quality assessment are discussed: quality assurance and quality improvement. Though similar regarding their emphasis on the process of providing health services, each approach differs in terms of its purpose and procedures. Quality assurance refers to "the formal and systematic exercise of identifying problems in medical care delivery, designing activities to overcome these problems, and carrying out follow-up steps to ensure that no new problems have been introduced and that corrective actions have been effective."[1] Quality improvement is "a management philosophy to improve the level of performance of key processes in the organization."[2]

An understanding of these approaches requires first placing them in the broader context of quality assessment, involving structures, processes, and outcomes of health services. Berwick[3] suggests that understanding quality requires that practitioners (*a*) know what works (efficacy or effectiveness), (*b*) use what works (appropriateness), (*c*) do well what works (execution), and (*d*) know the purpose for doing it (value assessment). A fifth perspective should be added to this list: knowing the resources needed to do what works. The approaches emphasized in this section, quality assurance and quality improvement, are related to the second and third of these issues. Before turning to a discussion of them, brief consideration is given to the first and fifth issues concerning the outcome and structure of health services.

Knowing the Resources for What Works

Operational and financial resources have been identified as essential for quality care in health services organizations. These are often viewed as structural concerns that are preconditions to the delivery of any services. Operational structures consist of physical facilities and personnel needed to accomplish the level of services that are desired. The earliest quality assessment procedures employed professional or organizational measures in developing licensure, certification, and accreditation for individuals, health care institutions, and educational programs. The evidence is now clear that these aspects of providing care are necessary but not sufficient to ensure high quality. For example, the major organizational accreditation agencies for health-related organizations, the Joint Commission for the Accreditation of Healthcare Organizations (JCAHO) and the National Committee for Quality Assurance (NCQA), emphasize process and outcome rather than structural measures.

Knowing What Works

Knowing what works requires information on the efficacy of specific technologies, pharmaceuticals, and clinical interventions under controlled conditions and on the effectiveness of medical and surgical treatments as well as diagnostic, preventive, and rehabilitative care in the course of practice.[4] These approaches provide assessments of the technical results of interventions or services as perceived by the developers or providers of the activity. The primary methodologies in the assessment of efficacy are clinical trials and sophisticated technology assessment techniques.[5] The benefits of control in these approaches are balanced with the lack of generalizability resulting from restricted study groups of patients, the restrictions on delivery protocols used, and the limited outcomes addressed. Investigations of effectiveness of practitioners and organizations are referred to generically as "outcomes research." These studies consider the long and short term and broad and narrow effects of services provided by specific practitioners or by specific types of organizations. The measures of these outcomes include mortality, morbidity, and patient health status indicators. Substantial attention has been given to the measurement of these factors,[6,7] but equal or greater focus needs to be placed on the process of improving quality in all types of health service organizations and in communities. A primary example of outcomes studies are the Patient Outcomes Research Teams (PORT) funded by the Agency for Health Care Policy and Research (AHCPR). These research programs are large-scale cohort studies using data drawn from routine practice settings.[8]

Knowing what works can also be assessed in terms of consumers' perceptions of the services that they receive. This assessment may be of the technical care provided or of interpersonal relationships or amenities experienced.[9] As health services organizations have experienced increased pressure to respond to consumer expectations, the distribution of patient or consumer satisfaction questionnaires has become routine and their methodologies increasingly diverse and sophisticated.[10–12] At the community level, evaluation of services is conducted through report cards that are "standardized, publicly released reports on the quality of care."[13] Report cards have been developed for specific areas of care and types of health care organizations.[14] A widely cited example of these instruments is the Health Plan Employer Data and Information Set (HEDIS), which was developed to assess managed care plans and is employed by the NCQA.[15]

Using What Works

Using what works, or quality assurance, implies a consideration of the process by which services are provided. The fundamental issue is the appropriateness of the care provided: (*a*) overuse of services when other or no intervention would have been beneficial, (*b*) underuse of the services that would benefit the patient, and (*c*) improper or incorrect use of beneficial care or prevention. The third issue will be discussed in the next segment of this section. Consideration of appropriateness leads directly to related questions of who determines what is appropriate care and who makes the judgment as to appropriateness in specific instances.

Appropriateness is the aspect of quality assessment with which health care professionals, especially physicians, are most comfortable if they maintain control of the process. Physicians are trained to determine what actions should be taken in specific situations and to take responsibility for their actions in each instance. Concurrent and post hoc assessment by committees in hospitals or other health services organizations are the routine means through which physicians and other professionals perform peer evaluation and discipline. State boards and hospital utilization review programs have also attempted to maintain appropriate care. Concerns regarding the effectiveness of peer evaluation of both providers and institutions have lead to more formal process assessment by external bodies such as Peer Review Organizations (PROs) at the state level, the Health Care Financing Administration at the federal level, and insurance companies.

Although there are many approaches to assessing the appropriateness of care, perhaps the most extensively examined recently is the use of standards of care. Standards of care are "statements describing specific diagnostic or therapeutic maneuvers that should or should not be performed in certain clinical circumstances."[16] Standards can be applied to a population of individuals in the community or to individual patients. The key question is do standards of care influence physician behavior and thus improve quality? There is limited evidence to date that this is the case.[17] Chassin argues, however, that standards can be effective in changing physician behavior if guidelines regarding their construction and use are followed. These include: (*a*) consensus and credibility concerning clinical content, (*b*) presentation in the context of a physician's performance, (*c*) the legitimacy and focus of the presentation, and (*d*) reinforcement of the initial education.[17]

How, then, should standards be developed and who should use them for what purposes? The dilemma in answering the first question is that efficacy research exists for a very limited number of clinical procedures, especially research applying the treatment in a clinical setting or linking it to specific effectiveness outcomes. Hence, although the best attempts to develop standards, such as those created by the RAND Corporation, begin with a careful evaluation of the existing empirical literature, other consensus methods must be used to establish a standard of care. The Delphi methods used by the RAND Corporation produce appropriateness ratings similar to those based on research studies; however, the use of such reliable and valid consensus techniques is not always present in the development of standards of care.[18] Although methods for assessing appropriateness based on judgments can be developed and used in clinical and research settings, e.g., the Appropriateness Evaluation Protocol,[19] substantial methodological study remains to be done.

Despite the lack of agreement on how to establish standards, there is increasing demand for them. Insurers, private and governmental, seek standards as a basis for determining what care they will pay for, which health care organizations they will use, and which treatments they will cover in their policies. In addition, they provide a basis for external regulation of physician and hospital practice and internal assessment of the clinical care provided by physicians and other practitioners. The concern expressed by physicians regarding these multiple uses of standards of care is that treatment and prevention are constantly evolving processes based on research evidence and practice experience. The standard set today may not be appropriate to the care given tomorrow. It is this concern that has led scholars, especially in the past 10 years, to study the question of how medicine can continually improve what it does.

Doing Well What Works

Doing well what works results from a process of continuous quality improvement (CQI) or total quality management (TQM), terms that are used interchangeably in this chapter. The concepts and principles of CQI are based largely on the works of three scholars in the United States (W. Edwards Deming,[20] Joseph Juran,[21] and Philip Crosby[22]) and two others from Japan (Genichi Taguchi and Kaoru Ishikawa).[23] Numerous applications of CQI have now been made in health services and public health organizations, perhaps the most significant of which was the National Demonstration Project on Quality Improvement in Health Care conducted by Donald Berwick and others.[24]

As a management philosophy, the aspects of CQI require a significant shift in management behavior. In Table 70–3, these changes in management approach are summarized in seven principles adapted from Berwick and his associates' work on the national demonstration project. In this approach, organizations emphasize the management of processes rather than the management of people. The vast majority of problems are said to result from failures in a process or the suppliers or inputs to it, while only a small minority occur from idiosyncratic events, including the behavior of individuals.

From a quality improvement perspective, problems occur most frequently across functions as work moves from one area to another or as materials or products enter or leave the organization. Because of this fact, customers and suppliers should not be viewed as problems but as partners in the process of service delivery.

The implementation of CQI in a health services organization results in a transformation that impacts all aspects of the organization. Deming described this change process as the integration of "profound knowledge" into management structures, policies, and procedures.[25] As depicted in Figure 70-1, traditional improvement is a function of professional knowledge comprised of information on discipline, subject matter, and values. In health care, quality assurance is a form of traditional improvement in which an individual's failure to perform appropriately is viewed as correctable through greater professional training or better judgment based on professional standards or values. Quality improvement requires both professional knowledge and improvement knowledge.

The first aspect of improvement knowledge, an appreciation for system, implies the ability to answer three questions: why do we make what we make, how do we make what we make, and how do we improve what we make? An answer to the first of these questions requires knowledge of customer preferences and community needs; the second, knowledge of processes, their inputs and suppliers, the services provided, and their customers; and the third, knowledge of

TABLE 70-3. THE PRINCIPLES OF CONTINUOUS QUALITY IMPROVEMENT

1. Productive work is accomplished through processes.
2. Sound customer-supplier relationships are absolutely necessary for sound quality management.
3. The main source of quality defects is problems in the process.
4. Poor quality is costly.
5. Understanding the variability of processes is key to improving quality.
6. The modern approach to quality is thoroughly grounded in scientific and statistical thinking.
7. Total employee involvement is critical.
8. New organizational structures can help achieve quality improvement.

Adapted from Berwick DM, Godfrey AB, Roessner J: Curing Health Care: New Strategies for Quality Improvement. San Francisco, CA: Jossey-Bass, 1991, Chapter 3.

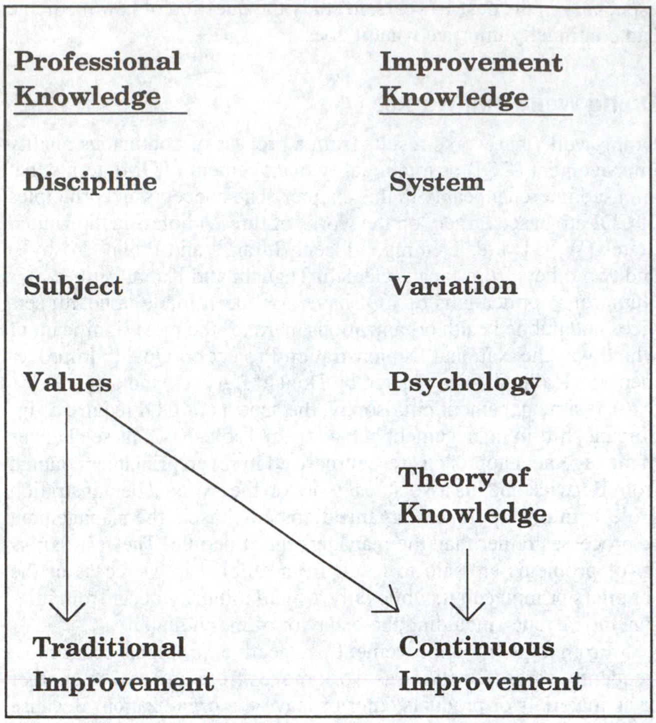

Figure 70-1. The aspects of Deming's "profound knowledge." (Adapted from Batalden PB, Nolan TW: Knowledge for the leadership of continual improvement in healthcare. In Taylor J (ed): Manual of Health Services Management. Gaithersburg, MD: Aspen, 1993.)

organizational vision, a plan for improvement, and an approach for design or redesign of key processes.

Knowledge of variation requires an understanding of two types of causes for variation in processes. The first are special causes that are identifiable as resulting from specific and idiosyncratic problems of individuals, machines, or events. These causes, if found, should be removed immediately without the need for greater knowledge of the process. Common causes produce variation, which is inherent to the elements of the process. In other words, to remove common causes of variation, the process must be studied thoroughly and the structure of the process, its inputs, and/or its suppliers must be changed. As outlined in Table 70-4, eight statistical procedures can be used to assist in the identification and resolution of process variation and, hence, to produce process improvement.[26]

The psychology of improvement is based on the power of intrinsic motivation. Goals may be achieved through competition, but also by working independently and in cooperation with others. The success and survival of an organization is more likely to be based on the work of cross-functional teams who understand how system processes work and are committed to a vision for the organization that advances it beyond its current reality.

The final aspect of Deming's profound knowledge is the use of a theory of knowledge. Improvement comes through the use of knowledge, which allows us to predict the impact of changes. The theory of knowledge advocated for quality improvement is fundamentally the scientific method. Based on planning and study of the process, hunches or hypotheses are developed as to the causes of process failures. These hunches are tested through small experiments based on existing or newly collected data. If a cause is identified, other experiments are attempted to continue the iterative process of improvement, and knowledge gained is distributed to everyone in the organization. This approach to quality improvement has been called the Shewhart, or the Plan, Do, Check, Act (PDCA), cycle.

Many health services organizations have developed unique approaches for the implementation of CQI. One of the most widely recognized is the FOCUS-PDCA procedure developed and used by the former Hospital Corporation of America. The steps in this process can be illustrated with an example of process improvement completed by the Springfield/Greene County Department of Health (DOH) in Missouri. First, the DOH identified a process for improvement (FIND). In the county, political concern had been expressed regarding the length of time needed to abate environmental hazards. Although many approaches had been used in the past to achieve the outcome of reduced abatement time, none had worked. A CQI approach was suggested and a team was organized, the members of which understood the process of hazard abatement from their participation in or supervision of it (ORGANIZE). To clarify their current knowledge of the process (CLARIFY), the team created a flowchart of its steps and found the number of days that each step in the process required. Having described the process, the team undertook further investigation to discover what the causes of the delay were and which causes were the most important for reducing abatement time (UNDERSTAND). The team used Pareto charts and cause-and-effect diagrams to assist with this part of their work. Using this approach, the team discovered that the preparation of formal abatement requests through a typing pool and the search of courthouse records for property ownership were the most significant causes of abatement delay. Focusing on the second issue, the team attempted a modem connection to the records of the county utility company rather than the search of courthouse records to establish property ownership (SELECT). Having selected a potential solution, appropriate contacts were made with the utility company, and a clerk was trained to make the modem connections and search the database (PLAN). Data was collected by the clerk on the length of time for discovery of ownership and presented in a simple bar graph comparing the length of time for utility company versus courthouse searches (DO). The analysis in this instance was simple and obvious, the average time for courthouse searches was 3 to 5 days, and for utility database searches it was 15 minutes (CHECK). Hence, approximately 4 days could be removed from each search. The DOH acted to train all clerks to do searches and expanded the investigation time of sanitarians, which was formerly wasted in courthouse searches (ACT). Although this presentation of the abatement case is oversimplified, continuous quality improvement provided a systematic approach to process improvement based on team knowledge rather than administrative authority.

How effective has continuous improvement been in improving quality and controlling costs? Although many scholars have described CQI implementation or presented normative explanations for its use, little systematic study of the impact of CQI on quality and costs has appeared in the health services literature. A prominent exception is the work of Shortell and others involving 61 western hospitals.[27] Their study found that participative, flexible, and risk-taking culture was significantly related to quality improvement implementation and that use of CQI produced better perceived clinical and human resource outcomes. In addition, larger hospitals had lower efficiency concerning charges and length of stay (LOS) because of their bureaucratic and hierarchical culture. Hence, the study supports the positive effect of CQI on clinical and financial outcomes, emphasizing the need for supportive and flexible cultures as a key aspect for success.

TABLE 70-4. SEVEN BASIC TOOLS FOR DATA ANALYSIS IN PROCESS IMPROVEMENT

1. Flow charts
2. Cause-and-effect (fishbone or Ishikawa) diagrams
3. Pareto charts
4. Frequency distributions (histograms)
5. Scatter diagrams or regression analyses
6. Run charts
7. Control charts

Knowing the Purpose for Doing It

Those involved in quality assurance and quality improvement must ultimately consider the purpose for quality assessment and the values underlying decisions. Unfortunately, this area has received little systematic attention in the literature. Berwick suggests that the issue can be addressed from an economic perspective. That is, to what extend is health care a social good, a product whose acquisition does not reduce one's wealth? The answer to this question Berwick believes is intertwined with the distribution of insurance in our society. Brodeur provides a second approach for considering the purposes of quality assurance or improvement, ethical analysis.[28] He believes that each management perspective has associated with it a set of more or less well-articulated values that provide the basis for an ethical analysis of how each approach views the nature of work. From this view, work as a group activity must not subjugate the value of the persons performing the work to organizational concerns for efficiency and productivity.

Conclusion

In this section, the conceptualization, implementation, and significance of quality assurance and quality improvement are discussed in the context of the range of approaches to quality assessment discussed in the literature. There is some evidence that quality assurance has not met expectations regarding its ability to change practitioner behavior although the concept has been implemented in several different ways and this variation is related to the inconsistency of results. Alternatively, although its detractors abound, research on quality improvement is beginning to demonstrate the potential of this approach for linking process and outcome of health services. Complete assessments of quality, however, require the several approaches of efficacy, effectiveness, appropriateness, and efficiency studies. In addition, these investigations must identify how the structural, process, and outcome components of quality are related in the delivery of preventive and treatment services.

Evaluation

Thomas G. Rundall

Evaluation of health programs and policies is fundamental for public health.[1,2] Building and maintaining an effective health care system requires programs and policies that promote health and prevent disease in an effective and efficient manner. Evaluation is a process designed to collect and analyze information to determine program performance and to improve it. This process involves a variety of concepts, methods, and analytic schemes to determine whether a given program is needed and likely to be used, whether it is appropriately designed to meet the targeted need, whether the program is implemented as planned, and whether the program actually does help people in need at a reasonable cost without undesirable side effects.[3] Hence, evaluation is used to assist in health program planning, program quality assurance and improvement, and policy development. In planning an evaluation, the evaluator collaborates with other stakeholders to decide (*a*) what is the purpose of the evaluation, (*b*) what will be the focus of the evaluation, and (*c*) what specific evaluation model will guide the data collection and analysis.

Purpose of the Evaluation

Evaluations can be conducted for *formative* or *summative* purposes.[4] Formative evaluation is done primarily for the purpose of providing program staff with information for making midstream alterations in the program to increase the likelihood of achieving desired outcomes. The primary purpose of summative evaluation is to provide information for decision-makers with respect to whether the program in its final form, refined through the use of formative evaluation, is sufficiently superior to existing alternatives to justify the allocation of resources to its continuation and/or its adoption in other settings.

Formative evaluation is most useful during the development of a new program or as a means of re-examining a program that may need modification. Formative evaluations usually have three major components: (*a*) assessment of participant and staff satisfaction with features of the program, such as relevance and clarity of information presented, structure of the program, qualifications and skill of staff, and interpersonal dynamics among participants and staff; (*b*) assessment of the short-term cognitive (knowledge and awareness), affective (attitudes, motivation, and beliefs), or behavioral effects of the program; and (*c*) assessment of the sustainability of the program, including an appraisal of current and future levels of participation in the program and an analysis of resource requirements.

Summative evaluation provides information about a health program's effectiveness over a defined period of time, with a defined population, in one or more settings. Decision-makers then use this information to help them decide whether to terminate a program, continue it, or expand it to new settings. Such evaluations should be conducted only when program managers are satisfied that the program is functioning as intended and that it is being properly delivered to participants.

Evaluation Focus

Evaluations may focus on assessing program *process, outcome, or impact*.[5] While the usage of these terms varies somewhat in the field, the following provides generally accepted descriptions of each type of evaluation.

Process evaluation documents what is going on in the program and examines the strengths and weaknesses of program components and activities. A process evaluation may include descriptions of the characteristics of those who use the program, patterns of use or attendance, characteristics of the program setting, satisfaction of participants and staff with the program, and the extent to which program components and activities are implemented as planned. Process evaluation is most useful as part of a formative evaluation. However, process evaluations are also useful in summative evaluations by helping the evaluator understand why certain effects were or were not observed.

Outcome evaluation assesses the effectiveness of a program in producing favorable cognitive, affective, and behavioral changes in the target population. While it is most commonly conducted as part of a summative evaluation, short-term assessments of outcomes are also used in formative evaluations.

Impact evaluation assesses the effect of the program on more distal goals such as changes in health status, perceived quality of care, and quality of life. Because change in these types of outcomes typically take a long time to achieve and to measure, the use of impact evaluation is normally restricted to summative evaluations.

Although clarifying whether the evaluation is for formative or summative purposes and whether it will focus on program processes, outcomes, or impacts are important steps in planning an evaluation, there is still one other another fundamental decision to be made: which model of evaluation practice is most appropriate for the program being evaluated?

Models of Evaluation

The modern era of program evaluation in the United States began in the early 1960s, when policymakers sought data on the effects of the huge federal investments that were made in health, education, and social programs. Since that time, numerous approaches to evaluation have been developed. Four prominent models of evaluation are described below. Each of these models emphasizes a valuable aspect of evaluation. The specific questions being addressed by an evaluation and the opportunities and constraints present in the program setting will determine which model, or combination of models, is appropriate.[6]

Social Science Research Model

In an attempt to develop a rigorous evaluation methodology, early evaluators borrowed heavily from the designs and methods used by social scientists to establish the causal effect of an independent variable on a dependent variable. Program evaluation was viewed as a specialized form of social science research. From this perspective, the success of a program is determined by forming two randomized groups, providing the service (treatment) to one group and using the second group as a control. In some cases more elaborate experimental and quasi-experimental designs are used to control for possible threats to internal or external validity.[7,8] After implementation of the program, data on the appropriate dependent variables are collected from the members of each group. Statistical tests developed for basic research are applied to these data. If the difference between treatment and control group mean scores on a selected outcome measure is in the predicted direction and statistically significant, the program is considered a success. If the means are not statistically significant, the program is determined to be a failure. While the strength of this approach for the purposes of making causal interpretations is widely accepted, over time many stakeholders criticized this approach on a variety of grounds. For example, the social science approach was: often judged to be so time-consuming that deadlines for making budgetary and political decisions about a program being evaluated could not be met, impractical to implement because randomization was not possible in many nonclinical settings, too focused on a small number of quantifiable outcomes, too reliant on statistical tests to determine program effectiveness, subject to incorrect interpretation, unable to provide information useful to managers for quality improvement purposes, and too costly.[9]

Goal-Based Evaluation

In an effort to make evaluations more sensitive to the full range of expected program outcomes, evaluators often work with program staff to clearly state the goals and objectives for the program and then measure the extent to which these are achieved. This approach provides program planners with the opportunity to establish the criteria and standards to be used to determine program success. Further, qualitative goals and objectives can be stated, explicitly incorporating qualitative methods to evaluation research. This approach also has its drawbacks. It focuses so much attention on the stated program objectives that evaluators sometimes fail to come to understand why programs may or may not have achieved those objectives. Further, goal-based evaluations often fail to consider unanticipated beneficial or harmful effects of program activities.

Goal-Free Evaluation

To avoid the pitfalls of goal-based evaluation, an evaluator might not build an evaluation's design and measurement strategies around the stated goals of the program. A goal-free evaluation studies the program activities, staff, clients, program settings, and records to determine all the positive and negative effects of the program, without regard to the program's stated objectives. This information is then communicated to program staff, clients, funding agencies, and other stakeholders, who decide whether the findings are compatible with the goals of the program and determine what adjustments should be made to improve the program.

Naturalistic Evaluation

Evaluations that attempt to understand the implementation and effectiveness of a program by observing it in its "natural" state are referred to as naturalistic evaluations. Such evaluations do not impose research designs or intrusive data collection strategies on interventions, but rather attempt to collect information on program performance in as unobtrusive a way as possible. Such evaluations are often heavily qualitative, using interviews, focus group discussions, observations, and record reviews to collect information. Naturalistic evaluations typically include extensive descriptions of the program and its participants. Some naturalistic evaluators build their method on the assumption that reality is socially defined.[10] From this perspective, evaluation is a process of constructing a shared understanding of a program's effectiveness. Moreover, this perspective emphasizes the empowerment and enfranchisement of relatively weak stakeholders, so that they may participate more equally in the evaluation. Multiple iterations of collecting data, providing stakeholders feedback, and assessing the understandings of stakeholders with regard to program accomplishments are performed until a mutually satisfactory understanding representing the program's performance at that moment in time is achieved.

There is no one right way to do an evaluation. Successful evaluators tailor each evaluation to the questions that are important to program stakeholders and the opportunities and constraints present in the program setting. The specification of the evaluation's purpose, focus, and data collection and analysis model must evolve from an evaluation planning process that will provide the evaluator with information essential to the design of the evaluation. There are six general steps in this process: (*a*) identification of stakeholders; (*b*) determination of the most important concerns of each stakeholder group; (*c*) assessment of the evaluability of the program (Is there sufficient agreement among stakeholders on the rationale for the program, the key evaluation questions, and the potential to make changes in the program to improve it, that justifies doing the evaluation?); (*d*) examination of the literature; (*e*) determination of the methodology to be used, including the research design, sampling, selection of criteria, data collection, and type of statistical analysis; and (*f*) preparation of a written proposal.[11]

The Special Case of Evaluations of Communitywide Interventions

Communitywide health promotion and disease prevention programs are at the core of public health. These types of programs are aimed at modifying health risk behaviors and the conditions that produce and reinforce them. These activities typically include communitywide health education programs and activities designed to change laws or regulatory policy in areas that affect health. Communitywide interventions are complex, using multiple theories of change and channels of communication, and often target healthy individuals as well as those in need. The distinguishing characteristic of communitywide interventions is that they attempt to improve health-related characteristics of the entire community. These interventions are typically implemented over several years, making it likely that non-program–related factors such as historical events and migration in and out of the community will affect program outcomes. These aspects of communitywide interventions make them difficult to evaluate. In recent years special research approaches have been developed to evaluate communitywide interventions, including random assignment of multiple communities to treatment and control conditions, combining cross-sectional and cohort research designs within communities, extensive monitoring of intervention processes, measurement of environmental variables, and utilization of multiple data collection methodologies.[12–16]

Evaluation is more than just research. It is fundamental to good management, and it is an essential part of the process of developing enlightened public policy. It is a complex enterprise, requiring researchers to balance the rigor of their research strategies with the relevance of their work for managers and policymakers. The challenge for the evaluation researcher is to understand the opportunities and constraints associated with a given program and to use the concepts and methods introduced above to tailor an evaluation in such a way that a defensible assessment of program performance is produced.

▶ REFERENCES

Planning

1. Blum HL: Planning for Health: Generics for the Eighties: 2nd ed. New York: Human Sciences Press, 1981
2. Pegels CC, Rogers KA: Strategic Management of Hospitals and Health Care Facilities. Rockville, MD: Aspen Publishers, 1987
3. Reeves PN, Cole R: Introduction to Health Planning. 4th ed. Arlington, VA: Information Resources Press, 1989
4. Shonick W: Government and Health Services: Government's Role in the Development of U.S. Health Services. New York: Oxford University Press, 1995
5. Sofaer S: Community health planning in the U.S.: a postmortem. Family and Community Medicine 10:1–12, 1988
6. Havens DM, Hannan C: Renewal of the Ryan White CARE Act. J Pediatr Health Care 9(5):230–233, 1995
7. Gray BH: The Profit Motive and Patient Care: The Changing Accountability of Doctors and Hospitals. Cambridge, MA: Harvard University Press, 1991
8. Bryson J: Strategic Planning for Public and Nonprofit Organizations. San Francisco: Jossey-Bass, 1988
9. Kaluzny AD, Warner MD, Warren DG, Zelman WN: Management of Health Services. Englewood Cliffs, NJ: Prentice-Hall, 1982
10. Kotler P, Clarke R: Marketing for Health Care Organization. 2nd ed. Englewood Cliffs, NJ: Prentice Hall, 1987
11. Juran JM: Juran on Planning for Quality. New York: Free Press, 1988
12. Green LW, Ottoson JM: Community Health. 7th ed. St. Louis: CV Mosby, 1994
13. Reeves PN: Introduction to Health Planning. 3rd ed. Arlington, VA: Information Resources Press, 1984
14. Teutsch SM, Churchill R: Principles and Practice of Public Health Surveillance. New York: Oxford University Press, 1994
15. Seidel LF, Gorsky RD: Applied Quantitative Methods for Health Services Management. Baltimore, Health Professions Press, 1995
16. Gold MR, Russell LB, Seigel JE, Weinstein MC: Cost-Effectiveness in Health and Medicine. New York: Oxford University Press, 1996
17. Mali P: Improving Total Productivity: MBO Strategies for Business, Government, and Not-for-profit Organizations. New York: Wiley, 1978
18. Worthley JA, Ludwin WG: Zero-Base Budgeting in State and Local Government: Current Experiences and Cases. New York: Praeger, 1979
19. US Department of Health and Human Services: Healthy People 2000 Review. Hyattsville, MD: National Center for Health Statistics, 1995
20. Sutocky J: Healthy People 2000: California's Experience in Achieving the National Health Promotion and Disease Prevention Objectives. 1995
21. National Commission on Quality Assurance. Health Plan Employer Data and Information Set (HEDIS) 2.5, 3.0. Annapolis Junction, MD: National Commission on Quality Assurance, 1996
22. American Public Health Association, Association of State and Territorial Health Officials, National Association of County Health Officials, United States Conference of Local Health Officers, and Centers for Disease Control: Model Standards: A Guide for Community Preventive Health Services. 2nd ed. Washington, DC: American Public Health Association, 1985
23. Ugarte CA, Duarte P, Wilson KM: PATCH as a model for development of a Hispanic health needs assessment: the El Paso experience. J Health Educ 23(3):153–156, 1992
24. Osborne DE, Gaebler T: Reinventing Government: How the Entrepreneurial Spirit Is Transforming the Public Sector. Reading, MA: Addison-Wesley, 1992
25. Institute of Medicine Committee for the Study of the Future of Public Health: The Future of Public Health. Washington, DC: National Academy Press, 1988

Public Health Leadership: Current Constraints and a Vision of the Future

1. Institute of Medicine: The Future of Public Health. Washington, DC: National Academy Press, 1990
2. Scutchfield FD, Spain C, Pointer DD, Hafey JM: The Public Health Leadership Institute: leadership training for state and local health officers. J Public Health Policy 16(3):304–323, 1995
3. Pointer D, Sanchez J: Leadership: A Framework for Thinking and Acting.
4. Lammers JC, Bhrany V: Applying systems thinking to public health leadership. Journal of Public Health Management & Practice 1997, in press
5. Wallack G: Media Advocacy and Public Health: Power for Prevention. Newbury Park, CA: Age Publishers, 1995
6. Kreps G, Thornton B: Health Communication: Theory and Practice. Prospect Heights, IL: Waveland Press, 1992
7. Senge P: The Fifth Discipline. New York: Doubleday, 1990
8. Chrislip D, Larson C: Collaborative Leadership: How Citizens and Civic Leaders Can Make A Difference. San Francisco: Jossey-Bass, 1995
9. Senge P, Kleiner A, Roberts C, Ross R, Smith B: The Fifth Discipline Fieldbook: Strategies and Tools for Building a Learning Organization. New York: Currency Doubleday, 1994
10. Nanus B: Visionary Leadership. San Francisco. Jossey-Bass, 1992
11. Schwartz P: The Art of the Long View. New York: Currency Doubleday, 1991
12. Gardner J: On Leadership. New York: Free Press, 1990

Policy Development

1. Cobb R, Ross J, Ross MH: Agenda building as a comparative political process. Am Polit Sci Rev 70:126–138,
2. Kingdon JW: Agendas, Alternatives, and Public Policies. New York: Harper Collins, 1984
3. Scutchfield FD, Keck (ed): The Principles of Public Health Practice. Delmar. Albany, NY, 1997
4. Washington State Department of Health: Public Health Improvement Plan. Olympia, WA: Washington Department of Health, November 29, 1994
5. US Department of Health and Human Services: For a Healthy Nation: Returns on Investment in Public Health. Washington, DC: Public Health Service, 1994
6. Schauffler HH: Disease prevention policy under Medicare: an historical and political analysis. Am J Prev Med 9(2):71–77, 1993
7. Wilson JQ: The Politics of Regulation. New York: Basic Books, 1980, pp 357–394
8. Schauffler HH, Rodriguez T: Exercising purchasing power for preventive care. Health Affairs 15:74–85, 1996
9. Omen GS: Prevention: Benefits, Costs and Savings. Washington, DC, Partnership for Prevention, 1994
10. US Public Health Service: Healthy People 2000: National Health Promotion and Disease Prevention Objectives. Washington, DC: US Department of Health and Human Services, 1990

11. US Preventive Services Task Force: Guide to Clinical Preventive Services: An Assessment of the Effectiveness of 169 Interventions. Baltimore: Williams & Wilkins, 1989
12. National Committee on Quality Assurance: Health Plan Employer Data and Information Set (HEDIS), Version 2.0. Washington, DC: National Committee on Quality Assurance, 1993
13. McGinnis J, Lee PR: Healthy People 2000 at Mid Decade. JAMA 273:1123–1129, 1995
14. Stone DA: Policy Paradox and Political Reason. Glenview, IL: Scott, Forseman, 1984
15. World Health Organization: Ottawa Charter for Health Promotion. An International Conference on Health Promotion. Ottawa, Ontario, Canada, November 17–21, 1986
16. Schauffler HH, Faer M, Faulkner L, Shore K: Health promotion and disease prevention in health care reform. Am J Prev Med 10(Suppl): 1–35, 1994

Quality Assurance and Quality Improvement

1. Brook RH, Lohr KN: Efficacy, effectiveness, variations and quality: boundary-crossing research. Med Care 23:710–722, 1985
2. Flood AB, Shortell SM, Scott WR: Organizational performance: managing for efficiency and effectiveness. In Shortell S, Kaluzny A (eds): Health Care Management: Organizational Design and Behavior. Albany, NY: Delmar, 1994
3. Berwick DM: Health services research and quality of care: assignments for the 1990s. Med Care 27:763–771, 1989.
4. Guadagnoli E, McNeil BJ: Outcomes research: hope for the future or latest rage? Inquiry 31:14–24, 1994
5. Fineberg HV: Technology assessment: motivation, capability, and future direction. Med Care 23:663–671, 1985
6. Iezzoni L: Risk Adjustment for Measuring Health Care Outcomes. Ann Arbor, MI: Health Administration Press, 1994
7. Ware J, Sherbourne C: The MOS 36-item short form health survey (SF-36): I. Conceptual framework and item selection. Med Care 30:473–483, 1992
8. Maklan CW, Greene R, Cummings MA: Methodological challenges and innovations in patient outcomes research. Med Care 23:JS13–JS21, 1994
9. Wyszewianski L: Quality of care: past achievements and future challenges. Inquiry 25:13–22, 1988
10. Ross CK, Steward CA, Sinacore JM: A comparative study of seven measures of patient satisfaction. Med Care 33:392–406, 1995
11. O'Connor S, Shewchuk R, Bowers M: A model of service quality perceptions and health care consumer behavior. Journal of Hospital Marketing 6:69–92, 1991
12. Babakus E, Mangold WG: Adapting the SERVQual scale to hospital services: an empirical investigation. Health Serv Res 26:767– 786, 1992
13. Epstein A: Performance reports on quality—prototypes, problems, and prospects. N Engl J Med 333:59–61, 1995
14. Green J, Wintfeld N: Report cards on cardiac surgeons. N Engl J Med 332:1229–1232, 1995
15. Health plan employer data and information set and user's manual, Version 2.0. Washington, DC: NCQA, 1993
16. Chassin MR: Standards of care in medicine. Inquiry 25:437–453, 1988
17. Luke RD, Krueger JC, Modrow RE: Organization and Change in Health Care Quality Assurance. Rockville, MD: Aspen, 1983
18. Fink A: Consensus methods: characteristics and guidelines for use. Am J Public Health 74:979–983, 1984
19. Gertman PM, Restuccia JD: The appropriateness evaluation protocol: a technique for assessing unnecessary days of hospital care. Med Care 19:855–871, 1981
20. Deming WE: Out of the Crisis. Cambridge, MA: M.I.T. Center for Advanced Engineering Study, 1986
21. Juran JM: Juran on Planning for Quality. New York: The Free Press, 1988
22. Crosby PB: Quality is Free: The Art of Making Quality Certain. New York: Mentor, 1979
23. Jaeger BJ, Kaluzny AD, McLaughlin CP: TQM/CQI: from industry to health care. In McLaughlin CP, Kaluzny AD (eds): Continuous Quality Improvement in Health Care: Theory, Implementations, and Applications. Gaithersburg, MD: Aspen, 1994
24. Berwick DM, Godfrey AB, Roessner J: Curing Health Care: New Strategies for Quality Improvement. San Francisco, CA: Jossey-Bass, 1991
25. Batalden PB, Nolan TW: Knowledge for the leadership of continual improvement in healthcare. In Taylor J (ed): Manual of Health Services Management. Gaithersburg, MD: Aspen, 1993
26. Plsek PE: Techniques for managing quality. Hospital and Health Services Administration 40:50–79, 1995
27. Shortell SM, O'Brien JL, Carman JM, et al.: Assessing the impact of continuous quality improvement/total quality management: concepts versus implementation. Health Serv Res 30:377–401, 1995
28. Brodeur D: Work ethics and CQI. Hospital and Health Services Administration 40:111–123, 1995

Evaluation

1. Institute of Medicine Committee for the Study of the Future of Public Health: The Future of Public Health. Washington, DC: National Academy Press, 1988
2. American Public Health Association: APHA's vision: public health a reformed health care system. The Nation's Health 23(6):9–11, 1993
3. Posavac EJ, Carey RG: Program Evaluation. 4th ed. Englewood Cliffs, NJ: Prentice Hall, 1992, p 1
4. Scriven M: The Logic of Evaluation. Inverness, CA: Edgepress, 1980
5. Rossi PH, Freeman HE: Evaluation: A Systematic Approach, 5th ed. Newbury Park, CA: Sage Publications, 1993
6. Shadish WR, Cook TD, Leviton LC: Foundations of Program Evaluation. Newbury Park, CA: Sage Publications, 1991
7. Campbell DT, Stanley JC: Experimental and Quasi-experimental Designs for Research. Chicago: Rand-McNally, 1963
8. Cook TD, Campbell DT: Quasi-experimentation. Chicago: Rand-McNally, 1979
9. Posavac EJ, Carey RG: Program Evaluation. 4th ed. Englewood Cliffs, NJ: Prentice Hall, 1992, p 25
10. Guba EG, Lincoln YS: Fourth Generation Evaluation. Newbury Park, CA: Sage Publications, 1989
11. Posavac EJ, Carey RG: Program Evaluation. 4th ed. Englewood Cliffs, NJ: Prentice Hall, 1992, pp 28–36
12. Jackson C, Altman DG, Howard-Pitney B, Farquhar JW: Evaluating community-level health promotion and disease prevention interventions. New Directions for Program Evaluation 43:19–33, 1989
13. Mattson MA, Cummings KM, Lynn WR, Giffen C, Corle D, Pechacek T: Evaluation plan for the Community Intervention Trial for Smoking Cessation (COMMIT). Int Q Community Health Educ 11(3):271–290, 1990–91
14. Wickizer TM, Von Korff M, Cheadle A., Maeser J, Wagner EH, Pearson D, Beery W, Psaty BM: Activating communities for health promotion: a process evaluation method. Am J Public Health 83(4): 561–567, 1993
15. The COMMIT Research Group: Community Intervention Trial for Smoking Cessation (COMMIT): I. Cohort results from a four-year community intervention. Am J Public Health 85(2):183–192, 1995
16. The COMMIT Research Group: Community Intervention Trial for Smoking Cessation (COMMIT): II. Changes in adult cigarette smoking prevalence. Am J Public Health 85(2):193–200, 1995

71

Categorical Public Health Sciences

Public Health Issues Associated with Disasters

Scott R. Lillibridge • Trueman W. Sharp

Disasters are catastrophic occurrences that invariably have profound implications for public health. The term "disaster" can be defined as a destructive event that results in the need for a wide range of emergency resources to assist and ensure the survival of the stricken population.[1] Critical public health actions following disasters include providing basic life-sustaining commodities, such as food, water, and shelter, and establishing essential curative and prevention-oriented medical services.[2] Besides emergency relief, disaster preparedness, prevention, and mitigation are increasingly important public health activities. Public health priorities for dealing with disasters should be determined by the predominant causes of morbidity and mortality in a particular disaster and the best methods of prevention for the population.[3]

Disasters encompass a wide variety of events with multiple causes and consequences. *Natural disasters* are precipitated by the forces of nature such as floods, earthquakes, fires, or hurricanes.[4–7] Such disasters may be slow developing, as in the case of the famine of 1977 in Ethiopia, which followed successive years of drought.[8] Most natural disasters occur suddenly, such as the earthquake in Kobe, Japan, in 1995, which caused 5,000 immediate deaths and created the need for an urgent and massive relief effort.[9]

Technological disasters refer to catastrophes associated with the industrial process or its by-products.[10] These disasters involve explosions, fires, and chemical or radiological releases into the environment.[11] Adverse health effects from technological disasters include acute effects, such as trauma, burns, and smoke inhalation injury, or indirect ones through environmental exposures from the soil, water, or food.[12,13] An example is the 1986 radionuclide release from disabled reactor number 4 at Chernobyl in the former USSR. This disaster resulted in acute injuries, but more importantly it exposed more than 2 million people to radiation.[14–16] Radiation exposures from this incident continue to result in a variety of adverse health effects, such as increased rates of thyroid cancer.[17]

Conflict-related disasters, or complex emergencies, are the result of interrelated social, economic, and political problems and almost always involve armed confrontation.[18,19] In these increasingly common and often prolonged disasters, there is typically extensive destruction of social and public health infrastructure, large-scale population displacement, epidemic disease, and food shortages.[19–21] Recent examples of complex emergencies include the humanitarian crises in Bosnia-Herzegovina, Rwanda, and Somalia.

Understanding the Public Health Consequences of Disasters

What is identified as a "disaster" is often better understood as a trigger event that exposes and exacerbates underlying societal problems and weaknesses. For example, in virtually every famine of the last 20 years drought has been an important contributing factor, but food shortages have been primarily the result of armed conflict, inadequate economic and social systems, failed governments, and other human-made factors.[17,22] The famine in Somalia in 1992–1993 highlights the dramatic amplification of drought by internecine clan warfare.[23] Understanding the consequences of disasters, and effectively coping with them, requires looking well beyond the event itself.

Natural Disasters

In the past 20 years, natural disasters have affected at least 800 million people and caused more than 3 million deaths.[24,25] Each week there is at least one natural disaster of sufficient magnitude to require external assistance from the international community.[24,25] The incidence of natural disasters appears to be increasing, and the number of highly vulnerable persons in disaster-prone areas, particularly in the developing world, is at least 70 million peoples and growing.[26,27] The devastating tropical cyclone in Bangladesh in 1991, in which more than 100,000 persons were killed, illustrates the potential impact of a natural disaster on a population residing in a hazardous coastal region.[28]

Natural disasters may be associated with a wide variety of acute and long-term health effects.[3,17] For example, volcanic eruptions may result in injury or death due to lava flow, falling debris, asphyxiating gases, mudflows, and blast injury from violent explosions.[29–31] Ash and other particulate matter vented from an active volcano may exacerbate respiratory illness in persons within the downwind population for many months following the eruption.[32] Volcanic ash may contaminate the soil or water, resulting in long-term toxic exposures to the population. One of the most unusual gas releases associated with volcanic activity occurred in 1986 in Cameroon.[17] In this disaster, asphyxiating carbon dioxide was released from an active volcano underneath Lake Nyos. The gas enveloped nearby villages and caused approximately 1,500 deaths.

Public health issues associated with floods extend beyond concerns for mortality due to drowning.[3,17] In Bangladesh, the flooding that followed the 1991 tropical cyclone reduced the potability of water from wells and caused widespread outbreaks of diarrheal disease.[28] Flooding may result in increased numbers of breeding sites for mosquitoes and their associated diseases, such as malaria or dengue fever.[17] Immediate public health actions following floods usually include the provision of potable water, food, vector control, and the restitution of vital environmental health services.[7,33,34] However, early warning systems, improved evacuation plans, and discouragement of settling in flood-prone areas may have much greater potential to save lives than activities associated with external emergency response to flood disasters.

Earthquakes typically cause destruction of structures and traumatic injuries and deaths.[3,17,35] The 1976 Tangshan earthquake, for example, caused more than 200,000 sudden trauma-related deaths.[36] In contrast to floods, the morbidity and mortality of earthquakes is much more immediate. Deaths are primarily due to crush injuries and other trauma resulting from unstable, collapsing, or crumbling buildings.[3,17,35] Earthquakes are not usually followed by long-term public health problems such as famine or epidemic diseases, although following the Northridge earthquake (1994) a wide range of external primary care services were required by the population for up to 4 weeks.[37] Other public health issues associated with earthquakes include concerns for the health of persons in shelters, occupational health protection for rescue workers, and the provision of mental services for survivors.[38]

Sudden onset natural disasters have been the traditional model for understanding and organizing emergency relief services for disaster-affected populations in this country. For example, external medical services may be urgently needed after earthquakes to treat injured persons and to extract survivors trapped in collapsed buildings.[35,37,39] This led to the development of specialized emergency services in many countries such as Urban Search and Rescue teams, which are designed to extract and treat entombed victims.[35,40] Disaster response at the federal level has included the development of Disaster Medical Assistance Teams (DMATs), designed to provide emergency curative medical services primarily in response to natural disasters.[41,42]

While this paradigm has been valuable, effectively coping with disasters involves much more than the timely delivery of external emergency resources. Local vulnerabilities in a community such as population density, lack of disaster planning, and poverty may enhance the risk to a population to disasters.[2] For example, the 1988 earthquake in Armenia resulted in more than 30,000 deaths, while an earthquake of similar force, the 1989 Loma Prieta earthquake in California, resulted in less than 500 deaths.[39,43] The low mortality associated with the Loma Prieta earthquake was thought to be due to enforcement of local building codes, better local emergency medical services (EMS), and superior local disaster management services, and other community-based prevention and mitigation activities.[3,17,44]

Conflict-Related (Complex) Emergencies

These disasters are largely a phenomenon of the post Cold War world. In the late 1970s there were approximately five conflict-related disasters per year, but by the late 1980s there were 10 to 15 per year, and today there are an average of 25 to 30 per year.[26,36] The increase in conflict-related disasters closely relates to the number of armed conflicts in the world, which also have increased dramatically in recent years, and particularly in this decade.[27,45] Since 1980, there have been over 150 major armed conflicts,[45] and in 1995, there were an estimated 26 ongoing wars.[45]

War has always been destructive, but in recent years the nature of armed conflict has become more devastating than ever before.[46–49] In many conflicts today, for every death in a combatant there are 8 to 9 deaths among civilians.[45,46] Toole and Waldman have described the insidious cycle of armed confrontation, famine, and population displacement.[19,50] In 1980 there were approximately 5 million refugees in the world, but largely as a consequence of this cycle, today there are approximately 23 million.[26,51] In addition, today there are another 25 million internally displaced persons.[26,51]

Many of the public health problems of refugees and displaced persons have been well described.[19–21,50] Crude mortality rates among refugees and displaced populations often rise dramatically above baseline levels, principally due to nutritional shortages, environmental problems, and preventable infectious diseases. Conflict-related disasters also have similar effects on those who do not flee when the infrastructure of society is destroyed or severely damaged, which causes problems in having access to food, potable water, refuse disposal, and basic medical services.[18]

International humanitarian law in many conflicts today is unknown or disregarded, and human rights abuses are common.[52] As a result, in some disasters, violence may be a direct, and the primary, cause of morbidity and mortality.[53,54] For example, in the former Yugoslavia, while morbidity and mortality due to infectious diseases increased to some extent, deaths due to fighting or so-called ethnic cleansing operations were by far the principal cause of death.[53,54] Areas of increasing focus in complex emergencies are mental health, womens' health issues, and coping with chronic medical conditions.

Coping with these disasters is one of the great public health challenges of our time.[55] There are a multitude of technical and logistical issues involved in providing life-sustaining services to large populations.[55,56] Events may not progress in a clear linear fashion; public health needs often evolve substantially.[53] For example, priorities for refugees who have just arrived in a location—usually shelter, food, water, basic medical care—are different from what this population may need a few months after a camp has been established, such as family planning, medical care for more chronic problems, and rehabilitation. As with natural disasters, increasing attention is devoted toward prevention, early warning, and preparation activities.[55–57] Because complex emergencies are the result of many years of deeply rooted social problems, effectively dealing with them requires that relief efforts be closely integrated with political, social, economic, military, cultural, and other activities.[18,55,56]

Technological Disasters

Public health problems resulting from technological accidents, or the unregulated and unsafe use of industrial technologies, are increasingly recognized as an important and increasingly common type of disaster.[3,9–14] The extensive environmental pollution in former Soviet block nations, the nuclear reactor accident at Chernobyl, and the toxic gas leak at Bhopal, India, are examples of the disastrous consequences that can ensue from these disasters. The potential for harm from improper management of industrial technologies is a major concern in developed nations where at any given moment there are a myriad of complex industries in operation and tons of hazardous materials in transit through populated areas. In developing countries, these problems are exacerbated when rapid industrialization exceeds the development of counterbalancing safety controls.

Technological disasters are usually the result of poor engineering, improper safety practices, or simple human error. However, natural disasters can be an important factor in precipitating a technological disaster. For example, the gasoline fires that killed over 500 persons in Durunka, Egypt, in 1994 were the result of flash flooding that ruptured a fuel storage tank and carried burning petroleum into the nearby town.[58] Such synergistic disasters have been termed NA-TECHs (natural-technological).[3] In many places in the world, chemical plants, nuclear reactors, or other potentially dangerous industry are seated in geological regions that are highly vulnerable to natural disasters.

Dealing with the consequences of a technological disaster or a NA-TECH presents many challenges. Recognizing the hazardous material involved, evacuating citizens after an accident, providing appropriate medical care for victims, and protecting emergency responders against hazardous exposures are a few of the many challenges to emergency responders.[59,60] In addition, because industrial disasters may leave toxic residues in the environment that pose ongoing threats to the health of populations, the initiation of chemical exposure and disease registries to track adverse health effects of disaster victims over time may be a fundamental component of the emergency response. Clinical investigations after technical disasters may require assistance from laboratory scientists, toxicologists, and environmental epidemiologists.[50,60] Public health prevention efforts include sound plant design and operation, safe disposal of waste products, thorough safety occupational programs, linkage to local emergency management operations, and proper site selection for industrial facilities.

Public Health Tools for Disaster Response

Prior to mobilizing an emergency response on behalf of a disaster-stricken population, the initial step is to obtain information regarding the extent of their immediate needs and the status of their supporting public health infrastructure. This task is accomplished through an organized needs assessment.[61,62] The purpose of initial assessments is to rapidly obtain objective, reliable, population-based information that describes a population's specific needs for emergency relief services. These assessments should identify the extent of the needed response and technical areas where specialized assistance is needed and should suggest other areas where more focused health surveys or surveillance should be conducted (e.g., the nutritional status of the population, status of water and sanitation).

It is often impractical to evaluate the needs of all affected persons at the disaster site due to the size of the population and resource limitations. Relief personnel must sample representative cross-sections from the affected population through a statistically valid sampling process using standardized assessment protocols.[61–63] Such an activity requires knowledge of the geographic distribution and size of the population, which may be obtained through census information, aerial photos, rapid surveys, and other sources. During sudden-impact disasters such as hurricanes the initial assessments of the affected population should be completed as soon as possible, ideally within 24 to 48 hours.[61,63] Slow-onset disasters such as endemic warfare and famines that persist for years may require repeated emergency health assessments.[62]

Public health surveillance is the logical continuum of the initial epidemiologic task of emergency health assessment. Surveillance systems need to be established after disasters in sentinel sites such as clinics to monitor the health of the population and gauge the effectiveness of ongoing relief programs, particularly during the implementation of emergency programs that are likely to continue beyond the immediate aftermath of the disaster.[21,64–66] New technologies such as e-mail, computers, and epidemiologic software permitted the rapid implementation of a statewide system surveillance in Iowa following the Great Flood of 1993.[67] Among refugees, in developing countries, critical public health events for surveillance include deaths, appearance of malnourished children, and the occurrence of vaccine preventable infectious diseases.[21,62] When establishing surveillance after a disaster, it is likely to be more effective to re-establish a pre-existing system than to build a new system with external resources.[68,69]

Targeted investigations and surveys complement initial assessments and surveillance. For example, in some situations, the rapid assessment of the nutritional status of a population is a critical aspect of developing appropriate relief programs.[70] Investigation of outbreaks, surveys of vaccine coverage, and surveys for the prevalence of certain diseases are other common areas of more focused investigation. As public health information is collected through assessment, surveillance, and special surveys, relief interventions should be modified accordingly. In the absence of current data to evaluate the health of the target population, relief priorities and resources may easily become skewed.[3,71–74]

Public Health Interventions in Disasters

Environmental Health Control

Populations affected by disasters often require emergency environmental health services. Potable water is often the most important immediate relief commodity necessary for ensuring the survival of disaster-affected populations. Some water is necessary for drinking and cooking, but decreased water supplies also lead to inadequate personal hygiene. As a baseline, persons should have access to at least 15 to 20 liters of potable water per day.[75,76] Heat stress and physical activity can substantially increase the human daily requirements for potable water to levels that are many times normal. Health authorities at disaster sites must plan for additional allotments of water to support clinical facilities and feeding centers, and other public health activities.

The proper management of human waste is also an important environmental health priority, particularly during disaster conditions.[77,78] The principal public health thrust of sanitation measures in emergency conditions is to reduce fecal contamination of food and water supplies.[56,75–78] Communicable diseases that can be transmitted through contact with human feces include typhoid fever, cholera, bacillary and amoebic dysentery, hepatitis, polio, schistosomiasis, various helminth infestations, and viral gastroenteritis. Temporary latrines can be established in a disaster site in a variety of ways, including pits and trenches, or more permanent methods.[56,75–78]

Apart from access to water and food, shelter is often the most immediate need of disaster-stricken populations, particularly in cold weather. High mortality rates, particularly among the young and elderly, can occur when displaced populations are suddenly subjected to severe cold stress.[79] In some situations, control of insect vectors can be an important measure to prevent or control infectious disease.[80] Other types of environmental measures may be necessary after disasters when, for example, in a technological disaster, industrial chemical compounds are swept into the water sources used for drinking or soil used for agriculture.[3,9–13,34]

Communicable Disease Control

When infectious diseases occur after a disaster, they were almost invariably endemic before the disaster occurred. However, disaster conditions often serve to facilitate disease transmission and increase individual susceptibility to infection. Infectious diseases sometimes occur in a population that moves to a new location where an unfamiliar disease is endemic. For example, devastating malaria epidemics have occurred in nonimmune populations who were displaced to a malaria endemic area.[81,82]

The principal infectious disease problems in conflict-related disasters have been measles, diarrheal diseases, acute respiratory infection, and malaria.[20,21,81,82] For example, during the Somali famine (1991–1992), measles and diarrheal diseases accounted for the vast majority of the deaths among persons in temporary camps.[23] Disease outbreaks in complex emergencies are usually the result of many factors, including breakdowns in environmental safeguards, crowding of persons in camps, lack of appropriate immunization programs, malnutrition, inadequate case-finding, and limited availability of appropriate curative medical services.

Despite the more limited potential for disease outbreaks following natural disasters, notable exceptions have occurred. For example, following Hurricane Flora in 1963 a malaria epidemic occurred within the Haitian population.[83] During the recent Northridge earthquake of 1995, the emergence of coccidioidomycosis infections among emergency responders as a result of environmental contamination was a public health concern.[84] Due to such threats and the propensity for epidemics to occur when the normal public health infrastructure has been damaged, following a natural disaster it may be necessary to expand surveillance for certain diseases and rapidly institute appropriate disease control efforts.

Coping with infectious diseases after disasters involves a number of fundamental public health strategies applied to disaster settings. For example, in some settings, emergency measles vaccination programs along with the administration of vitamin A are critical and highly effective measures to prevent cases of measles and to reduce morbidity and mortality caused by this infection.[85] In regard to diarrheal diseases, for which there are not effective immunizations, a combination of basic environmental measures to provide clean water and sanitation, plus rapid case-finding and aggressive treatment (rehydration and appropriate antibiotics) can substantially reduce the consequences of diarrhea outbreaks.[86]

Nutritional Rehabilitation

After some disasters, particularly conflict-related disasters, there may be substantially decreased availability of food, which can result in specific nutrient deficiencies, overall undernutrition, or outright starvation.[56,87–89] Poor nutritional status increases susceptibility to communicable diseases such as measles and diarrhea. Indeed, the immediate cause of death in most malnourished persons is not usually starvation per se but infectious diseases.[90]

Emergency nutritional rehabilitation efforts for a starving population may involve a number of different types of programs to distribute food.[56,75,89] In a food crisis, decisions must be made regarding whether emergency feeding programs should focus on widespread distribution of general food rations, targeting specific food supplements to select high-risk groups (such as pregnant or lactating women), or on preparing food for consumption on-site in feeding centers. The type of food distributed is an important concern as well. Food must be culturally acceptable and must be nutritionally balanced. Donor-provided food has resulted in iatrogenic micronutrient deficiencies in some long-term relief operations.[87] Sound program decisions should be based on information from rapid nutritional surveys as well as analyses of economic indicators that provide more detail on the nutritional status of the population and the context of the specific food shortage.

During emergency famine relief, it is not the mere delivery of food to the disaster site that saves lives. The most rapid reduction in morbidity and mortality will occur when improvements in environmental health and communicable disease control accompany the restoration of proper nutritional resources.[56,75,88] Because the lack of sufficient food in disasters is usually the result of many factors such as economic collapse, disruption of production, inadequate distribution, and other socioeconomic conditions, rather than a true lack of food, the long-term solution is in restoring an indigenous food economy, not in maintaining emergency feeding programs.

Public Health Challenges in Disaster Relief Today

Coping with Violence

Relief organizations that wish to be neutral and impartial can have tremendous difficulty operating in settings of armed confrontation. Unfortunately, the provision of humanitarian relief can easily be perceived as a partisan act, or it can be manipulated for the benefit of different warring factions.[71,91] In situations of conflict, traditional medical and public health interventions may not be very effective in preventing injury and death. Indeed, some have argued that in some situations emergency relief has served to exacerbate and prolong the conflict. Development initiatives, weapons control, conflict resolution, and other such measures may be more effective ways of preventing mortality in these situations.[55,57] The role of relief organizations in preventing and coping with human rights abuses, including torture and genocide, is still complex and uncertain. Also, increasingly today, the provision of emergency relief is very dangerous.[92] Many relief workers have been killed in recent years; how to adequately protect them is a major dilemma.

Improved Emergency Public Health Response

Many problems still remain in the effective implementation of emergency relief programs. In the Kurdish refugee crisis, despite a massive international relief effort, many deaths occurred due to preventable diarrheal disease.[70] This was in large part due to a failure to implement basic environmental health interventions and diarrhea control programs early enough in this crisis. During the 1994 Goma, Zaire, refugee emergency as many as 50,000 persons died from cholera within the temporary camp system in only a matter of weeks.[93] The Goma (Zaire) Epidemiology Group reported after the Rwanda refugee crisis that there is an urgent need for more intensive and focused training of relief workers to develop relevant expertise in the prevention and management of diarrheal diseases, as well as other essential elements of relief programs, such as measles immunization, public health surveillance, community outreach, and nutritional rehabilitation.[93] A review of public health assessments and surveys conducted in Somalia demonstrated a lack of consistency in methodology, which led to difficulties in interpreting and acting upon critical public health data.[94] Few training programs in schools of public health have curricula that cover the broad range of knowledge needed to cope with the public health issues associated with disaster-affected populations.[1,95,96]

Vulnerable Populations

Disasters do not affect all persons evenly; identifying and focusing on populations with special needs after disasters is a critical issue. For example, the unique concerns of women in disasters have become a greater focus in disaster relief in the last few years.[97–99] Recent data suggests that in some disasters women have less access to medical care and other relief services.[93] Additionally, while data is limited, pregnancy, sexually transmitted diseases, sexual abuse, and human immunodeficiency virus (HIV) infection are believed to be common issues among women in some disaster-affected populations, especially refugees. Few relief programs have sufficiently addressed these issues. The special problems of children in disasters are increasingly recognized.[100,101] Children are much more vulnerable to many of the adverse health effects of disasters, such as malnutrition and infectious diseases. Additionally, the plight of unaccompanied children in Rwanda illustrated a problem common to many complex emergencies today.[100,102] In disaster situations there are many other potentially vulnerable groups, such as members of a particular ethnic group, the elderly, and immigrants.

Land Mines

One of the most extensive public health catastrophes today is the extensive worldwide dissemination of land mines. It is estimated that 65 to 110 million land mines are scattered throughout more than 60 countries.[103,104] Land mines persist for decades. They impede the resettlement of displaced populations and serve to remove land from cultivation. Worldwide, land mines are responsible for more than 15,000 fatalities each year. However, many land mines are designed to maim. The survivors require emergency surgical services and prolonged rehabilitation largely related to lower limb amputation. This has had devastating impact on the individuals, the economy, and the health care system. Countries affected by severe land mine problems in the wake of endemic warfare include Afghanistan, Mozambique, former Yugoslavia, Angola, and Rwanda.

Terrorism

Terrorism is regarded by many as an increasing and evolving threat. Terrorists of today have unparalleled access to highly destructive technologies.[105–108] In addition to conventional explosives, nuclear devices, chemical weapons, and biological weapons are believed to have potential as terrorist weapons. The release of the nerve gas sarin in the Tokyo subway system illustrates the emerging threat from such weapons of mass destruction and the complex public health issues that arise from an intentional technological disaster.[108] Such issues include the need for rapid characterization of the offending agent, mass decontamination, ready access to antidotes, specialized medical training, and proper protective equipment for emergency responders.

Mental Health

In addition to traditional public health concerns, disasters may present medical responders with patients who are suffering from complaints that are predominantly psychological in nature. Consequently, mental health issues may predominate the health concerns during the acute phase of disaster response.[109] Such concerns may include the need for specialized psychological triage and treatment programs for victims. Emergency response personnel are also subject to short- and long-term effects as a result of stress imposed by the disaster, particularly among persons required to be involved in postdisaster management of decedents.[110] The psychological impact of disasters on children has only just begun to be documented but is clearly profound. The appalling use of children as soldiers in many countries of the world may have long-term mental health consequences of unprecedented proportions.[100,101]

Conclusions

The public health consequences of disasters are wide ranging, and their effects on populations are long lasting. Knowledge and experience from many health disciplines is needed for effective emergency response. Such skills include epidemiology, community health and primary care, environmental science, communicable disease control, and international health. Research is needed to develop standardized and valid assessment tools, reliable surveillance programs, low-technology environmental health interventions, and more effective intervention strategies. Unfortunately, the reality today is that many relief workers in the health sector, though well-intentioned, are often recruited and deployed on short notice with little public health preparation or training. Schools of public health must continue to expand their training in the emergency skills that practitioners will need to deal with the public health needs of disaster-affected populations if we are going meet this challenge.

Maternal and Child Health

Alan W. Cross

This chapter provides an overview of maternal and child health, highlighting the basic principles that make the health of women and children different from that of other segments of the population. Most of the details of specific aspects of maternal and child health are covered in other chapters.

History

The health of women and children began to receive separate attention early in this century, in recognition of their greater vulnerability, particularly to socioeconomic and environmental forces, and the interdependence of the child's health and that of the mother. In 1909 the first White House Conference on Child Health recommended the formation of the Children's Bureau, which proceeded to investigate the causes of infant mortality (then more than 100 per 1,000 live births). The first direct support of health services for mothers and children came with the Shepard-Towner Act of 1921, which resulted in complete birth registration and the establishment of maternal and child health divisions in state and local health departments.[1] Title V of the Social Security Act of 1935 extended services to handicapped children and further established the principle of public responsibility for the health of mothers and children.

In the 1960s and early 1970s a host of additional programs were initiated by Congress. These included Medicaid, Early Periodic Screening, Diagnosis and Treatment (EPSDT), Neighborhood Health Centers, Maternity and Infant Care, Family Planning, Children and Youth Projects, Head Start, Title I educational assistance, the Right to Education of the Handicapped (PL 94-142), and nutrition programs (WIC and School Lunch). While these laws expanded services at the state and local levels, the resultant programs were administered by a variety of different branches of government, diffusing responsibility and often leading to poor coordination and the undermining of maternal and child health (MCH) divisions.

MCH services were seriously weakened by the budget cuts of the Reagan years. Rather than cutting specific services, the programs were lumped into block grants that gave state governments greater freedom to apportion the reduced funds as they saw fit. This has begun the trend of providing greater local autonomy in the establishment and administration of health programs for women and children. This trend may hold promise for the creation of innovative programs that more precisely address the community's needs, making greater use of local resources.

Managed care has emerged from the multiple efforts to control health care costs, and this new structure for the delivery of medical care has had a significant impact on maternal and child health services. Medicaid recipients are rapidly being shifted into managed care plans that restrict access to all but primary care services, causing health departments to lose their base of clients for immunization, family planning, and other health care service programs. Meanwhile the managed care plans that have enrolled these high-risk populations are not held accountable in the same manner as was the health department for service delivery. Cost control efforts led to postpartum hospital stays being reduced to 1 day until Congress intervened with a rule that allowed at least a 48-hour stay at the discretion of the mother and her physician.

Progress in MCH has been driven by the dual forces of research and advocacy. Multidisciplinary studies over the last 20 years have shed important light on the health problems of women and children and provided numerous examples of effective means to ameliorate those problems.[2] Articulate and committed individuals and organizations have played a critical role in fostering public commitment to improve the lives of mothers and children. However, that support has been significantly reduced through the 1980s. As our knowledge of what to do has continued to grow, the political will to use that knowledge has shrunk.

Health Indicators

Various health indicators are used to assess the health status of mothers and children. The continuous monitoring of these indicators is an essential part of evaluating our progress in improving the health status of women and children.

Maternal mortality rates have reached such a low level that they are of little value now. Maternal health is better reflected in fertility rates and birth rates as well as in pregnancy-related morbidity rates. Pregnancy outcomes have become a more important measure of maternal health and quality of maternity services provided. Miscarriage, therapeutic abortion, stillbirth, and especially low–birth weight rates can be used to assess the success of the pregnancy. Prenatal care, place of delivery, attendant at delivery, type of delivery, complications, length of stay, and cost all measure the availability and quality of maternal health services.

The infant mortality rate remains an important though crude measure of MCH. Linking infant birth and death records has provided a far more precise way of assessing factors associated with pregnancy outcome, particularly when the causes of death are grouped by pregnancy-related conditions such as prematurity, rather than the organ system taxonomy of the ICD-9 codes.[3] The new birth certificate form that was adopted in 1989 includes a wider array of information on both the mother and the child, offering opportunities for future exploration of the relationships between more extensive socio-demographic and medical information and various pregnancy outcomes. Childhood morbidity is less easily measured. Birth defects registries, neonatal intensive care use, discharge diagnoses, and national health surveys provide some estimates of morbidity. Immunization rates, school-based health data, and the data from such programs as EPSDT are also helpful indicators of child health, although they are not systematically collected at either the state or national level.

Larger social and demographic changes are also important indicators of the status of mothers and children. Over the last 20 years there have been dramatic increases in the percentage of mothers in the workforce, the percentage of marriages that end in divorce, the numbers of homeless mothers and children, and the percentage of children living in poverty. These social problems contribute directly or indirectly to most of the health problems of women and children.

Service Delivery

The goals of MCH services are (*a*) to encourage desired pregnancy, achieving the best possible outcome for the baby and the mother; (*b*) to promote healthy relationships within the family to nurture the growing child; (*c*) to optimize the normal developmental processes to allow the child to achieve his or her fullest potential; (*d*) to prevent child health problems and reduce the risks of adult health problems; and (*e*) to provide early intervention in the health problems of women and children so as to minimize morbidity and mortality in a cost-effective manner. To achieve these goals, attention must be paid to several basic principles of MCH. These principles are a product of the nature of women and children and the problems from which they suffer and therefore are a bit different from the general principles that underlie all health service delivery.

Two Clients

Maternal services are unique in that they simultaneously provide care for two, equally important, clients, the mother and the fetus. Balancing the needs of both to achieve the best possible outcome requires a thorough understanding of the complex interdependence of the maternal/fetal unit and the implications of events and treatments for both mother and baby.

Family-Centered Services

Because of the extreme importance of the family in the nurturing of the pregnant woman and the young child, it is essential that MCH services be delivered with attention to the family circumstances of the clients. The family influences growth, development, health-related behaviors, and lifestyle habits. Family resources influence the use and availability of health services and the ability to provide the care needed, particularly in chronic disease. The child is not merely the passive recipient of the influences of the family, but, rather, plays an increasingly interactive role in the family, shaping in part the environment in which he or she lives.

Developmental Perspective

The fetus and child are being continuously shaped by the normal developmental processes that result in a reasonably predictable series of changes from conception through adolescence. Progress over this course is a sensitive measure of both health and disease. These developmental forces can be potent allies in the management of chronic health problems. However, continued disruption of normal development can have progressively magnifying adverse effects on the fetus or child. Because of the importance of development, the dimension of time and the continuity of care over time become critical elements in the provision of MCH services. Prompt identification of problems and early intervention, therefore, hold the greatest promise for achieving the best outcome.

Health Promotion and Disease Prevention

There is great potential in childhood for health promotion and disease prevention to benefit both the current child and the future adult. However, careful attention must be paid to the immediate implications of interventions that are aimed at preventing problems in the distant future, making sure that the desired long-term benefits are not counterbalanced by short-term hazards.

Timely, Cost-Effective Treatment

The early identification and proper treatment of common health problems is a critical dimension of reducing morbidity and mortality in women and children. Simple early treatments can often prevent very expensive and serious problems, such as adolescent pregnancy, a premature birth, or a handicapping condition.

Integration of Principles

Perhaps the greatest challenge to delivery of MCH services is trying to integrate all the principles articulated above into the care of each client. It is difficult for the provider to attend simultaneously to the treatment and prevention needs while considering the family and development issues in the care of both the mother and the child. However, the greatest success is achieved when all these concepts are addressed together.[4]

Trends and Innovations in Services

The United States lags way behind all other developed countries in the provision of most services to mothers and children. Western Europe and Japan offer extensive maternity benefits, prenatal care, day care, and well-child care to all women and children.[5] In infant mortality rates, the United States ranks 20th in the world, a fact that many attribute at least in part to the inadequate provision of maternal and infant services. The last decade has seen little progress in this arena, but some interesting innovations in the delivery of MCH services have recently emerged and warrant brief description. Many of these have not yet come into general practice but hold promise for the future, once they have been more carefully evaluated. Social trends of the last decade have also had an effect on MCH services and must be considered in the process of recommending improvements for the future.

Family Planning and Abortion

Optimum health for both mother and child has long been known to be related to maternal age, spacing of children, and the balance between family resources and family size. The ready availability of birth control and the option for abortion have provided means of achieving family planning. Norplant was hoped to be an easy means of contraception that required no action for 5 years after its insertion, but it has turned out to be unpopular due to its side effects. RU-487 will soon be available as an early pregnancy abortion pill. Having such a nonsurgical abortion option will make it very difficult to ever restrict abortion fully.

Preconceptional Health Promotion

Many of the critical phases of fetal development have already occurred before a woman is even aware that she is pregnant. Optimum fetal health, therefore, requires attention to maternal health and health-related behaviors even before conception. Efforts to counsel women before conception to avoid alcohol, drugs, tobacco, and other fetal hazards are currently being tested to determine the impact on pregnancy outcome.[6] The efficacy of periconceptional dietary folic acid in the prevention of neural tube defects will likely soon result in routine folic acid fortification of bread.

Prenatal Care

Improving access to and quality of prenatal services continues to be a challenge with no obvious solution. Expansion of Medicaid to include women up to 185 percent of the federal poverty level in comprehensive services has made prenatal care more accessible. Some states have developed innovative programs to improve quality and access for the poor, and many local community-based projects have also been created with these goals in mind.

Human Immunodeficiency Virus

The vertical transmission of human immunodeficiency virus (HIV) from infected women to their babies will infect approximately one-quarter of these babies. However, treatment with azidothymidine (AZT) during pregnancy can reduce this transmission to as low as 8 percent. This creates the dilemma of whether pregnant women should be required to be HIV tested and, if positive, treated for the sake of their baby or whether they should merely be given the information and the option.

Immunization

The recently approved acellular pertussis vaccine offers hope that some of the complications of the whole cell vaccine might be avoided.[7] The use of conjugated vaccine against *Haemophilus influenzae* in infants as young as 2 months of age has significantly reduced the incidence of meningitis in infants. The hepatitis B vaccine is now widely used in the prevention of both hepatitis and the consequent hepatic cancer—both major problems, particularly in developing countries. The eradication of polio from the Western Hemisphere has led to a recent switch from oral polio vaccine to a combination of oral and inactivated vaccines to reduce the incidence of paralytic reactions to the oral vaccine.[8]

Day Care

As maternal employment continues to rise, we are falling further behind in providing adequate, affordable day care for young children. Most states provide little regulation of day care facilities, particularly home-based centers with few children. This aggravates concerns about spread of infection, injury, and child abuse in day care facilities, as well as potentially being a poor substitute for parents.

Sexual Abuse

Over the last decade we have been forced to recognize that child sexual abuse occurs far more frequently than we would like to believe. As this problem has come out of the closet, innovative programs have been developed to teach children how to avoid sexual exploitation and to identify and treat more effectively those who are victims. Many school systems have adopted curricula in prevention of sex abuse for children as young as those in kindergarten, and the open discussion of this problem has made it easier to inquire about such incidents as a part of routine health care. Many states are also experimenting with creative ways of humanely dealing with the child witness in court without unduly infringing on the constitutional rights of the accused. However, we are probably still studying only the tip of this iceberg as we begin to explore the consequences of the more subtle forms of abuse and try to gain a better understanding of the abusers and the factors that lead to abuse in some families.

Community-Based Social Support

Pregnant women and young children thrive best when they are surrounded by friends and relatives who provide companionship and assistance. As unwed motherhood becomes more common and the extended family further disintegrates, more young families face isolation and inadequate social supports. To remedy this, several programs have utilized home visitors to befriend and work closely with pregnant women and young families, offering the assistance and social support that are so often inadequate. Some of these programs have been able to demonstrate benefits in health and well-being associated with participation in the program.[9,10]

Future Directions

The 1960s and 1970s produced a number of centrally funded programs to help mothers and children. Through the 1980s the support for these programs eroded, and control over spending priorities for the diminished funding was shifted to the state capitols through the block grants. Over the same period new initiatives for the elderly received increasing support. Despite renewed outcries about the plight of America's children, Congress was able to pass sweeping welfare reform, which is predicted to have significant negative impact on women and children.

As managed care appears to be cutting costs, there is a rising pressure for shifting MCH services from public sector provider systems into managed care plans where demand can be controlled. In those states where many of these services are provided by health departments, the work and the funding of these departments will be dramatically reshaped by this trend. Both the consumers and the managed care providers will need to make adjustments if this new system is to simultaneously save money and still meet the health needs of this population. The tightening of other welfare benefits for the poor will additionally compromise the basic well-being of poor women and their children. Over the next decade it will be increasingly important to monitor the well-being of women and children to ensure that the systems established to improve their health are indeed succeeding. A recently released report of the Institute of Medicine of the National Academy of Sciences addresses ways in which communities might improve health through performance monitoring.[11]

Desmotology: The Practice of Prison Health

Jonathan B. Weisbuch

The population confined in American jails, prisons, and juvenile detention facilities doubled between 1986, when 750,000 individuals were behind bars,[1] and the end of 1996, with more than 1.6 million individuals behind bars.[2] In early 1996, over 100,000 were in federal prisons, 1 million were in state correctional systems, 507,000 were in local jails awaiting trial or serving short sentences, and nearly 100,000 juveniles (under 18 years old) were held in juvenile detention facilities.[3] More than 11 million men, women, and adolescents were processed through correctional facilities in 1995; and, on any day, over 3.3 million people were on parole.[4] When admitted to a facility, each requires a screening health examination followed by a more complete history and physical examination from a physician, nurse practitioner, or physician's assistant within 14 days of incarceration. Every inmate has a right to medical care, and they use that right. When discharged, their ongoing medical needs, many of which may require follow-up, become problems for public health.

As the prison population grows, the demands upon prison health providers multiply. On any day, between 5 and 10 percent of those behind bars seek service; over 100,000 sick call visits occur each day in American correctional facilities. Sick call, counseling, referrals to specialists, hospitalizations, drug treatment, and continuing care cost an estimated \$3.0 billion per year. Prison health care is big—big medicine, big business, and unless managed well, a big problem for correctional officials. Managing and providing health care in correctional settings demands unique clinical, managerial, and social skills, not required in other health care settings. The term, *desmoteric medicine*, or *desmotology*, (from the Greek word, *desmoterion*, "prison") has been suggested by several authors[5–7] to define this special branch of medicine practiced behind steel and concrete. Desmotologists serve the unusual health needs of a unique population in distinct settings removed from the mainstream of medical care. As more and more individuals are incarcerated for longer and longer periods of time, the demands for specialists trained in prison health will grow apace.

Desmotologists must be expert in the most complex problems facing modern medicine: acquired immunodeficiency syndrome (AIDS), multiple drug–resistant tuberculosis (MDR-TB), hepatitis, neuropsychiatric illness and suicide, trauma and violence, the physiology and psychology of severe substance abuse, epilepsy, environmental stress, and, as sentences grow longer, all the chronic problems found in an aging population. The prison provider must deal with patients who use the medical encounter for secondary gain unrelated to their signs or symptoms; he or she must recognize that medical decisions often impact both the health of the patient and the security of the institution. Desmotologists care for litigious individuals who use both the legal system and individual or group violence to exert their will or express their anger. Prison providers have been injured, taken hostage, and involved in riots in prisons where inadequate medical care has been alleged. Prison providers must be prepared to play a central role when emergencies arise that affect individuals, groups, or the entire system.

Desmotology is intellectually and physically stimulating. It involves a balancing act between conflicting priorities in the prison environments: security, social rehabilitation, and medical service. Where these priorities overlap (*shaded areas* in Figure 71-1), frustrating dilemmas, described by Thornburn[8] and Prout and Ross,[9] confront the prison provider committed to serve the prisoner-patient and be responsible to the system. To overcome these frustrations and serve the medical needs of the prisoner, the practitioner must use skills not acquired in medical school or residency—medical administration, interpersonal diplomacy, and social anthropology. He or she must practice preventive medicine and health promotion, be able to apply epidemiology, create and manage clinical information systems, and be expert in quality improvement. The desmotologist must be able to recognize and reduce environmental hazards to reduce the risk of disease. He or she must also treat mental illness, substance abuse, violence, stress, the risk of suicide, and other dysfunctional behaviors manifested by prisoners as patients. Medical leadership in a prison health system must budget, plan, organize staff, lead, practice good clinical medicine, and show that the quality of care in the system is equal to that available in the outside community. Prison practitioners must be specialists in primary care, preventive medicine, and the sociology of health. They are preventionists in the broadest definition of the term. Prison medicine may be the most difficult and the most exciting practice area in modern medicine.

Prison health systems, which a generation ago were generally poorly managed with no quality standards and inadequate resources, are now legally obligated to provide quality care to inmates and are investing billions of dollars in the activity. This change occurred as a result of three independent forces coming together in the 1970s. The first was the pressure brought by the civil liberties bar challenging inadequate medical services across the country.[10–12] In 1976,

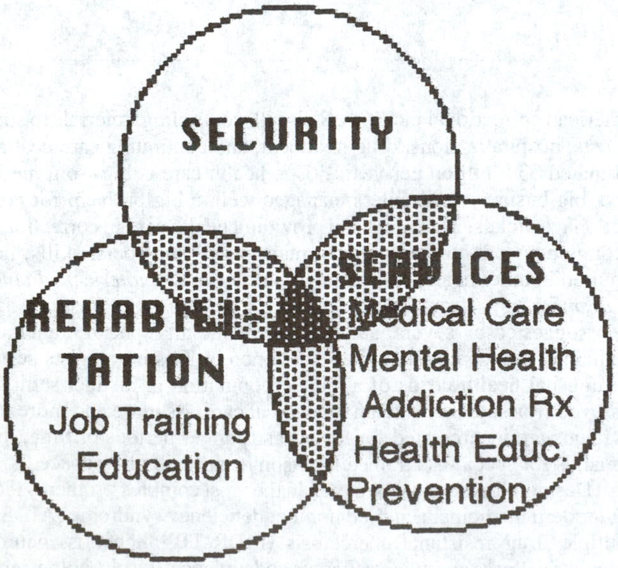

Figure 71-1. The overlapping priorities in corrections.

in the landmark Supreme Court decision, *Estelle v. Gamble*,[10] the legal ground rules under which prison health care was provided were changed. Prior to *Estelle*, medical care in prisons and jails was a responsibility of jail wardens and prison superintendents. A prisoner's *right to health care* was not a consideration. After *Estelle*, prisoners were recognized to have a constitutional right under the Eighth Amendment to a community standard of medical care. Many subsequent decisions[13] have bolstered these findings, obligating prison systems to provide care equal to that available in the outside community.

The second force helping to improve service in correctional facilities was that of organized medicine concerned that the quality of care provided to prisoners was deficient. The American Medical Association (AMA), following a survey of medical conditions in jails and prisons that identified deplorable conditions,[14] initiated a process to define standards for correctional health care. These standards, now promulgated by the National Center for Correctional Health Care (NCCHC), are a measure of acceptable care in jails,[15] prisons,[16] and juvenile halls.[17] By the end of 1996, 150 state prisons, 194 jails, and 32 juvenile facilities had adopted the NCCHC Standards in an effort to provide care that meets the mandate of the federal courts.

The third factor helping to change correctional health care is the recognition by public health authorities that prison health problems, untreated, have the potential for becoming community problems. In 1977, Weisbuch[18] urged public health professionals to join with those working in prisons to develop and improve the system of care available to prisoners. In the late 1970s and early 1980s, a few state and local health departments began working with prisons to improve quality and ensure that the care continued after discharge.[19,20] But it was not until the late 1980s when the AIDS epidemic and the resurgence of tuberculosis forced cooperation between correctional health and public health officials working to protect the health of the community.[21] Providers and managers of prison health services cannot resolve all the public health problems that enter prison gates, but in conjunction with health departments, prison providers can become a major link in the chain to improve community health status, reducing the burden of illness in society.[22]

This history, the response of the U.S. court system, U.S. medicine, and local public health to improve correctional health care, is well documented by Anno and others.[14,23,24] This history, and the published standards for correctional health care from the American Public Health Association (APHA, second edition),[25] the National Center for Correctional Health Care (NCCHC, third edition),[14–16] The Joint Commission for the Accreditation of Health Care Organizations (JCAHCO), and the American Correctional Association (ACA), should be read by all who enter the field.

The quality of care in prisons has improved since the mid-1970s. Private companies now provide quality health care for many prison systems under contract.[9] Several states (e.g., Texas, Massachusetts, Oregon) have developed managed care contracts with state medical schools or private health maintenance organizations in an effort to preserve clinical quality and lower cost. In virtually all prison systems that are under contract with private health delivery systems, the measure of quality is accreditation by either JCAHCO or NCCHC. Professionals in the field now receive recognition of excellence under the Certified Correctional Health Care Professional program managed by NCCHC. The number of certified professionals exceeds 1,000. The scientific literature relating to correctional health expands in volume and quality. All this augurs well for the preservation of quality care in the correctional setting.

One note of caution has sounded, however. The judicial mandate for better prison health care, well established under the several cases noted above, may be under pressure as the Supreme Court and Congress move to limit access to the federal court system by state jail and prison inmates. If access to the court system is restrained, correctional departments, always under budgetary pressure, may opt to lower quality to save resources. Accreditation will be dropped, health budgets reduced, and a lower standard adopted. A return to the dark ages of the past is a possibility, unless public health and correctional providers continue to assert that high-quality correctional health care helps to ensure a healthy environment for all citizens whether they are within a prison or not.

▶ PRISON ENVIRONMENT AND THE PUBLIC'S HEALTH

Prisons, jails, and juvenile halls are conduits through which significant public health problems and the social pathology of our society is funneled. Substance abuse, AIDS, hepatitis, trauma, violence, tuberculosis, suicide, mental illness, venereal diseases, and unwanted pregnancy are far more prevalent in jails and prisons than in the outside world.[26–28] This burden of illness among prisoners increases the demand for medical care, increases the need for specialty referral services, and increases the cost of prison health care above that which might be expected from other young, predominantly male, populations.

The burden of prison pathology requires that prison health providers maintain a close relationship with those in public health. Infectious diseases cross prison walls in both directions. Trauma prevention and the management of prison violence requires linkage to the community emergency system. Enforcement of environmental health regulations for jails and prisons requires public health involvement. Promoting health, reducing drug and alcohol abuse, controlling sexually transmitted diseases, and ensuring early prenatal care and high-quality health care are not tasks for jailers; nor can they be performed effectively by correctional health care providers working in isolation.

These tasks are public health responsibilities that do not cease when people are jailed any more than when children attend school or workers enter a factory. By coordinating their responsibilities with prison health professionals, whose primary task is to provide acute care to inmates, public health practitioners can improve the health of the public. Several examples of prison health problems that impact on the public's health are discussed below.

Substance Abuse: Alcohol and Drugs

Substance abuse—with its public and private medical, social, legal, and criminal ramifications is, according to the American Medical Association,[29] the most significant public health problem facing the United States. It is also the most significant problem in jails and prisons. In 1979, a nationwide survey of substance abuse among state prisoners, reported by Miller,[30] found that 33 percent of males and 29 percent of females were drunk when they committed their current offense and that 8.5 percent of males and 13.7 percent of females admitted to daily IV heroin use at the time of incarceration. The proportion of inmates with an addiction to drugs, alcohol, or both constituted 30 percent of the Cook County Jail population in 1982–1983;[31] by 1988–1989, Wiosh and O'Neil reported that 60 percent of arrested persons were using a drug other than alcohol when arrested;[32] by 1994–1995, the proportion of addicted inmates in California was reported to be 80 to 90 percent of the population (California Sheriffs Association, personal communication, October 1995). In 1994, drug law violators constituted 25 percent of all jail inmates; they are the most rapidly growing segment of the jail population.[33] Alcohol and the use of other addictive drugs in the general population of young adults is an important health problem; but it pales when compared to the frequency of substance abuse among the incarcerated.[34]

Substance abusers bring into prisons and jails all the infirmities associated with their addictions: AIDS, tuberculosis, hepatitis (B and C), withdrawal syndromes, injuries, emotional illness, and the potential for suicide. Each individual and each problem must be managed by prison clinicians. Treatment for the acute manifestations of disease takes precedence, but several studies have shown that rapid enrollment of jail and prison addicts into drug treatment programs reduces their prison stay and the rate of recidivism.[35–38] Even if the addiction is not completely abated by treatment, addicts in and out of prison are less prone to commit criminal acts when in remission.[39] Treatment begun in prison must continue when the patient is returned to the community, if the addictive lifestyle and its progression of human suffering, disease transmission, disability, and death is to be stopped.

The management and treatment of substance abusers and addicts constitutes one of the most complex aspects of desmotology: medical service, rehabilitation, and security all overlap on this issue. Initiating treatment programs within a correctional health system may involve the use of contraband substances, often will require linkage with community programs, and may conflict with other rehabilitation programs managed by the correctional system. Success can reduce recidivism, lower correctional costs, improve the health status of addicts, and reduce the burden of addiction-related problems in the community. In most prisons, however, initiating drug treatment is an extremely hard sell that will take every ounce of administrative skill, tact, and medical acumen of the desmotologist.

Quoting the AMA's Board of Trustees, ". . . substance abusers in the United States will not be reduced in number through the interdiction of supply nor the enforcement of tougher laws. Only through the expansion of treatment programs, and the education of users and potential users will addiction decline."[40] These public health functions should begin in the prison environment. Addicts are recognized upon admission, treatment is begun as soon as possible, and when discharged, inmates can be referred to community treatment as part of the requirement for parole.

AIDS

The AIDS epidemic created a growing crisis for an overburdened American correctional system in the early 1980s. By 1988, in state and federal prisons, the average prevalence of entering prisoners was 75 cases per 100,000, being as low as zero in Iowa and Nebraska, and as high as 536 per 100,000 in New York.[47] At that time the national prevalence was 13.7. These rates have continued to rise; in 1992–1993, the National Institute of Justice[42] reported an aggregated rate of 363 cases per 100,000, which has risen to 532 in 1994–1995.[43] These data are shown graphically in Figure 71-2. By 1994, 22,713 of nearly 1 million state and federal inmates were HIV infected, 4,849 of whom had full-blown AIDS. New York (8,295), Florida (1,986), Texas (1,584), and California (1,055) held the majority of HIV cases (12,920). From the beginning of the epidemic, the rate of confirmed AIDS cases in prisons, always eight to ten times the national rate, has risen sharply, as shown in Figure 71-2. By 1994, 955 deaths from AIDS were reported in American prisons. These deaths, over one-third of all fatalities reported in state prison systems, were nearly twice the 520 deaths recorded in 1991.[43]

Risk factors among inmates are also changing. In 1984 and 1985 homosexuality was the predominant HIV risk factor. By 1988, however, more than half of new AIDS cases in New York City and Baltimore were associated with IV drug abuse.[44–46] This phenomenon will decline only when public health activities are initiated that reduce the transmission of virus in contaminated needles.

Viral transmission within the prison environment also occurs.[45,47–49] The problem for the desmotologist is how to control viral spread within the prison while not conflicting with security needs of the prison administration. Should all new inmates be tested for HIV?[50–52] Should only those who are homosexual or IV drug users be tested? Should those at high risk who are found HIV negative by the standard enzyme-linked immunosorbent assay (ELISA) Western blot process be further evaluated for silent viral infection by lymphocyte culture? What housing arrangements are appropriate for HIV-positive inmates? Who should be informed of the prisoner's HIV status? Should contact tracing both inside the prison and in the outside community be initiated? By whom? Can confidentiality be maintained in the prison setting? What are the implications for the individual's health when his or her HIV status is known? Should patients with clinical AIDS be discharged from the jail or prison? Should zidovudine and other drugs be given, and who should pay the cost? Who should be responsible to provide counseling to the patients? Who shall attempt to allay fear of the disease among inmates and correctional staff? Should drug abusers regardless of their HIV status be enrolled in prison treat-

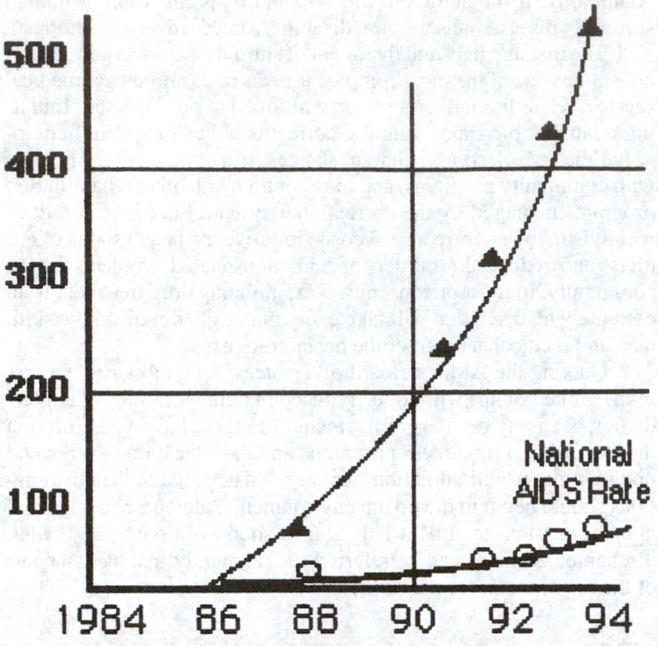

Figure 71-2. Confirmed AIDS rate per 100,000 admissions.

ment programs? Should condoms and sterile needles be distributed to reduce the risk of viral transmission? Should inmates who demonstrate the clinical findings of the HIV viremia be treated with antiviral drugs and protease inhibitors? The list goes on ad infinitum.

These questions have ramifications well beyond the prison walls. The public health implications deserve input from public health experts who manage the AIDS problem in the community. Decisions concerning the prison population at risk to HIV infection should not be made in a vacuum and should not be made only to satisfy narrow security requirements of the correctional system. Preventing HIV transmission in prison protects the community at large. Allowing prisoners to participate in antiviral drug testing could benefit the entire population.

Most prison systems do have a written AIDS policy to answer some or all of these questions. State or local health departments may have been consulted in the development of the policy; but without continuing support from these professionals, implementation and continuing revision of these policies remains problematic. Resources within prisons are limited. Isolation beds may not exist. In prison, confidentiality is impossible. AIDS phobia has declined since the 1980s, but where it exists, inmates who carry the virus are at risk to injury and even death. Desmotologists must stay abreast with the rapidly changing status of AIDS research; any medical intervention that reduces HIV prevalence, lowers the risk of HIV transmission within the walls, and lowers the morbidity and mortality from AIDS must be considered.

Optimal HIV policies serve the prison system and the public well. Voluntary HIV testing, pretest and posttest counseling, the education of inmates and correctional staff have been shown to be effective[46,53] and deserve the highest level of professional input available. Contact tracing, the protection of confidentiality,[54] the support of family and friends, the treatment of the terminal phase of the illness, and the referral of HIV-positive prisoners to appropriate community resources, upon discharge from prison, are functions best performed by health department personnel cooperating with their colleagues in corrections. In a system where public health and corrections services coordinate their activities toward prevention of HIV infection, the public at large will be maximally protected. Since HIV infection is often recognized first in the prison environment, correctional health providers must work with public health providers to create linked services to meet the needs of this population both within the prison walls and upon its return to the community.

Hepatitis

Hepatitis, A, B, and C are diseases whose high prevalence among prisoners is also related to IV drug use. Each poses a health threat to patients and to others in prison and in the community after discharge. Prevalence studies of inmates in the United States[55,56] and in Australia[57] indicate that 50 percent or more have used drugs, and in Australia 33 and 39 percent, respectively, have been exposed to hepatitis B and C prior to incarceration.

Hepatitis B and C are transmitted to those susceptible with the prison environment of the same mechanisms as HIV: intravenous drug use and homosexual sex. The incidence of prison transmission, a function of viral prevalence on admission and the frequency of contact within the facility, varies between 8 to 14 cases per 1,000 exposure-years.[40,58,59] Unlike the transmission of HIV within a prison environment, which may not become symptomatic as full-blown AIDS for 10 years or more, prison hepatitis infection may become manifest within a few weeks or months. Acute hepatitis requiring medical management, isolation, special diets, concern for carrier states, and other sequellae of the disease are a common prison health problem with high morbidity and a mortality of 1 to 2 percent.

Hepatitis is preventable. The Michigan State Correctional System has adopted a policy to vaccinate all inmates with the hepatitis B virus (HBV) vaccine,[60] a policy suggested by Anda[56] and his coworkers. Desmotologists should consider vaccination against HBV, needle and condom distribution, and the expansion of drug treatment programs to reduce both hepatitis and HIV transmission. These innovations promote community health both within the correctional setting and in the outside community by improving prisoner health status.

Desmotologists must consider the public health perspective of their work since prisoners generally return to their community. The current period of imprisonment may be the only chance society has to protect these individuals from infection with hepatitis B and C viruses. In prison, addicts who have not been exposed to HB_SAg can be identified and vaccinated; something that is unlikely to occur in the outside world. If half of all jail and prison admissions are IV drug users, and half of that number are unexposed to HB_SAg, the vaccination of susceptible individuals would cost less than $25 per prison admission. Whether this expense would reduce the treatment and the social costs associated with the annual incidence of 300,000 cases of hepatitis B in the nonprison community can be evaluated only when transmission rates in the community are known.

Working together, a prison system and a public health department can determine the appropriate plan for their community. Decisions should be based upon the needs of the outside community, the security requirements of the prison, *and* appropriate medical care. If the public benefits, the costs of vaccination should be assumed by the public health department.

Tuberculosis

Tuberculosis, another public health problem long recognized as a significant health problem among prisoners,[61] can be controlled and possibly eliminated as a threat to prisoners and correctional staff if public health and prison health authorities work together. Throughout the twentieth century, until the early 1980s, the incidence of active tuberculosis in the United States and in its prisons and jails had been declining. By 1985, the national TB death rate had dropped below 10 cases per 100,000 population. In state correctional systems, tuberculosis case rates, while still exceeding those for nonincarcerated adults 15 to 64 years old, often by 3-fold or more,[62] had been trending downward with the general decline in the disease.

In the mid-1980s, however, trends in tuberculosis changed. In 1985 the number of new cases in prisoners increased over the previous year. In the nation at large, the downward trend in TB incidence slowed in 1985–1986, and began to rise in 1987 (Fig. 71-3). Several factors contributed to this resurgence in tuberculosis. HIV infection in those with previous exposure to human tuberculosis

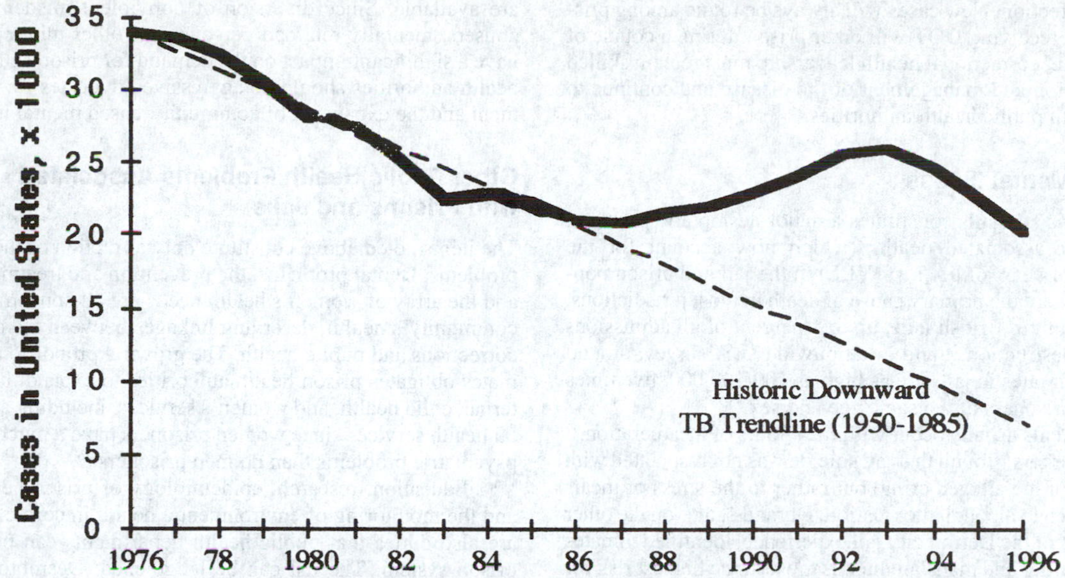

Figure 71-3. Total tuberculosis cases, United States.

were at great risk to active disease as their immune systems became more compromised; previously uninfected HIV-positive individuals are highly susceptible to the Mycobacterium for the same reason.[63–65] Changes in state and federal financial commitment to TB control in the late 1970s and early 1980s diminished the local public health infrastructure for TB control, resulting in inadequate follow-up and treatment of diagnosed cases. The increase in homelessness and the changing drug abuse culture brought high-risk populations together in shelters poorly designed to prevent transmission. And the increase in incarceration produced by the "war on drugs" increased crowding in jails and prisons, enhancing the potential for infection.[66]

Between 1985 and 1994, active TB in U.S. prison and jail populations escalated, becoming the most important epidemic problem facing correctional health systems. In 1987, TB case rates in California prisons were 80.3 per 100,000; in New York, 105.5; and in New Jersey, 109.9.[62] The national rate in that year was 9.4, slightly above the rate in 1986.[67] These rates continued upward until 1994–1995, when efforts in prevention and control began to have their effect. Across the nation and in its prisons and jails, tuberculosis has fallen sharply since 1994. The decline should continue, provided health professionals maintain their vigilance and their active programs to control and eliminate the disease.

The history of tuberculosis in prisons prior to 1985 and subsequently is a case history of the importance of maintaining constant surveillance over critical public health diseases and protecting the programs for their control. Prior to 1985, prison health policies focused on the identification of new inmates with a positive PPD who were then screened by x-ray. Those with positive films were given a course of antituberculosis therapy while in the institution. Little effort was made to ensure that a full course of treatment was maintained. Once the inmate left the facility, little if any follow-up occurred. One exception was the Los Angeles County Jail where new inmates were universally screened by small chest films; those with radiological evidence of active disease were placed under treatment and actively followed by the Health Department, even after discharge[68] (J Clark [Medical Director of the LA County Jail] and P Davidson [Director of the LA Health Department TB program], personal communication with the author, who during that period was the Medical Director of the LA County Department of Health Services). This activity proved of great value as the epidemic occurred; the number of cases with multiple drug–resistant strains of TB were minimal compared with those cases on the East Coast.

The rapid expansion of new active cases of tuberculosis in prisoners, among correctional staff, and in the communities from which the prison population arose stimulated a return to aggressive efforts to control the disease. The U.S. Public Health Service, Centers for Disease Control's *Manual on Control of Tuberculosis in Correctional Facilities*[69] was published in 1994. The third edition of the NCCHC's *Jail and Prison Standards for Correctional Health Care* includes several requirements for tuberculosis control. Both stress early identification of an active case upon admission, chest x-ray, isolation, identification of the offending organism, and the initiation of a full course of directly observed treatment (DOT) for 6 to 9 months using up to four drugs to which the bacillus is susceptible.

The appropriate management and control of tuberculosis in the correctional setting must be a joint program between the local public health authorities and the desmotologist. Factors for consideration include the local TB prevalence, the HIV prevalence, the daily admission rate, and the medical staff available for PPD or x-ray testing and follow-up. The specific problems of prisoner follow-up resulting from rapid transfer must be considered against the relative costs of mini–x-ray or PPD testing.[66] All TB cases must be tested for HIV infection, and all HIV-positive patients must be tested for tuberculosis. The protocols ensuring DOT while in prison *and* after discharge must be worked out between prison health and public health leadership. All prisons and jails today should have access to at least one negative pressure isolation room for the safe management of the active patient. Failure to adhere to this regimen has resulted in several TB epidemics in state prisons with deaths of both inmates and correctional officers.[70–72]

For tuberculosis, communication between public health and correctional health providers is a two-way street. Since continuity of prophylactic and therapeutic therapy is essential to reduce the spread of tuberculosis, patients who move between the community and the prison system in either direction must continue their medication. Active communication between local providers and prison health authorities will improve the registration of new cases, enhance contact tracing, reduce the failure rate in prophylaxis and treatment, diminish the development of MDR-TB, and reduce transmission. These linkages, built since 1985, have helped control the epidemic; but the return to previous morbidity levels will be short-lived if continued collaboration is neglected.

Tuberculosis in the United States will be controlled and possibly eliminated only if trained professionals continue to perform appropriate testing and treatment of converters, active cases, and those at high risk to infection. New cases will always be found among prisoners, and those receiving DOT will enter prison during a course of therapy; therefore, correctional health leadership must remain skilled in the identification and management of the disease and continue to work closely with public health authorities.

Suicide and Mental Illness

Suicide in prisons and jails constitutes a major desmoteric problem. Excluding AIDS-associated deaths (which now account for the largest number of years of life lost (YLL) in the jail and prison population), suicides are the primary cause of death in most jurisdictions. Estimates vary, but in British jails, up to 1 percent of all admissions attempted self-destruction,[73] and a nationwide U.S. survey[74] found that suicide death rates in jails are as high as 100/100,000, five times the rate for nonprisoners of the same age and sex.[75,76]

Suicides in jails usually occur within 24 hours of incarceration.[77] Jordan and coworkers[78] found that jail suicide was not associated with the seriousness of the alleged crime but rather to the stress of incarceration, and often to alcohol intoxication. Durand et al,[79] on the other hand, in a review of the Detroit city jail experience, identified inmates charged with murder and manslaughter as those at the highest risk for suicide, especially if they had a history of previous suicide attempts. The Detroit experience with suicides is more consistent with those that occur in prisons after sentencing. Prison suicides are associated with long sentences for serious crimes; they often occur months after confinement.[80]

Desmotologists are not expected to manage suicide prevention alone or in a vacuum. The problem requires input from mental health and public health professionals working as a team within the correctional system. Correctional officers can be trained for suicide prevention[81] under the direction of the mental health department. Mental health professionals should participate in the training of correctional employees, review protocols, and provide psychiatric backup for those inmates with profound emotional problems. Public health providers can integrate substance-abuse programs into the prevention process and create the reporting system necessary for management. Active suicide prevention programs, managed with support from prison authorities, trained professionals, and local mental health resources can lower suicide morbidity and mortality. The Detroit program lowered the suicide rate from 100 cases per 100,000 admissions in the 1970s to fewer than 13 cases per 100,000 between 1987 and 1992.

The prevention of suicides in both the jail and prison setting is achieved through early identification of those at risk, training of the correctional staff, and mental health intervention as soon as possible after incarceration. In the prison setting, those with a history of suicide attempt and those with long sentences for murder and manslaughter must be considered in the highest risk categories; mental health personnel must be available for this population.

Suicide is not the only mental health problem faced by desmotologists. In 1996, the largest repository for those with emotional illness in America was the prison system. The frequency of serious mental illness (psychoses) exceeds 6 percent of the inmate population, three to four times the rate in the population at large.[82] Individuals with serious emotional problems are often incarcerated for misdemeanors and other minor infractions. They spend an excessive amount of time behind bars, and while behind bars, are at increased risk of suicide, decompensation, and other mental disorders.[83] The lack of availability of community-based mental health services places these individuals under the charge of the desmotologists in the local jail. Diversion programs—programs that move the minor offender from the jail to community mental health programs—are not available in all jurisdictions. Where available, and when well managed, they may reduce incarceration of the mentally ill; full evaluation of their effectiveness has yet to be demonstrated, however.[84,85] The absence of community health services in many areas requires the desmotologist to expand mental health services within the correctional walls and create linkages with those community experts who are available. Since diversion of nonviolent misdemeanants, drug abusers, mentally retarded persons, and other minor offenders will have a significant impact on the demand for prison cells, correctional health authorities should be aggressive advocates for their development and the expansion of community-based mental health services.

Other Public Health Problems Associated with Prisons and Jails

The items noted above constitute only a fraction of the prison health problems. Dental problems, the prevention and treatment of injuries, and the array of women's health needs are all concerns affecting the community's health, deserving linkages between the departments of corrections and public health. The growing proportion of women inmates obligates prison health authorities to expand the array of maternal, child health, and women's services, including a need for mental health services since women prisoners have a much higher rate of psychiatric problems than do men prisoners.[86]

Education, research, epidemiology of prison health problems, and the monitoring of environmental health in correctional facilities are also duties that public health departments can perform for the prison system. The list can be lengthened. Desmotology will rely upon public health departments to ensure that its future is focused on preventing illness as well as providing first-rate care.

Regulation, Licensure, and Accreditation

If the gains in health care quality that jails and prisons have achieved over the past generation are to be preserved, prison health authorities should request state laws requiring licensure of their health facilities. Regulations, however, do not necessarily result in improvements in care in prison systems, but they are a first step. Regulation of correctional health systems by public health licensure authorities may be problematic since it requires agreement between two equal partners in government. Once established, however, it helps to ensure that prison health quality will not be subject to changes in court decisions or the vagaries of legislatures, often more concerned with budget shortfalls than with the health of inmates. To establish a licensure responsibility for public health over correctional health care, both parties must agree that quality care serves the needs of all aspects of prison management, security, rehabilitation, and service to the inmate.

Regulating the quality of care in prisons through licensure of the delivery process could be managed under the licensure authority of state and local departments of public health. The current process of voluntary accreditation by some state and county facilities will not ensure that correctional institutions will adhere to acceptable standards of care. These efforts may well be dropped as budgets become tighter and the protective eye of the Supreme Court dims. Services not regulated by law are subject to a diminution and decline in quality.

Since health problems in prisons overlap those in the community, a decline in prison health care will have a direct impact on the public's health. Maintaining correctional health quality through state licensure, continual surveillance, and public health oversight will protect inmates and the public. Achieving this objective, however, requires the initiation and preservation of the communication and linked services discussed in this chapter. Statutory licensure is certainly in the best interests of those prison health providers who have built credible systems over the years.

Accreditation by national agencies such as the NCCHC or the JCAHCO may be substituted for on-site examination of facilities by local public health inspectors; but the public health agency should require that a regular review process ensures that health services for inmates meet minimal standards. Correctional health leadership, which has been in the forefront of the development of prison and jail standards and the accreditation process, should now, in concert with their colleagues in public health, call for mandatory licensure of prison health services linked to the greater health community serving the general public.

▸ SUMMARY

Correctional health care problems currently exceed the boundaries of the prison systems. The major health problems confronted by health providers in American prisons overlap the major problems faced by society at large. These problems include substance abuse, HIV infection, hepatitis, trauma, violence, tuberculosis, suicide, mental illness, and venereal disease. These problems and the many others facing correctional health providers may well overwhelm the prison health systems, forcing a return to the inadequate levels of care that existed less then a generation ago.

To prevent a decline in quality, the correctional health leadership should develop close working relationships with local and state health and mental health departments, sharing professional and financial resources, with the combined objective being the improvement of health services for both prisoners and society at large. By making an effort to link with public health systems and providers, correctional providers will be taking advantage of the mission of public health providers to ensure that the conditions in which people live and work are healthy.[87] Solidifying these linkages through mandatory licensure of correctional health services will preserve the quality standards developed during the past 20 years.

The health of over 11 million citizens who pass through prisons annually and the well-being of those in close contact with them before, during, and after incarceration deserve a public commitment that the conditions in which they live and work are healthy. To neglect this population is perilous to society. Public health professionals, using their resources to ensure that prison health continues to improve, serve the community. Desmotologists who link their resources to the public health system also help to reduce the burden of preventable illness in U.S. society. By so doing they improve the health status of prisoners and reduce the problems faced by correctional administrators.

Preventive Medicine Support of Military Operations

Llewellyn J. Legters

> A corps of medical officers was not established solely for the purpose of attending the wounded and sick; the proper treatment of these sufferers is certainly a matter of a very great importance, and is an imperative duty, but the labors of Medical Officers cover a more extended field. The *leading idea*, which should be constantly kept in view, is to strengthen the hands of the Commanding General by keeping his army in the most vigorous health, thus rendering it, in the highest degree, efficient for enduring fatigue and privation and for fighting.
>
> ——Dr. Jonathan Letterman, Surgeon,
> Army of the Potomac, 1862 to 1864[1]

By congressional statute, military commanders are responsible for the health of their commands. The command "surgeon" serves as the commander's principal medical staff advisor, and in this role, he or she participates in the development of all command plans and policies. The command surgeon, usually with the assistance of a staff preventive medicine officer, advises the commander on the health status of the command, threats to the health of the command, and on policies and practices to protect the health of the command.

Preventive medicine programs for military units and personnel are designed to preserve and promote health and to prevent physical and mental diseases and disabilities. Knowledge of the environment in which the programs are to be effected is essential to assess the physical, chemical, and biologic hazards to which military personnel may be exposed. During military operations, besides the risk of injury from the weapons of war, principal hazards include accidents with machines, especially motor vehicles, explosives and fire; exposures to noise, smoke, and toxic fumes; extremes of altitude, heat, and cold; and a host of infectious diseases, many with the capacity to produce catastrophic morbidity in deployed forces (e.g., malaria, dengue fever, sand fly fever).

The dissolution of the Soviet Union has substantially altered the nature of the threat to global and U.S. national security, and along with it, the U.S. national military strategic response. U.S. military forces were formerly preoccupied with the potential for large-scale, high-intensity armed conflicts, especially in the defense of Europe. The primary strategic concern now appears to have shifted to the containment of various regional ethnic and religious conflicts and to the prevention of terrorist attacks against U.S. interests, both at home and abroad. The use of weapons of mass destruction (biological, chemical, and nuclear) among warring factions or by terrorists against U.S. targets is regarded as a distinct possibility. The effect of these trends has been to increase the mission diversity of the U.S. Armed Forces to include not only fighting war, but also peacekeeping, humanitarian assistance, and disaster relief missions, which, in turn, require the medical capacity to provide highly flexible and mobile support over long distances and in widely diverse environments.

Field Preventive Medicine Organization

In "Joint" Operations, such as Operations Desert Shield and Desert Storm, the deployed force will usually include combat elements from the Army, Navy, Marine Corps, and Air Force. The Joint Task Force (JTF) will be tailored with respect to the kinds of units and their size so as to be able to accomplish the mission articulated for it by the Joint Chiefs of Staff. Each combat unit (Army and Marine divisions; Air Force tactical fighter wings, etc.) has its own "organic" support elements (meaning support units that *belong* to the combat unit), including medical and preventive medicine units and personnel. At the combat unit level, preventive medicine capabilities include water testing for chlorine residuals and bacterial coliforms and limited vector control. Backing up the organic medical support units are additional medical units under the command and control of the JTF Commander, and under the technical supervision of the JTF Surgeon. These assets may include epidemiology, entomology, environmental sanitation, and environmental engineering capabilities. Since Operations Desert Shield and Desert Storm, the Army also has established a Theater Army Medical Laboratory (TAML), which performs the functions of a public health laboratory in the Theater of Operations. In addition, the Air Force maintains an aerial spray squadron, with three C-130 aircraft configured to spray insecticide over large areas, should it become necessary to control widespread vector-borne disease outbreaks in the deployed force.

Disease and Injury Prevention in Operating Forces

There are five key elements of the strategy for disease and injury prevention among forces deployed in field and combat operations:

1. Determining the nature and magnitude of the disease and injury threats in the planned area of operations before force deployment;
2. Identifying the principal countermeasures that must be emphasized to reduce the threats to an acceptable level and promulgating these countermeasures among the operating forces;
3. Training individuals in the use of these countermeasures;
4. Enforcing these countermeasures in the operational area;
5. Conducting medical surveillance to monitor the health of the deployed force and to identify events that require preventive medicine interventions.

Medical Threat Assessments

The threats to health from disease and nonbattle injury (DNBI) in a deployed military force depend principally on the mission and composition of the force, the geographical area of operations, including the diseases that are endemic in the area, the time of year, and the intensity of the conflict. DNBI rates in past conflicts have invariably exceeded rates due to battle injury and have resulted from naturally occurring infectious diseases (e.g., malaria, dengue fever, sand fly fever); environmental extremes of heat, cold, and altitude; motor vehicle accidents; athletic injuries; and psychological stresses. In peacekeeping operations in Bosnia, industrial chemical and radioactive wastes are also considered to be potential threat agents.

During Operations Desert Shield and Desert Storm, rates of hospitalization due to DNBI were extremely low in comparison with previous conflicts (Table 71-1) because of a unique set of favorable circumstances: (*a*) good medical intelligence about the area before the deployment, (*b*) sound preventive medicine policies that, for the most part, were rigorously subscribed to and enforced by unit commanders, (*c*) the seasonal ebb of insect vectors (e.g., sand flies), (*d*) the religious proscriptions of the host nation, (*e*) a slow and unimpeded buildup phase, and (*f*) a brief ground combat phase.[2]

As a general rule, naturally occurring infectious diseases are likely to remain the most important causes of preventable medical noneffectiveness in most future overseas deployments. In past wars involving U.S. forces, infectious diseases have produced higher morbidity rates than battle injuries, and until World War II, higher mortality rates as well.[3–5] The infectious diseases causing high morbidity among U.S. forces in past wars, arranged more or less in the relative order of their importance, are show in Table 71-2.[6] Because deployed troops usually must live and work under relatively primitive conditions, they are also at risk for "emerging" infectious diseases. As one example, hemorrhagic fever with renal syndrome due to Hantaan virus was first reported in Japanese and Soviet troops in Manchuria just before World War II, affected UN troops during the Korean War, and continues to be reported among Korean and United States soldiers in association with field operations along the demilitarized zone (DMZ) in South Korea.[7] As a second example, cutaneous leishmaniasis due to *Leishmania tropica* was known to be endemic in the Persian Gulf region before the deployment of U.S. troops on Operations Desert Shield and Desert Storm. However, the capacity of the parasite to "visceralize" (i.e., to invade liver, spleen, and bone marrow) was not well documented before its appearance in returning U.S. troops.[6] Experience during Operations Desert Shield and Desert Storm indicates that medical threat assessments in future deployments certainly must also include evaluation of the capability of enemy forces to employ biological and chemical agents as weapons.

TABLE 71-1. U.S. ARMY DNBI RATES[a] IN OPERATIONS DESERT SHIELD AND DESERT STORM COMPARED WITH PREVIOUS CONFLICTS

	Combat Troops	*Support Troops*
World War II	1.98	1.60
Korean War	1.67	2.14
Vietnam	0.89	0.92
Desert Shield	0.34	—
Desert Storm	0.41	—

Source: Preventive Medicine Division, Office of the Surgeon General, U.S. Army, 1991.

[a] Per 1,000 per day.

TABLE 71-2. INFECTIOUS DISEASES CAUSING HIGH MORBIDITY IN U.S. FORCES IN PAST CONFLICTS: WORLD WAR II, KOREA, VIETNAM, AND OPERATIONS DESERT SHIELD AND DESERT STORM

Acute respiratory disease and influenza	All
Acute diarrheal diseases	All
Malaria	WWII, Korea, Vietnam
Hepatitis	WWII, Korea, Vietnam
Sexually transmitted diseases	WWII, Korea, Vietnam
Arthropod-borne diseases[a]	WWII, Vietnam
Rickettsial diseases[b]	WWII, Vietnam
Leptospirosis	WWII, Vietnam
Leishmaniasis	WWII, Desert Storm
Schistosomiasis	WWII[c]

Source: L. J. Legters, Department of Preventive Medicine and Biometrics, Uniformed Services University of the Health Sciences, Bethesda, MD, 1992.
Abbreviation: WWII, World War II.

[a] Especially dengue fever, sand fly fever, hemorrhagic fevers, and encephalitides.

[b] Principally scrub typhus, whose distribution is limited to parts of Asia and northern Australia.

[c] Principally in engineer bridge-building units in Luzon, Philippines.

The purpose of medical threat assessments is to help decide on the specific disease and injury countermeasures that must be planned for use by the force. The information needed to develop such assessments for a particular country or region is available from a variety of sources, including statistical reports of national and international health agencies, publications in general medical literature, medical historical data from previous operations in the area, and the unpublished observations of health care personnel and epidemiologists working or visiting in the geographical areas of interest. In addition, in a number of widely dispersed geographical areas the U.S. Army and Navy maintain medical research laboratories dedicated to the study of the epidemiology and prevention of regional medical problems of potential military importance. The U.S. Navy also maintains a number of Environmental Preventive Medicine Units (EPMUs) with regional responsibility for updated assessments of current health risks in areas of possible deployment of Navy and Marine forces. The EPMUs publish "Disease Risk Assessment Profiles," which provide information about disease threats and countermeasures on all countries within their geographic areas of responsibility. The collection and evaluation of medical information from these various sources and the preparation of a variety of medical information products for particular countries and regions are accomplished by the Armed Forces Medical Intelligence Center (e.g., "Disease and Environmental Alert Reports" (DEARs)) and the Defense Pest Management Information and Analysis Center of the Armed Forces Pest Management Board ("Disease Vector Ecology Profiles" (DVEPs)). The Army and Navy overseas laboratories and the EPMUs are excellent sources of current information because they have people working "on the ground" in regions of interest, constantly updating the medical threat assessments. During Operations Desert Shield and Desert Storm, the Navy Medical Research Unit 3 in Cairo deployed a so-called "Joint Forward Laboratory" into Saudi Arabia to provide for the rapid diagnosis of infectious diseases among deployed troops. This small, but highly sophisticated laboratory, in concert with an established medical surveillance program, was able to provide continuous medical intelligence updates in the area of operations. In addition, satellite-based remote-sensing and associated geographic information systems technologies, though presently having only limited application, show promise for future use during deployments in the prediction, both in time and place, of vector-borne diseases of military importance.[8–10]

Identifying the Countermeasures and Promulgating the Force Preventive Medicine Program

In military operations there are two general kinds of disease and injury countermeasures: those taken by or applied to individual soldiers and measures taken by the unit and applied to the environment in which the unit is operating. Individual countermeasures are those that alter the individual in some way to increase refractoriness to the various risks, including immunizations, prophylactic drugs, insect repellents, protective clothing, and safety equipment. Environmental countermeasures are those directed at removal or attenuation of environmental risk factors, including measures directed at the provision of potable unit water supplies and sanitary food supplies, the sanitary disposal of wastes, and the control of disease vectors and animal reservoirs of disease. In addition, in the development and testing of major items of equipment (armored vehicles, artillery pieces, etc.), attention is paid to the design of the equipment so as to minimize the risk of injury from its use. For example, the ventilation system in the Bradley fighting vehicle (and other armored vehicles) is designed to rapidly remove from the troop compartment the smoke and gases generated by the combustion of ammunition propellants during weapons firing.

In the highly mobile tactical operations characteristic of modern warfare, it is frequently necessary to place nearly total reliance for disease and injury prevention on individual countermeasures applied under the direction of the lieutenants and sergeants at the platoon and squad level. In more stable tactical situations and in rear areas, it is possible to place heavier reliance on environmental controls applied by the units themselves or by combat service support units (engineer, quartermaster, and medical) on an area basis. Besides the function of disease vector control, which is accomplished by specialized medical units, most environmental controls are the responsibility of nonmedical personnel and units. For example, in the Army, quartermaster units are responsible for food and water procurement and distribution. Medical personnel and units retain responsibility for technical inspections to ensure compliance with prescribed sanitary standards.

Malaria is perhaps the best example of a highly significant military disease problem that would receive the careful attention of preventive medicine planners during preparations for deployment to known malaria-endemic areas. Decisions about the countermeasures to be employed by the force would be written into the medical annexes of the operations orders; these have the authority of command directives. These decisions would also represent the basis for procurement of medical supply items for use in the prevention and control of malaria, such as drugs for chemoprophylaxis and treatment, and insecticides and insecticide dispersal equipment for mosquito control.

A primary consideration would be the malaria chemoprophylactic regimen to be used by the force. Factors that would be taken into consideration in determining the malaria chemoprophylactic regimen include the malaria prevalence in the region, the predominant infecting species, and the prevalence of drug-resistant *Plasmodium falciparum* and *Plasmodium vivax*.

Besides the chemoprophylactic regimen, other individual countermeasures against malaria that would be addressed include use of the standard-issue insect repellent (diethyltoluamide (DEET)), which would be used on exposed skin surfaces in conjunction with the permethrin-impregnated battle dress uniform (BDU), the proper wearing of the uniform ("shirts on, collars buttoned, sleeves rolled down, from dusk to dawn"), and the use of bed nets in secure areas. Area malaria control programs in the operational area, including insecticide dispersal methods, would be devised based upon on-site professional entomological surveys conducted to determine the principal malaria vector species, their breeding sites, and adult mosquito biting and resting habits. Additional environmental controls that might be addressed include policies regarding campsite selection in relation to native villages, whose inhabitants might represent a reservoir of malaria infection, the use of indigenes in labor forces, and medical civic action programs directed at reduction of the size of the malaria reservoir though the identification and treatment of infected individuals.

Training Personnel to Use Countermeasures

As noted, it is frequently necessary to rely almost entirely on individual countermeasures for disease and injury prevention in the early stages of deployments and during other kinds of offensive operations. During these periods, the combat service support units responsible for the implementation of area environmental controls ordinarily will be given a lower priority for transport than the combat elements. The medical personnel present in the forward areas will be those who are assigned to the combat units, and they will be more preoccupied with the care of combat casualties at the time than with the institution of environmental countermeasures. Moreover, it is during this period, in the disorganization of battle and before the construction of any permanent facilities, such as barracks, latrines, and mess halls, that troops are most vulnerable to vector-borne disease transmission, including diseases with the demonstrated capacity to produce catastrophic morbidity in fighting forces (e.g., malaria, dengue fever, sand fly fever).

The individual countermeasures determined to be necessary for use by the force must be integrated into predeployment training programs (see Table 71-3).[11] Through repetition and constant reinforcement by the lieutenants and sergeants at platoon and squad level, it is to be expected that the application of individual countermeasures will become second nature among the troops. The principal prerequisite for ensuring that the desired health behaviors are incorporated into each individual soldier's repertoire is to convince the lieutenant and sergeant leaders of small tactical units that the countermeasures are important to the success of their unit's mission.

Rigorous Command Enforcement of Countermeasures

Enforcement of the use of countermeasures is a command function. The appearance in a unit of cases of a specific disease that should have been prevented by the application of the command-directed countermeasures (e.g., cases of malaria that should have been prevented with the prescribed chemoprophylaxis) should bring about an epidemiological investigation to determine if the outbreak is due

TABLE 71-3. INDIVIDUAL PREVENTIVE MEDICINE COUNTERMEASURES TO BE EMPHASIZED IN TROOP TRAINING EXERCISES

Safety first: be alert and be cautious.
Drink water frequently during the day.
Wash hands after using the latrine and before meals.
Take the malaria pills regularly.
Keep insect repellent on exposed skin.
Sleep under a bed net.
Follow work-rest cycles to prevent exhaustion.
Do not consume local foods or untreated water/ice.
Defecate only in constructed latrines or designated areas.
Avoid contact with all animals, large and small.
Wear hearing protection when exposed to combat noises.

Adapted from Walter Reed Army Institute of Research: Somalia: Preliminary Report. WRAIR Communicable Disease Report 3(4):11, 1992, Table 2.

to unexpected failure of the prescribed countermeasures to prevent the cases (e.g., the malaria parasites are resistant to the prescribed chemoprophylaxis) or the result of command failure to enforce the countermeasures (e.g., soldiers are not taking the prescribed chemoprophylaxis). If the investigation shows that the cases are the result of failure of the prescribed countermeasures, then better methods must be decided upon and put in place quickly. If due to the latter, command-directed disciplinary action may be warranted. In this connection, Field Marshall Sir William Slim, commander of the British Army in Burma in World War II, in his personal history of the period, stated:

> Good doctors are no use without discipline. More than half the battle against disease is fought, not by doctors, but by the regimental officers. . . . When mepacrine was first introduced . . . often the little tablet was not swallowed. An individual medical test in almost all cases will show whether it has been taken or not. . . . I, therefore, had surprise checks of whole units, every man being examined. If the overall result was less than ninety-five per cent positive I sacked the commanding officer. I only had to sack three; by then the rest got my meaning.[12]

Conducting Medical Surveillance

Medical surveillance of the deployed force is necessary to continuously monitor the health status of the force, ensure that preventive medicine countermeasures are working, rapidly identify disease and injury threats that have the potential to compromise the combat effectiveness of the units, and if necessary, develop and recommend preventive medicine interventions to the appropriate unit commanders. As noted above, it is the commander who is ultimately responsible for the health of the command and the implementation of disease and injury countermeasures.

Before Operations Desert Shield and Desert Storm, disease and injury surveillance programs during military operations were, for the most part, decentralized to brigade, regiment, and division level; were dependent upon the ad hoc, usually less than systematic observations of unit surgeons; and were frequently subject to reporting delays to higher headquarters, which prevented timely interventions from that level. During Operations Desert Shield and Desert Storm, U.S. Navy and Marine Corps medical personnel systematically recorded outpatient disease and injury data by category of illness or injury (heat and cold injury, diarrhea and gastrointestinal infections, dermatologic conditions, respiratory conditions, injury or orthopedic conditions, unexplained fever, sexually transmitted diseases, ophthalmologic conditions, psychiatric conditions, and other acute conditions) and reported these data weekly using a standard format. Unit strength figures were included in reports to permit the calculation of rates, by unit, location, and in the aggregate. The system is credited with the identification of a forcewide diarrheal disease outbreak early in the operation related to the serving of fresh lettuce in U.S. Marine Corps field messing facilities; the lettuce was being provided along with other fresh foods by indigenous contractors outside the network of sources approved by the U.S. military. Rates had increased simultaneously throughout the force, exceeding 8 percent per week in some locations. A command decision was made to ban the use of lettuce in Marine Corps field messing facilities, which was followed by a precipitous decline in rates of diarrheal disease in the force to around 1 percent per week.[13] The success of this centralized surveillance and reporting system during Operations Desert Shield and Desert Storm has resulted in adoption of a triservice system mandated for use in future Joint Force deployments.[1]

Public Health Nursing

Kristine M. Gebbie

For over 100 years public health nurses have been "promoting and protecting the health of populations using knowledge from nursing, social and public health sciences."[1] This effort has taken many forms and led practitioners to crowded urban tenements, to isolated farms, to suburban workplaces, to healthy children, to tubercular workers to the elderly seeking to maintain their independence. While it is difficult to say that there is a "typical" public health nurse, there are commonalities across many agencies of different sizes, serving diverse communities. Public health nurses are usually employed to work in those public health programs that require some contact with individuals, especially if that contact involves some aspect of "hands on" clinical practice. This includes the staffing of immunization clinics, sexually transmitted disease and tuberculosis control programs, child and maternal health services, senior health promotion programs, and workplace health clinics. Nurses are found staffing epidemiology programs and working to ensure quality health care in day care centers and hospital and long-term care facilities through licensing and certification. In large health departments, a nurse might work exclusively in one or two program areas, and even in a limited part of the jurisdiction served. In many middle-sized and most small departments, the nurse must be a generalist, moving day to day and hour by hour from program to program. Much of the apparent specialization and narrow targeting of work efforts is driven by the current approach to funding of public health, in which dollars are tied to very defined activities and population groups, rather than being available for more broad-based efforts to work with a population group or community to improve health overall.

While complex models to explain the experience of health in populations (such as the Evans and Stoddard Field Model[2]) have not been in use for any extended period of time, public health nurses have understood that to best serve any individual requires attention to family situation, economic circumstance, and community. As the turbulent decade of the nineties winds down, many public health nurses believe that this rich heritage is being forgotten, and that the rush to downsize government and control spending for health and illness services will inadvertently eliminate important community-based nursing services. On the other hand, nurses have some of the most flexible skills in public health, recognized as both providers of individual clinical care and as contributors to communitywide services. While it is too early to draw any firm conclusions, there is every reason to be optimistic that the skills and focus of public health nurses are very well suited to the challenges of public health and that their contributions will be sought rather than eliminated.

What Defines the Field?

The field of public health nursing can be distinguished from other areas of nursing practice by the combined impact of three foci: prevention, community, and systems. While none of these is unique to either nursing or public health, the combination is a particularly powerful one. Prevention is, of course, the historic defining feature of public health. As causal links and antecedents of disease have been understood, public health practitioners have taken steps to reshape exposure patterns, strengthen resistance, or eliminate causes of diseases. The earliest efforts were directed at infectious conditions, both before and after the introduction of protective immunizations and effective antibiotic treatment. More recently, prevention has extended to noninfectious diseases, such as cancer and heart disease, and to injury, both unintentional and intentional. The expanding science base for prevention practice has supported provision of services in a variety of settings (home, school, workplace, health clinic) using multiple media (brochures, audio and video tapes, games, drama) and multiple reinforcers (public policy on tobacco control being a prime example). Emerging approaches such as harm reduction (seeking to achieve at least some movement toward more healthful choices, even if full prevention of risk is not feasible) also play a part.

Some prevention activities, such as immunizations or prenatal care, are directly provided to specific individuals. Many others are provided to people at the population group or community level. In either case, public health is differentiated from the vast majority of health and illness care practice by the use of settings other than hospitals and doctors' offices as the site of intervention. Schools and work sites have already been mentioned; store-front clinics, homes, and shopping malls have also been used to ensure that services and messages are available to people at the times and places where the effort will have the greatest impact in promoting health. The term *community* may well be overused; the fact that a health-related service is outside the four walls of a hospital does not make it a community service. Changes in medical and nursing practice have meant that many procedures previously requiring a hospital operating room or nursing care unit are performed in clinics or homes. For someone thinking of public health, all activities are done in the context of community.

Community means more than place and may not occur in a single place. It also means relationship, whether one is considering an official geopolitical community, a neighborhood, or a community of affinity such as an advocacy or professional group. One widely used statement about public health in the United States[3] captures the importance of relationships in the vision of "healthy people in healthy communities." Supporting people to live healthy lives in their multiple relationships is a key part of public health nursing.

Related to the concept of community is that of systems, the notion that any one component of the community is tied in some way to all others, so that changes in any one component will lead sooner or later to some changes elsewhere. A focus on both prevention and community from a systems perspective pushes the practitioner to consider how the system relationships may be developed or strengthened or how illness-fostering, noncommunity system elements may be reduced. Working with this perspective means that any work with an individual can be the source of data regarding the functioning of systems within the community and lead to intervention at additional levels to promote healthy change. No one person can simultaneously work at all levels (individual, family, neighborhood, communitywide system), so that the system of workers collaborating to ensure that needed information flows among those performing different functions is an additional important part of the systems view.

Who Practices Public Health Nursing?

Most nurses, describing their field of study and practice, would include care for individuals and families and probably mention that a distinguishing feature is awareness of or attention to family impact on health and illness, and community impact on health or illness. This does not make all nurses public health nurses and neither does the site of practice. The nurses providing infusion therapy in the home may be doing no more public health practice than those doing the same acts in outpatient departments or inpatient units. The growing field of home health nursing has moved many nurses to new, mobile practices, but has not changed their focus.

Nor is public health nursing exclusively defined by the name on the employing agency door, though it is probable that the vast majority of public health nurses are employed by official public health agencies (local, regional, state, or federal).[a] Some community programs such as the not-for-profit community health centers and migrant health centers employ nurses to work with the community to improve health in ways that are clearly public health practice. And in areas where there are large numbers of individuals uninsured or lacking primary care, public health departments have hired large numbers of practitioners to provide personal care services. There is no indication that this care has automatically been given in ways that differ in content or focus from that provided in any other ambulatory care practice. Having said that, it is also important to say that many health department-based primary care programs are different in their attention to prevention, the special community needs of the populations seeking care, and the potential for building new, better systems of care and prevention.

Because of the myriad of entry routes to nursing practice, nurses with the same legal credential to practice may have widely differing education. Neither the associate degree nor diploma education include public health as a required curriculum component. Basic education about public health nursing practice is included in the baccalaureate curriculum, and some public health systems have attempted to reserve the job title "public health nurse" for baccalaureate graduates only. Whatever their entry education, nurses employed to work in public health agencies or other entities with a focus on public health and the community must master at least some content about population perspectives on health, epidemiology, health behavior, and environmental influences on health.

Advanced education for practice in communities is at least as confusing as entry-level education. Some public health nurses have studied in schools of public health, others in schools of nursing; some have degrees in both fields. As nursing has explored advanced practice, and health departments have increased their medical care-giving, public health nurses have obtained credentials as family and pediatric nurse practitioners and nurse-midwives. And as with entry-level education, the degrees and job titles alone do not identify whether the nurse is practicing public health nursing or not. The answer to that question must be sought in questions of focus and goal.

Given the issues identified above, it is no wonder that nurses in public health are concerned about improving their knowledge base. The statement about public health nursing cited above describes the practice of public health nursing as the process by which

1. The health and health care needs of a population are assessed to identify subpopulations, families, and individuals who would benefit from health promotion or who are at risk of illness, injury, disability, or premature death;
2. A plan for intervention is developed with the community to meet identified needs that takes into account available resources and the range of activities that contribute to health and the prevention of illness, injury, disability, and premature death;
3. The plan is implemented effectively, efficiently, and equitably;
4. Evaluations are conducted to determine the extent to which the interventions have an impact on the health status of individuals and the population;
5. The results of the process are used to influence and direct the current delivery of care.

To do this, any public health nurse would need to know, at least, the evaluation of individual health status, evaluation of community sys-

---

[a] *Because of the lack of clear definitions of public health positions and the minimal attention to public health within the overall health system, there is no good, recent enumeration of the public health workforce. Efforts now under way within the Bureau of Health Professions, Health Resources and Services Administration, U.S. Department of Health and Human Services should provide this needed data.*

tems, application of epidemiology and biostatistics, environmental health, and health systems. At the state and national level, public health nurses are reassessing what is known and taught in these areas and designing continuing education and on-the-job and academic preparation to ensure that both entering and currently employed public health nurses are prepared appropriately.[4]

As a framework for this education and reeducation, public health nurses are making increasing use of statements such as that of the Public Health Functions Steering Committee's enumeration of the essential services of public health. Beginning to make nursing-specific expansions of the basic listing assists the practitioner as well as the managers who employ them and the communities that benefit from their efforts understand their contributions. For example, in contributing to the essential service "monitor health status to identify community health problems," the public health nurse may contribute through developing population perspectives out of the cumulated individual observations from well-child encounters or senior hypertension control activities. To "mobilize community partnerships to identify and solve health problems," public health nurses may bring particular expertise in connecting disenfranchised groups (low-income mothers, immigrants, migrants, the homeless) with committees or task groups concerned about health or health-related issues.

What Are the Current Challenges?

The two most prominent challenges to public health nursing today are those associated with reinvention and reduction of governmental presence and the expansion of managed care, especially with Medicaid populations. These two often occur simultaneously, as the movement of care for publicly insured populations is moved to the private sector becomes a part of downsizing health agencies at the local level. However, they may occur separately, and are discussed individually.

A continuing feature of public life in the United States is concern that government has gotten "too big" and that a goal for all elected officials is to substantially reduce the presence of government. This is easily translated into a reduction in the size of governmental agencies, the major expense of which is usually the workforce. The most extreme instance of this may occur over the next 5 years, as the drive to reduce the federal deficit without major reduction in entitlement programs or defense would require a cut of 25 to 40 percent in all other activities. Public health programs and activities have never been designed as entitlements, that is, services to which people are ensured access by virtue of some identifying feature (e.g., Medicare for those over 65, Medicaid for those on Aid to Families with Dependent Children, Social Security to workers over 65). Each public health program is reauthorized and refunded year to year, or at best, in 5-year cycles. Few public health managers at any level of government have succeeded in presenting their programs as being exempt from cuts during recessions or from across-the-board reductions. Further, public health practitioners have generally failed to identify the conceptual basis of public health as being substantially different from the other "human service" programs with which they are often grouped organizationally. As welfare and other social services are reduced, assumptions are made that the need for public health is also diminishing. This is untrue, partly because people's health may be more threatened during periods when resources are low (as described above in the field model of health) and partly because all people are "clients" of public health agencies all of the time.

Public health nurses need to become more articulate in describing this *population focus* of public health and in making certain that their efforts are truly driven by epidemiology and an interest in community systems toward actions that will raise the level of health in the *whole community*. In the framework used by many quality improvement programs, this means not only looking for the worse health problems and reducing them, but looking at the average level of health and working to "raise the mean" of health for the whole population.

The provision of care to Medicaid populations is a substantial part of nursing activity in many health departments. This has been done with fee-for-service financing and driven by the difficulties that many Medicaid recipients have finding a primary care provider. Sometimes the care is very specialized, as in services for high-risk pregnant women and children; in other areas, it is general primary or comprehensive ambulatory care. As health maintenance organizations (HMOs) of various types have emerged in the private sector as an apparently successful approach to providing insured populations with care with a slower rate of cost increase, public purchasers of care have taken note and moved aggressively to use the same mechanisms. State after state has made managed care the major approach for Medicaid beneficiaries, citing not only the potential for cost savings, but the presumed advantage of establishing relationships with primary care providers. As these contracts have been written and patients are enrolled, there is less need for Medicaid-billed care in health departments.

These changes have a 2-fold impact on public health nurses. In some cases, their long-standing patients are being moved elsewhere for care, and the nurses are faced with decisions about marketing their services to managed care organizations as value-added staff members who can not only work with individuals but assist the managed care organization in developing a population focus on enrollees. To the extent that the HMO understands and values prevention and investment in improvements in the determinants of health, the addition of public health nurses to the staff will make sense and will allow an effective bridge between this new system and the long-established system of prevention and health promotion.

The second impact is often of greater concern, and that is the need for service capacity due to the continuing or rising numbers of the completely uninsured. Health departments have been a major source of primary care and prevention for these individuals, often supporting the services by quietly riding on the economic coat-tails of Medicaid or other special funding sources. A maternal-child health–focused public health nurse generating up to ⅔ or ¾ of salary costs through billable services may well be supported to invest the remaining ⅓ to ¼ of time in work with the uninsured, either providing community-based primary care or working on improved community health systems. Absent the Medicaid resource, the health department may be unable to find the resource to continue employing the nurse at even half time. Making the case for a community-funding base for this shift is an important challenge to public health nurses across the country. The challenge is to ask the correct question, which is "how will I ensure that care is available to those who lack it?", not "how can I be sure that I am still here to give the care?" It may be, in this case, that the most important impact that public health nurses will have is in assembling the data and framing options for the development of new services outside of the health department. Such a demonstration of the powerful contribution of nursing to the policy development process would indeed facilitate the continued contribution of public health nurses to the public's health.

Public health is by its nature the most interdisciplinary of practices. On a day-to-day or hour-to-hour basis, the activities of physicians, nurses, social workers, and sanitarians may appear identical. Yet each of these brings perspectives unique to a discipline, and each is important to the wide-ranging functions of public health. The challenges and opportunities of today are such that the public health nursing understanding of the health of individuals, families, and communities is essential to the accurate assessment of health concerns, the development of sound policy, and thus the assurance of continuing movement toward healthy people in healthy communities.

Family Planning Programs and Practices: An Epidemiological Viewpoint

Carl W. Tyler, Jr. • Herbert B. Peterson

▶ THE FAMILY PLANNING PROBLEM IN PUBLIC HEALTH

The World Health Organization (WHO) reports that an estimated 94 percent of the world's population lives in countries with policies that favor family planning. Despite these policies, five of every six couples of reproductive age do not use adequate measures of fertility regulation. Nonetheless, important advances have been made in family planning over the past three decades. As recently as the end of the 1960s, only four major countries in Africa and two in Latin America had official family planning policies. By the beginning of the 1980s, more than 80 percent of Africa's people and more than 90 percent of those in Latin America lived in countries that supported family planning programs.[1] Although family planning and the control of human fertility influence health and the quality of human life throughout the world as they never have before, the benefits from family planning services have yet to be fully realized. Some areas of family planning, birth prevention, and their effects on public health remain under careful scrutiny.

The rapid changes in family planning policies have led to similar changes in health programs and have presented health professionals with areas of responsibility with which many are not yet entirely comfortable. The first area involves human values. Another focuses on the need for scientific knowledge on personal fertility control. Although the elimination of disease and disability is accepted almost universally as the goal of health programs, the limitation of fertility is not accepted in the same way. We can agree that diseases such as smallpox, measles, and polio can and should be eliminated, but we clearly do not want to reduce fertility to zero. Nevertheless, what level is desirable or acceptable? What means should individuals and national policymakers be permitted to use to achieve this level? Although most societies limit fertility by some means, only recently has scientific information been found on the determinants of fertility and on the effectiveness and safety of methods for limiting fertility. These issues have become even more difficult to address in the presence three key contemporary world events: (*a*) the global epidemic of acquired immunodeficiency syndrome (AIDS); (*b*) the development of RU 486, an effective antiprogestational agent; and (*c*) worldwide concerns about side effects of widely used contraceptives, e.g., oral contraception and its possible relationship to breast cancer.

In this chapter, we identify some important issues related to family planning, health, and human values. After identifying the relevant basic values, discussing the practice of epidemiology in relationship to family planning, and reviewing the goals, policies, and laws related to family planning programs, we describe the effectiveness and safety of current methods of fertility control. Next, we focus on specific issues important to family planning, viz., teenage pregnancy, breast cancer and oral contraception, and AIDS. In closing we consider the factors that might influence personal decisions about family planning.

▶ FAMILY PLANNING AND HUMAN VALUES

We define family planning to be the voluntary use of methods and procedures intended to affect the number and timing of pregnancies. This definition includes all the proximate determinants of fertility, including age of a person at first sexual intercourse or marriage, postpartum lactation for spacing purposes, contraception, and sterilization. Induced abortion, although not a method of family planning by this definition, is widely used to influence the timing and number of births. This method will also be addressed in this chapter. Communities (and also states and nations) may select strategies that modify one or all these determinants to achieve their family planning goals.

Most human value systems respect life, place a high value on the family, are pronatalist, and have strong taboos and values related to sexuality and reproduction. Nonetheless, most of them have very little ethical tradition directly related to family planning and fertility control.

There are four major ethical justifications for making family planning a part of public policy and programs. Each is relevant to both community and individual decision-making, and none is based on any one system of values, religion, or philosophy. These four values, which are mentioned in the Preamble to the Constitution of the United States, are freedom, justice, general welfare, and security/survival.[2] The most acceptable policies might reflect all four. Controversy and debate surround family planning because of different opinions on the relative merits of these values and because some policies emphasize one value at the expense of another.

Freedom is identified in the U.S. Declaration of Independence as one of the "inalienable rights" of "life, liberty, and the pursuit of happiness." This goal provides one criterion for evaluating any public policies, including those dealing with family planning information and services. International documents establish a consensus that a right to family planning exists. In 1966, the United Nations General Assembly resolved that "the size of the family should be the free choice of each individual."[3] In 1974, a consensus of 136 countries meeting in Bucharest stated in the *World Population Plan of Action* that "all couples and individuals have the basic right . . . to decide freely and responsibility the number and spacing of their children" and went on to assert that these couples should exercise their rights in a way that takes account of the future needs of children and communities.[4] A decade later, in 1984 in Mexico City, the United Nations International Conference on Population reaffirmed the Bucharest plan of action but gave greater emphasis to child survival and primary health care.[5] Since the conference in Mexico City, new emphasis has been given to the study of the relation between birth intervals and child health by funding both organizations and researchers. In 1994 the conference, held in Cairo, Egypt, received the title "The International Conference on Population and Development," indicating the increased range of issues for discussion. For the first time, Vatican representatives attended. Human rights, most specifically those of women, received the greatest emphasis.

Justice means equality in law. Social justice requires mutual respect among members of society and nondiscrimination in relation to human life and worth. Distributive justice means reducing the differences in health and other social problems among people of different income levels, places of residence, and ethnic and cultural backgrounds. Distributive justice is the major rationale for public health programs in the United States. The objective of these programs is to reduce health problems among those lacking resources, skills, or motivation to use private health care services for preventing or resolving health problems.

General welfare involves two precepts related to family planning. The first is that regulating fertility is as important as controlling mortality and morbidity and is an essential component of personal, social, and economic development. General welfare also includes the health rationale for family planning, which can be described in several ways. The average potential number of live births per women in most societies is approximately 15.[6] A policy of limiting fertility to replacement levels or fewer benefits society by permitting existing resources to be distributed more equitably. If each couple had two children, 13 births would be prevented, as would 86 percent of the maternal and infant deaths that would occur at maximum fertility levels. Preventing these births would also permit a greater allocation of health resources per person and should, therefore, lead to further improvements in the quality of services provided to those children who are born. The specific methods for limiting fertility also influence the health rationale for adopting family planning.

Family planning can improve the health for women in their childbearing years and for their offspring. At least three approaches help achieve both health and family planning objectives: (*a*) postponing heterosexual activities for 5 to 10 years after reaching the age of potential childbearing, (*b*) breast-feeding for a lengthy interval, and (*c*) using birth control services provided by health professionals.

The final rationale related to family planning is security/survival. This issue relates both to the survival of individuals, families, and communities, and to the definition of the onset of life. The former includes concerns regarding maternal and infant welfare. The latter concerns the morality at the individual level of induced abortion and morality at the community level of having large families. The onset of human life has been variously defined as conception, quickening, birth, or viability. The definition one chooses affects one's perception of the morality of induced abortion.

► EPIDEMIOLOGY AND ITS APPLICATION TO FAMILY PLANNING

Family planning became part of everyday life around the world in a very short time. Despite this rapid change, epidemiologists have made important and timely contributions to scientific knowledge regarding the effectiveness, safety, and acceptability of family planning programs and birth prevention technology. The fundamental concepts of epidemiology and its practice apply as effectively in fertility and family planning methods and services as they can in other health problems and programs. Studies of oral contraception, intrauterine devices,[8] abortion,[9] and sterilization[10] all confirm this observation.

Definition of Epidemiology Applied to Family Planning

The definition of epidemiology has two fundamental elements: it is "the study of the distribution and determinants of health related states and events in populations and the application of this study to the control of health problems."[11] Epidemiology is, therefore, the scientific basis of and essential to the practice of public health and preventive medicine. As such, it can be applied to family planning and to family planning programs. Like all other fields of public health, the results of epidemiological studies in family planning must meet the criteria of direct, or causal, association, and those associations must not be because of chance, bias, or confounding.

Epidemiology As a Basis for Action

The basic tasks of epidemiological practice are (*a*) public health surveillance, (*b*) investigation, (*c*) analysis, and (*d*) evaluation. Each of these tasks can be applied to the problems of family planning. Surveillance, for instance, has documented changes in the practice of induced abortion in the United States.[12] Epidemiological investigations have shown that use of intrauterine contraception devices may be related to clusters of septic spontaneous abortion[13] and that oral contraceptive use protects against ovarian cancer.[14] Epidemiological analysis showed a causal association between oral contraceptive use and benign liver tumors.[15] Epidemiological evaluation showed the relative benefits and hazards of different kinds of intrauterine contraceptive devices[16] and evaluated the effects of community programs on fertility change.[17]

► FAMILY PLANNING PROGRAMS

Goals

The goals of national family planning programs reflect a country's aspirations. In some cases, these aspirations are conceived as a national need for improved economic development, improved general welfare, or enhanced rights for individuals. Beginning in the early 1960s, several Asian nations sought to improve their economic development.[18] Programs in Latin America, on the other hand, sought to improve the health of mothers and children. In Chile, for example, epidemiological studies of abortion emphasized the burden that this illegal practice placed, not only on the health of women, but on the nationalized health and hospital service system.[19] A contraceptive service program, therefore, became acceptable because it was viewed as a campaign against abortion. The few programs based on national policies in Africa sought to improve the health of mothers and children by improved child spacing.[20] The national family planning program in the United States seeks primarily to prevent unintended pregnancies.[21,22] By 1980, national goals to reduce population growth and to improve the health of women and children, or both, were recognized as crucial in nearly every country worldwide. Moreover, most nations agreed that couples and individuals had the right to control their own fertility.[22]

The United States set specific national health objectives to be achieved by 1990 and developed new objectives for the year 2000. The national objective that addresses family planning has specific components for preventing teenage pregnancies, reducing sexual activity, and increasing use of effective contraceptives among young and unmarried individuals.[21,23]

Policy and Law

How are these goals carried out regarding national policies and laws? Both social customs and family planning practices can influence fertility. Recognizing the importance of reducing the years during which an individual is at risk of pregnancy, many Asian countries have passed laws prohibiting child marriage and establishing a minimum age of wedlock (ranging from 12 to 25 years).[24] Paradoxically, most nations have overlooked how breast-feeding improves infant nutrition and curbs on fertility. They do not, therefore, have laws or policies that promote breast-feeding.

Historically, many countries, including the United States, have had laws that restrict the use of most approaches to fertility control, i.e., contraception, abortion, and sterilization. These restrictions on fertility control exist because of the complex deliberations intrinsic to the legislative processes. They are essential to developing laws that serve society's current needs and values. Legislators have great difficulty developing laws at a pace that matches technologic change.

The rapid global increase in the use of surgical sterilization has led to the enactment of legislation influencing its availability. Although some countries specifically permit voluntary surgical sterilization, the larger number of countries permitted this form of fertility control to be legal simply because no law prohibited it. Nonetheless, even where voluntary surgical sterilization is permitted, some legal constraints still exist. Among them are requirements for a minimum age, the establishment of specific medical indications, authorization by a spouse, or a minimum number of living children.

The legal status of voluntary induced abortion has changed substantially during the past 30 years and is likely to be further modified in the future. In 1959, the American Law Institute proposed a model penal code that justified abortion on the following grounds: (*a*) the risk of continuing pregnancy to the life, the physical, or the mental health of the women; (*b*) the likely occurrence of serious physical or mental impairment of a child born of the pregnancy; (*c*) pregnancy resulting from incest; (*d*) pregnancy resulting from rape.[25] Subsequently, as states in the United States and other countries enacted laws that permitted abortion, both followed the guidance of the American Law Institute and added additional legal grounds for the voluntary interruption of pregnancy. These grounds include the effects of childbirth on the health and welfare of the woman, her existing children, and the rest of the family; jeopardy to the social position of the woman or her family; failure of routinely used contraception; and/or on request (usually during the first trimester of pregnancy) of the pregnant woman. Some legislative changes included special constraints such as a minimum age, a minimum period of residence in the area of jurisdiction, or a maximum duration of pregnancy.[26]

Except in China, recent laws permitting abortions require that physicians carry out the procedure. Most legislation requires that the procedure be done in medically approved facilities such as hospitals or clinics. Moreover, these institutions may have additional requirements. Among them are, for example, concurrence by another physician or a committee decision. In addition, consent statements, or clauses that concern individuals who work in health facilities, addressing the voluntary nature of the procedure are required in some clinical centers.

In the United States, judicial action has led to important changes. In 1973, the cases of *Doe v. Bolton* and *Roe v. Wade* led to nationwide changes in the performance of legal abortion.[27] Fifteen years later, the United States Supreme Court decision in *Webster v. Reproductive Health* limited this practice. Further decisions are expected to continue this general trend. However, some cases have been settled by the disputants before reaching the United States Supreme Court. Moreover, advocates of the right to choose abortion may seek legislated rather than judicial action in support of their position.[28]

Four fundamental legal principals can be used in evaluating abortion laws and their related human values. The first is the right to privacy. Decisions related to fertility regulation are generally accepted to be private matters and not subject to the control of other individuals. This right of privacy conflicts with the countervailing argument that the fetus has its own right to exist. The second principle is necessity; that is, individuals who do abortions to preserve the life or health of others should not have to fear criminal liability. Third, laws should be applied equally. If only wealthy women can evade the limitations on the practice of abortion, then laws should be changed to permit poor women access to the same service. Fourth, the physician must act in the health interests of individual patients. The WHO defines health as a state of complete physical, mental, and social wellbeing, not merely the absence of disease or infirmity. The 1973 decisions made by the United States Supreme Court in *Roe v. Wade* and *Doe v. Bolton* relied on this WHO definition of health.[27]

Education on reproductive health and family planning, both formal and informal, is an essential component of any program for preventing unintended pregnancies. A WHO meeting on this subject declared that appropriate education on reproductive health for the public has the highest priority because of its importance in prevention and its potential influence on the largest possible number of people.[29] This concept received reinforcement in the recommendations that resulted from the International Conference on Population held in Mexico City in 1984.

Preventing pregnancy among teenagers is a high priority in many countries throughout the world, including the United States. If sexually active adolescents are to prevent pregnancies, then access to safe, effective fertility control must be permitted. In some countries, however, contraceptives may be distributed legally only to married persons.[24] In the United States notifying parents when adolescents plan to use contraceptive services is a topic of public debate. Right now, adolescents face serious problems in finding the information and skills needed to defer parenting.

Services and Methods

Family planning services may be provided through hospitals, clinics, individual health professionals, or commercial facilities such as drug stores. The services may include temporary contraception or permanent surgical sterilization. In considering services and methods of fertility control, both service providers and individuals needing service are influenced by certain key facts. These facts include the characteristics of service providers (for example, the gender of the examining physician) and facilities (for example, hospitals, public clinics, or private physician offices). In addition, they also include the effectiveness, prevalence, popularity, perceived risk, and scientific evidence for the safe use of each approach to limiting fertility.

Contraception

Widespread public service programs that enable individuals and couples to limit childbearing are relatively recent. In the mid-1930s, several states began to provide limited contraceptive counseling and services for poor women. In July 1969, President Nixon proposed creating a federal program to help poor women have the same access to effective contraceptive methods as the affluent. The legislation supporting that proposal, Title X of the Public Health Service Act, was passed in 1970. In 1991, 4.2 million women received family planning services at clinics receiving support under this legislation.[30]

Overall, where do women obtain family planning services? The answer depends heavily on income. Seventy-seven percent of women with family incomes that are one and one-half times the established level of poverty who make a family planning visit are more likely to see a private physician compared with 53 percent of lower income women. Teenagers are less likely to visit a private physician (48 percent) for family planning. By contrast, family planning clinic patients are largely poor; 83 percent have incomes below the established level of poverty. Twenty-six percent of family planning clinic patients are black and 11 percent are Hispanic.[31]

In the United States family planning services are provided primarily by physicians, nurse family planning practitioners, and pharmacists. In other countries, successful programs have marketed contraception through the commercial sector with appropriate advertising and distributed contraceptives through community-based family planning programs. Research shows that in at least one region—the United States-Mexico border region—most Mexican Americans and Anglos would accept family planning services from medically trained persons who are not physicians. Moreover, roughly half would accept them from trained nonmedical persons.[32]

Oral Contraception

Use. Oral contraception, the pill, is a popular, highly effective, and for most women, a safe method of contraception. An estimated 10.7 million U.S. women were using the pill in 1988, compared with 8.4 million in 1982.[33] Pills are the most popular method of birth control for never-married women and for all women less than 25 years old.

Effectiveness. The pill is a highly effective method of temporary contraception; currently available preparations containing both estrogen and progestin have an efficacy approaching 100 percent. Because they must be used consistently and correctly, however, the actual failure rate for combined (estrogen-progestin) pills is about 3 percent (Fig. 71-4).[34]

Progestin only, or so-called "mini-pills," may be less effective than pills that combine both progestin and estrogen because ovulation is not prevented as often. Studies on the efficacy of the mini-pill are less comprehensive than those of combined pills, and reliable estimates of efficacy are, therefore, lacking. Nevertheless, mini-pills are considered highly effective.[34]

Complications. The short- and long-term health effects of oral contraceptives have been studied more thoroughly than those of any other drugs currently prescribed. On balance, most such studies show that the pill is safe for most women. In fact, studies attempting to identify potentially harmful effects of oral contraceptives have documented important noncontraceptive health benefits. Oral contraceptive users are less likely to be hospitalized for pelvic inflammatory disease (PID), ectopic pregnancy, benign breast disease, and functional ovarian cysts. They are also less likely to have iron deficiency anemia, and they may

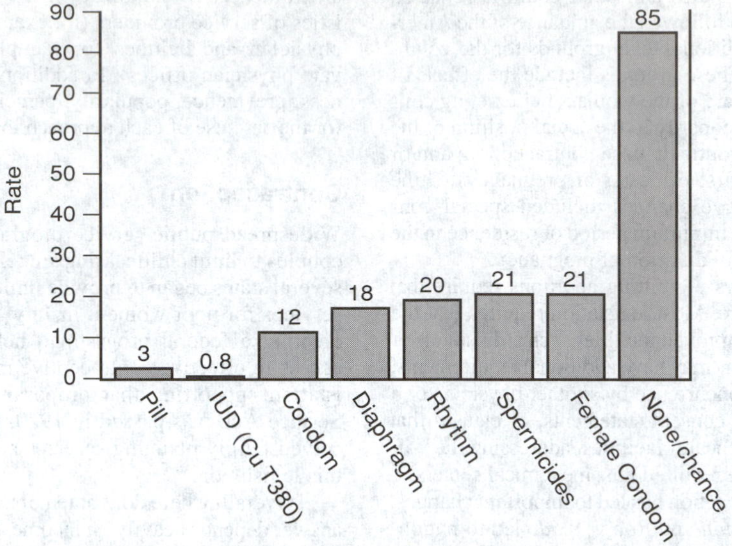

Figure 71-4. Typical unintended pregnancy rate during the first year of use by contraceptive method used in the United States. Rate is pregnancies per 100 women. (From Hatcher RA, Trussell J, Stewart F, et al: Contraceptive Technology. 16th ed. New York: Irvington Publishers, 1979, pp 637–653.)

be less likely to have uterine fibroids.[35] Finally, oral contraceptives have been shown to protect against both endometrial and ovarian cancer.[14,36] (Concerns about a potentially positive relationship between pill use and breast cancer are sufficiently controversial that this topic will be discussed in a separate section later in this chapter.)

Nonetheless, the pill is not without risk. Oral contraceptive use has been clearly associated with an increased risk of myocardial infarction, venous thrombosis, and stroke.[35] The increased risk is largely, but not exclusively, found among older women who smoke (Table 71-4).[37] Most studies report that past users have no increased risk; the increased risk appears attributable to current oral contraceptive use. Furthermore, the reported risk for cardiovascular diseases associated with oral contraceptive use may be overestimated because most reports include estimates based, in part, on use of oral contraceptive formulations no longer available. In 1988, the marketing of preparations containing more than 50 μg of estrogen was phased out because of a ruling by the U.S. Food and Drug Administration's Fertility and Maternal Health Drugs Advisory Committee. This committee concluded that such preparations did not have sufficient clinical advantage to warrant continued distribution. Only limited data are available to determine the risks associated with oral contraceptives that are currently used. Data regarding whether pills containing less than 50 μg carry a reduced risk of venous thromboembolism are contradictory. Recent reports from the Group Health Cooperative of Puget Sound[38] and the Oxford Family Planning Association[39] suggest that oral contraceptives now in use pose a lower risk of myocardial infarction than those previously studied. In the former report, no deaths from cardiovascular disease were identified in the period 1977 to 1981 after approximately 55,000 women-years of oral contraceptive use. In the latter report, no cases of myocardial infarction and only one case of angina were reported among women using oral contraceptives containing less than 50 μg of estrogen.

Gallbladder disease and rare, benign liver tumors are also occasionally associated with taking the pill. There is controversy regarding the relationship between pill use and development of malignant melanoma[40] and liver cancer (hepatocellular carcinoma).[41,42] Both tumors are rare in the United States, but any relationship between oral contraceptive use and malignant liver tumors could be important in developing countries where liver malignancies are more common.

The relationship between pill use and cervical cancer continues to be controversial. This is caused, in part, because bias related to sexual behavior complicates the study of this association. One recent report from a study in Costa Rica[43] has also highlighted the importance of detection bias in the study of this relationship. In this report from

TABLE 71-4. CURRENT USE OF ORAL CONTRACEPTIVES (OCs), CIGARETTE SMOKING, AND RISK OF MYOCARDIAL INFARCTION (MI)

		MIs per 100,000 Women per Year		MIs per 100,000 Current OC Users per Year	
Age (yr)	*Cigarettes per day*	*OC Users*	*Nonusers*	*Relative Risk*[a]	*Attributable Risk*
30–39	All women	11	4	3	7
	0–14	6	2	3	4
	15+	30	11	4	19
40–44	All women	89	22	4	67
	0–14	47	12	4	35
	15+	246	61	4	185

From Lee NC, Peterson HB, Chu SY: The health effects of contraception. In Parnell A (ed): Contraceptive Use and Controlled Fertility: Health Issues for Women and Children—Background Papers. Washington, DC: National Academy Press, 1989.
[a] Relative risk of MI for OC users compared with that for nonusers.

Costa Rica, when the effects of sexual activity were adjusted for statistically controlled, oral contraceptive users had no increased risk of cervical cancer. Although there was an increased risk of cervical carcinoma in situ, the risk was limited to those women in whom oral contraceptive use was strongly linked to Pap smear screening. This suggests that the finding may result from bias that is due to the way information was obtained on subjects with cancer in situ.

The United States Food and Drug Administration (FDA) considers the following conditions as absolute contraindications to oral contraceptive use: (*a*) thrombophlebitis or thromboembolic disorders; (*b*) a history of deep vein thrombophlebitis or thromboembolic disorders; (*c*) cerebrovascular or coronary artery disease; (*d*) known or suspected cancer of the breast; (*e*) known or suspected estrogen-dependent neoplasia; (*f*) undiagnosed, abnormal genital bleeding; (*g*) pregnancy; and (*h*) benign or malignant liver tumors that developed during the use of oral contraceptives or other estrogen preparations. Oral contraceptives are not usually prescribed for women who have not established a regular menstrual pattern, and estrogen-containing pills are not prescribed for women during the first 6 weeks that they are breast-feeding an infant.[44] Although no absolute upper age restriction for use has been determined, women over the age of 40 have generally been discouraged from using oral contraceptives. Recently, this age limit has been questioned. The American College of Obstetricians and Gynecologists now recommends that healthy, nonsmoking women ages 35 to 44 years may continue using oral contraceptives if they do not wish to or are unable to use another reversible method or undergo surgical sterilization.[45]

Intrauterine Devices

Use. Intrauterine contraceptive devices (IUDs) are an effective, safe method of birth control for most women. In 1982, an estimated 2.2 million women were wearing IUDs in the United States, but by 1988, only 0.7 million women were using them.[33] In other countries such as China, the IUD is the most popular form of contraception.[37] In the late 1980s, manufacturers voluntarily stopped the sale of most IUDs in the United States. Sales were stopped for marketing reasons largely attributable to the cost of litigating many lawsuits brought against manufacturers. Most such lawsuits allege that IUD use resulted in pelvic infection or infertility.[46] In 1989, a new copper IUD, the Copper T380A, was introduced to U.S. markets.

Effectiveness. The IUD is highly effective, with method failure rates of about 3 percent per year (Fig. 71-4). The user-effectiveness rate, including the risk of undetected IUD expulsion, is higher, at about 6 percent per year.

Complications. Unlike oral contraceptives, IUDs have no documented noncontraceptive health benefits. Although pregnancy rates are low for IUD users, women who do become pregnant have a greater risk of ectopic pregnancy and spontaneous, septic abortion of an intrauterine pregnancy.[47] If the IUD is removed as soon as the pregnancy is diagnosed, most cases of septic abortion can be prevented.

In particular, IUDs have been associated with an increased risk of PID. The Dalkon Shield IUD, which is no longer available, has been associated with a high risk of PID.[48] Modern IUDs, including the Copper T380A—which is currently the most widely used IUD in the United States—carry low risks of PID among women at low risk of sexually transmitted diseases (STDs). One large case-control study found that IUD users in some mutually monogamous sexual relationships had little or no increased risk of PID associated with IUD use[48] and another study found that IUD users who reported having only one sexual partner had no increased risk of tubal infertility.[37] Recently the WHO summarized data from 12 randomized studies and one nonrandomized study and concluded that the data suggest that IUD users selected for low risk of STD have little, if any, excess risk of PID. The overall rate of PID occurrence among 22,903 IUD insertions was 1.6 cases per 1,000 women-years of use. The risk of PID was highest (by greater than 6-fold) during the first 20 days after insertion; after that time, the risk of PID was consistently low for up to 8 years of use.[49] Research is under way to determine whether the use of prophylactic antibiotics at IUD insertion will reduce the risk of PID attributable to insertion. Taken together, available data suggest that, among women at low risk for STD, the risk of PID associated with IUD use is low and primarily related to the time of insertion.[50]

Wearing an IUD is absolutely contraindicated for women with active pelvic infection, including known or suspected gonorrheal infection, or for those with uterine or cervical malignancy. Women with abnormal uterine bleeding, dysmenorrhea, distortions or congenital malformations of the uterine cavity, or impaired resistance to infection should not use IUDs. Uterine perforation is more likely to occur when an IUD is inserted into the uterus of a lactating woman.[44]

Traditional Methods

The condom, vaginal diaphragm, and spermicidal creams, foams, jellies, and suppositories are the traditional contraceptive methods in the United States. Newer related methods include the cervical cap and the female condom. These methods require substantial user motivation and are likely influenced by user experience and skill at use.

Use. Traditional contraceptive methods have been used by millions of American couples, despite the widespread prevalence of the pill and IUD. Condoms were used by approximately 3.6 million United States couples in 1982; this number increased to 5.1 million (a 41 percent increase) in 1988.[33] The role of condoms for prevention of human immunodeficiency virus and other sexually transmitted diseases has likely led to this increased prevalence of use. In the United States during 1982, diaphragms were used by 1.9 million and spermicides by 1.5 million women; there were slight decreases in use in 1988.[33] Newly developed methods similar to the traditional methods include cervical caps and female condoms. The female condom was approved by the FDA in 1993 for protection against pregnancy and STDs. These approaches to fertility control are used less frequently now than are the more established traditional methods.

Effectiveness. Failure rates will be largely influenced by user determinants. Of the traditional methods, the condom is the most effective when used consistently and correctly. The estimated user failure rate for condoms in the first year is 12 percent (Fig. 71-4). The diaphragm (used with spermicides), vaginal spermicide (alone), and the female condom have a one and a half to two times greater risk of unintended pregnancy compared with that of the condom.

Complications. The risks associated with use of traditional contraceptives include the risk of unintended pregnancy and the usual minor and specific complaints associated with the method. These complaints include vaginal irritation by spermicidal jelly, discomfort from a poorly positioned diaphragm, or local response to condom lubricant. In addition, diaphragm users have a 2- to 3-fold increased risk of urinary tract infections compared with women who do not use contraceptives.[37] Although one report raised concern about a possible positive relationship between spermicide and the risk of congenital defects, several larger and better designed studies failed to confirm any association.[37] Both sponge and diaphragm users have a relative increased risk of toxic shock syndrome.[51] Because toxic shock syndrome is an extremely rare disease, however, the absolute risk associated with sponge or diaphragm use is small. Women immediately postpartum and women who have had toxic shock syndrome should not use either the sponge or diaphragm, and neither the sponge nor diaphragm should be left in the vagina for more than 30 hours.[52]

Rhythm and Fertility Awareness

Use. Rhythm and fertility awareness, or natural family planning methods, are not widely used in the United States, although they are more prevalent in other countries. Fewer than a million couples used these methods in the United States in 1988.[33]

TABLE 71-5. APPROVED REGIMENS USING ORAL CONTRACEPTIVES FOR EMERGENCY CONTRACEPTION

Trade Name	Formulation	Number of Pills Taken with Each Dose
Ovral	0.05 mg of ethinyl estradiol 0.05 mg of norgestrel	2
Lo-Ovral	0.03 mg of ethinyl estradiol 0.30 mg of norgestrel	4
Nordette	0.03 mg of ethinyl estradiol 0.15 mg of levonorgestrel	4
Levlen	0.03 mg of ethinyl estradiol 0.15 mg of levonorgestrel	4
Triphasil	(Yellow pills only) 0.03 mg of ethinyl estradiol 0.125 mg of levonorgestrel	4
Trilevlen	(Yellow pills only) 0.03 mg of ethinyl estradiol 0.125 mg of levonorgestrel	4

Adapted from American College of Obstetricians and Gynecologists: Emergency Oral Contraception. ACOG Practice Pattern No. 3, 1996.

Effectiveness. The reported method failure rates for periodic abstinence are 2 percent, but the user failure rate is 18 percent; the method failure rate for withdrawal is 10 percent, and the user failure rate is 20 percent. Clearly, methods of natural family planning depend largely on user determinants, such as motivation and skill.

Complications. Other than unintended pregnancy, which occurs more frequently than with most other methods mentioned thus far, no adverse health effects are associated with these methods.

Emergency Contraception

In 1997, the FDA determined that oral contraceptives are safe and effective for emergency contraceptive use. Likewise, in 1996, the American College of Obstetricians and Gynecologists (ACOG) determined that there was good evidence to support the offering of emergency contraception. Moreover, appropriate regimens will be at least 75 percent effective in preventing pregnancies that would otherwise have occurred.[53,54] Emergency contraception should be taken within 72 hours of unprotected intercourse. Approved regimens for emergency use of oral contraceptives are listed in Table 71-5. Nausea occurs in 30 to 66 percent of patients using emergency contraception; nausea may be reduced when antiemetics are administered 1 hour before the dose.[53]

Injectable and Implantable Hormonal Progestins

In 1990, the FDA approved an implant for sustained release of the progestin levonorgestrel (marketed in the United States as Norplant). The implant is highly effective for pregnancy prevention and is approved for 5 years of use. Since compliance during use plays no discernable role, the typical and perfect use failure rates are estimated to be the same at 0.09 percent for the first year of use.[34] Although the risk of pregnancy may increase slightly by the fifth year of use,[55] the implant remains approximately as effective as tubal sterilization as measured by the 5-year cumulative probability of pregnancy. Most women using the implant will experience menstrual cycle disturbances; some will also experience weight gain, breast tenderness, and headaches. Women discontinuing use of the levonorgestrel implant will experience a prompt return to fertility.

In 1992, the FDA approved use of injectable depo-medroxyprogesterone acetate (DMPA) (marketed in the United States as Depo-Provera). DMPA 150 mg, injected every 3 months, provides a high degree of protection from pregnancy—similar to that seen for the levonorgestrel implant and tubal sterilization. As with the implant, the main side effects are menstrual disturbances. While menstrual disturbances vary among implant users, DMPA users may become amenorrheic over time.[55] Although menstrual irregularities may be bothersome and are a frequent reason for discontinuation of implant and DMPA use, the irregularities are generally not associated with increased blood loss.[55] Besides menstrual disturbances, most DMPA users experience some weight gain; some have breast tenderness, and headaches have also been reported. In addition, a reversible loss of bone density during DMPA use has been reported.[56] In contrast to the implant, there is a delayed return to fertility with discontinuation of DMPA use. It has been estimated that up to 18 months delay in return to fertility can occur.[55]

Findings among beagle dogs led to concerns regarding the possibility that use of DMPA may increase breast cancer risk. However, a pooled analysis of data from the World Health Organization and from New Zealand[57] is largely reassuring. Overall, women who ever used DMPA had similar breast cancer risks as women who never used DMPA (relative risk 1.1; 95 percent confidence interval 0.97 to 1.4). However, the pattern of use made a difference; recent users of DMPA (use within 5 years) had an increased risk of breast cancer diagnosis, while past users (use more than 5 years previously) had no increased use. This distinction between recent and past users is similar to that seen for oral contraceptive use and breast cancer risk. The risk for recent DMPA users was similar for women having one injection or many injections. This argues for the possibility that DMPA users were more likely either to be under medical surveillance and to have existing tumors diagnosed. Alternatively, they might have accelerated growth in previous tumors, or they may have had enhancement of the late stages of tumor promotion.

Breast-Feeding

Breast-feeding is described as "nature's contraceptive," and it is asserted that on a worldwide scale more births are prevented by breast-feeding than by any other method of contraception. One relatively isolated society that has no other practices that limit fertility, such as delaying the age of marriage or having a taboo against intercourse during lactation, has breast-feeding as one of its most important means of limiting fertility. These people have an average completed family size of 4.7 children and an average birth interval of 4.1 years. Their use of breast-feeding differs, however, from practices in the Western world in that the mother and infant are together throughout the day and night. The infant suckles frequently (on average four times per hour) for brief intervals when being carried about by the mother during the day and while the mother is sleeping at night.[58] Because breast-feeding in the United States is a relatively infrequent practice, controlling fertility while lactating becomes a problem of choosing the right contraceptive during the time that a mother is breast-feeding her infant. Since oral contraceptives with estrogen suppress lactation, their use should be deferred until either lactation is well established (usually until the infant is 6 weeks old and gaining weight) or another method is chosen. Traditional contraceptives, progestational agents, intrauterine devices, and surgical sterilization do not inhibit lactation.

Sterilization

Surgical sterilization is estimated to be the most prevalent form of contraception in the world today. Globally, more than 100 million couples are using this form of birth control; an estimated 95 million women have undergone tubal sterilization—making it the most widely used contraceptive method in the world.[59] China, India, and the United States have the highest estimated numbers of sterilized couples. In 1988, an estimated 47 percent of United States women ages 35 to 44 were relying on surgical sterilization (including vasectomy of the spouse) for fertility control.[33]

Female Sterilization

Use. The prevalence of tubal sterilization in the United States increased dramatically during the 1970s. The number of tubal sterilizations performed in hospitals increased from approximately 200,000 in 1970 to approximately 702,000 in 1977. Thereafter, the number of procedures done in hospitals began to decline.[60,61]

This decline was at least in part attributable to an increased performance of tubal sterilization in out-of-hospital facilities. Because systematic national surveillance of outpatient tubal sterilization has not been conducted, we cannot accurately assess trends in outpatient tubal sterilization over time. A recent report, however, estimates that, in 1987, 640,000 tubal sterilizations were done in the United States, and an estimated 33 percent of these were performed out-of-hospital.[62]

The large number of tubal sterilizations continuing to be done in the United States is particularly remarkable given that the number of reproductive-age women who can bear children (and thus are candidates for tubal sterilization) is reduced by the practice of hysterectomy and also by tubal sterilization. About one of every three United States women will undergo a hysterectomy by the time she is 60 years old.[63] The prevalence rate for tubal sterilization in 1978 was adjusted for cumulative prevalences of hysterectomy and tubal sterilization among women of reproductive age in the United States. The corrected sterilization rates were appreciably higher than the uncorrected rates, particularly among older women.[64]

Effectiveness. Findings from the U.S. Collaborative Review of Sterilization—a large U.S. multicenter cohort study—show that, although tubal sterilization is highly effective, pregnancy after tubal sterilization occurs more often than previously thought.[65] A total of 10,685 women undergoing tubal sterilization was enrolled from medical centers in nine U.S. cities and followed for up to 14 years after sterilization. The six most popular methods of tubal sterilization were evaluated. The 10-year cumulative probability of pregnancy was highest among women having sterilization by clip application (36.5 per 1,000 procedures) and lowest after procedures with unipolar coagulation (7.5 per 1,000 procedures) and postpartum partial salpingectomy (7.5 per 1,000 procedures). Women sterilized at a young age (age 18 to 27) were 2.7 times as likely to become pregnant as women sterilized at older ages (age 34 to 44). This may be caused by younger women being more fecund and remaining fecund for a longer period than older women. Among women sterilized at a young age, the 10-year cumulative probability of pregnancy was nearly 5.0 percent with two methods (bipolar coagulation at 54.3/1,000 and clip application at 52.1/1,000).

One of the most remarkable findings of the U.S. Collaborative Review of Sterilization was that pregnancies may occur many years after sterilization. Moreover, the further removed from sterilization, the more likely the pregnancy is to be ectopic.[66] Among the cohort of 10,685 women, the 10-year cumulative probability of ectopic pregnancy for all methods combined was 7.3 per 1,000 procedures. The probability of ectopic pregnancy varied substantially by method among women sterilized at a young age. The cumulative probability of ectopic pregnancy among women sterilized by bipolar coagulation before age 30 was 27 times greater than that for women sterilized by postpartum partial salpingectomy before age 30 (31.9 versus 1.2 per 1,000 procedures). The proportion of pregnancies that were ectopic ranged from 65 percent (bipolar coagulation) to 15 percent (clip application). The risk that a pregnancy will be an ectopic gestation is sufficiently great, no matter what method of sterilization was used, that the possibility of ectopic pregnancy should be carefully evaluated as soon as feasible. Further, women of childbearing age who have signs or symptoms of ectopic pregnancy should be evaluated even if they had a tubal sterilization in the distant past.

Complications. The short-term safety of tubal sterilization, which has been extensively studied, shows that the risk of dying from tubal sterilization in the United States is estimated to be one to two deaths per 100,000 procedures.[67] Complications from general anesthesia cause most deaths attributable to sterilization. Hemorrhage, usually associated with abdominal penetration for laparoscopy, and infection, particularly associated with thermal bowel injury following unipolar electrocoagulation, are other important causes.[68] Although case-fatality rates in developing countries have been reported to be higher than those in the United States, the major causes of death are similar. For example, in Bangladesh a case-fatality rate of 19 per 100,000 tubal sterilizations was identified in 1982, and complications of anesthesia were also the leading causes of death; however, in this instance, oversedation with narcotic analgesics during local anesthesia was the problem.[69] A follow-up study revealed that the case-fatality rate dropped dramatically after recommendations for lower doses of analgesics and larger doses of local anesthetics.[70]

Major morbidity from tubal sterilization is also uncommon. In the World Health Organization's Multinational Study, approximately 1,600 women were randomly assigned to be sterilized by either minilaparotomy (i.e., abdominal entry via a 2- to 5-cm incision) or laparoscopy (i.e., insertion of a surgical endoscope through a 1-cm subumbilical incision). Major complications occurred in 1.5 percent of approximately 800 women who underwent minilaparotomy and 0.9 percent of approximately 800 women who underwent laparoscopy using electrocoagulation.[71] A multicenter follow-up study of laparoscopic tubal sterilization in the United States revealed that 1.7 percent of women had at least one of six intraoperative or postoperative complications.[72] The most frequent (1.1 percent) was unintended major surgery that sometimes occurred because of incidental pathology identified during laparoscopy or because of technical limitations of laparoscopy, not because of procedural complications per se. In that study the risk of complications increased at least 2-fold because of the following factors: obesity, pulmonary disease, diabetes mellitus, previous abdominal or pelvic surgery, or a history of pelvic inflammatory disease.

Although major complication rates are generally reported as less than 2 percent, these rates, nevertheless, indicate that sterilization-attributable complications can and do result in serious injury. The likelihood of serious injury apparently varies by surgical approach and method of tubal occlusion. Most minilaparotomy complications are not serious; minor bleeding, minor wound infections, and uterine perforations are the most frequently reported.[59]

By contrast, complications of laparoscopy are more likely to be life-threatening. Although rare, thermal bowel injuries may result during tubal occlusion by electrocoagulation. In addition, major vessel injury or viscus perforation may result from abdominal penetration before insertion of the laparoscope.[72] When such complications occur, early diagnosis and intervention can be critical for a patient's survival.

The long-term safety and acceptability of tubal sterilization are less completely studied, but recently published reports are mostly reassuring, although a longer period of follow-up will be needed. The existence of a so-called "postubal syndrome" has been debated since the early 1950s. The debate began when menstrual disturbances were reported at varying intervals after sterilization. Most recent data suggest that such changes are not likely attributable to sterilization per se, but to other factors, e.g., cessation of oral contraceptive use. Although studies that provide the most reassurance are based on only 1 to 2 years of poststerilization follow-up, two studies[73,74] with longer follow-up were less encouraging. Thus, an answer to the question of whether a "postubal syndrome" exists must await further studies with long-term follow-up.

Tubal sterilization and hysterectomy are both common surgical procedures. Tubal sterilization could potentially increase the risk of subsequent hysterectomy by at least three possible mechanisms: (*a*) the postubal syndrome, if real, may result in menstrual disturbances managed by hysterectomy; (*b*) the perception that the postubal syndrome exists may encourage the use of hysterectomy for managing poststerilization menstrual disturbances even if they are not attributable to sterilization per se; and (*c*) once a woman is sterilized, she or her physician may more quickly resort to surgical management of a gynecologic problem. A cohort study in the United Kingdom, however, identified no increase among sterilized women in hospital referrals for hysterectomy at 3 and 6 years after tubal sterilization compared with wives of men who had vasectomies.[73] By contrast, a population-based study in Canada found an increased likelihood of subsequent hysterectomy limited to women undergoing tubal sterilization at ages 25 to 29.[75] Beginning with a 2-year follow-up and increasing for up to 9 years, that group had a 60 percent statistically significant increased risk of subsequent hysterectomy.

Most data suggest that women are satisfied with their decisions to undergo tubal sterilizations; the range of estimated dissatisfaction across studies varies widely, however, from 2 to 13 percent.[59] This range likely reflects, to some extent, variations of definitions of regret used for study. For example, a survey of United States women found that 26 percent responded affirmatively when asked, "If it were possible for you to have another baby, would you, yourself, like to have one?"[76] No matter how a study defines younger women, being young at the time of sterilization is a key determinant of later regret. Most women who express regret attempt to have their sterilization reversed by surgical reanastomosis. In a United States follow-up study, approximately 2 per 1,000 sterilized women had undergone tubal reanastomosis by the fifth year of poststerilization follow-up.[77] Reversal surgery is expensive, requires laparotomy, and is not always available. In general, a reported 50 to 70 percent of women who undergo reversal surgery achieve intrauterine pregnancy, but many factors, including method of tubal occlusion used for sterilization, influence this rate of intrauterine pregnancy.[59] Most published reports are likely overestimates, for they usually represent the selected series of highly skilled surgeons using sophisticated techniques.

Male Sterilization

Use. More than 40 million men are currently using vasectomy for contraception worldwide; most of these men live in the United States, United Kingdom, China, and India.[78] Because vasectomy is rarely done in a hospital, the number of men who undergo this procedure each year in the United States can only be approximated. In 1987, an estimated 336,000 men in the United States underwent vasectomy.[79]

Effectiveness. Most studies of the effectiveness of vasectomy are case series done by individual physicians or institutions; they do not allow for a comparison of the methods of vas occlusion. Such studies report failure rates less than 1 percent with a range from 0 to 2 percent.[80] Those failures typically result either from unprotected coitus shortly after vasectomy or from spontaneous reanastomosis of the vas. To avoid pregnancy from unprotected coitus, clearance of sperm from the reproductive tract should be documented before intercourse is resumed. Without such documentation, additional contraception should be used for the first 15 ejaculations, or for 6 weeks, after vasectomy.[81] Most true vasectomy failures result from spontaneous reanastomosis of the vas via fistulous tracks within sperm granulomas.[80] The likelihood of spontaneous reanastomosis may vary by vasectomy technique, and coagulation occlusion is theoretically less likely than ligation to result in sperm granuloma and fistula formation at the vas occlusion site.[82] Coagulation occlusion may, however, result in a greater likelihood of epididymal sperm granuloma formation; this may impair any subsequent attempt at reversing a vasectomy.

Complications. Vasectomy is a minor surgical procedure that usually takes 5 to 20 minutes to do. Local anesthesia without premedication is used for most vasectomies. During the procedure, the vas deferens is isolated and then occluded, using either ligation, coagulation, or clip application. Ligation is the most widely used approach.

The risk of death attributable to vasectomy is quite low. The Association For Voluntary Surgical Contraception has identified only two vasectomy-attributable deaths associated with more than 160,000 procedures done in the international programs it has supported.[81] Major morbidity is also uncommon. Although as many as 50 percent of men may experience minor complications, such as swelling of the scrotal tissue, bruising, and pain, these generally subside without treatment within 1 to 2 weeks after vasectomy.[80] Hematoma formation and infection occur much less frequently and generally are not serious. A 1983 survey of United States physicians reported a hematoma rate of 2 percent.[83] Infection after vasectomy is generally reported as occurring in fewer than 2 percent of men. Epididymitis, which is manifested by swelling and tenderness of the epididymis, is usually reported in fewer than 1 percent of men undergoing vasectomy.[80] "Epididymitis" may be a misnomer because bacterial infection as a cause is unusual and much of the aching associated with epididymitis is likely to result from epididymal congestion caused by back pressure rather than infection or inflammation. Formation of sperm granulomas at the surgical site or in the epididymis is another complication of vasectomy. Most sperm granulomas are, however, small and asymptomatic. Nonetheless, their presence may complicate any future attempt at reversing sterilization.[80]

The long-term health effects of vasectomy are now well characterized. Reports of an increased risk of atherosclerosis among cynomolgus monkeys after vasectomy caused great concern regarding the risk of atherosclerosis among men after vasectomy. This concern led to many epidemiological investigations in men and further laboratory studies in monkeys. All strongly suggest that vasectomy does not increase the risk of myocardial infarction or coronary heart disease in men after vasectomy.[84]

The same reports that addressed the possibility of cardiovascular disease remote from vasectomy also studied the relationship between vasectomy and a variety of other diseases. In 1990, Rosenberg et al reported an association between vasectomy and prostate cancer. Subsequent studies have been inconsistent and inconclusive.[85] The associations in the studies showing a positive association between vasectomy and prostate cancer have been relatively weak ones and therefore, could be explained by chance, bias, or a true causal relationship.[86] A large, U.S., multiethnic case-control study[87] reported in 1995 found no association between vasectomy and prostate cancer. This prompted the accompanying editorial from the National Center Institute to state that, "... vasectomy appears either not to cause prostate cancer or to have only a relatively weak relationship to the disease. . . ."[85]

Program Effects

Family planning services and programs can have profound effects on fertility, health, and society.

Fertility Change

Family planning influences the fertility of countries and communities, as well as individuals. Taiwan was one of the first countries to undertake a nationwide family planning program, and one of the first to document a reduction in fertility. In this island nation, the crude birth rate declined 48 percent from 37.7 births per 1,000 population in 1961 to 19.6 per 1,000 population in 1984. The general fertility rate (live births per 1,000 women ages 15 to 44) and the total fertility, both of which allow for the age structure of the women in a population, decreased even more (58 and 63 percent).[88] Moreover, the use of effective fertility control measures increased strikingly as fertility declined. In 1965, 41 percent of women ages 35 to 39 years had used contraception at some time; by 1980, 92 percent of the women in this age group stated that they had used some form of contraception. The number of individuals who had undergone abortion, sterilization, or both also increased. Finally, responses to questions about the preferred number of children per family reflected a decline during these years.[89]

Similar effects have been found in other nations. South Korea, Singapore, China, and Chile are countries where IUD use has played an important role. In others, such as Brazil,[90] Colombia,[91] and Puerto Rico,[92] contraceptive sterilization has played a prominent role. The effect of induced abortion on fertility change is best documented in eastern Europe.[93] The influence of organized family planning programs is presumed to be important in Costa Rica, Panama, and Mauritius.

A worldwide assessment of family programs in developing countries has shown that, where programs make a strong effort, then a decline in fertility often follows. In regions where developing countries predominate, south and east Asia includes nations that make the greatest effort, while sub-Saharan African countries as a group make the least.[94] Nonetheless, even in countries with high fertility rates and national programs considered rather ineffective, areas can be found where contraceptive prevalence is comparatively higher and fertility is substantially lower than in the rest of the nation.[95]

Health Change

Family planning programs may influence health in at least four ways:

1. By permitting a woman to bear children at an age when the risk of health problems to her and her offspring is lowest;
2. By permitting a couple to choose the number of children they wish to have;
3. By permitting a couple to decide the spacing of their children;
4. By providing safe and effective measures of fertility control that are part of a service program that includes information, education, and comprehensive preventive health services.

The risk of health problems during pregnancy increases with age and with the number of pregnancies. A report from the United Kingdom states that toxemia of pregnancy is an important cause of maternal mortality for young women (less than 20 years of age) having their first child.[96] Thus, the use of family planning enhances maternal health by permitting women to delay the birth of their first child and to avoid childbearing in their later reproductive years, by using surgical sterilization, if so desired.[97]

Infant health will also be improved if women postpone the birth of their first child until they are at least 20 and avoid childbearing after they reach age 35. Recent data from the United States using linked birth and infant death records show high infant mortality for young mothers (ages 10 to 14) and for women in their later reproductive years (age 35 and older). In addition, the risk of infant death is lowest for infants of second and third live birth order, and highest for infants of birth order five and greater.[98] Birth defects, such as Down's syndrome and heart malformations—most likely to affect infants of mothers who are in their mid- and late 30s or older—are specific causes of death that cause particular concern. The incidence of Down's syndrome in the United States has declined by 50 percent in the past several decades. At least half of this decline has been attributed to the use of effective family planning by women in the later years of reproductive life.[99]

Family size also influences the health of children. Not only do infant death rates increase as the birth order of the pregnancy increases, but so do fetal death rates.[100,101] In addition, family size influences nutritional status; as the number of children per family increases, the per capita protein consumption declines, and the proportion of children who are malnourished increases.[102,103]

Birth spacing influences survival during the neonatal and postneonatal periods and throughout the years before the fifth birthday.[104] For births that occur fewer than 2 years apart, the risk of mortality may increase by more than 50 percent. Because breast-feeding is an important determinant of the birth interval, and because hormonal contraception may suppress lactation, the use of fertility control agents that may limit breast-feeding needs careful consideration. It may be desirable to postpone the use of methods such as the pill. Instead a woman might use an effective but nonhormonal method or consider voluntary postpartum sterilization to establish lactation and optimize family health.

Social Change

Family planning programs and services in some countries have social change as a goal. In the United States, for example, "family planning is based on the voluntary decisions and the actions of individuals. Its purpose is to enable individuals to make their own decisions regarding reproduction and to carry out their decisions. Family planning includes measures, both to prevent unintended fertility and to overcome unintended infertility."[21]

Can family planning programs and services actually attain such goals? Survey research permits the analysis of fertility to separate births into specific categories: mistimed, unwanted, and planned. A mistimed birth is one that did not exceed the total number a woman wanted but occurred at a time in the life cycle when it was not desired (e.g., before marriage). An unwanted birth is one that occurred after the last wanted birth. The sum of the mistimed and unwanted births may be termed unintended or unplanned.

In the United States, mistimed births increased between 1979–1982 and 1984–1988 for all ages except 30 to 34. Overall, the percent of mistimed births increased from 27 to 28 percent, and the percent for mothers whose age was between 15 and 19 years was 54 percent during the years 1979–1982 and 57 percent during 1984–1988. The percent unintended for 15 to 19-year-old mothers increased from 67 percent in 1979–1982 to 73 percent in 1984–1988.[105]

Demographers have analyzed the status of unwanted fertility for several countries. In the United States, family planning efforts have focused on reducing unwanted childbearing. The results of national surveys show that unwanted births declined in all race and marital status groups since 1968.[106] However, the 1988 National Survey of Family Growth (NSFG) showed an increase in unwanted births since the 1982 NSFG from 10 to 12 percent for mothers of all ages and from 14 to 16 percent for those younger than 20 years of age.[105] Analysis of these trends shows that, if unwanted fertility were prevented, the population increase in this country would be at replacement, assuming no changes in determinants other than fertility, i.e., mortality or migration.[107]

In an analysis of the demographic and health surveys done in a selected group of developing countries, the importance of increasing the prevalence of contraceptive use in reducing unwanted fertility was emphasized if unwanted births were to be prevented.[107]

As profound as these changes are in the United States, they may fall short of the goal, as stated in the national health objectives. Persistent differences in the proportion of unwanted and mistimed pregnancies between different racial groups for women of every marital status are associated with differences in contraceptive use, including the use of surgical sterilization. Comparing unplanned fertility and family planning services in the United States with those in other developed countries shows that family planning services in the United States are less likely to promote highly effective contraception. This approach to health promotion may help to explain the shortfall in meeting the nation's goal.

Women with a wanted pregnancy may be more likely to seek earlier prenatal care than those with an unwanted pregnancy.[108] In addition, married women with an unwanted pregnancy are less likely to stop smoking than are those whose pregnancy is wanted.[109]

Abortion

Use and Changes in Practice. The number of legal abortions reported to the Centers for Disease Control and Prevention (CDC) increased each year from 1969 through 1982. The number declined slightly the following year, and has remained near 1.3 million each year since. Data for 1994 show that 1.267 million abortions were done in 1994. Most of the women undergoing legal, voluntary termination of pregnancy were younger than age 25, non-Hispanic white, unmarried, and had no previous live births. Almost all of the procedures were suction curettage and were done in the first 12 weeks of pregnancy.[110,111]

Current trends in the medical practice of abortion in the United States continue to favor improved health for pregnant women. Since 1983, intrauterine saline instillation has been used for fewer than 2 percent of all abortions for which the procedure is known. This percent reached a level of 0.4 percent in 1994. Major surgical procedures, i.e., hysterotomy/hysterectomy, were used for fewer than

0.05 percent of all procedures (fewer than 200 each year) beginning in 1984. In the late 1970s, two trends that continued into the 1980s started: abortions were performed in the state where the woman lives and within the first 12 weeks of pregnancy.[110,111]

Complications. Legal abortion continues to be a safe surgical procedure for pregnant women. CDC reports that the death-to-case rate was less than 1 per 100,000 procedures for every year in the 1980s, and was less than 0.5 in 1985.[111] Beginning with the eighth menstrual week of gestation, the longer of pregnancy, the more likely a pregnant woman is to experience morbidity or mortality.

The risk of nonfatal complications from abortion, like the risk of mortality, increases with the length of pregnancy. In 1980, an estimated 4,530 hospitalizations occurred because of the complications of legal abortions. This is estimated to be half the number related to the use of oral contraceptives and IUDs.[112] Only six women died from these complications in 1985.[113]

Concern about abortion and continued differences in viewpoints on abortion in the United States have focused attention on the mental health, educational, and behavioral aspects of this approach. A review of available studies by the Surgeon General of the Public Health Service led Dr. C. Everett Koop to report that the evidence regarding adverse mental health effects was insufficient and of such poor quality as to provide no information.[114] Moreover, a study of black teenage women beginning at the time they sought pregnancy testing and lasting for 2 years of follow-up found higher rates of timely high school graduation, improved economic status, and no greater anxiety, stress, or psychological problems for those who underwent abortion compared with those who carried their pregnancy to term or those who had negative pregnancy tests.[115]

▶ KEY ISSUES

Teenage Fertility

Teenage pregnancy is an important issue to public health for at least three reasons: (*a*) pregnancies in very young women of reproductive age are often not intended; (*b*) teenage pregnancies may be at high risk of preventable health problems for both infant and mother; and (*c*) children born to young women may lead to unanticipated momentum in population growth by increasing total family size over a lifetime and by shortening the time between generations of future children.

The United States Department of Health and Human Services goals for 1990 and for 2000 highlight the problem of childbearing among teenagers.[21] Specifically, the 1990 national health objectives stated that: (*a*) there should be almost no unintended births to girls 14 years of age and under; (*b*) the fertility rate for girls 15 years of age should be reduced to 10 per 1,000; (*c*) the fertility rate for girls 16 years of age should be reduced to 25 per 1,000; and (*d*) the fertility rate for girls 17 years of age should be reduced to 45 per 1,000.

Survey data showed that in 1973 nearly 60 percent of births to women younger than age 20 were unplanned (i.e., unwanted or mistimed); more recent data showed that in 1982 that proportion had reached nearly 80 percent. The number of teenage births increased nearly 8 percent from an estimated 361,000 in 1973 to 389,000, yet the total number of births to women in this age group declined nearly 20 percent. The national birth rates for this age group did not decline substantially since 1982, and the percent of unintended births increased between the 1982 NSFG and the 1988 NSFG. Given these findings, there is no reason to believe this trend has changed in recent years.

This estimate deals only with live births. It does not include the legal abortions (232,000 in 1973 and 418,000 in 1982) that women in this age group underwent. In addition, it does not add in the births and abortions to those younger than age 15; these pregnancies accounted for more than 24,000 pregnancies in 1973 and in 1982.[33] Pregnancy rates for teenagers of a race other than white are double the rates for those who are white, though the proportion of unplanned pregnancies are not appreciably different for these two groups of young women.[116]

The Pill and Breast Cancer

A pooled analysis of 54 studies worldwide reported in 1996 by The Collaborative Group on Hormonal Factors in Breast Cancer[117] has shed important light on the relationship between oral contraceptive use and risk of breast cancer. The pooled analysis combined data on 53,297 women with breast cancer and 100,239 women without breast cancer from studies conducted in 25 countries. The pooled analysis, which included about 90 percent of all available data on the relationship between pill use and breast cancer risk, had four main findings. First, current or recent (within 10 years of stopping use) pill users have a small increase in risk of having breast cancer diagnosed (for current versus nonusers, RR was 1.24; 95 percent confidence interval 1.15 to 1.33). The increase for current users was seen for women with little pill use (less than 1 year) and did not increase with increasing durations of use.[118] Second, past users (10 or more years after stopping use) have no increased risk. Third, the additional cancers identified are less advanced clinically than those in never users. Fourth, no subgroups of women were at increased risk for pill use. In particular, women with a family history of breast cancer were not at additional risk from pill use relative to women without such a history. These four findings suggest that either oral contraceptive users are more likely than nonusers to have breast cancers detected; that existing tumors are identified at an earlier stage in pill users; or that pill use accelerates tumor growth.

These findings regarding pill use raise important questions regarding whether the relationship between pill use and breast cancer diagnosis is causal and, similarly, whether the effect is harmful or beneficial. Because oral contraceptives have been available only since 1960, all reports of the relationship between pill use and breast cancer risk have focused on women with breast cancers diagnosed at relatively young ages. Studies are now in progress to evaluate risks among women with breast cancers diagnosed at later ages.

AIDS and Family Planning

AIDS, first described in 1981, is now a worldwide epidemic. Since AIDS was first identified, more than 100,000 people in the United States have contracted this disease. An estimated 1 to 1.5 million people in the United States and an estimated 5 to 10 million people worldwide are currently infected with the human immunodeficiency virus (HIV).

AIDS is caused by the human immunodeficiency virus, which was first described in 1984. There are only three routes of HIV transmission: (*a*) sexual, by exposure to an infected person's genital secretions; (*b*) exposure to infected blood or blood products; and (*c*) mother-to-infant (vertical or perinatal) transmission before, during, or shortly after birth. Although treatment under development promises to improve the length and quality of life for many persons with AIDS, no cure is on the horizon and, therefore, prevention of AIDS remains paramount.

Family planning plays a key role in preventing AIDS because of its relation to both heterosexual and mother-to-infant transmission of HIV. Condom use has been considered by family planners primarily to be a method of family planning and by STD personnel primarily as a method for prevention of STD. In fact, the condom serves both important functions within the family planning–AIDS relationship.

The most effective strategies for preventing heterosexual transmission of HIV are abstinence or having sex with an uninfected partner in a mutually monogamous relationship. However, there is now compelling evidence that consistent and correct use of latex condoms is highly effective in preventing the sexual transmission of HIV infection. The strongest evidence for this assertion comes from studies of couples discordant for HIV infection, i.e., couples in which one member is known to be infected with HIV and the other is known to be initially uninfected. In one large European study[119] of discordant couples followed for about 2 years, 124 couples reported consistent condom use during about 15,000 episodes of intercourse. Among those couples, none of the seronegative partners became infected with HIV. By contrast, among inconsistent condom users, the rate of HIV transmission was similar to that of nonusers of condoms. In two other discordant couple studies, one conducted in Italy[120] and the other in Haiti,[121] findings were similar among consistent condom users except that the rate of transmission to the uninfected partner was approximately 1 percent per year of use.

The relationship between other methods of family planning and HIV transmission are unclear and controversial. Data regarding oral contraceptives, DMPA, and intrauterine devices are inconsistent and inconclusive. Because it must be assumed that none of these methods protect against HIV transmission, women at risk for HIV infection and other STD need a separate strategy for STD prevention. For individuals who choose to remain sexually active with partners who may be infected, consistent and correct latex condom use is the best strategy.[122]

Couples who cannot or will not use latex condoms should consider use of the female condom. Use of spermicides alone is not recommended for HIV prevention. Although nonoxynol-9 inactivates HIV in the laboratory, data in humans are insufficient to determine whether nonoxynol-9 use is harmful, beneficial, or does not affect HIV transmission. In sum, a condom, preferably a male latex condom, should be used consistently and correctly by all persons at risk for STD, even if they choose to use another contraceptive method for pregnancy prevention.

HIV infection among women of reproductive age represents a compound tragedy because of the potential for transmission of infection from mother to infant. The percentage of AIDS cases among women in the United States is increasing; among cases diagnosed in 1996, 20 percent occurred among women. Most pediatric AIDS cases result from mother-to-infant transmission. Therefore, preventing AIDS in children will largely depend on the prevention of HIV infection among women of reproductive age and unintended pregnancy among women already infected. Fortunately, in 1994, a randomized controlled trial[123] showed that the risk of mother-to-infant transmission could be reduced by as much as two-thirds by administering zidovudine (AZT or ZD) antepartum, intrapartum, and postpartum to the infant for 6 weeks after birth. Subsequent observational studies have confirmed that the regimen markedly reduces the risk of mother-to-infant transmission.

HIV-infected women who choose not to become pregnant because of this risk of transmission or for any other reason should have highly effective birth prevention methods available. In the United States, most HIV-infected women are members of minority groups and at substantial socioeconomic disadvantage. Often, such women have reduced access to family planning services. Even when such services are available, many women who are likely to be HIV-infected fail to use them. Thus, innovative outreach programs may be needed to ensure that HIV-infected women who choose not to become pregnant have the resources to support that decision.

▸ FACTORS INFLUENCING PERSONAL CHOICE

The prediction that there will be no fundamentally new approaches to fertility control before the next century[124] seems accurate. Thus, for the foreseeable future, individuals will make choices about fertility control from among existing options.[105] How does one make these choices, particularly in view of the need to balance personal health needs and values, on the one hand, with the health needs and values of the community, society, and future generations on the other? Given an individual's own sense of social responsibility, the prevalent diversity of career aspirations, and plans for childbearing and family lifestyles, decisions about reproduction are more complicated than ever. Despite this complexity, three general rules apply almost universally:

1. When pregnancy is not wanted, almost any method of fertility control is safer and more effective than no method.
2. Consistent, careful use of contraception will both increase pregnancy prevention and limit adverse side effects.
3. The better informed a person is about human reproduction and its control, the more likely the person is to make satisfactory decisions about the important issues related to fertility and his or her family.

In reflecting on personal values and responsibility to society, and in going beyond these general rules, there is a series of important personal questions one might ask;

1. How do I feel about being sexually active outside marriage?
2. Do I want children?
3. How do I feel about the importance of avoiding an unintended pregnancy?
4. Am I afraid to use birth control?
5. How do I feel about abortion?
6. How old do I want to be when I start my family?
7. Where do I want to be in terms of my career when I start my family?
8. If I have more than one child, how old do I want each to be when the next one is born?
9. How many children are enough for me and my family?
10. Do my partner and I agree on the answers to the key questions about fertility control?
11. After I have all the children I want, how do I feel about sterilization as a permanent method of fertility control, or would I prefer to continue using a method of contraception that is not permanent?
12. How does my partner feel about being sterilized, or using temporary contraception?

From now into the foreseeable future, choices and recommendations regarding methods of fertility control should include the need for protection against sexually transmitted diseases, including AIDS. For individuals who are at risk because of having sexual intercourse with partners who may be infected, consistent and correct use of condoms is the only approach that can be recommended, other than abstinence. Therefore, individuals at risk of infection who choose to use methods other than condoms to prevent pregnancy will need to use condoms, in addition, to avoid the transmission of infection.

One key factor that influences choice is an individual's own intentions. Women who wish to avoid any more pregnancies are consistently more effective users of the birth control method they choose, no matter what that method may be, than are those who are trying to only delay their next conception.

▸ REFERENCES

Public Health Issues in Disasters

1. Lillibridge SR, Burkle FM, Noji EK: Disaster mitigation and humanitarian assistance training for uniformed service medical personnel. Mil Med 159:397–403, 1994
2. SAEM Disaster Medicine White Paper Subcommittee: Disaster medicine: current assessment and blueprint for the future. Acad Emerg Med 12:1068–1076, 1995
3. Noji EK: Disaster epidemiology. Emerg Med Clin North Am 14:289–300, 1996
4. Centers for Disease Control and Prevention: Morbidity surveillance following the Midwest flood—Missouri. MMWR 42:797–798, 1993
5. Centers for Disease Control and Prevention: Public health consequences of a flood disaster—Iowa. MMWR 42:653–656, 1993
6. Noji EK, Kelen GD, Armenian HK, et al: The 1988 earthquake in Soviet Armenia: a case study. Ann Emerg Med 19:891–897, 1990

7. Centers for Disease Control and Prevention: Rapid health needs assessment following Hurricane Andrew—Florida and Louisiana. MMWR 41:696–698, 1992
8. Office of Foreign Disaster Assistance: Significant Disasters from 1990–1995—World Disaster Report. Washington, DC: Office of Foreign Disaster Assistance, 1996, p 84
9. Logue JN: Disasters, the environment, and public health: improving our response. Am J Public Health 86:1207–1210, 1996
10. Sanderson LM: Toxicologic disasters: natural and technologic. In Sullivan JB, Krieger GR (eds): Hazardous Materials Toxicology, Clinical Principles of Environmental Health. Baltimore: Williams & Wilkins, 1992, pp 326–331
11. Noji EK: Public health challenges in technological disaster situations. Arch Public Health 50:99–104, 1992
12. Baxter PJ: Review of major chemical incidents and their medical management. In Murray V (ed): Major Chemical Disasters—Medical Aspects of Management. London: Royal Society of Medicine Services Limited, 1990, pp 7–20
13. Binder S: Deaths, injuries, and evacuations from acute hazardous materials releases. Am J Public Health 79:1042–1044, 1989
14. Fong F, Schrader DC: Radiation disasters and emergency department preparedness. Emerg Med Clin North Am 14:349–370, 1996
15. Sidel VW, Onel E, Geiger JH, et al: Public health response to natural and human-made disasters. In Last J, Wallace R (eds): Public Health & Preventive Medicine. 13th ed. Norwalk, CT: Appleton & Lange, 1992, pp 1173–1186
16. Anspaugh LR, Catlin RJ, Goldman M: The global impact of the Chernobyl reactor accident. Science 242:1513–1519, 1988
17. Centers for Disease Control and Prevention: Public Health Consequence of Disasters. Atlanta: Centers for Disease Control and Prevention, 1989
18. Burkle FM: Complex, humanitarian emergencies: I. Concepts and participants. Prehospital and Disaster Medicine 10(1):36–42, 1995
19. Toole MJ, Waldman RJ: Refugees and displaced persons: war, hunger and public health. JAMA 260:2795–2796, 1993
20. Toole MJ, Waldman RJ: Prevention of excess mortality in refugee and displaced populations in developing countries. JAMA 263: 3296–3302, 1990
21. Centers for Disease Control and Prevention: Famine-affected, refugee, and displaced populations: recommendation for public health issues. MMWR 41;(RR-13):1–76, 1992
22. Macrai J, Zwi AB: Food as an instrument of war in contemporary African famines: a review of the evidence. Disasters 16:299–321, 1992
23. Moore PS, Marfin AA, Quenemoen LE, et al: Mortality rates in displaced and resident populations of central Somalia during 1992 famine. Lancet 341:935–938, 1993
24. National Research Council: Confronting Natural Disasters: an International Decade for Natural Disaster Reduction. Washington, DC: National Academy Press, 1987, pp 1–67
25. Wasley A: Epidemiology in the disaster setting. Current Issues in Public Health 1:131–135, 1995
26. United States Mission to the United Nations: Global Humanitarian Emergencies, 1996. New York: ECOSOC Section of the United States Mission to the United Nations, 1996
27. International Federation of Red Cross and Red Crescent Societies: World Disasters Report 1996. New York: Oxford University Press, 1996
28. Bilqis AH, Hoque R, Bradley S, et al: Environmental health and the 1991 Bangladesh cyclone. Disasters 17:143–152, 1993
29. Baxter PJ, Ing RT, Falk H, et al: Medical aspect of volcanic disasters: an outline of the hazards and emergency response measures. Disasters 6:268–276, 1982
30. Baxter PJ, Ing RT, Falk H, et al: Mount St. Helens eruptions: the acute respiratory effect of volcanic ash in a North American community. Arch Environ Health 38:38–43, 1983
31. Baxter PJ, Stoiber RE, Williams SN: Volcanic gases and health: Masaya Volcano, Nicaragua [Letter]. Lancet 2:150–151, 1982
32. Centers for Disease Control and Prevention: Surveillance for respiratory disease following eruptions of Mt. St. Helens. MMWR 29: 252, 1980
33. Sommer AS, Mosley WH: East Bengal Cyclone of November 1970. Lancet 1:1029–1036, 1972
34. Lillibridge SR: Managing the environmental health aspects of disasters: water, human excreta, and shelter. In Noji EK (ed): Public Health Consequences of Disasters. New York: Oxford University Press, 1997, pp 65–78
35. Noji EK: The medical consequences of earthquakes: coordinating the medical and rescue response. Disaster Management 4:32–40, 1991
36. Office of Foreign Disaster Assistance: World Wide Disasters from 1900–1996. Washington, DC: Office of Foreign Disaster Assistance, 1996
37. Papadatos Y, Nikou K, Potamianos G: Evaluation of psychiatric morbidity following an earthquake. Int J Soc Psychiatry 36:131–136, 1990
38. Teeter DS: Illnesses and injuries reported at disaster application centers following the 1994 Northridge earthquake. Mil Med 161:526–530, 1996
39. Noji EK, Armenian HK, Oganessian A: Issues of rescue and medical care following the 1988 Armenian earthquake. Int J Epidemiol 22:1070–1076, 1993
40. Barbera JA, Lozano M: Urban search and rescue medical teams: FEMA task force system. Prehospital Disaster Medicine 8:88–92, 1993
41. Henderson AK, Lillibridge SR, Salina C, et al: Disaster medical assistance teams: providing care to a community struck by Hurricane Iniki. Ann Emerg Med 23:726–730, 1994
42. Roth PB, Gaffney JK: The Federal Response Plan and Disaster Medical Assistance Teams in domestic disasters. Emerg Med Clin North Am 14(2):371–382, 1996
43. Thiel CC, Schneider JE, Hiatt D, et al: 9-1-1 EMS process in the Loma Prieta earthquake. Prehospital and Disaster Medicine October–December:348–358, 1992
44. Schultz CH, Koenig KL, Noji EK: A medical disaster response to reduce immediate mortality after an earthquake. N Engl J Med 334:438–444, 1996
45. Sivard RL: World Military and Social Expenditures 1996. Washington, DC: World Priorities, 1996
46. Fitzsimmons DW, Whiteside AW: Conflict, War, and Public Health. Conflict Study 276. London: Research Institute for the Study of Conflict and Terrorism, 1994
47. Van Crevald M: The Transformation of War. New York: The Free Press, 1991
48. Coupland RM: The effect of weapons on health. Lancet 347: 450–451, 1996
49. Coupland RM: The effects of weapons: surgical challenge and medical dilemma. J R Coll Surg Edinb 65–71, 1996
50. Toole MJ: The public health consequences of inaction: lessons learned responding to sudden population displacement. In Cahill KM (ed): The Framework for Survival: Health, Human Rights, and Humanitarian Assistance in Conflicts and Disasters. New York: Basic Books, 1993, pp 144–158
51. U.S. Committee for Refugees: World Refugee Survey. New York: Immigration and Refugee Services of America, 1996
52. Leaning J: When the system doesn't work: Somalia 1992. In Cahill KM (ed): A Framework for Survival: Health, Human Rights, and Humanitarian Assistance in Conflicts and Disasters. New York: HarperCollins, 1993, pp 103–120
53. Burkholder BT, Toole MJ: Evolution of complex disasters. Lancet 346:1012–1015, 1995
54. Toole MJ, Galson S, Brady W: Are war and public health compatible? Lancet 341:1193–1196, 1993

55. Toole MJ, Waldman RJ: Refugees, Displaced Persons and Relief Today. Public Health Rev 35–45, 1996
56. Perrin P: War and Public Health. Geneva: International Committee of the Red Cross, 1996
57. Findlay T: Armed conflict prevention, management and resolution. In Bielckus B, Borg JG, Johanson E, Odom D (eds): Stockholm International Peace Research Institute Yearbook 1996. New York: Oxford University Press, 1996, pp 31–74
58. Office of Foreign Disaster Assistance: Report of the Durunka Oil Fires. Washington, DC: Office of Foreign Disaster Assistance, 1994
59. Nadig R: Hazardous materials releases and decontamination. In Lewis R, Goldfrank LR (eds): Toxicologic Emergencies. 5th ed. Norwalk, CT: Appleton & Lange, 1994, pp 1265–1276
60. Lillibridge SR: Industrial disasters. In Noji EK (ed): Public Health Consequences of Disasters. New York: Oxford University Press, 1997, pp 354–372
61. Lillibridge SR, Noji EK, Burkle FM: Disaster assessment: the emergency health evaluation of a population affected by a disaster. Ann Emerg Med 22:1715–1720, 1993
62. Toole MJ: The rapid assessment of health problems in refuge and displaced populations. Medicine and Global Surveillance 1:200–207, 1994
63. Hlady WG, Quenemoen LE, Amenia-Cope RR, et al: Rapid needs assessment after Hurricane Andrew in South Florida using a modified cluster sample method. Ann Emerg Med 23:719–725, 1994
64. Glass RI, Noji EK: Epidemiologic surveillance following disasters. In Halpern WE, Baker I (eds): Textbook of Public Health Surveillance. New York: Van Nostrand Reinhold, 1992, pp 195–205
65. Marfin AA, Moore J, Collins C, et al: Infectious disease surveillance during emergency relief to Bhutanese refugees in Nepal. JAMA 272:377–381, 1994
66. Elias CJ, Alexander BH, Sokly T: Infectious disease control in a long term refugee camp: the role of epidemiologic surveillance and investigation. Am J Public Health 80:824–828, 1990
67. O'Carroll PW, Friede A, Noji EK, et al: The rapid implementation of a statewide emergency health information system during the 1993 Iowa flood. Am J Public Health 85:564–567, 1995
68. Armenian HK: Perceptions from epidemiologic research in an endemic war. Soc Sci Med 28:643–647, 1989
69. Weinberg J, Simmonds S: Public health, epidemiology and war. Soc Sci Med 40:1663–1669, 1995
70. Yip R, Sharp TW: Acute malnutrition and high childhood mortality related to diarrhea. JAMA 270:587–590, 1993
71. Cobey JC, Flanigin A, Foege WH: Effective humanitarian aid: our only hope for intervention in a civil war. JAMA 270:632–634, 1993
72. Hakewill PA, Moren A: Monitoring and evaluation of relief programmes. Trop Doct 21:24–28, 1991
73. Seaman J: Disaster epidemiology: or why most disaster relief is ineffective. Injury 21:5–8, 1990
74. Anonymous: Disaster epidemiology [Editorial]. Lancet 336:845–846, 1990
75. UNICEF: Assisting in Emergencies; A Resource Handbook for UNICEF Field Staff. New York: UNICEF, 1992, pp 34–365
76. United Nations High Commissioner for Refugees: Water Manual for Refugee Situations. Geneva: United Nations High Commissioner for Refugees, 1992
77. Pan American Health Organization: Environmental Health Management after Natural Disasters. Scientific Publication 432. Washington, DC: Pan American Health Organization, 1982
78. Cairncross S, Feachem R (eds): Environmental Health Engineering in the Tropics. 2nd ed. New York: John Wiley and Sons, 1993
79. World Health Organization: Health Principles of Housing. Geneva: World Health Organization, 1989
80. Pan American Health Organization: Emergency Vector Control after Natural Disasters. Scientific Publication 419. Washington, DC: Pan American Health Organization, 1982
81. Howard MJ, Brillman JC, Burkle FM: Infectious disease emergencies in disasters. Emerg Med Clin North Am 14:413–428, 1996
82. Aghababian RV, Teuscher J: Infectious diseases following major disasters. Ann Emerg Med 21:362–367, 1992
83. Mason J, Cavalie P: Malaria epidemic in Haiti following a hurricane. Am J Trop Med Hyg 14:533–539, 1965
84. Centers for Disease Control and Prevention: Coccidioidomycosis following the Northridge earthquake. MMWR 43:194–195, 1994
85. Toole MJ, Steketee RW, Waldman RJ, et al: Measles prevention and control in emergency settings. Bull World Health Organ 67:381–388, 1989
86. World Health Organization: Guidelines for Cholera Control. Geneva: World Health Organization, 1993
87. Toole MJ: Micronutrient deficiencies in refugees. Lancet 339: 1214–1215, 1992
88. Shears P: Epidemiology and infection in famine and disasters. Epidemiol Infect 107:241–251, 1991
89. Arbelot A (ed): Nutrition Guidelines. Paris: Medicins sans Frontiers, 1995
90. Hansch S: How Many People Die of Starvation in Humanitarian Emergencies? Washington, DC: Refugee Policy Group, 1995
91. Shawcross W: The Quality of Mercy. New York: Simon & Schuster, 1984
92. Sharp TW, DeFraites RF, Thornton SA, Burans JP, Wallace MR: Illness in journalists and relief workers during international relief efforts in Somalia, 1992–93. Journal of Travel Medicine 2:70–76, 1995
93. Goma Epidemiology Group: Public health impact of Rwandan refugee crisis: what happened in Goma, Zaire, in July, 1994? Lancet 345:339–344, 1995
94. Boss LP, Toole MJ, Yip R: Assessments of mortality, morbidity, and nutritional status in Somalia during the 1991–1992 famine. Recommendations for standardization of methods. JAMA 272:371–376, 1994
95. Waeckerle JF, Lillibridge SR, Burkle FM, Noji EK: Disaster medicine: challenges for today. Ann Emerg Med 23:715–718, 1994
96. Perrin P: Training medical personnel: HELP and SOS course. International Reviews of the Red Cross 284:505–512, 1994
97. Anonymous: Reproductive freedom for refugees [Editorial]. Lancet 341:929–930, 1993
98. Swiss S, Giller JE: Rape as a crime of war—a medical perspective. JAMA 270:612–615, 1993
99. Heise LL, Raikes A, Watts CH, Zwi AB: Violence against women: a neglected public health issue in less developed countries. Soc Sci Med 39:1165–1179, 1994
100. UNICEF: The State of the World's Children. New York: Oxford University Press, 1996
101. UNICEF: Children in War: A guide to the Provision of Services. New York: Oxford University Press, 1992
102. Manoncourt S, Doppler B, Enten F, et al: Public health consequences of the civil war in Somalia, April 1992. Lancet 340:176–77, 1992
103. Strada G: The horror of land mines. Sci Am 274:40–45, 1996
104. Stover E, McGrath R: Land Mines in Cambodia—The Coward's War. Boston: Physicians for Human Rights, 1991
105. Mobley J: Biological warfare in the twentieth century: lessons from the past, challenges for the future. Mil Med 160:547–553, 1995
106. Yeskey K: Susceptibility to terrorism. Presentation to The First Harvard Symposium on The Medical Consequences of Terrorism, April 24–25, Boston, MA
107. Laquer W: Postmodern terrorism. Foreign Affairs 75(5):24–36, 1996
108. Okumura T, Takasu N, Ishimatsu S, et al: Report on 640 victims of the Tokyo subway sarin attack. Ann Emerg Med 28:129–135, 1996
109. Burkle FM: Acute-phase mental health consequences of disasters: implications for triage and emergency medical services. Ann Emerg Med 28:119–128, 1996
110. Ursano RJ, McCarroll JE: The nature of a traumatic stressor: handling dead bodies. J Nerv Ment Dis 178:396–398, 1990

Maternal and Child Health

1. Schmidt WM: The development of health services for mothers and children in the United States. Am J Public Health 63:419–437, 1973
2. Schorr LB, Schorr D: Within Our Reach: Breaking the Cycle of Disadvantage. New York: Anchor Press/Doubleday, 1988
3. Dollfus C, Patetta M, Siegel E, Cross AW: Infant mortality: a practical approach to the analysis of the leading causes of death and risk factors. Pediatrics 86:176–183, 1990
4. Institute of Medicine: Health Services Integration: Lessons for the 1980's. Washington, DC: National Academy Press, 1982
5. Miller CA: Maternal Health and Infant Survival. Washington, DC: National Center for Clinical Infant Programs, 1987
6. Cefalo RC, Moos M-K: Preconceptional Health Promotion: A Practical Guide. Rockville, MD: Aspen, 1988
7. Blennow M, Granstrom M, Jaatmaa E, et al: Primary immunization of infants with an acellular pertussis vaccine in a double blind randomized clinical trial. Pediatrics 82:293–299, 1988
8. Miller M, Sutter RW, Strebel PM, Hadler SC: Cost-effectiveness of incorporating inactivated poliovirus vaccine into the routine childhood immunization schedule. JAMA 276:967–971, 1996
9. Chapman J, Siegel E, Cross A: Home visitors and child health: analysis of selected programs. Pediatrics 85:1059–1068, 1990
10. Olds DL, Kitzman H: Can home visitation improve the health of women and children at environmental risk? Pediatrics 86:108–116, 1990
11. Durch JS, Bailey LA, Stoto MA (ed): Improving Health in the Community: A Role for Performance Monitoring. Report of the Committee on Using Performance Monitoring to Improve Community Health. Institute of Medicine, National Academy of Sciences. Washington, DC: National Academy Press, 1997

Desmotology: The Practice of Prison Health

1. Bureau of Justice Statistics: Jail Inmates, 1986. NCJ 107123. Washington, DC: US Dept of Justice, 1987
2. Bureau of Justice Statistics: Jail Inmates, 1996. Washington, DC: US Dept of Justice, 1997
3. Prison and Jail Inmates 1995. NCJ 161132. Washington, DC: US Justice Department, 1995
4. Bureau of Justice Statistics: Probation and Parole Populations, 1995. NCJ-161722. Washington, DC: US Dept of Justice, 1996
5. Tauxe RV, Patterson CB: A word about prisons: "desmoteric." N Engl J Med 317:1669–1670, 1988
6. Weisbuch JB: Prison health. In Last JM, Wallace RB (eds): Public Health & Preventive Medicine. 13th ed. Norwalk, CT: Appleton & Lange, 1992, pp 1159–1163
7. Shansky R: Desmotology. [quarterly Newsletter of the American Society of Correctional Physicians]
8. Thornburn KM: Croaker's dilemma: should prison physicians serve prisons or prisoners? West J Med 134:457–461, 1981
9. Prout C, Ross RN: Care and Punishment: The Dilemmas of Prison Medicine. Pittsburgh: University of Pittsburgh Press, 1988, pp 117–126
10. Estelle v Gamble, 97 S.Ct. 285, 429 US 97 (1976)
11. Newman v Alabama, 349F. Supp278, 503 F2d 1320, 5th Cir (1974), cert denied 421 US 948 (1975)
12. Todaro v Ward, 565 F2d 48, 52 (2 Cir 1977)
13. Poster MJ: The Estelle medical professional judgment standard: the right of those in state custody to receive high-cost medical treatments. Am J Law Med 18(4):347–368, 1992
14. American Medical Association: Medical Care in US Jails—A 1972 Survey. Chicago: American Medical Association, 1973
15. National Commission on Correctional Health Care: Standards for Health Services in Jails. Chicago: National Commission on Correctional Health Care, 1996
16. National Commission on Correctional Health Care: Standards for Health Services in Prisons. Chicago: National Commission on Correctional Health Care, 1997
17. National Commission on Correctional Health Care: Standards for Health Services in Juvenile Detention and Confinement Facilities. Chicago: National Commission on Correctional Health Care, 1995
18. Weisbuch JB: Public health professionals and prison health care needs. Am J Public Health 67(8):720–722, 1977
19. Grantham EV, Sandler ES, Block MJ: Treatment of correctional center inmates at a public health department: a cooperative venture. J Public Health Dent 42(3):251–255, 1982
20. Rice D: Judicial involvement in Colorado prison health care reform. J. Health Polit Policy Law 6(2):315–320, 1981
21. Centers for Disease Control and Prevention: Control of Tuberculosis in Correctional Facilities—A Guide for Health Care Workers. Atlanta: Centers for Disease Control and Prevention, 1992
22. Weisbuch JB: The new responsibilities for prison health: working with the public health community. J Prison Jail Health 10(1):3–18, 1991
23. Anno BJ: The role of organized medicine in correctional health care. JAMA 247:2923–2925, 1982
24. Anno BJ: Prison Health Care: Guidelines for the Management of an Adequate Delivery System. Washington, DC: National Institute of Corrections, 1991
25. American Public Health Association: Standards for Health Care in Correction Institutions, Jails and Prisons, 1983. Washington, DC: American Public Health Association
26. Shapiro S, Shapiro MF: Identification of health care problems in a county jail. J Community Health 12(1):23–30, 1987
27. Sheps SB, Schechter MT, Prefontaine RG: Prison health services: a utilization study. J Community Health 12(1):4–22, 1987
28. Freeman RW, Gollub RE, Wolski M, Gschwend JA, Al-Ibrahim MS, Hawthorne PR, Fox LJ, Golden AS, Kamka G, Kelly GB: Planning health services for a city jail: impact of contractual services on men's sick call. Med Care 19(4):410–418, 1981
29. American Medical Association. Substance Abuse as a Public Health Hazard. AMA Policy, 95.975. House of Delegates Resolution 7, I-89, December 1989, Honolulu, Hawaii
30. Miller RE: Nationwide Profile of Female Inmate Substance Involvement. J Psychoactive Drugs 16(4):319–326, 1984
31. Teplin LA: Psychiatric and substance abuse disorders among male urban jail detainees. Am J Public Health 84:290–293, 1994
32. Wiosh ED, O'Neil JA: Drug Use Forecasting (DUF) Research Update, January to March, 1989. Washington, DC: National Institute of Justice, 1989
33. Perkins CA, Stephan JJ, Beck AJ: Jails and jail inmates 1993–94: census of jails and survey of jails. Bureau of Justice Statistics Bulletin April 1995
34. O'Malley PM, Bachman JG, Johnston LD: Period, age, and cohort effects on substance use among young Americans: a decade of change, 1976–86. Am J Public Health 78(10):1315–1321, 1988
35. Leukefeld CG, Tims FR: Drug Abuse Treatment in Prisons and Jails. J Subst Abuse Treat 10:77–84, 1993
36. Primm BJ: New component created within ADANHA to enhance drug treatment services. NIDA Notes 5(3):21, 1990
37. Inciardi JA, McBride DC, Weinerman BA: (1993) The assessment and referral of criminal justice clients: examining the Focused Offender Disposition Program. In Inciardi JA (ed): Drug Treatment and Criminal Justice. Newbury Park, CA: Sage, 1993, pp 149–164
38. Peters RH, Kearns WD: Drug abuse history and treatment needs of jail inmates. Am J Drug Alcohol Abuse 18(3):355–366, 1992
39. Nurco DN, Hanlon TE, Bateman RW, Kinlock TW: Drug abuse treatment in the context of correctional surveillance. J Subst Abuse Treat 12(1):19–27, 1995
40. American Medical Association: Drug Abuse in the United States: A Policy Report. In: Proceedings of the House of Delegates, 137th Annual Meeting, June 26–30, 1988, pp 236–250

41. Hammett TM: 1988 Update: AIDS in Correctional Facilities. NCJ-115522. Washington DC: US Department of Justice, National Institute of Justice, 1989
42. Hammett TM, Harrold L, Gross M, Epstein I: 1992 Update: HIV/AIDS in Correctional Facilities. Washington, DC: National Institute of Justice, 1994
43. Brien PM, Beck AJ: HIV in Prisons, 1994. Bureau of Justice Statistics Bulletin, 1996
44. Weisfuse IB, Greenberg BL, Back SD et al: HIV-1 infection among New York City inmates. AIDS 5:1133–1138, 1991
45. Brewer TF, Vlahov D, Taylor E, Hall D, Munoz A, Polk BF: Transmission of human immunodeficiency virus, type 1 (HIV-1) within a statewide prison system. AIDS 2:363–368, 1988
46. Behrendt C, Kendig N, Dambita C, Horman J, Lawlwor J, Vlahov D: Voluntary testing for human immunodeficiency virus (HIV) in a prison population with a high prevalence of HIV. Am J Epidemiol 139:918–928, 1994
47. Castro K, Shansky R, Scardino V, Narkunas J, Coe J, Hammett T: HIV transmission in correctional facilities. [abstract MC 3067]. VII International Conference on AIDS, Florence, 1991
48. Harnsbvurgh CR, Jones JQ, McArthur T, Ignacia T, Stock P: Seroconversion to HIV in prison inmates. Am J Public Health 80: 209–210, 1990
49. Taylor A, Goldberg D, Emslie J, et al: Outbreak of HIV infection in a Scottish prison. BMJ 130:289–292, 1995
50. National Commission on Correctional Health Care: Policy Statement on Intake Testing for HIV in Prisons and Jails. Chicago: National Commission on Correctional Health Care, April, 1988
51. American Medical Association: Board of Trustees Report UU. In: Proceedings of the House of Delegates, Chicago, June 1987
52. Diamond J: HIV testing in prison: what's the controversy? Lancet 344:1650–1651, 1994
53. Kendig N, Stough T, Austin P, et al: Profile of HIV seropositive inmates diagnosed in Maryland's State Correctional System. Public Health Rep 109(4):756–760, 1994
54. Vernon T: Partner notification. JAMA 260:3274, 1988
55. Bader TF: Hepatitis B in prisons. Biomed Pharmacother 40:248–251, 1986
56. Anda RF, Perlman SB, D'Alessio DJ, Davis JP, Dodson VN: Hepatitis B in Wisconsin male prisoners: considerations for serologic screening and vaccination. Am J Public Health 75(10):1182–1185, 1985
57. Crofts N, Stewart T, Hearne P, Xin YP, Breschkin AM, Locarnini SA: Spread of bloodborne viruses among Australian prison entrants. BMJ 310:285–288, 1995
58. Decker MD, Vaughn WK, Brodie JS, et al: Incidence of hepatitis B in Tennessee prisoners. J Infect Dis 152(1):214–217, 1985
59. Hull HF, Lyons LH, Mann JM, Hadler SC, et al: Incidence of hepatitis B in the penitentiary of New Mexico. Am J Public Health 75(10):1213–1214, 1985
60. Daneluk R, Elliot L, Welihan D: Hepatitis B virus vaccination program for prisoners. Presentation 21, 20th Annual Conference on Correctional Health Care, Nashville, Tennessee, October, 1996.
61. Stead WW: Undetected tuberculosis in prison: source of infection for the community at large. JAMA 240:2544–2547, 1978
62. Centers for Disease Control: Prevention and control of tuberculosis in correctional institutions: recommendations of the advisory committee for the elimination of tuberculosis. MMWR 38:313–320, 325, 1989
63. Selwyn PA, Hartel D, Lewis VA, Schoenbaum EE, Vermund SH, Klein RS, Walker AT, Friedland GH: A prospective study of the risk of tuberculosis among intravenous drug users with human immunodeficiency virus infection. N Engl J Med 320(9):545–550, 1989
64. Salive M, Brewer TF: Tuberculosis and human immunodeficiency virus infection: an emerging problem in inmates. J Prison Jail Health 7(2):80–89, 1988
65. Braun MM, Truman BI, Maguire B, DiFerninando GT Jr, Wormser G, Broaddus R, Morse DL: Increasing incidence of tuberculosis in a prison inmate population: association with HIV infection. JAMA 261(3):393–397, 1989
66. Skolnick AA: Some experts suggest the nation's "War on Drugs" is helping tuberculosis stage a deadly comeback. JAMA 268(22): 3177–3178, 1992
67. Reider HL, Cauthen GM, Kelly GD, Bloch AB, Snider DE Jr: Tuberculosis in the United States. JAMA 262(3):385–389, 1989
68. Skolnick AA: Correctional facility TB rates soar; some jails bring back chest roentgenograms. JAMA 268(22):3175–3176, 1992
69. Centers for Disease Control and Prevention: Manual on Contol of Tuberculosis in Correctional Faclities. Atlanta: Centers for Disease Control and Prevention, 1994
70. Schwartz F, Singh S, Small PM, Cashman D, Campbell R, Khoury N, Coulter S, Royce S, Roberto R, Rutherford GW: Epidemiological notes and reports: Tuberculosis transmission in a state correctional system—California 1990–91. MMWR 41: 927–928, 1992
71. Campbell R, Sneller VP, Khoury N: Probable transmission of multidrug-resistant tuberculosis in correctional facility—California. MMWR 42:48–51, 1993
72. Johnsen C: Tuberculosis contact investigation: two years of experience in New York City correctional facilities. Am J Infect Control 21(1):1–4, 1993
73. Wool RJ, Dooley E: A study of attempted suicides in prisons. Med Sci Law 27(4):297–301, 1987
74. National Center on Institutions and Alternatives: National Study of Jail Suicides: Seven Years Later. Alexandria, VA: National Center on Institutions and Alternatives, 1988
75. Tuskan JJ Jr, Thase ME: Suicides in jails and prisons. J Psychosoc Nurs Ment Health Serv 21(5):29–33, 1983
76. Burtch BE: Prisoner suicides reconsidered. Int J Law Psychiatry 2:407–413, 1979
77. Brackett SA: Suicide in Scottish prisons. Br J Psychol 151:218–221, 1987
78. Jordan FB, Schmeckpeper K, Strope M: Jail suicides by hanging: an epidemiological review and recommendations for prevention. Am J Forensic Med Pathol 8(1):27–31, 1987
79. DuRand CJ, Burtka GJ, Federman EJ, Haycox JA, Smith JW: A quarter century of suicide in a major urban jail: implications for community psychiatry. Am J Psychiatry 152:1077–1080, 1995
80. Salive ME, Smith GS, Brewer TF: Suicide mortality in the Maryland State prison system, 1979 through 1987. JAMA 262(3):365–369, 1989
81. Rowan JR, Hayes LM: Training Curriculum on Suicide Detection and Prevention in Jails and Lockups. 2nd ed. Marshfield, MA: Center on Institutions and Alternatives,1995
82. Teplin L: The prevalence of severe mental disorders among male urban jail detainees: comparison with the epidemiologic catchment area program. Am J Pub Health 80:663–669, 1990
83. Axelson GL, Wahl OF: Psychotic versus nonpsychotic misdemeanants in a large county jail: an analysis of pretrial treatment by the legal system. Int J Law Psychiatry 15(4):379–386, 1992
84. Steadman HJ, Morris SM, Dennis DL: The diversion of mentally ill persons from jails to community-based services: a profile of programs. Am J Public Health 85:1630–1635, 1995
85. Solomon P, Draine J, Meyerson A: Jail recidivism and receipt of community mental health services. Hospital and Community Psychiatry 45(8):793–797, 1994
86. Maden T, Swinton M, Hunn J: Psychiatric disorders in women serving a prison sentence, J Psychol 164:44–54, 1994
87. Institute of Medicine: The Future of Public Health. Washington, DC: National Academy Press, 1988, pp 223

Preventive Medicine Support of Military Operations

1. Letterman J: Medical Recollections of the Army of the Potomac. New York: D. Appleton and Co., 1866
2. Withers BG, Erickson RL, Petrucelli BP, Hanson RK, Kadlec RP: Preventing disease and non-battle injury in deployed units. Mil Med 159:39–43, 1994
3. Coates JB Jr, Hoff EC, Hoff PM (eds): Preventive Medicine in World War II. Volume IV. Communicable Diseases Transmitted Chiefly through Respiratory and Alimentary Tracts. Washington, DC: Medical Department, United States Army, 1958
4. Reister FA: Battle Casualties and Medical Statistics. US Army Experience in the Korean War. Washington, DC: The Surgeon General, Department of the Army, undated
5. Washington Headquarters Services Directorate for Information, Operations and Reports: Department of Defense. US Casualties in Southeast Asia. Statistics as of April 30, 1985. Washington, DC: Government Printing Office, 1985
6. Lederberg J, Shope RE, Oaks SC Jr (eds): Emerging Infections. Microbial Threats to Health in the United States. Committee on Emerging Microbial Threats to Health, Division of Health Sciences Policy, Division of International Health, Institute of Medicine, Washington, DC: National Academy Press, 1992
7. Benenson AS (ed): Control of Communicable Diseases Manual. Washington, DC: American Public Health Association, 1995
8. Beck LR, Rodriguez MH, Dister SW, Rodriguez AD, Rejmankova E, Ulloa A, Meza RA, Roberts DR, Paris JF, Spanner MA, Washino RK, Hacker C, Legters LJ: Remote sensing as a landscape epidemiologic tool to identify villages at high risk for malaria transmission. Am J Trop Med Hyg 51(3):271–280, 1994
9. Roberts DR, Paris JF, Manguin S, Harbach RE, Woodruff R, Rejmankova E, Polanco J, Wullschleger B, Legters LJ: Predictions of malaria vector distribution in Belize based on multispectral satellite data. Am J Trop Med Hyg 54(3):304–308, 1996
10. Cross ER, Newcomb WW, Tucker CJ: Use of weather data and remote sensing to predict the geographic and seasonal distribution of *Phlebotomus papatasi* in Southwest Asia. Am J Trop Med Hyg 54(5):530–536, 1996
11. Walter Reed Army Institute of Research: Somalia: preliminary report. WRAIR Communicable Disease Report 3(4):11, 1992
12. Slim W: Defeat into Victory. London: Cassell and Company, 1956
13. Hanson K: Surveillance in military medicine: the ultimate convincer. In Kelly PW (ed): Military Preventive Medicine: Mobilization and Deployment. Washington, DC: Walter Reed Army Institute of Research, in press

Public Health Nursing

1. American Public Health Association: The Definition and Role of Public Health Nursing: A Statement of APHA Public Health Nursing Section. Washington, DC: American Public Health Association, 1996
2. Evans, RG, Barer ML, Marmor TR: Why are Some People Healthy and Others Not? The Determinants of Health of Populations. New York: Aldine De Gruyter, 1994
3. Public Health Functions Steering Committee: Public Health in America Statement, Fall 1994. (Current members of this group include the American Public Health Association, the Association of Schools of Public Health, Association of State and Territorial Health Officers, National Association of County and City Health Officials, Environmental Council of the States, National Association of State Alcohol and Drug Abuse Directors, National Association of State Mental Health Program Directors, Partnership for Prevention, and the Public Health Foundation.)
4. Pope AM, Snyder MA, Mood LH, (eds): Nursing Health and Environment. Washington, DC: National Academy Press, 1995
5. McNeil C: Public Health Nursing within Core Public Health Functions. Olympia: Washington State Department of Health, 1993

Family Planning Programs and Practices: An Epidemiologic Approach

1. Nortman DL: Population and Family Planning Programs: A Compendium of Data Through 1981. 11th ed. New York: Population Council, 1982
2. Callahan D: Ethics and population limitation. Science 174: 487–494, 1972
3. United Nations Fund for Population Activities: The United Nations and population: major resolutions and instruments. Resolution 2211(xxi). New York: Oceana Publications, 1974, pp 81–82
4. United Nations: Report of the International Population Conference, Bucharest, August 19–30, 1974. New York: Oceana Publications, 1975
5. United Nations: Report of the International Conference on Population, Mexico City, August 6–14, 1984. New York: United Nations Publication, 1984
6. Freedman R, Whelpton PK, Campbell AA: Sterility and fecundity of American families. Family Planning, Sterility, and Population Growth. New York: McGraw-Hill, 1959, pp 17–56
7. Ory HW, Cole PT, MacMahon B, Hoover R: Oral contraceptives and reduced risk of benign breast tumors. N Engl J Med 294: 419–422, 1976
8. Cates W Jr, Ory HW, Rochat RW, Tyler CW: The intrauterine device and deaths from spontaneous abortion. N Engl J Med 295: 1155–1159, 1976
9. Centers for Disease Control: Abortion surveillance, 1977. Atlanta: Centers for Disease Control, 1979
10. Peterson HB, DeStefano F, Greenspan JR: Mortality risk association with tubal sterilization in United States hospitals. Am J Obstet Gynecol 143:125–129, 1982
11. Last JM: A Dictionary of Epidemiology. 3rd ed. Oxford, England: Oxford University Press, 1993
12. Ellerbrock TV, Atrash HK, Rhodenheiser EP, Hogue CJ, Smith JC: Abortion surveillance, 1982–1983. MMWR CDC Surveill Summ 36(1):11SS–42SS, 1987
13. Kafrissen ME, Grimes DA, Hogue CJR, Sacks JJ: Cluster of abortion deaths at a single facility. Obstet Gynecol 68:387–389, 1986
14. Lee NC, et al: The reduction in risk of ovarian cancer associated with oral contraceptive use. N Engl J Med 316:650–655, 1987
15. Rooks JB, Ory HW, Ishak KG, et al: Epidemiology of hepatocellular adenoma the role of oral contraceptive use. JAMA 242:644–648, 1979
16. Tietze C, Lewit S: Evaluation of intrauterine devices: ninth progress report of the cooperative statistical program. Stud Fam Plann 5:1–40, 1970
17. Warren CW: Fertility determinants in Puerto Rico. Stud Fam Plann 18:42–48, 1987
18. Berelson B, Freedman R: A study in fertility control. Sci Am May: 29–44, 1964
19. Requena M: Chilean program of abortion control and fertility planning: present situation and forecast for the next decade. In Behrman SJ, Corsa L, Freedman R (eds): Fertility and Family Planning: A World View. Ann Arbor: University of Michigan Press, 1969, pp 478–489
20. Omran AR, Standley CC (eds): Family Formation Patterns and Health: An International Collaborative Study in India, Iran, Lebanon, Philippines and Turkey. Geneva: World Heath Organization, 1976
21. US Department of Health and Human Services, Public Health Service: Family Planning. In Promoting Health/Preventing Disease: Objectives for the Nation. Washington, DC: Government Printing Office, 1990
22. Nortman DL: Government positions on population growth and family planning in less-developed countries, 1982 (map). In Population and Family Planning Programs: A Compendium of Data Through 1981. 11th ed. New York: Population Council, 1982

23. US Department of Health and Human Services, Public Health Service: The 1990 Health Objectives for the Nation: A Midcourse Review. Washington, DC: Government Printing Office, 1990
24. Paxman JM: Reproductive health, youth and the law. WHO Chronicle 38:199–207, 1984
25. American Law Institute: Model Penal Code: Proposed Official Draft: Section 230.3:189–192. Philadelphia: American Law Institute, May 4, 1962
26. Tietze C: Induced Abortion, a World Review, 1983. 5th ed. New York: The Population Council, 1983
27. Supreme Court of the United States: The abortion experience: Psychological and medical impact. Supreme Court of the United States. Syllabus number 70-18 (Roe et al v Wade: appeal from the United States District Court for the Northern District of Texas. Decided January 22, 1973) and number 70-40 (Doe et al v Bolton: appeal from the United States District Court for the Northern District of Georgia. Decided January 22, 1973)
28. Supreme Court of the United States: Syllabus Number 88-605 (Webster et al v Reproductive Health Services: appeal from the United States Court of Appeals for the Eighth Circuit. Decided July 3, 1989)
29. Magarick RH, Burkman RT (eds): Reproductive Health Education and Technology: Issues and Future Directions. Geneva: World Health Organization, 1988
30. Smith JC, Franchino B, Henneberry JF. Surveillance of Family Planning Services at Title X Clinics and Characteristics of Women Receiving These Services, 1991. In: CDC Surveillance Summaries, May 5, 1995. MMWR 4(No. SS-2):1–22, 1995
31. Forrest JD: The delivery of family planning services in the United States. Fam Plann Perspect 20:88–98, 1988
32. Smith JC, Warren CW, Nunez JG: Attitudes toward family planning services. In: The U.S. Mexico Border: Contraceptive Use and Maternal Health Care in Perspective. Atlanta: United States-Mexico Border Health Association, 1983, p 21
33. Mosher WD, Pratt WF: Contraceptive use in the United States, 1973–1988: Advance data from Vital and Health Statistics of the National Center for Health Statistics. March 20, 1990
34. Hatcher RA, Trussell J, Stewart F, et al: Contraceptive Technology. 16th ed. New York: Irvington, 1979, pp 637–653
35. Peterson HB, Lee NC: The health effects of oral contraceptives; misperceptions, controversies, and continuing good news. Clin Obstet Gynecol 32:339–355, 1988
36. Kendrick JS, Lee NC, Wingo PA, Rubin GL: Oral contraceptive use and the risk of endometrial cancer. JAMA 257:796–800, 1987
37. Lee NC, Peterson HB, Chu SY: The health effects of contraception. In Parnell A (ed): Contraceptive Use and Controlled Fertility: Health Issues for Women and Children—Background papers. Washington, DC: National Academy Press, 1989
38. Porter JB, Jick H, Walker AM: Mortality among oral contraceptive users. Obstet Gynecol 70:29–32, 1987
39. Mant D, Villard-Mackintosh L, Vessey MP, et al: Myocardial infarction and angina pectoris in young women. J Epidemol Community Health 41:215–219, 1987
40. Stadel B: Oral contraceptives and the occurrence of disease. In Gregoire AT, Blye RG (eds): Contraceptive Steroids—Pharmacology and Safety. New York: Plenum Press, 1986, p 3
41. Neuberger J, Forman D, Doll R, et al: Oral contraceptives and hepatocellular carcinoma. Br Med J 292:1355–1357, 1986
42. World Health Organization: Collaborative study of neoplasia and steroid contraceptives: combined oral contraceptives and liver cancer. Int J Cancer 43:254–259, 1989
43. Irwin KL, Rosero-Bixby L, Oberle MW, et al: Oral contraceptives and cervical cancer risk in Costa Rica: Detection bias or causal association? JAMA 259:59–64, 1988
44. Physicians Desk Reference. 44th ed. Oradell, NJ: Medical Economics Co., 1990
45. American College of Obstetricians and Gynecologists Committee on Gynecologic Practice: Contraception for women in their late reproductive years. ACOG Committee Opinion No. 41. Washington, DC: American College of Obstetricians and Gynecologists, 1985
46. Forrest JD: The end of IUD marketing in the United States: what does it mean for American women? Fam Plann Perspect 14:52–55, 1986
47. Ory HW: The Women's Health Study: ectopic pregnancy and intrauterine contraceptive devices: new perspectives. Obstet Gynecol 57:137–141, 1981
48. Lee NC, Rubin GL, Borucki R: The intrauterine device and pelvic inflammatory disease revisited: new results from the Women's Health Study. Obstet Gynecol 712:1–6, 1988
49. Farley TMM, Rowe PJ, Rosenberg MJ, Chen J-H, Meirik O: Intrauterine devices and pelvic inflammatory disease: an international perspective. Lancet 339:785–788, 1992
50. Burkman RT: Intrauterine devices and pelvic inflammatory disease: evolving perspectives on the data. Obstet Gynecol Surv 51:S35– S41, 1996
51. Schwartz B, Gaventa S, Broome CV, et al: Nonmenstrual toxic shock syndrome associated with barrier contraceptives: report of a case-control study. Rev Infect Dis (Suppl 1):S43–S49, 1989
52. Reingold AL: Toxic shock syndrome and the contraceptive sponge. JAMA 255:242–243, 1986
53. American College of Obstetricians and Gynecologists: Emergency Oral Contraception. ACOG Practice Pattern No. 3. Washington, DC: American College of Obstetricians and Gynecologists, 1996
54. Trussell J, Ellertson C, Steward F: The effectiveness of the Yuzpe regimen of emergency contraception. Fam Plann Perspect 28: 58–64, 1996
55. Speroff L, Darney PD: A clinical Guide for Contraception. 2nd ed. Baltimore: Williams & Wilkins 1996, pp 129–189
56. Cundy T, Cornish J, Evans MC, Roberts H, Reid JR: Recovery of bone density in women who stop using medroxyprogesterone acetate. BMJ 308:247–248, 1994
57. Skegg DLG, Noonan EA, Paul C, Spears GFS, Meirik O, Thomas DB: Depot medroxyprogesterone acetate and breast cancer: a pooled analysis of World Health Organization and New Zealand studies. JAMA 273:799–804, 1995
58. Short RV: Breast feeding. Sci Am 250:35–41, 1984
59. Liskin L, Rinehart W, Blackburn R, et al: Minilaparotomy and laparoscopy: safe, effective, and widely used. Popul Rep C 9:C125–C167, 1985
60. DeStefano F, Greenspan JR, Ory HW, et al: Demographic trends in tubal sterilization: United States, 1970–1978. Am J Public Health 72:480–484, 1982
61. Centers for Disease Control: Tubal sterilization among women of reproductive age, United States, update for 1979–1980. MMWR CDC Surveill Summ 32(3):9SS–14SS, 1983
62. Schwartz D, Wingo PA, Antarsh L, Smith JC: Female sterilizations in the United States, 1987. Fam Plann Perspect 21:209–212, 1989
63. Pokras R: Hysterectomy: past, present and future. Stat Bull Metrop Insur Co Oct–Dec: 12–21, 1989
64. Nolan TF, Ory HW, Layde PM, Hughes JM, Greenspan JR: Cumulative prevalence rates and corrected incidence rates of surgical sterilization among women in the United States, 1971–1978. Am J Epidemol 116:776–781, 1982
65. Peterson HB, Xia Z, Hughes JM, Wilcox LS, Tylor LR, Trussell J for the U.S. Collaborative Review of Sterilization Working Group: The risk of pregnancy after tubal sterilization: findings from the U.S. Collaborative Review of Sterilization. Am J Obstet Gynecol 174:1161–1170, 1996
66. Peterson HB, Xia Z, Hughes JM, Wilcox LS, Tylor LR, Trussell J for the U.S. Collaborative Review of Sterilization Working Group: The risk of ectopic pregnancy after tubal sterilization. N Engl J Med 336:762–767, 1997

67. Escobedo LG, Peterson HB, Grubb GS, Franks AL: Case-fatality rates for tubal sterilization in U.S. hospitals, 1979 to 1980. Am J Obstet Gynecol 160:147–150, 1989
68. Peterson HB, DeStefano F, Rubin GL, et al: Deaths attributable to tubal sterilization in the United States, 1977 to 1981. Am J Obstet Gynecol 146:131–136, 1983
69. Grimes DA, Peterson HB, Rosenberg MJ, et al: Sterilization-attributable deaths in Bangladesh. Int J Gynaecol Obstet 20:149–154, 1982
70. Grimes DA, Satterthwaite AP, Rochat RW, et al: Deaths from contraceptive sterilization in Bangladesh: rates, causes, and prevention. Obstet Gynecol 60:635–640, 1982
71. World Health Organization Task Force on Female Sterilization: Minilaparotomy or laparoscopy for sterilization: a multicenter, multinational, randomized study. Am J Obstet Gynecol 143:645–652, 1982
72. DeStefano F, Greenspan JR, Dicker RC, et al: Complications of interval laparoscopic tubal sterilization. Obstet Gynecol, 61:153–158, 1983
73. Vessey M, Huggins G, Lawless M, et al: Tubal sterilization: findings in a large prospective study. Br J Obstet Gynaecol 90:203–209, 1983
74. DeStefano F, Perlman JA, Peterson HB, et al: Long-term risk of menstrual disturbances after tubal sterilization. Am J Obstet Gynecol 152:835–841, 1985
75. Cohen MM: Long-term risk of hysterectomy after tubal sterilization. Am J Epidemiol 125:410–419, 1987
76. Henshaw SK, Singh S: Sterilization regret among U.S. couples. Fam Plann Perspect 18:238–240, 1986
77. Wilcox LS, Chu SY, Peterson HB: Characteristics of women who considered or obtained tubal reanastomosis: results from a prospective study of tubal sterilization. Obstet Gynecol 75:661–665, 1990
78. Gallen ME, Liskin L, Kak N: Men—new focus for family planning programs. Popul Rep J 33:J889–J919, 1986
79. Association for Voluntary Surgical Contraception: The 1987 estimate of U.S. sterilizations: trend to outpatient services continues. AVSC News 27(2):1–4, 1989
80. Liskin L, Pile JM, Quillin WF: Vasectomy—safe and simple. Popul Rep D 4:61–100, 1983
81. Ross JA, Hong S, Huber DH: Voluntary Sterilization—An International Fact book. New York: Association for Voluntary Sterilization, 1985
82. Schmidt SS: Vasectomy. JAMA 259:3176, 1988
83. Kendrick JS, Gonzales B, Huber DH, et al: Complications of vasectomies in the United States. J Fam Pract 3:245–248, 1987
84. Peterson HB, Huber DH, Belker AM: Vasectomy: an appraisal for the obstetrician-gynecologist. Obstet Gynecol 76:568–572, 1990
85. Hayes RB: Are dietary fat and vasectomy risk factors for prostate cancer? J Natl Cancer Inst 87:629–631, 1995
86. Howards SS, Peterson HB: Vasectomy and prostate cancer: chance, bias, or a causal relationship? JAMA 269:913–914, 1993
87. John EM, Whittemore AS, Wu AH, et al: Vasectomy and prostate cancer: results from a multi-ethnic case-control study. J Natl Cancer Inst 87:662–669, 1995
88. Chang C, Freedman R, Sun T: Trends in fertility, family size preferences and family planning practice: Taiwan, 1961–1980. Stud Fam Plann 18:320–337, 1987
89. Chang C, Freedman R, Sun T: Trends in fertility, family size preferences and family planning practice: Taiwan, 1961–1980. Stud Fam Plann 12:211–218, 1981
90. Rutenberg N, Ferraz EA: Measuring unmet need, female sterilization and its demographic impact in Brazil. Int Fam Plann Perspect 14:61–67, 1988
91. Prada E, Ojeda G: Fertility and contraception in Colombia: selected findings from the demographic and health survey in Colombia, 1986. Int Fam Plann Perspect 13:116–120, 1987
92. Warren CW, Westoff CF, Herold JM, Rochat RW, Smith JC: Contraceptive sterilization in Puerto Rico. Demography 23:351–365, 1986
93. David HP: Eastern Europe: pronatalist policies and private behavior. Popul Bull 36(6), 1982
94. Lapham RJ, Mauldin WP: Family planning program effort and birthrate decline in developing countries. Int Fam Plann Perspect 10:109–118, 1984
95. Goldberg HI, McNeil M, Spitz A: Contraceptive use and fertility decline, Chogoria, Kenya. Stud Fam Plann 20:17–25, 1989
96. Tomkinson J, Turnbull A, Robson G, et al: Report on confidential enquiries into maternal deaths in England and Wales, 1973–1975. Department of Health and Social Security, Report on Social Subjects 14. London: Her Majesty's Stationary Office, 1979
97. Fortney JA: The importance of family planning in reducing maternal mortality. Stud Fam Plann 18:109–114, 1987
98. Centers for Disease Control: National infant mortality weekly report. MMWR CDC Surveill Summ 38 (3), 1989
99. Smith RG, Gardner RW, Steinhoff P, Chung CS, Palmore JA: The effect of induced abortion on the incidence of Down's syndrome in Hawaii. Fam Plann Perspect 12:201–205, 1980
100. Lyle KC, Segal SL, Chang C, Ch'ien L: Perinatal study in Tientin: 1978. Int J Gynaecol Obstet 18:280–289, 1980
101. Puffer RR, Serrano CV: Birthweight, maternal age, and birth order: three important determinants in infant mortality. Scientific Publication No. 294. Washington, DC: Pan American Health Organization 1975
102. Rao KV, Gopalan C: Nutrition and family size: J Nutr Diet 6:258–266, 1969
103. Study Committee of the Office of the Foreign Secretary, National Academy of Science: Rapid Population Growth: Consequences and Policy Implications. Baltimore: Johns Hopkins University Press, 1971
104. Pebley AR, Millman S: Birthspacing and child survival. Int Fam Plann Perspect 12:71–79, 1986
105. Forrest JD, Singh S: The sexual and reproductive behavior of American women. Fam Plann Perspect 22:206–214, 1990
106. Weller RH, Heuser RL: Wanted and unwanted childbearing in the United States. Vital Health Stat (21), no. 32, 1978
107. Westoff CF et al: The demographic impact of changes in contraceptive practice. Popul Dev Rev 15:91–106, 1989
108. Joyce TJ, Grossman M: Pregnancy wantedness and the early initiation of prenatal care. Demography 27:1–17, 1990
109. Weller RH, Eberstein IW, Bailey M: Pregnancy wantedness and maternal behavior during pregnancy. Demography 24:407–412, 1987
110. Centers for Disease Control: Abortion surveillance, United States, 1982–1983. MMWR CDC Surveill Summ 36(1):11SS–42SS, 1987
111. Centers for Disease Control: Abortion surveillance, preliminary data—United States, 1994. MMWR 45(51 & 52):1123–1127, 1997
112. Ory HW, Forrest JD, Lincoln R: Making choices: evaluating the health risks and benefits of birth control methods. Washington, DC: Alan Guttmacher Institute, 1983
113. CDC Abortion Surveillance special tabulations, provided by Hani Atrash, M.D., 1990
114. Koop CE: The United States surgeon general on the health effects of abortion. Popul Dev Rev 15:172–175, 1989
115. Zabin LS, Hirsch MG, Emerson MR: When urban adolescents choose abortion: effects on education, psychological status and subsequent pregnancy. Fam Plann Perspect 21:248–255, 1989
116. Henshaw SK, Kenney AM, Somberg D, Van Vort J: Teenage pregnancy in the U.S.: The scope of the problem and state responses, New York: Alan Guttmacher Institute, 1989
117. Collaborative Group on Hormonal Factors in Breast Cancer: Breast cancer and hormonal contraceptives: collaborative reanalysis of individual data in 53,297 women with breast cancer and 100,239 women without breast cancer from 54 epidemiological studies. Lancet 347:1713–1727, 1996

118. Collaborative Group on Hormonal Factors in Breast Cancer: Breast cancer and hormonal contraceptives: further results. Contraception 54:1S–106S, 1996
119. DeVincenzi I, for the European Study Group on Heterosexual Transmission of HIV: A longitudinal study of human immunodeficiency virus transmission by heterosexual partners. N Engl J Med 331:341–346, 1994
120. Saracco A, Musicco M, Nicolosi A, et al: Man-to-woman sexual transmission of HIV: longitudinal study of 343 steady partners of infected men. J Acquir Immun Defic Syndr 6:497–502, 1993
121. Deschamps M-M, Pape JW, Hafner A, Johnson WD Jr: Heterosexual transmission of HIV in Haiti. Ann Intern Med 125:324–330, 1996
122. Centers for Disease Control and Prevention: Update: barrier protection against HIV infection and other sexually transmitted diseases. MMWR 42:(30), 1993
123. Connor EM, Sperling RS, Gelber R, et al: Reduction of maternal-infant transmission of human immunodeficiency virus type 1 with zidovudine treatment. N Engl J Med 331:1173–1180, 1994
124. Djerassi C: The bitter pill. Science 245:356–361, 1989

VII

Injury and Violence

Edited by Mark L. Rosenberg and Katie Baer

72

Injury Control: The Public Health Approach

Jess F. Kraus • Corinne Peek-Asa • Dushyanthi Vimalachandra

Injuries are a focus of public health practice because they pose a serious health threat, occur frequently, and are theoretically preventable. Thus, the reduction in the number and severity of injuries offers a cost-effective manner in which to improve the health status of populations. Injuries are a very broad group of afflictions, arising from many different activities and risk factors and can affect all organ systems of the body. Since injuries are so diverse in mechanisms of occurrence, formulating an organized and structured approach to studying their incidence and prevention is helpful.

Injuries affect people of all ages and range from minor cuts and bruises to major catastrophes that take thousands of lives. Some injuries may result in prolonged pain or life-long disabilities that restrict an individual from performing personal and work-related activities. Furthermore, injuries often affect more than a single individual, destroying families and devastating communities as seen in recent earthquakes, hurricanes, and plane crashes. These events can leave individuals and societies with enormous medical costs, extensive rehabilitation needs, major lifestyle adjustments, and depression—losses that cannot easily, if ever, be recouped.

However, the majority of injuries do not occur as a result of a catastrophic disaster; instead they are related to daily events. For example, the annual number of deaths from motor vehicle crashes in the United States far exceeds that from airline crashes and natural disasters combined. Injuries disproportionately affect the young, the frail, and the underserved populations. In fact, those in the youngest age groups are more in danger of sustaining injuries than they are of being affected by the more recognized threats to health such as infections, cancer, and cardiovascular disease. Hence, injuries account for the most years of premature productive life lost, number of school and work days missed, and have become one of the largest components of the medical care dollar expenditure per capita.

The public is largely unaware of the preventable nature of many injuries. The most common reference to injurious events, "accidents," evokes a feeling of chance, misfortune, and helplessness. Hence, the word "accident" should be avoided in discussing injury control, and instead, the focus should be on exposures to hazards and resulting injuries, as well as their preventability. In recent years, great strides have been made in injury prevention. Modifications in vehicle design and changes of hazardous behaviors, such as drunk driving, have been effective in reducing traffic-related injuries. Preventive measures have been successful in reducing the incidence of drownings, poisonings, falls, and fires. Despite successes in many areas of injury prevention, new risks and increasing population size constantly challenge the public health community. Development of effective injury prevention strategies warrants an interdisciplinary approach that draws on public health, biomechanics, engineering, behavioral sciences, law enforcement, medicine, and urban planning. Hence, future work should involve collaborative efforts of professionals from these various fields.

This chapter presents a short public health history of injuries, examines the magnitude and distribution of injuries in the United States, and outlines approaches to injury control measures. Unintentional injuries are the focus of this chapter, namely those that have no human intentional motivation behind them and include injuries from traffic-related events, falls, drownings, and most poisonings. Intentional injuries, on the other hand, have discernible human motivation and may be self-directed, such as suicide, or outwardly directed, such as homicide and assault. Although the number of intentional injuries is increasing more rapidly than unintentional injuries, unintentional injuries, currently and historically, have composed a greater share of deaths and nonfatal injuries.

▸ PUBLIC HEALTH HISTORY OF INJURIES

Injury prevention measures, such as the use of protective clothing in warfare, existed long before injuries were systematically studied. In the early 1940s, one of the first epidemiologic studies recognized the importance of studying defined populations using comparison groups. Cairns and his associates compared head injury incidence between helmeted and unhelmeted motorcycle riders in the military.[1,2] These studies demonstrated a decrease in head injuries among those riders wearing helmets.

In 1949, John Gordon[3] noted that injuries were patterned by age, gender, and other demographic factors, as well as by time and place. He recognized that "accidents" could be studied utilizing epidemiologic methods similar to those used in infectious or chronic disease prevention. In 1961, James Gibson[4] defined the agent of injury as energy in its many forms. William Haddon Jr. placed this theory into a framework, which identified vehicles and vectors of injury occurrence, analogous to the models used for the study of infectious diseases.[5,6] He recognized that injuries occur when energy delivered to a living host from a vehicle or vector exceeds human tolerance. He further categorized the energy-host interaction into (*a*) the energy delivered in excess of human tolerance, such as mechanical energy in motor vehicle crashes or in falls, and (*b*) interference with energy use in normal metabolic functions, such as occurs in drownings or poisonings. Using these basic ideas as a framework, Haddon created a comprehensive matrix of host-energy interactions, which is discussed later in this chapter.

Surviving the crash of his trainer aircraft, Hugh DeHaven found a connection between his abdominal injuries and the shape

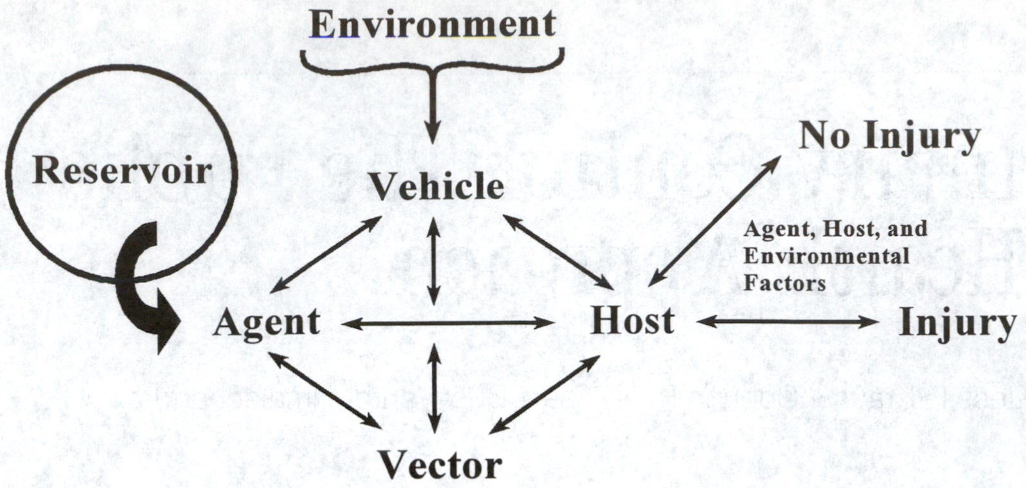

Figure 72-1. Epidemiologic model.

and riveting location of his safety belt. In 1941, DeHaven studied ways in which engineering could reduce the severity of injuries during motor vehicle crashes.[7] His work bred new studies on human tolerance to energy forces during many types of impacts. His approach using biomechanical principles coupled with epidemiologic evaluation is now prominent in motor vehicle crash research.

▶ INJURY CONTROL AND THE PUBLIC HEALTH MODEL

In the 1960s and 1970s, the traditional model used for infectious disease epidemiology provided the framework for epidemiologic studies of injuries. Hence, the underlying concepts of the model, such as exposure and outcome, are also being applied to injuries (Fig. 72-1).

Reservoir

Reservoir is that place in the environment where the agent is usually found. The concept of a "reservoir" may be explained by visualizing the scheme of an energy source and its transfer. For example, generators are the reservoirs of electricity, which is then transferred to a host via electrical wires. The gun is a reservoir of potential energy while holding bullets; this energy is released when a bullet is fired from the gun and then represents kinetic energy.

Agent

Energy (in the form of mechanical, electrical, chemical, thermal, and radiation) is the agent that causes injury to the host. The delivery mechanism of this energy causes damage to the host, ranging from blunt trauma to tissues and organs to penetrating wounds to these same organs. Understanding energy transfer to the body and the resulting damage will aid us in the development of preventive and treatment methods.

Vehicles and Vectors

Vehicles and vectors are mechanisms of energy transmission: they transport the energy from the reservoir to a susceptible host. Vehicles are inanimate objects, such as motor vehicles and bullets; vectors are animate, such as dogs and bees. Both vehicles and vectors may also be involved in energy transfer, as in the case of one individual (vector) stabbing another with a knife (vehicle).

Host Response

Not all, but some exposures to energy result in noticeable injury. However, measures such as exercise and the use of protective devices increases human resistance to injury-causing agents. On the contrary, changes in both intrinsic factors (medical conditions and increasing age) and extrinsic factors (fatigue and alcohol) can potentially reduce host response to these same energies.

The Haddon Matrix

The Haddon Matrix is a detailed model of the agent-host relationship in injury causation used as the foundation for the study of motor vehicle crashes and countermeasures for highway safety.[5,8] The Haddon Matrix divides the timing of the injury event into three phases: pre-event, event, and postevent (Table 72-1). The preinjury or pre-event phase refers to the period before the event occurs and includes all factors that influence potential exposure, for example, use of alcohol

TABLE 72-1. THE HADDON MATRIX WITH ILLUSTRATIONS

	Factors			
			Environment	
Phases	***Human***	***Vector (Vehicle)***	***Physical***	***Socioeconomic***
Preinjury	Alcohol intoxication	Instability in utility vehicles	Poor visibility of road hazards	Lack of knowledge regarding injury risks
Injury	Resistance to energy	Sharp or pointed edges and surfaces	Flammable building materials	Lack of enforcement of safety belt legislation
Postinjury	Existing conditions that affect energy tolerance	Rapidity of energy reduction	Emergency medical response	Lack of funding for emergency medical services and rehabilitation services

before driving a car. The injury phase involves factors that affect energy transmission during the event, such as the presence of energy-absorbing materials, and the postinjury phase is the host response to the event. Each of these phases is further influenced by human, vehicle or equipment, and environmental components. Table 72-1 presents the Haddon Matrix along with examples of each phase.

▶ INJURY OCCURRENCE

This section presents information on data sources available to study the magnitude and scope of the injury problem in the United States. A detailed review of the data sources is not provided here; however, a complete listing of national data sources can be found in Gable's article "A Compendium of Public Health Data Sources" in the *American Journal of Epidemiology*[9] and in Annest et al.[10]

Data Sources

Mortality

Most countries use death certificates to obtain an official mortality count. In this manner, deaths in developed countries have been accurately reported for many years. On the other hand, mortality counts in less developed countries are not as reliable and are often not recorded by cause of death. International comparisons of mortality statistics are routinely reported by the World Health Organization, yet limitations posed by differing age distributions and varying exposures reduce comparability of the data across countries. Differences in reporting, coding criteria, and data reliability also affect comparability and generalizability of the information obtained.

Since the 1900s, data on fatal injuries in the United States are available as Vital Statistics Records collected by the National Center for Health Statistics (NCHS). These data are collected from death certificates of all deaths occurring in the United States and are classified by the International Classification of Diseases External Cause of Death Codes (E-codes). The U.S. Vital Statistics Records are a good source of fatal injuries resulting from broadly defined causes, as well as those categorized by age, race, and gender. However, detailed information about events and types of injuries sustained is not available.

A complete United States database on motor vehicle crash-related fatalities is found in the Fatal Accident Reporting System (FARS), developed in 1975 and sustained by the U.S. Department of Transportation (DOT). Fatalities resulting from and occurring within 30 days of a crash are collected from reports recorded by state and local police agencies in the United States and assembled by the National Highway Traffic Safety Administration of the U.S. DOT. Beginning in 1988, the General Estimates System (GES) was added to the FARS database. The GES uses a nationally representative probability sample selected from all police-reported cases to estimate annual nonfatal crash injuries in the United States.

Work-related fatal injuries are collected by several sources. The National Traumatic Occupational Fatality System developed by the National Institute for Occupational Safety and Health uses United States death certificates for case identification. Work-related fatalities are determined by an item on the death certificate that asks whether or not the death in question occurred while the decedent was at work. The validity of this item to identify work-related fatalities varies by occupation, age, and gender. The specificity in correctly identifying all work-related fatalities may be low, leading to underestimates of this figure.[11] Since 1992, the Bureau of Labor Statistics has maintained the Census of Fatal Occupational Injury (CFOI) program, which may be the most accurate system currently in place, due to the use of multiple data sources in identifying and classifying work-related injuries. The National Safety Council is yet another source of work-related fatality counts. Though three sources of work-related fatal injury data exist, each uses a different definition of work, collects information from varying work populations, and uses different values as denominators for rate calculations.

Morbidity

Estimates of injury morbidity in the United States are available from the National Health Interview Survey, conducted among a sample of households. Responses obtained from this telephone interview survey are weighted to estimate the incidence of all injuries in the United States, regardless of any medical care received. Although this survey provides valuable prevalence information, it is also likely to undersample the severely injured individuals and those institutionalized with injury disabilities.

Hospital discharge information is a source of national and state estimates of injury incidence. The National Hospital Discharge Survey conducted by the NCHS collects discharge data from a national sample of nonfederal, short-stay hospitals and estimates the number of injuries requiring hospital admission. Many states also aggregate their discharge data to create the Uniform Hospital Discharge Data Sets (UHDDS). To calculate national estimates of emergency department visits, the NCHS conducts a survey of injury-related visits to hospital emergency departments. Among many other surveys, the NCHS conducts the National Ambulatory Medical Care Survey to estimate the number of office visits for several types of medical conditions and the National Nursing Home Survey to obtain information on injuries sustained by the elderly population residing in nursing homes.

In addition to determining work-related fatality rates, the Bureau of Labor Statistics conducts a mail survey of occupational injuries and illnesses on a sample of approximately 280,000 employers. This survey has been criticized for a number of technical and administrative reasons,[12] but is improving and becoming a more reliable source of information regarding work-related injuries and fatalities.

The Centers for Disease Control and Prevention conducts a telephone interview survey in diverse areas of the United States to determine changes in the population's perception of risk and the prevalence of behavioral risk factors such as helmet and seat belt use. Information from the Behavioral Risk Factor Surveillance System is then used to determine the various risk-taking behaviors that contribute to the 10 leading causes of death.

Regional surveillance systems, where they exist, provide the most comprehensive information on injury incidence, cause, and outcome. Surveillance systems use different sources of information based on both the needs of the community and the goals of the program. Comprehensive surveillance systems combine information from hospitals, police, and emergency medical services.

Many surveillance systems provide detailed information about specific types of injuries, exposures, and outcomes. The National Electronic Injury Surveillance System (NEISS), conducted by the U.S. Consumer Product Safety Commission, gathers information from a national sample of hospitals about product-related injuries requiring either hospital admission or emergency department treatment.[13] The NEISS includes fewer than 70 hospitals, which raises questions of representation and completeness of reporting resulting from small sample size. Such national surveillance systems also exist for burns, boating injuries, and high school athletic injuries.[14]

Surveillance of injuries has been an important development in injury research. Agencies such as the Bureau of Labor Statistics, the National Highway Traffic Safety Administration, and the Centers for Disease Control and Prevention have been instrumental in establishing national surveillance systems for particular injury mechanisms and situations. As the high incidence and cost of injuries are becoming better recognized, hospitals and communities are establishing local trauma registries and injury surveillance systems. The first documented computerized trauma surveillance system was introduced in 1969 at Cook County Hospital in Chicago.[15] Other areas, such as San Diego County in California, are combining information from hospitals, the Emergency Medical Service Authority, and police to form a comprehensive surveillance program. Furthermore, many states and regions have specialized surveillance programs targeting specific types of injuries, for example, brain and spinal cord injury. These surveillance systems follow models used by cancer registries and the like. Surveillance systems and registries are necessary to follow trends in injury occurrence, identify new injury mechanisms, and evaluate intervention strategies.

▶ INJURY INCIDENCE AND TRENDS

Mortality

In 1994, unintentional injuries were the fifth leading cause of death, with a mortality rate of 34.6 per 100,000 population.[16] Unintentional injuries, however, were the leading cause of death for all those age 1 to 24, the second leading cause for those age 25 to 44, and the third leading cause among those age 45 to 64. Up to age 24, the injury mortality rate is more than twice that for diseases of the heart, cancer, and chronic obstructive pulmonary disease.

The unintentional injury mortality rate shows a decline for ages 1 to 4 years compared with that for ages 5 to 14 and then increases sharply to a rate of 38.7 per 100,000 from ages 15 to 24 (Figure 72-2). Most of this increase can be attributed to motor vehicle crash-related injuries. The unintentional injury mortality rate remains between 30 and 40 deaths per 100,000 population until the increase at about age 65. Death rates by age group for heart disease, cancer, and chronic obstructive pulmonary disease remain below 10 per 100,000 population until the age of 35 and then increase steadily with increasing age. Thus, mortality rates that are not age-adjusted may not accurately reflect the role of injuries in killing the young. The leading causes of unintentional injury death from birth through age 5 are poisonings and drownings; the leading cause in the elderly is falls. Motor vehicle-related death rates are the highest of all injuries between the ages of 5 and 34 and peak between the ages of 15 and 24, the age group when young drivers are first licensed. Alcohol use is an important risk factor in motor vehicle crashes during these ages.

Injury mortality rates show characteristic patterns by age, gender, and race (Figs. 72-3 and 72-4). For all racial groups, males consistently have higher injury death rates than do females.[17] Figures 72-3 and 72-4 show mortality rates by age for African Americans and whites for males and females, respectively. The y axis is kept constant in Figures 72-3 (males) and 72-4 (females) to show contrasts between males and females. Among males, the black population has higher mortality rates for all ages except those between 15 and 24 years. Injury rates show the characteristic increase between ages 15 and 24, and then in black males, but not white males, increase with increasing age. Rates for white males decrease between the ages of 24 to 64, and then increase above age 64.

Through all age and race categories, males have higher unintentional injury rates than females. Increased injury death rates in males have been attributed to aggressive, risk-taking behavior, exposure to motor vehicles, drinking, and drug use. Motor vehicle crashes are responsible for about 25 deaths per 100,000 males, accounting for the largest single component of unintentional injury deaths. The death rate from unintentional injuries among white males is almost twice that of white females, and the rate for black males is almost three times that of black females.

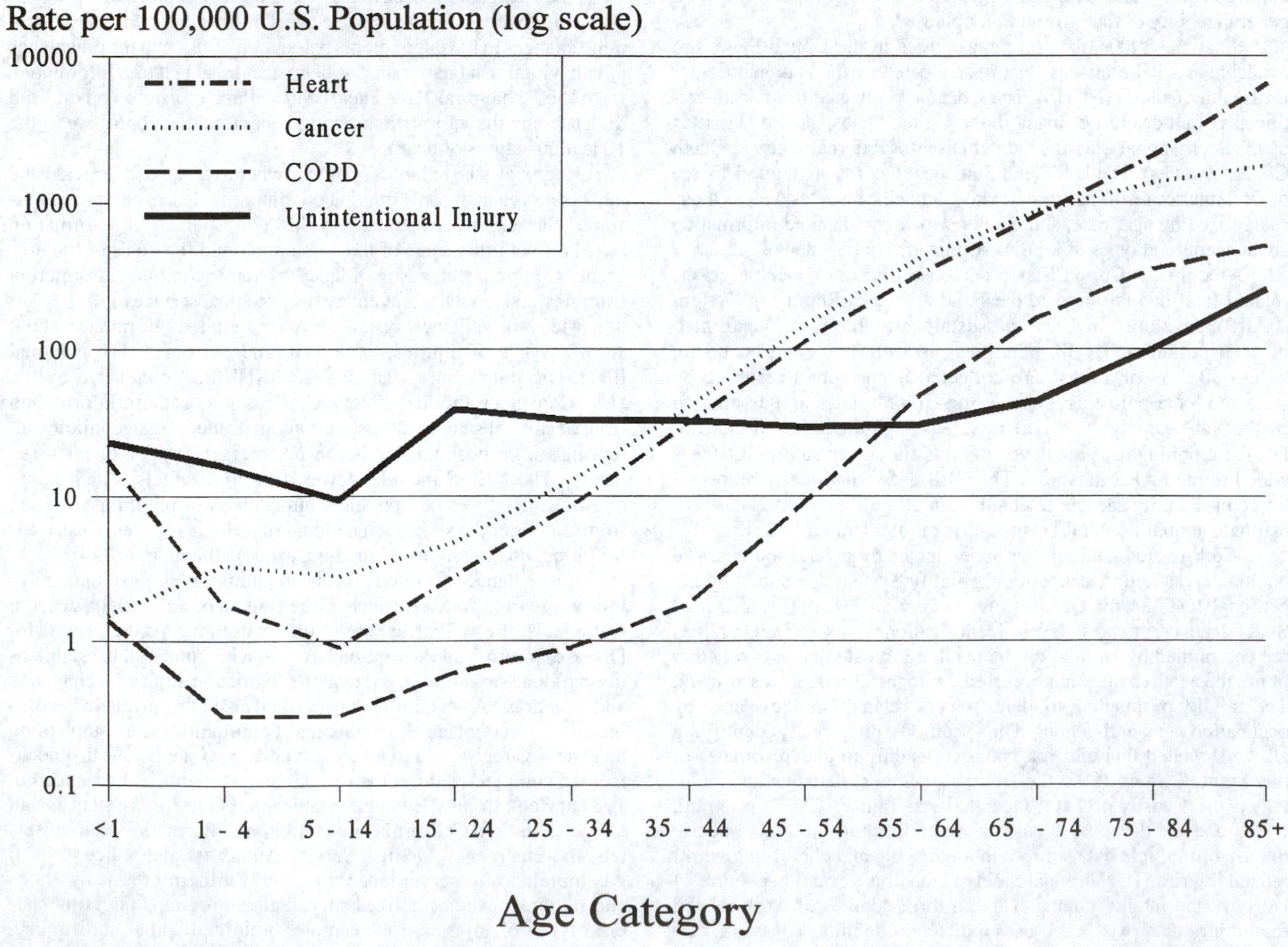

Figure 72-2. Mortality rates for leading casues of death, by age, United States, 1994. *COPD*, chronic obstructive pulmonary disease.

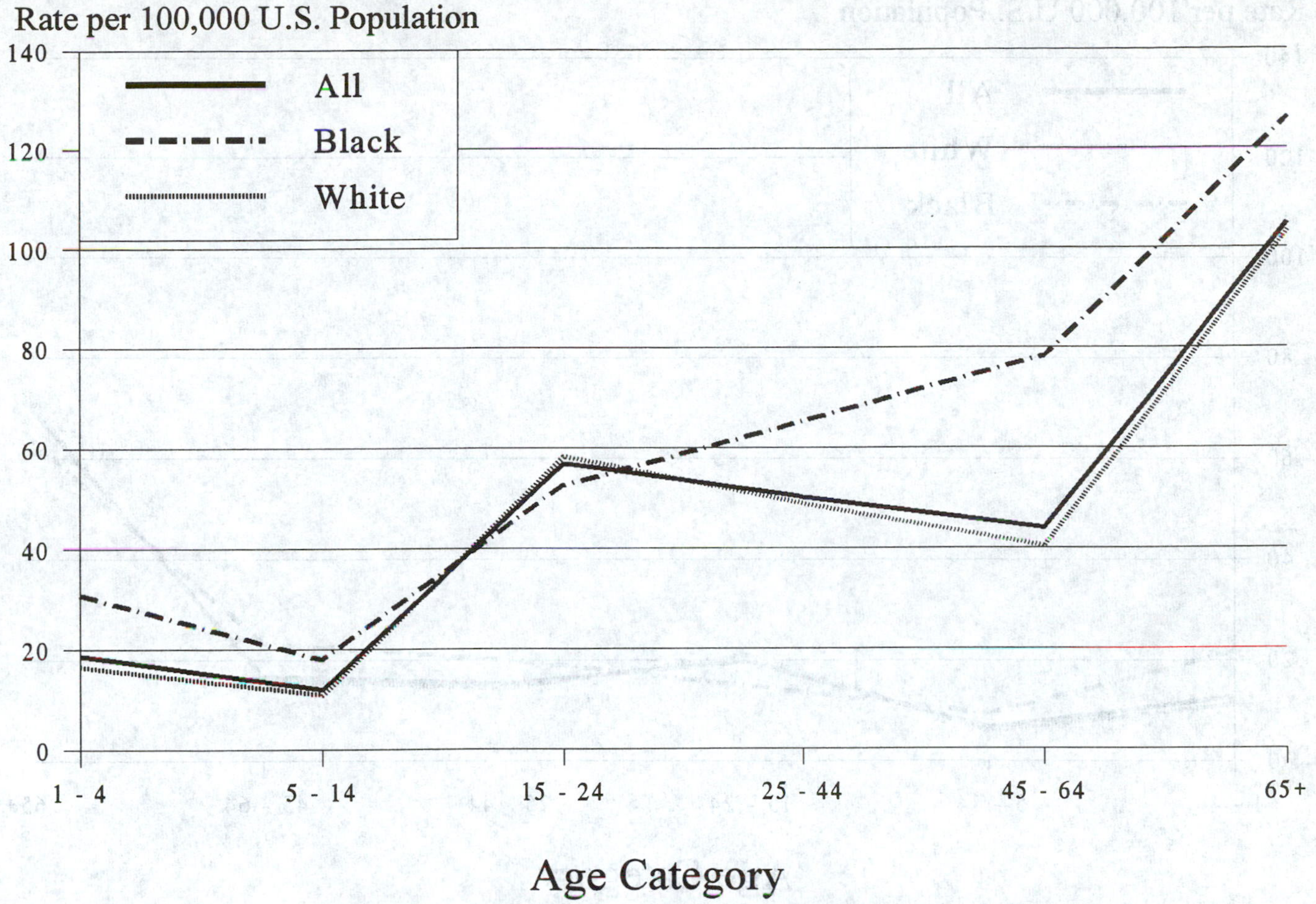

Figure 72-3. Rates of unintentional injury deaths among males, by age and race, United States, 1994.

Differences in injury death rates for African American and white females are much less disparate than those found among males. As with males, black females show higher injury mortality rates than do white females between the ages of 1 and 14 and then have lower rates between the ages of 15 and 24. Unlike rates for males, the rate for white females surpasses that of black females after age 64. This increase is almost exclusively attributed to fall-related injuries, and the discrepancy in mortality rates between races has yet to be fully explained.

Morbidity

Figure 72-5 shows the injury pyramid, which depicts the number of injury deaths and the estimated number of hospital admissions, emergency department visits, and office visits for injuries during 1992.[18] In 1992, almost 3 million people were hospitalized in the United States for injuries, as estimated by the National Hospital Discharge Survey.[18] This is a ratio of 19 admissions for every death. For every death, 233 injured individuals (almost 40 million annually) were treated and released from hospital emergency departments and 450 injured individuals were treated in physician's offices. Adding all levels of the injury pyramid yields over 100 million injuries requiring some level of medical care in 1992.

Emergency Department Visits

Of the 89.8 million emergency department visits in the United States in 1992, about 38 percent were for injuries.[19] Nonfatal injuries differ from injury deaths not only in magnitude but also in cause of injury (Fig. 72-6). In 1992, unintentional injuries accounted for almost 60 percent of all injury-related deaths and 65 percent of classifiable injury-related emergency department (ED) visits in the United States. Motor vehicle crashes accounted for 28 percent of injury fatalities but only 14 percent of ED visits. Falls represented 18 percent of fatal injuries and 27 percent of ED visits. The number of falls leading to fatality among the elderly, however, may be underestimated because deaths may be attributed to comorbid conditions.

Among emergency department visits for injuries in 1992, males had higher injury rates up to age 65 (Fig. 72-7). The greatest disparity between males and females was among those 15 to 24, in which 25 of every 100 males and 15.4 of every 100 females had an injury-related ED visit. This age group had the highest rates for both males and females. The lowest rates for both males and females was between ages 45 and 74.

Emergency department visits by cause of injury vary by race (Fig. 72-8). The rate of visits for falls was higher for whites than blacks; for motor vehicle injuries, higher for blacks than whites. Rates were approximately equal among races for injuries caused by accidentally being struck by an object or cut by an object.

Injury Diagnoses

Table 72-2 provides information on first-listed and all-listed injury diagnoses for U.S. hospital admissions in 1992. The first-listed diagnosis is usually but not necessarily the most severe injury sustained. First-listed diagnoses from the hospital discharge summary approximate the total number of individuals injured. However, first-listed diagnoses do not reflect multiple injuries and therefore underestimate the total number of individuals sustaining particular types of injuries each year, especially the less severe injuries. All-listed

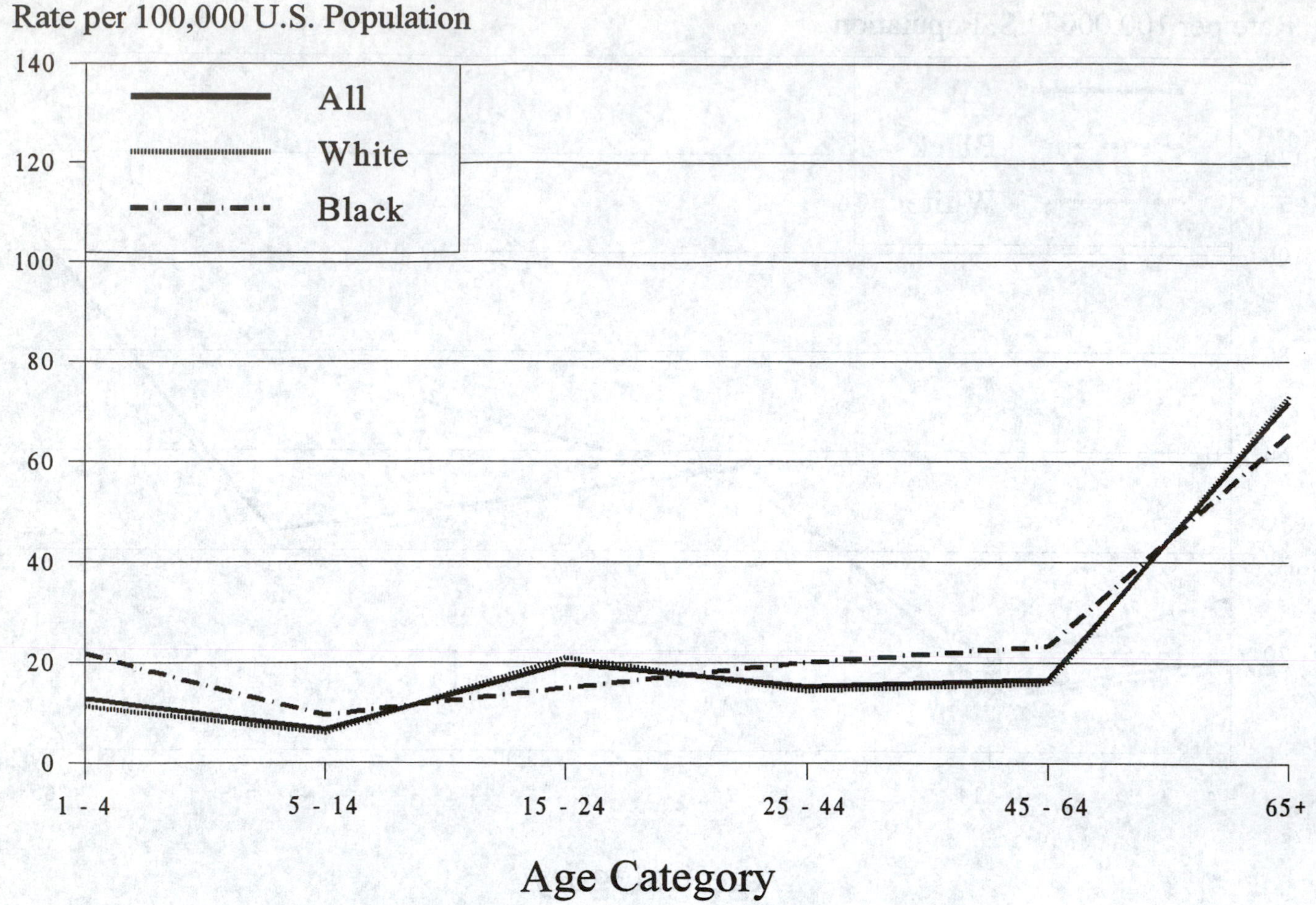

Figure 72-4. Rates of unintentional injury deaths among females, by age and race, United States, 1994.

diagnoses provide better estimates of the total number of individuals sustaining a given type of injury, but a single injured person may have several different injuries.

"Lower limb fractures and dislocations" are the most common first-listed diagnosis, composing almost 25 percent of all discharges with a rate of about 259 per 100,000 population in 1992. The rate of lower extremity injuries by all-listed diagnoses increases to about 344 per 100,000 population, indicating that lower extremity injuries often occur with other, more severe injuries, as in a motorcycle crash. Falls and motor vehicle crashes are the most common cause of lower extremity injuries. "Internal organ, blood vessel injuries, or open wounds" was the next most common diagnosis with a rate of about 85 per 100,000 population for first-listed and about 287 per 100,000 population for all-listed diagnoses. Skull fractures and brain injuries are sustained by about 401,000 individuals each year (a rate of 158 individuals per 100,000 population for all-listed diagnoses). Skull fracture with associated brain injury and brain injury without skull fracture, both of which almost always lead to some degree of disability, are sustained by approximately 180,000 individuals annually. Motor vehicle crashes and homicides are leading causes of head injuries, although head injuries in motor vehicle crashes have been reduced through the use of seat belts and air bags.

Diagnoses involving spinal cord, brain, and burn injuries account for the longest average lengths of hospital stay. Individuals diagnosed with vertebral fractures and skull fractures with brain injury have average hospital stays of over 15 days, and burn victims average over 10 days in a primary care hospital. In addition, many of these individuals are discharged to rehabilitation or nursing care facilities for extended stays.

Impairment and Disability

The average annual prevalence of physical impairments due to injuries in the United States between 1985 and 1987 was almost 19 million, or 80 per 1,000 persons.[13] Individuals with moderately severe motor vehicle crash injuries have an average of 6.5 years of resulting impairment and 2.7 years of lost productivity. Over 26 percent of all physical impairments are due to injuries, and impairments due to

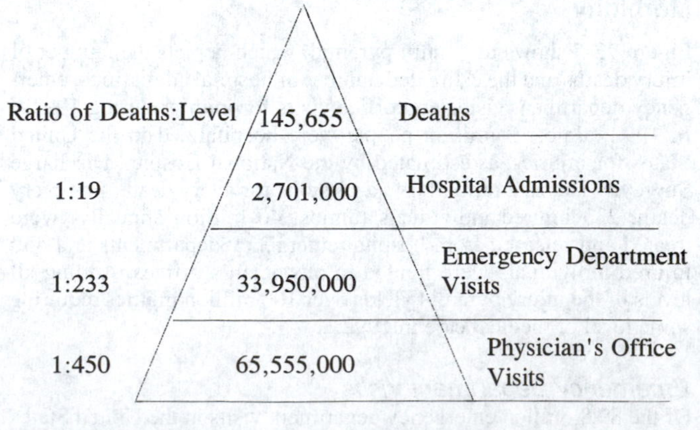

Figure 72-5. Numbers and ratios of injury deaths, hospital admissions, emergency department and office visits for injuries, United States, 1992.

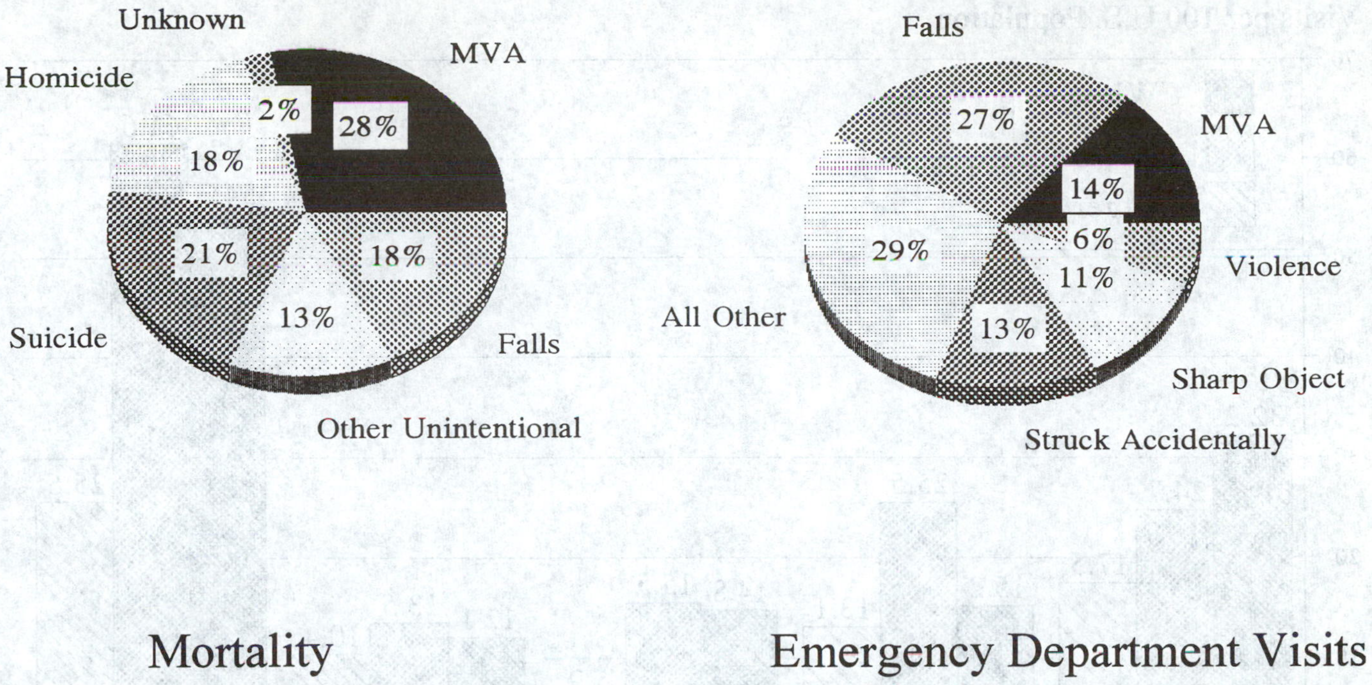

Figure 72-6. Proportionate causes of injury mortality and emergency department visits, United States, 1992. *MVA*, motor vehicle accidents.

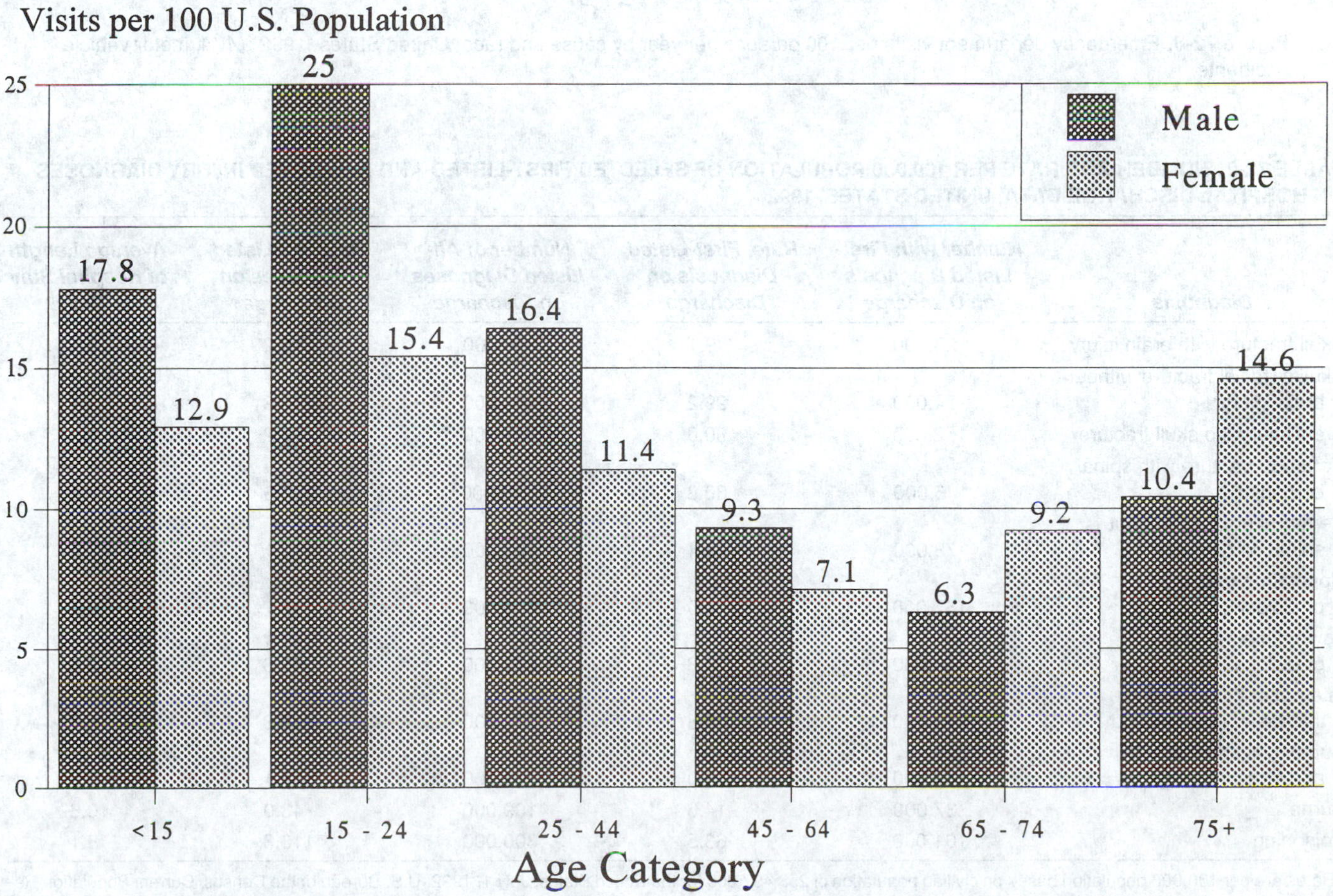

Figure 72-7. Emergency department visits per 100 persons per year by age and sex, United States, 1992.

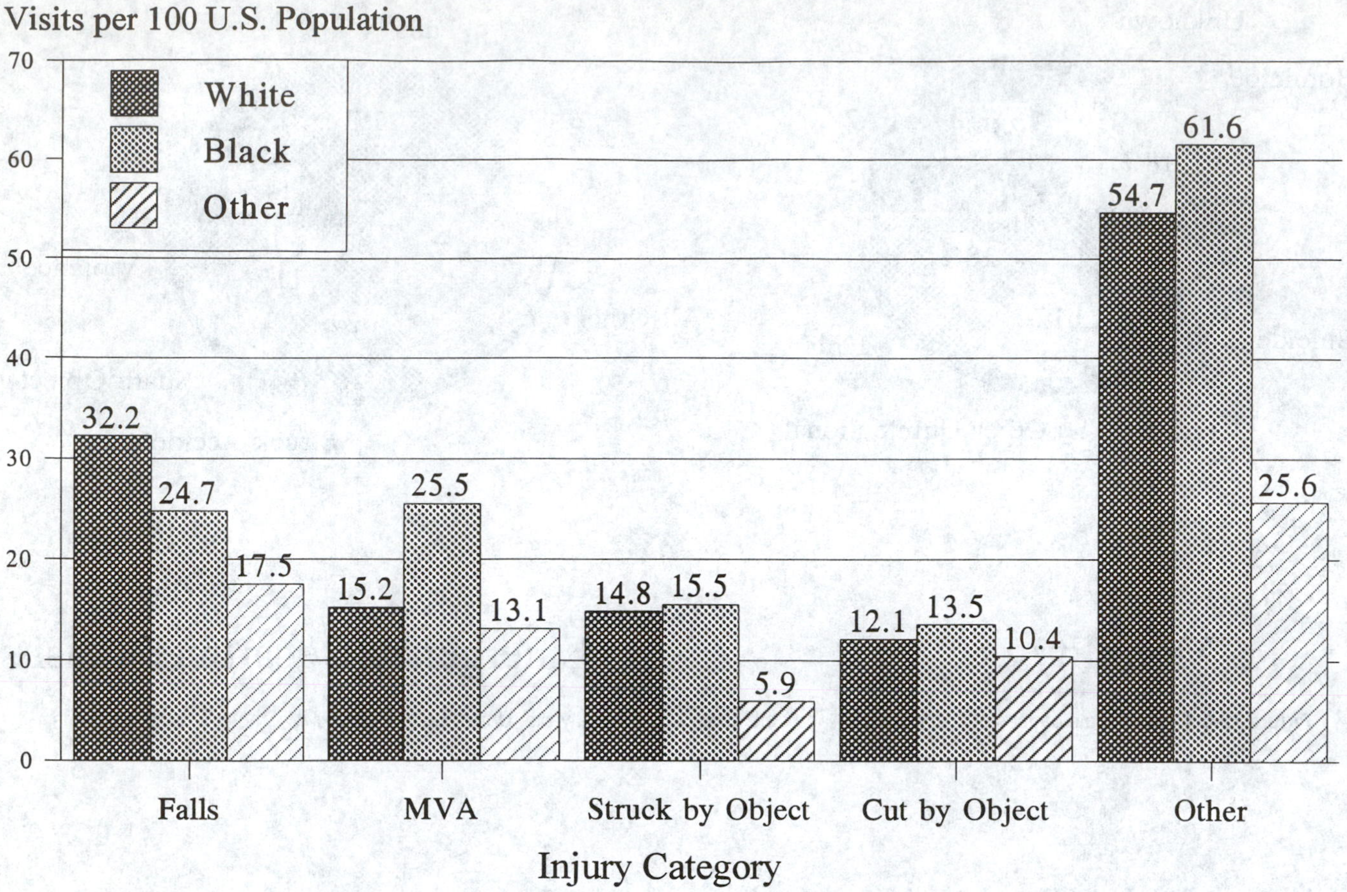

Figure 72-8. Emergency department visits per 100 persons per year by cause and race, United States, 1992. *MVA*, motor vehicle accidents.

TABLE 72-2. NUMBER AND RATE PER 100,000 POPULATION OF SELECTED FIRST-LISTED AND ALL-LISTED INJURY DIAGNOSES ON HOSPITAL DISCHARGE DATA, UNITED STATES, 1992

Diagnosis	*Number with First-Listed Diagnosis on Discharge*	*Rate, First-Listed Diagnosis on Discharge*[a]	*Number of All-Listed Diagnoses on Discharge*	*Rate, All-Listed Diagnoses on Discharge*[a]	*Average Length of Hospital Stay in Days*[b]
Skull fracture with brain injury	23,000	9.1	36,000	14.2	15.1
Skull or facial fracture without brain injury	74,000	29.2	144,000	56.8	3.7
Brain injury, no skull fracture	152,000	60.0	221,000	87.2	5.5
Vertebral fracture with spinal cord injury	6,000	30.8	9,000	3.6	15.5
Vertebral fracture without spinal cord injury	78,000	2.4	127,000	50.1	7.8
Upper limb fracture or dislocation	162,000	64.0	301,000	118.7	3.7
Lower limb fracture or dislocation	656,000	258.8	871,000	343.6	8.6
Internal or blood vessel injuries or open wound	215,000	84.8	727,000	286.8	5.0
Superficial sprains and strains	147,000	58.0	274,000	108.1	3.3
Burns	37,000	14.6	109,000	43.0	10.6
Poisoning	161,000	63.5	300,000	118.3	3.1

[a] Rates are per 100,000 population based on civilian population of 253,497,000 for the United States, July 1, 1992. U.S. Bureau of the Census, Current Population Reports, series P-25.
[b] Average length of hospital stay is based on first-listed discharge diagnosis.

injuries compared to impairments from other causes disproportionately affect younger people.[13]

According to the National Health Interview Survey (NHIS) for 1985–1987, over 70 percent of impairments reported were deformities or orthopedic impairments, which affect about 57 per 1,000 population per year.[13] Almost 43 percent of orthopedic impairments involve the back, and 40 percent involve the lower extremities. Amputations of extremities or parts of extremities, excluding tips of digits, represent about 7 percent of impairment (5/1,000 individuals), and paralysis represents 1.4 percent (1/1,000 individuals). Of the causes of impairments included in the NHIS, motor vehicle crash injuries are the most common cause of impairment, followed by work-related injuries and injuries occurring in the home.

Disabilities due to brain and spinal cord injuries are generally the most severe, long-lasting, and tragic. National estimates of the prevalence of permanently disabled persons due to brain and spinal cord injuries are not readily available. Because permanently disabled individuals often live in care-providing facilities, domestic telephone surveys underestimate the prevalence of disability. Based on brain injury incidence and outcome estimates, the rate of new disabilities from brain injuries each year could be as high as 33 to 45 per 100,000 population.[20]

Researchers are just beginning to measure the emotional trauma that impairment and disability have on loss of quality of life, self-esteem, and family structure. An increased public health focus on injury prevention will not only decrease the incidence of annual impairment and disability but improve quality of life for impaired individuals by increasing awareness about disabilities, modifying the environment to prevent injury, and increasing access and mobility for those with impairments.

Lost Productivity and Cost of Injuries

The person-years of productive life lost from injuries exceeds all other life-threatening conditions.[21] Injury mortality was responsible for over 5 million life-years lost, with an average of 36 years lost per death. Heart and cerebrovascular diseases and cancer account for more lost lives, but average less than half of the years lost per life compared with injuries. Injuries accounted for 6.8 percent of all deaths, but 15.4 percent of all life-years lost.

Years of life lost due to premature mortality in the United States vary by gender and racial group. For males, African Americans have the largest number of years of life lost before age 65, followed by American Indians, Hispanics, non-Hispanic whites, and Asians. Among females, whose years of life lost are much less than that for males, non-Hispanic white females had greater losses than did Hispanic females.[22]

Little is known about the degree of disability and quality of life for survivors of major trauma. Measuring years of functional life lost is complicated because so many factors must be considered, including functional status, preinjury and postinjury employment, and life satisfaction. The years of functional life lost are greatest for survivors of brain and spinal cord injuries. In one study, only 55 percent of patients who survived severe closed head injury and who were employed full-time before their injury could return to work.[23] However, the greatest toll on lost work days is probably from minor injuries, which, although they result in relatively short absences, are highly prevalent.

Motor vehicle deaths are responsible for 37 percent of life-years lost to injury, followed by firearms and falls, responsible for 22 and 19 percent of life-years lost to injury, respectively. While the number of life-years lost to motor vehicle crashes has decreased in the last several years, the number due to firearm injuries is rapidly increasing, especially among individuals living in the inner cities of large metropolitan areas.

The economic costs of injuries can be measured in direct costs, those resulting from medical care, and indirect costs, such as those resulting from years of life lost, lost productivity, or property damage. In 1985, 57 million injuries resulted in an estimated total cost of $157.6 billion: $44.8 billion in direct costs, $64.9 billion in lost productivity, and $47.9 billion due to premature death.[21]

Figure 72-9 shows the average total lifetime cost per fatality and hospitalized person by cause in 1985.[21] Hospitalizations from motor vehicle crash injuries were the most costly, averaging $43,409 per injured person. Falls, burns, firearm injuries, and drownings all averaged over $30,000 per hospitalization.

The cost of medical care increases with increasing injury severity. For motor vehicle-related injuries in 1990, the cost of medical care averaged $18,585 for a moderate injury, $57,030 for a serious injury, and $249,753 for a critical injury.[24] Indirect costs also increase with injury severity because extended treatment needs are greater, there is more loss of productivity, and disabilities are more common.

Although fatalities often do not result in high medical costs, indirect costs due to premature loss of life can be extensive. Deaths due to drownings and poisonings are very costly because of the large number of affected children. The total lifetime cost of injury deaths far exceeds those of cancer and cardiovascular diseases combined.

▶ CONCEPTUAL APPROACHES TO THE PREVENTION OF INJURIES

The main objectives of injury research are to prevent the occurrence of injuries and to reduce their level of severity. Limiting injury prevention strategies to any single aspect of the many causes of injuries is an ineffective and narrow approach; successful strategies will incorporate many countermeasures and involve many different professionals.[25] Rather than "accident prevention," the goal of injury prevention is better conceptualized by focusing on a general downshifting of severity over the entire spectrum of injuries. The phrase adapted by injury professionals to describe the desired effects of injury research is "injury control," which embodies the goal of decreasing injuries through increased knowledge about risk factors, predicting injury occurrence, and actively controlling of these factors.

Unlike many chronic diseases, the agent of injury is always known and can be measured, and the mechanism of energy transfer from reservoir to host can be described. With the exception of some poisonings and burns, injuries usually occur immediately after exposure, having very short "latent" periods unlike many infectious and chronic conditions. Within the framework of the public health model (Fig. 72-1), the primary focus of injury control is to identify sources of energy forces that cause injury, define mechanisms of human exposure, and identify precisely where interventions (countermeasures) may be introduced in the "natural history" of injury.

Given the many contributing factors to injuries, such as different types of energy forces or circumstances of exposure, human reactions, health status, and medical care, there are several areas in which to introduce prevention. Public health has defined three levels of prevention. *Primary prevention* aims to prevent the event that causes injury by eliminating the mechanisms of energy transfer or exposure. Traffic safety laws, fences around swimming pools, locking devices on guns, and safety caps on poisonous substances are all examples of primary prevention that reduce or eliminate the chance of exposure.

The goal of *secondary prevention* is to eliminate injuries or reduce injury severity once a potential injury-producing exposure has occurred. Motorcycle helmets, seat belts, life vests, and bulletproof vests are examples of secondary prevention. It is important to note that some of the most effective secondary prevention strategies do not eliminate all injuries. For example, the motorcycle helmet is very effective in reducing head trauma in motorcycle crashes, but is not effective in preventing trauma to other body regions.[26] Seat belts do not prevent *all* injuries in vehicle crashes; cuts, contusions, and extremity fractures are common among belted vehicle occupants because belts do not restrain the limbs. The crucial role of seat belts is to reduce severe injury to critical anatomic regions such as the head or chest, and for this purpose they are enormously effective. *Tertiary prevention* acknowledges that an injury has occurred, and aims to reduce the consequences of the injury. Physical, occupational, and speech therapists are dedicated to tertiary prevention.

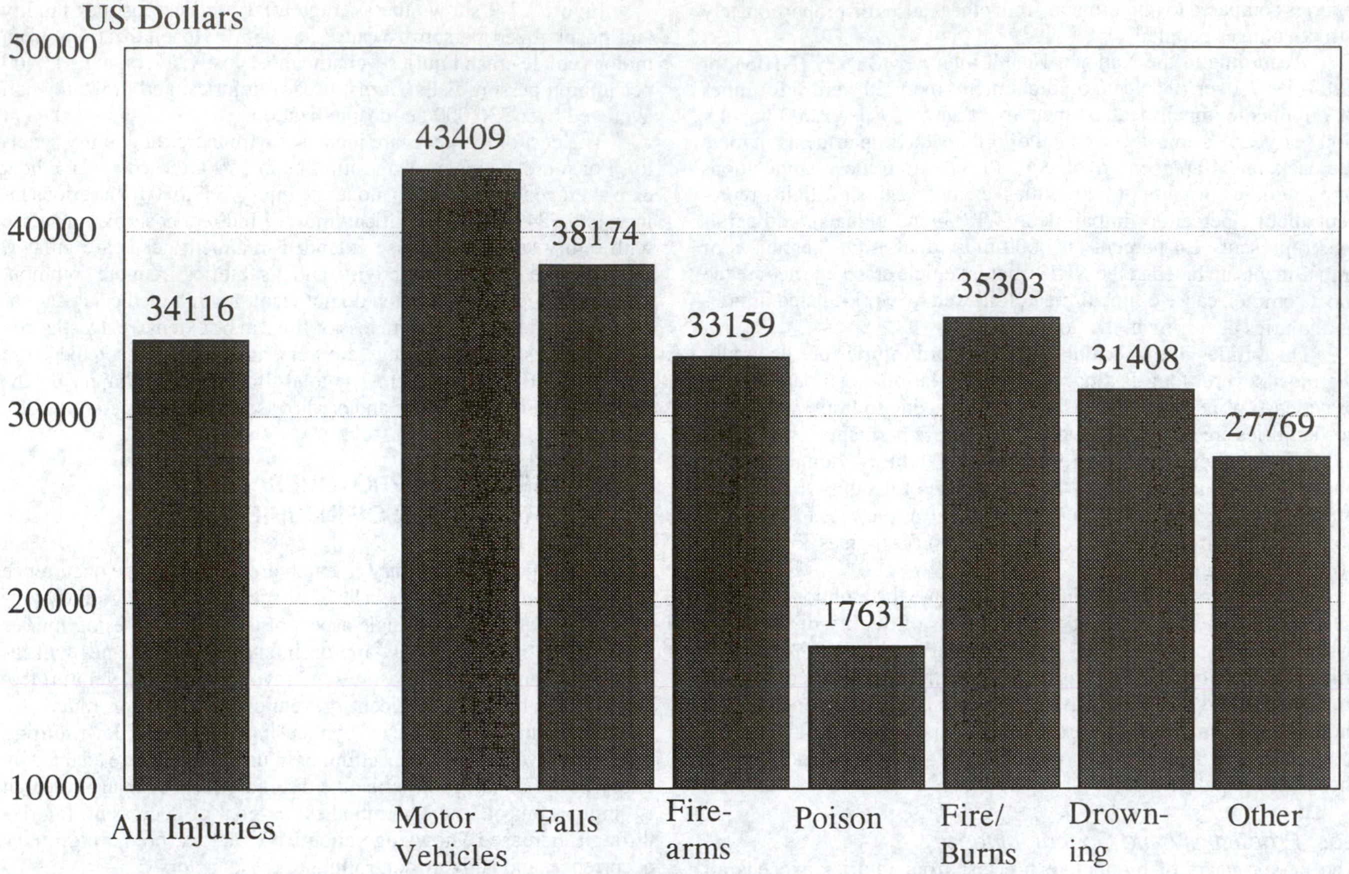

Figure 72-9. Average total lifetime cost of injuries by cause, United States, 1985 (From Rice D, MacKenzie E, et al: Cost of Injury in the United States. A report to Congress, 1989. San Francisco: Institute for Health and Aging, University of California, 1989.)

Specific injury prevention strategies can be divided into two very broad groups based on need for host actions. *Passive* intervention requires no input or action by the host and is usually accomplished by modifying the agent, vehicle, vector, or environment. Modifications in car design that improve brakes or increase energy absorption by the vehicle frame are two examples. *Active* intervention requires that the host take some type of action for the intervention to work. Seat belts and helmets are examples of active intervention. Just as effective injury control strategies must address multiple facets of injury occurrence, they should also incorporate active and passive intervention strategies to be fully effective. Passive intervention strategies are usually considered more effective, especially when compared to active interventions, which require frequent or time-consuming action.[27] Air bags, which require no driver action, will work in frontal crashes, whereas seat belts can be effective only if riders remember to fasten them. The most effective prevention, however, is the combination of both approaches. The circumstances of specific types of injury must be considered when identifying injury control approaches.

One framework for conceptualizing the many approaches to injury prevention is termed the "4 E's," which consist of education, environmental modification, enforcement, and engineering. Education refers to efforts using educational messages to increase safe behavior among the intended audience. Of the four approaches, education is perhaps the most difficult to implement. Successful educational messages must be clear, appropriate for the audience, and periodically repeated to maintain behavior change. Community-based efforts have shown some success in decreasing childhood injuries,[28,29] but these programs were not evaluated over extended periods of time. Many types of educational material has been introduced, the most recent being public service announcements stressing safe behavior. The effects of these programs is largely unknown, however, because few scientific evaluations have been undertaken.

The effectiveness of environmental modification has been demonstrated through reduction in motor vehicle crashes following changes in the driving environment. Examples include skid-free road surfaces, cross slopes on curved roadways in areas with heavy rainfall, separation barriers on freeways, and two-way roads. Environmental modification as simple as removing trees and adding guardrails can reduce traffic crashes in some areas by as much as 75 percent.[30] Another example of successful environmental modification includes the introduction of pool fencing barriers.

Enforcement refers to legislative regulations and the enforcement of these activities. While legislatively mandated prevention activities have been highly successful, they can be controversial. The introduction of a mandatory helmet use law in California in 1992 led to a decrease in motorcycle fatalities of over 35 percent and a decrease in severe head injuries among injured motorcycle riders of over 50 percent.[26] Efforts to repeal this law based on freedom of choice have continued since its inception. Another example of successful legislation has been the implementation of blood alcohol limits for drivers. The success of much legislation may be due in part to public recognition of the laws, and it is often this public recognition that leads to the legislation.

Engineering advancements have been highly successful in reducing injuries. The most notable examples are the seat belt and air bag, which have been attributed with decreasing injuries in frontal collisions by over 50 percent.[31] Many effective prevention measures have been introduced to motor vehicles without the consumer's knowledge, including improvements in brakes, collapsible steering columns, and stronger headrests. As consumers of automobiles have started to demand safety in vehicle design, these improvements will likely continue. Although engineering measures tend to be very effective, they must be followed to determine if the engineering strategy introduces new injury risks. An example of this phenomenon involves air bags, which have caused several fatalities among infants in car seats placed in the front passenger seat.

One of the most recognized frameworks for injury prevention was introduced by William Haddon. The next section introduces the 10 Haddon Countermeasures with examples of successful prevention strategies.

▶ SUCCESSFUL INJURY CONTROL STRATEGIES USING THE 10 COUNTERMEASURE APPROACH TO INJURY PREVENTION

Successful reduction of injuries incorporates many approaches and knowledge from many types of professionals because of the nature and elements in the chain of events leading to injury. The role of human behavior, which includes voluntary risk-taking, the use of behavior-altering substances, and lack of knowledge regarding safe behavior, coupled with physical limitations in perception, reaction time, and attention, which vary by individual, creates a complex set of conditions for host response. Agents of energy and environments in which energy is transferred to the host change constantly with a technologically expanding world. The interaction of the agent, host, and environment provides many opportunities for intervention, but experience has shown that introducing change into one injury element without considering the other components will rarely be effective.

Prevention strategies should be founded on an understanding of the hazard, its introduction into the human environment, and exposure to the host. This understanding needs to incorporate the state of the physical, sociocultural, and political climate in which the hazard interacts with the host. Of the many successful injury control strategies, the majority "control" rather than eliminate energy transfer. "Control" acts by reducing the magnitude of the energy transfer, thereby reducing the severity of the injury incurred. For example, neither seat belts nor helmets prevent all injuries, but they are very effective in reducing the amount of injury transferred to the host and therefore in reducing injury sustained.

In 1962, William Haddon Jr. defined the strategies for injury control into 10 logically distinct categories. However, the 10 countermeasures are not always mutually exclusive; for certain injuries a number of the countermeasures may point to the same intervention. The following is a list of the 10 countermeasures along with examples of successful injury-control strategies in use.[32]

1. Preventing Creation of the Agent

Preventing creation of the agent aims to stop the production of the agent before it can present a hazard. This approach is theoretically the most effective but is not often a realistic alternative. Although motor vehicles are known to be the cause of many fatalities and injuries, they are essential for modern living. Preventing the manufacture of motor vehicles would not only be difficult to implement but would have unfavorable economic consequences. However, it is feasible to control the production of dangerous vehicles with demonstrated mechanical failures or operating failures. An example of this approach is the recall of motor vehicles with significant hazards to safe operation.

2. Reducing the Amount of the Agent

Reducing the amount of the agent involves identifying a hazard and reducing its presence in the environment. One example of this intervention is seen in unintentional drug overdose among the elderly. In a study many years ago at the Maryland Poison Center, unintentional poisonings from oral medications were noted in the elderly population.[33] The interventions involved better packaging and labeling to reduce the chances of ingesting extra doses of medicine due to forgetfulness or failure to understand the purpose and interactions of all medications. The agent (pills) was reduced by limiting the number in each prescription so that taking them all at once would not kill or disable an individual. Another approach could include comprehensive review by physicians of all medications prescribed and taken voluntarily so that potentially harmful combinations or overmedication can be avoided.

3. Preventing Release of the Agent

Preventing release of the agent deters it from entering the environment and hence reduces exposure. Childproof safety caps on medicine dispensers is an example of this approach because the potentially harmful substance cannot be obtained by a child. The introduction of the Poison Prevention Packaging Act in the late 1970s played a significant role in reducing by over 50 percent poisonings in children ages 0 to 4.[34] This act incorporates engineering (through the design of the child-resistant container), education (through the need to identify and address the problem), and enforcement (through mandatory compliance by manufacturers).

Another example of this countermeasure involves falls. Among those 65 and older in the United States, 2.3 million are injured due to falls, leading to nearly 9,000 deaths, 370,000 hospitalizations per year, and aggregate lifetime costs of 9.8 billion dollars.[35] Providing the elderly with canes or walkers and installing handrails and traction strips in stairways and bathtubs decreases the number of falls in this population. One community-based program to reduce falls in senior citizens reported a 60 percent reduction in falls following this type of intervention.[35]

4. Modifying the Rate or Spatial Distribution of the Agent

Modifying the rate or spatial distribution of the agent involves altering the mechanism by which energy is transferred to the host. Use of child restraints and seat belts in automobiles reduces the risk of injury of drivers and passengers when crashes occur. Laws enforcing the presence of safety equipment in automobiles and their use by occupants are in effect, helping increase the number of people who benefit from this strategy. Seat belt use reduces motor vehicle fatalities and serious injuries by 40 to 55 percent.[14,36–38] The lap portion of the lap-shoulder belt protects against rider ejection from the motor vehicle and the shoulder harness portion reduces violent contact with the car interior.[39]

The effectiveness of seat belts in reducing large numbers of fatalities and injuries nationwide, however, rests with compliance to mandated laws requiring their use. The National Highway Traffic Safety Administration (NHTSA) estimates that for 1990 more than 5,770 fatal injuries would have been averted by lap/shoulder belts if at least half of all car occupants wore them.[31] NHTSA estimated in 1988 that 4,573 lives were saved and that 15,959 lives could have been saved if everyone had worn safety belts.[40] The cost of introducing and maintaining a mandatory seat belt law is only $69 per life-year saved, which is considerably smaller than the costs of treating injured drivers.[41]

5. Separating the Host and Agent, in Time or Space

Separation of the host and agent prevents an injurious event by eliminating contact between the energy source and the host. Road designs that separate vulnerable road users from potential hazards is one type of prevention using this approach. Removing pedestrians and bicyclists from vehicle traffic through signal control, overhead crossings, and bicycle trails are other examples.

This strategy can be, at times, inexpensive and easily implemented to protect children from toxic substances. One method of reducing poisonings from household cleaners and other toxic substances is placing toxic agents and poisonous substances in locked cabinets or out of children's reach.

Removing the host from the agent in time involves extracting the host from potential energy transfer before the exposure occurs or increases in extent. One example of this is the use of smoke detectors.

In 1980, 4,509 Americans died in home fires. In addition, fire caused 31,000 reported civilian injuries, 200,000 unreported injuries, and $6.5 billion in direct property losses. The residential smoke detector provides an early warning of home fires, thereby facilitating escape and reducing the number of fire deaths. Legislation to ensure installation of smoke detectors in homes is in effect in many states and appears to be successful.[42]

6. Separating the Agent from a Susceptible Host by Interposition of a Material Barrier

Interposition of a material barrier separates the agent from a host, preventing or minimizing damage to the host. Use of air bags in motor vehicles is an example of this countermeasure. It is estimated that air bags are 18 percent effective in mitigating serious driver injuries,[43] 18 percent effective in preventing fatalities to drivers, and 13 percent effective in reducing fatalities to right front-seat passengers.[44] Zador and Ciccone estimate that air bags reduce driver fatalities by 19 percent and driver fatalities in frontal crashes by 28 percent.[45] Based on this overall reduction, it is estimated that, if all vehicles had driver-side air bags, about 4,000 fewer people would have died from crashes in 1990. The average dollar savings from these injury reductions is 8.7 billion annually. At an estimated cost of 4 billion dollars to install front-seat air bags in all cars, the surplus savings is 4.7 billion dollars.[21]

Use of helmets by motorcycle and bicycle riders is yet another effective measure. The scientific literature on the effect of helmets to reduce injuries is compelling. Motorcycle riders who crash when wearing helmets sustain head injuries at a rate less than half that of nonhelmeted riders, yet only about half of all motorcycle riders voluntarily wear helmets.[46,47] Bicycle helmets reduce the risk of head injury by at least 60 percent and the loss of consciousness by up to 85 percent.[48,49] To reduce the burden and cost of motorcycle injuries, 25 states and the District of Columbia have increased helmet use by introducing legislation requiring all motorcycle riders to use them. Legislation has also been introduced in many states including Washington and California to increase use of bicycle helmets. After states were required to introduce mandatory motorcycle helmet use laws in 1976, fatalities decreased between 20 and 40 percent. In states that later repealed universal use laws, fatalities increased and approached the original rates.[46] Head injuries among both fatally and nonfatally injured motorcycle riders decreased over 50 percent after the introduction of mandatory helmet legislation.[26]

Helmet use is a cost-effective countermeasure because helmets are relatively inexpensive and they prevent head injuries, which are the most costly of all injuries because of their severity and long-term effects. In 1979, helmet use by motorcycle riders averted approximately 61 million dollars in hospital, physician, rehabilitation, and other health provider costs. Increasing helmet use through mandatory helmet use laws could have increased these savings by about $500,000 per 100,000 registered motorcycles. Repeals of state helmet laws during the 1970s were responsible for over $16 million in medical care and rehabilitation costs yearly in 1979 dollars.[50]

Using self-latching gates or fencing swimming pools and other aquatic environments have also proven effective. A study by Present showed between 50 and 90 percent of childhood pool drownings and near drownings could be prevented with widespread use of pool fencing.[51] Based on the effectiveness of pool fencing, many communities and some states have introduced mandatory pool fencing laws. Drownings among adolescents occur mostly in natural bodies of water and alcohol use is a contributing factor in 40 to 50 percent of the cases.[52] Therefore, limiting alcohol on or near recreational water areas is one way to control the number of related injuries in this age group.

One approach that has proven successful in preventing childhood fall injuries was demonstrated in New York City with the introduction of window gates to prevent fall fatalities in children. This effort led to a decrease from 57 fatalities in 1973 to 25 in 1974 and 19 in 1975.[53]

7. Modifying Relevant Qualities of the Agent

Injuries may be lessened through modification of agent characteristics. Modification of the transfer of thermal energy is an example of this approach. Burns are extremely painful, often resulting in severe physical and psychological damage. The current average hospital stay for a moderately severe burn is 17 days with a hospital cost of approximately $42,500. This does not include the costs for reconstructive surgery, physical therapy, and psychological counseling.[54] Clothing ignition, once a pronounced source of burn injury, has been reduced through the legislatively mandated use of flame-retardant materials for children's sleepwear.[55] However, the use of cotton fabrics in children's sleepwear is re-emerging without appropriate clothing warnings.

Many burns occurring among young or elderly populations result from high-temperature tap water. These scalds are easily prevented by regulating hot water heater levels to no more than 120°.[55] These antiscald devices are readily available and can easily be installed on existing plumbing.

8. Strengthening the Susceptible Host

Strengthening the host is also a possible means for preventing injuries. Alcohol consumption not only increases the risk of all types of injuries, including motor vehicle crashes and falls, but also significantly alters physiological response after head injury by promoting secondary injury processes.[56,57]

Strengthening the susceptible host can also occur through health promotion activities. Regular exercise helps strengthen muscles and improve balance and coordination, which reduces the potential for injury. Nutrition programs that increase bone density in older persons can help prevent falls and injury from falls.

9. Countering the Injury Already Caused by the Agent

This approach to injury prevention involves immediate intervention after energy transfer has occurred. Regional poison control centers are an effective approach in providing early care when poisonous substances have been ingested. Poison control centers provide a phone hotline with immediate advice on the appropriate action to take depending on the substance ingested. An evaluation of Massachusetts poison control centers found that 1 percent of parents who called the poison control center after ingestion of a hazardous substance by their child went to the emergency room, compared with 44 percent of those who did not call the centers. Furthermore, only 0.5 percent of those calling the center made unnecessary trips to emergency departments compared with 28 percent of those who did not call.[58]

Providing immediate resuscitation to injured individuals is essential to recovery.[51,59] In a study of children with submersion injuries, those who received immediate resuscitation were five times more likely to have a good outcome than those not receiving resuscitation.[60] Hence, cardiopulmonary resuscitation (CPR) certification should be required, especially of mothers with small children and others working with vulnerable populations.

Timely access to skilled medical treatment, especially in the case of severe injuries, has long been recognized as a crucial factor in determining whether an individual can survive and recover from serious injuries.[14] Kries estimated that approximately 20 percent of trauma deaths in Dade County, Florida, were preventable, and that the most important barrier to preventing these deaths was delay in access to treatment.[61] Since the Emergency Medical Services Act of 1973, many communities have developed very sophisticated systems of emergency medical response, transport, and trauma care. Although improvements in emergency response have been significant, many individuals in the United States still have inadequate access to emergency medical treatment.

10. Stabilizing, Repairing, and Rehabilitating the Injured Host

Once damage has occurred, stabilization, repair, and rehabilitation help restore function and aid in ensuring quality of life. In the event that an individual needs therapy or is disabled, his or her quality of life is dependent upon access to rehabilitation, assistance by equipment such as wheelchairs and personal attendants, and structural access to buildings and transportation. Successful rehabilitation involves a comprehensive approach to health care and a focus on returning the injured individual to a life of quality and not just subsistence. The team approach to rehabilitation developed in the 1930s involves treatment of patients by rehabilitation specialists in conjunction with other medical providers including orthopedists, neurologists, and psychiatrists.[14] Current efforts involve an even more comprehensive approach, which begins the process of rehabilitation soon after emergency care.

▸ REFERENCES

1. Cairns H: Head injuries in motor-cyclists: the importance of the crash helmet. Br Med J 2:465–471, 1941
2. Cairns H, Holbourn H: Head injuries in motor-cyclists: with special reference to crash helmets. Br Med J 1:591–598, 1943
3. Gordon J: The epidemiology of accidents. Am J Public Health 39:504–515, 1949
4. Gibson J: The contribution of experimental psychology to the formulation of the problem of safety: a brief for basic science. In: Behavioral Approaches to Accident Research. New York: Association for the Aid of Crippled Children, 1961
5. Haddon W Jr: A note concerning accident theory and research with special reference to motor-vehicle accidents. Ann N Y Acad Sci 107: 35–64, 1963
6. Haddon W Jr, Schuman E, Klein D: Accident Research. Methods and Approaches. New York: Harper & Row, 1964
7. DeHaven H: Beginnings of crash injury research. In Brinkhaus K (ed): Accident Pathology. FH 11-6595. Washington, DC: US Department of Transportation, 1968
8. Haddon W Jr: A logical framework for categorizing highway safety phenomena and activity. J Trauma 12:193–207, 1972
9. Gable CB: A compendium of public health data sources. Am J Epidemiol 131:381–394, 1990
10. Annest JL, Conn JM, James SP: Inventory of Federal Data Systems in the United States for Injury Surveillance, Research, and Prevention Activities. Atlanta: Centers for Disease Control and Prevention, National Center for Injury Prevention and Control, 1996
11. Kraus JF, Peek C, Silberman T, Anderson C: The accuracy of death certificates in identifying work-related fatal injuries. Am J Epidemiol 141(10):973–979, 1995
12. Pollack E, Keimig D (eds): Counting Injuries and Illnesses in the Workplace: Proposals for a Better System. Washington, DC: National Academy Press, 1987
13. National Center for Health Statistics: Impairments due to injuries: United States, 1985–87. Vital Health Stat 10(177):1–55, 1991
14. National Committee for Injury Prevention and Control: Injury prevention: meeting the challenge. Am J Prev Med 5(3):1–303, 1989
15. Pollock DA, McClain PW: Trauma registries: current status and future prospects. JAMA 262:2280–2283, 1989
16. National Center for Health Statistics: Annual summary of births, marriages, divorces, and deaths: United States, 1994. Monthly Vital Statistics Report, 43(13), 1995
17. Baker SP, O'Neill B, Ginsburg MJ, Guohua L: The Injury Fact Book. 2nd ed. New York: Oxford University Press, 1992
18. National Center for Health Statistics: National Hospital Discharge Survey: annual summary, 1992. Vital Health Stat 13(119):1–63, 1994
19. National Center for Health Statistics: (1995a). Injury-related visits to hospital emergency departments: United States, 1992. Hyattsville, MD: National Center for Health Statistics, 1995
20. Kraus JF: Epidemiology of head injury. In Cooper PR (ed): Head Injury. 3rd ed. Baltimore: Williams & Wilkins, 1993, pp 1–25
21. Rice D, MacKenzie E, et al: Cost of Injury in the United States. A Report to Congress, 1989. San Francisco: Institute for Health and Aging, University of California, 1989
22. Desenclos JC, Hahn RC: Years of potential life lost before the age 65, by race, Hispanic origin, and sex—United States, 1986–1988. MMWR CDC Surveill Summ 41(6):13–23, 1992
23. Stambrook M, Moore AD, Peters LC et al: Effects of mild, moderate and severe closed head injury on long-term vocational status. Brain Inj 4(2):183–190, 1990
24. National Highway Traffic Safety Administration: Economic Costs of Motor Vehicle Crashes 1990. US Department of Transportation Publication HS 807 876. Washington, DC: National Highway Traffic Safety Administration, 1992
25. National Center for Injury Control: Injury Control in the 1990's: A National Plan for Action. A Report to the Second World Conference on Injury Control. Hyattsville, MD: National Center for Injury Control, 1993
26. Kraus JF, Peek C, McArthur D, Williams A: The effects of the 1992 California mandatory motorcycle helmet use law on motorcycle crash fatalities and injuries. JAMA 272:1506–1511, 1994
27. Waller JA: Injury Control: A Guide to the Causes and Prevention of Trauma. Lexington, MA: DC Heath, 1985
28. Blomberg RD, Pruesser DF, Hale A, Leaf WA: Experimental Field Test of Proposed Pedestrian Safety Messages. vol 2, Child Messages. Washington, DC: US Department of Transportation, 1983
29. DiGuiseppi CG, Rivara FP, Koepsell TD, Polissar L: Bicycle helmet use by children: evaluation of a community-wide campaign. JAMA 262:2256–2261, 1989
30. McFarland WF, Griffin LI, Rollins JB, Stockton WR, Philips DT, Dudek CL: Assessment of Techniques for Cost-Effectiveness of Highway Accident Countermeasures. Washington, DC: Federal Highway Administration, 1979
31. National Highway Traffic Safety Administration: Final Regulatory Impact Analysis: Amendment to FMVSS 208 Passenger Car Front Seat Occupant Protection. US Department of Transportation Publication HS-805-572. Washington, DC: National Highway Traffic Safety Administration, 1984
32. Haddon W Jr: On the escape of tigers: an ecologic note. Am J Public Health 60:2229–2234, 1970
33. Klein-Schwartz W, Oderda GM, Booze L: Poisoning in the elderly. J Am Geriatr Soc 31(4):195–199, 1983
34. Rivara FP: Traumatic deaths of children in the United States: currently available prevention strategies. Pediatrics 75(3):456–462, 1985
35. Plautz MD, Beck DE, Selmar C, Radetsky M: Modifying the environment: a community-based injury-reduction program for elderly residents. Am J Prev Med 12(Suppl 1):33–38, 1996
36. Evans L: The Effectiveness of Safety Belts in Preventing Fatalities. Research Publication GMR-5088. Warren, MI: General Motors, 1985
37. Hedlund J: Casualty reductions resulting from safety belt use laws. Presentation to OECD meeting, Washington, DC, 1985
38. Mackay M: Seat belt use under voluntary and mandatory conditions and its effect on casualties. In: Human Behavior and Traffic Safety. New York: Plenum Press, 1985
39. Chorba TL: Assessing technologies for preventing injuries in motor vehicle crashes. Int J Technol Assess Health Care 7:296–314, 1991
40. Paryka SC, Womble KB: Projected lives saved from greater belt use. In: National Center for Statistics and Analysis Research Notes. Washington, DC: National Highway Traffic Safety Administration, 1989
41. Tengs TO, Adams ME, Pliskin JS, Safran DG, Siegel JE, Weinstein MC, et al: Five-hundred life-saving interventions and their cost-effectiveness. Risk Analy 15(3):369–390, 1995
42. McLoughlin E, Marchone M, Hanger SL, German PS, Baker SP: Smoke detector legislation: its effect on owner-occupied homes. Am J Public Health 75(8):858–862, 1985

43. Metz HJ: Restraint performance of the 1973–76 GM air cushion restraint system. Warrendale, PA: Society of Automotive Engineers, 1988
44. Evans L: Restraint effectiveness, occupant ejection from cars, and fatality reductions. Accid Anal Prev 22:167–175, 1990
45. Zador PL, Ciccone MA: Automobile driver fatalities in frontal impacts: air bags compared with manual belts. Am J Public Health 83: 661–666, 1993
46. US General Accounting Office: Motorcycle Helmet Laws Save Lives and Reduce Costs to Society. GAO/RCED-91-170. Washington, DC: U.S. General Accounting Office, 1991
47. Kraus JF, Peek C, Williams A: Compliance with the 1992 California motorcycle helmet use law. Am J Public Health 85:96–99, 1995
48. Thomas S, Acton, C, Nixon J, Battistutta D, Pitt WR, Clark R: Effectiveness of bicycle helmets in preventing head injury in children: case-control study. Br Med J 308:173–177, 1994
49. Maimaris C, Summers CL, Browning C, Palmer CR: Injury patterns in cyclists attending an accident and emergency department: a comparison of helmet wearers and non-wearers. Br Med J 308:1537–1540, 1994
50. Muller A: Evaluation of costs and benefits of motorcycle helmet laws. Am J Public Health 70(6):586–592, 1980
51. Present P: Child Drowning Study: A Report on the Epidemiology of Drowning in Residential Pools to Children under Age Five. Washington, DC: Consumer Product Safety Commission, Directorate for Epidemiology, 1987
52. Division of Injury Control, Center for Environmental Health and Injury Control, Centers for Disease Control: Childhood injuries in the United States. Am J Dis Child 144:627–646, 1990
53. Spiegel CN, Lindaman FC: Children can't fly: a program to prevent childhood morbidity and mortality from window falls. Am J Public Health 67(12):1143–1147, 1977
54. Crawley T: Childhood injury: significance and prevention strategies. J Pediatr Nurs 11(4):225–232, 1996
55. Wilson MH, Baker SP, Teret SP, Shock S, Garbarino J: Saving Children, a Guide to Injury Prevention. New York: Oxford University Press, 1991, pp. 1–247
56. Modell JG, Mountz JM: Drinking and flying—the problem of alcohol use by pilots. N Engl J Med 323:455–461, 1990
57. Waller PF, Stewart JR, Hansen AR, et al: The potential effects of alcohol on driver injury. JAMA 256:1461–1466, 1986
58. Chafee-Bahamon C, Lovejoy FH: Effectiveness of a regional poison center in reducing excess emergency room visits for children's poisonings. Pediatrics 72:164–169, 1983
59. Wintemute GJ, Kraus JF, Teret SP, Wright M: Drowning in childhood and adolescence: a population-based study. Am J Public Health, 77:830–832, 1987
60. Kyriacou DN, Arcinue EL, Peek C, Kraus JF: Effect of immediate resuscitation on children with submersion injury. Pediatrics 94:137–142, 1994
61. Kries DJ Jr, Plasencia G, Augenstein D, Davis JH, Echenique M, Vopal J, et al: Preventable trauma deaths: Dade County, Florida. J Trauma 26:649–654, 1986

73

Violence

The Problem of Violence in the United States and Globally

Mark L. Rosenberg • James A. Mercy • Joseph L. Annest

Violence Prevention As a Public Health Concern

Until recently, violence was not considered a traditional public health problem. That view is changing as people realize the extent to which violence meets traditional criteria as a threat to public health and the contribution that a public health approach can make to violence prevention.

First, the magnitude of the problem in terms of health consequences is great. For example, in 1994, suicide ranked as the ninth leading cause of death; and homicide, as the eleventh leading cause.[1] Further, violence affects so many young people that each homicide or suicide on the average results in many years of potential life lost. Homicide is the ninth leading cause of years of potential life lost and suicide is the eleventh leading cause.[2] For younger age groups, violence takes an even greater toll. For African Americans 15 to 24 years of age, homicide is the leading cause of death.[1] For all Americans in the 15- to 24-year age group, homicide is the second leading cause of death and suicide is the third leading cause of death. Moreover, these deaths represent only a fraction of the impact on the health and quality of life of the U.S. population. For every death from assaultive violence, there are probably 100 times as many nonfatal injuries.[5] Estimates also suggest that nearly 2 million women in the United States each years are assaulted by intimate partners, resulting in psychological as well as physical injury. The consequences of these assaults include fear, depression, and incapacitation, all of which greatly diminish the quality of the life of the women, their families, and their communities. In another example, firearm violence claims 18,000 lives from homicide and 17,000 from suicide each year.[4] In nine states and the District of Columbia, firearm-related deaths outnumber fatalities caused by motor vehicle crashes. Firearms are the most common cause of injury deaths in the United States overall for young people ages 15 to 34. Injuries and disabilities related to violence impose a tremendous economic burden on the health sector, exceeding $105 billion annually.[5] Firearm injuries are now the leading cause of death from traumatic brain injury (TBI), and to an ever-increasing degree, violence-related injuries are filling rehabilitation hospitals.

Second, no other sector takes responsibility for preventing these consequences of violence. The criminal justice sector has long acknowledged that, because most homicides occur among people who know each other and not in connection with any other felony, the police are not able to prevent most of these. Like suicide prevention, many violence-related injuries require societal interventions that can be planned and carried out by public health practitioners.

Third, the traditional tools of public health can be successfully applied to violence prevention, and public health practitioners can play an effective role in spearheading and coordinating prevention programs.

The traditional tools of public health are rooted in the notion that ours is a cause-and-effect world and that we can both understand these causes and change this world by controlling those causes to bring about the desired effects. Violence prevention follows the four steps of the public health approach, the same approach that guides public health efforts in prevention of infectious diseases, chronic diseases, and environmental and occupational health problems. Because a common approach runs through efforts in each of these areas, it is not difficult for public health workers in any discipline to understand and work on a public health approach to violence prevention.

The Public Health Approach to Violence Prevention

The public health approach to violence prevention is guided by three central concepts.

Prevention

Although treatment for victims of violence is important, public health aims to prevent people from becoming injured in the first place and to prevent the perpetrators from ever resorting to violence. For example, it is important to have an adequate number of shelters for battered women, but if battering could be prevented in the first place, these shelters would not be needed. This focus on prevention does not in any way diminish the importance of providing care for victims or the importance of arresting and prosecuting perpetrators. Rather the approach complements the contributions of other fields such as the criminal justice system and emergency medical care.

The prevention focus has several implications.

1. *Interventions should be developed earlier on the pathway toward violence.* In the area of domestic violence, for example, interventions could target women who are in relationships with a high risk for physical violence, but in which physical violence has not yet occurred. This could involve intervening with couples who are newly married, engaged but not yet married, or with young men and women just beginning to date. Or it could mean pushing the intervention even further back in time to school-age children and starting to educate them about the risks of violence and how to avoid it.
2. *Children should be involved in preventive programs.* Young children and youth may be more receptive to preventive interventions, and behaviors learned early tend to endure.
3. *New methods of delivering programs need to be developed.* Traditionally, the criminal justice and police sectors have conceptualized violent situations as having a perpetrator and a victim. They often targeted some programs at perpetrators

and others at victims. That approach makes sense *after* a violent incident has occurred. However, this way of identifying victims and perpetrators is not useful in the context of prevention programs that are designed to intervene *before* violence occurs scenarios.

4. *Programs need to target increasingly broad and larger groups at multiple levels.* After specific acts of violence have occurred, individual perpetrators and victims can be identified. If we wish to intervene preventively, then we can only say that a certain group is *at risk* for violence, and we need to focus our interventions at all members of this high-risk group, some of whom might otherwise become perpetrators or victims, but many of whom would not. Other interventions might be even more broadly targeted to a general population in an effort to achieve *universal* coverage. Still other intensive interventions could be targeted at people who are at *very high risk* for violence. For example, traditional programs to assist battered women have delivered services and information at shelters where women seek refuge after they leave a battering relationship. But with a focus on early intervention, an array of support services should be made available to women who are not yet ready to leave their relationships and go to a shelter—and this will be a much larger group.
5. *Very early intervention programs should try to reach young children.* All types of violence prevention programs will address the same universal target of all young children.

Science

The four steps of the public health approach characterize this scientific method and provide a rational framework for examining the problems of violence (Fig. 73-1). This approach is based on asking four questions.

1. *What is the problem?* The answer should include the elements that every reporter addresses: who, when, what, where, and how? And we ask this question and look for patterns not just in a single case, but for many cases—10, 100, 10,000, or even 100,000 cases.
2. *Why did it happen?* What are the risk factors? What characteristics increase the chance that the event would happen to a particular person? What characteristics decrease the chance and may be protective?
3. *What works?* Based on the patterns and the causes related to the answers to the first two questions, what interventions might work to prevent the event from happening in the future? This evaluation must be tough and is absolutely essential.
4. *How do you do it?* Once an intervention has been evaluated and found to be effective, how do we implement it? How do we work with the community, organize the communications, and develop the resources required?

Integrative Leadership or Teamwork

Violence prevention does not "belong" to any one field, domain, or discipline. It will require many disciplines and fields, and departments and agencies, all working together. It will require practitioners who implement programs into communities to work with researchers in designing and evaluating these programs.

Epidemiology of Firearm-Related Deaths and Injuries

This same public health approach is useful in understanding the role that firearms play in contributing to death and injury.

In 1994, firearm-related injuries were the eighth leading cause of death in the United States[1] accounting for 38,505 deaths, including 18,765 firearm suicides, 17,866 firearm homicides, 1,356 unintentional firearm deaths, and 518 firearm deaths with undetermined intentionality.[2] Compared to other causes of injury death in 1994, the number of firearm deaths are surpassed only by the number of motor-vehicle–related deaths (42,524).[3] From 1968 to 1994, the number of motor-vehicle–related deaths steadily cycled downward, while the number of firearm-related deaths increased (Centers for Disease Control and Prevention, unpublished data, 1996). If those trends continue, firearm injuries are predicted to replace motor-vehicle crashes as the leading cause of injury death in the United States by the year 2000. In 1994, this crossover had already occurred among persons ages 20 to 44 years in at least nine states and the District of Columbia (Centers for Disease Control and Prevention, unpublished data, 1996). Overall, firearm-related deaths are the leading cause of death for young people ages 15 to 34.

Although there is good historical data on fatal firearm-related injuries or deaths, long-term trends in national estimates of nonfatal firearm injuries have not been described.[4] In fact, nationally representative data for nonfatal firearm-related injuries have only recently become available. Studies[5,6] suggest that nonfatal firearm-related injuries treated in hospital emergency departments exceed fatal firearm-related injuries by about 2.6 to 1 (95 percent CI, 1.5:1 to 3.7:1), accounting for an estimated 100,000 injured persons treated each year. This estimate includes only those persons treated for a penetrating injury or gunshot wound from a weapon that used a powder charge to fire a projectile. Annually an additional 32,000 persons are treated for gunshot wounds involving BB and pellet guns.[7,8]

In firearm-related fatalities, suicide is the most common cause of death,[2] whereas most nonfatal firearm-related injuries are due to interpersonal violence.[5] Additionally, 4 percent of firearm-related deaths are unintentional, but 20 percent of nonfatal firearm-related injuries treated in hospital emergency departments resulted from unintentional shootings.[5,9]

Males ages 15 to 24 years are at highest risk of being shot by another person when compared to other age and sex groups.[2,5] While males in this age range compose 7 percent of the U.S. population, they are the victims of 35 percent of all firearm homicides and 44 percent of firearm-related assaults treated in U.S. hospital emergency departments.

Firearm death rates also vary by race, occupation, degree of urbanization, per capita income, and geographic area of residence, and internationally. Although firearm suicide rates are higher among Caucasians and American Indians/Alaskan Natives, firearm homicide rates are higher among African Americans.[10,11] Homicide is the leading cause of occupational injury death among females and a majority of these involve of a firearm.[12] Death rates from unintentional shootings and firearm suicide rates are higher in rural areas, but firearm homicide rates are highest in the largest cities.[13,14] Firearm death rates are higher in low-income areas[13] and in the Southeastern and Western regions of the United States.[15] Among children less than 15 years of age, firearm death rates among U.S. children are 12 times higher than their counterparts from 25 other industrialized countries.[16]

Definition of Violence and Brief Typology of Violence

In May 1996, the 190 member nations of the World Health Assembly passed a resolution (WHA 49.25) declaring violence "a public health priority world-wide." This resolution directed the World Health Organization (WHO) to develop a plan of action for a science-based public health approach to violence prevention. The first step is to develop an operational definition of violence, which must recognize the many different forms that violence may take. It may take different forms within a single culture, where it may present as child abuse, youth violence, sexual assault, domestic violence, elder abuse, or child sexual abuse. And it may present in very different forms or manners in different cultures or countries.

The definition of violence will continue to evolve, but a good starting point is the definition adopted by the World Health Organization in *Violence: A Public Health Priority*, a working paper developed by the WHO Global Consultation on Violence and Health in December 1996:

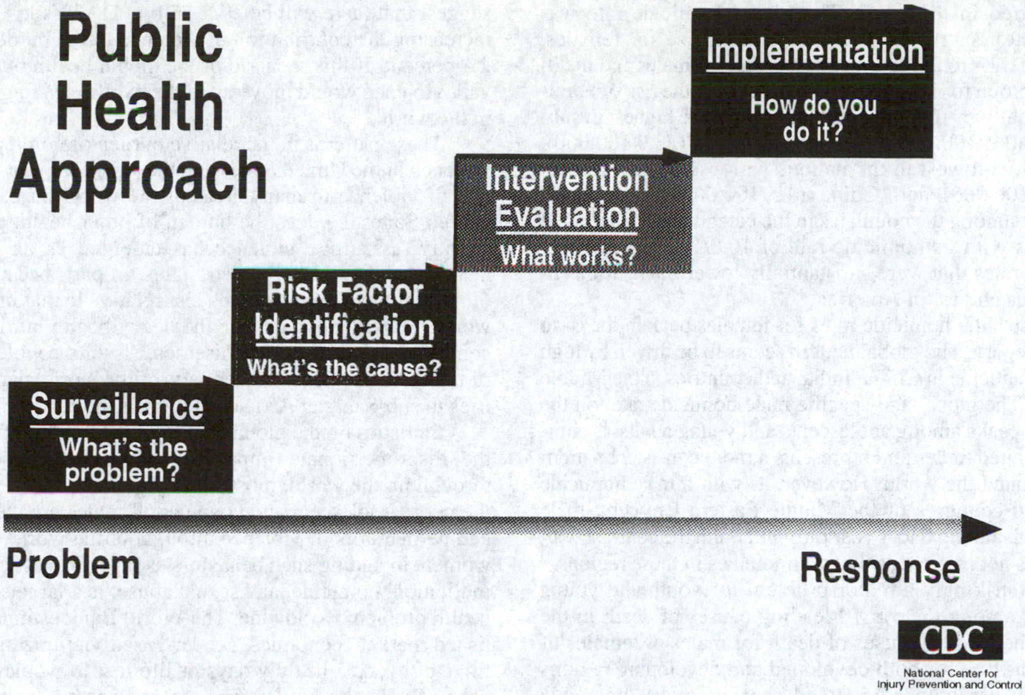

Figure 73-1. Public health approach to violence prevention.

Violence is the intentional use of physical force or power, threatened or actual, against oneself, another person, or a group or community, that results in or has a high likelihood of resulting in injury, death, psychological harm, maldevelopment, or deprivation.

The WHO working document identified three major types of violence:

- *Self-inflicted violence*, which encompasses intentional and harmful behavior directed at oneself, with suicide being the most severe manifestation. Other forms are suicide attempts, mutilation, and behavior whose intent is self-destructive but not lethal.
- *Interpersonal violence*, which consists of violent behavior that occurs between individuals, but is not organized or planned by social or political groups in which they participate. This type of violence can be classified by the victim-offender relationship, which distinguishes domestic violence (involving family and intimates) from violence among acquaintances and between strangers.
- *Organized violence* is behavior that is planned to achieve, or motivated by, specific political, economic, or social objectives of an organized social or political group. This includes, for example, political violence in which efforts to violently intimidate an opposing political faction may be carefully planned and executed. War may be considered the most highly organized type of violence, and gang or mob violence is another category of organized violence.

WHO is currently working with the Centers for Disease Control and Prevention to develop a set of definitions and data elements that will be compatible with the 10th edition of the *International Statistical Classification of Diseases and Related Health Problems* (ICD-10).[17] The next step in the WHO plan is understanding the patterns and characteristics of violence in each country by collecting surveillance data for the major types of violence.

Global Health Burden of Violence

In assessing the health impact of violence, it is useful to look at the problem globally. Although the United States has high rates of homicide and assaultive violence compared to those of other industrial countries, the problem of violence in many parts of the world greatly eclipses the dimension of violence in the United States. Estimates of the relative and absolute contribution of assaultive violence to the global health burden have recently become available through a project that provides a comprehensive assessment of mortality and disability from disease and injuries in 1990 and projected to 2020.[18] The burden of assaultive violence is quantified by measures of two general types of health consequences: (*a*) premature mortality as measured by numbers, rates, and years of life lost due to homicide, and (*b*) combined burden of fatal and nonfatal health outcomes, as indicated by a new measure called disability-adjusted life years lost (DALYs).

DALYs is a new method of measuring disease burden that is based on a quantification of years of potential life lost through death and years of life expected to be lived with disability. Disability is defined as the incidence, duration, and severity of the morbidity and complications associated with specific conditions.[19] This measure was developed by the World Health Organization and the World Bank to overcome the limitations of using mortality as the sole measure of health impact. Although the DALY measure represents a clear advance for assessing the burden of disease, its application is limited because the information needed to calculate the DALY is not complete, particularly in many developing countries and also because suitable indicators to measure such factors as the psychological consequences of violence have not yet been developed or made generally available. Nevertheless, DALYs do provide a crude indicator of the health impact of assaultive violence across different regions of the world and relative to other health problems.

In 1990, there were estimated to be 563,000 homicides throughout the world.[19] These deaths represent about 1.1 percent of all the deaths that occurred in that year. The global homicide rate was 10.7/100,000. Rates for males were 3.5 times those for females. Rates peaked in the 15- to 29-year-old age group for males and the 0- to 4-year-old age group for females. These patterns in the risk of homicide vary substantially by region. Homicide rates were highest in sub-Saharan Africa (40.2/100,000) and Latin America (23.0/100,000). Homicide rates were lowest in the nations with established market economies (3.8/100,000) and China (4.5/100,000). The United States is an outlier among the countries in the category of established market economies with its homicide rate of 10.0/100,000 in 1990, but had homicide rates that were substantially lower than nations in sub-Saharan Africa and Latin America.

Global, age-specific homicide rates for females peak in the 0- to 4-year-old age category. The global pattern seems to be driven by high rates of female infanticide in China, India, and countries in the Middle Eastern Crescent. The global age-specific male homicide rate, on the other hand, which peaks among adolescents and young adults, is similar to that of the United States and represents a more consistent pattern among regions around the world. However, as with female homicide rates in China and countries of the Middle Eastern Crescent, male homicide rates peak among 0 to 4 year olds, although the contrast with older age groups is not as great as that with females in those regions.

Homicide is strikingly a major problem for youth and young adults. It was not among the top 10 leading causes of death in the world or among the leading causes of death for males or females of all ages.[18] This was true for both developed and developing regions of the world. However, among 15- to 44-year-old males, homicide was the third leading cause of death in the world, accounting for 8.8 percent of all deaths among males in that age category. In contrast, in 1990 homicide was the tenth leading cause of death for the United States as a whole and for males specifically. Similar to the global pattern, homicide was the third leading cause of death among males 15 to 44 years of age. In the United States, but in contrast to the global pattern, homicide was the fourth leading cause of death among 15- to 44-year-old females. Homicide was the tenth leading cause of years of life lost in the world for males in both developed and developing regions. Based on knowledge of epidemiologic transition and the assumption that the ongoing secular increases in the rate of violence will continue, it is estimated that in the year 2020 more than 1 million homicides will occur, and the global homicide rate will increase from 10.7/100,000 in 1990 to 13.3/100,000. Given this scenario, homicide would become the tenth leading cause of death among males in the world in 2020.

In 1990 assaultive violence was estimated to account for 1.3 percent of the total global health burden, or 17.5 million DALYs worldwide. It is estimated that males lost about 13.7 million DALYs to violence compared with 3.8 million for females. Violence posed a relatively greater health burden in Latin America/Caribbean, sub-Saharan Africa, and in European countries with formerly socialist economies than in other regions of the world. This regional variation was similar for both males and females. In 1990, violence ranked as the nineteenth leading cause of DALYs. Projections to the year 2020 suggest that there will be 29.5 million DALYs lost to violence, thus increasing the contribution of violence to the burden of disability to 2.4 percent. If this scenario of the global health burden were to prevail, violence would move up to the twelfth leading cause of DALYs in the world.

These patterns in the relative burden of homicide and assaultive violence in the United States and the world suggest that, although the risk of violence in many areas of the world far exceeds that in the United States, so does the burden of other health problems. Consequently, assaultive violence has emerged as an important public health problem in the United States, in part, because the burden of other health problems is much less relative to that in other parts of the world. Nevertheless, despite the heavy health burden attributable to communicable and chronic diseases, assaultive violence remains a serious health problem in other parts of the world, particularly in countries in sub-Saharan Africa and Latin America.

Statistics on the global and regional burden of violence obscure the disproportionate impact of violence on specific subgroups throughout the world, most notably youth, women and children, and the poor. Adolescent and young adult males are the primary victims and perpetrators of violence throughout the world. Violence against women, including such behaviors as rape, domestic violence, genital mutilation, homicide, and sexual abuse, is a large and serious public health problem worldwide. The World Bank estimates that, in established market economies, gender-based victimization is responsible for 1 of every 5 healthy days of life lost to women of reproductive age.[20] The health burden imposed by rape and domestic violence in the industrial world is roughly equivalent to that in the developing world on a per capita basis, but because the total disease burden is so much greater in developing nations, the proportion of the health burden attributable to gender-based violence is smaller.[21] Children are particularly vulnerable to the ravages of violence, and they become unwitting agents in the perpetuation and amplification of the problem. Child abuse and neglect are worldwide problems, the dimensions and consequences of which are only beginning to be understood.

Violence has profound psychological implications for victims and witnesses that statistics do not capture. Victims of violence exhibit a variety of psychological symptoms that are similar to those experienced by victims of other types of trauma, such as motor vehicle crashes and natural disaster. Although a single victimization can lead to emotional scars, ongoing and repetitive violence such as that often associated with intimate partner violence and child abuse can have profound effects on psychological well-being.[22]

Clearly violence is a global health problem of major and increasing proportions. The magnitude of the health consequences of this problem and its social and economic sequelae point to the need for effective prevention strategies, as well as strategies to mitigate the severity of the physical and emotional consequences of violence. In recognition of the magnitude of this problem and the power of the public health approach, the World Health Assembly passed its resolution in May 1996, declaring violence to be a public health priority worldwide.

Assaultive Violence

Mark L. Rosenberg • James A. Mercy • W. Rodney Hammond

Definition of the Problem

In 1994, almost 25,000 people in the United States died from homicide, making this type of assaultive violence the eleventh leading cause of death and the fifth leading cause of premature mortality.[1] In 1994, homicide ranked as the second leading cause of death among persons 15 to 24 years of age and was the leading cause of death for black males 15 to 24 years of age. The lifetime risk of death from homicides is 1 in 28 for black males compared with 1 in 164 for white males.[2,3] And while homicide is the fatal outcome of assaultive behaviors, the ratio of nonfatal assaults to homicide is probably far greater than 100:1. There are about 60,000 firearm-related assaults treated in U.S. hospital emergency departments each year.[4]

Assaultive violence includes both nonfatal and fatal interpersonal violence in which physical force by one person is used with the intent of causing harm, injury, or death to another. Homicide is death caused by injuries inflicted by one person with intent to injure or kill another by any means. Homicide can be classified as criminal or noncriminal. Noncriminal homicide includes deaths caused by negligence and those committed in self-defense.

Four legal categories used to designate types of nonfatal assaultive violence are aggravated assault, simple assault, rape, and robbery. Aggravated assault is (*a*) an attack with a weapon, whether or not there is an injury; (*b*) an attack without a weapon, resulting in serious injury (e.g., broken bones, loss of teeth, internal injuries, or loss of consciousness) or an undetermined injury requiring 2 or more days of hospitalization; or (*c*) an attempted assault with a weapon.[4] Simple assault is an attack or attempted attack without a weapon, resulting either in minor injury (e.g., bruises, black eyes, cuts, scratches, or swelling) or in an undetermined injury requiring less than 2 days of hospitalization. Research literature generally presents assault and homicide as similar categories of behavior and considers homicide "completed" assault. Rape is carnal knowledge through the use of force or the threat of force, including attempts. Robbery is a completed or attempted theft of property or cash directly from a person by force or threat of force, with or without a weapon.

Assaultive violence can be categorized by different types of victim-offender relationship, setting, and circumstances. Categorizing by the nature of victim-offender relationship is helpful because both the etiology and prevention strategies vary by this relationship. Three general categories that are particularly useful are family, acquaintance, and stranger.

Assaultive violence has only recently been recognized as an important public health problem. During the past 30 years, assaultive violence was considered to be the domain of the criminal justice system alone, and control strategies focused primarily on deterrence through punishment and imprisonment. However, there have been dramatic increases in homicide rates in the United States over this same 30-year period.[5] The public health approach suggests that homicide and other types of assault are concerns to be addressed and remedied, not accepted as inalterable facts of life. As with other public health problems, a public health approach to the problem of assaultive violence is to establish a framework for developing relevant information through epidemiology and then to transfer that information into effective action. This approach has four steps: surveillance to collect, analyze, interpret, and disseminate relevant data; identification of risk factors and risk groups and the places, times, and other circumstances associated with increased risk; identification and evaluation of interventions; and program development and implementation (Fig. 73-1).

National Data Sources

Federal Bureau of Investigation Uniform Crime Reports

The Federal Bureau of Investigation Uniform Crime Reports (FBI-UCR) program receives monthly information from more than 16,000 city, county, and state law enforcement agencies. During 1994, the agencies active in the FBI-UCR program held jurisdiction over 97 percent of the U.S. population.[3] These law enforcement agencies report the number of actual offenses known for murder and nonnegligent manslaughter, justifiable homicide, negligent manslaughter, forcible rape, robbery, aggravated assault, burglary, larceny, motor vehicle theft, and arson. This program also uses the Supplementary Homicide Report (SHR) to collect information on the age, race, and sex of the victim and the offender; the relationship of the offender to the victim; and the crime circumstances. For cases that are "unsolved" at the time of reporting, the relationship of victim to offender is listed as "unknown." Unless specifically amended in a later report, the "relationship unknown" is counted in the final statistics for the year. Each year, data are incomplete for approximately 5 to 10 percent of the total number of murder and nonnegligent manslaughter cases.

A principal limitation of FBI-UCR data on aggravated assault, robbery, and rape is that these data represent only the violent offenses known to the police; however, the majority of nonfatal violent offenses do not come to the attention of law enforcement agencies.[6] In addition, the FBI-UCR program does not collect information on victim and offender characteristics or relationships for aggravated assaults, robberies, or rapes. Finally, these data are categorized by a crime hierarchy, so that if an incident occurs that includes several different types of assault, the system counts only the most serious act, with homicide ranked as the most serious, followed by rape, robbery, aggravated assault, burglary, larceny, and motor vehicle theft.

National Crime Victimization Survey

The National Crime Victimization Survey (NCVS) was developed by the Bureau of Justice Statistics of the U.S. Department of Justice to acquire detailed information about victims and consequences of crime, to estimate numbers and types of crimes not reported to police, and to establish uniform measures for selected types of crimes in order to permit reliable comparisons over time and between areas.[7] Focusing on rape, robbery, assault, burglary, larceny, and motor vehicle theft, these surveys collect information on physical injury, medical treatment, property loss, characteristics of the victim, relationship of the victim to the offender, and whether the police were notified.

Because it is based on interviews with victims and not on official law enforcement records, the NCVS is an excellent source of information on victimization and its consequences. However, the accuracy of information on injuries and victimization caused by spouse, child, and elder abuse is questionable because interviews with household members are not conducted privately, and subjects may be reluctant to speak openly in the presence of the person who victimized them. In addition, the survey asks about criminal assaults, and subjects may not perceive assaults by family members as "criminal." Groups at highest risk for serious injury from assault may be difficult to reach using the sampling and interviewing techniques of this survey. Finally, the survey uses the same crime hierarchy used in the FBI-UCR; therefore, serious crimes are more accurately estimated than crimes lower in the hierarchy.

National Center for Health Statistics Mortality Data

The Vital Statistics Program has compiled data from records of all death certificates filed in state vital statistics offices since 1933. The system provides annual data on homicide for the nation and each state, counties, and other local areas and monthly provisional data for the nation and each state. Rates, numbers, gender, and geographic detail for all deaths are published monthly,[8] but there is considerable delay in the publication of detailed reports on specific causes of death. Collection of data is based on the *International Classification of Diseases*, 9th revision (ICD-9)[9] with the Supplementary External Cause (E) code for homicide. Limitations of these data include the lack of information on the victim-offender relationship and the lack of distinction between criminal homicides and homicide committed in self-defense.

Problems and Limitations in Data Collection

These three national systems that collect data on violent crime count and classify elements in slightly different ways, thus complicating the task of describing a national pattern of violence.[10] For example, estimates of homicides reported by UCR and NCVS vary slightly, due partly to criteria used to define a case as a homicide and different reporting practices.[11,12] Moreover, NCVS does not report assaults on children under the age of 12, and its counts of violent victimization within families tend to be lower than special purpose surveys.[10]

Ensuring accuracy of data on ethnic minorities can be a problem. National surveys often exclude certain ethnic groups from data analysis because the numbers are too small or aggregate them in a category termed "other," which limits the potential for understanding unique problems associated with specific ethnic groups. Also, misclassification of ethnic groups can result in substantial underestimates of injury and death.[13] There are additional problems in *how* ethnicity is determined (e.g., self-identification versus next of kin), access to individuals to be surveyed, inappropriate study instruments, and analyzing the data within the cultural context of the violent behavior.[14]

Other Sources

Other national data sources could prove useful in surveillance and research on assaultive violence if modifications are made in the types of information collected. Currently the National Health Interview Survey (NHIS) staff interview persons in about 40,000 households sampled to be representative of the civilian, noninstitutionalized population in all 50 states and the District of Columbia each year. The survey collects data on a number of health issues including injury, but some of the information on injuries cannot be broken down by cause of injury (e.g., assaultive violence, suicidal behavior, unintentional injury) because of the small number of injuries in the sample. In addition, the considerable ambiguity in the way the questions are asked precludes detailed analysis.

National Hospital Discharge Survey. The National Hospital Discharge Survey (NHDS) collects information on discharge diagnosis and type of surgical procedure performed from approximately 275,000 records each year. These records represent a sample of about 500 short-stay, nonfederal hospitals. Information is available on traumatic injury, but is of limited value because data on the cause of injury are not completely reported and vary greatly by the type of injury. Also, the sample of hospitals is based only on those that agree to cooperate with the survey.

National Electronic Injury Surveillance System. The National Electronic Injury Surveillance System (NEISS) collects data on all injuries seen in the emergency rooms of 101 hospitals throughout the United States. These hospitals represent a stratified probability sample of all hospitals in the United States and its territories. The system collects information on all injuries seen at the emergency room that are "product related," but certain products such as automobiles, trains, boats, and planes are not included. Data are being obtained on nonfatal firearm-related injuries for the Centers for Disease Control and Prevention (CDC) to use for public health research purposes.[4]

State and Local Data Sources

Thirty-nine state criminal justice agencies have mandatory reporting requirements; data from these agencies are forwarded to the FBI-UCR program. The agencies in the other 11 states report voluntarily to the UCR program. The bases for the state- and national-level UCR data are detailed reports on crime from county and city law enforcement agencies, which are a potentially rich source of information on assaultive violence.

Coroners' and medical examiners' records are also potential sources of data, and the Centers for Disease Control and Prevention is assessing the feasibility of developing suicide and homicide surveillance systems based on these data. At present, these data are useful for state and local studies, but few coroners' or medical examiners' offices collect standardized information on homicide, and data from these offices are not collected or analyzed nationally. The quality of information varies considerably since few states have medical examiners in each county and records are often completed by persons without medical or forensic training who act as coroners. Data from these offices may be particularly useful for examining the relationship between alcohol and drug use and homicide victimization.

Data from medical and social service agencies such as hospitals, battered women's shelters, mental health clinics, and substance abuse treatment facilities may contain a tremendous amount of useful information concerning the circumstances and histories of persons who have been victims or perpetrators of assaultive violence. However, definitions and records have not been standardized, nor has there been any attempt to collect and analyze these data nationally. With the aim of standardizing data elements for emergency department–based information systems, the National Center for Injury Prevention and Control is heading a project called Data Elements for Emergency Department Systems (DEEDS) to identify uniform data elements.

At both the national and local levels, there is an urgent need for information on injuries resulting from nonfatal assaults and for systems that collect accurate information on the magnitude and nature of nonfatal assaultive violence between persons known to one another (e.g., family members, intimates, friends, and acquaintances). Present sources of such information have only limited use for epidemiological research and surveillance, but their utility will increase significantly when hospital discharge data routinely include information on external cause of injury (E-coding).

Causes and Risk Factors

There are many types of assaultive violence, and for each type the causes are complex and diverse. It is helpful to examine various disciplinary approaches to aspects of the problem because each contributes valuable perspectives. However, these separate approaches can obscure the complex interaction of different types of factors that contribute to assaultive violence. Ultimately, what is needed are "causal" explanations that combine biological, psychological, and sociological factors in ways that explain the occurrence of assaultive violence involving different perpetrators, victims, and circumstances. And, indeed, various disciplines have begun to converge in their quest for an explanation for assaultive violence, examining the issue from a multifactorial perspective.

Biological explanations of assaultive violence have examined sex, age, and certain psychiatric illnesses as important risk factors for homicide victimization and perpetration.[15] For example, greater numbers of males among perpetrators and victims may reflect the influence of male sex hormones on aggressive behavior, and the decreasing numbers of victims and perpetrators with increasing age may be a result of biological transformations associated with aging.[16]

Psychological approaches to violence address factors in four general areas.[17] *Biobehavioral factors* encompass the biological influences on a person's proclivity for violence, including neuroanatomy and brain chemistry. *Socialization factors* address the process by which children learn "rules" for social behavior. In this context, young children are believed to be influenced by aggressive and violent behavior of others in their environment, including family members, peers, and role models. *Cognitive factors* include the ideas, beliefs, and patterns of thinking that emerge as a child develops. Research suggests that aggressive and violent people process information and think about social situations in different ways than do nonviolent individuals, for example, tending to perceive hostility in others where it does not, in fact, exist. They also may be less adept at managing nonviolent ways to resolve conflict. *Situational factors* also contribute to a propensity for violent behavior. Aversive situations such as stressful life events, violence in the family or neighborhood, presence of the means to carry out violence, such as guns—all these may have a role in stimulating violent acts. Overall, through the perspective of these four conceptual groupings, psychology contributes to our understanding of violence by underlining that human aggression is learned behavior and thus can be prevented or minimized.[18]

Four major **sociological approaches** to understanding are cultural, structural, interactionist, and economic. The *cultural approach* views violent behavior as the result of learned and shared values and behavior specific to a given group that are applied in recognizable situations and transmitted across generations. Certain subgroups exhibit higher rates of assaultive violence because they are in a subculture that has violence as a norm. However, critics point to the frequency of violence in groups where violence is clearly not a norm (e.g., the middle class) and to the fact that this theory tends to "blame the victim."

The *structural approach* holds that rates of assaultive violence are largely influenced by broad-scale social forces, such as poverty or lack of opportunity. In one widely known formulation, violence and other "illegitimate" behaviors arise when persons are deprived of "legitimate" means and resources to realize culturally valued goals. This theory does not adequately explain, however, why conflicts arising from structural deprivation lead to violence in one situation and to other behaviors, passivity for instance, in other situations.[19]

The *interactionist approach* focuses on the nature of the interaction sequence as it escalates into violent behavior. For example, one investigator describes it as a series of offender and victim "moves" as they relate to each other and to the reaction of the audience. From this, he derived a set of time-ordered stages that most of the transactions followed.[20] Other research has shown that violence grows out of a series of provocative arguments that escalate to murder. The arguments often are threats to identity (especially sexual identity) and self-esteem. Still another team of investigators posits that people engage in violence to "control others' behavior, to achieve retribution, or to preserve self-image."[21,22] For example, a young person may resort to violence in retribution for a perceived wrong or to save face. This aspect of social intervention theory may help illuminate problems of violence among young minority youth who are "quick to fight over what many adults would consider to be trivial matters."[21]

The *economic approach* is the basis for many current policies aimed at reducing homicide and assault. This theory posits that decisions to engage in criminal behavior are based on a person's perception of what outcome appears more valuable.[23] Thus, some people commit assaults not because their motivation differs from that of other people but because their perceived benefits and costs differ. In order for the desired choices to be made, people must be aware of the benefits and costs of the alternatives available to them. This assumes that people have equal capability of making rational decisions under all conditions and circumstances, but the ability to make a rational judgment may be impaired, for example, if the person is under the influence of alcohol or drugs.

Specific structural factors that relate to homicide include poverty (associated with murders of friends and acquaintances, children, and spouses, and with robbery-associated murders of strangers);[24] belief in male dominance (spouse abuse); and racial discrimination (linked with killings of strangers and friends or acquaintances).[25,26]

An interactionist factor, consumption of alcohol and drugs, has been associated with all types of homicide except child homicide. Many studies have shown that about half of all victims and perpetrators of homicides had consumed alcohol. However, without control or comparison populations, these studies have not been able to demonstrate a causal role for alcohol.[27] The same situation applies to the association between alcohol use and family violence. Some researchers suggest that the disinhibiting effect of alcohol may be more psychological than physiological and that alcohol may serve as an excuse for behavior already decided on.[28]

It may be that alcohol and drug use contributes to homicide by influencing the risk of both victimization and perpetration, for example, if it has a physiological effect on the brain that reduces inhibitions against aggressive behavior. Alternatively, alcohol and drug use may be associated with homicide because their use is associated with specific situations, environments, or activities that place individuals at high risk of victimization. Moreover, individuals who take illicit drugs, distribute them, or do both may have higher risks for homicide victimization because of the high profits, criminal behaviors, and instability associated with drug dealing.[29]

Overall, it should be emphasized that a "reductionist" way of examining various approaches and factors provides some insight to help understand violent behavior; however, these are not independent of each other, but rather are interactive.

Outcomes

Mortality

In 1994, homicides in the United States accounted for the loss of at least 24,926 lives based on NCHS mortality data, of which 379 (1.5 percent) were perpetrated by law enforcement officials in the line of duty. The United States has one of the highest homicide rates among countries of the world reporting homicide statistics to the World Health Organization.[30] Reporting methods of individual countries may differ, and domestic and international wars may affect homicide rates in some areas.

Homicide is far more prevalent among minorities, males, and the young. Although homicide was the eleventh leading cause of death for the U.S. population, homicide was the leading cause of death for young people (15 to 24 years of age) who are black. Although the homicide rates for black males are much higher than those for all other races, it is difficult to determine the precise contribution of race to these high rates. Several studies suggest that socioeconomic status is a more important determinant than race.[31,32]

Ethnicity also appears to be an important determinant of homicide rates. In 1994, homicide was the sixth leading cause of death among persons of Hispanic origin. The overall homicide rate for Hispanics ages 15 to 24 years of age (36.6 per 100,000) was more than six times the non-Hispanic white rate (5.9 per 100,000). This difference was most striking in the young male age groups in which the Hispanic homicide rate was almost five times that for Anglos.[33]

Of the homicides committed in the United States in 1994 and reported to the FBI, 47 percent involved friends and acquaintances; 12 percent were within families; and 13 percent were between strangers.[3] The percentage of homicides with an unknown relationship was 40 percent.

Most family homicides involve spouses and occur in the home, frequently after many assaultive incidents.[20,28] In 38.4 percent of the cases, a handgun is used, followed by other guns (19.5 percent), knives (17.0 percent), and other means (25.1 percent).[32]

Victims of acquaintance homicide are typically younger than the victims of family homicide and are much more likely to be male and black. In 1986, 43.4 percent of the victims were black, and 37.3 percent were white. Offenders (median age, 23 years) are usually younger than their victims. Handguns were used in 44.7 percent of the cases; knives, in 19.5 percent. Acquaintance homicides are most likely to occur within a private residence, although one-third occur on the street, and a higher percentage occurs in bars than is true for other types of killings.[34]

In homicides among strangers, the victims and offenders are predominantly male and the median age of the victim (31 years) is higher than that of the offender (25 years). Most such killings are with firearms (49.1 percent with handguns, 12.2 percent with another type of gun). Nationally, 46.9 percent of killings of strangers are associated with another crime, often robbery, although the chance of being killed in a robbery remains relatively small.

In 1994, 70 percent of homicides were committed with firearms, with almost 83 percent of these victims being killed with handguns. After firearms, cutting and piercing instruments were the next most frequently used weapon (12.7 percent), followed by bodily force (5.3 percent) and blunt objects (4.1 percent). Other or undetermined weapons accounted for 7.9 percent of homicides.[3]

A relatively small proportion of homicides (18.4 percent in 1994) are committed during the perpetration of another felony or crime, such as robbery or narcotics offenses. Verbal arguments are the most frequently occurring circumstance associated with homicide (28.1 percent in 1994), while other nonfelony circumstances including brawls due to the influence of alcohol or narcotics, juvenile gang killings, and institutional killings accounted for 24.8 percent of the circumstances associated with homicide. In 28.1 percent of the cases, the circumstances leading to the killing were unknown.[3]

Morbidity

For Americans over the age of 12 years, 10.9 million incidents of violent crime (i.e., excluding homicide, but including simple and aggravated assault, robbery, and rape) occurred in 1994 (51 violent crimes per 1,000 people). Simple and aggravated assaults accounted for 83.5 percent of these incidents; attempted and completed robbery,

11.9 percent; attempted and completed rape, 3.7 percent. Males were 1.4 times more likely to be victims than were females, with men ages 16 to 19 years being at greatest risk (121.7 per 1,000). Blacks were at 1.3 times greater risk of being a victim of a violent crime than were whites, and Hispanics were about 1.2 more likely than non-Hispanics to have been a victim.[35]

Almost one-third of victims (30.2 percent) of robbery and assault sustained a physical injury. Given the severe emotional trauma associated with rape, all victims are considered to have been injured regardless of whether or not a physical injury was reported. Of all victims of violent crime, 7.8 percent received hospital care. Hospital costs (for those who survived assaults plus those who eventually died as a result of aggravated assault) totaled approximately $606 million. The cost of physician visits raised that cost to $638 million. No data are available for the costs of emergency room treatment, pharmaceuticals, extended care after initial hospitalization, or the treatment of offenders who were injured in aggravated assaults.

Aggravated assaults accounted for more than 8 million days lost from activities such as paid work (at least 4,718,200 days), school, or child rearing. The costs of disabilities, primarily psychological, sensory, and musculoskeletal, resulting from assaults cannot even be estimated.

Projections based on the National Crime Survey indicate that from 1982 to 1984 there were approximately 1.5 million incidents of assaultive violence (rape, robbery, aggravated assault, simple assault) among family members (213.8 per 100,000 U.S. population). Other estimates of the number of women beaten each year range from 1.8 million[30] to 3 to 4 million.[36] Assaults within families represent at least 21,000 hospitalizations, 99,800 hospital days, 28,700 emergency room visits, and 39,900 physician visits. Health care costs incurred for domestic assaults totaled at least $44,393,700.

Assaults within families accounted for at least 175,500 days lost from paid work in 1980. Medical resources are used by abused women to a greater extent than other groups. Battered women frequently use medical services instead of other refuge; of all the emergency room visits made by women seeking treatment for injury, 19 percent involve battering. Primary care sites such as maternity clinics or ambulatory care services are frequent sites of visits precipitated by battering. Research indicates that children who are victims of violence suffer delays in physical, social, and emotional development. Many who witness violence suffer from posttraumatic stress disorders, particularly if they must participate in the court process.[37] Battered women are at risk of alcoholism, drug abuse, attempted suicide, fear of child abuse, rape, and mental health problems, including severe depression and even psychosis.

Family violence is often cited as a reason for divorce, which can result in economic hardship for women and children even though it may solve the immediate problem. However, being divorced or single does not necessarily protect women from subsequent battering. At one large metropolitan hospital, 72 percent of the women who had battering injuries were single, separated, or divorced.[36]

Society as a whole also pays for violence through expenditures for police and criminal justice intervention, social service intervention, emergency room and trauma center services, and educational services in school systems that must cope with children with academic and social problems as a result of maltreatment at home.

Interventions to Prevent Assaultive Violence

Strategies to reduce or prevent the incidence of assaultive violence must involve both broad social changes in our overall approach to violence and specific interventions aimed at cases of potential or actual violence, assault, or abuse. These specific interventions may try to reach individuals before a pattern of victimization or interpersonal violence is established, or they may attempt to minimize the consequences and costs of interpersonal violence. The recommendations discussed here are grouped for consideration as changes in general public policy in the health and social services, in the criminal justice system, and in the environment.

Social and Cultural Services

1. Decrease the cultural acceptance of violence particularly among and against certain groups (blacks, teenagers, women, children) and promote the notion that violent individuals are responsible for their own behavior. Of special interest in this area is the portrayal of violence in children's television programming and the role of corporal punishment at schools and in homes.
2. Reduce racial discrimination and the effects of racism associated with the low self-esteem and low valuation of human life that have been linked with violence.
3. Reduce gender inequality and support male role models that emphasize flexibility, shared decision-making, and nonviolent means of self-development and expression.
4. Reduce the consumption of alcohol and other drugs through interventions directed toward adolescents and young adults, emphasizing the benefits of dependence-free development as well as the effects of harmful substances on self-control. Prevention can also focus on environmental changes such as raising the minimum drinking age, passing stricter laws against selling alcohol to individuals already intoxicated, limiting the hours and places where alcohol can be served, and regulating alcohol advertising.

Health and Related Social Services

1. Develop educational programs to teach social skills and conflict-resolution skills. Special programs in schools, churches, and health care and other community organizations could focus on (*a*) the magnitude of the threat that homicide and assault pose to lives and health, (*b*) how to recognize volatile situations before they escalate, and (*c*) how to diffuse or walk away from potentially homicidal fights.[38–40]
2. Increase education for family life, family planning, and child rearing to reduce family stress and violence.[41] Information and services that reduce the incidence of unwanted or unexpected children, that identify families at risk, and provide preventive education as well as education about reporting physical and sexual abuse could reduce violence in the home, thus reducing the amount of violence learned there and later perpetrated against acquaintances and strangers. Family education about developmental difficulties might help parents identify and seek appropriate treatments for children with aggressive and antisocial behaviors and children whose learning disabilities make it harder to learn appropriate social skills.[42,43]
3. Support families with community-based support services that help to integrate individuals into the community because research indicates that individuals and families embedded in kin and community groups are less likely to be abusive than individuals who are socially or physically isolated.[44,45] Tax, welfare, and business policies that promote isolation and divide families should also be reexamined.
4. Address problems in the recognition of cases of violence by the medical care system by making risk profiles and a history of victimization or perpetration of violence a part of every physical examination.
5. Decrease disincentives for medical personnel to become involved by addressing the legal entanglements that surround cases of child and woman abuse and by addressing the inhibitions and threats of violence that keep health care personnel from even questioning their patients about the cause of their injuries.
6. Improve the management and treatment of victims of violence, particularly for high-risk groups, such as infants or adolescents, who may be in danger of repeated attacks or homicide. Among the victims of violence should be included siblings, family members, and close friends of murdered and seriously injured persons.

7. Improve the ability of the health care system to recognize and treat consequences of violence other than injuries, including alcoholism, drug dependency, and psychiatric trauma. Intervention programs for children who are victims of violence as well as those who witness violence are urgently needed. Witnesses of violence also need help dealing with the criminal justice system since their experience as witnesses may traumatize them further.
8. Ensure that victims can receive medical care without being dependent on a spouse for adequate medical insurance.
9. Improve the identification and treatment by the health care system of perpetrators of violence; since perpetrators are often injured, they frequently require health services.
10. Improve record-keeping and reporting for victims of interpersonal violence by health care institutions and personnel.
11. Improve communication and cooperation among health care providers, police departments, social service organizations, and schools to improve identification of individuals at risk and documentation for victims who later may decide to prosecute.
12. Develop programs to train high-risk adolescents and to make jobs available for them to provide clear, positive roles for adolescents in our culture.
13. Emphasize prevention in the treatment of illness related to consumption of alcohol and other drugs. Health care personnel usually concentrate on immediate problems, such as bruises, overdoses, and detoxification, and fail to address prevention issues.
14. Develop health education curricula that address issues of self-directed and interpersonal violence.

Criminal Justice Changes

Changes in the criminal justice system focus on more active citizen interaction with the police and on changes that involve the courts, lawmakers, prosecutors, and prisons. Attempts to deal with homicide in this sector have usually taken two forms: deterrence (discouraging others by imposing sanctions) and incapacitation (preventing offenders from committing other crimes by physically restraining them). Despite many studies on deterrence and incapacitation, the effect of different sanctions on various crime types is mostly unknown.[3]

1. Train police to treat physical assaults among family members, intimates, and acquaintances as criminal behavior.
2. Train police and citizen intervention teams to mediate disputes and refer troubled people to other social service agencies. These teams need to be very sensitive to the concerns of women and minorities if they are going to reduce rather than potentially increase violence. Crisis intervention units that are not staffed by police may be even more effective. These units may be those located within the police complex although administered by civilian personnel; located within city hall and working in close conjunction with the police and other emergency services; or may be community-based with direct access to police and other emergency services. These groups can prevent situations from erupting into violence by providing backup to the police or support to victims.
3. Improve linkages between police and social services in response to violence.[24]
4. Initiate informal citizen surveillance and silent-witness programs.
5. Facilitate access of victims to legal services through protective orders, temporary restraining orders, and peace bonds to keep violent offenders from attacking partners or children.
6. Initiate victim- and witness-assistance programs that eliminate long waiting periods between the initial arrest and final disposition.

Environmental and Other Changes

1. Develop strategies to reduce injuries associated with firearms. Despite the magnitude and costs of injuries and mortality attributed to firearms, the role of firearms in producing injury and crime is an extremely contentious political and social issue in our society. However, if effective strategies are to be devised for preventing firearm injuries, a scientific perspective must be adopted toward this issue. Common approaches to the prevention of firearm injuries were addressed by the National Academy of Sciences in their report, *Understanding and Preventing Violence*.[10]

   We must establish a scientific basis for understanding the nature and patterns and causes of firearm injuries. This will help provide a common ground. There is no all-or-nothing solution for preventing firearm injuries. Instead, there is a wide array of diverse strategies and interventions that need to be evaluated. If scientific information on the health risks and possible benefits of firearm use is developed and disseminated, people will be empowered to understand the problem, assess the interventions, and make decisions to reduce risks for themselves, their families, and their communities in ways that support their own values. By reframing the debate, public health can help to engage many more people in this critically important issues creating a common ground on which people from both extremes, as well as the vast majority of people in the middle, can participate in constructive dialogue.

   There is a tremendous need for research in the area of firearm injury to determine the magnitude, characteristics, and costs of nonfatal firearm injuries; to estimate the risks of owning or carrying a firearm; and to evaluate the effectiveness of laws, regulations, and other strategies designed to prevent firearm injuries.
2. Create safe environments through architectural and social-planning principles.
3. Define high-risk settings and occupations and determine interventions specific for them, such as bulletproof vests for police and barriers for taxicabs.

Woman Battering

Evan Stark • Anne H. Flitcraft

Definition of the Problem

In addition to its impact on the public health of women and families, woman battering presents a challenge to public health because its parameters are not well defined, its severity is highly subjective, its causes are poorly understood, and its psychosocial consequences are often linked to physical events in very complex ways. Equally important, perhaps more than any other health problem, battering raises political concerns about which medical care and public health officials may have ambiguous feelings, including the implications of sexual inequality for health, the competing rights of husbands and spousal victims, and public intervention in private lives.

Definitional Issues

The terms *domestic violence, spouse abuse, partner or intimate violence, family violence*, and *woman battering* are often used interchangeably. State statutes and service providers often subsume battering under the category of domestic or family violence. It is useful to examine these terms separately.

Domestic violence, spouse abuse, and *partner or intimate violence* refer to the use of threats or physical force in family or other intimate relationships among adults.

Family violence is a broad term that encompasses domestic violence (the use of force among partners in marriage or other intimate relationships) and abuse of children, the elderly, or the disabled. Abuse is defined as the violent exploitation, mistreatment, or neglect of persons who are dependent because of their age or physical incapacity. Although state statutes define both domestic violence and abuse as criminal, state protective service agencies handle abuse of children, the frail elderly, or handicapped persons, except in the most severe cases. By contrast, in almost half the states—and the U.S. military—police are mandated to arrest offenders in cases of domestic violence.

Four characteristics differentiate family violence crimes from assaults between strangers or acquaintances. In family violence:

1. Force is used in close or blood relationships.
2. Perpetrators usually have continued access to their victims and repeat their assaults, often multiple times.[1]
3. The perpetrator controls numerous aspects of his victim's life.
4. Acts of force are rooted in norms about how certain persons (parents, males, lovers, husbands) *should* behave, given various occasions or provocations. For example, because of social norms that equate manliness with exclusive possession of a woman, many men may feel that they are not "macho" unless they use force to control or possess their partners.

These characteristics differentiate the experience of woman battering from the "trauma" suffered by victims of discrete or severe acts of stranger violence such as rape or wartime atrocities.

Domestic violence laws differ widely in the types of acts (assaults, threats, stalking, etc.) covered and the relationships that comprise a "domestic crime." However, the most effective operational definition for health settings relies on an inclusive notion of coercion and control, regardless of the severity of injury inflicted or whether the presentation involves injury, medical or psychosocial problems, or simply fear. Emphasizing "violence" or "domestic" may give the misleading impression that only physical injury is of interest or that concern is only for victims living in intact couple relationships.

Because the practitioner's central concern is with future health risks, the important distinction is between an anonymous incident, where future assault or control by the criminal is unlikely, and assault or control by a social partner, present or past, regardless of gender, age, or marital status. The term "partner" in reference to abuse includes males as well as females and situations in which both partners are equally abusive. Though far less frequently reported, assaults by homosexual partners and adolescent dating partners certainly do occur.[2]

As distinct from discrete acts of partner assault, the term *battering* is used to describe the *ongoing process of victimization* that accompanies domestic violence against women in an estimated 80 percent of all cases.[3]

Woman battering describes the most devastating context of domestic violence and encompasses the spectrum of strategies partners use to hurt, intimidate, coerce, isolate, control, or humiliate their victim. In a typical situation, these behaviors include, but are not limited to, repeated episodes of assault, sexual assault, threats, verbal abuse, the destruction of property, abuse, neglect or threats against the victim's children, stalking, degradation, isolation from friends and family, and a pattern of control over key aspects of the victim's life, including money, food, sexuality, physical appearance, social life, transportation, work, religion, and access to help. Battering compromises the victim's rights to physical safety, liberty, self-development, and self-expression.

In marked contrast to partner violence, in which women frequently hit men, battering appears to be gender-specific. Whereas partner violence and certain coercive acts by partners (such as stalking) are crimes, to date, the complex range of strategies employed to batter women has not received special legal recognition.

The battering syndrome is a process in which relationships pass through phases marked by increasing fear, isolation, and control, often accompanied by increasingly complex psychological and psychosocial adaptations. During this process, the victim's response to her situation alternates between hope (things will improve, he will change, the violence will end, she will escape) and mounting fear that she or the children will be hurt or killed if they leave or that she will not be able to survive on her own. Many victims believe, incorrectly, that if they change their behavior, the violence will stop. The battered woman feels repeatedly frustrated by the contradictory nature of the batterer's demands, the unpredictability of his impulsive behavior, and his refusal to accept responsibility for or change any part of the problem. In addition, she has a chronic fear of violence to herself and children. Thus, she may have little self-confidence as a mother, be suspicious and wary, and have little sense of control over her environment.

Scope of the Problem

Over time, according to state and national population surveys, almost a third of all couples experience one or more episodes of partner violence during their marriage. A national household survey in 1975 by Straus et al estimated that 3.9 million instances of partner violence occur annually in the United States, that 3.8 percent or 1.8 million wives are hit by husbands, and that 4.6 percent or 2.2 million husbands are hit.[4] Follow-up telephone surveys in 1985 and interviews in 1992 suggest a decline in "severe" violent acts by husbands (as reported by husbands and wives) possibly due to widespread intervention. But the same research shows a dramatic *increase* in "minor assaults" as reported by wives.[5–7] A 1992 Harris poll commissioned by the Commonwealth Fund estimated that 2 percent of the women interviewed had been "kicked, bit, hit with a fist or some other object" (1.1 million women) in the last year and an additional 2.9 million women had been "pushed, grabbed, shoved or slapped."[8] The risk to women who are single, separated, or divorced is even higher.[9,14] These surveys suggest that the prevalence of domestic violence is between 250 and 300 cases per 1,000 adult females.

Although general population surveys implicate both sexes equally in partner violence, official statistics on arrest or self-reported victimization indicate that partner violence is most often a gendered crime in which men typically are the offenders and women the victims. By contrast, if a man is assaulted, there is only approximately one chance in 40 that his wife or girlfriend is the assailant.[9]

Not surprisingly, partner violence is an enormous problem for women's health. A Harris poll of Kentucky housewives reported that 17 percent of the women who had been abused used emergency medical services.[10] A Texas survey found that 358,595 women required medical treatment at some point in their lives because of abuse.[11]

Based on a review of 3,676 medical charts, the Yale Trauma Studies found that 18.7 percent of female trauma patients had a history of domestic violence and that an even higher proportion of abused women could be identified among obstetrical patients, mothers of abused children, and patients in the psychiatric emergency service.[12,13] Studies using patient questionnaires report even higher proportions of battered women. For example, 30 percent of the women in a Philadelphia emergency department (ED) reported being abused and 28 percent of the women in a primary care clinic did, as well.[14]

Importantly, the Yale Trauma Studies also found that, in the typical case, violence is ongoing. In just 18 percent of the identified cases of battering, the current visit was the woman's first presentation of an at-risk injury, yielding an institutional incidence rate of 0.032. Thus, from the perspective of health care providers, domestic violence is a chronic health problem with a low spontaneous cure rate.

A better picture of the actual at-risk population is provided by a recent survey of 648 randomly sampled women who sought treatment at emergency departments in Denver. More than half (54.2 percent) had been threatened or physically injured by a husband or boyfriend at some time in their lives.[15]

Injury is the most dramatic consequence of ongoing domestic violence. The Yale studies concluded that domestic violence was the leading cause of injury for which women sought medical attention. Although abuse-related injuries were relatively minor, victims averaged more than one trauma visit a year, far more than nonbattered women. As important, compared to a baseline population of nonbattered patients, battered women were 5 times more likely to attempt suicide; 15 times more likely to abuse alcohol; 9 times more likely to abuse drugs; 6 times more likely to report child abuse; and 3 times more likely to be diagnosed as "depressed" or psychotic.[16]

Data from the National Crime Victim Survey (NCVS) indicate that between 25 and 30 percent of all abused women suffer "serial victimization," many beaten as frequently as once a week. In addition to repeated violence, batterers also employ strategies to intimidate, isolate, and control their partners, a pattern of "coercive control" that deprives the battered woman of material resources (such as food or money), access to family, friends, or helpers, and other basic rights and liberties.[17] Being subjected to coercive control elicits the syndrome of problems presented by battered women to the health system. No evidence of the battering syndrome has been reported among men. Battering relationships have been estimated to last, on average, 5.5 to 6 years, but continue far longer in many instances.[18]

Data Sources

General Population Data

There are no ongoing and updated standardized databases from which to reliably estimate the prevalence of partner violence and no population data that shed light on the complex of controlling behaviors involved in woman battering. Estimates of the most severe forms of partner violence—homicide and assault—can be gleaned from the Federal Bureau of Investigation (FBI), Uniform Crime Report (UCR) and the NCVS taken each year by the Department of Justice.

The UCR is particularly helpful in identifying aggravated assault and homicide. However, UCR data do not indicate whether or not the victim and perpetrator live together—a common criterion in distinguishing domestic violence—and only include problems reported to the police and the FBI, a small proportion of all spousal assaults.

By contrast, the NCVS, a general population survey, records many crimes not reported to the police and includes data on medical treatment, characteristics of the victim-offender relationship, and whether or not police are notified. NCVS estimates of partner violence must be considered extremely conservative, however, because respondents are often questioned in the presence of their spouses and because respondents may misinterpret the emphasis on "criminal" acts as excluding domestic violence. Still, the NCVS is particularly useful in detecting sex differences in how family members interpret the use of force, i.e., when they think an "assault" has occurred. Significantly, the NCVS and Straus et al report identical rates of severe violence against women (3.9 and 3.8 percent) but very different rates of violence by wives against husbands (0.03 versus 4.6 percent), suggesting that most incidents of "hitting" by wives are not considered assaultive by their husbands.

Alternative estimates are based on representative state and national surveys which use the Conflict Tactics Scale (CTS). Developed by Straus et al[4] for use with intact couples, the CTS includes any acts of force that partners employ during conflicts, ranging from a push or shove to the use of weapons. The scale provides a useful picture of the family members who employ physical force and of the relative frequency of different types of force. The resulting data from surveys using this scale exclude the large number of victims who are single, separated, or divorced at the time of their abuse, a group that is included in the NCVS; fail to differentiate violent acts according to their intent or physical consequences; and omit the large number of unilateral violent acts.[19]

The different ways that the NCVS and the CTS measure partner violence have important consequences for how we define the incidence, duration, and prevalence of the problem; whom we identify as victims and offenders; how we understand the dynamics involved and the extent and type of resources mobilized to address domestic violence. For instance, studies based on the CTS indicate that men and women in couples are equally likely to employ violence to resolve conflicts. By contrast, when injury is considered or only acts that partners consider criminal are counted (as in the NCVS), battering appears to be gender-specific, with women victimized 13 times more frequently than men. According to the Justice Department, in 1992 and 1993, "intimates"—boyfriends or husbands—accounted for more than 1 million of reported assaults against women, seven times the estimated 143,000 assaultive crimes that were committed against men by intimates.[9]

Problems in Measuring Battering

Violence directed against a partner is only one component of battering and not necessarily the one of greatest consequence for women's health or the most salient to victims. Unfortunately, there are no data on the range of coercive and controlling tactics used in battering. From a public health or medical standpoint, in which the prevention of future harm is a major concern, the population considered at risk for battering includes (*a*) women who have ever experienced violence, coercion, or control; (*b*) women who present with complaints or fear of battering, regardless of whether injury is involved; and (*c*) women who are experiencing intimidation, isolation, or control, even if violence has stopped. Existing surveys of partner violence offer little guidance in determining the size, risk, or service needs of these groups. Moreover, because battering has yet to be criminalized, the UCR and the NCVS do not collect data on battering.

Criminological data obscure the chronic nature of woman battering. Incidence (new cases of a problem) is normally figured separately from prevalence, or the cumulative burden a problem poses to the community because of its duration. Prevalence (P) is calculated by multiplying incidence (I) by duration (D) ($P = I \times D$). Secondary prevention aims to reduce the prevalence of a problem, whereas primary prevention aims to curtail its incidence as well. Most crimes, including stranger assaults, involve single, discrete episodes, making it unnecessary to calculate prevalence separately. While strategies of interdiction and prevention may differ, their common aim is to keep the crime from occurring.

Typically, surveys report the annual number of intimates assaulted by their partners as the "incidence" of domestic violence. But because battering is typically a chronic health problem, these data reflect neither true incidence (since most cases identified as new are actually ongoing) nor prevalence (since battering is also ongoing in many cases, although no assault occurred during the year). Thus, with currently available data, it is impossible to determine the average duration of cases or the cumulative burden that domestic violence poses in terms of suffering, service utilization, and cost. A recent London survey gives some sense of the actual annual burden that chronic battering places on the community. The approximately 12 percent of adult women victimized by domestic violence suffered an average of 7.1 assaults during the previous 12 months, resulting in an average of 4.3 injuries and an annual assault incidence rate of 85 per 100 women.[20]

Research and Identification in the Health System

Gathering data on woman battering in health care settings for case identification is important for clinical and epidemiologic reasons. This process begins with the patient encounter, but may extend to a complete review of the patient's medical history to determine the extent and consequences of abuse and to document the patient's previous attempts to find aid.

Because physicians rarely record abuse or list it as a diagnosis in medical records, data based on physician reporting consistently underestimate the magnitude of the problem. At a time when the extent of battering was unknown and few services were in place for identified victims, the critical screen of medical records developed by Flitcraft for the Yale Trauma Studies (YTS)[21] was the primary research tool. This method classifies patients as positive, probable, or suggestive for woman battering based on a review of each episode in their adult trauma history.

The most effective and least conservative means to identify the incidence, duration, and prevalence of battering in the health setting are anonymous questionnaires or simple screens administered at intake or during routine health examinations. These have been used successfully to garner data on domestic violence in a variety of health settings and could easily be expanded to elicit information on the range of coercive strategies employed in woman battering.[15,22]

Procedures to identify battered women are slowly being introduced in clinical settings and typically rely only on physical trauma presented in the emergency department. As recently as 1991, a survey of all emergency departments in Massachusetts revealed that 80 percent had no written protocol in place to identify domestic violence and 58 percent reported that they identify five or fewer battered women each month, a figure that is far below research estimates.[23] However, when simple, frank questioning about violence, fear, and control are incorporated into routine health interviews and screening procedures throughout the health system, battered women are forthright, cooperative, and willing to engage in joint safety planning for themselves and their children.[24,25]

Causes and Risk Factors

Vulnerability Factors and High-Risk Populations

Although there are statistical associations between a risk of battering and marital status, pregnancy, age, substance use, and exposure to violence in childhood, the only factors consistently linked to future risk of battering are a history of violence, fear of violence, and control.

The confusion that surrounds population-based research on battering means that all generalizations about battered women and offenders should be approached skeptically, including demographic profiles suggesting that some groups are more susceptible than others. Furthermore, research on domestic violence fails to establish the clear temporal sequence needed to show that personality or behavioral characteristics are risk factors, rather than outcomes of spouse abuse. Therefore it is best to view associations as vulnerability factors rather than as causal or risk factors for spouse abuse.[26] These factors may interact with the situational dynamics in domestic conflict to increase the likelihood that violence will result.

Demographic Factors

Research has failed to identify clear demographic patterns in domestic violence by race, social class, or age. Population surveys suggest that battering is two to three times more common among blacks than whites; however, among groups with similar income, blacks are less likely than whites to experience spousal violence.[4] There may be significant racial differences in outcome, however. Domestic violence appears more likely to prompt a suicide attempt in black than in white women for instance.[27] One survey also reported higher rates of abuse among poor, unemployed, or working-class groups and showed that drinking, approval of violence, and blue-collar status had a cumulative relation to violence, with the highest rates appearing when all three elements were present.[28] But occupational class itself was not predictive.[29] The difference between low-income and middle-income women may be smaller than for almost any other health problem, and extensive abuse has been identified in relatively affluent communities. For example, in a survey to which 786 medical students and faculty responded, 17 percent of the women and 3 percent of the men reported physical abuse or sexual abuse by a partner in their adult life.[30] As the control facets of battering are incorporated into research, its inverse relation to social class may disappear altogether.

Pregnancy is positively associated and marital status negatively associated with the risk of battering. Pregnancy is a high-risk period for abused women. Between 20 and 25 percent of obstetrical patients are abused women, an even higher percentage than seen in the emergency department.[31,32]

Married women are the least likely, and single, separated, and divorced women the most likely to experience partner assault, with separated women at highest risk.[33] Among women seeking medical assistance, 73 percent of the victims were separated, single, or divorced at the time they received abusive injuries.[12]

Personality and Behavioral Factors

Victims. Studies with the most reliable designs report few, if any, significant personality differences between battered and nonbattered women, and no personality profile identifies certain women as "violence prone."[34] A more controversial view suggests that battered women become trapped in abusive relationships by a "cycle of violence" (buildup of tension, explosion, and a "honeymoon" phase), which elicits a battered woman's syndrome (BWS) characterized by learned helplessness, depression, and delayed or reluctant help-seeking.[35] Although some victims evidence both the cycle and the BWS, in the majority of cases, battered women are aggressive help-seekers (with help-seeking increasing as abuse escalates) and employ a range of strategies, including frequent separations, to minimize or end abuse.[36]

Perpetrators. Based on offenders' self-reports on various psychological tests, researchers have identified a number of personality disorders among batterers, including borderline and schizoidal disorder, narcissistic/antisocial personality, and passive/dependent compulsive disorders.[37,38] A comparative study of batterers and nonbatterers established a strong correlation between abusive behavior (as measured by the CTS) and elevated scores on a measure of borderline personality organization, suggesting to some that woman battering is the result of psychopathology and casting serious doubt on the theory that all or most sexual violence against women is gender motivated.[39,40] Some form of childhood exposure to violence (child abuse, severe physical punishment as a child, or witnessing parental domestic violence) occurs in the background of 60 to 70 percent of batterers in treatment, leading many policymakers to support therapeutic intervention to break the cycle of violence. In contrast to clinical samples, population data fails to support the belief that most batterers were exposed to violence as children.[41] Meanwhile, other clinical studies show that batterers are psychologically indistinguishable from nonabusive men.[42]

Increasing evidence suggests that offenders are men with diverse personalities, family histories, and behavioral profiles who typically use several strategies, as well as physical abuse, to establish control, extract obedience, and secure such tangible benefits as sex, money, and feelings of power.

The Role of Alcohol. Although the reported violence rates among men who use alcohol are 2 to 15 times higher than rates among abstainers, a causal role for alcohol cannot be supported. Among women, alcohol is typically the consequence, rather than the cause of victimization. Although drinking is associated with higher rates of wife abuse, alcohol is not typically an immediate antecedent, nor does cessation of alcohol use appear to affect abusive behavior.[43] Alcohol appears to be involved in only 6 to 8 percent of the family disputes in which police are involved.[44] Moreover, abuse is unaffected by recovery. Neither length of sobriety nor membership in Alcoholics Anonymous (AA) are linked to any reduction in male violence.[45]

Violence in the Family of Origin. Childhood victimization increases the risk that a boy will abuse his adult partner. But, neither the typical batterer nor his victim come from a violent home. Survey and case-control studies report significant correlations between current victimization and a woman's abuse as a child. But two well-designed studies using multiple comparison groups and collecting data from men and women found no significant effect of childhood violence on later victimization.[46,47] Straus et al demonstrate that men from violent childhoods (5 percent of the population) are 10 times more likely to abuse their wives than are men who had nonviolent childhoods. However, a consideration of the relative size of the groups exposed and not exposed to childhood violence shows that a current batterer is seven times more likely to come from a nonviolent than a violent home.[48] Even 80 percent of the children from families classified as most violent do not become batterers. Kaufman and Zigler are more conservative in estimating that 70 percent of those abused as children do not become violent as adults.[41]

High-Risk Populations

Although the typical victim of battering is a young woman (under 30) with a child, battering is a problem at every point in the life cycle. It may be initiated during adolescence, escalate during pregnancy, present through problems among children, and continue into old age. Special treatment issues relate to the age, developmental stage, and lifestyle of the individuals and families involved in battering. Children, adolescents, and older women are often unrecognized as populations at high risk for battering. Additional high-risk populations about whom there is little research include disabled women, homeless women, and women with human immunodeficiency virus (HIV) infection.

Children. Children whose mothers are battered are exposed either to acts of violence, coercion, and control or to the consequences of these acts. As a result, children may be covictims who are also are at risk for severe injury as well as short- and long-term physical, medical, and psychological problems. As covictims, children are injured in an estimated 17 percent of all battering episodes. The estimated 68 to 80 percent of the children of batterers who witness their father's behavior may be more damaged psychologically than victims of child abuse.[49] The estimated 3.3 million to 10 million children who are exposed to battering each year are forced to cope with high stress, including fear of injury to their mother and themselves.[50] The medical and psychological effects of exposure flow directly from the developmental age of the child, the dynamics in particular relationships, and the nature and extent of exposure.[51,52]

Adolescents. Adolescent girls are also at high risk for battering. Nineteen to 31.5 percent of young women are threatened or assaulted during dating relationships, with 45 percent of these incidents resulting in injury.[53] Thirty-four percent of injuries brought to the emergency department by girls between the ages of 16 and 18 are the result of partner violence.[22] Partner violence also is a major context for sexual assault, unwanted pregnancy, depression, attempted suicide, addiction, and a range of somatic complaints among female adolescents. Presentations frequently associated with partner abuse among adolescents include injury, teen pregnancy, malnutrition, isolation, depression, anxiety or suicidality (among males as well as females), truancy, homelessness, and the use of addictive substances.[54,55] The battered adolescent may fall between the cracks, as she is too old for child protective services and too young for adult protective services, including domestic violence shelters.

Older Women. Partner violence poses a major threat to the health of older women, accounting for 18 percent of the injuries presented to the hospital by women over 60.[22] In addition to injury, partner violence also may account for depression and other psychiatric disorders among the elderly, as well as attempted suicide, physical disability, addiction, chronic pain syndromes, and a range of somatic complaints. In general, physical injury is a less prominent feature of battering among the elderly than is a complex psychosocial profile reinforced by chronic mental abuse, isolation, and control over social life and resources in the relationship. Common presentations of domestic violence among the elderly include recent onset of substance use, noncompliance with medical regimes, chronic anxiety, malnutrition, depressive symptoms with no supporting history, and complaints of pain with no clinical evidence of disease. This profile often subjects the older battered woman to the dual stigma associated with age discrimination and with pseudopsychiatric labels that obstruct her access to health and other services. Although most domestic violence among the elderly is long-standing, in certain cases, its onset or intensification is linked to developmental milestones such as aging, dependence on medication, retirement, loss of sexual function, or another sudden change in social, medical, or mental health status.

Health Outcomes

The health consequences of woman battering follow from its dynamics of violence, intimidation, isolation, and control. They include the direct consequences of these strategies, such as injury, child abuse, disability, unwanted pregnancy, sexually transmitted diseases (STDs), HIV disease, and the medical, behavioral, and mental health problems that result as victims adapt to living with chronic stress and trauma. Prominent among these problems are drug and alcohol addiction, depression, and attempted suicide.

Consequences of Violence. Violence is used in battering to subdue a partner, instill fear, appropriate material resources, and inflict pain. Violence may occur during conflicts. But in many abusive relationships, violence becomes routine or occurs without warning.

Partner violence is the leading cause of injury for which women seek medical attention[3] and is the leading cause of injury during pregnancy. Battered women are 13 times more likely than nonbattered women to be injured in the breast, chest, and abdomen and 3 times as likely to be injured while pregnant, an injury pattern suggesting the sexual nature of assault in woman battering.

The hallmarks of injury in woman battering are the frequency and ongoing nature of a woman's injury, not necessarily its severity. Almost 1 battered woman in 5 has presented at least 11 times with trauma, and another 23 percent have brought 6 to 10 abusive injuries to the attention of clinicians.[12] Still, abusive injuries are no more likely to result in hospitalization than nonabusive injuries, suggesting that in itself severity is not a good indicator of abuse. A woman who comes to a health facility three times with injuries has an 80 percent chance of being a battered woman, whether those injuries require sutures or not. Frequency and the central pattern of injury combine to constitute an adult trauma history typical of woman battering.

Sexual assault is also part of the pattern. A majority of domestic violence victims report that they have been forced to have sex without their consent. This is consistent with the reported findings that a third of all rapes—and almost half among women over 30—are committed by partners.

In addition to injury, medical problems indirectly related to partner assault comprise 14 to 20 percent of women's visits to ambulatory care or internal medicine clinics. The bulk of these presentations involve headaches from head trauma, joint pains from twisting injuries, abdominal or breast pain following blows to the torso, dyspareunia or recurrent genitourinary infections from sexual assault, dysphagia following choking, or chronic pain syndromes. As the result of forced sex, battered women are also at elevated risk for HIV infection. Repeated somatic complaints are a common presentation of battering at primary care clinics.

Complications of previous, repeated trauma are a second source of medical illness among battered women and include, for instance, recurrent sinus infections among those who have suffered fractured facial bones and hearing deficits following repeated blows to the ears.

Consequences of Intimidation. Intimidation includes threats, surveillance, and degradation or mental abuse and may extend to the health setting, where it can include indirect warnings that are invisible to the outsider.

As a result of intimidation, battered women live with chronic stress and anxiety. Women describe a life of "walking on eggshells." Outcomes of intimidation frequently presented to medical or mental health clinics include anxiety disproportionate to the situation, isolation from friends and family, unwanted pregnancy, and symptoms of posttraumatic stress disorder (including re-experiencing past trauma, inappropriate or dull affect, a "startle" response, "splitting," and loss of boundaries). Other somatic problems frequently associated with the stress of intimidation include gastrointestinal complaints; chronic pain syndromes; atypical chest pain; hyperventilation; sleep, mood, and eating disorders; noncompliance with medication; requests for tranquilizers and sleeping pills; anxiety disorders; agitation; disorganized activity state; and immobilization.

Isolation. A sudden constriction of social contacts is the most common sign of *isolation* in battering relationships. Women may somatize their isolation through various "pleas for help." These may be expressed medically in the presentation of vague complaints with no evidence of medical disease. They may be expressed more dramatically in suicidal gestures or other behaviors that can mimic frank psychiatric disease. These commonly include depressed mood, codependency, low self-esteem and self-blame, psychomotor retardation, constriction of thought or complete immobilization, sleep disorders, and rapid weight loss.

Traditional medical and mental health interventions frequently contribute to a woman's sense of isolation. In response to the pain, headaches, the multiple injuries and somatic complaints, battered women are often mistakenly given pain or sleep medications, anxiolytics, and frankly punitive referrals to psychiatry or child protective services.

Instead of viewing the woman who returns multiple times to the medical clinic as a persistent help-seeker, she is often misidentified as someone who is overusing health resources or using them inappropriately. In this situation, clinicians often resort to labels such as "frequent visitor," "hypochondriac," or "hysteric," to validate their lack of intervention. These relatively common medical practices isolate the woman from further health resources, reinforce the isolation imposed at home, and validate the batterer's claim that the victim is "crazy."[56]

Control. Control can extend from the details of everyday life to the material, sexual, and psychological moorings on which survival and identity rest. Rapid weight loss, malnutrition, and chronic fatigue may reflect attempts to cope with stress and also may be the direct result of an escalation of the batterer's control strategies in a relationship. Some women suffer extreme psychological reactions to control, including paralyzing depression alternating with homicidal rage, a sense of depersonalization (e.g., that one's body is not one's own), dissociative disorders, and regression to an almost childlike state of dependence.[57]

Substance Use. The use of licit and illicit substances often begins as a means of self-medicating injury that results from partner assault and often becomes abusive as the woman attempts to cope with the isolation and control aspects of battering. Substance use in the context of battering is a particular risk among pregnant women.

Battering appears to be the single most important context yet identified for female alcoholism. The risk that a battered woman will abuse alcohol increases 400 percent after the onset of domestic violence (from 4 to 16 percent).[58] This is 16 times the percentage found among nonbattered women. Abused women who abuse alcohol use emergency medical and psychiatric services more frequently than any other population of female patients.

There is also an overlap between partner violence and illegal drug use. Although battered women evidence no more drug abuse than nonbattered women before the onset of abuse, their risk becomes nine times greater than expected once an abusive episode has been presented to the hospital.[31]

Mental Health Problems. Mental health problems are another prominent feature of late-stage domestic violence. The prevalence of woman abuse among mental health clients is even greater than among medical patients, approaching half of all female inpatients.[59,60] Compared to nonbattered mental health patients, battered women are less likely to manifest psychotic illness, but are more likely to carry a diagnosis of situational or personality disorder and to exhibit impaired self-esteem. The most common diagnosis of abuse victims is depression (37 percent), but 1 abused woman in 10 suffers a psychotic break. Battered women are also far more likely than others to be given a pseudopsychiatric label such as "hysteric," "hypochondriac," and "crock."[16] Psychologically, the combination of ongoing assault and coercive control may evoke symptoms of posttraumatic stress disorder, characterized by flashbacks, nightmares, hypervigilance, loss of boundaries, numbing, and chronic fear and anxiety.[61,62] An extreme consequence of isolation and control is resignation to the situation (fatalism), a sense that "no one can help me" (learned helplessness), and a reluctance to ask for help even when viable options are available.[63]

Suicide Attempts. Attempted suicide—and particularly multiple attempts—is a significant outcome as abused women feel themselves trapped by isolation and controlled by the batterer. Descriptive studies of battered women report that between 35 and 40 percent attempt suicide.[35] Although suicide risk factors do not differ between battered and nonbattered women before the first reported episode of abuse, subsequently battered women experience a 4.8 relative risk of attempted suicide compared with nonbattered women. Of the 10 percent who attempt suicide, 50 percent do so more than once.[3] Overall, battering is the context for almost a third of all female suicide attempts (29.5 percent), half of those by black women and a majority of those by women who are pregnant. Importantly, 65 percent of the suicide attempts by battered women are within 6 months of a visit for abuse, and 36.5 percent occur on the same day as an abuse-related health visit. For most battered women, the suicide attempts are an adaptive reaction to an intolerably stressful situation. Although these women may evidence no underlying psychopathology, their situation should be considered an emergency, and advocacy and support services should be initiated.

Child Abuse. Batterers frequently use the children to extend their intimidation and control over the mother, particularly after a couple separates. This may extend from using children to spy on the victim, threatening to report the mother for child abuse, or hurting the child as a way to hurt the mother. In these cases, child abuse is part of the pattern of battering. Even if no injury is inflicted on the child, the use of children by the batterer represents an escalation in risk for the mother, in the way that the introduction of a gun into the household may represent a marked escalation of domestic violence.[63]

There are sharply discrepant findings about the frequency of child abuse among battered women, possibly due to definitional differences. Rates of child abuse reported by battered women range from 1.7 percent in a British medical practice[64] to a third of the children in a rural mental health practice, and 70 percent of the children of a volunteer sample.[65,66] By contrast, reports of woman battering as the background for child abuse are consistently high.[67] In a review of a year's sample of mothers whose children were suspected of physical abuse or neglect, Stark and Flitcraft[68] reported that 45 percent were battered women, the highest percentage of battered women identified among any client population. In these cases, it was typically the batterer who was also abusing the child. Bowker et al[66] reported a strong relationship between male dominance in the prevailing year and spousal child abuse, a finding that supports the gender-politics thesis.

Interventions

Health Interventions

The traditional public health division of primary, secondary, and tertiary prevention offers a useful way to conceptualize the merger of a preventive health perspective and a clinical perspective on woman battering. To effectively prevent woman battering, intervention must proceed at all three levels.

Primary Prevention: Professional Change. In traditional public health terms, primary prevention entails reducing the number of new cases by changing behavior or environmental factors. Physicians can address environmental factors by recognizing ways in which the medical profession may be helping to perpetuate a harmful environment.

Following the U.S. Surgeon General's 1985 conference and the recognition of battering as a problem for a significant number of pregnant women, the American College of Obstetricians and Gynecologists led the way among health professionals in recognizing domestic violence as a threat to women's health and mounted a campaign to educate its members. In 1991 the American Medical Association (AMA) launched a campaign to address family violence as a major health problem. The development of diagnostic and treatment guidelines on child abuse and neglect, child sexual abuse, domestic violence, and elder abuse and neglect formed the backdrop for the AMA's organizational efforts. The AMA also played a key role in the formation of the National Coalition of Physicians against Family Violence, with institutional membership from more than 75 major medical organizations. The American Medical Women's Association, the American Academy of Family Practice, and the American College of Emergency Physicians also have participated in creating a comprehensive medical response to family violence. The success of these and other professional organizations in bringing these issues to the attention of their membership is significant.

Today, the medical and public health response to domestic violence includes the Centers for Disease Control and Prevention; state health departments; the American Medical Association; other professional medical, public health, and nursing organizations; federally funded centers for information on health and domestic violence, such as those housed at the San Francisco–based Domestic Violence Prevention Fund and the Pennsylvania Coalition Against Domestic Violence; and state-funded health training organizations such as the Domestic Violence Training Project (DVTP) in Connecticut.

Further changes to the structure of medical practice are still needed if the environment surrounding woman battering is to be altered successfully. The structure of medicine with its traditional male bias and the hierarchical organization of medical training are barriers to physicians' participation in domestic violence intervention and pose even more formidable obstacles in the context of responding to coercion men employ in battering. Although the logic of managed care favors community prevention and early intervention to avoid costly emergencies, powerful financial incentives tend to exclude populations, such as battered women, that appear to place inordinate demands on health resources. To move medical care into the mainstream of political and community life where woman battering is unacceptable, primary prevention efforts must address both the substance of physician norms and their organizational context.[69,70] At present, such efforts are rare.

Secondary Prevention: The Doctor/Patient Encounter. Early claims that abused women delay or fail to report injuries have not been sustained. Indeed, abusive injury is reported promptly. Sensitive probing can evoke an accurate patient account of abuse as a source of injury. After staff training and the introduction of an identification protocol in the emergency department at the Medical College of Pennsylvania, the percentage of women found to be battered increased almost 6-fold, from 5.6 to 30 percent.[22] Protocols lose their efficacy, however, without ongoing staff training and quality assurance mechanisms to ensure compliance.

In screening for battering, frank questioning to elicit a history of assault (the adult trauma history) is the first step in patient identification. Equally important are questions focused on other aspects of battering such as fear ("Is there someone in your life who is making you afraid?"), isolation ("Is anyone in your life preventing you from seeing someone with whom you used to have regular contact?"), or control ("Is someone in your life controlling what you do?").

Integrating a brief screen for battering into the basic patient interview for all female patients helps identify abuse before the extent and nature of injuries escalates. Routine assessment for battering is a form of health education. A practitioner's acknowledgement of the problem validates the fact that coercion and control pose a threat to health. Just as routine questions about a patient's smoking habits identify smoking-related problems and reinforce a patient's decision not to smoke, routine questions about abuse identify the problems of abused women, assess current safety of women who were battered in the past, and heighten the awareness of women who have not been in an abusive relationship.

Most health visits by abused women are to nonemergent primary care sites. Thus, health care organizations should develop a protocol that outlines procedures to help identify battered women and delineates responsibilities for assessment and referral at all primary care and general medical and mental health clinics, as well as at emergency medical and psychiatric settings.

Secondary prevention includes appropriate early intervention. To date, specific elements of intervention generally include identification, validation, treatment of medical needs, assessment of mental health needs, clear documentation, safety assessment, and referral to law enforcement and/or community-based domestic violence services. Limited by the relative paucity of clinical experience with victims of domestic violence, health care organizations should update protocols to deal with woman battering.

It seems intuitively obvious that practitioner intervention in woman battering must be modeled after involvement in other abuse situations or in other criminal investigations such as homicide or rape. Given the chronic nature of woman battering, however, better models might come from the current approach to alcohol and drug use, HIV disease, tuberculosis and syphilis treatment, and family planning. In such an approach, health care providers integrate periodic crisis intervention with ongoing monitoring, patient-centered planning, and liaison with community-based service organizations such as battered women's shelters. Meanwhile, because of its emphasis on patient empowerment, domestic violence intervention converges with many contemporary challenges in public health and medical practice—including smoking cessation, cancer screening, HIV prevention, occupational and environmental health, and the care of terminally ill patients—where new models of practitioner/patient relationships are emphasized.

Developing appropriate intervention strategies involves the skills of many health professions, including nursing and social work, and will call on the expertise of a broad range of clinicians. Evaluation and research in this area is vital.

Tertiary Prevention: Health Care Organizations. The role of health care organizations in a comprehensive response to domestic violence is the least developed. In 1992, the Joint Commission on the Accreditation of Healthcare Organizations (JCAHO) expanded its guidelines on emergency departments and hospital-sponsored ambulatory care centers to encourage the development of staff education and protocols on domestic violence. Such protocols outline the responsibilities of clinical staff to identify abuse with referral to police, domestic violence services, child protective services, social services, and mental health treatment programs.

The JCAHO guidelines were part of a strategy to expand the identification of victims of domestic violence seen predominantly in emergency departments. To this extent, the current guidelines are based on an extremely limited notion of the essential components of medicine's response to woman battering. Protocols use the medical encounter largely for case finding and evidence gathering for subsequent criminal proceedings. Current protocols generally do not commit additional health care resources to victims of woman battering, nor do they contribute to shifting resources (in alcohol treatment, intensive care unit trauma admissions, or adverse birth outcomes) to include specific support or safety initiatives. Tertiary prevention of woman battering calls on health care organizations to incorporate and invest in crisis intervention, emergency hospitalization for shelter, counseling, support groups, and advocacy, rather than simple identification and referral. Such a comprehensive approach will require changes in medical practice that rival those seen in law and law enforcement practice.

Complex Social Prevention

Complex social prevention involves broad changes in the overall approach to woman battering and aims to reduce the use of coercion and control that perpetuate gender inequality in intimate relations.

The traditional model emphasizes physical harms, including those from violence-related injury, but greatly undervalues the psychological and social costs associated with inequality and the loss of liberty in woman battering. Only when these intangible costs are calculated can a full picture of woman battering emerge.

The traditional model also emphasizes individual behavior change, specifically, the propensity to use violence to resolve conflict. Cessation of violent and controlling behaviors is critical, but equally important is addressing structures of sexual inequality that increase women's vulnerability to becoming entrapped in a battering relationship. Because medical practice itself frequently contributes to a woman's dilemmas in a battering relationship, an important priority in prevention is to close what Reiker and Carmen[70] call the "gender gap" in medical and psychiatric services.

The traditional model also emphasizes public education as opposed to interdiction. In the case of woman battering, prevention requires much more than public education. It requires the coordinated and joint efforts of a broad range of providers, including the criminal justice system.

Coordinated Community Response

The most important change in how communities approach woman battering is the development of a coordinated response that links health and social service providers to develop and implement a comprehensive strategy of service development, policy change, and prevention. This approach is based on the reality that changing one facet of the service response without changing the system can actually worsen the situation. For example, a battered woman may be identified, but not protected, or an offender may be arrested, but not prosecuted. A coordinated response can be developed by an informal, community-based network or emerge from a formal family violence council facilitated by the public health or police departments or by the mayor, a judge, or other public figure. The initiating group provides a public forum so that agencies with very different levels of institutional power (large teaching hospitals, courts, and battered women's programs) can address each other as relative equals. This process also provides an opportunity for advocates and survivors of family violence to give crucial feedback on aspects of the system that are not easily apparent from official data or the perspective of institutions.

The coordinated community response allows the community to take ownership of the problem of woman battering and is a vehicle to move the service response from crisis management of violent episodes to prevention. The objectives are to address three broad areas: ensuring safety and support for victims and accountability for perpetrators; coordinating and evaluating existing services and developing new services where needed; and initiating efforts to promote "zero tolerance" for coercion and control, including public education, professional training, and policy change. Although professional staff assist in developing communitywide prevention strategies, often with the support of state or federal funding, volunteers and front-line service organizations provide the infrastructure of the coordinated community response.

As in the case of other health problems—HIV infection and alcoholism, for example—victims and their advocates have played a key role in bringing the scope and consequences of woman battering to the attention of public health. More than other branches of medicine, public health has a long tradition of working closely with community-based groups in prevention efforts. Moreover, without such alliances, the forceful political action and creative programming needed to challenge the entrenched beliefs and practices that give rise to woman battering will not materialize. Rather than respond defensively to these challenges, the appropriate response is to mobilize behind the view that liberating citizens from coercion and control is a vital part of the public health mission.

Rape and Sexual Assault

Judith M. Von • Dean G. Kilpatrick • Ann W. Burgess • Carol B. Hartman

Definition of the Problem

Part of the problem inherent in understanding rape and sexual assault is derived from its equivocal definition. From a legal perspective, rape is a criminal act. Old laws viewed rape as an act of illicit sex; more recent legislation defines rape as a type of assault. As defined by the Federal Bureau of Investigation (FBI) Uniform Crime Report (UCR), forcible rape "is the carnal knowledge of a female forcibly and against her will".[1] Although some variations among states exist, rape is generally legally defined as forced sexual penetration of a victim by an offender who is not the victim's spouse. Some state laws patterned after the FBI's definition limit the term "rape" to incidents in which the victim is female and vaginal penetration has occurred. Many statutes have a marital exclusion rule, which states that criminal sexual conduct cannot legally occur if the offender and victim are married. This rule stems from the historical legal theory that a wife is the property of her husband.[2]

Because the legal definition of forcible rape is so restrictive, the term "sexual assault" has been used to cover a wider range of sexual crimes, including any manual, genital, or oral contact with the victim's genitalia without consent and obtained by force, threat, or fraud. Most states define as illegal any type of sexual behavior with a child. Statutory rape may also be charged in cases where the victim cannot give consent because of mental deficiency, psychosis, or altered consciousness induced by sleep, drugs, illness, or intoxication. Reformed legislation with its increased emphasis on force, threat of force, and coercion comes closer to capturing the psychological dimension of rape.

The manner in which rape is defined affects incidence and prevalence rates. That is, the number of sexual assaults and rape incidents, both detected and reported, depends on the victim's and the authority's (e.g., police, researcher) perception of what occurred. The process involved in getting a rape reported can be arduous.[3] First, victims must perceive that a rape has occurred. Second, they must classify the event as an illegal activity. Third, they must decide whether to disclose it. Fourth, the police officer (or researcher) decides whether the disclosed event meets the definition of the illegal activity. Only if the authority's classification concurs with that of the victim does the incident become recorded. The process of definition, then, is important both at the victim's or respondent's level and at the inquirer's level. If there is substantial disagreement, considerable underrepresentation in victimization surveys will result. This is particularly true for women who have been defined as "unacknowledged" victims:[4] women whose experiences meet the legal definition of rape (i.e., forced sexual penetration obtained without consent), but who do not view the experiences as criminal and thus do not report them. Often the unacknowledged victim has been assaulted by someone known to her. The public perception that rape involves a brutal attack by a stranger in a remote setting is so firmly entrenched in our society that many individuals, including the victims themselves, do not apply the label "rape" to an assault that deviates from the commonly accepted stereotype. This problem highlights the importance of asking about sexual assault by using behavioral descriptions, thereby avoiding the subjective bias introduced by using the word *rape*.

Data Sources

Contrary to popular belief, rape is not a rare event, but rather affects the lives of thousands of people each year. It has been estimated[5] that the population of the United States includes 12.1 million adult women who have been the victims of rape. Yet in our society, rape victims remain relatively silent and invisible. Although all types of crime have harmful effects, rape is particularly damaging. Rape victims experience long-term psychological problems including fear, anxiety, depression, and problems with sexual functioning. Further, being a rape victim is associated with an increased risk of suicide and an increased risk of developing a substance abuse problem. In addition, the recovery rate from rape appears to be slower and may be less complete than researchers once thought. Sexual assault claims many indirect victims as well. Often marriages dissolve or victims are forced to leave their jobs or relocate to prevent retaliation after they have pressed criminal charges. Even women who have never been raped may restrict their daily mobility because of the fear of rape. Among urban women age 35 years and younger, rape is a greater fear than murder.[6]

The human suffering implied in these statistics indicates that rape is a problem of major public health importance. It is currently the most underreported violent crime, partly because of the way the criminal justice system often has responded.[7] However, without victim cooperation the criminal justice system cannot effectively prosecute offenders, which leaves them free to reoffend. If the treatment of rape victims is improved, more victims may seek help and report these crimes to authorities, thus improving the ability of the criminal justice system to prosecute offenders and ultimately prevent subsequent rapes.

Compared to other types of serious crime, rape has a number of unique characteristics. First, it is particularly difficult to know how frequently rape occurs because of the low reporting rate. Second, in contrast to other crimes, there is a subjective element in the determination of whether the sexual act occurred against the victim's will. If the victim is of unquestioned chastity and if considerable force is employed by the assailant, then the act is considered to be "real" rape. However, if a woman is forced to have sex with a man she has dated and originally met in a bar, many individuals may not construe the act as rape. Third, rape is the only serious crime in which victims are sometimes held responsible for their own assaults. Many individuals still believe that women like to be overpowered sexually and say "no" when they mean "yes." Rules of evidence accepted in the courtroom have been stringent; for example, signs of resistance are required as proof of nonconsent.

Data on rape and sexual assault are available at the national level from both the FBI-UCR and the National Crime Victimization Survey (NCVS).[8] Both these federal data sources provide information on rape incidence, that is, the number of rapes that occur within a 1-year period. A major limitation of both of these data sets is the degree of underreporting. The UCR provides statistics on the number of forcible rapes reported annually to the police. Yet, it is well known that only a small percentage of rapes are ever reported, and of those reported rapes, some proportion are deemed "unfounded" by the police and hence never become part of the UCR statistics. In addition, the UCR uses a restricted definition of rape ("carnal knowledge of a female forcibly and against her will"), thereby excluding cases involving oral or anal penetration, male victims, or wives assaulted by their husbands. Furthermore, the FBI employs a hierarchy of defining crimes in which events are classified according to the most serious crime. For instance, a case in which a victim is both raped and killed is recorded only as a homicide.

The NCVS reports annual victimization data on the basis of a continuing survey of a nationally representative sample of households.[8] In response to widespread criticism[9,10] that its wording and format resulted in significant underreporting, the NCVS was recently revised following a 10-year redesign project. A revised form of the questionnaire has been in use since January 1992, with changes phased into the survey over a period of years. The most recent report of the survey[8] cautions readers that the data based on the redesigned format are not comparable to survey data collected prior to 1993.

According to the data most recently available from the UCR,[1] rape accounted for 5 percent of the violent crime volume and 0.7 percent of the Crime Index total, with 97,464 forcible rapes reported to law enforcement agencies in 1995. An estimated 72 of every 100,000 females in this country were reported rape victims. Approximately 51 percent of these reported rapes were cleared by arrest in 1995, a 5 percent decline in clearance rate from 1994.

According to the NCVS,[8] there were two completed or attempted rapes for every 1,000 persons age 12 or older in the United States. This translated into 430,000 rapes/sexual assaults, of which two-thirds of the rape victims knew their assailants and almost two-thirds of the victims of completed rapes did not report the crime to the police. According to the 1994 data, 36 percent of the completed rapes, 20 percent of the attempted rapes, and 41 percent of the sexual assaults were reported to the police. There were no significant racial or ethnic differences among victimization rates for rape or sexual assault. However, individuals in households with incomes of less than $15,000 were three times more likely to be raped or sexually assaulted as compared to households with annual incomes greater than $15,000. Large differences in victimization rate was also found for age, with younger persons more likely to be victimized. The NCVS reports 4 rapes/sexual assaults per 1,000 for those under age 25, 2 per 1,000 for those 25 to 49 years old, and 0.1 for those age 50 or older.

With regard to other characteristics, two-thirds of the rapes/sexual assaults occurred between 6 P.M. and 6 A.M.; approximately 6 of 10 assaults occurred in the victim's or someone else's home with assailants using a weapon in 16 percent of all rapes/sexual assaults.

Prevalence rates reflect the number of individuals who have been raped at any time in their life. There are no available federal estimates of sexual assault, but individual researchers have estimated prevalence on the basis of victimization surveys. In a review of these studies, Koss[11] concluded that estimates of rape/sexual assault prevalence among adult women generally ranges between 14 and 25 percent. As in the federal databases, methodological differences between studies will affect the estimates.

One recently released independent study,[6] based on a national sample, estimated a 13 percent completed rape prevalence rate. This translates into an estimated 12.1 million adult U.S. women having been forcibly raped during their lifetime and over 680,000 adult women having been raped during a 1-year period.

Causes and Risk Factors

Broadly conceptualized, research on sexual offenders falls into two categories: studies that focus on offender characteristics and studies that view social/cultural factors as causative.

The first approach (i.e., the psychopathology model) focuses on known offenders, typically incarcerated rapists. Early research in this area resulted in a large number of descriptive studies that attempted to differentiate rapists from other non-sex–offending criminals.[12] Attempts to identify discriminating characteristics have been largely unsuccessful to date, with the general consensus that convicted rapists represent a heterogeneous group.[13] Research in this domain continues with the goal of developing typologies among rapists.[14]

Studies examining social or cultural factors have generally relied on male subjects (typically, college students) who self-report engaging in sexual violence. Available research indicates that between 15 and 25 percent of male college students admit to sexual aggression.[16]

The social/cultural model maintains that perpetrators adhere to a belief system that both allows them to engage in and justify rape. This belief system is viewed as the result of a society that legitimizes violence against women, of which sexual aggression is one form. Viewed from this perspective, sexual aggression is not the result of any diagnosable individual pathology, but rather is the result of acceptance of societal attitudes that foster male dominance and dehumanize females. The results of numerous studies have lent support to this model by showing a relationship between certain attitudes (e.g., acceptance of rape myths, sex role stereotyping) and various measures of aggression.[17,18]

Current research in this area appears driven by the view that neither approach adequately explains sexual violence and that there may not be just a single etiological factor. The recent literature encompasses the gamut from bisocial theorizing, including evolutionary and neurohormonal variables,[19] to quadripartite models,[20] incorporating physiological, cognitive, affective, and personality variables.

Outcomes

A considerable database documents the psychological aftermath of rape.[21] However, as the literature on crime victims has expanded, attention has shifted from simply describing symptoms to assessing symptom constellations consistent with major psychiatric diagnoses. Posttraumatic stress disorder (PTSD) has frequently been identified among victims of sexual assault.[22] In fact, rape victims may constitute the largest single group of PTSD sufferers.[23] It has been found that rape is more likely to result in PTSD than a host of other traumatic events including natural disasters and physical assaults.[24]

Criminal victimization has been linked to a lifetime of increased risk for mental disorders.[22,25] However, few studies have addressed the long-term physical health impact of criminal victimization.[26,27] Until very recently, research has focused almost exclusively on forensic studies and emergency care. Fortunately, recent studies have documented the effect of crime on women's health status.[28,29]

Victimized women differ from nonvictimized women on several dimensions including perceived health status, number of physician visits, and negative health behaviors such as less exercise, smoking, alcohol consumption, and failure to use seat belts.[30,31]

There also appear to be some differences in diagnosable conditions between victimized and nonvictimized women. Respondents in the 1990 study by Waigandt et al[31] reported a higher number of reproductive illness symptoms. Koss and Heslet[32] found that certain conditions disproportionately diagnosed among rape victims included headaches, chronic pelvic pain, premenstrual pain, and gastrointestinal disorders.

It has been estimated that rape results in a sexually transmitted disease in approximately 4 to 30 percent of victims.[33] Despite the research[5,34] documenting rape victims' fear of contracting the human immunodeficiency virus (HIV), the potential for contracting HIV from sexual assault has received scant attention in the literature.[35] More importantly, the victims themselves have received little attention. Based on a national sample, Kilpatrick et al[5] found that 60 percent of rape victims reported receiving no pregnancy testing or prophylaxis, and 73 percent reported no testing for exposure to HIV.

Interventions

Victims of rape and sexual assault require access to a comprehensive system of resources, including emergency clinical services and counseling. These important resources should include a 24-hour rape hotline staffed by trained personnel and available trained staff to accompany victims to the hospital following an assault. Accompaniment to the hospital can help ensure that rape victims are adequately informed about hospital procedures (including procedures for the collection of evidence). Because many initial police interviews are conducted at the hospital, accompaniment provides trained advocates to help victims make informed choices about prosecution.

However, the magnitude of the impact of sexual assault and the longevity of its damage are just beginning to be understood. To date, crisis intervention has been the most widely used intervention, although research makes clear that this is not enough. Moreover, even this resource appears threatened as limited funding has resulted in reduced or no services to many survivors, particularly in rural areas.[36]

Given the longevity of rape's effects, it is imperative that agencies work with victims to provide access to long-term treatment. Resick[21] has noted the importance of instituting outreach efforts to reach those victims whose persistent symptomatology may cause them to feel abnormal or abandoned. It is clear that more education about rape's serious and persistent effects is needed for both professionals and the lay public. Further, continued effort should be directed at developing effective treatments, particularly for long-term problems. Research documenting the young age of victims[5] suggests that treatment should be geared to the developmental stage of the victim and may be required at varying points in the victim's life span.

Data indicating that rape victims are more likely to visit a physician than a mental health professional[36] suggest that greater attention should be directed toward training physicians. Further research is also needed to examine the relationship between rape and subsequent illness.

Although prevention of rape is of utmost importance, this is probably the least understood and the most overlooked dimension of the problem. McCall[37] details the historical debate over whether sexual assault prevention should be viewed from a criminal justice or public health perspective. His review and the work of Sparks and Bar On[38] highlight the view that prevention efforts to date have emphasized curtailment of women's mobility through advocating avoidance of certain situations ("don't travel alone at night"), adherence to certain precautions ("lock your car doors"), and/or self-defense training. The result of this approach is that a rapist may choose one victim over another, but the overall problem of sexual aggression may remain untouched. McCall[37] clearly shows the need to move beyond victim control strategies to addressing the causes and prevention of sexual violence. As McCall concludes and the research on sex offenders demonstrates, we are nowhere near that point.

Child Abuse

Eli H. Newberger

Definition of the Problem

Definitions of child abuse have broadened significantly in the last two decades. The commonsense meaning of the term "child abuse" is a situation where a caregiver, generally a parent, sets out in a systematic way to harm a child. In 1962, Professor C. Henry Kempe and his associates published an article in the *Journal of the American Medical Association* entitled "The Battered Child Syndrome"[1] that drew great attention in the professional and lay media. One of the outcomes of increased public awareness was the drafting of a model child abuse reporting statute by the Children's Bureau, the lead federal agency for children. Child abuse came to be defined in the state reporting laws as injuries inflicted by caregivers, and many believed that it could be diagnosed by physicians and medical institutions. However, Kempe's perpetrator-victim model of etiology and the notion of a syndrome of physical examination findings in the child and psychopathology in the caregiver led to several problematic consequences.

Physicians are likely to confuse the task of diagnosis with investigation (to find out who did what to whom and how). Perceptions persist that all adults who harm children in their care are mentally ill, and agencies that receive the reports maintain a conflicted sense of responsibility. The perpetrator-victim model substantially inhibits the range of diagnostic and therapeutic possibilities in these agencies.

In the 1970s, laws concerning child abuse reporting were revised. Parents of abused children were seen as people who could be helped, and child abuse was perceived as related to other family disturbances with implications for the health and welfare of children. The government's role was to provide timely help to troubled families and prevent child abuse. Toward that goal, the National Center on Child Abuse and Neglect was created in 1973. At the same time, the definition of child abuse was broadened to include child neglect, emotional injury, deprivation of medical care, and factors injurious to a child's moral development. The draft statute proposing this new definition also lengthened the list of professionals required by law to report child abuse to include virtually anyone responsible for the care of children. However, the draft legislation included nothing about budgeting for services. Although a dramatic increase in reports was foreseen, the people drafting the legislation assumed that state legislators would contend with the cost implications.[2] Furthermore, unless states' statutes conformed to the new model reporting statute, they would not be eligible for their share of federal monies that were stipulated to go for improving state services.

One unforeseen consequence of that effort was a changing sense of government's responsibility for children and families in trouble. With new reporting legislation and media attention came a deluge of reports of child abuse. Child welfare agencies are now overburdened in every state.

In 1985, in the reauthorization of the National Center on Child Abuse and Neglect, child abuse was conceived still more broadly to include situations where handicapped infants may be denied medical care necessary to ensure their survival. Highly publicized cases of child sexual abuse in day care centers has led to yet another initiative to expand the concept of child abuse and the role of child protection agencies.

Physicians are trained not to make judgments about the people they treat. If they are obliged to make known abuse or risks of abuse, conforming to the ethical doctrines under which physicians practice will be difficult.

Practitioners oriented to the perpetrator-victim model may restrict their field of vision to major findings, such as fractures, bruises to portions of the body that would not ordinarily occur in play, scalds, collections of blood around, above, or beneath the dense lining of the brain, poisonings, lacerations, and contusion to internal organs. These injuries evoke greater concern when children are younger or when different forms of trauma occur simultaneously or over time.[3]

A medical concept of child abuse that goes beyond the perpetrator-victim model focuses on relationships among the "pediatric social illness" (i.e., maltreatment), unintentional injuries, poisonings, and failure to thrive.[4] The child's physical symptoms are placed in an ecological framework that includes many interacting elements: developmental qualities and risk, parents' adaptations to their children's needs, psychological attributes of the family, realities and exigencies of the nurturing environment; and the favorable and unfavorable qualities of professional personnel, service programs, and institutions with which they have contact. Physicians should focus on family strengths and on prevention of abuse rather than on pathologies to be treated.

Recent attention has also been focused on two other concerns to physicians and other medical workers: the Munchausen by proxy syndrome (MBPS) and the problem of sexual victimization of children by professionals, including physicians.[5,6] The Munchausen syndrome has been used to describe the adult patient who falsifies medical history and examination findings. In its application to child abuse, the syndrome relates to the parent—almost always the mother—who fabricates information about her child's health or intentionally makes the child gravely ill.[7] Physicians often perceive the child's mother as an ideal, concerned, and loving parent and prefer to perform diagnostic studies rather than question the validity of the proffered history. Although there are insufficient data to confirm the prevalence of MBPS, experts say it is far from rare and often missed by clinicians.[7]

Data Sources

There are few data sources on child abuse that permit inferences to be drawn on prevalence, incidence, risk factors, outcomes, and the effectiveness of interventions. This is a consequence of the selective nature of case ascertainment for clinical research, limitations of study design in nearly every clinical study, and of a reluctance in the formation of national policy on child abuse to make use of standard methods of measurement and program evaluation.

The major data sets on child abuse give some useful estimates of reported prevalence, and four studies demonstrate the utility of methodologies that do not rely on case reports. The first, established by David Gil,[8] is a systematic treatment of child abuse case reports to agencies mandated by the initial wave of reporting statutes in the early and mid-1960s. From respondents in a national probability sample, an incidence estimate of approximately 2.5 million cases per year was made. The study's conclusion that poverty is the principal determinant of abuse has been criticized on the grounds that demographic attributes of the reported cases reflect the class and other biases of the reporting process.

The American Humane Association (AHA) compiles official reports of child abuse and neglect;[9] however, the lack of standardized definitions, dependence on individual states' data aggregation methods, and inability to gauge the meaning of the case reports in reference to any sampling methodology hinders the usefulness of these data. As with data in the previous study, AHA describes children who get into the child protection system identified as abused or neglected. Most of these children come from indigent families, reflecting in part the bias of ascertainment that causes poor children to be reported to agencies of the state.

However, the AHA data do document how the problem of child abuse has grown. The Gil study in 1967 and 1968 documented only 6,000 to 7,000 cases a year; in 1986 the AHA survey yielded an estimated prevalence of 1,928,000 abused children. AHA data also document an increasing number of reported cases of child sexual victimization, perhaps prompted by media attention and increased public and professional awareness.

The first national survey of family violence by Murray Straus and his associates[10] used a scale to measure the techniques that family members used to resolve conflicts among themselves. In turn, this scale provided the entry point for a series of questions about violent practices. On the basis of a national sample of families with two adults and at least one child between the ages of 3 and 17, the researchers produced the first systematic and reliable projections of the frequency of particular incidents of violence, including the use or threat to use a knife or gun in resolving conflict. There were several limitations to this survey: the sample was not representative of U.S. families with children; infants were not represented because the investigators were interested in violence between adults and among children and adults; and neither neglect nor sexual abuse was explored.

However, the study yielded a prevalence estimate suggesting that in 1975 there were 1.4 million children ages 3 to 17 years who had been abused. Gelles and Straus[11] recently reported the findings of a second national family violence survey that yielded a much lower prevalence estimate, perhaps because their 1985 interviews were collected over the phone, thus excluding families without phones, a group more likely to experience social isolation and economic adversity. Respondents in 1985 also may have been more reluctant to report family violence than in 1975. However, the authors of the study believe that there has been a true decline in the rates of violence against children.

A national incidence study of child abuse and neglect was conducted through funding by the Children's Bureau to delineate the dimensions of the "iceberg" of child abuse, the tip of which was seen in child abuse case reports. Data were gathered from child protective agencies and other sources such as hospitals, police departments, and mental health agencies.[12] Systematic definitions were declared and a weighting system devised to generalize to the national experience. For the 26-county sample, 17,645 cases of child abuse were recorded between May 1, 1979, and April 30, 1980. It was projected that nationwide 1,151,600 cases were suspected by professionals. Of these, 562,000 were considered likely to meet the study's criteria and therefore to be true cases of child abuse and neglect.

This study methodology has been criticized because child sexual abuse was rarely reported at the time of the incidence study.[13] Other studies suggest a far greater frequency than the case reporting compilations would suggest. The first national incidence study data are available now and are useful for studies of agency practice.

A second national incidence study used similar methodology.[14] The data for 1986 are presented in the recently published report, along with perceived changes since the earlier study. The estimated 1986 national incidence of abuse and neglect was 1,584,700. There was a 74 percent increase in the incidence of abuse (to 657,000 cases), within which there was an increase of 58 percent for child physical abuse (to 358,300 cases) and over 300 percent for child sexual abuse (to 155,900 cases). No changes were noted in the incidence of emotional abuse or neglect. Physical abuse was the most frequent type of abuse identified in the study, followed by emotional abuse and by sexual abuse, with respective incidence rate estimates of 5.7, 3.4, and 2.5 cases per 1,000 children.

More recently, a survey of child abuse reporting and fatalities from all states found that the rate of *reported* child abuse and neglect increased 15 percent between 1990 and 1995, from 40 to 46 per 1,000 children, with more than 3 million children being reported to child protective service (CPS) agencies in 1995.[15] Overall, reports of child abuse have remained stable over that period, with an average annual increase of about 4 percent. Rates of substantiated reports of child maltreatment over that period remained level at about 15 of every 1,000 children. In 1995, neglect accounted for about half the cases; physical abuse, about a quarter; sexual abuse, about 10 percent; and emotional and other types of abuse constituting the balance. The survey also found that child deaths as a result of maltreatment rose by 5 percent between 1992 and 1995, suggesting that about three children died each day in 1995 as a result of parental maltreatment.[15]

Causes and Risk Factors

Early efforts to understand child abuse centered on psychological problems of the parents of the victims, focusing on distorted expectations of their children, frustrated dependency needs, personal isolation, and histories of having themselves been abused as children.[16] But many other social and cultural factors have been proposed as contributing to the causes of child abuse in addition to individual deviant behavior. The psychoanalytical approach posits that unconscious parental drives and conflicts determine abusive behavior.[17] Social learning theory suggests that abusers learn the behavior as abused children themselves. Environmental stress theory suggests that overwhelmingly stressful factors, such as poverty, unemployment, social isolation, and inadequate housing, help cause the violence or interfere with the parent's ability to care for the child. Cognitive-developmental theory suggests that immature parental understanding of the child and of the parental role are associated with abuse. By presuming social inequality, labeling theory suggests that the interests of dominant power groups are served by defining as deviant a class of socially marginal individuals (child abusers) whose problems are the concerns of helping professionals.[18]

All these theories individually explain some part of the problem, but all have clear limitations. Professionals and researchers have begun to integrate parts of these theories into interactive, multicausal theories that investigate how aspects of an individual's personality or environment interact with his or her particular experience.

Some researchers have attempted to integrate causal factors for child abuse from multiple levels: individual, family, and society.[19–22] At the individual level, one consistent finding has been the prevalence of acute or chronic illness in the abused children.[23] However, a number of long-held "causes" of child abuse are now viewed with skepticism; these include low–birth weight of the infant, young maternal age, and inadequate mother-infant bond formation.

A number of recent studies have pointed to the association between domestic violence and child abuse. For example, one report found that marital violence is a statistically significant predictor of physical child abuse. The greater amount of violence against a spouse, the greater likelihood of physical abuse to the child by the abusive spouse.[24]

Behavioral and social science research have not generally produced results that are applicable in clinical settings, mostly because the predominant research approach attempts to explain child abuse statistically, factor by factor, thus ignoring the complexity of individual cases. Those studies that have considered the complexity of family interactions have focused on the formation of universal rules that govern behavior, whereas the clinician is concerned with treatment appropriate to individual cases. Interaction among clinicians and researchers is needed to develop a body of knowledge concerning etiology, therapeutic interventions, and effective intervention programs.

Outcomes

Documented medical consequences of child abuse include injuries of every organ system, which can frequently cause chronic impairment.[25] Another outcome of child abuse is homicide, which is the fourth leading causes of death of children ages 1 to 9 and the third leading cause of death for children in the 10 to 14 age group.[26] Sexual abuse of children resulted in venereal disease in 13 percent of the 409 children in one study.[27]

Because of varying definitions of abuse and problems with differing methodologies and outcome criteria, studies of long-term psychological effects of child abuse have mixed descriptions of outcome, but most agree that there are profound and serious effects, including a propensity to aggression in adolescence, language disorders, and lower performance on standardized tests of intelligence. However, a sampling bias that favors selection of children from impoverished families makes it impossible to separate developmental attrition associated with low socioeconomic status from the presumed effects of abuse.[28]

Although there has been no systematic study of the immediate and long-term effects of child sexual victimization, changes that have been described from clinical case studies include hypervigilance, phobias, nightmares, feelings of guilt and shame, and changes in sleeping and eating patterns.[29–31] Psychosomatic disorders include abdominal pain, headaches, and loss of appetite. When force has been used in sexual acts, the subsequent symptoms are more severe. These behavioral outcomes may reflect several variables and their interactions, such as the presence of antecedent behavioral problems, the family's support after disclosure, how much the child is blamed or stigmatized, and the nature and quality of interventions used to help the child.

Sexual abuse of boys may be associated with a propensity toward violence toward others—perhaps allowing the victim the feeling of no longer being vulnerable. Sexual abuse during childhood is a frequent finding in studies of pedophiles, rapists, and murderers.[32] Women who have been sexually abused as children appear to have an unusual frequency of depression and self-destructive behavior, as well as disturbances in adult sexual functioning and in protecting themselves from other victimizing relationships.[33]

Interventions

There is much disagreement about the most effective intervention for preventing child abuse. Although many consider child abuse a crime and there is a strong impulse toward retribution of abusers, most social policy in the United States has inclined toward a human service model for victims. Compounding the problem are judicial systems that may further abuse a child in the process of prosecuting an abuser and child protective services that are seriously overburdened and underfunded. Decisions to remove children from their homes are often made in haste by personnel responsible for protecting children and without sufficient attention to the strengths of families that could be maintained by providing homemakers, child care, parent aides, self-help groups, or specialized medical or psychiatric services.

Interventions must provide protection, but should also develop support for the family. One study[34] of a child abuse program suggests that interdisciplinary review of individual cases with a systematic program to follow up cases with agencies designated to provide services to children and families is associated with a shorter duration of hospitalization, a lower dollar cost of treatment, and a reduction in the reinjury rate. Another study shows that lay interventional agents may be as effective as child welfare professionals.[35]

The National Clinical Evaluation Study[36] found that cost-effective treatment in child sexual abuse cases included a combination of family and group counseling for the victim, the victim's siblings, the perpetrator, and the perpetrator's spouse. In cases of child neglect, the most efficient interventions combine family counseling with parent education and basic care services such as babysitting, medical care, clothing, and housing assistance. The author of this study, noting the paucity of resources available for victims and the families of victims, also points out that treatment efforts are at best successful with only half of the clients. Given the risks of reinjury and the consequences of child abuse, the high cost of treatment services, the lack of funds, and the limited promise for remedying the consequences of maltreatment, prevention efforts may be the most efficient alternative.

Primary and secondary preventive initiatives may be organized in relation to the following theories of etiology:

Psychoanalytical Theory

- Include emotional health as well as biological health in our concepts. Train physicians and others to recognize and tend to emotional issues. Third party payers should support services that support mental health.

Leaning Theory

- Provide parents with access to information about child development and about nonviolent methods of socializing their children.

Attachment Theory

- Elevate the parent-child relationship to an appropriate position of respect and importance by preventing premature delivery through prenatal care, bringing fathers into the delivery room, emphasizing the father's supportive role, and encouraging paternity leaves as well as maternity leaves from work.[37]

Stress Theory

- Provide hotlines for parents to use at times of distress.
- Make mental health services available to all children.
- Make emergency homemaker and other child care services available to families in crisis.
- Reduce social isolation by ensuring access to telephones and public transportation to facilitate social interactions.
- Support existing community organizations that offer support, a sense of community, and feelings of self-worth for their members.
- Empower women. Acknowledge the extent to which male-dominated professions hold power compared with professions comprised mainly of women.

Labeling Theory

- Remove stigma associated with getting help by detaching protective services from public welfare systems.
- Expand public awareness of the prevalence of child abuse and domestic violence and emphasize that the potential for violence is in all of us, rather than attributing the problem to deviant and minority individuals.

Child Sexual Abuse

David Finkelhor

Definition of the Problem

Child sexual abuse is sexual contact with a child that occurs as a result of force or in a relationship where it is exploitative because of an age difference or caretaking responsibility. There is almost universal agreement that sexual contact between a child and the child's father, stepfather, mother, stepmother, another older relative, teacher, or baby sitter constitutes sexual abuse, as does sexual contact by any adult or older person, whether known or unknown. Also included are rape and forced sexual contact at the hands of anyone, even a peer.

However, not everyone uses this definition, nor is there universal agreement about the exact boundaries of various terms.

The National Center on Child Abuse and Neglect (NCCAN) and related child welfare agencies within individual states tend to restrict their definition to activity at the hands of caretakers,[1] which separates child welfare functions from criminal justice functions. Other researchers limit child sexual abuse to contacts with adults, excluding forced sex at the hands of other children.[2]

Other specific definitional disagreements include the age range of what constitutes childhood (persons up to age 16? or 18?),[3] what is an exploitative age difference,[3] and what sexual activities are included. Most definitions of child sexual abuse include the use of children in prostitution and pornography.

State statutes vary widely in defining sexual abuse, involving a mixture of offenses including rape, statutory rape, sodomy, indecent liberties, and incest, with terminology such as "carnal knowledge" and "lewd and lascivious acts." All states but one include sexual abuse in their laws requiring the reporting of child abuse and neglect, but sexual abuse is rarely defined in this context either.

This variation in reported rates of child sexual abuse reflects a variety of factors, including the use of different definitions of sexual abuse, differences in the extent of victimization in different geographic areas and population subgroups, and the way in which investigators select subjects and ask questions about an extremely sensitive subject. The best sense of the scope of child sexual abuse comes from community surveys of adults.[4–10] Researchers have found that at least 5 percent of adults report sexual abuse in their childhood, but the variation among the studies is great, with the reported incidence ranging from 6 to 62 percent for women and from 3 to 31 percent for men.[11,12] There were an estimated 300,000 cases of child sexual abuse identified by professionals in 1993, more than double the number in 1986.[13] However, research on this subject is difficult, scarce, and extremely variable in quality.

Data Sources

Police, protective services, and medical facilities are the main agencies that document reports of child sexual abuse. Numerous studies have been done on samples from all these sources.[14–18] The National Child Abuse and Neglect Data System collates state reports of child abuse and neglect including sexual abuse.[19,20] In addition, the NCCAN conducted three national incidence studies from counties selected to represent the country.[1,21] Another data source is mental health facilities where victims seek treatment.[22] Data on abusers come from studies mostly in prison settings,[23] and studies of adults in the "normal" population have identified individuals with histories of sexual abuse.[11]

All data sources on child abuse have serious limitations. Fear of prosecution and the shame and embarrassment associated with abuse make it difficult to obtain valid and reliable data. The national data collected by the National Child Abuse and Neglect Data System used uniform definitions and protocols, but there are relatively few variables relating to each case and the reported cases represent a fraction of all occurrences of child sexual abuse.[20] Three national incidence studies conducted by NCCAN have many of the same problems.

Data from the criminal justice system are limited by the variability of laws that define sexual abuse in the states, which makes it difficult to compare data across or even within states. The Federal Bureau of Investigation Uniform Crime Reports have not included the age of the victim, making it impossible to distinguish child sexual abuse from other sexual assaults. Also, cases that come to the attention of the system constitute only a small percentage of actual cases.

Although studies of offenders have suggested hypotheses about the motivations for sexual abuse, many of these studies are limited by the inclusion of only incarcerated offenders, which is a small and unrepresentative fraction of offenders.[23]

Community surveys are the most representative data collection efforts because they gather information on cases that are never reported to an agency. However, these surveys are very expensive to conduct; there are questions concerning reliability and validity of the data gathered; there may be distortion or withholding of information because of memory loss or embarrassment; and the data from adults may not be generalizable to the current generation of children because rates and circumstances of victimization may be very different.

Developing Better Data Sources

This field needs ongoing national data collection with uniform standards and mandated participation. In addition, other data sources that should be considered are large community surveys of young adults and adolescents who are old enough to be free from possible retaliation from their abusers but close enough to the experience to give accurate information; surveys of young dependent children (which must be combined with extremely sensitive efforts to screen for, and intervene in, cases of ongoing abuse discovered in the study); longitudinal studies of cohorts of children to determine which ones become victims and how this affects their development; and case-control studies of offenders and nonoffenders to discover risk sources for abusive behavior among representative samples of incarcerated and nonincarcerated abusers.

Causes and Risk Factors

Community studies are the best sources of information about the characteristics of different types of sexual abuse.[4,10] These studies suggest that abuse by fathers and stepfathers, even though it dominates reports from the child welfare system, actually constitutes no more than 7 to 8 percent of all abuse cases. Abuse by other family members (most frequently uncles and older brothers) make up an additional 16 to 42 percent. Other nonrelatives known to the child make up 32 to 60 percent of offenders. Abuse by strangers is substantially less common than abuse by family members or persons known to the child.

The largest category of abuse in most studies involves groping or fondling of children's bodies on top of or underneath the clothing. Only 16 to 29 percent of the abuse involves intercourse or attempted intercourse. Another 3 to 11 percent of the activities involve attempted or completed oral or anal intercourse; and 13 to 33 percent, manual touching of the genitals.

Community studies show that the frequency of child sexual abuse seems to occur when victims are between ages 9 and 12 and then declines somewhat during later adolescent years. Most studies show that a quarter of the incidents occur before the child is 8 years of age, and some clinicians insist that this percentage would be even greater if it were not for the occlusion of memories from these early years. Approximately 42 to 75 percent of experiences reported in the surveys are single events. Repeated abusive experiences occur at older ages and are associated with abuse within the family.

In addition to community surveys, compilations of cases known to professionals have been used to generate incidence estimates and describe other characteristics of child sexual abuse. For example, the Third National Incidence Study[13,21] projected that 300,000 new cases of sexual abuse became known to professionals in the United States in 1993. Incidence estimates based on reported cases such as these appear to overrepresent (*a*) abuse involving fathers and stepfathers, (*b*) abuse involving intercourse and other more intrusive acts, and (*c*) abuse perpetrated over an extended period. The ages of the victimized children also tend to be higher in these incidence studies because reported cases record the age at the time of the disclosure rather than the age at onset. Compared with the community studies, there seems to be an underreporting of the sexual abuse of boys.[6]

Community surveys also have provided information on the sociodemographic distribution of sexual abuse.[24,25] These studies consistently fail to find differences in rates among different social classes or races. However, other factors have been associated with risk of abuse: (*a*) living without one of the biological parents, (*b*) unavailability of the mother because of outside employment or disability or illness, (*c*) reports from the child stating that the parents' marriage is unhappy or full of conflict, (*d*) reports from the child of a poor relationship with the parents or of extremely punitive discipline or child abuse, and (*e*) report by the child of having a stepfather. Although few studies have examined why these factors increase risk, poor supervision, emotional turmoil, neglect, and rejection may make the child vulnerable to child molesters. With little help or support from parents, children may also find it hard to stop the abuse once it begins.

Research on Offenders

Offenders are predominantly males, which clearly distinguishes sexual abuse from other forms of child abuse and neglect. Studies of incarcerated offenders[5] have suggested a wide variety of theories that account for behavior of abusers: (*a*) they get powerful, developmentally induced emotional gratification from the acts; (*b*) they have deviant physiological sexual arousal patterns; (*c*) they are blocked in their capacity to meet their sexual needs in more conventional ways; and (*d*) they have problems in their capacity for behavioral inhibition.

Empirical support for these theories includes studies that show unusual levels of deviant sexual arousal to children among offenders,[26,27] histories of offenders who have been victims of sexual abuse (25 to 33 percent),[28] history of conflict over heterosexual relationships or disruption of normal adult heterosexual partnerships among offenders,[29] and use of alcohol related to the act in 19 to 70 percent of the offenses.

A review of studies of incestuous fathers[30] shows evidence that such men have difficulties in empathy, nurturing, and caretaking and are socially isolated and lacking in social skills. They frequently have histories of physical abuse, have poor relationships with their fathers, and are weakly identified with masculine roles. One study of incestuous fathers[31] found that these men had participated less actively in early care of their victim children than had a comparison group of normal fathers.

Another study found a much greater extent and variety of deviant sexual acts among child molesters and found that these histories of deviance and deviant fantasies go back to adolescence.[32]

Outcomes

Clinicians have noted many symptoms in children who have been sexually abused. These include fear, compulsivity, hyperactivity, phobias, withdrawal, guilt, depression, mood swings, suicidal ideation, fatigue, loss of appetite, somatic complaints, changes in sleeping and eating patterns, hostility, mistrust, sexual acting out, dissociative disorders, compulsive masturbation, and school problems.[33–35]

In contrast to these initial effects, the long-term impact of sexual abuse has been the subject of more sophisticated studies. Various surveys of sexually abused women in the general population have all found significant, identifiable mental health impairment in victims compared to nonvictims in the same samples.[33] One of the best studies was a survey of 344 women in Calgary using such epidemiological measures as the Middlesex Hospital Health survey and the CES-D depression scale.[36] This study found that sexually abused women, when compared with women without histories of abuse, have about twice the risk for depression, psychoneurosis, somatic anxiety, psychiatric hospitalization, and suicidal gesture. Moreover, sexual abuse was demonstrated to be a major risk for such outcomes even when controlling for other negative developmental and family background factors. However, severe levels of psychopathology were apparent in less than 25 percent of the sexual abuse victims. Another epidemiological survey[37] found two to three times the rate of morbidity for the *Diagnostic and Statistical Manual*, third edition, revised (DSM-III-R) category diagnoses among adults molested as children, men as well as women. Two other outcomes uncovered by studies in the general population are sexual problems—including frigidity, vaginismus, flashbacks, and other emotional problems related to sex—and a much higher risk of subsequent sexual victimization.[8,38]

Studies that have compared sexual abuse victims to other help-seekers in various clinical populations have also found sexual abuse victims to be more impaired on a number of dimensions:[21] victims experienced more isolation, lower self-esteem, fear of men, anxiety attacks, sleeping difficulties, nightmares, and alcohol and drug abuse; they also were more prone to suicide and self-mutilation. Additional research suggests connections between sexual abuse and prostitution,[39] multiple personality disorder, and eating disorders.[37] In short, these studies contribute to very rapidly mounting evidence of negative mental health outcomes for victims of child sexual abuse. None of the studies by themselves are definitive on this point, but the weight of the growing number of studies is impressive.

Given such evidence of serious effects on some individuals, researchers have now begun to look at whether certain aspects of the experience or the context of the experience may explain the degree of trauma. However, this research is still very tentative.[33] The weight of current evidence is that victims show more long-term symptoms when the abuse involves fathers and stepfathers, sexual intercourse, and force. On the other hand, studies have not been able to demonstrate consistently that abuse at any particular age is more traumatic. One study of initial effects in children[40] shows that the factors predictive of greater disturbance are (*a*) violence and physical injury in the abusive episode, (*b*) a mother's hostile attitude toward the child upon revelation of the abuse, and (*c*) removal of the child from his or her home subsequent to the abuse. Unfortunately, research to date does not yet provide a clear basis for designating those types of abuse that should receive priority for professional attention.

Interventions

Professional efforts to respond to the problem of sexual abuse can be grouped into five categories:

1. *Public awareness*: Broad campaigns to increase public and professional awareness have caused a rapid growth in the number of cases reported to authorities. This, in turn, has raised many questions about policy. No criteria exist for how to prioritize reported cases for investigation, and the cases are very difficult to confirm. There also have not been any studies assessing the reliability of various means of substantiating reports. Considerable controversy surrounds the issue of children's credibility, and although most information about sexual abuse urges disclosure, it is also true that disclosure is extremely stressful on victims and families. Studies are badly needed to better understand the effects of disclosure and to minimize these effects.
2. *Preventive education*: Various programs are aimed at enabling children to better protect themselves, explaining what sexual abuse is, informing children that they have the right and an obligation to refuse such activity, and encouraging them to tell someone about it. Research indicates that children do learn the concepts and report incidents, but it is not known if such programs reduce the amount of victimization.
3. *Treatment programs for victims and their families*: Specialized programs have been established to help victims and families deal with disclosure and reduce the potential for long-term trauma. The treatment outcome research is encouraging, but few true randomized designs have been used in evaluations.[41]
4. *Treatment programs for offenders*: Some specialized experimental child molester treatment programs exist around the country. These use a diversity of techniques such as individual and group psychotherapy, behavior modification, social skills training, and some drug treatment.[42] Although the programs exist both within and outside the criminal justice system, it has been generally found that the threat or reality of criminal sanctions must be used to ensure participation. There are many reports of successful treatment of child molesters,[43] but skepticism is still warranted because of the lack of long-term follow-up. Moreover, there are no techniques for identifying offenders who are not amenable to treatment.

5. *Reforms of the criminal justice system*: Changes that have been suggested include the use of videotaped testimony by children, victim advocates to assist victims and their families during the court process, diversion programs to encourage guilty pleas by offenders, restraining orders to remove offenders from the household to avoid removal of the child, expediting prosecution in sexual abuse cases, and redrafting of criminal statues and their associated penalties. Research is needed on how these criminal justice reforms actually affect the conviction, sentencing, and recidivism of offenders and on how often children are traumatized by the criminal justice process and which aspects of the process contribute to the trauma.

Elder Abuse

Karl Pillemer • Rosalie S. Wolf

Definition of the Problem

Wide variation exists in the way researchers have defined the term "elder abuse." The confusion surrounding exactly what constitutes elder abuse has made it difficult to interpret the results of studies on the subject. Researchers have included some or all of the following dimensions in describing maltreatment of the elderly: physical abuse, physical neglect, emotional abuse, emotional neglect, emotional deprivation, sexual exploitation and assault, verbal abuse, medical neglect, material abuse, and neglect of the elder's environment.

Despite definitional issues, researchers agree on certain points. For example, they concur that physical assault against an elder constitutes abusive behavior. Most of the research literature also includes in the terminology the following: psychological or emotional abuse; financial abuse (the misuse or theft of an elder's property or assets); and the intentional failure of a clearly designated caregiver to meet the needs of an elder (neglect). Beyond these generally accepted categories, however, there is little consensus on definitions.

Recently, attention has shifted to learning more about the older person's perception of mistreatment[1] and the role of culture and attitudes in defining the issue.[2] A study[3] of how various potentially abusive situations were perceived by African American, Korean American, and Caucasian American women revealed that African American women tended to interpret abuse more broadly; and Korean American women, least broadly. The reluctance of older Korean American women to label situations as abusive or to seek help was explained within the context of Korean culture, which "emphasizes, as desirable behavior, family harmony over individual well-being, denotes some degree of human suffering as a virtue, and dictates enduring and keeping one's problem to oneself, rather than exposing the problem to others." A study of Japanese Americans also reported similar findings of valuing group above self. Thus, cultural variations confound attempts to define elder abuse.

Data Sources

Research on the extent of elder abuse has been inconsistent because of the limited sources of data. Existing data come from three different approaches to the study of elder abuse: surveys, agency records and other secondary sources, and case-control studies.

Surveys

In the early years of research on this topic, surveys of professionals who had direct contact with elder abuse were the most common; researchers have continued to conduct such surveys over the years. The Pennsylvania state survey[4] on elder abuse funded by an Administration on Aging grant is an example. A sample of professionals, including administrators and direct service workers from 16 types of agencies, was surveyed in each of Pennsylvania's 67 counties. Half of the responding agencies reported encountering elder abuse, ranging from more than 90 percent of domestic violence agencies, to less than 30 percent for law enforcement, emergency services, medical clinics, and drug/alcohol agencies. A survey[5] of Alabama physicians and registered and licensed practical nurses reported that 38 percent of the physicians and 53 percent of the nurses had seen cases of elder abuse in the previous year.

Random sample community surveys provide more scientific estimates of the prevalence of elder abuse. A survey[6] of older persons living in the Boston metropolitan area found 63 elderly persons who had been maltreated out of a stratified random sample of 2,020 community-dwelling elderly persons age 65 years or older. This survey inquired about personal experiences of three types of maltreatment: physical violence, chronic verbal aggression, and neglect by family members and persons close to them. The findings translated into a rate of 32 maltreated elderly persons per 1,000, or between 8,647 and 13,487 abused and neglected elderly in the Boston area. The number of cases identified as occurring in the previous year was 14 times the number of cases that had been reported to the state's protective service agency from the same area in the same time period.

A random sample telephone survey[7] of 2,008 Canadians used instruments and methodology from the Boston survey, with the addition of questions on financial abuse. The Canada survey found a rate of 40 maltreated elders per 1,000 elders, 25 of whom were victims of financial abuse. In Britain, several questions from the Boston survey were added to an omnibus national survey of 2,000 adults.[8] The survey yielded a rate of 54 maltreated elderly persons per 1,000 elders for verbal abuse and 15 per 1,000 each for physical and financial abuse.

Another approach was used by a Finnish team of geriatric physicians in which they asked respondents to define whether they were abused.[9] Three elder abuse questions were added to a depression study questionnaire that was mailed to all persons born on or before 1923 in a semi-industrialized Finnish town. Respondents were asked: "Do you know some person who has been abused after the age of retirement?" and "Have you yourself been abused after the age of retirement?" The rate of self-reported abuse was 54 per 1,000 elders; psychological abuse was the most common form.

The findings from these studies are striking. Despite the different methods, the studies quite reliably suggest that the prevalence of elder abuse falls in the 3 to 5 percent range. In the United States, a national survey is greatly needed to estimate the prevalence of elder abuse in the general population, as well as in specific regions and subgroups.

Agency Case Records

Generally based on professional assessments rather than interviews with victims themselves, case records can be a rich source of data. In one study, case workers in three model projects[10] recorded comprehensive information on 328 cases of elder abuse. Three distinct profiles emerged.

1. *Physical and psychological abuse*: The perpetrator was more likely to have a history of psychopathology and be dependent on the victim. These types of abuse involved family members who were very intimately related and emotionally connected. The victims were apt to be in poor emotional health, but relatively independent in the activities of daily living. This form of maltreatment likely had its roots in long-standing, pathological family dynamics and interpersonal processes, which became more highly charged when the dependency relationship was altered, either because of illness or financial need.
2. *Neglect*: The victim typically was very old, widowed, with few social supports, and functionally impaired. In marked contrast to the cases of physical/psychological abuse, cases involving neglect appeared to be very much related to the dependency needs of the victim.
3. *Financial abuse*: Victims were generally unmarried with few social supports. The perpetrators had financial problems and histories of substance abuse. Rather than interpersonal pathology or victim dependency, the motivating factor appeared to be desire for money, often stemming from substance abuse.

Another source of data comes from records of persons reported to adult protective services systems. Because each state has its own tracking system, there is great variation in the amount and kind of data that are collected.[11] Thirty-six states receive detailed data on individual cases from local units, either through computerized client tracking systems or from reporting forms, and 13 states receive only summary data. Illinois is one of the few states to use a risk assessment form that can be scored to determine the extent to which the client is in danger of harm, injury, or loss.[12] The form is comprised of 23 items, including client characteristics, environmental factors, transportation and support systems, past/present mistreatment, and abuser characteristics.

In the mid-1980s, the U.S. Administration on Aging funded a study to gather information on reports of elder mistreatment from the 50 states and estimate the national incidence of elder abuse. Because state statutes vary considerably, attempts to make national estimates were limited. However, despite these limitations, the researchers concluded in 1986 that there were about 117,000 reports of domestic elder abuse in the nation.[13] This figure rose to 293,000 reports in 1996,[14] indicating a dramatic rise in reported cases. Of course, we do not know the proportion of actual cases that get reported, nor whether this proportion has changed over time.

In an attempt to ascertain the number of actual cases and under a mandate from the Congress to "make a complete study and investigation of the national incidence of abuse, neglect, and exploitation of elderly persons . . ." (Public Law 102-95), the Department of Health and Human Services in 1994 funded a National Elder Abuse Incidence Study.[15] Conducted by the National Center on Elder Abuse in collaboration with a survey research firm, the study is expected to furnish results by the end of 1997. The survey methodology, adapted from three national incidence studies of child abuse and neglect, involves collecting all reports received by adult protective services agencies in 20 representative counties in the United States over an 8-week period. Additionally, a selected group of persons ("sentinels") from a representative group of agencies within each of those counties (for example, hospitals, police departments, social service agencies, home health companies, and senior centers) will complete the same form for suspected or observed cases of elder abuse. Although the study lacks the rigor of a population survey, it is anticipated to provide numbers and characteristics of cases handled by protective services agencies (reported) and those seen by other community organizations and professionals (reported and nonreported).

Other Sources

Several secondary sources of data that may provide important information about domestic violence against the elderly include law enforcement agencies, health providers, and state agencies. The National Crime Victimization Survey and the Comparative Homicide File documented trends and patterns of both lethal and nonlethal forms of violent victimization against the elderly in comparison with that against younger Americans.[16] Over the past two decades, the elderly victims of nonlethal violence increasingly reported that their assailants were relatives rather than strangers. The elderly also appear to be proportionately more vulnerable than younger persons are to nonlethal forms of violence committed by strangers. Other sources of information about criminal behavior against the elderly are the police, courts, and prisons. All these sources are subject to underreporting, the extent of which is unknown.

Emergency room personnel and other health care providers have been sources of data on child and partner abuse and could provide information on elder abuse as well.[17] Only recently have efforts been made to collect data on elder mistreatment from health providers. The required implementation of an elder abuse protocol in hospital emergency rooms and the beginning of universal screening for domestic violence in some localities represent new potential sources of data, but, as with crime statistics, such reports will be subject to bias; only cases in which abuse results in injury are likely to be recorded.

Case-Control Studies

Several recent studies include interviews with the victims and a control group of nonabused elders. One study[18] focused only on physical abuse, which was verified by use of the Conflict Tactics Scale. A second study[6] in Boston compared elder abuse victims identified in a random sample survey of residents with a group of elderly control subjects randomly selected from the nonabused survey respondents. Two other studies focused on caregivers and care recipients in both abusive and nonabusive households.[19,20] The findings from these studies showed that abuser characteristics were more powerful predictors of elder mistreatment than were victim characteristics.

A more recent set of studies, which examined the relationship between dementia and elder abuse, also compared abusive families with nonabusive families' households, which were drawn from the same registry or survey sample.[21–23]

Causes and Risk Factors

Characteristics of Abuse Victims

Despite their methodological limitations, studies suggest fairly consistent findings about the abused elderly who come into contact with the human service systems. Although a number of studies based on agency samples suggest that abused individuals tend to be female, several prevalence studies have found roughly equal numbers of women and men in the victimized group. This apparent discrepancy may be due to women's greater likelihood of suffering injuries and emotional distress as a result of abuse.[6]

Many studies have found victims to be somewhat vulnerable because of illness or impairment, making it difficult for them to defend themselves or escape the situation. In addition, a shared living arrangement is strongly associated with abuse: most studies have found that the majority of physical abuse victims live with the abuser.

These, however, are the only findings that emerge reliably from the studies. Results relating to the frequency with which abuse occurs and the types of abuse most often found are virtually impossible to compare because of the widely varying definitions employed.

Causal Factors

Extensive research literature in the area of child and spouse abuse and on the relations between older persons and adult children can provide important insights into elder abuse, particularly in concert with the literature on domestic violence in younger populations and with the limited literature on elder abuse. Five primary risk factors have emerged from research: intraindividual dynamics (psychopathology of the abuser), intergenerational transmission of violent behavior, dependency and exchange relations between abuser and abused, external stress, and social isolation.

Intraindividual dynamics emphasizes pathological characteristics of the abuser as the primary cause of maltreatment. Some research has indicated that abusers of the elderly are more likely to be developmentally disabled, mentally ill, or alcoholic.[18,24,25]

A number of studies of child and wife abuse have provided evidence concerning *intergenerational transmission* of violent behavior; the findings indicate that people learn to be violent in the family setting. Research evidence shows that witnessing parental violence during childhood is a strong risk factor for wife abuse as an adult, and the amount of physical punishment experienced as a child is positively associated with the rate of abusive violence to one's own children. Given the strength of this connection in other forms of family violence, it is reasonable to postulate that abusers of the elderly will also be more likely to have been raised in violent homes. Studies of this issue are, unfortunately, still lacking, so this risk factor remains to be tested.

Two competing theories relate *dependency* to elder abuse. One emphasizes the role of "caregiver stress" as a risk factor for maltreatment, and the second suggests that increased dependency of the abuser on his or her victim leads to maltreatment. Based on the literature on family caregiving, some analysts have postulated that families experience "generational inversion" when the elderly person becomes dependent on the children for financial, physical, or emotional support,[26] which leads to stress on the caregiver. As economic pressures for the caregiver grow and rewards diminish, the change is perceived as unfair. If the caregivers do not have the ability to ameliorate the situation, they may become abusive. Although this theory seems plausible, there are few firm research findings to support it.

Several recent studies on dementia and elder abuse may provide some insight into dependency and family relationship.[20–22,27] However, the results are mixed. These studies view cognitive impairment as a measure of dependency. Two research groups[20,28] found no association between abuse and mental impairment in the patient sample, whereas two others[29,30] report a positive relationship. The inconsistent findings prompted one research team[28] to suggest that the triggering factor for abuse in families with a member with Alzheimer's disease may not be the cognitive impairment, but rather the disruptive behaviors exhibited by the patients. A study of caregivers who feared that they would become violent with elderly family members and those who actually did become violent also showed disruptive behavior of the care recipient to be a significant factor.

In contrast to the work on dependency of the victim, a number of other studies[10,23,24,26,28] have found that abusers were likely to be dependent on their victims financially and in a variety of other ways. The finding that continued dependence of an adult child or spouse on an elderly victim is related to physical violence may be explained by the *social exchange theory* and the concept of power.[31] It is possible that the feeling of powerlessness of an adult child who is still dependent on a parent is particularly acute because it violates society's expectation for normal adult behavior. The role of dependency—in either direction, parent or adult child—deserves serious attention as a potential risk factor for abuse. Further, some differences in findings may be explained by the type of abuse under consideration: dependency of the victim is more often associated with neglect, and dependency of the perpetrator, with physical abuse.

External stress caused by social-structural, macrolevel variables such as unemployment and economic conditions may play an important role in elder abuse, but the model alone does not explain why some families respond to stress with abuse and others do not. This area is an important one for future investigation.

Social isolation is characteristic of families in which other forms of domestic violence occur, although it is not clear whether social isolation precedes violence or is a consequence of it. Because behaviors considered to be illegitimate tend to be hidden, the presence of an active social network may be a particularly strong deterrent to elder abuse. Again, definitive studies of this risk factor remain to be conducted.

Outcomes

Beyond our concern about the long-term consequences of maltreatment for victims and abusers, elder abuse has important policy implications because abused victims may use health care services and depend on support services more than the nonabused elderly do. Although little is known about the health care consequences of elder abuse, some data do exist on the physical manifestations of abuse, such as bruises and sprains, abrasions, bone fractures, burns, and wounds.[10] Anecdotal evidence suggests that victimization also produces negative psychological outcomes. Several case-control studies have revealed a much higher level of depression among the abused group, even when the study controlled for other variables related to depression.[18,32,33] However, because of the cross-sectional nature of the studies, none can state with certainty whether the depression was an antecedent or consequence of the abuse.

The literature on partner abuse, especially with regard to the older battered woman, may be particularly relevant. Negative psychological consequences have included lowered self-esteem, confusion, a sense of powerlessness and helplessness, increased dependency on others, depression, disturbed eating and sleeping patterns, and a sense of isolation.[33] Posttraumatic stress disorder as a consequence of physical and sexual abuse in elderly patients has been suggested, although no empirical data are available. Withdrawal, vigilance, distrust, and dysphoria of elder abuse victims have been proposed[33] as symptoms stemming from posttraumatic stress disorder.

It is equally difficult to document the physical consequences of maltreatment because these effects may be confounded with normal physical changes that accompany aging and various physical ailments. An exception is a study[34] that compared data from one of the National Institute of Aging–funded Established Populations for Epidemiologic Studies of the Elderly (EPESE) sites with the reports filed with the local adult protective services agency over an 11-year period. The researchers tracked mortality rates for three groups: those who had been physically abused and/or neglected; those who had been investigated for other complaints, mainly self-neglect; and the rest of the cohort. No difference in rates were found in the first few years, but by the 13th year there was a significant difference with 36 percent of the noninvestigated group, 20 percent of the self-neglect group, and 11 percent of the abused group still alive. Further investigation is under way to begin to identify the variables that affect mortality.

Interventions

Although almost 20 years have passed since the problem of elder abuse and neglect first came to the public's attention, the ability to design prevention and intervention strategies and programs is still greatly handicapped by lack of knowledge about the extent, nature, and dynamics of elder abuse. In the absence of a comprehensive national policy, states and communities have designed their own programs, ranging from elder protective services to family counseling and legal intervention. The different strategies generally can be categorized as mandatory reporting laws, protective services, and direct services. Lack of evaluation data regarding the various types of interventions is a major gap in information.

Mandatory Reporting Laws

Forty-three states have mandatory reporting laws for cases of suspected elder mistreatment.[11] Several states that passed elder abuse legislation more recently have excluded mandatory reporting (Pennsylvania, 1987; Illinois, 1988; New Jersey, 1995). Proponents of mandatory reporting maintain that these laws are the best method for identifying cases of elder abuse. In contrast, opponents[35–37] argue that there is no evidence that mandatory reporting is effective. Some claim that an increased number of reports results from publicity and that penalties for not reporting are rarely enforced. Critics note that states have failed to provide sufficient funds for services to victims and abusers, and limited staff must attempt to handle a large number of referrals in response to the law.[35] Others claim that reporting interferes with the relationship and confidentiality between the professionals and clients.

Under mandatory reporting legislation, professionals are faced with a dilemma: either to violate the law or break trust with a client and possibly jeopardize a therapeutic relationship. Critics maintain that by extending a child abuse model to the elderly, states are adopting a set of assumptions that are not applicable to older people. Specifically, they infantalize the elder's position in society, foster negative stereotypes of the elderly, and limit the older persons' abilities to control their own lives. A General Accounting Office[38] survey of state officials concluded that reporting laws were not considered as effective in identification of elder abuse cases as a high level of public and professional awareness of elder abuse. This report, as well as testimony before the Select Committee on Aging of the House of Representatives, was responsible for the elimination of a federal mandatory reporting requirement from the Older Americans Act. However, the controversy continues. At a minimum, mandatory reporting must be accompanied by a substantial commitment of resources to the designated reporting agency.

Protective Services

If a state protective services program operates under an *adult protective service* statute, it is generally limited to "incapacitated" adults, leaving other agencies such as the police, legal services, and the criminal justice system to handle situations involving more competent and physically able persons. On the other hand, programs authorized under *elder abuse* legislation usually apply to *any* older individual who is at risk of abuse, neglect, or exploitation. Some states restrict their cases to persons living in their own homes; others include group and institutional settings as well.

Even though adult protective services has gained greater visibility and credibility in the past decade, it is still a controversial area of service. Some critics see such programs as an intrusion on the civil liberties of the elderly. They also argue that states define abuse too broadly and allow an intrusion into families with merely the normal range of human problems.[37] In all fairness, the emphasis on ensuring individual safety over client autonomy, which was evident a quarter of a century ago, is no longer the rule. Today, the client's right to self-determination is usually one of the basic principles of protective services. However, when the elderly person is judged to be incompetent, protective services will use legal surrogate options, such as guardianship or conservatorship.

Numerous changes have strengthened adult protective services, including the realignment of programs in state human services departments, amendments to the protective services statutes, education and training of workers and other professionals, improvement in their information management systems, participation in communitywide coalitions, and the formation of the National Association for Adult Protective Services Administrators. Underlying all these activities is the desire to bring adult protective services into closer working relationships with other service systems.[39]

Although protective services programs have investigated hundreds of thousands of cases, no program has been rigorously evaluated. In fact, the 1970s study of protective services demonstration projects, on which the original protective services legislation was based, revealed *negative* results.[40] A recent search of the literature on elder abuse program evaluation of any type produced only a handful of studies meeting the minimum quasi-experimental standard.[41] Generally, these programs had small numbers of clients and produced ambiguous results. Thus, systematic program evaluation should take place before continuing the proliferation of adult and elder protective services.

Service Options

Service options in communities tend to be based on one of two assumptions: that dependency of the victim causes maltreatment or that a relatively independent elder is abused by a dependent relative. Based on the first assumption, communities have emphasized health and service needs of the elderly that are not specific to abuse. Typically, services aim to relieve the burden of caregiving by providing housekeeping and meal preparation, respite care, and day care. However, research indicates that this dependency pattern of elder abuse occurs only in a minority of cases.

In contrast, the finding that many elders are abused by a dependent relative suggests that maltreated older persons may benefit from interventions found to be effective with victims of wife abuse. Options for the elderly that relate to the spouse abuse model are social support for the older person, self-help groups that contribute to consciousness-raising, "safe houses" or emergency shelters, and legal action. Earlier research on spouse abuse suggested that police arrests may reduce further episodes of abuse and that police can link victims with effective community services.[42] However, a reanalysis of the data from that research indicates that arrest was no better or worse than other police actions.[43,44] The role of police intervention in elder abuse cases remains to be studied.

The inclusion of elder abuse within federal family violence policy initiatives is bringing about a greater awareness of the problem among criminal justice, law enforcement, and health personnel. Many communities have created task forces of service providers and other interested individuals to raise awareness, identify needs, develop service programs, and advocate for legislation that will meet the needs of abused and neglected elders.

Recommendations

Given the lack of firm research findings in many areas, it is perhaps more appropriate to make proposals for future research than for practice and policy. The most critical need is information about the causes of elder abuse and effective methods of intervention. Suggestions for research are included below.

1. Emphasize direct interviews with abused elders in studies on elder abuse. Although assessment data compiled by competent professionals may accurately describe certain aspects of reported cases, understanding the family dynamics that produce maltreatment must ultimately rely on direct interviews with the people involved.
2. Institute a national voluntary reporting system using a minimum data set with standards accepted by all the states as the initial step in developing a national surveillance system for elder abuse.
3. Conduct control group studies, with attention to older battered women and other groups, to identify victim characteristics.
4. Study the effect of culture, traditions, and attitudes on definitions, intervention, and treatment.
5. Because perpetrator characteristics appear to be more predictive of abuse than the frailties of the victim, include a focus on perpetrator as well as the victim in studies.
6. Focus on the consequences of abuse as an area of research.
7. Examine the content of abusive acts, the specifics regarding the circumstances in which abuse occurs, and the pattern of abusive acts against the elderly.
8. Systematically evaluate intervention programs, emphasizing a partnership between researchers and practitioners. Sophisticated evaluation research techniques should be used to determine the impact of the treatment programs. Without such careful evaluation, funds may be wasted on inappropriate services that fail to help or may even harm elder victims and their families.

Suicide

Lloyd B. Potter • Patrick W. O'Carroll

Definition of the Problem

Suicide is the result of violence directed against self. In 1994 there were 31,142 deaths from suicide in the United States, making suicide the ninth leading cause of death in this country.[1] Unlike the rates for many diseases, suicide rates are substantial among both young and old people. As a result, in 1991, suicide was the sixth leading cause of premature death, as defined by years of potential life lost before age 65.[2] In past decades, the rate of suicide was relatively low among adolescents and young adults and increased steadily with age. However, in the last four decades, suicide rates among younger age groups have increased dramatically.[3] In particular, the suicide rate among persons 15 to 24 years of age has more that tripled. In 1950 the suicide rate for this age group was 4.5 per 100,000, and in 1994, this rate was 13.8.[1] Suicide has been the third leading cause of death among persons 15 to 24 years of age in recent years and the fourth leading cause of death among persons 10 to 14 years of age. Although most suicides occur among persons younger than 40, the highest rates occur among the elderly.[2]

In general, males are more than four times as likely to commit suicide than females; this is true across all age and race groups. White males are at the highest risk of suicide, followed by males of races other than white, white females, and females of races other than white. During the past decade, suicide rates among white males 10 to 19 years of age substantially increased. One of the most significant increases in suicide over the past decade—more than 300 percent—was among young black males 10 to 14 years of age.[4]

For both males and females, firearms are the most frequently used method of suicide; overall, approximately 60 percent of all suicides are committed with firearms. Among males, hanging is the second most common method of suicide, followed by poisoning by gases (chiefly carbon monoxide). Among females, ingestion of an overdose of drugs is the second most common method. The predominance of firearms as a method of suicide has been increasing among both males and females. In 1970, the number of female suicides by firearms were fewer than those completed by drug ingestion, yet by 1980, suicides by firearms surpassed drug-related suicides among women. In recent years, firearm suicides have accounted for an increasingly large proportion of all suicides among persons 10 to 19 and those older than 85 years of age. From 1980 to 1994 the proportion of suicides committed with firearms increased by 18 percent.[2]

Reliable information about morbidity from attempted suicide is sparse, although notable advances in collecting morbidity data have been made. For example, Oregon has implemented hospital-based surveillance of suicide attempts among persons younger than 18 years of age.[5] In one large, multisite survey of adults in the United States, approximately 3 of every 1,000 respondents reported having attempted suicide at some point during the preceding year.[6] This estimate, which is congruent with previous smaller surveys, suggests that approximately 750,000 adults attempt suicide each year in the United States and that there are approximately 25 suicide attempts for each completed suicide. Data from a 1994 nationally representative telephone survey of adults (ICARIS) estimated that 0.7 percent of the adult population of the United States, representing 693,974 people, had attempted suicide that required medical attention in the past 12 months (Crosby AE, Cheltenham MP, Sacks JJ: Incidence of Suicidal Ideation and Behavior in the United States, 1994, unpublished manuscript). The Youth Risk Behavior Survey estimates that in 1995, 3.4 percent of high school students reported suicide attempts that required medical attention.[7]

Data Sources

Suicide mortality data ultimately derive from death certificate data. The determination of suicide as a cause of death, however, is not necessarily a straightforward process. Suicide has been defined fairly succinctly as death from intentionally self-inflicted injury,[8] but it can be difficult to apply this definition. In particular, determining whether a decedent intended to commit suicide necessarily involves retrospective collection of data regarding the person's state of mind prior to death. The amount and quality of such information varies greatly from case to case. Moreover, until recently, there were no published guidelines explicitly describing what type of data ought to be collected in a death investigation in order to make an informed determination of manner of death.[8] The great variability across the United States in the qualifications of the coroner or official responsible for medicolegal certification raises additional questions about the validity and reliability of death certificate information.[9,10]

Against the backdrop of these structural problems in suicide certification is also the social stigma associated with suicide. For religious, financial, and even political reasons, coroners and medical examiners may sometimes be reluctant to certify suicide as a cause of death. Given these limitations in the way suicide is recorded as a cause of death, it is not surprising that many investigators believe that official suicide statistics substantially underestimate the true suicide rate. Estimates of the true suicide rate range from a low of 1.01 to 1.8 times the official rate, but it is likely that the true rate of suicide is no more than 1.25 times the official rate.[11]

There is essentially no information at the national level concerning the magnitude of the physical and mental health consequences of attempted suicide. Indeed, the incidence estimates from surveys of adults cited above are quite limited in what they tell us about attempted suicide. For example, because attempted suicide was self-defined in these surveys, it is unclear what proportion of these "suicide attempts" resulted in injury, in a visit to an emergency health facility, or in subsequent attempted or completed suicide. There also are no national estimates of the incidence of attempted suicide among persons younger than 18 years of age, although there are indications that the attempted suicide rate in this group may be even higher than in the adult population. Without such information on a national, longitudinal basis, it is difficult to accurately estimate suicide attempt morbidity and trends or to assess the efficacy of suicide prevention programs.

Causes and Risk Factors

Even though it is common to hear people say that a person committed suicide because he was mentally ill or because he could not cope with stressful events in his life, in reality, many factors contribute to the causal mechanism of suicide. Certain psychiatric illnesses are, of course, both extremely important and well-recognized as risk factors. In particular, affective disorders have been clearly shown, in both retrospective case-control studies and prospective cohort studies, to increase markedly the risk of suicide. For example, in a population-based cohort study of 3,563 males in Sweden who were observed for 15 to 25 years, the suicide rate among men with an initial diagnosis of any mental illness was almost 39 times higher than the rate for men with no mental disorder. Men with an initial diagnosis of a depressive disorder had a suicide rate 80 times higher than the rate for men with no mental disorder.[12]

Alcoholism is the second most commonly reported mental illness, after clinical depression, associated with suicide.[13-18] However, many studies have lacked a control group to help assess the contribution of alcohol use to suicide risk.[19–21] In addition, the independent effect of alcoholism on the suicide rate is rarely estimated; rather, the diagnosis of alcoholism among the case series is often reported, in addition to the prevalence of affective illness, social isolation, and other factors that might, in themselves, account for any observed increase in the risk of suicide. Because most of the studies have been carried out among special populations, such as psychiatric inpatients[22–24] or hospitalized alcoholics,[25–27] their findings are not necessarily applicable to alcoholics in general. Finally, little work has been done separately to assess the effects of acute exposure to alcohol (i.e., alcohol intoxication) and alcohol abuse on the risk of suicide. More research is needed to elucidate the mechanism(s) underlying the observed association between alcoholism and suicide.

Certain personality disorders (in particular, borderline and antisocial personality disorders) are correlated with suicidal behavior.[28] The interpretation of this correlation is problematic, however, because suicidal behavior is inherently part of the definition of certain of these disorders, such as borderline personality disorder. Future research should emphasize the strength and predictive value of personality disorders as risk factors for suicide, as well as the mechanisms explaining the observed association between certain of these disorders and suicide.

An increasing body of literature addresses putative genetic and biological risk factors for suicide.[29] Suicide has long been observed to "run in families" but such a phenomenon might either be caused by common exposure among family members to environmental-sociocultural risk factors for suicide or by genetic factors shared by family members. There is evidence of a genetic link for risk factors of suicide, such as depression.[30,31] Meta-analysis of twin studies, however, strongly suggests a genetically based risk for mental illness and suicide. Moreover, several Danish-American adoption studies suggest that this genetic risk may be inherited independently of major psychiatric illness, perhaps as an inability to control impulsive behavior.[32]

Certain neurotransmitter metabolites have been convincingly associated with an increased risk of suicide.[33–35] In particular, a clear relationship has been demonstrated between low concentrations of the serotonin metabolite 5-hydroxyindoleacetic acid (5-HIAA) in cerebrospinal fluid and an increased incidence of attempted and completed suicide in psychiatric patients. Most of the evidence for this relationship is based on studies of patients with major affective illness (particularly unipolar depression), but some evidence suggests that this relationship may hold for other diagnostic categories as well, particularly for personality disorders[36] and possibly for schizophrenia.[37] The mechanism that accounts for the relationship between a disturbed or inadequate serotonin system and suicidal behavior is not clear.

Recent suicide clusters among teenagers and young adults have suggested that suicides may sometimes be caused by exposure to the suicide or suicidal behavior of others.[38,39] This phenomenon is often referred to in the literature as "contagion." There is ample anecdotal evidence to suggest that, in any given suicide cluster, suicides occurring later in the cluster often appear to have been influenced by suicides occurring earlier in the cluster.[40] This contagion hypothesis has not been extensively tested at the individual level. However, several studies have identified elevated risk of depression in youth who have lost friends to suicide,[41,42] and one study found elevated risk for suicidal ideation and planning.[43] However, the strength and public health importance of contagion as a risk factor for suicide remains to be determined. Despite uncertainty about contagion as a risk factor for suicide, many believe it is prudent to recognize the possibility of a contagious effect of suicide and to institute measures to minimize potential contagion in the context of an apparent suicide cluster.[44,45]

Suicide contagion may not be limited to geographically localized clusters of suicides. A number of ecological studies have been done to assess whether the incidence of suicide in the general population is increased by exposure to television news stories and movies about suicide. Some investigators have reported an increase in suicide following such exposure,[46,47] but this finding has not been seen in all studies[48,49] and has been challenged in others.[50,51] Both the nature of the exposure to suicide and the hypothesized induction nod from exposure to outcome in these studies are quite different than is hypothesized for geographically localized suicide clusters. In the former the exposure is to stories, fictional or otherwise, of suicides by persons unknown to the study subjects; induction period implied in the study designs is 1 to 2 weeks. In the case of geographically localized suicide clusters, however, the suicides to which victims of the suicide cluster were exposed were frequently those of close or intimate friends; reported suicide clusters have typically occurred over the course of 1 to 4 months[52] but have ranged from several weeks to over 1 year.[53]

There is a variety of situational risk factors for suicide. Stressful life events, such as the death of a loved one or recent loss of employment, often appear to be clear precipitants of suicide.[54] In general, stressful life events may elevate the background risk of suicide by a factor of 5 to 10, although the duration of time after exposure to these stressful events during which suicide risk remains elevated has not been well characterized.[55] A loss or disruption of normal social support mechanisms also increases the risk of suicide. Divorce, unemployment, and migration from one community to another are but three examples of factors that may lead to some disruption of social support networks; all three have been shown to be related to increased suicide rates.[56,57] Youth in Oregon who had attempted suicide listed family discord, arguments with boyfriends/girlfriends, and school-related problems as the most common reasons they had attempted suicide.[4] Absent or inadequate social support networks presumably increase the risk of suicide through interaction with other suicide risk factors, such as clinical depression and recent stressful life events.

The suicide rate among children younger than 15 years of age in the United States is twice that of children in other industrialized countries, and the firearm suicide rate is almost 10 times as high.[58] Unlike drug ingestions, carbon monoxide poisoning, and many other suicide methods, a suicide attempt with a firearm is often immediately lethal, leaving little or no opportunity for postattempt rescue.[59,60] Easy access to a firearm may both limit the preattempt opportunity for intervention by others and facilitate impulsive suicidal acts.[61,62] Recent increases in U.S. suicide rates among both the young and the elderly have been largely the result of increases in firearm-related suicide. While increased access to firearms may lead to increases in firearm-related suicides, it is just as likely that these increases are largely a result of increased selection of firearms as a means to attempt suicide with little or no change in accessibility. The process by which persons select means to act out suicidal behavior is complex and poorly understood. There is a clear need for careful research to better understand how people select methods, an understanding that may lead to interventions that would move suicide attempters away from more lethal means.

Finally, several risk factors for suicide are useful for delineating high-risk groups, although these factors do not appear to be "causal" in the traditional sense. For example, being male or elderly identifies one as belonging to a high-risk group, and having a past history of attempted suicide has also been clearly shown to increase the risk of future completed suicide.[56] These markers for increased suicide risk presumably correlate with other causal risk factors for suicide. A past history of attempted suicide, for example, may correlate with impulsivity or with a vulnerability to affective illness.

Outcomes

In human and economic terms, the cost of suicide in the United States is enormous. In 1954 alone, suicide among persons younger than 65 years of age resulted in the loss of over 645,000 years of potential life.[63] Weinstein and Saturno[64] estimate that in 1980, suicide among persons 15 to 24 years of age alone resulted in the loss of 276,000 years of potential life and economic costs of $2.26 billion. Adding in attempted suicide among persons in this age group brought the estimated economic costs to $53.19 billion. At the individual level, one study in Washington state estimated that the average medical cost of one suicide death was $13,023 and the economic cost (including lost of lifetime earnings) was $737,600.[65,66] Medical costs of a nonfatal, hospitalized, suicide attempt (including follow-up and nonhospital medical charges) was estimated at $27,501.

The emotional trauma experienced by the "survivors" of suicide—family members and friends of the victims—is enormous.[67] The process of grief and bereavement over the death of a loved one is always painful and difficult, but when the decedent has committed suicide, this process is even more difficult and traumatic. Death from suicide is usually sudden and unexpected. In addition, suicide may engender feelings of guilt or rejection in the survivors. Because of the social stigma associated with suicide, traditional mourning rituals may be avoided, and the usual social supports for the decedent's family and friends may be withdrawn or attenuated. All of these factors increase the risk of disturbed or unresolved grief reactions among the survivors.[68]

Interventions

Although a wide variety of suicide prevention programs have been devised, the strategies underlying these programs may be considered under five broad conceptual categories.[69] The first such strategy is to improve the identification, referral, and treatment of persons at high risk of suicide by various caretakers and "gatekeepers" in the community. Increased training of primary care physicians in the recognition and treatment or referral of patients with clinical depression is one example of this approach; school-based screening programs designed to identify suicidal youth in the context of an evolving suicide cluster is another. A second suicide prevention strategy focuses on the treatment of underlying risk factors for suicide. Clinical depression, for example, is addressed through psychotherapeutic and pharmacological treatment of patients with this illness. Although alcohol rehabilitation programs are not traditionally thought of in terms of suicide prevention, they may nevertheless contribute to the prevention of suicide by addressing one of the most important risk factors—alcoholism.

A third general suicide prevention strategy is to decrease individual vulnerability to suicide through education of the general population. Effective education programs, for example, seek to help individuals understand and cope with the type of problems that can lead to suicide.[70] Other programs are designed to increase public awareness of helping resources in the community to facilitate help-seeking behavior by suicidal persons. A fourth, related suicide prevention strategy is to provide or expand the accessibility of self-referral resources for suicidal persons. Hotlines and walk-in crisis centers are the best-known examples of this strategy.

A final strategy for suicide prevention seeks to limit access to lethal means of suicide, such as high places, prescription drugs, or firearms.[51] This strategy derives from the hypothesis that, if substantial efforts are required by an individual to arrange for a lethal suicide method or if a less lethal method is substituted in its stead, the likelihood of a completed suicide will be diminished.

The above strategies have differing strengths and weaknesses, and each may be important in the prevention of suicide. Unfortunately, the effectiveness of many of these strategies has yet to be established. Eddy and colleagues[70] surveyed 15 suicide experts as to their judgments of the effectiveness of a variety of existing and proposed youth suicide prevention strategies. On the average these experts estimated that approximately 10 percent of potential youth suicides were being averted by existing prevention programs and that each of the proposed strategies to improve prevention might reduce the incidence of youth suicide by 6 to 16 percent, depending on the strategy. Even if all of the proposed strategies were simultaneously implemented, the expected reduction in youth suicide was estimated to range from 15 to no more than 50 percent. The uncertainty regarding program effectiveness and the relatively modest nature of the reduction in mortality that may be expected from our present array of interventions are not limited to youth suicide prevention programs but extend to suicide prevention in general. There is an urgent need to develop a better empirical base of information regarding the effectiveness of various prevention strategies so that policymakers can make the best use of limited suicide prevention resources.

▶ REFERENCES

The Problem of Violence in the United States and Globally

1. Centers for Disease Control and Prevention: 1994: 10 Leading Causes of Death. Atlanta: Centers for Disease Control and Prevention, 1997
2. Centers for Disease Control and Prevention: Injury Mortality: National Summary of Injury Mortality Data, 1987–1993. Atlanta: Centers for Disease Control and Prevention, 1996
3. Annest JL, Mercy JA, Gibson DR, Ryan GW: National estimates of nonfatal firearm-related injuries: beyond the tip of the iceberg. JAMA 273:1749–1754, 1995
4. Wintemute GJ: Firearms as a cause of death in the United States, 1920–1982. J Trauma 27:532–536, 1987
5. Miller TM, Cohen MA, Wiersema B: Victim Costs and Consequence: A New Look. Research Report NCJ 155282. Washington, DC: US Department of Justice, National Institute of Justice, Office of Justice Programs, and US Department of Health and Human Services, Maternal and Child Health Bureau, 1996
6. Zawitz MW: Firearm Injury from Crime. NCJ 160093. Washington, DC: Bureau of Justice Statistics, 1996
7. Centers for Disease Control and Prevention: BB and pellet gun-related injuries—United States, June 1992–May 1994. MMWR 44: 909–913, 1995
8. McNeill AM, Annest JL: The ongoing hazard of BB and pellet gun-related injuries in the United States. Ann Emerg Med 26:187–194, 1995
9. Sinauer N, Annest JL, Mercy JA: Unintentional, nonfatal firearm-related injuries: a preventable public health burden. JAMA 275: 1740–1743, 1996
10. Wallace LJD, Calhoun AD, Powell KE, O'Neil J, James SP: Homicide and Suicide Among Native Americans, 1979–1992. Atlanta: National Center for Injury Prevention and Control, 1993, pp 9, 18
11. Wallace LJD, Kirk ML, Houston B, Annest JL, Emrich SS: Injury Mortality Atlas of Indian Health Service Areas, 1979–1987. Atlanta: National Center for Injury Prevention and Control, 1993, pp 14–19
12. Jenkins EL: Occupational injury deaths among females. The US experience for the decade 1980 to 1989. Ann Epidemiol 4:146–151, 1994
13. Baker SP, O'Neill B, Ginsburg MJ, Li G: The Injury Fact Book. 2nd ed. New York: Oxford University Press, 1992, pp 39–88
14. Kachur SP, Potter LB, James SP, Powell KE: Suicide in the United States, 1980–1992. Atlanta: National Center for Injury Prevention and Control, 1997
15. Centers for Disease Control and Prevention: Injury Mortality Atlas of the United States, 1986–1994. Atlanta: National Center for Injury Prevention and Control, 1997
16. Centers for Disease Control and Prevention: Rates of homicide, suicide, and firearm-related deaths among children—26 industrialized countries. MMWR 46:101–105, 1997
17. World Health Organization: International Statistical Classification of Diseases and Related Health Problems. 10th ed. Geneva: World Health Organization, 1992
18. Murray C, Lopez A (eds): The Global Burden of Disease: A Comprehensive Assessment of Mortality and Disability from Diseases, Injuries, and Risk Factors in 1990 and Projected to 2020. Geneva: World Health Organization, 1996
19. Murray C: Rethinking DALYs. In Murray C, Lopez A (eds): The Global Burden of Disease: A Comprehensive Assessment of Mortality and Disability from Diseases, Injuries, and Risk Factors in 1990 and Projected to 2020. Geneva: World Health Organization, 1996, pp 1–98

20. World Bank: World Development Report 1993: Investing in Health. New York: Oxford University Press, 1993
21. Heise L: Violence Against Women: The Hidden Health Burden. World Bank Discussion Paper No. 255. Washington, DC: The World Bank
22. Follingstad DR, Brennen AF, Hause DS, Polek DS, Rutledge LL: Factors moderating physical and psychological symptoms of battered women. Journal of Family Violence 6:81–95, 1991

Assaultive Violence

1. Centers for Disease Control and Prevention: 1994: 10 Leading Causes of Death. Atlanta: Centers for Disease Control and Prevention, 1997
2. O'Carroll PW, Mercy JA: Patterns and recent trends in black homicide. In Hawkins DF (ed): Homicide Among Black Americans. Lanham, MD: University Press of America, 1986, pp 29–42
3. US Department of Justice: Crime in the United States, 1994: Uniform Crime Reports. Washington, DC: Federal Bureau of Investigation, 1995
4. Annest JL, Mercy JA, Gibson DR, Ryans GW: National estimates of nonfatal firearm-related injuries. JAMA 273(22):1749–1754, 1995
5. Centers for Disease Control: Homicide Surveillance, 1979–1988. MMWR CDC Surveill Summ, 41(3):ss1–ss34, 1992
6. Barancik JI, Chatterje BF, Greene YZ, McKenzie EM, Fife B: Northeastern Ohio Trauma Study. I. Magnitude of the problem. Am J Public Health 73:746–751, 1983
7. US Department of Justice, Bureau of Health Statistics: National Crime Surveys: National Sample, 1973–1979. Ann Arbor, MI: Inter-University Consortium Political and Social Research, 1981
8. National Center for Health Statistics: Technical notes. Mon Vital Stat Rep [monthly]
9. US Department of Health and Human Services: International Classification of Diseases. 9th Revision. Clinical Modification. Washington, DC: US Department of Health and Human Services, 1980
10. Reiss AJ, Roth JA (eds): Understanding and Preventing Violence. Washington, DC: National Academy Press, 1993, pp 42–43, 48
11. Zawitz MW: Firearm Injury from Crime: Bureau of Justice Statistics Selected Findings. Washington, DC: US Department of Justice, Office of Justice Programs, April 1996, p 6
12. Rokaw WM, Mercy JA, Smith JC: Comparing death certificate data with FBI crime reporting statistics on U.S. homicides. Public Health Rep 105:447–455, 1990
13. Sugarman JR, Soderberg R, Gordon JE, Rivara FP: Racial misclassification of American Indians: its effect on injury rates in Oregon, 1989 through 1990. Am J Public Health 83:681–684, 1993
14. Yung B, Hammond R. Antisocial behavior in minority groups: epidemiological and cultural perspectives. In Staff D, Breiling J, Maser J (eds): Handbook of Antisocial Behavior. New York: John Wiley, in press
15. Nlednick SA, Pollock V, Volavka J, Gabrielli J: Biology and Violence. In Wolfgang ME, Weiner NA (eds): Criminal Violence. Beverly Hills, CA: Sage Publications. 1982, pp 21–80
16. Wolfgang ME: Patterns in Criminal Homicide. New York: John Wiley & Sons, 1958
17. American Psychological Association: Reducing Violence: A Research Agenda. Washington, DC: American Psychological Association, 1996
18. Hammond WR, Yung B: Experience of violence: African Americans. In Eron LD, Gentry J, Schlegel P (eds): Reason to Hope: A Psychosocial Perspective on Violence and Youth. Washington, DC: American Psychological Association, 1995, pp 105–118
19. Wolfgang ME, Zahn MA: Criminal homicide. In Kadish SH (ed): Encyclopedia of Crime and Justice. New York: The Free Press, 1983
20. Luckenbill DF: Criminal homicide as a situated transaction. Social Problems 25:176–186, 1977
21. Yung B, Hammond R. Breaking the cycle: a culturally sensitive violence prevention program for African American children and adolescents. In Lutzker J (ed): Handbook of Child Abuse Research and Treatment. New York: Plenum, in press
22. Felson R, Tedeschi J: A social interactionist approach to violence: cross-cultural applications. Violence Vict 8:295–308, 1993
23. Rubin PH: The economics of crime. Atlanta Economic Review 29(4):38–43, 1978
24. Smith MD, Parker RN: type of homicide and variation in regional rates. Social Forces 136–147, 1980
25. Curtis LA: Violence, Race, and Culture. Lexington, MA: DC Heath, 1975
26. Riedel M, Zahn MA: The Nature and Patterns of American Homicide: An Annotated Bibliography. Washington, DC: National Institute of Justice, 1982
27. Goodman RA, Mercy JA, Loya F, Rosenberg ML, Smith JC, Allen NH, Vargas L, Kolts R: Alcohol use and interpersonal violence. Alcohol detected in homicide victims. Am J Public Health 76:144–149, 1986
28. Gelles RJ: The Violent Home: A Study of Physical Aggression Between Husbands and Wives. Beverly Hills, CA: Sage Publications, 1974
29. Goldstein PJ: The drugs-violence nexus: a tripartite conceptual framework. Drug Issues 15:493–506, 1985
30. World Health Organization: World Health Statistics Annual. Geneva: World Health Organization, 1994
31. Williams KR: Economic sources of homicide: reestimating the effects of poverty and unequality. Am Soc Rev 49:283–289, 1984
32. Centerwall BS: Race, socioeconomic status and domestic homicide, Atlanta, 1971–72. Am J Public Health 74:813–815, 1984
33. Singh GK, Kochanek MA, MacDorman MF: Advance report of final mortality statistics, 1994. Mon Vital Stat Rep 45 (Suppl 3), 1996
34. Riedel M, Zahn MA: The Nature and Patterns of American Homicide: An Annotated Bibliography. Washington, DC: National Institute of Justice, 1982
35. US Bureau of Justice Statistics: National Crime Victimization Survey, Criminal Victimization 1996. (NCJ 165812) Washington, DC: US Department of Justice, Office of Justice Statistics, November 1997
36. Stark E, Flitcraft A, Zuckerman D, et al: Wide Abuse in the Medical Setting: An Introduction for Health Personnel. Monograph No 7. Washington, DC: Office of Domestic Violence, 1981
37. Eth S, Pynoos RS: Bearing witness: a model of research and intervention. Presented to the American Psychiatric Association, Anaheim, California, May 10, 1984
38. Prothrow-Stith D: Primary prevention of homicide: preliminary report of a demonstration project investigating the value of health education in the high school on anger and violence. Presented at the NASW-NIMH workshop on prevention of black homicide, Washington, DC, June 1984
39. Prothrow-Stith D: Violence Prevention Curriculum for Adolescents. Newton MA: Education Development Center, 1987
40. Powell KE, Hawkins DF (eds): Youth violence prevention: descriptions and baseline data from 13 evaluation projects. Am J Prev Med 12(Suppl), 1996
41. Ross CH, Zigler E: An agenda for action. In Gerbna G, Ross CJ, Zigler E (eds): Child Abuse: An Agenda for Action. New York: Oxford University Press, 1990, pp 293–304
42. Grossman DC, Neckelman HJ, Koepsell TD, et al: Effectiveness of a violence prevention curriculum among children in elementary school: a randomized controlled trial. JAMA 277(20):1605–1611, 1997
43. Rosenberg ML, Powell KE, Hammond R: Applying science to violence prevention [Editorial]. JAMA 277(20):1641–1642, 1997
44. Straus MA, Gelles JR, Steinmetz SK: Behind Closed Doors: Violence in the American Family. Garden City, NY: Anchor Press/Doubleday, 1980

45. Garbarino I: The human ecology of child maltreatment. J Marriage Fam 39:412–427, 1977

Woman Battering

1. Klaus PA, Rand MR: Family Violence: Special Report. Washington, DC: Bureau of Justice Statistics, 1984
2. Lie G, Gentlewarrior S: Intimate violence in lesbian relationships: discussion of survey findings and practice limitations. J Soc Serv Res 15:41–59, 1991
3. Stark E, Flitcraft A: Women at Risk: Domestic Violence and Women's Health. Thousand Oaks, CA: Sage, 1996
4. Straus M, Gelles R, Steinmetz S: Behind Closed Doors: A Survey of Family Violence in America. New York: Doubleday, 1980
5. Straus MA, Gelles R: Societal change and change in family violence from 1975–1985 as revealed by two national surveys. J Marriage Fam 48:465–479, 1986
6. Straus MA, Gelles R: How violent are American families? Estimates from the National Family Violence Resurvey and other studies. In Hotaling G et al (eds): Family Abuse and Its Consequences. Thousand Oaks, CA: Sage Publications, 1988
7. Straus M, Kantor GK: Change in spouse assault rates from 1975 to 1992: a comparison of three national surveys in the United States. Paper presented at the 13th World Congress of Sociology, Bielefeld, Germany, July 19, 1994
8. Commonwealth Fund, Louis Harris and Associates: The Commonwealth Fund Survey of Women's Health. New York: Commonwealth Fund, 1993
9. Bachman R, Salzman LE: Violence against Women: Estimates from the Redesigned Survey. Bureau of Justice Statistics Special Report NCJ-154348. Washington, DC: US Department of Justice, 1995
10. Schulman MA: A Survey of Spousal Violence Against Women in Kentucky. Harris Study No. 792701. Washington, DC: Law Enforcement Assistance Administration, 1979
11. Teske RHC, Parker ML: Spouse Abuse in Texas: A Study of Women's Attitudes and Experiences. Huntsville, TX: Criminal Justice Center, Sam Houston State University, 1983
12. Stark E: The Battering Syndrome: Social Knowledge, Social Theory, and the Abuse of Women [Thesis]. Binghamton State University of New York, 1984
13. Stark E, Flitcraft A: Women and children at risk: a feminist perspective on child abuse. Int J Health Serv 18:97–118, 1988
14. Stark E, Flitcraft A: Spouse abuse. In Rosenberg M, Fenley MA (eds): Violence in America: A Public Health Approach. New York: Oxford University Press, 1991
15. Abbott J, Johnson R, Kozial-McLain J, Lowenstein SR: Domestic violence against women; incidence and prevalence in an emergency department population. JAMA 273:1763–1767, 1995
16. Stark E, Flitcraft A: Personal power and institutional victimization: treating the dual trauma of women battering. In Ochberg F (ed): Posttraumatic Therapy and Victims of Violence. New York: Brunner/Mazel, 1988
17. Stark E: Framing and reframing battered women. In Buzawa E (ed): Domestic Violence: The Criminal Justice Response. Westport, CT: Auburn House, 1992
18. Walker L, Edwall GE: Domestic violence and determination of visitation and custody in divorce. In Sonkin D (ed): Domestic Violence on Trial. New York: Springer, 1987
19. Berk RA, Berk SF, Loeske DR, Rauma D: Mutual combat and other family violence myths. In Finkelhor D et al (eds): The Dark Side of Families: Current Family Violence Research. Beverly Hills, CA: Sage Publications, 1983
20. Mooney J: Domestic Violence in North London. Middlesex, England: Middlesex University, Center for Criminology, 1993
21. Flitcraft AH: Battered Women: An Emergency Room Epidemiology with a Description of a Clinical Syndrome and Critique of Present Therapeutics [Doctoral dissertation]. New Haven, CT: Yale University, 1977
22. McLeer SV, Anwar R: A study of women presenting in an emergency department. Am J Public Health 79:65–67, 1989
23. Isaac NE, Sanchez RL: Emergency department response to battered women in Massachusetts. Ann Intern Med 23:855–858, 1994
24. Olson L, Anctil C, Fullerton L, Brillman J, Arbuckle J, Sklar D: Increasing emergency physician recognition of domestic violence. Ann Emerg Med 27:741–746, 1996
25. Freund KM, Bak SM, Blackhall L: Identifying domestic violence in primary care practice. J Gen Intern Med 11:44–46, 1996
26. Brown GW, Harris T: Social Origins of Depression: A Study of Psychiatric Disorder in Women. London: Tavistock Press, 1978
27. Stark E: Killing the beast within: women battering and female suicidality. Int J Health Serv 25:43–64, 1995
28. Kantor GK, Straus M: The drunken bum theory of wife beating. Social Problems
29. Peterson R: Social class, social learning, and wife abuse. Soc Serv Rev 54:390–406, 1980
30. deLahunta EA, Tulsky AA: Personal exposure of faculty and students to family violence. JAMA 275:1903–1906, 1996
31. Gelles, RJ: Violence and pregnancy: are pregnant women at greater risk of abuse? J Marriage Fam 50:841–847, 1988
32. McFarlane J, Parker B, Soeken K, Bullock L: Assessing for abuse during pregnancy: severity and frequency of injuries and associated entry into prenatal care. JAMA 267:3176–3178, 1992
33. Gauquin DA: Spouse abuse: data from the National Crime Survey. Victimology 2:632–643, 1978
34. Star B: Comparing battered and nonbattered women. Victimology 3:32–44, 1978
35. Walker L: The Battered Woman. New York: Harper and Row, 1979
36. Gondolph E: Battered Women as Survivors: An Alternative to Learned Helplessness. Lexington, MA: Lexington Press, 1988
37. Dutton D: The Domestic Assault of Women: Psychological and Criminal Justice Perspectives. Vancouver, British Columbia: University of British Columbia Press, 1995
38. Hamberger KL, Hastings JE: Personality characteristics of men who batter and nonviolent men: some continuities and discontinuities. J Family Violence 6:131–147, 1991
39. Hamberger LL, Hastings JE: Characteristics of abusive men suggestive of personality disorders. Hosp Community Psychiatry 39:763–770, 1988
40. Dutton D: Behavioral and affective personality correlates of borderline personality organization in wife assault. Int J Law Psychiatry 17:265–277, 1994
41. Kaufman J, Zigler E: Do abused children become abusive parents? Am J Orthopsychiatry 57:186–193, 1987
42. Caesar PL: Men who batter: a heterogeneous group. Paper presented at the American Psychological Association, Washington, DC, 1986
43. Coleman DH, Straus M: Alcohol use and family violence. In Gottheil EL et al (eds): Alcohol, Drug Abuse, and Aggression. Springfield, IL: Charles C Thomas, 1983, 104–124
44. Bard M, Zacker J: Assaultiveness and alcohol use in family disputes: police perceptions. Criminology 12:281–292, 1974
45. Richardson DC, Campbell JL: Alcohol and wife abuse: the effect of alcohol on attributions of blame for wife abuse. Pers Soc Psychol Bull 6:51–56, 1980
46. Arias I, O'Leary D: Factors moderating the intergenerational transmission of martial aggression. Paper presented at the 18th annual meeting of the Association for the Advancement of Behavior Therapy, Philadelphia, November 1994
47. Telch CP, Linquist CU: Violent versus nonviolent couples: a comparison of patterns. Psychotherapy 21:242–248, 1984
48. Stark E, Flitcraft A: Woman-battering, child abuse, and social heredity: what is the relationship? In Johnson N (ed): Marital Violence.

Sociological Review Monograph No. 31. London: Routledge & Kegan Paul, 1985
49. Jaffe PG, Wolf DA, Wilson SK: Children of Battered Women. Newbury Park, CA: Sage Publications, 1990
50. Carlson BE: Children's observations of interparental violence. In Roberts AR (ed): Battered Women and Their Families. New York: Springer, 1984, pp 147–167
51. Goodman GS, Rosenberg M: The child witness to family violence: clinical and legal consideration. In Sonkin DJ (ed): Domestic Violence on Trial. New York: Springer, 1987, pp 97–126
52. Hughes HM: Psychological and behavioral correlates of family violence in child witness and victims. Am J Orthopsychiatry 18:77–90, 1988
53. Makepeace JM: The severity of courtship violence injuries and the effectiveness of individual precautions. In Hotaling G, et al (eds): Family Abuse and Its Consequences: New Directions in Research. Beverly Hills, CA: Sage Publications, 1988, pp 297–311
54. Bogal-Albritten RB, Allbritten B: The hidden victims: Premarital abuse among college students. Paper presented at the meeting of the American Psychological Association, Anaheim, CA, 1983
55. Murphy JE: Date abuse and forced intercourse among college students. Paper presented at the Second National Family Violence Research Conference, 1984
56. Kurz D, Stark E: Not so benign neglect: the medical response to battering. In Yllo K, Bograd A (eds): Feminist Perspectives on Wife Abuse. Newbury Park, CA: Sage Publications, 1988
57. Herman JL: Trauma and Recovery. New York: Basic Books, 1992
58. Stark E, Flitcraft A, Frazier W: Medicine and patriarchal violence: the social construction of a private event. Int J Health Serv 9:461–493, 1979
59. Carmen EH, Rieker P, Mills T: Victims of violence and psychiatric illness. Am J Psychiatry 141:378–383, 1984
60. Post RD, Willet AB, Frank RD, House RM, Back SM, Weisberg, MP: A preliminary report on the prevalence of domestic violence among psychiatric inpatients. Am J Psychiatry 137:974–975, 1980
61. Koss, MP, Heslet L: Somatic consequences of violence against women. Arch Fam Med 1:53–59, 1992
62. Koss, MP, Koss PK, Woodruff WJ: Deleterious effects of criminal victimization on women's health and medical utilization. Arch Intern Med 151:342–347, 1991
63. Graff TT, 1980
64. Levine M: Intergenerational violence and its effect on the children: a sample of 50 families in general practice. Med Sci 15:172, 1978
65. Hilberman E, Munson K: Sixty battered women. Victimology: An International Journal 2:460–470, 1977–78
66. Bowker L, Arbitell M, McFerron JR: On the relationship between wife-beating and child abuse. In Yllo K, Bograd M (eds): Feminist Perspectives on Wife Abuse. Newbury Park, CA: Sage Publications, 1988, pp 158–175
67. McKibben L, Devos R, Newberger E: Victimization of mothers of abused children: a controlled study. Pediatrics 84:531–535, 1989
68. Stark E, Flitcraft A: Women and children at risk: A feminist perspective on child abuse. In Stark E, Flitcraft A (eds): Women at Risk: Domestic Violence and Women's Health. Thousand Oaks, CA, Sage Publications, 1996, pp 73–98
69. Warshaw C: Limitations on the medical model in the care of battered women. Gender and Society 3:506–517, 1989
70. Rieker PP, Carmen EH: The Gender Gap in Psychotherapy: Social Realities and Psychological Processes. New York: Plenum Press, 1984

Rape and Sexual Assault

1. Federal Bureau of Investigation: Crime in the United States 1995: Uniform Crime Reports. Washington, DC: US Department of Justice, 1995
2. Brownmiller S: Against Our Will: Men, Women and Rape. New York: Simon & Schuster, 1975
3. Sparks RF, Glenn HG, Dodd DJ: Surveying Victims. New York: John Wiley & Sons, 1977
4. Koss MP: The hidden rape victim: personality, attitudinal and situational characteristics. Psychol Women Q 9:193–212, 1985
5. Kilpatrick DG, Edmunds CN, Seymour AK: Rape in America: A Report to the Nation. Arlington, VA: National Victim Center, 1992
6. Warr M: Fear of rape among urban women. Soc Probl 32:239–250, 1985
7. Kidd RF, Chayet EF: Why victims fail to report? The psychology of criminal victimization. Social Issues 40:34–50, 1984
8. US Bureau of Justice Statistics: Criminal Victimization, 1994. Department of Justice Publication No. NCJ-158022. Washington, DC: Bureau of Justice Statistics, 1994
9. Biderman AD, Lynch JP: Understanding Crime Incidence Statistics. Secaucus, NJ: Springer-Verlag, 1991
10. Eigenberg HM: The national crime survey and rape: the case of the missing question. Justice Quarterly 655–672, 1990
11. Koss MP: Detecting the scope of rape: a review of prevalence research methods. Journal of Interpersonal Violence 8:98–122, 1993
12. Knight RA, Rosenberg R, Schneider BA: Classification of sexual offenders: perspectives, methods and validation. In Burgess AW (ed): Rape and Sexual Assault. New York: Garland, 1985, pp 222–292
13. Knight RA, Prentky RA: Classifying sexual offenders: The development and corroboration of taxonomic models. In Marshall WL, Laws DR, Barbaree HE (eds): The Handbook of Sexual Assault. New York: Plenum Press, 1990, pp 23–52
14. Prentky RA, Knight RA: Identifying critical dimensions for discriminating among rapists. J Consult Clin Psychol 59:643–661, 1991
15. Koss MP, Koss P, Woodruff WJ: Deleterious effects of criminal victimization on women's health and medical utilization. Arch Intern Med 151:342–357, 1991
16. Malamuth NM, Sockloskie RJ, Koss MP, Tanaka JS: Characteristics of aggressors against women: testing a model using a national sample of college students. J Consult Clin Psychol 59:670–681, 1991
17. Koss MP, Leonard KE, Beezley DA, Oros CJ: Nonstranger sexual aggression: a discriminant analysis of the psychological characteristics of undetected offenders. Sex Roles 12:981–992, 1985
18. Malamuth NM, Donnerstein E (eds): Pornography and Sexual Aggression. Orlando, FL: Academic Press, 1984
19. Ellis L: A synthesized (biosocial) theory of rape. J Consult Clin Psychol 59:631–642, 1991
20. Hall, GCN, Hirschman R: Toward a theory of sexual aggression: a quadripartite model. J Consult Clin Psychol 59:662–669, 1991
21. Resick PA: The psychological impact of rape. Journal of Interpersonal Violence 8:223–255, 1993
22. Kilpatrick, DG, Saunders BE, Veronen LJ, Best CL, Von JM: Criminal victimization: lifetime prevalence, reporting to police, and psychological impact. Crime Delinq 33:479–489, 1987
23. Foa EB, Rothbaum, BO, Steketee GS: Treatment of rape victims. Journal of Interpersonal Violence 8:256–276, 1993
24. Norris FH: Epidemiology of trauma: frequency and impact of different potentially traumatic events on different demographic groups. J Consult Clin Psychol 60:409–418, 1992
25. Burnam MA, Stein JA, Golding JM, et al: Sexual assault and mental disorders in a community population. J Consult Clin Psychol 56:843–850, 1988
26. Leymann H: Somatic and psychological symptoms after the experience of life threatening events: a profile analysis. Victimology 10:512–538, 1985
27. Sorenson SB: Health service utilization following sexual assault. Am J Consult Psychol 16:625–643, 1988
28. Council on Scientific Affairs: Violence against women: relevance for medical practitioners. JAMA 267:3184–3189, 1992

29. Hendricks-Mathews MK: Survivors of abuse: health care issues. Prim Care 20:391–406, 1993
30. Koss MP, Woodruff WJ, Koss P: Criminal victimization among primary care medical patients: prevalence, incidence, and physician usage. Behav Sci Law 9:85–96, 1991
31. Waigandt A, Wallace DL, Phelps L, Miller DA: The impact of sexual assault on physical health status. J Trauma Stress 3:93–102, 1990
32. Koss MP, Heslet L: Somatic consequences of violence against women. Arch Fam Med 1:53–59, 1992
33. Murphy SM: Rape, sexually transmitted diseases and human immunodeficiency virus infection. Int J STD AIDS 1:79–82, 1990
34. Baker TC, Burgess AW, Brickman E, Davis RC: Rape victims' concerns about possible exposure to HIV infection. J Interpersonal Violence 5:49–60, 1990
35. Gostin LO, Lazzarini Z, Alexander D, et al. HIV testing, counseling and prophylaxis after sexual assault. JAMA 271:1436–1444, 1994
36. Avner JI: Rape, Sexual Assault and Child Sexual Abuse: Working towards a More Responsive Society. Final Report of the Governor's Task Force on Rape and Sexual Assault. Albany: New York State Division for Women, 1990
37. McCall GJ: Risk factors and sexual assault prevention. J Interpersonal Violence 8:277–295, 1993
38. Sparks CH, Bar On BA: A Social Change Approach to the Prevention of Sexual Violence against Women. (Stone Center for Developmental Services and Studies, work in progress, Series No. 83-08.) Wellesley, MA: Wellesley College, Stone Center for Developmental Services and Studies, 1985

Child Abuse

1. Kempe CH, Silverman FN, Steele BF, et al: The battered child syndrome. JAMA 181:17–24, 1962
2. Cohen S, Sussman R: Reporting Child Abuse. Cambridge, MA: Ballinger, 1977
3. Bittner, S, Newberger EH: Pediatric understanding of child abuse and neglect. Pediatrics 2:197–207, 1981
4. Newberger EH, Hampton RL, Marx TI, White KN: Child abuse and pediatric social illness: an epidemiological analysis and ecological reformulation. Am J Orthopsychiatry 56:589–601, 1986
5. Meadow R: Munchausen syndrome by proxy: the hinterland of child abuse. Lancet 2:343–344, 1977
6. Newberger CM, Newberger EH: When the pediatrician is a pedophile. In Burgess AW, Hartman CR (eds): Sexual Exploitation of Patients by Health Professionals. New York: Praeger, 1986, pp 99–106
7. Schreier HA, Libow JA: Hurting for Love: Munchausen by Proxy Syndrome. New York: The Guilford Press, 1993
8. Gil DG: Violence Against Children: Physical Child Abuse in the United States. Cambridge, MA: Harvard University Press, 1970
9. American Humane Association: Annual Report of Official Child Abuse and Neglect Reporting. Denver: American Humane Association, 1986
10. Straus M, Gelles RI, Steinmetz SK: Behind Closed Doors: Violence in the American Family. New York Doubleday, 1980
11. Gelles RI, Straus MA: Intimate Violence. New York: Simon & Schuster, 1988
12. US Department of Health and Human Services: Study Methodology: National Study of the Incidence and Severity of Child Abuse and Neglect. DHHS Publication No (OHDS) 81-30326. Washington, DC: Government Printing Office, 1981
13. Finkelhor D, Hotaling GT: Sexual abuse in the national incidence study of child abuse and neglect: an appraisal. Child Abuse Negl 8:23–27, 1984
14. US Department of Health and Human Services: Study Findings; Study of National Incidence and Prevalence of Child Abuse and Neglect. DHHS Report of Contract 105-85-1702. Washington, DC: Government Printing Office, 1988
15. Lung CT, Daro D: Current Trends in Child Abuse Reporting and Fatalities: The Result of the 1995 Annual Fifty State Survey. Working Paper No. 808. Chicago: National Committee to Prevent Child Abuse, 1996
16. Steele BF, Pollock C: A psychiatric study of parents who abuse infants and small children. In Hefner RE, Kempe CH (eds): The Battered Child. Chicago: University of Chicago Press, 1974, pp 8–133
17. Galdston R: Violence begins at home. Am J Child Psychiatry 10: 336–350, 1971
18. O'Toole R, Turbett, Nalepka C: Theories, professional knowledge, and diagnosis of child abuse. In Finkelhor D, Gelles R, Hotaling GT, Straus MA (eds): The Dark Side of Families: Current Family Violence Research. Beverly Hills, CA: Sage Publications, 1983, pp 349–362
19. Starr RH: Controlled study of the ecology of child abuse and drug abuse. Child Abuse Negl 2:19–28, 1978
20. Burgess RL, Draper P: The explanation of family violence: the role of biological, behavioral, and cultural selection. In Ohlin L, Tonry M (eds): Family Violence. Chicago: University of Chicago Press, 1989, pp 59–116
21. Garbariano J, Gilliam G: Understanding Abuse Families. Lexington, MA: Lexington Books, 1980
22. Zuravin S: Fertility patterns: their relationship to child physical abuse and child neglect. J Marriage Fam 50:93–99, 1988
23. Sherrod KB, O'Connor S, Vietzze PNI, et al: Child health and maltreatment. Child Dev 55:1174–1183, 1984
24. Ross SM: Risk of physical abuse to children of spouse-abusing parents. Child Abuse Negl 20:589–598, 1996
25. Ellerstein NS: Child Abuse: A Medical Reference. New York: John Wiley, 1981
26. National Summary of Injury Mortality Data, 1988–1994. Atlanta: Centers for Disease Control and Prevention, National Center for Injury Prevention and Control, 1996
27. White ST, Loda FA, Ingram DL, et al: Sexually transmitted diseases in sexually abused children. Pediatrics 72:16–21, 1983
28. Elmer E: A follow-up study of traumatized children. Pediatrics 59: 273, 1977
29. Wyatt GE, Powell GJ: Lasting Effects of Child Sexual Abuse. Newbury Park, CA: Sage Publications, 1988
30. Sedney NI, Brooks B: Factors associated with a history of childhood sexual experience in a nonclinical population. J Am Acad Child Psychiatry 23:215, 1984
31. Summit R, Kryso J: Sexual abuse of children: a clinical spectrum. Am J Orthopsychiatry 48:237–251, 1978
32. Groth A, Bimbaum J: Men Who Rape: A Psychology of the Offender. New York: Plenum Press, 1979
33. Newberger CM, DeVos E: Abuse and victimization: a life-span developmental perspective. Am J Orthopsychiatry 58:505–511, 1988
34. Newberger EH, Hagenbuch JJ, Ebeling NB, et al: Reducing the literal and human cost of child abuse: impact of a new hospital management system. Pediatrics 51:840–848, 1973
35. Cohn AH: Evaluation of Child Abuse and Neglect Demonstration Projects. Washington, DC: National Center for Health Services Research, 1978
36. Daro D: Confronting Child Abuse: Research for Effective Program Design. New York: The Free Press, 1988
37. Garbarino J: Changing hospital childbirth practices: a developmental perspective on prevention of child maltreatment. Am J Orthopsychiatry 49:538–597, 1979

Child Sexual Abuse

1. National Center on Child Abuse and Neglect: National Study of Incidence and Severity of Child Abuse and Neglect. Washington, DC: National Center on Child Abuse and Neglect, 1981

2. MacFarlane K, Jones B, Jenstrom L: Sexual Abuse of Children: Selected Readings. Publication No 8-30161. Washington, DC: U.S. Department of Health and Human Services, 1980
3. Kocen L, Bulkley J: Analysis of criminal child sex offense statutes. In Bulkley J (ed): Child Sexual Abuse and the Law. Washington, DC: American Bar Association, 1981, pp 1–5
4. Bagley C, Ramsay R: Disrupted childhood and vulnerability to sexual assault: long-term sequels with implications for consulting. Soc Work Hum Sexuality 4:33–48, 1935
5. Committee on Sexual Offenses Against Children and Youth: Sexual Offenses Against Children. Ottawa: Canadian Government Publishing Centre, 1984, vol 1
6. Finkelhor D: Child Sexual Abuse: New Theory and Research. New York: The Free Press, 1984
7. Kercher G, McShane M: The prevalence of child sexual abuse victimization in an adult sample of Texas residents. Child Abuse Negl 8:495–502, 1984
8. Russell DEH: The Secret Trauma: Incest in the Lives of Girls and Women. New York: Basic Books, 1986
9. Wyatt G: The sexual abuse of Afro-American and white American women in childhood. Child Abuse Negl 9:507–519, 1985
10. Finkelhor D, Hotaling G, Lewis I, Smith C: Sexual abuse in a national survey of adult men and women: prevalence, characteristics and risk factors. Child Abuse Negl 14:19–28, 1990
11. Peters S, Wyatt G, Finkelhor D: The prevalence of child sexual abuse. In Finkelhor D, et al (eds): A Sourcebook on Child Sexual Abuse. Beverly Hills, CA: Sage Publications, 1986, pp 15–59
12. Finkelhor D: Current information on the scope and nature of child sexual abuse. Future Child 4:31–53, 1994
13. Sedlak AJ, Broadhurst DD: The Third National Incidence Study of Child Abuse and Neglect (NIS-3). Washington, DC: US Department of Health and Human Services, 1996
14. Burgess AW, Groth AN, Holstrom LL, Sgroi SM: Sexual Assault of Children and Adolescents. Lexington, MA: Lexington Books, 1978
15. DeFrancis V: Protecting the child victim of sex crimes committed by adults. Denver: American Humane Association, 1969
16. Griffith S, Anderson S, Bach C, Paperny D: Intrafamily sexual abuse of male children: an underreported problem. Presented at the Third International Congress of Child Abuse and Neglect, Amsterdam, 1981
17. Jaffe AC, Dynneson L, Ten Bensel R: Sexual abuse: an epidemiological study. Am J Dis Child 129:689–692, 1975
18. Queen's Bench Foundation: Sexual Abuse of Children. San Francisco: Queen's Bench Foundation, 1976
19. National Center on Child Abuse and Neglect: Child Maltreatment 1994: Reports from the States to the National Center on Child Abuse and Neglect. Washington, DC: Government Printing Office, 1996
20. American Association for Protecting Children, Inc: National Study on Child Neglect and Abuse Reporting. Denver: American Humane Association, 1984
21. National Center on Child Abuse and Neglect: Study Findings: Study of the National Incidence and Prevalence of Child Abuse and Neglect. Washington, DC: US Department of Health and Human Services, 1988
22. Briere J: The effect of childhood sexual abuse on later psychological functioning: defining a "post-sexual-abuse syndrome." Presented at the Third National Conference on Sexual Victimization of Children, Washington, DC, April 1984
23. Araji S, Finkelhor D: Explanations of pedophilia: review of empirical evidence. Bull Am Acad Psychiatry Law 13:17–38, 1985
24. Finkelhor D, Baron L: High risk children. In Finkelhor D et al. (eds). A Sourcebook on Child Sexual Abuse. Beverly Hills, CA: Sage Publications, 1986, pp 60–68
25. Finkelhor D: Epidemiological factors in the clinical identification of child sexual abuse. Child Abuse Negl 17:67–70, 1993
26. Abel GG, Becker JV, Murphy WD, Falanagan B: Identifying dangerous child molesters. In Stuart RB (ed): Violent Behavior. New York: Brunner/Mazel, 1981, pp 116–137
27. Freund K: Erotic preference in pedophilia. Behav Res Ther 5:209–228, 1967
28. Hanson R, Slater S: Sexual victimization in the history of sexual abusers: a review. Ann Sex Res 1:485–499, 1988
29. Langevin R: Sexual Strands: Understanding and Treating Sexual Anomalies in Men. Hillsdale, NJ: Erlbaum Associates, 1983
30. Williams LM, Finkelhor D: The characteristics of incestuous fathers: a review of recent studies. In Marshall W, Laws R, Barbaree H (eds): The Handbook of Sexual Assault: Issues, Theories and Treatment of the Offender. New York: Plenum Press, 1990
31. Parker H, Parker S: Father-daughter sexual abuse: an emerging perspective. Am J Orthopsychiatry 56:531–549, 1986
32. Abel GG, Cummingham-Rathner J, Becker JB, McHugh J: Motivating sex offenders for treatment with feedback of their psychophysiologic assessment. Presented at the World Congress of Behavior Therapy, Washington, DC, December 1983
33. Browne A, Finkelhor D: The impact of child sexual abuse: review of the research. Psych Bull 99(1):66–77, 1986
34. Gelinas DJ: The persisting negative effects of incest. Psychiatry 46:312–332, 1983
35. Kendall-Tackett K, Williams LM, Finkelhor D: The impact of sexual abuse on children: A review and synthesis of recent empirical studies. Psychol Bull 113:164–180, 1993
36. Oppenheimer R, Palmer RL, Braden S: A clinical evaluation of early sexually abusive experience in adult anorexic and bulimic females: implications for preventative work in childhood. Presented at the Fifth International Conference on Child Abuse and Neglect, Montreal, 1984
37. Stein I et al: Long-term psychological sequela of child sexual abuse: the Los Angeles Epidemiologic Catchment Area study. In Wyatt G, Powell G (eds): Lasting Effects of Child Sexual Abuse. Newbury Park, CA: Sage Publications, 1988
38. Herman JL: Father-Daughter Incest. Cambridge, Mass: Harvard University Press, 1981
39. Silbert MN, Pines AM: Sexual child abuse as an antecedent to prostitution. Child Abuse Negl 5:407–411, 1981
40. Tufts New England Medical Center, Division of Child Psychiatry: Sexually Exploited Children: Service and Research Project. Final Report for the Office of Juvenile Justice and Delinquency Prevention. Boston: US Department of Justice, 1984
41. Finkelhor D, Berliner L: Research on the treatment of sexually abused children: a review and recommendations. J Am Acad Adolesc Psychiatry 34:1408–1423, 1995
42. MacFarlane K, Bulkley I: Treating child sexual abuse: an overview of current program models. In Conte J, Shore D (eds). Social Work and Child Sexual Abuse. New York: Haworth, 1982, pp 69–81
43. Kelley RJ: Behavioral re-orientation of pedophiliacs: can it be done? Clin Psychology Rev 2:387–408, 1982

Elder Abuse

1. Gebotys RJ, O'Connor D, Mair KJ: Public perceptions of elder physical mistreatment. Journal of Elder Abuse and Neglect 4:151–172, 1992
2. Hudson MF: Elder abuse: its meaning to middle-aged and older adults. Part II: Pilot results. Journal of Elder Abuse and Neglect 6(1):55–82, 1994
3. Moon A, Williams O: Perceptions of elder abuse and help-seeking patterns among African-American, Caucasian American, and Korean-American elderly women. Gerontologist 33(3):386–395, 1993
4. Fiegener JJ, Fiegener M, Meszaros J: Policy implications of a statewide survey on elder abuse. Journal of Elder Abuse and Neglect 1(2):39–58, 1989

5. Clark-Daniels CL, Daniels RS, Baumhover LA: Physicians' and nurses' responses to abuse of the elderly: a comparative study of two surveys in Alabama. Journal of Elder Abuse and Neglect 1(4):57–72, 1989
6. Pillemer K, Finkelhor D: Prevalence of elder abuse: a random sample survey. Gerontologist 28:51–57, 1988
7. Podnieks E: National survey on abuse of the elderly in Canada. Journal of Elder Abuse and Neglect 4(1/2):5–58, 1989
8. Ogg J: Researching elder abuse in Britain. Journal of Elder Abuse and Neglect 5(2):37–54, 1993
9. Kivelä SL, Köngäs-Saviaro P, Kesti E, Pahkala K, and Ijäs ML: Abuse in old age: epidemiological data from Finland. Journal of Elder Abuse and Neglect 4(3):1–18, 1992
10. Wolf R, Pillemer K: Helping Elder Victims: The Reality of Elder Abuse. New York: Columbia University Press, 1989
11. Tatara T: An Analysis of State Laws Addressing Elder Abuse, Neglect, and Exploitation. Washington, DC: National Center on Elder Abuse, 1995
12. Quinn KM, Hwalek, M, Goodrich CS: Determining Effective Interventions in a Community-Based Elder Abuse System. Final Report. Springfield, IL: Illinois Department on Aging, 1993
13. Tatara T & Kuzmeskus L: Summaries of the statistics data on elder abuse in domestic settings for FY95 and FY96. Washington, DC: National Center on Elder Abuse, 1997
14. Tatara T: Understanding the Nature and Extent of Elder Abuse in Domestic Settings. Washington, DC: National Center on Elder Abuse, 1996
15. National Center on Elder Abuse: National Elder Abuse Incidence Study. Washington, DC: National Center on Elder Abuse, 1995
16. Bachman R: The double edged sword of violent victimization against the elderly: patterns of family and stranger perpetration Journal of Elder Abuse and Neglect 5(4):59–76, 1993
17. Lachs M, Pillemer K: Current concepts: elder Abuse. N Engl J Med 332:269–271, 1995
18. Pillemer K: Risk factors in elder abuse: results from a case-control study. In Pillemer K, Wolf RS (eds): Elder Abuse: Conflict in the Family. Dover, MA: Auburn House, 1986
19. Bristowe E, Collins JB: Family mediated abuse of non-institutionalized elder men and women living in British Columbia. Journal of Elder Abuse and Neglect 1(1):45–54, 1989
20. Phillips LR: Theoretical explanations of elder abuse. In: Pillemer KA, Wolf RS (eds): Elder Abuse: Conflict in the Family. Dover, MA: Auburn House, 1996
21. Paveza GJ, Cohen D, Eisdorfer C, et al: Severe family violence and Alzheimer's disease: prevalence and risk factors. Gerontologist 32:493–497, 1992
22. Coyne AC, Reichman WE, Bergib LJ: The relationship between dementia and elder abuse. Am J Psychiatry 150:643–646, 1993
23. Pillemer K, Suitor JJ: Violence and violent feelings: what causes them among family caregivers? J Gerontol 47:S165–S172, 1992
24. Anetzberger GJ: Etiology of Elder Abuse by Adult Offspring. Springfield, IL: Charles C Thomas, 1987
25. Pillemer K, Finkelhor D: Causes of elder abuse: caregiver stress versus problem relatives. Am J Orthopsychiatry 59:179–187, 1989
26. Hwalek M, Sengstock M, Lawrence R: Assessing the probability of abuse of the elderly. Presented at the Annual Meeting of the Gerontological Society of America, San Francisco, November 1984
27. Homer AC, Gilleard C: Abuse of elderly people by their carers. Br Med J 301:1359–1362, 1990
28. Pillemer K: The dangers of dependency: new findings on domestic violence against the elderly. Soc Prob 33:149–158, 1985
29. Godkin MA, Wolf RS, Pillemer KA: A case-comparison analysis of elder abuse and neglect. Int J Aging Hum Dev 28:207–225, 1989
30. Grafström M, Nordberg A, Winblad B: Abuse is in the eye of the beholder. Scand J Soc Med 21:247–256, 1994
31. Finkelhor D: Common features of family abuse. In Finkelhor D, Gelles RI, Hotaling G, Straus M (eds): Dark Side of Families: Current Family Violence Research. Beverly Hills, CA: Sage, 1983, pp 17–26
32. Pillemer K, Prescott D: Psychological effects of elder abuse: a research note. Journal of Elder Abuse and Neglect 1(1):65–74, 1989
33. Harris S: For better or for worse: spouse abuse grown old. Journal of Elder Abuse and Neglect 8(1):1–34, 1996
34. Lachs MS: The morbidity and morality of elder abuse. In American Federation for Aging Research: The Paul Beeson Physician Faculty Scholars in Aging Research Program 1995–1996. New York: American Federation for Aging Research, 1996
35. Crystal S: Social policy and elder abuse. In Pillemer K, Wolf RS (eds): Elder Abuse: Conflict in the Family. Dover, MA: Auburn House, 1986, pp 331–339
36. Faulkner LR: Mandating the reporting of suspected cases of elder abuse: an inappropriate, ineffective and ageist response to the abuse of older adults. Family Law Quarterly 16:69–91, 1982
37. Callahan JJ: Elder abuse programming: will it help the elderly? Urban and Social Change Review 15:15–19, 1982
38. US General Accounting Office: Elder Abuse: Effectiveness of Reporting Laws and Other Factors. Washington, DC: Government Printing Office, 1991
39. Wolf RS: Adult protective services. In Maddox G (ed): Encyclopedia of Aging. 2nd ed. New York: Springer, 1996
40. Blenkner M, Bloom M, Nielson M: A research and demonstration project of protective services. Social Casework 52:483–497, 1978
41. Wolf RS: Current trends in elder abuse research. In National Research Council/Institute of Medicine (eds): Service Provider Perspectives on Family Violence Interventions. Washington, DC: National Academy of Sciences, 1995, pp 52–56
42. Sherman LW, Berk RA: Minneapolis domestic violence experiment. Police Foundation Reports 1, 1984
43. Garner J, Fagen J, Maxwell C: Published findings from the spouse abuse replication project: a critical review. Journal of Quantitative Criminology 11:3–28, 1995
44. National Research Council: Understanding Violence against Women. Washington, DC: National Academy of Sciences, 1996, p 116

Suicide

1. Singh GK, Kochanek KD, MacDorman MF: Advance Report of Final Mortality Statistics, 1994. Mon Vital Stat Rep 45(3), 1996
2. Kachur SP, Potter LB, James SP, Powell KE: Suicide in the United States, 1980–1992. Violence Surveillance Summary Series, No. 1. Atlanta: National Center for Injury Prevention and Control, 1995
3. Rosenberg ML, Smith JC, Davidson LE, Conn JM: The emergence of youth suicide: an epidemiologic analysis and public health perspective. Annu Rev Public Health 8:417–440, 1987
4. Centers for Disease Control and Prevention: Suicide among Children, Adolescents, and Young Adults—United States, 1980–1992. MMWR 44(15):289–291, 1995
5. Centers for Disease Control and Prevention: Fatal and Nonfatal Suicide Attempts among Adolescents—Oregon, 1988–1993. MMWR 44(16):312–323, 1995
6. Moscicki EK, O'Carroll PW, Rae DS, Roy AG, Locke BZ, Regier DA: Suicidal ideation and attempts: The Epidemiologic Catchment Area study. In Alcohol, Drug Abuse and Mental Health Administration: Report of the Secretary's Task Force on Youth Suicide. vol. 4. Strategies for the Prevention of Youth Suicide. DHHS Publication No. (ADM)89-1624. Washington, DC: Government Printing Office, pp 115–128
7. Kann L, Warren C, Harris W, Collins J, Williams B, Ross J, Kolbe L: Youth Risk Behavior Surveillance—United States, 1995. MMWR CDC Surveill Summ, 45(4), 1996

8. Rosenberg NIL, Davidson LE, Smith JC, et al: Operational criteria for the determination of suicide. J Forensic Sci 33:1445–1456, 1988
9. Nelson FL, Farberow NL, MacKinnon DR: The certification of suicide in eleven Western states: an inquiry into the validity of reported suicide rates. Suicide Life Threat Behav 8:75–88, 1978
10. Kleck G: Miscounting suicides. Suicide Life Threat Behav 18(3):219–236, 1988
11. O'Carroll PW: A consideration of the validity and reliability of suicide mortality data. Suicide Life Threat Behav 19:1–16, 1989
12. Hagnell O, Lanke J, Rorsman B: Suicide rates in the Lundby study: Mental illness as a risk factor for suicide. Neuropsychobiology 7:248–253, 1981
13. Murphy GE: Problems in studying suicide. Psychiatric Dev (4):339–350, 1983
14. Miles CP: Conditions predisposing to suicide: a review. J Nerv Ment Dis 164(4):231–246, 1977
15. Roy A, Linnoila NI: Alcoholism and suicide. Suicide Life Threat Behav 16(2):244–273, 1986
16. Kendall RE: Alcohol and suicide. Subst Alcohol Actions Misuse 4(2–3):121–127, 1983
17. Murphy GE, Wetzel RD: The lifetime risk of suicide in alcoholism. Arch Gen Psychiatry 47(4):383–392, 1990
18. Roy A: Suicide among alcoholics. Int Rev Psychiatry. 4(2):211–216, 1992
19. Fernandez-Pol B: Characteristics of 77 Puerto Ricans who attempted suicide. Am J Psychiatry 143:1460–1463, 1986
20. Kost-Grant BL: Self-inflicted gunshot wounds among Alaska Natives. Public Health Rep 98(1):72–78, 1983
21. Roy A: Risk factors for suicide among adult alcoholics. Special issue: Alcohol, aggression, and injury. Alcohol Health Res World. 17(2):133–136, 1993
22. Morrison JR: Suicide in a psychiatric practice population. Clin Psychiatry 43(9):348–352, 1982
23. Robbins DR, Alessi NE: Depressive symptoms and suicidal behavior in adolescents. Am J Psychiatry 142:588–592, 1985
24. Black DW, Warrack G, Winokur G: The Iowa record-linkage study: I. Suicides and accidental deaths among psychiatric patients. Arch Gen Psychiatry 42(1):71–75, 1985
25. Shuckitt MA: Primary men alcoholics with histories of suicide attempts. J Stud Alcohol 47(1):78–81, 1986
26. Bacue LO, Epstein L: Suicide attitudes and experiences of hospitalized alcoholics. Psychol Rep 47:1233–1234, 1980
27. Berglund M: Suicide in alcoholism: a prospective study of 88 suicides: I. The multidimensional diagnosis at first admission. Arch Gen Psychiatry 41(9):888–891, 1984
28. Frances A, Blumenthal S: Personality as a predictor of youthful suicide. In Alcohol, Drug Abuse and Mental Health Administration: Report of the Secretary's Task Force on Youth Suicide. vol 2. Risk Factors for Youth Suicide. DHHS Publication No. (ADM)89-1624. Washington, DC: Government Printing Office, 1989, pp 160–171
29. Roy A: Genetics, biology, and suicide in the family. In Maris RW, Berman AL, Maltsberger JT, Yufit RI (eds): Assessment and Prediction of Suicide. New York: Guilford Press, 1992, pp 574–588
30. Rainer JD: Genetic factors in depression and suicide. Am J Psychother 38(3):329–340, 1984
31. Wender PH, Kety SS, Rosenthal D, Schulsinger F: Psychiatric disorders in the biological and adoptive families of adopted individuals with affective disorders. Arch Gen Psychiatry 43(10):923–929, 1986
32. Roy A: Genetics and suicidal behavior. In Alcohol, Drug Abuse and Mental Health Administration: Report of the Secretary's Task Force on Youth Suicide. vol 2. Risk Factors for Youth Suicide. DHHS Publication No. (ADM)89-1624. Washington, DC: Government Printing Office, 1989, pp 247–262
33. Nordstrom P, Asberg M: Suicide risk and serotonin. Int Clin Psychopharmacol 6(suppl 6):12–21, 1992
34. Nordstrom P, Samuelsson M, Asberg M, Traskman-Bendz L: CSF 5-HIAA predicts suicide risk after attempted suicide. Suicide Life Threat Behav 24(1):1–9, 1994
35. Kety SS: Genetic factors in suicide: family, twin and adoption studies. In Blumenthal SJ, Kupfer DJ (eds) Suicide over the Life Cycle: Risk Factors, Assessment, and Treatment of Suicidal Patients. Washington, DC: American Psychatric Press, 1990, pp 127–133
36. Traskman L, Asberg M, Bertulson L, Sjostrand L: Monoamine metabolites in CSF and suicidal behavior. Arch Gen Psychiatry 38: 631–636, 1981
37. van Praag HM: CSF 5-HIAA and suicide in non-depressed schizophrenics. Lancet 2:977–978, 1983
38. Robbins D, Conroy C: A cluster of adolescent suicide attempts: Is suicide contagious? J Adolesc Health Care 3:253–255, 1983
39. Davidson L, Gould MS: Contagion as a risk factor for youth suicide. In Alcohol, Drug Abuse and Mental Health Administration: Report of the Secretary's Task Force on Youth Suicide. vol 2. Risk Factors for Youth Suicide. DHHS Publication No. (ADM)89-1624. Washington, DC: Government Printing Office, 1989, pp 88–109
40. Centers for Disease Control: Cluster of suicides and suicide attempts—New Jersey. MMWR 37:213–216, 1988
41. Brent DA, Perper JA, Moritz G, Allman C: Bereavement or depression? The impact of the loss of a friend to suicide. J Am Acad Child Adolesc Psychiatry 32(6):1189–1197, 1993
42. Brent DA, Perper JA, Moritz G, Liotus L: Major depression or uncomplicated bereavement? A follow-up of youth exposed to suicide. J Am Acad Child Adolesc Psychiatry 33(2):231–239, 1994
43. Brent DA, Perper JA, Moritz G, Allman C: Psychiatric sequelae to the loss of an adolescent peer to suicide. J Am Acad Child Adolesc Psychiatry 32(3):509–517, 1993
44. O'Carroll PW, Mercy JA, Steward IA: CDC recommendations for a community plan for the prevention and containment of suicide clusters. MMWR 37(Suppl 56):1–12, 1988
45. O'Carroll PW, Potter LB: Suicide contagion and the reporting of suicide: recommendations from a national workshop. MMWR 43(RR-6):13–18, 1994
46. Phillips DP, Carstensen LL: Clustering of teenage suicides after television news stories about suicide. N Engl J Med 315:685–689, 1986
47. Gould MS, Shaffer D: The impact of suicide in television movies: evidence of imitation. N Engl J Med 315:690–694, 1986
48. Phillips DP, Paight DJ: The impact of televised movies about suicide: a replicative study. N Engl J Med 317:809–811, 1987
49. Berman AL: Fictional depiction of suicide in television films and imitation effects. Am J Psychiatry 145:982–986, 1988
50. Kessler RC, Stipp H: The impact of fictional television suicide stories on U.S. fatalities: a replication. AJS 90:151–167, 1984
51. Baron IN, Reiss PC: Same time. next year: aggregate analyses of the mass media and violent behavior. Am Sociol Rev 50:347–363, 1985
52. Gould MS: A Study of Time-Space Clustering: phase I report. Atlanta: Centers for Disease Control, 1985
53. Davidson LE, Rosenberg NIL, Mercy JA, et al: An epidemiologic study of risk factors in two teenage suicide clusters. JAMA 262: 2687–2692, 1989
54. Paykel ES, Prusoff BA, Myers JK: Suicide attempts and recent life events: a controlled comparison. Arch Gen Psychiatry 32:327–337, 1975
55. Paykel ES: Stress and life events. In Alcohol, Drug Abuse and Mental Health Administration: Report of the Secretary's Task Force on Youth Suicide. vol 2. Risk Factors for Youth Suicide. DHHS Publication No. (ADM)89-1624. Washington, DC: Government Printing Office, 1989, pp 110–130
56. Monk M: Epidemiology of suicide. Epidemiol Rev 9:51–69, 1987
57. Platt S: Unemployment and suicidal behavior: a review of the literature. Soc Sci Med 19:93–115, 1984

58. Centers for Disease Control and Prevention: Rates of Homicide, Suicide, and Firearm-Related Death Among Children—26 Indiustrialized Countries. MMWR 46(5):101–105, 1997
59. Card JJ: Lethality of suicidal methods and suicide risk: two distinct concepts. Omega (Westport) 5(1):37–45, 1974
60. Lee RK, Waxweiler RJ, Dobings JG, Paschetag T: Incidence rates of firearm injuries in Galveston, Texas, 1979–1981. Am J Epidemiol 134(5):511–21, 1991
61. Boyd IH: The increasing rate of suicide by firearms. N Engl J Med 308:872–874, 1983
62. Sloan JH, Rivara FP, Reay DT, Ferris IAI, Kellerman AL: Firearm regulations and community suicide rates: a comparison of two metropolitan areas. N Engl J Med 322:369–373, 1990
63. Centers for Disease Control: Premature mortality due to suicide and homicide—United States, 1984. MMWR 36:531–534, 1987
64. Weinstein MC, Saturno PJ: Economic impact of youth suicides and suicide attempts. In Alcohol, Drug Abuse and Mental Health Administration: Report of the Secretary's Task Force on Youth Suicide. vol 4. Strategies for the Prevention of Youth Suicide. DHHS Publication No. (ADM)89-1624. Washington, DC: Government Printing Office, 1989, pp 82–93
65. LeMier M: An Assessment of Suicide in Washington State. Olympia, WA: Washington State Department of Health, 1994
66. Miller T: Washington State Costs for Hospitalized Suicide Attempts and Fataltities. Landover, MD; Children's Saftey Network Economics and Insurance Resource Center, National Public Services Research Institute, 1994, unpublished data
67. Dunne EJ, Dunne-Maxim K: Suicide and Its Aftermath: Understanding and Counseling the Survivors. New York: Norton, 1987
68. Hauser MI: Special aspects of grief after a suicide. In Dunne EJ, Dunne-Maxim K, (eds): Suicide and Its Aftermath: Understanding Counseling the Survivors. New York: Norton, 1987, pp 57–70
69. O'Carroll PW, Potter LB: Programs for the Prevention of Suicide among Adolescents and Young Adults. MMWR 43(RR-6):1–7, 1994
70. Eddy DM, Wolpert RL, Rosenberg ML: Estimating the effectiveness of interventions to prevent youth suicides. In Alcohol, Abuse and Mental Health Administration: Report of the Secretary's Task Force on Youth Suicide. vol 4. Strategies for Prevention of Youth Suicide. DHHS Publication No. (ADM)89-1624. Washington, DC: Government Printing Office, 1989, pp 37–81

Index

Page numbers in *italics* denote figures; those followed by "t" denote tables.